Volume 1

TEXTBOOK OF VETERINARY INTERNAL MEDICINE

THIRD EDITION

DISEASES OF THE DOG AND CAT

STEPHEN J. ETTINGER, DVM
California Animal Hospital, Los Angeles, California

1989
W.B. SAUNDERS COMPANY *Philadelphia, London, Toronto, Montreal, Sydney, Tokyo*
Harcourt Brace Jovanovich, Inc.

[redacted]
Harcourt Brace Jovanovich, Inc.

The Curtis Center
Independence Square West
Philadelphia, PA 19106

Library of Congress Cataloging-in-Publication Data

Textbook of veterinary internal medicine.

Includes bibliographies and indexes.

1. Dogs—Diseases. 2. Cats—Diseases. 3. Veterinary internal medicine. I. Ettinger, Stephen J. [DNLM: 1. Cat Diseases—diagnosis. 2. Cat Diseases—therapy. 3. Dog Diseases—diagnosis. 4. Dog Diseases—therapy. SF 991 T355]

SF991.T48 1989 636.7′0896 87–31428

ISBN 0–7216–1944–4
0–7216–1942–8 (Vol. 1)
0–7216–1943–6 (Vol. 2)

Listed here is the latest translated edition of this book together with the language of the translation and the publisher.

Japanese *(first edition)*—Gakusosha Company, Tokyo, Japan

Italian *(second edition)*—Scientific Book Market, Via dei Mille 13, Parma, Italy

Italian translation, 1989

Editor: John Dyson
Production Manager: Frank Polizzano
Designer: Lorraine B. Kilmer
Manuscript Editor: Stephen J. Ettinger, DVM
Indexer: Alexandra Nickerson

Textbook of Veterinary Internal Medicine

ISBN 0–7216–1942–8 Vol. 1
0–7216–1943–6 Vol. 2
0–7216–1944–4 Set

Printed in the United States of America.

Last digit is the print number: 9 8 7 6 5 4 3 2 1

to NICOLE and ANDREW

I love you

Dad

TO MY MOTHER AND FATHER–
THANK YOU FOR YOUR LIFELONG INSPIRATION

TO ALL MY FELLOW VETERINARIANS AND FRIENDS–

We stand in awe of all created things,
the power within them that gives them form,
the ancient law that rules them all.

We stand in awe of courage:
Honor to those who endure:
the seeker, the giver, the one who loves:
all who sing and all who weep;
the one who makes his loss a gain;
the one who gives his heart to life.[1]

No man is an Iland, intire of it selfe; every man
is a peece the Continent, a part of the maine; if
Clod bee washed away by the Sea, Europe is the lesse,
as well as if a Promontorie were, as well as if a Mannor
of thy friends or of thine owne were; any mans death
diminishes me, because I am involved in Mankinde;
And therefore never send to know for whom the bell tolls;
It tolls for thee.[2]

[1]From the High Holy Day Liturgy, Wilshire Boulevard Temple, Los Angeles, CA.
[2]John Donne, 16th century poet quoted by Ernest Hemingway in *For Whom the Bell Tolls*, 1940.

EDITOR

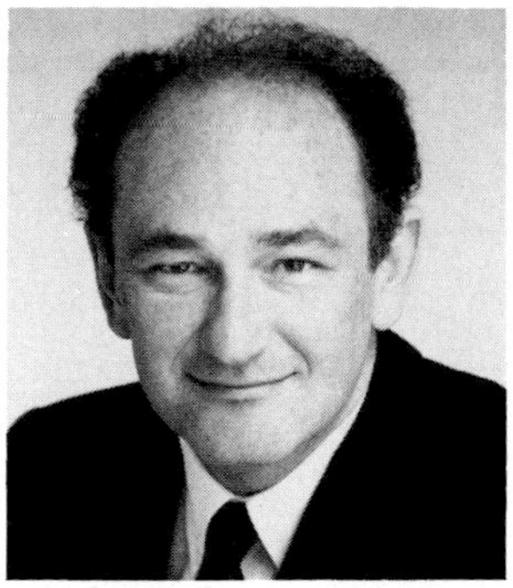

STEPHEN J. ETTINGER, D.V.M., F.A.C.C.

Diplomate, American College of Veterinary Internal Medicine (Internal Medicine and Cardiology); Fellow, American College of Cardiology (F.A.C.C.); Associate Fellow, Council on Clinical Cardiology, American Heart Association; Distinguished Veterinary Practitioner, National Academies of Practice; California Animal Hospital, Inc., 1736 S. Sepulveda Blvd., Los Angeles, CA 90025.

Formerly Clinical Professor of Medicine, School of Veterinary Medicine, University of California at Davis, Davis, California; Assistant Head of Medicine, Animal Medical Center, New York, New York.

Peripheral Edema; Weakness and Syncope; Changes in Body Weight; Coughing; Dyspnea and Tachypnea; Ascites, Peritonitis, and Other Causes of Abdominal Enlargement; Diseases of the Trachea; Diseases of the Lower Respiratory Tract (Lung) and Pulmonary Edema; Valvular Heart Disease; Cardiac Arrhythmias

CONTRIBUTORS

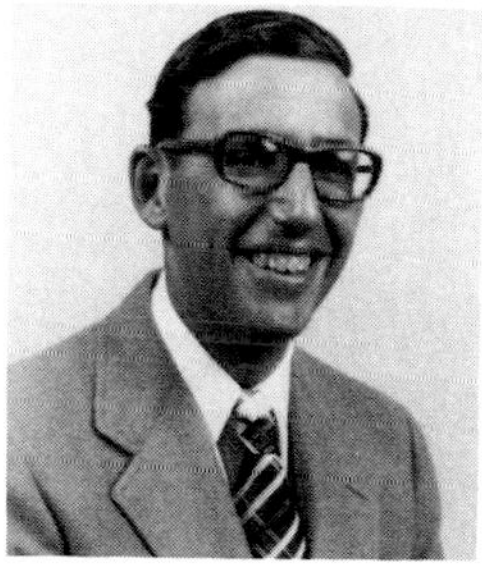

NORMAN ACKERMAN, D.V.M.

Diplomate, American College of Veterinary Radiology; Professor of Veterinary Radiology, Department of Veterinary Radiology, College of Veterinary Medicine, University of Florida, Gainesville, Florida.

Clinical Approach to the Patient with Respiratory Disease

TIMOTHY A. ALLEN, D.V.M.

Diplomate, American College of Veterinary Internal Medicine (Internal Medicine); Veterinary Nutritionist, Mark Morris Associates, Topeka, Kansas.

Specialized Nutritional Support

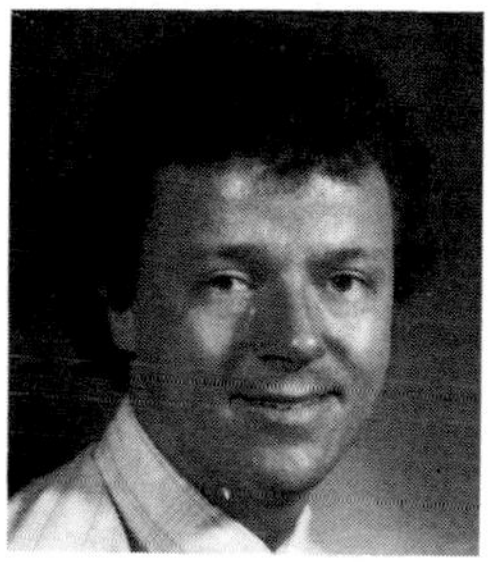

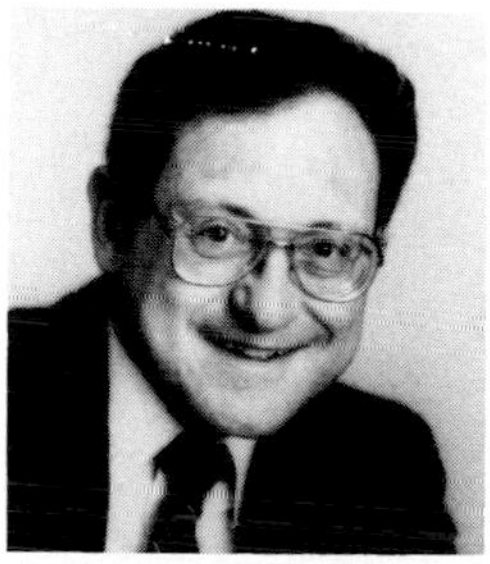

SHELDON ALTMAN, D.V.M.

Member, International Veterinary Acupuncture Society; Private Practice, M.S. Animal Hospitals, Inc., North Hollywood, California.

Acupuncture Therapy in Small Animal Practice

P. JANE ARMSTRONG, D.V.M., M.S.

Diplomate, American College of Veterinary Internal Medicine (Internal Medicine); Assistant Professor of Internal Medicine, Department of Companion Animal and Special Species Medicine, School of Veterinary Medicine, North Carolina State University, Raleigh, North Carolina.

Parathyroid Disease and Calcium Metabolism

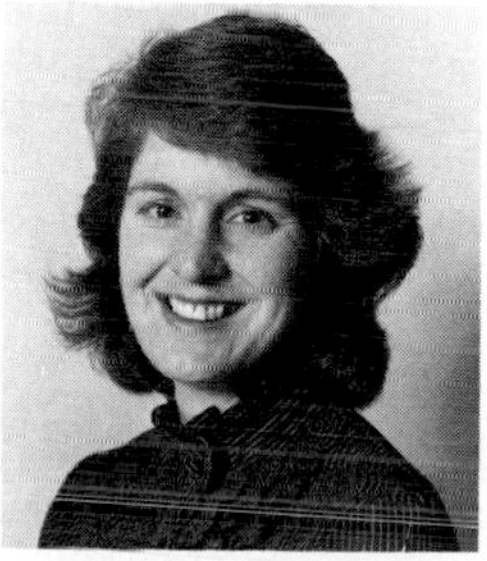

ARTHUR L. ARONSON, D.V.M., Ph.D.
Professor and Head, Department of Anatomy, Physiological Sciences and Radiology, College of Veterinary Medicine, North Carolina State University, Raleigh, North Carolina.
Antimicrobial Drugs

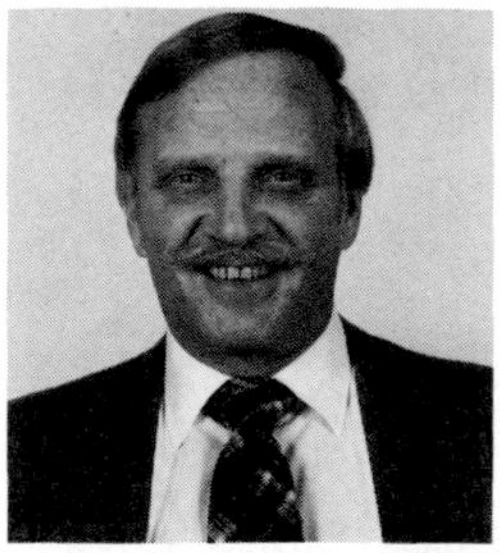

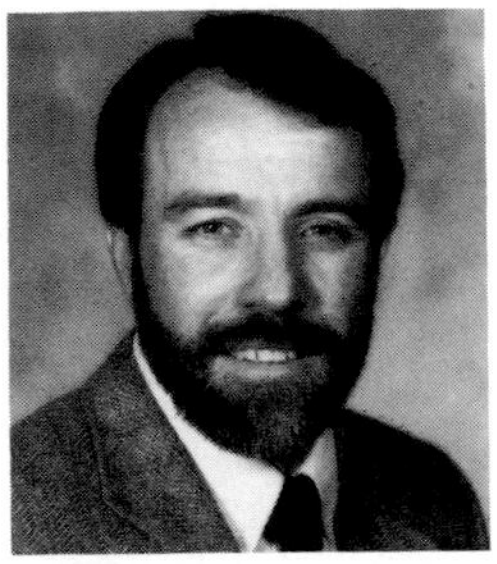

CLARKE E. ATKINS, D.V.M.
Diplomate, American Academy of Veterinary Internal Medicine (Internal Medicine); Associate Professor, College of Veterinary Medicine, Department of Companion Animal and Special Species, North Carolina State University, Raleigh, North Carolina.
Polyuria and Polydipsia

DAVID P. AUCOIN, D.V.M.
Assistant Professor, Clinical Pharmacology Unit, Department of Anatomy, Physiological Sciences and Radiology, College of Veterinary Medicine, North Carolina State University, Raleigh, North Carolina.
Antimicrobial Drugs

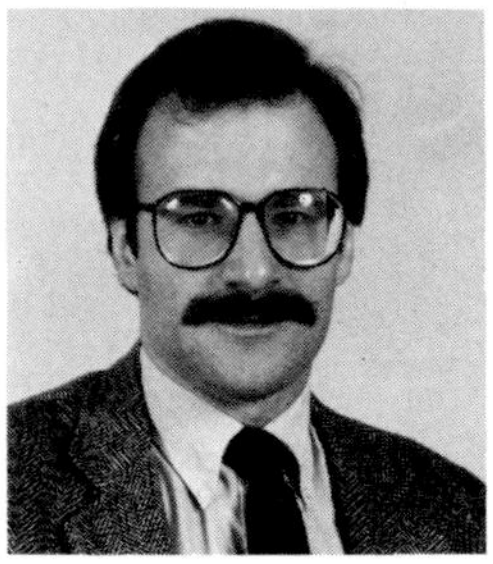

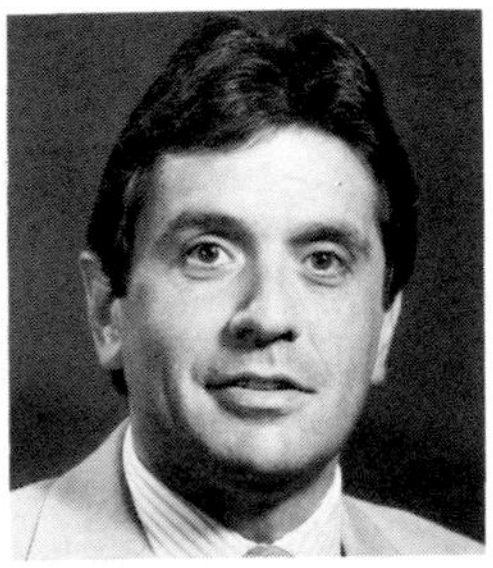

JOHN R. AUGUST, B.Vet.Med., M.S., M.R.C.V.S.
Diplomate, American College of Veterinary Internal Medicine (Internal Medicine); Professor and Head, Department of Small Animal Medicine and Surgery, College of Veterinary Medicine, Texas A and M University, College Station, Texas.
Food Hypersenstivity; Feline Viral Diseases

J. DESMOND BAGGOT, M.V.M., M.R.C.V.S., PhD., D.Sc.
Director, Irish Equine Centre, Johnstown, County Kildare, Ireland; Professor of Clinical Pharmacology, School of Veterinary Medicine, University of California, Davis, California.
Pharmacologic Principles in Therapeutics

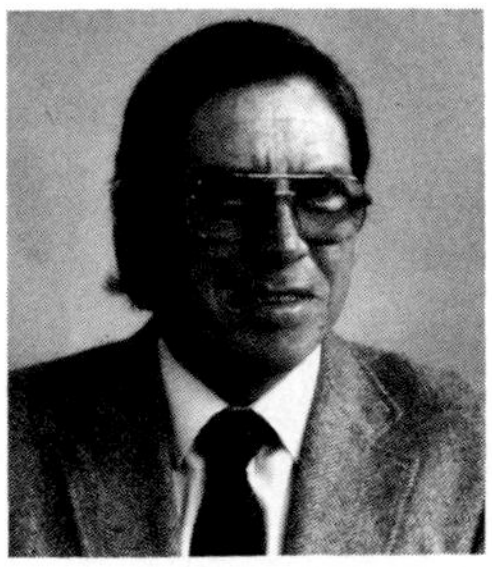

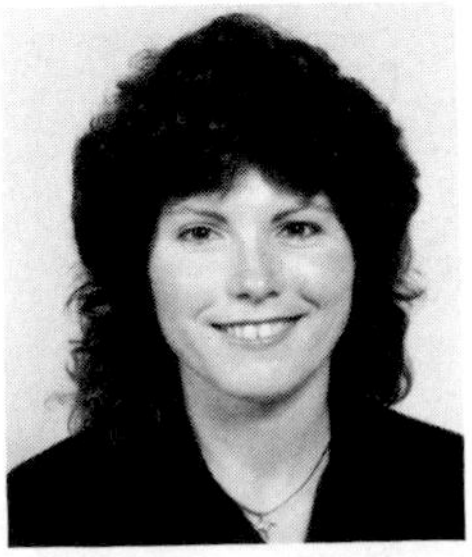

KAREN W. BANKEMPER, D.V.M.
Department of Microbiology, School of Veterinary Medicine, Auburn, Alabama.
Bacterial, Rickettsial, Protozoal, and Miscellaneous Infections

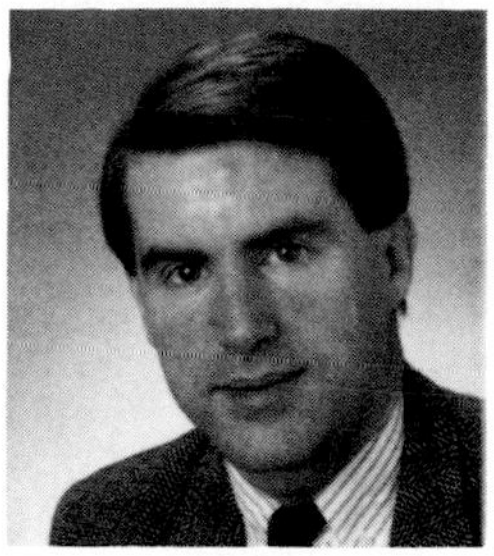

J. F. BARDET, Dr.Vet., M.S.

Surgeon, General and Orthopedic Surgery, Clinique Chirurgicale, 4, Rue François 1er, Paris, 75008 France.

Lameness in Dogs; Lameness in Cats

JEANNE A. BARSANTI, D.V.M., M.S.

Diplomate, American College of Veterinary Internal Medicine (Internal Medicine); Professor, Department of Small Animal Medicine and Department of Physiology, University of Georgia College of Veterinary Medicine, Athens, Georgia.

Canine Prostatic Diseases; Diseases of the Bladder and Urethra

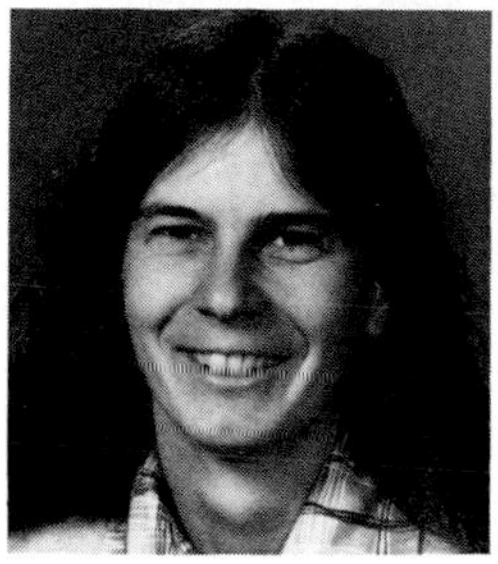

TIM BAUER, D.V.M.

Private Practice, Seattle, Washington.

Mediastinal, Pleural, and Extrapleural Diseases

PETER G. C. BEDFORD, B.Vet.Med., Ph.D., F.R.C.V.S., D.V. Ophthal.

Diplomate, Veterinary Ophthalmology (U.K.); Reader in Veterinary Ophthalmology, Department of Surgery, Royal Veterinary College; Department of Pathology, Institute of Ophthalmology, London, England.

Diseases of the Nose and Throat

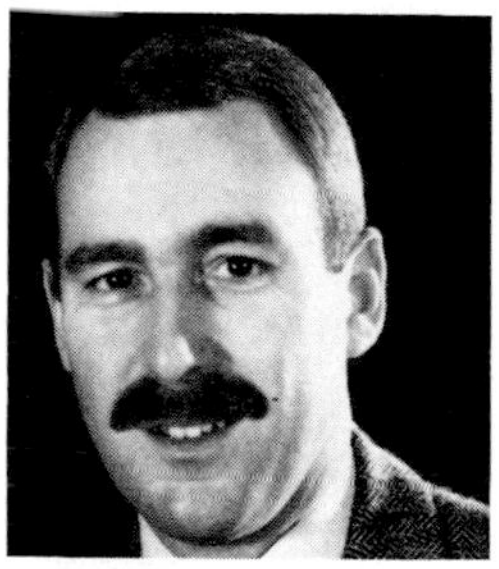

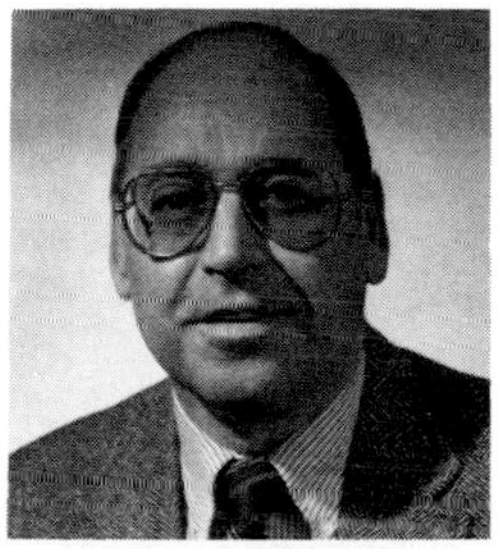

DARRYL N. BIERY, D.V.M.

Diplomate, American College of Veterinary Radiology; Professor of Radiology, School of Veterinary Medicine and Professor of Radiological Science, School of Medicine, University of Pennsylvania, Philadelphia, Pennsylvania.

Skeletal Diseases

KATHLEEN L. BOLDY, V.M.D.

Diplomate, American College of Veterinary Ophthalmology; Private Ophthalmology Practice, Los Angeles, California.

Ocular Manifestations of Systemic Disease

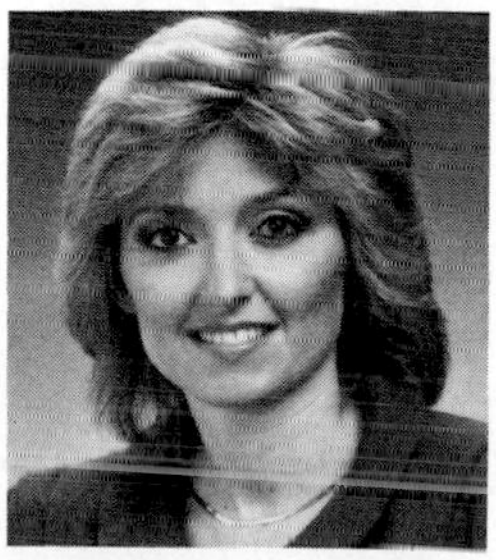

GARY R. BOLTON, D.V.M. (DECEASED)
Assistant Professor of Veterinary Medicine, Cornell University, Ithaca, New York.
Peripheral Edema

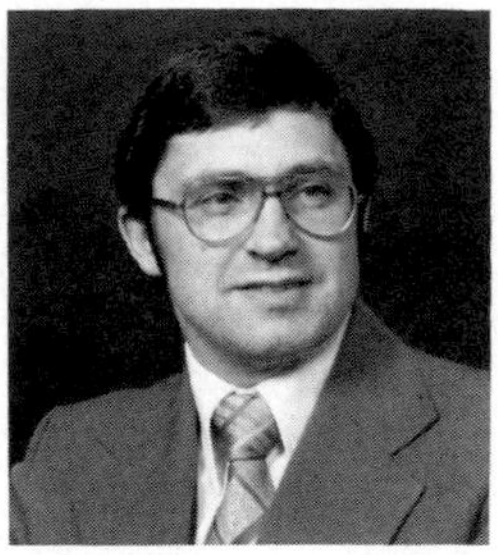

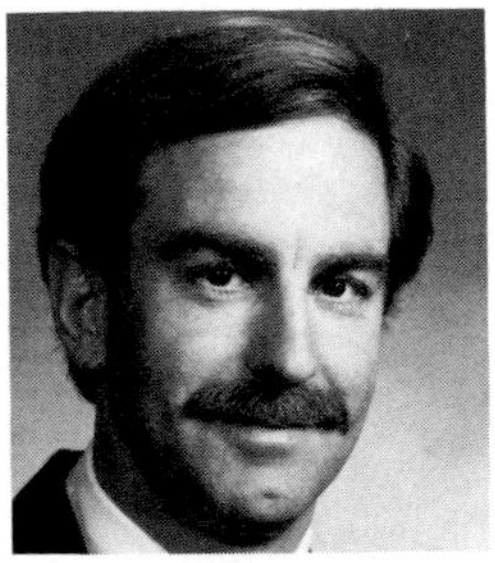

JOHN D. BONAGURA, D.V.M., M.S.
Diplomate, American College of Veterinary Internal Medicine (Cardiology and Internal Medicine); Professor, Department of Veterinary Clinical Sciences, Cardiologist, Veterinary Teaching Hospital, The Ohio State University College of Veterinary Medicine, Columbus, Ohio.
Congenital Heart Disease

G. DANIEL BOON, D.V.M., M.S.
Diplomate, American College of Veterinary Pathologists; Associate Professor, Purdue University School of Veterinary Medicine, West Lafayette, Indiana.
The Clinical Approach to Disorders of Hemostasis

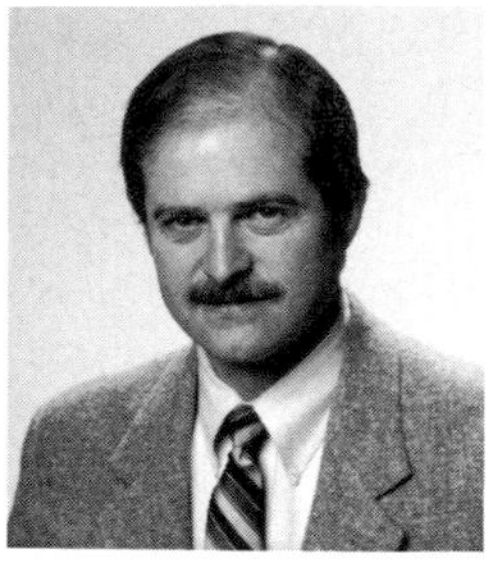

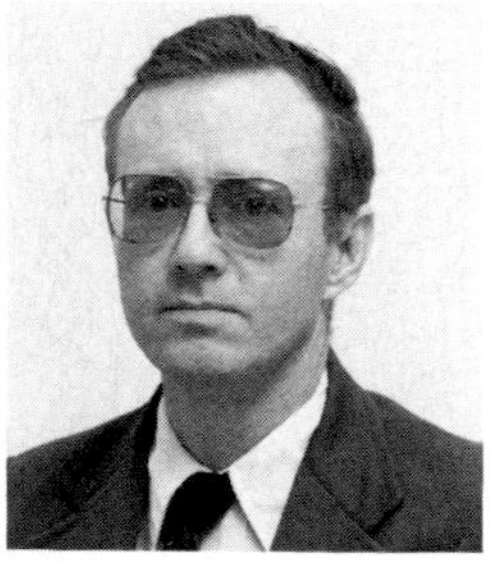

RICHARD A. BOWEN, D.V.M., Ph.D.
Assistant Professor, Animal Reproduction Laboratory, Colorado State University School of Veterinary Medicine, Fort Collins, Colorado.
Persistent Estrus in the Bitch

KYLE G. BRAUND, B.V.Sc., M.V.Sc., Ph.D.
Diplomate, American College of Veterinary Internal Medicine (Neurology); Professor and Director, Neuromuscular Research Unit, Scott-Ritchey Research Program; Consultant Clinical Neurologist, Department of Small Animal Medicine and Surgery, Auburn University College of Veterinary Medicine, Auburn, Alabama.
Diseases of the Brain

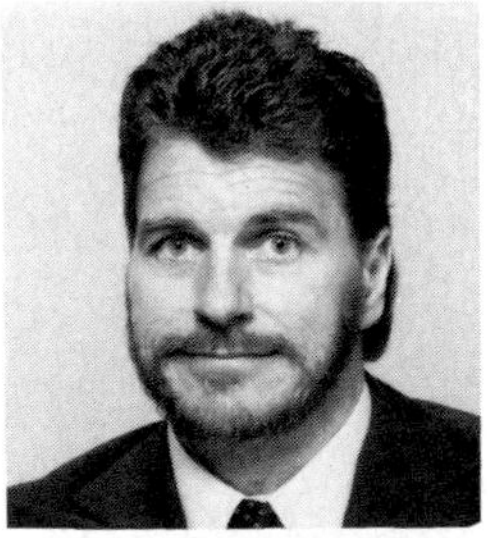

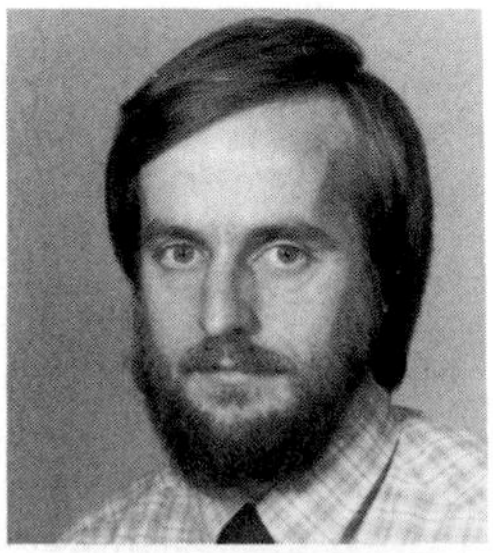

SCOTT A. BROWN, V.M.D.
Diplomate, American College of Veterinary Internal Medicine (Internal Medicine); Research Fellow, University of Georgia/Neurology Trainee, University of Alabama at Birmingham; Department of Physiology and Pharmacology, College of Veterinary Medicine, University of Georgia, Athens, Georgia; Department of Physiology, School of Medicine, University of Alabama at Birmingham, Birmingham, Alabama.
Diseases of the Bladder and Urethra

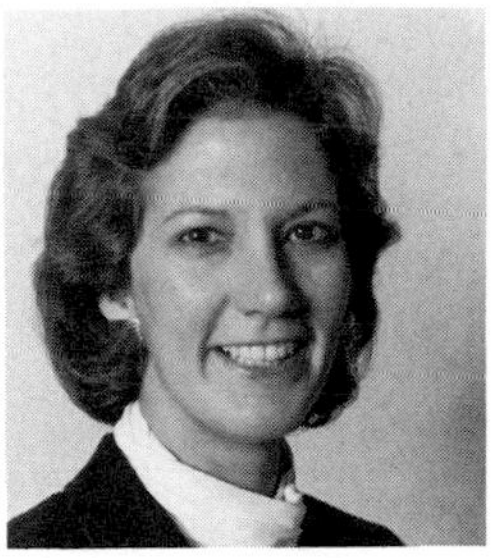

SUSAN E. BUNCH, D.V.M., Ph.D.
Diplomate, American College of Veterinary Internal Medicine (Internal Medicine); Associate Professor of Internal Medicine, North Carolina State University College of Veterinary Medicine, Raleigh, North Carolina.
Jaundice

COLIN F. BURROWS, B.Vet.Med., Ph.D., M.R.C.V.S.
Diplomate, American College of Veterinary Internal Medicine (Internal Medicine); Professor of Medicine, University of Florida, College of Veterinary Medicine, Gainesville, Florida.
Recto-Anal Disease

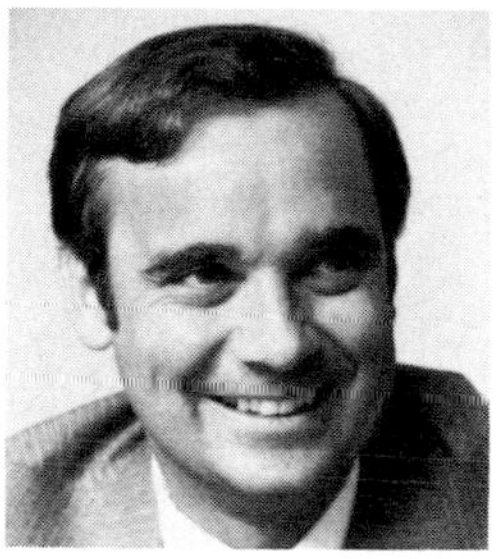

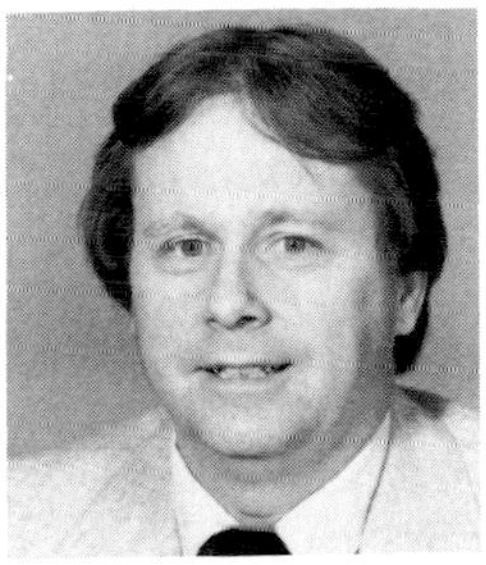

CLAY A. CALVERT, D.V.M.
Diplomate, American College of Veterinary Internal Medicine (Internal Medicine); Associate Professor, Department of Small Animal Medicine and Surgery, College of Veterinary Medicine, University of Georgia, Athens, Georgia.
Heartworm Disease

SHARON A. CENTER, D.V.M.
Diplomate, American College of Veterinary Internal Medicine (Internal Medicine); Associate Professor, New York State College of Veterinary Medicine, Cornell University, Ithaca, New York.
Pathophysiology and Laboratory Diagnosis of Liver Disease

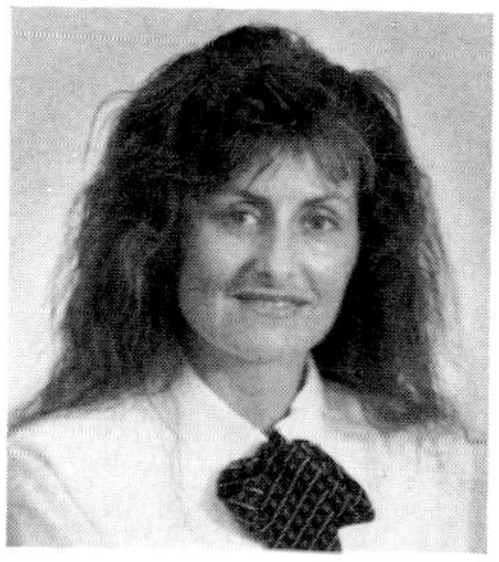

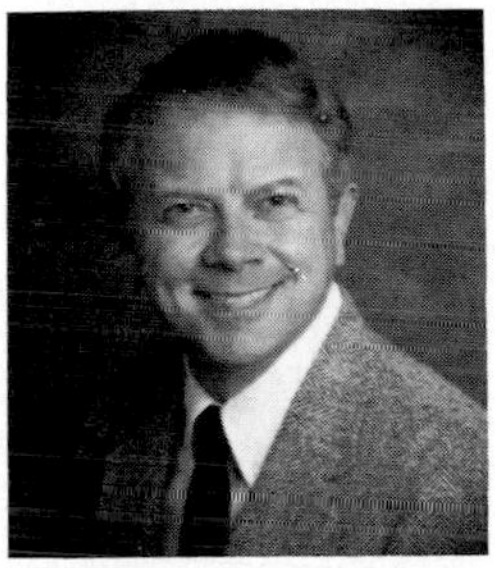

C. B. CHASTAIN, D.V.M., M.S.
Diplomate, College of Veterinary Internal Medicine (Internal Medicine); Professor and Section Head of Small Animal Medicine, Coordinator of the Small Animal Veterinary Medical Teaching Hospital, Department of Veterinary Medicine and Surgery, College of Veterinary Medicine, University of Missouri, Columbia, Missouri.
Use of Corticosteroids

DENNIS J. CHEW, D.V.M.
Diplomate, American College of Veterinary Internal Medicine (Internal Medicine); Associate Professor of Medicine, Department of Veterinary Clinical Sciences, College of Veterinary Medicine, Ohio State University, Columbus, Ohio.
Diagnosis and Pathophysiology of Renal Disease

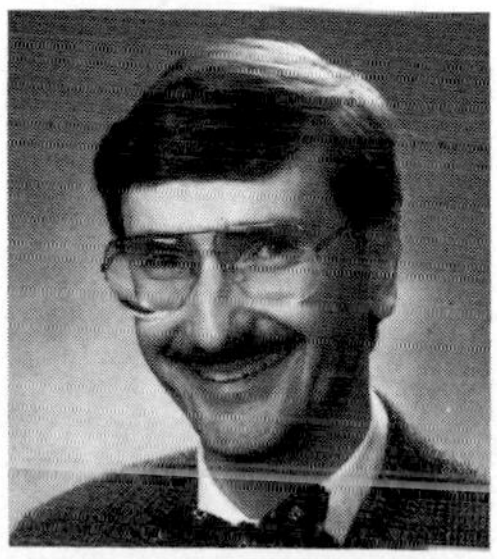

GEORGINA CHILD, B.V.Sc., M.R.C.V.S.
Diplomate, American College of Veterinary Medicine (Neurology); Research Associate, Veterinary Teaching Hospital, Colorado State University, Fort Collins, Colorado.
Diseases of the Spinal Cord

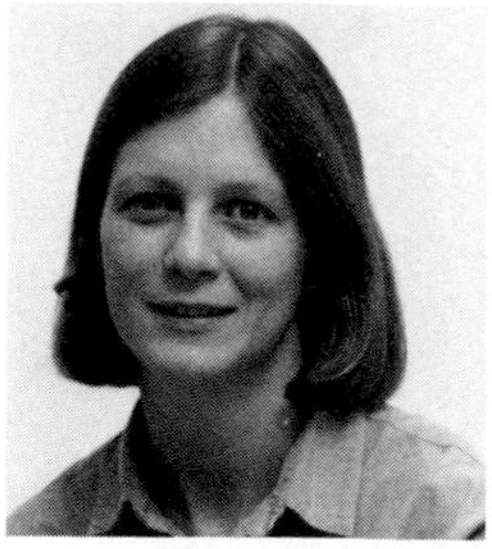

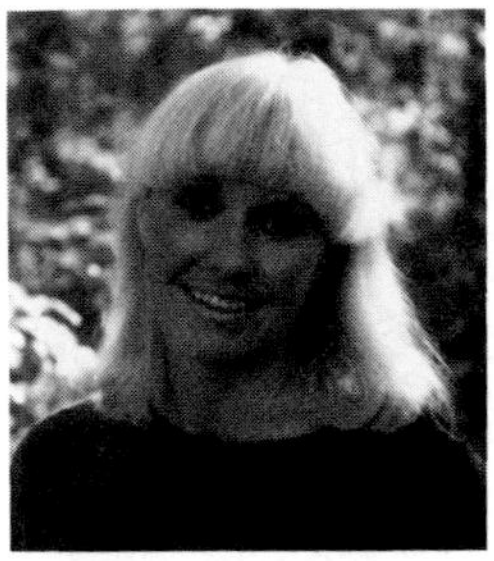

CHERYL L. CHRISMAN, D.V.M., M.S.
Diplomate, American College of Veterinary Internal Medicine (Neurology); Professor, Assistant Dean for Instruction, and Chief of Neurology Service, Veterinary Medical Teaching Hospital, University of Florida, Gainesville, Florida.
Peripheral Nerve Disorders

BERNARD CLERC, D.V.M.
Professeur de Pathologie Medicale, Ecole Nationale Veterinaire, Lyon, France.
Ocular Manifestations of Systemic Disease

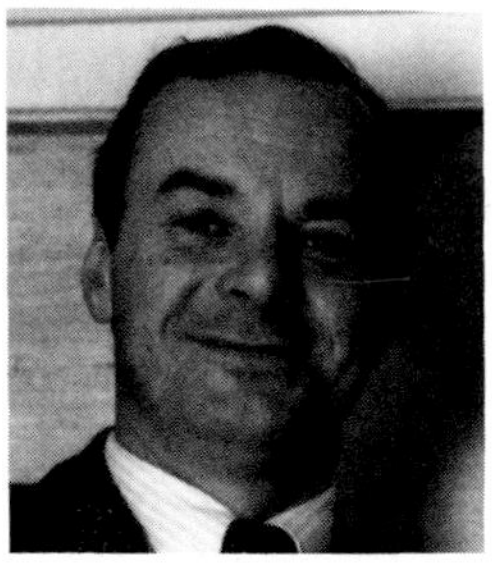

EMBERT H. COLES, D.V.M., Ph.D.
Professor Emeritus and Consultant, Veterinary Reference Laboratory, College of Veterinary Medicine, Kansas State University, Manhattan, Kansas.
Tables of Abnormal Blood Values as a Guide to Disease Syndromes

SUSAN M. COTTER, D.V.M.
Diplomate, American College of Veterinary Internal Medicine (Internal Medicine and Oncology); Associate Professor of Medicine and Head, Small Animal Medicine, Tufts University School of Veterinary Medicine, North Grafton, Massachusetts.
Anemia

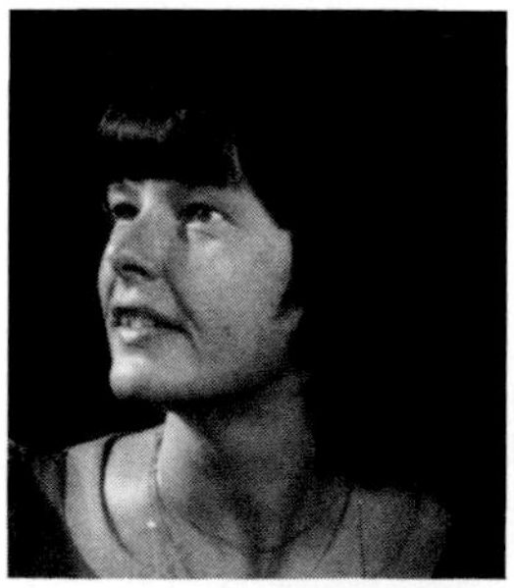

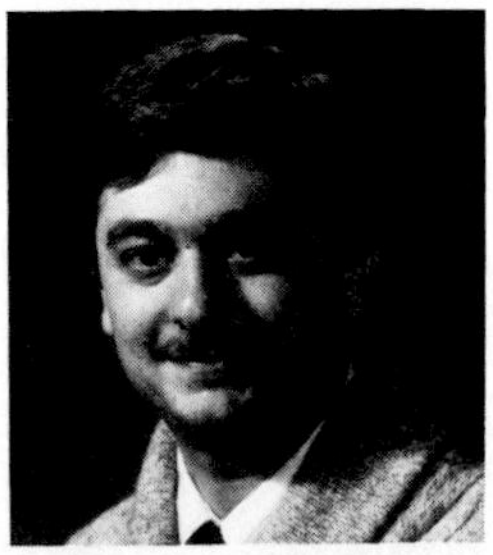

C. GUILLERMO COUTO, D.V.M.
Diplomate, American College of Veterinary Internal Medicine (Internal Medicine and Oncology); Assistant Professor, Department of Veterinary Clinical Sciences, College of Veterinary Medicine, The Ohio State University, Columbus, Ohio.
Diseases of the Lymph Nodes and Spleen

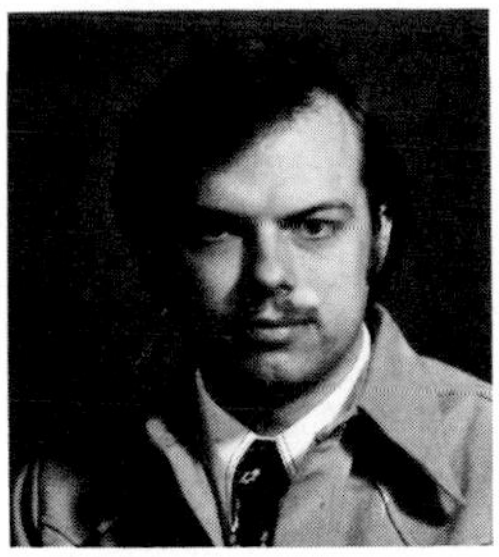

STEVEN E. CROW, D.V.M.

Diplomate, American College of Veterinary Internal Medicine (Internal Medicine and Oncology); Associate Professor of Internal Medicine and Oncology, Department of Small Animal Clinical Sciences, College of Veterinary Medicine, Michigan State University, East Lansing, Michigan.

Tumor Biology

LLOYD E. DAVIS, D.V.M., Ph.D.

Professor of Pharmacology and of Veterinary Clinical Medicine, College of Veterinary Medicine, University of Illinois at Urbana-Champaign, Illinois.

Adverse Drug Reactions

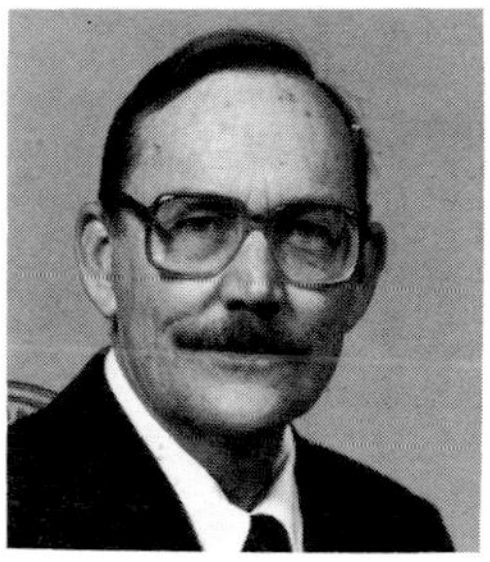

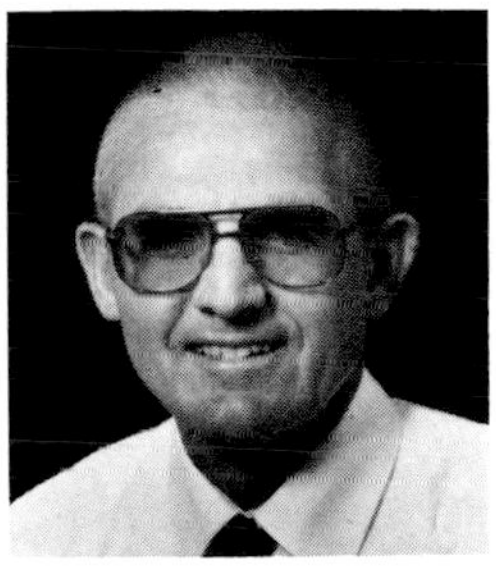

ALEXANDER de LAHUNTA, D.V.M., Ph.D.

Diplomate, American College of Veterinary Internal Medicine (Neurology); Professor of Anatomy and Chairman, Department of Anatomy, New York State College of Veterinary Medicine, Cornell University; Clinical Neurologist, Veterinary Medical Teaching Hospital, Ithaca, New York.

Neuro-ophthalmology

STANLEY MARK DENNIS, B.V.Sc., Ph.D., F.R.C.V.S., F.R.C.Path.

Diplomate, American College of Theriogenologists; Professor of Pathology, Kansas State University, College of Veterinary Medicine, Manhattan, Kansas.

Chromosomal and Genetic Disorders

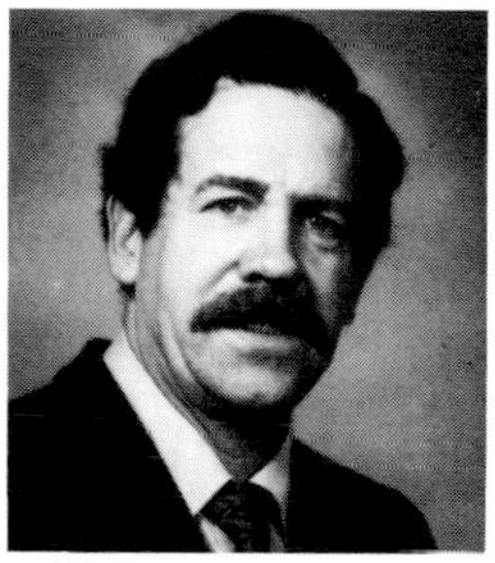

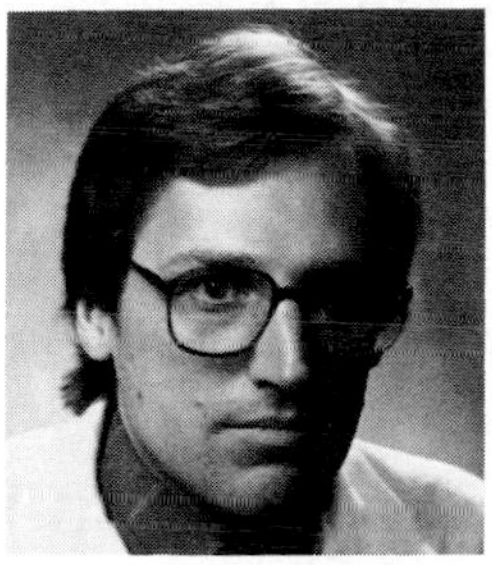

STEPHEN P. DiBARTOLA, D.V.M.

Diplomate, American College of Veterinary Internal Medicine (Internal Medicine); Associate Professor of Medicine, Department of Veterinary Clinical Sciences, College of Veterinary Medicine, Ohio State University, Columbus, Ohio.

Diagnosis and Pathophysiology of Renal Disease

FREDERICK HOWARD DRAZNER, D.V.M.

Diplomate, American College of Veterinary Medicine (Internal Medicine); Director of Medical Services, Wright Animal Hospital, Des Plaines; Chief of Staff, Animal Specialty Service of Cook County, Des Plaines; Consultant: Illinois Veterinary Laboratory, Elmhurst, Colorado, Veterinary Laboratories, Broomfield, Comparative Medicine, Rush Medical School, Chicago, Illinois.

Polycythemia

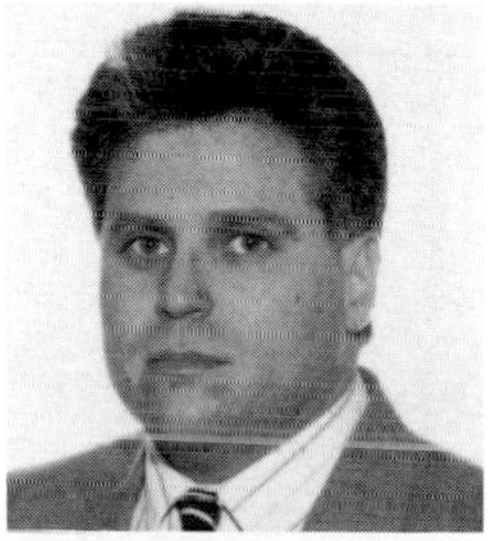

J. E. EIGENMANN, D.V.M., Ph.D.
Clinique Veterinaire, Boudevillers, Switzerland.
Pituitary-Hypothalamic Disease

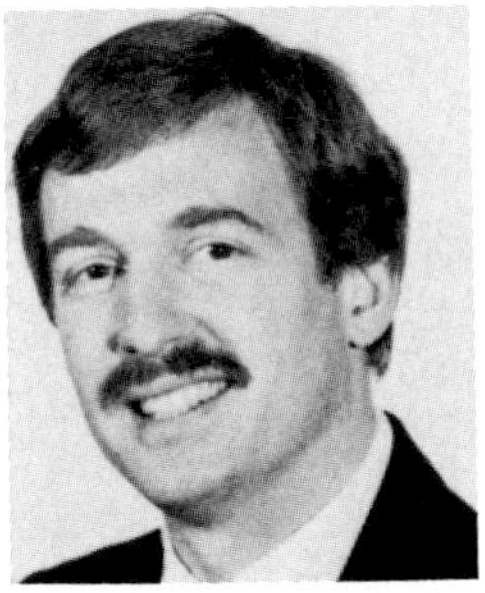

GARY W. ELLISON, D.V.M., M.S.
Diplomate, American College of Veterinary Surgeons; Assistant Professor, Department of Surgical Sciences, College of Veterinary Medicine, University of Florida, Gainesville, Florida.
Recto-Anal Disease

BERNARD F. FELDMAN, D.V.M., Ph.D.
Professor of Clinical Hematology and Biochemistry, Director, Comparative Hemostasis Laboratory, Chief, Bone Marrow Cytology Service, Veterinary Medical Teaching Hospital, School of Veterinary Medicine, University of California at Davis, Davis, California.
Platelet Dysfunction

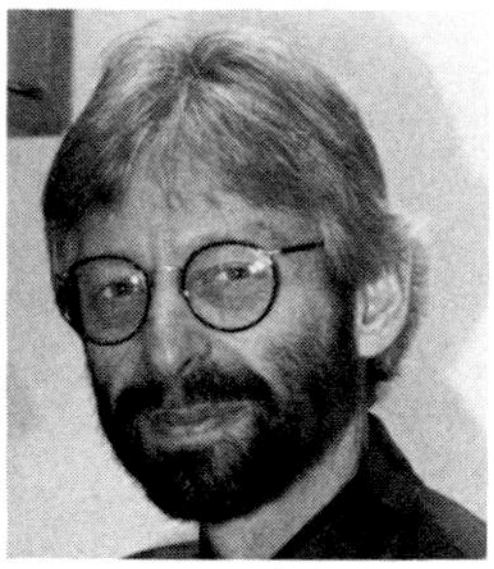

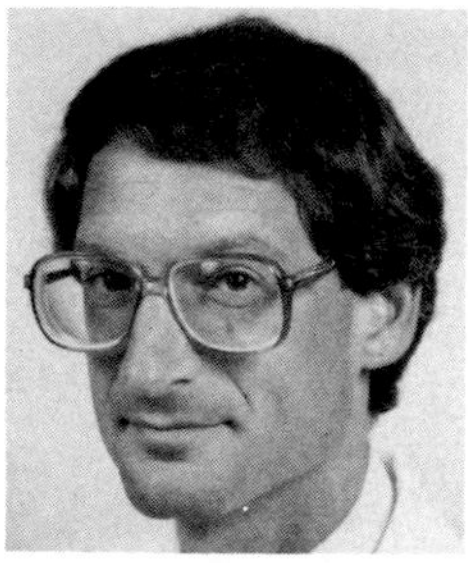

EDWARD C. FELDMAN, D.V.M.
Diplomate, American College of Veterinary Internal Medicine (Internal Medicine); Professor, Small Animal Medicine and Reproduction, Department of Reproduction, School of Veterinary Medicine, University of California at Davis, Davis, California.
Adrenal Gland Disease; Infertility

WILLIAM R. FENNER, D.V.M.
Diplomate, American College of Veterinary Internal Medicine (Neurology); Associate Professor, Department of Veterinary Clinical Sciences, College of Veterinary Medicine; Staff Neurologist, Veterinary Teaching Hospital, College of Veterinary Medicine, The Ohio State University, Columbus, Ohio.
The Neurologic Evaluation of Patients

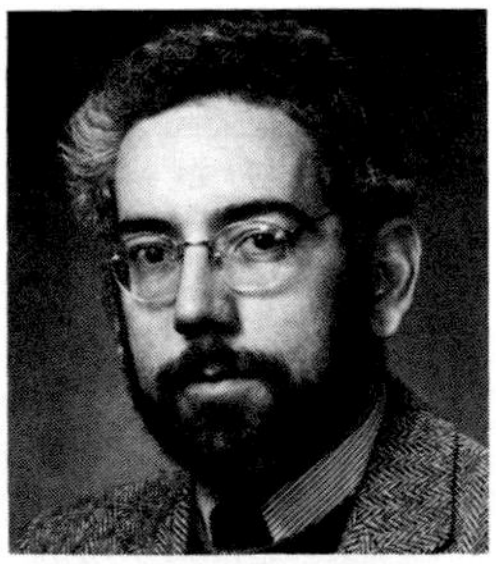

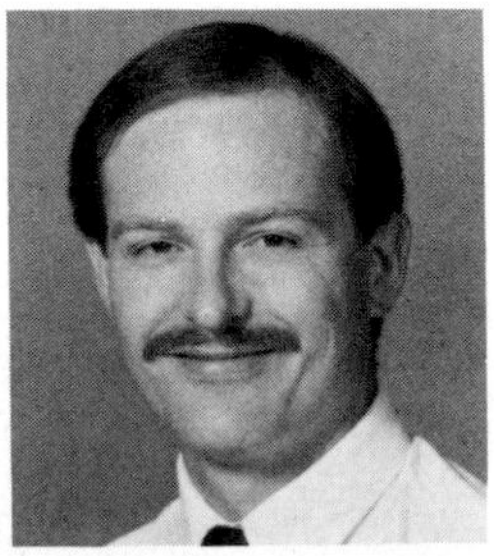

DUNCAN C. FERGUSON, V.M.D., Ph.D.
Diplomate, American College of Veterinary Internal Medicine (Internal Medicine); Assistant Professor of Physiology and Pharmacology, University of Georgia College of Veterinary Medicine, Athens, Georgia.
Thyroid Diseases

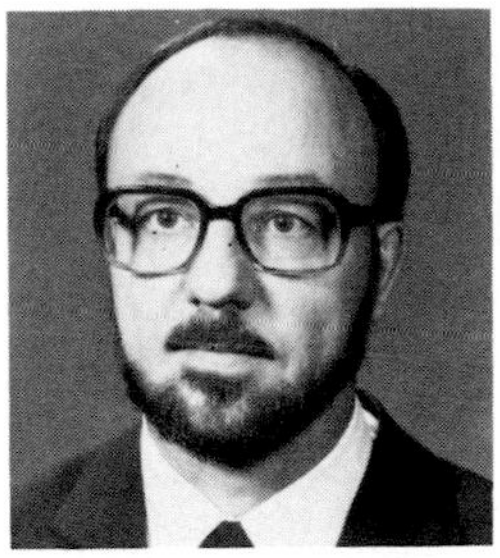

DELMAR R. FINCO, D.V.M., Ph.D.
Diplomate, American College of Veterinary Medicine (Internal Medicine); Professor of Physiology and Pharmacology, College of Veterinary Medicine, University of Georgia, Athens, Georgia.
Canine Prostatic Diseases

PHILIP R. FOX, D.V.M., M.Sc.
Diplomate, American College Veterinary Internal Medicine (Cardiology); Chairman, Department of Clinic Services and Staff Cardiologist, Animal Medical Center, New York, New York.
Myocardial Diseases

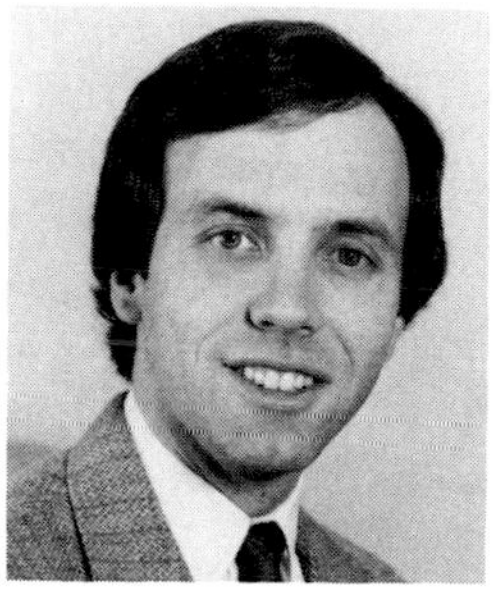

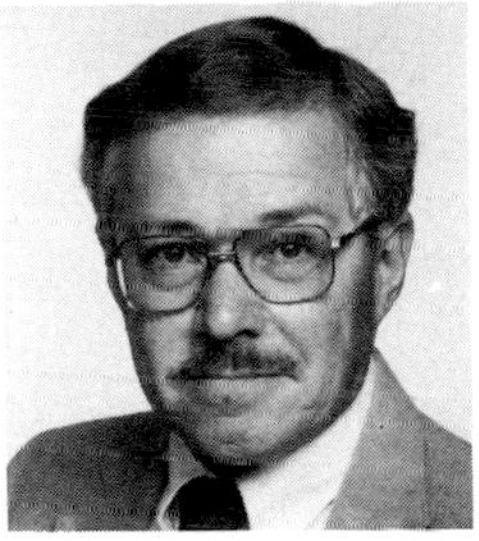

ROBERT A. GREEN, D.V.M., Ph.D.
Diplomate, American College of Veterinary Pathologists; Professor of Veterinary Pathology and Director, Clinical Pathology Laboratory, Veterinary Teaching Hospital, College of Veterinary Medicine, Texas A and M University, College Station, Texas.
Hemostatic Disorders: Coagulopathies and Thrombotic Disorders

CRAIG E. GREENE, D.V.M., M.S.
Diplomate, American College of Veterinary Medicine (Internal Medicine and Neurology); Professor of Small Animal Medicine, College of Veterinary Medicine, University of Georgia, Athens, Georgia.
Diseases of the Brain

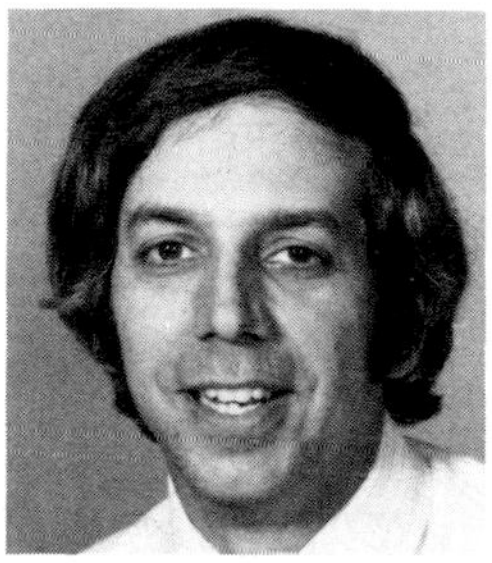

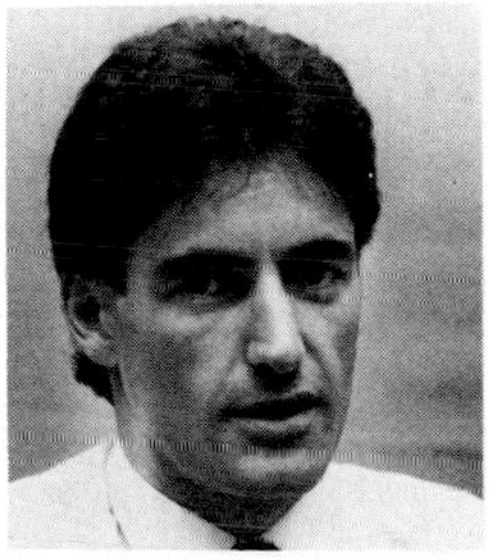

W. GRANT GUILFORD, B.Phil., B.V.Sc.
Diplomate, American College of Veterinary Internal Medicine (Internal Medicine).
Diseases of the Esophagus

DAVID A. HAGER, D.V.M.
Diplomate, American College of Veterinary Radiology; Radiology Consulting Service, Cardiff, California.
Diseases of the Gallbladder

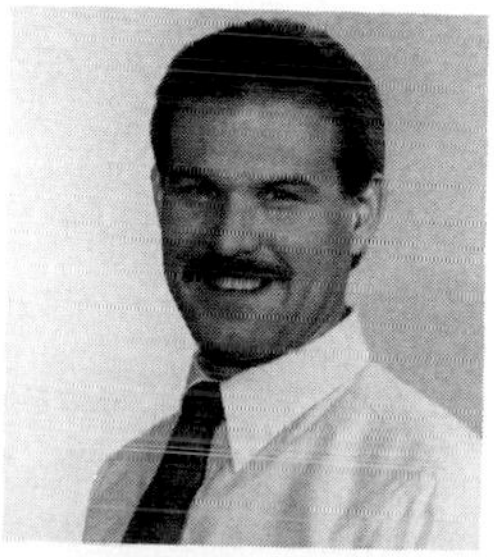

ROBERT M. HARDY, D.V.M.
Diplomate, American College of Veterinary Internal Medicine (Internal Medicine); Associate Professor, Department of Small Animal Clinical Sciences, College of Veterinary Medicine, University of Minnesota, St. Paul, Minnesota.
Diseases of the Liver and Their Treatment

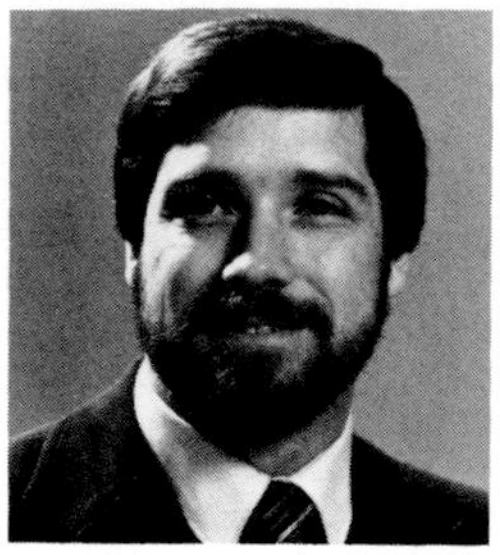

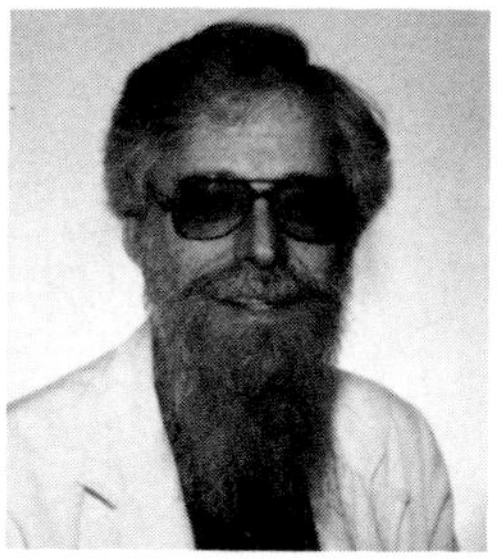

JAMES M. HARRIS, D.V.M.
Montclair Veterinary Hospital, Oakland, California; Chairperson, Human/Animal Bond Committee, C.V.M.A., Member, Human/Animal Bond Commitee, A.V.M.A.
Human-Animal Bond and Euthanasia—A Special Problem

COLIN E. HARVEY, B.V.Sc., F.R.C.V.S.
Diplomate, American College of Veterinary Surgeons; Diplomate, American Veterinary Dental College; Professor of Surgery, Department of Clinical Studies, School of Veterinary Medicine; Adjunct Professor, School of Dental Medicine, University of Pennsylvania, Philadelphia, Pennsylvania.
Oral, Dental, Pharyngeal, and Salivary Gland Disorders

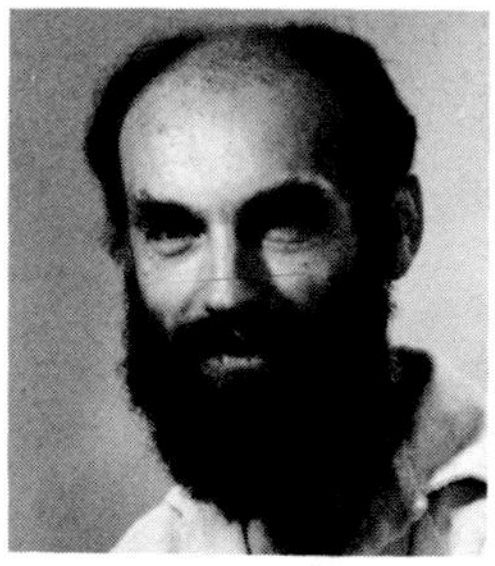

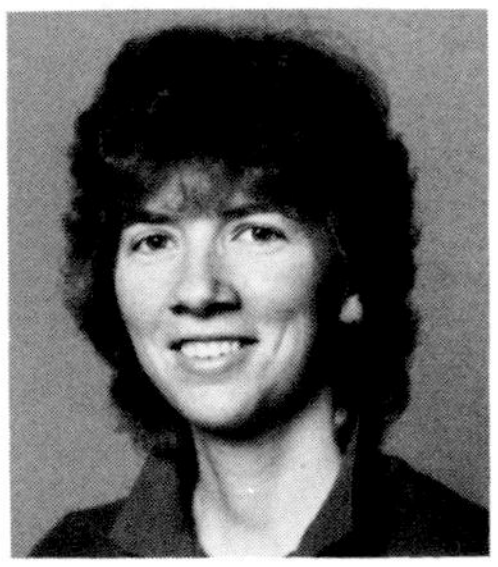

ELEANOR C. HAWKINS, D.V.M.
Diplomate, American College of Veterinary Internal Medicine (Internal Medicine); Assistant Professor, Department of Veterinary Clinical Sciences, School of Veterinary Medicine, Purdue University, West Lafayette, Indiana.
Diseases of the Lower Respiratory Tract (Lung) and Pulmonary Edema

ROSEMARY A. HENIK, D.V.M., M.S.
Internist, Peninsula Veterinary Service, Sturgeon Bay, Wisconsin.
Cardiopulmonary Arrest and Resuscitation

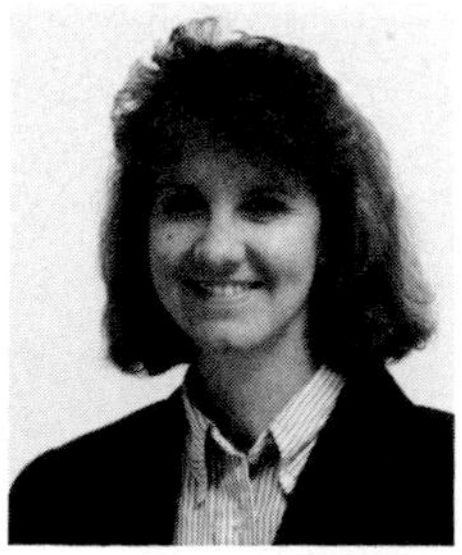

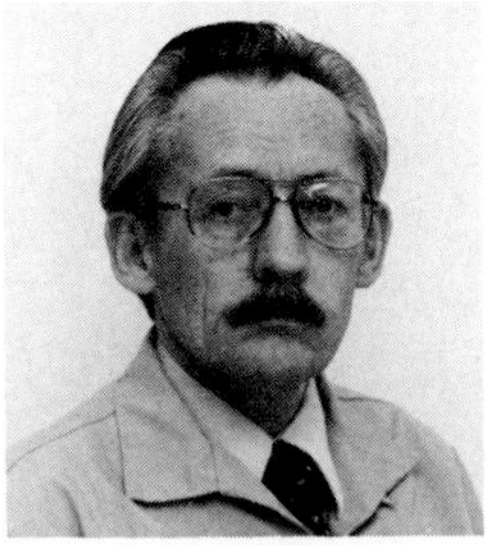

PAUL W. HUSTED, V.M.D., M.S.
Department of Reproduction, College of Veterinary Medicine, Colorado State University, Fort Collins, Colorado.
Persistent Estrus in the Bitch

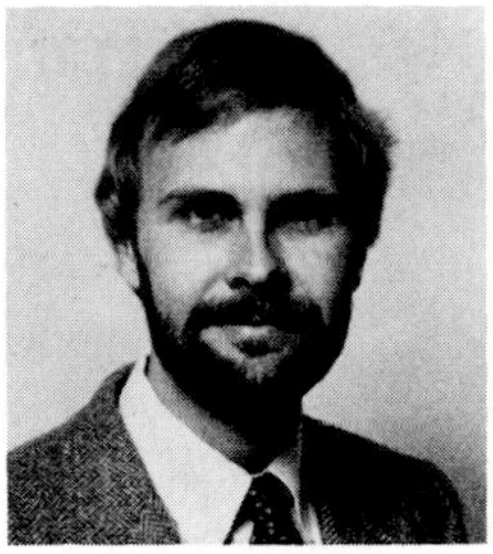

PETER J. IHRKE, V.M.D.
Diplomate, American College of Veterinary Dermatology; Associate Professor of Dermatology and Allergy, School of Veterinary Medicine, University of California at Davis; Chief, Dermatology Service, Veterinary Medical Teaching Hospital, Davis, California.
Pruritus

GILBERT JACOBS, D.V.M.
Diplomate, American College of Veterinary Internal Medicine (Cardiology); Assistant Professor of Medicine, Department of Small Animal Medicine, College of Veterinary Medicine, University of Georgia, Athens, Georgia.
Cyanosis

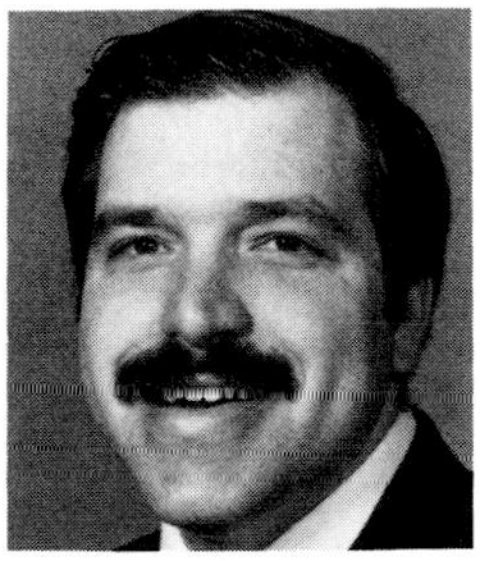

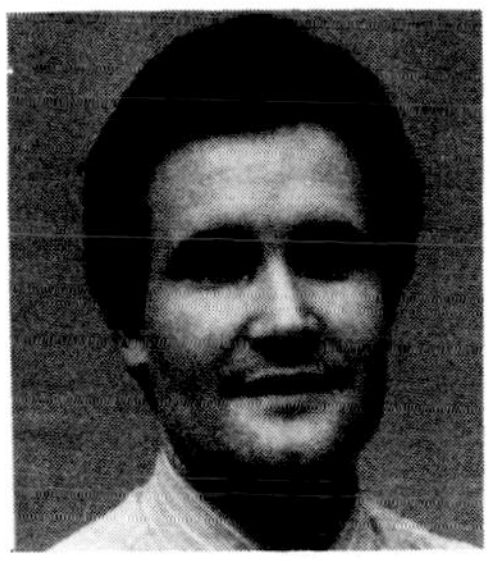

ALBERT E. JERGENS, D.V.M.
Diplomate, American College of Veterinary Internal Medicine (Internal Medicine); Angell Memorial Animal Hospital, Boston, Massachusetts.
Diseases of the Esophagus

CHERI A. JOHNSON, D.V.M., M.S.
Diplomate, American College of Veterinary Internal Medicine (Internal Medicine); Associate Professor, Department of Small Animal Clinical Sciences, Michigan State University, East Lansing, Michigan.
Uterine Diseases; Vaginal Disorders

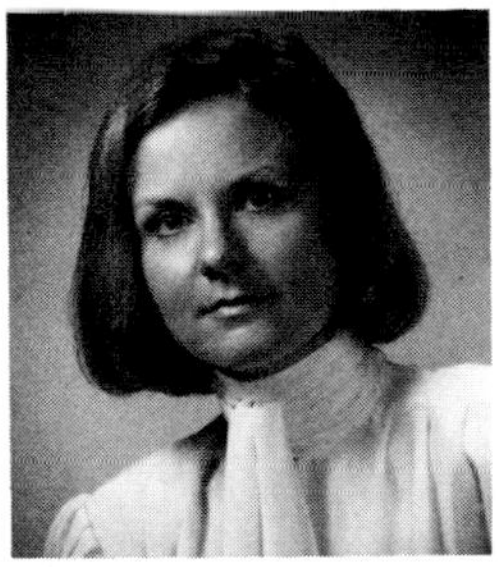

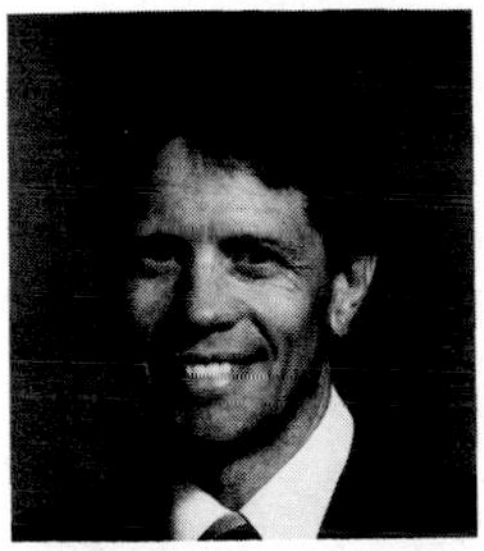

ROGER K. JOHNSON, D.V.M.
Diplomate, American College of Veterinary Internal Medicine (Internal Medicine); Encino Veterinary Hospital, Walnut Creek, California.
Canine Hyperlipidemia

GARY R. JOHNSTON, D.V.M., M.S.
Diplomate, American College of Veterinary Radiology; Associate Professor of Comparative Radiology, Department of Small Animal Clinical Sciences, College of Veterinary Medicine, University of Minnesota, St. Paul, Minnesota.
Feline Lower Urinary Tract Disorders; Canine Uroliths

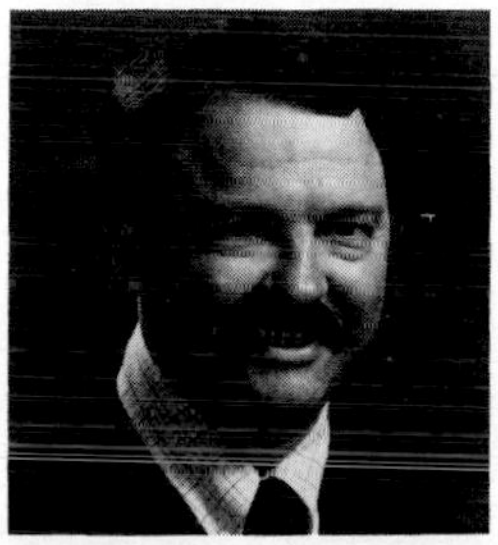

SHIRLEY D. JOHNSTON, D.V.M., Ph.D.
Diplomate, American College of Theriogenologists; Associate Professor, Small Animal Medicine, Department of Small Animal Clinical Sciences, College of Veterinary Medicine, University of Minnesota, St. Paul, Minnesota.
Disorders of the External Genitalia of the Male

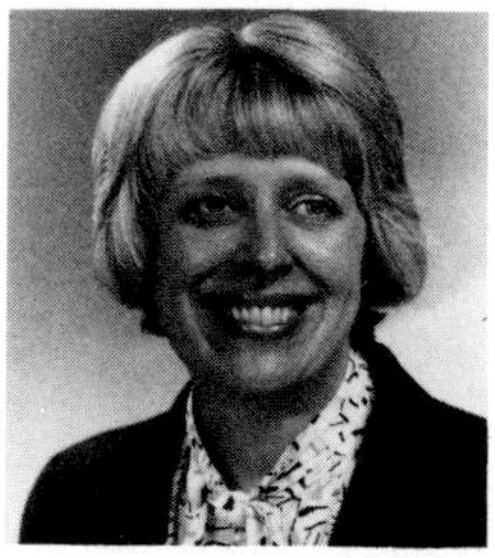

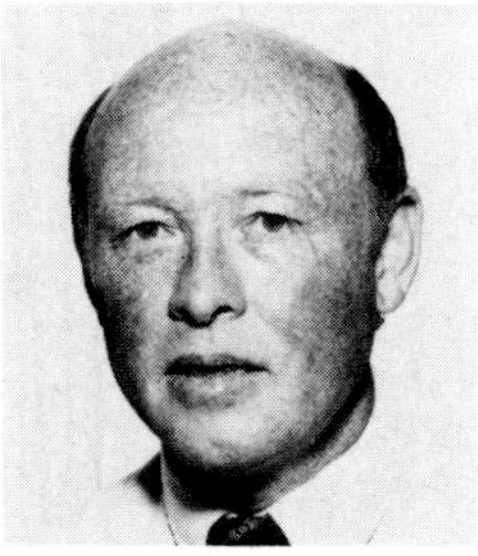

BOYD R. JONES, B.V.Sc., F.A.C.V.Sc.
Senior Lecturer in Small Animal Medicine, Massey University, Palmerston North, New Zealand.
Feline Hyperlipidemia

BRENT D. JONES, D.V.M.
Associate Professor, Department of Veterinary Medicine and Surgery, College of Veterinary Medicine, University of Missouri; Staff Gastroenterologist, Veterinary Medical Teaching Hospital, University of Missouri, Columbia, Missouri.
Diseases of the Esophagus

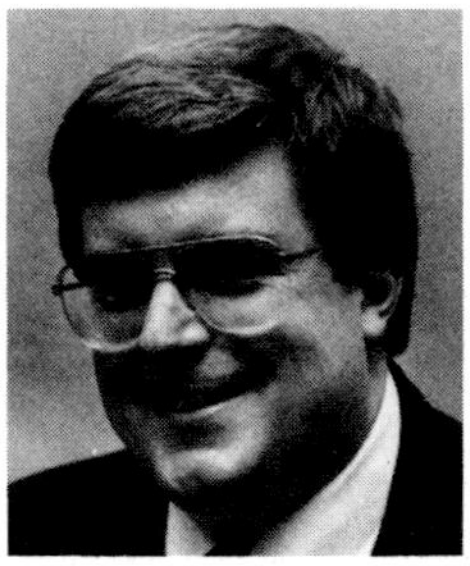

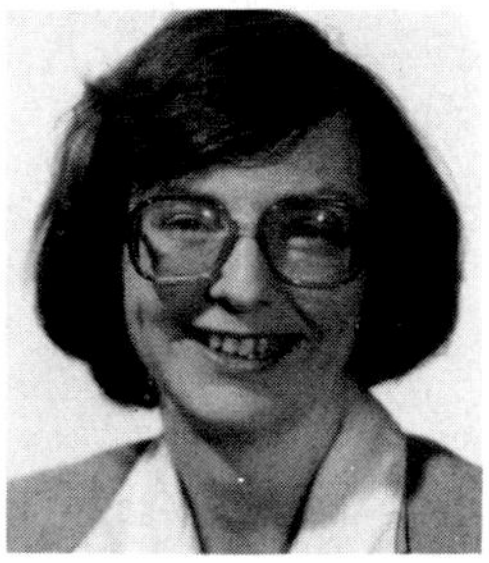

GERALDINE McCALL KAUFMAN, D.V.M.
Diplomate, American College of Veterinary Internal Medicine (Internal Medicine); Private Referral Practice, Bridgeton, New Jersey.
Hematuria–Dysuria

BRUCE W. KEENE, D.V.M., M.Sc.
Diplomate, American College of Veterinary Internal Medicine (Cardiology); Assistant Professor, College of Veterinary Medicine, Department of Companion Animal and Special Species, North Carolina State University, Raleigh, North Carolina.
Therapy of Heart Failure

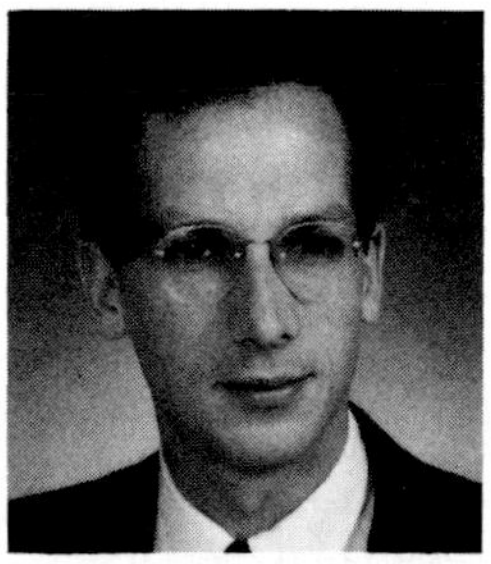

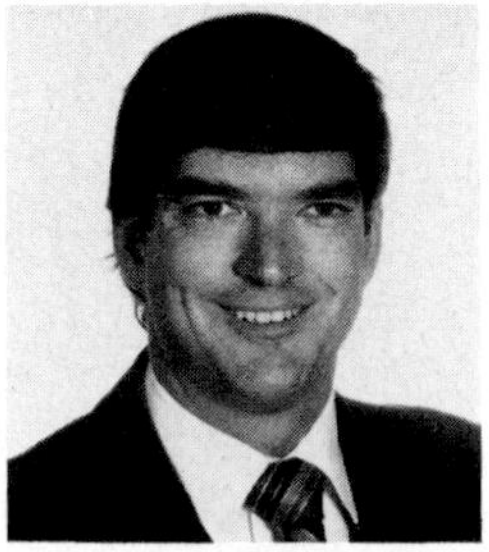

MICHAEL JOHN KELLY, D.V.M.
Diplomate, American College of Veterinary Internal Medicine (Internal Medicine); Head of Medicine, Main Street Small Animal Hospital, San Diego; Consultant, Veterinary Reference Laboratory, San Diego, California.
Pain (General, Back, Extremities, Abdomen)

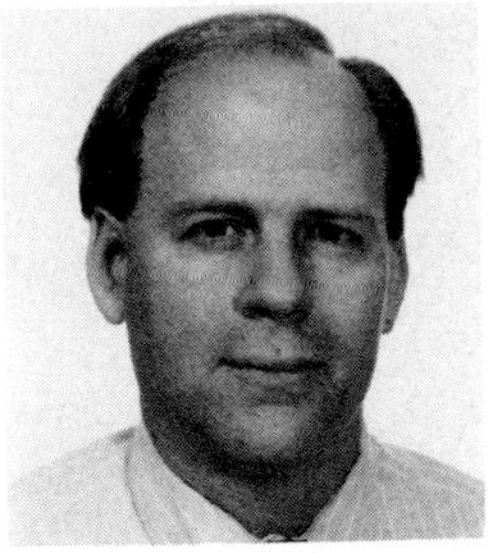

ROBERT R. KING, D.V.M., Ph.D.
Assistant Professor and Chief of Cardiopulmonary Service, University of Florida College of Veterinary Medicine, Gainesville, Florida.
Clinical Approach to the Patient with Respiratory Disease

BARBARA E. KITCHELL, D.V.M.
Diplomate, American College of Veterinary Internal Medicine (Internal Medicine); Staff Internist/Oncologist, Special Veterinary Services, Berkeley; Assistant Clinical Professor of Oncology, University of California, School of Veterinary Medicine, Davis, California.
Anorexia and Polyphagia

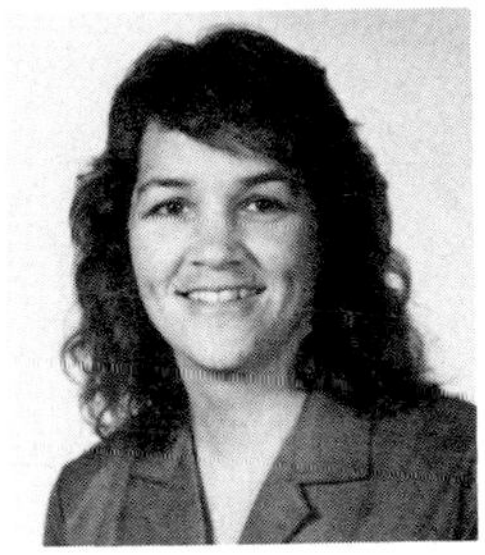

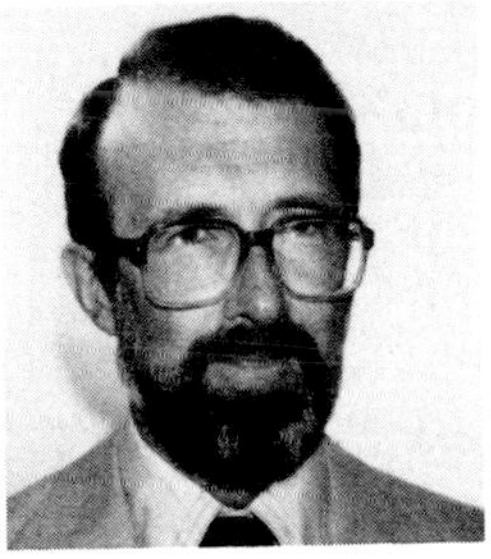

DAVID H. KNIGHT, D.V.M.
Diplomate, American College of Veterinary Internal Medicine (Cardiology); Associate Professor of Medicine and Cardiologist, Veterinary Hospital, University of Pennsylvania School of Veterinary Medicine, Philadelphia, Pennsylvania.
Pathophysiology of Heart Failure

LILLY I. KONG, D.V.M., M.S.
Hillcrest Biologicals, Cyrecs, California.
Bacterial, Rickettsial, Protozoal, and Miscellaneous Infections

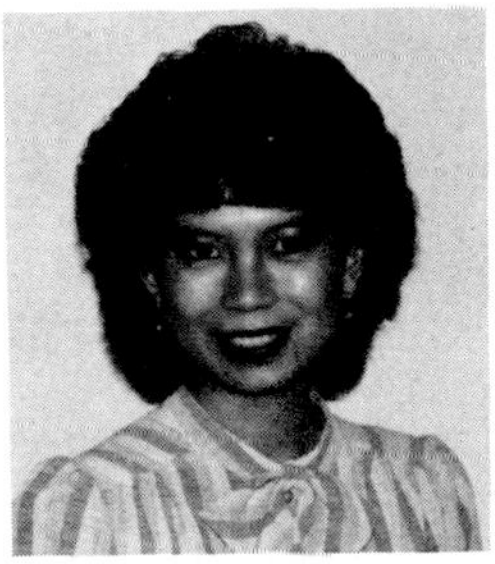

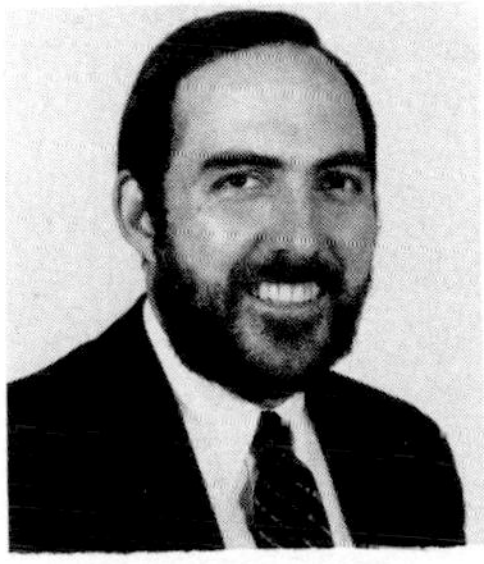

JOE N. KORNEGAY, D.V.M., Ph.D.
Diplomate, American College of Veterinary Internal Medicine (Neurology); Professor of Neurology, North Carolina State University College of Veterinary Medicine, Raleigh, North Carolina.
Trembling and Shivering; Seizures

JOHN M. KRUGER, D.V.M.
Veterinary Medical Associate, Department of Small Animal Clinical Sciences, College of Veterinary Medicine, University of Minnesota, St. Paul, Minnesota.
Feline Lower Urinary Tract Disorders

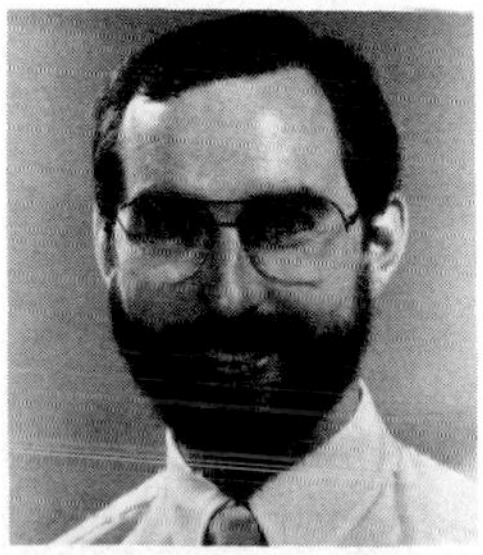

STEPHEN B. LANE, D.V.M.
Resident in Neurology, North Carolina State University, College of Veterinary Medicine, Raleigh, North Carolina.
Seizures

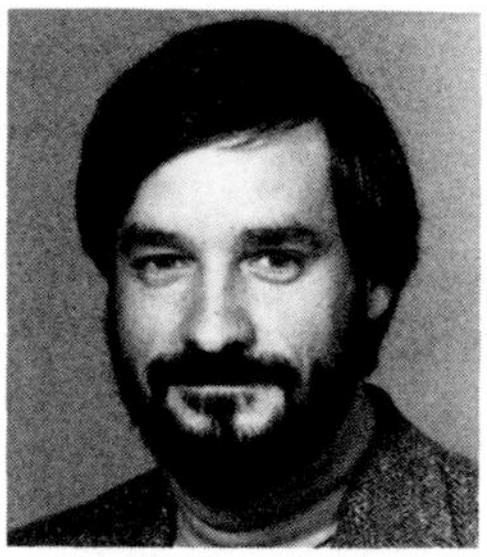

KENNETH S. LATIMER, D.V.M., Ph.D.
Diplomate, American College of Veterinary Pathologists (Clinical Pathology); Associate Professor of Pathology, Department of Veterinary Pathology, College of Veterinary Medicine, University of Georgia, Athens, Georgia.
Leukocytes in Health and Disease

RICHARD A. LeCOUTEUR, B.V.Sc., Ph.D.
Diplomate, American College of Veterinary Internal Medicine (Neurology); Associate Professor, Department of Clinical Sciences, College of Veterinary Medicine and Biomedical Sciences, Colorado State University, Fort Collins, Colorado.
Diseases of the Spinal Cord

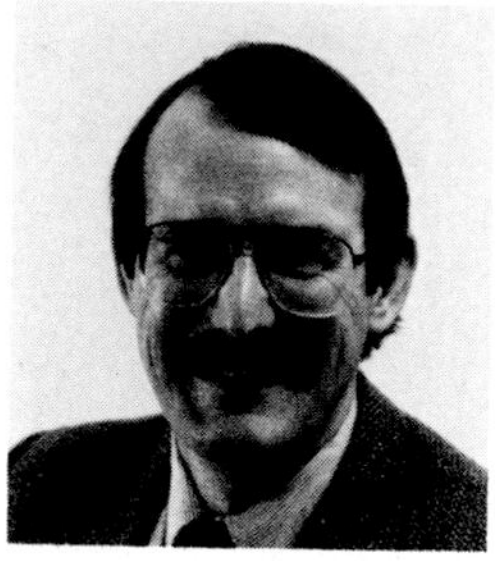

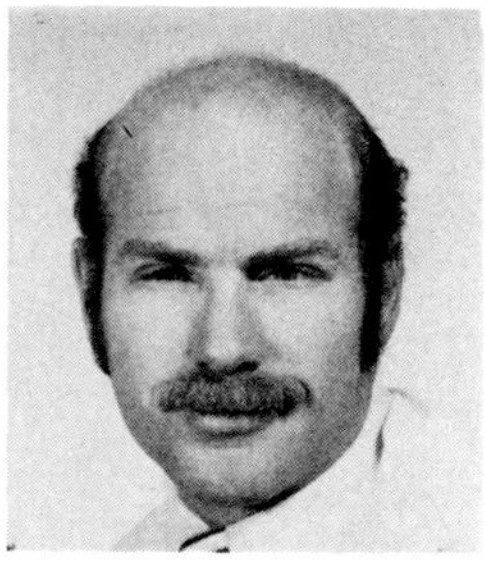

GEORGE E. LEES, D.V.M., M.S.
Diplomate, American College of Veterinary Internal Medicine (Internal Medicine); Professor and Chief, Small Animal Medicine Services, Department of Small Animal Medicine and Surgery, College of Veterinary Medicine, Texas A and M University, College Station, Texas.
Incontinence, Enuresis, and Nocturia; Urinary Obstruction and Atony

MICHAEL S. LEIB, D.V.M., M.S.
Diplomate, American College of Veterinary Internal Medicine (Internal Medicine); Associate Professor, Department of Small Animal Clinical Sciences and Chief, Small Animal Medicine, Veterinary Teaching Hospital Virginia-Maryland Regional College of Veterinary Medicine, Virginia Tech, Blacksburg, Virginia.
Food Hypersensitivity

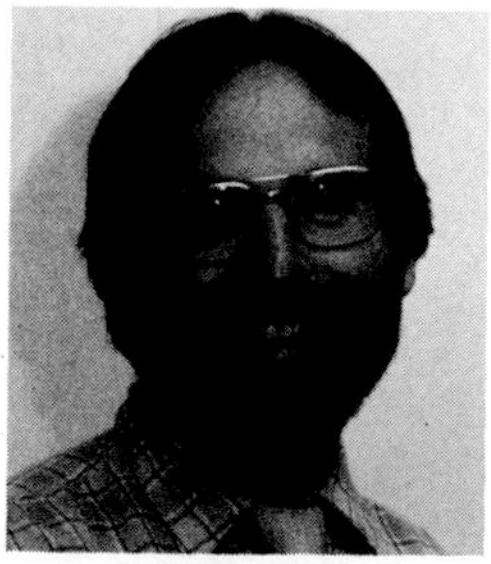

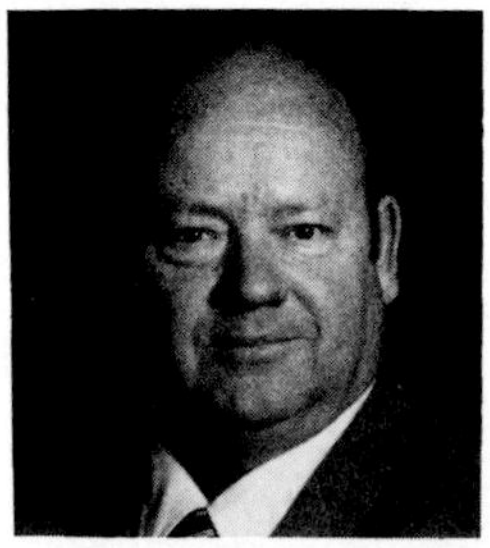

H. W. LEIPOLD, D.V.M., Ph.D.
Distinguished Professor, Department of Pathology, College of Veterinary Medicine, Kansas State University, Manhattan, Kansas.
Chromosomal and Genetic Disorders

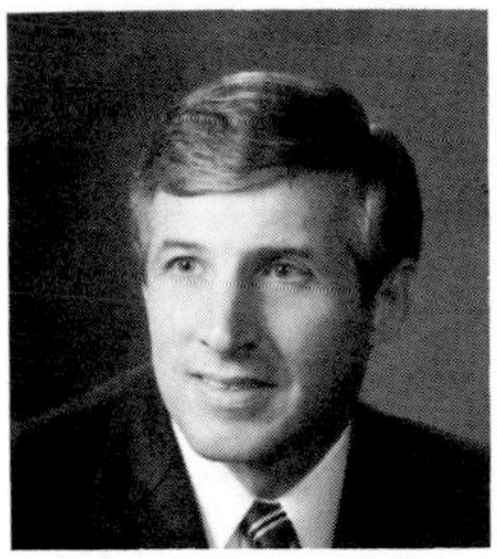

CHARLES L. LIPPINCOTT, D.V.M.
Diplomate, American College of Veterinary Surgeons; Head of Surgery, California Animal Hospital Corporation, West Los Angeles, California.
Gastric Dilatation-Volvulus-Torsion Syndrome

ANDREW S. LOAR, D.V.M.
Diplomate, American College of Veterinary Internal Medicine (Internal Medicine); Consultant, Veterinary Reference Laboratory, Anaheim; Oncology Referral Practice, San Diego; West Los Angeles Veterinary Medical Group, Los Angeles, California.
Tumors of the Genital System and Mammary Glands

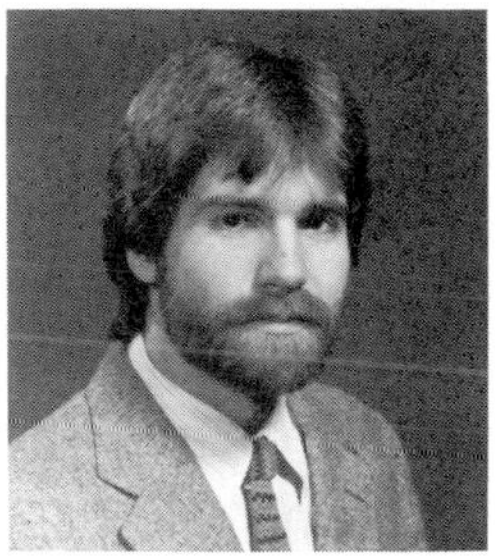

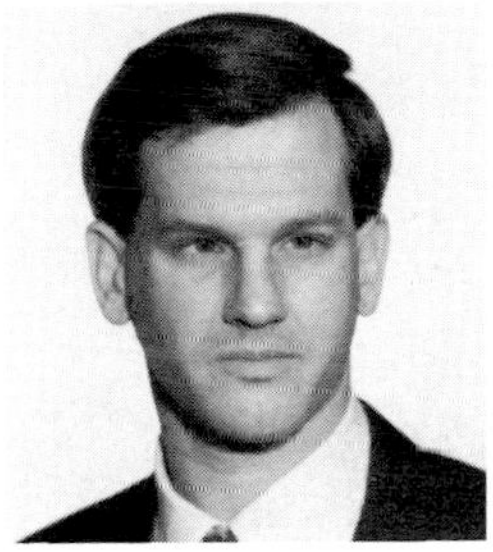

ROBERT H. LUSK, Jr., D.V.M.
Staff Member in Medicine, California Animal Hospital Inc., Los Angeles, California.
Thermoregulation

E. GREGORY MacEWEN, V.M.D.
Diplomate, American College of Veterinary Internal Medicine (Internal Medicine and Oncology); Professor of Medicine and Oncology and Associate Dean for Clinical Affairs; Interim Chairman, Department of Surgical Sciences, School of Veterinary Medicine; University of Wisconsin-Madison, Madison, Wisconsin.
Approach to Treatment of Cancer Patients

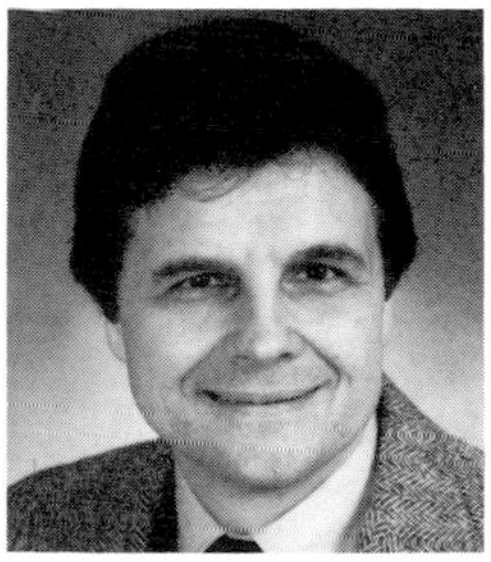

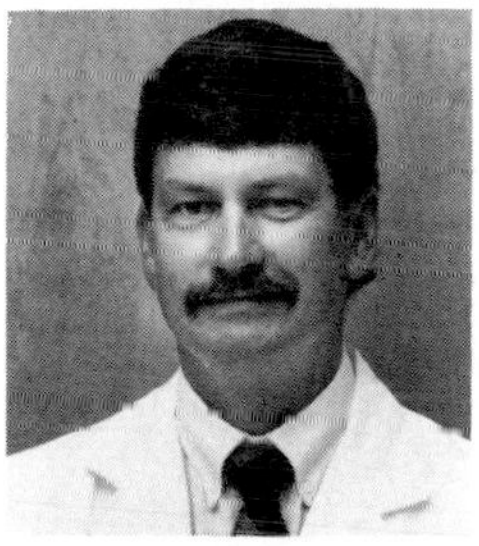

DENNIS W. MACY, D.V.M., M.S.
Diplomate, American College of Veterinary Internal Medicine (Internal Medicine and Oncology); Associate Professor of Medicine, Medical Oncology and Internal Medicine, Department of Clinical Sciences, College of Veterinary Medicine and Biological Sciences, Colorado State University, Fort Collins, Colorado.
Diseases of the Ear

MICHAEL L. MAGNE, D.V.M.
Diplomate, American College of Veterinary Internal Medicine (Internal Medicine); Staff Internist, Santa Rosa Veterinary Specialty Group, Rohnert Park, California.
Diseases of the Stomach

RICHARD K. MARTIN, D.V.M.
Diplomate, American College of Veterinary Internal Medicine (Internal Medicine); Staff Member, Brentwood Pet Clinic, Los Angeles, California.
Diarrhea

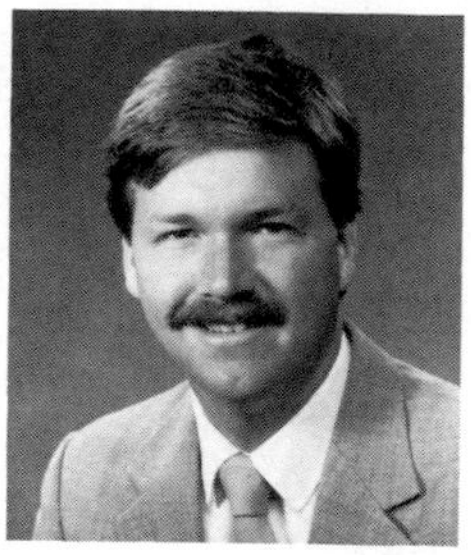

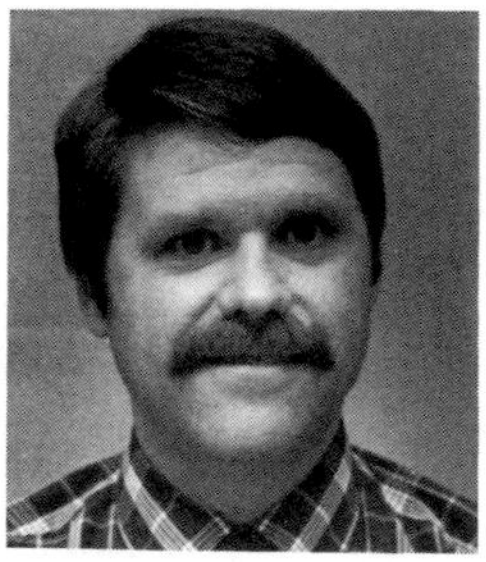

DUDLEY L. McCAW, D.V.M.
Diplomate, American College of Veterinary Internal Medicine (Internal Medicine); Assistant Professor, Department of Medicine and Surgery, College of Veterinary Medicine, University of Missouri, Columbia, Missouri.
Lumps, Bumps, Masses, and Lymphadenopathy

WILLIAM F. McCULLOCH, D.V.M., M.P.H.
Associate Dean, College of Veterinary Medicine and Biomedical Sciences, Colorado State University, Fort Collins, Colorado; Chairman, Committee for Human-Animal Bonding, AVMA.
Human-Animal Bond and Euthanasia—A Special Problem

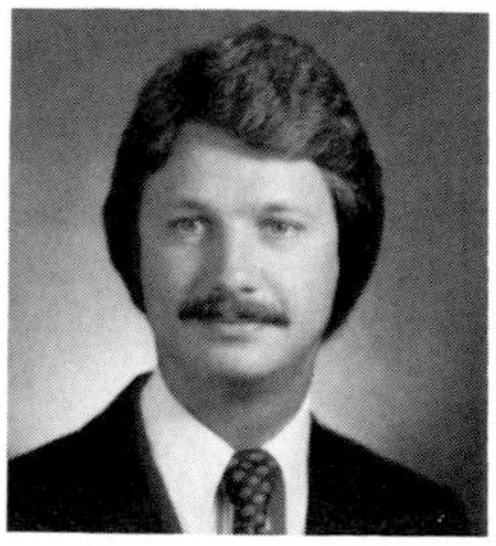

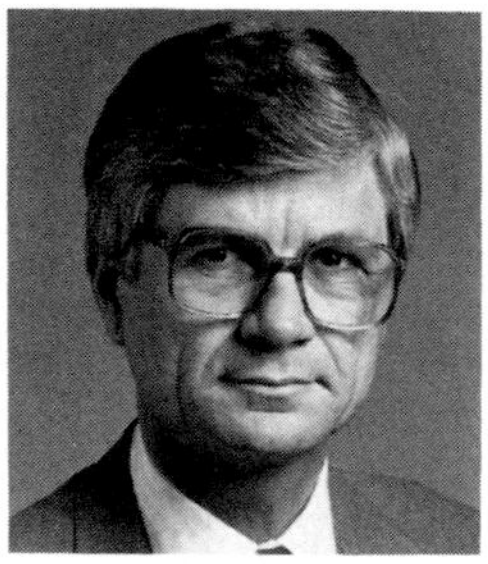

MICHAEL J. McCULLOCH, M.D. (DECEASED)
Associate Clinical Professor of Psychiatry in Veterinary Medicine, Oregon State University, School of Veterinary Medicine, Corvallis, Oregon; Practicing Psychiatrist, Northwest Psychiatric Associates, Portland, Oregon.
Human-Animal Bond and Euthanasia—A Special Problem

DONALD J. MEUTEN, D.V.M., Ph.D.
Diplomate, American College of Veterinary Pathologists; Associate Professor of Pathology, North Carolina State University School of Veterinary Medicine, Raleigh, North Carolina.
Parathyroid Disease and Calcium Metabolism

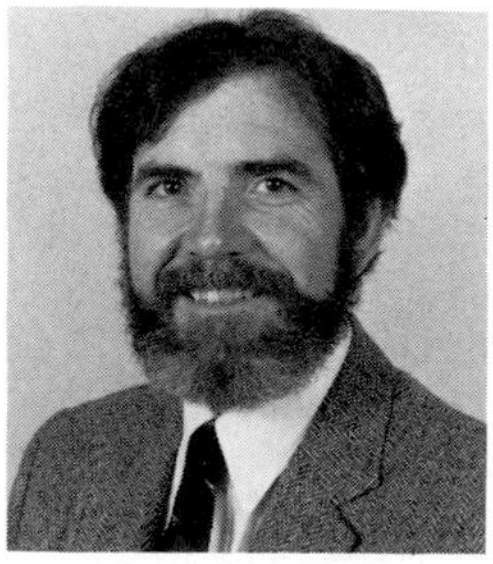

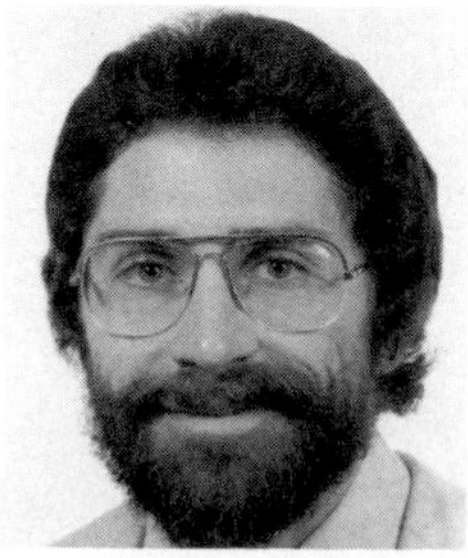

DENNIS J. MEYER, D.V.M.
Diplomate, American College of Veterinary Internal Medicine (Internal Medicine) and American College of Veterinary Pathology (Clinical Pathology); Associate Professor, Department of Medical Sciences and Department of Physiological Sciences, College of Veterinary Medicine, University of Florida, Gainesville, Florida.
Leukocytes in Health and Disease

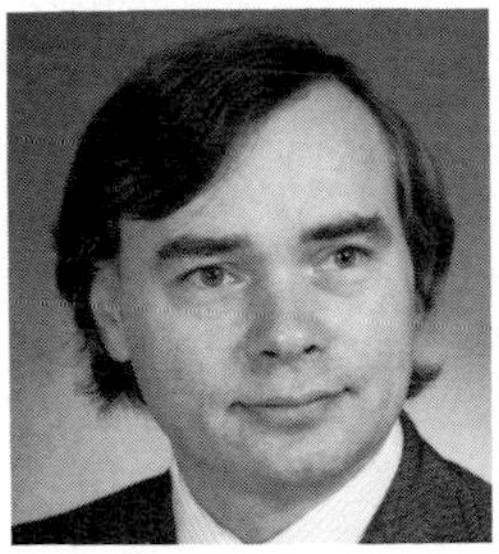

JAMES B. MILLER, D.V.M., M.S.
Diplomate, American College of Veterinary Internal Medicine (Internal Medicine); Clinical Associate Professor and Coordinator, Small Animal Medicine Service, University of Wisconsin-Madison School of Veterinary Medicine, Madison, Wisconsin.
Small Animal Zoonoses

PHILIPPE M. MOREAU, D.V.M.
Clinique Vétérinaire de Vanteaux, Limoges, France.
Incontinence, Enuresis, and Nocturia; Urinary Obstruction and Atony

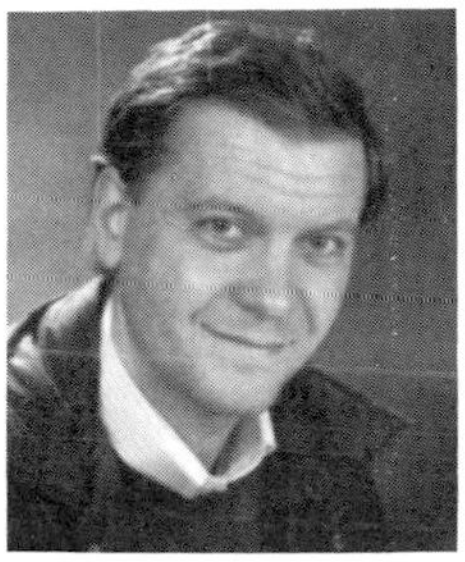

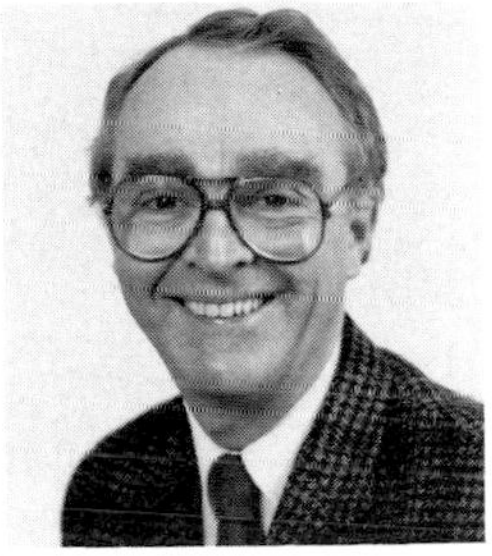

JOE P. MORGAN, D.V.M., V.M.D. (STOCKHOLM)
Diplomate, American College of Veterinary Radiology; Professor, Laboratory for Energy Related Health Research, University of California at Davis, Davis, California.
Joint Diseases of Dogs and Cats

JACOB E. MOSIER, D.V.M., M.S.
Diplomate, American College of Veterinary Internal Medicine (Internal Medicine); Professor of Veterinary Medicine, Kansas State University Veterinary Medical Center, Manhattan, Kansas.
Parturient and Post-parturient Diseases

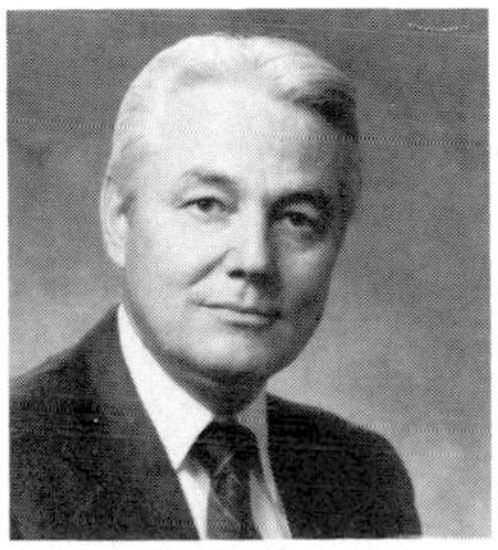

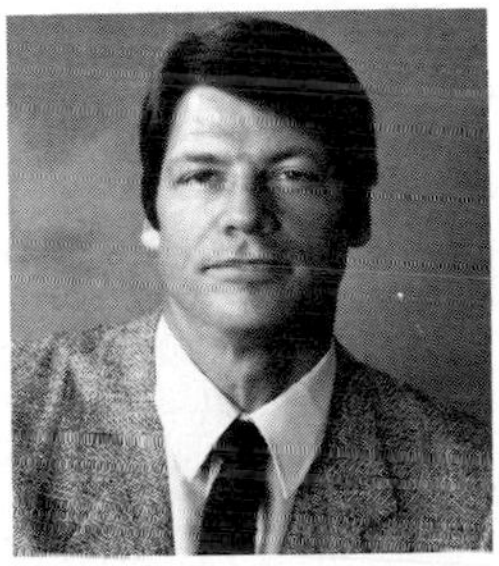

MICHAEL E. MOUNT, D.V.M., Ph.D.
Diplomate, American Board of Veterinary Toxicology; Associate Professor of Pharmacology and Toxicology, Clinical Toxicologist, School of Veterinary Medicine, University of California, Davis, California.
Toxicology

ROBERT J. MURTAUGH, D.V.M., M.S.
Diplomate, American College of Veterinary Internal Medicine (Internal Medicine); Assistant Professor and Co-Director, Critical Care Services, Department of Medicine, Tufts University School of Veterinary Medicine, North Grafton, Massachusetts.
Emergency Medicine

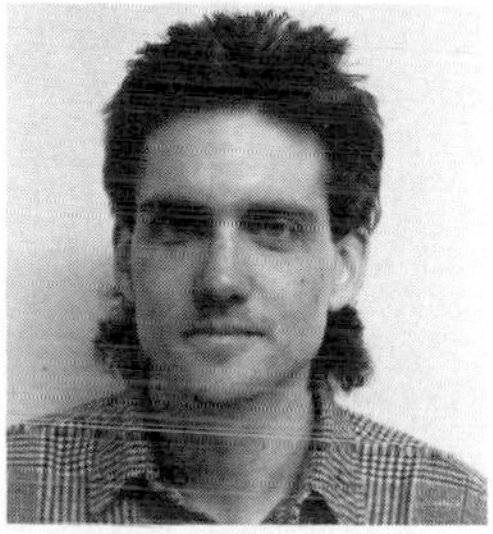

RICHARD W. NELSON, D.V.M.
Diplomate, American College of Veterinary Internal Medicine (Internal Medicine); Assistant Professor, Department of Medicine, University of California, Davis, California.
Disorders of the Endocrine Pancreas

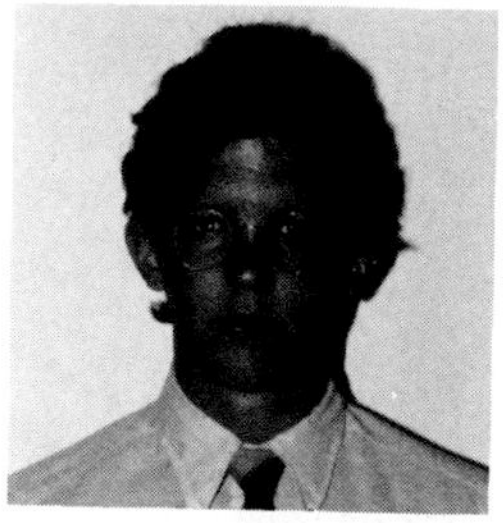

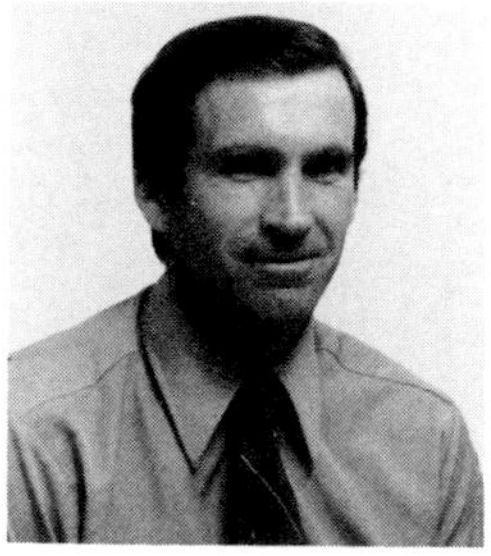

TERRY M. NETT, Ph.D.
Professor, Department of Physiology, College of Veterinary Medicine and Biomedical Sciences, Colorado State University, Fort Collins, Colorado.
Persistent Estrus in the Bitch

CHARLES D. NEWTON, D.V.M., M.S.
Diplomate, American College of Veterinary Surgeons, Professor of Orthopedic Surgery and Chief, Section of Surgery, School of Veterinary Medicine, University of Pennsylvania, Philadelphia, Pennsylvania.
Skeletal Diseases

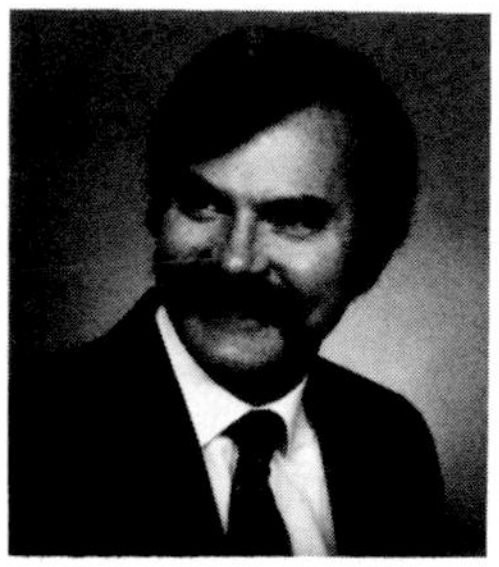

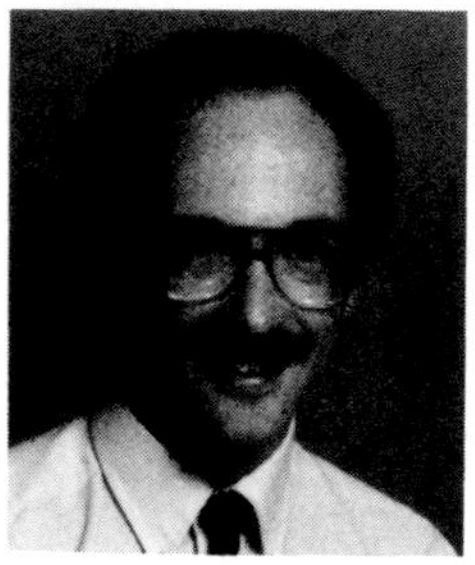

TIMOTHY D. O'BRIEN, D.V.M., Ph.D.
Diplomate, American College of Veterinary Pathologists; Assistant Professor of Veterinary Pathology, Department of Veterinary Pathobiology, College of Veterinary Medicine, University of Minnesota, St. Paul, Minnesota.
Diseases of the Kidneys and Ureters; Canine Uroliths

PATRICIA N. OLSON, D.V.M., Ph.D.
Diplomate, American College of Theriogenologists; College of Veterinary Medicine and Biomedical Sciences, Colorado State University, Fort Collins, Colorado.
Persistent Estrus in the Bitch

CARL A. OSBORNE, D.V.M., Ph.D.
Diplomate, American College of Veterinary Internal Medicine (Internal Medicine); Professor, Department of Small Animal Clinical Sciences, College of Veterinary Medicine, University of Minnesota, St. Paul, Minnesota.
Diseases of the Kidneys and Ureters; Feline Lower Urinary Tract Disorders; Canine Uroliths

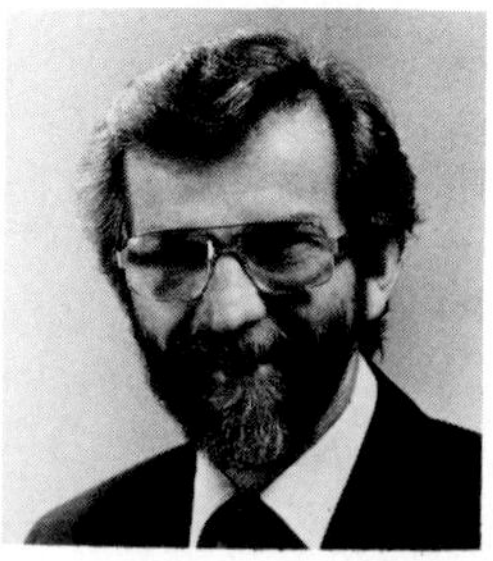

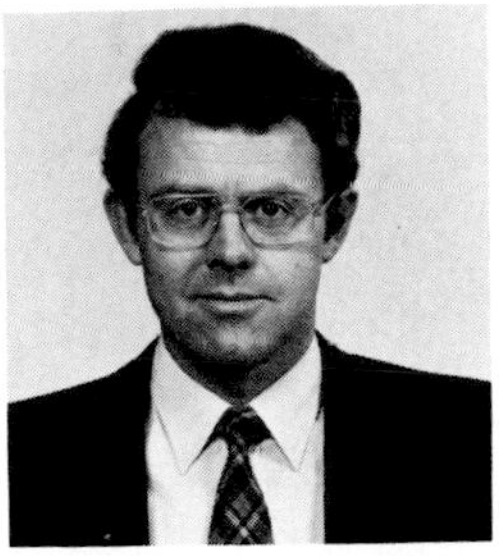

ALAN J. PARKER, M.R.C.V.S., Ph.D.

Diplomate, American College of Veterinary Internal Medicine (Neurology); Professor of Medicine, University of Illinois, College of Veterinary Medicine, Urbana; Consultant in Neurology, Berwyn Veterinary Associates Hospital, Berwyn, Illinois.

Behavioral Signs of Organic Disease

NIELS C. PEDERSEN, D.V.M., Ph.D.

Professor, Small Animal Internal Medicine, Department of Medicine, School of Veterinary Medicine, University of California, Davis; Clinician, Veterinary Medical Teaching Hospital, Davis, California.

Joint Diseases of Dogs and Cats

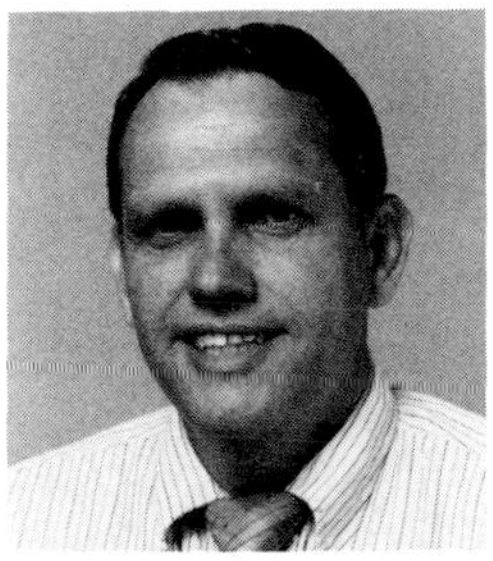

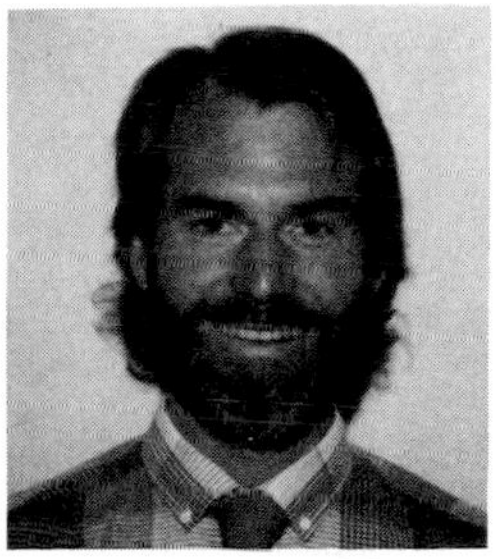

VINCENT G. PEDROIA, D.V.M., Ph.D.

Neurology and Neurosurgery, Special Veterinary Services, Berkeley, California.

Disorders of the Skeletal Muscles

MARK EARL PETERSON, D.V.M.

Diplomate, American College of Veterinary Internal Medicine (Internal Medicine); Adjunct Associate Professor of Medicine, The New York Hospital-Cornell Medical Center, New York; Adjunct Assistant Professor of Medicine, Department of Clincal Sciences, New York State College of Veterinary Medicine, Cornell University, Ithaca, New York.

Thyroid Diseases

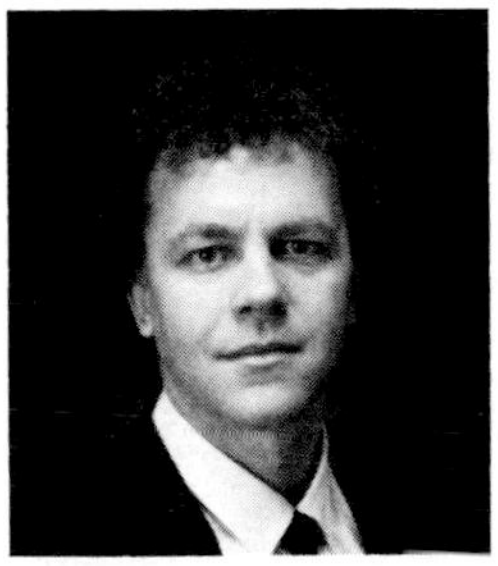

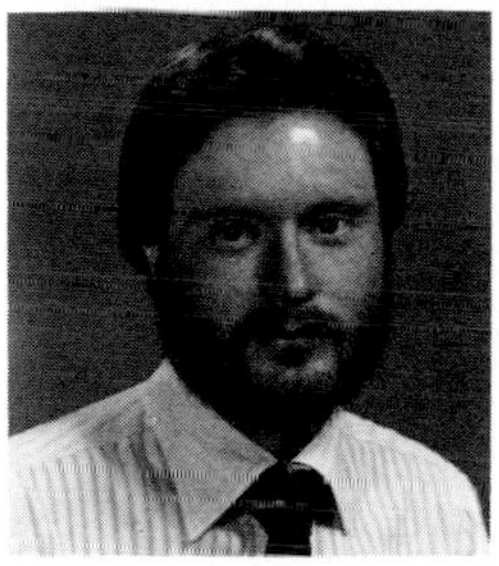

DAVID J. POLZIN, D.V.M., Ph.D.

Diplomate, American College of Veterinary Internal Medicine (Internal Medicine); Assistant Professor, Veterinary Internal Medicine, University of Minnesota, College of Veterinary Medicine, St. Paul, Minnesota.

Diseases of the Kidneys and Ureters; Feline Lower Urinary Tract Disorders; Canine Uroliths

ROY R. POOL, Jr., D.V.M., Ph.D.

School of Veterinary Medicine, University of California Davis, Davis, California.

Joint Diseases of Dogs and Cats

CLARENCE A. RAWLINGS, D.V.M., Ph.D.
Diplomate, American College of Veterinary Surgeons; Professor of Small Animal Medicine, and Physiology and Pharmacology; Chief of Staff, Small Animal Surgery, College of Veterinary Medicine, University of Georgia, Athens, Georgia.
Heartworm Disease

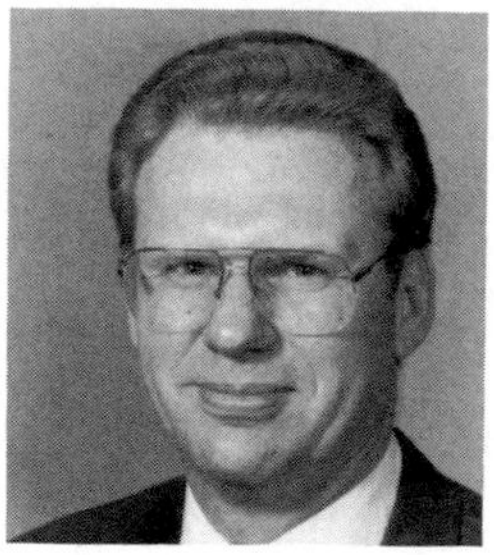

ALAN H. REBAR, D.V.M.
Diplomate, American College of Veterinary Pathologists (Clinical Pathology); Purdue University School of Veterinary Medicine, West Lafayette, Indiana.
The Clinical Approach to Disorders of Hemostasis

LON J. RICH, D.V.M., Ph.D.
Diplomate, American College of Veterinary Pathologists; ALL CARE Animal Referral Center, Mountain Valley, California.
Tables of Abnormal Blood Values as a Guide to Disease Syndromes

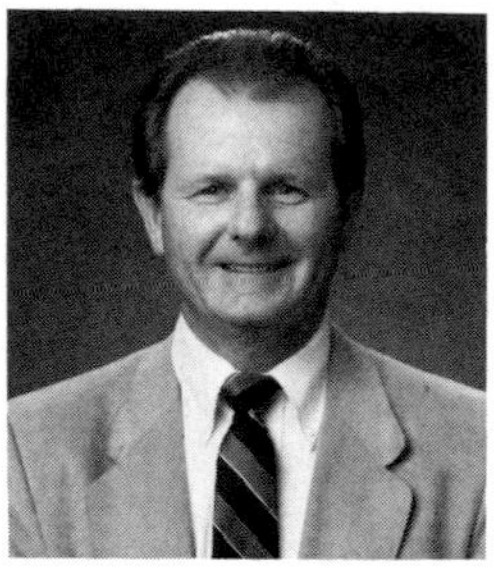

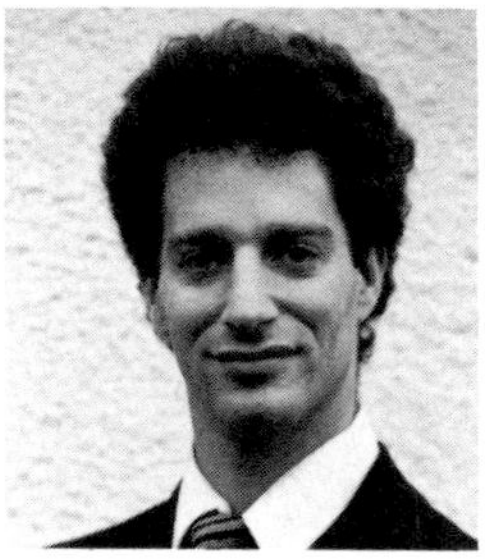

KEITH P. RICHTER, D.V.M.
Diplomate, American College of Veterinary Internal Medicine (Internal Medicine); Staff Clinician in Internal Medicine, Veterinary Referral Center, Helen Woodward Animal Center, Rancho Santa Fe, California.
Diseases of the Large Bowel

ROBERT C. ROSENTHAL, D.V.M., M.S., Ph.D.
Diplomate, American College of Veterinary Internal Medicine (Internal Medicine and Oncology); Assistant Professor of Medicine/Oncology, Department of Medical Sciences, School of Veterinary Medicine, University of Wisconsin-Madison, Madison, Wisconsin.
Approach to Treatment of Cancer Patients

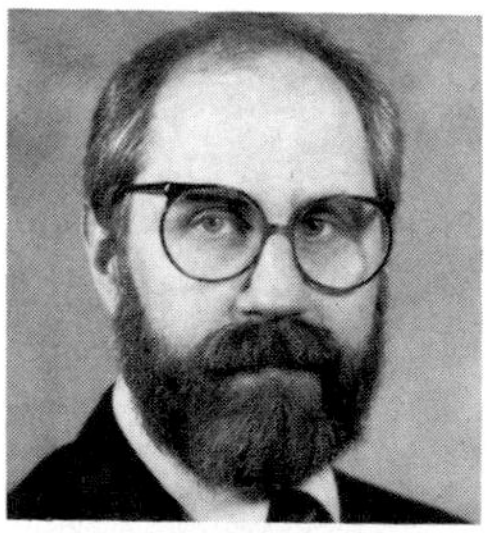

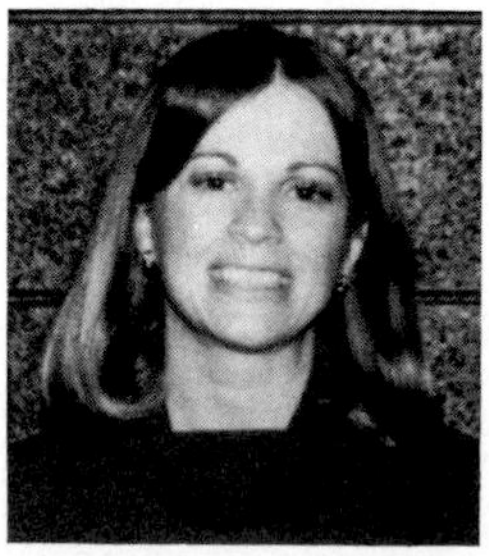

LINDA A. ROSS, D.V.M., M.S.
Diplomate, American College of Veterinary Internal Medicine (Internal Medicine); Assistant Pɪofessor, Department of Medicine, Tufts University School of Veterinary Medicine; Clinician, Foster Hospital for Small Animals, North Grafton, Massachusetts.
Hypertensive Diseases

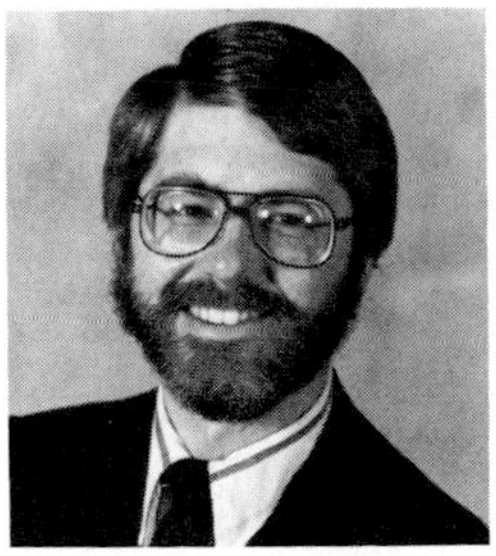

PHILIP ROUDEBUSH, D.V.M.

Diplomate, American College of Veterinary Internal Medicine (Internal Medicine); Associate Professor and Chairman, Department of Clinical Sciences, College of Veterinary Medicine, Mississippi State University, Mississippi State, Mississippi.

Ataxia, Paresis, and Paralysis; Altered States of Consciousness: Coma and Stupor

JOHN E. RUSH, D.V.M., M.Sc.

Diplomate, American College of Veterinary Internal Medicine (Cardiology); Assistant Professor, Department of Medicine; School of Veterinary Medicine, Tufts University, North Grafton, Massachusetts.

Therapy of Heart Failure

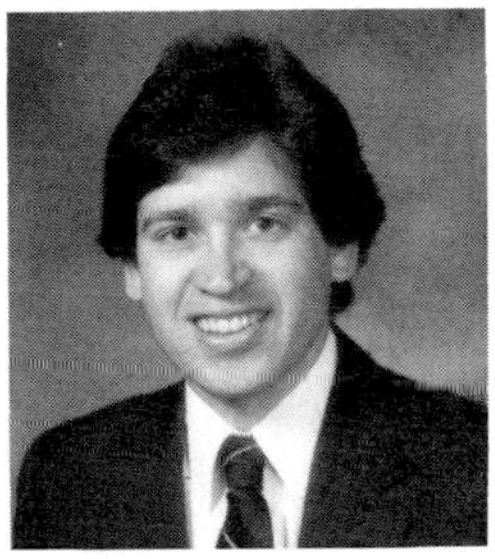

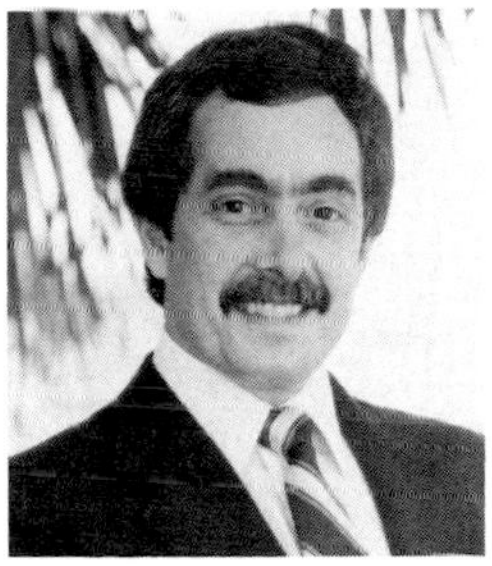

MICHAEL SCHAER, D.V.M.

Diplomate, American College of Veterinary Internal Medicine (Internal Medicine); Professor of Medicine, Associate Chairman; Department of Small Animal Clinical Sciences, University of Florida College of Veterinary Medicine, Gainesville, Florida.

Clinical Approach to the Patient with Respiratory Disease

LYNN P. SCHMEITZEL, D.V.M.

Diplomate, American College of Veterinary Dermatology; Assistant Professor of Dermatology, Department of Urban Practice, College of Veterinary Medicine, University of Tennessee, Knoxville, Tennessee.

Alopecia

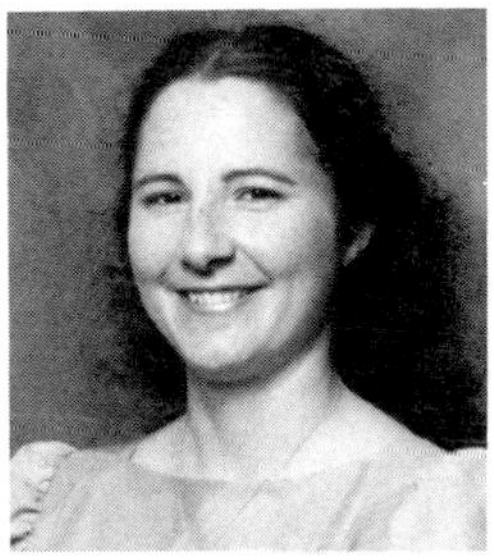

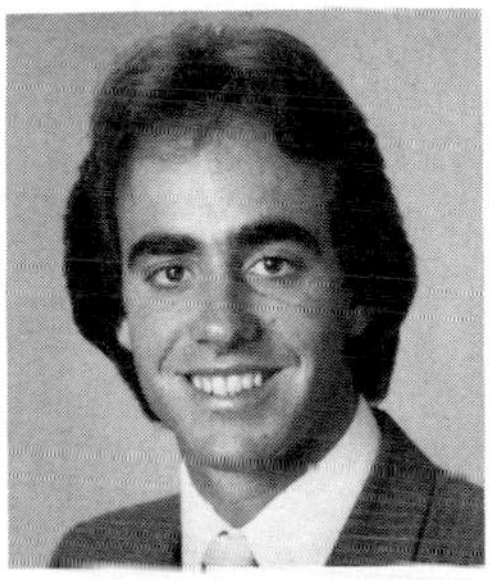

ALAN J. SCHULMAN, D.V.M.

Diplomate, American College of Veterinary Surgeons; Private Practice, Los Angeles, California

Gastric Dilatation-Volvulus-Torsion Syndrome

DAVID F. SENIOR, B.V.Sc.

Diplomate, American College of Veterinary Medicine (Internal Medicine); Associate Professor of Medicine, Department of Medical Sciences, College of Veterinary Medicine, University of Florida, Gainesville, Florida.

Fluid Therapy, Electrolyte and Acid-Base Control

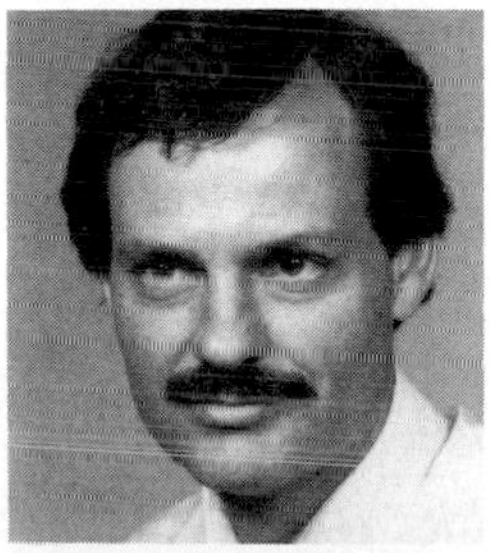

ROBERT G. SHERDING, D.V.M.
Diplomate, American College of Veterinary Internal Medicine (Internal Medicine); Associate Professor and Head of Small Animal Medicine, Department of Veterinary Clinical Sciences, Ohio State University College of Veterinary Medicine, Columbus, Ohio.
Diseases of the Small Bowel

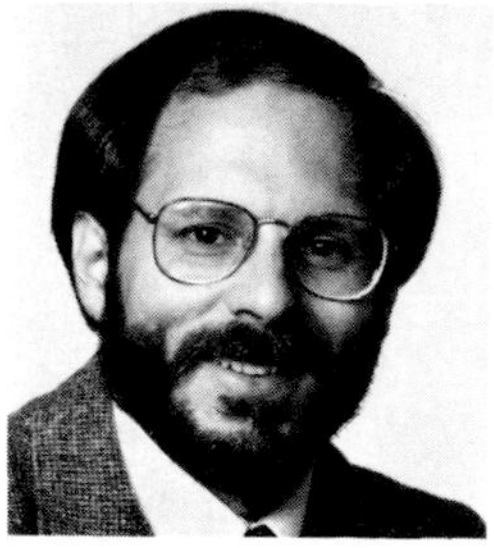

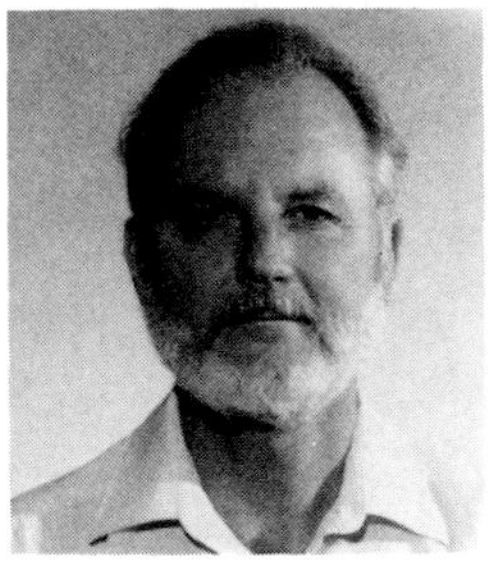

VICTOR M. SHILLE, D.V.M., Ph.D.
Diplomate, American College of Theriogenologists; Associate Professor of Theriogenology and Director, Florida Association of Kennel Clubs Laboratory for Studies in Canine Reproduction, University of Florida College of Veterinary Medicine, Gainesville, Florida.
Reproductive Physiology and Endocrinology of the Female and Male

ANDY SHORES, D.V.M., M.S., Ph.D.
Associate Professor, Neurology/Neurosurgery, Department of Small Animal Clinical Science, College of Veterinary Medicine, Michigan State University, East Lansing, Michigan.
Ataxia, Paresis, and Paralysis; Altered States of Consciousness: Coma and Stupor

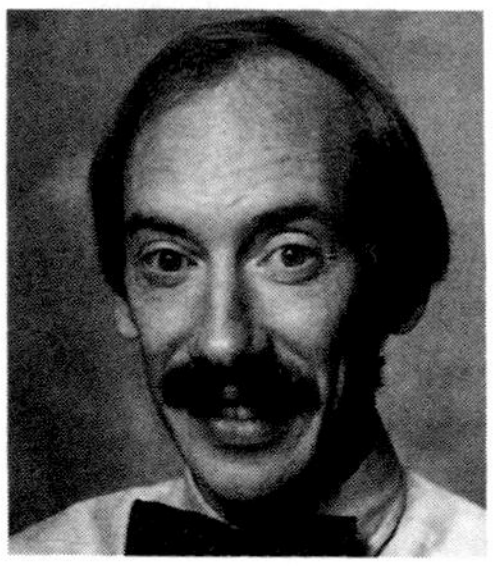

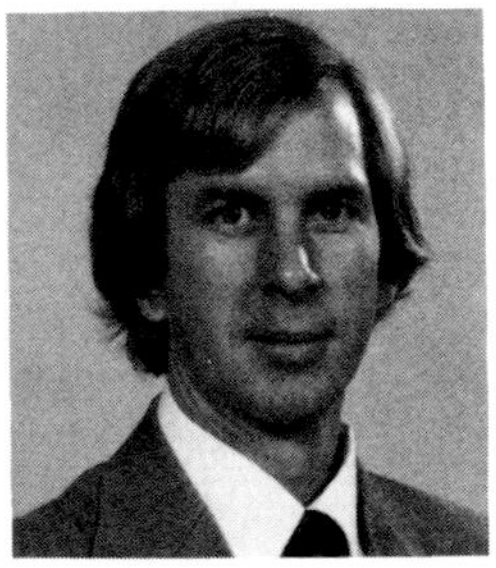

DAVID SISSON, D.V.M.
Diplomate, American College of Veterinary Internal Medicine (Cardiology); Assistant Professor and Staff Cardiologist, College of Veterinary Medicine, University of Illinois, Urbana, Illinois.
The Clinical Evaluation of Cardiac Function; Infective Endocarditis

GEOFFREY SUNSHINE, D.V.M., Ph.D.
Department of Surgery, Tufts University School of Veterinary Medicine, North Grafton, Massachusetts.
Principles of Immunology

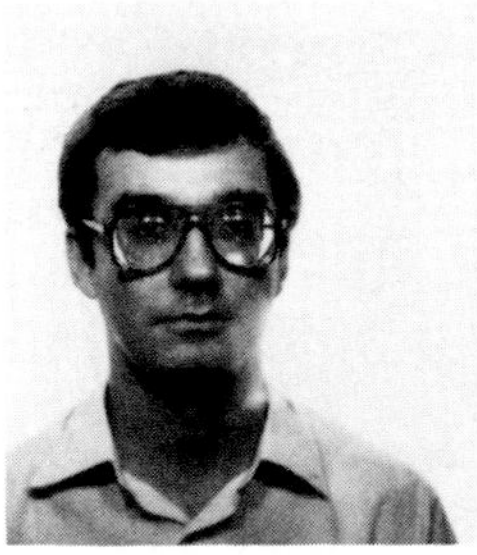

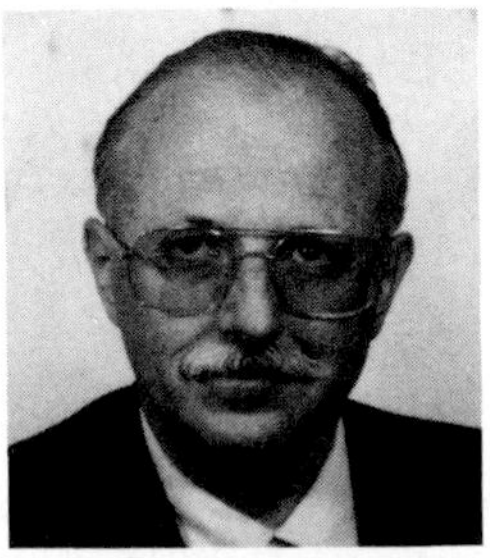

PETER F. SUTER, D.V.M., Ph.D.
Diplomate, American College of Veterinary Radiology; Dean, Veterinary Medical College, University of Zurich, Zurich, Switzerland.
Diseases of the Lower Respiratory Tract (Lung) and Pulmonary Edema; Peripheral Vascular Disease

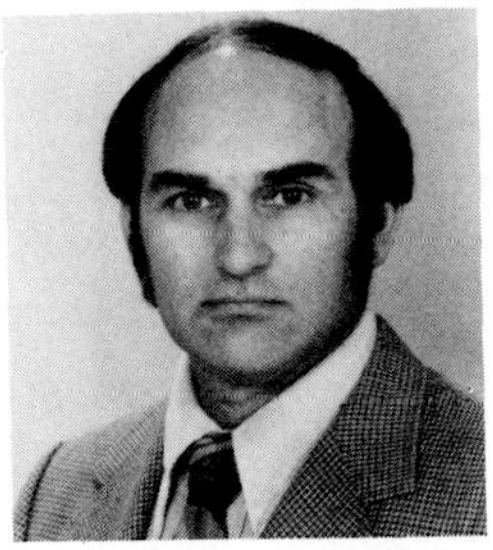

LARRY J. SWANGO, D.V.M., Ph.D.
Associate Professor of Virology in the Department of Pathobiology, College of Veterinary Medicine, Auburn University, Auburn, Alabama.
Bacterial, Rickettsial, Protozoal, and Miscellaneous Infections; Canine Viral Diseases

TODD R. TAMS, D.V.M.
Diplomate, American College of Veterinary Internal Medicine (Internal Medicine); Medical Director and Staff Internist, West Los Angeles Veterinary Medical Group, Los Angeles, California.
Vomiting, Regurgitation, and Dysphagia

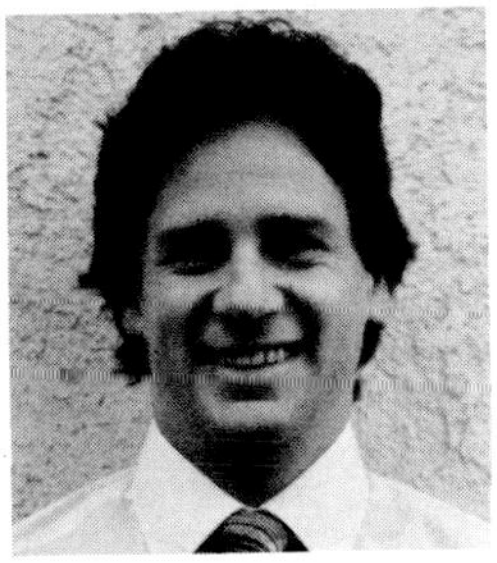

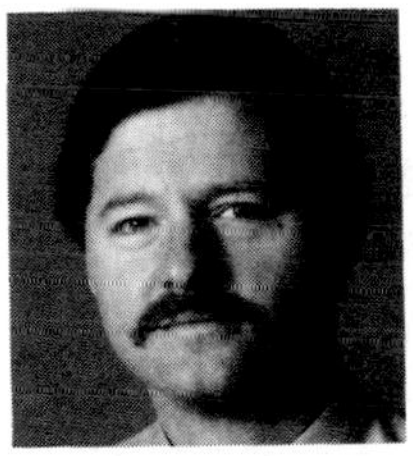

WILLIAM P. THOMAS, D.V.M.
Diplomate, American College of Veterinary Internal Medicine (Cardiology); Professor of Medicine (Cardiology), Department of Medicine, and Chief, Cardiology Service, Veterinary Medical Teaching Hospital, University of California Davis, Davis, California.
Pericardial Disorders

JAMES P. THOMPSON, D.V.M., Ph.D.
Diplomate, American College of Veterinary Internal Medicine (Internal Medicine); Assistant Professor, Department of Medical Services; Director, Clinical Immunology Laboratory; Chief, Clinical Oncology Service; College of Veterinary Medicine, University of Florida, Gainesville, Florida.
Immunologic Diseases

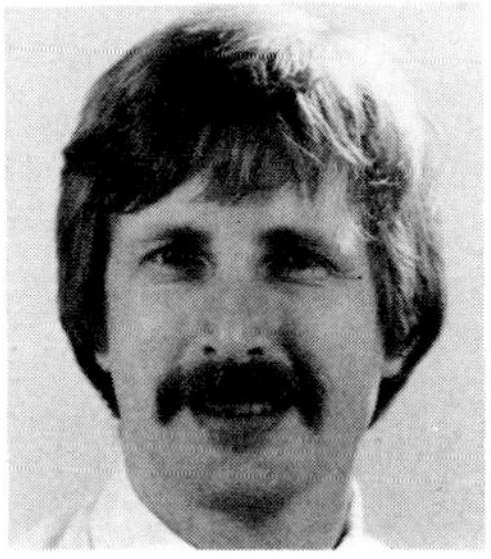

CHRISTINE E. THOMSON, B.V.Sc.
Resident in Neurology, North Carolina State University, College of Veterinary Medicine, Raleigh, North Carolina.
Trembling and Shivering

JAMES W. TICER, D.V.M., Ph.D.
Diplomate, American College of Veterinary Radiology; Associate Clinical Professor, Department of Radiological Sciences, School of Veterinary Medicine, University of California Davis, Davis; Private Veterinary Radiology Practice, Santa Cruz, California.
Diseases of the Trachea

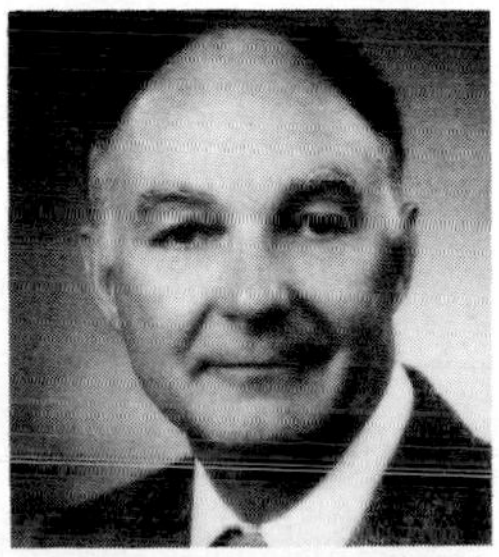

GREGORY C. TROY, D.V.M., M.S.
Diplomate, American College of Veterinary Internal Medicine (Internal Medicine); Professor, Department of Small Animal Clinical Sciences; Hospital Director, Veterinary Medical Teaching Hospital, Virginia-Maryland Regional College of Veterinary Medicine, Blacksburg, Virginia.
Deep Mycotic Diseases

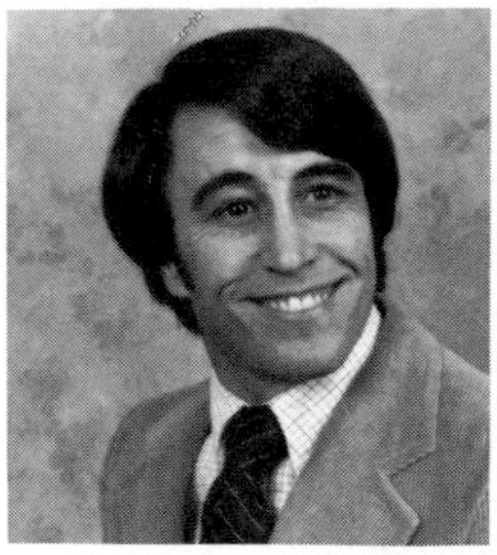

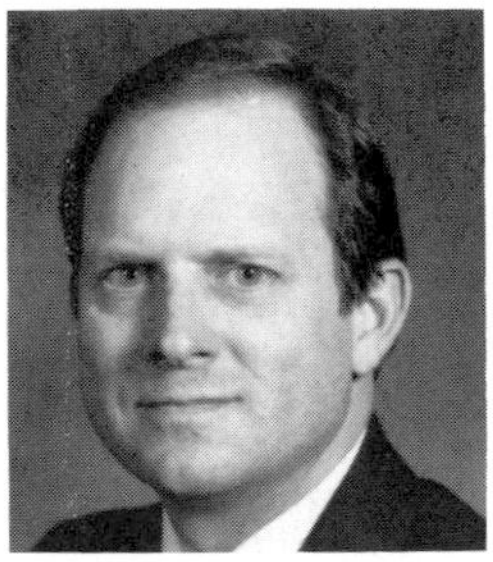

DAVID C. TWEDT, D.V.M.
Diplomate, American College of Veterinary Internal Medicine (Internal Medicine); Associate Professor, Department of Clinical Sciences, College of Veterinary Medicine and Biomedical Sciences, Colorado State University, Fort Collins, Colorado; Clinical Gastroenterologist, Veterinary Teaching Hospital, Fort Collins, Colorado.
Diseases of the Stomach

JOSEPH VAN HEERDEN, M.Med.Vet. (Medicine); B.Sc. (Hon)
Professor and Head of the Department of Companion Animal Medicine and Surgery, Faculty of Veterinary Science, Medical University of Southern Africa, Onderstepoort, South Africa.
Small Animal Problems in Developing Countries

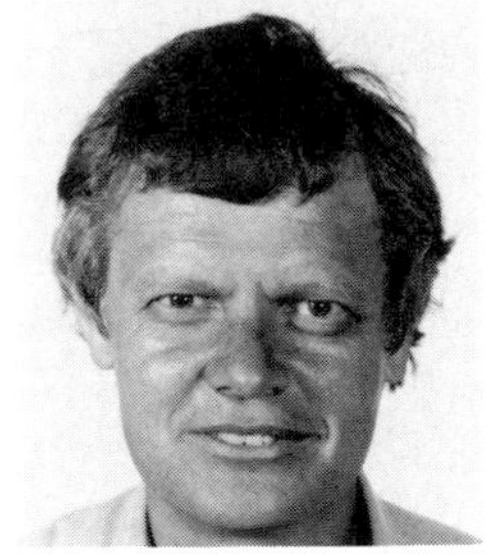

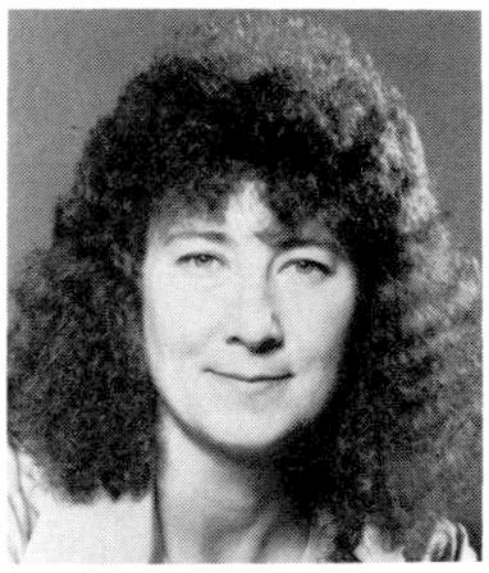

VICTORIA LEA VOITH, D.V.M., M.Sc., M.A., Ph.D.
Adjunct Assistant Professor, Clinical Studies, School of Veterinary Medicine, University of Pennsylvania, Philadelphia, Pennsylvania; Animal Behavior Consultants, San Antonio, Texas.
Behavioral Disorders

RICHARD WALSHAW, B.V.M.S.
Diplomate, American College of Veterinary Surgeons; Associate Professor, Small Animal Surgery, Department of Small Animal Clinical Sciences, College of Veterinary Medicine, Michigan State University, East Lansing, Michigan.
Constipation, Tenesmus, and Dyschezia

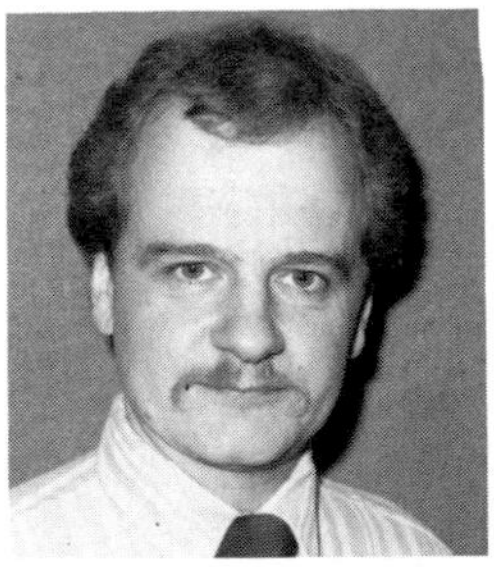

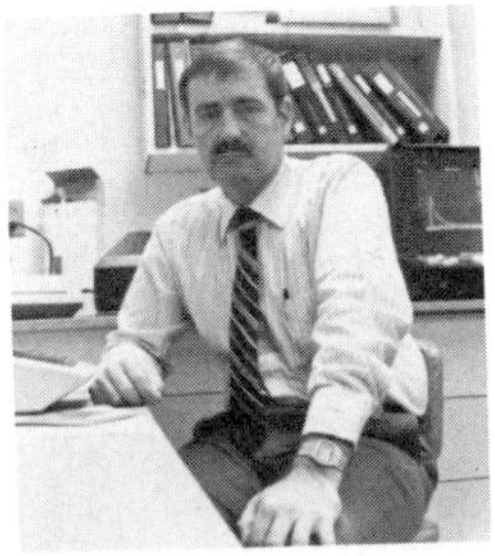

M. GLADE WEISER, D.V.M.
Diplomate, American College of Veterinary Pathologists (Clinical Pathology); Associate Professor, Department of Pathology, Colorado State University, Fort Collins, Colorado.
Erythrocyte Responses and Disorders

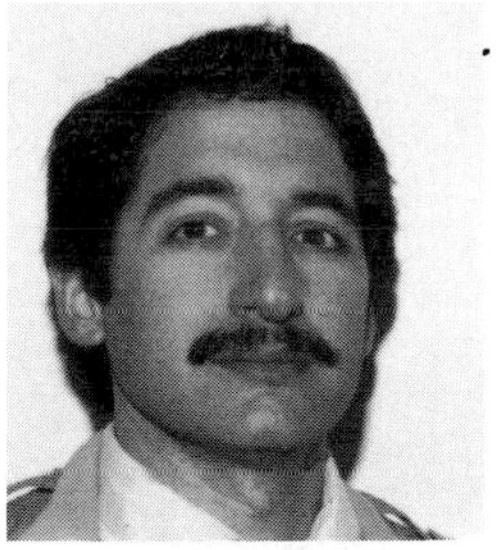

STEPHEN D. WHITE, D.V.M.

Diplomate, American College of Veterinary Dermatology; Assistant Professor, Department of Clincal Sciences, College of Veterinary Medicine and Biomedical Sciences, Fort Collins, Colorado.

The Skin as a Sensor of Internal Medical Disorders

MICHAEL D. WILLARD, D.V.M.

Diplomate, American College of Veterinary Internal Medicine (Internal Medicine); Professosr of Internal Medicine, Department of Small Animal Medicine, College of Veterinary Medicine, Texas A and M University, College Station, Texas.

Constipation, Tenesmus, and Dyschezia

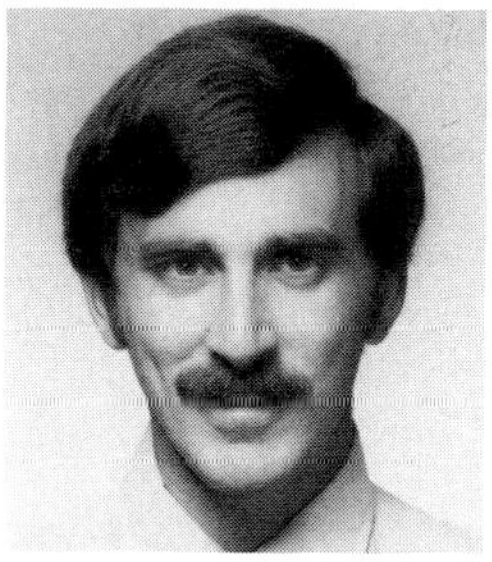

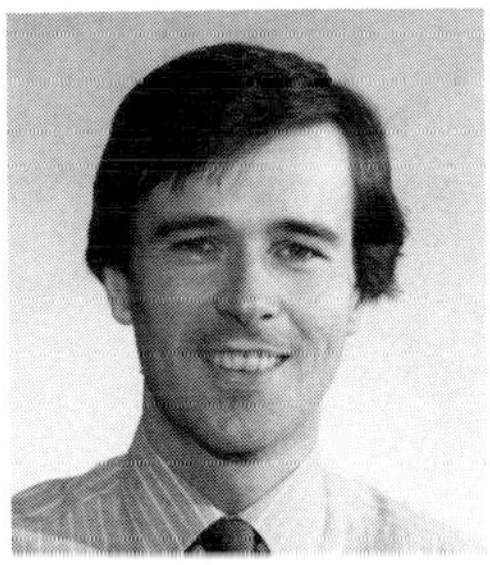

DAVID A. WILLIAMS, Vet.M.B., Ph.D., M.R.C.V.S.

Diplomate, American College of Veterinary Internal Medicine (Internal Medicine); Associate Professor of Medicine, College of Veterinary Medicine, Kansas State University, Veterinary Medical Center, Manhatten, Kansas.

Exocrine Pancreatic Disease

ALIDA WIND, D.V.M.

School of Veterinary Medicine, University of California Davis, Davis, California.

Joint Diseases of Dogs and Cats

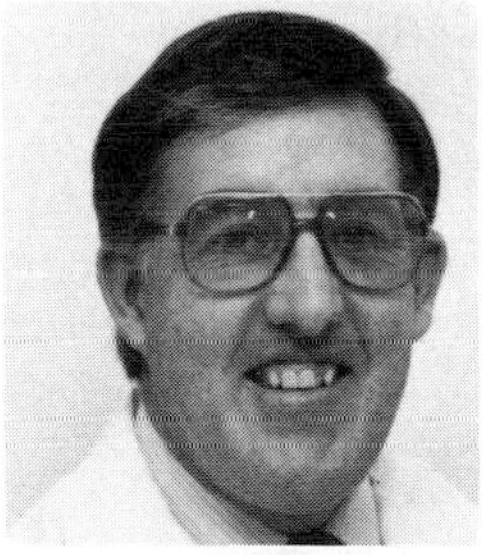

WAYNE E. WINGFIELD, D.V.M., M.S.

Diplomate, American College of Veterinary Surgeons; Professor of Medicine, Department of Clinical Sciences, College of Veterinary Medicine and Biomedical Sciences; Chief, Emergency Medicine and Intensive Care, and Staff Cardiologist, Veterinary Teaching Hospital, Colorado State University, Fort Collins, Colorado.

Cardiopulmonary Arrest and Resuscitation

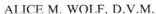

ALICE M. WOLF, D.V.M.

Diplomate, American College of Veterinary Internal Medicine (Internal Medicine); Associate Professor, Department of Small Animal Medicine and Surgery, College of Veterinary Medicine, Texas A and M University, College Station, Texas.

Deep Mycotic Diseases

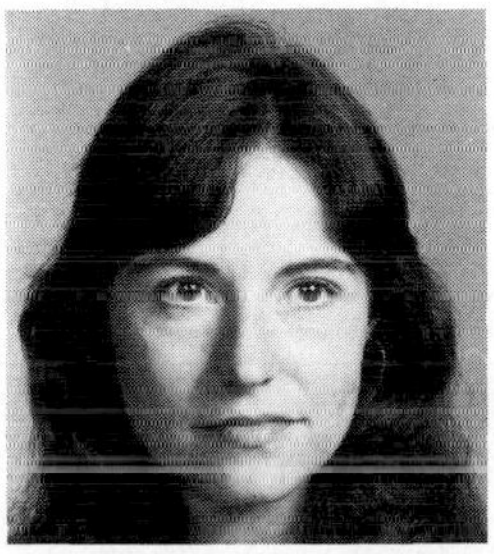

JERRY A. WOODFIELD, D.V.M.
Diplomate, American College of Veterinary Internal Medicine (Cardiology); Assistant Professor, Department of Small Animal Clinical Sciences, Staff Cardiologist, Veterinary Medical Teaching Hospital, Virginia-Maryland Regional College of Veterinary Medicine, Virginia Tech, Blacksburg, Virginia.
Infective Endocarditis

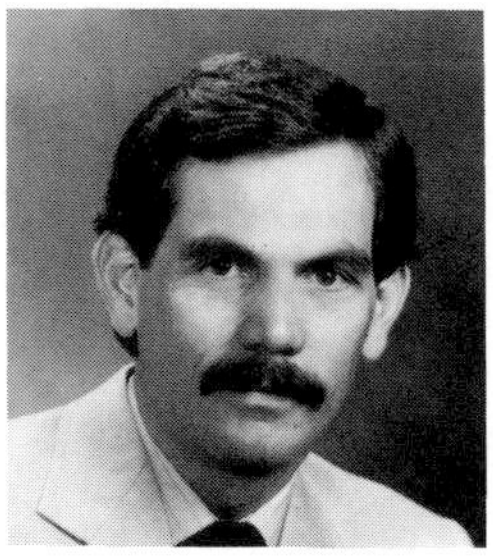

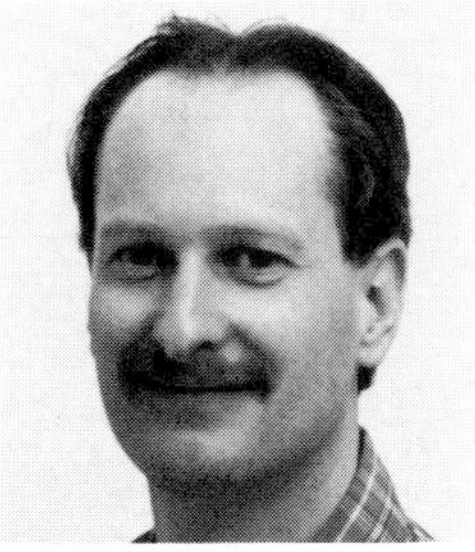

ROBERT H. WRIGLEY, B.V.Sc., M.S., D.V.R., M.R.C.V.S.
Colorado State University, College of Veterinary Medicine, Fort Collins, Colorado.
Persistent Estrus in the Bitch

CALIFORNIA EDITORIAL STAFF

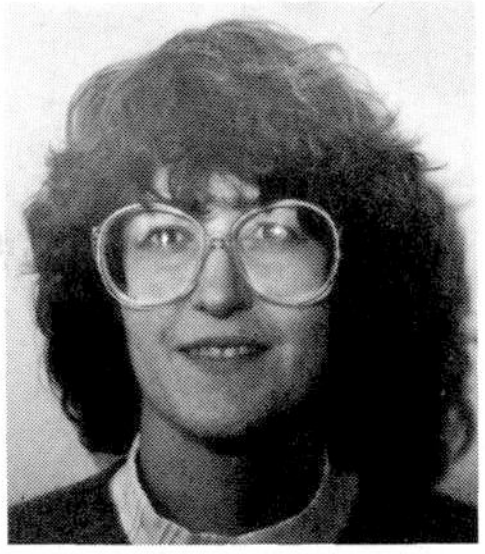

MELONIA MUSSER-BRAUNER
Technical Editor

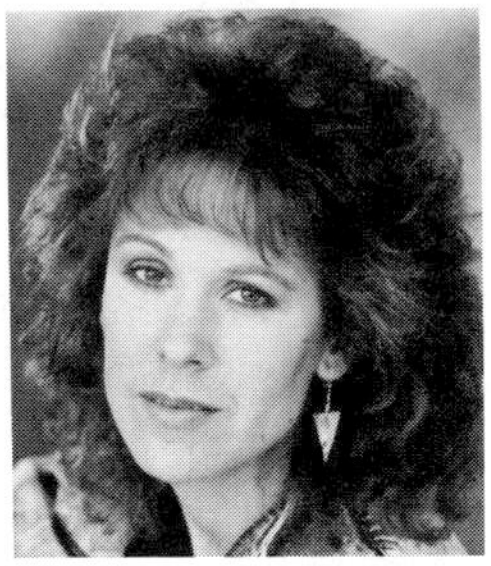

DANA ST. JOHN-BUXTON
Administration Coordinator

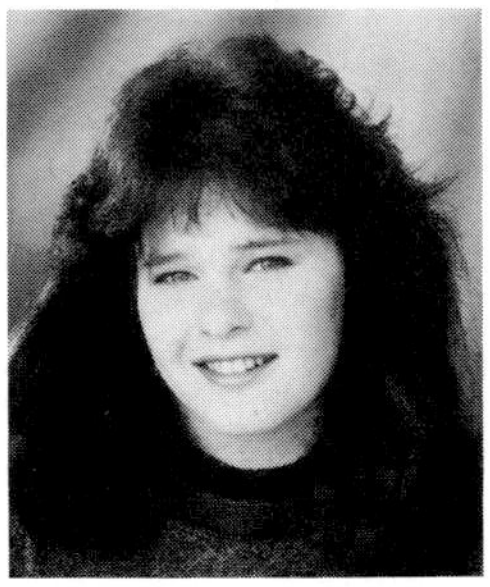

NICOLE L. ETTINGER
Clerical Assistant

W. B. SAUNDERS STAFF

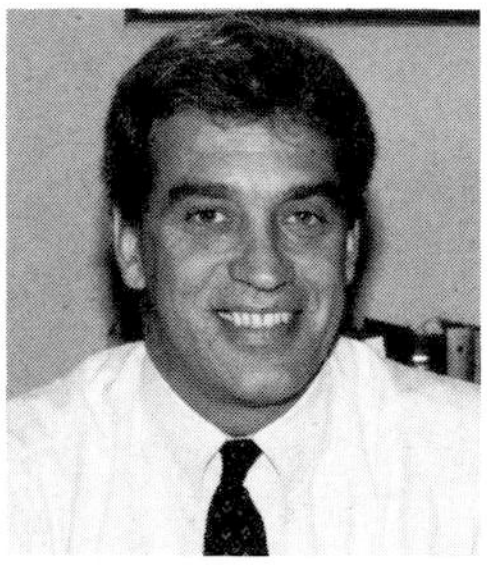

AL BERINGER
Manager, Typesetting Department

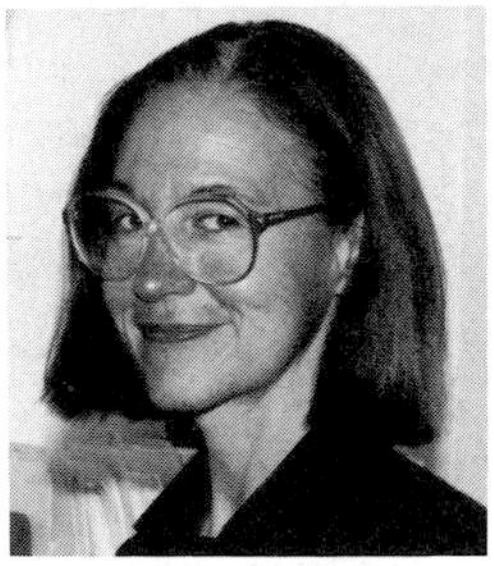

EDNA DICK
Senior Supervising Editor

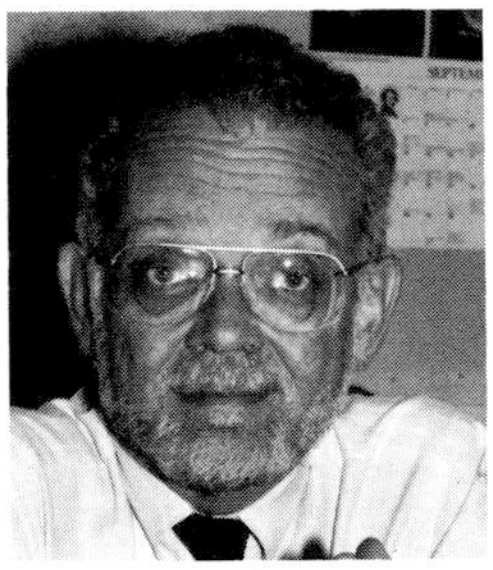

JOHN DYSON
Sponsoring Editor

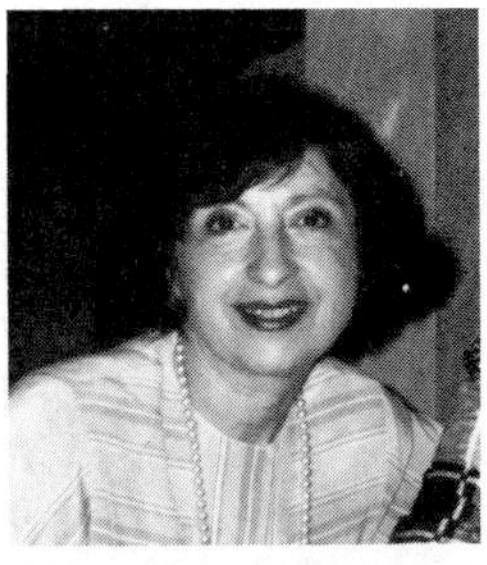

LORRAINE B. KILMER
Team Manager and Designer

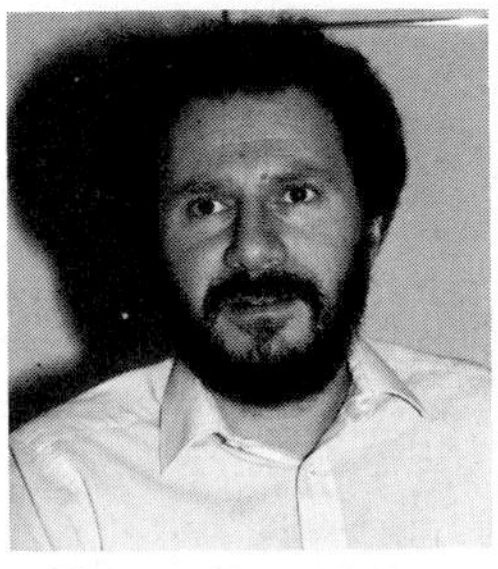

FRANK POLIZZANO
Production Manager

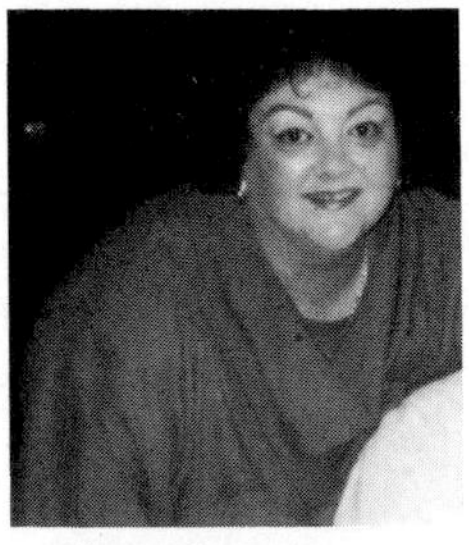

CASS STAMATO
Editorial Assistant

PREFACE
TO THE THIRD EDITION

It is not sufficient that we know, we must also apply;
It is not sufficient that we have good intentions, we must also act.

GOETHE

Since publication of the first edition of this textbook, a significantly increased body of knowledge has become available to the veterinary profession. This profusion of published data raised both the scientific level of our knowledge and our ability to practice. Keeping up with this material requires sorting and integrating applicable data with care and thought.

The third edition of this textbook proved in many ways the most difficult to produce. Providing modern and relevant information and references remains the goal of this text, but space constraints and efforts to control costs also had to be considered. Style changes, the use of numbered references, and the computerization of text have made possible an increase in the number of written words with only a modest increase in cost and size. Contributors have deleted outdated material and have prepared thorough, well-structured chapters. References remain extensive; to have reduced their number would have deprived the reader of one of the major advantages of an all-encompassing textbook.

The author pool continues to expand, and this edition benefits from over 150 contributors. Representing both academic and practice backgrounds, these highly qualified men and women come from all regions of the United States and from many other countries. More than 80 per cent of the contributors are board-certified in the United States or are recognized foreign specialists. All are well qualified in their respective fields. These veterinary scientists have been thorough but have coordinated their chapters with others to avoid unnecessary duplication. At times, of course, the restatement of certain concepts cannot be avoided. When feasible, authors have presented relevant controversies. Personal bias is identified as such.

This edition presents a significantly expanded initial section on the clinical manifestations of disease. The problem-oriented approach to medicine developed over the past decade represents a major advance in clinical veterinary medicine, and the clinician first identifies disease by signs. While this expanded section should continue to be relevant, the reader must also remember that no algorithm in medicine is final or complete. Always include a blank line for as yet unidentified information.

Laboratory testing by panel analysis is accepted as routine in the United States, but has yet to become established world-wide. The tables on abnormal laboratory values and their correlations should be very helpful. Abnormalities of the skin and eyes often reflect an internal medical problem. Thus, a discussion of these topics is included in this section.

Problems in veterinary medicine that cannot logically be placed in a specific section or that cut across multiple organ systems have been included. New sections on chromosomal and genetic disorders, hyperlipidemias, and food allergies will no doubt be expanded in future editions. Other topics of current concern in small animal practice include emergency medicine, diseases of the ear, small animal problems in developing countries, and small animal zoonoses. Behavioral disorders and the human-animal bond are increasingly important. The inclusion of all these topics will be helpful to the practicing veterinarian.

The infectious diseases section has expanded—particularly viral diseases. Reorganized and expanded sections on infectious disorders continue to include traditional concepts and principles involving drugs and antimicrobial agents. Therapy is discussed throughout the book. The appropriate uses of fluids, corticosteroids, and specialized nutritional support are covered in this section. Toxicology and adverse drug reactions are explored thoroughly. Acupuncture, an alternative modality, is presented to complete the review of therapeutics.

The section on cancer was written with the understanding that individual organ system presentations would review more specific information. This section was adapted to include the general biologic behavior of tumors and a review of their management.

The organ system approach remains the principal method of teaching the bulk of scientific knowledge in veterinary science. Neuro-ophthalmology has been added; peripheral neuropathies and muscular disorders have been separated and expanded. The cardiovascular system incorporates updated information provided by improved diagnostic study tools, such as Doppler ultrasonography. Recent studies have expanded our knowledge of esophageal disorders, the gastric dilatation-volvulus complex, and intestinal pathophysiology and diagnosis. There are thoroughly revised and expanded sections on the pathophysiology and treatment of both liver and pancreatic diseases. Endocrine disorders are a frequent clinical problem. These topics are presented in great detail, with new chapters on the pituitary-hypothalamic system and parathyroid disease.

I believe that the inclusion of uterine and vaginal disorders, reproductive oncology, infertility, parturient diseases, and prostatic disorders remains in the field of general medical practice. Their inclusion in this textbook indicates the importance of these subjects to veterinary internal medicine.

Urinary problems are given the extensive space they deserve, considering their frequent occurrence. Expanded knowledge of lower tract disorders has meant dividing topics into feline and canine chapters. The problem of systemic hypertension is included in this section.

Blood cell disorders, coagulopathies, and lymph node and splenic problems are widely encountered in both dogs and cats. Discussion of both diagnosis and treatment often overlaps with the chapters on cancer, immunology, and toxicology. Many conditions not covered in previous editions have been added to this section.

Knowledge of immunology expands at such a rapid rate that even a textbook revised as frequently as this one can hardly remain current. Subject overlapping has made cross-referencing chapters and sections necessary.

Often considered as surgical problems are joint and bone diseases. However, a cursory examination of these chapters reflects their importance as a medical topic. To ensure a thorough description, internists, radiologists, surgeons, and pathologists have worked together to coordinate the discussion. Surgical corrections are mentioned, and the reader is referred to appropriate surgical references.

Throughout the book I have endeavored to follow Pasteur's recommendation to keep my enthusiasm but to let strict verification be a constant companion. The references are very detailed except in the initial sections. The remainder of the book is heavily referenced and at times almost appears encyclopedic.

This textbook describes both canine and feline diseases. When one species suffers more than the other—or not at all—that point is clearly made. Occasionally chapters are specific to the dog or cat; this represents an overwhelming need for separate discussion of the topic.

Because veterinary clinicians in the United States continue to relate to ounces and pounds, drug recommendations are provided that way as well as in metric units. Laboratory values in the United States occasionally are stated in terms that are not in international units. I have encouraged the use of values that are readily interpretable by the vast majority of the readership. Normal values are best determined in each laboratory, and this textbook stresses deviations from the normal.

In what is a new concept for this book, contributors have been asked to include a table identifying the drugs recommended in the body of the text. Dosages and specific notations about such therapy are included in the table. Most of the clinical chapters have such a table at the beginning or the end of the chapter for easier reference.

This third edition is not really a revised book, but rather a new work. Some previous sections have been revised, but a careful comparison of all three editions will reveal that each chapter has been written specifically for this edition and that most chapters are entirely new. As the editor, I have read every chapter. I have also had the benefit of several qualified editorial assistants. Despite this intense editorial effort, some errors in grammar, style, and perhaps even content may remain. The contributors and I would appreciate your comments concerning errors that may be corrected in subsequent printings. A book of this size is an overwhelming editorial task, and I take complete responsibility for it. Because it is not possible to have expertise in every subject, I rely heavily on the contributing authors to carefully review and edit their own sections after my editorial comments are made.

The authors for each edition are carefully chosen from the ranks of our profession. I hope that many others, equally qualified, will have an opportunity to participate in future editions. New and expanded sections will be chosen as the need becomes apparent. Suggestions from readers are welcome as I aim to present to the profession a timely and current review of internal medical problems affecting the dog and the cat.

I particularly wish to express my appreciation to my colleagues for their encouragement in preparing this manuscript. The contributing authors have done a tremendous job in their individual chapters. The W. B. Saunders staff has skillfully coordinated the manuscript production. I am pleased to have had the opportunity to have worked with Lorraine Kilmer, John Dyson, Edna Dick, Al Beringer, and Frank Polizzano.

Words alone cannot express my gratitude to the members of my staff who have supported me during the difficult periods of the past two years. Dr. Bob Lusk, my associate, has consistently been there when I needed him. My partners, Doctors Dan Didden, Larry Lippincott, and Al Plechner, along with the entire staff at the California Animal Hospital, were encouraging when there was no light at the end of the tunnel. To my editorial staff, I can only say thank you again for the superb effort. Ms. Dana St. John has dealt courageously with me and has managed the production from the time manuscripts began to arrive. She handled production of the book with skill and a smile and has often kept me from attacking the computer. The IBM and its peripherals also deserve a note of thanks—how else could I keep so many authors and their manuscripts looking alike and in Word Perfect order? My daughter Nicole worked through her junior and senior years in high school feeding manuscript into the computer so that we would always have material to edit. Additionally, Melonia Musser-Brauner, Teena Heim, and Catherine Fix deserve a thank-you. My special thanks are extended to Lori O'Brien as well as to my special four-legged friends Mr. Buster, Ms. Alice, Fiji, and Puff.

It remains an honor for me to have so many of the contributing authors as past and present associates or trainees. We have had a significant effect on each other's lives. In particular I take enormous pride in the accomplishments of my special friends and colleagues, Doctors Ed Feldman and Peter Suter. Dr. Robert Kirk remains my mentor and friend.

The veterinary profession has seen a tremendous growth in the clinical specialties over the past ten years. Projections indicate that the need for practicing board certified internists is increasing by over ten per cent annually at this time. It is also important to remain aware that better and improved service to the public remains our principal purpose. I wish to express my hope that our specialty organizations will rise to the occasion by encouraging and implementing more training opportunities. Further, these men and women assured of a variety of practice and institutional quality programs must then have the opportunity to readily enter the specialty groups. We need to guard against becoming restrictive fraternities; at the same time it is essential that we maintain the high standards of academic professionalism developed to date.

To the entire profession at large, may I also re-emphasize that our primary function to the public remains service. It is time to acknowledge this responsibility to the public by adhering to the goal of continued competence. Many avenues need to be explored to implement this goal.

In conclusion, I sincerely hope that the student—and we are all students—will benefit from this textbook. An old Chinese proverb summarizes it nicely. . . I hear and I forget, I see and I remember, I do and I understand.

STEPHEN J. ETTINGER
Malibu, California 1989

CONTENTS

VOLUME 1

SECTION I: MANIFESTATIONS OF CLINICAL DISEASE

1 CHANGES IN BODY WEIGHT 3
Stephen J. Ettinger

2 THE SKIN AS A SENSOR OF INTERNAL MEDICAL DISORDERS 5
Stephen D. White

3 TABLES OF ABNORMAL BLOOD VALUES AS A GUIDE TO DISEASE SYNDROMES 11
Lon J. Rich and Embert H. Coles

4 ANOREXIA AND POLYPHAGIA 15
Barbara E. Kitchell

5 PAIN (GENERAL, BACK, EXTREMITIES, ABDOMEN) 18
Michael J. Kelly

6 THERMOREGULATION 23
Robert H. Lusk, Jr.

7 VOMITING, REGURGITATION, AND DYSPHAGIA 27
Todd R. Tams

8 DIARRHEA 33
Richard K. Martin

9 CONSTIPATION, TENESMUS, AND DYSCHEZIA 36
M. D. Willard and R. Walshaw

10 PERIPHERAL EDEMA 41
Gary R. Bolton and Stephen J. Ettinger

11 WEAKNESS AND SYNCOPE 46
Stephen J. Ettinger

12 TREMBLING AND SHIVERING 54
Joe N. Kornegay and Christine E. Thomson

13 ATAXIA, PARESIS, AND PARALYSIS 57
Andy Shores and Philip Roudebush

14 ALTERED STATES OF CONSCIOUSNESS: COMA AND STUPOR 61
Andy Shores and Philip Roudebush

15 SEIZURES 66
Joe N. Kornegay and Stephen B. Lane

16 BEHAVIORAL SIGNS OF ORGANIC DISEASE 70
Alan J. Parker

17 OCULAR MANIFESTATIONS OF SYSTEMIC DISEASE 75
Kathleen L. Boldy and Bernard Clerc

18 COUGHING 85
Stephen J. Ettinger

19 DYSPNEA AND TACHYPNEA 88
Stephen J. Ettinger

20 ANEMIA 91
Susan M. Cotter

21 CYANOSIS 95
Gilbert Jacobs

22 POLYCYTHEMIA 101
Frederick H. Drazner

23 THE CLINICAL APPROACH TO DISORDERS OF HEMOSTASIS 105
G. Daniel Boon and A. H. Rebar

24 JAUNDICE 108
Susan E. Bunch

25 ALOPECIA 113
Lynn P. Schmeitzel

26 PRURITUS 122
Peter J. Ihrke

27 LUMPS, BUMPS, MASSES, AND LYMPHADENOPATHY 126
Dudley L. McCaw

28 ASCITES, PERITONITIS, AND OTHER CAUSES OF ABDOMINAL ENLARGEMENT 131
Stephen J. Ettinger

29 POLYURIA AND POLYDIPSIA 139
Clarke E. Atkins

30 INCONTINENCE, ENURESIS, AND NOCTURIA 148
Philippe M. Moreau and George E. Lees

31 URINARY OBSTRUCTION AND ATONY 155
Philippe M. Moreau and George E. Lees

32 HEMATURIA–DYSURIA 160
Geraldine McCall Kaufman

33 LAMENESS IN DOGS 165
J. François Bardet

34 LAMENESS IN CATS 169
J. François Bardet

35 CARDIOPULMONARY ARREST AND RESUSCITATION 171
Wayne E. Wingfield and Rosemary A. Henik

SECTION II: PROBLEMS IN VETERINARY PRACTICE

36 CHROMOSOMAL AND GENETIC DISORDERS 183
H. W. Leipold and S. M. Dennis

37 SMALL ANIMAL ZOONOSES 188
James B. Miller

38 FOOD HYPERSENSITIVITY 194
Michael S. Leib and John R. August

39 FELINE HYPERLIPIDEMIA 198
Boyd R. Jones

40 CANINE HYPERLIPIDEMIA 203
Roger K. Johnson

41 EMERGENCY MEDICINE 209
Robert J. Murtaugh

42 SMALL ANIMAL PROBLEMS IN DEVELOPING COUNTRIES 217
Joseph Van Heerden

43 BEHAVIORAL DISORDERS 227
Victoria L. Voith

44 HUMAN-ANIMAL BOND AND EUTHANASIA—
A SPECIAL PROBLEM 239
Michael J. McCulloch, James M. Harris, and William F. McCulloch

45 DISEASES OF THE EAR 246
Dennis W. Macy

SECTION III: INFECTIOUS DISEASES

46 BACTERIAL, RICKETTSIAL, PROTOZOAL,
AND MISCELLANEOUS INFECTIONS 265
Larry J. Swango, Karen W. Bankemper, and Lilly I. Kong

47 CANINE VIRAL DISEASES 298
Larry J. Swango

48 FELINE VIRAL DISEASES 312
John R. August

49 DEEP MYCOTIC DISEASES 341
Alice M. Wolf and Gregory C. Troy

SECTION IV: THERAPEUTIC CONSIDERATIONS IN MEDICINE

50 PHARMACOLOGIC PRINCIPLES IN THERAPEUTICS 375
J. Desmond Baggot

51 ANTIMICROBIAL DRUGS 383
Arthur L. Aronson and David P. Aucoin

52 USE OF CORTICOSTEROIDS 413
C. B. Chastain

53 FLUID THERAPY, ELECTROLYTE AND ACID-BASE CONTROL 429
David F. Senior

54 SPECIALIZED NUTRITIONAL SUPPORT 450
Timothy A. Allen

55 TOXICOLOGY 456
Michael E. Mount

56 ACUPUNCTURE THERAPY IN SMALL ANIMAL PRACTICE 484
Sheldon Altman

57 ADVERSE DRUG REACTIONS 499
Lloyd E. Davis

SECTION V: CANCER NEOPLASIA

58 TUMOR BIOLOGY 513
Steven E. Crow

59 APPROACH TO TREATMENT OF CANCER PATIENTS 527
E. Gregory MacEwen and Robert C. Rosenthal

SECTION VI: THE NERVOUS SYSTEM

60 THE NEUROLOGIC EVALUATION OF PATIENTS 549
William R. Fenner

61 DISEASES OF THE BRAIN 578
Craig E. Greene and Kyle G. Braund

62 DISEASES OF THE SPINAL CORD 624
Richard A. LeCouteur and Georgina Child

63 NEURO-OPHTHALMOLOGY 702
Alexander de Lahunta

64 PERIPHERAL NERVE DISORDERS 708
Cheryl L. Chrisman

65 DISORDERS OF THE SKELETAL MUSCLES 733
Vincent G. Pedroia

SECTION VII: THE RESPIRATORY SYSTEM

66 CLINICAL APPROACH TO THE PATIENT WITH RESPIRATORY DISEASE ... 747

Michael Schaer, Norman Ackerman, and Robert R. King

67 DISEASES OF THE NOSE AND THROAT ... 768

Peter G. C. Bedford

68 DISEASES OF THE TRACHEA ... 795

Stephen J. Ettinger and James W. Ticer

69 DISEASES OF THE LOWER RESPIRATORY TRACT (LUNG) AND PULMONARY EDEMA ... 816

Eleanor C. Hawkins, Stephen J. Ettinger, and Peter F. Suter

70 MEDIASTINAL, PLEURAL, AND EXTRAPLEURAL DISEASES ... 867

Tim Bauer

SECTION VIII: THE CARDIOVASCULAR SYSTEM

71 PATHOPHYSIOLOGY OF HEART FAILURE ... 899

David H. Knight

72 THE CLINICAL EVALUATION OF CARDIAC FUNCTION ... 923

David Sisson

73 THERAPY OF HEART FAILURE ... 939

Bruce W. Keene and John E. Rush

74 CONGENITAL HEART DISEASE ... 976

John D. Bonagura

75 VALVULAR HEART DISEASE ... 1031

Stephen J. Ettinger

76 CARDIAC ARRHYTHMIAS ... 1051

Stephen J. Ettinger

77 MYOCARDIAL DISEASES ... 1097

Philip R. Fox

78 PERICARDIAL DISORDERS ... 1132

William P. Thomas

79 INFECTIVE ENDOCARDITIS ... 1151

J. A. Woodfield and David Sisson

80 HEARTWORM DISEASE ... 1163

Clarence A. Rawlings and Clay A. Calvert

81 PERIPHERAL VASCULAR DISEASE ... 1185

Peter F. Suter

VOLUME 2

SECTION IX: THE GASTROINTESTINAL SYSTEM

82 ORAL, DENTAL, PHARYNGEAL, AND SALIVARY GLAND DISORDERS 1203
Colin E. Harvey

83 DISEASES OF THE ESOPHAGUS 1255
Brent D. Jones, Albert E. Jergens, and W. G. Guilford

84 GASTRIC DILATATION-VOLVULUS-TORSION SYNDROME 1278
Charles L. Lippincott and Alan J. Schulman

85 DISEASES OF THE STOMACH 1289
David C. Twedt and Michael L. Magne

86 DISEASES OF THE SMALL BOWEL 1323
Robert G. Sherding

87 DISEASES OF THE LARGE BOWEL 1397
Keith P. Richter

88 PATHOPHYSIOLOGY AND LABORATORY DIAGNOSIS OF LIVER DISEASE 1421
S. A. Center

89 DISEASES OF THE LIVER AND THEIR TREATMENT 1479
Robert M. Hardy

90 EXOCRINE PANCREATIC DISEASE 1528
David A. Williams

91 DISEASES OF THE GALLBLADDER 1555
David A. Hager

92 RECTO-ANAL DISEASE 1559
Colin F. Burrows and Gary W. Ellison

SECTION X: THE ENDOCRINE SYSTEM

93 PITUITARY-HYPOTHALAMIC DISEASE 1579
J. E. Eigenmann

94 PARATHYROID DISEASE AND CALCIUM METABOLISM 1610
Donald J. Meuten and P. Jane Armstrong

95 THYROID DISEASES 1632
Mark E. Peterson and Duncan C. Ferguson

96 DISORDERS OF THE ENDOCRINE PANCREAS 1676
Richard W. Nelson

97 ADRENAL GLAND DISEASE 1721
Edward C. Feldman

SECTION XI: THE REPRODUCTIVE SYSTEM

98 REPRODUCTIVE PHYSIOLOGY AND ENDOCRINOLOGY OF THE FEMALE AND MALE 1777
Victor M. Shille

99 PERSISTENT ESTRUS IN THE BITCH 1792
Patricia N. Olson, Robert H. Wrigley, Paul W. Husted, Richard A. Bowen, and Terry M. Nett

100 UTERINE DISEASES 1797
Cheri A. Johnson

101 VAGINAL DISORDERS 1806
Cheri A. Johnson

102 TUMORS OF THE GENITAL SYSTEM AND MAMMARY GLANDS 1814
Andrew S. Loar

103 PARTURIENT AND POST-PARTURIENT DISEASES 1826
J. E. Mosier

104 INFERTILITY 1838
Edward C. Feldman

105 CANINE PROSTATIC DISEASES 1859
Jeanne A. Barsanti and Delmar R. Finco

106 DISORDERS OF THE EXTERNAL GENITALIA OF THE MALE 1881
Shirley D. Johnston

SECTION XII: THE URINARY SYSTEM

107 DIAGNOSIS AND PATHOPHYSIOLOGY OF RENAL DISEASE 1893
Dennis J. Chew and Stephen DiBartola

108 DISEASES OF THE KIDNEYS AND URETERS 1963
David J. Polzin, Carl A. Osborne, and Timothy D. O'Brien

109 HYPERTENSIVE DISEASES 2047
Linda A. Ross

110 FELINE LOWER URINARY TRACT DISORDERS 2057
Carl A. Osborne, John M. Kruger, Gary R. Johnston, and David J. Polzin

111 CANINE UROLITHS 2083
Carl A. Osborne, David J. Polzin, Gary R. Johnston, and Timothy D. O'Brien

112 DISEASES OF THE BLADDER AND URETHRA 2108
Scott A. Brown and Jeanne A. Barsanti

SECTION XIII: DISEASES OF BLOOD CELLS, LYMPH NODES AND SPLEEN

113 ERYTHROCYTE RESPONSES AND DISORDERS 2145
M. G. Weiser

114 LEUKOCYTES IN HEALTH AND DISEASE 2181
Kenneth S. Latimer and Dennis J. Meyer

115 DISEASES OF THE LYMPH NODES AND SPLEEN 2225
C. Guillermo Couto

116 HEMOSTATIC DISORDERS: COAGULOPATHIES AND THROMBOTIC DISORDERS 2246
Robert A. Green

117 PLATELET DYSFUNCTION 2265
Bernard F. Feldman

SECTION XIV: THE IMMUNOLOGIC SYSTEM

118 PRINCIPLES OF IMMUNOLOGY 2283
Geoffrey Sunshine

119 IMMUNOLOGIC DISEASES 2297
James P. Thompson

SECTION XV: JOINT AND SKELETAL DISORDERS

120 JOINT DISEASES OF DOGS AND CATS 2329
Niels C. Pedersen, Alida Wind, Joe P. Morgan, and Roy R. Pool

121 SKELETAL DISEASES 2378
Charles D. Newton and Darryl N. Biery

INDEX i

SECTION I

MANIFESTATIONS OF CLINICAL DISEASE

1 CHANGES IN BODY WEIGHT

STEPHEN J. ETTINGER

An alteration in body weight that is not deliberately induced is one reason for presentation of a pet to the veterinarian. Weight gain or loss may be quite obvious and disturbing to the owner, or it may go unnoticed. Recording the pet's weight at each annual vaccination or examination is useful in assessing such changes. Changes in body appearance, such as the loss of muscle and fat with the simultaneous accumulation of abdominal fluid, may be misinterpreted by the owner as insignificant or simply a redistribution of body weight. However, the clinician should consider the possibility that such discrepancies are indicative of disease that requires further study.

Normally, weight is maintained when caloric intake equals caloric expenditure. About half the caloric intake supports basal metabolic requirements, while a small percentage is required for food absorption. The remainder is available to supply energy for physical activity and other needs. Excessive caloric intake coupled with reduced activity may account for weight gain.

Weight loss or gain occurring over a short period (several days) usually represents a shift of body fluids. In contrast, weight change persisting for weeks to months indicates a change in tissue mass. Weight gain resulting from fluid retention in the presence of hepatic, cardiac, renal, or gastrointestinal disease may initially obscure the true picture of body mass loss.

Weight Gain

Few clinical states are responsible for weight gain in the dog and cat. Hypothyroidism, hypogonadism, insulin-secreting tumors, exogenous steroid administration, and rarely, Cushing's syndrome, should be ruled out. Hypothyroidism and insulin-secreting tumors may be differentiated by commonly available laboratory tests. The associated clinical signs in Cushing's syndrome of polyuria, polydipsia, hair coat or skin changes, and the typical hemogram as well as post adrenal gland stimulation blood cortisol determinations may aid in the differential diagnosis. Hypertensive patients and dogs with primary hyperlipidemias (cholesterol and/or triglycerides) may also demonstrate an otherwise unexplained weight gain.

Even when hypogonadism is ultimately responsible for weight gain following ovariohysterectomy or castration, the excessive intake of calories and the pet's reduced level of activity are likely to be the direct cause.

While a specific breed or line may be prone to weight gain, it is usually excessive caloric intake that is at fault. Older, less active pets require fewer calories. Younger, unspayed females may gain weight when pregnant. Fluid-retaining conditions need to be differentiated from an increase in body tissue mass. Dogs with chronic degenerative bone and joint disease may initially gain body mass, again as a result of maintaining their caloric intake while decreasing physical activity.

Weight Loss

The causes of weight loss are numerous, but there are usually clues that point to its etiogenesis. The owner or animal handler should be able to say whether the weight change is associated with an increased or decreased appetite. Weight loss with an increased appetite suggests diabetes mellitus, hyperthyroidism, chronic pancreatic insufficiency, or an intestinal malabsorption syndrome. Weight loss with decreased appetite suggests other causes.

Gastrointestinal symptomatology in the form of masticatory or swallowing difficulty, vomiting, and chronic diarrhea provides information regarding some causes of weight loss. Behavioral changes or psychosocial factors such as a new living environment, a new member of the family (pet or human), or the loss of a family member are also important points to consider. Dietary changes, variations in the formulation of the diet, or a reduction in the quantity or quality of food being fed is another area to explore. Occasionally, clients who favor food fads such as health foods or vitamins may inadvertently cause a state of malnutrition. Animals subjected to extreme stress such as a very cold climate, periods of rapid growth, gestation, lactation, and racing or prolonged exercise have higher caloric demands that may not be provided for at times.

General Pathophysiology

Pathophysiologic causes of weight loss include an increased rate of tissue metabolism, loss of calories through urine or stool, or a diminished intake of calories, usually due to a loss of appetite. The list of individual diseases that could be incriminated is far too lengthy for this chapter, but by categorizing the most likely conditions the veterinarian should be better able to establish a differential diagnosis.

Gastrointestinal Disease. Dysphagia due to painful oral lesions involving the mucous membranes, tongue, or teeth prevents the intake of adequate calories. Neurologic disease responsible for diminished prehension and/or swallowing of food results in a form of starvation. Many commonly used drugs cause nausea and anorexia.

Vomiting, when excessive, reduces true caloric intake. It may be transient, but when prolonged, weight loss may occur. Common gastrointestinal causes of vomiting are esophageal dilatation, gastritis, gastric neoplasia, gastric or intestinal foreign body, acute relapsing pancreatitis, and roundworm infestation. Diseases of the small and large bowel (enteritis and colitis) may, with prolonged diarrhea, result in a protein-losing enteropathy (examples are steatorrhea, malabsorption syndromes, chronic parasitic disease, and food- or drug-induced diarrhea).

Endocrine Diseases. Hyperthyroidism, hypopituitarism, and adrenal insufficiency are hormone-induced causes of anorexia and weight loss. In contrast, diabetes mellitus causes a weight loss associated with an increased intake of food. Exocrine pancreatic insufficiency is associated with a ravenous appetite, chronic diarrhea, and weight loss. It can be associated with diabetes mellitus, juvenile pancreatic acinar atrophy, and chronic fulminant pancreatic inflammation and destruction.

Hypoprotein States. Protein-losing nephropathies may be insidious early in the course of the disease, but are always associated with an increased quantity of protein in the urine. Hepatitis (both acute and chronic) and cirrhosis are related to weight loss as a result of decreased production and/or use of serum proteins. Chronic cardiac disease is associated with cachexia, weight loss, and hypoproteinemia. Cardiac cachexia may be due to increased body fluids as well as enzymatic changes in the liver and intestines.

Infections and Fever. Infectious and granulomatous diseases, chronic endometritis, chronic sepsis, localized abscess formation, feline infectious peritonitis (FIP), and feline leukovirus are examples of such disease states. These are often associated with anorexia. Inflammation induces fever, which increases the basal metabolic rate and protein metabolism responsible for weight loss. The differential diagnosis of fever is discussed in Chapter 6.

Malignancy. Tumors increase the metabolic processes even in the absence of overt anatomic or metabolic dysfunction. They may be responsible for fever, which also increases the metabolic rate. Weight loss of unexplained origin should include a careful evaluation of the gastrointestinal tract, liver, pancreas, lymph nodes, and bone marrow for suggestions of a neoplastic process.

Diagnostic Approach

The history and physical examination usually suggest the organ system(s) involved with weight loss. When the etiology remains obscure, a comprehensive evaluation of the blood count, blood chemistries, and urinalysis is indicated. Serum electrolytes should be included in the blood chemistry studies and thyroid (T_3 and T_4) studies should be evaluated. Fecal examinations for trypsin activity as well as ova and parasites using direct and flotation methods, are in order when chronic diarrhea is present. In the feline, leukovirus studies and FIP serology are indicated. When the cause is still obscure, contrast radiography (gastrointestinal and urinary), biopsy (bone marrow, muscle, liver), and special chemistry studies (protein electrophoresis) should be considered. Plasma cortisol levels and serology (ANA, LE, RA) should be considered if the signs suggest the possibility of such a problem.

Summary

While weight gain is occasionally associated with an endocrinopathy, it most commonly results from excessive caloric intake. Weight loss is usually more significant in terms of its serious medical implications. Thyrotoxicosis, diabetes mellitus, malabsorption syndromes, and inadequate caloric intake in the face of increased requirements are associated with weight loss and an increased intake of food. Malignancy, fever, endocrinopathies, renal and liver disease, infectious disease, and psychosocial factors usually are related to a decreased level of food intake and weight loss.

2 THE SKIN AS A SENSOR OF INTERNAL MEDICAL DISORDERS

STEPHEN D. WHITE

The knowledge of skin diseases in small animals has so increased in recent years that is difficult to describe a cutaneous condition that does *not* have some relation to internal medicine. Even the ubiquitous flea allergy dermatitis involves internal immunologic mechanisms more complex than a simple insect bite. However, the purpose of this chapter is to discuss those diseases having cutaneous manifestations that should alert the clinician to further investigation of other organ systems. The text is arranged by categories of diseases, while Table 2–1 is organized by clinical signs.

CONGENITAL-HEREDITARY SYNDROMES (GENODERMATOSES)

These diseases are present at birth or noted shortly thereafter. Affected animals should not be bred.

Dermatomyositis. This disease has been reported in collies and Shetland sheepdogs and their crosses. As its name implies, the disease affects both the muscles and the skin. Cutaneous changes include crusts, ulcerations, vesicles, and/or alopecia around the mucocutaneous junctions, front legs, ear tips, and tail, though other body areas may be affected. Muscular atrophy may be generalized or may be selective, often affecting the temporal and masseter muscles. Clinical manifestations vary, with some dogs showing only skin or muscular signs, while in others both systems are affected. Serum enzymes such as creatinine phosphokinase (CPK) are usually normal, and muscle involvement often may only be proven by biopsy or electromyography. Skin biopsies generally reveal intracellular edema of the basal cell layer of the epidermis, with subepidermal clefts. The onset of clinical signs usually occurs before six months of age. The severity of the disease varies greatly, with some dogs improving with age. Vitamin E at 100 to 400 IU q12h or immunosuppressive doses of prednisolone have been tried as therapy with inconsistent results. The inheritance is autosomal dominant. A disease formerly reported as epidermolysis bullosa probably represents the cutaneous manifestations of dermatomyositis.

Cyclic Neutropenia. This condition is primarily seen in gray collies, but is reported in other breeds. Affected dogs have a predisposition for developing infections of various organ systems, including the skin. Oral and lip ulcerations are common and may lead to severe necrotizing stomatitis. The condition occurs in the first six months of life, occurs in all gray (not merle) collies, and is uniformly fatal.

Enzyme Deficiencies. Mucopolysaccharidoses are storage diseases caused by a deficiency of either arylsulfatase B or alpha-L-iduronidase and the subsequent accumulation of mucopolysaccharides in various tissues. These diseases have been reported only in the cat. Affected kittens have broad flat faces, small ears, and corneal clouding. Occasionally cutaneous nodules, lameness, and pectus excavatum (depression of the sternum) may be seen. Clinical signs are evident at six weeks of age. The arylsulfatase B deficiency has an autosomal recessive mode of inheritance.

Tyrosinemia has been reported in a young dog with corneal opacities, ulceration and erosions of the foot pads and nose, and erythematous bullae of the ventral abdomen. The exact enzyme deficiency was not reported. Treatment in the form of dietary changes may be helpful in tyrosinemia.

Definitive diagnosis of these rare diseases is made by various biochemical tests usually performed at a research institution.

Chediak-Higashi Syndrome. This disease is an autosomal recessive disorder reported in Persian cats with yellow eyes and "blue-smoke" hair color. Affected cats have partial oculocutaneous albinism, a bleeding tendency, increased incidence of infection, and enlarged granules in many cell types, including melanocytes and leukocytes. No therapy is effective.

TABLE 2–1. DERMATOLOGIC SIGNS AND DIFFERENTIAL DIAGNOSES OF INTERNAL DISEASES

Sign	Differential Diagnosis
Alopecia without pruritus	Hypothyroidism
	Hyperadrenocorticism
	Growth hormone abnormalities
	Gonadal hormone-responsive syndromes
	Demodicosis
	Drug reaction
	Systemic lupus erythematosus
	Thallium toxicosis
Erythema without pruritus	Systemic lupus erythematosus
	Demodicosis
	Drug reaction
	Pheochromocytoma
	Thallium toxicosis
Mucocutaneous lesions	Systemic lupus erythematosus
	Demodicosis
	Staphylococcal pyoderma
	Zinc-responsive dermatosis
	Cyclic neutropenia
	Dermatomyositis
	Cold agglutinin disease
	Leishmaniasis
	Thallium toxicosis
	Renal disease
	Toxic epidermal necrolysis
	Erythema multiforme
Petechia	Ehrlichiosis
	Rocky Mountain spotted fever
	Babesiosis
	Systemic lupus erythematosus
	Hyperadrenocorticism
Pruritus	Staphylococcal pyoderma
	Demodicosis
	Food hypersensitivity
	Cutaneous lymphoma
	Sertoli cell tumor
	Neuter-responsive dermatoses
Persistent pyoderma	Demodicosis
	Hyperadrenocorticism
	Hypothyroidism
	Diabetes mellitus
	Food hypersensitivity
	Brucella canis pyoderma
	Zinc-responsive dermatosis
Seborrhea	Staphylococcal pyoderma
	Hypothyroidism
	Hyperadrenocorticism
	Gonadal hormone abnormalities
	Demodicosis
	Cutaneous lymphoma
	Zinc-responsive dermatosis
	Vitamin A–responsive dermatosis
	Food hypersensitivity
	Systemic lupus erythematosus
	Hepatic disease
Scrotal dermatitis	*Brucella canis* infection
	Rocky Mountain spotted fever
	Cold agglutinin disease

This table is not meant to be exhaustive and does not include such diseases as contact, flea, or inhalant allergies; scabies; or other skin diseases not usually associated with dysfunction of other organ systems.

ENDOCRINOPATHIES

These diseases are probably the most common internal diseases associated with cutaneous manifestations.

Hypothyroidism. Cutaneous lesions may consist of total or partial alopecia; seborrhea; hyperpigmentation; thick, cool, or puffy skin; easy bruising; a dry, easily epilated hair coat; secondary pyoderma or dermatophytosis; and otitis externa. Pruritus may be present, particularly in association with pyoderma or seborrhea (see Chapter 95).

Hyperadrenocorticism. Cutaneous lesions that may be seen are alopecia (usually truncal, but occasionally facial), hyperpigmentation, seborrhea, pyoderma, dermatophytosis or demodicosis secondary to immunesuppression, thin skin, comedones, easy bruising, and calcinosis cutis. Pruritus may be present in conjunction with pyoderma, seborrhea, demodicosis, or calcinosis cutis. Skin lesions may be the *only* abnormality noted by the client or the veterinarian, without polyuria, polydipsia, hepatomegaly, eosinopenia, or increased serum alkaline phosphatase (see Chapter 97).

Gonadal Hormone Abnormalities. Sertoli cell tumors of the testes in dogs may cause alopecia and feminization in approximately one-third of affected dogs. Both seminomas and interstitial cell tumors may (rarely) cause the same clinical signs. The cause (at least in the Sertoli cell tumors) is the increased levels of estrogen produced by the tumor. These dogs are occasionally quite pruritic with a papular eruption. Therapy consists of the removal of *both* testicles: not all tumors are palpable, and undescended testicles are at higher risk for developing the tumor. A thorough presurgical evaluation is indicated (complete blood and platelet count, thoracic and abdominal radiographs) as bone marrow suppression and malignancy with metastases have been reported, though not commonly.

Other gonadal hormonal abnormalities are much less common than Sertoli cell tumors. These include both testosterone- and estrogen-responsive alopecias, usually in castrated and spayed dogs, respectively, and castration- and spay-responsive dermatoses in intact male and female dogs, respectively. A clinical sign in the hormonally-responsive dogs is generally a diffuse to patchy alopecia beginning in the perineal area, usually with minimal or no pruritus. In the male, the clinical signs of the neutering-responsive dermatosis are similar to those caused by Sertoli cell tumors; in the female, alopecia (both ventral and perineal), seborrhea, pruritus, gynecomastia, and estrus cycle abnormalities occur. Diagnosis is made by clinical signs, ruling out other endocrine diseases, and response to therapy. Caution is advised in the administration of estrogen (1 mg diethylstilbestrol orally, once to twice weekly) or testosterone (0.5 mg/lb. orally, up to 30 mg, q48h for three months, then once or twice weekly) because of the risk of inducing bone marrow suppression or cholestatic liver disease, respectively. Owners should be informed of the advantages and disadvantages of using these drugs to treat abnormal-appearing, but usually otherwise healthy, dogs.

Growth Hormone Dependent Syndromes. Growth hormone deficiency in dwarf dogs is a hereditary disease usually seen in the German shepherd or Carnelian bear-dog. Cutaneous lesions are alopecia or retention of a "puppy-coat," seborrhea, and/or hyperpigmentation. Adult onset growth hormone deficiency usually occurs in mature dogs, with a seeming breed predisposition for Pomeranians, poodles, chow chows, and keeshonds. Alopecia and hyperpigmentation, often in a strikingly bilateral truncal pattern, are the clinical signs (see Chapter 93).

Diabetes Mellitus. Cutaneous lesions associated with this disease are uncommon, but have been reported as pyoderma, seborrhea, thin skin, alopecia, demodicosis, and xanthomatosis. An ulcerative dermatosis associated with diabetes mellitus in the dog has been reported. Erythema, crusts, and alopecia are found periorally, periocularly, and on the footpads. Both clinical signs and histopathology (inter- and intracellular edema in the upper half of the epidermis) resemble a condition in humans known as necrolytic migratory erythema. The human condition is usually associated with a glucagon-secreting neoplasm of the pancreas. However, in the dogs reported, either such a tumor could not be identified, or necropsy was refused by the owner. Diabetic animals are usually brought to the veterinarian for nondermatologic signs (see Chapter 96).

Pheochromocytoma. Like diabetics, dogs with pheochromocytomas are usually brought to veterinarians for other clinical problems. However, flushing or signs due to tumor thrombus of the posterior vena cava (rear limb edema, distention of caudal epigastric veins) may be features, and this disease should be included in the differentiation of erythema without pruritus. (See Chapter 97.)

BACTERIAL INFECTIONS

Staphylococcal Infections. Staphylococcal pyoderma is the second most common canine skin disease (after flea-related conditions) seen by the author. While many recurrent staphylococcal infections are (thus far) considered idiopathic, the veterinarian should always attempt to rule out an underlying cause, such as an allergy (food, fleas, inhalant), an endocrine disease (hypothyroidism, hyperadrenocorticism), or other immunosuppressive condition (neoplasia, administration of cortisone or antineoplastic drugs).

Brucellosis canis. Infections with this bacterium occasionally cause a scrotal swelling or dermatitis secondary to orchitis. A pyogranulomatous dermatitis has also been reported and was the first sign noted (see Chapter 104).

Lyme Disease. Lyme disease is a tick-borne disorder of dogs and humans caused by the spirochete *Borrelia burgdorfi*. In the United States this disease is transmitted by the tick *Ixodes dammini*. The cases reported in the dog have been from the northeastern United States, with arthritis and fever the prominent signs. Early disease in humans is often characterized by an expanding annular lesion called erythema chronicum migrans, which may precede other systems' involvement by days to months. While not yet documented in the dog, clinicians should be suspicious of any such lesion in a dog from an endemic area (see Chapter 46).

FUNGAL INFECTIONS

Sporotrichosis. *Sporothrix schenckii* causes a cutaneous infection characterized by nodular, draining, suppurative lesions. Usually introduced into the skin via trauma with plant material, such as thorns, it may infect humans from the scratches of an affected animal. While generally a cutaneous or subcutaneous disease, sporotrichosis may become generalized, affecting internal organs. Other subcutaneous fungal diseases such as phaeohyphomycosis and protothecosis may also affect other organ systems.

Deep or Systemic Mycoses. Infections such as those caused by *Blastomyces dermatitides*, *Histoplasma capsulatum*, *Cryptococcus neoformans*, and *Coccidioides immitis* may involve a number of organ systems. Cutaneous lesions may be varied, including nodules, plaques, draining tracts, alopecia, and seborrhea, and may be the first signs noted by the client. (See Chapter 49.)

PARASITIC DISEASES

Demodicosis. Generalized demodicosis is thought to occur in dogs with an underlying immune-suppressive disorder. In young dogs this has been hypothesized to be a specific T lymphocyte dysfunction. In older dogs that develop generalized demodicosis (or demodectic pododermatitis), hyperadrenocorticism, diabetes mellitus, or internal neoplasia should be considered as possible underlying etiologies. A thorough diagnostic evaluation, including a complete blood count, serum biochemical profile, thoracic and abdominal radiographs, and adrenal evaluation tests, is indicated. Therapy consists of the miticidal dips amitraz (Mitaban) or ronnel (Ectoral). The former is easier to use (once weekly versus once daily) but probably has a lower cure rate. Immunostimulants and ivermectin have not been therapeutically effective. Older dogs with demodicosis have a poorer chance of cure, but usually may be adequately controlled with intermittent amitraz dips and resolution of any underlying disease. Generalized demodicosis in cats is very rare, but when present is usually in association with diabetes mellitus, feline leukemia virus infection, or possibly hyperadrenocorticism.

Leishmaniasis. This protozoal disease has been reported in dogs in the United States both from an endemic focus in Oklahoma (species undetermined), and in dogs that have spent time in the Mediterranean area *(Leishmania donovani)*. The disease may cause skin lesions as the first signs noted by owner or clinician. Alopecia, erythema, and especially scaling and ulceration of the ears and mucocutaneous junctions may occur. These dogs often have hyperproteinemia, hyperglobulinemia, nonresponsive anemia, and proteinuria. Diagnosis is by demonstration of the organism in the skin, spleen, liver, bone marrow, or synovial fluid, by histology or culture. Therapy is usually intravenous antimony compounds. Practitioners with a suspected or confirmed case should contact the public health authorities, as the dog may serve as a reservoir of the disease via vectors (*Phlebotomus* or *Lutzomyia* sand flies), although the disease probably cannot be directly transmitted from dog to human. (See Chapter 46.)

Rickettsial Diseases. Ehrlichiosis and Rocky Mountain spotted fever may both present with petechiae of the mucous membranes or skin. These diseases may also cause edema of the extremities, and a scrotal dermatitis has been reported with Rocky Mountain spotted fever (see Chapter 46).

Heartworms. *Dirofilariasis immitis* has been isolated from cutaneous nodules, implicated in causing a scabies-like eruption, and mentioned as a possible underlying etiology for generalized demodicosis. While these manifestations of heartworm disease are rare, dogs from endemic areas should provoke a high index of suspicion if they exhibit these signs (see Chapter 80).

Intestinal Nematodes and Cestodes. Hookworms, whipworms, roundworms, and tapeworms may cause skin disease. Hookworms may cause a papular, inflammatory eruption on the parts of the body in contact with infected soil, as the third-stage larvae enter the dog's skin. Species of both *Ancylostoma* and *Uncinaria* have been implicated. Any of these intestinal parasites may rarely cause an allergic condition of uncertain pathogenesis, with pruritus, papules, erythema, and/or seborrhea present. Anthelminthic therapy is curative, with rapid clinical improvement.

Babesiosis. Babesiosis in dogs may be associated with edema, petechiae, urticaria, and erythema. While not a common sign of this tick-borne protozoal disease, it may be the first sign noted by the owners. To the author's knowledge, these cutaneous signs have been observed only in canine babesiosis seen in France (see Chapter 46).

NUTRITIONAL DISORDERS

While relatively uncommon, these conditions are important for their differential diagnoses as well as their usually excellent response to therapy.

Zinc-Responsive Dermatosis. This disease is seen as two syndromes. The first occurs primarily in Siberian huskies and Alaskan malamutes, though other breeds have been reported. Crusts, scale, erythema, and alopecia occur around the mucocutaneous junctions, face, footpads, and abdomen, and are not always bilateral. Pruritus is variable. These dogs are on balanced diets with adequate levels of zinc for normal dogs. The underlying etiology is thought to be a decreased ability to absorb zinc from the gut. Syndrome II occurs in pups of any breed fed an over-supplemented (especially a high-calcium) diet (calcium may interfere with gut absorption of zinc). Hyperkeratotic plaques and crusts may occur on the head, trunk, extremities, and footpads. Depression, fever, and anorexia may be present. A similar disease has been seen in dogs fed generic dog food.

Diagnosis is based on skin biopsy, which usually shows excessive follicular and/or epidermal parakeratosis. Therapy for syndrome I is zinc supplementation, either zinc sulfate 220 mg q12-24h for a standard size husky, or zinc methionine (Zinpro), 15 mg zinc (1 tablet)/20 lbs q24h. For syndrome II, changing to a balanced dog food with or without zinc supplementation is indicated.

A disease resembling a zinc deficiency with secondary pyoderma has been reported in bull terriers. Oral and parenteral zinc replacement was *not* therapeutic, and all dogs died at an early age.

Vitamin A-Responsive Dermatosis. This disease has been seen primarily in cocker spaniels. The dermatosis is characterized by a seborrhea with marked follicular plugging, hyperkeratotic plaques, and surface "fronds." Diagnosis is by elimination of other causes of seborrhea and by skin biopsy, revealing extreme follicular orthokeratotic hyperkeratosis. Affected dogs are healthy otherwise, with no signs of hypovitaminosis A. The therapeutic response seen with vitamin A is probably due to its various pharmacologic effects on epithelium. Recommended doses approximate to 300 IU/lb q12–24h.

Pansteatitis. This disease's etiology is a deficiency of vitamin E and its antioxidant property. The deficiency is either due to inadequate initial amounts in the diet or a relative deficiency associated with the consumption of highly unsaturated fatty acids, which destroy vitamin E. It has been reported only in cats, usually those eating diets containing red fish or excessive cod liver oil. Affected cats are usually depressed, febrile, anorexic, and sore or painful on palpation of the skin or abdomen. Subcutaneous and abdominal fat may feel firm or lumpy. Draining tracts may be present. Diagnosis is based on history and biopsy, with the latter showing on gross examination yellow to orange-brown fat nodules which, when formalin-fixed, fluoresce yellow-orange under ultraviolet light. Histopathology shows fat necrosis and a septal panniculitis, with a pink-yellow material seen within fat vacuoles and macrophages. This substance is termed ceroid, and is felt to be a intermediate product of lipids. Abdominal and omental fat is frequently involved. Therapy consists of changing to a proper diet, oral vitamin E (alpha-tocopherol) 25 to 75 IU q12h, and corticosteroids for their anti-inflammatory and appetite-stimulating effects (prednisolone 0.5 mg/lb q12h). Despite these measures, the author has seen cats with this disease that failed to improve.

Food Hypersensitivity. A hypersensitivity reaction to foods has been documented in the dog and the cat. Immunologic mechanisms have not been thoroughly delineated. Clinical signs in dogs are generally pruritus, papules, and erythema, but otitis, pododermatitis, and seborrhea may also occur. In cats, pruritus is often prominent on the face, head, and neck. Diagnosis is based on the feeding of a strict home-cooked diet containing one meat and one starch source not usually fed to the pet (the author prefers lamb and rice) for three weeks. If improvement is noted, the animal may be challenged with individual food stuffs to determine the offending allergen; alternatively, prescription or nonpreservative-containing diets may be used once the diagnosis is made. (See Chapter 38.)

AUTOIMMUNE DISORDERS

Systemic Lupus Erythematosus (SLE). This disease exhibits a great variety of clinical signs. Cutaneous lesions often are crusts, ulcers, or depigmentation affecting the mucocutaneous junctions and footpads. However, erythema, seborrhea, panniculitis, and vasculitis have all been reported. These lesions may be exacerbated by exposure to sunlight. Other clinical signs that may be noted are anemia, proteinuria, and polyarthritis. The etiology probably involves the deposition of antibody-antigen complexes in various tissues with subsequent activation of the complement cascade. In SLE involving the skin in humans, approximately 10 per cent of the people do not have a positive antinuclear antibody (ANA) test, but do have anticytoplasmic antibodies. The importance of this finding in dogs and cats is unknown. (See Chapters 118, 119, and 120.)

Cold Agglutinin Disease. This condition has been reported in dogs, and is due to a cold-reacting erythrocyte autoantibody, usually IgM. When these dogs are exposed to cold (usually 0 to 4°C), the antibodies are activated with subsequent agglutination and interference with blood flow and/or anemia. This is particularly evident at the extremities (paws, ears, nose, scrotum, tip of tail) and erythema, cyanosis, ulceration, and necrosis may all be present. Diagnosis is by demonstrating significant titers of cold agglutinins. Therapy is immunosuppressive drug regimens and avoidance of cold. (See Chapters 113 and 119.)

Drug Eruption. Cutaneous reaction to drugs may occur with long- or short-term usage or even after therapy is discontinued. Lesions may mimic almost any skin condition other than the genodermatoses. A thorough history of all medications is essential for accurate diagnosis.

Toxic Epidermal Necrolysis (TEN). This is a rare vesiculobullous and ulcerative disease of the skin and mucosa of dogs and cats. It is characterized by an acute onset of pyrexia, anorexia, lethargy, and/or depression, and a multifocal or generalized vesiculobullous eruption. The outer layer of the skin adjacent to lesions may be easily rubbed away (positive Nikolsky sign). Pain is moderate to severe. Histopathology includes intracellular edema (hydropic degeneration) of the basal epidermal cells, full-thickness epidermal necrosis, and minimal dermal inflammation. Dermoepidermal separation may be present. It is important to realize that TEN often seems to be associated with various diseases, such as neoplasia, bacterial infection, drug eruption, or liver disease. Therapy involves treating the underlying disease, symptomatic and supportive therapy, and corticosteroids (prednisolone, 0.5 to 1 mg/lb q12h).

Erythema Multiforme. Erythema multiforme, like TEN, is an acute eruption of the skin and mucous membranes. It is characterized clinically by annular ("target") lesions. Vesicles, maculae, and urticarial plaques may also be seen. The lesions are generally asymptomatic and self-limiting. Like TEN, the lesions may be secondary to another disease; in dogs erythema multiforme has been reported in association with staphylococcal folliculitis and drug eruption.

Graft-versus-Host Disease (GVHD). This condition has been reported in experimental dogs undergoing bone marrow transplantation. It is mediated by donor T lymphocytes, which react against the recipient's tissues. Clinical signs affecting the skin may be erythema of the ears, axilla, and groin as well as skin atrophy. Diagnosis is confirmed on skin biopsy; if the mucosa are involved, the lip is the best site for detection. Histopathologic changes are sclerodermoid and/or poikilodermatous, and are well described in the experimental literature. Treatment is directed at prevention by choosing donors and recipients with compatible major histocompatibility complexes, and immunosuppressive drug therapy.

MISCELLANEOUS DISEASE

Thallium Toxicosis. This is uncommon in the United States with a ban on its use; however, it is still used in other parts of the world as a rodenticide. Acute thallium poisoning generally kills the animal within four to five days with little time for skin lesions to occur. In chronic thallium poisoning, the animal may be ill for three to six weeks before death. Alopecia, erythema, crusts, and ulceration occur on the axillae, ears, genitalia, posterior abdomen, paws, and mucocutaneous junctions. "Brick-red" mucous membranes may be noted. Depression, vomiting, diarrhea, nephrosis, and polyneuritis may also be seen. Diagnosis is by a positive urine test for thallium. Gabriel's test with rhodamine B may give false positives in cats. Therapeutic recommendations consist of supportive care (especially fluids) and administration of Prussian blue 50 mg/lb orally q8h. This disease has a poor prognosis even with therapy.

Hepatic Disease. While hepatobiliary disease in humans often causes pruritus and other clinical signs, this seems to be relatively rare in small animals. Occasionally a cat with cholangiohepatitis or other liver disease is seen with a pruritic, generalized exfoliative dermatitis. The etiology of this is not understood. (See Chapters 88 and 89.)

Pancreatic Disease. Rarely in severe pancreatitis, subcutaneous fat necrosis with erythema and draining tracts may be noted. It has been hypothesized that this is due to the high circulating levels of lipase released from the inflamed pancreas (see Chapter 90).

Renal Disease. Uremia has been reported to cause oral ulcerations. Usually other signs of renal failure are also present. The etiology of the oral lesions is thought to be due to the toxic effects of urea and other waste products on the oral mucosa (see Chapters 107 and 108).

A generalized nodular dermatofibrosis syndrome in

German shepherds associated with renal cystadenocarcinomas has been reported. Histopathology of the nodules reveals dense collagen fibrosis.

Neoplasia. Internal neoplasia may cause nonspecific clinical signs related to the skin, such as a sparse, dull, or dry haircoat, mild seborrhea, or possibly pruritus. These animals are usually cachectic and have other clinical signs. Cutaneous lymphoma, especially the epitheliotrophic form (mycosis fungoides) may cause seborrhea, pruritus, erythema and alopecia, in its initial stages, without obvious tumors being present. Multiple biopsies may be needed for diagnosis. (See Chapter 58.)

3 TABLES OF ABNORMAL BLOOD VALUES AS A GUIDE TO DISEASE SYNDROMES

LON J. RICH and EMBERT H. COLES

If properly interpreted, clinical laboratory profiles provide a wealth of information regarding the health of dogs and cats. The following tables are designed to provide a summary of laboratory abnormalities and the disease conditions in which they occur.

The causes of the alterations in blood values are listed in descending order of frequency. The condition that, in our opinion, most commonly produces a change is first and the condition least likely to produce the change is last.

Laboratory profiling should be considered an aid to diagnosis. The veterinarian must use all available tools and information before arriving at a final diagnosis. These tables should be used as a guideline to assist in arriving at a logical diagnosis.

NEUTROPHILIA

Cause	Neutrophil Response	Other Leukocytes	Mechanism
Physiologic–exercise, hypoxia, excitement	Mature-moderate absolute increase	Lymphocytosis, particularly in cats	Marginal granulocyte pool (MGP) to circulating granulocyte pool (CGP)
Increased glucocorticoids (endogenous, exogenous)	Mature-moderate absolute increase	Lymphopenia, eosinopenia, monocytosis (dog)	Decreased removal of neutrophils from blood, increased removal from marrow storage pool
Early inflammation	Left shift with moderate increase in absolute neutrophil count	Little change unless stress. With stress, lymphopenia, eosinopenia, and monocytosis (dog)	Increased tissue demand, excess release from storage pool of marrow
Established inflammation (suppurative)	Left shift with marked increase in absolute neutrophil count	Monocytosis. If stress, lymphopenia, eosinopenia	Increased neutrophil production and release to meet tissue demand
Chronic inflammation (suppurative)	Marked left shift and increase, absolute mature neutrophils; often toxic neutrophils	Monocytosis, occasionally lymphocytosis if considerable antigenic stimulation. With stress, lymphopenia, eosinopenia	As above

NEUTROPENIA

Cause	Neutrophil Response	Other Leukocytes	Mechanism
Overwhelming bacterial infection	Marked neutropenia, usually with marked left shift	Normal, or if stress, lymphopenia eosinopenia, monocytosis (dog)	Increased tissue demand-depletion of peripheral pool; increased removal from marrow pools
Decreased production of neutrophils	Neutropenia with slight or no left shift	Normal, or if stress, lymphopenia eosinopenia, monocytosis (dog)	Decreased marrow production with normal tissue demand
Sequestration	Sudden neutropenia, no left shift	Frequent lymphopenia	CGP to MGP
Ineffective granulopoiesis	Neutropenia, no left shift	Increased marrow granulopoiesis; if stress, lymphopenia, eosinopenia	Improper release from marrow pools

MONOCYTES

Causes of Monocytosis
1. Increased glucocorticoids (dog)
2. Chronic inflammation (necrosis)
3. Internal hemorrhage
4. Hemolytic disease
5. Suppuration (body cavity)
6. Immune mediated disease
7. Granulomatous disorders
8. Monocytic leukemia (rare)

LYMPHOCYTES

Causes of Lymphocytosis

Physiologic: Cats and rarely other species
- Increased epinephrine activity, e.g., exercise, anxiety
- Temporary following some vaccinations

Pathologic:
- Chronic infection (prolonged Ag stimulation)
- Lymphosarcoma (not in all patients)

Causes of Lymphopenia

Excess glucocorticoids
1. Endogenous
   - Debilitating disease
   - Hyperadrenocorticism
   - Surgery
   - Shock
   - Trauma
   - Heat or cold exposure
2. Exogenous
   - Glucocorticoid or ACTH therapy

Lymphocyte loss
1. Protein-losing enteropathy (lymphangiectasia)
2. Chylothorax with repeated drainage

Reduced lymphopoiesis
1. Chemotherapy (cancer)
2. Irradiation
3. Prolonged corticosteroid therapy
4. Congenital T cell immunodeficiency (CID–horse)

EOSINOPHILS

Causes of Eosinophilia

Hypersensitivity:
1. Anaphylaxis
2. Parasitism in sensitized hosts: (dirofilariasis, ancylostomiasis, ascariasis, aeleurostrongylosis, demidocosis, and so on)

Specific eosinophilic diseases:
1. Eosinophilic enterocolitis
2. Eosinophilic granuloma (cat, dog)
3. Eosinophilic pneumonitis (dog, cat)
4. Staphylococcal dermatitis (dog, occasionally)
5. Eosinophilic leukemia
6. Mast cell leukemia

Other causes:
1. Metastatic carcinoma (rare)
2. Hypoadrenocorticism (not usual but seen occasionally)

Causes of Eosinopenia

Excess corticosteroids
1. Endogenous: Hyperadrenocorticism, inflammation with stress
2. Exogenous: Corticosteroid or ACTH therapy

BASOPHILS

Causes of Basophilia
1. Concurrent with eosinophilia in hypersensitivity (heartworm infection)
2. Hyperadrenocorticism
3. Hyperlipoproteinemia (diabetes mellitus, nephrosis, chronic liver disease)
4. Basophilic leukemia (rare)

SERUM ENZYMES

AMYLASE AND/OR LIPASE

Causes and Increases
1. Pancreatic inflammation, necrosis, and neoplasia
2. Renal disease
3. Occasionally with salivary lesions
4. Prostatitis
5. Intra-abdominal diseases
6. Diabetic ketoacidosis
7. Cancer (liver)

ALKALINE PHOSPHATASE

Causes of Increased Serum Activity

1. Induced isoenzymes by glucocorticoids (dog only); steroid therapy
2. Bone growth in young animals
3. Cholestasis secondary to liver disease such as inflammation, neoplasia, cirrhosis, lipidosis, or hyperadrenocorticism
4. Isoenzymes induced by anticonvulsants (phenobarbital)
5. Increased bone osteolytic activity (hyperparathyroidism, panosteitis)
6. Neoplasia–mixed mammary tumor, sarcomas, carcinomas

BILIRUBIN

Hyperbilirubinemia

1. Increased direct bilirubin is 40–50% of total = intrahepatic icterus with cholestasis
2. Increased direct bilirubin is 75% or more of total = intrahepatic plus posthepatic icterus
3. Increased indirect bilirubin with 80% or more of total with anemia = prehepatic icterus

CALCIUM

Causes of Hypercalcemia

1. Young growing animals
2. Hypercalcemia of neoplasia (pseudohyperparathyroidism)
3. Hypoadrenocorticism
4. Osteolytic bone disease
5. Renal disease (occasionally in horse and cow, rarely in dog)
6. Hypervitaminosis D (iatrogenic)
7. Primary hyperparathyroidism
8. Hyperalbuminemia (if Ca corrected for protein, Ca will be normal)
9. Hypocalcitonism
10. Lipemia

Causes of Hypocalcemia

1. Hypoalbuminemia (if Ca corrected for protein, Ca will be normal)
2. Secondary renal hyperparathyroidism
3. Eclampsia
4. Necrotizing pancreatitis
5. Dietary imbalance
6. Intestinal malabsorption
7. Hypoparathyroidism
8. Hypovitaminosis D
9. Hyperadrenocorticism
10. Hypercalcitonism
11. Chelation by EDTA

CHLORIDE

Causes of Hyperchloremia

1. Dehydration
2. Metabolic acidosis
3. Fluid therapy
4. Renal tubular acidosis
5. Mineralocorticoid insufficiency

Causes of Hypochloremia

1. Vomiting (monogastric animals)
2. Metabolic alkalosis
3. Mineralocorticoid excess
4. Salt-losing nephropathy

CREATININE KINASE

Causes of Increased Serum Activity

1. Muscle trauma–contusions, downer animals, intramuscular injections, convulsions, surgery, hemorrhage into tissue
2. Myositis–clostridial, purulent, eosinophilic
3. Nutritional myopathies
4. Degenerative myopathies
5. Myocardial infarctions

CHOLESTEROL

Causes of Hypercholesterolemia

1. Diet
2. Postprandial
3. Hypothyroidism
4. Diabetes mellitus
5. Pancreatitis
6. Hyperadrenocorticism
7. Extrahepatic biliary obstruction
8. Liver disease
9. Protein-losing enteropathy
10. Nephrotic syndrome
11. Glomerulonephritis
12. Starvation

GLUCOSE

Causes of Hyperglycemia

1. Postprandial (monogastric animals)
2. Exertional (very common in cats)
3. Increased glucocorticoids (stress, hyperadrenocorticism, administration of corticoids or ACTH)
4. Diabetes mellitus
5. Acute pancreatitis
6. Drug-induced (thiazide diuretics, morphine, intravenous fluids with glucose, Ovaban in some cats)

Causes of Hypoglycemia

1. Sample held on erythrocytes
2. Hepatic diseases including glycogen-storage disease and end-stage liver disease
3. Hyperinsulinism (islet cell neoplasm or insulin therapy)
4. Extrapancreatic tumors
5. Idiopathic in toy breeds
6. Bacterial infection
7. Endocrine hypofunction including hypopituitarism, hypoadrenocorticism, hypothyroidism
8. Intestinal malabsorption
9. Canine renal glycosuria (severe cases)
10. Drug-induced (salicylates, ethanol, sulfonyurea)

POTASSIUM

Causes of Hyperkalemia

1. Acidosis (diabetes mellitus)
2. Akita breed of dogs
3. Urethral obstruction (FUS-cat)
4. Hypoadrenocorticism
5. Severe renal disease (acute renal failure)
6. Increased potassium intake in animals with renal disease
7. Therapy (fluid infusions, K-sparing diuretics)
8. Crush syndrome (trauma, muscle necrosis)
9. KCl dietary substitute for animals on sodium restricted diet
10. Artifact if a thrombocytosis

Causes of Hypokalemia

1. Gastrointestinal loss (vomiting, neoplasia, laxatives, diarrhea)
2. Metabolic alkalosis
3. Parenteral administration of potassium-free fluids
4. Insulin therapy
5. Steroid treatment or hyperadrenocorticism
6. Urinary loss associated with renal tubular acidosis, postobstructive diuresis, chronic pyelonephritis, nephrotic syndrome
7. Decreased potassium intake with normal water intake
8. Diuretics (furosemide, thiazides)
9. Aldosteronism

LACTATE DEHYDROGENASE (LDH)

Causes of Increased Serum Activity

1. Handling artifact–serum standing on erythrocytes
2. Hemolysis of erythrocytes
3. Cell necrosis of liver, kidney, muscle, and other cells
4. Neoplasia

SERUM PROTEINS

Causes of Hyperproteinemia (usually globulins)
1. Dehydration from any cause (albumin and sometimes globulins)
2. Increased globulin production:
   a. Inflammation
   b. Chronic antigen stimulation as with ehrlichiosis, feline infectious peritonitis, chronic bacterial infection, and so on
   c. Neoplasia–particularly plasma cell myeloma and some cases of lymphosarcoma
3. Hyperfibrinogenemia during inflammatory disease
4. Lipemia–artifact that increases both albumin and globulin

Causes of Hypoproteinemia (usually hypoalbuminemia)

Decreased production
1. Intestinal malabsorption (primary or secondary)
2. Maldigestion (exocrine pancreatic insufficiency)
3. Malnutrition (parasitic or dietary)
4. Chronic liver disease (atrophy or fibrosis)

Increased loss
1. Renal disease with chronic proteinuria
2. Hypoadrenocorticism
3. Exudative skin lesion
4. External hemorrhage (also hypogammaglobulinemia)
5. Protein losing enteropathy (also hypogammaglobulinemia)

SODIUM

Causes of Hyponatremia
1. Severe diarrhea
2. Vomiting
3. Hypoadrenocorticism
4. Hypervolemia
5. Therapy (diuretics, fluids with low Na content)
6. Psychogenic water drinking with medullary washout
7. Metabolic acidosis
8. Ketonuria
9. Salt-wasting nephropathy
10. Inappropriate ADH secretion
11. Hypothyroidism

Causes of Hypernatremia
1. Dehydration or lack of water (i.e., coma, hypothalmic disease)
2. Osmotic diuresis
3. High salt diet with decreased water intake
4. Diabetes insipidus with inadequate water intake
5. Advanced chronic renal failure with very low glomerular filtration rate
6. Hyperadrenocorticism (rare)
7. Hyperaldosteronism (possible but not reported in dog and cat)
8. Iatrogenic–administration of hypertonic sodium-containing fluids

UREA NITROGEN AND/OR CREATININE

Causes of Azotemia
1. Renal disease
2. Any disease that reduces glomerular filtration rate (GFR)
3. Pre-renal
   a. Dehydration
   b. Cardiac insufficiency
   c. Shock (septic or hypovolemic)
   d. High protein diet (UN but not creatinine increase)
4. Postrenal
   a. Obstruction of urinary tract

PHOSPHATE

Causes of Hyperphosphatemia
1. Sample held too long before analysis (phosphorus is released from RBC)
2. Young animals
3. Decreased renal function (dogs and cats)
4. Dietary imbalance (high phosphate intake–oral, enema, or injection)
5. Hypervitaminosis D (iatrogenic)
6. Hypoparathyroidism
7. Tissue trauma or necrosis
8. Hemolyzed sample
9. Osteolytic bone lesions
10. Idiopathic and transient in anorectic or vomiting animals

Causes of Hypophosphatemia
1. Dietary imbalances (inadequate intake–dietary or malabsorption)
2. Primary hyperparathyroidism
3. Hypercalcemia of neoplasia (pseudohyperparathyroidism)
4. Hyperinsulinism (iatrogenic or endogenous with insulinoma)
5. Diabetes mellitus
6. Hypovitaminosis D
7. Translocation from extracellular to intracellular location due to administration of glucose or development of alkalosis
8. Eclampsia
9. Hypercalcitonism

TRANSAMINASES (ALT, AST)

Increased Serum AST (GOT) and ALT (GPT) Activity

Serum AST
1. Increase due to necrosis of:
   a. Skeletal muscle
   b. Cardiac muscle–usually accompanied by an increase in serum CK (creatinine kinase) activity
   c. Liver–but is not specific for liver
2. Increase (usually less than with necrosis) due to changes in cell membrane permeability of liver, skeletal muscle, and cardiac muscle caused by:
   a. Anoxia
   b. Toxins
   c. Inflammation
   d. Metabolic disorders

Serum ALT
1. Increase due to necrosis of
   a. Liver
2. Increase (usually less than with necrosis) due to increased cell membrane permeability of hepatocytes caused by:
   a. Anoxia
   b. Toxins
   c. Inflammation
   d. Metabolic disorder

4 ANOREXIA AND POLYPHAGIA

BARBARA E. KITCHELL

Changes in food consumption patterns in animals frequently prompt owners to seek veterinary care for their pets. A hearty appetite is viewed as a sign of robust health, while a poor or selective appetite indicates illness to most people. *Anorexia* can be defined as failure to intake food, even in the face of obvious nutrient depletion. Anorexia may be complete or partial, depending upon the underlying cause. The patient may show interest in food and appear hungry but fail to ingest food in adequate quantities. Other patients are completely unresponsive to stimuli that normally induce a feeding response.

Polyphagia is defined as excessive consumption of food. This response may be appropriate in certain physiologic conditions, such as lactation, gestation, extreme cold weather, and rigorous exercise. Polyphagia may also be inappropriate and may result in obesity, as seen in patients taking certain medications (anticonvulsants, glucocorticoids, megestrol acetate), and in rare patients with hypothalamic lesions. Polyphagia may represent a behavioral response to highly palatable, desired foods. Polyphagia may also be seen as the body attempts to compensate for diseases that induce significant weight loss, such as diabetes mellitus, hyperthyroidism, and malassimilation syndromes.

PATHOPHYSIOLOGY

The physiology of body weight balance and regulation of energy intake is an area of active, ongoing investigation, and complex metabolic and neural interactions are being uncovered. Traditionally, the hypothalamus has been considered the neural center for the control of food intake. Stimulation of the ventromedial hypothalamus (satiety center) results in cessation of eating; destruction of this center leads to polyphagia and obesity. The lateral hypothalamic (feeding) center is inhibited by activation of the satiety center, and destruction of this lateral center results in complete, though temporary, anorexia. Feeding is stimulated by alpha adrenergic mechanisms and inhibited by beta-adrenergic and dopaminergic input. Dietary levels of central neurotransmitter precursors can influence appetite control. Increased central serotonin turnover is associated with decreased appetite, and decreased turnover is associated with hyperphagia. Central nervous system levels of tryptophan (the serotonin precursor) have been shown to increase in tumor-bearing experimental animals with profound anorexia and cancer cachexia.

Other factors influencing central mediation of food intake include the gut peptides (particularly cholecystokinin, which is released during feeding and promotes satiety), insulin, glucagon, growth hormone, thyroid hormone, and estrogen. Low environmental temperature promotes increased food intake. Local effects of the gastrointestinal system may induce anorexia (e.g., pain associated with mastication or gastric ulceration) or polyphagia (e.g., pica and abnormal appetite associated with duodenal ulceration). Gastric effects are mediated by afferent vagal transmission to the satiety center. Cerebral input can cause changes in eating patterns associated with anxiety or depression. Food aversions can develop in animals, as when eating certain foods at the onset of an illness promotes association of the food with clinical signs. Altered taste sensation is known to influence the appetite of human cancer patients, who classically have impaired ability to taste sweets and taste bitter substances at lower concentrations than normal subjects. Presumably, the same process occurs in animal cancer patients.

Finally, anorexia is seen in a myriad of systemic disease states secondary to the effects of metabolic derangements such as fever and toxicosis with endogenous (uremia toxins, hepatic toxins, lactic acid) and exogenous (drugs, chemicals) substances. The exact pathophysiologic mechanisms in most of these cases are unknown.

HISTORY

As anorexia is generally a nonspecific sign of disease, an accurate medical history is essential to defining the problem. Polyphagia, on the other hand, is a more specific sign and may be physiologic (in response to increased energy needs) or pathologic.

Duration and Degree. The duration of anorexia or

polyphagia, as well as the degree (partial or complete anorexia; mild, moderate, or severe polyphagia), help to establish the severity of the underlying problem.

Diet. Changes in the quality of the diet may result in anorexia due to lack of palatability and food preferences or aversions. Conversely, polyphagia may result from a change to a highly palatable diet.

Environmental Stress. Many animals become temporarily anorexic in the face of psychological stress, such as boarding, moving, or the addition of new animals or people to the household. Polyphagia may be the result of cold temperature stress or competition for food.

Body Weight. The owner's assessment of the magnitude and rate of any weight loss is very important in evaluating the anorexic patient. Sudden, dramatic weight loss implies more serious disease. The polyphagic patient may gain weight, lose weight, or remain stable. Polyphagia with weight gain is seen in changes in palatability of the diet, drug-induced polyphagia (glucocorticoids, anticonvulsants, megestrol acetate) and rarely, with hypothalamic lesions. Polyphagia with weight loss is seen in association with malabsorption and maldigestion, and endocrine imbalances such as diabetes mellitus and hyperthyroidism.

Other Clinical Signs. Obviously, clinical signs seen in association with diseases of neurologic, gastrointestinal, genitourinary, or endocrine origin should be explored via a careful history.

PHYSICAL FINDINGS

Physical examination should be carefully performed in the evaluation of patients with anorexia and polyphagia. Evidence of fever, dehydration, anemia, and jaundice should be sought as indicators of underlying diseases associated with anorexia. The general condition (haircoat, body weight, attitude) of the animal should be evaluated.

Head and Neck. The head and neck should be carefully evaluated for evidence of oral, dental, and cervical lesions that might induce pain on mastication, or dysphagia. Patients with cricopharyngeal achalasia and vascular ring anomalies are often ravenous but are unable to use the food they ingest due to chronic regurgitation. The animal's ability to prehend, masticate, and swallow food should be evaluated. Lymphadenopathy may be seen in anorexic patients, as the result of neoplastic or inflammatory disorders. Thyroid nodules are often palpable in geriatric feline patients with hyperthyroidism. This disease usually induces polyphagia with weight loss, but occasionally anorexia is encountered.

Thoracic Cavity. The thoracic cavity should be auscultated and palpated. Cardiac and pulmonary diseases often result in severe anorexia in stressed and decompensated patients. Cranial mediastinal masses may impair the patient's ability to swallow.

Abdomen. Abdominal palpation is extremely important in evaluating these patients. Hepatomegaly and abdominal distention are seen in spontaneous or iatrogenic hyperadrenocorticism, with associated polyphagia. Pain on palpation of bowel loops, foreign bodies, masses, or thickened bowel loops are all significant findings. Pain or masses involving the spleen, kidneys, urinary bladder, or prostate should be identified.

Neurologic Evaluation. The neurologic evaluation may uncover signs of central nervous system disease that cause anorexia. Patients with hypothalamic masses may show profound weight loss in the face of polyphagia (diencephalic syndrome).

DIAGNOSTIC PLAN

Results of the history and physical examination direct the order of diagnostic testing. In patients with occult anorexia, broad general screening tests must be applied. *Complete blood counts* and *serum chemistry panels*, including liver and kidney function and electrolyte status, should be obtained. *Urinalysis* completes the assessment of renal insufficiency and protein-losing nephropathy, and uncovers diabetes mellitus.

Fecal examination for parasites is important, and fecal digestion studies for malassimilation syndromes may prove helpful in patients with gastrointestinal signs such as chronic weight loss and steatorrhea.

Specific *endocrine tests*, including serum thyroxine level and assessment of adrenal function, may be required to diagnose cases of polyphagia.

Tests for *infectious diseases*, such as feline leukemia virus, feline infectious peritonitis, and toxoplasmosis, are useful in evaluating anorexia in cats.

Radiographic evaluation of involved body systems should be carried out if laboratory findings fail to uncover a specific cause. Radiographs of the abdomen may disclose enteritis or occult masses. Radiographs of the thorax may uncover evidence of heart disease or pulmonary metastasis in anorexic patients.

GOALS OF THERAPY

The goal of therapy in managing the anorexic patient is to support the patient while correcting the underlying cause. Specific therapies for systemic and gastrointestinal diseases are discussed elsewhere in the text. Simple approaches to enhancing an animal's interest in food include providing a wide selection of foods, warming the food, or applying flavorful additives such as garlic to food. Food should be prepared in a form that the patient can easily ingest, such as soft or liquid diets for animals with oral lesions. In cases of mild enteritis, resting the gastrointestinal system for 24 hours followed by offering bland, easily digested foods may be all that is necessary. Correction of fever, dehydration, and electrolyte imbalances often results in a return of appetite.

In patients that require nutritional support because of prolonged anorexia and catabolic disease processes, use of nasogastric, pharyngostomy, gastrostomy, or jejunostomy tubes and commercially prepared liquid or elemental diets may be necessary. If the intestinal system is impaired, parenteral alimentation should be considered (see Chapter 54).

Drugs that stimulate the appetite are being evaluated for use in animals. The benzodiazepine derivative tranquilizers (i.e., diazepam, oxazepam, and elfazepam) may prove useful as clinical appetitive agents in the future. Diazepam given intravenously at a dose of .02 to .18 mg/lb (.05 to .4 mg/kg) has been reported to be useful in managing anorexia in cats. The higher dosage range may result in significant ataxia and sedation in debilitated animals, and is the dose-limiting toxicity. Agents with more specific central appetite stimulation and less sedative impact are being investigated. The serotonin antagonist cyproheptadine has not proven to be clinically useful as an appetite stimulant in humans.

Therapy for the polyphagic patient involves correction of underlying endocrine, metabolic, or systemic disorders. Restriction of food availability and caloric content may be necessary to control obesity.

5 PAIN (GENERAL, BACK, EXTREMITIES, ABDOMEN)

MICHAEL J. KELLY

Pain perception is a purely subjective phenomenon. It can be defined as the awareness or perception of a noxious stimulus that is potentially damaging to tissue. Such stimuli can be traumatic, chemical, mechanical, inflammatory, ischemic, or thermal (heat or cold). Although animals cannot verbally describe pain, we can infer pain exists by their actions: crying, whining, disuse of a particular limb, reluctance to move about, less activity than usual, or alteration in their normal behavioral patterns. Since animals are unable to communicate abstract concepts such as pain, it is up to the veterinary clinician to be alert to subtle behavioral changes that may indicate that an animal is suffering from some noxious pain stimulus. An important concept to bear in mind is that although the threshold of pain perception appears to be quite constant across the species, actual tolerance of a painful stimulus may vary widely even within a single species, i.e., we all (animal and human) have similar pain thresholds, but some individuals can tolerate a higher level of pain than others without showing clinical signs.

GENERAL PATHOPHYSIOLOGY

Two basic kinds of pain, superficial and deep, have been recognized. Superficial pain can be divided into pricking, bright, sharp, or fast pain (first pain). Deep pain can be divided into burning, aching, or slow pain (second pain). First and second pains are, respectively, produced by activation of A delta (myelinated) and C (unmyelinated) nerve fibers. The temporal lag between the two types of pain is due, in part, to their different peripheral conduction velocities. A simple example of the A delta (first) pain and C fiber (second) pain is cutting oneself with a sharp knife. Initially you feel sharp pain, an A delta response. A few seconds later you feel the throbbing dull pain caused by C fiber influence. This is known as double pain and is common after tissue injury. Before the A delta and C fibers can carry their impulses to the brain, pain receptors (nociceptors) in the affected organ or structure must be stimulated above their thresholds. In both acute and chronic pain, the inflammatory process causes firing of the pain receptors. Pain mediators such as histamine, serotonin, prostaglandins, and complement are released from various cellular structures during the course of the inflammatory process, and cause the initiation and continuation of pain.

Pain receptors have some special attributes. Structurally, they can be bare nerve endings or specialized structures, they have relatively small receptor fields, a high threshold to stimuli, and manifest persistent afterdischarges for any suprathreshold noxious stimulus. They are able to provide the central nervous system with a continuum of information about the presence of a high-intensity stimulus that is damaging to tissue.

Once a noxious stimulus has been applied to an organ, sufficient pain mediators are released to stimulate the pain receptors to produce the existence of pain. The pain receptors use the A delta and C fibers to transmit this information to the brain so that the organism is aware that it hurts somewhere.

Primary Afferent Neuron. A primary afferent (PA) neuron is a nerve cell whose processes conduct the nerve impulses from the periphery to the central nervous system. The primary afferents involved in the transmission of noxious nerve impulses that lead to the perception of pain are some of the smallest of the myelinated fibers (A delta) and some of the nonmyelinated fibers (C). The receptors are free nerve endings. Not all A delta fibers and C fibers function in the production of pain. The spinal cord structure involved in the experience of pain is the gray matter (dorsal horn).

The primary afferents enter the spinal cord by forming

the lateral division of the dorsal roots. When they enter the spinal cord they divide into ascending and descending branches.

The primary afferents from cutaneous areas of the head and face reach the brain via branches of the V (trigeminal), VII (facial), and X (vagus) cranial nerves. Primary afferents from the mucous membranes of the head reach the brain via the same cranial nerves, in addition to some branches of the IX (glossopharyngeal) nerve. Both A delta and C fibers, similar to those found in spinal nerves, are involved. These pain fibers terminate in the nucleus caudalis (spinal nucleus) of the trigeminal nerve in a manner similar to that in which spinal pain fibers terminate in the dorsal horn of the spinal cord. The afferents in the first cervical nerve use the nucleus caudalis along with pain fibers from the head and face. There are no cutaneous afferents present in the first cervical nerve of the dog.

Ascending Pathways. Traditionally, ascending pathways have been illustrated as in series linkage of nerve cells, including the first order neuron (primary afferent neuron), synapsing with a second order neuron in a relay nucleus formed by the cell body of the second order neuron, a fiber tract or pathway formed by the axon of the second order neuron, then a third order neuron, usually with its cell body in the thalamus and its axon entering the cerebrum via the internal capsule. Inhibition, both presynaptic and postsynaptic, as well as postsynaptic excitation, occur in relay nuclei. Relay nuclei are best thought of as processing stations because of the modification of neural activity that occurs in the synaptic relay nuclei.

In the dorsal horn, and in the nucleus caudalis of the trigeminal nerve, two types of pain second order responsive cells can be found. One type, the pain-specific cell, responds to primary afferents stimulated by noxious mechanical and thermal stimuli. The other type of second order neurons, the wide dynamic cells, respond slightly to innocuous mechanical stimuli, but respond maximally when a stimulus is noxious. All of these cells are subject to either excitatory or inhibitory activity from other dorsal horn cells acted upon by other primary afferents.

Five ascending pathways have received consideration as possible pain pathways in domestic animals. These are the lateral spinothalamic tract (LSTT), the ventral spinothalamic tract (VSTT), the spinocervicothalamic tract (SCTT), the spinoreticular tract (SRT), and the dorsal column postsynaptic system (DCPS).

It appears that no single entity within the nervous system serves as the pain perception center. The pain pathways are multiple, especially in animals; lesions in one pathway appear to be compensated for or even enhanced by activity within another pathway. The strongest evidence available suggests that the ventrobasal nuclei (or the ventrobasalventral lateral nuclear junction in the cat) serve as the sensory-discriminative components of pain.

Pain Theory. The currently accepted pain theory, the gate control theory, involves three major principles: (1) The key to the gating system is the substantia gelatinosa. This system modifies all afferent impulses to the cord before they influence the T cells, which are the first central transmission cells. (2) The T cells are responsible for stimulating the action system, which is the whole pain experience. (3) The dorsal column system acts as a central control trigger that activates selective processes within the brain, which in turn activate the gate control system.

The gate control theory suggests that the actual pain felt as a result of the stimulus depends not only upon the strength and nature of the stimulus, but also upon the ongoing activity that precedes the stimulus and the balance of large versus small fiber stimuli.

Large diameter A-alpha and A-beta (non-pain) fibers stimulate the T cells, but at the same time a negative feedback mechanism stimulates the substantia gelatinosa to inhibit the T cells. Small diameter pain fibers also stimulate the T cells and at the same time inhibit the substantia gelatinosa from modulating the T cells. Therefore, stimulation of non-pain fibers closes the substantia gelatinosa gating mechanism, while pain fiber stimulation keeps it open. It is the balance of the large versus small fiber stimuli that determines the strength of impulses that reach the T cells. When the barrage of impulses that have cleared the gate move the output of the T cell stimuli beyond a critical level, the experience of pain occurs.

There are midbrain analgesic areas which, when stimulated either electrically or by local administration of opiates, cause inhibition of pain pathways both in the spinal cord and anterior to the foramen magnum. The analgesic areas are stimulated by naturally occurring, opiate-like substances in the brain that have an analgesic neurotransmitter function. Substances called enkephalins have been isolated and synthesized. These enkephalins produce analgesia when injected intraventricularly in the rat. There is evidence for a neurotransmitter role for the morphine-like peptides. Endorphins are other morphine-like peptides that are found in the pituitary and have analgesic function. The enkephalins have been located in the brain and gastrointestinal tract of many species. The term "endorphin" is used as a generic term for the sequenced opiate peptides, including the enkephalin pentapeptides and alpha-, beta-, and gamma-endorphins, and endorphin has also been applied as a descriptive term designating substances with morphine-like activity but with unspecified structure found in pituitary extracts.

Ischemic Pain. It is proposed that the pain from ischemia is the net result of the following metabolic alterations: anoxia, changes in pH, lactic acid production, histamine release, and increased release of potassium from ischemic cells. When ischemia is compounded by increased metabolism of the ischemic organ, the time to onset of pain is decreased and the intensity of the pain is increased.

DIFFERENTIAL DIAGNOSIS OF PAIN

A firm understanding of general pain allows one to begin working on a differential diagnosis list based on anatomical location.

A differential list involving the back and head must

include trauma, congenital or genetic lesions, infectious or inflammatory lesions, neoplasms, dietary causes, and idiopathic causes.

Traumatic causes of pain include projectiles, intervertebral disc disease, cord contusion with dorsal route pain, and vertebral fracture or fracture dislocation. Congenital or genetic lesions include dens disease such as angulations with or without ligamentous damage, C1-2 subluxation, (odontoid-dens hypoplasia), and cervical vertebral instability. Infection and inflammation includes discospondylitis, vertebral osteomyelitis, spondylitis, spinal meningitis, intracranial meningitis, epidural abscess, myelitis, spondylosis, and spinal arthritis. Neoplastic etiologies are vertebral body tumors, cord tumor, and nerve root tumor. A possible dietary cause is hypervitaminosis A with its multiple exostoses causing nerve root entrapment syndrome.

The extremities involve a similar differential list. Trauma causes fractures, dislocations, and muscle contusions. Congenital and genetic lesions include aseptic necrosis, such as osteochondritis dissecans or Legg-Perthes disease. Infections and inflammations to be considered are panostitis, osteomyelitis, polyarthritis, polymyositis, neuritis, subcutaneous cellulitis, abscesses, and neuritis.

The differential diagnosis of abdominal pain must include trauma, projectiles, inflammation, pancreatitis, infection (peritonitis, hepatic abscess), ischemic disease such as a torsed testicle or splenic torsion and passing of ureteral or urethral calculi. Tumors are an uncommon cause of abdominal pain.

In all three categories, if the pain cannot be diagnosed, then it must be recorded as idiopathic.

HISTORICAL FINDINGS AND THEIR MEANINGS

Trauma. Trauma suggests an immediate etiology such as being struck by a car or shot while hunting. The clinician should concentrate on the degree of trauma. Are there single or multiple organs involved?

Disuse of a Particular Limb or Limbs. This localizes the area of immediate concern and allows the clinician to concentrate the physical examination and diagnostics in that area. It is important to do a complete physical with this historical finding, since other limbs may also be involved but not to such a degree that clinical pain exists. A historically important fact is the duration of the limb disuse. Does the patient have acute or chronic disease?

Acute Pain or Chronic Pain. Is the patient sore and slow-moving on rising in the morning but warms out of it as he/she begins to ambulate? A yes to this historical finding points in the direction of an arthritic problem rather than an acute, nonresponding disuse of a rear leg that might point one in the direction of a ruptured cruciate ligament or hip luxation.

Crying or Whining. Few animal patients provide their owners with this historical clue that pain exists. However, if it is present in the history, it is conclusive that the pain is very real. This sign alone should lead the clinician to do a thorough physical and workup to localize the source and etiology of the pain.

Alteration in Normal Behavioral Pattern. This provides an extremely subtle clue that pain is present. It does not help to localize the pain, or even suggest an etiology, but does challenge the clinician to look for the cause of the change in an otherwise normal behavioral pattern.

Age, Breed, Sex. A toy breed dog with anterior cervical pain should prompt the clinician to think of a C1-2 subluxation, while a Doberman pinscher or Great Dane with cervical pain and mild to severe posterior paresis brings to mind the diagnosis of cervical vertebral instability.

PHYSICAL FINDINGS AND THEIR INTERPRETATION

Observation. A most important aspect of the physical examination for localization of pain is observation of the patient at rest and when walking. Observation allows localization of the problem to a single limb or multiple limbs. It is important, however, not to jump to diagnostic conclusions based on observation. An obese, middle-sized dog dragging both the rear legs might just as easily have bilateral cruciate ruptures or multiple pelvic fractures as a spinal disc prolapse.

Reluctance to move the head and neck freely points to the cervical region. Roaching of the back and tucking of the abdominal muscles suggests that the clinician should look for abdominal or thoracolumbar disease. A reluctance of the patient to freely ambulate up and down stairs suggests spinal pain.

Palpation. The single most important part of pain evaluation is palpation. A systematic approach to palpation not only localizes the problem, but may provide the clinician with a diagnosis and prognosis. Begin by opening the mouth. If pain is present, search for the etiology, such as a foreign body, broken jaw, or retrobulbar abscess. Carefully palpate the temporomandibular joint and the bones of the skull. Next palpate and manipulate the cervical region. If pain exists and one takes into consideration the animal's signalment, then a working diagnosis is apparent. Examples are a toy breed with pain on manipulation of the region of the dens (the diagnosis could be C1-2 subluxation) or a Great Dane or Doberman pinscher with pain on ventral dorsal or lateral manipulation of the neck (the diagnosis might be cervical vertebral instability). Palpate each limb carefully looking for periosteal pain (panostitis). Manipulate each joint gently, extending and flexing each independent of all other joints. Pain on flexion of the shoulder joint in a large, rapidly growing dog under one year of age is strong evidence of osteochondritis dissecans. Palpate the shaft of all long bones, feeling for lumps and bumps. Painful areas that are warm relative to the surrounding tissue suggest a cellulitis, abscess, or underlying osteomyelitis. Feel for any crepitation of the joints; this suggests laxity and/or osteoarthritis. When palpating the hips, be careful to abduct the hips to see if pain is present. Good palpation in this case permits the clinician to distinguish between a luxated hip and one that has an aseptic necrosis of the femoral head. The lumbar sacral junction should be palpated very carefully, feeling for crepitation and pain. Pressure applied dorsally at the lumbosacral junction may cause severe pain and can be a good clue, leading to a diagnosis of cauda equina syndrome. The stifles should be palpated thoroughly to feel for patellar luxation or the anterior drawer syndrome characteristic of a ruptured anterior cruciate ligament. All joints should be evaluated individually and collectively to separate localized disease from a systemic problem such as polyarthritis. Muscle masses should be palpated to search for cellulitis, abscess, or a polymyositis.

Palpation of the abdomen must be gentle yet firm. Feel for splinting and/or discomfort. Localize the area of pain. The anterior right quadrant suggests pancreatitis. Diffuse abdominal pain with no palpable foreign body suggests peritonitis. A cryptorchid dog that has acute abdominal pain and a palpable, firm, round mass suggests a torsed ischemic testicle. Pain elicited while palpating the posterior abdominal quadrant in a male dog can be localized by doing a rectal simultaneously and checking for prostate enlargement and discomfort.

Neurologic Examination. The neurologic examination helps to localize the etiology of pain. It localizes the lesion to the peripheral area, spinal cord, or skull. By using the upper and lower motor neuron concept and looking for differences in symmetry, it is possible to isolate the lesion as lower motor neuron to the rear legs (L4-S1), upper motor neuron to the rear legs (anterior to L4), lower motor neuron to the forelegs (C5-T2), upper motor neuron to the forelegs (anterior to C5), or anterior to the foramen magnum (cranial nerve defects and/or seizures). Differences in symmetry detected during the neurologic examination enable localization of the main lesion to the right or left side of the body.

Temperature. Elevated temperature suggests an inflammatory and/or infectious process (abscess, myelitis, osteomyelitis, or meningitis).

DIAGNOSTIC PLAN

After a thorough history and physical examination, *radiographs* are the most important tool in the diagnosis of pain. Radiographs diagnose most cases of back and extremity related pain due to trauma, congenital, genetic, neoplastic, and dietary etiologies. Occasionally, *contrast radiology* such as the *myelogram* is indicated in order to make an accurate diagnosis (intervertebral disc syndrome, spinal cord tumors, or cervical vertebral instability). The infectious and inflammatory diseases require *clinical pathologic* help (vertebral osteomyelitis, discospondylitis, spinal meningitis, epidural abscess, myelitis, polyarthritis, polymyositis, neuritis, cellulitis, abscessation, and intracranial meningitis). Tests that need to be run include a *complete blood count*, *microbiology* (spinal meningitis, discospondylitis, vertebral osteomyelitis, or spondylitis), and *serology* (spinal meningitis, discospondylitis, vertebral osteomyelitis, spondylitis, and myelitis). A special procedure such as *cerebrospinal fluid analysis* may be necessary (spinal meningitis, epidural abscess, myelitis, and intracranial meningitis). *Biopsy* is indicated in polymyositis, neuritis, and neoplasms. *Electrophysiology*, such as EEG and EMG, is a valuable tool in the diagnosis of myelitis, polymyositis, neuritis, and intracranial meningitis.

The diagnostic plan of abdominal pain involves *radiographs*, *clinical pathology* (pancreatitis, peritonitis, prostatitis, and hepatic abscessation), *contrast radiology* (prostatitis, ruptured organ), *ultrasound* (solid or fluid masses), *microbiology* (septic peritonitis, hepatic abscessation, and ruptured organ) and/or *exploratory surgery*.

GOALS OF TREATMENT

Never consider pain a diagnosis; pain is only a sign. First diagnose and treat the etiology of the pain, in other words, treat and resolve the primary problem, and the treatment of the pain will often be unnecessary. The goals of treatment, when needed, are twofold: to bring about relief of pain and to restore function to the affected part or organ. Treatment modalities ranging from medical to surgical are used.

Analgesic drugs can be divided into three groups: narcotic analgesics, narcotic antagonists, and nonsteroidal anti-inflammatory drugs (mild analgesics). Both the narcotic analgesics and narcotic antagonists are potent analgesics that increase pain tolerance greatly. The mild analgesics or nonsteroidal anti-inflammatory drugs elevate the pain threshold but have little effect on pain tolerance. A list of dosages of these drugs occurs at the end of this chapter.

Acupuncture is a treatment modality that may have application in pain. Its mechanism of action is best explained by the gate theory of pain. A beta fibers, which are large, fast conducting myelinated fibers, have a voltage threshold of .02 to .04 volts. C fibers, which are nonmyelinated, small, slow conducting fibers, have a voltage threshold of 10 to 15 volts. The intensity of a stimulus is related to volts and cycles.

If a needle or needles are inserted and twirled or electrically stimulated at 105 cycles per minute, a barrage of A beta non-pain impulses ascend the peripheral nerves to the substantia gelatinosa and close the gate. The impulses from C pain fibers cannot pass the gate and cannot cause any pain (see Chapter 56).

OUTCOME

Surgery is curative in a number of pain-related diseases: fractures, foreign bodies, intervertebral disc disease, cauda equina syndrome, and abscesses. In most cases of traumatic acute disuse pain, involving the back and extremities (fractures, luxations, ligament rupture, projectile injuries, and intervertebral disc rupture), the proper use of analgesics plus surgery restores the patient to a pain and disease free state. Congenital and genetic lesions such as C1-2 subluxation, dens angulation, and

TABLE 5–1. MEDICATIONS FOR PAIN

Generic	Trade	Dosage Dog	Dosage Cat	Route	Frequency	Brief Description
Morphine sulfate		0.11 mg/lb	NR	IM/SQ	Q4H	Narcotic
Meperidine	Demerol	2.5 mg/lb	5 mg/lb	IM	Q4H D Q2H C	Narcotic
Codeine		0.68 mg/lb	NR	P.O.	Q8H	Narcotic
Methadone		0.05 to 0.25 mg/lb	NR	IM	Q4H	Narcotic
Oxymorphone	Numorphan	0.05 to 0.09 mg/lb	NR	IM		Narcotic
Pentazocine	Talwin (Winthrop)	0.32 mg/lb	NR	IM	Q4H	Narcotic antagonist
Butorphanol Tartrate	Stadol (Bristol)	1–4 mg/dog	NR	½IM½IV	Q6H–Q12H	Narcotic antagonist
Aspirin		5 mg/lb	4.5 mg/lb	P.O.	Q12H D Q48H C	Mild analgesic
Acetaminophen	Tylenol	5 mg/lb	NR-toxic	P.O.	Q12H	Mild analgesic
Flunixin* Meglumine	Banamine (Schering)	0.12 mg/lb	NR	IV	Q24H × 3	Mild analgesic
Phenylbutazone	Butazolidin	4 mg/lb	NR			
Ibuprofen*		2.5 mg/lb	NR	P.O.	Q8H	Mild analgesic

D = Dog.
C = Cat.
NR = Not recommended.
*Not approved for dogs.

cervical vertebral instability can be treated either medically or surgically with variable prognosis. The prognosis of the infectious and inflammatory causes of pain (vertebral osteomyelitis, spondylitis, discospondylitis, spinal meningitis, epidural abscesses, myelitis, spondylosis, and spinal arthritis) depends on the presence of acute or chronic disease and the specific etiology of the disease. Treatment involves antibiotics and steroidal anti-inflammatories, as well as the therapy mentioned previously. The management of chronic arthritis involves good weight control and diet in addition to the analgesic drugs. Dietary hypervitaminosis A can be arrested by dietary control. Many of the "poly" diseases (polyarthritis, polymyositis, and polyneuritis) lend themselves to control, if not total cure, if the exact etiologic agent can be found. Subcutaneous abscesses or cellulitis respond very well once the microbiologist isolates the causative agent and appropriate antimicrobial therapy is instituted.

Abdominal pain is surgically corrected with a good prognosis if a torsed organ such as a testicle or spleen is present. However, the outcome of a diffuse septic peritonitis, even with aggressive medical and surgical treatment, is very poor. Pancreatitis causing severe pain lends itself nicely to aggressive medical therapy, while hepatic abscessation carries a variable prognosis. A ruptured hollow organ such as the bowel or bladder, if diagnosed early and treated aggressively (both medically and surgically), carries a guarded prognosis. Bladder rupture, however, has a better prognosis than bowel rupture.

6 THERMOREGULATION

ROBERT H. LUSK, JR.

The body produces heat by muscular exercise, assimilation of food, and metabolic processes that contribute to the basal metabolic rate. Heat is lost from the body by radiation, conduction, and vaporization of water on the skin surfaces and in the respiratory passages. Small amounts of heat are lost in the urine and feces as well. The balance between heat production and heat loss determines the body temperature. Enzyme systems in the body have narrow temperature ranges for optimal function, and therefore normal body function depends upon a relatively constant body temperature.

In mammals, body temperature is controlled by the thermoregulatory center located in the preoptic region of the anterior hypothalamus. The thermoregulatory center establishes a body temperature, known as the set point, around which body temperature fluctuates very little. The thermoregulatory center in the hypothalamus interprets changes in body temperature through both peripheral and central temperature receptors. The thermoregulatory center moderates both behavioral and physiological mechanisms to return the body to its established set point temperature.

The temperature-regulating system is a negative feedback control system. It consists of receptors that sense the existing central temperature, effector mechanisms that permit adjustment in temperature, and integrative structures that determine whether the existing temperature is too high or too low and activate the appropriate physiological response. Thermoregulation is a negative feedback system because a rise in central temperature initiates mechanisms for losing heat, while a decrease in central temperature activates mechanisms of heat production and conservation.

Heat loss can be accomplished by postural changes, seeking a cool environment, cutaneous vasodilation, panting, and sweating (Table 6–1). Heat gain mechanisms include shivering, increased voluntary activity, increased thyroxine production, and increased catecholamine production. Mechanisms of heat conservation include environment changes, postural changes, piloerection, and cutaneous vasoconstriction.

An understanding of the thermoregulatory system is fundamental for the practicing clinician. Patient care must be based on the understanding of physiological principles. Treatments for true fever, hyperthermia, and hypothermia are outlined here. In disease, temperature is often a diagnostic, prognostic, and therapeutic barometer. The clinician should always strive to determine and eliminate the cause of thermoregulatory imbalance. In cases of hypothermia, hyperthermia, and extreme fever that threaten the patient's life, appropriate therapeutic and emergency measures must always be taken.

HYPERTHERMIA

Hyperthermia is a general term for the elevation of body temperature above the normal range. In hyperthermia (not true fever), the established thermoregulatory set point is not changed (Figure 6–1). Etiologies of hyperthermia in small animal practice include heat stroke, hypothalamic lesions, malignant hyperthermia, exercise, seizures, thyrotoxicosis, drug reactions, and heating pads.

Heat stroke is the most commonly encountered hyperthermia in small animals. It often results when animals are enclosed in a car on a warm day. Physiological mechanisms of heat loss are unable to prevent an increase in body temperature when overburdened by abnormally high environmental temperature. Lesions of the hypothalamus of inflammatory, neoplastic, or traumatic origin can impair the thermoregulatory center and result in an inappropriate response, allowing hyperthermia. Malignant hyperthermia

TABLE 6–1. TEMPERATURE-REGULATING MECHANISMS

Mechanisms activated by cold	
Shivering	Increase heat production
Increased voluntary activity	
Increased secretion of norepinephrine and epinephrine	
Increased thyroxine production	
Cutaneous vasoconstriction	Heat conservation
Postural changes	
Piloerection	
Environmental changes	
Mechanisms activated by heat	
Cutaneous vasodilatation	Increase heat loss
Sweating	
Postural changes	
Seeking cool places	
Increased respiration	
Panting	
Anorexia	Decrease heat production
Apathy and inertia	

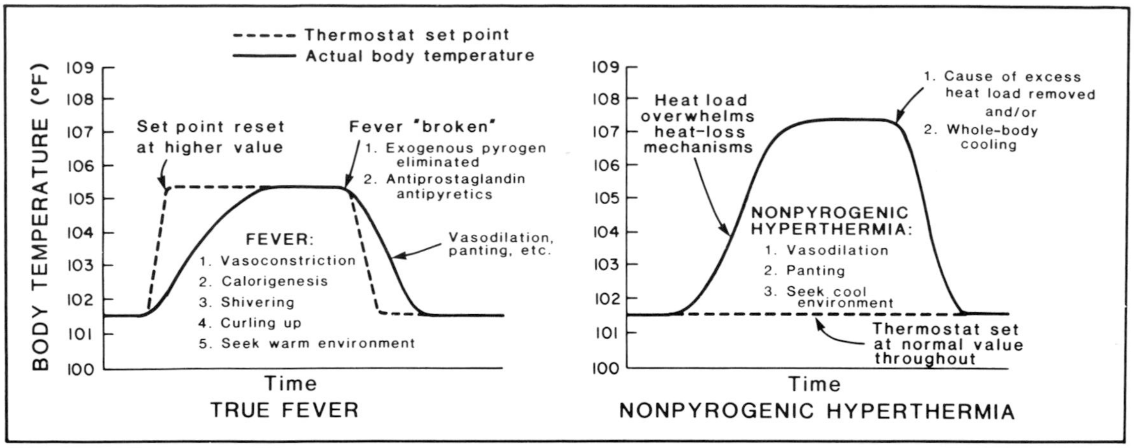

FIGURE 6–1. True fever versus nonpyrogenic hyperthermia. The relationship of thermostat setting to body temperature is illustrated. From McMillan, FD: The Compendium on Continuing Education for the Practicing Veterinarian. Oct. 1985.

is a unique, inherited condition that causes membrane disease and rapid heat production following exposure to inhalant anesthetics, skeletal muscle relaxants, or amide local anesthetics. It is rarely reported in the dog and cat. Physical movement and increased muscle activity can create increased body temperatures and result in hyperthermia during exercise. Seizures increase muscle contractions and generate hyperthermia secondary to the increased muscle activity. Thyrotoxicosis due to increased thyroid hormone may create hyperthermia by increasing the metabolic rate. Hyperthyroidism is often seen in the cat. Drugs may create hyperthermia by increasing the metabolic rate and/or impairing the ability of the thermoregulatory system to appropriately respond. Heating pads, in a manner similar to heat stroke, may overload the body's ability to dissipate heat, especially in a compromised patient.

FEVER

Fever is a specific type of hyperthermia. In all classes of hyperthermia the temperature is elevated above the normal range. However, in true fever the body's thermoregulatory set point is changed. The set point is raised and the appropriate physiological responses are initiated to elevate the body temperature to the new set point (Figure 6–1). During true fever there are four key points: (1) The elevation in body temperature during fever is a regulated rise generated by thermoregulatory mechanisms alone. (2) There is an increase in the desired body temperature. (3) The higher desired body temperature is attained and maintained by a fully functional thermoregulatory system. (4) Salicylate-like agents can intervene in the febrile process by altering the set point and returning body temperature to an afebrile state.

PATHOGENESIS OF FEVER

The introduction of an exogenous pyrogen or antigen into the body initiates a febrile response (Figure 6–2). Exogenous pyrogens indirectly cause fever by precipitating the release of endogenous pyrogens. Endogenous pyrogens are stored and released by bone marrow-derived phagocytes of the lung, liver, and spleen. Lymphocytes do not produce endogenous pyrogens but aid the febrile response by secreting lymphokine, which stimulates the release of endogenous pyrogens from macrophages. Cells of certain neoplasms also produce and secrete endogenous pyrogens (Figure 6–2). Several agents are known exogenous pyrogens, including viruses, Gram-positive bacteria, Gram-negative bacterial endotoxins, fungi, certain steroids, antigen-antibody complexes, antigens that produce delayed hypersensitivity, and some inorganic substances. The mechanism by which the exotoxin activates the leukocyte to synthesize and release endogenous pyrogens is unknown. The secreted endogenous pyrogens act directly on the preoptic area of the hypothalamus to elevate the thermoregulatory set point. Once the set point has been raised, physiological mechanisms of heat generation and heat conservation are initiated to obtain the new set point. The mechanisms by which endogenous pyrogens reset the thermoregulatory set point are unknown. There are several substances suspected as mediators in this process, including prostaglandins, monoamines, cholinergic mechanisms, and locally altered sodium and calcium ratios.

CLINICAL PRESENTATION

The small animal clinician is often presented with a patient that has an elevated temperature. Mild temperature elevations of two degrees or less have to be carefully evaluated. Normal body temperatures for the canine range from 100.2 to 102.8° F (37.8 to 39.3° C) and for the feline, from 100.5 to 102.5° F (38.0 to 39.2° C). The stress and anxiety related to the physical examination, waiting room, and car ride to the clinic often cause a mild temperature elevation. If the animal is clinically normal and not presented for a medical syndrome associated with fever/hyperthermia, the clinician should not be misled. When presented with an animal with clinical signs of any type, the temperature becomes much more meaningful. An almost invariable accom-

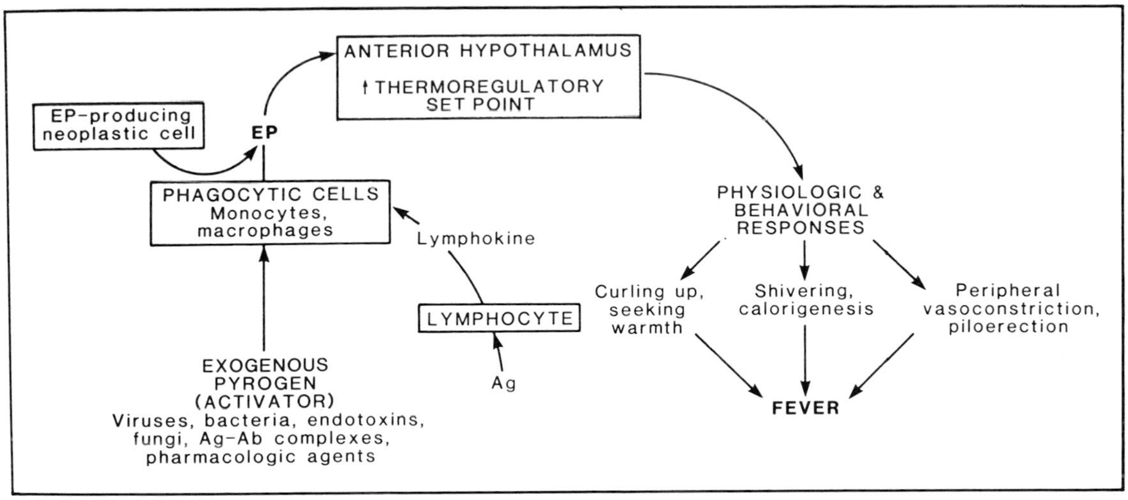

FIGURE 6–2. Postulated pathogenesis of fever. EP = endogenous pyrogen, Ag = antigen, Ab = antibody. From McMillan, FD: The Compendium on Continuing Education for the Practicing Veterinarian. Oct. 1985.

paniment of systemic illness is a disruption of temperature regulation, usually causing fever.

Temperatures greater than 104° F (40° C) require clinical correlation regardless of the presentation. Fever is never the sole manifestation of illness. When approaching a patient with fever, a complete physical examination and history, including drug therapy, animal exposure, and environmental conditions, should be performed. The degree of fever is often important. Temperatures of 103° F (39.4° C) or less, as previously mentioned, may be stress-related or clinically significant. Temperatures between 104° F (40° C) and 107° F (41.7° C) are almost always significant. Temperatures of greater than 107° F (41.7° C) are rare in small animal practice. Temperatures greater than 107° F (41.7° C) are usually not true fevers and relate to some other cause of hyperthermia. Temperature elevations of this magnitude require immediate treatment.

The majority of clinically significant fevers in small animal practice are caused by infectious agents. The clinician should always rule out bacterial, fungal, and viral etiologies. If the history and physical examination do not yield an etiology for the fever, then as with any clinical syndrome, the data base should be expanded. A complete blood count is mandatory and a complete blood chemistry and urinalysis are often extremely helpful in determining the fever etiology. If not, a systemic medical evaluation must be initiated to determine the cause of the fever. The workup should be extended to include feline infectious peritonitis and feline leukemia titers in the cat. Both thoracic and abdominal radiographs can be used to screen for infectious, as well as neoplastic, processes. If the etiology remains elusive, antinuclear antibody tests, toxoplasmosis titers, blood cultures, and fungal titers may be indicated. On occasion, the extended workup may include an echocardiogram to rule out valvular or mural endocarditis.

When evaluating the patient with fever of unknown origin, a specific etiology should be obtained before treatment is initiated. Fevers of less than 106° F (41.1° C) are rarely life-threatening and treatment may preclude elucidation of their true etiology and therefore delay correct treatment.

TREATMENT

Fever. The treatment of fever always begins with the specific treatment for the underlying disease that has initiated the pyrogenic response. The reader is directed to the specific chapter that deals with each disease syndrome. In some cases it is advantageous to treat the temperature elevation concurrently with the underlying disease process. Benefits to treating fever directly in small animal medicine include (1) protection against prolonged or further temperature elevation, which may have detrimental physiologic effects. Prolonged fevers of 105° F (40.5° C) and greater may cause metabolic drain, dehydration, anorexia, and depression. Small animals, especially cats that remain anorexic, often show poor clinical response regardless of the underlying disease process. Fevers of 106° F (41.1° C) or more, even of short duration, may lead to cerebral edema, tissue damage, bone marrow depression, and activation of disseminated intravascular coagulation, (2) reduction of patient discomfort, and (3) hastening of clinical response. The clinician must always weigh the benefits of treatment against the potential drawbacks of treatment intervention. Potential drawbacks to treatment include the following: (1) Fever may aid the body's response in fighting certain infections. (2) Fever promotes rest. (3) Fever is an important indication of treatment response. Interfering with fever may falsely indicate clinical response, affecting patient evaluation and prognosis. (4) Fever may be beneficial in some neoplastic diseases.

It is important to differentiate true fever from other causes of hyperthermia because their therapies differ greatly. The treatment of true fever is directed at the preoptic area of the hypothalamus. Agents are used that reset the thermoregulatory set point, which has been elevated by the endogenous pyrogens. Antipyretic agents used in small animal medicine include salicylates, acetaminophen, dipyrone, flunixin meglumine, and phenothiazines (Table 6–2). These are all inhibitors of prostaglandin synthesis. Corticosteroids may be used in certain cases to reduce circulating endogenous pyrogens. The use of steroids must be cautioned; however, steroids

TABLE 6–2. DOSAGES OF ANTIPYRETIC AGENTS USED IN DOGS AND CATS

Agent	Dogs	Cats
Acetylsalicylic acid (Aspirin)	11 to 16 mg/lb q8–24 h PO	6 to 11 mg/lb q24–48h PO (cautioned)
Sodium salicylate	4.5 mg/lb IV q8h	4.5 mg/lb IV q24–48h (cautioned)
Acetaminophen (Tylenol)	4.5 to 7 mg/lb q8–24h PO	contraindicated
Dipyrone (50% solution)	0.1 to 0.5 cc maximum SQ q8–24h 5 days or less	0.1 to 0.2 cc maximum SQ q8–24h (cautioned) 5 days or less
Flunixin meglomine (Banamine)	0.2 to 0.45 mg/lb IV or IM one dose only	not recommended
Prednisolone	0.2 mg/lb q12–24h PO (cautioned)	0.2 mg/lb q24h PO (cautioned)
Phenothiazines	dependent on agent	dependent on agent

are often helpful in cats with prolonged temperature elevations. Steroids also serve as an appetite stimulant. The salicylates are inexpensive and reasonably safe in the dog. Side effects of salicylate treatment include emesis, gastric ulceration, gastric hemorrhage, and rarely, central nervous system disturbances and acid-base imbalances. Cats have slow hepatic clearance of salicylates and they must be used with caution. Some authors advocate their use in cats at a much reduced dosage, but due to great individual variation, this should be done with care. Acetaminophen is also inexpensive and reasonably safe in the dog. The side effects are similar to those of salicylates. Acetaminophen is contraindicated in severe liver disease, as it may be hepatotoxic. The use of acetaminophen in the cat is contraindicated due to the formation of methemoglobin. Dipyrone is an extremely potent antipyretic agent that may be used in the dog and cat. Dosages needed for safe reduction of fever appear to be much lower than those suggested by the manufacturer. The use of dipyrone for more than five days is not suggested due to its potential bone marrow suppression. Side effects include hypothermia and bone marrow depression. Flunixin meglumine is a potent antipyretic and analgesic. Multiple doses are not suggested. It is not currently approved for use in small animal medicine. Possible side effects include muscle stiffness, vomiting, diarrhea, and gastrointestinal hemorrhage. Phenothiazines also possess some antipyretic properties. They act both centrally and peripherally. However, their hypotensive and sedative effects limit their use.

Fluid therapy is especially advantageous in the dehydrated or anorexic patient. Physically cooling the body with water baths and alcohol is of questionable use. Except in cases of extremely high fever (greater than 106° F (41.1° C)), this practice should be restricted. Whole body cooling opposes the body's effort to reach the new set point. Thus, cooling the body surface can cause metabolic stress as the patient strives to raise its body temperature to the new hypothalamic set point.

Hyperthermia. Treatment of hyperthermia often involves physically cooling the body surfaces with alcohol and/or water. The use of intravenous fluids may be indicated to reduce core temperature. Cool water enemas may also be used to reduce body heat. If shock is present, the use of corticosteroids for shock treatment is indicated. In these cases broad-spectrum antibiotics are used to protect against bacterial infection from damaged gastrointestinal mucosa. Furosemide (Lasix 1 to 2 mg/lb PO, SQ, or IV) may be indicated to promote urination and prevent renal shutdown. If laryngeal edema and secondary upper airway obstruction are present, sedation and/or anesthesia with intubation can be life-saving.

Hypothermia. Hypothermia occurs when the normal thermoregulatory system is unable to sustain body temperature by mechanisms of heat generation and heat conservation. A precise value at which hypothermia becomes clinically important has not been established. Patients with prolonged temperatures of 98.5° F (36.9° C) would benefit from treatment. Temperatures of 96° F (35.6° C) and below should always be treated. Hypothermia is most often diagnosed in the neonatal, geriatric, or compromised patient. Accidental hypothermia usually results from environmental exposure. Iatrogenic hypothermia may result from surgical intervention and immobilization. Sedatives and other drugs may induce hypothermia by their effects on the brain and/or periphery. Hypothermia may be seen in hypothyroidism related to decreased circulation of thyroid hormone. The most common clinical findings in the hypothermic patient are shivering (not present at extremely low temperature), depressed consciousness, weak pulses, bradycardia, muscle stiffness, and depressed respiration. Hypothermia may result in acidosis due to decreased respiration and hypotension. The treatment of hypothermia should include active rewarming of the body core, minimization of heat loss, correction of acid/base imbalance, increased caloric intake, and treatment of underlying or concurrent disease. Patient monitoring and patient support are imperative in the hypothermic patient. Special attention must be paid to the cardiovascular system, as ventricular fibrillation may occur during rewarming. Rewarming may be accomplished with warm water blankets, warm intravenous fluids, and peritoneal dialysis. Warm water baths may interfere with patient monitoring systems. Accurate and continuous temperature monitoring are required, as rewarming should be done at a rate of 0.9 to 1.8° F (0.5 to 1.0° C) per hour. Slower warming rates are associated with increased mortality. During the rewarming process, the torso should be warmed before the extremities. Warming the extremities before the body core can result in peripheral vasodilation and release of sequestered cold fluids and acid metabolites into the bloodstream.

7 VOMITING, REGURGITATION, AND DYSPHAGIA

TODD R. TAMS

VOMITING

Vomiting refers to a forceful ejection of gastric contents (and occasionally proximal small intestinal contents) through the mouth. This occurs during a forceful, sustained contraction of the abdominal muscles during which the cardia of the stomach is elevated and opened and the pylorus is contracted. The vomiting act includes three stages: nausea, retching, and vomiting. Changes in gastrointestinal motility occur with each stage. Serious consequences of vomiting include aspiration pneumonia, volume and electrolyte depletion, and acid-base imbalance.

Nausea is a state that defies precise definition in animals. A variety of stimuli (e.g., labyrinthine stimulation, visceral pain) may produce nausea, but the exact neural pathways mediating nausea are not known. It is recognized as a premonitory sign occurring prior to the more definitive stages of retching and vomiting and is clinically manifested in animals by a state of depression, salivation, licking of the lips, and increased swallowing motions. Although these are subtle signs, a keen clinician can recognize their presence and significance.

Retching results from a series of spasmodic respiratory movements that occur while the glottis is closed. It is characterized by repeated thoracic herniations of the abdominal esophagus and cardia, which coincide with negative intrathoracic pressure pulses mirrored by positive pulses in the abdomen. Retching seems to be a preparatory maneuver during which forceful respiratory movements overcome natural antireflux characteristics of the abdominal esophagus and cardia. During this stage the distal stomach (antrum and pylorus) contracts. Vomiting then occurs as the high intra-abdominal pressure expels gastric contents through a relaxed cardia.

It is essential that the clinician make a clear differentiation between *regurgitation* and *vomiting* at the outset. *Regurgitation* is defined as *passive*, retrograde movement of ingested material, usually before it has reached the stomach. Failure to recognize the difference between regurgitation and vomiting often leads to misdiagnosis. Regurgitation may occur immediately after uptake of food or fluids or may be delayed for several hours or more.

Dysphagia is defined as difficulty in swallowing and is usually due to a pharyngeal or esophageal motility disturbance, obstruction, or pain. *Odynophagia* refers to pain on swallowing or radiating chest pain manifested as reluctance to eat.

Pathophysiology of Vomiting

The mechanism of vomiting involves a complex set of activities that is under central neurologic control. The emetic mechanism consists of two anatomically and functionally separate units: a *vomiting center* located in the reticular formation of the medulla oblongata and a *chemoreceptor trigger zone* (CTZ) in the floor of the fourth ventricle. Regardless of the cause of vomiting, all stimuli are mediated through a reflex arc that must pass through the vomiting center, which then coordinates a patterned response. The vomiting center integrates efferent activity from a number of sources, including higher central nervous system centers (e.g., psychogenic vomiting), vestibular input arising from the semicircular canals (vomiting associated with motion sickness, vestibular disorders), the gastrointestinal tract, and the CTZ. A variety of receptors that respond to certain chemicals, inflammation, and changes in osmolality can invoke an afferent stimulus. Vomiting may also result from receptor response to distention of the pyloric end of the stomach (but not the fundus), small intestine, colon, and biliary ducts. In addition, there is evidence that the pharynx, heart, peritoneum, and mesenteric vasculature can be a source of afferent impulses that are transmitted directly to the vomiting center. Salivation occurs commonly in conjunction with nausea and vomiting because of the close proximity of the medullary centers that control these activities.

The CTZ is not able to cause vomiting without the mediation of an intact vomiting center. The CTZ is ***not*** responsive to the various electrical stimuli that activate the vomiting center but acts primarily in response to chemical substances in the blood, including a variety of drugs such as cardiac glycosides, emetic agents such as apomorphine and copper sulfate, general anesthetics, dopaminergic agonists, and antineoplastic agents. Blood-borne chemicals are able to exert a stimulus because the CTZ does not have a normal blood-brain barrier. The CTZ is also important in mediating nausea and vomiting associated with diabetic ketoacidosis, uremia, and bacterial toxins.

Clinical Features of Vomiting

Because of the wide variety of disorders and stimuli that can cause vomiting (Table 7–1), it can present the clinician with a major diagnostic challenge. Although vomiting does not always signify the presence of a serious disorder, it may be the first indication of intestinal obstruction, renal failure, pancreatitis, addisonian crisis, drug toxicity, neoplasia, or other causes. A complete historical review with emphasis on all body systems is essential for determining a realistic and effective initial work-up plan and treatment protocol. Concentration on only the gastrointestinal tract too often leads to a misdiagnosis and inappropriate treatment for the cause of the vomiting. Consideration of the following features is useful in assessing and diagnosing a patient with vomiting.

Duration of Signs and Systems Review. The first question to ask is "Is the vomiting a recent acute problem or is it chronic in nature?" The signalment, immediate signs, past pertinent history, and beneficial or deleterious effects of any drugs that may have been administered (either for the immediate symptoms or as treatment for another disorder) should be determined. At times, a chronic, previously asymptomatic disorder first presents with an acute onset of vomiting, which may then persist as either a frequent or sporadic problem until definitive treatment is begun. Feline inflammatory bowel disease is an example of a common disorder that may present in this way. Specific information regarding diet (type of food, any recent changes), vaccinations (consider systemic disorders such as distemper or parvovirus), travel history, and environment (exposure to toxins, ingestion of garbage or foreign bodies) is obtained in all cases. A thorough systems review with questions investigating any significant occurrence of signs not necessarily referable to the GI tract (e.g., polyuria-polydipsia, coughing and sneezing, dysuria or dyschezia) should also be addressed. This routine systematic approach helps to alleviate diagnostic "tunnel vision" on the part of the clinician.

Time Relation to Eating. A description of the vomiting episodes, including any association with eating or drinking, yields important information in some cases. Normally the stomach empties six to eight hours following meals. Vomiting shortly after eating most commonly

TABLE 7–1. CAUSES OF VOMITING

Dietary Problem	**Disorders of the Gastroesophageal Junction**
Sudden diet change	Hiatal hernia (axial, paraesophageal, diaphragmatic herniation, gastroesophageal intussusception)
Ingestion of foreign material (garbage, grass, plant leaves, etc.)	**Disorders of the Small Intestine**
Eating too rapidly	Parasites
Intolerance to specific foods	Enteritis
Food allergy	Intraluminal obstruction (foreign body, intussusception, neoplasia)
Drugs	Inflammatory bowel disease—idiopathic
Intolerance (e.g., antineoplastic drugs, cardiac glycosides, arsenical compounds)	Diffuse intramural neoplasia (lymphosarcoma)
Injudicious use of anticholinergics	Fungal disease
Accidental overdosage	Intestinal volvulus
Toxins	Paralytic ileus
Lead	**Disorders of the Large Intestine**
Ethylene glycol	Colitis
Others	Obstipation
Metabolic Disorder	Irritable bowel syndrome (IBS)
Diabetes mellitus	**Abdominal Disorders**
Hypoadrenocorticism	Pancreatitis
Renal disease	Zollinger-Ellison syndrome (gastrinoma of pancreas)
Hepatic disease	Peritonitis (any cause, including FIP)
Sepsis	Steatitis
Acidosis	Prostatitis
Hypokalemia	Pyometra
Heat stroke	Urinary obstruction
Disorders of the Stomach	Diaphragmatic hernia
Obstruction (foreign body, pyloric mucosal hypertrophy, external compression, etc.)	Neoplasia
Chronic gastritis (superficial, atrophic, hypertrophic)	**Neurologic Disorders**
Parasites (*Physaloptera* spp in the dog and cat, *Ollulanus tricuspis* in the cat)	Psychogenic (pain, fear, excitement)
Gastric hypomotility	Motion sickness
Bilious vomiting syndrome	Inflammatory lesions (e.g., vestibular)
Gastric ulcers	Edema (head trauma)
Gastric polyps	Autonomic or visceral epilepsy
Gastric neoplasia	Neoplasia
Gastric dilatation	**Miscellaneous Causes of Vomiting**
Gastric dilatation–volvulus	Heartworm disease (feline)
	Hyperthyroidism (feline)

suggests dietary indiscretion or food intolerance, overeating, stress or excitement, gastritis, or a hiatal disorder. Vomiting of undigested or partially digested food more than six hours after eating is an important clinical sign that usually indicates a gastric motility disorder or gastric outlet obstruction. Dogs with gastric hypomotility may vomit undigested food twelve to eighteen hours or more after eating and often exhibit a cyclic pattern of clinical signs. This disorder has been recognized much more frequently in recent years. Misconceptions commonly lead to misdiagnosis and mismanagement of such patients. It is often incorrectly assumed that gastric retention means gastric outlet obstruction, and unnecessary surgery such as pyloromyotomy may be performed. Diagnosis and management of gastric motility disorders may be found in Chapter 85.

Causes of gastric outlet obstruction include foreign bodies, hypertrophic gastritis, pyloric mucosal hypertrophy, and antral or pyloric neoplasia or polyps. All are characterized by chronic vomiting that may occur shortly or a number of hours after eating.

Content of the Vomitus. Significant information can often be obtained from a complete description of the color and consistency of the vomitus. As previously discussed, if food is present, the degree of digestion and time since the most recent meal should be determined. If either undigested food or clear fluid is present, determining the pH may be useful in differentiating regurgitation from the esophagus (alkaline pH) from vomiting of gastric content (acid pH). Bile is often present when vomiting is caused by inflammatory bowel disease, bile reflux syndromes, idiopathic or secondary gastric hypomotility (bile alone or bile with food), intestinal foreign bodies, and pancreatitis. Its presence helps to rule out a complete pyloric obstruction. Small amounts of fresh blood may be present in any case of gastric mucosal compromise with gastric erosions (e.g., hypovolemia, drug-induced gastric erosions, chronic gastritis, gastric ulceration, or neoplasia). Large clots of blood or "coffee grounds" (blood altered by and mixed with gastric juice) usually indicate a more significant degree of erosion or ulceration. A fecal odor suggests intestinal obstruction, peritonitis with ileus, ischemic injury to the intestine, or stasis with bacterial overgrowth.

Projectile Vomiting. Projectile vomiting is an imprecise term that is used to describe vomitus that is ejected forcefully from the mouth and that is expelled a considerable distance. Its occurrence suggests a significant degree of gastric or proximal small bowel obstruction (foreign body, antral or pyloric polyps or neoplasia, pyloric hypertrophy). This is an uncommon clinical sign in the author's experience.

Intermittent Chronic Vomiting. Chronic intermittent vomiting is a common presenting complaint in veterinary medicine. Often there is no specific time relation to eating, the content of the vomitus varies, and the occurrence of vomiting may be cyclic in nature. Depending on the disorder, other signs such as diarrhea, lethargy, inappetence, and salivation (nausea) may occur as well. When presented with this pattern of clinical signs, the clinician should strongly consider chronic gastritis, inflammatory bowel disease, irritable bowel syndrome, and gastric motility disorders as leading differential diagnoses. A detailed work-up including gastric and intestinal biopsies is often required for definitive diagnosis in these cases. It is important to note that chronic intermittent vomiting is a *common* clinical sign of inflammatory bowel disease in both dogs and cats (a complete review can be found in Chapters 86 and 87).

Vomiting from systemic or metabolic causes may be an acute or chronic sign, and generally there is no direct correlation with eating and no predictable vomitus content.

Physical Examination

It is important to stress the enormous significance that a complete physical examination plays in the evaluation of a vomiting patient. A frequent error in clinical practice is to make a diagnosis based on an incomplete history and cursory examination. This may lead to use of unnecessary diagnostic tests and inappropriate treatment. Essential early diagnosis of a serious disorder may be missed. A systematic approach should be both thorough and time efficient.

The mucous membranes are evaluated for evidence of blood loss, dehydration, sepsis, shock, and jaundice. An oral examination may reveal part of an oral or pharyngeal foreign body that may extend to the stomach or intestine. The best example of this is a string foreign body in a cat in which a portion of the foreign material is lodged under the tongue with the remainder causing intestinal plication with potential for perforation. It is extremely important that an oral examination be done in all vomiting cats. In some cases mild tranquilization is required so that a definitive examination can be done. The cervical soft tissues of vomiting cats should be palpated for thyroid nodules as hyperthyroidism commonly causes vomiting. Cardiac auscultation may reveal rate and rhythm abnormalities that can occur with metabolic disturbances such as hypoadrenocorticism (bradycardia, weak femoral pulses), infectious enteritis with septic shock (tachycardia, weak pulses), or gastric dilatation–volvulus (tachycardia, weak pulses, pulse deficits).

A careful assessment is made for abdominal pain, either generalized (e.g., GI ulceration, peritonitis, severe enteritis) or more localized (e.g., pancreatitis, foreign body, pyelonephritis, hepatic disease, regional inflammation in inflammatory bowel disease). Other abdominal factors to evaluate include abnormal organ size (e.g., hepatomegaly), small or large kidneys, presence of a mass (foreign body, intussusception, lymphadenopathy, neoplasia), degree of gastric distention (increased with gastric dilatation, dilatation-volvulus, gastric retention due to hypomotility or outflow obstruction), and altered bowel sounds. Bowel sounds are often absent in peritonitis and increased in acute inflammatory disorders. An increased pitch suggests distention of intestinal loops.

A rectal examination is always done to evaluate stool characteristics for fresh blood or mucus (approximately 30 per cent of patients with colitis present with concurrent vomiting), melena, presence of foreign material, and to obtain a fresh sample for parasite examination.

Serial rectal examinations are most important when GI bleeding is either suspected or has been identified.

Diagnostic Plan

Vomiting patients in some cases require an extensive work-up, but an organized approach helps to minimize the tests necessary for an early diagnosis. The most important initial considerations in determining what tests to perform are (1) signalment, (2) acute (less than three to four days) or chronic duration, (3) frequency of vomiting, (4) degree of symptoms (mild or moderate to severe illness, i.e., life threatening), (5) other clinical signs such as shock, melena, and abdominal pain, and (6) physical examination findings. If reasonable concern is established, then a minimum data base of *CBC*, *biochemical profile* (or specific tests for evaluation of liver, kidneys, pancreas, electrolytes), complete *urinalysis* (pretreatment urine specific gravity is extremely important for diagnosis of renal failure), and *fecal examination* is essential. *Survey abdominal radiographs* are indicated if thorough abdominal palpation is not possible or suggests an abnormality (e.g., foreign body, pancreatitis, pyometra). Unfortunately these tests are often not done early enough. Even if baseline results are unremarkable they are more than justified because they help to rule out serious problems at the outset (e.g., vomiting due to renal failure, diabetes mellitus, liver disease). Alternatively, abnormalities provide direction for initial treatment and further diagnostics.

The decision for performing more in-depth diagnostic tests is based on ongoing clinical signs, response to therapy, and initial test results. These tests include *ACTH stimulation* to confirm hypoadrenocorticism in a patient with an abnormal Na:K ratio or to investigate the possibility of this disorder if electrolytes are normal (see Chapter 97), *complete barium series* (for gastric or intestinal foreign body, gastric hypomotility, gastric outflow obstruction, partial or complete intestinal obstruction), and *serum bile acids assay* (to assess for significant hepatic disease). The many limitations of barium contrast radiography for diagnosis of mucosal disorders are described in Chapters 85 and 86. *Barium swallow with fluoroscopy* is often necessary for diagnosis of hiatal hernia disorders and gastroesophageal reflux disease (see Chapters 83 and 85). Because vomiting is a *frequent* presenting sign in cats with heartworm disease, *serologic tests* should be done to investigate this possibility (see Chapter 80). In endemic areas serologic tests should be considered part of the minimum data base. *Thyroid testing* should also be done on vomiting cats over five years of age to evaluate the possibility of hyperthyroidism. *Serum gastrin levels* are run if a gastrinoma (Zollinger-Ellison syndrome, see Chapter 85) is suspected.

One of the most reliable and cost-efficient diagnostic tools currently available for evaluation of vomiting is *fiberoptic endoscopy*. Endoscopy allows for direct gastric and duodenal examination, mucosal biopsy from these areas, and in many cases gastric foreign body retrieval. Endoscopy is considerably more reliable than barium series for diagnosis of gastric erosions, chronic gastritis, gastric neoplasia, and inflammatory bowel disease. It is stressed that biopsy samples always be obtained from stomach and whenever possible, small intestine, regardless of gross mucosal appearance. Normal gastric biopsies may support gastric motility abnormalities, psychogenic vomiting, irritable bowel syndrome (see Chapter 87), or may tell the clinician only to look elsewhere for the diagnosis. Many dogs and cats with vomiting due to inflammatory bowel disease have no abnormalities on gastric examination or biopsy. If gastric biopsies only are obtained, the diagnosis may be missed.

Abdominal exploratory surgery is indicated for a variety of problems, including foreign body removal, intussusception, gastric mucosal hypertrophy syndromes, procurement of biopsies, and for resection of neoplasia.

Treatment

Since vomiting is a clinical sign of many different disorders, treatment varies depending on the specific cause. The reader is referred to the section in the text that specifically deals with the disorder that has been diagnosed.

In general, goals of therapy include (1) removing the initiating cause, (2) controlling the vomiting episodes, and (3) correcting the fluid, electrolyte, and acid-base abnormalities that are a frequent consequence. Indiscriminate use of antiemetic agents cannot be recommended since they may mask the progression of a potentially life-threatening disorder such as intestinal obstruction. It is reasonable, however, to use antiemetics to maintain patient comfort and to minimize fluid and electrolyte loss as long as efforts are being made to make a diagnosis. Antiemetics that act on both the vomiting center *and* the CTZ (e.g., phenothiazines such as chlorpromazine) are the safest and most effective. Anticholinergics are *not* recommended except in selected psychogenic or irritable bowel syndrome vomiting cases.

Fluid therapy is frequently indicated for patients with disorders causing vomiting. Fluid administration is based not only on replacing daily maintenance and dehydration requirements, but also on the replacement of continued fluid losses that can occur with vomiting. Refer to Chapter 53 for specific recommendations regarding fluid therapy. Hyperalimentation (see Chapter 54) is indicated in some disorders characterized by marked weight loss and chronic anorexia.

REGURGITATION

Regurgitation refers to a passive, retrograde movement of ingested material to a level proximal to the upper esophageal sphincter. Usually this occurs before ingested material reaches the stomach. Regurgitation is a clinical sign of many disorders and should not be considered a primary disease. The term *reflux* refers to movement of gastric or duodenal contents into the esophagus without associated eructation or vomiting. This process may or may not produce symptoms.

Megaesophagus, which refers to a specific syndrome

characterized by a dilated hypoperistaltic esophagus, is one of the most common causes of regurgitation in dogs. By definition and for use in this discussion, megaesophagus is differentiated from other causes of esophageal dilation, such as esophageal foreign body, vascular ring anomaly, and neoplasia, which may or may not be characterized by abnormal peristalsis.

Table 7–2 provides a differential list for the problem of regurgitation. Significant complications of regurgitation include aspiration pneumonia and chronic wasting disease.

Pathophysiology

Regurgitation is usually a clinical sign of an esophageal disorder. The esophagus is a tremendously dilatable muscular tube that acts via a series of well-coordinated peristaltic contractions to move ingesta from the mouth to the stomach. Regurgitation in most cases results from abnormal esophageal peristalsis, esophageal obstruction, or asynchronous function of the gastroesophageal junction.

Normal esophageal motility is controlled via a centrally mediated nervous reflex pathway. Primary esophageal peristalsis is defined as the muscular waves of contraction initiated by a food bolus as it passes through the upper esophageal sphincter into the esophagus. These contractions may sweep the entire length of the esophagus or may subside in the upper to mid-esophageal area. Secondary peristaltic waves arise from reflexes stimulated locally within the esophagus and function to propel any ingesta not carried by the primary contractions. Primary and secondary contractions are manometrically and physiologically similar and are distinguished only by their points of origin. Synchronous function of the lower esophageal sphincter, a zone of high resting pressure that separates the gastric and esophageal lumens, requires a normal esophagus proximal to the sphincter to relay sensory information for mediating its relaxation and opening. A comprehensive review of esophageal function may be found in Chapter 83. Esophageal dysfunction and regurgitation may result from any abnormality along the peristaltic reflex pathway.

TABLE 7–2. CAUSES OF REGURGITATION

Megaesophagus—idiopathic
Megaesophagus—secondary
Myasthenia gravis
Polyneuropathy (giant axonal neuropathy—canine, Key-Gaskell syndrome—feline)
Systemic lupus erythematosus
Polymyositis
Hypoadrenocorticism
Hypothyroidism
Lead toxicosis
Thallium toxicosis
Foreign body
Stricture
Intraluminal lesion
Extraluminal compression (anterior mediastinal mass, hilar lymphadenopathy, abscess)
Vascular ring anomaly
Motility disorder—segmental
Neoplasia of esophagus
Primary
Metastatic
Granuloma (e.g., *Spirocerca lupi*)
Hiatal disorder
Esophageal diverticula

Clinical Features

Many animals with disorders causing regurgitation are presented by owners who incorrectly interpret the problem as vomiting. Regardless of the client's terminology, the clinician should review (1) the nature of the disorder (is it truly active and accompanied by retching (vomiting) or is it passive (regurgitation)?), (2) content of material expelled, and (3) time relation to eating (regurgitation often involves undigested food seconds to hours after eating, or quantities of thick saliva if no food is present in the esophagus). Dogs with megaesophagus are often incorrectly diagnosed and treated for chronic vomiting because the clinician failed to thoroughly review their history.

Recognition of the following associated clinical findings that may be present is extremely important.

Coughing and Dyspnea. Coughing and/or dyspnea suggest aspiration secondary to regurgitation. Many patients with megaesophagus have radiographic evidence of aspiration pneumonia at the time of initial diagnosis. Conversely, any patient that is initially diagnosed as having pneumonia should be investigated at least by history and detailed review of survey thoracic radiographs for evidence of a dilated esophagus. Puppies with congenital megaesophagus frequently present with coughing and nasal discharge.

Weakness. Weakness or collapse in association with regurgitation suggests the presence of a systemic disorder such as myasthenia gravis, hypoadrenocorticism, or polymyositis. These disorders can all cause esophageal motility abnormalities or megaesophagus. In some cases of myasthenia gravis, regurgitation may precede the clinical signs of muscle weakness.

Weight Loss. Weight loss in association with regurgitation indicates insufficient nutrient uptake to meet the body's needs. This is due to decreased intake (either inadequate amounts fed or anorexia secondary to esophageal discomfort or aspiration pneumonia), or decreased volume transfer to the stomach, as caused by megaesophagus or esophageal diverticulum.

Post-ingestion Distress. Discomfort or distress that occurs shortly (i.e., within seconds to several minutes) after eating and that is characterized by extension of the head, frequent swallowing attempts, and then regurgitation, most often indicates an acquired esophageal stricture. These signs are usually accompanied by a ravenous appetite. A puppy or kitten with vascular ring anomaly may show the same signs as soon as solid foods are initiated. A dilated, food-filled esophagus may cause respiratory distress due to partial compression of the lungs.

Ravenous Appetite. A ravenous appetite that occurs in conjunction with regurgitation indicates hunger due to inadequate nutrient transfer to the level of the stomach. This usually occurs in cases of esophageal stricture (any cause) or idiopathic megaesophagus.

Physical Findings

Physical examination findings may vary considerably. Animals with intraluminal esophageal strictures are often normal on examination. Many megaesophagus patients are thin and in poor condition. Thoracic auscultation may reveal pulmonary crackles secondary to aspiration pneumonia. Bulging of the cervical region adjacent to the thoracic inlet, secondary to an enlarged esophagus, may be seen on expiration. Other findings such as weakness (myasthenia gravis), weakness and bradycardia (hypoadrenocorticism), muscle pain (polymyositis), and signs that may include joint pain, shifting limb lameness, erosive glossitis, and others (systemic lupus erythematosus) often occur with systemic disorders. Cats that regurgitate secondary to an anterior mediastinal mass often have a noncompressible anterior chest cavity. Physical findings in cats with Key-Gaskell syndrome, a neurologic disorder characterized in part by regurgitation due to megaesophagus, include persistent pupillary dilation, decreased nasal and lacrimal secretions, bradycardia, and constipation (see Chapter 64).

Diagnostic Plan

Thoracic radiography for survey evaluation of the esophagus is the first and most important step in the diagnosis of a regurgitation disorder. Radiographs are evaluated for evidence of esophageal dilation and presence of a foreign body or thoracic mass. If survey radiographs fail to provide a definitive diagnosis, a *barium esophagram* (with fluoroscopy if available) should be performed to evaluate the cervical and thoracic esophagus. (See Chapter 83 for technique and interpretation.) If radiographs reveal any suggestion of esophageal stricture, foreign body, mass, or diverticulum then *fiberoptic endoscopy* provides the most rapid and cost-effective method of making a definitive diagnosis.

In an adult dog a careful *neurologic examination* should be performed to help rule out neuromuscular disease. Specific tests to evaluate for systemic disorders such as hypoadrenocorticism (*ACTH stimulation*), systemic lupus erythematosus (*antinuclear antibody*), and myasthenia gravis (*Tensilon test, acetylchlorine receptor antibody titer*) are done if the history and physical examination indicate that these primary disorders may exist. *Serum lead* levels are indicated if lead toxicity is considered a possibility.

The main objectives of treatment for regurgitation disorders are to (1) remove the initiating cause as early as possible, (2) minimize chances for aspiration of esophageal content, and (3) maximize nutrient intake to the GI tract. In most cases idiopathic megaesophagus is incurable and treatment involves an individually tailored feeding regimen with the patient eating in an elevated position. Esophageal foreign bodies and intraluminal strictures can often be managed successfully with fiberoptic endoscopy techniques and bougienage or balloon dilation, respectively. Medical management is indicated for such secondary causes of esophageal dilation as myasthenia gravis, hypoadrenocorticism, systemic lupus erythematosus, and anterior (cranial) mediastinal lymphosarcoma in cats. Surgery may be indicated for selected foreign body, stricture, granuloma, and tumor cases. For specific treatment details, the reader is referred to the appropriate chapter for the diagnosis that has been made.

DYSPHAGIA

The term *dysphagia* refers to difficulty in swallowing and may be due to obstruction, motility disturbance, or pain. If clinical signs are acute and persistent or progressive, a morphologic lesion such as a foreign body or mass should be suspected. Intermittent occurrence of clinical signs usually is consistent with a motility disturbance. The reader is referred to Chapter 83 for a review of the swallowing mechanism.

Clinical Findings

Clinical signs associated with disorders causing dysphagia include acute gagging, increased frequency of swallowing, salivation, ravenous appetite (hunger due to inability to ingest an adequate amount of calories), inappetence (rarely), and coughing due to laryngotracheal aspiration. Dysphagia and regurgitation often occur concurrently, especially when a proximal esophageal disorder is present. Abnormal eating habits such as prehending food in unusual positions, throwing the head back to initiate passage of a bolus, excessive chewing, and dropping food from the mouth may also be noted.

Diagnostic Plan

Following a thorough history and physical examination, which includes *observation of eating*, the initial diagnostic step involves *survey cervical and thoracic radiography* as a screen for gross pharyngeal and esophageal abnormalities (e.g., mass, foreign body, evidence of a penetrating wound). If no morphologic lesion is identified, then a *barium contrast study* with emphasis on the pharyngeal area and proximal esophagus should be performed. Many cases of dysphagia due to motility disturbances require a complete *fluoroscopic examination* of the swallowing process for diagnosis. Veterinarians should recommend referral for this procedure if morphologic pharyngeal and esophageal disorders and primary systemic disorders cannot be implicated as the cause of dysphagia. *Esophagoscopy* (for direct mucosal evaluation) and *manometry* (for diagnosis of upper or lower esophageal sphincter dysfunction) are recommended if radiographic studies are unremarkable. The differentiation and treatment of the various disorders causing dysphagia are described in Chapter 83.

8 DIARRHEA

RICHARD K. MARTIN

Diarrhea is an increase in fecal water. This manifests clinically as an increase in frequency and/or volume of bowel movements. The intestinal tract is a complex organ system with a variety of functions that revolve around the digestion and absorption of food. Diarrhea is one of the most common client complaints and can result from any insult to the gut that disrupts normal intestinal physiology. Diarrhea can be classified according to duration of disease, location in the intestinal tract, mechanism of diarrhea, or etiology.

PATHOPHYSIOLOGY

Enterosystemic Cycle. Changes in intestinal water balance have offered the major clues to our current understanding of the pathophysiology of diarrhea. An enterosystemic cycle of fluid absorption and secretion occurs each day in the gut. Under normal circumstances, although absorptive and secretory processes occur simultaneously in the intestine, the absorptive processes greatly predominate. The gastrointestinal tract of a normal 44 lb (20 kg) dog processes approximately three liters of water daily. Of this fluid volume, about 95 per cent is absorbed.

Diarrhea of small bowel origin occurs because the fluid volume presented to the colon is too large; it overwhelms the colonic absorptive reserve capacity. Diarrhea of large bowel origin occurs because the colonic absorptive capacity is decreased and the normal volume of water presented is not absorbed. Clinically, this is an important concept because the colonic absorptive capacity is large and the normal colon can increase its absorptive capacity three- to fivefold. Thus, pure small bowel disease must increase the volume of water presented to the normal colon significantly before diarrhea results. Conversely, relatively minor changes in colonic absorption routinely result in diarrhea.

Normal Intestinal Motility. The major movement of the small intestine is called segmentation. The circular muscle constricts, forming a series of rings. This produces mixing of chyme with digestive fluids as well as increased exposure to the absorptive surface of the intestine.

Peristalsis is due to contraction of a small segment of longitudinal smooth muscle that moves at a rate of a few centimeters per minute. The movement of intestinal contents distally is the net result of the braking effect of rhythmic segmentation and the acceleration effect of peristalsis. When the strength of segmentation is decreased in intestinal disease, very little peristalsis is needed to propel contents over a considerable length of "open pipe," and diarrhea results. Most diseases that alter motility produce clinical signs because of hypomotility (see Mechanisms).

Mechanisms of Diarrhea. Although the absorptive processes normally exceed the secretory processes in magnitude, in diarrhea the secretory processes predominate. All diarrheal diseases studied have had net intestinal secretion in some part of the gastrointestinal tract.

In different disorders the disease process can convert some portion of the gastrointestinal tract from an absorptive organ into a secretory organ by one of these four mechanisms: increased luminal osmolarity, hypersecretion, increased permeability, or motility alterations.

The net result is that either the absorptive processes are decreased or the secretory processes are increased.

Osmotic diarrhea occurs when an excess of water-soluble components remain in the intestinal lumen and hold water with them. Maldigestion or malabsorption of nutrients results in a hyperosmolar load. Some clinical conditions resulting in osmotic diarrhea are dietary overload, pancreatic exocrine insufficiency, bile-salt deficiency, and small intestinal mucosal disease.

Secretory diarrhea occurs when abnormal amounts of extracellular fluid are secreted into the intestinal lumen. The best clinical example of secretory diarrhea is that caused by enterotoxin produced locally in the gut by enteropathogenic *E. coli.* This enterotoxin, via cyclic AMP, stimulates increased secretion by the crypt cells.

A 48 to 72-hour fast can differentiate osmotic and secretory diarrhea. Secretory diarrhea continues in the fasting animal because the stimulus for increased secretion is still present. The fasting animal with osmotic diarrhea should improve since there is a decrease in the osmotic substances.

Increased permeability results from diseases that produce ulceration, inflammation, or infiltration. Mild lesions result in a slight increase in pore size and the loss of water and small molecules. More severe lesions result in larger molecule loss and protein-losing enteropathies.

Most diseases that alter motility produce clinical signs because of hypomotility due to a decrease in rhythmic segmentation. Hypermotility is uncommon, but occurs in certain diseases such as the severe tenesmus associated with colitis.

It is important to realize that combinations of pathophysiologic mechanisms are involved with most intestinal diseases. For example, parvoviral enteritis can produce diarrhea due to hyperosmolarity, hypomotility, hypersecretion, increased permeability, and changes in bacterial flora at various times during the course of the disease.

HISTORICAL FINDINGS

A thorough history should help localize the source of diarrhea in the intestinal tract, determine the chronicity of disease, and help determine whether diarrhea is a primary disorder, secondary to other organ dysfunction, or drug-related. The important historical findings are discussed below.

Duration of Diarrhea. The length of time the patient has had diarrhea helps differentiate simple diarrhea, which may be self-limiting, from chronic diarrhea.

Environment. The animal's environment may suggest possible exposure to infectious or parasitic agents. Animals in very stressful surroundings may be predisposed to diarrhea.

Diet. The nature of the diet and any recent diet changes are very important in the evaluation of the patient. Diarrhea that is corrected after fasting suggests a mechanism of increased osmolarity.

Character of the Stool. Loose to watery consistency with undigested food, fat droplets, or possible melena suggest small bowel disease. Loose to semi-formed consistency with increased mucus (and sometimes fresh blood) suggest large bowel disease.

Quantity of Stool. The quantity of stool is always increased with small bowel diarrhea. The quantity may be increased but is often normal with large bowel diarrhea.

Frequency. Defecation may be increased with small bowel disease but always is increased with large bowel disease.

General Body Condition. The animal with small bowel disease is often in a negative nutritional state. This may occur due to anorexia, vomiting, and fluid and electrolyte imbalances. The animal is often presented with a poor hair coat, lethargy, and loss of weight. The patient with large bowel disease has usually maintained a normal nutritional state.

Tenesmus. Tenesmus (straining) suggests large bowel disease. The clinician should consider inflammatory or obstructive diseases of the colon, rectum, or anus.

Dyschezia. Dyschezia (painful defecation) is associated with large bowel disease. Spastic colitis or rectal or anal lesions may produce noticeable discomfort.

Vomition. In the patient with diarrhea, vomiting usually reflects small bowel disease. However, it is thought that animals with colitis can experience vomiting approximately 30 per cent of the time. This vomiting is intermittent and does not contain bile or blood.

Polydipsia. Polydipsia may be observed in the patient with small bowel disease due to fluid and electrolyte depletion.

Drug Therapy. The clinician should be aware of any current drug therapy that could result in diarrhea (i.e., antibiotics, cardiac glycosides).

PHYSICAL FINDINGS

A thorough physical examination is necessary to help determine if the patient has simple diarrhea or diarrhea with complications. Diarrhea may be a complication of other organ dysfunction (i.e., renal failure, pancreatitis, hepatic disease). It is important to make this differentiation because therapy should always be directed at the primary disease process. Complications commonly result from the diarrheic state and are potentially fatal if not recognized and treated. The clinician must be able to differentiate a case of simple diarrhea from complicated diarrhea in order to accelerate the diagnostic and therapeutic approach to meet the patient's needs.

Hematochezia. Hematochezia (bloody stools) may be digested blood (melena) or fresh blood. It indicates loss of the mucosal defense barrier. Such animals are at risk of developing a septicemia.

Fever. Fever in the patient with diarrhea may indicate a septicemia secondary to the intestinal disorder. Both fever and hematochezia can be indications for antibiotic therapy.

Dehydration. Dehydration is a common complication of diarrhea and indicates fluid and electrolyte depletion. Fluid and electrolyte replacement therapy by the subcutaneous or intravenous route is the most important component of supportive care.

Weight Loss. Weight loss in the patient with diarrhea may reflect a state of anorexia, maldigestion/malabsorption syndrome, or a protein-losing enteropathy.

Abdominal Palpation. Abdominal palpation may reveal an intestinal nodule compatible with a granuloma, tumor, or foreign body. Fluidy bowel loops may be palpated, reflecting the diarrheic state. In small dogs and cats the small bowel may feel thickened due to infiltrative disease (i.e., chronic inflammatory bowel disease).

Rectal Examination. A rectal exam should be performed routinely, especially in patients with large bowel diarrhea. Rectal and anal tumors, strictures, and possible foreign bodies must be considered.

DIAGNOSTIC PLAN

A diagnostic plan should be formulated based on thorough history-taking and a complete physical examination. The clinician should try to determine if the diarrhea originates from the small or large bowel, is simple or complicated, and is primary or secondary to other organ dysfunction. This will help the clinician decide whether a conservative "step by step" approach is warranted or a more aggressive diagnostic plan is indicated (see Figure 8–1).

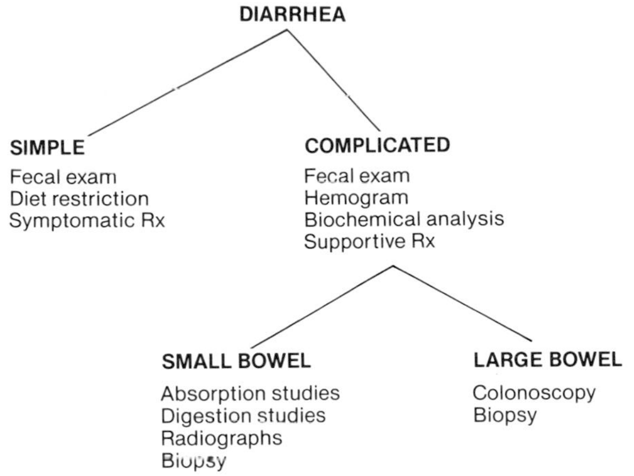

FIGURE 8–1. Diagnostic approach to diarrhea.

Fecal Studies. A complete fecal examination is indicated in all cases of diarrhea. The color and consistency of the feces and the presence of blood or mucus can help determine the source of diarrhea. *Microscopic examination* of the feces should include both a direct smear and fecal flotation to check for parasites and parasitic ova. Repeat examinations or special stains may be needed to identify some parasites. Examination for fecal fats following *Sudan III stain*, starch granules with *Lugol's iodine stain*, or *occult blood* by chemical analysis may be beneficial but are not always diagnostic. A 24-hour *quantitative fecal fat analysis* may be needed to document the presence of steatorrhea.

Gel digestion tests for trypsin activity using either gelatin or x-ray film are unreliable and are being replaced by more specific procedures.

Fecal examination following Wright's or new methylene blue stain may indicate fecal leukocytes (neutrophils or eosinophils) to help support a diagnosis of inflammatory bowel disease.

Fecal cultures for bacteria are indicated if there is a public health concern. Cultures should be performed for *Campylobacter jejuni*, *Salmonella* sp., and *Shigella* sp.

Function Tests. More complicated cases of diarrhea require specific function tests to determine the appropriate therapy. As more of these specific tests are developed in the future the clinician will be able to identify the pathophysiology much more accurately.

Pancreatic function tests include the *oral PABA test* and the *serum trypsin-like immunoreactivity* assay (TLI). Both of these tests are specific and reliable in the diagnosis of exocrine pancreatic insufficiency.

Absorption tests include the *oral glucose tolerance test* and the *D-xylose absorption test*. The *plasma turbidity test* is a simple in-office screening test but is not as reliable as the other absorption tests.

The *serum assay of folate and Vitamin B_{12}* may become useful in the diagnosis of bacterial overgrowth.

An *upper GI study* may indicate small bowel inflammation or a mass effect but may not provide enough diagnostic information to justify the effort and expense. *Barium enemas* are cumbersome and should not be performed in place of colonoscopy.

Intestinal biopsy is indicated in many cases of chronic diarrhea to document a specific disease condition. Fiberoptic endoscopy, a Quinton biopsy instrument, or exploratory celiotomy with full thickness biopsies are all useful. More basic diagnostic procedures should always be performed prior to biopsy to rule out common disease processes.

Hemograms and *biochemical analysis* are useful in determining if there is other organ involvement in addition to the diarrhea.

Anemia could indicate intestinal parasites; leukopenia, a viral enteritis; and eosinophilia, parasites or dietary allergy.

The clinician should formulate a diagnostic plan that considers the most common disease conditions in the area, the patient's comfort, and financial factors.

GOALS OF THERAPY

It is important to remember that the intestine is a multifunctional organ in a state of dynamic flux. The clinician should attempt to modify the ongoing pathophysiology and return the intestine to a normal physiologic state. Many of the time-honored medications used for diarrhea actually prolong the disease state.

Antibiotics should be used for a known intestinal pathogen (*Campylobacter jejuni*, *Salmonella* sp.), when there is a break in the mucosal defense barrier (leukocytosis, fever, hematochezia), or in cases of bacterial overgrowth. The routine use of most antibiotics can damage the normal microflora and delay the recovery of the normal mucosal defense barrier.

Motility modifiers should increase rhythmic segmentation. Those drugs that decrease both peristalsis and rhythmic segmentation help maintain an "open pipe" effect and prolong the diarrheic state. Motility modifiers should not be used in infectious diarrheas.

Fluid and electrolyte replacement is the most important part of supportive therapy. Dehydration and electrolyte imbalance is a common complication of severe diarrhea. Potassium depletion is especially critical due to its effects on intestinal motility.

Specific diagnostic procedures and treatment for various intestinal disorders are described in Chapter 86.

OUTCOME

The great majority of simple diarrheas are self-limiting and recover spontaneously without any clinical assistance. Confinement, inactivity, and dietary restriction for 24 hours are enough to "cure" many cases. Many patients with large bowel diarrhea respond well initially but develop a recurrent cyclic course of disease.

Patients with chronic diarrhea require a specific diagnosis. Some of these patients have advanced pathologic changes and may require long term maintenance therapy (i.e., corticosteroids, MCT oil, restricted diets). The prognosis for each specific disease entity is described in Chapter 86.

9 CONSTIPATION, TENESMUS, AND DYSCHEZIA

M. D. WILLARD and R. WALSHAW

Constipation is defined as a condition in which bowel movements are infrequent or incomplete. The feces are harder than normal. *Obstipation* refers to intractable constipation where defecation becomes impossible. Both constipation and obstipation may lead to megacolon. *Tenesmus* refers to straining, especially ineffectual or involuntary straining associated with defecation or urination. It generally indicates an urgent desire to evacuate the bowel or bladder. *Dyschezia* is defined as difficult and/or painful defecation. *Megacolon* is a condition in which there is extreme dilation of the colon with fecal impaction. The term itself does not refer to the cause of the problem. *Hematochezia* refers to the passage of bloody feces in contradistinction to melena or tarry stools. *Colitis* refers to inflammation of the colon. *Proctitis* refers to inflammation of the mucosa of the rectum.

PATHOPHYSIOLOGY

Constipation may be caused by foods; drugs; neuromuscular disease; metabolic disease; pelvic or perineal pain; obstruction of the colon, rectum, or anus; or miscellaneous factors (Table 9–1). Obstipation is the ultimate outcome of prolonged, severe constipation. Megacolon is a common consequence of uncorrected obstipation, especially when due to lower colonic, rectal, or anal obstruction.

Tenesmus may be alimentary or genitourinary in origin (Table 9–2). Alimentary tenesmus is caused by constipation, obstruction, or inflammatory disease. Obstruction may be due to abnormalities in anatomy, peristalsis, anal sphincter function, or feces (very hard feces or those containing foreign objects). Local inflammatory disease may be due to nonspecific inflammation, local infections, trauma, or neoplasia. *Dyschezia* can be the result of similar disease processes. Tenesmus of genitourinary origin can be secondary to urethral obstruction, cystitis, urethritis, vaginitis, neoplasia, or pregnancy. The diagnostic work-up for the dog or cat with constipation and obstipation is summarized in Figure 9–1, while that for tenesmus and dyschezia is outlined in Figure 9–2.

HISTORICAL FINDINGS

Constipation. The owner usually believes that constipation is occurring if stool has not been seen for two to five days. However, it is important to ascertain that the patient is eating, that the food has sufficient bulk to form feces, and that the patient (especially if a cat) is not defecating without the client's knowledge. Otherwise, failure to expel stool signifies an inability to evacuate feces (i.e., constipation) or an inflamed, empty colon. In the latter case, however, a small amount of feces is usually expelled. If constipation is present, one should seek evidence of iatrogenic causes such as drugs or foods, refusal to defecate, symptoms of neuromuscular dysfunction, and trauma.

Tenesmus. The history can help differentiate tenesmus of alimentary versus genitourinary origin. Tenesmus associated with alimentary tract problems may occur at different times relative to defecation. When tenesmus precedes defecation, it suggests constipation is a major problem. However, if it occurs after defecation, colitis or proctitis should be suspected. Constant tenesmus disassociated with defecation may indicate a colonic, rectal, or anal foreign object or neoplasm. Chronicity with progressive worsening of signs suggests an obstructive lesion.

The position that the dog or cat assumes during defecation is important. Squatting associated with tenesmus is suggestive of an inflammatory lesion, whereas a semi-squatting position is more often seen with an obstructive lesion.

Apparently unrelated signs may also be associated with tenesmus and can be helpful in diagnosis. For example, vomiting occurs in approximately one-third of patients with colitis, while regurgitation can be part of the presenting history in patients with neuromuscular disorders such as dysautonomia or myopathy.

TABLE 9–1. CAUSES OF CONSTIPATION/OBSTIPATION IN DOGS AND CATS

Food/liquids	Excessive indigestible bulk/fiber Foreign objects Dehydration
Drugs	Agents that add excess particulate matter (carafate, barium sulfate, antacids, kaopectate) Agents that inhibit peristalsis (narcotics, anticholinergics, vincristine, oral iron supplementation, antihistamines, phenothiazines, diuretics, chronic laxative abuse)
Neuromuscular disease	Ileus Paraplegia Spinal cord/sacral nerve disease CNS disease (lead intoxication, rabies) Dysautonomia Pseudo-obstruction Hypokalemia
Trauma	Pelvic fractures Hematoma Lacerations
Metabolic disease	Hypothyroidism Hyperparathyroidism/pseudohyperparathyroidism
Perineal/rectal pain	Septic/nonseptic inflammation Foreign object Pelvic fracture Rectal prolapse Perianal fistula Colonic/rectal/anal growth Colonic/rectal/anal stricture Anal sac impaction, infection, abscess
Colonic/rectal/anal obstruction	Neoplasia Granuloma Old malaligned pelvic fracture Cicatrix Rectal prolapse Foreign object Pseudocoprostasis Extramural compression (prostatomegaly, sublumbar lymphadenopathy, cystic uterus masculinus) Perineal hernia Congenital anomaly
Miscellaneous	Behavior (refusal to defecate/no litter box) Idiopathic, cystic uterus masculinus Persistent inactivity Inability to ambulate or squat (fractured pelvis or leg) Irritable bowel syndrome Pheochromocytoma

Dyschezia. Dyschezia can be due to foreign objects, obstruction, colitis, or proctitis, as well as inflammatory or infectious diseases of the perianal area. Pain associated with the positioning process may indicate musculoskeletal or neurologic problems or soft tissue injury.

TABLE 9–2. CAUSES OF TENESMUS AND/OR DYSCHEZIA IN DOGS AND CATS

Constipation	See Table 9–1
Colonic/rectal/anal pain	See Table 9–1 Colitis/proctitis Rectal spasm
Urogenital pain	Cystitis/urethritis/vaginitis Urethral obstruction Urethral or vaginal neoplasia
Miscellaneous	Pregnancy

A description of the feces may also prove helpful in diagnosis. A hard fecal mass is consistent with constipation. Foreign objects may have been noticed in the feces. Fecal discoloration can be due to digestive problems, drugs, or abnormal foods. Liquid feces suggests small bowel disease or colitis, however, constipation can result in small amounts of mucoid feces being passed due to colonic mucus secretion. Soft feces of a narrow diameter ("ribbon-like") imply a constrictive lesion. Bloody, mucoid feces are caused by colitis and rectal neoplasia. Hematochezia with discrete spots or lines of blood indicates a rectal or anal lesion (ulcer, granuloma, polyp, neoplasia).

PHYSICAL EXAMINATION

External Examination. The external examination should specifically look for evidence of trauma. Lacerations, bruises, bleeding, or hindlimb lameness indicate the need for a careful examination for evidence of orthopedic or soft tissue injury. *Neurologic deficits* to the hindquarters may be due to trauma, intervertebral disc disease, neoplasia, inflammation, and infectious causes. Weakness may suggest electrolyte imbalance, myopathy, or neuropathy. Dilated pupils and a dry rhinarium in a cat are consistent with dysautonomia. A poor hair coat and obesity in a dog may suggest hypothyroidism. Abdominal distension may indicate intestinal stasis or megacolon associated with these signs.

The Anal, Perianal, and Perineal Region. Next, there should be an examination of the anal, perianal, and perineal regions. Problems that may be found on examination of these areas include perineal hernia, perianal fistulae, anal sac disease, neoplasia, matting of hair over the anus (pseudocoprostasis), congenital anomalies, inflammatory disease, or protrusion of tissue from the anus (e.g., neoplasia, rectal prolapse). Soft tissue swelling, bruising, and/or laceration suggest trauma. The penis and prepuce or vulva should be examined to rule out urogenital causes of tenesmus.

Abdominal Palpation. Abdominal palpation should include an evaluation of the colon. Hard feces within the colon that cannot be indented by the clinician's fingers suggest constipation. A grossly enlarged colon impacted with hard feces may be diagnostic for megacolon. It is rarely possible to eliminate neoplasm in these patients. If colitis is present, an empty colon that is painful on palpation is often detected. *Posterior abdominal masses* may be due to prostatomegaly (due either to benign or malignant disease), sublumbar lymphadenopathy (due to metastatic disease), an enlarged, tense urinary bladder (due to obstruction), pregnancy, cystic disease, or neoplasia. A small, hard, painful urinary bladder may indicate cystitis as the cause of tenesmus.

Rectal Examination. Finally, the rectal examination often helps to define distal colonic disease. Pain may be elicited if one of the following problems is present: colitis, proctitis, anal sacculitis, abscess, perianal fistulae, prostatitis, rectal or anal neoplasia, rectal or anal stricture, or orthopedic problems. *Pelvic mass(es)* may be caused by the following: prostatomegaly, lymphade-

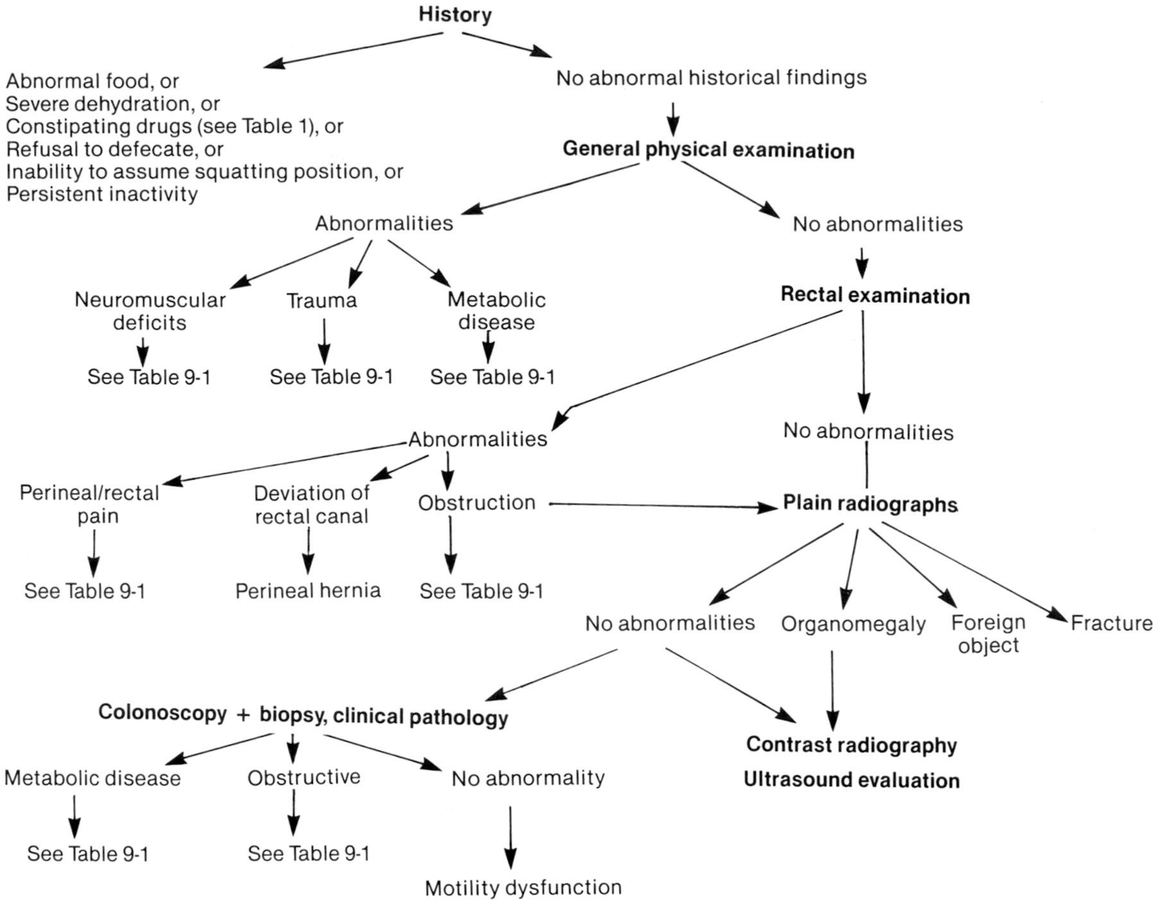

FIGURE 9–1. Diagnostic approach to the dog or cat with constipation, obstipation, or megacolon.

nopathy, and neoplasia of the anal sacs, circumanal glands, or other structures. *Obstruction* of the anal and rectal canals may be due to extramural masses (see above), mural lesions, or intraluminal problems. Mural lesions include neoplasia, inflammatory disease, and strictures. Intraluminal obstruction could be due to neoplasia, fecal impaction, or foreign objects. Deviation of the rectoanal canal is usually associated with perineal hernia. Frequently, fecal impaction is also present. Finally, *irregularities of the mucosal lining* may result from inflammatory disease or neoplasia.

ADDITIONAL DIAGNOSTIC PROCEDURES

The history, physical, and rectal examination should categorize if not diagnose the cause of constipation, tenesmus, or dyschezia in the majority of patients. However, additional testing may be required. *Plain abdominal and pelvic radiographs* confirm constipation and megacolon. In addition, abnormal masses in the posterior abdomen may be outlined. Plain radiographs are unlikely to detect mural lesions unless contrast (i.e., air or fecal material) is present in the lumen or the lesions are large. Obstruction may be visualized by an abrupt cessation of the fecal column. *Contrast radiographic studies* such as the barium enema are difficult to perform well in the dog and cat. They often do not demonstrate distal rectal lesions and can have many artifacts due to incomplete bowel preparation. Endoscopy is preferred to contrast radiography in most instances. Contrast radiographic studies of the lower urinary tract, however, may be helpful in deciding if a posterior abdominal mass is associated with this system, as in prostatomegaly. *Ultrasound examination* of the posterior abdomen can help differentiate the origin of posterior abdominal and pelvic masses. *Endoscopy* plus biopsy is a cost-effective diagnostic procedure for evaluating the lower intestinal tract. It is essential for evaluating mucosal diseases. Not only can an accurate diagnosis be made but optimal treatment methods can often be determined by evaluating the extent of the lesion (e.g., what surgical procedure would be best for a particular colorectal neoplasm). Endoscopy can also be therapeutic as when performed in conjunction with polypectomy or foreign body removal. *Exploratory celiotomy* of the abdomen may be necessary. In such cases the procedure should be approached as a possible treatment as well. Abdominal exploration is important in evaluating the problem and in accurately staging neoplasms.

GOALS OF TREATMENT

Constipation. The objective of symptomatic treatment of constipation is to prevent the formation of and/or to

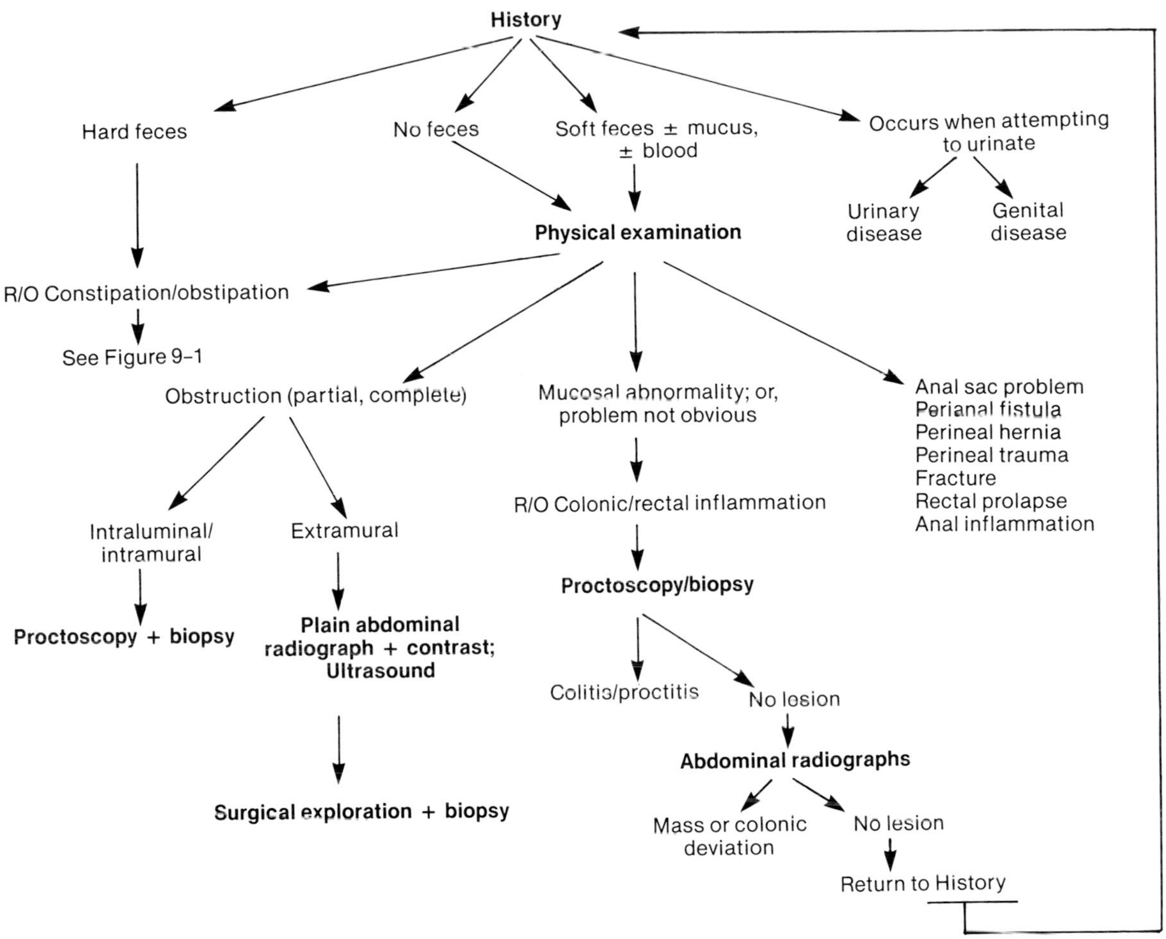

FIGURE 9–2. Diagnostic approach to the dog or cat with tenesmus and/or dyschezia.

remove hardened feces. This is done by maintaining adequate hydration and electrolyte balance plus using laxatives, cathartics, enemas, mechanical breakdown, and/or surgical removal (Figure 9–3). Maintaining adequate hydration is important, especially when fecal water loss is enhanced by laxatives and cathartics. The latter drugs, such as mineral oil, dioctyl sodium sulfasuccinate, and bisacodyl, with or without an enema are useful for mild constipation. In more severe cases, multiple warm water retention enemas with or without soap or wetting agents such as dioctyl sodium sulfasuccinate given over one to four days are safe and effective in all but the worst impactions. Hypertonic enemas must be avoided in obstipated or very small patients (i.e., most cats and small dogs). Mechanical breakdown of impacted feces is indicated if multiple retention enemas are inadequate, but this must be done carefully to avoid colonic damage. Surgical removal is reserved for megacolon or obstipation that is refractory to enemas and mechanical breakdown.

After removal of the feces, resolution of the underlying cause is indicated. If resolution is impossible or delayed, bulking agents and stool softeners added to the diet (e.g., psyllium, bran, dioctyl sodium sulfasuccinate) offer symptomatic control if there is no severe motility disorder present. Cholinergics such as urecholine can be given immediately prior to defecation to aid in evacuation, but must not be used if alimentary or urogenital obstruction is present. Megacolon must be prevented because of its guarded prognosis. If the colon has become nonfunctional secondary to prolonged megacolon, colectomy with anastomosis of the ileum to the rectum may be necessary.

Tenesmus and Dyschezia. Symptomatic treatment of tenesmus or dyschezia unassociated with constipation is difficult. Fasting can decrease the amount of feces, thereby lessening the pain due to colitis and proctitis. Removing perianal hair, gentle washing, and antibiotic-steroid ointments soothe an inflamed anus. Topical steroids with or without local anesthetics administered via retention enema may decrease colonic inflammation and irritability. Addition of fiber to the diet may decrease colonic myoelectrical activity and also help, although this is rarely successful by itself. Inflammatory bowel disease is common and a diagnosis derived from a biopsy is often required for specific treatment. Finally, patients with tenesmus or dyschezia of undeterminable origin may be empirically treated with antibacterial drugs (especially those effective against anaerobic bacteria), corticosteroids, or antispasmodics.

The reader is referred to Chapters 87 and 92 for a detailed description of the treatment of the various causes of constipation, tenesmus, and dyschezia.

Outcome. The outcome of treatment of constipated

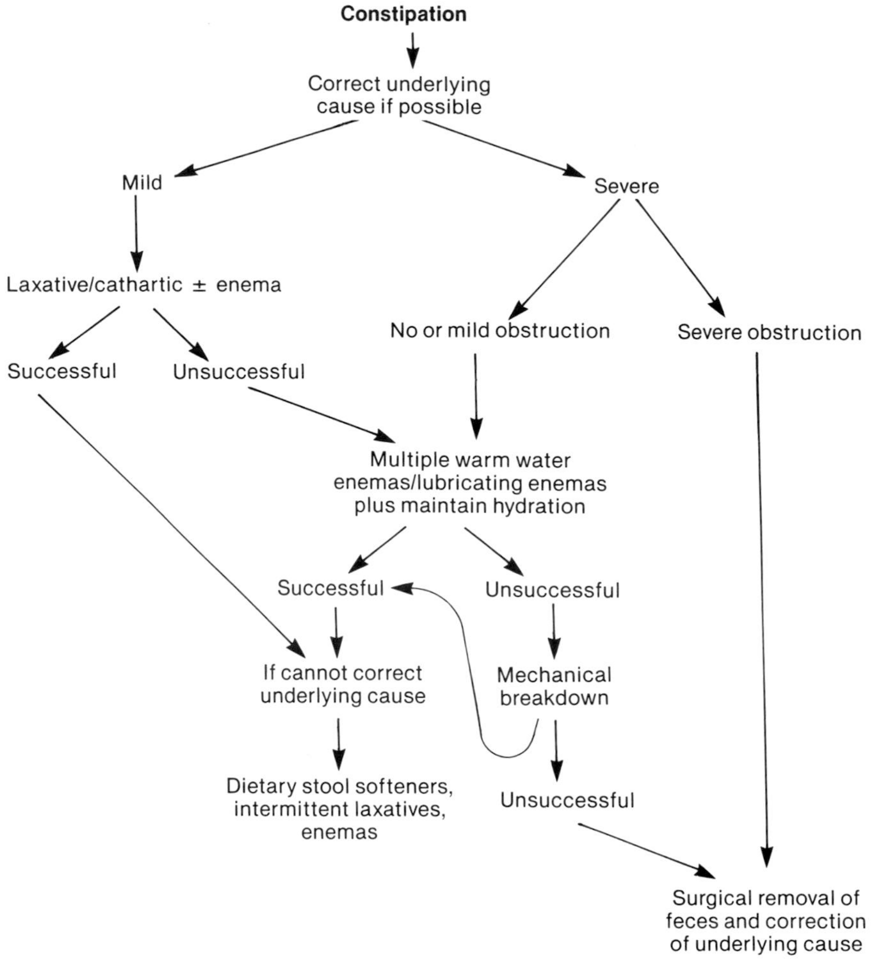

FIGURE 9–3. Therapeutic approach to the dog or cat with constipation.

patients depends upon the cause. Benign causes such as abnormal diet, drug therapy, and benign neoplasia can usually be treated successfully. Some diseases, such as idiopathic megacolon in the cat, may require extensive surgical intervention but still carry a good prognosis for recovery. Malignant neoplasms such as colorectal adenocarcinoma generally are associated with a poor to grave prognosis due to the difficulty in treating the primary lesion and metastatic disease. Neuromuscular diseases like dysautonomia are often associated with a poor prognosis for recovery unless there is specific surgical or medical therapy, as in spinal cord decompression.

Patients with tenesmus and/or dyschezia due to colitis and proctitis are usually manageable with appropriate medical therapy. However, failure to treat the underlying disease may lead to a chronically scarred lower bowel whose function is severely compromised. Surgical problems such as perianal fistula, perineal hernia, and congenital anomalies are potentially curable. Some of these problems (e.g., perianal fistula) carry a guarded prognosis due to the difficulty in resolving them. Finally, the potential for secondary problems such as anal sphincter incontinence must be considered.

10 PERIPHERAL EDEMA*

GARY BOLTON and STEPHEN J. ETTINGER

Edema is defined as excessive amounts of body fluid in the interstitial (extracellular) spaces. In this chapter, peripheral edema means subcutaneous edema, in order to differentiate it from central or intracavitary edema. Furthermore, localized edema is used to denote edema confined to a specific area. Generalized edema refers to edema of all four extremities, with or without ventral midline edema. Anasarca denotes severe, whole body, subcutaneous edema.

PHYSIOPATHOLOGY OF EDEMA FORMATION

Despite the fact that the interstitial fluid accounts for one-sixth of the total body fluids, the interstitial spaces are normally almost dry. This is because the interstitial fluid normally exists in a "gel" state. In this state it is viscid and nonmobile. If this were not so, it would be impossible to maintain even distribution throughout the body and gravity would continually shift the fluid to dependent regions. The interstitial fluid can also exist in a "free" or watery state, in which it is freely mobile. When edema is diagnosed clinically, most often it is due to accumulation of free interstitial fluid. It is important to understand the factors that play a role in maintaining "dry" tissues and to appreciate the wide margin of safety that exists between the edematous and the nonedematous states.

In the microcirculation, the significant factors that govern the state of interstitial fluid are hydrostatic pressure (HP or mean capillary pressure), plasma colloidal oncotic pressure (PCOP), tissue colloidal oncotic pressure (TCOP), interstitial fluid pressure (IFP), capillary permeability, and lymphatic flow (Figure 10–1). If all the forces tending to move fluid out of the capillaries are totaled (HP + TCOP + IFP), an outward force of 17 mmHg, plus 5 mmHg, minus −6.5 mmHg, or 28.5 mmHg, occurs. The major inward force tending to hold fluid within the capillaries is PCOP at 28 mmHg. Normally then, there is a slight pressure gradient of .5 mmHg acting to favor fluid (plasma) filtration into the interstitial spaces. The lymphatic system effectively returns this fluid to the circulation and maintains the tissues in their dry state.

Four dynamic abnormalities occur that cause edema formation. These are increased capillary pressure, decreased plasma colloidal oncotic pressure, increased capillary permeability, and blockage of lymphatic flow (Table 10–1). These may occur independently or in conjunction with one another. The crucial point at which

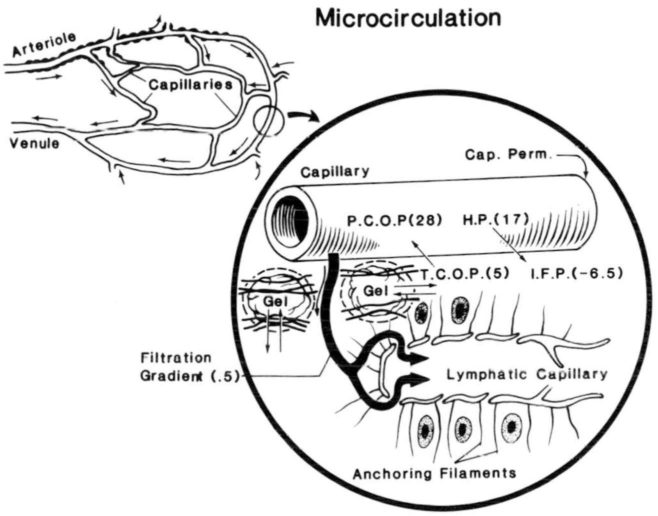

FIGURE 10–1. Diagram of the normal microcirculation depicting the factors that determine interstitial fluid formation. Plasma colloidal oncotic pressure (PCOP) is the main factor retaining plasma in the capillaries. Hydrostatic pressure (HP), tissue colloidal oncotic pressure (TCOP), and the negative interstitial fluid pressure (IFP) all draw plasma into the interstitial space. There is a resulting filtration gradient of .5 mmHg causing a net positive formation of interstitial fluid, which is effectively removed by the lymphatic capillaries. Disease states altering capillary permeability (cap. perm.) may also encourage interstitial fluid formation. Diagram adapted with permission from Zweifach: Factors Regulating Blood Pressure. Josiah Macy, Jr., Foundation, 1950, and from Guyton, A. C.: Integrated Dynamics of the Circulation and Body Fluids, Fig. 6–10. *In* Sodeman, W., and Sodeman, T. (eds.): Sodeman's Pathologic Physiology, W. B. Saunders Company, 1979.

*This chapter was prepared for the second edition of the textbook prior to Dr. Bolton's untimely death. Out of respect for our colleague, this chapter is re-presented by Dr. Ettinger. A donation to the Academy of Veterinary Cardiology–Bolton Memorial Lecture has been made.—The Editor.

TABLE 10–1. GENERAL CAUSES OF PERIPHERAL EDEMA

Increased Capillary Pressure	
	Venous hypertension
	Venous obstruction
	Arteriovenous fistula
	Overhydration
Decreased Plasma Colloidal Oncotic Pressure	
	Hypoproteinemia (hypoalbuminemia)
Lymphatic Obstruction	
	Inflammation
	Ablation by surgery
	Trauma
	Neoplasia
	Primary lymphedema
Increased Capillary Permeability	
	Burns
	Angioneurotic edema
	Inflammation
	Trauma

edema occurs is the point at which interstitial fluid pressure rises above 0 mmHg (atmospheric pressure). As the interstitial fluid pressure approaches this level, the gel fluid expands to a maximum of 30 per cent. When the pressure of the interstitial fluid rises above 0 mmHg, the gel has expanded to its limit and free interstitial fluid increases dramatically.

Safety factors provide a wide margin of protection against edema formation. Capillary pressure must double for edema to occur. Plasma colloidal oncotic pressure must fall from 28 mmHg to below 10 mmHg before edema begins. The interstitial fluid pressure must rise from −6.5 mmHg to above zero, and by the time it approaches zero, lymph flow has increased 20 to 25 times. The increased lymphatic flow washes protein from the interstitial space and lowers the tissue colloidal oncotic pressure. As long as the lymphatics can remove the excess interstitial fluid, edema does not occur. There is a maximum rate of lymphatic flow that cannot be exceeded, and by the time edema occurs, lymphatic flow is already maximal. When the safety factors are being used maximally but edema has not yet occurred, it is termed a pre-edematous stage. This pre-edematous stage can be clinically important. For example, fluid therapy given to a nephrotic patient in the pre-edematous stage may induce frank generalized edema.

More than simply a clinical sign, edema has medical significance. By increasing the diffusion distance between the blood vessels and the tissue cells, significant accumulations of edematous fluid interfere with cellular nutrition and metabolism. A chronically edematous area may eventually ulcerate and weep. These areas are also susceptible to infection and can result in the loss of a limb or in an uncontrollable infection.

TABLE 10–2. CAUSES OF GENERALIZED PERIPHERAL EDEMA

With Ascites	
	Hypoproteinemia
	Right-sided heart failure
	Pericardial effusion
Without Ascites	
	Hypoproteinemia

LOCALIZED VERSUS GENERALIZED PERIPHERAL EDEMA

To be considered generalized, edema must occur in both the front and rear quarters. Careful examination of all four limbs, as well as the entire ventral midline, is essential. Whole body edema (anasarca) is rare but is the most severe form of generalized edema. Most often the edema gravitates to the limbs and to the ventral midline. Edema can be bilateral but still considered local if it is restricted solely to the front or rear quarters.

If the edema is generalized, right-sided heart failure, pericardial effusion, or hypoproteinemia must be considered. The presence or absence of ascites is an important diagnostic clue. Heart failure and pericardial disease cause ascites before peripheral edema occurs in small animals. Generalized edema without ascites suggests hypoproteinemia (Table 10–2).

Four variations of localized edema may occur (Table 10–3). Edema may involve one extremity, the forelimbs may be edematous with normal hindlimbs, edema may be confined to the hindlimbs, or edema of the head and face may occur. In general, localized edema draws attention to that specific region, and examination of that region must include the regional blood and lymphatic supply.

When edema is confined to one extremity, four general causes must be considered: inflammation and/or infection, venous or lymphatic occlusion, arteriovenous fistula, and trauma. Inflammation, infection, and trauma may occur singly or together. They produce edema by impairing vascular integrity and altering capillary permeability. Large amounts of plasma leak into the interstitial spaces, and necrotic debris from tissue necrosis causes lymphatic plugging. Local swelling may cause lymphatic, as well as venous, collapse, trapping fluid in the tissues.

Edema due to venous occlusion tends to be severe, since two abnormalities occur. Hydrostatic pressure increases, favoring filtration of fluid into the interstitial spaces. At the same time, venous absorption is decreased. This combination of increased filtration and decreased absorption soon overwhelms the lymphatics, and edema occurs. Extensive examination may be required to determine the site of the obstruction.

An arteriovenous fistula is an open and abnormal communication of an artery and vein. This overloads

TABLE 10–3. CAUSES OF LOCALIZED PERIPHERAL EDEMA

Edema of One Extremity	
	Inflammation and/or infection
	Trauma
	Venous or lymphatic obstruction
	Arteriovenous fistula
Bilateral Forelimb Edema Without Hindlimb Edema	
	Cranial vena cava obstruction
Bilateral Hindlimb Edema Without Forelimb Edema	
	With ascites—caudal vena cava obstruction
	chronic portal hypertension
	Without ascites—sublumbar iliac venous obstruction
Facial Edema	
	Angioneurotic edema
	Juvenile pyoderma (initial phase)
	Myxedema

the venous system with arterial blood and causes local venous return and volume overloading of the right heart. The fistula may be congenital or acquired. Acquired fistulas are most often secondary to a severe inflammatory lesion, trauma, or a surgical procedure. In these instances an artery and a vein heal together and establish communication.

Lymphatic occlusion most often results from inflammation and plugging or from neoplastic processes and may accompany venous and/or arterial occlusion by neoplasms.

Bilateral forelimb edema unaccompanied by hindlimb edema almost always indicates occlusion of the cranial vena cava. Edema of the head and neck may also be present. Lymphatic tumors, heart base tumors, and right atrial hemangiosarcomas are the usual causes. Bilateral hindlimb edema exclusive of the forelimbs may also occur. When it does, the presence or absence of ascites is an important clue to the site of the vascular obstruction. If the site of venous occlusion is cranial to the renal veins, ascites will be present. Hindlimb edema without ascites confines the lesion to the pelvic canal region, with obstruction of the common iliac veins.

Sudden onset of edema confined to the head is typical of angioneurotic edema. The eyelids and lips are most severely affected. This form of edema is allergic in origin, resulting from increased capillary permeability and arteriolar dilatation. The initial phase of juvenile pyoderma may present as severe facial edema due to inflammation. Hypothyroid dogs may present with striking "fat faces" that do not pit and are referable to myxedema.

Occasionally, an animal with generalized disease may have local edema. The hypoproteinemic animal may be pre-edematous and on the verge of developing frank edema. In the prone or sitting position, the limb or limbs positioned underneath the animal may become edematous from interference with circulation. Attention may be called to that area when the problem is really a more generalized one.

Conversely, a localized condition that appears generalized is primary lymphedema, a congenital, imperfect development of the lymphatic system. It occurs in puppies and may present as an edematous swelling of one or all of the limbs. When it occurs in all of the limbs, it may mimic a generalized condition. This should be considered in such a puppy when no serum protein or cardiac abnormalities are found.

HISTORY AND PHYSICAL EXAMINATION

Animals with generalized edema should be evaluated for heart, kidney, liver, or gastrointestinal disease. Historical evidence of organ dysfunction such as coughing, exercise intolerance, fainting, vomiting, diarrhea, and polydipsia or polyuria may be of help. Murmurs, gallop rhythms, muffled heart sounds, distended jugular veins, arrhythmias, and abnormal femoral pulses may together or individually suggest cardiac disease. The abdomen is evaluated for fluid, masses, size and shape of the liver and kidneys, and consistency and tone of the intestine. Hypoproteinemia due to dietary indiscretion is rare today, but diet history should be obtained regardless of that.

When a single limb is involved, the entire limb and its blood supply are evaluated. Heat, pain, and redness denote inflammation. Cool, nonpainful swelling suggests vascular occlusion. The limb should be palpated for masses and auscultated for the presence of murmurs, since arteriovenous fistulas evoke a continuous murmur. If bilateral hindlimb edema is present without ascites, a rectal examination should be done and the caudal abdomen should be palpated carefully for sublumbar masses. A sublumbar mass might also occlude one or both of the femoral arteries, and the strengths of the right and left femoral pulse should be compared simultaneously.

The edema itself may provide a clue to an underlying etiology. The ability to pit the edematous area using digital pressure depends on the thickness or viscosity of the edematous fluid. The viscosity is determined by its protein content. The higher the protein, the more viscid the fluid. Hypoproteinemia usually implies a fluid with a protein content of less than 1 gm/L. Fluid in cases of heart failure contains 4 to 5 gm/L of protein. Fluid associated with inflammation and increased capillary permeability may contain over 10 gm/L of protein. The edematous fluid due to hypoproteinemia is watery and mobile. It pits easily and recovers within seconds of releasing pressure. Heart failure edema requires more pressure and the pit remains long after pressure is released. Edema due to inflammation tends to be nonpitting and is called "brawny edema."

ANCILLARY AIDS

Diagnostic aids that are often required to determine an etiology for peripheral edema include clinical pathology, electrocardiography, central venous pressure measurement, radiography, angiography, and exploratory surgery.

Clinical Pathology. With peripheral edema the clinician must establish whether the animal is hypoproteinemic. Since albumin provides the majority of the plasma colloidal oncotic pressure, the albumin value is critical, although the globulin level may also be important. Renal disease with urinary albumin loss results in a low serum albumin and a normal serum globulin. Hepatic disease with decreased albumin production results in low serum albumin with normal or elevated serum globulin. With gastrointestinal protein loss, both serum albumin and globulin levels are low (Table 10–4). In pure hypoalbuminemia such as that which occurs with renal or gastrointestinal disease, there are no congestive vascular phenomena and the albumin level must fall below 1 to 1.5 gm/dl before edema occurs. If congestive phenomena such as chronic portal hypertension are present, edema may occur at albumin levels as high as 1.5 to 2.0 gm/dl.

Persistent proteinuria must be documented to establish renal disease (nephrotic syndrome) as the cause of the hypoproteinemia. Bromsulphalein (BSP) clearance

TABLE 10–4. PROTEIN PATTERNS IN HYPOPROTEINEMIA

	Total Protein	Albumin	Globulin	A:G
Renal	↓	↓	Normal or ↑	↓
Hepatic	Normal or ↓	↓	Normal or ↑	↓
Gastrointestinal	↓	↓	↓	Normal
Chronic blood loss externally	↓	↓	↓	Normal
Malnutrition	↓	↓	↓	Normal

and prothrombin time are helpful indicators of advanced hepatic dysfunction, although BSP values may be falsely low when serum albumin content is below normal. BSP clearance is less commonly evaluated today and has been replaced by fasting bile acid assay. If gastrointestinal protein loss is suspected, parasitism must be ruled out, and occult blood tests are performed on the feces to determine if there is significant blood loss from the bowel. Radioactive-labeled albumin studies are available at many institutions to document gastrointestinal albumin loss.

Significant loss of protein, both albumin and globulin, can occur with chronic blood loss outside the body. Chronic loss through the urine or stool may be overlooked by the owner, whereas chronic hemorrhage from other areas is likely to be reported.

If ascites is present, laboratory evaluation of the ascitic fluid provides valuable information regarding the etiology of the edema formation (see Chapter 28).

Electrocardiography, Radiography, Central Venous Pressure. When ascites and generalized peripheral edema occur, heart disease must be considered in the differential diagnosis. Cardiomegaly may be a helpful clue and can be documented by ECG and thoracic radiology. The caudal vena cava should be examined on thoracic radiographs. Enlargement suggests elevated central venous pressure due to right-sided heart failure. Masses and pericardial effusion restrict venous return and these may also be visualized on radiographs.

The measurement of central venous pressure (CVP) is often helpful. Normally the CVP is less than 5 cm H_2O in dogs and cats. In most cases of right-sided heart failure, the CVP is between 8 and 15 cm H_2O. In severe cases it can range as high as 20 to 30 cm H_2O. A CVP greater than 30 cm H_2O suggests pericardial disease with restriction of venous inflow rather than right-sided heart failure.

Cardiac disease, particularly due to right-sided failure or obstruction, is effectively evaluated with cardiac ultrasonography. Pericardial effusion, severe tricuspid insufficiency, and venous obstruction are all readily recognized by ultrasound.

ANGIOGRAPHY. If venous occlusion is suspected, a radiograph following injection of contrast medium into a vein distal to the occlusion is often very effective in outlining the obstructed area. Delineation of an arteriovenous fistula requires an arterial injection of contrast medium, a procedure that is much more difficult. Lymphangiography may be helpful in outlining lymphatic channels but requires special equipment as well as special expertise. These procedures, however, are not unavailable to small animal practitioners, and venous angiograms are very easy to perform. Renografin-76 is an excellent injectable contrast medium and is given as a bolus at a dose 0.5 to 1.0 ml/lb.

SURGERY. Areas of vascular occlusion must be explored for diagnosis and correction. Arteriovenous fistulas must be surgically occluded or completely excised, depending on their location and their anatomic configuration. Abdominal exploratory surgery may be necessary for cases of intra-abdominal venous obstruction or for cases in which liver, kidney, or bowel biopsies are necessary. Liver and kidney biopsies are better and more safely determined via percutaneous biopsy, especially where low protein may reduce healing.

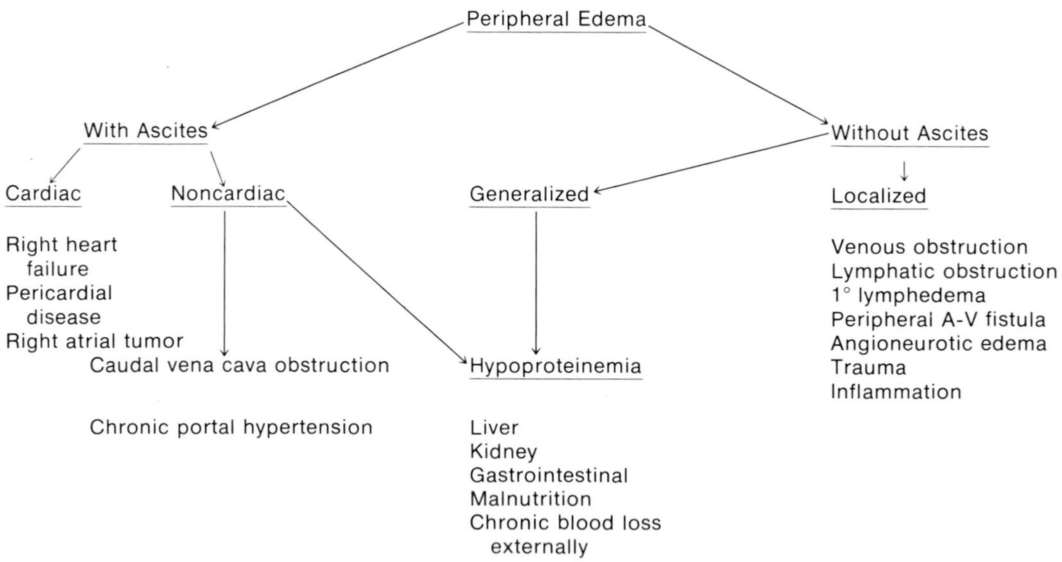

FIGURE 10–2. Use this flow chart to organize the diagnostic approach to cases of peripheral edema.

SUMMARY AND WORK PLAN

Use the flow chart (see Figure 10–2) to keep general causes of peripheral edema in mind.

Generalized Peripheral Edema. If generalized subcutaneous edema is present, evaluate the pitting properties of the fluid. Determine whether ascites is also present. If so, analyze a sample of ascitic fluid (see Chapter 28). Note the total protein and albumin-to-globulin ratio. If hypoproteinemia is present, pursue diet history, renal, hepatic, or gastrointestinal disease and evaluate for signs of chronic external blood loss. If the serum proteins are normal, examine the cardiac status and measure central venous pressure (Chapters 71 and 72).

Primary lymphedema is considered when generalized limb edema is present, without hypoproteinemia or demonstrable cardiovascular disease.

Localized Peripheral Edema. Even though the edema may appear to be confined to one area, serum proteins and cardiac function should be evaluated to rule out the possibility that the animal is pre-edematous due to a generalized problem and that positional changes have accentuated the edema in that area, as previously discussed. When right heart failure causes ascites and peripheral edema, the edema is often much more remarkable in the hindlimbs.

Thoracic radiographs, echocardiography, and cephalic or jugular vein angiography may be used to outline a cranial vena cava obstruction when bilateral forelimb edema occurs with or without facial and neck edema. Edema confined to the hindlimbs with no ascites suggests venous obstruction at the pelvic canal or sublumbar area. Radiography, palpation, abdominal ultrasound, and saphenous vein angiography help to determine the site of the obstruction. Obstruction of the caudal vena cava is suspected when the animal has normal serum proteins and a normal heart but is presented with ascites and bilateral hindlimb edema. Venous angiography prior to abdominal exploratory surgery is helpful in pinpointing the obstructed area.

11 WEAKNESS AND SYNCOPE

STEPHEN J. ETTINGER

WEAKNESS

Weakness as a clinical entity in veterinary practice is subdivided into lassitude, fatigue, generalized muscle weakness or asthenia, faintness or syncope, seizure disorders, and altered states of consciousness. This chapter deals only with lassitude, fatigue, asthenia, and syncope. A discussion of seizure disorders and epilepsy may be found in Chapters 15, 60, and 61. The causes and significance of altered states of consciousness may be found in Chapters 14 and 61.

Lassitude and *fatigue* both refer to a lack of energy. Other synonymous terms include lethargy, listlessness, weariness, languor, or without pep or interest. *Lethargy* further identifies a state of drowsiness, inactivity, or indifference in which there are delayed responses to external (auditory, visual, or tactile) stimuli. Overstimulation is necessary to evoke a normal response in these animals. Lethargy may progress to obtundation, which is a dull indifference displayed by the animal while still in an awake state. These states need to be distinguished from altered states of consciousness, such as stupor and coma, as well as from narcolepsy.

Generalized muscular weakness, or *asthenia*, refers to a true loss of strength, which is either continuous or occurs following repeated muscle contractions. Asthenia may proceed to the point of paresis, motor paralysis, loss of sensation, and ataxia, but does so without a loss of consciousness.

Syncope, or fainting, refers to a sudden, transient loss of consciousness due to a deprivation of energy substrates, either oxygen or glucose, that briefly impairs cerebral metabolism. The differences between lassitude, fatigue, and asthenia are really ones of degree; there are no clearly defined lines of distinction between the varying forms of weakness in dogs and cats. These terms are not synonymous and they do reflect progressive levels of disease or illness. Nevertheless, the owner usually ascribes clinical signs to weakness and relates that particular problem to the veterinarian. In cats, where clinical signs are often hidden, it is not unusual for the pet to pass surreptitiously into the more advanced stages. This is in contrast to very carefully observed toy breeds of dogs, in whom early signs of disease may be particularly evident. In the larger, more stoic breeds of dogs, disease is often not apparent until rather late in its course.

History (Data Base). The initial portion of the minimum data base required for the study of weakness or syncope begins with a thorough historical evaluation. Immediate signs, past pertinent history and surgical procedures, and whenever possible, a familial history, should be obtained. The clinician should also ask if any drugs have been prescribed in the past that have had a deleterious effect or if any drugs are currently being used. Exposure to drugs or chemicals should be identified.

Physical Examination. The physical examination may, in itself, identify the cause of the weakness. Weight loss, fluid in the abdomen, or limb edema may for example suggest a specific problem. The odor of the breath may suggest uremia or diabetes mellitus; a foul oral odor suggests an oral, dental, pharyngeal, or esophageal lesion. Evaluation of the mucous membranes for anemia, cyanosis, jaundice, and venous return, and the pulse for abnormal signs indicating cardiac disease, arrhythmias, anemia, hyperkinesis, or pulsus alternans may direct the clinician to the problem. Enlarged lymph nodes suggest lymphosarcoma or regional adenopathy associated with neoplasia or a septic process. Auscultation of the heart and lungs may identify cardiac arrhythmias, murmurs, or respiratory difficulty. Fever is associated with signs of generalized weakness in both dogs and cats (see Chapter 6). A complete description of the physical examination is not appropriate in this section but it is necessary to stress the enormous significance that the physical examination plays in the evaluation of the patient with signs of weakness and/or syncope.

Laboratory Tests. At a minimum, an animal with signs of weakness or syncope should have a complete blood count, a blood sugar analysis, and a blood urea nitrogen or serum creatinine determination, and the blood electrolytes (sodium, chloride, and potassium) and plasma carbon dioxide levels should be measured to evaluate the acid-base balance. A complete urinalysis is also indicated. If the problem warrants additional study, tests that may be in order and that are practical to run in most veterinary clinical situations include complete serum chemistry profiles, thyroid profiles, radiographs of the abdomen and thorax, and electrocardiography. More specialized laboratory techniques may be indicated as outlined in the chapters dealing with specific clinical diseases.

Most diseases at some point produce symptoms related to weakness. Table 11–1 lists the categories and major causes of weakness usually recognized in small animal veterinary practice. This chapter does not discuss individual causes of weakness but rather emphasizes important concepts regarding its clinical diagnosis. The reader is referred to the appropriate chapters in this textbook for further reading on specific subjects.

ANEMIA. When anemia occurs acutely, syncope is a more likely clinical finding than weakness. Weakness, when it occurs, is profound and rather sudden if there is acute blood loss. In contrast, long-standing anemia is associated with chronic weakness, usually intermittent and episodic. In chronic anemia, cardiomegaly may be apparent radiographically, whereas in severe acute anemia there is a microcardia.

Anemia in the dog usually does not present as weakness until hemoglobin levels drop below seven to eight grams per cent and the hematocrit levels are less than 22 to 25 per cent. In the cat, anemia is not clinically apparent until hemoglobin levels drop to four or five grams per cent and the hematocrit to 10 or 15 per cent (see Chapters 20 and 113). The differential diagnosis in acute and chronic blood loss includes the accelerated destruction of red blood cells as a result of hemolysis, and the loss of red cells by hemorrhage through the urinary or intestinal system, in the peritoneal or pleural fluid, in the subcutaneous tissue, or through the skin itself. Anemia may also be the result of insufficient production of red blood cells in the bone marrow.

ASCITES. The reader is referred to Chapter 28 for a complete discussion of the causes of acute and chronic accumulations of fluid in the abdominal cavity.

CARDIOVASCULAR SIGNS. Syncope may be the result of an acute decrease in cardiac output (see Chapter 71). In more chronic states with diminished cardiac output, both cardiac wasting and weakness can develop. Cardiac cachexia associated with chronic cardiac disease is described more fully in this chapter (see also Chronic Wasting, this chapter).

A reduction in cardiac output may be the result of hemodynamic consequences of a specific cardiac rhythm disturbance. Such hemodynamic consequences depend upon the ventricular rate, the duration of the abnormal rate, the temporal relationship between the atria and ventricles, the sequence of ventricular activation, the functional cardiac status, cycle length irregularities, associated cardiac drug therapy (see Drug-Induced Causes of Weakness, this chapter), concomitant medical diseases, the degree of preservation of the motor system, and the level of anxiety.

Tachycardia and bradycardia may cause signs of weakness and/or syncope as well as congestive heart failure and sudden death. Arrhythmias can reduce cerebral and coronary blood flow sufficiently to produce weakness or syncope (see Chapter 76).

Bacterial endocarditis is associated with signs of weakness, particularly when there is chronic infection or septicemia. Pericardial effusion, regardless of etiology, may diminish cardiac output and cause weakness. Cats and dogs with pericardial effusion often present first with signs of severe weakness, and congestive heart failure occurs later in the illness.

Unless congestive heart failure is incipient, valvular heart diseases and congenital heart diseases do not usually cause weakness. When heart failure does occur, weakness, along with congestive signs, is observed. The congestion and associated tissue hypoxia cause the weakness.

Heartworm disease is associated with weakness when heart failure, renal involvement, or pulmonary dysfunction is present.

CHRONIC INFLAMMATION OR INFECTION. One of the broadest and nonspecific categories of clinical conditions associated with weakness is the state in which a fever, white blood cell abnormality, and pain are present. Chronic diseases of inflammatory or infectious origin (e.g., liver, pancreas, prostate, skin, oral cavity, anal glands, ears, joints, bones, and muscles) all include weakness as a primary sign. In time, these diseases wear the patient (and the owner) down.

It is virtually impossible to describe all the clinical signs that may be associated with this category of disease. In most cases, the physical examination and laboratory analysis demonstrate abnormalities that permit the clinician to further investigate a specific problem.

CHRONIC WASTING. Another broad category of disease states that ultimately produces a loss of strength are those problems that result in chronic wasting; diseases of the liver terminating in cirrhosis and chronic cardiac cachexia are examples. Renal disease associated with prolonged elevation of the BUN level, electrolyte wasting, protein losses, and decreased red blood cell formation may also be associated with weakness.

Chronic gastrointestinal diseases in which electrolytes, protein, and body fluids are lost are a cause of wasting in dogs and cats. Biopsy of the affected tissue provides a pathologic diagnosis. Weakness due to loss of protein, fluid, and body heat through the skin results from cutaneous and subcutaneous diseases. Chronic cutaneous disease causes an irritable state, chronic wasting, lethargy, and fatigue. Many older patients also waste away and weaken as they age, without specific evidence of organ dysfunction.

TABLE 11–1. COMMON CATEGORIES OF CAUSES OF WEAKNESS IN SMALL ANIMALS

Anemia
Ascites
Cardiovascular signs
Chronic inflammation and infection
Chronic wasting diseases
Drug-related weakness
Electrolyte disorders
Endocrine disturbances
Fever
Metabolic dysfunction states
Neoplasia
Neurologic disorders
Neuromuscular diseases and polyneuropathies
Nutritional disorders
Overactivity
Psychological factors
Pulmonary diseases

DRUG-RELATED WEAKNESSES. Drugs thought to have beneficial therapeutic effects may also have adverse side effects. In some cases drugs do more harm than good. When patients fail to respond to medication or if the animal's condition deteriorates, it is reasonable to discontinue therapy and re-evaluate the condition.

The veterinarian should know the adverse effects of every drug used. Individual variations also occur. Commonly used drugs that are associated with signs of weakness and lethargy include the barbiturates, antidiarrheals with sedatives, anticonvulsant preparations, antihistamines, tranquilizers, antibiotics, diuretic agents, vasodilators, antiarrhythmic preparations, and inotropic agents such as digitalis.

ELECTROLYTE DISORDERS. Abnormalities of potassium, calcium, sodium, chloride, and magnesium, and acid-base imbalances are related to clinical signs of weakness in dogs and cats. Specific signs of weakness are associated with hyponatremia and hypokalemia and usually are associated with diuretic therapy, excessive fluid administration, or hormonal imbalances. Acid-base imbalances are seen in many medical situations as well as with drug therapy.

The most frequently recognized blood electrolyte abnormalities associated with signs of significant weakness are hypo- and hyperkalemia and hypo- and hypercalcemia. *Hyperkalemia* is associated with listlessness, severe asthenia, and bradycardia. The neuromuscular signs of hyperkalemia include weakness, paralysis, and loss of deep tendon reflexes, as well as confusion and mentation changes. The electrocardiogram provides an excellent method for assessing potassium levels while awaiting laboratory confirmation of a suspected hyperkalemic state. Table 11–2 lists the electrocardiographic changes commonly associated with hyperkalemia in the order of frequency in which the abnormalities are seen, beginning with mild increases in the serum potassium level to severe hyperkalemia associated with heart block and asystole. Table 11–3 lists the causes of hyperkalemia often recognized in small animal medicine.

Hypokalemia is recognized following excessive diuretic therapy, chronic vomiting, Cushing's syndrome, and reactions to insulin therapy. Table 11–4 lists the causes of hypokalemia in small animals. The associated electrocardiographic changes described in Table 11–2 are not as commonly observed as are the electrocardiographic changes with hyperkalemia.

Hypocalcemia is associated with the clinical signs of nervous excitability, tetany, and, in severe cases, convulsive seizures. Weakness is observed between periods of hyperexcitability. It is observed in eclampsia in the lactating bitch, in advanced cases of hypoparathyroidism, with calcium loss as a result of intestinal fluid loss with diarrhea, in hypoproteinemic states with decreased albumin levels, and when chronic renal failure occurs with increased phosphorus levels. Occasionally, hypocalcemia is also seen with paralytic ileus. The long-term treatment of hypocalcemia demands a knowledge of the primary cause. Electrocardiographic findings are outlined in Table 11–2.

Hypercalcemic states associated with either primary or secondary hyperparathyroidism, multiple myeloma, bony metastasis, and various sites of either carcinoma or lymphoma have been described in both the dog and cat. The signs are variable, but include depression, muscle weakness, and arrhythmias. The mechanism of hypercalcemia associated with carcinomas relates to the neoplastic destruction of bone and may be mediated by prostaglandins and an unknown osteoclastic activating factor. In lymphosarcoma, a parathormone-like substance is produced. The electrocardiographic findings associated with hypercalcemia are listed in Table 11–2.

ENDOCRINE DISTURBANCES. Weakness due to decreased neuromuscular excitability is a sign common to endocrine disturbances, including Cushing's syndrome (adrenocortical hyperplasia or neoplasia or pituitary neoplasia), hypothyroid disease, hypoadrenocortical activity (adrenal cortical insufficiency), hypoglycemia (insulinomas, mesenchymal tumors that release insulin-like substance, or, rarely, postprandial hypoglycemic episodes), hyperparathyroidism, hypoparathyroidism, the inappropriate secretion of antidiuretic hormone, and diabetes mellitus (both the ketoacidotic and hyperosmolar states).

The reader is referred to the section on endocrine dysfunctions in this textbook, which deals more specifically with the individual diseases. The clinical diagnosis usually requires a combination of the laboratory and radiographic studies described previously, as well as specific hormone analyses that are individually described for each specific endocrine dysfunction.

FEVER. The reader is referred to Chapter 6 for a complete discussion on the causes of hyperthermia and the differential diagnosis of weakness that occurs as a result.

METABOLIC DYSFUNCTION STATES. The diseases that fall in this category are related to endocrine diseases, chronic infections and chronic wasting problems, and those identified as nutritionally related (see Nutritional Disorders). This includes conditions in which there is either decreased protein production or use of protein substances, decreased production or use of glucose, and primary or secondary dyslipoproteinemia, which may induce sluggishness or weakness. Primary causes of

TABLE 11–2. ELECTROCARDIOGRAPHIC FINDINGS IN COMMON ELECTROLYTE DISTURBANCES

Hyperkalemia	Hypokalemia	Hypercalcemia	Hypocalcemia
Peaked T waves	Prolonged Q-T interval (U waves)	Short S-T segment	Prolonged S-T segment
Shortened Q-T	Sagging S-T segment	Tachycardia	Prolonged Q-T interval
Prolonged P-R	Depressed T wave amplitude	Premature beats	
Prolonged QRS	A.P.C. and V.P.C.		
P waves disappear			
Atrial fibrillation			
Sinus arrest			
Heart block and asystole			

TABLE 11–3. HYPERKALEMIA

- Excessive intake of potassium in face of renal failure
- Crush syndrome
  - Trauma
  - Muscle necrosis
- Adrenocortical insufficiency
- Acidosis
- Blood or fluid infusions with potassium
- Potassium-sparing diuretics
- Urethral obstruction

lipoprotein disorders are discussed in Chapters 39 and 40. Conditions that cause secondary elevation of lipid levels include diabetes mellitus, pancreatitis, myeloma, nephrosis, destructive liver disease, myxedema, dysgammaglobulinemia, glycogen storage disease, and pregnancy. Dietary indiscretions involving the excessive intake or metabolism of fats and carbohydrates may result in hyperlipoproteinemia.

NEOPLASTIC DISEASES. Neoplasia is frequently associated with episodic weakness resulting from an invasive, destructive, or obstructive mass. The tumor may produce substances that cause or exacerbate the clinical signs of weakness. Examples include the excessive production of insulin, estrogen, steroids, epinephrine, parathormone, and thyroid hormones. In other cases, the weakness is the result of acute episodes of bleeding due to the rupture of a tumor (e.g., hemangiosarcoma) or a secondary bleeding disorder such as disseminated intravascular coagulopathy (DIC), which is frequently associated with neoplastic processes. Tumor emboli or thrombi that lodge in the lung, brain, or peripheral vessels may produce specific organ signs or severe weakness due to organ dysfunction.

NEUROLOGIC DISORDERS. There are many central and peripheral nervous system disorders that are associated with signs of episodic weakness. Infections within the brain or spinal canal resulting from viral, bacterial, fungal, and rickettsial diseases are responsible for episodes of neurologic weakness. Space-occupying lesions such as hydrocephalus, neoplasia, or granulomas produce signs of weakness. Injury or trauma to either the brain or peripheral nerves can damage the nervous system, causing weakness, along with motor and/or sensory dysfunction. Vascular accidents or strokes have similar effects.

TABLE 11–4. HYPOKALEMIA

- NONRENAL CAUSES
  - Decreased Intake
  - GI Loss
    - Vomiting (alkalosis)
    - Neoplasms
    - Laxatives
    - Diarrhea (acidosis)
  - Insulin Therapy
- RENAL CAUSES
  - Potassium Wasting and Acidosis
    - Renal tubular acidosis
    - Postobstructive uropathy
    - Chronic pyelonephritis
    - Diuresis with acute tubular necrosis
  - Potassium Wasting and Alkalosis
    - Diuretics
    - Aldosteronism
    - Steroids—Cushing's syndrome

Epilepsy, regardless of the etiology (see Chapter 15), is likely to result in acute severe episodic weakness and may be associated with chronic weakness as well. The drugs used to treat epileptic-type conditions also frequently cause lethargy and weakness.

Central or peripheral vestibulitis or involvement of the inner ear is likely to cause clinical signs associated with head tilt, occasional nausea, weakness, and ataxia. Instability of the atlanto-occipital or atlantoaxial joints as well as cervical nerve root disorders and cervical myelopathies are a cause of weakness in small animals. Thoracic spinal cord problems are less common than thoracolumbar and sacral nerve root diseases such as intervertebral discs, myelopathies, infections, instabilities, and inflammations, which are other causes of neurologic episodic weakness.

The reader is referred to the section on central and peripheral neurologic diseases for a more complete description of these individual disease entities. Weakness is a primary sign associated with many neurologic states and this broad category should not be disregarded.

POLYNEUROPATHIES AND NEUROMUSCULAR DISEASES. Conditions such as tick paralysis, coonhound paralysis, and botulism are polyneuropathic diseases that classically present with signs of severe weakness in small animals. Other conditions causing generalized weakness and EMG abnormalities of the neuropathic potentials include the administration of drugs such as diphenylhydantoin, excessive accumulation of heavy metals (such as lead), some nutritional disturbances (avitaminoses), endocrine disturbances (such as diabetes mellitus), and immune disorders such as lupus erythematosus and periarteritis.

Myasthenia gravis is a condition that blocks myoneural functions and is associated with severe weakness. Polymyositis requires differentiation from the polyneuropathies and myasthenic states. Usually these conditions are differentiated on the basis of the neurologic examination, drugs that stimulate nerve terminals, and occasionally by electromyelographic (EMG) examination. Complete laboratory analyses may also provide additional, specific, differentiating information.

NUTRITIONAL DISORDERS. Primary nutritional disorders include inadequate diets that result in a starvation syndrome. Long-term nutritional deficiencies, either in general or specifically relating to individual vitamins, minerals, proteins, or carbohydrates, may result in generalized weakness. An owner's overindulgence of an animal's appetite may result in increased body weight and obesity, which prevents the animal from being able to exercise normally. In the "pickwickian syndrome," normal breathing is restricted and cor pulmonale, with signs of respiratory distress and weakness, occurs. Excessive caloric intake can induce a hepatic lipidosis with respiratory distress and weakness. In many cases, obesity restricts normal activity, which is then followed by specific weakness.

Diseases that result in secondary nutritional problems include parasitism, protein-losing diseases, hepatoencephalopathy-associated weakness as a result of abnormal breakdown of protein by the liver, cirrhosis, chronic diarrhea and steatorrhea, chronic pancreatic insufficiency, lymphangiectasia and similar neoplastic diseases, and, in young dogs, von Gierke-like syndrome. If underfed, animals performing high levels of work, such as hunting or working dogs, exhibit a starvation-like syndrome. These animals are likely to be receiving a poor-quality diet and as a result appear to be nutritionally weak.

OVERACTIVITY, OVERWORK, AND PSYCHOLOGICAL FACTORS. This important category in human medicine is one that should not be overlooked in veterinary practice. The cause of the vast majority of cases of weakness and lethargy in humans is psychological. Although psychological causes probably account for a very small percentage of the cases of weakness and lethargy seen in small animal veterinary practice, one should not disregard the signs of excessive stress. These may occur in animals being used for excessive racing or hunting, in those animals who are being deprived of normal rest, and occasionally in those animals being stressed by owners with excessive expectations of the animal. In some instances, animals become shy to the noise of a gun, firecrackers, and loud noises such as thunder. These problems often result in fear and weakness. Altered states of consciousness, such as narcolepsy, must also be considered in the differential diagnosis of weakness.

Pseudocyesis is a hormonal disorder, which is often not recognized on examination. It is associated with weakness, lethargy, and abnormal behavior. The dog is reported to hide, to fear normal people and experiences, and may even bite when approached. Unspayed female dogs may attempt to collect or hide toys and build nests. They often are anorexic. Usually, pseudocyesis occurs 45 to 90 days following the last heat cycle. Fever may be mild and there may or may not be milk in the engorged mammary glands.

PULMONARY DISEASES. Excessive weight results in restrictive pulmonary disease, respiratory distress, and weakness. The reader is referred to Chapter 70 for a more complete description.

Pulmonary emboli cause clinical signs associated with respiratory distress and weakness. This condition occurs not only with neoplastic diseases, but occasionally as a result of inflammatory diseases involving other organs and the showering of the pulmonary tree. Chronic coughing and chronic pulmonary infection are likely to weaken an animal, and the owner may complain of a generalized malaise in the pet. Heartworm disease may present initially as malaise and a lack of well-being and is associated with pulmonary infarction and right ventricular enlargement as a result of migration of the heartworms to the pulmonary arteries. The disease occurs in animals severely parasitized as well as in those with only a few worms. The actual mechanism of this condition relates not only to the physical obstructive properties of the heartworms, but also to the possible development of chemical abnormalities resulting from the heartworm infestation in the lungs.

SYNCOPE

Syncope or fainting refers to a sudden, yet transient, loss of consciousness due to a deprivation of energy substrate, either oxygen or glucose, that briefly impairs the cerebral metabolism. In contrast to that of all other organs, the metabolism of the brain is entirely dependent on the perfusion of oxygen. The storage of high energy phosphates in the brain is limited and energy supply depends on the oxidation of glucose extracted from blood. Cessation of cerebral blood flow for approximately ten seconds leads to a loss of consciousness. A syncopal event is transient and complete recovery occurs in seconds to minutes. Syncope should be considered a "symptom complex" rather than a primary disease.

Syncope includes the client-reported symptoms of lightheadedness, vertigo, and fainting in the animal. It is usually a reversible clinical state, but if not reversed, it can result in sudden death. Syncope may result from impaired cerebral circulation secondary to occlusive cerebrovascular disease, from a transient decrease in cardiac output, from diminished peripheral systolic pressure levels that are lower than those required to perfuse the brain, or from a shortage of energy substrates delivered to the brain through blood flow. Tables 11–5 and 11–6 identify the varying etiologies of syncope by categorizing the predominantly responsible physiologic mechanisms.

In small animals, syncope develops with generalized muscle weakness, progressing rapidly to ataxia, which may be followed by collapse and a brief period of loss of consciousness. Initially, the patient is motionless with relaxed skeletal muscles, but this may progress to uncoordinated muscular activity or jerks, giving the impression of seizure-like activity. Loss of control of muscle sphincters occurs in many cases, leading to involuntary urination and/or defecation. Often the animal cries out during the episode, and this release of central nervous activity is frequently interpreted by the owner as pain or fear. Recovery is usually rapid but the owner often reports that the episode is followed by a brief period of confusion. The differential diagnosis of syncope is discussed but the clinician must also consider nonsyncopal disorders, including neurogenic seizures, narcolepsy, and catalepsy. Episodic weakness, acute hemorrhage, and diseases associated with reduced alertness also need to be differentiated from syncope.

Clinical Summary. With a complete history and physical examination, most cases of syncope can be identified without further study. An electrocardiogram and simple blood chemical analyses are usually all that are required. In many cases the clinician can identify the type and cause of syncope from the history. Postural hypotension requires that the patient rise to an upright position, whereas syncope occurring when the animal is recumbent may be associated with hysterical fainting, hyperventilation, or vasovagal, cardiac, or hypoglycemic episodes. When exercise precipitates the fainting attack, outflow tract obstruction, tachycardia, and postural hypotension should be considered.

Heart block should be considered when the animal exercises and the heart rate is unable to rise sufficiently to maintain an adequate cardiac output for the patient's immediate needs. When fainting is continuously related to mealtime, the clinician should consider reactive or fasting hypoglycemic states. The use of antihypertensive

TABLE 11–5. SYNCOPE

DECREASED CEREBRAL PERFUSION
Peripheral or Neurogenic Dysfunction (Heart Structurally Normal)
Vasovagal
Postural hypotension
Hyperventilation
Carotid sinus sensitivity (vasodepressor type)
Glossopharyngeal neuralgia associated with syncope
Micturition syncope
Cardiac Dysfunction (Usually Structurally Abnormal)
Obstruction to flow
Aortic and pulmonary stenosis
Myxomas
Cardiac tamponade
Dirofilariasis—severe
Rhythm disturbances
Heart block
Tachyarrhythmia
Cardiopulmonary dysfunction
Pulmonary hypertension
Pulmonary emboli
Congenital heart disease (right-to-left shunt)
Myocardial infarction
METABOLIC DISTURBANCES
Hypoglycemia
IATROGENIC
Digitalis
Diuretics
Phenothiazine-Related Medications
Nitrates, Vasodilators, etc.
Quinidine Syncope
MISCELLANEOUS
Tussive Syncope
Pulseless Disease
Syncope Associated with Swallowing

Modified from Wright and McIntosh, 1971; and Noble, 1976.

agents, peripheral vasodilators, tranquilizers, nitrates, and nitroglycerin, as well as diuretics, quinidine, and digitalis are all possible causes for a syncopal episode.

Much can be determined by careful questioning. Syncopal episodes are usually brief and transient. When they are of a longer duration, outflow tract obstruction such as subvalvular aortic stenosis, hypoglycemia, and hysterical fainting should be considered.

Premonitory signs do not precede syncope due to arrhythmias or postural hypotension unless the patient feels the arrhythmia occurring. Since the latter is difficult to assess in small animals, most cases of cardiac-induced syncope do not have premonitory signs. In the rare case of cerebrovascular disease, the owner may report that the animal appears confused and has shown alterations in personality or mentation. Tussive syncope is preceded by bouts of hard, forceful coughing.

Auscultation of the heart, palpation of the pulses, and when indicated, palpation of the bilateral cerebral pulses, is required. Capillary refill time and the mucous membrane color should be evaluated. In some cases further evaluation is necessary to identify the cause or type of fainting episode. Most of the clinical studies required have been discussed and can be performed with the equipment usually available in a small animal veterinary practice. A full electrocardiogram is mandatory to detect arrhythmias, as well as ventricular and atrial abnormalities. If the cause of syncope is still unknown, the work-up is expanded to include an echocardiogram and 24-hour ambulatory electrocardiogram. Cardiac catheterization may be performed, but ultrasound is much to be preferred due to increased information yield and greatly reduced patient risk.

When blood pressure monitoring is available, indirect manometry for postural pressure measurements may yield valuable information in a small subset of patients.

Syncope in a Normal Heart but with Peripheral Vascular Dysfunction. With peripheral or neurogenic dysfunction and a normal heart, the primary problem is either an abnormal reflex or a physiological reflex initiated through a neuropsychiatric pathway. Vasovagal and vasodepressor syncope usually occurs in otherwise healthy individuals. In small animals it appears to be associated with a sudden incident of either fright or extreme excitement. Often the pet has been immobile for a period of time leading up to the incident. Respiration usually increases, both in rate and depth, and the animal may appear weak and confused. The pupils dilate just prior to the loss of consciousness. Hemodynamically, there is peripheral arterial vasodilation and venoconstriction. The cardiac output fails to rise despite a decrease in peripheral resistance and venoconstriction. Vagal overactivity results in a bradycardia. This can be blocked with atropine in humans but the fainting still occurs, suggesting that a decrease in the heart rate alone is not the cause.

Postural hypotension is also included in this category. Normal animals develop a slight fall in systolic blood pressure and a rise in diastolic pressure with only a slight elevation in the heart rate upon rising. In contrast, those with postural hypotension develop a fall in both systolic and diastolic pressures with variable changes in the heart rate. Postural hypotension can be a complication of a number of disease entities, including diabetes mellitus, hypoadrenocorticism, and severe intravascular volume depletion due to disease or intensive diuresis. Drug therapy, including the broad category of beta blocking agents, vasodilators, antihypertensives, and tranquilizers, are likely to induce similar side effects.

The hyperventilation syndrome belongs in the category of peripheral or neurogenic dysfunction. It is usually associated with anxious or hyperexcitable pets. The owner notes the patient's overbreathing, which, when continued, results in presyncopal symptoms up to and including a loss of consciousness. Such conscious episodes may occur while the animal is sitting, standing, or recumbent. Hyperventilation causes an overaeration of the alveoli and a subsequent fall in alveolar and arterial PCO_2 levels. Low PCO_2 levels have a profound effect on the vascular system and produce progressive cerebral arterial vasoconstriction along with peripheral vasodilation. With stable or decreased perfusion pressure there is a progressive decrease in oxygen delivery to the brain. The effects of hypoxia can be demonstrated on the electroencephalogram by diffuse slowing.

Carotid sinus sensitivity also belongs in the category of neurogenic dysfunction. The underlying reflex occurs as afferent impulses from the carotid sinuses are transmitted via the glossopharyngeal nerve to vasomotor and cardioinhibitory centers in the medulla. Vagal stimulation slows the heart by decreasing sinus and A-V nodal rates. This bradycardia and variable degree of A-V block decrease cardiac output and cerebral blood flow, and can cause cerebral anoxia. This chain of events can

TABLE 11–6. SYNCOPAL-ASSOCIATED DISEASE

Type of Syncope	Pathophysiology	Physiologic Event
1. Obstruction to Cerebral Blood Flow	Arteriosclerosis Thrombosis Embolus Neoplasia Trauma	Cerebral Vascular Accident Transient Ischemic Attack Tussive Syncope Hyperventilation
2. Cardiogenic	Heart Rate Rhythm: ↓ Heart Rate	Heart Block Tachycardia-Bradycardia Syndrome Vasodepressor Syncope Carotid Sinus Hypersensitivity
	Heart Rate Rhythm: ↑ Heart Rate	Supraventricular Tachycardia Ventricular Tachycardia
	Obstruction	Asymmetric Hypertrophy (IHSS) Myxoma Pulmonary Hypertension Ischemic Heart Disease Heartworm Disease
3. Blood Pressure: ↓ Cardiac Output: ↓ Heart Rate		Cardiogenic
3. Blood Pressure: ↓ Cardiac Output: ↓ Stroke Volume	Contractility	Cardiogenic
	↓ Filling: ↓ Volume	Blood Loss Adrenal Insufficiency Tussive Syncope
	↓ Filling: ↓ Venomotor Tone	Postural Hypotension Vasodilator Drugs
3. Blood Pressure: ↓ Peripheral Resistance	Vascular	Hyperventilation
	↓ Sympathetic Stimulation	Micturition Syncope Adrenergic Blocking Drugs Postural Hypotension Vasodepressor Syncope Carotid Sinus Hypersensitivity
4. Blood Constituency	↓ O_2	Cardiopulmonary
	↓ Glucose	Reactive or Fasting Hypoglycemia

cause vertigo, lightheadedness, and syncope. Atropine blocks this process, especially in brachycephalic dogs. Direct or indirect stimulation of the carotid sinus also causes sympathetic inhibition or vasodepressor effects that precipitate a fall in blood pressure. This syndrome is observed in cases where neoplasms, inflammatory processes, or tight collars stimulate the carotid sinuses. Afferent impulses associated with pain in the ear, soft palate, or pharynx are transmitted centrally via the glossopharyngeal and vagal nerves and may also give rise to reflex hypotension and syncope (glossopharyngeal neuralgia). Syncope or occasionally severe dysrhythmia without syncope may be provoked by swallowing, usually in association with an esophageal tumor, diverticulum, or spasm, but syncope may occur without overt esophageal disease (deglutition syncope). Postmicturition syncope, infrequently recognized, may occur in healthy patients during or immediately after micturition.

Syncope Due to Cardiac Dysfunction. A second major group of diseases resulting in decreased cerebral perfusion are those associated with cardiac dysfunction. Cardiac dysfunction for this purpose is divided into obstruction to blood flow, rhythm disturbances, cardiopulmonary dysfunction, and severely impaired myocardial contractility.

Subvalvular and valvular aortic stenosis are associated with syncope and a high incidence of sudden death. Exertional hypotension is a characteristic feature of virtually all forms of heart disease in which cardiac output is relatively fixed and fails to rise normally or declines during exertion. It is most characteristic of aortic stenosis and other forms of obstruction of left ventricular outflow in which cerebral ischemia occurs during exertion. Systemic vascular resistance ordinarily declines as a consequence of arteriolar dilation secondary to the accumulation of vasodilator metabolites during exercise. Normally this vasodilation is compensated for by the augmentation of cardiac output and arterial pressure during exertion. However, with outflow obstruction cardiac output rises proportionately less than vascular resistance falls and arterial pressure declines. The fixed, narrowed outflow tract is unable to accommodate the increased demands of cardiac output and oxygen requirements. In some cases syncope occurs at rest. Animals with severe pulmonic stenosis with or without right-to-left shunts may similarly (but less commonly) suffer syncope upon exertion. Atrial tumors may present with syncope, as the pedunculated tumor intermittently obstructs the valve orifice. In severe dirofilariasis, the obstruction in the pulmonary arteries impairs blood flow to the lung. Ball valve thrombi in the atrium may similarly obstruct flow. Herniation of the appendage of the left atrium through an opening within the pericardium is a rare cause of syncope.

In cardiac tamponade, pericardial effusion, and restrictive pericarditis, there is a delicate balance between the inflow of blood to the heart and the cardiac output. Sudden changes that decrease the return of blood to the heart or slow the rate may result in a decreased cardiac output and secondarily, in syncope. In all cases associated with obstruction to the outflow of blood, ventricular dysrhythmias or left ventricular failure following exercise should be considered as a possible cause of the syncope, as well as a simple reduction in the cardiac output. Obstructive cardiomyopathy in dogs and cats may reduce LV output enough to induce syncope. The heart rate increases but the left ventricular volume is decreased and the result is a total reduction in cardiac output. Echocardiographic studies also suggest movement of the anterior (septal) mitral valve leaflet toward the ventricular septum during systole.

Rhythm disturbances causing syncope may include bundle branch block irregularities as well as the bradyarrhythmias and tachyarrhythmias. In heart block, the animal is characteristically alert when it regains consciousness. Often the animal appears unconcerned about the event and appears unaware that a problem existed. Transient heart block is a difficult diagnosis to establish without 24-hour continuous electrocardiographic monitoring. Stokes-Adams syncope is a reference to the syndrome associated with incomplete or complete A-V heart block and also includes sinus arrest, sino-atrial pause and block, and the sick sinus syndrome. In addition to syncope, there may be urinary and/or fecal incontinence due to a temporary loss of sphincter control. Seizure activity of a transient nature may also occur, necessitating a differential diagnosis from diseases of the central nervous system. Seizures are usually brief, may be tonic-clonic, tonic only, or the animal may be flaccid only but reported as having had a seizure.

Tachyarrhythmias result in decreased systolic filling of the left ventricle, thereby resulting in a decreased cardiac output. Fainting may occur during the period of rapid heart beating or at the end of a paroxysm of atrial or ventricular tachycardia if asystole follows, the result of overdrive suppression.

In cardiopulmonary dysfunction, syncopal episodes usually occur with physical exertion or shortly thereafter. The duration of unconsciousness varies but is usually brief (one to two minutes). Cyanosis is often present with this type of syncope. In congenital heart disease with shunting of blood from right to left, syncope is not uncommon since the blood has a lowered PO_2 content, producing cerebral anoxia. In the unusual occurrence of true myocardial infarction in dogs and cats, syncope may be due to left ventricular dysfunction or significant pain. Dogs and cats with severe myocardial disease have diminished cardiac reserve. Acute demands for additional cardiac output associated with exercise, excitement, or activity may result in a syncopal episode. Arrhythmias may similarly result in a short-term, severe deficiency of blood flow.

Metabolic Disturbances Associated with Syncope. Syncopal episodes are associated with some metabolic disturbances. Hypoglycemic coma is the best example of this. Hyperventilation with its associated alterations in physiologic parameters, calcium imbalances, and renal dysfunction are other examples of metabolic disturbances that can cause fainting. Often the longer duration of the syncopal attack suggests to the clinician a metabolic rather than a cardiac problem. Dogs with portacaval liver shunts occasionally faint. The actual mechanism is not understood but may be either vascular or metabolic in nature.

Iatrogenic Causes of Syncope. Iatrogenic causes of syncope must be considered whenever drugs are being administered. Digitalis intoxication associated with heart block, A-V dissociation, or a slow junctional rhythm are examples. Ventricular tachycardia and ventricular fibrillation can also result from digitalis intoxication. Potent diuretics, including the thiazides and furosemide, when given in excess, produce intravascular volume depletion that may contribute to or cause hypotension. Phenothiazine derivatives may produce a profound postural hypotension, resulting in disorientation and/or syncope when the patient suddenly rises. Peripheral vasodilating agents such as nitroglycerin and long-acting nitrates, propranolol, and prazosin may be associated with a fall in blood pressure, resulting in postural hypotension. Quinidine has been incriminated in dogs as having the potential to produce arrhythmias and syncopal episodes, although the cause of these seizures has not been determined.

Miscellaneous Causes of Syncope. Another category of syndromes resulting in syncopal episodes includes problems associated with coughing, lack of pulse, and swallowing. When attacks accompany paroxysms of coughing, *tussive syncope* is the result of an alteration in the normal circulation. Fainting occurs in the recumbent or standing subject and consciousness is rapidly regained without serious sequelae. Coughing raises the intrathoracic pressure as well as cerebrospinal pressures. When the cerebrospinal fluid pressure is greater than the intracranial capillary perfusion pressures, there is a decrease in blood flow to the brain. The brain is then rapidly depleted of blood and oxygen, resulting in a syncopal attack. Therapy is directed toward the relief of the force and duration of the cough.

Pulseless disease is a cause of syncope when there are major obstructions to one or more major vessels supplying the head. The syncopal attack is usually precipitated by activity. Syncope associated with swallowing occurs with esophageal diverticula and other obstructive esophageal diseases. Various degrees of heart block develop upon initiation of the swallow reflex. The laryngeal nerves are sensitive to pressure and these nerves are anatomically related to the carotid sinus. This disease should be considered a form of carotid sinus syncope, which was described earlier.

12 TREMBLING AND SHIVERING

JOE N. KORNEGAY and CHRISTINE E. THOMSON

Tremor, an involuntary, regular, oscillatory movement of a body part or parts, often referred to as either *trembling* or *shivering*, is the most common movement disorder of human beings and also occurs relatively commonly in animals. The movement is caused by alternating contractions of opposing muscles and may take the form of rhythmic flexion-extension, pronation-supination, or abduction-adduction. The regular nature of tremor distinguishes it from a number of other involuntary body movements (chorea, myoclonus, athetosis, ballismus) seen in human beings. Similarly, tremor is distinguished from movements associated with nystagmus, convulsions, and muscle fasciculations because of its absence during sleep.

GENERAL PATHOPHYSIOLOGY

Tremor in human beings has been classified according to whether the involuntary movement is benign or affects normal daily function and whether it occurs at rest or during muscular activity. Those occurring during muscular activity (action tremors) are further categorized based on whether the movement is accentuated by holding the affected body part in an outstretched position (postural tremor), by maintaining an isometric contraction (contraction tremor), or by attempting a goal-oriented movement (intention tremor). The principal benign tremor of human beings is primarily postural in character and has been termed physiologic tremor. Physiologic tremor may be exaggerated to the point of being clinically significant because of catecholamine excess due to anxiety or drug/toxin ingestion (enhanced physiologic tremor). Both forms of physiologic tremor are accentuated locally by intra-arterial injection of a beta-adrenergic agent (isoproterenol) and both are reduced locally by injection of a beta-adrenergic blocker (propranolol). This suggests that peripheral beta-adrenergic receptors, perhaps at the skeletal muscle membrane, may have a role in inducing physiologic tremor. The most common pathologic tremor of human beings is termed essential tremor. The movement may occur in the limbs, hands, or head and often has both postural and intention components. There usually are no other neurologic signs. Essential tremor may be noted early in life but is most often seen in older individuals (senile tremor). An autosomal dominant mode of inheritance has been verified in some patients, particularly those with early onset. Essential tremor was not blocked locally by intravenous propranolol in one study, suggesting the tremor originates centrally as opposed to the presumed peripheral origin of physiologic tremor. However, contradictory results were obtained by another investigator and one author has suggested that essential tremor is simply an exaggerated form of physiologic tremor. The principal pathologic tremor occurring at rest in human beings is that of Parkinson's disease, a complex disorder in which there is neuronal loss in the substantia nigra and apparent altered dopamine metabolism. Loss of inhibitory input from the substantia nigra to the corpus striatum of the brain results in characteristic signs of Parkinsonism, such as akinesia (absence of movement) and rigidity, but the cause of the tremor is unknown. Cerebellar disease is the main cause of intention tremor in human beings, particularly when lesions involve the superior cerebellar peduncle. Cerebellar tremor presumably occurs because of loss of the cerebellum's modulating effect on motor function.

Trembling or shivering is seen in normal animals because of either nervousness or hypothermia. Syndromes in which the movement is pathologic have not been defined as well as in human beings. However, several conditions are now recognized and veterinarians are asked to evaluate affected animals fairly commonly. The following discussion concentrates on these conditions. Because mechanisms responsible for the tremor seen in some of these syndromes are poorly understood, correlations will be made with analogous syndromes in human beings when appropriate.

SENILE TREMOR

Trembling or shivering is noted occasionally in older dogs. The tremor usually is exaggerated by movement or when the dog is standing and is less pronounced or absent at rest. In the authors' experience, the pelvic limbs are most commonly affected; however, a single limb or all four limbs may be involved. While some dogs appear to be weak in the affected limb(s), there usually are no other signs of neurologic involvement. The etiology and pathogenesis of the tremor is unknown in most cases. Dogs with concomitant weakness may have underlying musculoskeletal or neurologic disease. Peripheral nerve or nerve root entrapment should be considered in those in which the tremor affects a single limb. Lesions affecting the spinal cord or cauda equina may be present in dogs with bilateral pelvic limb involvement. Dogs in which all four limbs are affected may have generalized neuromuscular disease or a lesion involving the brain or spinal cord cranial to the second thoracic segment. Several diseases that cause biochemical abnormalities, such as hypoglycemia and hypocalcemia, also have been said to cause tremor. However, care should be taken to distinguish tremor from muscle fasciculations that also may be seen in some of these diseases. The actual cause of the tremor cannot be defined in many affected dogs. Trembling and shivering occurring in older dogs without additional neurologic or metabolic disease could be analogous to the senile form of essential tremor, but physiologic studies that might support such an hypothesis have not been done. The tremor itself in many affected dogs does not cause significant clinical dysfunction, so treatment often is not warranted. Propranolol and primidone are the most effective drugs in the treatment of essential tremor in human beings and might have some value in managing older dogs with tremor. However, supportive clinical data in dogs is lacking.

HYPOMYELINATION

Reduced (hypo-) or abnormal (dys-) myelination of the central nervous system has been reported in chow chows, springer spaniels, Samoyeds, Weimaraners, a Dalmatian, and a mixed breed dog. Tremor is the characteristic sign seen in these dogs. The tremor occurs diffusely in the limbs, trunk, head, and eyes as early as ten days of age. It is most pronounced during goal-oriented activity (intention tremor), lessens at rest, and resolves during sleep. Mildly affected dogs have no other neurologic deficits, except for dysmetria demonstrable at gait and upon evaluation of postural reactions. Dogs that are affected more severely are unable to stand. Tremor in most affected chow chows and Weimaraners gradually resolves and is absent by one year of age.

The syndrome in springer spaniels appears to be inherited as a sex-linked recessive trait, with males being principally affected. Evidence of tremor and either proven or assumed hypomyelination in multiple litters of chow chows, Weimaraners, and Samoyeds suggests a heritable basis in these breeds as well, but there is no definite familial evidence to establish a pattern. Mechanisms responsible for the tremor are not known. The lack of myelin, presumably, results in an overall slowing of nerve impulse conduction centrally, which might cause a loss of coordinated motor control. Alternatively, nonmyelinated axons may discharge spontaneously (ectopic excitation), due possibly to high extracellular potassium that accumulates because of continuous conduction in nonmyelinated fibers. In speculating on the cellular basis for hypomyelination in affected dogs, the most striking feature is the relative sparing of the peripheral nervous system. Axons passing to and from the spinal cord often are normally myelinated in the nerve root, while being thinly myelinated or nonmyelinated in the spinal cord. Since peripheral myelin is produced by Schwann cells and central myelin is produced by oligodendrocytes, the basic lesion may involve altered function or delayed maturation of oligodendrocytes. Oligodendrocyte numbers, in fact, are reduced in springer spaniels, Samoyeds, and Weimaraners. Furthermore, the rough endoplasmic reticulum of oligodendrocytes in affected springer spaniels often is dilated, suggesting there may be defective protein synthesis or transport. A similar, but less pronounced, lesion has been seen in Weimaraners and Samoyeds. Delayed gliogenesis has been proposed to account for the reduction of oligodendrocytes in Samoyeds because there were relatively few mature oligodendrocytes in the dog studied. However, most oligodendrocytes in affected Weimaraners appear relatively mature. For this reason, it seems possible that the resolution of tremor in Weimaraners may occur subsequent to myelination of axons by existing oligodendrocytes rather than because of further oligodendrocyte differentiation from glioblasts. Treatment of dogs with tremor due to hypomyelination has not been described and usually is not necessary in mildly affected dogs. Severely debilitated dogs require extensive supportive care or malnutrition and death will occur.

TREMOR OF WHITE DOGS

Acute head and body tremor has been noted in adult dogs, particularly smaller breeds with white coat color such as Maltese terriers, West Highland white terriers, and beagles. Dogs with other coat colors also have been affected. Tremor in affected dogs is exaggerated by stress and excitement and lessens or resolves during relaxation and sleep. Most dogs have no other neurologic deficits, although the tremor may be sufficiently severe to cause difficulty in standing and walking. Seizures have been noted in some dogs. Diffuse, slow-wave activity has occasionally been noted on electroencephalography. Some dogs have had increased numbers of mononuclear inflammatory cells on cerebrospinal fluid evaluation and nonsuppurative meningoencephalitis has been seen at necropsy in a few dogs. The inflammatory nature of these changes suggests that infection or autoimmunity may be involved in the pathogenesis of this syndrome. In order to account for the common involvement of white breeds of dogs and the histopathologic evidence of nonsuppurative meningoencephalitis, one author suggested that there may be an immunologic attack against cells that metabolize tyrosine to produce melanin pigment and neurotransmitters such as epinephrine and norepinephrine. A somewhat analogous disease

(Vogt-Koyanagi-Harada syndrome) in which there is an immunologic attack against melanin-producing cells that results primarily in uveitis has been described in human beings and dogs. However, data to support any immunologic basis for the tremor syndrome seen in white dogs is lacking. Nevertheless, clinical signs in some dogs improve after administration of glucocorticoids at an immunosuppressive dosage (prednisone, 0.4 to 1 mg/lb (1 to 2 mg/kg), orally, q24h). Chronic alternate-day maintenance therapy at a smaller dosage may be necessary. Diazepam (Valium) also may reduce the tremor. Some dogs recover spontaneously after several weeks.

DRUG- AND TOXIN-INDUCED TREMOR

Some of the many drugs and toxins that have been said to cause tremor also cause muscle fasciculations and so may have been mistakenly classified as being tremorgenic. However, several agents appear to definitely cause tremor in dogs and cats. Hexachlorophene intoxication subsequent to bathing or ingestion causes intention tremor, with pups being particularly susceptible. Some dogs recover spontaneously within a week of intoxication, while others develop additional systemic and neurologic signs and die. Tremor presumably occurs because hexachlorophene causes separation of myelin at the intraperiod line in the central nervous system, resulting in intramyelinic accumulation of fluid.

The authors have seen several dogs and cats that developed tremor after having been treated topically with the organophosphorus compound fenthion (Spot-on) for flea control. Tremor in affected dogs usually occurred after multiple doses, applied according to established dosage regimens. The tremor affected the entire body and was more pronounced during activity. Some of the affected animals were also depressed, while others were normal except for the tremor. Mechanisms responsible for the tremor are not clear but may relate more to the neuropathic effect of chronic organophosphorus exposure than the anticholinesterase effect at the neuromuscular junction. The effect of fenthion on serum cholinesterase concentrations is dose-dependent. Serum cholinesterase concentrations have been decreased in some affected animals and others have had normal levels. Red blood cell levels are a less sensitive indicator of toxicity. Considering the chronic nature of the organophosphorus exposure and the relatively benign nature of the tremor, the authors generally have only bathed affected animals in the hope of reducing further absorption. Some of the animals, however, had received atropine prior to the authors' evaluation, without benefit. The tremor usually resolved over a period of several weeks. Use of organophosphorus compounds in previously affected animals must be questioned because of their apparent idiosyncratic response to such agents.

One of the authors has seen several dogs develop tremor after sedation with a combination of droperidol and fentanyl citrate (Innovar Vet). Tremor in these dogs was particularly pronounced in the muscles of mastication and usually resolved in one to three weeks. Interestingly, human beings given this combination occasionally develop extrapyramidal signs of Parkinson's disease, shivering, and twitching. Other neuroleptic drugs akin to droperidol sometimes cause lip smacking and tongue and masticatory movements. Reasons for the abnormal movements are unclear, but they presumably relate to the dopaminergic blocking effects of the neuroleptic drug group. Some of the many other drugs shown to cause tremor in human beings are isoproterenol, phenothiazines, and sodium valproate.

CEREBELLAR TREMOR

Cerebellar disease is the most common cause of intention tremor in dogs and cats. The tremor is usually particularly pronounced in the head, but also may involve the limbs. Tremor resulting from cerebellar disease is not nearly as diffuse or pronounced as that seen subsequent to hypomyelination. The presence of truncal ataxia and dysmetria in dogs with cerebellar lesions further distinguishes this form of tremor from those due to other causes. Specific diseases that may affect the cerebellum are discussed in Section VI.

13 ATAXIA, PARESIS, AND PARALYSIS

ANDY SHORES and PHILIP ROUDEBUSH

Ataxia, paresis, and paralysis are gait alterations associated with dysfunction of the central or peripheral nervous systems. Table 13–1 outlines the diagnostic evaluation of the ataxic, paretic, or paralyzed small animal. Ataxia is defined as a failure of muscle coordination, paresis is partial loss or impairment of motor function in a body part, and paralysis is complete loss or impairment of motor function in a body part.

TABLE 13–1. DIAGNOSTIC EVALUATION FOR ATAXIA, PARESIS, OR PARALYSIS

1. Minimum Data Base
   a. Signalment and history
   b. Physical examination
2. Neurologic Examination
   a. Mental status
   b. Locomotion
   c. Cranial nerves
   d. Postural reactions
   e. Spinal reflexes
   f. Sensory perception
   g. Localization of lesion
3. Differential Diagnosis List
4. Ancillary Tests
   a. Clinical pathology (hematology, serum chemistries, urinalysis, CSF analysis)
   b. Radiology
   c. Electrodiagnostics
   d. Additional diagnostics (e.g., biopsy)
5. Diagnosis, Prognosis, Client Education
6. Therapy

ATAXIA

The ataxic animal is characterized by a broad-based stance and may exhibit incoordination of the head, trunk, or limbs. Ataxia has been classified into three major categories (sensory, vestibular, and cerebellar) and is associated with sensory dysfunction of the spinal cord, vestibular system, or cerebellum, respectively.

Sensory Ataxia. Sensory ataxia results from a disruption of proprioceptive pathways from the limbs, and, occasionally, the trunk (*truncal ataxia*). Several spinal cord diseases produce sensory ataxia and can be associated with varying degrees of paresis.

Vestibular Ataxia. Vestibular ataxia results from lesions involving the central or peripheral portions of the vestibular system. Table 13–2 describes neurologic findings with central and peripheral vestibular diseases. The vestibular system is composed of the cristae ampulares, the maculae, the vestibular division of cranial nerve VIII, the vestibular nuclei, and the associated efferent and afferent pathways. It maintains position of the head, eyes, and trunk relative to gravity, and receives sensory input reflecting rotational movements of the head and linear acceleration. Although this system does not initiate motor function, its input to other brain stem centers, the cerebellum, and the cerebral cortices serves to coordinate muscles associated with maintaining equilibrium, head position, and eye movements. The vestibular system's influence on coordination is mediated through efferent pathways from the vestibular nuclei to the cerebellum via the middle and caudal cerebellar peduncles. The cerebral cortices receive proprioceptive information from the vestibular nuclei. Vestibulospinal pathways influence the antigravity muscles of the limbs, usually by stimulation of ipsilateral extensors.

Ataxia resulting from a unilateral vestibular lesion can be characterized by an ipsilateral head tilt, tight circling toward the side of the lesion, nystagmus with a fast phase away from the site of the lesion, and a tendency to fall to the ipsilateral side. The latter results

TABLE 13–2. NEUROLOGIC SIGNS ASSOCIATED WITH CENTRAL AND PERIPHERAL VESTIBULAR DISEASE

Central	Signs	Peripheral
+	Head tilt	+
++	Circling	+
++	Falling, rolling	+
+	Postural deficits	–
+	Spontaneous or positional nystagmus	+
+	Horizontal	+
+	Rotary	+
+	Vertical	–
+	Positional change of direction	–

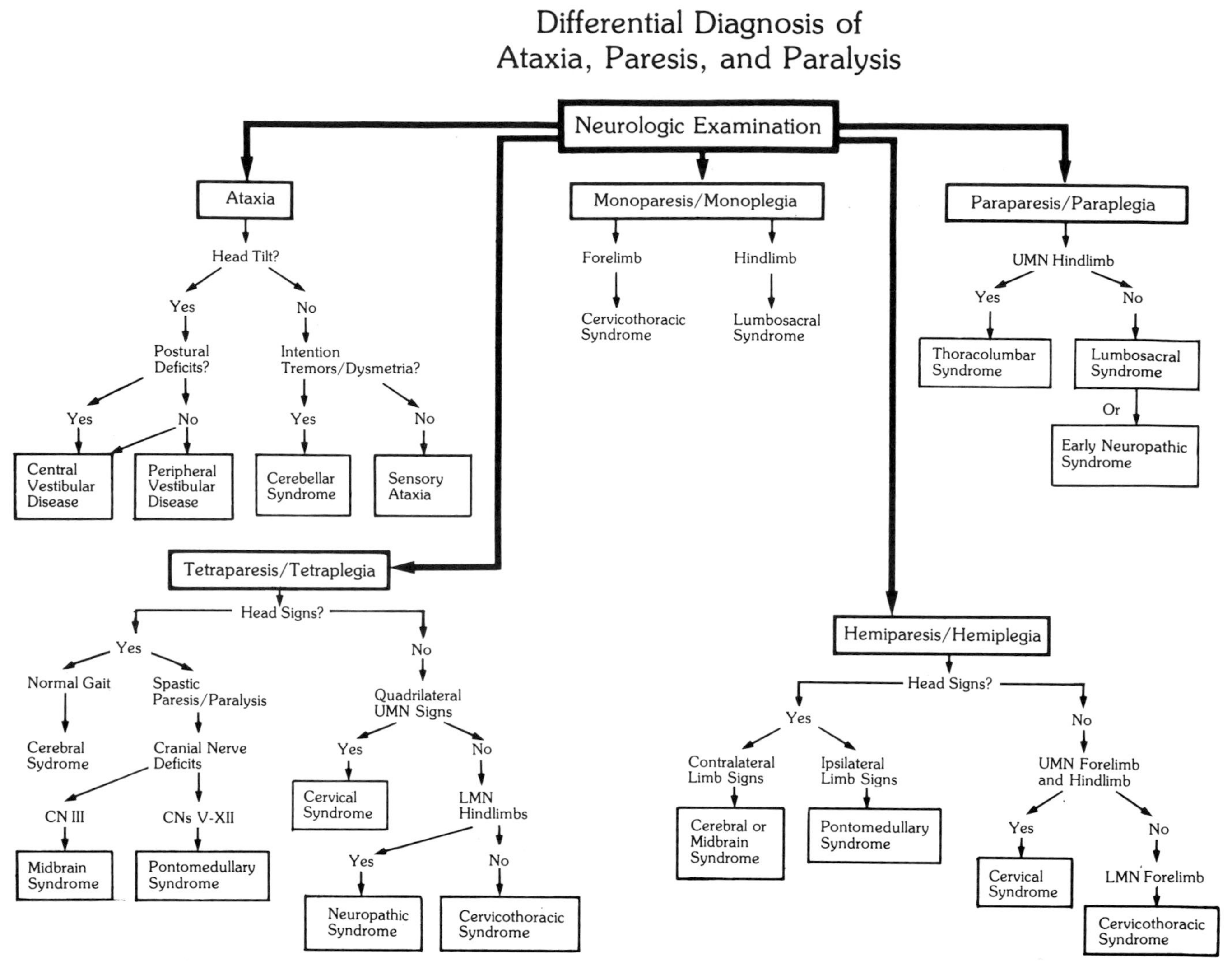

FIGURE 13–1. Algorithm for the differential diagnosis of ataxia, paresis, and paralysis in small animals.

from reduced ipsilateral extensor tone in opposition to normal contralateral extensor tone.

The most frequently observed diseases that produce vestibular ataxia include otitis media/interna, canine and feline idiopathic vestibular syndromes, cranial trauma, granulomatous meningoencephalitis, aminoglycoside toxicity, and neoplasia.

Cerebellar Ataxia. Cerebellar diseases are typically diffuse, producing a symmetrical syndrome characterized by a broad-based stance, ataxia in all limbs with preservation of strength, dysmetria (usually hypermetria), truncal ataxia, intention tremors of the head and eyes, delayed postural reactions with exaggerated responses, and menace deficits with normal vision.

The cerebellum receives sensory input from the spinal cord, vestibular system, brain stem, and cerebral cortex through the caudal and middle cerebellar peduncles. The information is integrated and relayed through the rostral and caudal cerebellar peduncles. The cerebellum coordinates, but does not initiate, muscle activity. Paresis, therefore, is not associated with cerebellar disease. Animals with severe cerebellar disease may be unable to stand, but voluntary muscle activity can be initiated.

Unilateral cerebellar disease is rare and produces ipsilateral signs. Involvement of the vestibular components of the cerebellum may produce a paradoxical vestibular syndrome. Central vestibular and cerebellar signs can result from lesions affecting the caudal brain stem.

Cerebellar ataxia can result from degenerative disease (cerebellar abiotrophy, globoid leukodystrophy), congenital and developmental anomalies (cerebellar hypoplasia, hypomyelinogenesis), neoplasia, inflammatory diseases (canine distemper, rabies, and toxoplasmosis), cranial trauma, or toxins (hexachlorophene).

PARESIS AND PARALYSIS

Paresis and paralysis as defined earlier imply voluntary motor dysfunction and can result from disease above the foramen magnum, of the spinal cord, peripheral nerves, or myoneural junction. The terms paresis and paralysis must also be qualified when describing a patient. Quadriparesis/plegia or tetraparesis/plegia describes the animal with voluntary motor dysfunction in all four limbs and therefore a lesion involving the central

TABLE 13–3. RULE-OUT CATEGORIES FOR NEUROLOGIC SYNDROMES THAT PRODUCE ATAXIA, PARESIS, AND PARALYSIS

Ataxia

Central Vestibular Syndrome	Peripheral Vestibular Syndrome
neoplasia	neoplasia
inflammatory disease	inflammatory disease
infarction	idiopathic syndromes
trauma	trauma
toxicity	toxicity
Cerebellar Syndrome	**Sensory Ataxia**
degenerative disease	degenerative disease
anomalies	anomalies
neoplasia	neoplasia
inflammatory disease	inflammatory disease
trauma	infarction
toxicity	trauma

Tetraparesis/Tetraplegia

Cerebral Syndrome	Midbrain Syndrome
degenerative disease	anomalies
anomalies	neoplasia
metabolic disease	inflammatory disease
neoplasia	infarction
inflammatory disease	trauma
infarction	
trauma	
toxicity	
Cervical Syndrome	**Cervicothoracic Syndrome**
degenerative disease	degenerative disease
anomalies	anomalies
neoplasia	neoplasia
inflammatory disease	inflammatory disease
infarction	infarction
trauma	trauma
Neuropathic Syndrome	
degenerative disease	
metabolic	
neoplastic	
inflammatory disease	
immune mediated	
ischemia	
trauma	
toxicity	

Paraparesis/Paraplegia

Thoracolumbar Syndrome	Lumbosacral Syndrome
degenerative disease	degenerative disease
anomalies	anomalies
neoplasia	neoplasia
inflammatory disease	inflammatory disease
infarction	ischemia
trauma	trauma

Hemiparesis/Hemiplegia

Cerebral Syndrome	Midbrain Syndrome
degenerative disease	anomalies
anomalies	neoplasia
inflammatory disease	inflammatory disease
infarction	infarction
trauma	trauma
Pontomedullary Syndrome	**Cervical Syndrome**
degenerative disease	degenerative disease
anomalies	anomalies
neoplasia	neoplasia
inflammatory disease	inflammatory disease
infarction	infarction
trauma	trauma
Cervicothoracic Syndrome	
degenerative disease	
anomalies	
neoplasia	
inflammatory disease	
infarction	
trauma	

Monoparesis/Monoplegia

Cervicothoracic Syndrome	Lumbosacral Syndrome
neoplasia	neoplasia
inflammatory disease	inflammatory disease
infarction	infarction
trauma	trauma

nervous system cranial to the T3 spinal segment, involvement of the peripheral nervous system, or multifocal disease affecting the cervical and lumbar intumescences. Paraparesis/plegia describes the animal with a partial or complete loss of voluntary motor function in the hind limbs. This indicates involvement of the spinal cord between the T3 and S1 segments or the peripheral nerves to the hindlimbs. Monoparesis/plegia indicates involvement of one limb (e.g., right forelimb monoparesis). Hemiparesis/plegia involves the right or left side and indicates an ipsilateral spinal cord or brain stem lesion. Hemiparesis (but not hemiplegia) can result from a contralateral cerebral lesion. In veterinary terminology, the suffix -plegia does not address sensory function. A sensorimotor paraplegia defines paralysis of the hindlimbs with loss of sensory function.

Cerebral Dysfunction. Cerebral cortex or diencephalon dysfunction produces circling to the affected side, contralateral amaurosis, and contralateral postural deficits. The gait, however, is normal since the motor cortex does not maintain locomotion in domestic animals. For this same reason, hemiplegia does not occur with cerebral dysfunction in animals as it does in humans. Diffuse, bilateral cerebral involvement produces depression, cortical blindness, and quadrilateral postural deficits. An animal with a neoplasm of the left cerebral cortex may present with wide circling to the left, right visual field deficits, and right forelimb and hindlimb postural deficits. Examples of diseases affecting the cerebral cortex are cranial trauma, distemper encephalitis, neoplasia, rabies, granulomatous meningoencephalitis, feline ischemic encephalopathy, and hepatic encephalopathy.

Brain Stem Dysfunction. Brain stem dysfunction can be accompanied by hemiparesis or tetraparesis. Unilateral involvement above the pons (e.g., midbrain syndrome) produces contralateral spastic hemiparesis; bilateral involvement produces a spastic tetraparesis. Accompanying signs include depression or coma and oculomotor nerve deficits (ventrolateral strabismus, unresponsive dilated pupils with normal vision).

An ipsilateral spastic hemiparesis results from a unilateral brain stem dysfunction in pontomedullary syndrome. Spastic tetraparesis with bilateral involvement may also occur. The motor deficits are ipsilateral because the motor tracts decussate rostral to this level. Additional signs may include involvement of cranial nerves V through XII.

Paresis resulting from brain stem dysfunction can be caused by a number of disorders, including neoplasia, cranial trauma, and encephalitis.

Cervical Spinal Cord or Lower Motor Neuron Disease. Tetraparesis or tetraplegia without evidence of abnormalities above the foramen magnum indicates cervical spinal cord or generalized lower motor neuron disease. Focal lesions within the C1 to C5 spinal cord segments can produce spastic tetraparesis/plegia with exaggerated reflexes, normal to increased muscle tone in all limbs, and reduced postural reactions in all limbs. Caudal cervical involvement (spinal cord segments C6 to T2) results in reduced forelimb reflexes, normal to increased muscle tone in the forelimbs, normal to increased muscle tone in the hindlimbs, and increased hindlimb reflexes. When the brachial plexus is involved on only one side, a monoparesis may occur. Generalized lower motor neuron diseases result in flaccid tetraparesis/plegia and reduced or absent reflexes in all limbs.

Cervical spinal cord diseases encountered in veterinary practice include intervertebral disk disease, trauma, cervical vertebral malformation/malarticulation syndrome, fibrocartilaginous emboli, and neoplasia. Generalized lower motor neuron syndromes are discussed later.

Thoracolumbar spinal cord dysfunction (spinal cord segments T3 to L3) produces paraparesis or paraplegia with normal to increased muscle tone in the hindlimbs. Hindlimb reflexes are characteristically exaggerated and postural deficits are present. Examples of diseases affecting the thoracolumbar spinal cord are intervertebral disk disease, neoplasia, and trauma.

Spinal cord segments L4 to S3 comprise the lumbosacral intumescence and contain the cell bodies of origin for the femoral, sciatic, and sacral plexus nerves. Paraparesis that results from focal involvement of the spinal cord segments that contribute to the femoral nerve (L4 to L5) also produce an inability to support weight in the hindlimbs. The L6 to S1 spinal cord segments contain the sciatic nerve cell bodies of origin and focal dysfunction results in paraparesis/paraplegia with decreased sciatic reflexes (cranial tibialis, gastrocnemius, flexor). Unless the L4 to L5 segments are also involved, patellar reflexes are not affected. Conscious proprioception is reduced or absent. If the sacral segments are injured, a flaccid bladder and anal sphincter result. Animals with lesions affecting only the sacral spinal cord segments usually have normal function of the hindlimbs.

Generalized lower motor neuron diseases include tick paralysis, polyradiculoneuritis (coon hound paralysis), metabolic polyneuropathies, botulism, and dysimmune polyneuropathies. The lower motor neuron consists of the spinal motor neuron in the ventral gray column, the ventral root, the efferent neuron, and the myoneural junction. Involvement of any of these components results in lower motor neuron signs (hyporeflexia or areflexia, flaccid paralysis/paresis). Initial signs may be restricted to the hindlimbs, but these disorders eventually involve the forelimbs (ascending paresis/paralysis). Autonomic functions (e.g., micturition) are usually not affected and sensory function is usually intact with these disorders, although most motor nerves in the dog and cat contain some sensory fibers. There are certain diseases that are classified as pure sensory neuropathies.

Certain muscular diseases also produce weakness that can be interpreted as paresis, for example, toxoplasmosis and steroid myopathy. Myopathies are usually bilaterally symmetrical and are often associated with exercise intolerance. Reflexes are preserved and muscular atrophy is seen.

Diseases that produce paresis or paralysis can also originate in the cardiovascular system. Aortoiliac thromboembolic disease (*saddle thrombi*) has been associated with feline cardiomyopathy and produces an acute onset paraplegia. Disorders of the forelimb can also occur with embolic disease. Aortoiliac thromboembolism is less common in the dog and is usually a sequel to left ventricular mural thrombi, bacterial endocarditis or neoplastic emboli. Weakness or syncope associated with cardiovascular disease is discussed in Chapter 11.

DIFFERENTIAL DIAGNOSIS

The differential diagnosis of ataxia, paresis, or paralysis encompasses a long list of disease entities. Figure 13–1 is an algorithm outlining this approach. Table 13–3 is a list of *rule-out* categories for the different neurologic syndromes that result in ataxia, paresis, or paralysis. The differential diagnoses require an accurate history and assessment of the historical findings, thorough physical and neurologic examinations, localization of the lesion, and the proper design of a diagnostic plan. Ancillary diagnostics include radiological studies, electrodiagnostics, cerebrospinal fluid analysis, muscle and nerve biopsies, and serology. Therapy is discussed in other chapters of this text.

14 ALTERED STATES OF CONSCIOUSNESS: COMA AND STUPOR

ANDY SHORES and PHILIP ROUDEBUSH

An altered state of consciousness can result from many diseases that affect the reticular activating system or cerebral cortex. Diagnostic evaluation of animals with an altered state of consciousness includes the history, physical examination, neurological examination, and ancillary diagnostic aids. Therapy for the comatose or stuporous patient is based on etiology. Prognosis is based on the suspected course of the disease process or the response to appropriate therapy.

FUNCTIONAL STATES OF THE BRAIN

Normal consciousness is represented by a patient who is bright, alert, and responsive to all environmental and external stimuli. *Delirium* implies a disoriented, incoherent, irritable, or fearful animal. The delirious animal is capable of responding to environmental or external stimuli but the response may be inappropriate. *Depression* connotes a lethargic, despondent individual who is capable of responding to the environment in a normal manner. This can be characteristic of any ill animal. *Stupor* is a semicomatose state in which the animal responds only to noxious stimuli. Dementia and unconscious vocalization may be present or a stuporous animal may appear asleep when undisturbed. *Coma* is an unconscious state where the animal is unresponsive to repeated noxious stimuli.

MAINTENANCE OF WAKEFULNESS

Wakefulness, the normal state of consciousness, is characterized by a bright and alert animal that exhibits an expected response to visual, auditory, and tactile stimuli. Wakefulness is maintained by the ascending reticular activating system (ARAS). The ARAS consists of a portion of the reticular formation's diffuse network of neurons in the central portion of the brain stem and receives sensory input from spinal somatosensory pathways and all cranial nerve afferents. These major special sensory and somatic pathways transmit impulses from auditory, visual, touch, pain, and thermal stimuli, vision, and proprioception. A diffuse network of neuronal projections from the diencephalic portion of the ARAS stimulates the cerebral cortex to initiate and maintain consciousness. A positive feedback mechanism from cholinergic cortical neurons to the ARAS assists in the maintenance of an "awake" state, allowing the ARAS to balance itself against the adrenergic system. The adrenergic system projects to the cerebral cortex from nuclei in the midbrain and diencephalon, which are considered the sleep system.

Consciousness and wakefulness are initiated by sensory stimuli that act on the cerebral cortex through the ARAS and they are maintained by continued sensory input and the positive feedback mechanism. Decreasing levels of consciousness indicate abnormal cerebral cortex function or interference with cortical activity by the ARAS. The level of consciousness may be altered by disease processes involving the cerebral cortex or the rostral brain stem.

RULE-OUTS FOR COMA AND STUPOR

The rule-outs for coma and stupor can be characterized by historical information (acute, chronic, progressive, nonprogressive) and by neurologic signs (focal, lateralizing, diffuse, multifocal).

Head Trauma. The most frequent cause of coma or stupor in animals is motor vehicle trauma. These animals are frequently presented with multiple injuries and require emergency care. Other causes of cranial trauma present similarly but seldom have accompanying injuries.

Terms used to describe pathologic alterations associated with cranial trauma include concussion, a transient loss of consciousness without structural brain damage; brain contusion, injury from blunt trauma accompanied by edema, petechial hemorrhage, and parenchymal damage; and cerebral edema, interstitial fluid accumulation that occurs (to varying degrees) with all cranial trauma. These terms are useful in describing the injury, but are not used in determining the therapeutic regime. Of the intracranial hemorrhages, subarachnoid and intramedullary hemorrhage occur most frequently in dogs and cats. Epidural hemorrhage consists of bleeding between the dura and the calvarium and is usually the result of laceration of a meningeal artery or its branches. Subdural hemorrhage (bleeding between the arachnoid and dura) is rare in animals and develops slowly as a result of hemorrhage into the subdural space from bridging veins.

Vascular Diseases. Nontraumatic vascular compromise that results in coma or stupor is uncommon in animals but is considered when the history suggests an acute, nonprogressive syndrome. Cerebrovascular accidents (CVAs), arteriovenous anomalies, and coagulopathies are rule-outs. The terms CVA and stroke are synonymous with cerebral infarction, which can be ischemic or hemorrhagic. Spontaneous intracranial hemorrhage, coagulopathies, thromboembolic disease, cerebral arteriovenous anomalies, or cerebral vasospasm can result in CVAs.

Neoplasia. Neoplasms within the cranial vault can produce coma or stupor as a result of their location, rate of growth, circulatory embarrassment, or cerebral edema. Neoplasms usually result in a chronic, progressive syndrome, but the onset of stupor or coma can be acute and result from alterations in intracranial pressure or a CVA. The signs are determined by the location of the mass.

Metabolic Encephalopathies. A wide variety of metabolic abnormalities can affect the cerebrum, causing diffuse or multifocal lesions. Normal glucose homeostasis is critical for optimal cerebral function; hypoglycemia or hyperglycemia can result in CNS signs. Endogenous toxins associated with uremia (uremic encephalopathy) and hepatic insufficiency (hepatic encephalopathy) can serve as false neurotransmitters and result in similar signs. Hyperosmolality associated with hyperglycemia or exogenous factors (e.g., ethylene glycol) also adversely affects cerebral function. Hyperlipidemia, heat stroke, and hypoxia are less common metabolic abnormalities that can result in stupor or coma.

Toxicity. Certain toxins can directly or indirectly affect cerebral function. Hypoxia is induced by carbon monoxide and cyanide poisoning. Generalized depression of cerebral function results from alcohol and barbiturates. Heavy metals, especially lead, can cause CNS signs. Ethylene glycol directly affects the brain but can contribute to hyperosmolality. Most plant toxins affecting small animals do not result in CNS signs but mushroom poisoning is one toxin that does cause stupor or coma. Hallucinogens and cannabinoids must also be considered in stuporous animals.

Inflammatory Lesions. Inflammatory lesions can produce acute or chronic, progressive, and local or diffuse clinical signs. Pathogenic organisms enter the CNS by either direct extension from adjacent structures, ascension of cranial or peripheral nerves, or hematogenous spread. Neurotropic microorganisms primarily affect the neural parenchyma (encephalitis) with secondary meningeal involvement. Neurotropic infections include viral encephalitis (canine distemper, rabies, pseudorabies) and protozoal encephalitis (toxoplasmosis). Non-neurotropic infections usually result in meningoencephalitis, intracranial abscesses, or granulomas. Organisms that cause meningitis, intracranial abscess, or granuloma formation enter the subarachnoid space hematogenously from external foci of infection. Bacterial meningoencephalitis, fungal meningoencephalitis (especially cryptococcosis and blastomycosis), rickettsial infection (ehrlichiosis, Rocky Mountain spotted fever), and some viral infections (feline coronavirus) can result in stupor or coma.

Granulomatous meningoencephalitis (GME) is a sporadic, idiopathic inflammatory or immunoproliferative disorder. Lesions of GME may be disseminated (granulomatous or inflammatory reticulosis) or focal (neoplastic reticulosis). The onset of disseminated GME is usually acute with a progressive course over a one- to eight-week period. The focal form of GME has a more insidious onset and slowly progresses over a period of months.

Congenital Abnormalities. Congenital or developmental abnormalities can result in stupor or coma. These abnormalities result in decreased cerebral parenchyma or cerebral degeneration. Hydrocephalus, lissencephaly, otocephaly, and storage disease (lipofuscinosis, and so on) are examples of these problems.

EVALUATION OF THE STUPOROUS OR COMATOSE ANIMAL

Minimum Data Base

HISTORY

Vaccination History. Canine distemper and rabies are unlikely, but still rule-outs in a patient with proper and current vaccinations.

Description of Environment. Toxicosis is suggested by a history of potential or known exposure to a toxin in the animal's environment. Heat stroke and trauma can also be suspected based on the environmental history. Blastomycosis commonly infects the CNS and is endemic in the Mississippi, Ohio, and Tennessee river basins and in the central Atlantic states.

Signalment. Congenital, developmental, and toxic problems occur most commonly in young animals, while an increased incidence of neoplasia occurs in older animals.

Bleeding Disorder. Historical evidence of recent epistaxis, hematuria, melena, petechia, ecchymoses, or contusions should increase the suspicion of a bleeding disorder leading to cerebral hemorrhage.

Previous Illnesses. A history of previous renal disease, hepatic disease, diabetes mellitus, hypothyroidism, hyperadrenocorticism, or hyperlipidemia should increase the suspicion of metabolic abnormalities contributing to stupor or coma.

Loss of Consciousness. Acute brain stem injuries result in immediate loss of consciousness, while subdural or tentorial herniation results in loss of consciousness over a period of hours.

Seizure Description. Many neurologic disorders causing stupor or coma may be preceded by, or be superimposed on, seizures. The seizure should be described (prodromal, ictal, and postictal phases) with the frequency and total number of seizures. The age when the first seizure occurred and any alteration in personality should be noted.

Cranial Trauma Description. A description of the animal's behavior immediately following trauma can assist in determining the site(s) of injury. Seizure activity immediately following trauma indicates intraparenchymal cerebral hemorrhage. An immediate loss of consciousness often accompanies rostral brain stem injuries.

PHYSICAL EXAMINATION

Pupil Size and Pupillary Light Response. Alterations in pupil size and pupillary light responses usually indicate brain stem disease. The neurologic alterations that occur with midbrain disease and their prognostic implications are listed in Figure 14–1. Normal pupillary light responses require a functional retina, optic nerve, optic tract, pretectal area, parasympathetic nucleus of the oculomotor nerve, oculomotor nerve, and ciliary body. Midbrain lesions result in dysfunction of the parasympathetic nucleus of the oculomotor nerve. Unilateral lesions of this nucleus, except during impending tentorial herniation, are rare since the paired nuclei are in close apposition near the midline of the midbrain.

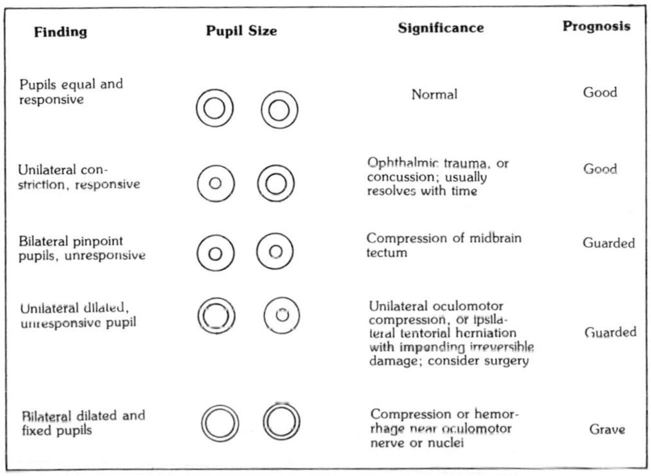

Finding
Pupil Size
Significance
Prognosis
Pupils equal and responsive
Normal
Good
Unilateral constriction, responsive
Ophthalmic trauma, or concussion; usually resolves with time
Good
Bilateral pinpoint pupils, unresponsive
Compression of midbrain tectum
Guarded
Unilateral dilated, unresponsive pupil
Unilateral oculomotor compression, or ipsilateral tentorial herniation with impending irreversible damage; consider surgery
Guarded
Bilateral dilated and fixed pupils
Compression or hemorrhage near oculomotor nerve or nuclei
Grave

FIGURE 14–1. Pupillary light responses.

BLOOD AND URINE ANALYSIS

Complete Blood Count. Neutrophilic leukocytosis often accompanies inflammation. Basophilic stippling and nucleation of erythrocytes may accompany lead toxicosis.

Serum Biochemical Profile. Metabolic abnormalities can be quickly ruled out by screening with a complete serum biochemical profile.

Urinalysis. Renal failure, urinary tract infection, and certain metabolic diseases such as diabetes mellitus can be ruled out based on urinalysis in conjunction with the complete blood count and serum biochemical profile.

NEUROLOGIC EXAMINATION

A complete neurologic examination should be performed with the goals of determining the state of consciousness and localizing the CNS lesion.

Mental Status. See definitions given previously.

Pupil Size and Pupillary Light Responses. See the section on Physical Examination and Figure 14–1.

Menace Response. Cranial nerve II function (menace response) is evaluated in view of the animal's mental status since stuporous or comatose patients do not react to visual menace. Vision is not affected by focal midbrain or pontine injuries, but cerebral injuries may result in contralateral menace deficits.

Nystagmus. Vestibular (physiologic) nystagmus, a normal finding, is elicited by moving the animal's head from side to side or up and down. The eyes should move in the direction of the head movement. Reduced vestibular nystagmus results from damage to the midbrain, pons, or cranial nerves III, IV, VI, or VIII. Complete absence of vestibular nystagmus indicates midbrain and pontine injuries or involvement of cranial nerves III, IV, VI, or VIII.

Eye Position. Midbrain injuries can alter eye position. A slight dorsomedial strabismus can occur with oculomotor nucleus or nerve damage and an ipsilateral ventral or ventrolateral strabismus can occur with central or peripheral vestibular disease.

Postural Changes. Postural changes occur with severe CNS injury. Decerebrate rigidity, manifested by opisthotonos and quadrilateral limb rigidity, results from brain herniation or severe midbrain disease and constitutes a grave prognosis. This posture should be differentiated from the Schiff-Sherrington posture seen in animals with severe injuries between the T-2 and L-3 spinal segments.

Decorticate Behavior. A decorticate animal may be blind, is unaware of surroundings and confused. Wide circling, propulsive pacing, paddling, head pressing, or other similar activities may be exhibited. Decorticate animals usually resist restraint.

ANCILLARY DIAGNOSTICS

Blood Coagulation Profile. Activated clotting time (ACT), activated partial thromboplastin time (APTT), prothrombin time (PT) and platelet count are indicated when clotting disorders, disseminated intravascular co-

TABLE 14–1. COMA SCALE

Motor Activity	
Normal gait, normal spinal reflexes	6
Hemiparesis, tetraparesis or decorticate activity	5
Recumbent, intermittent extensor rigidity	4
Recumbent, constant extensor rigidity	3
Recumbent, constant extensor rigidity with opisthotonos	2
Recumbent, hypotonia of muscles, depressed or absent spinal reflexes	1
Brain Stem Reflexes	
Normal pupillary light responses and oculocephalic reflexes	6
Slow pupillary light responses and normal to reduced oculocephalic reflexes	5
Bilateral miosis with normal to reduced oculocephalic reflexes	4
Pinpoint pupils with reduced to absent oculocephalic reflexes	3
Unilateral, unresponsive mydriasis with reduced to absent oculocephalic reflexes	2
Bilateral, unresponsive mydriasis with reduced to absent oculocephalic reflexes	1
Level of Consciousness	
Occasional periods of alertness and responsive to environment	6
Depression or delirium, capable of responding to environment but response may be inappropriate	5
Semicomatose, responsive to visual stimuli	4
Semicomatose, responsive to auditory stimuli	3
Semicomatose, responsive only to repeated noxious stimuli	2
Comatose, unresponsive to repeated noxious stimuli	1
Prognosis	
3–8 Grave	
9–14 Poor to fair	
15–18 Fair to good	

agulopathy, or severe liver dysfunction are suspected. See Chapter 116.

Radiography. Skull radiography is important in cases of known or suspected cranial trauma, since many skull fractures cannot be palpated.

Cerebrospinal Fluid Analysis. Cerebrospinal fluid (CSF) collection is contraindicated in acute brain trauma and is performed with caution if elevated intracranial pressure is suspected. When intracranial pressure is elevated the sudden loss of small amounts of CSF from the cisterna magna can precipitate brain herniation and death. When indicated, CSF should be removed from the cisterna magna for cytological and chemical analysis. Pressure measurement is performed using a manometer with a three-way stopcock valve. Pressures of CSF are always measured with the patient in lateral recumbency and under barbiturate or neuroleptic-analgesic restraint only. Culture of CSF is indicated when bacterial or fungal diseases are suspected.

Electrodiagnostics. The electroencephalogram (EEG) is a graphic record of the electrical activity of the cerebral cortex, which is also influenced by subcortical structures. The EEG can help determine if the disease is focal or diffuse and acute or chronic. The EEG does not provide a specific diagnosis but it may indicate the general category of disease (e.g., inflammatory vs. degenerative). The brain stem auditory evoked response (BAER) may be altered with lesions of the brain stem caudal to the midbrain.

MONITORING

Serial Examinations. The stuporous or comatose animal should be monitored continuously and reevaluated every 15 to 60 minutes, depending on the initial patient status. Monitoring should include vital signs, pupillary size and response, other cranial nerve reflexes, mental status, postural reactions, and spinal reflexes. Continued deterioration of signs indicates progressive cerebral edema, hemorrhage, or both and warrants aggressive therapy.

Coma Scale. A coma scale is used in evaluating and monitoring stuporous or comatose patients. The scale is an adaptation of the Glasgow Coma Scale used in human neurology (see Table 14–1). Low scores (3 to 8) represent a grave prognosis, moderate scores (9 to 14) represent a poor to fair prognosis, while higher scores (15 to 18) represent a favorable prognosis. The animal is examined periodically and the coma scale score is recorded. Improved scores represent patient response to therapy, while decreasing scores may dictate additional therapy. Many factors are involved in patient response to therapy and this scale is intended as a guideline for patient monitoring.

TREATMENT OF THE COMATOSE OR STUPOROUS ANIMAL

INITIAL EMERGENCY TREATMENT

The "ABCs" (establishing patent Airway, proper Breathing, Cardiac function) are evaluated first (see also

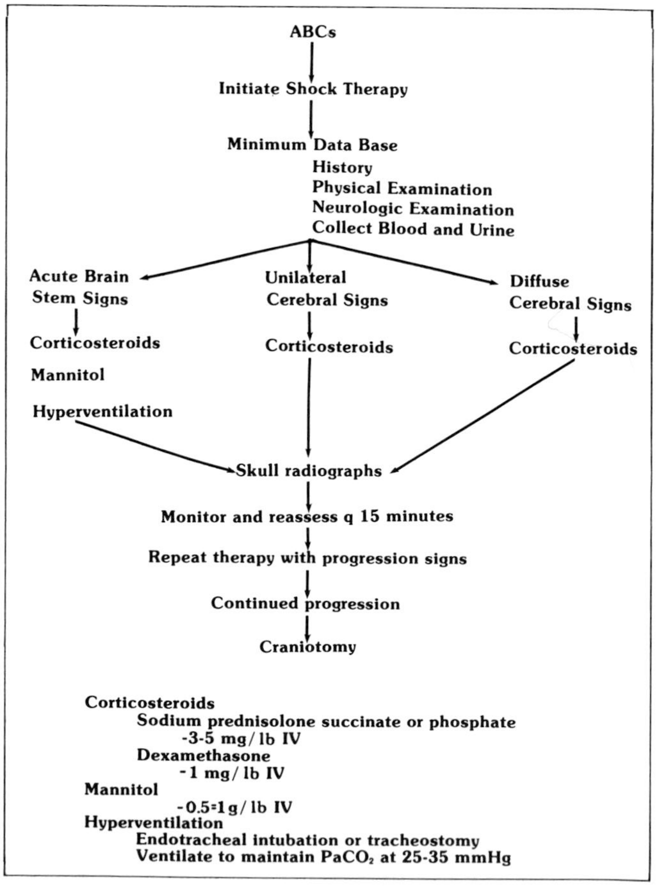

FIGURE 14–2. Emergency management for cranial trauma.

Figure 14–2). Appropriate therapy is initiated if shock is present (Chapter 35). Intravenous fluids are restricted to maintenance once shock is controlled since they can contribute to cerebral edema. Monitoring central venous pressure is helpful.

ADDITIONAL EMERGENCY MEASURES

Corticosteroids, osmotic diuretics, and hyperventilation have been advocated for control of cerebral edema. The use of mannitol is controversial, especially when the differentiation between hemorrhage and edema has not been made. Mannitol is efficacious with an intact vascular system, but may seep into an area of hemorrhage, drawing more fluids into the area. Reducing brain edema in the presence of epidural or subdural hemorrhage may create more room for hemorrhage and result in deterioration of signs.

Hyperventilation can be performed with conventional tracheal intubation in the comatose patient or through a tracheostomy. When blood gas analysis is available, the arterial PCO_2 should be maintained between 25 and 35 mmHg.

A craniotomy is advised in the presence of subdural hemorrhage or uncontrolled cerebral edema. Surgical management of the cranial trauma patient is indicated for evacuation of the hematoma, hemostasis, providing decompression for uncontrollable cerebral edema, skull fracture reduction, or removal of bone fragments from the brain parenchyma. In the absence of progressive clinical signs, surgery is warranted during the first 24 to 48 hours for depressed skull fractures, compound skull fractures, or removal of bone fragments imbedded in the brain parenchyma.

MAINTENANCE THERAPY

If the animal remains in a comatose state for more than 48 hours, in spite of medical or surgical therapy, a grave prognosis is warranted since this usually indicates brain stem hemorrhage or malacia. Maintenance of a comatose patient requires good nursing care, including frequent turning to prevent hypostatic lung congestion, adequate cage padding to prevent decubital ulcers, maintenance of fluid and electrolyte balances, maintenance of urinary and bowel functions, and proper nutrition. A pharyngostomy or gastrostomy tube can be placed for feeding a gruel and continued nursing care for two to four weeks may be rewarding in rare instances.

15 SEIZURES

JOE N. KORNEGAY and STEPHEN B. LANE

The term *seizure* (convulsion, ictus, fit) refers to an involuntary, paroxysmal disturbance of the brain usually manifested as uncontrolled muscular activity. Seizures characteristically are unprecipitated, stereotypic, and cease spontaneously. *Epilepsy* refers to the recurrence of seizures, particularly if the underlying cause cannot be identified. When seizures occur continuously with minimal periods of intervening normalcy, the condition is referred to as *status epilepticus*. The site of the seizure's origin in the brain is called the *seizure focus*.

Seizures may be broadly subdivided into *generalized* and *focal* (partial) forms. *Generalized seizures* may originate within the cerebral cortex, thalamus, or brain stem, and are associated with symmetric clinical and electroencephalographic dysfunction.

The principal generalized seizure affecting dogs and cats is the grand mal (major motor, tonic clonic) seizure. Petit mal (absence) seizures, manifested by transient loss of consciousness and muscle tone, are a second relatively common generalized seizure of human beings but rarely occur in animals. *Focal seizures* characteristically include clinical features that allow more precise localization of the seizure focus. Temporolimbic seizures (psychomotor seizures, limbic system or temporal lobe epilepsy) are characterized by behavioral changes such as aggression, biting at imaginary objects (fly-biting), and tail-chasing. Focal motor seizures are usually manifested clinically by tonic movements on the side of the body contralateral to the seizure focus. These tonic movements may remain confined to this side, but often generalize within a few seconds.

GENERAL PATHOPHYSIOLOGY

Seizure foci have been identified in individuals who have never had clinical evidence of seizures. In fact, seizures can be generated by pharmacologic and electrical changes in any individual; however, the threshold for seizure activity varies widely among individuals, implying an inherent susceptibility to seizure disorders. Any disease that affects the brain either primarily (intracranial cause) or secondarily (extracranial cause) may alter the seizure threshold.

The principal intracranial diseases that can cause seizures include encephalitis, neoplasia, and congenital lesions such as hydrocephalus (see Section VI, Diseases of the Nervous System). Most of these disorders are themselves progressive, however, some potential intracranial causes of seizures (trauma, brain infarction) are nonprogressive. Nevertheless, in either case seizures often eventually increase in frequency and severity.

Extracranial diseases cause seizures by altering the biochemical homeostasis of the brain. The insult may be exogenous, as with toxins (organophosphates, strychnine, chlorinated hydrocarbons) or endogenous, in which case the abnormality arises because of dysfunction of another organ system (hepatic encephalopathy, hypoglycemia, hypocalcemia).

When neither a primary brain lesion nor an extracranial cause that accounts for the seizures can be identified, a diagnosis of idiopathic (functional) epilepsy is made. Idiopathic epilepsy may be inherited in certain dog breeds, including beagles, Belgian Tervuren shepherds, German shepherds, Irish setters, and keeshonds.

Cellular Mechanisms. Cellular mechanisms responsible for epilepsy are not completely defined. Neurons maintain resting membrane potentials of approximately −70 mV through active sodium-potassium pumps, membrane ionic channels, and electrochemical gradients. The generation and conduction of changes in this resting membrane potential (excitability) is the basis of neurologic function. A change in membrane potential may lead to release of either excitatory or inhibitory neurotransmitters from the neuron. Excitatory neurotransmitters cause an influx of sodium, leading to a decrease in the resting membrane potential and a state of depolarization. If the potential decreases to −60 mV, the membrane potential shifts dramatically to +35 mV and an action potential results. In contrast, release of an inhibitory neurotransmitter leads to an efflux of potassium and an influx of chloride; the membrane becomes hyperpolarized so as to be refractory to excitatory input.

The basic physiologic phenomenon seen at the time of seizures is a prolonged period of depolarization, called the paroxysmal depolarization shift (PDS). This dramatic depolarization may occur because of an excess of excitatory synaptic input or because of an increase in the intrinsic excitability of the neuron itself. In either case, the hyperexcitable state of the neurons involved can arise either because of an actual increase in excitation or because of a decrease in inhibition (disinhibition). Increased excitation or disinhibition might, in turn, occur subsequent to an increase in either the neurotransmitters involved (excitatory, acetylcholine; inhibitory, gabba-aminobutyric acid) or their receptors. Considerable attention has recently been focused on the role of disinhibition, in that several convulsants have been shown to interfere with inhibitory neurotransmitters.

While these mechanisms explain the origin of the PDS, a clinical seizure does not occur unless the neuronal hyperexcitability is propagated to adjacent cortical and subcortical structures. Fortunately, spread of the PDS is normally prevented by an area of inhibition surrounding the seizure focus. Intense neuronal discharge may overcome this zone of surrounding inhibition and a clinical seizure results. The spread of the discharge may occur either synaptically or because of a change in the extracellular environment. An increase in extracellular potassium due to repetitive neuronal discharge is one environmental factor that has been incriminated in the spread of seizures. As normal neurons are repeatedly exposed to spontaneous discharges, their inherent excitability is increased and they also may contribute to the seizure focus. This phenomenon of increased cortical excitability occurring subsequent to electrical stimulation or seizures themselves is called *kindling*. It probably accounts, in part, for the increased refractoriness to anticonvulsants of some seizures. The number and location of neurons that become incorporated into the seizure focus and the structures to which the PDS spreads determines the clinical character of the seizure.

HISTORICAL FINDINGS

In obtaining the history of an animal with seizures, the clinical features of the seizure and its duration and frequency must be established before collecting information that may determine the underlying cause. The fact that seizures are unprecipitated, stereotypic, and cease spontaneously should distinguish them from other conditions. As an example, syncope generally is precipitated by exercise rather than occurring spontaneously. Animals with seizures often are historically nervous or disoriented prior to the seizure. This *preictal phase* is followed by the actual seizure, which is usually characterized by loss or derangement of consciousness and by alteration of muscle tone or movement (tonic-clonic limb movements). Owners should be questioned closely to determine if the initial motor movements of the seizure are seen consistently on one side of the body. Such a pattern is typical of focal motor seizures that often occur subsequent to primary brain disease. Some affected animals also have evidence of autonomic dysfunction (urination or defecation, salivation). Others have behavioral changes, particularly in the case of psychomotor seizures in which aggression or abnormal behavior such as fly-biting may predominate. After the actual seizure, for a period ranging from several minutes to days (*postictal phase*), the affected animal may be either overly excited or depressed and exhibit additional neurologic deficits.

When the seizure has been characterized, information relative to potential underlying causes must be collected. The importance of different historical details varies considerably, depending on the clinical character of the seizure, the age of the animal being evaluated, and results of the physical examination. As an example, information regarding the affected animal's vaccination history and whether seizures also occurred in its parents and littermates is more critical in young animals. Similarly, questions relative to potential exposure to toxins or underlying metabolic disorders are more important when results of the physical examination include other features of toxicity or additional organ dysfunction. However, certain information should be determined in each case. This includes the age of the affected animal at the time of seizure onset, its vaccination history, the health status of its littermates and parents, potential exposure to toxins, and whether there was prior cranial trauma or neurologic disease.

PHYSICAL FINDINGS

Abnormalities identified during the general physical examination that indicate involvement of organs other than the brain suggest possible polysystemic disease (infectious, toxic, metabolic, and others). Animals with seizures due to primary brain lesions (neoplasia, encephalitis) often also have neurologic deficits of unilateral cerebrocortical or thalamic involvement, including contralateral postural reaction and visual deficits, compulsive walking or circling to the side of the lesion, and depression or altered attitude. When there are additional signs that indicate the brain stem, cerebellum, or spinal cord is affected, diseases that typically cause multifocal central nervous system involvement such as the encephalitides and certain congenital disorders should be considered more strongly. Results of the neurologic examination must be interpreted relative to the animal's condition at the time of the examination. Animals examined during the postictal phase of the seizure may have significant neurologic deficits as a function of the seizure rather than as an indicator of a primary intracranial lesion. Depression or confusion, loss of visual acuity, and conscious proprioception deficits may persist until at least 24 hours after the seizure. Consistently asymmetric deficits such as circling or turning to one side are more meaningful, particularly if they persist during the interictal period.

DIAGNOSTIC PLAN

The extent of the evaluation recommended for an animal with seizures varies, depending on the results of the history and physical examination. A neurologic examination and serum chemistry panel should be done in every affected animal. Additional tests to more specifically measure organ function may be indicated if evidence of liver disease or another potential metabolic cause of the seizures is identified. When the animal has had only a single seizure and results of the neurologic examination and serum chemistry panel are normal, additional tests usually are not indicated. However, if the seizures persist and are refractory to anticonvulsant medication or if there are additional deficits indicating intracranial disease, a thorough neurologic evaluation should be done. This should include electroencephalography, cerebrospinal fluid examination, and computed tomography, if available.

GOALS OF TREATMENT

Treatment should be directed at the underlying cause of the seizures, if possible. When there is no specific treatment for the causative disease or a diagnosis of idiopathic epilepsy is made, chronic anticonvulsant therapy may be indicated. However, while even occasional seizures conceivably may render the brain more susceptible to further seizures (see previous discussion of kindling), there is no specific time at which anticonvulsants should be initiated. Some owners will insist that therapy be instituted when seizures are occurring relatively infrequently and others will refuse medication for various reasons even though their animals have frequent seizures. As a rule, anticonvulsants should be considered when single seizures are occurring more than once every six weeks or clusters of seizures are occurring more than once every eight weeks. Prior to recommending chronic anticonvulsant therapy, owners should be made aware that the medication is not a cure and may be required throughout the affected animal's life. The fact that the animal will probably continue to have occasional seizures despite medication must be stressed. Potential side-effects of the drug to be used and its expense also should be discussed.

Factors determining the potential efficacy of an anticonvulsant include its degree of absorption, half-life, and margin of safety relative to toxicity. To maintain steady state, the dosage interval of a drug cannot be greater than the half-life. By administering a drug at intervals of one-half of its half-life, steady state should be reached in five half-lives. Even at steady state, the blood level of the drug still fluctuates considerably, generally being greatest within one to two hours of the time of administration (*peak level*) and lowest just prior to the next dose (*trough level*). Phenobarbital is the only anticonvulsant with proven efficacy in controlling seizures in dogs. While primidone (Mylepsin, Mysoline) often is also effective, its anticonvulsant effects in dogs appear to be due largely to its metabolite, phenobarbital. The other metabolite of primidone, phenylethylmalonamide (PEMA), apparently contributes little to the overall efficacy of primidone in dogs and serum levels of unmetabolized primidone are negligible in most cases. For this reason and because primidone appears to potentially be more toxic than phenobarbital in dogs, primidone should be given only when phenobarbital fails to control seizures. Diphenylhydantoin (Dilantin) is poorly absorbed in dogs and has a considerably shorter half-life in them (three to seven hours) than in human beings (22 to 24 hours). It has been largely ineffective in controlling seizures in dogs at the dosages that have been routinely used. A higher dosage (18 mg/lb, q8h) might be effective in some dogs. None of the other anticonvulsants evaluated thus far in dogs such as valproic acid (Depakene) and carbamazepine (Tegretol) achieve therapeutic serum concentrations at dosages routinely used in human beings. However, valproic acid might still have some value since it is less protein-bound in dogs than in man and may therefore pass more freely across the blood-brain barrier. Phenobarbital is also preferred for chronic anticonvulsant therapy in cats. The use of diphenylhydantoin in cats is precluded because of potential toxicity due to its long half-life (42 hours). While clinical data is lacking, one recent study suggested that primidone may be an effective anticonvulsant in cats.

Serum levels of any anticonvulsant must be measured to determine the proper dosage. Phenobarbital should initially be given at a dosage of 2.5 mg/lb daily divided into two or three equal oral doses. Assuming there is seizure control without toxicity, the trough serum level should be determined after two weeks. When there is evidence of toxicity, the peak serum level should be measured. In either case, the dosage should then be adjusted at two-week intervals to achieve a serum level between 15 and 45 μ/ml. An even higher serum level may be necessary to control seizures in some dogs; however, toxicity may occur. When seizures consistently are noted just prior to the next dose of phenobarbital, the dosage interval should be decreased so as to maintain a more consistent serum concentration. Serum drug levels should be monitored at least every six months after steady state and seizure control have been achieved. When seizures cannot be controlled with phenobarbital, the use of primidone should be considered. The recommended initial dosage of primidone is 20 mg/lb divided into three equal oral doses. Serum levels of phenobarbital may be monitored as described above to adjust the primidone dosage. If seizures cannot be controlled with either phenobarbital or primidone, concomitant use of valproic acid or a long-acting benzodiazepine such as clonazepam (Clonapin) should be considered. The potential interactions of anticonvulsants with other drugs must be considered before instituting treatment for unrelated disorders. As an example, chloramphenicol inhibits metabolism of both diphenylhydantoin and phenobarbital.

Animals receiving anticonvulsants frequently have polyuria-polydipsia and increased serum concentrations of hepatic enzymes. Some will be depressed, particularly during the initial days of medication before hepatic microsomal enzymes are activated. Primidone appears to be hepatotoxic in some dogs. Other potential adverse reactions, such as blood dyscrasias, also may occur subsequent to the use of anticonvulsants in animals but are not well documented.

Single seizures usually are transient and have little noticeable lasting effect. When concerned owners seek immediate veterinary care, the affected animal often is normal except for postictal confusion or depression. However, animals in status epilepticus must be evaluated and treated as soon as possible or death may occur. A venous catheter should be placed to obtain blood for measurement of serum biochemical parameters such as glucose and calcium and to initiate anticonvulsant therapy. Diazepam (Valium) alone given IV at 0.12 to 0.25 mg/lb controls seizures in many animals. However, because of the short half-life of diazepam, there may be seizure recurrence within 10 to 15 minutes. When seizures are not controlled or recur subsequent to diazepam administration, the same dose may be repeated every five minutes for a total of three doses. Phenobarbital should be given IV at 1 to 2 mg/lb if seizures are not controlled with diazepam. A similar dose may be repeated every 30 minutes until a maximum of 10 mg/lb has been given. Oral phenobarbital also should be instituted as discussed above as soon as possible. Pentobarbital may be required in animals when seizures cannot be controlled with either diazepam or phenobarbital.

OUTCOME

Seizures often cannot be completely eliminated regardless of the cause. However, most affected animals can have relatively normal lives if appropriate anticonvulsant medication is given. Seizure control is defined as a 50 per cent decrease in seizure frequency without drug intoxication. One study suggested that seizure control can be achieved with phenobarbital in approximately 60 per cent of affected dogs. A slightly higher rate of control may be achieved with primidone, presumably due to the added anticonvulsant effects of PEMA and unmetabolized primidone. The prognosis for dogs in which phenobarbital or primidone is not effective must be guarded. Seizures in certain large dog breeds with idiopathic epilepsy are particularly difficult to control.

16 BEHAVIORAL SIGNS OF ORGANIC DISEASE

ALAN J. PARKER

This chapter deals primarily with the diagnosis of organic diseases of the nervous system and other body systems that produce behavioral changes in the cat or dog.

A behavioral change such as lethargy or withdrawal from contact is exhibited by most sick or injured animals. One client may perceive normal estrus behavior in a cat as the cat being demented. Another client may dismiss the extreme personality loss associated with a brain tumor, as the normal changes of aging. If a clinician is told that a cat is urinating outside its litter box, the initial differential diagnosis might focus on a possible "behavioral problem." If the cat had already been diagnosed as having acute urinary cystitis, then the inappropriate urination would likely be dismissed as a clinical sign that is not "behavioral" in origin. These examples demonstrate that the terms behavioral "changes," "problems," and "signs" are present with most diseases, are hard to define adequately, do not necessarily mean the same thing to everyone, and may be ignored or focused upon.

Making lists of which organic diseases are to be expected with which behavioral changes is not likely to help the reader. This chapter uses one, all-inclusive table (Table 16–1), which ignores most nonorganic behavioral problems. More specific lists are useful for the diagnosis of nonorganic behavioral diseases, such as elimination problems, aggression, or vocalization. These nonorganic behavioral problems are discussed in Chapter 43.

DIAGNOSIS OF BEHAVIORAL SIGNS

A behavioral "sign" in an animal is recognized either by an owner or a clinician when the animal behaves in a way considered abnormal for a given environment or event. An important diagnostic goal is to ascertain if the behavioral change is the result of an organic disease, of a nonorganic "true mental" nature, or a combination.

The word *dementia* is often used by a clinician, if the behavioral signs are severe or disorientation is involved, but it can be logically applied to virtually any abnormal behavior. Neurosis and psychosis are terms rarely used in veterinary medicine. To aid diagnosis, it is preferable to attempt to describe the signs exhibited by the animal rather than use any such general terms. Associating the signs with the environment, events, and past medical history and searching for current disease are vital diagnostic steps. At least a simple neurologic examination is mandatory on any animal with a behavioral sign. Any association of events with feeding or periods of refusal of food must be identified. Depending on the sign shown and the organic diseases suggested by Table 16–1, serum chemistry tests are indicated and perhaps hematology, radiography, and others.

In general, whatever the behavioral sign, the clinician not only examines the patient systemically and neurologically but obtains a wider history and environmental background than is usual with most presenting signs. This is essential to categorize the cases into "true" nonorganic behavioral, organic systemic disease, organic brain, spinal or peripheral nervous system disease, or a combination of organic disease with environmental stress and learnt attention-getting aspects. Effective client education and treatment is built on this foundation.

TYPE OF BEHAVIORAL SIGNS

Aggression. Aggression is a common behavioral sign, and is rarely of pure organic origin. In the initial approach to the patient, aggression should be further defined. The clinician should find out against whom the aggression is directed, under what circumstances it takes place, how often, for how long, and what event triggers it. Does the animal attack, stand its ground, or try to

TABLE 16–1. ORGANIC CAUSES OF BEHAVIORAL CHANGES

(This table ignores most neurotic or relationship causes of behavioral problems seen either in or between the animal and its owner. The relationships between the animal, other animals or humans, and the owner should always be considered before an organic lesion is diagnosed. Past or present organic lesions anywhere in the body may be the initiators or excitors of true behavioral changes.)

I. Brain Lesions and Diseases with Largely Intracranial Signs
- Brain tumor (primary, metastatic, local invasion, multicentric)
- CNS reticulosis/chronic granulomatous meningoencephalitis
- Feline hyperesthesia syndrome. Many cases seem stress-induced and are thus not organic. Multiple etiologies/exciting factors are probable. Also known as psychogenic alopecic dermatitis or neurodermatitis.
- Post-ictal (post-seizure) effects
- Convulsive episodes (especially psychomotor, e.g., some fly-snappers, few tail-chasers)
- Toxicity, e.g., lead poisoning, ethylene glycol, organophosphates, chlorinated hydrocarbons, agene-bleached flour and bleached rawhide dog chews, chocolate, ivermectin, levamisole, or other toxicities. Some food preservatives may produce excitation in some animals.
- Thiamine deficiency/thiaminase toxicity
- Acute or post-encephalitis (canine distemper, FIP, FeLV, toxoplasmosis, pseudorabies, rabies, parainfluenza, migrating parasites, vaccinial encephalitis, systemic lupus erythematosus, immune system reactions, babesia, encephalitozoon and other viruses or rickettsia)
- Intracranial or spinal meningitis (bacterial, fungal, viral, or algal)
- Hepatic encephalopathy (cirrhosis, portacaval shunt, urea cycle enzyme deficiency)
- Sedatives, tranquilizers, anticonvulsants, and other mood-altering drugs
- Hallucinogenic (therapeutic or recreational) drugs (especially amphetamines or morphine overdose in cats and marijuana)
- Acute brain trauma at post-trauma (including projectile)
- Acute or post-cerebral anoxia of respiratory, cardiac or vascular origin with or without anesthetic (even if the anesthesia period was "uneventful")
- Acute cerebrovascular accident (CVA), residual effects of CVA. Also known as stroke, feline ischemic encephalopathy, or polioencephalomalacia. Known causes include thrombocytopenia, coagulopathy, atherosclerosis, vasculitis, thrombosis, embolus, and hemorrhage.
- Hydrocephalus (juvenile, decompensating, occult, acquired)
- Idiopathic "senile" brain degenerations or generalized chronic encephalopathies, e.g., old dog encephalitis, unknown degeneration
- Face-rubbing syndrome (with front paws or on floor) cranial fifth sensory neuropathy or "attention-getting" (more common in small dogs)
- Lysosomal enzyme deficiency diseases or other inherited CNS degenerations
- True hyperkinesis (not just hyperexcitable), diagnosed by paradoxical response to amphetamines
- Various unprovoked aggression syndromes not of a dominance, sexual, or territorial nature, i.e., not a simple behavior problem (mental lapse or sleep disorientation aggression syndromes)

II. Diseases with PNS Spinal Cord Lesions
- Tumor, inflammation, vasculitis, trauma, necrosis, granuloma, disk compression, and immune-mediated, viral, toxic, and post-inflammatory conditions of the PNS (nerve root tumor especially) and spinal cord or even brain (inflammation or stroke) in which a pain, dysesthesia, or hyperesthesia is produced so that the animal licks, scratches, or chews a limited area. These are all rare except for tumor and disk nerve root entrapment; most cases of "neuritis" are a true behavioral mutilation, e.g., attention-getting, stress effect.
- $L_{6-7}S_{1-3}$ nerve root lesions (bowel habit changes and pain), e.g., fractures, infections, tumors, instability, disk
- Dancing Doberman syndrome (possibly a sensory/motor myoneuropathy of the hind legs)

III. Some Potentially Confusing "Behavior Problems" (real or misinterpretation) **and Diseases with Non-Nervous System Lesions** (most likely signs are specified)
- Estrus behavior (especially cats)—client interpretation
- Owner's misinterpretation of normal cat or dog activities (play, aggression, territoriality, sexual behavior)
- Puberty (physical and mental maturation)
- Feline hyperesthesia syndrome (see CNS above)—many cases seem primarily nonorganic in origin
- Lick granuloma, flank-sucking, head-bobbing, jaw-champing, most tail-chasers, self-mutilation, some fly-snappers, for behavioral reasons such as attention-getting, vice, boredom, obsession, exteriorization of inner tensions or stress, relief of unreachable or generalized pruritus
- Hyper- or hypothyroidism (cholesterol elevation) (lethargy, disorientation, excitement, hyperactive, pica, polydipsia)
- Hyper- or hypoadrenocorticism (lethargy, pica, polydipsia, withdrawal)
- Hypoglycemia, hypocalcemia, diabetes mellitus, diabetes insipidus, medullary washout (weakness, lethargy, disorientation, tremors, seizures, inappropriate bowel habits)
- Any organic cause of change in bowel or urinary habits (e.g., cystitis, prostatitis, female hormone-dependent incontinence, any cause of polyuria or polydipsia) (inappropriate urination/defecation)
- Arthritis, polymyositis, temporo-masseter myositis (eosinophilic/atrophic forms) (pain, withdrawal, anorexia, tremors, lethargy)
- Vitreous degeneration of eye (possibly rare cases of fly-snapping, visual hallucinations)
- Fleas or any pruritic skin disease (self-mutilation)
- Old age (lethargy)
- Body trauma (lethargy, pain)
- Steatitis (pain)
- Any systemic disease, pyrexia, or other cause of depression/withdrawal
- Pain of undiagnosed cause
- Abscess (depression, anorexia, pain)
- Anal gland inflammation/impaction (tail-chasing, self-mutilation)

back away? Animals *mutilating* themselves (exhibiting self-aggression) by *licking*, *chewing*, *scratching*, and *rubbing* a part of their body can be similarly characterized. The clinician should verify the part of the body involved, stress in environment, presence of owner while the activity occurs (attention-getting), evidence of pain or limp or sudden cries, and present (tumor PNS or cord, disk problems) or previous diseases (otitis, anal gland irritation, fleas, strokes, disk problems, canine distemper).

Fear, Disorientation, Lethargy. Animals hiding, cowering, exhibiting tremors, being unresponsive, disoriented, lethargic, or dull should be palpated for a pain focus, examined for systemic disease signs, and have their senses of hearing and sight examined. The frequency and duration of these events is significant; most focal and diffuse brain diseases can cause these nonspecific signs. This group of signs is frequently caused by systemic metabolic diseases listed in Part III of Table 16–1.

Personality Changes. Changes of personality may be either to or from being friendly, aggressive, dominant, solitary, gregarious, irritable, and so on. Descriptions of the signs and their frequency, progression, or acute nature are necessary. Diffuse and focal CNS diseases and systemic metabolic diseases must all be considered; these are nonspecific signs.

Changes in Urinary or Bowel Habits. Urinary and bowel habits should be described in the following terms: Does the animal dribble or void in its sleep (female hormone incontinence)? Try to get to the appropriate place to relieve itself (polyuria)? Does it even get close to the place? Is it done in front of the owner (attention-getting), on the owner's personal property or furniture, or anywhere the animal happens to be at the time? Does the animal adopt an elimination posture (true behavioral) or does it drip or drop stool (organic)? Does it eliminate in a particular spot (territory), or after a seizure? Are there other animals in the house (territory marking)? If so, when did they arrive or are they sick?

Repetitive Behaviors. Fly-snapping, head-bobbing, tail-chasing, and flank-sucking activities must be correlated with environmental and family emotional events or changes, especially of a stressful nature. They are usually nonorganic in origin. Animals may react rapidly to emotional changes in their owners, perhaps even before the owner realizes there has been a change. Evidence that these might be "motor release" or "attention-getting" events should be looked for. *Excessive amounts of normal activities* such as hissing, back twitching, and running about need to be similarly correlated with the environment.

Pacing and Circling. Pacing and circling are likely to be acute or progressively more constant activities accompanied by neurologic deficits or signs (e.g., conscious proprioception loss, head tilt, seizure). Diffuse degenerative CNS diseases or focal brain lesions such as tumor, stroke, or encephalitis are likely. *Aimless vocalization*, not of the separation anxiety type, may be caused by similar diseases or even deafness.

Severe Disorientation or Hysteria. Animals severely out of touch with their environment, *totally disoriented*, or *hysterical* usually do not present a diagnostic challenge because evidence of organic diseases (brain tumor, encephalitis, hepatitis) or historical suspicion (toxicity, seizures, trauma) is usually obtained in such extreme cases.

CLIENT RELATIONS

Apart from the extent of the history-taking in cases with behavioral signs, some other aspects of diagnosis and client relations must be emphasized. The clinician must become accustomed to using the expression, "*We don't know why* an animal does this" (e.g., head bob) or "*We can't explain* how an animal starts or learns this activity" (e.g., fly-snapping). Suggestions can be made such as a "stress-induced motor release similar to finger nail chewing in humans" or "inherited motor pattern being exhibited inappropriately," but these are only opinions.

The clinician should not be surprised by any behavioral sign. A logical explanation for all aspects of a sign will not always be apparent. The client's description of a sign is generally accurate, even if the clinician cannot believe that such a sign could occur in such circumstances. It is essential to respect the client's description and opinion initially, even if the opinion later proves to be inaccurate (e.g., the mutilation is a classic attention-getting phenomenon rather than a neuritis). Respect enhances client confidence, which makes client education easier.

The clinician should never underestimate the ability of stress (environmental, population, emotional, pain, irritation, disease) to produce or affect the frequency of any behavioral sign. Just because the mechanism of the stress effect cannot be easily explained does not mean the behavioral sign did not occur or there is no connection. Stress may increase seizure frequency in epileptics, precipitate colitis episodes, cause polydipsia, polyuria and pica, as well as urine marking, roaming, self-mutilation, destruction of property, and aggression.

Learned attention-getting phenomena (tail chasing, paw chewing) can develop rapidly in some dogs if the client provides adequate reinforcement, after even a short-duration organic lesion of the tail, anal glands, or paw. The vice of carpal-lick granuloma may quickly follow even one episode of general pruritus. Thus, the superimposition of a true behavioral syndrome can quickly follow an organic lesion in some dogs. These phenomena may also start without any identifiable precipitating circumstances. The severity of the self-inflicted injury or the ferocity of the vocalization does not rule out a nonorganic behavioral process.

Aggression episodes usually involve a complete performance of the animal's threat display with all its sympathetic nervous system components. The pupil dilation and intense, nonblinking stare often make clients describe the animal as "glassy-eyed" and "not itself." This is often attributed to a seizure rather than a simple behavioral change. Even if the client describes the animal as being apologetically friendly immediately after the episode, it should not generally be interpreted as a seizure.

Clients tend to interpret most *mutilation, tail-chasing*, and *excessive grooming* activities as a response to a sensation of pain or pruritus. They look for a diagnosis of a focal lesion such as a disc rupture or a neuritis. It is hard for them to accept that a dog might chew a toe or its tail off just to get attention, or that a cat licks all its hair off because of stress. Most severe self-mutilation cases are not attributable to organic disease; most are behavioral responses even if originally set up or triggered by a temporary organic lesion (e.g., anal glands, fleas). Complications in treatment, diagnosis, and client education arise if such a behavioral mutilator is affected again by any pruritic process, such as fleas. Appropriate drug treatment may have to be added to that of a behavioral approach. Without adequate explanation, this causes the client to doubt your original diagnosis of a nonorganic behavioral problem.

Many clients do not like to hear that their animal has a *stress-related disease* or a behavioral problem not explainable in terms of an organic disease; they think it reflects a failing on their part. Diplomacy is required, but the following points can help if your diagnosis involves stress or a lack of organic disease. Emphasize that the stress need not be unpleasant stress; any change of routine is stressful to some animals. Explain that some animals seem more affected by minor stresses than others. Explain that some animals seem inherently more aggressive (dominant) and the animal training methods used by most people will not be effective for such animals; only experienced trainers may ever be able to handle such animals. Point out that urine marking, learned attention-getting, and separation anxiety do not necessarily result from a deprived home life; more likely they represent an overreaction by the animal to what are normal events in most animals' lives. In general, it achieves little to blame anything directly on the client. The client's emotional state may be partly to blame for the animal's problem; making the client feel worse about himself or herself is unlikely to help. Any treatment suggestions, for a case with a behavioral sign of an organic and/or nonorganic origin, should begin with a joint shouldering of the burden by simply using the pronoun "we," e.g., "We are going to have to work at this and see how well we can do."

DIAGNOSTIC GOALS

Although a primary goal in the diagnosis and treatment of behavioral signs is to decide if the case has an organic and/or nonorganic cause, this is not always possible. The final diagnosis of the cause of behavioral signs is often inexact and may leave the clinician frustrated at the lack of hard data and complexity of possible alternative interpretations of events. The clinician may be confused because certain aspects of the case indicate organic disease while others imply a learned response or nonorganic disease. It is easier to live with this frustration when one views the diseases in question as a continuous spectrum and the animal's behavioral responses to events as exactly what they are: an individual's unusual responses that are not always easily explained. In such situations, client education and therapy have to involve suitable behavioral training as well as appropriate drugs.

The spectrum of diseases causing behavioral signs begins with "true" nonorganic, sexual, dominance, or other relationship entities and blends into stress-induced responses, self-mutilation responses triggered by organic disease, or learned responses. Next come poorly understood entities such as hyperkinesis and mental lapse aggression syndrome, perhaps caused by minimal brain damage (e.g., at birth) or a catecholamine dysfunction. This leads into true organic diseases of the nervous and other body systems (e.g., tumor, stroke, infection, toxicity). This spectrum is similar to that of epilepsy, other seizure disorders, dreams, sleep disorders, and narcolepsy. Some cases seem to fall somewhere between specific named disease states.

SPECIFIC DISEASE STATES

Each of the diseases listed in Table 16–1 has a tendency to produce a certain group of behavioral signs. The most likely behavioral signs caused by each of these diseases is outlined here. Most other neurologic deficits and clinical signs are not discussed.

A *brain tumor* and *CNS reticulosis* usually produce a slow progression from dulling of the personality, aimless and constant pacing, circling, nonrecognition of familiar people and objects, to lethargy, obtundation, and seizures. Signs tend to be constant. Aggression is an unusual sign. The *feline hyperesthesia syndrome* is characterized by episodes of either excessive grooming, sometimes to the point of virtual baldness from the neck caudally (psychogenic alopecic dermatitis, PAD) and/or excessive twitching of the back, hissing, sudden body jerks, running wildly, apparent disorientation and fear, irritability, intolerance of being petted, and occasionally, attacking the owners. Epileptic *seizures* can produce wild postictal signs, ranging from fear, disorientation, pacing, thirst, hunger, and nonrecognition of the owner to depression and withdrawal. Signs are episodic. Aggression is rarely seen unless the animal is cornered. Some psychomotor seizures produce only behavioral signs, e.g., cases with disorientation episodes, some fly-snappers, a few tail-chasers, and rare cases with unexplained aggressive episodes. *Toxic agents* can collectively cause any behavioral sign(s) either episodic or continuous. Worthy of note are lead and some rawhide dog chews (if bleached by agene). Both are capable of producing hysterical episodes, often leading to seizures. Other toxic agents can occasionally cause self-mutilation.

Encephalitis can also produce the entire spectrum of behavioral signs from aggression to withdrawal, loss of any social or bowel habit, nonrecognition of the owner, self-mutilation and wild hysteria. Signs may be episodic or constant. *Hepatic encephalopathy* tends to lead to episodes of several hours of depression, pacing, disorientation, blindness, coma, and seizures rather than aggression. These episodes may develop within a few hours of a high protein meal. In terminal cases with cirrhosis, signs may become constantly progressive. *Drugs* tend to produce depression or seizures but some *hallucinogens* can produce wild behavior, including howling, pacing, and the following of imaginary objects on the walls or floor.

Brain trauma and episodes of *cerebral hypoxia* do not usually present as a diagnostic problem, but clients should be warned that changed bowel habits, disorientation, and loss of owner recognition may be permanent deficits even in cases where the animal makes a rapid motor recovery. *Strokes* occur in the cat from six months of age and in the dog from two years of age. Profound, constant, and often long-term or permanent behavioral changes may follow a stroke even if a good motor recovery occurs rapidly. A calm animal may become vicious or vice versa, all social habits and owner recognition may be lost, or the animal may just remain disorientated. *Hydrocephalus* usually produces dullness, lethargy, disorientation, and coma rather than aggression. Signs may be acute and progressive at any age or insidious. "Senile" *brain* and *inherited CNS degenerations* can mimic the signs of a brain tumor but rarely cause seizures. *Facial rubbing syndrome* is self-explanatory mutilation/pruritic syndrome. It is usually bilateral. It is often aggravated by stress and the presence of the owner but usually responds to corticosteroids; hence, it may be an attention-getting phenomenon and/or a sensory neuropathy. True *hyperkinesis* is rare in dogs, unreported in cats, and characterized diagnostically by a paradoxical calming response to amphetamines. Excitable, nervous animals should not be automatically diagnosed as hyperkinetics.

Mental lapse aggression syndrome is a behavioral, and perhaps catecholamine dysfunction-induced syndrome, characterized by unprovoked and unexplained attacks on companion animals or people with whom the dog is normally on good terms. *Sleep disorientation aggression* is characterized by the animal waking in an aggressive threat display. Both are highly dangerous syndromes; euthanasia should be recommended. Sometimes they may be diagnosed as a psychomotor seizure. There is no evidence of their being forms of epilepsy. *Dancing Doberman syndrome* is said to occur when a dog, usually a Doberman, constantly picks up one hind leg in turn while standing still. It can usually sit and move normally and does not lick or mutilate the limbs. The activity may suggest a hyperactive syndrome to some observers.

Among other diseases in Table 16–1, only a few require specific explanation here. Most are self-explanatory or can be read about in later chapters of this text. *Flank-sucking*, *head-bobbing*, and *jaw-champing* are common Doberman behavioral traits, aggravated by stress and usually unresponsive to medical treatment, except tranquilizers or sedatives. Behavioral modification may help.

The metabolic diseases listed in part III of Table 16–1 are the ones most likely to present with signs interpretable as behavioral. Changes in body glucose, calcium, sodium, potassium, and hormones can have surprising effects on alertness, personality, orientation, and response to the environment or people, as well as appetite, thirst, and elimination habits.

17 OCULAR MANIFESTATIONS OF SYSTEMIC DISEASE

KATHLEEN L. BOLDY and BERNARD CLERC

The eye provides the astute clinician with a noninvasive method of observing internal mechanisms. The purpose of this chapter is to encourage complete ocular assessment with every physical examination and to provide guidelines for correlating ophthalmic abnormalities with systemic disease.

DIAGNOSTIC PRINCIPLES

Knowledge of techniques for ophthalmic exam and of normal ophthalmic variations provides a foundation for the evaluation of ocular structures. To identify whether an ocular abnormality is related to internal disease, additional testing procedures such as blood panels, urinalysis, and radiography are often necessary. Breed and hereditary predispositions offer valuable clues for distinguishing primary and secondary ocular conditions.

Inflammation and hemorrhage are important heralds of systemic dysfunction. Inflammation can occur in periocular tissue, representing immune-mediated or infectious dermatopathies, or in uveal tissue, reflecting many types of internal trouble. Granulomatous inflammation should be distinguished from nongranulomatous disease, since awareness of these different pathologic processes can help pinpoint etiology. Hemorrhage not associated with a history or signs of trauma should be fully evaluated, as ocular findings may be the first indication of clotting defects, systemic hypertension, or neoplasia.

THERAPEUTIC PRINCIPLES

It is beyond the scope of this chapter to discuss particular ocular treatment regimens. The ability to recognize the systemic disease allows the reader to find details of general therapeutic management in other chapters of this text. However, the eye often requires specific therapy or localized intensive medication. A few basic principles provide a template for action.

The anterior segment (i.e., external eye, anterior chamber, iris, and ciliary body) benefits from topical medication. Although systemic therapy is often indicated, therapeutic levels of topically administered drugs aid in assuaging anterior ocular disease. Posterior ocular abnormalities (those involving the vitreous, retina, and optic nerve) do not benefit from topically-applied drugs unless they are applied frequently enough to provide systemic therapeutic concentrations. For posterior abnormalities, subconjunctival or systemic treatment is indicated.

Effective ocular therapy preserves vision. The requirement for clarity dictates that inflammation be effectively controlled. Concurrent anti-inflammatory medications (preferably nonsteroidal) may be indicated in the course of treating ocular infections that threaten function by destroying clarity, apposition of the retina and choroid, or iridal movement. Resolution of an infection may be followed by anti-inflammatory therapy (steroidal) to decrease scarring and preserve visual acuity. Topical atropine may be administered to relieve ciliary spasm and pain, and to prevent development of synechiae in many diseases, with the important exception of most glaucomas. Notations are made in this chapter following discussion of diseases that require definitive ocular treatment that is not found elsewhere in the text or applications that are not easily inferred from these rudimentary ocular principles.

DERMATOLOGIC DISEASE

Ocular abnormalities associated with disease of the skin and mucous membranes may involve any part of the eye or its adnexa. Integumentary disorders are often breed-related, and can have systemic consequences (see Chapter 2).

Allergic and Immune-Mediated Skin Conditions

Immediate Reactions. The immediate type lesion (histamine and IgE-mediated disease) is seen after food absorption, insect bites, and drug administration. Swelling of eyelid and conjunctival tissue is rapid and impressive. It usually resolves spontaneously but may be helped by the parenteral administration of antihistamine and corticosteroids.

Delayed Reactions. Delayed ocular allergic reactions may occur in sensitized animals. A higher incidence is noted in certain breeds, the American cocker spaniel, for example. Allergens are pollens, dust, and bacterial toxins. Eyelids and conjunctiva may appear red and swollen in dogs with atopic disease. Chronic blepharoconjunctivitis may be complicated by infection. Diagnosis is thus difficult and may require allergy skin testing. Routine management is achieved with topical and general corticosteroids; superinfection can only be controlled by antibiotics. Effective disease control requires at least two weeks of therapy.

Blepharitis. Blepharitis may be part of a generalized or of an extensive immunologic disease with pemphigus-like lesions, discoid lupus lesions, and lupus erythematosus disseminated (LED) lesions. Although commonly associated with nose lesions, the blepharitis itself is not specific and exact diagnosis is made after biopsy using pathologic examination and immune fluorescence. Treatment is that of the generalized disease (i.e., immunosuppressive drugs).

Keratoconjunctivitis Sicca (KCS). This is also, in most cases, an immune-mediated disease and part of a sicca syndrome. A breed predilection for the miniature schnauzer, cocker spaniel, and West Highland white terrier has been reported. However, the disease can be seen in every breed and age. Pathology indicates the lymphoplasmocytic infiltration of lacrimal glands and labial glands. It has been shown that there is a general immunologic reaction in a high percentage of dogs: antinuclear antibody 41 per cent, rheumatoid factor 32 per cent, antisalivary glands 27 per cent. An equivalent of the Sjögren syndrome, characterized by keratoconjunctivitis sicca–xerostomia and a connective tissue disease, or of the sicca syndrome (dry eye and dry mouth), has been identified in the dog. Etiologic treatment is use of systemic immunosuppressive drugs; the disease is usually not severe enough to justify such treatment.

Dry eye syndrome may also be the consequence of long-term medical treatment for other systemic diseases. Salicylazosulphapyridine, phenazopyridine, sulfadiazine, sulfasalazine, and other sulfonamides can be responsible for KCS, and the authors have observed other cases associated with pheneturide, or phenytoin administration. Susceptibility of animals is variable and disease may be regressive after cessation of treatment.

Uveitis. Uveitis may just be a local reaction (i.e., traumatic uveitis, lens-induced uveitis) or the reaction of an immunocompetent tissue when antigens in the eye are processed in distant sites. Sensitized lymphocytes migrate toward the antigen, enter the uvea, and produce antibodies with immune complex formation in the eye or sensitized cell reaction.

Some of the generalized infectious diseases that cause a local reaction of uveitis are listed in Table 17–1. Therapy comprises both the suppression of the immunostimulating agent and the nonspecific treatment of uveitis (i.e., immunosuppressive therapy and atropine).

Uveodermatologic Syndrome. A uveodermatologic syndrome characterized by chronic or recurrent uveitis and dermal depigmentation has been described in several breeds of dogs, including the Akita, Samoyed, Irish setter, Siberian husky, Shetland sheep dog, Ainu, and Shiba. The canine disease has been compared to the Vogt-Koyanagi-Harada syndrome in humans, in which granulomatous uveitis is coupled with poliosis (whitening of the hair), vitiligo (whitening of the skin), dysacousia, and meningitis. Meningitis has not been recognized in the reported canine cases, but the other findings are very similar to the disease affecting humans. Retinal detachment, secondary glaucoma, and cataracts are seen in a high percentage of both canine and human patients. The exact etiology of the diseases has not been identified. Intensive immunosuppressive therapy is necessary.

INFECTIOUS DERMATOLOGIC DISEASE

Staphylococcal Infections. Cutaneous staphylococcal infection of young pups often involves the eyelids. Intense, edematous blepharitis is observed. Staphylococcal skin infections can be generalized or localized in young dogs. Pyoderma can cause blepharitis with swelling and pustule formation. Hot packs, drainage of lid abscesses, and systemic antibiotics are recommended therapy. Nonresponsive cases may be due to immune abnormalities in which systemic anti-inflammatory therapy or staphylococcal bacterins can be used to alter immune responses.

Parasitic Skin Infections. Parasitic skin infections include the demodectic, notoedric, or sarcoptic manges. Dermatophytosis involving the eyelids causes hyper-

TABLE 17–1. INFECTIOUS AND PARASITIC CAUSES OF UVEITIS IN THE DOG

Piroplasmosis	*Babesia canis*
Cryptococcosis	*Cryptococcus* spp.
Blastomycosis	*Blastomyces* spp.
Coccidioidomycosis	*Coccidioides immitis*
Leptospirosis	*Leptospira* spp.
Toxoplasmosis	*Toxoplasma gondii*
Histoplasmosis	*Histoplasma capsulatum*
Leishmaniosis	*Leishmania icterohemorrhagiae*
Canine hepatitis	Canine adenovirus type 1
Tuberculosis	*Mycobacterium tuberculosis*
Brucellosis	*Brucella canis*
Ehrlichiosis	*Ehrlichia canis*
Rocky Mountain spotted fever	*Rickettsia rickettsii*
Ocular filariasis	*Dirofilaria immitis*
Visceral larval migrans	*Toxocara canis*
Geotrichosis	*Geotricha* spp.
Protothecosis	*Prototheca* spp.

emia, and often alopecia, pruritus, and a crusty appearance. Diagnosis is made by the observation of lesions and skin scrapings. Treatment is that of generalized forms. The only precaution is to avoid irritating solutions on the eye.

CONGENITAL AND HEREDITARY INTEGUMENTARY DISORDERS

Pigmentary disorders such as partial or complete albinism can affect the eyes. Cats with white fur and deafness exhibit blue irides. This syndrome is inherited as a dominant autosomal gene with complete penetrance for white fur, and incomplete penetrance for deafness and blue iris. Dogs with partial albinism and deafness can exhibit more serious ocular disorders such as microphthalmia, cataracts, and colobomas of the iris, optic disc, and retina, in addition to the more benign, lightly pigmented irides. The white or merle Australian Shepherd dog also exhibits a syndrome of ocular dysgenesis that can include the problems listed above as well as retinal dysplasia, scleral ectasia, staphyloma, optic nerve hypoplasia, and spherophakia.

The *Chediak-Higashi syndrome* (CHS) has been described in cats (see Chapter 2). Clinical ocular manifestations of CHS include photophobia, partial oculocutaneous albinism, congenital cataracts, nystagmus, and hyperreflectivity of the tapetum. Enlarged cytoplasmic granules have been found in the pigment epithelium, in the choroid, and also in the central nervous system retinal projections. Clinical diagnosis may be confirmed by microscopic studies.

Other rare congenital integumentary abnormalities that can affect eyelid skin include *acanthosis nigricans*, *ichthyosis*, and *Ehlers-Danlos syndrome*.

METABOLIC DISEASES

Diabetes mellitus, a common endocrine disorder in dogs and cats, is associated with a high incidence of bilateral cataracts. Even though small retinal aneurysms are occasionally seen, these animals are spared the blindness associated with retinal neovascular and proliferative changes frequently observed in humans.

The pathogenesis of cataract formation is not completely understood, but current evidence points to osmotic imbalance as the underlying cause. Glucose enters the lens from the aqueous humor, facilitated by transport. Under normal conditions, the majority of lens glucose is converted to lactic acid via the anaerobic glycolytic pathway. High levels of glucose saturate the glycolytic enzymes, notably hexokinase. The usually inactive sorbitol pathway becomes the primary means of glucose metabolism. Aldose reductase converts the sugar to sorbitol, a hydrophilic alcohol that cannot exit the lens. The presence of sorbitol increases intralenticular osmotic pressure. The resultant influx of water leads to swelling, rupture of lens fibers, and cataract formation. In a similar fashion, high plasma levels of galactose or xylose cause the buildup of dulcitol and xylitol, respectively.

Diabetic cataracts exhibit three distinguishing clinical features. The first is rapid development, within a few days in some cases. The second is subepithelial cortical vacuoles apparent in the equatorial region in the early developmental stages of cataract formation. The third is the presence of lens intumescence with clefting of lens sutures in a mature cataract. These characteristics are strongly suggestive of, but not pathognomonic for, diabetes.

Cataract surgery in diabetic patients is highly successful. This elective procedure should be considered only after the diabetes is well-controlled and the animal is exhibiting visual deficits from diffuse, bilateral cataracts. The owner of a diabetic dog should be informed that there is a high probability of cataract development, but that cataract surgery can restore vision if the animal should become blind.

DISORDERS OF LIPID METABOLISM

Hyperlipemia and hyperlipoproteinemia may be associated with *corneal lipodystrophies, lipid-laden aqueous humor,* and *lipemia retinalis*. These ocular signs are clinically striking, may cause disturbance of vision, and aid in the diagnosis of systemic abnormalities.

Lipid deposits in the canine cornea can present as crystalline gray-white lesions in the superficial cornea, which later may extend into the deeper stroma (see Figure 17–1*A*). These deposits should be differentiated from calcium band keratopathy, which can occur secondary to hypercalcemia or chronic severe ocular inflammation. A blood panel identifies hypercalcemia, and ocular examination provides evidence of uveitis or other inflammatory conditions. Lipodystrophies occur frequently as a result of localized ocular disease, but have been reported in dogs with hypercholesterolemia for which hypothyroidism is often the underlying cause. Suspicion of hypothyroidism should be aroused when a rapidly progressing lipid keratopathy occurs in an obese, lethargic dog. Hypothyroidism has also been associated with KCS, and the multiple ocular signs occurring secondary to systemic hypertension.

Lipid-laden aqueous humor has been observed in dogs and a cat with type V chylomicronemia and triglyceride levels elevated to ten times their normal values. Anterior uveitis usually accompanies the anterior chamber lipid. Dietary restriction of fat, and topical application of mydriatics and corticosteroids usually result in clearing of the aqueous humor in five to seven days.

Lipemia retinalis is an uncommon clinical presentation that has been associated with hypercholesterolemia in a dog and iatrogenic diabetes mellitus and Cushing's disease in a cat. Retinal blood vessels appear pink or creamy rather than bright red, and may seem distended (see Figure 17 1*B*). The condition is usually asymptomatic, but its incidental finding should trigger a diagnostic work-up for precipitating metabolic disorders.

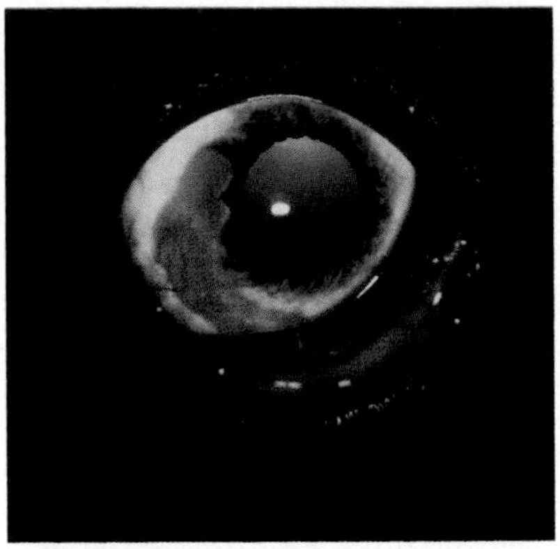

FIGURE 17–1. *A,* Degenerative crystalline superficial keratopathy in a ten-year-old dog with hyperlipidemia secondary to chronic hypothyroid.

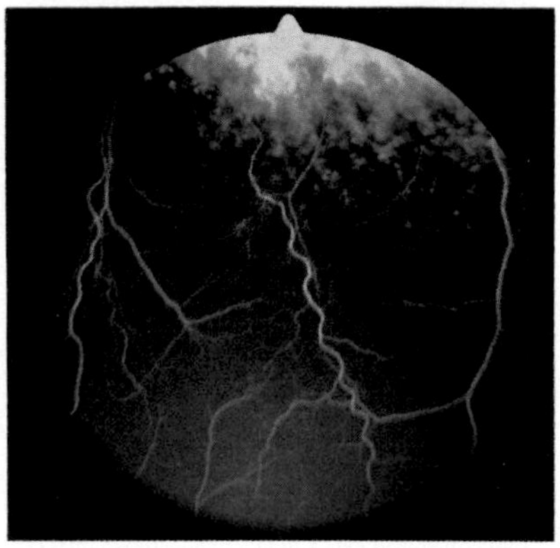

B, Lipemia retinalis.

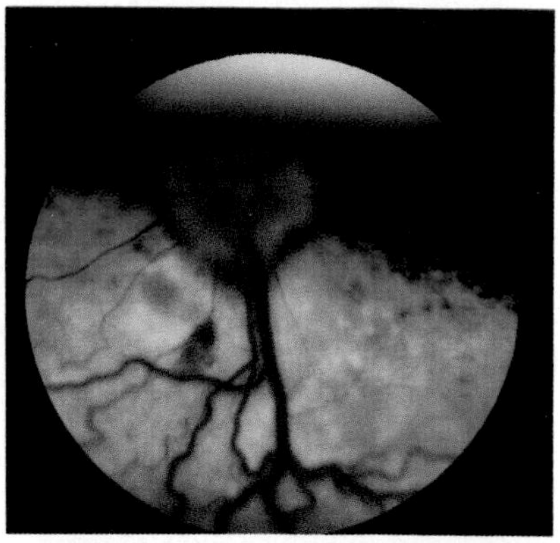

C, Retinal hemorrhage (flame-shaped) and adjacent choroidal ischemia ("cotton spot") in an 11-year-old dog with severe renal failure and systemic hypertension.

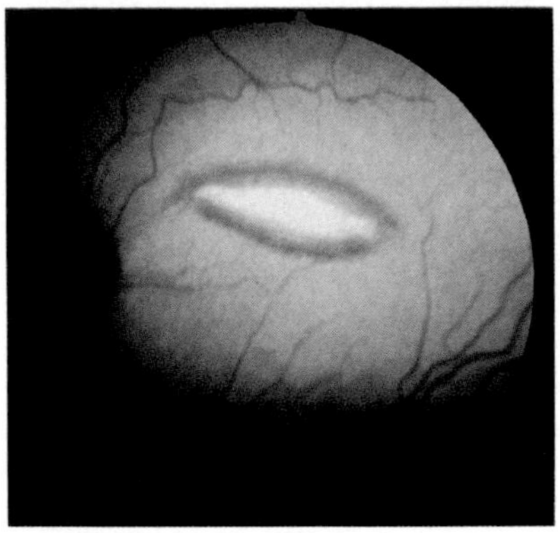

D, Feline central retinal degeneration in a two-year-old cat that was fed dog food as a primary diet.

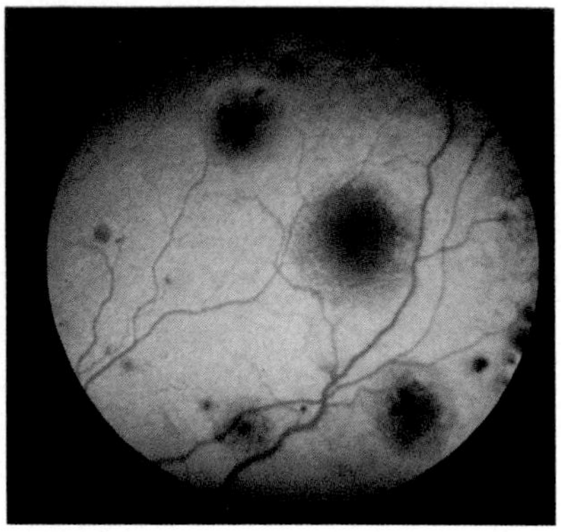

E, Cryptococcosis chorioretinitis in a four-year-old cat exhibiting seizures, lethargy, weight loss, and some visual deficits.

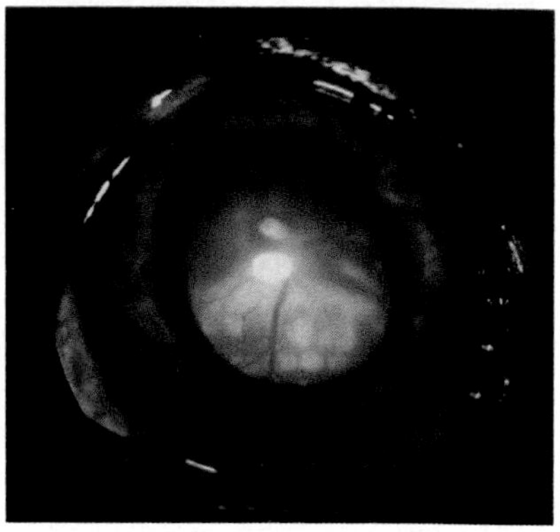

F, Granulomatous retinal detachment in a dog with systemic blastomycosis.

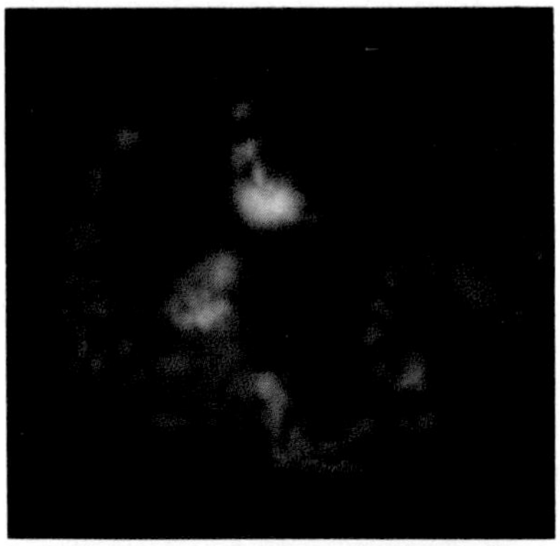

G, Active granulomatous chorioretinitis in a five-year-old dog with protothecosis.

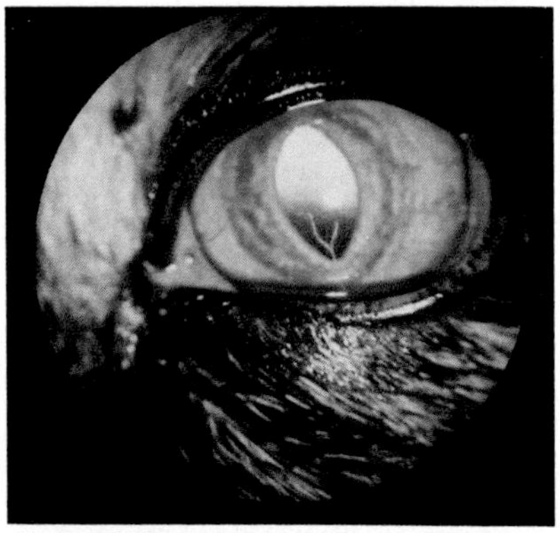

H, Dendritic ulceration in the superficial cornea of a cat with feline herpesvirus.

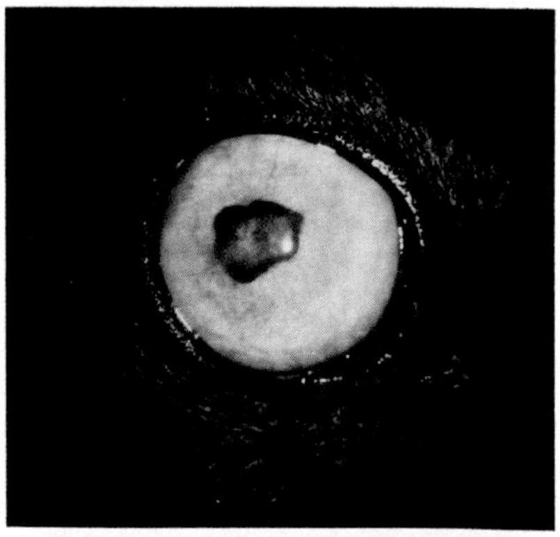

I, Anterior uveitis, cataract, posterior synechia, ansd secondary glaucoma in a ten-year-old cat with feline lymphosarcoma.

INBORN ERRORS OF METABOLISM

Inherited metabolic disorders occur in most domestic species and are models of comparable diseases in humans. Most of these rare disorders are progressive, degenerative conditions of the nervous system. No treatment is effective. Two of the more well-known syndromes are described, and additional storage diseases are listed in Table 17–2.

LIPID STORAGE DISEASE

Neuronal Ceroid Lipofuscinosis. This a genetic syndrome characterized by juvenile amaurosis and central nervous system symptoms, due to the biochemical deficiency of phenylene-diamine-mediated peroxidase. There is a high incidence in setters; the disease is sometimes called "Idiopathic Amaurosis of the English Setter." Clinical signs begin at one year of age, with a decrease in visual acuity, followed by behavioral abnormalities. Nervous symptoms appear with depression, ataxia, muscular pain, and masseter muscle hypersensitivity; convulsions are then observed and animals die approximately one year after the onset of clinical signs. Pathology shows mainly central nervous system lesions–cortical degeneration due to the deposit of ceroid and lipofuscin in the neurons. The same lesions are seen in the ganglion cells of the retina.

Gangliosidosis GMI. This disease is found in the Siamese cat and is inherited as a simple autosomal recessive trait. The enzymatic deficiency is a lack of beta-galactosidase. Visual deficits, multiple opacities in the cornea, and small, gray, multifocal retinal lesions may be observed. Polysaccharide accumulation appears in the corneal endothelium and keratocytes. Glycolipid deposits and subsequent degeneration occur in neurons of the central nervous system, sympathetic ganglia, and the ganglion cells of the retina. Involved neurons appear plump and swollen due to the intracytoplasmic accumulation of the abnormal metabolic products.

VASCULAR DISEASE

Systemic Hypertension. This condition occurs more frequently as a clinical entity in dogs and cats than has been identified previously. Many animals with elevated blood pressure are brought to the veterinarian with suspected primary ocular disease. Newer methods of blood pressure analysis and increased awareness have linked blindness from retinal detachment and intraocular hemorrhage to systemic hypertension. Recognition of the etiology for ophthalmic problems is critical to proper patient management.

Retinal hemorrhage is the hallmark of ocular hypertensive disease. Other ocular signs include nongranulomatous chorioretinitis, exudative retinal detachment, "cotton wool spots" (areas of retinal ischemia in the nerve fiber layer), sclerosis of retinal vasculature, vitreous hemorrhage, secondary uveitis, and glaucoma (see Figure 17–1*C*). Ocular lesions may regress with systemic treatment.

Anemia. Anemia may cause retinal hemorrhages, which are more frequently reported in the cat than in the dog. Low hemoglobin levels (usually less than 5g per 100 ml) are primarily associated with posterior segment hemorrhage; anterior uveal hemorrhage is much less common.

Clotting Disorders. These can initiate ocular signs that may alert the owner and clinician to serious internal problems. Subcutaneous eyelid, subconjunctival, uveal, and retinal hemorrhages have been associated with immune-mediated thrombocytopenia, coumarin toxic-

TABLE 17–2. STORAGE DISEASES OF OPHTHALMIC SIGNIFICANCE

Breed	Syndrome	Clinical Signs
Cairn and West Highland white terrier	Globoid cell leukodystrophy/Krabbe's disease	Ascending paresis and ataxia at 3–6 months of age; cerebellar ataxia and visual deficit. Death before 12 months.
English setter	Lipodystrophy, neuronal ceroid lipofuchsinosis/ juvenile amaurotic familial idiocy	Ataxia and visual deficit at 6–12 months; "dummy" attitude, convulsions. Death by 2 years.
German short hair pointer	Lipodystrophy, GM_2 gangliosidosis	As for English setter.
Chihuahua	Neuronal ceroid lipofuchsinosis/Kuf's disease	Incoordination, restlessness, progressing blindness to 24 months.
Dachshund	Neuronal ceroid lipofuchsinosis/Kuf's disease	Cerebellar ataxia, onset at 3 years, still progressing at 4–5 years.
Bluetick hound	Globoid cell leukodystrophy/Krabbe's disease	Ascending paresis, tremors, proprioceptive deficit and death by 8 months of age.
Beagle	Globoid cell leukodystrophy/Krabbe's disease	Paraparesis and dysmetria at 4 months.
Australian silky terrier	Neurovisceral glucocerebroside storage disease/ Gaucher's disease	Incoordination, hyperkinesis, exaggeration of spinal reflexes at 8 months.
Lapland	Glycogen storage disease type II/Pompe's disease	Dysphagia and vomiting at 1½ years.
Siamese	Mucopolysaccharidosis	Facial joint and skeletal deformities, multifocal spinal cord disease, cloudy cornea, and retinal atrophy.
Domestic short hair	GM_1 gangliosidosis	Ataxia and tremor at weaning; lethargy, gross ataxia and hypermetria, intention tremor, and visual deficit at 2–3 months; corneal opacity and retinal lesions.
Siamese	Sphingomyelin lipidosis/Niemann-Pick disease	Cerebellar disturbance at 4 months progressing to death at 9 months.
Siamese	GM_1 gangliosidosis	Tremors, progressive paresis, and ataxia at 4 months; tetraplegia at 6 months.

ity, disseminated intravascular coagulation (DIC), and other diseases that disrupt normal clotting activity. Vacuolar disruption of the pigment epithelium and thrombotic occlusion of the choriocapillaris have been reported with DIC.

Polycythemia. Polycythemia or other secondary hypoxic conditions that elevate packed cell volume may cause retinal vessels to be visibly distended, tortuous, and dark. Retinal or vitreal hemorrhage and retinal detachment have been reported.

Other Problems. Hyperviscosity syndromes, hypergammaglobulinemia, and specific canine monoclonal gammopathies (plasma cell myeloma) have been associated with retinal hemorrhage and detachment or in association with immune-mediated bleeding tendencies.

NUTRITIONAL DISORDERS

Taurine Deficiency. This is an important diagnostic consideration in cats with central retinal or panretinal degeneration. Affected animals show bilateral elliptical hyperreflective lesions in the area centralis in early stages of the disease (see Figure 17–1*D*). If taurine remains deficient in the young feline diet, retinal degeneration can be diffuse and blindness may result. Clinical cases have been identified in cats fed purified casein, vegetarian, or dog food diets. Experimental disease has been reported in animals receiving taurine-free diets.

Taurine is an aminosulfonic acid that is necessary for normal retinal function and structure. Cats appear to be incapable of producing taurine adequately from precursors. The histologic findings include loss of photoreceptor outer segments.

Thiamin Deficiency. Thiamin deficiency may occur in cats after prolonged anorexia. The condition is associated with eating raw fish that contains thiaminase and with eating commercial pet foods in which the thiamin was destroyed during processing. The pupils of an affected animal become dilated and fixed, although vision is retained. Papilledema and retinal neovascularization have been observed.

Vitamin A Deficiency. Vitamin A deficiency is a very rare disorder in dogs and cats, but if it occurs, ophthalmic manifestations may be apparent. Night blindness can be observed; retinal changes are characterized by altered reflectivity of the tapetal retina. Xerophthalmia (literally, "dry eye") is a common presentation in people of Third World countries where nutrition is poor and malabsorption may be found from high loads of intestinal parasitism. An entire spectrum of disease is seen, including retinopathy, conjunctival and corneal xerosis, corneal ulceration and melting, and less obvious changes in the epithelial structure of a number of organs. The process is reversible if diagnosis is made and treatment is instituted early in the course of the disease. Research was recently undertaken to identify localized vitamin A deficiencies in dogs with keratoconjunctivitis sicca. Such deficiencies can be caused by abnormal metabolism of the vitamin.

Vitamin E Deficiency. This condition in the dog has been accompanied by the development of ocular lesions similar to central retinal atrophy. The first change is a fine mottling in the central retina. This mottling increases and affected animals become night blind, then eventually completely blind. The syndrome rarely has been reported clinically. Advanced histologic findings are extensive retinal degeneration involving the outer rod and cone segments and the outer nuclear and plexiform layers. Retinal pigment epithelium may migrate through the degenerated retina.

Other Deficiencies. Deficiencies associated with milk replacements have been described in newborn puppies. Replacements for bitch's milk may be associated with the development of cataracts, which usually occur in the posterior cortical area and do not cause blindness. After the affected animals are fed solid food, the new lens growth is normal. Although the pathogenesis is uncertain, amino acid deficiency or galactose excess may be responsible.

INFECTIOUS DISEASES IN THE DOG

In the dog, there are two main manifestations of ocular diseases in relationship with an infectious disease. Either the agent has a special tropism for one part of the eye, where it replicates (e.g., distemper virus in the neuroretina), or the uvea of the eye (highly immune-reactive) is sensitized to a foreign agent after the breakdown of the blood-aqueous barrier. In the latter case, the eye reacts in a singular manner—uveitis (canine hepatitis virus, *Brucella canis*, *Mycobacterium tuberculosis*) in reaction to the stimulus of an infectious agent (see Table 1–1).

PARASITIC DISEASES

Toxoplasmosis. Toxoplasmosis is a disease caused by a widespread coccidial protozoa, *Toxoplasma gondii*, in which the cat is the definitive host. The focus of the disease can be the digestive or respiratory apparatus, the muscles, the central nervous system, or the eye.

Ocular lesions in toxoplasmosis may be anterior and/or posterior. Anterior uveitis can be exudative or granulomatous in the cat; generally granulomatous inflammation is seen in the dog. Chorioretinitis, retinal detachment, and retinal necrosis have been reported. Nonspecific lesions include cell perivascular cuffings and granulomatous retinal infiltration around toxoplasmic pseudocysts. In dogs, distemper and toxoplasmosis can occur together in young immunodeficient animals.

Since 60 per cent of all cats and 25 per cent of all dogs have been in contact with *Toxoplasma gondii*, and show positive IgG- and IgM-specific serum antibody, diagnosis by serology is difficult. A rising antibody titer is indicative of current disease. Granulomatous uveitis or retinal lesions associated with a dye test value above 1024 suggests recent infection. Ocular antibody formation can also be studied by aqueous examination. A positive response indicates an ocular infection.

Clinical disease requires medical treatment, but the response of animals is inconsistent. Pyrimethamine and sulfonamide are used (see Chapter 46).

Leishmaniasis. Leishmaniasis is an endemic disease affecting human beings and mammals in Southern Europe (around the Mediterranean), Africa, Asia, and South America. The causative organism is *Leishmania donovani* var. infantum, a hemoflagellate protozoa. The dog is an important reservoir for the parasite. Transmission of the parasite is due to a sandfly, genus *Phlebotomus.*

The parasite first develops in the reticulo-histiocytic system, but lesions are prominent in lymph nodes, spleen, skin, nose, and eye (see Chapters 2 and 46).

Ocular signs can be associated with general disease or seem apparently isolated. Chronic keratoconjunctivitis and keratouveitis are the prominent signs. "Spectacle blepharitis" with squamosis and loss of hair is characteristic. Acute conjunctivitis is the rule, although nodular conjunctivitis has been described. Chemosis and keratitis occur very frequently. Granulomatous and nongranulomatous uveitis are observed; anterior uveitis is the most frequent. Fundus lesions associate hyalitis and chorioretinitis with retinal hemorrhages. Long-term keratouveitis leads to blindness. Complicating immunologic reactions in the eye can continue for years. Clinical diagnosis is confirmed by indirect immunofluorescence, or the organisms can be identified in the bone marrow. An amastigot form is detected in the cells after May-Grünwald and Giemsa staining.

Current treatment with ethylstibamine and pentamidine does not cure the disease. It offers a remission, but animals must be treated when serologic reactions turn positive again.

Ehrlichiosis. Ehrlichiosis (tropical canine pancytopenia) is associated with ocular signs that include conjunctivitis, corneal opacities, conjunctival hemorrhage, and hyphema. In the early stages of experimentally induced disease, retinal vascular engorgement accompanies the initial febrile response. Horseshoe-shaped gray, perivascular lesions characteristic of nongranulomatous chorioretinitis develop and later regress, resulting in focal or diffuse retinal atrophy. Extensive subretinal hemorrhage can lead to retinal detachment. Anterior uveitis, hyphema, and corneal opacities from the deposition of cellular precipitates occur frequently (see Chapter 46).

Ophthalmomyiasis. Ophthalmomyiasis is the presence of parasitic larval stages of certain dipterous flies in the orbit and accessory organs of the eye (ophthalmomyiasis externa) or within the globe (ophthalmomyiasis interna). Ophthalmomyiasis interna may be anterior when the larvae are found in the anterior segment and posterior when larvae are found posterior to the lens. There have been reports of ophthalmomyiasis interna occurring in four cats and a dog. Clinical abnormalities included uveitis, multiple curvilinear tracks involving both tapetal and nontapetal fundi, and low-grade chorioretinitis.

Other Diseases. *Rocky Mountain spotted fever* is a rare rickettsial infection that can cause scleral vascular congestion, conjunctivitis, chemosis, and mucopurulent ocular discharge. Petechial retinal hemorrhages, anterior uveitis with deep corneal vascularization, corneal edema, aqueous flare, and miosis have been described.

Visceral larval migrans, caused by the migratory stages of *Toxocara canis*, may result in ocular granulomatous inflammation. Rare instances of chorioretinal granulomas, endophthalmitis with exudative retinal detachments, and optic neuritis have been reported. The ocular reaction associated with larval infestation may be acute or chronic, depending upon the location of the parasite and the foreign body reaction elicited.

Ocular filariasis results from invasion of the anterior chamber and vitreous by immature heartworms, *Dirofilaria immitis*. Chronic, low-grade anterior uveitis may be associated with the worm and/or a toxic effect of its metabolic products. Diagnosis is based on clinical observation and treatment is surgical removal of the offending worm in conjunction with appropriate systemic therapy (see Chapter 80).

BACTERIA AND MYCOBACTERIA

Intraocular inflammation can be induced by primary foci of bacterial infection elsewhere in the body. Endophthalmitis, intraretinal hemorrhage, and toxic anterior uveitis have been reported in dogs with endocarditis and pyometra. Systemic infection with *Brucella canis* may cause chronic anterior uveitis or endophthalmitis, and *Leptospira icterohaemorrhagiae* has been associated with episcleral injection, yellowing of the sclera, conjunctival petechiae, and anterior uveitis. The severity of the ocular signs depends upon the extent and virulence of the infectious organism. Any intraocular hemorrhage or inflammation of undetermined etiology should alert the clinician to possibilities of metastatic bacterial infection (see Chapter 46).

Tuberculosis has been reported to cause ocular granulomatous inflammation in the cat. Primary conjunctival lesions, nodular choroiditis with associated retinal detachment, and anterior uveitis have been identified with the bovine strain of *Mycobacterium tuberculosis*. Direct contact, hematogenous dissemination, and congenital infection are the proposed routes of ocular entry (see Chapter 46).

FUNGUS AND ALGAE

Granulomatous inflammation characterizes the ocular response to mycotic and algal pathogens. Hematogenous spread accounts for ocular infection in most cases; the well-vascularized uvea is often the target.

Cryptococcosis is a worldwide pansystemic disease, which can produce subretinal granulomas, retinal detachments, hyphema, anisocoria, papilledema, papillitis, and orbital cellulitis. Choroidal granulomas appear gray-white, but can become hyperpigmented as they regress to chorioretinal scars in the course of medical therapy (see Figure 17–1*E*). The organisms have a predilection for the meninges and brain, and can migrate via direct anterior extension from the brain to the eyes.

Systemic *blastomycosis* can be associated with severe granulomatous chorioretinitis with retinal detachment, optic neuritis, anterior uveitis, and secondary glaucoma (see Figure 17–1*F*). Multiple organism-containing granulomas in the optic nerve, and lesions in iris, ciliary body, sclera, and peripheral cornea have been described. Ocular histopathology may include extensive subretinal exudate containing fibroblastic elements, neutrophils and mononuclear cells.

Ocular manifestations of *coccidioidomycosis* include granulomatous panuveitis with infiltration of inflammatory cells into the cornea and iridocorneal angle. A severe interstitial keratitis may accompany the anterior uveitis.

Histoplasmosis infrequently produces ocular signs in the dog and cat. Focal granulomatous anterior and posterior uveitis occur with disseminated disease. *Geotrichosis*, a rare mycosis, can generate panuveitis with focal inflammatory infiltration of uveal tissue and exudative retinal detachment (see Chapter 49).

Prototheca is a colorless algae that has caused systemic and ocular disease in the dog. Granulomatous necrotizing chorioretinitis with retinal detachment and hemorrhagic gastroenteritis characterize the pathology (see Figure 17–1*G*).

VIRUSES

Infectious Canine Hepatitis. The typical ocular lesion of infectious canine hepatitis is unilateral or bilateral anterior uveitis called "blue eye" or "blue keratitis." The corneal edema responsible for "blue eye" is caused by damage to corneal endothelium. Approximately 20 per cent of dogs infected with canine hepatitis and one per cent of dogs vaccinated with live canine hepatitis virus (canine adenovirus type 1 = CAV-1) also exhibit such a lesion. It was hypothesized and then demonstrated that the lesions were a manifestation of ocular hypersensitivity rather than a direct effect of viral growth.

Mild signs of inflammation appear five days after infection and a very marked inflammation and deposit of immune complexes begins at seven days during the rise of antibody titer. The visible reaction occurs usually 9 to 14 days after vaccination or infection. Resorption of immune complexes begins at ten days after inoculation. In most cases of the disease, the lesions regress spontaneously after a short period of time.

Certain breeds such as Afghan hounds, basset hounds, and Saint Bernards are especially sensitive to this type of uveitis. If lesions are severe, regression does not occur and certain cases can be complicated by glaucoma (see Chapter 47).

Canine Distemper. Ocular manifestations are, by decreasing frequency, conjunctivitis, chorioretinitis, keratoconjunctivitis sicca (KCS), and optic nerve lesions.

Conjunctivitis is always present in an acute form. Eyes have a serous and then heavy mucopurulent or purulent discharge; in some cases, tear secretion is evidently diminished and mucopurulent discharge adheres to the cornea. Acute keratoconjunctivitis sicca can result in an epithelial breakdown, corneal ulceration, and perforation. The cause of KCS in this disease is attributed to a viral-induced dacryoadenitis. Cytologic examination of the conjunctiva reveals a predominantly mononuclear reaction. After some days, cellular population is progressively replaced by polymorphonuclear cells. Inclusion bodies (Lentz inclusions) may be found in the epithelial cells after six days. Although a positive finding is conclusive, a negative one is inconclusive. Superior diagnostic results have been reported with the use of a fluorescent antibody technique that uses macrophages.

Acute conjunctivitis responds well to local application of broad spectrum antibiotic eye drops, following routine ocular cleansing. If KCS is present, it is necessary to replace the tears by artificial wetting solutions. Tear secretion usually returns in three to six weeks.

Chorioretinitis or optic nerve or optic tract lesions result from the neurotropism of the distemper virus. These can occur in conjunction with the general disease or be apparently isolated, as occurs in older dogs. Reported incidence of clinically active retinitis is variable, although it has been stated that 60 per cent of dogs with distemper may exhibit signs of retinitis. Active retinal inflammatory lesions can be observed in both the tapetal and nontapetal zones. Acute distemper retinal lesions are characterized by hazy areas of retinitis and perivascular infiltration. After several weeks, this area becomes atrophic and is marked by bright, hyperreflective lesions in the tapetal retina. In the nontapetal area, depigmented patches and areas of light-gray color appear. Optic nerve edema and papilledema are seldom observed. Optic tract lesions are not seen ophthalmoscopically.

The histopathology of acute retinitis is characterized by congestive edema of the optic fiber layer and inner plexiform layer. Perivascular cuffing of the veins and optic neuritis with gliosis and degeneration are present in few cases (see Chapter 47).

INFECTIOUS DISEASES OF THE CAT

Chlamydia, Mycoplasma, and Viruses

FELINE UPPER RESPIRATORY INFECTION (URI)

External ocular diseases frequently accompany feline URI. A triad of signs is often present: ocular discharge, nasal discharge, and sneezing. The agents responsible for the upper respiratory/ocular syndrome may infect singly, but mixed infections are more common.

Chlamydia psittaci. These infections, previously known as feline pneumonitis, reflect an acute but generally benign, conjunctival disease. Initially, the conjunctiva is chemotic, hyperemic, and covered by a seromucous discharge that becomes mucopurulent after a few days. Chronic cases exhibit thickened conjunctiva, minimal exudate, and occasional follicles. Adhesions between the palpebral and bulbar conjunctiva (symblepharon) may occur infrequently in long-standing disease. Early infections are often unilateral, but progression to bilateral involvement is common. In the typical neonatal syndrome, selected animals in a litter are affected. Diagnosis is based upon the presence of typical inclusions in the epithelial cells of conjunctival scrapings. The inclusion bodies are dark blue when stained with Giemsa stain and are typically found in groups or clusters appearing in focus at the same plane as the epithelial cell nucleus.

Mycoplasma felis and M. gatae. *Mycoplasma felis* and *M. gatae* are the agents previously classified as pleuropneumonia-like organisms causing conjunctivitis in cats. There is usually a monocular purulent ocular discharge with a mildly hyperemic conjunctival surface. In more severe infections, the conjunctiva may be covered with a gray pseudohyperdiphtheritic membrane. Usually the cornea is spared, but the infection readily spreads to the opposite conjunctiva. Giemsa-stained conjunctival scrapings reveal the presence of numerous dust-blue coccoid or coccobacillary bodies in the periphery of the epithelial cytoplasm. Inclusions are in focus near the epithelial cell wall, not at the plane of the nucleus.

Feline Herpesvirus. Feline herpesvirus can produce three different ocular forms, which appear to be age-dependent. Neonatal ophthalmia in kittens two to four weeks old is part of a severe systemic disease. In contrast to *Chlamydia* infections, the entire litter is usually affected. Intense chemosis, conjunctival vascular injection, partial prolapse of the nictitans, and mucopurulent ocular discharge characterize the fulminant viral disease. Keratitis can occur with secondary infection. An acute conjunctivitis affects cats four weeks to six months of age. These animals exhibit a more benign disease that is usually self-limiting in 10 to 14 days. Older cats develop a keratoconjunctivitis with very mild, short-lived respiratory signs. Ulcerative keratitis is remarkable for early punctate or dendritic (branching) superficial corneal ulcers (see Figure 17–1*H*), although geographically deeper ulcers and interstitial keratitis can occur. Bilateral descemetoceles have been described and feline herpesvirus was isolated from the affected eyes. Cats that recover from feline herpesvirus infection periodically excrete the virus and remain reservoirs of infection.

Diagnosis is based on history, signs, conjunctival scrapings, or virus isolation. Cellular conjunctival response is initially mononuclear, but polymorphonuclear cells become more numerous later in the course of the disease. Typical intranuclear inclusion bodies that are seen in tissue sections from feline herpesvirus cases have not been identified in the conjunctival scrapings. However, a specific fluorescent antibody test has been developed to provide cytologic identification of herpesvirus.

Therapy for viral conjunctivitis may be symptomatic and/or specific. Gentle ocular cleansing and broad spectrum antibiotics are adequate if self-limiting disease is suspected. Currently, effective specific antiviral treatment is available only for topical application. Idoxuridine, vidarabine, trifluridine, and acyclovir have been used clinically. *In vitro* studies indicate that trifluridine is the most effective viricidal agent for feline herpes. Frequent topical therapy (6 to 12 times daily) may also provide some systemic benefit. Corticosteroids should be administered only with great caution and concurrent antiviral treatment.

Feline Infectious Peritonitis. Clinically, *feline infectious peritonitis* (FIP) has been categorized in three forms: those with abdominal and/or thoracic signs, those with neural and/or ophthalmic signs, and a combination of these forms.

Cats with ocular signs of FIP may be presented initially without signs of systemic illness, although eventually other systemic signs usually develop. A typical ocular lesion is pyogranulomatous anterior uveitis, although both anterior and posterior segments may be involved. The uveitis is usually severe with aqueous flare, inflammatory cells, and hemorrhage. The iris becomes edematous and infiltrated, and posterior synechia develop. When the fundus is visible, focal retinal hemorrhages, perivascular edema, chorioretinitis, and sometimes retinal detachment can be noted. Histologic study indicates a granulomatous vasculitis and panuveitis with a predominance of mononuclear and plasma cells. Uveal pathology includes edema and necrotizing foci with vasculitis. The vitreous may contain inflammatory cells. The retina may exhibit similar lesions with proteinaceous exudates between the neural retina and the retinal pigment epithelium (see Chapter 48). Definitive diagnosis and treatment are difficult.

CANINE OCULAR TUMORS

Primary ocular melanomas are the most common ocular tumors in dogs. In contrast to ocular melanomas in humans, they very seldom metastasize. It is generally accepted that canine epibulbar melanomas have local development and a more favorable prognosis (see Chapters 58 and 59).

Adenocarcinomas are the most common nonpigmented anterior uveal tumors. These are invasive as well as proliferative, and are known for their pulmonary and liver metastases.

Metastatic Ocular Neoplasms. *Malignant lymphoma* is the most common secondary intraocular tumor in the dog. Ocular or periocular structures can be involved, although the uvea is the most frequently affected intraocular tissue. Frequently, bilateral ocular disease is the primary presenting complaint.

Clinical signs of ocular involvement are variable. Conjunctivitis is common, and corneal infiltration with cells and vessels is often seen. Anterior uveal infiltration results in mild uveitis, flare, and hypopyon with keratic precipitates. Choroidal involvement is less frequent and occurs primarily adjacent to the optic disc. Retinal involvement is characterized by increased vascular tortuosity, papilledema, intraretinal hemorrhage, and localized or complete retinal detachment. The earliest changes in the fundus are altered color in the tapetal and nontapetal areas, superficial flame-shaped hemorrhages, and small, deep, round hemorrhages. Malignant lymphoma may also invade the orbit.

As in all cases of uveitis, complications such as synechiae, glaucoma, hyphema, and complete retinal detachment may occur. Diagnosis of canine lymphosarcoma should be considered any time uveitis with hypopyon or cell infiltration is identified.

Focal diagnosis is established by paracentesis of the anterior chamber or of the vitreous cavity of the eye. Differential diagnosis includes bleeding and clotting disorders. There is no special treatment for the ocular lymphoma. Chemotherapy used for generalized lymphomas is also the treatment of choice for the localized forms.

Involvement of the uvea in metastatic disease from distant or adjacent sites has been infrequently reported in the dog. Secondary adenocarcinomas occur most frequently with metastases reported from kidney, thyroid, pancreas, nasal cavity, uterus, and mammary gland. Secondary ocular tumors have been described as occurring also with hemangiosarcoma, giant cell sarcoma, fibrosarcoma, and transmissible venereal tumors.

The uvea is the major site of involvement of ocular metastatic carcinoma; common clinical signs include intraocular hemorrhage, iridocyclitis, nonpigmented uveal nodules, and secondary glaucoma. Evaluation of tumor extension by ophthalmoscopy, transillumination of the globe, gonioscopy, radiographs, ultrasound, computerized tomography, and careful examination of the thorax and abdomen are essential for the detection of the primary disease.

The intraocular extension from optic nerve tumors is seen with meningiomas, astrocytomas, gliomas, gangliogliomas, and reticulosis. These cases may appear clinically as optic neuritis (i.e., blindness with a dilated, unresponsive pupil). Reticulosis of the CNS in dogs and cats can cause severe visual defects from involvement of the optic tracts and/or the optic nerves. Optic neuritis progressing to optic atrophy is a fairly common finding in affected animals. Clinical signs associated with the disease include circling, abnormal reflexes, poor postural reactions, and blindness. Reticulosis can mimic other types of neurologic pathology, such as encephalitis and neurovegetative disorders (see Chapters 61 and 63).

FELINE OCULAR TUMORS

Metastatic Ocular Tumors of the Cat. Secondary intraocular tumors of the eye of the cat include the feline lymphosarcoma leukemia complex (FeLLC), reticulosis, plasma cell myeloma, and intraocular extension of tumors of the orbit, optic nerve, and adjacent tissues. Carcinoma metastases to the anterior and posterior uvea from primary sites in the lung, uterus, and mammary gland have been known to occur.

Intraocular tumors may present with a variety of signs and should be suspected in all cases of otherwise inexplicable inflammation, uveitis, hyphema, and/or glaucoma. Suspicion warrants a thorough systemic evaluation for primary and metastatic sites. When enucleation is warranted, final diagnosis may depend upon histopathological interpretation.

Feline lymphosarcoma leukemia complex (FeLLC) is the most frequent ophthalmic neoplasm in the cat. The orbit eyelid, nictitating membrane, conjunctiva, cornea, anterior uvea, iridocorneal angle, and ocular fundus can be involved. Cats presented with ocular FeLLC exhibit clinical signs varying from isolated ocular lesions to severe systemic illness. The ocular signs may differ from one eye to the other. The lesions are typically cell infiltration of tissues. The anterior uvea is the most commonly affected intraocular structure and the disease produces the well-known signs of anterior uveitis (see Figure 17–1*I*). Posterior segment changes may occur, but they are often masked by the anterior uveal and corneal opacities.

Diagnosis requires a blood evaluation and an ELISA test for FeLLC virus infection. Confirmation of the FeLLC ocular involvement is obtained by paracentesis of the aqueous (anterior lesions) or of the vitreous (posterior lesions). Cytology reveals neutrophils and lymphocytes. Presence of abnormal leukocytes is significant, but their absence cannot exclude the occurrence of FeLLC.

Chemotherapy is the treatment of choice for FeLLC, even for the ocular disease. Topical corticosteroids and atropine may reduce the uveitis.

Primary Intraocular Tumors. Intraocular malignant melanoma is the most common primary ocular tumor of cats. These tumors tend to metastasize. Study of the globes of 12 cats with histories suggesting metastatic disease indicates extensive ocular involvement with replacement of the iris stroma and ciliary stroma, and invasion of the sclera. Early surgical removal of the globe seems beneficial to prevent metastasis.

Primary ocular sarcomas other than malignant melanomas are uncommon. Affected animals are mainly old cats (7 to 15 years) with a mean of 12 in the Peiffer series; 12 of 13 cats were male. In the history of these cats, 11 had either a trauma of the eye or previous chronic inflammation. Some have emphasized the tendency of the post-traumatic tumor to invade the posterior portion of the globe, retina, optic nerve, and posterior lens capsule. In one series, 6 of 13 cats were euthanized because of blindness and neurologic signs caused by tumor infiltration of the CNS structures. Ocular neoplasia is suspected in chronically inflamed, enlarged eyes with or without direct observation of a proliferative process. The potential malignancy of these tumors warrants careful enucleation.

18 COUGHING

STEPHEN J. ETTINGER

Coughing and respiratory distress are terms often misused or misunderstood by the layman. *Coughing* is an expiratory effort producing a sudden, noisy expulsion of air from the lungs, usually in an effort to free the lungs of foreign material (real or imagined). A description of the nature of the cough is helpful in identifying its origin. *Respiratory distress* is a general term referring to difficulty, or a change for the worse, in breathing habits (see Chapter 19). Coughing may be associated with respiratory distress but is not necessarily a sign of the same. Coughing and respiratory distress need to be distinguished from each other. Animal owners unfamiliar with pet medical problems often confuse coughing with panting, difficult or labored breathing, forceful breathing, wheezing, reversed sneezing, gagging, retching, or attempted vomiting. Occasionally, an animal retches or actually vomits following a forceful bout of coughing. This should not be misinterpreted as a gastrointestinal problem. The presence of a terminal retch, either productive or nonproductive, is significant, as will be discussed later.

The causes of coughing in small animals may be divided into the following major categories (see Table 18–1): inflammation, neoplasia, cardiovascular disease, allergy, trauma, physical causes, and parasites. This division provides the clinician with a familiar grouping of etiologies within which he or she may differentiate the coughing pet's problem.

DIAGNOSTIC APPROACH

General Approach. The approach to the coughing patient should include a review of past medical problems and all current medical activity, not just the cough. Dosages and frequency of treatments given in the past and those currently being administered should be listed. A complete physical and radiographic examination of the thorax and cervical region is part of the evaluation of the coughing patient. Radiographs are not necessary in every case but certainly are indicated when there is failure of response to initial conservative treatment. Auscultation of heart sounds for murmurs and arrhythmias and the lungs for abnormal breath sounds, as well as palpation of the larynx, trachea, and thorax for physical deformities or pain, are essential in all cases. A complete blood count, fecal flotation examination, and heartworm examination (in endemic areas) should be considered in appropriate situations. Specific testing of the blood chemistry profile, electrocardiogram, and bronchial wash, as well as culture, bronchoscopy, pleural tap, and blood gas analysis may, in the more chronic or advanced cases, provide the clinician with specific information relevant to the diagnosis and treatment of the malady.

Nature of the Cough. Careful questioning regarding the nature of the cough should precede the physical examination. Specific information requested should include when the cough occurs, what, if anything, brings it about, whether it is moist or dry, whether it is productive or nonproductive, and a description of the coughing sound itself.

Nocturnal coughing is generally associated with cardiac disease, psychogenic causes, and collapsing of the trachea. Pulmonary edema, due to a variety of causes, is also likely to result in nocturnal coughing. The cardiac cough is most prominent at night initially but later is progressively heard throughout the day. Pneumonia is likely to be worse initially during the day. Coughing principally due to infectious disease, parasites, and allergic or neoplastic disease most commonly occurs in the daytime during the earlier phases of the disease.

Coughing due to tracheal irritation and trauma is initiated by excitement or pulling on the collar and chain, thereby stimulating the trachea. Coughing due to collapse of the trachea and bronchi is stimulated by drinking water. These coughing episodes occur both day and night, but may be particularly stressful to the owner when the typical "goose-honk" sound occurs continuously during the night. A pet may also learn through experience that paroxysmal coughing yields it immediate attention, suggesting a psychogenic component as well in some cases.

Pneumonia, bronchitis, and bronchiectasis are initially daytime coughing syndromes that do not require stimulation to start, although excitement and pulling on the collar may bring about severe paroxysms of coughing.

Patients with cardiac disease are likely to begin coughing without apparent cause; however, following exercise, tracheal pressure, or excitement, they are also likely to experience paroxysms of coughing. Cardiac coughing does occur at rest because of pathophysiologic alterations in pulmonary interstitial fluid. These pathophysi-

TABLE 18–1. CAUSES OF COUGHING IN DOGS AND CATS

INFLAMMATION
Pharyngitis
Tonsillitis
Tracheobronchitis
Chronic bronchitis
Bronchiectasis
Pneumonia—bacterial, viral, fungal
Granuloma
Abscess
Chronic pulmonary fibrosis
Collapsed trachea
Hilar lymph node enlargement
Secondary to achalasia
Inhalation
NEOPLASIA
Primary
Mediastinal
Metastatic
Tracheal
Laryngeal
Ribs, sternum, muscle
Lymphoma
CARDIOVASCULAR
Left heart failure
Enlarged heart (esp. left atrium)
Heart failure (pulmonary signs)
Pulmonary emboli
Pulmonary edema (vascular origin)
ALLERGIC
Bronchial asthma
Eosinophilic pneumonitis
Eosinophilic pulmonary granulomatosis
Pulmonary infiltrate with eosinophilia (PIE)
Other immune states
Sinusitis (?)
Reverse sneeze (postnasal drip?)
TRAUMA AND PHYSICAL
Foreign body—esophageal, tracheal
Irritating gases
Trauma
Collapsed trachea
Hypoplastic trachea
Hepatomegaly
Inhalation—liquid, solid
PARASITES
Visceral larval migans
Filaroides osleri (lung worm)
Aelurostrongylus (feline lung worm)
Paragonimus kellicotti (lung fluke—dog; cat)
Dirofilaria immitis (dog; cat)
Pneumocystis
Capillaria aerophilia (dog; cat)
Crensoma vulpis (dog)
Filaroides milksi (dog)

ologic changes also result in an inability to breathe while in a recumbent position (*orthopnea*).

Sound of the Cough. When attempting to determine the etiology of the cough there is value in describing its sound. Moist coughing suggests free alveolar or bronchial pulmonary fluid. Soft, moist coughing is often a sign of pneumonia, or parasitic or allergic (with fluid) disease. Inhalation pneumonia, pulmonary emboli, and pulmonary edema are usually characterized by soft, moist coughing.

Dry coughing sounds suggest a cardiac origin (without cardiac failure), bronchitis, tracheobronchitis, tonsillitis, most allergic coughs, and those associated with neoplasia where free alveolar fluid accumulation is not present. Physical deformities of the trachea are initially characterized by dry coughing. Metastatic neoplastic disease, tracheal irritation, and pulmonary foreign bodies cause a cough of similar quality unless there is fluid accumulating in the lower lung. Often this type of cough is associated with terminal nonproductive retching, i.e., nothing is brought up.

Coughing sounds resembling a goose's "honk" are typically associated with the collapsing trachea, hypoplastic trachea, collapsing main stem bronchi (which are also associated with sibilant rales), and segmental tracheal injury. These coughing episodes are usually dry.

Wheezing and rattling are noisy types of sounds often heard with bronchiectasis, chronic obstructive lung disease, and some allergies. The sounds represent passage of air though spastic airways that are narrowed or obstructed with mucus or pus.

Terminal Retch. A terminal retch associated with the cough is often reported. It tends to be nonproductive in early cardiac disease, tracheitis, bronchitis, and with irritating but noninfectious lesions of the pulmonary tract. In cardiac disease it remains nonproductive until pulmonary edema develops. Then the fluid brought up is pink or blood-tinged. Earlier in the course of the disease, the owner may report attempts at gagging with only a small amount of white or clear phlegm produced. This is often the case in tracheitis and bronchitis before excessive fluid develops. In diseases in which mucus, edema, mucopurulent materials or hemorrhage accumulates in the pulmonary tree, there is likely to be material expectorated following the coughing episode. Regardless, in veterinary patients, the owner often reports that the material coughed up is swallowed rather than coughed out of the mouth and therefore the owner may not be able to describe its appearance.

Environmental Factors Related to Coughing. Urban animals are more likely to develop chronic respiratory disease as a result of the increased pollutants in the environment in which they live. Rural animals, on the other hand, if living outside, exposed to the elements and an inclement environment, may be more susceptible to pneumonia, respiratory foreign bodies, and grass-related allergies. Indoor animals have a lower frequency of heartworm disease than do those living outside. Dogs and cats in contact with the intermediate hosts of parasites likewise have a higher incidence of such diseases. Cats maintained indoors and those kept isolated from other cats are less likely to experience upper respiratory viral or parasitic diseases. Those in large catteries or with frequent exposure to other outdoor creatures have a greater incidence of infectious or parasitic pulmonary diseases.

The presence of a damp environment is a factor to consider in the history of animals suspected of having airway disease. Similarly, those experiencing coughing and living in a hot, dry region may have inflamed bronchial linings. Exposure to noxious gases and smoke is a definite predisposing factor to irritated pulmonary linings and coughing.

Environmental factors must be considered when evaluating an animal with respiratory-related signs. Careful questioning regarding other specific habits may prove useful. For example, is there a change in diet, environment, walking habits, or exercise? The clinician may

TABLE 18–2. ANTITUSSIVE AND BRONCHODILATOR-ANTITUSSIVE COMBINATION MEDICATIONS

Generic Name and Preparation		Trade Name	Dosage
Aminophylline 1½ gr (100 mg) tablets		—	5 mg/lb q6-12h as needed.
Theophylline (elixir 80 mg/Tbls) (capsules 100 and 200 mg)		Elixophyllin, Theolixir	5 mg/lb q6-12h as needed.
Oxtriphylline 400 or 600 mg SA tablets		Choledyl SA	Similar to aminophylline; reported to cause fewer GI problems.
Theophylline with glyceryl guaiacolate: 150 mg theophylline + 90 mg glyceryl guaiacolate per capsule or Tbls		Quibron	1 capsule q8-12h for larger dogs. ¼ to 1 Tbls elixir q8-12h for smaller dogs and cats.
Aminophylline with ¼ or ½ gr phenobarbital		—	½ to 1 tablet q6-12h.
Theophylline 130 mg Ephedrine HCl 24 mg Phenobarbital 8 mg		Tedral tablets	¼ to 1 tablet q8-12h.
Hydrocodone bitartrate 5 mg Homatropine methylbromide 1.5 mg	per tablet or per 5 cc	Hycodan	½ to 1 tablet (or teaspoon) q6-24h as needed. May increase dosage if sedative effect does not occur.
Hydrocodone 5 mg Phenyltoloxamine 10 mg	per tablet or per 5 cc	Tussinex	½ to 1 tablet (or teaspoon) q6-24h as needed. May increase dosage if sedative effect does not occur.
Butorphanol tartrate 5, 10, 25 mg tabs		Torbutrol	0.25 mg/lb q6-12h. May cause sedation.
Prednisone 2 mg Trimeprazine 5 mg	per tablet or spansule	Temaril-P	1 tablet per 20 lbs q12h. Good for allergic and noninfectious inflammatory coughing (i.e., tracheal collapse).
Guaifenesin 100 mg Dextromethorphan 15 mg	per 5 cc	Robitussin-DM	Non-narcotic; OTC preparation; for temporary antitussive effect. Dosage similar to that for adults and children.

ask a general question about changes in the environment or management to seek specific direction. Dogs known to cough only with excitement or when pulling on a collar or leash are likely to have a collapsing trachea, the signs of which may be avoided by using a harness rather than a collar. Obese animals are more likely to experience signs of restrictive lung disease and those with an enlarged liver appear to be more prone to restrictive lung disease, tracheal collapse, and coughing episodes.

TREATMENT GOALS

Knowledge of the history and environmental factors in a pet's life may be very useful in identifying the cause or etiology of a specific respiratory problem. This information alone may allow the veterinarian to begin a schedule of modification that reduces the frequency or severity of the coughing. This does not negate the need for a thorough physical examination but it facilitates the proper approach to the diagnosis and treatment of a specific clinical malady.

Accurate knowledge of the frequency, sound, and nature of the cough usually permits reasonable and accurate classification of the problem into one of the categories identified in Table 18–1.

A description of the treatment plan for the coughing dog or cat is unrealistic without a working, preliminary diagnosis. To treat a cough without knowing why it is present is akin to worming a dog without evidence of intestinal parasites.

In general, drugs that are used to treat the coughing pet include antibiotics for infectious disease, corticosteroids for allergic conditions, cardiac agents such as digitalis, diuretics and vasodilators for congestive heart failure, and antispasmodic or antitussive agents for inflammatory, noninfectious lung and tracheal problems. Specific disease problems usually require specific therapy. Antitussive agents are discussed in Chapters 68 and 75. Table 18–2 outlines antitussive agents generally used in nonspecific or specific coughing episodes. The patient requires a thorough evaluation when the cough is severe or when there is failure to respond to nonspecific symptomatic medication. Thoracic radiographs, a total body blood profile panel and a fecal parasite examination are required at a minimum in such situations. Additional testing as outlined in this chapter should enable the clinician to at least identify the category or cause of the coughing, thereby enabling specific therapy to be instituted.

19 DYSPNEA AND TACHYPNEA

STEPHEN J. ETTINGER

Dyspnea is a state of labored, difficult, or painful breathing, which is recognized as being abnormally uncomfortable. It may be exertional, paroxysmal, or continuous. Dyspnea, especially in animals, is difficult to define and essentially impossible to quantify. Orthopnea indicates difficulty breathing while in a recumbent position (typically associated with pleural fluid accumulation, any form of diaphragmatic hernia, and congestive heart failure). Paroxysmal nocturnal dyspnea is a sign of both cardiac and pulmonary disease. Stridor, rhonchi, and wheezing may accompany any form of dyspnea. Tachypnea (polypnea) refers to an increased rate of breathing, but it need not be an indication of distress. It may be an independent sign or it may accompany dyspnea. The differentiation between tachypnea with and without dyspnea is important because in many cases tachypnea is not an indication of disease, but is rather a physiologic function associated with exertion, exercise, fever, heat, anxiety, or other stress.

GENERAL PATHOPHYSIOLOGY

Upper Airway Problems. Dyspnea is a syndrome associated with several major clinical categories of disease (Table 19–1). Obstruction of the upper airways due to either external compression or intraluminal restriction is frequently associated with dyspnea and respiratory stridor. *Upper airway obstruction (UAO)* in general is

TABLE 19–1. CAUSES OF DYSPNEA

Upper Airway Disease (Obstructive or Compressive)	**Disease of the Pleural Space and Lining**
1. Stenotic nares	1. Pneumothorax
2. Nasal and sinus obstruction (infection, neoplasm, inflammation)	2. Pleural effusions
3. Edematous soft palate	a. hydrothorax (heart failure, neoplasm, lymphosarcoma)
4. Laryngeal edema, paralysis, collapse, or spasm	b. hemothorax (trauma, coagulopathy)
5. Intraluminal tracheal-bronchial obstruction (foreign body, neoplasm)	c. pyothorax
6. Extraluminal tracheal-bronchial obstruction	d. nonseptic exudates (neoplasms, infectious feline peritonitis)
Mediastinal mass	e. chylothorax
Main stem bronchus collapse from enlarged left atrium	3. Diaphragmatic hernia
Hilar lymphadenopathy (neoplasm, systemic mycosis)	4. Displacement of the diaphragm
7. Traumatic rupture of airway	5. Peritoneal-pericardial diaphragmatic hernia
Disease of the Lower Airways or Pulmonary Parenchyma	6. Neoplasia of the mediastinum and thoracic wall
1. Bronchial disease	7. Trauma to the thoracic wall and spine
2. Pulmonary edema (cardiogenic and noncardiogenic)	**Reduced Hemoglobin**
3. Pneumonia (infectious, parasitic, inhalation)	1. Anemia
4. Allergic or immunologic pulmonary disease	2. Methemoglobinemia
5. Pulmonary neoplasia	3. Cyanosis
6. Pulmonary embolism (heartworm disease, pulmonary embolus)	**Miscellaneous Causes of Dyspnea-Tachypnea**
7. Pulmonary artery thrombosis	1. Head trauma
8. Pulmonary hemorrhage	2. Neuromuscular weakness or denervation of muscles of respiration
9. Restrictive lung disease (pulmonary fibrosis)	3. Abdominal masses—restrictive diaphragm
10. Inhalation (pneumonia, pollutants, suspended allergens or particles)	4. Pain
11. Pulmonary emphysema	5. Fever
12. Bronchial asthma	6. Electrical shock
	7. Acidosis (metabolic, diabetic, uremia)
	8. Central nervous system disease
	9. Anxiety-fear
	10. Heat stroke
	11. Ascites
	12. Hepatomegaly
	13. Obesity
	14. Megaesophagus

TABLE 19–2. APPROACH TO THE EVALUATION OF THE DYSPNEIC ANIMAL

	Clinical Parameters
Patient Medical History	
Observation of Patient	
1. Psychic component	Determine level of anxiety, ability to handle
2. Degree of dyspnea	Determine need for immediate therapy, ability to obtain diagnostic information
3. Pattern of ventilation	Helps demonstrate origin of dyspnea
a. Chest excursion	r/o Rib fractures, flail chest, tension pneumothorax
b. Inspiratory dyspnea	r/o Pleural effusion, pneumothorax, pulmonary edema, upper airway obstruction
c. Expiratory dyspnea	r/o Lower airway diseases, pulmonary edema
4. Mucous membranes	
a. Cyanosis	r/o Airway obstruction, diffusion barrier (edema), ventilation/perfusion mismatch (atelectasis, shunt)
b. Pallor	r/o Anemia, decreased cardiac output, shock
c. Brownish	r/o Methemoglobinemia
Physical Examination	
1. Body temperature	r/o Infection, sepsis, heat stroke, increased work of breathing
2. Oral examination (sedation may be needed)	r/o Pharyngeal-laryngeal obstruction (dyspnea relieved by tracheal intubation)
3. Cardiac auscultation	r/o Murmurs, gallops, arrhythmias, muffled sounds (may be obscured by respiratory noises)
4. Pulmonary auscultation	Evaluate level of abnormality
a. Increased sounds (obstructive noises, rales, and rhonchi)	r/o Obstruction of large airways, pulmonary infection, bronchitis, asthma, pulmonary edema
b. Decreased sounds	r/o Pleural effusion, pneumothorax, mass lesions
5. Other findings	r/o Other signs of heart failure and abnormalities that accompany disorders causing acute dyspnea
Thoracic Radiographs	
1. Cardiac chambers and great vessels	r/o Heart disease—congenital and acquired
2. Pulmonary vasculature and parenchyma	r/o Extracardiac signs of heart failure and other primary or secondary pulmonary disorders
3. Pleural space	r/o Pleural effusion, pneumothorax, diaphragmatic hernia; r/o restriction due to obesity
Electrocardiogram	
1. Cardiac rhythm	r/o Cardiac arrhythmias; define their significance
2. Voltage criteria	r/o Cardiac chamber enlargement
3. Other criteria	r/o Evidence for pericardial disease, myocardial disease, or ischemia
Other Tests	
1. Routine laboratory tests	r/o Anemia, polycythemia, methemoglobinemia, acidosis, uremia, diabetes, hypothyroidism, heartworm disease

characterized by inspiratory, stridulous (noisy) breathing. Excitement, exercise, and stress tend to exaggerate the symptoms. Tachypnea need not be present and the animal often appears otherwise normal. Cyanosis is an unusual complication.

Lower Airway Problems. Lower airway diseases commonly are characterized by dyspnea. Coughing and/or tachypnea frequently accompany the dyspnea. A fever is associated with an infectious disease, orthopnea with heart failure, and wheezing or rhonchi are likely to be associated with lower airway diseases. Respiratory symptoms are likely to be worsened by stress, and paroxysmal or nocturnal symptoms may occur, depending upon the cause (e.g., cardiac, allergic, or asthmatic states).

Pleural Diseases. Disease of the pleural space may be acute or chronic. With chronic fluid accumulation, the symptoms of dyspnea or tachypnea are likely to be slowly progressive, whereas an acute fluid build-up stresses the ventilatory state and is one cause of rapid onset of both dyspnea and tachypnea. Pneumothorax is an acute condition where air enters the pleural space, restricts lung volume and expansion, and causes both painful and rapid respiration, which requires immediate attention. Pleural diseases are aggravated by stress, are usually less intense while at rest, and are not likely to be associated with stridulous or wheezy-type breathing, although the breathing sounds may be harsh and tracheal due to transmission of the tracheal sounds into the thorax. Heart and lung sounds may be diminished if pleural fluid is present or if there is an occupying lesion in the pleural space. The animal may attempt to seek a specific position to lessen the respiratory discomfort and enhance ventilation.

Reduced Hemoglobin States. Reduced hemoglobin states such as anemia, cyanosis, and methemoglobinemia are associated with mucous membrane discoloration. The pulse, if thready and rapid, reflects the degree of anemia; the animal is quiet and weak. Dyspnea occurs only when the blood oxygen level falls below a critical point, which varies with each animal. Exertion accentuates the need for oxygen and can cause dyspnea. Associated disease problems and the acuteness of the anemia are factors that affect the severity of the clinical signs.

Miscellaneous Causes. In addition to the disease categories already outlined, there are a number of other conditions that may be associated with difficult breathing. Ascites, hepatomegaly, and other abdominal masses are often recognized causes of respiratory distress. By reducing ventilatory space by compression and prevention of full lung volume expansion, abdominal disease states and obesity may cause rapid, shallow, and dyspneic breathing (see Chapter 28).

Other potential causes of dyspnea include severe pain, anxiety, overexertion, brain and spinal cord trauma, heat prostration, and acidosis.

DIAGNOSIS AND TREATMENT

The approach to the patient with dyspnea involves first an overall understanding of the disease states possibly related to such a clinical condition. The first step taken in the differential diagnosis is to obtain a thorough history. Observation and physical examination alone may permit the clinician to make a specific diagnosis or to identify the rule-outs. Table 19–2 provides the clinician with a basic design for evaluating dyspnea. It provides the clinician with a logical and sequential approach to this problem, although it alone may not identify every form of dyspnea. Therapy must be directed entirely at the inciting cause. There is no single category of medicine for the relief of dyspnea or tachypnea. Sedation alone may lessen the signs but aggravate the disease or prevent the rapid breathing required to satisfy the oxygen demands of the patient.

20 ANEMIA

SUSAN M. COTTER

Anemia may be defined as a decreased red cell mass resulting in insufficient oxygen delivery to the tissues. Anemias may be classified into *regenerative*, with increased red cell production to compensate for increased losses, and *nonregenerative*, with decreased production. They may also be classified by red cell morphology into *macrocytic, normocytic*, and *microcytic* with increased, normal, or decreased cell size (*mean corpuscular volume*); and *normochromic* or *hypochromic* with a normal or decreased hemoglobin level (*mean corpuscular hemoglobin concentration*).

GENERAL PATHOPHYSIOLOGY

Anemia is a clinical sign, not a diagnosis. Classification into regenerative and nonregenerative is helpful in understanding pathophysiology and narrowing the list of causes in a given case. In regenerative anemias, young anucleated red cells (*reticulocytes*) are released into the circulation in numbers that correlate with the rate of effective erythropoiesis in the marrow. The reticulocyte count represents the most important means for classification (see Chapter 113).

REGENERATIVE ANEMIA

Regenerative anemia results when red cells are lost through hemorrhage or hemolysis. The marrow can expand its output up to ten times the normal rate, so that low grade blood loss may be associated with reticulocytosis without anemia. It is only when the loss exceeds the rate of production that anemia results.

Acute Blood Loss. Acute blood loss results in loss of both red cells and plasma, so the major problem is hypovolemia, and the packed cell volume (PCV) remains normal. For this reason the PCV is not an accurate indicator of severity of ongoing bleeding. Twelve to 24 hours after blood loss, fluid shifts occur and the PCV drops. Reticulocyte counts do not increase significantly for three to four days after acute blood loss.

Chronic Blood Loss. Chronic blood loss results in depletion of red cells and nutrients, especially iron, with circulatory volume remaining normal. Reticulocytosis gradually subsides and a microcytic, hypochromic nonregenerative anemia results. Occult blood loss may occur with blood-sucking external parasites in pups or kittens or with intestinal loss from parasites, tumors, or ulcers.

Internal hemorrhage may be harder to detect. Some red cells are reabsorbed and those that are damaged give rise to a clinical picture more closely resembling hemolysis than hemorrhage. Iron is conserved so deficiency does not occur. Some causes of internal bleeding are trauma or tumors such as hemangiosarcomas. Coagulopathies can cause either internal or external blood loss. Platelet abnormalities cause petechiae or mucosal bleeding. Factor deficiencies are more likely to cause hematomas or bleeding into body cavities or joints.

Hemolysis. Hemolytic anemia may be associated with icterus and other signs of systemic disease. Chronic hemolysis is less likely to be associated with other signs. Red cell destruction may occur in the circulation (intravascular hemolysis) and results in hemoglobinemia and hemoglobinuria. Some of the hemoglobin is bound to haptoglobin and metabolized to unconjugated bilirubin. Hemolysis may also occur when red cells are phagocytized by the fixed macrophages in the spleen and other organs (extravascular hemolysis). Hemoglobin is metabolized and released as unconjugated bilirubin. Intravascular hemolysis tends to be a more severe disease than extravascular hemolysis. Those conditions associated primarily with intravascular hemolysis are IgM mediated autoimmune hemolytic anemia, large red cell parasites (e.g., *Babesia*), oxidant toxicity (acetaminophen, onions), and microangiopathic hemolysis (e.g., splenic torsion or vena caval syndrome).

Conditions associated primarily with extravascular hemolysis are most autoimmune hemolytic anemias, small red cell parasites (e.g., *Haemobartonella*), intrinsic red cell disorders (e.g., pyruvate kinase deficiency), and drugs (e.g., propylthiouracil, gold salts, modified live virus vaccines).

In dogs, the most common form of anemia is immune-mediated hemolysis. Occasionally a predisposing cause such as a drug or a recent vaccination is present, but most cases are idiopathic. In severe cases, icterus, hemoglobinemia, hemoglobinuria, or autoagglutination are present. The onset may also be insidious, and anemia may be the only presenting sign. Reticulocytosis is usually present at the time of initial examination.

NONREGENERATIVE ANEMIA

Nonregenerative anemia results from decreased production of red cells that usually have a normal appearance and lifespan. This may occur with primary marrow failure or when erythropoiesis is suppressed from an extramedullary cause. Primary marrow disorders include the following conditions.

Myelophthisic Anemia. Myelophthisic anemia is infiltration of the marrow by neoplastic cells. Neoplastic hematopoietic cells fill the marrow and inhibit normal hematopoiesis. These malignant cells may or may not appear in the blood, but neutropenia, anemia, and thrombocytopenia are usually present.

Feline Leukemia Virus (FeLV)-related Red Cell Aplasia in Cats. The mechanism of myelosuppression by FeLV is unknown but any or all cell lines may be suppressed. This is the most common form of anemia in cats, with 70 per cent of all anemic cats being viremic. Some FeLV-negative cats with red cell aplasia have been found to have latent infections. In these cats foci of nonreplicating virus are detectable on *in vitro* marrow cultures, but not detectable by routine ELISA or IFA testing.

Hormones, Drugs or Chemicals. Cytotoxic antineoplastic drugs, chloramphenicol, endogenous or exogenous estrogen, benzene, and phenylbutazone are mylosuppressive. Granulocytopenia and thrombocytopenia occur before anemia because red cells have the longest lifespan.

Deficiency Syndromes. Iron deficiency and hypothyroidism cause suppression of red cell production. Rarely, macrocytic anemia occurs with decreased folate or B_{12} levels in chronic intestinal disease.

Renal Failure. Anemia occurs because of decreased erythropoietin.

Anemia of Chronic Disease. A mild nonregenerative anemia may occur with any chronic, debilitating disease. Cats, because of their normally short red cell lifespan, are more at risk than dogs. Anemia of chronic disease is associated with sequestration of adequate iron stores, primarily in the marrow. The serum iron and total iron-binding capacity are both decreased. Iron supplementation is not necessary because the anemia is seldom serious and resolves if the underlying disease improves.

Canine Ehrlichiosis. Anemia in ehrlichiosis may be partially hemolytic but is primarily nonregenerative. Decreases of white cells and/or platelets may also be seen.

Idiopathic Red Cell Aplasia. In dogs, immune-mediated destruction of red cell precursors may be a cause. If reticulocytes are destroyed as well as mature red cells, the anemia appears nonregenerative. If the marrow is examined, increased erythropoiesis is usually evident. In some cases, very early precursors are destroyed in the marrow, so even a marrow aspirate appears nonregenerative. Here the immune-mediated cause is substantiated only in retrospect if a clinical response occurs with immunosuppressive drug therapy. If the marrow fails to produce granulocytes and platelets as well as red cells, pancytopenia (aplastic anemia) results. Animals with aplastic anemia have an increased risk of sepsis and bleeding.

HISTORICAL FINDINGS AND THEIR MEANING

Except for acute hemolysis or blood loss, the onset of anemia is often insidious. Clinical signs may be limited to lethargy and anorexia. Careful attention may be directed to the points described in the following sections.

Breed, Age, Environment. Initial observations can lead one to consider congenital disorders (e.g., pyruvate kinase deficiency in basenjis and beagles, and phosphofructokinase deficiency in springer spaniels). Boxers are prone to neoplasia, German shepherds to hemangiosarcoma, poodles, cocker spaniels, and old English sheepdogs to immune-mediated hemolytic anemia. Old animals are more likely to have tumors, middle-aged dogs are likely to have immune-mediated anemia, and young animals are likely to have congenital disorders. Animals allowed outdoors may suffer trauma, have parasites, or ingest toxins. Cats from multiple cat households are more likely to be exposed to FeLV.

Drug or Travel History. Any medication or recent vaccination should be considered as a possible cause of anemia until proven otherwise. Drugs have caused either hemolysis or marrow suppression. Certain infections such as babesiosis, ehrlichiosis or dirofilariasis are more likely in some geographic areas than others.

Diet. Dietary deficiencies are uncommon with today's commercial diets. Young animals have low iron stores and become deficient more quickly than adults if iron is lost or missing from the diet. Additives such as onions or excessive copper can cause hemolysis.

Changes in Urine or Feces. Owners may notice dark urine (bilirubinuria or hemoglobinuria) indicative of hemolysis, or dark feces indicative of upper GI blood loss.

In addition to specific signs, any other abnormality reported by the owner should be considered as possibly relevant. Respiratory signs could indicate cardiac or pulmonary disease or dirofilariasis instead of just hypoxia secondary to anemia. Gastrointestinal signs could indicate a bleeding intestinal lesion.

PHYSICAL FINDINGS AND THEIR INTERPRETATION

Most anemic patients have pale mucous membranes, tachycardia, sharp pulses, and tachypnea. An assessment of the strength of the patient relative to the degree of anemia may provide subjective clues. A slow onset of anemia, as in marrow failure, is associated with compensation so that the clinical signs may be minimal despite severe depletion of red cell mass. More specific findings and their interpretation are listed here.

Icterus. Icterus in the presence of anemia suggests acute hemolysis. A rough estimate is that the destruction of four grams of hemoglobin (a drop of 12 points in the PCV) in a 24-hour period may cause icterus even in the presence of normal liver function. If the rate of destruction slows, then the icterus should subside. Persisting icterus indicates primary or secondary hepatic or biliary disease. Severe liver dysfunction may cause microangiopathic hemolysis, or severe anemia may cause centrilobular necrosis, so it may be difficult to distinguish the primary problem. Icterus is comparably more severe with extravascular than intravascular hemolysis since hemoglobin lost in the urine is not metabolized to bilirubin.

Fever. Temperature deviations may occur in acute hemolytic anemia of any cause, in infectious anemias, and in infections secondary to granulocytopenia in aplastic anemia.

Hemorrhage. Petechiae or ecchymoses may be seen on the skin and mucous membranes and are most likely caused by thrombocytopenia. Accompanying anemia may be hemolytic or from blood loss from mucosal hemorrhages throughout the gastrointestinal tract. If thrombocytopenia has been caused by marrow failure, then anemia may be nonregenerative. Myeloma can cause bleeding from immunoglobulin coating of platelets and decreased production of red cells because of marrow invasion. Neoplasia or sepsis may cause anemia from disseminated intravascular coagulopathy with hemorrhage.

Muffled heart sounds or abdominal distention may accompany bleeding into the pericardium, pleural cavity, or abdomen. These lead one to consider factor deficiencies or a bleeding tumor such as hemangiosarcoma. Dark feces indicate upper GI bleeding. This may be obvious, but bleeding may be intermittent, and repeated observation and quaiac testing may be necessary for detection. Fresh blood in the feces from lower GI bleeding is more easily observed.

Lymphadenopathy or Splenomegaly. Lymphadenopathy may indicate lymphoma with anemia resulting from myelophthisis. Lymphadenopathy may also be reactive from FeLV, FTLV, or other infections in the cat, or from ehrlichiosis or systemic granulomatous infections in dogs. Splenomegaly may occur but is not a specific sign. It may occur in hemolytic or nonregenerative anemias or from hematopoietic neoplasia.

Systemic Disease. Oral ulcers or a uremic odor to the breath indicate renal failure. The signs of uremia are usually more severe than the anemia. Any severe illness may cause anemia of chronic disease. In dogs, a testicular tumor (sertoli cell tumor) or signs of feminization may indicate hyperestrogenism as a cause of marrow failure.

DIAGNOSTIC PLAN

Complete Blood Count (CBC) and Reticulocyte Count. Information is gained as to the severity of anemia and initial classification. When blood is drawn, a drop should be placed on a slide and observed for autoagglutination. If it is present, a drop of saline is added to disperse rouleaux, which may simulate autoagglutination in situations of elevated serum proteins. If the autoagglutination remains in the presence of saline, this is evidence of immune-mediated hemolysis. Indicators of regenerative anemia are reticulocytosis (see Chapter 113), polychromasia, anisocytosis, and elevated white blood count. Spherocytes (small red cells without central pallor) may be seen in immune-mediated hemolysis. Fragmented red cells (schistocytes, helmut cells) may be seen in microangiopathic hemolysis. Heinz bodies (denatured hemoglobin) or brown blood (methemoglobin) are indicative of oxidant toxins or drugs. Red cells should be examined for the presence of parasites. Nucleated red cells in the absence of reticulocytosis are *not* indicative of regenerative anemia.

Red cell indices either calculated or obtained from an automated counter are helpful. An increased mean corpuscular volume (MCV) is usually associated with reticulocytosis. In cats, an increased MCV without reticulocytosis may be seen in FeLV infection and probably represents skipped mitoses. A decreased MCV is usually indicative of iron deficiency but has also been seen in some dogs with portal-systemic shunts. The mean corpuscular hemoglobin concentration (MCHC) may be decreased in the presence of severe reticulocytosis. With new models of automated cell counters the red cell distribution width (RDW), sometimes with a histogram, may be reported. The RDW represents one standard deviation from the MCV, and provides specific information as to the variability of red cell size. The RDW is increased in reticulocytosis but the histogram may show additional populations of cells such as spherocytes or microcytic cells. For example, the MCV could be normal if both macrocytic and microcytic red cells are present. A normal RDW is 15.

Other Tests. Depending on the history, physical findings, and initial classification of the anemia, other tests are selected to narrow the list of rule-outs. In the dog, a *direct antiglobulin test* (Coombs test) is indicated in both regenerative and nonregenerative anemias since a positive result may be present even in immune-mediated red cell aplasia. Immune-mediated hemolysis is less common in cats so the direct antiglobulin test is run in cases of idiopathic regenerative anemias. A *FeLV test* should be run on every anemic cat regardless of the classification of the anemia. In both dogs and cats, a minimum data base should include a *chemistry profile*, *urinalysis*, and *examination of the feces* for color, consistency, and parasites.

If chronic blood loss is suspected, a fecal *quaiac test* for occult blood is done as well as measurement of *serum iron* and *total iron binding capacity*. If fecal blood loss is substantiated and parasites are not found, then a *barium study* may be done to look for a bleeding intestinal lesion. *Clotting tests* (see Chapter 116) are indicated if bleeding is present and a cause is not evident. In endemic areas dogs should be tested for *microfilaria* and for serologic evidence of *ehrlichiosis*. *Thoracic and abdominal radiographs* and *ultrasound* can be helpful in detection of malignancy.

Examination of the Marrow. Bone marrow examination is indicated if nonregenerative anemia is present.

The marrow should also be examined in cases of unexplained abnormal circulating cells or monoclonal gammopathy. The marrow is not likely to add information in the presence of regenerative anemia. A bone marrow aspirate is the best preparation for evaluation of cytology. Hematopoietic malignancies tend to invade the marrow diffusely and are best detected by an aspirate. A marrow core biopsy is needed only if the aspirate is hypocellular, since the biopsy gives information on cellularity or presence of myelofibrosis.

Bone marrow aspirates are done most frequently in cats because of the variety of hematopoietic disorders related to FeLV infection. Most cats with leukemias and myeloproliferative disorders present with nonregenerative anemia and a normal or low white blood count. Malignant cells may be in the blood, but it is possible for the marrow to be replaced with malignant cells with none in the circulation. Not all anemic, FeLV-positive cats have leukemia. The marrow may show decreased production of hematopoietic cells or may even be normal. The prognosis varies with findings on the marrow aspirate.

In dogs, marrow aspirates are also helpful in differentiating between causes of nonregenerative anemia, leukopenia, or thrombocytopenia, and to rule out hematopoietic malignancy. Myeloma may be diagnosed by finding increased immature plasma cells in the marrow when monoclonal gammopathy is present. Ehrlichiosis may also show a monoclonal gammopathy and increased marrow plasma cells, usually of normal morphology. Sequential examinations of marrow are occasionally performed to determine prognosis during treatment of hematopoietic disorders.

OUTCOME

The prognosis for recovery in anemic animals varies with cause. In general the prognosis is better in regenerative than in nonregenerative anemias. Acute and chronic blood loss can be treated successfully if the cause is removed. Hemorrhage from coagulopathies varies as to prognosis (see Chapter 116). Immune-mediated thrombocytopenia may be either transient or refractory. Postvaccine thrombocytopenia in young animals has the best prognosis. Immune-mediated hemolytic anemia may respond readily to immunosuppressive therapy and never recur. In other cases, particularly those with intravascular hemolysis, the disease may be rapidly progressive and refractory to all therapy. Some dogs have a good response to therapy but experience relapses periodically.

Hemolysis from exogenous causes such as parasites and toxins has a relatively favorable prognosis after removal of the cause. Microangiopathic hemolysis is a sign of serious disease such as vascular tumor, splenic torsion, or disseminated intravascular coagulation. The prognosis depends upon the underlying disease.

Nonregenerative anemias from nutritional deficiencies, or secondary to certain toxins or treatable chronic or infectious diseases, are most likely to be correctable. Marrow failure from hyperestrogenism may be irreversible. Cats with red cell aplasia from FeLV sometimes improve, particularly if a treatable coexisting infection is present. The prognosis is poor for most FeLV-positive cats with severe nonregenerative anemia and especially for those with pancytopenia.

Nonlymphocytic leukemias and myeloproliferative disorders are rarely treated successfully in dogs or cats. Dogs with well-differentiated lymphocytic leukemia usually respond well for long periods of time. Acute lymphoblastic leukemia (ALL) in dogs and cats sometimes responds to aggressive therapy (see Chapters 59 and 114). The prognosis for ALL is not as good as for lymphoma. Granulocytopenia is usually present, adding to the risk of infectious complications. A systematic approach to the anemic patient allows for proper classification and results in accurate diagnosis, treatment, and prognosis.

21 CYANOSIS

GILBERT JACOBS

Cyanosis refers to the bluish color of the skin or mucous membranes that is usually the result of an increased amount of reduced hemoglobin in the blood circulating in those areas. (*Reduced hemoglobin* is synonymous with deoxygenated hemoglobin, deoxyhemoglobin, or desaturated hemoglobin.) *Arterial hypoxemia* is a reduction in the partial pressure of oxygen in arterial blood (PA_{O_2} below the normal range of 85 to 100 mmHg), which results in decreased oxygen saturation of hemoglobin and an increased amount of reduced hemoglobin. *Partial pressure* of a gas is the pressure exerted by the molecules of that gas in a volume of mixed gases (as in lung alveoli) or dissolved in liquid (as in blood). The partial pressure of O_2 in alveoli and that of CO_2 in tissues provide the driving force for the dissolution of those gases in the blood.

GENERAL PATHOPHYSIOLOGY

In general, about 5 gm/dl of deoxygenated hemoglobin is required to detect cyanosis, and the degree of cyanosis is determined by the absolute amount of deoxygenated hemoglobin. A cyanotic condition can be obscured for a number of reasons. Cyanosis is generally less apparent in patients with severe anemia since the absolute amount of hemoglobin is reduced. Recognition of cyanosis is also dependent upon external variables such as lighting conditions and skin pigmentation. Cyanosis may also be *more* apparent, when the hemoglobin content of blood is higher, as occurs in polycythemic patients. This is because in patients with polycythemia and normal oxygen saturation, the relative amount of reduced hemoglobin is unchanged from normal but since the absolute hemoglobin concentration is higher, so is the absolute amount of reduced hemoglobin.

The basic cause of cyanosis is an increased amount of deoxygenated hemoglobin in the blood of the cyanotic tissue. The mechanisms responsible are (1) hypoxemia of arterial and thus capillary blood, (2) increased extraction of oxygen in capillary blood, or (3) an increase in the amount of oxygen-poor venous blood in the skin due to dilatation or congestion of the venous system. Cyanosis can also be produced (4) by an increase in circulating abnormal hemoglobin pigments.

Clinically, cyanosis may be classified as either central or peripheral (Table 21–1). *Central cyanosis* implies that the cyanosis is generalized, involving both mucous membranes and skin; it is due to arterial hypoxemia or abnormal circulating hemoglobin pigments. *Peripheral cyanosis* is localized, usually involving the extremities, and is due to increased extraction of oxygen in capillary blood or to an increase in the amount of venous blood in the skin.

Central Cyanosis

Oxygen saturation of arterial blood in normal individuals is generally between 95 and 97 per cent. This is maintained by a partial pressure of oxygen in arterial blood (PA_{O_2})between 85 to 100 mmHg. The oxygen dissociation curve reminds us of the relationship between PA_{O_2} and oxygen saturation in arterial blood. At PA_{O_2} above 60 mmHg the curve is relatively flat and oxygen saturation changes little. At these levels, cyanosis is generally undetectable. Thus, hypoxemia can occur without cyanosis.

Arterial Hypoxemia. There are five causes of arterial hypoxemia: (1) reduced inspired oxygen concentration (2) alveolar hypoventilation, (3) diffusion impairment, (4) ventilation-perfusion mismatch, and (5) anatomic shunt. More than one cause may be responsible for hypoxemia in some diseases.

Reduced inspired oxygen. Reduction of inspired

TABLE 21–1. CAUSES OF CYANOSIS

Central Cyanosis
Hypoxemia
Reduction of Inspired PO_2
Impaired Respiratory Function
Alveolar hypoventilation
Diffusion impairment
Ventilation-perfusion mismatching
Anatomic Shunts
Congenital heart disease
Intrapulmonary shunts
Methemoglobinemia
Peripheral Cyanosis
Vasconstriction
Cold Exposure
Heart Failure
Shock
Arterial Obstruction
Venous Obstruction

oxygen concentration lowers the partial pressure of oxygen in alveoli and is encountered only under special circumstances, such as at high altitudes or when breathing a mixture of low oxygen concentration (e.g., a failure in the oxygen source during anesthesia).

Alveolar hypoventilation. Alveolar hypoventilation occurs when the volume of fresh inspired air going to the alveoli per unit time is reduced. Alveolar hypoventilation is always associated with an increase in the partial pressure of CO_2 in arterial blood (PA_{CO_2}). Indeed, more important than the hypoxemia in alveolar hypoventilation is the increase in PA_{CO_2}. In practice hypoxemia is generally not marked as a result of pure alveolar hypoventilation unless hypoventilation is severe. Even then, respiratory acidosis and acidemia as a result of CO_2 retention dominate the clinical picture. Causes of alveolar hypoventilation include (1) depression (morphine, barbiturates, or anesthesia) or disease (trauma, hemorrhage, or inflammation) of the central nervous system (brain stem) involving respiratory control centers, or (2) severe damage to spinal cord conducting pathways as a result of cervical spinal cord disease. These disorders impair the centrally mediated drive to respiratory muscles (see Chapters 61 and 62). Other causes are (3) failure of the muscles of respiration as a result of chest wall damage or paralysis of the respiratory muscles from neuromuscular diseases (see Chapters 64 and 65), or (4) severe airway obstruction such as laryngeal paralysis, tracheal collapse, or tracheal foreign body (see Chapters 67 and 68).

Diffusion impairment. Diffusion impairment means that equilibration does not occur between alveolar oxygen and pulmonary blood because of an increase in the barriers through which the oxygen must pass to reach hemoglobin. In order for oxygen in alveoli to reach hemoglobin, diffusion must occur across the alveolar epithelium, interstitium, capillary basement membrane, and endothelium. Normally at rest, equilibration between alveolar and capillary oxygen partial pressures occurs after about one third of the total contact time available in the capillary. Thus, there is considerable reserve and even with exercise, when contact time is reduced, equilibration is virtually complete. Diffusion impairment may occur in diseases in which the normal diffusion barriers are thickened, such as with pulmonary interstitial diseases (fibrosis, pneumonia, edema, and other infiltrative diseases). In practice, diffusion impairment is probably a less important cause of hypoxemia than other mechanisms because of the large amount of reserve in diffusion time. Diseases in which impaired diffusion may occur generally also have ventilation-perfusion mismatching, which is a more powerful cause of hypoxemia. However, with diminished contact time in the pulmonary capillaries associated with exercise, equilibrium between alveolar and capillary oxygen is incomplete and diffusion impairment may contribute to hypoxemia. With diffusion impairment PA_{CO_2} is usually not elevated and may, in fact, be reduced due to hyperventilation stimulated by hypoxemia.

Ventilation-perfusion mismatch. Ventilation-perfusion mismatching or inequality means that alveolar ventilation and perfusion in various regions of the lung are not properly matched so that gas transfer is inefficient. This is a common cause of hypoxemia and occurs in most pulmonary parenchymal diseases. Ventilation-perfusion mismatch is responsible for the hypoxemia in interstitial/alveolar lung disease such as pneumonia and pulmonary edema, severe chronic bronchitis, chronic obstructive lung diseases, asthma, and pulmonary embolism (see Chapter 69).

Anatomic shunts. Anatomic shunts in which some blood reaches the arterial system without passing through ventilated regions of lung result in the addition of mixed venous blood with arterial blood and are an important mechanism of hypoxemia in veterinary medicine. The addition of deoxygenated venous blood to arterial blood can alter the oxygen saturation of hemoglobin in arterial blood and markedly diminish PA_{O_2}. In congenital heart disease unoxygenated blood from the right heart shunts directly to the left heart without passing through the pulmonary circulation. This is the most common cause of shunts (see Chapter 74). Intrapulmonary anatomic shunts are produced by pulmonary artery to pulmonary venous fistulas or from lung lobe consolidation due to pneumonia in which a large portion of lung is completely unventilated but is perfused. Some readers may argue that lung lobe consolidation is an extreme example of ventilation-perfusion mismatching. However, as will be discussed later, a shunt causes a characteristic pattern of gas exchange in response to breathing 100 per cent oxygen and it is convenient to include this example under shunts.

Methemoglobinemia. Methemoglobinemia occurs when there is an increased amount of the circulating abnormal hemoglobin pigment, methemoglobin. Methemoglobin is produced when heme iron is oxidized to the ferric state and consequently is unable to bind oxygen. Methemoglobin is normally produced daily by the oxidation of hemoglobin, however, enzyme systems within the red blood cell reduce the iron in methemoglobin to keep circulating methemoglobin at a very low level. Clinical methemoglobinemia can be (1) acquired due to the presence of oxidant chemicals that increase the rate of oxidation of heme iron or (2) congenital due to an enzyme deficiency that decreases the normal rate of methemoglobin reduction. Individuals with congenital enzyme deficiency are especially sensitive to oxidant drugs. Oxidants that have been responsible for methemoglobinemia include topical benzocaine, nitrates, nitrites, methylene blue, acetaminophen, phenazopyradine, and cetacaine. Congenital enzyme deficiency (methemoglobin reductase deficiency) has been described in the dog (see Chapters 55 and 113).

Peripheral Cyanosis

Peripheral cyanosis is associated with circulatory abnormalities of the peripheral vascular beds and usually involves the extremities. Depending on the cause, cyanosis may involve only one or a few extremities or may involve all extremities. The PA_{O_2} is usually normal. One mechanism is increased oxygen extraction at the capillary level because of diminished or sluggish blood flow, which results in reduced partial pressure of oxygen at the venous end of the capillary. Peripheral cyanosis can also occur from an increased amount of venous blood in the skin due to venous congestion.

Blood flow in the peripheral vascular beds can be altered by vasoconstriction in response to cold exposure, heart failure, or shock. In heart failure and shock, compensatory mechanisms redistribute the blood flow, favoring vital organs. Consequently, blood flow to the skin is often diminished (see Chapter 71).

Peripheral cyanosis can also be produced by arterial or venous obstruction (see Chapter 81). Acute arterial obstruction to an extremity as a result of thromboembolism or thrombosis can occur with feline cardiomyopathy, bacterial endocarditis (septic emboli), hypercoagulable conditions, such as nephrotic syndrome, and cold hemagglutinin disease. Venous obstruction can be generalized, as occurs in right-sided heart failure. In this case, cyanosis occurs because of venous congestion and because oxygen extraction is increased as a result of sluggish capillary blood flow. Localized venous obstruction can occur from thrombophlebitis or from restrictive devices, such as a rubber band around a limb.

HISTORICAL FINDINGS

SIGNALMENT

An important clue to aid in the diagnosis of cyanosis can often be found in the patient signalment.

Age. Central cyanosis in a young patient (less than one year) is very suggestive of congenital heart disease. Congenital methemoglobinemia can also be responsible in young animals, but this disorder is rare. Congestive heart failure, chronic pulmonary disease (chronic bronchitis, pulmonary fibrosis) or neoplasia of the respiratory tract are usually associated with adult or aged patients.

Breed. Chronic cardiopulmonary diseases (tracheal collapse, chronic bronchitis, and chronic mitral valve disease with congestive heart failure) are most often diagnosed in small or toy breeds. Several cases of laryngeal paralysis have been described in the Bouvier des Flandres.

PATTERN OF RESPIRATION

The pattern of respiration must not be overlooked in the history, as it can help determine not only whether cardiopulmonary disease is present but if so, at what anatomic level (lower versus upper airway disease).

Stridor. Stridor is a harsh, high-pitched inspiratory sound. Its presence suggests upper airway obstructive diseases such as laryngeal paralysis, tracheal foreign body, or neoplastic obstruction of the larynx or trachea. Stridorous sounds are often intermittent and exacerbated by exercise.

Dyspnea. Dyspnea is difficult or labored breathing and is usually characterized by an increase in the rate and depth of breathing, abdominal breathing, neck extension, and open-mouthed breathing. A history of dyspnea provides strong evidence of severe respiratory disease, usually of the lower airway (pulmonary edema, asthma, pneumonia) or pleural space (pleural effusion).

Cough. A cough is a sudden explosive forcing of air through the glottis. Persistent coughing is a common manifestation of cardiac (e.g., pulmonary edema) or pulmonary disease (e.g., chronic bronchitis, tracheal collapse) in the dog. Cough is also a common complaint with respiratory disease (e.g., asthma) but not cardiac disease in cats.

GAIT

Alveolar ventilation requires central neurological input and appropriate respiratory skeletal muscle function. Thus questions regarding the neurologic and musculoskeletal systems in the cyanotic patient may elicit answers that direct the clinician appropriately to extrapulmonary causes of the cyanosis. Cyanosis in these patients is likely due to alveolar hypoventilation because of decreased ventilatory drive or skeletal respiratory muscle weakness.

Episodic Weakness. Episodic (intermittent) weakness should alert the clinician to consider neuromuscular disorders.

Tetraparesis/Tetraplegia. Tetraparesis and tetraplegia mean weakness (paresis) or paralysis (plegia) of all four limbs and indicates severe brain stem or cervical spinal cord disease or injury, peripheral nerve disease, or neuromuscular disorders. In addition, a history or clinical evidence of head trauma may also be present.

Hindlimb Paralysis. Hindlimb paralysis with cyanosis and pain of the affected limb(s) suggests arterial obstruction. In cats, this is most often associated with cardiomyopathy. Arterial obstruction can affect individual limbs in both the front and rear.

OTHER HISTORICAL SIGNS

Other historical findings also offer important diagnostic information.

Syncope. Syncope (fainting) in cyanotic patients suggests congenital heart disease, low-output heart failure, or obstructive respiratory disorders such as tracheal collapse or laryngeal paralysis.

Pain. Pain localized to an extremity in association with cyanosis of that extremity is suggestive of arterial or venous obstruction.

Drug Use. Methemoglobinemia as the cause of cyanosis should be considered if drugs with the potential to cause methemoglobinemia have been administered.

PHYSICAL FINDINGS

Since cyanosis is most often due to cardiac or respiratory disorders, the physical examination related to these systems deserves the clinician's special attention.

AUSCULTATION

Heart Murmur. Heart murmurs are prolonged audible vibrations that occur during a normally silent period of the cardiac cycle. Patients with cyanotic heart disease usually have a murmur. The presence of a murmur in a young cyanotic patient should alert the clinician to the possibility of congenital heart disease. In adult dogs, congestive heart failure can cause cyanosis because of pulmonary edema (central cyanosis) or low-cardiac output (peripheral cyanosis). These patients almost always have a cardiac murmur, especially if the cause is chronic mitral valve disease. Similarly, cats with cardiomyopathy frequently have a murmur.

Pulmonary Crackles. Pulmonary crackles are discontinuous, intermittent sounds that resemble the sounds produced by Velcro or crumpling cellophane. Its detection in the cyanotic patient is very informative since it suggests lower airway diseases such as pulmonary edema, pneumonia, pulmonary fibrosis, or chronic bronchitis.

PALPATION

Palpation of the thoracic wall and other respiratory structures should be performed.

Cough. Coughing easily elicited by tracheal palpation is frequent in patients with tracheal collapse or other tracheobronchial diseases (foreign body).

Stridor. Stridor may be elicited from palpation of the larynx in patients with laryngeal paralysis or other causes of laryngeal obstructions.

Subcutaneous Emphysema. Subcutaneous emphysema is the accumulation of air within the subcutaneous tissues. When detected along the thoracic wall or neck, it suggests a rent in the airways (tracheal or bronchial tears). Trauma is often the cause; rib fractures may be palpable.

PATTERN OF RESPIRATION

In addition to the history regarding the patient's pattern of respiration, the clinician must also carefully observe the patient in order to document historical abnormalities in respiratory pattern.

Stridor. Stridor is the hallmark of upper airway obstruction and its presence should prompt a thorough upper airway examination, including observation of the motion of laryngeal structures during spontaneous breathing.

Dyspnea. Dyspnea usually indicates severe lower airway or pleural disease.

Other. Finally, poor excursions of the thoracic wall during breathing in a cyanotic patient may indicate respiratory muscle weakness from neuromuscular disease. If neuromuscular disease is present, other nonrespiratory signs of neuromuscular disease should be conspicuous.

EXAMINATION OF THE EXTREMITIES

Cool extremities in association with peripheral cyanosis indicate diminished blood flow to those regions. When generalized, causes of decreased cardiac output or vasoconstriction should be considered. Syncope or signs of heart failure may also be present. Pain and edema of the extremities are not present. When localized, causes of local arterial or venous obstruction should be considered. In such cases *pain* and/or *edema* of the extremity is usually present.

NEUROLOGIC EXAMINATION

General neurologic examination (see Chapter 60) of the cyanotic patient has critical importance not only in diagnosis but in developing the correct initial therapeutic plan (see Section VI). Cyanosis in patients with neurologic disorders is usually due to alveolar hypoventilation.

Weakness. Persistent or episodic weakness, especially when aggravated by exercise, is frequently observed with neuromuscular disorders.

Tetraplegia. Weakness may progress to tetraplegia in severely affected patients with neuromuscular, peripheral nerve, or cervical spinal cord disorders. Tetraplegia due to brain-stem disease or injury may be associated with altered consciousness (stupor or coma).

DIAGNOSTIC PLAN

The order in which laboratory data is acquired and the extent of the preliminary diagnostic plan are dictated by clinical assessment of the patient. Often, cyanotic patients are presented in a life-threatening condition and a complete diagnostic work-up should be delayed. In such cases the category of disease causing cyanosis often can be surmised on the basis of signalment, brief history, and a cursory physical examination. For example, pulmonary damage from thoracic trauma versus pulmonary edema due to congestive heart failure should be easy to differentiate on the basis of signalment, history, and physical examination. Pursuing a specific diagnosis can be delayed while appropriate life-saving measures are instituted.

Central and peripheral cyanosis also are differentiated on the basis of the history and physical examination. Subcategories of disease such as upper airway obstruction versus primary pulmonary disease can often be distinguished.

HEMOGRAM

A venous blood sample for a hemogram should be taken. *Gross inspection* of the venous blood can be helpful since with methemoglobinemia the blood is usually very dark with a brownish tinge, or in some cases chocolate-colored. The brown color of the blood may be more easily appreciated by placing a drop of blood on white filter paper. Further, shaking an aliquot of the venous blood exposed to room air will not result in a bright red color, because methemoglobin impairs the oxygen binding ability of heme. Normal venous blood exposed to room air will bind oxygen.

From the hemogram, the *hematocrit* is determined and is very important in the diagnosis of patients with central cyanosis. As mentioned previously, polycythemia often accompanies severe chronic hypoxemia (see Chapter 22). In veterinary medicine polycythemia accompanied by hypoxemia is most marked and common in cyanotic congenital heart diseases.

TABLE 21–2. TREATMENT OF CYANOSIS

Generic	(Trade)	Dosage	Route	Frequency	Brief Description
Oxygen		30–40% by volume	inhalation	as needed	improve oxygen saturation of hemoglobin
Methylene Blue		1–2 mg/kg	IV	once	*treatment of methemoglobinemia in dogs
N-Acetylcysteine	(Mucomyst)	140 mg/kg initial dose then repeat every 6 hours at 70 mg/kg	orally or IV	5–7 total treatments	treatment of acetaminophen toxicity in dogs and cats

*Caution—can cause Heinz hemolytic anemia and probably should not be used if Heinz body formation is present.

Examination of *red blood cell morphology* may reveal Heinz bodies when methemoglobinemia is the cause of cyanosis. Heinz body formation can also result in hemolytic anemia (see Chapter 113).

THORACIC RADIOGRAPHY

Since most causes of central cyanosis and some causes of peripheral cyanosis involve disease of the cardiopulmonary system, thoracic radiography is critical to the diagnosis of cyanotic disorders. Cyanotic congenital heart diseases generally demonstrate radiographic abnormalities of cardiac size and/or shape, and abnormalities of the pulmonary circulation (see Chapter 74). The pulmonary parenchyma is usually radiographically unremarkable. Likewise, cardiac causes of peripheral cyanosis are almost always associated with radiographic abnormalities of cardiac size and/or shape. Pulmonary edema (heart failure) may also be present. Central cyanosis due to pulmonary disease generally results in conspicuous radiographic abnormalities of the pulmonary parenchyma (see Chapter 69).

ARTERIAL BLOOD GAS ANALYSIS

Important information can be derived from arterial blood gas analysis. If you are unsure whether it is central or peripheral cyanosis, determining the PA_{O_2} is helpful. Decreased PA_{O_2} (hypoxemia) is associated with all causes of central cyanosis, whereas PA_{O_2} is generally normal in patients with peripheral cyanosis. Hypoxemia can be further categorized on the basis of arterial blood gas analysis. Arterial partial pressure of CO_2 is always elevated (hypercarbia) in alveolar hypoventilation. Consequently, most of these patients will be acidemic with respiratory acidosis. Hypercarbia is not present with the other causes of hypoxemia except for severe ventilation-perfusion mismatching, which decreases the efficiency of gas transfer for all gases. However, most patients with ventilation-perfusion mismatching are able to maintain a normal PA_{CO_2} by increasing ventilation in response to hypercarbia. Similarly, the PA_{CO_2} is usually not raised in anatomic shunts, because although the shunted blood is rich in CO_2, central chemoreceptors sense the increase in PA_{CO_2} and ventilation is increased, enhancing CO_2 elimination.

Additional information can be obtained by evaluating arterial blood gases while the patient is *breathing 100 per cent oxygen*. Hypoxemia associated with most respiratory conditions (alveolar hypoventilation, diffusion impairment, or ventilation-perfusion mismatching) is usually eliminated by breathing 100 per cent oxygen. (The exception is severe ventilation-perfusion mismatching.) Indeed, the PA_{O_2} may nearly reach levels seen in normal subjects breathing 100 per cent O_2 ($PA_{O_2} \approx 500$ mmHg). With an anatomic shunt (e.g., congenital heart disease), hypoxemia cannot be eliminated by raising the inspired oxygen concentration to 100 per cent, because shunted blood continues to bypass ventilated alveoli and thus is never exposed to the high alveolar oxygen concentration.

ELECTROCARDIOGRAPHY

Electrocardiography may provide important information to aid in the diagnosis of a patient with cyanosis. Because most cyanotic congenital heart diseases involve pulmonary outflow tract obstruction or pulmonary hypertension, a right ventricular hypertrophy pattern is most consistent with congenital heart disease in young cyanotic patients. A right ventricular hypertrophy and/or right atrial enlargement pattern may be seen occasionally with chronic pulmonary disease. Electrocardiographic abnormalities may be present in cats with cardiomyopathy.

GOALS OF TREATMENT

Appropriate and specific treatment depends on an accurate diagnosis. Cyanosis can be caused by many different pathophysiologic conditions, each of which may demand individual treatment directed at correcting the underlying pathophysiologic state. Nevertheless, in the *hypoxemic patient*, symptomatic treatment in the form of *increasing inspired oxygen concentration* is appropriate and often life-saving. The rise in PA_{O_2} during oxygen administration is greatest in patients with impaired respiratory function (alveolar hypoventilation, diffusion impairment, or ventilation-perfusion mismatching). However, if the cause of cyanosis is alveolar hypoventilation, the clinical significance of hypoxemia is usually minimal compared to the CO_2 retention. In these patients, *increasing alveolar ventilation* (relieving airway obstruction or intubating and ventilating) is mandatory in order to eliminate retained CO_2.

Although shunts respond less remarkably to oxygen administration than do the other causes of hypoxemia, administration of oxygen in these patients is still helpful. This is because the additional amount of dissolved oxygen that can be achieved at high alveolar partial pressure of oxygen can be appreciable. Practically, however, most veterinary patients with cyanotic congenital heart disease are stable at rest and oxygen treatment is usually unnecessary. The administration of oxygen is potentially hazardous. High concentrations of oxygen administered over prolonged periods can damage the lungs. The lowest inspired oxygen concentration that provides clinical benefit or an acceptable PA_{O_2} should be used. In general, no more than 40 per cent oxygen concentration is recommended and the patient should be weaned from the enriched oxygen environment as soon as clinically possible.

Relatively few clinical signs may be associated with moderate *methemoglobinemia*. If drug-induced methemoglobinemia is suspected then removing the offending drug may be sufficient. In certain instances when methemoglobinemia is severe and life-threatening, methylene blue has been advocated in dogs. This drug must be used with caution as it can cause or enhance Heinz body hemolytic anemia in dogs and cats. In some clinical reports whole blood transfusion has been helpful in severe cases. Acetaminophen toxicosis in cats can result in life-threatening methemoglobinemia. Gastric lavage and oral administration of activated charcoal to reduce absorption soon after acetaminophen ingestion and N-acetylcysteine orally or intravenously have been advocated as treatments (see Chapters 55 and 113).

Treatment of *peripheral cyanosis* depends entirely upon the cause. Symptomatic treatment of the cyanosis is not indicated and efforts should be directed at identifying and correcting the underlying cause.

22 POLYCYTHEMIA

FREDERICK H. DRAZNER

The term polycythemia refers to a syndrome characterized by an increase in the red blood cell count and its associated parameters (hemoglobin concentration and hematocrit). The increase may or may not be associated with an increase in the total quantity of red blood cells in the body.

Polycythemia may be subdivided into relative polycythemias, characterized by a normal red cell mass, and absolute (true) polycythemias, characterized by an expanded red cell mass.

Relative polycythemias occur as a result of a marked loss of body fluids associated with persistent vomition, profound diarrhea, hyperventilation due to hyperthermia, or abnormally diminished fluid intake. In certain instances loss of electrolytes from the extracellular compartment, when not associated with a corresponding loss of water, results in a diminished osmotic pressure in the extracellular fluid. The resultant shift of water into the intracellular compartment may cause a marked relative polycythemia. Certain types of peripheral circulatory failure states may produce a relative polycythemia due to a loss of plasma into the interstitial fluid. Finally, dogs and cats that are stressed may exhibit a relative polycythemia due to splenic contraction.

Absolute polycythemias may result from the abnormal proliferation of red cell precursors within the bone marrow (polycythemia vera) or from various syndromes associated with an increased synthesis and release of erythropoietin.

ETIOPATHOGENESIS

The pathophysiologic events responsible for the development of relative polycythemia (i.e., fluid loss, peripheral circulatory failure, and splenic contraction) have previously been mentioned. Absolute (true) polycythemias may be further classified according to the plasma erythropoietin levels of affected dogs and cats. See also Table 22–1.

Primary polycythemia (polycythemia vera) is a myeloproliferative disorder thought to be related to an acquired stem cell dysfunction. In this rare syndrome affected dogs and cats exhibit markedly low to undetectable erythropoietin levels. The hematopoietic overproduction exhibited in polycythemia vera is thought to be the result of the development of abnormal, autonomous clones of multipotential stem cells. The event responsible for the emergence of these autonomous clones is unknown, although a viral etiology is suspected based on the fact that several viruses can cause polycythemia in certain strains of mice.

Secondary polycythemias are associated with elevated plasma erythropoietin levels, which may or may not be physiologically appropriate. Normally, plasma erythropoietin levels increase as a response to tissue hypoxia. Thus, dogs and cats with chronically low PO_2 levels as the result of pulmonary disease, cardiovascular disease, or high altitude habitation may exhibit polycythemia.

APPROPRIATE SECONDARY POLYCYTHEMIA

Tissue hypoxia stimulates increased synthesis and release of REF (renal erythropoietic factor, erythropoietin) from the kidney. REF is converted to active erythropoietin upon linkage to a hepatic-derived alphaglobulin. Erythropoietin increases the rate of erythropoiesis in the bone marrow and enhances the oxygen-carrying capacity of the blood. In addition, accelerated erythropoiesis results in an increase in blood volume with subsequent dilatation and opening of vessels, causing enhanced tissue perfusion.

TABLE 22–1. PATHOPHYSIOLOGIC AND CLINICAL CLASSIFICATION OF POLYCYTHEMIA

- Relative
  - Diminished Plasma Volume
    - Profound vomition
    - Severe diarrhea
    - Peripheral circulatory failure
  - Splenic contraction
- Absolute
  - Normal or Diminished Erythropoietin Levels
    - Bone marrow proliferation (polycythemia vera)
  - Elevated Erythropoietin Levels
    - Appropriate production
      - Chronic pulmonary disease
      - Chronic congestive heart failure with cyanosis
      - High altitude (above 10,000 feet)
      - Obesity (pickwickian like syndrome)
    - Inappropriate Production
      - Renal neoplasia
      - Hydronephrosis
      - Polycystic renal disease
      - Hyperadrenocorticism
      - Pheochromocytoma

High Altitude. Dogs living at or above the timber line (above 10,000 feet) may have hematocrits and hemoglobins exceeding 65 per cent and 22 gm/per cent, respectively. At these altitudes the pressure gradient for oxygen transport from the air to the venous end of tissue capillaries becomes quite diminished. To compensate for the reduced oxygen diffusion gradient, acclimatized dogs rely upon hyperventilation and polycythemia.

Pulmonary Disease. Chronic obstructive pulmonary disease (COPD) with hypoxemia and hypercapnia as the result of emphysema and bronchiectasis may cause polycythemia, although it is not as severe as that caused by high altitude. The erythropoietic response may be quite variable in dogs with chronic disease, possibly due to an increased production of 2,3-diphosphoglycerate (2,3- DPG) with an increase in arterial desaturation and a shift of the oxygen dissociation curve to the right. Dogs with COPD and polycythemia may have deteriorating clinical signs due to the resultant hyperviscosity, adding to the already excessive cardiac workload present (especially right ventricular) and pulmonary hypertension.

Alveolar Hypoventilation. Impairment of ventilatory function, either central (cerebral vascular accident, encephalitis) or peripheral (marked obesity, i.e., pickwickian-like syndrome) in origin causes erythropoiesis due to arterial hypoxia.

Cardiovascular Disease. Dogs and cats with congenital heart disease and right-to-left shunting (tetralogy of Fallot reversed ventricular septal defect with Eisenmenger's complex) exhibit polycythemia. Often patients with acquired left-sided congestive heart failure exhibit an increased red cell mass, which may be obscured by the simultaneous expansion of plasma volume.

Testosterone. Testosterone (in both natural and synthetic forms) occasionally causes a marked secondary polycythemia by stimulating the synthesis of erythropoietin and by augmenting the effects of erythropoietin upon erythroid precursor cells in the bone marrow.

INAPPROPRIATE SECONDARY POLYCYTHEMIA

Erythropoiesis is said to be inappropriate when no evidence of circulatory or pulmonary dysfunction is found. In this setting polycythemia occurs as a result of an unregulated secretion of erythropoietin in the absence of general tissue hypoxia. Inappropriate secondary polycythemia is caused by both renal and extrarenal disorders.

Renal Disorders. The most common cause of inappropriate secondary polycythemia in small animal practice is the presence of space-occupying renal lesions, which may be cysts, hydronephrotic lesions, or renal neoplasms (adenocarcinoma, lymphosarcoma, and fibroma). Since the assay of erythropoietin from tumor extracts or cystic fluid is tedious, it is not commonly performed. Thus, there is speculation that many renal tumors associated with polycythemia are not actively secreting excessive quantities of erythropoietin but that polycythemia occurs as a result of the space-occupying effects of the tumor, which induce hypoxia by pressuring the adjoining renal parenchyma. In contrast, however, nephrectomy has resulted in the normalization of the red blood cell count in affected patients and in certain instances, the emergence of metastatic foci has caused the recurrence of polycythemia. This phenomenon gives credence to the existence of an orthoendocrine paraneoplastic syndrome.

In humans, polycythemia has been associated with many non-renal tumors, including uterine leiomyoma, pheochromocytoma (the only nonrenal tumor causing polycythemia identified thus far in the dog), pulmonary squamous cell carcinoma, and cerebellar hemangioblastoma. In some instances assay of the tumor reveals erythropoietin, thus documenting ectopic hormone production (paraendocrine paraneoplastic syndrome). It can be argued, especially in the case of large tumors of the uterus, adrenal glands, and lungs that the direct compressive effect of the tumor may create hypoxia in the kidney or lung, respectively.

Hyperadrenocorticism. Hypercortisolemia due either to pituitary adenoma, negative feedback defect, or functional adrenal tumor sometimes results in polycythemia due to the compensatory effect of cortisol on erythropoietin in the bone marrow.

PATHOPHYSIOLOGY

The clinical signs exhibited by polycythemic dogs and cats are the result of increased blood viscosity and expanded blood volume. An increase in blood viscosity has an effect upon the cardiovascular system owing to an increase in peripheral resistance and a decrease in cardiac output, ultimately resulting in diminished oxygen transport to the tissues, which in turn stimulates the synthesis and release of additional REF. In addition, sluggish blood flow may lead to thrombotic episodes. An increase in blood volume causes vascular expansion and venous engorgement. It is obvious that the high incidence of dizziness, headache, and tinnitus associated with human polycythemic patients is unknown in small animal practice, but these symptoms may account for the lethargy, anorexia, restlessness, and reluctance to ambulate seen in affected dogs and cats. Venous engorgement is also responsible for frequent bilateral epistaxis and for hematemesis associated with polycythemia.

HISTORICAL FINDINGS

Lethargy, Reluctance to Ambulate. The hyperviscosity and venous engorgement in the circulation of the brain may produce headache, tinnitus, and dizziness in affected dogs and cats, causing them to be reluctant to move about in their environment.

Coughing, Dyspnea. Dogs and cats with polycythemia due to chronic respiratory disease are usually presented for cough and exercise intolerance.

Hematuria. Malignant renal tumors associated with polycythemia may cause hematuria that is unresponsive to antibiotic therapy.

TABLE 22–2. DRUGS USED IN TREATMENT OF POLYCYTHEMIA

Generic name	Trade name	Dosage	Route of Administration	Frequency	Description
Chlorambucil	Leukeran	0.2 mg/kg	oral	sid	alkylating agent (chemotherapy)
Busulfan	Myleran	4.0 mg/m^2	oral	sid	alkylating agent (chemotherapy)

Stunting, Failure to Thrive in a Puppy or Kitten. The owner of a puppy or kitten with congenital heart disease and polycythemia due to right-to-left shunting often seeks veterinary help because of concern that the pet is not growing and is not playful.

Epistaxis. Polycythemic dogs and cats occasionally exhibit a bilateral epistaxis. In contrast, animals with nasal tumors usually exhibit a unilateral epistaxis.

Miscellaneous Historical Findings. The clinician suspicious of polycythemia in the pet of the new client should question the owner regarding a recent move from a high altitude location or the recent administration of androgen compounds.

PHYSICAL FINDINGS

Hyperemia With or Without Cyanosis. Polycythemic dogs and cats, especially those with severe chronic respiratory disease or cardiac disorders associated with right-to-left shunting, display both hyperemia and cyanosis. Animals with polycythemia not associated with generalized hypoxic conditions will obviously not be cyanotic.

Cardiac Murmur. Puppies or kittens with polycythemia due to congenital heart disease and right-to-left shunting exhibit a holosystolic murmur associated with ventricular septal defect and tetralogy of Fallot in which the crescendo-decrescendo murmur of pulmonic stenosis may also be detected. Murmurs are not heard in all cardiac diseases if the right- and left-sided pressures are equal.

Obesity, Expiratory Harsh Lung Sounds. Examination and auscultation of polycythemic dogs with COPD and/or pickwickian-like syndrome often reveal an animal that is grossly overweight and has dry rales.

Splenomegaly and Ecchymoses. These clinical findings are often detected in animals with polycythemia vera.

Palpable Retroperitoneal Masses. In cats and small, thin dogs with large renal tumors it may be possible for the clinician to palpate these masses.

DIAGNOSTIC PLAN

CBC. A complete blood count is necessary to establish the existence of a polycythemic state. A red blood cell count, hematocrit and hemoglobin of greater than 10,000,000/mm^3, 65 per cent, and 22 gm per cent, respectively, documents the presence of an increased red blood cell mass. Relative polycythemia can be excluded by the presence of a normal total plasma protein level, the absence of clinical dehydration, and a calm, unstressed patient. Occasionally dogs with polycythemia vera exhibit accompanying leukocytosis and thrombocytosis.

Radiology. Thoracic x-rays reveal signs of chronic bronchitis, bronchiectasis, or emphysema. In young puppies or kittens with suspected congenital cardiac disease, selective angiography and/or ultrasonography are necessary to identify the defect. Often abdominal radiographs reveal a retroperitoneal mass in dogs and cats with large erythropoietin-secreting renal tumors or splenomegaly in dogs with polycythemia vera. Abdominal ultrasonography and/or intravenous pyelography further delineates the tumor.

Measurement of Erythropoietin. Although it is a difficult and expensive diagnostic test that is performed by only a handful of laboratories, the measurement of erythropoietic activity (employing an exhypoxic polycythemic mouse assay) is useful in documenting absolute secondary polycythemia. The presence of elevated erythropoietin levels in a polycythemic dog or cat in the absence of severe cardiopulmonary disease is considered inappropriate. Animals with polycythemia vera have low or undetectable levels of erythropoietin.

Bone Marrow Aspirate. Polycythemia vera is documented via bone marrow aspiration. The bone marrow is hyperplastic with a decrease in fat cells, marked erythropoiesis, and clumps of megakaryocytes.

THERAPEUTIC PRINCIPLES

Polycythemia Vera. Often periodic phlebotomies (to lower the hematocrit to less than 55 per cent) are all that is necessary for the long-term management of dogs and cats with polycythemia vera. The removal of 20 ml/kg of blood at three-day intervals until the desired hematocrit is achieved appears to be the desired protocol. In resistant cases the use of the alkylating agents busulfan or chlorambucil may be indicated.

Chronic Pulmonary Disease. The use of bronchodilators, antibiotics when indicated, and drastic weight reduction in obese dogs and cats occasionally improves pulmonary oxygenation, thereby reducing the excessive synthesis and release of erythropoietin. However, often it is necessary to perform occasional phlebotomies to normalize red blood cell indices.

Cardiac Disease. Surgical correction of tetralogy of Fallot or medical therapy of acquired left-sided congestive heart failure with cardiac glycosides, vasodilators,

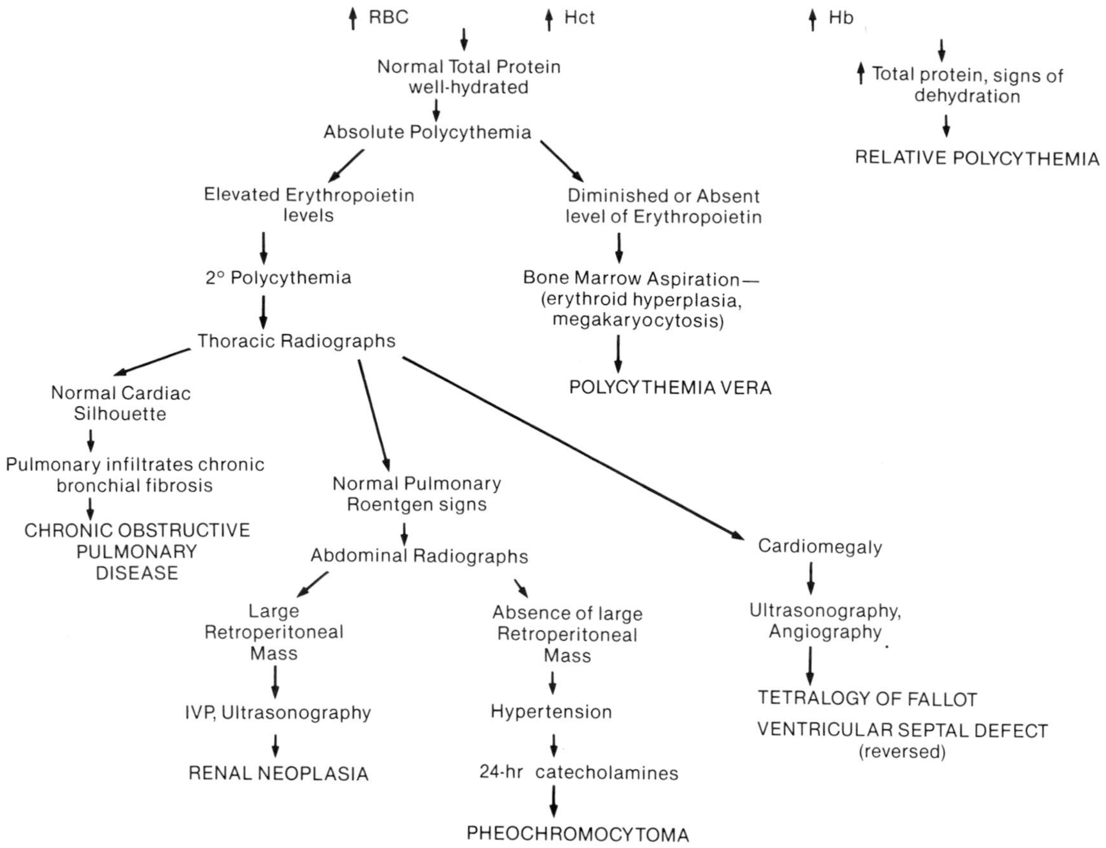

FIGURE 22–1. Algorithm of the diagnostic plan for polycythemia.

and diuretics improves pulmonary oxygenation and thus normalizes the hematocrit.

Renal Tumors. Nephrectomy of the causative renal tumor usually reduces the hematocrit.

Adrenal Disease. Adrenalectomy for pheochromocytoma or functional adrenal tumor associated with Cushing's syndrome or the administration of O'P-DDD (Mitotane) for pituitary-dependent hyperadrenocorticism lowers the RBC indices due to the normalization of plasma cortisol levels.

PROGNOSIS

Aside from polycythemia vera (primary polycythemia), the prognosis for other diseases associated with polycythemia depends upon the degree of success in the management of the primary disorder. Patients with chronic obstructive pulmonary disease rarely have a favorable long-term prognosis due to widespread irreversible destruction of pulmonary parenchyma. Dogs with acquired left-sided congestive heart failure may enjoy a considerable period of functional survival with proper medical and dietary therapy. Surgical extirpation of renal or adrenal tumors is often curative, however, this depends upon the histologic character of the tumor and its metastatic potential.

Polycythemia vera may be managed for many months with periodic phlebotomies, with or without adjunctive chemotherapy. Potential sequelae encountered in affected humans include acute myelogenous leukemia, myelosclerosis, and massive splenomegaly. The incidence of the above complications in dogs and cats is unknown because of the extremely limited number of reported cases of polycythemia vera in small animal practice.

23 THE CLINICAL APPROACH TO DISORDERS OF HEMOSTASIS

G. DANIEL BOON and A. H. REBAR

The maintenance of hemostasis is a complex and amazing process. Upon contact with almost anything other than an endothelial surface, blood converts from a liquid that carries gases and nutrients to a solidified jelly. However, hemostasis depends on more than the simple gelling of blood. The proper functioning of vessels, platelets, and plasma coagulation factors, all interacting in an integrated way, is necessary if blood loss is to be terminated after vessels have been breached. Some of these interactions have only been elucidated in the last few decades. Much has been learned, but our knowledge of the mechanisms involved is still imperfect. For example, there is still no exact explanation for the lack of clinical bleeding in patients with deficiencies of factor XII.

The complexity of the coagulation mechanism can be somewhat intimidating. It is easy to get lost in the roman numeral system of nomenclature, especially since the order of reaction sequence does not follow the numerical sequence. In a field as difficult as hemostasis, it might be successfully argued that diagnostic problems should be left to "specialists" and this might be true in the clarification of congenital abnormalities. However, every practitioner is occasionally faced with a presurgical patient with a vague history of bleeding. A logical approach and a few simple screening tests allow these patients to be quickly and efficiently evaluated. This chapter presents such an approach to the clinical evaluation of the bleeding patient.

Perhaps the most important rule to keep in mind when evaluating the bleeding patient is that blood can be lost from vessels for reasons other than hemorrhagic tendencies. The animal that has been hit by a car and is bleeding does not need a hemostatic profile. Likewise, the pet which has just had an ovariohysterectomy that bleeds postoperatively has a greater chance, by orders of magnitude, of having a slipped ligature than of having a bleeding tendency. Obviously, the proper care of such patients seldom requires a hemostatic evaluation.

GENERAL CONCEPTS OF ABNORMAL BLEEDING

Levels of Platelets. Thrombocytopenia is the most common cause of abnormal bleeding in both humans and animals. The degree of bleeding associated with thrombocytopenia is highly variable and often does not correlate with the platelet count. The reasons for this variation are not completely clear, but may involve the mechanism by which the thrombocytopenia is produced. If platelets are being destroyed peripherally with a compensatory increase in marrow production, the resulting circulating population of relatively young platelets probably functions better than an older population and prevents bleeding at low concentrations. Conversely, if thrombocytopenia is the result of decreased production, the remaining circulating platelets comprise a relatively old population with proportionately poorer function that allows bleeding to occur at higher concentrations. There also appears to be a species variation in platelet concentrations associated with bleeding. In the experience of one of the authors (GDB), cats can withstand severe episodes of thrombocytopenia with little or no bleeding problem.

The commonly quoted concentrations of 40,000 to 50,000 platelets per microliter (μl) at which bleeding may become apparent are probably good rules of thumb, but the following ranges are more appropriate. Spontaneous bleeding is likely to occur at platelet counts below 20,000/μl, bleeding following trauma is possible at platelet counts between 20,000 and 100,000/μl, and spontaneous bleeding is unlikely at platelet counts between 50,000 and 100,000/μl.

Levels of Coagulation Factors. The association between clotting factor concentrations and a clinical tendency to bleed is much better than that between platelet concentrations and tendency to bleed. To prevent bleeding after surgery or trauma, the minimum level of all coagulation factors necessary is generally accepted to be 25 per cent of normal. This is in contrast to the concentrations of 50 per cent needed for most screening tests of coagulation to be within normal limits.

CLINICAL APPROACH TO THE PATIENT

History. Historical information can be a most effective way to diagnose bleeding disorders. In life there are many challenges to hemostasis and those challenges are better and more realistic tests of hemostasis than any laboratory evaluation. When taking a history, specific questions must be asked about the appropriateness of bleeding in trauma, and in surgery such as ovariohysterectomy and castration. Age of onset is an obviously essential piece of information to be elicited. It is very important to get specific details because many pet owners may overestimate the amount of blood lost. A negative history, of course, does not guarantee freedom from disease. Several classes of disorders may not be revealed in the history. These include disorders that are acquired or mild, or that involve the contact activation pathway (see Chapter 116).

When the clinician considers that a congenital bleeding disorder is likely, an examination of the pedigree can be beneficial in diagnosing the specific problem. Deficiencies of factors VIII and IX are sex-linked, while factor XI deficiency and von Willebrand's disease are autosomal. A more complete hereditary listing is found in Chapter 116.

The presence of underlying diseases is important to note for two reasons. Bleeding is a direct result of many conditions such as leukemias, uremia, and liver disease. Also, any drug therapy that has been instituted subsequent to a disease process may affect hemostasis. Examples of drugs that affect hemostasis are coumarin derivatives, heparin, and many prostaglandin inhibitors such as aspirin.

Physical Examination. The physical examination primarily provides diagnostic information regarding types of bleeding, discussed below. An additional major benefit of the physical examination is the ruling out of underlying diseases. Such abnormalities as splenomegaly, lymphadenopathy, jaundice, and bone tenderness are indicative of primary diseases that may be associated with bleeding diatheses.

The appearance of the bleeding in a patient often suggests the underlying cause. In all cases this judgment must be tempered by the clinical information available, that is, bleeding is expected in trauma, but is the bleeding appropriate to the degree of trauma?

Petechiae are pinpoint-sized subepithelial hemorrhages associated with both thrombocytopenia and vascular defects. There can be a subtle difference between the petechiae in these two disorders, however. Petechiae due to vascular defects are often raised due to the associated increase in capillary permeability. Petechiae due to thrombocytopenia are flat and often concentrated in areas of trauma or increased hydrostatic pressure. Other areas where petechiae are commonly found in patients with thrombocytopenia are the gingiva, respiratory mucosa, gastrointestinal mucosa, and urinary mucosa. The result is often epistaxis, melena, and hematuria, respectively.

Ecchymoses are small hemorrhagic spots in the skin or mucous membranes that are larger than petechiae. They are often considered to be confluent petechiae and therefore caused by thrombocytopenia or vascular disorders. While this is often true, ecchymoses can also be caused by defects of coagulation.

Bleeding into tissues resulting in hematomas or hemarthroses are most often associated with deficiencies of coagulation factors. The most common by far is factor VIII deficiency (hemophilia A).

Prolonged bleeding from minor trauma such as venipuncture is associated with defects of primary hemostasis (thrombocytopenia, defective platelet function, or vascular disorders). It must be emphasized that this is probably the most overinterpreted of all bleeding signs. Puncture of a vein causes bleeding of variable duration in even the most normal animal.

Rebleeding after a lag phase of apparently normal hemostasis is the hallmark of coagulation factor deficiencies. This usually takes place within 24 hours after the occurrence of the trauma. This delay is present because the platelet plug, which forms normally, is not stabilized by fibrin formation. The degree of hemorrhage associated with such rebleeding episodes can be very large and life-threatening.

LABORATORY APPROACH TO THE PATIENT

Principles of Laboratory Examination. Normal hemostasis is a complex interaction of a large number of factors, making it impractical to test for each one individually in every bleeding patient. For this reason the initial screening tests must be designed to measure

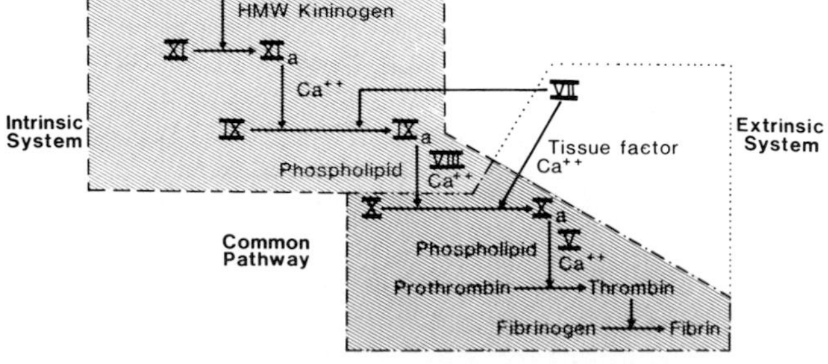

FIGURE 23–1. The coagulation cascade.

groups of hemostatic mechanisms. In this way the defect can be localized to allow a more efficient use of specific tests. Since special tests are not available in most practices, this approach also allows intelligent ordering of specific tests when a sample is mailed to a reference laboratory. Complete discussion of hemostatic testing is found in Chapters 116 and 117. Here we discuss a basic approach that allows at least a tentative diagnosis in most cases.

Platelets. Because thrombocytopenia is so common and evaluation of platelet numbers is simple, we recommend that platelets be evaluated in all cases of bleeding. Evaluation can be accomplished by several methods. Regardless of the method used, it is important to pay special attention to sample collection. Difficult venipuncture results in contamination with tissue fluid, causing platelet aggregation and a falsely decreased count. The quickest and probably most efficient means of platelet evaluation for the general practitioner is simply examining the peripheral blood smear. In the absence of platelet clumps at the feathered edge, six to seven platelets per oil immersion field represents about 100,000 platelets per microliter. Fewer than three or four platelets per oil immersion field is a serious thrombocytopenia. Alternatively, if platelets are counted in ten oil immersion fields and the total number multiplied by 2000, the result closely approximates the platelet count by other techniques. The reference method for platelet enumeration is the method of Brecher and Cronkite, which uses ten per cent ammonium oxalate as the diluent, a Neubauer hemacytometer, and phase-contrast microscopy. It is the basis for the Unopette method. Interestingly, all methods of platelet counting must be supplemented by examining a well-made and well-stained peripheral blood smear as a check on technique.

Evaluation of platelet function is beyond the scope of this brief discussion. A thorough treatment can be found in Chapter 117.

TABLE 23–1. TESTING FOR COAGULATION ABNORMALITIES WITH THE ACTIVATED PARTIAL THROMBOPLASTIN TIME (APTT) AND THE PROTHROMBIN TIME (PT)

Pattern of Test Abnormality	Location of Coagulation Abnormality	Possible Factor Deficiencies
1. APTT–normal PT –normal	Normal or mild deficiency	Any
2. APTT–normal PT –prolonged	Extrinsic system deficiency	VII
3. APTT–prolonged PT –normal	Intrinsic system deficiency	VIII, IX, XI, or XII
4. APTT–prolonged PT –prolonged	Common pathway or multiple deficiencies	X, V, II, I or combinations of patterns 2 and 3

Coagulation Factors. The coagulation cascade can be conveniently divided into three parts (Figure 23–1): the intrinsic system, the extrinsic system, and the common pathway. Most defects of coagulation can be localized to one of these areas using only two routine tests of coagulation. These are the activated partial thromboplastin time (APTT) and the (one stage) prothrombin time (PT). The APTT assesses the intrinsic system and the common pathway, while the PT assesses the extrinsic system and the common pathway. As can be seen in Figure 23–1, both tests evaluate a rather large number of factors, so they are not specific. However, this does have the advantage of allowing screening so that specific tests can be performed appropriately. The localization process is illustrated in Table 23–1.

It is important to note that these are not particularly sensitive tests. If the patterns in Table 23–1 are detected, a coagulation deficit is assured, and can be definitively diagnosed with appropriate follow-up tests. If these tests are normal, however, the patient is not guaranteed to be free of such a deficit. If a situation arises where there is historical or other evidence that a bleeding problem exists and these initial screening tests show no abnormality, further testing or referral is indicated.

24 JAUNDICE

SUSAN E. BUNCH

Jaundice or *icterus* may be defined as the clinical state in which hyperbilirubinemia is detectable as yellowish discoloration of the plasma (biochemical) or tissues, e.g., mucous membranes, sclerae, and skin (clinical). The terms *jaundice* and *cholestasis* cannot be used interchangeably, since not all causes of jaundice are associated with bile secretory failure. Deposition of bile pigments must be distinguished from yellowish staining of the skin and urine by certain therapeutic agents, such as quinacrine hydrochloride, or consumption of inordinate amounts of carotene-containing substances, principally carrots. In such instances, the skin and urine are stained, but the sclerae usually remain free of color. Though these conditions have been recognized in human patients, they have not been documented in companion animals.

METHODS OF DETECTION

The intensity and distribution of staining of tissues by bile pigments depend upon several factors, including total plasma bilirubin concentration and predominant form (which are directly related to the underlying disease process), capillary perfusion, and tissue composition. Subtle jaundice may not be detectable in tissues with rich capillary beds, since the color of hemoglobin tends to obscure the faint yellow hue. Differences in tissue affinity for bile pigments account for the deposition of water-soluble conjugated bilirubin in tissues high in elastic fibers, such as skin and sclerae, whereas lipid-soluble unconjugated bilirubin has a propensity for deeper-lying fat depots. Likewise, the form of bile pigment found in urine is water-soluble conjugated bilirubin.

It is generally accepted that hyperbilirubinemia becomes clinically detectable when the total plasma concentration exceeds 2 mg/dl. Sites where jaundice is likely to be discovered early include the sclerae, areas of nonpigmented thin skin such as the inner pinnae, and, in the cat, the caudal aspect of the palate.

Though in general the intensity of jaundice is proportional to the plasma level of bilirubin, the appearance and disappearance of tissue jaundice do not necessarily coincide with the onset and resolution of the causative disease process, and jaundice may resolve more slowly than hyperbilirubinemia. For example, jaundice is not clinically evident both in dogs and in cats with experimentally created complete extrahepatic bile duct obstruction until three to four days after surgery.

When clinically evident jaundice is not present, yellow staining of the plasma may be apparent as bilirubin levels approach 1.5 mg/dl. Owing to species differences in the role of the kidney in bilirubin metabolism, bilirubinuria may or may not be indicative of hyperbilirubinemia. Bilirubin should not be present in the urine of healthy cats, in which the renal threshold for conjugated bilirubin is seven to nine times higher than that of the dog. Because the canine kidney is able to synthesize and conjugate bilirubin and has a low threshold for conjugated bilirubin, the finding of low concentrations of bilirubin in urine of specific gravity greater than 1.025 is considered normal in dogs. Progressive increases in urine bilirubin in the dog, however, may precede hyperbilirubinemia and the onset of tissue jaundice.

PATHOPHYSIOLOGY

Hyperbilirubinemia occurs when the rate of production of bilirubin exceeds the rate of elimination. Under normal conditions, bilirubin has no physiologic function, and is only a waste product of heme catabolism. Normal senescent erythrocytes are the primary source of heme to be degraded (60 to 70 per cent of the total in dogs), with other heme-containing proteins, e.g., myoglobin and cytochrome enzymes, and defective erythrocytes from ineffective erythropoiesis in the bone marrow, amounting to approximately 35 per cent. After phagocytosis by cells of the monocyte-macrophage system or release directly into the bloodstream by intravascular hemolysis, the protoporphyrin ring of the hemoglobin molecule is opened by heme-oxygenase, forming biliverdin. Heme-oxygenase is found primarily in the liver, spleen, and bone marrow, and to some extent, renal tubules in the dog. The final product, bilirubin IX a, is formed when biliverdin is reduced by biliverdin reductase in the liver and spleen. Released from the monocyte-macrophage cells into the circulation, bilirubin is bound to albumin (2:1) for transport to the hepatic sinusoidal membrane for uptake. At this point, the albumin molecule is removed, and the bilirubin molecule is taken up by means of a bidirectional, carrier-mediated, competitively inhibited process into the hepatocyte, is reversibly bound intracellularly to Y and Z proteins, which, by facilitated diffusion, transport bilirubin to microsomes for conjugation to carbohydrates. The purpose of conjugation is to render the bilirubin molecule water-soluble so that it may be excreted into the bile, and not absorbed by the intestine. Diconjugates (80 per cent) of glucuronide (59 per cent) predominate in both dogs and cats, with xylosyl (31 per cent) and glucosyl (10 per cent) conjugates produced in addition in dogs. It has been shown in rats that hepatic conjugation is the rate-limiting step in the overall removal of bilirubin, since the efficiency of clearance of conjugated bilirubin is three times greater than that of unconjugated bilirubin.

The final phase of bilirubin elimination is accomplished by carrier-mediated excretion into the bile canaliculus, where it is incorporated into micelles in the bile. Conjugated bilirubin is deconjugated, then reduced to urobilinogen in the large intestine after discharge into the duodenum. Most urobilinogen is absorbed to complete an enterohepatic circulation, a fraction escapes recycling to be excreted in the urine, and the remainder is oxidized to stercobilin, which imparts normal fecal color.

Hyperbilirubinemia may be classified as *extrahepatic* or *intrahepatic* (Figure 24–1), according to the location of the disturbance in bilirubin metabolism. Increased production of bilirubin (Figure 24–1*A*), one of the two major causes of extrahepatic hyperbilirubinemia, is usually caused by greatly accelerated erythrocyte destruction, associated with either intra- or extravascular hemolysis of normal or abnormal cells, incompatible blood transfusion, or absorption of a large hematoma. The magnitude of hyperbilirubinemia usually is mild in such cases, as long as hepatic clearance remains normal. Studies of bilirubin clearance in dogs with severe Coombs' positive hemolytic anemia, however, have shown that increased production of bilirubin is accompanied by reduced hepatic clearance, perhaps because of hepatocellular hypoxia. The maximal plasma bilirubin level attainable in human patients with sustained, severe hemolysis has been determined to be approximately four mg/dl. Review of clinical cases of canine hemolytic anemia supports this observation in general, with total bilirubin levels usually less than ten mg/dl. Bacterial degradation products of blood lost into the gastrointestinal tract are not absorbed to provide additional heme substrate for bilirubin synthesis, so hyperbilirubinemia does not occur even when there is major gastrointestinal hemorrhage.

Intrahepatic hyperbilirubinemia results when there is interference at any step along the normal pathway of hepatocellular transport of bilirubin. Impaired hepatic uptake of unconjugated bilirubin (Figure 24–1*B1*) may occur as a result of competition with other organic anions, excluding bile acids, as a congenital multiple enzyme defect in human patients with Gilbert's syndrome and in mutant Southdown sheep, or in severe hepatic dysfunction, as has been suggested in human patients with cirrhosis.

Congenital deficiencies in enzymes responsible for conjugation of bilirubin (Figure 24–1*B2*) have been known in human patients with Crigler-Najjar syndrome, types I and II, for many years. A similar condition is known to occur in homozygous Gunn rats, but not in companion animal species. It is possible that the feline species, because of its susceptibility to protein catabolism during anorexia and inherent low activity of glu-

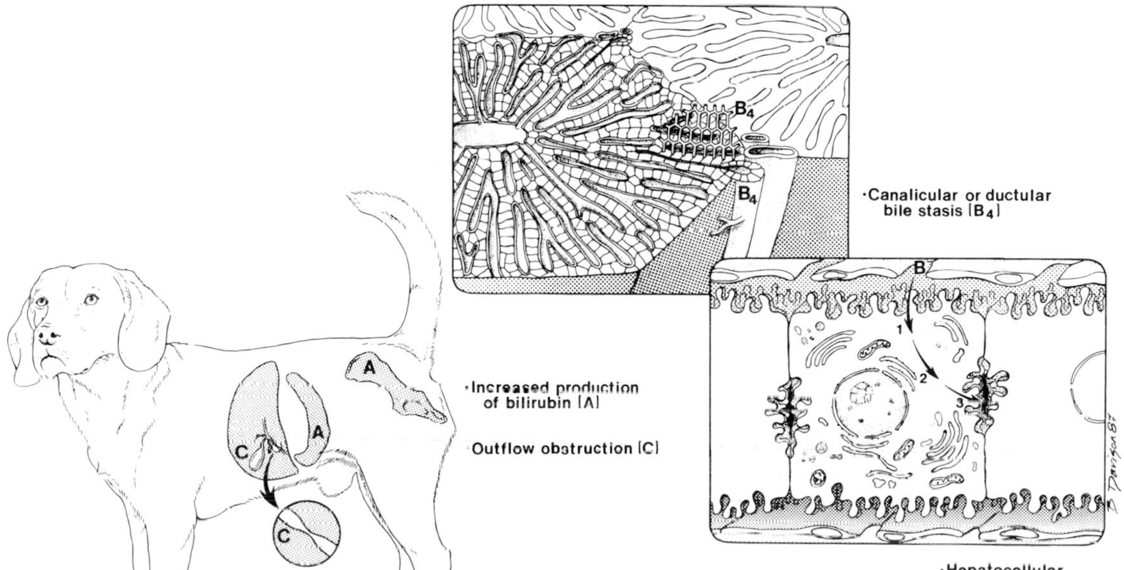

FIGURE 24–1. Schematic representation of mechanisms of hyperbilirubinemia, divided into extrahepatic and intrahepatic causes. A = Increased production of bilirubin within the monocyte-macrophage system. B = Reduced elimination of bilirubin within the liver. C = Obstruction to outflow of bile.

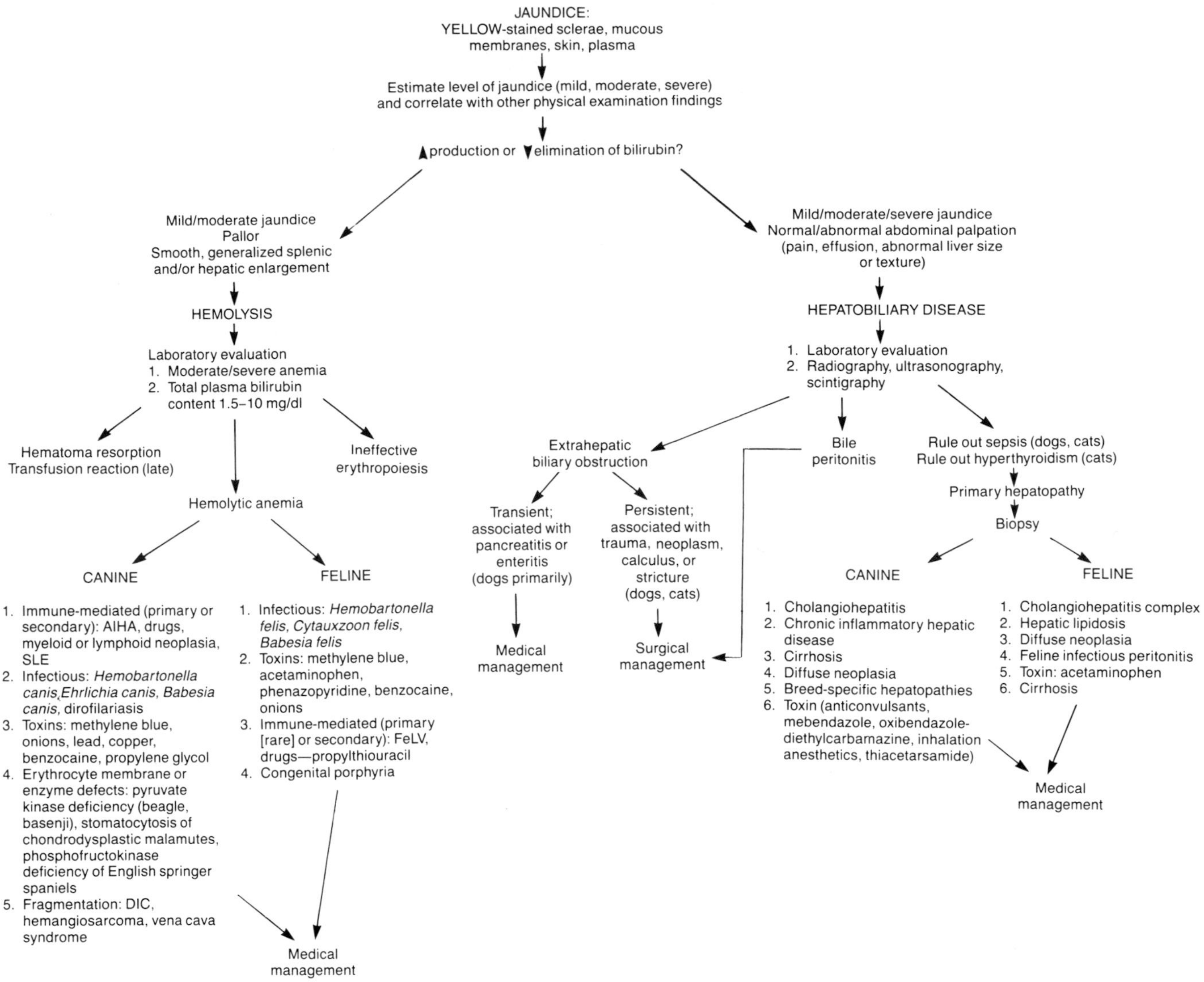

FIGURE 24–2. Rational diagnostic approach to the companion animal with jaundice. (Research for this material supported by Berkeley Veterinary Research Foundation.)

curonyl transferase conjugating enzymes, may develop fasting unconjugated hyperbilirubinemia, but this has not been proven.

Altered excretion of conjugated bilirubin into the bile canaliculus (Figure 24–1*B3*) is the cause of jaundice induced by certain therapeutic agents, e.g., norethandrolone, in human patients, and by circulating bacterial endotoxins. Rare inherited defects in the transport of conjugated forms of both bilirubin and sulfobromophthalein (BSP) from the hepatocyte into the bile canaliculus may also cause mild conjugated hyperbilirubinemias in human patients and in mutant Corriedale sheep with Dubin-Johnson syndrome.

Acquired hepatobiliary diseases (Figure 24–1*B1* through 4, 24–1*C*) may impair the removal of both unconjugated and conjugated bilirubin as well as other bile constituents, resulting in cholestasis. All steps in the elimination of bilirubin from uptake to discharge into the duodenal lumen may be affected, which may explain why mixtures of unconjugated and conjugated bilirubin are detected in the plasma. Bilirubin conjugates are believed to enter the systemic circulation after regurgitation directly from hepatocytes via the sinusoidal membrane or paracellularly from bile canaliculi. The theory that hepatic deconjugation of bilirubin conjugates may contribute to the total plasma bilirubin pool has been confirmed using histochemical staining techniques on human cholestatic liver tissue; this mechanism deserves consideration in companion animal hepatobiliary disease. Partial or complete occlusion of the common bile duct, the other major cause of extrahepatic hyperbilirubinemia, may be associated with either primary diseases of the biliary tract (trauma leading to bile duct rupture or to blood clot formation within the extrahepatic biliary tract, neoplasm, congenital malformation, cholelithiasis, inspissated bile), or peribiliary tract diseases such as inflammatory or neoplastic conditions of the pancreas and duodenum.

In summary, since heritable defects in bilirubin metabolism are not known in companion animals, hyperbilirubinemia might be expected to result in these species from massive overproduction of erythrocyte degradation products (hemolysis) complicated by diminished hepatic clearance of bile pigments. Hyperbilirubinemia from acquired hepatobiliary disease may be anticipated when bilirubin is produced in excess from degradation of both erythrocytic and hepatic heme-containing proteins and its elimination is impaired by hepatocellular and/or biliary tract dysfunction.

DIAGNOSTIC APPROACH

History. A rational diagnostic approach to the dog or cat with clinical or biochemical jaundice is offered in Figure 24–2. Typical features in the history of an animal with marked hemolytic disease may include anorexia, weakness, and, if the hemolysis is intravascular, port wine-colored urine. Jaundice caused by occlusion of the common bile duct may be preceded by a history of vomiting and diarrhea one to three weeks earlier, or no other signs except anorexia, weight loss, and depression. The finding of acholic feces signifies complete interruption of bile flow to the duodenum. The histories of animals with primary hepatobiliary disease may be extremely variable.

Hematologic Tests. Occasionally, a distinction between hemolysis and hepatobiliary dysfunction as the major cause of hyperbilirubinemia can be made only after thorough laboratory evaluation. In the absence of blood loss, there should be strong evidence of marked hemolysis in the results of hematologic tests (a decline in erythrocyte numbers, high mean cell volume, pronounced reticulocytosis, poikilocytosis, anisocytosis, regenerative leukocytosis, and enlarged platelets) before hemolysis may be implicated as the sole cause of mild to moderate hyperbilirubinemia (total bilirubin less than ten mg/dl). Spherocytes may be observed in large numbers in the peripheral blood of dogs with primary immune-mediated hemolytic anemia, and, to a lesser extent, with fragmentation anemias. The duration of hemolysis and timing of hematologic evaluation must be taken into consideration when interpreting the regenerative response of the erythron, since immune-mediated anemias may occasionally be characterized by delayed regeneration. Though low-grade hemolysis associated with alterations in erythrocyte membrane composition is often a component of hepatobiliary disorders in companion animals, the rate and magnitude of cell destruction in such cases usually are not sufficient to cause severe anemia and a disproportionate contribution of bilirubin to the total plasma pool. Except for morphologic changes in erythrocytes, e.g., target cells, spur cells, microcytes, and schistocytes, the erythron usually is minimally affected in hepatobiliary diseases.

Serum Biochemical Analysis. Serum biochemical analysis, incorporating tests that specifically evaluate hepatocellular integrity and reactivity (hepatic enzyme activities and globulins), synthetic ability (urea, proteins, ammonia, cholesterol, coagulation factors), and excretory capacity (bile acids, total bilirubin, BSP excretion) is necessary to tentatively classify the cause of jaundice as either extrahepatic cholestasis or a primary hepatopathy. The results of these tests may vary according to the histologic characteristics of the lesion and duration of the disease process, and, in fact, may overlap considerably. For example, separation of total bilirubin content into conjugated and unconjugated fractions does not reliably discriminate hemolytic from extrahepatic obstructive from primary hepatobiliary disease in the dog. Readers are encouraged to refer to the discussion on pathophysiology and diagnosis of liver disease in Chapter 88 of this text for further details.

Noninvasive Assessment. Noninvasive assessment of the hepatobiliary tract and adjacent cranial abdominal organs using two-dimensional ultrasonography and scintigraphy has recently been explored in veterinary medicine. This additional information may provide sound justification for diagnostic or therapeutic surgical intervention.

Invasive Assessment. If sepsis, hyperthyroidism, and uncomplicated pancreatitis can be ruled out as the causes of jaundice, in which case surgery is not indicated, then exploratory celiotomy is the next logical step, either to repair a ruptured biliary tract and reestablish bile flow, to decompress the biliary tract and remove the underlying source of obstruction, if possible, or to obtain specimens for histologic study and definitive diagnosis in the case of primary hepatopathy. Other, less involved methods for hepatic biopsy may be selected, e.g., blind percutaneous or laparoscopic, based on individual case considerations. Though hepatic lesions involving the portal and periportal regions of the hepatic lobule generally are associated with marked hyperbilirubinemia, and those affecting hepatocytes adjacent to the central vein frequently result in normal to mildly elevated plasma bilirubin content, there is no substitute for the objective information gained from histologic examination of a hepatic tissue specimen to enable an accurate diagnosis and prognosis to be made.

TREATMENT

The specific goal of treatment of an animal with jaundice is resolution of the underlying cause, if possible. Selection of the appropriate treatment depends on the predominant form of bilirubin circulating, and the causative lesion. Since unconjugated bilirubin levels in the plasma of jaundiced companion animals rarely reach 20 mg/dl, the level at which bilirubin deposition in the basal ganglia, brain stem, and cerebellum (kernicterus) is known to cause neuronal death in human neonates, central nervous system injury is improbable, though this has been reported in a newborn kitten. A hypoactive glucuronyl transferase enzyme system combined with excessive hemolysis in such infants leads to severe unconjugated hyperbilirubinemia. Likewise, the danger of bilirubin papillary necrosis, in which unconjugated bilirubin chronically accumulates in the outer renal medulla, is remote. Specific efforts to reduce the blood levels of unconjugated bilirubin by use of, for example, phototherapy or exchange plasmapheresis, are generally not indicated. There is reason to believe, however, that severe, likely primarily conjugated hyperbilirubinemia (total bilirubin content greater than 20 mg/dl), may be associated with decreased glomerular filtration rate and proximal renal tubular dysfunction, based on results from experimental models of obstructive cholestasis in dogs. Prompt resolution of obstructive or traumatic lesions of the extrahepatic biliary tract would be of most benefit in such cases. Whether the severity of jaundice may be improved in an animal with hepatic parenchymal disease is contingent upon the character of the hepatobiliary disease and the probability that it will respond to appropriate drug therapy, e.g., *E. coli*-induced cholangitis, hepatic lymphosarcoma, steroid-responsive chronic active hepatitis, copper-retention hepatopathy of Doberman pinscher and Bedlington terrier dogs, or drug-induced hepatic injury.

Symptomatic treatment of animals with persistent or progressive cholestatic disorders is aimed at stimulation of forward bile flow. Surgical removal of inspissated bile plugs may be necessary, followed by hydrocholeretic therapy. Systemic fluid therapy to restore and maintain hydration and fluidity of the bile is essential. Use of synthetic bile acids, e.g., dehydrocholic acid, to increase the volume and water content of bile is of questionable value in human patients with cholestasis, and may even interfere with bilirubin excretion, but is reported to be of some benefit in cats with inspissated bile and bile sludging. The reported dosage is quite variable, ranging from 4.5 to 7 mg/lb (10 to 15 mg/kg) every eight hours to 28 mg (62.5 mg total dose) every eight hours given orally.

25 ALOPECIA

LYNN P. SCHMEITZEL

The term *alopecia* refers to the partial or complete absence of hair where it is normally present. Scarring of the skin with destruction of hair follicles results in permanent hair loss called *cicatricial* (scarring) alopecia. Whenever the hair bulb is destroyed, the alopecia will be cicatricial. *Noncicatricial* (nonscarring) alopecia is caused by transient disruption of hair follicle physiology, resulting in nonpermanent hair loss and eventual regrowth of hair. *Hypotrichosis* refers to the presence of less than the normal amount of hair. The distribution of alopecia may be *focal*, *multifocal*, *patchy*, or *generalized*.

NORMAL HAIR GROWTH AND STRUCTURE

Hair is a keratinized structure produced by an epidermal appendage, the hair follicle. Hair is composed of "hard" keratin, which is higher in sulfur and cystine than the "soft" keratin of the epidermis. The strength of hair is determined by disulfide bonds.

Hair is divided into three main sections, the shaft, root, and bulb. The shaft protrudes from the skin surface. The root lies within the hair follicle. The bulb surrounds a group of mesenchymal cells in the dermis called the dermal papilla.

The cells within the hair bulb are called matrix cells. Matrix cells produce the inner root sheath of the hair follicle that surrounds the hair root; the hair cuticle, the outermost portion of the hair; the hair cortex, the middle layer of the hair; and the medulla, the core of the hair. Surrounding the inner root sheath is the outer root sheath of the hair follicle, which is contiguous with the epidermis.

There are three stages of hair growth: anagen, catagen, and telogen. During the growth phase or anagen, cells of the outer root sheath grow down to the dermal papilla. Catagen is the transition phase, between the growing and resting phases. Telogen phase is the resting phase. The length of hair is determined by the growth rate and the time spent in the anagen phase. In dogs and cats the length of the growth stage of contiguous follicles varies.

Dogs and cats have compound hair follicles with one primary or guard hair surrounded by several secondary hairs (undercoat), all emerging from one opening in the skin.

PATHOPHYSIOLOGY OF ALOPECIA

Many skin disorders affecting hair growth result in alopecia (see Tables 25–1, 25–2, 25–3, and 25–4).

Genetic Causes. Genetics are important in determining the type and length of coat. Hereditary alopecias may affect hair follicles alone or they may affect other ectodermal structures, such as sebaceous and apocrine glands, and teeth, as well. Hereditary hair loss may be associated with coat color such as color mutant alopecia associated with a coat color dilution gene (e.g., blue Doberman) and canine black hair follicle dysplasia.

Hereditary alopecias may be congenital and recognized at or near birth or may not develop until several months later. Hereditary alopecias recognized near birth include hereditary hairless breeds such as the Chinese crested dog and Sphinx cat, feline hypotrichosis, canine black hair follicle dysplasia, and aplasia cutis. Hereditary alopecias not recognized until several months after birth include canine color mutant alopecia, dermatomyositis, generalized demodicosis, pattern baldness, and pinnal alopecia.

Metabolic Causes. Metabolic causes of alopecia include the endocrinopathies and telogen effluvium. Imbalances of pituitary, thyroid, adrenal, or gonadal hormones frequently result in pathologic hair loss (see Section X, Endocrine Diseases). Hormonal imbalances may affect the hair growth rate or the amount of time the hair follicle spends in different phases (anagen, catagen, telogen). Through hormones, light naturally causes nonpathologic, seasonal shedding.

Hormonal changes after giving birth may cause all of the hairs to enter telogen abruptly, resulting in postpartum telogen effluvium. Telogen effluvium may also occur after a high fever or severe illness.

Malnutrition. Malnutrition causes an abnormal hair coat. Though vitamin and mineral deficiencies are rare in small animals, they may cause alopecia. Fatty acid and protein and calorie deficiencies result in dry brittle coats and subsequent hair loss.

Neoplasia. Neoplasia causes alopecia when tumor

TABLE 25–1. FOCAL ALOPECIA

Disease	Lesion Distribution	Other Cutaneous Lesions	Pruritus	Diagnostic Tests
Infectious/Parasitic				
Dermatophytosis	Face, extremities	Scales, nodules (kerion)	–	Wood's lamp (*M. canis* only), KOH prep, Histopathology, Fungal culture*
Subcutaneous, systemic mycoses	Extremities, anywhere	Nodules, draining tracts, abscesses, ulcers, grains in exudates	–, + +	Histopathology, Fungal culture
Localized demodicosis				
Canine	Face, extremities (esp. feet)	Papules, pustules (secondary pyoderma), scales	None unless pyoderma present	Skin scrapings
Feline	Eyelids, periocular, head, neck	Scales	–	Skin scrapings
Miscellaneous Inflammatory				
Acute moist pyotraumatic dermatitis	Rump, anywhere	Papules, crusts, ulcers, excoriations	+ + +	Not usually required Scrape to R/O demodicosis
Rabies vaccination injection reactions	Usually hindlegs	Fibrosis of underlying tissues	–, +	Histopathology
Alopecia areata	Anywhere	Leukotrichia	–	Histopathology
Stud tail (feline)	Dorsal tail	Comedones, oily exudate	–	Histopathology
Preen body alopecia (canine)	Proximal dorsal tail	Comedones; oily exudate; nodule ("tail gland hyperplasia"); papules and draining tracts (secondary pyoderma)	–	Histopathology
Neoplasia	Anywhere	Nodules, scales, ulcers, crusts	–, +	Histopathology
Physical/Chemical				
Psychogenic				
Lick granuloma	Extremities	Ulcers; papules and draining tracts if secondary pyoderma	+ + +	Histopathology
See Multifocal Alopecia				
Physical/Chemical/Toxic				
Radiation	Anywhere	Scar, leukotrichia	–	Histopathology
Thermal	Anywhere	Scar	–	Histopathology
Frostbite	Extremities, ear and tail tip	Scar, leukotrichia	–	Histopathology
Contactants	Axilla, groin, ventral feet, muzzle	Macules, papules (allergic); ulcers, exudation (irritant), scars	–, +	Patch test*, Histopathology
Steroid injection reactions	Anywhere	Cutaneous atrophy	–	Histopathology

– None; + Mild; + + Moderate; + + + Severe.
*Most diagnostic test; KOH prep = potassium hydroxide preparation; R/O = rule out.

cells damage the hair follicle. Neoplastic disease may also cause alopecia through cachexia.

Inflammation. Most inflammatory dermatoses of small animals cause alopecia. The hair follicle may be directly attacked by the inflammatory response, as in alopecia areata and bacterial or fungal folliculitis, or the follicle may be destroyed by inflammation directed elsewhere, as occurs in a subcutaneous mycotic infection or foreign body reaction. In immune-mediated skin disease the hair follicle may be directly attacked by inflammation or may be an "innocent bystander" that is subsequently destroyed. The inflammation of allergic and many parasitic dermatoses causes pruritus that results in self-induced alopecia.

Physical or Chemical Causes. Other causes of alopecia include the physical/chemical dermatoses. Boredom or a severe psychological disturbance can cause psychogenic dermatoses such as flank-sucking, lick granulomas, and tail-biting. Drugs and chemicals may also cause alopecia after systemic administration converts hairs to the telogen phase. Topical chemicals cause alopecia by causing allergic or irritant reactions. Radiation, burns, and frostbite cause direct damage to the hair follicles.

SIGNALMENT

Age. Early age of onset often suggests a genodermatosis (e.g., hereditary hairlessness). Demodicosis usually affects young dogs before puberty. Allergic dermatoses usually develop after puberty. Hormonal and neoplastic dermatoses tend to occur in mature to older dogs and cats.

Breed. There are several hairless breeds of dogs and cats (e.g., Chinese crested dog, Sphinx cat). Pattern baldness and pinnal alopecia is common in dachshunds. Atopy is common in terriers.

Sex. Sex hormone imbalances occasionally cause alopecia in dogs (e.g., Sertoli cell tumor in males, ovarian imbalance type I in intact females, ovarian imbalance type II in spayed females). Feline endocrine alopecia is suspected to be a sex hormone imbalance in cats.

TABLE 25–2. MULTIFOCAL ALOPECIA

Disease	Lesion Distribution	Other Cutaneous Lesions	Pruritus	Diagnostic Tests
Infectious/Parasitic				
Dermatophytosis	Face, extremities, anywhere	Scales, nodules (kerion)	–	Wood's lamp (*M. canis* only), KOH prep, Histopathology, Fungal culture*
Subcutaneous, systemic mycoses	Extremities, anywhere	Nodules, draining tracts, abscess, ulcers, grains	–	Histopathology, Fungal culture
Pyoderma	Axilla, groin, anywhere	Pustules, papules, draining tracts, scars, epidermal collarettes, crusts, ulcers, excoriations	Usually absent except some superficial pyodermas ("bacterial hypersensitivity")	Bacterial culture and sensitivity, Histopathology
Demodicosis				
Canine	Face, extremities (esp. feet)	Scales, papules, pustules, draining tracts	None unless pyoderma present	Skin scrapings
Feline	Periocular, head, neck	Secondary pyoderma, scales	–	Skin scrapings
Miscellaneous Inflammatory				
Subcorneal pustular dermatosis	Head, trunk	Pustules, scales, epidermal collarettes	–, + + +	Histopathology
Dermatitis herpetiformis	Trunk, head, feet	Papules, crusts	+ + +	Histopathology
Seborrheic dermatitis	Anywhere	Scales	+ +	Histopathology
Vitamin A responsive dermatosis	Anywhere	Scales	–, +	Histopathology, Response to vitamin A
Sterile nodular panniculitis	Anywhere	Draining tracts with oily exudate, nodules, scars	–	Cytology, culture, Histopathology*
Neoplasia	Anywhere	Nodules, scales, ulcers, crusts	–, +	Histopathology
Physical/Chemical				
Psychogenic				
Lick granuloma	Extremities	Ulcers, papules and draining tracts if secondary pyoderma	+ + +	Histopathology
Physical/Chemical/Toxic				
Radiation	Anywhere	Scars, leukotrichia	–	Histopathology
Thermal burns	Anywhere	Scar	–	Histopathology
Frostbite	Extremities, ear and tail tips	Scar, leukotrichia	–	Histopathology
Contactants	Axilla, groin, ventral feet, muzzle	Macules, papules (allergic); ulcers, exudation (irritant)	+ + –, +	Patch test*, Histopathology

– None; + Mild; + + Moderate; + + + Severe.
*Most diagnostic test; KOH prep = potassium hydroxide preparation.

Coat Color. Color mutant alopecia occurs in many breeds having coat color dilution (e.g., blue Doberman pinscher).

HISTORICAL FINDINGS

An accurate dermatological case history is paramount in evaluating an animal with skin disease. A thorough history narrows the list of differential diagnoses, thus helping the clinician to decide which tests to perform.

Past History. Past history includes information not directly related to the animal's dermatosis.

Diet. Determine all dietary items. Determine if the animal is on a balanced diet; if not, a nutritional deficiency may be causing the alopecia. Note if an exacerbation of pruritus or gastrointestinal signs occurs after the feeding of a particular food, since these signs may result from a food allergy.

Sexual History. A reproductive history should be obtained for intact animals. If an intact bitch is not cycling normally, hypothyroidism or ovarian imbalance type I should be suspected. If she recently whelped, postpartum telogen effluvium could be causing the alopecia. If a male dog is no longer interested in females or has stopped lifting his leg to urinate, hypothyroidism, male feminizing syndrome, or Sertoli cell tumor should be suspected. If the bitch was spayed before her first heat cycle, then ovarian imbalance type II should be considered.

Environment. Determine whether the animal is kept indoors, outdoors, or both. What does the pet contact indoors, such as bedding or carpets? Are inhalant allergens such as wool, tobacco, or feathers in the environment? Are contact allergens such as cedar, redwood, wool, rubber, and vinyl in the environment? Is the yard fenced? If the animal runs free, he is more likely to be exposed to contagious ectoparasites such as scabies or fleas.

Other Pets in the Household. The presence of other, similarly affected pets in the household may indicate a contagion, such as dermatophytes, scabies, or fleas.

Persons in the Household. If a family member has a skin disease, a zoonosis such as dermatophytosis, scabies, or cheyletiellosis should be suspected.

TABLE 25–3. PATCHY ALOPECIA

Disease	Lesion Distribution	Other Cutaneous Lesions	Pruritus	Diagnostic Tests
Genetic				
Ectodermal defects and hypotrichosis	Anywhere	Dentition abnormalities	–	Histopathology
Black hair follicle dysplasia	Only black-haired areas affected	Scales	–	Histopathology
Pattern baldness (dachshunds)	Ears, ventrum	Scales	–	Histopathology
Pinnal alopecia (dachshunds, miniature poodles)	Ears	Scales	–	Histopathology
Aplasia cutis	Anywhere	Ulcers, scars	–	Histopathology
Dermatomyositis (*see* immunologic)				
Nutritional				
Zinc responsive	Mucocutaneous junctions, pressure points, footpads, anywhere	Thick crusts	–	Histopathology, Response to zinc supplementation
Generic dog food dermatosis	Mucocutaneous junctions, pressure points, anywhere	Crusts, scales, papules, pustules, (secondary pyoderma)	–	Change to balanced diet
Biotin deficiency	Periorbital, anywhere	Crusts, miliary dermatitis (cats)	–	Change to balanced diet
Riboflavin deficiency	Head (cats), lips	Erythema, scales	–	Change to balanced diet
Inflammatory				
Allergic				
Flea bite allergy	Dogs–rump, groin, hindlegs	Papules, excoriations, erythema, lichenification	+ + +	Intradermal skin test, Histopathology,
	Cats–rump, abdomen, head, and neck	Small crusts (miliary dermatitis), Excoriations	+ + +	Response to therapy*
Atopy	Face, feet, anywhere	Scales, lichenification, erythema, hyperpigmentation	+ +, + + +	Intradermal skin test
Food allergy	Face, feet, anywhere	Scales, lichenification, erythema, hyperpigmentation, papules, urticaria	+ +, + + +	Elimination diet
Parasitic				
Canine demodicosis	Face, feet, anywhere	Papules, pustules (secondary pyoderma), scales	None unless pyoderma present	Skin scrapings
Feline demodicosis	Head, neck, legs	Scaling, erythema, hyperpigmentation, crusting papules	–	Skin scrapings
Canine scabies (*Sarcoptes*)	Ears, face, legs	Papules, excoriations, erythema	+ + +	Skin scrapings, Response to therapy*
Feline scabies (*Notoedres*)	Ears, head, neck, feet	Papules, excoriations, miliary dermatitis, erythema	+ + +	Skin scrapings
Cheyletiellosis	Dorsal midline	Scales	–, + +	Acetate tape preparation, Skin scrapings
Pelodera dermatitis	Ventrum, feet, legs	Papules, excoriations, erythema, scales, crusts	+ + +	Skin scrapings
Pediculosis	Anywhere	Papules, crusts	+, + + +	Acetate tape preparation
Hookworm dermatitis	Feet, legs, ventrum	Papules, lichenification, erythema	+, + + +	Skin scrapings, Histopathology
Bacterial				
Skin fold dermatitis	Skin folds	Erythema, exudation	–, + +	Histopathology (usually not necessary)
Superficial pyoderma	Anywhere (esp. trunk)	Papules, pustules	–, + + +	Bacterial culture, Histopathology
Pressure point pyoderma	Pressure points	Papules, draining tracts, scars	–	Bacterial culture, Histopathology
Folliculitis/furunculosis	Anywhere	Papules, draining tracts, scars	–, + +	Bacterial culture, Histopathology
Fungal				
Dermatophytosis	Anywhere	Scales	–	Wood's lamp, KOH prep, Histopathology, Fungal culture*
Subcutaneous, systemic mycoses	Extremities, anywhere	Nodules, draining tracts, abscesses ulcers, grains in exudate	–	Histopathology, Fungal culture
Immunologic				
Discoid lupus erythematosus	Nasal planum, bridge of nose, mucocutaneous junctions, mucous membranes	Ulcers, erythema, crusts, hypopigmentation	–	Histopathology, DIF

TABLE 25–3. PATCHY ALOPECIA *Continued*

Disease	Lesion Distribution	Other Cutaneous Lesions	Pruritus	Diagnostic Tests
Systemic lupus erythematosus	Nasal planum, bridge of nose, mucocutaneous junctions, mucous membranes	Polymorphic (scales, ulcers, erythema, crusts, hypopigmentation, bullae, nodules, scars), multisystemic disease	–, +	Histopathology, DIF, ANA
Pemphigus	Face, mucocutaneous junctions, mucous membranes, foot pads	Crusts, erythema, erosions, ulcers, epidermal collarettes, pustules, vesicles, bullae	–, +	Histopathology, DIF
Bullous pemphigoid	Axilla, groin, mucocutaneous junctions, mucous membranes	Ulcers, bullae, erythema, epidermal collarettes	–, +	Histopathology, DIF
Dermatomyositis (collies, shelties)	Face, ears, bony prominences, tail tip	Atrophy, scars, erythema, hyper/hypopigmentation, ulcers, crusts, vesicles, muscular atrophy	–, +	Histopathology, DIF (negative)
Miscellaneous/Inflammatory				
Drug reactions	Anywhere	Polymorphic	–, + + +	Histopathology
Eosinophilic granuloma complex	Lips, ventral abdomen, caudal hindlegs, oral cavity	Nodules, plaques, ulcers	–, + + +	Histopathology
Acanthosis nigricans	Axilla, groin, medial hindlegs, pinnae	Hyperpigmentation, scales, oily exudate	–, + + +	Histopathology
Physical				
Psychogenic				For these diseases rule out other causes of pruritus
Flank sucking (Doberman pinscher)	Flanks	Lichenification, hyperpigmentation	+ + +	
Foot licking (toy breeds)	Feet	Lichenification, hyperpigmentation	+ + +	
Tail biting/sucking	Tail	Lichenification, hyperpigmentation, ulcers	+ + +	
Feline psychogenic alopecia, dermatitis	Dorsal back, ventral abdomen, legs	Excoriations (not always)	+ + + (may not be observed by owner)	
Physical/Chemical/Toxic				
Radiation	Anywhere	Scars, leukotrichia	–	Histopathology
Thermal burns	Anywhere	Scars	–	Histopathology
Frostbite	Extremities, ears and tail tips, scrotum	Scars, leukotrichia	–	Histopathology
Contactants	Axilla, groin, ventral feet, muzzle	Macules, papules (allergic), ulcers, exudation, scars (irritant)	–	Histopathology
Solar dermatitis	Nasal planum, bridge of nose, ear tips, periocular	Erythema, scales, crusts	–	Histopathology

– None; + Mild; + + Moderate; + + + Severe.
*Most diagnostic test; KOH prep = potassium hydroxide preparation; DIF = direct immunofluorescence; ANA = antinuclear antibody titer.

Related Animals. If the sire, dam, or siblings were similarly affected, a genodermatosis such as juvenile onset generalized demodicosis should be suspected.

Onset and Progression. The onset and progression of the dermatosis should be determined. Dermatophytosis and most endocrinopathies have a gradual onset and slow progression. Most drug eruptions have an acute onset and rapid progression.

Pruritus. Is there pruritus? If so, when did it develop in relation to the alopecia? If the pruritus occurred prior to the alopecia, allergic or ectoparasitic diseases should be considered. If the pruritus developed after the alopecia and pustules are also present, a pruritic superficial pyoderma could be causing the hair loss. Is the pruritus seasonal or nonseasonal? Seasonal pruritus may indicate atopy or flea allergy; nonseasonal pruritus may indicate food allergy.

Medications. Determine all medications used. Response to therapy may help determine the cause of the alopecia. On the other hand, the medication may be causing the dermatosis or making it worse.

PHYSICAL EXAMINATION

Skin lesions are divided in two categories, primary and secondary.

Primary Skin Lesions. Primary skin lesions are directly caused by the disease process. A *macule* is a flat circumscribed area (up to one cm) of color change in the skin caused by increased melanin pigment, depigmentation, erythema, or hemorrhage. A *patch* is a macule greater than one cm in diameter. A *papule* is a solid elevation in the skin up to one cm in diameter. Papules are frequently caused by ectoparasites (especially fleas) and pyodermas. A *plaque* is a flat-topped, solid elevation in the skin greater than one cm in diameter. Plaques may be caused by a coalition of papules. A *nodule* is a circumscribed solid elevation in the skin greater than one cm in diameter. Nodules are commonly associated with neoplasia or severe inflammation. A nodular form of dermatophytosis is called a kerion. A *tumor* is a neoplastic enlargement in the skin.

TABLE 25–4. BILATERALLY SYMMETRICAL GENERALIZED ALOPECIAS

Disease	Lesion Distribution	Other Cutaneous Lesions	Pruritus	Diagnostic Tests
Genetic				
Canine hereditary hairlessness	Generalized; head and feet may have hair	Comedones	–	Histopathology
Canine color mutant alopecia	Generalized	Comedones, scales, papules, pustules (i.e., secondary pyoderma)	–, + + +	Histopathology
Feline alopecia universalis (Sphinx cat)	Generalized	Comedones, oily exudate	–	Histopathology
Feline hypotrichosis	Generalized	—	–	Histopathology
Generalized demodicosis	Generalized	Scales, papules, pustules, crusts, draining tracts (i.e., secondary pyoderma)	–, + + +	Histopathology
Infectious				
Dermatophytosis	Generalized	Scales, pustules (rare)	–, +	Wood's lamp (*M. canis* only), KOH prep, Histopathology, Fungal culture*
Metabolic				
Endocrine				
Hypothyroidism	Trunk, neck, tail, legs (giant breeds)	Scales, hyperpigmentation, myxedema, pustules, papules (i.e., secondary pyoderma)	–	Thyroid function tests, Histopathology
Hyperadrenocorticism	Trunk	Calcinosis cutis, comedones, cutaneous atrophy, hyperpigmentation	–	Adrenal function tests, Histopathology
Growth-hormone responsive	Trunk	Severe hyperpigmentation	–	Growth hormone function tests, Histopathology
Pituitary dwarfism	Trunk—generalized	Severe hyperpigmentation, short stature	–	Growth hormone, thyroid, adrenal function tests
Sertoli cell tumor	Perineal, ventral abdomen, chest, flanks, neck	Gynecomastia, pendulous prepuce, testicular mass	–	Estrogen levels, Histopathology (testicle, skin)
Male feminizing syndrome	Perineal, ventral abdomen, flanks, neck	Scales, oily exudate, gynecomastia	–, + + +	Response to castration or testosterone
Testosterone-responsive dermatosis of male dogs	Perineal, ventral abdomen, flanks	Scales, cutaneous atrophy	–	Response to testosterone
Ovarian imbalance Type I	Ventral abdomen, ventral thorax, flanks	Gynecomastia, enlarged vulva, scales, oily exudate	+ +	Response to ovario-hysterectomy
Ovarian imbalance Type II	Entire ventrum, pinnae	Small vulva and nipples, scales, atrophy	–	Response to estrogen
Feline endocrine alopecia	Perineal, caudomedial thighs, ventral abdomen	—	–	Histopathology, Response to progestational compounds, sex hormones, thyroxine
Telogen effluvium (postpartum, stress, fever, etc.)	Generalized	—	–	Histopathology
Nutritional				
Vitamin A deficiency	Generalized	Scales	–	Response to supplementation
Vitamin E deficiency	Generalized	Scales, oily exudate, pansteatitis	–	Response to supplementation
Protein deficiency	Generalized	Hyperpigmentation, leukotrichia, scales	–	Response to supplementation
Essential fatty acid deficiency	Generalized	Scales, oily exudate, lichenification	–, +	Response to supplementation
Neoplasia				
Mycosis fungoides	Generalized	Scales, erythema (early); plaques, nodules, tumors (later)	–, + + +	Histopathology
Physical/Chemical				
Cancer chemotherapeutic agents	Generalized	—	–	—
Thallium	Mucocutaneous junctions, feet, generalized	Erythema, erosions, ulcers, crusts, scales	–	Histopathology, Urine thallium levels
Heparin	Generalized	—	–	—
Mercury	Generalized	Papules, erythema, scales	+ +	Blood mercury levels
Arsenic	Generalized	Hypo/hyperpigmentation	–	Arsenic levels, urine, hair, nails
Copper	Generalized	—	–	Blood copper levels
Lead	Generalized	—	–	Blood lead levels
Contactants (irritant)	Anywhere	Ulcers, exudation, scars	–	Histopathology

– None; + Mild; + + Moderate; + + + Severe.
*Most diagnostic test; KOH prep = potassium hydroxide preparation.

A *cyst* is an epithelial-lined cavity filled with fluid or solid material. A *pustule* is a circumscribed elevation in the skin, filled with pus. Pustules are the hallmark of pyodermas. Pemphigus foliaceous and subcorneal pustular dermatosis are less common diseases that result in sterile pustules. A *wheal* is a circumscribed, raised erythematous lesion consisting of dermal edema. Wheals are infrequent spontaneous lesions and are usually the result of insect bites (stings). Allergic reactions to drugs, foods, inhalant allergens, and allergy skin tests may result in wheals. Wheals frequently cause severe pruritus. *Angioedema* is edema involving the dermis and subcutaneous tissues caused by an allergic reaction. A *vesicle* is a circumscribed lesion up to one cm in diameter, filled with clear fluid. Vesicles are rare lesions caused by immune-mediated dermatoses, irritants, or viral diseases. A *bulla* is a circumscribed lesion greater than one cm in diameter, filled with clear fluid. Bullae are caused by the same conditions as vesicles.

SECONDARY LESIONS

Secondary lesions develop from primary lesions or are caused by self-trauma or medications. Secondary lesions are less helpful than primary lesions in determining the cause of the dermatosis. *Scale* is an accumulation of epidermal keratin fragments on the surface of the skin. Scales develop in seborrhea, hormonal dermatoses, dermatophytosis, and demodicosis. *Epidermal collarettes* are scale arranged in an annular ring. Epidermal collarettes usually represent a ruptured pustule, vesicle, or bulla. *Crust* is dried exudate formed from pus and blood. A *scar* is an area of fibrous tissue replacement of dermis or subcutaneous tissue. Scars are usually depigmented and alopecic and result from burns, traumatic wounds, and deep pyodermas. An *erosion* is a shallow break in the epidermis that does not penetrate the basement membrane zone (dermoepidermal junction). Erosions do not heal with scars. Erosions may develop from ruptured pustules, vesicles or trauma. An *ulcer* is a deep break in the epidermis that penetrates the basement membrane zone. Ulcers heal with scars. Ulcers develop in indolent (eosinophilic) ulcers, deep pyodermas, and bullous pemphigoid. An *excoriation* is a self-induced ulcer or erosion. Excoriation is the hallmark of pruritus. *Lichenification* is a thickening of the epidermis characterized by an "elephant hide" appearance. Lichenification indicates chronicity. *Hyperpigmentation* is increased melanin pigment in the skin. Hyperpigmentation occurs after inflammation and in endocrine dermatoses. A *comedo* is keratin plugging a hair follicle. Comedones develop in seborrheic and endocrine dermatoses. *Alopecia* is loss of hair from normally hair-covered skin. Alopecia may be partial or complete. Alopecia is caused by any disorder affecting hair or hair follicles or by self-trauma.

DIAGNOSTIC PLAN

Most tests used to diagnose skin diseases are easily performed. These tests include skin scrapings, Wood's lamp examination, potassium hydroxide preparation, fungal culture, cytology, bacterial culture and antibiotic sensitivity, skin biopsies, elimination diets, intradermal skin testing, patch testing, hormone function testing, and response to therapy.

A skin scraping is the most important test to diagnose skin disease and should be performed on all patients. Multiple skin scrapings should always be done. Although most ectoparasites can be demonstrated on skin scrapings, *Sarcoptes scabei* var. *canis* is frequently missed. Therefore, response to insecticidal dips is often used to diagnose canine scabies.

In cases of localized demodicosis, normal as well as lesional skin should be scraped to determine if the disease is becoming generalized. Baseline ratios of live to dead and immature to mature mites should be performed in all cases of demodicosis. These ratios should be determined every two to four weeks and compared to prior ratios to monitor response to therapy.

A Wood's lamp examination is useful as a screening test for dermatophytosis. The only dermatophyte of veterinary importance that fluoresces (yellow-green) is *Microsporum canis*; only 50 per cent of the strains fluoresce.

A potassium hydroxide (KOH) preparation may demonstrate arthroconidia and hyphae of dermatophytes in hairs or scales. However, these fungal elements may be difficult to observe.

If multiple skin scrapings, Wood's lamp examination, and KOH preparation are negative, a fungal culture is generally indicated.

Cytology of intact pustules, exudates, and aspirates may yield a definitive diagnosis. For example, the presence of neutrophils and cocci bacteria from a pustule or draining tracts indicate a pyoderma. Neutrophils, acantholytic keratinocytes, and the absence of bacteria in a pustule is indicative of the autoimmune skin disease pemphigus foliaceous. *Blastomyces dermatitidis* may be found on cytology of exudates from draining tracts in cases of blastomycosis.

Bacterial cultures and antibiotic sensitivity testing are indicated in cases not responding to empirical antibiotic therapy, deep pyodermas, and most pyodermas in large breed dogs where cost is usually a factor. If intact pustules or draining tracts are not present, culture a biopsy of a papule with a centrally protruding hair follicle (folliculitis).

Skin biopsies are usually performed when other tests are negative or if there is minimal response to empirical therapy. Several biopsies should be submitted. Primary skin lesions (see above), if present, yield the best results. In addition to routine formalin fixation, biopsies from suspected immune-mediated skin diseases should be submitted in Michel's media for direct immunofluorescence testing.

Elimination diets are used to diagnose food allergies (see Chapter 38).

Intradermal skin testing is used to confirm atopy and flea bite allergy. Complete intradermal testing is time consuming and costly.

Patch testing is used to confirm contact dermatitis. Since contact allergies are rare in animals, patch testing is seldom performed. Furthermore, the animals frequently remove the patch before the proper time has elapsed (24 to 72 hours).

Hormone function testing is necessary in suspected cases of endocrinopathies. Baseline hormone levels are not helpful, so stimulation or suppression tests are preferred. (See Section X, Endocrine Diseases.) Gonadal endocrinopathies may result from hard to document alterations of sex hormone ratios or local metabolism of these steroids. Diagnosis of a sex hormone aberration is usually made by response to therapy.

Response to therapy is useful in making certain diagnoses. Diagnosis of most cases of canine scabies is made by response to insecticidal dips. Response to removal of a contact allergen is usually used to make a diagnosis of contact allergy. Diagnosis of a gonadal endocrinopathy is usually made when the dermatosis responds to neutering or hormonal supplementation.

TREATMENT GOALS

Genetic Causes. Therapy is only symptomatic for most genodermatoses. Mild antiseborrheic shampoos and emollient rinses prevent excessive dryness of the alopecic skin. Antibiotics may be needed for secondary pyodermas. (For generalized demodicosis, see Parasitic Causes; for dermatomyositis, see Immunologic Causes).

Metabolic Causes. Diagnose and correct the underlying disorder.

Endocrine Causes. Give replacement hormone therapy or reduce hormone production/secretion when indicated. Response to therapy should be observed in six to eight weeks. (See Section X, Endocrine Diseases.)

Telogen Effluvium. Correct the underlying cause and in a few weeks the hair follicles should enter anagen phase again.

Nutritional Causes. Place the animal on a diet that meets the requirements established by the National Research Council. Give additional supplementation when indicated.

Neoplasia. Surgically remove the neoplasm when possible. Treat mycosis fungoides with topical nitrogen mustard.

Inflammatory Causes. The key in treating inflammatory dermatoses is to find and correct the underlying cause of the inflammation rather than merely treat the signs.

Bacterial Causes. Skin fold dermatitis is usually controlled with topical antibacterial shampoos. Surgical excision of the skin fold is necessary for cure. Superficial pyodermas require three to four weeks, whereas deep pyodermas require six to eight weeks of systemic antibiotics and topical antibacterial therapy. Corticosteroids should be avoided even if the pyoderma is pruritic. Provide soft bedding for cases of pressure point pyodermas. Since most pyodermas are secondary to another problem (allergies, hypothyroidism, demodicosis), the underlying cause of any pyoderma should be determined, otherwise the pyoderma will recur.

Fungal Causes. Dermatophyte cases should be treated with both systemic and topical antifungals. Treat for two weeks beyond clinical cure or until fungal cultures are negative. Subcutaneous and systemic mycoses may require surgical excision in addition to long-term, systemic antifungal medication.

Immunologic Causes. Treat immune-mediated skin diseases with immunosuppressive doses of short-acting corticosteroids (prednisone, prednisolone) until the disease is in remission. Then gradually determine the minimal alternate day maintenance dose. If the disease is not easily controlled with corticosteroids, then cytotoxic drugs such as cyclophosphamide, azathioprine, or chlorambucil may be used. Chrysotherapy (gold salt therapy) may also be used in refractory cases. Serious adverse side effects are common with these drugs, so close patient monitoring is necessary. Sunscreens, reducing sunlight exposure, and vitamin E therapy are useful in both types of lupus erythematosus.

Allergic Causes. The best mode of therapy for allergic skin disease is to eliminate exposure to the allergen. In atopy (allergic inhalant dermatitis), hyposensitization is beneficial. If exposure to the allergen cannot be eliminated, low-dose, short-acting corticosteroid therapy may be necessary. Antihistamines have limited effectiveness but may allow reduction of the steroid dose.

Parasitic Causes. Appropriate insecticidal shampoos, sprays, powders, or dips should be used until the disease completely resolves. Cases of generalized demodicosis should be treated for one month after negative skin scrapings. For scabies, all contact animals of the same species must be treated. Remove decaying organic bedding materials to successfully treat *Pelodera strongyloides* dermatitis. Systemic steroids may be needed for pruritus. Clean up environmental fecal contamination to treat hookworm dermatitis. Systemic corticosteroids are frequently necessary in pruritic parasitic dermatoses.

Miscellaneous/Inflammatory Causes. Acute moist pyotraumatic dermatitis (hotspots) usually responds to topical cleansing, astringents, and short courses of low-dose corticosteroids. Some cases require systemic antibiotics.

For drug reactions, remove the offending drugs. Systemic corticosteroids may also be helpful.

Treat the eosinophilic granuloma complex with high doses of corticosteroids until the lesions completely resolve.

Antiseborrheic shampoos may control acanthosis nigricans. Melatonin may be helpful in some cases. Corticosteroids may be necessary in severe cases. Antibiotics are indicated for secondary pyodermas.

Sterile nodular panniculitis is responsive to high doses of corticosteroids. Do not use steroids if the panniculitis is secondary to a pancreatitis.

Alopecia areata may spontaneously resolve. Some cases may respond to steroids.

Antiseborrheic shampoos and gels control stud tail and preen body alopecia.

Dermatitis herpetiformis and subcorneal pustular dermatosis are rare diseases and respond only to dapsone.

Traumatic (Physical/Chemical) Causes. Therapy for physical/chemical dermatoses involves removal of the offending agent.

Psychogenic Causes. If possible, treat psychogenic dermatoses by correcting the underlying cause. For cats the underlying cause is usually a disturbing influence. For dogs the underlying cause is usually boredom. Mechanically preventing the animal from licking and chewing (e.g., Elizabethan collars) works temporarily, until the device is removed. Use tranquilizers or progestational compounds until the lesions are completely resolved. The animal may require maintenance therapy with these drugs.

Physical/Chemical/Toxic Causes. Remove agents when possible. Treat solar dermatitis with topical sunscreens and by reducing sunlight exposure. Corticosteroids may reduce inflammation if present.

OUTCOME

The outcome of an alopecic dermatosis depends on the clinician's ability to determine and correct the underlying cause. The outcome is also dependent on whether the dermatosis causes cicatricial or noncicatricial alopecia.

Noncicatricial alopecias include endocrinopathies, telogen effluvium, nutritional dermatoses, feline psychogenic alopecia, most dermatophyte infections, surface/superficial pyodermas, and alopecia areata.

Cicatricial alopecias include severe dermatophyte infections, subcutaneous/systemic mycoses, neoplasia, deep bacterial folliculitis, and furunculosis.

Inflammatory and physical/chemical dermatoses may be cicatricial or noncicatricial, depending on the duration and depth of the inflammation or injury. Self-trauma in allergic skin disease may result in severe yet noncicatricial alopecia. Self-trauma causing lick granulomas may or may not be cicatricial. Radiation burns, caustics, and frostbite likewise may or may not cause severe cicatricial alopecia. If the hair bulb is destroyed, the hair loss will be permanent.

26 PRURITUS

PETER J. IHRKE

Pruritus is defined as a sensation that elicits the desire to scratch, or more subjectively, an uneasy sensation of irritation within the skin. As a characteristic sensory feature of many skin diseases, pruritus is one of the most common dog and cat owner complaints in small animal practice. Pruritus or itching is also one of the more frustrating manifestations of skin disease because of the visual similarity of self-traumatized lesions.

PATHOPHYSIOLOGY

Itching is accepted as a primary skin sensation along with touch, pain, heat, and cold. The skin has no specialized itch receptors. Naked nerve endings located predominantly at the dermal-epidermal junction transmit the itch sensation. These naked nerve endings may increase in number and respond to a lower threshold of stimulation after skin damage, such as excoriations, have occurred.

Proteolytic enzymes, other proteases, and vasoactive polypeptides currently are believed to be the most important mediators of pruritus in dogs and cats. Histamine is less important as a mediator of pruritus in domestic animals than was previously assumed. Endopeptidases elaborated by bacteria and fungi may be important in producing pruritus seen with skin infection.

The concept of threshold is important in understanding pruritus. The threshold theory states that a certain pruritic load may be tolerated by an individual without disease manifestations. However, a small increase in that load may push the individual over the threshold and initiate clinical signs of pruritus. Experimental evidence in humans has shown that the itch threshold is lower at night, and with increased skin temperature, decreased skin hydration, and increased psychic stress. Similar factors are probably important in veterinary medicine. A summation of effect often occurs, whereby the additive pruritus from various skin diseases may raise an animal above its individual pruritic threshold. For example, in certain geographic areas, pruritus from even mild flea allergy may complicate many other skin diseases. Itch-scratch cycles are perpetuated, since pruritus from a variety of underlying causes is additive, the pruritic threshold is lowered by skin damage, and excoriations created by self-trauma release more mediators of pruritus.

HISTORICAL FINDINGS

A good clinical history may offer more direct clues to the final diagnosis than the physical examination, since many pruritic dermatoses are visually similar due to superimposed self-trauma.

SIGNALMENT

The signalment of a patient may be useful in directing an index of suspicion toward certain diseases.

Age. Age is important in prioritizing differential diagnoses. Canine scabies, demodicosis, flea allergy, and endoparasitic larval migration are all common causes of pruritus in puppies. Canine scabies may be seen in dogs of any age but greater contact with other dogs increases the likelihood of contagion in puppies. Conversely, atopy, food allergy, pyoderma, and seborrhea are more frequent causes of pruritus in adult dogs. Flea allergy is common in all age groups.

Breed. Certain breeds of dog, such as wirehaired fox terriers, Dalmatians, and golden retrievers, have a genetic predilection for atopy. The Chinese Shar Pei appears to have a breed predilection for demodicosis, pyodermas, and food allergy. Foot-licking in miniature poodles is often attributed to psychogenic reasons.

Sex. Few pruritic diseases show any sex bias. Atopy has been reported to be slightly more common in female dogs. Pruritus can be seen in conjunction with chronic skin changes from Sertoli cell tumors or male feminizing syndrome.

GENERAL HISTORY

The term general history may be used to refer to the general health of the animal and information not directly referable to the presenting complaint of pruritus.

Diet. Diet may be important in the diagnosis of various pruritic dermatoses. It is important to record the type of food, brand name, and approximate percentages of various foods in any history of a pruritic dog or cat. Fat-deficient diets may contribute to seborrhea. Food allergy in both dogs and cats is probably more common than previously thought.

Sexual Data. Reproductive and behavioral sexual data are occasionally valuable. Pruritus may be seen as a complicating factor with hypothyroidism, Sertoli cell tumors, ovarian imbalances, and pseudocyesis.

Environment. Environment is extremely important in diagnosing the causes of pruritus. The likelihood of ectoparasitic diseases such as flea allergy, canine scabies, feline scabies, cheyletiellosis, pelodera dermatitis, and hookworm dermatitis are all influenced by the animal's primary environment (indoor, outdoor, roams free) and geographic region.

Exposure. Recent exposures, such as a new pet in the household or the sheltering of a stray animal, increase the likelihood of ectoparasitic disease. Exposure to other animals at grooming establishments, kennels, or veterinary hospitals provides additional opportunity for contagion.

Other Household Pets. Pruritus or lack of pruritus in contact animals may offer clues to contagion. However, it must be remembered that even though dogs and cats share fleas as common ectoparasites, flea allergy is much more common in dogs. A seemingly unaffected "indoor/outdoor" cat may be an asymptomatic carrier for fleas. Since a hypersensitivity is critical to the development of symptomatic canine scabies, it should be remembered that asymptomatic carriers do exist.

Human Contacts. Canine scabies and feline dermatophytosis are the two most common pet-related zoonoses. The presence of a pruritic papular rash (canine scabies, feline scabies, cheyletiellosis) or annular erythematous lesions (dermatophytosis) in the human contacts of a pruritic pet may suggest one of these zoonoses (see Chapter 37).

SPECIFIC HISTORY

History referable to the presenting complaint is an often overlooked critical step in the diagnosis of the pruritic animal. Since the owner's definition of itching or pruritus may differ substantially from the veterinarians, common ground must be reached. The subjective manifestations of pruritus most commonly reported by pet owners include licking, chewing, and the rubbing of the body on rugs or furniture. Animals may harass the owner or even exhibit an irritability or personality change. Frequency of pruritic episodes may be crudely quantitated by asking the owner how many times the dog will scratch (or chew, or lick) if left to its own devices for one hour while the owner is reading or watching television.

Onset. A rapid onset most often signifies a contagious ectoparasitic disease such as flea allergy, canine scabies, or feline scabies. A more gradual onset is commonly seen with atopy, pyodermas, and seborrhea.

Progression. Disease progression and site of initial lesions may be important, since the owners have seen the disease from the onset. For example, generalized canine scabies commonly begins with hair loss and itching of the margins of the pinna.

Duration. Duration of the disease is important, since in general, the longer a disease has been present, the more likely it is that secondary changes have obscured the initial lesion.

Intensity. The intensity of the pruritus may be useful information. Few diseases are as pruritic as canine and feline scabies.

Pattern. Canine atopy and flea allergy are often *seasonal* diseases in many areas of the world. Alternatively, a cyclical pruritus with no seasonality associated with a vacation home, might signify a contact dermatitis.

Predictability. If cyclical bouts of pruritus occur, are they in any way predictable by the owner? Pets with psychogenic pruritus may have chewed, licked, or scratched as an attention-getter before the action became a constant vice.

General Home Skin Care. Any shampoo, rinses, powders, sprays, or deodorizers should be noted since generalized pruritus has been reported with the use of all these product groups.

PHYSICAL FINDINGS

Proper lighting is mandatory for a dermatologic examination. The evaluation of the skin, mucocutaneous junctions, oral cavity, ears, genitals, and lymph nodes should be emphasized in the examination of the pruritic animal. During the taking of the history, the clinician should observe the animal for general demeanor and signs of pruritus. Both the haircoat and the underlying skin should be examined. The objective cutaneous signs of pruritus include excoriations, broken hairs, postinflammatory pigment changes and, occasionally, worn incisors.

Pruritus in the dog and cat may occur with or without any primary skin lesions. If present, primary skin lesions such as papules, pustules, and macules may be quite helpful in establishing a diagnosis. Unfortunately, secondary self-trauma often obscures the nature or presence of primary lesions.

Diagnostic primary lesions are seen most often with ectoparasitic disease. When lesions are located in particular sites, this may suggest a specific disease (Tables 26–1 and 26–2). Identifiable primary lesions may be seen in pyodermas and seborrhea. In general, primary lesions are most often evident in diseases of an exogenous nature.

Atopy and food allergy are endogenous causes of pruritus with infrequent primary lesions. Self-trauma at predisposed sites may be the only clue. Endogenous causes of pruritus are less likely to cause primary skin lesions. Drug allergy is an exception.

Endogenous causes of pruritus associated with other organ systems need further clarification (see Chapter 2).

The distribution of lesions and major foci of pruritus are valuable aids. In some diseases, pruritus may be localized to the face, feet, or the dorsal lumbosacral area.

DIAGNOSTIC PLAN

A diagnostic plan should be formulated based on the most likely differential diagnoses. Differential diagnoses

TABLE 26–1. PRURITIC CANINE DERMATOSES

Disease	Site	Lesions
Flea allergy dermatitis A, E, F	Symmetric, dorsal lumbosacral, caudal thighs, groin, axilla, caudal half of body	Papules, macules, alopecia, erythema, lichenification, hyperpigmentation, excoriations
Canine scabies A	Ventral, ear margins, elbows	Macules, papules, erythema, alopecia, crusts, excoriations
Demodicosis A	Periorbital, commissures of mouth, forelegs, generalized	Alopecia, erythema, crusts, follicular plugging, hyperpigmentation, secondary deep pyoderma
Pyoderma A	Groin, axilla, ventrum, interdigital, generalized, pressure points	Pleomorphic, pustules, crusted papules, erythema, alopecia, target lesions coalescing collarettes, hyperpigmentation
Seborrhea A, E, F	Dorsum, ears, preen body	Pleomorphic, scales, crusts, alopecia, erythematous plaques
Atopy A, F	Face, feet (dorsum), ears, axilla, generalized	Erythema, alopecia, excoriations
Food allergy B	Face, feet, ears, generalized	Pleomorphic, erythema, alopecia, excoriations
Contact dermatitis B	Hairless areas, feet (ventrum), genitals, groin, axilla, generalized	Erythema, exudation, lichenification, hyperpigmentation, papules
Drug eruptions B	Anywhere, localized or generalized	Pleomorphic
Endoparasitic migration in puppies B	Face, feet, generalized	Erythema, alopecia, excoriations, scales
Cheyletiellosis B, E	Dorsum of thorax	Large scales, crusts, alopecia
Chiggers B, E, F	Ventrum, legs, anywhere	Erythema, scales, crusts
Psychogenic pruritus C	Carpi, feet (one or more, especially forelegs), perianal, generalized	Erythema, alopecia, excoriations
Pediculosis C, E, F	Dorsum	Scales, crusts, alopecia
Pelodera dermatitis C, E, F	Ventrum, legs, groin	Erythema, papules, alopecia, scales, crusts
Subcorneal pustular dermatosis D	Generalized, especially face and ears	Pleomorphic, papules, pustules, vesicles, crusts, alopecia
"Diabetic dermatosis" D	Face, genitals, feet, footpads	Erythema, ulcers, crusts, excoriations
Sterile eosinophilic pustulosis D	Generalized, ventrum	Erythema, papules, pustules, alopecia, scales, crusts

Key: A—Common, B—Less common, C—Uncommon, D—Rare or controversial, E—Regional, F—Seasonal.

TABLE 26–2. PRURITIC FELINE DERMATOSES

Disease	Site	Lesion
Flea allergy dermatitis A, E, F	Neck, dorsum, lumbosacral, caudal and medial thighs, groin, ears, generalized	Miliary dermatitis, alopecia, erythema
Food allergy A	Head, neck, ears, generalized	Miliary dermatitis, excoriations, alopecia, erythema
Self-induced psychogenic hair loss A	Symmetric, stripe(s) on dorsal thorax, caudal and lateral thighs, ventral abdomen, perineum, forelegs	Alopecia, hair stubbles, normal underlying skin
Self-induced pruritic hair loss	Symmetric, caudal and lateral thighs, ventral abdomen, perineum	Alopecia, hair stubbles, underlying skin can be normal
Eosinophilic plaque A, E, F	Ventral abdomen, medial thighs, anywhere	Raised, ulcerated, erythematous plaques, seen with flea allergy
Otodectic ascariasis A	Ears, head, neck, rarely generalized	Otitis externa, excoriations, miliary dermatitis
Cheyletiellosis B, E	Dorsum of thorax	Large scales, crusts, seborrhea, miliary dermatitis
Endoparasitic migration in kittens B	Face, feet, generalized	Erythema, alopecia, excoriations, miliary dermatitis
Pediculosis C, E, F	Dorsum	Scales, crusts, alopecia
Feline scabies C, E	Head, neck, generalized	Erythema, scales, crusts, alopecia, excoriations
Psychogenic dermatitis C	Legs, abdomen, flank	Erosion, ulceration
Dermatophytosis with pruritus C	Head, neck, ears, thorax	Erythema, alopecia, miliary dermatitis, hyperpigmentation
Atopy C?	Head, neck, ears, generalized	Miliary dermatitis, erythema, alopecia

Key: A—Common, B—Less common, C—Uncommon, D—Rare or controversial, E—Regional, F—Seasonal.

are generated by the clinician's clinical judgment, taking into account general history, specific history, and physical findings.

Skin Scrapings. Multiple skin scrapings should be part of the minimum data base for any pruritic dog or cat. The affected area must be clipped prior to scraping. A number ten scalpel blade is dipped in mineral oil and scraped perpendicular to the skin surface in the direction of hair growth. The acquired debris is spread on a slide and examined microscopically with low light. Since scabies mites are documented in fewer than 50 per cent of strongly suspected cases, negative scrapings should not preclude a tentative diagnosis of scabies and trial therapy. With proper technique including clipping, demodectic mites are readily demonstrable.

Pustular Smears. A Gram stain or Difquik stain of pustular contents is an invaluable aid in the diagnosis of pustular diseases. Smears are not used frequently enough. The presence of bacteria and activated neutrophils confirms the presence of a pyoderma. Smears are frequently as valuable as bacterial cultures and are more cost-effective. *Bacterial cultures* are more useful in the selection of a proper antibiotic than in making a diagnosis.

Skin Biopsy. The skin biopsy is another valuable tool used too infrequently in the diagnosis of pruritus. A biopsy may either give a definitive diagnosis or rule out unlikely differential diagnoses. The biopsy of early primary lesions free of self-trauma is most rewarding. Specimens should be handled gently and useful clinical information should be sent with the specimen. Results will be substantially better if specimens are sent to veterinary dermatopathologists.

Fungal Cultures. Most animals with dermatophytosis are not markedly pruritic. However, since most cases of dermatophytosis are not visually diagnostic, fungal culture is frequently warranted. Fungal culture is the only consistently accurate method of diagnosing dermatophytosis. Unfortunately, misinterpretation of results due to faulty technique is common. The *Wood's lamp* is the most abused tool in veterinary practice. Its value is severely limited by nonfluorescing pathogenic strains and the frequent interpretation of false positives.

Elimination Diet. Elimination diets are used to determine food allergy. Since all commercial pet foods share common protein sources, dyes, preservatives, and stabilizers, they cannot be used as elimination diets. The animal must be fed a single protein and carbohydrate source as the exclusive ration for three weeks. Mutton, cottage cheese, or whitefish with either rice or potatoes is used for dogs, and cats are fed either mutton or pork, sometimes with rice cereal baby food. Lamb or pork baby food is economically feasible for cats and small dogs. There is no scientific evidence that *cytotoxic* testing may be used as a substitute for elimination diets.

Intradermal Skin Testing. Intradermal skin testing is used to definitively diagnose atopy in dogs and cats. Although it is an accurate, practical testing procedure, extensive training is needed to properly choose antigens and interpret test results. RAST and ELISA testing may prove to be a useful adjunct, but will not replace intradermal skin testing.

Environmental Restriction. If allergic contact dermatitis is suspected, the animal may be housed in a markedly different environment (water-rinsed kennel) for ten days.

Trial Therapy. Occasionally trial therapy may be indicated if other diagnostic tests have proven fruitless. The trial use of parasiticidal agents to eliminate the possibility of canine scabies or flea allergy is commonly indicated. Since pyodermas are frequently not obvious clinically, antibiotic therapy is frequently successful in idiopathic pruritic dogs. Response to parenteral corticosteroids indicates the likelihood of an allergic or other corticosteroid-responsive disease.

Cost Containment. Skin scrapings, pustular smears, and fungal cultures are the most cost-effective diagnostic procedures for evaluating the pruritic dog or cat. Somewhat surprisingly, skin biopsy is also relatively cost-effective when unnecessary re-examinations and medications are factored in. Elimination diets are time-consuming and sometimes expensive for the owners. However, they enjoy wide acceptance by owners, perhaps because the owners feel that they are contributing to the diagnostic plan. Intradermal skin testing should only be considered if more cost-effective diagnostic tests have proven fruitless and if historical and physical findings are supportive of atopy.

GOALS OF THERAPY

Obviously, the successful management of the pruritic dog or cat is contingent upon reaching an accurate diagnosis.

Ectoparasitic diseases require repetitive parasiticidal therapy. Long-term therapy is needed with flea allergy to prevent recurrences. Corticosteroids may be used adjunctively; preferably using prednisolone, prednisone, or methyl-prednisolone on an alternate day basis in the initial management. Demodicosis is a notable exception since glucocorticoids are contraindicated because of their immunosuppressive effect. Pyodermas may require long-term antibiotic therapy if underlying causes are not identified or in animals susceptible to recurrences. Idiopathic seborrhea requires long-term topical management with shampoos and rinses.

When the causes of pruritus cannot be identified, referral to a veterinary dermatologist is recommended. Long-term corticosteroid therapy should be considered an admission of defeat.

27 LUMPS, BUMPS, MASSES, AND LYMPHADENOPATHY

DUDLEY McCAW

Most lumps, bumps, and masses encountered in small animals are tumors, abscesses, cysts, hematomas, granulomas, or excessive fibrous scar tissue. Tumor in the strictest definition means a swelling; therefore, all lumps, bumps, and masses could be referred to as tumors regardless of the cause. A more specific and commonly used definition of *tumor* is a new growth of cells or tissues that resembles normal cells but proliferates without control. This term is used synonymously with neoplasm, and is the definition used in this chapter.

An *abscess* is a localized collection of pus. When well developed it has a wall of fibrous tissue separating it from surrounding tissue. A *cyst* is a sac with a distinct wall, which contains fluid or other material (air, saliva, a foreign body, a parasite, or blood). Any focal extravasation of blood is commonly referred to as a *hematoma*. A *granuloma* is a lump or mass composed of capillaries and fibroblasts.

Lymphadenopathy means any disease of the lymph nodes. Most lymphadenopathies lead to enlargement of the lymph nodes, but diseases that cause atrophy of lymph nodes must be included under the term lymphadenopathy. The common usage of *lymphadenopathy* means lymph node enlargement and that connotation is used in this chapter. *Lymphadenectasis* is really the proper term for enlarged lymph nodes. The following discussion is confined to diseases that produce lymph node enlargement.

GENERAL PATHOPHYSIOLOGY

The causes of lumps, bumps, and masses include anomalous (cysts), metabolic (hematomas), neoplastic (tumors), inflammatory (abscesses, granulomas, scar tissue, and cysts), and traumatic (hematomas). Lymphadenopathy is the result of inflammatory or neoplastic conditions.

Tumors. Tumors usually have an unknown etiology. Some have a viral etiology, such as papillomas in dogs and fibrosarcomas in cats. Chronic irritation, trauma, and sunlight exposure have been implicated in some neoplasms. *Spirocerca lupi* has been associated with tumors of the esophagus.

Once tumors begin to grow, the expansion seems to be relentless with few or no constraints upon the size attained. Malignant tumors exhibit invasive growth. Their growth is characterized by infiltration between normal cells, which are robbed of nutrients, causing the death and necrosis of the normal cells. Malignant tumors are so invasive that they can destroy any tissue except cartilage. Malignant cells are also able to enter the blood or lymph system. Once within the circulation, they are carried to other organs and continue to proliferate. This is known as metastasis. Benign neoplasms are not as destructive. They grow by expansion, which means they push normal cells away but they do not invade or grow between normal cells. The destructive powers of benign tumors are related to their size and pressure that they put upon normal structures.

Inflammation. Acute inflammation is often caused by bacteria, although parasites, foreign material, or trauma are other possible causes. All of these etiologies produce the classic signs of inflammation: redness, swelling, pain, heat, and loss of function. In the inflammatory process, initially there is an increased blood flow to the area. Vessel dilatation allows neutrophils, fluid, and red blood cells to pass through the vessel wall. An abscess forms when purulent exudate collects in the tissues as a result of neutrophils dying in an attempt to digest the bacteria or foreign material. This exudate consists of dead neutrophils and tissue cells that are killed by the enzymes released from the neutrophils. A pyogenic membrane forms around the focus of inflammation. The portion of the membrane nearest the abscess consists of necrotic tissue and fibrin. The more external portion of the membrane is granulation tissue. The pressures within abscess are increased and uneven. This results in the abscess bursting through the pyogenic membrane and draining. Once draining occurs the tissue usually heals.

Sometimes an abscess may heal without draining if the inflammatory stimulus has been neutralized. The pus is removed by enzymatic digestion. The remaining watery substance is resorbed. If the suppurative process is prolonged, the fibroblasts in the pyogenic membrane can proliferate, and a lump composed of dense fibrous tissue forms.

Cysts. Cysts can be the end result of an abscess. This occurs if the pyogenic membrane is complete and the fluid that is present after the pus is digested is not resorbed. Cysts may also form as the result of plugging of the duct of a gland, or as an anomaly.

Granulomas. Tumor-like masses of granulation tissue, called granulomas, can form as the result of chronic inflammation. The stimulus for the chronic inflammation can be bacteria, viruses, or parasites. The stimulus exists in tissues for long periods and evades the body's immune system, thus failing to produce acute inflammation and abscess. Other causes of chronic inflammation include irritants, prolonged mechanical irritation, and hypersensitivity to chemical substances. The body is unable to overcome the stimulus of the chronic inflammation. Rather than an acute response by neutrophils, the substance stimulates fibroblasts, epithelioid cells, and giant cells that encapsulate the offending agent.

Hematomas. Hematomas can be the result of local trauma causing extravasation of blood from the rupture of a vessel. The problem of hemostasis must also be considered. Hemophilia or the absence of clotting factors commonly produces hematomas, especially after minor trauma, which under normal circumstances would go unnoticed.

Lymph Nodes. Lymph nodes can enlarge due to primary or metastatic neoplasia, or infectious, immune-mediated, or inflammatory diseases. Hyperplasia of lymph nodes caused by septicemia results in a proliferation of the lymphoid and reticular structures of the nodes. Exudation and hemorrhage can also contribute to the increase in size. If an infection is overwhelming, the node can abscess, with the capsule of the lymph node serving as the pyogenic membrane of the abscess. Immunologic stimulation of the lymph nodes produces an increase in node size as the result of an increase in the number of lymphocytes. The germinal centers, filled with lymphoblasts, become numerous.

Primary neoplasia of the lymph nodes (lymphosarcoma) causes an increase in node size because of an increase in the number of lymphocytes, the result of uncontrolled cell division. In metastatic neoplasia the increase in size is not only caused by growth of the neoplastic cells within the node but also by the node's reaction to it. An inflammatory reaction with an increase in macrophages and lymphoid cells commonly occurs in an attempt to kill the neoplastic cells.

HISTORICAL FINDINGS

Attempting to gather historical information about a lump can at times be futile. Many masses, even large ones, go unnoticed by the owners for long periods of time. Hence, they give a history stating that the lump appeared overnight. Although it is not always possible, the clinician should attempt to obtain a good history because the events that have occurred since the lump appeared can be of help in differentiating the type of lesion present. Hematomas develop rapidly when the extravasation of blood occurs. If the owners noticed a hematoma and did not seek veterinary attention, they may report that the mass became firmer as the hematoma organized and possibly even reduced in size as the clot contracted and fluid was resorbed.

Abscesses appear quickly and owners may notice the signs of inflammation. Pain and loss of function are clues that the mass is an abscess. The owners may report an injury to the animal two to three days prior to presentation. A hard mass that has softened in the center is suggestive of an abscess that has organized. The history of a cyst that formed from a resolving abscess should indicate that signs of inflammation were observed, then abated as the mass reduced in size. Cysts can also be the result of an anomalous formation of tissue. In this case the cyst will have been present since the animal was young. Granulomas also form after inflammation. The owners may report the signs of inflammation followed by a firm mass.

Sometimes neoplasms seem to appear suddenly, according to the owners; this is related to a number of factors. Unless a tumor is in an area that is readily visible or frequently petted, such as the eyelid or head, clinical detection of a tumor does not occur until it reaches about one cm in diameter. A thick hair coat or occurrence in an area that is seldom seen or touched can allow masses to become quite large before detection. The growth pattern of tumors frequently gives the impression they have suddenly appeared and are growing rapidly. Tumor growth is generally considered to be a factor of doubling time. Assuming that the neoplasm begins as one malignant cell and all daughter cells survive, 30 doublings occur before that tumor is one cm in diameter (a tumor this size contains about 10^9 cells). If the doubling time is two weeks, then the neoplasm will be present for over a year before it is clinically detectable. Once a noticeable size is reached, the growth appears to be rapid because each doubling greatly increases the size of the tumor. The growth of most tumors actually slows as the size increases. Another factor that gives the appearance of sudden growth of a tumor is an inflammatory reaction around the mass of neoplastic cells.

Generalized lymph node enlargement in the absence of systemic illness is most likely the result of lymphosarcoma. A sick animal with generalized lymph node enlargement may have an infectious or autoimmune disease, or lymphosarcoma.

The owner should be asked about previous tumor removal in the case of single lymph node enlargement, as this could be the metastasis from a previous removal. Lymphosarcoma can be limited to one node or region but this is not as common as generalized lymph node enlargement.

PHYSICAL FINDINGS

All superficial lumps, whether neoplasms or not, should be approached in the manner in which tumors are staged. Although many clinicians are reluctant to use the tumor, node, metastasis (TNM) system, it assures that the proper information is observed and placed in the record. The T refers to the physical properties of the tumor that should be recorded, such as size. The information can then be passed along to the pathologist if a biopsy is submitted or used for reference during future exams. Attachment to underlying structures and overlying skin should also be noted.

The following general characteristics of masses can help distinguish the different types. Hematomas are unattached to tissues, are not encapsulated, and initially appear to be fluid-filled. Once organization of the hematoma has occurred, the mass is firm. Abscesses may be attached to deeper structures or skin. Their consistency varies with the stage of organization, being either firm or fluctuant. Pain upon palpation occurs with abscesses because of associated acute inflammation. Granulomas and scar tissue are the result of chronic inflammation; signs of pain are absent. These masses are firm and can be attached to underlying structures or skin.

The presentation of neoplasms varies, depending upon tumor type and degree of malignancy. Tumors of connective tissue tend to be firm, whereas those of vascular tissue can be variable, at times possessing soft areas similar to abscesses. Malignant neoplasms have broad attachments, invade underlying structures, can be fixed to the skin, and may ulcerate. Benign tumors may be pedunculated. Since benign tumors grow by expansion, they are not attached to underlying structures and are sometimes encapsulated.

Evaluation of the lymph nodes (N) should be a routine part of the physical examination of every lump. First, the regional lymph node draining the area of the lump should be checked for enlargement. If enlarged, the node should be measured. It should also be noted whether the node is movable or fixed to surrounding tissue and whether it is painful or warm. The texture of the node should be assessed. Nodes draining an inflammatory lesion become enlarged as a result of the normal filtering, resulting in an increase in lymphocytes and macrophages. Lymph nodes draining a tumor may be enlarged because of inflammation or because the tumor has metastasized to the node. After the regional node is assessed, all nodes should be palpated for enlargement. Generalized lymph node enlargement could result from septicemia, a generalized immune response, or lymphosarcoma.

Metastasis (M) refers to spread of the tumor to sites other than the lymph nodes. With malignant neoplasms, this is often the lungs or abdominal organs. Radiographs are necessary to fully assess metastasis. If the clinician has a high index of suspicion that the lump is malignant, radiographs should be obtained because the spread of the tumor to distant sites greatly alters the therapeutic plan. With a benign neoplasm or a non-neoplastic mass, the check for metastasis is really a check for other lumps that might be present. The clinician should palpate all areas of the animal by running his or her hands over the skin to detect other superficial lumps. If other lumps are found then one must determine if they are the same type as the initial lump.

Physical examination of lumps in the abdominal cavity is more difficult than examination of superficial masses. If abdominal palpation is a part of every physical examination, lumps will be detected prior to any abnormalities noted by the owner. This is best accomplished by standing behind the animal, placing one hand on each side, and gently moving the hands together. The examination should start at one end of the abdomen and work toward the other end. When examining the posterior abdomen, a rectal examination should be performed. To determine the positional relation of structures to the descending colon, a probe such as a fecal loop can be inserted into the colon as a reference point. Performing the examination with the animal in lateral recumbency as well as standing helps to differentiate structures. Sedation may be required in some animals to facilitate a good examination. If the animal is sedated or anesthetized for another procedure, abdominal palpation should be repeated.

When one enlarged lymph node is present the animal should be examined for other enlarged lymph nodes. If other peripheral nodes are found to be enlarged, the abdomen should be palpated for enlarged nodes and possibly an enlarged spleen or liver. The finding of only one enlarged node should prompt an examination of the area drained by that node for possible disease, which may have been filtered by the node or caused an inflammatory reaction in the lymph node.

DIAGNOSTIC PLAN

After the physical examination, tests and procedures that should be considered are serum biochemical profiles, complete blood cell counts, urinalyses, radiographs, ultrasonography, cytology, and histopathology. If the animal is a cat, a test for feline leukemia virus should be performed.

Serum biochemical profiles, complete blood cell counts, and urinalyses help in diagnosis but they are also an important part of the evaluation of the patient prior to anesthesia or treatment. If the animal has other medical problems such as renal failure, the therapeutic plan should be altered. The total white blood cell count and differential white blood cell count can aid in separating inflammatory conditions from neoplastic ones. In the case of lymphadenopathy, the presence of neoplastic lymphocytes in the peripheral blood aids in diagnosis.

Radiology. Radiographs are used to evaluate the primary mass and to detect metastasis if the mass is a tumor. If a mass appears to be attached to underlying tissue and is on a limb where the bones are fairly superficial, a radiograph should be obtained to detect bone involvement. In cases of lymphadenopathy, thoracic and abdominal radiographs are necessary to assess the nodes in those areas.

Radiographs are an essential part of the examination of an abdominal mass. Proper preparation of the patient is necessary if diagnostic radiographs are to be obtained. The gastrointestinal system must not contain large amounts of digestive material, which easily obscures abdominal structures. Fasting and enemas prior to the examination may be necessary to obtain quality films.

Contrast radiography, pneumoperitoneogram, or excretory urogram may be used to outline masses. The abdominal radiographs should be examined for areas of involvement in addition to the primary mass. Enlarged lymph nodes, areas of bone involvement, or abnormal shadows in the portion of the lung field present in the film give evidence that the mass is a malignant neoplasm.

Prior to any invasive procedure, radiographs of the thorax to assess the presence of metastases should be completed. When looking for lung metastases, a ventrodorsal view and two lateral views, one with the animal in right lateral recumbency and one with the animal in left lateral recumbency, should be taken. Metastases in the upper lung are more visible because that lung is better aerated; the contrast between a gas-filled lung and a water-dense mass is enhanced. In most situations, these do not reveal any metastasis even with malignant neoplasms. However, the presence of metastatic disease so drastically alters the therapeutic plan that it is imperative to have this information.

Ultrasonography. The use of ultrasonography is becoming widespread in veterinary medicine and it greatly increases the clinically useful information that can be obtained in the assessment of abdominal masses. An ultrasound examination can determine whether the mass is solid or cystic. Unlike radiographs, which are obscured by fluid in the abdominal cavity, ultrasound examinations are enhanced by the presence of fluid.

Cytology. After the patient has been thoroughly evaluated for the extent of the disease, cytology of the mass or lymph node should be performed to attempt identification of the cell type.

FINE NEEDLE ASPIRATION. A fine needle aspiration is an easy and safe procedure. It is performed by using a 22-gauge or smaller needle attached to a 12 ml (or larger) syringe. The area is clipped and surgically prepared. While immobilizing the structure, the needle is inserted and the plunger of the syringe withdrawn. The needle should be moved to different areas of the structure, but care should be taken to assure that the end of the needle does not exit the mass or node. The plunger is released. After the pressure within the syringe has equalized, the syringe and needle are withdrawn. The needle is removed from the syringe and the syringe filled with air. After the needle is reattached, the contents of the needle are blown onto the slide. The material is smeared onto the slide by using another slide held at a 45-degree angle if the material is liquid; if the material is solid it is smeared by placing the two slides together and then pulling them apart. When the specimen is seen in the needle hub or syringe, aspiration should be stopped to prevent diluting the sample. With solid lumps material may not be seen in the syringe but enough sample is present in the needle for cytology. If material is seen in the syringe, the sample is probably contaminated with blood or fluid. Visual inspection may be enough to determine if the fluid is saliva, blood, pus, or fluid from a cyst. However, a cytologic exam should still be performed since it may detect neoplastic cells.

Fine needle aspirates of intra-abdominal masses can be accomplished if the mass can be immobilized and moved close to the body wall so that other intra-abdominal structures do not have to be penetrated to reach the mass. The technique is the same as described previously, however, sedation of the animal may be required to prevent movement while the needle is within the abdominal cavity. There are few contraindications to fine needle aspiration. Even the most vascular tissue is unlikely to bleed from the small needle puncture wound. Cystic structures that may be abscesses should be aspirated with caution, if at all. The potential complication of introducing bacteria of unknown pathogenicity into the abdominal cavity should be avoided.

Biopsy. A more definitive diagnosis can be obtained by tissue biopsy, which is formalin-fixed and submitted for histopathology. Biopsies can be obtained using a variety of biopsy instruments or a scalpel. In the case of lymphadenopathy, a lymph node can be removed. If the lump is surgically removed, a portion of it should be submitted for histopathology. A representative sample of the lump that also incorporates normal tissue at the edges of the surgical wound should be submitted to determine if all the diseased tissue has been removed. The advisability of a biopsy prior to surgical removal of a mass should be considered. The logical solution to this question is to ask whether or not a biopsy will alter the treatment. If so, a presurgical biopsy is indicated. If not, then the biopsy should be obtained at surgical removal. No matter how benign a mass appears, a portion should be submitted for histopathological diagnosis. Arguments that the cost of histopathology cannot be justified are weak. The expense of histopathology is minor compared to the overall expense of surgically removing a mass. Prognosis after treatment is important, and without an accurate diagnosis, the prognosis has no validity.

Abdominal masses can be accomplished using most biopsy instruments. These can be inserted blindly into the mass if it can be immobilized and moved close to the body wall. For masses where this cannot be performed, the instrument can be guided with a laparoscope or by ultrasound. Biopsies can also be obtained by using laparotomy. The technique to be used must be determined by the degree of health and additional problems present in each particular case, as well as the availability of equipment. Laparoscopy has the advantages of being rapid, requiring a minimal surgical wound, and allowing good visualization of the abdominal structures. Its disadvantage is that it does not allow for the removal of masses to the extent that might be "curative." It does, however, allow biopsies to be obtained with visual guidance of the biopsy needle.

Ultrasound guidance of the biopsy needle has the advantages of not requiring a surgical wound and needing only narcotic analgesia and local anesthesia. Although direct visualization is not possible, ultrasound allows the clinician to visualize both the biopsy instrument and the organ being biopsied. Unlike other methods, it allows for accurate biopsy of a mass within an organ. The procedure does not allow removal of lumps.

Laparotomy is the preferred technique in many situations. It is the one procedure that affords the opportunity to remove abnormal masses as well as obtain biopsies. The other advantages include the fact that special equipment is not required, it is a procedure with which most veterinarians are familiar, and it allows good inspection of other structures (organs and lymph nodes) in the abdominal cavity. Disadvantages include cost, discomfort involved, poor patient risk, anesthetic risk, and in some cases damage to the patient when surgical stress complicates a solely medical problem.

GOALS OF TREATMENT

Abscesses should be treated by surgical drainage and antibiotic therapy. Granulomas, cysts, and scar tissue are all treated by surgical removal. Benign neoplasms benefit from surgical removal, while malignant neoplasms may require a combination of surgery, radiation, and chemotherapy.

Lymphadenopathy caused by infectious diseases should be treated with the appropriate antibacterial agents. Immune-mediated diseases are treated with corticosteroids and immunosuppressive agents. Lymphosarcoma can be treated with chemotherapy.

OUTCOME

The results of treatment for infectious and inflammatory diseases should be complete cure. If surgical removal is complete, then benign neoplasms, cysts, granulomas, and scar tissue should cause no further disease. The outcome for malignancies and immune-mediated diseases is rarely curative, but treatment can produce long remissions and therefore should be offered to pet owners.

28 ASCITES, PERITONITIS, AND OTHER CAUSES OF ABDOMINAL ENLARGEMENT

STEPHEN J. ETTINGER

THE PERITONEAL SURFACE

The peritoneal surface is a serous membrane that lines the abdominal cavity and covers the visceral surfaces of the abdominal organs. The peritoneal surface is of mesodermal origin and is composed of a single layer of flat, serrated cells with underlying layers of connective tissue, blood vessels, and lymphatic channels.

The purposes of the peritoneum are protection and absorption. It protects the peritoneal cavity by walling off areas of inflammation and permits the absorption, exudation, or transudation of fluids. Usually, the peritoneal cavity contains little free fluid. The presence of free fluid in the abdominal cavity is considered pathologic. The absorbent quality of the peritoneal surface allows peritoneal dialysis to be performed, as all elements of the blood pass freely across the serosal surface.

In the male, the peritoneal cavity is a closed cavity covered by the peritoneum. In the female, the peritoneal cavity is that space enclosed by the peritoneum but that remains open to the outside through the female reproductive system.

In general, increased abdominal and peritoneal pressures result in the cranial displacement of the diaphragm, resulting in increased respiratory activity. In addition, increased abdominal pressures produce venous stasis in the abdomen, diminished arterial blood pressures, and a decrease in renal blood flow.

RECOGNITION OF PERITONEAL DISEASE

There are three signs, which, presented independently or in association with each other, suggest peritoneal disease. These signs are abdominal pain, abdominal enlargement, and/or a history of acute trauma to the abdomen. Rarely, the peritoneal disorder is a primary disease; more likely, it is a sign of a primary disease. The signs associated with peritoneal disease are characterized here to permit an orderly approach to both the recognition and treatment of abdominal disorders.

Abdominal pain is a commonly encountered clinical entity. It may reflect a disease process involving the peritoneal lining or may be due to a specific process affecting an abdominal organ. It is beyond the scope of this chapter to discuss the entity of abdominal pain other than to comment on some of the peritoneal diseases in which pain is a clinical feature. Peritonitis, acute abdominal hemorrhage, free urine in the abdominal cavity, abdominal organomegaly, and ascites, especially when associated with hepatomegaly and referred neurologic pain, are the most common conditions to consider when pain is evident during abdominal palpation.

Abdominal enlargement usually develops slowly and insidiously, except when due to traumatic hemoperitoneum or rupture of the urinary bladder. Abdominal enlargement is also associated with such common clinical entities as pregnancy; hydrometra; pyometra; hepatomegaly and renomegaly; growths involving the spleen, liver, lymph nodes, or other abdominal organs; intermittent engorgement of vascular tumors; and ascites due to heart failure, hypoproteinemia, and venous obstruction of the posterior vena cava.

In addition, the slowly enlarging abdomen is associated with Cushing's syndrome, peritonitis, and fluid collection associated with feline infectious peritonitis. Chronic urinary bladder distention or obstruction, obstipation, and gastric torsion are also reasons for an enlarging abdomen.

Acute traumatic lesions, resulting in a hemoperitoneum or a ruptured bladder, may cause sudden abdominal enlargement. In such cases, an associated peritonitis usually develops, producing abdominal pain. Warfarin poisoning may produce intra-abdominal hemorrhage associated with painful enlargement of the abdomen.

ABDOMINAL ULTRASONOGRAPHY

A noninvasive technique of great value in the differential diagnosis of abdominal fluid collection and the enlarged abdomen is clinical ultrasound. This relatively new method of visualizing the interior of the abdomen has improved and facilitated the examination of the abdomen. Ultrasound (U/S) uses the concept of reverberating sound waves produced by the transducer. The waves are transmitted into the abdomen and then the echoes, or reflected sound waves, are recorded by the receiving transducer unit. Sound waves are absorbed and reflected to variable degrees by the different abdominal structures. Each parenchymal organ has specific echo patterns based on its cellularity and stromal composition. These echo patterns are distinct relative to the echogenicity of the surrounding tissue. Echoes penetrate highly reflective surfaces such as gas, air, bone, and barium poorly. As a result, when U/S is visualized on the recording screen, fat appears densely white, bone and air are white, and fluid and blood are black (see Table 28–1 and Figure 28–1).

The specific structural appearance of each organ permits the experienced clinician to look at the abdominal contents without surgically interrupting the abdominal wall. Whereas radiography permits visualization of the abdominal global structures, U/S identifies gross organ enlargement and irregularities, internal dilation, abscessation, and structural changes within the organ. Additionally, free abdominal fluid, ruptured neoplasms or abscesses, peritonitis, and lack of abdominal fat often preclude a successful abdominal radiographic examination. In contrast, such features may be specifically diagnosed, suggested, or identified using U/S.

Figure 28–1 shows abnormal U/S recordings from dogs and cats with enlarged abdomens. Table 28–1 is a summary outline of different U/S findings in abdominal enlargement.

TABLE 28–1. ULTRASOUND CHARACTERISTICS OF ABDOMINAL FLUID ACCUMULATIONS

Ascites
- Anechoic*
- Hypoechoic-mixed to black-appearing fluid outlines of abdominal organs†

Abdominal Masses
- (neoplasms, hematoma, granuloma, and abscess)
- Hypoechoic or hyperechoic‡
- Indistinct, irregular, ill-defined borders
- Poor far wall (back wall) definition
- Poor through transmission

Abdominal Cysts
- Anechoic or hypoechoic
- Sharp, well-defined borders
- Sharp, far wall definition
- Good through transmission
- Peripheral refractory and reflective zones

*Anechoic means without internal echoes typical of nonviscid fluid (black appearing).

†Hypoechoic means reduced internal echoes typical of viscid filled lesions having a mixed black and white to white appearance on the echo screen.

‡Hyperechoic patterns have increased internal echoes and acoustic shadows and appear densely white.

TECHNIQUES OF ABDOMINAL PARACENTESIS

Abdominal paracentesis is usually performed after ultrasound and radiographic examinations confirm the clinical suspicion of free peritoneal fluid. Depending upon the amount of fluid present and the nature of the examination that the clinician wishes to perform on the abdominal fluid, the form of paracentesis varies.

The simplest form of abdominal paracentesis is midline centesis using a needle and syringe. This technique is performed after radiographic examination of the abdomen reveals the presence, if any, of organ enlargement. The urinary bladder should be evacuated prior to paracentesis. If the liver does not extend too far posteriorly, the ventral midline abdomen at the level of the umbilicus is clipped and prepared in a sterile manner. Then, midline paracentesis may be safely performed.

A small amount of lidocaine may be instilled into the cutaneous, subcutaneous, and muscular regions; however, in most cases, a simple paracentesis does not require local infiltration with anesthetic agents. A standard short, 20- or 22-gauge needle is thrust into the abdominal cavity and a small amount of fluid (about 10 cc) is removed. In general, it is best to perform this operation with the animal in either a standing or a lateral recumbent position. The patient should be held firmly without moving about, thereby preventing the pushing of organs against the needle. The fluid sample should be withdrawn and the examination terminated as quickly as possible. Fluid is taken for culture, cytology, and chemical analysis as well as for red and white cell counts.

An alternative procedure that is somewhat safer in terms of preventing accidental organ laceration is to use a short, polyethylene, indwelling IV catheter. After just penetrating the abdominal wall, the plastic catheter is advanced into the peritoneal cavity and the needle stylet is removed. A syringe is attached to the hub and the sample withdrawn. This technique is useful for pneumoperitonography and peritoneal contrast dye studies.

Another technique that is occasionally used for diagnostic abdominal paracentesis and lavage makes use of a standard human dialysis catheter. Usually, a small midline stab incision is required to penetrate the abdominal wall. The catheter, directed toward the pelvis and urethral column, is longer than an IV catheter and is more likely to collect free fluid. Lavage with saline also permits fluid collection for analysis. This is a particularly

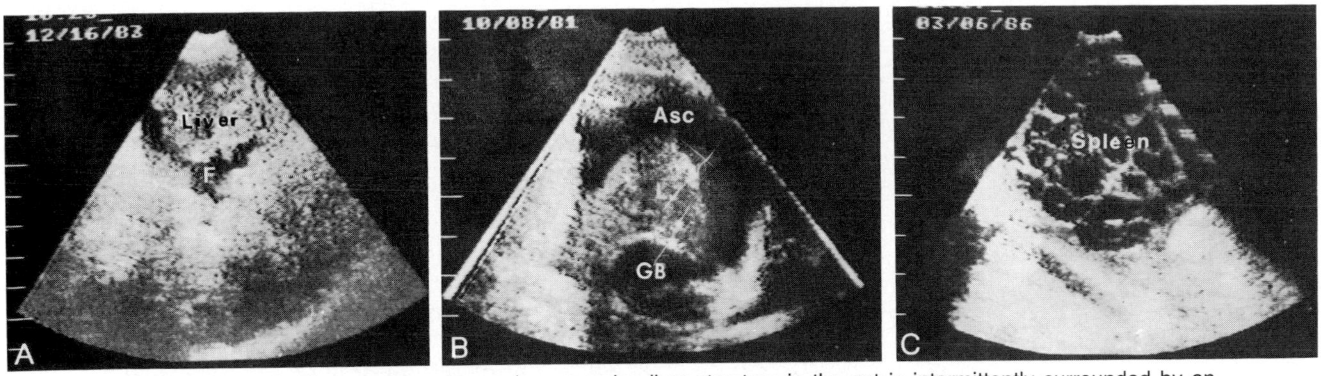

FIGURE 28–1. *A,* The coarse and granular appearing liver structure in the cat is intermittently surrounded by an irregular black area (F) which represents ascitic fluid. The liver was homogeneous in appearance. On percutaneous biopsy the pathologist identified adenocarcinoma of the liver. *B,* In a dog with ascites, the abdominal fluid (Asc) surrounds the liver (L) and outlines the gallbladder (GB). The ascitic fluid in this case was the result of congestive heart failure. Often the hepatic veins are dilated, but this is not shown in this view. *C,* Splenic hemangiosarcoma was detected in this dog presented for weakness, syncope, and acute abdominal distention. The area below the xiphoid in the midabdomen was echoed and a mixed hyper- and hypoechoic lesion typical of a cystic mass was noted. On exploratory surgery the diagnosis was confirmed and the spleen was removed.

useful technique in the evaluation and management of acute abdominal trauma.

Regardless of the method used, any sanguineous fluid removed is divided into two samples; one is stored in an anticoagulant, the other is permitted to clot. The latter provides the clinician with valuable information about the presence of whole blood in the peritoneal cavity. Bloody fluids should be compared with venous blood with respect to clotting time and cell counts. High white counts suggest peritonitis, as do fluids containing bile, urine, and foreign materials.

For cases that require removal of larger quantities of abdominal fluid, the abdomen is prepared in a similar manner after the bladder has been drained. Only occasionally is mild sedation required. After sterile preparation and instillation of a local anesthetic agent, a number 11 or 15 scalpel blade is inserted into the abdominal wall, just off the midline. A small incision into the peritoneal cavity is made, and a sterile *soft* catheter (a Brunswick-type feeding tube may be used) is then inserted into the abdominal cavity through the incision site and muscular layers by blunt perforation with a hemostat. Prior to inserting the catheter, small holes should be added to the distal end of the tube. These holes must be small to prevent the catheter from folding in on itself.

The catheter is introduced far enough into the abdominal cavity to freely drain the fluid. To prevent accidental slippage, a tag is attached to the catheter, which is then attached to the abdominal wall with a purse string suture. The suture should go through the drain to guarantee its position and prevent it from slipping into the abdomen. Drainage of the abdomen may be performed over a period of several hours to a day by allowing the fluid to drain slowly through the catheter. It is imperative to use an Elizabethan collar to prevent chewing and then accidental loss of the tube. In cases where a pneumoperitoneum is desired, after removal of the ascitic fluid, air may be instilled into the abdominal cavity. Often, after enough fluid is drained, air is sucked into the abdomen through the tube. This can yield an excellent double contrast study. In general, after the catheter is removed from the abdominal cavity, the incision site closes rapidly. Occasionally, a single suture is placed in the cutaneous tissue.

Table 28–2 lists the common causes of abdominal effusions.

Removal and collection of abdominal fluid either in small or large quantities may temporarily relieve discomfort or distress of the patient. The primary benefit, however, is that it allows the clinician to make a diagnosis and thereby choose a mode of therapy for long-term effects. Radiography after fluid removal may assist in the diagnosis. Laboratory evaluation of the fluid is similarly important. Fluid should be collected and a sterile sample saved if culture is deemed necessary after cell counts and microscopic exams are complete. Samples should be saved in EDTA tubes (for cell counts), in heparinized tubes (for cytology), and in plain tubes (for chemistry and cytology, if a nonclotting fluid). Slides should be prepared immediately after withdrawal in accordance with the preference of the pathologist (in alcohol, spray fixed, or air dried).

ASCITES

Ascites refers to a collection of serous fluid within the peritoneal cavity. The definition is broad and encompasses the collection within the abdominal cavity of bile, chyle, urine, and blood, as well as exudative and transudative fluids.

Ascites is a secondary sign of disease rather than the primary cause of the disease. Consequently, the correct approach to patients with ascitic fluid is to determine the nature of the primary problem.

Ascites develops in only a limited number of disease conditions. The more frequently encountered causes of ascites include abdominal carcinomatosis; congestive heart failure (right-sided or right- and left-sided); venous stasis at the level of the liver or within the thoracic cavity; abdominal trauma with the spilling of blood, urine, chyle, or bile into the abdomen; starvation; portal

TABLE 28–2. COMMON CAUSES OF ABDOMINAL EFFUSION

- **Transudate**
  - Hypoproteinemia
    - Intestinal malabsorption
    - Intestinal protein loss
    - Glomerular disease
  - Lymphangiectasia
  - Neoplasia
  - Obstructing lymph drainage
- **Modified Transudate**
  - Congestive heart failure
  - Portal venous obstruction
  - Hepatopathies
    - Postnecrotic cirrhosis
    - Hepatoma
    - Bile-duct carcinoma
  - Abdominal neoplasia obstructing lymphatics and blood vessels
    - Carcinoma
    - Sarcoma
- **Serosanguineous Exudate**
  - Feline infectious peritonitis
  - Urine peritonitis
  - Bile peritonitis
  - Pancreatic peritonitis
  - Steatitis
  - Hepatopathies
    - Chronic active hepatitis
  - Diaphragmatic hernia
  - Abdominal neoplasia
    - Carcinoma
    - Sarcoma
    - Lymphosarcoma
- **Purulent Exudate**
  - Intestinal perforation
  - Penetrating wounds
  - Ruptured pyometra
  - Ruptured abscess
  - Extension of infection
- **Hemorrhagic Effusion**
  - Traumatic injury to major vessel, spleen, liver
  - Neoplasm
    - Hemangiosarcoma
    - Vascular tumor
  - Bleeding disorders
    - Warfarin toxicity
    - Thrombocytopenia
  - Thrombosis
  - Torsion
    - Stomach
    - Spleen
  - Tumor eroding a vessel
    - Pheochromocytoma

hypertension; and hypoproteinemia secondary to parasitism, the nephrotic syndrome, and other renal disease. Hepatic cirrhosis, chylothorax (traumatic or obstructive), warfarin poisoning with hemorrhage into the abdominal cavity, and peritonitis (infectious and parasitic) are also causes, as is parasitic ascites due to *Mesocestoides* sp.

History and Physical Examination. The histories of patients with ascites vary from acute trauma to chronic, insidiously developing problems. The physical examination usually reveals findings that are specific or suggestive of the cause. In many cases, the fluid has collected slowly, often without being noticed by the owner. Where fluid collection has been rapid, clinical signs of weakness and dyspnea are more likely to be apparent.

Clinical signs such as a cardiac cough or jaundice may be associated with the primary disease. Massive ascites results in the cranial displacement of the diaphragm, causing reduced ventilatory capacity and compromised respiratory exchange. In addition to respiratory distress, patients may be weak, and, with chronic fluid collection, debilitated. The patient has a distended ventral abdomen, yet there is simultaneous loss of muscle and flesh along the vertebral column. This classic wasting situation occurs with the cardiomyopathies, hypoproteinemic syndromes, and chronic neoplastic diseases. Often, the owner is unaware of the loss of flesh because the body weight is nearly maintained by the increased abdominal size.

Palpation of the fluid-filled abdomen reveals a dense abdomen, often with organs that cannot be discretely palpated but that can be balloted. Tapping the abdominal wall with one's fingers sets in motion a physical wave that is transmitted to the opposite side of the abdomen. In cases with advanced fluid collection, the femoral pulse becomes thready in character, as a result of diminishing arterial flow to the periphery. Dependent subcutaneous edema of one or both hindlimbs and subcutaneous tissue of the abdomen and scrotum may develop.

Abdominal paracentesis is indicated on the basis of physical examination findings and the radiographic findings described below. The techniques used for abdominal paracentesis, drainage, and pneumoperitoneum have already been described.

Radiographic Examination. Radiographic examination provides little in the way of specific information in most instances. A generally hazy, opaque abdominal cavity with the classic "ground-glass" appearance is recognized. The serosal surfaces throughout the abdomen are nonexistent. Occasionally, ileus is recognized. Because of excessive fluid density, recognition of specific abdominal organs may not be possible. Occasionally, neoplastic or enlarged organs may be suggested by the radiographic examination. *Abdominal ultrasonography* is a useful technique in identifying ascitic fluid, as previously described (see Figure 28–1 *A* and *B*).

Differential Diagnosis. The differential diagnosis of ascitic fluid requires both chemical and cytologic analysis of the fluid. It is first necessary to differentiate those diseases known to produce ascites from conditions that could clinically be confused with abdominal enlargement. Radiographic and ultrasound examinations of the abdomen are always in order prior to stating that free fluid is present. This is important before performing an abdominal paracentesis because of the possible dangers associated with paracentesis of an abdominal organ.

Hepatomegaly, splenomegaly, obesity, abdominal muscle flaccidity (as occurs with Cushing's syndrome), malignant neoplasms, pyometra (or hydrometra), pregnancy, atonic bladder, urethral obstruction with bladder enlargement, and advanced obstipation all may initially be misinterpreted as fluid collection. Gastric torsion may be similarly misdiagnosed.

Treatment. The treatment of ascites varies with the nature of the primary disease state. The reader is referred to the sections in the text that specifically deal with the abnormality that has been diagnosed.

The clinician should not assume that diuretic therapy is indicated or helpful whenever ascites is present.

Diuretic therapy in cirrhosis with ascites may compromise plasma volume, causing a decrease in circulation that results in renal decompensation. Hypoalbuminemia in nephrotic patients is associated with a shift of fluid into the interstitial spaces from the plasma. Loss of further plasma volume may then reduce glomerular filtration and aggravate the azotemic state. Overzealous therapy in right heart failure may reduce filling pressure in the right heart, resulting in a reduction in cardiac output.

Abdominal fluid, when present and causing respiratory distress or abdominal discomfort, should be removed. Otherwise, the presence of fluid in the abdomen should lead the clinician to search for the cause rather than to concentrate on immediate removal of the fluid.

PERITONITIS

Peritonitis is an inflammatory process that involves all, or a portion of, the peritoneal cavity. Peritonitis can be caused by the introduction of microorganisms into the serosal-lined peritoneal cavity. This may result from traumatic incidents, surgically induced lesions, gangrenous obstruction of the gastrointestinal tract, perforation of the bowel, gastrointestinal tract ulcers, incarcerated hernias, or volvulus of a portion of the gastrointestinal tract.

Inflammation of the peritoneal cavity may result from release of neoplastic tissues, blood, urine, or bile into the abdominal cavity, or may occur secondary to a disease such as pancreatitis, where irritating acid products are released into the abdominal cavity. Abscess of any abdominal organ or periabdominal tissue may result in the release of microorganisms into the abdominal cavity with a secondary inflammatory response.

Physical Examination. Local or generalized tenderness may be recognized in peritonitis, although in general, the pain is diffuse and the abdomen is acutely tender and tympanic. Splinting of the abdominal wall is often apparent initially. Following the acute attack, abdominal distention develops. Pyrexia, tachycardia, hypotension, and vomiting develop, and ultimately there is an inability to pass gas or stool. Increased peristalsis initially gives way to ileus. Where primary diseases such as gastric torsion, pancreatitis, or prostatitis are present, specific signs referable to these illnesses may be apparent.

Radiographic and Ultrasound Examinations. The radiographic examination in peritonitis demonstrates loss of serosal surfaces with the "ground-glass" appearance of part or all of the abdominal cavity. Distention of the intestinal tract with gas- and/or fluid-filled loops of bowel occurs, with secondary edema of the bowel wall. Free fluid in the peritoneal cavity may be apparent in more advanced cases. Where rupture of a viscus has occurred, free air in the abdomen may also be apparent. Free air is best recognized from radiographs taken with a horizontal beam, allowing the free air to rise to the most dorsal position in the abdomen. When peritonitis is associated with pancreatitis, a fixed and dilated duodenum is anticipated, with areas of localized peritonitis in the periduodenal regions. Pulmonary edema may be a complicating associated finding. Localized pelvic peritonitis with prostatitis may obscure the normal serosal surfaces separating the colon, bladder, and prostate. Clinical ultrasound often localizes the area of fluid accumulation and may provide additional data regarding the etiology.

Laboratory Examination. Blood counts usually reveal a marked leukocytosis, with the predominant cell type being polymorphonuclear leukocytes, a large percentage of which are juvenile forms. Abdominal paracentesis with a fine needle is likely to result in aspiration of a small amount of a pus-like fluid, which microscopically reveals numerous white blood cells, especially of the immature series. Suspected inflammatory fluids should be examined cytologically and cultured aerobically, anaerobically, and for fungi. Bile, blood, or urine obtained by tapping the abdomen suggests specific causes to be investigated.

Differential Diagnosis. The problem associated with the diagnosis of peritonitis is not the difficulty in recognizing the disease, but rather the difficulty in determining the nature or cause of the disease. Since peritonitis is an inflammatory response within the peritoneal cavity, it is necessary for the clinician to determine the nature and cause of the irritation rather than to attempt to treat only the irritation. In general, sudden insults result in a localized peritonitis and the process is self-limiting unless continued contamination occurs.

Treatment. The goal in the treatment of peritonitis is to remove the prime source of contamination and to restore lost plasma volume. The loss of free fluid into the abdominal cavity accounts for only a portion of the total fluid lost in peritonitis. A large amount of fluid may also be lost in the gastrointestinal tract, which remains in a state of adynamic ileus.

In addition to replacing fluid, it may be necessary to supplement potassium and sodium electrolytes by venous infusion. Serum electrolyte determinations may be difficult to interpret properly in the presence of hemoconcentration.

The maintenance of normal pulmonary function is also an important consideration in the treatment of the disease process, since the respiratory apparatus is generally compromised by the cranial displacement of the diaphragm by large quantities of abdominal fluid.

Ultimately, peripheral vasoconstriction and increased peripheral resistance develop, with a subsequent decrease in organ perfusion and venous return. Of paramount importance in the latter stages of peritonitis is the maintenance of adequate cardiac output. To combat sepsis, antimicrobial therapy is recommended initially while awaiting the results of specific culture and sensitivity testing from samples obtained by prior peritoneal cavity centesis. Gram stain of a small sample of fluid is suggested initially to aid in the choice of antimicrobials.

In some cases, the cause of the peritonitis cannot be determined. In cases of bowel rupture, incarceration of the bowel, or other forms of obstruction, surgical exploration of the abdomen is necessary. It is appropriate to surgically explore nonresponsive cases of peritonitis in patients where thorough medical evaluation cannot determine the nature of the disease process.

PNEUMOPERITONEUM

Pneumoperitoneum results when free air collects in the abdominal cavity. It is often associated with traumatic stab wounds, rupture of a viscus, gastric dilatation with rupture, or ulceration of the gastrointestinal tract. The disease occurs only rarely as a spontaneous process because peritonitis is more likely to result from a rent in the gastrointestinal tract than is pneumoperitoneum. Pneumoperitoneum results from iatrogenic injection of air into the abdominal cavity and after abdominal laparotomy. After surgery, it may persist for ten or more days. Another possible cause is pneumothorax and pneumomediastinum with peritoneal dissection of gas.

HEMOPERITONEUM

Hemoperitoneum develops secondary to penetrating or nonpenetrating abdominal trauma. Such trauma may be associated with rupture of the spleen and/or liver. Perforation of gastric or intestinal ulcers and abdominal tumors also results in hemoperitoneum. Warfarin poisoning may result in the release of free, nonclotting blood into the abdominal cavity.

Initially, when bleeding into the peritoneal cavity occurs, signs of peritoneal inflammation develop. Weakness, pallor, diminished hematocrit levels, and shock develop. When bleeding is severe, syncopal episodes may be associated with it. Abdominal distention develops as fluid collection progresses. If reabsorption occurs and the trauma is not extensive, the symptoms regress rapidly. Reabsorption of blood from the peritoneal cavity occurs over a period of several weeks. Icteric serum obtained from the peritoneal centesis is commonly associated with blood loss into the abdominal cavity.

CHYLOUS PERITONITIS

Chylous peritonitis results from trauma to the abdominal cavity; tumors, especially lymphoma, involving lymphatic channels within the abdominal cavity; intestinal obstruction that results in rupture of a major lymph channel; and lymphangiectasia. The recognition of chylous peritonitis in dogs and cats is uncommon. The abdominal fluid in cases of chylous peritonitis reveals the classic chyle-like, milky fluid containing numerous fat globules. Chemically, the fat content of the fluid is extremely high in lipoproteins and chylomicrons. The diagnosis is confirmed by measuring triglyceride levels or by ether or chloroform solvent extraction that results in clearing of the fluid. Pseudochylous fluids that fail to clear after mixture with solvents are usually associated with neoplasms or infection.

Therapy may include surgical exploration of the abdomen to ligate a ruptured duct. Specific therapy requires identification of the etiology. Patients with an unknown cause are good candidates for intestinal biopsy when malabsorption is present.

ABDOMINAL CARCINOMATOSIS

Abdominal carcinomatosis refers to the widespread dissemination of cancer throughout the abdominal cavity. This involves the peritoneal and/or omental surfaces. Some authorities limit the condition to those tumors arising only from epithelial or glandular tissues. Others consider any generalized neoplastic involvement of the abdominal cavity to fall within this category.

In veterinary medicine, primary abdominal carcinomatosis (mesothelioma) is unusual. However, with secondary abdominal carcinomatosis, the peritoneal effusion is due to secretions from neoplastic glandular cells as well as from inflammatory effusions associated with irritated serosal surfaces.

History and Physical Examination. Patients with abdominal carcinomatosis usually have a history of chronic, progressive abdominal distention. The history can include weakness, debilitation, cachexia, and pallor. The owners may indicate that the animal responded satisfactorily to treatment initially but that a more progressive, uncontrollable problem followed. Diuretic therapy is usually of little or no benefit in controlling the ascitic fluid.

The most prominent feature of the physical examination is an enlarged abdomen. Debilitation may be present; ascites is usually apparent. Occasionally, it is possible to ballot or palpate a mass involving one of the major organs. In other cases, the history and physical examination reveal little except the presence of ascites. In all cases, radiographic examination of the abdomen and laboratory evaluation of the ascitic fluid are essential to confirm the clinical suspicion. Ultrasonography (see Table 28–1) may be helpful in the differential diagnosis of the etiology.

Radiographic Examination. Abdominal carcinomatosis is associated with areas of increased radiodensity within the abdomen and generalized ascites. The "ground-glass" appearance of the abdomen with concomitant loss of serosal surfaces confirms the presence of fluid in the abdominal cavity. Occasionally, specific masses may be recognized. Following removal of the abdominal fluid and the instillation of air into the abdominal cavity, the resultant pneumoperitoneum may demonstrate one or more neoplastic masses. The cranial ventral abdomen may appear nodular and patchy with irregular densities in a diffuse pattern throughout.

Laboratory Examination. In abdominal carcinomatosis, the ascitic fluid removed by paracentesis has a high specific gravity, a large quantity of protein, and a quantity of red blood cells. Occasionally, frank blood is present. Cytology demonstrating "signet ring" cells is presumed to be evidence of glandular, neoplastic cells. Anaplastic epithelial cells also suggest carcinoma. Some pathologists classify abdominal carcinomatosis as any generalized abdominal cavity malignancy. Cytologic examination of the fluid in such cases is likely to reveal malignant cell types other than glandular or epithelial.

Differential Diagnosis. Unless a definitive diagnosis of abdominal carcinomatosis is made by radiographic or cytologic examination before surgery, exploratory laparotomy may be required.

If one categorized abdominal carcinomatosis as a tumor of glandular or epithelial cells only, it would be necessary to consider such common malignancies as lymphosarcoma, metastatic splenic and hepatic hemangiosarcoma, and other tumors that metastasize to the abdomen in the differential diagnosis. If one uses a more liberal definition to indicate neoplastic disease involving the peritoneal cavity, then the diagnosis by cytology would be less difficult. Chronic fluid accumulation results in very reactive mesothelial lining cells, which should not be misinterpreted as carcinomatous.

In addition to other forms of malignancy, it is also necessary to exclude free fluid accumulation or generalized peritoneal adhesions that result from bowel perforation and peritonitis.

Feline infectious peritonitis (FIP) should be considered in the differential diagnosis in cats with proteinaceous ascites (see below). FIP generally does not result in a diffuse nodular pattern radiographically before or after the fluid has been removed.

FELINE INFECTIOUS PERITONITIS (FIP) WET FORM

Feline infectious peritonitis is a chronic debilitating disease in cats that is often associated with peritoneal and/or pleural cavity fluid accumulation. Nonperitoneal forms occur far more frequently than originally thought. Etiologically, it is due to infection by a member of the coronavirus family (see Chapter 48).

The disease affects cats of all ages, although it is most frequently seen in felines under five years of age. The disease is known to develop insidiously and become rampant in catteries.

Clinical Signs. The outstanding clinical feature of the "wet form" of the disease is peritoneal effusion. Other clinical features often seen are anorexia, depression, wasting, dehydration, persistent or recurrent fever, unresponsiveness to antibiotics, anemia, and nonspecific gastroenteritis, as well as dyspnea or jaundice. Nonperitoneal forms reported include ocular lesions (uveitis, iritis, hypopyon), CNS signs, pyogranulomatous renal disease, uremia, and pleural effusion among their clinical features.

Radiographic Examination. The "ground-glass" appearance of a fluid-filled abdomen is recognized with FIP when the peritoneal form occurs. Serosal surfaces are absent and specific organ recognition is not usually possible. Even after large quantities of the fluid are removed by centesis, it is difficult to recognize organ lines in the abdomen.

Pleural effusion with rounding of the costophrenic angles, disappearance of the borders of the cardiac silhouette, and pleural lines between the lung lobes may occur in conjunction with, or independent of, peritoneal effusions.

The radiographic features of this disease are not diagnostic. However, when such findings are evident, FIP should be included in the differential diagnosis.

Laboratory Examination. The effusion produced in this disease has a characteristic thick and tenacious appearance with a golden color. Strands of a white flocculent fibrin material may develop after the fluid is allowed to stand, and its appearance may be hastened by refrigerating the fluid. The fluid, which is abundant, has a specific gravity greater than 1.030 and contains large quantities of protein and few cells. Serum fibrinogen levels are elevated over 400 mg/dl in about half the cases and serum protein electrophoresis reveals a hyperglobulinemia. The peritoneal fluid, like the serum protein, usually has a polyclonal increase in the alpha-2, beta-2, and gamma-1 and gamma-2 globulin fractions.

The urine in patients with FIP is normal. White blood cell counts are often elevated with an absolute neutrophilia and lymphopenia. Terminal leukopenia may occur. A low normal to low hematocrit and red blood cell count is expected and a nonregenerative depression anemia is common. Simultaneous infection with *Hemobartonella felis* and the virus of feline leukemia may be present, and subclinical cases of FIP may be exacerbated by the leukovirus.

The recently introduced immunofluorescent antibody tests for recognition of the myeloproliferative diseases and leukemias are positive in many cats with FIP. The antibody titer rises during the active disease process.

Differential Diagnosis. The clinical course must be differentiated from the feline anemias, toxoplasmosis, chylothorax, exudative peritonitis, neoplastic processes, and cardiovascular or hepatic disease.

When fluid collection occurs, the diagnosis may be made presumptively based on its examination and the presence of increased gamma globulin serum protein levels.

OTHER CAUSES OF ABDOMINAL ENLARGEMENT

Hepatomegaly, Splenomegaly, and Renomegaly. The specific diseases associated with enlargement of the liver, spleen, and kidney are not discussed in this chapter. The reader is referred to the individual sections on those organs for a detailed review of the causes of enlargement. It is germane, however, to note that many patients presented for examination have a generalized abdominal enlargement alone, or in addition to other signs. Prior to performing abdominal paracentesis for fluid collection, the clinician should be aware that only organ enlargement may be present, and this may be evaluated by a thorough physical examination as well as radiographic and ultrasound examinations.

Patients with generalized abdominal enlargements may be presented for many complaints. One sign is respiratory distress, i.e., dyspnea, tachypnea, wheezing, or coughing (see Chapters 18 and 19). Hepatomegaly may produce increased cranial pressure on the diaphragm, thereby reducing ventilatory capacity and diminishing respiratory exchange. Patients presenting with respiratory distress syndromes and abdominal enlargement should be evaluated for pulmonary function as well as for abdominal disorders such as hepatomegaly.

Canine Cushing's Syndrome. In addition to the cutaneous manifestations of canine Cushing's syndrome and polydipsia and polyuria, cases with an advanced disease process develop marked muscle weakness. Marked abdominal muscle weakness with flaccidity may falsely lead the clinician to a tentative diagnosis of abdominal fluid collection. The abdominal distention may be confused with ascitic fluid collection or other peritoneal disease. The differential diagnostic features of Cushing's syndrome are discussed in Chapter 97.

29 POLYURIA AND POLYDIPSIA

CLARKE E. ATKINS

Polyuria, the production of a large volume of urine in a period of time, and polydipsia, or excessive thirst, are defined in the cat and dog as urine production of more than 25 ml/lb (50 ml/kg) body weight per day and water consumption of more than 50 ml/lb (100 ml/kg) body weight per day, respectively. Increased urine production and thirst may, however, exist in an individual animal whose urine output and water intake are within the normal range. Although not specific, once confirmed, these clinical signs are useful to the clinician, allowing for a specific diagnostic approach to a relatively limited number of differential diagnoses. For this reason, the clinical findings of polyuria and polydipsia (PU-PD) warrant specific consideration. Like fever, anemia, and hypoglycemia, the syndrome of PU-PD is a manifestation of disease and not a definitive diagnosis. Both polyuria and polydipsia can occur normally. While not hazardous in itself, polyuria may cause dehydration, hypotension, and cardiovascular collapse if urine output exceeds water intake. In a survey of final diagnoses from academic veterinary institutions, the relative frequency of PU-PD was 2.5 cases per 1000 canine accessions and one case per 1000 feline accessions (Figure 29–1). The incidence is, of course, much higher in diseased animals. The relative frequencies of disease processes associated with PU-PD for dogs and cats are displayed in Figures 29–2 and 29–3.

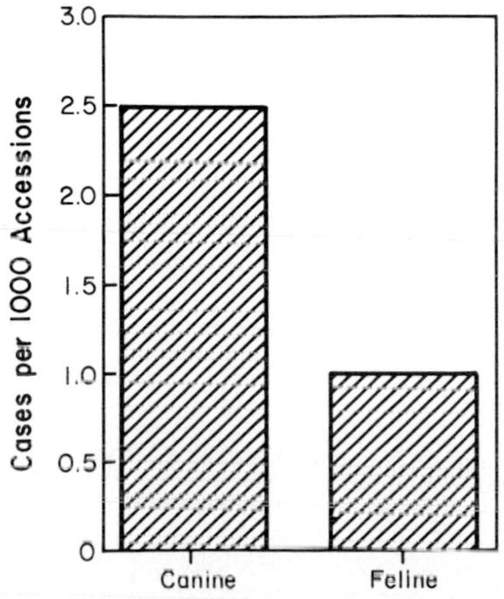

FIGURE 29–1. The relative frequency of PU PD expressed as number of cases per 1000 accessions in dogs and cats.

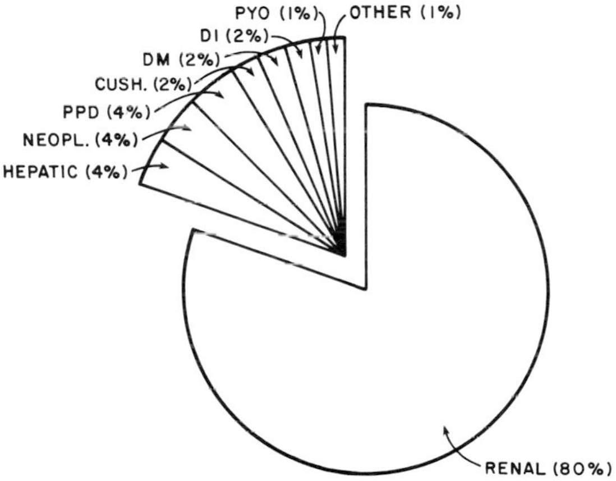

FIGURE 29–2. The relative frequency of diagnoses associated with PU-PD in 280 dogs. Most cases are associated with renal disease. It should be kept in mind that these data were the result of a retrospective survey and caution must be used in their interpretation. Diabetes insipidus, for example, does not occur with equal frequency with diabetes mellitus. This finding likely resulted from CDI and NDI being coded as diabetes insipidus and by the fact that data were derived from referral centers, meaning that an accurate cross-section of expected cases may not be seen in all instances. NEOPL. = polyuric syndromes associated with neoplastic processes and/or hypercalcemia; CUSH. = hyperadrenocorticism; DM = diabetes mellitus; DI = diabetes insipidus; PYO = pyometra. The category OTHER includes hyperthyroidism, hypoadrenocorticism, and renal glycosuria.

PATHOPHYSIOLOGY

Although polydipsia is more commonly recognized by owners than is polyuria, it is usually secondary to polyuric states. Excessive urine production occurs with renal tubular dysfunction, osmotic diuresis, and inadequate antidiuretic hormone concentration or action. When, for any reason, urinary and insensible water loss exceeds intake, compensatory increases in water intake and renal water retention occur. More specifically, changes in plasma osmolality stimulate osmoreceptors in the thirst center, located in the hypothalamus, anterior to the supraoptic nuclei. When the sodium concentration rises 2 mEq/liter or osmolality rises 4 mOsm/liter above normal, the thirst mechanism is triggered. In addition to increasing water intake, compensatory mechanisms reduce water lost as urine. Osmoreceptors in the

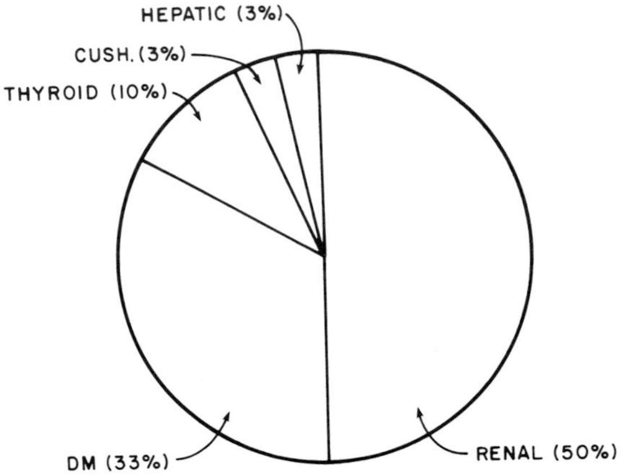

FIGURE 29–3. The relative frequency of diagnoses associated with PU-PD in 32 cats is depicted. Abbreviations are the same as those in Figure 29–1. THYROID = hyperthyroidism.

hypothalamic supraoptic nuclei are excited, stimulating the posterior pituitary gland to release antidiuretic hormone (ADH). Falling blood pressure and diminished cardiovascular volume, which are sensed by aortic, carotid, and pulmonary arterial baroreceptors and by atrial volume receptors, also trigger ADH release. Antidiuretic hormone acts on the terminal distal tubules and collecting ducts to increase passive water reabsorption without sodium, thus diminishing plasma osmolality and therefore, the stimulation of osmo- and baroreceptors. Although ADH is very important in maintaining normal plasma osmolality, its effect on blood volume is negligible. The vasoactive octapeptide, angiotensin II, produced when blood pressure falls and renin is released from the kidney, may be more important in increasing blood volume by decreasing salt and water excretion, stimulating aldosterone secretion, and producing thirst. Aldosterone has little effect on the maintenance of cardiovascular volume because its effect of reducing urine volume by enhancing sodium and water retention at the terminal distal tubules and collecting ducts is offset by the concomitant elevation in blood pressure and glomerular filtration rate. The role of atrial natriuretic factor in the maintenance of body water is undetermined.

The kidney is ultimately responsible for fluid and electrolyte homeostasis. To effect concentration of urine due to ADH release, one-third of the nephron mass of both kidneys must be functional and the medullary interstitium must be hypertonic. Water and solute are filtered through the glomerulus, which is freely permeable to molecules with weights of less than 5000. Molecules smaller than this are found in equal concentrations in glomerular filtrate and in plasma. Approximately one per cent of the filtrate is normally excreted as urine. Sixty per cent of transluminal volume is reabsorbed in the proximal tubule. Water passively follows sodium, potassium, glucose, amino acids, and phosphate, which are actively reabsorbed. In the loop of Henle, which is freely permeable to solute and water in the descending limb, urine becomes more hypertonic as it nears the medulla. Since the ascending limb is impermeable to water, while allowing active chloride transport, urine becomes hypotonic to plasma by the time it reaches the distal convoluted tubule. The selective permeability and active transport capabilities of the loop of Henle, coupled with the countercurrent exchange function of the vasa recta, maintain the interstitial concentration gradient from the cortex to the medulla. The final urine concentration is determined in the distal convoluted tubule and collecting ducts and depends on the state of hydration, renal function, and the mechanisms of plasma volume and osmolality control discussed previously.

The most important factor in the maintenance of body water and, therefore, cardiovascular volume is thirst. For this reason, the obligate, polyuric patient can become quickly and profoundly dehydrated if a source of water is not available.

Polydipsia may be the primary factor in PU-PD. Psychogenic polydipsia, in which excessive thirst increases total body and cardiovascular fluid volumes, results in secondary polyuria. The increase in blood volume and reduction in plasma osmolality reduce ADH release, while increased blood volume and pressure increase glomerular filtration rate. This results in an increased production of dilute urine. In primary polydipsia, the risk of patient dehydration is markedly less than in primary polyuria.

HISTORY

Polyuria and polydipsia occur together but, depending on the severity of PU-PD, the owner's observational powers, and the patient's habits, either or both may go unreported. In a study of historical findings in dogs with diabetes mellitus, excessive thirst was reported by owners in virtually all cases, while polyuria, the primary problem, was noted in only half of the cases. Information regarding the existence of PU-PD is often derived only with prompting from the clinician. This requires careful questioning, as most clients respond to the poorly phrased question "Does your pet drink a lot of water?" with an enthusiastic "yes." Taken literally, this answer could result in needless laboratory tests and expense. The veterinary historian should strive rather to establish whether *changes* in urinary and drinking habits have occurred. This requires careful distinction of polyuria from pollakiuria. Other historical findings, such as stranguria and/or hematuria, lead the clinician away from polyuria and toward pollakiuria, although the latter findings are not mutually exclusive. Polyuria is manifested most often in the dog by nocturia, inappropriate urination, increased need to be let out, or incontinence. In the cat, an excessively moist litter box is often noted. Polydipsia is evident in an ever-empty water bowl and by a pet's drinking from standing water, eating snow, drinking from toilets, or, in extreme cases, drinking urine. Other historical findings, such as current medications or supplements, presence of weight or appetite change, whether the female is intact, the duration of signs and relationship to estrus, or whether the pet is exhibiting gastrointestinal signs may give specific information as to the cause of PU-PD.

The signalment may be of use in determining the cause of PU-PD. For example, large dogs are more apt to suffer psychogenic polydipsia, while poodles are predisposed to diabetes mellitus, Doberman pinschers to hepatic disease, Lhasa apsos and Shih Tzus to congenital renal disease, and of course, intact females to pyometra. Young pets are more apt to have congenital kidney disease and portosystemic shunts, while older animals are more likely to suffer from diabetes mellitus, acquired renal failure, hyperthyroidism, and PU-PD associated with neoplastic processes. Cats exhibiting PU-PD probably have renal disease, diabetes mellitus, or hyperthyroidism (Figure 29–3). Physical findings such as painful, large, or small kidneys (renal disease), hepatomegaly and/or ascites (liver disease), emaciation and cataracts (diabetes mellitus), the presence of endocrine alopecia, comedones, and diminished abdominal musculature (hyperadrenocorticism), a thyroid mass (thyroid neoplasia), lymphadenopathy (lymphosarcoma), and bradycardia and/or shock (hypoadrenocorticism), also provide useful adjunctive information.

ETIOLOGY

The recognized list of causes of PU-PD in dogs and cats is relatively short (Table 29–1). A definitive diagnosis, therapeutic plan, and accurate prognosis is possible in most cases. The following discussion of PU-PD emphasizes the diagnostic effort and is ordered in approximate frequency of diagnosis. Information provided refers to the dog unless otherwise stated. More information on diagnosis, therapy, and prognosis can be obtained in specific sections of this text.

Renal Tubular Disease. Renal tubular disease (see Chapters 107 and 108), a syndrome with multiple etiologies, is the underlying cause in the majority of cases of PU-PD (Figure 29–2). Nephron loss results in diminished ability of the organism to adapt to various changes in fluid, electrolyte, and acid/base status. Renal compensatory mechanisms include anatomic and functional adaptations of glomeruli and tubules that are effective until the glomerular filtration rate is diminished by 75 per cent. At that point, retention of solutes (urea, creatinine, and phosphorus) occurs and signs of uremia may develop. Failure to adequately concentrate and dilute urine occurs at an earlier stage of renal dysfunction and patients may therefore present with no signs other than PU-PD and the inability to appropriately alter urine concentration. Polyuria in chronic renal failure results from solute diuresis, as remaining nephrons are called upon to handle a greater amount of solute and water. Other mechanisms, including alterations in medullary hypertonicity, altered intrarenal blood flow, and reduced responsiveness of the renal collecting ducts may also play as yet undefined roles. Polydipsia occurs secondarily. Diverse etiologies for renal tubular disease and failure include congenital defects, toxins, neoplastic processes, and infectious agents. Tubular disease may also occur secondarily to obstructive processes and immune-mediated and degenerative glomerular disease. The classical presentation for such a patient includes historical and physical signs of inappetence, dehydration, and vomition, accompanied by azotemia and isosthenuria. A definitive diagnosis can generally be made from renal biopsy. In pre-azotemic renal disease, the diagnostic challenge is greater but the diagnosis may be made by means of a water deprivation test, measuring creatinine clearance and/or serum phenolsulfonphthalein (PSP) clearance, or by renal biopsy.

TABLE 29–1. DIFFERENTIAL DIAGNOSES FOR POLYURIA AND POLYDIPSIA

Renal tubular disease or failure
Hyperadrenocorticism
Psychogenic polydipsia
Liver disease
Diabetes mellitus
Central diabetes insipidus
Hypercalcemia
Pyometra
Hypoadrenocorticism
Hyperthyroidism
Primary renal glycosuria/Fanconi syndrome
Nephrogenic diabetes insipidus
Hypokalemia
Iatrogenic (drug-induced)
diuretics
corticosteroids
methoxyflurane
lithium
sodium bicarbonate
fluid therapy
amphotericin B
thyroid hormones
Pheochromocytoma

Acute renal failure is usually thought of as being associated with oliguria and anuria. This is not, however, always the case. Acute renal failure is associated with azotemia, metabolic acidosis, hyperphosphatemia, hyperkalemia, and urine inadequately concentrated in the presence of azotemia and for the degree of dehydration. Clinical signs are those of uremia as described previously. Profound solute diuresis may occur during the recovery phase of acute renal failure.

After the relief of urinary obstructive syndromes, a severe solute and water diuresis may occur and, if untreated, can result in extreme dehydration. On rare occasions, this diuresis is protracted and is thought to be due to renal tubular defects with or without ADH unresponsiveness.

Hyperadrenocorticism. A common cause of PU-PD is hyperadrenocorticism (Cushing's syndrome, see Chapter 97). Polyuria and polydipsia are recognized in over 80 per cent of cases. Hypercortisolemia results from cortisol overproduction by neoplastic or hyperplastic adrenal cortices. The majority of cases are secondary to adrenocorticotropic hormone-producing (ACTH) pituitary adenomas resulting in bilateral adrenal hyperplasia. From 15 to 20 per cent of cases are due to benign or malignant adrenal gland neoplasia. Hyperadrenocorticism is a disorder of middle-aged and aged dogs and is only rarely recognized in the cat. Other signs of hyperadrenocorticism include polyphagia, lethargy, a pendulous abdomen, endocrine alopecia with comedones and calcinosis cutis, hepatomegaly, and muscle weakness.

Features of the minimum data base that suggest hyperadrenocorticism include eosinopenia, mature leucocytosis, erythrocytosis, lymphopenia, increased serum alkaline phosphatase (SAP), increased serum alanine aminotransferase (ALT), hyperglycemia, and hypophosphatemia. Hypercholesterolemia is observed in approximately 50 per cent of cases. The exact cause of polyuria is unclear but likely involves interference with the action of ADH on the renal collecting ducts. Urine analysis frequently reveals evidence of infection and urine specific gravity is usually less than 1.025 but ranges from less than 1.005 to more than 1.030. A modified water deprivation test has been used to distinguish hyperadrenocorticism with hyposthenuria from psychogenic polydipsia (PPD), central diabetes insipidus (CDI), and nephrogenic diabetes insipidus (NDI).

Ancillary tests are necessary to confirm clinical suspicions of hyperadrenocorticism. The ACTH stimulation and low-dose dexamethasone suppression tests are used to confirm the diagnosis, while the high-dose dexamethasone suppression test is used to differentiate adrenal hyperplasia from neoplasia.

Psychogenic Polydipsia. The majority of dogs diagnosed as having this syndrome are of large breeds (more than 30 kg), and the German shepherd may be predisposed (see Chapter 93). The owner's complaint is usually extreme PU-PD. Frequently, an inciting cause for PPD can be elicited with careful questioning of the owner. Physical examination is usually unremarkable, although affected dogs may be excessively nervous. Quantitation of water intake and urine production reveals a four- to six-fold increase over normal. Urine specific gravity ranges from 1.001 to 1.003, with low urine osmolality (approximately 100). Serum osmolality is in the low normal range (285 to 295 mOsm/kg) and serum sodium concentrations range from subnormal to normal. The ratio of urine to plasma osmolality (U:P osmolality) is less than one. Compulsive drinking in dogs is diagnosed by exclusion of other causes of PU-PD and by demonstrating that the dog can concentrate its urine after water deprivation. In some dogs, hospitalization alone may markedly reduce water consumption, presumably by diminishing or altering causal psychological stresses. The diagnosis can be confirmed with the water deprivation test in approximately two thirds of cases. In the remaining cases, renal medullary washout prevents urine concentration, making it necessary to perform the hypertonic saline infusion test (Hickey-Hare test). Alternatively, renal medullary hypertonicity can be reestablished by the gradual restriction of water consumption and by providing supplementary salt and a high protein diet. The water deprivation test is then repeated.

Liver Disease. As is evident from Figure 29–2, PU-PD is often associated with hepatic disease due to inflammatory, degenerative, neoplastic, or vascular causes (see Chapter 89). The exact mechanism of this sign is unknown but may involve hypokalemia, loss of medullary hypertonicity secondary to altered renal blood flow, and/or PPD. Although in most instances other signs of liver disease (anorexia, lethargy, vomiting, diarrhea, jaundice, ascites, alteration in liver size, CNS dysfunction) are evident, the primary complaint may be that of PU-PD. Laboratory abnormalities may include liver enzyme elevation (SAP and ALT), low blood urea nitrogen (BUN), hypoglycemia, hypoalbuminemia and hyperglobulinemia, increased serum and urine bilirubin, and hyposthenuria. Ancillary diagnostic tests that may be useful in diagnosing the exact etiology, extent, and prognosis of liver disease include serum bromsulphalein (BSP) retention, ammonia tolerance test, fasting and postprandial bile acid determination, portal angiography, and biopsy.

Diabetes Mellitus. Diabetes mellitus has multiple etiologies in the dog (see Chapter 96). The most commonly recognized cause is chronic, relapsing pancreatitis, but congenital islet aplasia or hypoplasia, insulin-resistant states (hyperadrenocorticism and growth hormone excess during the luteal phase of the estrous cycle), neoplasia, and toxins are also associated with diabetes in the dog. In the cat, the cause or causes are even less well defined. Feline diabetes has been associated with megestrol acetate administration and amyloidosis of the pancreatic islets. The clinically diabetic dog and cat are invariably polyuric and secondarily polydipsic, although this is not always recognized. For glucosuria to be responsible for sustained solute diuresis (by overwhelming the ability of the proximal tubule to reabsorb filtered glucose), urine sugar should register 3 to 4+ by semiquantitative measurement, and must comprise a minimum of 50 per cent of the urinary osmoles. The degree of PU-PD associated with diabetes is determined by the degree and persistence of glycosuria, which is determined, in part, by the degree and persistence of hyperglycemia, by renal function, and by the renal threshold for glucose. The renal threshold for glucose varies with species, individuals, and with time in the same individual. The thresholds reported for normal dogs and cats are 175 to 220 and 270 to 310 mg/dl, respectively. The urine specific gravity in diabetic dogs ranges from 1.007 to 1.068 with a mean value of 1.034. The effect of glycosuria on urine specific gravity is nominal; 4+ glycosuria (2.5 mg/dl) produces an increase in urine specific gravity of only 0.010.

The diagnosis of polyuric diabetes mellitus is not problematic and can usually be made from information derived from the minimum data base. Consistent fasting hyperglycemia of more than 150 mg/100 ml with the appropriate signs is diagnostic in the dog. Usually the blood glucose concentration is much higher than this and is accompanied by glycosuria and, in some cases, ketonuria. Physical findings may include weight loss or obesity, cataracts, dehydration, hepatomegaly, and ketotic breath.

Even though the incidence of diabetes in the cat is less than that of the dog, it is the second most common disorder producing PU-PD in the cat. Presenting signs may include polydipsia, polyuria, obesity or weight loss, anorexia or polyphagia, and icterus. The cat frequently suffers from an underlying disease process that exacerbates and/or confuses the signs of diabetes mellitus. The diagnosis of diabetes in cats is complicated by the potential for stress-induced hyperglycemia, which is observed in ill or stressed cats. If hyperglycemia persists after the cat has been rested, if clinical signs are appropriate, or if hyperglycemia is accompanied by ketosis, the diagnosis of diabetes mellitus can be assumed.

Central Diabetes Insipidus. CDI is due to an absolute or relative deficiency in ADH activity (see Chapter 93). Supraoptic and paraventricular nuclear or pituitary gland dysfunction may be idiopathic or secondary to

CNS trauma, infection, parasitic migration, neoplasia, or diminished blood flow. The ADH deficiency results in profound polyuria (three to ten times normal) and compensatory polydipsia. Complete CDI is characterized by hyposthenuria (1.001 to 1.005 with osmolality ranging from 50 to 200 mOsm/kg). In CDI, unlike PPD, plasma osmolality tends to be normal or slightly increased. The U:P osmolality is less than one. Other clinical signs are usually minimal unless dehydration has occurred due to water restriction. In some instances, neurological signs related to underlying CNS disease may be apparent. The diagnosis of CDI is made using the water deprivation test, followed by vasopressin administration. With water deprivation there is no increase in urine specific gravity or osmolality, while plasma osmolality increases. With vasopressin administration, urine concentration increases from 50 to 500 per cent and urine production falls. When medullary washout exists, the response to ADH may be suboptimal. Medullary washout can be corrected as described under PPD or by repeated administration of repositol ADH. Further confusing the issue is the potential for only partial destruction or dysfunction of the hypothalamic-neurohypophyseal axis. This results in suboptimal ADH concentrations with the ability to concentrate urine to more than 1.010 (urine osmolality of 300 to 1000) with the U:P osmolality greater than one.

Nephrogenic Diabetes Insipidus. Another syndrome characterized by extreme polyuria, secondary polydipsia, and hyposthenuria is NDI. This syndrome results from a failure of the kidney to concentrate urine despite appropriate ADH release. This may be congenital or acquired. Acquired (or partial) NDI has been classified as metabolic (hyperadrenocorticism, hypercalcemia, and hypokalemia), due to intrinsic renal disease (pyelonephritis, *E. coli* endotoxin inhibition of ADH activity, amyloidosis, polycystic kidney disease), and drug-induced (corticosteroids, lithium, vinblastine). While acquired NDI is relatively common, congenital NDI is rare. Clinical signs may be those of the underlying disease, stunted growth in congenital disease, dehydration, or vomiting due to gastric overdistention. The diagnosis is made using the modified water deprivation test. Initial urine specific gravity ranges from 1.001 to 1.007 (U:P osmolality less than one) and urine is neither concentrated with water deprivation nor with vasopressin administration in congenital cases. Acquired cases vary in severity and, with water deprivation, urine concentration may increase, with U:P osmolality reaching as high as 2.5. There is no further increase after ADH administration.

Hypercalcemia. Hypercalcemia may result from paraneoplastic disease (most frequently associated with lymphosarcoma, an anal sac adenocarcinoma), hypervitaminosis D, osteolytic disease, hyperparathyroidism, hypoadrenocorticism, and, uncommonly, from acute and chronic renal failure. The polyuric state is actually a form of NDI due to calcium-induced collection duct insensitivity to ADH with resultant hyposthenuria. Eventually calcium precipitation and calcium's direct toxic effect on tubular cells result in renal failure with attendant azotemia and isosthenuria. Polydipsia is secondary. Clinical signs may include anorexia, behavioral change, gastrointestinal signs, dehydration, weakness, and cardiac arrhythmias. The diagnosis is made by finding persistent, significant hypercalcemia (greater than 12 mg/dl). Ancillary tests that prove useful in elucidating the underlying cause of the hypercalcemia include careful examination of the rectum, thyroid and parathyroid glands (usually unrewarding), and lymph nodes; thoracic, abdominal, and skeletal radiographs; serum parathyroid hormone assay; and tumor biopsy.

Pyometra. Another form of NDI frequently accompanies pyometra (see Chapter 98). The mechanism of this reversible polyuria is thought to be the inhibition of ADH activity by renal deposition of *E. coli* endotoxins. Secondary polydipsia is noted by owners in 63 per cent of cases, while polyuria is noted in 39 per cent, reflecting the relative insensitivity of polyuria as a historical finding. Anorexia, depression, and gastrointestinal signs are also noted. The diagnosis of pyometra is usually not difficult. Physical findings of uterine enlargement and possibly vaginal discharge in an older bitch (usually more than six years) within two to three months post-estrus, are strongly suggestive. Laboratory abnormalities evident from the minimum data base may include leukocytosis, left shift, monocytosis, elevations in total protein, nonresponsive anemia, azotemia (in less than 20 per cent of cases), and proteinuria with an inactive urine sediment (30 per cent of cases). The latter two findings suggest that organic renal disease accompanies pyometra in some cases. Urine concentration varies with the degree of renal disease, renal ADH unresponsiveness, and the state of hydration. Urine specific gravity was less than 1.007 in 20 per cent, 1.008 to 1.024 in 52 per cent, and greater than 1.024 in 27 per cent of cases studied. Abdominal radiography, vaginal cytology, and bacterial culture of uterine contents provide additional diagnostic and therapeutic information.

Hypoadrenocorticism. Hypoadrenocorticism (Addison's disease) is a syndrome of diminished adrenal production of glucocorticoid and mineralocorticoid hormones (see Chapter 97). Adrenocortical destruction may be immune-mediated, iatrogenic (OP'DDD), or due to inflammatory processes, neoplasia, or infarction. In most cases, the etiology remains unknown. Young to middle-aged females are most frequently affected. The paucity of adrenal cortical hormones may result in hyponatremia, hyperkalemia, lymphocytosis, eosinophilia, pre-renal azotemia, muscular weakness, metabolic acidosis, gastrointestinal signs, dehydration, bradycardia, and shock. Although not usually the primary complaint, polyuria is associated with 20 per cent to 40 per cent of cases of hypoadrenocorticism. Urine specific gravity may range from 1.006 to 1.056 (with a mean value of approximately 1.020). The pathogenesis of polyuria is unclear, but may involve renal sodium loss and medullary washout. In addition, hypercalcemia (usually mild, but it may reach more than 15 mg/dl) is present in approximately 20 per cent of cases and may contribute to PU-PD. The cause of this latter biochemical aberration is likely increased renal tubular reabsorption of calcium. The correct diagnosis of hypoadrenocorticism is imperative because without appropriate therapeutic intervention, death may ensue. Once correctly diagnosed, this disease is readily treatable. Because of the presence of azotemia and potential for isosthenuria, primary renal failure may be inappropriately diagnosed in these patients. Hypoadrenocorticism is suspected when suggestive clinical signs and laboratory abnormalities are noted. The diagnosis is confirmed with an ACTH stimulation test.

Hyperthyroidism. As can be seen from Figures 29–2 and 29–3, hyperthyroidism is relatively more important in the cat than the dog (see Chapter 95). Hyperthyroidism is characterized by the presence of thyroid mass in an aged animal displaying PU-PD, polyphagia, tachycardia, vomition, weight loss, soft, voluminous stools, and hyperactivity. The mechanism for PU-PD is unclear, but may involve medullary washout and/or thyrotoxic PPD. In the dog, thyroid tumors are unilateral, uncommonly functional (fewer than 25 per cent) and are usually malignant, while in the cat, bilateral, functional adenomas prevail. In many cases, a thyroid mass is palpable in the ventral cervical region. Heart murmurs are frequently audible in hyperthyroid cats. Although mild to moderate elevations in serum liver enzyme concentrations, mature leucocytosis, and erythrocytosis are observed in cats, the minimum data base reveals little specific diagnostic information. Such ancillary tests as T3 and T4 assay, excisional biopsy, and nuclear imaging may provide both diagnostic and prognostic information. In cats, cardiac disease and failure have been observed secondary to hyperthyroidism. Thoracic radiography, electrocardiography, and echocardiography are useful in determining the degree of cardiac involvement.

Renal Glycosuria. Two disorders of the renal tubules, resulting in glycosuria and PU-PD, are recognized in the dog (see Chapter 108). Renal glycosuria has been recognized in Norwegian elkhounds, Scottish terriers, and mixed breeds. The primary tubular defect, thought to be hereditary in Norwegian elkhounds, prevents normal reabsorption of filtered glucose. Persistent glycosuria, evident in a dilute urine, produces polyuria and secondary polydipsia. A second syndrome, similar to Fanconi syndrome in humans, has been described in basenjis, Norwegian elkhounds, Shetland sheepdogs, and schnauzers. The onset of signs occurs between one and six years of age with glycosuria and moderate weight loss being noted in addition to PU-PD. The primary defect in renal tubular transport of glucose, phosphate, potassium, uric acid, amino acids, sodium, and bicarbonate results in osmotic diuresis. The serum chemical profiles are most often normal, although 50 per cent of the affected dogs die in acute renal failure within 90 days of diagnosis. Urine specific gravity ranges from 1.005 to more than 1.035. The diagnosis is made by the presence of clinical signs, persistent glycosuria without hyperglycemia, and aminoaciduria (demonstrated with paper chromatography).

Miscellaneous Causes. Hypokalemia can result from polyuric renal failure, anorexia, vomiting, diarrhea, potassium-deficient fluid therapy, diuretic therapy, diabetic ketoacidosis, and metabolic alkalosis. Polyuria with hypokalemia has been associated with adrenal adenocarcinomas in dogs and cats and is suspected to be caused by hyperaldosteronism. Clinical signs include muscular weakness, intestinal ileus, and electrocardiographic abnormalities. In some species, by reducing medullary solute concentration, hypokalemia may render the terminal portion of the nephron less responsive to ADH, producing NDI. The importance of this cause of polyuria in the dog has been questioned.

Iatrogenic (drug-induced) causes of polyuria and polydipsia are frequent but usually present little diagnostic challenge. Most difficulties in this regard come in determining the effects of various drugs on laboratory results obtained while the patient is on medications that can alter thirst or urine-concentrating ability. For this reason, blood and urine samples should be obtained prior to the onset of therapy. This is especially true with fluid, diuretic, and corticosteroid therapies. Drugs known to produce PU-PD are listed in Table 29–1.

Pheochromocytoma, a rare tumor of the adrenal medulla, is associated with PU-PD. Excessive catecholamine concentrations, either constant or intermittent, produce hypertension, restlessness, epistaxis, retinopathy, panting or dyspnea, cardiac arrhythmias, weakness, collapse, and diarrhea. Functional or nonfunctional tumors may produce signs of ascites or rear leg swelling if the posterior vena cava is involved. Pheochromocytoma is suspected when clinical signs are suggestive, especially if accompanied by proven hypertension. Neutrophilia, hematuria, and proteinuria may be present in some cases. The diagnosis can be made by measuring urine catecholamine concentrations, by vena caval venography, and by provocative or suppression tests while observing changes in blood pressure.

DIAGNOSTIC APPROACH

Although useful in determining the cause of PU-PD, the history and physical examination are usually inadequate to allow definitive diagnosis. Laboratory tests are used to further a diagnosis. A minimum data base is obtained (Table 29–2). From this, either a diagnosis is made or further tests are indicated. Certain ancillary tests that may be of use in formulating a diagnosis in PU-PD are listed in Table 29–3. It is emphasized that not all tests are required in a given patient. To provide the safest and most cost-effective diagnostic approach, care must be taken to choose only the appropriate ancillary procedures. To this end, Figure 29–4 outlines a diagnostic approach to the patient with PU-PD. Prior to specific laboratory testing, the presence of PU-PD

TABLE 29–2. MINIMUM DATA BASE FOR PATIENTS WITH POLYURIA AND POLYDIPSIA*

Urine analysis
Complete blood count
Blood glucose concentration
Serum alanine aminotransferase
Serum alkaline phosphatase
Serum potassium
Serum sodium
Serum calcium
Serum phosphorus
Serum urea nitrogen
Serum creatinine

*This minimum data base is in addition to a complete history and physical examination, as well as confirmation of polyuria and polydipsia.

TABLE 29–3. ANCILLARY LABORATORY TESTS FOR EVALUATION OF PATIENTS WITH POLYURIA AND POLYDIPSIA

1. Plasma and urine osmolality
2. Water deprivation test
   a. Vasopressin response test
3. Gradual water restriction/NaCl supplementation
4. Hickey-Hare test (hypertonic saline infusion test)
5. BSP retention
6. Blood ammonia/Ammonia tolerance test
7. Portal angiography
8. Serum PSP retention
9. Creatinine clearance
10. Urine chromatographic amino acid analysis
11. Serum cortisol concentration
    a. ACTH stimulation
    b. Dexamethasone suppression
12. Serum T3 and T4
13. Radiography
    a. Thoracic
    b. Abdominal
    c. Skeletal
14. Cytology of cervix/culture
15. Biopsy
16. Blood pressure measurement
    a. Provocative tests
17. Posterior caval venography
18. Urine catecholamine assay
19. Parathyroid hormone assay
20. Aldosterone assay

should be confirmed and, preferably, quantified. Certain pet owners may be able to supply reliable information as to water consumption. In most instances where PU-PD is the primary complaint and other disease processes are not evident, it is preferable to measure water intake and, if possible, urine production. This is generally accomplished in the clinic, using a metabolism cage, with simultaneous measurement of water intake and urine output over a 24-hour period. Such quantitation may provide specific diagnostic information in addition to confirming (or denying) the owner's complaint. Extreme PU-PD is most often associated with CDI, NDI, or PPD. Also, the nonazotemic dog, which is known to be polydipsic at home and not polydipsic in the clinic, is most likely to be diagnosed as psychogenically polydipsic.

Minimum Data Base. The *urinalysis*, while usually not rendering a definitive diagnosis, is the first and single most valuable test in the evaluation of polyuria and polydipsia. It is also useful in "confirming" the presence of polyuria in equivocal cases. Finding a urine specific gravity of more than 1.030 argues against the likelihood of polyuria, while a consistently isosthenuric or hyposthenuric urine suggests it. It must be emphasized that concentrated urine can be observed in polyuric states and unconcentrated urine can be observed in normal animals on occasion. Hyposthenuria of less than 1.005 allows a tentative diagnosis of CDI, NDI, or PPD, while glycosuria suggests diabetes or renal glycosuria, and urine with a specific gravity of more than 1.030 in proven PU-PD suggests hypoadrenocorticism, diabetes mellitus, or renal glycosuria. It is now apparent that neither are all dogs with renal tubular impairment isosthenuric, nor does a urine specific gravity of 1.025 ensure that adequate renal tubular function exists. A urine specific gravity of at least 1.030 in dogs and 1.035 in cats is considered necessary to eliminate the possibility of clinically significant renal tubular dysfunction. This same degree of concentration must be obtained by the kidneys of azotemic and/or dehydrated animals before prerenal azotemia with normal tubular function can be diagnosed. Urine for analysis should be obtained prior to initiation of fluid or other therapy to avoid alteration of the results.

The *hemogram* and *serum chemistry and electrolyte determinations* provide useful information in the diagnosis of PU-PD syndromes. Details are found in sections on specific diseases and in Figure 29–4. Serum electrolyte concentrations can be used to estimate serum osmolality by the formula:

$$\text{mOsm} = 1.86(\text{Na} + \text{K}) + \text{Glucose}/18 + \text{BUN}/2.8 + 9.$$

In certain instances laboratory data may be normal or otherwise noncontributory. Nonazotemic renal failure, PPD, CDI, and NDI, hyperthyroidism, and pheochromocytoma are disorders in which the lack of specific findings makes the diagnostic challenge greater, requiring careful appraisal of physical and historical findings and the use of ancillary laboratory tests (Table 29–3).

Ancillary Tests. An increase in plasma osmolality of two to five per cent stimulates osmoreceptors and promotes ADH release, resulting in the production of smaller volumes of more concentrated urine. If endogenous ADH is not produced or if the kidney cannot respond, no change in urine concentration or production results. In ADH deficiency, exogenous ADH administration usually results in the concentration of urine.

Provocative testing, using *water deprivation* and *vasopressin administration*, evaluates the patient's ability to produce and respond to ADH, allowing the diagnosis and differentiation of PPD, CDI, NDI, and nonazotemic renal failure. Water deprivation should not be performed in dehydrated or azotemic patients nor prior to obtaining a minimum data base and body weight. Prolonged water deprivation in dogs suffering extreme polyuria may be dangerous. The total testing period lasts from less than 4 to over 24 hours. The following description of the water deprivation test is modified only slightly from the method of Hardy and Osborne. The dog is deprived of water but may be allowed dry food. Body weight, urine specific gravity, skin turgor, PCV, total protein, and BUN are determined at two- to four-hour intervals. To ensure accurate assessment of urine concentrating ability, the bladder is evacuated approximately one hour prior to sampling. The test is terminated when the urine is concentrated to more than 1.025, weight loss of over five per cent is noted, azotemia develops, or clinical dehydration is apparent from examination of skin turgor and/or PCV and total protein.

Urine is concentrated to more than 1.030 in PPD without medullary washout. If the test is terminated and urine has not been concentrated, exogenous ADH (aqueous vasopressin) at five milliunits per pound body weight is administered intravenously in five per cent dextrose in water (5 units/liter, administered at 1 ml per pound over a 60-minute period). Water restriction continues and urine samples are obtained 30, 60, and 90 minutes after the onset of ADH administration. An

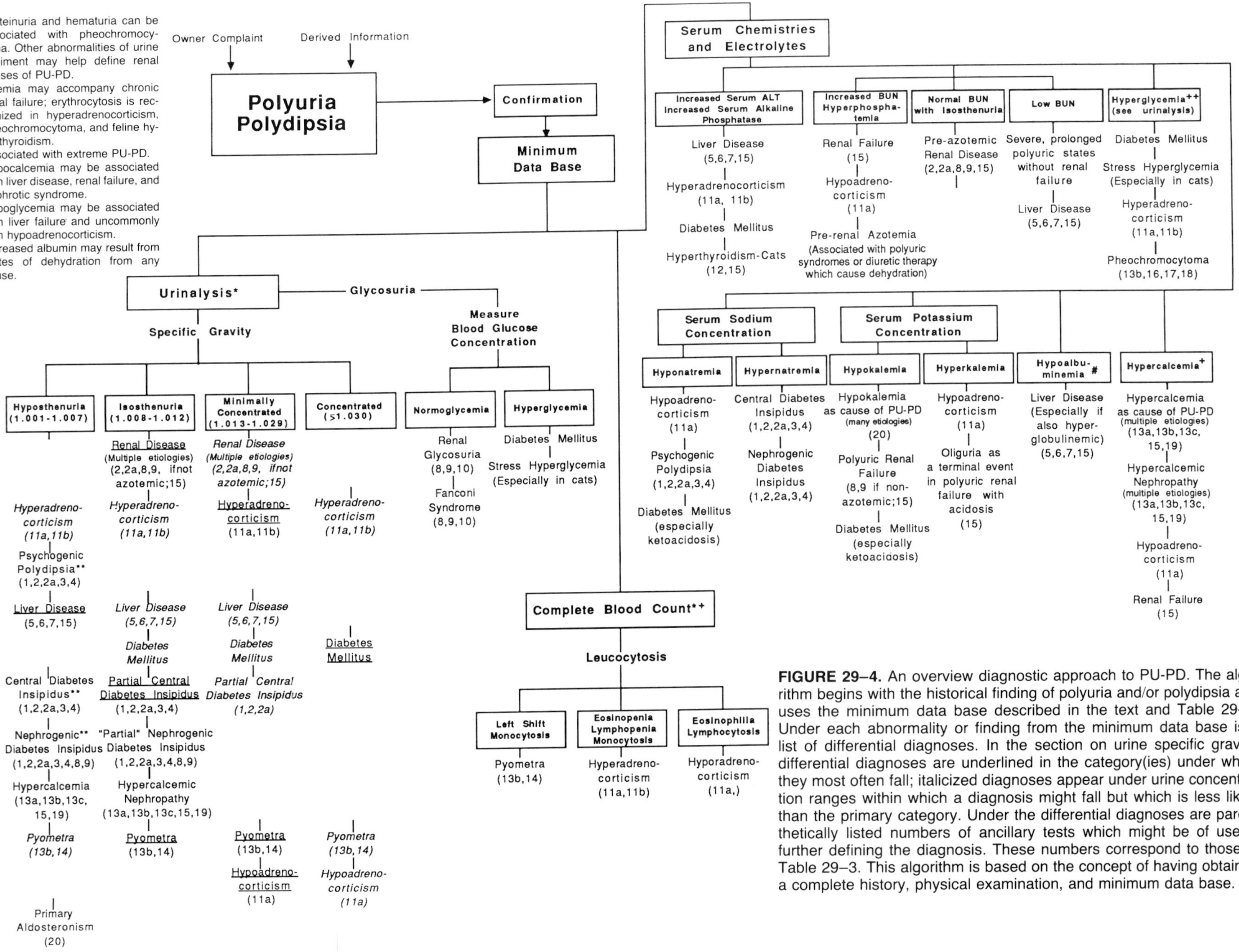

* Proteinuria and hematuria can be associated with pheochromocytoma. Other abnormalities of urine sediment may help define renal causes of PU-PD.

*+ Anemia may accompany chronic renal failure; erythrocytosis is recognized in hyperadrenocorticism, pheochromocytoma, and feline hyperthyroidism.

** Associated with extreme PU-PD.

\+ Hypocalcemia may be associated with liver disease, renal failure, and nephrotic syndrome.

\++ Hypoglycemia may be associated with liver failure and uncommonly with hypoadrenocorticism.

\# Increased albumin may result from states of dehydration from any cause.

FIGURE 29–4. An overview diagnostic approach to PU-PD. The algorithm begins with the historical finding of polyuria and/or polydipsia and uses the minimum data base described in the text and Table 29–2. Under each abnormality or finding from the minimum data base is a list of differential diagnoses. In the section on urine specific gravity, differential diagnoses are underlined in the category(ies) under which they most often fall; italicized diagnoses appear under urine concentration ranges within which a diagnosis might fall but which is less likely than the primary category. Under the differential diagnoses are parenthetically listed numbers of ancillary tests which might be of use in further defining the diagnosis. These numbers correspond to those of Table 29–3. This algorithm is based on the concept of having obtained a complete history, physical examination, and minimum data base.

increase in urine specific gravity to as little as 1.012 in previously hyposthenuric patients suggests complete or partial CDI. Dogs with isosthenuria or minimally concentrated urine usually have generalized renal disease and hyposthenuric dogs with no response either have NDI or medullary washout secondary to the prolonged PU-PD of CDI or PPD.

Medullary washout, the depletion of renal medullary hypertonicity resulting in the inability of the kidneys to concentrate maximally, must be differentiated from NDI. The hypertonic saline infusion test may be performed to make this distinction. Dogs with medullary washout respond by decreasing urine formation, while those with CDI or NDI show no decrease in urine production. The hypertonic saline infusion test is cumbersome and the following alternative approach may be taken. Gradual water deprivation of five to ten per cent per day of the previously measured, unrestricted, daily intake is made while supplementing with salt and protein to allow reconstruction of the medullary solute gradient with sodium and urea. Total water provided should be divided throughout the day and should never total less than 20 ml/lb/day (40 ml/kg/day). Dogs should be carefully weighed twice daily to allow detection of impending dehydration. Patients with CDI and NDI are not able to reduce their urine formation and quickly dehydrate. Dogs with CDI do, however, respond to ADH administration after gradual water deprivation, while dogs with PPD gradually increase urine concentration (to greater than 1.030) and reduce urine formation over a period of several days. Dogs with NDI can do neither.

A modification of this test has been described in which the osmolality of serum and urine are determined prior to water deprivation. Urine and plasma osmolalities are determined at one- to two-hour intervals until the urine osmolality between two testing periods has increased no more than five to ten per cent, more than five per cent of body weight is lost, plasma osmolality increases to over 350 mOsm/kg, or serum sodium concentration exceeds 165 mEq/liter. At that point, aqueous vasopressin (100 mU/kg) is administered subcutaneously and sampling is continued for two additional hours. In normal, water-deprived dogs, the urine osmolality exceeds 1000 mOsm/kg and the U:P osmolality exceeds four. In CDI and severe NDI, the plasma osmolality rises but urine osmolality does not, leaving the U:P osmolality less than one. Partial CDI is characterized by U:P osmolality greater than one but submaximal urine concentration. Partial NDI varies greatly with U:P osmolality reaching as high as 2.5. The post-ADH response with severe NDI is characterized by U:P osmolality of less than one, while with partial NDI and PPD, there is no further increase in urine osmolality. This test allows definitive diagnosis in most cases but does not allow differentiation of partial CDI from partial NDI in the form of hyperadrenocorticism.

Intramuscular repositol ADH (three to five units) can be used as an alternative to the aqueous vasopressin test. The peak response occurs at 9 to 12 hours after administration and urine should be sampled at those times. The patient may be released and the owner instructed to observe thirst and urine volume. A marked decrease in urine production and thirst suggests CDI, while continued PU-PD suggests NDI or medullary washout.

The measurement of *plasma and urine osmolality* is more useful than the measurement of urine specific gravity because the latter is affected by not only the number of solute particles, but the type of solute as well. It is evident that measurement of plasma and urine osmolality increases the safety of, and information obtained from, the water deprivation and vasopressin challenge tests discussed above. The finding of a resting U:P osmolality of more than 3:1 indicates normal renal concentrating ability, U:P osmolality equal to 1:1 indicates defective renal function, and U:P osmolality of less than one suggests CDI, NDI, or water loading (usually PPD).

The usefulness of other tests in the diagnosis of PU-PD, such as biopsies, radiographic procedures, blood pressure measurement, and less commonly used laboratory tests (Table 29–3) is put forth in Figure 29–4. A more complete description is found in the appropriate section on individual diseases that present with PU-PD.

30 INCONTINENCE, ENURESIS, AND NOCTURIA

PHILIPPE M. MOREAU and GEORGE E. LEES

Micturition is the entire physiologic process that accomplishes normal storage of urine in the urinary bladder and complete voiding of urine on appropriate occasions. *Urination* is the normal act of emptying the bladder by discharging urine through the urethra. Normal voiding of urine is produced by smooth muscle activity that is controlled by the autonomic nervous system. However, urination is ordinarily a conscious act and largely under voluntary control. *Urinary incontinence* refers to lack of voluntary control over the flow of urine from the body and is a problem that often occurs in animals with disorders of micturition. *Enuresis* is a term that may be used to refer to urinary incontinence that occurs while the animal is asleep, whether at night or during the day. Such apparently unconscious passage of urine from a somnolent animal must be distinguished from *nocturia*, which is occurrence of the urge or need to urinate during ordinary periods of nighttime sleep.

Urinary incontinence must be differentiated from abnormal elimination behavior (Chapter 43) and inadequate house-training. Additionally, pet owners may misinterpret their observations and confuse such clinical problems as polyuria (Chapter 29), pollakiuria, or dysuria (Chapter 32) with urinary incontinence.

GENERAL PATHOPHYSIOLOGY

Normal Micturition. Normal micturition can be divided into two phases: a storage (filling) phase and a voiding (emptying) phase. Actions of the bladder and urethra are coordinated to produce both these phases. During the storage phase, the bladder relaxes, forming a low pressure reservoir where urine can accumulate gradually as it is formed. Simultaneously, the urethra contracts to maintain sufficient pressure (outlet resistance) to prevent urine flow. During the voiding phase, these pressure relationships are reversed by simultaneous contraction of the bladder and relaxation of the urethra to produce urination.

Smooth muscle fibers in the proximal urethra form the internal sphincter, and striated muscle fibers in the urethra form the external sphincter. Anatomically, the external sphincter is located predominantly in the midurethral region in females and in the membranous urethra in males. However, striated muscle fibers are spread throughout the entire length of the urethra. Although the muscular components regulating outlet resistance are called sphincters, they are not distinct anatomic structures. Distinction between them is more functional than anatomic.

Micturition depends on a complex neural control system that coordinates autonomic and somatic afferent activities to the smooth muscle (detrusor) of the bladder wall and of the internal urethral sphincter, as well as to the skeletal muscle of the external urethral sphincter. Sympathetic innervation is from the lumbar spinal cord (L1-L2) via the hypogastric nerve, and parasympathetic innervation is from the sacral spinal cord (S1-S3) via the pelvic nerve. Somatic innervation is also supplied by the sacral spinal cord (S1-S3) via the pudendal nerve. Cholinergic and adrenergic receptors normally predominate in certain portions of the bladder and urethra. Cholinergic and beta-adrenergic neuroreceptors predominate in the bladder body, but they also exist in the bladder outlet and urethra. Alpha-adrenergic neuroreceptors predominate in the trigonal area (bladder neck) and in the proximal urethra, but they are absent in the bladder body.

The storage phase of micturition is dominated by sympathetic autonomic neurologic activity. As the bladder fills, beta-adrenergic effects on detrusor smooth muscle fibers maintain relaxation of the bladder, allowing the volume of the bladder to increase without substantially increasing intravesical pressure. Simultaneously, alpha-adrenergic effects cause contraction of the smooth muscle components of the internal urethral sphincter to sustain a resting outlet resistance sufficient to maintain continence. If needed, an additional increment of outlet resistance can be added by either voluntary or reflex stimulation of the striated muscle fibers of the external urethral sphincter.

The occurrence of the micturition reflex causes the transition from the storage phase to the voiding phase. When the normal bladder capacity and pressure threshold are reached, efferent (motor) discharges initiate the voiding phase. During the voiding phase of micturition, parasympathetic autonomic impulses stimulate detrusor depolarization and contraction. The wave of depolarization and contraction spreads from one cell to another through tight junctions, which represent specialized areas of fusion of the cell membranes. Simultaneously with detrusor muscle contraction, inhibition of both sympathetic and somatic activities to the urethral sphincters normally facilitates complete bladder emptying. When the bladder is empty, detrusor contraction and urethral relaxation are terminated, and the micturition cycle returns to the storage phase.

Abnormal Micturition. The signs exhibited by animals with disorders of micturition correlate with the phase of micturition that is abnormal. Storage phase disorders are generally manifested by urinary incontinence, whereas emptying phase disorders usually produce some degree of incomplete bladder emptying and urinary retention, although urinary incontinence may also occur. Urinary incontinence has both neurogenic and non-neurogenic causes.

Neurogenic Disorders. Neurologic disorders are common causes of urinary incontinence in dogs and cats. The pathophysiology of neurogenic urinary incontinence varies with the location and with the severity of the lesion. Neurologic lesions that disrupt the upper motor neuron segments of the micturition reflex arc impair voluntary control of urination and produce a spastic neuropathic bladder (Chapters 13, 61, and 62). Because lower motor neurons are intact, detrusor contraction can be stimulated, but disruption of upper motor neuron control causes bladder and urethral function to be abnormal. Injury to the pyramidal tracts causes loss of cortical inhibition; therefore, as the bladder fills with urine, contractions occur more frequently and vesical capacity is decreased. Furthermore, reflex detrusor contraction is generally not coordinated with urethral sphincter relaxation. Voiding is interrupted, involuntary, and incomplete. Functional urinary obstruction and urinary retention are often present. The preferred term for upper motor neuron bladder dysfunction is spastic neuropathic bladder, but reflex or automatic bladder are other terms that have been used.

Neurologic lesions that disrupt the lower motor neuron segment of the micturition reflex arc preclude detrusor contraction and produce a flaccid or atonic neuropathic bladder (Chapters 13, 62, and 64). Absence of a sensation of fullness and lack of detrusor contraction allow excessive bladder distention and may damage tight junctions between smooth muscle fibers. Thus, the capacity of the bladder is progressively increased. The bladder fills with urine until intravesical pressure exceeds outlet resistance, whereupon an overflow of urine occurs. In this circumstance, urine flow is influenced by the tone of the urethral sphincters. When urethral tone is minimal, even small increments of intravesical pressure produce some discharge of urine. When urethral tone is sufficient, however, the flow of urine is restrained and partial continence may exist. The preferred term for lower motor neuron bladder dysfunction is flaccid neuropathic bladder, but atonic, nonreflex, or autonomous bladder are other terms that have been used.

Non-neurogenic Disorders. A variety of anatomic abnormalities of the lower urinary tract may cause urinary incontinence. The most common congenital disorder is ectopic ureter, which is usually seen in young female dogs (Chapters 108 and 112). Ectopic ureters terminate in abnormal locations bypassing normal sphincters, and affected animals tend to dribble constantly. Other congenital anatomic abnormalities that have been described in dogs and cats with urinary incontinence include exstrophy of urinary bladder, female pseudohermaphroditism, patent urachus, ureterocele, urethral diverticulum, urethral fistula (rectal or vaginal), and vestibulovaginal stenosis. Acquired anatomic abnormalities also have been associated with urinary incontinence. Inflammatory or infiltrative diseases of the bladder or urethra may impair function of these organs. Chronic cystitis and urethritis, neoplasia, urolithiasis, and prostatic diseases are frequent causes of such problems (Chapters 105, 110, 111, and 112). Urinary incontinence caused by inflammation, infection, and postsurgical adhesions also have been described following abdominal operations such as ovariohysterectomy, cystotomy, and prostatic surgery. Traumatic or postsurgical urethral fistula also may impair normal sphincter function and cause urinary incontinence.

Functional abnormalities are identified when the bladder and urethra appear to be structurally normal, but they do not perform properly (Chapter 112). Some animals are unable to maintain sufficient outlet resistance to prevent urine flow during the storage phase, even when bladder function is apparently adequate and intravesical pressure is not excessive. Urinary incontinence because of such insufficiency of outlet resistance during the storage phase indicates urethral incompetence, and usually occurs when the animal is resting or sleeping. At these times, outlet resistance depends mainly on the resting tone of the internal urethral sphincter; resistance provided by the external urethral sphincter is minimal. However, when the animal is awake and ambulatory, continence usually is maintained and micturition appears normal, presumably because the bladder and the external urethral sphincter function adequately. One form of urethral incompetence occurs in some spayed female dogs. Administration of low doses of estrogens to these dogs controls the incontinence, and obtaining this therapeutic response identifies the syndrome as estrogen-responsive urinary incontinence. A similar condition that responds to testosterone administration has been observed occasionally in castrated male dogs.

Diseases of the urinary bladder that increase stimulation of the micturition reflex may cause "urge incontinence" (Chapter 112). In this condition, the sensation of bladder fullness and need to urinate is increased. Voiding is basically normal, but the storage phase is shortened because the micturition reflex is initiated more frequently. The animal becomes unable to wait as long as usual between urinations. However, the urge to urinate may develop so rapidly and intensely that it becomes impossible to control. Voiding is involuntary, but the animal is conscious, usually demonstrates some discomfort, and attempts to remain continent. Additionally, polyuria may cause urge incontinence because the bladder fills more rapidly than normal (Chapter 29).

A number of disorders of micturition are associated with excessive outlet resistance during voiding efforts. Such obstruction to urine flow typically produces stranguria and urinary retention rather than incontinence (Chapters 31 and 32). However, conditions that cause partial obstructions of the urethra may allow leakage of urine past the obstruction as pressure increases within the bladder (Chapters 110, 111, and 112). This type of paradoxic or obstructive incontinence may be caused by intraluminal or extraluminal diseases of the urethra. Intraluminal abnormalities simply produce mechanical obstructions, whereas extraluminal abnormalities produce functional obstructions because they prevent adequate relaxation of the urethra during voiding. Intramural lesions may damage the muscular components of the urethra and produce a myogenic functional obstruction. Neurologic lesions may disrupt reflex arcs that relax urethral sphincters during detrusor contraction and produce neurogenic functional obstruction (Chapters 62 and 112). Reflex dyssynergia is the term used to describe lack of synchrony between detrusor and sphincter function when the lesion is centrally located in the nervous system (Chapter 31).

Complications of Urinary Incontinence. The most common complication of urinary incontinence is development of urinary tract infection. Indeed, many of the disorders that cause urinary incontinence also impair urinary tract defenses against infection by bypassing important anatomic and functional barriers to the ascent of microbes (Chapter 112). Except in instances of urge incontinence, urinary tract infection is more likely to be a complication of urinary incontinence than it is to be the cause of incontinence. However, severe or longstanding inflammatory diseases of the bladder or urethra may induce sufficient fibrosis to cause functional disability. Additionally, disruption of tight junctions between smooth muscle fibers may occur as a sequela to bladder overdistention and produce further detrusor malfunction (Chapter 31).

Incontinent animals tend to soil themselves and lie in their urine, especially when paralysis or paresis is also present. Consequently, development of skin disorders such as rashes or decubital ulcers often is a problem. Animals with urinary incontinence often require extensive nursing care and tremendous patience on the part of their owners. Euthanasia of the pet may be requested if the problem is not rapidly controlled.

RECOGNITION OF URINARY INCONTINENCE

History. When obtaining the history of an animal with urinary incontinence, the owner's description of the animal's pattern of urination should be carefully reviewed. Indications of polyuria, pollakiuria, stranguria, dysuria, and nocturia may be mistaken for urinary incontinence (Chapters 29 and 32). Additionally, any of these signs could be a manifestation of a disorder of micturition, and urinary incontinence should be considered in the differential diagnosis of any of them. For example, polyuria may be associated with, or partially responsible for, urinary incontinence in animals with urethral incompetence. Animals with pollakiuria, stranguria, or dysuria may be incontinent because of disturbances of their micturition reflex or may have paradoxic incontinence.

The signalment may suggest possible causes of incontinence. Young animals are more likely to be affected by congenital disorders, whereas older animals are more likely to have acquired disorders. Incontinence due to ureteral ectopia usually occurs in young females, while older neutered female or male dogs are more likely to have hormone-responsive incontinence. The origin and breed of the animal is also important because some congenital abnormalities are known for their breed predilection (Chapter 112).

The history obtained regarding an incontinent animal should include a description of the onset and the chronologic progression of the problem. Whether urination is voluntary also should be established. Ability to voluntarily initiate and maintain urination suggests that the detrusor muscle is capable of normal reflex activity. When urine fills the bladder properly, absence of the micturition reflex suggests a neurogenic disorder of micturition. When an animal has intermittent dribbling of urine, stranguria, and incomplete bladder emptying, excessive outlet resistance is suggested. Intermittent dribbling of urine may also be present in animals with neurogenic disorders of micturition. Leakage of urine during recumbency or sleep is suggestive of urethral incompetence, including the hormone-responsive forms of this problem. Continuous dribbling of urine may be produced by a variety of anatomic or functional abnormalities.

The animal's past medical and surgical history also should be reviewed. Traumatic incidents might be the cause of nerve or spinal cord injuries. Previous abdominal or urogenital surgery might be responsible for lower urinary tract damage leading to urinary incontinence.

Physical Examination. A complete physical examination should always be performed, but special attention should be given to the urogenital system. Abdominal palpation combined with digital rectal palpation and vaginal or male external genitalia examination may disclose a non-neurogenic cause for incontinence. Palpation of the bladder should be performed before and after urination. Finding that the bladder is large, distended, and has thin walls suggests that it is flaccid and hyporeflexive. Alternatively, finding that the bladder is small, contracted, and has thick walls suggests that it is spastic and hyperreflexive. Manual expression of the bladder should then be performed to induce bladder emptying and to evaluate outlet resistance. Expelling urine easily during bladder palpation suggests decreased outlet resistance. A difficult or unsuccessful manual expression of the bladder suggests either normal or increased outlet resistance.

The animal's urination efforts should be observed to assess whether voluntary control is exhibited and whether detrusor contraction occurs and is accompanied by sphincter relaxation. Measurement of postmicturition residual urine volume is performed by urethral catheterization (normal values are 0.2 to 0.5 ml/kg). An excessive residual urine volume reveals incomplete voiding, which suggests either detrusor hyporeflexia or outflow obstruction. Passing a urinary catheter also helps to detect mechanical obstructions of the urethral lumen.

A complete neurologic examination should be performed with special emphasis given to sacral reflexes. The bulbospongiosus reflex, perineal reflex, anal tone, and sensation over the caudal portion of the back and tail should be carefully evaluated (Chapters 13 and 60). When these functions are normal, the sacral reflex arc and pudendal nerve function (to the urethra) are probably intact.

DIAGNOSTIC PLAN

On the basis of the aforementioned historical and physical findings, an algorithm for the diagnosis of urinary incontinence can be used to categorize the probable causes of the problem (Figure 30–1).

Laboratory Testing. Results of a routine hemogram, serum biochemical profile, and complete urinalysis should be evaluated. Results of a routine hemogram and serum biochemistry tests generally do not indicate the cause of incontinence, but they help determine the animal's overall physiologic status. Metabolic complications (e.g., azotemia, electrolyte disorders, and acid-base imbalances associated with urethral obstruction and paradoxic incontinence) may require immediate medical attention or modify the prognosis. Laboratory test results may also provide evidence of conditions that might alter bladder contractility or the rate of urine formation.

In the investigation of urinary incontinence, urinalysis findings are especially important because they may indicate urinary tract disease. Identification of hematuria, proteinuria, and/or pyuria suggests presence of pathologic changes in the urinary tract. Discovery of significant bacteriuria is also important because it indicates the presence of urinary tract infection. Although bacteria may be seen during examination of urine sediment, reliance upon the results of urine culture is preferred for evaluation of bacteriuria. Urinary tract inflammation and infection are found frequently in animals with urinary incontinence. Whether such changes are primary or secondary is often difficult to determine, but their diagnosis and management are always important. Severe or long-standing inflammatory diseases of the bladder and urethra may cause sufficient fibrosis to produce functional disability.

When planning further diagnostic investigation of animals with urinary incontinence, two general principles should be considered. First, priority should be given to alterations requiring immediate therapeutic intervention. Second, diagnostic procedures that are noninvasive, safe, simple, and inexpensive should be used before proceeding with others.

Radiography and Ultrasonography. Radiography is an important diagnostic aid for patients with urinary incontinence. Spinal radiographs, sometimes including myelography, often are necessary to identify the cause of a neurogenic disorder of micturition. Evaluation of the size, shape and position of the bladder, ureters, urethra, uterus, and prostate, as well as measurement of the thickness of the bladder wall, detection of structural anomalies of the lower urinary tract, and identification of neoplasms or uroliths, are also accomplished using radiography. Survey abdominal radiographs may detect radiodense calculi and some neoplasms or prostatic disorders, but contrast radiographic studies are usually necessary to diagnose anatomic abnormalities contributing to urinary incontinence. Positive contrast urethrography and double contrast cystography are ordinarily the most informative studies. However, excretory urography is used to investigate suspected ureteral ectopia and may also be used to evaluate the bladder.

Fluoroscopy or ultrasonography may be used to evaluate the bladder, urethra, and surrounding structures. The major advantage of these diagnostic methods is that they can be used to produce dynamic studies yielding data regarding function as well as structure. Also, these studies can be recorded for subsequent review either on videotape or with a few spot films. Although noninvasive diagnostic technologies are increasingly available, clinical experience with use of these techniques for diagnosis of urinary incontinence in animals is still limited.

Endoscopy and Biopsy. Invasive methods may be required for definitive diagnosis of some lesions of the bladder and urethra. A cystoscopic examination can be performed in some dogs. Using rigid endoscopes (in females) or small diameter flexible endoscopes (in males), visualization and biopsy of lesions in the bladder and urethra are possible. These procedures require special equipment, and they are technically easier to perform in female dogs of medium to large size. Without endoscopy, bladder wash and catheter biopsy techniques can be used to acquire specimens containing cells or small fragments of tissue for microscopic examination. Exploratory laparotomy also may be performed to examine and obtain biopsies of portions of the urinary tract. These invasive diagnostic methods are used primarily to characterize the pathologic features of lesions in the urinary tract that are detected using other diagnostic methods of investigation.

Electromyography. In animals with neuropathic bladders, electromyography may be used to substantiate the results of neurologic examination when lesions of the sacral spinal cord segments are suspected. Activity of the anal sphincter may be recorded when visual evidence of its normal function is not obtained during the neurologic examination. Recording needles are inserted in the anal sphincter, and the muscle's activity is measured during stimulation of the perineal and bulbospongiosus reflexes. Additionally, measurement of the electrical activities of muscles and nerves may aid detection of disruptions of dorsal back and tail innervation.

Electromyography may also be used with various urodynamic studies to evaluate coordination of detrusor contraction with sphincter activities. The anal sphincter works in synchrony with the external urethral sphincter and electrical activity of the anal sphincter can be used as a crude index of external urethral sphincter function. Another technique uses a urinary catheter equipped

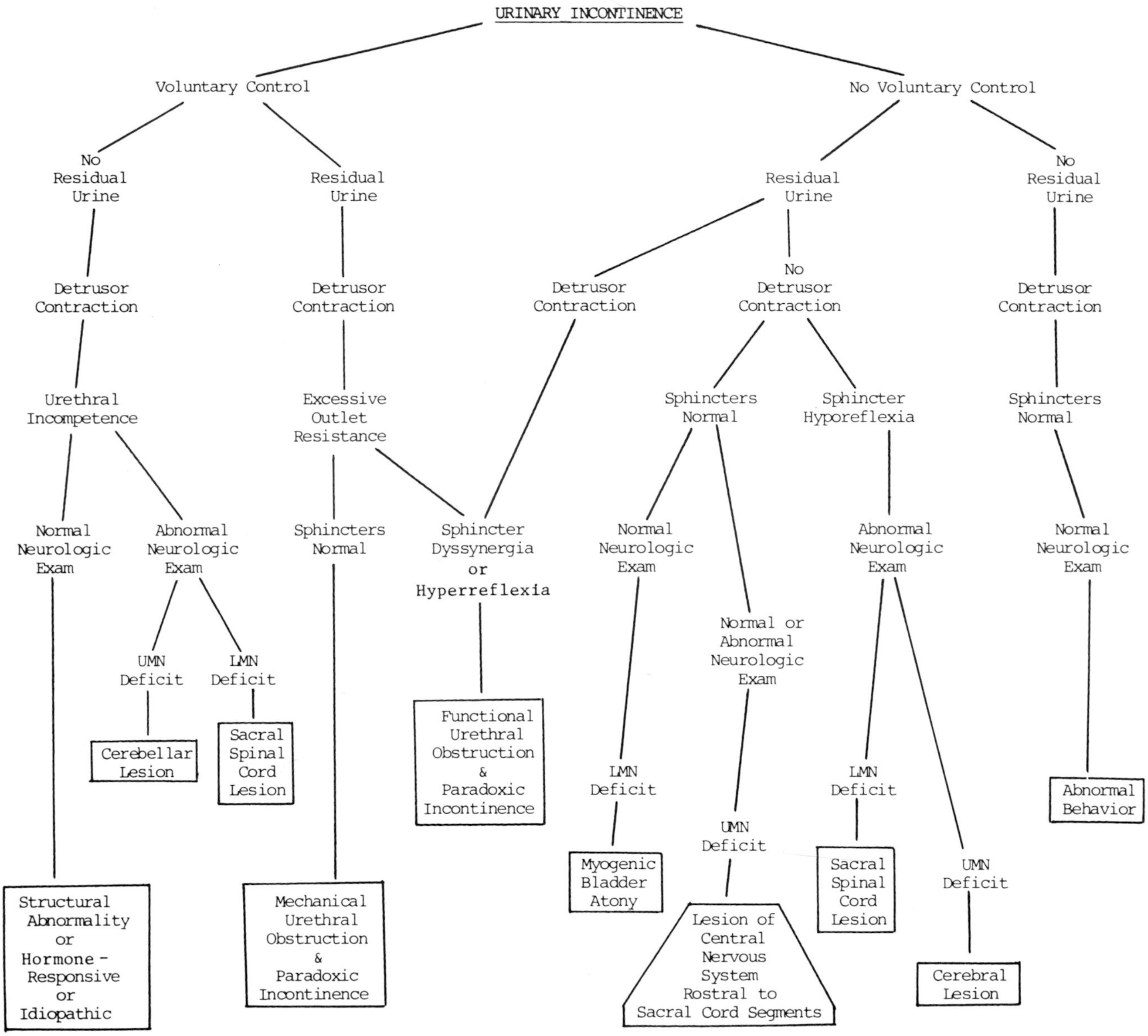

FIGURE 30–1. An algorithm for the diagnosis of urinary incontinence in dogs and cats. UMN = Upper motor neuron, LMN = Lower motor neuron.

with surface electrodes to directly record the electrical activities of muscular components of the urethra.

Urodynamic Studies. Urodynamic studies measure pressure, volume, and flow relationships within the bladder and urethra during various phases of micturition. They provide objective data regarding bladder and urethral function that may aid diagnosis, prognosis, and treatment of disorders of micturition. Urodynamic tests that have been performed in dogs and cats include cystometrograms, urethral pressure profiles, and simultaneous cystometry and uroflowmetry studies.

A cystometrogram is a recording of intravesical pressure and volume during bladder filling and detrusor contraction. This test provides measurements of bladder tone, bladder capacity, and bladder compliance during filling, as well as determining threshold volume and threshold pressure for the micturition reflex. Cystometry is especially helpful in evaluating bladder function during filling, to detect the presence of a micturition reflex, and to measure the elastic and contractile properties of the bladder wall. Urethral function during bladder filling is not measured and may even be altered by the catheter that is positioned within the urethral lumen during the test.

A urethral pressure profile is a recording of the pressure measured at the tip of a catheter as it is slowly withdrawn through the urethra. Measurement of intraluminal pressure along the length of the urethra provides a graphic record of urethral tone and resistance. This aids in identifying and localizing areas of excessive outlet resistance (increased urethral pressure) or urethral incompetence (decreased urethral pressure). The urethral pressure profile evaluates urethral tone only during the storage phase of micturition. Even for investigation of storage phase disorders, this test has limited value because adequacy of urethral function is not assessed relative to intravesical pressure or volume. Urethral activity during detrusor contraction and coordination with the micturition reflex are not measured by the urethral pressure profile.

Simultaneous cystometry and uroflowmetry also has been called a micturition study. Catheters placed in the bladder lumen through the abdominal wall are used to fill the bladder and to measure intravesical pressure without interfering with urethral function during the test. As urine escapes from the urethra during micturition events, its rate of flow is also measured. This procedure evaluates the bladder and urethra as a single functional unit during both the storage and voiding phases of the micturition cycle. Intravesical pressure measurements characterize detrusor activity, while urine flow rates determine urethral function during bladder contraction. A micturition study may be necessary for definitive diagnosis of reflex dyssynergia. Although it can also be used to evaluate the micturition reflex, excessive outlet resistance, or urethral incompetence, the micturition study procedure is more invasive and requires more expertise and equipment than the other tests.

For many clinical cases, these urodynamic tests are not available, but often they are not needed. Valid functional assessments can be based on observations of pressure and flow relationships indicated by clinical and physical findings, although the variables are estimated rather than measured precisely.

MANAGEMENT OF URINARY INCONTINENCE

Goals of Treatment. Two major principles should be considered when managing patients with urinary incontinence. First, priority should be given to alterations requiring immediate care, such as fluid deficits, electrolyte disturbances, acid-base imbalances, and azotemia. Second, normal micturition should be restored as soon as possible, regardless of the cause. Delays in treating disorders of micturition may lead to severe complications such as decubital ulcers and urinary tract infection (secondary to urethral incompetence) or azotemia, electrolyte disorders, bladder overdistention, and bladder atony (secondary to excessive outlet resistance).

Medical or surgical management of the problem causing incontinence usually is initiated along with treatment of complications such as urinary tract infections. However, when urge incontinence associated with urinary tract infection is diagnosed, antibiotic treatment alone might be sufficient to resolve the incontinence. When morphologic abnormalities are responsible for urinary incontinence, surgical correction is usually indicated. Surgery is also the treatment of choice at times for paradoxic (obstructive) incontinence. When the cause of excessive outlet resistance is functional rather than mechanical, however, medical management usually is indicated.

Pharmacologic agents are selected for management of urinary incontinence when urinary tract infection, morphologic abnormalities, and mechanical types of excessive outlet resistance have been excluded as possible causes of the problem.

Pharmacotherapy of Disorders of Micturition. Urethrovesical function can be altered by various pharmacologic agents. However, their use is mostly palliative, and they should be administered only for short periods of time. The essential purpose of drug treatment is to assist micturition until normal function is restored. In addition to drug therapy, general nursing care of the patient often is required until sufficient function is obtained.

When selecting drugs for treatment of disordered micturition, categorizing the micturition disorder on the basis of whether it primarily affects the storage or voiding phase is usually helpful. However, this classifi-

TABLE 30–1. TABLE OF DRUGS RECOMMENDED FOR INCONTINENCE, ENURESIS, AND NOCTURIA

Generic Name	Trade Name	Dosage*	Route	Frequency	Description
Bethanechol	Urecholine	5 to 15 mg (Dogs)	PO	q 8 h	Cholinergic agent
		1.25 to 5 mg (Cats)	PO	q 8 h	
Propantheline	Pro-Banthine	5 to 30 mg (Dogs)	PO	q 8 h	Anticholinergic agent
		5 to 7.5 mg (Cats)	PO		
Butyl hyoscine	Buscopan	2 to 5 mg (Dogs)	PO	q 12 h	Anticholinergic agent
		1 to 2 mg (Cats)	PO	q 12 h	
Aminopromazine	Jenotone	1 mg/lb (Both)	PO	q 12 h	Smooth muscle relaxant
Phenoxybenzamine	Dibenzyline	5 to 15 mg (Dogs)	PO	q 24 h	Alpha-adrenergic antagonist
		2.5 to 7.5 mg (Cats)	PO	q 24 h	
Nicergoline	Sermion	1 to 5 mg (Both)	PO	q 8 h	Alpha-adrenergic antagonist
Moxisylyte	Carlytène	5 to 30 mg (Both)	PO	q 8 h	Alpha-adrenergic antagonist
Dantrolene	Dantrium	0.25–0.5 mg/lb (Dogs)	PO	q 8 h	Skeletal muscle relaxant
		0.25–0.5 mg/lb (Cats)	PO	q 12 h	
Baclofen	Lioresal	0.5–1 mg/lb (Dogs)	PO	q 8 h	Skeletal muscle relaxant
Diazepam	Valium	2 to 10 mg (Dogs)	PO	q 8 h	Skeletal muscle relaxant
		2 to 5 mg (Cats)	PO	q 8 h	
Phenylpropanolamine	Propagest	12.5 to 50 mg (Dogs)	PO	q 8 h	Alpha-adrenergic agonist
Imipramine	Tofranil	5 to 15 mg (Dogs)	PO	q 12 h	Alpha- & beta-adrenergic
		2.5 to 5 mg (Cats)	PO	q 12 h	agent
Diethylstilbestrol	for 3 to 5 days	0.1 to 1.0 mg	PO	q 24 h	Estrogen hormone
	then continue	1.0 mg	PO	q 7–14 d	
Testosterone cypionate		1.0 mg/lb	IM	q 30 d	Hormone
proprionate		1.0 mg/lb	IM	q 2–7 d	

*Begin treatment at lower dosage, raising dosage by small increments as needed to obtain an adequate response, without exceeding the maximum dosage listed.

cation is difficult or confusing in some cases because both the storage and emptying phases may be affected simultaneously. It is also helpful to classify incontinent patients on the basis of whether the bladder is hypocontractile or hypercontractile and whether urethral sphincters are hyporeflexive or hyperreflexive and acting in synchrony with detrusor activity.

Dogs and cats with bladder hypocontractility may have an inability to generate sufficient intravesical pressure caused by loss of bladder innervation. Alternatively, the condition may be caused by impairment of detrusor smooth muscle function, such as occurs when tight junctions are damaged by excessive bladder distention. To increase intravesical pressure with pharmacologic agents, however, the same drugs are used for both neurogenic and myogenic disorders. Cholinergic agents such as bethanechol are used to stimulate smooth muscle activity and detrusor contraction.

Dogs and cats with bladder hypercontractility may lack inhibitory control of cholinergic receptors and experience frequent stimulation of the micturition reflex even when intravesical volume is small. In animals with bladder hypercontractility, drugs such as propantheline or butyl hyoscine that block cholinergic receptors may be used effectively. Smooth muscle relaxing agents such as aminopromazine also have been recommended.

Urethral hyperreflexia may be associated either with internal urethral sphincter or external urethral sphincter dyssynergia. Drugs that have been used to decrease smooth muscle activity of the urethra include alpha-adrenergic blocking agents such as phenoxybenzamine and nicergoline. Drugs that have been used to decrease striated muscle activity of the urethra include myorelaxing agents such as dantrolene and baclofen or tranquilizing agents such as diazepam.

Urethral hyporeflexia (urethral incompetence) is usually associated with abnormal smooth muscle function. Drugs that have been recommended to increase smooth muscle activity of the urethra include alpha-adrenergic agonists such as phenylpropanolamine. Sympathomimetic agents that block reuptake of norepinephrine, such as imipramine, also have been used successfully in dogs with internal sphincter incompetence. Hormone-responsive urinary incontinence is a particular form of urethral incompetence that is identified principally by observing response to therapy. Presumptive diagnosis may be based on the signalment, history, lack of physical or laboratory abnormalities, and characteristic pattern of incontinence, but the diagnosis can only be confirmed by therapeutic trial. Estrogen (diethylstilbestrol) is given to spayed female dogs, and testosterone is given to castrated male dogs.

Management of Complications. The most common complication of urinary incontinence is urinary tract infection, and appropriate antimicrobial therapy should be administered when urinary tract infection is present (Chapter 112). Decubital ulcers also develop frequently and often require devoted nursing care, including cleaning, drying, wound dressing, padding, and bandaging. Severe bladder distention due to excessive outlet resistance may disrupt tight junctions and produce further detrusor malfunction. In this circumstance, bethanechol administration is used to improve contraction of the bladder.

31 URINARY OBSTRUCTION AND ATONY

PHILIPPE M. MOREAU and GEORGE E. LEES

Urinary retention refers to inappropriate accumulation of urine within the bladder. Disorders that are characterized by, or associated with, urinary retention are those diseases that impair urination, the normal act of emptying the bladder. Urination is normally accomplished by smooth muscle activity that is controlled by voluntary, as well as involuntary, nervous activity. Following normal urination, the residual volume of urine remaining in the bladder of dogs and cats is 0 to 0.25 ml/lb. Discovery of an excessive amount of residual urine within the bladder following urination identifies urinary retention. The severity of urinary retention varies and usually correlates with the degree of bladder distention and with the prevailing residual volume of the bladder.

Bladder atony refers to lack of detrusor muscle tone and contractile function of the bladder. Excessive urinary retention leads to bladder atony because severe, sustained distention of the bladder produces deleterious effects on its neuromuscular contractile mechanisms.

Other clinical signs or problems may be either confused or associated with urinary retention. Most of these are abnormalities of the voiding phase of micturition, such as anuria, dysuria, and stranguria (Chapter 32), but abnormalities of the storage phase of micturition, such as urinary incontinence (Chapter 30), are sometimes involved.

GENERAL PATHOPHYSIOLOGY

CAUSES OF URINARY RETENTION

Normal micturition is divided into a storage phase and a voiding phase (Chapter 30). During storage, urine accumulates within the bladder; during voiding, the bladder is emptied by urination. Clinically, voiding phase disorders are usually manifested by urinary retention, whereas storage phase disorders are usually characterized by urinary incontinence. Animals with voiding phase disorders may exhibit both urinary retention and paradoxic incontinence. Additionally, both the storage and emptying phases are affected by some neurogenic disorders. Causes of urinary retention can be classified into two categories: abnormal detrusor activity and excessive outlet resistance.

Abnormal Detrusor Activity. Abnormal detrusor contraction can be neurogenic or myogenic. Neurogenic disorders are caused by lesions involving the micturition reflex arc. Both upper motor neuron lesions and lower motor neuron lesions may be responsible for an abnormality of the micturition reflex, producing urinary retention.

Neurologic lesions that disrupt the upper motor neuron segments of the micturition arc impair voluntary control of urination and produce a spastic, neuropathic bladder (Chapters 13, 61, and 62). When the lower motor neuron loop is intact, voiding may occur, but it is typically interrupted, involuntary, and incomplete because cortical inhibition and sphincter synergism are disrupted (Chapter 30). Bladder distention usually is not excessive, vesical capacity may even be decreased, but postmicturition residual urine volume is increased. This type of urinary retention is usually accompanied by pollakiuria because of frequent detrusor contractions. When sphincter dyssynergia is present because of bladder-urethral incoordination, animals may exhibit functional urinary obstruction and paradoxic incontinence. Animals with sphincter dyssynergia usually have urinary retention as well as stranguria, pollakiuria, and urinary incontinence.

Neurologic lesions that disrupt the lower motor neuron loop of the micturition reflex arc preclude detrusor contraction (Chapters 13, 62, and 64). Absence of the sensation of bladder fullness and disruption of efferent motor activity to induce detrusor contraction produce a flaccid, neuropathic bladder. Excessive bladder distention damages tight junctions between smooth muscle fibers of the detrusor and further impairs bladder contractility. Urinary retention may become severe, and bladder distention and capacity increase progressively. The bladder fills with urine until intravesical pressure exceeds outlet resistance, whereupon urine overflows through the urethra. The animal does not demonstrate a desire to urinate, but involuntarily dribbles urine or empties its bladder partially and passively. The status of urethral sphincter function is an important variable. When urethral tone is minimal, even small increments of intravesical pressure cause the discharge of urine. However, detrusor contraction does not actually occur and the bladder remains greatly distended. When urethral tone is sufficient, the flow of urine is restrained even further.

Myogenic causes of abnormal detrusor contraction are either primary or secondary. Primary myogenic disorders have not been described in dogs and cats. Secondary myogenic disorders are acquired lesions that occur frequently. They are usually associated with outlet obstruction and subsequent disruption of tight junctions between smooth muscle fibers, producing a decrease in detrusor contraction strength. During the emptying phase of micturition, parasympathetic autonomic impulses stimulate depolarization and contraction of smooth muscle fibers. The wave of depolarization and contraction normally spreads from one cell to another through tight junctions, which represent specialized areas of fusion of the cell membranes. Disruption of these close contacts owing to long-standing bladder overdistention impairs normal propagation of the wave of depolarization and contraction through the bladder smooth muscle. Consequently, detrusor contraction stimulated by the micturition reflex is weaker than normal. Other causal mechanisms of secondary myogenic detrusor malfunction include disorders that contribute to generalized muscular weakness, such as electrolyte imbalances and metabolic disorders.

Excessive Outlet Resistance. Excessive outlet resistance is caused either by mechanical or functional obstructions to urine flow. Mechanical obstructions are physical impediments such as amorphous plugs or uroliths located in the urethral lumen (Chapters 110 and 111). Functional obstructions are caused by failure of the urethra to dilate appropriately as the bladder contracts. Intramural lesions such as inflammation, hemorrhage, edema, fibrosis, prostatic enlargement, or neoplasia may damage muscular components of the urethra, producing myogenic functional obstruction (Chapters 105 and 112). Neurologic lesions also may disrupt sphincter relaxation during detrusor contraction, producing neurogenic functional obstruction (Chapters 62 and 112). This lack of bladder-sphincter coordination is also called reflex dyssynergia. Smooth muscle components of the internal sphincter and striated muscle components of the external sphincter can be involved separately or together.

Animals with urinary retention associated with excessive outlet resistance may display a variety of other clinical signs related to lower urinary tract disease, such as dysuria, hematuria, pollakiuria, stranguria, and urinary incontinence (Chapters 30 and 32).

COMPLICATIONS OF URINARY RETENTION

Many of the complications of urinary retention depend on the etiology, rate of onset, and severity of the underlying obstructive disorder. Abrupt, complete urinary obstruction produces postrenal azotemia and uremia, a set of metabolic and clinical abnormalities that is fatal in three to five days if the problem is not corrected. In contrast to complete obstructions, partial obstructions can be chronic. When a chronic partial obstruction causes excessive pressure in the excretory pathway, the urinary tract may dilate progressively, producing hydroureter and hydronephrosis. Damage to renal parenchyma in such instances may be sufficient to cause chronic renal failure. When a chronic partial obstruction is less severe, gradual increase of bladder capacity may prevent development of excessive pressure in the excretory pathway. Nonetheless, excessive distention of the bladder may disrupt tight junctions and lead to further detrusor weakness and malfunction. Urinary retention also predisposes the animal to develop a urinary tract infection.

RECOGNITION OF URINARY RETENTION

Diagnosis of urinary retention is usually based on observation and physical examination of the patient. When urinary retention is mild or moderate, repeated measurement of postmicturition residual urine volume may be required to document the problem. Radiographic examinations and other diagnostic techniques are often needed to determine specific underlying causes. In animals with urinary obstruction, however, diagnosis of excessive urinary retention and bladder overdistention is readily made on the basis of history and physical examination (Figure 31–1).

History. The signalment may suggest possible causes of urinary retention. Young animals are more likely to exhibit congenital disorders, whereas older animals are more likely to develop acquired disorders. Male animals are much more likely to experience mechanical urethral obstructions than are females. Knowledge of the origin and breed of the animal also may be important because some disorders are known for their breed predilection.

When evaluating a patient with a suspected disorder of micturition such as urinary retention, the clinician should obtain a precise description of the animal's pattern of urination. Indications of anuria, dysuria, hematuria, nocturia, pollakiuria, stranguria, and urinary incontinence may be misleading and erroneously interpreted by the owners. Conversely, these signs also may be clinical manifestations of disorders that produce urinary retention as well.

One important aspect to determine during the history is whether the animal makes voluntary attempts to urinate. Ability to voluntarily initiate and maintain urination suggests that the detrusor muscle is capable of normal reflex activity. Assuming proper bladder filling, absence of an effective detrusor contraction suggests a neurogenic disorder of micturition or bladder atony. An animal that demonstrates intermittent dribbling, stranguria, pollakiuria, and excessive postmicturition residual urine volume is likely to have excessive outlet resistance, which could be mechanical or functional in origin. However, intermittent dribbling of urine may also be

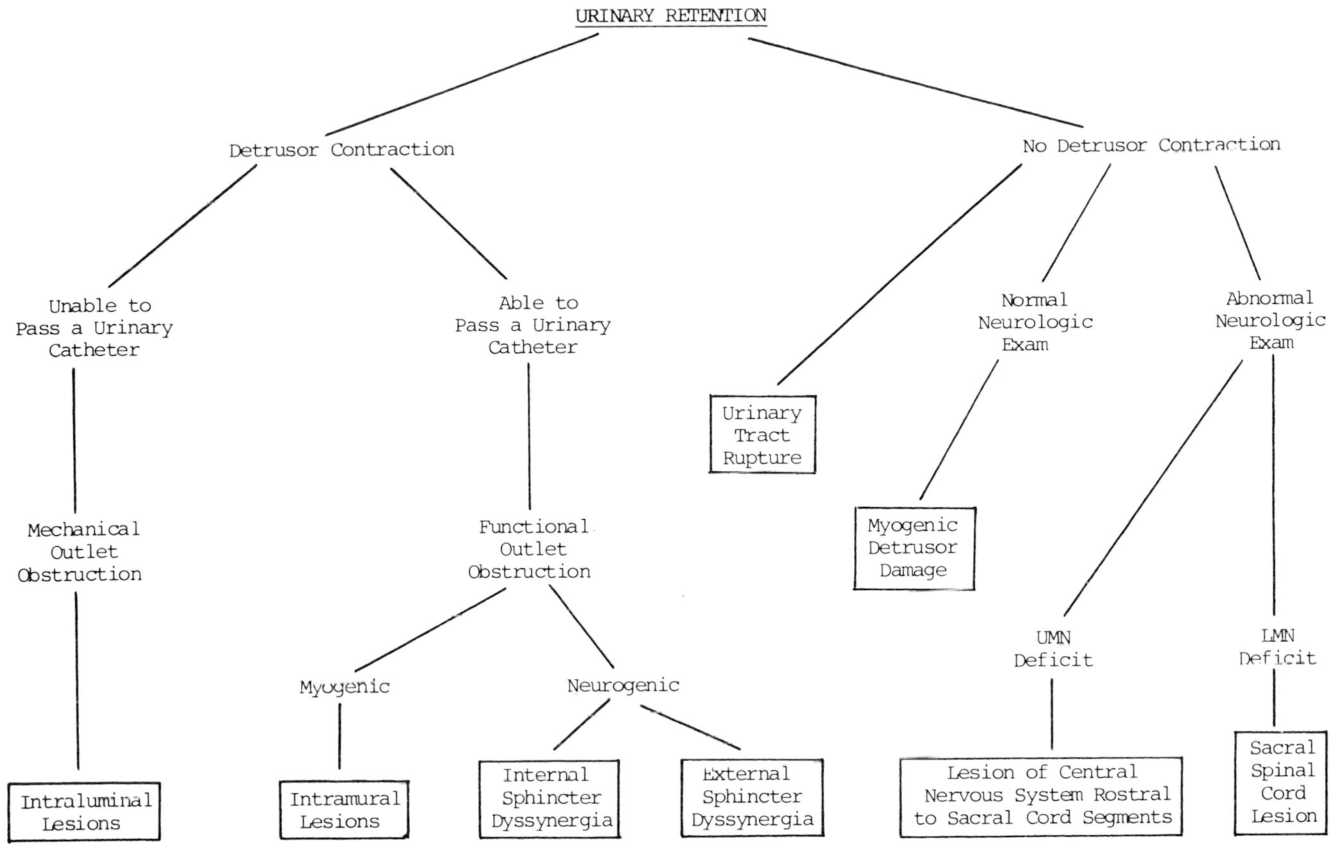

FIGURE 31–1. Algorithm for the diagnosis of urinary retention in dogs and cats. UMN = Upper motor neuron; LMN = Lower motor neuron.

present in animals with either spastic or flaccid neuropathic bladders.

The type of onset and the chronologic progression of urinary retention should be determined. Urethral obstruction caused by urolithiasis often has an abrupt onset, whereas urinary obstruction caused by neoplasia usually has an insidious onset. The past medical and surgical history should be obtained. Previous urogenital surgery, episodes of urolithiasis, and traumatic incidents that might have produced nerve or spinal cord injury should be identified.

Physical Examination. The veterinarian should observe the animal urinating and check for ineffective voiding efforts. A complete physical examination should always be performed, with special attention given to the urogenital system. Abdominal palpation of the bladder and surrounding organs before and after urination often is sufficient for diagnosis of urinary retention.

Animals with excessive outlet resistance are characterized by an excessive postmicturition residual urine volume and inability to generate an adequate urine stream during voiding efforts produced spontaneously or by manual compression of the bladder. When evaluating animals with bladder distention associated with urethral obstruction, it is essential to avoid using excessive force, which might produce bladder rupture. Fluid accumulations in the peritoneal cavity or periurethral tissues of animals with signs of urinary obstruction may indicate a rupture or laceration of the bladder or urethra. The external genitalia of males and the vulva and vagina of females should be carefully examined and palpated to detect structural abnormalities and causes of obstruction. Digital rectal palpation of the prostate and the pelvic portion of the urethra is also important.

Discovery of severe urinary retention associated with complete urethral obstruction is a medical emergency and measures should be taken to correct the problem immediately. Urinary catheterization and hydropropulsion techniques usually are sufficient for removal of the obstruction. When these efforts are not successful, cystocentesis or percutaneous transabdominal catheterization of the bladder should be performed before proceeding with other diagnostic and therapeutic steps. Metabolic complications of urinary obstruction should be evaluated and treated at the same time.

Unusual or unexplained difficulty in attempting to pass a urinary catheter is an indication for additional diagnostic investigations, such as contrast radiography. Conversely, finding that a catheter can be passed easily through the urethra of an animal with urinary retention is an indication that a functional obstruction might be present. Catheterization of the bladder after urination allows measurement of postmicturition residual urine volume as a basis for objective evaluation of bladder emptying and detrusor activity.

When urinary retention is due to impaired detrusor activity, manual bladder compression usually generates an adequate urine stream. The force of bladder compression that is required varies as much with patient cooperation as with sphincter function. Animals with abnormal detrusor activity may have incomplete bladder emptying because of the impairment of detrusor contractile strength as a manifestation of generalized muscle weakness, lack of micturition reflex initiation, or myogenic bladder dysfunction. Muscle weakness is often associated with electrolyte imbalances, and concomitant impairment of gastrointestinal tract function may indicate that muscular weakness is a generalized problem. Gastrointestinal problems that could indicate muscular weakness include vomiting, gas formation, and lack of intestinal motility. A complete neurologic examination should also be performed, with particular attention given to evaluation of reflexes involving the sacral spinal cord segments (see Figure 31–1).

DIAGNOSTIC PLAN

Laboratory Testing. Results of a routine hemogram, serum biochemical profile, and complete urinalysis should be evaluated. Results of these tests generally do not indicate the cause of urinary retention. However, the metabolic abnormalities that may develop in animals with urinary retention are important, sometimes life-threatening, problems. They may require immediate medical attention, modify prognostic judgments, or alter therapeutic strategies for the patient's other problems. Additionally, these laboratory test results may provide evidence for metabolic disturbances that can alter bladder or urethral function.

In the investigation of urinary retention, urinalysis findings are particularly important because they may indicate urinary tract disease. Identification of hematuria, proteinuria, and/or pyuria suggest the presence of pathologic changes in the lower urinary tract. Crystalluria may provide a clue to the existence or character of uroliths. Discovery of significant bacteriuria is also important. Although bacteria may be seen during examination of urine sediment, reliance should be placed on the results of urine culture for the diagnosis of urinary tract infection. Animals with urinary retention frequently have a urinary tract infection or develop infection as a complication of their primary problem. Although urinary tract infection is more likely to be a consequence than a cause of most forms of urinary retention, discovery and treatment of infection is always important.

Severe or long-standing inflammatory diseases or neoplastic involvement of the bladder and/or urethra may cause sufficient fibrosis and tissue damage to produce functional disability. Cytologic examination of the urine sediment may identify distinctive cells associated with such pathologic processes. Bladder wash or prostatic massage techniques may be used to increase the cellularity of specimens obtained for cytologic examination.

When planning further diagnostic investigation of animals with urinary retention, two general principles should be considered. First, priority should be given to abnormalities requiring immediate attention. Second, diagnostic procedures that are safe, simple, and noninvasive should be used before proceeding with others.

Radiology and Ultrasonography. Radiography and ultrasonography are imaging techniques that may be used effectively to identify the cause of urinary retention, especially when excessive outlet resistance is the problem. The size, shape, and position of the bladder, urethra, and prostate should be evaluated. Survey abdominal radiographs may demonstrate radiodense calculi and prostatic enlargement. However, special radiographic studies, such as positive contrast urethrography and double contrast cystography, are frequently necessary to demonstrate lesions of the wall of the bladder and/or urethra and some intraluminal abnormalities. Retrograde cystography and urethrography procedures are the radiographic tests of choice for the diagnosis of obstructive disorders of the bladder and urethra.

Endoscopy and Biopsy. Invasive techniques are sometimes required for definitive diagnosis of disorders causing urinary retention. Cystoscopic examination can be performed in some dogs and provides a method for inspecting the bladder and urethra for abnormal contents or mural lesions. During cystoscopy, tissue specimens may be obtained for microscopic examination. Exploratory laparotomy also may be performed to examine and biopsy lesions of the urinary tract. Invasive diagnostic methods are used mainly to characterize the pathologic features of lesions of the urinary tract that have been discovered by other diagnostic methods. However, surgical procedures often are needed to correct some of the problems that produce urinary retention, so diagnostic and therapeutic objectives may be accomplished simultaneously.

Electrodiagnostic and Urodynamic Studies. Special electrophysiologic techniques can be used to evaluate patients with functional urinary retention. Urodynamic studies measure pressure, volume, and flow relationships within the bladder and urethra during various phases of micturition (Chapter 30). Electromyography can be used to evaluate coordination of detrusor contraction with sphincter activities and to verify results of the neurologic examination when lesions of the sacral spinal cord segments are suspected (Chapter 30). These diagnostic techniques provide objective data regarding the function of the bladder and urethra that may aid diagnosis, prognosis, and treatment of urinary retention caused by abnormalities of detrusor activity and functional outlet obstruction.

MANAGEMENT OF URINARY RETENTION

Goals of Treatment. Two main principles should be considered when managing patients with urinary retention. First, priority should be given to correcting life-threatening abnormalities, such as complete urethral obstruction and the azotemia, hyperkalemia, and acidosis it produces. Second, complete bladder emptying should be restored as soon as possible. Delays in treating urinary retention may produce potentially severe complications such as urinary tract infections, metabolic disorders, bladder atony, hydroureter, and hydronephrosis.

Relief of intraluminal obstruction is usually accom-

TABLE 31–1. DRUGS RECOMMENDED FOR URINARY OBSTRUCTION AND ATONY

Generic Name	Trade Name	Dosage*	Route	Frequency	Description
Bethanechol	Urecholine	5 to 15 mg (Dogs) 1.25 to 5 mg (Cats)	PO PO	q 8 h q 8 h	Cholinergic agent
Phenoxybenzamine	Dibenzyline	5 to 15 mg (Dogs) 2.5 to 7.5 mg (Cats)	PO PO	q 24 h q 24 h	Alpha-adrenergic antagonist
Nicergoline	Sermion	1 to 5 mg (Both)	PO	q 8 h	Alpha-adrenergic antagonist
Moxisylyte	Carlytène	5 to 30 mg (Both)	PO	q 8 h	Alpha-adrenergic antagonist
Dantrolene	Dantrium	0.25 to 1 mg/lb (Dogs) 0.25 to 1 mg/lb (Cats)	PO PO	q 8 h q 12 h	Skeletal muscle relaxant
Baclofen	Lioresal	0.5 to 1 mg/lb (Dogs)	PO	q 8 h	Skeletal muscle relaxant
Diazepam	Valium	2 to 10 mg (Dogs) 2 to 5 mg (Cats)	PO PO	q 8 h q 8 h	Skeletal muscle relaxant

*Begin treatment at lower dosage, raising dosage by small increments as needed to obtain an adequate response, without exceeding the maximum dosage listed.

plished by urethral catheterization combined with hydropropulsion techniques. When the obstruction cannot be dislodged, cystocentesis should be performed to decompress the bladder. After cystocentesis, repeated efforts to relieve the obstruction are usually successful, but a urethrotomy may be required to remove the obstruction in some cases. Appropriate fluid therapy should also be initiated for treatment of the metabolic complications of urinary retention. In most animals with abnormal detrusor activity and/or functional outlet obstruction, and in some animals after relief of mechanical obstruction, urinary retention is a continuing problem that must be managed with intermittent or indwelling catheterization. Generally, intermittent catheterization is preferred over indwelling catheterization when repeated insertion of the catheter can be accomplished without substantial difficulty. Use of indwelling catheterization maximizes the risk of catheter-induced urinary tract infection.

Pharmacotherapy of Urinary Retention. Pharmacologic agents alter urethrovesical function by acting on autonomic or somatic receptors to modify smooth or striated muscle activity. Drugs may be used to relax urethral sphincters in animals with functional urethral obstruction and to promote a more vigorous detrusor contraction in patients with abnormal detrusor activity (see Table 31–1). In addition to pharmacotherapy, nursing care often is required to aid bladder emptying until bladder and urethral function are adequately restored. Manual compression or intermittent sterile catheterization of the bladder may be required several times a day to avoid excessive urinary retention and further bladder distention. However, spontaneous emptying of the bladder and response to therapy cannot be evaluated if the bladder is continuously emptied passively with the veterinarian's or owner's help. Therefore, animals should be given the opportunity to initiate spontaneous bladder emptying at increasing intervals after drug treatment has been initiated.

Various drugs that stimulate smooth muscle activity by acting as agonists on cholinergic receptors have been used to treat bladder atony. Drug therapy is the same whether the cause is a neurogenic or a myogenic problem. Bethanechol is the cholinergic agent that is most often recommended for treatment of bladder hyporeflexia or atony.

Functional outflow obstruction may be associated with internal urethral sphincter hyperreflexia or with external urethral sphincter hyperreflexia. Drugs that are used to decrease smooth muscle activity of the urethra include alpha-adrenergic blocking agents such as phenoxybenzamine, nicergoline, and moxisylyte. Drugs that have been used to decrease striated muscle activity of the urethra include myorelaxing or tranquilizing agents such as dantrolene, baclofen, and diazepam.

Management of Complications. Urinary tract infections are the most common complications of urinary retention and bladder atony. Appropriate antimicrobial therapy should be administered when urinary tract infection is present (Chapter 112). Additionally, precautions against inducing urinary tract infection should always be taken because animals with urinary retention are greatly predisposed to the development of infection.

The metabolic complications of urethral obstruction are azotemia and potentially fatal fluid, electrolyte, and acid-base disturbances. Immediate care of these abnormalities involves fluid therapy to correct extracellular fluid volume deficits, hyperkalemia, and metabolic acidosis (Chapter 53). Following restoration of urine flow, continued fluid therapy and supportive care are needed until azotemia and other metabolic abnormalities are resolved.

32 HEMATURIA-DYSURIA

GERALDINE McCALL KAUFMAN

HEMATURIA

Hematuria refers to the presence of blood mixed with urine. It is usually recognized by the obvious discoloration of urine when contaminated by large quantities of blood (gross hematuria). However the term also applies to urine that is grossly normal but has abnormal numbers of erythrocytes upon microscopic examination (microscopic hematuria).

Pathologic hematuria must be differentiated from *normal red cell loss* in the urine of healthy individuals. This population is defined by the paucity of red cells (usually fewer than five per high-powered field in the dog and cat), the absence of proteinuria and dysuria, and the finding of normal red cell morphology. This is generally an incidental finding from a routine urine analysis.

Pathologic hematuria must also be differentiated from *iatrogenic hematuria*. This is defined as blood loss into the lower urinary tract after instrumentation or during use of an invasive collection technique. Catheterization (particularly in the bitch and cat) and cystocentesis may result in hematuria unrelated to disease. The risk of iatrogenic hematuria increases with repeated or difficult catheterizations or if the catheter remains in place for several hours.

Iatrogenic hematuria confuses urine analysis and subsequent diagnostics. It is usually distinguished by occurring only after catheterization, by discrete spots or swirls of blood in the urine sample, and by resolution within 24 hours. Finally, pathologic hematuria must also be differentiated from *pigmenturia*. There are many pigments that can discolor urine. Drugs (phenytoin, sulfas, tranquilizers), infectious agents (*Pseudomonas*), and endogenous products (myoglobin, hemoglobin, bilirubin) must be differentiated from hematuria. History and laboratory examination support the diagnosis of hematuria. Unlike pigmenturia, in hematuria there are red cells in the urine and the color of spun urine and spun serum is clear (unless hemolyzed). Hemoglobin and myoglobin are the most frequent pigments seen.

The following discussion of hematuria excludes these three differentials.

General Pathophysiology

Hematuria may arise from lesions in the kidneys or in the lower urinary tract (i.e., distal to the renal pelvis). Lesions may be single or multiple, and may manifest as primary urinary tract disease or be part of a wider systemic disease. Localization of the source of hematuria provides significant information as to the further diagnostic approach, etiology, therapy, and prognosis (Table 32–1).

Renal parenchymal hematuria may be caused by blood loss across any part of the nephron from the glomerulus to the collecting duct. Erythrocytes may be seen free in the urine or trapped in a protein gel. The latter are called red cell casts. The protein that incorporates the red cells (Tamm-Horsfall mucoprotein) is produced in the medullary and cortical ascending limbs of the nephrons. Therefore, red cell casts are only seen in renal parenchymal blood loss. Red cell casts do not differentiate between the intrarenal sites of hemorrhage: glomerular, tubulointestinal, and vascular (Table 32–1). Glomerular blood loss is generally differentiated from other renal parenchymal hematuria by protein loss disproportionate to that expected from the contaminating blood itself. Otherwise, only massive urinary tract bleeding can account for heavy proteinuria (Dipstick +3 or +4; daily loss greater than 18 mg/lb body weight).

Lower urinary tract hematuria reflects the loss of the endothelial-epithelial barrier somewhere along the urine collecting system from the renal pelvis to the urethral orifice. The urine from these patients does not contain red cell casts. These patients frequently show clinical signs associated with abnormal urination (see the following section on dysuria). This reflects the inflammatory or obstructive nature of most etiologies of lower tract hematuria (calculi, cystitis, and malignancy). Infections should be differentiated from other sources by the presence of infectious and inflammatory patterns (leukocytosis, fever, bacteriuria), physical examination, and laboratory tests.

Hematuria secondary to systemic disease in the dog and cat can be divided into bleeding disorders due to platelet deficiencies or disorders, bleeding disorders due to coagulation disorders, hypercatabolic states (fever

TABLE 32–1. THE CAUSES OF HEMATURIA

I. Renal Parenchymal Disease
- A. Glomerular
  - Acute glomerulonephritis
  - Chronic glomerulonephritis (not as common as acute)
  - Immune complex disorders (*Dirofilaria immitis,* pyometra)
  - SLE
  - Amyloidosis (rare)
- B. Tubulointestinal and vascular
  - Neoplastic, usually primary
    - Renal carcinoma
    - Hemangiosarcoma
  - Hypersensitivity
    - Acute interstitial nephritis (drugs, especially antibiotics–rare)
  - Idiopathic
  - Hereditary polycystic kidneys
  - Papillary necrosis (rare), analgesics
  - Vascular–benign vascular ectasia of Welsh Corgis, renal infarcts, fistulae
  - Trauma and postradiation intoxication
  - Infections
    - Leptospirosis
    - Acute bacterial pyelonephritis
    - Lower urinary tract diseases (renal pelvis to distal urethra)
    - Neoplasia–transitional cell carcinoma
    - Trauma
    - Severe hydronephrosis
    - Dioctophyma renale
- C. Lower urogenital tract
  - Urinary
    - Neoplasia of ureters, bladder, urethra
    - Transitional cell carcinoma of the bladder
    - Polypoid cystitis
  - Chemical cystitis–cyclophosphamide
  - Calculi–renal pelvis to urethral orifice
  - Trauma including iatrogenic
  - Infection–viral, especially FUS, bacterial, possibly fungal, Capillaria plica
  - Genital
    - Prostatic disorders (prostatitis, prostatic cysts, tumor)
    - Proestrus
    - Vaginal disorders (polyps, neoplasia, foreign bodies, vaginitis)
    - Subinvolution of placental sites
    - Transmissible venereal cell tumor (dog and bitch)

II. Systemic Disturbances
- A. Platelet deficiency or defect
  - Idiopathic bone marrow disease (tumor, fungal infiltration)
  - Drug-induced
  - Immune-associated (systemic lupus erythematosus, infection such as ehrlichiosis)
- B. Coagulation disorder
  - Congenital (hemophilia, von Willebrand's disease)
  - Acquired (warfarin or salicylate intoxication, disseminated intravenous coagulopathy)
- C. Other
  - Hypercatabolic states (fever, systemic infections)
  - Exercise
  - Heart failure and cardiomyopathy

and systemic infections), and miscellaneous disease states. This last group is rare in small animals and consists of chronic heart failure, exercise-induced hematuria, renal infarcts from cardiomyopathy and subacute bacterial endocarditis, and benign hematuria.

Genital disorders, especially prostatitis, may be associated with hematuria.

Diagnostic Approach

An overview of the approach to the patient with hematuria can be found in Table 32–2.

History. Historical findings may be difficult to elicit from the owner if the only problem is hematuria. Hematuria, in itself, is usually asymptomatic and the elimination habits of most small animals do not lend themselves to careful observation of urine color. Nevertheless, hematuria is frequently associated with other problems that a thorough and complete history is able to elicit. Information regarding the last normal voiding and the degree and consistency of hematuria should always be sought.

DYSURIA. Dysuria refers to any abnormality of urination: urgency, difficulty, or frequency (see the subsequent section on dysuria). Its presence, therefore, localizes pathology to the bladder, urethra, and genital structures. It is associated with discrete lesions (calculi, tumors) and infections of the lower urinary tract.

WEIGHT CHANGES. Weight loss may be associated with malignancy, chronic renal failure, or chronic infections. Weight gain may be seen in nephrotic syndrome (see Chapters 107 and 108) and is due primarily to third-space fluid (edema, ascites).

ABDOMINAL PAIN AND FEVER. Abdominal pain and fever may be described or documented by astute owners. A "hunched" stance, characteristic of renal pain, is occasionally associated with acute renal parenchymal disease. Prostatic pain may present with an ataxic gait. Signs associated with fever are panting, listlessness, and polydipsia (see Chapter 6). Moderate to severe fevers

TABLE 32–2. APPROACH TO THE EVALUATION OF HEMATURIA

1. Renal Loss
   - a. Microscopy of urinary sediment
     - + RBC casts
     - dystrophic erythrocytes
   - b. Hematologic evaluation
     - ± elevated creatinine, BUN
     - CBC–leukocytosis, anemia (usually regenerative)
   - c. Radiographic examination
     - Intravenous pyelogram (excretory urogram)–tumors, calculi, obstruction, polycystic disease
     - Arteriography
     - Ultrasonography
   - d. Evaluation if massive proteinuria is present–Quantitation of protein loss, protein electrophoresis, renal biopsy, ANA, LE prep
2. Lower Urinary Tract
   - a. Microscopy of urinary sediment
     - WBC, bacteria–inflammation, infection
     - Crystals–calculi
     - Cytology–tumor cells
     - Normal red cell morphology
   - b. Hematologic evaluation
     - Frequently unrewarding
     - + anemia (usually regenerative)
     - + leukocytosis (rare)
   - c. Radiographic evaluation
     - Survey and contrast studies
     - Ultrasonography
   - d. Cystoscopy–urethral lesions, calculi, tumors, diverticuli, bleeding
3. Systemic
   - a. Platelet count (thrombocytopenia)
     - Platelet function tests (thrombocytopathia)
   - b. Clotting profile–prothrombin time, partial thromboplastin time, activated clotting time (coagulopathies)
   - c. Von Willebrand's disease
   - d. Cardiac evaluation

are associated with infections, immune disorders, and neoplasia.

MISCELLANEOUS FACTORS. The history must also include thorough questioning of the owner regarding previous surgery, trauma, infection, dental care, or drug ingestion that may precipitate or cause hematuria (Table 32–1).

Breeds that are frequently associated with coagulation defects, especially von Willebrand's disease, may have previously been screened for the appropriate coagulopathy. If not previously done, this testing should be incorporated into the work-up.

Physical Findings. The physical examination should include a thorough evaluation of all organ systems, emphasizing those associated with hematuria.

SKIN AND MUCOUS MEMBRANES. The skin and mucous membranes should be examined for petechiation or hemorrhage suggestive of bleeding or vasculitic disorders. The *heart and lungs* should be evaluated for murmurs and rales, respectively, that may be associated with hematuria due to congestive heart failure. *Joint pain* (systemic lupus erythematosus) and *gait abnormalities* (prostatitis, acute renal disease) may provide valuable clues.

ABDOMINAL EXAMINATION. Abdominal examination must be particularly meticulous. Gentle palpation of the normal kidney should not elicit pain. In acute renal disease, the renal parenchyma swells and stretches Glisson's capsule, which contains nerve fibers specific for pain. The kidneys should be of normal *size*. Large, tender kidneys are associated with acute disease (acute pyelonephritis, acute glomerulonephritis); large, nonpainful kidneys are associated with chronic disease (hydronephrosis, amyloidosis, neoplasia, polycystic disease). Small kidneys, found only in chronic disease, are not often the source of hematuria. Kidney size, as evaluated from radiographs, should span approximately one to two lumbar vertebrae in small animals. The kidney should be regular in outline. Neoplasia, abscesses, and cysts may cause rough, irregularly shaped kidneys.

The *bladder* is the only part of the lower urinary tract that is easily palpated. It should be palpated and percussed to determine size and texture. Distention may be normal, indicate muscle atony, or be associated with impaired emptying (neurogenic obstruction). Expressing the bladder should be easy in the first two and difficult in the last. A small, firm bladder usually indicates inflammatory disorders such as cystitis. Calculi are often palpated as irregular, hard, mobile masses and may produce "crepitation" when moved against one another. Neoplasia gives rise to a firm, palpable mass that may be fixed or mobile.

RECTAL EXAMINATION. A rectal examination must be done on all male dogs to evaluate the prostate and on females to evaluate the uterus. This is most effective if done bimanually with abdominal palpation. The external genital organs should be examined for signs of trauma (bruising), infection (discharge), physical abnormalities (tumors, ulcers), and coagulopathy (petechiation).

OBSERVATION OF URINATION. One of the most important aspects of the physical examination is the *observation of urination* and the characterization of hematuria during micturition. Dysuria localizes the lesion to the lower urogenital system. Normal micturition supports a renal or systemic cause.

The location of blood in the urine stream implicates specific anatomic sources for the blood. Blood present only early in the urine stream implies urethral bleeding. If blood is found mainly in the final (end voiding) sample, this indicates bladder bleeding. Hematuria throughout the stream is found in renal hematuria. There are definite logistic problems in obtaining these data in veterinary medicine, and one must be cautious about overinterpreting them.

Laboratory Data. A careful *urinalysis* should be carried out. In order to evaluate the urine sediment appropriately, the urinalysis should be done promptly (less than 20 minutes) as casts deteriorate and contaminating bacteria multiply. Urine should be evaluated for the presence of significant proteinuria (glomerular origin renal disease). See Chapters 107 and 108 for the discussion of the assessment of proteinuria, for increased white blood cell numbers in excess of the number expected due to hematuria (cystitis, infections, neoplasia), for crystals (calculi, infections), and for casts (red blood cell - renal hematuria, white blood cell - pyelonephritis). Red cell morphology may differentiate lower urinary tract hematuria (normal red cells) from renal hematuria (dystrophic erythrocytes).

A *minimum data base* includes CBC, chemistry screen, and if the cause of hematuria is not immediately obvious (e.g., palpable cystic calculi), a coagulation profile should be added. The presence of leukocytosis suggests infection, immune disease, neoplasia, or marrow stimulation of other origin. An elevated serum creatinine or serum urea nitrogen level points to renal dysfunction if the animal is well-hydrated and if no obstruction is present. In patients with hypoalbuminemia concurrent with proteinuria, efforts should be directed toward evaluating and characterizing the protein loss (creatinine to protein ratio, 24-hour urine protein loss, protein electrophoresis of urine and serum, and renal biopsy). If the clinician suspects an immune disorder, then an ANA or LE prep is appropriate. Anemia is generally mild in hematuria unless there is a coagulation defect. Otherwise, it is a nonspecific feature associated with all forms of hematuria. Regenerative characteristics of the red cell line are to be expected.

Radiography and Other Techniques. If history, physical examination, and initial laboratory screens are unrewarding, or if the veterinarian needs to further investigate the specific cause at a given location, then *radiographic studies* are indicated. Survey radiographs (renal silhouette abnormalities, neoplasia, polycystic disease), intravenous urography (intravenous pyelograms [IVP] outline renal masses, nonlucent calculi, hydronephrosis), ultrasonography, arteriography, and computerized tomography can further delineate renal lesions as to specific location and probable cause (malignancy, abscess). Radiographic evaluation of the lower urogenital tract is much easier and may require only survey radiographs (radiopaque calculi, some tumors, prostatic lesions). Contrast studies, fluoroscopic voiding studies, and ultrasonography can localize and define lesions.

Cystoscopic examination permits direct visualization and biopsy of lesions.

Exploratory laparotomy is not usually rewarding if the primary location of the lesion is unknown. Tissue biopsies, correction of anatomic abnormalities, drainage of abscesses, and removal of stones are indications for surgery. Calculi that are removed should be analyzed (see Chapter 111).

Goals of Treatment

The etiologies of hematuria are varied to such a degree that once the diagnosis is made the reader should refer to the appropriate chapter on oncologic, immunologic, lower urinary tract, renal, genital, or coagulation disorders. There are two sequelae of hematuria that can be potentially life-threatening and should be described here.

Massive blood loss, although infrequent, may require transfusions (less than 15 per cent hematocrit) or fluid support. *Renal insufficiency or failure* may be associated with systemic coagulopathies, renal bleeding, primary renal disease, or obstructive disease of the lower urinary tract. Management of renal parenchymal dysfunction is reviewed in Chapter 108.

DYSURIA

Dysuria is defined as any abnormality related to urination and includes increased frequency (pollakiuria), urgency, hesitancy, and difficulty in urination (stranguria). It must be differentiated from two conditions that overlap in etiology and clinical signs. Many authors include both of the above as forms of dysuria. Because they are discussed elsewhere in this text, they will not be described in detail here.

Incontinence. Incontinence is defined as loss of voluntary control of micturition due to inappropriate or incomplete voiding and storage of urine. Hesitancy in starting or maintaining urination and straining to urinate may be associated with both incontinence and dysuria. Examples are reflex dyssynergia of the urethra, post-obstruction atonic bladder, neurologic dysfunction due to lumbosacral trauma (discussed in Chapters 30 and 31).

Polyuria. Polyuria is considered to be an increased volume of urine, which may or may not be associated with urgency and increased frequency. When it is associated, it may be confused with dysuria. Examples of conditions causing polyuria are diabetes mellitus and renal insufficiency (discussed in Chapter 29).

General Pathophysiology

A detailed description of the pathophysiology of micturition is presented in Chapters 30 and 31. The abnormalities of dysuria can be divided into two categories by the specific urination abnormality (Table 32–3).

Pollakiuria. Pollakiuria is an increase in frequency

TABLE 32–3. CAUSES OF DYSURIA

Associated with Pollakiuria/Urgency
Urinary tract infections
Cystitis (bacterial, viral–FUS, aspergillosis)
Urethritis (bacterial, viral)
Vaginitis, vulvitis (rare)
Bladder-Filling Disorders
Chronic interstitial cystitis
Neurogenic bladder
Cystic calculi
Associated with Stranguria
Enlarged prostate (prostatitis, prostatic neoplasia, cysts, hypertrophy, abscess)
Cystic or urethral calculi
Neurogenic bladder
Cystic uterus masculinus
Feline dysautonomia

with or without urgency, and is associated with decreased bladder capacity and compliance, or with increased pain on bladder distention. The mechanism responsible for the latter is not fully understood, but bladder and urethral irritation and inflammation are significant components of premature urination.

Stranguria. Stranguria is defined as difficulty in initiating or maintaining urine flow. In humans, this is frequently associated with pain. Conditions that may cause stranguria include urethral compression (enlarged prostate) and cystic calculi. Neurologic dysfunction must be eliminated as a cause of stranguria (see Chapters 30 and 31).

Lesions of the lower urinary tract are most frequently responsible for the signs of dysuria. Compression and distortion of the tract from other systems (gastrointestinal and genital) may occur.

Diagnostic Approach

History. The approach to defining the relevant history is similar to that described in hematuria. Because many of the etiologies of dysuria are recurrent, an additional history should emphasize diagnosis of previous episodes and their response to therapy.

The owner's chief complaint may often be misleading. Polyuria, constipation, and spraying are frequently confused with dysuria. A thorough, often imaginative, history-taking is required to confirm or appropriately describe an animal's condition. All descriptions should be confirmed by personal observation. Pollakiuria may be associated with urgency, hematuria, and inappropriate urination. There may be some straining after urination if bladder irritation is present. Urine volume may vary, but unless polyuria is present, urine volume is generally small. There may be a history of fever or lethargy if infection is the cause.

The hallmark of stranguria is straining. Hesitancy, marked by a delay between assuming the urination position and urination, is often present. The urine stream may be interrupted or weak.

Physical Examination. The overall health status of the animal should be reviewed. A neurologic examination (see Chapter 60) is essential to confirm appropriate innervation of the bladder and sphincter muscles (see Chapters 30 and 31). The essentials of the lower urinary tract examination were described in the previous section on hematuria. Specific attention should be paid to the following points in evaluating dysuria.

BLADDER SIZE. Small, firm bladders are palpated in conditions in which bladder irritation occurs. Pollakiuria and urgency are the clinical manifestations. Pain on palpation and hematuria are expected if cystitis or cystic calculi are present. Calculi often feel "gritty" on palpation. Large calculi may be palpated and may even distend the bladder.

Large, firm bladders that are difficult to express should be palpated with care. Outflow obstructions may cause significant bladder distention. These bladders may be necrotic and rupture easily on palpation. Stranguria, often with unproductive straining, is observed. A large, hard bladder may contain a stone; pollakiuria and hematuria are seen in such cases.

Enlarged, easily expressible bladders with a history of dribbling are associated with muscle atony or lower motor neuron disease. They may be seen after trauma (especially after pelvic trauma involving spinal nerves) or after an outflow obstruction has been relieved.

EXTERNAL GENITALIA. Signs of self-trauma, hemorrhage, sexual receptivity, or inappropriate discharge should be noted. If stranguria is present, a catheter should be passed through the urethra into the bladder. Obstruction and compressions of the urethra make passage difficult at the site of the lesion.

MICTURITION. If at all possible the animal should be observed during urination by a trained technician or a veterinarian. The events recorded by the owner in the history should be supported or refined.

Laboratory Data. *Urinalysis*, including careful evaluation of urine sediment, may show *hematuria*, which may occur in the presence of calculi, tumors, cystitis, or it may show *pyuria* (leukocytes in large numbers imply an infectious or inflammatory etiology). Pyuria in the absence of bacteria indicates inflammatory lesions or nonbacterial infections (viral, fungal).

Bacteria may be seen in voided urine in normal animals because of contamination from the prepuce or vulva, or in normal urine that has stood unrefrigerated. Urine for evaluation of infection should be obtained by cystocentesis or catheterization. Urine with pathologic bacteriuria should be Gram stained, if possible, and cultured. A positive culture confirms the diagnosis of bacterial infection and provides antimicrobial sensitivity.

Casts and massive proteinuria are atypical in dysuric patients and imply a renal component to the problem, for example, an ascending infection from an infected bladder.

Crystals may help to identify stones if present (see Chapters 110 to 112). They may also be normal components of urine or canine urolithiasis present during infections.

Neoplastic cells may be present in urine sediment. *Hematology and chemistry screens* are useful only for indicating systemic infection and renal function.

Survey radiographs are unremarkable unless gross neoplasia, prostatic disease, or radiopaque stones are present. Contrast radiology, including intravenous pyelography, double contrast cystography, retrograde urethrocystography, and positive contrast vaginourethrography, can show radiolucent stones, tumors, ectopic ureters, and overdistended bladder. Ultrasonography and computerized tomography generally do not provide much additional information.

Direct visualization of the urethra and bladder (cystourethroscopy), voiding cystourethrography, and cystometric studies are done at referral centers. These studies are most useful for definition of dysfunctional voiding and for biopsy for pathologic diagnosis of lower urinary tract lesions.

Goals of Treatment

Treatment regimens for specific diagnoses are described in detail in the appropriate chapters. Measures must be taken to prevent some of the untoward sequelae of dysuria as they may create severe and irreversible damage.

Detrussor Atony. Acute or chronic bladder distention can be caused by partial or full obstruction. Atony is seen clinically as incontinence that may persist after therapy of the primary disorder. Prevention includes decreasing bladder size and preventing overdistention by frequent catheterizations or bladder expressions.

Urinary Tract Infection. Malposition of the bladder, outflow obstructions, and ectopic ureters can lead to cystitis, urethritis, and pyelonephritis. If the initiating cause is reversed early, the prognosis is good. Cultures and sensitivities of the urine allow for optimal efficacy of antibiotic choice. If the initiating cause is not reversed, or if pyelonephritis is present, long-term antibiotic therapy (months) may be required.

33 LAMENESS IN DOGS

J. FRANCOIS BARDET

Lameness is an indication of a structural or functional disorder in one or more limbs. The term lameness signifies some alteration in the quality of movement during progression but must be extended to include the quality of stance. Lameness is divided into weightbearing lameness and nonweightbearing lameness. A weightbearing lameness is one in which the dog may place the limb and attempt to bear weight on his leg. A nonweightbearing lameness is one in which the dog may advance the limb but refuses to bear weight on it.

A complete assessment of history, a thorough and organized examination, and some ancillary tests are mandatory to an accurate diagnosis of lameness.

PATHOPHYSIOLOGY

Many disease states at some point produce symptoms of lameness. Table 33–1 lists the diseases and causes of lameness recognized in dogs. This chapter discusses the general causal mechanisms of lameness and presents an outline of concepts regarding the clinical diagnosis. The reader is referred to the appropriate chapters for further reading.

Most lameness is pain-related. Other forms are associated with mechanical, metabolic, and neurologic disorders. Pain may be cutaneous or deep. *Cutaneous pain*, caused by superficial injury, is induced by the release of bradykinin, serotonin, histamine, and prostaglandins. The intensity of *deep pain* appears to be related to the density of the innervation of the involved area. The periosteum has the densest nerve supply of the deep tissues and therefore has the lowest pain threshold, followed by the joint capsule, tendon, fascia, and muscle body. Most deep pain is secondary to tissue trauma causing structural alterations, edema, and signs of inflammation. Circulatory obstruction to a tissue, ischemia, and increased metabolism of an area are responsible for other types of deep pain.

A *mechanical lameness* results from an abnormal limb conformation such as shortening, angulation, rotational abnormalities, or from an abnormal joint motion seen with muscle contracture and myositis.

TABLE 33–1. CAUSES OF LAMENESS IN DOGS

CONGENITAL DISORDERS	Radial agenesis Ectrodactyly; syndactyly Chondrodysplasia Congenital hyperextension of the stifle Vertebral abnormalities Spina bifida
DEGENERATIVE DISORDERS	Degenerative joint disease Degenerative myelopathy
DEVELOPMENTAL DISORDERS	Physeal disorders Limb shortening Congenital elbow luxation Osteochondrosis Hip dysplasia Patellar luxation Legg-Perthes disease
GENETIC DISORDERS	Hemophilic arthropathy Mucopolysaccharidosis Periarticular calcinosis
INFECTIOUS DISORDERS	Bacterial, viral, fungal, mycoplasmal and protozoal arthritis Bacterial and fungal osteomyelitis Infectious polymyositis Cellulitis and soft tissue abscess Bacterial or mycotic granulomas of the footpads
IMMUNOLOGIC DISORDERS	Canine rheumatoid arthritis Idiopathic nondeforming polyarthritis Systemic lupus erythematosus Pemphigus of the footpads Polyneuropathies
METABOLIC DISORDERS	Hyperparathyroid bone diseases Rickets Osteomalacia Polymyopathies Polyneuropathies
NEOPLASIA	Bone: primary and secondary Synovium Spinal cord Nerve roots and peripheral nerves Connective tissues of a limb
TRAUMATIC DISORDERS	Fracture Luxation Contusion Strain Sprain Muscular contusion, laceration, rupture, and contracture Tendinous laceration avulsion Traumatic neuropathy Intervertebral disc herniation
VASCULAR DISORDERS	Fibrocartilaginous infarct of the spinal cord Bone infarct
UNKNOWN ETIOLOGY	Panosteitis Multiple cartilaginous exostoses Myositis ossificans Hypertrophic osteodystrophy
OTHERS	Bone cyst Hypertrophic osteoarthropathy

Signs of *weakness* are often confused with lameness. A discussion of weakness disorders may be found in Chapter 11. The causes and significance of *paraplegia, paraparesis, ataxia* of the rear limbs and *paresis or paralysis of one limb* may be found in Chapters 13, 60, 62, 64, and 65.

EVALUATION OF THE LAME DOG

MINIMUM DATA BASE

History. The history of the patient should precede any physical examination. The medical and surgical background, activity level of the dog, diet, and chronology of the lameness should be obtained. The acuteness of onset, progression of the lameness, and duration or shifting of the condition are critical. Acute and major lameness tend to be constant while chronic lameness due primarily to degenerative joint disease often worsens with exercise and following periods of rest. Peripheral nerve tumors cause unilateral progressive lameness, unresponsive to medical therapy.

Signalment. The age, sex, breed, and size of the lame patient are extremely important in establishing a diagnosis and selecting the appropriate therapy. Immature dogs in small breeds are more commonly affected by Legg-Perthes disease and patellar luxation. Osteochondritis dissecans, ununited anconeal process, fragmented coronoid process, hip dysplasia, avulsion of the long digital extensor, panosteitis, and hypertrophic osteodystrophy are seen most often in immature dogs of large and giant breeds.

Physical Examination, Blood, and Urine Analyses. While very few causes of lameness are part of generalized diseases, a complete physical examination should be performed and the dog should have a complete blood count and a urine analysis.

Orthopedic Examination. The goal of an orthopedic examination is to localize the cause(s) of lameness. The examination must be thorough and systematic and the clinician should not focus only on the main complaint and overlook other problems. The clinician should first observe the patient and then proceed to a local examination.

OBSERVATION. The dog is observed in a normal standing position at rest. The conformation and posture, signs of atrophy, swelling, and gait should be noted.

CONFORMATION AND POSTURE. Conformation is the shape of the animal that is dictated by inherited characteristics of the skeleton. Acquired changes in shape resulting from disease are usually reversible when associated with changes in stance or posture. In a normal stance, the dog bears 60 per cent of its weight on its front limbs. When severe pathologic problems develop in the hind limbs, such as painful hip dysplasia, the dog shifts its center of gravity as far forward as possible and may carry up to 90 per cent of its weight on its forelimbs. When evaluating posture, the general appearance of the limb may give an indication of the problem. Special characteristics of the posture may be referable to specific orthopedic problems, although not pathognomonic (Table 33–2).

MUSCLE ATROPHY AND EDEMA. Marked muscle atrophy is indicative of chronic painful conditions such as an old ruptured cranial cruciate ligament. Localized edema of one extremity may be caused by inflammation and/or infection, trauma, and venous or lymphatic obstruction.

GAIT. The dog is observed when walking on a leash and at a slow trot from the front, side, and rear. In a weightbearing lameness the dog shifts his weight away from the affected limb and therefore extends the stance phase of a stride on the sound limb. The stride of the affected limb is usually shortened as compared to the opposite, normal limb. Lesions of the shoulder and hip may result in a markedly shortened stride, as these joints have the greatest range of motion. Normal gait requires use of almost the entire nervous system. A disturbance of gait may be either sensory or motor. Sensory disturbances causing abnormalities in gait are seen clinically as ataxia of one, two, or all four limbs. Motor disturbances of gait may be voluntary motor disturbances, causing paresis or paralysis of one, two, or four limbs. With mild neurologic dysfunction, the clinical signs may suggest lameness, or pain from musculoskeletal disease. Neurologic types of lameness may be regional, affecting either the front legs (intervertebral disc disease and cervical myelopathy) and/or the rear legs (degenerative myelopathy, intervertebral disc disease, tumor, cauda equina syndrome). Paresis or paralysis of one limb suggests fibrocartilaginous infarction of the spinal cord, traumatic neuropathy, or peripheral nerve neoplasia. Finally, stiffness and a short and choppy gait may indicate focal or multifocal myopathy. The dog may be lame because of pain or lack of proper mobility of the limb(s). Congenital, traumatic, endocrine, infectious, and idiopathic causes of myopathies should also be suspected.

TABLE 33–2. CHARACTERISTIC POSTURAL ABNORMALITIES

Gait Abnormality	Characteristic of
Circumduction of the forelimb	Infraspinatus contracture
Adduction, external rotation of hindlimb	Coxofemoral luxation
Hyperextension of the hock	Hip dysplasia, OCD of tarsus
Dropped hock	Achilles tendon rupture, calcaneal fracture
"Winging" (abduction) of elbow	Ununited anconeal process
Abduction, external rotation of the forelimb	Elbow luxation
Weightbearing with partial flexion of stifle	Patellar luxation
Dropped carpus	Rupture of deep flexor tendons

From Arnoczky, S. P., and Tarwin, G. B.: Physical examination of the musculoskeletal system. Vet. Clin. North Am. *3*:575, 1981.

SUMMARY. The objective of observation is to localize the most probable site of lameness. A thorough local examination must always be conducted in spite of an obvious lesion.

LOCAL EXAMINATION. Once the affected limb(s) is identified, a thorough examination of the affected limb(s) is necessary to further localize the problem. The examination must be systematic, starting at one end of the limb and proceeding in an orderly, step-by-step fashion. Each portion of the limb is palpated as gently as possible without tranquilization until the painful area is located. Each joint is isolated and flexed, extended and rotated through the entire range of motion while feeling for pain, restriction of motion, instability, swelling, crepitus, and proper relationship. Signs of pain elicited by hyperextension or hyperflexion of a joint is the most reliable test of joint disease although not pathognomonic of any disorder. Abnormal laxity may

TABLE 33–3. DIAGNOSTIC APPROACH TO THE EVALUATION OF LAMENESS IN DOGS

MINIMUM DATA BASE	
1. History	Acuteness, progression, duration of lameness Influence of exercise
2. Signalment	Age, sex, breed, size of the patient
3. Physical examination	
Body temperature	R/O infection, sepsis, abscess, cellulitis Acute osteomyelitis and septic arthritis Immune-mediated polyarthritis
Cardiac auscultation	R/O causes of weakness
Neurologic examination	R/O tetraparesis, paraparesis, monoparesis
Other major functions	
ORTHOPEDIC EXAMINATION	
1. Observation	Helps localize probable site of lameness
Comformation and posture	R/O hyperextension, hyperflexion of joint, torsional and rotational abnormality, limb length
Muscle atrophy	R/O chronic causes of lameness
Gait	Number of affected limbs Nonweightbearing lameness: fracture, luxation, septic arthritis versus weightbearing lameness
2. Local examination	
Joints	R/O luxation, fracture, sprain, degenerative joint disease, septic arthritis, mass lesions
Bones	R/O fracture, mass lesions, pain
Tendons, muscles, soft tissues	R/O infection, laceration, mass lesions
Foot	R/O infection, laceration, abrasion, foreign body, tumors
ANCILLARY DIAGNOSTICS	
1. Radiographs	R/O fracture, luxation, nonunion tumor, osteomyelitis, degenerative joint disease, OCD, panosteitis, multiple cartilaginous exostosis, hypertrophic osteodystrophy, bone cyst, myositis ossificans
2. Bacterial and fungal cultures	R/O septic disorders
3. Arthrocentesis and synovial fluid analyses	R/O inflammatory vs noninflammatory disorders Septic vs nonseptic disorders
4. Arthrotomy and/or exploratory surgery and biopsy	R/O tumors, tissue of unknown origin
5. Synovial biopsy	R/O nonseptic inflammatory polyarthritis, protozoal arthritis, bacterial infection
6. Electromyographic studies	Help evaluate neurologic causes of lameness
7. Arthroscopy	R/O evaluate cartilage, ligament, menisci, joint capsule

be indicative of ligamentous injury. Laxity medially or laterally suggests insufficiency of the medial or lateral collateral ligaments. Increased rotatory movements are also indicative of laxity of the collateral ligaments and joint capsule. Restricted or excessive movements, crepitus, pain, and abnormal relationship of bony structures are the hallmarks of fracture and luxation. A hot, swollen joint with synovial effusion indicates inflammation, possibly of an infectious origin. The bones are palpated deeply for thickening or pain. Large muscle groups commonly atrophy following prolonged lameness. Local muscle tenderness, swelling, and subcutaneous ecchymosis suggest partial or complete muscle rupture. Finally, all soft tissues should be examined and palpated for wounds, draining tracts, heat, swelling, and pain.

Ancillary Diagnostics. Certain diagnostic procedures are used routinely in the evaluation of the lame patient. Radiographic examination, bacterial and fungal cultures, arthrocentesis examination of the joint fluid, arthrotomy, and biopsy are commonly performed in dogs. Other procedures such as immune profiles, synovial membrane biopsy, and electromyographic studies are done less frequently. More involved procedures such as arthroscopy can be performed if the patient is referred to an orthopedic surgeon.

Radiography. Once the affected bone and/or joint is localized, the area should be radiographed if bony lesions are suspected or must be ruled out. Radiographic examinations often require adequate sedation to obtain the necessary positioning of the animal. True caudal and lateral views are the minimum necessary for diagnostic evaluation. Often multiple oblique views are also necessary to demonstrate the lesion.

Bacterial and fungal cultures. Aerobic and anaerobic cultures are more useful in the selection of a proper antibiotic than in making a diagnosis. They are commonly carried out in open fractures, osteomyelitis, septic arthritis, and extensive soft tissue injuries of a limb. Blood culture should be taken in septic patients suspected of having hematogenous osteomyelitis or arthritis. Mycoplasmal and fungal arthritis and osteomyelitis, although infrequent, can be diagnosed by appropriate cultures.

Arthrocentesis and synovial fluid analyses. Arthrocentesis should be performed whenever joint effusion is present. The color, viscosity, mucin clot test, and cytologic and bacterial analyses may identify etiologic factors and characterize the joint fluid as inflammatory or noninflammatory and septic or nonseptic.

Arthrotomy, exploratory surgery, and biopsy. Arthrotomy may be indicated to identify intra-articular lesions such as a partial tear of the cranial cruciate ligament or for a synovial biopsy. Exploratory surgery may be performed for any unidentified mass and chronic draining tracts. Biopsy samples are routinely taken from tumors and any abnormal tissue.

Immune tests. Immune tests such as rheumatoid factor, LE preparation, ANA titer, and Coombs' test often provide helpful diagnostic information in animals with immune-mediated polyarthritis.

Synovial membrane biopsy. A synovial membrane biopsy is a useful diagnostic tool in the detection of nonseptic inflammatory polyarthritis as well as with protozoal arthritis (*Leishmania donovani*). The biopsy can also be cultured for microbial infection.

Electromyographic studies. Electromyographic studies help to differentiate neurologic and orthopedic causes of lameness. The muscles of the hindlimbs and forelimbs may be individually examined to evaluate the health of the muscles themselves, the peripheral nerves of the lumbosacral or brachial plexus, and the nerve roots from spinal cord segments L4 to S2 and C6 to T2. The details of such studies are discussed in Chapter 62.

Arthroscopy. Arthroscopy provides an effective diagnostic technique with minimum invasiveness and tissue morbidity, and it permits rapid postoperative recovery. Future clinical applications of arthroscopy in dogs include diagnosis and curettage of osteochondritis dissecans lesions of the humeral head and femoral condyle, biopsy of synovial membrane, diagnosis of tears in ligaments, tendons, or joint capsule and visualization, retrieval, and removal of the free bodies in joints. Table 33–3 summarizes a diagnostic approach to the evaluation of lameness in dogs.

34 LAMENESS IN CATS

J. FRANCOIS BARDET

Cats have many fewer orthopedic problems than dogs, with the exception of those caused by trauma. Some of the problems are so rare that they have no clinical significance. The anatomy of the domestic cat's locomotor system has changed little from that of its ancestors, which may explain the low incidence of orthopedic diseases. However, lesions of the musculoskeletal system are possible in cats. The diagnosis of lameness in cats does not differ from that of dogs. Only characteristics specific to the feline patient are given in this chapter. The reader should refer to Chapter 33 for the general discussion of lameness.

PATHOPHYSIOLOGY

The pathophysiologic mechanisms of lameness in cats are identical to those in dogs. Table 34–1 lists the diseases and causes of lameness recognized in cats.

Congenital Disorders. Only a few reports of congenital disorders in cats have appeared in the veterinary literature. Radial or tibial agenesis and congenital hyperextension of the stifle may be recognized early as angular deformities of the affected limbs.

Longitudinal splitting of the extremities (ectrodactyly), presence of one or more extra digits (polydactyly), and bony and/or tissue fusion of two digits (syndactyly) may cause only slight dysfunction. Spina bifida is most common in Manx cats; kittens are presented for chronic paraparesis, constipation, and fecal and urinary incontinence. Most cases are presented with bilateral, exaggerated flexion of the hocks, giving the cat a rabbit-like stance.

Degenerative Disorders. Although uncommon in cats, degenerative joint disease (DJD) may affect any joint. The majority of cases of DJD that occur in cats are the result of a traumatic condition such as articular fractures or ligament instability. DJD resulting from hip dysplasia may have no clinical significance. The reader is referred to Chapter 62 for a discussion of degenerative myelopathy in cats.

Developmental Disorders. Angular, torsional, and rotational abnormalities and limb shortening resulting from physeal disorders are exceptional causes of lameness in cats. Although patellar luxation is not rare in cats, few animals exhibit signs of lameness.

Genetic Disorders. Mucopolysaccharidosis results from inborn errors of aminoglycoside metabolism. Affected cats are often presented for lameness associated with epiphyseal dysplasia of the long bones, osteoarthritis of major joints, severe hip dysplasia, and spinal deformities. This disorder is also characterized by growth retardation, corneal clouding, and hepatosplenomegaly. Cats may exhibit signs of spinal or cerebral dysfunction. Mucopolysaccharidosis should be differentiated from hypervitaminosis A.

Infection. Infection is an important cause of lameness in cats. Many disorders are associated with fever, leukocytosis, and pain. The physical examination and joint fluid analysis usually identifies the nature of the problem.

Immunologic Disorders. Two clinically recognizable forms of feline polyarthritis have been described: the more common periosteal proliferative form and a deforming type that resembles rheumatoid arthritis. The periosteal-proliferative type tends to occur in younger cats. Initial clinical signs include fever, generalized stiffness, lameness, swollen joints, and periarticular edema. After several weeks, periosteal proliferation occurs, sometimes resulting in palpable exostoses around the joints. The less common, deforming type tends to occur in older cats. The clinical signs of this form include a slowly developing lameness and stiffness, joint instabilities with luxations, and subluxations of distal joints. The arthritis of feline systemic lupus erythematosus (SLE) is a nonerosive arthritis. Serologic abnormalities are the sole basis for classifying the condition as SLE.

Metabolic Disorders. Hypervitaminosis A and primary or secondary hyperparathyroidism often result in lameness. Hypervitaminosis A in cats is also associated with lethargy, anorexia, neck stiffness, and evidence of spinal exostoses. In young cats, bone growth may be severely retarded, while bony exostoses are the predominant lesions in mature animals. There is a subperiosteal proliferation of new woven bone around the joints. The process can bridge the joint. It may be confused with degenerative joint disease. Lameness resulting from primary or secondary hyperparathyroidism results from bone pain and pathologic fractures. Kittens fed exclu-

TABLE 34–1. CAUSES OF LAMENESS IN CATS

CONGENITAL DISORDERS
Radial and tibial agenesis
Ectrodactyly
Polydactyly
Syndactyly
Congenital hyperextension of the stifle
Spina bifida
DEGENERATIVE DISORDERS
Degenerative joint disease
Degenerative myelopathy
DEVELOPMENTAL DISORDERS
Physeal disorders
Limb shortening
Hip dysplasia
Patellar luxation
GENETIC DISORDERS
Mucopolysaccharidosis
INFECTIOUS DISORDERS
Bacterial, viral, fungal, and mycoplasmal arthritis
Bacterial and fungal osteomyelitis
Infectious myositis
Cellulitis and soft tissue abscess
Feline osteochondromatosis
IMMUNOLOGIC DISORDERS
Feline progressive polyarthritis
Feline chronic progressive polyarthritis
Systemic lupus erythematosus
METABOLIC DISORDERS
Hypervitaminosis A
Hyperparathyroid bone diseases
Primary or secondary
NEOPLASIA
Bone
Synovium
Connective tissue of a limb
Spinal cord
TRAUMATIC DISORDERS
Fracture
Luxation
Contusion
Strain
Sprain
Intrameniscal calcification
Muscular contusion, laceration, rupture, and contracture
Tendinous laceration, avulsion
Traumatic neuropathy
Intervertebral disc herniation
VASCULAR DISORDERS
Thromboembolism of caudal aorta and/or its branches
Necrotizing myelopathy
UNKNOWN ETIOLOGY
Fibrodysplasia ossificans
OTHERS
Hypertrophic osteoarthropathy

sively on meat become orthopedically demineralized. The cat may refuse to walk. Chronic constipation and retention of urine are the result of pelvic obstruction due to fracture and abnormal healing of the pelvic canal.

Neoplasia. Neoplasia is frequently associated with lameness as a result of a destructive or obstructive mass. Any tumor of the musculoskeletal tissues, spinal cord, nerve roots, or peripheral nerve may result in lameness.

Traumatic Disorders. Traumatic disorders include a broad category of disease states that produce lameness. Most orthopedic cases are traumatic, caused by falls, automobile accidents, dog bites, and cat fights. The physical and local orthopedic examination and radiographs help to differentiate the traumatic causes of lameness.

Vascular Disorders. The clinical signs associated with aortic thromboembolism vary with the location of the embolus. Brachial artery embolization causes forelimb paresis and pain. Aortic thromboembolism is one of the most common causes of hindlimb paresis in cats. The clinical signs of an embolus at the aortic trifurcation are the "five Ps:" pain, paresis, pulselessness, poikilothermy, and pallor. The severity of pelvic dysfunction is associated with the extent of vascular obstruction. Some cats present with unilateral paresis or with a slight neurologic deficit in both pelvic limbs. With complete obstruction, cats are paralyzed and in severe pain (see Chapters 77 and 81).

The clinical signs and significance of necrotizing myelopathy in cats may be found in Chapter 62.

Unknown Etiology. Fibrodysplasia ossificans, known as generalized myositis ossificans, is a rare musculoskeletal disorder. It manifests clinically as a progressive alteration of gait over periods of weeks to several months. The cat is stiff and awkward in its movements and may cry out in pain when attempting to walk. The affected muscles are swollen and firm. Fibrodysplasia ossificans is a non-neoplastic form of heterotopic ossification that affects connective tissue and skeletal muscle. The disease appears as a defect of fibroblasts in collagenous connective tissue. Treatment is palliative and is often ineffective.

Hypertrophic osteoarthropathy was described in a cat. There were firm massive swellings of the forelimbs from the proximal humerus to the carpus. Periosteal proliferation was most prominent in the forelimbs and stopped at the carpus and tarsus. There was an associated large benign thoracic thymoma.

EVALUATION OF THE LAME CAT

The minimum data base required for the study of lameness in cats includes a complete historical evaluation, signalment, physical examination, complete blood count, and urine analysis.

Orthopedic Examination. As in dogs, observation and local examination are mandatory in order to localize the cause or causes of lameness in cats.

Observation. Cats are difficult patients to observe in a standing position as they tend to lie on the examination table. Their small size and stealthy nature make the observation of conformation, posture, and signs of atrophy or swelling difficult. Since cats are not used to being walked on a leash, it may be useful to leave them in the center of the examination room. They will generally walk to get to a corner or their box. The clinician may have to repeat this to determine the abnormal leg or gait abnormality. Some patients refuse to move. In that instance, the clinician refers to the chief complaint expressed by the owner and proceeds to a local examination.

Local Examination. Each position of the limb is palpated as gently as possible. Each joint is isolated, flexed, extended, and rotated throughout the entire range of motion. Bones, muscles, and tendons are individually palpated. The local examination helps in localizing the painful area. Since this examination is the same as that for dogs, the reader should refer to Chapter 33.

Ancillary Diagnostics. Diagnostic procedures used in the evaluation of lameness in cats are described in Chapter 33.

35 CARDIOPULMONARY ARREST AND RESUSCITATION

WAYNE E. WINGFIELD and ROSEMARY A. HENIK

Cardiopulmonary arrest (CPA) is a sudden and unexpected cessation of ventilation and effective circulation that results in a loss of consciousness and requires emergency intervention to avoid a fatal outcome. CPA may occur as a result of either primary cardiac or primary respiratory dysfunction, or secondary to abnormalities that lead to circulatory and ventilatory impairment.

RECOGNITION OF CARDIOPULMONARY ARREST

PATIENTS AT RISK

Cardiopulmonary arrest in the small animal patient occurs infrequently. The prevalence rate of CPA is 0.46 per cent of cats and 0.45 per cent of dogs presented for examination at the Colorado State University Veterinary Teaching Hospital (CSU VTH).

Primary respiratory arrest is associated with a higher resuscitation rate than primary cardiac arrest. CPA is associated with a poor chance for long-term survival in veterinary medicine. A major reason for unsuccessful resuscitation is a delay in the diagnosis of CPA and a subsequent delay in therapy. The small animal patient often has multiple medical abnormalities prior to the arrest, including traumatic injuries and systemic disease processes. A study of CPA in cats and dogs at CSU VTH shows that the most common etiology of CPA in cats is trauma, while primary respiratory disease is the most common etiology of CPA in dogs.

Any clinical condition that ultimately leads to cellular hypoxia predisposes the patient to CPA. This can include either primary cardiac disease resulting from inadequate cardiac output and peripheral vasoconstriction or primary pulmonary pathology leading to ventilation-perfusion imbalance, shunting, or a diffusion barrier at the level of the alveoli. Other factors that may cause tissue hypoxia include airway obstruction, hypoventilation, a decreased concentration of inspired oxygen, anemia, and peripheral vasoconstriction secondary to shock.

Vagal stimulation in a healthy animal does not induce a cardiac arrest; however, in the face of hypoxia, hypercarbia, or hyperkalemia, it can precipitate ventricular asystole. Common procedures that stimulate the vagus nerve include the following: surgical manipulation of abdominal, thoracic, and cervical tissues, ophthalmic procedures, proctoscopic examination, endotracheal intubation and extubation, and tracheal suction.

Acid-base and electrolyte imbalances predispose an animal to CPA. Hypoxia, hypercarbia, and acidemia stimulate the release of catecholamines, which increase cardiac automaticity and metabolic rate. The resulting sinus tachycardia leads to ventricular tachycardia or fibrillation in the presence of metabolic abnormalities. Acidemia lowers the fibrillation threshold of the myocardium.

Pre-anesthetic and anesthetic agents decrease cardiorespiratory function and may induce CPA. Certain anesthetic agents sensitize the myocardium to circulating catecholamines and precipitate the development of ventricular arrhythmias. CPA is also triggered indirectly through brain stem stimulation (i.e., head trauma) or directly by myocardial irritation (i.e., myocardial contusions, cardiac catheterization, electrical shock, or cardiac surgery).

CLINICAL SIGNS OF CARDIOPULMONARY ARREST

The most crucial factor in determining the success of resuscitation is the *time interval* between onset and diagnosis of CPA. Early warning signs of impending CPA include changes in respiration, cyanosis, hypotension, and a weak, irregular pulse. CPA may be preceded by a change in atrioventricular or intraventricular conduction patterns or an unexplained change in the level of anesthesia. *Hypothermia* (rectal temperature less than 100°F (37.8°C)) was noted in 80 per cent of cats and 34 per cent of dogs prior to the onset of arrest in a study at the CSU VTH and may be a good indicator of circulatory failure and impending arrest.

Obvious signs of CPA include *cyanosis* (present when reduced hemoglobin exceeds 5 gm/deciliter of whole blood), the *absence of ventilations*, or the *absence of a palpable pulse*. A peripheral pulse is absent in the dog once the systolic pressure falls below 60 torr. Heart sounds in the dog cease at 50 torr systolic pressure. The absence of heart sounds may indicate inadequate cardiac output, not necessarily cardiac arrest.

Pupillary dilatation begins within 20 seconds of circulatory arrest, and is maximal by 45 seconds. Knowledge of prior drug administration is necessary to evaluate pupil size during cardiopulmonary resuscitation (CPR). Administration of ganglionic-blocking agents, epinephrine, or atropine may lead to dilation of the pupils. Pupillary dilatation is not a reflection of irreversible neurologic damage; pupillary size must be interpreted as an indicator of effective therapy rather than as an indicator of when to abandon resuscitative efforts. The constriction of the pupils in closed chest CPR in dogs nearly always predicts effective CPR technique and survival is more likely.

The electroencephalogram begins to show changes within 20 seconds of arrest, and is isoelectric by 30 seconds. Capillary refill time is a poor indicator of the circulatory status of the animal. Normal refill has been observed up to 30 minutes after the heart has stopped.

Electrocardiography of Arrest Patients

The animal requiring resuscitative therapy will have one of several electrocardiographic patterns. *Ventricular asystole, electromechanical dissociation (EMD), ventricular fibrillation*, or *severe brady-* or *tachyarrhythmias* all lead to an inadequate cardiac output and necessitate immediate intervention.

Ventricular Asystole. Ventricular asystole is characterized by the absence of both electrical and mechanical activity from the ventricles. Electrocardiographically, it appears as a straight line, or as P waves without QRS complexes (Figure 35–1).

Ventricular asystole may occur as the end result of ventricular fibrillation, EMD, or heart block. It is usually the result of extensive myocardial ischemia from prolonged periods of inadequate coronary perfusion. Other abnormalities, such as severe hyperkalemia, severe pre-existing acidosis, or high parasympathetic tone, may also contribute to the development of asystole. In the presence of ventricular asystole, the prognosis for resuscitation is poor.

Electromechanical Dissociation. Electromechanical dissociation (Figure 35–2) is the continuation of organized electrical impulses after mechanical cardiac activity has ceased. The pathophysiology of EMD is unknown, but probably represents a failure of myocardial contractility resulting from the depletion of myocardial high energy phosphate compounds, in part due to inadequate myocardial perfusion. EMD carries a grave prognosis. It is important to recognize that hypoxemia, severe acidosis, pericardial tamponade, tension pneumothorax, hypovolemia, vagotonia, and pulmonary embolus can induce EMD. Thus, a search for correctable causes is mandated. Be aware that EMD may lead to the erroneous conclusion that therapy is effective and that cardiac function is returning.

Ventricular Fibrillation. Ventricular fibrillation is characterized by irregular and disorganized ventricular activity that results in an immediate cessation of effective cardiac output (Figure 35–3). Fibrillation may develop as a result of a single ectopic focus that rapidly discharges, or through a re-entrant excitation pathway. The process of re-entrant excitation is often termed "circus movement" due to the circling pathway of the depolarizing wave. A premature beat arriving during the "vulnerable period" of the cardiac cycle (when ventricular cells are repolarized to various degrees), sometimes called "R on T," may trigger an abnormal depolarization pathway and lead to ventricular fibrillation. Depolarization waves creating large re-entrant circuits are seen electrocardiographically as "coarse" fibrillation, while smaller depolarization pathways produce "fine" fibrillation waves, and may eventually be seen as ventricular asystole. Early experiments showed that a critical myocardial mass (greater than 4 cm^2) is necessary to sustain fibrillation. This phenomenon explains why ventricular fibrillation occurs more commonly in larger animals, and why smaller animals, such as cats, may spontaneously revert to normal sinus rhythm. Ventricular fibrillation increases myocardial oxygen demands three to five times above resting values, as it simulates sustained systole, and therefore impedes coronary blood flow and myocardial oxygen delivery.

Arrhythmias. Cardiovascular collapse may occur during any episode of brady- or tachyarrhythmias, necessitating resuscitative efforts. Bradycardia may result in

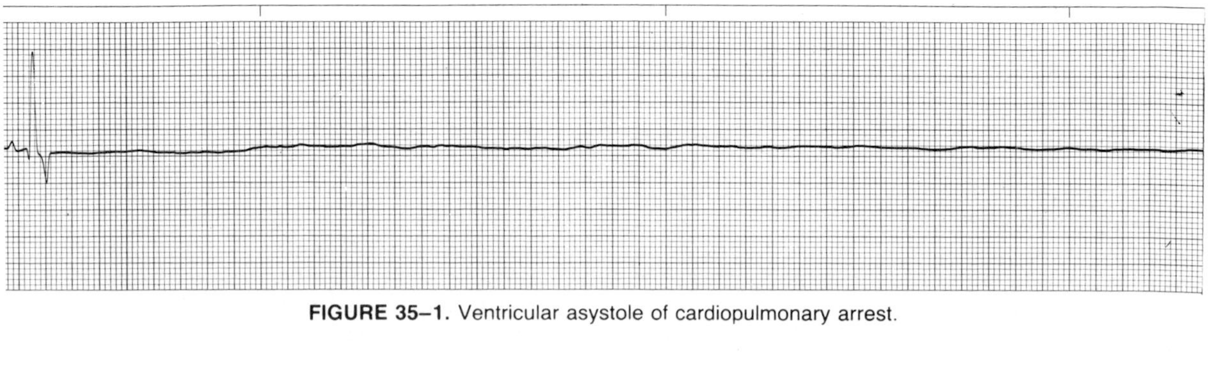

FIGURE 35–1. Ventricular asystole of cardiopulmonary arrest.

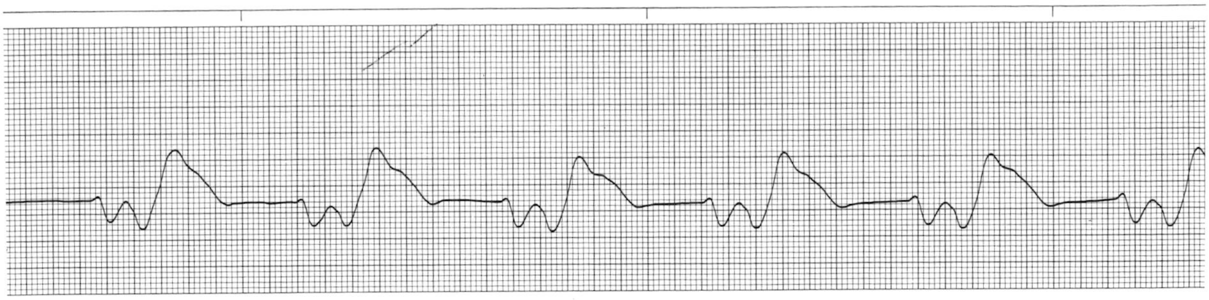

FIGURE 35–2. Electromechanical dissociation of cardiopulmonary arrest. Note the bizarre electrocardiographic pattern with indistinguishable P-QRS-T complexes.

inadequate cardiac output and peripheral oxygen delivery, while tachycardia prevents adequate diastolic filling of the ventricles and cardiac output falls secondarily.

Common ventricular arrhythmias include frequent ventricular premature contractions, multifocal premature ventricular contractions, ventricular tachycardia, atrioventricular dissociation and ventricular flutter. In veterinary medicine, many of these arrhythmias occur as sequelae to diseases of organs other than the heart. It is imperative to attempt to find the cause and provide appropriate therapy.

Other tachyarrhythmias predisposing to CPA include atrial fibrillation in congestive cardiomyopathy, atrial tachycardia, extreme sinus tachycardia, and, occasionally, junctional tachycardia. Again, recognition of the cause of the arrhythmia and appropriate treatment may avert development of CPA.

Bradycardias that become symptomatic include sinus bradycardia, sinus arrest, sinus block, junctional blocks, and third degree AV block. Rarely is a cause for these arrhythmias identified and therefore, therapy is directed to increasing heart rate and cardiac output.

An animal with the sick sinus syndrome exhibits episodes of bradycardia and tachycardia. Either may lead to signs of inadequate cardiac output and CPA. No causes have been identified in veterinary patients and therapy usually requires electrical cardiac pacing.

PHASES AND STEPS OF CARDIOPULMONARY RESUSCITATION

Basic life support (BLS) is the phase of emergency care that either (1) prevents circulatory or respiratory arrest or insufficiency through prompt recognition and intervention or (2) externally supports the circulation and ventilation of a patient with respiratory or cardiac arrest through cardiopulmonary resuscitation (CPR). The major objective of CPR is to provide adequate oxygen to the brain, heart, and other organs until definitive medical treatment (advanced cardiac life support) can restore normal cardiac and ventilatory function. Speed is critical and is the key to success.

Primary respiratory arrest usually allows the heart to continue to pump oxygenated blood for several minutes. Early intervention for patients in whom respirations have ceased can prevent cardiac arrest. When there is a primary cardiac arrest, oxygen is not circulated, and oxygen stored in vital organs is depleted in a few seconds.

The original ABCs of CPR are still valuable to remind one of the priorities of therapy in resuscitation: establish a patent *Airway, Breathe* for the animal, and maintain circulation through *Cardiac Compression*. Once these basic life support measures have been instituted, advanced and prolonged life support measures should be addressed. Advanced life support measures include *D*efinitive *D*iagnosis of the cardiac abnormality with electrocardiography, administration of *E*mergency drugs and *F*ibrillation treatment. Finally, prolonged life support measures include: *G*auging patient response to resuscitative efforts, instituting measures for neurologic recovery, and *Intensive care* monitoring of the post-arrest patient.

Basic Life Support

The *assessment* phases of BLS are crucial. No patient should undergo any one of the more intrusive proce-

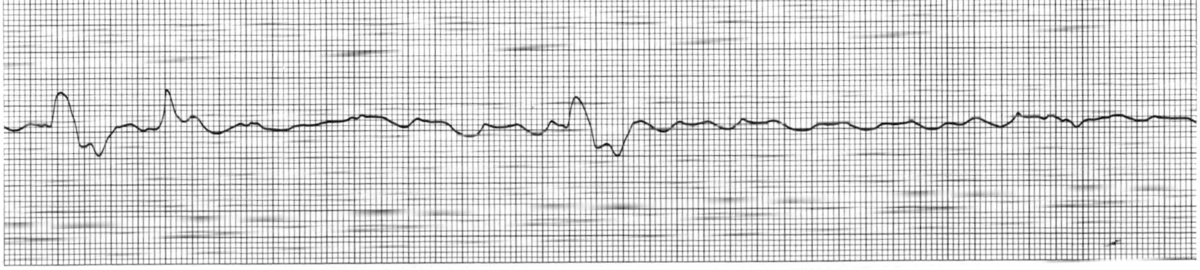

FIGURE 35–3. Fine ventricular fibrillation of cardiopulmonary arrest.

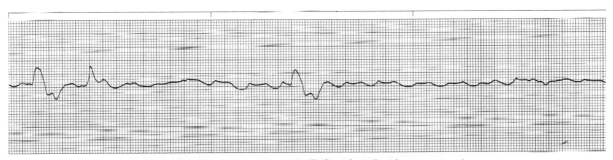

dures of CPR until the need for it has been established by appropriate assessment. Each of the ABCs of CPR, *A*irway, *B*reathing, and *C*irculation, begins with an assessment phase: determine lack of responsiveness, breathlessness, and pulselessness, respectively. Assessment also involves a more subtle, constant process of observing patient responses.

Basic life support techniques have been standardized in humans for one and two rescuers (American Heart Association guidelines). One person performing both external compression and ventilation gives 15 thoracic compressions followed by two ventilations, for a total of 80 to 100 external cardiac compressions per minute. The ratio changes to 5:1 (compressions:ventilations) if two rescuers are available.

Step A: Airway

1) Assessment—determine unresponsiveness of the patient.
2) Call for help from co-worker.
3) Position the patient in an oblique lateral recumbency in cats and dogs less than 15 lbs (7 kg) or in a dorsal recumbency in dogs greater than 15 lbs (7 kg).
4) Open the airway to assure its patency. The mouth, pharynx, and trachea should be suctioned if there is vomitus, blood, mucus, or pulmonary edema fluid in the airway.

Step B: Breathing

5) Assessment—determine breathlessness. Watch for the chest to rise and fall, listen for air escaping during exhalation, and feel for air flow. The assessment procedure should take no more than three to five seconds.
6) Breathe for the patient. Artificial ventilation should begin when there is clinical evidence of hypoxia. Tracheal intubation and ventilation with 100 per cent oxygen from an anesthetic machine, room air with an AMBU bag, or even mouth-to-tube or mouth-to-nose breathing should be the first step of resuscitation. An emergency tracheostomy may be necessary if trauma prevents access to the larynx for intubation. Tissue hypoxia and acidosis will be minimized if artificial ventilation is performed immediately.

Extrapolation of CPR techniques for humans to veterinary patients does not take into account the faster respiratory rates of animals. The American Heart Association (AHA) technique permits 16 to 20 ventilations per minute, yet the normal respiratory rate of dogs and cats may exceed 30 breaths per minute. Many of the newer techniques, such as simultaneous compression and ventilation, which increase intrathoracic pressure, also increase the ventilatory rate. However, more than one rescuer is necessary when ventilation is given simultaneously with external cardiac compression (see section titled Circulation below).

When CPA occurs in the anesthetized patient, all anesthetic gases should be immediately turned off. The system should be flushed with 100 per cent oxygen, and positive pressure ventilation should be provided for the animal.

The "four quick" initial ventilations formerly recommended in one-rescuer CPR have been changed to two initial breaths of one to one and a half seconds each. This prolonged ventilation cycle is continued throughout CPR.

Step C: Circulation

7) Assessment—determine pulselessness. Check either the carotid or femoral arteries for evidence of a pulse. This should require no more than five to ten seconds. If a pulse is present but there is no breathing, rescue breathing should be initiated at a rate of 12 to 15 times per minute after the initial two breaths of one to one and a half seconds each. If no pulse is palpated, the diagnosis of cardiac arrest is confirmed.

Cardiac compression in dogs weighing over 15 lbs (7 kg) is performed with the patient in a dorsal recumbency. This position maximizes the increase in intrathoracic pressure due to the larger ventrodorsal dimension of the thorax. Chest compression is applied over the distal one third of the sternebrae and with enough force to compress the thorax 25 to 30 per cent of its dimension.

In cats and small dogs less than 15 lbs, studies at the CSU VTH have shown an increased oxygenation with the patients in lateral recumbency. In these patients, compression is applied over the heart (4th to 5th intercostal space). The thorax is compressed 30 to 40 per cent of its lateral dimension.

8) CPR in animals requires a rapid compression rate (80 to 120 per minute). The time of release should equal the time required for compression. Rescue breathing and cardiac compression must be combined for effective resuscitation in cats and dogs. In dogs weighing over 15 lbs, cardiac compression is applied while the animal is positioned in a dorsal recumbency. With one-person CPR, the rate continues at 80 to 100 and two ventilations are given after every 15 compressions of the chest.

Theories of Blood Flow During Cardiopulmonary Resuscitation

Once artificial ventilation is instituted, circulation must be maintained to the brain and heart, the two organs of major concern during CPA. The original theory of forward blood flow during CPR stated that the heart was compressed between the sternum and the spine (humans) or between the ribs (animals) and that blood was forced antegrade from the heart due to direct cardiac compression and valvular closure. This premise is termed the "Cardiac Compression Theory" and is probably true for infants, cats, and small dogs with narrow, compliant chest cavities.

However, in human adults and dogs greater than 44

pounds, the heart acts as a passive conduit and blood moves forward by an increase in intrathoracic pressure. The "Thoracic Pump Theory" was formed when it was noted that human patients in ventricular fibrillation could remain conscious by coughing continuously, which elevated intrathoracic pressure. Measurements obtained during thoracic compression in CPR demonstrate an identical and almost simultaneous increase in intrathoracic, right atrial, left ventricular, and aortic pressures.

During external thoracic compression, the transmission of increased pressure to the thin-walled intrathoracic veins causes venous collapse. The presence of venous valves also aids in preventing venous retrograde blood flow.

The thin-walled right ventricle and atria may be compressed during artificial systole, but the left ventricle acts as a conduit, with only a three per cent reduction in size noted by echocardiography during thoracic compression. Studies show that the mitral and tricuspid valves remain open during both compression and relaxation. Blood flows out of the lungs during both the compression and relaxation phases of CPR.

The increased pressure generated in the heart during compression is transmitted to the thick-walled intrathoracic arterial vessels, which resist collapse and permit blood flow out of the thorax with a minimal drop in pressure. An arteriovenous pressure gradient is created in the extrathoracic vessels and forward blood flow occurs across the resistance vessels and capillary beds.

The relaxation phase of CPR (artificial diastole) allows intrathoracic pressures to return to near atmospheric, thus creating a pressure difference between extrathoracic and intrathoracic venous vessels. The result is the forward flow of blood into the intrathoracic veins.

The coronary arteries are perfused during diastole in CPR, as under normal conditions. Diastolic pressure is slightly higher in the aorta than in the right atrium, thus permitting forward coronary blood flow.

Closed Chest Cardiopulmonary Resuscitation

Research into more effective mechanisms of forward blood flow have combined methods of increasing intrathoracic pressure with thoracic compression. Simultaneous ventilation and compression, in which the lungs are inflated while the thorax is compressed, increases systolic pressure and carotid artery flow. Airway pressure reaches 60 to 110 cm H_2O with this method, and overinflation of the lungs is actually prevented by the simultaneous compression of the thorax. Studies comparing CPR techniques in cats demonstrate that arterial oxygenation is significantly increased when simultaneous ventilation and compression is used as opposed to "standard" AHA CPR. Arterial oxygenation is increased even further when simultaneous compression and ventilation plus an interposed ventilation after every tenth compression is used during CPR (a combination of AHA CPR and simultaneous ventilation and compression).

Interposed abdominal compression, which requires three rescuers, uses cranial abdominal compression between thoracic compressions to increase venous return to the heart. Pressure intermittently applied to the cranial abdomen is found to increase arterial systolic and diastolic pressures, increase cardiac output, and increase cerebral perfusion. Interposed abdominal compression requires no special equipment and can easily be instituted with basic life support measures.

Open Chest Cardiopulmonary Resuscitation

Since closed chest CPR was introduced in 1960, opening the thorax in order to directly compress the heart has not been frequently used as a resuscitative technique. However, certain conditions do not allow adequate forward blood flow unless direct cardiac compression is performed—specifically, massive chest trauma with rib fractures, hemothorax, pneumothorax, or pericardial effusions. If adequate perfusion is not obtained with closed chest cardiac massage, the thorax should be incised at the left fifth to sixth intercostal space, and internal cardiac massage should begin immediately. Poor response to closed-chest CPR may occur in large breed dogs (more than 50 lbs) and studies support that most successful resuscitations in dogs occur in those animals who weigh less than 20 lbs (9 kg). The use of open chest CPR after 20 minutes of arrest is shown to have no effect on improved resuscitation, therefore the clinical conditions that dictate the institution of open-chest CPR should be recognized early in the course of resuscitation.

Advanced Life Support

The basic life support measures of artificial ventilation and compression can be augmented by advanced life support, which includes oxygen therapy, defibrillation if necessary, and drugs, in order to restore normal sinus rhythm and improve cardiac output.

Step D: Diagnosis and Defibrillation

Cardiac arrest should be diagnosed if no peripheral pulses are palpable, heart sounds are absent, and respirations have ceased. Electrocardiographic recordings show the cardiac arrhythmia underlying cardiac arrest to be ventricular fibrillation, asystole, electromechanical dissociation, or brady- or tachyarrhythmias. *Do not delay* initiation of resuscitation to obtain an electrocardiogram.

The diagnosis of cardiac arrest during a cardiac or thoracic operation is easy because the heart is either exposed or available to palpation. It may occur completely without warning, but in most instances there are premonitory signs, such as bradycardia, tachycardia, or premature beats.

If ventricular fibrillation is present, electrical *defibrillation* should be performed at this time. The success of defibrillation is directly dependent upon the duration of fibrillation. When electrical defibrillation is applied within 30 seconds of the onset of fibrillation, a 98 per cent successful defibrillation rate is reported. Allowing fibrillation to proceed for more than two minutes decreases the success rate to 27 per cent (see the section titled Step F, below, for further discussion of fibrillation).

Step E: Emergency Drugs

CARDIOPULMONARY RESPONSE TO ADRENERGIC STIMULATION

Pharmacologic agents given during CPR act at specific adrenergic receptor sites to bring about vasodilation or vasoconstriction of selective vascular beds. Certain organs, especially the brain and the heart, are more dependent on autoregulatory mechanisms to control blood flow than the adrenergic receptors of their vessels. The coronary vessels, for instance, dilate in response to the build-up of adenosine from ATP breakdown, even in the face of potent alpha-adrenergic vasoconstrictor agents.

The use of alpha-agonists in CPR augments the normal reflex response to hypotension. Alpha stimulation constricts the arterioles of the vascular beds of the skin, kidneys, skeletal muscle, and gut, leading to an increase in diastolic pressure. A diastolic pressure of greater than 40 torr increases coronary blood flow and myocardial oxygen delivery, and has been correlated with the resumption of spontaneous pacemaker activity.

Beta stimulation was once thought to be desirable in CPR in order to increase inotropic response, automaticity, excitability, and coronary blood flow. However, these responses lead to increased oxygen demand and potentiate ischemia in ventricular fibrillation by impeding subendocardial blood flow.

Resuscitation studies using epinephrine, which has potent alpha and beta effects, prove the benefits of alpha stimulation in CPR by selective blockade of either alpha or beta receptors prior to arrest. Animals given a beta blocker and those not given any blocking agent were all resuscitated, while only 27 per cent of animals given an alpha blocker were successfully resuscitated.

Epinephrine. Epinephrine has both alpha and beta effects, however, its usefulness in CPR has been questioned due to beta effects, which can worsen myocardial ischemia by increasing oxygen consumption and impeding coronary blood flow. Recent work has supported epinephrine's ability to significantly increase cerebral and myocardial perfusion pressures and blood flows. These effects have been shown to occur in different age groups of different species under variable CPR techniques. In addition, epinephrine benefits cerebral and coronary blood flow even with delayed onset or prolonged CPR, which are associated with profound anoxia and acidosis. Epinephrine may precipitate ventricular fibrillation, especially when hypoxia has not been corrected by adequate artificial ventilation. Recent experimental evidence suggests that undiluted epinephrine (1:1,000) allows better *cerebral perfusion* during CPR than pure alpha agonists.

Methoxamine. Methoxamine is a pure alpha agonist which is used to increase diastolic pressure without perpetuating myocardial ischemic hypoxia and cardiac arrhythmias. Its pressor effects decrease blood flow to the kidneys, gut, skin, and skeletal muscle.

Atropine. Atropine is a parasympatholytic agent that abolishes the protective vagally mediated effects on ventricular irritability. It is used intravenously or endotracheally in CPA associated with bradyarrhythmias, but may potentiate ventricular arrhythmias, including premature ventricular contractions, ventricular tachycardia, and ventricular fibrillation, by increasing myocardial oxygen demands. There are some data to suggest atropine's efficacy in the therapy of ventricular asystole.

Calcium Chloride. Beneficial effects of calcium in CPR are presently in question. It does not assist resuscitation in humans with ventricular asystole, but is of benefit in one subset of EMD associated with wide QRS complexes induced by ischemia. Calcium enhances the excitability of the ventricles and suppresses sinus impulse formation. The conversion of "fine" to "coarse" fibrillation with calcium is not recommended prior to defibrillation due to the concomitant increase in myocardial oxygen consumption.

Studies in successfully resuscitated dogs have shown a zero cerebral blood flow within 90 minutes of restoration of blood flow. This has been termed the "no flow" phenomenon, and can be reversed by the administration of calcium antagonists.

Calcium causes coronary vasospasm and subsequently enhances myocardial ischemia. It has been shown that calcium diffuses rapidly into all hypoxic cells and results in the generation of arachidonic acid. The subsequent production of prostaglandins, thromboxanes, leukotrienes, and endoperoxides leads to metabolic alterations, which are especially important in neural tissues. Endoperoxides and leukotrienes may have free radical oxidant characteristics, leading to disruption of neuronal DNA and permanent damage to the central nervous system.

Current American Heart Association recommendations suggest except when hyperkalemia, hypocalcemia, or calcium channel blocker toxicity is present, calcium should not be employed in CPR.

Sodium Bicarbonate. Ensuring adequate alveolar ventilation is the basis of the control of acid-base balance in CPA. Sodium bicarbonate administration has been recommended in the past to counteract the metabolic acidosis seen in CPA. Respiratory acidosis results from inadequate ventilation and metabolic acidosis results from tissue hypoxia as a consequence of inadequate blood flow. Studies of dogs that were fibrillated and held hypoxic for three minutes before mechanical ventilation was started, demonstrated that the arterial pH did not fall below 7.35 until more than 15 minutes of artificial ventilation and chest compression. In a model of asphyxial arrest in cats, the arterial bicarbonate concentration did not fall below 10 mEq/L until more than 15 minutes of airway obstruction.

Infusion of sodium bicarbonate in previously recommended doses has been correlated with rapid increases in serum osmolality and $PaCO_2$ due to the immediate conversion of bicarbonate to water and carbon dioxide. Carbon dioxide readily crosses the blood-brain barrier, leading to paradoxical cerebrospinal fluid acidosis, and diffuses into myocardial cells, resulting in exacerbation of intracellular acidosis and decreased myocardial cell function. Cardiac output has been shown to transiently decrease after bicarbonate administration. Ventricular arrhythmias that do not respond to antiarrhythmic therapy have been associated with an arterial pH of greater than 7.55.

Alkalosis causes the oxyhemoglobin dissociation curve to shift to the left. This effect results in increased oxygen binding by hemoglobin, and thus less oxygen is delivered to the peripheral tissues. The use of bicarbonate should be based on the objective measurements of pH, serum osmolality, and $PaCO_2$. Currently, bicarbonate is used only after techniques such as defibrillation, cardiac compression, support of ventilation, and pharmacologic therapies, such as epinephrine and antiarrhythmics, have been employed. Bicarbonate may be used at a dosage of 0.5 mEq/lb as the initial dose and no more than one-half this dosage after every ten minutes.

Isoproterenol. Isoproterenol is a pure beta agonist that was used in CPR in the past for its direct effects on myocardial contractility and conduction. Its use in CPR is now contraindicated; it has been shown to shunt blood away from the brain and heart in the face of maintaining a normal cardiac output. The only indication for isoproterenol is for the immediate control of hemodynamically significant bradycardia that is refractory to atropine in a patient with a pulse.

Lidocaine. Lidocaine increases the electrical stimulation threshold of the ventricle during diastole, and increases the threshold to ventricular fibrillation. It is effective in suppressing ventricular tachyarrhythmias induced by epinephrine and other catecholamines. Lidocaine is of no value in asystole or EMD, but has been used occasionally to successfully treat ventricular fibrillation when electrical defibrillation is not available.

After successful resuscitation, a continuous infusion of lidocaine should be initiated at a dosage of 45 μg/lb/minute to suppress the development of arrhythmias. Should toxic reactions occur, they are generally manifested as seizures or muscle twitching. Treatment is then directed at changing the lidocaine dosage and, possibly, the use of diazepam.

Intravenous Fluids. The rapid administration of intravenous fluids during CPR has been recommended to increase fluid volume. Although an increased total forward blood flow has been documented, a disproportionate rise in right atrial pressure and resting intracranial pressure decreases coronary perfusion pressure and cerebral perfusion pressure, respectively. Fluid therapy should not be aggressively administered unless hypovolemia is a precipitating factor in CPA. The administration of an alpha-agonist causes a relative increase in blood volume by constricting nonessential vascular beds.

ROUTES OF DRUG ADMINISTRATION

Four routes of administration are commonly used for drugs given in CPR. The intravenous and intracardiac routes were recommended, but recently the endotracheal route and the intraosseous route have become popular due to their safety, efficacy, and accessibility.

Intravenous Route. The intravenous route of drug administration is usually available only if an intravenous catheter has been placed prior to or early during the arrest. Delivery of drugs into the right atrium from a jugular catheter is desirable in CPR, since the uptake of drugs from peripheral veins is poor due to vasoconstriction and poor blood flow.

Intracardiac Route. Intracardiac administration of drugs has inherent dangers in the delivery of the medication. Possible laceration of a coronary vessel with resultant pericardial tamponade, as well as possible airway laceration or intramyocardial delivery of the drug, which may incite ventricular arrhythmias, make this an unsafe route of administration. In addition, the heart is usually inaccessible in CPR due to external thoracic compression.

Endotracheal Route. The endotracheal route of drug administration has been found to be extremely efficacious due to the tremendous surface area for exchange between the alveoli and pulmonary capillaries, as well as the proximity to the left side of the heart. Drugs can easily be injected into a sterile urinary catheter or venous extension line placed inside the endotracheal tube. The drug is forced deep into the pulmonary tree by blowing into the end of the catheter or by artificially ventilating the animal. This procedure requires that artificial ventilation be interrupted for approximately ten seconds.

Drugs that have been effectively administered via the endotracheal route include atropine, epinephrine, lidocaine, and methoxamine. Experiments with endotracheal administration of epinephrine have demonstrated a faster uptake time when epinephrine was diluted with water than with no dilution or dilution with isotonic saline. Epinephrine was also found to have a longer duration of action when administered by the endotracheal route rather than intravenously. Sodium bicarbonate has deleterious effects when given by the endotracheal route. It inactivates surfactant and causes pulmonary atelectasis.

Studies using epinephrine show the endotracheal (ET) dosage must be much higher than the intravenous (IV) dosage to achieve the same results during resuscitation from EMD. When an effective dosage is given, no difference exists between the ET and IV routes in the time required to elicit a blood pressure response or in the time to establish circulatory recovery. The hypertension following recovery is more severe and lasts longer with the higher ET dosage.

Intraosseous Route. Since the intramedullary space is confluent with the vascular system, the intraosseous route can be used for drug administration and fluid replacement. A bone marrow needle or other needle with a stylet (i.e., spinal needle) may be inserted into the proximal tibia in less than 15 seconds. Studies have shown that the following substances can be given by the intraosseous route: epinephrine, dopamine, dobutamine, sodium bicarbonate calcium gluconate, atropine, lidocaine, insulin, digitalis heparin, dexamethasone, 50 per cent dextrose, blood, and colloids. A controlled study of the intraosseous technique compared with peripheral IV administration of diazepam and phenobarbital in dogs showed no significant differences in the serum levels of the two drugs over time.

TABLE 35–1. EMERGENCY DRUGS IN CARDIOPULMONARY RESUSCITATION (CPR)

Drug	Dosage and Route	Action	Indications
Acetylcholine Cl + Potassium Cl	0.45 mEq/lb Ach + 2.7 mEq/lb KCl IC	Chemical defibrillation	Ventricular fibrillation
Amrinone	0.45–1.4 mg/lb bolus IV 13.6–45.5 μg/lb/min CRI	Nonadrenergic cardiotonic agent	Low cardiac output
Atropine	0.02 mg/lb IV or ET	Parasympatholytic	Sinus bradycardia A-V block at nodal level Ventricular asystole
Bretylium tosylate	4.5 mg/lb IV 1–2 mg/min CRI	Antifibrillatory	Ventricular fibrillation Ventricular tachycardia
Calcium chloride	1–2 ml 10% solution IV or ET	Positive inotrope	Hyperkalemia Hypocalcemia Calcium-channel blocker toxicity
Dexamethasone	1 mg/lb IV	Anti-inflammatory	Cerebral edema post-CPA
Dobutamine hydrochloride	1.1–9.1 μg/lb/min CRI	Beta agonist	Low cardiac output
Dopamine hydrochloride	0.9–4.5 μg/lb/min CRI	Dopaminergic, beta agonist (alpha agonist at higher doses)	Low cardiac output Low renal and mesenteric blood flow
Electrical therapy	0.23–4.5 watt sec/lb	Simultaneous myocardial depolarization	Ventricular fibrillation Ventricular tachycardia Supraventricular tachycardia
Epinephrine	0.1 mg/lb (1:1,000) q 5 min IV (0.2 mg/lb ET)	Alpha and beta agonist	Asystole EMD Refractory ventricular fibrillation
Furosemide	0.25–1.0 mg/lb IV	Loop diuretic	Acute pulmonary edema Cerebral edema post-CPA
Isoproterenol hydrochloride	0.0045 μg/lb/min CRI (increase to effect)	Beta agonist	Atropine-refractory bradycardia
Lidocaine	1.0 mg/lb bolus IV or ET 45.5 μg/lb/min CRI	Antiarrhythmic	Ventricular tachycardia Premature ventricular contractions Ventricular fibrillation resistant to electrical defibrillation
Methoxamine	0.18 mg/lb IV (1.8 mg/lb ET)	Alpha agonist	Asystole EMD Refractory ventricular fibrillation
Morphine	0.02–.045 mg/lb IV, IM, SQ (dogs and cats)	Analgesic Vasodilator	Acute pulmonary edema Anxiety
Norepinephrine	8–16 μg/ml dilution Slow IV infusion to effect	Alpha and beta agonist	Severe refractory hypotension Low total peripheral resistance
Propranolol	0.02–0.03 mg/lb IV	Beta blocker	Supraventricular tachycardia
Sodium bicarbonate	0.45 mEq/lb IV after 10 min of CPR (subsequent doses 0.23 mEq/lb) not for ET use	Alkalinizing agent	Pre-existing acidosis Prolonged CPA
Sodium nitroprusside	0.45–2.3 μg/lb/min CRI	Direct peripheral vasodilator	Heart failure Hypertension Fulminant pulmonary edema
Verapamil	0.02 mg/lb IV over 5 min	Calcium-channel blocker	Paroxysmal supraventricular tachycardia

Abbreviations: CPA = cardiopulmonary arrest; EMD = electromechanical dissociation; ET = endotracheal; IV = intravenous; CRI = constant rate infusion; IC = intracardiac; IM = intramuscular; SQ = subcutaneous.

Step F: Fibrillation Treatment

The treatment of choice for ventricular fibrillation is immediate electrical cardioversion. The most important factor determining ease and success of defibrillation is the time delay between onset of fibrillation and the administration of the electrical countershock. Ventricular fibrillation of greater than two to three minutes duration must be accompanied by artificial circulatory support, or spontaneous circulation will not be restored by electrical countershock.

Electrical Countershock. The optimal *delivered* energy for direct current electrical defibrillation is between .9 to 2.3 joules/pound. In the dog, at least 28 per cent of the myocardium (termed the critical myocardial mass) must be depolarized for electrical defibrillation to be successful.

Proper electrode placement allows the depolarization wave to pass through the thick-walled left ventricle, which comprises the greatest portion of the myocardium. One electrode should be placed to the left of the sternum in the 6th intercostal space, and the other dorsal to the costochondral junction in the right 3rd to 4th intercostal space.

A reduction in transthoracic impedance allows more current to be delivered to the heart. Factors that influence impedance include the electrode surface area, the number of previous shocks, the electrode-skin interface material, the pressure on the electrodes, and the phase of ventilation. Shocks given in succession (less than three-minute intervals) lower transthoracic impedance. The power setting should not be increased if the previous shock has even a minimal effect on the fibrillation pattern. A variety of commercial interface materials have become available, however, not all lower impedance to the same degree. Saline-soaked gauze offers the highest resistance to electrical flow of the commonly used interface materials, while several gels and pastes have low impedance values. Care should be taken when applying alcohol to the ECG leads of the patient to be electrically defibrillated in order to avoid combustion at the time of the electrical discharge. Increased pressure on the paddles decreases transthoracic impedance by forcing air out of the chest. Likewise, a patient being ventilated creates less electrical resistance if the shock is delivered during expiration.

Chemical Defibrillation. An efficacious chemical defibrillator would be invaluable in a veterinary practitioner's drug inventory, since electrical defibrillators are often not available. Drugs that have been recommended include potassium, bretylium tosylate, and an acetylcholine-potassium mixture. Only the acetylcholine-potassium cocktail was shown to have a significant defibrillation rate in experimentally induced fibrillating dog hearts. Unfortunately, acetylcholine is only available as a chemical grade reagent and cannot be recommended for clinical usage. Recently the use of lidocaine as a defibrillating agent has been experimentally evaluated.

Prolonged Life Support

Step G: Gauging Patient Response to Therapy

Cardiopulmonary resuscitation should not be undertaken when the patient is in the terminal stages of an incurable disease or when there is no reasonable chance to regain central nervous system function. When, after the start of emergency resuscitation, it becomes known the patient is in the terminal stage of an incurable disease or that the patient is unlikely to regain central nervous system function (proven pulselessness at normothermia without CPR), all resuscitation efforts should be discontinued.

After restoration of spontaneous circulation, reactive pupils, increased responsiveness, spontaneous movements, and resumption of spontaneous breathing efforts are strong indicators that there is cerebral oxygenation. Dilated, fixed pupils can occur in the absence of cerebral hypoxia, as a result of brain trauma, intracranial hemorrhage, catecholamines, or parasympatholytic drugs given for resuscitation. Neurologic signs suggesting cerebral or brain death are not reliable prognostic indicators during and immediately after CPR. A useful observation is the fact that patients with no midbrain reflexes 6 to 12 hours after restoration of circulation will suffer variable degrees of permanent brain damage.

Step H: Hopeful Measures for Brain Resuscitation

Previously it was felt that irreversible neurologic damage occurred after four minutes of global ischemia had passed. Emphasis in CPR research is now being placed on cerebral resuscitation. The use of calcium antagonists after successful resuscitation can reverse iatrogenically administered calcium-induced vasospasm and prevent the massive influx of calcium into cells. Experimentally, the infusion of certain calcium antagonists after resuscitation from circulatory arrest results in improved neurologic function when compared to nontreated controls. Barbiturates have been recognized in some studies for their protective effect on the CNS during periods of global ischemia. The barbiturates are mild calcium antagonists, and decrease arachidonic acid and free fatty acid levels in neurons. They also have free radical scavenging activity, and therefore may prevent neuronal DNA damage.

Measures that decrease intracranial pressure following circulatory arrest allow cerebral perfusion pressure to be maintained, and permit acid metabolites to be removed from the cerebral circulation. Cerebral edema may necessitate the use of diuretics such as furosemide or mannitol, and corticosteroids aid in reducing postresuscitation cerebral edema.

Step I: Intensive Care

Successful resuscitation of the veterinary patient is frequently associated with subsequent respiratory or cardiac arrests in the immediate postresuscitative period. Dogs that were initially resuscitated at the CSU VTH were most likely to have a second CPA three to six hours after the initial event. It is of greatest importance to expect secondary arrests, and to closely monitor the patient's ECG, ventilatory pattern, electrolytes, acid-base status, central venous pressure, body temperature, and urinary output in the postresuscitative period.

Inotropic agents in the postresuscitative period are indicated, since depressed ventricular function is common following cardiac arrest. Also, peripheral vasodilators may be useful after successful resuscitation to reverse pharmacologically elevated afterload (via alpha agonists) and to improve low cardiac output. Adequate fluid volume should be maintained to avoid hypovolemia during the postresuscitative period, and some researchers recommend overexpanding the vascular volume in order to maximally perfuse capillary beds and decrease the concentrations of metabolites generated during anaerobic cellular metabolism.

Conclusions

Because prognosis for recovery is so poor once CPA occurs, the best therapy is prevention of its occurrence. Attention to patients at risk for CPA, and the ability to recognize circulatory collapse or respiratory compromise, can avert the disastrous effects of arrest.

All patients in an intensive care area should have proper emergency drug dosages calculated and readily available on the patient's hospital chart. Those animals who are classified as "high risk" should have an appropriately-sized endotracheal tube attached to the animal's cage, where it will be immediately accessible. Laryngoscopes should be available in the intensive care area.

The maintenance of a "crash cart" or "crash box" is of benefit in order to decrease time prior to the administration of therapy for CPA. The cart or box should contain endotracheal tubes, a laryngoscope, emergency drugs (see Table 35–1), syringes, needles, and diluents.

The cart may also contain the electrical defibrillator and ECG oscilloscope, and should always be brought *to the patient* in order to decrease response time.

The decision to abort (or not even begin) resuscitative efforts should be based on the underlying disease process (irreversible versus potentially reversible) and the owner's wishes. Most successful resuscitations are quickly accomplished and require few drugs. Respiratory arrest requiring only oxygen therapy and without cardiac involvement has the most favorable prognosis.

SECTION II

PROBLEMS IN VETERINARY PRACTICE

36 CHROMOSOMAL AND GENETIC DISORDERS

H. W. LEIPOLD and S. M. DENNIS

Many structural and functional defects have been described in puppies and kittens, ranging from variant through blemish, imperfection and deviant, to malformation and monstrosity. Many are obvious at birth, but detection of the others depends on the nature and extent of the defect. Congenitally defective neonates pose a diagnostic challenge to veterinarians. They also may act as sentinels of human environment and are of comparable significance for other animal species. Defective development may manifest as embryonic mortality, fetal death, abortion, stillbirth, or nonviable or viable neonates.

Defects are being reported more frequently as a cause of neonatal mortality because practitioners are increasingly being asked the question, "Is the defect inherited?" Dog and cat breeders are becoming aware of genetic defects and the need for reducing their incidence. It is important to recognize congenital defects and to recommend control measures. Some breed associations have programs for controlling specific, undesirable traits and genetic defects. Such programs include sharing the names of dogs or cats known to transmit defects with breeders. This approach allows dog and cat owners to seek advice from their veterinarians for genetic control programs.

The cause, nature, effect, and diagnosis of canine and feline congenital defects are covered in this chapter.

FREQUENCY

The frequency of canine or feline congenital defects is not a fixed proportion of all births, but rather varies because they are caused by hereditary and environmental factors, or their interactions.[1] The frequency of individual defects varies among breeds.[2] Furthermore, purebred dogs express genetic defects more frequently than mixed breed dogs.[1–5] Frequencies of canine or feline congenital defects, as well as those of individual structures or functions, are difficult to obtain because many are identified only by necropsy. Many defects go unnoticed, others are not reported for economic reasons, and some occur so rarely as to defy accurate accounting. Frequent reporting of some defects may reflect the individual interest of the observer rather than high incidence of the defect. A total of 137,717 patients in veterinary college clinics in the United States and Canada included 6,455 animals with congenital defects.[6] Incidence of congenital canine defects is estimated to be 0.5 to 1 per cent of all puppies and 1.0 to 1.5 per cent of all kittens born.[7, 8] Naturally occurring congenital defects afflicted 0.17 per cent of 2,184, 2.1 per cent of 1,157, 1.1 per cent of 1,360, and 0.27 per cent of 737 beagle pups.[9–11] The range of defects observed is wide; the most common defects involve the central nervous, ocular, muscular, skeletal, and cardiovascular systems.[1, 2, 5]

NATURE AND EFFECT

Congenital defects are abnormalities of structure, formation, or function present at birth. All body structures and functions may be affected. They may affect a single anatomical structure or function, an entire body system, parts of several systems, may involve several body systems, or combine functional and structural defects to form syndromes. Most defects are obvious grossly, but some are not recognized without radiologic, clinicopathologic, or necropsy examination.

A defective neonate is an adapted survivor from a disruptive event at one or more stages in the complexly integrated process of embryonic and fetal development. If the disruptive event is not immediately lethal, normal developmental sequences follow that must accommodate the defective event and its sequelae. Often this is not possible and the affected embryo or fetus dies and is resorbed or aborted, often undetected.

Susceptibility to injurious environmental or genetic agents varies with the stage of development and decreases with fetal age. Before implantation, the zygote is resistant to teratogens but susceptible to genetic mutations and chromosomal aberrations. The embryo is highly susceptible to teratogens but this decreases with age as the critical developmental periods for the various organs or organ systems are passed. The fetus becomes increasingly resistant to teratogenic agents with age, except for later differentiating structures such as cerebellum, palate, and urogenital system.

Developmental defects may be lethal, semilethal, or compatible with life; they may impair viability, have little effect, or may be aesthetic and thus lower an animal's economic value. Additional economic losses occur when congenital defects are only one manifestation of a syndrome that also includes embryonic and fetal mortality. Genetic improvement is lessened through loss of replacements and consequent reduction in selection potential.

Congenital defects result in fewer losses than those caused by nutritional deficiencies, infectious agents, or neoplasia. Defects, however, may cause considerable economic losses to individual breeders by increasing perinatal mortality. Furthermore, loss of value of relatives of genetically defective animals can be serious. Congenital defects may also confuse the diagnosis of other diseases. Knowledge or suspicion that a defect is genetic influences the advice given.

CAUSES

Many congenital defects have no clearly established cause; others are caused by environmental or genetic factors, or from environmental-genetic interactions. The concept of genetic defects as basically structural is changing as an increasing number involving formation and function are being identified in dogs and cats.

Environmental Factors. Although toxins, viruses, drugs, trace elements, and physical agents have been shown to be teratogenic in various species of domestic animals, few have been incriminated in dogs and cats.[1, 12–15] Natural and experimental infection of pregnant cats with feline panleukopenia virus has caused cerebellar hypoplasia and other brain defects in newborn kittens.[16, 17] Although difficult to identify, teratogens often follow seasonal patterns or known stressful conditions, may be linked to maternal disease, and do not follow familial patterns like genetic causes.

Genetic Factors. Hereditary defects are the pathologic or pathophysiologic results of mutant genes or chromosomal aberrations. Chromosomal aberrations have been demonstrated in dogs and cats, but as yet, have not gained the diagnostic prominence they have in humans. Cytogenetic studies, however, have resulted in discovery of a number of sporadic and familiar chromosomal abnormalities in dogs and cats.

Chromosomal Abnormalities. The dog has a diploid number of chromosomes (2n = 78,XY or 78,XX), 76 of which are telocentric or acrocentric and two of which are metacentric sex chromosomes. The canine X chromosome is one of the largest and the Y chromosome, one of the smallest. Chromosomal aberrations in general may take different forms, such as single and double gaps, breaks, ring chromosomes, and fragmentation.[18] Fragments of chromosomes and ring chromosomes without centromeres are eliminated at meiosis. Furthermore, there are deletions, deficiencies, duplications, inversions, and translocations. There are two theories regarding the pathogenesis of chromosomal defects: breakage-reunion and exchange. The breakage-reunion theory states that chromosome breakage is healed either by the original breaks healing (restitution) or by wrong unions (repair). The exchange theory contends there are no breaks, but chromatids or chromosomes are exchanged at predetermined places of contact.

Changes in chromosomal numbers atypical for the species (species-specific homoploidy) may involve entire sets or only single chromosomes. It is referred to as *heteroploidy*. Heteroploidy, in turn, may be seen as euploidy or aneuploidy. *Euploidy* is defined as cells or individuals characterized by changes in entire sets of chromosomes such as alloploidy, haploidy, or polyploidy. *Alloploidy* represents occurrence of structural and genetic nonidentical sets of chromosomes as encountered in species hybridization. *Haploidy* reveals only one set of chromosomes in a cell. *Polyploidy* is caused by spontaneous or induced disturbances of mitosis or meiosis due to nondisjunction, polyandry such as polyspermia, polygeny due to two or more female pronuclei participating at fertilization, and aneugamy due to aneuploidy of one gamete or disturbance of the first cell division. Polyploidy results in lethal blastopathies and embryopathies, followed by embryonic resorption and early abortion. Polyploidy was seen (3n = 117, XXY and 4n = 156,XXYY) in puppies affected with internal hydrocephalus, agyria, cryptorchidism, and hypospadias.[19] Progesterone injections may induce polyploidy as well as aneuploidy.[20]

Aneuploidy does not involve the entire set of chromosomes and may result in *hyperploidy* (increased number) and *hypoploidy* (decreased number). The cause of aneuploidy is nondisjunction and may involve autosomal or sex chromosomes. In dogs, 79,XXY trisomy has been described, resulting from a female gamete 40,XX and a male gamete 39,Y. It is referred to as Klinefelter syndrome and is characterized by testicular hypoplasia and hypoplasia of tubular and accessory reproductive organs, as well as sterility.[21] A karyotype of 79,XXX was reported in a four-year-old airedale terrier with a history of primary anestrus. The bitch had ovarian dysplasia.[22] Chimeras of XX/XY have also been reported in dogs. Prenatal postzygotic chimeras in female dogs were sterile and examination revealed gonadal hypoplasia, arrested müllerian duct development, clitoris hypertrophy, and development of parts of the Wolffian ducts.[23] There is a spectrum merging into intersex. Male pseudohermaphrodism in miniature schnauzers is characterized by persistence of müllerian duct derivatives, unilateral or bilateral cryptorchidism, and Sertoli cell tumors or endometritis, or both. Chromosomal studies in one dog revealed an XXY constitution.[24] A male, miniature rough-haired dachshund with a history of hematuria was diagnosed as pseudohermaphroditic with XX/XY mosaicism in various tissues. A littermate also had a urogenital tract defect. Their bitch had been implanted with progesterone during pregnancy.[25] Hermaphrodism occurs in three forms: unilateral (one gonad is an avotestis and the other, an ovary or testis), bilateral (both gonads are ovotestes), and lateral (a testis and an ovary). Most studies report hermaphroditic dogs as phenotypic females with XX karyotype.[26, 27]

Serologic analysis of white blood cells from cocker spaniels indicates that a form of abnormal sexual development, in which individuals with a female karyotype have testes or ovotestes, is caused by anomalous transmission of male-determining H-Y genes.[28]

Chromosomes may fuse, as occurs in Robertsonian translocation, where two acrocentric chromosomes fuse to form a metacentric chromosome (centromere fusion). The phenotypic picture is variable, ranging from normal to involvement in sarcomas of the reproductive area, lymphosarcoma, various congenital heart defects, cleft lip and jaw, ectopic ureters, inguinal hernias, and other problems.[29–34] The inheritance pattern is autosomal dominant. However, the pathogenetic mechanism is not quite clear. The affected dog has a 2n=77,XY or 2n=77,XX karyotype. Cell division may be disturbed and result in nonviable zygotes. There are no established control measures at present.

Centric fusion of autosomal chromosomes number 13 and 17 was described in a golden retriever crossbred bitch. She had four subsequent litters, a total of 16 pups; seven were identified as carriers, however, none revealed any structural or functional abnormalities.[33] A new Robertsonian translocation (1/31) was described recently in poodles. The translocation had a high frequency in the population studied, was well-tolerated, and had little effect on fertility.[34]

Clonal chromosomal aberrations have been described in a case of canine fibrosarcoma; the karyotype was hypoploid with 54 and 56, with many biarmed chromosomes.[35]

A nine-and-a-half-year-old Labrador retriever with disseminated lymphosarcoma had hypodiploidy ranging from 56 to 68 chromosomes. The number of metacentric chromosomes in the neoplastic cells ranged from 14 to 36, with an average of 24.[36] The chromosomal defects included centric fusion and aneuploidy.[37, 38]

Cytogenetic observation of canine venereal tumors reported a modal number of 59, containing 17 to 19 abnormal metacentric chromosomes. Cytogenetic studies in many parts of the world have found remarkably similar karyotypes.[39]

The cat has a diploid number of chromosomes (2n = 38,XY or 38,XX). With few exceptions, this area has received little attention in cats, but sporadic and familiar chromosomal aberrations have been reported.[40]

In cats, gene O for orange hair coat is transmitted as sex-linked. The gene is located on the X-chromosome and it reveals an effect in the single dose in the hemizygous state. If orange O and O^+ (not orange) occur in a female cat, they are manifested in a coat pattern referred to as tortoiseshell.[41] Tricolored cats are usually females. White is autosomal, however, the codominant gene O for orange and its normal codominant allele O+, are located on X chromosomes. Therefore, tricolored cats are females with two different X chromosomes. The exceptions are tricolored males who must have two X chromosomes. These aneuploidic cats have a XXY chromosomal picture and are further characterized by testicular hypoplasia.[42–44]

In two feline littermates with spina bifida and meningocele, the phenotypic male had a normal 38,XY chromosome complement and the phenotypic female had a 37,XO chromosome complement.[45] It was concluded that spina bifida was due to Manx ancestry and not to the 37,XO karyotype.

A feline runt considerably smaller than his littermates had 39 chromosomes with trisomy of an autosome.[46] A X-chromosome monosomy (37,XO) was detected in a Burmese cat affected with gonadal dysgenesis.[47] Bone marrow of two female cats with acute lymphoblastic leukemia revealed cytogenetically marked aneuploidies.[48]

A recent report described a genetic map of 31 biochemical loci located on 17 feline syntenic groups. It was derived by somatic cell genetic analysis of cat-rodent hybrids.[49] Chromosomal location for endogenous sequence (RDV1-4) was determined by correlating the occurrence of specific feline chromosomes using viral DNA fragments of cat x rodent somatic cell hybrid. The endogenous RD-114 sequences are located on multiple cat chromosomes.[50]

GENETIC DEFECTS. Diagnosis of genetic defects is based on the rule that genetic diseases run in families in typical intergenerational and intragenerational patterns, requiring enumeration of normal and abnormal offspring and identification of their familial relationships. Various statistical methods are used to analyze such data, and breeding trials may be necessary to confirm inheritance patterns. Many congenital diseases follow simple Mendelian inheritance, mostly simple autosomal recessive. Other monofactorial inheritance patterns described are characterized as overdominant, dominant, incompletely dominant, and polygenic. Only a few reports describe sex-linkage in dogs and cats.

Genes are chemical entities that control growth and development within environmental limits. They are present in pairs (alleles) located on chromosomes. Dogs have 39 pairs of chromosomes; cats have 19 pairs. All pairs but one (sex chromosomes) are exactly the same size and shape. Gene pairs are located on the same location (locus) of homologous chromosomes. Such genes on the given locus may be mirror-like and are referred to as homozygous for that locus. A gene has the property to mutate while the other allele remains unchanged. If the mutation has no visible effect in its carrier (heterozygote), it is *recessive*. Mating recessive heterozygous animals results in three genotypic states; only the homozygous state of the defective gene results in disease or defect. However, recessive mutation may be carried along for several generations until by chance, two carriers are mated and the defect is exposed. If the mutation modifies the heterozygote, it is *dominant*.

The recessive inheritance pattern involves only two kinds of animals, normal or defective. Only a few normal carriers or heterozygotes can transmit the disease. Although two heterozygous parents produce defectives, most defective animals do not reproduce, hence most defectives are born to normal parents. Each normal heterozygous parent transmits one of the two abnormal genes necessary to produce a defective offspring (homozygous abnormal). Normal animals cannot transmit the disease (homozygous normal). When nondisease-carriers are mated with other noncarriers, or even with normal carriers, they produce only normal offspring.

When normals (carriers or heterozygotes) that produced a defective offspring are mated repeatedly, 25 per cent of their progeny should be defective and 75 per cent normal. Two of every three normal animals from such parents carry a hidden recessive gene that they may transmit to their progeny, just as their parents transmitted the abnormal gene to them. Thus, recessive defects are "carried" generation after generation by normal phenotypic animals (carriers or heterozygotes), resulting in insidious spread of undesirable recessive genes.

Eliminating defective progeny usually keeps recessive defects at low frequencies. Breeds in which there are only a few foundation breeding animals or in which many animals are closely related to some outstanding animal, are vulnerable to a startlingly increased frequency of genetic defects. This may happen when the foundation animals carry an unidentified recessive gene. The recessively inherited defects are exposed when descendants of such animals are mated. Inbreeding, therefore, is one way of exposing abnormal recessive genes.

Dominance, a less common pattern, is the reverse of the recessive inheritance pattern. Dominant genes are passed from one generation to the next and do not skip generations as recessive genes may do. They are usually found in parents and offspring. With dominant inheritance, normal, unaffected animals breed true, but defective animals may produce both normal and abnormal offspring. Dominant defects are easily controlled by eliminating all defective animals.

Incomplete dominance creates three types of animals: normal, slightly defective, and severely deformed. Both normal and severely deformed animals breed true. Slightly abnormal animals, when mated together, produce one quarter normal, one half slightly defective, and one quarter severely deformed offspring. Incomplete dominant defects are easily controlled by eliminating all defective progeny.

Overdominance is similar to incomplete dominance in that three types of animals are produced: normal, superior, and deformed. Normal and deformed breed true. The superior animals, mated with other superiors, produce one quarter normal, one half superior, and one quarter defective offspring. Superior animals are usually selected as breeders in preference to normal animals. The cost of mating is a 25 per cent loss of offspring from like mates because they are defective. Overdominant traits are difficult to control because superior dogs also carry the undesirable gene and owners are reluctant not to breed them.

Genetic analysis usually proceeds from the simpler modes of inheritance to the more complex. Modes based on two alleles at a single autosomal or sex-linked locus are tested first, then their modification caused by the variable expressivity–incomplete penetrance phenomenon, or by sporadic cases occurring as phenocopies, spontaneous mutations, or other sources of confusion. Such occurrence may be due to incomplete penetrance resulting when genetically defective but clinically normal animals are mated.

To summarize, genetically caused diseases run in families, in typical intergenerational patterns and intragenerational family frequencies. Most defects are inherited as simple autosomal recessives. The goal of studies should be frequency of genetic defects, mode of transmission, and economic significance. Furthermore, there is a need to find families with fewer or none of the genetic traits.

The primary importance of diagnosis of transmission patterns is prevention, particularly of defects impairing structure or function and hence, usefulness. Undesirable inherited traits that do not impair usefulness should also be listed on the pedigree, or in any advertisement of breeding animals.

CONCLUSIONS

Breeders and veterinarians are involved daily with producing quality pets or working animals. Many different congenital defects due to genetic, environmental, or unknown causes, or to environmental-genetic interaction, have been identified. A concerted effort is needed to identify environmental agents that are teratogenic in dogs and cats. The highly complex and poorly understood interaction between environmental and genetic factors also requires clarification in both species. It is important to recognize that congenital defects are economically significant. Accurate diagnosis of defects, partly or wholly caused by genetic factors, is necessary before appropriate control measures can be recommended. Diagnosis involves understanding hereditary patterns of defects. Not only is diagnosis important but methods to control genetically induced defects should be understood. Many dog and cat breed associations have programs for monitoring and controlling undesirable traits and genetic defects. Surgical correction of defects should not be performed on breeding animals.

It is recommended that practitioners do the following:

1. Take greater interest in perinatal puppy and kitten mortality.
2. Become familiar with the common gross findings in dead perinates.
3. Encourage clients to consult them concerning perinatal problems.
4. Monitor perinatal problems by routinely necropsying dead puppies and kittens.
5. Take an interest in canine and feline teratology.
6. Become familiar with the common congenital defects in dogs and cats.

References

1. Leipold HW and Dennis SM: Congenital defects of domestic and feral animals. Issues and Reviews Teratology, 1984. In Kalter, H(ed): Vol II. New York, Plenum Press, 1984, p 91.
2. Patterson DF: Congenital defects of the cardiovascular system of dogs: studies in comparative cardiology. Adv Vet Sci Comp Med 20:1, 1976.
3. Hodgman SFG: Abnormalities and defects in pedigree dogs. I. An investigation into the existence of abnormalities in pedigree dogs in the British Isles. J Sm Anim Pract 4:447, 1963.
4. Johnston DE and Cox B: The incidence in purebred dogs of abnormalities that may be inherited. Aust Vet J 46:465, 1970.

5. Padgett AG, et al.: Genetic disorders affecting reproduction and the parturient. Vet Clinics N Am: Sm Anim Pract 16:577, 1986.
6. Priester WA, et al.: Congenital defects in domesticated animals: general considerations. Am J Vet Res 31:1871, 1970.
7. Bailie NC, et al.: Teratogenic effect of acetophydroxamic acid in clinically normal Beagles. Am J Vet Res 47:2604, 1986.
8. Nelson NS, et al.: Developmental Abnormalities. In Benirschke K, Garner FM, and Jones TC (eds) Pathology of Laboratory Animals. Vol. II. New York, Springer-Verlag, 1978, p 1887.
9. Smalley HE, et al.: Teratogenic action of carbaryl in Beagle dogs. Toxicol Pharmacol 13:392, 1968.
10. Marsboom R, et al.: Incidence of congenital abnormalities in a Beagle colony. Lab Anim 5:41, 1971.
11. Earl FL, et al.: Teratogenic research in Beagle dogs and miniature swine. In: Spiegel H (ed) The laboratory animal in drug testing: 5th symposium internal committee lab animals. Stuttgart: Fisher 1973, p 233.
12. Weldman WH, et al.: The effect of thalidomide on the unborn puppy. Staff Meet Mayo Clin 38:518, 1963.
13. Schardein JL, et al.: Canine teratogenesis with an estrogen antagonist. Teratology 7:199, 1973.
14. Robertson RT, et al.: Aspirin: teratogenic evaluation in the dog. Teratology 20:313, 1979.
15. Scott IW: Teratogenesis in cats associated with griseofulvin therapy. Teratology 11:79, 1974.
16. Kilham L and Margolis G: Viral etiology of spontaneous ataxia of cats. Am J Pathol 48:991, 1966.
17. Greene CE, et al.: Hydranencephaly associated with feline panleukopenia. JAVMA 80:767, 1982.
18. Epstein CJ: The Consequences of Chromosome Imbalance. Principles, Mechanisms and Models. New York, Cambridge University Press, 1986.
19. Herzog A and Höhn H: Chromosomenanomalien mit letaler Wirkung bei Welpen. Kleintier-Prax. 17:176, 1972.
20. Williams DL, et al.: Chromosome alterations produced in germ cells of dogs by progesterone. J Lab Clin Med 77:417, 1971.
21. Clough E, et al.: An XXY sex-chromosome constitution in a dog with testicular hypoplasia and congenital heart disease. Cytogenetics 9:71, 1971.
22. Johnston SD, et al.: X Trisomy in an Airedale bitch with ovarian dysplasia and primary anestrus. Theriogenol 24:597, 1985.
23. Hare WCD: Intersexuality in the dog. Canad Vet J 17:7, 1976.
24. Marshall LS, et al.: Persistent mullerian duct syndrome in miniature Schnauzers. JAVMA 181:798, 1982.
25. Weaver AD, et al.: Phenotypic intersex (female pseudohermaphroditism) in a dachshund dog. Vet Rec 105:230, 1979.
26. Thomas TN, et al.: Lateral hermaphroditism and seminoma in a dog. JAVMA 189:1596, 1986.
27. Seldon JR, et al.: Genetic basis of XX male syndrome and XX true hermaphroditism: evidence in the dog. Science 201:644, 1978.
28. Seldon JR: Intersexuality in the dog: classification, clinical presentation, and etiology. Compend Cont Educ Pract Vet 1:435, 1979.
29. Larsen RE, et al.: Centric fusion of autosomal chromosomes in a bitch and offspring. Am J Vet Res 39:861, 1978.
30. Larsen RE, et al.: Breeding studies reveal segregation of a canine Robertsonian translocation along Mendelian proportions. Cytogenet Cell Res 24:95, 1979.
31. Shive RJ, et al.: Chromosome studies in dogs with congenital cardiac defects. Cytogenetics 4:340, 1965.
32. Mann SF and Gilmore CE: Chromosomal abnormality in a phenotypically and clinically normal dog. Cytogenetics 10:254, 1971.
33. Larsen RE, et al.: Centric fusion of autosomal chromosomes in a bitch and offspring. Am J Vet Res 39:861, 1978.
34. Mayr B, et al.: A new type of Robertsonian translocation in the domestic dog. J Hered 77:727, 1986.
35. Sonoda M, et al.: A case of canine fibrosarcoma with abnormal chromosomes. Jap J Vet Res 18:145, 1970.
36. Idowu L: Observations on the chromosomes of a lymphosarcoma in a dog. Vet Rec 99:103, 1976.
37. Miles LP, et al.: Chromosome analysis of canine lymphosarcoma: Two cases involving probable centric fusion. Am J Vet Res 31:783, 1970.
38. Benjamin SA and Noronha F: Cytogenetic studies in canine lymphosarcoma. Cornell Vet 57:526, 1967.
39. Adams EV, et al.: Cytogenetic observations on the canine venereal tumor in long-term culture. Cornell Vet 71:336, 1981.
40. Berepubo NA and Long SE: A study of the relationship between chromosome anomalies and reproductive wastage in domestic animals. Theriogenol 20:177, 1983.
41. Robinson R: Genetics for Cat Breeders. New York, Pergamon Press, 1971, pp 105.
42. Centerwall ER and Benirschke K: Animal male tortoiseshell and calico (T-C) cats: animal models of sex chromosome mosaics, aneuploids, polyploids and chimerics. J Hered 64:272, 1973.
43. König H, et al.: Hodenhypoplasie (Fehlen von Spermiogonien) und linksseitige Nebenhodenaplasie bei einem dreifarbigen Kater vom 39/xxy-Karyotyp. Dtsch Tierärztl Wschr 90:341, 1983.
44. Long SE, et al.: Male tortoiseshell cats: an examination of testicular histology and chromosome complement. Res Vet Sci 30.274, 1981.
45. Long SE and Amaitar Berepubo N: A 37XO chromosome complement in a kitten. J Sm Anim Pract 21:627, 1980.
46. Benirschke K, et al.: Trisomy in a feline fetus. Am J Vet Res 35:257, 1974.
47. Johnston SD, et al.: X-Chromosome monosomy (37,XO) in a Burmese cat with gonadal dysgenesis. JAVMA 182:986.
48. Goh K, et al.: Chromosomal aberrations in leukemic cats. Cornell Vet 71:43, 1981.
49. O'Brien SJ, et al.: Genetic mapping in mammals: Chromosome map of domestic cat. Science 216:257, 1982.
50. Reeves RH, et al.: Genetic mapping of endogenous RD-114 retroviral sequence of domestic cats. J Virol 56:303, 1985.

37 SMALL ANIMAL ZOONOSES

JAMES B. MILLER

The small animal clinician is confronted with many tasks, including the prevention, diagnosis, and therapy of disease in the dog and cat. As a health care provider for animals, it is also the responsibility of the veterinarian to have knowledge of diseases that may be transmitted from dogs and cats to human beings (zoonoses) and, when necessary, to inform the pet-owning public of potential risks from these diseases, as well as explaining ways to minimize the chance of exposure to themselves and their children. Several texts and review articles have recently been devoted to the subject of zoonoses.[1–3]

In recent years, human organ transplantation and advances in chemotherapy for neoplastic processes have led to a significant increase in the number of human beings taking therapeutic agents that are potent suppressors of the immune system. In addition, the spread of acquired immune deficiency syndrome (AIDS) has also contributed to the number of persons with suppressed immune systems. These patients are, in general, more susceptible to a variety of disease processes, including many of the zoonoses to be discussed in this chapter. Although no correlation has been established between pet ownership and an increased incidence of disease in a immune-suppressed person, consultation with an owner's health care provider is always indicated when a zoonotic or potentially zoonotic disease is diagnosed in the owner's pet.

In many instances, spending time with pet owners explaining parasite control, vaccination programs, and simple sanitation with regards to dog and cat feces and urine reduces the risk of zoonotic disease. This chapter deals with many, but certainly not all, of the zoonoses transmitted, directly or indirectly, by small pet animals to humans (Table 37–1). It includes modes of transmission to human beings and practical approaches to their prevention. Therapy of specific diseases is, in general, not discussed and the reader should refer to other portions of this book for more specific details concerning clinical signs, diagnosis, and therapy of diseases discussed in this chapter.

PARASITIC DISEASES

VISCERAL LARVAL MIGRANS

Visceral larval migrans may occur following human ingestion of the infective ova of the roundworm *Toxocara canis*. Larvae of ingested ova may penetrate the intestinal wall of human beings and, although they cannot complete their life cycle, migrate through many tissues before being destroyed by the body's immune system. Although the disease is probably subclinical in most cases, the migration of larvae occasionally can cause significant eosinophilic granulomatous reactions in the myocardium and central nervous system. In addition, larval migration in the eye (ocular larval migrans) may lead to blindness. Most clinical cases of visceral larval migrans occur in young children (one to four years) with the ocular form being more common in slightly older children.

Dogs are more commonly infested with roundworms and appear to be the primary source of visceral larval migrans.[4] A majority of dogs acquire *Toxocara canis* in utero and begin shedding ova in their feces at about 21 days of age. Some of the larvae obtained by the pup in utero are passed in the pup's feces and are ingested by the bitch when licking the neonate. Consequently, many bitches also begin passing ova at 21 days or more following parturition. Once the ova reach the outside environment, there is a period of one to two weeks before they become infective. Some immunity does develop to *T. canis* but it is frequently not sufficient to protect the animal from future infestation. As many as 15 per cent of all adult dogs are infested.[5]

Prevention. Due to the *in utero* infestation of most puppies, all newborn dogs and mothers should be treated for *Toxocara canis*, beginning when the pups are two to three weeks old. The treatment should be repeated every two weeks for at least three treatments. Many dogs are not presented to a veterinarian until they reach six to eight weeks of age. These dogs should be treated twice for roundworms at a two-week interval. The use of new anthelmintics that can kill the larval stage of *T. canis* in the tissue phase, if given during gestation, may decrease *in utero* infestation of pups.

Owners should be informed of the life cycle of the parasite and be told that prompt disposal of fecal material before ova can become infective is important in the prevention of human disease. Adult dogs should be tested yearly for the presence of *T. canis* and treated appropriately. Veterinarians should support laws prohibiting the fouling of public parks and playgrounds with dog feces. Such laws may prevent potential exposure of children to infective ova.

TABLE 37–1. ZOONOSES ASSOCIATED WITH DOGS AND CATS

Disease	Source of Infection	Mode of Transmission
Parasitic Diseases		
Visceral larval migrans	dogs (primary), cats	contamination of soil (feces)
Toxocara canis		
Cutaneous larval migrans	dogs (primary), cats	contamination of soil (feces)
A. caninum,		
A. braziliense		
Dipylidiasis	dogs, cats	intermediate host (flea)
Echinococcosis	dogs	direct (feces)
E. granulosus		
Dirofilariasis	dogs, cats (rare)	intermediate host (mosquito)
D. immitis		
Toxoplasmosis	cats	direct (feces)
T. gondii		
Giardiasis	dogs, cats	no direct transmission has been proven
G. lamblia		
Cryptosporidiosis	dogs, cats	direct
Cryptosporidia spp.		
Diseases Transmitted by Ectoparasites		
Rocky Mountain spotted fever	dogs	ticks
Rickettsia rickettsii		
Plague	dogs, cats	fleas (dog, cat); direct (cat bite, scratch)
Y. pestis		
Tularemia	dogs, cats	ticks (dog, cat); direct (cat bite, scratch)
F. tularensis		
Lyme disease	dogs	ticks–no direct transmission has been proven
Borrelia burgdorferi		
Bacterial Infections		
Brucellosis	dogs	direct (urogenital secretions)
B. canis		
Leptospirosis	dogs	direct (urine)
several species of leptospira		
Campylobacteriosis	dogs, cats	direct (feces)
Campylobacter jejuni		
Salmonellosis	dogs, cats	direct (feces)
Salmonella spp.		
Cat scratch disease	cats, dogs (rare)	direct (scratch, bite)
gram-negative bacillus		
Mycotic Infections		
Dermatomycosis	cats, dogs	direct (hair)
Microsporum canis		
Sporotrichosis	cats	direct (skin lesion)
Sporothrix schenckii		
Miscellaneous		
Bites	dogs, cats	direct
Rabies	dogs, cats	direct (bite)
Flea and mite dermatitis	dogs, cats	

CUTANEOUS LARVAL MIGRANS

Cutaneous larval migrans occurs following the penetration of the infective larvae of *Ancylostoma caninum* (dogs) or *A. braziliense* (dogs, cats, other carnivores) through the intact skin of human beings.[6] The parasite is unable to migrate beyond the dermoepidermal junction in humans, but causes intense pruritus as it migrates through the dermal tissue before being destroyed by the immune system.

Many puppies are infested with hookworms neonatally through the ingestion of infective larvae in the bitch's milk and, less commonly, by *in utero* transplacental transmission. Older dogs and, occasionally, cats, are infested through oral ingestion of infective larvae. Puppies can begin shedding ova in their feces as early as 21 days. The incidence of hookworm infestation in dogs varies greatly in different parts of the United States.

Prevention. In regions where the rate of hookworm infestation in dogs is high, preventative measures described for control of roundworms should be used. As with roundworms, early treatment of pups, yearly fecal evaluation, prompt disposal of feces, and prevention of fouling of parks and playgrounds will decrease soil contamination and help decrease human exposure to infective larvae. In nonendemic areas, treatment should be based on fecal evaluation.

DIPYLIDIASIS

Tapeworm infestation is extremely common in dogs and, to a lesser extent, in cats. Human beings may become infested with the adult tapeworm *Dipylidium caninum* following ingestion of the intermediate host, the flea. Human infestation usually shows no clinical signs and occurs most frequently in young children.

Prevention. The prevention of human dipylidiasis is best accomplished through flea control. The treatment of dogs and cats for adult tapeworms when proglottids are observed in the feces is probably of little benefit in preventing human disease without good flea control.

ECHINOCOCCOSIS

The dog is a definitive host for the tapeworm *Echinococcus granulosus*. Human ingestion of the ova of *E. granulosus* allows the parasite access to the portal circulation, where it can lead to cyst formation in the liver, lungs, and other organs. It is a potentially fatal disease in humans, and at one time echinococcosis led to the killing of virtually all the dogs in Iceland. The disease is occasionally reported in sheep ranching areas of the United States.[7] Sheep act as the primary intermediate host for the parasite and most dogs are infested through the ingestion of sheep entrails.

Prevention. In areas where dogs are used extensively in the herding of sheep, veterinarians should be cognizant of the potential risks to themselves and to the public. Checking with local public health officials about any reported cases of echinococcosis and routine fecal evaluation for tapeworm ova helps to direct the veterinarian toward appropriate measures to prevent human exposure. If *E. granulosus* is diagnosed in a dog, the animal should be treated appropriately and the owner should be informed of the public health significance. In addition, all dogs in that household should be treated. In areas where *E. granulosus* has been diagnosed, it may be appropriate to treat all dogs that work with sheep in that area on a routine basis for the parasite.

DIROFILARIASIS

The canine heartworm, *Dirofilaria immitis,* is common in many areas of the United States. Although far less common, the cat may also serve as a definitive host for the parasite. The transmission of the parasite to human beings can occur via the intermediate host, the mosquito. Human dirofilariasis is rarely recognized and is caused by emboli of dead larvae of the parasite in the lung.[8] The larval emboli appear as nodules radiographically and, although the disease is frequently asymptomatic, requires surgical biopsy and histologic evaluation to confirm the diagnosis and rule out more serious conditions.

Prevention. The prevention of human dirofilariasis depends, in part, on decreasing the incidence of canine dirofilariasis. The treatment of all dogs with microfilaremic heartworm disease for both adult worms and microfilaria is indicated. The use of preventative medications in endemic heartworm areas may decrease the incidence of canine heartworm disease and, consequently, decrease the number of mosquitoes carrying infective larva.

TOXOPLASMOSIS

Infection with the protozoan parasite *Toxoplasma gondii* occurs in a variety of warm-blooded animals, but the cat family appears to be the only definitive host (only host where the sexual cycle of the parasite occurs). Cats become infected following the ingestion of prey or raw meat that contains trophozoites. Following infection, cats excrete oocysts in their feces for one to two weeks. The oocysts become infective in two to three days and may survive in the environment for several months. Human infection occurs with ingestion of trophozoites in raw or undercooked meat, ingestion of oocysts from cat feces, and by the transplacental route.[9] The infection rarely causes clinical disease in adult humans unless they are immunocompromised. Congenital infection of the human fetus through transplacental transmission presents the greatest threat to human beings. Congenital infection can lead to severe clinical disease at birth and ocular disease later in life.

Prevention. The veterinarian is most frequently questioned about toxoplasmosis when a member of the household is pregnant or anticipating pregnancy. The significance of the cat as the cause of human exposure to toxoplasmosis is questionable. Since human infection can occur as a result of exposure to oocysts in cat feces, pregnant women should not clean cat litter boxes. Litter boxes should be cleaned daily in order to prevent oocysts from becoming infective. Cats should not be fed raw meat or allowed to hunt for prey when there is a pregnancy or anticipated pregnancy in the household. Serologic testing of cats is of no value because a positive titer does not prove active infection or shedding of oocysts. When discussing toxoplasmosis with an owner, it should be explained that human infection can also be contracted through ingestion of raw or undercooked meat and not only from cat feces.

GIARDIASIS

The protozoan parasite *Giardia lamblia* can cause enteric disease in a variety of species, including dogs, cats, and human beings. The role, if any, of dogs and cats in the transmission of giardiasis to humans has not been established, consequently, the treatment of all pets with giardiasis may or may not be significant in the prevention of human infection.

CRYPTOSPORIDIOSIS

Species in the genus *Cryptosporidia* have been incriminated in the cause of diarrhea in domestic animals and humans. Infection in humans is often asymptomatic or self-limiting, except in immunosuppressed patients where the disease may be fatal. Although cattle appear to be the primary reservoir and have been shown to have zoonotic potential,[10] the protozoan has been found in the feces of both dogs and cats and there exists the possibility of direct transmission from them to human beings. The risk of transmission from dogs or cats to humans appears very small, although special precautions might be taken if the pet owner is immunosuppressed. In the case where the owner is at higher risk of severe disease, the infected pet should be hospitalized or boarded and weekly fecal evaluations should be performed. Although there is no available therapy for cryptosporidiosis, the disease does appear to be self-limiting in the dog and cat.[11] Consequently, once several negative fecal samples have been obtained, the animal probably does not pose a risk to the owner.

DISEASES TRANSMITTED BY ECTOPARASITES

ROCKY MOUNTAIN SPOTTED FEVER

Rocky Mountain spotted fever (RMSF) is a rickettsial disease caused by *Rickettsia rickettsii*. The disease is transmitted by ticks and the primary reservoir for the disease is wild rodents and rabbits. The two species of ticks that have been incriminated in the transmission of RMSF are *Dermacentor andersoni* (wood tick), found primarily in the western United States, and *Dermacentor variabilis* (dog tick), found primarily in the southeastern United States. Dogs are susceptible and can act as a reservoir or as a transient host for the tick vector. Although the disease may be subclinical in the dog, experimentally produced canine RMSF causes signs of vasculitis similar to those that occur in human disease.[12]

Ticks frequently become infected as larvae or nymphs while feeding on rodents or rabbits. If they are heavily infected, they may transmit the rickettsial infection to their progeny by transovarian means. When infected adult ticks are inactive and not feeding (usually during winter months), the rickettsiae become "avirulent." Transmission of disease to dogs or humans is possible, but requires the tick to feed on the host for 5 to 20 hours before the rickettsia is activated and becomes virulent.[13]

Prevention. In order to reduce the risk of transmission of RMSF from dogs to humans, the veterinarian should have knowledge of the incidence of the disease in human beings in the area. Serologic testing of dogs in areas where human RMSF is more common usually reveals a high incidence of exposure in dogs. In such regions, the veterinarian should be especially vigilant in explaining to the owner the need for good tick control. Dogs should be checked daily for the presence of ticks during time of the year when ticks are abundant. Since it may require 5 to 20 hours of feeding by the tick before transmission is possible, early discovery and prompt removal of ticks may reduce the chance of canine infection. Dogs with severe or recurring tick infestation should be dipped or shampooed with an appropriate medication on a routine basis.

PLAGUE

Infection with the bacterium *Yersinia pestis* causes plague in human beings, dogs, and cats. Wild rodents serve as the primary reservoir for the disease, which is endemic in these animals throughout portions of the southwestern United States. Transmission to dogs and cats occurs when the animal is bitten by a flea from an infected rodent. Dogs usually have mild clinical signs of lymphadenopathy but cats frequently have severe systemic disease, leading to death.[14] Direct transmission of the disease from cats to humans has been reported through scratches or bites, while the dogs may act only to disseminate the flea vector.[15]

Prevention. Although flea control in the dog and cat may decrease the number of vectors present, effective prevention of transmission from dogs and cats to humans is best accomplished by not allowing pets' exposure to wild rodents in endemic areas. In endemic areas or when cases of plague have been reported in wild rodents in the region, the veterinarian should warn pet owners not to allow their cats to hunt wild prey and to avoid taking their dogs to parks, campgrounds, or other areas where they may contact wild rodents and their accompanying fleas. If *Y. pestis* is confirmed in a dog or cat, the appropriate public health officials should be contacted since early therapy is important in the treatment of human plague.

TULAREMIA

The bacterium *Francisella tularensis* causes tularemia in a variety of mammals including humans, dogs, and cats. It is endemic in certain portions of the southeastern and north central United States and sporadic cases have been reported throughout the country. Rabbits and rodents appear to be the primary reservoir for the disease. The disease is transmitted by ticks and other blood-sucking arthropods or by handling or ingestion of infected meat. Both dogs and cats can show pulmonary signs and lymphadenopathy. As with plague, the cat may transmit the disease directly to human beings by scratches or bites, while dogs appear to act only to disseminate the vector.

Prevention. Prevention of the direct or indirect transmission of tularemia from pets to humans depends primarily on prevention of pet exposure to the wild reservoir of the disease. Recommendations similar to those described in the prevention of plague transmission from pets to humans also apply to tularemia.

LYME DISEASE

Lyme disease is caused by the spirochete *Borrelia burgdorferi* and the common vector for transmission is the deer tick, *Ixodes dammini*, although *Ixodes pacificus* has also been incriminated as a vector.[16] Both dogs and human beings are susceptible to the disease.[17] In the dog a variety of clinical signs may occur, but acute lameness due to polyarthritis appears to be the most commonly recognized sign. It is still unclear whether the dog can act as a reservoir for the disease or if there should be concern for zoonotic potential from dogs to humans. Because of its zoonotic potential, all dogs with proven Lyme disease should be treated.

BACTERIAL INFECTIONS

BRUCELLOSIS

Dogs infected with *Brucella canis* may be asymptomatic, have reproductive problems, or show systemic disease such as discospondylitis. Human infection with *B. canis* is rare but is possible by direct transmission from genitourinary secretions, especially the aborted fetuses or placenta of infected dogs.[18] Human illness is characterized by fever, headache, and myalgias.

Prevention. No effective therapy is available for the

treatment of canine brucellosis. Although killing all dogs that test positive for *B. canis* might reduce the risk of dog-to-human transmission, it is more reasonable to recommend that all positive dogs be neutered.

LEPTOSPIROSIS

Infections with a variety of species of *Leptospira* occur in most mammals, including dogs and humans. The dog may act as a vector for human disease. Serologic testing has shown that stray dogs in urban areas have a much higher incidence (40 per cent) of previous leptospiral infection than do household dogs (5 per cent).[19] Human infection may occur following exposure to urine, blood, or tissues from infected dogs. In addition, contamination of the environment by infected canine urine may lead to human infection.

Prevention. The role of the veterinarian in the prevention of dog-to-human transmission of leptospirosis consists primarily of vaccinating dogs against the disease. The bacterins used to immunize against several species of *Leptospira* in the dog usually prevent clinical disease, but may allow subclinical infection.[20] These subclinical infections involve shedding of the infective organism in the urine, making current vaccines less than ideal in helping prevent dog-to-human transmission.

CAMPYLOBACTERIOSIS AND SALMONELLOSIS

Both dogs and cats may harbor *Campylobacter jejuni* and a variety of nontyphoidal *Salmonella* species. Infections with these bacteria in dogs and cats do not always cause clinical disease and have been isolated from the feces of healthy animals. Most cases of human enteric disease caused by these bacteria are not associated with pet exposure. The veterinarian should advise pet owners that all feces, especially those associated with diarrhea, be handled with care and disposed of in a manner that avoids potential human exposure.

CAT SCRATCH DISEASE

Cat scratch disease is an infectious disease that occurs in human beings following cat scratches or handling of cats. The disease is thought to be caused by a small gram-negative bacillus that has been demonstrated in tissues of persons with the disease.[21] The disease is usually characterized by a primary papule or pustule, followed in several weeks by regional lymphadenopathy. The lymphadenopathy may last for weeks to months but is usually self-limiting. Occasionally the disease has occurred following exposure to a dog rather than a cat.[22]

Prevention. Since there is no known way to test for the presence of the causative organism in the cat, prevention is best accomplished by advising cat owners of ways to avoid exposure. Teaching children to avoid rough handling of cats or declawing cats in households that have children may reduce the risk of transmission. Cats should not be allowed to lick open wounds or sores, since this has also been incriminated in the transmission of the disease. Although no therapy is available to treat cats that have been incriminated as the vector for human disease, the ability to transmit the organism appears to be transient, making isolation or euthanasia of the animal unnecessary.[23]

MYCOTIC DISEASES

The systemic fungal diseases blastomycosis, coccidioidomycosis, histoplasmosis, and cryptococcosis are generally not considered direct zoonoses. Pets affected with these fungal diseases frequently shed the organisms, leading to increased contamination of the environment. This could lead to increased human exposure to the infective forms of the fungi. The advisability of treating a pet infected with one of these systemic fungal diseases in a household with children or immunosuppressed individuals may be questioned.

DERMATOMYCOSIS

Direct transmission of *Microsporum canis* from dogs and cats does occur. As many as 30 per cent of human ringworm cases in urban areas have been associated with direct animal contact. Owners should be advised to wash their hands well following handling an infected dog or cat and to not allow their children to play with the pet until therapy has resolved the disease.

SPOROTRICHOSIS

Sporotrichosis is a chronic cutaneous or lymphocutaneous fungal disease caused by *Sporothrix schenckii*. Dogs, cats, and humans are susceptible to the disease, which is usually associated with traumatic, penetrating wounds. Recent reports indicate that infected cats can transmit the infection directly to human beings.[24, 25] Because of these findings, cats with sporotrichosis should be handled with gloves until the disease is resolved.

MISCELLANEOUS DISEASES

BITES

Bites inflicted by dogs and cats pose a serious threat for both physical trauma and the introduction of infectious agents. Dogs account for the majority of approximately 500,000 bites that occur annually in the United States.[26] Although many bite wounds go unreported, they still account for one per cent of emergency room visits.[27] The majority of dog and cat bites are inflicted on the pet owner or a person familiar with the animal. The rare fatalities associated with bite wounds are usually children. Aside from the physical trauma caused by the bite, a variety of bacteria normally found in the oral cavity of the dog and cat may lead to secondary infection. Puncture wounds, especially from cats, frequently become infected with *Pasteurella multocida*, which causes acute swelling and pain within 24 hours of the bite.[28]

Prevention. The role of the veterinarian in helping

prevent bite wounds should begin when a puppy or kitten is first presented. Owners should be informed of the importance of early socialization and training. Leaving infants or young children unattended with a pet should always be discouraged. Restraint of pets by owners while the veterinarian performs potentially painful procedures should not be allowed for both safety and legal reasons.

RABIES

Human rabies is a rare disease in the United States.[29] Although the incidence of rabies in dogs and cats accounts for less than ten per cent of laboratory confirmed cases of rabies in the United States, bites from these species are the major reason for administering post-exposure rabies vaccination in man.[30] Despite the low incidence of human rabies in this country, the near 100 per cent mortality rate in human beings makes the prevention of this zoonosis of particular importance.

Prevention. Many effective vaccines are available for use to protect both dogs and cats from rabies. Most of these are inactivated viral products, although modified live virus vaccines are available. These vaccines have contributed to the tremendous decrease in the incidence of rabies in dogs over the past 40 years. It is important to have owners understand that there is still a large reservoir of endemic rabies, especially in skunks and bats. Veterinarians should encourage all pet owners to have their dog or cat vaccinated against this disease and support local and state laws that require rabies vaccination of dogs and cats. Although some vaccines are available for subcutaneous administration, most require intramuscular injection in the thigh muscle to assure adequate immune response. Failure to follow recommendations concerning route of administration (giving an intramuscular vaccine subcutaneously) may lead to inadequate or no protection.

The veterinarian should be aware of the current status of rabies in both wild and domestic species in their area. In regions where a large number of rabies cases are present, pre-exposure rabies vaccination should be considered not only for veterinarians but animal handlers employed by the veterinarian.

FLEAS AND MITES

Canine and feline scabies (*Sarcoptes scabiei* var. *canis* and *Notoedres cati*), cheyletiellosis (*Cheyletiella* spp.), and fleas (*Ctenocephalides* spp. and *Pulex* spp.) all have zoonotic potential. The dermatosis associated with fleas or mites in humans is usually self-limiting but can recur if the offending pet and, in the case of fleas, the environment, is not adequately treated. The veterinarian should always inquire about any dermatologic problems in family members when evaluating a dog or cat with skin disease.

References

1. Elliot, DL, et al.: Pet-associated illness. N Engl J Med 313:985, 1985.
2. Greene, CE: Clinical Microbiology and Infectious Diseases of the Dog and Cat. Philadelphia, W B Saunders, 1984.
3. August, JR and Loar, AS: Zoonotic Diseases. Vet Clin North Am Jan 1987.
4. Glickman, LT and Schantz, PM: Epidemiology and pathogenesis of zoonotic toxocariasis. Epidemiol Rev 3:230, 1981.
5. Glickman, LT and Schantz, PM: Canine and human toxocariasis: review of transmission, pathogenesis, and clinical disease. JAVMA 175:1265, 1979.
6. Cypress, RH: Cutaneous larva migrans. In: Steele, JH, et al., eds. CRC handbook series in zoonoses. Section C. Boca Raton, FL, CRC Press, 1982, p 213.
7. Grove, DI, et al.: Algorithms in the diagnosis and management of exotic diseases. X. Echinococcis. J Infect Dis 133:354, 1976.
8. Tsung, SH, et al.: Pulmonary dirofilariasis in man. Am J Med Sci 283:106, 1982.
9. Ganley, JP and Comstock, GW: Association of cats and toxoplasmosis. Am J Epidemiol 111:238, 1980.
10. Wolfson, JS, et al.: Cryptosporidiosis in immunocompetent patients. N Engl J Med 312:1278, 1985.
11. Willard, MD, et al.: Gastrointestinal zoonoses. In: August, JR, Loar AS, eds. Vet Clin North Am: Zoonotic diseases. 17:145, 1987.
12. Green, CE and Phillips, RN: Rocky Mountain spotted fever. In: Green, CE, ed. Clinical Microbiology and Infectious Diseases of the Dog and Cat. Philadelphia, W B Saunders, 1984, p 562.
13. Spencer, RR and Parker, RR: Rocky Mountain spotted fever: infectivity of fasting and recently fed ticks. Public Health Rep 38:333, 1923.
14. Rust, JH, et al.: The role of domestic animals in the epidemiology of plague. I. Experimental infection of dogs and cats. J Infect Dis 124:522, 1971.
15. Weniger, BG, et al.: Human bubonic plague transmitted by a domestic cat scratch. JAMA 251:927, 1984.
16. Ryan, CP: Selected arthropod-born diseases. In: August JR, Loar AS, eds. Vet Clin North Am: Zoonotic diseases. 17:179, 1987.
17. Kornblatt, AN, et al.: Arthritis caused by *Borrellia burgdorferi* in dogs. JAMA 186:960, 1985.
18. Polt, SS, et al.: Human brucellosis caused by *Brucella canis*. Ann Intern Med 97:717, 1982.
19. Theirmann, AB: Canine leptospirosis in Detroit. Am J Vet Res 41:1659, 1982.
20. Schultz, RD: Theoretical and practical aspects of an immunization program for dogs and cats. JAVMA 181:1142, 1982.
21. Wear, DI, et al.: Cat scratch disease: A bacterial infection. Science 221:1403, 1983.
22. Margileth, AM: Cat scratch disease. In: August, JR, Loar AS, eds. Vet Clin North Am: Zoonotic diseases. 17:91, 1987.
23. Warwick, WJ and Good, RA: Cat-scratch disease in Minnesota. II. The family epidemics. Am J Dis Child 100:236, 1960.
24. Dunstan, RW, et al.: Feline sporotrichosis. JAVMA 189:880, 1986.
25. Read, SI and Sperling, LC: Feline sporotrichosis. Arch Dermatol 118:429, 1982.
26. Moore, RM, et al.: Surveillance of animal-bite cases in the United States, 1971-1972, Arch Environ Health 32:267, 1977.
27. Douglas, LG: Bite wounds: Am Fam Physician 11:93, 1975.
28. Callaham, ML: Treatment of common dog bites: infection risk factors. JACEP 7:83, 1978.
29. Anderson, IJ, et al.: Human rabies in the United States, 1960 to 1979: epidemiology, diagnosis, and prevention. Ann Intern Med 100:728, 1984.
30. Helmick, CG: The epidemiology of human rabies postexposure. Prophylaxis, 1980 1981. JAMA 250:1900, 1983.

38 FOOD HYPERSENSITIVITY

MICHAEL S. LEIB and JOHN R. AUGUST

Food hypersensitivities comprise a group of imprecisely defined, poorly understood, and controversial disorders of dogs and cats. Although food hypersensitivity manifested primarily by cutaneous changes has been well described in the veterinary literature, the prevalence and pathogenesis of this disorder is disputed. Reports indicate that food hypersensitivity may cause one per cent of all clinical dermatoses seen in general practice and may contribute to the pruritus in up to 62 per cent of dogs with nonseasonal allergic skin disease.[1–7]

The pathogenesis of several human primary gastrointestinal diseases may involve dietary hypersensitivity. Therefore, it is possible that food hypersensitivity in dogs and cats could also cause primary gastrointestinal syndromes. The infiltration of plasma cells and lymphocytes into the small intestinal lamina propria that occurs in several primary enteric disorders of dogs and cats suggests that food hypersensitivity could be involved in the pathogenesis. Also supporting this role is the occurrence of vomiting, mucoid, and hemorrhagic diarrhea, and abdominal discomfort in up to 15 per cent of animals affected with the cutaneous syndrome of food hypersensitivity.

In humans, the following diagnostic criteria have been established for food hypersensitivity: (1) the signs are caused by a specific substance that is innocuous to most other people, (2) lesions or functional changes in the gastrointestinal tract exist, (3) other causes of gastrointestinal disease can be excluded, (4) offending substances are tested under controlled conditions, and (5) a true food hypersensitivity results from an immunologic reaction.[8, 9] Few cases of food hypersensitivity in the veterinary literature satisfy the above criteria.[10]

Many veterinary cases diagnosed as food hypersensitivity might better be defined as "food intolerance." Food intolerance describes an abnormal physiologic response (idiosyncratic, metabolic, pharmacologic, or toxic) to a food that is not an immune-mediated process.[9] Lactase deficiency, an inherited disorder in man, is a food intolerance; failure of normal lactose assimilation results in osmotic diarrhea.[11] Lactase deficiency has often been suspected but rarely described in dogs and cats,[12] however, decreased brush border enzymes occur secondary to many types of small intestinal mucosal disease, resulting in lactose intolerance.[13] Another type of food intolerance is food toxicity; clinical signs are caused by the direct toxic action of a food or food additive. Food toxicity is not immune-mediated and involves the release of chemical mediators, toxins, or microorganisms.[9] The "garbage can" acute gastroenteritis syndrome of dogs and cats is a common example of food toxicity.

CUTANEOUS MANIFESTATIONS OF FOOD HYPERSENSITIVITY

After atopy and flea bite allergic dermatitis, food hypersensitivity is the most common cause of canine allergic skin disease. The disorder probably accounts for no more than five to ten per cent of all feline allergic dermatitides.[5, 14] Although food hypersensitivity may cause only one per cent of all dermatoses seen in small animal practice, the disease is an important cause of severe refractory pruritus. There are no pathognomonic signs to allow early diagnosis.

Pathogenesis. The immunologic mechanisms causing food hypersensitivity in dogs and cats are incompletely understood. Overt clinical hypersensitivities to multiple dietary antigens are rare,[1, 6] suggesting that affected animals do not develop a nonselective, exaggerated immunologic response to commonly encountered dietary components. However, most basic food ingredients (especially those weighing more than 10,000 daltons) have the potential to induce a hypersensitivity response: lipoproteins, glycoproteins, lipopolysaccharides, carbohydrates, artificial food additives, and possibly metals that leach out of cans.[2]

Food hypersensitivity in the dog and cat may involve both immediate (type I and/or type III) and delayed (type IV) hypersensitivity responses.[3, 6, 14] These different responses may partially explain the variable delay in onset of signs between patients after ingestion of the offending antigen, and the failure of the intradermal test as a reliable diagnostic aid for the disease.

Hypersensitivity to beef and/or cow's milk accounts for approximately 80 per cent of the cases of food hypersensitivity seen by the authors. About five per cent of cases result from cereals (wheat and soy), five per cent from artificial food additives, and sporadic hypersensitivities to pork, horse meat, chicken, egg, fish, and fungal contaminants in drinking water account for the remaining cases.[6]

Historical Findings. There are no established breed or sex predispositions in canine or feline food hypersensitivity. Signs are usually abrupt in onset, nonseasonal, and poorly responsive to anti-inflammatory dosages of corticosteroids. Signs in dogs and cats may develop at any age, however, food hypersensitivity is an important cause of severe pruritus in dogs less than nine months old.[6] Many affected animals have been exposed to the offending antigen for two years or more before signs develop.

Cutaneous Manifestation. The cutaneous signs of food hypersensitivity in dogs and cats are characterized by severe pruritus, erythema, and evidence of self trauma. In dogs, the pruritus is usually generalized, although the face, feet, and external ear canals are often preferentially affected.[1–3, 6] A papular eruption may be present.[2] However, the rapid development of alopecia, hyperpigmentation, lichenification, and dyskeratinization in repeatedly traumatized areas usually prevents observation of primary lesions. Recurrent pruritic superficial or deep pyodermas occasionally may be the only overt signs of food hypersensitivity. In some affected dogs, the pattern of lesions may mimic those caused by other, more common pruritic dermatoses, such as flea bite allergic dermatitis, scabies, or atopy. Urticaria or angioedema are occasionally observed. Concurrent hypersensitivity dermatoses are commonly seen in dogs with food hypersensitivity. Gastrointestinal signs occur in less than 15 per cent of affected dogs.

Food hypersensitivity in cats may appear as a pruritic ulcerative dermatitis of the head and neck, generalized pruritus without lesions, a pruritic miliary eruption, or pruritic urticaria or angioedema.[1, 3, 5, 14] Self-induced alopecia, seborrhea, and cutaneous hyperesthesia may be present. In one study, food hypersensitivity was responsible for 10.6 per cent of all cases of miliary dermatitis.[15] Superficial inguinal lymphadenopathy and other cutaneous lesions, such as eosinophilic plaques or indolent ulcers, were present in some cats with miliary eruptions. Peripheral eosinophilia may be present.[15, 16] Concurrent gastrointestinal signs are common.

Diagnosis. The cutaneous signs of food hypersensitivity in dogs and cats must be differentiated from those caused by other hypersensitivity disorders and the ectoparasitic dermatoses. For patients suspected of having food hypersensitivity, it is necessary to demonstrate that pruritus decreases while a hypoallergenic diet is being consumed, and that reinstitution of the patient's original diet causes a resumption of signs.[1–3, 6]

In dogs with dietary hypersensitivity uncomplicated by severe secondary changes or concurrent dermatoses, the hypoallergenic diet trial is ideally initiated with a 48-hour period of hospitalization. The patient should be fasted during this time and offered only distilled water to drink. Enemas should be given three times at 12-hour intervals. Response to the introduction of a hypoallergenic diet is considerably slower if residual dietary antigens are not removed from the intestinal tract in this manner.

When the dog returns home, the owner should be asked to continue assessing the extent of pruritus. Choice of hypoallergenic diet depends on the size of the dog, previous eating habits, and local availability of ingredients for a home-cooked diet. By definition, the hypoallergenic diet must contain ingredients not previously encountered by the patient. Because beef and pork are often included as meat by-products, meat meal, and bone meal in many commercial diets, they should not be used. For small dogs, the authors prefer a mixture of cooked lamb (four oz.) minced into boiled brown rice (one cup). This mixture, to which nothing else is added, provides about 550 kcal. For convenience, some small dogs may accept lamb-based, preservative-free baby food mixed into brown rice.

The authors find the commercially prepared mutton and rice-based Prescription diet d/d (Hill's Pet Products) to be a reliable hypoallergenic food. Metals leaching from cans have been incriminated as sensitizing agents in human beings. Whether the same phenomenon occurs in dogs and cats is unknown. Such a reaction may explain the failure of Prescription diet d/d as a hypoallergenic diet in certain patients with food hypersensitivity.[2] Disadvantages of this diet include poor acceptance by some smaller dogs (a problem that is usually overcome on the second or third day) and the development of diarrhea in about 30 to 50 per cent of patients. The latter problem may be corrected by the addition of boiled brown rice to the prescription diet.

Owners should be advised that all other potential sources of dietary antigens should be excluded, including rawhide chew toys, table scraps, vitamin and mineral supplements, and access to food and feces of other dogs and cats in the household. Dogs receiving a chewable, flavored heartworm preventive wafer should be placed on a plain diethylcarbamazine tablet during the trial. Access to other water sources in the household should be minimized.

Most patients with uncomplicated dietary hypersensitivity have a distinct decrease in pruritus in the second or third trial week. Owners should be requested on days 14 and 21 of the trial to give a progress report, expressing the severity of signs of pruritus (scratching and discomfort) as a percentage of the original intensity. By day 21, dogs with uncomplicated dietary hypersensitivity usually have residual pruritus less than 25 per cent of that originally observed.

Many dogs with severe, chronic dietary hypersensitivity have secondary complications that exacerbate the extent of pruritus, so it is often necessary to address these problems first. These patients should be placed on three weeks of appropriately chosen antimicrobial therapy, weekly antiseborrheic and antibacterial shampoos with moisturizing rinses, and otic preparations as necessary. The hypoallergenic diet should be started on day one of therapy. Owners should reassess the extent of pruritus at the start of antimicrobial therapy and on days 14, 21, 28, and 35 by the method described previously. In this manner, nonspecific reductions in pruritus resulting from supportive therapy and specific improvements resulting from dietary alteration can be assessed independently in a sequential manner.

It is not uncommon for dietary hypersensitivity to appear concomitantly with other pruritic dermatoses, especially atopy and flea bite allergic dermatitis. The success of dietary alteration may have to be assessed on the basis of an observed reduction in corticosteroid maintenance therapy while the patient is on the hypoallergenic diet, and a need to increase the corticosteroid dose when the original diet is reintroduced.

At the end of the dietary trial, the entire original diet and regular drinking water of the patient can be reintroduced. Patients with dietary hypersensitivity usually have an exacerbation of pruritus within 12 to 72 hours. This may be controlled by immediately placing the dog back on the hypoallergenic diet and distilled water, and administering a short course of corticosteroids (0.5 mg/lb of prednisolone for three to five days). In most cases, pruritus ceases within five to seven days. Most clients are more willing to investigate which specific antigen is the cause of the problem when they have observed the beneficial effects of the hypoallergenic diet, and have witnessed the immediate adverse signs induced by reintroduction of the original diet.

Introduction of individual dietary antigens is now based on examination of the list of ingredients in the patient's original commercial dog food. Ground beef should be added to the commercial hypoallergenic diet, or substituted for the lamb in the home-cooked recipe. If there is no resumption of pruritus within seven days, dried powdered milk (one-half to two tbsp) should be added to the basal diet. Dogs that react adversely to beef should also be evaluated for milk sensitivity and vice versa because cross-reactivity is not uncommon, and affects the final choice of a maintenance diet.

If neither of the previously mentioned ingredients induces pruritus, wheat flour (one-half to two tbsp daily) and then soy meal may be added to the basal diet. Cross-reactivity between cereal antigens is observed. If the patient's history suggests that other, less common antigens are involved, they should be introduced in a similar manner. Finally, plain tap water can be substituted for the distilled drinking water being offered. If there is still no resumption of pruritus, the patient may be placed on a commercial diet free of additives, artificial flavors and colors, and preservatives. Failure to develop clinical signs on this diet confirms that artificial additives are at fault.

Long-Term Nutritional Management. Avoidance of the offending antigen is the only specific and practical treatment of food hypersensitivity[1–3, 5, 6] because the disorder is usually poorly responsive to corticosteroid treatment. The ultimate goal of therapy is to return the patient to an economical and nutritionally complete commercial diet that does not contain the offending antigen. Strict attention must be paid to proper treatment of secondary bacterial and seborrheic complications and concurrent pruritic dermatoses. In uncomplicated patients, corticosteroid therapy is rarely necessary after the offending antigen has been identified and removed from the patient's diet.[6]

GASTROINTESTINAL SYNDROMES THAT MAY BE ASSOCIATED WITH FOOD ALLERGY

Gluten-induced enteropathy is a malabsorption syndrome well documented in humans and believed to occur in the dog.[17–19] Gliadin is a toxic mixture of proteins extracted from glutens, found in cereals such as wheat, barley, rye, buckwheat, and oats. Ingestion by susceptible individuals results in small intestine villous flattening, cuboidal epithelial cells, and infiltration of the lamina propria with plasma cells and lymphocytes. Although the pathogenesis is not completely established, immune mechanisms are believed to be involved. In affected human beings, circulating anti-gluten antibodies, mucosal anti-gluten antibodies, elevated serum immunoglobulin (Ig) A levels, and deposition of immune complexes into the lamina propria have been demonstrated. It is believed that both humoral and cell-mediated immune mechanisms participate in the pathogenesis.

Recently a wheat-sensitive enteropathy of Irish setter dogs has been described.[20–22] Affected dogs had small intestinal diarrhea with weight loss or failure to thrive. Villous atrophy and altered activity of intracellular enzymes occurred. Although the pathogenesis remains unknown, a type I hypersensitivity reaction is suspected.[22]

Eosinophilic gastroenterocolitis is an uncommon disorder in humans, dogs, and cats that could be a manifestation of food hypersensitivity. Eosinophilic infiltrates occur in the small intestinal mucosa, and less commonly in the stomach and colon.[23–28] Eosinophils may extend throughout all layers of the alimentary tract wall, and on rare instances produce a scirrhous mass.[29, 30] The infiltration of eosinophils may be the end result of an immediate hypersensitivity response involving IgE antibodies to food allergens, cell-mediated chemotaxis, or an immediate hypersensitivity reaction to immune complex activation of the complement system with subsequent eosinophil chemotaxis.[25] In humans, a mechanism involving food hypersensitivity is supported, as affected individuals have elevated serum IgE levels that increase with specific food challenge, symptomatic responses to food challenges, and positive radio-allergo-sorbant tests.[25] However, evidence of food hypersensitivity is not present in all patients and some individuals fail to improve clinically after the removal of incriminated food antigens. In addition, visceral larval migrans has also been pinpointed in dogs as a possible cause.[27]

Plasmacytic-lymphocytic enterocolitis causes vomiting, small bowel and large bowel diarrhea, and weight loss in dogs and cats.[31, 32] Infiltration of the lamina propria by plasma cells and lymphocytes suggests an immunologic mechanism.[32] In a small group of cats with plasmacytic-lymphocytic colitis, dietary modification produced clinical improvement, suggesting a possible etiologic role of food hypersensitivity.[33] Cats with inflammatory bowel disease with infiltration of plasma cells and lymphocytes into the small intestinal mucosa clinically improved with dietary modification.[24] A cat with cow's milk hypersensitivity had a great increase in plasma cells in the small intestinal lamina propria.[10] We have successfully treated a small group of dogs and cats with plasmacytic-lymphocytic enteritis and colitis with a hypoallergenic diet.

Lymphocytic-plasmacytic enteritis has been reported in basenjis.[34, 35] This disease appears to have a genetic basis and is influenced by stressors. The role of dietary antigens in the pathogenesis of this condition remains unknown,[35] but the presence of immunocytes in the small intestinal wall suggests a hypersensitivity response.

Summary. Although a commonly described syndrome of food hypersensitivity resulting in severe cutaneous changes exists in veterinary medicine, further immunologic investigation is necessary to determine if it is a true allergy or a form of food intolerance. The gastrointestinal syndromes discussed in this chapter were presented to broaden the reader's perspective on these perplexing diseases. The role of dietary antigens in these disorders remains speculative. However, trial treatments with hypoallergenic diets seem warranted. Further immunologic study is needed to elucidate the potential relationship between food hypersensitivity and the pathogenesis of these disorders. Further information concerning the clinical signs, differential diagnosis, diagnostic planning, and current treatment of these gastrointestinal syndromes can be found in Chapters 85 to 87.

References

1. Walton GS: Skin responses in the dog and cat to ingested allergens. Vet Rec 81:709, 1967.
2. White SD: Food hypersensitivity in 30 dogs. JAVMA 188:695, 1986.
3. Baker E: Food allergy. Vet Clin North Am 4:79, 1974.
4. Scott DW: Immunologic skin disorders in the dog and cat. Vet Clin North Am 8:644, 1978.
5. Scott DW: Feline dermatology 1900-1978: A monograph. JAAHA 16:380, 1980.
6. August JR: Dietary hypersensitivity in dogs: Cutaneous manifestations, diagnosis, and management. Comp Cont Educ Pract Vet 7:469, 1985.
7. Baker E: Food allergies in the cat. Fel Pract 5:18, 1975.
8. Greenberger N: Allergic disorders of the intestine and eosinophilic gastroenteritis. In Sleisenger MH and Fordtran JS (eds), *Gastrointestinal Disease*. WB Saunders, Philadelphia, 1983, p 1069.
9. American Academy of Allergy and Immunology Committee on Adverse Reactions to Foods. National Institute of Allergy and Infectious Diseases. *Adverse Reactions to Foods*. NIH Publication 84-2442, 1984, pp 1–6.
10. Walton GS, et al.: Spontaneous allergic dermatitis and enteritis in a cat. Vet Rec 83:35, 1968.
11. Hammond JB and Littmann A: Disaccharide malabsorption. In Berk JE (ed), *Gastroenterology*. WB Saunders Co, Philadelphia, 1985, p 1703.
12. Hill FWG: Malabsorption syndrome in the dog: A study of thirty-eight cases. J Small Anim Pract 13:575, 1972.
13. Hill FWG and Kelly DF: Naturally occurring intestinal malabsorption in the dog. Dig Dis 19:649, 1974.
14. Scott DW: The skin. In Holzworth J (ed): *Diseases of the Cat, Volume I*. Philadelphia, WB Saunders Co, 1986, p 619.
15. Scott DW, et al.: Miliary dermatitis: A feline cutaneous reaction pattern. In Feline Medicine II (Proceedings of the 2nd Kal Kan Seminar), Lawrenceville, Vet Learning Syst Inc, 1986, pp 11–18.
16. Medleau L, et al.: Food hypersensitivity in a cat. JAVMA 189:692, 1986.
17. Falchuk ZM: Update on gluten-sensitive enteropathy. Am J Med 67:1085, 1979.
18. Kaneko JJ, et al.: Malabsorption syndrome resembling nontropical sprue in dogs. JAVMA 146:463, 1965.
19. Vernon DF: Idiopathic sprue in a dog. JAVMA 140:1062, 1962.
20. Batt RM, et al.: Wheat sensitive enteropathy in Irish Setter dogs: possible age-related brush border abnormalities. Res Vet Sci 39:8083, 1975.
21. Batt RM, et al.: Morphological and biochemical studies of a naturally occurring enteropathy in the Irish setter dog: A comparison with coeliac disease in man. Res Vet Sci 37:339, 1984
22. Batt RM: Chronic small intestinal disease in the dog. Proc Kal Kan Sym 8:93, 1985.
23. McEwen SA, et al.: Hypereosinophilic syndrome in cats: A report of three cases. Can J Comp Med 49:248, 1985.
24. Tams TR: Chronic feline inflammatory bowel disorders. Part II. Feline eosinophilic enteritis and lymphosarcoma. Comp Cont Educ Pract Vet 8:464, 1986.
25. Cello JP: Eosinophilic gastroenteritis: A complex disease entity. Am J Med 67:1097, 1979.
26. Hendrick M: A spectrum of hypereosinophilic syndromes exemplified by six cats with eosinophilic enteritis. Vet Pathol 18:188, 1981.
27. Hayden DW and Van Kruiningen HJ: Eosinophilic gastroenteritis in German Shepherd dogs and its relationship to visceral larva migrans. JAVMA 162:379, 1973.
28. Quigley PJ and Henry K: Eosinophilic enteritis in the dog: A case report with a brief review of the literature. J Comp Path 91:387, 1981.
29. Hayden DW and Fleischman RW: Scirrhous eosinophilic gastritis in dogs with gastric arteritis. Vet Pathol 14:441, 1977.
30. Van Der Gaag I, et al.: Eosinophilic gastroenteritis complicated by partial rupture and a perforation of the small intestine in a dog. J Sm Anim Pract 24:575, 1983.
31. Hayden DW and Van Kruiningen HJ: Lymphocytic plasmacytic enteritis in German shepherd dogs. JAAHA 18:89, 1982.
32. Tams TR: Chronic feline inflammatory bowel disorders. Part I. Idiopathic inflammatory bowel disease. Comp Cont Educ Pract Vet 8:371, 1986.j
33. Nelson RW, et al.: Lymphocytic-plasmacytic colitis in the cat. JAVMA 184:1133, 1984.
34. Breitschwerdt EB, et al.: Clinical and laboratory characterization of basenjis with immunoproliferative small intestinal disease. Am J Vet Res 45:267, 1984.
35. Breitschwerdt EB, et al.: Clinical and epidemiologic characterization of a diarrheal syndrome in basenji dogs. JAVMA 180:914, 1982.

39 FELINE HYPERLIPIDEMIA

BOYD JONES

Lipemia and hyperlipidemia are general terms for elevated concentrations of any or all of the lipids in plasma. Hyperlipoproteinemia is an excess of lipoproteins in blood due to a disorder of lipoprotein metabolism. The hyperlipoproteinemias that are widely recognized in humans are disturbances of lipid transport that result from primary defects in the metabolism of lipoprotein particles and those that are secondary to an underlying metabolic abnormality such as insulin deficiency or resistance or thyroid hormone deficiency.

The primary lipoproteinemias are inherited in humans; therefore a familial disease incidence is often seen. In recent years knowledge of lipoprotein and lipid metabolism has increased as a result of the use of animals as experimental models for lipid metabolism in humans. In addition, primary hyperlipoproteinemias have been identified in dogs and, more recently, in the cat. Primary hyperlipoproteinemias are rare in the cat but are important because they must be considered in the differential diagnosis of the more common secondary hyperlipoproteinemia in this species.

PHYSIOLOGICAL ROLE OF LIPOPROTEINS IN LIPID TRANSPORT

The lipoprotein particles are complexes of triglyceride, cholesterol, and phospholipid united with apoproteins. Apoproteins are synthesized in the liver or in intestinal cells and at least four major groups (termed A, B, C, and E) have been identified. Apoproteins play an essential role in lipid metabolism in that they provide an important structural component of the lipoprotein particle, they act as activators of metabolic enzymes, and they provide recognition sites for cell surface receptors.[1]

The cat has four major lipoprotein classes. On the basis of their differences in density and electrophoretic mobility, these are classified as chylomicrons (CM), very low density lipoproteins (VLDL), low density lipoproteins (LDL), and high density lipoproteins (HDL). The characteristics of these major classes of lipoproteins in human plasma have been identified, and similar data have been published for many animal species, including the cat.[2]

In normal cats HDL is the major lipoprotein class and is the major vehicle for cholesterol transport, whereas in humans LDL is responsible for the major proportion of this lipid.[3,4] Cat and human HDL have a similar composition but cat LDL contains the AI apoprotein, while human LDL does not. Feline HDL consists of two distinct subfractions, HDL_2 and HDL_3, and the apoprotein AII is absent from this lipoprotein subfraction.[5] Full data on the apoprotein concentrations in cats are not available at this time.

LIPOPROTEIN METABOLISM

The roles of the different lipoprotein classes in lipid metabolism are well known in humans and it is presumed that lipid metabolism in the cat is somewhat similar. CM and VLDL are the predominant carriers of exogenous and endogenous triglyceride, respectively, and LDL and HDL are predominantly involved with cholesterol transport to and from tissues and the liver.

There are also important enzymes involved with lipid transport. Lipoprotein lipase (LPL), which is located in the vascular endothelium, is responsible for hydrolyzing the triglyceride of CM and VLDL, thus releasing free fatty acids (FFA) and monoglycerides. Hepatic lipase (HL) located in the liver in the cat also appears to have a function in hydrolyzing CM and VLDL.[4,5] Lecithin cholesterol acyltransferase (LCAT) is an enzyme responsible for the esterification of cholesterol, by which cholesterol is returned to the liver.

Lipid and lipoprotein metabolism is complex, and a defect in one or more steps in the pathway can result in abnormalities in lipoprotein concentrations. An abundance or deficiency of a particular lipoprotein class may indicate where a metabolic defect may be present. In addition, lipid metabolism is dependent on the normal secretion of a variety of hormones, especially insulin and thyroxine.

Hyperlipidemia is not a common finding in cats, but occasionally the cause of persistent fasting lipemia must be investigated.

DIAGNOSTIC TESTS FOR CHOLESTEROL AND TRIGLYCERIDES

Serum cholesterol and triglycerides can be measured, but if levels are elevated they give no indication of the cause of the elevation or the underlying disease process. The laboratory values for cholesterol and triglyceride in normal fasting cats are cholesterol, 38 to 130 mg/dl (1.5 to 5.0 mmol/l), triglyceride, 17 to 50 mg/dl (0.2 to 0.6 mmol/l). If secondary causes of hyperlipemia are eliminated, then it is important to identify which of the lipoprotein classes are elevated. This can be investigated by using the following four methods.

Chylomicron Test. Because of their large size and tendency to aggregate in the cold, CM form a cream layer on the surface of the serum sample after overnight storage at 40° F (4° C). The other lipoprotein classes remain in the infranatant.

Ultracentrifugation. The other three classes of lipoproteins can be separated by ultracentrifugation since the differing proportions of lipid and protein in each lipoprotein complex produce a different density.

Electrophoresis. In addition to its specific density, each lipoprotein class can be separated on the basis of electrophoretic mobility. Following electrophoresis, CM remain at the origin, VLDL migrate to a pre-beta position, LDL migrate to a beta position, and HDL migrate to an alpha position analogous to the alpha and beta globulins of serum.

Lipoprotein Lipase Activity. CM and VLDL triglycerides are hydrolyzed and FFA are delivered to the tissues by the interaction at the endothelial surface with activated LPL; LPL activity is measured *in vivo* after the administration of heparin 5 to 20 IU/lb intravenously, which activates the enzyme *in vivo*. Basal blood samples are collected and lipase activity should be measured ten minutes after heparin administration. Alternatively, concentrations of lipoprotein can be measured before and afterward. No change in the lipoprotein pattern suggests defective LPL activity.

DIAGNOSIS OF HYPERLIPEMIA

If lipemic plasma is detected, three alternatives should be considered: that the sample is a nonfasting sample, that the lipemia is secondary to an underlying metabolic disorder, or that the lipemia is due to a primary disorder of lipid metabolism. The case history may provide clues to underlying diseases that may cause secondary hyperlipemia, especially diabetes mellitus and drug-induced lipemia (megestrol acetate). Physical examination can detect abnormalities associated with diseases causing secondary hyperlipemia. Serum triglyceride and cholesterol levels should be measured in a fasting sample and plasma should be examined after refrigeration overnight for the presence of a cream layer (CM) and infranatant turbidity (other lipoprotein classes, especially VLDL). Appropriate serum biochemistry and urinanalyses are essential to rule out the causes of secondary hyperlipemia (Table 39–1). If a cause for hyperlipemia is found, lipoprotein electrophoresis or ultracentrifugation to determine the abundance of the different lipoprotein fractions becomes unnecessary. However, if the condition is still undiagnosed in spite of the above data, then a hereditary disease should be suspected and lipoprotein electrophoresis and/or ultracentrifugation is essential to define the nature of the defect. Further details of littermates and relations should be sought, as some of these animals may also be affected.

TABLE 39–1. CAUSES OF HYPERLIPEMIA IN THE CAT

Postprandial hyperlipemia
Secondary hyperlipemia
Diabetes mellitus
Drug induced, e.g., megestrol acetate
Nephrotic syndrome
Primary hyperlipemia
Idiopathic hyperchylomicronemia
Lipoprotein lipase deficiency

SECONDARY HYPERLIPIDEMIA

Hypothyroidism. Although hypothyroidism is a common cause of hyperlipidemia in the dog, naturally occurring acquired hypothyroidism has not yet been definitely diagnosed in the feline.

Nephrotic Syndrome. Plasma cholesterol levels are usually raised in feline nephrotic syndrome, although the reasons for this elevation are not clearly understood (see Chapter 108).

Diabetes Mellitus. Diabetes mellitus occurs either when pancreatic B cells no longer produce and/or secrete sufficient insulin to maintain carbohydrate homeostasis,

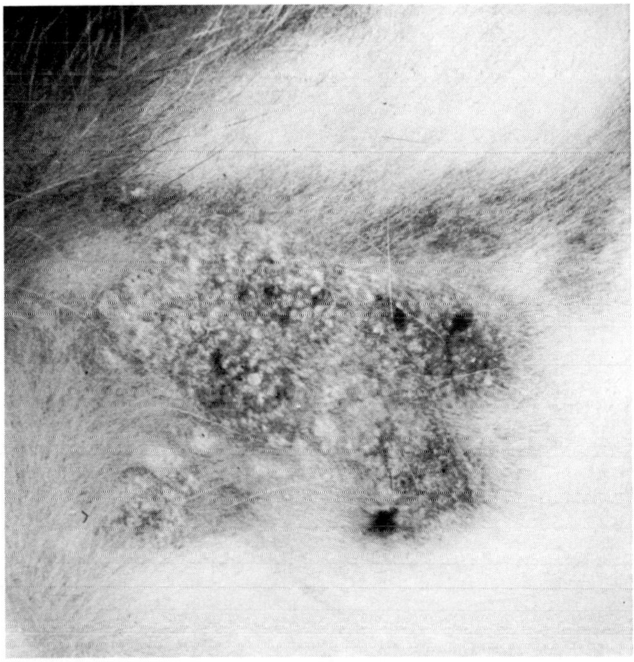

FIGURE 39–1. Skin xanthoma in the axilla of a cat with diabetes mellitus. (From Jones, BR, et al.: Cutaneous xanthoma associated with diabetes mellitus in a cat. J Sm Anim Pract 26:33, 1985. Published with permission of the Journal of Small Animal Practice.)

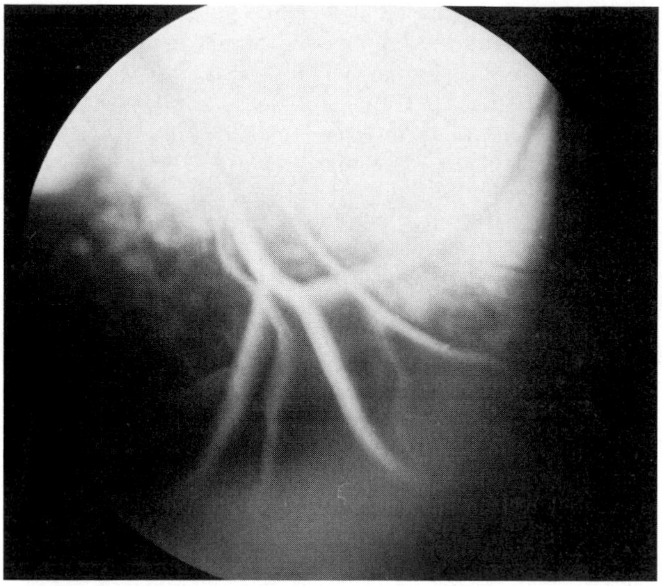

FIGURE 39–2. Lipemia retinalis. (From Jones BR: Inherited hyperchylomicronemia in the cat. Feline Pract 16:17, 1986. Published with permission of Feline Practice.)

or when there is a diminished responsiveness by target cells to the action of insulin (see Chapter 96).

LPL is the enzyme responsible for the breakdown and removal of triglyceride-rich chylomicrons from the plasma and insulin is necessary for its normal activity. Thus, patients with diabetes mellitus and insulin insufficiency have low LPL activity, which in some cases results in triglyceride-rich diabetic hyperlipemia, especially of CM and VLDL fractions.

Cutaneous xanthomas have been diagnosed in a cat found to be affected with naturally occurring diabetes mellitus[6] (Figure 39–1).

Insulin therapy causes the lipoprotein lipase activity to return to normal, accompanied by clearing of triglycerides and hyperlipemia and rapid resolution (three to six weeks) of xanthomas. Dietary modification also helps to restore blood lipid levels to normal.

Drug-Induced Hyperlipemia. Diabetes mellitus has been reported in cats receiving long-term progestogen therapy using megestrol acetate.[7, 8] Drug withdrawal, with or without insulin therapy in cats with megestrol acetate–induced diabetes mellitus, results in resolution of the diabetic condition over periods ranging from ten days to eight months.[7] Occasionally, some cats require insulin therapy indefinitely. Resistance to insulin associated with increased levels of the insulin antagonist growth hormone is thought to be the major cause of the diabetes and concurrent hyperlipemia. In one reported case[8] cutaneous xanthomatosis was present in addition to hyperlipidemia and hyperglycemia. This author has also observed cutaneous xanthomas in cats receiving megestrol acetate.

TABLE 39–2. CLINICAL MANIFESTATIONS OF PRIMARY FAMILIAL HYPERCHYLOMICRONEMIA IN 24 CATS

Manifestation	Prevalence
Hyperchylomicronemia	24
Lipemia retinalis	10
Cutaneous xanthomas	3
Granulomas palpable in liver, kidney, spleen, intestine	3
Peripheral neuropathy*	9
Horner's syndrome	3
Facial nerve paralysis	1
Tibial nerve paralysis	4
Peroneal nerve paralysis	2
Femoral nerve paralysis	1
Trigeminal nerve paralysis	1
Recurrent laryngeal nerve paralysis	1
Radial nerve paralysis	3
Splenomegaly	1

*Some cats had more than one nerve affected.

PRIMARY HYPERLIPIDEMIAS

INHERITED HYPERCHYLOMICRONEMIA

In 1983 a persistent-fasting lipidemia in related cats was described and subsequent breeding of these cats

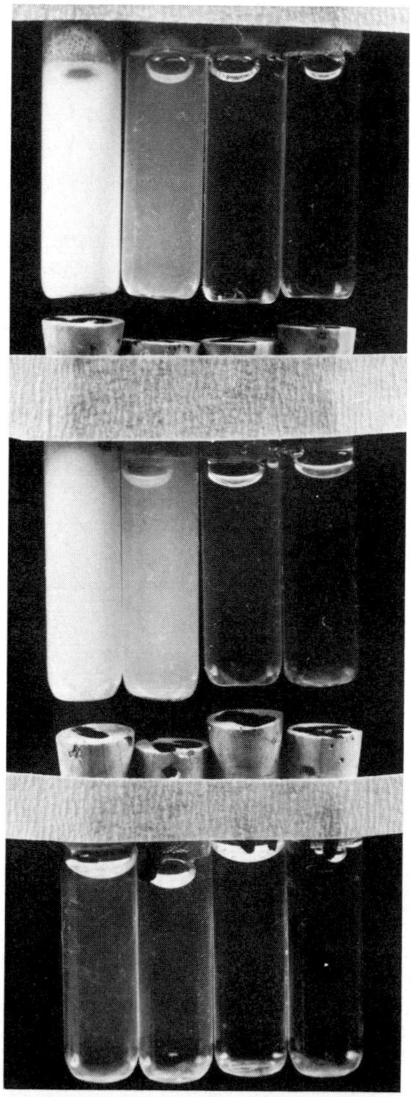

FIGURE 39–3. The physical appearance of the four main lipoprotein fractions (chylomicrons, VLDL, LDL, and HDL) for three serum samples from two hyperlipidemic cats and from a control cat (bottom row). (From Jones, BR: Inherited hyperchylomicronemia in the cat. Feline Pract 16:17, 1986. Published with permission of Feline Practice.)

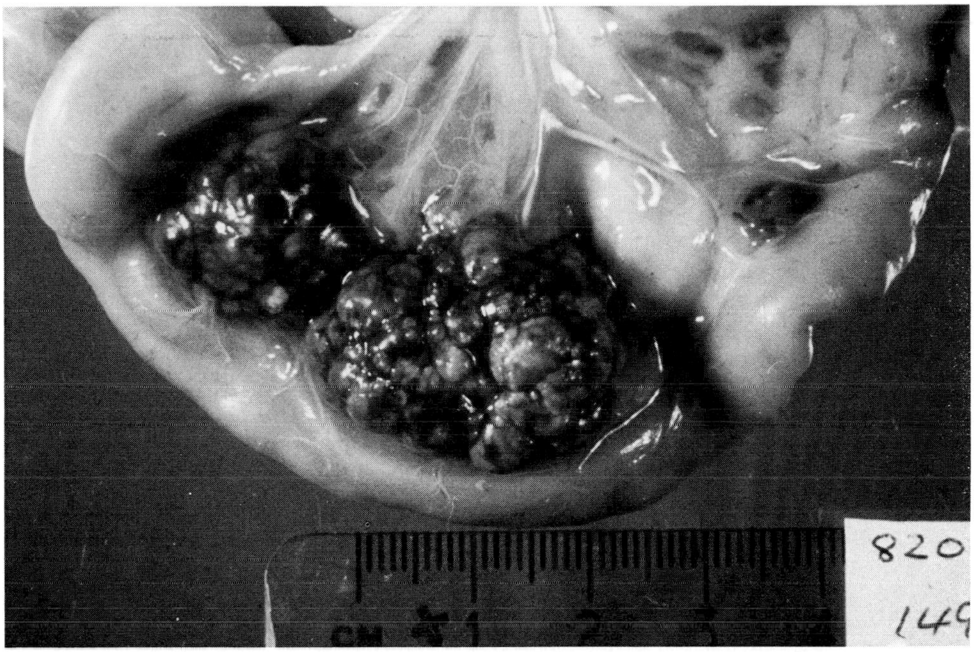

FIGURE 39–4. Multiple xanthomatous nodules in the mesentery of an affected cat. (From Jones BR: Inherited hyperchylomicronemia in the cat. Feline Pract 16:17, 1986. Published with permission of Feline Practice.)

confirmed that the condition was familial and inherited.[3, 9–11] In another report, fasting lipemia in two kitten siblings was described.[12] In both these investigations low post-heparin lipoprotein lipase activity was demonstrated in plasma. The findings in both cases were similar to those found in human Type I hyperlipoproteinemia, which is caused by reduced or lowered activity of LPL. The metabolic basis for the condition in cats has not been determined.

Clinical Signs. Affected cats may not show any clinical signs other than the presence of fasting hyperlipemia; the blood has the appearance of "cream of tomato soup." Examination of the ocular fundus reveals lipemia retinalis in some cats (Figure 39–2). In such cases, the retinal arterioles and venules develop a pale color that is due to light scattering by the large CM, which are present in excess in the blood.

Kittens that display clinical signs in addition to hyperlipemia often do not do so until eight to nine months of age. The clinical manifestations shown by 24 affected cats examined by the author are listed in Table 39–2.

Cutaneous nodules (xanthomas) may be palpable in the skin over bony prominences or at pressure points, e.g., the ventral tarsus. Firm, painless granulomas or xanthomas may be detected by palpation of other organs, e.g., the kidney, liver, or intestine. In one animal, massive splenomegaly and subsequent rupture was detected. The most consistent clinical sign shown by affected cats is the development of peripheral nerve paralyses. Cats with these nerve signs develop a slow-onset unilateral paralysis with loss of conscious proprioception and motor function. Where mixed nerves are affected, sensation to painful stimuli is retained. The nerves most commonly affected are the cervical sympathetic nerves (Horner's syndrome) and the sciatic nerves. One cat died as a result of paralysis of the recurrent laryngeal nerve, which prevented the vocal cords from being abducted during inspiration. The peripheral nerve paralyses are caused by pressure from the xanthomas on the nerves. Xanthomas form at spinal foramina where the nerves exit from the spinal cord and also at bony prominences, i.e., areas where nerves are susceptible to trauma and hence to the development of xanthomas.

The fat content of the diet does influence the severity of the lipidemia. Thus, cats on a high fat diet are more likely to show clinical signs.

Laboratory Findings. Affected cats show no hematological abnormalities; serum chemistry, urinalysis, glucose tolerance, and serum thyroxine measurements are also normal. The plasma of the affected cats is lactescent, with marked elevation of both cholesterol and triglyceride levels. Overnight refrigeration of plasma at 40° F (4° C) allows a cream supernatant to develop, indicating CM elevation, together with a slightly turbid infranatant, indicating slight elevation of VLDL. Cholesterol levels (mean for 24 affected cats = 25.5 mg/dl (6.6 mmol/l)) and triglyceride levels (mean for 24 affected cats = 899.7 mg/dl (10.02 mmol/l)) are raised. The physical appearance of the four main lipoprotein fractions in serum samples separated by ultracentrifugation shows a significant increase in CM and a smaller increase in VLDL (Figure 39–3).

In affected cats CM represents the major proportion of triglyceride. Cholesterol is carried predominantly in HDL but is also elevated in CM compared to values for normal cats.

Lipoprotein Lipase Measurement. Affected cats show reduced (but not absent) LPL activity in plasma after heparin administration. Presumably, the remaining activity is due to other plasma lipases, e.g., hepatic lipase.

Inheritance. The condition in cats is inherited. An autosomal recessive trait is suspected, in a pattern of inheritance similar to the equivalent disease in humans.

Pathologic Findings. The outstanding feature in affected cats is the presence of disseminated, usually multiple, nodular granulomas and organizing hematomas in many tissues (Figure 39–4). The granulomas range in size from a few millimeters to five centimeters in diameter. Granulomas were shown to compress some peripheral nerves, particularly at sites where the nerves were most susceptible to trauma, e.g., at spinal foramina and over bony prominences.

The clinical signs of peripheral neuropathy can be explained by the presence of granulomas that compress these nerves not only externally, but also within the perineurium. Histologically, there is evidence of axonal degeneration with loss of myelinated fibers. The nodular lesions in tissues are organizing hematomas with a granulomatous reaction elicited by the extravasated lipid. There are many large, multinucleated macrophages with vacuolated cytoplasm ("foam cells") scattered among a coagulum of blood, degenerating blood components, fibrin, serum, and lipids. Lipofuscin, hemosiderin, and crystals of triglycerides and cholesterol are also present. Older lesions have an outer zone of fibrosis and granulation tissue.

Therapy. Feeding the animal a low fat diet results in a reduction in plasma lipid levels, and all the clinical manifestations of hyperchylomicronemia are reversible provided the plasma triglyceride levels are lowered.[13] *The peripheral nerve paralysis can be expected to resolve in affected cats after two to three months on a low fat diet.*

Summary. Familial hyperchylomicronemia due to LPL deficiency is a new condition in the cat and must be considered in the differential diagnosis of not only hyperlipidemia, but also of peripheral nerve paralyses, especially when these two signs occur together. There is also a possibility that other primary disorders of lipid metabolism occur in the cat. Clinicians should be aware of this possibility when interpreting blood lipid profiles of cats with fasting hyperlipidemia.

References

1. Hancock, WS, et al.: Fats for the Future. Proc. International Conference on oils, fats, waxes. Duromark Publishing, 1983. p 156.
2. Chapman, MJ: Animal lipoproteins: Chemistry structure and comparative aspects. J Lipid Res 21:189, 1980.
3. Jones, BR, et al.: Occurrence of idiopathic familial hyperchylomicronaemia in a cat. Vet Rec 12:543, 1983.
4. Demacker, PNM, et al.: Accumulation of chylomicrons and B VLDL during inhibition of hepatic lipase in cats. Biochem Biophys Acta. In Press.
5. Demacker, PNM, et al.: A study of the lipid transport system in the cat, felis domesticus. Artherosclerosis. In Press.
6. Jones, BR, et al.: Cutaneous xanthomata associated with diabetes mellitus in a cat. J Sm Anim Pract 26:33, 1985.
7. Middleton, DJ: Megestrol acetate in the cat. Vet Annual 26:341, 1986.
8. Kwochka, KW and Short, BG: Cutaneous xanthomatosis and diabetes mellitus following long term therapy with megestrol acetate in a cat. Compend Cont Educ 185, 1984.
9. Jones, BR, et al.: Peripheral neuropathy in cats with inherited primary hyperchylomicronaemia. Vet Rec 119:268, 1986.
10. Jones, BR, et al.: Inherited hyperchylomicronaemia in the cat. Feline Pract 16:17, 1986.
11. Jones, BR, et al.: Inherited hyperchlomicronaemia in the cat. Vet Annual 26:330, 1986.
12. Bauer, JE and Verlander, JW: Congenital lipoprotein lipase deficiency in hyperlipidemic kitten siblings. Vet Clin Path 13:7, 1984.
13. Brunzell, JD and Bierman, EL: Chylomicronemia syndrome. Med Clin North Am 66:455, 1981.

40 CANINE HYPERLIPIDEMIA

ROGER K. JOHNSON

Hyperlipidemia or hyperlipoproteinemia can be divided into two major categories, *hypertriglyceridemia* (lipemia, hyperlipemia) and *hypercholesterolemia.* The not uncommon observation of milky (lactescent) serum in the fasted canine patient is a result of excess circulating triglyceride molecules that are large enough to refract light, whereas even with severe elevations of cholesterol and other lipids, the serum remains clear. Perhaps because the incidence of canine atherosclerosis is negligible, hypercholesterolemia is but a diagnostic clue, whereas hypertriglyceridemia has major clinical and therapeutic significance as well as diagnostic importance.

PHYSIOLOGY OF LIPIDS

Types of Lipids

Cholesterol, which is available from dietary sources and can be synthesized by virtually all nucleated mammalian cells, is an essential constituent of plasma membranes and myelin sheaths and is required for the production of bile acids as well as adrenal and gonadal steroidogenesis.[1] Free cholesterol, the metabolically active form, is esterified with a fatty acid by the enzyme lecithin cholesterol acyltransferase (LCAT) to form esterified cholesterol, which is the predominant form in which cholesterol is transported and stored. *Phospholipids* are also important structural components of cell membranes and play an important role in phosphorylative and energy-linked transport of ions across cell membranes.[2] *Triglycerides* are glycerol esterified with three fatty acids; their function is to transport and store energy-rich *fatty acids*.

LIPOPROTEINS

Since plasma lipids are insoluble in water, they are transported in association with protein. Free fatty acids are bound to albumin, however, phospholipids, cholesterol, and triglycerides are combined with carrier "apoproteins" to form soluble macromolecules called lipoproteins.[3] All of the major lipoproteins transported in the plasma are spherical; each has a core of varying amounts of triglyceride and cholesterol esters, which are hydrophobic or nonpolar. Surrounding that core is a monolayer coating of varying thickness consisting of polar lipids (phospholipids and unesterified cholesterol) and apoproteins (A, B, C, D, and E), which renders the lipoproteins soluble in plasma (Figure 40–1). The apoprotein combination is specific to each lipoprotein and among its responsibilities is the task of directing the lipoprotein to its site of metabolism.[1]

Five distinct types of lipoproteins have been identified in the serum of healthy dogs: chylomicrons, very low density lipoprotein (VLDL), low density lipoprotein (LDL), high density lipoprotein-1 (HDL_1), and high density lipoprotein-2 (HDL_2). Their classification is based on size, density as determined by ultracentrifugation, and by electrophoretic mobility (Table 40–1). The size is directly proportional and the density is inversely proportional to the triglyceride content. The electrophoretic mobility is predominantly a function of the type of apoprotein on the surface membrane.

Chylomicrons. Dietary triglycerides are hydrolyzed by pancreatic lipase and absorbed by intestinal epithelial cells where fatty acids are re-esterified to form triglyceride, which combines with a very small amount of esterified dietary cholesterol to form the core of this, the largest lipoprotein molecule. Phospholipid then combines with a small amount of unesterified cholesterol and apoproteins B, and to a lesser extent, A and E, to form its solubilizing membrane. The chylomicron is then released into intestinal lymphatics, where its predominant function is to transport "exogenous" triglyceride.[1]

Chylomicrons are the largest (150 nm ±) and least dense lipoproteins, consisting predominantly of triglyceride. Owing to their larger size and small amount of apoprotein, they do not migrate past the point of origin with agarose gel electrophoresis. Chylomicrons are not found in serum from normal dogs who have been fasted for 12 hours.[4]

Very Low Density Lipoprotein. Triglycerides are formed in the liver from circulating or hepatically synthesized free fatty acids derived from catabolism of carbohydrate and amino acids. They are combined with a small amount of cholesterol to form the core of the second largest (26 to 90 nm) lipoprotein, VLDL, whose

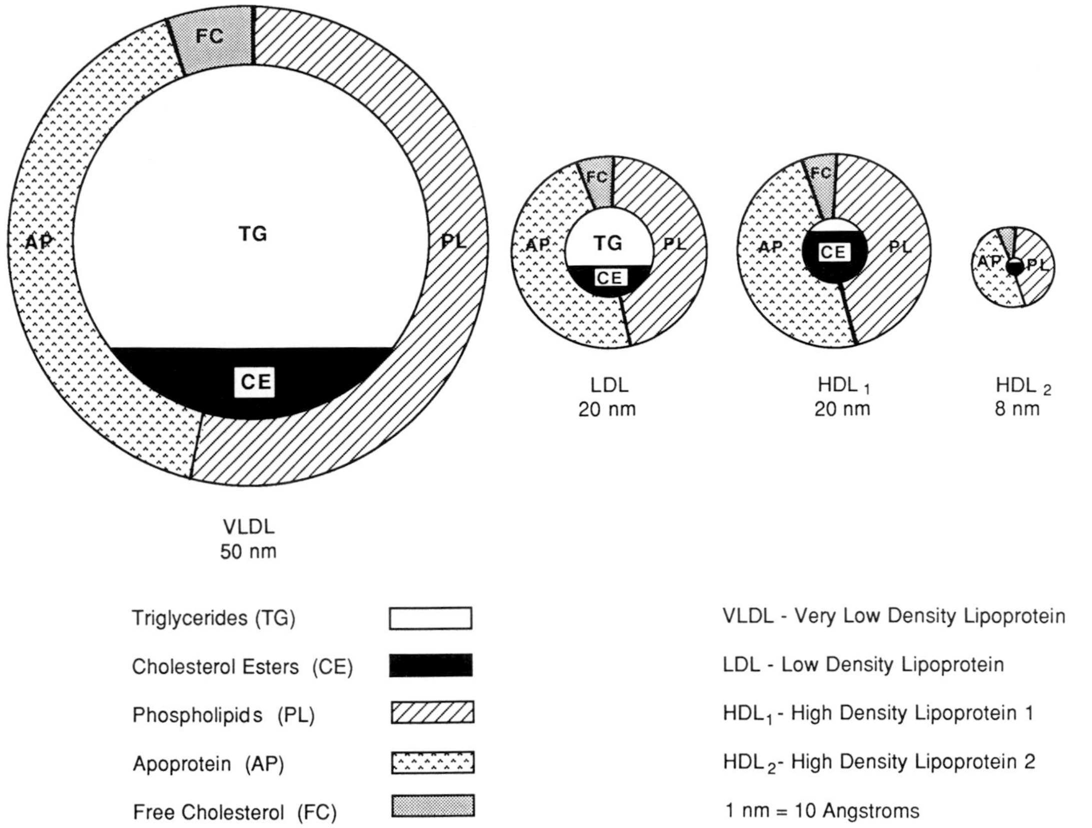

FIGURE 40–1. A diagrammatic representation of normal serum lipoproteins of fasted dogs showing an inner "hydrophobic" lipid core and an outer coating. The coating, consisting of polar lipids (phospholipid and free cholesterol) and apoprotein, causes the lipoprotein to be soluble in plasma. Note that the coating is roughly the same thickness even though the overall size varies greatly. The hydrophobic core contains varying amounts of triglyceride and cholesterol esters. The larger lipoproteins generally contain more triglyceride and smaller ones a higher percentage of cholesterol esters. Not shown is the chylomicron, which is roughly three times the size of VLDL.

major function is to transport endogenous triglyceride. The solubilizing membrane contains beta apoproteins, which causes its electrophoretic mobility to be in the "pre-beta" range, which is faster than beta and slower than alpha.[4]

Fatty acids derived from the two triglyceride-rich lipoproteins (chylomicrons and VLDL) are delivered to tissues after hydrolysis by *lipoprotein lipase* (LPL), which is found in high concentration on the endothelium of the capillaries of cardiac and skeletal muscle, as well as adipose tissue. To a lesser extent, triglycerides can be directly metabolized in peripheral tissue, a pathway that increases in importance in hypertriglyceridemic states. The predominant cause of elevation in triglyceride-rich lipoproteins is clearly diminished LPL activity. However, increased production of VLDL has long been recognized in humans consuming excessive calories in the form of simple carbohydrates.[3]

Low Density Lipoprotein. Hydrolysis of VLDL by LPL causes the progressive depletion of the triglyceride from the VLDL core, resulting first in the formation of a relatively cholesterol-rich "VLDL remnant," which is then catabolized by the liver to form LDL. This smaller (20 nm) lipoprotein migrates in the beta electrophoretic band, owing to the high concentration of beta protein in its outer membrane. In contrast to humans, where LDL contains very little triglyceride, 50 per cent cholesterol, and is the major cholesterol-containing (atherosclerogenic) lipoprotein, canine LDL functions to carry both triglyceride (30 per cent) and cholesterol (20 per cent).[4]

High Density Lipoprotein. In humans, a single HDL arises from two sources. The liver secretes nascent HDL, which is essentially the HDL coating in a bilayered disc shape. Unesterified cholesterol is converted by LCAT to the esterified form, which is then inserted between layers, transforming it into a sphere. HDL is also formed during the catabolism of chylomicrons and VLDL.[1] Two distinct high density lipoproteins have been described in the sera of normal dogs.

HDL_1. HDL_1 is equal in size to LDL (10 to 35 nm), is impossible to separate from LDL by ultracentrifugation, and migrates electrophoretically between LDL and HDL in the alpha 2 band. While it only contains 20 per cent cholesterol, it is the predominant carrier of cholesterol in the hypothyroid cholesterol-fed dog.[4]

HDL_2. The most abundant lipoprotein in the dog is HDL_2, which is the smallest (8 nm), densest, and fastest migrating (alpha 1) electrophoretically because of its high concentration of apoprotein A (42 per cent). HDL_2 contains almost no triglyceride, 20 per cent cholesterol, and carries most of the cholesterol in the normal dog.[4]

An extraordinary amount of research into the metabolism of cholesterol-containing lipoproteins in humans

TABLE 40–1. COMPOSITION AND CHARACTERISTICS OF CANINE LIPOPROTEINS

Lipoprotein Class*	Composition (%) (Core + Coating)				Diameter nm	Major Apoprotein	Electrophoretic Mobility	Ultracentrifugation Density Range qm/ml
	Triglyceride	*Cholesterol*	*Phospholipids*	*Protein*				
Chylomicron	80–95	2–7	3–6	1–2	80–200	Apo A Apo B Apo C	Origin	—
VLDL	59	15	16	10	26–90	Apo B Apo C Apo E	Pre-beta	>1.006
LDL	30	22	24	23	20	Apo B	Beta	1.006–1.087
HDL_1	2	35	40	22	10–35	Apo A	Alpha 2	1.025–1.100
HDL_2	1	20	36	42	5.5–8.5	Apo A	Alpha 1	1.070–1.210

*Very low density lipoprotein = VLDL; low density lipoprotein = LDL; high density lipoprotein = HDL.
(Modified from Zerbe, 1985.)

has shown that LDL, and to a lesser extent, HDL, are responsible for transporting esterified cholesterol and phospholipid from the liver as well as circulating chylomicrons and VLDL to extrahepatic cells for cell membrane and steroid synthesis. Surplus cholesterol is then transferred from those cells to HDL molecules, which in turn "hand them off" to LDL and remnants of chylomicrons and VLDL to be returned to the liver.[1] This cycle of LDL delivery and HDL return of cholesterol to and from extrahepatic cells may prove to be true in the dog as well.

Abnormal Lipoproteins. Two additional abnormal lipoproteins have been observed in dogs with hyperlipidemia. Dogs fed high cholesterol diets may produce an alpha-migrating HDL whose major apoprotein is E rather than A, termed HDL-cholesterol (HDL_C); this is thought to be simply HDL_2 overloaded with cholesterol. Also recognized in cholesterol-fed dogs is a VLDL molecule that contains apoprotein E and has normal density characteristics. It is termed beta-VLDL. Electrophoretically, it migrates in the beta range, is slower than the pre-beta of normal VLDL, and is suspected to be triglyceride- and cholesterol-rich.[2]

CLINICAL RECOGNITION OF HYPERLIPIDEMIA

CLINICAL SIGNS

The vast majority of canine hyperlipidemias are secondary to other endocrine or metabolic diseases. The clinician is well trained in recognition of clinical signs of such common diseases as diabetes mellitus, acute pancreatitis, and hypothyroidism. However, hypertriglyceridemia may, whether secondary to other disease or primary from an inborn error of metabolism, produce such signs as acute abdominal pain, seizures, vomiting, diarrhea, hepatosplenomegaly, lipid-laden aqueous humor, cardiovascular embarrassment, lethargy, and anorexia. Isolated hypercholesterolemia may be responsible for atherosclerosis[5] (rarely), lipemia retinalis,[6] and arc-like patterns of lipid opacification in the cornea.[7]

CLINICAL LABORATORY TESTS

Serum chemistry profiles routinely include cholesterol assays, which should be interpreted as total (esterified plus free) cholesterol. Normal values may vary with laboratory techniques. Representative values are presented in Table 39–2. The author is using 193 ± 13 mg/dL as normal, 250 to 500 mg/dL as mild elevation, 500 to 750 mg/dL as moderate elevation, and greater than 750 mg/dL, severe elevation.

Triglyceride assay is almost always available. Triglyceride values of 55 ± 8.1 mg/dL are considered normal, 200 to 400 mg/dL mild elevation, 400 to 1000 mg/dL moderate elevation, and greater than 1000 mg/dL severe elevation.

Particularly annoying to clinicians is the inability of a laboratory to perform certain routine chemistry tests accurately when the serum is lipemic. Depending on the severity of lipemia, the serum bilirubin, total protein, albumin, calcium, phosphorus, and glucose will be falsely increased, and, depending on methodology, the amylase may be falsely decreased. Serum sodium and to a lesser extent, potassium, may be falsely decreased in severe hypertriglyceridemia. There is an increased (nonsodium-containing) lipid phase of plasma and a normal (sodium-containing) aqueous phase that result in a decreased estimation of total plasma sodium concentration.[2] Furthermore, lipemia renders red blood cells more fragile, predisposing them to iatrogenic hemolysis.

Chylomicrons may persist in the serum for 14 hours, therefore, it is important to evaluate serum only from fasted patients.

Severe elevations in triglycerides may cause freshly drawn whole blood to present with a lactescent appearance, especially if the elevation is due to hyperchylomicronemia. Whole blood lactescence (cream of tomato soup appearance) may also be observed with only moderate lipemia if the dogs are also anemic. More typically, however, lipemia may first be appreciated by inspection of serum when triglyceride levels reach 300 to 400 mg/dL. Determination of which triglyceride-rich lipoprotein (chylomicron or VLDL) is responsible for lipemia may be accomplished by inspecting the serum after it is refrigerated for six to eight hours. Chylomicrons rise to the surface, forming a cream layer, whereas

VLDL molecules are homogeneously distributed beneath. This so-called "*chylomicron test*," combined with measurement of serum cholesterol and triglyceride concentrations, provides the clinician who understands the basics of lipoprotein metabolism with all clinically relevant information in a vast majority of cases.

Elevation in triglyceride levels with normal or mildly elevated cholesterol is the result of increases in chylomicrons or VLDL. If cholesterol is elevated and triglycerides are normal or mildly elevated, increased levels of HDL_2, LDL, and to a lesser extent, HDL_1, can be anticipated. However, if moderate or severe elevations of both triglyceride and cholesterol are observed, it results from a combination of triglyceride-rich and cholesterol-rich lipoproteins or occasionally from abnormal lipoproteins beta-VLDL or HDL_C.

Lipoprotein electrophoresis has been employed to separate graphically the classes of lipoproteins in humans and has been reported in dogs.[8, 9] However, in the author's experience most veterinary laboratories do not provide this test in a timely manner, it contributes little clinically useful information, and is usually not cost-effective.

CLINICAL INVESTIGATION TOOLS

The study of the pathogenesis of canine hyperlipidemia may be enhanced by the indirect assay of LPL activity by injection of heparin. When given intravenously, heparin releases LPL from the capillary endothelium, which in turn causes hydrolysis of the triglycerides of chylomicrons and VLDL. Serum for triglyceride and cholesterol concentrations and lipoprotein electrophoresis determination should be collected prior to, and 15 minutes after, the intravenous administration of heparin (45 IU/lb body weight). If there is no change in the serum lipid concentrations or the lipoprotein electrophoretic pattern, an absent or defective LPL enzyme system should be suspected. Direct assays of canine lipoprotein lipase are being investigated but are not presently available.[2] The most complete characterization of a patient's lipoproteins is achieved in a research laboratory by quantitative measurement of cholesterol and triglyceride content and electrophoretic behavior of individual lipoprotein fractions, separated by sequential preparative ultracentrifugation and other more sophisticated means.[1] Analysis of lipoprotein electrophoretic patterns may provide some qualitative information when quantitative tests are not available to determine if hyperlipidemia is caused by inborn errors of metabolism or if abnormal lipoprotein fractions are present in the diseased states.

DISEASES ASSOCIATED WITH HYPERLIPIDEMIA

DIABETES MELLITUS

The serum from diabetic dogs is frequently lactescent with or without a chylomicron layer after refrigeration and there is moderate to severe elevation in triglyceride and mild to moderate increase in cholesterol. Absence or marked insufficiency of insulin results in a deficiency of LPL activity and, therefore, an accumulation of the triglyceride-rich lipoproteins, chylomicrons, and VLDL. Cholesterol elevations in diabetic dogs have been associated with increased staining in the alpha 2 (HDL_1) and beta regions (LDL and VLDL) on electrophoresis; the mechanism for this abnormality remains speculative.[4]

ACUTE PANCREATITIS

Acute pancreatitis may be characterized by clear serum with mild to moderately elevated cholesterol or by lipemic serum with or without a cream layer, hypertriglyceridemia, and mild or moderate cholesterol elevation. Although clinicians disagree and actual data are lacking, the author's impression is that pancreatitis occurs with lipemia about as often as it does with clear serum.

Published pathophysiologic mechanisms for hyperlipidemia in acute pancreatitis are unavailable; however, it is inviting to speculate that diminished LPL activity will someday be proven. Of interest is the absence of pancreatitis from the list of causes of hyperlipidemia in the human literature. There is, in fact, a considerable amount of data to suggest that the hyperlipidemia seen in human subjects with acute pancreatitis precedes the onset of that disease. Although the mechanism remains unknown, it is speculated that high levels of triglyceride meet with increased concentrations of pancreatic lipase in the pancreatic capillaries, releasing large quantities of free fatty acids that exceed the albumin binding capacity. They are, therefore, free to induce toxic vascular injury and acute pancreatitis. This theory is so widely held that humans with severe hypertriglyceridemia are considered medical emergencies due to pending pancreatitis and are hospitalized without food until their levels fall below 1000 mg/dL. Continued, vigorous efforts are then made to cause the triglycerides to return to below 500 mg/dL.[10] Ingestion of a fatty meal frequently precedes the onset of acute pancreatitis in dogs, yet in most instances it is unknown whether hyperlipidemia was pre-existing. However, there does appear to be an increased prevalence of pancreatitis in dogs known to have unresolved lipemia. In order to prevent recurring pancreatitis, clinicians are well advised to monitor serum lipid concentrations in dogs recovering from pancreatitis.

HYPOTHYROIDISM

The serum of dogs with documented hypothyroidism varies from clear with normal to moderately elevated cholesterol to lipemic with or without a chylomicron layer and with severe cholesterol elevation greater than 750 mg/dL. The dogs who develop hypertriglyceridemia and severe elevation in cholesterol have clearly been shown to be predisposed to clinically significant atherosclerosis and should be treated vigorously.[5] Thyroid hormones are known to regulate cholesterol synthesis and enhance the hepatic degradation of cholesterol to bile acids, but the mechanism is not clear. Thyroid hormone may be necessary for the activation of lipoprotein lipase.[9]

CORTICOSTEROID EXCESS

In both hyperadrenocorticism and exogenous steroid administration, hyperlipoproteinemia may occur. It is reported to be somewhat proportional to the amount of peripheral insulin resistance induced, which in turn depresses LPL activity, resulting in increased triglyceride-rich lipoproteins.[1]

CHOLESTATIC LIVER DISEASE

In humans, serum cholesterol concentrations exceeding 400 mg/dL may be associated with an abnormal lipoprotein X (LPX) or hypertriglyceridemia from lipoprotein Y (LPY).[1] Elevations in serum cholesterol are frequently observed in dogs with cholestasis; however, the resulting abnormal lipoprotein has not been characterized and its significance is limited to diagnostic information.

Other diseases that cause hyperlipidemia in humans, many of which are presumed to do so in dogs, are nephrotic syndrome, uremia, estrogen administration, immunoglobulin-lipoprotein complex disorders, hypopituitarism, and acromegaly.

IDIOPATHIC HYPERLIPOPROTEINEMIA

A presumably inherited disease of miniature schnauzers with signs of abdominal distress and/or seizures, and occasionally overt pancreatitis, is now well recognized. Hyperlipidemia with this condition is characterized by lactescent serum with chylomicrons and usually marked hypertriglyceridemia and moderate cholesterol elevation. Decreased activity of lipoprotein lipase has been demonstrated as a major mechanism,[9] and it has been speculated that the triglyceride is carried in an abnormal beta-VLDL similar to familial dysbetalipoproteinemia in humans.[2]

IDIOPATHIC HYPERCHYLOMICRONEMIA

The refrigerated serum from two reported cases[8] demonstrated a significant chylomicron layer, clear serum below and marked elevation in triglycerides, yet with normal cholesterol values. Both dogs responded to dietary fat restriction.

TREATMENT

The goal of treatment of canine hyperlipidemia is to reduce the triglyceride level in order to decrease clinical signs directly attributable to hypertriglyceridemia and to reduce the risk of pancreatitis. Additionally, specific cholesterol-lowering measures should be employed if serum concentrations are near the atherogenic level of 750 mg/dL.

Whether treating an idiopathic hyperlipidemia or hyperlipidemia persisting after appropriate therapy of underlying disease, the therapy is the same. If hypertriglyceridemia exists, strict compliance to a commercial (R/D, Hill Pet Products) or home-cooked low fat and low calorie diet is very often successful. In the unlikely event that chylomicronemia persists in the face of low fat diet, medium chain triglyceride oil (MCT Oil, Mead Johnson 0.25 ml/lb/day), which contains fatty acids with not more than ten carbons, may be substituted for what little fat is in the above-mentioned diet. If cholesterol levels exceed 500 mg/dL, appropriate doses of thyroid supplementation (Synthroid, 0.25 mg/10lb/q12hr) should be administered, even if T_4 assays are in the normal range. In the event that counseling of the owner results in strict compliance to the above therapy and persisting moderate or severe hypertriglyceridemia is determined to pose a significant health hazard, some clinicians have elected to use lipid-lowering drugs intended for similar use in humans. Clofibrate (Atromid-S) and gemfibrozil (Lopid) decrease hepatic VLDL synthesis, and niacin, a B vitamin, lowers both triglycerides and cholesterol. These drugs are renowned for side effects in humans and they cannot be recommended for use in dogs until their safety and efficacy have been demonstrated.

Editor's Note: We have successfully employed niacin (Nicolar tablets) in low dosage schedules with apparent clinical results. Usually the drug is given one to two times daily beginning with ¼ to ½ tablet per dose, depending on the dog's size. Gemfibrozil (Lopid) is similarly used, dispensing the product in ¼ capsule size for most 20-pound dogs. This requires refilling smaller capsules or having the client administer only a portion of a full capsule for each dose. (See Table 40–2.)

Recently, dietary fish oils rich in Omega-3 fatty acids have been shown to reduce plasma triglycerides by 64 per cent and cholesterol by 27 per cent in humans with hypertriglyceridemia.[11] Human subjects with familial hyperchylomicronemia who are taking fish oils have been observed to produce markedly fewer chylomicrons after ingesting fatty meals. It is inviting to speculate that

TABLE 40–2. PHARMACEUTICAL AGENTS

Generic	Trade	Dosage	Route	Frequency	Brief Description
Med. Chain Triglyceride Oil	MCT Oil	0.25 ml/lb	PO	divided	Dietary fatty acid supplement
Thyroid Supplement	Synthroid	0.25 mg/10 lb	PO	q12h	Synthetic thyroid hormone
Marine Lipid Concentrate	Formula Plus	15 to 30 mg/lb	PO	q24h	Lipid lowering agent
Niacin	Nicolar	¼ to ½ tab	PO	q12h	Lowers cholesterol and triglycerides. May need to vary dosage
Gemfibrozil	Lopid	¼ to ½ caps	PO	q12h	Lowers triglycerides and occasionally cholesterol. Must reduce capsule size. Begin low dosage and adjust with time based on results

feeding of fish oils would similarly augment fat tolerance in dogs predisposed to pancreatitis. Preliminary studies by the author, using dogs with idiopathic hyperlipoproteinemia who have incompletely responded to dietary therapy, have shown reduced triglyceride levels when the dogs were given a marine lipid concentrate (Formula Plus) at the dose of 15 to 30 mg/lb daily. No clinical or biochemical side effects have been observed.

References

1. Kane, JP and Malloy, MJ: Disorders of lipoprotein metabolism. *In* Greenspan, FS, et al. (eds): Basic and Clinical Endocrinology. Lange Medical Publ, Los Altos, CA, 1983, p 557.
2. Zerbe, CA: Canine hyperlipemias. *In* Kirk, RW (ed): Current Veterinary Therapy IX. WB Saunders, Philadelphia, 1986, p 1045.
3. Fredrickson, DS, et al.: Fat transport in lipoproteins—an integrated approach to mechanisms and disorders. N Engl J Med 276:34, 1967.
4. Mahley, RW and Weisgraber, KH: Canine lipoprotein and atherosclerosis. I. Isolation and characterization of plasma lipoproteins from control dogs. Circ Res 35:713, 1974.
5. Manning, PJ: Thyroid gland and arterial lesions of beagles with familial hypothyroidism and hyperlipoproteinemia. Am J Vet Res 40:820, 1979.
6. Olin, DD, et al.: Lipid-laden aqueous humor associated with anterior uveitis and concurrent hyperlipemia in two dogs. JAVMA 168:861, 1976.
7. Crispin, SM and Barnett, KC: Arcus lipoides corneae secondary to hypothyroidism in the Alsatian. J Sm Anim Pract 19:127, 1978.
8. Rogers, WA, et al.: Idiopathic hyperlipoproteinemia in dogs. JAVMA 166:1087, 1975.
9. Rogers, WA, et al.: Lipids and lipoproteins in normal dogs and in dogs with secondary hyperlipoproteinemia. JAVMA 166:1092, 1975.
10. Consensus Development Panel in Consensus Conference: Treatment of hypertriglyceridemia. JAMA 251:1196, 1984.
11. Phillipson, BE, et al.: Reduction of plasma lipids, lipoproteins, and apoproteins by dietary fish oils in patients with hypertriglyceridemia. N Engl J Med 312:1210, 1985.

41 EMERGENCY MEDICINE

ROBERT J. MURTAUGH

Emergency and critical care medicine have become increasingly important in the practice of veterinary medicine. People are requesting and are increasingly willing to pay for these services for their pets. Enhanced public awareness of the importance of pets and of the services veterinarians can provide has encouraged this trend. This public awareness has been created through client education by the profession, publicity from the media, and efforts by society to explore and understand the importance of the human-animal bond. The veterinary profession faces the obligation of meeting the increasing demands for emergency and critical care services. Important issues regarding quality and sophistication of service, costs of these services, and medicoethical concerns need to be addressed by veterinarians involved in this practice specialty.

CLASSIFICATION OF EMERGENCIES

Veterinarians define an emergency as a situation where the institution of medical or surgical treatment cannot wait, e.g., a potentially life-threatening condition in an animal. An owner's definition of an emergency can be quite different. Veterinarians frequently encounter animals presented for emergency services that are not "true" emergencies. These instances include cases ranging from flea allergy dermatitis and chronic diarrhea to an owner's first experience with a cat in heat or an owner's need for vaccination and examination of a pet prior to travel. The emergency practice veterinarian must be prepared to deal with a broad scope of veterinary care, ranging from emergencies of true medical need in the animal to "emergencies" of ignorance, procrastination, and lack of foresight on the part of an owner. A veterinarian confronted with these situations must have the experience, training, and aptitude necessary to properly triage and manage cases presented simultaneously for the variety of reasons listed.

Principles of Evaluation and Triage

Evaluation of the emergency patient must be approached in a logical fashion. Initial evaluation of the animal must be rapid, but complete. The severity of the animal's condition must be determined. Shock, severe hemorrhage, respiratory compromise, and cardiopulmonary arrest are presentations of animals that require immediate and vigorous approaches to treatment. A complete history and physical examination of the animal and accompanying dialogue with an owner must be undertaken as soon as stabilization of the crisis in the animal is achieved.

The approach to a medical or surgical emergency in an animal should incorporate the following principles: (1) introduction and development of rapport with owner, (2) discussion of the animal's medical history and physical examination of the animal, (3) categorization and prioritization of patient injury, and (4) definitive treatment and monitoring. The order in which these principles are realized varies, depending on the condition of the animal at the time of presentation.

Client Relations in the Emergency Practice

The successful practice of emergency medicine does not depend wholly on providing the best in medical and surgical care to the animal, but depends greatly on the rapport and communication developed between clients and clinicians. The clinician must recognize that the client bringing an animal to an emergency clinic needs understanding and support for emotional and psychological trauma just as his or her animal may require treatment for physical illness or injury.[1, 2] The veterinarian, receptionist, and technical staff must be prepared to handle misdirected anger and the stress caused by demanding clients seeking assistance for their animal. Members of the emergency clinic team should do the following: (1) communicate concern for the animal, (2) allow owners to express their fears (potential for death of the animal, personal guilt related to the pet's illness), and (3) allay these fears through accurate and complete communication to the owner about the animal's condition.

A sign stating that animals are treated in order of severity of injury, not order of arrival, should be placed in the waiting room. Should a client have to wait to be seen, an initial evaluation of the animal by the doctor in the waiting area helps calm the client's anxieties. Receptionist and technical staff should continue to check back with the client every 10 to 15 minutes until the animal can be examined. Placing clients and animals into examination rooms is an interim step that assures people they are not being ignored. Veterinarians must fully discuss fees and medical options for the pet with the owners. This can be time-consuming and may be delayed in situations where life-saving treatment must be instituted. The client should not be dismissed until the veterinarian has addressed all pertinent issues, and answered all questions or has arranged a specific time to undertake a more detailed discussion over the phone, should this discussion be impossible at the time of an animal's admission. Prompt communication to the owner of changes in the animal's condition and detailed instructions to the owner (in writing and verbally) at the time of discharge are also vital parts of proper client relations in emergency practice. If the emergency practice operates during "off-hours" only, clients need to be informed that they must return to pick up their pet the following morning for transport to their regular veterinarian if extended care is required.

Considerable effort is required to establish and maintain communication with clients. The practice of emergency medicine requires that this effort be expended. Failure to communicate to clients and referring veterinarians results in dissatisfaction with the services provided by an emergency practice and, subsequently, a diminished caseload. Plans to address these issues must be established when an emergency facility is started and stringently applied during its operation.

History and Physical Examination of the Emergency Patient

Determination of the presence or absence of a life-threatening condition(s) in an animal at time of presentation is first priority. Respiratory compromise, hemorrhage, or shock requires immediate treatment. Complete history taking and physical examination of the patient are temporarily postponed. Baseline measurements of vital parameters such as temperature, weight, pulse, respiration, and capillary refill time should be determined in all patients prior to treatment. Blood and urine samples should be obtained in all patients prior to treatment, and determination of packed cell volume (PCV), total solids (TS), urine specific gravity, BUN (Azostick), and blood glucose (chemstrip BG) is essential to planning initial therapy. Respiratory compromise can occur secondary to airway obstruction, intrapulmonary disease (edema, inflammation), or pleural disease (pneumothorax, pleural effusion). Life-saving procedures to correct respiratory compromise may include O_2 administration, tracheal intubation or tracheostomy, thoracocentesis or chest tube placement, mechanical ventilation, or pharmacologic interventions, depending on the cause of respiratory distress.

Hemorrhage should be controlled immediately by direct pressure bandages or, in some instances, by tourniquets and ligation of bleeding vessels.

Shock should be treated quickly through placement of a large-bore intravenous catheter(s) and rapid administration of one blood volume of crystalloid fluids. Determination of the cause of shock must be obtained in order to plan administration of ancillary treatments of corticosteroids, catecholamines, antibiotics, and possibly colloids or whole blood. Following initial resuscitation, continuous monitoring of cardiovascular parameters determines the amount of fluid, type of fluid, and drug administration required for continued treatment of the animal.

Following initial resuscitation of an animal presented with a life-threatening condition, and at the time of initial evaluation of all other patients presented for examination, a complete medical history and physical examination of the patient should be obtained. Owners should be asked for a brief description of circumstances leading to development of the medical emergency in their pet. Specific, but nonleading, questions should be asked of clients to aid in determining differential diagnoses and the formulation of diagnostic and therapeutic plans. Questions concerning medication usage and prior illnesses in the pet may be extremely useful in understanding an animal's condition. Physical examination of the cardiovascular, pulmonary, central nervous, urogenital, gastrointestinal, skeletal, and integumentary systems should be completed as soon as possible. Examination of the various organ systems should be detailed and pointedly geared to early detection of primary disease, extension of disease, or sequelae of injury that might be associated with the animal's presentation for emergency care.[3]

In addition to shock and respiratory compromise, other examples of conditions with first priority for treatment and intensive monitoring include anaphylaxis, severe head injury, sepsis, hypoglycemia, heat stroke, and gastric dilatation-volvulus. These patients will die unless immediate action is undertaken by an emergency clinician.

CATEGORIZATION AND PRIORITIZATION OF PATIENT INJURY

Animals presented in shock or respiratory distress are easy to categorize with respect to severity of the medical emergency. These animals require immediate therapeutic intervention and continuous vigilant monitoring in order to ensure recovery and survival. The limited resources (personnel, equipment, and time) of most emergency clinics require a veterinarian to categorize new arrivals with respect to severity of disease. This procedure allows prioritization of diagnostic tests and treatments among animals and determination of the extent of monitoring required for each animal. This allocation of resources based on need is the practice of triage. Correct application of triage is crucial to the practice of emergency medicine.

Animals with minor, noncritical, or self-limiting disease are generally stable, compensating well for their injury, and do not require intensive monitoring. Mild pneumothorax, minor lacerations and abrasions, and simple pelvic fractures are injuries found in this category.

Animals with severe, non-life-threatening injury or

illness include, but are not limited to, animals with thoracic trauma, gastrointestinal obstruction, and spinal cord injury. These animals require treatment and monitoring sufficient to correct or compensate for altered homeostasis and prevent development of serious, life-threatening sequelae. The timing of surgical intervention can be a significant dilemma in the management of many animals in this category. These animals require prompt identification and correction of cardiac arrhythmias, hypovolemia, hypoxia, and other alterations in homeostasis in order to maximize chances for survival. Resources must be committed to treating these animals as next order of priority once animals with life-threatening emergency situations have been attended to.

Clinicians must rely on knowledge, experience, intuition, and common sense to properly triage animals presented for emergency care. Triage may be difficult to perform in various cases, as well-established guidelines for determining when a patient's condition becomes life-threatening do not exist. In these situations, a high priority must be given to monitoring that patient until its injury status is established. *All* patients require some monitoring, since an animal's condition can progress to more serious levels.

STANDARDS OF PRACTICE

PHYSICAL PLANT

An emergency clinic should be located in an area with access to major roads. The building should be clearly identified by signs. The parking area and entrance should be well lit. The client waiting area should be clean and pleasant. Attention to these simple details greatly minimizes client stress. Emergency clinics must be designed to accommodate the full range of needs of clients and their pets. Emergency clinics must incorporate a reception area; examination rooms; treatment area; intensive care ward; surgery, radiology, and laboratory facilities; and an isolation ward. The floor plan should centralize the intensive care/treatment area with easy access and close proximity of patients to other service areas (Figure 41–1). Cages should be arranged in a fashion that allows visualization of all patients from any location in the intensive care/treatment area. Floors and walls should be designed to allow easy cleaning. Electrical outlets should be properly grounded and screened to avoid electrical interference that might inhibit monitoring devices. An emergency generator should be incorporated into the design of a facility. Environmental control should allow for 9 to 12 air changes per hour, with a separate ventilation system for any isolation ward, humidity of approximately 55 per cent, and a temperature of 65°F to 75°F (18°C to 24°C). The treatment areas, operating room, and intensive care ward must be well lit. Ceiling tracks for intravenous fluids and wall-mounted sources of O_2 and vacuum suction must be placed in treatment and cage areas.

PERSONNEL

Emergency medicine is a team effort requiring esprit de corps and cohesiveness to meet the objectives of patient care and client communication. A veterinarian, surgeon on call, receptionist, two technicians, and possibly a ward attendant are required to ensure proper emergency care in a busy emergency practice.

Receptionists form the front line and represent a client's first contact with a practice, both over the phone and in person. Front desk personnel must be educated in triage of patients and the art of client relations.[1, 2] These individuals must ensure smooth flow of clients through clinic area, handling admissions, discharges, phones, pharmacy, records, and fee collection. Technicians serve as reception personnel in many emergency practices. This provides continuity between front office and other hospital functions, but stretches personnel limitations if that technician also has responsibility for patient monitoring and treatment. Separation of front desk functions from hospital functions appears in the best interest of patient care, but front desk personnel should be trained in recognition of life-threatening emergencies, animal restraint, and cardiopulmonary resuscitation.

The success of the critical care team does not depend as much on electronic monitoring devices as it does on diligent hands-on monitoring and nursing care from highly trained technical staff. Technicians must be able to make clinical observations and recognize changes in patients that require attention, must be able to respond automatically in emergency situations, and must be able to use all equipment at their disposal. The pace of an emergency clinic is demanding and individuals must be willing to work long hours and be open to change, new ideas, and new techniques developed to enhance patient care. Intellectual curiosity and continual willingness to learn must be motivating forces for technicians and doctors involved in emergency medicine; continuing education programs are an essential element. Emergency medicine is a demanding specialty where correct split-second decisions and reactions spell the difference between life and death. Trained animal health technicians are a necessity in emergency clinics. Employers should train and pay these technicians well, as the team approach required for efficient practice of emergency medicine is hampered by personnel turnover. A pool of part-time technicians provides a buffer against short staffing on the holidays, vacations, and sick leave of full time staff. The efficient, high quality operation of an emergency clinic requires a minimum of two technicians per shift. This ensures one technician is always observing animals in intensive care and another technician is available to help the doctor receive clients, to assist in performing diagnostic and surgical procedures, and to perform laboratory testing of samples. Animals housed in an emergency clinic should be under observation at all times to assure proper medical care.

Veterinarians staffing emergency clinics may be full-time employees, owners/operators, or part-time personnel that staff the facility as part of a rotation with members of other practices that participate in the emergency facility. Ideally, full-time employees offer the best alternative from the standpoint of team approach (continuity), management, and development of a noncompetitive clinic. This approach is expensive during the initial period of development, but can be rewarding if

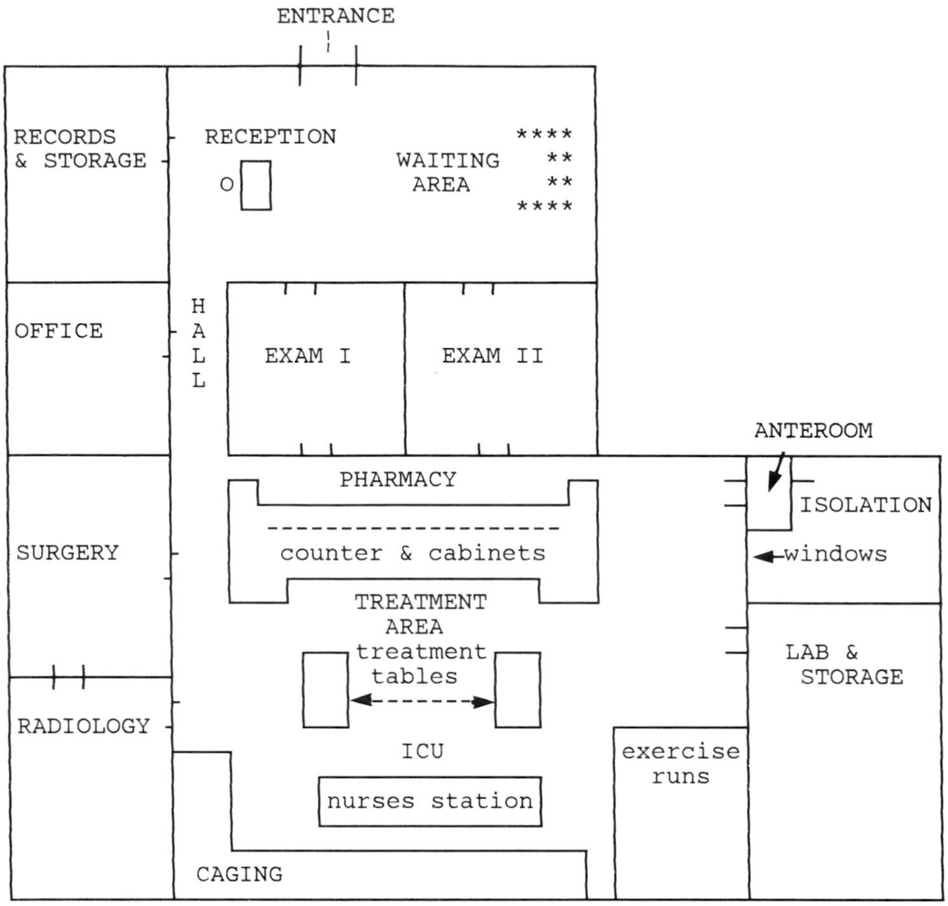

FIGURE 41–1. Floor plan for an emergency clinic incorporating easy access to service areas with easy visualization of hospitalized animals from treatment area and nurses' station.

established as part of the setup. Presently, veterinarians involved in practice of the emergency medicine specialty have received their specialized training through self-education and experience. This suggests that the practice of emergency medicine incorporates individuals with varied interests, experience, backgrounds, and training. The lack of uniformity in an area of practice where the life of the animal hangs in the balance is a deficiency in the specialty at this time. It is hoped that this deficiency in uniformity of training will change as veterinary schools and large animal hospitals answer the demand for veterinarians trained in critical care medicine. The veterinarian must be all things to all people involved in emergency practice: administrator, policy maker, client relations expert, educator, internist, surgeon, anesthesiologist, and an omnipresent force that maintains the enthusiasm and team spirit of the critical care team.

EQUIPMENT, DRUGS, AND SUPPLIES

Emergency clinics must be equipped and stocked with essential material (Tables 41–1, 41–2, and 41–3). Economics may dictate the sophistication of laboratory, radiology, and monitoring equipment available. If budget constraints are tight, expenditure of funds for full-time technical and veterinary staff should be of priority as long as basic equipment needs are met. The practice of emergency medicine depends directly on the observational, technical, and intellectual skills of the clinician and technicians. Hands-on monitoring, good nursing care, and sharp interpretative skills with regard to patient trends determine successful resuscitation and management of animals to a greater degree than does the extent of sophisticated diagnostic testing and monitoring. However, the more trends or parameters that are monitored and correctly interpreted in a patient, the better the level of emergency care provided to individual patients. The public and professional demand for emergency services and 24-hour critical care facilities dictates an increasing need to provide increased sophistication of service and to address the associated economic and ethical concerns.

SUPPORT SERVICES

Emergency clinics must be equipped with complete radiology units capable of performing myelography and other contrast studies. Fluoroscopy and two-dimensional ultrasound capabilities are features to consider when establishing or updating a facility. An automatic film processor is imperative in a busy emergency practice in order to maximize efficiency.

Surgical support must be available and capable of handling multiple trauma injuries, such as diaphragmatic hernia, penetrating abdominal and thoracic injury, gastric dilatation-volvulus, and acute intervertebral disc prolapse that causes paralysis. Presurgical evaluation and resuscitation, careful anesthetic management, and

TABLE 41–1. ALPHABETICAL LIST OF EQUIPMENT RECOMMENDED IN VETERINARY EMERGENCY CLINICS

Ambu bag, face mask, humidified oxygen source (wall-mounted)
Anesthetic machine(s)
Autoclave
Bird cage(s)
Blender
Blood donor animals
Blood gas analyzer
Catheter cart
Ceiling-mounted clippers
Centrifuges (blood tubes, hematocrit, for separation of blood components)
Clinical laboratory equipment (spectrophotometer, flame photometer, Coulter counter)
Crash cart (see Chapter 35)
Defibrillator with assorted external and internal paddles
ECG recorder
ECG oscilloscope monitor(s)
Endotracheal tubes
Enema equipment
Fluid infusion pump(s)
Fluid-warming chamber
Freezer
Gurney and stretcher
Hall air drill
Heat block
Heat lamps and circulating warm water heating blankets
Incubator(s)
Indirect blood pressure–measuring equipment
IV stands
Laryngoscope and blades
Microscope
Ophthalmoscope/otoscope
Osmometer
Oxygen cage(s)
Portable cage(s)
Pressure cuffs for fluid infusion
Radiograph machine and film processor
Refractometer
Refrigerator
Reptile tank(s)
Respirator(s)
Sandbags and wedges for positioning
Scales
Stethoscopes
Stomach tubes and pump
Suction apparatus (wall-mounted) and catheters
Surgical instrument packs (general, orthopedic, laminectomy, ophthalmology, chest, laceration)
Swan-Ganz balloon catheters
Temperature and pulse monitors
Tonometer
Transvenous cardiac pacing catheters/equipment
Ultrasonic nebulizer
Ultrasound machine
Waterbed(s)
Wood's lamp

postoperative monitoring are crucial factors in successful treatment of patients requiring emergency surgery. The timing of surgical intervention is critical and should not be undertaken without stabilization of the animal. Very few animals are in need of emergency surgery. Gastric dilatation-volvulus, severe unrelenting internal hemorrhage, and acute presentations of spinal fractures or disc prolapses with loss of deep pain sensation represent the few examples where uniform agreement exists concerning the need for emergency surgery. Animals with pyometra, diaphragmatic hernia, intervertebral disc disease, gastrointestinal obstruction, and many other "surgical" emergencies are primarily in need of aggressive medical management and stabilization. Surgical correction of these conditions is often best delayed until response to medical treatment can be accurately assessed. Nighttime surgical procedures, with limited facilities or staff support, are not in the best interest of these patients.

Laboratory support is essential to the practice of emergency medicine. The minimum laboratory data base needed prior to treatment of animals includes determination of packed cell volume and total solids, chemistry determinations of blood glucose and blood urea nitrogen, complete urinalysis (including determination of urine specific gravity), blood smear evaluation, and fecal examination.[4] Blood samples should be collected at admission and held for later submission for complete hematologic and serum biochemical profiles, if indicated. Appropriate culture specimens should be collected from patients with sepsis or localized infections. Gram stain evaluation of exudates is recommended in order to plan initial antibiotic administration. Many emergency clinics have limited laboratory capabilities and this severely handicaps a clinician's ability to diagnose and treat animals properly.

TABLE 41–2. ALPHABETICAL LIST OF SUPPLIES RECOMMENDED IN VETERINARY EMERGENCY FACILITIES

Baby food
Bags (large, heavy plastic) for handling animal remains
Bandage, tape, and splint materials
Blood collection and administration sets (transfusions)
Blood culture media
Blood syringes for irrigation
Chemistry strips for urine, blood glucose, blood urea nitrogen
Chest drain units (continuous suction collection devices)
Containers for disposal of biohazardous waste
Cotton-tipped applicators
Culture media and broth for transport and maintenance of specimens for bacterial and fungal cultures
Diagnostic peritoneal lavage catheters
Disposable plastic gloves
Fluid administration sets (including microdrip and burettes)
Fluorescein stain
Glass slides, assorted stain preparations
Gray-topped blood collection tubes for activated clotting time test
Hydrogen peroxide
Intravenous catheters (assorted length, gauge, type), catheter caps, extension tubing
Laboratory reagents and supplies
Microhematocrit tubes
Paper coveralls for isolation
Pediatric feeding tubes
Petrolatum
Prescription diets
Radiographic film/screens and contrast agents
Sample collection tubes (blood, urine, culture, tissue)
Schirmer tear test strips
Sterile aqueous lubricant
Sterile gloves, gowns, masks, shoe covers
Surgical scrub and disinfectant solutions (chlorhexidine, iodinated)
Suture material (assorted sizes)
Syringes, needles (assorted sizes)
Syringes, 60 cc catheter-tip
Thermometers
Three-way stopcocks
Tongue blades
Tracheostomy tubes
Trocar chest drain cannulas (assorted sizes)
Urinary catheters (including Foley catheters)
Urine collection bags (for use with indwelling urinary catheters)

TABLE 41–3. ALPHABETICAL LIST OF DRUGS RECOMMENDED FOR USE IN VETERINARY EMERGENCY FACILITIES

- Fluids
  - Blood (A-negative)
  - Dextrans
  - 5% dextrose
  - 2.5% dextrose and 0.45% saline
  - 50% dextrose in water
  - Lactated Ringer's solution
  - Mannitol
  - Potassium chloride
  - 0.9% and 5–7.5% saline
  - Sodium bicarbonate
  - Sterile water for injection
- Acepromazine
- Acetylcysteine
- Activated charcoal
- ADE vitamins, injectable
- Aminophylline
- Amrinone
- Antibiotics (assorted types, dosage forms)
- Antihistamine(s)
- Apomorphine
- AquaMEPHYTON
- Ascorbic acid
- Assorted eye and ear medications
- Atropine
- B vitamins, injectable
- Butorphanol (analgesic)
- Calcium gluconate and chloride
- $CaNa_2$ EDTA
- Captopril
- Carbonic anhydrase inhibitor
- Chlorpromazine
- Desoxycorticosterone
- Dexamethasone
- Digoxin (injectable and oral)
- Dimercaprol (other antidotes, based on type of practice caseload)
- Dipyrone
- Dobutamine
- Dopamine
- Doxapram
- Emerald II (birds)
- Ensure plus
- Epinephrine
- Ethanol
- Euthanasia solution
- Fenbendazole
- Flourinef
- Flunixin meglumine
- Furosemide
- Heparin
- Hydralazine
- Hydralazine, injectable
- Inhalation anesthetic
- Isoproterenol
- Ketamine
- Lactulose
- Lidocaine
- Magnesium sulfate
- Metoclopramide
- Morphine
- Nalorphine
- Naloxone
- Neostigmine
- Neuromuscular blocking agent
- Nitroglycerin ointment
- Oxymorphone
- Oxytocin
- Pepto-Bismol
- Phenobarbital
- Phenylephrine
- Pralidoxime (organophosphate antidote)
- Prednisolone succinate
- Procainamide
- Propranolol
- Quinidine
- Sodium nitroprusside
- Sulfadimethoxine
- Thiobarbiturate
- Valium
- Verapamil
- Vinegar (for neutralization of alkali)
- Xylazine (emetic in cats)

Ideally, emergency clinical laboratories should be equipped to do complete blood counts, platelet counts, clotting screens, reticulocyte counts, specimen preparations for cytologic evaluation, microbiologic techniques, various serum chemistry analyses, and blood gas analysis.

RECORDS

Records should follow the problem-oriented medical record format.[5, 6] Attention to accurate and complete medical records is important for proper patient care, accurate communications to client and referring veterinarians, and for legal reasons. Flow sheets charting various parameters should be used to allow accurate assessment of trends in critical patients. All treatment orders should be written in the record as well as verbalized to technicians. Discharge forms should be in triplicate (medical record, client, referring veterinarian copies) and must contain detailed instructions to owners along with information on diagnosis and treatment of the patient for the referring veterinarian's records. All entries in medical records, discharge instructions, and referral letters should be legible, complete, signed, and detailed enough to allow a person unfamiliar with the case to obtain all necessary information. Detailed medical records represent the best witness and defense in instances of litigation.

PATIENT CARE

Quite often in a busy emergency practice, individuals become wrapped up in the mechanization of patient monitoring and sophistication of medical/surgical approaches. Clinicians often forget the psychological aspect of an animal's condition and concentrate on diagnosis and treatment. The importance of concern for the overall well-being of patients cannot be underestimated. Cleanliness of animals and cages, comfortable padding for recumbent animals, attention to individual and environmental temperature control, appropriate use of physical therapy, walking of animals outside if possible, hand feeding of animals, soothing words of comfort, and petting of patients are important factors to be considered by emergency clinic staffs. The actual impact of attention to these details on successful outcome of treatment cannot be easily measured, but ensuring comfort of sick pets enhances overall patient monitoring and minimizes complications.

RELATIONSHIP WITH REFERRING VETERINARY COMMUNITY

Continuous attention must be devoted to maintaining good relationships with referring veterinarians. Their ideas and suggestions should be solicited. Communication to referring veterinarians on animals treated by an emergency clinic must be considered a priority by the veterinary staff. Invariably, all problems with the referring veterinary community have their basis in miscommunication or lack of communication. A successful emergency practice has the communication channels to referring veterinarians open and working well.

PRINCIPLES OF MONITORING AND SUPPORTIVE CARE IN CRITICAL PATIENTS

Many parameters should be monitored in seriously injured or sick animals presented to emergency clinics (Table 41–4).[7, 8] The number of and frequency with which various parameters need measurement depends on the trend in a particular patient and the seriousness of the animal's condition.[3] Electrocardiograms should be obtained on all animals as part of the initial data base. The use of self-adherent electrode pads on the chest wall and/or use of telemetry devices can minimize problems associated with continuous electrocardiographic monitoring. Indirect blood pressure measurements, coupled with central venous pressure measurements, can provide valuable information with respect to an animal's hemodynamic status. The changes in these parameters are more valuable than are values of isolated measurements. Urine output should be assessed during treatment of shock or when acute renal failure is suspected. Urine output provides an indirect measure of

TABLE 41-4. LIST OF PARAMETERS THAT SHOULD BE MONITORED IN ANIMALS TREATED AT EMERGENCY CLINICS

Temperature (rectal/toe-web)
Pulse
Respiration
Capillary refill time and mucous membrane color
Total solids, packed cell volume
Urine specific gravity
Weight/hydration status
Chemstrip blood urea nitrogen and blood glucose
Electrocardiogram
Urine output
Central venous pressure
Indirect arterial blood pressure
Serum electrolytes
pH/blood gases
Clotting mechanisms
Pulmonary capillary wedge pressure

tissue perfusion and blood pressure (normal output, 0.5 to 1 ml/lb/hr). Indwelling urinary catheters should be removed as soon as adequate urine flow is assured or oliguria is confirmed. Intermittent urinary catheterizations can be performed to follow trends in urine output once a baseline has been established. Maintenance of unnecessary indwelling urinary catheters needlessly predisposes the animal to nosocomial bacterial colonization and infection. Measurement of body weight is an often-overlooked parameter that can be of great value in determining fluid needs, overhydration, and caloric requirements. Baseline weight measurement at time of admission and continued reassessment of repeated measurements provide an accurate means of assessing response to fluid treatment.

Good supportive care of critical patients requires proper selection, usage, placement, and management of intravenous catheters, urinary catheters, tracheostomy/endotracheal tubes, and chest drains. Short, large-bore intravenous catheters are indicated for treatment of animals in shock. All indwelling tubes should be placed using sterile surgical technique. Closed collection or administration systems should be used with all indwelling tubes. Tracheostomy tubes should have disposable inner liners and double cuffs to allow easy cleaning and alternating inflation/deflation at different tracheal sites to minimize tracheal injury. Tracheostomy tubes must be suctioned with sterile technique as frequently as necessary (every 30 minutes to several hours). Nebulization to humidify airways is important in patients with tracheostomy tubes in place. All indwelling tubes should be removed as soon as they are no longer critical to the medical management of the animal. The chances of acquiring nosocomial infections is directly related to the length of time catheters and tubes are maintained in patients. Intravenous catheters should be changed every 48 to 72 hours.

EXTENDED MANAGEMENT OF THE CRITICAL PATIENT

Most emergency clinics do not need to concern themselves with extended care of their patients, as animals are discharged to referring veterinarians the following day. Many of these animals are still in need of intensive care monitoring and the practice of emergency medicine should begin to strive for development of 24-hour critical care facilities to benefit clients, patients, veterinarians, and the specialty of emergency practice.

Veterinarians involved in emergency medicine, especially those treating animals in transition from emergency to convalescence, should be concerned with factors such as nutrition, nosocomial disease prevention, and prevention of late post-trauma sequelae.

The metabolic response to injury and surgery coupled with presence of anorexia in most sick animals leads to significant protein and calorie deficits in these animals.[9] Early nutritional support decreases catabolic tissue losses, increases wound healing and immunologic competence, and improves patient survival.[3] Considerations for use of enteral and parenteral nutritional support will become increasingly important in management of animals presented to emergency clinics.

Critically ill animals have an increased susceptibility to infection, related to the stress of their disease, a catabolic metabolic state, and invasive diagnostic and monitoring techniques employed. Sterile technique in placement of indwelling tubes, hand washing between animals, the use of disposable gloves when handling patients (changed between patients), appropriate antibiotic administration, shortening the duration of hospitalizations, and minimizing the use of indwelling tubes will help decrease the chance of nosocomial disease in critical care patients.[3] Following the initial resuscitation of critically injured or ill patients, supportive care, specific treatments, and careful monitoring must continue in order to prevent organ dysfunction from occurring. Respiratory distress syndrome, cardiac arrhythmias, disseminated intravascular coagulation, sepsis, and acute renal failure are potential sequelae to trauma and other conditions for which patients are treated in an emergency clinic. Careful attention to prevention and early identification of these complications is extremely important in the extended management of the emergency patient.[10]

ANESTHESIA AND RADIOLOGY IN CRITICAL CARE PATIENTS

Anesthesia. Use of general anesthesia may be required during the course of diagnosis and treatment of seriously compromised patients in emergency situations. Whenever possible patients should be fasted prior to anesthesia in order to minimize their chances of vomiting and aspirating gastric contents into the airways during anesthetic induction. Preoperative and intraoperative treatments to maintain cardiopulmonary and renal function must be used. Anesthesia protocols should be individualized to minimize problems of metabolism associated with hepatic or renal impairment that may exist in an animal; minimize stresses of anesthetic induction; maximize control of the patient during anesthesia induction and maintenance; and ensure smooth, rapid recovery following termination of the diagnostic or surgical procedure. Intraoperative monitoring of the patient is critical and a separate person should be charged with anesthetic management. This person should have no other responsibilities during the period in which the patient is anesthetized. There is no such thing as a minor general anesthetic.[3]

Radiography. Radiography is a valuable tool in the diagnostic armamentarium of the emergency clinician; it supplements or confirms findings based on a good, thorough clinical examination. Radiographs of the chest and abdomen should be obtained in all trauma patients. The presence of occult critical injuries such as a ruptured diaphragm and ruptured urinary bladder should be detected early in patients with musculoskeletal injuries. When radiographs are obtained as a part of the initial data base, they provide another means of objectively reassessing individual patients, e.g., as with laboratory tests, radiographs can be repeated and results compared with previous findings to enable more accurate diagnosis.

Contrast studies should be performed when clinical signs and preliminary radiographic findings suggest compromise or rupture of the diaphragm, gastrointestinal tract, or urinary tract. Lateral and dorsoventral or ventrodorsal views should be taken in all instances when radiographing the thorax and abdomen. This procedure prevents missed diagnoses such as diaphragmatic hernia or pulmonary contusion, which can occur if only single views are obtained. Radiographs must be interpreted in a systematic, careful manner in order to avoid overlooking subtle findings such as vertebral fractures or loss of retroperitoneal detail that could be missed when concentrating on obvious abnormalities, e.g., pelvic fractures. Radiographs represent a significant practice standard in diagnostic workups and are legal documents that can be used to defend positions should litigation occur.

Ultrasonography. Ultrasonography represents an additional imaging modality that is of great use in the evaluation of cardiac, pericardial, hepatobiliary, uterine, prostatic, and other organ system diseases. Ultrasonography will probably be indispensable to the emergency clinician in the future.

ETHICOLEGAL CONCERNS IN PRACTICE OF EMERGENCY MEDICINE

The unique factors involved in emergency practice (highly charged, emotional, life and death situations) require veterinarians in this specialty to be familiar with and prepared to act on issues of client relations, death and dying, the grief process, the ethics of clinical decision making and triage, and the ethics of euthanasia and animal rights when confronted with stray animals or clients unable to afford the care required by their pets. These problems are complicated and require reading and thinking about approaches to the situations involving these issues that are encountered daily.[11, 12]

DIRECTIONS FOR THE FUTURE

Emergency medicine is becoming a major part of the professional services expected of veterinarians. Training programs in critical care medicine are being established at several veterinary schools across the United States. A specialty board to set standards of practice and training programs and to administer specialty board examinations is in the planning stages. Clinicians in emergency practice will be expected to upgrade standards of personal training and expertise, technical staffing, laboratory capabilities such as blood gas analysis, monitoring capabilities such as indirect blood pressure measurement, and diagnostic capabilities such as ultrasound over the next few years. Development of 24-hour critical care facilities to improve extended management of critical care patients has become essential. The increased professional and public attention focused on the psychological and nutritional needs of veterinary patients will impact heavily on individuals providing emergency medicine services. The economics of a critical care practice that becomes increasingly sophisticated will result in increasing discussion of ethical issues in veterinary circles, currently hotly debated in human medicine, concerning appropriate allocation of the limited resources available.[13] The challenges and opportunities in veterinary emergency medicine are vast.

References

1. Silverman, B: Public Relations in Emergency Medicine: Practice in a Glass House. J Vet Crit Care 8:5, 1985.
2. Milligan, JA: Care of the traumatized client. J Vet Emerg Crit Care 3:18, 1986.
3. Haskins, SC: Overview of Emergency and Intensive Care. *In* Sherding RG (ed): Medical Emergencies. New York, Churchill Livingstone, 1985, p 1.
4. Greene, RT: An Emergency Laboratory Data Base: Simple In-hospital Tests. Comp Cont Ed Pract Vet 7:197, 1985.
5. Zaslow, IM: Personnel and Physical Requirements. *In* Sattler FP, Knowles, RP, Whittick, WG (eds): Veterinary Critical Care. Philadelphia, Lea and Febiger, 1981, p 3.
6. Kirk, RW and Bistner, SI: Medical Records. *In* Kirk RW, Bistner, SI (eds): Handbook of Veterinary Procedures and Emergency Treatment, 3rd edition. Philadelphia, WB Saunders, 1981, p 320.
7. Wingfield, WE: Monitoring of Patients in the Emergency Clinic. Vet Clin North Am 11(1):23, 1981.
8. Burrows, CF: Intensive Care of the Critically Ill Dog and Cat. Part I. Philosophy, Organization of the Intensive Care Unit, and Monitoring Techniques. Comp Cont Ed Pract Vet 4:875, 1982.
9. Burrows, CF: Intensive Care of the Critically Ill Dog and Cat Part II. Fluid Therapy, Respiratory Care, and Nutrition. Comp Cont Ed Pract Vet 4:1008, 1982.
10. Rodkey, WG: Transition from Emergency. *In* Sattler, FP, et al. (eds): Veterinary Critical Care. Philadelphia, Lea and Febiger, 1981, p 474.
11. Quackenbush, J and Voith, VL: The Human-Companion Animal Bond. Vet Clin North Am 15(2):1, 1985.
12. Irwin, RS and Pratter, MR: Making Clinical Decisions for the Critically Ill: A View From Critical Care Physicians. J Int Care Med 1:63, 1986.
13. Engelhardt, HT and Rie, MA: Intensive Care Units, Scarce Resources and Conflicting Principles of Justice. JAMA 255:1159, 1986.

42 SMALL ANIMAL PROBLEMS IN DEVELOPING COUNTRIES

JOSEPH VAN HEERDEN

Developing countries are those countries of the world characterized by a shortage of food and a Gross National Product considerably lower than those of developed countries such as the United States of America and West Germany. Lack of training, schooling, and equipment, and disease conditions are major factors responsible for their poor economic performance. These countries usually have an increasing population characterized by decreasing death rates and increasing birth rates among humans. About three quarters of the world's human population reside in the developing countries of Africa, Asia, and Latin America.[1] However, such a one-sided economic approach to the classification of the countries of the world loses sight of important features of populations such as social characteristics and predominant animal uses within societies. This may perhaps explain why massive aid by developed countries has often not achieved the expected results in developing countries.[2]

The ever-changing milieu within many developing countries is characterized in many instances by massive urbanization of people, which may be accompanied by favorable increases in per capita income. This is usually reflected in changing social structures and changing attitudes toward animals. The dog, for example, once regarded as solely a hunter, now becomes a protector of property and/or a household pet.

The veterinarian involved in veterinary services in developing countries is invariably employed by "the State" and is primarily involved in preventive and production medicine, as well as veterinary public health. In many instances, the policy and manpower resources of the state make minimal provision for the health and care of small animals. Veterinarians employed by the state therefore have to be alerted to the needs of the society for small animal health services, which may range from simple preventive medicine to the relatively more sophisticated needs that are likely to originate from the more affluent portions of these ever-changing societies. Although the growing need for veterinary services to companion animals has been identified but described as in low demand,[3] it is the author's opinion that the dire need of a developing country's society for veterinary services for small animals is only illustrated once the service becomes readily available to the community.

SOCIOECONOMIC FACTORS

The personal income of people in a third-world country is low and, in general, communities cannot afford even moderate veterinary fees. Most veterinary services to small animals such as dogs and cats have to be provided by sponsored or state-supported institutions such as state-employed veterinarians or university-affiliated small animal clinics.

Transportation, which is almost taken for granted in developed countries, is a major problem in developing countries.

Patients may be transported to a small animal clinic by various methods such as walking the animal (sometimes over considerable distances), on an improvised stretcher, on a wheelbarrow, on a bicycle carrier, on an animal-powered cart, and in a taxi. The great difficulty and expense that owners manage to overcome to get a small animal to a clinic make it essential at times to admit an animal for hospitalization rather than to insist on a repeat visit the following day. This, in itself, creates further problems in that it usually results in unnecessarily prolonged periods of hospitalization due to an inability to contact the animal owner. Telephones are often nonexistent and surface mail very erratic. The strain on the limited space of an already stretched facility is further complicated by the fact that dogs in developing societies are usually relatively large because of their role as hunter/gatherers or protectors of property. The majority of first visit patients also have had no previous inoculations against infectious diseases, which may pose a potential risk for hospitalization.

Lack of knowledge and illiteracy are usually responsible for suboptimal small animal care, often resulting in severe malnutrition as well as endo- and ectoparasitism. In the author's experience, effective communication usually results in praiseworthy improvements in general pet care and health. Mobile clinics, which would take the veterinarian to the doorstep of people, would render an invaluable clinical and preventive medicine service. The combination of a mobile clinic with mobile exhibits, as has been used in Kenya,[4] would contribute tremendously towards the general improvement of pet care, human health, and the well-being of the community. Illiteracy demands clearly illustrated and/or demonstrated instruction. In the author's experience, a copy of all details of a visit to the clinic (veterinary consultation) has facilitated treatment of the patient at home (there is often someone that can read) and future follow-up consultations.

In a developing society, nothing should be taken for granted. Basic needs like water are often very hard to come by and limited quantities often have to be bought and collected on foot over considerable distances. This limitation may directly influence activities of the veterinarian. The ability of dog owners to dip dogs at home, for example, should never be assumed and the veterinarian therefore often has to provide dipping facilities for small animals. Dispensing concentrated insecticidal agents for ectoparasite control under these circumstances may often impose considerable demands on already limited water supplies.

PET-OWNER RELATIONSHIPS

Stray dogs are a major problem in most developing countries.[5–8] Among traditional African peoples in rural areas, dogs may lead an almost self-sufficient existence.[9] Although traceable to particular properties, they enjoy the freedom of a community with either limited or no borders between properties. Within these communities dogs may act as hunters, guards, or sanitary agents for the removal of children's excreta. In the urban environment, the situation is often the same, with the result that a large number of free-ranging dogs seems to be a prominent feature of the urban scene in Africa.[7, 10] With urbanization and development, however, a progressively larger percentage of dogs seems to be regarded as guard dogs[9] and pets.

The attitudes of different populations toward dogs and cats are probably largely determined by culture and development. Schwabe's[2] societal types, with their respective predominant animal uses, are well demonstrated by individual dog and cat owners in various stages of development in a developing country. Regardless, however, of whether the owner attaches a financial value to the animal because of its usefulness or whether the animal is simply kept as a pet, the author has found owners equally unwilling to part with their small animals. Tremendous expectations are often encountered in dog owners visiting veterinary clinics. The concept of euthanasia, for example, is often ill-understood and should be explained in detail before it is executed.

NUTRITIONAL DISORDERS

Developing countries are "have not" countries where protein/calorie malnutrition of the people and their animals is extremely common. The erratic and insufficient production of food means that either food is not available or cannot be afforded by those who are in need. The problem is further compounded by lack of knowledge of proper nutrition. This results in starvation despite the presence of adequate supplies of proteins and calories.

Dogs and cats compete with humans for the same resources and it is therefore no wonder that they often receive very little food, the wrong food, or no food at all. Their chances of survival are probably better when they join the ranks of stray dogs. These, at least, may survive on the offal from fish markets and abattoirs, for example.[6, 10] The underfed scavenger dog is at far greater risk of becoming infected with ecto- and endoparasites,[7] as well as various infectious agents. The coprophagous and free-ranging habits of the underfed dog possibly explain the not too infrequent occurrence of salmonellosis and spirocercosis in dogs in the author's clinic and elsewhere.[11]

Underfed pregnant bitches may whelp pups that are essentially starved from birth due to her often insufficient milk production. The problem of the malnourished, underfed, disease-prone pup is further compounded by the premature weaning and selling of pups.

The protein/calorie malnutrition problem in developing countries is not likely to be solved by foreign aid in the form of capital and food. Although temporary alleviation of the problem may be achieved by such aid, it may in fact be counterproductive. Education and population control, the overriding needs of developing countries, apply equally well to the dog and cat problem. We have found dog owners often totally ignorant of the most basic aspects of dog nutrition such as hygienic aspects, frequency of feeding, volume of food, type of food, and the need for fresh drinking water. In general, owners have been enthusiastic in learning about these basics and when within their means, keen to implement them (like feeding their dogs commercially available rations). Improvement of dog and cat nutrition in developing countries cannot be divorced from proper nutrition for the people of the household and should be part of a community development plan. It is highly unlikely that dog nutrition will improve if the community at large is still suffering from severe protein/calorie malnutrition.

PARASITIC INFESTATIONS

Parasites are probably of major veterinary importance in all countries of the world where parasite control is

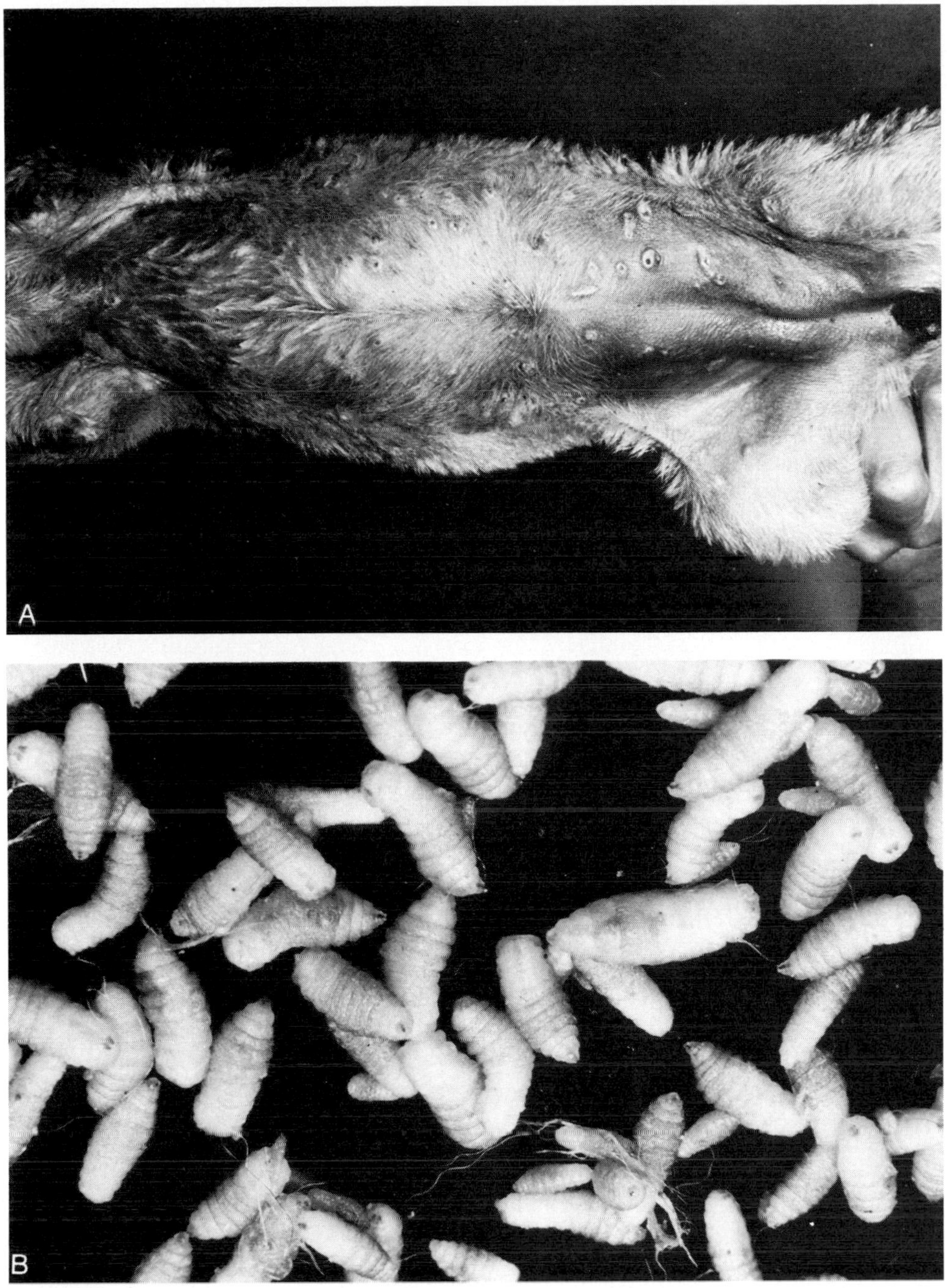

FIGURE 42–1. Ventral abdomen of a puppy *(A)* showing small crater-like lesions after expulsion of numerous larvae of *Cordylobia anthropophaga* *(B)*.

minimal or non-existent, where the level of care for small animals is suboptimal, and where these animals are allowed to roam and scavenge freely. Most reports in developing countries, however, deal with the parasite situation in production animals or parasite infestation in dogs and cats from a public health point of view.

A summary of the effects of tick infestation on livestock production[12] is equally applicable to the canine population. Results include irritation, allergic reactions, blood loss, paralysis or toxicosis, skin lesions, debilitating disease, deaths, predisposition of animals to infection, and transmission of pathogenic organisms. All these are adequately illustrated in mild to very severe ectoparasitism that is regularly encountered in dogs in developing countries.

The survival of *Rhipicephalus sanguineus* and *Haemaphysalis leachii*, perhaps the most important ticks of dogs in Africa, is facilitated by the presence of large numbers of scavenging dogs and by the presence of ticks in human dwellings and/or dog kennels. Both species can be encountered on dogs throughout the year.[13] In a survey of ectoparasites of dogs in Maboloka, Bophuthatswana,[14] the large majority of ticks (99.18 per cent) were found to be *Rhipicephalus sanguineus*, the remainder (0.82 per cent) being *R. appendiculatus, R. sinus*, and *Amblyomma* spp. Apart from ticks, the stable fly, *Stomoxys calcitrans*, the tumbu fly, *Cordylobia anthropophaga*, and fleas were important causes of ectoparasitism in dogs. Fleas, mainly *Echidnophaga gallinacea*, were responsible for massive infestations of the skin of the head, mainly around the eyes and on the ears. *C. anthropophaga*, which thrive under hot, humid, unhy-

TABLE 42–1. DISEASES DIAGNOSED IN A RANDOM SAMPLE OF 1000 DOGS PRESENTED FOR TREATMENT*†

	% of Total	% Tick-Borne	Different Conditions	% of Total
Infectious diseases	63.6	50	Canine ehrlichiosis	30.9
			Canine babesiosis	18.2
			Canine distemper	8.6
			Parvovirus enteritis	4.6
			Hepatozoonosis	
			Encephalitozoonosis, infectious canine hepatitis	1.3
			Salmonellosis	
Ecto- and endoparasitism and related disorders‡	19.2	2.7	Endoparasitism	11.8
			Ticks	2.6
			Tumbu-fly	1.8
			Demodicosis	1.1
			Fleas	
			Stomoxys calcitrans, sarcoptic mange	1.9
			Myiasis, tick toxicosis, ringworm	
Organ diseases	12.4		Gastrointestinal	4.2
			Urogenital	2.0
			Dermatologic	1.7
			Respiratory	1.3
			Oropharyngeal	0.9
			Hepatic	0.6
			Ophthalmologic	0.6
			Cardiac	0.4
			Neurologic	0.4
			Musculoskeletal	0.2
			Endocrine	0.1
Trauma/bite wounds/ fractures/abscessation/ hernia/dislocations	13.4			
Neoplasia	3.5		Transmissible venereal tumor	2.3
			Other	1.2
Congenital abnormalities	0.3			

*All owners belonged to a very low income group.
†A diagnosis of malnutrition was ignored.
‡Probably underdiagnosed as a diagnosis of ectoparasitism and endoparasitism was only made if this was severe and/or the only problem.

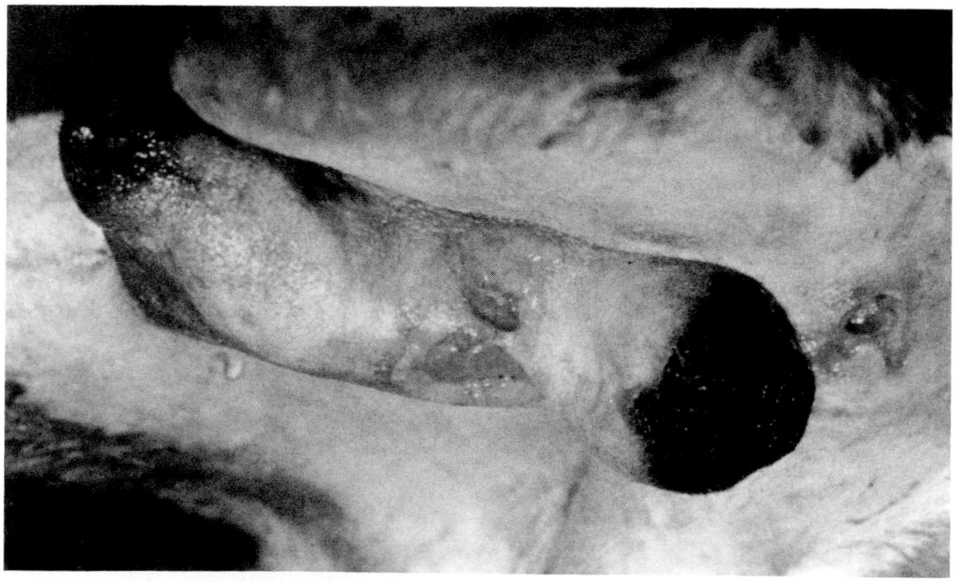

FIGURE 42–2. Perineal and sheath area of a dog showing well-demarcated ulcers where the animal was bitten by the bont-legged tick *Hyalomma rufipes.*

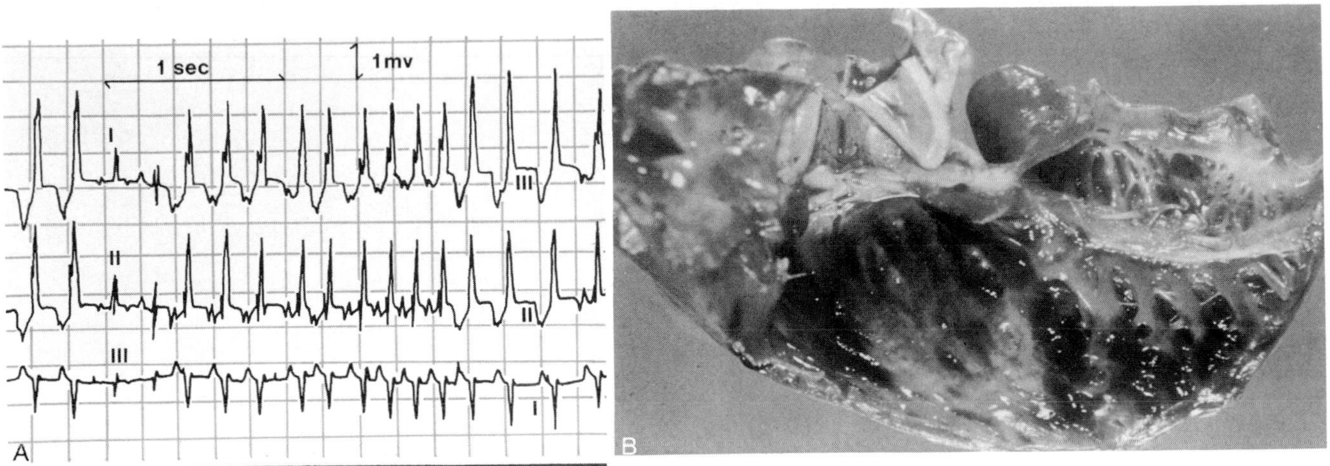

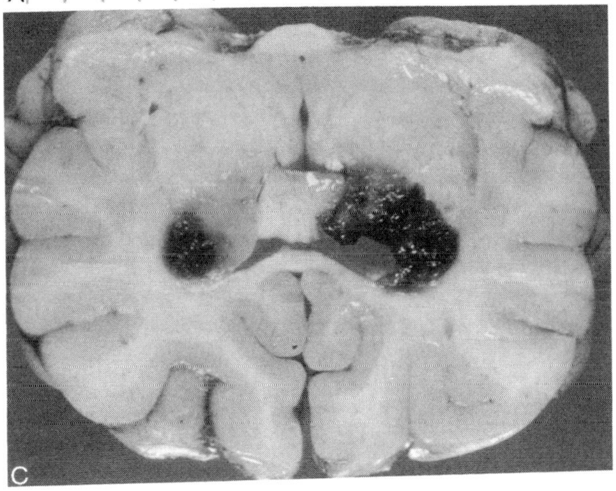

FIGURE 42–3. An electrocardiogram demonstrating a bizarre rhythm *(A)* obtained from a dog with peracute babesiosis. On postmortem examination, severe myocardial hemorrhages *(B)* as well as brain hemorrhage *(C)* were observed.

gienic conditions, are especially important in young puppies where massive infestations (Figure 42–1) may result in painful skin disease. The author's own survey supports these findings (Table 42–1). The bont-legged tick, *Hyalomma rufipes*, can cause severe localized pain as well as subsequent well-demarcated areas of skin necrosis (Figure 42–2) and is another example of ectoparasite-induced disease in areas where ticks abound.

Apart from their localized and systemic effects on the body of the animal, ectoparasites also act as important vectors of disease. Ticks, for example, may transmit *Babesia canis, Hepatozoon canis, Eperythrozoon canis,* and *Ehrlichia canis*; tsetse flies may transmit trypanosomes.

Among the endoparasites, hookworms seem to be a very important cause of malaise in dogs in developing countries. In most surveys of endoparasites of dogs and cats, *Ancylostoma caninum, Dipylidium caninum,*[15, 16] *Toxocara* sp., *Taenia hydatigena,*[10] and *Spirocerca lupi*[17] are important infestations.[14, 18–20] In the author's clinic, severe helminth infestations in dogs have been associated with a variety of clinical syndromes such as convulsions, muscle weakness, diarrhea, and anemia.

Ancylostomiasis, which is very common, is usually associated with loss of body condition and severe anemia. To complicate the clinical picture further, puppies are often presented in severe states of malnutrition, heavily infested with ecto- and endoparasites, and infected with one or more infectious agents, such as canine distemper virus or *Ehrlichia canis*. These patients, which suffer from a multitude of disease conditions, often present with very low packed cell volumes and albumin concentrations that may be very low. The treatment of such patients is often a futile exercise.

Whereas it is generally possible to treat the other helminth infestations, advanced spirocercosis in the dog is usually difficult to impossible to treat. Manifestation of clinical signs of spirocercosis usually occurs only in the advanced stages of infestation when extensive involvement of the esophagus and/or carcinomatous involvement of the lungs may be present.

Hydatidosis control programs may result in large-scale dog elimination programs such as those in Chipre.[21] More than 40,000 dogs of a canine population with an alleged infection rate of 48 per cent were exterminated.

INFECTIOUS DISEASES

Most reports on infectious diseases in small animals in developing countries deal with the zoonotic implications of some of these diseases.

Rabies continues to be of major public health and economic significance on all continents except Australia and Antarctica.[7, 8, 22] Large numbers of stray dogs, shortages of trained personnel,[8] sociocultural reasons such as reluctance to have dogs and cats vaccinated,[23] vaccination failures due to poor storage and transport facilities, and political events[24] are some of the factors that have complicated effective control in developing countries. In Africa the disease is well known[25] and it is often one of the only dog diseases recognized and named by locals. For example, it is called "kichaa cha mbwa" (dog madness) in Kiswahili.

Despite only occasional reports of canine distemper in developing countries,[26] it probably remains the most important viral disease of dogs wherever preventive immunization of dogs is neglected. In the author's experience, the condition is very common and all the different manifestations of the disease are regularly encountered. Dogs are often presented with advanced neurological signs such as myoclonus of muscles of the head and forequarters, posterior paresis, and posterior paralysis. It is not unusual to see entire litters of puppies that are affected. Treatment failures are often ill-understood by owners, who fail to comprehend the etiology of the condition. The clinician practicing in an area rife with canine distemper should, however, beware of the pitfall of diagnosing every patient presented with neurological signs as suffering from canine distemper.

Reports from Nigeria,[27, 28] India,[29, 30] Madagascar,[31] and South Africa[32] suggest that canine parvovirus infection is probably an important cause of mortality of pups in developing countries. In the author's clinic, canine parvovirus enteritis is commonly seen in puppies and usually necessitates intensive sustained supportive therapy. The intensive treatment required in these puppies, which may also suffer from babesiosis, verminosis, and ectoparasitism at the same time, for example, makes this condition one of the most expensive (and therefore most subsidized) medical conditions to treat. It also necessitates hospitalization of the patient. Intensive care with 24-hour medical supervision of patients in developing countries is, however, seldom feasible because of financial limitations.

There are relatively few reports on bacterial diseases in dogs and cats in developing countries. Brucellosis has been reported in dogs in Nigeria.[33, 34] The many different serotypes of *Salmonella* isolated from both healthy and sick dogs in various countries may reflect the relatively poor animal care extended to these animals.[11, 35] Salmonellosis is usually a fatal disease, especially of young dogs in the author's clinic.

Protozoal parasites like *Babesia canis, Trypanosoma cruzi, T. vivax, Hepatozoon canis, Haemobartonella canis, Toxoplasma gondii,* and *Encephalitozoon cuniculi* have been reported in dogs in developing countries.[15, 34, 36–41] Confirmation of the presence of one or more of these parasites does not necessarily imply a disease condition, as they are often encountered in physically healthy animals. However, patients are often infected with more than one of these parasites. Infections with *Babesia* sp. may, in especially young dogs, result in severe to fatal disease. Dogs are often presented in an advanced stage of disease with severe anemia and icterus and in a general state of collapse. Patients are also often victims of syndromes such as shock lung, nephrosis, myocardial hemorrhage, and cerebral necrosis (Figure 42–3). These, apart from the fact that treatment is intensive and expensive, carry a poor prognosis. In the author's experience, specific babesiacidal therapy with either imidocarb, diminazene azeturate, phenamidine isethionate, or trypan blue is usually effective. Care should be taken not to repeat treatment with the diminazene group of drugs, however. A fair number of babesiosis cases require supportive therapy, which often necessitates a blood transfusion. Blood transfusions in dogs in babesiosis-endemic areas are therefore a routine and standard procedure often limited only by the inability to locate a suitable donor.

Trypanosomiasis is an important cause of chronic debilitating disease in countries like Zaire and Argentina, where there is inadequate control of the vector.[37, 41] In a survey conducted in Uganda, a relatively large percentage of dogs was found to be infected with *Trypanosoma vivax* and *T. brucei.* All infected animals developed signs of acute disease.[42] Rapid recovery after treatment is possible.[26]

Hepatozoon canis, although commonly encountered on examination of peripheral blood smears, is less commonly implicated as the cause of disease in dogs.[40, 43] Further investigations of hemobartonellosis,[36] toxoplasmosis,[44, 45] and encephalitozoonosis[46] (Figure 42–4) may well demonstrate that these diseases are more common than is presently believed.

The rickettsial disease canine ehrlichiosis is a major disease of dogs in third world countries such as Zimbabwe, Botswana, Namibia/South West Africa, and the

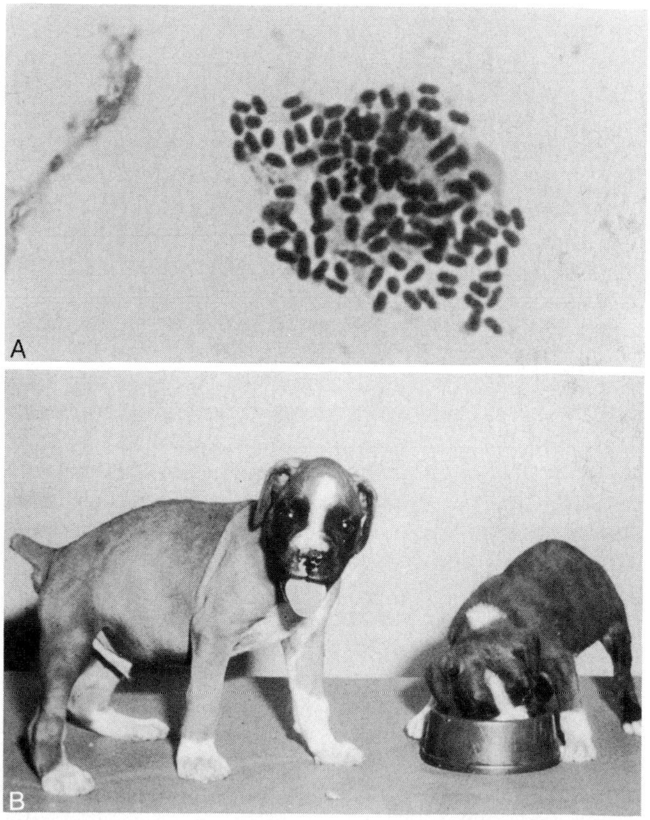

FIGURE 42–4. Gram-stained urinary sediment revealed numerous *Encephalitozoon cuniculi* organisms *(A)* in this puppy with a history of poor growth. The puppy is considerably smaller than its littermate *(B)*.

Republic of South Africa. Infection with *E. canis* usually results in chronic debilitating disease. The acute phase of the disease, which is usually of a transient nature, often goes unnoticed by the owner. This results in dogs being presented in an advanced stage of the disease when the prognosis is often guarded to unfavorable. The clinical signs of the disease are usually[43] nonspecific. Confirmation of the infection, in the absence of a serologic diagnostic technique, depends on demonstration of morulae in a blood smear, which may be a frustrating and time-consuming exercise. Diagnosis of the disease in the author's clinic is augmented by complete blood counts and serum protein electrophoresis. In the author's experience, patients presented with a total white cell count of less than 2,000 cells/mm^3 have a hopeless prognosis. It is not unusual to encounter patients with total white cell counts as low as 300 cells/mm^3. Specific therapy with either oxytetracycline or doxycycline is effective in most cases with the proviso that the total white cell count is above 2,000 cells/mm^3. Contrary to reports elsewhere, imidocarb dipropionate has been found to be totally ineffective.[47] The most important supportive treatment is a transfusion of fresh blood. In the author's opinion, corticosteroid therapy has never resulted in long-term clinical improvement and may result in a more rapid deterioration of the patient's condition.[46]

Very little has been published about feline diseases in developing countries. The most common infectious diseases are probably feline panleukopenia and feline leukemia.

MEDICAL, DERMATOLOGIC, AND SURGICAL DISORDERS

The diagnosis of the entire range of medical, dermatologic, and surgical conditions in developing countries is probably limited only by lack of investigation, facilities, and finance. In the author's experience, patients from developing countries present with as wide a range of medical and surgical disorders as those from more affluent societies (Table 42–1). Interesting differences have been encountered, however; allergic skin disorders are far less commonly encountered. Most of the allergic skin conditions encountered may be attributable to flea infestations. The incidence of mitral valve insufficiency, with or without congestive heart failure, is very low. This aspect needs further investigation but it should be

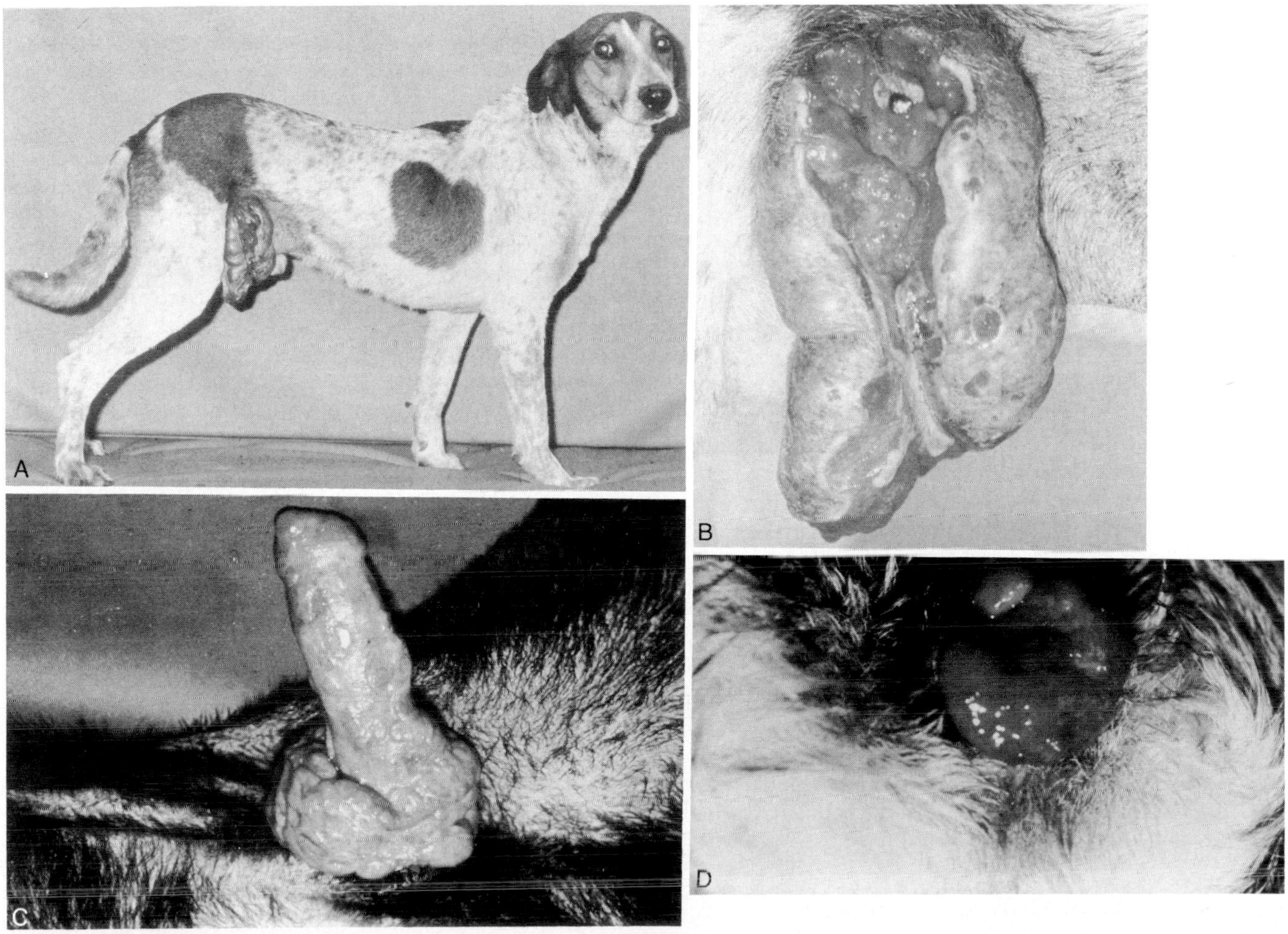

FIGURE 42–5. Transmissible venereal tumor affecting the skin (*A* and *B*). Penis of a male *(C)* and vulva of a female *(D)* dog.

recognized that very few dog owners own small to medium-sized dogs. Obesity is very rarely encountered. The incidence of endocrine disorders is also very low. Patients with conditions requiring surgical intervention, such as bite wounds and fractures of long bones, are often presented with lesions of several days' standing. Due to difficulties the owners experience in making return visits to the animal hospital, these patients often have to be hospitalized for long periods.

NEOPLASIA

Surveys on the incidence and nature of neoplasms in the dog and cat in developing countries have been published.[15, 48, 49] A wide range of tumors have been revealed by these surveys. Transmissible venereal tumor (TVT) is probably an important condition of dogs in countries with high populations of stray dogs[50] and where relatively small proportions of the animals are sterilized. The relatively high incidence of TVT in the author's survey is in accordance with the findings of others,[14] who also found a relatively high incidence rate in a study where 57.7 per cent of animals surveyed were allowed to roam freely. In the author's clinic, dogs are seen with a variety of clinical signs attributed to TVT, ranging from severe depression and other nervous signs to very large to small growths on the penile sheath/vulva (Figure 42–5), and nodules on the skin. Tumors are also encountered in the brain and on the eyelids, skin, vulva, penis, and uterus. Treatment with vincristine in combination with sterilization of the patient has been very successful. Cyclophosphamide/vincristine combination therapy was successful in the treatment of TVT in Nigeria.[51]

DIAGNOSTIC AIDS

In the pioneering days of veterinary science in Africa, the light microscope was one of the most important diagnostic aids of the veterinarian. The examination of a peripheral blood smear is still one of the most important diagnostic tools in a developing country where blood parasites are often major causes of disease in animals.

Specimen transport over considerable distances may limit specimen analyses to those tissues that can be adequately preserved prior to transport to diagnostic centers. The ability of veterinary clinics, university departments, and state institutions to perform a wide range of special diagnostic investigations such as hematology, blood chemistry, serology, microbial cultivation and identification, histopathology, endoscopy, and electrocardiography usually encourages and attracts veterinary scientists to work at these centers. These facilities, which are important centers of research, would help to create and promote job-satisfaction among veterinary scientists.

The veterinarian working in a developing country has to acquaint him- or herself not only with the norms of the local laboratory but also with the norms of the particular local population. In the author's experience, range values for blood chemical parameters of apparently normal dogs from a developing country may differ considerably from those of an apparently normal population from a more affluent society. Significant differences between two such populations have been demonstrated.[14]

DRUGS IN DEVELOPING COUNTRIES

Due to insufficient control by authorities, among other causes, markets in developing countries may be flooded with preparations for which no guarantee for safety or efficacy exists. At the same time there may be a complete absence of basic lifesaving drugs.[52] An international system of registration conforming to basic standards has been proposed by Gimeno and Vilches.[53]

PREVENTIVE MEDICINE

Societies in developing countries are usually in need of the basic commodities of life. The dog and/or cat often come last with regard to food, care, and protection. Preventive medicine in the sphere of production animals has become highly fashionable and absolutely essential. It appears, however, as if preventive medicine of the dog and cat has been limited to conditions of these animals that may endanger the life and productivity of other members of the community, namely humans and production animals. Preventive medicine of small animals could, with relatively minimal input, achieve major results in these societies. In the process, further doors could be opened to education and development of the community. Preventive medicine in developing countries should include instruction in feeding of the dog and cat, general hygienic principles, adequate endo- and ectoparasite control, vaccination, and control of reproduction. A healthy, good-looking dog is probably the best advertisement for the veterinarian in a developing society.

VETERINARY EDUCATION

The veterinary instructor in a developing country constantly has to marry the needs of the country or region with international academic standards. This is by no means an easy task, especially when these needs are ill-defined and everchanging. It has been stressed that in veterinary training in Africa, particular emphasis should be placed on animal production, veterinary public health, and preventive medicine.[3] The increasing demand for veterinary services for pets in many developing countries should not, however, be ignored. Undergraduate veterinary training in developing countries should thus include sound instruction in common disorders of all domestic animals. The student should not be trained in such a way as to become completely dependent on the use of sophisticated diagnostic aids. Greater emphasis should be placed on the role of the veterinarian as an instrument of positive reform and to the uplifting of the community as a whole.

The creation of diagnostic and animal health centers of excellence, adequately equipped and staffed to handle a variety of investigative techniques, would allow and stimulate research. This would increase the level of postgraduate studies and help to prevent the emigration of highly-trained scientists elsewhere.

References

1. Coleman, JR: Developing country. *In* The World Book Encyclopedia Vol 9. Chicago, World Book Childcraft International Inc, 1986, p 40.
2. Schwabe, CW: Veterinary Medicine and Human Health. Third Ed. Baltimore, Williams and Wilkins, 1984, p 1.
3. Report of the fourth meeting of the FAO/WHO expert consultation on veterinary education. Rome, Food and Agricultural Organization of the United Nations, 1978, p 7.
4. Mann, I: Mobile animal health and industry extension service. Bull Epiz Dis Afr 12:345, 1964.
5. Botros, BAM and Moch, RW: Rabies in Egypt: A report of four cases showing some deviation from classical rabies. Bull Epiz Dis Afr 24:29, 1976.
6. Ayanwale, FO, et al.: The incidence of *Echinococcus* infection in dogs, sheep and goats slaughtered in Ibadan, Nigeria. Int J Zoon 9:65, 1982.
7. Okoh, AEJ: Canine diseases of public health significance in Nigeria. Int J Zoon 10:33, 1983.
8. Turner, GS: A review of the world epidemiology of rabies. Trans Royal Soc Trop Med Hyg 70:175, 1976.
9. Hayles, LB, et al.: Observations on the epizootiology of rabies in Zambia, 1970-1974. Bull Anim Hlth Prod Afr 25:9, 1977.
10. Shamsul Islam, AWM, et al.: Prevalence of helminth parasites of dogs in Lusaka, Zambia. Trop Anim Hlth Prod 15:234, 1983.
11. Brit, DP, et al.: Salmonellae from dogs in Vom, Northern Nigeria. Trop Anim Hlth Prod 10:215, 1978.
12. Aliu, YO: Tick-borne diseases of domestic animals in Nigeria: current treatment procedures. Vet Bull 53:233, 1983.
13. Dipeou, OO, et al.: Scavenging dogs and the spread of tick infestation in Nigeria. Int J Zoon 9:90, 1982.
14. Rautenbach, GH: A cross-sectional, descriptive study of the health status of a canine population in the town of Maboloka, Bophuthatswana. Med Vet Thesis, University of Pretoria, 1987.
15. Murray, M: A survey of diseases found in dogs in Kenya. Bull Epiz Dis Afr 16:121, 1968.
16. Idowu, L, et al.: A three-year analysis of parasitic disease of dogs and cats in Ibadan, Nigeria. Bull Anim Hlth Prod Afr 25:166, 1977.
17. Fabiyi, JP: Gastro-intestinal helminths of dogs on the Jos Plateau, Nigeria. Trop Anim Hlth Prod 15:137, 1983.
18. Morsy, TA, et al.: Intestinal parasites of stray cats in Cairo, Egypt. J Egypt Soc Paras 2:331, 1981.
19. Kamara, JA: The incidence of canine spirocercosis in the Freetown area of Sierra Leone. Bull Epiz Dis Afr 12:465, 1964.
20. Williams, MO: The intestinal helminths of dogs in Freetown, Sierra Leone. Bull Epiz Dis Afr 12:471, 1964.
21. Morini, EG: En Chipre se sacrificaron millares de perros en relacion al control de la hidatidosis. Gaceta Veterinaria 39:486, 1977.
22. Okoh, AEJ: Canine rabies in Nigeria, 1970–1980 Reported cases in vaccinated dogs. Int J Zoon 9:118, 1982.
23. Oboegbulem, SI: Rabies: Human exposure potential in Africa. Int J Zoon 5:80, 1978.
24. Aruo, SK: Progress and problems of rabies control in Uganda. Bull Epiz Dis Afr 22:321, 1974.
25. Rweyemamu, MM, et al.: Observations on rabies in Tanzania. Bull Epiz Dis Afr 21:19, 1973.
26. Schillhorn van Veen, TW, et al.: Common diseases of pet animals in West Africa. Tijd Diergenees 104 suppl:163, 1979.
27. Kamalu, BP: Canine parvovirus infection in Nigeria. J Sm Anim Pract 26:663, 1985.
28. Ezeokoli, CD, et al.: Parvovirus enteritis in Nigerian dogs. J Sm Anim Pract 26:669, 1985.
29. Nayak, BC, et al.: An enteric disease of dogs simulating parvovirus infection—a clinicopathological study. Indian Vet J 61:165, 1984.
30. Rao, VNA, et al.: An outbreak of acute haemorrhagic enteritis in dogs. Cheiron 12:165, 1983.
31. Rajaonarison, JJ, et al.: Identification de la parvovirose canine à Madagascar. Rev Elev Med Vet Pays Trop 35:135, 1982.
32. Van Rensburg, IBJ, et al.: Parvovirus as a cause of enteritis and myocarditis in puppies. J S Afr Vet Assoc 50:249, 1979.
33. Adesiyun, AA, et al.: Prevalence of *Brucella abortus* and *Brucella canis* antibodies in dogs in Nigeria. J Sm Anim Pract 27:31, 1986.
34. Okoh, AEJ, et al.: Brucellosis in dogs in Kano, Nigeria. Trop Anim Hlth Prod 10:219, 1978.
35. Monteverde, JJ, et al.: Salmonelas en perros con y sin transtornos entericos. Revista de Medicina Veterinaria. Buenos Aires 49:357, 1968.
36. Leeflang, P, et al.: The occurrence of *Haemobartonella canis* in Nigeria. Bull Epiz Dis Afr 22:51, 1974.
37. Pandey, VS, et al.: Parasitic diseases of animals in the Republic of Zaire. Bull Epiz Dis Afr 24:308, 1976.
38. Leeflang, P, et al.: Prevalence and significance of blood parasites in dogs in Zaria, Northern Nigeria. Bull Anim Hlth Prod Afr 24:181, 1976.
39. Bansal, SR, et al.: Prevalence of *Babesia canis* and *Hepatozoon canis* infection in dogs of Hissar (Haryana) and Delhi and attempts to isolate *Babesia* from human beings. Indian Vet J 62:748, 1985.
40. Ezeokoli, CD, et al.: Clinical and epidemiological studies on canine hepatozoonosis in Zaria, Nigeria. J Sm Anim Pract 24:455, 1983.
41. Bakos, E: Epidemiologia de la enfermedad de Chagas en la Provincia del Chaco y prevalencia en el Noroeste argentino. Gace Vet 44:69, 1982.
42. Okuna, NM, et al.: The incidence of trypanosomiasis in domestic animals and their role in the sleeping sickness epidemic in Busoga. Seventeenth meeting of the International Scientific Council for Trypanosomiasis Research and Control, Arusha, Tanzania, 19–24 October 1981. Nairobi, Kenya. OAU/Scientific, Technical and Research Commission 163, 1983.
43. Van Heerden, J: A retrospective study on 120 natural cases of canine ehrlichiosis. J S Afr Vet Assoc 53:17, 1982.
44. Van Heerden, J, et al.: Toxoplasmosis in a dog. J S Afr Vet Assoc 50:211, 1979.
45. Aganga, AG, et al.: A serological survey of *Toxoplasma gondii* in pet dogs in Nigeria. Br Vet J 140:207, 1984.
46. Botha, WS, et al.: Canine encephalitizoonosis in South Africa. J S Afr Vet Assoc 50:135, 1979.
47. Van Heerden, J and Van Heerden, A: Attempted treatment of canine ehrlichiosis with imidocarb dipropionate. J S Afr Vet Assoc 53:173, 1981.
48. Mugera, GM: Canine and feline neoplasms in Kenya. Bull Epiz Dis Afr 16:367, 1968.
49. Bastianello, SS: A survey on neoplasia in domestic species over a 40 year period from 1935 to 1974 in the Republic of South Africa. VI Tumours occurring in dogs. Onderstepoort J Vet Res 50:199, 1983.
50. Kimeto, A and Mugera, GM: Transmissible venereal tumour of dog in Kenya. Bull Epiz Dis Afr 22:327, 1974.
51. Idowu, AL, et al.: Cyclophosphamide and vincristine chemotherapy for canine transmissible venereal tumour. Trop Vet 2:159, 1984.
52. Richards, T: Drugs in developing countries: inching towards rational policies. Br Med J 292:1347, 1986.
53. Gimeno EJ, Vilches: Benefits to be derived from establishing a veterinary product approval process in developing countries. Rev Sci Tech Off Int Epiz 3:883, 1984.

DRUG INDEX

Generic (Trade)	Dosage	Route	Frequency	Brief Description
Diminazene (Berenil)	3.5 mg/kg 1.6 mg/lb	IM	Once only	Babesiacide
Phenamidine isethionate (Phenamidine)	12.5 mg/kg 5.7 mg/lb	SQ	Once only	Babesiacide
Trypan blue (Trypan Blue)	10 mg/kg 4.5 mg/lb	IV	Once only	Babesiacide
Imidocarb dipropionate (Forray-65)	6 mg/kg 2.7 mg/lb	SQ	Once only	Babesiacide
Oxytetracycline (Oxytetracycline capsules)	100 mg/kg 45.5 mg/lb	Orally	Divided dosages q 8 h or q 12 h	Antibiotic
(Liquamycin)	10 mg/kg 4.5 mg/lb	IV	q 24 h	Antibiotic
Doxycycline (Doxycycline)	3–10 mg/kg 1.4–4.5 mg/lb	Orally, IV	q 24 h	Antibiotic
Vincristine (Pericristine)	0.025 mg/kg 0.01 mg/lb	IV	Three treatments at weekly intervals	Antineoplastic

43 BEHAVIORAL DISORDERS

VICTORIA L. VOITH

The behaviors of animals range from simple reflexes to complex sequences and are the result of a multitude of variables, such as genetics, early experience, learning, the physiologic state of the animal, and concurrent environmental stimuli. A behavior problem may reflect an underlying pathologic disorder or may be a normal, healthy behavior that is undesirable from the owner's perspective.

When an animal's behavior changes or becomes disruptive, the owner expects the veterinarian to be able to distinguish or identify the variables that are influencing the pet's behavior and, in particular, to determine whether or not surgical or pharmacologic intervention will change the behavior. Even if the client is referred to a specialist in animal behavior, the referring veterinarian may still prescribe drug therapy to be used in conjunction with behavior modification procedures; if so, the veterinarian would be responsible for monitoring and evaluating the patient during drug therapy.

In a brief chapter it is impossible to cover all of the normal behaviors of dogs and cats, interviewing and observation techniques, complete lists of differential diagnoses, and detailed descriptions of all of the behavior modification procedures that can be used to treat animals. The reader is therefore referred to other sources that cover these topics in greater detail.[1–3] This chapter is primarily devoted to brief descriptions of behavior modification techniques and drug or physiologic interventions that may work in specific behavior disorders (Table 43–1).

The clinician should keep in mind that the behavior of an animal is rarely the result of a single factor. Multiple factors generally act additively or synergistically to trigger a particular behavior. For example, cats possess the genetic predisposition to spray. Whether or not a specific cat sprays is influenced by factors such as its age, hormonal status, and environmental stimuli. It should also be kept in mind that any one particular behavior, such as spraying, is part of a larger behavioral system.

Behavior systems are composed of many types of behaviors and sequences of behavior patterns that serve a common function. An analogy is that of organ systems, which are composed of many different types of tissues that are organized to perform a common function. For example, the elimination behavior system of cats and dogs involves not only the processes of urination and defecation to rid the body of wastes, but also the search for a specific location and/or surface, pre-elimination behaviors such as sniffing and circling, and post-elimination behaviors such as scratching the ground. Urine and feces can also be used for communication among animals. The clinician must explore the behaviors and behavioral needs of the animal in all of the behavior systems suspected to be involved when analyzing a behavior problem, rather than focus on a specific behavioral complaint. Take, for example, the case of a dog presented for eliminating in the house, assuming that pathophysiologic disorders have been ruled out. If the dog is engaging in normal elimination behaviors in the home, then is the dog taken out frequently enough? What is the relationship between being taken out and its feeding schedule? Does the dog have a strong preference for specific locations and surfaces in the home as opposed to outdoors? Has it ever had the opportunity to develop locations and surfaces outdoors? If the dog is an intact male, is it urine marking in the home? Is the amount of urine deposited usually small? If the dog is distressed when left alone and eliminates as a consequence, it is experiencing separation anxiety and behaviors related to attachment should be explored. How does the dog interact with the owners when they are home and how does the dog greet them upon return? How does the dog act as the owners prepare to depart? How long is the dog left alone each day? Are there any other animals in the household? If the dog appears to be afraid to venture outdoors and is reluctant to walk on a leash, it may be afraid of traffic noises or crowds of people. How does it behave outdoors? All of the behavior systems suspected should be examined and analyzed to determine whether or not they are contributing to a specific behavior problem.

The major behavior systems, all of which can influence an animal's behavior, are ingestive, eliminative, reproductive, care-of-body surface, sleep and rest, attachment, aggressive (intra- and interspecific aggression), anti-predator, play, and explorative or investigative. The behavior systems are interrelated and influence each other, much as organ systems in the body affect each other. Veterinarians who wish to develop expertise in clinical animal behavior should learn as much as possible about the particular species that interest them as well as trying to understand general theories about why animals behave as they do.

TABLE 43–1. PHARMACEUTICAL AGENTS

Generic	Trade	Dosage	Route	Frequency	Behavioral Applications
		Dogs			
Diazepam	Valium	¼ to 1 mg/lb	orally	as needed	Noise phobias
Amitriptyline hydrochloride	Elavil	1 to 2 mg/lb	orally	variable schedules	Antianxiety, separation anxiety
Megestrol acetate	Ovaban Megace	1 to 2 mg/lb	orally	variable schedules	Antianxiety, typically masculine behaviors
Dextroamphetamine	Dexedrine	.1 to .6 mg/lb	orally	?	Hyperkinesis
Medroxyprogesterone	Depo-Provera	5 mg/lb	IM, SQ	as needed	Typically masculine behaviors
Phenylpropanolamine HCl		¼–2 mg/lb	orally	BID	Excitement, submissive urination
		Cats			
Diazepam	Valium	1 to 3 mg/cat	orally	BID or TID	Spraying, antianxiety
Amitriptyline HCl	Elavil	5 to 10 mg/cat	orally	SID	Antianxiety, displacement grooming

Another concept clinicians should keep in mind is that a behavioral complaint is not a diagnosis. Urinating in the house is no more a diagnosis than is polyuria or diarrhea. There is no all-embracing effective treatment for urinating in the house any more than there is a completely effective treatment for polyuria. The behavioral complaint is best viewed as a sign; it is the clinician's obligation to determine the underlying reason for the animal's behavior.

Clinical animal behavior is an important as well as exciting new area in veterinary medicine. Dissatisfaction with behavior is one of the most common reasons for owners to abandon or euthanize their pets.[4, 5] Treating a behavior problem can save an animal's life. As the public becomes more aware that behavior problems can be treated, veterinarians are increasingly expected to know how to deal with behavior problems themselves or to refer clients to trained colleagues. The interrelationship between behavior and disease (e.g., overactivity and excessive vocalization in many hyperthyroid cats, restlessness in older dogs with cystitis) and the use of drugs to treat behaviors unrelated to disease (e.g., phobias, spraying, aggression) necessitate the involvement of veterinarians. Clinical animal behavior is a new and developing area in veterinary medicine with potential for growth in the area of basic research as well as application.

COMMON BEHAVIOR PROBLEMS IN DOGS

Fears and Phobias

Fear is a complex system involving the interactions of behavioral, emotional, and physiologic components.[6, 7] Fearful behavior is generally an adaptive response that removes or protects an animal from immediate or impending dangers or a noxious stimulus. Animals may startle, withdraw, escape, avoid, or take a defensive aggressive position when afraid. Stimuli that usually evoke fear responses are predators, physical and environmental dangers, situations and events associated with risks of predation or danger, and the behaviors of conspecifics or companions.[8, 9]

When afraid or defensive, cats and dogs exhibit species-specific facial and body expressions and behavior. Veterinarians should be familiar with these signs.[10–13] Most of the fearful behaviors displayed by companion animals involve such responses as freezing, trembling, panting, increased heart rate, digging, biting, or fleeing. A response to a fearful stimulus that is out of proportion to the real threat of the stimulus is classified as a phobia. Phobias may be self-destructive. Dogs are most often presented for fear of noises such as thunderstorms, firecrackers, traffic sounds, and/or fear of people, usually strangers.

Behavioral therapy for fears and phobias involves identifying the stimuli that elicit the fears and then exposing the animal to these stimuli in such a way that the animal does not experience fear. The techniques include *systematic desensitization* (gradual exposure to the stimuli), *counterconditioning* (conditioning the animal to respond in an opposite manner to the fear-eliciting stimuli), and *flooding* (leaving the animal exposed to fear-eliciting stimuli until the animal is no longer afraid). When the eliciting stimuli can be identified and controlled, behavior modification techniques are highly successful in treating fears and phobic responses. Between treatment sessions, the fear-eliciting stimuli should be avoided or treatment will be retarded.

A phobic animal should be treated with an effective antianxiety drug whenever exposure to a fear-eliciting stimulus cannot be avoided. Ideally, the dog should be treated before it begins manifesting the fear response, but an appropriate drug can be helpful even if administered after the onset of the stimulus. It may be necessary to try several drugs and different doses before an effective medication is found. Theoretically, *consistent* treatment with an antianxiety drug can lead to successful treatment of a dog's fear response. If chronic drug therapy is used, the dose should be *gradually reduced* while the animal is exposed to the stimulus before the drug is eventually discontinued. The owner should be advised that lasting positive effects of drug therapy are more likely to occur if the animal is continuously protected from any phobic response during the course of therapy and that the positive effects of drug therapy are more likely to transfer to the nondrug state if the drug dose is gradually reduced. There is always the possibility that even though the animal is not afraid or anxious while on medication, the effect will not transfer to the nondrug state.

The fear-eliciting stimulus of thunderstorms cannot usually be avoided. Phenothiazines and phenobarbital sometimes appear to calm a noise-phobic dog, but often they merely suppress the dog's motor responses and not the emotional response to the noises. Diazepam (Valium), 0.25 to 1.0 mg/lb orally, does appear to suppress the dog's fear responses to noises without rendering it ataxic. Dogs that are afraid of thunderstorms or are periodically exposed to noises to which they have a phobic response should be treated with an antianxiety drug every time there is potential for exposure to these sounds. Usually, dogs should not be given diazepam while undergoing behavior modification sessions, as diazepam may interfere with memory storage of new information.

In the author's experience, as well as in that of other behavioral therapists, diazepam can increase aggressive behavior in fearful dogs. Perhaps diazepam does reduce fear, but it also lowers the inhibition of aggression. The author recommends that diazepam not be given to dogs that are fearful of people, particularly if they have shown any signs of aggression in any context.

Some dogs become more active or excited under the influence of diazepam. Such dogs, obviously, do not benefit from diazepam. Diazepam is not a general CNS suppressant and sometimes can lead to an increase in behaviors including aggression.[13]

Sometimes a dog is presented for what appears to be fearful behavior (e.g., shivering or shaking), but the dog is suffering from a metabolic disorder such as hypoglycemia. If it is difficult to identify stimuli that reliably elicit the "fearful" behavior, a pathophysiologic etiology should be vigorously sought.

Separation Anxiety

Approximately one third of the dogs presented to the Veterinary Hospital of the University of Pennsylvania Behavior Clinic are presented for complaints related to separation anxiety. The most common presenting signs of separation anxiety are vocalization, elimination, and destructive behavior, which occur as soon as or shortly after the owner leaves the dog alone. Most dogs with separation anxiety are anorectic when left alone. Some dogs also exhibit psychosomatic signs of diarrhea, vomiting, or excessive grooming when left alone and excessive greeting behaviors when the owner returns, constantly following the owner around the home. Sometimes these dogs are presented for hyperactivity because of relentless attention-seeking. Occasionally, a dog with separation anxiety is presented with a complaint of aggression exhibited toward the owner at the time of departure. The dog is described as trying to "prevent the owner from leaving." A detailed description of the event usually reveals that the dog is really trying to accompany the owner and when the owner physically restrains the dog, the dog becomes aggressive. A thorough history almost always reveals that these dogs exhibit aggression toward their owners in other circumstances compatible with dominance aggression. The dog's aggression at the time of departure is really precipitated by physical manipulation by the owner; the motivation for the dog to accompany the owner is, however, related to separation anxiety.

The underlying principle of separation anxiety treatment is to accustom the dog to being alone without experiencing anxiety. The behavior modification technique involves habituating the dog's anxiety to the owner's predeparture behaviors (e.g., picking up car keys, moving towards the door, straightening magazines) and then accustoming the dog to progressively longer intervals of being alone.[14] In the beginning, the animal should be left alone for only a few minutes. This is later extended to several hours. Generally, when the dog is comfortable being alone for a few hours, it will be fine all day.

Crates are usually contraindicated in extreme cases of separation anxiety because confinement does not address the motivation or underlying emotional disorder of the animal. The dog usually engages in the same behaviors in the crate that it does outside of the crate; it will eliminate, destroy whatever is available, or howl and bark. Many dogs have been severely injured in frantic attempts to escape from crates.

Punishment, since it usually increases anxiety, is generally contraindicated for dogs with separation anxiety. Even if punishment were not contraindicated in principle, it would be difficult for most owners to meet the criteria for effective punishment. To be effective, punishment must be applied while the dog is engaging in the behavior and administered each time the dog engages in the behavior. Specific aversive techniques such as the placement of mouse traps or balloons to keep dogs away from specific items or the delivery of an electric shock when the dog barks may suppress that particular behavior, but the underlying distress caused by being left alone is not addressed and the dog is likely to exhibit other signs.

Ideally, during the course of treatment the dog should not be left alone for periods of time longer than it is known to be able to tolerate. Otherwise, the dog experiences anxiety and treatment will be retarded or, if this occurs repeatedly, treatment will be unsuccessful. Owners might take the dog to a boarding kennel until it can tolerate being alone for several hours, hire a dog sitter, use a companion dog, or "dog-proof" one room in the house so that the dog cannot injure itself while the problem is being treated. In the author's experience, treatment of separation anxiety is not likely to be successful if the pet is kept in a "dog-proof" room, where it continues to experience anxiety, while the owners attempt to treat the problem at other times.

ANTIANXIETY MEDICATION

Antianxiety drugs sometimes can be helpful in the treatment of dogs with separation anxiety. Dogs with mild separation anxiety may respond to the medication without necessarily implementing behavior modification techniques. Dogs that must be left alone at home during the course of treatment may have their anxiety attenuated if they are on drug therapy.

A good antianxiety drug should not sedate the dog. In fact, sedation may interfere with the dog's learning abilities. There are a wide range of doses and several antianxiety drugs that can be used for this syndrome. Some experimentation may be necessary to find a drug or combination of drugs that affects a particular dog. The first time a particular drug is tried, the owner should stay home with the dog for several hours to observe any potential side effects. Drugs that are potentially useful in suppressing separation anxiety are tricyclide antidepressants, progestins, barbiturates, phenothiazines, and benzodiazepines. If an effective drug is found, the dog should be medicated every time it is left alone (except during behavior-modification sessions) for 15 to 20 absences; the dose can then be gradually reduced over subsequent absences. A suggested reduction schedule is to progressively halve the dose after 15 to 20 successful absences. When the dose is so low that it is probably ineffective, medication should cease. Amitriptyline hydrochloride (Elavil), 1 to 2 mg/lb, administered orally one hour prior to departure, is the most effective drug for suppressing the separation anxiety response of dogs in the author's experience. Although the human medical literature indicates that tricyclide antidepressants require two to three weeks of administration before therapeutic effects are achieved in people, it is the author's impression that these drugs often produce an immediate reduction of anxiety in dogs.

The tricyclide antidepressants have been reported to produce cardiac arrhythmias and sinus tachycardia and to prolong conduction time. Other potential side effects are hypotension, excitement, and anticholinergic effects such as dry mouth, blurred vision, and constipation. Clinicians should familiarize themselves with contraindications and side effects of the tricyclide antidepressants, as well as other drugs, particularly of those not specifically marketed for dogs.

Synthetic progestins such as megestrol acetate (Ovaban, MegAce), 1 to 2 mg/lb orally, produce tranquilizing effects without rendering the dog ataxic and may be beneficial in treating dogs with separation anxiety. Some practitioners have reported that diazepam is effective in reducing separation anxiety. The clinician should, of course, be aware of contraindications and side effects of these drugs.

Obedience school is not an effective way of dealing with separation anxiety. Many dogs that are highly trained still exhibit separation anxiety. Separation anxiety is not the result of disobedience or the lack of training, but is a distress response.

Because separation anxiety is such a common problem, one of the greatest services a clinician can offer a client is instruction in ways to prevent its development. It is helpful to explain that a puppy should not always accompany the owner but that it should gradually become accustomed to being alone and thereafter periodically be left alone for several hours each week. Separation anxiety more often occurs in households that have only one dog and a prophylactic measure might be to keep at least two pets. The addition of a dog or cat after a dog has developed separation anxiety, however, is not very likely to correct the problem. Besides, few owners are receptive to getting a second pet when they already have one that is destroying the house.

The prognosis for treatment of separation anxiety is very good with properly implemented behavior modification techniques and/or if effective drug therapy can be found. Dogs that are left alone for prolonged periods of time (12 to 14 hours) day after day are not often treated successfully. Owners who must repeatedly leave a dog alone for prolonged amounts of time should consider placing the dog in another home.

Problems Related To Play

Play problems can manifest themselves as high activity levels, destructive behaviors, and aggression. Typically, the dog with a play problem is young (generally under one year of age), of either sex, and the only dog in the household. These dogs are also often left alone or are restricted in the house or a cage for much of the day. Unfortunately, the response of many owners to an active, playful dog is to confine it without allowing sufficient opportunity to engage in play. Consequently, when the pet is released, it is even more active. Many owners inadvertently reward playful exuberance by chasing the dog or intermittently trying to swat it, both of which the dog interprets as play.

The overactive, playful dog must be allowed to play and expend energy. The dog should be encouraged to exercise and play games such as catching flying disks or Frisbees, chase and run, or even tug-of-war. These activities can take place in the house (if a small dog), a fenced backyard, or a large area with the dog on a long line or leash. Only dogs that reliably come when called should be allowed to run loose in unfenced areas. One of the best forms of exercise for a playful dog is to play with another dog.

Sometimes long walks help to alleviate a playful dog's overactive behavior. Dogs should not be expected or required to heel constantly on a walk. Leashes with a retractable line allow dogs to investigate and explore several feet from the owner. Some owners do not walk active dogs because they are unruly, but several aids now available, such as the K-9 Kumalong* and Gentle Leader,** are somewhat like a horse halter and provide the owner with excellent control of the dog.

Normal play, particularly in young mammals, often comprises segments of aggressive behaviors. Aggressive play usually involves inhibited bites and species-typical signals that indicate this is play and not serious aggression. However, dogs should not be allowed to engage in excessively rough play or to grab the owner's hands or feet directly. Owners should play with intermediary objects such as a thick, soft cotton rope or toys specifically sold for shaking by dogs. If the dog does grab the owner's arm, leg, or body during play, a quick abrupt punishment is appropriate. A loud startling noise is usually effective. The author generally recommends that owners buy a foghorn and carry it with them constantly for several days so that each time the dog leaps at them they can sound it immediately. As most aggressive vocalizations among animals are of a lower pitch than other vocal communication[15, 16] foghorns meet this criterion well. A loud, deep voice may also work. Regard-

*K-9 Kumalong, Altru, P.O. Box 340, Sandia Pard, NM 87047.

**Gentle Leader, 1450 Energy Park Drive Suite 117B, St. Paul, MN 55108.

less of the means of punishment used, the owner must be consistent and prepared to startle the dog each time it grabs at a body part.

Both overly active and aggressively playful dogs should be taught to inhibit themselves on command. This first requires that the dog be taught to sit-stay or lie down-stay when the dog is not highly aroused. Gradually the dog is accustomed to remaining immobile in more arousing situations and then is periodically asked to inhibit itself for progressively longer intervals during active periods.

Chewing and destructive behaviors are normal forms of play often seen in puppies. Puppies should have toys of their own. If chewing occurs when the puppy cannot be supervised, the puppy can be put in a "puppy-proof" area (large crate or specific room) until it demonstrates that it will leave valued objects alone. If the dog attacks specific items, these items might be "booby trapped" or made to taste aversive. However, the dog should always have access to something it finds attractive and acceptable for play.

Punishment by itself should never be the sole approach to coping with a play problem. Play is a normal behavior in which young animals are highly motivated to engage. The play needs of an animal must be met or it will find ways of its own to meet these needs. Owners must provide the animal with opportunities and appropriate objects with which to play. Punishment, however, is not contraindicated if it is properly implemented and used in conjunction with other approaches.

Elimination Behavior Problems

URINATION AND DEFECATION

Behavior problems involving both urination and defecation generally stem from separation anxiety or fear of a particular stimulus (e.g., thunder or noises) or are housebreaking problems (e.g., the dog is not inhibited about eliminating in the house).

Separation Anxiety. The profile and treatment of a dog with separation anxiety has been described previously. This syndrome is very treatable when approached properly.

Fear Reactions. If fear is diagnosed as the cause of an elimination behavior problem, the stimuli that elicit the fear must be carefully identified. Behavior modification techniques and/or appropriate antianxiety drugs can be used to treat the dog's fearful behavior.

Housebreaking. Urination and defecation problems due to lack of inhibition of eliminating in the house usually occur whether or not a dog has access to the owner, although the problem may occur less frequently when the owner is home because the dog is allowed out more often. The history of a dog with a housebreaking problem generally reveals that it was never well housebroken from the time it was a puppy.

Housebreaking techniques for puppies and older dogs involve the establishment of location and surface preferences for elimination outdoors or in areas that are acceptable to the owner. Simultaneously, the tendency to eliminate in an inappropriate area must be reduced or prohibited. First, the dog should be frequently taken to the area where the owner wants the dog to urinate and defecate. When the dog is in the house it should be kept under the supervision of the owner or in a small area that will inhibit its desire to eliminate. Housebreaking is a function of not allowing a dog to eliminate in the wrong place and instead setting up situations in which the dog will eliminate and develop a location and surface preference for a desired area.

Punishment is not an effective way of treating housebreaking problems because in most cases the owner cannot meet the criteria for effective punishment.

Some dogs develop firmly entrenched habits of eliminating in the house and refuse to eliminate outdoors even if kept there for 24 hours. Some of these dogs have an underlying fear of traffic noises, a possibility that must be explored and then treated. Cases in which the dog has a strong inhibition about eliminating outdoors may be helped by the administration of a diuretic and/or laxative shortly before taking the dog outside. After the dog has eliminated outdoors several times, drug therapy should be discontinued. Of course, the dog must be closely monitored when inside.

URINATION PROBLEMS

Possible causes for dogs urinating in the home include disease, pathophysiologic disorders, separation anxiety, housebreaking problems, fear-eliciting stimuli, urine marking, excitement-related urination, and submissive urination.

Urine Marking. Urine marking is generally exhibited by intact male dogs after they reach sexual maturity. The amount of urine is usually small and is regularly deposited in a few specific locations, generally on vertical objects. Castration has been reported to be approximately 68 per cent effective in suppressing urine marking in the house in male dogs neutered for that behavior.[17] Castration does not change the posture that the dog uses, but should lessen the frequency of urine marking.[18]

If urine marking occurs in only a few locations, the practice of placing food, water, or the dog's bed in those locations may inhibit the dog from marking there. The areas of urine marking should, of course, be thoroughly cleaned. If stimuli that elicit the marking behavior can be identified (e.g., entering visitors or delivery of mail), the dog may be counterconditioned to assume a different behavior when these stimuli appear or may be punished when it begins urine marking.

Some male dogs, even if neutered, may be stimulated to urine mark when estrous bitches are in the vicinity. In these cases, a short course of progestin therapy may be helpful.

Submissive Urination. Submissive urination is sometimes exhibited by puppies and young adults during greeting responses or when scolded. As the dog matures, this behavior usually ceases.

Specific treatment of submissive urination can take many forms. One form involves the owner identifying exactly what stimuli elicit this behavior, for example, staring at or petting the dog or raising one's voice, and then avoiding these behaviors until the dog matures to the age at which it gains control of its bladder. Alternatively, the owner can change the dog out of the greeting behavior system or submissive mood by engaging it in play or eating before it begins to urinate. Adult dogs that persist at submissive urination can be specifically counterconditioned.[19] Such dogs can be conditioned to assume a standing posture when the eliciting stimuli occur. This treatment procedure usually involves the help of a person skilled at teaching owners how to implement behavior modification techniques.

Physical punishment of dogs with submissive urination problems is contraindicated at any time because such discipline is likely to intensify the dog's submissive tendencies. Methods other than punishment can usually be used to treat most behavior problems.

Excitement Urination. Excitement urination often occurs in young dogs in highly arousing circumstances such as during greeting and play. The dog does not necessarily assume a submissive posture but may urinate while standing or walking. The exciting stimuli that elicit the urination can be identified, and the dog can be counterconditioned or taught to relax in these circumstances. Another way to cope with this particular problem is to avoid exposing the dog to the eliciting stimuli when its bladder is likely to be full. Drugs that increase the tone of the bladder sphincter or decrease the tone of the bladder may also prove helpful. Phenylpropanolamine HCl, ¼ to 2 mg/lb BID orally, increases the tone of the bladder sphincter and often prevents urination related to excitement and submission.

DEFECATION BEHAVIOR PROBLEMS

Defecation behavior problems can be caused by the same factors that result in urination problems. Occasionally dogs appear to mark by depositing feces on vertical objects. Fecal marking, however, is not a common behavior problem in dogs.

Excessive Vocalization

Excessive vocalization is usually either related to separation anxiety or elicited by extraneous stimuli. The diagnosis and treatment of separation anxiety was discussed previously. Barking at extraneous stimuli can be treated by counterconditioning or with a bark-activated, or preferably, a vibration-activated, shock collar. Such collars must be used with discretion. Unless there is a built-in delay period after shock, a vicious circle of shock-bark/shock-bark can ensue. Owners should be aware that when they attempt to take the collar off, while the dog is being shocked, the dog may direct aggression toward them.

Overactivity

Overactive behaviors can be either normal behaviors of a dog that are more than the owner can tolerate or an actual above-normal activity level. Restricted play, excessive confinement, separation anxiety, and direct reinforcement from the owner are some perpetuating causes of overactivity in dogs. Some breeds have been selected for high activity levels. In addition to having vigorous periods of exercise, these dogs should have access to either a large backyard or a run.

Physiologic disorders, such as hyperthyroidism, are a possible cause of restlessness and nervousness in dogs. There should be concurrent signs of disease to support this diagnosis, as well as confirming laboratory tests. Hyperkinesis is a rare physiologic disorder in which dogs are overactive, have short attention spans, are difficult to train to inhibit themselves, resist restraint, and do not respond to tranquilizers that usually suppress activity.[20–23] Approximately 50 per cent of dogs meeting the criteria for physiologic hyperkinesis have been reported to respond to the oral administration of 0.1 to 0.6 mg/lb of dextroamphetamine or 0.5 to 2.0 mg/lb of levoamphetamine.[20, 21, 23] It must be emphasized, however, that this is an uncommon disorder in the household pet.

An overdose of amphetamines in either a normal or hyperkinetic dog results in an increase in activity level, elevated heart and respiratory rates, and an increase in oxygen consumption. The animal may also become anorexic and exhibit stereotypic behaviors (nonsensical repetitive movements such as running in circles), hyperthermia, and convulsions. Treatment of amphetamine poisoning includes reduction of absorption (e.g., emesis, gastric lavage, activated charcoal, cathartics), acidification of urine, sedation, and supportive care.[24, 24a]

Aggression

Aggression (growling, baring teeth, threatening barks, nipping, snapping, and biting) is the most common complaint of owners presenting dogs to animal behavior therapists.[25] Although some aggressive conditions can be treated, owners should always be advised that there is never a guarantee that treatment will completely attenuate the dog's aggressive behaviors. Appropriate treatment often can reduce, but will not always eliminate, the frequency and intensity of aggression. Owners must carefully assess whether or not the benefits outweigh the risks.

Dominance Aggression. Dominance aggression is generally presented as sudden, unprovoked aggressive attacks by intact, pure-bred male dogs at approximately two years of age.[26, 27] Detailed questioning usually reveals the following circumstances under which the dog manifests aggression: (1) while being physically manipulated, i.e., being petted, restrained, pushed against; having collars, leashes, or muzzles put on or taken off; during grooming, bathing, or towel drying, (2) when disturbed while resting or sleeping (some of these dogs are presented for sleep disorders and because they are aggressive "upon awakening"), (3) when a person approaches food, an estrous bitch, a favorite person, or the dog's resting area even if the dog is not in it, and/or (4) while being stared at, scolded, disciplined, or threatened in some way.

At times these dogs assume dominant postures, such as bracing their feet against the owner's shoulders or lap, or even pressing their chins down on top of the owner's shoulder, and staring at the owner until the owner looks away. The dog may not be aggressive to all family members and often shows no aggression toward strangers.

The primary goals of managing a dominant aggressive dog are to avoid having a person injured and to get the dog to assume submissive and unaggressive behaviors in circumstances that previously elicited aggression. Megestrol acetate (Ovaban), 1 to 2 mg/lb/day orally for two weeks, then progressive reduction of the dose over several weeks, or medroxyprogesterone acetate (Depo-Provera) at 5 mg/lb/IM or SQ can dramatically suppress dominance aggression in some dogs. These progestins can also suppress dominance aggression exhibited by female dogs. However, unless the owner also implements behavior modification techniques and new ways of interacting with the dog, the aggression may return. The side effects and contraindications of using progestin therapy must always be taken into consideration.

Castration, but not spaying, may reduce but not eliminate dominance aggression directed toward people. Many dogs are not affected at all.

In theory, physically confronting these dogs in an aggressive manner could reverse the dominance hierarchy. In reality, however, many of these dogs escalate their aggression when physically confronted by the owners and the owners may be injured. It is a mistake to assume that dominance hierarchies are always settled without serious injury when confrontations occur between animals in the wild. A major cause of death among wolves in dense populations is the result of intraspecific fighting.[28]

This author generally takes the approach of identifying all the stimuli or situations known to elicit the aggressive behavior and advising the owners to initially avoid these circumstances. Over subsequent weeks the owners should begin to restructure their daily interactions with the dog. For example, the dog should never receive anything, such as being allowed out, allowed in, or being petted, without being required to sit or lie down. Gradually it may become accustomed to accepting more dominant gestures from the owner, such as being petted more firmly, pushed against, and having its neck or muzzle grabbed, before it is allowed to get what it wants. Because physical manipulation such as hugging and petting can elicit aggression, small children who cannot be relied upon to avoid these behaviors should not be allowed access to such a dog. Elderly people who might stumble and accidentally step on a dog are also at great risk for injury.

Electroconvulsive therapy may reduce or eliminate dominance aggression for a few months to several years.[29] The effectiveness of the treatment may be based on memory loss and the dog subsequently being relegated to a lower social status or the therapeutic effects may involve neurotransmitter changes.

The treatment of dominance aggression cases should not be taken lightly. As the interaction between owner and dog changes, the situations that elicit aggression and the form of aggression may change. The course of treatment of this problem is dynamic, and frequent communication with the owner is usually necessary. Assuming responsibility for treating these cases can involve prolonged commitment on the part of the clinician.

Intermale Aggression. Intraspecific intermale aggression is a common complaint of dog owners. Of 391 owners of intact male dogs in a survey conducted in Britain, 30 per cent indicated that their dogs fought with other males.[30]

A retrospective survey reported that castration was effective in stopping or reducing intermale fighting in five of eight dogs castrated for this behavior.[17] Megestrol acetate (Ovaban), 1 to 2 mg/lb/day orally for two weeks, followed by half of the original dose for another two weeks and medroxyprogesterone acetate at a dose of 5 to 7.5 mg/lb IM or SQ can be effective in suppressing intermale aggression in male dogs for varying lengths of time.[30, 31]

Behavior modification is another method of treating intermale aggression in dogs. A systematic program using positive reinforcements and response prevention can be effective in training dogs to sit or stand immobile next to their owners in the presence of other male dogs. Since many male dogs are the sole pet in the household and encounter other males only when outdoors with their owners, the technique is valuable in enabling owners to control their dogs. This technique depends upon the presence of the owner and is not effective in preventing intermale aggression between dogs which are left together without supervision. Progestin therapy is often a helpful adjunct while owners are training their dogs to inhibit aggressive tendencies.

Environmental stimuli, such as the presence of a bitch in heat, can influence intermale fighting. Manipulating these stimuli should be considered as a means of managing the problem. Finally, if the aggression involves two dogs in a home, then finding one of the dogs another home should be considered. Dogs that are aggressive to other dogs are not necessarily aggressive to people and can be excellent pets in a household without other male dogs.

Interfemale Aggression. When interfemale aggression occurs it usually is between two females in the same household. It is often of gradual onset and begins when the younger dog or both dogs reach behavioral maturity, usually between 18 and 24 months of age. Spaying is unlikely to affect this behavior unless the aggression is related to the estrous cycle. Drug therapy, including progestins, usually does not suppress interfemale aggression. Sometimes owners can achieve excellent verbal control over both dogs, requiring them to remain immobile in situations that otherwise might lead to an aggressive encounter. The owner can also contribute to the development of a stable dominance hierarchy among the dogs by supporting the dog most likely to be dominant. That dog should be petted, greeted, and fed first, and the more subordinate dog should be discouraged from intruding until a specific invitation is given. Even if the owners can control the dogs' behaviors when they are present, the dogs may fight and one may even kill the other when unsupervised. Dogs that persist in fighting should be kept separated when unsupervised. Sometimes the easiest and safest solution to the problem is to place one of the dogs in a home that has no other female dog. Such a dog is not necessarily aggressive to people and can be an excellent pet in another home.

Fear-Induced Aggression. The history, the facial and body expressions, and the circumstances in which the pet exhibits aggression are the means of diagnosing fear-induced aggression. Dogs that exhibit fear-induced aggression usually do not go out of their way to bite anyone and usually bite only when someone reaches for them. The facial expressions and body postures of the animal are indicative of fear. Desensitization and counterconditioning techniques, covered elsewhere in this chapter, generally can successfully ameliorate fear-induced aggression.

Castration and spaying are not effective in ameliorating fear-induced aggression. Amygdalectomies have been reported as an effective treatment of fear-induced aggression in dogs.[32]

This author and other behavior therapists believe that diazepam therapy is contraindicated in dogs with fear-induced aggression. Propranolol has been reported to successfully treat fear-induced aggression in dogs[33] and has been used to treat temper outbursts in humans.[34]

Pain-Induced Aggression. Pain should always be considered as a possible cause of aggressive behavior. Pain cannot be ruled out as a possible cause simply because an animal demonstrates aggression toward specific individuals. An uncomfortable animal may suppress an aggressive display toward an adult or dominant animal in a household, yet threaten a child or a submissive member of the family. Physical examination, history, and breed predispositions to specific disorders should help identify pain as a possible etiology.

The treatment involves correction of the physical disorder, possible use of analgesics, avoidance of evoking the aggressive behavior, and perhaps counterconditioning the animal so that it does not respond with fright to approaches toward the painful area. The pet can be rewarded for a nonaggressive attitude first while people approach it, then as reached for, and then when areas progressively closer to the painful area are touched. Eventually the painful areas can be touched and, if necessary, even manipulated for treatment.

Parental Aggression. It is quite normal for a mother who has offspring to react aggressively toward approaching individuals. Since dogs are social animals whose ancestors and wild relatives engage in communal rearing of offspring, it should not be surprising that other dogs in the household may also act protectively toward puppies. If people cannot avoid eliciting parental aggressive behavior, counterconditioning may prove to be effective in suppressing this behavior.

Pseudocyesis. Pseudocyesis may be the rule rather than the exception in the nonpregnant bitch following estrus.[35–37] A bitch manifesting pseudocyesis may show one or all of the following signs: distention of the abdomen, engorgement of the uterus and development of the mammary glands, lactation, and behaviors such as nervousness, nesting, guarding of enclosed areas, and mothering of objects. The behavioral signs usually begin to manifest themselves six to eight weeks after estrus. The bitch may exhibit one or all of the behavioral signs yet be without observable physiologic changes, such as lactation. Occasionally a bitch may guard "surrogate puppies" or exhibit aggression in enclosed areas that she treats as nest sites. Sometimes other dogs in the household aggressively protect the bitch.

A variety of therapeutic courses are available. The owner can treat the bitch as though she were a pregnant or lactating mother and simply leave her alone and try to avoid eliciting aggression. If it is necessary to approach her, her aggressive behavior can be counterconditioned. Mibolerone is the current drug of choice, but estrogens, androgens, and progestins have all been reported to suppress the pseudocyesis syndrome.[37] Megestrol acetate at 1 mg/lb (2 mg/kg) orally for five to eight days given early in the course of false pregnancy is reportedly effective, but when the drug is withdrawn, 10 to 15 per cent of the dogs may again experience a false pregnancy.[38]

The use of phenothiazines probably should be avoided during pseudocyesis because these drugs inhibit or antagonize dopamine, which is prolactin-inhibiting factor. Prolactin, in addition to facilitating lactation, may be partially responsible for maternal behaviors. Dopaminergic agonists such as bromocriptine, which is used to treat hypergalactemia in humans, may prove to be an effective drug therapy for pseudocyesis of the dog. Emesis is, however, a side effect.[36, 37]

Probably the best course of therapy is to let nature take its course without interference, unless the behavioral signs are causing the dog discomfort or are a danger to the owner. Although there have been no controlled clinical studies regarding the effect of spaying a bitch during pseudocyesis, many practitioners believe that doing so will prolong the syndrome.[37]

Territorial/Protective Aggression. Animals of either sex may aggressively protect their house, yard, or any area they consider their territory. Neutering reportedly has little effect on reversing territorial aggression,[17] as is also the case with progestins or other drugs. Diagnosis of this type of aggression is made according to the history; the therapeutic approach is counterconditioning or preventative measures, e.g., keep the dog away from potential targets.

A dog can usually be taught that one or two barks when a stranger approaches is acceptable and to become quiet and immobile when asked to do so. It is unreasonable to expect the dog to distinguish between the owner's friends and foes. If the owner wants the dog to act as a guard dog in the owner's absence, the owner should be prepared for the dog to threaten friends and strangers alike.

Predatory Behavior. Predatory behavior is not uncommon in domestic dogs. In fact, the hunting and herding behaviors of dogs were selected from predatory sequences.[39]

The most effective way to prevent a dog from engaging in predatory behavior is to not allow the dog to run loose. Livestock killing is often performed by dogs that have homes and are allowed to roam. An individual dog may not be motivated to hunt livestock, but when in the company of other dogs will engage in the chase. Unfortunately, humans (particularly children) can also elicit predatory behavior from a pack of dogs. Individually, dogs may be relatively unaggressive and afraid of people, but as a pack they are capable of killing a human being.[40]

If used consistently, strong punishment, such as electric shock, at the onset of chasing behavior may be effective in preventing hunting behavior. Although the treatment of meat with an emetic to induce vomiting after eating may suppress an appetite for specific foods,[41] this approach may not be effective in suppressing chasing and killing behaviors.[42] None of these aversive procedures is as effective as confinement.

Pathophysiologic Aggressive Disorders. Differentiating pathophysiologic disorders from normal behavior is important. In general, the history of a pathophysiologically based disorder is not consistent with descriptions of a normal aggressive behavior. The presence of other abnormal neurologic and physiologic parameters supports a diagnosis of an abnormal aggressive behavior.

Aggressive behaviors have occasionally been correlated with neurologic impairment. Unprovoked, aggressive attacks on family members in a household have been reported to be correlated with cardiac disease and cerebral and hippocampal neuronal degeneration.[43] Dextro- and levo-amphetamine (0.1 to 0.6 mg/lb orally) have been reported to suppress aggressive behaviors.[20] One dog extensively handled while behaving amicably under the influence of amphetamine remained unaggressive when the drug therapy was discontinued.[20]

Psychomotor epilepsy is another possible etiology of aberrant aggressive behavior. The aggressive behavior may occur spontaneously or be elicited by excitement or by specific stimuli such as noise or food.[43a] The aggression may be directed toward a person, the animal itself, or an object. The diagnosis of epilepsy can be tentatively supported by an abnormal electroencephalogram, presence of other abnormal neurologic signs, cessation of the behavior when the animal is treated with antiepileptic medication, or precipitation of the behavior when treated with phenothiazines or other epileptogenic drugs.

Unpredictable aggressive attacks have been reported as a syndrome in Bernese mountain dogs,[44] English cocker spaniels,[45] springer spaniels, and St. Bernards. To date, no pathophysiologic findings have been reported associated with these behaviors in these breeds. The histories available concerning such dogs closely resemble dominance-related aggression patterns. The aggressive behavior is generally directed toward family members and is precipitated by petting or by ordering the animal to do something. Dogs genetically predisposed to being extremely aggressive can be equally dangerous whether the aggression is a normal aggressive pattern or a pathophysiologically based disorder.

Neurologic disorders stemming from conditions such as infection, trauma, and infestations of parasites can cause abnormal behaviors, including aggression. The resultant behavior may be caused by irritative neuronal lesions or ablative lesions. Generally, ablative neural lesions must be bilateral in order to produce any effect on behavior.

COMMON BEHAVIOR PROBLEMS IN CATS

Eliminatory behaviors are the most common problems of cats presented to behavior therapists. The cause of the behavior may be disease, anxiety, urine marking, or simply a preference for eliminating on surfaces other than the litter provided or in locations other than where the owner wishes the cat to eliminate.[46]

Spraying Problems

Spraying, a urine marking behavior, is performed in a standing position. The cat's tail is erect and urine is voided backwards, usually onto a vertical object. Spraying is more likely to occur in intact cats than in neutered ones and males are more likely to spray than females. It is estimated, however, that spraying is a behavior of ten per cent of castrated males, regardless of the age at which they are neutered and is a behavior of five per cent of neutered females.[17]

Androgens facilitate spraying. Castration is effective in suppressing spraying in 90 per cent of cats neutered for that behavior.[48] Anabolic steroids, often used to treat older and debilitated cats, may evoke spraying behavior. Withdrawal of such drugs coincides with the cessation of spraying. Incompletely ovariectomized female cats may exhibit estrous behavior and may spray. These cats should have cornified vaginal epithelial cells and respond to a complete ovariectomy.[49]

Environmental stimuli play a significant role in eliciting spraying behavior. If eliciting stimuli, such as the sight of another cat or foreign objects brought into the house, can be identified, steps can be taken to prohibit the cat's access to these stimuli. Antagonistic encounters among cats in the household may elicit spraying. Solving this problem or reducing the number of cats in the household may resolve or decrease the spraying behavior.

Occasionally, changing the significance of the spraying site inhibits spraying. Placing food, water, toys, or bedding material in the location the cat sprays may stop spraying. If spraying occurs only in a few locations, prohibiting the cat access to or repelling the cat from those areas may suffice. Commercial pet repellents are available in many grocery stores or pet shops. The citrus odor found in the rinds of oranges or lemons or a citrus room deodorizer stick also may act as a repellent.

Diazepam (Valium) at 1 to 3 mg/orally/BID, dramatically reduces spraying behavior.[50] In a series of 24 cats treated with diazepam, 43 per cent stopped spraying completely and 75 per cent either stopped or reduced spraying by 75 per cent of the initial frequency. Cats may be slightly ataxic for a few days and then accommodate this side effect. Cats experience a temporary increase in appetite and may retain some impairment of perception, which is most noticeable when the cat jumps onto a raised surface.

The efficacy of megestrol acetate (Ovaban) and medroxyprogesterone acetate (Depo-Provera) in suppressing spraying in cats has been estimated at 30 per cent;[51] these drugs are more likely to cause serious side effects than diazepam.

Regardless of the drug used to suppress spraying, it is wise to take a cat off medication periodically to determine if the environmental factors that facilitated the spraying behavior are still present.

Olfactory tractotomies have been reported to suppress spraying and urine marking in approximately 50 per cent of cats that did not respond to neutering or progestin therapy.[52]

Urination and Defecation Problems

Urination and defecation are performed in squatting postures for the purpose of eliminating body waste. These behaviors are usually preceded by scratching in the dirt and followed by covering up the urine or excrement after elimination. Such scratching behavior usually does not accompany urine marking.

Aversive Box Area. A cat may avoid using a litter box for any number of reasons: the box is used by other cats, it is an undesirable shape, it is not cleaned frequently, it contains an aversive litter, it has a substance incorporated in the litter that is aversive, or the cat repeatedly experiences an aversive event there, such as being caught to be medicated, played with by rambunctious children, or startled by a noisy washing machine or dryer. The most common reason for a cat to stop using a litter box is that the box is not cleaned frequently enough.

Obviously once an instigating cause has been discovered, steps must be taken to remedy the situation. Sometimes this is sufficient but, in the interim, the cat frequently develops a new location or surface preference and these factors must also be dealt with.

Location Preference. If the cat is eliminating in a specific spot because it seems to prefer that location to the litter box, the owner has several options. The cat may be discouraged from eliminating in that location by cleaning the area well with a product that neutralizes or counteracts the urine and fecal odors. Compounds containing ammonia should be avoided because they may attract the cat to these areas. If necessary, the owner can cover the area with aluminum foil or simply prohibit access to the room where the cat has been eliminating. Pet repellents or citrus odors may keep the cat from walking to that area. The significance of the location can be changed from an elimination site to a feeding station, play area, or resting spot by placing appropriate items in that area. Obviously, the owner must address problems with the litter or litter box simultaneously with the application of these techniques.

Substrate Preference. Some cats appear to develop preferences for specific substrates, such as carpet or linoleum. In the case of a carpet preference, all of the areas in which the cat eliminates should be cleaned well, allowed to dry, then covered with another substrate that the cat does not find attractive. Heavy plastic, such as that used to cover windows, is usually effective. A roll of plastic can be put around the perimeter of a room, along a carpeted hallway or, if necessary, on the entire floor of a room. Plastic allows the owner and cat to walk in this area and use the room but usually inhibits the cat from scratching, which is the first part of the elimination behavior sequence. After the cat has resumed the use of the litter box, the plastic can be taken up slowly over a period of months. It should first be removed from the area in which the cat is least likely to eliminate. If the cat prefers to eliminate in tubs and sinks, a small amount of water can be put in these receptacles. Tile and linoleum can be covered with newspaper or an inexpensive rug.

Altering the surfaces where a cat is eliminating will not always result in the cat using a litter box it has been avoiding. The litter box and its material also must be examined and experiments conducted to determine what type of litter or shape of box the cat will use. Usually a cat that does not use a litter box has both a location and a surface preference, and both factors must be manipulated.

A persistent location preference may be treated by putting the litter box in that location and gradually moving it over a period of weeks to the location the owner prefers.

Aggressive Behavior Problems

Intraspecific. Aggression between intact cats of the same sex is often reduced by neutering the animals. Sometimes, however, aggression between cats in a household involves neutered animals. Aggression of sudden onset between two cats in the household in which both cats appear frightened, that is, they assume defensive postures (ears back, body arched, dilated pupils, piloerection), is *fear-induced or defensive aggression*. This can occur between cats of either sex and of any age. Such cats do not seek each other out, but when they see each other both immediately assume defensive postures. Often the initiating cause leading to the aggression is a frightening event such as a loud noise or an incident of redirected aggression. This type of aggressive behavior among cats is usually readily treatable using desensitization, counterconditioning, or flooding procedures.

Territorial aggression is manifested by one cat in the household persistently seeking out and relentlessly attacking another. The aggression may be of sudden or gradual onset. It often develops slowly among cats that have lived together for several years when one or both reach approximately 18 months of age. In the author's experience, this is not a highly treatable behavior problem, and it is usually recommended that owners find one of these cats a home without another cat. A cat that is aggressive to other cats is not necessarily aggressive to people and can usually be an excellent pet in a household where it is the only cat.

Aggression Toward People. Not infrequently, cats direct aggression toward people. *Play-induced aggression* is usually exhibited by young cats that are the only cat in a household. The behavior may be directed toward one or more persons, but it is often limited to attacks on the cat's "favorite person." The behavior of the cat includes predatory-like behaviors (stalking, hiding, and rapid attacks). Although the bites hurt, they are usually inhibited and are not severe unless the person's skin is fragile.

This is a readily treatable problem. The owners need to initiate active play with the cat several times a day, and if necessary, redirect the aggressive attacks before they are completed. For example, if the owners know that the cat attacks before descending the stairs, when they walk down the steps, they can throw a toy that the cat will run after rather than attack the owners. Punishment is also appropriate as one of the methods for halting playful aggression. A startling noise such as a foghorn or a compressed air siren is usually effective. The device should be carried around constantly for several days so that whenever the cat begins an attack the noise can be sounded. To be effective, the punishment must be administered immediately and consistently. If used correctly, a punishment need only be used two or three times. However, owners should not be advised to punish the cat for any playful aggressive behavior. The owners must also allow the cat sufficient exercise and allow the cat to play in acceptable ways. An excellent approach to solving a playful aggression problem is to get another cat of the same age for the problem cat to play with.

A serious form of aggression that is directed toward owners is *redirected aggression*. The bites are not inhibited and are often quite severe. When a cat is aroused, such as by another cat or a frightening event, it may become defensively aggressive and remain so for several hours. If the owner approaches the cat or tries to pick it up, the owner may be attacked. This type of aggression is often presented as a sudden, unprovoked aggressive behavior, but a detailed history reveals an arousing stimulus that brought the cat into the defensive state. If the eliciting stimuli can be identified and the owners cautioned not to reach for or pick up the aroused cat, many owners are able to live safely with their cats without suffering recurring attacks.[53]

Occasionally, cats are aggressive toward people because they are *afraid* of people in general or specific individuals. These cats assume defensive aggressive postures and show signs indicative of fear. Desensitization and counterconditioning are successful ways of treating this problem. Occasionally, cats exhibit *territorial aggression* toward strangers. The author does not know of an effective means of treating this particular type of problem. If a cat is known to be territorially aggressive to strangers, the owners' only recourse is to keep the cat away from visitors. Any time cats become aggressive out of character, CNS diseases, such as those caused by toxins, cerebral infarcts, or rabies, should be considered.[54–56]

Excessive Vocalization and Overactivity

Excessive restlessness, pacing, and vocalization in a cat should always prompt a physical examination and consideration of cystitis and, particularly if the cat is old, hyperthyroidism. Cats also pace and vocalize unrelated to disease states. Sometimes this may be to engage the owner in social interactions or to be fed. In these latter cases, extinction should be implemented, that is, the cat should not be rewarded by playing with or feeding it. The owners can also try to decrease the cat's motivation to engage in those behaviors by playing with it more during the day, feeding the cat a high-protein meal just before going to bed, and/or punishing the cat for these behaviors. For example, if the cat insists on rattling the bedroom door to get in, the owner could contrive a punishment that can immediately be implemented, such as a vacuum cleaner placed at the crack in the door with the air exhaust going out.

Ingestive Behavior Problems

It is a peculiarity of some Siamese and Siamese-crosses to eat wool and cloth materials. There is no reliably effective treatment procedure for this problem.

Excessive Grooming

Dermatologic conditions should always be the first consideration when cats engage in behaviors resulting in hair loss. However, when cats are in conflict or anxiety-provoking situations they may groom excessively. Prolonged conflict may lead to self-mutilation. Grooming is a common displacement activity in many species of animals. Displacement activities are behaviors exhibited by animals in a conflict situation.[57] Displacement activities have nothing to do directly with the conflict situations, but are irrelevant behaviors such as grooming.

In these cases, situations that can be identified as inducing conflict or anxiety should be addressed and dealt with. Antianxiety medication such as amitriptyline hydrochloride (Elavil) 5 to 10 mg orally SID, diazepam (Valium) 1 to 2 mg orally BID, or chlorpheniramine maleate 2 to 4 mg orally BID, may be helpful for excessive grooming. Megestrol acetate and medroxyprogesterone are also anxiety-reducing drugs.

Destructive Behavior

"Claw-sharpening," a normal feline species-typical behavior, serves to remove old sheaths from the claws as well as to leave a visual mark. Ideally the cat's scratching behavior should be redirected to objects that are acceptable to the owner, e.g., bark or scratching posts. The owner may have to experiment to find what the cat likes to scratch. Most cats that are allowed to spend some time outdoors do not engage in excessive scratching behavior in the house. Whenever the cat is caught scratching, the owner could punish it by startling it with a loud noise or a squirt of water. This should at least reduce the incidence of scratching when the owner is present.

Declawing is another option. There is no evidence that indicates that declawing is psychologically harmful to cats. Declawed cats continue to engage in scratching behaviors and do not appear to be distressed or "frustrated" while doing so. Declawed cats do not become more aggressive or bite more than cats that have their claws.[58]

References

1. Voith, VL and Borchelt, PL (eds): Vet Clin North Am 12:4, 1982.

2. Voith, VL and Borchelt, PL: History taking and interviewing. Comp Contin Educ Pract Vet 7(5):432, 1985.
3. Rimm, DC and Masters, JC: Behavioral Therapy. Academic Press, New York, 1975.
4. Stead, A: Euthanasia in the cat and dog. Report to Br Sm Anim Vet Assoc, 1979.
5. Arkow, P: The humane society and the human-companion animal bond: Reflections on the broken bond. Vet Clin North Am 15(2):455, 1985.
6. Mayes, A: The physiology of fear and anxiety. *In* Sluckin, W (ed): Fear in Animals and Man. Van Nostrand Reinhold Co, New York, 1979, p 24.
7. Ratner, SC: Animals' defenses: Fighting in predator-prey relations. *In* Pliner, P, et al. (eds): Advances in the Study of Communication and Affect: II. Nonverbal Communication of Aggression. Plenum, New York, 1976.
8. Russell, PA: Fear-evoking stimuli. *In* Sluckin, W (ed): Fear in Animals and Man. Van Nostrand Reinhold Co, New York, 1979.
9. Voith, VL and Borchelt, PL: Fears and Phobias in Companion Animals. Comp Contin Educ Pract Vet 7(3):209, 1985.
10. Schenkel, R: Ausdrucks-studien an wolfen. Behaviour 1,2:81-129, 1947.
11. Schenkel, R: Submission: Its features and functions in the wolf and dog. Am Zool 7:319, 1967.
12. Leyhausen, P: Cat Behavior. STPM Press, New York, 1979.
13. Fox, MW: Behaviours of wolves, dogs, and related canids. Harper and Row, New York, 1971.
13a. Davis, LE: General care of the patient. *In* Davis, LE (ed): Handbook of Small Animal Therapeutics. Churchill Livingstone, New York, 1985, p. 17.
14. Voith, VL, and Borchelt, PL: Separation anxiety in dogs. Comp Cont Educ Vet Pract 7(1):42, 1985.
15. Collias, NE: An ecological and functional classification of animal sounds. *In* Lanyon, WE and Tavolga, WN (eds). Animal Sounds and Communication, Am Inst Biol Sci, Washington, DC, 1960, p 368.
16. Harrington, FH: Aggressive howling in wolves. Anim Behav 35(1):7, 1987.
17. Hopkins, SG, et al.: Castration of adult male dogs: effects on roaming, aggression, urine marking, and mounting. JAVMA 168:1108, 1976.
18. Beach, FA: Effects of gonadal hormones on urinary behavior in dogs. Physiol Behav 12:1005, 1974.
19. Voith, VL: Animal behavior: Submissive urination. Methods III, (4):5, 1980.
20. Corson, SA, et al.: Animal Models of Violence and Hyperkinesis. Interaction of Psychopharmacologic and Psychosocial Therapy in Behavior Modification. *In* Suban, G and Kling, A (eds): Animal Models in Human Psychology. Plenum Press, New York, 1976.
21. Corson, S A, et al.: Interaction of genetics and separation in canine hyperkinesis and in differential responses to amphetamine. Pavlov J Biol Sci 15:5. 1980.
22. Ginsburg, BE, et al.: Genetic variation in drug responses in hybrid dogs: a possible model for the hyperkinetic syndrome. Behav Genet 6:107, 1976.
23. Bareggi, SR, et al.: Paradoxical effects of amphetamine in an endogenous model of the hyperkinetic syndrome in a hybrid dog: Correlation with amphetamine and p-hydroxyamphetamine blood levels. Psychopharmacology 62:217, 1979.
24. Stowe, CM, et al.: Amphetamine poisoning in dogs. JAVMA 168:504,1976.
24a. Graver, GF, and Hjelle, JJ: Household drugs. *In* Morgan, RV (ed): Handbook of Small Animal Practice, Churchill Livingstone, New York, 1988.
25. Borchelt, PL and Voith, VL: Aggressive behavior in dogs and cats. Comp Contin Educ Pract Vet 7(11):949, 1985.
26. Borchelt, PL: Aggressive behavior of dogs kept as companion animals: classification and influence of sex, reproductive status and breed. Applied Animal Ethology, 10:45, 1983.
27. Line, S and Voith, VL: Dominance aggression of dogs towards people: Behavior profile and response to treatment. Appl Anim Behav Sci 16:77, 1986.
28. Mech, LD: Productivity, mortality, and population trends of wolves in northeastern Minnesota. J Mammal 58:559-574, 1977.
29. Redding, RW and Walker, TL: Electroconvulsive therapy to control aggression in dogs. Med Vet Pract 57:595, 1976.
30. Evans, JM: Current thoughts concerning hypersexuality in dogs, with particular reference to the role of progestins. Proc Refresher Course for Veterinarians No. 37, Post-Graduate Committee in Veterinary Science. University Press, Sydney, 1978.
31. Voith, VL: Intermale aggression in dogs. Modern Veterinary Practice, 1980.
32. Andersson, B, and Olsson, K: Effects of bilateral amygdaloid lesions in nervous dogs. J Sm Anim Pract 6:301, 1965.
33. Paegt: Behaviour Troubles: Behaviour Speciality Meeting, Pre-Congress, 11th World Congress W.S.A.V.A., Paris, 1986.
34. Mattes, JA: Psychopharmacology of temper outbursts: A review. J Nervous Metab Dis 174:464–470, 1986.
35. Voith, VL: Proposed functional significance of pseudocyesis. Am Assoc Zoo Pract, 1977.
36. Voith, VL: Effects of castration on mating behavior. Mod Vet Pract 60:1041, 1979.
37. Allen, WE: Pseudopregnancy in the bitch: the current view on etiology and treatment. J Sm Anim Pract 27:419, 1986.
38. Anon: A Glaxorat guide to ovarian function. Glaxo, England, 1984, p 17.
39. Coppinger, R, et al.: Degree of behavioural neoteny differentiates canine polymorphs. Ethology, 75:89, 1987.
40. Borchelt, PL, et al.: Attacks by packs of dogs involving predation of human beings. Public Health Reports, 98:57, 1983.
41. Garcia, J, et al.: Conditioning food illness aversions in wild animals: Caveant Canonical. *In* Davis, H, Hurwitz, HMB (eds): Operant-Pavlovian Interactions. Lawrence Erlbaum, Hillsdale, NJ, 1977.
42. Lehner, PN and Horn, SW: Research on forms of conditioned avoidance in coyotes. Appetite, 6:265, 1985.
43. Meierhenry, EF and Liu, S: Atrioventricular bundle degeneration associated with sudden death in the dog. JAVMA 172:1418, 1978.
43a. Voith, VL: Behavioural problems. *In* Chandler E.A., et al. (eds): Canine Medicine and Therapeutics, 2nd ed. Blackwell Scientific Publications, Oxford, 1984.
44. Van der Velden, NA, et al.: An abnormal behavioral trait in Bernese Mountain Dogs (Berner Sennenhund). Tijdschr Diergeneesk 101(8), 1976.
45. Mugford, RA: Aggressive behavior in the English cocker spaniel. Vet Annual 24:310, 1984.
46. Borchelt, PL and Voith, VL: Elimination behavior and problems in cats. Comp Cont Edu Vet Pract 8, 1986.
47. Hart, BL and Cooper, L: Factors relating to urine spraying and fighting in prepubertally gonadectomized cats. JAVMA, 184(10):1255, 1984.
48. Hart, BL and Barrett, RE: Effects of castration on fighting, roaming, and urine spraying in adult male cats. JAVMA, 163:290,j1973.
49. Stein, BS: Feline reproductive dysfunction. Am Assoc Feline Pract Meeting, Barbados, 1986.
50. Marder, AR and Voith, VL: Effectiveness of diazepam for the treatment of spraying in cats, paper presented at Animal Behavior Society Meeting, Raleigh, NC, 1985.
51. Hart, BL: Objectionable urine spraying and urine marking in cats: evaluating progestin treatment in gonadectomized males and females. JAVMA, 177:529, 1980.
52. Hart, BL: Olfactory tractotomy for control of objectionable urine spraying and urine marking in cats. JAVMA, 179:231, 1981.
53. Chapman, B and Voith, VL: Sudden aggressive behavior of cats directed toward owners. Submitted to JAVMA
54. DeLahunta, A: Veterinary Neuroanatomy and Clinical Neurology, 2nd ed. WB Saunders, Philadelphia, 1983, p 144.
55. Shepard, DE, and deLahunta, A: Central Nervous System Disease in the Cat. Comp Cont Edu Vet Pract 2:306, 1980.
56. Burridge, WJ: Wildlife rabies in the United States. Aviary Exotic Practice, 1(1):17, 1984.
57. Eible-eiblesfelt: Ethology, the Biology of Behavior.
58. Borchelt, PL and Voith, VL: Aggressive behavior in cats. Comp Cont Ed Pract Vet, 9:49, 1987.

44 HUMAN-ANIMAL BOND AND EUTHANASIA—A SPECIAL PROBLEM

MICHAEL J. McCULLOCH,
JAMES M. HARRIS, and
WILLIAM F. McCULLOCH

It has long been known that companion animals play an important role in the lives of individuals and families, but only in recent decades have scientific efforts been made to understand and describe the complex nature of the human-animal bond.[1–4] Veterinarians are linked to companion animals and their owners in a complex triangular relationship.

By virtue of the complicated nature of the bond between people and their pets, veterinarians are concerned with matters that ultimately have the potential to directly affect the owner's health.[5] The utmost sensitivity and understanding of the strength of the attachment that people have with their pets is required, so that deleterious advice is not given.[6]

To appreciate the level of the veterinarian's involvement in human health matters, it is essential to understand what is currently known about the human-animal bond, especially concerning patterns of pet ownership, dynamics of the pet-owner relationship, motives for keeping pets, functions pets serve, and the nature of the physical interaction with pets. The ways animals are currently being used in the treatment of human health problems (animal-facilitated therapy) are explored and the various roles that the veterinarian can fulfill are examined.

PET OWNERSHIP

Pet ownership is widespread in the United States. Fifty-four per cent of all households have dogs and/or cats; 28.4 per cent of American households have cats and 42.5 per cent have dogs. There are 55.7 million dogs and 52.2 million cats.[7]

Owner Attitudes. Cat owner attitudes were classified into three groups.[8] Low-involvement owners comprise 59 per cent. They chose cats because of the minimal attention required to care for them. For these owners, the cat's company is not valued and there is little emotional attachment. A second category consists of quality/status-conscious owners, comprising 21 per cent. They take pride in their cat's appearance and are especially conscious of pedigrees. These animals are generally very well cared for. High-involvement owners represent 20 per cent of the total of all cat owners. The primary difference between this group and the status-conscious group is that love fulfillment needs take high priority.

Five common attitudes of dog owners were noted in the study: companionship (27 per cent), enthusiastic (27 per cent), worried (24 per cent), valued object (19 per cent), and dissatisfied (19 per cent). The companionship and enthusiastic groups both report important psychological benefits from their dogs and consider them members of the family. The small difference between the companionship and enthusiastic owners is the degree to which they include the animals in all family activities. Worried owners are very concerned over the liability of their pet and are especially concerned about physical harm to others or property damage. Virtually no companionship need is fulfilled. Valued object owners maintain their animals primarily for their aesthetic value but have some psychological commitment to them. The dissatisfied owners view their animal as a nuisance and are overtly unhappy with the presence of the dog in the household. These categories are not fixed and owners may shift from one category to another over the course of animal ownership. The dissatisfied owner struggling with the problems of housebreaking a pet may later shift to an enthusiastic category as the pet matures. Although more than 40 per cent of owners report important psychological benefits from pet ownership, an equal number report being dissatisfied or worried.

It is especially troubling to note the large number of

dissatisfied owners when an estimated 13 to 18 million dogs and cats are euthanized in this country each year.[9] It has been suggested that a significant percentage is being euthanized because of behavior problems that may be treatable. A study in the United Kingdom indicated that 17 per cent of all dog euthanasia is performed for behavior problems.[10] The etiology of these behavior problems is a major problem of public health importance.

It is estimated that practicing veterinarians participate in over 55 million pet visits per year. Office surveys have indicated that approximately 1.7 people accompany each pet, making nearly 100 million human contacts by the profession each year. If only a small percentage of these involve clients who are emotionally upset or struggling with a very difficult decision regarding care of their pet, the potential consequences of the veterinarian's acts are significant.[11]

THE PET'S ROLE IN SOCIETY

No single explanation accounts for the extent of pet ownership. Motives for owning pets and functions pets serve vary by age and interest. Noncritical acceptance by pets is believed to improve the self-image of many owners. Play, attachment and love, and emotional security have also been described.[12, 13] Pets frequently play the role of child substitute or substitute for other human relationships, although it is currently believed that relationships with animals are unique and should not be considered just an analogue of human relationships.[14] Seven functions of companion animals have been listed and are summarized in Table 44–1.

The influence of pets on child development has been discussed in literature that reflects primarily anecdotal material.[15–19] It is believed that pets can provide a "dress rehearsal" for later life. This includes the opportunity to learn a sense of responsibility by daily feeding, grooming, and care and to become aware of the life cycle. Since the life cycle of the pet is frequently completed while a child is growing up, it is important to recognize that the developing child has differing capacities to understand these events at different ages. The relationship with the pet can be used as a learning opportunity, contingent upon the parents' willingness to encourage questions and to assist the child in working through problems that may occur with the pet. What the parents expect from the pet and the child is exceedingly important, as this can represent a point at which serious animal behavior problems can develop and lead to dissatisfaction and eventual removal of the pet. Studies have established that there are developmental tasks of adult life that must be mastered, just as there are tasks of childhood and adolescence.[20] It is not known, however, whether positive interactions with pets in any way signal the capacity for completion of adult maturational stages.

TABLE 44–1. FUNCTIONS OF COMPANION ANIMALS

Function	Suitable Animals
Companionship	Any responsive animal (cats, dogs, birds)
Something to care for	Any animal
Something to touch	Any furry animal or caged bird
Something to keep one busy	Any animal or group of animals that require routine daily care
Focus of attention	Any active animal
Exercise	Dog of any size
Safety	Dog

From Katcher, A and Friedman, E: Potential health value of pet ownership. Comp Cont Ed Pract Vet 2(2):117, 1980.

Allergy to animal dander is a common human health problem, although its actual incidence is not known.[21] It is also believed that cat dander may be more allergenic than dog dander. The intensity of attachment between families and pets has not been appreciated by human allergists, since 32 per cent stated they would recommend removal of the pet without skin tests.[22] It has been suspected that noncompliance with allergists' recommendations is high. In one study, 73 per cent of families stated they would not remove pets, even with a positive skin test.[23]

It has been known that persons who are widowed, divorced, or single have a higher age-specific death rate than those who are married.[24] Holmes and others[25] have described the impact of life change on physical and emotional health. It has been observed that persons undergoing a large degree of life change may rely more heavily on pets for social support and are more vulnerable to the loss of pets. This may be expressed as a fear for the pet's safety and well-being.

A recent study of survival following discharge from a coronary care unit revealed that out of 92 subjects, 78 survived after one year. Eleven of the 39 non-pet owners died, whereas only three of 53 pet owners died. These findings appear to be independent of age, physiologic severity, and type of pet. It is suggested that differences in the personalities of pet-owning persons may be the factor determining survival and not the mere presence of the pets; however, this requires further study.[26]

A study of 31 pet owners suffering from a medical illness and depression examined the perceived impact of illness on their lives, their support system, and the perceived influence of pets on their lives and their ability to cope with illness.[27] Most of those interviewed enjoyed an adequate support system in the form of significant family relationships; two were living alone. When true/false questionnaires were administered, an interesting discrimination developed when it was determined if the subject was his/her pet's "closest companion" (Table 44–2).

Even for the 52 per cent of patients who reported that the pet belonged to someone else in the household, the perceived benefits were still quite high, such as promoting humor and play, and helping to cope with loneliness and isolation. The role of humor as a healing force has been eloquently described by Norman Cousins.[28]

The social facilitating role of pets has been a subject of considerable interest. Previous reports suggest that pet owners like people less than do non-pet owners and are less healthy psychologically.[29, 30] More recent data indicate the opposite. In a Swedish study it was found that 63 per cent of dog owners believed that their dog helped initiate opportunities to interact with people.[31]

TABLE 44–2. EMOTIONAL SUPPORT PROVIDED BY PETS

Influence of Pet	Patient Has Primary Bond with Pet	Other Has Primary Bond with Pet	Average %
1. Pets have been an important part of my life.	93	81	87
2. Pet was important source of companionship during illness.	87	56	71
3. Pet made me feel needed.	80	56	68
4. Felt more secure with pet around.	80	63	71
5. Pet distracted me from worrying about problems.	80	50	65
6. Pet improved my morale.	73	56	65
7. Pet's affection greatly appreciated.	93	88	94
8. Pet's playfulness improved my spirits.	80	69	74
9. Pet helped me cope with isolation and loneliness.	87	81	84
10. Pet helped me to laugh and maintain a sense of humor.	100	88	94
11. Pet's needs stimulated me to be more physically active.	93	38	68

From McCullough, M: The pet as prosthesis—defining criteria for the adjunctive use of companion animals in treatment of medically ill, depressed outpatients. In Fogle, B (ed): Interrelations Between People and Pets. Springfield Il, Charles C Thomas, 1981.

Brown concluded that people's affection for others varied as a function of their affection for dogs and stated that "Man's emotional involvement with others is mirrored in his reported emotional involvement with dogs."[32] Lee concluded that pet owners who interacted frequently with their pets had significantly higher desire for affiliations with others than did non–pet owners and went on to state that "this disproves the view that dogs substitute for human relationships to the point of exclusion and supports the view that pets may be owned by persons who are unable to satisfy affiliative needs."[33]

Basic physiologic effects of people's interactions with pets are being studied and are providing valuable insights into the nature of the human-animal bond. It is known that stroking an animal lowers its pulse and blood pressure. Conversely, greeting an animal with words and stroking also has the effect of lowering the person's blood pressure. The character of touch between people and their pets has also been explored. It revealed a broad range of physical contact, from rough play to gentle caressing, but significantly, there was no difference in the frequency or kind of contact among owners of dogs of different sizes, nor was there any difference in the frequency, amount, and kind of touching by men and women.[14] This finding appears to refute the notion that men are by nature less affectionate and less expressive tactually than women. Idle play, distracted petting, and fondling are other activities that have been observed and frequently associated with a person's being in a very relaxed state. The data accumulated strongly imply that the relationship between people and pets is unique and not simply analogous to relationships with other human beings.[34]

ANIMAL-FACILITATED THERAPY

The term "animal-facilitated therapy" refers to the use of companion animals as therapeutic agents in the treatment of various human problems. Its history dates back as far as 1792, when patients at the York Retreat, an asylum for the mentally ill, were encouraged to care for rabbits, poultry, and other small animals. In 1867, in Bielefeld, Germany, Bethel was founded along similar lines; this facility has more recently included horses.[35] Unfortunately, no systematic study of the use of animals in these settings has ever been undertaken. Levinson was the first psychotherapist to document the way in which pets could greatly hasten the development of rapport and increase patient motivation.[16] Others have reinforced this notion.[36] Corson[37–40] attempted to employ programs of pet-facilitated therapy systematically in a psychiatric ward at Ohio State University and also at a nursing home. In both places the effect was to increase the interest and participation of many previously withdrawn and uncommunicative patients. Bietostolen, in Norway, was established in 1966 to rehabilitate handicapped persons and uses dogs and horses as adjunctive therapy to the intense program of physical therapy.[41] David Lee, a psychiatric social worker, has established a unique pet therapy program at the State Hospital for the criminally insane in Lima, Ohio.[42] Here, after a trial period, inmates are permitted to have caged birds or rodents on an incentive system and must make certain sacrifices in order to maintain their animals. This novel approach decreased the violence in the institution, increased the participation of staff with patients, and increased patient cooperation with therapy. Unfortunately, no quantitative data have been gathered from this unique program. Other animal-facilitated therapy programs include guide dogs for the blind and hearing dogs for the deaf. Hearing dogs are currently achieving the same legal status as seeing eye dogs in many states. Therapeutic horseback riding programs for the handicapped are widespread in America and Europe and are greatly assisting therapy efforts of those who suffer from physical handicaps. Many smaller community programs are currently being established to use the known data and to develop animal-facilitated therapy programs tailored to their community needs.[33] Developing placement criteria for pets is an essential element in any program.[43] Recent studies have also emphasized the need to develop scientific criteria to guide clinicians in the use of prescription pets to treat emotional problems.[27]

The actual benefits and/or problems of animal-facilitated therapy have not been subjected to adequate scientific study. How benefit is mediated is also unclear. It is possible that in institutional settings the presence of animals may improve the morale of staff and thereby act as a catalyst to more staff involvement with patients. The ultimate effect may have the highly desirable outcome of creating a more humane treatment environment in nursing homes, prisons, mental hospitals, halfway houses, and elderly persons' homes.

VETERINARIANS' INVOLVEMENT

The inherent nature of the human-animal bond causes the veterinarian to be drawn into matters that affect human health and emotional well-being.[44, 45]

MAKING BONDS

Traditionally, clients arrive at the veterinarian's office having already obtained a companion animal. Whether the animal is well-established or a new addition, there is an opportunity to provide information to the client. This effort at educating clients is one of the veterinary profession's primary tasks. If the visit is an initial pediatric service, the practitioner can assist the family by providing appropriate information on husbandry, nutrition, training, and health care. Building and reinforcing this on subsequent visits hopefully assists in forming a long-term, satisfying bond between the family unit and the companion animal.

Very often clients choose animals with little thought or preparation. The selection may be made on impulse or as a well-meaning act of rescue of a stray. These bonds may last, but are often broken, resulting in the animals being turned in to shelters for placement or euthanasia or simply being abandoned. Adult size, temperament, behavior problems, change in life style, medical conditions, and animal care requirements are but a few of the reasons for failure to maintain the bond.

The veterinarian is in a unique position to facilitate successful human-animal bonds. Ideally, the place to start with clients is prior to the acquisition of the animal. Veterinarians need to provide their time to clients to counsel them on the selection process. This time is well spent, appreciated by clients, and further increases the chances for a successful long-term human-animal (and veterinarian) relationship. Areas that should be covered at this time include type of animal, breed, size, temperament, care requirements, previous experiences of the family, special family medical problems, special animal problems such as genetic diseases and life expectancy of the animal, and alternative choices. Clients are often unaware that the animal in the magazine ad will grow to weigh 150 pounds, has an abbreviated life expectancy, has a tendency to bond with only one family member, needs a long exercise period daily, has special nutritional requirements, is nocturnal, and/or has special housing needs. The American Veterinary Medical Association's "Pet Selection Brochure" would certainly be a useful aid at this time and could be provided to the client prior to the consultation visit. A carefully prepared client questionnaire providing information on the family is an invaluable aid to the veterinarian at this consultation. More and more clients are requesting preplacement counseling and as a profession veterinarians should promote and encourage this service.

MAINTAINING BONDS

Once established, the veterinary practitioner can play a vital role in maintaining a high-quality relationship between client and animal and helping to realize the fullest promise in human-animal interactions. Veterinarians are qualified professionals, providing information on companion animals, defining problems, and facilitating decision-making on the part of our clients. A good "bedside manner" is paramount for success. The art of listening is essential. "Big ears, eye contact, and a small mouth" are appropriate. Clients almost always verbalize their perceptions of the status of the patient and problems if encouraged to talk and discuss the issues at hand. A comfortable, pleasant, nonhostile setting aids this process. When appropriate, records should be tagged to alert staff to potential physical danger and/or aberrant behavior on the part of both client and patient. The veterinarian must constantly strive to maintain good communication with clients, making the process as easy as possible for all involved. Well-trained support staff, both receptionists and assistants, as well as adequate records, promote a high level of communication and trust in a veterinarian's service on the part of the clients. Pets are sometimes used as a "ticket of admission."[23, 46] The owner wants to talk to the veterinarian about matters that may be quite unrelated to the health of the pet. For example, an anxious woman brings in her cat for the third visit in two months. The animal has been completely well at each examination. During the course of each visit the client discusses her difficult family situation and requests advice.

Because of veterinarians' professional stature and rapport with clientele, they are viewed as counselors also. Indeed, many pet owners see their veterinarian more frequently than their family doctor. It is essential to note that many clients' emotional problems are entirely coincidental to pet ownership but are very apparent to the practitioner. These can include anxiety, depression, senile changes, and even psychotic disturbances. Interventions here must be very limited unless there are responsible family members or friends whose help can be enlisted. Relatively few referrals are made to mental health professionals, partly to avoid offending clients. Veterinarians are placed in a difficult position when asked to render counsel on matters for which they have had no specialized training and when the request may be for marriage counseling, psychotherapy, or personal financial advice. This requires tactful limit-setting and redirection, for example, "I appreciate your sharing this with me, but I haven't really been trained to handle these concerns."

It is essential to establish limits as early as possible, or clients come to expect additional time from the veterinarian for matters quite unrelated to their animal's health. Having office staff members that are sensitive to and aware of behavioral problems in clients can be of great assistance in alerting the veterinarian to potential problems. Staff can frequently observe clients in the waiting room and make valuable observations regarding the pet-owner interaction and the client's emotional state. For example, "Mrs. Jones is here with Fifi again and is complaining to us about how lonely she has been since her husband died last year. She's crying and probably just wants to talk. You had better plan to spend a little more time with her today. It would probably be a good idea to let her son know that she has come in again."

Increasingly, evidence has shown that health professions and the public are becoming more aware of the nature of attachments between people and pets. Legal pressures are mounting to change the "animal as chattel" laws and to permit clients to recover damages for mental anguish in veterinary malpractice litigation.[47] The increased sophistication of the public will lead to increased expectations of all health professions.

BREAKING BONDS

Terminal illness and death require the greatest sensitivity from veterinarians and their staff. As an example, an elderly couple bring a terminally ill pet terrier that is being treated for a malignancy to the veterinary clinic. The wife is upset and very tearful. Her husband tries to console her, but in the end they request that everything possible be done to extend the pet's life.

The veterinarian is faced with numerous client emotional problems in daily practice, but none as frequent as involvement in discussions involving euthanasia of pets. The practitioner is usually the only member of the human health team to interact with a client and family at this difficult time and his or her contribution can be crucial.[48, 49] A study was done to determine the frequency of euthanasias performed in clinical practice.[50] Ten practices were analyzed over a four-week period. The total number of inpatient and outpatient contacts was tabulated and the number of euthanasias performed and alternatives to euthanasia discussed was recorded. One hundred forty euthanasias were performed out of 7917 patient contacts, for an average of 1.8 per cent. The range was 0.3 per cent to 4.1 per cent in the practices sampled. Thus, the practitioner can expect to perform approximately one euthanasia for every fifty patients seen. An additional 1.2 per cent of patient contacts involved discussion of euthanasia and alternatives where euthanasia was not performed. The veterinarian can therefore expect to encounter opportunities for discussing euthanasia and euthanasia alternatives in three per cent of patient contacts.

Clients may react in a wide variety of ways to the news of a pet's terminal condition or death, from acceptance to acute grief.[51, 52] Grief is a normal psychological and physiologic reaction to loss and should be encouraged as a healthy expression of loss.[53] Recommendations for obtaining another pet should be undertaken with great caution, as the grieving process requires at least four to eight weeks and frequently as long as a year.[54] Fifteen per cent of former pet owners say they will not obtain another pet because they cannot bear to go through another loss.[8]

The various roles that the veterinarian can play include identification of high risk factors in the pet owner, such as a history of difficulty with loss and a recent, superimposed loss in an elderly person. Additional roles include facilitating decisions for clinical management, including euthanasia. Dispensing information and educating and counseling at the time of loss are important functions for the veterinarian to perform. Comforting pet owners in their time of need remains essential, for as previously emphasized, the veterinarian is often the only health professional who interacts with a person during this difficult time. Giving clients permission to express grief or upset openly is important, for many are embarrassed by the intensity of their feelings.[23, 54]

Another example is a family of four—mother, father, 14-year-old son, and 10-year-old daughter. They enter the veterinarian's office with their beagle, which has just been struck by a car. Following assessment, the nature and cost of treatment are discussed. The dog has been the boy's pet for eight years, but it is also greatly loved by the 10-year-old sister. Father says that euthanasia is necessary because of cost. Mother breaks down and cries.

Problems like this can occur with multiple-owner pets. Because cost is a significant factor in the treatment of pets, the veterinarian must tactfully determine who has the emotional attachment and who makes the decisions. Marked variations in emotional attachment and attitudes toward pets among family members make this task very challenging. In this case, the veterinarian asked to speak to the boy alone and was impressed with the boy's deep concern for his pet. After discussing the necessary treatment, the boy indicated his willingness to do odd jobs to help pay for treatment. The veterinarian then asked to speak with the parents alone and explained how attached their son was to the dog and outlined the boy's offer to do additional chores to pay half the cost. The father hesitated, but then agreed; the mother appeared very relieved. By separating family members, one can frequently mediate and facilitate difficult treatment decisions in an effective manner. In other cases, when just one family member brings the animal to the clinic, it is not clear whether other family members have been consulted, especially if the request is for euthanasia. The veterinarian in these instances can be an unwitting accomplice, because one can never be certain what the pet owner tells the remaining family members about the practitioner's recommendations. It is not unusual for the practitioner to be asked to fabricate a clinical reason for euthanasia for the benefit of those family members not present. Whenever there is a question about the attitudes and feelings of absent family members, it is perfectly appropriate to ask if they have been consulted or to refuse a request such as euthanasia if there is doubt.

EUTHANASIA— A SPECIAL PROBLEM

As mentioned earlier, three per cent of patient contacts involve euthanasia. A follow-up study in one of the practices revealed that 76 per cent of all animal loss was from euthanasia.[55] The act of taking life must never be taken lightly and "convenience euthanasia" must be discouraged, but when there is intractable pain or poor quality of life for the animal, a decision to euthanize on the part of the client is appropriate.

Every effort must be made to make this process as comfortable as possible for all involved. As with any predictable death, some preparatory efforts on the part of the practitioner will be of invaluable aid to the family. In the case of euthanasia service, the moment can also be determined. Discussions of euthanasia should include, in addition to the appropriateness of the decision, the options that are available to the client. The time, place, presence or absence of the family, special requests, disposition of the remains, and exploring the possible need for a service or ritual, should all be included in the list of decisions that the family needs to consider and discuss. Decisions on these matters are not only of value to the family, but are of great use to the veterinarian in arranging the euthanasia procedure.

Grief and bereavement counseling has indeed come of age in the field of companion animal medicine. In recent years a number of excellent guides have been published.[56, 57]

CONCLUSION

It is increasingly apparent that veterinary medicine shares considerable common ground with psychiatry, psychology, and the social sciences. Because of this, the profession faces many challenges. Among them are (1) understanding the psychology of pet ownership, including a basic knowledge of child and adult development, of the ways in which people cope with loss, and of the uniqueness of relationships between people and pets (i.e., that they are not simply a distortion of human relationships), (2) awareness of the many facets of animal-facilitated therapy and the opportunities for involvement of veterinarians, (3) willingness to adjust undergraduate and postgraduate education to reflect new knowledge about the human-animal bond, and (4) recognition that veterinarians play an integral part in maintaining and promoting human health through their interaction with people and their companion animals. In this capacity veterinarians perform many important services, including counseling, mediation, facilitation of difficult decisions, limit-setting, and above all, comforting in time of need.

As a member of the human health care team, the veterinarian is guided by the maxim that all health professions share: "Cure when possible, but comfort always."

References

1. Fox, M: Pet-owner Relations. *In* Anderson, RS (ed): Pet Animals and Society. Bailliere Tindall, London 1975, p 37.
2. Heiman, M: Man and His Pet. *In* Knight, JA, and Slovenko, R (eds): Motivation in Play, Games and Sports. Springfield IL, Charles C Thomas, 1967, p 329.
3. Leigh, D: The Psychology of the Pet Owner. J Sm Anim Pract 7:517, 1966.
4. Levinson, B: Interpersonal Relationships Between Pet and Human Being. *In* Fox, MW (ed): Abnormal Behavior in Animals. Philadelphia, WB Saunders, 1968.
5. McCulloch, M: Contributions to Mental Health. *In* Anderson, RK, et al. (eds): A Description of the Responsibilities of Veterinarians as They Relate Directly to Human Health. Report for the Bureau of Health Manpower, Dept HEW, US Govt contract #231-76-0202, 1976.
6. Antelyes, J: The troubled pet-owner visits the veterinarian. VM SAC 64:38, 1978.
7. Charles, Charles and Associates: The Veterinary Services Market Study. Prepared for AVMA, July 1983.
8. Wilbur, R: Pet ownership and animal control, social and psychological attitudes. Report to the national conference on dog and cat control, Denver, 1976.
9. Beck, A: The public health implications of urban dogs. Am J Pub Health 65:1315, 1975.
10. Stead, A: Euthanasia in the cat and dog. Report to Br Sm Anim Vet Assn, 1979.
11. McCulloch, M: The pet-owner relationship—dealing with the difficult client. Paper presented to the AVMA. Anaheim, CA, July, 1975.
12. Mugford, R: Basis of the normal and abnormal pet/owner bond. Proceedings of group for the study of human/companion animal bond. Dundee, Scotland, University of Dundee, March, 1979.
13. Mugford, R: The Social Significance of Pet Ownership. *In* Copera, SA (ed): Ethology and Non-verbal Communication in Mental Health, London, Pergamon Press, 1979.
14. Katcher, A: Interactions Between People and their Pets—Form and Function. *In* Fogle, B (ed): Interrelations Between People and Pets. Springfield, IL, Charles C Thomas, 1981.
15. Condoret, A: Pour une biologie du comportement de l'enfant: Sa relation a l'animal familier. Bul Acad Vet de France 50:481, 1977.
16. Levinson, B: Pet-oriented Child Psychotherapy. Springfield, IL, Charles C Thomas, 1969.
17. Levinson, B: Pets and Human Development. Springfield, IL, Charles C Thomas, 1972.
18. MacDonald, A: Review: children and companion animals. Child Care Health Dev 5:347, 1979.
19. Van Leeuwen, J: A Child Psychiatrist's Perspective on Children and their Companion Animals. *In* Fogle, B (ed): Interrelations between People and Pets. Springfield, IL, Charles C Thomas, 1981.
20. Vaillant, G, et al.: Natural history of male psychological health: IX. Empirical evidence for Erikson's model of the life cycle. Am J Psychiatry 137:1348, 1980.
21. Ohman, J: Allergy in man caused by exposure to mammals. JAVMA 172:1403, 1978.
22. Baker, E: A veterinarian looks at the animal allergy problem. Ann Allergy 43:214, 1976.
23. McCulloch, M: Educational programme methods for teaching pet-owner relationships to health care professionals. Proceedings of the group for study of the human companion animal bond. University of Dundee, Dundee, Scotland, March, 1979.
24. Lynch, J: The Broken Heart: The Medical Consequences of Loneliness. New York, Basic Books, 1977.
25. Holmes, T, et al.: The social readjustment rating scale. J Psychosom Res 11:312, 1967.
26. Friedmann, E and Katcher, A: Animal companions and one-year survival of patients after discharge from a coronary care unit. Pub Health Rep 95(4):307, 1980.
27. McCulloch, M: The Pet as Prosthesis—Defining Criteria for the Adjunctive Use of Companion Animals in the Treatment of Medically Ill, Depressed Outpatients. *In* Fogle, B (ed): Interrelations Between People and Pets. Springfield, IL, Charles C Thomas, 1981.
28. Cousins, N: Anatomy of an Illness As Perceived by the Patient: Reflections of Healing and Regeneration. New York, WW Norton and Co, 1979.
29. Cameron, P, et al.: Pet ownership and sex as determinations of stated affect towards others and estimated others' regard of self. Psychol Rep 19:884, 1966.
30. Cameron, P, et al.: Psychological correlates of pet ownership. Psychol Rep 30:286, 1972.
31. Bath, M: Is the dog needed? A study of the dog's social importance to man. Unpublished thesis, School of Social Studies, University of Gothenburg, Gothenburg, Sweden, 1976.

32. Brown, L, et al.: Affection for people as a function of affection for dogs. Psychol Rep 31:957, 1972.
33. Lee, R: The pet dog: interactive correlates of a man-animal relationship. Prog Rep, Dept of Psychology, University of Hull, 1976.
34. Katcher, A and Friedmann, E: Potential health value of pet ownership. Comp Cont Ed Pract Vet 2(2):117, 1980.
35. Bustad, LK: The veterinarian and animal facilitated therapy. LaCroix lecture. In Proceedings of Am Anim Hosp Assn, 47th Annual Meeting, 1980, p 269.
36. Siegal, A: Reaching the severely withdrawn through pet therapy. Am J Psychiatry 118:550, 1962.
37. Corson, S, et al.: Pet-facilitated Psychotherapy. *In* Anderson, RS (ed): Pet Animals and Society. London, Bailliere Tindall, 1975, p 19.
38. Corson, S, et al.: The Socialising Role of Pet Animals in Nursing Homes: An Experiment in Non-verbal Communication Therapy. *In* Society, Stress and Disease: Aging and Old Age. Oxford University Press, 1977.
39. Corson, S, et al.: Pet dogs as nonverbal communication links in hospital psychiatry. Compr Psychiatry 18:61, 1977.
40. Corson, S, et al.: Pets as Mediators of Therapy in Custodial Institutions for the Aged. *In* Masserman, JD (ed): Current Psychiatric Therapies 18, New York, 1979.
41. Bustad, LK: The Contribution of Companion Animals to Human Well-being. *In* Animals, Aging, and the Aged. University of Minnesota, 1980, p 116.
42. Lee, D: Hi Ya., Beautiful. Documentary film on pet therapy at Lima State Hosp, The Latham Foundation, Alameda, CA, 1978.
43. Bustad, LK: Profiling animals for therapy. West Vet 17(1):2, 1979.
44. Levinson, B: The veterinarian and mental hygiene. Mental Hygiene, July, 1965, p 40.
45. Proceedings of the group for the study of the human companion animal bond. Univ of Dundee, Dundee, Scotland, March, 1979.
46. McCullough, M: The Veterinarian in the Human Health Care System: Issues and Boundaries. *In* McCullough, L and Morris, J (eds): Implications of History and Ethics to Medicine—Veterinary and Human. College Station, TX, Texas A & M University, 1978.
47. Morris, W, et al.: Damages for mental anguish in veterinary malpractice litigation. Comp Cont Ed Pract Vet 2(7):579, 1980.
48. Hopkins, A: Ethical Implications in Issues and Decisions in Companion Animal Medicine. *In* McCullough, L and Morris, J (eds): Implications of History and Ethics to Medicine— Veterinary and Human. College Station, TX, Texas A & M University, 1978.
49. Speck, R: Mental health problems involving the family, the pet, and veterinarian. JAVMA 145:2, 1964.
50. McCullough, M and Bustad, LK: Incidence of Euthanasia and Euthanasia Alternatives in Veterinary Practice. *In* Katcher, A and Beck, A (eds): New Perspectives on our Lives with Companion Animals. Philadelphia, University of Pennsylvania, 1983, p 366.
51. Brodey, R: The pet animal with cancer. JAVMA 162:403, 1973.
52. Edney, A: Management of euthanasia in small animal practice. JAAHA 15(5):645, 1979.
53. Lindemann, E: Symptomatology and management of acute grief. Am J Psychiatry 101(2):141, 1944.
54. Katcher, A and Rosenburg, M: Euthanasia and management of the client's grief. Comp Cont Ed Pract Vet 1(12):887, 1979.
55. Harris, JM: A Study of Client Grief Responses to Death or Loss in a Companion Animal Veterinary Practice. *In* Katcher, A and Beck, A (eds): New Perspectives on our Lives with Companion Animals. Philadelphia, University of Pennsylvania, 1983, p 370.
56. Nieburg, H and Fischer, A: Pet Loss: A Thoughtful Guide for Adults and Children. New York, Harper & Row, 1982.
57. Rosenberg, MA: Companion Animal Loss and Pet Owner Grief. Viewpoints in Veterinary Medicine, Alpo Pet Center, Allentown, PA, 1986.

45 DISEASES OF THE EAR

DENNIS W. MACY

In 1633, published reports indicate otitis ranked only behind rabies in importance in diseases of the dog.[1] Diseases of the ear are still extremely common in small animal clinical practice. They are the primary complaint in 8 per cent of all cases presented in small animal clinics and are found to exist in 18 to 20 per cent of all canine patients admitted for other conditions.[2–5] The prevalence of ear disease in the cat is significantly lower and is observed in only 2 to 6.6 per cent of hospitalized patients.[4]

Historical Information of Importance

Historical information can be especially beneficial in the diagnosis and management of ear disease. The breed of dog or cat can be important in interpreting the likelihood of a particular etiology when certain breed-related alopecias of the pinnae are observed. Breed and coat color are often helpful in assessing the likelihood of congenital deafness and vestibular disease or of neoplasia of the pinnae.

The animal with ear disease frequently shakes its head and scratches at or near the ears. Determining the duration of ear disease is sometimes helpful in that dogs with acute otitis externa due to infections more frequently have gram-positive infections, while dogs with chronic otitis externa usually have gram-negative infections.

Discharges may vary in odor and consistency, depending on the etiology and stage of the disease. A history of stumbling, rolling, or head tilt is often helpful in localizing the extension of the disease from the external ear canal to the inner ear. Medical histories of hypothyroidism or hyperadrenocorticism may suggest a reason for recurrent bacterial otitis externa. Histories of skin disease or clinical signs associated with skin disease, such as scratching or chewing at the flank, are especially important since many animals with integumentary disease such as atopy, endocrinopathies, or immune-mediated diseases have some component that will be exhibited in a portion of the ear.

Questions regarding the animal's environmental husbandry are important when considering etiologies such as fly strike, frostbite, or ear mites. A history of systemic or topical drug use is also valuable since drug reactions may be confused with other etiologies of ear disease.

Physical Examination

A good general physical examination is a mandatory basic component of a thorough examination of the ear. It should start with observation of the animal's movements in the examination room, head carriage, eye movements, and evidence of circling.

The symmetry of the eyes should be examined to rule out the presence of Horner's syndrome associated with disruption of the sympathetic nerve that passes between the tympanic bulla and the petrous temporal bone. The presence of nystagmus and head tilt indicates eighth cranial nerve involvement. The direction of the head tilt and the fast and slow component of the nystagmus should be noted because they are helpful in localizing the lesion.

The oral cavity should be examined for the presence of inflammation or swelling. Cats with upper respiratory viral diseases may develop secondary otitis media. Ear polyps are the most common growth found in the ear canals of cats; they frequently grow down the eustachian tubes into the oral pharynx, causing dysphagia and even dyspnea. Infections of the middle ear may result in various neurological abnormalities, especially those associated with the facial and sympathetic nerves. Clinicians should examine the external nares for excessive crusting and the eye for keratoconjunctivitis sicca, both of which may be the result of interruption of the parasympathetic component of the facial nerve caused by inflammation in or around the middle ear.

The patient's general skin condition should be evaluated for clinical signs associated with hyperadrenocorticism, hypothyroidism, seborrhea, atopy, and parasitic infestation, as these conditions frequently become symptomatic when they involve the ear. Three lymph nodes drain the ear: retropharyngeal, submandibular, and prescapular. These should be evaluated in all ear disease patients.

THE PINNAE

ANATOMIC CONSIDERATIONS

The ear can be divided into four parts: auricle or pinna, external auditory meatus, middle ear, and internal ear.[6]

The pinna of the external ear is a funnel-like plate of cartilage that receives air vibrations and transmits them via the ear canal to the tympanic membrane (eardrum). The pinnae are highly mobile and can be controlled independently. A total of 19 separate muscles control the movement of the external ear, all of which are innervated by the auriculopalpebral branch of the facial nerve (VII), which departs from the main branch of the facial nerve as it curves forward beneath the ear canal.[6] Animals with facial nerve paralysis have abnormal carriage of the pinna.

The shape of the pinna is characteristic of the breed, but may be abnormally large or small in animals with multiple genetic defects.[7]

The erect pinna is generally assumed to be standard for description purposes. The convex surface of the erect ear faces medially and slightly caudally and the concave surface faces laterally and slightly rostrally.

Macroscopically, the external ear is composed of three elastic cartilages: the annular, the scutiform, and the auricular. The annular cartilage is a portion of the horizontal canal and conjoins the osseous meatus of the temporal bone and the auricular cartilage. The annular cartilage is not usually involved in surgery of the external ear. The scutiform cartilage is boot-shaped and lies medial to the auricular cartilage, adjoining its convex surface; it is within the auricular muscles and assists in the attachment of the auricular cartilage to the head.[6] This cartilage is important in correcting ear carriage but not in reconstructive procedures.

The auricular cartilage is the largest cartilage of the ear and the most complicated anatomically. It is cone-shaped at its origin at the annular cartilage and flares distally to form the pinna. It is heavily convoluted, which gives it a more intricate appearance. The six important surgical landmarks of the auricular cartilage are the helix, the anthelix, the tragus, the antitragus, the scapha, and the cavum conchae.

The large auricular cartilage has skin on both sides. Generally, the inner surface contains fewer hairs than the outer surface, but the number and distribution of adnexal structures are breed-dependent.[6]

The skin lining the inner surface of the peripheral part of the pinna contains hairs, sebaceous glands, and a few apocrine (tubular) glands.

The principal arteriovenous system of the external ear is the great auricular arborization of the external carotid artery and the internal maxillary vein. The lateral, intermediate, and medial vascular rami course along the convex surface and wrap around the helicine margins; they also directly penetrate the scapha to supply the concave epithelium. The maxillary artery is closely associated with the rostral medial aspect of the ventral canal and it branches from the external carotid artery. It is, therefore, a potential surgical hazard. The vessels on the ear margins in cats may be used to collect small amounts of blood for laboratory evaluation.[8]

EXAMINATION OF THE PINNA

Examination of the ear should start with the pinna. It should be examined for the presence of alopecia, scale, crusts, bullae, and exudates. The ear margin should be checked closely for thickening, erythema, or increased temperature. Plucked hair and skin scrapings from the pinna may be helpful in the diagnosis of dermatophytes or parasitic infestation such as sarcoptic mange. The presence of auricular hematomas on the concave side of the ear almost always indicates inflammation of the external ear canal.

CONGENITAL DEFECTS

Anotia. Anotia (lack of the external ear) is a rare congenital condition and is usually associated with anophthalmia and other severe anatomic deformities. Cats with four pinnae have been described several times in the literature; this is reported to be inherited as a simple recessive trait.[8–10]

Congenital Alopecia of the Pinna. Several hereditary and congenital alopecias have been described in the dog and cat. These conditions may affect other parts of the body as well as the head. The breeds most frequently affected include Chihuahuas, dachshunds, whippets, and Siamese cats.[11, 14] Congenital alopecia of the pinna usually starts around one year of age but because of its insidious onset may not be noticed by the owner until the animal is several years old. The alopecia may be partial or complete. The ease with which hairs may be epilated is considered normal but hairs are fine and short. Lesions may progress to complete pinnal alopecia. The condition does not appear to be associated with underlying disease and is of little consequence to the animal but is frequently of concern to the pet owner. The owner should be informed of the benign nature of the condition.

ACQUIRED DISEASES

The anatomic distribution of acquired pinnal lesions is shown in Figure 45–1.

Marginal Auricular Dermatosis. Marginal seborrhea of the pinna is characterized by numerous small gray plugs adhering to the skin and hairs of the medial and lateral margins of the ear. It is most common in dachshunds, springer spaniels, cocker spaniels, and basset hounds, but also occurs in other breeds with pendulous ears.[3] The small particles can be removed easily with the thumbnail or a flat instrument for diagnosis. Occasionally the particles resemble the nits of lice but are softer, more irregular, and greasy. Histopathologically, these lesions show marked orthokeratotic and parakeratotic hyperkeratosis.[3] In dachshunds, the condition is frequently accompanied by partial alopecia of the pinna. In severe cases, inflammation, necrosis, ulceration, vascular thrombosis, and permanent deformities may occur. This condition must be differentiated from the more pruritic parasitic condition, sarcoptic mange, which fre-

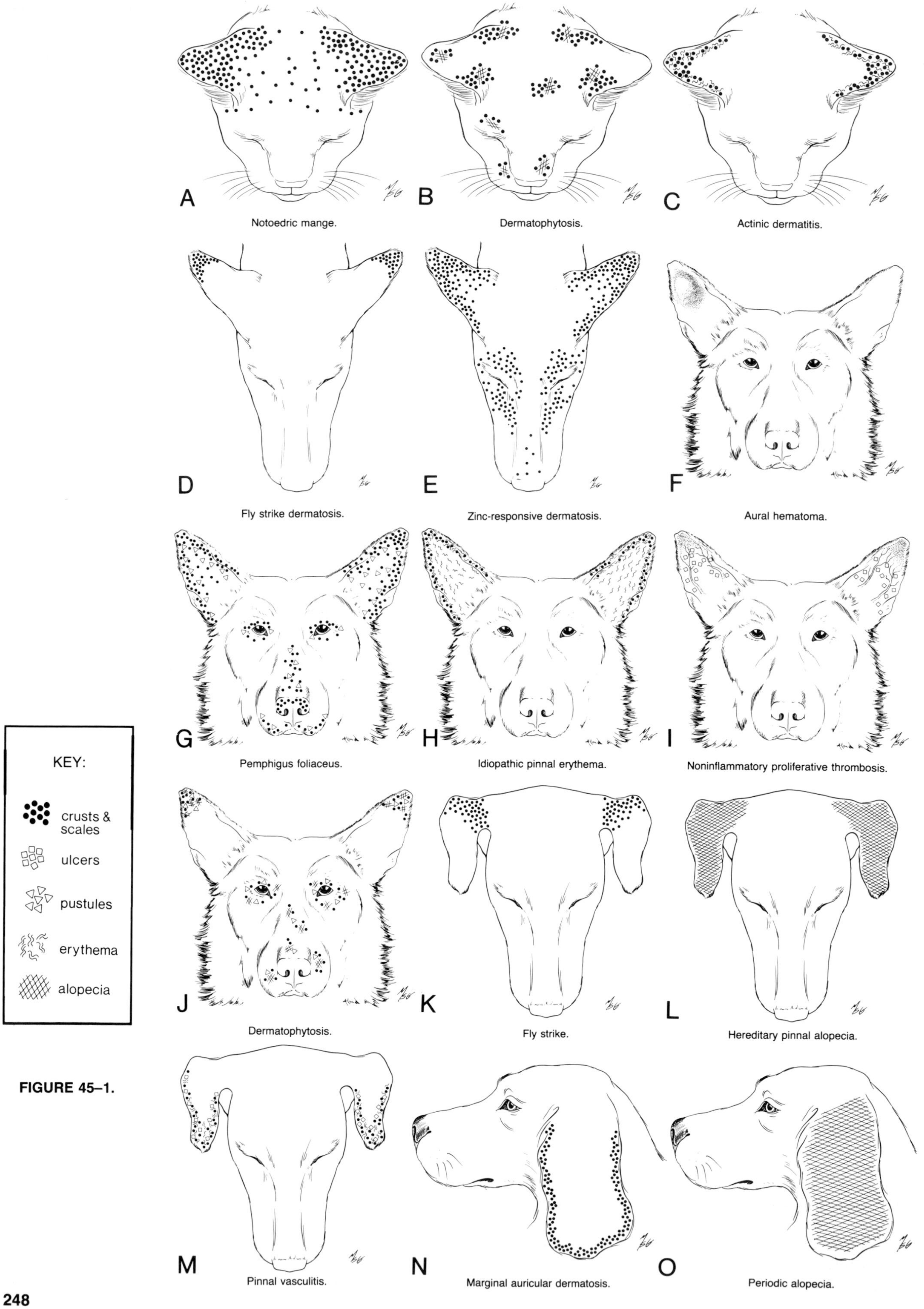
A
Notoedric mange.
B
Dermatophytosis.
C
Actinic dermatitis.
D
Fly strike dermatosis.
E
Zinc-responsive dermatosis.
F
Aural hematoma.
G
Pemphigus foliaceus.
H
Idiopathic pinnal erythema.
I
Noninflammatory proliferative thrombosis.
J
Dermatophytosis.
K
Fly strike.
L
Hereditary pinnal alopecia.
M
Pinnal vasculitis.
N
Marginal auricular dermatosis.
O
Periodic alopecia.
KEY:
crusts & scales
ulcers
pustules
erythema
alopecia

FIGURE 45–1.

quently involves the ear margins. Treatment of ear margin seborrhea consists of removing the accumulation of material and treating the underlying dermatologic condition. Ceruminolytic agents are useful in partially dissolving the cutaneous debris. Ceruminolytic agents should be massaged into the lesions and allowed 10 to 15 minutes of contact time before application of antiseborrheic shampoos. This sequence facilitates more complete removal of the scales. Treatment should be repeated three to four times weekly initially, then as needed.

After the shampooing, an antibiotic steroid preparation may be applied to counteract the inflammation and infection that may be associated with these conditions.

Dermatophytosis. *Microsporum* and *Trichophyton* infections of the pinna are most common in young cats, although it is occasionally seen in dogs. This must be differentiated from solar dermatitis in older white cats. Skin scraping for KOH preparation, Wood's lamp evaluation, and fungal cultures are helpful in making a definitive diagnosis. Although many *M. canis* infections are considered self-limiting by some,[3] the public health considerations and potential for spread to other cats make treatment advisable. Clipping the areas of the lesions and topical application of clotrimazole, cuprimyxin, miconazole, or thiabendazole is indicated. Systemic therapy with either ketoconazole or griseofulvin should also be instituted.[3, 11]

Actinic Dermatitis. Solar dermatitis or actinic dermatitis is a chronic dermatitis of white-eared cats and occasionally, dogs,[3, 12] caused by repeated sun exposure. If left unattended, it may eventually develop into carcinoma in situ or squamous cell carcinoma. Blue-eyed, white cats appear to be the most susceptible. Solar ultraviolet rays in the wavelengths of approximately 300 Å are the most damaging. The condition occurs most frequently in sunny climates such as Florida, California, Hawaii, and Australia, or higher altitudes, such as Colorado. The earliest clinical signs are usually associated with erythema of the ear margins and hair loss. The condition is chronic and worsens each year, developing into nonhealing and crusting lesions. Squamous cell carcinomas of the pinna are usually of low grade but on rare occasions metastasize to regional lymph nodes. Feline solar dermatitis must be differentiated from severe ear mite infestation, fight wounds, frostbite, pemphigus foliaceus, and systemic lupus erythematosus. Treatment consists of keeping cats out of the sunlight between the hours of 10 AM and 4 PM, when ultraviolet light is most damaging. During the summer months the ears may be protected by topical application of a sunscreen that contains PABA. Recently beta carotene and canthaxanthin have been successfully used to treat feline solar dermatitis.[13] Carotinoids are thought to quench the triple state of the signet oxygen and free radicals and to possibly form a lipid-carotene complex in the skin that absorbs the damaging solar radiation.[13] If caught early, lesions may be treated surgically by cosmetic amputation of the ear tips (rounding off of the ear tips), replacing the thinly haired tips with more heavily haired skin. Radical amputation of the ear is usually curative in most cases of even advanced squamous cell carcinoma.[3]

Periodic Alopecia. Periodic alopecia is a noninflammatory condition of the pinna that occurs in mature miniature poodles.[3] The disease is characterized by acute onset of hair loss in one or both pinnae, which usually progresses over a period of one to two months to complete alopecia. Hair starts to return in several months without therapy. Diagnosis must be based on the breed, clinical course, and the ruling out of other diseases such as telogen effluvium or drug reactions.

Fly Strike Dermatitis. Adult male and female stable flies *(Stomoxys calcitrans)* are particularly adapted for attacking the skin of the host and sucking blood. The rasping teeth and blades of the labia tear open the skin. This is highly irritating to the host. The flies usually attack the face or ears of dogs. Multiple bites are commonly found on the tips of the ears or on the folded edge of the skin in dogs whose ears are pendulous, such as collies and shelties. Erythema, hemorrhage, and crusts from oozing blood and serum are typical of the lesions. Affected dogs are always housed outdoors and often confined where they cannot escape fly attacks. Fly repellents or fly sprays are helpful when the dog cannot be removed from the environment. If ulceration is seen, a protective ointment such as zinc oxide or petroleum jelly may be mixed with repellents and applied to lesions to prevent fly attack and provide a mechanical barrier to both flies and irritating sunlight.[11] Commercial products containing corticosteroids should be avoided in cases where there are breaks in the skin surface, since they tend to impede skin epithelialization.[3] The source of the flies should be investigated and straw piles, manure piles, and other likely areas removed or sprayed with insecticides every three weeks to help decrease the fly population.

Frostbite. Frostbite affects the tips of the ears of cats and erect-eared dogs.[3] Other areas of the body that are frequently involved include the tail and scrotum, where the hair covering is sparse and the circulation is poor. Most affected are nonacclimated animals that have been exposed to subzero temperatures for many hours. While frozen, the skin appears pale and is hypostatic and cool to the touch. After thawing there may be a mild erythema, pain, and eventual scaling of the skin. Later the tips and the margins of the pinna may curl. In severe cases, the skin becomes necrotic and sloughs. Healing proceeds slowly. If the tips of the ears are lost, the remaining pinna has a rounded contour that is cosmetically acceptable and often goes unnoticed. The lesion may appear similar to a burn in mild cases. Pinna deformity associated with chronic frostbite must be differentiated from an autosomal dominant condition in cats that is characterized by bilateral inward folding of the pinna.[8, 15, 16]

When presented with cases of possible frostbite, the pinna should be rapidly thawed by gently applying warm water. Tissue at this stage must be handled gently. With mild frostbite resulting in erythema and scaling, a bland protective ointment such as vaseline or cod liver oil ointment should be applied. In severe cases with necrosis, amputation of affected tissue should be performed. Once frozen, tissue may be more susceptible to subsequent damage by the cold. Ear tips that are permanently scarred and alopecic can benefit from a cosmetic partial amputation. The objective of the surgery is to remove the hairless portion and leave remaining pinna well covered with hair for protection from the cold; it is identical to the surgery described for solar dermatitis.[3] Every effort should be made to keep these patients indoors during severe cold snaps to prevent further damage.

Scabies (sarcoptic mange, notoedric mange). Canine and feline scabies are similar. Lesions associated with scabies in both the dog and cat are frequently located at the edge of the pinna as well as at other locations on the body. Scabies is intensely pruritic in both species.[3]

In dogs, rubbing the apex pinnal margins or folding the pinna and rubbing the margins together results in the hind leg scratch reflex. This is sometimes referred to as the "pinnal femoral reflex." Although it is not specific for scabies and can be elicited by conditions such as atopy or food allergies, its absence reduces the probability of scabies.

The life cycle of the *Sarcoptes* mite is 17 to 21 days. The female burrows through the epidermis to lay its eggs. The mites' activity causes the skin to react with acanthosis and hyperkeratosis. The intense pruritus caused by the burrowing of the mite causes a self-inflicted excoriation. Scraping of the ear margins is frequently rewarding in making the diagnosis. A negative scraping does not rule out a *Sarcoptes* infestation, however, and a therapeutic trial with a scabicide is a medically reasonable approach in dogs with crusting or scaling of the ear margins that are intensely pruritic. In contrast to the dog, *Notoedres* mites are usually found in large numbers in skin scrapings from cats.

Treatment should include the ears and the entire animal as well as any other animals living in the same environment. Amitraz (Mitaban), chlordane, lindane dips, or organophosphate dips such as Paramite are effective scabicides in dogs. Because of low toxicity, four weekly lime/sulfur baths provide the best treatment for cats with scabies.[3] Ivermectin has recently been reported as being effective in the treatment of sarcoptic mange in the dog and cat, but it has been reported to be toxic in sight hounds and is not approved for this use in dogs or cats.[17]

Drug Reactions. Drug reactions that result in ear lesions are uncommon, but can occur as the result of either systemic or topical application of medications. This may result from local irritation or Type I, Type II, Type III, or Type IV allergic reactions. Reaction to topical application of medications is most frequently observed. Propylene glycol, five per cent DSS, neomycin, insecticides for ear mites, and topical anesthetics are the most frequently incriminated topical preparations.[11, 18, 19] Reactions to systemically administered erythromycin, trimethoprim sulfa, and other antibiotics have also been observed.[11] In addition to the ears, drug reaction lesions are frequently noted on the head, dorsal spine, and mucocutaneous junctions. Erythema, easily epilated hair, edema, and occasional vesicle or papule formation are the most frequently reported lesions. The diagnosis depends upon confirming an appropriate history of recent drug use and the resolution of lesions after discontinuing the offending drug. Ancillary treatment should include corticosteroid therapy (approximately 0.5 to 1 mg/lb [1 to 2 mg/kg] prednisolone orally for ten days).

Pinna Erythema. There are a number of clinical entities that may present with patchy or diffuse erythema of the pinna. These patients may be intensely pruritic and have bulla or pustules on the concave surface of their ears. Often such ears become very thickened and even warm to the touch. In the later stages of the disease, the lesions start to crust and scale. Diagnostically it is important to determine the extent of involvement of other parts of the body. A complete history of diet, topical or parenteral drug therapy, and the possibility of insect exposure are all important considerations in trying to determine the etiology of pinna erythema. Etiologies for pinna erythema include atopy, food allergy, juvenile cellulitis, dermatomyositis, immune-mediated diseases, or idiopathic pinna erythema.

Idiopathic pinna erythema (IPE) is an acute condition observed in dogs in which there is marked swelling and erythema of both pinnae. Both ears are warm to the touch and intensely pruritic; patients are often very uncomfortable. Dogs with this disease do not have histories of insect bites or dietary allergies or symptoms suggestive of juvenile cellulitis, nor do they have lesions on other parts of the body that suggest an etiology. These patients respond to a five-to-ten-day course of glucocorticoid such as prednisolone. Recurrence is rare. Canine juvenile cellulitis presents with signs and lesions similar to idiopathic pinna erythema, but is usually associated with lymphadenopathy and facial lesions.[20, 21] Food allergies in cats may mimic some of the clinical signs seen with idiopathic pinna erythema in dogs in that erythema is present but is almost always associated with facial lesions secondary to excoriation due to pruritus. If facial edema is present, it must be differentiated from acute Tylenol toxicity in this species.

Pustular and Ulcerative Immune-Mediated Diseases. Immune-mediated diseases in dogs and cats may be accompanied by lesions on the pinna.[11] The lesions are usually characterized by ulcerative erythematous alopecia and crusting vesicles and bullae may be seen. They may be caused by pemphigus foliaceus, pemphigus discoid lupus erythematosus, systemic lupus erythematosus, or bullous pemphigoid diseases. Lesions almost always involve other parts of the body in addition to the pinnae, although cases of pemphigus foliaceus involving only the ears have been reported.[22] The diagnosis depends upon history, lesion morphology, distribution, histopathology, and immunohistopathology and must be differentiated from pyodermas, dermatitis herpetiformis, and subcorneal pustular dermatosis. Treatment is directed at the underlying immune-mediated disease.

Vasculitis. Lesions of the pinna associated with vasculitis, regardless of the etiology, are similar and are characterized by circular or oval lesions.[3] These lesions are initially erythematous but usually progress to a purpuric macule. These eventually develop areas of scarring and sometimes deformity of the pinna. Vasculitis may have multiple etiologies but the underlying mechanism is usually a Type III hypersensitivity reaction. Drug reactions, rickettsial diseases, and systemic lupus erythematosus have all been identified as etiologies of vasculitis, although in most cases the causes are not determined.[3] A cryoglobulin-induced vasculitis is produced by a Type II allergic reaction[20] and has a lesion similar, in terms of distribution, to other forms of vasculitis; it should be considered in animals that have had recent exposure to moderate cold. Vasculitis affecting the pinnae, however, usually exhibits lesions on other parts of the body. Involvement of the lips, tail, tongue, nailbeds, pads, and lower extremities are most frequently reported.[3] Although lesions are histologically characterized by an inflammatory vasculitis and degenerative changes affecting vessel walls, a definitive diagnosis of the underlying etiology depends on good history, serology, and other physical findings. Treatment depends on the specific etiology. In the case of infectious causes, specific antimicrobial therapy, such as tetracycline for rickettsial diseases, is indicated. For immune-mediated diseases, corticosteroids or other immunosuppressive therapy is the treatment of choice.[20]

A noninflammatory vascular disorder that affects the ears in Chihuahuas, terrier crosses, Labrador retrievers, dachshunds, and Rhodesian ridgebacks has been reported.[20] The initial lesion in this disease is characterized by a proliferative disorder of the lumina of the arterioles of the ear, which eventually results in an obstructive thrombosis. The lesions are noted at the apex margins and over the concave surface of the pinna. Although discoloration and necrosis occur in association with the thrombosis like other vasculitides, no inflammation is present in this disorder. Vessels around the lesion may be prominent and the clinical course of this disease is usually slower than that observed with the immune-mediated vasculitides. No medical therapy has been reported to be effective and aggressive surgical removal of the ear has been reported to be the only successful treatment for the disease.

Dermatomyositis. Dermatomyositis may present with alopecia as crusting lesions of the pinna. The disease is seen in Shetland sheepdogs and collies two to four months old and is inherited as an autosomal dominant trait.[23, 24] Lesions usually begin as small erythematous vesicles on the concave surface of the pinna and progress to scaling and crusting. These lesions are associated with lesions on other parts of the body, such as the bridge of the nose, around the eyes, and the distal extremities. This is frequently accompanied by atrophy of the temporal musculature.

Another disease that may present with lesions similar to immune-mediated disease occurs in spaniels.[25] It has been described as a patchy, erythematous plaque lesion, found usually in young springer spaniels. These lesions have a rough, scaly appearance. Histologically they exhibit lichenoid changes in the epithelium; however, lesions are noted on other parts of the body in many cases.

Zinc-Responsive Dermatoses. Zinc-responsive dermatoses may look similar to immune-mediated disease but usually affect other parts of the body. However, affected animals may be presented for pinnal lesions. Lesions on the pinnae are located on the convex surface and are characterized by crusting and minimal alopecia, which may help to differentiate them from other diseases of the pinnae.[26]

Endocrine Abnormalities. Animals with various endocrine abnormalities may be presented with ear disease as the primary complaint. Ovarian imbalance type I and type II, the idiopathic male feminization syndrome, hypothyroidism, Sertoli cell feminization, and acanthosis nigricans are the most frequently encountered conditions.[3, 14, 27] All are usually associated with some degree of hyperpigmentation, lichenification, and alopecia. Lesions are usually not confined to the pinnae and involve other parts of the body.

Neoplasms. Neoplasms of the ear arise from the skin and its adnexal structures. Sebaceous gland adenomas and adenocarcinomas, basal cell carcinomas, mast cell tumors, chondromas, chondrosarcomas, tricoepitheliomas, ceruminous gland adenocarcinomas, and fibrosarcomas have been reported. Squamous cell carcinomas occur less frequently in the dog than in the cat. In general, ear tumors in the dog are more common, but less malignant, than those observed in the cat. Clinical signs are usually associated with those of otitis externa.[3, 28, 29]

Tumors of the auricle can be treated by excision, cryosurgery, or amputation (partial or complete). If the tumor is located on the convex surface of the auricle, wide excision is facilitated by the freely movable skin, allowing primary closure. Tumors located on the concave surface of the pinna are generally treated with cryosurgery due to the adherent skin-cartilage interface. Care must be taken not to damage the cartilage when freezing begins. Tumors close to the helical margin can be treated by partial amputation. Generally, malignant tumors should be handled by wide excision. This may require amputation of the entire pinna in some cases.

Parasites of the Pinna. One parasite of the pinnae is the larval form of the chigger (harvest mite), which is most frequently seen on the concave surface of the ear margins of the cat. These may be difficult to see and may require magnification. *Otobius megnini,* or the spiny ear tick of the dog (and occasionally the cat), is noted at the base of the ear.[3] *Demodex* may cause lesions in the pinna and are usually located on the convex side of the ear.

Auricular (Aural) Hematoma. The etiology of auricular hematomas is unknown. It is thought to be a self-inflicted injury caused by scratching and head shaking; however, many dogs that are known to be aggressive head shakers and ear scratchers never develop the problem. Another possible etiology is an external ear infection, which helps trigger the shaking-scratching cycle; however, there are reports of dogs that present with aural hematomas with no concurrent ear disease. The problem is more common in the pendulous eared breeds than in the erect-eared dogs, but some erect-eared dogs have been reported to develop hematomas. The problem is recognized in both dogs and cats. One author suggests the possibility of an increased vascular fragility, predisposing patients to hematoma formation.[30] Others suggest that autoimmunity may be the underlying etiology.[31]

It is generally agreed that the anatomic location of the hematoma is between the skin and the auricular cartilage on the concave surface of the pinna. Because the skin is so firmly attached to the auricular cartilage on the concave surface, the hematoma actually develops subparachondrally or intrachondrally, not subcutaneously.

Aural hematomas can be treated conservatively or surgically. Some of the conservative methods include aspiration, aspiration and steroid injection, and aspiration and enzyme injection. The fluid is aspirated with a syringe and an 18 to 20 gauge needle, the steroid or enzyme preparation is injected, and the ear taped firmly to the head. The bandage must remain in place for a minimum of two weeks. The advantages of this form of management are that (1) no anesthetics are necessary, (2) it can be done on an outpatient basis, (3) it is relatively quick and easy, and (4) it causes minimal ear disfigurement secondary to scar formation. The disadvantages of this procedure include the facts that (1) clots in the hematoma often cannot exit through the small needle, (2) patient cooperation with the bandaged ear is necessary, (3) owner compliance for bandage care is necessary, and (4) recurrence of the hematoma after bandage removal is frequent.[11]

Approximately 50 per cent of hematomas treated in this fashion recur after the first treatment and about 30 per cent of those treated for a second time recur.[11]

An important part of any treatment regimen, conservative or surgical, includes treating the cause. Ear cleansing and management of otitis, removal of ear canal foreign bodies, or resection of sensitive tumors in the ear canal must be done at the time of management of the aural hematoma.

THE EXTERNAL EAR CANAL

ANATOMIC CONSIDERATIONS

The external ear canal is both cartilaginous and osseous. It extends from the external acoustic orifice to the tympanic membrane. The first part of the canal is formed by the rolled auricular cartilage, which is continued medially by the annular cartilage, a narrow sheet rolled into a tube. The latter partially telescopes into the auricular cartilage. The annular cartilage is attached to the auricular cartilage and to the temporal bone by ligamentous tissue.[6]

The external auditory meatus presents a cutaneous lining that includes stratified squamous epithelium (three to five cells thick), sebaceous and tubular glands, and hair. The sebaceous glands form a superficial glandular bed immediately below the epithelial surface, whereas the tubular apocrine (ceruminous) glands are found in the deeper connective tissue layers. Normal ear wax is made up of secretions from both sebaceous and apocrine glands in addition to desquamating epithelium. In the cartilaginous part of the external auditory meatus, the skin is structurally very similar to that of the pinna, but it becomes progressively thinner as it passes into the bony meatus. Likewise, the lining membrane becomes less glandular and only occasional hairs may be present in the deeper parts of the canal. The normal ear secretion, cerumen, is a product of both types of glands. The vagus nerves provide sensory innervation to the external auditory meatus. Motor supply is via the facial nerve.[6]

The tympanic membrane (eardrum) separates the external ear from the middle ear. It is a thin, semitransparent sheet, oval in shape, and concave when viewed from the external aspect. Its long axis is horizontal. The tympanic membrane is thin centrally and becomes thicker near its periphery. The membrane may be divided into two parts: the pars flaccida and pars tensa. The pars flaccida is a small, triangular portion that lies between the lateral process of the malleus and the margins of the tympanic incisure. The remainder of the membrane is composed of the pars tensa. The external aspect of the tympanic membrane is concave owing to traction on the medial surface by the manubrium of the malleus. A light-colored streak, the stria malleolaris, may be seen running dorsocaudally from the umbo toward the pars flaccida when viewed from the external side. This is caused by the manubrium being partly visible through the tympanic membrane along its attachment.[6]

PATHOPHYSIOLOGY OF OTITIS EXTERNA

The macroscopic changes that take place in the external ear canal are usually the result of inflammatory changes. In long-standing cases of otitis there may be significant hyperplasia of the epidermis and dermis, resulting in constriction of the lumen of the external ear canal, ulceration, and secondary bacterial infection with pyogenic bacteria, yeast, and fungi. Otoscopic examination of the tympanic membrane reveals that it becomes increasingly opaque, assuming a gray to gray-white appearance. Later the pars tensa is a dense gray-white opaque wrinkled membrane, the clefts of which become darker and even black in color. Once the tympanic membrane becomes necrotic, rupture occurs easily. Microscopically, most otitis externa shows hyperplastic changes in the epidermis up to 40 cell layers thick. In almost all cases, numerous aggregates of inflammatory cells are found in the deeper layers of the epithelium and dermis and there is usually some degree of hyperplasia of these tissues. In clinically infected ears, especially those infected with gram-negative bacilli, there is hyperemia and frequently numerous extensive areas of ulceration of the lining epithelium. Fibroplasia of the dermis is also often seen and thus thickening of the subcutaneous tissue can result in total occlusion of the external auditory meatus. An important difference between the tissues of healthy ears and infected ears is the appearance and distribution of the glandular structures along the length of the external ear canal. In the healthy ear, sebaceous glands are usually numerous, large, and actively secreting. In chronic otitis externa, they are less active, much smaller, and appear to be displaced in the superficial dermal layers by the grossly dilated ducts of the apocrine glands. In healthy ears, the thin straight tubular secreting ducts of the apocrine gland are usually difficult to distinguish; in infected ears they appear to be enormous sac-like diverticuli, distended with eosinophilic homogeneous colloidal material. The great increase in size, distribution, and state of activity of apocrine glands, together with inflammatory reaction and possible presence of pyogenic bacteria, accounts for the changes in the appearance of the ear secretions.[32–34]

OTITIS EXTERNA EPIZOOLOGY

History and clinical signs of otitis externa occur more frequently in some breeds than others, due to a number of breed anatomic or physiologic differences. Thus, in the assessment and management of the individual patient, it becomes important to know various breed predilections for ear disease. Miniature poodles, cocker spaniels, and other pendulous-eared breeds account for 80 per cent of reported cases of otitis externa.[4, 35] Although many authors suggest that breed conformation that prevents aeration of the ear canal is responsible for the increased incidence in these dogs,[4] other studies suggest another reason for the high prevalence. The incidence of otitis externa in dogs of the same breed with cropped ears is essentially the same as its incidence in those with noncropped ears. Recent histologic comparisons of ear canal microscopic anatomy of different breeds of dogs indicate differences in the number and distribution of adnexal structures, which may provide a better explanation for the observed breed predilections.[36] Otitis externa is seen in dogs most frequently between five and eight years of age,[37] perhaps reflecting a peak development of co-factors, such as allergic conditions, and keratinization disorders, such as seborrhea, which occur in this species. Cats are not as frequently affected by allergic disease or keratinizing disorders and have a peak incidence of otitis between one and two years of age, 50 per cent of which are directly associated with ear mites.[28] Therefore, the presence of other carnivores in the house becomes an important part of the history for that individual patient. Peak incidence of otitis externa usually occurs in the summer months.[38] In areas where grass awns or foxtails (*Hordeum jubatum*) are prevalent, otitis externa is more prevalent in dry seasons when they are easily dislodged.[39] Moisture is considered a predisposing factor. Factors such as high humidity or swimming increase the moisture content of the stratum corneum, reducing its normal protection. Given enough time, it results in maceration of the epithelium and provides an excellent medium for bacterial or yeast growth.[40, 41] No sex predilection has been described for either species for ear disease. The clinical signs of otitis externa include head shaking and scratching at the periauricular region. The excoriation associated with scratching may result in alopecia, ulceration, and secondary infections in the periauricular region. Exudates of varying types are frequently present and their consistency in color and odor may aid in the diagnosis of ear disease. Animals with acute otitis externa may be head-shy due to pain or swelling and may develop inappetence secondary to fever in rare situations.

THE EXAMINATION

Visual examination of the ear canal begins with noting the presence or absence of exudate and its color and odor. A dark brown, crumbly exudate is characteristic of *Otodectes cyanotes*. A brown, waxy adherent exudate is characteristic of yeast infection, a light brown, creamy exudate suggests staphylococcus or streptococcus infections, and a yellow exudate is usually characteristic of gram-negative infections such as *Proteus, Pseudomonas,* or *E. coli*.[42] A sweet, odoriferous exudate is often noted in dogs with keratinizing disorders such as seborrhea. An otoscopic examination may or may not be possible, depending on the amounts and characteristics of the exudate and the degree to which the ear canal has narrowed secondary to inflammatory response. A cytologic examination of material collected on a swab from the ear canal is the single most valuable procedure in evaluating ear canal disease. The slide is prepared by rolling the swab onto the slide and staining it with a modified Wright's stain. If bacteria are seen, gram stain is indicated. The preparation should be evaluated on both low- (LPF) and high-powered (HPF) magnification for the following:

1. Microorganisms such as bacteria or yeast. Both the type and number per HPF should be noted.
2. Parasites such as *Otodectes*. These are usually seen on low or scanning powers.
3. Cellular components present and their relative numbers. Cellular components such as leukocytes and the amount of keratin provide insight into the type of response the patient has made to the primary disease. The relative numbers of each of these are important since most body orifices have some bacteria or yeast growing in them that can be isolated on culture. Since most bacteria and yeasts are sensitive to standard combination ear preparation, culture and sensitivity testing is only recommended when rod-shaped organisms are seen.[4] These are characteristic of *Proteus* or *Pseudomonas* infections, which are frequently resistant to antimicrobial agents found in standard ear medications.[19]

EXAMINATION OF THE EXTERNAL EAR CANAL

The external ear canal requires special equipment and restraint of the animal for proper examination. The equipment necessary for proper otoscopic examination includes a good otoscope and an appropriately sized specula.

The Otoscope. The light source of an otoscope should be as brilliant as possible without producing excessive heat. A halogen light source is ideal for the veterinary otoscope because of the long ear canal and the need for bright illumination. However, the halogen light source may not be ideal for veterinary ophthalmologic examination because of the reflective nature of the tapetum in domestic animals.[11]

Specula. Cones should be selected in a variety of lengths, diameters, and shapes to accommodate the different species and sizes of patients that are seen in veterinary medicine. Cones designed for human use are unsatisfactory because they are too short for adequate viewing of the tympanic membrane in most dogs. Cones must be long enough and narrow enough to reach within one half inch of the tympanic membrane. Cones should be firmly attached to the otoscope because of the substantial lateral pressure exerted during examination of the canine ear canal. Unfortunately, some otoscopes on the market have cones that are too easily dislodged from the body of the instrument to be practical for veterinary use. Cones may be metal or plastic. The metal are more durable, although they are not tolerated as well as the plastic by the patient because they are cold to the touch. Disposable plastic cones are unsatisfactory because they lack the stability necessary for examining the external ear canal of the dog.[11]

Other Equipment. Serrated alligator forceps are often helpful for removing foreign bodies and debris from the external ear canal during its examination. Curved hemostats are of value in removing hair from the external ear canal and thus facilitating the examination.[11]

Restraint. Examination of the external ear canal also requires proper restraint for the examiner's protection and for proper visualization of the ear canal and tympanic membrane. Physical restraint is relatively easy with long-nosed dogs. Chemical restraint (tranquilizers, general anesthesia) may be required for fractious cats and brachycephalic breeds of dogs. Proper physical restraint in examination of the external ear canal of the dog requires two people. The person restraining the dog should place the fingers of one hand between the rami of the mandible and the thumb on the bridge of the nose (built-in handle) (Figure 45–2*A*, 45–2*B*). The other hand should be placed over the dog's elbow, locking the elbow and forcing the leg against the table (Figure 45–2*C*). The patient can be further restrained by drawing one's elbow toward one's body. The external ear canal may normally contain a small amount of wax that is yellowish-brown in color. Some breeds normally have hair growing in the external ear canal (e.g., wirehair, fox, and Airedale terriers, and poodles). The ear canal should then be straightened out by grabbing the pinna and pulling it up and away from the dog. Next, the otoscope cone should be placed down the vertical portion of the ear canal. While looking in the ear, one should gradually lower the otoscope angle to visualize the horizontal ear canal and tympanic membrane. It should then be rotated slowly so that a panoramic inspection can be made. The tympanic membrane is a thin, glistening membrane that appears gray in color. It may have opaque radiating strands in it. This membrane is frequently ruptured in cases of chronic otitis externa.

CAUSES OF OTITIS EXTERNA

Otitis externa is often considered a multifactorial disease, thus it is important to identify as many of the components as possible before treatment to insure successful managment. Although a clinician may be successful in treating the staphylococcus infection, recurrence is probable if he or she fails to diagnose and treat a predisposing hypothyroid condition.

TREATMENT

Cleaning the Ear Canal. After diagnosis is made, the essential first step in medical management of otitis externa is a thorough cleansing of the ear canal. Topical ear medication may not be effective when applied to an ear full of exudate. Ceruminous material may inactivate some medications in addition to acting as a mechanical barrier to the infected skin surfaces. In mild cases of otitis externa, this may be accomplished by repeated application (two to four times daily) of combination ear medications having ceruminolytic properties as well as antibacterial or antimycotic properties. In such patients most of the exudative material has been dissolved and flushed from the ear canal within two to three days. After this period of intensive drug administration, application of medications may be reduced to once or twice daily for an additional 10 to 14 days.

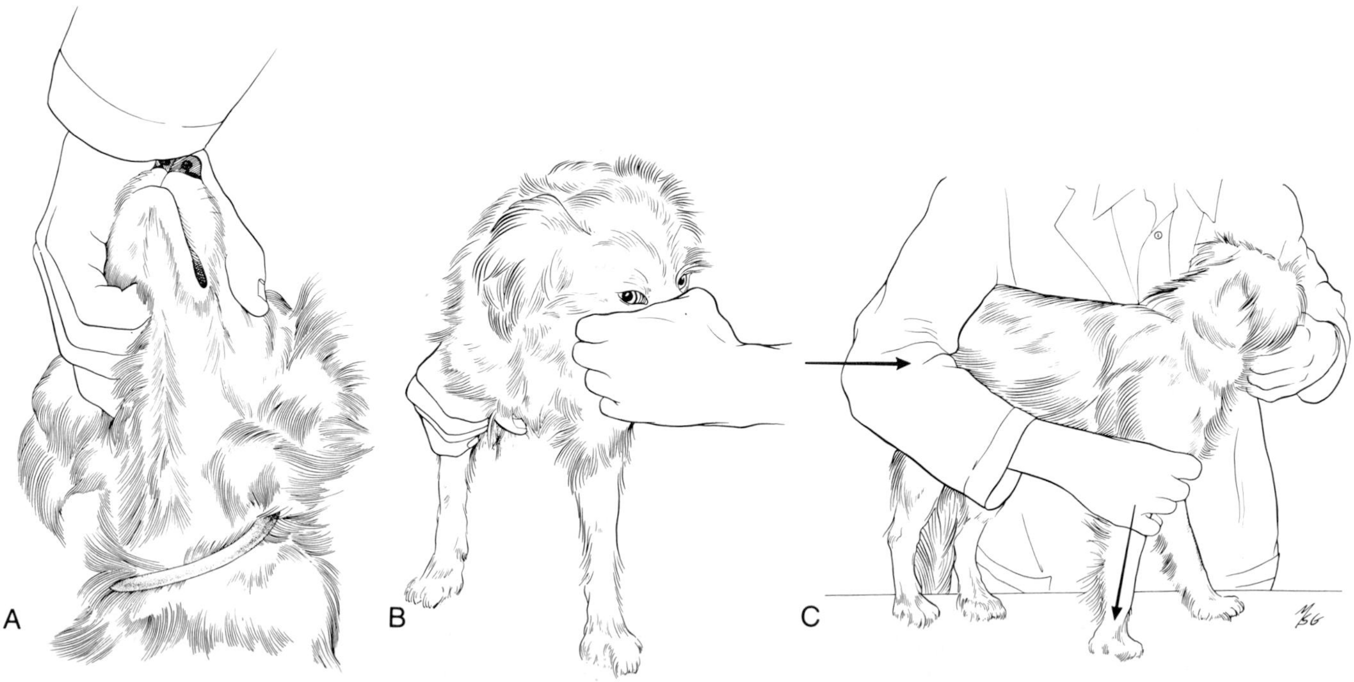

FIGURE 45–2. Physical restraint for external ear examination.

In patients with more severe otitis externa or when owner compliance is questionable, patients should be sedated or placed under general anesthesia for a thorough cleansing. While under general anesthesia, the external ear canal should be examined for the presence of the tympanic membrane. Hair should be plucked or trimmed from the ear canal. Debris is removed by gentle irrigation of the canal with a warm antiseptic solution (0.5 per cent chlorhexidine, 10 per cent betadine solution). A ceruminolytic agent should be applied to ears 10 to 15 minutes before irrigation, depending on the character of the exudative material, to facilitate its removal. A warm sterile saline solution should be used if there is any indication of ruptured tympanic membrane, since chlorhexidine and other flush solutions have been known to cause labyrinthitis.[44] A small catheter, polyethylene tubing, or Water Pik may be used to irrigate the external ear canal effectively. If a Water Pik is used in the procedure, only low pressure irrigation should be used to prevent rupture of the tympanic membrane. Cotton swabs should not be used routinely in cleaning ear canals because they tend to pack material against the tympanic membrane. Swabs are effective in wiping out the external portion of the ear canal and cleaning parts of the convex portion of the pinna. Gentle drying of the ear canal with suction and reexamination of the ear canal with an otoscope is then initiated. If large ulcers are present in the external ear canal, they may be chemically cauterized at this time with a 5 per cent silver nitrate solution or a 5 per cent tannic acid or alcohol solution.[11] If the dog has pendulous ears, the concave aspect of the pinnae may be clipped and/or the ears taped above the head for 7 to 10 days to promote increased air movement in the ear canal. Following proper cleansing and drying of the external ear canal, application of specific antimicrobial and drying agents should be instituted. This is usually done by applying a thin film of medication to the entire ear lining.

Application of Medicants. It is important to instruct the owner in the proper method of application of external medicants. This is done by extending the pinna and introducing the drug applicator into the external ear canal, depositing a small amount of drug and then lightly massaging the external ear canal. The excess medication is then wiped from the opening of the external ear canal with a small cotton swab. Aminoglycosides and oil-based products should not be used in cases of otitis externa when the tympanic membrane has been ruptured.[11]

Medication. Selection of specific ear medication is based on the etiologic agent causing the otitis externa, the status of the eardrum, and the body's response to the disease process. In animals in which the tympanic membrane is ruptured, use of ceruminolytic agents, antiparasitic agents, detergents, disinfectants, and topical aminoglycosides is discouraged because of their potential to produce toxicity.[43, 44] Most topical ear medications are combinations containing one or more of the following general categories of agents: antiparasitic, antibacterial, antimycotic, anti-inflammatory, local anesthetic, ceruminolytic, and drying and cleaning agents.

ANTIPARASITIC AGENTS. Antiparasitic agents contain either pyrethrins, rotenone, thiabendazole, or carbamates as active ingredients and are effective in the treatment of ear mites.

ANTIBACTERIAL AGENTS. Antibacterial agents are usually in the form of antibiotics. Neomycin, polymyxin, gentamicin, and chloramphenicol are most commonly used alone or in combination and are effective against most ear bacterial isolates. Because of their ototoxicity, aminoglycosides should be avoided in patients with ruptured tympanic membranes.

ANTIMYCOTIC AGENTS. Antimycotic ingredients usually include nystatin, thiabendazole, cuprimyxin, or miconazole and are effective against the common ear yeast (*Malassezia*).

ANTI-INFLAMMATORY AGENTS. Anti-inflammatory ingredients include various glucocorticoids, some of which are extremely potent. Glucocorticoids decrease inflammation, ceruminous secretions, swelling, pain, and proliferation seen with ear conditions of many etiologies. Topical corticosteroids can produce iatrogenic Cushing's. Consideration of the potency and duration of therapy is in order when selecting combination preparations containing glucocorticoids.

LOCAL ANESTHETICS. Local anesthetics may be used alone or may be contained within ear preparations. They are effective in aiding the examination of the ear canal, in the removal of foreign bodies, and in combination preparations. Local anesthetic allows for more complete application of topical ear medications. Lidocaine, proparacaine, and tetracaine are most frequently used.

CERUMINOLYTIC AGENTS. Ceruminolytic agents may be used alone or in combination with other ingredients. They act to facilitate the cleaning of the ear canal by acting as surfactants or detergents in emulsifying the waxes. New ceruminolytic carbamide peroxide reacts with the exudate and creates a bubbling action. Docusate sodium solution (DSS), squalene, and dioctyl calcium sulfosuccinate are common active ingredients. These work best if applied 15 minutes before cleaning or two to three times a day.

DRYING AND CLEANING AGENTS. Drying and cleaning agents are used to help prevent maceration of epithelial surfaces that predispose the animal to bacteria or yeast overgrowth. Thus, they are helpful in cases of swimmer's ear and ceruminous otitis. They may be used alone or in combination with other active ingredients. Malic, benzoic, acetic, and salicylic acids are frequently used. Alcohol, aluminum acetate, and dimethyl sulfoxide (DMSO) are also used for this purpose.

GENERAL MEDICATION CONSIDERATIONS. It is important to consider the vehicle or base in which the active ingredients of all topical medications are contained. Oil or ointment bases help moisturize the skin and are effective in dry, scaly, or crusty lesions. Oil bases should be avoided in animals with ruptured eardrums. Solutions or lotions are most frequently used in exudative ear lesions. Pastes or cream bases are difficult to apply and are not suitable for ear application.

Treatment Considerations. The veterinarian should select, based on knowledge of the etiology and the response of the patient to the disease process, the appropriate product or combination product for the disease condition. Systemic therapy may be indicated in addition to topical therapy in certain conditions. Prednisone (1/4 mg/lb for 3 to 5 days) is often indicated when severe inflammation is present. Systemic antibiotics may also be indicated in febrile patients. The oral administration of ketoconazole is indicated for recurrent yeast infection or where owner compliance is doubtful.[11] Therapy of the external ear may be facilitated by plucking or trimming of hair in the ear canal. Buckets and Elizabethan collars may be needed to prevent excoriation while healing is taking place. Eighty-five per cent of all cases of otitis externa of bacterial origin are resolved in 7 to 14 days. A higher percentage may be cured if the clinician takes care to make an accurate diagnosis and prescribe the appropriate treatment. Chronic otitis externa is usually associated with underlying skin conditions such as seborrhea, hypothyroidism, or improperly treated or neglected ear disease. Such chronic cases require more prolonged therapy and in some cases (i.e., idiopathic seborrhea) the treatment may be lifelong. Clinicians should try to identify and treat the underlying problems whenever possible.

TREATMENT OF BACTERIA AND YEAST INFECTIONS

Small numbers of bacteria and yeast can usually be isolated from clinically normal ears. Therefore, cytologic evaluation is important in establishing the relative numbers of these organisms to determine their role, if any, in the ear disease. In one study, 73 per cent of the cases of otitis externa had a significant bacterial component. About half of these were associated with a single pathogen, while others had two or more pathogens. Although gram-positive organisms such as *Staphylococcus intermedius* (both coagulase-positive and coagulase-negative forms) are cultured from normal ears, gram-negative organisms such as *Pseudomonas, Proteus*, and *E. coli* are usually found in diseased ears.[45] Serotyping of gram-negative organisms has traced them to the GI tract of the individual patients. This accounts for speculation that fecal contamination of the ear is the source of the patients' infections.[11] Gram-positive infections are most frequently associated with acute otitis externa.[45, 46] *Staphylococcus intermedius* is the most common isolate and can be found in 30 to 50 per cent of the cases of otitis externa. *Streptococcus* is isolated in only four to nine per cent of the cases of otitis externa in the dog. Gram-negative organisms are rarely isolated from normal ears and are most frequently observed in chronic otitis externa or recurrent ear disease.[47] The most common gram-negative isolates are *Proteus mirabilis*, which is found in 3 to 20 per cent of the cases, *Pseudomonas* sp. in 5 to 34 per cent, and *E. coli* and *Pasteurella* represent a smaller percentage.[5] *Pasteurella* is the most frequent gram-negative isolate in cats with otitis externa of bacterial origin.[11] Gram-negative infections are often associated with ulceration and epithelial erosion and can significantly weaken or destroy the tympanic membrane, resulting in otitis media.[44]

Malassezia canis (also known as *Pityrosporum pachydermatis*) is a 12-micron, bottle-shaped gram-positive budding yeast that may be found in 20 to 49 per cent of the ears of normal dogs and cats.[38, 48, 49] As with commensal bacteria, once the environment of the ears is changed in such a way that the organism causes an opportunistic infection, this may be secondary to chronic topical antibacterial therapy or keratinization disorders due to maceration following continual moistening of the ear following swimming. Yeast may be found alone or with bacteria, thus reinforcing the importance of cytologic evaluation of all patients presenting for otitis externa. Studies suggest that more than ten organisms per HPF is consistent with yeast infections,[50] although the author feels that more than five organisms per HPF is significant and represents yeast overgrowth that requires treatment. Although other fungal elements have occasionally been reported from the ear canal (*Candida* sp., *Aspergillus, Microsporum, Trichophyton,* and *Sporotrichosis*), they make up a very small portion of cases of otitis externa.[2, 19, 42, 51, 52]

In the cat, the two most common pathogens are *Staphylococcus* and *Pasteurella*. Topical antibiotic selection for bacterial infections need not depend on culture and sensitivity studies. Gram-positive and gram-negative infections are susceptible to the antimicrobials contained in combination ear products. Although studies indicate bacterial isolates from the ear have become more resistant over the last decade, the fact that antimicrobial concentrations obtained through topical applications are 10 to 100 times those obtainable in the blood through systemic administration accounts for their continued successful use clinically. The exception to this statement is the occasional *Pseudomonas* and *Proteus* isolates from the ear.[11, 19] *Pseudomonas* isolates from the ear are frequently found to demonstrate both in vitro and clinical resistance to topical gentamicin therapy.[11] This therapeutic problem can be overcome by making up a .5 to 1 per cent Tobramycin or Amikacin solution, usually in Synotic.[11] Coly-mycin Otic (Parke-Davis) is a commercially available human ear medication that contains colistin sulfate, which is effective against resistant *Pseudomonas* strains. Treatment of yeast infections may be topical or systemic. Topical preparations containing miconazole (Conofite lotion), nystatin (Panalog), and thiabendazole (Tresaderm) are all effective topically.[43] However, when owner compliance is in doubt or inconsistent, oral ketoconazole is a very effective agent in controlling yeast infection in both the dog and cat.[11]

EAR MITES

Otodectes cyanotis is an obligatory parasite that does not burrow into the epidermis like *Sarcoptes* but lies on the surface of the skin. Adult mites are large, white, and free-moving and are easily seen during otoscopic examination.[53] The life cycle of the ear mite is three weeks. Mites cause intense irritation and are characterized by thick, reddish-brown crust in the ears of dogs and cats. Ears become filled with a mixture of loose crusts and cerumen. Lesions most commonly are restricted to the external ear canal but mites may be found on other parts of the body. Ear mites are the single most frequent cause of otitis externa in the cat (more than 50 per cent) but may also affect other species of carnivores such as dogs, in which they are responsible for ten per cent of otitis externa. The mites are highly contagious. Mites are usually more numerous in the young kitten or puppy than in the adult. Various immune mechanisms have been proposed to explain this clinical observation.[54] Control is especially difficult in kennels or catteries. Suggestions for environmental flea control are appropriate for control of mites in these situations. Individual animal treatment requires local ear treatment. Several products appear to be effective in the treatment of the local condition. Rotenone (Canex), pyrethrins (Cerumite), and thiabendazole (Tresaderm) are effective but may cause local irritation.[3, 18] Any treatment should be continued for at least three weeks, considering the life cycle of the mite, and should include all susceptible animals whether symptomatic or not. Animals affected should be treated with a flea spray, powder, or shampoos to remove mites that may be present on parts of the body other than the ear. Ivermectin has been recently reported effective against *Otodectes* in the dog.[17]

TICKS

The spinous ear tick *(Otobius megnini)* is found in the external ear canal of dogs and cats.[3, 11, 28] Its range is limited primarily to the Southwestern portion of the United States. The larvae and nymphs infest the ear canal of the host, producing acute otitis externa accompanied by pain. Frequently the ear canals become packed with immature ticks. Adults are not parasitic; however, larvae engorge on the lymph from the ear canal and are yellow-pink in color. Damage done by the spinous ear tick results from loss of blood and lymph in addition to the severe irritation and secondary bacterial infections caused by the vigorous head shaking and scratching. Treatment involves mechanical removal of ticks with a pair of forceps or hemostats. Spraying or dipping the coat with insecticide material such as lindane or malathion and the treatment of local otitis with a combination antibiotic-corticosteroid product is usually satisfactory for the individual canine patient.

MISCELLANEOUS PARASITIC INFESTATIONS

Occasionally, other parasites are isolated from the pinna or the external ear canal. The list includes fleas, *Demodex*, chiggers, and *Cheyletiella*. The diagnosis and proper treatment depends upon identification of the parasite.[3]

CERUMINOUS OTITIS

Ceruminous otitis is a condition that usually reflects a generalized skin disease such as a keratinization disorder like seborrhea.[44, 55] Seborrheic or ceruminous otitis is frequently misdiagnosed as a purulent otitis. Its clinical appearance may vary from an oily golden-yellow film or large, soft flakes (particularly in spaniels) to dry flakes (particularly in old German shepherds). The ear canal usually contains a heavy, almost sweet-smelling material. Cytologically, large amounts of keratin without significant numbers of microorganisms are seen.[11] If examined thoroughly, dogs usually have an underlying generalized seborrheic condition. However, the most severe lesions frequently are localized in the ear. Ceruminolytic and drying agents are helpful in controlling the accumulation of exudative material. Drying and cleaning agents such as HB101, Burrows solution, hydrocortisone propylene glycol, OtiClens, malic acid, benzoic plus salicylic acids, alcohol, otic Domeboro, and acetic acid in aluminum acetate solution work well. Products containing potent glucocorticoids should be avoided because of their potential to produce signs of Cushing's syndrome. Owners should be advised that control, not cure, is the norm for the condition and that lifelong therapy on either a daily or weekly basis may be required. If generalized seborrhea is present, treatment with seborrheic shampoo should be instituted at the time of diagnosis. Clinicians should try to determine the cause of the seborrhea (e.g., nutritional or hormonal) and eliminate it.

ALLERGIC OTITIS

Atopy, food allergies, and contact sensitivities can all cause otitis externa.[11, 19]

Allergic otitis occurs in 50 per cent of the cases of atopy in dogs and dogs with food allergies.[11, 19] Dogs may be presented for head shaking or ear scratching as a primary complaint. Examination of the ear canal may fail to reveal the presence of exudative material or other forms of pathology. However, in chronic cases, erythema and some mild exudative material are frequently present. The clinician must take a careful history and do a thorough physical examination to determine if generalized atopy is the underlying cause of ear pruritus. Atopic otitis is treated in the same manner as other forms of atopy. In the absence of exudative material, systemic corticosteroids are usually effective in controlling the pruritic condition. Those associated with food usually respond to dietary changes. Allergic reactions to topical or parenteral drugs may also be seen as mentioned in the section on the pinnae.

NEOPLASMS OF THE EXTERNAL EAR CANAL

Ear tumors of the cat are of three primary types: squamous cell carcinoma of the pinna, ceruminous gland tumors of the ear canal, and polypoid masses of the nasopharynx.[28] Other types occur less frequently and include basal cell carcinoma, hemangioendothelioma, mastocytoma, and malignant melanoma.[3, 28] Squamous cell carcinoma in the cat has already been described. The majority of the ceruminous gland tumors in the cat are malignant and 50 per cent have metastasized by the time of diagnosis. Metastases are frequently found in the regional lymph nodes and lungs. The clinical presentation of these tumors mimics otitis externa. Careful examination of the ear canal with an otoscope usually reveals the mass. Histologic evaluation must be done to differentiate hyperplastic changes (polyps) and ceruminous gland adenomas from adenocarcinomas. Careful palpation of the local nodes and thoracic radiographs may reveal disseminated disease. Occasionally the regional lymph node involvement outgrows the primary tumor in the ear canal, resulting in the client presenting the cat because of a mass in the parotid gland area.

Careful examination of the ear reveals the primary tumor in such cases.

The fibroma or inflammatory polyp of the ear canal of the cat deserves special attention. These lesions are considered the most common tumors in the ears of cats and are reported most frequently in young cats three months to five years old.[8] These growths are thought to originate from the epithelial lining of the external ear canal and/or middle ear. The clinical signs are generally associated with chronic otitis externa or chronic otitis media and include ear discharge, head shaking, head tilt, disequilibrium, nystagmus, respiratory distress, dysphagia, and coughing. The surgical management of these polypoid growths is dictated by the location of the polyp. Growths originating in the external canal tend to grow toward the horizontal and vertical canal. They are often seen during otoscopic examination for chronic otitis externa.[56] These polyps can be effectively treated by tonsil snare and gentle traction. Lateral ear resection may be necessary to enhance visualization. Growths that originate in the middle ear may grow toward the external ear canal or into the nasopharynx via the eustachian tube. Those growing into the nasopharynx can cause dysphagia, dyspnea, or chronic cough. These growths are approached via ventral bulla osteotomy.[11] Occasionally, growths will be visible in the external ear canal and the nasopharynx. In such cases a combined approach, bulla osteotomy and lateral ear resection, may be necessary for removal.

The prognosis after treatment of polyps by resection is guarded. Approximately one-third of resected polyps recur. Presenting neurological signs generally take several weeks to resolve and may not resolve completely. The condition occurs in dogs, but less frequently than in cats.

SURGICAL MANAGEMENT OF CHRONIC OTITIS EXTERNA

Although surgical intervention is clearly indicated with neoplasms of the ear, surgical management of cases of chronic proliferative otitis that have failed medical therapy is not always successful.[57] Recent evaluation of lateral ear resection for the treatment of chronic otitis indicates resolution of the problem was only seen in 41 per cent of the cases, improvement in 12 per cent, and response was considered poor in 47 per cent of the cases.[58] Poor response rate has been attributed to the failure to recognize otitis media and to endocrine, allergic, and autoimmune disorders in these patients.[42, 59]

THE MIDDLE EAR

Anatomic Considerations

The tympanum of the dog is a somewhat pear-shaped cavity situated in the petrosal portion of the temporal bone. The tympanic cavity is filled with air and is lined primarily with a columnar, ciliated epithelium that is continuous with that of the internal auditory canal (eustachian tube) and the nasopharynx.[60]

There are several nerves that pass through the middle ear, but only two, the facial nerve and sympathetic trunk, appear to be clinically significant. The facial nerve leaves the brain stem in close association with the eighth cranial nerve, travels in the facial canal of the petrosal portion of the temporal bone, then enters the middle ear cavity. The sympathetic nerve leaves the cranial cervical ganglion, which is located just caudal to the tympanic bulla, and enters the middle ear cavity.[3] The clinical signs associated with involvement of these nerves may be significant.

Otitis Media

Otitis media is an inflammation of the middle ear. The middle ear consists of the tympanic cavity and its contents and the auditory or eustachian tubes. Otitis media is most frequently a sequela to otitis externa. In one study 16 per cent of otitis externa cases had concurrent otitis media. The incidence of otitis media is as high as 50 per cent in cases of chronic otitis externa.[2, 5, 11]

ETIOLOGY AND PATHOGENESIS

The most common cause of otitis media is bacterial infection. The common pathogens cultured from the middle ear include *Staphylococcus*, *Streptococcus*, *Pseudomonas, Escherichia coli*, and *Proteus mirabilis*. *Staphylococcus* and *Streptococcus* are the most common.[60]

Inflammation of the middle ear can be initiated through three routes. First, inflammation can proceed across the tympanic membrane. In these cases, a primary otitis externa infection progresses to secondary otitis media. The second route is through the eustachian tube. The incidence of infection via this route is much lower in animals than it is in humans. It has been reported that cats can develop otitis media through this route as a sequela to upper respiratory disease, but this also occurs infrequently. In one study exploring the effects of eustachian tube obstruction, it was found that obstruction or malfunction evoked middle ear effusion in cats and that the tube can function as a middle ear drainage conduit if the tympanic membrane is perforated.[60] The third route is via blood-borne pathogens that invade the middle ear. Most authors agree that otitis media in dogs and cats most commonly occurs secondary to otitis externa and that many cases are overlooked because examination of the ear is not carried far enough when otitis externa is obvious. This is certainly the case in the patient presented with unilateral otitis externa in which a thorough search for a foreign body is not undertaken; at a later date, the animal develops otitis media secondary to foreign body migration.

The middle ear defense mechanisms include a mucociliary system and a cellular defense system. For decades it was accepted that a ciliated respiratory epithelium lined the eustachian tube and, in the last few years, this epithelium was described as lining important parts of the middle ear as well. The epithelium in the middle ear can function actively in clearing foreign material, as demonstrated experimentally by the rapid clearance of radiopaque material and as observed directly through tympanic membrane perforations.[60]

A substance that lowers surface tension has been found in the auditory tube of dogs. This substance may play an important role in otitis media. An infection may diminish production or antagonize the presence of the surface tension-lowering substance. This decrease would result in a greater cohesive force between the coapting walls of the auditory tube. With the auditory tube more resistant to opening during the act of swallowing, a lack of aeration of the middle ear may occur.

Bacteria are the primary causative agents in otitis media, but other agents such as yeast infections *(Malassezia, Candida)* and *Aspergillus* should be considered. In unilateral cases, foreign bodies, trauma with intratympanic hemorrhage, and tumors such as polyps, fibromas, squamous cell carcinomas, and primary bone tumors should be considered.

Dentigerous cysts and temporal odontoma are rare. The ectopic incomplete development of a tooth within the cyst is most commonly located near the mastoid process of the petrous temporal bone. This cyst is recognized because of the sinus tract that forms at the base of the ear. The treatment involves incision over the tract followed by blunt dissection and removal of the cyst.[60]

CLINICAL SIGNS AND FINDINGS

Many of the signs of otitis media also occur with otitis externa. The irritation caused by these changes is manifested by the dog's shaking its head and pawing and rubbing the affected ear(s). Some animals may show evidence of pain when petted on the affected side, even without obvious external ear changes. This may be the primary reason that the animal is presented to the veterinarian. Signs of facial nerve involvement may be seen and include a lack of or diminished palpebral reflex, a wide palpebral fissure, drooping of the ear and lips, and excessive drooling. Horner's syndrome may also occur secondary to damage of the sympathetic nerve as it passes through the middle ear. Ptosis, myosis, enophthalmos, and protrusion of the third eyelid are the clinical signs that are diagnostic of Horner's syndrome. These nerve palsies may be seen on presentation, or postoperatively, after curettage of the tympanic bulla.[11, 60]

DIAGNOSTIC PROCEDURES

On otoscopic examination, foreign bodies, neoplasms, and polyps can usually be seen, and appropriate biopsies can be taken if needed. If the tympanic membrane is ruptured, aerobic, fungal, and yeast cultures can be taken directly from the middle ear for identification and susceptibility testing. A smear of the exudate can be stained with new methylene blue or Wright's stain and examined for yeasts or fungal agents such as *Malassezia, Candida*, and *Aspergillus*. If the disease condition is controlled, regrowth of the tympanic membrane can be expected in two weeks.

If the tympanum is intact and there appears to be fluid in the middle ear cavity, myringotomy can be performed to obtain samples for culture. This is done by using a blunt probe and passing it through the ventral half of the tympanum. A spinal needle of adequate length is passed through the perforation, a syringe is attached, and fluid is aspirated. This technique is only necessary with ascending otitis media since with otitis media secondary to otitis externa, the tympanum has usually already been ruptured.[11]

Radiographic examination of the tympanic bulla is extremely helpful in establishing a diagnosis of otitis media. Radiography often reveals a fluid-filled osseous bulla or a sclerotic bone around the bulla. X-ray computed tomography (CT) may reveal lesions that are not evident on plain radiographs. The most useful views in evaluation of the middle ear are dorsal ventral projection, frontal projection, lateral projections, and right and left oblique views.[11]

MEDICAL TREATMENT

The essential treatment in most cases of otitis media consists of removing the infected, inflammatory, or foreign material from the bulla and providing ventilation and free exit for discharges (drainage). Because most cases of otitis media are accompanied by chronic otitis externa and since each condition contributes to the other, there is little purpose in attempting to effect a remedy for otitis media without treating the otitis externa, and vice versa. This can be accomplished by medical and/or surgical means.

Medical therapy should be evaluated before surgical procedures are performed, but with the realization that surgery may eventually be needed to provide drainage.

Systemic antibiotic therapy should be based on cytology and culture and susceptibility, if indicated. Because of potential toxicity, topical antibiotics should be used sparingly, if at all, after thoroughly cleansing and flushing the external ear canal and middle ear cavity with warm saline and then drying it.

The ear canal can be dried with a cotton swab and by aspirating it with a syringe and feeding tube or a low-vacuum suction. Topical drying agents should not be used in patients with ruptured tympanic membranes. Anti-inflammatory doses of systemic corticosteroids may be used in animals with neurologic dysfunction. Animals should be professionally evaluated twice weekly and have warm saline flushes as needed. Systemic antibiotics and corticosteroids should be continued for two to three weeks.[11, 60]

The most common indication for middle ear surgery is lack of a satisfactory response to the treatment of bacterial otitis media with proper aggressive medical therapy. When dealing with these patients, an adequate drainage procedure (lateral ear resection) and/or bulla osteotomy must be done to resolve the disease process. Animals with chronic sclerotic bony otitis media often do not benefit from surgery. Other indications for middle ear surgery include foreign bodies that have migrated into the middle ear and neoplasms of the middle ear, most commonly polypoid growth.

THE INNER EAR

Anatomy and Considerations

The inner ear consists of three parts: the cochlea, vestibule, and semicircular canals. These are communicating excavations of the petrosal portion of the temporal bone known as the osseous labyrinth. The osseous labyrinth is lined with membranes that form the membranous labyrinth, which is a closed duct system filled with endolymph. The labyrinth is made up of three parts: the vestibule (saccule and utricle), cochlea, and three semicircular canals.[3]

The cochlea of the inner ear is concerned with hearing, while the saccule, utricle, and semicircular ducts are important in maintaining equilibrium. Inner ear nerve supply is via the cochlear and vestibular branches of the acoustic or eighth cranial nerve. The cochlear component passes to the cochlea and the vestibular branch is related to the saccule, utricle, and semicircular canals.[3]

The ear, specifically the membranous labyrinth, serves as the sensory end organ for the vestibulocochlear nerve and vestibular mechanism (equilibrium). This mechanism consists of receptors in the labyrinth (semicircular canals, sacculus, utriculus), the vestibular nerve, and the vestibular nuclei and their tracts. It is a proprioceptive apparatus stimulated by changes in position of the head and is used to control the tone of the muscles used in maintaining posture.[3]

If part of the vestibular mechanism is damaged on one side, there is unequal influence on the opposite mechanism. Depending on the degree of damage, the dog may tilt its head and circle toward the affected side or may show a horizontal nystagmus with the fast component away from the affected side (peripheral involvement only). If damage to this apparatus is severe, the dog may not be able to walk, may walk with an ataxic gait, or may continually roll over toward the affected side. Connections between the vestibular nuclei and cranial nerves III, IV, VI through pathways within the brain stem account for nystagmus in conditions affecting the vestibular system.[11]

Hearing and Deafness

Hearing in dogs and cats is considered more sensitive than in humans. Humans have an upper range of around 20,000 cycles per second (Hz), while the upper range of dogs and cats is 50,000 to 60,000 Hz, inaudible to humans. Some sounds in the inaudible range for humans, such as those emitted by electronic pest repellent devices, have been reported to irritate cats and dogs.[8] A rare condition called "objective tinnitus," which has also been reported in dogs, can be annoying to humans. Objective tinnitus results in the production of an audible high-pitched tone about 15 dB from the affected ear. The condition has been reported in humans but the pathogenesis is unknown.[62]

Whether deafness is congenital or acquired, testing of hearing is difficult because animals can detect low frequency sounds by the movement of air around their whiskers. Hearing in dogs and cats can be definitively evaluated using electrodiagnostic procedures that selectively assess the integrity of the peripheral and CNS structures. The two procedures most frequently used are the acoustic reflex (AR) and the brain stem auditory-evoked response (BAER). Both tests evaluate components of the external ear canal, middle and inner ear cavities, selected sections of the brain stem, and cranial nerves. When these procedures are used in combination with tympanometry, conductive and neural hearing disorders can be differentiated and characterized in pet animals.[63–66]

Congenital deafness is associated with incomplete pigmentation of the hair coat and uvea in dogs and cats. Hearing deficits are also associated with inheritance of the merling gene. All homozygotes and many of the heterozygotes are deaf.[11] The breeds most frequently affected include Dalmatians,[65] Old English sheepdogs,[67] cocker spaniels,[68] and bull terriers.[69] Deafness may be partial, complete, unilateral, or bilateral in affected animals.[65] In cats, a single pair of alleles determines if an individual white cat will be blue-eyed, yellow-eyed, or "odd-eyed" heterochromic.[70] Blue-eyed cats are more often deaf than odd-eyed cats but deafness need not be on the same side as the blue eye.[8] Odd-eyed cats are more frequently deaf than yellow-eyed cats. Congenital deafness in both dogs and cats is permanent. It results from postnatal degeneration of structures derived from the neural crest, which are usually detectable histologically four to six days after birth. The fully developed lesion is characterized by cochleosaccular degeneration, composed of atrophy of sensory and supporting cells of the organ of Corti and the saccula macula, collapse of the dorsal or lateral walls of the cochlear and saccular membranous labyrinth, and secondary degeneration of neurons within the spiral ganglion.[71]

Acquired deafness is common in older dogs as they reach ten years of age. This phenomenon, called presbyacusis, is most noticeable in this species because voice command is frequently used in dogs; however, cats are also affected.[72] The lesions are characterized by degradation of epithelial tissues within the cochlea and spiral ganglion. Acquired deafness can be produced experimentally in dogs and cats by loud noises, but such cases are rarely reported in the clinical setting.[73] Drug-induced deafness has been reported with aminoglycoside antibiotics and diuretics in dogs and cats, cats being the most sensitive.[72] Ototoxicity is associated with absolute blood levels and duration of exposure, thus overdosing or continued dosing of these drugs in patients with impaired renal function predisposes them to ototoxicity. Fortunately, clinical signs of vestibular dysfunction often precede evidence of hearing impairment. The lesions are first noted in the apical portion or cochlear hair cell. The early lesions are reversible but chronic exposure results in permanent loss.

Otitis Interna

Inflammatory vestibular disease is most frequently caused by extension of otitis media to otitis interna. In contrast to signs associated with otitis media that may be overlooked, clinical signs of otitis interna are prominent enough that veterinary care is frequently sought.[11] Clinical signs may appear suddenly or have a gradual onset. They may appear acutely following ear cleaning or the application of ear medications. Inflammation of the external ear canal and middle ear can result in head tilts associated with pain rather than vestibular dysfunction. The clinical signs most frequently observed are head tilt, nystagmus, and falling and rolling toward the side of the affected ear. Nystagmus may be present and is usually horizontal, unchanging with the fast component away from the affected ear. If the disorientation is severe, an asymmetric ataxia may be exhibited by a wide stance and crouching walk. In addition to auditory and vestibular abnormalities, the neurological dysfunctions associated with otitis media may also be present: dropped ear, drooped lip, miotic pupil, ptosis, enophthalmos, and an inability to close the eyelids.

With these signs there is a possibility that a brain stem abscess will develop, since the meninges follow the 8th nerve into the inner ear and infection may proceed through this route. If an abscess does develop, motor deficits to the limbs and other cranial nerves become apparent. If the inflammation extends into the brain stem, the trigeminal nerve is frequently involved, resulting in significant motor deficit. Additionally, animals may be depressed due to inflammatory changes affecting the reticular activating system near this portion of the brain stem. Treatment of otitis interna is essentially the same as for otitis media, with the addition of anti-inflammatory drugs such as corticosteroids (0.5 mg/lb or 1 mg/kg). Otitis interna is associated with an inflammatory process and does not necessarily represent an infectious process of the brain or brain stem. Systemic antibiotics that cross the blood-brain barrier, such as chloramphenicol, should be used concurrently with corticosteroids since inflammation and infections are not easily separated.

Animals with peripheral vestibular disease signs that have normal external ear, tympanic membrane, and radiographic examinations suggest etiologies other than inflammatory otitis. In young purebred dogs and cats, congenital vestibular disease should be considered. Most animals with congenital vestibular abnormalities develop clinical signs by three months of age, some soon after birth. Reported congenital vestibular diseases vary in severity and onset and have been reported in German shepherds,[74] Siamese and Burmese[74] cats, Doberman pinschers,[61, 75] Shetland sheepdogs,[61] beagles,[74] and English cockers.[68] The reader is referred to a review[61] and specific references for more detailed descriptions.

Other acquired vestibular abnormalities must be differentiated from those associated with ear disease. Vestibular diseases associated with nutritional, traumatic, toxic, neoplastic, or idiopathic etiologies should be considered. Thiamine deficiency may result in ataxia in addition to other neurologic dysfunctions in cats.[74] Blunt trauma to the head often results in acute vestibular disease.[61] Toxic vestibular disease has been reported with aminoglycoside use in dogs and cats, with cats being the most susceptible.[75] A wide variety of both primary (most common) and metastatic tumors have been associated with acquired vestibular disease in older animals.[61] The most frequent cause of noninflammatory vestibular disease in dogs and cats is idiopathic vestibular syndrome.[61] Idiopathic vestibular syndrome in cats is characterized by acute onset of crying, severe head tilt, rolling, falling to one side, and nystagmus. The syndrome occurs in adult cats of any age, most frequently in the summer months. The etiology is unknown and recovery can be expected in two to four weeks with the possible exception of a residual head tilt. Idiopathic old dog vestibular syndrome in dogs is similar to the disease described in cats except that it occurs in geriatric dogs. No etiology is routinely found; however, vascular infarcts sometimes observed with hypothyroidism have been implicated. Recovery takes somewhat longer than in cats (four to six weeks).

References

1. Mascal, L: The government of Cattell. London, John Harrison, 1633, p 295.
2. Wilson, JF: A practitioner's approach to complete ear care. Derm Rep 4:1, 1985.
3. Muller, GH, et al.: Small Animal Dermatology, 3rd ed, Philadelphia, WB Saunders Co, 1983.
4. Priester, WA: A summary of diagnosis in the ox, horse, dog and cat from 12 veterinary school clinics in the US and Canada. Vet Rec 86:654, 1970.
5. Grono, LR: Otitis externa. *In* Kirk RW (ed): Current Veterinary Therapy VII, Philadelphia, WB Saunders Co, 1980, p 461.
6. Miller, ME, et al. (ed): Anatomy of the Dog. Philadelphia, WB Saunders Co, 1964, p 847.
7. Field, B and Wanner, RA: Cerebral malformation in a manx cat. Vet Rec 96, 1975, p 42.
8. Holzworth, J: The ear. *In* The Diseases of the Cat, Medicine and Surgery, Philadelphia, WB Saunders, 1987, p 724.
9. Fasnacht, DW: Four-eared cat. JAVMA 154:1145, 1969.
10. Little, CC: Four-ears, a recessive mutation in the cat. J Hered 48:57, 1957.
11. Macy, DW and Seim, HB: Medical and surgical aspects of the ear. Parts I and II. Proc AAHA 53rd Annu Meet, 1985, p 120.
12. Hargis, AM: A review of solar-induced lesions in domestic animals. Comp Cont Ed Pract Vet 3:287, 1981.
13. Irving, J, et al.: Porphyrin values and treatment of feline solar dermatitis. Am J Vet Res 43:2067, 1982.
14. Kunkle, GA: Hereditary alopecias and haircoat abnormalities of the dog. Derm Rep 4:6, 1985.
15. Dyte, CE: Further data on folded-ear cats. Carnivore Genetics Newsletter 2:112, 1973.
16. Todd, NB: Folded eared cats: further observations. Carnivore Genetics Newsletter 2:64, 1972.
17. Yazwinski, TA, et al.: Efficacy of ivermectin against *Sarcoptes scabiei* and *Otodectes cyanotis* infestation of the dog. VM SAC 76:1749, 1981.
18. Scott, DW: Drug eruption in a cat due to miticide. Feline Pract 3:47, 1977.
19. August, JR: Diseases of the ear canal. *In* The Complete Manual of Ear Care. Veterinary Learning Systems Co, Inc, 1986, p 35.
20. Griffin, C: Pinnal diseases. *In* The Complete Manual of Ear Care. Veterinary Learning Systems Co, Inc, 1986, p 21.
21. Scott, DW: Observations on canine atopy. JAAHA 17:91, 1981.
22. Ihrke, PJ, et al.: Pemphigus foliaceus in dogs: a review of 37 cases. JAVMA 186:59, 1985.
23. Haupt, KH, et al.: Familial canine dermatomyositis; clinical electrodiagnostic and genetic studies. Am J Vet Res 46:1861, 1985.
24. Hargis, AM, et al.: A skin disorder in three Shetland sheepdogs. Comparison with familial canine dermatomyositis of collies. Comp Cont Ed Pract Vet 7:306, 1985.
25. Gross, TL, et al.: Psoriasiform lichenoid dermatosis in springer spaniels. Vet Path 23:76, 1986.

26. Kunkle, GA: Zinc responsive dermatosis in dogs. *In* Kirk RW (ed): Current Veterinary Therapy VII, Philadelphia, WB Saunders Co, 1980, p 472.
27. Rosenkrantz, WS and Griffin, C.: Alopecia in dogs and cats. Derm Rep 3:1, 1984.
28. Scott, DW: External ear disorders. JAAHA 16:426, 1980.
29. Legendre, AM and Krahwinkel, DJ: Feline ear tumors. JAAHA 17:1035, 1981.
30. Dubielzig, RR, et al.: Pathogenesis of canine aural hematoma. JAVMA 185:873, 1984.
31. Kuwakara, J: Canine and feline aural hematoma: clinical, experimental and clinicopathologic observations. Am J Vet Res 47:2300, 1986.
32. Fraser, G: The histopathology of the external auditory meatus of the dog. J Comp Pathol 71:253, 1961.
33. Weisbroth, SH, et al.: Immunopathology of naturally occurring otocariasis in the domestic cat. JAVMA 165:1088, 1974.
34. Fernando, SD: Certain histopathologic features of the external auditory meatus of the cat and dog with otitis externa. Am J Vet Res 28:278, 1967.j
35. Baba E, et al.: Incidence of otitis externa in dogs and cats in Japan. Vet Rec 108:393, 1981.
36. Stout, M: Personal communication, 1987.
37. Grono, LR: Otitis externa. *In* Kirk RW (ed): Current Veterinary Therapy VII, Philadelphia, WB Saunders Co, 1980, p 461.
38. Sharma, VD and Rhoades, HE: The occurrence and microbiology of otitis externa in the dog. J Sm Anim Pract 16:241, 1975.
39. Brennan, KE and Ihrke, PJ: Grass awn migration in dogs and cats. A retrospective study of 182 cases. JAVMA 182:1201, 1983.
40. Senturia, BH and Carr, CD: Studies of factors considered responsible for diseases of the external ear. Laryngoscope 68:2052, 1958.
41. Blank, H: The skin as an organ of protection against the external environment. *In* Fitzpatrick TB, Eisen AZ, et al. (eds): Dermatology in General Medicine, 2nd ed, San Francisco, McGraw-Hill, 1978, p 102.
42. Griffin, G: Otitis externa. Comp Cont Ed Pract Vet 3:741, 1981.
43. Griffin, G: Principles for treatment of the diseased ear canal. *In* The Complete Manual of Ear Care, Veterinary Learning Systems, 1987, p 61.
44. Haagen, AJ: Managing diseases of the ear. *In* Current Veterinary Therapy VIII, Kirk RW (ed): Philadelphia, WB Saunders, 1983, p 48.
45. Dickson, DB and Love, DN: Bacteriology of the horizontal ear canal of dogs. J Sm Anim Pract 24:413, 1983.
46. Blue, JL and Wooley, RE: Antibacterial sensitivity patterns of bacterial isolates from dogs with otitis externa. JAVMA 171:362, 1977.
47. Fraser, G: An etiology of otitis externa in the dog. J Sm Anim Pract 6:445, 1965.
48. Smitka, CM, et al.: Isolation and characterization of pityrosporum species isolated from dog ears. Can Vet J 25:110, 1984.
49. Baxter, A: The association of pityrosporum pachydermatis with normal external ear canal of dogs and cats. J Sm Anim Pract 17:231, 1976.
50. Rausch, FP and Skinner, GW: Incidence and treatment of budding yeast in canine otitis externa. Mod Vet Pract 53:914, 1978.
51. Rose, WR: Otitis externa 4: Otomycosis. VM SAC 71:1025, 1976.
52. Dion, WM and Speckmann, G: Canine otitis externa caused by the fungus *Sporothrix schenkii*. Can Vet J 19:410, 1978.
53. Thoday, KL: Canine pruritus: An approach to diagnosis stage II infestations and infections. J Sm Anim Pract 21:449, 1980.
54. Weisbroth, W, et al.: Immunopathology of naturally occurring otodectic otacariasis in the domestic cat. JAVMA 165:1088, 1974.
55. Halliwell, RE: Seborrhea in the dog. Comp Cont Ed Pract Vet 2:227, 1981.
56. Harvey, C and Goldschmidt, MH: Inflammatory polypoid growths in the ear canal of cats. J Sm Anim Pract 19:669, 1978.
57. Tutvesson, G: Operation for otitis externa in dogs according to Zepp's method. Am J Vet Res 16:565, 1955.
58. Gregory, CR and Vasseur, PB: Clinical results of lateral ear resection in dogs. JAVMA 182:1087, 1983.
59. Bojrab, WV and Renegar, WR: The ear. *In* Bojrab MJ (ed): Pathophysiology in Small Animal Surgery, Philadelphia, Lea & Febiger, 1981, p 70.
60. Neer, TM and Howard, PE: Otitis media. Comp Cont Ed Pract Vet 4:410, 1982.
61. Simpson, S: Diseases of the Vestibular System. *In* Kirk RW (ed): Current Veterinary Therapy VIII, Philadelphia, WB Saunders 1983, p 726.
62. Decker, TN: Objective tinnitus in the dog. Philadelphia, WB Saunders, JAVMA I80:74, 1984.
63. Sims, MH and Shull-Selcer, E: Electrodiagnostic evaluation of deafness in two English setter littermates. JAVMA 187:398, 1985.
64. Bodenhamer, RD, et al.: Brain stem auditory-evoked responses in the dog. Am J Vet Res 46:1787, 1985.
65. Marshall, EA: Use of brain stem auditory-evoked response to evaluate deafness in a group of Dalmatian dogs. JAVMA 189:718, 1986.
66. Forsythe, WB: Tympanographic volume measurements of the canine ear. Am J Vet Res 46:1351, 1985.
67. Anniko, M, et al.: Deafness in an Old English sheepdog. A case report. Arch Oto-Rhino-Laryngol 218:1, 1979.
68. Bedford, PG: Congenital vestibular disease in English cocker spaniel. Vet Rec 105:530, 1979.
69. Hayes, HM, et al.: Canine congenital deafness: epidemiologic study of 272 cases. JAAHA 17:473, 1981.
70. Todd, NB, et al.: The inheritance of blue eyes and deafness in the domestic cat. Carnivore Genetics Newsletter 5:100, 1968.
71. Main, IW: Hereditary cochleosaccular degeneration. *In* Spontaneous Animal Models of Human Diseases, Andrew EJ (ed): 1:86, New York Academic Press, 1979.
72. Wilcock, BP: The eye and ear. *In* Pathology of Domestic Animals, 3rd ed, Jubb KV, et al. (eds): New York, Academic Press, vol 1, 1985, p 395.
73. Liberman, MC and Kiang, NY: Acoustic trauma in cats. Cochlear Pathology and Auditory Nerve Activity. Acta Otolaryngol S358:1, 1978.
74. deLahunta, A (ed): Vestibular System—Special Proprioception. *In* Veterinary Neuroanatomy and Clinical Neurology, Philadelphia, WB Saunders, 1977, p 221.
75. Chrisman, CL: Vestibular diseases. Vet Clin North Am 10:103, 1980.

SECTION III

INFECTIOUS DISEASES

46 BACTERIAL, RICKETTSIAL, PROTOZOAL, AND MISCELLANEOUS INFECTIONS

LARRY J. SWANGO, KAREN W. BANKEMPER, and
LILLY I. KONG

BACTERIAL DISEASES

BACTERIAL INFECTIONS OF THE RESPIRATORY TRACT

Bacterial infections of the respiratory tract in dogs and cats are usually secondary to viral infections, trauma, or surgical intervention. The normal bacterial flora of the nasal passages and pharynx is diverse, with many species of bacteria capable of causing rhinitis, sinusitis, or pharyngitis as secondary invaders.[1–4] Staphylococci, streptococci, *Pasteurella multocida*, *Escherichia coli* and other gram-negative organisms are the most commonly isolated bacteria from the upper respiratory tract, but secondary infections with *Pseudomonas aeruginosa* are among the most problematic, due in part to its marked resistance to antibiotics but also due to the inability to achieve adequate concentrations of antibiotics in secretions of the respiratory tract.[5] Parenterally administered antibiotics may fail to eliminate bacterial infections of the upper respiratory tract and persistently recurring or chronic infections may develop. *Bordetella bronchiseptica* colonizes the nasal mucosa of dogs and may cause rhinitis as a primary pathogen, although it is more commonly associated with infectious tracheobronchitis, "kennel cough."[6–9]

The respiratory tract below the epiglottis is usually sterile. Bacterial infections of the lower respiratory tract in dogs and cats are usually secondary to viral infections. Primary bacterial pneumonias in both dogs and cats have been caused by *B. bronchiseptica*, *Pasteurella multocida*, and *Streptococcus zooepidemicus*. Bacterial pneumonia is less common in cats than in dogs due in part to a greater prevalence of infections with *B. bronchiseptica* in dogs.[8] Tuberculosis occurs as a primary disease in both dogs and cats. The prevalence of canine and feline tuberculosis correlates with the frequency of tuberculosis in humans and cattle.

Bordetellosis. Bordetellosis is caused by *Bordetella bronchiseptica,* a gram-negative, rod-shaped bacterium. It has been established as a primary cause of canine infectious tracheobronchitis or kennel cough.[6, 7, 9, 10] Although kennel cough is the most common clinical manifestation of bordetellosis, fatal bronchopneumonia may occur as a result of primary or secondary infections.[2, 6, 11] Since *B. bronchiseptica* is a gram-negative rod, endotoxins may play a role in its pathogenicity. The organism attaches to the cilia of respiratory epithelium at all levels of the respiratory tract resulting in ciliostasis within five minutes after attachment.[12] Pathologic changes characterized by loss of cilia, necrosis of epithelial cells, and infiltration of the mucosa with polymorphonuclear leukocytes occur in the respiratory epithelium.[7, 11, 13] A viscous, purulent exudate occurs in the more severe infections, resulting in rhinitis with purulent nasal discharge in the upper respiratory tract and in tracheobronchitis with plugging of bronchi and bronchioles by cellular exudate in the lower respiratory tract.[7, 10] Primary infection of nursing puppies with *B. bronchiseptica* can result in death due to hypoxia resulting from obstruction of bronchi and bronchioles with purulent exudate. Affected puppies have "rattling" or "gurgling" respiratory sounds. Bronchopneumonia may occur in dogs of any age, occasionally resulting in acute death from primary infection, but more commonly as a secondary infection to canine distemper or other respiratory virus infections.[4] *B. bronchiseptica* has been isolated from the lungs of cats with pneumonia.[14]

The classic kennel cough manifestation of bordetellosis is usually a mild, self-limiting infection. The disease is characterized by episodes of paroxysmal coughing that are usually exacerbated by exercise, excitement, or pressure on the trachea. The cough may be harsh and dry or soft, moist, and pulsating; it may or may not be productive but it often terminates with gagging. Affected dogs are usually active, alert, and afebrile with normal blood cell counts. The incubation period varies from four to ten days, the morbidity ranges from 25 to 75 per cent, and affected dogs usually recover in seven to ten days. The clinical signs are not unique to bordetellosis. Specific etiologic diagnosis depends upon isolation and identification of the organism. *B. bronchiseptica* can be isolated from nasal swabs early in the course of the disease. It persists in the lower respiratory tract after it is no longer present in the nasal passages, and transtracheal washings often yield pure cultures.[15, 16] Recovered dogs continue to harbor and shed the organism for three months or longer after cessation of clinical signs; some dogs may become persistently infected carriers.[16] The shedding of organisms by asymptomatic dogs serves as the source for transmission to susceptible dogs.

Antibiotics administered by parenteral routes are not effective in eliminating *B. bronchiseptica* from the trachea and bronchi due to inadequate concentrations of the antibiotics in tracheobronchial secretions.[5, 16] Administration of antibiotics directly into the respiratory tract either by nebulization or intratracheal injection is effective in eliminating *B. bronchiseptica* from the tracheobronchial area.[16] Gentamicin and kanamycin are the antibiotics of choice for aerosol or intratracheal treatment of bordetellosis. Aerosol treatment or intratracheal injection should be done at 12-hour intervals on the first day and once daily for five to seven days. The aerosol or intratracheal dose is 50 mg per treatment for gentamicin or 200 mg per treatment for kanamycin.

Antibiotics administered parenterally or orally can be effective in treatment of pneumonia caused by *B. bronchiseptica*, provided that high dosages are used for a period of 10 to 14 days or longer.[8, 17, 18] Concentrations of antibiotics are greater in bronchioalveolar secretions than in tracheal and upper respiratory secretions, and there is some evidence that the concentrations of antibiotics in bronchioalveolar secretions may be greater in patients with pneumonia than in normal patients.[8, 19] Ideally, antibiotic therapy should be based on isolation, identification, and testing for antibiotic sensitivity of the organism. When the clinical signs indicate pneumonia and systemic illness, antibiotic therapy should be started using a broad-spectrum antibiotic and changed as necessary when the results of isolation and antibiotic sensitivity testing become available. Based on the reported spectrum of *in vitro* antibiotic effectiveness against isolates of *B. bronchiseptica*, gentamicin, kanamycin, chloramphenicol, or tetracycline would be antibiotics of choice.[14] A combination of trimethoprim-sulfadiazine has also been found to be effective in treatment of bordetellosis but relapses may occur if treatment is not continued for at least 14 days.[18]

Dogs that have persistent harsh, dry, hacking coughs that do not clear up within seven to ten days may require additional diagnostic evaluations and treatments. In addition to antibiotic therapy, treatments may be necessary to suppress inflammation and to maintain patency of the bronchi. Corticosteroids can be used to reduce inflammation of the respiratory tract that may be enhanced by persistent coughing.[13, 20] Corticosteroids may be administered directly into the respiratory tract by aerosol or intratracheal injection concurrently with antibiotics at a dosage of 0.1 to 0.2 mg/lb of body weight. Treatment with corticosteroids may be necessary for two weeks by parenteral or oral administration at daily dosages of 0.5 to 1.0 mg/lb. Bronchodilating drugs may be needed to relieve bronchospasms and expectorants may be beneficial in helping to facilitate clearance of secretions from the lower respiratory tract by a functional mucociliary escalator. Antitussive therapy should be used with discretion and restricted to periods of intense exacerbations because complete suppression of coughing may allow for retention and accumulation of bronchial mucus and exudates with further enhancement of the problem.

Two types of vaccines are available for immunizing against *Bordetella*: killed bacterins for IM or SQ administration and avirulent strains of live *B. bronchiseptica* for intranasal administration.[21–24] Both types of vaccine provide immunity that results in decreased morbidity and in reduced severity of clinical signs of disease, but neither type of vaccine completely prevents infection when vaccinated dogs are exposed to *B. bronchiseptica*.[21–23] The addition of attenuated parainfluenza virus and/or canine adenovirus type 2 to the intranasal *Bordetella* vaccine significantly decreased clinical signs of kennel cough in both experimental studies and in clinical trials.[21, 22, 24]

The "first-generation" killed bacterins contained inactivated whole bacterial cells. Since *B. bronchiseptica* is a gram-negative rod, endotoxins in the first-generation bacterins caused inordinate postvaccinal reactions, both localized swelling and induration, as well as occasional systemic signs of endotoxic shock. A "second-generation" of *Bordetella* bacterins are now available containing antigens extracted from the bacterial cell. The second-generation bacterins have greatly reduced the postvaccinal reactions while providing a measure of protection. Immunity to bordetellosis may last for 10 to 12 months following vaccination with either the intranasal vaccine or the bacterins containing extracted *Bordetella* antigens.[22, 24] Annual revaccination is recommended, except in boarding kennels, where revaccination semiannually provides maximal protection. Since maternal antibody does not interfere with intranasal vaccines,[9] it is recommended that nursing pups be vaccinated intranasally prior to weaning.[25] Immunization of pups prior to or at the time of weaning is most beneficial in kennels where bordetellosis has been a major problem.

Pasteurellosis. *Pasteurella multocida* is common as a commensal in the oral cavity of dogs and cats.[26, 27] It may cause disease as a secondary invader, but it has been found to occasionally cause pneumonia as a primary pathogen.[15, 28, 29] Clinical signs of *Pasteurella* pneumonia are not unique and include coughing, tachypnea, dyspnea, abnormal sounds of respiration (wheezing, crackling, and rhonchi), fever, and leukocytosis with left shift.[8, 30] Specific etiologic diagnosis depends on isolation and identification of the organism. *Pasteurella multocida* does not grow on MacConkey agar, which can be an aid in distinguishing *Pasteurella* from *Bordetella* and Enterobacteriaceae. Treatment is directed at resolution of the pneumonia and requires antibiotic therapy. Antibiotic therapy should be based upon results of culture and testing for antibiotic sensitivity.[31] A trimethoprim-sulfadiazine combination, amoxicillin, ampicillin, chloramphenicol, or gentamicin are antibiotics of choice for initial treatment, pending the results of testing for antibiotic sensitivity of isolated organisms.[31]

Streptococcal Pneumonia. Lancefield group C *Streptococcus zooepidemicus* has been reported to cause an acute necrotizing hemorrhagic pneumonia in dogs.[32, 33] A remarkable feature of streptococcal pneumonia in dogs is sudden death without prior signs of illness.[33] This occurs in a small percentage of dogs, but clustering of cases may occur. Interconcurrent infection with canine distemper virus may be important in the development of this syndrome.[33] Necropsy examination reveals hemorrhagic necrosis of the lungs with ecchymotic hemorrhages in various tissues in the thoracic cavity and excessive amounts of nonclotted, hemorrhagic fluid in the thoracic cavity. Except for the acute hemorrhagic pneumonia in some cases, streptococcal pneumonia in both dogs and cats is clinically similar to other bacterial pneumonias.[8, 34] Specific etiologic diagnosis depends upon isolation and identification of the organism. Antibiotic therapy is essentially the same as for *Pasteurella* pneumonia; ampicillin, amoxicillin, gentamicin and trimethoprim-sulfadiazine are the drugs of choice.[8, 34] Cephalosporins are generally effective against streptococci although they are not drugs of choice for treatment without the results of culture and antibiotic sensitivity testing.[35]

Tuberculosis. Tuberculosis in dogs and cats involves infection with primarily either *Mycobacterium tuberculosis*, the human tubercle bacillus, or *M. bovis,* the bovine tubercle bacillus. These organisms are gram-positive, acid-fast rods. Dogs can be infected by both species, whereas cats appear to be relatively resistant to *M. tuberculosis*.[36]

Transmission is by two routes: inhalation of infected aerosols or ingestion of infected materials.[37] The portal of entry determines which manifestation of the disease is present. Dogs more frequently have a pulmonary form of disease, while the intestinal form predominates in cats.[37]

Tuberculosis is usually a subclinical infection in cats and dogs.[38] When clinical signs occur they are nonspecific and can include coughing; depression; emaciation; polyuria; polydipsia; loose, malodorous feces; icterus; vomiting; and dehydration.[39, 40]

The characteristic lesion is the tubercle, which is a granulomatous reaction to the organism in tissues. Tubercles are gray in color and circumscribed; they resemble neoplasms grossly. Although the initial lesions develop around the site of entry, secondary lesions can develop in local and regional lymphatics. A disseminated form can occur if the organisms escape the lymphatics and reach the bloodstream. As the tubercle grows, a necrotic center forms and becomes surrounded by more macrophages. Caseation and dystrophic calcification of the lesion can occur. Necrosis allows the organism to spread from the lesion site. In the pulmonary form, bacilli can reach the bronchi and be expectorated into the environment or swallowed to be shed in feces or urine.[41] Diagnosis is usually made at necropsy where generalized icterus, lymphadenitis, and the characteristic tubercles are seen. Demonstration of the tubercle bacilli in specimens is confirmative. Intradermal skin testing, although useful in human diagnosis, is unreliable in dogs and cats.[37] Radiography may be helpful. Differential diagnoses include chronic hepatitis, neoplasia, and pancreatitis.[39]

Treatment is usually not instituted due to the public health significance of this disease.[42] Dogs contract the infection mainly from humans and, to a lesser degree, from cattle. Transmission back to humans and cattle is possible. Cattle are the major source of disease in cats, although humans can also be a source. Diagnosis in the pet may be the first sign that tuberculosis exists in an owner's household. State and local health officials should be notified.[39] Infected dogs and cats must be considered as potential reservoirs of tuberculosis for humans and cattle.[38]

BACTERIAL INFECTIONS OF THE INTESTINAL TRACT

Colibacillosis. Colibacillosis refers to enteritis with systemic illness due to septicemia with *Escherichia coli*, a gram-negative, rod-shaped, ubiquitous bacterium that is part of the normal flora of the intestinal tract. Colibacillosis in dogs and cats is primarily a problem in neonatal puppies during the first week of life as part of the fading puppy syndrome; neonatal kittens are affected less frequently. It is also a contributing factor to severe fatal hemorrhagic gastroenteritis associated with enteric viral infections in dogs of all ages.[43–45] Disruption of the integrity of the intestinal mucosa by viral infection seems to be an important factor, allowing for invasion of *E. coli* and septicemia in dogs and puppies beyond weaning age. Inadequate absorption of antibody from colostrum and inadequately developed immune functions of newborn puppies are important factors in the susceptibility of neonatal puppies to colibacillosis. Enterotoxigenic strains of *E. coli* have been associated with vomiting and diarrhea in dogs as possible primary pathogens, similar to the effects of virulent strains of *E. coli* in pigs and cattle.[43, 46]

Clinical signs of colibacillosis are primarily those of endotoxic shock. They include depression, deficits of central nervous system functions, anorexia, diarrhea, weakness, cyanosis, hypothermia, and death. Acute death may occur from endotoxic shock. Definitive diagnosis depends on isolation of *E. coli* from blood or tissues at necropsy. Grossly, post-mortem lesions are not pathognomonic but usually consist of congestion of blood vessels in the intestines, liver, and lungs, with hemorrhages that involve both the serosal and mucosal surfaces present in the lungs and intestines. Gram-negative rods can be seen microscopically in impressions or sections of tissues.

Treatment involves replacement of electrolytes and

fluids, administration of antibiotics, and measures aimed at combating shock.[47] Corticosteroids used in conjunction with antibiotics have been shown to be therapeutically beneficial in cases of colibacillosis with signs of endotoxic shock.[48] Transfusions with plasma replace proteins lost from the circulation and also provide protection against the lethal effects of endotoxin in dogs.[49] Antibiotics or antimicrobial agents are mandated in *E. coli* septicemia. The antibiotic of choice should be based on isolation and testing for antibiotic sensitivity. However, antibiotic therapy should be initiated with gentamicin and ampicillin while waiting for the laboratory results, after which treatment can be modified as indicated.[50] Therapy is often unsuccessful in dogs with signs of endotoxic shock. Antibiotics may enhance the severity of the endotoxic shock by causing increased release of endotoxins as bacteria are being killed by the antibiotics. Flunixin meglumine and corticosteroids may be indicated to combat shock.[45, 47]

Campylobacteriosis. Campylobacteriosis is an acute enteritis caused by *Campylobacter jejuni*, a leading cause of acute enteritis in humans.[51] It has recently been implicated as an enteropathogen in dogs and cats and as a cause of zoonotic disease in humans.[52–54] *C. jejuni* is a small, motile, gram-negative, curved, spiral-shaped rod. Isolation of *C. jejuni* requires the use of special selective media and controlled atmospheric conditions for incubation. Because these special techniques are required, the organism can commonly be overlooked during routine microbiologic examination of feces.[55] *C. jejuni* is isolated more frequently from young animals housed in kennels, strays, and dogs and cats with concurrent enteric infection with parasites, bacteria, or viruses.[55–57] Transmission of infection is by the fecal/oral route directly from the ingestion of feces or indirectly through the ingestion of contaminated food or water. The organism can survive outside the host for two to five weeks in milk or water and for up to a month in infected feces.[51, 58] Houseflies have been shown to be mechanical vectors.[59]

Canine campylobacteriosis is characterized by lassitude and a watery diarrhea that may or may not contain blood or mucus; tenesmus and vomiting have also been observed.[60] The incubation period varies from one to seven days and the course of the illness ranges from seven to ten days. Gnotobiotic dogs developed a superficial erosive colitis after experimental infection, whereas involvement of the jejunum and ileum has been reported in normal dogs.[61] *C. jejuni* is known to produce two exotoxins: an enterotoxin and a cytotoxin. The role of the enterotoxin in humans appears to be similar to that of the cholera toxin, which mediates a secretory diarrhea.[62] In contrast to dogs, cats seem to experience milder clinical signs and have lower rates of infection. The reported prevalence of *C. jejuni* ranged from 4 per cent in the U.S. to 45 per cent in England in cats housed in humane shelters and animal pounds.[63, 64]

Although no clinical efficacy trials have been conducted in animals, it has been reported that erythromycin (which is the drug of choice in humans) or tylosin eliminated infection in dogs and cats.[54, 55] Since the disease is usually self-limiting, pets may only need treatment if clinical signs persist and they become dehydrated. In these animals, fluid and/or antibiotic therapy is recommended. The oral route of administration may be used since vomiting usually does not occur with campylobacteriosis. Feces should be cultured from one to four weeks post-therapy to confirm the effectiveness of treatment. It should be noted that the duration of excretion in untreated pets can vary from one to four months.[65]

Recently pet-to-human transmission has been recognized as an important route for the spread of infection. Most human cases are associated with newly acquired diarrheic puppies and kittens.[66–68] Veterinarians should advise owners of infected animals to practice appropriate hygienic measures, i.e., thorough hand washing, to prevent transmission of infection to themselves.

Salmonellosis. Salmonellae are gram-negative, nonspore forming rods. They colonize the villous lining of the ileum and multiply intracellularly. The release of endotoxins accounts for many of the clinical signs, while some strains of *Salmonella* increase adenyl cyclase activity in the gut, which leads to secretory diarrhea. Of the more than 148 serotypes isolated from dogs, *S. typhimurium* and *S. anatum* are recovered most frequently.[69, 70] In cats, the former species predominates.[71]

Infection is through the oral route and usually involves direct contact with the organism. Sources of infection in pets are ingestion of contaminated, raw, or commercial foods,[72, 73] scavenging,[74] unsanitary environment, or coprophagia. Cats appear to be more resistant to infection than dogs, as evidenced by their lower isolation rates.[75, 76] In dogs, the prevalence of *Salmonella* infection ranges from 4 to 28 per cent.[74, 77–81] There have been several reports of a seasonal prevalence for salmonellosis, with increased rates of isolation of *Salmonella* spp in the late fall and early winter.[82, 83] The actual fecal shedding of the organism may be quite sporadic and precipitated by stress.[81, 84]

Clinical salmonellosis is uncommon in mature dogs and cats. Young animals are more susceptible to infection.[83] Clinical signs are typical of endotoxemia with severe gastroenteritis and include vomiting; bloody, malodorous diarrhea; fever; anorexia; dehydration; depression; and incoordination. Severe leukopenia is a striking clinicopathologic finding. Septicemia may occur, with subsequent localization in the lung, kidney, liver, and uterus. Pneumonia, pyelonephrosis, necrotizing hepatitis, abortion, and stillbirth have all been associated with *Salmonella*.[85–87] The acute phase of the illness lasts four to ten days but intermittent diarrhea for up to one month can occur. Fecal shedding of the organism occurs on average for about six weeks in dogs and four weeks in cats.[71] Diagnosis is confirmed by isolation of the organism from fecal or tissue specimens or by serologic testing. Differential diagnosis includes intestinal parasitism, colibacillosis, canine distemper, infectious canine hepatitis, canine parvovirus, enteric coronavirus, and feline panleukopenia. At necropsy, gross lesions include mucoid, hemorrhagic enteritis, dehydration, pallor, petechial or ecchymotic hemorrhages on various organs, pneumonia, and mesenteric lymphadenopathy. Specimens to be submitted for culture include lymph nodes, bone marrow, spleen, liver, heart, blood, and intestine.

Therapy depends upon the severity of illness. Parenteral fluid replacement is indicated with acute *Salmonella* gastroenteritis. Indomethacin, a prostaglandin inhibitor, has been used experimentally to combat the effects of endotoxin and prevent increased intestinal secretion of fluids.[88] Antimicrobial therapy should be reserved only for those animals that show signs of systemic illness and only after culture and testing for antibiotic sensitivity have been completed. Routine use of antimicrobials may potentiate drug resistance mediated by the transfer of plasmids.[84, 89] Also, such therapy may prolong fecal shedding of the organism and precipitate a carrier state. Many *Salmonella* organisms are sensitive to chloramphenicol and trimethoprim but are resistant to ampicillin and streptomycin.[71, 84]

Prevention involves isolation of infected animals and good sanitation and hygiene. Salmonellosis is a zoonotic disease. Humans have acquired the disease from pets.[90, 91] Most human cases occur in children who have had contact with contaminated pet feces. Diarrheic young animals are believed to present a greater risk to their owners than clinically normal mature animals. Organisms are shed in higher numbers in feces from diarrheic animals. Aborted fetuses also represent a health hazard.

Tyzzer's Disease. The intracellular, gram-negative, spore-forming rod *Bacillus piliformis* is the etiologic agent of Tyzzer's disease. Although originally described as a disease in laboratory animals, it has been diagnosed in cats and dogs, usually of weaning age.[92, 93] The organism is part of the normal intestinal flora of rodents, in which disease is usually associated with stress. It is thought that dogs and cats acquire infection from contact with rodent feces. Depression, weakness, abdominal pain, hypothermia, and anorexia are clinical signs observed in cats and dogs.[92, 93] A small amount of dry, pasty feces is more a consistent finding than diarrhea. Death occurs 24 to 48 hours after clinical signs appear. Treatment has not been successful because animals die before therapy can take effect. Tyzzer's disease should be considered in the differential diagnosis of liver disease, especially in the young animal that has been stressed.

Diagnosis is made primarily at necropsy. The principal lesion consists of diffusely distributed, circular, white-to-grayish necrotic foci in the liver. The mesenteric lymph nodes may be enlarged and contain small abscesses. Thickening and congestion may also be apparent in the terminal ileum and proximal colon. Microscopically, focal areas of hepatic and ileal necrosis are evident.[94] Long, slender rods may be observed in the cytoplasm of hepatic and intestinal epithelial cells when the tissues have been stained by Giemsa, Gomori, or Warthin-Starry techniques. Since methods for the reliable cultivation of the organism on artificial media have yet to be developed,[95] inoculation of specimens directly into embryonating chicken eggs or mice is used for isolation and is confirmatory.

Yersiniosis. The organism *Yersinia enterocolitica* is a gram-negative, small rod or coccobacillus. It has been isolated from the feces of a variety of clinically normal animals, including dogs and cats, in which it is thought to be a commensal. However, in young dogs *Y. enterocolitica* has been associated etiologically with persistent diarrhea of several weeks' duration, characterized by frequent defecation of soft stools with streaks of blood and mucus, tenesmus, and absence of systemic illness. Human cases of yersiniosis have been linked to infected household pets, wherein dogs were suspected of transmitting the disease to humans.[99] Although yersiniosis has been identified as a zoonosis, dogs appear not to be a major source of infection for humans. Isolation of the organism from feces is suggestive of the disease, but since it is often isolated from feces of clinically normal dogs, caution should be exercised in making a diagnosis based only on isolation of the organism from feces. Because of zoonotic potential, antibiotic therapy should be implemented in dogs or cats with positive fecal cultures with or without signs of disease. Trimethoprim-sulfamethoxazole, tetracycline, and gentamicin have been used with success to treat the disease and eliminate fecal shedding of the organism.[96, 97]

Bacterial Overgrowth. A chronic diarrhea in German shepherds older than eight months of age has been described in which there is overgrowth of bacteria in the proximal portion of the small intestine.[98–100] Normal flora of the intestinal tract grow to excessive numbers in the duodenum, apparently due to a decrease in the production of gastric acid and an increase of pH of the proximal portion of the small intestine.[98] Excessive numbers of *E. coli*, enterococci, and *Clostridium perfringens* have been found in duodenal secretions.[99] The bacteria produce excessive amounts of folic acid, which enters the circulation and is detected as an increased concentration in the serum of affected dogs. There is a concurrent decrease in serum concentration of vitamin B_{12}, apparently due to binding of the vitamin by the excessive numbers of bacteria in the intestine. Clinical signs observed in affected dogs include chronic weight loss and persistent or recurrent diarrhea that may be watery and fetid. Affected dogs improve with antimicrobial therapy, vitamin supplements, and restriction of diet to bland foods.[99, 100] The diarrhea can be expected to recur, with periodic antimicrobial therapy required to manage the condition.

SYSTEMIC BACTERIAL DISEASES

Leptospirosis. Leptospirosis is a zoonotic disease caused by spirochetes, which are long, slender, spiral-shaped bacteria that may have hooked ends. They are actively motile and are difficult to stain and culture. All pathogenic strains of *Leptospira* belong to one species, *Leptospira interrogans*, of which there are many serovars. In the United States, the majority of cases of canine leptospirosis are caused by *Leptospira canicola* and *L. icterohaemorrhagiae*. Clinical leptospirosis is rare in cats.[101] Rats and mice are susceptible to infection and they serve as a primary reservoir of infection for *L. icterohaemorrhagiae*.[102] Dogs are the primary reservoir of infection for *L. canicola*.[101]

Infected animals shed spirochetes in their urine, which contaminates water, soil, and animal feed if these are not protected from urine contact. Moist, alkaline soils favor the survival of these organisms in the environment. Disease incidence appears to be seasonal, with more cases being reported in summer and early fall. The principal mode of transmission is indirect, through exposure to contaminated food, water, or soil, but it can be direct, by contact with infected urine. Infection occurs by penetration of the skin or mucous membranes by the spirochetes. After penetration by the spirochete, leptospiremia occurs, with dissemination to the kidneys, liver, and other organ systems where colonization occurs. Infected animals as carriers may shed leptospires in the urine for long periods of time. Various toxins are thought to cause tissue necrosis.

The disease may be latent or acute. Clinical signs, when present, are related to disorders of the liver, kidney or vasculature.[103] Anorexia, vomiting, and fever are often the first observed signs. Hemorrhagic gastroenteritis, myalgia, polyuria, polydipsia, necrotic stomatitis, and icterus occur later in the disease process. Hematologic abnormalities include thrombocytopenia, leukocytosis with a left shift, and increased plasma fibrinogen.[104–106] Biochemically, blood urea nitrogen (BUN), serum alanine aminotransferase (ALT, formerly SGPT), serum lactic dehydrogenase (LDH), serum aspartate aminotransferase (SGOT), serum alkaline phosphatase (SAP), and serum bilirubin may be increased.[105] Urinalysis may show pyuria, proteinuria, and/or bilirubinuria. Differential diagnoses include acute toxic nephrosis or hepatopathy, distemper, infectious hepatitis, and erlichiosis. Definitive diagnosis is by culture of the organism from fresh urine or blood or by direct visualization of leptospires in urine under a darkfield microscope. Serologic testing on paired serum samples can provide a definitive diagnosis if there is a tenfold or greater rise in titer between the first and second serums. Guinea pig inoculation may also be used to isolate the organism.

Pathologic changes include petechial and ecchymotic hemorrhages on many serosal surfaces; the lungs may be edematous. Focal ulcerations of the buccal cavity or tongue may be seen. Hepatomegaly and icterus are common findings with *L. icterohaemorrhagiae* infections, while enlarged, pale kidneys are associated with *L. canicola* infections.

Massive doses of penicillin (50,000 units/lb) and dihydrostreptomycin (5 mg/lb) used in combination intramuscularly for seven to ten days is the recommended therapeutic regimen.[106] Dihydrostreptomycin is necessary to keep the organism from being harbored in the kidney and causing a carrier state. Unless the animal is properly treated with dihydrostreptomycin, a carrier state lasting one to four years may develop, with organisms continuing to be shed in the urine.[101] When treating infected animals, gloves should be worn and all materials that come in contact with infected animals should be disinfected, autoclaved, or incinerated. Supportive therapy involves correction of dehydration and electrolyte disturbances. Blood transfusions may be needed when the patient's hematocrit is very low. Because of the zoonotic potential of the disease, owners should be advised to take precautions against exposure by avoiding contact with urine and by disinfection of premises.

Canine Brucellosis. During the mid to late 1960s *Brucella canis* was recognized as a new species of *Brucella* and was linked to abortions and reproductive disorders of dogs.[107, 108] It is a gram-negative coccobacillus that is difficult to grow on ordinary bacteriologic media. It is antigenically related to *B. ovis*, but it differs from most species of *Brucella* by the absence of a lipopolysaccharide antigen in its cell wall that has endotoxic properties. *B. canis* has a limited host range. Ruminants and swine are resistant to infection. Wild canids and cats are susceptible to experimental infections. Cats inoculated orally developed bacteremia but pregnant queens did not abort. Human infections with *B. canis* have been documented; they are generally milder than human infections with other species of *Brucella*.[109, 110]

Transmission of *B. canis* involves direct contact with the organism, which is capable of penetrating mucous membranes. Infections usually begin through oronasal, conjunctival, or venereal routes of entry.[111, 112] Intrauterine infections occur, often leading to abortion. Vaginal discharges, placental tissues, and aborted fetuses contain large numbers of organisms. Contact with postparturient or postabortion discharges and tissues is the most common source of infection by the oronasal route. Infected bitches apparently shed the organism only in postgestational vaginal secretions, in milk, or in vaginal secretions during estrus. Congenital infection of pups is common from either vaginal secretions or milk. Susceptible males are more likely to become infected from infected females during estrus by oronasal contact with vaginal secretions than by venereal transmission. Venereal transmission occurs readily from infected males to susceptible females. Infected males shed large numbers of organisms in seminal fluid for several weeks after initial infection. The organism localizes in the prostate and epididymis of infected males, resulting in intermittent shedding in semen and urine for two or more years. Venereal transmission by carrier males is of major concern in breeding kennels, where the disease can be devastating.[112, 113] Transmission among male dogs housed together is probably the result of shedding of *B. canis* in urine and entry through oronasal or conjunctival routes.[114]

Most infections with *B. canis* in dogs are inapparent.[111–113, 115] After the organism penetrates a mucous membrane, it may be taken to regional lymph nodes by lymphatic drainage or it may be phagocytized by macrophages, in which it multiplies as an intracellular parasite.[116, 117] Bacteremia follows and may persist for more than two years if the dog is not treated with antibiotics.[111] Although infection with *B. canis* becomes systemic, infected dogs are not usually systemically ill. Infertility in either males or females, abortions, and the birth of stillborn or weak puppies are the most common manifestations of canine brucellosis. Male dogs may have scrotal dermatitis, testicular atrophy, epididymitis, and/or prostatitis.[114, 118, 119] Infertility in bitches is usually due to early embryonic death. In rare cases either sex may develop lymphadenopathy, discospondylitis, splenitis, anterior uveitis, glomerulopathy, or meningoencephalitis.[113, 120–122]

Diagnosis can be confirmed by isolation and identification of the organism or by serologic testing to determine the titer of antibody to *B. canis*.[114, 123] The organism can be isolated from aborted fetuses, placenta, vaginal discharge, semen, biopsy specimens, or blood. A variety of serologic test procedures have been used in laboratories to detect antibody to *B. canis*.[114] A rapid slide agglutination test (RSAT) is available commercially as an in-office procedure. It is inexpensive, sensitive, and provides results rapidly. It is lacking in specificity and many positive test results are due to cross-reacting antibody to other organisms. Positive test results should always be confirmed by a specific test procedure in a diagnostic laboratory before definitive conclusions are made. In spite of its lack of specificity, the RSAT is a valuable screening procedure since a negative test indicates a very low probability of infection with *B. canis*. Negative test results can occur if the serum sample is collected too soon after initial infection with *B. canis*. When infection with *B. canis* is suspected or there has been known exposure, a dog with a negative RSAT should be retested in a month, since antibody titers may not become detectable until four weeks after infection. All breeding animals should be tested regularly for antibody to *B. canis*, especially within one month of mating. All positive dogs should be eliminated from breeding kennels. An infected stud should not be returned to service even after treatment with antibiotics. If a valuable bitch is infected, isolation, antibiotic therapy, and strict hygiene may allow her to produce healthy puppies. The puppies should be tested to determine that they are free of infection and to eliminate carriers. Maternally derived antibody may cause puppies to test positive until they are several weeks of age. It is necessary to do repeat testing of the puppies to demonstrate declining titer of antibody to a sero-negative status. Pups should remain sero-negative over a period of six months before they are regarded as free from infection.

Because of the intracellular nature of *B. canis*, antibiotic treatment is difficult and all infected animals should be regarded as potential carriers for life. There is a lack of information from controlled studies that have been done to confirm the long-term benefits of antibiotic treatment in eliminating *B. canis*. Titers of antibody decline after treatment but may remain at significant levels for six weeks after the organism has been cleared from the blood. Titers of antibody increase again if relapse of infection occurs after treatment is completed. It is recommended that pet dogs be neutered before treatment with antibiotics to decrease the risk of human exposure to genital secretions and to decrease the risk of transmission to susceptible dogs.[110, 111, 117] The most effective treatment regime described has been the use of minocycline (12 mg/lb or 25 mg/kg orally q12h for 14 days) concurrently with streptomycin (5 mg/lb or 10 mg/kg IM q12h for 7 days).[114, 123] This regime with gentamicin in place of streptomycin has been used to treat pregnant dogs successfully.[114] Unfortunately, it is an expensive treatment regime and the cost may be prohibitive in many instances. Sequential therapy with tetracycline (10 mg/lb or 20 mg/kg orally q8h for 14 days) followed by dihydrostreptomycin (5 mg/lb or 11 mg/kg orally q12h for 14 days) and then trimethoprim-sulfadiazine (7 mg/lb or 15 mg/kg orally q12h for 14 days) was used to prevent abortion due to experimental *B. canis* infection during pregnancy, but bacteremia recurred after whelping.[124] It is because of documented relapses of this type after treatment that dogs should *not* be regarded as free of infection because of having been treated with antibiotics.

Borreliosis. Borreliosis, commonly referred to as Lyme disease, is caused by the tick-borne spirochete, *Borrelia burgdorferi*. Originally described as a human disease in Europe, the disease was first recognized in the U.S. in 1975 in Lyme, Connecticut.[125] The first canine case was diagnosed in New York in 1984.[128]

Borreliosis in dogs is characterized by sudden onset of lameness with hot, swollen joints and possibly a history of exposure to ticks. The lameness initially lasts only a few days but may be recurrent, with the time between episodes ranging from 1 to 23 months.[127] Accompanying the lameness are myalgia, fever, and weakness. Humans exhibit similar symptoms; however, expanding red annular lesions called erythema chronicum migrans appear at the site of the tick bite prior to the onset of lameness. Humans may develop neurologic and cardiac abnormalities.[128]

The primary tick vector is *Ixodes dammini*.[129] Other tick vectors have been implicated and include *Amblyomma americanum*, *Ixodes pacificus*, and *Ixodes scapularis*. White-footed mice and white-tailed deer are probable reservoirs of tick infection.[129–131]

In the United States there are three endemic areas for borreliosis: the Northeast (Massachusetts to Maryland), the Midwest (Wisconsin and Minnesota), and the West (California and Oregon). Clustering of cases have been reported recently in Georgia, North Carolina, Florida, Arkansas, and Texas, which suggests that *B. burgdorferi* has spread from the three endemic areas.

Diagnosis can be accomplished through serology, radiology, immunofluorescence tests, or the direct examination of blood and synovial fluid. Serologic results can be supportive but need to be interpreted with caution since some dogs have subclinical infections. Also, there appear to be serologic cross-reactions with leptospires.[129] Radiologic results should reveal no abnormalities. Microscopic examination of synovial fluid and bacteriologic culturing may provide a definitive diagnosis, but they often yield negative results. Differential diagnoses include Rocky Mountain spotted fever, leptospirosis, rheumatoid arthritis, septicemia, systemic lupus erythematosus, and idiopathic arthritis.

Antibiotic therapy is curative in humans, so the use of penicillin, tetracycline, or erythromycin appears logical in the canine disease.[132] Lissman used 500 mg ampicillin orally every eight hours for ten days to treat the originally reported canine case.[126]

It is not believed that humans are infected directly from dogs, but instead that unattached ticks in the pet's haircoat transfer to people. Cats have also been shown to be a risk factor in that they bring ticks inside their owners' homes. Tick removal from pets and people is the most important method of disease prevention.[130]

Actinomycosis. Actinomycosis is an infection caused by *Actinomyces* spp, which are ubiquitous, gram-positive, filamentous, branching bacilli or coccobacilli.[133] These organisms are microaerophilic to anaerobic, non-acid fast, and appear to be commensals in the mouths of many animals.[134, 135] Infected cats and dogs may present with varying clinical syndromes but usually there is a history of trauma.[136] Young dogs of the hunting breeds are commonly affected. Abscesses with draining tracts, osteomyelitis, respiratory infections with pleuritis, and abdominal masses have all been reported.[136–140] Infections are mainly localized; however, a disseminated form of the disease can occur.[140] Lesions are pyogranulomatous and contain yellow granules ("sulfur granules"), which are actual colonies of the organism.[133] Clinical signs depend on which organ is involved and include fever, emaciation, dyspnea, abdominal distention, and lameness.[136] Clinicopathologic abnormalities are leukocytosis, monocytosis, decreased packed cell volume, toxic neutrophils, hypoglycemia, and hypoalbuminemia.[136] Diagnosis is based on staining and culture of the organism to differentiate it from nocardiosis, a disease it closely resembles. Antibiotic therapy with penicillin is the treatment of choice. Dosages of up to 50,000 IU/lb given IM once daily are required and therapy should be continued until cultures are negative.[133] Debridement and drainage of lesions is also important. Povidone-iodine lavage is advocated when the lesions are localized. The prognosis is good for localized infections.

Nocardiosis. Nocardiosis refers to chronic disease processes caused by one of the three species: *Nocardia asteroides*, *N. brasiliensis*, and *N. caviae*. These are responsible for the majority of canine and feline infections.[141] These organisms are primarily saprophytic and found worldwide in soils. Like the *Actinomyces*, they are opportunistic, gram-positive, filamentous branching bacilli or coccobacilli. Unlike the *Actinomyces*, they are aerobic and may be partially acid-fast.[142] Nocardiosis may be localized or systemic. Localized infection is acquired through injury. Grass awns have been frequently associated with tissue inoculation.[143] The systemic form appears to be more common in this disease than in actinomycosis and is acquired from either ingestion or inhalation.[144] There is a tendency for hematogenous spreading. Cats reportedly have a decreased incidence of disease, with the majority of clinical cases being seen in young dogs. Lowered host resistance may predispose to infection.[145] The disease is not contagious to humans or other animals.[141]

In dogs there may be cutaneous, subcutaneous, abdominal, bone, pulmonary, or central nervous system involvement.[144–149] Clinical signs are referable to the affected organ. With brain involvement, convulsions and incoordination occur. Cutaneous disease is characterized by ulcerative, suppurative lesions with draining tracts. Dyspnea, coughing, and rales occur with pulmonary infection. Other signs are nonspecific and include fever, depression, and dehydration. Differential diagnoses are distemper, neoplasia, chronic abscess, and actinomycosis. Confirmation of the diagnosis is aided by the use of radiology, cytology, and bacteriology. Pleural effusion, lung consolidation, osteomyelitis, and metastatic nodules may be visible radiographically.[141] Cytologic examination of exudates may reveal yellow granules that are actual colonies of organisms; granules are not produced by *N. asteroides*.[145] Aerobic culture of exudates on blood agar or Sabouraud-dextrose agar at 25°C to 37°C reveals adherent, granular colonies with varying pigmentation. Plates should be incubated for at least two weeks before being considered negative.[141] Organisms from colonies should be Gram-stained and tested for acid-fastness by the Hank's method. Pleural and abdominal effusions, lung congestion, cerebral granulomas, lymphadenopathy, and disseminated abscesses are among the gross pathologic findings. Microscopic lesions are necrotic and granulomatous, containing the characteristic organisms.

Treatment involves debridement of granulomatous lesions, drainage and lavage, and antimicrobial therapy. The sulfonamides are the drugs of choice and both the oral and injectable types have been used successfully. Triple sulfa is given intravenously at 60 mg/lb initially, followed by 30 mg/lb twice daily until clinical signs regress and cultures are negative, which may require several months of therapy.[141] Testing for antibiotic sensitivity *in vitro* revealed that minocycline, amikacin, and lincomycin were effective.[150] An *in vitro* synergy existed between erythromycin and ampicillin.[151] In cases with concurrent empyema, chest drains should be employed both to drain and flush the thoracic cavity. Lactated Ringer's solution containing antimicrobials and proteolytic enzymes may be used to lavage the cavity.[141] Failure to treat aggressively results in a poorer prognosis in the systemic disease. The localized cutaneous form of nocardiosis has a better prognosis than the systemic disease.

Tularemia. Tularemia is a naturally occurring disease of wild animals, particularly rodents and rabbits. Humans, and less frequently, dogs and cats, become infected. The etiologic agent is *Francisella tularensis*, a small, gram-negative coccobacillus. The disease has been reported in all 50 states, with the highest incidence in Kansas, Missouri, Oklahoma, Texas, and Utah.[152] The most important reservoirs appear to be rabbits and ticks. Transmission usually occurs through biting arthropods or direct contact with infected animals or their carcasses. Animal bites or scratches, aerosol inhalation, and ingestion of contaminated food or water are all reported routes of infection.[153–155] The organism has also been shown to penetrate intact skin.[156] There have been several reports where humans contracted the disease directly from domestic cats.[153, 155]

Clinical signs in dogs include ulcerative dermatitis, lymphadenopathy, pneumonia, and hindleg paralysis.[157, 158] Cats may present with weight loss, fever, depression, generalized lymphadenopathy, and pneumonitis.[153, 155] The pathogenesis initially involves a localized infection that progresses to a bacteremia with the development of granulomatous necrotic foci in the lymph nodes, liver, lungs, and spleen. Miliary, white to yellow foci appear in the liver, spleen, and lymph nodes, and they can be observed grossly at necropsy. Care should be taken when performing a necropsy because of the ease of transmission to humans. The organism can be isolated from lesions by guinea pig inoculation or on special media that contains cystine.[154] Fluorescent antibody techniques can be used to detect the organism in tissues. Testing suspected clinical cases for rising titer of antibody in paired serums collected two weeks apart can be helpful in confirming a diagnosis.

Treatment with antibiotics, tetracycline, chloramphenicol, streptomycin, or gentamicin is usually effective. Streptomycin is the drug of choice in treating human cases of tularemia; relapses occur more frequently when tetracycline or chloramphenicol has been used.[152] Prevention of tick infestation and of contact with carcasses of diseased animals are important in the prevention and control of tularemia.

Anthrax. Anthrax is one of the oldest recorded infectious diseases. It is caused by *Bacillus anthracis*, a gram-positive, encapsulated rod that has a tendency to form chains during vegetative growth as a facultative anaerobe in the host.[158] Sporulation occurs under aerobic conditions with the formation of centrally located spores that are responsible for resistance to heat and chemical and environmental changes and for the organism's ability to survive in the environment for many years. Certain regions of the United States are known as "incubator areas," where anthrax is endemic: the Mississippi Delta, the California Valley, and the Northern Plains.[159] Spores of *B. anthracis* can survive almost indefinitely in these areas of neutral to slightly alkaline, calcareous soils. Outbreaks of anthrax usually occur after periods of drought followed by heavy rains.

Anthrax occurs in humans and many species of mammals, but swine, dogs, and cats are relatively resistant to infection and disease.[160] Infection occurs from spores entering the host by inhalation, ingestion, or cutaneous penetration. Ingestion of contaminated carcasses is the principal route of entry in dogs and cats.[161] Deaths have occurred in large Felidae fed horse meat from a horse that died from anthrax.[162] After ingestion, spores are carried by phagocytes to local lymph nodes, where vegetation and multiplication occur. The capsule of the vegetative form of the organism provides an antiphagocytic barrier that allows uncontrolled growth. Dissemination occurs via the lymphatics and bloodstream, with invasion occurring in many tissues.[163] Direct tissue necrosis and edema result from the production of a lethal toxin. Anthrax in dogs begins as a localized pharyngitis and gastrointestinal illness. As the infection progresses edema occurs, affecting the lips, face, head, and neck.[161] If septicemia occurs, the dog will become febrile and acute death may occur due to shock, renal failure, and respiratory distress. The disease can be treated successfully if large doses of penicillin or ampicillin are given early enough in the infection to prevent the uncontrolled growth and subsequent toxin production by the organism. Chemical toxicity, acute septicemia, endotoxemia caused by other organisms, and allergic reactions must be considered in the differential diagnosis.

If anthrax is suspected as the cause of death, necropsy should not be performed. Opening of the carcass allows environmental oxygen to stimulate sporulation. Lack of rigor mortis and blood-tinged fluid exuding from body orifices are characteristics suggestive of anthrax. Examination of smears prepared from peripheral blood, blood-tinged fluids, or edema fluid may reveal characteristic rod-shaped bacilli with centrally located spores when stained by gram stain. Fluorescent antibody examination of smears prepared from blood or body fluids can be used to confirm the diagnosis. In the laboratory isolation of the organism is often done by inoculation of guinea pigs since spores may not readily undergo vegetation and multiplication on artificial media. Once growth is established, colonies on blood agar have a "ground glass" appearance with irregular or "Medusa head" margins.[164] All specimens submitted for laboratory diagnosis should be handled with extreme care.

Tetanus. A neurotoxin produced by *Clostridium tetani* is responsible for the disease tetanus. *C. tetani* is a gram-positive, anaerobic rod that produces a terminal, spherical spore that causes the bacterial cell to swell, giving it a "drumstick-like" appearance. These spores are highly resistant to adverse environmental conditions. The organism is found in soil and in the intestinal tracts of animals and humans. Tetanus is rare in dogs and cats because they appear to be relatively resistant to the toxin.[162, 165] Wound contamination is by far the most common mode of infection. The organism may also spread from the intestinal tract and invade tissues following trauma or intestinal surgery.[166] Tetanus has occurred postpartum and in neonates from umbilical infections. Once spores contaminate an area, an anaerobic environment is necessary for their sporulation. Tissue necrosis within a wound creates the proper conditions. Bacterial cells multiply and eventually lyse. Two exotoxins are elaborated upon lysis: tetanospasmin and tetanolysin. It is the former that is responsible for the majority of the clinical signs associated with tetanus. The toxin travels intraneurally, as well as hematogenously.[167] The spinal cord, brain, skeletal muscle motor end-plates, and sympathetic nervous system are all affected. As a result of this toxin, polysynaptic reflexes are disrupted, cerebral gangliosides are bound, release of acetylcholine at the neuromuscular junction is inhibited and sympathetic stimulation occurs.[168, 169] Primary motor neuron damage results in the clinical sign of rigidity.[170]

Stiffness is one of the earliest clinical signs of tetanus. Hyperesthesia with clonic/tonic muscle spasms, which can be elicited by the slightest stimulus, follows. Spasms of the facial masticatory muscles result in the production of "sardonic grin" and "lockjaw," respectively. Muscle spasms may pull the ears closer together on top of the head with the skin folding into wrinkled ridges. A "sawhorse stance" with an erect tail is due to extensor rigidity. Additional signs include prolapse of the membrana nictitans, fever, opisthotonos, and respiratory distress. Tetanus may be localized or generalized, depending on the amount of toxin present.[171] The prognosis is less favorable if the clinical signs progress rapidly. The incubation period ranges from days to months and is related to the distance between the wound and the central nervous system.[172] For example, head injuries have shorter incubation periods than leg wounds. Differential diagnoses include strychnine toxicosis, rabies, eclampsia, cerebrospinal meningitis, and spinal trauma. Laboratory diagnosis involves culture of the organism from specimens placed in anaerobic transport media. Gram stains taken directly from wound exudates may reveal the characteristic gram-positive rods. However, diagnosis is based primarily on the characteristic clinical signs.

The objectives in the treatment of tetanus are to neutralize unbound toxin, prevent further replication of *C. tetani*, and maintain vital functions through the use of sedatives, muscle relaxants, and supportive therapy. Antitoxin should be administered early in the disease to neutralize any free toxin. Once toxin reaches the peripheral nerve fibers or passes through the blood-brain barrier, antitoxin is unable to work.[173] The recommended dosage of antitoxin is 50 to 500 units/lb (100 to 1000 units/kg) of body weight.[165, 166] The animal's sensitivity to the antitoxin should first be tested by injecting 0.1 to 0.2 ml intradermally. If after 30 minutes nothing abnormal is noted, antitoxin can be administered safely by slow intravenous injection.[174] If the site of infection is a localized wound, it should be debrided and flushed to disrupt the anaerobic environment necessary for multiplication of the organism. Large doses of penicillin, ampicillin, or tetracycline should be given to destroy any actively growing bacteria.[175] Sedatives, muscle relaxants, and tranquilizers are all used to reduce clinical signs since there appears to be no single ideal drug. Phenobarbital given either IV or IM at 1 to 3 mg/lb (2 to 6 mg/kg) q6 to 12h is useful for sedation.[167] Diazepam and methocarbamol are the most commonly used central-acting muscle relaxants. Acepromazine given at 0.10 to 0.25 mg/lb (0.25 to 0.5 mg/kg) intravenously every four to eight hours has also been advocated.[167] Supportive care is also important. The animal should be kept in a dark, quiet room or cage to minimize the stimuli that induce spasms. Decubital ulcers should be prevented by laying the animal on heavy padding and turning frequently. Adequate hydration, electrolyte balance, and caloric intake must be maintained. Since tetanus toxoids are not routinely given to small animals, proper wound management and aseptic surgery are necessary in disease prevention.

Botulism. Neurotoxins produced by *Clostridium botulinum*, a gram-positive, anaerobic, spore-forming rod, are responsible for the noncontagious disease botulism. There are eight antigenically different types of neurotoxins: A, B, C1, C2, D, E, F, and G.[176] Types C and D are associated with most cases of animal disease.[177]

Naturally occurring intoxications have been reported in dogs but not in cats.[178–180] Both dogs and cats appear to be relatively resistant to disease. Toxins are usually ingested pre-formed in carrion. There is a direct relationship between the severity of clinical signs and the quantity of toxin ingested.[180] Ingested toxin is absorbed from the gastrointestinal tract and into systemic circulation, where it eventually reaches cholinergic neuromuscular junctions. Neuromuscular blockage results from a decreased release of acetylcholine from the presynaptic nerve fibers.[181] The incubation period in dogs can range from hours to several days after the ingestion of the toxin.[178, 182]

The major presenting problem is that of a lower motor neuron disorder with a progressive, symmetric, ascending weakness that can result in complete quadriplegia. This paralysis is flaccid in nature. Dogs remain mentally alert and can still wag their tails. Cranial nerve function can also be altered with decreased palpebral, gag, and pupillary light reflexes. Bradycardia and decreased respiratory rates are also noted. There are no abnormalities found in hematology or serum chemistry with routine lab work.[178, 179] Differential diagnoses to be considered include polyradiculoneuritis ("coon hound paralysis"), tick paralysis, and myasthenic disorders. A definitive diagnosis involves the demonstration of toxin in ingested materials, vomitus, serum, or feces through neutralization tests in laboratory rodents. Isolation of the organism from feces is difficult but may lend support to the diagnosis. Electromyography is helpful in the differentiation of botulism from polyradiculoneuritis, tick paralysis, and myasthenia gravis.[183] There are no gross or microscopic lesions with botulism.[183] Treatment is primarily supportive. Adequate hydration and nourishment should be maintained. Enemas and emetics given at first recognition of the disease may help to remove any toxins left in the gastrointestinal tract. Decubital ulcers may be prevented by the use of padding and frequent turning of the patient. Ophthalmic ointments may be necessary to prevent exposure keratitis, which results from inability to close the eyelids. Oral and parenteral penicillin have been used but their efficacy is doubtful since signs are due to ingested toxins rather than replicative organisms. Antitoxins are available but should be administered during onset of signs because once toxin becomes bound, antitoxins will not help to regress signs. The use of neuromuscular potentiators such as guanidine hydrochloride or 4-aminopyridine, to increase acetylcholine release, has yielded variable therapeutic results.[180, 184, 185]

MISCELLANEOUS BACTERIAL INFECTIONS

Pyoderma. Bacterial infection of the skin is commonly referred to as pyoderma. The condition occurs more frequently in dogs than cats and is usually secondary to other dermatologic problems, e.g., ectoparasitism, allergic dermatitis, or hormonal imbalances.[186] There are three categories of pyoderma based on the degree of dermal involvement: surface, superficial, and deep. Coagulase-positive strains of staphylococci are the most important primary pathogens; however, secondary invaders include the gram-negative rods *Proteus*, *Pseudomonas*, and *Escherichia coli*.[187] Clinically, the characteristic primary skin lesions (pustules and papules) may be seen only early in the course of the infection. More commonly excoriations, erosions, and crusts are seen. Diagnosis involves cytology and aseptic culture of an intact pustule. Skin biopsies may also be useful in differentiating pyoderma from subcorneal pustular dermatosis, demodecosis, dermatophytosis, and pemphigus. Systemic antibiotic therapy is needed to resolve pyoderma. Selection of a proper antibiotic ideally should be based on the results of culture and testing for antibiotic sensitivity; however, lincomycin (10 mg/lb orally q12h), erythromycin (5 to 8 mg/lb orally q8h PO), trimethoprim-sulfadiazine (14 mg/lb orally once daily), cephalothin (10 to 15 mg/lb orally twice daily), and gentamicin (2 mg/lb IM or SQ q12h) have all been used with success.[187] The minimum length of treatment should be seven days. Additionally, the affected areas should be clipped and hydrotherapy performed to remove crusts and scabs. Daily bathing with povidone iodine or benzoyl peroxide shampoos may also be beneficial. Elimination of the primary cause of the pyoderma is the key to successful treatment. Persistent chronic pyoderma may occur in immunosuppressed patients.

Conjunctivitis. The bacteria isolated from the majority of cases of canine conjunctivitis are similar to the normal conjunctival flora, i.e., coagulase-positive staphylococci, beta-hemolytic streptococci, *E. coli*, and *Proteus mirabilis*.[188] Disease is most often secondary to infections with canine distemper virus, herpesviruses, *Chlamydia*, or *Rickettsia*. Clinical signs include lacrimation, purulent ocular discharge, and photophobia. Specimens for bacteriologic culture should be collected on moist swabs that were rolled over the most affected portion of the conjunctiva. Cytology may also be a valuable aid. Topical therapy is usually sufficient with a broad-spectrum antibiotic such as triple antibiotic ointment (neomycin-polymyxin-bacitracin). Every effort should be made to uncover a primary cause for the disease.

Otitis Externa. Otitis externa is an infection of the external ear canal and is a common problem in dogs and cats. The bacteria most commonly associated with the condition are *Staphylococcus aureus*, *Staphylococcus intermedius*, *Streptococcus* spp., *Pseudomonas aeruginosa*, *Proteus* spp., and *Pasteurella multocida*.[189] Staphylococci and streptococci are part of the normal ear flora.[190] Predisposing factors to infection are pendulous ears, parasites, moisture, and hair in the ear canal. The color of the exudate can be valuable in making a presumptive etiologic diagnosis. Brown exudate is most often associated with a gram-positive bacterial infection while a yellow exudate may be indicative of a gram-negative infection. Microscopic examination of exudate is helpful in differentiating bacterial infections from infections with yeasts or ear mites. Before starting therapy, the ears should be cleaned thoroughly with a ceruminolytic agent. Topical therapy is usually effective. Antibiotic otic preparations containing neomycin, polymyxin, gentamicin, or chloramphenicol are useful in the treatment of gram-positive infections. Gentamicin otic preparations are indicated when a gram-negative rod is involved. To decrease inflammation, topical corticosteroids are useful. To normalize ear pH, 1 to 2 per cent acetic acid solutions are valuable. Treatment should be continued for a minimum of two weeks. In chronic conditions, culture and sensitivity is indicated. Lateral ear canal resection may also have to be performed as a last resort.

Otitis Media and Interna. Otitis media and interna usually result from a chronic otitis externa.[191] Clinical signs vary from pawing at the ears to signs of brain stem involvement: ataxia, head tilt, nystagmus, circling, and facial nerve paralysis. Radiographs are useful in making a diagnosis. Osteomyelitis of the tympanic bulla may be present. An otoscopic examination should be performed to determine whether or not the tympanic membrane is intact. If it is intact and bulging, a myringotomy with subsequent dilute povidone-iodine flushes may be helpful. Broad-spectrum antibiotics applied topically and given systemically should be used, based on results of culture and sensitivity. In cases of experimental *Pseudomonas* infection, lavage with EDTA, trimethamine, TRIS buffer, and lysozyme increased the effectiveness of antibiotics.[192] Surgical intervention may be a last resort. Lateral ear canal resection and bulla osteotomy are two frequently used procedures.

Abscesses. The majority of abscesses result from bite or other puncture wounds. *Pasteurella multocida*, streptococci, coliforms, and anaerobic fusiform bacteria are the most common isolates from abscesses.[193, 194] Clinical signs are nonspecific and include fever, depression, and anorexia. Swelling, pain, heat, and skin discoloration over the puncture site may not always be present; undetectable abscesses may be part of the fever of unknown origin syndrome in cats. Most of the bacteria involved are susceptible to the penicillin derivatives ampicillin and amoxicillin; however, systemic administration may fail to diffuse into walled-off abscesses.[194] Therefore, hot-packs are used to help the abscess mature so that it may be lanced. Flushing of the cavity with hydrogen peroxide, povidone-iodine solution, or antibiotics has been successful.

Vaginitis. Vaginitis is more common in the bitch than the queen. The presenting complaint is that of a purulent vaginal discharge or that the dog licks or chews around her vulva. Upon physical examination the vaginal mucosa appears inflamed but signs of systemic illness are absent. Metritis, pyometra, or cystitis must be ruled out as causes of the discharge. Diabetes mellitus tends to predispose female dogs to vaginitis. A nonspecific vaginitis is fairly common in puppies prior to their first estrus and usually clears up after the estrus cycle is completed. An abundance of neutrophils and bacteria is found on cytologic examination. Cultures taken through a sterile vaginal speculum may indicate the causative bacteria. Interpretation of culture results may be difficult because the normal vaginal flora can be potential pathogens.[195] In general, gram-negative organisms are most often associated with infections.[196, 197] Systemic antibiotic therapy can be used and should be based on results of bacterial culture and testing for antibiotic sensitivity. Vaginal antibiotic suppositories or povidone-iodine douches used daily have also been advocated.

Metritis. Metritis is an inflammation of the endometrium and myometrium. Usually it is a disease of the postpartum period and is associated with retained placentas and/or fetuses or difficult labor and delivery. Systemic signs of illness, as well as a malodorous, mucopurulent vaginal discharge are observed. In severe cases shock may be a presenting sign. A thickened, enlarged uterus is apparent on physical examination. Diagnosis is by a history of recent whelping or queening and clinical signs. Vaginal cytology reveals a septic process with the presence of neutrophils, erythrocytes, and bacteria. Hematologically, a neutrophilic leukocytosis occurs, followed by a leukopenia in more advanced cases.[198] Bacterial culture and testing for antibiotic sensitivity should be performed in order to determine the proper selection of antibiotics for systemic therapy. Uterine lavage with dilute povidone-iodine may be warranted. Fluid therapy may be indicated in cases with a shock component. Ovariohysterectomy may be necessary in severe, life-threatening, or chronic cases of metritis.

Cystitis. In the healthy animal the bladder is a sterile environment. The usual cause of cystitis is the ascending of bacteria through the urethra.[199] Bacterial cystitis is more frequent in dogs than cats and is more common in females than males.[200] Hematuria, pollakiuria, and dysuria are the characteristic signs of cystitis. Signs of systemic illness are usually not evident unless reflux from the bladder into the ureters results in pyelonephritis. The bladder is thickened and painful to physical examination. Diagnosis is through bacterial culture of the urine, urinalysis, and clinical signs. Cystocentesis is the method of choice for urine collection; catheterization and midstream collection may also be used but contamination with normal flora is more likely to occur. The bacteria most often involved in canine urinary tract infections in dogs are *Escherichia coli*, *Staphylococcus aureus*, *Proteus mirabilis*, streptococci, *Pseudomonas* spp, and *Klebsiella pneumoniae*.[200, 201] Therapy involves the use of antimicrobial agents that reach the urine in high concentrations. Effective antimicrobials include chloramphenicol (15 mg/lb or 33 mg/kg orally q8h), trimethoprim-sulfadiazine (6 mg/lb or 13 mg/kg orally q12h), and ampicillin (10 mg/lb or 26 mg/kg orally q8h). Therapy should be continued for a minimum of seven days. Urine should be recultured three days after therapy is terminated to determine the efficacy of treatment and to monitor the possibility of chronic infection.

RICKETTSIAL AND CHLAMYDIAL DISEASES

Rickettsia and *Chlamydia* are gram-negative, obligate intracellular organisms that, except for one rickettsial agent, have not been cultured on artificial media. They have cell walls and intracellular organelles similar to bacteria. Although *Chlamydia* have many characteristics in common with *Rickettsia* and were once classified as a family of the order *Rickettsiales*, the *Chlamydia* are now recognized as a distinct group of organisms and have been assigned to the order *Chlamydiales* based on biochemical and morphologic differences from *Rickettsia*.[202] Three families of rickettsia are recognized in the order *Rickettsiales*: *Rickettsiaceae*, *Bartonelleaceae*, and *Anaplasmataceae*.[202] Diseases in dogs and cats are caused by members of the *Rickettsiaceae* and *Anaplasmataceae* families. *Hemobartonella felis* and *H. canis* are classified in the family *Anaplasmataceae* and they are the etiologic agents for feline and canine hemobartonellosis, respectively. There is only one genus of *Chlamydia*, which contains two species: *Chlamydia psittaci* and *Chlamydia trachomatis*. With the exception of a few isolates from rodents, all strains of *C. trachomatis* are human isolates. In contrast, there are many biologically different strains of *C. psittaci* that infect both birds and mammals (including humans). *Chlamydia* have not been associated with disease in dogs.[203]

Feline Chlamydiosis (Feline Pneumonitis). In cats, a feline strain of *C. psittaci* causes a relatively mild, persistent upper respiratory disease referred to as feline pneumonitis. Persistent and recurrent chlamydial infections occur in cats due to inadequate immune responses to the chlamydial infection. Topical treatment with tetracycline ophthalmic ointment for two to four weeks is often necessary to clear up conjunctivitis in cats. Treatment should be continued for two weeks after clinical signs have disappeared. Chlortetracycline and oxytetracycline given orally provide temporary improvement but signs return within two to three weeks after therapy is terminated. Administration of low doses for two months may prevent recurrence of disease.[204] Attenuated chlamydial feline pneumonitis vaccines are available for use in cats, but vaccine-induced immunity provides limited protection against infection with the feline pneumonitis agent. Vaccinated cats become infected with the feline pneumonitis agent following challenge with feline *Chlamydia*, but morbidity and severity of signs are decreased in vaccinated cats when compared to controls.[205] Feline pneumonitis is discussed in greater detail in Chapter 69 in conjunction with feline respiratory disease complex.

Hemobartonellosis. The clinical signs of feline hemobartonellosis are manifestations of acute to chronic anemia and include weight loss, pale mucous membranes, weakness, depression, anorexia, and occasionally splenomegaly and icteric mucous membranes. Mortality may exceed 30 per cent in untreated cats.[206] *Hemobartonella felis* replicates epicellularly on the surface of erythrocytes, resulting in parasitemia. Parasitemia usually occurs in a recurring cyclic pattern correlating with alternating decreases and increases in packed cell volume (PCV). Parasitized erythrocytes are bound by macrophages in the spleen, resulting in splenic sequestration of erythrocytes with decreases in PCV and in the level of parasitemia. The organisms are destroyed or removed from erythrocytes by macrophages. Previously parasitized erythrocytes return to the circulation with a resultant increase in PCV. Organisms undergo new cycles of replication, with another increase in parasitemia and the initiation of another cycle of fluctuating parasitemia and changing PCV.[207] The primary mechanism in the development of anemia appears to be erythrophagocytosis of infected erythrocytes by macrophages in the spleen. With persistent infection and recurrent fluctuating levels of parasitemia, erythrocytes become more fragile and have shortened life span. Immune responses to the organism may be accompanied by immune responses to altered or unmasked antigens on the surface of erythrocytes and result in immune-mediated destruction of erythrocytes. Infected cats become Coombs' positive.

Transmission of *H. felis* requires the transfer of infected blood from an infected cat to a susceptible cat. Natural transmission is primarily by fleas, but other blood sucking arthropods may also transmit the infection. Four stages in the course of feline hemobartonellosis have been defined: preparasitemic, acute, recovery, and carrier.[206] The preparasitemic stage averages about two weeks in length and can be regarded as the incubation period from time of initial infection to the onset of clinical signs associated with the recurring cyclic parasitemias that occur during the acute stage of the disease. The acute stage lasts from one to two months and is the period from the first to the last major episode of parasitemia.[206] Clinical signs of disease become evident during the acute stage. It is during the acute stage that cats die; some die quickly from marked parasitemia and anemia. Cats that develop adequate immune responses to the organism and are able to overcome the anemia with adequate bone marrow hematopoiesis enter the recovery stage of the disease. The recovery stage is the period of time from the last cycle of parasitemia and anemia until the PCV has returned to normal and becomes stabilized.[206] Treatment of cats with oxytetracycline (10 mg/lb or 20 mg/kg orally q8h to q12h for 3 weeks) is beneficial in effecting recovery, but it does not eliminate the carrier status.[206] Glucocorticoids, e.g., prednisolone at 1 mg/lb or 2 mg/kg orally q12h, are indicated for treatment of severely anemic cats to suppress erythrophagocytosis and immune-mediated hemolytic anemia.[208] Blood transfusions may be indicated when the PCV decreases to 15 or less. Clinical hemobartonellosis in dogs has been successfully treated with oxytetracycline (20 mg/lb or 40 mg/kg orally q12h for 2 weeks).[209]

Natural transmission of *H. canis* to susceptible dogs is by the brown dog tick, *Rhipicephalus sanguineus*, which is an important reservoir because of transstadial and transovarial passage of the organism.[206] Experimentally, *H. canis* has been transmitted by transfusion of infected blood and by oral administration of infected blood. Clinical signs of disease are rare in dogs infected with *H. canis* unless there is a concurrent disease process that is immunosuppressive. Splenectomy has been necessary to produce clinical signs of disease experimentally with *H. canis*.[206] Inapparent infection or carrier status has been found in as many as 50 per cent of dogs in some surveys.[210]

The diagnosis of hemobartonellosis in either dogs or cats depends on detection of the organism on the surface of erythrocytes in thin smears of peripheral blood. Wright-Giemsa stain reveals *H. felis* as cocci, ring, or rod-shaped organisms 0.5 to 1.0 microns in diameter on the surface of an erythrocyte from infected cats. There may be as many as 15 to 20 individual organisms on the surface of an erythrocyte or as few as one or two organisms. Individual organisms of *H. canis* are similar in appearance to *H. felis* but there is tendency for *H. canis* to form chains of organisms across the surface of erythrocytes from infected dogs.[206] *Hemobartonella* organisms must be differentiated from Howell-Jolly bodies and cytauxzoon organisms in feline erythrocytes. Due to the cyclic nature of *Hemobartonella* parasitemia, the absence of organisms in a stained blood smear does not necessarily rule out hemobartonellosis. Hematologic and biochemical changes are nonspecific and are of limited value in diagnosing hemobartonellosis.

Salmon Poisoning Disease. Salmon poisoning disease (SPD) is a highly fatal rickettsial disease of dogs and wild canids.[211, 212] It is caused by *Neorickettsia helminthoeca*, which is transmitted by the trematode *Nanophyetus salmincola*. The etiologic agent of SPD is found in all stages of the life cycle of the trematode, from egg to adult fluke.[212] The essential first intermediate host for the trematode is a small pleurocerid snail, *Oxytrema silicula*, which is found only in streams along the coastal areas of Washington, Oregon, and California. Salmon poisoning disease occurs only in the limited geographic areas where the snail is found along the Pacific Northwest coast of the United States on the western slopes of the Cascade Mountains, from northwestern California to southwestern Washington.

The snail is the essential first intermediate host in the complex life cycle of the trematode. Eggs of the trematode are shed in the feces of definitive hosts that are infected with the adult fluke. The eggs undergo change into miracidiae, which are ingested by the snail, the first intermediate host. The miracidiae develop into cercariae, which leave the snail and penetrate the second intermediate host, usually a salmonid fish, where further development occurs into metacercariae, which become encysted in tissues of the fish with a tendency for localization in the kidneys. Development into mature flukes occurs in the intestines of the definitive host, usually raccoons, bears, or canids, that eat metacercaria-infected raw fish. Clinical signs of SPD occur only in dogs and wild canids that become infected with *N. helminthoeca* by transfer of the rickettsial organisms from the adult flukes to the intestinal epithelium and intestinal lymphoid tissue. The rickettsial organism enters the blood and is disseminated to many organ systems. The incubation period is usually about seven days, but may be as long as a month after eating parasitized fish.

Sudden onset of high fever, greater than 104°F (40°C), accompanied by anorexia is the first sign of SPD. Depression, weakness, and weight loss occur as the disease progresses. Vomiting and diarrhea may occur, with the diarrhea getting progressively worse and often consisting primarily of blood terminally. Death usually occurs seven to ten days after the onset of clinical signs in untreated dogs. There is marked enlargement of lymph nodes and aspirates from lymph nodes often contain cells with characteristic intracytoplasmic inclusion bodies revealed by Giemsa stain. The clinical signs of SPD are similar to those of canine distemper and canine parvovirus disease, which must be considered in the differential diagnosis. Hematology is of limited value in diagnosing SPD, since the total white cell counts vary greatly, from leukopenia to leukocytosis. The disease can be treated successfully provided that antibiotic therapy and supportive fluid therapy are started early in the course of the disease. Tetracyclines are the antibiotics of choice, although penicillin, chloramphenicol, and sulfonamides are also effective.[211] Due to vomiting and diarrhea, antibiotics should be administered by parenteral routes rather than orally. Oxytetracycline at 10 mg/lb (20 mg/kg) IV or IM q12h for 5 to 7 days is a recommended antibiotic treatment schedule. Fluids and electrolytes, antiemetics, and antidiarrheals are indicated in most cases. In severe cases of bloody diarrhea, whole blood transfusions may be necessary.

Canine Ehrlichiosis. Canine ehrlichiosis refers to a variety of clinical syndromes in dogs and wild canids caused by infection with *Ehrlichia canis* or *E. equi*, rickettsial organisms transmitted in nature by the brown dog tick, *Rhipicephalus sanguineus*.[213–215] Canine ehrlichiosis occurs in temperate, tropical, and subtropical countries of the world in accordance with the geographic range of the brown dog tick, except for Australia, where canine ehrlichiosis has not been reported.[213] The brown dog tick is the only known vector for *E. canis*.[213] In addition to *E. canis* and *E. equi*, dogs are also infected by *E. platys*, which causes infectious cyclic thrombocytopenia.[216, 217] The vector for *E. platys* has not been definitely established although it is presumed to be tick-borne.[215]

Ehrlichia canis was first recognized in the United States in 1962.[218] The role of *E. canis* as a significant pathogenic *Rickettsia* in dogs came to light in the late 1960s when it was established as the etiology of tropical canine pancytopenia.[219, 220] *Ehrlichia equi* infection in dogs was first recognized as an unusual form of *E. canis* due to the replication and formation of morula primarily in the cytoplasm of neutrophils rather than primarily in lymphocytes.[221, 222] The host range for *E. canis* is limited to dogs and wild canids, whereas *E. equi* is capable of infecting many species of mammals.[222] Although the patterns of infection are similar, *E. equi* causes less severe disease in dogs than *E. canis*.

Ticks become infected with *E. canis* while feeding on dogs that are rickettsemic during the first two weeks after the dog became infected. The organisms replicate in hemocytes, midgut cells, and salivary gland cells of infected ticks. The organisms can persist in ticks for more than five months. Ticks transmit *E. canis* transstadially but not transovarially. Ticks are the primary reservoir of infections, with both male and female ticks capable of transmitting the infection to dogs. Transmission from ticks to dogs occurs when an infected tick ingests a blood meal and its salivary secretions containing the organism contaminate the feeding site.[214] *E. canis* can be transmitted by transfer of blood from an infected dog to a susceptible dog. Transmission has occurred by blood transfusion from dogs chronically infected for more than five years.[214] However, the chronically infected dog does not serve as a reservoir for natural transmission to other dogs. The ecology and epizootiology of *E. equi* are not as well defined as for *E. canis*, but it is assumed that they are similar to those of *E. canis*.

The incubation period for the acute phase of canine ehrlichiosis is 8 to 20 days following either natural or experimental infection.[215] Clinical signs during the acute phase of canine ehrlichiosis are usually mild, consisting of nonspecific pyrexia, anorexia, lymphadenopathy, oculonasal discharge, and dyspnea.[213–215, 223] Most dogs recover after one to two weeks without treatment, although they remain persistently infected and some will develop chronic disease one to six months later. Inapparent infections are common. *E. canis* enters the bloodstream or lymphatics and localizes in reticuloendothelial cells of the liver, spleen, and lymph nodes where it replicates primarily in mononuclear macrophages and lymphocytes; lymphoreticular hyperplasia occurs in these organs. Infected mononuclear cells disseminate the infection to other organ systems, where they apparently interact with endothelial cells of small vessels and induce vasculitis or perivascular inflammatory cell response after migration into subendothelial tissue.[214, 215] Hematologic changes are variable during the acute phase of canine ehrlichiosis. Slight leukopenia is common during the period of clinical signs and is usually followed by leukocytosis. Thrombocytopenia is a consistent finding in canine ehrlichiosis. Anemia develops in some dogs during the acute phase.

Following the acute phase of infection, a subclinical phase occurs during which the persistence of antigen in infected cells serves as a stimulus to the immune system. Antibody titers continue to rise and immunocompetent dogs usually eliminate *E. canis* during this phase of infection.[214, 215] Dogs that do not eliminate the infection with *E. canis* progress to the chronic phase of disease. The subclinical phase of infection usually occurs six to nine weeks after initial infection and lasts from one to four months. Clinical signs are absent, but hematologic changes persist, consisting of thrombocytopenia, nonregenerative anemia, and variable white blood cell responses from leukopenia to lymphocytosis and monocytosis. Regenerative anemia may occur in dogs with concurrent babesiosis.[214, 215]

Chronic ehrlichiosis occurs in dogs that fail to develop an effective immune response to the organism. Hypergammaglobulinemia results from persistent antigenic stimulation and is suggestive of an ineffective immune response, probably an ineffective cell-mediated immune response, since both specific antibody and immune cells are essential for immunity.[224–227] Chronic weight loss, poor appetite or anorexia, pale mucous membranes due to anemia, weakness, and depression are the most common clinical findings in chronic canine ehrlichiosis.[213–215, 223] The clinical signs are a reflection of pathophysiologic changes resulting from severe anemia and from perivascular infiltration of many organ systems with lymphoreticular and plasma cells.[213–215] Hypoplasia of bone marrow occurs, leading to pancytopenia and increased destruction of platelets.

Bleeding tendencies with hemorrhages in mucous membranes, retina, abdominal skin, or almost any organ system are common manifestations of severe chronic ehrlichiosis due to persistent thrombocytopenia and marked decrease in platelets.[213, 214] Epistaxis in dogs that have general signs of chronic ehrlichiosis is regarded as distinctly characteristic of the disease, although epistaxis occurs in only a small proportion of cases.[213, 215, 223] Severe pancytopenia and hemorrhage secondary to thrombocytopenia occur primarily in German shepherds with chronic ehrlichiosis and were first recognized during the Vietnam war. This resulted in the disease's being named tropical canine pancytopenia.[219, 220] Dogs with the chronic phase of canine ehrlichiosis may have signs of interstitial pneumonia, renal failure, reproductive disorders, arthritis, and meningoencephalitis.[213, 215, 223, 228]

A presumptive diagnosis of canine ehrlichiosis can be made, usually on the basis of history and clinical signs. However, the signs of acute ehrlichiosis are similar to those of Rocky Mountain spotted fever, from which it must be differentiated. Thrombocytopenia and nonregenerative anemia are the most consistent hematologic findings in both acute and chronic cases. Anemia may be regenerative when there is concurrent infection with *Babesia canis*. Laboratory diagnosis by detection of *E. canis* in smears of peripheral white blood cells is not efficient in clinical practice because of the variable presence of the organism in peripheral blood. Pancytopenia and hypoplasia of bone marrow are usually found in chronic cases. Laboratory confirmation of suspected canine ehrlichiosis is best done by serologic testing for antibody to *E. canis*. An indirect fluorescent antibody (IFA) test provides specific results using infected cell cultures as the antigen. Antibody to *E. canis* can be detected between two and three weeks after infection. Titers of antibody equal to or greater than 1:10 by the IFA test are regarded as positive. Titers increase to maximal levels by about three months after infection and may become as high as 1:10,240.[229] Titers of antibody persist at high levels as long as infection with *E. canis* is present. After *E. canis* is eliminated by tetracycline therapy or by an effective immune response of the dog, titers of antibody decline over a period of 6 to 9 months and often become undetectable within 12 months after treatment.[230] The IFA test is a useful aid for detecting healthy carriers of infection in that titers of antibody persist at high levels. A second course of therapy is indicated in dogs that have persistent titers of antibody or that have recurrence of clinical signs.

Tetracyclines are effective in treating the acute phase of ehrlichiosis, with improvement in clinical condition often occurring within 24 to 48 hours after therapy is initiated. The response is less favorable in dogs with chronic ehrlichiosis. Tetracycline or oxytetracycline (10 mg/lb or 22 mg/kg q8h for 14 to 21 days) eliminates *E. canis* in about 75 per cent of dogs. Doxycycline is effective orally or IV at dosages of 2.5 mg/lb (5 mg/kg) once daily for seven to ten days in acute infections and 5 mg/lb (10 mg/kg) once daily for seven to ten days in chronic infections. Doxycycline is less nephrotoxic than tetracyclines and is the drug of choice in chronic infections with evidence of renal insufficiency. Imidocarb dipropionate has been found to eliminate infection in about 80 per cent of dogs with a single intramuscular injection at a dosage of 2.5 mg/lb (5 mg/kg).[231]

Supportive fluid therapy and blood transfusions may be required in dogs with severe chronic ehrlichiosis. Corticosteroids, e.g., prednisolone (2 mg/lb or 5 mg/kg daily for 3 to 5 days) or methylprednisolone acetate (1 mg/lb or 2 mg/kg IM once only), are beneficial in combating the effects of thrombocytopenia and bleeding disorders. Other anti-inflammatory or immunosuppressive drugs may be used. Treatment with immunosuppressive drugs should last a few days only, since prolonged use may further compromise an already immunosuppressed, leukopenic dog and interfere with elimination of the organism during antibiotic therapy.

It should be noted that *E. canis* has been confirmed as causing disease in a human.[229] The patient had clinical symptoms and signs resembling those of Rocky Mountain spotted fever in humans, except that there was no cutaneous rash. The diagnosis was confirmed by the IFA test for antibody to *E. canis* and by the morphologic appearance of infected peripheral blood lymphocytes. Subsequent serologic surveys have revealed that about eight per cent of humans with tick-associated illnesses in a ten-state region tested positive for antibody to *E. canis*; in one state 11 per cent of patients who tested negative for Rocky Mountain spotted fever were positive for antibody to *E. canis*.[232] Further studies may indicate that *E. canis* should be considered as another tick-borne zoonotic rickettsiosis.

Infectious Cyclic Thrombocytopenia of Dogs. Infectious cyclic thrombocytopenia of dogs is caused by *Ehrlichia platys*, a rickettsial organism that is antigenically unrelated to *E. canis* or *E. equi*.[216, 217] The organism replicates only in platelets of dogs and can be transmitted by IV inoculation of blood from infected dogs into dogs negative for antibody to *E. platys*. The natural mode of transmission probably involves ticks, but this has not been clearly established. Platelets containing basophilic inclusions appear in the blood seven to twelve days after experimental inoculation.[216, 233] Most infected platelets contain only a single compact inclusion, but two or three inclusions in a single platelet are not uncommon in Giemsa-stained smears. By day four after the initial appearance of infected platelets, 30 to 60 per cent of platelets may contain inclusions with the total platelet count remaining normal. Within the next three to four days there is a marked decrease in the platelet count to less than 20,000/μl.[216] Infected platelets are not usually detectable during the period of minimal platelet count. Platelet counts return to normal within three to four days after the disappearance of the organism from platelets. Organisms reappear in platelets followed by another decrease in platelet count. This cyclic pattern of parasitemia followed by thrombocytopenia has a periodicity of one to two weeks. With each succeeding cycle the percentage of infected platelets decreases until eventually platelets with inclusions are found only sporadically and thrombocytopenia becomes less pronounced. The hematologic changes eventually cease to occur. There are no consistent changes in other leukocytes of infected dogs.

Except for a transient elevation in rectal temperature, signs of illness are not usually evident in dogs infected with *E. platys*.[216] There has been one case report of uveitis in a dog with nonregenerative anemia and thrombocytopenia.[233] Platelets contained one to three densely basophilic inclusions. The dog was negative for antibody to *E. canis* but had a titer of 1:100 to *E. platys*. The dog responded to therapy with oral tetracycline (10 mg/lb or 22 mg/kg q8h for 14 days) and topical ophthalmic ointment.[233] Although infections with *E. platys* are usually asymptomatic, *E. platys* would probably enhance concurrent infections with *E. canis* or *Babesia canis*.[214, 215]

The diagnosis of *E. platys*–induced infectious cyclic thrombocytopenia can be made by detection of characteristic basophilic inclusions in platelets stained with Giemsa, or by demonstrating antibody to *E. platys* in serum. Detection of inclusions in platelets is not reliable because of the cyclic nature of the parasitemia and the declining percentage of platelets that are infected with time. An indirect fluorescent antibody (IFA) test has been developed that provides a reliable specific diagnosis.[217] Antibodies to *E. platys* appear in serum of infected dogs within two to three weeks after infection and immediately after the peak of the first parasitemia or concurrently with the initial thrombocytopenia.[217] The antibody is specific for *E. platys* and does not cross react with *E. canis* or *E. equi*. The results of a serologic survey using the IFA test indicated that infection with *E. platys* was widely distributed but at a low rate (5 per cent) in healthy, random-source dogs, whereas 35 per cent of thrombocytopenic dogs had antibody.[217] The highest prevalence of antibody to *E. platys*, 50 per cent positive, was found in dogs that were positive for antibody to *E. canis*, suggesting that concurrent infections are relatively common.

Rocky Mountain Spotted Fever. Rocky Mountain spotted fever (RMSF) is a tick-borne, zoonotic, rickettsial disease of humans, dogs, and small mammals in the Western hemisphere. It is caused by *Rickettsia rickett-*

sii.[202, 234–236] The geographic occurrence of RMSF is determined by the distribution and ecology of ticks that are the vectors of *R. rickettsii*.[236] In the United States, the American dog tick, *Dermacentor variabilis*, is the primary vector from the central plains states and Texas to the East coast; the woodtick, *Dermacentor andersoni*, is the primary vector from the Rocky Mountain states to the West coast. The Lone Star tick, *Amblyomma americanum*, has been implicated in transmission of RMSF to humans in the United States.[234] The brown dog tick, *Rhipicephalus sanguineus*, has been implicated in transmission of RMSF in Mexico and South America.[236] In the Mediterranean region of southern Europe and North Africa, the brown dog tick is the primary vector in transmission to humans and dogs of *R. conorii*, the causative agent of Mediterranean spotted fever (MSF), which is similar to RMSF in humans and dogs.[237]

Many species of small mammals are susceptible to infection with either *R. rickettsii* or *R. conorii*, and they serve as the primary mammalian reservoirs of the agents in nature. Ticks become infected when larvae and nymphs ingest large numbers of *Rickettsia* while feeding on small mammals that are rickettsemic.[234] If the magnitude of infection in the immature ticks is adequate, the infection persists and progresses during maturation into adult ticks. Transovarian transmission is a major mechanism for maintaining an infected population of ticks.[234, 236] Infected adult ticks transmit the disease to humans and dogs during attachment and feeding. Contact with or handling of infected ticks can result in human infections in the absence of tick attachment.[236] Removal of engorged, infected ticks from pets can result in human infections. The role of dogs in the maintenance of the agents of RMSF or MSF in nature is primarily as carriers of infected ticks, since only adult ticks feed on dogs and the level of rickettsemia in dogs is too low to result in infection of ticks.

The portal of entry into the body for *R. rickettsii* is usually through the bite of an infected tick. Endothelium is the target cell system for infection with *R. rickettsii*. An obligate intracellular parasite, *R. rickettsii* invades and replicates in endothelial cells, resulting in necrosis of cells and increased vascular permeability.[234–236] The endothelial necrosis extends to cells of the intima, media, smooth muscle of arterioles, and occasionally venules, with the occurrence of perivascular cuffing. Loss of fluids and electrolytes from the vascular pool to extravascular spaces results in edema and vascular collapse. Vascular necrosis allows for extravasation of blood, which leads to the characteristic skin rash and petechial hemorrhages in RMSF. Vascular thrombosis and microinfarction occur systemically, resulting in clinical signs related to pathophysiologic changes in many organ systems.[236] Vascular collapse and death may occur within a few days of the onset of clinical signs, which emphasizes the importance of an early diagnosis and therapy with tetracyclines or chloramphenicol.

Most infections with *R. rickettsii* in dogs are inapparent.[238–242] However, clinical signs of RMSF in dogs may be mild and transient or they may be severe and fatal.[243–245] The clinical signs of RMSF in dogs are similar to those of acute canine ehrlichiosis and canine distemper.[234, 235, 246] The most common clinical findings in dogs are depression, listlessness, fever (greater than 104° F (40° C) in more than 80 per cent of cases), anorexia, vomiting, and diarrhea.[234–236, 244, 245, 247] Conjunctivitis with scleral injection, mucopurulent oculonasal discharge, nonproductive cough, and lymphadenopathy are frequently observed. As the disease progresses, petechial and ecchymotic hemorrhages may occur in mucous membranes and nonpigmented skin; edema occurs in the extremities and dependent areas, anterior uveitis and retinal hemorrhage occur frequently, and bleeding disorders with hematuria, melena, and epistaxis may occur.[234–236] Extravasation of blood and fluid loss can lead to shock, cardiovascular collapse, renal failure, and death. Death may be preceded by signs of meningoencephalitis and myelitis. The signs of multisystemic disease usually develop within one to two weeks after onset of clinical signs. Necrosis of skin on extremities and dependent areas may occur in dogs that survive the acute phase of the disease.

The incubation period ranges from two to three days after experimental inoculation to as long as one to two weeks after the attachment of ticks in naturally acquired infections.[245, 247] The length of the incubation period and the severity of signs of acute disease vary according to the dose of *R. rickettsii* at the time of initial infection. Transient, slight leukopenia occurs early in the disease, followed by leukocytosis, which becomes more pronounced with increasing duration of clinical signs. Leukocytosis may be the initial hematologic finding when dogs with RMSF are presented, depending upon how long the dog has been ill before it is examined. Toxic neutrophils may be observed. Thrombocytopenia occurs in most dogs with RMSF and is believed to be due to platelets being consumed by damage to vascular endothelium.[234, 236] Synovial fluid from dogs with joint pain and swelling usually contains inflammatory cells, predominantly neutrophils. Biochemical changes reflect tissue damage and are not diagnostically specific for RMSF.[236, 247]

Because the clinical signs of RMSF in dogs are similar to those of acute canine ehrlichiosis and canine distemper, confirmation of the diagnosis depends on the results of laboratory tests. Thrombocytopenia has been regarded as an indicator of either ehrlichiosis or RMSF[235]; however, thrombocytopenia has been found to occur also during infection with canine distemper virus.[237] Thrombocytopenia concurrent with leukocytosis would be suggestive of RMSF, since leukopenia is more common with ehrlichiosis and canine distemper. It is recommended that dogs presenting with signs suggestive of RMSF or acute distemper in spring and summer months from geographic areas of endemic RMSF (South Atlantic, southeastern, and south central states in the United States) be treated with tetracycline (10 mg/lb or 22 mg/kg orally q8h for 14 days). Chloramphenicol (7 mg/lb or 15 mg/kg orally q8h for 14 days) is an alternative antibiotic, especially in young dogs less than six months of age (to avoid staining of teeth), but it should be used with caution if the dog is anemic. Dramatic improvement in clinical condition should occur within 48 hours in dogs with acute RMSF or acute ehrlichiosis. Antibiotic treatment should be continued for at least two weeks in order to increase the chance for elimination of the

RMSF organism. Complete recovery from RMSF depends on the immune response of the dog. Supportive therapy is important in dogs with signs of shock and bleeding disorders, but IV fluid therapy must be used with caution because of the increased vascular permeability.[236]

Isolation and identification of *R. rickettsii* provides the most definitive diagnosis but it is time consuming, expensive, and not routinely performed by most laboratories. Rickettsial organisms may be detected intracellularly in endothelial cells from impressions or sections of tissues using the Giemsa stain.[248] The organisms stain red with the cellular background staining green. The presence of such organisms is supportive of a diagnosis of RMSF but it is not specific for *R. rickettsii* since all *Rickettsia* and *Chlamydia* stain similarly. Specific identification of the organism in tissue impressions or biopsies can be done by direct immunofluorescent or immunochemical methods, which provide a definitive diagnosis.[236] Direct fluorescent antibody (FA) testing can be done by human or veterinary laboratories that have conjugated antibody specific for *R. rickettsii*. Biopsies of skin taken from edematous, reddened areas of vascular damage are preferred, but biopsies of normal skin from the vascular-rich inguinal area have been found to yield positive FA results for the organism.[236] Negative results with the FA test do not categorically rule out RMSF. Negative results may occur if the dog has been on tetracycline or chloramphenicol therapy for 48 hours or longer before the biopsy is taken. Positive findings early in the course of the disease facilitate implementation of appropriate antibiotic therapy. Incorrect diagnosis and delay in treatment are contributing factors to fatal disease in human cases of RMSF and have similar adverse effects in dogs.[236]

A definitive diagnosis of RMSF can be made by serologic testing for a rising titer of antibody in paired serums collected two to four weeks apart. It is advisable to collect a serum sample when the dog is first examined in the event that it should be needed as the first sample for paired serums. The first serum should be stored frozen until the second serum is collected two to four weeks later. Both serums should be submitted and tested at the same time. Antibody titers to *R. rickettsii* do not become detectable until two to three weeks after infection and, therefore, should be undetectable or at a low level during acute illness when the first serum is collected. A titer of antibody four times greater in the second serum compared to the first serum, i.e., a fourfold rise in titer of antibody, indicates recent infection concurrent with the clinical signs and is the basis for confirmation of the diagnosis serologically.

The most useful serologic test, and the test being used by essentially all laboratories that do serologic testing for RMSF, is an indirect fluorescent antibody (IFA) test commonly referred to as microscopic immunofluorescence (Micro-IF). Dilutions of serum from the patient are added to a slide containing fixed cells infected with *R. rickettsii*. After a period of incubation, the slides are washed to remove the serum proteins and a conjugate of anti-species-specific immunoglobulin is added to the slide to detect specific antibody that has bound to *R. rickettsii*. Laboratories equipped to test human serums for antibody to *R. rickettsii* are not usually capable of testing canine serums because they require anti-canine IgG conjugates. Most state veterinary diagnostic laboratories or veterinary schools in RMSF-endemic areas do testing for antibody to *R. rickettsii*. The IFA or Micro-IF has been used for serologic surveys as well as for diagnosis of individual cases.[240–245] Titers less than 1:64 are regarded as negative. Recently infected dogs usually have titers greater than 1:128, with many dogs developing titers greater than 1:30,000.[236] Titers decline after recovery from infection but may remain above the 1:128 level for a year or longer. Titers greater than 1:128 indicate prior infection with *R. rickettsii*, which is the basis for serologic surveys using single serums.[242] However, demonstration of a rising titer of antibody in paired serums is required for serologic diagnosis of RMSF or suspected active infections in dogs.[245]

PROTOZOAL DISEASES

COCCIDIAL DISEASES

The coccidia that infect dogs and cats are classified into six genera: *Besnoitia*, *Cryptosporidium*, *Cystoisospora*, *Hammondia*, *Sarcocystis*, and *Toxoplasma*, under the families Cryptosporidiidae and Sarcocystidae.[249] They are basically intestinal parasites of dogs and cats, with *Toxoplasma* causing disease due to disseminated extraintestinal stages of infection. Some species of *Cystoisospora* may penetrate the intestinal wall and form monozoic cysts in extraintestinal tissues, where they become arrested without further replication or development. Coccidia that were formerly in the genus *Isospora* are now included in the genus *Cystoisospora*, which are the most commonly recognized coccidia infecting dogs and cats. Coccidia in the genus *Eimeria* have not been documented as infecting dogs or cats, although ingested oocysts may pass through the intestinal tract unaltered and they may be detected in feces of dogs or cats.

Intestinal coccidial infections in dogs and cats are usually asymptomatic except in young puppies or kittens or in animals that are immunosuppressed or concurrently infected with other agents.[250–252] Coccidial infections may predispose to increased severity of enteric viral infections. The patterns of infection and "disease-causing potential" are similar for all the genera of coccidia in dogs and cats except *Toxoplasma*, which differs considerably. In general the factors that affect the pathogenicity of intestinal coccidia are the number of oocysts ingested, the location of the infection in the intestine, the depth of penetration in the intestinal mucosa by the replicating organisms, the size of developing endogenous stages, strain differences of the same species, and the age and immunologic status of the host.[251]

Cystoisospora. Coccidia in the genus *Cystoisospora* are the most common cause of intestinal coccidiosis in dogs and cats.[249, 251] They are species specific, with *Cystoisospora canis*, *C. ohioensis*, *C. burrowsi*, and *C. neorivolta* infecting dogs and *C. felis* and *C. rivolta* infecting cats. Dogs and cats are definitive hosts and become infected by ingestion of sporulated oocysts or small rodents that serve as paratenic hosts. Ingested oocysts excyst in the presence of bile and free sporozoites infect epithelial cells of the small intestine, where two to four generations of asexual reproduction occur before gametogony results in the development of microgamonts and macrogamonts. After fertilization, a zygote is formed and enclosed in a cyst wall. Oocysts are released from infected cells and shed in feces unsporulated. In the external environment the oocysts undergo sporulation and become infective for the initiation of another cycle of infection and replication. The prepatent period ranges from five to eleven days, depending on the species of *Cystoisospora*.[249] Free sporozoites may penetrate the intestinal wall and form monozoic cysts in extraintestinal tissues of either the definitive host or the paratenic host. Ingestion of monozoic cysts in a paratenic host shortens the prepatent period.

Besnoitia. Cats are the only definitive hosts for members of the genus *Besnoitia*, which are naturally heteroxenous coccidias. Intermediate hosts for this genus include ruminants, small rodents, opossums, snakes, and lizards. Only *B. wallacei* and *B. darlingi* have been reported in the United States; *B. besnoiti* has been found only in Africa and the Middle East. Cats become infected by ingesting tissue cysts in mice and other small vertebrates. Unsporulated oocysts are shed in feces after a prepatent period of 11 to 13 days; patency lasts about one week. Sporulated oocysts are not infective for cats. Cats do not shed oocysts upon reinfection. Clinical disease has not been associated with *Besnoitia* infections.

Hammondia. Hammondial infections are regarded as uncommon in dogs and cats. However, the prevalence may be underestimated because of the small size of the oocyst, the relatively short period of patency, and the absence of clinical signs.[253] Three species of *Hammondia* have been recognized: *H. heydorni* which infects dogs, foxes, and other wild canids, and *H. hammondi* and *H. pardalis* which infect cats. The first two were once known as the "small part" of *Isospora bigemina*.[249] Like *Besnoitia*, the life cycle of *Hammondia* is heteroxenous; sporulated oocysts do not infect the definitive host. Dogs, cats, and related carnivores are definitive hosts. Many species of animals, including herbivores and rodents, serve as intermediate hosts.[253] Upon ingestion of infected meat, dogs and foxes shed unsporulated oocysts in the feces after a prepatent period of five or more days. Patency lasts only about three days. Cattle, goats, sheep, and other ruminants are intermediate hosts for *H. heydorni*. Muscle, but not visceral organs, contains infective stages of *H. heydorni*.[253] *H. hammondi* infects cats only. Mice, rats, and other rodents serve as intermediate hosts. Cats become infected by ingesting cyst-infected mice, and start shedding unsporulated oocysts in six to nine days. The patent period is usually seven to 14 days. Cats may periodically shed oocysts for several weeks. Reinfection may occur.[249] Felidae are definitive hosts for *H. pardalis,* and mice are the only known intermediate hosts. The prepatent period is five to eight days, and the patent period is five to 13 days.

Sarcocystis. Coccidia of the genus *Sarcocystis* have been found in the musculature of fish, reptiles, birds, and mammals. Carnivores serve as definitive hosts and herbivores or omnivores serve as intermediate hosts. There are at least 14 species of *Sarcocystis* that can infect dogs and 11 other species that infect cats as definitive hosts.[249] *S. horvathi* is the only species that infects both dogs and cats.

The definitive host becomes infected by ingesting bradyzoites contained within muscle cysts of intermediate hosts. Oocysts or free sporocysts are not infective for the definitive host. Upon ingestion of the infected intermediate host by a suitable definitive host, bradyzoites undergo sexual reproduction; asexual reproduction does not occur with sarcocystis. The resultant zygote then matures into an oocyst. Oocysts sporulate within the intestine to an isosporoid type. Both oocysts and free sporocysts are shed in the feces and are infective for the intermediate host. Shedding lasts 60 days or longer.[254] No immunity occurs to prevent reinfection. Clinical enteric disease has not been documented in dogs and cats with natural infections of sarcocystis.[249]

The intermediate host becomes infected by ingestion of sporocysts or sporulated oocysts which undergo excystation with release of sporozoites that penetrate the intestinal mucosa and invade endothelial cells, where they undergo several generations of merogony in vascular endothelium in many organs. The resultant merozoites subsequently enter muscle cells and develop into bradyzoite-containing cysts, which are infective for the definitive hosts.[249] The tissue forms of many genera of coccidia may be nonpathogenic in their intermediate hosts. However, when normal animals receive large numbers of oocysts or prenatal, neonatal, or immunodeficient hosts are infected, some of these extraintestinal replicative forms are quite pathogenic. For example, acute sarcosporidiosis in cattle and swine causes widespread proliferation of endothelial cells, resulting in generalized lymphadenopathy, hemolytic anemia, abortions, edema, and hemorrhagic diathesis.[249] Although coccidia may be pathogenic for the intermediate herbivorous hosts, they are usually considered nonpathogenic for the definitive carnivorous hosts with the exception that they have been reported to be pathogenic for neonates and severely immunosuppressed dogs and cats. Mild diarrhea or soft stools, occasionally with spots of blood, may be observed in infected puppies and kittens.

Since most coccidial infections are subclinical, the primary cause of diarrhea in animals may be another agent, with the coccidia being found as an incidental or secondary infection. When extraintestinal forms of coccidia occur in infected definitive hosts, granulomatous dermatologic disease can occur, but rarely.[255] More likely, extraintestinal monozoic cysts cause clinical signs in hosts with immunodeficiency syndromes. Dogs have been found to develop conjunctivitis, facial edema with congestion of the eyelids and the commissures of mouth, oculonasal discharge, and hyperemia of skin on the abdomen after oral administration of oocysts of *Caryospora*. Diagnosis of intestinal coccidial infection of dogs and cats is made by identification of the oocysts in feces. Some coccidians can be distinguished by the size and morphologic appearance of the oocysts. Other coccidians can be identified by the inoculation of oocysts into the proper intermediate host and examining this host for the clinicopathologic features of the resulting disease and the location and structure of the cysts that are produced in tissues.

Sulfonamides have been the drugs of choice for the treatment of coccidiosis in puppies and kittens.[249] The initial dose of sulfadimethoxine should be 25 to 30 mg/lb (50 to 60 mg/kg) orally as a single dose on the first day of treatment with the dosage reduced to 10 to 15 mg/lb (25 to 30 mg/kg) orally once daily for 10 to 14 days. Sulfadiazine has been reported to be effective at a dosage of 50 mg/lb (100 mg/kg) daily with 15 mg/lb (33 mg/kg) orally q8h for 5 days.[256] Nitrofurazone at a daily dosage of 10 mg/lb (20 mg/kg) orally for 7 days has also been effective. Nitrofurazone can be administered in drinking water by adding 2 gm of 4.59 per cent powder to one gallon of water as the sole source of drinking water for 7 days. Amprolium has been found to be an effective treatment of coccidiosis in kenneled puppies.[249, 250] Amprolium is not yet approved for use in dogs, but it is approved for use in treating coccidiosis in cattle and is marketed under the trade name Corid.* A convenient method for treatment of kenneled research puppies has been to provide amprolium in water as the sole source of drinking water for ten days. Corid* solution (9.6 per cent amprolium) is added to water at the rate of 22 to 25 ml (5 teaspoons or 1½ tablespoons) per gallon of water. Treatment with amprolium for longer than 10 to 12 days can result in signs of thiamine deficiency. Treatment should be discontinued after ten days, but can be repeated in two weeks if evidence of coccidial infection is still present. Treatment of bitches soon after whelping has been found to be beneficial in preventing the spread of coccidiosis to newborn puppies.[257] Good sanitation is essential in preventing coccidiosis in puppies and kittens. Contact with intermediate or paratenic hosts must be prevented and uncooked meat should not be fed to dogs or cats.

Cryptosporidium. Cryptosporidium is a genus of coccidia in the suborder Eimeriina, family Cryptosporididae; there are four species: *Cryptosporidium baileyi*, *C. maleagridis*, *C. muris*, and *C. parvum*.[258, 259] The first two, *C. baileyi* and *C. meleagridis*, infect birds, but neither infects humans or other mammals. The last two species, *C. muris* and *C. parvum*, infect mammals. *C. parvum* has a broad host range and has been associated with severe gastroenteritis in animals and humans.[258, 259] Cryptosporidiosis has become a major problem in humans with immunodeficiency syndromes. In recent years, public health concern about cryptosporidiosis has heightened because of documented transmission from animals to humans.[258] Dogs and cats are relatively resistant to cryptosporidiosis but naturally occurring infections and disease have been reported. Cryptosporidiosis was reported in an adult cat with clinical signs of persistent diarrhea, weight loss, and anorexia.[260] *Cryptosporidium* has been associated etiologically with diarrhea in neonatal puppies and in dogs with immunodeficiency secondary to canine distemper.[261, 262] Experimental infections in healthy pups resulted in asymptomatic infection with shedding of oocysts in feces.[258] Asymptomatic infections in cats have been reported.[249] Cryptosporidial infections are usually self-limiting in immunocompetent humans and animals. The prognosis is poor in immunodeficient patients, in which treatment is usually ineffective. Cryptosporidiosis is diagnosed by detecting oocysts in fecal samples using Sheather's sugar flotation medium or by demonstration of the organism in intestinal tissue by microscopic examination of intestinal biopsies or specimens collected at necropsy.[249] The oocysts are very small and range in size from four to eight microns in diameter, depending on the species.

Toxoplasmosis. Toxoplasmosis is caused by the ubiquitous *Toxoplasma gondii*, with essentially a worldwide distribution that correlates with the presence of cats throughout the world.[249, 263, 264] Cats and other Felidae are the only definitive hosts for *T. gondii*, and they may serve also as intermediate hosts due to encystment of extraintestinal replicating forms of the organism in tissues of many organs.[265] Many species of vertebrates serve as intermediate hosts, including amphibians, fish, reptiles, birds, and mammals.[263, 264, 266] Cats become infected by ingestion of sporozoites in sporulated oocysts or by ingestion of extraintestinal cysts of bradyzoites or tachyzoites in tissues of intermediate hosts. Two different patterns of replication occur in cats after infection: an enteroepithelial cycle and extraintestinal cycle.[249, 264] The enteroepithelial or intestinal cycle of infection occurs only in cats and other Felidae, whereas the extraintestinal cycle of infection is the pattern that occurs in all species that serve as intermediate hosts.

The enteroepithelial cycle of infection with *T. gondii* in cats differs considerably from the pattern of infection and replication of other coccidia. The exact mechanisms of early stages of infection and replication are not known when infection results from ingestion of sporozoites or tachyzoites. When infection results from ingestion of encysted bradyzoites, three stages of replication and development of the organisms are recognized: the multiplying merozoite stage, the gametocyte stage, and the oocyst stage.[266] The time from ingestion of bradyzoites until oocysts are shed in feces, the prepatent period, is about three to five days. The prepatent period after ingestion of tachyzoites is usually five to ten days, but it may be longer, and the prepatent period after ingestion of sporozoites is a minimum of 20 days but it may be 4 weeks or longer.[249, 264] Cats usually shed oocysts for less than two weeks. Shedding of oocysts may recur during periods of severe stress and immunosuppression from debilitating diseases or from chemotherapeutic drugs.

The extraintestinal or systemic cycle of infection with *T. gondii* occurs when the organisms penetrate the intestinal mucosa and multiply by asexual budding in cells in the submucosa.[249, 264, 266] The rapidly multiplying organisms are referred to as tachyzoites.[264] Infected cells rupture after becoming filled with tachyzoites, allowing the infection of other cells to occur. Tachyzoites infect and multiply in almost any type of cell. They invade gut-associated lymphoid tissue and become disseminated by lymphatics, blood, and infected macrophages to essentially all organ systems, with liver, lungs, and lymphoid tissue being the tissues where the greatest concentration of tachyzoites occurs. Within two weeks

*MSD Agvet, Division of Merck & Co., Inc., P.O. Box 2000, Rahway, NJ 07065.

the host begins to develop immunity, which causes the rate of multiplication to decrease. The slowly multiplying organisms are referred to as bradyzoites, which become enclosed within an elastic cyst wall in the cytoplasm of infected cells. The immune response of the host destroys tachyzoites but the bradyzoites are protected by the intracellular cyst and remain viable for years in an arrested state. Encysted bradyzoites can be found in most organ systems, but especially in neural, muscular, and retinal tissues.[249, 264, 266] Immunosuppression from chemotherapeutic agents or debilitating diseases such as canine distemper or feline leukemia may effect reactivation of multiplication, with bradyzoites reverting to proliferating tachyzoites.[249, 264]

Clinical toxoplasmosis may occur in intermediate hosts, including cats, during the acute phase of extraintestinal infection or during reactivation of proliferating tachyzoites from arrested bradyzoites in immunosuppressed hosts with chronic infections.[249, 264] The clinical manifestation depends upon the degree of cellular necrosis that occurs in various organ systems. The most common clinical syndromes include neurologic deficits, retinochoroiditis, myositis, lymphadenopathy, cholangiohepatitis, pancreatitis, intestinal granuloma, abortion, and neonatal disease.[249, 264, 267–271] Puppies and kittens may develop gastroenteritis, pneumonia, encephalitis, hepatitis, myositis, retinitis, or nonspecific signs of a febrile illness. Intrauterine infections are less common in cats; queens rarely abort because of infection with *T. gondii*.[249, 272]

Clinical signs have not been observed in cats resulting from the enteroepithelial cycle of naturally acquired infection with *T. gondii*.[249, 264] Newborn kittens experimentally infected with bradyzoite cysts developed diarrhea that became fatal within seven to ten days if not treated.[265] The diarrhea was milder when kittens were two to four weeks of age at the time of infection. Diarrhea did not occur in weanling kittens or adult cats similarly infected; however, weanlings and young cats occasionally died an acute death from neurologic toxoplasmosis resulting from extraintestinal infection.[265] Laboratory confirmation of suspected clinical cases of toxoplasmosis can be made by microscopic identification of *T. gondii* or by serologic testing. Oocysts may be detected in feces of cats during the one- to two-week period of active shedding from the enteroepithelial cycle of infection. However, since most cats are asymptomatic during this stage, fecal examinations are not normally done unless there are clinical signs of systemic toxoplasmosis due to concurrent extraintestinal cycle of infection. Oocysts range from 8 to 12 microns in diameter, they are unsporulated when shed, and they cannot be distinguished morphometrically from oocysts of *Hammondia hammondi* and *Besnoitia darlingi*, which also occur in cats.[249] Because of the public health significance of *T. gondii*, the finding of coccidian oocysts 8 to 12 microns in diameter should be regarded as *Toxoplasma* until proven otherwise. Sheather's sugar solution for flotation by centrifugation facilitates detection of the small oocysts.

Tachyzoites or bradyzoite cysts may be detected in tissues taken by biopsy or at necropsy. Microscopic lesions are characteristic and the presence of cysts permits definitive diagnosis.[266] Aspirates from enlarged lymph nodes and from the thoracic or abdominal cavities may allow the detection of tachyzoites; however, negative findings do not rule out toxoplasmosis.

Toxoplasmosis can be diagnosed serologically by demonstrating a rising titer of antibody to *T. gondii* in paired serums or by demonstrating a high titer of antibody in a single serum. Historically many different serologic tests have been used but the serologic tests commonly used today are indirect hemagglutination (IHA), indirect latex agglutination (ILA), enzyme-linked immunosorbent assay (ELISA), and indirect fluorescent antibody (IFA). The IHA, ILA, and ELISA tests are available commercially in kit form for in-office use.* They are practical and the results are dependable when tests are done according to the test kit instructions.[1] The ELISA test is a qualitative test and does not yield a titer. Some diagnostic and research laboratories have developed in-house ELISA tests that provide titers for both IgG and IgM antibodies.[249]

Antibody titers equal to or greater than 1:512 usually indicate recent active infection in dogs and cats; titers of 1:128 to 1:256 usually indicate recent but arrested infection; titers of 1:32 to 1:64 usually indicate past inactive infections; and titers equal to or less than 1:16 usually are regarded as negative. A low titer of 1:16 to 1:32 may be found early in the course of acute disease because titers may not become detectable for four to six weeks after initial infection or one to two weeks after the onset of clinical signs. The finding of a low titer in dogs or cats with clinical signs suggestive of toxoplasmosis should not be regarded as negative until results are available from a second serum collected two to four weeks later. Demonstration of a fourfold or greater rise in titer of antibody confirms a currently active infection.

Sulfonamides, with or without pyrimethamine and clindamycin, are the antimicrobial drugs of choice for treating toxoplasmosis.[249, 273] Near toxic doses must be given in order to be effective. Sulfadiazine is recommended at 30 mg/lb (60 mg/kg) orally q12h for 10 to 14 days. The dosage can be reduced to 15 mg/lb (30 mg/kg) orally q12h when sulfadiazine is used in combination with pyrimethamine at 0.5 mg/lb/day (1 mg/kg/day) orally in dogs and 0.25 mg/lb/day (0.5 mg/kg/day) orally in cats for 7 to 10 days. Pyrimethamine is an inhibitor of folic acid and has a greater effect on tachyzoites than on host cells. Cats are quite sensitive to the effects of pyrimethamine and signs of toxicity often appear within a week after starting treatment. Supplementation of the cat's diet with folic acid (5 mg/day) or folinic acid (0.5 mg/lb/day or 1 mg/kg/day) aids in ameliorating the toxic effects in the cat without compromising the effectiveness of pyrimethamine against tachyzoites of *T. gondii*.[249] Because of the inhibitory effect on folic acid metabolism, pyrimethamine should not be used in continuous therapy for more than two weeks. Clindamycin has been shown

*Commercial sources in the United States for kits are as follows: (1) Indirect hemagglutination test (TPM-TestR, Wampole Laboratories, Cranbury, NJ, and Toxoplasmosis Passive (Indirect) Hemagglutination Test Kit, Burroughs Wellcome, Research Triangle Park, NC), (2) Indirect latex agglutination test (Toxotest-MT, Tech America Diagnostics, Elwood, KS), and (3) ELISA (Toxoplasma Gondii Antibody Test Kit, Pitman-Moore, Washington Crossing, NJ).

to be effective against *T. gondii* and is the drug of choice in treating pregnant animals (20 mg/lb or 40 mg/kg orally q12h for 10 to 14 days).[249, 273]

Clindamycin, sulfadiazine, and pyrimethamine at the highest therapeutic doses for extraintestinal infections decreased shedding of oocysts from the enteroepithelial cycle of infection.[273] The shedding of oocysts was only partially controlled and therefore these drugs should not be regarded as totally effective in preventing the risk of transmission from an exposed or infected cat. The anticoccidial drug monensin used as a feed additive in preventing and treating coccidial infections in poultry and cattle was found to be effective in suppressing shedding of oocysts by infected cats.[274] Monensin was incorporated in dry cat food at a concentration of 0.02 per cent by weight and fed to cats for several months without inducing signs of toxicity. Although not yet licensed or approved for use in cats, monensin has potential for long-term use as a preventive of oocyst shedding in cats, which could be of great benefit in reducing the risk of exposure of humans, especially pregnant women.[249]

Extraintestinal infections with *T. gondii* occur in humans and clinical signs of disease are similar to those in dogs and cats. Most human infections are asymptomatic but intrauterine infections of fetuses in asymptomatically infected women can result in fetal death and abortion from infections early in pregnancy or neurologic and visual deficits from infections during the last trimester of pregnancy. Human infections result from ingestion of bradyzoite cysts in improperly cooked meat or from ingestion of sporulated oocytes. Oocysts are unsporulated when shed in feces of cats; sporulation requires a minimum of one to three days under ideal conditions of warm temperature and high humidity. Sporulated oocytes can survive in the environment for months and years. Contact with any area contaminated with cat feces carries a risk of human infection, e.g., sand boxes, garden soil, litter boxes. Since sporulation requires up to three days or longer, daily cleaning and disinfection of litter boxes greatly reduces the risk of human infection. Pregnant women should take extreme measures to avoid contact with fecal material from cats. Handling of raw meat results in increased risk of exposure as shown by the fact that slaughterhouse workers have a high prevalence of antibody to *T. gondii*.[249]

ENTERIC PROTOZOAL DISEASES

Giardiasis. Giardiasis is an infection of the small intestine caused by *Giardia lamblia*, a flagellated protozoan, which has both a trophic and cystic stage. The pyriform trophozoites are dorsoventrally flattened and bilaterally symmetrical, measuring 9 to 21 μ long by 5 to 15 μ wide by 2 to 4 μ thick. They are motile by means of eight flagella, and they have a unique adhesive disc that helps them attach to the intestinal epithelial surface.[275, 276] The cysts are nonmotile and infectious. Transformation to the cystic form is believed to occur in the distal small intestine. Cysts are observed more commonly than trophozoites in feces of infected dogs, unless the dog has profuse watery diarrhea in which the rapid transit of intestinal contents does not allow time for encystation.[275, 276]

Infection with *G. lamblia* begins with ingestion of cysts, followed by excystation of trophozoites. Excystation is initiated in the stomach by gastric acid, which "activates" the cysts, and it is completed in the duodenum. The acid environment of the stomach, a pH of 2.0 or less, and the nearly neutral pH of the duodenum are essential for excystation of trophozoites.[277] The excysted trophozoite undergoes cell division and the daughter trophozoites migrate to the microvillus surface. Colonization with trophozoites is limited to the distal duodenum and proximal jejunum.[278] Once they are in the milieu of the intestinal contents and fecal stream, environmental changes cause the trophozoites to encyst. Cysts are passed in feces after a prepatent period in dogs of from 6 to 14 days; the prepatent period in cats is unknown.[275] After ingestion by an appropriate host, the cycle repeats. Giardiasis is transmitted by ingestion of cyst-contaminated food and water. Outbreaks of waterborne gastrointestinal disease have been increasing in the United States and other developed countries, and *Giardia lamblia* is the most frequently encountered pathogen of waterborne diseases.[279, 280] Experimental infection of mongrel dogs has been achieved by oral inoculation with either cysts or cultured trophozoites of *G. lamblia*.[281]

The mechanism by which *Giardia* causes diarrhea and malabsorption is unclear. Several hypotheses have been proposed: (1) blanketing of the intestinal epithelium by numerous trophozoites with physical hinderance of nutrient absorption, (2) toxic substances secreted by the parasite, (3) competition between parasite and host for nutrients, (4) excessive mucous secretion due to mucosal irritation by the parasites, (5) associated bacterial overgrowth, and (6) bile salt abnormalities.[282–285] Invasion of the intestinal lamina propria by trophozoites has been observed occasionally but has been considered to be unimportant in the pathogenesis of the disease.[286]

Most giardial infections are asymptomatic and self-limiting. However, clinical giardiasis can occur in animals of any age, but it is more common and more severe in immature animals.[275, 276] Clinical signs of giardiasis are referable to the gastrointestinal tract. The most prominent sign is diarrhea, usually with the history of continuous or intermittent chronic diarrhea.[275, 276, 287] The stool is usually soft, pale, and mixed with mucus. Steatorrhea is frequently reported. Weight loss usually accompanies diarrhea, sometimes despite a good appetite and adequate food intake. Puppies and kittens may experience stunted growth due to malabsorption of nutrients. A secondary deficiency of the fat-soluble vitamins results in dry skin and a deterioration of hair coat quality. Giardiasis has been reported in association with chronic ulcerative colitis, but the cause and effect relationship with *Giardia* was unclear.[287]

Like many parasitic infections, giardiasis is only definitively diagnosed by demonstrating the causative organisms in the host or in its excretions. However, a negative fecal examination does not rule out giardial infection, because the prepatent period may be longer than the incubation period, and the host often sheds the parasites intermittently. Examination of fecal samples daily for three consecutive days is necessary to support statistical confidence that giardiasis can be eliminated from diagnostic consideration.[288] At present, the best way to detect trophozoites is by microscopic examination of direct fecal smears. Zinc sulfate centrifugal flotation facilitates detection of cysts in fecal samples. A drop of iodine solution added to the slide can help to reveal the characteristic organelles of giardial cysts.[287]

Three drugs are commonly used for treatment of giardiasis in humans and animals: quinacrine (Atabrine, Mepacrine), metronidazole (Flagyl), and furazolidone (Furoxone).[276, 280] The first two are the drugs of choice to treat canine giardiasis. Quinacrine is given at a total dosage of 100 mg, q8h for five or six days. The dose should be reduced to 50 mg q8h in puppies and toy breeds. Some dogs may vomit and dark urine may appear due to the side effects of quinacrine. Metronidazole is given at a dosage of 12 mg/lb or 25 mg/kg, q12h for five to seven days. Occasionally the course of therapy may have to be repeated, or increased dosage or a different drug may be necessary to resolve the clinical condition and eliminate shedding of cysts. Metronidazole is carcinogenic, teratogenic, and mutagenic; its use is thus contraindicated in pregnant animals.[276] Cats have been treated successfully with metronidazole, 5 mg/lb (10 mg/kg), orally q12h for five days, or with furazolidone, 2 mg/lb (4 mg/kg), q12h for five days.[276]

Since giardiasis is a zoonosis transmitted primarily by ingestion of food or water contaminated by giardial cysts, all dogs and cats infected with *Giardia* should be treated, including asymptomatic carriers. Outbreaks of human giardiasis in family groups have been traced to a newly acquired puppy that was shedding giardial cysts.[278] A high level of sanitation must be practiced. Measures should be taken to prevent fecal contamination of food. Water from nontreated municipal water systems should be boiled, filtered, or treated with disinfectants approved for potable water before it is used for drinking or other consumption. Private wells may become contaminated with *Giardia* and be a continuing source of infection. Disinfectants commonly used for potable water are sodium hypochlorite, calcium hypochlorite, chlorine gas, trichloroisocyanuric acid, and hydantoin derivatives. They should be used according to manufacturers' recommendations and concentrations of residual disinfectant must be monitored regularly to assure that adequate, but safe, concentrations are being used. A new class of potential water disinfectants shows promise for future use.[289, 290]

Trichomoniasis. *Pentatrichomonas hominis* occurs in the cecum and colon of humans, lower primates, various monkeys, rodents, cattle, dogs, and cats.[276, 291, 292] The trophozoite is a pyriform flagellate measuring 4 to 6.5 μ by 6 to 14 μ, and contains five anterior flagella, a prominent nucleus, undulating membrane, and axostyle. The existence of cysts has not been proven. Transmission is believed to be through a fecal-oral route. The prevalence of the organism in dogs and cats is unknown.[276]

At present, whether *P. hominis* is pathogenic remains unknown. Some authors think that because the organisms tend to multiply in fluid feces, many cases of diarrhea are mistakenly attributed to them. In fact, their abundance in fluid feces is often the effect, but not the cause of the diarrhea.[291] Other authors suggest that *P. hominis* is the cause of canine diarrhea, especially in immature dogs, although other concurrent infections may be necessary for disease to occur.[276] Microscopic examination of direct saline smears of fresh feces reveals the trophozoites. *P. hominis* infection can be eliminated by treatment with metronidazole at the dosages given for the treatment of giardiasis.[276, 292]

Amebiasis. *Entamoeba histolytica* is a pathogenic ameba that resides in the large intestine of humans, dogs, cats, and other mammals.[276, 293] The motile trophozoites, measuring 12 to 50 μ, may be found in loose or watery stools. The cysts are 10 to 12 μ in diameter. Cysts are more often found in formed stools and are also infective. Trophozoites are commonly observed in feces from infected dogs and cats, whereas cysts are rarely found. Transmission of amebiasis is through the fecal-oral route, and it seems that most canine and feline *E. histolytica* infections are acquired from human sources.[276, 294]

E. histolytica can lyse target cells following direct contact. Because of their lytic actions, the trophozoites not only reside in the lumen of large bowel, but they can also invade the mucosa, submucosa, and even the muscularis layer and serosa. This invasiveness often results in flask-shaped ulceration and bleeding in the colon.[293] Extraintestinal dissemination of amebae occurs in humans occasionally, but is rarely reported in dogs and cats.[276] Infection of dogs or cats with *E. histolytica* may be clinically apparent or inapparent. Weight loss, chronic diarrhea or fulminant dysentery, anorexia, and mucus in the feces are signs of clinical amebiasis.[276] If acute dysenteric amebiasis remains untreated, death may occur.

The definitive diagnosis of *E. histolytica* infection is based on the identification of the organisms in tissues or in the feces. Metronidazole is the drug of choice and should be given at a dosage of 11 mg/lb (25 mg/kg) orally q12h for 7 to 10 days. Furazolidone at a dose of 2 mg/lb (4 mg/kg) q12h for 7 days can be used as an alternate drug and is the preferred drug in pregnant animals.

Balantidiasis. *Balantidium coli* is a normal component of the intestinal fauna of the pig and rat. Although harmless to pigs and usually harmless to humans, *B. coli* occasionally causes diarrhea that may progress to severe dysentery and ulcerative colitis in humans.[295] Balantidiasis occurs less frequently in dogs than in humans, and the disease has not been reported in cats.[276] There have been very few reported descriptions of balantidiasis in dogs, but severe dysentery has been the most common manifestation. Most infections in dogs are probably asymptomatic. It has been suggested that concurrent infection with whip worms, *Trichuris vulpis*, may enhance the pathogenicity of *B. coli* for dogs.[276, 296]

Infection with *B. coli* is acquired by ingestion of the cyst. After the cyst wall is dissolved by action of gastric acid and enzymes in the small intestine, a trophozoite emerges and invades the mucosa of the large intestine. Extraintestinal infections are rare, although ulcers may occur in the large intestine, with perforation and secondary peritonitis having been reported in severe human balantidiasis.[295]

The diagnosis of balantidial infection depends on the identification of cysts in feces processed by the zinc sulfate centrifugal flotation or sedimentation techniques or the identification of cysts and trophozoites from direct smears of fecal samples.[295] The cysts of *B. coli* are spherical to ovoid, 40 to 60 μ in diameter, and the trophozoites are ovoid, 100 to 200 μ in length and 30 to 100 μ in width. The trophozoites are completely covered by short cilia. A prominent, bean-shaped macronucleus is present in both the cyst and the trophozoite. A drop of acidic methyl green dye solution helps to reveal the characteristics of either cysts or trophozoites in fecal smear preparations.[276]

Specific therapy for canine balantidiasis is still inconclusive at present because of the infrequency of occurrence. However, it is suggested that metronidazole at dosages used for giardiasis or amebiasis should be considered as the drug of first choice. Oxytetracycline and chlortetracycline are recommended as effective drugs in human balantidiasis.[295]

CARDIOVASCULAR AND VISCERAL PROTOZOAL DISEASES

Babesiosis. Babesiosis is a tick-borne hematozoal disease with progressive anemia as the primary factor in the development of clinical signs of disease.[297, 298] Canine babesiosis occurs in tropical and subtropical regions around the world, according to the geographic distribution of vector ticks. Feline babesiosis has a more limited geographic distribution, with naturally acquired infections occurring in countries on the continents of Asia, Africa, and South America. Feline babesiosis has not been reported in cats indigenous to North America.[297]

There are three species of *Babesia* known to infect dogs and wild canids: *B. canis*, *B. gibsoni*, and *B. vogeli*. *Babesia canis* is the most common worldwide. *Babesia vogeli* is the least common and has been recognized only in African and Asian countries. *Babesia vogeli* may be a strain of *B. canis* rather than a distinct species.[297] The organisms of *B. canis* and *B. vogeli* are similar in size and morphologic appearance; they are usually observed as paired, piriform trophozoites in infected erythrocytes. The organism of *B. gibsoni* is smaller in size and is usually observed as a single oval or annular trophozoite in infected erythrocytes. The brown dog tick, *Rhipicephalus sanguineus*, is the principal vector in the transmission of *B. canis* and *B. vogeli*, and it may also transmit *B. gibsoni*, although the principal vector for *B. gibsoni* is *Haemaphysalis bispinosa*. Other ticks, including species of *Dermacentor*, *Hyalomma plumbeum*, and *Haemaphysalis leachi*, may transmit *B. canis*. A reservoir of infected ticks is maintained by both transovarial and transstadial transmission of *B. canis* and *B. gibsoni*.[297, 298]

There are four species of *Babesia* that are known to infect cats: *B. cati*, *B. felis*, *B. herpailuri*, and *B. pantherae*. The specific tick vectors for feline *Babesia* are not known. The biologic characteristics of feline *Babesia* and the pathogenesis of feline babesiosis are less well defined than for canine babesiosis, but they are similar. In general, feline babesiosis is a less severe disease than canine babesiosis, although severe fatal disease may occur in cats, especially in kittens.[297, 299–301]

Naturally acquired infection of dogs with babesial organisms occurs via the attachment of infected ticks. Transplacental transmission has been reported and transfusion of infected blood is commonly used for experimental transmission.[297, 302] An initial parasitemia develops within a day or two after infection and lasts for about four days.[303] Organisms then disappear from peripheral blood for a period of 10 to 14 days, after which a more intense second parasitemia occurs. Thereafter, alternating periods of parasitemia and dormancy occur at variable and unpredictable intervals. Dogs that survive acute babesiosis or that have asymptomatic infections usually become chronic carriers unless they are treated to eliminate the babesial organisms.

Replication of *B. canis* occurs by binary fission of trophozoites in erythrocytes. This intra-erythrocytic parasitemia causes both intravascular and extravascular hemolysis. When hypoxia occurs as a result of hemolysis, microvascular damage leads to the development of disseminated intravascular coagulation, which may involve smaller vessels and capillaries of many organs, including the brain, and may result in neurologic manifestations of canine babesiosis.[297] Trophozoites of *B. canis* are also found in endothelial cells of the lungs and liver and in macrophages and neutrophils.[304] Splenic and hepatic enlargement occur due to passive congestion and hyperplasia of the mononuclear-phagocyte system. Mildly pathogenic strains of *B. canis* may induce only a chronic carrier state without clinically apparent disease in adult dogs, but the same mildly pathogenic strain may cause acute clinical babesiosis in young puppies.

Many infections with *Babesia* in dogs and cats are inapparent. In some instances clinical signs become apparent only after stress from strenuous exercise, surgery, or concurrent infections. Clinical findings in cases of typical canine babesiosis include pyrexia, icterus, weakness, depression, anorexia, pale mucous membranes, and splenomegaly.[297, 298] Mucopurulent oculonasal discharge may be observed with signs similar to canine ehrlichiosis; concurrent infection with *Ehrlichia canis* is a common occurrence.[298] Hemoglobinemia, hemoglobinuria, and bilirubinuria occur early in the infection and are followed by bilirubinemia and icterus. The Coombs' test becomes positive in most dogs with babesiosis.[305] Young dogs often develop peracute babesiosis and are presented in a state of shock with history of an illness of short duration. Heavy tick infestation is frequently found in young dogs with peracute disease. The prognosis is guarded to poor for cases of peracute babesiosis.[298] Chronic infections are characterized by intermittent fever, emaciation, variable appetite, weakness, lethargy, mild anemia, and mild icterus.[297, 298] Splenomegaly and lymphadenopathy may be present in chronic infections.[298]

In canine babesiosis, early laboratory findings include hemolytic anemia, bilirubinemia, bilirubinuria, and hemoglobinuria. Peripheral blood smears usually reveal anisocytosis, poikilocytosis, polychromasia, and nucleated erythrocytes consistent with a regenerative anemia. Most dogs are positive for Coombs' test, and thrombocytopenia often occurs.[305] Diagnosis is confirmed by identification of organisms in erythrocytes in Giemsa-stained blood smears. The babesial organisms may be detected more readily in blood smears prepared from the microcapillary system, such as the margins of the ears, toenails, or edge of foot pads.[297] However, parasites cannot always be demonstrated in blood smears and in those cases animal inoculation or serological testing may be necessary to confirm the diagnosis. Animal inoculation involves the IV injection of blood from a dog suspected of having babesiosis into a splenectomized dog, followed by the daily preparation of blood smears and their examination for organisms in erythrocytes from the splenectomized dog.[297] An indirect fluorescent antibody (IFA) test can be used to demonstrate antibody to *B. canis*, with titers greater than 1:40 being considered positive for either *B. canis* or *B. gibsoni*.[297]

Feline babesiosis is characterized clinically by inappetence, lethargy, weakness, pale mucous membrane, and rough hair coat. This disease usually affects cats younger than two years.[300] Fever and icterus are rarely seen in cats, which differs from babesiosis in dogs.[297] A macrocytic hypochromic anemia is often found in cats with feline babesiosis.[301] A rapid drop in hematocrit may occur after infection. Identification of parasites in erythrocytes confirms the diagnosis. When organisms are not found in erythrocytes, animal inoculation may be necessary to confirm the diagnosis. Nonsplenectomized cats should be used as recipients for transfusion with blood from a cat suspected of having feline babesiosis, since splenectomy does not appear to facilitate the transmission of *B. felis*. An IFA or other serologic tests have not been developed for practical application in the clinical diagnosis of feline babesiosis.

Therapy of canine and feline babesiosis involves supportive therapy and antibabesial chemotherapy to eliminate the organism. Supportive therapy is most important in severe, acute, and peracute babesiosis and has the objectives of combating shock and correcting severe anemia and metabolic acidosis. Transfusions with packed erythrocytes or whole blood are indicated in cases with severe anemia (hematocrit less than 15 per cent).[297, 298] Following transfusion, the hematocrit should be at least 30 per cent in the recipient. Care must be taken to minimize stress in severely anemic patients, especially cats, to prevent iatrogenic death.[297] Glucocorticosteroids (prednisolone sodium succinate, 5 mg/lb or 11 mg/kg IV q3h as needed) and broad-spectrum antibiotics (ampicillin, chloramphenicol, or clindamycin) IV are recommended for dogs presented in shock.[298] Metabolic acidosis is an important factor affecting the survival of dogs with anemic shock in severe babesiosis. Rapid IV administration of sodium bicarbonate at a dosage of 1 mEq HCO_3^-/lb of body weight is recommended in dogs with severe anemic shock. The IV injection of bicarbonate ion may need to be repeated in 24 hours; ideally, further administration of bicarbonate should be based on analysis of HCO_3^- in serum.[297] Treatment with an antibabesial drug should be initiated as soon as the severely affected patient is stabilized by emergency treatment.

At least three drugs have been found to be effective in treating babesiosis with a single dose: diminazene aceturate (1.6 mg/lb or 3.5 mg/kg IM or SQ), phenamidine isethionate (7 mg/lb or 15 mg/kg SQ), or imidocarb dipropionate (2.2 mg/lb or 5 mg/kg IM or SQ). Imidocarb is the drug of choice because it is the least toxic and it has a high curative rate against *B. canis*.[298] It is not as effective against *B. gibsoni*, which is more difficult to eliminate by chemotherapy. Imidocarb is also effective against *Ehrlichia canis* and *Hepatozoon canis*, both of which may occur concurrently with babesiosis. A second dose of imidocarb 14 days after the initial dose is recommended in treating the mixed infections.[297]

Protective immunity does not develop against babesial organisms, and animals are susceptible to reinfection after the organism is eliminated by chemotherapy. In areas with endemic canine and feline babesiosis, the objective of treatment is to decrease the replication of the organism without complete elimination.[297, 298] A state of premunition develops in chronically infected asymptomatic animals, which are resistant to further infection as long as the persistent infection is under control and in balance with the immune response of the host. Stress or immunosuppression results in relapses and reactivation of chronic infections. Blood donors should be tested periodically to assure that they are not chronically infected, since transfusion is an effective means of transmission of babesial organisms. Control of ticks is essential in the prevention of babesioses.

Cytauxzoonosis. Cytauxzoonosis, a fatal blood protozoal disease in domestic cats, is caused by *Cytauxzoon felis*, classified in the order Piroplasmid and family Theileriidae. The life cycle of *Cytauxzoon* is not clear. Ticks may be involved in the transmission of cytauxzoonosis. The organisms develop primarily within mononuclear phagocytes first; then after rupture of the cells, they invade uninfected erythrocytes. The cat is most likely an accidental or dead-end host because of the relatively short course of illness and the uniformly fatal outcome of the disease.[306]

Clinical signs in infected cats are anorexia, lethargy, dyspnea, dehydration, icterus, depression, pallor, and high fever (39.4 to 46.6° C, 103 to 107° F).[306] The incubation period for naturally infected cats is unknown, but for experimentally induced feline cytauxzoonosis, it ranges from five to 20 days.[307] Cats usually die two or three days after the temperature peaks, and the entire course of clinical illness usually takes less than one week.[306]

Diagnosis is made by demonstrating the erythrocyte phase (piroplasms) and the tissue phase in impression smears of spleen. The piroplasms within erythrocytes appear as round "signet ring"-shaped bodies 1 to 1.5 μ in diameter, bipolar oval "safety pin" forms 1 by 2 μ, or anaplasmoid round "dots" less than 1 μ in diameter. A single cell usually contains one parasite; however, pairs and tetrads are observed occasionally.[306] Therapeutic parasiticidal drugs are not currently available. Supportive therapy with fluids and broad-spectrum antibiotics may prolong the course of illness but do not effect a cure.

American Trypanosomiasis. American trypanosomiasis (Chagas' disease) is caused by a hemoflagellated protozoan, *Trypanosoma cruzi*, which is classified in the class Zoomastigophorea and family Trypanosomatidae. Naturally acquired infection with *T. cruzi* occurs in humans and a large number of domestic and wild animals, including dogs and cats. In the blood of the vertebrate host, *T. cruzi* is a 16 to 20 μ long, spindle-shaped parasite with a pointed posterior end, a large subterminal kinetoplast, a nucleus, a well-developed, undulating membrane, and a free flagellum.[309] *T. cruzi* is transmitted by hematophagous insects of the family Reduviidae, often known as kissing bugs. Infection occurs through contamination of the bite site with the insect's feces, or after the trypomastigotes penetrate the mucous membranes and enter macrophages of the skin. The trypomastigotes then transform into amastigotes, which contain a large nucleus and a rod-like kinetoplast but no free flagellum or undulating membrane. This intracellular form occurs primarily in muscle, especially heart muscle. Here they multiply and form pseudocytes. The host cell and pseudocyst rupture, releasing the organisms as trypomastigotes, which invade macrophages or reach the bloodstream, where they may spread throughout the host.[309] In addition to being transmitted by reduvii insects, transmission of infection may occur congenitally through the milk of lactating animals during mating, the eating of raw meat, and by blood transfusion.[309, 310] Several mechanisms for the pathogenesis have been proposed, which include mechanical destruction of cardiac fibers, cell-mediated hypersensitivity, destruction of cardiac fibers by toxic products of the parasite, and destruction of cardiac adrenergic innervation by the parasite.[311] However, the exact mechanism is still unknown. The clinical signs in dogs are mostly related to cardiac dysfunction, and include tachycardia, ascites, weak pulse, pale mucous membranes, and hepatomegaly.[306] Some dogs may develop systemic disease characterized by lymphadenopathy, diarrhea, anorexia, and weight loss.[312] Other dogs die suddenly without developing prior clinical signs of disease.

A definitive diagnosis of Chagas' disease is based on the demonstration of the parasite in the blood or other tissues of the patient. Protozoa can be isolated when the number of parasites in the patient's blood is low. Isolation of the organism by inoculation of mice is a useful, but time-consuming procedure. Serologic tests such as complement-fixation, indirect fluorescent antibody, or direct hemagglutination tests are commonly used to detect antibodies to *T. cruzi*. Demonstration of a rising titer of antibody in paired serums is necessary to confirm infection.[306]

Chagas' disease does not respond well to chemotherapeutic agents.[313] Since canine Chagas' disease is an often fatal disease that may be transmitted to humans, euthanasia of the dog is recommended.[306] Experimental nifurtimox drugs have shown promise in treating Chagas' disease in dogs. Lampit (4 to 15 mg/lb/day or 8 to 30 mg/kg/day given orally for 3 to 5 months) has been reported to be effective in treating both experimental and naturally acquired infections.[314]

To prevent infections with *T. cruzi*, protection of humans and animals from contact with infected vectors is important. Blood donors should be subjected to serologic testing to determine their possible exposure to *T. cruzi* before blood transfusion.

Leishmaniasis. Infections of humans and animals with protozoan organisms of the genus *Leishmania* occur in tropical and subtropical countries with humid, warm climates. *Leishmania* is classified in the family Trypanosomatidae. Various local names can be grouped together on the basis of their common characteristics. Four species of *Leishmania* are recognized as important pathogens: *Leishmania donovani* causes visceral leishmaniasis, kala azar, or dum dum fever; *L. tropica*, *L. braziliensis*, and *L. mexicana* cause cutaneous leishmaniasis, Oriental sore, or Delhi sore; additionally, *L. braziliensis* has been associated with disseminated mucocutaneous or American leishmaniasis, or espundia.[315, 316]

Leishmania occurs in vertebrate hosts in the leishmanial form, which is a small, ovoid protozoan about 1 to 2 μ wide by 2 to 4.5 μ long, with neither flagellum nor undulating membrane. In their invertebrate or immediate host and in culture medium, the organisms assume shapes varying from the leishmanial to the leptomonad form, the latter being slender and spindle-shaped, from 14 to 20 μ in length and 1.5 to 4 μ in width. This latter form is motile by means of a flagellum that arises from the blepharoplast and projects from the anterior pole of the organism.[315] *Leishmania* reproduces in the vertebrate host by longitudinal binary fission, but the complete life cycle and maintenance of virulence depend upon an intermediate host or vector. Several species of sandflies serve as intermediate hosts and biological vectors in the transmission of *Leishmania* and are necessary for their perpetuation, but certain other flies, such as *Stomoxys calcitrans*, may mechanically transmit the infection.[315, 316]

Leishmaniasis is acquired through the bite of infected sandflies as biological vectors or the bite of other flies as mechanical vectors. The infection varies from mild and self-limiting to fatal disease. Visceral leishmaniasis usually starts as a primary nonulcerating skin lesion. The incubation period is three to seven months or longer, and parasites are found in liver, bone marrow, spleen, and lymph nodes. In visceral leishmaniasis, phagocytic cells multiply and harbor large numbers of amastigotes, resulting in enlargement and dysfunction of organs. Visceral leishmaniasis occurs naturally in dogs, cats, humans, and other animals. It is observed usually as a chronic debilitating disease with periods of fever, gradual weight loss, and lymphadenopathy, with anemia appearing in the terminal stages.[315] The disease has a wide geographic distribution throughout tropical and subtropical areas of the world but is most prevalent in countries bordering the Mediterranean, large areas of Africa, India, and China.[315] Dogs are especially appropriate reservoirs because they offer the insect vector direct access to the parasitized macrophages of cutaneous lesions.[317] In cutaneous and mucocutaneous leishmaniasis, the dermis becomes filled with large numbers of macrophages, lymphocytes, plasma cells, and rarely, eosinophils. Numerous parasites are present within the macrophages. The lesions progress to well-defined, deep ulcers.[315] Ulcers may be seen on the skin of the nose, earflap, and back and in the nasal and oral mucosae. The dog may be anorectic, lethargic, have episodes of epistaxis, and show pain or weakness in one or more legs.[316]

Normocytic normochromic anemia is characteristic of canine visceral leishmaniasis.[316] Leukopenia is often present and total serum proteins are increased. The erythrocyte sedimentation rate is accelerated. Serologic tests, such as complement fixation and indirect immunofluorescence, aid the diagnosis. However, final determination must be based on demonstration and identification of the causative organisms in tissue sections, smears, or cultures. Tissues taken by biopsy are most useful to demonstrate the organisms in a living animal.[315]

Curative agents or drugs are not currently available. The pentavalent antimonials, sodium stibogluconate and meglumine antimoniate, are currently the drugs of choice for the treatment of leishmaniasis although both drugs are cardiotoxic and nephrotoxic. Treatment for 10 to 12 days, with 15 to 25 mg/lb/day or 30 to 50 mg/kg/day of antimony administered intravenously or intramuscularly, is the usual therapeutic regimen for either of these compounds in dogs with leishmaniasis.[318] Because of the side effects, drugs must be used with caution. The treatment may need to be repeated several times for permanent recovery. In case of treatment failure, second-line agents such as pentamidine and amphotericin B have been used with varying degrees of success.[316] Other antileishmanial agents, including liposomes and 8-aminoquinoline, may also be effective for treatment.[316] Supportive therapy and blood transfusion should be given when needed. Prevention of the disease depends on the control of the vectors, elimination of animal reservoirs, and early diagnosis and treatment of infected patients.

Hepatozoonosis. Hepatozoonosis in dogs and other carnivores is caused by *Hepatozoon canis*, which is transmitted by the brown dog tick, *Rhipicephalus sanguineus*. Ticks become infected by ingestion of gametocytes in monocytes and neutrophils during the taking of a blood meal from an infected carnivore.[320] The organisms replicate in the tick and develop into sporozoites in the hemocele. Sporozoites do not migrate to salivary glands or mouth parts; transmission from infected ticks does not occur by the bite of ticks. Natural infections in dogs occur by ingestion of infected ticks. After ingestion, the sporozoites of *H. canis* are released from the tick, penetrate the intestinal wall, and are carried by blood or lymph to mononuclear phagocytes or endothelial cells where schizogony results in the development of macroschizonts and subsequent release of macromerozoites. The macromerozoites penetrate cells in skeletal muscle, myocardium, lungs, spleen, lymph nodes, and liver, where further cycles of schizogony result in the development of microschizonts. Microschizonts may persist in cells as cyst-like structures for varying periods without inciting an inflammatory response. Eventually micromerozoites are released from the microschizonts, at which time a granulomatous inflammatory response occurs with neutrophils, macrophages, and eosinophils as the predominant cell types; intense infiltrations with neutrophils occur in skeletal muscles.[321] Neutrophils and monocytes become infected either by phagocytosis or direct penetration by micromerozoites, which develop into gametocytes. This is the form of *H. canis* found in the leukocytes of infected dogs.[320]

Infections with *H. canis* in dogs have been reported in southeast Asia, Africa, the Middle East, Europe, Brazil, and the Gulf Coast region of Texas in the United States.[320] It is anticipated that the distribution of *H. canis* in the United States will eventually extend to other areas because of the widespread distribution of the brown dog tick. The clinical syndrome of hepatozoonosis in dogs in the United States differs somewhat from the disease in other parts of the world, suggesting that there may be differences in strains of *H. canis*.[322]

The hepatozoonosis syndrome is complex. In general, the only dogs that develop clinical signs of hepatozoonosis are those that are concurrently infected with some other agent, are immunosuppressed, have genetically defective neutrophil function, or are younger than four months of age.[320] The incubation period after experimental infection orally with suspensions of infected ticks is three to seven days with diarrhea, sometimes bloody, occurring three to four days before pyrexia is detected. The most common clinical signs in dogs with naturally acquired infections are intermittent or persistent fever and emaciation even though the dog's appetite often remains normal until the terminal stages before death.[320, 322–324] Other signs that have been reported include muscular hyperesthesia with lumbar pain and reluctance to move, depression, diarrhea (which may be bloody), mucopurulent ocular and nasal discharge, leukocytosis, regenerative anemia, and cachexia and anorexia terminally.[320, 321, 325] The leukocytosis is primarily a neutrophilia with a left shift and occasionally, an eosinophilia. The total white blood cell count may range from 20,000 to 200,000. The muscular hyperesthesia seems to be related to inflammatory cell infiltration of muscles when merozoites are released from infected muscle cells, as well as to periosteal bone proliferation at origins and insertions of skeletal muscles. Antibody to *H. canis* can be detected in serum from clinically affected dogs but there is no evidence for protective immunity.[320]

A definitive diagnosis of hepatozoonosis is made by finding the organism in neutrophils or monocytes in freshly prepared blood smears or in biopsies of skeletal muscle. Blood smears should be prepared immediately after collection of the blood and they should be stained with Giemsa or Leishman's stain.[320] Gametocytes in the cytoplasm of neutrophils or monocytes stain uniformly light, "ice" blue and may be present in only 1 or 2 cells/1000 leukocytes. Cysts with a central nucleus or developing microschizonts are found in biopsies of skeletal muscle.

Antiprotozoal and antimicrobial drugs are not effective against *H. canis*. Apparently successful treatments have not been reproducible by other investigators. The complexity of the hepatozoonosis syndrome has made it difficult to evaluate chemotherapeutic agents. Palliative therapy with nonsteroidal anti-inflammatory drugs, e.g., aspirin, phenylbutazone, or flunixin meglumate, has resulted in temporary improvement in clinical signs.[322]

Prevention of hepatozoonosis depends on control of the brown dog tick vector. Regular spraying of kennels, dog houses, and home environments, as well as treatment of dogs by dipping and the use of acaricidal sprays or powders, are essential for control of brown dog ticks.[320]

Pneumocystosis. A protozoan organism of uncertain taxonomic classification, *Pneumocystis carinii* commonly inhabits the pulmonary alveoli of humans and animals without causing pathophysiologic dysfunction; however, under certain conditions it causes severe pneumonia. Clinical pneumocystis pneumonia has been reported in dogs, humans, goats, pigs, horses, and nonhuman primates.[315, 326–328] Human beings and animals suffering from disorders of the lymphoreticular system or immune mechanisms or who undergo immunosuppressive therapy are at greatest risk for developing pneumocystosis. The primary mode of transmission is by aerosol.

The organisms localize in alveoli adjacent to the surface of alveolar lining cells.[315] The entire life cycle of the parasite is completed within the alveolar spaces, where they form clusters and adhere to cells lining the alveoli. *Pneumocystis carinii* has both trophozoite and cyst forms. The trophozoite is a small (2 to 5 μ), thin-walled pleomorphic organism with a reticular cytoplasm and an eccentric nucleus. They replicate by binary fission or by an ascospore-like process within a thick-walled cyst (4 to 7 μ in size).[326] The mature cyst contains complete organisms in even multiples of two to eight. In the normal, subclinically infected hosts, the pneumocystis organisms replicate slowly and rarely increase in numbers to a pathologic density. When the overgrowth of pneumocystis clusters is sufficient to decrease gaseous exchange, or when the body mounts a massive inflammatory response to the parasite, clinical signs of respiratory distress become apparent. The organisms may cause some thickening of alveolar septa, but they do not invade the lung tissue.[315, 326]

Clinical disease in humans and dogs is similar. Clinical disease has not been reported in cats even though *Pneumocystis carinii* has been found in cats. Infected dogs usually show gradual weight loss and increasing respiratory difficulty progressing over one to four weeks. Reduced exercise tolerance is commonly seen in dogs, and coughing is occasionally reported. Dyspnea, tachycardia, and increased dry respiratory sounds on thoracic auscultation are often present. Affected dogs are usually afebrile, remain alert, and have a good appetite. They may have diarrhea and occasionally vomit. Dry lung sounds, a nonproductive cough, and lack of fever are the clinical features that differentiate pneumocystis pneumonia from respiratory disease caused by other infectious agents. Hematologic changes are usually nonspecific; neutrophilia with a left shift suggesting inflammation is the most common finding. Findings on thoracic radiography include diffuse bilateral alveolar and interstitial lung disease, with compensatory emphysema in severely affected animals.[326] Finding the organism in biopsy samples or aspirates confirms the diagnosis of pneumocystic infection. Percutaneous needle aspiration of lung parenchyma is the most rapid and simplest procedure to confirm a diagnosis.[329] The aspirated material is air dried on slides and stained with methenamine silver to reveal cysts or Giemsa stain to detect trophozoites. Pneumocystis has not been cultured successfully on artificial media.[330]

Trimethoprim combined with sulfadiazine or sulfamethoxazole is the drug of choice for treating pneumocystosis in dogs.[326] An oral dosage of 30 mg/kg q12h for 2 weeks is recommended. Dogs should be observed closely for signs of toxicity to the drug, which are usually manifested as ataxia or other impairment of neurologic function. Signs of toxicity usually disappear within 48 hours of withdrawal of the drug. Anemia and leukopenia may occur and hematograms should be done at weekly intervals, especially if therapy is continued for more than two weeks. Although treatment of pneumocystis pneumonia may be successful, the prognosis is guarded since pneumocystis is indicative of impaired immune functions. Trimethoprim-sulfadiazine can be used for long-term prophylactic therapy at a dosage of 7 to 15 mg/lb (15 to 30 mg/kg) once daily in immunosuppressed dogs or dogs scheduled for immunosuppressive therapy. Oxygen therapy, mucolytic drugs or aerosols, and supportive care are often needed in dogs with pneumocystosis.

Antiprotozoal drugs of the aromatic diamidine type may prove to be useful in treating pneumocystosis in dogs. In general, aromatic diamidines are more toxic than trimethoprim-sulfadiazine and they are no more effective. Pentamidine isethionate has been used successfully to treat pneumocytosis in a dog with minimal side effects.[327]

Encephalitozoonosis. Encephalitozoonosis is a disease caused by the microsporidian *Encephalitozoon cuniculi. E. cuniculi* is a small (1.5 by 2.5 μ) intracellular parasite found in renal tubular epithelial cells, endothelial cells, tissue macrophages, and less frequently, glial cells, hepatocytes, and myocytes.[331] The organisms are found within vacuoles of host cell origin. *E. cuniculi* undergoes asexual division within the host cell. Natural infection with *E. cuniculi* has been reported sporadically in dogs, domestic cats, foxes, leopards, and suricates, but is frequently reported in lagomorphs and rodents, such as rabbits, rats, guinea pigs, hamsters, and mice.[315] Unless laboratory animals are markedly stressed or immunosuppressed, the disease is clinically inapparent. Arctic blue foxes appear to be particularly susceptible to *E. cuniculi*, with high mortality in blue fox cubs resulting in major economic loss on fox farms.[332, 333] The mechanism for transmission is unknown. The most likely route of natural infection, especially in canine and feline encephalitozoonosis, is oronasal.[334] Vertical transmission has been postulated in blue foxes, rabbits, and mice.[331, 336]

In dogs, the most common clinical signs are stunted growth and general unthriftiness.[331, 334, 335] Other signs that may develop include depression, ataxia, blindness, convulsions, and signs of renal failure. Signs of aggressive behavior may develop, including biting, abnormal vocalization, and viciousness. Encephalitozoonosis should be considered in young puppies when signs of both encephalitis and renal failure are found. Clinical signs in feline encephalitozoonosis are variable.[331] Severe muscle spasms, depression, paralysis, and death have been reported in natural infections.

A normochromic, normocytic anemia is a consistent finding in animals infected with *E. cuniculi*.[335] The diminished erythropoietic activity is manifested by significant decreases in both hemoglobin and erythrocyte numbers, with corresponding decrease in hematocrit. Blood leukocytes, especially the lymphocytic and monocytic elements, are increased. Spores shed into the urine from parasitized renal tubular epithelial cells are readily identifiable in urine sediment with Gram stain.[331] Experimentally, dogs can mount antibody directed *E. cuniculi* by three days after inoculation. This can be detected using an indirect fluorescent antibody test. Titers greater than 1:40 are regarded as indicative of current active canine encephalitozoonosis.[331] Antibody responses in cats are slower to develop and titers are generally low. Currently, no specific treatment exists for either canine or feline encephalitozoonosis.

References

1. Smith, JD: The anaerobic bacteria of the nose and tonsils of healthy dogs. J Comp Pathol 71:428, 1961.
2. Clapper, WE and Meade, GH: Normal flora of the nose, throat, and lower intestine of dogs. J Bacteriol 85:643, 1963.
3. Snow, HD, et al.: Canine respiratory disease in an animal facility—viral and bacteriological survey. Arch Surgery 99:126, 1969.
4. Brennan, PC and Simkins, RC: Throat flora of a closed colony of beagles. Proc Soc Exp Biol Med 134:566, 1970.
5. Permington, JE and Reynolds, HF: Concentrations of gentamicin and carbenicillin in bronchial secretions. J Infect Dis 128:63, 1973.
6. Wright, NG, et al.: *Bordetella bronchiseptica*: a reassessment of its role in canine respiratory disease. Vet Rec 93:486, 1973.
7. Thompson, H, et al.: Experimental respiratory disease in dogs due to *Bordetella bronchiseptica*. Res Vet Sci 20:16, 1976.
8. Thayer, GW: Infections of the respiratory system. *In* Greene, CE (ed): Clinical Microbiology and Infectious Diseases of the Dog and Cat. Philadelphia, WB Saunders, 1984, p 238.
9. Appel, MJ: Canine infectious tracheobronchitis (Kennel cough): A status report. Comp Cont Ed Pract Vet 3:70, 1981.
10. Batey, RG and Smith, AF: The isolation of *Bordetella bronchiseptica* from an outbreak of canine pneumonia. Aust Vet J 52:184, 1976.
11. Bemis, DA, et al.: Pathogenesis of canine bordetellosis. J Infect Dis 135:753, 1977.
12. Bemis, DA and Kennedy, JR: An improved system for studying the effect of *Bordetella bronchiseptica* on the ciliary activity of canine tracheal epithelial cells. J Infect Dis 144:349, 1981.
13. Thayer, GW: Canine infectious tracheobronchitis. *In* Greene, CE (ed): Clinical Microbiology and Infectious Diseases of the Dog and Cat. Philadelphia, WB Saunders, 1984, p 430.
14. Roudebusch, P and Fales, WH: Antibacterial susceptibility of *Bordetella bronchiseptica* isolates from small companion animals with respiratory disease. JAAHA 17:793, 1981.
15. Creighton, SR and Wilkins, RJ: Bacteriologic and cytologic evaluation of animals with lower respiratory disease using transtracheal aspiration biopsy. JAAHA 10:227, 1974.
16. Bemis, DA and Appel, MJG: Aerosol, parenteral and oral antibiotic treatment of *Bordetella bronchiseptica* infections in dogs. JAVMA 170:1082, 1977.
17. Bolton, GR: Aerosol Therapy. *In* Kirk, RW (ed): Current Veterinary Therapy VI. Philadelphia, WB Saunders, 1977, p 12.
18. McCandlish, IAP and Thompson, H: Canine bordetellosis: Chemotherapy using sulfadiazine-trimethoprim combination. Vet Rec 105:51, 1979.
19. Alexander, MR, et al.: Bronchial secretion concentrations of tobramycin. Ann Rev Respir Dis 125:208, 1982.
20. Amis, TC: Chronic bronchitis in dogs. *In* Kirk, RW (ed): Current Veterinary Therapy IX. Philadelphia, WB Saunders, 1986, p 306.
21. Goodnow, RA and Shade, FJ: Control of canine bordetellosis. Mod Vet Pract 61:587, 1980.
22. Bey, RF, et al.: Intranasal vaccination of dogs with live avirulent *Bordetella bronchiseptica*: correlation of serum agglutination titer and the formation of secretory IgA with protection against experimentally induced infectious tracheobronchitis. Am J Vet Res 42:1130, 1981.
23. Chladek, DW, et al.: Canine parainfluenza *Bordetella bronchiseptica* vaccine: Immunogenicity. Am J Vet Res 42:266, 1981.
24. Shade, FJ and Rapp, VJ: Studies of bacteria incorporating an extracted *Bordetella bronchiseptica* antigen for controlling canine bordetellosis. VM/SAC 77:1635, 1982.
25. Swango, LJ: Canine immunization. *In* Kirk, RW (ed): Current Veterinary Therapy VIII, Philadelphia, WB Saunders, 1983, p 1123.
26. Buxton, A and Faser, G: *Pasteurella, Yersinia* and *Francisella*. *In* Animal Microbiology. Philadelphia, JB Lippincott, 1977, p 124.
27. Gillespie JH and Timoney, JF: The genus *Pasteurella*. *In* Hagan and Bruner's Infectious Diseases of Domestic Animals, 7th ed. Ithaca, NY, Cornell University Press, 1981, p 107.
28. Snyder, SB, et al.: Respiratory tract disease associated with *Bordetella bronchiseptica* in cats. JAVMA 163:193, 1973.
29. Hirsch, DC: Bacteriology of the lower respiratory tract. *In* Kirk, RW (ed): Current Veterinary Therapy IX. Philadelphia, WB Saunders, 1986, p 247.
30. McKiernan, BC: Lower respiratory tract diseases. *In* Ettinger, SJ (ed): Textbook of Veterinary Internal Medicine. Philadelphia, WB Saunders, 1983, p 795.
31. Jenkins, WL: Respiratory tract—dog, cat. *In* The Bristol Veterinary Handbook of Antimicrobial Therapy. Syracuse, NY, Veterinary Learning Systems, 1982, p 52.
32. Buxton, A and Fraser, G: Animal Microbiology. Philadelphia, JB Lippincott, 1977, p 171.
33. Garnett, WI, et al.: Hemorrhagic streptococcal pneumonia in newly procured research dogs. JAVMA 181:1371, 1982.
34. Carter, GR: Essentials of Veterinary Bacteriology and Mycology. Philadelphia, Lea and Febiger, 1986, p 93.
35. Harpster, NK: The effectiveness of the cephalosporins in the treatment of bacterial pneumonias in the dog. JAAHA 17:7666, 1981.
36. Karlson, AG: Tuberculosis of animals. JAVMA 119:108, 1951.
37. Snider, WR: Tuberculosis in canine and feline populations: Review of the literature. Am Rev Respir Dis 104:877, 1971.
38. Snider, WR, et al.: Tuberculosis in canine and feline populations; Study of risk populations in Pennsylvania, 1966-1968. Am Rev Respir Dis 104:866, 1971.
39. Ferber, JA, et al.: Tuberculosis in a dog. JAVMA 183:117, 1983.
40. Liu, S, et al.: Canine tuberculosis. JAVMA 177:164, 1980.
41. Gillespie JH and Timoney, JF: Hagan and Bruner's Infectious Diseases of Domestic Animals, 7th ed. Ithaca, NY, Cornell University Press, 1981, p 247.
42. Carter, GR: Veterinarian's guide to the laboratory diagnosis of infectious diseases. Lenexa, KS, Veterinary Medicine Publishing Company, 1986, p 274.
43. Olson, P, et al.: Enterogenic *Escherichia coli* infection in two dogs with acute diarrhea. JAVMA 184:982, 1984.
44. Kreeger, TJ, et al.: Bacteremia concomitant with parvovirus in a pup. JAVMA 184:196, 1984.
45. Brunner, CJ and Swango, LJ: Canine parvovirus infection: effects on the immune system and factors that predispose to severe disease. Comp Cont Ed Pract Vet 12:979, 1985.
46. Janke, BH, et al.: Attacking and effacing *Escherichia coli* infections in calves, pigs, and dogs. Proceed 30th Annual Mtg Am Assoc Vet Lab Diagnosticians, October, 1987.
47. Greene, CE: Host-microbe interactions. *In* Greene, CE (ed): Clinical Microbiology and Infectious Diseases of Dogs and Cats. Philadelphia, WB Saunders, 1984, p 84.
48. White, GL, et al.: Therapeutic effects of prednisolone sodium succinate vs. dexamethasone in dogs subjected to *E. coli* septic shock. JAAHA 18:639, 1982.
49. Walker, RI, et al.: Protection of dogs from lethal consequences of endotoxemia with plasma transfusions. Cir Shock 6:190, 1979.
50. Calvert, CA and Greene, CE: Cardiovascular infections. *In* Greene, CE (ed): Clinical Microbiology and Infectious Diseases of Dogs and Cats. Philadelphia, WB Saunders, 1984, p 232.

51. Blaser, MJ and Reller, LB: *Campylobacter* enteritis. New Engl J Med 305:144, 1981.
52. Fox, JG, et al.: The prevalence of *Campylobacter jejuni* in random-source cats used in biomedical research. J Infect Dis 151:743, 1985.
53. Prescott, JF and Munroe, DL: *Campylobacter jejuni* enteritis in man and domestic animals. JAMA 181:1524, 1982.
54. Holt, PE: The role of dogs and cats in the epidemiology of human *Campylobacter* enterocolitis. J Sm Anim Pract 22:681, 1981.
55. Fleming, MP: Incidence of Campylobacter infection in dogs. Vet Rec 107:202, 1980.
56. Bernie, AG, et al.: The excretion of *Campylobacter*, *Salmonellae*, and *Giardia lamblia* in the feces of stray dogs. Vet Res Comm 6:133, 1983.
57. Sandstedt, K and Wierup, M: Concomitant occurrence of Campylobacter and parvovirus in dogs with gastroenteritis. Vet Res Commun 4:271, 1981.
58. Blaser, MJ, et al.: Survival of *Campylobacter fetus* spp. *jejuni* in biological milieus. J Clin Microbiol 11:309, 1980.
59. Rosef, O and Kapperud, G: Houseflies (*Musca domestica*) as possible vectors of *Campylobacter fetus* subsp. *jejuni*. Appl Environ Microbiol 45:381, 1983.
60. Fox, JG, et al.: *Campylobacter jejuni* associated diarrhea in dogs. JAVMA 83:1430, 1983.
61. Dillon, AR and Wilt, GR: Campylobacter species in the dog and cat: a cause for concern? Vet Clinics N Amer 13:647, 1983.
62. Walker, RI, et al.: Pathophysiology of *Campylobacter* enteritis. Microbiol Rev 50:81, 1986.
63. Blaser, JJ, et al.: Reservoirs for human campylobacteriosis. J Infect Dis 141:665, 1980.
64. Bruce, D, et al.: *Campylobacter jejuni* in cats and dogs. Vet Rec 190:200, 1980.
65. Greene, CE: Enteric bacterial infectious—campylobacteriosis. *In* Greene, CE (ed): Clinical Microbiology and Infectious Diseases of the Dog and Cat. Philadelphia, WB Saunders, 1984, p 624.
66. Skirrow, MB: *Campylobacter* enteritis in dogs and cats: a "new" zoonosis. Vet Res Commun 5:13, 1981.
67. Blaser, M, et al.: Campylobacter enteritis associated with canine infection. Lancet 88:979, 1978.
68. Svedham, A and Nokrans, G: *Campylobacter jejuni* enteritis transmitted from cat to man. Lancet 1:713, 1980.
69. Morse, EV and Duncan, MA: Canine salmonellosis; Prevalence, epizootiology, signs, and public health significance. JAVMA 167:817, 1975.
70. Khan, AQ: *Salmonellae* infections in dogs in the Sudan. Br Vet J 126:607, 1970
71. Timoney, JF: Feline salmonellosis. Vet Clin North Am 6:395, 1976.
72. Galton, MM, et al.: *Salmonella* isolation from dehydrated dog meals. JAVMA 126:57, 1955.
73. Thornton, H: The public health danger of unsterilized pet foods. Vet Rec 91:430, 1972.
74. Frost, A, et al.: The incidence of *Salmonella* infection in the dog. Aust Vet J 45:109, 1969.
75. Shimi, A and Barin, A: Salmonellosis in cats. J Comp Path 177: 87:315.
76. Fox, JG and Beaucage, CM: The incidence of *Salmonella* in random-source cats purchased for use in research. J Infect Dis 139:362, 1979.
77. Vos, P: The dog as a symptomless carrier of *Salmonella typhimurium*. Vet Rec 85:565, 1969.
78. Kaufmann, AF: Pets and *Salmonella* infection. JAVMA 149:1655, 1966.
79. Shimi, A, et al.: Salmonellosis in apparently healthy dogs. Vet Rec 98:110, 1976.
80. Ball, MR: Salmonella in dogs and cats of the Los Angeles, Honolulu, and Bermuda areas. JAVMA 118:164, 1951.
81. Day, WH, et al.: Salmonellosis in the dog. Am J Vet Res 24:156, 1963.
82. Carway, CT, et al.: Salmonellosis in the dog. II. Prevalence and distribution in greyhounds in Florida. J Infect Dis 91:6, 1952.
83. Borland, ED: *Salmonella* infection in dogs, cats, tortoises and terrapins. Vet Rec 96:401, 1975.
84. Beaucage, CM and Fox, JG: Transmissible antibiotic resistance in *Salmonella* isolated from random-source cats purchased for use in research. Am J Vet Res 40:849, 1979.
85. Thompson, H and Wright, NG: Canine salmonellosis. J Sm Anim Pract 10:579, 1969.
86. Crow, SE, et al.: Pyonephrosis associated with *Salmonella* infection in a dog. JAVMA 169:1324, 1976.
87. Redwood, DW and Bell, A: *Salmonella panama* isolation from aborted and newborn canine fetuses. Vet Rec 112:362, 1983.
88. Giannella, RA, et al.: Effect of indomethacin on intestinal water transport in *Salmonella*-infected rhesus monkeys. Infect Immunol 17:136, 1977.
89. Pocurull, DW, et al.: Survey of infectious and multiple drug resistance among *Salmonella* isolated from animals in the United States. Appl Microbiol 21:358, 1971.
90. Madewell, BR and McChesney, AE: Salmonellosis in a human infant, a cat and two parakeets in the same household. JAVMA 167:1089, 1975.
91. Morse, EV, et al.: Canine Salmonellosis: A review and report of dog to child transmission of *Salmonella enteritidis*. Am J Pub Health 66:82, 1976.
92. Oureshi, SR, et al.: Tyzzer's disease in a dog. JAVMA 168:602, 1976.
93. Kovatch, RM and Zebarth, G: Naturally occurring Tyzzer's disease in a cat. JAVMA 162:136, 1973.
94. Ganaway, JR, et al.: Tyzzer's disease. Am J Pathol 64:717, 1971.
95. Greene, CE: Enteric bacterial infections. *In* Greene, CE (ed): Clinical Microbiology and Infectious Diseases of Dogs and Cats. Philadelphia, WB Saunders, 1984, p 628.
96. Wilson, HD, et al.: *Yersinia enterocolitica* infection in a four-month-old infant associated with infection in household dogs. J Pediatr 89:767, 1976.
97. Papageorges, M, et al.: *Yersinia enterocolitica* enteritis in two dogs. JAVMA 182:618, 1983.
98. Hoenig, M: Intestinal malabsorption attributed to bacterial overgrowth in a dog. JAVMA 176:533, 1980.
99. Batt, RM, et al.: Bacterial overgrowth associated with a naturally occuring enteropathy in the German Shepherd dog. Res Vet Sci 35:42, 1983.
100. Carman, RJ and Lewis, JCM: Recurrent diarrhea in a dog associated with *Clostridium perfringens* type A. Vet Rec 112:342, 1983.
101. Schnurrenberger, PW and Hubbert, WT: Leptospirosis. *In* An Outline of the Zoonoses. Ames, Iowa: Iowa State University Press, 1981, p 18.
102. Fessler, JF and Morter, RL: Experimental feline leptospirosis. Cornell Vet 54:176, 1964.
103. Higgins, R: A minireview of the pathogenesis of acute leptospirosis. Can Vet J 22:277, 1964.
104. Navarro, CEK and Kociba, GJ: Hemostatic changes in dogs with experimental *Leptospira interrogans* scrovar *icterohaemorrhagiae* infection. Am J Vet Res 43:904, 1982.
105. Keenan, KP, et al.: Pathogenesis of experimental *Leptospira interrogans* serovar *bataviae* infection in the dog; microbiological, clinical, hematologic, and biochemical studies. Am J Vet Res 39:449, 1978.
106. Gourley, IMG: Canine leptospirosis. *In* Kirk, RW (ed): Current Veterinary Therapy V. Philadelphia, WB Saunders, 1974, p 971.
107. Carmichael, LD and Bruner, DW: Characteristics of a newly-recognized species of *Brucella* responsible for infectious canine abortions. Cornell Vet 58:579, 1968.
108. Munford, RS, et al.: Human disease caused by *Brucella canis*: A clinical and epidemiologic study of two cases. JAMA 231:1267, 1975.
109. Polt, SS, et al.: Human brucellosis caused by *Brucella canis*; clinical features and immune response. Ann Intern Med 97:717, 1982.
110. Pickerill, PA: Comments on epizootiology and control of canine brucellosis. JAVMA 156:1741, 1970.
111. Currier, RW, et al.: Canine brucellosis. JAVMA 180:132, 1982.
112. Carmichael, LE: Canine brucellosis: an annotated review with selected cautionary comments. Theriogenology 6:105, 1976.
113. Barton, CL: Canine brucellosis. Vet Clin North Am 7:705, 1977.
114. Greene, CE and George, LW: Canine brucellosis. *In* Greene, CE (ed): Clinical Microbiology and Infectious Diseases of the Dog and Cat. Philadelphia, WB Saunders, 1984, p 646.
115. Lewis, GE: A serological survey of 650 dogs to detect titers for *Brucella canis*. JAAHA 8:102, 1972.

116. McCullough, NB: Microbial and host factors in the pathogenesis of brucellosis. *In* Mudd, S (ed): Infectious agents and host reaction. Philadelphia, WB Saunders, 1970, p 324.
117. Carmichael, LE and Kenney, RM: Canine brucellosis: The clinical disease, pathogenesis and immune response. JAVMA 156:1726, 1970.
118. Moore, JA and Kakuk, TJ: Male dogs naturally infected with *Brucella canis*. JAVMA 155:1352, 1969.
119. Schoeb, TR and Morton, R: Scrotal and testicular changes in canine brucellosis: A case report. JAVMA 172:598, 1978.
120. Carmichael, LE and Keenney, RM: Canine abortion caused by *Brucella canis*. JAVMA 152:605, 1968.
121. Henderson, RA, et al.: Discospondylitis in three dogs infected with *Brucella canis*. JAVMA 165:451, 1974.
122. Riecke, JA and Rhoades, HE: *Brucella canis* isolated from the eye of a dog. JAVMA 166:583, 1975.
123. Flores-Castro, R and Carmichael, LE: Canine brucellosis: current status of methods for diagnosis and treatment. *In* Proceedings 27th Gaines Symposium. Texas A & M, 1977.
124. Johnson, CA, et al.: Effect of combined antibiotic therapy on fertility and brood bitches infected with *Brucella canis*. JAVMA 180:1330, 1982.
125. Steere, AC, et al.: Lyme arthritis: An epidemic of oligoarticular arthritis in children and adults in three Connecticut communities. Arthritis Rheum 20:7, 1977.
126. Lissman, BA, et al.: Spirochete associated arthritis (Lyme disease) in a dog. JAVMA 185:219, 1984.
127. Kornblatt, AN, et al.: Arthritis caused by *Borrelia burgdorferi* in dogs. JAVMA 186:960, 1985.
128. Steere, AC, et al.: Lyme carditis: cardiac abnormalities of Lyme disease. Ann Intern Med 93:8, 1980.
129. Magnarelli, LA, et al.: Borreliosis in dogs from Southern Connecticut. JAVMA 186:955, 1985.
130. Schulze, TL, et al.: *Ambylomma americanum*: A potential vector of Lyme disease in New Jersey. Science 224:601, 1984.
131. Burdorfer, W and Keirans, JE: Ticks and lyme disease in the United States. Ann Intern Med 99:121, 1983.
132. Steere, AC, et al.: Treatment of the early manifestations of Lyme disease. Ann Intern Med 99:76, 1983.
133. Attleberger, MH: Mycoses and mycosis-like diseases. *In* Kirk, RW (ed): Current Veterinary Therapy VIII. Philadelphia, WB Saunders, 1983, p 1184.
134. Saphir, DA and Carter, GR: Gingival flora of the dog with special reference to bacteria associated with bites. J Clin Microbiol 3:344, 1976.
135. Davenport, AA, et al.: *Actinomyces viscosus* in relation to the other actinomycetes and actinomycosis. Vet Bull 45:313, 1975.
136. Hardie, EM and Barsanti, JA: Treatment of canine actinomycosis. JAVMA 180:537, 1982.
137. Davenport, AA, et al.: Canine actinomycosis due to *Actinomyces viscosus*: report of six cases. VM/SAC 69:1442, 1974.
138. Dunbar, M and Vulgamott, SC: Thoracic and vetebral osteomylities caused by actinomycosis in a dog. VM/SAC 76:1159, 1981.
139. Lotspeich, M: Actinomycosis in a cat. VM/SAC 69:571, 1974.
140. Swerczek, TW, et al.: Canine actinomycosis. Zentralbl Veterinaermed [B] 15:955, 1968.
141. Attleberger, MH: Actinomycosis, nocardiosis, and dermatophilosis. *In* Kirk, RW (ed): Current Veterinary Therapy VIII. Philadelphia, WB Saunders, 1983, p 1184.
142. Jungerman, PF and Schwartzman, RM: Veterinary Medical Mycology. Philadelphia, Lea and Febiger, 1972, p 171.
143. Macy, DW and Small, E: Deep mycotic diseases. *In* Ettinger, SJ (ed): Textbook of Veterinary Internal Medicine, 2nd ed. Philadelphia, WB Saunders, 1983, p 261.
144. Walton, AM and Libke, KG: Nocardiosis in animals. VM/SAC 69:1105, 1974.
145. Swerczek, TW, et al.: Canine nocardiosis. Zentralbl Veterinaermed [B] 15:171, 1968.
146. Neal, JE and Heath, MK: Nocardiosis in dogs. Auburn Vet 11:112, 1955.
147. King, CB, et al.: Systemic nocardiosis with bone lesions in a dog. Auburn Vet 11:115, 1955.
148. Rhoades, HE, et al.: Nocardiosis in a dog with multiple lesions of the central nervous system. JAVMA 142:278, 1963.
149. Brodey, BS, et al.: Nocardial mycetoma in a dog. JAVMA 127:433, 1955.
150. Lerner, PI and Baum, GL: Antimicrobial susceptibility of *Nocardia* species. Antimicrob Agents Chemother 4:85, 1973.
151. Bach, MC, et al.: Susceptibility of *Nocardia asteroides* to 45 antimicrobial agents in vitro. Antimicrob Agents Chemother 3:1, 1973.
152. Boyce, JM: *Francisella tularensis* (tularemia). *In* Mandell, et al. (eds): Principles and Practice of Infectious Diseases. 2nd ed. New York, John Wiley and Sons, 1985, p 1290.
153. Packer, RM, et al.: Tularemia associated with domestic cats—Georgia, New Mexico. MMWR 31:39, 1982.
154. Bell, JF: Tularemia. *In* Steele, JH, (ed): CRC handbook series in zoonoses. Vol II. Boca Raton, Florida: CRC Press Inc, 1980, p 161.
155. Evans, ME, et al.: Tularemia transmitted by a cat. JAVMA 246:1343, 1981.
156. Quan, SF, et al.: Infectivity of tularemia applied to intact skin and ingested in drinking water. Science 123:942, 1956.
157. Hamilton, HB and Greene, CE: Zoonoses. *In* Greene, CE (ed): Clinical Microbiology and Infectious Diseases of the Dog and Cat. Philadelphia, WB Saunders, 1984, p 878.
158. Klemm, DM and Klemm, WR: A history of anthrax. JAVMA 135:458, 1959.
159. Van Ness, GB and Stein, CD: Soils of the United States favorable for anthrax. JAVMA 182:7, 1956.
160. Blood, DC, et al.: Diseases caused by *Bacillus* sp. *In* Veterinary Medicine. 6th ed. London: Balliere Tindall, 1983, p 531.
161. Farrow, BRH and Love, DH: Bacterial, viral and other infectious problems. *In* Ettinger SJ, (ed): Textbook of Veterinary Internal Medicine. 2nd ed. Philadelphia, WB Saunders, 1983, p 299.
162. Foster, JW, et al.: Animal anthrax associated with pack saddle pads. Morb Mortal Weekly Report, CDC, September 28, 1974, p 339.
163. Gillespie, JH and Timoney, JF: The genus *Bacillus*. *In* Hagan and Bruner's infectious diseases of domestic animals. 7th ed. Ithaca, NY. Cornell University Press, 1981, p 190.
164. Whitford, HW and Nelson, C: Anthrax: a review of the disease and its occurrence in Texas in 1974. Southwestern Vet 28:35, 1975.
165. Maxon, JH: Tetanus in the dog and cat. J S Afr Vet Med Assoc 35:209, 1964.
166. Greene, CE: Tetanus. *In* Clinical Microbiology and Infectious Diseases of the Dog and Cat. Philadelphia, WB Saunders, 1984, p 608.
167. Rubin, S, et al.: Tetanus following ovariohysterectomy in a dog: a case report. JAAHA 19:293, 1983.
168. Ryer, KA: Tetanus in a dog. VM/SAC 74:830, 1979.
169. Brooks, VB, et al.: Mode of action of tetanus toxin. Nature 175:120, 1955.
170. Stoll, BJ: Tetanus. Ped Clin N Amer 26:415, 1979.
171. Killingsworth, C, et al.: Feline tetanus. JAAHA 13:209, 1977.
172. Mally, KV and Rao, PM: Localized tetanus in a dog as a wound complication—diagnosis and successful treatment. Indian Vet J 52:807, 1975.
173. Webster, RA and Lawrence, DR: The effect of antitoxin on fixed and free toxin in experimental tetanus. J Pathol Bacteriol 86:413, 1963.
174. Catcott, EJ: Canine Medicine. 4th ed. Santa Barbara, California, American Veterinary Publishing, 1979, p 50.
175. Hoerlein, BF: Canine Neurology. 3rd ed. Philadelphia, WB Saunders, 1978, p 286.
176. Sugiyama, H: *Clostridium botulinum* neurotoxin. Microbiol Rec 44:419, 1980.
177. Rosen, MN: Clostridial infections and intoxications. *In* Hubbert, WT, et al. (eds): Diseases Transmitted from Animals to Man. Springfield, Ill, Charles C Thomas, 1975, p 257.
178. Barsanti, JA, et al.: Type C botulism in American foxhounds. JAVMA 172:809, 1978.
179. Richmond, RN, et al.: Type C botulism in a dog. JAVMA 173:202, 1978.
180. Barsanti, JA: Botulism. *In* Greene, CE (ed): Clinical Microbiology and Infectious Diseases of the Dog and Cat. Philadelphia, WB Saunders, 1984, p 599.
181. Kao, I, et al.: Botulinum toxin: mechanism of presynaptic blockade. Science 193:1256, 1976.
182. Marlow, GR and Smart, JL: Botulism in foxhounds. Vet Rec 111:252, 1982.

183. Chrisman, CL: Differentiation of tick paralysis and acute idiopathic polyradiculoneuritis in the dog using electromyography. JAAHA 11:455, 1975.
184. Cherington, M and Ryan, DW: Treatment of botulism with guanidine. N Engl J Med 282:195, 1970.
185. Oh, SJ: Botulism: Electrophysiologic studies. Ann Neurol 1:481, 1977.
186. Muller, GH, et al.: Small Animal Dermatology. 3rd ed. Philadelphia, WB Saunders 1983, p 197.
187. Kunkle, GA: Canine pyoderma. Comp Cont Ed Sm Anim Pract 1:7, 1979.
188. Murphy, JM, et al.: Survey of conjunctival flora in dogs with clinical signs of external eye disease. JAVMA 172:66, 1978.
189. Woody, BJ and Fox, SM: Otitis externa: Seeing past the signs to discover the underlying cause. Vet Med 81:616, 1986.
190. Griffin, CE: Otitis externa. Comp Cont Ed Pract Vet 3:741, 1981.
191. Neer, TM and Howard, PE: Otitis media. Comp Cont Ed Pract Vet 4:410, 1982.
192. Blue, JL, et al.: Treatment of experimentally induced *Pseudomonas aeruginosa* otitis externa in the dog by lavage with EDTA-trimethamine (Tris)-lysozyme. Am J Vet Res 35:1221, 1974.
193. Joshua, JO: Abscesses and their sequelae in cats. Feline Pract 1:9, 1971.
194. Scott, FW: Etiology and treatment of cat abscesses. Feline Pract 1:13, 1971.
195. Barton, CL. Canine vaginitis. Vet Clin N Am 7:711, 1977.
196. Ling, GV, et al.: Bacterial pathogens associated with urinary tract infections. Vet Clin N Am 9:617, 1979.
197. Weaver, AD and Pillinger, R: Lower urinary tract pathogens in the dog and their sensitivity to chemotherapeutic agents. Vet Rec 101:77, 1977.
198. Wheeler, SL, et al.: Postpartum disorders in the bitch. Comp Cont Ed Prac Vet 6:493, 1984.
199. Kivisto, AK, et al.: Canine bacteria. J Sm Anim Pract 18:707, 1977.
200. Ling, GV, et al.: Bacterial pathogens associated with urinary tract infections. Vet Clin North Am 9:617, 1979.
201. Finco, DR: Urinary tract infections. *In* Kirk, RW (ed): Current Veterinary Therapy VII, Philadelphia, WB Saunders, 1980, p 1158.
202. Weiss, E and Moulder, JW: The *Rickettsias* and *Chlamydias*. *In* Krieg, NR (ed): Bergey's Manual of Systematic Bacteriology. Baltimore, Williams and Wilkins, 1984, p 686.
203. Wills, JM: Chlamydia zoonoses. J Sm Anim Pract 27:717, 1986.
204. Schaefer, J and Keller, F: The control of feline pneumonitis. Speculum 15:11, 1962.
205. Kolar, JR and Rude, TA: Duration of immunity in cats inoculated with a commercial feline pneumonitis vaccine. VM/SAC 76:1171, 1981.
206. Harvey, JW: Haemobartonellosis. *In* Greene, CE (ed): Clinical Microbiology and Infectious Diseases of the Dog and Cat. Philadelphia, WB Saunders, 1984, p 576.
207. Meade, Y: Sequestration and phagocytosis of *Hemobartonella felis* in the spleen. Am J Vet Res 40:691, 1979.
208. Harvey, JW and Gaskin, JM: Feline hemobartonellosis: attempts to induce relapses of clinical disease in chronically infected cats. JAAHA 14:453, 1978.
209. Middleton, DJ, et al.: Hemobartonellosis in a dog. Aust Vet J 59:29, 1982.
210. Pryor, WH and Bradbury, RP: *Hemobartonella canis* infection in research dogs. Lab Anim Sci 25:566, 1975.
211. Gorham, JM and Foreyt, WJ: Salmon poisoning disease. *In* Greene, CE (ed): Clinical Microbiology and Infectious Diseases of the Dog and Cat. Philadelphia, WB Saunders, 1984, p 538.
212. Knapp, SE and Millemann, RE: Salmon poisoning disease. *In* Davis, JW (ed): Infectious Diseases of Wild Mammals. Ames, Iowa State University Press, 1981, p 376.
213. Price, JE and Sawyer, PD: Canine ehrlichiosis. *In* Kirk, RW (ed): Current Veterinary Therapy VIII—Small Animal Practice. Philadelphia, WB Saunders, 1983, p 1197.
214. Greene, CE and Harvey, JW: Canine ehrlichiosis. *In* Greene, CE (ed): Clinical Microbiology and Infectious Diseases of the Dog and Cat. Philadelphia, WB Saunders, 1984, p 545.
215. Hibler, SC, et al.: Rickettsial Infections in Dogs. Part II. Ehrlichioses and Infectious Cyclic Thrombocytopenia. Comp Cont Ed Pract Vet 8:106, 1986.
216. Harvey, JW, et al.: Cyclic thrombocytopenia induced by a *Rickettsia*-like agent. J Infect Dis 137:182, 1978.
217. French, TW and Harvey, JW: Serologic diagnosis of infectious cyclic thrombocytopenia in dogs using an indirect fluorescent antibody test. Am J Vet Res 44:2407, 1983.
218. Ewing, SA: Observations on leukocytic inclusion bodies from dogs infected with *Babesia canis*. JAVMA 143:503, 1963.
219. Huxsoll, DL, et al.: *Ehrlichia canis*—The causative agent of hemorrhagic disease in dogs? Vet Rec 85:587, 1970.
220. Nyindo, MBA, et al.: Tropical canine pancytopenia: In vitro cultivation of the causative agent—*Ehrlichia canis*. Am J Vet Res 32:1651, 1971.
221. Ewing, SA: A new strain of *Ehrlichia canis*. JAVMA 159:1771, 1971.
222. Madewell, BR and Gribble, DH: Infection in two dogs with an agent resembling *Ehrlichia equi*. JAVMA 80:512, 1982.
223. Troy, GC, et al.: Canine ehrlichiosis: A retrospective study of 30 naturally occurring cases. JAAHA 16:181, 1980.
224. Lewis, GE and Ristic, M: Effect of canine immune macrophages and canine immune serum on the growth of *Ehrlichia canis*. Am J Vet Res 41:1266, 1980.
225. Burghen, GA, et al.: Development of hypergammaglobulinemia in tropical canine pancytopenia. Am J Vet Res 32:749, 1971.
226. Buhles, WC, et al.: Tropical canine pancytopenia: clinical, hematologic, and serologic response of dogs to *Ehrlichia canis* infection, tetracycline therapy, and challenge inoculation. J Infect Dis 130:357, 1974.
227. Nyindo, M, et al.: Cell-mediated and humoral immune responses of German shepherd dogs and beagles to experimental infection with *Ehrlichia canis*. Am J Vet Res 41:250, 1980.
228. Bellah, JR, et al.: *Ehrlichia canis*—related polyarthritis in a dog. JAVMA 189:922, 1986.
229. Maeda, K, et al.: Human infection with *Ehrlichia canis*, a leukocytic rickettsia. N Engl J Med 316:853, 1987.
230. Ristic, M: Canine ehrlichiosis. Lab Communic 10:3, 1986.
231. Price, JE and Dolan, TT: A comparison of the efficacy of imidocarb dipropionate and tetracycline hydrochloride in the treatment of canine ehrlichioses. Vet Rec 107:275, 1980.
232. Fishbein, D, et al.: Canine tick-borne disease found in humans. ASM News 53:671, 1987.
233. Glaze, MB and Gaunt, SD: Uveitis associated with *Ehrlichia platys* infection in a dog. JAVMA 188:916, 1986.
234. Hibler, SC, et al.: Rickettsial infections in dogs. Rocky Mountain spotted fever and *Coxiella* infections. Comp Cont Ed Pract Vet 7:856, 1985.
235. Greene, CE: Rocky Mountain spotted fever and ehrlichiosis. *In* Kirk, RW (ed): Current Veterinary Therapy IV. Philadelphia, WB Saunders, 1986, p 1080.
236. Greene, CE and Philip, RN: Rocky Mountain spotted fever. *In* Greene, CE (ed): Clinical Microbiology and Infectious Diseases of the Dog and Cat. Philadelphia, WB Saunders, 1984, p 562.
237. Raoult, D, et al.: Mediterranean spotted fever in South of France: serosurvey in dogs. Trop Geograph Med 37:258, 1985.
238. Badger, LF: Rocky Mountain spotted fever: susceptibility of the dog and sheep to the virus. Public Health Rep 48:791, 1933.
239. Sexton, DJ, et al.: Rocky Mountain spotted fever in Mississippi: survey for spotted fever antibodies in dogs and for spotted fever group rickettsiae in dog ticks. Am J Epidemiol 103:192, 1976.
240. Kelley, DJ, et al.: Rocky Mountain spotted fever in areas of high and low prevalence: survey for canine antibodies to spotted fever rickettsiae. Am J Vet Res 43:1429, 1982.
241. Smith, RC, et al.: Rocky Mountain spotted fever in an urban canine population. JAVMA 183:1451, 1983.
242. Brietschwerdt, EB, et al.: Antibodies to spotted fever—group rickettsiae in dogs in North Carolina. Am J Vet Res 48:1436, 1987.
243. Lissman, BA and Benach, JL. Rocky Mountain spotted fever in dogs. JAVMA 176:994, 1980.
244. Rutgens, C, et al.: Severe Rocky Mountain spotted fever in five dogs. JAAHA 21:361, 1985.
245. Brietschwerdt, EB, et al.: Canine Rocky Mountain spotted fever: a kennel epizootic. Am J Vet Res 46.2124, 1985.
246. Greene, CE, et al.: Rocky Mountain spotted fever in dogs—

differentiation from canine ehrlichiosis. JAVMA 186:465, 1985.
247. Kennan, KP, et al.: Studies on the pathogenesis of *Rickettsia rickettsii* in the dog: clinical and clinicopathologic changes in experimental infection. Am J Vet Res 38:851, 1977.
248. Giminez, DF: Staining rickettsiae in yolk sac cultures. Stain Technol 39:135, 1964.
249. Greene, CE and Prestwood, AK: Coccidial infections. *In* Greene, CE (ed): Clinical Microbiology and Infectious Diseases of the Dog and Cat. WB Saunders, 1984, p 824.
250. Dubey, JP: Life cycle of *Isospora rivolta* (Grassi, 1879) in cats and mice. J Protozool 26:433, 1979.
251. Long, PL: Pathology and pathogenicity of coccidial infections. *In* Hammond, DM and Long, PL: The Coccidia: Eimeria, Isospora, Toxoplasma, and Related Genera. Baltimore, University Park Press, 1973, p 253.
252. Dubey, JP: Pathogenicity of *Isospora ohioensis* infection in dogs. JAVMA 173:192, 1978.
253. Dubey, JP and Williams, CSF: *Hammondia heydorni* infection in sheep, goats, moose, dogs and coyotes. Parasitology 8:123, 1980.
254. Levine, ND: Nomenclature of Sarcocystis in the ox and sheep and of fecal coccidia of the dog and cat. J Parasitol 63:36, 1977.
255. Shelton, GC, et al.: A coccidia-like organism associated with subcutaneous granulomata in a dog. JAVMA 152:263, 1968.
256. Correa, WM, et al.: Canine isosporosis. Canine Pract 10:44, 1983.
257. Smart, J: Amprolium for canine coccidiosis. Mod Vet Pract 52:41, 1971.
258. Current WL, et al.: Human cryptosporidiosis in immunocompetent and immunodeficient persons. N Engl J Med 308:1252, 1983.
259. Current, WL, et al.: The life cycle of *Cryptosporidium baileyi* n. sp. (Apicomplexa, Cryptosporidiidae) infecting chickens. J Protozool 33:289, 1986.
260. Poonacha, KB and Pippin, C: Intestinal cryptosporidiosis in a cat. Vet Pathol 19:708, 1982.
261. Sisk, DB, et al.: Intestinal cryptosporidiosis in two pups. JAVMA 184:835, 1984.
262. Turnwald, GH, et al.: Cryptosporidiosis associated with immunosuppression attributable to distemper in a pup. JAVMA 192:79, 1988.
263. Wallace, GD: The role of the cat in the natural history of *Toxoplasma gondii*. Am J Trop Med Hyg 22:313, 1973.
264. Jones, SR: Toxoplasmosis: a review. JAVMA 163:1038, 1973.
265. Dubey, JP and Frenkel, JK: Cyst-induced toxoplasmosis in cats. J Protozool 19:155, 1972.
266. Frenkel, JK: Pathology and pathogenic mechanisms in tissue infection. *In* Mettrick, DF and Desser, SS: Parasites; Their World and Ours. New York, Elsevier-North Holland Biomedical Press, 1982, p 258.
267. Koestner, A and Cole, CR: Neuropathology of canine toxoplasmosis. Am J Vet Res 83:831, 1960.
268. Vainsi, CJ and Campbell, LH: Ocular toxoplasmosis in cats. JAVMA 154:141, 1969.
269. Smart, ME, et al.: Toxoplasmosis in a cat associated with cholangitis and progressive pancreatitis. Can Vet J 14:313, 1973.
270. Hagiwara, T, et al.: Experimental feline toxoplasmosis. Jpn J Vet Sci 43:329, 1981.
271. Averill, DR and deLahunta, A: Toxoplasmosis of the canine nervous system: clinicopathologic findings in four cases. JAVMA 159:1134, 1971.
272. Dubey, JP and Hoover, EA: Attempted transmission of *Toxoplasma gondii* infection from pregnant cats to their kittens. JAVMA 170:538, 1977.
273. Dubey, JP and Yeary, RA: Anticoccidial activity of 2-sulfamoyl-4, 4-diaminodiphenylsulfone, sulfadiazine, pyrimethamine and clindamycin in cats infected with *Toxoplasma gondii*. Can Vet J 18:51, 1977.
274. Frenkel, JK and Smith, DD: Inhibitory effects of monensin on shedding of Toxoplasma oocysts by cats. J Parasitol 68:851, 1982.
275. Kirkpatrick, CE and Farrell, JP: Giardiasis. Compend Cont Ed 4:367, 1982.
276. Kirkpatrick, CE: Enteric protozoal infections. *In* Greene, CE: Clinical Microbiology and Infectious Diseases of the Dog and Cat. WB Saunders, 1984, p 806.
277. Bingham, AK and Meyer, EA: Giardia excystation can be induced in vitro in acid solution. Nature 277:301, 1979.
278. Craft, JC: Giardia and giardiasis in childhood. Ped Infect Dis 1:196, 1982.
279. Tartakow, IJ and Vorperian, JH: Foodborne and Waterborne Diseases: Their Epidemiologic Characteristics. Westport, Connecticut, AVI Publishing Company, 1981, p 1.
280. Erlandsen, SL and Meyer, EA: Giardia and giardiasis—biology, pathologenesis, and epidemiology. New York, Plenum Press, 1984.
281. Hewlett, EL, et al.: Experimental infection of mongrel dogs with *Giardia lamblia* cysts and cultured trophozoites. J Infect Dis 145:89, 1982.
282. Morecki, R and Parker, JG: Ultrastructural studies of the human *Giardia lamblia* and subjacent jejunal mucosa in subjects with steatorrhea. Gastroenterology 52:151, 1967.
283. Alp, MH and Hislop, IG: The effect of *Giardia lamblia* infestation on the gastro-intestinal tract. Australasian Annals of Medicine 18:232, 1969.
284. Cowen, AE and Campbell, CB: Giardiasis—a cause of vitamin B_{12} malabsorption. Am J Digest Dis 18:384, 1973.
285. Yardly, JH, et al.: Epithelial and other mucosal lesions of the jejunum in giardiasis. Jejunal biopsy studies. Bulletin Johns Hopkins Hosp 115:389, 1964.
286. Smith, JW and Wolfe, MS: Giardiasis. Annu Rev Med 31:373, 1980.
287. Barlough, JE: Canine giardiasis: a review. J Sm Anim Pract 20:613, 1979.
288. Kirkpatrick, CE, et al.: Giardiasis in a cattery. JAVMA 187:161, 1985.
289. Worley, SD, et al.: New halamine water disinfectants. *In* Janauer, GE (ed): Progress in Chemical Disinfection, State Univ. of New York, Binghamton, 1986, p 61.
290. Kong, LI, et al.: Inactivation of *Giardia lamblia* cysts by combined and free chlorine. Appl Environ Microbiol. Submitted December, 1987.
291. Levine, HD: The Flagellates. *In* Textbook of Veterinary Parasitology. Burgess Publishing, 1978, p 11.
292. Honigberg, BM: Trichomonads of importance in human medicine. *In* Kreier JP: Parasitic Protozoa. New York, Academic Press, 1978, p 275.
293. Connor, DH, et al.: Amebiasis. *In* Binford, CH and Connor, DH: Pathology of Tropical and Extraordinary Diseases. Washington, DC, Armed Forces Institute of Pathology, 1976, p 308.
294. Wittnich, C: *Entamoeba histolytica* infection in a German shepherd dog. Can Vet J 17:259, 1976.
295. Zaman, V: *Balantidium coli*. *In* Kreier, JP: Parasitic Protozoa, New York, Academic Press, 1978, p 633.
296. Ewing, SA and Bull, RW: Severe chronic canine diarhea associated with *Balantidium-Trichuris* infection. JAVMA 149:519, 1966.
297. Breitschwerdt, E: Babesiosis. *In* Greene CE: Clinical Microbiology and Infectious Diseases of the Dog and Cat. WB Saunders, 1984, p 796.
298. Abdullahi, SU and Sannusi, A: Canine babesiosis. *In* Kirk, RW (ed): Current Veterinary Therapy IX. Philadelphia, WB Saunders, 1986, p 1096.
299. Futter, GJ, et al.: Studies on feline babesiosis: Chemical pathology; macroscopic and microscopic postmortem findings. J S Afr Vet Assoc 52:5, 1981.
300. Futter, GJ and Belonje, PC: Studies on feline babesiosis: Clinical observations. J S Afr Vet Assoc 51:143, 1980.
301. Futter, GJ, et al.: Studies of feline babesiosis: Hematological findings. J S Afr Vet Assoc 51:271, 1980.
302. Correa, WM: Canine babesiosis: transplacental transmission. Biologico 40:321, 1974.
303. Ewing, SA: Method of reproduction of *Babesia canis* in erythrocytes. Am J Vet Res 26:727, 1965.
304. Simpson, CF: Phagocytosis of *Babesia canis* by neutrophils in the peripheral circulation. Am J Vet Res 35:701, 1974.
305. Farwell, GE, et al.: Clinical observations on *Babesia gibsoni* and *Babesia canis* infections in dogs. JAVMA 180:507, 1982.
306. Kier, AB: Cytauxzoonosis. *In* Greene, CE: Clinical Microbiology and Infectious Diseases of Dog and Cat. WB Saunders, 1984, p 791.

307. Bendele, RA, et al.: Cytauxzoonosis-like disease in Texas cats. Southwest Vet 29:244, 1976.
308. Wagner, JE, et al.: Experimentally induced cytauxzoonosis-like disease in domestic cats. Vet Parasitol 6:305, 1980.
309. Chapman, WL, Jr and Hanson, WL: American trypanosomiasis. *In* Greene, CE: Clinical Microbiology and Infectious Diseases of Dog and Cat. WB Saunders, 1984, p 757.
310. Lushbaugh, CC, et al.: Intrauterine death from congenital Chagas' disease in laboratory-bred marmosets (*Saguinus fuscicollis lagonotus*). Am J Trop Med Hyg 18:662, 1969.
311. Anselmi, A and Moleiro, F: Pathogenic mechanisms in Chagas' cardiomyopathy. *In* Ciba Foundation Symposium No. 20: Trypanosomiasis and Leishmaniasis with Special Reference to Chagas' Disease. Amsterdam, Associated Scientific Publishers, 1974, p 125.
312. Williams, GD, et al.: Naturally occurring trypanosomiasis (Chagas' disease) in dogs. JAVMA 171:171, 1977.
313. Steck, EA: The Chemotherapy of Protozoan Disease. Washington, DC, Walter Reed Army Institute, 1972, p 8.
314. Tippit, TS: Canine trypanosomiasis (Chagas' disease). Southwest Vet 31:97, 1978.
315. Jones, TC and Hunt, RD: Diseases due to protozoa. *In* Veterinary Pathology. Philadelphia, Lea and Febiger, 1983, p 719.
316. Chapman, WL, Jr, and Hanson, WL: Leishmaniasis. *In* Greene, CE: Clinical Microbiology and Infectious Diseases of Dog and Cat. WB Saunders, 1984, p 764.
317. Acha, PN and Syfres, B: Zoonoses and Communicable Diseases Common to Man and Animals. Washington, DC, PAHO/WHO Scientific Publication No. 354, 1980, p 388.
318. Garett, A: Visceral leishmaniasis. Southwest Vet 31:125, 1978.
319. Berman, JD and Wyler DJ: An in vitro model for investigation of chemotherapeutic agents of leishmaniasis. J Infect Dis 142:83, 1980.
320. Craig, TM: Hepatozoonosis. *In* Greene, CE: Clinical Microbiology and Infectious Diseases of Dog and Cat. WB Saunders, 1984, p 771.
321. Gaunt, PS, et al.: Extreme neutrophilic leukocytosis in a dog with hepatozoonosis. JAVMA 182:409, 1983.
322. Barton, CL, et al.: Canine hepatozoonosis: a retrospective study of 15 naturally occurring cases. JAAHA 21:125, 1985.
323. Ezeokoli, CD, et al.: Clinical and epidemiologic studies on canine hepatozoonosis in Zaria, Nigeria. J Sm Anim Pract 24:455, 1983.
324. Craig, TM, et al.: Hepatozoon canis infection in dogs: clinical, radiographic and hematologic findings. JAVMA 173:967, 1978.
325. El Hindaway, MR: Studies on the blood of dogs. Haematological findings in some diseases caused by specific blood parasites. (a) *Babesia canis;* (b) *Hepatozoon canis.* Br Vet J 107:303, 1961.
326. Greene, CE and Chandler, FW: Pneumocystosis. *In* Greene, CE: Clinical Microbiology and Infectious Diseases of Dog and Cat. WB Saunders, 1984, p 859.
327. Farrow, BRH, et al.: Pneumocystitis pneumonia in the dog. J Comp Pathol 82:447, 1972.
328. Gajdusek, DC: *Pneumocystis carinii*—etiological agent of interstitial plasma cell pneumonia of premature and young infants. Pediatrics 19:543, 1957.
329. Chaudhary, S, et al.: Percutaneous transthoracic needle aspiration of the lung. Diagnosing *Pneumocystis carinii* pneumonitis. Am J Dis Child 131:902, 1977.
330. Pifer, LL, et al.: Propagation of *Pneumocystis carinii* in vitro. Pediatr Res 11:305, 1977.
331. Szabo, JR, et al.: Encephalitozoonosis. *In* Greene, CE: Clinical Microbiology and Infectious Diseases of Dog and Cat. WB Saunders, 1984, p 781.
332. Nordstoga, K, et al.: Nosematosis (encephalitozoonosis) in a litter of blue foxes after intrauterine infection of Nosema spores. Acta Vet Scand 19:150, 1978.
333. Mohn, SF, et al.: Encephalitozoonosis in the blue fox. Identification of the parasite. Acta Pathol Microbiol Scand 89:117, 1981.
334. Shadduck, JA, et al.: Isolation of the causative organism of canine encephalitozoonosis. Vet Pathol 15:449, 1978.
335. Botha, WS, et al.: Canine encephalitozoonosis in South Africa. J S Afr Vet Med Assoc 50:135, 1979.

47 CANINE VIRAL DISEASES

LARRY J. SWANGO

RABIES

Rabies is a virus-induced neurologic disease of warm-blooded animals that, with rare exceptions, is fatal. Except for selected island countries and states, rabies occurs worldwide. The recorded history of rabies extends to the twentieth century B.C. in the form of an ordinance in the Eshnunna code of Mesopotamia, which defined penalties for the owner of a mad dog if a bite from the dog resulted in a person's death.[1]

The infectious nature of rabies was demonstrated in the early 1800s by transmission of the disease by experimental injection with saliva from a rabid dog.[1–3] The work of Louis Pasteur, starting in 1881, was the beginning of understanding of rabies as an infectious disease that could be prevented by treatment with rabies virus that had been altered by serial passage in rabbits. Historically, this became known as the Pasteur treatment for humans after exposure to rabies. Rabies is regarded as a fatal disease although survivors of rabies have been documented, including dogs and humans.[3–6] As a fatal disease, rabies is generally regarded as not treatable but it is preventable by immunization of domestic animals and humans in groups at high risk of exposure and by postexposure treatment of humans with known exposure to rabies virus. Because of its fatal nature, rabies is a most important zoonotic disease.

ETIOLOGY

Rabies virus is classified in the Rhabdoviridae family and is a member of the genus *Lyssavirus*.[3, 7] Rhabdo means rod; members of the Rhabdoviridae family are rod-shaped, with one flat end and one rounded end, giving a bullet-shaped appearance. Rabies virus is about 75 × 180 nm in size; it possesses a lipid envelope and a genome of RNA. Rabies virus is a labile virus that does not persist in the environment. Sunlight, warm temperatures, drying, heat, and common disinfectants all destroy the infectivity of rabies virus. It is somewhat more resistant to phenolic disinfectants than to other chemical disinfectants. Rabies virus is generally regarded as being of one antigenic type, although rabies-like viruses have been isolated from various parts of the world. Although there is basically only one antigenic type of rabies virus, antigenic differences have been established with the use of monoclonal antibodies. These differences have been correlated with animal species of origin and monoclonal antibodies have been used to biotype isolates of rabies virus.[8–10]

EPIZOOTIOLOGY

All species of warm-blooded animals are susceptible to infection with rabies virus, although there are differences in susceptibility. Opossums and birds are among the most resistant species[1, 3]; skunks, wild canids, raccoons, bats, and cattle are among the most susceptible species. Dogs, cats, horses, sheep, goats, nonhuman primates, and humans are intermediate in susceptibility to rabies. Wild animals are the primary reservoirs for rabies in many parts of the world but domestic animal pets are the principal source for transmission of rabies to humans. When rabies in dogs and cats is controlled, the occurrence of rabies in humans is reduced to a very low level. In the United States, decreased occurrence of rabies in humans has paralleled the decline in dog rabies following the implementation of rabies vaccination programs for dogs and cats beginning in the early 1950s.[1, 11] Vaccination of at least 70 per cent of the dog population controls epizootics of dog rabies and provides a barrier for reducing the risk of human exposure to rabies.[12]

Rabies virus must contact nerve endings and enter nerve fibers before infection occurs that leads to the development of rabies. Infection occurs primarily by infected saliva from a rabid animal making contact with nerve endings or damaged nerve fibers as a result of a bite from a rabid animal. Contamination of a fresh wound with saliva containing rabies virus, or rabies virus making contact with the conjunctivum or olfactory mucosa can also result in the transmission of rabies. Aerosol transmission has been documented in caves with large populations of infected bats and has been performed experimentally in the laboratory. Transmission by ingestion has been accomplished experimentally.[1, 3]

The incubation period for rabies from the time of exposure to the onset of clinical disease is usually from three to eight weeks, but it can vary from a time as short as a week to more than a year.[1, 3, 7] The location of the bite or exposure and the amount of virus present at the exposure are the two most important factors affecting the incubation period. Bites that occur on the face, head, and neck result in shorter incubation periods. After infection occurs, rabies virus migrates centripetally in peripheral nerve fibers to the central nervous system and eventually affects neurons, leading to abnormal behavior and paralysis. After rabies virus reaches the brain and multiplies in neurons, it migrates centrifugally in nerve fibers from the central nervous system to salivary glands, allowing for shedding of virus in the saliva and further transmission. Rabies virus may be found in other peripheral tissues and organs but they are not important in transmission of the virus.

CLINICAL SIGNS

Three clinical stages of rabies have been defined: the prodromal, excitative, and paralytic stages of the disease.[1, 3, 7] The prodromal stage of the disease is characterized by change in behavior and is indicative that the rabies syndrome is to follow. Change in behavior is the basis for the expression, "mad dogs and friendly foxes." Wild animals lose their fear of humans and they may be observed during the day in locations that are not normal, i.e., nocturnal animals are observed during the day in locations where they normally would be afraid to go. Friendly, affectionate pets become apprehensive, unusually alert to changes in their surroundings, and may hide out of fear. The prodromal stage of the disease may last for one to three days and is followed by the excitative or hyperreactive stage of the disease. Animals that manifest a prominent hyperreactivity to external stimuli or that are easily excited may attempt to bite anything close by, including solid objects such as wood, metal, and fences, and they may snap at imaginary objects. It is this stage of the disease that typifies the association of rabies with a "mad dog." If the manifestations of hyperreactivity are prominent, the animal is regarded as having "furious" rabies. Some animals with rabies may not manifest signs of hyperreactivity or it may be of very short duration; they may be oblivious to their surroundings and appear to be in a state of stupor. Such animals are regarded as having "dumb" rabies. The excitative stage of the disease may be nonexistent, as in dumb rabies, or it may last as long as three to four days and be followed by the paralytic stage of the disease. Viral-induced damage to motor neurons results in paralysis, which is usually an ascending ataxia of the back legs. Incoordination is often one of the first signs of the paralytic stage of rabies. Animals with unexplained paralysis should be regarded as possibly rabid even though there may have been no antecedent signs suggestive of rabies. Paralysis of muscles of deglutition is responsible for drooling of saliva and inability to swallow. The paralytic stage of the disease may last for one to two days and is followed by death due to respiratory arrest. Death from rabies in domestic animals usually occurs within two to seven days after the onset of clinical signs. Survival or recovery from rabies has been documented in dogs as well as in rare cases in human patients.[4–6] Recovery from rabies in dogs has implications for possible exposure to rabies virus from dogs that appear to recover from lower motor neuron diseases that resemble polyradiculoneuritis.[3] The lack of reliable methods for the antemortem diagnosis of rabies necessitates a cautious approach to minimize the risk of human exposure to rabies virus in cases that are misdiagnosed.[7]

DIAGNOSIS

Rabies should be suspected based on the clinical signs. Confirmation of the diagnosis depends on postmortem examination for rabies virus in portions of the brain and brain stem. The fluorescent antibody test is the primary method used in the postmortem diagnosis of rabies; it is more than 99 per cent accurate in diagnosing rabies based on correlations with mouse inoculation. If rabies virus is found in the brain, there is potential for the virus to be in salivary glands and saliva. If rabies virus is not found in the brain, it is concluded that there would be no virus in the salivary glands and saliva because rabies virus reaches the salivary glands by migration through nerve fibers from the brain. If there has been possible human or animal exposure from an animal with clinical signs suggestive of rabies, mouse inoculation is usually done to verify negative fluorescent antibody results. A disadvantage of the mouse inoculation test is that a period of two to three weeks may be required to make final conclusions about the presence or absence of rabies virus in the brain. The presence of intracytoplasmic inclusion bodies (Negri bodies) in neurons is pathognomonic for rabies in dogs, but Negri bodies are not always present and their absence does not rule out rabies.

Fluorescent antibody and immunoperoxidase techniques have been applied to biopsies of skin, especially the sensory vibrissae, in an attempt to develop a suitable procedure for antemortem diagnosis of rabies.[3, 13, 14] Positive results were achieved in several species of animals; however, negative results are not reliable in ruling out rabies in the diagnosis. It is now generally concluded that immunologic examination of skin biopsies is not reliable for antemortem diagnosis of rabies.[7]

TREATMENT AND PREVENTION

Treatment is not recommended for animals with rabies because of the risk of human exposure.[3] Dogs that present clinical signs consistent with rabies should be placed in strict isolation to prevent possible exposure of animals or humans, or they should be euthanatized and the brain examined for rabies virus. Rabies is preventable by immunization of dogs and cats and by control of stray animals. Vaccination of dogs on a widespread basis has been one of the most effective programs in decreasing the occurrence of human rabies. With the implementation of rabies vaccination programs in dogs in the United States in the early 1950s, the number of cases of human rabies declined from more than 40 per year in the 1940s to only one to two per year in the 1960s.[11] During the same period, cases of rabies in dogs declined from more than 8,000/year to about 300/year in the 1960s.

Excellent rabies vaccines are currently available in the United States for use in dogs and cats, and, in some instances, for use in horses, cattle, and sheep. Most of the vaccines contain inactivated rabies virus of tissue culture origin. They are safe and effective, with many of them providing immunity for three years. A list of licensed animal rabies vaccines is revised annually as part of a Compendium of Animal Rabies Control that is published in the Journal of the American Veterinary Medical Association.[15] It is recommended that dogs and cats be vaccinated at three to four months of age, again one year later, and either annually or triennially thereafter, depending upon whether a one-year or three-year rabies vaccine is used. It is recommended that three-year vaccines be used, since they are more effective in increasing the percentage of immunized dogs and cats.[15] Three-year vaccines are recommended even in areas where state or local laws require annual vaccination for rabies. There are no rabies vaccines approved for use in wild or exotic animal pets.

HUMAN RABIES VACCINATION

Recommendations for immunization of humans are promulgated by an Advisory Committee on Immunization Practices (ACIP) for the Centers for Disease Control (CDC) of the United States Public Health Service and by the World Health Organization (WHO). The rabies vaccine licensed for use in humans in the United States is prepared from rabies virus propagated in human diploid cell cultures and it is referred to as human diploid cell vaccine (HDCV). The vaccine contains inactivated rabies virus and it is approved for use in both pre-exposure and post-exposure immunization using a 1.0 ml dose intramuscularly, or for pre-exposure immunization only using 0.1 ml intradermally.[16, 17] It is marketed in two separate dosage formulations, 1.0 ml for intramuscular use and 0.1 ml for intradermal use.

The ACIP recommendations for pre-exposure immunization are based on defined categories for risk of exposure to rabies virus.[16] Four risk categories are defined: continuous, frequent, infrequent, and rare. The rare risk category includes the human population at large and pre-exposure rabies immunization is not recommended for this group of people. Pre-exposure immunization is recommended for persons in the other three risk categories. The continuous risk category includes laboratory workers in research and biologics production who work with virulent rabies virus in high concentrations on a regular basis. The frequent risk category includes rabies diagnostic laboratory workers, spelunkers, veterinarians, veterinary technicians, and animal control and wildlife workers in areas with epizootic rabies. The infrequent risk category includes the same population groups as the frequent risk of exposure category except in areas of low rabies endemicity, in addition to certain travellers or workers in foreign countries with epizootic rabies.

Pre-exposure immunization consists of primary immunization with a three-dose series of HDCV given on a schedule of days 0, 7, and 21 or 28.[16] Essentially, everyone who takes HDCV either IM or ID according to this schedule develops a primary immune response to rabies virus.[16, 17] Persons in the continuous and frequent risk of exposure categories are advised to have their titer of antibody to rabies virus determined periodically and to take a single injection booster dose of HDCV when their titer has dropped to an insignificant level. Routine boosters on a regular schedule of every two or more years could be taken in lieu of having titers determined, but about 7 per cent of previously immunized persons develop systemic allergic reactions to booster doses of HDCV.[18] Booster doses of HDCV are not recommended for persons in the infrequent risk of exposure category.

Post-exposure treatment with HDCV is recommended for persons with known or probable exposures to rabies virus.[16] For persons who have had pre-exposure immunization, post-exposure treatment consists of only two doses of HDCV taken three days apart regardless of how long it has been since they were vaccinated. For persons who have not had pre-exposure immunization to rabies, post-exposure treatment consists of five doses of HDCV given on a schedule of days 0, 3, 7, 14, and 28, in addition to rabies immune globulin at a dosage of 9 IU/lb (20 IU/kg) on day 0.

MANAGEMENT OF DOGS AND CATS THAT HAVE BITTEN A HUMAN

Dogs showing signs of neurologic disease at the time of biting a human and unwanted or stray dogs or cats that have bitten a person should be euthanatized immediately and their brain examined for rabies virus to determine if the bitten person was possibly exposed to rabies.[15] Healthy dogs or cats that are owned pets should be confined for ten days of observation after the bite for signs of rabies. The purpose of the ten-day observation is to determine if the bitten person was exposed to rabies. This determination is based on the knowledge that dogs and cats do not shed rabies virus in their saliva for more than a few days before the onset of rabies. Six days before the onset of clinical signs of rabies is the earliest that rabies virus has been detected in the saliva of either dogs or cats. Therefore, if the dog or cat remains healthy for ten days after the bite, the person was not exposed to rabies. There are no provisions for confinement and observation of other species due to lack of information on the length of time that they may shed virus before the onset of clinical signs of rabies. As a result all "biters" except owned, healthy dogs and cats should be euthanatized immediately after the bite and examined for rabies virus to determine if the person was exposed to rabies. If rabies virus is not detected in the brain of the animal, the person was not exposed to rabies virus. If the animal is found positive for rabies, post-exposure immunization should be initiated as soon as possible since there is no safe waiting period before treatment is started.

MANAGEMENT OF DOGS AND CATS EXPOSED TO RABIES

Dogs or cats that are currently immunized to rabies according to recommendations for rabies vaccination and that are bitten by a proven rabid animal, or that are bitten by a wild animal in a rabies endemic area should be revaccinated immediately and observed for

90 days.[15] Unvaccinated dogs or cats that have known exposure to rabies virus should be euthanatized or confined in strict isolation for six months if the owner is unwilling to consent to euthanasia. The dog or cat should be vaccinated at the fifth month of isolation and if they are healthy at the end of six months, they may be released to the owner. The purpose of these requirements for management of dogs or cats that are exposed to rabies is to prevent secondary exposure of other animals or humans if the bitten dog or cat should develop rabies as a result of the known exposure.

CANINE DISTEMPER

Canine distemper is a highly contagious febrile disease of dogs and other carnivores with a worldwide distribution. It is the most prevalent viral disease of dogs; there are only a few isolated dogs that have not been exposed to or infected with the virus. Canine distemper virus (CDV) causes more morbidity and mortality than any other virus that infects dogs. The incidence of disease is greatest in young dogs three to six months of age, after maternally derived passive immunity has waned. The morbidity ranges from 25 to 75 per cent and the fatality to case ratio is often as high as 50 to 90 per cent, depending on the strain of virus. Only rabies has a higher fatality rate in dogs than canine distemper.

ETIOLOGY

Canine distemper virus is classified in the Paramyxoviridae family and it is closely related antigenically and biophysically to measles virus of humans and rinderpest virus of ruminants.[19, 20] The three viruses are grouped together in the *Morbillivirus* genus. The morbilliviruses are relatively large RNA viruses (150 to 250 nm in diameter) with helical symmetry; they possess a lipoprotein envelope. They are relatively labile viruses, with infectivity being destroyed by heat, drying, detergents, lipid solvents, and disinfectants.[20, 21] Routine cleaning and disinfection procedures are effective in destroying CDV on hard surfaces and inanimate objects in veterinary clinics and kennels. In warm climates CDV does not persist in kennels after infected dogs have been removed.[21] The virus survives longer in colder environments and during winter months. It can remain viable for a few weeks at temperatures slightly above freezing and it is stable for months to years in the frozen state at ultracold temperatures.[20, 21] Although CDV is susceptible to ultraviolet light, germicidal lamps are of limited value in controlling the spread of canine distemper in veterinary hospitals and kennels.

EPIZOOTIOLOGY

Canine distemper virus is transmitted primarily by aerosol and infective droplets from body secretions of infected animals, and infection spreads rapidly among susceptible young dogs.[21, 22] The recurring supply of puppies throughout the year maintains the infection in the population of young dogs. There is only one serotype of CDV, but there are biologically different strains of virulent CDV.[20, 22, 23] Some strains of CDV are mildly virulent and usually cause inapparent infections. Some strains cause acute disease with a high frequency of encephalitis and high mortality. Other strains are more viscerotropic and cause a debilitating disease with high mortality but with a low frequency of encephalitis. A common feature of all virulent strains of CDV is immunosuppressive effects in dogs.[21, 22]

Immunosuppression from viral replication in lymphoid tissue during the incubation period is an important factor in determining the outcome of infection with CDV.[21] Signs typical of acute distemper usually occur only in dogs that are immunosuppressed by CDV.[21, 22, 24] Dogs that win the battle between the virus and the host develop immunity and overcome the inapparent infection without developing signs of acute distemper except for the occurrence of encephalitis in a relatively small percentage of dogs.[24] Secondary bacterial infections due to the immunosuppressive effects of CDV are often responsible for many of the clinical signs associated with distemper, and they contribute to increased mortality. In addition to secondary bacterial infections, toxoplasmosis, coccidiosis, viral enteritis, and mycoplasmal infections are enhanced by the immunosuppressive effects of concurrent CDV infection.[21, 23, 25]

CLINICAL SIGNS

The incubation period for the onset of clinical signs of acute distemper is usually 14 to 18 days.[24] After exposure and infection with CDV, a transient fever and leukopenia occur between the fourth and seventh days without overt signs of disease.[21, 22, 23] The temperature returns to normal for a period of 7 to 14 days, after which there is a second rise in body temperature accompanied by conjunctivitis and rhinitis. Coughing, diarrhea, vomiting, anorexia, dehydration, and weight loss with debilitation are commonly observed in dogs with acute distemper. Mucopurulent oculonasal discharges and pneumonia often result from secondary bacterial infections. *Bordetella bronchiseptica* is commonly found in dogs with distemper. A skin rash progressing to pustules may occur, especially on the abdomen. It is thought that the initial rash may be immune-mediated; dogs that develop skin lesions often recover.[21, 22] Signs of acute encephalitis may develop with a variety of manifestations. Myoclonus or involuntary twitching of muscles, "chewing gum" seizures, ataxia, incoordination, circling, hyperesthesia, muscle rigidity, vocalization as if in pain, fear responses, and blindness are among the more commonly observed signs of neurologic complications in acute distemper.[21, 22, 26] The magnitude of neurologic involvement has a major influence on the prognosis of canine distemper.

Neurologic signs may occur with delayed onset weeks or months after recovery from inapparent infections or after recovery from acute distemper.[21, 22, 26] Dogs that develop late onset neurologic signs usually have immunity to CDV, which suggests that the virus may have escaped elimination by the immune response due to the protective effects of the blood-brain barrier. The clinical signs observed in subacute distemper encephalitis are similar to those in acute distemper encephalitis; the most characteristic sign is myoclonus or flexor spasm, but any of the signs listed may appear.[21, 22, 26] Canine distemper virus is regarded as the most common cause of convulsions in dogs less than six months of age.[26] Pathologically, demyelination is a consistent finding in acute and subacute distemper encephalitis, in addition to neuronal changes, gliosis, tissue necrosis, edema, and macrophage infiltration.[26] Dogs that survive may have permanent neurologic deficits involving flexor spasms and visual and olfactory dysfunction.[21, 22, 26, 27]

In addition to acute and subacute encephalitis, CDV has also been associated etiologically with two different forms of chronic encephalitis in mature dogs.[26, 28, 29] One form of chronic distemper encephalitis is referred to as a multifocal encephalitis.[26, 28] It is a slowly progressive disease that may have a clinical course of more than a year. It usually occurs in dogs four to eight years of age. The clinical signs include incoordination, weakness in pelvic limbs, unilateral or bilateral menace deficits, head tilt, nystagmus, facial paralysis, and head tremors without myoclonus.[26] Affected dogs may occasionally fall and the condition may progress to eventual paralysis. There may be intermittent periods of clinical and pathologic plateau followed by further progression of the disease. Affected dogs remain mentally alert. Generalized seizures and personality changes are not features of this disease.[26]

The other form of chronic distemper encephalitis is referred to as "old dog encephalitis." It is a progressive disorder of rare occurrence found usually in dogs over six years of age. Initial clinical signs are generally visual impairment and bilateral menace deficit.[26] As the disease progresses, affected dogs become mentally depressed, develop compulsive circling or head pressing, and manifest personality changes of a stupor or dumb status and fail to recognize owners or respond to normal stimuli in their environment. The clinical course may be subacute in progression and the pathologic changes have been described as subacute diffuse sclerosing encephalitis.[26]

DIAGNOSIS

The diagnosis of canine distemper in the acute or subacute form is usually based on history and clinical signs. A combination of fever, respiratory signs (rhinitis, coughing, and pneumonia), mucopurulent oculonasal discharges, diarrhea, hyperkeratosis of footpads, and neurologic signs is highly indicative of distemper, especially in unvaccinated young dogs or mature dogs with inadequate vaccination history.[21–23, 26, 30] Ophthalmoscopic examination may detect chorioretinitis with gray-to-pink irregular areas of degeneration on either the tapetal or nontapetal fundus in the acute disease and evidence of retinal atrophy and scar formation characterized by areas of hyperreflectivity of light, appearing as brightly colored "gold medallion" lesions in dogs that have chronic infection with CDV or that have recovered from a previous infection.[21, 26] Irregularities in the surface of teeth may be present due to hypoplasia of enamel, resulting from direct CDV injury to the ameloblastic layer of the developing tooth.[26] Lymphopenia is a consistent finding in acute distemper and may be supportive of a clinical diagnosis. Thrombocytopenia may be present early in the course of the disease.[31] A definitive diagnosis can be made by detection of CDV in epithelial cells by fluorescent antibody examination or by isolation of the virus.[22, 32] Serologic testing may or may not be helpful in diagnosing acute distemper because dogs with distemper usually fail to respond immunologically.[22, 33] Dogs that recover from acute distemper have lower titers of antibody than dogs with inapparent infections or with vaccine-induced immunity, but the ratio of CDV-specific IgM to IgG is higher in the recovering dog.[33, 34]

The fluorescent antibody test is usually done on epithelial cells collected from the conjunctivum or other mucous membranes or on smears of blood or buffy coat cells, since CDV infects lymphocytes and thrombocytes. Cells can be collected by gently scraping the mucous membrane with the blunt end of a sterile scalpel handle or other blunt instrument and transferring the cells to a clean slide by imprint touching of the slide. Care must be taken to avoid a smearing or streaking effect, which would disrupt intact cells. Cells can be collected from mucous membranes with a sterile, dry cotton or Dacron-tipped applicator and applying the cells to a clean slide by rolling the applicator on the slide; again, smearing or streaking must be avoided. When collecting conjunctival epithelial cells, it is important to first clean the eye to remove exudate, which can complicate the collection and examination of epithelial cells. Interpretation of the FA test is based on detection of CDV antigen only within intact epithelial cells. The success of the FA test in detecting cells positive for CDV is good during the first few days of acute signs of distemper.[22, 32] The FA test is usually negative in cases of subacute, delayed onset, or chronic distemper encephalitis because dogs with these disorders usually have neutralizing antibody that has eliminated the virus or that blocks the FA reaction.[22] Viral antigen persists longer in macrophages and epithelial cells in the lower respiratory tract and in epithelial cells of footpads in dogs that have recovered from systemic distemper.[22, 32, 35] A negative FA test for CDV does not categorically rule out distemper in the diagnosis. A positive test for CDV indicates that CDV antigen was detected in the cells observed, and the results should be interpreted in conjunction with the clinical signs. Attenuated strains of CDV used in MLV vaccines are not disseminated from lymphoid tissue to epithelial cells and are not detected by the FA test.[22, 36] Positive FA for CDV has been detected in dogs without clinical signs of distemper and in some instances in dogs that have titers of neutralizing antibody that would be regarded as protective. Exposure to aerosols of CDV may result in localized infection with limited replication of virus when inadequate levels of antibody are present in mucous or lacrimal secretions. Systemic immunity prevents dissemination of the virus while local immunity is developing to eliminate the virus. It is this type of limited replication and immune response that maintains immunity in adult dogs with frequent exposure to CDV.

TREATMENT AND PREVENTION

There are no antiviral drugs or chemotherapeutic agents of practical value for specific treatment of distemper in dogs. Broad-spectrum antibiotics are indicated to control secondary bacterial infections, and fluids, electrolytes, B vitamins, and nutritional supplements are indicated for supportive therapy. The prognosis is guarded for most cases of acute distemper, especially if neurologic signs are present, but control of secondary infections and supportive therapy improve the chances for recovery. Vitamin C and diethyl ether have been claimed to be of benefit in the treatment of distemper but there is a lack of controlled studies to substantiate such claims. In the author's opinion, they are of no value. Dexamethasone has been reported to be of some value in treating dogs with postdistemper neurologic signs.[21] Administration of MLV distemper vaccine IV has been claimed to have therapeutic value but there is a lack of data from controlled studies to support such claims.

The currently available MLV vaccines for CDV induce effective immunity to distemper.[37] A single dose of MLV distemper vaccine usually immunizes dogs that are free of antibody and are susceptible to distemper. Maternally derived immunity to CDV interferes with immunization of puppies. The age at which puppies become susceptible to distemper is proportional to the titer of antibody of their mother and varies according to the colostral transfer of antibody to the puppies. Approximately 50 per cent of puppies are immunizable to distemper by 6 weeks of age, about 75 per cent by 9 weeks of age, and more than 95 per cent by 13 weeks of age. Because of the variable age at which puppies become immunizable to distemper, a series of vaccinations are given to puppies according to schedules that are practical but that maximize the probability of inducing immunity (Table 47–1). Vaccination of puppies every 2 weeks from 6 weeks of age through 14 weeks of age optimizes the chances of immunization and minimizes the risk of infection with CDV during the period of vaccination, but the expense and inconvenience of vaccination every two weeks cause such a schedule to be regarded as impractical. More commonly recommended vaccination schedules start puppies with the first dose of vaccine at five to seven weeks of age, with additional doses at three- to four-week intervals until puppies are 14 weeks of age. This schedule is more practical and results in immunization of 95 per cent or more of puppies. Annual revaccination is recommended in that the titer of antibody will have declined to levels that are generally not protective within one year in up to one-third of young dogs. Titers last longer after a booster response; however, booster responses do not occur in dogs that have protective titers of antibody.

Attenuated strains of measles virus induce "heterotypic" immunity to distemper.[22, 37] Measles virus is not neutralized by low levels of antibody to CDV and stimulates cell-mediated and humoral immunity to distemper in the presence of maternally derived immunity that would interfere with CDV vaccines. The immunity stimulated by measles in young pups is primarily cell-mediated immunity with low titers of antibody that provide temporary protection against CDV. Older pups and dogs develop higher titers of antibody to measles virus. Female dogs with high titers of antibody to measles transfer antibody to their puppies, which then interferes with immunization using measles virus. Measles virus vaccine is not recommended in pups over ten weeks of age and it is contraindicated in breeding bitches. Measles vaccine given singly or in combination with distemper vaccine is indicated only in pups four to ten weeks of age. If a pup is ten weeks of age or older when first vaccinated, MLV canine distemper vaccine is preferred to measles vaccine. Measles virus vaccine used in dogs is not the same as measles vaccine for humans; the latter should not be used in dogs.

Different strains of CDV are used in the manufacture of MLV distemper vaccines, and there are differences in the degree of attenuation of virulence among the MLV distemper vaccines. Attenuation of virulence is usually based on safety testing in young dogs or puppies of weaning age. Evidence suggests that some strains of MLV canine distemper vaccines may occasionally induce disease in susceptible puppies vaccinated at less than four weeks of age.[38] Egg-adapted CDV vaccines should be used in orphaned puppies that may need to be vaccinated before five weeks of age. Only egg-adapted CDV vaccines are safe for use in gray foxes; other MLV canine distemper vaccines are virulent in gray foxes.[39] Egg-adapted CDV vaccines are indicated for vaccination of wild and exotic animals for distemper.

INFECTIOUS CANINE HEPATITIS

Infectious canine hepatitis (ICH) was recognized as a specific viral disease entity of dogs in 1947.[40] Previously it was regarded as part of the canine distemper complex. It was also found to be the cause of fox encephalitis, which had been recognized previously as a specific infectious disease of foxes.[41] Most infections with ICH virus in dogs are inapparent, but occasionally it causes acute, fatal disease that clinically resembles distemper and canine parvovirus disease. It is distributed worldwide.

ETIOLOGY

Infectious canine hepatitis virus is classified in the Adenoviridae family and is recognized as canine adenovirus type-1 (CAV-1). It is a medium-sized (75 nm in diameter) DNA virus without a lipoprotein envelope. It is moderately resistant and survives in the environment for days to months, depending upon the temperature and humidity. The infectivity of CAV-1 is destroyed by heating to 132° F (56° C), which allows for disinfection of kennels and contaminated areas with steam. It is moderately resistant to disinfectants, but quaternary ammonium compounds inactivate its infectivity within ten minutes. There is antigenic relatedness between CAV-1 and CAV-2 and they provide cross-protective immunity.[43, 44, 45]

EPIZOOTIOLOGY

Infection of dogs with CAV-1 occurs by the oronasal route of entry. The virus infects the tonsils and regional lymph nodes where primary replication occurs. Virus

TABLE 47–1. SUMMARY OF SUGGESTED VACCINATION PROTOCOLS FOR IMMUNIZATION OF DOGS TO VIRAL AND BACTERIAL INFECTIONS

Rabies	Due to the public health aspects of rabies, vaccination of dogs for rabies is regulated by local, municipal, and state laws. Young dogs should be vaccinated at 3 to 4 months of age with a single injection of rabies vaccine, revaccinated 1 year later and at 1- to 3-year intervals thereafter, depending upon the licensed approval for the vaccine used and the legal requirements in the area. Killed virus vaccines with 3-year duration of immunity are recommended.
Distemper	Vaccination schedules for distemper are the basis for immunization for other canine viruses except that additional doses may be required for canine parvovirus immunization. MLV distemper in combination with other canine vaccine viruses should be given to pups starting at 5 to 7 weeks of age with subsequent doses at 3- to 4-week intervals until the pup is 13 to 15 weeks of age. At least two doses of combination distemper MLV vaccine are recommended for initial immunization of dogs regardless of age when first presented for vaccination. Annual revaccination is recommended. MLV measles vaccine may be used instead of MLV distemper vaccine in pups less than 9 weeks of age.
Hepatitis	Vaccinate according to schedule for distemper using combination vaccine. Either CAV-1 or CAV-2 provides effective immunity.
Parvovirus	Vaccinate according to schedule for distemper using combination vaccine. An additional dose of CPV vaccine should be given at 16 to 18 weeks of age after the distemper vaccination series has been completed. In selected cases, additional doses of CPV vaccine may be indicated up to 6 months of age. Annual revaccination is recommended. Both killed virus and MLV vaccines are available for parvovirus; the MLV vaccines are preferred by this author.
Coronavirus	Killed virus vaccines are currently available for CCV. Two doses of vaccine are required for initial immunization regardless of the age of the dog when first presented, revaccination with a single dose of vaccine at 6-month intervals is recommended. Due to a lack of data on the importance of CCV as a pathogen of dogs and the lack of information on the efficacy of killed CCV vaccines in protecting dogs against disease, CCV vaccine is recommended by this author only for use in dogs that have frequent contact with dogs from varied sources, e.g., show dogs and dogs in kennels with frequent movement of dogs in and out of the kennel. If CCV should be confirmed by laboratory procedures to be a contributing factor to clinical disease in dogs, CCV vaccine should be used regularly. CCV vaccine should not be given concurrently with distemper vaccine.
Tracheobronchitis	Vaccinate according to schedule for distemper using combination vaccine containing CAV-1 or CAV-2 and CPI. Revaccinate annually.
Bordetellosis	Bordetella bacterin is recommended for dogs that have frequent contact with dogs from varied sources, e.g., show dogs and dogs in kennels with frequent movement of dogs in and out and for dogs confined to veterinary hospitals and in animal shelters. Two doses of bordetella bacterin are required for initial immunization; revaccination with a single dose every 6 to 12 months is required to maintain adequate immunity. Avirulent, live *Bordetella bronchiseptica* singly or in combination with canine parainfluenza virus is recommended as a single dose intranasal vaccine; it can be used in pups as young as 4 weeks of age. Vaccination for bordetellosis is indicated during epizootics of bordetellosis.
Leptospirosis	Two doses of bacterin containing *Leptospira canicola* and *Leptospira icterohaemorrhagiae* serovars are recommended beginning at 9 to 12 weeks of age in combination with distemper and other vaccine viruses; revaccinate annually.

Canine vaccines have limited therapeutic value and are recommended for prophylactic immunization only.

released from infected cells causes viremia with virions free in the plasma. The virus infects hepatic parenchymal cells and reticuloendothelial cells in most organ systems as the target cells for secondary replication of virus. Clinical signs of disease caused by CAV-1 are due to cellular damage as a result of direct effects of viral replication. Damage to endothelial cells may lead to hemorrhagic diathesis. During the acute stage of the infection, CAV-1 is present in all bodily secretions and fluids. It can be isolated readily from feces, urine, oropharyngeal secretions, and blood. There is a tendency for CAV-1 to localize in renal tubules, from which viral shedding in the urine may occur for up to a year after apparent recovery from the infection.[42, 43, 46] Contamination of the environment by CAV-1 shed in feces and urine is the source of virus for further transmission. CAV-1 is not readily transmitted by aerosol. Recovery from infection confers life-long immunity.

CLINICAL SIGNS

Clinical signs of disease are most frequently observed in young dogs, but seronegative dogs of all ages can be affected. The incubation period is from four to seven days. Fever with rectal temperature from 103° to 106° F (39.5° to 41.0° C) occurs at the onset of the clinical signs, which may be accompanied by depression and lethargy. The temperature usually declines within 24 hours and in mild cases the dog may recover after a brief illness of only one to two days. In dogs with moderate disease, the temperature declines but often fails to return to normal. After one to two days of low-grade fever, the temperature increases again with the development of more pronounced depression, lethargy, reluctance to move, abdominal tenderness, pale mucous membranes, and anorexia. Tonsillitis, pharyngitis, and cervical lymphadenopathy are common findings.[42, 43, 46] Dogs with uncomplicated cases of moderately severe hepatitis usually recover after an illness of three to five days' duration. Corneal opacity due to immune-mediated corneal edema may occur during convalescence. In more severely affected dogs, hemorrhagic diathesis with petechial and ecchymotic hemorrhages may occur. The bleeding time is prolonged and coagulation abnormalities typical of disseminated intravascular coagulation occur.[42] Coughing may develop as a result of bronchitis and bronchiolitis, which occasionally progress to pneumonia. Bloody diarrhea may occur with or without vomiting. Neurologic signs related to vascular damage may occur. Abdominal distention may result from serosanguineous ascites. Hepatomegaly occurs and in some cases the liver can be palpated along the posterior border of the rib cage. The prognosis becomes guarded in dogs with multisystemic involvement from CAV-1 infection. Dogs may develop hepatic coma and die or they may die suddenly of shock.[42] The exact cause of death from CAV-1 infection is not known. In addition to the typical clinical finding with infectious canine hepatitis, peracute disease with sudden death may occur. The peracute disease must be differentiated from poisoning.

DIAGNOSIS

Combined neutropenia and lymphopenia occur during the early stages of the disease. The total white blood cell count may be less than 2500 in severe cases, especially in cases with bloody diarrhea, which necessitates differentiation from canine parvovirus disease. Leukocytosis occurs during recovery from the disease. Thrombocytopenia usually occurs, except in very mild cases. Prolonged bleeding time and coagulation abnormalities occur in the more severe cases. Serum alanine aminotransferase is a liver-specific enzyme in dogs and may become elevated in moderate to severe cases of ICH.[42] CAV-1 can be isolated in canine cell cultures from swabs of the oropharynx during the early stages of disease. Antibody titers to CAV-1 rise sharply in response to the infection and eliminate the virus, allowing for recovery. Demonstration of rising titer of antibody in paired serums confirms the diagnosis. Enlargement and mottling of the liver with fibrinous exudate in the interlobular fissures, edema and hemorrhage of the gallbladder, and hemorrhages on the serosal surface of the stomach are common gross findings at necropsy. Characteristic intranuclear inclusion bodies may be detected in hepatic parenchymal cells by staining of imprint impression slides.

TREATMENT AND PREVENTION

Therapy for ICH is symptomatic. Most dogs recover without supportive therapy. Prevention is afforded by immunization with vaccines containing either attenuated CAV-1 or CAV-2.[43–45, 47] Immunity to CAV-1 is highly effective due to the pathogenesis of ICH involving viremia with virions free in the plasma. Any detectable level of virus-neutralizing antibody is protective against ICH. Convalescent immunity is life-long; immunity induced by MLV CAV-1 vaccines often lasts for three to five years; and immunity induced by MLV CAV-2 vaccines is effective for one to two years. Most vaccines currently marketed in the United States contain MLV CAV-2 in combination with other canine viruses. Vaccines containing MLV CAV-2 provide effective immunity and are essentially free of postvaccinal reactions or complications.[45, 48] Vaccination schedules for immunization of puppies against CAV-1 are the same as those for immunization against distemper (Table 47–1).[37]

INFECTIOUS TRACHEOBRONCHITIS (KENNEL COUGH)

Several viruses, bacteria, and *Mycoplasma* have been determined to be involved in the etiology of kennel cough. *Bordetella bronchiseptica* is perhaps the single most important cause of kennel cough (see Chapter 46). Viruses involved in kennel cough include CDV, CAV-1, CAV-2, and canine parainfluenza virus. Canine herpesvirus and reoviruses have been isolated from dogs with respiratory disease but they have a relatively insignificant role in the etiology of kennel cough. Canine distemper virus and CAV-1 have been considered in the sections above. Canine parainfluenza virus and CAV-2 are considered together, since both are associated only with respiratory infections in dogs.

ETIOLOGY

Canine parainfluenza (CPI) virus is classified in the Paramyxoviridae family and is regarded as parainfluenza type 2 in the *Paramyxovirus* genus.[49] It is a relatively large (200 to 250 nm) RNA virus with a lipoprotein envelope. It is relatively labile and does not survive long in the environment. It is easily inactivated by chemical disinfectants. Canine adenovirus type 2 is classified in the Adenoviridae family. It is a medium-sized (75 nm) DNA virus without a lipoprotein envelope.[43] It is moderately resistant and can survive for months in the environment, depending on temperature and humidity. It is relatively sensitive to heat and can be inactivated by heating to 132°F (56°C); steam cleaning is effective in disinfecting kennels and utensils. Quaternary ammonium disinfectants are effective against both CAV-2 and CPI virus.

EPIZOOTIOLOGY

Both CAV-2 and CPI virus are highly infectious and are transmitted readily by aerosols. Both viruses cause localized infections of the respiratory tract without dissemination to other organ systems. They replicate in both the upper and lower respiratory tract and are shed in respiratory secretions. Bronchioles are the primary target site for infection with CAV-2.[48, 50] The characteristic lesion caused by CAV-2 is described as a proliferative, necrotizing bronchiolitis.[50, 51] Peribronchiolar inflammatory cell infiltration occurs followed by interstitial pneumonia.[50] Most infections with CAV-2 are mild or inapparent, with morbidity ranging from 25 to 75 per cent; deaths in uncomplicated CAV-2 infections are rare. The inflammatory reaction to CAV-2 provides an ideal environment for secondary bacterial infections, which can result in fatal disease. Canine parainfluenza virus has greater affinity for alveolar macrophages and causes a more uniformly distributed interstitial pneumonia.[52] Infections with CPI virus are usually inapparent, with morbidity ranging from 10 to 50 per cent; deaths are rare. Secondary bacterial infection may occur and contribute to a more severe disease, with occasional deaths.

CLINICAL SIGNS

The primary manifestation of CAV-2 or CPI virus infection is paroxysmal coughing of varying frequency and intensity. Fever is variable, with rectal temperature ranging from normal to more than 105° F. The coughing results from irritation at the tracheobronchial-bronchiolar level of the respiratory tract. Infectious tracheobronchitis is pathologically a disease of the lower respiratory tract. The concept that kennel cough is an upper respiratory disease does not agree with the anatomic location of lesions with CAV-2 or CPI infections. Dogs usually recover from CAV-2 or CPI virus-induced tracheobronchitis within three to seven days after the onset of clinical signs. Coughing may be elicited by palpation or manipulation of the trachea for a longer period of time. Recovery corresponds to the development of immunity to the virus infection. The immune response brings viral replication under control, with a cessation of virus shedding. Experimentally, it has been difficult to reproduce respiratory disease with CPI virus.[53] Experimental studies with CAV-2 revealed an inverse relationship of magnitude of the febrile response and duration of clinical signs of disease. Dogs that developed a rectal temperature greater than 104.5° F recovered more quickly than dogs that had a low-grade fever.

DIAGNOSIS

An etiologic diagnosis of viral-induced tracheobronchitis can not be made based on clinical signs. Etiologic diagnosis depends on isolation and identification of the virus or demonstration of a rising titer of antibody to a specific virus in paired serums. There are no consistent clinicopathologic changes that are helpful in establishing the cause. Practically speaking, it is not necessary to establish the etiology since management of clinical cases is the same regardless of the viral cause.

TREATMENT AND PREVENTION

There are no specific antiviral drugs or chemotherapeutic agents for treatment of either CAV-2 or CPI virus infections. Most animals recover spontaneously without complications or sequelae. Treatment with broad-spectrum antibiotics is indicated when there is evidence of secondary bacterial infection. Attenuated virus vaccines are available for both CAV-2 and CPI virus. Vaccines induce immunity that aids in preventing infection and disease. Immunologic protection of the respiratory tract against infection depends on the presence of antibody in respiratory secretions. Antibodies of the IgG class are present in secretions of the lower respiratory tract in proportion to the titer of humoral antibody. Very little antibody is present in secretions of the upper respiratory tract unless there has been infection and stimulation of secretory antibodies of the IgA class (S-IgA). Recovery from an infection confers immunity of long duration. Memory cells effect an anamnestic response to exposure and reinfection that extends the duration of immunity. The MLV CAV-2 vaccine given by IM or SC routes of inoculation reaches the respiratory tract and undergoes replication, resulting in the stimulation of local secretory immunity in addition to humoral or systemic immunity.[45, 48] Vaccines for CAV-2 and CPI virus are available in combination with other attenuated canine viruses. Attenuated CPI virus is available in combination with attenuated *Bordetella bronchiseptica* for intranasal administration.[54] The intranasal CPI virus vaccine induces more effective immunity than the MLV vaccine given by IM or SC routes of inoculation. When an endemic kennel cough becomes a serious problem in a kennel, intranasal vaccines are recommended for use in puppies as young as three to four weeks of age. Generally, CAV-2 and CPI virus vaccines are given in combination with other canine viruses according to the schedule used for MLV distemper vaccine (Table 47–1).[37]

VIRAL GASTROENTERITIS

Viral gastroenteritis became of great importance with the emergence of canine parvovirus in 1978 as a new virus infection in dogs. Canine coronavirus had been described in 1971 but it had not been associated with naturally occurring disease in dogs until about the same time that canine parvovirus was discovered. Canine distemper virus and ICH virus both cause diarrhea and vomiting in some dogs but they are associated primarily with other manifestations of disease. Canine rotavirus has been shown to cause diarrhea in newborn puppies but it has not been associated with naturally occurring enteric disease in older puppies or mature dogs.[55, 56] Rotavirus is of minor importance as a cause of canine gastroenteritis but it should be considered as a possible cause of diarrhea in newborn puppies. Canine parvovirus and canine coronavirus are discussed here.

CANINE PARVOVIRUS

Canine parvovirus (CPV) was first identified in 1978 as a new virus infecting dogs. It was found to be associated with hemorrhagic gastroenteritis of dogs in which the fatality to case ratio was high. The knowledge of canine parvovirus and its effects in dogs expanded exponentially. A vaccine was developed and put into use within three years from the time CPV was first isolated and identified. Although a wealth of information has been learned about canine parvovirus, a considerable amount of confusion also occurred and there is still misunderstanding about certain aspects of canine parvovirus pathogenicity and immunology.

Etiology. Canine parvovirus is a small (20 to 25 nm) DNA virus without lipoprotein envelope. It is classified in the Parvoviridae family and it is closely related antigenically to feline panleukopenia and milk enteritis viruses.[57–59] Canine parvovirus is among the most resistant viruses known. It survives in the environment for months and years and it is not affected by most commercially available disinfectants. Sodium hypochlorite (common household bleach) is the only disinfecting agent that is effective against CPV. It is transmitted by fecal shedding and the oral route of entry into susceptible dogs. Parvoviruses replicate only in cells undergoing mitosis. CPV replicates initially in lymphoid tissue and is disseminated to the crypts of the small intestine by means of viremia. There is only one antigenic type of pathogenic canine parvovirus, although slight changes in CPV have occurred since it first emerged.[60]

Epizootiology. Dogs become infected by ingestion or inhalation of CPV into the oropharynx. The virus is taken up by the tonsils, regional lymph nodes, and gut-associated lymphoid tissue, where primary replication occurs. Viremia (as free virions in the plasma) occurs after the primary replication of CPV in lymphoid tissue, with dissemination of virus to the crypt cells in the small intestine, which is the target organ for secondary replication.[61, 62] The pathologic changes that lead to the development of clinical disease occur in the crypt cells, resulting in mucosal collapse.[61–64] CPV is capable of replicating in cells in other organ systems, including bone marrow, heart, and endothelial cells. CPV-induced neurologic disease has been described due to virus-induced damage to vascular endothelium in the brain.[65]

There is marked variation in the clinical response of dogs to infection with CPV, ranging from inapparent infections to acute fatal disease.[25] Inapparent infections occur in most dogs. The morbidity is less than 20 per cent and the mortality is less than 5 per cent, perhaps less than 1 per cent. The fatality/case ratio may vary from 10 to 90 per cent. Factors that predispose to severe disease include age, stress, genetics (with breed differences in susceptibility), and concurrent infections with intestinal parasites or bacteria.[25] There are significant differences among breeds of dogs in response to CPV infection, with Rottweilers and Doberman pinschers being more severely affected by canine parvovirus than other breeds.[25–66] Black Labrador retrievers are also more severely affected than most other breeds. It has been suggested that von Willebrand's disease in Dobermans and Rottweilers may be an important factor in their increased susceptibility.[25, 66] Concurrent infection with a mildly virulent strain of CDV or with intestinal parasites resulted in more severe disease experimentally. There have been claims about immunosuppression caused by CPV but most reports lacked definitive data from controlled studies to substantiate the claims. More recently, the results from controlled studies have revealed that dogs infected with virulent or attenuated strains are not immunosuppressed and respond immunologically to other antigens no differently than uninfected littermates.[67–69]

Clinical Signs. Most infections with CPV are clinically inapparent. In dogs that develop clinical disease, vomiting and diarrhea are the first signs observed.[25, 57] Affected dogs become lethargic and depressed. Anorexia develops as the disease progresses. Fever is variable, but leukopenia is a consistent finding. Leukopenia with total white blood cell counts decreasing to less than 2,000 are common; lymphopenia is more pronounced than neutropenia. Mildly affected dogs recover in one to two days without treatment. More severely affected dogs may require symptomatic and supportive therapy but most recover after an illness of three to five days' duration. If the vomiting is protracted and if severe hemorrhagic diarrhea occurs, the prognosis is less favorable and dogs may die even with supportive therapy. Some dogs may die acutely within 24 hours after onset of clinical signs. The acute fatal disease is more common in young pups, some of which may have myocarditis if infected at less than eight weeks of age.[25, 61, 62]

Diagnosis. Not all cases of bloody diarrhea, with or without vomiting, are caused by canine parvovirus.[25, 57, 70] Canine distemper and ICH viruses both cause bloody diarrhea in some dogs. Textbooks published prior to the emergence of CPV contain descriptions of hemorrhagic gastroenteritis in dogs caused by agents other than CPV; those same agents continue to cause hemorrhagic gastroenteritis. Young dogs presenting signs of vomiting and diarrhea should be regarded as possibly infected with canine parvovirus, but the differential diagnosis must include other possible causes. Finding of leukopenia may be supportive of the diagnosis, but CDV and CAV-1 both cause leukopenia associated with hemorrhagic diarrhea. A definitive diagnosis is made on detection of viral antigen in feces or by demonstrating a rising titer of antibody to CPV.

Commercially available diagnostic test kits based on enzyme-linked immunosorbent assays (ELISA) are available for in office use. Controlled studies in the author's laboratory comparing results from these tests to other procedures for detection of CPV indicate that they are specific for CPV and relatively sensitive. All of the test kits are based on detection of CPV in fecal samples. Positive results are confirmatory; negative results may or may not rule out CPV. If dogs have been sick for more than three days, they usually have a high titer of antibody that will be entering the intestinal tract along with blood.[25] The newly formed antibody can bind with CPV in the intestinal tract and inhibit its detection with ELISA tests or by hemagglutination. The immune response to CPV infection is quick, with antibody detectable within four to five days after exposure and titers attaining very high levels by day seven after exposure.[25, 70] With an incubation period of four to seven days, many dogs have high titers of antibody soon after the onset of clinical signs of disease. The presence of a high titer (hemagglutination inhibition titer of 1:10,240 or greater) in a single serum collected after the dog has been sick for three or more days is diagnostic of CPV even though CPV may not be detectable in feces.[25, 71, 72] Serologic tests that reveal a high ratio of CPV specific IgM to IgG are diagnostically significant.[34]

Treatment and Prevention. Treatment for gastroenteritis caused by CPV is symptomatic and supportive. Fluids and electrolytes are indicated based on evaluation of the clinical condition. Broad-spectrum antibiotics may be indicated to guard against secondary bacterial infections. If the dog is not vomiting, aminoglycosides (neomycin, gentamicin, or kanamycin) may be given orally to aid in reducing the bacterial flora of the intestinal tract as a precautionary measure against systemic invasion of normal intestinal coliforms, which may cause endotoxic shock. High dosages of penicillin derivatives and aminoglycosides administered IV together are indicated when there is evidence of septicemia.[58] Incorporation of corticosteroids and/or flunixin meglumine is indicated in the therapeutic regimen to combat endotoxic shock in CPV disease.[25]

Antiemetics are indicated in dogs with persistent

vomiting. Antidiarrheal drugs should be used with caution since slowing of the movement of ingesta may increase the absorption of endotoxins.[58] Transfusion with plasma or whole blood may be indicated in dogs with hypovolemia due to severe intestinal loss of serum proteins. Plasma or serum with high titer of antibody to CAV has therapeutic benefits when administered IV at the rate of 0.5 to 1.0 ml/lb (1 to 2 ml/kg) of body weight.[25, 73] High-titered serum also provides passive immunity to CPV when administered to healthy pups at the rate of 1 to 2 ml/kg of body weight.[25, 72] This is of particular value in pups or young dogs scheduled for elective surgery when the immune status is unknown. Discretion must be used in selecting a donor for the serum since there are inherent risks associated with the injection of serum.

The currently available vaccines for CPV are safe and effective. A transient lymphopenia occurs 4 to 6 days after the administration of some MLV vaccines. The lymphopenia occurs during the initiation of the active immune response and it is not due to immunosuppression by the vaccine virus.[25, 68, 69] The MLV of some CPV vaccines replicates in the intestinal tract and is shed in the feces. Although concern has been expressed about the possibility of MLV vaccine virus undergoing reversion of virulence and causing disease, the results from controlled studies indicate that MLV vaccines are safe.[74, 75] Vaccine-induced CPV disease has not been documented in either field or uncomplicated, controlled experimental studies.[25] The primary cause of failure of CPV vaccines is interfering levels of maternally derived antibody to CPV.[72, 76] The age at which pups become immunizable is proportional to the titer in the dam and the efficacy of colostral transfer of antibody. Pups from dams with low protective titers of antibody to CPV are immunizable by 6 weeks of age, but maternally derived antibody may persist at interfering levels to 18 weeks of age or longer in pups from dams with very high titers of antibody.[70, 72] Approximately 25 per cent of puppies will be immunizable by six weeks of age, 40 per cent by nine weeks, 60 per cent by 13 weeks, 80 per cent by 16 weeks, and more than 95 per cent by 18 weeks of age.[25, 37, 70] Without knowing the antibody status of each litter of puppies, it is difficult to recommend a practical vaccination schedule that will result in immunity of nearly all pups.[37] There is the additional problem of pups becoming susceptible to infection with virulent CPV two to three weeks before they become immunizable. There are no vaccines that completely eliminate this "window" of susceptibility before the animals become immunizable.[70, 72] The most immunogenic vaccines will not immunize in the presence of interfering levels of maternally derived antibody which may persist in some pups beyond 16 to 18 weeks of age. The MLV vaccines are preferred over inactivated CPV vaccines.[37]

In order to maximize the probability of immunizing the individual pup, it is recommended that pups of unknown immune status be vaccinated at six, nine, 12, 15, and 18 weeks of age followed by revaccination annually (Table 47–1).[37] It is recognized that some dogs with high titers of maternally derived antibody may not be immunized by vaccine given through 18 weeks of age. In selected cases it may be advisable to give a sixth dose of vaccine at six months of age. A practical, but possibly less effective, vaccination schedule would be to give CPV vaccine in combination with distemper, adenovirus, parainfluenza, and leptospira vaccine for the first three doses beginning at six to seven weeks of age and repeating the vaccination at three to four week intervals through 13 to 14 weeks of age followed by a fourth dose of CPV vaccine at 16 to 18 weeks of age and revaccination annually. The combination vaccines are equally as effective as CPV vaccine by itself.[25, 70, 74, 75] Regardless of the vaccination schedule used, there is always the risk of exposure and development of disease during the "window" of susceptibility when pups are not yet immunizable.[70, 72] Immunity induced by the currently available MLV vaccines for CPV lasts for one to three years. There is no need for booster vaccination more frequent than annually. Dogs that have recovered from infection with virulent CPV appear to have lifelong immunity.

CANINE CORONAVIRUS

Canine coronavirus (CCV) was first isolated in 1971 from adult dogs with diarrhea.[77] In early 1978, it was again isolated from adult dogs with diarrhea.[57] Experimental infections of seronegative adult dogs were usually inapparent or resulted in mild diarrhea after an incubation period of 24 to 36 hours.[57, 58] Experimental infection of neonatal pups resulted in moderate to severe diarrhea in all pups after an incubation period of 24 to 48 hours.[78] Diarrhea persisted for seven to ten days after which pups generally recovered.[78] The virus spread rapidly to uninoculated litter mates that also developed diarrhea. Bitches became infected from their experimentally inoculated pups but they did not develop signs of disease.[78]

Etiology. Canine coronavirus is a pleomorphic, medium to large (60 to 180 nm) RNA virus with an outer envelope of lipoprotein. It is classified in the Coronaviridae family and is antigenically related to transmissible gastroenteritis virus of swine and feline infectious peritonitis virus.[57, 58, 79] Coronaviruses are relatively labile and, unlike parvoviruses, can be inactivated by most commercial disinfectants.

Epizootiology. Canine coronavirus is highly contagious and spreads rapidly through kennels of susceptible dogs.[57] The virus is shed in the feces of infected dogs for two weeks or longer and fecal contamination of the environment is the primary source for transmission of CCV.[57, 78, 80] The ingestion of virus is the primary route of entry for infection resulting in a fecal-oral pattern for spread of infection. Most infections with CCV are inapparent or result in mild, self-limiting signs of disease. There is lack of information to determine the significance of CCV as a pathogen of dogs. It is generally thought that the morbidity and mortality are both low. Neonatal pups are more severely affected than pups of weaning age and adult dogs.[57, 78] There may be breed differences in susceptibility to CCV-associated disease.[78]

Clinical Signs. Difficulty in reproducing clinical disease experimentally with CCV has necessitated the description of clinical signs associated with CCV based on field observations of cases that may have concurrent infections with other agents. Sudden onset of diarrhea with or without vomiting is the most commonly reported characteristic of CCV disease in field cases.[57, 58] Vomiting usually subsides within 24 to 36 hours. Diarrheic fecal material often has an orange-tinted color and has an unusually fetid odor. The diarrhea may vary from a soft or loose stool to a frothy orange-colored semisolid material to projectile watery diarrhea with mucus and blood.[57] Fever is variable. Leukopenia has not been recognized as a feature of CCV infection. Dogs generally recover spontaneously, although treatment may be necessary in the more severe cases. Stools usually return to normal in seven to ten days but soft stools or intermittent diarrhea may occur for three to four weeks.[57, 58] The mortality rate is low, with death more likely to occur in young pups although a few deaths in adult dogs have been attributed to CCV disease.[57]

Diagnosis. It is difficult to make a definitive diagnosis of CCV-induced disease. The clinical signs attributed to CCV infection are variable and similar to signs of gastroenteritis caused by other viruses, and CCV-induced disease cannot be differentiated clinically from other etiologies. The lack of leukopenia may be supportive of probable CCV infection.[57] The detection of CCV in feces must be evaluated with caution since CCV can be detected in feces of clinically normal dogs and since concurrent infections with other agents may be present. Concurrent infection with CCV enhances the severity of CPV infection. A definitive diagnosis is not essential when therapy is needed because treatment is nonspecific and supportive based on clinical findings.

Treatment and Prevention. Treatment of dogs with CCV-associated gastroenteritis is symptomatic and supportive. The approach to therapy is the same as for parvovirus disease. Fluids and electrolytes may be indicated if dehydration, electrolyte imbalance and acidosis occur.[58] Antibiotics are rarely indicated due to the mild nature of CCV infections.

Inactivated virus vaccines are currently marketed for use in preventing CCV infection. Two doses three to four weeks apart and annual revaccination are recommended for immunization of dogs regardless of age (Table 47–1). They provide incomplete protection against infection due to the localized superficial infection of CCV in the intestinal tract of dogs.[78] It is difficult to assess the role of the CCV vaccines in protection against disease since CCV infections experimentally are usually inapparent or cause only mild signs of disease.

CANINE HERPESVIRUS INFECTION

Canine herpesvirus (CHV) has been isolated from dogs with various clinical syndromes in several countries of the world.[81] Its primary role as a pathogen of dogs is in causing a generalized, fatal, hemorrhagic disease in newborn puppies less than two weeks of age.[82] In adult dogs CHV causes infections of the reproductive tract with persistent, latent infection that can be reactivated with periodic shedding of virus and venereal transmission to adult dogs or to pups at the time of birth.[83] CHV has been isolated from dogs with kennel cough but it is a minor component in the etiology of the kennel cough complex.[84, 85]

Newborn pups usually become infected with CHV during passage through the birth canal of an infected bitch that is shedding virus, or by contact with infectious vaginal or nasal secretions of the dam. Horizontal transmission occurs among pups in a litter, and intrauterine transmission has been documented. The incubation period varies from three to six days in puppies less than three weeks of age. Affected puppies cease sucking, cry persistently, become weakened and depressed, often pass soft, yellow-green feces, and develope a nasal exudate.[81] Petechial hemorrhages often occur in mucous membranes and the abdominal-inguinal skin may become erythematous.[81] Death usually occurs in 24 to 48 hours after onset of clinical signs. Mortality is high in pups less than three weeks of age. Between three and five weeks of age, CHV infections cause less severe signs and many pups survive. Pups that survive usually have persistent latent infections and some may develop signs of neurologic disease characterized by ataxia and blindness.[81] Naturally occurring hypothermia is an important factor in the increased susceptibility of puppies less than three weeks of age.

Multifocal petechial and ecchymotic hemorrhages are consistent findings in fatal cases in neonatal pups. Hemorrhages are most commonly observed in kidneys, liver, lungs, and the gastrointestinal tract.[82] Intranuclear inclusion bodies may be present in affected organs, and foci of necrosis are observed microscopically in the areas of hemorrhage.

Treatment of affected puppies is usually unrewarding except that intraperitoneal injection of serum (1 to 2 ml) containing antibody to CHV lessens the mortality in a litter of affected pups.[83] Serum containing antibody can be collected from dogs known to have recovered from CHV infection. There is no specific antiviral therapy of practical value, and there are no vaccines for use in prevention of infections. Bitches may lose a litter of pups to CHV and raise litters subsequently due in part to colostral transfer of antibody.

Infection of the genital tract is the most important problem of CHV in adult dogs. Most infections are inapparent with occasional mild vaginitis or balanoposthitis. Adult bitches often have raised vesicular lesions of a focal to diffuse distribution in the vaginal mucosa without overt discharge. Abortions, stillbirths, and infertility may occur in bitches. Adult males often have similar lesions on the base of the penis and the preputial mucosa accompanied by a preputial discharge. Virus is shed by adult dogs during periods of active infection with lesions and venereal transmission occurs readily. Lesions regress with apparent recovery but the virus persists as a latent infection without active replication and shedding. Recrudescence of lesions with virus replication and shedding of CHV can occur during stress. In bitches, lesions tend to recur during proestrus and regress during anestrus.[81] There are no effective curative treatments for CHV. Spread of infection can be controlled by not breeding dogs known to have been infected. The overall incidence of CHV in adult dogs is less than 20 per cent based on prevalence of antibody to CHV.

PSEUDORABIES

Pseudorabies is caused by a herpesvirus that usually causes disease in swine; however, many mammalian species are susceptible. Pseudorabies in dogs occurs only in areas where pseudorabies virus (PRV) is endemic in the swine population. Naturally acquired infections in dogs occur following ingestion of the virus. Dogs with pseudorabies have sudden onset of clinical signs usually characterized by sudden change in behavior and intense pruritus of the head.[86] The disease progresses rapidly with death usually occurring within 48 hours after onset of clinical signs. Intense scratching of the face and head result in self-mutilation. Generalized convulsions often follow an episode of frantic scratching. Paresis and paralysis may occur shortly before death. The diagnosis of pseudorabies should be suspected based on the clinical signs. Rabies must be considered at the onset of the change in behavior. Definitive diagnosis is dependent upon histopathologic examination of the brain and/or by virus isolation.

References

1. Sikes, RK: Rabies. *In* Hubbert, WT, et al (eds): Diseases Transmitted from Animals to Man. Springfield, Charles C Thomas, 1975, p 871.
2. Steele, JJ: History of Rabies. *In* Baer, GM (ed): The Natural History of Rabies, Vol 1. New York, Academic Press, 1975, p 1.
3. Greene, CE, et al.: Rabies. *In* Greene, CE (ed): Clinical Microbiology and Infectious Diseases of the Dog and Cat. Philadelphia, WB Saunders, 1984, p 356.
4. Fekadu, M and Baer, GM: Recovery from clinical rabies of two dogs inoculated with a rabies virus strain from Ethiopia. Am J Vet Res 41:1632, 1980.
5. Blendon, DC and Breitschwerdt, EB: Recovery of a dog from an experimental rabies infection. *In* Baer, GM (ed): Rabies Information Exchange 2:9, 1980.
6. Hattwick, MA, et al.: Recovery from rabies. A case report. Ann Intern Med 76:931, 1972.
7. Fenner, F, et al.: Veterinary Virology, New York, Academic Press, 1987, p 534.
8. Smith, JS, et al.: Antigenic characteristics of isolates associated with a new epizootic of raccoon rabies in the United States. J Inf Dis 149:769, 1984.
9. Whetstone, CA,et al.: Use of monoclonal antibodies to confirm vaccine-induced rabies in ten dogs, two cats, and one fox. JAVMA 185:285, 1984.
10. Webster, WA, et al.: Antigenic variants of rabies virus in isolates from eastern, central, and northern Canada. Canad J Comp Med 49:186, 1985.
11. Hattwick, MAW and Gregg, MB: The disease in man. *In* Baer, GM (ed): The Natural History of Rabies, Vol II. New York, Academic Press, 1975, p 281.
12. Kelly, VP, et al.: Control of 2 rabies epizootics. Mod Vet Pract 64:380, 1983.
13. Blendon, DC and Bell, JF: Summary of results of immunofluorescence staining on skin and brain taken at all stages of infection: a blind coded study on multiple species. *In* Baer, GM (ed): Rabies Information Exchange 1:41, 1979.
14. Tsao, AT and Blendon, DC: Detection of rabies virus in the skin by immunofluorescence and immunoperoxidase staining and virus isolation: a blind study. *In* Baer, GM (ed): Rabies Information Exchange 4:23, 1981.
15. Compendium of Animal Rabies Control, 1988. JAVMA 192:18, 1988.
16. Rabies Prevention—United States. 1984. Recommendations of the Advisory Committee on Immunization Practices for the Centers for Disease Control of the US Public Health Service. Morb Mort Wkly Rep (CDC) 33:393, 1984.
17. Rabies Prevention: Supplementary Statement on the Preexposure use of Human Diploid Cell Rabies Vaccine by the Intradermal Route. ACIP, CDC. USPHS, Morb Mort Wkly Report (CDC) 35:768, 1986.
18. Schnurrenberger, PR, et al.: Systemic allergic reactions following immunization with human diploid cell rabies vaccine. Morb Mort Wkly Report (CDC) 33:185, 1984.
19. Imagawa, DT, et al.: Immunological relationship of measles, distemper, and rinderpest viruses. Proc Natl Acad Sci 46:1119, 1959.
20. Appel, MJG and Gillespie, JH: Canine distemper virus. Virol Monogr 11:1, 1972.
21. Greene, CE: Canine distemper. *In* Greene, CE (ed): Clinical Microbiology and Infectious Diseases of the Dog and Cat. Philadelphia, WB Saunders, 1984, p 286.
22. Appel, M: Canine distemper. *In* Kirk, RW (ed): Current Veterinary Therapy VI. Philadelphia, WB Saunders, 1977, p 1308.
23. Fenner, F, et al.: Veterinary Virology. New York, Academic Press, 1987, p 499.
24. Appel, MJG: Pathogenesis of canine distemper. Am J Vet Res 30:1167, 1969.
25. Brunner, CJ and Swango, LJ: Canine parvovirus infection: Effects on the immune system and factors that predispose to severe disease. Comp Cont Ed Pract Vet 7:979, 1985.
26. Braund, KG: Clinical Syndromes in Veterinary Neurology. Baltimore, Williams & Wilkins, 1986, p 92.
27. Myers, LJ, et al.: Anosmia associated with canine distemper. Am J Vet Res, In press, 1988.
28. Vandevelde, M, et al.: Chronic distemper virus encephalitis in mature dogs. Vet Pathol 17:17, 1980.
29. Imagawa, DT, et al.: Isolation of canine distemper virus from dogs with chronic neurologic diseases. Proc Soc Exp Biol & Med 164:355, 1980.
30. Lauder, IM, et al.: A survey of canine distemper. Vet Rec 66:606, 1954.
31. Axthelm, MA and Krakowka, S: Canine distemper virus-induced thrombocytopenia. Am J Vet Res 48:1269, 1987.
32. Kristensen, B and Swango, LJ: Evaluation of the fluorescent antibody test in diagnosis of canine distemper in naturally infected dogs. *In* Proceed 56th Conf Res Workers Anim Dis 1: 1975.
33. Winters, KA, et al.: Immunoglobulin class response to canine distemper virus in gnotobiotic dogs. Vet Immunol Immunopath 5:209, 1983/1984.
34. Black, JW: Single serum-sample diagnosis of canine viral diseases. VM/SAC 78:1393, 1983.
35. Miry, C, et al.: Immunoperoxidase study of canine distemper virus pneumonia. Res Vet Sci 34:145, 1983.
36. Lisiak, JA and Swango, LJ: Studies on the shedding of vaccine viruses by dogs vaccinated with modified live virus (MLV) vaccines. *In* Proceed 60th Conf Res Workers Anim Dis 5, 1979.
37. Swango, LJ: Canine immunization. *In* Kirk, RW (ed): Current Veterinary Therapy VII. Philadelphia, WB Saunders, 1983, p 1123.
38. Krakowka, S, et al.: Canine parvovirus infection potentiates canine distemper encephalitis attributable to modified live-virus vaccine. JAVMA 180:137, 1982.
39. Halbrooks, RD, et al.: Response of gray foxes to modified live-virus canine distemper vaccines. JAVMA 179:1170, 1981.
40. Rubarth, S: An acute virus disease with liver lesions in dogs (hepatitis contagiosa canis): a pathologico-anatomical and etiological investigation. Acta Pathol Microbiol Scand Suppl 69:1, 1947.
41. Gillespie, JH and Timoney, JF: Hagan and Brunner's Infections Diseases of Domestic Animals, 7th ed. Ithaca, Cornell University Press, 1981, p 507.
42. Greene, CE: Infectious canine hepatitis. *In* Greene, CE (ed): Clinical Microbiology and Infectious Diseases of the Dog and Cat. Philadelphia, WB Saunders, 1984, p 406.
43. Fenner, F, et al.: Veterinary Virology. New York, Academic Press, 1987, p 334.
44. Swango, LJ, et al.: Serologic comparisons of infectious canine hepatitis and Toronto A26/61 canine adenoviruses. Am J Vet Res 30:1381, 1969.
45. Bass, EP, et al.: Evaluation of a canine adenovirus type-2 strain

as a replacement for infectious canine hepatitis vaccine. JAVMA 177:234, 1980.
46. Poppensiek, GC and Baker, JA: Persistence of virus in urine as a factor in spread of infectious canine hepatitis. Proc Soc Exp Biol Med 77:279, 1951.
47. Emery, JB, et al.: Cross-protective immunity to canine adenovirus type-2 by canine adenovirus type-1 vaccination. Am J Vet Res 39:1778, 1978.
48. Appel, M, et al.: Canine adenovirus type 2–induced immunity to two canine adenoviruses in pups with maternal antibody. Am J Vet Res 36:1199, 1975.
49. Fenner, F, et al.: Veterinary Virology. New York, Academic Press, 1987, p 491.
50. Swango, LJ, et al.: A comparison of the pathogenesis and antigenicity of infectious canine hepatitis virus and the A26/61 virus strain (Toronto). JAVMA 156:1687, 1970.
51. Kelly, DF: Canine proliferative and necrotizing tracheobronchitis, with intranuclear inclusion body and hyaline membrane formation. Pathol Vet 6:227, 1969.
52. Thayer, GW: Canine infectious tracheobronchitis. *In* Greene, CE (ed): Clinical Microbiology and Infectious Diseases of the Dog and Cat. Philadelphia, WB Saunders, 1984, p 430.
53. Lazar, EC, et al.: Serologic and infectivity studies of canine SV-5 virus (35012). Proc Soc Exp Biol Med 135:173, 1970.
54. Chladek, DW, et al.: Canine parainfluenza-Bordetella bronchiseptica vaccine: Immunogenicity. Am J Vet Res 42:266, 1981.
55. Fulton, RW, et al.: Isolation of a rotavirus from a newborn dog with diarrhea. Am J Vet Res 42:841, 1981.
56. Johnson, CA, et al.: Inoculation of neonatal gnotobiotic dogs with a canine rotavirus. Am J Vet Res 44:1682, 1983.
57. Appel, MJG, et al.: Canine viral enteritis. I. Status report on corona- and parvo-like viral enteritides. Cornell Vet 69:123, 1979.
58. Greene, CE: Canine viral enteritis. *In* Greene, CE (ed): Clinical Microbiology and Infectious Diseases of the Dog and Cat. Philadelphia, WB Saunders, 1984, p 437.
59. Fenner, F, et al.: Veterinary Virology. New York, Academic Press, 1987, p 415.
60. Parrish, CR, et al.: Natural variation of canine parvovirus. Science 230:1046, 1985.
61. O'Sullivan, G, et al.: Experimentally induced severe canine parvoviral enteritis. Austral Vet J 61:1, 1983.
62. Meunier, PC, et al.: Pathogenesis of canine parvoviral enteritis: The importance of viremia. Vet Pathol 22:60, 1985.
63. Cooper, BJ, et al.: Canine viral enteritis. II. Morphologic lesions in naturally occurring parvovirus infection. Cornell Vet 69:134, 1979.
64. Macartney, L, et al.: Canine parvovirus enteritis I: Clinical, hematological, and pathological features of experimental infection. Vet Rec 115:201, 1984.
65. Johnson, BJ and Castro, AE: Isolation of canine parvovirus from a dog brain with severe necrotizing vasculitis and encephalomalacia. JAVMA 184:1398, 1984.
66. Glickman, LT, et al.: Breed-related risk factors for canine parvovirus enteritis. JAVMA 187:589, 1985.
67. Swango, LJ, et al.: The effect of experimental infection with canine parvovirus on the antibody response to MLV canine distemper and adenovirus type-2 vaccines. *In* Proc 65th Annual Mtg, Conf Res Workers in Anim Dis 10:51, 1984.
68. Brunner, CJ, et al.: Effect of infection or vaccination with canine parvovirus on leukocyte function in young dogs. *In* Proc 65th Annual Mtg, Conf Res Workers in Anim Dis 10:52, 1984.
69. Phillips, TR and Schultz, RD: Failure of vaccine or virulent strains of canine parvovirus to induce immunosuppressive effects on the immune system of the dog. Viral Immunol (In press), 1987/1988.
70. Swango, LJ: Frequently asked questions about CPV disease. Norden News 58:4, 1983.
71. Carmichael, LE, et al.: Hemagglutination by canine parvovirus: serologic studies and diagnostic applications. Am J Vet Res 41:784, 1980.
72. Pollock, RVH and Carmichael, LE: Maternally derived immunity to canine parvovirus infection: Transfer, decline and interference with vaccination. JAVMA 180:37, 1982.
73. Ishibashi, K, et al.: Serotherapy for dogs infected with canine parvovirus. Jap J Vet Sci 45:59, 1983.
74. Carmichael, LE, et al.: A modified live canine parvovirus vaccine. II. Immune response. Cornell Vet. 73:13, 1983.
75. Kahn, DE, et al.: Safety and efficacy of modified-live canine parvovirus vaccine. VM/SAC 78:1739, 1983.
76. O'Brien, SE, et al.: Response of pups to modified-live canine parvovirus component in a combination vaccine. JAVMA 188:699, 1986.
77. Binn, LN, et al.: Recovery and characterization of a coronavirus from military dogs with diarrhea. *In* Proc, 78th Ann Meeting, US Livestock Health Assoc, Roanoke, VA Oct. 1974 (1975): 359.
78. Keenan, KP, et al.: Intestinal infection of neonatal dogs with canine coronavirus 1-71: Studies by virologic, histologic, histochemical, and immunofluorescent techniques. Am J Vet Res 37:257, 1976.
79. Fenner, F, et al.: Veterinary Virology. New York, Academic Press, p 511, 1987.
80. Carmichael, LE and Binn, LN: New enteric viruses in the dog. Adv Vet Sci Comp Med 25:1, 1981.
81. Greene, CE and Kukak, TJ: Canine herpesvirus infection. *In* Greene, CE (ed): Clinical Microbiology and Infectious Diseases of the Dog and Cat. Philadelphia, WB Saunders, p 419, 1984.
82. Fenner, F, et al.: Veterinary Virology. New York, Academic Press, p 359, 1987.
83. Poste, G and King, N: Isolation of a herpesvirus from the canine genital tract: Association with infertility, abortion, and stillbirths. Vet Rec 88:229, 1971.
84. Binn, LN, et al.: Viruses recovered from laboratory dogs with respiratory disease. Proc Soc Exp Biol Med 126:140, 1967.
85. Wright, NG, et al.: Canine herpesvirus respiratory infection. Vet Rec 87:108, 1970.
86. Vandevelde, M: Pseudorabies. *In* Greene, CE (ed): Clinical Microbiology and Infectious Diseases of the Dog and Cat. Philadelphia, WB Saunders, 1984, p 381.

48 FELINE VIRAL DISEASES

JOHN R. AUGUST

FACTORS PREDISPOSING CATS TO INFECTIOUS VIRAL DISEASES

Widespread vaccination of cats for viral diseases has significantly decreased the number of sick cats presented for veterinary care. However, even though vaccination programs are usually in place, infectious diseases continue to be the major cause of morbidity and mortality in young cats. This failure to effectively eliminate viral diseases in multiple cat populations is largely due to an overdependence on vaccination, without proper attention to sound management principles.[1]

The host, agent, and environmental factors that predispose cats to infectious diseases are shown in Table 48–1.[2] When one or more of these factors influence a population of animals, the severity of clinical illness worsens, the mortality rate increases, and the number of cats affected with chronic symptomatic illness or the subclinical carrier state rises.[2]

The factors that contribute most frequently to enzootic infectious disease in multiple cat households include the mixing of cats of different age groups and susceptibilities, the presence of unrecognized carriers, the accumulation of pathogens due to inadequate ventilation and sanitation, the frequent introduction of new cats into the group, the retention of minimally affected cats, and high population density. The clinician's ability to control the prevalence of viral infections in these populations is complicated by the practical difficulty of achieving a rapid viral diagnosis, the unavailability of effective antiviral agents to treat symptomatic patients, and the common occurrence of the subclinical carrier state found with many viral infections.[3] Several viruses, including feline herpesvirus I, feline leukemia virus, and feline infectious peritonitis virus, induce latent carrier states that may, on occasion, recrudesce as a result of stressful stimuli.[1]

High population density causes a build-up of pathogens, increased chance of exposure to a larger challenge dose of virus, and competition for food that may result in nutritional deficiencies in younger and weaker members of the group.[2] The detrimental effects of infectious diseases and overt or subclinical malnutrition tend to be synergistic.[4] Clinical infections may be more severe in undernourished animals and the infections subsequently cause a marginal nutritional plane to progress to a state of overt malnutrition. Cell-mediated immune (CMI) responses are often damaged in states of malnutrition, with total numbers of lymphocytes, especially T-cells, being depleted. During acute and chronic malnutrition, dysfunctions of the complement system, phagocytosis, and opsonization occur.[5]

The effects of malnutrition and infectious disease in young animals may be exacerbated by concurrent gastrointestinal disease.[5] The debilitating effects of anorexia, pyrexia, and dehydration, coupled with malabsorptive or protein-losing enteropathies, rapidly decrease the plane of nutrition, thus worsening the immune dysfunction.

Immunologic competence varies with the life stage of the normal dog; a similar situation probably occurs in cats.[6] Immune function appears to increase during the fetal and early neonatal periods and peaks after puberty. The responsiveness of B- and T-lymphocytes decreases in older animals, and thus older cats may be more susceptible to infectious diseases than younger adult animals. Annual revaccination is therefore of great importance for the older cat. Since proper nutrition may slow the age-associated decline in immune function, the special nutritional needs of the geriatric cat should be addressed.[6]

General Principles of Disease Control in Cat Populations

Practical control of infectious viral diseases in the feline population depends on five procedures:[7] (1) Vaccination programs must be tailored to the specific needs of the group. Most vaccines protect cats against the development of severe clinical disease, but do not protect the animal against infection. (2) Cats manifesting clinical signs of infectious disease, however mild, should be removed from the group. (3) Using available diagnostic tests, asymptomatic carriers should be identified and removed from the population. (4) Young, susceptible cats should be isolated from any remaining uniden-

TABLE 48–1. FACTORS INFLUENCING OUTCOME OF INFECTIONS

Host Factors
1. Developmental and heritable anomalies of the immune system
2. Undefined heritable resistance factors
3. Maternal immunity
4. Age at time of exposure
5. Intercurrent illness
6. Nutrition

Environmental Factors
1. Population density
2. Sanitation
   a. Ventilation
   b. Accumulation of excretions
3. Interchange of animals from one population to another

Agent Factors
1. Virulence
2. Dosage
3. Route of inoculation

Reproduced with permission from Pedersen, NC: Feline infectious diseases. *In* Proceedings of the American Animal Hospital Association 45th Annual Meeting, 1978, p. 125.

tified carriers until fully immunized. (5) The concentration of infectious agents in the environment should be minimized through attention to sanitation and ventilation.

Controlling Infectious Diseases in Catteries

Maintenance of general and reproductive health in animals living in catteries or breeding colonies requires careful attention to environmental and host factors.[8] Variations in ambient temperature and relative humidity may precipitate outbreaks of viral respiratory disease, especially in environments with a high animal density and with a constantly changing population. A temperature of 72°F (22°C), with a relative humidity of 40 to 60 per cent is considered appropriate. Ventilation providing 17 air exchanges per hour and a light-dark cycle of 14:10 hours is ideal.[9] Animal handling should be performed on an age-priority schedule, with the youngest kittens handled first, then the weaned kittens, pregnant females, and finally the remaining adult cats.[8] Separate facilities should be available for quarantining new arrivals and for isolating animals with overt signs of infectious disease.[1] All deaths within the group, especially neonatal losses, should be investigated thoroughly through necropsy and histopathologic and microbiologic examinations.[8]

Planned sanitation programs are necessary to reduce enzootic infectious disease in catteries. The routine use of a disinfectant does not replace other management procedures.[8] No single disinfectant reliably kills all of the major infectious pathogens of cats; however, sodium hypochlorite, used at a final concentration of 0.175 per cent, was shown to be the best overall virucidal agent for disinfection of cages, floors, and food dishes.[10] The disinfectant used should be nonirritating and nontoxic to human beings and cats. Treated surfaces should be completely dry before cats are reintroduced to the area. Disposable food and water bowls and litter pans, although expensive, reduce disinfection procedures and the chance for cross-contamination. The specific husbandry procedures designed to reduce infectious disease in feline populations have been reviewed.[1, 8, 11]

Principles of Vaccination

The ideal goal of a vaccination program is to induce complete immunity against viral diseases, with minimal complications or side effects.[12] Since most available vaccines protect the animal from serious disease but not from infection, a more realistic goal might be the prevention of overt clinical disease in susceptible animals by the limitation of viral replication.[13]

The type of vaccine used, route of administration, effect of maternal antibody derived from colostrum, and the age of the cat all affect the immune response that occurs following vaccination.[14] The degree of protection afforded by vaccination often depends on the level of antigen-specific antibodies produced, including immunoglobulin (Ig)M, IgA, and IgG.[15] However, in some diseases such as feline calicivirus and feline herpesvirus I infections, the serum antibody titer does not correlate well with protection, because CMI and local immunity both play a greater role than systemic antibodies in disease protection.[16]

Strong early protection should be afforded to the young susceptible cat by vaccinating the queen before breeding and by isolating the weaned kitten from all adult cats until at least two weeks after the initial vaccination series is properly completed.[1] The time at which the young animal becomes susceptible to infection and the time at which it is able to mount an active response to vaccine antigen are not the same.[16] Vaccination is contraindicated in most situations for cats that are overtly sick, for pregnant queens, and for those cats undergoing cytotoxic chemotherapy.[15] A preventive health care schedule for cattery cats and pet cats is shown in Table 48–2.[1]

TABLE 48–2. PREVENTIVE HEALTH CARE SCHEDULE FOR CATTERY CATS AND PET CATS

3 weeks	Fecal examination
6 weeks	Fecal examination
9–10 weeks	FHV–1/FCV/FPV vaccine
	ELISA test for FeLV
	FeLV vaccination
	Fecal examination
12–14 weeks	FHV–1/FCV/FPV vaccine
	FeLV vaccination
	Rabies vaccination
	Fecal examination
6 months	FeLV vaccination
	Fecal examination
12 months	Fecal examination
15–16 months	FHV–1/FCV/FPV vaccine (repeated annually)
	FeLV vaccine (repeated annually)
	Rabies vaccine (repeated according to manufacturer's instructions)
	Fecal examination (repeated every 6 months)

Reproduced with permission from August, JR: Feline preventive health care and infectious disease control. *In* Sherding, RG (ed): Diseases of the Cat: Diagnosis and Management. New York, Churchill Livingstone Inc, In Press.

TYPES OF VACCINES

The most effective vaccines are those that most closely mimic the route and type of infection they are designed to prevent. Thus, modified live virus (MLV) vaccines that replicate in the host are usually superior to inactivated or subunit products.[17]

Inactivated vaccines do not replicate in the host, precluding any possibility of reversion to virulence. Compared to MLV vaccines, they are safer for very young or old cats, and may be administered, when absolutely necessary, to debilitated or pregnant cats, and to colostrum-deprived neonatal kittens.[12] The efficacy of inactivated products depends on the antigenic mass present.[17] Since inactivated vaccines usually induce a shorter duration of immunity than MLV products, multiple inoculations are normally required.[12] Since no replication occurs in the cat at the time of the first vaccination, solid protection usually does not occur until after a second dose of vaccine.

Subunit vaccines contain viral capsid or envelope antigens, rather than intact virions.[12] These products have safety characteristics similar to inactivated vaccines and may be used, when necessary, in pregnant, immunosuppressed, or debilitated animals.[12] Smaller amounts of foreign antigenic material are included in these vaccines, thus decreasing the risk of adverse reactions.[17]

Modified live virus vaccines are attenuated so that they retain antigenicity and the continued ability to replicate in the host, without causing illness.[17] The ideal MLV vaccine should not be shed by the animal, revert to virulence, or persist in the animal after active immunity is established.[12]

Replication of virus after the first vaccine usually produces a marked protective response, compared to the inactivated products, which require two or more inoculations before an anamnestic response is observed. Thus, MLV products may offer more rapid protection in the face of an outbreak of infectious disease. Protection is usually of longer duration and stimulation of CMI is better with MLV vaccines. The ability of MLV products to stimulate CMI and the formation of local secretory antibody (IgA) is used in the intranasal vaccines for feline viral respiratory disease.[17] Disadvantages of MLV vaccines include their ability to cause vaccine-induced illness in neonatal cats or those cats on cytotoxic chemotherapy and the development of malformations, fetal deaths, and abortions in queens that are vaccinated during pregnancy.

PANLEUKOPENIA

Panleukopenia is a highly infectious viral disease, characterized by an abrupt onset of clinical signs, leukopenia, pyrexia, anorexia, depression, and vomiting and diarrhea. The disease is often associated with a high mortality rate in susceptible populations.[18] Although feline panleukopenia virus (FPV) is still considered the most important viral gastrointestinal pathogen of cats, other viruses that have been isolated from the feces of diarrheic cats include rotavirus, astrovirus, enteric coronavirus, calicivirus, and feline leukemia virus (FeLV).[19]

ETIOLOGIC AGENT

The causative agent of panleukopenia is a small, serologically homogeneous parvovirus belonging to the family Parvoviridae.[20] These viruses are isometric, nonenveloped particles, with single-stranded linear DNA.[21] The absence of an envelope is responsible for their resistance to environmental and chemical inactivation. Feline panleukopenia virus is resistant to ether and chloroform[21] and is not inactivated by alcohols, iodines, phenols, or quaternary ammonium compounds.[18] However, the virus is reliably destroyed by a 1:32 dilution of a commercial sodium hypochlorite solution (Clorox). The virus resists freezing and drying and can survive for one year at room temperature on solid fomites in organic matter.[20]

FPV replicates in the cell nucleus, requiring the presence of certain cellular factors that are expressed during the G2 and S phases of the cell cycle.[21] Thus, FPV needs actively dividing cells for replication, explaining the localization of virus to mitotically active tissues in the infected cat. However, not all rapidly dividing tissues are equally affected, suggesting that there is viral tropism for certain tissues.[21] Only one serotype of FPV exists, although there is some variation in virulence among strains.[18]

EPIZOOTIOLOGY

Infections with FPV occur in domestic and wild Felidae, raccoons, ferrets, and mink.[21] FPV is ubiquitous in the environment, due to its highly contagious nature and its ability to persist on fomites. Most free-roaming cats are exposed to FPV or become infected within the first year of life.[20] The incidence of clinical cases of panleukopenia in any feline population varies with the percentage of immune cats, virulence of the infecting strain, and the virulence of the intestinal bacteria in infected cats.[18] Presently, the incidence is low to nonexistent, except in circumstances where proper vaccination of kittens is not practiced.[19] Seasonal variations in the incidence of panleukopenia have been reported, associated with the appearance of a population of kittens that is losing its maternal immunity.

Feline panleukopenia virus is spread by direct contact with infected cats and their secretions. During the acute phase of infection, virus is shed in all body secretions and excretions.[18] Fomites contaminated with vomitus or diarrheic feces are potent sources of infection. Aerosol transmission may occur, especially if concurrent upper respiratory infections are present. Hematophagous ectoparasites, such as fleas, may also be capable of spreading the disease.[18] Virus may be shed in the urine and feces for up to six weeks after recovery from clinical illness.[20]

PATHOGENESIS

Since FPV requires actively dividing cells for effective replication, the most severely damaged tissues are those undergoing the most rapid mitotic activity. The clinical syndromes observed in feline panleukopenia vary, depending on the stage of development of the cat at the time of exposure. This is due to differences in organ development and bacterial flora between fetal, neonatal, adolescent, and mature cats.

In-utero Infections. FPV readily crosses the uterus and placenta of the queen to infect the fetuses.[18] Virus spreads throughout the fetus, crossing the blood-brain barrier. The distribution and severity of teratologic changes in the fetus depend on its stage of development at the time of infection.

Infections in the first half of gestation usually result in early fetal deaths, with abortion or resorption of fetal tissues. Fetuses infected in the second half of gestation may die and undergo subsequent abortion or mummification, or may be born alive, with a variety of teratologic defects. During this latter stage of gestation, the greatest mitotic activity is occurring in the central nervous system, and to a lesser extent, in the lymphoid tissues and bone marrow. Due to an absence of an established gut flora, the mitotic activity of the intestinal tract is low at this time, thus sparing this organ from viral damage. In cats, cerebellar development is most active during late gestation and the early neonatal period. Cerebellar infections during this time result in interference with the normal inward migration of the actively mitotic external germ cell layer, which passes the Purkinje cell layer to form the granular cell layer. The cell layers become reduced in size or may be distorted, in some cases resulting in cerebellar hypoplasia. Other central nervous system lesions observed from in-utero infection include spinal cord damage, hydrocephalus, hydranencephaly, and retinal dysplasia characterized by discrete gray foci with darkened margins and retinal folding or streaking.[20]

Early Neonatal Infections. Following oral inoculation, FPV first infects the oropharynx of the neonatal kitten. Viremia develops quickly, with the virus being found in every tissue within 48 hours.[18] The amount of virus recovered from most tissues is of the order of magnitude that can be accounted for by the viral content of the blood and does not indicate that replication is occurring in each of these tissues.[21] The virus continues to have an affinity for those tissues with high mitotic activity, including the cerebellum, thymus, and mesenteric lymph nodes. Cerebellar damage may occur with infections acquired up to nine days of age.

Infections in Older Kittens. When kittens more than two weeks old are infected orally with FPV, initial viral replication occurs in the lymphoid tissue of the oropharynx, with subsequent spread to the regional lymph nodes. Within 24 hours, the kitten becomes viremic.[18] Due to their high mitotic activity, the epithelial cells of the small intestine, particularly the ileum and jejunum and the stem cells of the bone marrow, the thymus, and lymph nodes, may all be damaged by viral replication. The cytolytic replication of virus in the basal cells of the intestinal crypts results in a lack of replacement of normal senescent cells at the tip of the villus, with eventual villus collapse and atrophy.[19] Viremia persists until circulating antibodies appear, usually about seven days after infection.[18]

CLINICAL SIGNS

Kittens Infected In-utero. Kittens surviving fetal infection with FPV may be born weak and succumb to opportunistic infections early in life or may appear normal at birth. Signs of cerebellar damage usually become apparent when affected kittens first start to walk, at about two to three weeks of age.[18] Hypermetria, intention tremors that disappear at rest, symmetrical incoordination, rolling and tumbling, and ataxia are noticed and persist for life.

Older Kittens and Adult Cats. Depending upon host, agent, and environmental factors, signs of feline panleukopenia may vary from asymptomatic infections to sudden death. In most cats, the incubation period is four to five days. Shorter incubation periods may occur in young, highly susceptible cats.

Peracute panleukopenia is often confused with accidental poisoning, since sudden death usually occurs without any characteristic gastrointestinal signs. The young kitten appears depressed for several hours before becoming comatose and dying. Emesis is occasionally observed, but diarrhea and dehydration are absent.

Acute panleukopenia is the most common manifestation seen in young cats. Sudden depression and anorexia are associated with the development of pyrexia. The rectal temperature varies from 104°F (40°C) to 106.8°F (41.6°C). Persistent emesis is an early sign, causing rapid dehydration, as evidenced by decreased skin elasticity and a dull hair coat. A severe, fetid diarrhea usually follows and the feces may contain blood and fibrin casts.[18] Diarrhea is a result of an absence of normal crypt cells that secrete water, an absence of water and nutrient absorption at the villus tip, and villus collapse and atrophy.[19] The affected cat often crouches near its water bowl, but refuses to drink. Although once considered pathognomonic for panleukopenia, this posture may be seen in cats suffering from other severe visceral diseases. The patient usually resents abdominal palpation due to the painful enteritis. Intestinal loops may be thickened and rope-like, or may be distended with gas and fluid. The mesenteric lymph nodes are palpably enlarged.

The mortality rate in acute panleukopenia ranges from 25 to 90 per cent. Those patients that survive five days or more of clinical illness usually recover gradually from the disease. Some recovered animals are left with a malabsorptive syndrome due to fusion of the intestinal villi and mucosal scarring.[18] The more severely affected patients become progressively weak and hypothermic, appearing comatose before death. Death is usually due to the complications of severe dehydration, gram-negative endotoxemia, or disseminated intravascular coagulation (DIC).

Other less common signs that have been reported in cats with acute panleukopenia include mild icterus, ulcerative or necrotic stomatitis, iritis with an aqueous flare, secondary infections (including purulent otitis externa), cutaneous hemorrhages, sloughs at injection sites, and necrosis and sloughing of the ear tips.[18]

Subacute panleukopenia causes a vague illness of one to three days' duration, characterized by anorexia, mild pyrexia, and discomfort upon abdominal palpation. Overt gastrointestinal signs are usually absent and recovery is rapid and uneventful.

Subclinical panleukopenia may be quite common in the adult cat population. Antibodies to FPV are present in the majority of free-roaming cats and asymptomatic queens may give birth to congenitally infected kittens.

DIFFERENTIAL DIAGNOSIS

Feline panleukopenia must be differentiated from other diseases that cause acute gastroenteritis, abdominal pain, or leukopenia. These include the panleukopenia-like syndrome caused by FeLV,[22] other viral enteritides, acute bacterial enteritides such as salmonellosis or campylobacteriosis, toxoplasmosis, cryptosporidiosis, toxicoses, linear foreign bodies, and pancreatitis.

DIAGNOSIS

An accurate diagnosis of panleukopenia depends on information derived from an accurate history, a physical examination, and laboratory data. Panleukopenia should be strongly considered in any cat less than 12 months of age that is presented with acute gastroenteritis and that has a history of incomplete or no vaccination against FPV.

LABORATORY DIAGNOSIS

Hematology. Leukopenia occurs in most cats with panleukopenia, even in those patients with mild or absent gastrointestinal signs. The total white blood cell (WBC) count drops progressively before emesis appears, being lowest on the fourth to sixth day after infection.[21] In most cases of acute panleukopenia, the leukopenia is due to an absolute neutropenia. However, in severely affected cats, an absolute lymphopenia may become evident. Total WBC counts of less than 4000 cells/μl are commonly observed in acute panleukopenia and counts of less than 2000 cells/μl are associated with a poor prognosis.[18]

Following recovery from FPV infection, a rebound leukocytosis may occur that is characterized by a marked left shift and the presence of many bizarre immature neutrophils.[18] The transient nature of the leukopenia in FPV infections may be helpful in differentiating FPV infections from disorders due to FeLV, which are often associated with a more persistent leukopenia. Additionally, concurrent lymphopenia is a more common finding in FeLV-associated diseases.[20]

Thrombocytopenia is occasionally observed in cats with acute panleukopenia complicated by DIC. A nonregenerative anemia may be found in those patients that have survived acute infection and are undergoing a slow recovery.[18]

Serum Biochemistries. Biochemical changes in feline panleukopenia are usually nonspecific. Prerenal azotemia may result from the severe dehydration due to persistent emesis and diarrhea. Biochemical icterus, defined as an elevated total serum bilirubin in the absence of clinically detectable icterus, may be present; it reflects a state of protein deficiency due to prolonged anorexia. In spite of severe dehydration, the total serum proteins may be normal because serum proteins may be lost through the damaged intestinal mucosa. Hypoproteinemia may become evident following rehydration.[20]

Serology. Serologic tests that are available for the diagnosis of feline panleukopenia include serum neutralization, complement fixation, and hemagglutination inhibition. Serum samples should be taken during the acute phase of the disease and again two weeks later.

Virus Isolation. Feline panleukopenia virus may be recovered from pharyngeal or rectal swabs from cats in the acute phase of the disease. In autopsied animals, the spleen, thymus, ileum, and mesenteric lymph nodes provide the best results.[18] Cytopathic effects are most readily observed when the feline cell cultures contain a large number of young, rapidly dividing cells.[20]

Electron microscopic examination of feces collected during the early acute phase of the disease may reveal typical parvovirus particles.

Pathologic Findings. In congenitally infected kittens, cerebellar hypoplasia is usually present, associated with a disorientation and paucity of cells in the granular and Purkinje cell layers.[20] Hydrocephalus may occur, as evidenced by thinning of the cerebral cortex and dilation of the lateral and third ventricles.[18]

In kittens with neonatal infections, thymic atrophy is usually present. Other gross or microscopic changes are usually absent.

In older kittens and adult cats with acute or peracute panleukopenia, the most remarkable lesions are found in the gastrointestinal tract, with the most severe changes occurring in the jejunum and ileum. The bowel wall is usually thickened and turgid, with gas being present in some bowel loops. The serosal surface of severely affected areas may be hyperemic, with notable ecchymotic or petechial hemorrhages.[20]

The intestinal crypts are usually dilated and contain debris consisting of sloughed necrotic epithelial cells. Blunting and fusion of villi may be present. The mesenteric lymph nodes, Peyer's patches, spleen, and thymus contain decreased numbers of lymphocytes.

Eosinophilic intranuclear inclusion bodies may develop transiently in tissues hosting viral replication.

THERAPY

Treatment for feline panleukopenia depends on supportive management until natural defenses return, and excellent nursing care. Unfortunately, the mortality rate in acute panleukopenia is high; however, those cats that survive for five or seven days will probably recover.[18] Due to the highly contagious nature of the disease, affected animals should be kept in strict isolation and special care must be taken to prevent accidental infection of other patients with contaminated hands or fomites.

Food or water should be withheld until antiemetics are no longer necessary to control vomiting. Phenothiazine-derivative antiemetics are preferable.[20] Parenteral fluid therapy should be administered through an indwelling intravenous catheter. The goals of fluid therapy are to replace electrolyte deficits, counteract dehydration, and provide daily maintenance requirements.[20] The fluid of choice is a balanced electrolyte solution such as lactated Ringer's. A multi B-vitamin complex supplement should be added to the daily parenteral fluids, ensuring that the brand chosen does not contain phenol as a preservative.

Early treatment with plasma or whole blood from healthy immune donors is indicated for moribund patients or for cats with severe anemia or hypoproteinemia. The platelet count and activated coagulation time should be evaluated before blood products are administered, in case DIC is present.

A parenteral antimicrobial such as gentamicin should be administered to the hydrated patient for five days to prevent gram-negative sepsis and endotoxemia, which are major causes of death in cats with acute panleukopenia. Antimicrobial treatment may be extended beyond five days if there are no signs of nephrotoxicity. Anticholinergic antiemetic-antidiarrheal agents are contraindicated, since they may cause sustained ileus.[20]

Excellent nursing care is necessary for the critically ill patient. Vomitus, feces, and spilled oral medications should be removed from the coat frequently. The rectal temperature should be checked regularly and a heating pad used if early hypothermia is detected. Concurrent opportunistic infections such as viral respiratory disease should be treated specifically.

After food and water have been withheld for 48 to 72 hours and emesis is no longer present, the patient may be offered frequent small amounts of bland, easily digestible foods, such as chicken-based baby food or a home-prepared mixture of boiled chicken and rice. The return to a normal commercial diet and feeding schedule should be gradual to avoid inducing dietary gastroenteritis. Since FPV may be shed in the urine and feces for up to six weeks after recovery from clinical illness, it is recommended that the convalescing patient be isolated from susceptible cats during this time.

PREVENTION

As with most infectious agents, kittens become susceptible to vaccination with FPV when passive immunity acquired through the colostrum wanes. The level and duration of passive immunity following nursing depends on the antibody titer of the queen at parturition, assuming that the kittens nurse properly.[14] In most kittens, maternal immunity for FPV can be broken through by 9 to 12 weeks; however, on rare occasions, it may be 16 to 18 weeks before vaccination is successful.

Kittens should receive their first FPV vaccine at eight to ten weeks of age. A second vaccine is given at 12 to 14 weeks and repeated annually. The initial vaccination series should never be terminated before 12 weeks of age. In areas of high concentration of street virus, a third vaccine may be recommended at 16 to 18 weeks, especially if inactivated products are being used. When vaccination of queens, severely immunosuppressed or sick cats, or kittens less than four weeks of age is indicated, inactivated products must be used.[17]

The parenteral administration of homologous antiserum provides rapid passive immunity for unvaccinated cats exposed to FPV or for colostrum-deprived kittens. Active immunization must be withheld for two to four weeks following antiserum therapy. Healthy colostrum-deprived kittens that do not receive antiserum may be vaccinated at seven to ten days of age with an inactivated product, which is repeated two to three weeks later.

VIRAL RESPIRATORY DISEASE

Since the introduction of commercial vaccines for feline viral respiratory disease, the number of pet cats presented with signs of upper respiratory disease (URD) has decreased substantially. However, URD continues to be a major cause of morbidity and mortality in young cats in multiple cat households or open catteries.[1]

Two distinct forms of URD are seen in the feline population. An acute form is associated with upper respiratory signs of abrupt onset, pyrexia, anorexia, and dehydration of widely varying severity and constitutes the traditional manifestation of the syndrome. A chronic form is also seen because most recovered cats become carriers of the causative viruses, usually manifesting few clinical signs, yet being capable of shedding virulent virus for months or years.

Etiologic Agents

Feline herpesvirus I (FHV-I) and feline calicivirus (FCV) are responsible for more than 80 per cent of the cases of viral respiratory disease in cats. Other viruses, including feline reovirus and possibly some coronaviruses, may be responsible for sporadic mild cases of URD.

FHV-I causes feline viral rhinotracheitis (FVR), the most severe URD of cats.[23] FHV-I is a large virus with double-stranded DNA and since it possesses a lipoprotein envelope, it is quite susceptible to chemical destruction and inactivation by desiccating environmental conditions. At room temperature, FHV-I is usually inactivated within 18 to 24 hours.[24] All known isolates belong to a single serotype and all field isolates are considered to be pathogenic.

FCV causes a highly contagious URD in cats. The virus contains a single-stranded, nonsegmented RNA molecule and exists as a single major antigenic type with multiple subtypes that have varying degrees of antigenic cross-reactivity.[24] Since it is a nonenveloped virus, FCV is resistant to lipotrophic solvents and disinfectants and is moderately resistant to environmental conditions. The 68/40 strain survives for up to eight days in dry environments, and up to ten days in damp locations.[25]

Factors Predisposing Cats to URD

Numerous factors appear important in predisposing cats to infection with FHV-I and FCV, the most critical of which is the age of the cat. High titers of colostrally derived maternal antibody protect the young kitten from challenge early in life. As passive immunity wanes, the young kitten becomes highly susceptible to challenge from exposure to cats undergoing acute infections or to carrier cats. Most fatal cases of URD occur in eight to ten week old kittens and outbreaks often occur in the spring and summer, when the spring crop of kittens starts to lose its passive immunity.[26]

Other significant factors include the virulence of virus strains, quality of ventilation and sanitation in the environment, population density, presence of intercurrent illnesses such as FeLV infection, nutritional status, and the natural bacterial flora of the cat at the time of infection.

Modes of Transmission

FHV-I and FCV are maintained in the feline population by a variety of mechanisms. Under epizootic conditions in unvaccinated populations, viruses pass by direct contact from acutely infected animals to susceptible cats. The viruses also persist on fomites for a variable period of time, necessitating careful cleaning of the environment to prevent cross-infection. Of major importance is the persistence of virus in carrier cats, which may be capable of shedding virulent virus.[27] Infection of susceptible queens with FHV-I may cause in utero infection of kittens.

Clinical Findings

FELINE VIRAL RHINOTRACHEITIS

Acute FHV-I Infections. The severity of clinical signs is widely variable, depending on the level of previously acquired specific immunity, the age and general health of the exposed cat, duration of exposure, and challenge dose of the virus. The most severe cases are seen in recently weaned kittens.[26]

Replication of FHV-I is most effective at temperatures slightly below the normal body temperature of the cat, thus predisposing the cooler superficial epithelial cells of the nasal turbinates and conjunctiva to viral infection.[24] Virus also replicates in the epithelium of the cornea, soft palate, and tonsils, and to a lesser extent, in the tracheal epithelium. FHV-I causes necrosis and ulceration of the nasal turbinate epithelium and induces marked osteolytic effects on the turbinate bones.[24] In most cases, FHV-I remains as a superficial infection; however, viremia may occur in severe cases.

Active shedding of FHV-I in oculonasal and oropharyngeal discharges continues for one to three weeks in primary infections.[28] Infrequently, virus may be recovered for up to seven weeks from the oropharynx of cats recovering from primary infections.

The incubation period is usually between two and six days, but may be shortened by severe challenge. In most uncomplicated cases, clinical signs last for five to seven days. The earliest sign of FVR is an acute paroxysmal attack of sneezing.[24] Pyrexia, anorexia, and depression are variable, depending on the severity of the infection. Serous conjunctivitis and rhinitis are early signs; however, the ocular and nasal exudates rapidly become mucoid and finally mucopurulent in nature as secondary bacterial infection occurs (Figure 48–1). The tenacious discharges obstruct the nares, inducing mouth breathing, and may cause the eyelids to adhere. Ulcerative glossitis is an uncommon finding. When tracheal or bronchial involvement occurs, coughing and rales may be heard.[24]

The ulcerative keratitis associated with FVR infection is characterized by the presence of numerous small punctate lesions or linear zig-zag dendritic ulcers, which eventually coalesce.[24]

Kittens with in-utero infections may shown signs of a generalized infection at birth or may appear normal for several days before signs of URD appear. Affected kittens cry continuously and usually die before two to three weeks of age.[24] Death is usually caused by dehydration and malnutrition, resulting from pneumonia and liver necrosis.

Chronic Sequelae to Acute FHV-I Infection. The necrosis and ulceration of the turbinate mucosa and the turbinate bone resorption that may occur during severe FHV-I infection predispose the cat to recurrent opportunistic bacterial and mycoplasmal infections. Affected cats with chronic rhinitis and frontal sinusitis often develop bouts of sneezing, which are temporarily responsive to antimicrobial therapy. Such animals are commonly known as "snufflers" (Figure 48–1). Exacerbation of snuffling may be due to new infections with secondary opportunists, reinfections with FHV-I, or recrudescences of viral shedding.[26]

Chronic infection of the lacrimal ducts may result in fibrosis and stenosis, causing chronic epiphora. Transient keratoconjunctivitis sicca is an unusual complication.[24]

The Carrier State of FHV-I. FHV-I is similar to several other herpesviruses that produce a carrier state characterized by a latent phase, punctuated by episodes of virus-shedding that are inconsistently accompanied by a recrudescence of clinical signs.[29] Virus replication and shedding are often preceded by some stressful episode. During the latent phase, FHV-I is undetectable by routine oropharyngeal or nasal swabbing and is in a quiescent, nonreplicating state.

Cats may remain infected with FHV-I for years, in

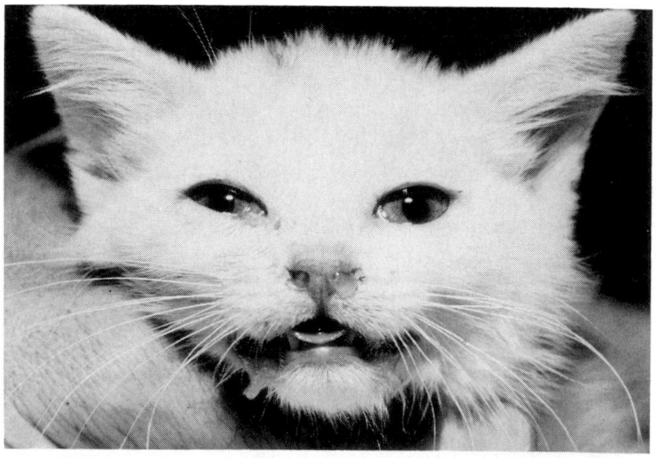

FIGURE 48–1. Mucopurulent conjunctivitis and rhinitis in an 8-week-old kitten with viral rhinotracheitis. (From August, JR: Feline viral respiratory disease. Vet Tech 7:88, 1986. Reprinted with permission.)

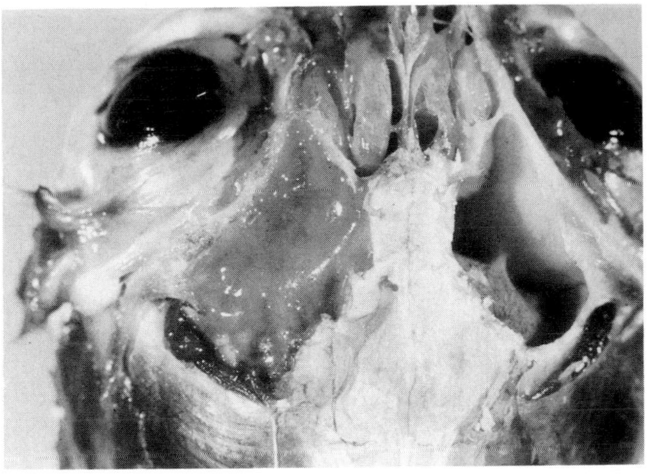

FIGURE 48–2. An opened frontal sinus showing gelatinous purulent exudate in an FeLV-infected cat with frontal sinusitis secondary to viral rhinotracheitis. A pure culture of *Pseudomonas aeruginosa* was isolated from the exudate. (From Bradley, RL: Selected oral, pharyngeal, and upper respiratory conditions of the cat. Vet Clin North Am 14:1173, 1984. Reprinted with permission.)

spite of the presence of serum neutralizing antibody acquired through natural exposure or vaccination. The integrity of local secretory IgA and CMI function may be important in the prevention of reinfection.[30] Following primary infection with FHV-I, 82 per cent of unvaccinated cats became chronic carriers.[31] Spontaneous shedding or shedding associated with natural stresses was observed in 45 per cent of all cats, suggesting that not all carriers are important in the spread of infection.

Examination of a wide range of tissues from latently infected cats has failed to reveal a consistent site of viral persistence. Due to the predilection of FHV-I for the turbinate mucosa during both acute and recrudescent infections, and the predilection of herpesviruses for nervous tissue, the olfactory bulbs and tracts (with their proximity to, and neurologic connections with, the turbinate region) are considered one possible site of latent infection.[28] Recently, FHV-I was isolated from the trigeminal ganglia of 18 per cent of a population of latently infected cats.[32]

Recrudescence of virus-shedding may be induced naturally by a variety of stressful stimuli, including rehousing, parturition and lactation, and concurrent illness. Kittens with declining maternal antibody are particularly susceptible to contact with lactating queens that start spontaneous shedding four to six weeks after parturition. Depending on the challenge dose of virus and the level of passive immunity remaining, exposed kittens may develop overt clinical disease or asymptomatic infections, subsequently becoming latent carriers themselves and efficiently perpetuating the presence of the virus in the group.[33]

Shedding is initiated most consistently by the administration of glucocorticoids.[31] Following administration of these drugs or rehousing, a delay of about seven days occurs before virus excretion is detected. Shedding lasts for about seven days. Occasional bouts of shedding that lasted 40 to 68 days have been observed.[31]

Close contact is required for successful transmission of FHV-I from shedding carriers to susceptible cats. Although the quantity of virus produced is essentially similar in acutely infected cats and shedding carriers, the copious oropharyngeal discharges of the former group allow more efficient spread.[33] Recrudescent shedding may be asymptomatic or may be accompanied by mild conjunctivitis and nasal discharge with sneezing.[11]

FELINE CALICIVIRUS INFECTION

Acute FCV Infection. The pathogenicity of FCV subtypes varies markedly. Some isolates are essentially nonpathogenic, causing minimal clinical signs, whereas others induce a marked cellular destruction of the epithelium of the buccal cavity and tongue and of the pulmonary interstitium. Kitten mortality may approach 30 per cent following infection with pneumotropic strains.

Acute FCV infections may take one or more of the following clinical manifestations: an upper respiratory infection, pneumonia, an ulcerative disease, enteritis, or acute arthritis. Calicivirus-like particles have been observed by electron microscopy in the feces of cats with diarrhea, but have not been grown in cell culture.[24] The etiologic significance of these particles remains unclear.

Acute FCV disease is observed most frequently in young unvaccinated cats that are housed in large groups, such as in humane shelters, pet shops, and research colonies.[34]

In general, FCV infections are milder than those caused by FHV-I, although the signs induced by some highly pathogenic strains may be indistinguishable from those seen in FVR. After an incubation period of three to five days, pyrexia occurs, accompanied by anorexia, malaise, and a mild serous oculonasal discharge. Superficial ulcers appear on the dorsum of the tongue, hard palate, and nasal philtrum, and less commonly, on the lips and footpads. The oral ulcers induced by FCV, which arise as a transient vesicular eruption, typically have a "punched out" appearance, in contrast to the more ragged and extensive ulcers occasionally noted in severe FHV-I infections. On occasion however, FCV may produce a large, horseshoe-shaped, necrotic ulcer on the anterodorsal surface of the tongue.[24]

Cats with experimentally induced FCV infections shed virus for no longer than 21 days. Excretion of virus from the oropharynx for 30 days or more suggests that the cat has become a chronic virus carrier.[35]

Many strains of FCV are capable of producing some degree of pneumonia.[24] In most cases, the lung involvement is transient without any overt signs of respiratory distress. Occasionally, FCV infection may cause severe dyspnea by inducing an interstitial pneumonia that later becomes proliferative.[36] FCV is considered to be the most common cause of interstitial pneumonia in the cat.[24] Sudden illness associated with depression, emesis, and death has been observed in kittens affected with pneumotropic strains of FCV. The presenting signs closely resemble those seen in peracute panleukopenia.

Other signs that are occasionally observed in FCV infections include tracheobronchitis, diarrhea, myalgia, stiff gait, and hyperesthesia. Localization of ulceration to the mouth and footpads may cause a "paw and mouth" syndrome with lameness. The 2280 and LLK strains of FCV have been associated with a transient febrile limping syndrome. The role of these strains of FCV in the pathogenesis of the generalized hyperesthesia, arthralgia, and cutaneous erythema over the tarsal joints seen in this syndrome has yet to be determined.[37]

The Carrier State of FCV. With certain strains of FCV, an asymptomatic period of virus-shedding is the natural sequel to acute primary infections. This carrier state is characterized by continuous excretion of virus from the oropharynx for weeks, months, or occasionally, for the life of the cat, irrespective of stressful episodes.

Complicating our understanding of the FCV carrier state and its prevalence is the knowledge that caliciviruses may be isolated from the oropharynx of some clinically healthy cats without prior evidence of overt respiratory disease. Identification of FCV in a single oropharyngeal swab from a healthy cat may indicate that the cat is (1) incubating an early primary infection with virulent virus, (2) an asymptomatic carrier of a virulent strain, (3) undergoing early reinfection with a virulent strain, (4) undergoing a primary infection or reinfection with an avirulent strain, or (5) a carrier of an avirulent strain.[38]

Persistent mild conjunctivitis, gingivitis, and periodontal disease have been observed in some FCV carriers. FCV was isolated in the oropharyngeal swabs of 80 per cent of cats with chronic stomatitis, compared to a healthy group of cats from which no isolations were made.[39] However, the association of FCV and stomatitis in the cat remains unclear, since there is presently no conclusive evidence that FCV is the primary cause of chronic oral lesions in the cat.

In most surveys of healthy cats, FCV is isolated more frequently than FHV-I. This discrepancy reflects the different nature of the carrier state of each virus rather than their prevalence in the population or their importance in feline URD.[38]

Using the A3, 68/40, and M8 strains of FCV, persistent viral replication was found consistently in oral tissues and, to a minimal extent, in the tissues of the upper and lower airways.[40] Virus was found most frequently and abundantly in the tonsils, which may be the preferred site of replication of FCV in both the acutely infected cat and the carrier cat.

Chronic FCV infections persist in the presence of serum neutralizing antibody. Virus production fluctuates around a mean for each individual carrier cat, with certain cats excreting virus at high levels and others at intermediate or low levels.[35] High level excretors are more important epizootiologically. Because the level of virus production in some low-level excretors may be below the sensitivity of some virus isolation techniques, a single negative oropharyngeal swab should not be used to confirm that a cat is free of FCV.[35]

Using three strains of FCV, cats were found to be persistently infected for 34 to 186 days. The proportion of persistently infected cats decreases logarithmically with time, with virus shedding usually terminating abruptly.[41] Following complete elimination of FCV, the recovered cat appears quite resistant to reinfection.

Differential Diagnosis

Signs of URD in cats may be induced by a variety of infectious and noninfectious causes. The following guidelines may be useful to differentiate clinically the diseases of infectious etiology.[24]

A presumptive diagnosis of FVR is justified if the examiner is investigating an acute outbreak of URD in which severe acute conjunctivitis and frequent paroxysmal sneezing are prominent signs. The concurrent presence of ulcerative keratitis adds further credence to the diagnosis.

FCV infection should be suspected when acute URD is associated with ulcerative glossitis in the absence of severe rhinitis and conjunctivitis or with acute pneumonia.

Chlamydiosis, caused by a feline strain of *Chlamydia psittaci*, should be suspected when URD in cats is characterized by recurrent or persistent follicular conjunctivitis. Rhinitis, an unusual finding, is mild when present.

Nasal infections with the yeast *Cryptococcus neoformans* may cause chronic sneezing and may be associated with the development of ulcerating lesions around the external nares. Some breeders are presently concerned that certain outbreaks of URD in catteries are due to primary infections with *Bordetella bronchiseptica*. The role of this organism in feline URD is presently unclear.

Noninfectious causes of acute or chronic sneezing in cats include irritant rhinitis, allergic rhinitis, severe dental disease, oronasal fistulae, nasal foreign bodies, nasal tumors, and nasopharyngeal polyps.

Laboratory Diagnosis

Hematology. A moderate neutrophilic leukocytosis and mild lymphopenia may be observed in cats with acute FVR. Hematologic changes are absent in uncomplicated FCV infections.[23]

Virus Isolation. Although virus isolation is usually unnecessary to confirm the diagnosis of viral URD in individual patients, the technique has value for the investigation and control of recurrent respiratory disease in populations of valuable cats. However, the recovery of FCV or FHV-I from a cat with signs of URD does not confirm conclusively that the virus is the primary cause of the respiratory disease. Some cats with signs of URD due to FHV-I may be carriers of FCV. Since FCV produces rapid cytopathic effects in cell cultures, the slower changes due to FHV-I may be missed, leading to an erroneous interpretation of the test results.

For the isolation of FHV-I in acutely infected cats, swabs should be taken from the pharynx, nares, or conjunctiva. For the detection of FCV, swabs should be taken from the oropharynx, tonsillar crypts, or from the lungs of kittens dying acutely.[24]

Samples for virus isolation should be taken as aseptically as possible. Swabs should be placed in individual sterile vials without preservative, stored at −4°F (−20°C), and transported to the diagnostic laboratory on Dry Ice.[42] Since virus isolation is an expensive and time-consuming diagnostic process and because the interpretation of results in feline patients with URD is fraught with difficulties, the procedure should be used only in carefully selected situations. Good communication between practitioner and diagnostic laboratory is needed before the exercise is initiated.

Immunofluorescent Testing. The preferred method for confirming FHV-I as the cause of acute URD in cats is the direct immunofluorescent examination of scrapings taken from the medial septum of the nasal cavity.[24] Unfortunately, this method does not detect latently infected carriers that are not actively shedding virus.

Serology. In some feline populations, viral URD continues to be a problem in spite of traditional vaccination programs. The use of serologic tests to investigate the importance of FHV-I and FCV as pathogens in these cats is complicated by prior vaccination.

Cats recovering from acute FCV infection often develop a high serum neutralizing antibody titer, whereas those cats recovering from acute FVR produce a small and slow increase in antibody titer.[42] When indicated, a serum sample should be taken during the acute phase of disease and again two weeks later.

Pathologic Findings. Postmortem examination of cats dying of FVR usually reveals dehydration, decreased body fat, and crusted exudates around the eyes and external nares. The mucosal surfaces of the nasal cavity and frontal sinuses are inflamed and a purulent exudate is often present (Figure 48–2). Focal areas of ulceration and necrosis may be observed. In severe cases, the inflammation may spread down the tracheobronchial tree and pulmonary lesions may be found. The tonsils are usually enlarged and may have areas of hemorrhage and necrosis on their surface. Generalized mild lymphadenopathy may be present. In young kittens with generalized infections, areas of focal hepatic necrosis may be observed. Histopathologic examination of affected tissues reveals the presence of intranuclear type A inclusion bodies and pyknotic cells.

Most deaths from FCV infection occur as a result of acute interstitial pneumonia. Patchy or diffuse consolidation may be seen in one or several lung lobes. Early histopathologic findings include edema, hemorrhage, leukocyte infiltration, and necrosis of the pneumocytes of the alveolar walls. In more chronic cases, proliferative changes are noted. Necrosis of the epithelium of the tonsillar crypts may be observed. No inclusion bodies are present.[24]

Treatment

As in feline panleukopenia, therapy for viral URD in cats depends on supportive care, excellent nursing, and the prevention of secondary bacterial complications. In most cases of the acute ulcerative form of FCV infection, no specific therapy is necessary unless the patient is dehydrated. In these cases, however, special attention should be paid to cleaning serous oculonasal discharges and saliva from the face of the patient and providing a soft appetizing diet while oral ulcers are present.

Whenever possible, cats with viral URD should be treated as outpatients, in order to prevent nosocomial infections in other hospitalized patients. Hospitalization should be reserved for those cats that show signs of dehydration, depression, hypothermia, dyspnea, severe secondary complications, or the need for artificial hyperalimentation.

The patient with severe URD should be kept in a warm environment, since viral replication in the upper respiratory tract is reduced at higher temperatures. Crusted exudates around the eyes and nose should be removed gently at frequent intervals. Correction of dehydration and warm humidification of inspired air decrease the tenacity of purulent oculonasal discharges. When these discharges are copious and serous or mucoid in nature, the intranasal administration of topical decongestants twice daily for no longer than 48 hours may improve the patient's sense of smell and stimulate appetite. In severely depressed or chronically inappetant cats, hydration and caloric intake may be maintained through the use of a pharyngo-esophagostomy tube.[43]

Oral antimicrobials should be used for a minimum of seven days in those patients with any evidence of secondary bacterial complications. Failure to address these opportunistic infections may predispose the cat to chronic bacterial rhinitis or frontal sinusitis at a later time. A palatable and well-tolerated antimicrobial such as amoxicillin is preferred. Ophthalmic antimicrobial preparations without corticosteroids are indicated for patients with conjunctivitis. Oxygen therapy and bronchodilators may be needed for cats with dyspnea due to pneumonia caused by FCV.

Several antiviral agents have been used in the management of feline herpetic keratitis. Idoxuridine, which suppresses viral DNA synthesis, is administered as a 0.1 per cent solution that is applied at a dosage of one drop in the affected eye q1h while the cat is awake.[44] Trifluridine is administered as a one per cent solution, at a dosage of one drop q2h in the affected eye during waking hours. This dosage frequency is continued until reepithelialization has occurred and then treatment is continued q4h for two more weeks.[30]

Management of cats with chronic rhinitis and sinusitis should include microbiologic, cytologic, and radiologic examinations to exclude noninfectious diseases. In addition, the cat should be tested for FeLV infection, since opportunistic bacterial and mycoplasmal infections are more likely to follow viral URD in FeLV-infected cats. *Pasteurella multocida* and *Mycoplasma* sp. are often isolated in abundance from nasal washings of cats with chronic rhinitis and sinusitis. The choice of antimicrobial for these patients should take into consideration the sensitivity patterns of the bacterial flora and the antimycoplasmal activity of the drug. Suitable antimicrobials for these patients include tetracycline, chloramphenicol, and erythromycin.

Control of URD in the Feline Population

Effective control of URD in populations at risk depends on a combination of strategically applied vaccination programs, minimization of exposure of susceptible cats to potential shedders, and maintenance of a physical environment designed to minimize concentration of virus.[26]

Vaccination for URD

Parenteral Vaccines. The routine use of parenteral MLV vaccines has substantially reduced the incidence of severe URD in pet cats and cattery cats. Intranasal MLV vaccines have not been widely accepted for routine use by the practitioner.

The ideal respiratory virus vaccine should be safe, induce no undesirable side effects, provide complete protection against clinical disease upon challenge with field virus, and prevent the development of the carrier state when administered before natural exposure has occurred.[1] Unfortunately, no such vaccine presently exists and vaccination against upper respiratory infections must be regarded as protection against serious disease rather than protection against infection.[45]

Maternal immunity may last no longer than five to six weeks for FHV-I and seven to eight weeks for FCV. Most kittens become susceptible to vaccination with parenteral vaccines against these viruses at nine to ten weeks of age.[14] A second vaccine should be administered four weeks later, ensuring that parenteral vaccination is not terminated before 12 weeks of age. Annual revaccination is necessary. Accurate subcutaneous vaccination with MLV products is needed, since cats licking a contaminated injection site may develop ulcerative stomatitis.

Using parenteral MLV products, vaccinated cats receive good protection against the development of clinical signs, but may later become carriers of field FHV-I after natural exposure.[46] There is no evidence that vaccination with parenteral or intranasal MLV products terminates the established carrier state of FHV-I or FCV.

Early vaccination may be useful in preventing clinically severe URD in young kittens. Two doses of an adjuvanted inactivated vaccine given at five and seven weeks of age provided an effective means of reducing morbidity in this situation.[47]

Experimental vaccination of cats with a subunit vaccine composed of the 15S component of FCV was effective in preventing disease.[48] In the future, subunit vaccines may provide an effective, safe, and inexpensive means of protection against viral URD.

Intranasal Vaccines. Intranasal vaccines use attenuated strains of FHV-I and FCV that are incapable of replicating outside the conjunctiva and turbinate mucosa. There is preliminary evidence that intranasal vaccination may protect against the development of the FHV-I carrier state if administered before the virus is first encountered. However, it is unclear whether cats vaccinated in this manner could withstand repeated challenge with virulent field strains over a protracted period of time.[45]

Intranasal vaccines appear especially useful for decreasing the severity of disease in susceptible cats in the face of an outbreak. Taking into account an incubation period of one to two days, intranasal vaccination four days before challenging protected the cats against clinical disease. In fact, attenuation of clinical signs may occur if vaccination precedes challenge by only 24 hours. Five to six days are required following vaccination for solid immunity to develop.[49]

Intranasal vaccination has been used to reduce kitten losses in catteries with enzootic URD. Vaccinating queens intranasally prior to breeding, combined with intranasal vaccination of kittens at eight to ten days of age and again at nine weeks of age, has reduced the prevalence of URD in some problem catteries. The dose of intranasal vaccine used for neonatal kittens is one drop into each nostril. This vaccination schedule remains controversial and in order to be effective must be combined with sound management techniques.[7]

A thorough understanding of the epizootiology of FHV-I and FCV is essential when implementing control measures in premises with enzootic URD. Failure to remove known carriers, properly segregate cats, reduce fomite contamination, or implement a vaccination schedule most suited to that population undoubtedly fosters perpetuation of the disease.[1, 7]

RABIES

In the days when rabies was poorly controlled in dogs and cats, the ratio of dog to cat cases was about 10:1. However, since 1981 the number of cases of rabies reported annually in cats has exceeded that in dogs and the ratio is now 1:1.4.[50, 51] The cat is now the most common rabid animal of all the domestic species. In continental Europe, the prevalence of rabies is twice as high in cats as in dogs.[52] The roaming and nocturnal tendencies of cats facilitate their contact with wild animals and their inquisitive nature makes them prone to interaction with the demented, moribund, or dead rabid animal.

The incidence of rabies in dogs declined by more than 95 per cent in the third quarter of this century, mainly due to the efforts of local health officials and veterinarians in appealing to the public to have their dogs vaccinated. It is now estimated that 40 per cent of pet dogs are regularly vaccinated for rabies. In contrast, little concerted effort has been made to increase the vaccination rate for cats. Presently, it is estimated that only four per cent of all cats are immunized against rabies.

ETIOLOGY

Rabies is an infectious viral disease characterized by encephalitis. Rabies virus (RV) is a rhabdovirus containing negative strand RNA, which measures approximately 180 × 70 nm.

The virus is neurotropic, being found primarily in nervous tissue and the salivary glands. The receptor for RV in mammalian tissues may be the acetylcholine receptor. This may explain the universal susceptibility of mammals to the virus and its tropism for nervous tissue. The virus is quite fragile in the environment and becomes inactivated in dried saliva within a few hours.

EPIZOOTIOLOGY

For decades the incidence and geographic distribution of rabies in domestic animals have shown close association with that of the disease in wildlife. This is clearly illustrated by comparing the prevalence of rabies in the raccoon and skunk with the geographic location of reported cases in cats. In general, the disease persists as a silent enzootic in wildlife and the disease in the cat and other domestic animals merely reflects the distribution of the disease in wildlife.[53] The danger of spread from silent cat or silent dog carriers appears remote or nonexistent.[54] Wherever rabies is eradicated in foxes, dogs, or other species, rabies in cats disappears spontaneously.[55]

Enzootic domestic animal rabies is now uncommon. Most domestic animals become infected through the bite of a rabid wild animal. The major wildlife species presently responsible for the maintenance of rabies in the United States are, in order of importance, skunks, raccoons, bats, and foxes. Terrestrial wildlife rabies tends to be localized to certain geographic regions of the country, based on the habitat and density of population of these species. The exception is bat rabies, which is considered to be ubiquitous.[56] Rabies virus isolated from bats differs from the virus isolated from terrestrial mammals in the incubation period and clinical signs that it causes in other species. Cats infected with the bat strain of RV may develop rabies and produce infective saliva during aggressive behavior.[57] It is recommended that any bat caught by a cat should be considered rabid and submitted for testing.[55]

PUBLIC HEALTH ASPECTS

Worldwide, the World Health Organization reports about 700 deaths from rabies each year. The number of deaths from rabies in the United States has fallen from about 40 annually in the 1940s to an average of less than two each year since 1980.

About one million persons are reported to have been bitten by animals each year in the United States. These bites result in about 25,000 persons receiving post-exposure prophylaxis for rabies annually. Although cases of human rabies resulting from exposure to rabid animals within the United States are now predominantly of wildlife origin, the administration of post-exposure prophylaxis to human beings is currently more likely to be a result of exposure to a rabid or potentially rabid domestic pet. Because of the frequent and prolonged contact that people have with their pets and the exposure of numerous human beings that often occurs when pets become rabid, the domestic pet currently provides the greatest risk of infecting human beings with rabies.[51]

The present low incidence of rabies in human beings in the United States is due to a number of factors, including the declining incidence of rabies in companion animals, the infrequent contact of most persons with the wildlife reservoir of the disease, the relatively low susceptibility of humans to infection with RV (only 15 per cent of human beings who are bitten by proven rabid dogs and who do not receive post-exposure prophylaxis develop clinical illness), and the high efficacy of post-exposure immunization and wound management.

TRANSMISSION

Cats and dogs usually become infected with RV as a result of the deep bite of a wild animal that is shedding virus in its saliva. Less commonly, infection may result from a nonbite exposure such as contamination of an open wound or scratch.

Wild animals may become infected through the ingestion of infected carrion, since the virus may remain viable for seven to ten days after death in salivary glands and nervous tissue. Transmammary and transplacental transmission may occur in some feral species.

PATHOGENESIS

In a deep bite wound, RV first replicates in local myocytes of striated muscle. The virus probably enters the peripheral nervous system through neuromuscular spindles and motor end plates. Passive transport of the virus in perineural structures results in ascending infection of the peripheral nerves.

During centripetal spread of RV, little stimulation is provided to the host's immune response, possibly due to the small amounts of initial inoculum or sequestration of the virus from the host's immune system.[56]

Once the virus reaches the spinal cord, spread of infection throughout the central nervous system takes only two to five days. Early preferential involvement of the limbic system results in signs of aggression, changes in character, and aberrant sexual behavior. Eventual widespread infection of the neocortex causes terminal depression and coma, with death usually resulting from respiratory arrest.

Centrifugal spread of rabies virus from the brain to nonneural tissues occurs via the peripheral nerves. The virus appears in the saliva coincidental with or slightly before the onset of clinical signs. Occasionally, the rabid cat may shed virus in the saliva for five days before overt clinical signs appear.[55] Effective transmission of the virus is ensured, since virus is present in the saliva during the furious phase of the disease.[56]

Virus-neutralizing antibodies and inflammatory cells are usually absent from the central nervous system at the time of appearance of encephalitic signs and only increase significantly at the time of death.

CLINICAL SIGNS

The incubation period of feline rabies ranges from two weeks to two months.[55] In most cases, clinical signs appear within 15 to 25 days of exposure.

Three classical phases of the disease have been described: the prodromal, furious, and paralytic phases. These phases are less sharply defined in cats than in dogs with rabies.[55]

Prodromal Phase. This phase usually lasts one to three days and is characterized by subtle changes in temperament, mild pyrexia, slow palpebral and corneal reflexes, and self-mutilation at the bite site. The cat may become unusually affectionate or may turn unexpectedly reclusive. Agitation and restlessness may be noted. Anorexia or polyphagia may occur.

In some rabid cats, these changes in temperament may go undetected and the first signs to appear are posterior weakness and ataxia, which precede a progressive ascending paralysis.[55]

Furious Phase. Cats tend to show furious signs more consistently than dogs and aggression is a common feature in the rabid cat. In fact, the rabid cat may be more dangerous than the rabid dog, often springing out from dark corners and attacking its victims around the head and neck.[54]

Episodes of aggression and hyperesthesia, which may progress to violent spasms, are often induced by visual or auditory stimuli. Later in this phase, muscular incoordination, disorientation, and generalized grand mal seizures may develop.

Paralytic Phase. Signs of paralysis usually appear within two to four days of the onset of clinical signs and last a similar length of time. Laryngeal and pharyngeal paralysis are usually the first signs of this phase, resulting in drooling of saliva, an inability to swallow food and water, dyspnea, and vocal changes. An ascending paralysis of the hind limbs that spreads to involve the whole body is usually noted. The cat becomes progressively comatose and usually dies from respiratory arrest.[55]

DIFFERENTIAL DIAGNOSIS

Rabies in cats must be differentiated from (1) other microbial diseases causing inflammatory or infiltrative lesions in the central nervous system, including the noneffusive form of feline infectious peritonitis, FeLV infection, toxoplasmosis, and cryptococcosis, (2) metabolic causes of altered mentation such as thiamine deficiency, lead poisoning, or portosystemic shunts, and (3) psychogenic aberrations such as those seen in severe neurodermatitis.

LABORATORY DIAGNOSIS

The reader is referred to Chapter 47 for a complete discussion of the laboratory diagnosis of rabies in companion animals.

MANAGEMENT OF SUSPECTED CASES

It is beyond the scope of this chapter to discuss this critical issue. The reader is referred to two recent reviews for further information on this subject.[51, 58]

CONTROL

Since control of rabies virus in wildlife species is not presently feasible, protection of the human population currently depends on the creation of an immune barrier of cats and dogs between the wildlife reservoir and human beings, reduction of contact between wildlife and companion animals through stringently enforced leash laws, and preexposure immunization of persons at risk, such as veterinarians, veterinary hospital employees, animal control officers, and wildlife control officers.

Vaccination. Practitioners should follow the guidelines of the Compendium of Animal Rabies Vaccines, prepared annually by the National Association of State Public Health Veterinarians. Concerted efforts must be made to vaccinate as many cats as possible, even in those states where vaccination is not required by law. Cats living in cities should be vaccinated, as the urban environment provides an excellent habitat for raccoons.[51]

Some inactivated rabies vaccines now provide protection for cats for at least three years.[52] The author prefers the use of a killed product with a three year duration of immunity, since the use of these vaccines precludes the possibility of vaccine-induced disease and increases the proportion of immunized cats at any single time.[58]

Using an inactivated vaccine that is licensed for use in cats with a three year duration of immunity, cats should be immunized between three and six months of age. The cat should be revaccinated one year later and then annually or triennially depending on state laws and the vaccine manufacturer's recommendations. It must be remembered, however, that cats and dogs that bite human beings and that are currently immunized against rabies, must not be presumed free of the disease.

FELINE LEUKEMIA VIRUS

Etiologic Agent

Feline leukemia virus (FeLV) was first associated with lymphoid malignancies in cats in 1969.[59] The virus is a contagiously transmitted retrovirus of pet cats, which originated millions of years ago through cross-species transmission of a rat endogenous retrovirus into the ancestors of the present day cat.[60] When traumatic injuries are excluded, FeLV-associated diseases become the leading cause of death in pet cats in the United States.

Exogenous retroviruses, like FeLV, are transmitted horizontally as infectious agents. These retroviruses are often oncogenic and exhibit a consistent pattern of induction of leukemia and/or lymphoma as their primary disease process.[61]

A new exogenous retrovirus, feline T-lymphotropic lentivirus (FTLV), has been identified in pet cats.[62] FTLV is considered to be a highly species-adapted lentivirus that has existed in cats for some time and may be widespread in the general feline population. Clinical signs in FTLV-infected cats included chronic rhinitis, cachexia, anemia, and a predisposition to opportunistic infections. Infected cats test negative for FeLV p27 antigen on the immunofluorescent antibody (IFA) or enzyme linked immunosorbent assay (ELISA) tests.

The clinical importance of FTLV is presently unknown. However, FTLV infections may explain some of the anemias, neurologic signs, and chronic infections that are seen in FeLV-negative cats.[62]

Feline syncytium-forming virus (FeSFV) is an exogenous retrovirus of unknown disease-producing potential. FeSFV has been statistically linked to chronic progressive polyarthritis and myeloproliferative disorders of cats. However, it is not clear what role the virus plays in the pathogenesis of these disorders.

Endogenous retroviruses, like the feline RD-114 virus, are present as an integral part of the genetic information of all cells of the species and are transmitted vertically to the next generation. Genes for these viruses are normally repressed, preventing the formation of whole virus particles.[61, 63]

FeLV is a replication-nondefective retrovirus, indicating that its RNA is complete and that it is capable of replicating successfully on its own without the assistance of a helper virus.

Cats are also hosts to a defective retrovirus, the feline sarcoma virus (FeSV), which is formed by recombination of the genes of FeLV and the host cell.[64] FeSV, which is isolated relatively rarely as a natural occurrence, cannot synthesize viral envelope proteins and uses the envelope supplied by its helper virus, FeLV.[64] FeSV is an acutely transforming retrovirus containing oncogenes, which rapidly causes multiple fibrosarcomas in cats younger than three years, and on rare occasion may induce malignant melanomas. In contrast, FeLV is a chronically transforming retrovirus, inducing tumors after a long latency period.[63] Three major FeLV subgroups (A, B, and C) are known to occur in nature.

Thus, pet cats are hosts to at least five groups of retroviruses, including (1) the nondisease-producing RD-114 virus, (2) feline syncytium-forming virus, (3) the leukemogenic FeLV, which also causes a variety of nonneoplastic diseases, (4) the sarcoma-inducing FeSV, and (5) the newly discovered FTLV.[62, 63]

The FeLV genome contains a single strand of RNA, which, like other retroviruses, contains signals for starting, stopping, and enhancing gene expression.[61] FeLV possesses three internal genes that code for core proteins (gag), envelope protein (env), and the enzyme reverse transcriptase (pol). This enzyme is a RNA-directed DNA polymerase, which copies the RNA of FeLV into complementary DNA, which is inserted into the chromosomal material of the infected cell as a provirus.[63, 64] This cell-integrated information is transmitted to daughter cells along with the other genes. The provirus codes for messenger RNA, initiating the production of new virus RNA in the cytoplasm of the infected cell and eventual budding of virus particles from the cell membrane. This results in horizontal spread of virus to other cells.[64] Thus, FeLV infects cells both vertically and horizontally.

The viral genome of FeLV does not contain an oncogene and induces neoplastic transformation by unknown mechanisms.[63] Participation of oncogenes does not appear to be an absolute requirement in retroviral oncogenesis.[61]

Structural Proteins

Within the FeLV virion, the single-stranded RNA molecule and the enzyme reverse transcriptase are enclosed in a capsid consisting of p27 antigen.[65] p27 is known as a group-specific antigen, since it is present in all other mammalian C-type oncornaviruses except bovine leukemia virus.[66] The ELISA and the IFA tests used to detect FeLV infection both detect p27 antigen. Antibodies produced against p27 antigen do not protect against viremia, and immune complexes containing p27 antigen may play a role in the pathogenesis of the glomerulonephritis seen in some persistently viremic cats.

The p27 core is surrounded by a lipid envelope that contains knoblike projections of gp70 antigen.[65] This envelope antigen is required for attachment of the virus to the membrane receptors of susceptible cells and contains the epitopes recognized by virus-neutralizing antibodies.[67] gp70 antigen is anchored in the viral envelope to intramembranous p15E antigen. The intact gp70/p15E complex is known as gp85.[65]

p15E antigen, a nonglycosylated envelope gene product, plays a major role in the pathogenesis of the profound immunosuppression seen in cats persistently infected with FeLV, by abrogating T-lymphocyte responses to interleukin 2.[68] In addition, p15E binds to the first component of complement, activating the classical pathway. This results in complement depletion and ineffective virolysis in infected cats.[69] There is also evidence that p15E plays a role in the pathogenesis of the nonregenerative anemia of FeLV infection.[70]

The feline oncornavirus cell membrane antigen (FOCMA) is a FeLV- and FeSV-induced, tumor-specific antigen found on the cell membranes of FeLV-induced lymphosarcoma, erythroleukemia, and myelogenous leukemia cells, and on the surface of FeSV-induced fibrosarcoma cells. FOCMA is found on the surface of lymphosarcoma cells from both FeLV-positive and FeLV-negative cats, but is absent on nontransformed cells infected with FeLV subgroups A and B.[63]

FOCMA appears to be a truncated or altered form of FeLV-C gp70.[69, 71] Complement-dependent antibodies produced against FOCMA are effective in preventing tumor development. However, anti-FOCMA antibodies do not protect the persistently viremic cat against the more common nonneoplastic diseases caused by FeLV.[71]

FeLV Subgroups

FeLV subgroups A, B, and C result from polymorphism in envelope antigen gp70.[67] Viruses of subgroups A and B are isolated in most naturally occurring FeLV infections, whereas viruses of subgroup C have apparently arisen by recombination of viruses of subgroups A and B with the apathogenic endogenous retroviruses of cats.[65]

FeLV-A is the predominant form and is isolated alone or in combination with other subgroups from all field cases.[64] By itself, FeLV-A is not particularly pathogenic, and infections in adult cats usually result in transient viremia with or without a subsequent period of latent infection. In young kittens, this subgroup may cause transient hemolytic anemia and eventual lymphosarcoma or leukemia after a long latency period.[67] Like the other subgroups, FeLV-A replicates in feline cell cultures. Its host range in the cells of other species is the most limited of the three subgroups, replicating only in canine and some human cells.[63]

FeLV-B, once engrafted, may cause myeloproliferative or myelosuppressive disease and profound immunosuppression. Its host range is the widest of all three subgroups, replicating in dog, mink, hamster, pig, cattle, monkey, and human cells.[63]

FeLV-C is rarely detected in nature. It is infectious only for neonates and adult cats that have been made viremic with FeLV-A.[67] FeLV-C causes erythroblastopenic anemias and is capable of replicating in dog, mink, guinea pig, and human cells.

Since it is evident that the three subgroups of FeLV are capable of causing different clinical syndromes, the combination of subgroups in an area may influence the manifestations of FeLV infection in the local cat population.[64] In order to fully protect cats against viremia, a vaccine against FeLV must induce virus-neutralizing antibodies against the envelope gene products of all three subgroups. The production of antibodies against FeLV-A gp70 is probably most important.[67]

Transmission

The natural reservoir of FeLV in nature is the asymptomatic persistently viremic cat, which may shed as many as one million viral particles in each ml of saliva—levels that equal or exceed those found in the plasma.[64] Infection of other cats usually requires prolonged close contact and results from infectious saliva acquired through grooming, fighting, and contamination of food and water bowls. Successful transmission is most likely under conditions of close intermingling. Asymptomatic viremic cats have mean salivary titers five to ten times higher than viremic cats with FeLV-induced neoplastic disease.[72] Cats undergoing transient infections may shed small amounts of virus in their saliva and represent another, less important source of infection. Small amounts of FeLV are shed in the urine of persistently viremic cats; however, the virus has not been cultured from the feces of these animals or from fleas removed from them.[72]

Transplacental transmission may occur in viremic queens.[69, 73] Neonatal kittens that escape in-utero infection may acquire transmammary infections or become contaminated with the infectious saliva of the viremic queen during grooming.

FeLV is inactivated by desiccation within a few hours in a dry environment, although it may remain viable for several days in moisture.[64] The virus is rapidly killed by most common disinfectants and its lipid envelope renders it susceptible to inactivation by detergents.

Prevalence of FeLV in Pet Cats

It is estimated that one to three per cent of the total cat population in the United States is persistently infected with FeLV. Two distinct patterns of FeLV infection are observed in the feline population.[72] In the free-roaming population of cats in the urban environment, persistent infections are uncommon in spite of the fact that the majority of cats show serologic evidence of prior transient infection. Most free roaming cats in this environment are mature animals that have acquired age-associated resistance to FeLV and usually do not intermingle closely enough with viremic cats to acquire a large challenge dose of virus. Within urban areas, cats living in high rise apartments have a lower infection rate than their more free-roaming suburban counterparts.

The second pattern is seen in the multiple cat household in which FeLV is enzootic and is known as an "exposure household." In these populations, 70 to 100 per cent of the cats show serologic evidence of infection. Cats that show no evidence of prior infection are thought to be the antisocial members of the group, which escape infection by not intermingling with the other cats. About 30 per cent of the group will be persistently infected and the remaining 40 to 70 per cent of the cats will have experienced transient infections.

Pathogenesis of FeLV Infections

STAGES OF INFECTION

Within weeks after exposure to FeLV, cats exhibit one of two major host-virus relationships: either a self-limiting regressive infection or, less commonly, a progressive and persistent infection.[69, 71]

Factors that determine the outcome of exposure to FeLV include the challenge dose of virus, the duration of exposure, age, immunocompetence, and poorly defined genetic factors.[73] Kittens that are nursing queens with protective antibodies are protected from challenge until two weeks of age by antibodies acquired in the colostrum. By two to three months of age, antibody levels are undetectable in these kittens, rendering them susceptible to infection.[64] Seronegative kittens exposed during the neonatal period are very likely to develop persistent infections, whereas cats infected after four months of age usually undergo transient viremia. However, the age-related resistance of adult cats to FeLV can be abrogated by the administration of corticosteroids.[64]

Following exposure to FeLV, six stages of infection may occur (Table 48–3).[66] The virus first enters the cat via tonsillar lymphocytes and macrophages in the oro-

TABLE 48–3. PATHOGENESIS OF FeLV INFECTION

Stage	Disease Progression
I (2–4 days)	Replication of FeLV occurs in lymphoid tissues surrounding the site of exposure (tonsils and pharyngeal lymph nodes via oronasal exposure)
II (1–14 days)	Small numbers of circulating lymphocytes and monocytes are infected
III (3–12 days)	FeLV replication is amplified in the spleen, lymph nodes, and gut-associated lymphoid tissue
IV (7–21 days)	Replication progresses to include bone marrow neutrophils, platelets, and intestinal crypt epithelial cells
V (14–28 days)	Peripheral viremia occurs once FeLV has been incorporated into bone marrow–derived neutrophils and platelets
VI (28–56 days)	Widespread epithelial infection causes excretion of virus in saliva and urine

From Beck, ER, Harris, CK, Macy, DW: Feline leukemia virus: Infection and treatment. Compend Contin Ed Pract Vet 8:567, 1986. Reproduced with permission.

pharynx, subsequently repopulating the draining submandibular lymph nodes. Macrophages play an important role in containing FeLV infection immediately after exposure.[66] From this point, the infection enters the recirculating lymphocyte pool for hematogenous spread to the sites of secondary viral replication and amplification. These include the B-lymphocyte areas of the visceral lymphoid tissue, Peyer's patches and spleen, the rapidly dividing precursor cells of the bone marrow (principally the myelomonocytic cells), and the crypt epithelial cells of the intestine.[74] Cats undergoing transient infections usually develop a virus-neutralizing antibody response by this stage of viral dissemination.

Failure to control virus replication at this stage allows a peripheral viremia, associated with the appearance of infected bone marrow–derived neutrophils and platelets, and widespread infection of mucosal or glandular epithelia, resulting in virus shedding.[73] During persistent viral infection, high titers (10^4 to 10^5/ml) of FeLV are found in the serum. Persistent submandibular lymph adenopathy may be noted in some viremic cats. The enlargement may be due to an excessive but ineffective stimulation of the lymphoid system in an attempt to escape persistent retrovirus infection.[74] Fewer than five per cent of persistently viremic cats are eventually able to mount a virus-neutralizing antibody response and recover from infection.[73]

CONSEQUENCES OF PERSISTENT VIREMIA

Recognizable signs of disease that are attributable to infection with FeLV are varied and appear only after an extended induction period.[72] For the retroviruses in general, the induction period before tumor appearance is approximately 15 to 20 per cent of the animal's life span.[61] About 50 per cent of persistently viremic cats will die within six months of detection of infection and 80 per cent will succumb within three years.[72]

ONCOGENIC PROPERTIES OF FELV

The mechanisms by which FeLV causes neoplastic transformation are not clearly understood. The virus may become incorporated into the genome of the cell, functioning as a promoter of endogenous oncogenes.[69]

Only about 70 per cent of cats with malignant lym phoid tumors are actively viremic at the time of diagnosis. There is epizootiologic evidence that the lymphoid tumors in the remaining cats are associated with past exposure to FeLV and FOCMA is found on the surface of the tumor cells. There is, however, one report of alimentary lymphosarcoma arising in a specific pathogen-free cat derived from stock that had been free of FeLV for many generations.[75] Cats that have virus-negative lymphosarcomas are usually older than seven years and have B-lymphocyte tumors. In contrast, cats with virus-positive tumors are usually younger than seven years and develop T-cell tumors.[63]

Lymphosarcoma cells from virus-negative cats show no evidence of integration of FeLV sequences in the host cell genome.[64] However, tumors that develop are many cell divisions away from the original transformed cell. As a result, the fraction of the virus genome remaining in the fully developed tumor cell may be so small as to be undetectable by currently available techniques.[61] FeLV has been reactivated from the bone marrow of cats with virus-negative lymphosarcoma, but not from their tumor cells.

Unlike the herpesviruses or the coronaviruses, FeLV is a nonlytic virus, budding from the cell membranes without killing the host cell. An infected cell produces virus for its normal lifespan and cell lysis must be induced in order to prevent cell transformation or division.[76] Clearance of virus-infected transformed cells is probably mediated by cytotoxic complement-dependent antibodies to both virion antigens and FOCMA.[71]

FeLV-INDUCED IMMUNOSUPPRESSION

Immunosuppression accompanies the onset of marrow origin viremia in cats with progressive FeLV infections and precedes detectable neoplastic transformation by months. The resulting immune dysfunction predisposes the viremic cat to infection with a variety of intercurrent and opportunistic organisms.[69] Immunosuppression associated with FeLV has been associated with a replication-defective FeLV mutant, "FeLV-FAIDS," that arises during natural infection with replication-competent FeLV.[77]

p15E antigen abrogates the response of T-lymphocyte helper cells to interleukin 2 (T-cell growth factor) and also causes complement depletion. Viremic cats often have high levels of circulating immune complexes that contain FeLV proteins and antiviral antibodies.[74] Neutrophils from viremic cats with signs of FeLV-associated disease have significantly lower chemotactic responses than those from healthy viremic cats.[78]

Other immunologic abnormalities seen in viremic cats include thymic atrophy, paracortical lymphoid depletion in lymph nodes, persistent lymphopenia, delayed allograft rejection, and decreased suppressor T-cells.[79] Successful therapeutic termination of FeLV-induced immunosuppression will most likely require reversal of viremia and cessation of production of virus by B-lymphocytes and macrophages.[74]

LATENT INFECTIONS

In 30 to 80 per cent of cats undergoing transient viremia, FeLV is not immediately eliminated from the cat and remains in an unexpressed form in monocytic precursor cells in the bone marrow and in certain T-lymphocytes in lymph nodes.[73, 80] It has been suggested that this latently infected state is a normal phase of recovery. Cats that become infected with FeLV soon after exposure are more likely to develop latent infections or persistent viremias. Those animals that become infected only after protracted exposure are more likely to undergo complete recovery.[80]

Latent FeLV infections probably are maintained by virus-neutralizing antibodies[81] and there is no significant difference in antibody titers between cats with latent infections and cats that have completely recovered from infection.[79, 80, 82] The duration of latency is short, with the majority of cats completely eliminating virus from the bone marrow within 30 months of exposure to FeLV.[83] Clones of hematopoietic or lymphoid cells harboring the latent virus may differentiate to extinction, leaving the cat genuinely free of FeLV.[64] Cats with true latent infections test negative on the ELISA and IFA tests for p27 antigen in blood.[71] Latent infections may be responsible for the persistently high anti-gp70 and anti-FOCMA antibody titers seen in some cats.[66] The relationship between latent infections and virus-negative lymphosarcomas remains unclear.

On occasion, latent infections may be reactivated naturally by stress, complement depletion, or intercurrent bacterial or viral diseases.[74] Exogenous corticosteroids reactivate latent infections more easily than natural stressors.[64] Reactivated latent infections may result in relapsing or persistent viremia, with subsequent shedding of virus in the saliva. Such recrudescences of virus shedding may be responsible for the unexpected outbreaks of FeLV-associated disease that occasionally occur in populations considered free of the virus. Virus neutralizing antibody levels may be high at the time of reactivation of a latent infection and virus particles released into the serum of these cats may become incorporated into immune complexes that are phagocytized and removed from the circulation. Under these circumstances, the ELISA test for p27 antigen may be negative, while the IFA test may give positive results.[73]

Cats with true latent infections that have not undergone reactivation do not appear to be infectious to susceptible cats that come in contact with them. However, the latent state is a fragile phase of the recovery process from FeLV infection and the cat with a latent infection becomes infectious if reactivation occurs. Procedures to decrease the risk of contagion from latently infected cats include the isolation for six months of cats that have undergone transient FeLV infections, the cautious use of corticosteroids in cats that have recently recovered from FeLV infection, the avoidance of natural stresses in these cats, and the isolation of queens that have recently recovered from FeLV until their kittens are weaned. In these circumstances, the kittens should be tested for FeLV before being placed back in the main colony.[64]

A subgroup of cats has been identified that are nonviremic, yet remain persistently positive on the ELISA test for p27 antigen (Table 48–4). These discordant cats are thought to be immune carriers of FeLV, maintaining a sequestered focus of infection in an epithelial tissue in the absence of virus-expressing leukocytes and platelets.[64, 73] Transmammary transmission of infectious FeLV has been reported in a discordant queen that had low virus-neutralizing antibody titers and that later reverted to a viremic state.[82] It is presently considered inadvisable to allow these discordant cats to live communally with uninfected cats.[1, 64]

TABLE 48–4. CLASSIFICATION OF CATS FOLLOWING EXPOSURE TO FELINE LEUKEMIA VIRUS

Classification	Blood *Virus*	Blood *Antigen*	Marrow *Virus*	Neutralizing Antibodies	Transmission of Virus
Viremic	+	+	+	None	Yes
"Discordant"		+	+	Low	Possible
Latent			+	High	No
Recovered				High	No

From Jarrett, O: Feline leukemia virus. In Pract 7:125, 1985. Reproduced with permission.

FeLV-Associated Diseases

Persistent infection with FeLV results in three different clinical syndromes that may occur alone or in combination: (1) uncontrolled proliferation of virally transformed cells, resulting in lymphosarcoma, or leukemia of the erythroid, lymphoid, or myeloid cell lines, (2) degeneration of progenitor (blast) cells, resulting in nonregenerative anemia, leukopenia, and/or thrombocytopenia, and (3) generalized immunosuppression, predisposing the cat to intercurrent or opportunistic infections (Table 48–5).[79]

Diagnostic Tests for FeLV

Presently, two tests are available to detect FeLV infection, both of which identify the group-specific core antigen of the virus. The IFA test detects antigen in infected leukocytes and platelets in fixed blood smears and positive results indicate that bone marrow cells are actively producing virus.[73, 79] There is a strong correlation between positive IFA results and the ability to recover infectious virus from the patient's blood and saliva.[67]

TABLE 48–5. FELINE LEUKEMIA VIRUS-ASSOCIATED DISEASES

Cell Type	Proliferative Diseases (Neoplastic)	Degenerative Diseases (Blastopenic)
Lymphocytes	Lymphosarcoma	Thymic atrophy Lymphopenias Feline acquired immune deficiency syndrome (FAIDS)
Bone marrow cells		
Primitive mesenchymal	Reticuloendotheliosis	—
Erythroblast	Erythremic myelosis Erythroleukemia	Erythroblastosis Erythroblastopenia Pancytopenia
Myeloblast	Granulocytic leukemia	Myeloblastopenia
Megakaryocyte	Megakaryocytic leukemia	Thrombocytopenia
Fibroblast	Myelofibrosis	—
Osteoblast	Medullary osteosclerosis Osteochondromatosis	— —
Kidney	—	FeLV immune complex glomerulonephritis
Uterus	—	Abortions and resorptions
Fibroblasts, skin	Feline sarcoma virus–induced multicentric fibrosarcomas	—

Reproduced with permission from Hardy, WD: Feline leukemia and sarcoma viruses. *In* Feline Medicine I. Lawrenceville, New Jersey, Veterinary Learning Systems Inc, pp. 4–11.

About 97 per cent of IFA-positive cats remain viremic for life and never reject the virus.[63] False-negative IFA tests may occur if peripheral blood or bone marrow smears are prepared poorly or if low numbers of infected cells are present on the smears.[73] False-positive tests occasionally result from nonspecific immunofluorescence in eosinophils and platelet clumps.[79] A subgroup of FeLV-infected cats has been identified that has negative results on IFA and ELISA tests on blood samples, yet shows strongly positive IFA test results on bone marrow smears.[70]

The ELISA test uses an antibody-linked enzymatic color change to detect p27 antigen.[66] Most of the plasma antigen detected by the ELISA test is in a soluble form and is not incorporated in whole virus particles. Compared to the IFA test, the ELISA test is more likely to detect weak, early, or transient infections when viral antigens are often not present in leukocytes.[84] Healthy ELISA-positive cats should be evaluated with the IFA test before a long-term prognosis is given.

Noninvasive ELISA tests (ClinEase-VIRASTAT™, Norden Laboratories) for the detection of FeLV p27 antigen in saliva provide the clinician with a convenient method of screening cats for FeLV. An ELISA test that detects p27 antigen in tears has been introduced, allowing sample collection at home by the owner.[84]

Healthy cats that test ELISA-positive and IFA-negative on a single examination may be undergoing a transient regressive infection or be in the early stages of a progressive infection (before the bone marrow has become infected), or may be immune carriers of a localized infection. Differentiation of the immune carrier cat from the animal with a transient or early persistent infection is accomplished by repeating both the ELISA and the IFA test 12 weeks after initial detection of the discordant state.[1] False-positive ELISA reactions are usually due to a failure to properly wash out reagents at each stage of the test and may occur more frequently when whole blood or badly hemolyzed serum is used.[84] Concentration immunoassay tests that use a bioreactive filter to detect p27 antigen may decrease technical problems encountered with the traditional ELISA test.

Cats with true latent FeLV infections test negative on the ELISA and IFA tests and the infections are undetectable without bone marrow explant cultures. IFA tests on the bone marrow of these cats are routinely negative.

Antibodies to gp70 antigen may be measured by serum neutralization tests. Maintenance of protective levels of serum neutralizing antibodies in the natural environment requires periodic exposure to FeLV, therefore a single serum neutralizing-antibody titer is of little value for the long-term prediction of a cat's susceptibility to FeLV infection. Serologic evaluation of cats may be useful to detect seroconversion associated with recent infection or to identify cats with low titers that are susceptible to infection.[79] Cats with anti-FOCMA antibody titers of more than 1:32 may be protected against the neoplastic effects of FeLV.[64] However, high levels of anti-FOCMA antibodies do not protect the cat against viremia or the development of the more common non-neoplastic diseases caused by FeLV.

Treatment of FeLV Infections

Treatment of FeLV infections at the present time is palliative and symptomatic, since there are no readily available and reliable methods to reverse the persistent viremia. Experimental treatments that have been used with variable success to terminate viremia include extracorporeal removal of immune complexes by treatment of the plasma with staphylococcal protein A, administration of feline plasma constituents such as fibronectin, and specific immunotherapy with anti-gp70 or anti-FOCMA antibodies.[73, 74] Monoclonal antibody therapy may hold more promise than polyclonal antibody treatment, which is not effective in reversing chronic viremias.[74] Suramin, a drug that competitively inhibits the activity of reverse transcriptase, had no long-term antiviral effect on persistently viremic cats.[85]

The decision whether to initiate supportive treatment depends on the severity of clinical signs associated with the particular FeLV associated disease and whether the cat is a potential hazard to susceptible cats in its immediate environment. Unfortunately, it is impossible to predict how long a cat has been infected before viremia is first detected and how each individual patient will respond to FeLV infection.[66]

In addition to specific therapy for any neoplastic or degenerative disorders that may be present, the viremic cat should receive aggressive treatment for opportunistic microbial infections as soon as they are noted. Bactericidal antimicrobials are preferred over bacteriostatic drugs due to the underlying immunosuppression. Corticosteroids should be used with great caution in viremic cats, unless specifically indicated in the treatment of neoplastic or immune-mediated diseases caused by FeLV infection. Natural stresses should be minimized.[66]

Control of FeLV

Control of FeLV in the general feline population depends on accurate identification and removal of persistently infected cats, reducing the exposure of susceptible cats to potentially infectious animals, and vaccination of cats that may be exposed to the virus.[1]

Test and removal programs using the IFA test have proven effective in greatly reducing the number of infected cats in populations where FeLV is enzootic.[63, 86] Cats that are IFA-positive are removed from the group. The remaining cats are retested after three months and those with positive tests are removed.[63] The author uses the blood ELISA test in this same situation, confirming the status of ELISA-positive cats with an IFA test. In this manner, cats with transient or persistently discordant infections may be identified.

The introduction of a soluble tumor cell subunit vaccine (Leukocell) has provided the practitioner with an additional means of reducing the prevalence of FeLV in the general feline population.[87] The inactivated vaccine contains a multiplicity of partly processed gag- and env-encoded products derived from FeLV subgroups A, B, and C, and soluble FOCMA. The vaccine is intended to protect FeLV-naive cats against viremia and the development of tumors and other FeLV-associated diseases. Subcutaneous vaccinations are given at 9, 12, and 24 weeks of age, and then annually.[67]

Considerable controversy has arisen over the efficacy of this vaccine.[88–90] Independent studies noted that the vaccine failed to induce adequate titers of virus-neutralizing antibodies directed against gp70 envelope antigen and that the vaccine had no protective effect against latent infections.[88] Countering these observations, the manufacturers defended the immunizing potency of the vaccine, stressing the importance of complement-dependent cytotoxic antibodies in the protection against FeLV and the effectiveness of the vaccine in preventing latent infections.[89, 91] Perceived problems with this vaccine include the presence of too many FeLV and cat cell products and the need for adjuvant coadministration to ensure effective immunogenicity.[67] The practical effectiveness of the vaccine will only be ascertained by evaluating its protective effects after widespread use in the field. Future generations of FeLV vaccines may consist of a synthetic oligopeptide that represents an immunogenic fragment of the surface glycoprotein gp70.[65]

Differing from the opinion of others, the author recommends that vaccination for FeLV be included in the routine health care program of all healthy cats and not limited to those cats at high risk for exposure to the virus. The efficacy of FeLV vaccination is easier to assess if the FeLV status of the cat is determined before vaccination is initiated. For this purpose, a screening ELISA test is taken before or at the time of the first vaccine. Peripheral blood or buffy coat smears are taken for IFA testing in case the ELISA test is positive. The vaccination of persistently viremic cats offers no benefits.

CORONAVIRAL INFECTIONS

Domestic cats are susceptible to infection with several coronaviruses.[92] Depending on which coronavirus is involved, clinical signs range from asymptomatic infections to gastrointestinal signs of varying severity to a syndrome of widespread fibrinous serositis and vasculitis known as feline infectious peritonitis (FIP).

The development of FIP may involve numerous predisposing factors including age, genetic susceptibility, general physical condition, presence of concurrent disease (especially FeLV infection), challenge dose and strain of FIP virus (FIPV), route of infection, previous sensitization with nonprotective coronaviral antibody, macrophage function, and cell-mediated immunocompetence. It is not surprising, therefore, that FIP is a sporadic disease that appears unpredictably in the feline population.[116]

Coronaviral infections in cats are among the most frustrating infectious diseases encountered by the small animal practitioner.[93] Some coronaviruses produce disease by unique methods, many are difficult to isolate or diagnose in the laboratory, the clinical diseases that they produce may closely resemble other disorders, there are no effective treatments or vaccines available at the time of writing, and generalized disease usually results in the death of the cat.

The Coronaviruses

Coronaviruses are pleomorphic, enveloped particles that average 100 nm in diameter and contain a single strand of RNA.[94, 95] Characteristic petal-shaped projections called peplomers protrude from the viral surface.[96] In many species of animals, coronaviruses have a relatively restricted organ tropism, infecting the respiratory and/or gastrointestinal systems.[97] The viruses are important causes of respiratory and enteric disease, vasculitis, serositis, hepatitis, and encephalomyelitis in several avian and mammalian species.[98] Following oral infection, the viruses have an affinity for the mature apical columnar epithelium of the villi in the duodenum, jejunum, and ileum.[99] Younger members of any species tend to develop overt signs of infection, whereas the asymptomatic carrier state is more common in adult animals. In the cat and mouse, however, coronaviral infections may involve several organs and persistent and chronic diseases often occur in these two species.[97]

Similar to other coronaviruses, FIPV replicates in enterocytes, but also uncharacteristically replicates in macrophages, budding from the endoplasmic reticulum. Tissues that have extensive reticuloendothelial components, such as the spleen, liver, and lymph nodes, are preferentially infected with FIPV.[100]

FIPV is a heat-labile virus, being inactivated at room temperature within 24 to 48 hours. Infectivity is destroyed by most household disinfectants and detergents.[101] In organ homogenates, however, FIPV remains stable for many months at −94°F (−70°C), resisting repeated freezing and thawing.[102]

FIPV, transmissible gastroenteritis virus (TGEV) of swine, canine coronavirus (CCV), and human respiratory tract coronaviruses of the 229E group comprise an antigenic cluster of closely related viruses within the Coronaviridae group. The major structural polypeptides of FIPV, TGEV, and CCV are so similar antigenically that some consider these three viruses as host range mutants rather than individual viral species.[98]

The Coronaviruses Infecting Cats

The coronaviruses that infect cats have been divided into those that cause FIP (FIPVs) and those that induce subclinical to severe enteritis – the feline enteric coronaviruses (FECVs).[103] The FIPVs differ from the FECVs in their ability to escape from the gastrointestinal tract and spread to replication sites in distant tissues.[104] FIPVs and FECVs may represent pathogenetic variants of a single coronavirus type.[98] Alternatively, FIPVs may arise periodically as mutants of FECV strains.[104] Classification of the known strains of feline coronavirus has been based on their morphologic, structural, and antigenic relationship to TGEV and CCV, the nature of the disease that they cause, their growth characteristics in cell culture, and their degree of relatedness to CCV in virus neutralization tests (Table 48–6).[103]

TABLE 48–6. CLASSIFICATION OF THE FELINE CORONAVIRUSES

Feline Coronaviruses

A. Non TGEV-like (theoretical existence)
B. TGEV-like
  1. Type I
    Difficult to grow in cell culture
    Grow best in selective cell lines
    Cell-associated growth
    Low level of virus production in cell culture
    Antiserum to these strains reacts weakly in VN tests with heterologous viruses such as CCV
    a. FIP inducing
      i. FIPV-UCD1
      ii. FIPV-UCD3
      iii. FIPV-UCD4
      iv. FIPV-TN406 (Black)
    b. Enteritis inducing
      i. FECV-UCD
  2. Type II
    Easily isolated in cell culture
    Grow in many different cell lines
    Produce large amounts of non cell-associated virus
    Cytopathic effect resembles that of CCV
    Antiserum to these strains reacts strongly in VN tests with heterologous viruses such as CCV
    a. FIP inducing
      i. FIPV-79-1146
      ii. FIPV-UCD2
    b. Enteritis inducing
      i. FECV-79-1683

Data from Pedersen, NC: Coronavirus diseases (coronavirus enteritis, feline infectious peritonitis). *In* Holzworth, J (ed): Diseases of the Cat, Vol. 1. Philadelphia, W. B. Saunders Co., 1987, p. 193; and Pedersen, NC, et al.: Pathogenic differences between various feline coronavirus isolates. Adv Exp Med Biol 173:365, 1984.

FELINE INFECTIOUS PERITONITIS VIRUS

The spectrum of virulence of FIPVs is shown in Table 48–7. The most virulent strains (FIPV-79-1146 and FIPV-Nor15) cause fatal disease in a high percentage of cats inoculated oronasally, while strains of intermediate virulence, for example FIPV-UCD1, cause FIP in a percentage of cats undergoing prolonged exposure. Finally, strains of low virulence, such as FIPV-UCD2 and FIPV-UCD3, may establish themselves as chronic asymptomatic infections, with clinical signs of FIP occurring only if the host's immunologic responsiveness later becomes compromised.[104]

Most clinical cases of FIP are a result of infection with strains similar to FIPV-TN-406 (Black) and not with those FIPVs that are closely related to CCV.[104] Most asymptomatic cats with coronavirus antibody have been infected previously by an FECV, or a strain of FIPV such as FIPV-UCD3 or FIPV-UCD4, which does not usually cause fatal disease by natural routes of infection. These two groups of cats may succumb later if challenged with a more virulent strain of FIPV. Those coronavirus antibody–positive cats that resist later challenge probably underwent prior seroconversion as a result of a systemic infection with a virulent strain of FIPV.[105]

TABLE 48–7. SPECTRUM OF VIRULENCE OF FIPVs

Most virulent	FIPV–NOR 15
	FIPV–79–1146
	FIPV–TN406 (Black)
	FIPV–UCD1
	FIPV–UCD3
	FIPV–UCD4
Least virulent	FIPV–UCD2

From Pederson, NC and Floyd, K: Experimental studies with three new strains of feline infectious peritonitis virus: FIPV-UCD2, FIPV-UCD3, and FIPV-UCD4. Comp Cont Ed Pract Vet 7:1001, 1985. Reproduced with permission.

FELINE ENTERIC CORONAVIRUSES

About 25 per cent of free-roaming cats have been or remain infected with FECVs.[105] Infections are especially prevalent in catteries and multiple cat households.

FECVs such as FECV-UCD and FECV-79-1683 are highly infectious by the oral route and have an affinity, like many coronaviruses, for the apical columnar epithelium of the intestinal villi from the mid-duodenum to cecum.[106] Most adult cats undergo subclinical infections; however, low grade fever, neutropenia, vomiting, and diarrhea may be observed in recently weaned kittens.

Infection with FECVs results in the production of coronaviral antibody that is, at present, serologically indistinguishable from that induced by infection with FIPVs, CCV, or TGEV.[105] Most cats that undergo infection with FECV remain persistently infected with the virus, shedding virus in the feces. FECV-infected cats with persistently high coronavirus antibody titers appear to be more infectious.[105]

Antibody formed as a result of FECV infection does not protect the cat from later challenge with a virulent strain of FIPV. In fact this antibody sensitizes the cat to later challenge, accelerating the disease process induced by the virulent FIPV. Coronaviral antibody induced by mildly pathogenic strains of FIPV has a similar sensitizing effect.[104]

CORONAVIRUS-LIKE PARTICLES

Coronavirus-like particles (CVLPs) have been identified by electron microscopy in the feces of human beings and a number of animal species, including cats. However, CVLPs are morphologically and antigenically distinct from the established coronaviruses. CVLPs do not cause detectable seroconversion or disease in cats when inoculated oronasally, intraperitoneally, intraduodenally, or intravenously. Natural infection may require prolonged close contact with shedding carrier cats.[107, 108]

Transmission of FIPV

It is unlikely that cats with FIP are the only source of FIPV in nature.[105] Similarly, contaminated fomites are an unlikely source of infection, due to the short stability of FIPV outside the host.[109]

In most cases, transmission of virus probably occurs via the feces and less commonly, the urine or oronasal secretions of asymptomatic carriers. However, such asymptomatic cats are probably very uncommon and shed very small amounts of virus at any given time.[105]

Queens that are asymptomatically infected with FIPV may infect their offspring in-utero or in the neonatal period. Kittens infected in-utero may be born sick or may show no signs of disease. However, some asymptomatic infected kittens may develop FIP at a later time if their immune responsiveness becomes impaired. Paradoxically, infection of kittens with FIPV at an early age appears to lead to a higher rate of immunity than infection with the same FIPV at a later date.[105]

Pathogenesis of FIP

Following experimental aerosol exposure, initial localization and replication of virus beyond the epithelium takes place in large mononuclear cells in regional lymphoreticular tissue or in subepithelial layers. The initial target cells for FIPV may be the dendritic macrophages, located in the cortex of lymph nodes.[100] One can speculate that similar internalization of FIPV might occur through the intestinal epithelium following oral exposure. It is recognized that certain strains of FIPV cause enteritis and/or fibrinous serositis after intragastric inoculation.[110, 111] Some naturally occurring strains of FIPV have a rather severe gastrointestinal infection and mesenteric lymphadenopathy as principal early signs. These infections usually progress to fatal disseminated FIP.[93]

A primary viremia occurs within one week of exposure, with free virus or FIPV-infected mononuclear cells eventually reaching organs such as the spleen, liver, and lymph nodes, which contain large populations of macrophages—the primary target cells for FIPV replication.[108]

If an effective CMI response is mounted at this stage of infection, it is likely that the cat will terminate viremia and will be protected against clinical disease.[96] Under these circumstances, most cats show no clinical signs. However, some cats may develop a transient pyrexia and localized mesenteric lymphadenopathy.[103] If the cat is unable to mount an effective CMI response and begins to develop anti-FIPV antibodies that are not virus-neutralizing, the infection progresses rapidly. A similar situation occurs if the cat already has coronaviral antibodies acquired through previous infection with FECV or a FIPV of low virulence.[109]

In the absence of an effective CMI response, a strong nonprotective humoral response results in the most fulminating form of the disease, effusive FIP. Cats that are capable of mounting a partial CMI response may ultimately develop the noneffusive form of FIP, which is considered a partially controlled or smoldering form of the disease. The intensity of inflammation and amount of virus is considerably less in lesions of noneffusive FIP, when compared to the effusive form.

An effective CMI response does not always result in total elimination of FIPV from the body. In some recovered cats, the infection may persist in a sequestered or latent form in the gastrointestinal tract or its associated lymph nodes.[103] Factors that depress CMI responsiveness, such as FeLV infection, concurrent disease, or advanced age, may allow recrudescence of this sequestered infection with subsequent shedding and/or disseminated disease.

An exaggerated and nonprotective humoral response results in antibody excess, causing the formation of large immune complexes that are rapidly phagocytized by cells of the reticuloendothelial system.[100] Immune complexes deposited in small blood vessels fix and activate complement, resulting in the release of the third component of complement (C3). Phagocytosis of aggregates containing FIPV, Ig, and C3 is aided by the presence of receptors for Ig and C3 on the macrophage surface.[112] The majority of immune complexes found in cats with FIP do not contain intact virions.[113]

Macrophages in perivascular locations that ingest aggregates of intact FIPV, Ig, and C3 foster replication of virus, degenerate, and release new virions and complement components.[114] Uptake of FIPV into macrophages appears to be enhanced by impaired T-lymphocyte function.[98] A vicious circle of complement-mediated damage ensues, resulting in the release of chemotactic complement components and the attraction of neutrophils. Release of proteolytic enzymes from degenerating neu-

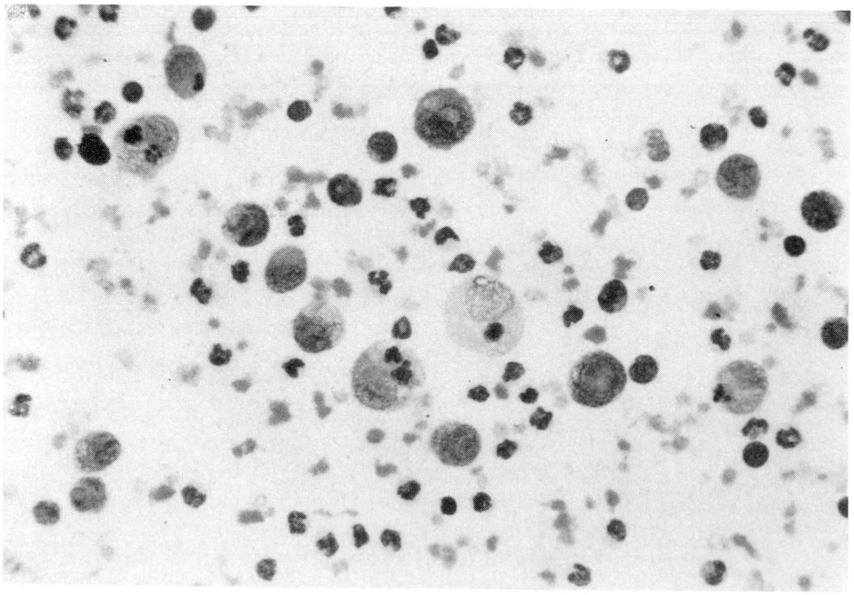

FIGURE 48–3. Nondegenerate neutrophils, macrophages, and erythrocytes in the abdominal exudate of a cat with effusive FIP. (From August, JR: Feline infectious peritonitis: An immune-mediated coronaviral vasculitis. Vet Clin North Am 14:971, 1984. Reprinted with permission.)

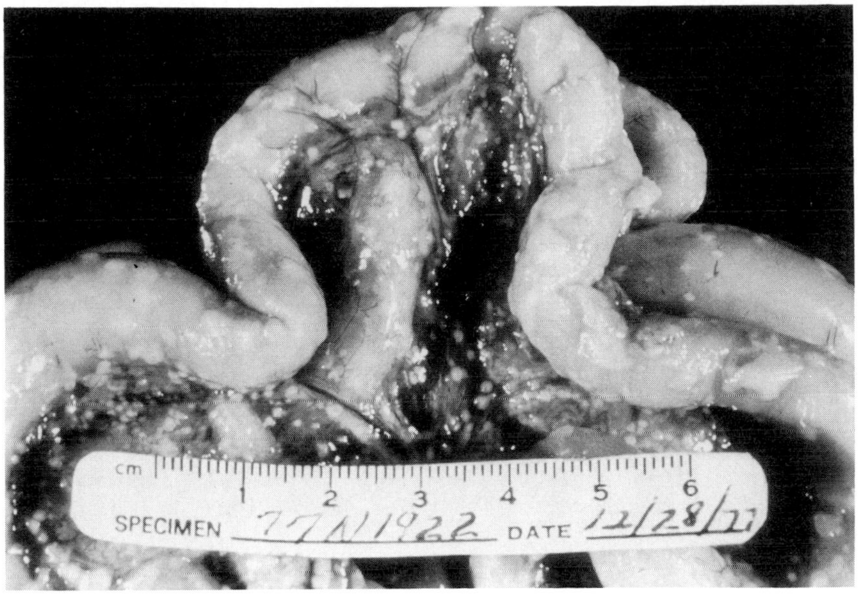

FIGURE 48–4. Multifocal fibrinous plaques on the intestinal serosa of a cat with effusive FIP. Mesenteric lymphadenopathy is also present. (From August, JR: Feline infectious peritonitis: An immune-mediated coronaviral vasculitis. Vet Clin North Am 14:971, 1984. Reprinted with permission.)

trophils exacerbates tissue damage. In naturally occurring cases, degenerative and proliferative changes occur in blood vessels, particularly in the endothelial and medial layers of small veins and arteries in the peritoneal and pleural serosa and in the interstitial connective tissue of parenchymatous organs.[115]

The vascular lesion of FIP is an Arthus-type reaction, resulting in a pyogranulomatous response. In fulminant cases, complement-mediated damage to the vascular endothelium results in increased vascular permeability and the outpouring of a nonseptic exudate that is rich in fibrin and immunoglobulin (Figure 48–3). In the light of our present knowledge of FIPV and the basic pathologic lesions it induces in terminally ill cats, FIP might be more accurately named feline coronaviral vasculitis.[116]

Under experimental conditions, damage to the vascular endothelium produced multiple in vitro clotting abnormalities.[117] The development of thrombocytopenia, hyperfibrinogenemia, increased quantities of fibrin-fibrinogen degradation products, and depression of factors VII, VIII, IX, XI, and XII plasma activities suggested that DIC might be an important terminal complication of FIP. Coagulopathies have been noted in naturally occurring cases of the disease.[101] Thrombosis and blood stasis in small veins may enhance seeding of virus and dissemination through vessel walls at these sites.[117]

Clinical Manifestations of FIP

CATS AT RISK

Both domestic and wild cats are susceptible to infection with FIPV. In domestic cats, the disease occurs predominantly in young animals, although cats of all ages are susceptible. A peak incidence occurs between 6 and 12 months of age. A decline in incidence is noted from 5 to 13 years of age, followed by an increased incidence in cats 14 to 15 years old.[96] Male and female cats are affected equally.

FIP occurs more frequently in purebred cats, probably because these cats are kept more commonly in catteries or multiple cat households. Young, susceptible cats in these environments may undergo prolonged exposure to a high concentration of coronaviruses and FeLV.[96] Several siblings in a litter, often the smaller and weaker kittens, may become affected.

FORMS OF FIP

Three forms of the disease have been recognized: (1) effusive FIP, characterized by fibrinous serositis and abdominal and/or thoracic effusions, (2) noneffusive FIP, characterized by marked pyogranulomatous lesions in parenchymatous organs, the central nervous system, and/or eyes, and (3) combinations of these two.[101] In nature, effusive FIP occurs about four times more frequently than the noneffusive form of the disease.[105]

As noted previously, the qualitative and quantitative nature of the humoral and CMI responses of the cat determine the severity of the inflammatory response that follows infection. Changes in immune response may take place during the development of lesions, since cats with noneffusive FIP always undergo an initial brief period of effusive disease.[105]

EFFUSIVE FIP

Clinical Signs. In the early stages of disease, cats with effusive FIP may be presented with nonspecific signs, including chronic fluctuating antibiotic-resistant fever, anorexia, lethargy, and progressive weight loss. Mucous membrane pallor is often present, and in severe cases icterus due to hepatic involvement may be noted.[101] Recurring bouts of diarrhea and constipation are occasionally observed.

Progressive abdominal distention develops as a result of accumulation of exudate in the peritoneal cavity. The

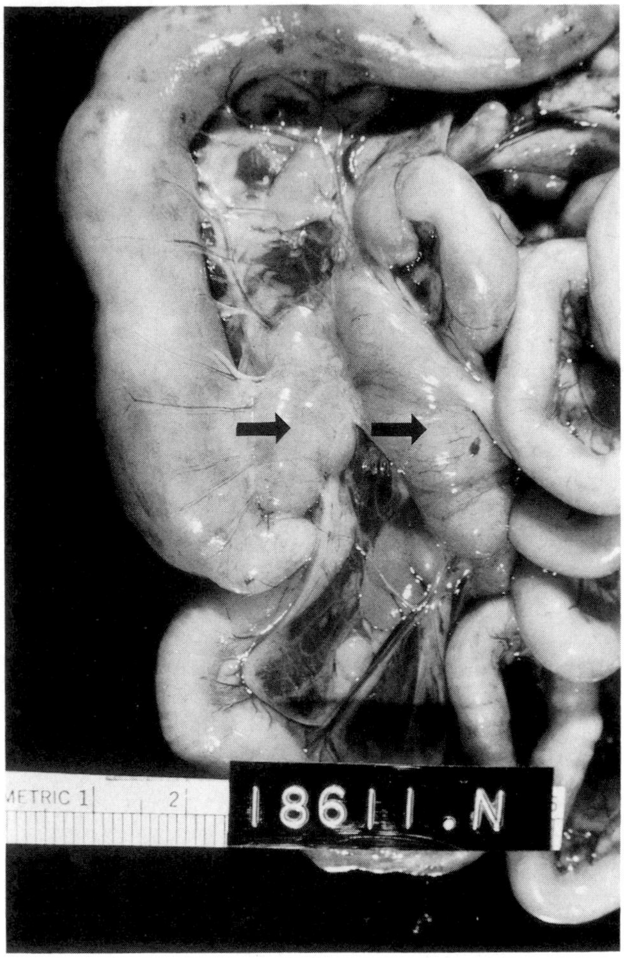

FIGURE 48–5. Enlarged ileocolic lymph nodes (arrows) in a cat with noneffusive FIP. (From August, JR: Feline infectious peritonitis: An immune-mediated coronaviral vasculitis. Vet Clin North Am 14:971, 1984. Reprinted with permission.)

volume of fluid varies, being greatest in chronic cases, in which a liter or more may be present.[101] Abdominal palpation usually elicits no signs of pain. In some cats, the omentum may be palpated as a contracted fibrinous mass in the cranioventral abdomen.

In about 25 per cent of cats with effusive disease, exudate may be present in the pleural cavity. These cats are presented with decreased exercise tolerance, dyspnea (especially upon handling), and muffled heart and lung sounds. Pericardial effusion may also be present.[118] In intact male cats, scrotal enlargement may occur, resulting from a direct extension of the fibrinous serositis from the peritoneal cavity. Ocular and central nervous signs are seen infrequently in effusive FIP.[96] The rare cat that recovers from effusive FIP undergoes a phase of noneffusive disease before complete recovery.[105]

Pathologic Lesions. The visceral, and to a lesser extent parietal, peritoneum is covered by a diffuse or multifocal plaque-like, white, necrotic, fibrinous exudate that is often most evident on the liver and spleen (Figure 48–4).[95] In chronic cases, fibrinous adhesions may develop between abdominal viscera. Mesenteric lymph nodes are often enlarged (Figure 48–4). The mesentery is often thickened and may have a watery, gelatinous consistency.[119] The omentum may appear as a contracted mass of adhesions in the cranial abdomen. In cases with thoracic effusion, a similar fibrinous exudate affects the pleura and pericardium.

The exudate on serosal surfaces is mainly composed of fibrin with some nuclear debris, necrobiotic neutrophils, histiocytes, lymphocytes, neocapillaries, and fibroblasts.[95] Mesothelial hyperplasia is also present.

NONEFFUSIVE FIP

Clinical Signs. Nonspecific signs of weight loss, antibiotic-resistant pyrexia, and malaise may last for several weeks before organ-specific manifestations appear. The early diagnosis of noneffusive FIP is hindered by a lack of localizing signs. Clinical signs reflecting involvement of the peritoneal cavity, central nervous system, or eyes are most common.

Abdominal palpation may reveal mesenteric lymphadenopathy (Figure 48–5) and nodular irregularities caused by surface-oriented pyogranulomas on the viscera, especially the kidneys (Figure 48–6).[116] Pyogranulomatous pneumonia occurs infrequently and dyspnea is uncommon. Pulmonary lesions consist of peribronchiolar mixed inflammatory cell infiltrates and appear radiographically as ill-defined, patchy, interstitial and peribronchiolar densities.[118]

Pathologic Lesions. Pyogranulomas, usually appearing as raised, white foci from 1 to 20 mm in diameter, characterize the lesions of noneffusive FIP. Lesions tend to be subcapsular and surface-oriented, but extend into the parenchyma of involved organs. Renal pyogranulomas may be large enough to be confused with nodular lesions of renal lymphosarcoma. Smaller renal lesions may have an arborescent pattern as a result of their association with large subcapsular blood vessels.[119] Pyogranulomas are also found in mesenteric lymph nodes, liver, spleen, pancreas, omentum, and serosal membranes. Omental and serosal lesions are more focal, fibrinous and organized, and less edematous than those occurring in effusive FIP.[120]

Histopathologic examination of pyogranulomas reflects the immune-mediated basis of the disease and

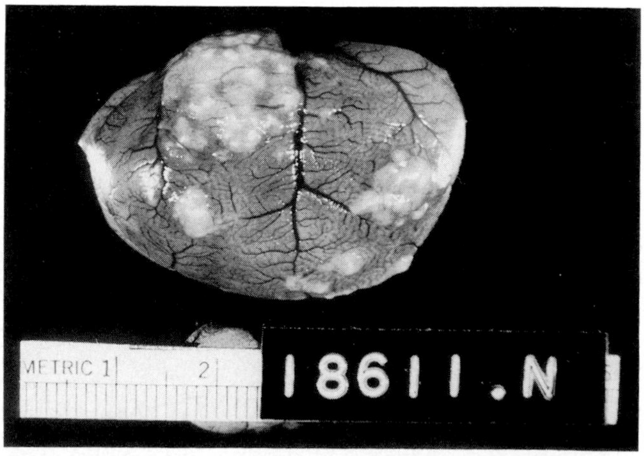

FIGURE 48–6. Multiple, small, subcapsular pyogranulomas in the kidney of a cat with noneffusive FIP. (From August, JR: Feline infectious peritonitis: An immune-mediated coronaviral vasculitis. Vet Clin North Am 14:971, 1984. Reprinted with permission.)

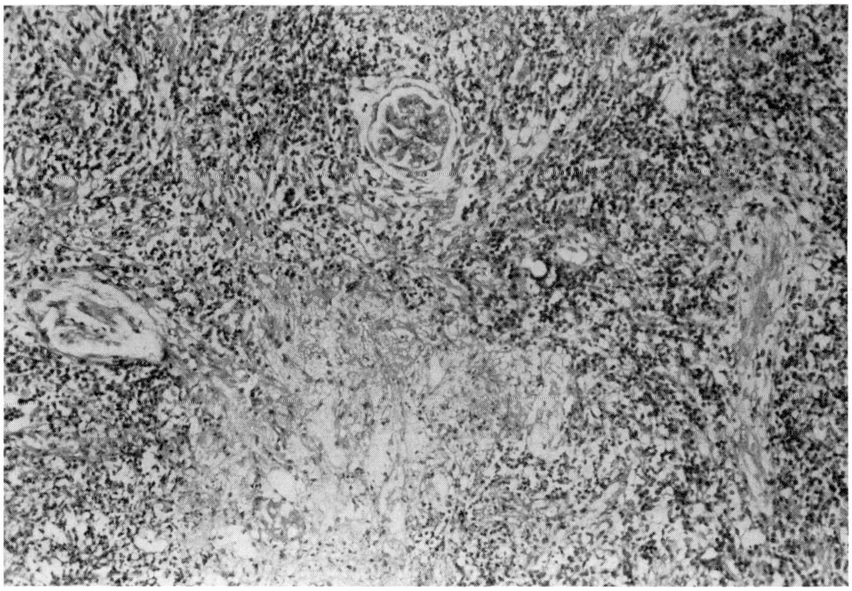

FIGURE 48–7. Focal necrosis with fibrin deposition and pleocellular infiltration of lymphocytes, neutrophils, and macrophages in a renal pyogranuloma of a cat with noneffusive FIP. (From August, JR: Renal diseases of the cat. In Feline Medicine I. Lawrenceville, Veterinary Learning Systems, 1985, p 16. Reprinted with permission.)

reveals a necrotizing vasculitis and perivasculitis. Variable coagulative necrosis may be present, associated with intense perivascular infiltrations of neutrophils and, to a lesser extent, macrophages, plasma cells, and lymphocytes (Figure 48–7).[102]

OCULAR MANIFESTATIONS OF FIP

Ocular signs usually occur in association with other signs of noneffusive FIP, but may be present in the absence of systemic signs.[96] Lesions develop as a result of a necrotizing and pyogranulomatous uveitis, which is localized around vascular structures. Changes in the anterior chamber include corneal edema, aqueous flare, hypotony, iritis, hyphema, hypopyon, and the presence of keratic precipitates.

On fundic examination, flame- or boat-shaped hemorrhages may be evident. Engorgement of retinal veins and perivascular cuffing are often noted. Choroidal inflammation may cause subretinal fluid exudation and secondary bullous or linear retinal detachments.[121] Histopathologic changes are found primarily in the iris, ciliary body (Figure 48–8), choroid, and retina.

NEUROLOGIC MANIFESTATIONS OF FIP

Neurologic signs in cats with noneffusive FIP are variable and include progressive incoordination, posterior paresis, nystagmus, convulsions, intention tremors, cranial and peripheral nerve paralysis, hyperesthesia, generalized ataxia, head tilt, behavioral changes, and urinary incontinence.[122]

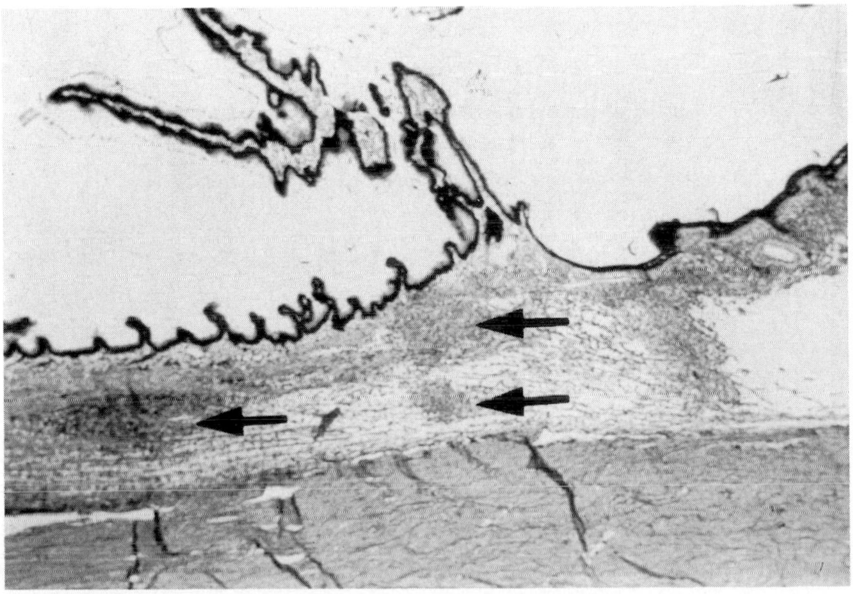

FIGURE 48–8. Multiple pyogranulomas (arrows) in the ciliary body of a cat with uveitis due to noneffusive FIP. (From August, JR: Feline infectious peritonitis: An immune-mediated coronaviral vasculitis. Vet Clin North Am 14:971, 1984. Reprinted with permission.)

Pathologic changes are typically multifocal or diffuse, and surface-oriented, affecting primarily the choroid plexus, meninges (Figure 48–9), and ependyma. These regions of the central nervous system may be prone to immune complex and/or cell-mediated tissue injury.[123] Gelatinous masses of fibrinous exudate may obstruct the normal flow of cerebrospinal fluid, resulting in hydrocephalus. Histologically, the lesions are characterized as a pyogranulomatous meningoencephalomyelitis. Lesions, as expected, are often oriented around small blood vessels, especially venules.[123] Many cats with noneffusive FIP that are not manifesting overt neurologic signs have histopathologic evidence of central nervous system involvement.[122]

LABORATORY FINDINGS

Hematology. The hemogram of cats with clinical FIP may show a mild to moderate normocytic normochromic anemia and a leukocytosis associated with a regenerative left shift. Lymphopenia is commonly observed, being more profound in those cats with concurrent FeLV infections.[124]

Biochemical Findings. Elevations in serum urea nitrogen and serum creatinine may be present in cats with effusive and noneffusive FIP and may reflect both a state of dehydration and the presence of inflammatory lesions in the kidneys. Similarly, elevations in hepatic enzymes reflect hepatic parenchymal damage. Hyperbilirubinemia may be present, resulting from chronic anorexia and the presence of hepatic lesions.

Total plasma proteins exceed 7.8 gm/dl in 55 per cent of cats with effusive disease and in 75 per cent of cats with noneffusive FIP, due to variable increases in alpha-2, beta, and gamma globulins. This polyclonal gammopathy is not pathognomonic for FIP and reflects the chronic inflammatory nature of the disease.[105] The hyperglobulinemia found in FIP may not result only from stimulation by viral antigen. Cell damage resulting from the intense tissue inflammation may stimulate an autoimmune humoral response to self antigens released in the process.[113]

Fluid Analysis. The peritoneal or pleural fluid is pale yellow to golden, clear or slightly opaque, sticky, and viscous. A stable foam often develops after shaking, probably reflecting the high protein content. Fibrin strands and flakes may be present, which settle with time. Fluid specimens may clot upon exposure to air.

The specific gravity of the fluid is usually between 1.018 and 1.047, with white blood cell counts of 1000 to 10,000 cells/μl. Stained smears reveal a mixture of intact neutrophils, macrophages, plasma cells, lymphocytes, and a few erythrocytes (Figure 48–3). A pink granular background composed of protein aggregates may be mistaken for bacteria. The fluid is characterized as a nonseptic exudate.

DIFFERENTIAL DIAGNOSIS

FIP must be differentiated from other feline diseases that may cause chronic pyrexia, lymphadenopathy, peritoneal or pleural effusions, uveitis, and central nervous system signs.

Diseases that may closely resemble effusive or noneffusive FIP include lymphosarcoma and visceral tumors, cardiomyopathy, pyothorax, chylothorax, diaphragmatic hernia, chronic bacterial peritonitis, the cholangiohepatitis complex, pansteatitis, toxoplasmosis, cryptococcosis, and tuberculosis.[98, 105]

DIAGNOSIS OF FIP

A presumptive diagnosis of FIP is made through a careful evaluation of the patient's history, physical findings, laboratory results, coronaviral antibody titer, and the exclusion of "look-alike" diseases. Unfortunately, none of these diagnostic procedures provides conclusive evidence that the cat has FIP, especially in cases of

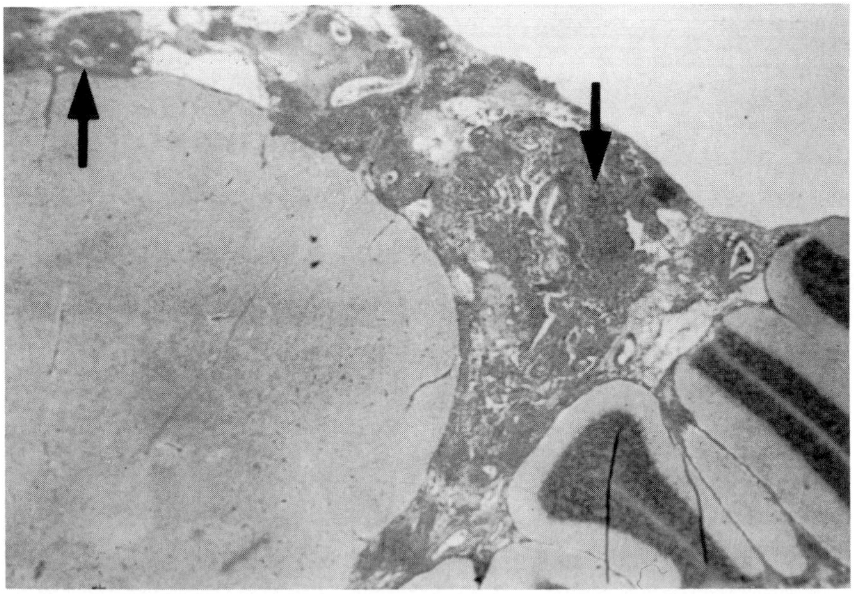

FIGURE 48–9. Pyogranulomatous meningitis in a cat with noneffusive FIP. Multiple pyogranulomas are present within a mass of exudate overlying the cerebral cortex and cerebellum. (From August, JR: Feline infectious peritonitis: An immune-mediated coronaviral vasculitis. Vet Clin North Am 14:971, 1984. Reprinted with permission.)

noneffusive disease where no exudate is available for examination.

Organ biopsy is the only diagnostic procedure that can be used to confirm the presence of FIP in the living cat, especially the patient with noneffusive disease. Any diagnosis of FIP made in the absence of biopsy or eventual necropsy examinations must be considered presumptive in these cases.[98]

Coronaviral Serology. Several laboratory tests are available for the detection of coronaviral antibody in cats, including biological assays such as virus neutralization, and nonbiological assays such as IFA, ELISA, and kinetics-based ELISA (KELA) methodologies.[98] The target antigen used in these tests may be FIPV (in liver sections of experimentally infected cats or in cell culture), or one of the other coronaviruses in the FIPV antigenic cluster, such as TGEV or CCV.[93]

Coronaviral antibody may be found in the serum of healthy cats, cats with diseases other than FIP, and cats with FIP. From 10 to 40 per cent of the general feline population (excluding those cats in catteries and in multiple cat households) have coronaviral antibody in their serum. Where cats are congregated in large groups, the rate of seropositivity will either be 80 to 90 per cent or 0 per cent, depending on whether coronaviruses are enzootic in that population.[98]

Unfortunately, the serologic tests for coronaviral antibody available at the time of writing do not identify which coronavirus was responsible for seroconversion in a particular cat and the presence of coronaviral antibody merely indicates that the cat has been infected with one of the viruses in the FIPV antigenic cluster (FIPV, FECV, TGEV, or CCV).[98] Most healthy cats with coronavirus antibody probably have been infected with FECVs, with nonFIP-producing strains of FIPV such as FIPV-UCD2, or with weakly FIP-producing strains of FIPV such as FIPV-UCD4. Most healthy coronavirus antibody-positive cats are probably not immune carriers of highly virulent FIPV.[104] It is impossible, at the present time, to predict with accuracy the long-term prognosis of the healthy coronavirus antibody-positive cat. A positive titer does not indicate that the cat (1) is protected against the future development of FIP, (2) will develop FIP at a later time, or (3) is a proven hazard to other cats.

Bovine serum components found in some commercial feline vaccines may induce antibody production in cats immunized with those products. These antibodies may react with antigenically similar bovine serum components in cell cultures used to propagate target viruses of the FIPV antigenic cluster for immunochemical assays. The resulting reactivity may be mistaken for coronavirus antibody in the recently vaccinated cat. Because of this potential interference, it is recommended that elective serotesting of healthy cats for evidence of exposure to coronavirus should be delayed until at least three to four months after the last parenteral vaccine has been given.[98]

At the present time, serologic testing for feline coronaviruses should be confined to use as a screening test to determine if coronaviruses are enzootic in any given cat population, and as an aid, and only an aid, in the diagnosis of feline infectious peritonitis.[98]

Most cats with histopathologically confirmed FIP have high titers of coronavirus antibody.[98] Titers of more than 1:3200 are usually associated with noneffusive FIP, while titers of 1:100 to 1:3200 may be found in cats with effusive FIP, some cats with noneffusive disease, and cats with FECV infection.[105] In some cats with FIP, a falling titer may be seen in the terminal stages of the disease and is a poor prognostic sign. In addition to correlating the titer with all other pertinent information about the patient, the clinician should be aware that different laboratories vary in the tests that they perform for the detection of coronaviral antibody and in the interpretation that they place on any given titer.

Some cats with histopathologically confirmed FIP may have negative coronavirus antibody titers.[98] Reasons for this phenomenon include (1) a disappearance of antibody in the terminal stages of disease, (2) the formation of immune complexes, leaving little or no free antibody to react in the assay, (3) the use of assay systems that are not sensitive enough to detect low levels of antibody, (4) the presence of small amounts of antibody in peracute fulminating cases of effusive FIP, and (5) the possibility that more than one serotype of FIPV may be present, resulting in low or negative titers in current assays.[93]

Treatment of FIP

The prognosis for cats with FIP is poor, since there is currently no effective treatment to terminate the viral infection. Some treatment regimens allow short-term remissions in carefully selected patients. The best patients for palliative therapy are those cats with FIP that are not infected with FeLV, are in good physical condition, maintain a good appetite, and have no evidence of severe anemia or neurologic signs.[108] Unfortunately, few cats with FIP are presented early enough in the course of disease to meet these criteria.

Present therapies rely on the use of corticosteroids and cytotoxic drugs to decrease the intense antibody-mediated inflammation.[108] While these drugs may provide a temporary palliative effect, their long-term use appears contraindicated in a patient whose disease has arisen as a result of a defective CMI response.

Cats with detectable lesions confined to the eye(s) may respond relatively well to the subconjunctival injection of 4 to 5 mg of triamcinolone acetonide.[93] If ocular inflammation is severe and sight has been lost, enucleation is probably indicated.

Control of FIP in Catteries

The incidence of new cases of FIP in catteries and multiple cat households may be decreased by prompt isolation of all cats with suspected signs of the disease, the removal of all cats infected with FeLV, decreasing the amount of stress in the group by reducing overcrowding and improving overall hygiene and nutrition, selecting queens that have good mothering instincts and the ability to raise large healthy litters, and the admission of cats that are coronavirus antibody–negative.[105]

There is no justification for the use of coronaviral antibody testing as part of a "test-and-removal" program to control FIP, similar to the programs used successfully to reduce the prevalence of FeLV. This is because of the poor specificity of the serologic tests used to detect coronaviral antibody compared to the high accuracy of ELISA or IFA tests used to detect FeLV antigen. Removal of healthy coronaviral antibody–positive cats from the group is justified only if there is strong epizootiological evidence that the cat is a source of infection of FIPV for other cats; for example, the seropositive queen that repeatedly produces litters of kittens in which FIP occurs.[1]

At the present time, there is no vaccine available to protect cats against FIPV. The antibody-mediated pathogenesis of the disease poses particular challenges for the vaccine manufacturer. The vaccine must produce long-lasting CMI, which may require persistence of vaccine virus in a chronic or latent infection. The ideal vaccine of the future may be made of a strain of FIPV that has been attenuated to prevent the induction of FIP in vaccinates, yet has retained its invasiveness and its ability to persist in the body. Overattenuation of the vaccine virus carries the danger of the induction of sensitizing antibodies.[104]

References

1. August, JR: Feline preventive health care and infectious disease control. *In* Sherding, RG (ed): Diseases of the Cat: Diagnosis and Management. New York, Churchill Livingstone Inc, In Press.
2. Pederson, NC: Basic and clinical immunology. *In* Holzworth J (ed): Diseases of the Cat, Vol 1. Philadelphia, WB Saunders Co, 1987, p 146.
3. Ford, RB and Greene, RT: The influence of host factors on the outcome of a viral infection. Vet Clin North Am 16:1041, 1986.
4. Sheffy, BE: Nutrition, infection, and immunity. Comp Cont Ed Pract Vet 7:990, 1985.
5. Sheffy, BE and Williams, AJ: Nutrition and the immune response. JAVMA 180:1073, 1982.
6. Schultz, RD: The effects of aging on the immune system. Comp Cont Ed Pract Vet 6:1096, 1984.
7. August, JR: Feline viral respiratory disease. The carrier state, vaccination, and control. Vet Clin North Am 14:1159, 1984.
8. Lawler, DF and Bebiak, DM: Nutrition and management of reproduction in the cat. Vet Clin North Am 16:495, 1986.
9. Lawler, DF and Monti, KL: Morbidity and mortality in neonatal kittens. Am J Vet Res 45:1455, 1984.
10. Scott, FW: Feline infectious diseases—Practical virucidal disinfectants. In Proc AAHA, 1979, p 105.
11. Gaskell, RM and Wardley, RC: Feline viral respiratory disease. A review with particular reference to its epizootiology and control. J Sm Anim Pract 19:1, 1977.
12. Pearson, RC, et al.: Vaccines and principles of immunization. Vet Clin North Am 16:1205, 1986.
13. Schultz, RD: Theoretical and practical aspects of an immunization program for dogs and cats. JAVMA 181:1142, 1982.
14. Scott, FW: Feline immunization. *In* Kirk RW (ed): Current Veterinary Therapy VIII. Philadelphia, WB Saunders Co, 1983, p 1127.
15. Scott, FW: Current canine and feline immunization guidelines. *In* Kirk, RW (ed): Current Veterinary Therapy VIII. Philadelphia, WB Saunders Co, 1983, p 1134.
16. Dhein, CR and Gorham, JR: Host response to vaccination. Vet Clin North Am 16:1227, 1986.
17. Greene, CE: Immunoprophylaxis and immunotherapy. *In* Greene CE (ed): Clinical Microbiology and Infectious Diseases of the Dog and Cat. Philadelphia, WB Saunders Co, 1984, p 321.
18. Scott, FW: Panleukopenia. *In* Holzworth J (ed): Diseases of the Cat, Vol 1. Philadelphia, WB Saunders Co, 1987, p 182.
19. Baldwin, CA: Feline viral enteritis. *In* Scott FW (ed): Contemporary Issues in Small Animal Practice, Vol 3. New York, Churchill Livingstone Inc, 1986, p 81.
20. Greene, CE: Feline panleukopenia. *In* Greene CE (ed): Clinical Microbiology and Infectious Diseases of the Dog and Cat. Philadelphia, WB Saunders Co, 1984, p 479.
21. Pollock, RVH: The parvoviruses. Part I. Feline panleukopenia virus and mink enteritis virus. Comp Cont Ed Pract Vet 6:227, 1984.
22. Reinacher, M: Feline leukemia virus-associated enteritis—A condition with features of feline panleukopenia. Vet Pathol 24:1, 1987.
23. Hoover, EA: Viral respiratory diseases and chlamydiosis. *In* Holzworth J (ed): Diseases of the Cat, Vol 1. Philadelphia, WB Saunders Co, 1987, p 214.
24. Scott, FW: Feline viral respiratory infections. *In* Scott FW (ed): Contemporary Issues in Small Animal Practice, Vol 3. New York, Churchill Livingstone Inc, 1986, p 155.
25. Povey, RC and Johnson, RH: Observations on the epidemiology and control of viral respiratory disease in cats. J Sm Anim Pract 12:233, 1971.
26. August, JR: Feline viral respiratory disease. Vet Tech 7:88, 1986.
27. Gaskell, RM: An update on feline upper respiratory disease (URD). In Grunsell CSG, Hill FWG, Raw R-E (eds): The Veterinary Annual, 26th Issue. Bristol, Scientechnica, 1986, p 318.
28. Gaskell, RM and Povey, RC: Feline viral rhinotracheitis: Sites of virus replication and persistence in acutely and persistently infected cats. Res Vet Sci 27:167, 1979.
29. Povey, RC: A review of feline viral rhinotracheitis (feline herpesvirus 1 infection). Comp Immun Microbiol Infect Dis 21:373, 1979.
30. Nasisse, MP: Manifestations, diagnosis and treatment of ocular herpesvirus infection in the cat. Comp Cont Ed Pract Vet 4:962, 1982.
31. Gaskell, RM and Povey, RC: Experimental induction of feline viralrhinotracheitis virus reexcretion in FVR-recovered cats. Vet Rec 100:128, 1977.
32. Gaskell, RM, et al.: Isolation of felid herpesvirus 1 from the trigeminal ganglia of latently infected cats. J Gen Virol 66:391, 1985.
33. Gaskell, RM and Povey, RC: Transmission of feline viral rhinotracheitis. Vet Rec 11:359, 1982.
34. Studdert, MS: Caliciviruses: Brief review. Arch Virol 58:157, 1978.
35. Wardley, RC: Feline calicivirus carrier state: A study of the host/virus relationship. Arch Virol 52:243, 1976.
36. Povey, RC: Persistent viral infection. The carrier state. Vet Clin North Am 16:1075, 1986.
37. Pedersen, NC, et al.: A transient febrile "limping" syndrome of kittens caused by two different strains of feline calicivirus. Fel Pract 14(2):32, 1984.
38. Wardley, RC, et al.: Feline respiratory viruses—their prevalence in clinically healthy cats. J Sm Anim Pract 15:579, 1974.
39. Thompson, RR, et al.: Association of calicivirus infection with chronic gingivitis and pharyngitis in cats. J Sm Anim Pract 25:207, 1984.
40. Wardley, RC and Povey, RC: The pathology and sites of persistence associated with three different strains of feline calicivirus. Res Vet Sci 23:15, 1977.
41. Wardley, RC and Povey, RC: The clinical disease and patterns of excretion associated with three different strains of feline calicivirus. Res Vet Sci 23:7, 1976.
42. Ott, RL: Diagnosis of feline viral infection. Vet Clin North Am 16:1157, 1986.
43. Sanford, TD, et al.: Tube pharyngo-esophagostomy and liquified diet in the treatment of feline upper respiratory disease. Fel Pract 15(6):35, 1985.
44. Gustafson, DP: Antiviral therapy. Vet Clin North Am 16:1181, 1986.
45. Gaskell, RM: The natural history of the major feline viral diseases. J Sm Anim Pract 25:159, 1984.

46. Goddard, LE: Feline viral rhinotracheitis—host versus herpes. Fel Pract 16(2):36, 1986.
47. Johnson, RP and Povey, RC: Vaccination against feline viral rhinotracheitis in kittens with maternally-derived feline viral rhinotracheitis antibodies. JAVMA 186:149, 1985.
48. Komolafe, OO and Jarrett, O: Feline calicivirus subunit vaccine—a prototype. Antiviral Res 5:241, 1985.
49. Cocker, FM, et al.: Responses of cats to nasal vaccination with a live, modified feline herpesvirus type 1. Res Vet Sci 41:323, 1986.
50. Centers for Disease Control Rabies Surveillance. Annual Summary, 1984. Atlanta, 1985.
51. Perry, BD: Rabies. Vet Clin North Am 17:73, 1987.
52. Soulebot, JP, et al.: Experimental rabies in cats. Immune response and persistence of immunity. Cornell Vet 71:311, 1981.
53. August, JR and Loar, AS: Zoonotic diseases of cats. Vet Clin North Am 14:1117, 1984.
54. Christie, AB: Rabies. J Infect 3:202, 1981.
55. Abelseth, MK: Rabies. *In* Holzworth J (ed): Diseases of the Cat, Vol 1. Philadelphia, WB Saunders Co, 1987, p 238.
56. Report on Rabies. Princeton, Veterinary Learning Systems Inc, 1983. Copyright, Fromm Laboratories.
57. Trimarchi, CV, et al.: Experimentally-induced rabies in 4 cats inoculated with a rabies virus isolated from a bat. Am J Vet Res 47:777, 1986.
58. August, JR: Rabies. *In* Barlough JE (ed): Manual of Small Animal Infectious Diseases. New York, Churchill Livingstone Inc, In Press.
59. Jarrett, WFH, et al.: A virus-like particle associated with leukemia (lymphosarcoma). Nature 202:567, 1969.
60. Hardy, WD: Feline leukemia and sarcoma viruses. *In* Feline Medicine 1. Lawrenceville, Veterinary Learning Systems Inc, 1985, p 4.
61. Mackowiak, PA: Microbial oncogenesis. Am J Med 82:79, 1987.
62. Pedersen, NC, et al.: Isolation of a T-lymphotropic virus from domestic cats with an immunodeficiency-like syndrome. Science 235:790, 1987.
63. Hardy, WD: Oncogenic viruses of cats: The feline leukemia and sarcoma viruses. *In* Holzworth J (ed): Diseases of the Cat, Vol I. Philadelphia, WB Saunders Co, 1987, p 246.
64. Barton, CL: The feline leukemia virus: Pathogenesis of disease. *In* Scott FW (ed): Contemporary Issues in Small Animal Practice, Vol. 3. New York, Churchill Livingstone Inc, 1986, p 109.
65. Moennig, V: Feline leukemia prophylaxis. J Sm Anim Pract 27:344, 1986.
66. Beck, ER, et al.: Feline leukemia virus: Infection and treatment. Comp Cont Ed Pract Vet 8:567, 1986.
67. Rojko, JL: Feline leukemia virus vaccines. Semin Vet Med Surg (Small Anim) 1:61, 1986.
68. Horohov, DW and Rouse, BT: Virus-induced immunosuppression. Vet Clin North Am 16:1097, 1986.
69. Olsen, RG, et al.: Oncogenic viruses of domestic animals. Vet Clin North Am 16:1129, 1986.
70. Legendre, AM: Feline leukemia: The disease. *In* Feline Leukemia: Virus and Vaccine. Lawrenceville, Veterinary Learning Systems Inc, 1986, p 3.
71. Olsen, RG: Feline leukemia: The virus. *In* Feline Leukemia: Virus and Vaccine. Lawrenceville, Veterinary Learning Systems Inc, 1986, p 7.
72. Gerstman, BB: The epizootiology of feline leukemia virus infection and its associated diseases. Comp Cont Ed Pract Vet 7:766, 1985.
73. Cockerell, GL: Unifying concepts of feline leukemia virus infection. *In* Kirk RW (ed): Current Veterinary Therapy IX. Philadelphia, WB Saunders Co, 1986, p 1055.
74. Rojko, JL and Mathes, LE: Feline acquired immunodeficiency syndrome (FAIDS) induced by the feline leukemia virus. *In* Kirk RW (ed): Current Veterinary Therapy IX. Philadelphia, WB Saunders Co, 1986, p 436.
75. Jarrett, O, et al.: Feline leukemia virus-free lymphosarcoma in a specific pathogen free cat. Vet Rec 115:249, 1984.
76. Sharpee, RL: Recent developments in the Leukocell™ feline leukemia vaccine. *In* Feline Leukemia: Virus and Vaccine. Lawrenceville, Veterinary Learning Systems Inc, 1986, p 13.
77. Mullins, JI, et al.: Disease-specific and tissue-specific production of unintegrated feline leukemia virus variant DNA in feline AIDS. Nature (London) 319:333, 1986.
78. Kiehl, AR, et al.: Effects of feline leukemia virus infection on neutrophil chemotaxis in vitro. Am J Vet Res 48:76, 1987.
79. Kiehl, AR and Macy, DW: Feline leukemia virus: Testing and prophylaxis. Comp Cont Ed Pract Vet 7:1038, 1985.
80. Madewell, BR and Jarrett, O: Recovery of feline leukemia virus from non-viraemic cats. Vet Rec 112:339, 1983.
81. Jarrett, O: Feline leukaemia virus. In Pract 7:125, 1985.
82. Pacitti, AM, et al.: Transmission of feline leukaemia virus in the milk of a non-viraemic cat. Vet Rec 118:381, 1986.
83. Pacitti, AM and Jarrett, O: Duration of the latent state in feline leukaemia virus infections. Vet Rec 117:472, 1985.
84. Hawkins, EC, et al.: Use of tears for diagnosis of feline leukemia virus infection. JAVMA 188:1031, 1986.
85. Cogan, DC, et al.: Effect of suramin on serum viral replication in feline leukemia virus-infected pet cats. Am J Vet Res 47:2230, 1986.
86. Weijer, K, et al.: Control of feline leukemia virus infection by a removal programme. Vet Rec 119:555, 1986.
87. Olsen, RG: Feline leukemia vaccine: Its role in the management of feline leukemia disease. Comp Cont Ed Pract Vet 7:998, 1985.
88. Pedersen, NC, et al.: Evaluation of a commercial feline leukemia virus for immunogenicity and efficacy. Fel Pract 15(6):7, 1985.
89. Olsen, RG and Sharpee, RL: Letter to the editor. Fel Pract 16(1):4, 1986.
90. Sharpee, RL, et al.: Feline leukemia vaccine: Evaluation of safety and efficacy against persistent viremia and tumor development. Comp Cont Ed Pract Vet 8:267, 1986.
91. Olsen, RG: New information on feline leukemia vaccination. In Proc 11th WSAVA Congress. Paris, France, 1986.
92. Barlough, JE: Serodiagnostic aids and management practices for feline retrovirus and coronavirus infections. Vet Clin North Am 14:955, 1984.
93. Scott, FW: The real and unreal feline coronaviruses. *In* Feline Medicine II. Lawrenceville, Veterinary Learning Systems Inc, 1986, p 27.
94. Barlough, JE, et al.: Feline coronaviral serology. Fel Pract 13(3):25, 1983.
95. Horzinek, MC and Osterhaus, ADME: The virology and pathogenesis of feline infectious peritonitis. Brief review. Arch Virol 59:1, 1979.
96. Pedersen, NC: Feline infectious peritonitis and feline enteric coronavirus infections. Part 2. Feline infectious peritonitis. Fel Pract 13(5):5, 1983.
97. Wege, H, et al.: The biology and pathogenesis of coronaviruses. Curr Top Microbiol Immunol 99:164, 1982.
98. Barlough, JE: Cats, coronaviruses and coronavirus antibody tests. J Sm Anim Pract 26:353, 1985.
99. Pedersen, NC, et al.: An enteric coronavirus of cats and its relationship to feline infectious peritonitis. Am J Vet Res 42:368, 1981.
100. Weiss, RC and Scott, FW: Pathogenesis of feline infectious peritonitis: Pathologic changes and immunofluorescence. Am J Vet Res 42:2036, 1981.
101. Barlough, JE and Weiss, RC: Feline infectious peritonitis. *In* Kirk RW (ed): Current Veterinary Therapy VIII. Philadelphia, WB Saunders Co, 1983, p 1186.
102. Ott, RL: Multisystemic viral infections. In Pratt PW (ed): Feline Medicine. Ed 1. Santa Barbara, American Veterinary Publications, 1983, p 85.
103. Pedersen, NC, et al.: Pathogenic differences between various feline coronavirus isolates. Adv Exp Med Biol 173:365, 1984.
104. Pedersen, NC and Floyd, K: Experimental studies with three new strains of feline infectious peritonitis virus: FIPV-UCD2, FIPV-UCD3, and FIPV-UCD4. Comp Cont Ed Pract Vet 7:1001, 1985.
105. Pedersen, NC: Coronavirus diseases (coronavirus enteritis, feline infectious peritonitis). *In* Holzworth J (ed): Diseases of the Cat, Vol 1. Philadelphia, WB Saunders Co, 1987, p 193.
106. Pedersen, NC: Feline infectious peritonitis and feline enteric coronavirus infections. Part 1. Feline enteric coronaviruses. Fel Pract 13(4):13, 1983.
107. Stoddart, CA, et al.: Experimental studies of a coronavirus and coronavirus-like agent in a barrier-maintained feline breeding colony. Arch Virol 79:85, 1984.

108. Barlough, JE and Stoddart, CA: Feline infectious peritonitis. *In* Scott FW (ed): Contemporary Issues in Small Animal Practice, Vol 3. New York, Churchill Livingstone Inc, 1986, p 93.
109. Barlough, JE: Do feline coronavirus antibody tests provide a conclusive diagnosis? VMSAC 79:1027, 1984.
110. Hayashi, T, et al.: Enteritis due to feline infectious peritonitis virus. Jpn J Vet Sci 44:97, 1982.
111. Hayashi, T, et al.: Role of circulating antibodies in feline infectious peritonitis after oral infection. Jap J Vet Sci 45:487, 1983.
112. Weiss, RC and Scott, FW: Pathogenesis of feline infectious peritonitis. Nature and development of viremia. Am J Vet Res 42:382, 1981.
113. Horzinek, MC, et al.: Virion polypeptide specificity of immune complexes and antibodies in cats inoculated with feline infectious peritonitis virus. Am J Vet Res 47:754, 1986.
114. Jacobse-Geels, HEL, et al.: Antibody, immune complexes and complement activity fluctuations in kittens with experimentally induced feline infectious peritonitis. Am J Vet Res 43:666, 1982.
115. Hayashi, T, et al.: Systemic vascular lesions in feline infectious peritonitis. Jpn J Vet Sci 39:365, 1977.
116. August, JR: Feline infectious peritonitis: An immune-mediated coronaviral vasculitis. Vet Clin North Am 14:971, 1984.
117. Weiss, RC, et al.: Disseminated intravascular coagulation in experimentally induced feline infectious peritonitis. Am J Vet Res 41:663, 1980.
118. Sherding, RD: Feline infectious peritonitis. Comp Cont Ed Pract Vet 1:95, 1979.
119. Holmberg, CA and Gribble, DH: Feline infectious peritonitis: Diagnostic gross and microscopic lesions. Fel Pract 3(4):11, 1973.
120. Pedersen, NC: Feline infectious diseases. Proc Meet AAHA, 1981, p 83.
121. Kern, TJ: Intraocular inflammation in cats as a manifestation of systemic diseases. Cornell Feline Health Center News, Winter 1984, p 4.
122. Kornegay, JN: Feline infectious peritonitis. The central nervous system form. JAAHA 14:530, 1978.
123. Barlough, JE and Summers, BA: Encephalitis due to feline infectious peritonitis virus in a twelve-week-old kitten. Fel Pract 14(1):43, 1984.
124. Stoddart, M: Feline infectious peritonitis. *In* Grunsell CSG, Hill FWG, Raw R-E (eds): The Veterinary Annual, 26th Issue. Bristol, Scientechnica, 1986, p 324.

DRUGS USED IN TREATING FELINE VIRAL DISEASES

Generic	Trade	Dosage	Route	Frequency	Brief Description
1. Gentamicin	Gentocin	1.5 mg/lb	SQ, IM, IV	q8h	Aminoglycoside antimicrobial
2. Amoxicillin	Amoxidrops Amoxi-Inject	5 mg/lb	PO SQ, IM	q12h	Antimicrobial
3. Oxymetazoline hydrochloride	Afrin Pediatric Nose Drops 0.025%	1 drop in each nostril	Intranasally	q12h	Nasal decongestant
4. Idoxuridine	Stoxic 0.1% Solution	1 drop in affected eye	Topically	q1h during waking hours	For feline herpetic keratitis
5. Trifluridine	Viroptic 1% Solution	1 drop in affected eye	Topically	q2h during waking hours	For feline herpetic keratitis
6. Tetracycline	Panmycin	10 mg/lb 7 mg/kg	PO IM, IV	q8h q12h	Antimicrobial
7. Chloramphenicol	Chloromycetin	25 mg/lb	PO, IV IM, SQ	q12h	Antimicrobial
8. Erythromycin	Erythrocin	5 mg/lb	PO	q8h	Antimicrobial

49 DEEP MYCOTIC DISEASES

ALICE M. WOLF and GREGORY C. TROY

BLASTOMYCOSIS

ETIOLOGY

Blastomyces dermatitidis is a thermal dimorphic fungus and the etiologic agent of blastomycosis in dogs and cats. The first naturally occurring canine case was described by Meyer in 1912.[1–3] Cases of feline blastomycosis were reported in 1961 and 1966 with descriptions of cutaneous and pulmonary lesions.[4, 5] Synonyms that have been used for blastomycosis include: Gilchrist's disease, Chicago disease, and North American blastomycosis.[3, 6–10]

The yeast form of *B. dermatitidis* is found in tissues. Microscopically, yeast cells have thick, refractile walls and are 8 to 20 μm in diameter.[3, 10, 13, 14] Reproduction of the organism occurs by broad-based budding.[6, 10–12, 15] The buds have wide pores, are usually single, and are approximately one-half the width of the parent organism.[3, 10, 12] Cultures of the yeast phase are whitish-brown to yellowish-brown in color.[10, 12]

The mycelial phase exists in soil and when the organism is grown at room temperature. The organism also reproduces sexually and in a perfect stage in soil. This sexual stage has been named *Ajellomyces dermatitidis*.[16] Both forms of the organism can produce disease. Hyphae are finely branched and septate, possessing spherical-to-oval smooth conidia, 3 to 5 μm in diameter. The colonial growth is white, with woolly mycelia found on a white leathery membrane.[3, 10, 15]

EPIZOOTIOLOGY

Blastomyces dermatitidis is a soil saprophyte; however, attempts to isolate the organism from this medium have been inconsistent. Rapid lysis of *Blastomyces* by mycolytic organisms may be a reasonable explanation for this occurrence. The organism has been isolated from cedar trees and pigeon droppings.[3, 17] *Blastomyces* survives only for short periods in soils, unless the soil is refrigerated or sterilized.[3, 6, 16, 17] Animal to animal or animal to human transmission via soil contamination thus seems remote.

Geographically, the organism is endemic in certain regions of the United States. These areas include most of the eastern seaboard, southern Canada, the Great Lakes region, and the Mississippi, Ohio, and St. Lawrence river valleys (Figure 49–1).[18–20] These areas are similar to the enzootic regions for canine histoplasmosis. States that have the highest incidence of canine blastomycosis are Kentucky, Illinois, Tennessee, Mississippi, Indiana, Iowa, Ohio, Arkansas, and North Carolina.[2, 3, 18] Two reports have suggested a seasonal occurrence of canine blastomycosis from June through September.[21, 22]

PATHOGENESIS

Three clinical forms of blastomycosis have been identified: the primary pulmonary infection, disseminated disease, and local cutaneous infection. Routes of infection for blastomycosis include inhalation of windborne or soilborne spores and direct inoculation of spores into the skin.[10, 11, 14, 23, 24] The inhalation of infective spores from the environment results in a primary focus of infection within the lung.[14] Experimentally, the disease can be reproduced by intratracheal inoculation or exposure of dogs to sterilized soil infected with the organism.[25–28] Incubation periods varied from 5 to 12 weeks in these experimental studies.[26–28] Young animals were found to be more susceptible to experimental infections.[28]

Once spores are inhaled, they are deposited in the alveoli, where they are phagocytized by macrophages.

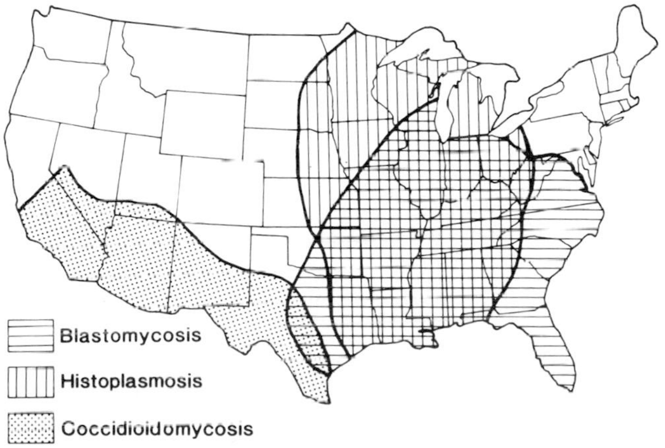

FIGURE 49–1. Major endemic areas for blastomycosis, coccidioidomycosis, and histoplasmosis in the United States.

Transformation from the mycelial phase to the yeast phase results, and multiplication of the organism occurs within the macrophage. Release of the yeast cells from macrophages results in an accumulation of organisms in the alveoli and a marked inflammatory reaction. Phagocytized organisms are moved into the interstitium of the lung to the lymphatics and vascular systems. If the host's immune system is able to respond appropriately, the disease may be limited to the pulmonary parenchyma and associated draining lymph nodes.[3, 10–12, 17] Dissemination to other organs may result in cutaneous, lymphatic, ocular, skeletal, urogenital, and central nervous system lesions.[1, 6, 8–10, 29–36] Hematogenous or lymphatic routes are the primary modes of dissemination. Direct inoculation of *Blastomyces* into the subcutaneous tissue has been reported in the dog and in humans.[23, 24, 37]

CLINICAL MANIFESTATIONS

The clinical signs of blastomycosis depend upon whether or not the disease remains localized to the pulmonary tissue or becomes disseminated. The disease is more prevalent in the dog, with limited reports in the cat. The localized pulmonary form in the dog may go unrecognized, with only patients with the disseminated form of the disease being presented for veterinary care.

In dogs, young males of the larger breeds are more commonly at risk of infection.[19, 22, 33, 38] Peak or mean ages of dogs were from 2.00 to 4.80 years of age.[19, 22, 33, 38, 39] Male animals represented 67 per cent to 72 per cent of animals in three studies.[19, 33, 39] Breed predispositions have not been identified; however, the beagle, Doberman pinscher and German shepherd breeds have been overrepresented.[20, 33] In the cat, the majority of cases have been reported in the Siamese breed.[4, 5, 8, 29, 40–43]

Dogs with localized pulmonary disease usually exhibit anorexia, depression, exercise intolerance, weight loss, fever, cough, and/or dyspnea.[7, 9, 20, 33, 38, 44] Spontaneous remission may occur or there may be mild clinical improvement until disseminated lesions appear. Systems affected with disseminated blastomycosis in dogs are the skin, lymphatic system, ocular, skeletal, male genital, and the central nervous systems.[2, 3, 6, 7, 9, 10, 31, 40, 45, 46] (Tables 49–1 and 49–2). Fever (greater than 103°F or 39.4°C) was noted in approximately 45 per cent of dogs in one study.[33]

TABLE 49–1. CLINICAL FINDINGS IN CANINE BLASTOMYCOSIS[20, 33, 38]

Clinical or Physical Finding	Percentage of Animals
Skin lesions (cellulitis, masses, or dermatitis)	43
Weight loss	42
Respiratory problems (dyspnea, cough)	39
Anorexia	30
Weakness	29
Ocular disease/blindness	26
Lameness	25
Depression	25
Fever	22
Ocular/nasal discharges	6
Lymphadenopathy	5
Testicular enlargement	1
Regurgitation	1
Seizures	0.5

Number of animals from which data is extracted is 192.

TABLE 49–2. DISTRIBUTION OF LESIONS IN DOGS WITH BLASTOMYCOSIS[20, 22, 33]

Location of Lesions	Percentage of Dogs
Lungs	65
Lymph nodes	36
Skin	32
Eyes	24
Bone or joints	15
Liver	8
Urogenital tract	6
Spleen	4
Kidney	4
Pleura	3
Brain	1
Nasal cavity	0.5

Number of dogs from which data extracted is 178.

Respiratory signs noted in affected dogs include cough, dyspnea, and ocular and nasal discharges. The cough is usually nonproductive and is the result of pulmonary interstitial disease, tracheal compression due to tracheobronchial lymphadenopathy, or pleural involvement. If tracheobronchial lymphadenopathy becomes severe, esophageal compression may result, causing regurgitation. Pleuritis and pleural effusions may be found on physical and radiographic examinations. Dyspnea results from both pulmonary parenchymal and pleural cavity involvement.

Cutaneous signs may be observed in approximately 40 per cent of dogs with naturally occurring disseminated disease and in 70 per cent of experimentally infected dogs.[28, 33] Multiple skin lesions are usually present; however, single lesions have been reported. The lesions are usually small, slightly raised, with central ulcers and fistulous tracts. Exudates from skin lesions may be serosanguineous to purulent and are often in various stages of healing. Generalized lymphadenopathy is commonly present.

Ocular disease is a frequent finding in dogs with disseminated blastomycosis, which is the most common form of oculomycosis in dogs.[38, 45] Uveitis, glaucoma, subretinal granuloma formation, or retinal detachment is frequently found on ophthalmologic examination.[45, 47–50] The disease may affect one or both eyes. Twenty to 46 per cent of dogs were reported to have ocular disease, with the choroid being most commonly involved.[20, 38, 47] Corneal edema, scleritis, iritis, ocular neuritis, exophthalmia, and conjunctivitis may be present. Blindness can result from optic neuritis, panophthalmitis, retinal detachment, chronic uveitis, and glaucoma.

Osseous involvement may occur in 7 to 24 per cent of dogs with disseminated blastomycosis.[7, 20, 33, 35] Lesions are usually single and involve the long bones of the appendicular skeleton.[7, 30, 35] The osteomyelitic lesions are characterized by periosteal reactions and osteolysis and most commonly affect the epiphyseal region.[35] Lesions from blastomycosis are suggestive of neoplastic diseases; however, they do not often arise in areas above the stifle or elbow joints.[7, 35]

Urogenital tract involvement with blastomycosis is

common in male animals. Clinical signs include hematuria, dysuria, nocturia, and tenesmus, which may result from urinary bladder or prostatic involvement. Organisms can be observed in urine and preputial exudates.[9, 46, 51, 52] Lesions can also be found in the testicles.

Involvement of the central nervous system with blastomycosis is uncommon. Direct extension from the nasal or sinus cavities, or hematogenous dissemination to the meninges, can produce lesions.

Most reports of blastomycosis in the cat have described disseminated lesions.[4, 5, 40–43, 53, 54] Respiratory, cutaneous, ocular, and central nervous system signs have been reported. Why the cat is not as commonly infected with blastomycosis as dogs and human beings is unknown.

DIAGNOSIS

Blastomycosis should be considered in animals located in certain geographic areas if the signalment and clinical signs or findings are compatible. A lack of appropriate response to antibiotic or glucocorticoid therapy should also alert the clinician to consider a diagnosis of systemic fungal disease.

Hematologic and Biochemical Findings. Hematologic and biochemical findings in blastomycosis are not specific or definitive. Nonregenerative anemia, considered due to chronic inflammatory disease, is frequently observed.[33, 55] The anemia is usually mild and is responsive to the treatment of the fungal disease. Leukocytosis with a left shift, monocytosis, and lymphopenia are usually present.[33] Forty per cent of dogs in one study were lymphopenic.[56] This may correlate with the depressed cell-mediated immunity that occurs in affected dogs. Total protein levels can be increased with blastomycosis. The distribution of the different serum proteins may involve decreased albumin levels and increased inflammatory proteins and immunoglobulins.

Blastomycosis should be considered in the differential diagnosis of hypercalcemia. Seven of 114 confirmed cases of blastomycosis have demonstrated hypercalcemia.[33, 57] Suggested pathogenetic mechanisms for this phenomenon include extensive granulomatous disease with increased extrarenal calcitriol production by the inflammatory reaction and/or the development of concomitant renal insufficiency.[33, 57] Calcium levels returned to normal in dogs treated appropriately by diuresis and specific antifungal therapy.

Cytologic and Histopathologic Findings. Cytologic evaluation of specimens obtained by aspiration or impression smears yields a definitive diagnosis in the majority of animals. In studies involving a total of 100 dogs, cytologic confirmation of blastomycosis was achieved in 84 animals.[33, 39, 55] Suitable specimens for cytologic examination include lymph node, tracheobronchial secretions, bone, fine-needle lung and ocular aspirates, and impression smears of cutaneous lesions, bronchoscopic brushings, urine specimens, bone biopsies, pleural fluids, and cerebrospinal fluid.[3, 10, 12, 17, 33, 44, 45, 58] Potassium hydroxide (KOH) (10 to 20 per cent), Wright's, Giemsa, new methylene blue (NMB), India ink, and phenol-cotton blue preparations have been used for identification (Figure 49–2). Skin lesion impres-

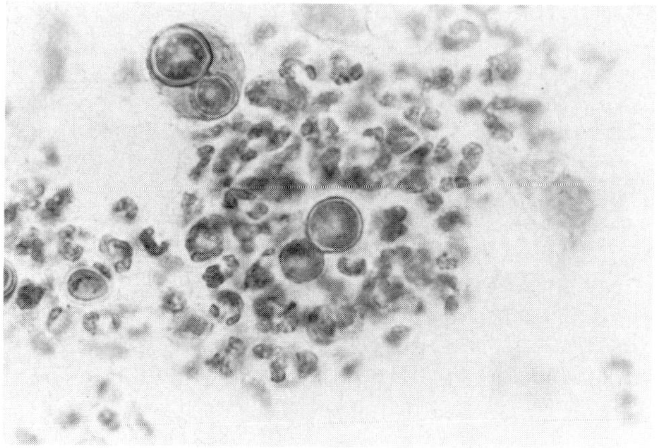

FIGURE 49–2. Impression smear from a dog with cutaneous draining tracts, revealing thick-walled, budding yeasts typical of *Blastomyces dermatitidis* (new methylene blue, 100 ×).

sion smears and lymph node aspiration should always be performed in any animal suspected of having blastomycosis, as these methods are highly diagnostic and relatively noninvasive.

Histopathologic examination of affected tissue reveals a mixed granulomatous to suppurative inflammatory reaction. Blastomycosis usually incites a more intense polymorphonuclear response than histoplasmosis.[10, 11, 59] Lesions may be found in lung, skin, bone, prostate, epididymis, urinary bladder, brain, meninges, and spinal cord (Table 49–2). Hematoxylin-eosin stain (HE) does not demonstrate the organism in tissue as efficiently as periodic acid–Schiff (PAS), Gridley methenamine silver (GMS), or Gomori stains (GS).[1, 3, 10, 11, 60, 61] Retraction of the protoplasm from the cell wall may cause difficulty in differentiating *Blastomycoses* from *Cryptococcus*. Mayer's mucicarmine stain can help differentiate *Blastomyces* from *Cryptococcus* by demonstrating the carmine-stained mucopolysaccharide capsule of cryptococcus. Special stains such as PAS, GMS, or GS cause the cell wall and contents of *Blastomyces* to stain, making identification of the cells more apparent in tissue specimens.

Radiographic Findings. Radiographic lesions in blastomycosis are observed most frequently in the lung and bone (Figure 49–3*A-C*). The most common pulmonary change observed in dogs with blastomycosis was a generalized, diffuse, miliary nodular interstitial pattern.[39] Mixed lung patterns or mixed interstitial-bronchovascular patterns were also observed frequently. Mediastinal and tracheobronchial lymphadenopathy were observed in 25 per cent of the cases. Mixed interstitial, alveolar, or peribronchial patterns can also be observed radiographically. Osseous lesions are usually confined to one bone and more commonly affect the epiphyseal region of long bones below the stifle and elbow. Multiple osseous lesions are infrequent.

Cultural Characteristics. Isolation of the organism is not performed often, due to the ease of identification of the organism in cytologic or histological specimens. Sabouraud's dextrose agar with antibiotics is used most frequently for isolation of the mycelial form of the organism. Cultures are usually apparent in one to four weeks. Yeast forms may be cultured on blood or brain-

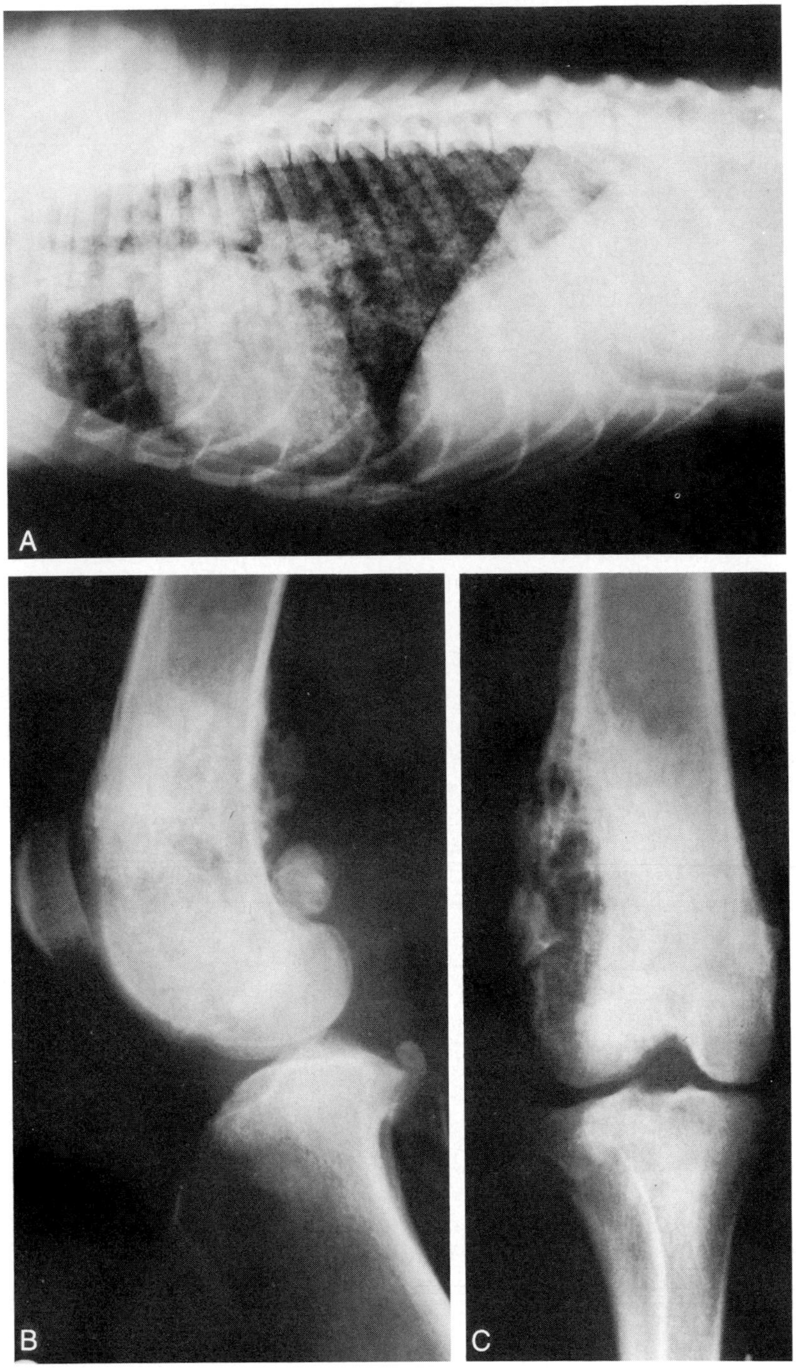

FIGURE 49–3. *A,* Lateral thoracic radiograph of a dog with blastomycosis, demonstrating a generalized, diffuse, miliary-nodular interstitial pattern and hilar lymphadenopathy. *B* and *C,* Lateral and caudocranial radiographs of the stifle in a dog with blastomycosis, illustrating an osteolytic, osteoblastic bone lesion in the distal femur. (Reprinted by permission, Roberts, RE: Vet Radiol 20:128, 1979.)

heart infusion media in approximately 10 to 14 days. Transformation of the organism from yeast to mycelial or from mycelial to the yeast phase is not as important as with other deep mycoses.

Serology. A variety of serologic methods are available to aid in the diagnosis of blastomycosis, including complement fixation (CF), agar gel immunodiffusion (AGID), counterimmunoelectrophoresis (CIEP), fluorescent antibody (FA), fluorescent immunoassay, antiglobulin hemagglutination (AGHA), and enzyme-linked immunosorbent (ELISA) tests.[1, 25, 26, 62–68] Presently, the AGID and CIEP tests possess similar sensitivities.[64, 65] The AGID test has an accuracy of greater than 90 per cent and is the serologic test used most frequently. The CIEP method possesses similar accuracy, but is less sensitive to the anticomplementary effects of canine serum.[12] The ELISA test using yeast antigens had a 100 per cent sensitivity and a 97 per cent specificity in a study of 37 dogs, when a cutoff point of 1:8 was used.[67]

TREATMENT AND PROGNOSIS

All animals infected with *Blastomyces* and demonstrating clinical signs warrant medical therapy. The notable exception is the rare case of primary cutaneous or isolated ocular blastomycosis that may be amenable to surgical excision.[33, 41, 69] Drugs that have been used in the treatment of blastomycosis are the iodides, hydroxystilbamidine, amphotericin B, and ketoconazole.[3, 8, 29, 30, 33, 45, 70–76] Currently, the drug of choice for blastomycosis is amphotericin B. Concurrent use of ketoconazole may help to manage animals with amphotericin B-induced nephrotoxicity or provide an outpatient treatment program.[72–74]

Amphotericin B is a polyene antifungal agent derived from a strain of *Streptomyces nodosus*.[77] This therapeutic agent is effective, in decreasing order of susceptibility, against *Blastomyces*, *Histoplasma*, *Cryptococcus*, *Candida*, *Sporothrix*, and *Coccidioides*.[77] Amphotericin B is commercially available as a colloidal suspension that is solubilized by the addition of sodium desoxycholate buffered with sodium phosphates.[76–79] Common routes of administration are intravenous and subconjunctival. Additional routes of administration include intrathecal, topical, intraocular, and intraperitoneal. Penetration across the blood-brain barrier, joint spaces, and ocular tissues is poor.

Following intravenous injection, amphotericin B is rapidly cleared from serum, with a plasma half-life of approximately 24 hours.[77, 78, 80] In vivo, the drug is strongly bound to lipoprotein sites on cell membranes and is metabolized at local tissue sites.[76] Concentrations of amphotericin B in tissues are highest, in decreasing order, in the kidney, liver, spleen, adrenal gland, lung, thyroid gland, somatic muscle, brain, and bone.[81] Approximately 2.5 per cent to 13 per cent of one intravenous dose is excreted in the urine within the first 24 hours. Forty per cent of an injected dose is excreted in the urine within seven days.[78] Amphotericin B can be found in blood and urine for up to four weeks after one intravenous injection.[82]

The mechanism of action of amphotericin B depends upon binding to ergosterol, the primary sterol in fungal cell membranes.[29, 30, 76–79] This binding induces a structural reorganization of the fungal cell membrane with a subsequent increase in permeability, resulting in a leakage of intracellular molecules and eventual cell death. The antifungal effects of amphotericin B are maximal within a pH range of 6 to 7.5.[77] In addition to the antifungal effects of amphotericin B, immunoadjuvant potentiation has also been observed in the humoral and cell-mediated immune systems.[30, 77]

The clinical use of amphotericin B is not without potential complications. Many toxic signs have been reported as a result of amphotericin B therapy. Anorexia, nausea, vomiting, chills, seizures, fever, thrombophlebitis, hypokalemia, anemia, cardiac arrest or arrhythmias, and renal impairment or dysfunction are a few of the more common side effects of amphotericin B.[74, 76–81]

Nephrotoxicity is the major reason for interruption or cessation of antifungal therapy with amphotericin B.[29, 30, 70, 74, 83] Toxicity may become evident as early as one hour after administration of a normal therapeutic dose. Amphotericin B results in an intense renal vasoconstriction with concomitant decreases in renal blood flow and glomerular filtration rates, which are responsible for increases in blood urea nitrogen and creatinine.[83] Amphotericin B may also cause distal renal tubular dysfunction. The drug binds to cholesterol in the distal tubular cells, causing a back diffusion of intraluminal hydrogen ions and loss of intracellular potassium. This induced renal tubular dysfunction accounts for the production of defects in urinary concentration ability, decreases in urine acidification, metabolic acidosis, and hypokalemia and hyperkaluria.[29, 30, 76, 84–86] Renal dysfunction may persist for long periods after cessation or termination of amphotericin B therapy.

Mannitol, sodium bicarbonate, saralasin, dopamine, furosemide, and salt loading have been used to decrease the frequency and severity of the nephrotoxicity.[87–92] Heparin, glucocorticoids, antiemetics, antihistamines, and phenobarbital may help decrease side effects other than the nephrotoxicity.

Mannitol did prevent the development of azotemia in studies in humans and dogs treated with amphotericin B.[87, 91, 92] Dogs treated concurrently with mannitol had increases of only 20 per cent and 25 per cent in serum creatinine and blood urea nitrogen, respectively, when compared with control dogs.[91] Excretion of amphotericin B in dogs treated with mannitol was 0.2 per cent greater in 24 hours. One study with mannitol showed that a greater dosage of amphotericin B could be given in an abbreviated period to dogs with some alleviation of nephrotoxicity.[74] Benefits from this more rapid administration of amphotericin B dosage were not noted. At present, the use of mannitol should be reserved for animals that demonstrate renal insufficiency during the course of antifungal therapy.

The use of sodium bicarbonate in conjunction with amphotericin B has been recommended, based on a study in mice.[85] A controlled study in dogs did not show any advantages from sodium bicarbonate administration. In fact, dogs treated with bicarbonate developed more severe nephrotoxicity.[93] This is also in agreement with an unpublished study by one of the authors.

Dopamine and saralasin, when used in combination, decreased the severity of amphotericin B nephrotoxicity. This combination is specific for decreasing the renal vasoconstriction associated with amphotericin B.[91] Controlled studies in clinical cases are lacking.

Salt loading and/or furosemide administration in dogs attenuated the reductions in renal blood flow and glomerular filtration rate produced by amphotericin B.[89, 90] This experimental study concluded that the renal nephrotoxicity associated with amphotericin B administration is consistent with the hypothesis that the acute response to this drug is mediated by the tubuloglomerular feedback system. The increase in delivery of chloride ions to the distal tubule in the region of the macula densa can lead to profound decreases in glomerular filtration rate. Salt repletion in humans revealed a decrease in nephrotoxicity associated with amphotericin administration.[90] Further consideration of these modalities for use in animals with systemic mycotic infections is needed.

Varying treatment regimens and dosages have been reported for amphotericin B. The manufacturer recommends that amphotericin B be reconstituted with sterile water, without preservatives or electrolytes that may result in precipitation of the antibiotic. Once amphotericin B is reconstituted, it should be refrigerated; a loss of potency is not evident for up to one week. Aliquots of amphotericin B have been frozen and later used for treatment. If the solution is cloudy after thawing, it should not be used. Intravenous administration of amphotericin B is preferred. Thrombophlebitis is commonly associated with its use or inadvertent extravasation.

Two intravenous methods of amphotericin B administration are used most frequently in animals.[3, 22, 29, 33, 74, 76, 77, 94] A slow drip method is recommended for use in debilitated animals. Amphotericin B is added to a quantity of five per cent dextrose solution (500 to 1000 ml) and is given over three to six hours. A rapid bolus technique, with the amphotericin B added to a small quantity (20 ml) of five per cent dextrose, is used in animals that are treated on an outpatient basis or do not require additional supportive care.

Doses of amphotericin B recommended for treatment of systemic fungal infections are numerous.[3, 8, 22, 29, 30, 33, 59, 74, 76, 77, 94] Daily doses range from 0.04 mg/lb (0.1 mg/kg) to 0.44 mg/lb (1.0 mg/kg). In the cat, doses should remain at the lower end of the suggested range, since this species appears more sensitive to the side effects of amphotericin B. Amphotericin B is administered three times weekly, unless toxicity results. Biweekly or once weekly doses have also been recommended.[22, 33, 74, 78]

Studies in dogs, using 0.22 mg/lb (0.5 mg/kg) on an initial dose, followed by 0.44 mg/lb (1.0 mg/kg) on consecutive doses, resulted in clinical cures in 65 per cent and 68 per cent of animals treated. Total accumulative dosages of amphotericin B for treatment of blastomycosis vary from 1.82 mg/lb (4 mg/kg) to 5 mg/lb (11.0 mg/kg) body weight.[3, 22, 29, 30, 33, 74, 76, 77]

Subconjunctival injection of 125 μg of amphotericin B has been recommended in the treatment of ocular disease.[70, 71] One study indicated that parenteral amphotericin B coupled with topical or systemic corticosteroids gave better clinical response with ocular blastomycosis than the subconjunctival route.[45] Clinical signs usually abate before the total accumulative dosage is achieved. In cases where amphotericin B nephrotoxicity occurs, ketoconazole may be an alternate choice.

Because of the nephrotoxicity that results from amphotericin B use, renal function should be assessed frequently. Blood urea nitrogen (BUN) and creatinine determination should be performed prior to each dose. If BUN concentrations are greater than 50 mg/dl, therapy should be discontinued until there is improvement in renal function. This usually occurs within one or two weeks. Urinalysis usually reveals tubular dysfunction, as indicated by isosthenuria and cast formation prior to azotemia.

Ketoconazole is a substituted imidazole that is becoming frequently used in the treatment of the systemic mycoses of dogs and cats.[3, 34, 72–75] The antifungal effects of ketoconazole include increased membrane permeability, inhibition of the uptake of RNA and DNA, changes in fatty acid and triglyceride synthesis, and disturbances in oxidative and peroxidative enzyme systems within the fungal cell.[3, 74, 95–99] Controlled studies are lacking in veterinary medicine. The use of ketoconazole at 4.4 mg/lb/day (10 mg/kg/day), orally, for 60 days in cases of canine blastomycosis resulted in a cure rate of 33 per cent, as compared to 65 per cent of animals treated with amphotericin B.[74] Combination therapy with amphotericin B and ketoconazole resulted in cure rates comparable to amphotericin B alone. Presently, a dose of 4.4 to 8.8 mg/lb (10 to 20 mg/kg) q8 or 12 hours is suggested for use in the dog. Dosages for the cat are 8.8 mg/lb (20 mg/kg) every other day or 50 mg once daily.[75] Higher doses of ketoconazole may be required when central nervous system involvement is present, as its concentration in cerebrospinal fluid is less than 0.1 per cent that of serum. High doses (800 mg q24h) in human beings provided better clinical responses than doses of 400 mg q24h. In animals treated with ketoconazole, clinical response is slower than with amphotericin B; however, side effects from ketoconazole are few. Anorexia, vomiting, fever, diarrhea, reversible elevation in liver enzymes, reversible alopecia and lightening of the hair coat, and teratogenesis have resulted from its use. Cessation of therapy for several days or a reduction in dose is usually required.[74, 75] Ketoconazole should be administered with food, as it is optimally absorbed in an acidic environment.

Prognostic factors have been identified in dogs with blastomycosis. Severity of lung lesions, absolute nonsegmented neutrophil numbers, and gender of the canine patient can realistically help in advising the clients about survival rates.[74] Most animals that die from blastomycosis do so in the first week of the treatment period.[33, 74] Death is usually attributable to respiratory failure or neurologic involvement. Animals with more severe lung lesions and higher absolute nonsegmented neutrophil numbers have the worst prognosis. Female animals have higher survival rates but are more likely to suffer relapses.[74] If animals survive the first week of treatment, cure rates approach 65 per cent. One study in dogs treated with amphotericin B showed an 88 per cent survival rate over a period of six years.[22] Relapses commonly occur within the first six months after the initiation of therapy. In certain instances, localization of the infection occurs that is not responsive to conventional periods of treatment. These cases may require intermittent or long-term management with medications.

PUBLIC HEALTH CONSIDERATIONS

Blastomycosis is not likely to be transmitted from animal to animal or animal to humans. Human beings have contracted blastomycosis following dog bites.[23, 24, 37] This is related to mechanical transfer of the agent to broken or abraded skin. Cases of canine blastomycosis do provide an environmental sentinel. Care should be exercised when contact is made with infected animals, especially in the presence of open draining wounds.

COCCIDIOIDOMYCOSIS

ETIOLOGY AND EPIZOOTIOLOGY

Coccidioides immitis is a geophilic, dimorphic fungus.[100, 101] The free-living mycelial phase in the soil produces arthroconidia, which are the source of infection for mammals.[101, 102] Animals are infected following inhalation of the small arthroconidia (2 by 5 μm),[101–104] although direct inoculation through the skin has resulted in infection in some cases.[101–103, 105] Once inside the mammalian host, the arthroconidia are transformed at 37°C to the spherular phase.[101, 103] These large spherules (20 to 100 μm)[101, 103] grow, mature, and divide internally to produce endospores.[100–103, 105] When released, the endospores spread the infection locally or to distant sites via the lymphatics or blood.[100, 101, 103, 104, 106]

The environmental distribution of *C. immitis* is restricted to the lower Sonoran life zone.[100–104, 107] This area is defined by semi-arid conditions, sandy alkaline soil, moderate winter temperatures, and low geographic elevation.[101, 103, 104, 107] Active mycelial growth occurs following winter rains.[100, 102] Mammalian infection is most likely to occur in the summer months when hot, dry conditions favor inhalation of arthroconidia spread by wind or by physical disturbance of infected soil.[102, 107, 108] In the United States, the endemic area for *C. immitis* includes parts of California, Nevada, Utah, Arizona, New Mexico, and Texas (Figure 49–1).[100–103] *Coccidioides immitis* is also widespread in parts of Mexico and in Central and South America.[100–102] Obtaining a detailed travel history is essential because the clinical signs of coccidioidomycosis may not appear for weeks to years following infection.[102, 104, 109, 110]

Because many *C. immitis* infections in animals are probably subclinical,[107, 110] it is difficult to determine the true incidence of infection. Cats rarely develop clinical coccidioidomycosis;[105, 107, 111, 112] dogs may develop severe disease.[103, 105, 107] The mean age of incidence for coccidioidomycosis in dogs has been reported as 1.5 years[103] and 4.0 years;[21] males are more likely to be affected than females.[21, 104, 110] One study suggests that sporting dogs (hounds) have a slightly increased risk of developing coccidioidomycosis,[21] another report indicates that the Boxer and Doberman pinscher breeds are more likely to develop severe disseminated disease.[103]

PATHOGENESIS

The sequence of fungal replication and spread is similar to that previously described for blastomycosis. Following inhalation of arthroconidia, the infection may be limited to a focal area of the lung (primary pulmonary coccidioidomycosis).[104, 107] The immune system may terminate the infection at this point, with clinical signs mild or absent.[104, 107, 113] If the dose of infecting arthroconidia is large or the immune system is impaired, the infection may spread locally throughout the pulmonary tree and/or to distant organs (disseminated coccidioidomycosis).[101, 107, 113] Direct cutaneous inoculation of arthroconidia (primary cutaneous coccidioidomycosis) is rare and the infection usually remains localized near the site of inoculation.[105, 106]

CLINICAL MANIFESTATIONS

Acute, primary pulmonary coccidioidomycosis usually occurs within one to three weeks following infection.[101, 107] Early clinical signs may be absent or include a mild, nonproductive cough, low-grade fever, partial anorexia, and weight loss.[104, 107] This form of disease is often self-limiting but may progress to more disseminated infection.[114] Primary cutaneous coccidioidomycosis usually results in a regional lymphadenitis and lymphangitis.[105, 106] Dissemination is possible but has not been definitively associated with primary cutaneous disease in animals.

Disseminated pulmonary coccidioidomycosis causes a more severe, productive cough due to widespread lung involvement and tracheobronchial lymphadenopathy.[104, 107, 110] Systemic signs include a fluctuating fever that is unresponsive to antibiotic treatment, depression, weakness, anorexia, and weight loss.[107, 110, 115, 116]

Coccidioides immitis may spread beyond the pulmonary tree to affect any organ or system in the body.[107] Dissemination may occur early in the course of infection.[117] Significant respiratory tract signs may not be observed prior to the development of other systemic involvement.[109, 110, 116]

Bone is a common site for *C. immitis* dissemination.[104, 107, 109, 110, 115] Most lesions occur in the metaphyseal regions of long bones; the vertebrae and flat bones are less frequently affected.[104, 110, 115, 116] Most dogs have multiple bone involvement, but the joints are usually spared.[104, 110, 115, 116] Coccidioidal osteomyelitis causes lameness, soft tissue swelling, and pain over affected bones.[104, 110, 116] Variable findings include fever, regional lymphadenopathy, and superficial draining tracts.[104, 110, 115] Vertebral involvement associated with nerve root entrapment or myelopathy may cause paresis or paralysis.[110]

Dissemination to other sites is less common. Infection of the heart and pericardium results in granulomatous myocarditis[118] and effusive or constrictive pericarditis.[103, 104] Clinical signs may include congestive heart failure (usually right-sided), cardiac arrhythmias, and ascites.[103, 107] Lesions associated with ocular involvement include granulomatous retinitis, uveitis, and keratitis.[111] Skin lesions include superficial nodules and chronic draining tracts.[110] All cutaneous lesions should be considered to be the result of systemic dissemination until proven otherwise. Infection of the reproductive tract has produced prostatitis, epididymitis, and orchitis.[110, 118] Central nervous system infection is associated with encephalitis and meningitis and may result in ataxia, seizures, or coma.[107] Signs of infection in the gastrointestinal system or liver include vomition, diarrhea, and icterus.[110] Kidney involvement may cause renal insufficiency and uremia.[110]

DIAGNOSIS

Hematologic parameters may be normal or reveal nonspecific changes that depend on the chronicity and severity of the disease.[107, 110] Mild, nonregenerative anemia,[107, 110, 119] mild to moderate neutrophilic leukocytosis with or without a left shift,[107, 109, 110, 115, 119] and an increased erythrocyte sedimentation rate are the most common findings.[107] Hypoalbuminemia and hyperglobulinemia are the most consistent biochemical changes and are usually associated with chronic disease.[107, 110, 115, 119] Other abnormal biochemical findings may reflect internal organ/system involvement.

Thoracic radiographs reveal a wide spectrum of pulmonary parenchymal changes.[104] Coccidioidomycosis usually causes lesions with an interstitial or mixed interstitial/bronchovascular distribution; alveolar involvement is unusual.[104, 110] The pulmonary changes may be localized or generalized and have an amorphous, linear, or miliary-nodular pattern (Figure 49–4). Hilar lymphadenopathy is a prominent feature of all forms of pulmonary coccidioidomycosis (Figure 49–5); involvement of the sternal and mediastinal lymph nodes is suggestive of disseminated pulmonary disease and must be differentiated from lymphoma.[104] There is no pathognomonic radiographic pattern for coccidioidal osteomyelitis. Bone lesions are usually more productive than destructive and frequently show evidence of both types of osseous change[104, 110, 115] (Figures 49–5 and 49–6). The endosteal, cortical, and periosteal portions of bone may be affected. Major differential diagnoses include other forms of osteomyelitis and osseous neoplasia.[104] Other radiographic findings may reflect associated organ and/or system involvement.

Direct observation of the *C. immitis* organism is the most definitive method of diagnosis.[107, 120] Unfortunately, recovery of spherules may be difficult because there are usually few organisms present in affected tissues.[107] Exfoliative cytology is useful to evaluate tracheal and bronchial wash specimens, lung, lymph node, or tissue aspirates.[59, 107, 120, 121] Spherules appear as refractile, double-walled bodies on direct wet mounts prepared with normal saline or ten per cent potassium hydroxide[107, 110, 120, 121] (Figure 49–7). With routine hematologic stains, the spherules stain blue with a surrounding unstained capsule. Biopsy procedures do not appear to encourage dissemination of coccidioidomycosis. Lung biopsy is rarely needed to establish a diagnosis of coccidioidomycosis; other organs or tissues may be sampled as indicated by clinical or laboratory findings. Bone specimens should be taken from several sites because it is particularly difficult to find organisms in this tissue.[110] Special fungal stains such as Gomori's methenamine silver (GMS) and periodic acid–Schiff (PAS) may improve diagnostic accuracy in examining aspirates or biopsy specimens containing few fungal organisms[101, 120] (Figure 49–8).

Serologic testing is a useful adjunct in diagnosis and an aid in monitoring the response to therapy. The tube precipitin (TP) test detects IgM antibody that develops early in the course of infection.[100, 101, 106, 110] IgM antibodies directed against *C. immitis* are usually present within two to four weeks following infection but levels often decrease rapidly even if the disease becomes chronic.[106, 110, 111] The TP test may be negative if infection is not present or if it is early in the course of infection, prior to IgM antibody production.[68, 107] Fulminating and rapidly progressive acute infections and chronic infections may also test TP-negative.[68] The TP test may be negative in cases of primary cutaneous disease.[105, 106]

Complement-fixing (CF) antibodies of the IgG class develop slowly following infection.[68, 100, 101, 106, 110] The CF titer generally increases with the severity and chronicity of the disease, therefore this test is useful in assessing the patient for possible dissemination and for monitoring response to treatment.[68, 100, 101, 106, 122] Agar gel immunodiffusion (AGID) is usually used as a qualitative screening test for CF antibodies.[68] If the AGID test is positive, a quantitative CF test is performed. Dog serum may have nonspecific anticomplementary antibodies that can interfere with accurate quantitative CF test results.[59, 68, 110] Low CF titers (less than 1:16) may be found early in the course of infection, with chronic localized disease, or may persist for months after resolution of the active infection.[68, 106, 107, 110] Titers of CF antibodies greater than 1:16 to 1:32 are suggestive of active, disseminated disease.[68, 106, 110, 123] Animals with primary cutaneous coccidioidomycosis should not develop CF antibodies or will have a very low CF titer.[105, 106] Skin testing is an unreliable method for the clinical diagnosis of coccidioidomycosis in the dog and cat.[107, 109, 110]

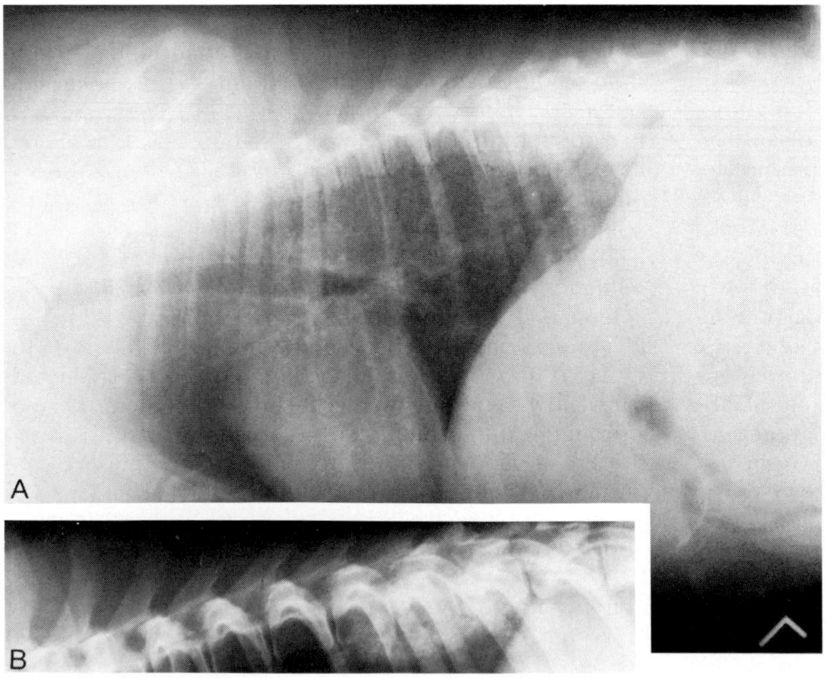

FIGURE 49–4. *A* and *B*, Thoracic radiograph of a four-year-old Walker hound with coccidioidomycosis, demonstrating miliary-nodular pulmonary infiltrate, and osteomyelitis of vertebral bodies T9 to T13.

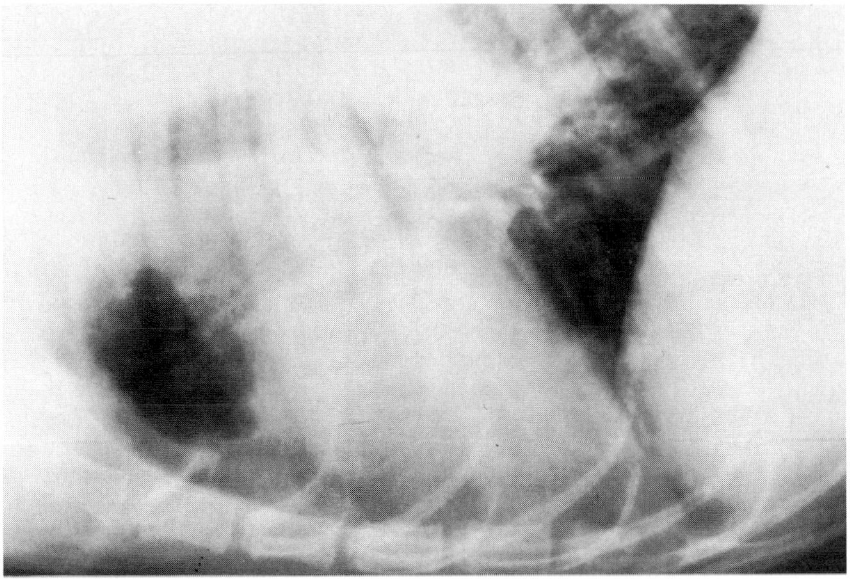

FIGURE 49–5. Lateral thoracic radiograph of a two-year-old English pointer with severe hilar lymphadenopathy associated with pulmonary coccidioidomycosis.

Coccidioides immitis returns to the mycelial phase and grows well on blood agar or routine fungal culture media incubated at room temperature.[121, 124, 125] Fungal colonies usually appear in three to four days and aerial hyphae are evident within ten days.[121, 125] Hyphae are typically cottony and white; however, other colors and colony types have been described.[121, 124, 125] *Coccidioides* colonies growing on dermatophyte test medium produce a red color change in the medium in seven days and may be confused with more common dermatophytes.[126] Because mycelial cultures are producing infectious arthroconidia, they should be sealed and handled carefully.[101, 106, 121, 124, 125] Due to the risk of human exposure, attempts to culture this organism in a routine practice setting are not recommended.

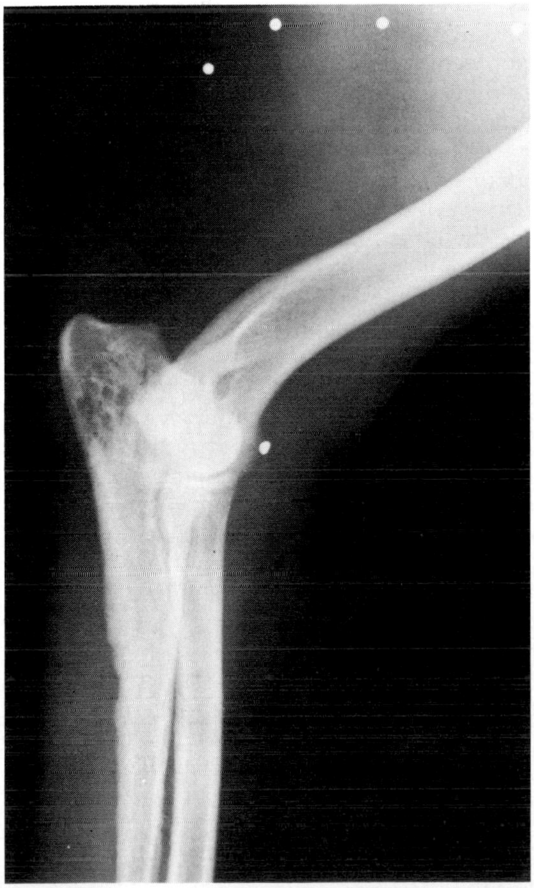

FIGURE 49–6. Lateral radiograph of the elbow of an eight-year-old English pointer with osseous coccidioidomycosis. Lytic areas are present in the proximal ulna; productive periosteal and endosteal change is seen in the ulna metaphysis. Metallic densities present in the soft tissue are lead-shot that was acquired while hunting.

TREATMENT

Because of the danger of dissemination, systemic antifungal chemotherapy is recommended for all forms of coccidioidomycosis except primary cutaneous disease.[107] Ketoconazole and amphotericin B are the two agents currently recommended for the treatment of coccidioidomycosis in the dog and cat.[107] The therapeutic mechanisms and indications for the use of these drugs have been discussed in the previous section. Two second generation imidazole compounds, itraconazole and fluconazole, are currently under investigation. Preliminary clinical studies with itraconazole suggest that this agent may be useful in the treatment of canine coccidioidomycosis in the future.[127] Fluconazole was more efficacious than ketoconazole but less effective than amphotericin B in prolonging survival in an experimental model of coccidioidal meningitis in mice.[128]

Ketoconazole has been recommended by some as the drug of choice for the treatment of coccidioidomycosis.[107, 129] This drug is fungistatic at therapeutic dose levels and the onset of action is slow.[75] Ketoconazole is administered orally at a dose of 4.4 mg/lb (10 mg/kg) q12h.[75, 107] Treatment should continue for at least two months following the resolution of clinical signs in localized pulmonary disease and for 8 to 12 months in animals with disseminated disease.[75, 107]

Patients with severe or disseminated coccidioidomycosis may respond slowly to treatment with ketoconazole alone and relapses often occur when the drug is discon-

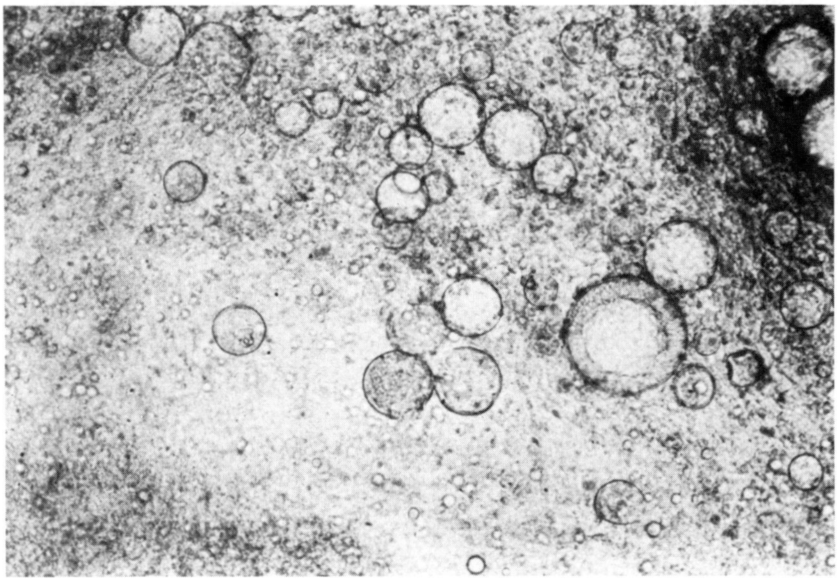

FIGURE 49–7. Potassium hydroxide wet mount of *Coccidioides immitis* spherules present in exudate from a draining cutaneous lesion, demonstrating the distinctive double-walled appearance of the large, variably sized spherules (40 ×).

tinued.[122, 129–131] Amphotericin B may be used concurrently with ketoconazole in these patients.[114, 123] The recommended dose and regimen for amphotericin B are the same as discussed for blastomycosis. Ketoconazole administration is continued for as long as necessary after the course of amphotericin B is completed. Serial radiographic studies and physical examinations should be used to monitor the response to treatment and determine when therapy may be safely terminated.[107] Hematologic, biochemical, and serologic studies may also be helpful in detecting amphotericin B nephrotoxicity and following resolution of abnormalities previously observed.

Patients that relapse following termination of treatment should receive an additional course of therapy until the disease is again in remission.[107] Remission can then be maintained with ketoconazole at a reduced oral dose of 0.9 to 2.2 mg/lb (2 to 5 mg/kg) q24h.[107] This regimen should suppress active fungal replication and spread, yet be of sufficiently low toxicity and cost to be safe and practical. The low dose protocol should not be used for initial management of active disease.

PROGNOSIS

Except for rare cases of primary cutaneous disease, dogs with confirmed coccidioidomycosis should be treated. Primary pulmonary coccidioidomycosis usually responds well to antifungal chemotherapy.[107, 132] Disseminated canine coccidioidomycosis carries a guarded prognosis. Many patients respond well initially but some relapse when treatment is discontinued.[110, 118, 122, 127] It may be possible to maintain these dogs with long-term, low-dose ketoconazole. Of seven reported cases of coccidioidomycosis in cats, one cat with primary cutaneous disease recovered without treatment and another was

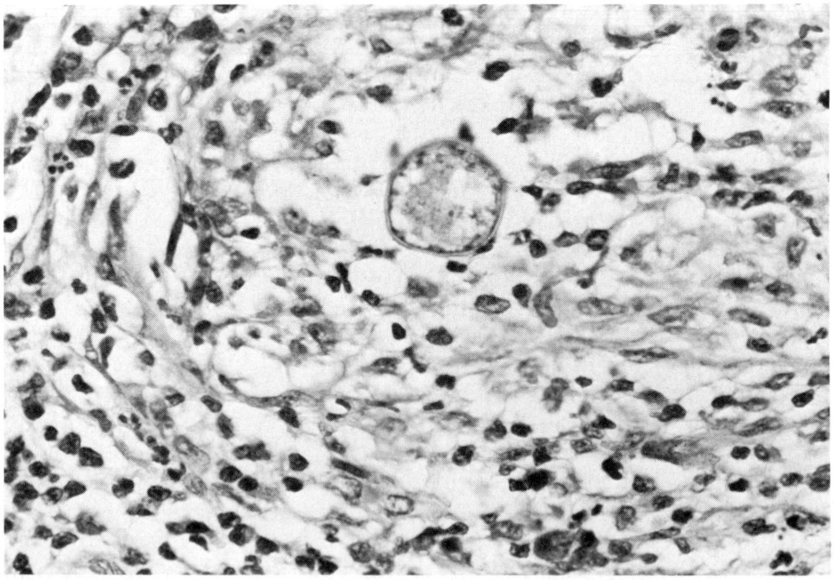

FIGURE 49–8. Coccidioidal granuloma within a prostatic biopsy from a seven-year-old cocker spaniel (H&E, 40 ×).

apparently cured following enucleation of an affected eye.[105, 111] Only two cats were treated and both of these apparently responded well to ketoconazole.[107] It is not known whether dogs and cats develop solid, protective immunity following recovery from coccidioidomycosis or whether they are susceptible to reinfection if they remain in endemic areas.[103, 122]

PUBLIC HEALTH SIGNIFICANCE

There is no known risk of direct transmission of *C. immitis* from companion animals to humans.[101, 104] Caution should be used in handling animals with draining cutaneous wounds. Dressings should be changed frequently because fungal spherules present in the exudate may revert to the mycelial phase and produce infectious arthroconidia on the surface of the bandages.[101, 123] Contact with mycelial growth in fungal cultures should be avoided.[101, 106, 121, 124]

HISTOPLASMOSIS

ETIOLOGY AND EPIZOOTIOLOGY

American histoplasmosis is a systemic mycotic infection caused by the soil-borne, dimorphic fungus *Histoplasma capsulatum*.[133–136] The mycelial stage in soil produces microaleuriospores (2 to 5 μm) and macroaleuriospores (5 to 18 μm), which are the source of infection for mammals.[133, 135–138]

Histoplasma capsulatum has a wide distribution throughout temperate and tropical regions of the world.[133, 136, 138] Thirty-one of the 48 continental United States have been shown to be endemic areas for this agent.[136] The majority of cases occur in the region comprising the drainage and tributary system of the Ohio, Missouri, and Mississippi rivers[133, 136, 138–140] (Figure 49–1). This organism prefers moist, humid soil conditions with nitrogen enrichment from decaying organic matter[133, 134, 136, 141] and can survive over a wide range of environmental temperatures (−18°C to 37°C).[134, 136] The association of *H. capsulatum* with bird and bat guano results, in part, from the nitrogen-rich nature of these excrements.[133, 136, 140]

As with other systemic mycoses, it is difficult to determine the true infection rate for *H. capsulatum* in companion animals because most infections are subclinical.[134, 140, 142–144] At one time, cats were considered less likely than dogs to develop clinical disease following infection by *H. capsulatum*.[143] Recent reports suggest that clinical histoplasmosis is at least as common in cats as in dogs.[137, 141, 145, 146]

PATHOGENESIS

It is generally believed that histoplasmosis is acquired by inhalation of the more abundant microaleuriospores, which are small enough to reach the lower respiratory tree.[136, 138, 147] In the lung, *H. capsulatum* aleuriospores convert to the yeast phase (2 to 4 μm), which then reproduces by budding.[133–135, 140, 148] The yeast cells are engulfed by macrophages and undergo intracellular replication.[135, 148] Involvement of the regional lymph nodes and systemic hematogenous dissemination occur early in the course of the infection.[141, 147–149] As with other systemic mycoses, activation of the cellular immune system rapidly brings the infection under control in most patients.[133, 148] If the immune system is overwhelmed or compromised, severe clinical disease may develop.[133, 147, 148]

The occurrence of gastrointestinal histoplasmosis in the absence of detectable pulmonary involvement[147, 150, 151] has led to speculation that the gastrointestinal tract might also be a primary portal of entry for *H. capsulatum*. Larger macroaleuriospores that are filtered out in the upper respiratory tract and swallowed could be the source for enteric infection;[150] however, experimental studies have failed to reliably produce clinical disease via this route.[134, 152]

CLINICAL MANIFESTATIONS

Histoplasma capsulatum disseminates rapidly and widely early in the course of the infection.[133] Cats tend to show more evidence of pulmonary involvement,[137, 139, 145, 146, 153, 154] while dogs frequently develop severe gastrointestinal signs.[140, 147] Nevertheless, it is important to remember that most animals have widely disseminated disease in spite of apparent localizing signs.

Feline Histoplasmosis. Feline histoplasmosis occurs most commonly in cats less than four years of age;[137, 145, 155] the age range of reported cases is from 0.3 to 13.5 years.[137] The domestic shorthair or longhair cat of mixed breeding is most frequently affected[137, 145, 146] but this may reflect population prevalence and the likelihood that purebred cats are not allowed access to the environment, rather than a true breed predisposition. There is no sex predilection.[145]

Histoplasmosis in the cat is usually an insidious disease characterized by nonspecific signs, including depression, weight loss, fever, anorexia, and pale mucous membranes.[139, 141–143, 145, 146, 150, 153, 156, 157] Dyspnea and abnormal lung sounds are found in about one half of the reported cases, but coughing is uncommon.[137, 139, 146, 153, 154, 156, 158, 159] Other frequent clinical findings include hepatomegaly and visceral or peripheral lymphadenopathy.[137, 142, 143, 150, 154, 160] Ocular lesions are uncommon but can include conjunctivitis, anterior uveitis, granulomatous chorioretinitis, retinal detachment, and optic neuritis.[142, 143, 146, 153, 156, 157] Several cats have had lameness due to osseous involvement.[143, 160, 161] Nodular or ulcerated skin lesions have been seen in a few cats.[137, 143, 156] Splenomegaly, oral ulcers, nasal polyps, vomiting, and diarrhea have been reported, but are rare findings.[143, 146, 150]

Histopathologic examination demonstrates granulomatous inflammation with *Histoplasma* organisms in many organs and systems. The lung, bone marrow, liver, spleen, and lymph nodes are most frequently affected.[137, 139, 141, 143, 145, 153, 156, 157, 159] Lesions have also been observed in the eyes, kidney, intestine, adrenal gland, thyroid gland, skin, bone, and brain of some cats.[137, 143, 150, 153, 156, 157, 160, 161]

Canine Histoplasmosis. Canine histoplasmosis is also a disease of young animals, with most cases occurring in dogs less than four years old;[149, 162] the age range of reported cases is from 0.2 to 14 years.[140, 163] Clinical disease occurs in both sexes with equal frequency.[149] Pointers, Weimaraners, and Brittany spaniels are reported to have an increased risk of infection;[21] however, the latter two breeds are notably absent from two large studies.[149, 162]

Clinical signs referable to gastrointestinal dysfunction are the most common manifestation of histoplasmosis in the dog.[134, 140, 151, 162, 164–168] Weight loss and diarrhea are the most frequent findings.[140, 147, 151, 162, 164–167, 169] Diarrhea is often "large bowel" in character, with mucus, tenesmus, and fresh blood.[140, 151, 167, 170] More extensive intestinal infiltration produces a profuse, watery stool with an accompanying protein-losing enteropathy.[140, 147, 151, 162, 165, 169] Pulmonary involvement is a fairly common finding and may cause dyspnea, coughing, and abnormal lung sounds.[137, 140, 156, 162, 169] Pale mucous membranes and a low grade fever are present in many cases.[140, 164, 169] Hepatomegaly, splenomegaly, icterus, and ascites have been reported;[140, 147, 151, 156, 166, 167, 169] vomiting is a relatively uncommon finding.[140, 164, 168] Unusual signs include peripheral lymphadenopathy, ocular lesions, skin lesions, lameness, and neurologic dysfunction.[140, 156, 162–164, 168, 170, 171] The clinical signs caused by these lesions are similar to those described for the cat.

In dogs with gastrointestinal signs, histopathologic examination reveals moderate to severe granulomatous enteritis with *Histoplasma* organisms.[141, 151, 164, 170] The mesenteric lymph nodes, liver, and spleen are often concurrently affected.[140, 147, 151, 163, 164, 170] Lesions in other organs and tissues are similar to those described for the cat.

DIAGNOSIS

Normocytic, normochromic, nonregenerative anemia is the most common hematologic abnormality associated with histoplasmosis in both dogs and cats.[55, 142, 147, 150–152, 160–163, 166, 167, 169, 170, 172] Anemia may be caused by a combination of *Histoplasma* infection of the bone marrow and chronic inflammation.[55, 141, 145, 147, 166] Leukocyte counts are variable; leukocytosis with neutrophilia, monocytosis, and eosinopenia is found most frequently.[55, 140, 145, 147, 151, 166, 169] Leukopenia and thrombocytopenia have also been reported.[141, 142, 147, 152, 160, 163, 166] *Histoplasma* organisms may occasionally be seen in monocytes or neutrophils during a routine blood film examination.[140, 141, 146, 147, 162, 163] Examination of buffy coat smears increases the chance of finding infected cells in peripheral blood.[140, 141] Most cats tested have been negative for feline leukemia virus infection.[139, 141, 142, 145, 146, 150, 154, 157]

Biochemistry profiles in most cats, and in dogs with pulmonary histoplasmosis, are often normal.[141, 145, 158] A few cats have had hyperproteinemia, hyperglobulinemia, or hypoalbuminemia.[145, 154, 157] Dogs with gastrointestinal involvement may have hypoproteinemia and profound hypoalbuminemia associated with a protein-losing enteropathy.[147, 151, 162, 166, 167] Liver dysfunction may cause hypoalbuminemia, increased serum alkaline phosphatase levels, hyperbilirubinemia, and abnormal liver function test results.[55, 147, 151, 162, 163, 166, 169, 170]

The most common radiographic finding in active pulmonary histoplasmosis is a diffuse or linear pulmonary interstitial pattern.[149, 154, 155, 158, 162, 173] Alveolar involvement has been seen in a few cases but is rare.[149, 155, 162, 173] The pulmonary infiltrates are often coalescing or nodular in appearance (Figure 49–9).[137, 149, 154, 155, 158, 159] Hilar lymphadenopathy is a prominent finding in some dogs[141, 147, 149, 169, 173] but is not common in cats.[149, 155] Calcified pulmonary nodules, indicative of inactive pulmonary histoplasmosis, have been found in dogs but not cats.[141, 149, 172, 173]

In gastrointestinal histoplasmosis, the emaciated condition of many animals and the presence of abdominal fluid may make interpretation of abdominal radiographs difficult.[147, 167, 169] Plain film abdominal examinations may demonstrate hepatomegaly, splenomegaly, and ascites.[162, 169, 173] Barium contrast studies may reveal thickened intestinal walls or irregularities of the mucosal surface.[140] Osseous lesions are rare; radiographic findings include osteolysis, periosteal new bone formation, and subperiosteal bone proliferation[143, 161, 163, 164, 171–173] (Figure 49–10).

Histoplasma organisms are usually numerous in affected tissues and a definitive diagnosis can usually be

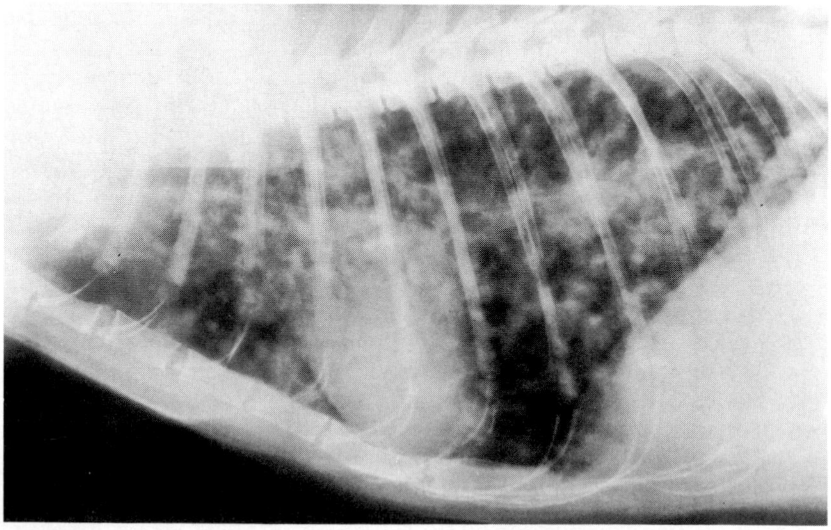

FIGURE 49–9. Lateral thoracic radiograph of an eight-year-old Siamese cat with a two-week history of dyspnea caused by *Histoplasma capsulatum* infection. This coalescing pattern of interstitial infiltrates is commonly seen in cats with pulmonary histoplasmosis.

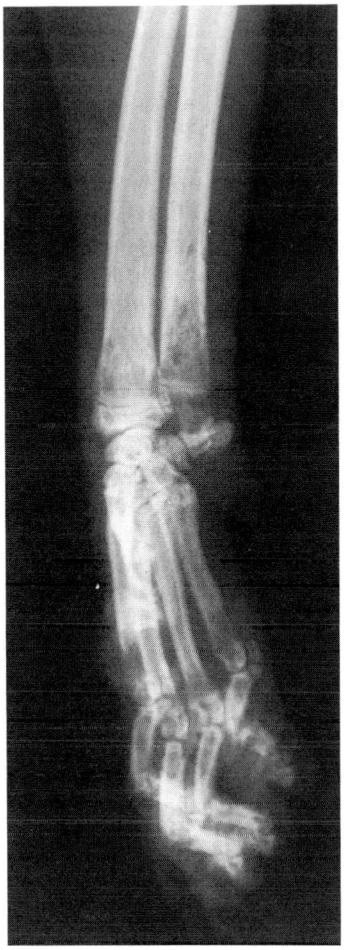

FIGURE 49–10. Lateral radiograph of the distal forelimb of a two-year-old domestic shorthair cat with osseous histoplasmosis. Lytic areas caused by fungal involvement are most prominent in the distal radial and ulnar metaphyses and the distal metacarpal bones.

made by cytologic or histopathologic examination.[55, 137, 140, 142, 146, 151, 166] With routine hematologic stains, *Histoplasma* appear as small (2 to 4 μm) round bodies with a basophilic center and surrounding light halo due to shrinkage of the yeast during staining.[135] Many of the organisms are contained within cells of the macrophage-monocyte system; one or many organisms may be present within each phagocytic cell.[135, 142, 154] In the cat, *Histoplasma* organisms are most likely to be found in bone marrow, lung, and lymph node aspirates.[55, 141, 142, 145, 146, 154] Rectal scrapings, imprints of colon biopsies, aspirates of liver, lung, spleen and bone marrow are most productive in the dog (Figure 49–11).[140, 147, 151, 162, 166, 167, 169, 170, 172] Aspirates or imprints of other tissues or body fluids may be examined as directed by the clinical signs in each case.[55, 146, 154, 166]

Biopsy specimens may be needed if cytologic examinations are not diagnostic. Histopathologic examination reveals granulomatous inflammation in affected organs and tissues. *Histoplasma* organisms are difficult to see with routine hematoxylin and eosin stain; fungal stains (PAS, GMS) provide better definition of the yeast cells.[135]

The results of intradermal skin tests[134, 140] and serologic evaluations for precipitin and complement-fixing antibodies are often falsely negative in dogs and cats with naturally occurring histoplasmosis.[139, 145, 146, 164, 168] *Histoplasma capsulatum* may be cultured from tissues, aspirates, and body fluids.[140, 154, 163] The yeast phase grows best on blood agar incubated at 30° C;[135, 138] the mycelial phase develops on routine fungal culture media incubated at room temperature.[135] Because microconidia produced by mycelial growth are infectious to human beings, attempts to culture this organism in a routine practice setting are not recommended.

TREATMENT

Pulmonary histoplasmosis in the dog can be self-limiting and may resolve without treatment.[133, 134, 140, 169] However, because of the risk of dissemination, antifungal therapy is recommended. Early or mild cases may respond to ketoconazole alone.[174, 175] Combination therapy with amphotericin B and ketoconazole is preferred in patients with severe or fulminating disease because

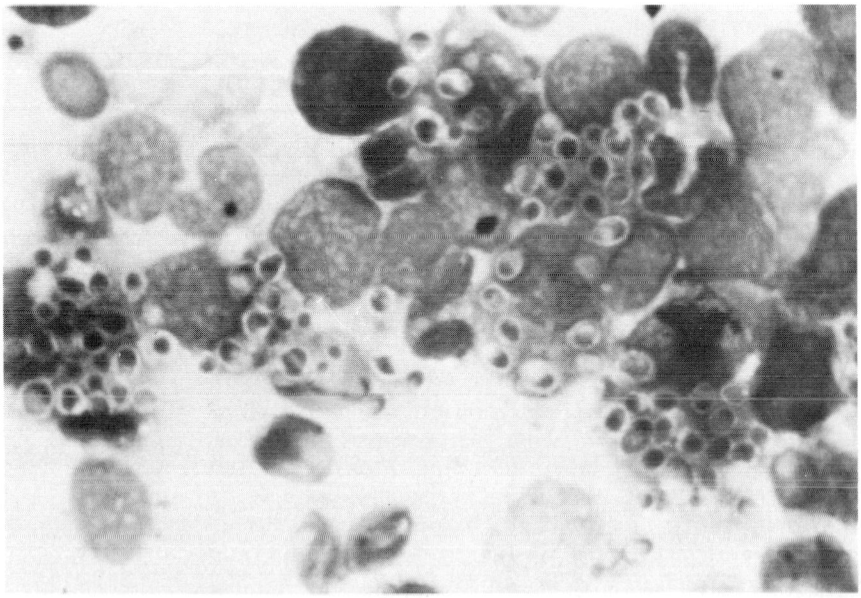

FIGURE 49–11. Colon scraping from a dog with gastrointestinal histoplasmosis, demonstrating numerous fungal organisms associated with a granulomatous inflammatory response (Difco Quick Stain, 100 ×).

more rapid control of the fungal infection may be possible with this regimen.[174–176] The dosage and administration schedule for these drugs has been previously described for blastomycosis. The duration of drug treatment required for each patient is variable and should be determined by monitoring the resolution of clinical signs, hematologic and biochemical abnormalities, and radiographic lesions. In most cases, treatment with ketoconazole should be continued for at least six months.[96, 142, 174, 175, 177] A new imidazole, fluconazole, has been at least as effective as ketoconazole in the treatment of experimental histoplasmosis in mice.[178] This drug may be useful in the treatment of naturally occurring histoplasmosis in companion animals in the future.

Dogs with intestinal involvement, and most cats, have extensive fungal dissemination at the time their disease is recognized.[137, 141–143, 145–147, 151, 153, 154, 156, 157, 160–162, 164, 166, 169, 170] Aggressive antifungal therapy with ketoconazole alone or in combination with amphotericin B is suggested for these patients. Unfortunately, because these animals are often severely debilitated and have widespread fungal involvement, treatment is frequently unrewarding.[137, 139, 146, 147, 154, 156, 162, 166, 169, 170] The patient response to antifungal therapy should be evaluated as previously discussed.

PROGNOSIS

The prognosis for dogs with pulmonary histoplasmosis is fair to good depending on the severity of fungal involvement. The prognosis for all cats, and for dogs with disseminated histoplasmosis, is guarded to grave.

CRYPTOCOCCOSIS

ETIOLOGY AND EPIZOOTIOLOGY

Cryptococcus neoformans is a saprophytic, budding yeast with a worldwide distribution.[179–182] The organism is small (1 to 7 μm) and is usually surrounded by a mucoid, polysaccharide capsule of variable size (1 to 30 μm).[180–182] The capsule apparently helps prevent desiccation of *Cryptococcus* in the soil and serves as a virulence factor, enabling the yeast to escape detection by the immune system of a mammalian host.[179–182]

Two sexual stages of *C. neoformans*, *Filobasidiella neoformans* var. neoformans and var. bacillospora or gattii, have been produced under experimental conditions but have not yet been found in nature.[179–181] This mycelial stage produces basidiopores, which acquire a capsule and revert to the yeast phase when incubated in tissue or on appropriate culture media.[179, 181] The basidiospores are produced in large numbers and are small enough (1.8 to 2.5 μm) to reach the lower respiratory tree if inhaled.[179, 181, 182] Definition of the role of *Filobasidiella* in the pathogenesis of cryptococcosis awaits further study and identification of a natural environmental source of this organism.

Growth of *C. neoformans* is enhanced in creatinine nitrogen-enriched environments associated with avian excreta, particularly pigeon droppings.[179, 180, 182] Unlike other deep mycotic diseases, cryptococcosis occurs more commonly in cats than in dogs.[182, 183]

PATHOGENESIS

The primary portal of entry for *C. neoformans* is the respiratory tract.[179, 181, 182, 184, 185] Once inhaled, larger organisms are filtered out in the upper respiratory tree, but smaller forms (1 to 2 μm) may be deposited in alveoli.[179, 181] Extension of infection from the respiratory tract occurs by local invasion and hematogenous or lymphatic dissemination.[181, 182, 184–187] Experimental attempts to establish cryptococcal infection via ingestion or direct cutaneous inoculation have been unsuccessful.[181, 183, 186] However, several cats have been reported that had cutaneous cryptococcosis without clinical or histopathologic evidence of systemic disease.[182, 188, 189]

The majority of cryptococcal infections in human beings occur in immunocompromised individuals.[179–181, 184] Although anticryptococcal factors have been found in human sera, the cellular immune system is the primary mechanism of host defense against this agent.[180, 181] Concurrent feline leukemia virus infection, which is known to cause immunosuppression, has been found in some cats with cryptococcosis.[186, 190–192] A temporal relationship with corticosteroid therapy was reported in two dogs with central nervous system (CNS) cryptococcosis;[193, 194] however, clinical signs of CNS infection were present prior to drug administration and corticosteroid therapy probably exacerbated, rather than precipitated, the infection. In most cases of cryptococcosis in companion animals, an underlying immunosuppressive disorder has not been identified.[185, 189, 195–199]

CLINICAL MANIFESTATIONS

Feline Cryptococcosis. Cryptococcosis is probably the most common systemic mycosis in cats.[182, 183, 186] The age range of affected cats is from 1 to 13 years with an average of approximately five years.[179, 189] There is no apparent breed or sex predilection.[182]

Cryptococcus neoformans most commonly affects the nasal cavity and sinuses of cats.[182, 183, 190–192, 197, 199–206] Clinical signs include sneezing, stertorous breathing, and chronic nasal discharge.[182, 183, 190, 191, 197, 199–206] The nasal discharge may be unilateral or bilateral and ranges in character from serous to mucopurulent to hemorrhagic.[182, 183, 191, 200–202, 204, 206] Granulomatous lesions in the nasal passages associated with the fungal infection may protrude from the external nares or cause swelling over the facial bones[182, 183, 190–192, 199, 201, 203–207] (Figure 49–12). Local extension of infection from the nasal cavity via lymphatics may cause regional lymphadenopathy.[182, 183, 199, 202, 204, 206] Signs of CNS involvement may result from direct invasion through the cribriform plate into the brain.[182, 183]

Skin lesions are fairly common in cats with cryptococcosis, occurring in about one-third of the reported cases.[182, 183, 188, 189, 197, 199, 200, 205–210] They occur as single or multiple, rapidly enlarging nodules that may ulcerate and exude a slimy serous material.[182, 183, 188–190, 199, 205–207, 209, 210] Regional lymphadenopathy is a common associated finding.[183, 199, 200, 208, 209] Most of these skin lesions

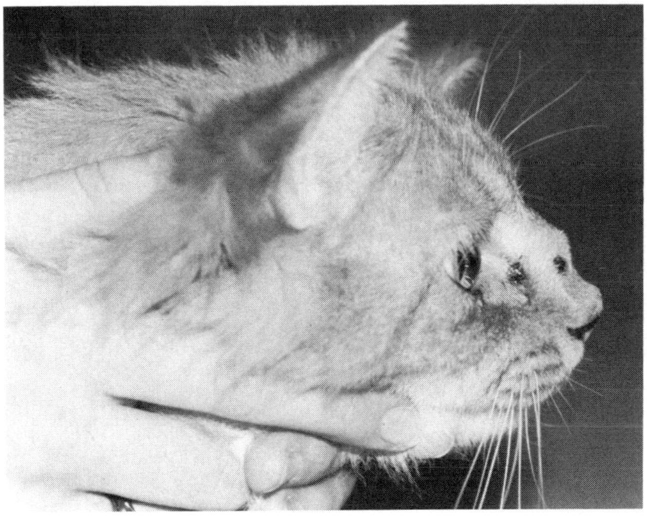

FIGURE 49–12. Lateral view of facial swelling and cutaneous granulomas associated with nasal cryptococcosis in a cat.

are the result of disseminated disease. As previously discussed, solitary skin nodules without evidence of other organ involvement have been seen in a few cats.

Cryptococcal infection of the CNS occurs in about one-fourth of the reported cases in cats and usually results from hematogenous dissemination of the fungus.[182–184] Diffuse meningoencephalitis occurs most commonly; granulomatous mass lesions of the brain and spinal cord have also been reported.[182, 183] Clinical signs can be quite variable and include depression, amaurotic blindness, ataxia, circling, paresis, paralysis, and seizures.[182, 183]

Cryptococcus neoformans occasionally affects the eye, and ocular lesions are often seen in cats with concurrent CNS infection.[182, 183, 190, 197, 198] Clinical signs include ocular discharge, optic neuritis, granulomatous chorioretinitis, retinal detachment, and anterior uveitis.[182, 183, 190, 196–198, 206] Other, less common sites of cryptococcal involvement in the cat include peripheral lymph nodes, lung, bone, and kidney.[182, 183, 195, 196, 207]

Signs of systemic illness are uncommon in cats with cryptococcosis but may include low-grade fever, malaise, anorexia, and weight loss.[182, 196, 204, 207, 208] It has been suggested that the yeast capsule protects the organism from the host's immunologic recognition and defense mechanisms.[184]

Canine Cryptococcosis. Cryptococcosis occurs less commonly in the dog than in the cat. The age range of reported cases is from 11 months to 10 years of age, with an average of 3.1 years.[182, 190, 211] Males and females are affected equally.[182] There is no specific breed predisposition; however, large breeds of dogs are more frequently affected than small breeds.[182, 187, 190, 193, 194, 197, 211–214]

The CNS is the most common site for *Cryptococcus* infection in the dog.[182, 185, 187, 193, 194, 211, 213–216] Neurologic derangements are usually caused by granulomatous meningoencephalitis[182, 185, 193, 213–215] and ocular lesions are common associated findings.[182, 185, 213–216] The clinical signs caused by the CNS and ocular involvement are similar to those previously described for the cat. In dogs, signs of vestibular system dysfunction are especially prominent, including head tilt, nystagmus, and gait abnormalities.[182, 185, 187, 193, 194, 211, 214–216]

Skin lesions are found in about one-fourth of the reported cases of canine cryptococcosis.[182, 197, 212, 214, 215, 217] Other sites of involvement are less frequent, but can include lymph nodes, bone, lung, kidney, heart, spleen, nasal cavity, pancreas, thyroid gland, and adrenal gland.[182, 185, 190, 193, 194, 197, 212–217]

DIAGNOSIS

Erythrocyte indices are usually within normal limits.[183, 185, 186, 191, 212, 216] Leukocyte counts are often normal but may vary from a degenerative left shift to a neutrophilic leukocytosis.[182, 183, 185, 196, 197, 212–214, 216] Biochemistry profiles occasionally reveal hyperproteinemia but are generally unremarkable unless there is extensive disseminated disease with internal organ involvement.[182, 183, 185, 191, 197, 199, 212–214] In nasal cryptococcosis, radiographs of the nasal cavity and frontal sinuses usually reveal increased soft tissue density on one or both sides; however, bone destruction is uncommon.[183, 190–192, 197] Although the pulmonary tree is the suspected portal of entry for disseminated cryptococcal infections in dogs and cats, thoracic radiographs rarely demonstrate significant changes.[183, 196, 199, 202, 214] Nodular pulmonary lesions, interstitial infiltrates, pleural effusion, and hilar lymphadenopathy have been recognized in some cases[185, 190, 192, 195, 205, 213, 217] (Figure 49–13). Examination of the cerebrospinal fluid (CSF) of animals with CNS involvement often reveals *Cryptococcus* organisms, increased cellularity, neutrophilia, and elevated protein concentrations.[182, 183, 185, 194, 214, 215]

Cryptococcus organisms are usually numerous in aspirates or impression smears prepared from affected tissues or body fluids[180, 182, 189, 190, 197, 199, 204, 214] (Figure 49–14). Organisms can be identified with routine hematologic stains, but Gram's stain, periodic acid–Schiff

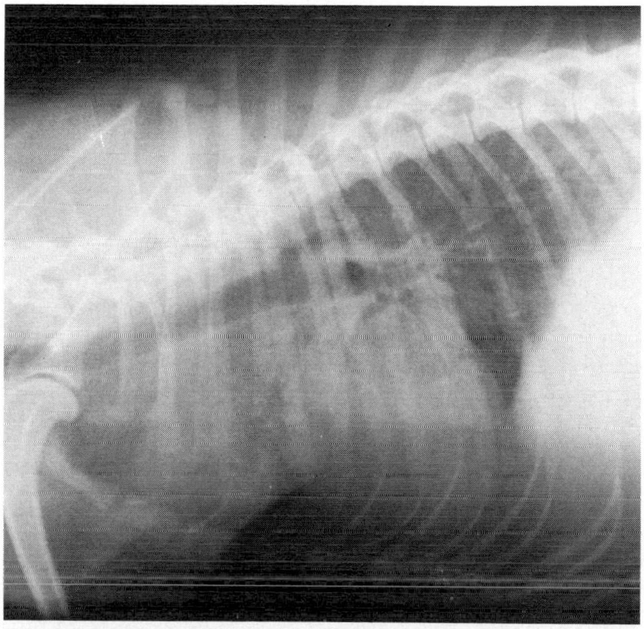

FIGURE 49–13. Lateral thoracic radiograph of a three-year-old beagle with disseminated cryptococcosis, demonstrating widespread, diffuse interstitial infiltrate in the pulmonary parenchyma.

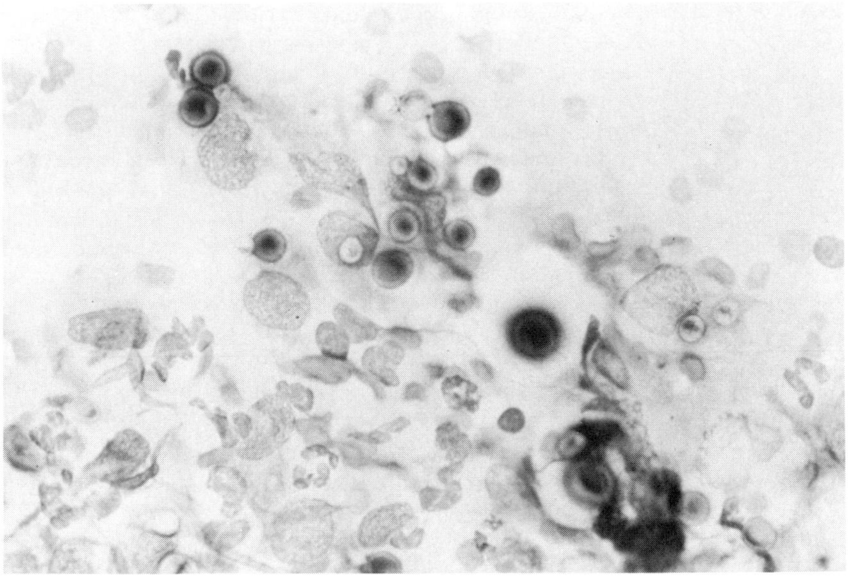

FIGURE 49–14. Periodic acid–Schiff stain of material aspirated from the nasal cavity of a cat with cryptococcal rhinitis. *Cryptococcus neoformans* organisms vary in size and are usually surrounded by an unstained capsular "halo" (100 ×).

(PAS), and new methylene blue are recommended because they provide better contrast.[180, 182] Tissue biopsy specimens may be stained routinely or with special fungal stains.[180, 182] Mayer's mucicarmine stain is particularly useful in identifying *C. neoformans* because it produces intense pink-red staining of the yeast capsule.[180, 182, 196, 213]

Fungal culture media without cycloheximide may be used to culture *C. neoformans* from tissue specimens or fluids.[180, 182, 183, 189, 200, 201, 208] Smooth, slimy, cream to white yeast colonies appear within two weeks in cultures incubated at 30°C.[180, 190]

The latex cryptococcal antigen test (LCAT) is a sensitive and rapid method for detecting capsular polysaccharide antigen in serum, urine, and CSF.[179, 180, 182, 184, 192, 197, 199, 201, 202, 204, 205] Cryptococcal antigen titers parallel the severity of infection and sequential samples may be used to monitor the patient's response to therapy.[179, 180, 197, 199, 201, 205] The LCAT test is available at some medical and veterinary laboratories, state diagnostic laboratories, and the Centers for Disease Control in Atlanta, Georgia.[182]

TREATMENT

Two cats with solitary cutaneous cryptococcal lesions were apparently successfully treated with surgery alone.[182, 189] However, because other lesions are present in most cases, antifungal chemotherapy is recommended. Amphotericin B and 5–flucytosine have been used successfully to treat some cases of cryptococcosis.[182, 186, 200–202, 204, 205] At this time, however, ketoconazole appears to be the treatment of choice for nasal and cutaneous cryptococcosis.[189, 191, 197, 199, 209] Ketoconazole is given orally at a dose of 4.4 mg/lb to 6.8 mg/lb (10 mg/kg to 15 mg/kg), q12h or q24h depending on the severity of disease, response to therapy, and the occurrence of drug-associated side effects.[75, 182, 187, 191, 199, 209] The duration of treatment should be based on the response of the patient, negative follow-up cytology or culture results, and changes in the serum LCAT.[182, 189, 197, 199] In general, therapy should be continued for at least two months following resolution of clinical signs of disease.

Treatment of CNS cryptococcosis in dogs and cats has been unrewarding.[182, 190, 212, 213] Combination therapy with intravenous amphotericin B at 0.13 mg/lb (0.3 mg/kg) q24h and oral 5–flucytosine at 68 mg/lb (150 mg/kg) q24h remains the treatment of choice in human beings with cryptococcal meningitis.[179, 184] This drug regimen is given for six weeks. Two of the newer imidazole compounds, itraconazole and fluconazole, have been effective in treating experimentally induced cryptococcal meningitis in rabbits.[218] Fluconazole appears particularly promising because of its ability to easily cross the blood-brain barrier and persist in high concentrations in the CSF.[218] Further studies are needed to assess the clinical efficacy of these compounds in the treatment of naturally occurring cryptococcal infections in animals.

PROGNOSIS

The prognosis for nasal and cutaneous cryptococcosis is fair to good. Cryptococcal meningoencephalitis warrants a grave prognosis at this time.

SPOROTRICHOSIS

ETIOLOGY

Sporotrichosis is a chronic pyogranulomatous infectious disease of dogs and cats caused by the dimorphic fungus *Sporothrix schenckii*. The organism was identified by Schenck in 1898 and from a naturally occurring case in the dog in 1908.[1, 11, 219–222] *Sporothrix schenckii* var. *luriei* has been isolated from humans but has not been identified in the dog and cat.[10, 222, 223]

Sporothrix schenckii, like other dimorphic fungi, exists in the mycelial form in soil and when cultured at room temperature. The yeast phase exists in tissues and when grown in vitro at 98.6°F (37.0°C) in the laboratory. Microscopically, the mycelia have thin, finely branched, septate hyphae with clusters of conidia (from 2 μm to 6 μm in diameter) arising from conidiophores.[1, 10, 11, 219, 224] Macrospores are produced by some strains of *Sporothrix* spp. and are considered characteristic of the organism.[10, 11, 219, 222, 224] Yeast forms are pleomorphic; round, ovoid or "cigar-shaped" cells (from 2 by 3 μm to 3 by 10 μm in diameter) can be observed microscopically (Figure 49–15).[1, 10, 219, 222] Identification of *Sporothrix schenckii* should be based on transformation of the mycelial form to the yeast form, or vice versa, or by inoculation of laboratory animals to demonstrate pathogenicity. Nonpathogenic strains of *Sporothrix* spp. exist.[1, 219, 222, 224]

EPIZOOTIOLOGY

Sporothrix schenckii is a ubiquitous saprophyte with a worldwide distribution. Moderate temperate zones with high humidity are conducive to organism growth.[1, 10, 30, 219, 220, 222] This is in contradiction to most reported cases, which originate from the north or central portions of the United States.[1, 224] The organism can be found in high organic content soils, vegetable debris, wood, the bark of certain trees, and spaghnum moss.[1, 10, 220, 221, 224–226] The organism has also been isolated from healthy animals, air, and water.[219]

PATHOGENESIS

Infection with *Sporothrix schenckii* is usually the result of accidental or traumatic inoculation of the fungus into the skin by thorns or plant materials.[1, 30, 219, 222, 224–230] Contamination of open wounds or broken skin by exudates from infected animals or laboratory materials are other routes of infection. Inhalation, ingestion, and mechanical vectors (animal bites) are also means by which infection can be established.[10, 30, 229, 231] Large numbers of organisms are required to initiate infection in experimental animals.[228, 232]

Once infection is established, it is usually localized to the cutaneous tissues; however, involvement of the lymphatics draining the area may occur. Papular or nodular lesions developed after three to five weeks at the sites of inoculation in experimental animals.[232] The papules ulcerate centrally and drain a reddish-brown or purulent exudate.[1, 219, 220, 227, 232–234] Scabs and crusts may form sequentially or spontaneous healing may result. In one experimental study, approximately one-third of the infected feline cases healed spontaneously.[235] Most infections remain localized to the cutaneous or cutaneous-lymphatic areas.

Dissemination of infection with *Sporothrix schenckii* can occur but is considered rare in the dog and cat. Experimentally, 50 per cent of cats infected with *Sporothrix schenckii* developed disseminated disease, as documented by culture of the organism from tissues.[232] Histopathologic lesions were not present in many of the tissues harboring organisms. Lymphatic or hematogenous spread may be the major routes of dissemination.[30, 219, 220, 229] Immunosuppression in humans and animals may predispose to dissemination; however, few naturally occurring cases of disseminated disease have been reported in animals.[228, 230, 234, 236] In cases of disseminated disease, organisms have been found in bone, eyes, gastrointestinal tract, central nervous system, and other visceral organs.[30, 230]

CLINICAL MANIFESTATIONS

The cutaneous and cutaneous-lymphatic forms of sporotrichosis are the most common.[1, 29, 30, 220, 224, 225, 237–242] Reported cases in the dog and cat have mainly described the cutaneous form.[220, 227, 236, 237, 241–243] The classically described lesions on extremities with involvement of ascending lymphatics appears to be less frequent in the dog and cat than in humans.[1, 10, 219, 222, 224] Age and sex predispositions have not been reported for the dog and cat. In 18 feline cases reported in the veterinary literature, all infected animals were males, except one, with an average age of 3.52 years.[230, 231, 236, 237, 242–246] Reports show equal numbers of female and male dogs affected by sporotrichosis, with an average age of 3.97 years.

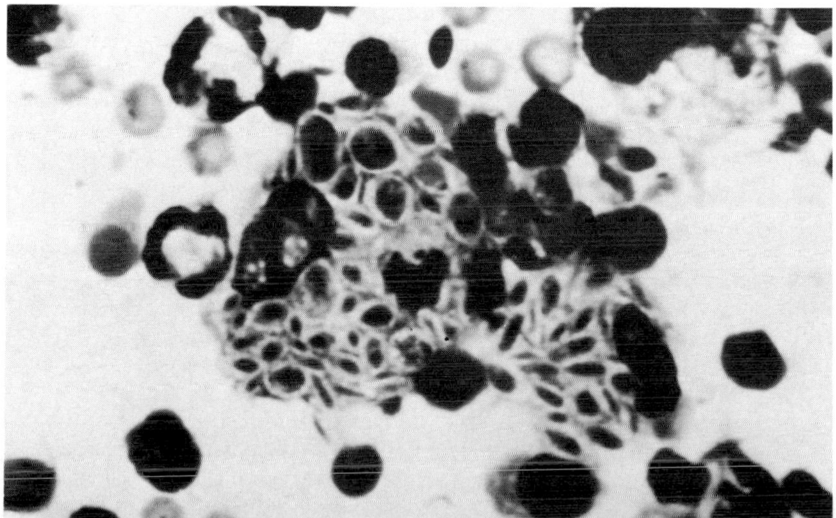

FIGURE 49–15. Impression smear made from an ulcerative skin lesion on a Siamese cat, demonstrating the many pleomorphic organisms characteristic of sporotrichosis (Difco Quick Stain, 100 ×).

Breed predispositions have not been recognized in the dog or cat.

Lesions of sporotrichosis are usually confined to the dorsal aspects of the head and trunk.[1, 30, 220, 224, 225, 241, 242, 247] Extremities may or may not be affected concurrently. Multiple, raised, circular lesions characterized by alopecia, crusts, and central ulceration are typical. These papular or nodular lesions may be linear in nature, usually indicative of a concurrent lymphangitis. Involved areas are usually nonpainful and nonpruritic. Disseminated sporotrichosis in the dog and cat usually has dermatologic lesions as well as clinical signs associated with a variety of affected organ systems. Ocular, central nervous, osseous, and lymphatic abnormalities may be present with disseminated disease.

DIAGNOSIS

The diagnosis of sporotrichosis can be made by demonstrating the organism in exudates or tissue specimens, isolation of the organism by culture techniques, or by laboratory animal inoculation with suspected infected materials. Direct visualization of the organism in exudates is uncommon, as the numbers of organisms present are few.[10, 30, 219, 220, 222, 237, 239, 248] Histopathologic examination of tissues may reveal organisms; however, routine hematoxylin-eosin stain (HE) does not allow reliable demonstration.[10, 11, 219, 220, 222, 224] Gomori's methenamine silver, periodic acid–Schiff, Gram's, Giemsa, or the Gomori-Grocott stain methodologies yield more consistent results.[10, 219, 220, 221] Fluorescent antibody techniques or pretreatment of tissues with diastase enhances visualization of the organism on formalin-fixed tissue specimens.[11, 224, 241, 243, 249, 250] Certain stains produce a "halo" effect or "asteroid body" surrounding the organism at times. This effect is called the "Splendore-Hoeppli phenomenon" and is due to a glycoprotein antigen-antibody reaction on the surface of the yeast cell.[222, 233, 251]

The inflammatory reaction resulting from all forms of sporotrichosis is a mixed purulent and granulomatous reaction.[10, 220, 222, 224, 230, 252] Epidermal ulceration, acanthosis, pseudoepitheliomatous hyperplasia, parakeratosis, and intraepidermal microabscesses are typical of the dermatologic changes.[10, 219, 222, 251] Granuloma formation with central microabscessation may be observed in the epidermis, dermis, subcutaneous, or in other tissues with disseminated disease. Epithelioid cells, giant cells, and lymphocytes encapsulated by fibrous connective tissue are classical cellular infiltrates within granulomas.[1, 10, 252]

Culture of exudates, tissues, or aspirates from unopened lesions provides the most reliable method of diagnosis of sporotrichosis.[11, 29, 30, 219–221, 224, 227, 237, 241] Sabouraud's dextrose agar with antibiotics and blood-heart infusion media are appropriate culture media for the isolation of the mycelial and yeast forms, respectively.[1, 10, 29, 30, 219, 220, 224] Mycelial growth occurs rapidly within three to five days at room temperature. Colonial morphology of the mycelial form is highly variable. Intraperitoneal inoculation of laboratory animals such as mice, rats, or hamsters can also be used to demonstrate pathogenicity of the organism.[1, 10, 29, 30, 219, 222, 224] Organisms can be identified in the testes, spleen, and liver of experimentally inoculated animals after two to three weeks.

Serologic tests are not currently available for use in animals to aid in the diagnosis of sporotrichosis. The latex agglutination, tube agglutination, and immunodiffusion tests, using a variety of antigens, need further investigation and evaluation prior to their use in animals.[219, 241]

THERAPY

The drugs of choice for treatment of cutaneous or cutaneous-lymphatic sporotrichosis are the inorganic iodides.[1, 11, 30, 220, 224, 227, 241, 243] Potassium and sodium iodides have been used in the dog and cat. Dosages for use in the dog have varied; however, 20 mg/lb (44 mg/kg) of a 20 per cent sodium iodide solution, used orally, q8h for seven to eight weeks did not produce toxic signs in treated dogs and resulted in clinical cures.[220, 253] One-half of this dosage (10 mg/lb or 22 mg/kg, q8 or q12h) has been recommended for cats.[224, 225, 231] Because of the marked sensitivity of the feline species to iodide preparations, cats should be monitored closely for evidence of toxicity. Signs of iodide toxicity include fever, ptyalism, anorexia, hyperexcitability, dry hair coat, and vomiting or diarrhea. Therapy with iodides should be continued for 30 days after clinical cure.

Ketoconazole, a substituted imidazole, has been used in a cat at 2.3 mg/lb (5 mg/kg) q12h for two months with only partial resolution of clinical signs.[231] An experimental study using ketoconazole in cats at a dosage of 2.3 mg/lb/day (5 mg/kg/day) for six weeks resulted in clinical and mycologic cure of skin lesions. However, regional lymph nodes still yielded *Sporothrix schenckii* on culture after the completed course of therapy.[228]

Amphotericin B, alone or in combination with iodides or ketoconazole, should be used in the treatment of animals with disseminated disease.[224, 229] Too few naturally occurring cases have been treated with amphotericin B to suggest a possible response rate. One case of disseminated sporotrichosis in a dog treated by one of the authors did not respond after four weeks of amphotericin B therapy. Dosage regimens should be the same as blastomycosis in the dog and for cryptococcosis in the cat.[225] Because of the extreme nephrotoxic effects of amphotericin B, renal function should be assessed frequently.

The use of applied heat in the treatment of sporotrichosis has also been suggested in humans. Low ambient temperatures have been shown to result in more severe disease. Application of heat and rubescents have resulted in cure of human cases.[254, 255]

PROGNOSIS

Generally, the response to treatment of cutaneous or cutaneous-lymphatic forms of sporotrichosis is excellent. An experimental study in cats has demonstrated the occurrence of spontaneous cures. One-third of the cats in this study resolved clinically.[232] In the disseminated form of sporotrichosis, the prognosis should be guarded. The immunologic status of patients with disseminated disease should not be compromised.[228, 233, 234] Immunologic dysfunction in humans is commonly associated with disseminated disease and a poor prognosis. Few cases in animals have been reported in regard to treatment outcome of disseminated sporotrichosis.

PUBLIC HEALTH ASPECTS

Persons that have come into contact with material from infected animals have acquired infections[221, 230, 244–246] as a result of contamination of open or broken skin with the organism. The animal is merely a mechanical vector. Care should therefore be exercised in the handling of infected animals and materials.

ASPERGILLOSIS

ETIOLOGY AND EPIZOOTIOLOGY

Several species of *Aspergillus* have been associated with disease in animals. *Aspergillus fumigatus* is commonly found in animals with primary respiratory tract involvement;[256–264] *Aspergillus terreus* and *A. deflectus* have been isolated from dogs with disseminated aspergillosis.[257, 258, 265–267]

Members of the genus *Aspergillus* are ubiquitous saprophytes with worldwide distribution.[257, 264, 268–271] *Aspergillus fumigatus* grows most abundantly in decaying vegetation, sewage sludge compost, decomposing wood chips, moldy hay, and organic compost piles; *A. terreus* is commonly found in soil, decaying vegetation, and grains.[264–267, 270, 271] *Aspergillus deflectus* has only been isolated from soil.[258] The *Aspergillus* species produce large numbers of small spores (less than 8 μm), which are the source of infection for animals.[261, 270, 271]

PATHOGENESIS

The respiratory tract is the primary portal of entry for *Aspergillus* spores.[261, 266, 270, 271] In most mammals, the respiratory phagocytic defense and mechanical clearance mechanisms prevent fungal colonization.[264, 270] The role and importance of the humoral and cellular immune systems in resistance to aspergillosis is unclear.[264] In human beings, aspergillosis is primarily an opportunistic infection associated with an immunocompromised host.[257, 264, 266, 268, 270–274] Although immune system defects have been demonstrated in some dogs with aspergillosis,[264, 265, 273] there is not a consistent association with a specific immunodeficient state.[257–259, 264, 267] Aspergillosis in cats is rare and has usually been reported in immunocompromised animals with concurrent feline parvovirus (panleukopenia) or feline leukemia virus infection.[264, 274–276]

Nasal cavity infection is the most common manifestation of aspergillosis in the dog.[257–259, 261, 262, 264–266, 273, 277 280] This form of disease is usually caused by *A. fumigatus*.[257, 261, 264] Fungal colonization is usually limited to the nasal passages and paranasal sinuses.[259, 261, 262, 264, 278–280]

Disseminated aspergillosis in dogs is caused by infection with *A. terreus* and *A. deflectus*.[257, 258, 265–267] The increased pathogenic potential of these two species is apparently due to their production of highly infective aleuriospores in tissue and their ability to invade blood vessels.[257, 258, 265, 266, 275] The respiratory tract is believed to be the primary portal of entry for these species; however, not all dogs with disseminated aspergillosis had nasal cavity or lung lesions at postmortem examination.[257, 258, 265, 267, 281] Other suggested routes of infection include invasion of the vasculature of the nasal or gastrointestinal mucosa and direct cutaneous inoculation.[258, 266] Whatever the portal of entry, the distribution of lesions suggests a hematogenous route for dissemination of the fungus.[257, 258, 265, 266]

Three cases of unifocal *Aspergillus* osteomyelitis or discospondylitis without other organ involvement have been reported in the dog.[277, 282] *Aspergillus fumigatus* was isolated from one of these dogs;[282] the species of *Aspergillus* was not identified in the others.[277] The portal of entry and route of fungal invasion in these cases is unknown.

CLINICAL MANIFESTATIONS

Canine Nasal Aspergillosis. Dogs affected with nasal aspergillosis are typically young to middle-aged; males predominate in reports in which the sex is recorded.[259, 261, 267, 273, 279] There is no specific breed predisposition, however, dolichocephalic breeds have a higher incidence of this disease than brachycephalic breeds.[259, 261, 262 264, 272, 273, 279, 280]

Nasal aspergillosis in the dog is an erosive disease that causes chronic nasal discharge.[259, 261, 262, 273, 279, 280] The nasal discharge is usually serous initially, later becomes purulent, and is often hemorrhagic.[259, 261, 264, 278–280] Sneezing, stertorous breathing, and facial pain are occasional associated clinical findings.[259, 261, 264] Most infections are unilateral initially but often spread to involve both sides of the nasal cavity.[262] Signs of systemic illness are not usually present.[259, 261, 264, 278, 280] In rare cases, the infection may erode through the cribriform plate and produce signs of central nervous system involvement.[261, 264]

Canine Disseminated Aspergillosis. Twenty-one dogs with disseminated aspergillosis have been reported.[257, 258, 265–267, 281, 283, 284] Eighteen of these 21 dogs were German shepherds.[257, 258, 265–267, 283] The predominance of this breed in disseminated aspergillosis is significant but attempts to define a specific breed-associated immunodeficiency have been inconclusive.[257, 267] The average age of affected animals was 3.4 years, with a range of one to seven years; females slightly outnumbered males.[257, 258, 265–267, 281, 283, 284]

The most common clinical signs in dogs with disseminated aspergillosis were weight loss, anorexia, depression or lethargy, weakness, fever, lameness, back pain, and paresis or paralysis.[257, 258, 265–267, 281, 283, 284] Ocular signs, including anterior uveitis, enophthalmitis, or chorioretinitis, were present in approximately half of the dogs and often preceded evidence of generalized illness.[257, 258, 265–267, 283] Other, less frequent findings were lymphadenopathy, cutaneous swellings or draining tracts, oral ulcers, and abdominal pain.[257, 258, 267, 283] Unusual signs included scrotal swelling, vomition, diarrhea, urinary incontinence, seizures, and cardiac arrhythmias.[257, 258, 266, 267]

Aspergillus Osteomyelitis. Three German shepherd

dogs have been identified with unifocal *Aspergillus* osteomyelitis or discospondylitis not associated with histopathologic evidence of disseminated disease.[277, 282] The major clinical signs were progressive lameness or paresis.[277] Vague generalized signs of systemic illness such as weight loss, inappetence, and malaise were present in two cases.[277]

Feline Aspergillosis. One case of nasal aspergillosis has been reported in a four-year-old cat with concurrent feline leukemia virus infection.[274] The clinical findings were similar to those described for the dog.[274] Another cat had bilateral sinusitis and orbital cellulitis caused by *Aspergillus*.[272] Systemic aspergillosis has been reported in nine cats, affecting the lung, intestinal tract, and/or kidneys.[275, 276, 285, 286, 288] Clinical signs included fever, dyspnea, anorexia, lethargy, vomiting, and diarrhea.[275, 274, 285, 286, 288] *Aspergillus* is suspected as an opportunistic secondary invader in these cats because most had concurrent feline parvovirus disease (or panleukopenia-like syndrome).[264, 276, 275] Unfortunately, because the test was not available at the time most cases were reported, evaluation for feline leukemia virus infection was not performed.[264, 275, 276, 286] Fungal involvement was not as widespread as is seen in dogs and many of the clinical signs reported in these cats may have been due to primary viral disease rather than aspergillosis.

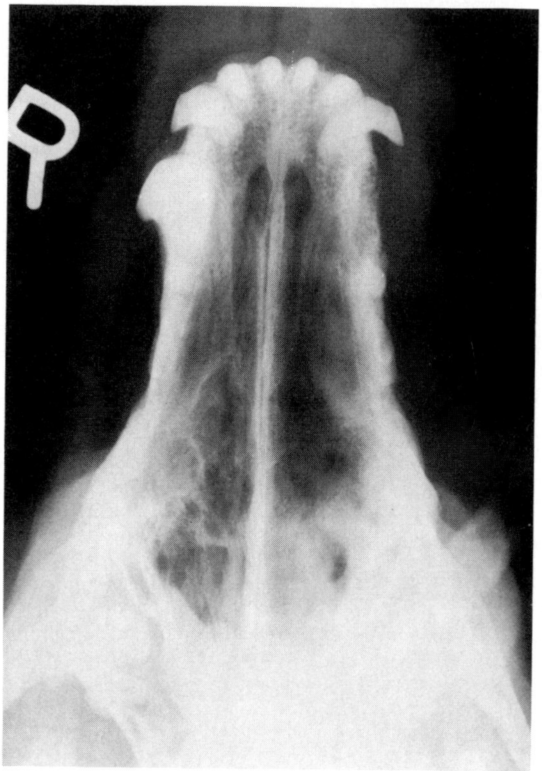

FIGURE 49–16. Ventrodorsal, open-mouth radiograph of an eleven-year-old mixed breed dog with unilateral nasal aspergillosis. The left side of the nasal cavity demonstrates loss of the normal turbinate pattern and punctate bone lysis anteriorly; increased soft tissue density is seen in the posterior part of the nasal cavity.

DIAGNOSIS

Nasal Aspergillosis. Routine hematology and serum biochemistry profiles are usually normal.[273, 278, 280] Peripheral eosinophilia and lymphopenia were reported in a few cases.[261, 264, 273]

Characteristic findings on radiographs of the nasal cavity include nasal turbinate loss, causing increased lucency rostrally, and a mixed density pattern in the caudal portion of the nasal cavity.[259, 261, 273, 279] Punctate erosions of the frontal bones and roughening of the vomer are frequently present[263, 279] (Figure 49–16). These erosions are believed to be due to pitting or focal bone destruction by the fungus or fungal toxins.[279] Radiographs should be examined carefully because up to 50 per cent of cases with clinical signs of unilateral disease demonstrate radiographic changes in both nasal cavities.[279] Increased opacity in the frontal sinuses may be due to either direct fungal involvement or accumulation of secretions due to obstruction of drainage.[279] Increased thickness or punctate lysis of bone suggests the former.[279]

Nasal endoscopy may be obscured by exudate and exploratory rhinotomy, and biopsy is most likely to provide a definitive diagnosis of nasal aspergillosis.[259, 273, 278, 280] *Aspergillus* lesions usually appear as yellow-green to gray-black fungal plaques and granulation tissue on the nasal mucosa and in the sinuses.[259, 261, 263, 264] Material may be collected for cytologic examination from nasal swabs, flushes, or imprints of biopsy specimens.[259, 261, 273, 280, 284] Branching, septate fungal hyphae can be seen on direct, 10 to 20 per cent KOH or new methylene blue stained wet mounts and with routine hematologic stains.[264, 273, 277] Hematoxylin and eosin stains usually reveal fungal hyphae in biopsy specimens; however, Gomori's methenamine silver stain improves detection if few organisms are present[264, 277, 279] (Figure 49–17).

Aspergillus spp. grow well on most fungal culture media incubated at room temperature or 35°C and on blood agar at 37°C.[264, 271] Isolation of *Aspergillus* from nasal swabs or wash specimens should be interpreted with caution because it is a normal contaminant in the upper respiratory tract.[260, 261, 271, 277, 280] Alternatively, failure to culture this organism does not rule out a diagnosis of aspergillosis.[260, 261, 271, 280]

Agar gel double diffusion (AGDD) and counterimmunoelectrophoresis (CIE) are used to detect the presence of systemic antibody directed against *A. fumigatus*.[256, 257, 263, 264, 271, 274, 280, 286] A positive result with either AGDD or CIE strongly supports the presence of active *Aspergillus* infection;[256, 259, 263, 264] however, CIE cross-reactivity with *Penicillium* spp. was reported in one study.[263] As with fungal cultures, negative serologic tests do not preclude the presence of fungal infection.[280]

Canine Disseminated Aspergillosis and Aspergillus Osteomyelitis. The most common hematologic abnormality in dogs with disseminated aspergillosis is leukocytosis with a mature neutrophilia.[257, 258, 265–267, 283, 284] One-third of the dogs had elevations of blood urea nitrogen, serum alkaline phosphatase, and total serum protein levels, but other biochemical abnormalities were inconsistent.[257, 258, 265, 267, 284] Persistent isosthenuria was present in many dogs and *Aspergillus* was seen in the urine sediment or cultured from the urine in about one-third of the reported cases.[257, 258, 265, 267] Two dogs with central nervous system infection had increased protein levels

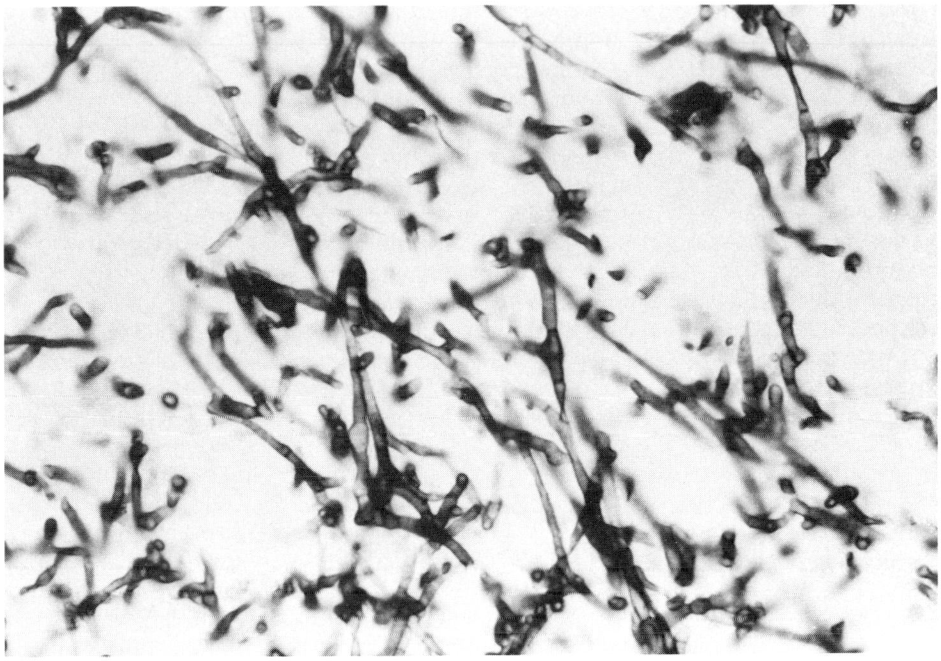

FIGURE 49–17. Biopsy specimen from a one-and-a-half-year-old Rottweiler with nasal aspergillosis, demonstrating branching fungal hyphae.

and a neutrophilic leukocytosis of the cerebrospinal fluid.[258, 266]

Little clinical pathology data are available from dogs with *Aspergillus* osteomyelitis alone.[277, 282] One dog had a peripheral leukocytosis;[277] however, because of the focal nature of the lesions, few other abnormalities would be expected.

Radiographs are useful in demonstrating fungal osteomyelitis and discospondylitis in focal disease and in nearly all cases of disseminated disease.[257, 258, 265, 267, 277] Osseous lesions are primarily lytic, with some periosteal new bone formation and overlying soft tissue swelling.[257, 258, 265, 267, 277] Other radiographic findings in some dogs with disseminated disease include visceral lymphadenopathy, hepatosplenomegaly, and pulmonary parenchymal changes.[258]

On histopathology, disseminated aspergillosis is characterized by widespread fungal vascular invasion and infarction in multiple organs and tissues.[257, 258, 265–267] The kidney, spleen, and bones are most commonly and severely affected.[257, 258, 265–267, 281, 284] Other sites of involvement include the liver, heart, eye, and visceral and peripheral lymph nodes.[257, 258, 265–267, 281, 283, 284] Lesions are less frequently found in lung, stomach, pancreas, mouth, and brain.[257, 258, 265–267, 281, 283] Fungal organisms are numerous in affected tissues and are easily seen with routine histopathologic and special fungal stains.[257, 258, 265–267, 277, 281–284]

Aspergillus terreus and *A. deflectus* may be cultured from urine, blood, or tissue specimens, using methods previously described.[257, 258, 265, 267] Serodiagnostic tests using *A. fumigatus* antigens have been negative in the few cases evaluated.[258] Precipitin antibody to *A. terreus* was present in 6 of 12 dogs in one group of cases.[257]

Feline Aspergillosis. The results of hematology and biochemistry profiles performed on cats with aspergillosis are difficult to evaluate because of the scarcity of reported cases and the presence of concurrent diseases in affected cats.[272, 274–276, 285, 286, 288] Mild anemia was present in a number of cats;[264, 275, 276] leukocyte counts were extremely variable, ranging from severe leukopenia to moderate leukocytosis.[275, 276] Biochemistry data are not available from most cases. The approach to diagnosis of aspergillosis in the cat should be the same as for the dog.

TREATMENT

Treatment of canine nasal aspergillosis has been difficult. Surgery alone usually results in incomplete excision of affected tissue and recurrence of disease.[264] Various antifungal agents, including amphotericin B, flucytosine, sodium iodide, and thiabendazole have been used alone or as adjunctive agents following surgery with some improvement in clinical cure rates.[260, 264, 273, 287] Ketoconazole has been used alone or following surgery at a dosage of 4.5 to 9 mg/lb (10 to 20 mg/kg) orally q12h with complete resolution of the fungal infection in about half the reported cases.[259, 260, 278, 280] Enilconazole is another imidazole compound that is very effective against *A. fumigatus* and *Penicillium* spp. and appears to have promise in the treatment of *Aspergillus* rhinitis.[256] Enilconazole was used in five dogs at a dose of 2.3 mg/lb (5 mg/kg) q12h instilled into the nasal cavities and sinuses via indwelling catheters for seven to ten days.[256] Follow-up therapy with ketoconazole at 4.5 mg/lb (10 mg/kg) orally q24h was given for six weeks after enilconazole treatment was completed.[256] All of the dogs responded with remission of clinical signs and negative fungal cultures.[256] The contribution of ketoconazole to the clinical response in these patients must be considered; however, two of the dogs had previously failed to respond to treatment with ketoconazole alone.[256]

Treatment of disseminated aspergillosis in dogs has been uniformly unsuccessful.[257, 258, 265] Amphotericin B, amphotericin B methyl ester, thiabendazole, and ketoconazole have been used without effect on the progression of the disease.[257, 258, 265] Some of the newer imidazole compounds may have a better spectrum of activity against *Aspergillus* and may be useful in the future. The treatment of choice in human beings with aspergillus osteomyelitis is surgical debridement, followed by amphotericin B given intravenously at 0.23 to 0.3 mg/lb (0.5 to 0.7 mg/kg) q24h for 6 to 12 weeks.[268] Treatment of dogs with focal aspergillus osteomyelitis has not been attempted.[277, 282]

The diagnosis of aspergillosis in most cats was made on postmortem examination; therefore, treatment was not attempted.[264, 275] One cat with only nasal and sinus involvement apparently responded to rhinotomy, curettage, and local iodine therapy.[274]

PROGNOSIS

The prognosis for nasal aspergillosis is fair to good, depending on the extent of the disease. Use of the newer antifungal agents is likely to improve our ability to treat many of these cases. Disseminated aspergillosis in dogs or cats and *Aspergillus* osteomyelitis have yet to be treated successfully. They carry a grave prognosis at this time.

PHYCOMYCOSIS

ETIOLOGY

Phycomycosis is a nonspecific term denoting infection with a group of saprophytic, poorly septate or nonseptate, filamentous organisms. The taxonomy regarding the Phycomycetes has resulted in a great deal of confusion about its terminology in the veterinary literature. Currently, phycomycosis describes infection caused by two families in the kingdom Fungi, Entomophthoraceae and Mucoraceae, and one family, Pythiaceae, in the kingdom Protista.[1, 10, 11, 124, 289–299] Individual genera that have been isolated from naturally occurring cases in the dog and cat are *Basidiobolus*, *Conidiobolus*, *Absidia*, *Rhizopus*, *Rhizomucor*, *Mucor*, *Mortierella*, and *Pythium*.[1, 225, 292, 293, 297, 299–305] At present, the *Pythium* species appears to be the most common isolate affecting the gastrointestinal system and subcutaneous tissues of the dog.[292, 297, 303, 304] The first report of phycomycosis in the dog was in 1885.[305, 306] The canine species is more often infected than the feline species.

The Phycomycetes are ubiquitous molds found in water, soil, decaying matter, feces, and substrates high in carbohydrate content.[10, 11, 124, 225, 291, 307] All genera produce large airborne spores with the exception of *Pythium* species. This species reproduces asexually by zoospores that are biflagellate and motile.[292, 299] Specific species of the organisms can only be identified by culture. However, the morphologic and histologic appearance of organisms in tissues appears to be satisfactory for identifying the involved genus in clinical cases without definitive culture of the organism.[292]

EPIZOOTIOLOGY

Phycomycosis is reported most frequently from the Gulf Coast regions, with the largest number of cases reported from Louisiana and Texas.[292, 297, 304] Miller described a seasonal occurrence of infection in dogs during the warm summer period, similar to a pattern of infection with *Pythium* in horses.[308] The highest incidence of cases in dogs occurred between the months of March through December.[292] The disease is rare in the cat.[297, 309]

PATHOGENESIS

The primary route of infection with phycomycosis has not been positively identified, but inhalation, ingestion, and contamination of wounds are suspected.[292, 297, 304, 307] Inhalation of spores into the nasal cavity with movement into the pharyngeal area and subsequent swallowing has been proposed as one route of infection in humans. The ingestion of *Pythium* zoospores seems the most feasible, because gastrointestinal lesions predominate in affected animals. Mucosal lesions of the gastrointestinal tract may not be required to establish an infection, as motile zoospores may directly penetrate the mucosa and invade the lymphatics. This may help to explain the finding of mesenteric lymph node involvement in some cases, without the presence of definitive gastrointestinal lesions.[292] Certain species of the Phycomycetes have a predilection for invasion of blood vessels, resulting in infarction and thrombosis.[289, 292, 310] Dissemination to other organ systems may result from this vascular invasion. Several cases of subcutaneous phycomycosis have also been reported after traumatic injury.[31, 297, 304]

Predisposing factors were once thought to be important in the acquisition of phycomycosis. This is now being disputed, especially with regard to the *Pythium* species. Trauma, diabetes mellitus, panleukopenia, distemper, and feline leukemia virus infection have been reported in animals with phycomycosis.[1, 297, 298, 300, 311] Cases of canine mucormycosis in Europe and the northern United States have been associated with debilitating and immunodeficient states.[292, 300]

CLINICAL MANIFESTATIONS

Clinical signs of phycomycosis are usually associated with the gastrointestinal tract and subcutaneous tissue. Of 138 reported cases in dogs, 128 animals had gastrointestinal lesions; subcutaneous involvement was present in only 14 dogs.[289, 290, 292, 297–305, 311–323] The duration of illness in either form varies but most are chronic. Additional organs affected include the lung, spleen, kidney, uterus, central nervous system, liver, heart, pancreas, and lymphatics.[292, 297, 300, 304] Disseminated disease appears to be rare in both the dog and cat.

Dogs appear to be more commonly infected with phycomycosis than cats. Young males (less than three years) of the medium to large breeds are overrepresented in case studies.[292, 297, 304] The average age of 93 reported cases of gastrointestinal phycomycosis was 2.05 years. Breed predisposition has not been identified, but the Labrador retriever and German shepherd breeds comprised 20 per cent of cases in several studies.[292, 297, 304]

Subcutaneous lesions in dogs are characterized by alopecia, nodules, ulceration, granulation tissue, serosanguineous to purulent exudates, and draining fistulous tracts.[31, 225, 290, 303] Lesions are usually single; multiple subcutaneous areas may be involved. Local lymphadenopathy is usually present.

Gastrointestinal or visceral involvement is the more common presentation of canine phycomycosis. Clinical signs depend upon the affected area of the gastrointestinal tract. Vomiting, weight loss, small or large bowel diarrhea, palpable abdominal masses, and anorexia are common clinical findings.[292, 297, 304] Oral and esophageal lesions are unusual.[292, 297, 315] The stomach and cranial small bowel are the areas of the gastrointestinal tract that are most frequently affected.[292, 297] Ileal and colonic lesions were more prevalent in one study.[304] Therefore, it appears that no specific area of the gastrointestinal tract is spared with phycomycosis.

The affected region of the gastrointestinal tract is firm, with transmural thickening of the bowel wall. Attenuation of the bowel lumen is often grossly visible and in some cases total obstruction is present. If lesions are extensive and penetrate the serosa, contiguous areas may become affected (pancreas, omentum, liver). Mucosal irregularities and ulceration are common, accounting for the melena observed in many patients. Yellow to yellowish-gray nodules may also be present on the serosal surfaces of the gastrointestinal tract.

DIAGNOSIS

Hematology and Biochemical Findings. Hematologic changes in phycomycosis are nonspecific and usually reflect the chronicity of the disease. A mild nonregenerative anemia was observed in 33 to 50 per cent of affected animals.[293] The anemia is associated with chronic inflammation or chronic gastrointestinal blood loss.[293, 297] Neutrophilia with a left shift also may be evident. Persistent eosinophilia was found in approximately 50 per cent of dogs with phycomycosis in one study.[304] This finding was considered to be significant, as other common causes of eosinophilia were excluded. Eosinophilia may be a reaction of the animal to certain antigenic substances contained in the cell wall of the organism. Eosinophilic infiltrates in tissue specimens can also be supportive of phycomycosis, especially with certain genera.

Biochemical findings have not been reviewed in a significant number of animals. Hypoalbuminemia, hyperproteinemia, azotemia, aciduria, and proteinuria were biochemical abnormalities noted in animals infected with phycomycosis.[225, 292, 293, 297, 304]

Radiographic Findings. Radiographic lesions compatible with phycomycosis can usually be demonstrated by positive contrast techniques.[292, 304] Plain film abdominal radiographs may not detect gross gastrointestinal lesions accurately, as most animals are thin and emaciated, precluding good radiographic contrast. Large abdominal masses may be documented by plain film radiography. Positive contrast findings in canine gastrointestinal phycomycosis include mucosal thickening and irregularities, luminal narrowing with obstruction and stricture formation, displacement of normal abdominal contents, and abnormal gas pattern accumulation.[297, 299, 304] Differential diagnosis for these radiographic findings in animals includes regional enteritis, infiltrative bowel diseases, foreign bodies, and intestinal obstructive disease. In cases of subcutaneous phycomycosis, only soft tissue swelling is present. Osseous involvement has not been reported.

Cytologic and Histopathologic Findings. Cytologic examination of exudates or tissue aspirates are not very rewarding for demonstrating the hyphae of Phycomycetes.[31, 225, 291, 293, 295] In fact, the isolation of the organism without evidence of tissue invasion or demonstration of the hyphae in a direct potassium hydroxide smear of tissue is insufficient for a diagnosis.[298] Potassium hydroxide or India ink stain may be used on exudates, tissue aspirates, or tissue scrapings.

Most cases of phycomycosis require histopathologic examination of tissues obtained by a variety of biopsy techniques for definitive diagnosis.[31, 225, 248] Hematoxylin eosin-stain (HE) does not always allow identification of fungal hyphae.[11] Foil et al. state that Zygomycetes are usually demonstrated by HE stain in contrast to the *Pythium* species.[303] Gridley's fungal stain, Gomori-silver stain, and periodic acid-Schiff (PAS) allow identification of fungal elements in tissue specimens with better efficacy and detail.[10, 11, 291]

Phycomycetes organisms range from 2.5 to 20 μm in diameter. The cell walls are smooth, parallel, and broad. Branching of hyphae is common but may be irregular (Figure 49–18). Fungal hyphae are usually nonseptate. A cuff of eosinophilic material 5 to 20 μm in width may be demonstrated in tissue samples surrounding fungal elements. This cuff, also termed the Splendore-Hoeppli phenomenon, represents an antigen-antibody complex that is frequently observed with certain species of Entomophthoromycetes in humans and dogs.[10, 11, 292, 307]

Histologically, the affected subcutaneous tissue contains a severe ulcerative pyogranulomatous dermatitis.[31, 290] Multifocal areas of necrosis within the superficial and deep dermis are typically present, with infiltration by neutrophils and macrophages. Granuloma

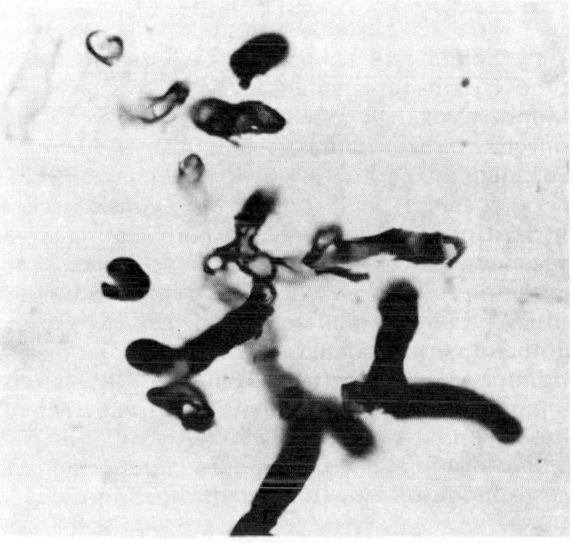

FIGURE 49–18. Gastric biopsy from a dog with phycomycosis. The hyphae are broad, nonseptate, and branching (GMS stain 100 ×).

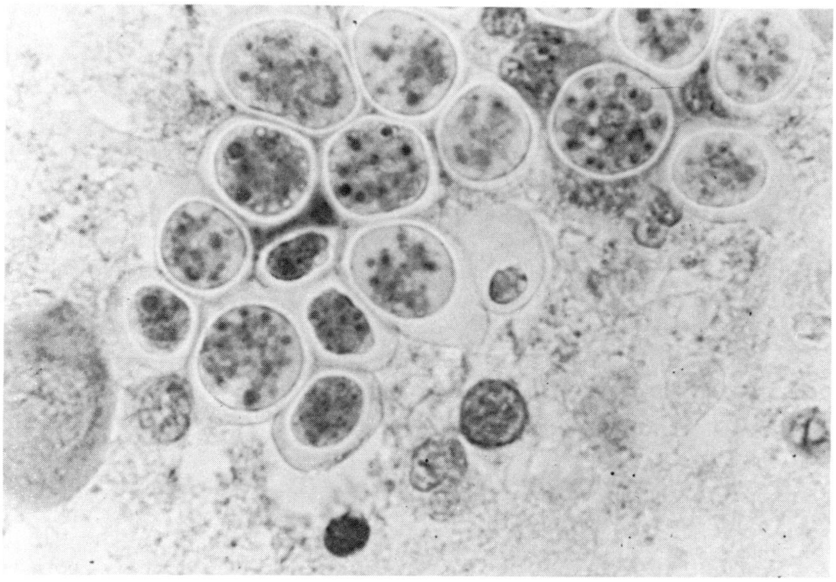

FIGURE 49–19. Impression smear from a nasal mass in a dog with rhinosporidiosis, illustrating the characteristic organism (new methylene blue stain, 100 ×).

formation may be dramatic. Vascular invasion by hyphae with concurrent thrombus formation may occasionally be observed.

Miller has described three histologic patterns of inflammation in canine gastrointestinal phycomycosis.[292] The most prevalent was that of large areas of liquefaction necrosis surrounded by macrophages, epithelioid cells, and giant cells. Additional histopathologic patterns were focal granulomas and areas of liquefaction and focal, well-differentiated granulomas. Mucosal lesions varied, with ulceration, atrophy, and fusion of villi and epithelial cell hyperplasia being present. The submucosa and muscularis mucosae of the gastrointestinal tract were the most severely affected areas.[292, 297, 289] Fungal organisms are found most frequently within areas of liquefaction necrosis.

Cultural Characteristics. Isolation of the etiologic agent from animals with phycomycosis has been inconsistent. However, in light of recent information about the growth characteristics of *Pythium* species, prior culture results may be have been misleading.[296, 299] Tissue specimens should be used as culture material. Sabouraud dextrose agar without cycloheximide is preferred.[1, 10, 11, 124, 225, 291] Specimens should not be refrigerated, as some species can be destroyed by this method of preservation. Most species grow rapidly and best at 98.6°F (37°C).[1, 10, 11, 124, 225, 291]

TREATMENT AND PROGNOSIS

Various therapies have been tried with both the subcutaneous and gastrointestinal forms of phycomycosis. Surgical excision of affected areas, amputation of affected limbs, excision with skin flaps, oral potassium iodide, intravenous and topical amphotericin B, ketoconazole, and a combination of these modalities have not significantly improved the outcome of animals infected with phycomycosis.[289, 290, 297, 298, 302, 304, 315] This is due mainly to the extensive involvement of the skin or gastrointestinal tract when animals are initially presented to veterinarians for diagnosis and treatment. If diagnoses are made early in the disease process and the affected area is amenable to removal, surgical excision seems to be the most effective means of therapy.[297, 298, 304, 307]

Prognosis for the subcutaneous and gastrointestinal forms of phycomycosis is poor. Local recurrence at the surgical site due to inadequate removal is the most common problem associated with subcutaneous involvement.[304] In one study, fewer than 5 per cent of dogs survived while 16 per cent of surgically treated cases were alive in another review.[292, 304] It appears that unless additional treatment regimens are identified for phycomycosis, poor response and high mortality rates are to be expected.

RHINOSPORIDIOSIS

ETIOLOGY AND EPIZOOTIOLOGY

Rhinosporidiosis is a rare, chronic infection involving the mucous membranes of the nasal cavity. The etiologic agent is *Rhinosporidium seeberi* (Figure 49–19). The organism has recently been grown on living cells and maintained for seven months.[324] The disease has been reported in dogs but not in cats.[1, 225, 294, 324–328]

Environmental sources of the agent have not been positively identified. The agent has a worldwide distribution, with endemic regions in India, Ceylon, and Argentina.[1, 225] Stagnant fresh water and arid conditions have been associated with infection; however, this has not been fully documented. Most cases in the dog have been reported from the southern United States.[324–328]

R. seeberi undergoes a maturation process in tissues. Juvenile sporangia are unilamellar and nucleated; intermediate stages are bilamellar. Mature sporangia are unilamellar and are 100 μm to 400 μm in diameter. The organism can be demonstrated by hematoxylin-eosin, Gridley's, or periodic acid–Schiff stains. Large numbers of spores may be observed within mature sporangia.

CLINICAL MANIFESTATIONS

Rhinosporidiosis usually affects the mucous membranes of the nasal cavity (Figure 49–20). Involvement of the vagina, penis, subconjunctival sac, and the ears has been reported in human beings.[1, 225] The infection usually involves the anterior nares and is unilateral. Sneezing, epistaxis, and stertorous breathing are the major clinical signs associated with rhinosporidiosis.[1, 225, 324–328] In the dog, 13 cases have been reported, including 7 males and 3 females.

The mass is usually single, polyoid, and located at the anterior nares. The mass may protrude from the nasal orifice and be pedunculated or sessile. The surface is often lobulated and can contain white or yellowish superficial specks on its surface, which are fungal sporangia.[225]

DIAGNOSIS

The diagnosis of *Rhinosporidium* infection is established by demonstration of the organism in nasal exudates or tissue specimens.[1, 225, 294] Histologic examination of tissues reveals a papillomatous hyperplasia of the epithelium with ulceration, and a fibrovascular stroma. An intense inflammatory reaction is usually present surrounding sporangia that have released spores into tissues.[324]

TREATMENT AND PROGNOSIS

Treatment for rhinosporidiosis is usually surgical. The mass can be removed through the external nasal orifice or by rhinotomy. If excision is incomplete, regrowth of the mass may occur. Dapsone has been used to treat rhinosporidiosis in humans. One canine case treated with dapsone had a favorable response but was not clinically cured.[327] The use of this drug is not without potential complications.

PROTOTHECOSIS

ETIOLOGY AND EPIZOOTIOLOGY

The *Prototheca* spp. are colorless algae related to the green alga *Chlorella*.[329–338] Because they lack chlorophyll, the *Prototheca* have a saprophytic, fungus-like mode of nutrition.[329] The cells are spherical to ovoid bodies ranging from 1.3 to 20 μm in diameter.[30, 332, 336, 339, 340] *Prototheca* reproduces by endosporulation and internal cleavage planes may be observed in some larger cells.[330, 331, 335–337, 341] Two species, *Prototheca wickerhamii* and *P. zopfii*, are pathogenic for mammals.[330–332, 335–338, 341–344] *Prototheca wickerhamii* is isolated most commonly from localized cutaneous infections;[332–334, 340–342, 345] *P. zopfii* is usually associated with disseminated disease.[330, 335, 338, 343, 344, 346, 347]

Prototheca are ubiquitous in the environment and have a worldwide distribution.[329, 330, 336, 346] Organisms can be isolated from slime flux from tree wounds, feces of normal animals and human beings, domestic and municipal sewage, soil and water sources contaminated with human or animal wastes, and chlorinated tap water.[329, 330, 334, 336]

The *Prototheca* spp. possess a natural organic polymer, sporopollenin capsule, which is extremely resistant to degradation.[329] This allows them to pass unharmed through the mammalian digestive tract and to survive sewage treatment and water purification procedures.[329] The capsule may also be antigenically relatively inert and protect the organism from host defenses. This may account in part for the minimal inflammatory response associated with many *Prototheca* lesions.

PATHOGENESIS

Animals are probably constantly exposed to *Prototheca* in the environment, yet clinical disease is rare.[329, 330] The rarity of clinical *Prototheca* infections suggests that it is of low virulence or that animals possess a high level of natural resistance to this organism.[329, 330] Depressed

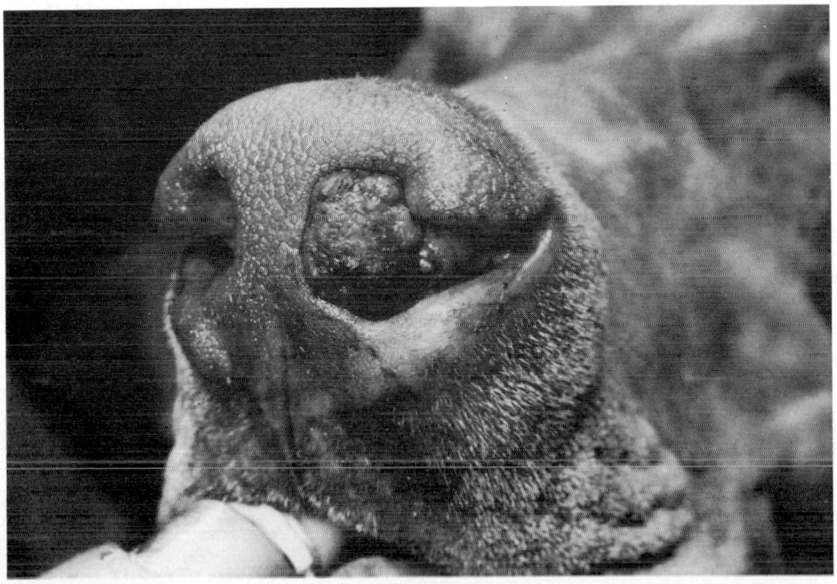

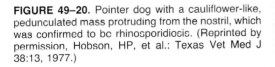

FIGURE 49–20. Pointer dog with a cauliflower-like, pedunculated mass protruding from the nostril, which was confirmed to be rhinosporidiosis. (Reprinted by permission, Hobson, HP, et al.: Texas Vet Med J 38:13, 1977.)

T-cell function and inhibition of neutrophil chemotaxis have been demonstrated in one dog with protothecosis.[343] Whether these immunologic defects were the cause or the result of the *Prototheca* infection is unclear.

The route of infection for *Prototheca* spp. is uncertain. Percutaneous inoculation via trauma or wound contamination is the most likely source of localized cutaneous infections.[329, 341] The frequency and severity of colonic lesions in dogs with protothecosis suggests that this might be an important portal of entry in this species.[329, 330, 335, 336, 338, 343, 344, 346, 348, 349] However, in experimental studies, *Prototheca* infection was not established by ingestion alone in dogs, rodents, or monkeys.[329]

CLINICAL MANIFESTATIONS

In the cat, three cases of the cutaneous form of protothecosis have been reported.[330, 332, 339, 342] The disease produced solitary, soft or firm, mass lesions on the limbs or head.[330, 332, 339, 342] Affected animals were over eight years of age; no breed or sex predilection has been established.[332, 339, 342]

Canine protothecosis is usually a disseminated disease that produces a variable spectrum of clinical signs.[330, 335, 336, 338, 343, 344, 346–351] The age range of affected dogs is from 1.5 to 10 years with no apparent age predilection.[330, 338, 350] Seven of 25 reported cases have occurred in collies; the occurrence in other breeds is sporadic.[330, 331, 338, 344, 346, 349, 351] Females outnumber males (12:6) in reports in which the sex is recorded.[330, 331, 335, 336, 338, 344, 346, 348–350]

Colonic involvement occurs in many dogs, causing a chronic, intermittent, bloody diarrhea.[330, 331, 335, 336, 338, 343, 344, 346, 348, 349] Ocular lesions are frequently present, including chorioretinitis, exudative retinitis with retinal detachment, anterior uveitis, and panophthalmitis.[330, 335, 343, 344, 346, 347, 349–351] Central nervous system (CNS) infection has been seen in a number of dogs, causing paresis, vestibular deficits, seizures, and deafness.[330, 333, 335, 338, 346] Kidney involvement may produce signs of renal insufficiency.[343, 348] Myocardial lesions are present in some dogs, but clinical evidence of cardiac dysrhythmias or failure has not been reported.[331, 343, 346–348, 350] Cutaneous protothecosis involving the skin or footpads has been reported in three dogs.[330] The lesions were deeper and more extensive than those reported in cats, affecting large areas of skin, subcutaneous tissue, and some regional lymph nodes.[330]

DIAGNOSIS

Hematologic parameters are often normal;[335, 338, 346, 347, 349, 350] neutrophilic leukocytosis has been seen in several dogs.[343, 344, 348] Biochemical profiles may be normal or reveal only minimal changes.[331, 335, 343, 344, 346, 347, 349, 350] Moderate increases in serum liver enzymes, blood urea nitrogen, or creatinine levels have been reported in a few cases.[330, 338, 343] The cerebrospinal fluid (CSF) revealed an eosinophilic pleocytosis and elevated protein level in a dog with CNS involvement.[330, 335]

Proctoscopic examination may reveal diffuse thickening, reddening, and hemorrhage in the colonic and rectal mucosa.[348] Radiographic examinations have not been performed in most cases; a barium contrast gastrointestinal study demonstrated thickening of the large and small intestinal walls in one dog[331] and shortening and thickening of the colon in another.[348]

The diagnosis of protothecosis is made most readily by identification of the organism on cytologic or histopathologic examination.[331, 335, 336, 338, 343, 348, 350] Tissues should be selected for evaluation on the basis of the clinical signs exhibited by the patient. *Prototheca* have been recovered from rectal scrapings and biopsies, aspirates of cutaneous masses, CSF, the vitreous or aqueous humor of the eye, and biopsies of other affected tissues.[331, 335, 336, 338, 343, 348, 350] *Prototheca* organisms may stain poorly with hematoxylin-eosin but are more clearly defined by Giemsa, GMS, or PAS techniques[332, 333, 338, 339] (Figures 49–21 and 49–22). In some lesions, the organisms may be surrounded by a mixed inflammatory exudate with plasma cells, lymphocytes, and macrophages predominating.[330, 333, 338, 339] Often there is little cellular response associated with the masses of infiltrating organisms.[330, 347, 348, 350]

Definitive diagnosis and speciation of *Prototheca* can be determined by fluorescent antibody techniques performed on formalin-fixed tissues or unstained tissue sections at the Centers for Disease Control in Atlanta, Georgia.[330, 338, 343] Pathogenic *Prototheca* spp. grow well on blood agar incubated at 37°C, producing small, flat, nonhemolytic, gray-white colonies within 72 hours.[335, 337, 340] On Sabouraud's agar incubated at 25°C, light tan to white, waxy, yeast-like colonies appear within 72 hours.[335, 337, 340, 344] Organisms taken from cultures can be readily identified with Gram's iodine stain.[335, 337, 338]

TREATMENT

The treatment of choice for cutaneous protothecosis in human beings or animals is surgical removal of affected tissues.[333, 340] One of three cats apparently responded to excision of a well-circumscribed cutaneous lesion; however, long-term follow-up was not reported.[339] In human beings with cutaneous disease, cure was also achieved in several patients with amphotericin B alone, amphotericin B in combination with tetracycline, or ketoconazole alone.[330, 333, 340, 341, 345]

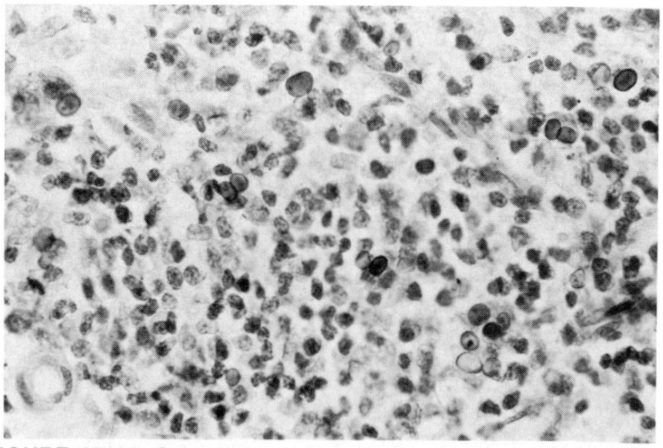

FIGURE 49–21. Colon biopsy specimen from a three-year-old boxer with protothecal colitis, demonstrating numerous organisms widely distributed throughout the lamina propria and muscularis. Inflammatory cellular infiltrate is sparse and consists of scattered mononuclear cells (H&E, 40 ×).

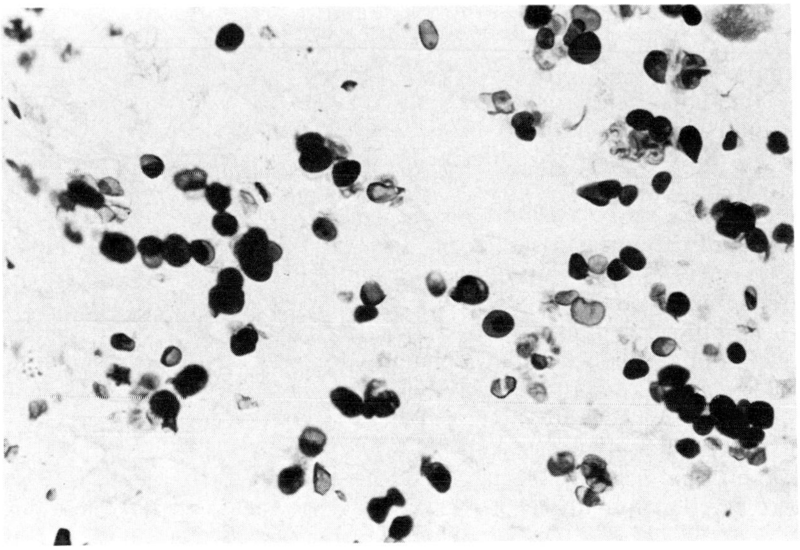

FIGURE 49–22. Similar section to Figure 49–21 stained with GMS provides better definition of the extent of the *Prototheca* invasion (40 ×).

Disseminated protothecosis is extremely rare in human beings. One person with disseminated protothecosis was reported to have responded to treatment with amphotericin B and transfer factor.[330] In reports of in vitro susceptibility studies of *P. zopfii* isolates from animals, about one-third to one-half of the strains were susceptible to gentamicin sulfate, amphotericin B, or polymyxin B, and all isolates were susceptible to nystatin.[352, 353] However, to date, amphotericin B, ketoconazole, oral nystatin with tetracycline, and simazine (a fishtank algicide) have not been effective in the treatment of disseminated protothecosis in dogs.[127, 330, 347]

PROGNOSIS

The prognosis for cutaneous protothecosis is guarded and depends on the extent and depth of the lesions. Disseminated protothecosis in dogs has not been responsive to treatment and the prognosis for this form of the disease is grave.

References

1. Jungerman, PF, Schwartzman, RM: Veterinary Medical Mycology. Philadelphia, WB Saunders, 1972.
2. Savage, A, et al.: North American blastomycosis in a dog. Can Vet J 3:260, 1962.
3. Barsanti, JA: Blastomycosis. *In* Greene, CE (ed): Clinical Microbiology and Infectious Diseases of the Dog and Cat. Philadelphia, WB Saunders, 1984, p 675.
4. Easton, KL: Cutaneous North American blastomycosis in a Siamese cat. Can Vet J 2:350, 1961.
5. Sheldon, WF: Pulmonary blastomycosis in a cat. Lab Anim Care 16:280, 1966.
6. Ajello, L: Comparative ecology of respiratory mycotic disease agents. Bacteriol Rev 31:6, 1967.
7. Ausherman, RJ, et al.: Clinical signs of blastomycosis in the dog. JAVMA 130:541, 1957.
8. Neunzig, RJ: Epidemiology, diagnosis and treatment of canine and feline blastomycosis. VM/SAC 78:1081, 1983.
9. Soltys, MA, Sumner-Smith, G: Systemic mycosis in dogs and cats. Can Vet J 12:191, 1971.
10. Chandler, FW, et al.: *In* Color Atlas and Text of the Histopathology of Mycotic Disease. Chicago, Yearbook Medical Publishers, 1980, p 39.
11. Rippon, JW: Medical Mycology. 2nd ed, Philadelphia, WB Saunders, 1982, p 125.
12. Shadomy, S and Dixon, DM: *Blastomyces* and *Paracoccidioides*. *In* Braude, AI (ed): Infectious Diseases and Medical Microbiology, 2nd ed, Philadelphia, WB Saunders, 1986, p 589.
13. Tuttle, JG, et al.: Systemic North American blastomycosis. Report of a case with small forms of blastomycosis. Am J Clin Path 23:890, 1953.
14. Schwarz, J and Baum, L: Blastomycosis. Am J Clin Pathol 21:999, 1951.
15. Madsen, DE: Some studies of three pathogenic fungi isolated from animals. Cornell Vet 32:383, 1942.
16. McDonough, ES: Blastomycosis—epidemiology and biology of its etiologic agent *Ajellomyces dermatitidis*. Mycopathol Myco Appl 41:195, 1970.
17. Attleberger, MH: Systemic Mycoses. *In* Kirk, RW (ed): Current Veterinary Therapy VIII. Philadelphia, WB Saunders, 1983, p 1180.
18. Furcolow, ML, et al.: Prevalence and incidence studies of human and canine blastomycosis. II. Yearly incidence studies in 3 selected states, 1960–1967. Am J Epidemiol 92:121, 1970.
19. Furcolow, ML, et al.: Prevalence and incidence studies of human and canine blastomycosis. I. Cases in the US, 1885–1968. Am Rev Respir Dis 102:60, 1970.
20. Menges, RW: Blastomycosis in animals. Vet Med 55:45, 1960.
21. Selby, LA, et al.: Epidemiologic risk factors associated with canine systemic mycoses. Am J Epidemiol 113:133, 1981.
22. Foster, RC and Dunn, TJ: Blastomycosis: A practical therapeutic approach. VM/SAC 2:200, 1981.
23. Gnann, JW, et al.: Human blastomycosis after a dogbite. Ann Intern Med 98:48, 1983.
24. Jaspers, RJ: Transmission of blastomyces from animals to man. JAVMA 164:8, 1974.
25. Ebert, JW, et al.: Experimental canine histoplasmosis and blastomycosis. Mycopathol Myco Appl 45:285, 1971.
26. Furcolow, ML, et al.: Supportive evidence by field testing and laboratory experiment for a new hypothesis of the ecology and pathogenicity of canine blastomycosis. Sabouraudia 12:22, 1974.
27. Smith, CD, et al.: Distribution of *Blastomyces dermatitidis* in dogs with skin test and serologic results following airborne infections. Sabouraudia 13:192, 1975.
28. Turner, C, et al.: Experimental histoplasmosis and blastomycosis in young pups. Sabouraudia 12:188, 1971.
29. Small, E: The Mycoses. *In* Ettinger, SJ (ed): Textbook of Veterinary Internal Medicine. Philadelphia, WB Saunders, 1975, p 181.

30. Macy, DW, Small, E: Deep Mycotic Infections. *In* Ettinger, SJ (ed): Textbook of Veterinary Internal Medicine. Philadelphia, WB Saunders, 1983, p 237.
31. Fadok, VA: Dermatologic manifestations of the subcutaneous and deep mycoses. Comp Cont Ed Pract Vet 2:506, 1980.
32. Higgins, RJ: Experimental canine blastomycosis with particular reference to lesions in the central nervous system and eye. Master's Thesis. Auburn, Alabama, Auburn University, 1978.
33. Legendre, AM, et al.: Canine blastomycosis: A review of 47 clinical cases. JAVMA 178:1163, 1981.
34. Pyle, RL, et al.: Canine blastomycosis. Comp Cont Ed Pract Vet 3:963, 1981.
35. Roberts, RE: Osteomyelitis associated with disseminated blastomycosis in nine dogs. J Am Vet Radiol Soc 20:124, 1979.
36. Maksia, D, et al.: Canine blastomycosis and canine histoplasmosis. Vet Scope 7:10, 1962.
37. Scott, MJ: Cutaneous blastomycosis: report of a case following a dog bite. Northwest Med 54:245, 1955.
38. Menges, RW, et al.: Clinical and epidemiologic studies on seventy-nine canine blastomycosis cases in Arkansas. Am J Epidemiol 81:164, 1965.
39. Walker, MA: Thoracic blastomycosis: A review of its radiographic manifestations in 40 dogs. Vet Rad 22:22, 1981.
40. Alden, C and Mohan, R: Ocular blastomycosis in a cat. JAVMA 164:527, 1974.
41. Campbell, KL, et al.: Cutaneous blastomycosis. Feline Pract 10:28, 1980.
42. Hatkin, JM, et al.: Two cases of feline blastomycosis. JAAHA 15:217, 1979.
43. Jasmin, AM, et al.: Systemic blastomycosis in Siamese cats. VM/SAC 64:33, 1969.
44. Ditchfield, J and Fischer, JB: North American blastomycosis in the dog. Can Vet J 2:103, 1961.
45. Albert, RA, et al.: Ocular blastomycosis in the dog. Comp Cont Ed Pract Vet 3:303, 1981.
46. Wilson, RW, et al.: Urogenital and ocular lesions in canine blastomycosis. Vet Pathol 10:1, 1973.
47. Bistner, S, et al.: Diseases of the uveal tract. Part III. Comp Cont Ed Pract Vet 2:46, 1980.
48. Simon, J and Helper, LC: Ocular disease associated with blastomycosis in the dog. JAVMA 157:922, 1970.
49. Nasissee, MP, et al.: Ocular changes in a cat with disseminated blastomycosis. JAVMA 187:629, 1985.
50. Buyukmichi, N: Ocular lesions of blastomycosis in the dog. JAVMA 180:426, 1982.
51. Savage, A, et al.: North American blastomycosis in a dog. Can Vet J 3:260, 1962.
52. Stubb, WJ, et al.: Blastomycosis in a hunting dog. Can Vet J 13:125, 1972.
53. McEwen, SA and Hulland, TJ: Cerebral blastomycosis in a dog. Can Vet J 25:411, 1984.
54. Welsh, RD: Feline blastomycosis. Southwest Vet 35:13, 1982.
55. Carakostas, MC, et al.: Clinical laboratory evaluation of deep mycotic diseases in dogs. J Sm Anim Pract 25:687, 1984.
56. Legendre, AM and Becker, PU: Evaluation of the agar-gel immunodiffusion test in the diagnosis of canine blastomycosis. Am J Vet Res 41:2109, 1980.
57. Dow, SW, et al.: Hypercalcemia associated with blastomycosis in dogs. JAVMA 188:706, 1986.
58. Nafe, LA, et al.: Central nervous system involvement of blastomycosis in the dog. JAAHA 19:933, 1983.
59. Roudebush, P: Mycotic pneumonias. Vet Clin North Am 15:949, 1985.
60. Nielson, SW: Laboratory diagnosis of systemic mycoses in dogs. Mod Vet Pract 60:210, 1979.
61. O'Hara, M: Histopathologic diagnosis of fungal diseases. Infect Control 7:78, 1986.
62. Barta, O, et al.: Counterimmunoelectrophoresis (immunoelectroosmosis) and serum electrophoretic pattern in serologic diagnosis of canine blastomycosis. Am J Vet Res 44:218, 1980.
63. Khansari, N, et al.: Diagnosis of blastomycosis by an antiglobulin hemagglutination test. Am J Vet Res 43:2279, 1982.
64. Legendre, AM and Becker, PU: Evaluation of the agar-gel immunodiffusion test in the diagnosis of canine blastomycosis. Am J Vet Res 41:2109, 1980.
65. Phillips, WE and Kaufman, L: Cultural and histopathologic confirmation of canine blastomycosis diagnosed by an agar-gel immunodiffusion test. Am J Vet Res 41:1263, 1980.
66. Porter, BM, et al.: Correlation of fluorescent antibody histopathology and culture on tissues from 372 animals examined for histoplasmosis and blastomycosis. J Bacteriol 89:748, 1965.
67. Turner, S, et al.: Diagnostic assessment of an enzyme-linked immunosorbent assay for human and canine blastomycosis. J Clin Microbiol 23:294, 1986.
68. Jackson, JA: Immunodiagnosis of systemic mycoses in animals: A review. JAVMA 188:702, 1986.
69. McMurray, TS: Successful clinical treatment of localized blastomycosis in a dog. VM/SAC 62:341, 1967.
70. Ausherman, RJ: Treatment of blastomycosis and histoplasmosis in the dog. JAVMA 163:1048, 1973.
71. Ausherman, RJ: Amphotericin B dosage for ocular diseases. JAVMA 164:438, 1974.
72. Dunbar, M and Pyle, RL: Ketoconazole treatment of osseous blastomycosis in a dog. VM/SAC 76:1593, 1981.
73. Dunbar, M, et al.: Treatment of canine blastomycosis with ketoconazole. JAVMA 182:156, 1983.
74. Legendre, AM, et al.: Treatment of canine blastomycosis with amphotericin B and ketoconazole. JAVMA 184:1249, 1984.
75. Moriello, KA: Ketoconazole: Clinical pharmacology and therapeutic recommendations. JAVMA 188:303, 1986.
76. Greene, CE, et al.: Antimicrobial Chemotherapy. *In* Greene, CE (ed): Clinical Microbiology and Infectious Diseases of the Dog and Cat. Philadelphia, WB Saunders, 1983, p 172.
77. Pyle, RL: Clinical pharmacology of amphotericin B. JAVMA 179:83, 1981.
78. Hermans, PF and Keys, TF: Antifungal agents used for deep seated mycotic infections. Mayo Clin Proc 58:223, 1983.
79. Medoff, G and Kobayashi, GS: Strategies in the treatment of systemic fungal infections. N Eng J Med 302:145, 1980.
80. Bindschadler, DD and Bennett, JE: A pharmacologic guide to the clinical use of amphotericin B. J Infect Dis 120:427, 1969.
81. Hoeprich, PP: Chemotherapy of systemic fungal disease. Ann Rev Pharmacol Toxicol 18:205, 1978.
82. Feldman, HA, et al.: Amphotericin B therapy in an anephric patient. Antimicrob Agents Chemother 4:302, 1973.
83. Butler, WT, et al.: Amphotericin B renal toxicity in the dog. J Pharmacol Exp Ther 143:47, 1963.
84. McCurdy, DK, et al.: Renal tubular acidosis due to amphotericin B. N Eng J Med 278:124, 1968.
85. Gouge, TH and Andriole, VT: Experimental model of amphotericin B nephrotoxicity with renal tubular acidosis. J Lab Clin Med 78:713, 1971.
86. Patterson, RM and Ackerman, GL: Renal tubular acidosis due to amphotericin nephrotoxicity. Arch Int Med 127:241, 1971.
87. Oliverio, JJ, et al.: Mitigation of amphotericin B nephrotoxicity by mannitol. Br Med J 1:550, 1975.
88. Hellenbusch, AA, et al.: The use of mannitol to reduce the nephrotoxicity of amphotericin B. Surg Gyn Obst 134:241, 1972.
89. Gerkens, JF and Branch, RA: The influence of sodium status and furosemide on canine acute amphotericin B nephrotoxicity. J Pharmacol Exp Ther 214:306, 1980.
90. Heidemann, HT, et al.: Amphotericin B nephrotoxicity in humans decreased by salt repletion. Am J Med 75:476, 1983.
91. Reiner, NE and Thompson, WL: Dopamine and saralasin antagonism of renal vasoconstriction and oliguria caused by amphotericin B in dogs. J Inf Dis 140:564, 1979.
92. Bullock, WE, et al.: Can mannitol reduce amphotericin B nephrotoxicity? Antimicrob Agents Chemother 10:555, 1976.
93. Macy, DW: The effects of bicarbonate and mannitol on amphotericin B nephrotoxicity in the dog. Master's Thesis, University of Illinois, Urbana, 1978.
94. Butler, WT and Hill, GJ: Intravenous administration of amphotericin B in the dog. JAVMA 144:399, 1964.
95. Bradsher, RW, et al.: Ketoconazole therapy for endemic blastomycosis. Ann Intern Med 103:872, 1985.
96. Treatment of blastomycosis and histoplasmosis with ketoconazole. Results of a prospective randomized clinical trial. Ann Intern Med 103:861, 1986.
97. Van Den Bossche, H, et al.: In vitro and in vivo effect of the antimycotic drug ketoconazole on sterol synthesis. Antimicrob Agents Chemother 17:922, 1980.

98. Sud, IJ and Feingold, DS: Mechanisms of action of the antimycotic imidazoles. J Invest Dermatol 76:438, 1981.
99. Heel, RC, et al.: Ketoconazole, a review of its therapeutic efficacy in superficial and systemic fungal infections. Drug 23:1, 1982.
100. Swatek, FE: The epidemiology of coccidioidomycosis. *In* Al-Doory, Y (ed): The Epidemiology of Human Mycotic Diseases. Springfield, Charles C Thomas, 1975, p 74.
101. Pappagianis, D: Coccidioidomycosis. *In* Di Salvo, A (ed): Occupational Mycoses. Philadelphia, Lea & Febiger, 1983, p 13.
102. Pappagianis, D: Epidemiology of Coccidioidomycosis. *In* Stevens, DA (ed) Coccidioidomycosis: A Text. New York, Plenum Medical Book Co, 1980, p 97.
103. Maddy, KT: Disseminated coccidioidomycosis of the dog. JAVMA 132:483, 1958.
104. Millman, TM, et al.: Coccidioidomycosis in the dog: its radiographic diagnosis. J Am Vet Radiol Soc 20:50, 1979.
105. Wolf, AM: Primary cutaneous coccidioidomycosis in a dog and a cat. JAVMA 174:504, 1979.
106. Pappagianis, D: Serology and Serodiagnosis of Coccidioidomycosis. *In* Stevens, DA (ed) Coccidioidomycosis: A Text. New York, Plenum Medical Book Co, 1980, p 97.
107. Barsanti, JA, Jeffery, KL: Coccidioidomycosis. *In* Greene, CE (ed): Clinical Microbiology and Infectious Diseases of the Dog and Cat. Philadelphia, WB Saunders, 1984, p 710.
108. Drutz, DJ: Urban coccidioidomycosis and histoplasmosis. N Engl J Med 301:381, 1979.
109. Martorana, FS: Coccidioidomycosis (San Joaquin valley fever) in a dog in central New York. VM/SAC 78(2):185, 1983.
110. Armstrong, PJ and DiBartola, SP: Canine coccidioidomycosis: a literature review and report of eight cases. JAAHA 19:937, 1983.
111. Angell, JA, et al.: Ocular coccidioidomycosis in a cat. JAVMA 187:167, 1985.
112. Schwartz, W: *Coccidioides immitis* infection in a cat. Southwest Vet 34:94, 1981.
113. Stevens, DA: Immunology of Coccidioidomycosis. *In* Stevens, DA (ed): Coccidioidomycosis: A Text. New York, Plenum Medical Book Co, 1980, p 87.
114. Drutz, DJ: Amphotericin B in the treatment of coccidioidomycosis. Drugs 26:337, 1983.
115. Owens, J, et al.: Polyostotic coccidioidomycosis in a dog. Vet Radiol 22:83, 1981.
116. Stowater, JL: Canine coccidioidomycosis: A case report. VM/SAC 75:627, 1980.
117. Stevens, DA: Coccidioidal meningitis. In Braude, AI, et al. (eds): Infectious Diseases and Medical Microbiology. Philadelphia, WB Saunders, 1986, p 1074.
118. Marks, DL: Treatment of coccidioidomycosis with ketoconazole. Canine Prac 10(4):35, 1983.
119. Schalm, OW: Coccidioidomycosis-myelomatosis complex in a dog. Canine Prac 6(3):52, 1979.
120. Warlick, MA, et al.: Rapid diagnosis of pulmonary coccidioidomycosis. Arch Int Med 143:723, 1983.
121. Huppert, M and Sun, SH: Mycological Diagnosis of Coccidioidomycosis. *In* Stevens, DA (ed): Coccidioidomycosis: A Text. New York, Plenum Medical Book Co, 1980, p 47.
122. Jackson, JA, et al.: Treatment of canine coccidioidomycosis with ketoconazole: serological aspects of a case study. JAAHA 21:572, 1985.
123. Kirkland, TN: Coccidioidomycosis. In Braude, AI, et al. (eds): Infectious Diseases and Medical Microbiology. Philadelphia, WB Saunders, 1986, p 867.
124. Al-Doory, Y: Laboratory Medical Mycology. Philadelphia, Lea & Febiger, 1980, p 213.
125. Huppert, M and Sun, SH: Overview of Mycology and the Mycology of *Coccidioides immitis*. *In* Stevens, DA (ed): Coccidioidomycosis: A Text. New York, Plenum Medical Book Co, 1980, p 21.
126. Jacobs, P H: Cutaneous coccidioidomycosis. In Stevens, DA (ed): Coccidioidomycosis: A Text. New York, Plenum Medical Book Co, 1980, p 213.
127. Wolf, AM: Unpublished observations.
128. Graybill, JR, et al.: Treatment of murine coccidioidal meningitis with fluconazole (UK 49,858). J Med Vet Mycol 24:113, 1986.
129. Stevens, DA, et al.: Experience with ketoconazole in three major manifestations of progressive coccidioidomycosis. Am J Med 70:58, 1983.
130. Varkey, B: Oral antifungal therapy: current status of ketoconazole. Postgrad Med 73:52, 1983.
131. Galgiani, JN: Ketoconazole in the treatment of coccidioidomycosis. Drugs 26:355, 1983.
132. Wolf, AM and Pappagianis, D: Canine coccidioidomycosis. Treatment with a new antifungal agent: ketoconazole. Calif Vet 35:25, 1981.
133. Domer, JE and Moser, SA: Histoplasmosis—a review. Rev Med Vet Mycol 15:159, 1980.
134. Barsanti, JA: Histoplasmosis. In Greene, CE (ed): Clinical Microbiology and Infectious Diseases of the Dog and Cat. Philadelphia, WB Saunders, 1984, p 687.
135. Larsh, HW and Hall, NK: *Histoplasma capsulatum*. *In* Braude, AI, et al. (eds): Infectious Diseases and Medical Microbiology. Philadelphia, WB Saunders, 1986, p 580.
136. Larsh, HW: The Epidemiology of Histoplasmosis. *In* Al-Doory, Y (ed): The Epidemiology of Human Mycotic Diseases. Springfield, Charles C Thomas, 1975, p 52.
137. Kabli, S, et al.: Endemic canine and feline histoplasmosis in El Paso, Texas. J Med Vet Mycol 24:41, 1986.
138. Larsh, HW: Histoplasmosis. *In* Di Salvo, A (ed): Occupational Mycoses. Philadelphia, Lea & Febiger, 1983, p 29.
139. Breitschwerdt, EB, et al.: Feline histoplasmosis. JAAHA 13:216, 1977.
140. Ford, RB: Canine histoplasmosis. Comp Cont Ed Pract Vet 2:637, 1980.
141. Gabbert, NH, et al.: Pancytopenia associated with disseminated histoplasmosis in a cat. JAAHA 20:119, 1984.
142. Noxon, JO, et al.: Disseminated histoplasmosis in a cat: successful treatment with ketoconazole. JAVMA 181:817, 1982.
143. Mahaffey, E, et al.: Disseminated histoplasmosis in three cats. JAAHA 13:46, 1977.
144. Forjaz, MH and Fischman, O: Animal histoplasmosis in Brazil. Mykosen 28:191, 1985.
145. Clinkenbeard, KD, et al.: Disseminated histoplasmosis in the cat: 12 cases (1981-1986). JAVMA 190:1445, 1987.
146. Wolf, AM and Belden, MN: Feline histoplasmosis: a literature review and retrospective study of 20 new cases. JAAHA 20:995, 1984.
147. Stickle, JE and Hribernik, TN: Clinicopathological observations in disseminated histoplasmosis in dogs. JAAHA 14:105, 1978.
148. Sarosi, GA and Davies, SF: Histoplasmosis. *In* Braude, AI, et al. (eds): Infectious Diseases and Medical Microbiology. Philadelphia, WB Saunders, 1986, p 863.
149. Burk, RL, et al.: The radiographic appearance of pulmonary histoplasmosis in the dog and cat: a review of 37 case histories. J Am Vet Radiol Soc 19:2, 1978.
150. Stark, DR: Primary gastrointestinal histoplasmosis in a cat. JAAHA 18:154, 1982.
151. Dillon, AR, et al.: Canine abdominal histoplasmosis: a report of four cases. JAAHA 18:498, 1982.
152. DaCosta, EO, et al.: Experimental histoplasmosis. I. Puppies exposed to a natural reservoir of *H. capsulatum*. Int J Zoonoses 8:77, 1981.
153. Percy, DH: Feline histoplasmosis with ocular involvement. Vet Pathol 18:163, 1981.
154. Blass, CE: Histoplasmosis in a cat. JAAHA 18:468, 1982.
155. Wolf, AM and Green, RW: The radiographic appearance of pulmonary histoplasmosis in the cat. Vet Radiol 28:34, 1987.
156. Gwin, RM, et al.: Multifocal ocular histoplasmosis in a dog and cat. JAVMA 176:638, 1980.
157. Peiffer, RL, Jr, and Belkin, PV: Ocular manifestations of disseminated histoplasmosis in a cat. Feline Pract 9:24, 1979.
158. Lenarduzzi, RF and Jones, L: Diagnosing pulmonary histoplasmosis despite nonspecific signs. Vet Med 81:412, 1986.
159. Weissman, S and Acampado, EE: Primary pulmonary histoplasmosis in a cat. Feline Pract 5:28, 1975.
160. Aronson, E, et al.: Disseminated histoplasmosis with osseous lesions in a cat with feline lymphosarcoma. Vet Radiol 27:50, 1986.
161. Goad, MEP and Roenigk, WJ: Osseous histoplasmosis in a cat. Feline Pract 13:32, 1983.
162. Mitchell, M and Stark, DR: Disseminated canine histoplasmosis: a clinical survey of 24 cases in Texas. Can Vet J 21:95, 1980.

163. Shelton, GD, et al.: Disseminated histoplasmosis with bone lesions in a dog. JAAHA 18:143, 1982.
164. Echols, JT: Histoplasmosis in a dog. Mod Vet Pract 61:1009, 1980.
165. Hoffman, D, et al.: Suspected *Histoplasma capsulati* of the intestine in a dog. Aust Vet J 62:390, 1985.
166. VanSteenhouse, JL and DeNovo, RC, Jr: Atypical *Histoplasma capsulatum* infection in a dog. JAVMA 188:527, 1986.
167. Dunbar, M Jr and Taylor, CE: Histoplasmosis in a dog. Canine Pract 8:9, 1981.
168. Olson, GA and Wowk, BJ: Oral lesions of histoplasmosis in a dog. VM/SAC 76:1449, 1981.
169. Ackerman, N, et al.: Respiratory distress associated with *Histoplasma*-induced tracheobronchial lymphadenopathy in dogs. JAVMA 163:963, 1973.
170. Schaer, M, et al.: Central nervous system disease due to histoplasmosis in a dog: a case report. JAAHA 19:311, 1983.
171. Lau, RE, et al.: *Histoplasma capsulatum* infection in a metatarsal of a dog. JAVMA 172: 1414, 1978.
172. Burk, RL and Jones, BD: Disseminated histoplasmosis with osseous involvement in a dog. JAVMA 172:1416, 1978.
173. Ackerman, N and Spencer, CP: Radiologic aspects of mycotic diseases. Vet Clin North Am 12:175, 1982.
174. Slama, TG: Treatment of disseminated and progressive cavitary histoplasmosis with ketoconazole. Am J Med 70:70, 1983.
175. Dunlap, MD and Goodpasture, HC: Histoplasmosis therapy. Kans Med 87:127, 1986.
176. Graybill, JR, et al.: Combination therapy of experimental histoplasmosis and cryptococcosis with amphotericin B and ketoconazole. Rev Infect Dis 2:551, 1980.
177. Shadomy, S, et al.: Treatment of systemic mycoses with ketoconazole: studies of ketoconazole serum levels. Mykosen 29:195, 1986.
178. Kobayashi, GS, et al.: Comparison of in vitro and in vivo activity of the bis-triazole derivative UK 49,858 with that of amphotericin B against *Histoplasma capsulatum*. Antimicrob Agents Chemother 29:660, 1986.
179. Gordon, MA: Cryptococcosis. *In* Di Salvo, A (ed): Occupational Mycoses. Philadelphia, Lea & Febiger, 1983, p 1.
180. Davis, CE: Cryptococcosis. *In* Braude, AI, et al. (eds): Infectious Diseases and Medical Microbiology. Philadelphia, WB Saunders, 1986, p 564.
181. Cohen, J: The pathogenesis of cryptococcosis. J Infect 5:109,1982.
182. Barsanti, JA: Cryptococcosis. *In* Greene, CE (ed): Clinical Microbiology and Infectious Diseases of the Dog and Cat. Philadelphia, WB Saunders, 1984, p 700.
183. Medoff, G: Cryptococcal Meningitis. *In* Braude, AI, et al. (ed): Infectious Diseases and Medical Microbiology. Philadelphia, WB Saunders, 1986, p 1072.
184. Jergens, AE, et al.: Cryptococcosis involving the eye and central nervous system of a dog. JAVMA 189:302, 1986.
185. Barrett, RE and Scott, DW: Treatment of feline cryptococcosis: literature review and case report. JAAHA 11:511, 1975.
186. Palmer, AC, et al.: Cryptococcal infection of the central nervous system of a dog in the United Kingdom. J Sm Anim Pract 22:579, 1981.
187. Wilkinson, GT: Feline cryptococcosis: a review and seven case reports. J Sm Anim Pract 20:749, 1979.
188. Brown, RJ, et al.: Dermal cryptococcosis in a cat. Mod Vet Pract 59:447, 1978.
189. Medlau, L, et al.: Cutaneous cryptococcosis in three cats. JAVMA 187:169, 1985.
190. Willard, MD: Cryptococcosis. Calif Vet 12:13, 1982.
191. Legendre, AM, et al.: Treatment of feline cryptococcosis with ketoconazole. JAVMA 181:1541, 1982.
192. Madewell, BR, et al.: Lymphosarcoma and cryptococcosis in a cat. JAVMA 175:65, 1979.
193. MacDonald, DW and Stretch, HC: Canine cryptococcosis associated with prolonged corticosteroid therapy. Can Vet J 23:200, 1982.
194. Sawchuk, SA: Apparent iatrogenic precipitation of CNS cryptococcosis in a dog. Canine Pract 9:43, 1982.
195. Moore, R: Treatment of feline nasal cryptococcosis with 5-flucytosine. JAVMA 181:816, 1982.
196. Rosenthal, JJ, et al.: Ocular and systemic cryptococcosis in a cat. JAAHA 17:307, 1981.
197. Noxon, JO, et al.: Ketoconazole therapy in canine and feline cryptococcosis. JAAHA 22:179, 1986.
198. Gwin, RM, et al.: Ocular cryptococcosis in a cat. JAAHA 13:680, 1977.
199. Pentlarge, VW and Martin, RA: Treatment of cryptococcosis in three cats using ketoconazole. JAVMA 188:536, 1986.
200. Thrall, MA, et al.: Feline cryptococcosis treatment with amphotericin B. Feline Pract 6:15, 1976.
201. Weir, EC, et al.: Short-term combination chemotherapy for treatment of feline cryptococcosis. JAVMA 174:507, 1979.
202. Moore, DR and Bullmore, CC: Pulmonary cryptococcosis in a cat. Feline Pract 14:14, 1984.
203. Ryer, K and Ryer, J: A case of feline mycotic rhinitis caused by *Cryptococcus neoformans*. VM/SAC 76:1150, 1981.
204. Wilkinson, GT, et al.: Successful treatment of four cases of feline cryptococcosis. J Sm Anim Pract 24:507, 1983.
205. Prevost, E, et al.: Successful medical management of severe feline cryptococcosis. JAAHA 18:111, 1982.
206. Buchanan, CA: Feline cryptococcosis: case report and review. Southwest Vet 35:41, 1982.
207. Rutman, MA, et al.: Feline cryptococcosis. Feline Pract 5:36,1975.
208. Sisk, DB and Chandler, FW: Phaeohyphomycosis and cryptococcosis in a cat. Vet Pathol 19:554, 1982.
209. Schulman, J: Ketoconazole for successful treatment of cryptococcosis in a cat. JAVMA 187:508, 1985.
210. Pal, M and Mehrothra, BS: Occurrence and etiologic significance of *Cryptococcus neoformans* in a cutaneous lesion of a cat. Mykosen 26:608, 1983.
211. Pal, M and Mehrothra, BS: Studies on the occurrence of cryptococcal meningitis in small animals. Mykosen 28:607, 1985.
212. Rebhun, WC and Edwards, NJ: Cryptococcosis involving the orbit of a dog. VM/SAC 73:1447, 1977.
213. Carlton, WW, et al.: Disseminated cryptococcosis with ocular involvement in a dog. JAAHA 12:53, 1976.
214. Sutton, RH: Cryptococcosis in dogs: a report on six cases. Aust Vet J 57:558, 1981.
215. Edwards, NJ and Rebhun, WC: Generalized cryptococcosis: a case report. JAAHA 14:439, 1979.
216. Gelatt, KN, et al.: Ocular and systemic cryptococcosis in a dog. JAVMA 162:370, 1973.
217. Browning, JW and Montgomery, J: Cryptococcosis in a dog. Aust Vet J 57:202, 1981.
218. Perfect, JR, et al.: Comparison of itraconazole and fluconazole in the treatment of cryptococcal meningitis and *Candida* pyelonephritis in rabbits. Antimicrob Agents Chemother 29:579, 1986.
219. Mariat, F and Garrison, RG: *Sporothrix schenckii*. *In* Braude, AI (ed): Medical Microbiology and Infectious Diseases. 2nd ed, Philadelphia, WB Saunders, 1986, p 577.
220. Scott, DW, et al.: Sporotrichosis in three dogs. Cornell Vet 64:416, 1974.
221. Thompson, DW and Kaplan, W: Laboratory acquired sporotrichosis. Sabouraudia 15:167, 1977.
222. Emmons, CW: Sporotrichosis. *In* Medical Mycology. 3rd ed, Philadelphia, Lea & Febiger, 1977, p 406.
223. Ajello, L and Kaplan, W: A new variant of *Sporothrix schenckii*. Mykosen 12:633, 1969.
224. Barsanti, JA: Sporotrichosis. *In* Greene, CE (ed): Clinical Microbiology and Infectious Diseases of the Dog and Cat. Philadelphia, WB Saunders, 1984, p 722.
225. Attleberger, MH: Subcutaneous and Opportunistic Mycoses. *In* Kirk, RW (ed): Current Veterinary Therapy VIII. Philadelphia, WB Saunders, 1983, p 1177.
226. Maddy, KT: Epidemiology and ecology of deep mycoses of man and animals. Arch Dermatol 96:409, 1967.
227. Berry, JM, et al.: Sporotrichosis in a dog: a case report. VM/SAC 66:226, 1971.
228. MacDonald, E, et al.: Reappearance of *Sporothrix schenckii* lesions after administration of Solu-Medrol to infected cats. Sabouraudia 18:295, 1980.
229. Lynch, PJ, et al.: Systemic sporotrichosis. Ann Int Med 73:23, 1970.
230. Dunstan, RW, et al.: Feline sporotrichosis: A report of five cases with transmission to humans. J Am Acad Dermatol 15:37, 1986.

231. Burke, MJ, et al.: Successful treatment of cutaneolymphatic sporotrichosis in a cat with ketoconazole and sodium iodide. JAAHA 19:542, 1983.
232. Barbee, WC, et al.: Sporotrichosis in the domestic cat. Am J Pathol 86:281, 1977.
233. Carrada-Bravo, T: New observations on the epidemiology and pathogenesis of sporotrichosis. Ann Trop Med Parasitol 69:267, 1975.
234. Hackisuka, H and Sasai, Y: Development of experimental sporotrichosis in normal and modified animals. Mycopathologia 76:79, 1981.
235. Raimer, SS, et al.: Ketoconazole therapy of experimentally induced sporotrichosis infection in cats: A preliminary study. Curr Therapeut Res 33:670, 1983.
236. Kier, AB, et al.: Disseminated sporotrichosis in a cat. JAVMA 175:202, 1979.
237. Anderson, NV, et al.: Cutaneous sporotrichosis in a cat. A case report. JAAHA 9:526, 1973.
238. Lindley, JW: *Sporotrichum schenckii* in the dog. Southwest Vet 18:234, 1965.
239. Londero, AT, et al.: Two cases of sporotrichosis in dogs in Brazil. Sabouraudia 3:272, 1964.
240. Scott, DW: Sporotrichosis. *In* Kirk, RW: Current Veterinary Therapy VI. Philadelphia, WB Saunders, 1977, p 557.
241. Koehne, G, et al.: Sporotrichosis in a dog. JAVMA 159:892, 1971.
242. Freitas, DC, et al.: Esporotricose em caes e gatos (Sporotrichosis in dogs and cats). Rev Fac Med Vet 7:381, 1965.
243. Werner, RE, et al.: Sporotrichosis in a cat. JAVMA 159:407, 1971.
244. Nusbaum, BP, et al.: Sporotrichosis acquired from a cat. J Am Acad Dermatol 8:386, 1983.
245. Read, SI and Sperling, LC: Feline sporotrichosis transmission to man. Arch Dermatol 118:429, 1982.
246. Dunstan, RW, et al.: Feline sporotrichosis. JAVMA 189:880, 1986.
247. Dion, WM and Speckman, G: Canine otitis externa caused by the fungus *Sporothrix schenkii*. Can Vet J 19:44, 1978.
248. Attleberger, MH: Practical Diagnostic Procedures for Mycotic Diseases. *In* Kirk, RW (ed): Current Veterinary Therapy VIII. Philadelphia, WB Saunders, 1983, p 1157.
249. Kaplan, W and Ivans, MS: Fluorescent antibody staining of *Sporotrichum schenckii* in cultures and clinical materials. J Invest Dermatol 35:151, 1960.
250. Kaplan, W: Application of the fluorescent antibody technique to rapid diagnosis of Sporotrichosis. J Lab Clin Med 62:835, 1963.
251. Garrison, R, et al.: Spontaneous feline sporotrichosis: a fine structural study. Mycopathologia 69:57, 1979.
252. Lurie, HI: Histopathology of sporotrichosis. Arch Pathol 75:92, 1963.
253. Woodard, DC: Splenic sporotrichosis in a dog. VM/SAC 75:1011, 1980.
254. Kwon-Chung, KJ: The relationship between temperature in vitro and type of disease produced in humans by strains of *Sporothrix schenckii*. Abst Ann Mtg Am Soc Microbiol 75:88, 1975.
255. Galina, J and Conti-Diaz, IA: Healing effects of heat and a rubefacient on nine cases of sporotrichosis. Sabouraudia 3:64, 1963.
256. Sharp NJH and Sullivan, M: Treatment of canine nasal aspergillosis with systemic ketoconazole and topical enilconazole. Vet Rec 118:560, 1986.
257. Day, MJ, et al.: Disseminated aspergillosis in dogs. Aust Vet J 63:55, 1986.
258. Jang, SS, et al.: *Aspergillus deflectus* infection in four dogs. J Med Vet Mycol 24:95, 1986.
259. Sharp, N, et al.: Canine nasal aspergillosis: serology and treatment with ketoconazole. J Sm Anim Pract 25:149, 1984.
260. Harvey, CE: Therapeutic strategies involving antimicrobial treatment of the upper respiratory tract in small animals. JAVMA 185:1159, 1984.
261. Goring, RL, et al.: A contrast rhinographic diagnosis of nasal and sinusoidal aspergillosis in a dog: a case report. JAAHA 19:920, 1983.
262. Cervantes, R, et al.: Aspergillosis nasal canina: informe de un caso. Veterinaria Mexico 16:101, 1985.
263. Richardson, MD, et al.: Rapid serological diagnosis of *Aspergillus fumigatus* infection of the frontal sinuses and nasal chambers of the dog. Res Vet Sci 33:167, 1982.
264. Barsanti, JA: Opportunistic Fungal Infections. In Greene, CE (ed): Clinical Microbiology and Infectious Diseases of the Dog and Cat. Philadelphia, WB Saunders, 1984, p 728.
265. Wood, GL, et al.: Disseminated aspergillosis in a dog. JAVMA 172:704, 1978.
266. Mullaney, TP, et al.: Disseminated aspergillosis in a dog. JAVMA 182:516, 1983.
267. Day, MJ, et al.: Immunologic study of systemic aspergillosis in German Shepherd dogs. Vet Immunol Immunopath 9:335, 1985.
268. Tack, KJ, et al.: *Aspergillus* osteomyelitis: report of four cases and review of the literature. Am J Med 73:295, 1982.
269. Glimp, RA and Bayer, AS: Pulmonary aspergilloma: diagnostic and therapeutic considerations. Arch Int Med 143:303, 1983.
270. Sinski, JT: Aspergillosis. *In* Al-Doory, Y (ed): The Epidemiology of Human Mycotic Diseases. Springfield, Charles C Thomas, 1975, p 210.
271. Joseph, JM: Aspergillosis in Composting. *In* Di Salvo, A (ed): Occupational Mycoses. Philadelphia, Lea & Febiger, 1983, p 123.
272. Wilkinson, GT, et al.: *Aspergillus* spp infection associated with orbital cellulitis and sinusitis in a cat. J Sm Anim Pract 23:127, 1982.
273. Barrett, RE, et al.: Treatment and immunological evaluation of three cases of canine aspergillosis. JAAHA 13:328, 1977.
274. Goodall, SA, et al.: The diagnosis and treatment of a case of nasal aspergillosis in a cat. J Sm Anim Pract 25:627, 1984.
275. Fox, JG, et al.: Systemic fungal infections in cats. JAVMA 173:1191, 1978.
276. Bolton, GR and Brown, TT: Mycotic colitis in a cat. VM/SAC 67:978, 1972.
277. Weitkamp, RA: Aspergilloma in two dogs. JAAHA 18:503, 1982.
278. Bauck, LB: Treatment of canine aspergillosis with ketoconazole. VM/SAC 78:1713, 1983.
279. Sullivan, M, et al.: The radiological features of aspergillosis of the nasal cavity and frontal sinuses in the dog. J Sm Anim Pract 27:167, 1986.
280. Hargis, AM, et al.: Noninvasive nasal aspergillosis (fungal ball) in a six-year-old standard poodle. JAAHA 22:504, 1986.
281. Isoun, TT: Disseminated aspergillosis in a dog. J Niger Vet Med Assoc 4:45, 1975.
282. Oxenford, CJ and Middleton, DJ: Osteomyelitis and arthritis associated with *Aspergillus fumigatus* in a dog. Aust Vet J 63:59, 1986.
283. Marks, DL: Systemic aspergillosis in a dog. Canine Prac 10:49, 1983.
284. Peet, RL and Robertson, ID: Suspected aspergillosis in a dog. Aust Vet J 52:539, 1976.
285. Pakes, SP, et al.: Pulmonary aspergillosis in a cat. JAVMA 151:950, 1967.
286. Sautter, JH, et al.: Aspergillosis in a cat. JAVMA 127:518, 1955.
287. Harvey, CE: Nasal aspergillosis and penicilliosis in dogs: results of treatment with thiabendazole. JAVMA 184:48, 1984.
288. Mutinelli, F: A case of disseminated aspergillosis in a cat. Atti Del Convegno Nazionale/Societa Italiana Delle Scienze Beterinarie 38:590, 1984.
289. Pavletic, MM, et al.: Intestinal infarction associated with canine phycomycosis. JAAHA 19:913, 1983.
290. Pavletic, MM and MacIntire, D: Phycomycosis of the axilla and inner brachium in a dog: Surgical excision and reconstruction with a thoracodorsal axial pattern flap. JAVMA 180:1197, 1982.
291. Mohr, JA: Mucormycosis. *In* Dietschy JM: The Science and Practice of Clinical Medicine, Vol 8, New York, Grune and Stratton, 1981, p 355.
292. Miller, RI: Gastrointestinal phycomycosis in 63 dogs. JAVMA 186:473, 1985.
293. Barsanti, JA: Miscellaneous Fungal Infections. *In* Greene, CE. Clinical Microbiology and Infectious Diseases of the Dog and Cat. Philadelphia, WB Saunders, 1984, p 738.
294. Martinson, FD: Phycomycosis (Zygomycosis). *In* Braude, AI: Medical Microbiology and Infectious Diseases. Philadelphia, WB Saunders, 1986, p 743.
295. Taber, WA: Classification of Fungi. *In* Braude, AI: Medical

Microbiology and Infectious Diseases. Philadelphia, WB Saunders, 1986, p 124.
296. Austwick, PK and Copland, JW: Swamp cancer. Nature 250:84, 1974.
297. Ader, PL: Phycomycosis in fifteen dogs and two cats. JAVMA 174:1216, 1979.
298. Barsanti, JA, et al.: Phycomycosis in a dog. JAVMA 167:293, 1975.
299. Miller, RI, et al.: Gastrointestinal phycomycosis in a dog. JAVMA 182:1245, 1983.
300. Gleiser, CA: Mucormycosis in animals. JAVMA 123:441, 1953.
301. English, MP and Lucke, VM: Phycomycosis in a dog caused by unusual strains of *Absidia corymbifera*. Sabouraudia 8:126, 1970.
303. Foil, CS, et al.: A report of subcutaneous pythiosis in five dogs and a review of the etiologic agent *Pythium* spp. JAAHA 20:959, 1984.
304. Troy, GC: Canine phycomycosis: A review of twenty-four cases. Calif Vet 39:12, 1985.
305. Rivolta, G: Cited by Christiansen, M: Mucormykose beim schwein I Mitteilung. Virchows Arch, 273:829, 1929.
306. Christiansen, M: Mucormycosis beim schwein. Virchow Arch Pathol Anat Physiol 273:829, 1929.
307. Braude, AI: The Zygomycetes. *In* Braude, AI: Medical Microbiology and Infectious Diseases. Philadelphia, WB Saunders, 1986, p 597.
308. Miller, RI and Campbell, RS: Clinical observation on equine phycomycosis. Aust Vet J 58:221, 1982.
309. Fox, JG, et al.: Systemic fungal infections in cats. JAVMA 173:1191, 1978.
310. Myerowitz, RL: The Zygomycoses. *In* The Pathology of Opportunistic Infections with Pathogenic, Diagnostic and Clinical Correlations. New York, Raven Press, 1983, p 129.
311. Gleiser, GA: Mucormycosis and distemper in a dog. JAVMA 127:337, 1955.
312. Howard, EB: Acute mycotic gastritis in a dog. VM/SAC 61:549, 1966.
313. Dawson, CO, et al.: Canine phycomycosis: A case report. Vet Rec 84:633, 1969.
314. Lucke, VM, et al.: Phycomycosis in a dog. Vet Rec 84:645, 1969.
315. Heller, RA, et al.: Three cases of phycomycosis in dogs. VM/SAC 66:472, 1971.
316. Gaunt, PS: Intestinal phycomycosis in a dog: A case report. Southwest Vet 35:51, 1982.
317. Gleiser, CA: Phycomycosis beim hund berl much. Tieraetztl Wochenschr 82:464, 1955.
318. Lee, GC, et al.: Mycotic gastritis in a dog. Vet Rec 85:487, 1969.
319. Rudel, JA: Gastric phycomycosis in a dog. Southwest Vet 27:274, 1974.
320. Dawson, CO and Wright, NG: Canine phycomycosis. A case report. Vet Rec 84:633, 1969.
321. Lee, CG, et al.: Phycomycosis in the ileum of a dog. Aust Vet J 52:388, 1976.
322. Osborne, AD and Wilson, MR: Mycotic gastritis in a dog. Vet Rec 85:487, 1969.
323. Mezza, LE, et al.: A new manifestation of canine zygomycosis: Zygomycotic pancreatitis. Vet Med 5:34, 1985.
324. Easley, JR, et al.: Nasal rhinosporidiosis in the dog. Vet Pathol 13:50, 1986.
325. Stuart, BP and O'Malley, N: Rhinosporidiosis in a dog. JAVMA 167:941, 1975.
326. Mosier, DA and Creed, J: Rhinosporidiosis in a dog. JAVMA 185:1009, 1984.
327. Allison, N and Willard, MD: Nasal rhinosporidiosis in two dogs. JAVMA 188:869, 1986.
328. Hobson, HP, et al.: Rhinosporidiosis in the canine. Texas Vet Med J 39:13, 1977.
329. Pore, RS, et al.: *Prototheca* ecology. Mycopathologica 81:49, 1983.
330. Tyler, DE: Protothecosis. *In* Greene, CE (ed): Clinical Microbiology and Infectious Diseases of the Dog and Cat. Philadelphia, WB Saunders, 1984, p 747.
331. Holscher, MA, et al.: Disseminated canine protothecosis: a case report. JAAHA 12:49, 1976.
332. Coloe, PJ and Allison, JF: Protothecosis in a cat. JAVMA 180:78, 1982.
333. Thianprasit, M, et al.: Protothecosis: a report of two cases. Mykosen 26:455, 1983.
334. Heitzman, HB, et al.: Protothecosis. South Med J 77:1477, 1984.
335. Tyler, DE, et al.: Disseminated protothecosis with central nervous system involvement in a dog. JAVMA 176:987, 1980.
336. Font, RL and Hook, SR: Metastatic protothecal retinitis in a dog. Electron microscopic observations. Vet Pathol 21:61, 1984.
337. Berkhoff, HA, et al.: Differential diagnosis of protothecosis from non-human sources. Am J Med Technol 48:609, 1982.
338. Migaki, G, et al.: Canine protothecosis: review of the literature and report of an additional case. JAVMA 181:794, 1982.
339. Finnie, JW and Coloe, PJ: Cutaneous protothecosis in a cat. Aust Vet J 57:307, 1981.
340. Pegram, PS, et al.: Successful ketoconazole treatment of protothecosis with ketoconazole-associated hepatotoxicity. Arch Int Med 143:1802, 1983.
341. McAnally, T and Parry, EL: Cutaneous protothecosis presenting as recurrent chromomycosis. Arch Dermatol 121:1066, 1985.
342. Kaplan, W, et al.: Protothecosis in a cat: first recorded case. Sabouraudia 14:281, 1976.
343. Rakich, PM and Latimer, KS: Altered immune function in a dog with disseminated protothecosis. JAVMA 185:681, 1984.
344. Gaunt, SD, et al.: Disseminated protothecosis in a dog. JAVMA 185:906, 1984.
345. Venezio, FR, et al.: Progressive cutaneous protothecosis. Am J Clin Pathol 77:485, 1982.
346. Cook, JR Jr, et al.: Disseminated protothecosis causing acute blindness and deafness in a dog. JAVMA 184:1266, 1984.
347. Moore, FM, et al.: Unsuccessful treatment of disseminated protothecosis in a dog. JAVMA 186:705, 1985.
348. Van Kruiningen, HJ: Protothecal enterocolitis in a dog. JAVMA 157:56, 1970.
349. Buyukmihci, N, et al.: Protothecosis with ocular involvement in a dog. JAVMA 167:158, 1975.
350. Merideth, RE, et al.: Systemic protothecosis with ocular manifestations in a dog. JAAHA 20:153, 1984.
351. Carlton, WW and Austin, L: Ocular protothecosis in a dog. Vet Pathol 10:274, 1973.
352. Segal, E, et al.: Susceptibility of *Prototheca* species to antifungal agents. Antimicrob Agents Chemother 10:75, 1976.
353. McDonald, JS, et al.: Susceptibility of *Prototheca* to antimicrobial agents. Am J Vet Res 45:1079, 1984.

SECTION IV

THERAPEUTIC CONSIDERATIONS IN MEDICINE

50 PHARMACOLOGIC PRINCIPLES IN THERAPEUTICS

J. DESMOND BAGGOT

PHARMACOLOGIC BASIS OF DRUG ACTION

Drugs act by affecting the functioning of physiological systems or the activity of biochemical processes in the body. In most but not all cases a physical interaction takes place between the drug and receptors. This interaction triggers a series of events, which are frequently complex, and culminates in a pharmacologic response. The response obtained is a function of both time and the concentration of the drug in the immediate vicinity of the receptor sites (biophase), which is related to its concentration in the plasma.

Drugs that interact with receptors and produce pharmacologic effects are termed agonists. The maximal effect that an agonist can produce is referred to as its efficacy, which may be determined by its inherent properties, or those of the receptor-effector system, or both. Only drugs that have the same mechanism of action can be compared with respect to potency, which is defined as the ratio of the plasma drug concentration that yields 50 per cent of the maximal response (ED50) of an agonist to that of the drug adopted as the standard for the class. Potency is influenced by the systemic availability and disposition (i.e., distribution and elimination) of a drug, as well as being determined by its inherent ability to combine with receptors and the functional relationship between the receptor and the effector tissue. Low potency is a disadvantage only if the effective dose is so large that it is cumbersome to administer. Efficacy and potency are not necessarily correlated; these two characteristics of a drug should not be confused.

SITE AND MECHANISMS OF ACTION

Drugs can act at various sites in the body and their effects can be either widespread or local. The effects produced by parenteral atropine sulfate (atropine) are widespread, while cimetidine has a localized action (it inhibits gastric acid secretion). Yet these drugs are specific—each has a single mechanism of action; atropine is an antimuscarinic agent and cimetidine is an H_2 receptor antagonist. It is the widespread distribution of muscarinic receptors that determines the multiplicity of effects produced by atropine. The formulation of a drug preparation and route of administration can influence the selectivity of a drug (the plasma concentrations at which primarily the effects desired are produced). Atropine, or rather its quaternary ammonium derivative, ipratropium, is present in some aerosol preparations of isoproterenol. It is intended to prolong the bronchodilator effect in addition to decreasing bronchial secretions. The most selective drugs that are available for treatment of bronchial asthma are the adrenergic agonists (salbutamol, metaproterenol, and terbutaline). The action of these drugs is specific.

The effects produced by a nonspecific drug result from its interaction with a variety of receptors. The phenothiazine-derivative tranquilizers, such as acetylpromazine, cause sedation (increase the turnover rate of dopamine in the brain), produce a broad spectrum antiemetic action (depress activation of the chemoreceptor trigger zone of the medulla), and can prevent morphine-induced excitement in cats (both effects are attributed to blockade of central dopaminergic receptors). In addition, the phenothiazine tranquilizers exert peripheral actions, prominent among which are hypotension (α-adrenoceptor blockade), an antispasmodic effect on gastrointestinal smooth muscle (anticholinergic action), and hypothermia (interference with hypothalmic control of temperature regulation). The hypotensive effect of these drugs can have serious consequences in hypovolemic animals.

In a pharmacodynamic sense penicillin is a good example of a specific drug that is selective in action. Even though penicillin has an extraordinarily wide margin of safety in the majority of animals, it can unpredictably produce an adverse response (hypersensitivity reaction) in some individual animals. The more specific a drug and the greater its selectivity of action, the less likely it is to cause unwanted systemic effects.

VARIATIONS IN DOSE-RESPONSE RELATIONSHIP

The variability in response to the usually recommended dose level (mg/lb) of a drug can be an important problem in therapy. It can be caused by individual or, more importantly, species differences in the relationship between dose and plasma drug concentration-time profiles (pharmacokinetics) and between plasma drug concentrations and the effect(s) produced by the drug (pharmacodynamics). When a drug is given orally, wide variations in plasma drug concentrations can be anticipated among individual animals, due largely to differences in systemic availability. It could be concluded that safe and effective drug therapy requires individualized drug dosing. An extreme view perhaps, but one that may be justified when consideration is being given to treating a sick animal with a drug that has a narrow margin of safety (such as digoxin).

There are notable pharmacodynamic differences between dogs and cats in the response to certain drugs such as morphine and certain drug formulations such as althesin. The interspecies difference in response to morphine can be offset by using a substantially lower dose level in the cat (0.04 mg/lb or 0.1 mg/kg). Due to a deficiency in microsomal glucuronyl transferase activity in cats the dosing rate for aspirin must be lower in this species (4.4 mg/lb or 10 mg/kg at 24-hour intervals) than in dogs (4.4 mg/lb or 10 mg/kg at 8-hour intervals). The longer dosing interval in cats is required to avoid salicylate toxicity.

DRUG ABSORPTION AND DISPOSITION

ROUTES OF ADMINISTRATION

The formulation of a drug preparation largely determines its route of administration and ultimately the plasma concentration-time profile. Oral dosage forms must dissolve in the stomach before the drug substance can be absorbed. Dissolution is generally the rate-limiting step in determining absorption. The absorption process, which takes place by passive diffusion, occurs mainly in the upper part of the small intestine. It is influenced by the stability of the drug in the acidic gastric fluid and upper intestinal environment and the combination of physicochemical properties that govern passage across mucosal barriers (i.e., pK_A of the drug, degree of ionization, and lipid solubility). Sustained-release oral preparations designed for use in humans may not produce therapeutic effects for a correspondingly extended duration in animals.

The majority of parenteral preparations (solutions or suspensions, for the most part aqueous) can be administered by slow intravenous injection, intramuscularly, or subcutaneously. There are exceptions in that some parenteral solutions such as diazepam and phenytoin sodium, due to their irritant character, should be given by intravenous injection only, while certain suspensions (even an aqueous one such as procaine penicillin G) should never be administered intravenously.

Intravenous infusion is the only technique for drug administration that allows precise control over the plasma concentrations attained, and intensity as well as duration of the effects produced. While the rate of infusion determines the steady-state concentration achieved in the plasma, the time taken to reach steady-state is determined solely by the rate of elimination (half-life) of the drug. For practical purposes it can be assumed that continuous infusion achieves a steady-state concentration of the drug in four times the half-life. Unique features associated with intravenous administration are that the dose is completely available systemically and that by varying the size of the dose and the rate of its introduction into the circulation, this route allows "dosing to effect."

BIOAVAILABILITY

When a drug product is administered by an extravascular route (particularly oral), its dosage should take bioavailability of the drug substance into account. This term is defined as the rate and extent to which the drug, administered as a particular dosage form, enters the systemic circulation unchanged.

An estimate of the rate of absorption can be obtained from the peak height and the time after drug administration at which a peak concentration in the plasma is attained. The usual technique for estimating the systemic availability (extent of absorption) employs the method of corresponding areas:

$$\text{Systemic availability} = \frac{(\text{AUC})_{\text{po}}}{(\text{AUC})_{\text{iv}}} \times \frac{\text{Dose}_{\text{iv}}}{\text{Dose}_{\text{po}}} \qquad \text{(Equation 1)}$$

where AUC is the total area under the plasma concentration-time curve following drug administration by the intravenous or extravascular route indicated. Since application of this technique is based on the assumption that body clearance of the drug is not changed by the route of administration, it is best to determine systemic availability in a group of six to ten animals using a crossover design. The systemic availability of a drug administered as an oral preparation is often incomplete (less than 100 per cent), which may be due either to incomplete absorption or metabolism of the drug prior to its entry into the systemic circulation. Presystemic metabolism can take place in the gut lumen or epithelium or in the liver; this is referred to as the first-pass effect (Table 50–1). It can substantially decrease the systemic availability of drugs that undergo extensive hepatic metabolism, such as propranolol. Lidocaine is not effective as an antiarrhythmic agent when administered orally because of presystemic metabolism. Sublingual administration avoids the first-pass effect and thereby the loss of what could be a large fraction of the dose, depending on the drug. Glyceryl trinitrate has been shown to be equally effective in humans when given orally or sublingually at one-tenth the oral dose.

TABLE 50–1. DRUGS THAT UNDERGO PRESYSTEMIC METABOLISM IN THE DOG

Drug	Dosage	Systemic Availability (per cent)	Site of Metabolism
Lidocaine	4.5 mg/lb	15	Liver
Levodopa	11 mg/lb	44	Gut lumen or wall (or both)
Flunitrazepam	1 mg/lb	0	Gut wall and liver
Aspirin	250 mg (total)	45	Gut wall and liver
Propranolol	80 mg (total)	2–17	Liver

Unfortunately, it is not feasible to use the sublingual route for administering drugs to animals. The use of medicated patches (such as scopolamine for preventing motion sickness), which rely on percutaneous absorption for drug uptake, is also not feasible for dogs and cats. It is worthy of mention that the absorption of an organophosphorus cholinesterase inhibitor, based on its rate of penetration through the excised skin of the dorsal thorax, was almost twice as rapid in cats as in dogs.[1] This difference in percutaneous absorption between the two species could influence the relative toxicity of organophosphates and other well-absorbed compounds when applied topically.

Cumulative urinary excretion data can be used as an alternative to area under the plasma concentration-time curves to estimate systemic availability. The technique is to compare the total amount of drug excreted unchanged in the urine after extravascular administration with the amount excreted unchanged after intravenous dosage. This approach is based on the assumption that the fraction of the dose excreted unchanged remains constant.

DRUG DISTRIBUTION

Drug molecules in the systemic circulation bind reversibly to plasma proteins (mainly albumin) or can be distributed to extravascular tissues. The rate at which a drug distributes can be limited either by perfusion (lipophilic drugs) or by diffusion (ionized and polar compounds). The pattern of distribution that is attained is determined largely by blood flow to the various tissues and by the capacity of the drug to penetrate cellular barriers. It is influenced to a lesser extent by binding to plasma proteins and extravascular tissue components.

Drugs with high lipid solubility are generally absorbed well in the gastrointestinal tract and become widely distributed throughout most tissues of the body. Examples include morphine, diazepam and other CNS acting drugs, digoxin, and erythromycin. The distribution of drugs with low lipid solubility (e.g., salicylates) and polar substances (e.g., aminoglycoside antibiotics) is limited and often confined largely to extracellular fluids. Extensive binding to plasma proteins (greater than 80 per cent) and a high degree of ionization in the plasma decrease accessibility to transcellular fluids, i.e., the aqueous humor and cerebrospinal and synovial fluids. Apart from the direct relationship between the plasma concentration and that attained in the immediate vicinity of the receptor sites, which is most important in determining drug action, the pattern of distribution is irrelevant. Only a small fraction of the amount of drug in the body (systemically available dose) reaches the site of action, while the major fraction distributes elsewhere, including the organs of elimination. Certain disease states such as hypoalbuminemia or uremia and competition between drugs for albumin binding sites can decrease protein binding of extensively bound drugs. The effect on pharmacologic response is likely to assume clinical importance only for drugs that bind extensively and have limited distribution (such as phenytoin, warfarin, and phenylbutazone). The decreased binding assumes greater significance when the drug has a narrow margin of safety.

ELIMINATION PROCESSES

There are two distinct processes for elimination of drugs. Both processes are involved in the elimination of the majority of drugs, in that they simultaneously undergo hepatic metabolism (biotransformation) and renal excretion. The precise mechanism of elimination is determined by the structure of the drug molecule and the physicochemical properties that influence its passage across lipoidal membranes.

Biotransformation is largely responsible for terminating the action of lipid-soluble drugs. The hepatic microsomal enzyme systems mediate a variety of oxidative reactions and glucuronide conjugation (synthesis). Many drugs undergo oxidative metabolism by more than one reaction and their elimination is a function of the sum of the rates of the oxidative reactions (enzyme activities). In addition to the liver, other tissues and organs, including the plasma, kidney, lung, and the gut microorganisms, can contribute to the metabolism of drugs. Hydrolysis is an important metabolic pathway for compounds with an ester linkage, such as procaine and succinylcholine, or those with an amide bond such as lidocaine. The rates of hydrolytic and microsomal-mediated oxidative reactions may differ between dogs and cats, while the rate of glucuronide synthesis is notably slower in cats. The inability of dogs to acetylate aromatic amino groups does not appear to have a toxicologic significance, since alternative metabolic pathways appear to compensate for the deficiency.

Polar drugs such as gentamicin and compounds that are highly ionized in the plasma (e.g., penicillins, cephalosporins, and sulfisoxazole) are eliminated largely unchanged in the urine. The renal mechanisms involved in the excretion of drugs and drug metabolites include glomerular filtration and, depending on the physicochemical properties of the compound, may include carrier-mediated proximal tubular excretion (ionized compounds, including glucuronide conjugates) or pH-dependent passive tubular reabsorption (nonionized, lipid-soluble compounds). Although extensive binding to plasma proteins decreases the availability of drugs for glomerular filtration, it does not delay carrier-mediated excretion of organic ions. The renal tubular excretion of ionized drugs (e.g., penicillins, phenylbutazone, and salicylates) can be delayed by competition for the carrier substances. Competitive inhibition provides the only conclusive evidence that a transport process is carrier-mediated, since delayed excretion (based on increased half-life) could be attributed to altered distribution. The effect of modifying urinary pH on the excretion rate of organic electrolytes is greatest for drugs with pK_A values between 5 and 8, and a prerequisite is that a significant fraction (at least 20 per cent) of the dose is eliminated unchanged by renal excretion.

Certain polar drugs, diagnostic reagents, and glucuronide conjugates of a variety of drugs and endogenous substances are excreted by the liver in the bile. Examples include clindamycin, bromsulphalein, iopanoic acid, and glucuronide conjugates of chloramphenicol, morphine, bilirubin, and steroid hormones. Low lipid solubility and a molecular weight exceeding 300 appear to be prerequisites for the excretion of a compound in the bile and the process involved is carrier-mediated. The compound enters the small intestine, where glucuronide conjugates may be hydrolyzed (by β-glucuronidase in the intestinal microorganisms) and the active drug can be reabsorbed. This cycle constitutes the enterohepatic circulation of a drug. When a significant fraction of the dose undergoes enterohepatic circulation, the elimination of the drug, particularly when it occurs mainly by renal excretion (e.g., tetracyclines), is slower than might be expected.

The overall rate of drug elimination is determined mainly by the mechanisms involved in the process. It may be influenced by the systemically available dose and its rate of absorption, extent of distribution and binding to plasma proteins, the activity of drug-metabolizing enzymes for the metabolic pathways involved, and the efficiency of the excretion (mainly renal) mechanisms.

CLINICAL PHARMACOKINETICS

Pharmacokinetics is defined as the study of the time course of change in concentration of drug in various sites (based on plasma concentrations) and includes knowledge of drug absorption, distribution, metabolism, and excretion. It provides a mathematical approach to predicting optimal dosage of drug preparations for different species of animals. The "usual" dosage regimen as recomended by the pharmaceutical manufacturer can be modified for an individual animal to make therapy more effective. The clinical utility of pharmacokinetics relies on the premise that the therapeutic range of plasma concentrations can be at least tentatively defined for the drug and this appears (or is assumed) to be the same in different species.

Pharmacokinetics provides a basis for explaining an important aspect of species variation in drug response and the mechanism of drug interactions.

DISPOSITION CURVE

The disposition curve, plotted on semilogarithmic paper, expresses graphically the decline in plasma concentration of a drug after intravenous injection of the dose. The curves for the majority of therapeutic agents (including the antimicrobials) show a biphasic decline that can be described mathematically by a biexponential equation (Figure 50–1). The coefficients (A, B) and exponents (α, β) that characterize the equation of the curves are best calculated by nonlinear least squares regression analysis.

The initial steep decline in plasma drug concentration is due mainly to distribution of the drug from the systemic circulation to the extravascular (peripheral) compartment. After distribution has taken place, a pseudoequilibrium is established between drug concentrations in the plasma and in the tissues. During the elimination (linear terminal) phase, the rate of decline in plasma concentration is slower, parallels the fall in tissue levels, and reflects elimination (metabolism and excretion) of the drug. Most drugs are eliminated by a first-order process, which implies that a constant fraction of the amount in the body is eliminated in each equal interval of time (i.e., 50 per cent is eliminated each half-life). For practical purposes first-order elimination can be considered to reach completion (actually 90+ per cent) after four half-lives have elapsed.

The pharmacokinetic behavior of drugs that bind selectively or accumulate in particular locations (such as adipose tissue) may be more appropriately described by a three-compartment model. Thiopental and oxytetracycline in some individuals are examples of such drugs. The number of compartments in the model selected is equal to the number of exponents in the equation describing the disposition curve. The objective is to select the model with the smallest number of compartments that adequately interprets the experimental

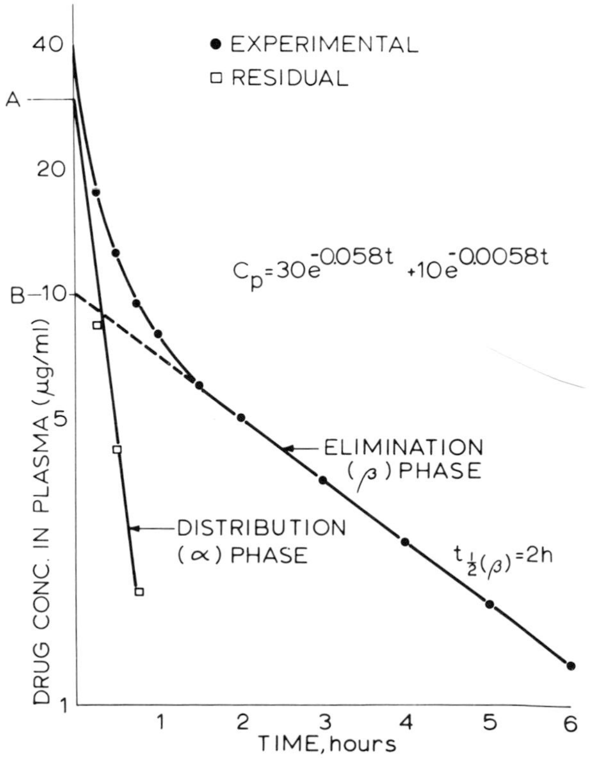

FIGURE 50–1. Semilogarithmic graph depicting the time course of drug concentrations in the plasma (disposition curve) following intravenous administration of a single dose. The data points represent measured (●) and residual (□) plasma drug concentrations. The equation of the biexponential disposition curve is shown.

plasma drug concentration-time data. The most important pharmacokinetic parameters are volume of distribution, half-life, and body (systemic) clearance. When the drug is administered by an extravascular route, its systemic availability, which is the fraction of the administered dose that reaches the systemic circulation unchanged, should be determined. The formulation of the preparation may influence both the rate and extent of drug absorption.

VOLUME OF DISTRIBUTION

The volume of distribution (V_d) of a drug provides an estimate of the extent of distribution, which is the apparent space in the body available to contain the drug. After pseudoequilibrium is established, there is usually a constant relationship between the concentration of drug in plasma and the amount in the body. The calculated value of the volume of distribution varies with the equation used (Table 50–2). The "extrapolation" method, which neglects the distribution phase of the disposition curve, generally gives a larger value than that given by the "area" method. Although the latter method is satisfactory in dosage calculations, it is influenced by changes in the elimination rate constant for the drug even when the distribution space remains unchanged. The steady-state distribution volume does not show this discrepancy and is probably the method of calculation that should be used when interpreting the influence of a physiological condition or disease state on the disposition of a drug.

For some drugs the apparent volume of distribution resembles the plasma volume (e.g., Evans Blue) or the extracellular fluid volume (e.g., penicillins, salicylates), while for other drugs (e.g., digoxin) it can exceed the actual volume of the body tissues (greater than 1L/kg). It is important to realize that distribution volumes are not related to physiological compartments and inferences should not be made on the distribution pattern of a drug based on its volume of distribution. Definitive information on the distribution pattern can be obtained only by measuring levels of the drug in the various organs and tissues of the body, such as kidney, liver, lung, heart, skeletal muscle, skin, and fat.

Drug access to certain tissues, such as the central nervous system, eye, or prostate, is limited to lipid-soluble compounds. The blood-brain barrier restricts drug access to the central nervous system, except the area postrema in the roof of the fourth ventricle, which contains the chemoreceptor trigger zone where central emetics (apomorphine in dogs, xylazine in cats) or excessively high plasma concentrations of certain drugs (digoxin) and antiemetic agents (some phenothiazine derivatives, metoclopramide) exert their action. In the treatment of ophthalmic disease, the limited drug access from the systemic circulation can be circumvented by either topical application or subconjunctival injection of appropriately formulated ophthalmic drug preparations. Since drugs enter saliva by passive diffusion, their concentration in this fluid may correlate well with the unbound concentrations in the plasma. The salivary drug concentrations may be influenced by pH of the saliva, which varies in different species.

HALF-LIFE

The half-life of a drug is the time required for the plasma concentration, as well as the amount in the body, to decrease by 50 per cent through the process of elimination. The half-life of the majority of therapeutic agents (including the antimicrobials) is independent of the dose administered, since overall elimination obeys first-order kinetics. There is, however, considerable species variation in the half-life of drugs that undergo extensive hepatic metabolism. The half-life of a small number of drugs is dose-dependent (follows zero-order kinetics) in certain species. This can generally be attributed to saturation of the principal metabolic pathways for these drugs. Examples include salicylates in cats and phenylbutazone and phenytoin in dogs and cats. For drugs that undergo zero-order elimination, an increase in the dose rate produces a longer half-life and a disproportionately greater accumulation of drug in the body.

Since for most drugs the duration of pharmacologic

TABLE 50–2. APPARENT VOLUMES OF DISTRIBUTION (ml/kg) OF SOME ANTIMICROBIAL AGENTS IN DOGS

Method of Calculation:	Extrapolation	Area	Steady-State
Drug	$V_{d(B)} = \frac{Dose}{B}$	$V_{d(area)} = \frac{Dose}{AUC \cdot \beta}$	$V_{d(ss)} = \left(\frac{k_{12} + k_{21}}{k_{21}}\right) V_c$
Penicillin G	273	156	115
Kanamycin	278	255	236
Gentamicin	448	335	260
Amikacin	292	245	214
Chloramphenicol	491	474	442
Trimethoprim	2097	1849	1675
Sulfadiazine	459	422	392
Sulfadimethoxine	523	410	342
Bay Vp 2674*	2512	2454	2409
Oxytetracycline†	3100	2096	1508

In the steady-state method, k_{12} and k_{21} are first-order rate constants for drug transfer between the central and peripheral compartments of the two-compartment open model; V_c is the apparent volume of the central compartment.

*Fluoroquinolone antimicrobial drug (CFPQ)

†Based on three-compartment open model.

Adapted from Baggot, 1977.

effect is directly related to the half-life, this parameter is most important in designing dosage regimens. In this context it is used, in conjunction with the range of therapeutic plasma concentrations, in selecting the dosing interval. Anticonvulsant drugs are assumed to have the same range of therapeutic plasma concentrations in humans and in dogs, but have considerably shorter half-lives in dogs (Table 50–3). This makes dosing of most potentially effective anticonvulsants impractical in the treatment of canine epilepsy.

The half-life of a drug is related to the volume of distribution and the clearance by the expression:

$$t^{1/2} = \frac{0.693 \times V_d}{Cl_B} \qquad \text{Equation 2}$$

Since the volume of distribution and clearance are independent variables, it follows that half-life depends on their values. A change in either parameter results in a change in the half-life of a drug, while proportionately equal, independent changes in both parameters leave the half-life unchanged. Because of this, half-life is not a reliable indicator of the effect of drug interactions (including anesthetic premedication) or disease states on the disposition of a drug.

CLEARANCE

The clearance of a drug indicates the volume of biological fluid (plasma, blood) from which the drug would have to be removed per unit of time (ml/min/lb) to account for its elimination. Body or systemic clearance is a measure of the ability of the body to eliminate a drug and represents the sum of individual clearances of the drug by the mechanisms of elimination. It can be calculated by dividing the systemically available dose by the area under the curve:

$$\frac{Cl_B = F \times Dose}{AUC} \qquad \text{Equation 3}$$

where F is the fraction of the dose that enters the systemic circulation unchanged and AUC is the total area under the plasma drug concentration-time curve. The concept of clearance is extremely useful in clinical pharmacokinetics, since the clearance of most therapeutic agents is constant over the clinically useful range of plasma drug concentrations.

The contribution of an elimination organ (or mechanism) to the body clearance of a drug can be determined, if the fraction of the intravenous dose that is cleared by the particular organ (or mechanism) is known. For the kidney

$$Cl_R = f_{ex} \times Cl_B \qquad \text{Equation 4}$$

where Cl_R represents renal clearance and f_{ex} is the fraction of the dose that is excreted unchanged in the urine. An estimate of nonrenal clearance, which is usually assumed to represent metabolic (hepatic) clearance, can be obtained by subtracting the renal clearance from body clearance of the drug. If nonrenal clearance is significantly greater than liver blood flow, at least some nonhepatic elimination is taking place. The hepatic clearance of a drug, which indicates the intrinsic ability of the liver to metabolize the drug, is the product of liver blood flow and the hepatic extraction ratio.

TABLE 50–3. THERAPEUTIC PLASMA CONCENTRATIONS AND HALF-LIVES OF ANTICONVULSANT DRUGS IN HUMANS AND DOGS

Drug	Therapeutic Range of Plasma Concentrations (μg/ml)	Average Half-Life (hours)	
		Human	*Dog*
Phenobarbital*	10–25	86	41
Primidone	10–25	8	2
Phenytoin†	10–20	24	6
Sodium valproate	40–100	16	2.5
Carbamazepine*	3–12	24	1.5
Diazepam	0.6–?	24–36	8

*Chronic medication induces hepatic microsomal oxidative activity.
†Half-life is dose-dependent.

DOSING RATE

The dosing rate of a drug can be defined as the systemically available dose divided by the dosing interval. It can be calculated from the expression

$$\frac{F \times D}{\tau} = C_{p(ss)} \times Cl_B \qquad \text{Equation 5}$$

which requires knowledge of the desired steady-state plasma concentration, the systemic availability (following extravascular administration), and the body clearance of the drug. This equation is valid only for drugs adequately described by linear pharmacokinetic models, i.e., drugs that have first-order absorption and disposition kinetics.

For example, the therapeutic range of plasma concentrations for theophylline, a phosphodiesterase inhibitor, is 5 to 20 μg/ml. The calculated dosing rate aims at maintaining a steady-stage plasma theophylline concentration of 10 μg/ml. Based on the desired steady-state plasma concentration, the systemic availability, and body clearance of theophylline, the calculated oral dosing rates for regular aminophylline tablets are 5 mg/lb (10 mg/kg) at 8 hour intervals for dogs and 2.5 mg/lb (5 mg/kg) at 12 hour intervals for cats (Table 50–4). Formulation of the oral theophylline dosage form affects the rate of absorption and systemic availability of theophylline.[2]

When a drug is administered by intravenous infusion, the righthand side of Equation 5 gives the infusion rate (μg/min/lb) that will gradually achieve the desired steady-state (plateau) concentration of the drug. After infusing the drug solution for a period corresponding to four times the half-life, the plasma concentration is within 90 per cent of the eventual steady-state concentration.

TABLE 50–4. COMPARISON OF ORAL DOSING RATES FOR AMINOPHYLLINE TABLETS

Species	Systemic Availability (%)	Clearance (ml/h•kg)	Dosing Rate	
			Dose (mg/lb)	*Interval (h)*
Dog	91	100	5	8
Cat	96	40	2.5	12

When the time required to reach the desired steady-state concentration is considered to be unacceptably long, therapeutic plasma concentrations can be attained more rapidly by the administration of a loading dose. This may be accomplished by administering the loading amount of drug as a single dose, or in the case of drugs with low therapeutic indices (such as digoxin), the loading dose can be given as a series of fractions of the total loading amount. The latter permits better individualization of the loading amount and avoids adverse effects that might occur during the distribution phase after a large single intravenous dose. The size of the average loading dose required to achieve the desired steady-state concentration can be determined from the fraction of drug eliminated during the dosing interval and the usual maintenance dose (in the case of intermittent drug administration):

$$\text{Loading dose} = \frac{100}{f_{el}} \times \text{maintenance dose}$$

Equation 6

where f_{el} is the fraction (per cent) of dose eliminated during the dosing interval.

MONITORING OF THERAPEUTIC PLASMA CONCENTRATIONS

Optimal individualization of therapy is assisted by measuring the concentration of certain drugs, such as digoxin, phenobarbital, and gentamicin, in the plasma. Monitoring can be justified for drugs that have a narrow range between the plasma concentrations yielding therapeutic and adverse effects, particularly since bioavailability (particularly oral dosage forms), rate of elimination, and steady-state plasma concentrations are difficult to predict in sick animals. Since increasing trough plasma concentrations are indicative of accumulation, blood samples should be collected immediately preceding the administration of maintenance doses. The first sample can be collected after the steady-state concentration has been achieved. Therapeutic drug monitoring should always be accompanied by clinical assessment of the response to therapy and is never a substitute for the latter.

ALTERATIONS IN DRUG DISPOSITION

The disposition kinetics of drugs can be altered by certain physiological conditions (pregnancy or during the neonatal period) or the presence of some disease states (uremia, fever, dehydration). Impaired renal function, including decreased glomerular filtration rate, or the capacity of the liver to metabolize drugs can decrease their rate of elimination. Certain types of drug interactions, such as displacement from albumin binding sites, induction or inhibition of major metabolic pathways, or competition for carrier-mediated (renal or biliary) excretion can affect the steady-state plasma concentrations and intensity of pharmacologic response obtained with multiple doses. It is exceedingly difficult to predict adjustments of dosage to offset the effect of altered drug disposition. The best approach is to individualize therapy based on clinical assessment of the patient in conjunction with monitoring the steady-state plasma drug concentration. When the usual dosage of a drug produces an adverse effect or lack of response, the possibility of altered disposition should be considered. How to modify dosage depends on the mechanism responsible for the altered disposition. Impaired renal function, for example, decreases the elimination rate of drugs that are excreted mainly unchanged in the urine. In this situation an appropriate lengthening of the dosing interval may be adequate dosage adjustment (as with gentamicin, for example). Knowledge of the fraction of normal renal function remaining, based on endogenous creatinine clearance, and of the fraction of drug usually excreted unchanged in the urine is required for determining the dosage adjustment. Other situations are less straightforward, as marker substances for systemic clearance of drugs by other elimination mechanisms or for altered distribution have not been studied.

The mechanism of some drug interactions is difficult to interpret, for example, the prolongation of thiopental anesthesia by acetylpromazine and of ketamine anesthesia by xylazine. Whether the premedicating drug prolongs the effect of the intravenous anesthetic agent by altering its disposition kinetics or has a pharmacodynamic basis is not clear. Pharmacokinetic interactions result from alterations in the delivery of drugs to their sites of action, whereas pharmacodynamic interactions are those in which the responsiveness of the target organ or system has been modified by other agents.

PRINCIPLES OF ANTIMICROBIAL THERAPY

BASIS OF SELECTION

An antimicrobial preparation is selected on the basis of microbial susceptibility, mechanism of antibacterial action, pharmacokinetic characteristics, convenience of administration, and cost of treatment with the preparation. The success of therapy depends on maintaining an effective level of the antimicrobial drug at the focus of infection for an adequate period of time. This requires the repeated administration of a drug that can reach the infection site. Drug access is determined by the location of the site of infection, the route of administration and formulation of the drug preparation, and the physicochemical properties of the drug substance that influence its disposition (i.e., distribution and elimination). It has been shown that only the lipid-soluble, nonionized moiety of organic acids (penicillins, cephalosporins, sulfonamides) and bases (aminoglycosides, macrolides, lincomycins, and trimethoprim) that is free (unbound) in the plasma can penetrate cell membranes and diffuse into transcellular fluids, for example, the cerebrospinal, synovial and ocular fluids. The concentration of drug attained in any location, whether tissue or biological fluid, depends not only on the systemically available dose, but also on drug access and degree of accumulation (either concentration or binding) at the particular location.

APPROACH TO THERAPY

The clinician must first determine whether a bacterial infection is present and establish its character. Specimens for bacterial culture and susceptibility testing should be collected before initiating antimicrobial therapy. Even though identification of the causative organism assists in selecting the most effective drug, it is advisable to commence treatment at the time of specimen collection. The initial choice of drug is based on broad experience in treating similar types of infections. The justification for empiric selection is that infections respond better when treated early in their course.

When culture results show coagulase-positive staphylococci or enteric bacteria *(E. coli, K. pneumoniae, Proteus mirabilis, Salmonella)* as the causative organisms, it is desirable to determine minimum inhibitory concentrations (MICs) of potentially useful antimicrobial agents, because the susceptibility of these microorganisms is unpredictable.

Knowledge of the quantitative susceptibility of the pathogenic microorganism together with information on the bioavailability and disposition of the antimicrobial agent of choice can be used to calculate an optimal dosage regimen. Dosage calculations of this type aim at maintaining plasma concentrations of the antimicrobial agent that provide effective concentrations at the site of infection and minimum toxicity in the sick animal. The usual dosage regimen differs from the optimal in that the former is based on maintaining plasma drug concentrations that exceed the average minimum inhibitory concentration of the majority of susceptible microorganisms. The duration of therapy and activity of the host's defense mechanisms are variables not directly included in dosage calculations, but can influence the response to treatment. Lack of response can sometimes be attributed to failure by the owner to comply with instructions to administer the drug preparation at the recommended dosing interval.

In many cases the drug selected empirically will be the same as that selected on the basis of susceptibility testing and pharmacokinetic considerations but, in some cases, the use of another drug may be preferable or an alternative dosage form of the drug initially selected may be more effective.

CANINE URINARY TRACT INFECTIONS

The treatment of bacterial infections of the canine urinary tract can be used to illustrate the application of microbiologic and pharmacologic principles in antimicrobial therapy.

Selection of the most suitable antimicrobial preparation for the treatment of urinary tract infections should be based on sensitivity pattern of the microorganism(s) causing the infection and convenience afforded by the dosage regimen. It must be kept in mind that urinary pH influences activity of some antimicrobial agents and dehydration or furosemide administration increases the toxicity of aminoglycosides.

The approach is to select an antimicrobial agent to which the infecting microorganisms are susceptible, which can be administered orally, and which is excreted largely unchanged in the urine. A unique feature of urinary tract infections is that exceedingly high concentrations of certain antimicrobial agents can be attained at the site of infection. Oral penicillin, for example, may be effective in the treatment of *E. coli* infection and oral tetracycline can be used to treat *Pseudomonas* infections of the lower urinary tract. The susceptibility of the pathogenic microorganisms to these drugs is conditional, in that susceptibility is related to the unusually high concentrations attained at the site of infection. Oral preparations of trimethoprim-sulfonamide (either sulfadiazine or sulfamethoxazole) could be considered the treatment of choice for *E. coli* and mixed infections. Severe infections caused by *Pseudomonas aeruginosa* or *Proteus mirabilis* may necessitate parenteral therapy with gentamicin. Microorganisms that have become resistant to gentamicin may remain susceptible to amikacin, under which circumstance the use of amikacin is indicated. The concurrent use of gentamicin and carbenicillin (or ticarcillin) can produce synergistic enhancement of bactericidal activity against some strains of *Pseudomonas aeruginosa.*

Impaired renal function decreases the urinary excretion rate of the drugs that are useful in the treatment of urinary tract infections. This not only decreases their accessibility to the site of infection but can lead to accumulation in the body with attendant toxic effects, depending on the drug. Accumulation can be prevented by adjusting dosage, either the size of maintenance doses or the dosing interval, so that plasma drug concentrations remain within the therapeutic range. The amount of drug excreted unchanged in the urine over a fixed period of time, say 24 hours, will be decreased by an amount proportional to the decreased dosing rate. This can influence the effectiveness of a drug in treating urinary tract infections.

References

1. McCreesh, AH: Percutaneous toxicity. Toxicol Appl Pharmacol 7 (Suppl 2):20, 1965.
2. Koritz, GD, et al.: Bioavailability of four slow-release theophylline formulations in the Beagle dog. J Vet Pharmacol Therap 9:293, 1986.
3. Baggot, JD: Principles of Drug Disposition in Domestic Animals. Philadelphia, WB Saunders Co, 1977.

51 ANTIMICROBIAL DRUGS

ARTHUR L. ARONSON and DAVID P. AUCOIN

ROLE OF ANTIMICROBIAL DRUGS IN TREATING INFECTIOUS DISEASE

The importance of antibacterial drugs in the treatment of infectious disease is well established. Nevertheless, experience has shown that there are instances in which these drugs are not successful in eradicating an infection. Failure may occur even when antimicrobial sensitivity tests are carried out and an appropriate antimicrobial agent is selected and administered according to a recommended dosage schedule. Several physiologic and pharmacologic factors have been identified that can affect the action of these drugs. An appreciation of these factors may suggest reasons for treatment failures when they occur and a rational basis for dealing with the situation. Even when the organism is sensitive to the drug, antimicrobial agents often do not work in areas of necrotic tissue, abscess formation, or suppurative lesions with foreign bodies. Surgical drainage may be required so that the antimicrobial drug can diffuse to the area of infection, exert its pharmacodynamic effect, and aid the host defense mechanisms in eradicating the infection.

The goal of antimicrobial therapy is to help the body eliminate infectious organisms. Burke[1] emphasized that the natural defense mechanisms of the patient are of primary importance in preventing and/or controlling infection. Once microbial invasion has occurred there are several host responses that serve to combat the invading organisms. These include the inflammatory response, cellular migration and phagocytosis, the complement system, and antibody production. These responses are most efficient if the homeostatic mechanisms of the body are maintained. Thus, procedures designed to maintain or improve normal physiologic processes (fluid and electrolyte balance, acid-base balance, and nutritional status) demand the highest priority. After appropriate attention has been given to supporting the normal physiology of the patient, the judicious use of an antimicrobial agent may be appropriate to supplement its natural defense mechanisms. The difficulty of controlling infections in the immunocompromised patient emphasizes the validity of viewing antimicrobial drugs as supplements rather than as "magic bullets" in antimicrobial chemotherapy.

FACTORS AFFECTING THE ACTION OF ANTIMICROBIAL DRUGS IN THE BODY

There are a number of microbial and host factors that can affect the action of an antimicrobial drug in the body. Most of these factors can be considered within the context of three fundamental criteria that must be satisfied for an antimicrobial drug to exert its effect. The fundamental criteria include (1) bacterial sensitivity to the drug, (2) drug distribution to the site of infection in adequate concentration and for sufficient duration (pharmacokinetic phase), and (3) favorable environmental conditions at the site of infection for drug action (pharmacodynamic phase). These, of course, are not the only factors involved in the treatment of infectious disease: host factors, such as hepatic and renal function and the integrity of the host defense mechanisms, play an important role as well. However, an appreciation of these three conditions serves to emphasize factors involved in administering an antimicrobial drug and the ability of that drug to exert its action against infecting organisms.

Bacterial Sensitivity to the Drug

Antimicrobial drugs are unique among drugs in that their effect is not directed toward modifying the physiologic processes of the host, but rather is directed specifically against the invading microorganism. Of course, one must take into account how the host disposes the drug in vivo; nevertheless, the purpose of administering an antimicrobial drug is to inhibit the growth of or kill invading pathogenic microorganisms.

The first criterion to be met in selecting an antimicrobial drug is that the pathogenic organism be sensitive to its action. It may be necessary to initiate treatment before the results of microbiologic confirmation are available. A valuable procedure for immediate identification of bacteria consists of using a gram stain on a smear of infected body fluid. With a presumptive diagnosis, clinical experience often is helpful in deciding which drug to use. A culture for antimicrobial sensitivity testing should be taken prior to therapy. Antimicrobial sensitivity tests are an important guide in determining whether or not the organism is sensitive to a particular drug at concentrations approximating those in vivo.

ANTIMICROBIAL SENSITIVITY TESTING

Are sensitivity tests always required? Hirsh and Ruehl[2] emphasize that certain organisms, including obligate anaerobes, β-streptococci, corynebacteria, *Pasteurella*, actinobacilli, *Actinomyces*, and *Haemophilus*, are almost uniformly sensitive to penicillin G. In these cases, rational therapy with penicillin G could proceed on the basis of an etiologic diagnosis alone. However, these organisms probably account for less than ten per cent of small animal infections. Sensitivity tests should be applied when organisms showing considerable variation in sensitivity are involved. These include staphylococci, Enterobacteriaceae (*Escherichia coli*, *Salmonella* spp., *Klebsiella* spp., *Proteus* spp.), *Pseudomonas* spp., and *Bordetella* spp. Sensitivity tests also may be indicated during the course of therapy to determine any changes in sensitivity.

The antimicrobial susceptibility test is perhaps one of the more frequently used laboratory tests in veterinary medicine. However, no test performed in clinical medicine is more misunderstood, yet more commonly employed to direct therapy. It is often misinterpreted to the point where some clinicians suggest the test not be used.[3] A complete discussion of these tests is not possible here, however, a few of their salient features should help clear up some confusion.

There are two different tests commonly employed in veterinary microbiology laboratories. The most commonly employed is the disc diffusion test.[4] This test is designed to correlate a concentration of an antibiotic with the distance the drug diffuses from a paper disc containing a standardized amount of a given antibiotic. Diffusion occurs through an agar medium that has been inoculated with the bacterial pathogen. Growth of the organism occurs at a distance from the disc where drug concentration is not inhibitory. This produces a zone of inhibition around the disc, which is read by measuring the radius of the zone. The radius corresponds to the drug's concentration where growth inhibition first occurred and is approximately equivalent to the minimum inhibitory concentration (MIC). This relationship between zone size and drug concentration was first demonstrated by Bauer and Kirby[4] and thus simplified antibacterial testing by replacing the serial tube dilution assay with a quick, simple, disc diffusion assay. The critical step is interpreting the zone size. Although the zone size relates back to a drug concentration, the test was designed to correlate the zone size with a qualitative determination of whether or not the bacteria is "Sensitive" (S) or "Resistant" (R) to the given antibiotic. These arbitrary terms are determined by the National Committee for Clinical Laboratory Standards (NCCLS). The designations of "Sensitive" or "Resistant"[5] reflect human clinical data accumulated in people; given the standard therapeutic dose of that drug, the treatment is likely to be successful if the zone is such a size or greater, or treatment should not be attempted if the zone is smaller than a certain size. Different drugs have different zone size criteria, since drugs diffuse from the disc at different rates and distances and, more importantly, at different concentrations. Therefore, one cannot just look at a plate and determine which drug is more sensitive by finding the largest clear zone. This relationship between zone size and likelihood of clinical efficacy is highly dependent on standard dosing regimes, rigorous assay conditions and quality control, and the understanding of the antibiotic disposition in humans. Veterinary microbiology laboratories use this relationship for all species of animals where clinicians do not use standard dosing regimens and where drug disposition may vary from humans. A critical fault with disc diffusion is the lack of quantitative information on the degree of susceptibility. For instance, lower urinary tract infections (UTI) can be successfully treated with many drugs that are reported as resistant due to the fact that many drugs achieve ten- to one hundredfold increase over serum concentrations in the urine, whereas the susceptibility is based upon achievable serum concentrations. Additionally, the disc diffusion does not indicate how susceptible an organism is to the drug. This information would help determine which drug to choose, what dose to use, and even which route of administration to use. For example, cephalosporins are used to treat *Klebsiella pneumoniae* respiratory infections and often require concentrations of 8 to 16 μg/ml to inhibit growth. A standard oral dose of cephalexin produces peak serum concentrations of 10 to 15 μg/ml or less in respiratory secretions, therefore, the oral route would probably be ineffective. An intravenous injection of cefazolin produces peak serum concentrations of 100 to 150 μg/ml, which would provide adequate concentrations in lung bronchi. This information is lacking in disc diffusion assays but is available from microdilutional susceptibility assays. These assays give quantitative information on antibiotic sensitivities, which are reported as minimum inhibitory concentrations (MIC).

MICs are becoming routine for most human hospitals and commercial laboratories.[6] The MIC is then used to determine probable Sensitivity or Resistance using NCCLS guidelines. The word "Resistance" should be more accurately interpreted as less sensitive, for no bacteria is totally resistant to an antibiotic if any concentration can be used. More importantly, the R and S designation is again based on human data of dose and drug disposition and therefore caution is urged in using just the R and S to determine therapy. If the clinician knows the average serum concentrations achieved in that species of animal over a dosage range by different routes of administration, then MIC data can be better used and the drug can be dosed more rationally. This chapter supplies some of this needed information so that clinicians can use it in conjunction with MIC data to arrive more rationally at appropriate antibiotic treatment. The authors hope the misconceptions of antibiotic sensitivity reports will be clarified in this chapter, and until more data in small animal medicine are obtained, the NCCLS guidelines should function very well, as they were intended to serve as guidelines, not absolutes, on antibiotic use.

Generally speaking, if an organism is resistant to a

drug in vitro, it is also resistant in vivo, although there are some exceptions in the urinary tract. If an organism is susceptible in vitro, the drug may be effective in vivo. For a drug to be effective in vivo, it must be able to distribute to the site of infection in the body and be effective there.

Distribution to the Site of Infection (Pharmacokinetic Phase)

An antimicrobial drug must be distributed to the site of infection in adequate concentration and come into intimate contact with the infecting organism in order to exert its antimicrobial effect. Thus, a knowledge of intracellular versus extracellular distribution of both drugs and infectious agents is crucial to rational antibacterial therapy.

Whereas most bacteria remain extracellular while causing systemic infections, there are notable exceptions, for example, *Salmonella*, *Brucella*, *Listeria*, and the tubercle bacillus. The ability of staphylococci to remain viable in an intracellular environment after being engulfed by macrophages has been reported.[7] Thus, these organisms may be protected from those antimicrobial drugs that are limited in distribution to the extracellular space. This is noteworthy because many antimicrobial drugs indicated for infections caused by these organisms are limited in distribution to the extracellular space (penicillins, cephalosporins, and aminoglycosides). This is an important consideration in understanding and managing, for example, recurring staphylococcal infections.

Infections can occur almost anywhere in or on the body. Whether the route of drug administration is topical, oral, or parenteral depends upon the site of infection, the severity of the infection, and the particular drug selected. If an animal is vomiting, oral administration is of necessity ruled out. Some drugs are not absorbed to any appreciable extent following oral administration (the aminoglycosides and polymyxins, for example); such drugs must be administered parenterally if the infection is systemic.

Drugs distribute in the body from their site of absorption via the blood and tissue fluids. An infectious process can alter the distribution of a drug in vivo by altering blood flow and increasing diffusion distances. This often occurs in the presence of inflammation, pus, abscesses, foreign bodies, or edema fluid.

In some cases the distribution of the drug to the site of infection may be enhanced. For example, this has been shown to occur with penicillin G in cases of meningitis.[8] The inflamed meninges offer a less effective barrier to many drugs that normally would permeate the cerebrospinal fluid with difficulty. On the other hand, an infectious process usually affects the distribution of a drug in vivo adversely. This is strikingly illustrated in the treatment of bacterial endocarditis in humans. In this condition, the invading bacteria become localized within fibrinous material. An antimicrobial drug must be capable of diffusing through this material in order to reach the bacteria responsible for the condition. Enterococci, *Streptococcus viridans* and *S. faecalis* are common etiologic agents in bacterial endocarditis. The organisms are susceptible to both penicillin G and sulfonamides in vitro. However, penicillin G is effective in treating the disease, but the sulfonamides are ineffective. This prompted studies of the diffusion of both drugs through fibrinous material characteristic of the lesion.[9, 10] It was demonstrated that penicillin G was capable of diffusing through the fibrin material and that the sulfonamides were not. Thus, it appears that the sulfonamides are ineffective in vivo because they do not distribute to the site of infection. This is another explanation for a lack of correlation between the effectiveness of an antimicrobial in vitro and its effectiveness in vivo.

Favorable Environmental Conditions (Pharmacodynamic Phase)

Infectious disease conditions may alter the distribution of drugs (pharmacokinetic phase) in the body. Infectious disease conditions also can create an unfavorable environment for antimicrobial drug action (pharmacodynamic phase) in an infectious process. Obstructed drainage routes, collections of purulent exudates, or abscess formations can create unfavorable conditions, and thereby result in slowing bacterial growth, binding or inactivating the drug, lowering oxygen tension, reducing pH, and facilitating the production of L-forms.

Bacteria must be actively growing for cell wall synthesis inhibitors (e.g., penicillins and cephalosporins) to exert their antibacterial effect. These drugs are most active against bacteria in the logarithmic phase of growth; there is no effect on bacteria in the lag phase.[11] Lack of growth of bacteria sequestered within abscesses may, in part, explain the lack of clinical efficacy of penicillins in conditions associated with abscess formation. Studies with radioactive penicillin G clearly demonstrate passage of the drug across the walls of abscesses.[12] Others have shown that penicillin G and several other antibiotics also penetrate abscess walls.[13–15] Findings such as these underscore the importance of surgical drainage, when practical, and emphasize some of the limitations of antibacterial drugs in effecting cures, even when organisms are sensitive to the drug.

The aminoglycoside group of antibiotics, although poorly bound by blood proteins, are markedly bound by intracellular constituents.[16] This binding occurs with insoluble intracellular components, including nucleic acids and perhaps acidic proteins.[17] Since these drugs penetrate mammalian cells poorly, this binding probably is of no consequence except in the kidney, where active transport mechanisms facilitate accumulation of the drug.[18] This drug accumulation underlies the nephrotoxic potential of this group of drugs and also the persistent residues found in food-producing animals. However, this proclivity to bind to intracellular constituents might be expected to assume significance in infectious disease states where the breakdown products of cellular destruction would, in part, constitute pus. It has been shown that a quantity of one milliliter of pus is capable of binding more than 700 μg gentamicin and 1500 μg polymyxin B or colistin sulfate.[19] The figure of 700 μg per milliliter becomes quite impressive when one considers that therapeutic concentrations of gentamicin in serum are in the order of 1 to 10 μg per milliliter. It is reasonable to assume that drugs so bound to constituents in pus would be unable to come into contact with bacteria and exert an antibacterial effect. The importance of surgical drainage and cleansing of wounds as much as possible in order to create an environment conducive to wound healing, as well as antibacterial drug action, cannot be overemphasized.

It also has been shown that aminoglycosides are markedly (between 44 and 90 per cent) bound to or adsorbed by fecal material.[20] Fortunately, in the treatment of intestinal infections, one can compensate for this binding by administering relatively large doses of drug orally.

Other conditions in the environment of infection may militate against aminoglycoside drug action. The transport of aminoglycosides across the cell membranes of susceptible bacteria depends on electron transport. This transport can be blocked by hyperosmolality, reduced pH, and anaerobiosis. Thus, the antibacterial activity of aminoglycosides is reduced, for example, in the anaerobic environment of an abscess, in concentrated urine, or urine of low pH.[21] This is an important point to keep in mind in the management of urinary tract infections. Procedures to acidify the urine should not be instituted when using an aminoglycoside to treat a urinary tract infection.

Low pH in leukocytic phagolysosomes (pH 5.0 to 5.4) may, in part, explain the inability of cloxacillin to kill intraleukocytic *Staphylococcus aureus*; the lethal action of penicillins depends upon autolytic enzyme activity in bacteria, which is impaired under conditions of low pH.[21]

In certain situations, environmental conditions at the site of infection can be modified to enhance the effectiveness of antimicrobial drugs. The antimicrobial activity of some drugs is enhanced by an acidic environment and others, by an alkaline environment. Thus, in urinary tract infections, it is highly desirable for the urine to be acidic when using nitrofurantoin or the tetracyclines and for the urine to be alkaline when using the aminoglycosides.

Antimicrobial drugs that work best in an acidic environment are weak organic acids and those that work best in an alkaline environment are weak organic bases. Consider the case of nitrofurantoin, a weak organic acid with a pK_A of 7.2. When nitrofurantoin is in solution at the same pH as its pK_A, 50 per cent of the molecules are electrostatically charged. If the pH is increased, more molecules become charged as they lose protons. Conversely, if the pH is decreased below the pK_A, fewer molecules are charged because of the addition of protons from the aqueous milieu. The significance of these physicochemical events is that lipid solubility of a molecule increases with decreasing electrostatic charge. Thus, more drug molecules are lipid-soluble at low pH and a higher percentage of the total number of drug molecules present are able to cross the lipid-rich, bacterial membranes to the site of antimicrobial action in susceptible bacteria.

When one considers some of the factors involved in antimicrobial drug action in vivo, it is no wonder that at times there is a poor correlation between clinical response and predictions based solely upon a sensitivity test.

INHIBITORS OF CELL WALL SYNTHESES

β-Lactam Antibiotics: Penicillins

Mechanism of Action. All β-lactam antibiotics exhibit similar modes of action.[22] Almost all bacteria have cell membrane-bound enzymes, called penicillin binding proteins (PBP), which act as catalysts in the final reactions in the synthesis of the cell wall.[23] β-lactams act as substrates for PBPs, binding essentially irreversibly to their catalytic site, resulting in the inhibition of cell wall synthesis. Cell lysis and death usually, but not always, follow. The ability of a given β-lactam to stop growth, kill, or lyse the bacterium depends in large part on the PBP with which it binds, its binding affinity, and the type and amount of inhibition it causes. Lysis is still not well understood, but is likely to involve either a direct or indirect effect of PBP binding. Gram-negative bacteria have five to seven different PBPs on their cell membrane. Each is involved in different catalytic reactions, some of which are vital to cell viability, some which are not. The cross-linking of the peptidoglycan in the cell wall is vital to the bacterium and this reaction is facilitated by a transpeptidase enzyme (PBP 1 in *E. coli* and PBP 3 in *Staphylococcus aureus*). However, other enzymes, carboxypeptidases and endopeptidases, are also sites of β-lactam binding and interference with their function may also play a part in the mechanism of β-lactam action. The scope of this chapter precludes a detailed discussion of this topic, but this is a very active area of research both for developing new β-lactam antibiotics and in understanding intrinsic β-lactam resistance.

Spectrum of Activity. Despite the attractiveness of classifying these antibiotics as narrow- or broad-spectrum, the reality of the situation has become more complicated by the emergence of resistant populations in what once were sensitive organisms. Therefore, the spectrum of the β-lactams is discussed on an individual drug basis that indicates the impact that resistant bacteria are making in clinical veterinary practice.

Resistance Mechanisms. Resistance to β-lactam antibiotics is mediated either by β-lactamase production or by intrinsic means. β-lactamases are a diverse group of bacterial enzymes whose function in the bacteria is probably not protection from β-lactam antibiotics, since they were isolated from bacteria before β-lactam antibiotics were ever used. Rather, they function to break transitory intermediate structures in bacterial peptidoglycan metabolism.[24] The Richmond-Sykes classification of β-lactamases describes six different types. The typing is both functional (differences in substrates, inducible or constitutive) and biochemical (size, plasmid versus chromosomal, and isoelectric point).[25] The complexity of the classification can be simplified by noting that all staphylococcal β-lactamases are essentially the same and that 80 per cent of the β-lactamases produced by Enterobacteriaceae (*E. coli*, *Proteus*, *Klebsiella*) are plasmid-mediated type III enzymes.[26] Of the remainder, only type I, chromosomal-mediated cephalosporinases, are of a major clinical concern, since they are commonly found in *Enterobacter* and *Pseudomonas* spp. However, new emerging resistant pathways involving intrinsic means are becoming evident among human pathogens and probably veterinary pathogens as well. It is important to note that the so-called β-lactamase–resistant penicillins (i.e., methicillin) are only resistant to staphylococcal β-lactamase, but not to many of the gram-negative ones. Similarly, the first generation cephalosporins exhibit increased resistance to some of these β-lactamases, but such stability in any given antibiotic is seldom universal. The spectrum of any given β-lactam is in large part determined by its stability against bacterial β-lactamases. It also is a function of two other properties; penetrability to the PBP on the cell membrane and its binding affinity for the target PBP. As can be seen in Figure 51–1, the major difference between gram-negative and gram-positive bacteria is the make-up of the structure outside the cell membrane.

Staphylococcal β-lactamase (penicillinase) is an inducible exocellular enzyme. Gram-negative β-lactamases are either inducible or constitutive, and are secreted into the periplasmic space of bacteria. The antibiotic has only a few layers of peptidoglycan wire structure to penetrate to get to its PBP in gram-positive bacteria; however, secretion of large amounts of this enzyme into the microenvironment often occurs when β-lactam binding occurs. The antibiotic needs to survive this inhospitable milieu to bind to its PBP and inactivate it. It cannot be overemphasized that induction of staphylococcal β-lactamase occurs during treatment. This may account for treatment failure in a patient with an in vitro penicillin-sensitive strain of *S. intermedius*. Selection of a β-lactamase–producing strain may occur during therapy; as its population increases it will inactivate penicillin before it can kill even the penicillin-sensitive strains.[27]

Natural Penicillins

Spectrum of Activity. In spite of the extensive resistance seen with clinical veterinary pathogens, the natural penicillins continue to be effective agents in selected clinical situations. Unlike some of the important pathogens of humans and food-producing animals, most small animal veterinary pathogens are not sensitive to natural penicillins. However, the drugs exhibit excellent activity (less than 1.0 μg/ml) against most nonenterococcal streptococcal infections (Group A, B, and G) and most, if not all, anaerobic bacteria. They are still the drugs of choice for *Actinomyces* infections. However, this organism requires a much higher concentration of the drug, necessitating use of the intravenous route and a much higher dose than is used for streptococcal infections. They also are the drugs of choice for oral spirochete infections (trench mouth). Aerobic gram-negative bacteria are resistant at achievable serum concentrations at high intravenous doses, but the drugs are effective against many *E. coli* and *Proteus* spp. at the high concentrations achieved in urine.[28]

Clinical Pharmacology. Benzylpenicillin G and phenoxmethyl-penicillin (penicillin V) are the two most commonly employed natural penicillins used in veterinary medicine. Both penicillins are available in oral and parenteral formulations. Most β-lactams are acid-labile to some degree, resulting in poor and sometimes erratic absorption. Oral absorption of acid-stable penicillin V is almost twice that of penicillin G (20 to 30 per cent versus 40 to 50 per cent); however, penicillin G is more active than penicillin V. Penicillin G is available in both sodium and potassium salts for parenteral use. Both the procaine and benzathine esters of penicillin G have slow, incomplete absorption following intramuscular or subcutaneous administration. Serum and tissue concentrations with procaine penicillin G are sufficient for most penicillin-sensitive organisms, but only the most sensitive of bacteria are inhibited by the benzathine formulation. Use of both these slow-absorbing products for prophylactic reasons and "diseases of unknown diagnosis" is irrational in that most veterinary pathogens are not sensitive to these agents. Moreover, the indiscrimi-

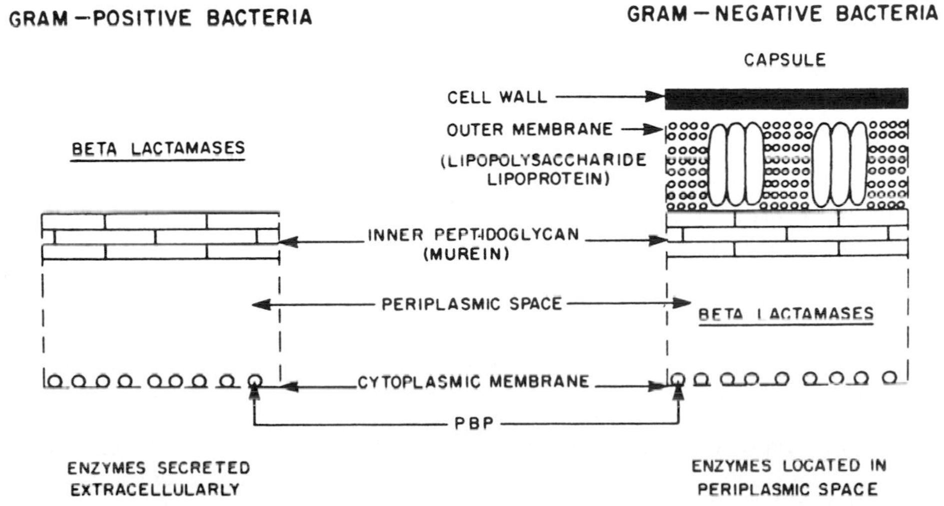

FIGURE 51–1. Schematic comparative outer cell structures of a gram-positive and gram-negative bacterium. Mechanism for β-lactam activity and resistance is (1) the presence of inactivating β-lactamases, (2) decreased penetration to the cell membrane, or (3) alteration in the binding affinity or structure of the target PBP.

nate use of these β-lactams has unquestionably resulted in selecting resistant organisms in the companion animal population.[29]

Penicillins distribute well into most body tissues (except the CNS and prostate) with concentrations in noninflamed tissues lagging only slightly behind those in serum.[30] Concentrations in inflamed tissues can actually eclipse serum concentrations. Inflammation of any tissue enhances penetration, but high doses are still needed to treat meningitis caused by susceptible organisms.[31]

Elimination in the dog and cat is rapid and occurs mainly through renal tubular secretion and filtration. Elimination half-lives are short, with averages being 20 to 40 minutes.[32] Typical intravenous and oral dosing frequencies of q 4 to 8 hours for the sodium or potassium salt reflect the rapid elimination of these products.

Antistaphylococcal Penicillins

The sensitivity of the natural penicillins to coagulase-positive staphylococci (*Staphylococcus aureus* and *Staphylococcus intermedius*) quickly fell after their introduction in 1944. Presently, only 10 to 20 per cent of human pathogenic staphylococcal infections are sensitive to penicillin G.[30] At two veterinary hospitals from 1983 to 1987, the percentage of coagulase-positive staphylococci (*S. intermedius*, *S. aureus*) sensitive to penicillin was only 26 per cent.[33] This emerging resistance was countered with the introduction of methicillin in 1957 as the first β-lactamase–stable penicillin. Since then a number of antistaphylococcal penicillins have been introduced. They are very similar in spectrum and clinical pharmacology. They have only minor differences in their resistance to hydrolysis by staphylococcal β-lactamases, but all are readily inactivated by most gram-negative β-lactamases. As a group, they all are less potent against penicillin-sensitive bacteria and, unlike penicillins, show little or no activity against enterococci.

This group can be divided into three groups, based on structure and metabolism: methicillin, the isoxazolyl penicillins, and nafcillin.

Spectrum of Activity. These agents are similar to the natural penicillins with the exception of their resistance to staphylococcal β-lactamases. They are less potent than penicillin G against any of the penicillin-sensitive organisms, including penicillin-sensitive staphylococci. This is of questionable clinical significance in staphylococcal infections, since even the small number of penicillin-sensitive staphylococci are effectively treated with the antistaphylococcal penicillins. These agents also differ from the natural penicillins in having little activity against enterococci (*S. faecalis* and *S. faecium*). Their use is restricted accordingly to the treatment of all staphylococcal infections in small animal practice.

Clinical Pharmacology. Methicillin was the first antistaphylococcal penicillin developed; however, because it must be given parenterally, it has had little use in veterinary medicine. It is the isoxazolyl penicillins that have received the most attention. In humans, oral absorption of these penicillins ranges from 30 to 80 per cent.[34] As with most penicillins, absorption is best on an empty stomach. Recent studies in the fasted dog indicate that oral absorption of both oxacillin and dicloxacillin dosed at 22 to 36 mg/kg is poor (16 and 22 per cent respectively), with much lower serum peak concentrations than obtained in humans. The half-life of these two penicillins is shorter in the dog than in humans, with dicloxacillin (16 minutes) being even shorter than oxacillin (22 minutes). These penicillins have the greatest degree of protein binding (more than 90 per cent in dog serum). Despite the great degree of binding, distribution into tissues appears similar to that of other penicillins. In spite of poor oral availability and rapid elimination half-life, these two penicillins have been successfully used for treating superficial and deep canine and feline pyodermas.[35] However, larger doses than previously reported may enhance efficacy (see Table 51–10). The rapid elimination of these penicillins may be indicative of hepatic metabolism. Up to 30 per cent of oxacillin is eliminated as metabolites, primarily the inactive penicillinoic derivative. It is possible that in the dog oxacillin and dicloxacillin metabolites may be active and contribute to the overall good clinical efficacy seen with these penicillins.

Nafcillin pharmacokinetics have not been reported for dogs or cats. Oral availability in humans is poor and erratic and treatment by this route is not recommended. It is unusual for a penicillin in that it is almost completely eliminated by hepatic metabolism, with little active drug being excreted in the urine.[30]

There are no solid data to recommend one antistaphylococcal penicillin over another in treating infections caused by staphylococci. However, it probably is more rational to use the isoxazolyl penicillins orally due to proven clinical efficacy in animals and to use either oxacillin or nafcillin intravenously in serious systemic staphylococcal infections.

Aminopenicillins

Spectrum of Activity. Ampicillin is the prototypic drug of this entire group. These penicillins were introduced in the 1960s and referred to as broad-spectrum penicillins. At the time, gram-negative infections were increasing in frequency with mainly *E. coli*, *Proteus* spp., and *Salmonella* spp. as pathogens. Ampicillin demonstrated excellent activity against these organisms and was quickly preferred over parenteral high-dose penicillin G therapy. Its increased activity against selected gram-negative organisms is due mainly to its increased binding affinity to the PBP 1b, and possibly PBP 3.[30] However, it is as sensitive to hydrolysis by gram-positive or gram-negative β-lactamases as is penicillin G. The spread of plasmids producing β-lactamases has resulted in many resistant strains of what once were ampicillin-sensitive bacteria. This, coupled with the increasing prevalence of *Klebsiella pneumoniae*, *Pseudomonas aeruginosa*, and *Enterobacter* spp. as pathogens, which were always ampicillin-resistant, has rendered the classification of "broad-spectrum" penicillins misleading. The prevalence of these plasmid-bearing Enterobacteriaceae may vary from one geographical location to another. At the Animal Medical Center (AMC) in New York City, 40 per cent (43/108) of *E. coli* isolated from dogs with urinary tract infections were resistant to ampicillin (MIC greater than 16 μg/ml), and 50 per cent (54/108) were resistant at achievable urinary concentrations of 64 μg/ml.[33] Similar resistance is seen at the School of Veterinary Medicine at North Carolina State University (NCSU) where 41 per cent (32/77) of *E. coli* isolated from similar patients were resistant to ampicillin (MIC greater than 16 μg/ml). It is important to keep in mind that dogs with uncomplicated acute urinary tract infections often have very sensitive *E. coli* infections that should respond to ampicillin and that the data from veterinary schools are often biased by the fact that referral cases often have chronic, relapsing infections where resistant organisms are expected to be more prevalent.

In general, ampicillin is as clinically effective against gram-positive organisms as are the natural penicillins. (One important exception is its greater activity against enterococci.) Ampicillin and other aminopenicillins are the drugs of choice for infections caused by *S. faecalis* and *S. faecium*.

Clinical Pharmacology. All the aminopenicillins are acid-stable and may be given orally. However, oral absorption is a problem. Ampicillin has 30 to 50 per cent oral bioavailability which decreases in the presence of food.[36, 37] In contrast, amoxicillin has excellent absorption (greater than 80 per cent), which is not affected by food.[38] Like all penicillins, aminopenicillins are widely distributed throughout extracellular fluids and exhibit increased penetration into inflamed areas. Unlike penicillin, a greater fraction of elimination is due to glomerular filtration rather than tubular secretion. As with other anions, biliary excretion occurs, but not in animals with biliary stasis due to cholecystitis.

Amoxicillin differs structurally from ampicillin in having a hydroxyl group in the para position of the benzene side chain. This structural alteration markedly enhances oral absorption, while having essentially no effect on antibacterial activity.[38] Although in vitro studies demonstrate subtle changes in bactericidal activity, these changes are of doubtful clinical significance. A two- to threefold increase in peak serum concentrations compared to ampicillin following a similar dose translates into a less frequent dosing schedule for highly susceptible organisms. However, with many moderately sensitive organisms (MIC = 4 μg/ml), a more frequent dosing interval is recommended.

Hetacillin. The condensation product of ampicillin and acetone, hetacillin is converted to ampicillin upon oral absorption by bowel mucosa and in the serum. This pro-drug has the advantage of improved oral bioavailability compared to ampicillin. However, no clinically important difference between ampicillin and hetacillin has been documented, and its usefulness is questionable.

Antipseudomonal Penicillins

These compounds were developed in an effort to improve the gram-negative spectrum of the semi-synthetic penicillins, especially against the increasingly more common pathogen, *Pseudomonas aeruginosa*.

Spectrum of Activity. Like the aminopenicillins, the enhanced gram-negative activity of the antipseudomonal penicillins is due to increased binding affinity for PBP 3 and to improved penetration through the porins of the bacterial cell wall. However, these compounds are susceptible to hydrolysis by β-lactamases secreted by the majority of pathogenic staphylococci, rendering them ineffective. Similarly, they are susceptible to the same plasmid-mediated TEM β-lactamases, which are responsible for most of the non-*Pseudomonas* ampicillin resistance.[26] Therefore, they show no advantage over ampicillin in the treatment of ampicillin-resistant organisms. These observations have been confirmed at NCSU, where most *E. coli*, *Proteus* spp., and *Klebsiella* spp. that are resistant to ampicillin appear resistant to these compounds (Table 51–1).

The differences in these compounds are in their potency, not in their efficacy. Ticarcillin demonstrates a two- to fourfold increase in anti-*Pseudomonas* activity over carbenicillin. However, no increase in efficacy for the other gram-negative species is seen. The introduction of clavulinic acid, a β-lactamase inhibitor, to this compound should improve its spectrum dramatically. Ticarcillin is more active than carbenicillin against *Pseudomonas aeruginosa*. However, high doses are still needed for antipseudomonal activity with ticarcillin since its antipseudomonal MIC (8 to 64 μg/ml) is higher than its MIC for other gram-negative bacteria. It is reported that unlike carbenicillin and ticarcillin, the newer members of this group, mezlocillin, piperacillin, and azlocillin, show activity toward *K. pneumoniae* and *K. oxytoca*.[30] However, this has not been the authors' experience. Of 30 isolates of *K. pneumoniae* from dogs at NCSU, only one demonstrated in vitro sensitivity to any of these newer penicillins (Table 51–1). More data need to be obtained prior to making any definitive statements regarding the role these newer penicillins may play in the treatment of ampicillin-resistant infections in veterinary medicine. However, there does not seem to be any advantage to selecting any of the newer antipseudomonal penicillins over ticarcillin or carbenicillin. Despite these cautions, these agents have demonstrated a useful purpose in both human and veterinary medicine. These penicillins are among drugs of choice in the treatment of serious systemic infections due to *P. aeruginosa*. However, it has been reported in human patients that using these agents as the sole therapy for *P. aeruginosa* infections has resulted in initial success but with a high degree of relapse.[30] One possible reason for these results is that the correlation between in vitro sensitivity and in vivo efficacy can be very discordant in this group. The number of bacteria present at the site of infection (inoculum) has a profound effect on how effective the in vivo response to the antibiotic will be. Most penicillins suffer from this inoculum effect and the antipseudomonal penicillins seem particularly affected.[39] Therefore, since in vitro tests are usually performed with 10^5 organisms and infections usually involve many times that number of bacteria, failure with an antipseudomonal penicillin when it demonstrated in vitro sensitivity may be due to this effect. Additionally, an infection with this organism often implies a degree of local or systemic immune suppression and the success of any antibacterial therapy depends on functional host defense

TABLE 51–1. SENSITIVITY OF ANTIPSEUDOMONAL PENICILLINS IN PERCENTAGE OF ISOLATES

	Ampicillin	Carbenicillin	Mezlocillin	Piperacillin	Ticarcillin
E. coli (n = 153)	59	60	53	50	41
Klebsiella pneumoniae (n = 32)	1	1	1	1	0
Proteus mirabilis (n = 67)	65	43	65	71	91
Pseudomonas aeruginosa (n = 40)	7	43	80	66	66

mechanisms. Therefore, therapy is often improved using combinational antibiotic therapy where a synergistic effect is achieved and a greater percentage of organisms are killed, thus depending less on the host defenses to eradicate the residual bacterial population that can be left from conventional monotherapy.[40] An aminoglycoside is recommended along with an antipseudomonal penicillin in any serious *Pseudomonas aeruginosa* infection. The synergism of this combination has been demonstrated by several combinations of these drugs in human patients with granulocytopenia secondary to cancer therapy.[41]

Clinical Pharmacology. Carbenicillin is not orally stable and must be administered parenterally. Due to the large MIC for *Pseudomonas aeruginosa* (32 to 128 μg/ml), high doses of carbenicillin must be given. Following an intravenous dose of 45 mg/lb (100 mg/kg), peak serum concentrations are greater than 500 μg/ml, which quickly decline as carbenicillin is both excreted renally and filtered with a half-life of 45 to 60 minutes. An oral formulation of a carbenicillin ester is available. The indanyl ester of carbenicillin is absorbed moderately well and has the distinction of being the only orally available antipseudomonal penicillin. However, with only moderate availability and doses of 22 mg/lb (50 mg/kg) producing less than 20 μg/ml peak serum concentrations, most *Pseudomonas* infections are not treatable by this drug unless they are located in the lower urinary tract.[42] Experience using this compound as the sole therapy, even in lower urinary tract infections, has resulted in a high rate of relapse or lack of cure.[30] This reinforces the earlier statements concerning use of these agents alone.

Ticarcillin produces peak serum concentrations similar to those of carbenicillin, following equivalent intravenous dosing. It is well distributed into noninflamed tissues (except for the CNS) following intravenous dosing. The drug is eliminated by renal secretion and filtration, with 60 per cent of the drug being recovered in the urine in 24 hours. The elimination half-life following intravenous administration is 45 to 60 minutes.[43] The half-life is prolonged in patients with renal disease; however, reduction of the dose is not indicated since the therapeutic index of ticarcillin is very large.

There is little clinical experience with the newer antipseudomonal penicillins, mezlocillin, piperacillin, and azlocillin. The pharmacokinetic disposition of these compounds is similar to other penicillins in the dog. Following an intravenous dose of piperacillin at 22 mg/lb (50 mg/kg), peak serum concentrations are 300 μg/ml, with a rapid elimination half-life of 30 to 40 minutes.[44] However, these agents are sufficiently different from carbenicillin and ticarcillin to indicate that they may have a therapeutic advantage. They are more active against ampicillin-sensitive gram-negative bacteria, requiring smaller doses to kill *Pseudomonas aeruginosa* and other Enterobacteriaceae. However, this enhanced potency with non-*Pseudomonas* bacteria is seen, at least in vitro, only in strains already sensitive to ampicillin. Like carbenicillin and ticarcillin, they are susceptible to the same β-lactamases. An interesting observation is that they seem to show a smaller decrease in activity in the presence of β-lactamases than carbenicillin or ticarcillin. The clinical significance of this relative resistance is unknown. Like the other antipseudomonal penicillins, they also exhibit an inoculum effect. This effect indicates that the combination with an aminoglycoside is probably still warranted with these newer penicillins.

β-Lactamase Inhibitors

The rapid emergence of resistance in the once ampicillin-sensitive Enterobacteriaceae family has led to the development of a new approach to overcoming this pathway of resistance. It has been difficult to create a β-lactamase–stable penicillin that is resistant to all types of this enzyme yet retains an excellent spectrum of activity. Instead, a different approach has been used to rescue the usefulness of older drugs by eliminating the β-lactamase–using competitive inhibitors. One such recently marketed β-lactamase inhibitor is clavulinic acid.

Spectrum of Activity. This compound is a β-lactam that lacks significant antibacterial properties but irreversibly binds and thus inactivates many different β-lactamases.[26] Addition of clavulinic acid to amoxicillin in a fixed combination has enhanced the in vitro spectrum of activity of amoxicillin considerably.

Amoxicillin/clavulinic acid was tested in a combined study at six universities and indicated that 47 per cent (840/1793) of the isolates of *E. coli* were ampicillin-resistant (MIC greater than 16 μg/ml). The combination of amoxicillin (which has a spectrum of activity identical to ampicillin) with clavulinic acid resulted in only a six per cent (106/1772) resistance. Similarly, many organisms that were never sensitive to ampicillin (*Klebsiella pneumoniae*) were sensitive in vitro. Preliminary data at NCSU indicates that the decrease in MIC with this combination in ampicillin-resistant organisms is four- to sixfold. This decrease is sufficient to indicate that therapy at conventional doses will be effective (i.e., the organism is labeled sensitive). However, the MIC for these gram-negative organisms is still usually higher than the MIC for ampicillin-sensitive organisms. Therefore, the authors recommend using higher doses of this combination in the treatment of nonurinary tract infections caused by ampicillin-resistant gram-negative infections. In contrast, the addition of clavulinic acid enhances the activity toward ampicillin-resistant *Staphylococcus intermedius* and *S. aureus* to the same degree as ampicillin-sensitive staphylococci.

A combination of ticarcillin/clavulinic acid is even more activity-enhancing than amoxicillin/clavulinic acid. The excellent binding affinity of ticarcillin to PBP, coupled with clavulinic acid to inactivate the major resistance pathway for the gram-negative bacteria, has resulted in a truly "broad spectrum" penicillin. At NCSU a consistent eightfold decrease in MIC is seen in ticarcillin-resistant organisms. This, combined with the high concentrations obtained with intravenous administration, makes this combination attractive to use as the sole therapy for serious gram-negative infections. However, such studies have yet to be performed in clinical veterinary medicine and enthusiasm for this product must await some clinical evidence of its place in the therapeutic armamentarium.

Clinical Pharmacology. Unlike humans, the disposition of clavulinic acid in the dog does not quite parallel that of amoxicillin. Clavulinic acid, like any other β-lactam, is well distributed into tissues and eliminated by renal secretion and filtration. Clavulinic acid also undergoes extensive metabolism, unlike amoxicillin, which accounts for its more rapid elimination half-life of 35 minutes compared to 60–70 minutes for amoxicillin.[38] This difference is accentuated in animals with renal dysfunction where both compounds exhibit increased half-lives, amoxicillin more so than clavulinic acid. The clinical significance of these differences in dogs is not known and may not be important. The spatial relationship of inhibitor and active drug at the site of infection is a very dynamic and complex situation and one that may not need constant ratios of the two products.

Studies of the absorption of ticarcillin/clavulinic acid following subcutaneous injections indicate that absorption is rapid and complete (80 to 90 per cent bioavailable). Following a 45 mg/lb (100 mg/kg) subcutaneous dose, peak serum concentrations of 100 μg/ml were seen at one hour. The effective half-life was only slightly longer (70 rather than 60 minutes) than the elimination half-life, again indicating rapid and complete absorption. These concentrations, together with the MIC of many non-*Pseudomonas* organisms, indicate that this route of administration may be effective in the treatment of serious gram-negative infections.

Cephalosporins

The cephalosporins are a family of primarily parenteral antibiotics. They are classified into arbitrary "generations" based on their spectrum of activity. The first generation has predominately gram-positive activity, with some gram-negative activity; the third generation is predominately effective against gram-negative organisms, with variable gram-positive efficacy. As β-lactam compounds, they exhibit the pharmacokinetic and toxicity profiles of the penicillins. Their use in clinical veterinary medicine has been primarily limited to the oral and parenteral first-generation compounds. However, with the degree of bacterial resistance now seen in veterinary medicine, there are potential uses for the second- and perhaps even some of the long-acting third-generation compounds. The following discussion of cephalosporins is not intended to be complete, but instead focuses on those cephalosporins that have been used in clinical practice or that have features which make them potential candidates for clinical practice.

FIRST-GENERATION CEPHALOSPORINS FOR PARENTERAL USE

Spectrum of Activity. The spectrum of activity of the first-generation cephalosporins is very similar. For this reason, the guidelines of the National Committee for Clinical Laboratory Standards (NCCLS) uses cephalothin sensitivity as an indicator of all first-generation cephalosporins' sensitivity.[5] Cefalothin, like all cephalosporins, has excellent resistance to inactivation by staphylococcal β-lactamases, which makes it an excellent antibiotic for infections caused by *Staphylococcus intermedius* and *Staphylococcus aureus*. However, cephalothin is sensitive to many of the gram-negative β-lactamases and thus its spectrum of activity with regard to gram-negative bacteria does not tend to be significantly different from ampicillin, with the exception of an increased activity toward *Klebsiella* spp., *Proteus vulgaris*, and *Proteus mirabilis*. Table 51–2 shows the in vitro sensitivities of these organisms to cephalothin and ampicillin. In addition, these spectrum similarities and differences depend on geographical location.

Even these differences would not make cephalothin a drug of choice in any gram-negative infection. It is widely held by clinicians that cephalosporins have improved gram-negative activity and are used in the very ill patient for this reason. There is no logical or rational justification for this feeling. The major, and only clinically important, difference between the first generation cephalosporins and the aminopenicillins is in the excellent sensitivity of cephalosporins to staphylococci, not to the common enterics.

Clinical Pharmacology. Although all first-generation cephalosporins have similar spectrums, their pharmacokinetic properties are sufficiently different to warrant discussion on a drug by drug basis.

Cefalothin is well absorbed following intramuscular or subcutaneous administration, with a 4.5 mg/lb (10 mg/kg) dose producing 10 μg/ml peak concentrations.[45] Following an intravenous dose of 4.5 mg/lb (10 mg/kg) peak concentrations of 50 to 75 μg/ml are achieved and urinary concentrations can be 100 to 200 times higher than peak serum concentrations. These differences in peak concentrations should be kept in mind when choosing a route of administration as well as a dose. Tissue penetration lags behind serum concentration in most tissues but is equal to or greater than serum concentration in inflamed tissue. Like most β-lactams, penetration into the CSF or prostate is poor, even when they are inflamed. Cephalothin is 50 per cent protein-bound in canine serum and exhibits a faster total body clearance than most of the penicillins. About 33 per cent of the drug undergoes hepatic metabolism to form O-desacetylcephalothin, which has some minor antibacterial activity, and the remainder is eliminated by renal filtra-

TABLE 51–2. COMPARATIVE SENSITIVITY PROFILE OF CEPHALOTHIN VS. AMPICILLIN AT TWO DIFFERENT GEOGRAPHIC LOCATIONS*

	Percentage of sensitive Isolates				
	Staphylococcus intermedius 138/66†	*E. coli* 153/108	*Klebsiella pneumoniae* 32/23	*Proteus mirabilis* 67/83	*Enterobacter* spp. 18/22
Cephalothin					
NCSU-SVM	98	41	53	91	12
AMC	90	26	74	30	32
Ampicillin					
NCSU-SVM	55	54	0	36	11
AMC	44	40	0	12	15

*North Carolina State University School of Veterinary Medicine (NCSU-SVM) and The Animal Medical Center, New York City (AMC). Cephalothin and ampicillin sensitivity based on MIC < 16 μg/ml.
†Number of isolates at NCSU/AMC.

tion.[46] The resulting mean elimination half-life is 45 minutes.

Cefazolin produces higher serum and tissue concentrations than cephalothin when given at the same dose. A 4.5 mg/lb (10 mg/kg) dose given intramuscularly gives a peak concentration of 20 μg/ml and intravenous peak concentrations of 100 to 150 μg/ml.[45, 47] The potency of these two antibiotics is equal for most organisms, making these differences in serum concentration potentially significant. However, clinical trials have failed to demonstrate any difference in efficacy in these two compounds in human patients where this same distinction in pharmacokinetics prevails. Cefazolin is less protein-bound than cephalothin and has a longer elimination half-life. These differences are due to the lack of any significant metabolism of cefazolin through an elimination pathway. The drug is eliminated primarily by renal filtration, with a half-life of 60 to 70 minutes.

Cephapirin has a disposition very similar to that of cephalothin. It undergoes hepatic metabolism to form the desacetyl cephapirin, but to a greater extent than cephalothin, such that only one-third of the dose is recovered in the urine as the intact drug.[48] The mean elimination half-life of 25 minutes is the shortest of the cephalosporins.

Although there are pharmacological differences between these products, as yet no clinical trial has proven any one of them superior to another.

FIRST-GENERATION CEPHALOSPORINS FOR ORAL USE

Members of this group include cephalexin, cepadroxil, and cefaclor.

Spectrum of Activity. All oral cephalosporins have an identical phenylglycine side group. This side group facilitates their absorption orally but also alters their potency. All orally available cephalosporins are first-generation products, although some include cefaclor in the second generation due to some enhanced activity toward *Hemophilus influenzae*. As a group they are as effective as the first-generation parenteral cephalosporins and are useful in treating infections caused by *Staphylococcus intermedius*, nonenterocococcal streptococci, ampicillin-sensitive *E. coli*, and some *Klebsiella* spp. However, cephalexin, cephadroxil, and cefaclor, although bactericidal, have a slower killing time than the parenteral first-generation cephalosporins. This slowness of killing may be due to a poorer binding affinity to PBP in general and to a higher affinity for PBP 3, which is not associated with autolysis, but rather causes long filamentous forms of bacteria to form.[30]

Clinical Pharmacology. These compounds are all well absorbed, with oral bioavailabilities of 65 to 100 per cent.[49] Cephalexin peak serum concentrations of 15 to 20 μg/ml occur in one to two hours following a 4.5 mg/lb (10 mg/kg) dose. These products display little protein-binding (ten per cent) and their tissue penetration is similar to the parenteral first-generation cephalosporins. As would be expected, the oral half-life of these cephalosporins is longer than the parenteral cephalosporins; it averages 80 to 90 minutes.[47]

There is no difference in the rate of elimination between cephalexin and cephadroxil, which in the dog display disposition kinetics virtually identical to cephalexin. This is not true in humans.

Cefaclor is well-absorbed orally, with a bioavailability of 80 to 100 per cent.[47] Peak serum concentrations of 10 μg/ml occur one to two hours following a dose of 7 mg/lb (15 mg/kg). These concentrations are smaller than those achieved by either cefalexin or cefadroxil at equivalent doses. The drug is eliminated by renal filtration and secretion, with an effective half-life of 80 to 90 minutes.

SECOND-GENERATION CEPHALOSPORINS

Second-generation cephalosporins include cefoxitin, cefamandole, cefonicid, cefuroxime, and cefoteten.

Spectrum of Activity. These compounds exhibit greater stability against the gram-negative β-lactamase, especially against the TEM plasmid-mediated β-lactamases responsible for most of the resistance seen in the Enterobacteriaceae.[26] This is especially true for the cephamycins included in this grouping (cefoxitin, cefoteten). This increased stability extends the gram-negative spectrum to include indole-positive *Proteus* and certain *Enterobacter* spp. The cephamycins also display excellent anaerobic activity. The differences within this group, as with the first generation, are primarily pharmacokinetic differences; however, unlike the first-generation cephalosporins, this group also has major differences in its spectrum of activity. The two members of this group that best illustrate this are cefoxitin and cefamandole.

Cefoxitin, a cephamycin, differs from the cephalosporins in that it has a methoxy group at the 7 carbon in the β-lactam ring. This methoxy group greatly enhances the stability of this compound against gram-negative β-lactamases and, therefore, increases its activity against these organisms. Cefoxitin has excellent activity against the ampicillin-resistant *E. coli* isolated from patients at NCSU-SVM (more than 98 per cent susceptible at MIC less than 8 μg/ml). It has become a drug of choice in renal-compromised patients with infections caused by these organisms. It is less active against gram-positive organisms than cephalothin or cephalexin. However, at doses administered it achieves sufficient concentrations to be effective. Cefamandole demonstrates poor activity against the ampicillin-resistant enterics and is especially poor against *E. coli*. This drug behaves more like a first-generation cephalosporin than a second-generation one against veterinary pathogens. Its classification is based on its enhanced sensitivity to *Hemophilus influenzae* and *Neisseria* species of bacteria that are not small animal pathogens. Cefonicid and cefuroxime have a spectrum similar to cefamandole.

Clinical Pharmacology. Cefoxitin is well absorbed following intramuscular dosing; however, it is irritating. The authors recommend using 0.5 per cent lidocaine in the diluent to reduce the pain of injection. Serum concentrations following intramuscular and intravenous dosing are similar to cefazolin. Cefoxitin is well distributed into tissues but does not reach therapeutic concentrations in the CNS. The drug is eliminated by renal filtration and secretion with more than 80 per cent of the drug recoverable in the urine. Its elimination half-life is 45 to 60 minutes. Cefoteten, another cephamycin, has a spectrum of activity very similar to cefoxitin. In humans the drug has a longer half-life than cefoxitin and twice-a-day dosing is recommended. However, in dogs this product has a half-life similar to cefoxitin (55 minutes) and therefore has no advantage over it.[50] Cefonicid has a longer half-life in humans (4.6 hours) and has been used effectively at one dose per day. The disposition of this drug has not been described in the dog or cat and it is not known whether the elimination is prolonged. Regardless of this, it is unlikely this drug would be of any major advantage in clinical veterinary medicine, since the spectrum of activity for cefonicid is similar to cefamandole.

THIRD-GENERATION CEPHALOSPORINS

Third-generation cephalosporins include cefotaxime, cefoperazone, moxalactam, ceftizoxime, ceftazidime, and ceftriaxone.

Spectrum of Activity. These compounds have had little reported clinical use in veterinary medicine. However, veterinarians may need to use these agents more frequently as resistant organisms become more prevalent. The third generation implies a broader gram-negative spectrum, including organisms with chromosomal type I β-lactamase enzymes such as *Enterobacter cloacae* and *Pseudomonas aeruginosa*. As a rule, these cephalosporins have reduced gram-positive activity, although this is not true of ceftazidime. As is true with cephalosporins, they are ineffective against enterococci (*Streptococcus faecalis*, *Streptococcus faecium*). As a group, they exhibit the greatest stability against both staphylococcal β-lactamases and the plasmid and chromosomal β-lactamases found in gram-negative species. In vitro testing against veterinary pathogens indicates excellent activity against many of the resistant Enterobacteriaceae species (Table 51–3).

Cefoperazone has shown the least amount of activity against the ampicillin-resistant gram-negative bacteria of the third-generation cephalosporins. Other than that major distinction, the group displays fairly similar in vitro sensitivities and no choice can be made between them based on spectrum differences. However, other, less expensive agents are still available in most cases, and no clinical trials on potential usefulness have been reported.

Clinical Pharmacology. Cefotaxime was the first third-generation cephalosporin introduced in this country. Its distribution kinetics in dogs and cats are similar to those of humans.[51, 52] Following a 23 mg/lb (50 mg/kg) intravenous dose of cefotaxime, peak serum concentrations are greater than 500 μg/ml and 90 μg/ml at one hour after dosing. The drug is well distributed (as are most of the β-lactams); however, unlike most β-lactams, it penetrates the CNS at sufficient concentrations to be a drug of choice for gram-negative meningitis. The drug is metabolized in the liver to desacetylcefotaxime and other minor metabolites, which accounts for 30 per cent of the eliminated drug. In this respect, its elimination is similar to cephalothin and cephapirin. The drug and its metabolites are excreted into the urine and bile; its elimination half-life is 45 to 60 minutes.

Moxalactam kinetics have been described for the dog.[47] Perhaps not surprisingly, the kinetics of this cephalosporin are different in humans than in the dog. In humans the drug is excreted primarily by renal filtration, with an elimination half-life of 2.3 hours.[30] In the dog, however, the drug has a smaller volume of distribution (0.114 rather than 0.220 l/kg) and a shorter elimination half-life of 60 minutes. This is the third example of a cephalosporin having a longer elimination half-life in humans than in the canine. Insufficient kinetic information exists on the pathways of elimination to determine what causes this difference; however, it is logical to assume that drugs that are eliminated primarily by renal filtration have a shorter half-life in the dog due to the dog's faster glomerular filtration rate. This observation is very important since some of the newer third-generation cephalosporins, such as ceftriaxone (half-life of 8 hr), have prolonged elimination times in humans, which makes their dosing less frequent and therefore less expensive. There is no doubt, given the expanded gram-negative spectrum of the third-generation cephalosporins, that if the cost of delivering these agents could be reduced by less frequent dosing they could have a valuable impact in clinical veterinary medicine. However, before clinicians can take advantage of these drugs, detailed pharmacokinetic studies will have to be performed to determine if any of the longer-acting cephalosporins are in fact longer-acting in the dog and/or cat.

β-Lactam Antibiotics: Nonclassical

CARBAPENEMS

Spectrum of Activity. Imipenum is the first of a newly developed β-lactam antibiotic family that differs from

TABLE 51–3. COMPARATIVE SENSITIVITIES OF VETERINARY PATHOGENS ISOLATED FROM DOGS AT NCSU-SVM TO THIRD-GENERATION CEPHALOSPORINS

	Percentage of sensitive Isolates				
	E. coli N = 153*	*Klebsiella pneumoniae* N = 32	*Proteus mirabilis* N = 67	*Pseudomonas aeruginosa* N = 40	*Enterobacter* spp. N=18
Cefotaxime	97	100	91	60	75
Cefaperazone	64	25	44	73	50
Moxalactam	97	97	36	62	89

Cefotaxime and moxalactam were determined sensitive if MIC < 32 μg/ml and cefaperazone at < 64 μg/ml.
*N = number of isolates.

the classical β-lactams in structure but retains a similar therapeutic margin of safety.[53] This antibiotic exhibits a very broad and potent spectrum of activity toward both gram-positive and gram-negative organisms. Carbapenems are uniformly resistant to all β-lactamase inactivation and demonstrate extensive binding affinity for PBP 3. Previously resistant *Pseudomonas aeruginosa*, *Enterobacter cloacae* and aminoglycoside-resistant Enterobacteriaceae are sensitive to this drug, with MICs less than 1 μg/ml. Imipenum has been used at NCSU for the treatment of *P. aeruginosa* infections resistant to all the antipseudomonal penicillins, aminoglycosides, and in three cases, to a combination of these two antibiotics. Seven of the eight dogs recovered clinically, with negative cultures following ten days of treatment with imipenum. Resistance is very infrequently encountered; however, an imipenum-resistant *P. aeruginosa* was cultured from the urine of a dog one week following treatment, indicating that it is possible to develop resistance during treatment.

The drug is marketed with cilastatin in a 1:1 ratio. Cilastatin has no antimicrobial activity and is used to inhibit the metabolism of imipenum by inhibiting dehydropeptidase-1 enzymes located in the basement membrane of the proximal tubular cells of the kidney. Inactivating this enzyme by competitive inhibition allows the accumulation of imipenum in the urine without changing its serum pharmacokinetics.[54] Nephrotoxicity has been seen in rabbits with high doses of imipenum given alone; however, this toxicity is eliminated when imipenum is combined with cilastatin. Presumably, a metabolite of imipenum is potentially nephrotoxic.

Clinical Pharmacology. Imipenum, like most β-lactams, is widely distributed into most tissues, except for the CNS. It has low protein binding in dogs (less than 20 per cent) and is eliminated largely by renal filtration, secretion, and metabolism. Imipenum is not very soluble in aqueous solutions and must be dissolved in a minimum of 50 ml of diluent. Therefore, the only route of delivery is by intravenous infusion. Following an intravenous dose of 2.3 mg/lb (5 mg/kg), peak serum concentrations of more than 50 μg/ml are obtained. The elimination half-life of imipenum in the dog is 30 minutes, with less than ten per cent of the active drug found in the urine.[55] When cilastatin is added to the formulation, the elimination half-life remains the same but more than 70 per cent of the administered imipenum is found intact in the urine.

MONOBACTAMS

Aztreonam is the first member of a new group of monocyclic β-lactam antibiotics that exhibits excellent resistance to gram-negative β-lactamase inactivation.[56] Like imipenum, its antibacterial activity is from binding with and interfering in the function of PBP 3, resulting in long filamentous forms of bacteria.

Unlike the carbapenems, this new addition to the β-lactam family acts against aerobic gram-negative bacteria only. In vitro studies on human pathogens have indicated excellent activity (greater than 95 per cent) against all the Enterobacteriaceae. In fact, in normal human volunteers treated with a standard 300 mg dose, no Enterobacteriaceae could be isolated from their fecal cultures.[56]

No data are available on the spectrum of activity or clinical pharmacology in companion animals. However, this family of monocyclic β-lactams will be enlarging and, given the rate of resistance developing in the companion animal population, they could find a useful place in the clinician's armamentarium.

Miscellaneous Cell Wall–Active Antibiotics

There remain two other antibiotics that do not fit into the previous classifications but that interfere in bacterial cell wall synthesis or function. These include bacitracin and vancomycin.

Bacitracin is really a mixture of ten different bacitracins, only some of which have been structurally identified. Bacitracin A is the major component; its spectrum of activity is confined to gram-positive organisms. Bacitracin A interacts with undecaprenylpyrophosphate, which is critical for cell-wall glycan polymerization, preventing it from dephosphorylating and thus preventing peptidoglycan formation and cell wall synthesis. This drug also disrupts lipid membranes, which is lethal to bacteria but also causes nephrotoxicity and limits its use to topical applications.

Vancomycin is an older parenteral antibiotic with an exclusively gram-positive spectrum. Its excellent activity against penicillin-resistant staphylococci and its obvious resistance to any β-lactamase has resulted in this drug being a drug of choice in methicillin-resistant staphylococcal infections. This organism is becoming a more common problem in most human hospitals but has yet to be described as a serious veterinary pathogen. Vancomycin inhibits the same step in cell wall synthesis as β-lactams, but not by competitive inhibition of the PBP, rather by directly binding to the d-alanyl-D-alanyl peptides that are involved in the cross-linking of the peptidoglycans. This drug is relatively expensive and its use is restricted to the last resort in very selected serious staphylococcal infections.

LABILIZERS OF MICROBIAL CELL MEMBRANES

Antimicrobials that act by labilizing cell membranes, that is, changing their permeability, and causing the cells to lose their osmotic integrity, do so by simple detergent action. These agents have hydrophilic and lipophilic regions in their structure and work by penetrating through the bacterial cell wall down to the cell membrane, where they penetrate easily into this lipid structure. They increase its surface area by bringing in water until it collapses. Their effectiveness depends on the amount of phospholipid in the cell membrane and on their being able to penetrate through the cell wall. Unfortunately, mammalian cells are also composed of phospholipid-containing cell membranes and therefore all these agents have varying degrees of toxic effects that limit many of them to nonsystemic routes of administration. The exceptions are some of the antifungal agents, which take advantage of the unique cell membrane structure of fungi.

Polymyxins

These agents are largely of more historical interest, since their extreme nephrotoxicity and the advent of aminoglycosides have reduced their role to only topical applications. Polymyxin B and colistin (polymyxin E) are the two most commonly used polymyxins.

Spectrum of Activity. These products are restricted to gram-negative bacteria, where most of the Enterobacteriaceae, *Enterobacter* spp., and *Pseudomonas aeruginosa* are sensitive to less than eight μg/ml of polymyxin B. Resistance is uncommon. These products are restricted to topical and ophthalmic applications, where they are very effective. They are not absorbed, even when applied to denuded skin or mucous membranes, and have been successfully used in the treatment of corneal ulcers caused by *P. aeruginosa*.

Polyene Antifungal Drugs

This group includes amphotericin B and nystatin.

Mechanism of Action. Unlike the simple detergent action of the polymyxins, the polyenes bind specifically to a sterol component (ergosterol) of the fungus cell membrane. Once bound, their amphoteric nature causes formation of channels through the membrane, which results in leakage of small cytoplasmic molecules. These agents can be fungistatic or fungicidal, depending on the dose and the fungus.[57]

Spectrum of Activity. These agents demonstrate excellent activity against *Histoplasma capsulatum*, *Cryptococcus neoformans*, *Coccidioides immitis*, *Blastomyces dermatitidis*, *Candida* spp., and many strains of *Aspergillus*. In vitro MICs for these organisms are on the order of 0.03 to 1.0 μg/ml for amphotericin B and 1.5 to 6.5 μg/ml for nystatin.[58] Amphotericin B is one of the drugs of choice for a patient with a systemic mycosis. Due to excessive toxicity, nystatin is restricted to topical use in infections caused by *Candida* spp.

Clinical Pharmacology. Nystatin is not administered parenterally and is not appreciably absorbed following oral administration. It is used to treat candidiasis of the skin, mucous membranes, and intestinal tract. Applications in veterinary medicine have been few, since candidiasis is usually an infection of immunosuppression or extended spectrum antibiotics. However, it is used extensively by avian practitioners in treating psitticines undergoing broad-spectrum antibiotic treatment.

Amphotericin B is used as a parenteral antifungal agent. It is administered by the intravenous route only since it is poorly absorbed orally. The drug binds to lipoproteins in the blood and extensively to cholesterol-containing membranes in the tissues. It has a prolonged distribution half-life of 1.5 hours and an elimination half-life of 45 to 50 hours. The drug's metabolism (if any) is unknown. Only 25 per cent of the administered dose is recovered in the urine nine days after a single dose, with another 20 per cent excreted in the feces and the remaining 65 per cent unaccounted for.[59] The drug does not accumulate in patients with renal dysfunction, which indicates that extensive storage of this drug occurs. Human patients still have measurable quantities seven to eight weeks following treatment. No antimicrobial has a more elaborate dosage regimen. Currently, the drug is administered once every other day by intravenous infusion or a slow diluted bolus, with a total administered dose of 3.5 to 4.0 mg/lb (8 to 9 mg/kg).[60] The current dose of 0.23 mg/lb (0.5 mg/kg) is expected to produce peak steady-state concentrations of 0.3 μg/ml and a trough of 0.13 μg/ml. This gives an average steady-state concentration of 0.2 μg/ml, which is close to that achieved in human patients (0.5 μg/ml).

Toxicity. Nystatin has few untoward effects unless given orally when vomiting and diarrhea are present. It apparently tastes terrible, which may make oral compliance difficult. Amphotericin B has serious toxic side effects, including renal toxicosis, fever, and nausea. The renal toxicity may be lessened, but not eliminated, by concurrent administration of mannitol. This, however, does not seem to increase the efficacy of amphotericin B.[60] Most dogs receiving this drug have mild to moderate fevers lasting up to 36 hours following dosing. The renal toxicity has been reported to be quickly reversible following discontinuation of the drug in human patients, but in the canine it appears to be more permanent.

Imidazole Antifungal Drugs

Substituted imidazoles used in the treatment of systemic mycoses are being actively investigated. One such drug, ketoconazole, has been available since 1983. The mechanism of action of these agents is slightly different than the polyenes. The imidazoles do not bind to ergosterol; they inhibit its formation by inhibiting a cell membrane–bound enzyme, lanosterol demethylase, which functions to demethylate lanosterol, a precursor of ergosterol. This difference in mechanism means that their fungicidal activity is slower (five to ten days) than the immediate action of polyenes.

Spectrum of Activity. The in vitro spectrum of these agents is very broad. However, the in vitro MIC deter minations are highly erratic and are so dependent on assay conditions that extrapolation to in vivo efficacy is difficult. Notwithstanding, these agents have been shown in clinical cases to be effective against the major systemic mycotic infections, histoplasmosis, blastomycosis, cryptococcosis, and coccidiomycosis. They are also effective against dermatophytes such as *Microsporum* and *Trichophyton* and are becoming a drug of choice for *Candida* infections.[61]

Clinical Pharmacology. Ketoconazole is well absorbed in the dog, with peak serum concentrations occurring within two hours after a standard oral dose of 4.5 mg/lb (10 mg/kg).[61] Maximum absorption occurs in an acidic environment, which is best in the fasted patient. Elimination is biexponential, with a prolonged distribution half-life of two hours and an elimination half-life of ten hours. In humans, less than five per cent of the drug is excreted unchanged in the urine, which is consistent with its extensive hepatic microsomal oxidation. However, in humans the elimination of this drug is dose-dependent; it may also be so in the dog and cat.[62] The relationship of serum concentration and efficacy and/or toxicity is not clear and dosing in the canine has been based more on empirical success.

Toxicity. Dogs have been given four times the recommended dose 18 mg/lb/day (40 mg/kg/day) for one year with few adverse effects. It is only at 27 to 36 mg/lb (60 to 80 mg/kg) that hepatotoxicity, consisting of increased liver enzymes and cholangiohepatitis, is seen.[61] Cats have experienced more gastrointestinal signs than dogs but the drug has still been used widely and safely in this species. A more immediate problem is the effect that ketoconazole has on mammalian steroid production. Dogs receiving 4.5 to 13.6 mg/lb/day (10 to 30 mg/kg/day) show a significant decrease in resting and post-ACTH cortisol concentrations, as well as a decrease in testosterone and an increase in progesterone.[63] These effects were dose-dependent and were described after the first dose. In contrast, cats given 13.6 mg/lb/day (30 mg/kg/day) for 30 days had no significant change in any of these hormones. No clinical effects have been noted in these dogs, in spite of lower plasma cortisols. However, caution is indicated in the use of these products in breeding animals. The significance of these findings will become more apparent as use of this and other imidazoles increases.

BACTERICIDAL INHIBITORS OF PROTEIN SYNTHESIS: AMINOGLYCOSIDES

Despite the advent of third-generation cephalosporins, carbapenems, and monobactams, the aminoglycosides remain the drugs of choice in serious gram-negative bacterial infections. The understanding of their toxicity along with improvement in therapeutic monitoring of these compounds has significantly reduced their nephro- and ototoxicity. In addition, a better appreciation of the mechanisms of bacterial resistance makes appropriate selection among these compounds more rational.

Mechanism of Action. The majority of an aminoglycoside's effect is due to binding to, and consequently distorting, bacterial ribosomes. More specifically, the individual aminoglycosides appear to do one or more of the following: they bind to one or more sites on the 30S ribosome unit, causing misreading of the RNA codon; they block the initiation process between the ribosome and the mRNA; they stabilize the peptidyl-tRNA binding to the ribosome so that it cannot translocate.[64] The end result is extensive loss of protein synthesis. Despite this and other cell surface–labilizing properties exhibited by these antibiotics, the reason for their bactericidal activity remains unclear.

Spectrum of Activity. Remarkably, almost all aerobic and facultative anaerobic bacteria growing under aerobic conditions are sensitive to aminoglycosides. Only the streptococcal species does not show any appreciable degree of sensitivity. Aminoglycosides are the drugs of choice in systemic infections caused by *Pseudomonas aeruginosa* and *Klebsiella pneumoniae*. Significantly, group D enterococci (*Streptococcus faecium*, *Streptococcus faecalis*) are resistant due to lack of a drug transport mechanism in their cytoplasmic membrane. The aminoglycosides are highly hydrophilic and penetrate poorly into bacteria. Their uptake into gram-negative species occurs by two mechanisms. The first uses small, water-filled channels called porins, located in the polysaccharide outer coating. The size of these channels allows small hydrophilic compounds to penetrate down to the cytoplasmic membrane. The second mechanism takes place here, for unlike the β-lactams, which work on the surface of the cell membrane, the aminoglycosides must be internalized. This internalization step is an active process that depends on oxygen. Thus anaerobic growing bacteria are resistant to the aminoglycosides due to lack of uptake. This is of critical importance when realizing that many of the Enterobacteriaceae are facultative anaerobes. Thus in abscesses, where oxygen tension is low, these organisms can grow. The in vitro sensitivity tests are performed under aerobic conditions and most likely will indicate the bacteria is sensitive. However, treatment failure is likely to occur in this situation due to the anaerobic condition of the infection.

The aminoglycosides can be empirically broken into two categories. The first category is limited-use compounds, including neomycin, streptomycin, dihydrostreptomycin, and kanamycin. Neomycin is restricted to nonsystemic uses by its nephrotoxicity and streptomycin and dihydrostreptomycin are restricted by the degree of bacterial resistance to them that has developed over the years. Kanamycin was introduced to overcome the resistance seen with these earlier compounds; however, it was never effective against *Pseudomonas aeruginosa* and is inferior in activity to every member of the second group. For these reasons it cannot be recommended for use.

The second group is composed of the most frequently used aminoglycosides and includes gentamicin, amikacin, and tobramycin. Newer aminoglycosides with which there is little veterinary experience include netilmicin and dibekacin. The difference in spectrum of these aminoglycosides is an important criterion in the selection of which to use. Ten years ago, little, if any, resistance to gentamicin existed and it was the drug of choice for all gram-negative infections. Now, however, in some centers resistance is unacceptably large. The reason for the resistance is discussed below; however, it is selection pressure caused by antibiotic usage that accelerates the appearance of these organisms.[29] The resistance in a given geographical locale most likely depends on the frequency of use of a given aminoglycoside. The in vitro activities of three aminoglycosides from NCSU (a hospital where gentamicin is frequently used) are shown in Table 51–4. As can be seen, gentamicin is the worst of the three in the overall activities. Its (and tobramycin's) activities toward *E. coli* are striking. This degree of resistance has not been reported before. The AMC in New York reported a 96 per cent sensitivity of *E. coli* from 1980 to 1983[33] and the University of California at Davis reported 97 per cent of their *E. coli* tested prior to 1982 were sensitive.[28] However, by 1985 the sensitivity of *E. coli* isolated from canine patients at the AMC had decreased to 86 per cent. These data are consistent with data reported from large referral human hospitals, where the more frequent use of gentamicin has resulted in an increase in resistance.[29] Again, it is important to note that the degree of resistance seen is probably greater at a veterinary teaching institute than will be encountered in private hospitals. However, most of the patients with resistant organisms presented to NCSU were already infected with these organisms prior to referral, meaning that these resistant strains for the most part do not represent nosocomial hospital strains. Therefore, across-the-board statements that a particular antibiotic is effective against a particular type of bacteria is becoming increasingly more difficult to make.

Mechanism of Resistance. Plasmid-mediated drug-modifying enzymes are responsible for the majority of bacterial resistance to the aminoglycosides.[65] Unlike the β-lactams, where all the different enzymes simply open the β-lactam ring, these enzymes are more diverse in the type of drug modification they cause. They are identified based on which portion of the molecule they modify. Basically, there are three types: phosphotransferases (APH), acetyltransferases (AAC), and adenyltransferases (AAD).

Clinical Pharmacology. All the aminoglycosides have essentially identical pharmacokinetics. These drugs are not orally absorbed and therefore are restricted to parenteral routes of administration. However, the oral route is used, usually with neomycin, in the therapy of hepatic encephalopathy, where a reduction in aerobic enterics decreases the production of ammonia. In addition, aerosolation of aminoglycosides provides a more logical approach to the therapy of gram-negative lower respiratory infections by getting the drug to the site of infection without systemic absorption.[66] Basically, the disposition of parenterally administered aminoglycosides best fits a three compartment model.[67] There is rapid tissue distribution confined to the extracellular fluid compartment. Aminoglycosides are highly hydrophilic and penetrate tissues poorly. This volume of distribution is increased during septicemia, causing a decrease in predicted serum concentrations at a given dose. Aminoglycosides are eliminated almost exclusively by renal filtration, with a half-life of 40 to 60 minutes and a drug clearance corresponding to the patient's glomerular filtration rate (GFR) (3.0 to 4.0 ml/min/kg). Obviously, any decrease in renal GFR causes a similar change in drug clearance, resulting in higher and more prolonged serum drug concentrations. The importance of these observations is discussed later.

These drugs also have a long terminal elimination phase, with a greater than 30 hour half-life.[68, 69] It is this terminal phase that is best correlated with nephrotoxicity, for it represents the release of drug from the proximal renal tubular cells where aminoglycosides are actively taken up against a concentration gradient.[70]

Toxicity. The important differences between these compounds lie in their intrinsic toxicity. The three possible toxicities exhibited to varying degrees by all members of this group are nephrotoxicity, ototoxicity, and neuromuscular synaptic dysfunction. The mechanisms of toxicity for each of these are not completely clear; however, they appear to operate independently to some degree.

The intrinsic potential for nephrotoxicity appears to be correlated with two factors of drug disposition. First is the amount of drug reabsorbed in the proximal tubules and second is the tendency to damage intracellular organelles. The uptake of aminoglycosides into the tubular cells depends on binding to acidic phospholipid receptors on the brush border of their proximal renal tubular cell. The drug is taken into the cell by endocytosis and then into the lysosomes, where it interferes with phospholipid metabolism.[71] Alteration in the phospholipase metabolism ultimately causes an increase in lysosome permeability and a leakage of proteolytic enzymes into the cytoplasm. Gentamicin, which exhibits the greatest degree of tubular reabsorption and is the most potent at interfering with phospholipase metabolism, has the greatest nephrotoxic potential. Amikacin and netilmicin show the smallest amount of net tubular uptake, poorly inhibit phospholipase metabolism, and are the least nephrotoxic aminoglycosides in human and animal studies.[72, 73] This difference between gentamicin- and netilmicin-induced nephrotoxicity has been con-

TABLE 51–4. COMPARISON OF THE IN VITRO SENSITIVITIES OF FIVE COMMON VETERINARY PATHOGENS TO THREE DIFFERENT AMINOGLYCOSIDES

	Percentage of sensitive Isolates				
	Staphylococcus intermedius N = 138*	*E. coli* N = 153	*Klebsiella pneumoniae* N = 32	*Proteus mirabilis* N = 67	*Pseudomonas aeruginosa* N = 40
Gentamicin	92	85	56	90	60
Amikacin	85	97	100	91	90
Tobramycin	87	83	66	90	88

Sensitivity for gentamicin and tobramycin determined at MIC < 8 μg/ml and for amikacin at < 32 μg/ml.
*N = number of isolates.

firmed in the dog and cat.[74, 75] However, it is important to point out that in the clinical patient studies done to determine which aminoglycosides are the most toxic, conflicting results have been obtained. In a review of over 10,000 human patients treated with aminoglycosides, the following incidences of nephrotoxicity were reported: 14 per cent for gentamicin, 12.9 per cent for tobramycin, 9.4 per cent for amikacin, and 8.7 per cent for netilmicin.[76]

The applicability of the research studies and this clinical study to veterinary medicine is that gentamicin is probably more intrinsically toxic than netilmicin and amikacin. Conversely, amikacin and netilmicin are still nephrotoxins and must be used with the same degree of care as gentamicin.

Dosage Modification. No group of antibiotics generates a more intense debate on the role of dose and frequency of dosing than does the aminoglycosides. This is obviously due to their inherent toxicity. However, the dosing rationale generated for these drugs can be applied to other antibiotics where toxicity is not a concern but improved efficacy is of concern. It is clear from experimental work that normal healthy animals with normal renal function are fairly resistant to the major toxic effects using standard clinical doses.[68] However, patients frequently have associated risk factors, clearly identified in humans, which potentiate the toxicity of these drugs. These risk factors are renal dysfunction, age, dehydration, fever, and sepsis. Obviously, these factors may occur together or separately, with the greatest potential for toxicity occurring in the patient in whom all of these factors are present. In renal dysfunction, particularly compensated chronic renal disease, the hypertrophied remaining nephrons filter and reabsorb a greater amount of drug than the nephrons of normal kidneys.[70] This situation is very commonly encountered in older dog and cat patients, where normal values for serum creatinine tell little regarding a patient's renal status. For these reasons treating patients with standard dosages of aminoglycosides can lead to nephrotoxicity.[77] However, it is important to keep in mind that renal tubular cells regenerate and that the dysfunction is reversible, given a situation where only a moderate amount of damage has been done before the toxicity is recognized. Therefore, dosage modification must be undertaken to prevent or minimize toxicity while assuring optimum efficacy.

Unfortunately, the veterinary clinician does not have the algorithms and formulas for more accurate dosage modifications based on a patient's risk factors, and due to the diversity in the dog population this information is unlikely to be developed. However, the clinician can improve therapy by the following measures. First, use a dosing range and dose according to the animal's size and associated risk factors. The larger the animal, the smaller the dose. The more risk factors the patient has, the smaller the dose. In an old patient or one with suspected renal disease, increasing the dosing interval from every eight hours to every 16 or 24 is less toxic than decreasing the dose and keeping the interval the same.[68] To monitor for renal toxicity, determine a serum creatinine concentration prior to therapy. A serum creatinine of 1.2 mg/dl may be in the normal range but if that patient started therapy with a value of 0.6 mg/dl then the GFR has decreased by 50 per cent and the drug should be discontinued. Monitoring the urine for changes in concentrating ability or sediment analysis is an excellent way to determine toxicity, but in a patient with a urinary tract infection it is not very useful. Toxicity is much easier to avoid than maximum efficacy is to achieve. The efficacy of these drugs in human patients is best correlated with peak serum concentrations, particularly the ratio of peak serum concentration to the MIC.[78] Since treatment starts before cultures are taken, the MIC is not known. Therefore, the highest safe peak concentration should be achieved. For gentamicin and tobramycin, 10 to 15 μg/ml is recommended and 40 to 60 μg/ml is recommended for amikacin. The dosages listed in Table 51–10 give those peak values if the drug is administered intravenously and the animal is "normal." However, patients are not always "kinetically" normal and desired concentrations are not always produced. Therefore, serum drug concentrations can be used to monitor therapy and more accurately modify the dosage. Therapeutic drug monitoring is easily accessible through most community hospitals or large commercial laboratories. New technology has made these tests very rapid and relatively economical. Blood samples drawn 30 minutes after dosing can be used to determine peak serum concentrations. Even without a full description of that patient's pharmacokinetics, dosages can be modified by less precise but still applicable dose-serum concentration relationships. If peak concentrations are 25 per cent lower than required, then the dose can be increased by 25 per cent. Similarly, if the peak concentration is 50 per cent higher than desired, the dose should be cut in half, or if renal disease is suspected, the dose should be kept constant and the dosing interval doubled. These simple relationships between a drug's concentration and serum concentrations apply to many drugs and should be used until more sophisticated methods of dosage modification are available.

BACTERIOSTATIC INHIBITORS OF PROTEIN SYNTHESIS

The antibiotics in this category share the mechanistic action of impairing protein synthesis, which impedes bacterial cell division. The effect is reversible in vitro, where the drug can be removed and bacterial function returned. In vivo, the effect is probably less reversible since the host's immune system can effectively remove these nondividing bacteria via phagocytic action. The clinical importance placed on bacteriostatic versus bactericidal action is often an academic exercise, since many of the so-called bactericidal agents are bacteriostatic in a given infection and vice versa. These terms relate to in vitro effects and with only a few exceptions, the choice of an antibiotic should not depend on this variable characteristic.

TETRACYCLINES

This group of antibiotics includes seven different congeners of the basic tetracycline structure. Tetracycline, oxytetracycline, doxycycline, and minocycline are discussed because they are the agents most likely to be used clinically.

Mechanism of Action. These agents, like aminoglycosides, inhibit protein synthesis by binding to the 30S ribosome and interfering in RNA-to-protein translation. More specifically, these drugs must first be actively taken into the cell by a periplasmic protein carrier.[79] Unlike aminoglycosides, this energy-dependent step does not depend on the membrane potential, which allows these drugs to work in anaerobic and hyperosmolar environments. Upon binding to the 30S ribosome, they interfere in the translocation of the amino acid carrying tRNA to the mRNA-ribosome complex, preventing addition of amino acids to the peptide chain being formed. Tetracyclines also bind to the 80S mammalian ribosome and inhibit protein synthesis. However, they do so with much less affinity. Nevertheless, the higher the dose of tetracyclines, the more host protein synthesis in rapidly dividing cells is impaired and the more catabolic the drug is.

Spectrum of Activity. Originally these agents were very efficacious against a very extensive group of microorganisms. The spectrum has not changed over the years but their efficacy has. With the advent of newer drugs in the 1960s and the emergence of resistance, these drugs have been less commonly used. However, they do inhibit growth of both aerobic and anaerobic gram-positive and gram-negative bacteria. Doxycycline and minocycline exhibit the greatest antimicrobial potency of the group. However, in vitro potency does not necessarily translate into more clinical efficacy, at least not in human patients, and the justification for using the newer, more expensive tetracyclines is sometimes lacking.

While their efficacy against these organisms in systemic infections may not be very good, they do seem to have a place in the treatment of simple lower urinary tract infections, where concentrations are much higher than in serum.[28] These agents are best used in infections caused by nonbacterial species such as *Rickettsia* (Rocky Mountain spotted fever) and *Borrelia* (Lyme disease), where they are very effective. They also are very effective in infections caused by *Mycoplasma pneumoniae* and *Chlamydia*. In humans, they are a drug of choice in the treatment of brucellosis and minocycline has been used successfully for canine brucellosis.[80]

Mechanism of Resistance. Resistance of the common bacterial pathogens to the tetracyclines has become a major problem. Resistance to *E. coli* and probably other organisms is caused by an R plasmid that does not cause modification of the drug, but rather changes the proteins in the inner cell membrane responsible for tetracycline uptake.[79] Resistance to nonbacterial pathogens such as *Rickettsia* and *Borrelia* has been reported but is not yet a major problem.

Clinical Pharmacology. All tetracyclines are sufficiently absorbed following oral dosing. However, oral absorption can be very erratic.[81] Oxytetracycline has the worst absorption, doxycycline and minocycline the best. Food, dairy products, and antacids impair absorption. These drugs' ability to chelate calcium ions correlates with their bioavailability. These drugs are well distributed into tissue, including the CNS, in accordance with their lipid solubility. Both minocycline and doxycycline achieve a higher percentage of drug in most tissue than do oxytetracycline and tetracycline. However, the lipophilicity of minocycline and doxycycline means that more is excreted into the bile than is filtered into urine, while oxytetracycline and tetracycline undergo more extensive renal filtration and achieve a high concentration of drug in the urine. Nevertheless, all these agents are concentrated in the liver and have significant biliary excretion. Doxycycline is different from the others in that it is eliminated by intestinal excretion as an inactive product, either conjugated or chelated by fecal products. Its elimination is not affected by renal disease and it is the tetracycline of choice in any patient with renal dysfunction. The elimination half-life of the tetracyclines in dogs is not as dramatically different as in humans. Oxytetracycline has the shortest half-life of five to six hours, while doxycycline has the longest (ten hours).[82] Minocycline, the longest-acting tetracycline in humans, does not appear to be so in dogs. Following intravenous injection the drug is eliminated as rapidly as oxytetracycline, with a half-life of six to seven hours.[83]

Toxicity. Species variation in the toxicity of the drugs is clear.[80] Cats, like horses, can exhibit severe gastrointestinal disorders following oxytetracycline administration. Vomiting, diarrhea, fever, and anorexia have been reported in cats receiving this product. Minocycline causes hypotension when given as an intravenous bolus.[83] There have been no reports on the other tetracyclines and the effects that these agents might have are unknown. The major toxicities of these drugs are seen in patients with azotemia, where the catabolic effects of these drugs can exacerbate the disease and precipitate uremia. Doxycycline can be given safely to azotemic human patients and probably should be used in dogs with renal disease. The drugs chelate with calcium pyrophosphate in teeth and bone, resulting in discoloration of puppies' teeth and more importantly, slowing of bone development. These drugs are not recommended in young growing dogs or in pregnant bitches due to their catabolic effects.

CHLORAMPHENICOL

Spectrum of Activity. The spectrum of chloramphenicol is very similar to the tetracyclines in its breadth. However, in almost all cases it excels them in efficacy. Aerobic and anaerobic gram-positive and gram-negative bacteria, Rickettsiae, *Chlamydia*, and *Mycoplasma* are all part of this drug's activity spectrum. Its efficacy against most bacterial pathogens is greater than tetracyclines; however, drugs of greater efficacy are available. In general, its efficacy against the Enterobacteriaceae is less than cephalothin. It is most efficacious against *E. coli*. It is not the drug of choice for any gram-positive infections, with similar or less activity than ampicillin against staphylococci and streptococci. In vitro MIC determinations conducted at the AMC and NCSU have shown that chloramphenicol's sensitivity to most gram-negative bacteria occurs at the upper range of sensitivity, 8 μg/ml. Its use in bacterial infections is as a second line drug, particularly in urinary tract infections, where in spite of the fact that only ten per cent of the drug is excreted unchanged, urine concentrations are in excess of 100 μg/ml following standard dosing.[84] Its major efficacy is against obligate anaerobes, where virtually 100 per cent in vitro sensitivity toward *Clostridium* and *Bacteroides* spp. is reported. It is a drug of choice in anaerobic infections, along with metronidazole. Chloramphenicol is also effective in the treatment of rickettsial infections and is given to patients not responding to tetracycline.

Mechanism of Action. Chloramphenicol is essentially a un-ionized, highly lipophilic compound that enters cells by passive, or perhaps facilitated, diffusion. Its binding site is primarily the bacterial 50S ribosome (same as the macrolides) but it may also bind to the 30S subunit as well. Once bound, the drug interferes in the elongation of the growing peptide by preventing the binding of the amino acid end of the aminoacyl tRNA to the ribosome.[85] Mammalian mitochondria contain ribosomes that resemble bacterial ribosomes. Chloramphenicol can bind to this 70S complex and interfere in mitochondrial protein synthesis. This is particularly evident in erythropoietic cells of the bone marrow and is the basis for chloramphenicol's major toxic effect, nonregenerative anemia.

Clinical Pharmacology. Oral formulations of chloramphenicol include capsules, tablets, and suspensions. Capsules and tablets are rapidly absorbed following a 15 mg/lb (33 mg/kg) dose in both dogs and cats, with peak serum concentrations of 20 to 25 μg/ml occurring in 30 minutes. However, chloramphenicol suspensions (palmitate ester) produce significantly lower serum concentrations in fasted cats.[86] The parenteral formulation consists of the sodium succinate salt. This salt is rapidly hydrolyzed in the liver to form chloramphenicol. This formulation is rapidly and completely absorbed from intramuscular and subcutaneous injections, producing peak concentrations in excess of 20 μg/ml following a 9 mg/lb (20 mg/kg) dose.[87, 88] The drug is well distributed throughout the body, achieving tissue concentrations equal to or exceeding serum concentrations. Concentrations in the CNS display a concentration-time profile similar to serum except for a substantial four to six hour delay.[89] Chloramphenicol does achieve significant concentrations across the inflamed or noninflamed meninges; however, its spectrum of activity may not make it the drug of choice in meningitis and one should not select it merely because it can pass the blood-brain barrier. In the dog, the drug is eliminated primarily by hepatic glucuronide conjugation, with only five to ten per cent of the intact drug excreted into the urine. Its elimination half-life is four to five hours. In contrast, the cat excretes in excess of 25 per cent of the intact drug into the urine, making the cat with renal dysfunction more susceptible to drug accumulation and toxicity.[90] The cat has little ability to glucuronidate drugs, which accounts for the greater amount of intact drug in the urine. However, the elimination half-life is similar to the dog, four hours following intravenous administration and seven to eight hours following oral administration.

Since toxicity precludes concentrations greater than 25 μg/ml, which can be achieved by the oral route, the parenteral route is used only in patients unable to take medication orally. This is in marked contrast to other antibiotics discussed, where the parenteral route is used to achieve greater serum concentrations and thus enhance tissue concentrations.

Toxicity. Chloramphenicol is a very bitter-tasting compound and oral dosing can be difficult in animals who discover this by breaking a capsule or tablet while being dosed. At doses exceeding 70 mg/lb/day (150 mg/kg/day), dogs can become anorexic. This happens in cats at much lower doses, which has prompted one clinician to propose a dose of 50 mg/cat/twice daily.[91] One author has found that this dose is less prone to produce anorexia in cats already inappetent from disease.

The most serious toxicity seen with chloramphenicol is a reversible, nonregenerative anemia. The anemia is not the idiosyncratic aplastic anemia seen in humans, but is due to a dose-dependent pharmacodynamic action of the drug inhibiting protein (enzymes) synthesis in erythropoietic cells. General bone marrow suppression can also be seen, particularly in cats receiving high doses of chloramphenicol. In humans this effect is correlated with serum concentrations greater than 25 μg/ml. Cats receiving the "dog" dose of 70 mg/lb/day (150 mg/kg/day) would be expected to have peak concentrations in excess of 70 μg/ml.[92] It is not surprising that the cat has been unfairly labeled as being "sensitive" to the drug when in actuality it is only sensitive if given toxic doses.

MACROLIDES AND LINCOSAMIDES

The agents in these two groups, although structurally different, share common activities, mechanisms of activity, and therapeutic uses. Of all the macrolides available outside the United States, only erythromycin and tylosin are used in small animal practice. Lincomycin and clindamycin are the two lincosamides that are commonly used in clinical veterinary medicine.

Spectrum of Activity. All these drugs have a primarily gram-positive spectrum of activity. They are extremely active against common streptococcal human pathogens such as *Streptococcus pneumoniae* and *Streptococcus pyogenes*. However, against veterinary pathogens, they are second-line antibiotics, displaying their greatest activity toward coagulase-positive staphylococci. Table 51–5 shows the sensitivities of pathogens isolated at NCSU to two representatives of this group compared with ampicillin. Clearly, they have better activity than ampicillin against *Staphylococcus intermedius*. However, any of the antistaphylococcal penicillins or oral cepha-

TABLE 51–5. PERCENTAGE OF ISOLATES FROM NCSU-SVM SENSITIVE IN VITRO TO ERYTHROMYCIN AND CLINDAMYCIN COMPARED TO AMPICILLIN

Antibiotic	*Staphylococcus intermedius* N = 138	*Streptococcus faecalis* N = 36	*Streptococcus faecium* N = 26
Erythromycin	70	50	28
Clindamycin	70	25	25
Ampicillin	55	100	40

Sensitivity determined for all three antibiotics at a MIC < 4 μg/ml.
N = number of isolates.

losporins exhibit greater activity. They are not as effective because they do not penetrate well into gram-negative bacteria. Notable exceptions are *Pasteurella multocida* and *Bordetella*. These compounds also show excellent activity against gram-positive and gram-negative obligate anaerobic bacteria, with clindamycin being the most active of the group.

Erythromycin is the drug of choice for infections caused by *Campylobacter jejuni* and can be used as a third drug of choice in the treatment diseases caused by *Rickettsia* and *Borrelia*. Clindamycin is more potent than lincomycin against all pathogens and should be used in its place.

Mechanism of Action. All members of these groups have mechanisms of action similar to chloramphenicol. Binding to the 50S ribosomal subunit causes the cessation of the development of larger polymerized peptides, but not smaller ones. Erythromycin penetrates better into bacteria in its nonionized state, which occurs in an alkaline environment (pH greater than 8). A five- to tenfold reduction in MIC can occur by changing the pH from 5.5 to 8.0.[89] Resistance to these drugs, at least in *Staphylococcus aureus*, is caused by R-plasmids encoding for enzymes that methylate the ribosomal binding site for these drugs. Resistance to one usually means resistance to all members of these groups.

Clinical Pharmacology. Oral absorption of these products is reasonably complete and rapid. All produce higher tissue concentrations than serum concentrations; therefore, serum concentrations should be interpreted with caution.

Erythromycin produces peak serum concentrations of 1 to 2 μg/ml following a 7 mg/lb (15 mg/kg) dose. The drug is distributed well into the tissues, including the prostate (where the drug unfortunately is not active due to the low pH). The drug is extensively metabolized in the liver, with less than five per cent excreted unchanged into the urine. Elimination is primarily through metabolism and biliary excretion with an elimination half-life of 60 minutes.[93]

Tylosin is virtually identical to erythromycin.

Lincomycin given orally at 11.5 mg/lb (25 mg/kg) produces peak serum concentrations of 3 μg/ml, with almost equivalent concentrations occurring in the skin. The elimination is by hepatic metabolism, with an oral elimination half-life of three hours.

Clindamycin is more rapidly absorbed following oral administration than the others and therefore produces the highest peak serum concentration (5 μg/ml after a 5 mg/lb or 11 mg/kg dose). This drug penetrates well into all tissues, including bone and white blood cells. The drug is eliminated by hepatic metabolism, with an elimination half-life of three to four hours.[93] Following subcutaneous administration of the phosphate salt of clindamycin, the elimination half-life is 1.5 hours, but a longer terminal half-life of 13 hours was noted.[94] This terminal phase may represent a slower release of the clindamycin from the injection site. Regardless, the peak concentration after a 5 mg/lb (11 mg/kg) subcutaneous dose was 8 μg/ml, with a trough of 0.5 μg/ml at 24 hours. Thus, a daily injection of clindamycin phosphate is probably sufficient.

INHIBITORS OF MICROBIAL NUCLEIC ACID SYNTHESIS

QUINOLONES

No group of antibiotics is generating more interest or holding more promise than the quinolones. They comprise a group of oral antibiotics with an extended spectrum of activity, including a gram-negative sensitivity profile unmatched by any other orally available antibiotic. Structurally, all quinolones are derivatives of nalidixic acid. Currently, the older quinolones, nalidic acid, and cinoxicin are available but not recommended for use in the dog. Nalidic acid is the prototype of this group; it suffers from unacceptable CNS toxicity in the dog and rapidly emerging resistance during treatment. Norfloxacin is the first commercially available new quinoline. It is limited to the treatment of urinary tract infections. However, ciprofloxacin and enrofloxacin should be available in 1988 and over a dozen others are in early phase I or phase II clinical trials. These newer quinolones should be able to treat systemic, as well as urinary tract, infections.

Spectrum of Activity. Against human pathogens, norfloxacin is bactericidal toward virtually all Enterobacteriaceae (*E. coli*, *Klebsiella pneumoniae*, *Enterobacter* spp., *Proteus* spp.), most with MICs less than 1 μg/ml. It is also very active toward *Pseudomonas aeruginosa*, with an incredible MIC of 1.0 μg/ml.[95, 96] The drug is effective toward staphylococcal species but not against the streptococci. It is also not effective against obligate anaerobes. Ciprofloxacin is more potent than norfloxacin against all these bacteria and in addition it is effective against all streptococci (except enterococci) and shows excellent activity against obligate anaerobes. This drug even has excellent activity against *Mycobacterium* spp. Preliminary in vitro studies performed on dog and cat pathogens at NCSU indicate similar sensitivity profiles.

Mechanism of Action. The quinolones are DNA gyrase inhibitors. Gyrases, or more properly, topoisomerases, are responsible for maintaining DNA in a negative supercoiled helical state to allow an enormous amount of DNA to fit into the tiny nucleus. Topoisomerases II consist of four subunits. Without this enzyme the DNA could not be transcribed, for in order to undergo transcription or replication, DNA sections must be unfolded (relaxed) and then refolded (negative supercoiling). Loss of either function results in bacterial cell death.[96] The drugs are specific for bacterial topoisomerases, with little binding affinity for the mammalian equivalent.

Resistance to norfloxacin has been reported, most commonly in regard to *Pseudomonas aeruginosa*. It is probably due to a change in membrane permeability. The extent of the resistance is small but the drug has only been in widespread use for a short time.

Clinical Pharmacology. Norfloxacin disposition in dogs is different from the disposition of nalidixic acid, which may explain its improved therapeutic safety. Oral bioavailability studies have not been performed in the dog or cat; however, it is well absorbed in humans, with peak serum concentrations greater than 1 μg/ml following a 400 mg oral dose. The drug is only moderately protein-bound (30 per cent) and is well distributed into tissue, including the prostate, where it achieves a two- to fourfold increase over serum concentrations.[95] The drug is eliminated in the dog primarily by renal filtration, with an elimination half-life of three hours. Urinary concentrations are in excess of 100 μg/ml.[97] In comparison, nalidixic acid is highly protein-bound (greater than 90 per cent), has poor tissue penetration, especially into the prostate, and undergoes extensive hepatic metabolism.

These differences in disposition may be the reason for the lower incidence of toxic side effects seen in human patients and the reason why these drugs, unlike nalidixic acid, may be useful in veterinary medicine.

Toxicity. The major untoward effect of these drugs seen in human patients and in dogs is gastrointestinal upset. CNS toxicity, including seizures seen in dogs taking nalidixic acid, has not been identified as yet. Thousands of human patients have been treated; however, experience with dogs is small and in cats, even smaller. The clinician must be cautious in using any product not approved for veterinary use that has toxic potential and for which there is little clinical experience. This experience will certainly grow over the next few years. Until then, doses of 4.5 mg/lb (10 mg/kg) q 12 hours have been used safely and efficaciously in both dogs and cats with chronic UTIs. At NCSU, three dogs and one cat with UTI were treated with norfloxacin for up to 30 days without any major toxicity. Anorexia was seen in two dogs but was temporary and resolved without stopping the drug.

METRONIDAZOLE

Spectrum of Activity. Metronidazole was first marketed as an antitrichomonal agent and it does have excellent activity against *Trichomonas* spp. More important to veterinary medicine is its efficacy toward protozoans, notably *Giardia lamblia*, *Entamoeba histolytica*, and *Balantidium coli*. It also is very active against obligate anaerobic bacteria, against which the drug is bactericidal. The drug has no effect on aerobic bacteria.

Mechanism of Action. Metronidazole is a nitroimidazole that is readily accumulated intracellularly under anaerobic conditions. The microbial enzyme, nitroreductase, reduces the nitro group and this reduced product binds to DNA, causing strands to break and the disruption of the helical structure.[98] The drug is both mutagenic and carcinogenic in long-term murine studies. The reduced products, acetamide and N-(2-hydroxethyl)-oxamic acid, are implicated. Mammalian cells do not contain nitroreductases and the risk of carcinogenicity in patients is questionable. Resistance has not been described for any of the susceptible microbes, making it an extremely useful antimicrobial.

Clinical Pharmacology. The oral bioavailability of metronidazole in dogs is high but variable (60 to 100 per cent). The absorption is improved when it is given in conjunction with food, with peak concentrations of 40 μg/ml occurring one hour following a dose of 20 mg/lb (44 mg/kg). Distribution is rapid for this lipophilic compound and the rate of elimination following intravenous or oral administration is similar, with a half-life of 4.5 hours.[99] The metabolic disposition is unknown in the dog but it is believed to undergo hepatic metabolism. The elimination half-life is twice as fast in the dog as in humans (4.5 hours compared to 7.8 hours) so it is possible that metabolism is more rapid in the dog. The MICs for over 200 anaerobic pathogens isolated at the University of Illinois indicated that 88 per cent could be inhibited by less than 6.2 μg/ml.[99] Therefore, a dosing schedule of 20 mg/lb (44 mg/kg) q 12 hours would be expected to have peak concentrations of more than 40 μg/ml and trough concentrations of 10 μg/ml, keeping the serum concentrations above MIC during the entire dosing interval. The calculated dosage for treatment of giardiasis was found to be similar to what has been recommended, 11.5 mg/lb (25 mg/kg) twice daily.

GRISEOFULVIN

This fungistatic drug is used primarily for the treatment of dermatophytosis caused by the common dermatophytes of dogs and cats, *Trichophyton* and *Microsporum* spp. The drug has no effect on other fungi, yeast, or bacteria. The drug's action is unique in that it is concentrated at the site of infection (keratin cells), where it inhibits dermatophyte mitosis, arresting their growth. Then, through the normal desquamation process, new uninfected epidermis replaces the older infected epidermis. The exact mechanism of action is not clear, although it is thought to affect microtubular function and disrupt the mitotic spindle. However, that assertion has been challenged.[100]

The disposition of the drug has not been fully described in the dog or cat although it has been used in these species for decades. The drug is insoluble in water and is therefore better absorbed with a high-fat diet. Additionally, the microparticle formulation (2.7 μ rather than 10 μ particle size) is absorbed twice as well as the older formulation. Thus dosing should be based on which formulation is used. It is known that the drug is extensively metabolized and that the rate of metabolism is six times faster in the dog than in humans, which accounts for the higher doses used in the dog.

The reported toxicity of this compound in dogs has been gastrointestinal upsets, although the drug is teratogenic and not recommended in breeding animals. In cats, the drug is implicated as a cause of leukopenia, anemia, lethargy, anorexia, ataxia, and depression, particularly in kittens.[101] Care should be taken when deciding to treat a kitten with griseofulvin. If treated, kittens should be monitored closely.

INHIBITORS OF MICROBIAL INTERMEDIATE METABOLISM

Two groups of antibiotics fall into this category: the sulfonamides and the nitrofurantoins. The sulfonamides are the oldest group of chemotherapeutic agents used for infectious diseases, preceding penicillin by three years. Following the advent of modern antibiotics and the development of extensive bacterial resistance, the sulfas have played a decreasing role in the treatment of infectious diseases. However, the potentiated sulfonamides have provided a renaissance for these agents and their uses are now ubiquitous in current therapeutic applications.

Sulfonamides

Spectrum of Activity. Few bacteria are uniformly sensitive to any of the sulfonamides at achievable serum concentrations. However, they have established if not restricted uses. Sulfisoxazole and sulfadimethoxine are bacteriostatic against staphylococci, streptococci, and some *E. coli*. Use of these drugs in systemic infections is seldom indicated due to the availability of more potent and efficacious drugs. However, they are sometimes effective against these pathogens at achievable urinary concentrations and are thus used in the treatment of lower urinary tract infections.[102] Topically, mafenide is effective in preventing colonization by gram-positive or gram-negative bacteria on severe burns; however, it is ineffective in treating infected burns. A poorly absorbed sulfa, sulfasalazine, is used in ulcerative and chronic colitis. In addition, long-acting agents such as sulfadimethoxine are used as coccidiostats in the treatment of coccidiosis in puppies and kittens. Sulfadiazine is combined with trimethoprim, a diaminopyridine, to form a potentiated sulfa. Trimethoprim alone has excellent gram-positive and gram-negative efficacy. The addition of a sulfa results in a synergistic antibacterial effect. This formulation is much more active than either drug alone, so much so that this combination has largely replaced use of sulfonamides in systemic infections. It is also effective against bacteria resistant to both drugs alone; however, the synergism in such a situation is not as dramatic as when both are sensitive.[103] Although there has been conflict over whether the potentiated sulfas are antianaerobic, it appears that they are effective against obligate anaerobes.[104] Although trimethoprim/sulfadiazine has been used in the treatment of *Toxoplasma gondii*, this organism is better treated by another diaminopyridine, pyrimethamine, in combination with sulfadiazine.

Mechanism of Action. The mechanism of these agents is known better than any other chemotherapeutic agent. Sulfonamides are structural analogs of para-aminobenzoic acid (PABA) and thus act as competitive antagonists. PABA is needed in microbial cells to form dihydrofolic acid, which is converted into tetrahydrofolic acid (folic acid) by the enzyme dihydrofolic acid reductase. Folic acid is required for purine and pyrimidine synthesis and thus for normal growth in both microbes and mammalian cells. Sulfas prevent the use of PABA, resulting in a deficiency of tetrahydrofolic acid and cessation of bacterial growth. Sulfas not only block the use of PABA in the formation of dihydrofolic acid but also are themselves incorporated into the precursors, forming a pseudometabolite. This condensation product is reactive and antibacterial.[105] Mammalian cells are not affected by these drugs, since they absorb and use preformed folic acid. Therefore, these drugs enjoy a wide therapeutic index. Resistance to the sulfas is caused by a variety of mechanisms, including plasmid-mediated changes in dihydrofolate syntheses, alternative metabolic pathways, and drug-modifying enzymes.[105] Trimethoprim works by binding to bacteria and inhibiting bacterial dihydrofolic acid reductase. This enzyme, in the presence of NADPH, converts dihydrofolic acid to tetrahydrofolic acid; its function is rapidly and irreversibly destroyed by trimethoprim. The binding affinity to the bacterial reductase is 10,000 to 100,000 times greater than binding affinity to the mammalian equivalent, giving trimethoprim a selective toxicity. The distinct actions of the sulfas and trimethoprim on the same metabolic pathway account for their synergistic antibacterial action.[103] The combination is so effective that it is often bactericidal.

Clinical Pharmacology. Sulfisoxazole, sulfadimethoxine, and sulfadiazine are the most common systemic sulfonamides currently used in practice. All are well-absorbed following oral dosing but have different distributions. Like the aminoglycosides, sulfisoxazole is confined to extracellular spaces, while sulfadiazine and to some extent, sulfadimethoxine, diffuses throughout the total body water. These drugs are eliminated in the dog by glucuronidation and renal filtration, with the majority of the drug being excreted as the intact parent drug. This differs from many mammalian species, where the drug undergoes N-deacetylation prior to renal elimination. Therefore, large amounts of these drugs accumulate in the urine. Following a 10 mg/lb (22 mg/kg) oral dose, sulfisoxisole urinary concentrations are in excess of 1000 μg/ml.[102] Sulfadiazine administered with trimethoprim at 4.5 mg/lb (10 mg/kg) (sulfadiazine dose) achieves urinary concentrations greater than 200 μg/ml.[106] Sulfadimethoxine has the longest elimination half-life of the group since it undergoes appreciable absorption following renal filtration.

Sulfadiazine is potentiated with the addition of trimethoprim in a 5:1 ratio (sulfadiazine/trimethoprim). Trimethoprim is a more lipid-soluble compound than sulfadiazine and achieves high tissue to serum concentrations of 6:1 in the lungs and 3:1 in the prostate, while sulfadiazine has tissue to serum ratios less than 1.[103] In the dog, trimethoprim is eliminated four times more rapidly as sulfadiazine. Elimination half-lives for trimethoprim and sulfadiazine are 2.5 hours and 10 hours, respectively. The tissues act as a deep compartment from which trimethoprim is slowly released and eliminated by renal filtration and secretion. Urine concentrations following a 2.2 mg/lb (5 mg/kg) dose (trimethoprim) peak at more than 80 μg/ml and are still around 10 μg/ml 24 hours after dosing. Sensitive bacteria MIC are less than 4 μg/ml of trimethoprim and 10 μg/ml of sulfadiazine,[5] which indicate that once-a-day dosing should be adequate for lower urinary tract infections.

The optimal synergistic ratio between these two drugs is not a well-defined static function. It depends on which organism is tested over a wide range of drug ratios. The serum-time concentration time profiles do not take into account the very different tissue distribution of these compounds.[106] Therefore, the difference in disposition between these drugs is not a major factor in this combination's efficacy.

Urinary Tract Anti-infectives

NITROFURANTOIN

The nitrofurans are a large group of antimicrobials, of which nitrofurantoin is the most common. The use of this product is restricted to the urinary tract since serum and tissue concentrations obtained following standard oral dosing are below the MIC for most organisms.

Spectrum of Activity. The gram-negative bacteria isolated from dogs and cats at NCSU indicate that the spectrum of activity is similar to that seen among human pathogens. Nitrofurantoin is very active against a wide variety of gram-negative bacteria, including *E. coli*, *Klebsiella pneumoniae*, and *Enterobacter* spp., while nearly always ineffective against *Proteus* spp. and *Pseudomonas aeruginosa*. The MICs for these organisms tend to be less than 16 μg/ml, a level exceeded tenfold in the urine.

Mechanism of Action. The actual mechanism for the bactericidal activity of the nitrofurans is not clear. However, they do inhibit a number of bacterial enzymes, which may be the source of their activity.[107]

Clinical Pharmacology. Nitrofurantoin is formulated in two sizes. Both are completely absorbed following oral dosing, with the macrocrystalline form (macrodantoin) being absorbed more slowly, prolonging its urinary concentrations. Therapeutic serum concentrations are not achieved since this agent is quickly eliminated. Its half-life in humans is 30 minutes. Urinary concentrations depend on urine pH. About 40 per cent of the drug is eliminated unchanged in the urine by renal filtration, secretion, and reabsorption. The more acidic the urine, the smaller the amount of drug reabsorbed and the greater the urinary concentration. The rate of elimination is correlated with GFR; patients with renal disease eliminate a smaller amount of drug and accumulate the drug systemically.[108] Since this drug does not reach therapeutic concentrations and is potentially toxic in patients with renal disease, it cannot be recommended for patients with pyelonephritis or prostatitis. However, in patients with chronic relapsing cystitis, once-a-night therapy may be effective in preventing relapses.

Toxicity. Toxicity, including chronic active hepatitis, neuropathies, and pneumonitis, has been reported in human patients. Toxicity has not been described in dogs or cats, but from personal experience, gastrointestinal disturbances and hepatopathy are not uncommon.

METHENAMINE

This antiseptic owes its antibacterial properties to its ability to decompose in acid solutions to form formaldehyde. The decomposition proceeds as follows:

$$N_4(CH_2)_6 + 6H_2O + 4H^+ \longrightarrow 4NH_4^+ + 6HCHO$$
$$\text{Methenamine} \longrightarrow \text{formaldehyde}$$

The reaction is pH-dependent, with optimal physiological production occurring at pH 5 or less. All bacteria are killed by concentrations of more than 20 μg/ml of formaldehyde; they cannot develop a resistance to this effect.[109] The production of ammonia precludes use of this drug in animals with hepatic encephalopathy or even hepatic disease. The drug is formulated with a urinary acidifier such as mandelate or hippuric acid. This agent is used to suppress urinary bacterial growth in human patients with chronic relapsing cystitis and not for primary treatment of urinary tract infections. It has been used in dogs for the same purpose. It is sometimes difficult to keep the urine pH low enough for long periods, lessening the usefulness of this product.

CLINICAL APPLICATIONS

Rational Approach to Therapeutics

Antimicrobial therapy is a paradox. On one hand, the objectives of therapy are the simplest of any chemotherapeutic agent. However, because they are simple, the common approach to therapeutics has been reduced to simply choosing the correct antibiotic. This simplistic approach deteriorates further when therapy is unsuccessful, since it implies that failure was the result of using the wrong antibiotic. Thus, the simple objective of antimicrobial therapy fails to convey the complex environment in which some infections exist. Despite this, antimicrobial therapy often is successful. This is possible only because the patient uses a number of intrinsic defenses that greatly facilitates recovery. When, for whatever reason, the patient fails to bring these factors into play or the pathogen has developed mechanisms against the antibiotics, the therapy is unsuccessful. By definition these are serious and/or chronic microbial infections, where the proper selection and use of an antimicrobial is crucial. They represent a therapeutic challenge and must be approached in a rational manner in order to optimize the therapeutic objectives.

Too often the response to treatment failure in these cases is to reach for a new and more "potent" antibiotic without first defining both the nature of the infection and the therapeutic objectives.

The nature of an infection begins with defining its primary location, the organ system involved, and the extent to which the pathogen resides within that system. The conditions at the site of infection that affect the pharmacodynamic phase of drug action should be anticipated and the competency of the patient to help in therapy evaluated. Once an infection has been diagnosed, the infection must be placed into the context of the patient's overall condition. Is the infection primary (the only disease present) or secondary to another disease (i.e., a UTI in a patient with diabetes mellitus)?

Therapeutic objectives are necessary to modify treatment efficiently. What clinical or laboratory signs will indicate successful treatment and how long into therapy are they expected? When should therapy be reevaluated and what criteria should be used to decide when to change antibiotics and to which antibiotic? Finally, antimicrobial therapy is sometimes expected to do more than kill pathogens. It is sometimes easy to forget that a patient's clinical signs may not all be attributed to the pathogen and that successful therapy does not ensure an improvement in a patient's clinical status. Thus, the clinician must develop a rational therapeutic approach to bacterial and fungal infections to insure that therapy is optimized and that decision making regarding changes in antimicrobials is based on failure to meet predetermined therapeutic goals. It is hoped that approaching antimicrobial therapy in a more rational and logical manner will improve the use and lessen the misuse of antibiotics.

Systematic Approach to Antimicrobial Selection

It is often axiomatic that diagnosis of the disease must precede treatment. Nevertheless, the common misuse of antibiotics, based on the sole premise that no harm is done if an infection is not present, negates that axiom. Diagnosis of a bacterial or fungal infection is based on clinical signs and/or laboratory tests indicating a pathogen's presence. These criteria are absolutely necessary if rational antibiotic therapy is to be used. They form the basis for answering the questions that determine the infection's nature, that are used to choose which antibiotic to administer, by what route, how frequently, and for how long. Additionally, these criteria are used in monitoring the response to antimicrobial therapy.

Any patient diagnosed as having a primary or secondary infection should have the following questions answered:

1. What organ system(s) is involved?
2. What pathogen is most likely present in that organ system(s)?
3. What antibiotic is most likely to be efficacious against that pathogen?
4. What drug concentration is required at the site of infection?
5. What dose and route of administration are most likely to achieve that concentration?

The MIC breakpoint, or the maximum concentration at which an organism would be considered sensitive, is given for each antibiotic in Table 51–10. If an MIC is not available for a particular pathogen, then the chosen antibiotic should be dosed and delivered to obtain at least this value at the site of infection. This value does not apply to uncomplicated urinary tract infections, since urinary concentrations are often 10- to 20-fold higher than serum and many resistant organisms can be overcome if enough antibiotic is present. However, it is important to keep in mind that the MIC merely reflects the degree of sensitivity an organism has to an antibiotic. For example, most *E. coli* sensitive to ampicillin are sensitive at concentrations less than 4 μg/ml and its gram-negative breakpoint is greater than 16 μg/ml. In order to even moderately increase the percentage of susceptible isolates, concentrations of 64 μg/ml must be achieved.[28] Thus, an *E. coli* infection that required 64 μg/ml of ampicillin to be inhibited would be considered resistant if in the lung but could be successfully treated in the urine because ampicillin concentrations greater than 250 μg/ml are achieved. Yet this MIC indicates that this organism has resistant mechanisms (most likely β lactamase production) and should be labeled as relatively insensitive. One can use MIC data in this fashion in selecting not only a sensitive antibiotic but the most sensitive one. An *E. coli* pneumonia with a cephalothin MIC of 8 μg/ml and an ampicillin MIC of less than 0.5 μg/ml would both be reported as sensitive. However, ampicillin would be expected to be more sensitive than cephalothin and would be the drug of choice. It is logical to assume that it would be easier to achieve the former MIC at the infection site than the latter and response to therapy should favor the former.

Table 51–10 also provides both the peak serum and urine concentrations obtainable by different routes of administration. This table should help answer questions 4 and 5.

UROGENITAL SYSTEM

Infections of the urogenital system comprise the largest group of infections seen in human or veterinary medicine. Over 40 per cent of bacterial isolates cultured at the microbiology laboratories of the AMC and NCSU are from this system.[33] Rorich has determined the most frequently isolated bacteria from urine of canine patients at the University of California at Davis[28] and Garvey from The Animal Medical Center in New York.[33] These findings, along with those from NCSU, are presented in Table 51–6.

Table 51–6 illustrates two important points regarding urinary tract infections. First, unlike human patients, the canine has a greater variety of pathogens causing UTI. Second, the diversity of organisms isolated from different geographical locations is fairly uniform. However, their sensitivities to antibiotics are not necessarily so similar.

As can be seen, 60 to 70 per cent of the pathogens are comprised of *E. coli*, *Staphylococcus* spp. and either *Streptococcus faecalis* or *Streptococcus faecium*. Therefore, obtaining a culture for primary UTI on the first occurrence is unnecessary since therapy can be directed at these organisms. Dogs or cats with either secondary UTI or recurring or relapsing infections should be cultured to determine at least the bacterial species. The antibiotic chosen should be one that is likely to be effective against these organisms. In simple lower UTI, the ability of most antibiotics to concentrate in the urine is a great advantage since many otherwise resistant bacteria are susceptible to the high concentrations these antibiotics achieve. Amoxicillin and trimethoprim/sulfadiazine are drugs of choice, since at achievable urinary

TABLE 51–6. PERCENTAGE OF ISOLATES COLLECTED FROM CANINE CYSTOCENTESIS PATIENTS AT UNIVERSITY OF CALIFORNIA AT DAVIS (UC-DAVIS), THE ANIMAL MEDICAL CENTER (AMC), NEW YORK, AND NORTH CAROLINA STATE UNIVERSITY (NCSU)*

	UC-DAVIS n >2000	AMC n = 659	NCSU n = 229
E. coli	46	41	38
Staphylococcus spp.	17	23	14
Enterococci	12	7	12
Proteus mirabilis	10	9	10
Klebsiella pneumoniae	7	6	10
Pseudomonas aeruginosa	5	5	?

*Percentage of total isolates recovered from urinary tract infections.

concentrations these organisms are virtually 100 per cent sensitive.[28] Penicillin V and ampicillin are also excellent choices.[110] The concentration of drug required in the urine (more than 64 μg/ml for amoxicillin and more than 16 μg/ml for trimethoprim) is easily achieved at standard oral doses. The frequency of dosing is more a function of rationalized justification than the pharmacodynamics of drug action. Amoxicillin can be given q 12 to 8 hours, depending on the frequency of urination and trimethoprim/sulfadiazine q 12 to 24 hours.[106, 110] Interestingly, many reports of human patients with UTI indicate that a single dose is often as effective as multiple dose therapy. This experience is not reported in veterinary medicine and therapy is recommended for 10 to 21 days. Clinical signs of dysuria and pollakiuria should resolve within a few days. A culture taken four to five days into treatment should be negative. If not, the antibiotic should be changed according to the susceptibility report. If pyelonephritis or prostatitis is suspected or determined, the choice of antibiotic, its dose, and route of administration now depends on predictable sensitivities at achievable serum, not urine, concentrations. A culture and susceptibility report are indicated to direct therapy in these situations. Chronic pyelonephritis is usually asymptomatic and only a negative urine culture indicates successful treatment. Reculturing within the first ten days of treatment is important to ensure appropriate therapy since therapy is prolonged (more than 30 days). Suppurative prostatitis, like any other abscess, requires surgical drainage. It also requires castration, along with antibiotic therapy for successful therapy.

RESPIRATORY SYSTEM

Nothing is more frustrating to a clinician than a case of chronic rhinitis/sinusitis. The frustration comes from the difficulty in making a causative diagnosis and in having unrealistic therapeutic expectations as to the role of antimicrobial therapy. The reason for the nasal discharge is often unclear. Nasal swabs used to identify a pathogen are often misleading, since it would be most surprising to find nares in which no bacteria could be isolated. Aspergillosis is a common airborne fungus and streptococci and staphylococci are common commensal organisms. One function of the nares is to filter these organisms without becoming infected. Therefore, if infection exists, the rational approach indicates finding why this organ has failed in its function. In one author's experience, very few cases of chronic rhinitis are primary in origin. Removing the pathogen permanently is difficult at best and even when successful, does not cure the primary pathology that allowed the infection to occur in the first place. Before antimicrobial therapy is started, a deep nasal culture and biopsies are recommended since simple swabbing is misleading.

If antibiotic therapy is to be used, expectations of outcome should be realistic. If the nature of the infection is unknown, then antibiotic therapy consisting of a series of multiple antibiotics only leads to a multiresistant organism, such as *Pseudomonas aeruginosa*, as resident bacteria. Almost 25 per cent of nasal sinus infections cultured at the AMC contain this organism. Treatment for these infections is ineffective, since aminoglycosides either alone or with an antipseudomonal penicillin are ineffective in the face of purulent material. Therefore, if exhaustive testing does not indicate the primary cause of chronic rhinitis, antibiotic therapy is unlikely to be effective except as a temporary measure.

TABLE 51–7. PERCENTAGE OF ISOLATES COLLECTED FROM TRANSTRACHEAL WASHES OF CANINE AND FELINE PATIENTS AT THE ANIMAL MEDICAL CENTER (AMC), NEW YORK AND NORTH CAROLINA STATE UNIVERSITY (NCSU)*

	AMC n = 174	NCSU n = 56
E. coli	19	17
Staphylococcus intermedius	14	8
Enterococci	9	8
Bordetella	2	11
Pasteurella multocida	10	11
Klebsiella pneumoniae	8	6
Pseudomonas aeruginosa	7	6

*Percentage of total isolates recovered from lower respiratory infections.

Lower respiratory infections, however, are more likely to be primary in origin and rational antimicrobial therapy is critical to the outcome. The bacteria most likely to be present in lower respiratory infections are very unpredictable (Table 51–7).

Unlike urinary tract infections, where 60 to 70 per cent of the bacterial isolates come from three species, seven species account for less than 70 per cent of the lower respiratory pathogens. It is therefore very important to obtain a tracheal or bronchial culture for bacterial identification and susceptibility testing prior to initiating therapy. Since the probable bacterial pathogens are not predictable, a combination antibiotic regimen consisting of an aminoglycoside and β-lactam is recommended. With β-lactam antibiotics, the MIC needed for gram-negative bacteria is usually higher than for gram-positive bacteria. This is illustrated for cephalothin in Table 51–8 and is applicable to most β-lactams. This is important in determining a dose and route of administration.

In many human therapeutic trials and experimental canine studies, successful therapy of lower respiratory infections depends on the antibiotic reaching at least its MIC in the lung parenchyma.[111] Both drugs penetrate into the lung parenchyma by concentration-dependent passive diffusion. Interstitial and alveolar drug concen-

TABLE 51–8. QUANTITATIVE ASSESSMENT OF THE DIFFERENCE IN GRAM-POSITIVE AND GRAM-NEGATIVE BACTERIA SUSCEPTIBILITY TO CEPHALOTHIN*

	Quantitative Sensitivity (μg/ml)			
	< 2	*2–4*	*8–16*	Total
Staphylococcus intermedius n = 66	89	3	2	94
Enterococci n = 32	38	9	6	53
E. coli n = 108	1	8	17	26
Klebsiella pneumoniae n = 23	4	34	35	74

*As determined by an in vitro microdilutional MIC assay. NCCLS Guidelines used to determine susceptible concentrations.

trations are similar to serum concentrations; however, bronchial concentrations are usually much lower.[111] Bronchial concentrations for most β-lactams and aminoglycosides are 10 to 20 per cent and 25 to 65 per cent of the peak serum concentrations, respectively. Therefore, to ensure tissue concentrations for cephalothin (or any other first-generation cephalosporin or aminopenicillin) or the aminoglycosides, the high end of the dose range is required and the route of administration should be intravenous. For example, a 4.5 mg/lb (10 mg/kg) dose of cefalothin produces a 75 μg/ml peak concentration, of which 10 per cent or 7.5 μg/ml is expected in the bronchiole secretions. Increasing the dose two- or threefold similarly increases the concentration at the site of infection. Thus, an intravenous dose of 14 mg/lb (30 mg/kg) is a rational dose of cefalothin in a lower respiratory infection.

In uncomplicated bacterial pneumonia, clinical improvement is used to assess therapy since radiographic changes are too insensitive to use in monitoring therapy. Improvement should be noted in 48 hours. Too often antibiotics are changed during the first 24 hours because of continuing patient decline. However, it is difficult in these infections to assess any antibiotic in fewer than 24 hours and no information is immediately available from the tracheal wash with which to make an informed decision as to which antibiotic should be administered instead. Since the duration of therapy often exceeds two weeks, a suitable oral antibiotic is often needed. It is important to note that response to intravenous cephalothin does not mean equal success with oral cefadroxil, since peak serum concentrations are five to eight times smaller. If possible, an MIC should be available in these cases in order to dictate which oral antibiotic, if any, would most likely reach its MIC in bronchial secretions. The dose chosen for this antibiotic should be at the high end of the dosing range.

DERMATOLOGIC INFECTIONS

Dermatologic infections are the most common in small animal practice.[35] They are also the most predictable as to type of bacterial pathogen. *Staphylococcus intermedius* is the coagulase-positive staphylococcus responsible for essentially all the superficial pyodermas and most of the deep pyodermas. Of 165 isolates from dogs with deep pyodermas, 55 per cent were staphylococci and 22 per cent consisted of *E. coli*, *Pseudomonas aeruginosa*, and *Proteus* spp.[33] However, many dogs with gram-negative bacteria also have staphylococci and these dogs respond well to treatment directed against the staphylococci, indicating it is the primary pathogen.[35]

There are many antibiotics that are effective against β-lactamase-producing staphylococci (Table 51–9). The isoxazolyl penicillins (oxacillin, dicloxacillin) dosed at 20 mg/lb (44 mg/kg) produce peak skin concentrations of 1 to 2 μg/gm for dicloxacillin and 0.2 to 0.8 μg/gm for oxacillin, which is in agreement with dicloxacillin's better oral absorption. The oral cephalosporins (cephalexin, cephadroxil) produce peak skin concentrations of 4 to 20 μg/gm following a 14 mg/lb (30 mg/kg) dose, with cephalexin producing the higher concentrations. Skin concentrations for erythromycin and clindamycin

TABLE 51–9. PERCENTAGE SUSCEPTIBILITY OF *STAPHYLOCOCCUS INTERMEDIUS* ISOLATED FROM CANINE PYODERMAS TO VARIOUS ANTIBIOTICS

	Staphylococcus intermedius N = 138	MIC* μg/ml
Oral Cephalosporins	97	< 2
Isoxazolyl Penicillins	90	< 1
Chloramphenicol	79	< 8
Trimethoprim/Sulfadiazine	70	< 2/38
Clindamycin	70	< 1
Erythromycin	70	< 2

*Minimum inhibitory concentration necessary to inhibit that percentage of isolates.

are similar to peak serum concentrations of 1 μg/ml and 5 μg/ml, respectively, following standard dosing.[93] Trimethoprim, and to a lesser extent, sulfadiazine, accumulates in inflamed tissues, producing trimethoprim tissue concentrations of more than 4 μg/ml following a 14 mg/lb (30 mg/kg) combined dose.[112] Skin concentrations of chloramphenicol are not reported for the dog but should be at least equivalent to obtainable serum concentrations. These obtainable peak skin concentrations indicate that if the bacteria is sensitive in vitro it will be sensitive in vivo, and the selection of which drug to use is one of personal preference and cost factors. The dosage recommended for oxacillin and dicloxacillin is higher than previously reported and reflects the new information on achievable skin concentrations.

Response to antimicrobial therapy should be seen within one week of treatment.[35] If no clinical improvement is seen, a deep culture should be taken and the pathogen and its susceptibility (preferably by MIC) determined. There is no need for the patient to be taken off antibiotics if there is no response prior to the culture. Any residual antibiotic present has not interfered with growth in vivo and should not in vitro.

ORTHOPEDIC INFECTIONS

Osteomyelitis is most frequently caused by open fractures and/or internal fixation of fractures.[113] Many cases of osteomyelitis are polymicrobial infections, with bacteria coming from the patient or the surgeon. The most frequently isolated bacteria are *Staphylococcus aureus* (humans) and *Staphylococcus intermedius* (animals) with gram-negative enterics such as *E. coli*, *Proteus* spp. and *Pseudomonas aeruginosa* also frequent pathogens.[114] Additionally, facultative and obligate anaerobes have been found to be an important component of osteomyelitis.[115] The very nature of chronic osteomyelitis makes antibiotic therapy alone highly unsuccessful. Bone necrosis, fracture instability, and metal implants are all at the root of infection and must be dealt with first before antibiotic therapy has any chance of success.[113] The selected antibiotic must be able to penetrate into cancellous tissue, producing concentrations equal to or exceeding the MIC of the pathogen(s). Fortunately, the β-lactams readily penetrate into the interstitial spaces of cortical bone, achieving concentrations almost equivalent to those in serum. Concentrations of β-lactams in the cortical bone itself are 10 to 20 per cent of concurrent serum concentrations.[116] Cephalosporins have been studied more than the others because of their excellent antistaphylococcal and anaerobic activity. Due to the polymicrobial nature of many cases of osteomyelitis, therapy should be initiated with a combination regimen, consisting of a β-lactam (i.e., oxacillin) and an aminoglycoside. The high end of the parenteral dose range is used to maximize the penetration gradient into the infected area. Once a culture and susceptibility are obtained, the antibiotic may be reduced to a single agent. However, a seven- to ten-day course of parenteral antibiotics seems a minimum amount of time to use parenterals since human patients are treated for four to six weeks in this manner. An excellent oral antibiotic in gram-positive osteomyelitis is clindamycin, which has a more reliable anaerobic activity than the cephalosporins and can reach 40 to 50 per cent of its average serum concentration in cancellous tissue.[98] However, none of the antibiotics can be effective against an osteomyelitis caused by avascular bone fragments or foreign material (plates, pins, or wires). Treatment in the face of these factors often is unsuccessful; even when using very sensitive antibiotics, foreign bodies act as a physical barrier to the antibiotic, which cannot reach the site of infection.

Therefore, the authors do not recommend treating cases of osteomyelitis with antibiotics until the infected sequestered bone and/or orthopedic hardware are removed, unless the infection is disseminating into distal soft tissues. In this case the antibiotic only helps to contain the infection and does not cure it.

Swelling and/or discharge should improve within several days and therapy should be continued for a minimum of 30 to 42 days. If no response is noted, reculturing is indicated. Culture of the draining tract is contraindicated, since it is not a reliable indicator of the bone pathogen. Instead, a deep needle aspirate or surgical biopsy is recommended. Failure to respond to appropriate antibiotics dosed and delivered properly is indicative of other factors, suggested above, preventing a response. Unless these factors are dealt with, the infection is unlikely to respond to any of the other antibiotics showing in vitro sensitivity.

SYSTEMIC INFECTIONS

In no disease situation is the expedient use of appropriate antibiotic therapy more beneficial than in human patients with disseminated bacterial infections, where mortality is reduced by 25 per cent.[33] In a disease with a 25 to 80 per cent mortality figure, that is considerable. The bacterial pathogens causing disseminated infections depend on their primary source. Urinary tract infections are the leading cause of septicemia in the dog, and thus *E. coli*, *Staphylococcus intermedius*, and enterococci are frequent systemic pathogens.[117] However, any bacteria from any organ system can cause disseminated infections. Blood cultures are recommended but are frequently used more as a confirmation of the diagnosis than as a tool to direct therapy. Results are frequently negative or take days to develop, due to the paucity of bacteria in the blood. Therefore, in a patient with septicemia it is imperative that antibiotic therapy be started soon and provide full, four-quadrant coverage (gram-positive and gram-negative, aerobes and anaerobes). A combination using an aminoglycoside and a β-lactam is recommended. Aminoglycoside efficacy in human patients with sepsis is correlated with the ratio of peak serum concentration to the MIC of that organism.[78] Therefore it is crucial that maximal safe peak concentrations be obtained. Sepsis can expand the extracellular fluid space by enhancing capillary fragility, leading to increases in interstitial fluid content and in the volume of distribution of gentamicin. One author has seen the consequence of this in 12 canine patients at NCSU receiving gentamicin during early acute sepsis. Peak serum concentrations were 22 to 50 per cent less than in nonseptic patients following a 1.0 mg/lb (2.2 mg/kg) dose. Therefore, in the early treatment of sepsis, gentamicin is dosed at 2 mg/lb (4 mg/kg) q 8 hours in order to achieve 15 μg/ml peak serum concentrations. Intramuscular injections, due to their lower peak serum concentrations, are inappropriate in acute sepsis unless no alternative exists. The dose is then usually decreased as the dog improves. Therapeutic drug monitoring is very helpful in sepsis since physiological changes in drug distribution sometimes occur daily and the dose can be adjusted accordingly. A therapeutic response should be noted in 12 to 24 hours and sometimes much sooner. Clinical signs of lethargy, depression, and/or fever are good markers of therapeutic response. If no response is noted, an alternative aminoglycoside should be used. Amikacin is dosed at 5 to 7 mg/lb (10 to 14 mg/kg) in the septic animal, producing 40 to 60 μg/ml peak serum concentrations. The β-lactam antibiotic is seldom changed unless cultures obtained from possible primary sites, such as the urinary tract, indicate a better choice. Therapeutic expectations for recovery are guarded, especially if the patient develops subacute bacterial endocarditis.[33]

PROPHYLACTIC USE OF ANTIMICROBIAL DRUGS

It has been established in human hospitals and veterinary hospitals that prophylactic antibiotic use is unnecessary in clean surgical procedures.[118] A clean surgical procedure has been defined as one where no inflammation is present, the gastrointestinal or respiratory system has not been invaded, and aseptic technique is not broken.[118] However, it is unclear whether this finding is true in private practice, where aseptic technique for elective surgeries is not as elaborate as at a veterinary teaching hospital. Regardless, the use and misuse of antibiotics appear to be very prevalent in this area and deserve discussion.

The appropriate use of prophylactic antibiotics is in clean but contaminated surgeries (spillage from an entered viscus) and contaminated and dirty surgeries (gross contamination from ruptured viscus or external invasion).[119] Contamination implies bacterial presence but not an established infection. Copious flushing with warm isotonic saline provides the mechanical action necessary to depopulate bacterial presence. Addition of antibiotics into the lavage fluid is unnecessary since they are ab-

TABLE 51–10. GUIDE TO USE OF ANTIMICROBIAL DRUGS

	Route	Dosage Range (mg/lb)	Dosage Interval (hr)	Elimination Half-Life	Achievable Peak Concentrations (μg/ml) Blood	Urine	Breakpoint MIC (μg/ml) Gram-Neg.	Gram-Pos.
Beta-Lactam Antibiotics								
Penicillins								
Penicillin								
(Na and K)	IV, IM	10–25,000	q 6–8	30–45 min	100–150	> 1000	ND	<1.0
Penicillin V								
(K salt)	PO	2.5–5	q 6–8	45–60 min	1–3	> 500	ND	< 1.0
Ampicillin								
(trihydrate)	IM, SC	2.5–5	q 8	45–60 min	20–40	> 500	< 16	< 4
(Na salt)	IV, SC	2.5–5	q 8	45–60	40–80			
	PO	10–15	q 8	60–80	2–4	> 250		
Amoxicillin								
(salt)	IM, SC	2.5–5	q 8	45–60 min	20–40	ND	< 16	< 4
(trihydrate)	PO	5–10	q 8–12	60–80	6–8	> 250		
Oxacillin								
(Na salt)	IV	2.5–5	q 8	20–30 min	25–40	NA	NA	< 1
	PO	12.5–15	q 8	20–30	1–3	NA		
Dicloxacillin	PO	12.5–15	q 8	20–30 min	1–4	NA	NA	< 1
Carbenicillin								
(Na salt)	IV	25–50	q 8	45–60 min	250–500		< 32 (512)	NA
Indanyl ester	PO	25	q 8		NA	> 1000		
Ticarcillin								
(Na salt)	IV	25–50	q 8	45–60 min	250–500	NA	< 256	NA
	IM, SC	25–50	q 8	60–80	75–250	NA		
Piperacillin	IV	25–50	q 8	30–40 min	250–500	NA	< 512	NA
Cephalosporins								
Cephalothin								
	IV	5–15	q 8	40–50 min	50–150	NA	< 32	< 32
	IM, SC	10–15	q 8	40–50	20–30	NA		
Cephapirin								
	IV	5–15	q 8	25–30 min	50–150	NA	< 32	< 32
	IM, SC	10–15	q 8	25–30	20–30	NA		
Cefazolin								
	IV	5–15	q 8	60–70 min	100–300	NA	< 32	< 32
	IM, SC	10–15	q 8	60–70	40–60	NA		
Cephalexin	PO	5–15	q 8	80–120 min	10–25	> 250	< 32	< 32
Cefadroxil	PO	5–15	q 8	80–120 min	10–25	> 250	< 32	< 32
Cefoxitin	IV	5–10	q 8	45–60 min	50–100	NA	< 32	< 32
Cefoteten	IV	5–10	q 8	50–60 min	50–100	NA	< 32	< 32
Cefotaxime								
	IV	12.5–25	q 8	45–60 min	50–100	NA	< 32	< 32
	IM, SC	12.5–25	q 8	45–60	15–35	NA		
Moxalactam	IV	12.5–25	q 8	60–70 min	200–400	NA	< 64	< 64
Beta-Lactamase Inhibitors								
Amoxicillin/								
Clavulinic acid	PO	5–10	q 8–12	60–80 min	6–8	> 250	< 16	< 4
Ticarcillin/								
Clavulinic acid	IV	25–50	q 8	45–60 min	250–500	NA	< 256	NA
	IM, SC	25–50	q 8	60–80	75–250	NA		
Carbapenems								
Imipenem/								
cilastatin	IV	1.5–2.5	q 8	20–30 min	25–50	> 70	< 64	< 64
Cell Wall Labilizers								
Amphotericin B	IV	.24	q 48	45–50 hr	0.2–0.3	NA	NA	NA
Ketoconazole	PO	5	q 8–12	4–6 hr		NA	NA	NA
Protein Synthesis Inhibitors								
Aminoglycosides								
Gentamicin	IV, IM	1–2	q 8	40–60 min	10–15	> 100	< 8	< 8
Amikacin	IV, IM	4–8	q 8	40–60 min	40–60	> 400	< 32	< 32
Tobramycin	IV, IM	1–2	q 8	40–60 min	10–15	> 100	< 8	< 8
Tetracyclines								
Oxytetracycline	PO	25–37.5	q 8	4–6 hr	0.5–1.0	ND	< 16	< 16
Tetracycline	PO	10–15	q 8	4–6 hr	ND	> 100	< 16	< 16
Doxycycline	PO	2.5–5	q 8	ND	2–6	ND	< 16	< 16

Table continued on following page

TABLE 51–10. GUIDE TO USE OF ANTIMICROBIAL DRUGS *Continued*

	Route	Dosage Range (mg/lb)	Dosage Interval (hr)	Elimination Half-Life	Achievable Peak Concentrations (μg/ml) Blood	Urine	Breakpoint MIC (μg/ml) Gram-Neg.	Gram-Pos.
Macrolides and Lincosamides								
Erythromycin	PO	5–10	q 8	60–80 min	1–3	NA	NA	< 8
Clindamycin								
	PO	2.5–5	q 12	3–4 hr	2–5	NA	NA	< 8
	SC	5–7.5	q 24	10–13 hr	8–12	NA		
Lincomycin	PO	10–15	q 12	3–4 hr	3–4	NA	NA	< 8
Others								
Chloramphenicol								
	PO	16.5–25	q 8	4–5 hr	20–30	> 100	< 16	< 16
	IM, SC	7.5–10	q 8	4–5 hr	20–30	> 100		
Metronidazole	PO	20–25	q 12–24	4–5 hr	40–50	NA	ND	ND

Dosing ranges, frequency interval, and disposition parameters were rounded to the nearest integer for sake of simplicity and readability. The table is a composite of previous published values and new data presented in the text. The breakpoint MICs are defined by the NCCLS Guidelines M7-T and are used to determine when an organism will be reported as resistant by most clinical microbiology laboratories. As a rule of thumb, the breakpoint is two dilutions higher than reported for sensitive organisms. Organisms susceptible between these dilutions are reported as moderately sensitive: for example, an organism requiring more than 32 μg/ml of cephalothin is resistant but is moderately susceptible at 16 μg/ml and sensitive at 8 μg/ml or less. MIC in parentheses refers to breakpoint for *Pseudomonas aeruginosa* only. The breakpoints for the antipseudomonal penicillins, ticarcillin, and piperacillin are also only for *P. aeruginosa*. Lower concentrations are adequate for other sensitive gram-negative species.

Key to abbreviations: NA, Not applicable for therapeutic purposes; ND, Not determined.

sorbed rapidly. Instead, a single dose of a β-lactam, such as ampicillin or cefoxitin, assists in removing whatever vestigial population of microbes remain following lavage. Unless the surgeon feels that infection was present (established before surgery), continued use of antimicrobials following surgery is unnecessary.[120]

The misuse of antibiotics by either indiscriminate use in clean surgeries or protracted use following surgery surely contributes to the emergence of resistant organisms. In an excellent review on this subject, McGowan lays out the full scope of this problem, which has been well documented in human medicine.[29] Although no reports in the veterinary literature have indicated that the indiscriminate use of antibiotics has caused resistance, it is clear that many veterinary pathogens are multiresistant. It is also clear that on the human side, the clinicians are keeping up with resistance by using newer and more expensive antibiotics. This tactic cannot be followed in veterinary medicine for long. Therefore, it is the responsibility of the veterinary clinician to not only use antibiotics more rationally in order to improve their effectiveness, but to use them less frequently in order to maintain their effectiveness.

References

1. Burke, JF: Preventative antibiotics management in surgery. Ann Rev Med 24:289, 1973.
2. Hirsch, DC and Ruehl, WW: A rational approach to selection of an antimicrobial agent. JAVMA 185:1058, 1984.
3. Woolcock, JB and Mutimer, MD: Antibiotic susceptibility testing: caeci caecos ducentes. Vet Rec 113:125, 1983.
4. Bauer, AW, et al.: Antibiotic susceptibility testing by a standardized single disc method. Am J Clin Pathol 45:493, 1966.
5. Jones, RN: NCCLS guidelines: Approved methods for dilutional antimicrobial susceptibility test. Antimicrob Newslett 3:1, 1986.
6. Sanders, CS: Failure to detect resistance in antimicrobial susceptibility tests: A "very major" error of increasing concern. Antimicrob Newslett 1:27, 1984.
7. Mandell, GL: Interaction of intraleukocytic bacteria and antibiotics. J Clin Invest 52:1673, 1973.
8. Karvounis, P, et al.: Antibiotic prevention of experimental staphylococcal meningitis. J Neurosurg 28:45, 1968.
9. Nathanson, MH and Liebhold, RA: Diffusion of sulfonamides and penicillin into fibrin. Proc Soc Exp Biol Med 62:83, 1946.
10. Nathanson, MH and Liebhold, RA: Studies relative to chemotherapy of bacterial endocarditis. Ann Intern Med 33:1224, 1950.
11. Eagle, H: Experimental approach to the problem of treatment failure with penicillin. I. Group A streptococcal infections in mice. Am J Med 13:389, 1952.
12. Ullberg, S: Studies on the distribution and fat of S35-labeled benzylpenicillin in the body. Acta Radiol Suppl 1:118, 1954.
13. Ure, W, et al.: Antibiotic-bacterial contact as a factor in persistence of antibiotic-sensitive staphylococci during treatment of infected hematomas in rabbits. Clin Res 9:25, 1961.
14. Garagusi, VF and Ritts, RE: Tritiated erythromycin in tissues and abscesses. Arch Pathol 77:587, 1964.
15. deLouvois, J and Hurley, R: Antibiotic concentrations in intracranial pus: A study from a collaborative project. *In* Williams JD, Geddes AM (eds): Chemotherapy Vol 4, Pharmacology of Antibiotics. New York, Plenum Press, 1976, pp 61.
16. Kunin, CM: Binding of antibiotics to tissue homogenates. J Inf Dis 121:55, 1970.
17. Craig, WA and Kunin, CM: Significance of serum protein and tissue binding of antimicrobial agents. Ann Rev Med 27:287, 1976.
18. Hsu, CH, et al.: In vitro uptake of gentamicin by rat renal cortical tissue. Ann Rev Med 27:287, 1977.
19. Bryant, RE and Hammond, D: Interaction of purulent material with antibiotics used to treat *Pseudomonas* infections. Antimicrob Agents Chemother 6:702, 1974.
20. Wagman, GH, et al.: Binding of aminoglycosides to feces. Antimicrob Agents Chemother 6:415, 1974.
21. Bryan, LE and Kwan, S: Mechanisms of aminoglycoside resistance of anaerobic bacteria and facultative bacteria grown anaerobically. Chemother Suppl D 8:1, 1981.
22. Ghuysen, JM, et al.: The D-alanyl-D-alapeptidases. Mechanism of action of penicillins and cephalosporins. *In* Salton M, Shockman GD (eds): β-lactam Antibiotics. New York, Academic Press, 1981, p 32.
23. Tomasz, A: Penicillin-binding proteins and the antibacterial effectiveness of β-lactam antibiotics. Rev Inf Dis 8:Suppl 3, S260, 1986.
24. Bauernfeind, A: Classification of β-lactamases. Rev Inf Dis 8:Suppl 5, S470, 1986.

25. Richmond, MH and Sykes, M: The β-lactamases of gram-negative bacteria and their possible physiological role. Adv Microb Physiol 9:31, 1973.
26. Neu, CH: β-lactamases: A perspective on the contribution of these enzymes to bacterial resistance. Post Grad Med (Custom Comm) Sept/Oct:7, 1984.
27. Neu, HC: β-lactam antibiotics: Structural relationships affecting in vitro activity and pharmacological properties. Rev Inf Dis 8(Suppl 3): S237, 1986.
28. Rorich, PJ, et al.: In vitro susceptibilities of canine urinary tract bacteria to selected antimicrobial agents. JAVMA 183:863, 1983.
29. McGowan, JE: Antimicrobial resistance in hospital organisms and its relation to antibiotic use. Rev Inf Dis 5:1033, 1983.
30. Actor, P and Lentnek, A: β-lactam Antibiotics. *In* Verdame M (ed): CRC Handbook of Chemotherapeutic Agents. Boca Raton, Florida, CRC Press, 1986, pp 31.
31. Hieber, JP and Nelson, JD: A pharmacological evaluation of penicillin in children with purulent meningitis. N Engl J Med 297:410, 1977.
32. Powers, TE, et al.: Pharmacotherapeutics of newer penicillins and cephalosporins. JAVMA 176:1054, 1980.
33. Garvey, MS and Aucoin, DP: Therapeutic strategies involving antimicrobial treatment of disseminated bacterial infection in small animals. JAVMA 185:1185, 1984.
34. Macy, SM and Klein, JO: The isoxazolyl penicillins: oxacillin, cloxacillin and dicloxacillin. Med Clin N Am 54:1127, 1970.
35. Ihrke, PJ: Therapeutic strategies involving antimicrobial treatment of the skin in small animals. JAVMA 185:1165, 1984.
36. Cabana, BE, et al.: Pharmacokinetic evaluation of the oral absorption of different ampicillin preparations in beagle dogs. Antimicrob Agents Chemother 35, 1969.
37. Mercer, HD, et al.: Bioavailability and pharmacokinetics of several dosage forms of ampicillin in the cat. Am J Vet Res 38:1353, 1977.
38. Bywater, RJ, et al.: Clavulanate-potentiated amoxycillin: Activity in vitro and bioavailability in the dog. Vet Rec 116:33, 1985.
39. Eliopoulos, GM and Moellering, RC: Azlocillin, mezlocillin, and piperacillin: New broad-spectrum penicillins. Ann Int Med 97:755, 1982.
40. Young, LS: Antimicrobial synergism and combinational therapy. Antimicrob Newslett 1:1, 1984.
41. Anderson, et al.: Antimicrobial synergism in the therapy of gram-negative rod bacteremia. Chemotherapy, 24:45, 1978.
42. Knirsch, et al.: Pharmacokinetics, toleration, and safety of indanyl carbenicillin in man. J Inf Dis 127(Suppl):105, 1973.
43. Tilmant, L, et al.: Pharmacokinetics of ticarcillin in the dog. Am J Vet Res 46:479, 1985.
44. Batra, VK, et al.: Pharmacokinetics of piperacillin and gentamicin following intravenous administration to dogs. J Pharmaceut Sci 72:894, 1983.
45. Fare, LR: Comparative serum level and protective activity of parenterally administered cephalosporins in experimental animals. Antimicrob Agents Chemother 6:150, 1974.
46. Brusch, JL, et al.: Comparative pharmacokinetics of thirteen antibiotics in dogs with especial reference to concentrations in liver, kidney, bile and urine. Infection 4(Suppl 2):82, 1976.
47. Thompson, TD, et al.: Cephalosporin group of antimicrobial drugs. JAVMA 185:1109, 1984.
48. Cabana, BE, et al.: Comparative pharmacokinetics and metabolism of cephapirin in laboratory animals and humans. Antimicrob Agents Chemother 10:307, 1976.
49. Wells, JS: Toxicology and pharmacology of cephalexin in lab animals. Antimicrob Agents Chemother 1968:489, 1969.
50. Komiya, M, et al.: Pharmacokinetics of new broad-spectrum cephamycin, YM09330, parenterally administered to various experimental animals. Antimicrob Agents Chemother 20:176, 1981.
51. Guerrini, H, et al.: Pharmacokinetic evaluation of a slow release cefotaxime suspension in the dog and in sheep. Am J Vet Res 47:2057, 1986.
52. McElroy, D, et al.: Pharmacokinetics of cefotaxime in the domestic cat. Am J Vet Res 47:86, 1986.
53. Birnbaum, J, et al.: Carbapenems, a new class of β-lactam antibiotics. Am J Med 78(Suppl 6A):3, 1985.
54. Norrby, SR: Imipenum/cilastatin: Rationale for a fixed combination. Rev Inf Dis 7(Supp 3):S447, 1985.
55. Kahan, FM, et al.: Thienamycin: development of imipenum-cilastatin. J Antimicrob Chemother 12:(Suppl D) 1, 1983.
56. Sykes, RB and Bonner, DP: Aztreonam: The first monobactam. Am J Med 78(Suppl 2A):2, 1985.
57. Hamilton-Miller, JT: Fungal sterols and the mode of action of the polyene antibiotics. Adv Appl Microbiol 17:109 1974.
58. Sande, MA and Mandell, GL: Antimicrobial agents: Antifungal and antiviral agents. *In* Gilman AG, Goodman LS (eds): The Pharmacological Basis for Therapeutics. New York, Macmillan, 1985, p 1219.
59. Kim, H, et al.: Comparative pharmacokinetics of SCH 28191 and amphotericin B in mice, rats, dogs and cynomolgus monkeys. Antimicrob Agents Chemother 26:446, 1984.
60. Legendre, AM, et al.: Treatment of canine blastomycosis with amphotericin B and ketoconazole. JAVMA 184:1249, 1984.
61. Moriello, KA: Ketoconazole: Clinical pharmacology and therapeutic recommendations. JAVMA 188:303, 1986.
62. Heel, RC, et al.: Ketoconazole: a review of its therapeutic efficacy and in superficial and systemic fungal infections. Drugs 23:1, 1982.
63. Willard, MD, et al.: Ketoconazole-induced changes in selected canine hormone concentrations. Am J Vet Res 47:2504, 1986.
64. Carbon, C, et al.: Aminoglycosides (aminocyclitols). *In* Peterson PK, Verhoef J (eds): Antimicrob Agents Annual I. Amsterdam, Elsevier, 1986, p 1.
65. Bryan, LE: Aminoglycoside resistance. *In* Bryan LE (ed): Antimicrobial Drug Resistance. New York, Academic Press 1984, p 41.
66. Riviere, JE, et al.: Gentamicin aerosol therapy in 18 dogs: Failure to induce detectable serum concentrations of the drug. JAVMA 179:166, 1981.
67. Baggot, JD, et al.: Clinical pharmacokinetics of amakacin in the dog. Am J Vet Res 46:1793, 1985.
68. Riviere, J, et al.: Pharmacokinetics and comparative nephrotoxicity of fixed-dose versus fixed interval reduction of gentamicin dosage in subtotal nephrectomized dogs. Toxicol Appl Pharmacol 75:496, 1984.
69. Riviere, JE and Carver, MP: Effect of familial hypothyroidism and subtotal surgical nephrectomy on gentamicin pharmacokinetics in beagle dogs. Chemotherapy 30:216, 1984.
70. Riviere, J, et al.: Decreased fractional renal excretion of gentamicin in subtotal nephrectomized dogs. J Pharmacol Exp Ther 234:90, 1985.
71. Hoestetler, KY and Hall, LB: Inhibition of kidney lysosomal phospholipase A and C by aminoglycoside antibiotics: possible mechanism of aminoglycoside toxicity. Proc Natl Acad Sci USA 79:1663, 1982.
72. Brion, et al.: Gentamicin, netilmicin, diebakacin and amikacin nephrotoxicity and its relationship to tubular reabsorption in rabbits. Antimicrob Agents Chemother 25:168, 1984.
73. Contrepois, A, et al.: Renal disposition of gentamicin, debakacin, tobramycin, netilmicin, and amakacin in humans. Antimicrob Agents Chemother 27:520, 1985.
74. Luft, FC: Netilmicin: A review of toxicity in laboratory animals. J Int Med Res 6:9, 1978.
75. McCormick, GC, et al.: Comparative ototoxicity of netilmicin, gentamicin, and tobramycin in cats. Toxicol Appl Pharmacol 77:479, 1985.
76. Kahlmeter, G and Dahlager, JI: Aminoglycoside toxicity: a review of clinical studies published between 1975 and 1982. J Antimicrob Chemother 13:(Suppl A)9, 1984.
77. Brown, SA, et al.: Gentamicin-associated acute renal failure in the dog. JAVMA 186:686, 1985.
78. Moore, RD, et al.: Clinical response to aminoglycoside therapy: Importance of the ratio of peak concentration to minimal inhibitory concentration. J Infect Dis 155:93, 1987.
79. Chopra, I, et al.: The tetracyclines: prospects at the beginning of the 1980's. J Antimicrob Chemother 8:5, 1981.
80. Aronson, AL: Pharmacotherapeutics of the newer tetracyclines. JAVMA 176:1061, 1980.
81. Cooke, KG, et al.: Bioavailability of oxytetracycline dihydrate tablets in dogs. J Vet Pharmacol Ther 4:11, 1981.
82. von Wittenau, MS and Yeary, R: The excretion and distribution

in body fluids of tetracyclines after intravenous administration to dogs. J Pharmacol Exp Ther 140:258, 1963.
83. Wilson, RC, et al.: Compartmental and noncompartmental pharmacokinetic analyses of minocycline hydrochloride in the dog. Am J Vet Res 46:1316, 1985.
84. Ling, GV and Ruby, AL: Chloramphenicol for oral treatment of canine urinary tract infections. JAVMA 172:914, 1978.
85. Watson, AJ and Middleton, DJ: Chloramphenicol toxicosis in cats. Am J Vet Res 39:1199, 1978.
86. Watson, AJ: Effect of ingesta on systemic availability of chloramphenicol from two oral preparations in cats. J Vet Pharmacol Ther 2:117, 1979.
87. Watson, AJ: Plasma chloramphenicol concentrations in cats after parenteral administration of chloramphenicol sodium succinate. J Vet Pharmacol Ther 2:123, 1979.
88. Davis, LE, et al.: Pharmacokinetics of chloramphenicol in domesticated animals. Am J Vet Res 33:2259, 1972.
89. Watson, AJ and McDonald, PG: Distribution of chloramphenicol in some tissues and extravascular fluids of dogs after oral administration. Am J Vet Res 37:557, 1976.
90. Watson, AJ: Oral chloramphenicol dosage regimens in cats. J Vet Pharmacol Ther 3:145, 1980.
91. Watson, AJ: Further observations on chloramphenicol toxicosis in cats. Am J Vet Res 41:293, 1980.
92. Watson, AJ: Systemic availability of chloramphenicol from tablets and capsule in cats. J Vet Pharmacol Ther 3:45, 1980.
93. Burrows, GE: Pharmacotherapeutics of macrolides, lincomycins and spectinomycin. JAVMA 176:1072, 1980.
94. Weber, DJ, et al.: Pharmacokinetics of clindamycin following subcutaneous administration of clindamycin phosphate in the canine. J Vet Pharmacol Ther 3:133, 1980.
95. Neu, HC: Quinolones revisited: Where are we. Antimicrob Newslett 4:9, 1987.
96. Piddock, LJV and Wise, R: The antibacterial action of the 4-Quinolones. Antimicrobic Newslett 2:1, 1985.
97. Shimada, J, et al.: Mechanism of renal excretion of AM-715, a new quinolonecarboxylic acid derivative, in rabbits, dogs and humans. Antimicrob Agents Chemother 23:1, 1983.
98. Gerding, DN: Metronidazole. *In* Peterson PK, Verhoef J (eds): The Antimicrobial Agents Annual I. Amsterdam, Elsevier, 1985, p 127.
99. Neff-Davis, CA, et al.: Metronidazole: a method for its determination in biological fluids and its disposition in the dog. J Vet Pharmacol Ther 4:121, 1981.
100. Grisham, LM, et al.: Antimicrobic action of griseofulvin does not involve disruption of microtubules. Nature 244:294, 1973.
101. Helton, KA, et al.: Griseofulvin toxicity in cats: Literature review and report of seven cats. JAAHA 22:453, 1986.
102. Ling, GV, et al.: Urine concentrations of chloramphenicol, tetracycline, and sulfisoxasole after oral administration to normal adult dogs. Am J Vet Res 41:950, 1980.
103. Bushby, SRM, et al.: Sulfonamide and trimethoprim combinations. JAVMA 176:1049, 1980.
104. Indiveri, MC and Hirsch, DC: Susceptibility of obligate anaerobes to trimethoprim-sulfamethoxazole. JAVMA 188:46, 1986.
105. Cates, LA: Sulfa drugs. *In* Verdame M (ed): Handbook of Chemotherapeutic Agents. Boca Raton, Florida, CRC Press, 1986, p 1.
106. Siegle, CW, et al.: Pharmacokinetics of trimethoprim and sulfadiazine in the dog: Urine concentrations after oral administration. Am J Vet Res 42:996, 1981.
107. Vosti, KL: Nitrofurantoin. *In* Peterson PK, Verhoef V (eds): The Antimicrobial Agents Annual I. Amsterdam, Elsevier, 1986, p 132.
108. Sachs, J, et al.: Effect of renal function on urinary recovery of orally administered nitrofurantoin. N Engl J Med 278:1032, 1968.
109. Mandel, GL and Sande, MA: Sulfonamides, Trimethoprim-sulfamethoxazole, and agents for urinary tract infections. *In* AG Gilman, LS Goodman (eds): The Pharmacological Basis of Therapeutics. New York, Macmillan, 1985, p 1108.
110. Ling, GL: Management of urinary tract infections. *In* RW Kirk (ed): Current Veterinary Therapy IX. Philadelphia, WB Saunders, 1986, p 1174.
111. Pennington, JE: Penetration of antibiotics into respiratory secretions. Rev Infec Dis 3:67, 1981.
112. Piercy, DWT: Distribution of trimethoprim/sulfadiazine in plasma, tissues and synovial fluid. Vet Rec 102:523, 1978.
113. Caywood DD: Osteomyelitis. Vet Clin N Am 13:43, 1983.
114. Hirsch DC, Smith TM: Osteomyelitis in the dog. Microorganisms isolated and susceptibility to antimicrobial agents. J Small Anim Prac 19:679, 1978.
115. Walker RD, et al.: Anaerobic bacteria associated with osteomyelitis in domestic animals. JAVMA 182:814, 1983.
116. Hall BB, et al.: The pharmacokinetics of penicillin in osteomyelitic canine bone. J Bone Joint Surg 65A:526, 1983.
117. Hirsch DC, et al.: Blood culture of the canine patient. JAVMA 184:175, 1984.
118. Vasseur PB, et al.: Infection rates in clean surgical procedures: A comparison of ampicillin vs a placebo. JAVMA 187:825, 1985.
119. Riviere JE, et al.: Prophylactic use of systemic antimicrobial drugs in surgery. Comp Cont Ed Prac Vet 3:345, 1981.
120. Padilla SL, et al.: Single-dose ampicillin for cesarean section prophylaxis. Obstet Gynecol 61:463, 1983.

52 USE OF CORTICOSTEROIDS

C. B. CHASTAIN

The medical use of corticosteroids began in 1949 when humans with rheumatoid arthritis were treated with cortisone and were reported to experience marked improvement.[1] In the years that have followed, corticosteroids have become one of the most frequently used and prescribed classes of drugs in veterinary medicine. Extraordinary corticosteroid-induced improvements have been documented in a wide range of diseases, especially those in which inflammation is severe or cell damage is immunologically mediated.

The beneficial effects of corticosteroid therapy have been accompanied by adverse effects. In 1952, the first case of fatal iatrogenic adrenocortical atrophy was reported in a human who had been treated with cortisone.[2] Corticosteroid-induced adrenocortical atrophy was described in dogs in 1961.[3] Although the first death in a dog caused by withdrawal from corticosteroids was reported in 1968,[4] the clinical significance of iatrogenic problems from corticosteroid administration was not well appreciated until 1974.[5] It is now thought that fifty per cent of cases in dogs with corticosteroid excess are iatrogenic in origin. These dogs, and many more dogs treated with corticosteroids without abnormal external signs, develop marked adrenocortical atrophy.

The use of corticosteroids should be rational. They should not be excluded from a clinician's pharmacologic options, nor should they be used indiscriminately without thought or knowledge of their potential and wide-ranging adverse effects. A proper balance of maximum desired effect with minimum adverse effect necessitates knowing corticosteroids' relative potency and duration of action, recommended initial dosages, conditions that require special consideration, and how to monitor for early indications of adverse effects.

NATURAL CORTICOSTEROIDS

Corticosteroids are hormones secreted by cells of the adrenal cortex. Synthesis requires a series of reactions that converts cholesterol to mineralocorticoids (those that promote sodium retention and potassium loss from the body), glucocorticoids (those that inhibit the inflammatory response and promote gluconeogenesis), or adrenal sex hormones. More than 95 per cent of the secreted corticosteroids in the dog are considered glucocorticoids (Table 52–1).[6] Exogenous glucocorticoids are the corticosteroids used by clinicians to treat inflammatory, pruritic, and immunologically mediated diseases. As a result, the term "corticosteroids" is generally assumed to mean glucocorticoids.

The conversion of cholesterol to pregnenolone, the precursor of secreted corticosteroids, is greatly facilitated by adrenocorticotropic hormone (ACTH).[7] ACTH is the only direct stimulus for the secretion of glucocorticoids. ACTH secretion is stimulated by low plasma cortisol levels. The secretion of ACTH from the adenohypophysis is, in turn, directly and indirectly (through inhibition of hypothalamic corticotropin-releasing hormone) suppressed by elevated plasma levels of corticosteroids, especially cortisol (see Figure 52–1). Plasma levels of secreted corticosteroids fluctuate during the day as a result of normal episodic bursts of ACTH secretion. These bursts may be of greater magnitude in the morning in dogs and in the evening in cats, but such diurnal rhythm in companion animals is difficult to assess or may not exist.[8–11] A wide variety of stresses can also cause ACTH secretion and even override the usually inhibitory effects of elevated plasma cortisol levels on ACTH secretion.[12, 13]

Glucocorticoids are products of the inner zones, the zonae fasciculata and reticularis, of the adrenal cortex. ACTH not only stimulates the secretion of these zones, but also maintains their normal microstructure by controlling adrenocortical cell replication. In the absence of

TABLE 52–1. APPROXIMATE CORTICOSTEROID SECRETION RATES IN THE DOG

Hormone	Secretion Rate (μg/lb) (μg/kg) (body weight/day)
Glucocorticoid	
Cortisol	350–400 (700–800)
Corticosterone	150–200 (300–400)
Deoxycortisol	40–45 (80–90)
Mineralocorticoid	
Deoxycorticosterone	2.5–5 (5–10)
Aldosterone	2.5–5 (5–10)
Total	0.5 mg/lb (1.2 mg/kg) body weight/day

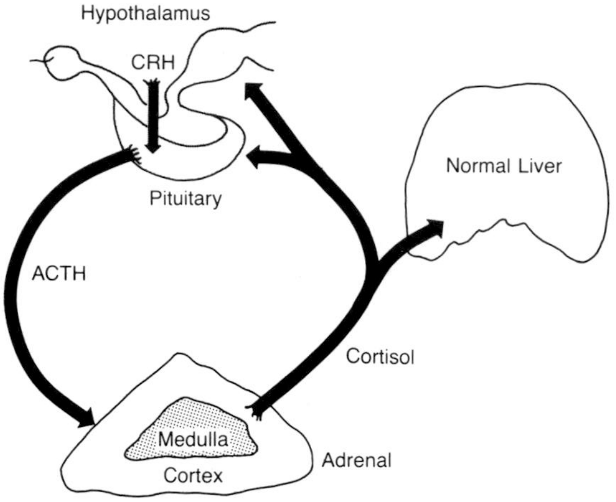

FIGURE 52–1. The normal hypothalamic-pituitary-adrenal (H-P-A) axis. CRH, corticotropin-releasing hormone. ACTH, adrenocorticotropic hormone (corticotropin).

ACTH, the inner zones of the adrenal cortex first become functionally inactive and then eventually atrophy.

All adrenocortical hormones are derivatives of the cyclopentanoperhydrophenanthrene nucleus.[14] C-21 compounds have carbons at the C-18, C-19, and C-21 positions (Figure 52–2). C-21 compounds may show glucocorticoid, mineralocorticoid, or progestogen activity. Natural C-21 compounds have actions that overlap in the three possible effects of C-21 compounds, but either mineralocorticoid, glucocorticoid, or progestogen effects predominate. Synthetic C-21 compounds have more exclusive effects as a glucocorticoid, mineralocorticoid, or progestogen than natural C-21 compounds.

Natural glucocorticoids, cortisol and corticosterone, have a strong affinity for the corticosteroid-binding alpha globulin called transcortin. Binding to albumin also occurs, but only weakly.[15, 16] In the dog, the primary circulating corticosteroid is cortisol, which has normal plasma concentrations of about 1 to 4 mg/dl.[9, 17] It is thought that 40 per cent of plasma cortisol is bound to transcortin, 50 per cent to albumin, and 5 to 10 per cent is free.[18] The plasma half-life of cortisol is one to two hours.

It is the free corticosteroid that enters target cells and mediates biological effects. Corticosteroid receptors are present in virtually all cells of the body. After passively penetrating the cell membrane, corticosteroids bind reversibly to the cytoplasmic receptors. The hormone-receptor complex then migrates to the cell nucleus, where it modulates DNA gene expression and messenger RNA (mRNA) formation. Messenger RNA codes for cell enzyme and other protein production responsible for the expression of corticosteroids' effects.[15]

TABLE 52–2. RELATIVE ANTI-INFLAMMATORY AND MINERALOCORTICOID POTENCY OF COMMON NATURAL AND SYNTHETIC CORTICOSTEROIDS ADMINISTERED SYSTEMICALLY

Glucocorticoid	Mineralocorticoid Potency (per mg)	Anti-inflammatory Potency (per mg)	Equivalent Dose (mg)
Cortisone	0.8	0.8	25.0
Hydrocortisone	1.0	1.0	20.0
Prednisone	0.25	4.0	5.0
Prednisolone	0.25	4.0	5.0
Methylprednisolone	0.0	5.0	4.0
Triamcinolone	0.0	5.0	4.0
Paramethasone	0.0	10.0	2.0
Flumethasone	0.0	15.0	1.5
Dexamethasone	0.0	30.0	0.75
Betamethasone	0.0	35.0	0.6

Corticosteroids are removed from the circulation by the liver. Natural corticosteroids are converted to water-soluble conjugates of glucuronic acid or sulfates for excretion in the urine of dogs. Other hormones and drugs that use the glucuronyl transferase system can competitively inhibit corticosteroid excretion. The steroid nucleus cannot be catabolized. In the cat, steroids are excreted in the bile.[19] Inactivation or excretion of corticosteroids can be impaired by some liver diseases. Decreased serum albumin resulting from liver disease, parasitism, or the nephrotic syndrome decreases serum binding capacity and can worsen adverse effects of corticosteroid therapy.[14] Enzyme inducers such as phenytoin and phenobarbital may speed corticosteroid clearance.[20]

COMMONLY USED NATURAL AND SYNTHETIC CORTICOSTEROIDS

There are ten generic corticosteroids commercially available in the United States. These are sold under more than a hundred proprietary names, as a single item preparation or in combination with antibiotics or various other drugs.

RELATIVE POTENCY

The potency of corticosteroids is assessed by their anti-inflammatory activity in experimental animals on granulomas induced by subcutaneous injection of tur-

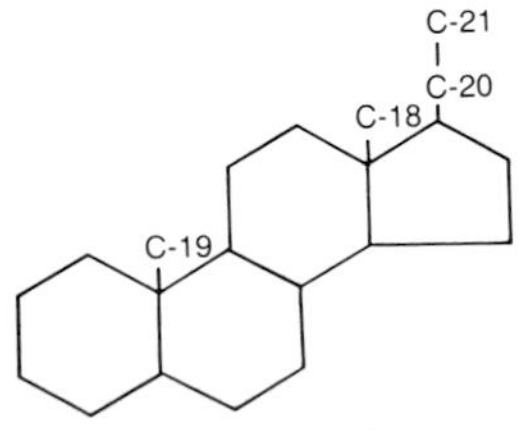

FIGURE 52–2. The basic structure of C-21 derivatives of the cyclopentanoperhydrophenanthrene nucleus, which includes corticosteroids, i.e., glucocorticoids.

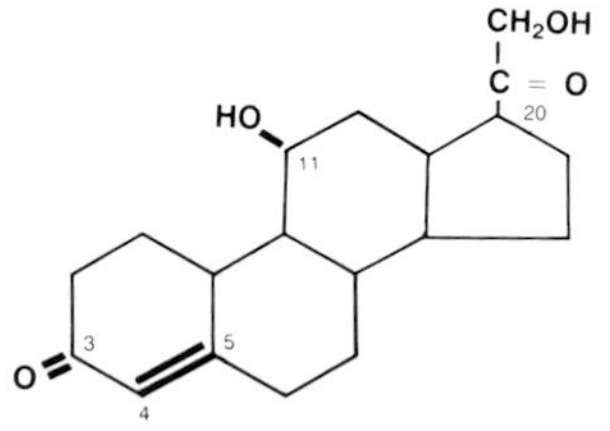

FIGURE 52–3. Essential anti-inflammatory groups (bold letters and lines) on the basic C-21 compound.

pentine or croton oil or by implantation of cotton pledgets. Hydrocortisone is used as a standard with an arbitrary value of one. The relative potencies of several corticosteroids are listed in Table 52–2. The essential anti-inflammatory groups needed on the cyclopentanoperhydrophenanthrene nucleus are shown in Figure 52–3. Corticosteroids with a keto group at C-11, such as cortisone and prednisone, do not have anti-inflammatory activity until the keto group is reduced by the liver to a hydroxy group, making prednisone into prednisolone and cortisone into hydrocortisone. Severe liver disease can impair this conversion. C-11 keto compounds are not effective topically.[14]

A great number of synthetic corticosteroids have been developed in an attempt to increase glucocorticoid potency while decreasing or eliminating the mineralocorticoid effects of natural corticosteroids. Glucocorticoid activity can be increased by the addition of a double bond at C-l to C-2, hydroxylation of C-16 or C-17, methylation of C-6 or C-16, or fluorination of C-6 or C-9.[14] Representative structures appear in Figure 52–4. Mineralocorticoid activity is decreased by hydroxylation or methylation of C-16.

Synthetic corticosteroids have greater anti-inflammatory and lesser mineralocorticoid effects per mg than natural corticosteroids. They bind less avidly to plasma proteins, have a longer duration of biologic action because of increased corticosteroid receptor affinity and more resistance to hepatic degradation, and are usually more expensive than natural corticosteroids.[14] Prednisone and prednisolone are the least expensive synthetic corticosteroids, have an intermediate duration of action, can be administered on an alternate-day program to successfully minimize hypothalamic pituitary-adrenal (H-P-A) axis suppression, and have relatively little mineralocorticoid effect.[21] For the preceding reasons, prednisone and prednisolone are the most frequently prescribed oral forms of corticosteroid. There is rarely a justifiable reason to use more potent and expensive corticosteroids for systemic effects. There is no qualitative difference in anti-inflammatory action among synthetic corticosteroids.[22]

The risk of adverse effects from corticosteroid therapy is directly related to the corticosteroid's potency, dosage, duration of action and dosage interval, duration of administration, and rate of systemic absorption. Potency is an inherent quality of each corticosteroid, based on its structure and a reflection of the dose used.[14] The duration of action is affected by the body's ability to metabolize and eliminate the corticosteroid, the dose used, and the rate of absorption. The amount and rate of systemic absorption varies with the route of administration.

DURATION OF ACTION

The plasma half-life of corticosteroids does not reflect the metabolic duration of their effects. Plasma half-lives of all corticosteroids in humans are from 30 minutes to approximately five hours when standard anti-inflammatory doses are used.[14] Based on the plasma half-life of prednisolone in dogs,[23] other corticosteroid half-lives in dogs are probably similar to humans. Corticosteroids do not mediate their effects while in the plasma. Their biologic effects begin after cytoplasmic receptors are bound, the receptor hormone complex moves to the cell nucleus, and mRNA transmits the message for modification in protein synthesis to ribosomes in the cytoplasm. Although this process requires only minutes, the modified cell function continues long after the corticosteroid disappears from the plasma.[14] For practical purposes, corticosteroids used for systemic effects are classified into three categories: short-, intermediate-, and long-acting, based on the duration of their metabolic effects (Table 52–3).[14, 24] Four to five biologic half-lives must elapse before more than 95 per cent of an administered dose is eliminated from the body.[25]

The rate of corticosteroid absorption is slowed and its own inherent duration markedly prolonged if it is bound to a poorly soluble ester for intramuscular injection. Examples include methylprednisolone acetate, which in a dose of 1.1 mg/lb (2.5 mg/kg) body weight in the dog suppresses the adrenal cortex for at least five weeks,[26, 27] and triamcinolone acetonide, which in a dose of 0.11 mg/lb (0.22 mg/kg) body weight in the dog suppresses the adrenal cortex for about four weeks.[28] Steroid esters, their relative solubility in water, and the estimated duration of the steroid's release are listed in Table 52–4.

Some drugs, if used concurrently with corticosteroids, can speed corticosteroid clearance by the induction of hepatic enzymes. Hepatic enzyme-inducing drugs include phenobarbital, organochlorines, phenylbutazone, and phenytoin.

PHYSIOLOGIC AND PHARMACOLOGIC EFFECTS OF CORTICOSTEROIDS

Corticosteroids affect virtually every mammalian cell, producing numerous diverse effects on the body. However, the physiologic effects are not as varied as the pharmacologic effects.

Significant physiologic effects of corticosteroids include a permissive effect on the lipolytic, pressor, and

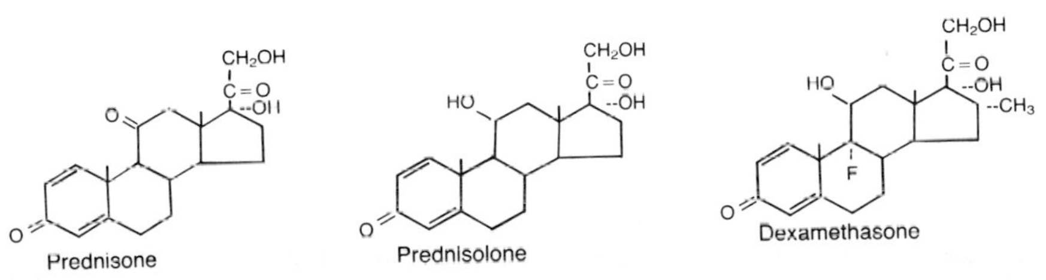

FIGURE 52–4. Structures of common synthetic corticosteroids.

TABLE 52–3. RELATIVE METABOLIC DURATION OF EFFECTS FOR COMMON CORTICOSTEROIDS

Duration	Corticosteroids	Appropriate Use: Replacement	Appropriate Use: Alternate Day
Short-acting (less than 12 hours)			
	Cortisone	+	–
	Hydrocortisone	+	–
Intermediate-acting (12 to 36 hours)			
	Prednisone	+	+
	Prednisolone	+	+
	Methylprednisolone	+	+
	Triamcinolone*	–	–
Long-acting (more than 48 hours)			
	Paramethasone	–	–
	Flumethasone	–	–
	Dexamethasone	–	–
	Betamethasone	–	–

*Duration can be up to 48 hours.

TABLE 52–4. CORTICOSTEROID ESTERS, SOLUBILITY (IN WATER), AND DURATION OF STEROID RELEASE FROM INTRAMUSCULAR INJECTION

Very soluble–released for minutes
Succinate
Hemisuccinate
Phosphate
Soluble–released for minutes to hours
Polyethylene glycol
Moderately insoluble–released for days to weeks
Acetate
Diacetate
Isonicotinate
Tebutate
Poorly soluble–released for weeks
Acetonide
Hexacetonide
Pivalate
Diproprionate

bronchodilating actions of catecholamines. Corticosteroids must also be present in small quantities to permit glucagon's glycogenolytic action and to form phenylethanolamine-N-methyl transferase, an enzyme in the adrenal medulla that converts norepinephrine to epinephrine.[15] Other physiologic effects of corticosteroids include maintenance of normal cardiac and skeletal muscle strength, maintenance of normal brain activity, maintenance of normal water compartment distribution in the body, and preparation of various organs to withstand the deleterious effects of certain stresses. Small quantities of corticosteroids, 0.2 to 0.5 mg/lb (0.5 to 1.1 mg/kg) body weight/day of hydrocortisone, are necessary for normal physiologic effects in unstressed dogs.[6]

CARBOHYDRATE, FAT, AND PROTEIN METABOLISM

Corticosteroids promote gluconeogenesis, which is the production of blood glucose at the expense of muscle and adipose tissue. Corticosteroids induce gluconeogenesis by promoting the formation of hepatic gluconeogenic enzymes such as glucose-6-phosphatase, tyrosine aminotransferase, tryptophan pyrrolase, fructose-6-diphosphatase, and phosphoenolpyruvate carboxykinase.[16] Increased secretion of insulin normally counters the tendency toward hyperglycemia.[29, 30] Protein, particularly the amino acid alanine, is mobilized from most of the body with the notable exception of the liver.[16] In the liver, protein synthesis is promoted.[15] Serum alpha-2 globulins are increased.[26] Corticosteroids also mobilize fatty acids and enhance their oxidation. Plasma levels of cholesterol, triglyceride, and glycerol are increased, and ketogenesis occurs if insulin's countereffects are exceeded.[15] Corticosteroids are not lipolytic in all adipose tissue. Lipogenesis is enhanced in the abdomen. In fact, adipose tissue tends to be redistributed from the extremities to the pelvis, neck, thorax, and omentum.[16]

WATER DISTRIBUTION, ELECTROLYTES, AND TRACE MINERALS

Corticosteroids promote diuresis, inhibit the water shift into cells, increase potassium excretion in urine, increase urinary and fecal losses of calcium, and decrease levels of serum zinc.[16] Proposed mechanisms for corticosteroid-induced diuresis include increased glomerular filtration rate, inhibition of the action of antidiuretic hormone (ADH) on the renal tubules, and increased ADH inactivation.[31, 32] Hypokalemia from corticosteroid administration is not likely because hydrocortisone is only 1/1000 as potent per mg as aldosterone. All synthetic corticosteroids, except fludrocortisone, have weaker mineralocorticoid effects than hydrocortisone.[16] Hypocalcemia does not develop as a result of corticosteroid administration as long as the parathyroids respond normally. However, secondary hyperparathyroidism and depleted bone mineralization may result.

GASTROINTESTINAL TRACT AND THE LIVER

Corticosteroids increase gastric acid and pepsin secretion, decrease mucosal cell proliferation, and stimulate pancreas secretions.[33] Hepatic changes in dogs caused by high dose corticosteroid administration are vacuolization of hepatocytes with glycogen or fat, a decrease in the number of mitochondria, and induction of an alkaline phosphatase isoenzyme.[34–38] Increased serum levels of alanine aminotransferase and gamma-glutamyl transpeptidase, which are also caused by corticosteroids, are not of the magnitude or the duration of serum alkaline phosphatase elevations.[26] Minor increased retention of bromsulphalein is also caused by corticosteroids.[37] Pancreatic secretions are made more viscous and the pancreatic ductal epithelium becomes hyperplastic.[39]

CARDIOVASCULAR SYSTEM

Corticosteroid use produces vasoconstriction by the permissive effect on responses to catecholamines and by an antagonistic effect on responses to kinins and histamine.[40] Capillary permeability and resulting edema is decreased.[16, 40] Corticosteroids also have a weak inotropic effect on the myocardium, which is probably insignificant in vivo.[15, 16]

MUSCULOSKELETAL SYSTEM

Pharmacologic doses of corticosteroids can cause physical weakness, muscular atrophy, and osteoporosis.[14, 15] Additional potential corticosteroid effects that affect the skeletal system are inhibition of growth hormone and somatomedin release, inhibition of fibrocartilage growth, catabolism of collagenous bone matrix, increased calcium excretion in urine and feces, and inhibition of vitamin D activation.[15, 41]

NERVOUS SYSTEM

Potential pharmacologic effects of corticosteroids on the nervous system include decreased seizure threshold, psychoses, decreased response to pyrogens, somnolence, and stimulation of the appetite.[15] At least some of these effects may be due to depletion of gamma-amino butyric acid, a neurotransmission inhibitor.[15] Induced psychoses in dogs have been manifested as aggression, paranoid behavior, amaurosis, disorientation, ataxia, vomiting, and depression.[42]

HEMATOLYMPHATIC SYSTEM

Corticosteroid use can cause neutrophilia, resulting from stimulated production, release from the bone marrow, decreased egress from the circulation, and release from the marginated pool of neutrophils.[15, 40] Lymphopenia, eosinopenia, and basopenia result from sequestration of cells in the spleen and lungs, decreased efflux from the bone marrow, and decreased lymphocyte mitosis.[15, 26, 40] Red blood cell (RBC) production is augmented by corticosteroids, whereas removal of old RBCs is suppressed. Target cells and Howell-Jolly bodies may increase. Platelets and monocytes may also increase in the circulation, but platelet aggregation is inhibited.[15]

IMMUNITY

At doses that exceed those commonly used to suppress inflammation, corticosteroids can cause immunosuppression. Corticosteroids can induce lymphocytes to disappear from the circulation, primarily because of redistribution into the bone marrow and other sites. Their DNA synthesis can also be inhibited as demonstrated by depletion of cortical areas of lymph nodes by two weeks of 0.4 mg prednisolone acetate/lb (1 mg/kg) body weight twice per day.[35] Mice, rats, hamsters, and rabbits are much more susceptible to immunological impairment by corticosteroids than are dogs, cats, and humans. Yet much of our knowledge of the effects of corticosteroids on immunity has been based on studies done on small laboratory animals. This has led some to overestimate the ability of conservative doses of corticosteroid to adversely affect immunity.

Thymic-derived (T) lymphocytes and therefore, cell-mediated immunity, are more affected by corticosteroids than bursa-equivalent (B) lymphocytes and humoral immunity.[16, 40] In addition to decreasing T cells in number, corticosteroids also inhibit the effects of lymphokines produced by sensitized T cells. The production of lymphokines is not directly inhibited. High doses of corticosteroids can decrease antibody production, even serum levels of beta and gamma globulins,[26] but the amnestic response is relatively resistant compared to the initial response.[15, 40]

Corticosteroids inhibit neutrophil, macrophage, and monocyte migration; chemotactic response; diapedesis; interferon production; processing of antigens; phagocytosis; and intracellular killing.[15, 16, 40] Nonspecific immune defenses are affected more than specific acquired immunity. Antigen-antibody reactions are not prevented, but the subsequent inflammatory response is suppressed.[16] The complement cascade is antagonized.[40] Serum iron levels are increased, promoting bacterial growth.[26] Fibroblastic proliferation to sequester infectious agents (especially those of granulomatous diseases) and to repair tissue is suppressed.[15] Clinical signs of infection, such as pain and leukocytosis, are masked by high doses of corticosteroids. The formation of the mediators and products of inflammation that are derivatives of cell membrane phospholipids, such as thromboxane, leukotrienes, prostacyclin, and prostaglandins, are inhibited.[43] The febrile response is lessened because the effects of endotoxins are decreased, the release of endogenous pyrogen (interleukin I) from monocytes is decreased, and neutrophil migration is decreased.[40, 44]

DETOXIFICATION

Corticosteroids have detoxifying actions such as stabilization of lysosomal membranes, reduction of capillary permeability, reduced endothelial swelling, suppression of the effects of vasoactive amines, and maintenance of cell membrane integrity.[16] Mast cell numbers are decreased and the synthesis of histamine is suppressed.[15]

PREGNANCY AND LACTATION

Unbound corticosteroids freely pass through the placenta. The administration of corticosteroids in early pregnancy may cause teratogenic effects.[45] The administration of corticosteroids in late pregnancy may induce premature parturition or cause adrenocortical atrophy in the neonate. Unbound corticosteroids also pass into the milk and, if administered during lactation, can cause suppression of growth and adrenocortical atrophy in nursing puppies or kittens.

ENDOCRINE SYSTEM

In unstressed animals even the smallest dose of corticosteroids suppresses ACTH secretion, which in turn inhibits endogenous corticosteroid production. Prolonged corticosteroid-induced suppression of ACTH secretion results in adrenocortical atrophy (see Figures 52–5 and 52–6). Stresses such as chronic renal failure, severe liver disease, and diabetes mellitus can sometimes override the inhibiting effects of circulating corticosteroids by stimulating ACTH secretion via suprahypothalamic neural stimuli.[12, 13] At pharmacologic doses, corticosteroids also adversely affect the secretion of thyroid-stimulating hormone (TSH), follicle-stimulating hor-

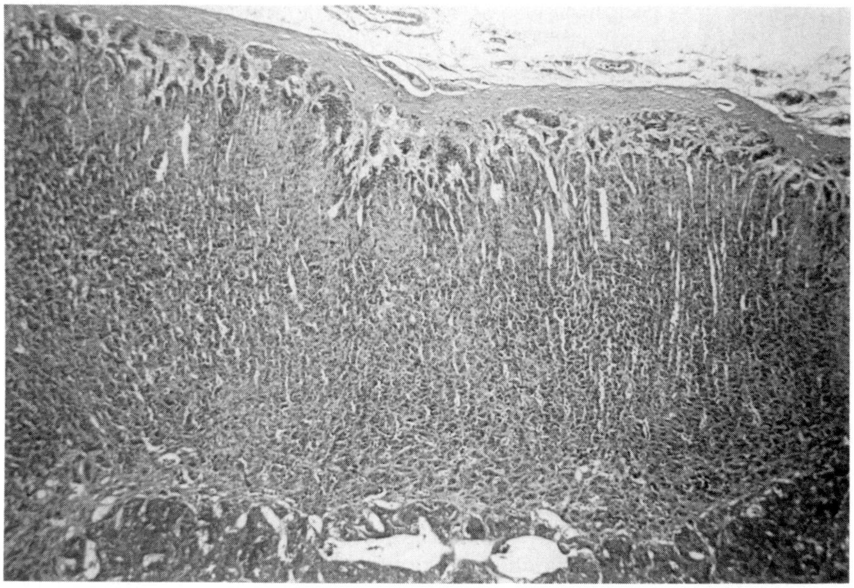

FIGURE 52–5. Photomicrograph of a normal canine adrenal cortex.

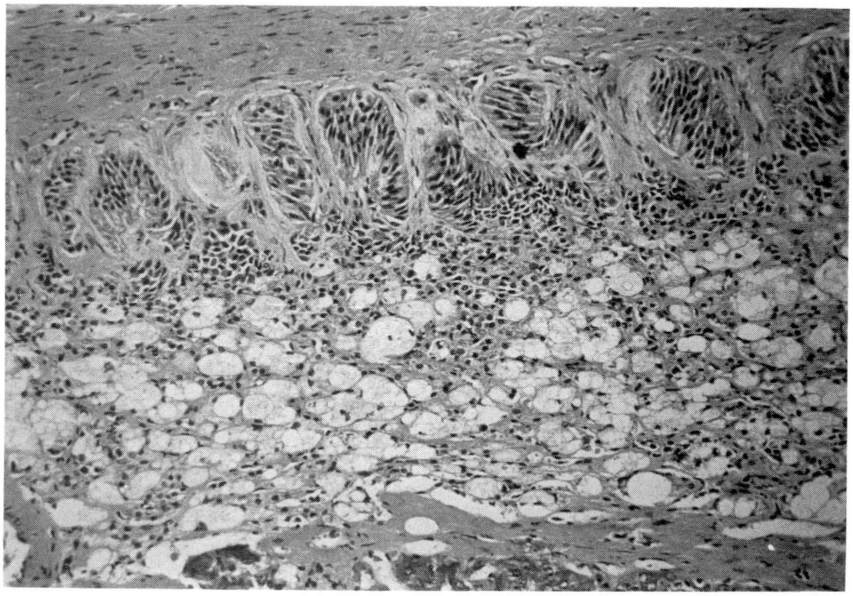

FIGURE 52–6. Photomicrograph of a canine adrenal cortex after 0.55 mg/kg body weight/day of prednisone for four weeks, demonstrating atrophy, vacuolization, cytoplasmic swelling, and disruption of the zonae fasciculata and reticularis.

mone (FSH), luteinizing hormone (LH), prolactin, and growth hormone.[15, 16, 32, 46] In addition to a deficiency of their tropic hormones, functions of the thyroids, testes, and ovaries may be directly inhibited by corticosteroids.[32, 46] Other effects on thyroid hormone metabolism include suppression of thyroxine's (T4) peripheral conversion to tri-iodothyronine (T3) and reduction of thyroxine-binding globulin levels. Insulin's binding to receptors and post-receptor effects are inhibited by corticosteroids.[32] The effects of ADH on renal tubules are also suppressed.[31] Plasma levels of parathyroid hormone are increased by corticosteroids due to corticosteroid-induced inhibition of calcium's absorption from the digestive tract and due to corticosteroid-promoted calciuria. Osteoblast activity may be directly inhibited by corticosteroids.[32]

SKIN

Prolonged pharmacologic doses of corticosteroids cause atrophy of the skin.[34] more specifically, the skin's surface develops fine scales, the dermis becomes thin and inelastic, and the hair growth cycle is inhibited, eventually leading to alopecia of the trunk and points of wear. Blood vessels are friable and bruising occurs easily. Hair follicles become distended with follicular debris.[34]

FETAL DEVELOPMENT

Fetal corticosteroids may be necessary for normal in utero development of myelin, surfactant in the lungs, the retinas, the pancreas, and mammary tissue.[15]

CLINICAL INDICATIONS AND RECOMMENDED DOSAGES

There are five general indications for corticosteroid use, each requiring a different dosage. The five basic indications are treatment of endogenous corticosteroid deficiency, anti-inflammation, immunosuppression, antineoplastic chemotherapy, and reduction of cerebrospinal edema.

Under experimental conditions, corticosteroid therapy for shock has shown some beneficial effects.[47–49] Corticosteroid use in the treatment of septic shock has improved survival rates by decreasing activation of complement, binding with endotoxin, decreasing beta-endorphin (a vasodilator), and inhibiting platelet aggregation.[49–52] The benefits of corticosteroid use in the treatment of other forms of shock are less evident. However, in 1981 the Food and Drug Administration removed septic shock (the only form of shock listed) as an indication for methylprednisolone sodium succinate because of insufficient proof of efficacy.[51] To be effective in the treatment of shock, corticosteroids must be administered as early as possible after the onset of shock, and they must be administered with other forms of therapy, especially fluids.[52] Such stipulations make the evaluation of corticosteroid usefulness in the treatment of shock under routine clinical conditions difficult.

Recommended dosages of corticosteroids for the treatment of shock are very large. For example, 18 mg of prednisolone sodium succinate or 2.2 mg dexamethasone/lb (40 and 5 mg/kg, respectively) body weight has been recommended.[49] There is risk that such large doses may increase the likelihood of bacteremia from infected sites.[51]

TREATMENT OF ENDOGENOUS CORTICOSTEROID DEFICIENCY

Glucocorticoid therapy is necessary to treat hypoadrenocorticism. Treatment of primary hypoadrenocorticism also requires replacement of mineralocorticoids. To replace glucocorticoids in the dog, about 0.2 to 0.5 mg/lb (0.5 to 1.1 mg/kg) body weight/day of hydrocortisone is required. An equivalent dose of prednisone or prednisolone is 0.05 to 0.1 mg/lb (0.11 to 0.22 mg/kg) body weight/day. If a replacement dose of glucocorticoid is administered to normal dogs, inhibition of the H-P-A axis and eventual adrenocortical atrophy of the zonae fasciculata and reticularis results. Adverse effects on cells outside the H-P-A axis do not occur. However, in stressed animals, decreased ACTH levels and adrenocortical atrophy do not necessarily occur because of adaptation and refractoriness to the usual inhibitory effects of elevated plasma corticosteroid levels. Atrophy of the adrenal cortex resulting from the administration of replacement or greater dosages of glucocorticoids is called iatrogenic secondary hypoadrenocorticism.

ANTI-INFLAMMATION

Dosages of corticosteroids that exceed replacement doses are referred to as pharmacologic (supraphysiologic) doses. Pharmacologic doses affect cells outside the H-P-A axis and these higher doses are required to suppress inflammation, to suppress immunity, to treat cerebrospinal fluid, and perhaps to treat shock. Anti-inflammation doses are smaller than those necessary to suppress immunity or to treat cerebrospinal edema or shock. Initial anti-inflammatory dosages of prednisone or prednisolone are approximately 0.2 to 0.45 mg/lb (0.5 to 1.0 mg/kg) body weight/day. If such dosages are administered for more than two weeks, tissues outside the H-P-A axis can become adversely affected.[34] Corticosteroid-induced extra-adrenal tissue alterations in function and morphology are collectively called iatrogenic hyperadrenocorticism-like disease. Iatrogenic secondary hypoadrenocorticism nearly always precedes iatrogenic hyperadrenocorticism-like disease, but occasionally stressed patients treated with glucocorticoids develop corticosteroid-induced extra-adrenal tissue alterations while the H-P-A axis is not inhibited owing to adaptive refractoriness of the hypothalamus and adenohypophysis to high circulating levels of corticosteroids.[13]

IMMUNOSUPPRESSION AND ANTINEOPLASTIC CHEMOTHERAPY

Suppression of immunity can be desirable. Corticosteroids are often used to control immune-mediated diseases such as systemic lupus erythematosus, idiopathic thrombocytopenia, pemphigus complex, and others. Various aspects of immunity are suppressed by different doses of corticosteroids. Nonspecific immune mechanisms such as trapping and processing of bacteria by macrophages are suppressed by dosages intended for anti-inflammation.[16] The release of neutrophils from the bone marrow is stimulated, but their margination, diapedesis, and oxidative metabolism is inhibited.[40] Corticosteroids at anti-inflammation doses during short-term therapy have little effect on cell-mediated immunity, complement action, and humoral immunity.[16] To suppress these aspects of immunity, a dose of 1 to 2 mg/lb (2 to 4 mg/kg) body weight/day of prednisone or prednisolone is necessary.

Corticosteroids are used as chemotherapy for lymphoreticular neoplasia because of their antimitotic effects on lymphoid tissue. There may be palliative benefits from corticosteroids in the treatment of nonlymphoreticular neoplasms, especially intracranial neoplasms, since corticosteroids pass the blood-brain barrier and relieve associated vasogenic cerebral edema.

REDUCTION OF CEREBROSPINAL EDEMA

In doses that exceed amounts necessary for anti-inflammation and immunosuppression, corticosteroids reduce some forms of cerebrospinal edema. Short-term corticosteroid therapy is efficacious for interstitial cerebral edema such as that occurring with hydrocephalus and tumor-associated vasogenic cerebral edema. The benefits of corticosteroid therapy for traumatic cerebral edema or cytotoxic cerebral edema are questionable. The recommended dosage of dexamethasone for cerebrospinal edema is 1 mg/lb (2 mg/kg) body weight, which is repeated every eight hours until improvement is apparent.[53] Although other corticosteroids are effective at doses equivalent to the anti-inflammatory effects of 1 mg/lb (2 mg/kg) body weight of dexamethasone, dexamethasone is preferable because of its potency per mg, cost, and lack of sodium retention effects. The recommended dosages for replacement, anti-inflammation, immunosuppression and antineoplasia, and anticerebrospinal edema therapies are summarized in Table 52–5.

SELECTION OF AN APPROPRIATE METHOD OF CORTICOSTEROID USE

The critical question facing clinicians is rarely whether or not corticosteroids will have a beneficial effect. That answer is usually an obvious yes or no. The critical question is what is the best method of use when they are indicated. There are potential hazards no matter what type, dose, or duration of corticosteroid is used.

The first consideration before instituting corticosteroid therapy is whether the disease to be treated has more potential hazards than the potential hazards of the corticosteroid therapy being considered. In other words, consider the risk-to-benefit ratio. The risks of therapy should never exceed the risk of the disease being treated.

METHOD OF ADMINISTRATION AND TYPE OF CORTICOSTEROID

The local administration of corticosteroids (topical, intralesional-sublesional, intra-articular, or subconjunctival) is always preferable to oral or injectable (intramuscular, subcutaneous, or intravenous) administration if systemic effects are not required to adequately treat the patient's disease. The systemic absorption and deleterious effects of corticosteroids used topically, intralesionally, or by intra-articular injection are slight when appropriate products, conservative doses, and short durations are used.

Local Administration Methods. A wide variety of topical corticosteroids are available. The selection of the type of topical corticosteroid, its concentration, its vehicle, and its frequency of administration are based on cosmetic considerations, relative expense, and clinical trial and error. Corticosteroid delivery rates to the tissues are affected by their vehicles. In increasing order of delivery rates are the following topical vehicles: ointments, creams, lotions, foams, gels, and solutions such as sprays. Absorption is also affected by the integrity of the skin or mucous membrane treated with a topical corticosteroid. Dermal application should be preceded by clipping of hair and cleansing of the skin. Fluorinated corticosteroid creams or ointments are appropriate only for short-term use. Chronic topical dermal corticosteroid ointments or creams should be the lowest effective concentration of 0.25 to 2.5 per cent hydrocortisone.[24] Treatment of ulcerative colitis with steroid enemas or intrarectal foam is especially likely to result in the systemic absorption of corticosteroids. Plastic gloves should be dispensed for owners to wear when applying corticosteroids to their pet's skin to eliminate the unlikely but unnecessary risk of adverse effects to the owner.

TABLE 52–5. BASIC INDICATIONS FOR CORTICOSTEROIDS AND REQUIRED DOSAGES

Indication	Initial Required Doses of Prednisone or Prednisolone
Glucocorticoid replacement	0.1 mg/lb (0.25 mg/kg) body weight/day
Anti-inflammatory (anti-allergic) treatment	0.2–0.5 mg/lb (0.5–1 mg/kg) body weight/day
Immunosuppression and antineoplastic chemotherapy	1–2 mg/lb (2–4 mg/kg) body weight/day
Reduction of cerebrospinal edema	6–8 mg/lb (15 mg/kg) body weight as necessary*

*Dexamethasone is more frequently used at an equivalent dose of 1 mg/lb (2 mg/kg) body weight.

Topical corticosteroid absorption can be facilitated as much as 100-fold by occluding the area with plastic wraps. If a chronic localized dermal lesion can be lightly wrapped and the wrap is tolerated by the patient, occlusive bandaging over corticosteroid cream should be considered. A plastic wrapping used to store food is adequate. After clipping, cleaning, and applying a topical corticosteroid cream, such as triamcinolone acetonide 0.1 per cent, the plastic is held in place over the lesions by a light gauze and tape bandage. Occlusive bandages should be replaced daily with periods of drying and exposure to light between bandaging, such as 12 hours on, 12 hours off, to reduce the risk of occlusion folliculitis and bacterial infection. Acetonide and valerate esters used in many topical dermatologic corticosteroid preparations bind to affected skin tissue, enhancing the effects of the corticosteroids.

Topical corticosteroids can cause adverse systemic effects in some circumstances. One study in 7.5- to 15-lb (3.5- to 7-kg) dogs treated with 1 per cent prednisolone acetate ophthalmic solution showed that the adrenal cortex was suppressed in its response to ACTH after two weeks of treatment using 4 mg prednisolone (0.35 mg/lb or 0.75 mg/kg body weight) in four divided doses daily.[54] Excessive storage of hepatic glycogen was also detected with the glucagon stimulation test, indicating extra-adrenal adverse effects had occurred in addition to adrenocortical suppression. Acetate as a topical ester is lipid-soluble and is readily absorbed by the cornea and conjunctiva. Alcoholic ophthalmic solutions are absorbed even more readily, while succinate or phosphate esters are not absorbed as well as acetate esters.[55] Significant adrenal suppression has also been shown to occur in dogs by the second week of treatment with ophthalmic 0.1 per cent dexamethasone sodium phosphate suspension administered to each eye four times per day.[56]

Intralesional or sublesional corticosteroid administration is indicated whenever the effect of corticosteroids is desired in a few small external lesions. Intralesional administration can be performed by using a relatively insoluble corticosteroid, tuberculin syringe, and intradermal gauge (23 to 25 gauge) needle. The injected volume should be no more than 0.1 ml per injection site. Sublesional injections should be considered if lesions are too fibrous to allow intralesional injection or when larger volumes of corticosteroids and fewer injections than those required for intralesional injections are desired. Highly concentrated corticosteroids should not be used because of the risk of systemic effects and cutaneous atrophy at the injection site. One method is to use up to 0.1 ml/cm^2 of the lesion of 6 mg/ml triamcinolone acetonide. Administration may be repeated every two weeks until remission or until beneficial effects are no longer observed.

Relatively insoluble corticosteroids should also be employed for intra-articular injections. Otherwise, the duration of the corticosteroid effects is no longer than if administered orally or injected intramuscularly and the risk-to-benefit ratio does not justify intra-articular injection. Joints to be injected should have no radiographic evidence of erosion or suggestive signs of infection. Potential hazards of intra-articular corticosteroid use are iatrogenically induced infections, arthropathy, and crystal-injection synovitis. An example of a commonly used form and dose of corticosteroid for intra-articular therapy is 10 mg/ml triamcinolone acetonide in a dose of 2.5 to 5.0 mg/joint.

Subconjunctival injection of relatively insoluble corticosteroids can be preferable to topical ocular, oral, or systemic parenteral administration of corticosteroids for some inflammatory ocular diseases. Small volume, relatively insoluble forms are the most practical. For example, injected quantities are usually less than 0.25 ml, delivering 2.5 to 10 mg of triamcinolone acetonide. Granulomas from relatively insoluble vehicles can form at the site of subconjunctival corticosteroid injections.[57]

Systemic Administration Methods. Systemic effects of corticosteroid therapy are generally achieved by oral, IM, subcutaneous, or IV administration. Selection of the form of oral or parenteral corticosteroids to be used requires the decisions of which route is necessary, which form of corticosteroid is least expensive, and whether inherent mineralocorticoid properties could create a problem. If the patient's condition allows oral administration, the least expensive oral corticosteroid should be chosen since there is no appreciable difference in the degree or rate of gastrointestinal absorption. Prednisone and prednisolone are the least expensive oral corticosteroids. The inherent mineralocorticoid effects of prednisone and prednisolone are rarely a problem. They may cause problems if very large doses (immunosuppressive or greater) are necessary or if edematous disease is present. Prednisone and prednisolone may be used interchangeably at identical dosages except possibly in the presence of severe hepatic disease, where prednisolone, which is the biologically active form of prednisone, is preferable.

In circumstances where the need for corticosteroid effects is urgent, intravenous administration is required. Corticosteroids for IV administration are those with a water-soluble ester in a water-soluble vehicle. Water-soluble forms of corticosteroids may be given IM or subcutaneously if the patient's condition is not critical and if the patient's condition or temperament rules out oral administration.

Repositol or depot corticosteroids are injectable corticosteroids that have been made moderately to markedly insoluble by combining them with a poorly soluble ester in order to produce prolonged effects. In spite of their widespread use, these products have few justifiable indications in veterinary medicine. Their risk-to-benefit ratio is too high. For example, a 1.2 mg/lb (2.5 mg/kg) body weight IM injection of methylprednisolone acetate much more effectively suppresses the H-P-A axis than does the daily oral administration of 2 to 4 mg of methylprednisolone.[58] In addition, depot IM corticosteroids lose their beneficial effects when used repeatedly, possibly because of tachyphylaxis, an adaptive decrease in target cell hormone receptors or post-receptor adaptation of effects.

Depot corticosteroid injections are ideal for intra-articular, intralesional, or subconjunctival methods of local administration because the required dose is small, the corticosteroid is released in high concentration into the area in need of treatment, and systemic effects are minimal. However, when depot corticosteroids are deposited into a vascular tissue such as skeletal muscle and when dosages are great enough to produce systemic effects, there is the potential for maximal and constant suppression of the H-P-A axis. Furthermore, there is no control over its rate or frequency of release into the systemic circulation. For example, if methylprednisolone acetate is given orally to dogs, 83 per cent is eliminated in the feces and urine in 48 hours. When methylprednisolone acetate is given intramuscularly, it takes 45 days to eliminate 86 per cent of the drug.[59] Yet at 0.5 to 2 mg/lb (1 to 4 mg/kg) body weight IM, beneficial suppression of signs of inflammation only persist for one to three weeks.[24, 26]

The duration of effects are affected by dosage. Dexamethasone 21-isonicotinate given once IM at 0.04 mg/lb (0.1 mg/kg) body weight suppresses plasma cortisol levels for ten days. When given at 0.4 mg/lb (1 mg/kg) body weight plasma, cortisol is suppressed for one month. The absorption is not rapid enough to produce detectable plasma dexamethasone levels.[60] A single IM administration of 20 mg methylprednisolone acetate to an adult Basenji resulted in corticosteroid hepatopathy and H-P-A-axis suppression for 7 to 11 weeks.[38]

The only reasonable justifications for the use of repositol corticosteroids for systemic effects are the lack of owner compliance with other forms of administration or a fractious patient. They should never be used solely for their convenience and should never be given subcutaneously.[61] Subcutaneous administration reduces the beneficial systemic effects, while prolonging the risk of adrenocortical suppression. Subcutaneous corticosteroid injections can cause local subcutaneous tissue atrophy because of vasoconstriction that impairs nutrition of tissues at injection site, a decrease in elastin, a decrease in acid mucopolysaccharides, and homogenization of collagen connective tissue.[61]

FREQUENCY AND DURATION OF ADMINISTRATION

The most appropriate frequency of administration of corticosteroids depends on their duration of effects. Their duration of effects varies with the type of corticosteroid; its ester, compound, or vehicle; the patient; and the patient's condition.

The duration of corticosteroid therapy should always be as short as possible. Anticipated duration of treatment is a subjective judgment based on the clinician's experience and the patient's condition. The dose interval for locally administered corticosteroids is empirical. Dose intervals for systemic therapy can be categorized as burst or intermittent, daily, or alternate-day.

Burst (Pulse) or Intermittent Therapy. Burst therapy can be defined as the use of non-depot, parenteral corticosteroids for systemic effects for up to three days at the equivalent dosage of 0.5 mg/lb (1.0 mg/kg) prednisone/day or greater. No lasting suppression of the H-P-A axis is expected,[28] but acute extra-adrenal adverse effects such as gastrointestinal ulceration or acute pancreatitis are possible.[16] Burst therapy is recommended for some forms of cerebrospinal edema, acute allergic reactions, and possibly septic or hypovolemic shock. Methylprednisolone or dexamethasone are recommended because of their potency and relative lack of sodium-retaining activity.

Daily Oral Therapy. Except during some very stressful diseases, any dose of systemically absorbed corticosteroid will suppress the H-P-A axis within one week of continuous treatment.[34] However, suppression of the ability of the H-P-A axis to rapidly recover requires more than one week of treatment.[14]

Extra-adrenal adverse (toxic) effects should not occur unless doses of corticosteroids exceed physiologic amounts. Using anti-inflammation doses, extra-adrenal adverse effects become evident with two weeks of continuous treatment.[34]

The likelihood of serious H-P-A axis suppression and extra-adrenal adverse effects is directly related to the duration of exogenous corticosteroids in the circulation and bound to cell receptors. Therefore, unless immunosuppressive doses are to be used and there is also concern about sodium retention, prednisone and prednisolone are the corticosteroids of choice because of their relatively short duration of action and low cost. Administering the recommended daily dose of prednisone in divided doses throughout the day causes more adverse effects than a single daily dose.[14] Once per day administration of dexamethasone has similar adverse effects as equivalent doses of prednisone divided throughout the day because of dexamethasone's long plasma and metabolic half-lives. Divided daily doses of prednisone are appropriate when attempting to put a corticosteroid-responsive disease into remission. Divided daily doses are not appropriate to maintain remission. Once a day administration of prednisone or prednisolone should be instituted as soon as possible. This is generally possible within the first week of treatment for inflammatory diseases.

Once per day dosing is recommended for mornings in humans since they have a marked diurnal variation in ACTH secretion, with the highest secretion of endogenous corticosteroids and the most profound negative feedback on ACTH secretion normally occurring in the mornings.[14] Although once per day oral corticosteroids administration in the morning to dogs and evenings to cats has been recommended, there is currently no evidence that such timing of administration causes less suppression of the H-P-A axis.[62] Objective evidence of the beneficial effects of dose tapering when withdrawing dogs and cats from short-term corticosteroid therapy is also lacking, but it has become a conventional practice. When the duration of daily oral therapy exceeds two weeks it is prudent to taper the dosage during withdrawal.[14, 16, 34] Fifty per cent reduction in dosage at weekly intervals is a commonly used method.

Alternate-Day Therapy. For more than 20 years it has been known that the risk of suppression of the H-P-A axis could be minimized by administering oral corticosteroids after the metabolic duration of effects of the last dose has dissipated and there has been a short period of recovery of the H-P-A axis. Fortunately, there is a discordance between the H-P-A axis recovery and the recurrence of many corticosteroid-responsive diseases. Using prednisone, prednisolone, or methylprednisolone in anti-inflammatory doses once every 48 hours produces little suppression of the H-P-A axis.[14] For example, a dose of 10 mg of prednisone given every other day for two weeks in a 22 lb (10 kg) dog produces much less suppression of the H-P-A axis than 5 mg every day for two weeks.[34] Alternate-day oral prednisone, prednisolone, or methylprednisolone should be considered in every case that requires systemic corticosteroid therapy longer than two weeks.[34] Attempts should be made not to administer 0.5 mg/lb (1.1 mg/kg) or more of prednisone or its equivalent every other day. Alternate-day dosages that meet or exceed 0.5 mg/lb (1.1 mg/kg) every other day saturate the dog's ability to fully metabolize the last dose before the next dose is given, therefore negating the primary advantage of alternate-day therapy.[34, 46]

Conversion of once per day therapy to alternate-day therapy should be gradual. This can be achieved by tapering the daily dose to the minimal effective dose, then doubling and administering it every other day while discontinuing or gradually tapering the dose on the "off" day.[24] Consideration should be also given to the possible benefits of adjunctive therapy such as nonsteroid anti-inflammatory agents or antihistamines that could aid in controlling the disease process.

PRECAUTIONS

Several conditions require special consideration of the risk-to-benefit ratio of corticosteroid therapy. Corticosteroid use is probably detrimental if administered to immature patients or to patients with bone healing, protein-losing nephropathies or enteropathies, diabetes mellitus, and muscle-wasting diseases because corticosteroids inhibit growth and reconstructive anabolism.[14]

Corticosteroid elimination from the body can be impaired if hepatic disease is present.[14] Corticosteroids can also directly cause hepatopathy or aggravate an existing hepatopathy.[34, 35, 38]

Inhibition of the inflammatory process by corticosteroids can be undesirable. Suppression of the inactivation, phagocytosis, sequestration, and other immunologic processing of infectious agents may allow them to become exacerbated, particularly fungal or viral keratitis, generalized demodectic mange, or chronic bacterial, viral, and deep fungal infections. The administration of corticosteroids for more than six months to control skin diseases in dogs has been associated with more than double the expected occurrence of urinary tract infection, especially in female dogs.[63] Rupture of prostatic abscesses in dogs has been apparently precipitated by corticosteroid administration.[64] Corticosteroid use can cause increased intravascular volume, thereby aggravating congestive heart failure because of facilitation of extracellular shifts of water, sodium retention, and polydipsia.

Large doses of corticosteroids may cause or aggravate psychoses in humans and dogs.[24] Psychotic manifestations of aggression and paranoid behavior have been observed in a dog that ingested a large number of prednisolone tablets.[42]

Precaution should be taken when considering corticosteroid use in pregnancy. Fetal adrenocortical atrophy is likely and cleft palate, as reported in rodents and rabbits, is possible.[45] Synthetic corticosteroids methylated at C-16 (dexamethasone, flumethasone, and betamethasone) administered during late gestation can induce premature parturition in horses, cows, sheep, and humans. One should assume that premature parturition, abortion, and fetal resorption are possible hazards of corticosteroid use in gravid dogs and cats.

The use of dexamethasone at doses recommended for spinal cord edema has caused gastrointestinal hemorrhage in 15 per cent of treated dogs and 2 per cent may die with perforation of the colon.[65] Fatal colonic perforations, usually occurring at the antimesenteric border of the proximal descending colon, have been attributed to dexamethasone treatment of spinal edema in dogs with intervertebral disk disease.[44, 66, 67] Similar perforations have occurred with neurologically normal dogs which have undergone surgery and dogs treated with corticosteroids other than dexamethasone. Major surgery seems to be a fairly consistent, but not a required, predisposing factor.[68] Most of the affected dogs have

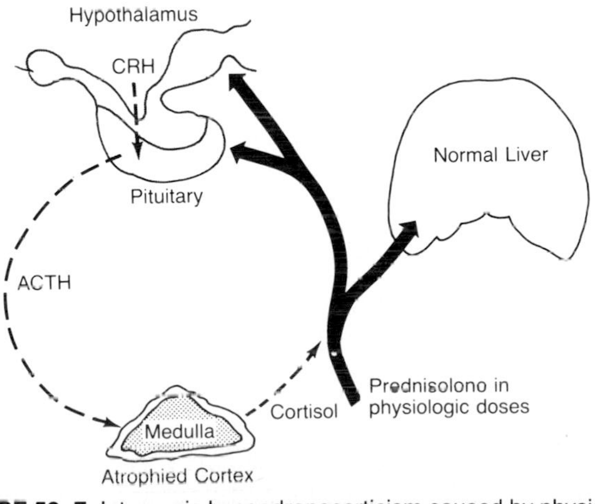

FIGURE 52–7. Iatrogenic hypoadrenocorticism caused by physiologic doses of corticosteroid administration that cause no adverse effects on extra-adrenal tissue such as the liver.

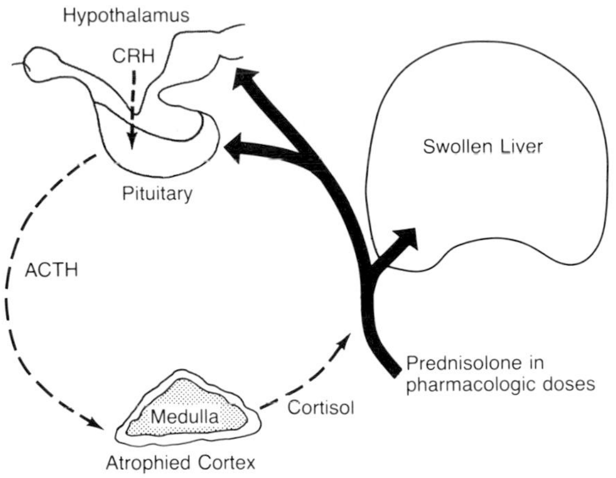

FIGURE 52–8. Iatrogenic hyperadrenocorticism-like disease (and hypoadrenocorticism) caused by pharmacologic doses of corticosteroid administration and resulting adverse effects on extra-adrenal tissue such as the liver.

been male dachshunds over five years old, but other breeds have also been affected.[44, 68] The risk of perforation of the colon parallels the severity of the spinal cord injury and duration of treatment. It is not correlated with the dexamethasone dose.[65] The mean dosage of dexamethasone and duration of treatment associated with perforations has been 3 mg/lb (6.4 mg/kg) over five days.[68] Spinal cord injury may alter autonomic balance, resulting in decreased colonic mucosal perfusion.[44]

Gastric ulcers are also possible because of corticosteroid-induced increases in plasma gastrin levels, gastric acid and pepsin secretion, decreased gastrointestinal production and viscosity of mucus, and decreased proliferation of mucosal cells.[66, 69] Pancreatic secretions increase in viscosity with corticosteroid therapy, causing or exacerbating acute pancreatitis.[39, 65]

Short term anti-inflammatory doses of corticosteroids do not significantly alter the ability of a dog to respond to canine distemper vaccinations. Resulting protection withstands challenge with virulent distemper virus.[70] Normal serum titers to rabies vaccinations occurs in dogs being treated with anti-inflammatory doses of corticosteroids,[71] but the ability to withstand challenge by virulent rabies virus may not be adequate. It is prudent to avoid treatment with corticosteroids in patients also

TABLE 52–6. POTENTIAL ADVERSE EFFECTS ASSOCIATED WITH IATROGENIC HYPERADRENOCORTICISM-LIKE DISEASE

Poor wound healing	Suppressed growth
Excessive appetite	Glucose intolerance
Diarrhea	Fasting hyperlipidemia
Polyuria and polydipsia	Seizures
Alopecia	Acute pancreatitis
Obesity	Immunosuppression and superinfections
Acne	Colonic perforations
Muscle weakness and atrophy	Infertility
Edema	Birth defects
Hepatomegaly	Abortion
Psychoses and changes in temperament	Osteoporosis
Easy bruising	

receiving or having recently received vaccinations whenever possible.

ADVERSE SYSTEMIC IATROGENIC EFFECTS

Hyperadrenocorticism-like systemic adverse iatrogenic corticosteroid effects are possible from pharmacologic doses, and secondary hypoadrenocorticism from pharmacologic or physiologic doses is also possible.

IATROGENIC SECONDARY HYPOADRENOCORTICISM

Inhibition of ACTH secretion is governed by corticosteroids in the circulation. In unstressed animals, any exogenous corticosteroid administration has an additive effect to endogenous glucocorticoid inhibition of ACTH secretion (see Figure 52–7). Subsequent ACTH deficiency results in failure to maintain endogenous corticosteroid secretions from the zonae fasciculata and reticularis. The zona arcuata, which is the primary source of mineralocorticoids, rarely atrophies.[34] The daily oral administration of corticosteroids that have prolonged plasma half-lives or that have relatively short plasma duration but are administered in divided daily doses particularly suppresses ACTH secretion. Repositol IM injections of corticosteroids are constantly released into the systemic circulation for days or weeks, causing the maximum possible suppression of the H-P-A axis.

Clinical signs of iatrogenic secondary hypoadrenocorticism are lethargy, weakness, anorexia, hypotension, and weight loss. These signs may be difficult to assess, and they do not appear until the treatment is withdrawn or the repositol injection is fully absorbed.[16, 58] Under basal conditions, signs may not be evident or may be mild because only minute amounts of corticosteroids are necessary for permissive effects on metabolism. If corticosteroids are readministered during the withdrawal corticosteroid-deficient period, marked transient diuresis due to intracellular to extracellular fluid shifts may occur. During stressful conditions, such as moderate hemorrhage, corticosteroid deficiency caused by iatrogenic secondary hypoadrenocorticism can lead to impaired blood volume reconstitution, vascular collapse, and shock.[72]

The diagnosis of iatrogenic secondary hypoadrenocorticism can be based on a history of corticosteroid administration plus an inadequate elevation of plasma cortisol values in response to exogenous ACTH stimulation. Routine laboratory examinations may be normal. Normal plasma cortisol values should be 6 μg/dl or more after ACTH administration, although this can vary among different laboratories. Response to ACTH (cosyntropin) can be indirectly evaluated by performing absolute neutrophil, lymphocyte, and eosinophil counts before and four hours after IV cosyntropin administration. Normal response is a rise of at least 30 per cent in the neutrophil to lymphocyte ratio and a decrease in eosinophils of at least 50 per cent.[73] Failure to achieve a normal response on the basis of neutrophil to lymphocyte ratios and eosinophil counts is suggestive of hypo-

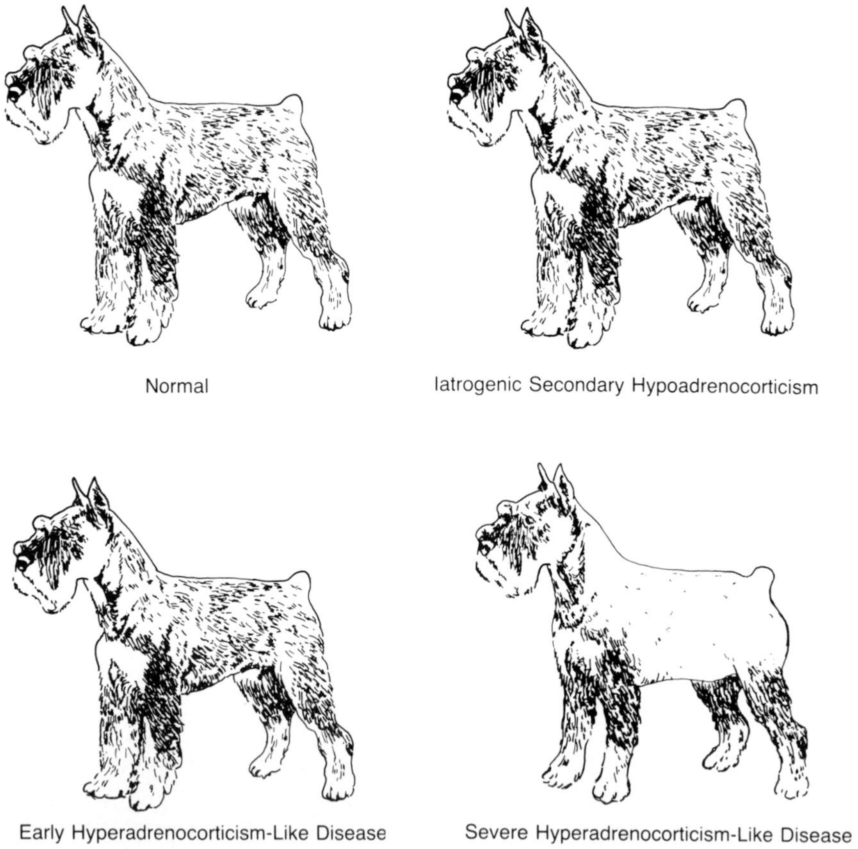

FIGURE 52–9. Clinical appearance of dogs treated with corticosteroids. Dogs with iatrogenic secondary hypoadrenocorticism and early hyperadrenocorticism-like disease appear normal. Dogs with severe hyperadrenocorticism have thinning of the truncal haircoat, enlargement of the abdomen, and an increase in fat depots on the torso.

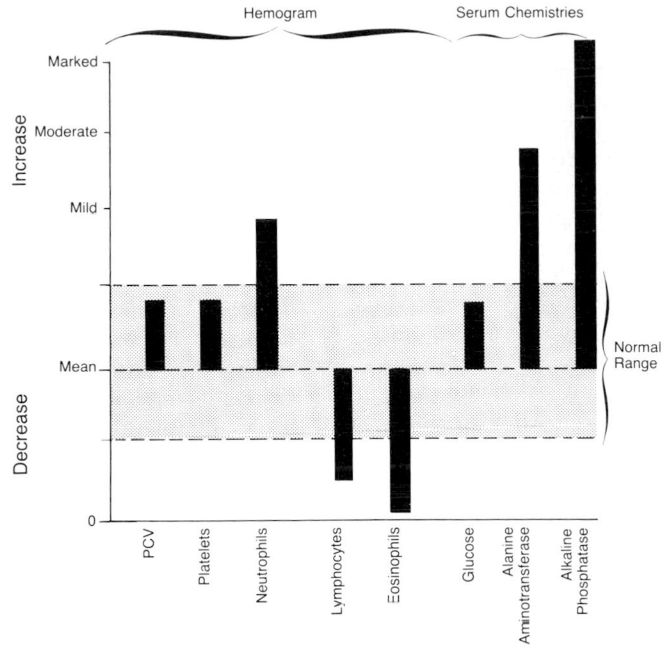

FIGURE 52–10. Characteristic changes in routine hemograms and serum chemistry values produced by corticosteroid administration.

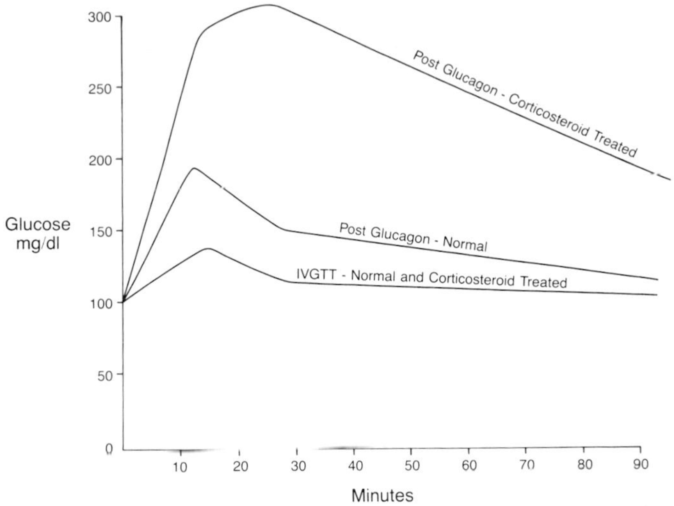

FIGURE 52–12. Typical blood glucose concentrations before and for 90 minutes after intravenous glucose (0.55 g/kg body weight) and intravenous glucagon (1 mg) in a normal and a corticosteroid-treated dog with iatrogenic hyperadrenocorticism-like disease. IVGTT, intravenous glucose tolerance test.

adrenocorticism and should be verified by assaying plasma cortisol values. In special cases, an endogenous ACTH assay may be indicated.

IATROGENIC HYPERADRENOCORTICISM-LIKE DISEASE

Prolonged corticosteroid use in pharmacologic doses can cause a disease resembling hyperadrenocorticism, since organs like the liver are bathed by abnormally high concentrations of corticosteroids (see Figure 52–8). For example, corticosteroid hepatopathy occurs in dogs given 2 mg/lb (4.4 mg/kg) body weight/day of prednisone for two weeks.[36, 37] Potential adverse extra-adrenal effects of corticosteroids are listed in Table 52–6. Cats are currently thought to be less susceptible than dogs to developing iatrogenic hyperadrenocorticism-like disease.[10, 62] For example, cats that receive corticosteroid therapy do not develop alopecia as readily as dogs that receive prolonged corticosteroid therapy. Also, cats may not develop polyuria until hyperglycemia and glycosuria occur from secondary steroid-induced diabetes mellitus.[35, 62] Since cats do not have a specific isoenzyme of alkaline phosphatase induced by corticosteroids, elevations of serum alkaline phosphatase are not as reliable an indication of iatrogenic hyperadrenocorticism-like disease as they are in dogs.[62] Clinical signs of iatrogenic hyperadrenocorticism-like disease do eventually develop in cats, however, and include in addition to polyuria and polydipsia, thinning of the skin, curling of the ear tips, decreased muscular mass, ecchymoses, and skin tears.[62]

Some adverse effects of corticosteroid use can be masked by other effects of corticosteroids. To illustrate, corticosteroid use may allow certain sequestered infectious agents to disseminate while the pain, fever, and visual signs of inflammation that are normally expected are concurrently suppressed by the administered corticosteroid.[44]

Characteristic physical examination findings of advanced iatrogenic hyperadrenocorticism-like disease in dogs are thinning of the hair coat on the caudal aspects of the hind legs and on the lateral area of the abdomen. Other common clinical findings include a pendulous abdomen, semisolid feces, lethargy, polyuria, polydipsia, inelasticity of the abdominal skin, and enlarged fat depots on the caudolateral gluteal area near the base of

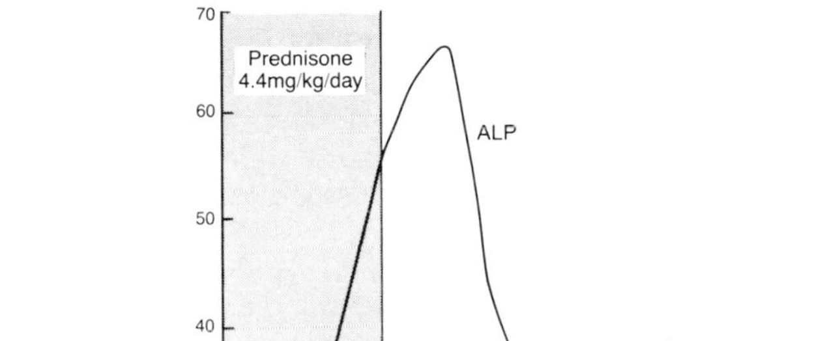

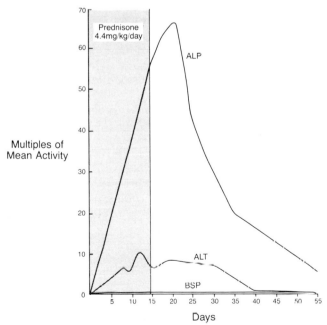

FIGURE 52–11. Multiples of mean activity of serum alkaline phosphatase (ALP), serum alanine aminotransferase (ALT), and Bromsulphalein (BSP) retention in dogs during and after two weeks of 4.4 mg/kg body weight/day of prednisolone. (Redrawn from Badylak, SF and Van Fleet, JF: Sequential morphologic and clinicopathologic alterations in dogs with experimentally induced glucocorticoid hepatopathy. Am J Vet Res 42:1310, 1981.)

the tail (see Figure 52–9).[36] Less commonly, synthetic corticosteroids, particularly those fluorinated at the 9-alpha position, may cause myopathy.[20]

Laboratory findings most consistent with iatrogenic hyperadrenocorticism in dogs are lymphopenia and abnormally elevated serum alkaline phosphatase values (see Figure 52–10). Serum levels of alkaline phosphatase and less often, alanine aminotransferase and Bromsulphalein retention, become elevated within two to six days and remain elevated for at least six weeks after the withdrawal of two weeks of 2.0 mg/lb (4.4 mg/kg) body weight of prednisone administration in the dog (see Figure 52–11).[36, 37, 74] Mild serum elevations of gamma glutamyl transpeptidase and bile acids may also occur.[36, 74] Plasma concentrations of tri-iodothyronine (T3) and less frequently, thyroxine (T4), are lowered by corticosteroid use.[75] Serum cholesterol is often elevated.

Another assessment of extra-adrenal adverse effects is based on the liver being induced by corticosteroids to store excessive glycogen. The amount of stored hepatic glycogen can be assessed practically by a dosage modification of a previously reported glucagon response test.[54, 76] The modified test is performed by injecting 1 mg glucagon IV and determining the blood glucose values at 0, 15, 30, and 90 minutes. Normal response is blood glucose levels that do not exceed 200 mg/dl at 15 and 30 minutes and a return to baseline levels by 90 minutes (see Figure 52–12). The 30-minute post-glucagon administration sample is the most useful. An intravenous glucose tolerance test is recommended prior to glucagon tolerance to verify adequate insulin secretion in response to increased blood glucose levels.

MANAGEMENT OF IATROGENIC ADVERSE EFFECTS

Restoration of the normal H-P-A axis after prolonged corticosteroid use must be attempted with caution. Restoration essentially requires discontinuation of corticosteroid use. Whenever daily corticosteroid use has occurred for two weeks or more, the administered doses of corticosteroids should be gradually reduced in a way that does not leave the patient deficient in both exogenous and endogenous corticosteroids.[14, 34] Recovery of the H-P-A axis may begin once administered corticosteroid doses fall below physiologic replacement levels so that endogenous ACTH may be secreted. If prolonged pharmacologic doses have caused extra-adrenal adverse effects in addition to adrenocortical atrophy, any other corticosteroid being used should be replaced by prednisone or prednisolone and gradually reduced to replacement levels, 0.1 mg/lb (0.22 mg/kg) once per day. One to two months at replacement dosages may be necessary for recovery of extra-adrenal adverse effects. Maintenance doses must be doubled or tripled during acute stress such as major surgery or serious illnesses.

After recovery from extra-adrenal adverse effects (iatrogenic hyperadrenocorticism-like disease), daily replacement doses of prednisone should be converted to alternate-day therapy. Alternate-day doses should be gradually reduced so that complete withdrawal can be tentatively completed after one month. Complete withdrawal depends on whether or not the plasma cortisol value response indicates satisfactory recovery of the H-P-A axis. If signs of a corticosteroid-responsive disease reappear during the withdrawal, withdrawal should be discontinued and the patient left on the least minimally effective dose.

Recovery of the H-P-A axis occurs in the following order: supranormal ACTH secretion, adrenocortical basal secretion of corticosteroids, and normal adrenocortical stress responsiveness and endogenous ACTH plasma levels.[14] Early during recovery the adrenal cortices may become hypersensitive to an ACTH stimulation test and the H-P-A axis refractory to low dose dexamethasone suppression.[13] Recovery depends upon plasma corticosteroid levels initially being allowed to become subnormal to permit maximal uninhibited ACTH secretion. Treatment with exogenous ACTH administration is not practical since twice per day injections of ACTH gel would be necessary. It is also not desirable because of the risks of developing ACTH hypersensitivity and possibly undesirable effects of mineralocorticoid or androgen secretion. Stimulation of adrenocortical recovery with exogenous ACTH administration also inhibits the first stage of permanent H-P-A axis recovery by prolonging inhibition of endogenous ACTH secretion with premature endogenous corticosteroid secretion.[14, 16]

References

1. Hench, PS, et al.: The effects of a hormone of the adrenal cortex (17-hydroxy-11-dehydrocorticosterone. Compound E) and of the pituitary adrenocorticotropic hormone on rheumatoid arthritis. Proc of Staff Meet Mayo Clin 24:181, 1949.
2. Fraser, CG, et al.: Adrenal atrophy and irreversible shock associated with cortisone therapy. JAMA 149:1542, 1952.
3. Black, WC, et al.: Inhibitory effect of hydrocortisone and analogues on adrenocortical secretion in dogs. Am J Physiol 201:1057, 1961.
4. Anderson, DC: Corticosteroid overdosage in dogs. N Z Vet J 16:18, 1968.
5. Scott, DW and Greene, CE: Iatrogenic secondary adrenocortical insufficiency in dogs. JAAHA 10:555, 1974.
6. Mulnix, JA: Corticosteroid therapy in the dog, in Proceedings, 44th Annu Meet AAHA p 173, 1977.
7. Ganong, WF, et al.: ACTH and the regulation of adrenocortical secretion. N Engl J Med 290:1006, 1974.
8. Rijnberk, A, et al.: Investigations on the adrenocortical function of normal dogs. J Endocrinol 41:387, 1968.
9. Johnston, SD and Mather, EC: Canine plasma cortisol (hydrocortisone) measured by radioimmunoassay: Clinical absence of diurnal variations and results of ACTH stimulation and dexamethasone suppression tests. Am J Vet Res 38:1766, 1978.
10. Scott, DW, et al.: Some effect of short-term methylprednisolone therapy in normal cats. Cornell Vet 69:104, 1979.
11. Kemppainen, RJ and Sartin, JL: Evidence of episodic but not circadian activity in plasma concentrations of adrenocorticotrophin, cortisol and thyroxine in dogs. J Endocrinol 103:219, 1984.
12. Keller-Wood, ME and Dallman, MF: Corticosteroid inhibition of ACTH secretion. Endocrine Reviews 5:1, 1984.
13. Chastain, CB, et al.: Evaluation of the hypothalamic pituitary-adrenal axis in clinically stressed dogs. JAAHA 22:435, 1986.
14. Axelrod, L: Glucocorticoid therapy. Medicine 55:39, 1976.
15. Baxter, JD and Forsham, RH: Tissue effects of glucocorticoids. Am J Med 53:573, 1972.

16. Melby, JC: Clinical pharmacology of systemic corticosteroids. Ann Rev Pharmacol Toxicol 17:511, 1977.
17. Chen, CL, et al.: Serum hydrocortisone (cortisol) values in normal and adrenopathic dogs as determined by radioimmunoassay. Am J Vet Res 39:179, 1978.
18. Plager, JE, et al.: Cortisol binding by dog plasma. Endocrinology 73:353, 1963.
19. Taylor, W: The excretion of steroid hormone metabolites in bile and feces. Vitam Horm 29:201, 1971.
20. Mendel, S: Steroid myopathy. Postgrad Med 72:207, 1982.
21. Schalm, SW, et al.: Development of radioimmunoassay for prednisone and prednisolone. Mayo Clin Proc 51:761, 1976.
22. Thorn, GW: Clinical consolidations in the use of corticosteroids. N Engl J Med 274:775, 1966.
23. Hankes, GH, et al.: Pharmacokinetics of prednisolone sodium succinate and its metabolites in normovolemic and hypovolemic dogs. Am J Vet Res 46:476, 1985.
24. Scott, DW: Dermatologic use of corticosteroids. Systemic and topical. Vet Clin North Am 12:19, 1982.
25. Coppoc, GL: Relationship of the dosage form of a corticosteroid to its therapeutic efficacy. JAVMA 183:1098, 1984.
26. Braun, JP, et al.: Haematological and biochemical effects of a single intramuscular dose of 6-methylprednisolone acetate in the dog. Res Vet Sci 31:236, 1981.
27. Kemppainen, RJ, et al.: Adrenocortical suppression in the dog after a single dose of methylprednisolone acetate. Am J Vet Res 42:822, 1981.
28. Kemppainen, RJ, et al.: Adrenocortical suppression in the dog given a single intramuscular dose of prednisone or triamcinolone acetonide. Am J Vet Res 42:204, 1982.
29. Magne, JL, et al.: Serum insulin and glucose concentrations in normal, stressed, and hyperadrenocorticism dogs. Proc of ACVIM p 42, 1984.
30. Wolfsheimer, KJ, et al.: Effects of prednisolone on glucose tolerance and insulin secretion in the dog. Am J Vet Res 47:1011, 1986.
31. Joles, JA, et al.: Studies on the mechanism of polyuria induced by cortisol excess in the dog. Vet Quart 2:199, 1980.
32. Kemppainen, RJ: Effects of glucocorticoids on endocrine function in the dog. Vet Clin North Am 14:721, 1984.
33. Watson LC, et al.: Effect of hydrocortisone on gastric secretion and serum gastrin in dogs. Surg Forum 24:354, 1973.
34. Chastain, CB and Graham, CL: Adrenocortical suppression in dogs on daily and alternate-day prednisone administration. Am J Vet Res 40:936, 1979.
35. Dillon, AR, et al.: Prednisolone induced hematologic, biochemical, and histologic changes in the dog. JAAHA 16:831, 1980.
36. Badylak, SF and Van Fleet, JF: Sequential morphologic and clinicopathologic alterations in dogs with experimentally induced glucocorticoids hepatopathy. Am J Vet Res 42:1310, 1981.
37. Badylak, SF and Van Fleet, JF: Tissue gamma-glutamyl transpeptidase activity and hepatic ultrastructural alterations in dogs with experimentally induced glucocorticoid hepatopathy. Am J Vet Res 43:649, 1982.
38. Meyer, DJ: Prolonged liver test abnormalities and adrenocortical suppression in a dog following a single intramuscular glucocorticoid dose. JAAHA 18:725, 1982.
39. Kimura T, et al.: Steroid administration and acute pancreatitis: Studies with an isolated, perfused canine pancreas. Surgery 85:520, 1979.
40. Fauci, AS, et al.: Glucocorticosteroid therapy: Mechanisms of action and clinical considerations. Ann Int Med 84:304, 1976.
41. Collins, EJ, et al.: Effect of adrenal steroids on radio-calcium metabolism in dogs. Metabolism 11:716, 1980.
42. Knecht, CD, et al.: Central nervous system depression associated with glucocorticoid ingestion in a dog. JAVMA 173:91, 1978.
43. Higgs, GA: Effects of anti-inflammatory drugs on arachidonic acid metabolism and leukocyte migration. Adv Inflammation Res 7:223, 1984.
44. Toombs, JP, et al.: Colonic perforation following neurosurgical procedures and corticosteroid therapy in four dogs. JAVMA 177:68, 1980.
45. Rowland, JM and Hendrickx, AG: Corticosteroid teratogenicity. Adv Vet Sc Compar Med 27:99, 1983.
46. Kemppainen, RJ, et al.: Effects of prednisone on thyroid and gonadal endocrine function in dogs. J Endocrinol 96:293, 1983.
47. Ferguson, JL, et al.: Dexamethasone treatment during hemorrhagic shock: Blood pressure, tissue perfusion, and plasma enzymes. Am J Vet Res 39:817, 1978.
48. Ferguson, JL, et al.: Dexamethasone treatment during hemorrhagic shock: Effects independent of increased blood pressure. Am J Vet Res 39:825, 1978.
49. Bowen, JM: Are corticosteroids useful in shock therapy? JAVMA 177:453, 1980.
50. White, GL, et al.: Increased survival with methylprednisolone treatment in canine endotoxic shock. J Surg Res 25:357, 1978.
51. Sheagren, JN: Septic shock and corticosteroids. N Engl J Med 305:456, 1981.
52. Sprung, CL, et al.: The effects of high-dose corticosteroids in patients with septic shock. A prospective, controlled study. N Engl J Med 311:1137, 1984.
53. Franklin, RT: The use of glucocorticoids in treating cerebral edema. Comp Cont Ed Pract Vet 6:442, 1984.
54. Roberts, SM, et al.: Effect of ophthalmic prednisolone acetate on the canine adrenal gland and hepatic function. Am J Vet Res 45:1711, 1984.
55. Brightman, AH: Ophthalmic use of glucocorticoids. Vet Clin North Am 12:33, 1982.
56. Crawford, MA, et al.: Systemic effects of ocular topical corticosteroids in dogs. Proc ACVIM :138, 1985.
57. Fischer, CA: Granuloma formation associated with subconjunctival injection of a corticosteroid in dogs. JAVMA 174:1086, 1979.
58. Spencer, KB, et al.: Adrenal gland function in dogs given methylprednisolone. Am J Vet Res 41:1503, 1980.
59. Buhler, DR, et al.: Absorption, metabolism and excretion of 6 α-methylprednisolone-3-H, 21-acetate following oral and intramuscular administrations in the dog. Endocrinol 76:852, 1965.
60. Toutain, PL, et al.: Pharmacokinetics of dexamethasone and its effect on adrenal gland function in the dog. Am J Vet Res 44:212, 1983.
61. Jacobs, MB: Local subcutaneous atrophy after corticosteroid injection. Postgrad Med 80:159, 1986.
62. Scott, DW, et al.: Iatrogenic Cushing's syndrome in the cat. Feline Pract 12:30, 1982.
63. Ihrke, PJ, et al.: Urinary tract infection association with long-term corticosteroid administration in dogs with chronic skin diseases. JAVMA 186:43, 1985.
64. Bauer, MS: Prostatic abscess rupture in three dogs. JAVMA 188:735, 1986.
65. Moore, RW and Withrow, SJ: Gastrointestinal hemorrhage and pancreatitis associated with intervertebral disk disease in the dog. JAVMA 180:1443, 1982.
66. Crawford, LM and Wilson, RC: Melena associated with dexamethasone therapy in the dog. J Sm Anim Pract 23:91, 1982.
67. Bellah, JR: Colonic perforation after corticosteroid and surgical treatment of intervertebral disk disease in a dog. JAVMA 183:1002, 1983.
68. Toombs, JP, et al.: Colonic perforation in corticosteroid-treated dogs. JAVMA 188:145, 1986.
69. Sorjonen, DC, et al.: Effects of dexamethasone and surgical hypotension on the stomach of dogs: Clinical, endoscopic, and pathologic evaluations. Am J Vet Res 44:1233, 1983.
70. Nara, PL, et al.: Effects of prednisolone on the development of immune responses to canine distemper virus in beagle pups. Am J Vet Res 40:1742, 1979.
71. Enright, JB, et al.: Effects of corticosteroids on rabies virus infections in various animal species. JAVMA 156:765, 1970.
72. Kemppainen, RJ, et al.: Restitution of blood volume after hemorrhage in dogs with adrenocortical suppression. Dom An Endocrin 3:217, 1986.
73. Osbaldiston, GW and Greve, T: Estimating adrenal cortical function in dogs with ACTH. Cornell Vet 68:308, 1978.
74. DeNovo, RC and Prasse, KW: Comparison of serum biochemical and hepatic functional alterations in dogs treated with corticosteroids and hepatic duct ligation. Am J Vet Res 44:1703, 1983.
75. Woltz, HH, et al.: Effect of prednisone on thyroid gland morphology and plasma thyroxine and triiodothyronine concentrations in the dog. Am J Vet Res 44:2000, 1983.
76. Kaufman, J and Macy, DW: The glucagon tolerance test as a screening method for canine hyperadrenocorticism. Proc ACVIM, p 30, 1984.

DRUG INDEX

Generic	(Trade)	Dosage	Route	Frequency	Brief Description
Cosyntropin	(Cortrosyn)	0.25 mg	IV	N/A	Synthetic subunit of ACTH used for assessment of adrenocortical function
Dexamethasone	(Azium Solution)	1 mg/lb 2 mg/kg	IM	q8h, if necessary	Effective for cerebral edema associated with some cases of hydrocephalus and intracranial tumors
Dexamethasone 21-Isonicotinate	(Voren)	0.125 to 1 mg	IM	N/A	Do not repeat within 3 months
Hydrocortisone Cream	(Hytone)	N/A	Topical	q6–12h	Preferred topical corticosteroid for chronic use
Methylprednisolone Acetate	(Depo-Medrol)	5 to 40 mg	IM	N/A	Do not repeat within 3 months
Prednisone	Common generic	0.12–2 mg/lb 0.25–4 mg/kg (see Table 52–5)	Oral	qod to q12h	Preferred systemic corticosteroid
Prednisolone	Common generic	0.12–2 mg/lb 0.25–4 mg/kg (see Table 52–5)	Oral	qod to q12h	Interchangeable with prednisone; preferred in severe liver disease
Triamcinolone Acetonide	(Kenalog–10 Injection)	2.5–5 mg/joint	Intra-articular	N/A	Do not repeat
Triamcinolone Acetonide	(Vetalog Parenteral)	0.6 mg/cm^2	Intralesional	Weekly	—
Triamcinolone Acetonide	(Vetalog Cream)	N/A	Topical	q24h to q6h	Use less potent topical corticosteroid after 10 days

53 FLUID THERAPY, ELECTROLYTE AND ACID-BASE CONTROL

DAVID F. SENIOR

PHYSIOLOGY OF BODY FLUID COMPARTMENTS

Water constitutes 55 to 80 per cent of the weight of the canine and feline body, with higher values in neonates and lower values in obese adults.[1] Body water is distributed between two major compartments: extracellular fluid (ECF) and intracellular fluid (ICF) (Figure 53–1). The ECF (20 to 30 per cent of body weight) is divided into the plasma space (5 per cent of body weight)

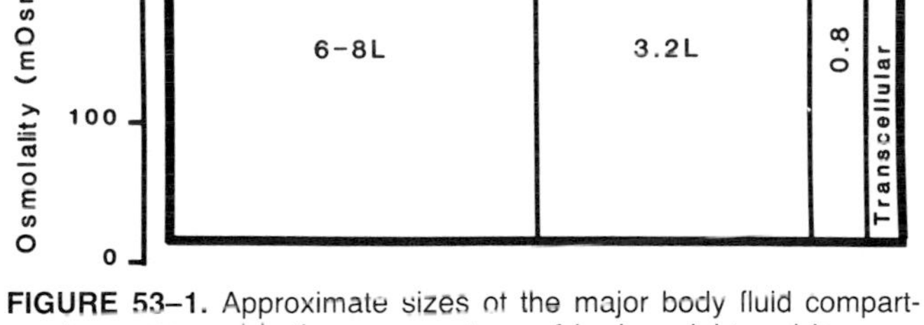

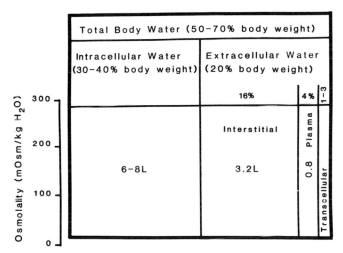

FIGURE 53–1. Approximate sizes of the major body fluid compartments, expressed both as percentage of body weight and in mean absolute values for an adult dog weighing 20 kg (44 lb). The normal range among individuals is considerable and thus no one value should be taken too rigidly; a good rule of thumb is "20, 40, 60," referring to the percentage of the body weight that is constituted by extracellular (ECW), intracellular (ICW), and total body water (TBW), respectively. The plasma has a very slightly higher osmolality than the intracellular and interstitial compartments; this small difference can be ignored when dealing with problems of fluid balance. (Adapted and reprinted with permission from Valtin, H: Renal Function: Mechanisms Preserving Fluid and Solute Balance in Health, 2nd ed, Little, Brown and Company, 1983, p 24.)

and the interstitial space (16 per cent of body weight). Plasma circulates rapidly in blood vessels separated from interstitial fluid by the vascular endothelium. Interstitial fluid bathes the cell membranes; enlargement of the interstitial fluid volume is recognized clinically as edema. The ICF (30 to 40 per cent of body weight) can be considered as a single space even though it is composed of many islands surrounded by cell membranes and the water content and chemical composition of cells with different functions vary tremendously.

The electrolyte solutes of ECF and ICF are quite different (Figure 53–2). In ECF the major cation is sodium (Na^+), while the major anions are chloride (Cl^-) and bicarbonate (HCO_3^-). In ICF the major cations are potassium (K^+) and magnesium, while the major anions are organic phosphates and protein.[2]

The vascular endothelium provides a selectively permeable barrier between the plasma space and interstitial fluid. The capillary basement membrane is highly permeable to water and small solutes but relatively impermeable to plasma protein. The intravascular retention of protein results in a slightly higher osmotic pressure in the plasma space than in the interstitial space, due to the Gibbs-Donnan effect.[3] The small difference in osmolality is known as the plasma oncotic pressure.

The forces involved in fluid movement between the plasma space and the interstitial space through capillary walls are known as Starling forces (Figure 53–3).[4] The intracapillary hydrostatic pressure fluctuates with precapillary sphincter tone, according to autonomic and humoral stimuli. Constriction occurs in hemorrhage and shock and relaxation occurs in inflammation. In the proximal segment of a normally functioning capillary, hydrostatic pressure exceeds plasma oncotic pressure and ultrafiltration of relatively protein-free plasma occurs out of the capillary into the interstitium. Toward the distal portion of the capillary, resistance to blood flow causes intracapillary hydrostatic pressures to drop; plasma oncotic pressure exceeds intracapillary hydro-

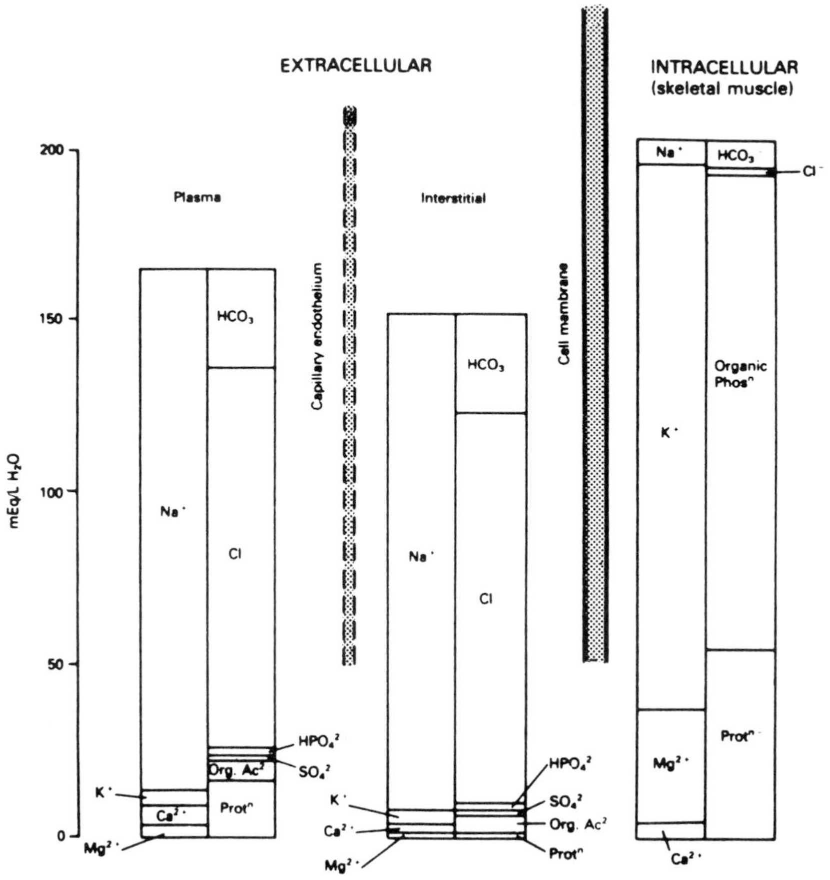

FIGURE 53–2. The main solute constituents of the major body fluid compartments. The concentrations are expressed as chemical equivalents to emphasize that the compartments are made up mainly of electrolytes and that within any one space the total number of negative charges is neutralized by the positive charges. The values depicted for intracellular fluid are rough approximations for skeletal muscle cells. The diagram serves to emphasize important and typical differences between intracellular and extracellular fluid. Organic phosphates include AMP, ADP, and ATP, glycerophosphate, and creatine phosphate. (Slightly modified from Gamble, JL: Chemical Anatomy, Physiology and Pathology of Extracellular Fluid. 6th ed, Cambridge: Harvard University Press, 1954. Reprinted with permission from Valtin, H: Renal Function: Mechanisms Preserving Fluid and Solute Balance in Health, 2nd ed, Little, Brown and Company, 1983, p 28.)

static pressure and fluid is reabsorbed from the interstitium back into the plasma space. Under normal circumstances the quantity of fluid lost from the plasma space in the proximal capillary is almost offset by reabsorption in the distal capillary. The small excess of ultrafiltrate is returned to the plasma space via lymphatics. Lymphatic flow is aided by muscular activity and the negative

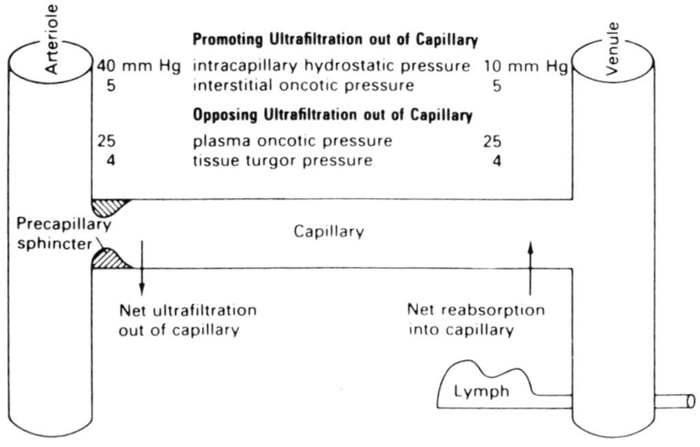

FIGURE 53–3. The Starling hypothesis of fluid exchange between plasma and interstitium. The four factors that determine this exchange are known as Starling forces. (Reprinted with permission from Valtin, H: Renal Function: Mechanisms Preserving Fluid and Solute Balance in Health, 2nd ed, Little, Brown and Company, 1983, p 34.)

intrathoracic pressure generated by inspiration. Thus, the distribution of ECF between the plasma space and the interstitial space is controlled by Starling forces active across the capillary endothelium. Adequate plasma protein is essential to maintaining normal plasma volume.

The strikingly different composition of the ICF is maintained by selective permeability of the cell membrane and the activity of energy-dependent membrane-bound Na, K-ATPase pumps, which take in K^+ and extrude Na^+ against a large electrochemical gradient. The cell membrane is relatively impermeable to intracellular organic phosphates and protein, which causes a large intracellular oncotic pressure due to Gibbs-Donnan effects. The tendency to draw interstitial fluid into the cells is offset by active ionic extrusion. Loss of active ion transport in the cell membrane due to hypoxia or metabolic poisons causes an influx of solutes and water, with cell swelling and ultimate lysis. The cell membrane is usually freely permeable to water, so most cells are not able to generate an osmotic pressure significantly different from the ECF. As a result, changes in ECF osmolality are able to change the size of the ICF. When ECF osmolality is high, water is drawn out of cells and cells shrink, whereas low ECF osmolality leads to cell enlargement.

Total body fluid size is maintained by two major mechanisms: one assesses plasma and interstitial volume and controls Na^+ excretion, the other senses body fluid osmolality and controls thirst and water excretion. External fluid balance in an adult requires that the daily dietary intake equals combined cutaneous, gastrointestinal, pulmonary, and renal output. As dietary intake may vary and nonrenal losses are poorly controlled, thirst and renal control of sodium and water excretion play a major role in maintaining external fluid balance.

GENERAL GUIDELINES FOR FLUID THERAPY

The goal of fluid therapy is to restore the volume and composition of body fluids to normal and, once this is achieved, to maintain external fluid and electrolyte balance so that treatment input matches fluid losses. Careful clinical assessment of the patient is required to accurately determine the nature and degree of fluid imbalance prior to treatment. Assessment should include history, physical examination, and laboratory tests.

Useful historical information includes food and water intake, gastrointestinal losses by vomiting and diarrhea, urine output, recent exercise, exposure to heat, trauma, hemorrhage, excessive panting, fever, and diuretic use.

Careful physical examination can determine fluid status and regular reassessment during fluid therapy is extremely important to determine the effectiveness of treatment and to guard against fluid excesses, particularly when the rate of administration is high.

Laboratory tests are useful to establish the nature and extent of fluid imbalance and to monitor progress in treatment. Appropriate information and samples should be collected prior to beginning treatment. The most frequently performed analyses are packed cell volume, total plasma protein, urine specific gravity, blood urea nitrogen (BUN), blood glucose, and an ECG, because they can be performed rapidly with equipment available in veterinary hospitals. Other tests not so readily available on an immediate basis include serum and urine creatinine (P_{Cr}, U_{Cr}), serum and urine Na^+ (P_{Na+}, U_{Na+}), serum potassium, chloride and bicarbonate (or total CO_2), serum calcium and inorganic phosphorus, blood gas values, and serum and urine osmolality.

From these values the anion gap, osmolar gap, and fractional excretion of sodium (FE_{Na+}) can be calculated as follows:

$$\text{Anion gap} = Na^+ - (HCO_3^- + Cl^-)$$

$$\text{Osmolar gap} = \text{Measured osmolality} - \left(2Na^+ + \frac{\text{glucose}}{18} + \frac{\text{BUN}}{2.8}\right)$$

$$FE_{Na+} = \frac{U_{Na+}}{P_{Na+}} \times \frac{P_{Cr}}{U_{Cr}} \times 100$$

An indwelling urinary catheter connected to a closed collection system allows an accurate measurement of urine output to aid in the calculation of fluid requirements, determine renal function, and assess the response to diuretics. Central venous pressure, a measure of right atrial pressure, is useful in determining excessive plasma volume expansion. Measurement of pulmonary artery wedge pressure with a Swan-Ganz catheter determines pulmonary venous pressure, which can be used to assess most accurately the risk of pulmonary edema. However, Swan-Ganz catheters are expensive, difficult to place, difficult to maintain, and carry some risks, so they have not been used regularly in clinical veterinary medicine.

Intravenous fluid administration is preferred, especially when rapid volume expansion is required. Both intraperitoneal and subcutaneous routes can also be used, but absorption from subcutaneous tissue may be unreliable and too slow in severe dehydration. Oral fluid administration is useful, provided the gastrointestinal tract is sufficiently functional. Fluids can be given by syringe into the mouth, by gavage, via a nasogastric tube, or via a gastrostomy tube.

The major parenteral fluids can be divided into colloidal solutions, electrolyte solutions, and five per cent dextrose in water (Table 53–1). The colloidal solutions, plasma and dextran, are given intravenously only. They cause an immediate and sustained increase in plasma volume because their volume of distribution is limited to the plasma space and they are metabolized slowly. The electrolyte solutions can be divided into replacement and maintenance solutions. Replacement electrolyte solutions provide 130 to 147 mEq/L of Na^+, similar to the values in ECF. The maintenance electrolyte solutions provide 40 to 77 mEq/l of Na^+, about one half or less of the values in ECF. Five per cent dextrose in water contains no Na^+. The dextrose enters ICF and is metabolized, so this solution provides free water.

A number of supplements can be added to the basic electrolyte solutions to provide more precise treatment tailored to the special needs of individual patients (Table 53–2).

DISORDERS OF TOTAL BODY SODIUM

Physiology of Sodium

Total body Na^+ is controlled by several extremely complex mechanisms, some of which remain poorly understood. The mechanisms can be divided into afferent sensors, which sense intravascular pressure,[5] vascular distention and plasma Na^+ concentration,[6–8] and efferent pathways that directly affect various aspects of Na^+ excretion by altering peritubular hydrostatic and oncotic pressure,[9] sympathetic tone in renal nerves,[10] and by activating various humoral factors, including the renin-angiotensin-aldosterone system,[11] prostaglandins,[12] and the atrial natriuretic factor.[13] When total body Na^+ losses cause decreased ECF volume, reduced intravascular and interstitial volume activate the afferent mechanisms, causing the CNS to initate a variety of effector mechanisms that alter renal Na^+ handling. Changes caused by efferent factors in the kidney result in a decrease in renal Na^+ excretion in an attempt to return ECF volume to normal. An increase in Na^+ content in the ECF results in changes opposite to those seen with Na^+ loss.

TABLE 53–1. SOLUTIONS FOR FLUID THERAPY

	Electrolyte Concentration (mEq/L)					Buffer mEq/L	pH	Osmolality mOsm/L	Caloric Value kcal/L
	Na^{+}	*K*$^{+}$	*Ca*$^{++}$	*Mg*$^{++}$	*Cl*$^{-}$				
Colloidal Solutions									
Dextran 70 6% w/v in 0.9% saline	154	—	—	—	154		4.5–7	300–303	
Plasma (average values, dog)	145	4.2	5	2.5	108	20	7.4	290	
Electrolyte Solutions									
Replacement Solutions:									
Lactated Ringer's	130	4	3	—	109	Lactate 25	6.5	273	9
Ringer's solution	147	4	5	—	156	—	5.8	310	—
Normal saline	154	—	—	—	154	—	5.4	308	—
Normosol R	140	5	—	3	98	Acetate 27 Gluconate 23	6.2	295	18
Maintenance Solutions									
2½% dex/0.45% saline	77	—	—	—	77	—	4.8	280	85
2½% dex/½ str lactated Ringer's	65	2	1	—	54	Lactate 14	5.0	263	89
Normosol M	40	13	—	3	40	Acetate 16	6.0	112	0
Normosol M in 5% dextrose water	40	13	—	3	40	Acetate 16	5.2	363	175
Other Solutions									
5% dextrose in water	—	—	—	—	—	—	5.0	252	170

Volume Contraction

ETIOLOGY

Volume contraction can involve simultaneous loss of both Na^{+} and water with reduced ECF volume while ICF volume is relatively spared, or pure-water loss where fluid depletion is distributed throughout the total body water. Reduced fluid intake or nonrenal and renal Na^{+} and water loss can cause volume contraction (Table 53–3).

CLINICAL SIGNS

In animals deprived of water, the first clinical signs of dehydration become evident when body weight is reduced by five to eight per cent. The signs are obvious at ten per cent and animals with 15 per cent loss of body weight show all the signs of hypovolemic shock (see Table 53–4).[14] However, the nature and severity of clinical signs vary with the type and manner of fluid loss. Rapid blood loss of five per cent of body weight causes extremely severe signs of hypovolemic shock because the loss is confined to the plasma space and represents more than 50 per cent of plasma volume. For a short period during rapid plasma volume contraction, skin elasticity may remain relatively normal prior to fluid equilibration between the plasma and interstitial space. When gastroenteritis causes fluid loss equal to five per cent of body weight, signs of plasma volume depletion are marked. As gastroenteritis causes loss of both Na^{+} and water, the loss is mostly confined to the ECF. So plasma volume and interstitial volume are reduced equally by 25 per cent. When reduced water intake and insensible water loss cause a five per cent reduction in body weight, the loss is shared evenly between all fluid spaces, plasma volume is reduced only by about eight per cent, and hypovolemia is barely perceptible. Only when pure water loss causes a 15 per cent loss of body weight and plasma volume is reduced by 25 per cent will the patient exhibit the signs of hypovolemic shock.

TABLE 53–2. SPECIAL SOLUTIONS FOR SUPPLEMENTATION OF PARENTERAL FLUIDS

	Concentration/ml
Potassium chloride	2 mEq K^{+}
Calcium gluconate 10%	0.465 mEq Ca^{++}
Calcium chloride 10%	1.36 mEq Ca^{++}
Sodium bicarbonate 5%	0.59 mEq HCO_3^{-}
Sodium bicarbonate 8.4%	1 mEq/ml HCO_3^{-}

TREATMENT

Volume. Fluid therapy for volume contraction must replace current deficits, provide maintenance requirements equivalent to normal insensible losses, and take into account ongoing extraordinary losses such as those incurred by continued vomiting and diarrhea or through burns. The general formula for calculation of fluid requirements is:

Fluid required (ml) = deficit:
BW (kg) × per cent dehydration × 1000
+ insensible losses (40 to 60 ml/kg/day)
+ extraordinary losses

The volume of the fluid deficit should be determined from the available history, physical examination, and laboratory test results. The amount usually is expressed as a percentage of body weight and is often an educated guess at best. For example, skin elasticity may overestimate the extent of dehydration in emaciated and older animals and underestimate it in obese and juvenile

TABLE 53–3. CAUSES OF VOLUME CONTRACTION

Nonrenal	Renal
Vomiting	Osmotic diuresis
Diarrhea	diabetes mellitus
Small bowel obstruction	mannitol
Pancreatitis	radiographic contrast
Peritonitis	diuretics
Burns	Hypoadrenocorticoidism
Hemorrhage	Polyuric phase of acute renal failure
Paracentesis	Postobstructive diuresis
Thoracentesis	
Insensible water loss in water deprivation	

animals. A more precise calculation of volume contraction can be determined from the body weight, packed cell volume (PCV), and total plasma protein if prevolume contracted values are known. The reduction in body weight in kilograms equals the volume of fluid lost in liters and when there is no loss of red blood cell mass (bleeding or hemolysis), the hematocrit rises by a percentage increment equivalent to the decrease in ECF volume. Thus, a 20 per cent decrement in ECF volume results in a 20 per cent increase in PCV and total plasma protein. These calculations are limited in value when red blood cell and protein losses occur concomitantly with fluid loss. In hypovolemic shock, the volume of fluid required for treatment may be two to four times the volume of blood lost because of vasodilation and increased volume of distribution of fluid.[15]

Maintenance fluid requirements are the sum of urinary and insensible fluid losses, which include pulmonary, cutaneous, and fecal losses. Urinary losses can be measured by an indwelling urinary catheter connected to a closed collection system, although this is not recommended unless very accurate measurement of urine output is required. Urine volume can be estimated, but the volume varies with body size, the solute load to be excreted, and renal concentrating capacity. A reasonable guess is 10 ml/lb/day (20 ml/kg/day). Normal fecal losses are usually about 2.5 ml/lb/day (5 ml/kg/day). Combined respiratory and cutaneous fluid loss usually amounts to about 7.5 ml/lb/day (15 ml/kg/day). However, the rate of fluid loss via the respiratory tract may greatly increase with fever and hyperventilation. Combined urinary, fecal, and insensible losses usually amount to about 20 ml/lb/day (40 ml/kg/day) and most clinicians calculate daily maintenance fluid requirements as 20 to 30 ml/lb/day (40 to 60 ml/kg/day), using the lower value for large dogs and the higher value for small dogs and cats.[14]

The magnitude of extraordinary fluid losses due to vomiting, diarrhea, burns, surgery, and centesis can be measured or estimated and these must be added to the daily fluid requirements.

Quite often the calculated volume of fluid overestimates the actual fluid deficit to some extent. In patients with normal renal function, excessive fluid administration is of little consequence because urine production increases rapidly once the animal is fully hydrated. However, animals with acute renal failure may be oliguric and continued rapid fluid administration results in overhydration and the risk of pulmonary edema. All patients receiving parenteral fluids should be assessed at regular intervals during treatment and adjustments in calculated deficits made as required.

Rate. The rate of fluid loss and the severity of clinical signs are important in determining the rate of fluid administration. Patients with sudden severe blood loss and hypovolemic shock require immediate rapid intravenous fluid treatment to restore intravascular volume and tissue perfusion. If fluid administration is too slow, tissue perfusion may remain inadequate for a prolonged period of time, exacerbating hypovolemic shock and predisposing the animal to acute renal failure. In the absence of cardiopulmonary disease, intravenous fluids can be safely administered to dogs and cats at 45 ml/lb/day (90 ml/kg/hr).[16,17] Patients with mild volume depletion require much less aggressive treatment, so intravenous fluids should be given more slowly. The fluid deficit can be corrected over a four-to-six-hour period. However, even with this reduced rate, the patient's cardiopulmonary status should be assessed carefully prior to treatment and regularly monitored during treatment. Intravenous fluids are delivered into the plasma space, from which they diffuse out into the interstitial and intracellular fluid. When intravenous fluid administration is very rapid, the plasma space may become overloaded even though a total body fluid deficit may still exist. For example, patients with mitral insufficiency are at particular risk for developing pulmonary edema. Central venous pressure and pulmonary artery wedge pressure can provide accurate information about fluid overload, if such measurements are available. Other consequences of rapid intravenous fluid administration include CNS signs due to rapid shifts in osmolality and acid-base balance.

Composition. Fluids available for treatment can be divided into several categories, including colloidal solutions, replacement and maintenance electrolyte solutions, and five per cent dextrose in water (Table 53–1). The choice of fluids should be based on the degree of volume depletion and the nature of the fluid loss. For a patient in shock, the treatment goal is to restore the intravascular volume as soon as possible. To accomplish this it is best to use a replacement fluid with a volume of distribution limited to the intravascular space. When plasma volume depletion is secondary to hemorrhage, the best replacement fluid is cross-matched whole blood. When volume depletion is not due to blood loss or if blood is unavailable, a colloidal solution, such as plasma or dextran, should be used initially. Isotonic electrolyte solutions may be used for plasma volume expansion, but Na^+ distributes throughout the ECF space, so only 20 to 25 per cent of the infused volume remains in the intravascular space. Thus, isotonic electrolyte solutions should be used as initial treatment for shock only until plasma or another colloidal solution is available. Colloidal solutions should also be given to patients with hypoalbuminemia secondary to ongoing losses such as those that occur in nephrotic syndrome and protein-losing enteropathy. Reduced plasma oncotic pressure leads to reduced plasma volume and blood pressure is maintained by alpha-adrenergically stimulated contraction of large venous capacitance vessels. Under anesthesia or sedation with tranquilizers, capacitance vessels may relax, causing the systemic blood pressure to fall precipitously. Intravenous administration of colloidal solutions can prevent and treat hypotension in this setting, while replacement with electrolytes is often inadequate to restore plasma volume because administered fluid tends to leave the plasma space and pool in the interstitium, leading to pulmonary and generalized edema.

Provided the patient does not require treatment with a colloidal solution, fluid deficits should be replaced with a fluid that most closely matches the type of fluid lost. Generally, replacement solutions should be used to replace deficits caused by balanced ECF losses, maintenance solutions can be used to replace normal urinary and insensible fluid losses, and sodium-free solutions should be used to replace deficits in patients suffering from insensible or pure water losses.

Animals dehydrating due to vomiting, diarrhea, or burns tend to lose fluids that closely match the composition of ECF, so replacement electrolyte solutions closely resembling ECF should be used to correct the deficit (Table 53–1). Five per cent dextrose in water is relatively ineffective in replacing balanced electrolyte losses because water distributes throughout total body fluids and only about 30 per cent remains within the ECF.

Further supplementation of replacement fluids may be required to correct acid-base imbalance and K^+ deficits, depending on the cause of fluid loss. Vomitus is fairly high in Na^+ and Cl^-, but net hydrogen ion (H^+) or HCO_3^- loss depends on the location of the lesion. Vomiting due to pyloric outflow obstruction causes metabolic alkalosis due to H^+ loss, leading to renal K^+ wasting under the combined effect of dehydration and metabolic alkalosis.[18] In such cases replacement electrolyte solutions containing no bicarbonate or bicarbonate precursors, such as Ringer's solution and 0.9 per cent NaCl, should be used and K^+ supplementation may be required. However, most causes of vomiting in the dog other than pyloric outflow obstruction have a minimal effect on acid-base balance except for a mild metabolic acidosis.[19] Thus, a replacement electrolyte solution containing a bicarbonate precursor, such as Ringer's lactate or Normosol R, can be used. Fluid losses due to diarrhea are usually high in Na^+, K^+, and HCO_3^-, so replacement fluids may need to be supplemented with K^+ and HCO_3^- (Table 53–2).[20]

Maintenance fluids do not need to match ECF composition because urinary and normal fecal losses are generally low in Na^+ and insensible loses via the respiratory tract and through the skin are virtually sodium-free. Thus, maintenance electrolyte solutions with reduced Na^+ such as 2.5 per cent dextrose in half-strength lactated Ringer's solution or 2.5 per cent dextrose in 0.45 per cent NaCl are recommended.

Animals with normal renal function that dehydrate due to insensible fluid losses and failure to drink water because of dementia have a pure water loss and should receive five per cent dextrose in water as the main replacement fluid.

Volume Expansion

ETIOLOGY

Extracellular fluid volume expansion can occur when Na^+ and water intake exceeds renal excretion, as occurs when excessive fluids are administered to patients with acute renal failure and when chronic renal failure patients are supplemented with too much dietary Na^+. ECF volume expansion induces the afferent and efferent pathways controlling total body Na^+ to maximize Na^+ excretion. If the kidneys are capable of sufficient Na^+ excretion, the signs are limited to a mild increase in body weight. However, increased Na^+ intake in the face of reduced renal function eventually causes interstitial fluid expansion to the point of overt edema, with a tendency toward hypertension.[21]

Cardiac failure, hepatic disease, and hypoalbuminemia due to protein-losing enteropathy and nephropathy also cause ECF volume expansion, where the predominant manifestation is interstitial volume expansion, leading to edema. The pathogenesis of edema in this setting appears to develop in two steps.[22] Altered transcapillary Starling forces, such as increased intracapillary hydrostatic pressure in cardiac failure and reduced plasma oncotic pressure in hypoalbuminemia, cause redistribution of ECF from the plasma space to the interstitium. Reduced effective arterial blood volume then initiates the afferent and efferent mechanisms to retain Na^+ in an effort to increase tissue perfusion. Sodium retention and transfer of intravascular fluid into the interstitium eventually causes edema. Hepatic disease may induce edema by a slightly different mechanism because renal Na^+ retention seems to develop before the onset of hypoalbuminemia, suggesting that hepatopathy may initiate inappropriate afferent mechanisms of Na^+ control.[23]

CLINICAL SIGNS AND DIAGNOSIS

Signs of overhydration due to excessive fluid administration are shown in Table 53–4. In cardiac failure, vascular engorgement may accompany ascites and generalized edema; in liver failure, ascites may precede development of generalized peripheral edema; and in hypoalbuminemia due to any cause, poor peripheral vascular perfusion may be evident and generalized peripheral edema usually occurs without overt ascites. Generalized edema without altered Starling forces suggests altered capillary permeability with leakage of plasma proteins into the interstitium, as would occur in vasculitis. Localized edema suggests venous or lymphatic obstruction.

Diagnosis of edematous conditions involves a systematic consideration of factors affecting fluid distribution between the plasma and interstitial fluid spaces, including Starling forces, capillary permeability, and venous and lymphatic integrity. The history, location of fluid, cardiac assessment, and serum albumin estimation are vital. Once the mechanism of edema formation has been identified, an appropriate list of differential diagnoses is apparent. For example, differential diagnoses of hypoalbuminemia include glomerulonephropathy, protein-losing enteropathy, liver failure, extensive burns or

TABLE 53–4. CLINICAL SIGNS OF ECF VOLUME DEPLETION AND OVERLOAD

Depletion	Overload
Increased temperature	Restlessness, coughing
Weak, rapid pulse	Increased respiration rate
Pale, dry mucous membranes	Subcutaneous edema
Slow capillary refill time	Ascites
Poor skin elasticity	Chemosis
Cool distal extremities	Exophthalmos
Sunken orbits	Vomiting
Reduced urine output	Serous nasal discharge
Microcardia on thoracic radiographs	Increased urine output (assumes normal kidney function)

other skin lesions, peritonitis, and excessive abdominal and thoracic drainage.

TREATMENT

Treatment of volume expansion in fluid overload and Na^+ retention should always include correction of the primary cause. Volume expansion in acute and chronic renal failure requires restriction of sodium and water intake. Judicious use of diuretics may alleviate the problem more quickly. Care must be taken to avoid overtreatment and volume contraction because this may precipitate further azotemic crises.

Edema due to sodium retention is treated using a low sodium diet combined with diuretics. Progress can be assessed by repeated body weight measurements. Edema should be reduced slowly when effective arterial blood volume is already reduced because rapid volume contraction can lead to hypovolemic shock.

DISORDERS OF WATER METABOLISM

Physiology of Water

The osmolality of body fluids is controlled by regulation of renal water excretion through the action of antidiuretic hormone (ADH) and regulation of thirst.[24] Antidiuretic hormone production and release is controlled by hypothalamic osmoreceptors that sense ECF osmolality and by peripheral low-pressure and high-pressure volume receptors that sense vascular fullness. Minor changes in ECF osmolality induce rapid changes in ADH release from the posterior pituitary gland. Plasma ADH levels control renal excretion of solute-free water by altering the water permeability of the cortical and medullary collecting tubules. Maximum and minimum responses in renal free water clearance (urine osmolality) occur over an ECF osmolar range of less than 20 mOsm/kg H_2O in humans, so body fluid osmolality is maintained very precisely.[24] Control of urine concentration alone cannot maintain ECF osmolality because the need to excrete the solute products of digestion and metabolism mandates an obligatory renal water loss. Balance is maintained by water intake and thirst is controlled by hypothalamic osmoreceptors separate from, but nearby, the osmoreceptors that control circulating levels of ADH.[24] The normal range for serum Na^+ concentration is 140 to 154 mEq/L in dogs and 150 to 162 mEq/L in cats, while the normal range for serum osmolality is 283 to 312 mOsm/kg H_2O in dogs and 280 to 310 mOsm/kg H_2O in cats.

As well as the hypothalamic osmoreceptors, peripheral vascular volume receptors can also modify ADH release in response to volume expansion and contraction. During volume contraction, the baroreceptor pathway lowers the ECF osmolality threshold for ADH release and sensitizes the ADH secretory response to changes in plasma osmolality.[25] Consequently, during volume contraction, ECF osmolality may reset at a lower level until normal ECF volume is restored. A variety of other processes, including beta-adrenergic stimulation,[26] decreased cardiac output,[27] left atrial distention,[28] and atrial tachycardia[29] result in alterations in ADH release via the baroreceptor pathway in humans. Nausea and pain promote ADH release,[30, 31] while a variety of drugs stimulate or inhibit ADH release in humans, including narcotics[32] and vincristine,[33] which stimulate ADH release, and ethanol[34] and diphenylhydantoin,[35] which inhibit ADH release.

As the number of solutes in ICF is relatively fixed and water moves freely across cell membranes, changes in water balance regulate ICF volume. Cells shrink in hyperosmolar states and cells expand in hyposmolar states. Expansion and contraction of CNS cells with major changes in body fluid osmolality can cause permanent or even fatal neurologic damage. The cells of the CNS are able to offset changes in cell volume to some extent by the generation of poorly identified intracellular solutes called "ideogenic osmoles."[36] Provided changes in body fluid osmolality are relatively slow, changes in the intracellular concentration of ideogenic osmoles confer some degree of protection against excessive CNS contraction or expansion.

Hyponatremia

ETIOLOGY

Hyponatremia occurs frequently in human patients but has not been recorded often in veterinary medicine. The more commonly recognized causes in animals are shown in Table 53–5.

Isotonic hyponatremia (pseudohyponatremia) occurs when the volume of dissolved substances in plasma is significantly increased. Sodium concentration usually is expressed as mEq/L of plasma volume even though seven to eight per cent of plasma volume is not water but dissolved solutes. Usually the small nonaqueous component does not significantly affect the value. In extreme hyperlipidemia and hyperglobulinemia due to multiple myeloma, plasma solutes may represent 30 per cent of the plasma volume.[37,38] Although Na^+ concentration of plasma water remains normal, clinical laboratories may measure and report serum (or plasma) Na^+ concentrations in mEq/L of plasma, not mEq/L of plasma water, so the stated plasma Na^+ concentration

TABLE 53–5. CAUSES OF HYPONATREMIA AND HYPERNATREMIA

Hyponatremia	Hypernatremia
Isotonic	Pure water loss
(pseudohyponatremia)	diabetes insipidus
hyperlipidemia	dementia
hyperglobulinemia	
Hypertonic	Hypertonic $NaHCO_3$ administration
diabetes mellitus	cardiac arrest
mannitol treatment	feline urethral obstruction
Hypotonic	Inappropriate Na^+ administration
hypoadrenocorticoidism	acute renal failure
postobstructive diuresis	
diuretic treatment	
postoperative	
SIADH	

is artificially low. Estimations using more recently available ion-specific electrode methodology avoid this error. The condition can be diagnosed readily by inspection of the plasma, which is milky-white in hyperlipidemia and extremely viscous in hyperglobulinemia.

Hypertonic hyponatremia occurs when large amounts of solutes incapable of diffusing across the cell membrane accumulate in ECF. Such substances draw water from the ICF, thereby diluting the Na^+ concentration in ECF. Hyperglycemia in uncontrolled diabetes mellitus and mannitol after intravenous infusion are the most common examples.[39,40] Serum Na^+ can be expected to fall by 1.3 to 1.6 mEq/L for every 100 mg/dl rise in serum glucose.[39] The decrease in ECF Na^+ concentration is not associated with an alteration in total body water but rather is due to altered distribution of water between ICF and ECF. The abnormal water distribution and hyponatremia correct spontaneously when the accumulated solute is reduced.

Hypotonic hyponatremia is seen in hypoadrenocorticoidism. Renal Na^+ loss is due to impaired aldosterone-dependent Na^+ reabsorption in the distal tubule. When ECF volume decreases, GFR drops and a larger than normal proportion of the filtered load is reabsorbed in the proximal tubule. As reduced tubular fluid delivery to the diluting segment impairs free water clearance, water is retained.[41] Also, hypovolemia stimulates ADH release at a lower ECF osmolality and lack of glucocorticoids tends to facilitate continued production of ADH.[42] During postobstructive diuresis, rapid elimination of urea and other solutes, as well as impaired collecting duct Na^+ handling, leads to a large urine output accompanied by a natriuresis.[43, 44] Hyponatremia can be observed in cats during postobstructive diuresis if sodium-free solutions are used to replace urine output. Vigorous long-term diuretic treatment in animals fed a low Na^+ diet also can cause hypotonic hyponatremia.[45] Volume contraction induces ADH production at lower ECF osmolality. Some animals exhibit hypotonic hyponatremia for a brief period postoperatively. Pain and stress are thought to enhance ADH production independent of ECF osmolality, with resultant water retention.[30]

In human medicine, hypotonic hyponatremia occurs quite commonly in the syndrome of inappropriate secretion of ADH (SIADH), so called because there is a sustained or intermittently elevated level of ADH inappropriate to any osmotic or volume stimuli that normally affect ADH secretion.[46] Criteria for diagnosis include hypotonic hyponatremia, inappropriate antidiuresis, normal glomerular filtration rate, normal adrenal and thyroid function, excretion of appreciable quantities of Na^+ when the patient is normovolemic, absence of clinical signs of hypovolemia, dehydration, and absence of a condition associated with generalized edema or ascites.[47] Both the hypotonic hyponatremia and natriuresis may be corrected by strict fluid restriction.[47] In humans, SIADH has been recognized in association with a number of malignant tumors, several disorders of the CNS, and pulmonary infections.[48] Tumors produce a variety of ADH-like substances,[49] CNS diseases probably directly affect endogenous ADH secretion,[47] and pulmonary diseases may cause ADH release via neural input from the lung via the CNS.[47] A dog with a condition resembling SIADH has been described.[50]

CLINICAL SIGNS AND DIAGNOSIS

Major signs are usually those of the underlying condition that is causing hyponatremia rather than those due to hyponatremia per se. Hyponatremia causes weakness, depression, vomiting, muscle fasciculations, seizures, and coma. The CNS signs are due to enlargement of the ICF with cerebral swelling. Signs are much more marked when hyponatremia develops rapidly because brain cells have insufficient time to attenuate cell swelling by dissipation of their ideogenic osmoles. In acute hyponatremia in human patients, signs begin once the plasma Na^+ concentration is less than 125 mEq/L and progress to maximum severity when the plasma Na^+ is less than 110 mEq/L.[47] In most cases, the cause of hyponatremia is apparent from the history, physical examination, direct examination of the serum, total plasma protein level, blood glucose estimation, and serum electrolyte values.

TREATMENT

Often hyponatremia spontaneously resolves once the underlying condition is adequately treated. Replacement electrolyte solutions (sodium concentration 130 to 154 mEq/L) should be given to correct hypotonic hyponatremia if the serum Na^+ concentration is above 120 mEq/L. Hypertonic saline solutions (3 per cent NaCl) and potent diuretics (furosemide 0.5 to 2 mg/lb (1 to 4 mg/kg) PO or IV q8-12h) may be necessary when the serum Na^+ concentration is less than 120 mEq/L or if the neurologic status is unstable.[47] Extremely rapid correction of chronically reduced ECF osmolality may cause dangerous brain shrinkage because ideogenic osmoles cannot be rapidly regenerated.[36] Gradual restoration of normal values over a 24 to 48 hour period is preferable if the pretreatment serum Na^+ concentration is very low.[47]

Hypernatremia

ETIOLOGY

Hypernatremia is observed frequently in small animal medicine and the cause is often iatrogenic. The most common causes are shown in Table 53–5.

Patients with diabetes insipidus have an obligatory renal water loss. During water deprivation, they conserve Na^+ but continue to excrete large volumes of water. Animals with dementia due to CNS disease may fail to drink adequately, causing dehydration due to pure water loss. Renal Na^+ conservation is maximal but obligatory insensible fluid losses via the respiratory tract and skin are virtually sodium-free. Excessive hypertonic $NaHCO_3$ is frequently given intravenously during cardiopulmonary resuscitation. Even animals that are not hypernatremic at the onset of cardiac arrest are often hypernatremic on recovery. A similar phenomenon can be observed in cats with urethral obstruction where the basic fluid loss is hypotonic and rapid administration of replacement solutions combined with hypertonic $NaHCO_3$ are used to correct volume contraction and metabolic acidosis. Animals with oliguric renal failure have continuous sodium-free insensible fluid losses. As they are unable to excrete excessive Na^+ loads, continued administration of replacement electrolyte solutions (Na^+ concentration 130 to 154 mEq/L) can lead to hypernatremia.

CLINICAL SIGNS AND DIAGNOSIS

The signs of hypernatremia include weakness, thirst, muscle fasciculations, depression, seizures, and coma. Clinical signs are likely to become apparent when plasma osmolality exceeds 350 mOsm/kg H_2O (Na^+ concentration greater than 170 mEq/L) and coma generally occurs above 400 mOsm/kg H_2O (Na^+ concentration greater than 190 mEq/L).[51] Hyperosmolality causes contraction of ICF volume and as intracellular dehydration develops, the brain shrinks and cerebral vessels tear. Rapidly increasing osmolality is more likely to induce CNS signs because brain cells are unable to develop ideogenic osmoles sufficiently fast to prevent severe brain cell shrinkage.[47] In most cases, the cause of hypernatremia is obvious from the patient history and record of previous medications.

TREATMENT

Hypernatremia due to pure water loss is treated either with oral water replacement or intravenous five per cent dextrose in water. Hypernatremia due to excessive administration of hypertonic saline and $NaHCO_3$ may be treated the same way, but more rapid reduction in serum Na^+ concentration can be achieved by simultaneous treatment with the diuretic furosemide given at 0.5 to 2 mg/lb (1 to 4 mg/kg) PO or IV q8-24h. Urinary volume should be replaced by equal volumes of oral or intravenous sodium-free fluids.

When treating chronic hypernatremia, plasma osmolality should not be reduced too rapidly. Ideogenic osmoles that develop in brain cells to prevent intracellular dehydration cannot dissipate rapidly. If ECF osmolality is decreased too fast, cerebral edema can occur with muscle fasciculations, seizures, coma, and death.[36, 51] In chronic hypernatremia, serum osmolality should not be reduced faster than 2 mOsm/kg H_2O/hour over the first 48 hours.[47]

Hypernatremia caused by excessive Na^+ administration in patients with oliguric renal failure often fails to respond to diuretic treatment. If ECF volume expansion with edema and hypertension is life-threatening, excess Na^+ can be removed by peritoneal dialysis. After correction of hypernatremia, five per cent dextrose in water should be continued to replace insensible losses, and urinary fluid losses, if any, should be replaced with a maintenance electrolyte solution (Na^+ concentration 40 to 77 mEq/L).

POTASSIUM IMBALANCE

Physiology of Potassium

The normal range for serum K^+ concentration in dogs is 4.0 to 5.8 mEq/L; in cats it is 3.7 to 5.5 mEq/L.[1] Potassium plays a major role in neuromuscular function of the heart, skeletal muscles, and gastrointestinal tract.

Potassium is the most abundant cation within cells and most body K^+ is located in the ICF of skeletal muscle cells because they constitute the largest portion of cellular tissue. About five to ten per cent of K^+ is in ECF, but only 1.4 per cent is contained in ECF water, with the rest located principally within bone.[52]

Potassium enters the body via the gastrointestinal tract and most is excreted through the kidneys. Gastrointestinal entry depends on dietary K^+ intake with no control on enteric K^+ absorption, so K^+ homeostasis is maintained by renal control of K^+ excretion. In the kidney, plasma K^+ is filtered by the glomerulus and about 70 per cent of the filtered load is reabsorbed by the proximal tubule regardless of whether the animal is K^+ replete or deplete.[53] The distal tubule is able to adapt K^+ handling to the needs of the animal with tremendous variation in K^+ reabsorption and secretion, so the fractional excretion of K^+ can vary from less than 10 per cent to more than 150 per cent.[53] Distal tubular K^+ handling and therefore K^+ excretion is closely matched to dietary K^+ intake; however, many other factors can alter this balance, including mineralocorticoid hormone levels, acid-base balance, Na^+ diuresis, and diuretic treatment.[53] In the dog, the kidneys are not able to reduce K^+ excretion to zero, so in anorectic patients there is an obligatory K^+ requirement of 2 to 40 mEq/day, depending on body size.[54]

The major determinant of resting membrane potential of muscles is the ratio of intracellular K^+ concentration to extracellular K^+ concentration, $[K^+]_I/[K^+]_E$.[52] Several factors other than total body K^+ can induce translocation of K^+ between ICF and ECF to affect this ratio and induce clinical signs, including H^+ balance, catecholamine hormones, insulin and glucagon, and changes in ECF osmolality due to nonpermeable solutes.[52] An alteration of 0.1 in plasma pH causes a reciprocal change in plasma K^+ levels of 0 to 0.7 mEq/L, with the magnitude of the shift depending on the primary cause of the change in plasma pH (Figure 53–4).[55]

Disorders of K^+ balance resulting in hypokalemia and hyperkalemia are relatively common in small animals. Serum K^+ levels do not always reflect total body K^+

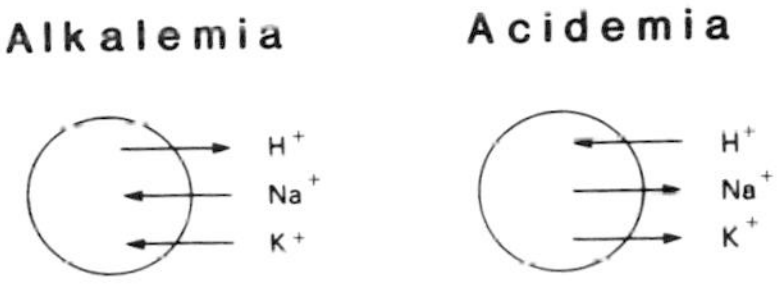

FIGURE 53–4. Reciprocal movement of H^+, Na^+, and K^+ during disturbances of H^+ balance. The circles represent body cells surrounded by extracellular fluid. In epithelial cells, such as those lining renal tubules, these shifts take place across the peritubular membrane. (Reprinted with permission from Valtin, H: Renal Function: Mechanisms Preserving Fluid and Solute Balance in Health, 2nd ed, Little, Brown and Company 1983, p 259.)

status because of factors that affect K^+ translocation between ICF and ECF. Because the ECF K^+ pool is so much smaller, relatively trivial shifts between ICF and ECF can alter serum K^+ levels greatly. However, if the clinical history suggests K^+ loss, then serum K^+ concentration gives a rough guide to the degree of K^+ depletion, provided other factors, particularly concurrent H^+ balance, are kept in mind. Thus, hypokalemia usually represents a negative external balance of K^+ that is often modified by changes of internal balance.

Hyperkalemia usually does not represent a great excess of total body K^+, because minor increases of plasma K^+ lead to fatal cardiotoxicity. Healthy kidneys can readily excrete excessive loads of K^+, so increased total body K^+ only occurs when urinary K^+ excretion is impaired, with or without increased K^+ release from injured and dying tissue. Thus, hyperkalemia is a poor indicator of external K^+ balance and rather represents a diminished ability of the kidneys to excrete K^+ and a decreased cellular mass to hold the K^+.[56]

Hypokalemia

ETIOLOGY

Hypokalemia usually arises from a negative external balance caused by reduced intake or excessive losses via renal or extrarenal routes. On occasion, total body K^+ is normal and hypokalemia is the result of ECF to ICF translocation of K^+. The most common causes of hypokalemia in dogs and cats are shown in Table 53–6.

Hypokalemia develops in fasted animals and the process is hastened by solute diuresis caused by saline intravenous fluids that enhance renal K^+ loss.[57] Nonrenal losses can occur via the intestinal tract, where diarrhea and repeated enemas can lead to marked K^+ depletion.[20] Loop and thiazide diuretics enhance renal K^+ excretion and may lead to hypokalemia if the diuresis is very large or the patient is not eating.[58] Renal K^+ wasting may be excessive during the polyuric phase of acute renal failure and during the postobstructive diuresis that follows relief of urethral obstruction.[52, 59] In intravenous saline administration, diuretic use, polyuric acute renal failure, and postobstructive diuresis, the renal K^+ loss appears to be due to increased delivery of salt and water to the distal nephron.

TABLE 53–6. CAUSES OF HYPOKALEMIA AND HYPERKALEMIA

Hypokalemia	Hyperkalemia
Reduced K^+ Intake	*Increased Intake*
Anorexia	Rapid infusion of K^+ salts
Potassium-poor fluid infusion	High doses of potassium penicillin G
Nonrenal K^+ Losses	*Decreased Renal Elimination*
Diarrhea	Oliguric acute renal failure
Enemas	Terminal stages of chronic renal failure
Renal K^+ Losses	Urethral obstruction
Diuretic use	Uroabdomen
Polyuric phase of acute renal failure	Hyperadrenocorticoidism
Postobstructive diuresis	*Translocation*
Vomiting with metabolic alkalosis	Metabolic acidosis
Renal tubular reabsorption defects	
glucose	
amphotericin B treatment	
Hyperadrenocorticoidism	
Translocation	
Metabolic alkalosis—any cause	
Insulin treatment	

Chronically vomiting animals frequently become hypokalemic, particularly if the vomiting induces metabolic alkalosis.[20] Although gastric secretions contain some K^+, most of the deficit is caused by renal K^+ loss. ECF volume contraction leads to secondary hyperaldosteronism, which stimulates distal tubular K^+ secretion. Metabolic alkalosis increases HCO_3^- delivery to the distal tubule and alkalemia causes H^+ to exit cells and K^+ to enter. Thus the stage is set for enhanced K^+ secretion to be excreted as an accompanying cation with HCO_3^-.

Hyperglycemia with glucosuria in diabetes mellitus induces an osmotic diuresis with enhanced renal K^+ loss so that fairly severe total body K^+ depletion occurs.[60] At presentation, affected animals are usually acidemic due to accumulation of ketoacids and the total body K^+ depletion can be masked by translocation of ICF K^+ into the ECF in exchange for H^+, so that plasma K^+ levels may be normal.[61] However, once insulin treatment begins the acidemia rapidly resolves as ketoacids are metabolized and glucose and potassium transfer into ICF, often leading to hypokalemia.[60]

In human patients, hypokalemia accompanies distal renal tubular acidosis (RTA) and bicarbonate-treated proximal RTA.[52] The renal K^+ loss in distal RTA is thought to be due to ECF volume depletion with secondary hyperaldosteronism and enhanced Na^+-H^+ exchange in the distal tubule. Proximal RTA patients supplemented with HCO_3^- have massive bicarbonaturia, which enhances distal K^+ secretion. Hypokalemia occurs in dogs treated with amphotericin B, a form of proximal RTA.[62] Renal K^+ wasting has been described in a disease in basenji dogs similar to the Fanconi syndrome[63] and hypokalemia has been described in two dogs with renal glycosuria.[64] Hypokalemia also has been observed in 45 per cent of dogs with hyperadrenocorticoidism due to adrenocorticoid tumors, where the exact cause of K^+ wasting is not known.[65]

CLINICAL SIGNS AND DIAGNOSIS

The signs of hypokalemia begin to develop once serum K^+ levels drop below 3.0 mEq/L. Signs include impaired gastrointestinal motility with ileus and constipation, generalized skeletal muscle weakness, and ECG abnormalities. ECG abnormalities in dogs are quite variable and include prolonged Q-T interval, sagging S-T segment, depressed T wave amplitude, and atrial and ventricular premature contractions.[66] As hypokalemia develops, the ratio $[K^+]_I/[K^+]_E$ becomes larger and both the resting membrane potential and the difference between the resting membrane potential and the threshold potential become greater. Consequently, muscles become less excitable than normal. This phenomenon probably explains some of the alterations in neuromuscular function. However, the paralysis observed in dogs with severe hypokalemia probably is associated with a fall in transmembrane voltage, with a deviation from the predicted value of $[K^+]_I/[K^+]_E$ mediated by altered Na^+ permeability of the sarcolemmal membrane.[67,68] The cause of hypokalemia usually is apparent from the history, physical examination, and routine diagnostic tests.

TREATMENT

Correction of K^+ deficits involves treating the underlying disease and providing K^+ supplementation. Several precautions should be taken to prevent fatal hyperkalemia during treatment. These include making sure there is adequate renal function, giving K^+ slowly and in dilute concentrations, and using the oral rather than the parenteral route of administration whenever possible.

The only clinical parameter available to determine the extent of K^+ depletion is serum K^+; if all other factors are constant there is a predictable relationship between the two.[69] Of other factors affecting the relationship, pH is the most important and to some extent changes in plasma pH have a somewhat consistent effect.[55] From these relationships, a nomogram can be developed to calculate total body potassium deficits from plasma K^+ and pH (Figure 53–5).[70,71] The effect of factors such as glucose, insulin, and cathecholamine hormones is not clinically quantifiable, so the nomogram only provides a rough estimation of K^+ deficits. During K^+ supplementation, plasma K^+ concentration should be checked routinely and deficits reestimated to monitor progress toward normokalemia.

Several different K^+ salts are available for supplementation, including potassium chloride, potassium phosphate, and potassium bicarbonate, or the metabolic precursors of bicarbonate such as gluconate, citrate, or acetate. The phosphate and bicarbonate salts are suitable for K^+ supplementation with concurrent hypophosphatemia and metabolic acidosis, respectively, but neither will correct K^+ depletion adequately in metabolic alkalosis.[52] The chloride salt is appropriate for treatment of metabolic alkalosis, the most common acid-base disturbance associated with hypokalemia, and is also adequate for all other disturbances, so if only one salt is to be stocked, it should be potassium chloride.

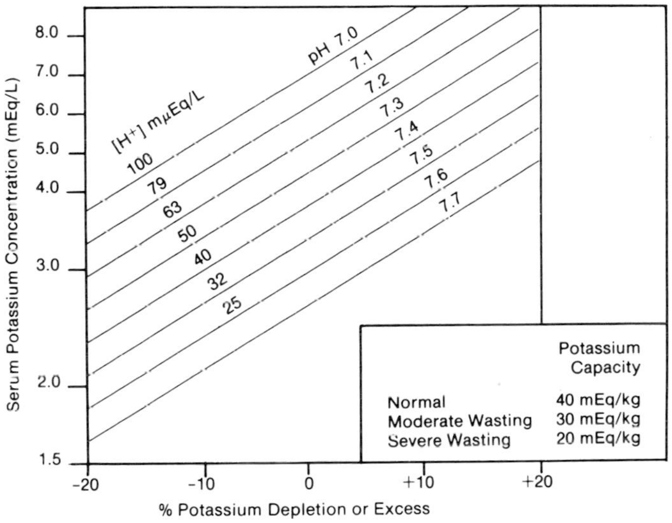

FIGURE 53–5. Relationship between serum potassium concentration, blood pH, and percentage change in content capacity. A potassium deficit is determined by drawing a horizontal line from the point of the serum potassium measurement to the diagonal isopleth of the measured pH. By following a vertical line from that point down to the x-axis, one can determine the percentage depletion or excess of potassium. Multiply that factor by the estimated body potassium capacity. For example, the potassium deficit in a severely wasted 15-kg patient with a measured potassium concentration of 2.5 mEq/L and a pH of 7.6 is approximately 30 mEq. (Reprinted with permission from Haskins, SC: Fluid and Electrolyte Therapy. Comp Cont Ed Pract Vet 6(3):244, 1984 Adapted from Schribner, BH (ed): Fluid and Electrolyte Balance. Seattle, University of Washington, 1969.)

Potassium salts can be given orally, subcutaneously, or intravenously. The oral route of administration is best if this is clinically feasible. Liquid, wax matrix tablet, and microencapsulated forms are available but as the liquid form is unpalatable, the wax matrix tablet and microencapsulated forms are preferred in small animals because they are the least irritating.[52] If the subcutaneous route is used, the concentration of K^+ should not exceed 30 mEq/L. Intravenous fluids should never exceed 40 mEq/L and such high concentrations should not be delivered intravenously into a central catheter placed in or near the heart.[52]

When calculating the rate of K^+ administration, it is better to err on the slow side than the fast side. With oral supplementation, 0.5 to 1.5 mEq/lb/day (1 to 3 mEq/kg/day) is a reasonable dose range. Intravenous K^+ can be given at 0.063 mEq/lb/hr (0.125 mEq/kg/hr) in mild hypokalemia. In severe K^+ depletion, the rate can be increased as high as 0.25 mEq/lb/hr (0.5 mEq/kg/hr), but this rate never should be exceeded and constant ECG monitoring is advisable during rapid treatment.[71]

The optimal way to manage K^+ depletion is to recognize clinical situations where hypokalemia may develop and provide preventive K^+ supplementation on a maintenance basis. In the face of normal kidney function, maintenance K^+ should be provided in the same quantities as usual dietary intake, 0.25 to 0.5 mEq/lb/day (0.5 to 1 mEq/kg/day). If parenteral routes of administration must be used, this corresponds to adding 12.5 to 25 mEq/L to a maintenance solution given at 20 ml/lb/day (40 ml/kg/day).

The main complication of K^+ supplementation is hyperkalemia and care should be taken to prevent cardiotoxicity, particularly with intravenous treatment. Oral K^+ salts can cause gastrointestinal irritation with vomiting, diarrhea, and melena; medication should then be discontinued.[52]

Hyperkalemia

ETIOLOGY

Hyperkalemia can be caused by excessive K^+ administration, but more commonly results from reduced renal K^+ excretion and a decreased cellular mass to hold the K^+. The most common causes of hyperkalemia in dogs and cats are shown in Table 53–6.

Increased K^+ intake can cause hyperkalemia, but this is very uncommon if renal function is normal—unless the intake is massive, such as in inappropriately high intravenous K^+ administration and with large doses of K^+ penicillin G.

Reduced GFR due to oliguric acute renal failure, very

low GFR in terminal chronic renal failure, urethral obstruction, and traumatic rupture of the urinary tract with peritoneal or retroperitoneal accumulation of urine all induce hyperkalemia due to reduced K^+ excretion. Translocation of K^+ from ICF to ECF may be enhanced due to hypercatabolism in acute renal failure, causing the plasma K^+ concentration to rise very rapidly. Hypoadrenocorticoidism induces hyperkalemia because K^+ secreting pumps in the distal tubule are less active and hyponatremia leads to volume depletion, reduced GFR, and reduced delivery of tubular fluid to distal K^+ secretory sites.

Acidemia due to any cause can increase the plasma K^+ concentration by translocation between the ICF and ECF (Figure 53–4).

CLINICAL SIGNS AND DIAGNOSIS

The signs of hyperkalemia usually develop once plasma K^+ exceeds 6.5 mEq/L. Signs include weakness and cardiac conduction abnormalities usually associated with bradycardia. When ECF K^+ rises, the ratio $[K^+]_I/[K^+]_E$ decreases, the resting membrane potential falls, and muscles, including the myocardium, become hyperexcitable.

Hyperkalemia also slows the pacemaker and conducting functions of the heart and the combined effects may lead to ventricular arrest or fibrillation when plasma K^+ exceeds 8 mEq/L. Typical early ECG changes include tall, peaked T waves, loss of P waves, and wide QRS complexes.[66] Hyperexcitability is not observed in skeletal muscles because when $[K^+]_I/[K^+]_E$ is low, the resting membrane potential decreases to the level of the threshold potential, so repolarization cannot occur and the muscle is no longer excitable.[56] The diagnosis of hyperkalemia is usually apparent from an assessment of the history, physical examination, and routine diagnostic tests.

TREATMENT

In most cases of hyperkalemia, excessively high concentrations of K^+ are confined to the ECF fluid and a total body excess of K^+ does not exist. Treatment strategies serve to antagonize the effects of hyperkalemia on the cell membrane potential, cause translocation of K^+ from the ECF to ICF, and enhance excretion of K^+.

The urgency of strategies used to counteract hyperkalemia should match the severity of ECG abnormalities as well as the degree of hyperkalemia. With severe abnormalities, the ECG should be monitored while calcium, insulin combined with dextrose, and bicarbonate are given intravenously.[72]

A ten per cent solution of calcium gluconate should be given by slow intravenous infusion to provide 0.25 ml/lb (0.5 ml/kg). Raising the ECF calcium concentration reduces the threshold potential to match the reduced membrane potential, thereby restoring the difference between the two potentials necessary for normal function. This effect begins within minutes and lasts about 30 minutes. Regular insulin combined with glucose causes transfer of K^+ from the ECF into the ICF.

TABLE 53–7. NORMAL ARTERIAL AND VENOUS BLOOD GAS VALUES IN DOGS AND CATS

	Canine		Feline	
	Arterial[73]	*Venous*[74]	*Arterial*[73]	*Venous*[75]
pH	7.407 ± 0.028	7.405 ± 0.0097	7.386 ± 0.038	7.300 ± 0.087
PCO_2 (mm Hg)	36.8 ± 3.0	36.6 ± 1.21	31.0 ± 2.9	41.8 ± 9.12
PO_2 (mm Hg)	92.1 ± 5.6	52.1 ± 2.11	106.8 ± 5.7	38.6 ± 11.44
HCO_3^- (mEq/L)	22.2 ± 1.7	22.3 ± 0.43	18.0 ± 1.8	19.4 ± 4.0

Insulin should be given intravenously to dogs at 2.5 U/lb/hr (5 U/kg/hr) and to cats at 0.25 U/lb (0.5 units/kg). Insulin should be combined with glucose at 2 g/unit of insulin. The onset of action takes about 30 minutes and can last several hours. Sodium bicarbonate given at 0.5 to 1 mEq/lb (1 to 2 mEq/kg) also induces transfer of K^+ to the ICF and the effect lasts as long as the effect of insulin combined with glucose.

The above measures are only transient and further treatment is required to enhance excretion of K^+ if the primary cause of hyperkalemia is not corrected. Volume contraction should be corrected and ECF expansion will both dilute ECF K^+ levels and increase renal perfusion, possibly leading to better K^+ excretion. The cation exchange resin, sodium polystyrene sulfonate (Kayexalate), can be given orally or by retention enema at 0.12 to 0.5 g/lb/day (0.5 to 1 g/kg/day) to extract K^+ via the gastrointestinal tract. One gram of the resin removes approximately 1 mEq K^+ in exchange for 1 mEq Na^+.[52] If hyperkalemia persists, dialysis represents the only alternative to further reduce ECF K^+ levels; however, peritoneal dialysis is not so effective in this respect because most reductions in ECF K^+ levels achieved by peritoneal dialysis are due to ICF translocation induced by bicarbonate and glucose in the dialysate.[57]

ACID-BASE IMBALANCE

PHYSIOLOGY OF ACID-BASE

In dogs and cats, the concentration of hydrogen ion (H^+) in ECF is maintained at around 40 mEq/L (pH 7.4), a level necessary for the normal function of many enzyme systems. Values of pH 6.9 and pH 7.8 represent the life-threatening extremes of acid-base imbalance. Control of ECF H^+ concentration is maintained by buffer systems, respiratory regulation of arterial carbon dioxide ($PaCO_2$), and renal regulation of plasma HCO_3^-. The normal values of arterial and venous blood gas for dogs and cats are shown in Table 53–7.[73–75]

Buffer Systems in ECF. A buffer is a weak acid with its conjugate base in solution:

$$\underset{\text{weak acid}}{HA} \rightleftarrows \underset{\text{proton}}{H^+} + \underset{\text{conjugate base}}{A^-}$$

By definition, a weak acid is only partially dissociated and the degree of dissociation in water or strength of an acid can be represented by the constant K, where:

$$K = \frac{[H^+][A^-]}{[HA]} \qquad \text{Equation (1)}$$

$$\text{then: } -\log K = -\log [H^+] - \log\frac{[A^-]}{[HA]}$$

$$\text{and: } -\log [H^+] = -\log K + \log\frac{[A^-]}{[HA]}$$

This expression can be converted into the clinically useful logarithmic form, the Henderson-Hasselbalch equation:

$$pH = pK + \log\frac{[\text{base}]}{[\text{acid}]} \ (\text{where } p = -\log)$$

Thus when pH equals pK, the concentration of base equals the concentration of acid. Buffers are most effective within 1 pH unit of their pK.

The major buffers in ECF are the bicarbonate-carbonic acid system, hemoglobin, and bone. Hemoglobin is not actually present in ECF, but being in red blood cells, it works rapidly in concert with bicarbonate ECF buffer. Other very powerful buffer systems in intracellular fluid include organic phosphates and protein. In the steady state, all buffers are in equilibrium with each other, so measurement of one system indicates the status of all buffers according to the following formula:

$$pH = pK_1 + \log\frac{[B_1^-]}{[HB_1]} = pK_2 + \log\frac{[B_2^-]}{[HB_2]} = pK_3 + \log\frac{[B_3^-]}{[HB_3]}$$

The relative contribution of each buffer system to the total buffering capacity varies with the pK and the concentration of the buffer. When a strong acid is infused into ECF, the bicarbonate system contributes to 42 per cent of the buffering, hemoglobin to 6 per cent, and intracellular protein and organic phosphates to 51 per cent.[76] However, the bicarbonate system is more important initially because it is readily available in ECF, while the ICF buffers and bone take several hours to be fully activated due to the time required for the H^+ load to diffuse evenly throughout the body. Two other factors contribute to the bicarbonate system being the most important buffer in ECF: large quantities of HCO_3^- exist in ECF and the bicarbonate system has both pulmonary and renal control of excretion.

$$\underset{\text{pulmonary control}}{CO_2} + H_2O \leftrightarrows H_2CO_3 \leftrightarrows H^+ + \underset{\text{renal control}}{HCO_3^-} \qquad \text{Reaction (1)}$$

The Henderson-Hasselbalch equation relative to the bicarbonate system is as follows:

$$pH = pK + \log\frac{[HCO_3^-]}{[H_2CO_3]}$$

Carbonic acid is difficult to measure directly, but at the pH of ECF there is a fixed relationship between $PaCO_2$ and $[H_2CO_3]$ such that $[H_2CO_3] = 0.03\ pCO_2$ and the Henderson-Hasselbalch equation can be rewritten in the clinically useful form:

$$pH = 6.1 + \log\frac{[HCO_3^-]}{0.03\ PaCO_2} \qquad \text{Equation (2)}$$

Thus, pulmonary control of $PaCO_2$ and renal control of plasma HCO_3^- are able to control ECF pH.

Respiratory Control of Carbon Dioxide. Oxidative metabolism in normal dogs and cats produces 150 to 250 mM CO_2/kg/day, which generates large amounts of acid by driving reaction (1) to the right. As CO_2 production leads to H^+ formation, it is called volatile acid.

At the tissue level the reaction $CO_2 + H_2O \leftrightarrows H_2CO_3 \leftrightarrows H^+ + HCO_3^-$ is driven to the right, catalyzed by red blood cell carbonic anhydrase. The H^+ formed is buffered by hemoglobin, while most of the HCO_3^- is carried to the lungs in plasma. Respiratory tidal volume and rate are controlled by many factors, the most important of which are the extremely sensitive medullary receptors that respond to CSF pCO_2 and pH. Also, the carotid body chemoreceptors respond to hypoxia, hypercarbia, and reduced ECF pH. So pulmonary function is controlled based on ECF $PaCO_2$ and pH and increases or decreases from the normal values result in immediate changes in ventilation.

Renal Control of Plasma Bicarbonate. Dogs and cats usually eat a diet rich in meat protein from which there is a net production of 0.5 to 2 mM/kg/day of organic and inorganic acids that are not derived from CO_2. For example, sulfuric acid is produced from metabolism of sulfur-containing amino acids including methionine:

$$\underset{\text{methionine}}{2\ C_5H_{11}NO_2S} + 15O_2 \leftrightarrows 4H^+ + 2SO_4^{2-} + \underset{\text{urea}}{CO(NH_2)_2}$$

These acids are neither volatile nor in equilibrium with a volatile component, so they are known as nonvolatile or fixed acids. On occasion, endogenous production of fixed acids can be excessive, as in lactic acid production during muscular work and acetoacetic acid and beta-hydroxybutyric acid production in uncontrolled diabetes mellitus. The H^+ generated by fixed acids entering ECF is buffered by bicarbonate driving reaction (1) to the left, so that buffer tends to become depleted. However, the kidneys are able to excrete H^+ and reclaim HCO_3^- consumed in the buffering process. Renal control of plasma HCO_3^- is mediated by control of HCO_3^- reabsorption, titratable acid excretion, and ammonium excretion (Figure 53–6).

In the normal kidney of a healthy animal, almost all filtered HCO_3^- is reabsorbed. However, virtually total reabsorption or massive excretion can occur in response to alterations of plasma HCO_3^-, $PaCO_2$, and plasma pH. Renal excretion of the titratable acid orthophosphate allows simultaneous excretion of H^+ according to the following reaction: $HPO_4^{2-} + H^+ \leftrightarrows H_2PO_4^-$. The extent to which this reaction is driven to the right depends on tubular fluid pH, which is in part a reflection of the ECF H^+ concentration. Intracellular generation of H^+ for secretion into the tubule is accompanied by formation of HCO_3^- that transfers into the peritubular capillary. In this manner, HCO_3^- that is consumed when

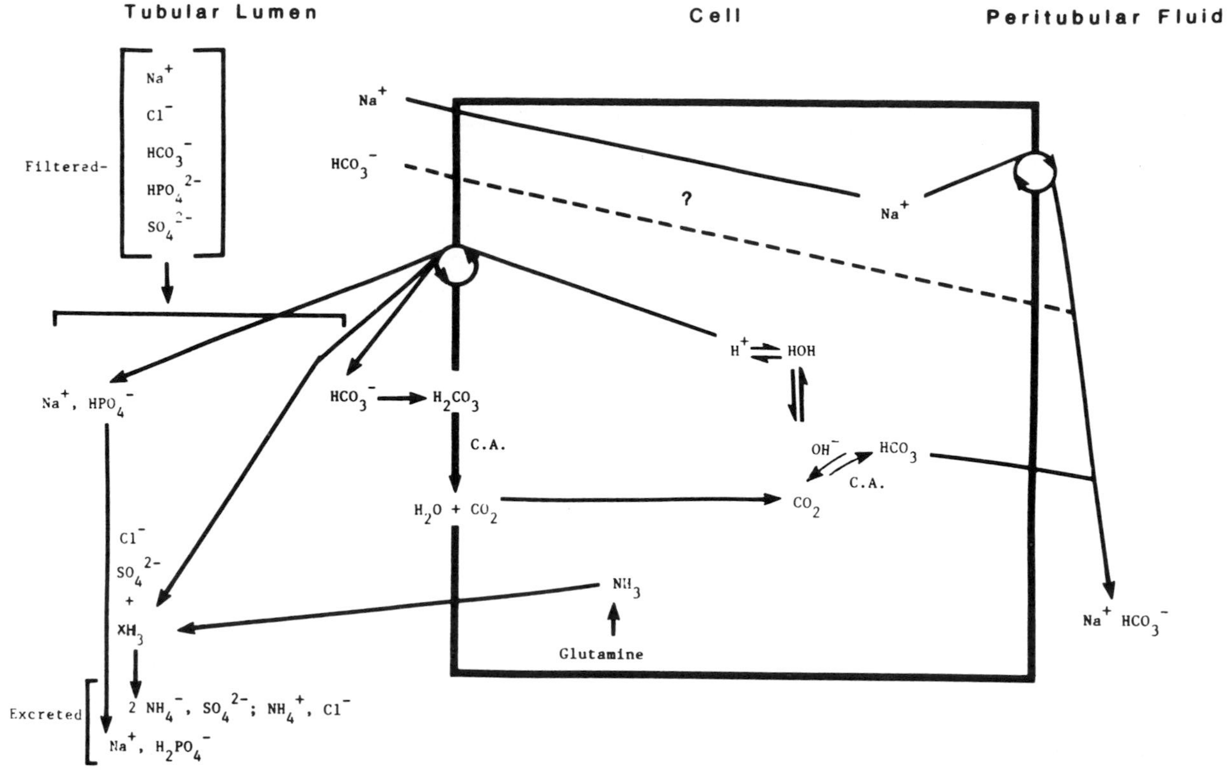

Figure 53–6. The various means by which the kidneys help maintain H^+ balance. Although each mechanism occurs in virtually all parts of the nephron, some processes predominate in one part (e.g., titration of filtered HCO_3^- in the proximal tubule), while others predominate in another part (e.g., titration of NH_3 in the collecting duct). (Reprinted with permission from Valtin, H: Renal Function: Mechanisms Preserving Fluid and Solute Balance in Health, 2nd ed, Little, Brown and Company, 1983, p. 241.)

buffering phosphates and other acids in the diet is reclaimed when orthophosphate undergoes renal excretion. The renal tubules are also capable of generating NH_3 from glutamine and after diffusion into the tubular lumen, NH_3 can accept secreted H^+ according to the following reaction: $NH_3 + H^+ \leftrightharpoons NH_4^+$. Thus, NH_3 acts as a urinary buffer. As tubular NH_3 production can adapt to altered acid-base balance and maximum production is enormous, the NH_3 buffer system is the most adaptive and important mechanism of H^+ excretion in the kidney. The system demonstrates "ion-trapping," whereby lipid-soluble NH_3 readily diffuses across the apical renal tubular cell membrane into the lumen. Once NH_3 is converted to poorly lipid-soluble NH_4^+, back diffusion cannot take place. Once again, as with excretion of titratable acid, intracellular H^+ production is associated with generation of HCO_3^- that reenters the ECF pool via the peritubular capillary. Therefore, NH_4^+ excretion is able to reclaim HCO_3^- that was consumed buffering strong acids that entered the ECF from the diet and metabolism. As the three mechanisms of renal control are influenced by ECF HCO_3^-, $PaCO_2$, and pH, renal control of ECF HCO_3^- concentration is appropriate to overall acid-base homeostasis.

Collection of Blood Samples. Arterial blood from dogs and cats can be collected from the femoral artery, while venous blood can be collected from any vein. Care must be taken to collect venous samples from free-flowing veins that have not been tourniqueted for a prolonged period. Arterial blood is preferred to venous blood because it is more consistent, more suitable for complete interpretation of blood gas values, and better for assessment of pulmonary function. Arterial blood is higher in O_2, slightly lower in pCO_2 and HCO_3^-, and slightly higher in pH than venous blood.

Acid-Base Disturbances. The bicarbonate buffer system is used to determine acid-base status in clinical medicine for several reasons: It is a major ECF buffer, it is in equilibrium with all other buffer systems, the volatile component CO_2 allows direct assessment of pulmonary function, and $PaCO_2$ is convenient to measure. Variations in plasma pH, HCO_3^-, and $PaCO_2$ constitute disturbances of acid-base balance and terms to describe changes in each variable are well established in clinical medicine.

alkalosis

metabolic

alkalemia

acidosis

$$pH = 6.1 + \log \frac{[HCO_3^-]}{0.03\ PaCO_2}$$

acidemia

acidosis

respiratory

alkalosis

Acidemia refers to reduced plasma pH and animals in this condition are said to be acidotic. Alkalemia refers to increased plasma pH and animals in this condition are said to be alkalotic.

Metabolic acidosis means a primary decrease in plasma HCO_3^-. Metabolic alkalosis means a primary increase in plasma HCO_3^-. Respiratory acidosis means a primary increase in plasma $PaCO_2$. Respiratory alkalosis means a primary decrease in plasma $PaCO_2$. The term primary denotes that the disturbance referred to is

TABLE 53–8. RELATIONSHIP BETWEEN HCO_3^- AND $PaCO_2$ IN SIMPLE ACID-BASE DISTURBANCES

Primary Disturbance	Expected Compensatory Responses
Metabolic acidosis	Δ $PaCO_2$ mm Hg = 1.2 × Δ HCO_3^- mEq/L
Metabolic alkalosis	Δ $PaCO_2$ mm Hg = 0.6 × Δ HCO_3^- mEq/L
Respiratory acidosis	
(acute)	Δ HCO_3^- mEq/L = 0.1 × Δ $PaCO_2$ mm Hg
(chronic)	Δ HCO_3^- mEq/L = 0.4 × Δ $PaCO_2$ mm Hg
Respiratory alkalosis	
(acute)	Δ HCO_3^- mEq/L = 0.1–0.3 × Δ $PaCO_2$ mm Hg
(chronic)	Δ HCO_3^- mEq/L = 0.2–0.5 × Δ $PaCO_2$ mm Hg

the initiating event and the pH is shifted, at least initially, in the same direction. So a primary metabolic acidosis refers to decreased plasma HCO_3^- as an initiating event that tends to cause acidemia or reduced pH. When a primary disturbance occurs there is always a secondary or compensatory response that tends to return plasma pH toward, but not completely back to, normal. So a primary metabolic acidosis (decrease in HCO_3^-) leads to a compensatory respiratory alkalosis (decrease in $PaCO_2$). The plasma pH initially falls (acidemia) but the compensatory response almost corrects it back to normal (mild acidemia). The expected compensatory responses for each primary disturbance have been established in human medicine and variations from these responses represent mixed acid-base disturbances in which both metabolic and respiratory disturbances are involved. The expected compensatory responses to primary disturbances of acid-base balance are shown in Table 53–8.[77]

METABOLIC ACIDOSIS

Metabolic acidosis is a primary reduction in plasma HCO_3^- to less than 17 mEq/L in dogs and 15 mEq/L in cats. Influx of a fixed acid consumes bicarbonate and other buffers, drives reaction (1) to the right, and causes acidemia according to equation (1).

COMPENSATION

The normal responses to an acid load involve buffers, respiratory compensation, and renal correction. The buffer response is extremely rapid. The bicarbonate system accounts for about 40 per cent of the buffering within minutes, while intracellular buffers such as hemoglobin, protein, and organic phosphates account for the rest within hours.[76] Reduced HCO_3^- and elevated $PaCO_2$ reduce ECF pH, leading to activation of chemoreceptors that stimulate respiration. Hyperventilation with reduced $PaCO_2$ is the compensatory response that tends to return ECF pH back to normal. In humans, normal respiratory compensation after 12 to 24 hours is a 1.2 mm Hg decrease in $PaCO_2$ for every 1.0 mEq/L decrease in plasma HCO_3^- (Table 53–8).[77] A greater or lesser response suggests the presence of a mixed acid-base disorder. Following rapid activation of buffers and respiratory compensation, metabolic acidosis due to an acid load can be corrected by renal H^+ excretion. The main adaptive renal mechanism of H^+ excretion is the generation of NH_3. After infusion of a large acid load, renal production of NH_3 takes at least five days to reach a maximum level, and at this point, renal H^+ excretion can be five to ten times normal levels.[78,79] Once the acid load is excreted, ECF pH returns to normal and renal NH_3 production returns to an appropriately low level.

ETIOLOGY

Metabolic acidosis can be caused by the addition of a strong acid to ECF, loss of HCO_3^- from ECF, or ECF expansion with a bicarbonate-poor solution. The more common causes of metabolic acidosis are shown in Table 53–9.

In diabetes mellitus, an absolute or relative lack of insulin can lead to hepatic overproduction of acetoacetic and beta-hydroxybutyric acids from acetyl-CoA, which is derived from fatty acid precursors.[80] The increased acid production leads to metabolic acidosis and acidemia. Concurrent hyperglycemia and glucosuria cause renal K^+ wasting and the total body K^+ level may be reduced. However, plasma K^+ concentration is usually normal because of H^+ exchange for K^+ between the ECF and the ICF (Figure 53–4). Lactic acidosis usually results from increased production of lactic acid during tissue hypoxia, as occurs in shock. Azotemia is associated with metabolic acidosis because of reduced tubular ability to produce ammonia and thus secrete H^+.[78] In renal failure, retention of fixed acids leads to an elevated anion gap, but the gap is not generally very high. Ethylene glycol ingestion enhances production of several acids, including glycolic acid, glyoxylic acid, and oxalic acid, leading to fairly severe metabolic acidosis with a very wide anion gap and osmolar gap.[81,82]

Severe acute and chronic diarrhea can lead to simultaneous loss of Na^+, K^+, and HCO_3^- with normal anion gap metabolic acidosis. Renal tubular acidosis (RTA), both proximal and distal, leads to metabolic acidosis because of impaired tubular H^+ secretion. Proximal RTA usually is associated with other transport defects for glucose, phosphate, and amino acids, as in the Fanconi syndrome of basenji dogs.[63] Excessive ammonium chloride administration for urinary acidification in cats causes mild metabolic acidosis and individual cats can develop severe metabolic acidosis (HCO_3^- less than 12 mEq/L) with hypokalemia.

CLINICAL SIGNS AND DIAGNOSIS

In most conditions causing metabolic acidosis, the clinical signs are those of the initiating disease rather

TABLE 53–9. CAUSES OF METABOLIC ACIDOSIS

Normal Anion Gap	Increased Anion Gap
Diarrhea	Azotemia
Renal tubular acidosis	acute renal failure
proximal—Fanconi syndrome	chronic renal failure
distal—amphotericin B	Diabetic ketoacidosis
Drugs	Lactic acidosis
acetazolamide	cardiac arrest
NH_4Cl administration	shock
	hypoxemia
	Toxins
	ethylene glycol
	metaldehyde

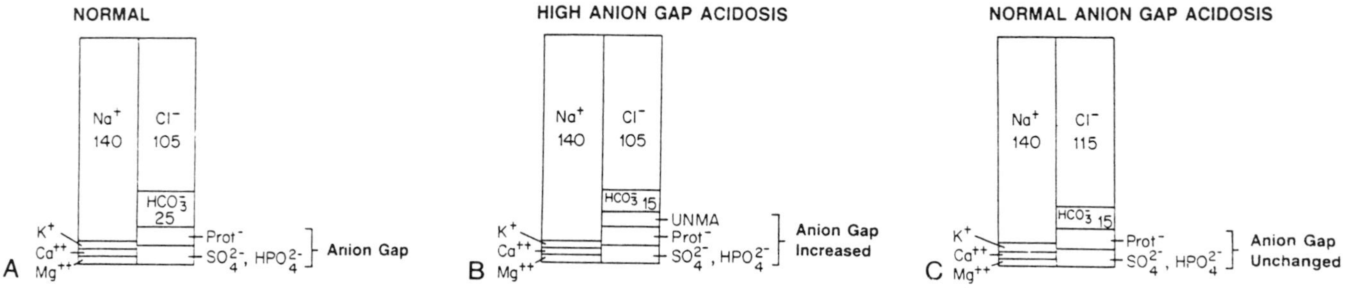

Figure 53–7. *A,* Normal plasma cation and anion composition. *B,* High anion gap acidosis as non-HCl acid titrates ECF bicarbonate (e.g., lactic acid), bicarbonate is stoichiometrically replaced with the acid anion, resulting in an increase in the calculated anion gap. *C,* Normal anion gap acidosis. When ECF bicarbonate is titrated by HCl, bicarbonate consumed is stoichiometrically replaced by chloride, resulting in hyperchloremic acidosis. (Reprinted with permission from Toto, RD: Metabolic acid-base disorders. *In* Kokko, JP and Tannen, RL: Fluids and Electrolytes. WB Saunders Company, 1986, p. 249.)

than those due to metabolic acidosis per se. However, the signs of severe metabolic acidosis may include hypotension and deep, rapid respiration (Kussmaul breathing). Laboratory findings include reduced plasma pH, reduced plasma HCO_3^- and pH with reduced $PaCO_2$ as compensation. Plasma K^+ may be normal or increased even if total body K^+ is depleted because of a shift of K^+ from ICF to ECF due to acidemia (Figure 53–4).

Serum electrolyte values allow calculation of the anion gap as follows:

$$\text{Anion gap} = [Na^+] - ([Cl^-] + [HCO_3^-]).$$

The anion gap allows differentiation of some causes of metabolic acidosis (Table 53–9).[83] Production of organic acids causes depletion of HCO_3^- stores with a subsequent increase in anion gap, whereas loss of HCO_3^- in diarrhea or renal tubular acidosis is matched by an equivalent renal retention of Cl^- and the anion gap remains unchanged. The normal anion gap is 5 to 20 mEq/L in dogs and 10 to 30 mEq/L in cats.[73] The cause of metabolic acidosis usually can be determined from careful review of the history, physical examination, and laboratory test results.

TREATMENT

The first priority in treating metabolic acidosis is accurate identification and treatment of the primary cause. No further treatment is usually required and in many instances intravenous alkali treatment should be considered only if plasma pH is less than 7.1 to 7.2.

The organic acidoses, such as ketoacidosis in diabetes mellitus and lactic acidosis in shock, rarely require HCO_3^- treatment except for a small initial dose to raise the plasma pH to 7.1 if the patient is extremely acidemic.[84] Once the primary cause is corrected, both ketoacids and lactate are rapidly converted to bicarbonate and metabolic acidosis corrects itself.[84] The deficit of HCO_3^- is extremely difficult to calculate because the distribution of HCO_3^- and the rate of acid production are variable. In those few cases where the plasma pH is less than 7.1, it is best to empirically treat with 0.5 mEq/lb (1 mEq/kg) HCO_3^- intravenously and then recheck the acid-base status. If too much HCO_3^- is given, rapid metabolism of ketoacids or lactate can lead to metabolic alkalosis and severe overshoot alkalemia once excessive organic acid production is stopped.

When metabolic acidosis is caused by a process other than an excess of organic acids, such as in diarrhea, renal tubular acidosis, and ammonium chloride intoxication, bicarbonate needs can be crudely calculated. The bicarbonate distribution varies between 30 per cent and 80 per cent of body weight, depending on the degree of acidemia.[85,86] As acidemia worsens, intracellular buffering of the increased acid load increases, so that administered alkali appears to be distributed in a space much larger than the ECF space. Calculated bicarbonate need based on a bicarbonate distribution of 30 per cent of body weight is:

$$\text{Bicarbonate deficit} = \text{BW (kg)} \times 0.3 \times (\text{desired} - \text{observed plasma } HCO_3^-).$$

If plasma pH is less than 7.1, the bicarbonate distribution may have to be increased to as high as 80 per cent. In making the calculation, it is wise to aim at a plasma HCO_3^- of 15 mEq/L to avoid overshoot alkalemia.[87] In severe acidemia (pH less than 7.1), 25 per cent of the calculated dose may be given by bolus over 10 to 15 minutes so that plasma pH rises above 7.1. Then the balance can be given over the following 12 to 18 hours. In less urgent circumstances, the deficit should be corrected gradually over 12 to 24 hours. Interstitial HCO_3^- distribution takes 30 minutes, while ICF distribution requires up to 18 hours.[88] If accurate blood-gas or total HCO_3^- estimations are unavailable but metabolic acidosis is strongly suspected based on clinical history and signs, a total dose of 0.5 to 1 mEq/lb (1 to 2 mEq/kg) HCO_3^- may be given empirically.

Several HCO_3^- precursors, such as lactate, gluconate, and acetate, are available but they all require metabolism to HCO_3^- to be effective. Lactate is converted to HCO_3^- by the liver, a process that is impaired by severe acidemia and reduced hepatic perfusion.[14] So isotonic $NaHCO_3^-$ is the best replacement solution because it requires no metabolism to convert it into the active form.

Several precautions must be taken to avoid serious complications associated with alkali treatment. Careless use of hypertonic $NaHCO_3^-$ solutions can easily cause excessive ECF fluid expansion and dangerous hyperosmolality. Rapid HCO_3^- infusion can lead to hypocalcemic tetany because a large proportion of plasma calcium can be converted to the inactive nonionized form bound to plasma proteins.[14] Paradoxical CSF acidosis with seizures may occur when rapid HCO_3^- treatment corrects plasma pH and inhibits compensatory hyperventilation. When plasma $PaCO_2$ increases toward normal, CO_2 rapidly diffuses into the CSF.[89] However, HCO_3^- cannot diffuse into the CSF at such a fast rate and the CSF can become dangerously acidic until HCO_3^- diffusion reaches equilibrium. Rapid HCO_3^- infusion can cause hypokalemia as K^+ enters ICF in exchange for H^+ (Figure 53–4), so simultaneous K^+ supplementation may be necessary.[84] Alkali treatment increases plasma pH, shifting the oxygen-hemoglobin dissociation curve to the left so that O_2 release from hemoglobin is reduced.[84] This may be a significant factor in lactic acidosis in shock where tissue O_2 requirements are poorly met to begin with.

METABOLIC ALKALOSIS

Accumulation of ECF HCO_3^- consumes H^+, drives reaction (1) to the left, and causes alkalemia according to equation (1). Metabolic alkalosis is due to an increase in plasma HCO_3^- above 24 mEq/L.

COMPENSATION

The normal response to an alkaline load involves buffers, respiratory compensation, and renal correction. Almost all of the H^+ used to buffer ECF HCO_3^- comes from ICF protein and organic phosphates. Respiratory compensation involves hypoventilation with an increase in $PaCO_2$. Hypoventilation is mediated by interstitial H^+ receptors in the CNS, but the extent to which hypoventilation can increase $PaCO_2$ and compensate for metabolic alkalosis is limited by the need for adequate PaO_2. In humans, a normal response results in a 0.6 to 0.7 mm Hg increase in $PaCO_2$ for every 1.0 mEq/l increase in plasma HCO_3^- (Table 53–8).[77] The renal response to metabolic alkalosis is rapid excretion of excess HCO_3^- to return plasma HCO_3^- to normal. However, metabolic alkalosis can persist when the normal renal response is prevented by ECF volume depletion. In ECF volume depletion, tubular sodium reabsorption necessitates concurrent anion reabsorption, including HCO_3^-, so metabolic alkalosis is maintained until ECF volume depletion is corrected.[84] This situation is exacerbated by concurrent K^+ depletion because sodium is reabsorbed in the distal tubule in exchange for K^+ or H^+. In K^+ depletion, intracellular K^+ is less readily available, so H^+ is preferentially secreted in exchange for Na^+ reabsorption. Secreted H^+ is associated with HCO_3^- entry into the ECF, which maintains the metabolic acidosis.[90] Thus, the kidneys appear to sacrifice acid-base balance and maintain metabolic alkalosis in an effort to maintain ECF volume. Hypokalemic ECF volume depletion with enhanced H^+ secretion in the distal tubule causes so-called "paradoxical aciduria" in the face of metabolic alkalosis.[14] Although K^+ depletion may contribute to the maintenance of metabolic alkalosis, it is unlikely to be a primary cause of metabolic alkalosis in dogs.[91,92]

ETIOLOGY

Vomiting, diuretic use, and excessive alkali administration are the most common causes of metabolic alkalosis. Vomiting associated with pyloric outflow obstruction causes loss of H^+ from the body with addition of HCO_3^- to the ECF. As vomiting is associated with ECF volume depletion, renal secretion of H^+ in exchange for Na^+ reabsorption in the distal tubule is enhanced, thus maintaining metabolic alkalosis.[84] Diuretic treatment with loop diuretics such as furosemide and thiazide diuretics causes loss of Cl^- in disproportionate amounts to the loss of HCO_3^-.[93] Thus, ECF volume depletion occurs in the face of relative HCO_3^- retention. Once again, avid distal Na^+ reabsorption in the face of ECF volume causes the metabolic alkalosis to be maintained.

CLINICAL SIGNS AND DIAGNOSIS

The signs of metabolic alkalosis are nonspecific and patients usually manifest signs characteristic of the disease process, causing metabolic alkalosis. In severe metabolic alkalosis muscle twitches and tetany may occur and affected animals are much more likely to have ventricular arrhythmias. The usual laboratory findings include elevated plasma pH, elevated plasma HCO_3^-, elevated $PaCO_2$, reduced plasma Cl^-, and often, reduced plasma K^+. Clinical circumstances may suggest metabolic alkalosis but the diagnosis is confirmed by the presence of an elevated plasma HCO_3^- level.

TREATMENT

When kidney function is normal, metabolic alkalosis rapidly responds to ECF fluid expansion with the replacement electrolyte solution 0.9 per cent NaCl. Provision of adequate Cl^- allows reabsorption of Cl^- instead of HCO_3^- with Na^+ in the proximal tubule. Bicarbonate retained in the renal tubule overwhelms distal reabsorptive sites and is excreted in the urine. Furthermore, as NaCl treatment reduces the need for avid distal Na^+ reabsorption, continued secretion of H^+ in exchange for Na^+ is reduced, so tubular cell generation of HCO_3^- is suppressed. With concurrent hypokalemia, intravenous fluids may need to be supplemented with K^+.

RESPIRATORY ACIDOSIS

Respiratory acidosis occurs when $PaCO_2^-$ rises above the normal level of 40 mm Hg. Hypercapnia results from decreased effective alveolar ventilation so that CO_2 production transiently exceeds CO_2 excretion. The $PaCO_2$ rises until a new steady state is reached where excretion equals production. Elevated $PaCO_2$ drives reaction (1) to the right and causes acidemia according to equation (1).

COMPENSATION

The defenses against respiratory acidosis include rapid buffering, renal compensation, and final correction by improved respiratory function. As increased $PaCO_2$ leads to elevated H_2CO_3 levels, the bicarbonate system cannot contribute to rapid buffering. Protein in ECF makes a small contribution to buffering, but most H^+ (about 97 per cent) combines with protein, organic phosphates, and hemoglobin in the ICF.[76] Renal compensation consists of tubular H^+ excretion and HCO_3^- retention stimulated by decreased pH and elevated $PaCO_2$. The excess H^+ secretion is buffered in the tubular lumen by NH_3 formed in renal tubular cells. Final correction of respiratory acidosis occurs when effective alveolar ventilation returns to normal.

During the first 12 to 24 hours after the onset of respiratory acidosis, buffers offer the entire defense against altered pH. In humans, the usual compensation is a 1 mEq/L increase in plasma HCO_3^- for every 10 mm Hg increase in $PaCO_2$ (Table 53–8).[77] In chronic pulmonary disease the compensatory changes in plasma HCO_3^- reflect both renal and buffer defense against pH change. Appropriate compensation is approximately a 4 mEq/L increase in plasma HCO_3^- for every 10 mm Hg increase in $PaCO_2$ (Table 53–8). Renal compensation requires about five days.[94]

CLINICAL SIGNS

The signs of respiratory acidosis are those of the primary respiratory disease, which may include dyspnea, tachypnea, restlessness, and stupor, ultimately leading to coma. Typical laboratory findings include decreased plasma pH, elevated $PaCO_2$, slightly elevated plasma HCO_3^-, and reduced PaO_2. The causes of respiratory acidosis are discussed in Chapters 68, 69, and 70 (Table 53–10).

TREATMENT

Treatment of acute respiratory acidosis should be aimed at restoring effective ventilation. Aminophylline may assist alveolar ventilation in some patients and mechanical ventilation may be necessary. If correction of the pulmonary disturbance is to be delayed, sufficient HCO_3^- to increase pH above 7.2 may be given, but further HCO_3^- treatment should be avoided because correction of the respiratory problem can induce severe alkalemia if HCO_3^- treatment has been excessive.[95] Treatment of chronic respiratory acidosis also involves treatment of the primary cause. However, this is frequently impossible because chronic pulmonary diseases are often irreversible. Oxygen supplementation without ventilation may induce life-threatening respiratory acidosis because animals with chronic hypercapnia maintain ventilation by hypoxic drive.[96] When increased O_2 is delivered without ventilation, the PaO_2 rises, the stimulation for ventilation decreases, and $PaCO_2$ can increase to very high levels, leading to severe acidemia, cardiac arrhythmias, coma, and death.

TABLE 53–10. CAUSES OF RESPIRATORY ACIDOSIS AND ALKALOSIS

Respiratory Acidosis	Respiratory Alkalosis
Neuromuscular Disturbances	*Central Stimulation*
Tick paralysis	Anxiety
Polyradiculoneuritis	CNS disease
Narcotic, sedative, or tranquilizer overdose	Fever
	Pain
Myasthenia gravis	*Peripheral Stimulation*
Organophosphate intoxication	Pneumonia
Severe hypothyroidism	Interstitial lung disease
Respiratory Disorders	*Other*
Airway obstruction	Gram-negative septicemia
Pneumothorax	Mechanical hyperventilation
Pleural effusion	
Severe pneumonia	
Severe pulmonary edema	
Diffuse metastatic disease	
Massive pulmonary embolism	
Cardiopulmonary arrest	

Respiratory Alkalosis

Respiratory alkalosis refers to reduced $PaCO_2$ below the normal level that occurs when CO_2 excretion by the lungs exceeds tissue production. Hyperventilation reduces $PaCO_2$, driving reaction (1) to the left and causing alkalemia according to equation (1).

COMPENSATION

The defense against respiratory alkalosis involves rapidly acting buffers, renal compensation, and correction of hyperventilation. Intracellular hemoglobin, protein, and phosphate buffers contribute to 97 per cent of the buffer activity, giving up H^+ to the ECF.[76] Buffer defenses are complete within 30 minutes to two hours and plasma HCO_3^- can decrease by 1 to 3 mEq/L for every 10 mm Hg reduction in $PaCO_2$ (Table 53–8).[77] Renal compensation is mediated by reduced tubular reabsorption of HCO_3^- and reduced secretion of H^+ in the distal tubule. Full renal compensation is complete within one to two days, and plasma HCO_3^- can decrease by 2 to 5 mEq/L for every 10 mm Hg decrease in $PaCO_2$ (Table 53–8). Final correction of respiratory alkalosis requires reestablishment of normal ventilation.

The signs of respiratory alkalosis are usually those of the underlying condition causing hyperventilation. If alkalemia is severe, tetany, seizures, and cardiac arrhythmias may be seen. Laboratory evaluation reveals elevated plasma pH, reduced $PaCO_2$, reduced plasma HCO_3^-, and slightly elevated plasma Cl^-. Causes of respiratory alkalosis are shown in Table 53–10. Treatment requires correction of hyperventilation.

MIXED ACID-BASE DISORDERS

Mixed acid-base disturbances occur when two conditions that affect acid-base balance occur concurrently in the same patient, such as metabolic acidosis and respiratory acidosis.[77] Mixed disturbances can be diagnosed when the expected compensation for a suspected primary disturbance fails to develop (Table 53–8). For example, in a dog with ethylene glycol intoxication, the following blood gas values are found: pH 7.15, HCO_3^- 15 mEq/L, and $PaCO_2$ 45 mm Hg. The drop in HCO_3^- below normal is $22-15 = 7$ mEq/L. The expected respiratory response for this drop in HCO_3^- should cause a $PaCO_2$ decrease by 1.2 times HCO_3^- to 25 mm Hg. The measured $PaCO_2$ is 45 mm Hg, so the dog has concurrent metabolic acidosis and respiratory acidosis. When the compensatory changes fail to fall within the expected range, the patient must be evaluated for possible causes of the second acid-base disturbance. In this case, the respiratory acidosis should be pursued diagnostically with thoracic radiographs and could be due to aspiration pneumonia. Even if the $PaCO_2$ or HCO_3^- values fall within the normal range, they still may represent an acid-base disturbance if the expected compensation means the value should be much higher or lower. In the case example given, a $PaCO_2$ of 37 mm Hg would still represent respiratory acidosis because the expected compensated value is 25 mm Hg.

When mixed disturbances alter pH in the same direction, for example, metabolic acidosis combined with respiratory acidosis, extremely dangerous plasma pH values may develop. However, when disturbances alter pH in different directions, for example, metabolic alkalosis combined with respiratory acidosis, the plasma pH may be nearly normal.

Mixed acid-base disturbances often require that both conditions be treated at once. When the disturbances have a concurrent effect on lowering or raising plasma pH, dangerous values inconsistent with survival often develop and immediate treatment is required to return plasma pH toward normal by whatever means are available. When the disturbances have a disparate effect, plasma pH may be near normal but treatment of one condition without the other will cause plasma pH values to deviate from normal. That is, the second disturbance will be unmasked.

References

1. Altman, PL and Dittmer, DS: Biology Data Book. 2nd ed, Bethesda Federation of American Societies for Experimental Biology Vol 3, 1974.
2. Gamble, JL: Chemical anatomy, physiology and pathology of extracellular fluid. 6th ed, Cambridge, Harvard University Press, p 5, 1967.
3. Donnan, FG: Theorie der membrangleichgewichte und membranpotentiale bei vorhandensein von nicht dialysierenden elektrolyten. Ein beitrag zur physikalisch-chemischen physiologie. Z Elektrochem 17:572, 1911.
4. Starling, EH: Physiological factors involved in the causation of dropsy. Lancet 1:1407, 1896.
5. Guyton, AC, et al.: Effects of pressoreceptor reflex and Cushing's reflex on urinary output. Fed Proc 11:61, 1952.
6. Davis, JO and Howell, DS: Mechanisms of fluid and electrolyte retention in experimental preparations in dogs. II. With thoracic inferior vena cava constriction. Circ Res 1:171, 1953.
7. Andersson, B: Central control of body fluid homeostasis. Proc Aust Physiol Pharmacol Soc 5:139, 1974.
8. Passo, SS, et al.: Hepatic receptors in control of sodium excretion in anesthetized cats. Am J Physiol 224:373, 1972.
9. Brenner, BM, et al.: The relationship between peritubular capillary protein concentration and fluid reabsorption by the renal proximal tubule. J Clin Invest 48:1579, 1969.
10. Bello-Reuss, E, et al.: Effect of renal sympathetic nerve stimulation on proximal water and sodium reabsorption. J Clin Invest 57:1104, 1976.
11. Schwartz, GJ and Burg, MB: Mineralocorticoid effects on cation transport by cortical collecting tubules in vitro. Am J Physiol 235:F576, 1978.
12. Stokes, JB and Kokko, JP: Inhibition of sodium transport by prostaglandin E_2 across the isolated perfused rabbit collecting tubule. J Clin Invest 59:1099, 1977.
13. Maack, T, et al.: Effects of auriculin (atrial natriuretic factor) on blood pressure, renal function and the renin-aldosterone system in dogs. Am J Med 77:1069, 1984.
14. DiBartola, SP: Disorders of fluid, acid-base and electrolyte balance. *In* Sherding, RG (ed): Medical Emergencies. New York, Churchill Livingstone p 137, 1985.
15. Brasmer, TH: Fluid therapy in shock. JAVMA 174:475, 1979.
16. Cornelius, LM, et al.: Physiologic effects of rapid infusion of Ringer's lactate solution into dogs. Am J Vet Res 39(7):1185, 1978.
17. Bjorling, DE and Rawlings, CA: Relationship of intravenous administration of Ringer's lactate solution to pulmonary edema in halothane-anesthetized cats. Am J Vet Res 44(6):1000, 1983.
18. Schwartz, WB, et al.: Role of anions in metabolic acidosis and potassium deficiency. N Engl J Med 279:630, 1968.
19. Cornelius, LM and Rawlings, CA: Arterial blood gas and acid-base values in dogs with various diseases and signs of disease. JAVMA 178(9):992, 1981.
20. Weinberg, JM: Fluid and electrolyte disorders and gastrointestinal diseases. *In* Kokko, JP, Tannen, RL (eds) Fluids and Electrolytes. Philadelphia, WB Saunders Co, p 742, 1986.
21. Cowgill, LD: Acute renal failure. *In* Bovee, KC (ed): Canine Nephrology. Media, PA, Harwal Publishing Co, p 405, 1984.
22. McKeown, JW: Disorders of total body sodium. *In* Kokko, JP, Tannen, RL (eds): Fluids and Electrolytes. Philadelphia, WB Saunders Co, p 63, 1986.
23. Levy, M and Allotey, JB: Temporal relationships between urinary salt retention and altered systemic hemodynamics in dogs with experimental cirrhosis. J Lab Clin Med 92:560, 1978.
24. Robertson, GL, et al.: Development and clinical application of a new method for the radio-immunoassay of arginine vasopressin in human plasma. J Clin Invest 52:2340, 1973.
25. Robertson, GL and Athar, S: The interaction of blood osmolality and blood volume in regulating plasma vasopressin in man. J Clin Endocrinol Metab 42:613, 1976.
26. Berl, T, et al.: Effects of alpha- and beta-adrenergic stimulation on renal water excretion in normal subjects and patients with diabetes insipidus. Kid Int 6:247, 1974.
27. Anderson, RJ, et al.: Mechanism of effect of thoracic inferior vena cava constriction on renal water excretion. J Clin Invest 54:1473, 1974.
28. DeTorrente, A, et al.: Mechanism of diuretic response to increased left atrial pressure in the anesthetized dog. Kid Int 8:355, 1975.
29. Boykin, J, et al.: Mechanism of diuretic response associated with atrial tachycardia. Am J Physiol 229:1486, 1975.
30. Robertson, GL: The regulation of vasopressin function in health and disease. *In* Pincus, G (ed): Recent Progress in Hormone Research: Proceedings, Laurentian Hormone Conferences, Vol 23, New York, Academic Press, p 333, 1977.
31. Hayward, JN and Jennings, DP: Influence of sleep-walking and nociceptor-induced behavior on the activity of supraoptic neurons in the hypothalamus of the monkey. Brown Res 57:461, 1973.
32. Duke, HN, et al.: The antidiuretic action of morphine: its site and mode of action in the hypothalamus of the dog. Q J Exp Physiol 36:149, 1951.
33. Stuart, JM, et al.: Syndrome of recurrent increased secretion of antidiuretic hormone following multiple doses of vincristine. Blood 45:315, 1975.
34. Kleeman, CR and Vorherr, H: Water metabolism and the neurohypophysial hormones. *In* Bondy, PK, (ed): Duncan's Diseases of Metabolism, 7th ed, Philadelphia, WB Saunders Co, 1974.
35. Guzek, JW, et al.: Inhibition by diphenylhydantoin of vasopressin

release from isolated rat neurohypophyses. Acta Pharmacol 34:1, 1974.
36. Arief, AL and Guisado, R: Effects on the central nervous system of hypernatremic and hyponatremic states. Kid Int 10:104, 1976.
37. Taral, R, et al.: Misleading reduction of serum sodium and chloride association with hyperproteinemia in patients with multiple myeloma. Proc Soc Exp Biol Med 110:145, 1962.
38. Albrink, MJ, et al.: The displacement of serum water by the lipids of hyperlipemic serum. A new method for the rapid determination of serum water. J Clin Invest 34:1481, 1955.
39. Katz, M: Hyperglycemia-induced hyponatremia-calculation of expected serum sodium depression. N Engl J Med 289:843, 1973.
40. Aviram, A, et al.: Hyperosmolality with hyponatremia caused by inappropriate administration of mannitol. Am J Med 42:648, 1967.
41. Ufferman, RI and Schrier, RW: Importance of sodium intake and mineralocorticoid hormone in the impaired water excretion of adrenal insufficiency. J Clin Invest 51:1639, 1972.
42. Boykin, J, et al.: Persistent plasma vasopressin levels in the hyposmolar state associated with mineralocorticoid deficiency. Mineral Electrolyte Metab 2:310, 1979.
43. Wilson, DR and Honrath, U: Cross-circulation study of natriuretic factors in postobstructive diuresis. J Clin Invest 57:380, 1976.
44. Klotman, PE, et al.: Postobstructive diuresis in the absence of significant elevated urea. Clin Res 30:453A, 1982.
45. Schrier, RW and Berl, T: Disorders of water metabolism. *In* Schrier, RW (ed): Renal and electrolyte disorders. Boston, Little, Brown and Co, p 1, 1980.
46. Bartler, FC and Schwartz, WB: The syndrome of inappropriate secretion of antidiuretic hormone. Am J Med 42:790, 1967.
47. Humes, HD: Disorders of water metabolism. *In* Kokko, JP, et al. (eds): Fluids and Electrolytes. Philadelphia, WB Saunders Co, p 118, 1986.
48. Hays, RM and Levine, SD: Pathophysiology of water metabolism. *In* Brenner, BM, et al. (eds): The Kidney, 2nd ed, Philadelphia, WB Saunders Co, p 777, 1981.
49. Vorherr, H, et al.: Localization and origin of antidiuretic principle in paraendocrine-active malignant tumors. Oncology 29:201, 1974.
50. Breitschwerdt, EB, et al.: Inappropriate secretion of antidiuretic hormone in a dog. JAVMA 175(2):181, 1979.
51. Arieff, AL, et al.: Pathophysiology of hyperosmolar states. *In* Andreoli, TE, et al. (eds): American Physiology Society. Disturbances in Body Fluid Osmolality. Baltimore, Williams and Wilkins, p 227, 1977.
52. Tannen, RL: Potassium disorders. *In* Kokko, JP, et al. (eds): Fluids and Electrolytes. Philadelphia, WB Saunders Co, p 150, 1986.
53. Malnic, G, et al.: Micropuncture study of renal potassium excretion in the rat. Am J Physiol 206:674, 1964.
54. Harrison, JB, et al.: Fluid and electrolyte therapy in small animals. JAVMA 137:637, 1960.
55. Adroguaa, HJ and Madias, NE: Changes in plasma potassium concentration during acute acid-base disturbances. Am J Med 71:456, 1981.
56. Valtin, H: Disorders of K^+ balance. *In* Renal Dysfunction: Mechanisms Involved in Fluid and Solute Imbalance. Boston, Little, Brown and Co, p 89, 1979.
57. Gabow, PA and Peterson, LN: Disorders of potassium metabolism. *In* Schrier, RW (ed): Renal and Electrolyte Disorders. Boston, Little, Brown and Co, p 183, 1985.
58. Tannen, RL and Gerrits, L: Response of the renal K^+ conserving mechanism to kaliuretic stimuli: evidence for a direct kaliuretic effect of furosemide. Clin Res 31:752A, 1983.
59. Hsu, CH and Weller, JM: Fluid and electrolyte abnormalities in obstructive uropathy and following urinary tract diversion. *In* Kokko, JP and Tannen, RL (eds): Fluids and Electrolytes. Philadelphia, WB Saunders Co, p 619, 1986.
60. Grekin, RJ: Ketoacidosis, hyperosmolar states, and lactic acidosis. *In* Kokko, JP and Tannen, RL (eds): Fluids and Electrolytes. Philadelphia, WB Saunders Co, p 688, 1986.
61. Adroguaa, HJ, et al.: Plasma acid-base patterns in diabetic ketoacidosis. N Engl J Med 307:1603, 1982.
62. Macy, DW and Small, E: Deep mycotic diseases. *In* Ettinger, SJ (ed): Textbook of Veterinary Internal Medicine. Philadelphia, WB Saunders Co, p 237, 1983.
63. Boveé, KC, et al.: Characterization of renal defects in dogs with a syndrome similar to the Fanconi syndrome in man. JAVMA 174(10):1094, 1979.
64. Easley, JR and Breitschwerdt, EB: Glucosuria associated with renal tubular dysfunction in three Basenji dogs. JAVMA 168(10):938, 1976.
65. Meijer, JC, et al.: Biochemical characterization of pituitary-dependent hyperadrenocorticism in the dog. J Endocrinol 77:111, 1978.
66. Ettinger, SJ: Weakness and syncope. *In* Textbook of Veterinary Internal Medicine. Philadelphia, WB Saunders Co, p 76, 1983.
67. Knochel, JP: Neuromuscular manifestations of electrolyte disorders. Am J Med 72:521, 1982.
68. Bilbrey, GL, et al.: Skeletal muscle resting membrane potential in potassium deficiency. J Clin Invest 52:3011, 1973.
69. Sterns, RH, et al.: Internal potassium balance and the control of the plasma potassium concentration. Medicine 60:339, 1981.
70. Schribner, BH (ed): Fluid and Electrolyte Balance. Seattle, University of Washington Bookstore, 1969.
71. Haskins, SC: Fluid and electrolyte therapy. Comp Cont Educ Pract Vet 6(3):244, 1984.
72. Cohen, JJ, et al.: Disorders of potassium balance. *In* Brenner, BM and Rector, FC (eds): The Kidney. Philadelphia, WB Saunders Co, p 908, 1981.
73. Haskins, SC: Blood gases and acid-base balance: clinical interpretation and therapeutic implications. *In* Kirk, RW (ed): Current Veterinary Therapy VIII, Philadephia, WB Saunders Co, 1980.
74. Rodkey, WG, et al.: Arterialized capillary blood used to determine the acid-base and blood gas status of dogs. Am J Vet Res 39(3):459, 1978.
75. Middleton, DJ, et al.: Arterial and venous blood gas tensions in clinically healthy cats. Am J Vet Res 42(9):1609, 1981.
76. Valtin, H: H^+ balance. *In* Renal Function: Mechanisms Preserving Fluid and Solute Balance in Health. 2nd ed, Boston, Little, Brown and Co, p 195, 1977.
77. Hamm, L and Jacobson, HR: Mixed acid-base disorders. *In* Kokko, JP and Tannen, RL (eds): Fluids and Electrolytes. Philadelphia, WB Saunders Co, p 382, 1986.
78. Pitts, RF: Renal regulation of acid-base balance. *In* Physiology of Kidney and Body Fluids. 3rd ed, Chicago, Yearbook Medical Publishers, p 198, 1974.
79. Warnock, DG and Rector, FC: Renal acidification mechanisms. *In* Brenner, BM and Rector, FC (eds): The Kidney. 2nd ed, Philadelphia, WB Saunders Co, p 440, 1981.
80. Foster, DW and McGarry, JD: The metabolic derangements and treatment of diabetic ketoacidosis. N Engl J Med 309:159, 1983.
81. Grauer, GF and Hull-Thrall, MA: Ethylene glycol (antifreeze) poisoning. *In* Kirk, RW (ed): Current Veterinary Therapy IX. Philadelphia, WB Saunders Co, p 206, 1986.
82. Feldman, BF and Rosenberg, DP: Clinical use of anion and osmolal gaps in veterinary medicine. JAVMA 178(4):396, 1981.
83. Polzin, DJ and Osborne, CA: Anion gap—diagnostic and therapeutic applications. *In* Kirk, RW (ed): Current Veterinary Therapy IX. Philadelphia, WB Saunders Co, p 52, 1986.
84. Toto, RD: Metabolic acid-base disorders. In Kokko, JP and Tannen, RL (eds): Fluids and Electrolytes. Philadelphia, WB Saunders Co, p 229, 1986.
85. Adroguaa, HJ, et al.: Influence of steady-state alterations in acid-base equilibrium on the fate of administered bicarbonate in the dog. J Clin Invest 71:867, 1983.
86. Garella, S, et al.: Severity of metabolic acidosis as a determinant of bicarbonate requirement. N Engl J Med 289:121, 1973.
87. Kaehny, WD and Gabow, PA: Pathogenesis and management of metabolic acidosis and alkalosis. *In* Schrier, RW (ed): Renal and Electrolyte Disorders. 2nd ed, Boston, Little, Brown and Co, p 115, 1980.
88. Haskins, SC: An overview of acid-base physiology. JAVMA 170:423, 1977.
89. Posner, J and Plum, F: Spinal fluid pH and neurologic symptoms in systemic acidosis. N Engl J Med 277:605, 1967.
90. Fuller, GR, et al.: Influence of administration of potassium salts on the renal tubular reabsorption of bicarbonate. Am J Physiol 182:111, 1955.
91. Burnell, JM, et al.: Metabolic acidosis accompanying potassium deprivation. Am J Physiol 227:329, 1974.
92. Hulter, HN, et al.: Pathogenesis of renal hyperchloremic acidosis resulting from dietary potassium restriction in the dog: role of aldosterone. Am J Physiol 238:F79, 1980.

93. Bosch, JP, et al.: Effect of chronic furosemide administration on hydrogen and sodium excretion in the dog. Am J Physiol 232:F397, 1977.
94. Schwartz, WB, et al.: The response of extracellular hydrogen ion concentration to graded degrees of chronic hypercapnia. The physiologic limits of the defense of pH. J Clin Invest 44:291, 1965.
95. Lakshminarayan, S, et al.: Bicarbonate therapy in severe acute respiratory acidosis. Scand J Resp Dis 54:128, 1973.
96. Flenley, DC and Millar, JS: Ventilatory response to oxygen and carbon dioxide in chronic respiratory failure. Clin Sci 33:319, 1967.

DRUG INDEX

Species	Generic	Trade	Dosage	Route	Frequency	Used to Treat
Dog and cat	Furosemide	Lasix	0.5–2.0 mg/lb 0.5–2.0 mg/lb	PO SQ, IM, IV	q 8–24 h q 8–24 h	Hypernatremia Hyponatremia Volume expansion
Dog and cat	Potassium chloride	Micro-K Extencaps; many forms	0.5–1.5 mEq/lb/day 0.06 mEq/lb/hr (usual) 0.25 mEq/lb/hr (max)	PO IV	q 12 h Continuous	Hypokalemia
Dog and cat	Calcium gluconate 10%	Many forms	0.25 ml/lb	IV slowly	Once	Hyperkalemia
Dog	Regular insulin 50% dextrose	Iletin I; many forms	2.5 U/lb/hr 2 g/U of insulin	IV	In combination	Hyperkalemia
Cat	Regular insulin 50% dextrose	Iletin I; many forms	0.25 U/lb 2 g/U of insulin	IV	In combination	Hyperkalemia
Dog and cat	Sodium bicarbonate	Many forms	0.5–1.0 mEq/lb	IV slowly	Usually once	Hyperkalemia
Dog and cat	Sodium polystyrene sulfonate	Kayexalate	0.12–0.5 g/lb	PO, rectally	q 6–24 hr	Hyperkalemia
Dog and cat	Sodium bicarbonate	Many forms	Empirical: 0.5–1 mEq/lb Calculate: BW (kg) × 0.3 × (desired − observed HCO_3^-)	IV	PRN	Metabolic acidosis

54 SPECIALIZED NUTRITIONAL SUPPORT

TIMOTHY A. ALLEN

Specialized nutritional support consists of providing specially formulated and/or delivered intravenous or enteral nutrients to prevent or treat malnutrition.[1] Enteral nutrition is the provision of protein, carbohydrates, lipids, vitamins, electrolytes, minerals, and water via the gastrointestinal tract. Enteral nutrition may be administered by mouth or by tubes that deliver nutrients distal to the oral cavity. In parenteral nutrition, nutrients are delivered into either a central, large diameter vein or a smaller peripheral vein.

Malnutrition is any disorder of nutrition, usually a deficiency of nutrient intake relative to requirements or impaired nutrient metabolism. Malnutrition may result in a clinical sequel such as immune dysfunction[2, 3] that increases the morbidity and mortality associated with the primary disease.[4–6] The immune dysfunction associated with malnutrition may initiate a vicious cycle of infection, sepsis, and persistent malnutrition.

EFFECTS OF BRIEF, NONSTRESSED STARVATION

During brief, nonstressed starvation, there is a decrease in glucose, amino acids, and fatty acids in the portal blood.[7] Insulin levels decrease and glucagon levels increase. As the concentration of glucose decreases, the liver stops removing glucose from the portal circulation and begins producing glucose by glycogenolysis and gluconeogenesis. Glycogen stores are rapidly exhausted. Although during early starvation other tissues can rapidly adapt to fatty acids as an energy substrate, the brain absolutely requires glucose. Consequently, gluconeogenesis accelerates to meet the glucose needs of the brain. Amino acids become the primary gluconeogenic substrate. Resting energy expenditures are decreased during periods of nonstressed starvation. This decrease in energy use is due to loss of cellular mass, decreased metabolic rate, decreased physical activity, and decreased conversion of T4 to T3. Adaptations to conserve protein occur and are evidenced by a decrease in urinary nitrogen excretion, decreased hepatic gluconeogenesis, increased ketone production, decreased plasma concentration of amino acids, and amino acid efflux from muscle.

RESPONSE TO STRESS

The metabolic response to sepsis, trauma, and severe illness is quite different from the response to brief, nonstressed starvation.[8] The stressed patient is hypermetabolic rather than hypometabolic and adaptations to conserve protein do not occur.[9] The increase in metabolic rate and protein catabolism is approximately proportional to the severity of the insult.[10] The mechanisms of this hypermetabolic response are not known, however, during infection, the release of acute phase proteins acts directly on organs and indirectly on the neuroendocrine system to increase the metabolic rate.

Increased protein catabolism is evidenced by increased urinary nitrogen losses. Increased nitrogen loss is primarily due to breakdown of skeletal muscle and may be five times greater than the nitrogen loss observed during nonstressed starvation.

In sepsis, trauma, and severe illness, there is a marked increase in plasma glucocorticoids, catecholamines, and glucagon and an inappropriately low insulin concentration for the degree of hyperglycemia. Although inappropriately low, the plasma insulin concentration is sufficient to inhibit lipolysis and ketone formation. Thus, proteins are the major energy substrate. This is different from the metabolic response to brief, nonstressed starvation, where fat is the major source of energy and proteins are spared.

In summary, the metabolic response to sepsis, trauma, or severe illness is hypermetabolism, hyperglycemia, glucose intolerance, and use of skeletal proteins as energy substrate.

NUTRITIONAL ASSESSMENT

Specialized nutritional assessment is a comprehensive evaluation of nutritional status, which includes clinical and dietary histories, physical examination, and laboratory evaluation.[11] The purpose of this assessment is to objectively identify malnourished patients.

A nutritional history includes the following information: 1) weight and if possible, change in weight over time, 2) diet at home and proportion of each type of food in the diet, 3) diet in the hospital, 4) duration of inappetence or anorexia, 5) gastrointestinal abnormalities such as diarrhea and vomiting, and 6) administration of drugs that may alter nutrient use or dietary intake (e.g., cancer chemotherapeutic agents or corticosteroids).

A quantitative evaluation of the nutrient needs of the patient should be performed prior to the start of specialized nutritional support.[12] Estimation of these nutritional requirements should include consideration of the specific disease process, the patient's current nutritional status, and the projected duration of inadequate nutrient intake or hypermetabolism.[1]

There is no practical, proven method of accurately defining nutritional status. However, to aid in the nutritional assessment of hospitalized patients, several techniques are suggested.

FAT RESERVES

Measurement of body fat serves mainly to estimate the duration and severity of inadequate dietary intake.[13] Changes in subcutaneous fat occur slowly and do not reflect acute nutritional changes; however, when subcutaneous fat is markedly depleted the problem is severe and chronic. Although distribution of subcutaneous fat varies, losses in subcutaneous fat with inadequate intake of calories is presumed to occur proportionately throughout the body. Estimation of body fat by skin-fold measurement requires standardization of technique and site of measurement. The clinician should determine the midpoint between the acromion and olecranon and make a mark on the caudal aspect of the foreleg. The skin and subcutaneous tissues are gently pinched at this midpoint and the thickness is measured with skin-fold calipers. This process is repeated three times and the average thickness is recorded. Subsequent body fat measurements should be performed by the same examiner with the patient in the same position. Repetitive measurements by one examiner are relatively reproducible; measurements by different examiners are not.

PROTEIN STATUS

Approximately 60 per cent of total body protein is contained in muscle. Skeletal muscle is the major site of protein hydrolysis and is the primary source of amino acids during protein malnutrition. For these reasons, measurement of muscle mass provides a reasonable estimate of protein reserves.

The most widely used estimate of body mass protein in humans is the 24-hour urinary creatinine excretion.[13] Creatine is an energy storage compound found primarily in muscle. Creatine spontaneously dehydrates at a relatively constant rate to form creatinine, which is excreted unchanged in the urine. Measurement of creatinine in a 24-hour urine specimen approximates the level of total body creatine and therefore, total body muscle mass. A single 24-hour urine creatinine excretion is of limited value. However, carefully performed serial studies may be used for comparisons in an individual patient.

In humans, the mid upper arm circumference and arm muscle area are anthropometric indicators of skeletal muscle protein mass.[11] Breed and individual variation reduce the applicability of these measurements in animals. Serial measurements by one observer may be of value in assessing trends in protein status.

BIOCHEMICAL PARAMETERS

Albumin is the major protein synthesized by the liver. Albumin is a relatively poor indicator of early protein malnutrition because serum levels change slowly.[11] This delayed response is due to the relatively long serum half-life and the large body pool of albumin.

Transferrin, a glycoprotein that transports iron, has a shorter half-life and smaller body pool than albumin. Consequently, transferrin is presumed to more accurately reflect acute changes in visceral protein.[11] Serum transferrin levels are best measured by radioimmunodiffusion, although an estimate can be obtained by measuring total iron binding capacity (TIBC). The relationship between transferrin and TIBC may vary depending upon technique, therefore each laboratory must validate formulas used for converting TIBC to transferrin.

MEASURES OF IMMUNE STATUS

Since malnutrition is associated with multiple defects in the immune system, the clinician must select a battery of immunologic tests in order to assess nutritional status. The immunologic tests should be simple, inexpensive, noninvasive, and both sensitive and specific for malnutrition. The present recommendation in humans is to perform total lymphocyte counts and intradermal skin testing.[6]

ENERGY METABOLISM

An animal in the resting state produces little or no work. Under these conditions, the intensity of energy metabolism can be estimated either by calculating the heat produced from the exchange of respiratory gases (indirect colorimetry) or by measuring the heat that is lost from the body by radiation, conduction, convection, and evaporation (direct colorimetry).[14]

A variety of techniques are available for the measurement of respiratory exchange; all measure oxygen consumption and carbon dioxide production per unit time.[15, 16] To make these measurements, it is necessary to either confine the animal to a chamber where changes in the ventilating air can be determined or to use a face mask connected to some analytical device. The effluent air is exhausted from the chamber or mask and is either collected or metered and analyzed for estimation of energy consumption.

INDICATIONS AND CONTRAINDICATIONS FOR SPECIALIZED NUTRITIONAL SUPPORT

Although there are no controlled clinical studies, the following general guidelines for the implementation of specialized nutrition are proposed.[17] Specialized nutrition should be implemented in animals that have lost more than 20 per cent of their body weight in less than 14 days and in animals exhibiting prolonged anorexia. The definition of prolonged anorexia varies, depending upon the circumstances. For example, in neonates one to two days without nursing is prolonged; for adult animals three to five days is required. Specialized nutrition should also be implemented in animals with increased metabolic requirements, such as those suffering from severe trauma, sepsis, or severe illness, in animals that will be unable to eat for more than five days due to mechanical problems, such as a fractured mandible or maxilla, and in animals with immediate specific nutritional needs (e.g., acute renal failure, hepatic encephalopathy, and ketoacidotic diabetes mellitus).[18]

The contraindications to nutritional support are unnecessary expense and the risk of complications.

THE NUTRITIONAL PLAN

A specific nutritional plan should be formulated prior to the onset of treatment. The goal of nutritional support may be to decrease the rate of weight loss and protein catabolism or to increase body weight and protein anabolism. The nutritional goals must be integrated into the overall medical and surgical management of the patient. The ability to achieve nutritional goals is influenced by such things as the control of sepsis, maintenance of feeding tubes and vascular access, fluid and electrolyte balance, and the concurrent use of catabolic drugs such as corticosteroids.

Maintenance energy requirements are calculated by the following formula:

$$\text{metabolizable kcal/day} = 2(30 \times \text{body weight(kg)} + 70)$$

The calculation of energy requirements is further refined by considering the difference between the patient's observed and ideal body weight, an estimation of the weight loss since the onset of the problem, and an estimation of the hypermetabolic response to trauma or illness. Quantification of the magnitude of the hypermetabolic response is highly subjective; however, the following stress factors have been used: minor surgery, 20 per cent; skeletal trauma, 35 per cent; and sepsis, 60 per cent. Finally, the caloric requirements are adjusted upward an additional 25 per cent to account for the stress associated with hospitalization and treatment.

Establishing energy requirements is the first step in determining protein requirements since protein metabolism and energy metabolism are closely related.[19] The relationship between energy and protein requirements varies, depending upon whether the patient is normal, nutritionally depleted, or hypermetabolic. Hypermetabolic patients have a pronounced inefficiency in handling dietary protein. In humans, branched chain amino acid supplementation appears to have several desirable effects:[20] branched chain amino acids serve as an energy source to spare endogenous protein, branched chain amino acids may decrease catabolism of skeletal protein, and branched chain amino acids appear to stimulate protein synthesis, especially in the liver. Protein needs can be approximated by collecting a 24-hour urine specimen and determining the urine urea nitrogen.[14] The urine urea nitrogen may be adjusted to approximate total nitrogen by dividing by 0.85.

The two possible routes for specialized nutritional support are parenteral (intravenous) and enteral.[1] The clinical dictum is that "if the gut works, use it." Enteral feeding is simpler, faster, cheaper, and more physiologic than parenteral feeding. Specific forms of enteral tube feeding include orogastric, nasogastric, pharyngostomy, gastrostomy, and jejunostomy.

The mode of nutritional support depends on the underlying medical problem, specific nutrient requirements, and economic considerations.

TUBE FEEDING

Orogastric tube feeding can be performed in the dog and cat several times a day to meet protein and calorie requirements. The principal limitation of this technique is patient tolerance.

Nasogastric tube feeding has not been used extensively in companion animals until recently. Cats and small dogs seem to tolerate nasogastric tubes for long periods of time. Compared with orogastric tube feeding, nasogastric feeding is more convenient and less time-consuming.

The technique for placing a nasogastric tube in the dog and cat has been well described.[21] A 3.5 to 8 French polyvinyl, Silastic, or polyurethane plastic tube is used. An advantage of the polyvinyl tubes is that they are sufficiently rigid to allow passage without the use of a stylette. The distance from the animal's external nares to the eighth rib is measured and the tube is marked with tape. Placement of the distal end of the tube in the midesophagus theoretically prevents gastric acid reflux in cats.[22] Ketamine sulfate may be used for chemical restraint in cats. If the cat is severely debilitated and chemical restraint is not necessary, proparacaine hydrochloride (0.5 per cent) can be instilled into the external nares. The tube is lubricated with lidocaine viscous (2 per cent) or proparacaine hydrochloride solution. In dogs, the tube is initially directed dorsally and in cats, it is directed in a ventral, medial direction. The tube is gently passed into the nasal cavity and advanced after the cat has been observed to swallow. Proper placement of the tube should be confirmed radiographically. The tube is reflected caudally and sutured to the forehead, taking care that the tube does not touch the whiskers. An Elizabethan collar is secured after recovery from anesthesia to prevent accidental removal of the tube.

In dogs and cats intolerant of a nasogastric tube, an alternative technique is the use of a pharyngostomy tube. The tube is placed into the caudodorsal portion of the pharynx as close to the entrance of the esophagus as possible.[23] The tube must be placed using blunt dissection in order to prevent damage to the carotid and lingual arteries, the lingual-facial and maxillary veins, and the hypoglossal and glossopharyngeal nerves. By placing the tube in this manner, there is less chance of the tube interfering with the movement of the glottis or patency of the airway. Tape and nonabsorbable sutures are used to secure the proximal end of the tube. The tube is capped when not in use in order to prevent aerophagia or reflux of esophageal contents.

Tube gastrostomy is useful in many patients requiring specialized nutritional therapy.[24, 25] Gastrostomy tube placement can be performed under light general anesthesia. A two to three cm incision is made just caudal to the last rib. The external abdominal fascia is incised and the abdominal oblique muscles are separated in the direction of their fibers. The peritoneal cavity is entered and the fundus of the stomach is located. The wall of the stomach is grasped with Allis tissue forceps and exteriorized. A full thickness purse-string suture of 2-0 nylon is placed in the gastric wall. Several simple interrupted sutures of 2-0 nylon are placed in the stomach and omentum and sewn to the subcutaneous tissues and skin. A stab incision is then made in the center of the purse-string suture to accommodate a Foley catheter. The abdominal muscles, subcutaneous tissue, and skin are closed with simple interrupted sutures. The tube is secured to the skin with nonabsorbable sutures. Local peritonitis and generalized peritonitis from leakage of gastric contents are the major complications of this technique.[26]

Needle catheter jejunostomy is another form of tube feeding.[27, 28] Jejunostomy is indicated in situations where nasogastric or gastrostomy tube feeding is contraindicated (e.g., severe persistent vomiting, partial gastric resection, and gastroenteric anastomosis) and the distal intestinal tract functions normally. The appropriate size needle (12-, 14-, or 16-gauge, 1.5 inch needle for large, medium, and small dog or cat, respectively) is introduced into the jejunal wall approximately four inches from the duodenocolic ligament on the antimesenteric border. The needle is inserted its full length in the seromuscular wall of the jejunum. After traversing the seromuscular layer, the needle is then directed into the lumen and an 18-inch Silastic or polyurethane cathcter of appropriate diameter is passed through the needle. The catheter is secured to the jejunum with a purse-string suture. The needle is then used to penetrate the peritoneum, abdominal wall, and skin. The catheter is passed through the needle and the needle is withdrawn and the catheter secured to the skin. The jejunum is then attached to the peritoneum. Omentum should be interposed between the jejunum and the peritoneum. A jejunostomy feeding tube is removed by pulling the tube and allowing the seromuscular tunnel to act as a seal. The complications associated with the use of needle catheter jejunostomy are jejunal perforation, peritonitis, subcutaneous leakage, and obstruction of the bowel.

DIETS

Many products are available for tube feeding of human patients. These products are formulated so as to be balanced and complete for human beings. The adequacy of these diets for dogs and cats is unknown. Cats require an amino acid, taurine,[29] the fatty acids linoleate and arachidonic[30, 31] and the vitamins niacin and vitamin A, which are not required by either human beings or dogs. The products designed for the enteral hyperalimentation of human patients use soy and casein as protein sources and corn oil as a source of fatty acids. Unfortunately, soy- and casein-derived protein is deficient in taurine and corn oil is deficient in arachidonic acid. Consequently, it is likely that the commercially available products are inadequate for maintenance nutrition in the cat. Since egg yolk contains arachidonic acid, arginine, and taurine, it can be used to supplement these commercial products. Although there have been few controlled studies in dogs, it is presumed that the commercial products are adequate for use in the dog. Enteral hyperalimentation diets can be classified as meal replacement, elemental, special formulations, or modular. Meal replacement formulations are used in patients with normal gastrointestinal function. These products contain high molecular weight proteins, carbohydrates, and fats, and have an osmolality of approximately 350 mOsm/L. Elemental diets contain amino acids, peptides, oligosaccharides, monosaccharides, and medium-chain triglycerides and are more hyperosmolar. Because these nutrients do not require digestion and are readily absorbed, they can be used in inflammatory bowel disease and pancreatic exocrine insufficiency.

In normal dogs and cats, the capacity of the stomach is about 80 ml of fluid/kg body weight. However, patients who have been anorectic can comfortably handle only approximately one-half of this volume at one feeding. The volume fed can be gradually increased to normal over a two to three day period. At least three feedings daily are recommended and if an infusion pump is available, constant infusion is preferred. If a jejunostomy catheter is used, the volume administered is even more critical. The patient's caloric needs should be calculated and one-fourth the calculated volume should be administered the first day, one-half the second day, three-quarters the third day, and full volume the fourth day. If the solutions are administered too rapidly or if they are hypertonic, rapid fluid and electrolyte influx into the intestinal lumen will occur, with resultant diarrhea and severe cramping.

TOTAL PARENTERAL NUTRITION

The major indication for total parenteral nutrition (TPN) is functional failure of the gastrointestinal tract. It is only undertaken when oral or tube feeding is impossible or inadequate.[32] Normally, the portion of nutrients reaching the systemic circulation is modified by the bowel and liver, but in TPN all of the nutrients infused are delivered directly to systemic circulation.[33]

If TPN is properly performed, adequate energy, nitrogen, vitamins, and trace elements are provided.

The problem of supplying adequate amounts of energy in TPN has been solved in two ways.[2] One approach has been to use fat emulsions. Since fat emulsions are not only a concentrated source of energy but are also isotonic, it is possible to administer them via a peripheral vein. The second approach is to supply all of the required energy in the form of carbohydrates. If the carbohydrate solutions are isotonic, the volume required to meet the energy requirements of the patient may produce overhydration and hypertonic carbohydrate solutions cause thrombophlebitis. Consequently, if carbohydrates are the sole energy source, it is necessary to administer concentrated carbohydrate solutions (20 to 30 per cent glucose) into a central vein in which the blood flow is sufficiently great to dilute the infused solution so that the vascular endothelium is not injured.

Glucose is generally the preferred carbohydrate for parenteral nutrition. Glucose is required by the brain, red blood cells, and nervous tissue. Glucose stimulates insulin secretion and thus has anabolic effects. However, under stressful conditions, the secretion of epinephrine and norepinephrine is associated with reduced levels of insulin and glucose intolerance may develop.

The advantage of using glucose as the main carbohydrate energy source is that glucose can be metabolized by all body cells and metabolism can be easily monitored by measuring blood glucose.[34] When glucose intolerance occurs, insulin can be readily added to the regimen and the dose of insulin adjusted based upon the blood glucose.

Two major problems can occur when carbohydrates are the main source of calories. If a patient has abnormal pulmonary function, the increased CO_2 produced may further stress the respiratory system. The other problem is that carbohydrate infusions may contribute to the development of fatty liver.

It is comparatively easy to meet energy requirements by infusing small volumes of isotonic fat emulsions into peripheral veins. The advantages of using fat emulsions as the main energy source are that thrombophlebitis is rare, diuresis does not occur, and essential fatty acids are provided. The essential fatty acids are linoleic and linolenic acids. If these fatty acids are not provided, immunocompromise, erythrocyte abnormalities, and dermatopathies may be observed.

Fat emulsions for parenteral nutrition contain a vegetable oil in water and emulsifiers to stabilize the emulsion. Intralipid contains soybean oil and purified egg-yolk phospholipids as emulsifiers. Isotonicity is achieved by adding glycerol. After the infusion of a fat emulsion, transient hyperlipidemia invariably occurs.

Adequate intravenous protein nutrition occurs if the amino acid mixture infused permits optimal protein synthesis by the patient. The ratio of essential amino acids to total nitrogen appears to be important; however, the optimal ratio has not been established for the various clinical situations encountered in companion animals. From the available information it appears that the optimal amino acid preparation for TPN should contain both the essential and nonessential amino acids in the L-form and in the approximate proportion found in proteins of high biological value, such as egg. Recent studies have shown that in critically ill human beings, modified branched chain amino acid solutions have a favorable influence on the patient's response to stress.[35] The branched chain amino acids, leucine, isoleucine, and valine, are used as a fuel source in severely stressed patients.

It is very difficult to predict vitamin and trace element requirements for the patient on TPN. Consequently, estimates of requirements are based on normal oral administration.

Central venous catheters are indicated if TPN is expected to continue for more than two weeks. Complications can arise when placing a central venous catheter or following long-term use.[36] Insertion problems include faulty positioning of the catheter[37] and hemorrhage. Long-term problems include thromboembolic disease[38] and sepsis.[39] The placement of a central venous catheter is a surgical procedure and should be performed in the operating room. The proper positioning of the central venous catheter should be confirmed radiographically. The central venous catheter should be used only for infusion of parenteral nutrition solutions; the catheter must not be used for infusing drugs or for obtaining blood specimens. Catheter-associated infection can be reduced by tunneling the end of the catheter subcutaneously, using meticulous technique when handling the catheter, changing administration sets daily, and covering the catheter site with a sterile dressing every other day.

References

1. Mitchel, I, et al.: Nutritional support of hospitalized patients. N Engl J Med 304:1147, 1981.
2. Louie, N and Niemiec, PW: Parenteral nutrition solutions. *In* Rombeau JL, Caldwell MD (eds): Parenteral Nutrition. Philadelphia, WB Saunders Company, 1986, p 272.
3. Law, DK: The effects of protein-calorie malnutrition on immune competence of the surgical patient. Surg Gynecol Obstet 139:257, 1974.
4. Cannon, PR, et al.: The relationship of protein deficiency to surgical infection. Ann Surg 120:514, 1944.
5. Mullen, JL, et al.: Reduction of operative morbidity and mortality by combined preoperative and postoperative nutritional support. Ann Surg 192:604, 1980.
6. Harvey, KB, et al.: Hospital morbidity-mortality risk factors using nutritional assessment. Clin Res 26:518, 1978.
7. Cahill, GR, Jr, et al.: Hormone-fuel interrelationships during fasting. J Clin Invest 45:1751, 1966.
8. Black, PR, et al.: Mechanisms of insulin resistance following injury. Ann Surg 196:420, 1982.
9. Kudsk, KA, et al.: Nutrition in trauma. Surg Clin N Am 61:671, 1981.
10. Moore, FD: Endocrine changes after anesthesia, surgery and unanesthetized trauma. Recent Prog Horm Res 13:511, 1957.
11. Buzby, GP and Mullen, JL: Nutritional assessment. *In* Rombeau JL, Caldwell MD (eds.): Parenteral Nutrition. Philadelphia, WB Saunders Company, 1986, p 331.
12. MacBurney, M and Wilmore, DW: Rational decisionmaking in nutritional care. Surg Clin N Am 61:571, 1981.
13. Grant, JP, et al.: Current techniques of nutritional assessment. Surg Clin N Am 61:437, 1981.
14. Long, CL, et al.: Metabolic response to injury and illness: Estimation of energy and protein needs from indirect calorimetry and nitrogen balance. J Parenter Enterol Nutr 3:452, 1979.

15. Feurer, ID, et al.: Measured and predicted resting energy expenditure in clinically stable patients. Clin Nutr 3:27, 1984.
16. Head, CA, et al.: A simple and accurate indirect calorimetry system for assessing resting energy expenditure. J Parenter Enterol Nutr 8:45, 1984.
17. Page, CP, et al.: Safe, cost-effective postoperative nutrition. Am J Surg 138:939, 1979.
18. Feinstein, EI, et al.: Clinical and metabolic responses to parenteral nutrition in acute renal failure: a controlled double blind study. Medicine 60:124, 1981.
19. Solomons, NW and Allen, LH: The functional assessment of nutritional status; principles, practice, and potential. Nutr Rev 41:33, 1983.
20. Cerra, FB, et al.: Nitrogen retention in critically ill patients is proportional to the branched chain amino acid load. Crit Care Med 11:775, 1983.
21. Crowe, DT: Enteral nutrition for critically ill or injured patients—Part I. Comp Cont Educ Pract Vet 8:603, 1986.
22. Lantz, GC, et al.: Pharyngostomy tube induced esophagitis in the dog: an experimental study. JAAHA 19:207, 1983.
23. Crowe, DT and Downs, MD: Pharyngostomy complications in dogs and cats and recommended technical modifications: experimental and clinical investigations. JAAHA 22:493, 1986.
24. Crane, SW: Placement and maintenance of a temporary feeding tube gastrostomy in the dog and cat. Comp Contin Educ Pract Vet 2:770, 1980.
25. Crowe, DT: Enteral nutrition for critically ill or injured patients—Part II. Comp Cont Educ Pract Vet 8(10):719, 1986.
26. Bernard, M and Forlaw, L: Complications and their prevention. *In* Rombeau JL, Caldwell MD (eds): Enteral and Tube Feeding. Philadelphia, WB Saunders Company, 1984, p 542.
27. Orton, EC: Enteral hyperalimentation administered via needle catheter jejunostomy as an adjunct to cranial abdominal surgery in dogs and cats. JAVMA 188:1406, 1986.
28. Crowe, DT: Enteral nutrition for critically ill or injured patients—Part III. Comp Cont Educ Pract Vet 8(11):826, 1986.
29. Rogers, QR and Morris, JG: Protein and amino acid nutrition of the cat. Am Anim Hosp Assoc 50th Annual Meeting Scientific Proceed.
30. MacDonald, ML, et al.: Role of linoleate as an essential fatty acid for the cat independent of arachidonate synthesis. J Nutr 113:1422, 1983.
31. Rivers, JPW: Essential fatty acids in cats. J Sm Anim Pract 23:563, 1982.
32. Goodgame, JT: A critical assessment of the indications for total parenteral nutrition. Surg Gyn Obst 151:433, 1980.
33. Stein, TP: Protein metabolism and parenteral nutrition. *In* Rombeau JL, Caldwell MD (eds): Parenteral Nutrition. Philadelphia, WB Saunders Company, 1986, p 100.
34. Ang, SD and Daly, JM: Potential complications and monitoring of patients receiving total parenteral nutrition. *In* Rombeau JL, Caldwell MD (eds): Parenteral Nutrition. Philadelphia, WB Saunders Company, 1986, p 331.
35. Mizock, BA: Branched chain amino acids in sepsis and hepatic failure. Arch Int Med 145:1284, 1985.
36. Ladefoged, K, et al.: Long-term parenteral nutrition. II, Catheter-related complications. Scand J Gastroenterol 16:913, 1981.
37. Gatti, JE and Mullen, JL: The malpositioned subclavian catheter. Surg Gynecol Obstet 153:91, 1981.
38. Firor, HV: Pulmonary embolization complicating total intravenous alimentation. J Pediatr Surg 7:81, 1972.
39. Colley, R, et al.: Fever and catheter-related sepsis in total parenteral nutrition. J Parenter Enterol Nutr 3:32, 1979.

55 TOXICOLOGY

MICHAEL E. MOUNT

Veterinary toxicology is a tremendously broad area that encompasses many specialty areas. Diagnosis is difficult since poisonings occur less frequently than common medical problems. There are five approaches to making a confirmatory diagnosis. Circumstantial and symptomatic evidence are the major routes taken. Applying clinical laboratory tests can provide supportive evidence that strengthens the former two. Response to antidotal therapy provides diagnostic support and, finally, chemical identification of the toxin confirms all suspicions. This treatise attempts to pull these five approaches together to enable the clinician to handle toxicological problems effectively. Toxic gases,[1] drugs of abuse, and various miscellaneous toxic substances such as fertilizers[2] are not addressed. Informational resources should be sought as previously presented.[3]

PRINCIPLES OF TREATMENT

A phone call from a panicked owner provides an opportunity for the veterinarian to give wise counsel. Instructing the owner to induce vomiting is *not* recommended. Contact of the animal's skin with a poison calls for immediate rinsing with soap and water. The owner should bring the animal in for evaluation. The presentation of an acutely poisoned animal commonly calls for emergency treatment. The principles outlined apply to individual poisons as discussed later.

Control of Life-Threatening Conditions

When faced with a life-threatening condition, remember the ABC's of therapy (airway, breathing, and circulation). Seizures that interfere with breathing must be controlled with anticonvulsant drugs such as pentobarbital or Valium. Endotracheal intubation insures proper airway maintenance and prevention of inhalation pneumonia. Positive pressure artificial respiration must be established to maintain breathing if respiratory paralysis is present. Medical drugs and/or surgical procedures to manage bronchospasm, pulmonary edema, or a space-occupying condition (e.g., hemothorax) are important considerations in reestablishing proper breathing. Cardiac dysrhythmias, tamponade, or vascular collapse require medication with cardiac drugs and/or surgical corrective measures to reestablish normal sinus rhythm for proper circulation to maintain life. Routine patient care for anesthetized animals must be applied since long periods of sedation may occur with these situations.

Removal of the Poison

This encompasses three aspects of therapy: physical removal, delay of absorption, and enhanced excretion of the poison. This is very important in providing proper therapy.

Physical removal should be performed within two hours of ingestion and can be achieved by one of two methods, emesis or gastric lavage. However, neither removes more than 80 per cent of the ingested poison. Induction of emesis is the most direct method. The animal must be conscious, alert to mildly depressed, have an intact gag reflex, and be known not to have ingested a caustic or petroleum product. Animals presented with nausea, vomiting, and diarrhea are not candidates for this procedure. Animals showing early signs of strychnine poisoning should also not be induced to vomit.

Apomorphine (0.02 mg/lb or 0.04 mg/kg IV; 0.04 mg/lb or 0.08 mg/kg IM, SQ) is the drug of choice to induce emesis in the dog. The intravenous route is the most accurate and effective manner to administer the drug. The tablet can be crushed and dissolved in a measured volume of sterile, distilled water and dosed accordingly. It is best to use a millipore filter (e.g., Ivex, Abbot) to remove any solid particles. Placement of an apomorphine tab into the conjunctival sac is satisfactory but conjunctivitis and excessive dosing can occur. The eye should be rinsed with sterile saline once emesis is achieved. Respiratory depression and protracted emesis are adverse effects. Commonly used narcotic antagonists such as naloxone (Narcan) 0.02 mg/lb (0.04 mg/kg) IV or levallorphan (Lorfan) 0.01 mg/lb (0.02 mg/kg) IV, can be used once or as necessary (PRN) to reverse these adverse reactions. Apomorphine is not recommended in cats. Xylazine administered at 0.25 mg/lb (0.5 mg/kg) IV (or 1 mg/kg IM) is an effective emetic in cats, but the sedative effect lasts for several hours. Administration of syrup of ipecac undiluted (3.0 ml/lb or 6.6 ml/kg PO) is effective in inducing vomiting within 15 minutes.[4]

However, follow-up therapy with activated charcoal is made less effective by the presence of ipecac.

A "through-and-through" enema[7] can be used immediately following known ingestion of highly toxic material (e.g., Compound 1080/1081) when the entire removal of unabsorbed poison is desired. After light anesthesia and stomach lavage, the stomach tube is kept in place and a high warm-water enema is performed, followed by continued enema fluid flow until clear fluid exits the stomach tube. This can be performed in an alert dog using only the enema; vomition can provide elimination of the intestinal contents.

A gastric lavage should be performed in cases where induction of emesis is not recommended or where the use of general anesthesia is anticipated. This is accomplished following light anesthesia by placing a cuffed endotracheal tube so that the cuff is pulled high in the trachea to prevent any inhalation of lavage fluid. The anterior end should be lower than the abdominal region. A large-bore stomach tube is lubricated and inserted after premeasurement to the xiphoid cartilage. In humans, a 36 French or larger tube is recommended even in one-year-old children in order to allow recovery of intact tablets.[5] Approximately 10 to 15 washings should be performed. Each washing is calculated at 3 to 5 ml/lb (5 to 10 ml/kg). Lavage solutions can vary from water to any combination of solutions imaginable. Basically a water/activated charcoal combination is fairly universal. Combination of the saline cathartic solution with the activated charcoal is also acceptable. Certain lavage solutions that aid in degradation of the toxic agent are recommended for specific poisons.

Whether physical removal was performed or not, the administration of a slurry of activated charcoal is highly recommended. A good quality, pharmaceutical grade charcoal should be used as previously specified,[6] and dosed orally at 1 to 4 gm/lb (2 to 8 gm/kg) body weight. The slurry is made by placing the charcoal into a screw cap jar (canning jar) and adding water at five to ten ml for every one gm of charcoal. Some commercial packets are already mixed with water. The administration of a saline cathartic as 40% solution (sodium sulfate, 0.5 gm/lb or 1 gm/kg orally) should follow within 30 minutes. Lower doses (0.25 gm/lb or 0.5 gm/kg) of activated charcoal given q3h for 72 hours are recommended for slowly excreted substances. A cathartic should be administered following the first and second treatments only.

Removal of the absorbed toxin is enhanced by supporting the renal system. Diuresis can be induced by saline solution administration, but mannitol and furosemide administration is favored. Following rehydration of the animal, mannitol (3 to 5 per cent at 2.5 ml/lb/h or 5.5 ml/kg/h infusion rate IV) and dopamine (1 to 3 μg/lb/min or 2 to 5 μg/kg/min) for 24 hours should be administered. If no effect is observed within one hour, administer furosemide at 1 mg/lb (2 mg/kg) IV. Hydration status and electrolytes should be monitored carefully. Acidification of urine (ammonium chloride, 100 mg/lb or 200 mg/kg PO for dog and 20 mg/lb or 40 mg/kg PO for cat q8h) enhances excretion of basic compounds, while alkalinizing (sodium bicarbonate, 2.5 mEq/lb or 5 mEq/kg IV q12h) the urine increases excretion of acid compounds.

Administration of the Antidote

A tentative diagnosis is crucial to apply this therapeutic feature. Specific antidotes are discussed under the respective poison. General detoxicants such as glucose, calcium gluconate, and sodium thiosulfate may demonstrate beneficial effects when no antidote is available.

Supportive and Symptomatic Care

Various conditions require these same treatments to provide support for proper hydration, electrolyte balance, hypothermia, cardiovascular integrity, and respiratory and renal function. Corrective symptomatic measures to control pain, depression, hyperactivity, pyrexia, acidosis, anemia, diarrhea, vomiting, and hypersalivation are needed periodically during the course of therapy. Follow-up care may be indicated for the coagulation, hepatic, renal, gastrointestinal, and cardiac systems.

Observation of the Poisoned Patient

Observation is a must when caring for acutely poisoned animals. Administration of drugs that have alleviated the signs does not waive observation. Signs will recur if the therapeutic drug has fallen below its therapeutic concentration when the poison is still present. Therefore, the clinician should make it a rule to always keep an animal under close surveillance until the life-threatening phase of poisoning has passed.

CHEMICAL POISONS

Ethylene Glycol

Circumstantial and General Information. This is a very common poisoning that is easily misdiagnosed due to the traditional mindset of "renal failure." More than 90 per cent of antifreeze is ethylene glycol (EG); it accounts for the majority of poisonings. Special preparations such as photographic solutions contain EG and can present a hazard. This substance is persistent in the environment, since an area once contaminated and then remoisturized can contain resuspended EG residue. The taste of EG is not objectionable to animals and both dogs and cats will consume it under most conditions. The hazard of poisoning in cats is much greater than in dogs because of their habits and lower tolerance to EG. Thus, 6.5 tablespoons of radiator fluid containing 50 per cent EG is lethal to a 25 lb dog, while only 0.9 tablespoon is lethal if consumed by a ten lb cat. History of ingestion strongly supports confirmation, while no history affords a diagnostic challenge.

Clinical Signs. Poisoning with EG is confusing since clinical signs vary considerably depending on the time of presentation and dose of EG consumed. The initial phase of poisoning is roughly the clinical period of time from 0 to 12 hours following exposure to EG, with three to six hours being the peak time of EG absorption. Signs of poisoning during this phase are predominately nausea and a progressive acidosis. Vomiting may be observed shortly after ingestion. Ataxia develops within one hour due to the effect of increasing blood levels of EG on the central nervous system. Within one to three hours, depression is the predominant clinical finding. Polydipsia/hyperpnea and dehydration commonly accompany the depression. The clinical condition can worsen (seizures/coma) or wane (temporary recovery) over a 12- to 48-hour period, leading to the classic acute renal failure syndrome. Renal azotemia is not a characteristic finding during the initial phase of poisoning.[8] The early clinical signs can be very nonspecific and easily overlooked by the owner.

In the final phase of poisoning, the animal shows clinical signs of acute renal failure and the client is more aware that a problem exists than during the milder signs of the initial phase. The presence of gastrointestinal and neurological signs and an empty bladder are classic findings. Because of this, most practitioners associate EG poisoning with renal failure.

Clinical Laboratory Information. Laboratory diagnostic tests are vitally important for recognition of the initial phase of poisoning, since the earlier the diagnosis is made and treatment initiated, the greater the chances for recovery. Results of laboratory tests that are characteristic of the initial three hours of poisoning are stress leukogram, normochloremic acidosis, and hyperosmolemia. Hyperphosphatemia may also be observed due to a dietary source of phosphate from the rust inhibitor in the antifreeze. Of these parameters, calculation of the osmolar gap using a formula such as the one given below is the most diagnostic test:[9]

$$\text{Calculated mOsm/kg} = 1.86(\text{Na} + \text{K}) + \text{glucose}/18 + \text{BUN}/2.8 + 9$$

$$\text{Osmolar gap} = \text{Measured serum mOsm/kg} - \text{Calculated mOsm/kg}$$

The unmeasured osmolarity is primarily due to EG, and 100 mg EG/dL accounts for a 16 mOsm/kg increase. Practitioners should make arrangements with a local hospital and provide them with a similar formula that the practitioner desires so that a STAT request can be made at any time, allowing for a turn-around time of one hour or less. The osmolar gap remains markedly wide (normal $\approx$ 10 mOsm/kg versus more than 50 mOsm/kg in early poisonings) for the first six hours following exposure and gradually decreases toward normal reference ranges as 24 hours following exposure approaches. In general, the osmolar gap remains highly suggestive of EG poisoning for 12 hours after exposure. Measurement of the anion gap also reflects the presence of unmeasured anions due to acid products. Hypocalcemia is not a feature of the initial phase of poisoning.

The urine is also extremely useful for diagnosis. Polyuria with a decrease in osmolality occurs within an hour and continues until oliguria/anuria develops, which is quite variable. The urine becomes acid and may contain protein, glucose, and blood cells, and cells of the urinary tract (including casts) that become more pronounced as the clinical course lengthens. Specific gravity is generally within the isosthenuric range.

By far the most direct diagnostic finding is crystalluria, containing both di- and monohydrate calcium oxalates, which can be observed as early as six hours following exposure. These crystals differ morphologically; dihydrate crystals are the classic maltese cross form, while monohydrate crystals are entirely different. Monohydrate crystals take on various forms, such as sheaf forms (dumbbell), hempseed forms, and six-sided and four-sided with budding bullet forms, which are mistaken for hippuric acid crystals.[10] Storage of urine results in dissolution of the dihydrate form, followed by recrystallization in the monohydrate form.

Following the initial phase of poisoning, the acute renal failure phase ensues due to renal tubular damage. Prerenal azotemia may occur earlier in the course of the disease. Azotemia, hyperphosphatemia, and hyperkalemia can all be seen, depending on the degree of oliguria. This generally occurs anywhere from 24 to 72 hours following exposure. Oxalate crystals may not be observed during this phase, since the kidney may be functioning as filter due to the heavy load of crystals. Hypocalcemia can be very pronounced during this phase. Many causes of acute renal failure could be responsible for these findings. Thus, a renal biopsy is the diagnostic test of choice. In the event of death, a cytologic examination of a renal cortex scraping is sufficient to verify EG poisoning by observation of masses of birefringent crystals.

Toxicological Analysis. Ethylene glycol determination of serum and urine samples collected prior to 48 hours after ingestion contain detectable concentrations. Stomach contents should also be submitted if the initial phase of poisoning is suspected.

Differentiation. The initial phase presents a diagnostic challenge and conditions causing depression and/or nausea must be considered. Other disease conditions to consider when presented with an animal showing clinical signs of the initial and acute renal failure phases of poisoning are presented in Tables 55–1 through 55–4.

Therapy. Therapy is worthwhile if initiated during the initial phase of poisoning. The goals of therapy are to alter the metabolism of EG and to correct the metabolic acidosis. Two basic methods are employed to alter the metabolism of EG by the hepatic enzyme, alcohol dehydrogenase (ADH). Administration of ethanol (vodka or the like can be used) is recommended at doses given in Table 55–5. An alternative method is administration of an alcohol dehydrogenase (ADH) inhibitor, 4-methylpyrazole (4-MP), which has been effective in dogs only.[11] This method has advantages over the ethanol method. Acidosis is best controlled by calculating the bicarbonate deficit (0.5 x body weight (kg) x (24 − patient's bicarbonate) every four to six hours (Table 55–5 gives a prescribed dosage).

Immediate presentation of an animal seen to have just ingested EG calls for induction of the basic procedures for acute poisoning and administration of ADH

TABLE 55–1. DISEASE CONSIDERATIONS WHEN DEPRESSION TO COMA IS THE PRIMARY CLINICAL FINDING THAT SHOULD BE RULED OUT WHEN NO OTHER CAUSES ARE OBVIOUS

Toxic Agent	Other Associated Findings for Differentiation
Acetaminophen	cyanosis, hemolysis, hepatic
Anticoagulant rodenticides	internal hemorrhage, shock
Anticholinesterase insecticides	nicotinic phase, weakness
Aspirin	acidosis, ketonuria
Cigarettes (tobacco products)	coma
Diabetic ketoacidosis	Kussmaul breathing, Glucostix
Drugs of abuse and antiaction (convulsive, depressive, psychotic)	
Amphetamines	coma
Barbiturates	sleeping to coma
Benzodiazepines	coma
Opiates	coma, respiratory depression
Phencyclidine (PCP)	coma, psychosis
Phenothiazines	coma
Tricyclic antidepressants	coma
Ethanol	whining, coma, hyperosmolality
Ethylene glycol	acidosis, initial stage
Fleet-like enema	hypocalcemic tetany
Hypoglycemia	coma to seizures, Glucostix
Iron	GI effects, shock
Mushroom (Group 5)	psychoactive
Phenolic products	renal and hepatic effects
Salt (dehydration; salt water)	coma, bright red mucous membrane
Shock	varied causes
Snakebite (neurotoxins)	little local swelling
Snakebite (pit-viper type)	obvious local swelling
Spider bite (black widow)	muscle spasms to paralysis
Toxic gases	
Methane (propane)	gas stove, asphyxiation
Hydrogen sulfide	rapid death, tachypnea to apnea
Carbon monoxide	cherry-red blood, cardiac, CNS
Traumatic injury	head injury

inhibitors. Ethanol is best given at a lower dosage level to avoid excessive CNS depressive effects. Ethanol given at 36 per cent of the recommended dose of 2.5 ml/lb (5.5 ml/kg) by a continuous drip method[12] proved effective when administered one hour following exposure as a 30 per cent solution in saline with one per cent sodium bicarbonate. The therapeutic regimen given in Table 55–5 for 4-MP could be followed in place of low-dose ethanol treatment. Oral administration of an alcoholic beverage to an animal immediately following exposure is advised if the owner is unable to present the dog immediately.

Pesticides Affecting the Central Nervous System

Rodenticides, molluscicides, and insecticides contain causative agents that produce marked central nervous system (CNS) manifestations. All these substances can produce sudden onset of illness and can be difficult to differentiate. An accurate history can provide diagnostic information.

Circumstantial and General Information. The two CNS rodenticides commonly encountered are strychnine and sodium fluoroacetate (Compound 1080) or a derivative, sodium fluoroacetamide (Compound 1081).[13] Access to baits (primary) or ingestion of poisoned target or nontarget species (secondary) results in the poisoning of dogs or cats. Ingestion of two g of 0.5 per cent strychnine bait can kill a 30 lb dog. Strychnine is commonly used as a malicious poison. Ingestion of 0.34 g of bait containing Compound 1080/1081 (0.2 per cent) can be lethal to a 30 lb dog.

Metaldehyde is one of the most common molluscicides used in the United States. Many homeowners use this for control of slugs and snails. The hazard for exposure

TABLE 55–2. GASTROINTESTINAL DISORDERS FOR DIFFERENTIAL CONSIDERATION

Toxic Agent	Other Associated Findings for Differentiation
1. Acute onset of vomiting, nausea, and/or diarrhea that commonly is self-limiting	
Garbage poisoning	can be serious
Mushroom (Group 4)	—
Fleet-like enemas	tetany, seizures
Plants	
Narcissus bulbs, etc.	—
Walnut hulls, other parts	can be serious
Intestinal parasites (roundworms)	radiographs, fecal
Viral enteritis	
2. Acute onset of vomiting, nausea, and/or diarrhea that progresses to weakness, prostration, and shock or other problems within 24 h.	
Arsenic	hemorrhagic, common
Iron	pills, hepatic
Phosphorus	smoking stool
Petroleum solvents	aspiration pneumonia
Zinc phosphide	commonly neurologic effects
Paraquat/diquat	oral ulcers, pulmonary
Caustics	GI/oral burns
Plant	severe GI effects
castor bean	
jequirity bean	
black locust seed	
oleander and others	cardiac effects
Jellyfish ingestion	—
3. Acute to subtle abdominal disorders associated with vomiting, abdominal pain, and diarrhea/constipation followed by icterus, marked dehydration leading to shock, and/or other problems that develop over several days.	
Lead	painful bowel, CNS
Ethylene glycol	initial signs of uremia
Acetaminophen (dog)	hepatic, Heinz body anemia
Zinc	AIHA, pancreatitis, hepatic
Mushroom (Groups 1, 2)	hepatic, sometimes renal
Phosphorus	hepatic effects
Thallium	many systems, especially integumentary
Phenolic disinfectants/products	hepatic, renal, ulcers
Aflatoxin	hepatic effects
(Nontoxic considerations for 2 and 3)	
Pancreatitis	radiographs, ultrasound, lipase
Foreign body	radiographs, ultrasound
Gastric torsion	acute, radiographs, ultrasound
Intussusception	radiographs, ultrasound
Other abdominal disorders	same, cytology, culture
Canine/feline viral diseases	viral panel
Salmon poisoning	lymphadenopathy
Bacterial diseases (Salmonella)	culture, previous debilitation
Campylobacter (cats)	culture
Parasitism (Giardia, Coccidia, Whips)	fecal
Adrenal cortical insufficiency	electrolytes, bradycardia

TABLE 55–3. DISEASE CONSIDERATIONS IF ACUTE RENAL DAMAGE IS SUSPECTED

Toxic Agent	Other Associated Findings for Differentiation
Acute nephritis (Leptospirosis)	febrile, culture
Aminoglycoside antibiotics	overzealous treatment
Congenital condition	—
Ethylene glycol	final stage
Hemolytic agents (see Table 55–8)	secondary to hemolysis
Hypercalcemia	primary problem
Hypotensive conditions (varied)	—
Mercury	primary site
Mushroom (Group 1)	GI signs 24 to 48 h prior
Pancreatitis	hepatorenal effects
Paraquat	pulmonary effects
Phenolic disinfectants/products	other general signs, hepatic
Septic nephritis	febrile, culture
Thallium	acute, other significant signs
Vasculitis and/or thrombosis	—
Zinc phosphide	other significant signs

is extremely high in those locations where it is used. Cats appear less attracted to the material. Other molluscicides contain the carbamate insecticide methiocarb.

The toxic insecticides include the anticholinesterase (AI; organophosphate and carbamate) and organochlorine (OCI; chlorinated hydrocarbon) insecticides. Many types of AI are available for pet exposure. Home treatments by owners are by far the most common cause of poisoning. Various drugs potentiate toxicity. Therapeutic baths of AI are commonly used in veterinary practices. Unusual events may precipitate problems even when treatments were performed as long as three months before owing to lingering residues in hair. Fewer OCI are currently used but many sources remain and certain chemicals such as chlordane have useful applications in special instances. In general, animals that exude a foul petroleum odor or that harbor an oily substance should be suspected of insecticide poisoning.

Clinical Signs. Signs of poisoning occur within two hours after ingestion of strychnine. Ingestion of massive doses may result in one fatal seizure shortly ($\approx$ 15 min) after ingestion. More commonly, the animal is initially apprehensive, nervous, and anxious. It shows stiffness along with a developing abdominal and cervical rigidity. The animal develops a "sawhorse stance" due to extensor rigidity. Continuous nervous input leads to grand mal tetanic seizures. These seizures may occur spontaneously or can be induced by tactile, auditory, or visual stimuli. Seizures are followed by periods of relaxation. Hyperthermia is expected immediately following a seizure, but subsides with relaxation. However, the seizures become more powerful and frequent as the course of disease progresses. Respiratory failure and exhaustion ensue, leading to death. The animals are generally semicomatose with dilated pupils during the course of this disorder.

Onset of clinical illness is delayed for at least two hours with Compound 1080/1081 and may be delayed for as long as 24 hours. Signs occur suddenly with initial vomition, urination, and/or defecation. Uneasiness leading to wild behavior can follow. Running fits, which are characteristic, may be evidenced by bizarre events such as jumping through a glass window. Periodic seizures

TABLE 55–4. DISEASES WITH PROMINENT NEUROLOGICAL EFFECTS REQUIRING DIFFERENTIAL CONSIDERATION

Toxic Agent	Other Associated Findings for Differentiation
1. Signs characterized by respiratory distress associated with neurologic deficits, ataxia, ptosis, facial/ocular paralysis, salivation/drooling, dry eye, paresthesias (e.g., pain in anterior abdominal cavity), posterior weakness, and/or paralysis. Vomiting may occur and depression of deep tendon reflex, withdrawal, gagging and/or pupillary reflexes are common.	
Organophosphate insecticides	nicotinic phase, tremors
Carbon monoxide	cherry-red blood
Snakebite (neurotoxin)	rapid progression of signs
Botulism	slow progression
Blue-green algae	rapid course, hepatic damage
Mercury (organic)	loss of proprioception, other
Ethanol	predominant neurologic effects
Tick paralysis	—
Polyradiculoneuritis	—
Rabies	variable
Trauma	—
Spinal disorders	—
Myasthenia gravis	—
Tetanus	dysphagia, ears, third eyelid
2. Nervous excitation characterized by seizures, muscle fasciculations, recumbency, hypoxia, hyperthermia, and/or status epilepticus. Hypersalivation, defecation (diarrhea), urination, miosis or mydriasis, tachycardia, and/or vomiting are additional.	
Strychnine	inducible tetanic seizures
Compound 1080/1081	running fits
Zinc phosphide	variety of seizure types
Organochlorine insecticides	seizures to depression
Anticholinesterase insecticides	SLUD, CNS effects, miosis
Metaldehyde	fasciculations, progressive
Moldy walnuts (or the like)	similar to metaldehyde
Avitrol	similar to metaldehyde
Lead	variety of neurologic signs
Phenoxyacetate herbicides	GI, tremors, paralysis
2,4-D	
MCPP	
MCPA	
Ethylene glycol	uremia, hypocalcemia
Chocolate (theobromine/caffeine)	nervousness
Mushroom (Group 3)	SLUD, little CNS
Moth crystals	ataxia, fasciculation, seizure
Cigarettes (tobacco products)	excitation to paralysis
Fleet-like enemas	hypocalcemic tetany, seizures
Salt (dehydration; salt water)	dementia to seizures, bright red mucous membranes
Thallium	tremors, develop dermatitis
Portal systemic vascular shunt	repeated bouts, esp. after meals
Hepatic disease	similar
Hypoglycemia	commonly comatose, Glucostix
Neoplasia	
Exercise	
Insulin overdose	
Hepatic disorder	
Epilepsy	historic progression
Brain lesion	variety of seizure types
Encephalitis	
Neoplasia	
Hemorrhage	anticoagulants
Hypocalcemia (endocrine/metabolic)	tetany, prolonged Q-T interval
Hypoparathyroidism	
Pseudohypoparathyroidism	
Acute pancreatitis	
Acute renal failure associated with hyperphosphatemia	
Transfusion using large volume of citrated blood	
Eclampsia (puerperal tetany)	
Idiopathic vestibular syndrome	cats, once called blue-tailed lizard poisoning
3. Psychoactive effects, including dissociation, delirium, dystonia, sleeping, coma, and/or staring into space.	
Plants	delirium to coma
morning-glory	
jimsonweed, etc.	
Mushroom (Group 6)	dissociation
Petroleum solvents	GI, pulmonary, cardiac
Drugs of abuse and antiaction (convulsive, depressive, psychotic)	
Amphetamines	mydriasis, delirium to coma
Benzodiazepines	drowsiness to hypotensive coma
Cocaine	mydriasis, cardiac, seizures
Marijuana	drowsiness, hypotension
MA oxidase inhibitors*	hyperthermia, seizures
Opiates	miosis/mydriasis, GI, seizures
Phencyclidine	nausea, seizures, psychosis
Phenothiazines	dystonia, hypotensive, dyspnea
Tricyclic antidepressants	confusion to seizures

*Monoamine oxidase inhibitors.

TABLE 55–5. DRUGS AND DOSAGES USED IN TEXT

Generic	(Trade)	Dosage/lb Body Weight	Route	Frequency	Description
Acepromazine	(PromAce)	0.5 mg	IV, IM	q8h	Sedative
		0.5–.75 mg	IV	q10min; PRN	Metaldehyde poisoning
N-Acetylcysteine	(Mucomyst) (10%, 20%)	70 mg	PO	once	Antidote for acetaminophen; give 3 to 5 times
		35 mg	PO	q4h	
Activated charcoal	(various)	1–4 gm	PO	once or q6–8h	Adsorbent, acute poisoning; give for 1 to 3 treatments
		0.25 gm	PO	q3h (≈72h)	Enhance excretion of slowly excreted poisons
Aminophylline	(various)	5 mg	IV, PO	q8h	Dog: pulmonary edema; hypersensitivity
		25–50 mg/trt	IV, PO		
		2–3 mg	PO	q12h	Cat: same
Ammonium chloride	(various)	100 mg	PO	q8h	Dog: acidification of urine
		20 mg	PO	q8h	Cat: same
Amoxicillin	(various)	5 mg	IM, PO	q12h	Antibiotic; snakebite
Ampicillin	(various)	2.5–5 mg	IV, IM	q6h	Antibiotic; snakebite
		5–10 mg	PO	q6h	
Antivenin $40/v	Pit viper (Crotalid) Polyvalent Antivenom	1 vial	IV	q 0.5–1h to effect	Snakebite; Wyeth Laboratories Philadelphia, PA (215)688-4400
$75/v	Micrurus (coral snake)	1 vial	IV	q 0.5–1h to effect	Snakebite; Wyeth (see above)
$12/v	Lactodectus (black widow) antivenom	1 vial	IV	q 0.5–1h to effect	Snakebite; Merck, Sharpe, & Dohme West Point, PA (215)699-5311
	Centuroides (scorpion) antivenom	1 vial	IV	q 0.5–1h to effect	Snakebite; Iatrics Laboratory Arizona State Univ. Tempe, AZ
Apomorphine hydrochloride	(——)	0.02 mg	IV	once	Induce emesis (dog only)
		0.04 mg	IM, SQ	once	
Aspirin	(various)	10–20 mg	PO	q8h	Dog: mild analgesic for stings or bites
		10 mg	PO	q24h	Cat: same
Atropine	(various)	0.1–0.2 mg	IV/SQ	PRN	Antidote: anticholinesterase insecticides
		0.02 mg	IV, IM, SQ	PRN	Preanesthetic dose
Bentonite, clay	(——)	0.5–1.5 gm	PO	once	Adsorbent, esp. paraquat
Bismuth subsalicylate	(Pepto-Bismol) (1.75%)	5–15 ml/dog (not established in cat)		q4–6h	Intestinal protectant; demulcent
CaEDTA[2]	(calcium disodium versenate)	15 mg	SQ	q6h (5 days; repeat)	Antidote: heavy metals same
		25 mg	SQ	q12h (5 days; repeat)	
Calcium chloride, 10%	(——)	2.5–5 ml	IV	PRN	Compound 1080/1081 poisoning
Calcium gluconate, 10%	(——)	25–75 mg (0.25–.75 ml)	IV	infusion over 20–30 min	Hypocalcemia; detoxification agent for neuro/muscular disorders[1]
		5–7.5 ml	IV	over 24 hr	General detoxicant and for maintenance of hypocalcemia
Captopril	(Capoten)	0.25–1 mg	PO	q6–8h	Dog: vasodilator for hypertension, e.g., scorpion stings
		6.25 mg/trt	PO	q8–12h	Cat: same
Cephalexin	(Keflex)	4–15 mg	PO	q8h	Broad-spectrum antibiotic
Cephalothin	(Keflin)	10–15 mg	IV, IM, SQ	q6–8h	Broad-spectrum antibiotic

Table continued on following page

TABLE 55–5. DRUGS AND DOSAGES USED IN TEXT *Continued*

Generic	(Trade)	Dosage/lb Body Weight	Route	Frequency	Description
Cimetidine	(Tagamet)	2 mg	PO	q8h	Decrease HCl in stomach
Chloramphenicol	(various)	10–25 mg	IV, IM, PO	q8h	Broad-spectrum antibiotic
Chlorpromazine	(various)	0.25 mg	IV, IM	q12h	Sedative esp. with psychoactive agents
		1.5 mg	PO	q12h	
Deferoxamine mesylate	(Desferal)	20 mg	IV	loading	Antidote for iron poisoning
		10 mg	IV	q4–12h	Infusion rate 15 mg/kg/hr
		10 mg	IM, SQ	q3–12h	Treat until response
Dexamethasone	(various)	2–4 mg	IV	loading	Snakebite
		0.5–3 mg	IV, IM, SQ	loading	Arthropod venomous sting or bite
		0.125–1.0 mg/animal	PO	q12–24h	Maintenance
Diazepam	(Valium)	0.5–2 mg	IV	as needed	Central nervous activity for anxiolytic purposes
		0.125 mg	PO	q8h	
Dimenhydrinate	(Dramamine)	4 mg	PO	q8h	Motion sickness
		0.5–.75 mg	IV, IM, SQ	once	Antiemetic
Dimercaprol	(BAL)	2.5 mg	IM	loading	Antidote for heavy metals
		1 mg	IM	q4h (2 days)	
		1 mg	IM	q6h (1 day)	
		1 mg	IM	q12h (1–10 days)	
Diphenhydramine	(Benadryl)	0.5 mg	IV, IM	PRN	Antivenin hypersensitivity and Hymenoptera stings
		2 mg	PO	q8h	
		0.25–1 mg	IV, IM, SQ	once	Antiemetic
Diphenylthiocarbazone	(Dithizone)	25–35 mg	PO	q8h for 1–5 days	Thallium-chelating agent
Dobutamine	(Dobutrex)	2.5–20 μg	IV	infusion/min	Positive iono/chronotropic effect for shock
Dopamine	(Intropin)	1–5 μg	IV	infusion/min for 24 h	Positive iono/chronotropic effect for shock
Epinephrine	(various)	5 μg	IV	PRN	Ventricular fibrillation; anaphylaxis
		0.05 ml	IV, IM	q5–15 min	1:10,000 solution[3]
Ethanol–95%[5]	(——)	2 ml	IV	q4h (5×); q6h (4×)	For EG in dogs
		2 ml	IP	same	For EG in cats
Ferric-cyanoferrate	(prussian blue)	50–100 mg	PO	q8h for 1–30 days	Recommended drug for thallium chelation
Fuller's earth, clay	(——)	0.5–1.5 gm	PO	once	Adsorbent, esp. paraquat
Furosemide	(Lasix)	1–4 mg	IV	q1–6h	Diuretic agent
		1–2 mg	PO	q8–24h	
Glycerol monoacetate	(Sigma Chem Co., Monacetin)	0.25 ml	IV, IM	q1h	Antidote: Compound 1080/1081
Guiafenesin 5%–10%	(——)	50 mg	IV	PRN	Muscle relaxant
Haloperidol	(Haldol)	0.01 mg	IM	q12h	Sedative esp. with psychoactive toxicosis (dog)
Hydralazine	(various)	0.5 mg	PO	q12h	Vasodilator for hypertension, e.g., scorpion stings
Hydrocortisolone sodium succinate	(Solu-Cortef)	4–10 mg	IV	once	Arthropod venomous sting or bite (short-acting corticosteroid)
Kaolin-pectin	(Kaopectate)	2.5 ml	PO	q1–6h	Intestinal protectant
Lactulose	(Cephulac)	2.5–15 ml/trt	PO	q6–8h	Acidify intestinal content[4]
Levallorphan	(Lorfan)	0.01 mg	IV	once	Reverse apomorphine overdose
Lidocaine	(various)	2 mg	IV	bolus	Cardiac dysrhythmia; repeat if needed
		25 μg	IV	continuous infusion/min	Initial infusion rate; 2 mg/kg bolus given if needed
		12.5–50 μg	IV	continuous infusion/min	Final infusion rate needed depending on severity
		3 mg	IM	q1.5h	(control less effective)
Magnesium hydroxide suspension	(milk of magnesia)	0.5–20 ml/trt	PO	once	Iron poisoning–binding agent
		0.5–10 ml/trt	PO	PRN	Indigestion
Magnesium sulfate	(——)	0.25–0.5 gm	PO	PRN	Cathartic and binding (Pb)

TABLE 55–5. DRUGS AND DOSAGES USED IN TEXT *Continued*

Generic	(Trade)	Dosage/lb Body Weight	Route	Frequency	Description
Mannitol 12.5% (0.5–2.0 gm/kg/24 hr)		2–8 ml	IV	infusion/24h	Diuresis
20–25% (0.25–0.5 gm/kg/ injection)		0.5–1 ml	IV	q4–6h	Renal failure; over 5–10 min; Repeat 1 to 2 times monitor electrolytes
3–5%		5.5 ml	IV	infusions/hr	Infusion rate for establishment of urine flow for 1 or more days
Meperidine HCl	(Demerol)	5 mg	IM	PRN	Narcotic analgesic, dog
		1–3 mg	IM	PRN	Narcotic analgesic, cat
Methocarbamol	(Robaxin)	75 mg	IV	loading	Central nervous activity
		45 mg	IV	PRN	same
		20–100 mg	IV	PRN	Therapeutic range
4-Methylpyrazole (4-MP)	(Aldrich Chemical Co)	10 mg	IV, IM	loading	For EG in dogs
		7.5 mg	same	q12h (2×)	
		2.5 mg	same	30h post	
Metoprolol	(Lopressor)	0.05–.15 mg	IV	q8h	Dysrhythmias in methylxanthine poisoning (equivalent to propranolol)
			(rate = <1 mg/2 min)		
Mineral oil	(——)	1 ml	PO	once	Cathartic
Morphine sulfate	(various)	0.125–.5 mg	IM	PRN	Narcotic analgesic, dog
		0.5 mg	IM	PRN	Narcotic analgesic, cat
		0.1 mg	IM	q5h	Antidiarrheal in dog
		0.05 mg	IM	q6h	Antidiarrheal in cat
Naloxone	(Narcan)	0.02 mg	IV	once	Reverse apomorphine overdose
Penicillamine	(Cuprimine)	12–15 mg	PO	q6–8h	Antidote: heavy metals[1]
Pentazocine lactate	(Talwin-V)	0.15–0.3 mg	IM	PRN	Mild analgesic; arthropod stings and bites (dogs only)
Pentobarbital	(various)	5–15mg	IV	PRN	Control of seizures; sedation (e.g., toad poison)
		0.5–3 mg	IV	PRN	
Phenobarbital	(various)	1–3 mg	IV, IM	q6–8h	Control of seizures
Phentolamine	(Regitine)	0.25 mg	IV	PRN	Cardiac; reduce primary hypertension; scorpion stings
Phenytoin	(Dilantin)	5 mg	IV	q8h	Dog: Anticonvulsant; cardiac antidysrhythmia
		15 mg	PO	q8h	Dog: used in toad poisoning
		1–2 mg	PO	q24h	Cat: same
Potassium acetate	(——)	35 mEq/L			
acetate		0.25–1.5 mEq	SQ	q24h	Severe hypokalemia with acidosis
chloride[6]	(——)	0.25–1.5 mEq	SQ	q24h	Severe hypokalemia with alkalosis
		0.5–1 gm	PO	q8–12h	Thallium poisoning
	(elixir, 10%)	2.5–7.5 mEq/day	PO	q24h	Dog: maintenance in a hypokalemic state
gluconate	(elixir, 10%)	2.5–7.5 mEq/day	PO	q24h	Cat: same
Pralidoxine chloride	(Protopam chloride)	25 mg	IV, IM	q8h	Dog: organophosphate; insecticide poisoning
		10 mg	same	same	Cat: same
Prednisolone sodium succinate	(Solu-Delta-Cortef)	5–15 mg	IV	PRN	Arthropod venomous sting/bite (short-acting corticosteroid)
		15 mg	IV	PRN	Snakebite therapy
		0.5–25 mg/trt	IV	PRN	Varied applications
Procainamide	(various)	3 mg	IV	bolus	Cardiac dysrhythmias; hydrocarbon toxicity
		5–20 μg	IV	continuous infusion/min	
		4–5 mg	IM	q4h	
		3 mg	PO	q4h	
Propranolol	(Inderal)	0.75–2.5 mg	IV	loading	Toad poisoning cardiac; β-blocker dose given for methylxanthine poisoning
		0.25–0.75 mg	IV	PRN	
		0.05–0.15 mg	IV	q8h (rate = <1 mg/2 min)	

Table continued on following page

TABLE 55–5. DRUGS AND DOSAGES USED IN TEXT *Continued*

Generic	(Trade)	Dosage/lb Body Weight	Route	Frequency	Description
Sodium Bicarbonate[8]	(——) 5%	4.0 ml	IP/IV	q4h(5×); q6h(4×)	For EG in dogs
		3.0 ml	IP/IV	same	For EG in cats
		2.5–20 ml	Lavage	once	For acid catalysis toxins
	3.75%	2 ml	IV	q1–12h	Alkalinization of urine[9]
	50%	Lavage solution		once	Iron poisoning
Sodium Chloride 0.9% or 0.45%	(——)	40–60 ml IV		q24h	Saline diuresis[7]
Sodium Sulfate	(——)	0.5 gm	PO	once	Osmotic cathartic
	1.6% in water	25 mg	IV	q4h	Alternative antidote for acetaminophen poisoning
	isotonic[10]	40–60 ml	IV	q24h	For hypercalcemic diuresis, monitor for hypernatremia
Sodium Thiosulfate	(——) 10%	≈30 mg	PO	q8–12h	General detoxicant
		≈15 mg	IV	same	same
Trihexyphenidyl	(Artane)	0.05–5 mg/trt	PO	q24h	Control of tremors
Trimethoprim and sulfamethoxazole	(various)	1 mg	PO, SQ	q12h	Broad-spectrum antibiotic
Tripelennamine	(various)	12.5–50 mg/trt	PO	q6–8h	Hymenoptera stings[11]
Vitamin B_6 pyridoxine hydrochloride	(various)	12.5 mg/kg	IM, IV, SQ	q12h	Antidote for *Gyromitra* spp mushroom poisoning
Vitamin C		100 mg/trt	IV, SQ	q4h	Correct methemoglobinemia
		60 mg/trt	PO	q6h	Used in cats
Vitamin K_1	(Veta-K_1)	2.5 mg	SQ	loading	Antidote: Anticoagulants
		1.25 mg	PO	q12h	
		1.25 mg	PO	q12h	same
Xyalzine	(Rompun)	0.25–0.5 mg	IV	PRN	Sedative; emetic in cats
		0.5–1 mg	IM	PRN	
		1 mg	IM	PRN	Seizure control of avitrol poisoning

1. Monitor for development of bradycardia and stop infusion.
2. Calcium disodium ethylenediaminetetraacetate.
3. Prepare by putting 1 ml of 1:1000 in 10 ml sterile saline.
4. Decrease ammonia production; used in mushroom poisoning and other hepatotoxic poisonings.
5. Dilute to 20% in sterile saline. Vodka and the like can be used as long as the proof is known so that proper dilution can be made.
6. Kay Ciel and Kaon are examples.
7. Monitor for fluid overload and electrolyte imbalances and stop if encountered. Once rehydrated, furosemide can be given (1–3 mg/lb q12h).
8. Baking soda.
9. Parenteral sodium bicarbonate ampule is 50 ml of 3.75% (44.6 mEq); dose to alkalinize the urine is 5 mEq/kg body weight divided over 12 h in humans.
10. 38.9 g sodium sulfate decahydrate/L water.
11. An antihistamine lotion for Hymenoptera stings used in humans.

develop that are tetanic in nature. Running-like motions may be observed during the seizures. Periods of relaxation follow the seizures. Hyperthermia is similar and seizures follow a course similar to that of strychnine poisoning. Cardiac abnormalities may be noted. Seizures are not inducible and muscle fasciculations are not characteristic, although tetany can develop.

The clinical syndrome of metaldehyde poisoning is commonly referred to as the "shake and bake" presentation. Initial signs develop within one hour following ingestion of a toxic amount. Uneasiness and apprehension accompanied by fine muscle fasciculations appear first. Muscle twitches and body tremors develop progressively, leading to seizure activity. Handling the animal may intensify the seizure activity. Tetanic seizures identical to those caused by strychnine can occur, but are not characteristically inducible in nature. The pupils are usually unresponsive and dilated. Animals can become markedly hyperthermic.

Onset of clinical signs with anticholinesterase insecticides (AI) generally occurs within an hour but can be delayed for a longer period, especially if exposure occurs through the skin. Salivation, lacrimation, urination, and/or defecation (SLUD) can occur in animals acutely poisoned with AI. Cats are particularly sensitive to these compounds and will salivate profusely, particularly if exposed by mouth contact. Muscle fasciculations are prominent, as are miotic pupils unless the animal is in shock. Concomitant with or following abatement of the acute signs are marked depression, weakness, and respiratory distress, and/or paralysis can develop (the nicotinic phase). Depending upon time of presentation following exposure, a combination of the above can be seen. The degree of depression is a good monitor for evaluating the overall toxic effect. Seizures are uncommon with AI.

On the contrary, seizures are the most common presenting sign with organochlorine insecticides (OCI). Neurologic excitation resulting in muscle fasciculations, salivation, tremors, and tonic-clonic seizures can be seen following acute exposure. Bouts of depression and strange behavioral actions and/or postural stances can be intermixed with seizure activity. Hyperthermia is characteristic of some of the OCI. Onset of clinical signs with OCI are more variable than with AI.

The less toxic pyrethrins and rotenone insecticides

cause nervous excitation similar to AI.[14] Pyrethrins are capable of causing nausea, vomiting, diarrhea, hyperexcitability, incoordination, tremors, convulsions, muscle paralysis, and respiratory failure. In addition, severe allergic reactions have resulted from exposure to these compounds in humans. Rotenone ingestion can produce nausea and protracted vomiting episodes. Direct contact can cause local irritation.

Clinical Laboratory Information. Stress response and a degree of metabolic acidosis are generally detected in all these disorders, depending upon the length and severity of the disorder. Hypertension, increased heart rate, and elevation of the rate of rise of right ventricular pressure can be observed in strychnine-poisoned dogs. Marked hyperglycemia and metabolic acidosis are highly probable findings in Compound 1080/1081 poisoning due to the metabolic lesion. Total blood calcium is normal but ionized calcium is chelated by citrate, identified by prolongation of the Q-T interval[15] leading to cardiac ventricular fibrillation. Marked metabolic acidosis commonly accompanies metaldehyde poisoning due to the toxic byproducts and lactic acid production. No characteristic findings accompany the insecticidal poisonings. Whole brain, serum, heparinized blood, plasma, and/or separated red blood cells are recommended samples for submission for cholinesterase measurement, which can provide diagnostic information. Bradycardia is generally anticipated with AI poisonings, but tachycardia commonly develops.

Toxicological Analysis. The stomach and/or its contents should be submitted for analysis of any of the above poisons. A colored dye such as green, blue, or red may be observed with strychnine poisoning. Gastric contents from metaldehyde-poisoned animals commonly have a sweet smell. Gastric contents containing rodent remains strongly implicates secondary poisoning. Strychnine is readily detected in veterinary toxicology laboratories. Few laboratories have the analytical expertise to detect metaldehyde or Compound 1080/1081.

A petroleum odor is highly suggestive of insecticidal poisoning. Hair (if exposure is external), urine, brain, liver, and blood may be useful samples for confirmatory diagnosis in veterinary laboratories.

Differentiation. Tables 55–4 and 55–6 (for AI) illustrate significant clinical aspects characteristic of these poisons and other diseases to be considered.

Therapy. Control of life-threatening situations is of major consideration with these types of poisonings. Intubation with establishment of ventilation and control of seizure activity is foremost. Establishment of fluid therapy for control of metabolic acidosis is also appropriate.

STRYCHNINE POISONING. Pentobarbital (30 mg/kg) given IV to effect is the first line of defense with strychnine seizure activity, and alternative methods are recommended.[16] Tachycardia associated with strychnine poisoning[17] can be treated with diazepam (0.05 to 0.1 mg/lb or 0.1 to 0.2 mg/kg IV) or phentolamine (alpha-adrenergic blocker, 0.5 mg/kg IV) for vasopressor effects and propranolol therapy (0.5 to 1.0 mg/kg IV) to reduce inotropic and chronotropic effects. Phenolamine and propranolol IV have only an effect for a few minutes, thus limiting their usefulness. Maintenance of dark, quiet quarters is essential if animals are not under general anesthesia. Additional therapy includes oral or IV administration of ammonium chloride to acidify the urine. Gastric lavage solutions of 1:2000 potassium permanganate or one to two per cent tannic acid (strong tea) are recommended.

COMPOUND 1080/1081 POISONING. The control of seizures with Compound 1080/1081 poisoning is similar to that used for strychnine poisoning. An antidote, glycerol monoacetate (Monoacetin), has been shown effective if administered early in the course of poisoning at 0.25 ml/lb or 0.5 ml/kg hourly IV or IM as needed. If unavailable, a 50 per cent ethanol/5 per cent acetic acid solution dosed at 4.5 ml/lb or 8.8 ml/kg orally can

TABLE 55–6. CAUSES OF PULMONARY EDEMA AND/OR RESPIRATORY DISTRESS

Toxic Agent	Other Associated Findings for Differentiation
1. Pulmonary hypertension	
Left heart failure	physical
Bicuspid valve obstruction	cardiac examination
Mediastinal masses	radiographs, cytology
2. Hypoalbuminemia	
Protein-losing enteropathy	body system workup
Renal disease	same
Hepatic disease	same
Chronic hemorrhage	same
3. Increased pulmonary secretions and/or damage to capillary-alveolar membrane resulting in increased permeability.	
ANTU	primary
Paraquat, diquat	progressive, GI
Anticholinesterase insecticides	SLUD
Petroleum solvents	GI, CNS, cardiac
Zinc phosphide	GI, CNS
Iron	second crisis
Phosphorus	smoking stool
Snake venom	local swelling
Thallium	other effects
Toxic gases	primary
Nitrogen oxide	
Sulfur dioxide, etc.	
Septic pneumonia	febrile
Pulmonary thrombosis	radiographs
Allergic reactions	epinephrine response
Aspiration pneumonia	radiographs
Smoke inhalation	history
Uremia	Azostix
Electrocution	burns: lip or palate
4. Hypoxia related to space occupying lesion and/or decreased or defective red cell mass.	
Anticoagulant rodenticides	pallor
Acetaminophen	methemoglobinemia
Nitrite	same
Cyanide	cherry-red blood
Pulmonary neoplasia	radiographs, cytology
Pneumonia/pleuritis	radiographs, cytology
Tamponade (chronic: neoplasia)	cytology
Pulmonary thrombosis	clear radiographs, blood gas
Cushing's disease	
Amyloidosis	
Heartworms	
5. Acidosis or other problems associated with increased respirations.	
Metaldehyde	hyperthermia, CNS
Aspirin	initial respiratory alkalosis
Compound 1080/1081	hyperglycemia, CNS
Diabetic ketoacidosis	Kussmaul breathing, Glucostix
Renal failure	Kussmaul breathing, Azostix
Pain (injury, disc problem)	localize area of pain

be substituted, but is far less effective. These preparations serve as acetate donors, which compete with the toxin at vital biochemical steps. In addition, continuous slow IV infusion of a one per cent solution of calcium chloride or administration of five to ten ml (ten per cent) with monitoring protects the heart from developing ventricular tachycardia/fibrillation. This replaces the free calcium believed chelated by the elevated citrate concentrations. Bicarbonate administration is vital to combat the severe metabolic acidosis. Generally, the prognosis is considered to be grave.

Metaldehyde poisoning. Metaldehyde poisoning is treated similarly to strychnine poisoning for seizure or nervous activity. Methocarbamol or diazepam is a convenient drug of choice. Acepromazine has also been found to provide good control at 0.5 to 1.0 mg/lb or 1 to 1.5 mg/kg IV PRN and to offer some advantages over the commonly used drugs.[18] However, this drug may cause seizures and may be contraindicated. Anesthesia with thiamalyl sodium or pentobarbital is often necessary. A tepid water bath helps reduce the hyperthermia. Fluid and bicarbonate therapy is highly recommended to enhance excretion of toxic products and to combat metabolic acidosis. Occasionally, respiratory alkalosis is concomitant with the metabolic acidosis and requires control of tachypnea and procedures to increase atmospheric CO_2. Hepatopathy has been observed in dogs within a week following poisoning with metaldehyde, which must be considered during the course of therapy.[19]

Anticholinesterase poisoning. Anticholinesterase insecticidal poisonings call for administration of one or two antidotes. Atropine is the pharmacologic antidote of choice and is diagnostic if a therapeutic response is observed at the high doses employed. Severely poisoned animals with cyanosis may require stabilization to correct hypoxia by intubation or by exposure to high oxygen concentrations prior to aggressive atropine therapy to avoid possible ventricular fibrillation. Atropine is administered (0.1 to 0.2 mg/lb or 0.2 to 0.4 mg/kg) slowly over five minutes IV, dosed at approximately ten times the preanesthetic dose. Response to therapy is observed within three to five minutes or longer after initiation of administration. Dryness of mucous membranes in the mouth, establishment of normal to increased sinus rhythm, and relief of bronchospasm are desired endpoints of atropinization. Repeated administration of atropine SQ or IV at lower dosages is usually required, particularly in cats. Development of tachyarrhythmias, delirium, and pyrexia are indications of excessive atropinization.

Organophosphate poisoning. Pralidoxime chloride (2-PAM; Protopam chloride) should be administered at 10 mg/lb or 20 mg/kg for cats and at 25 mg/lb or 50 mg/kg for dogs IV slowly or with fluids over a 30-minute period when poisoning is caused by organophosphate insecticides. Response to 2-PAM is observed within 30 minutes and includes disappearance of muscle fasciculations and muscle weakness. It should be repeated within an hour if these clinical signs persist and then administered every eight hours for 24 to 48 hours. Intensification of clinical signs may occur following rapid administration of 2-PAM; however, these are transient. The author recommends 2-PAM administration to animals that are severely depressed, weak, and anorectic one or more days after exposure, and were not previously treated with 2-PAM. Clinical signs such as respiratory distress may develop or intensify. Therefore, reduction of the dose and repeated one-hour infusions of 2-PAM in fluids every four to eight hours is a better method to follow in combination with atropine administration (0.02 to 0.2 mg/lb or 0.04 to 0.4 mg/kg) once or as needed. Poisoning with carbamate insecticides does not require 2-PAM administration. Activated charcoal should be administered orally in all cases of poisoning in combination with a saline cathartic.

Other insecticides. Chlorinated hydrocarbon insecticidal poisoning is treated similarly to strychnine or metaldehyde poisoning. Fluid therapy, with administration of glucose if indicated, is recommended. Activated charcoal is recommended even if the route of exposure was external, since enterohepatic circulation may occur.

Symptomatic and supportive therapy is required for intoxication with pyrethrins or rotenone insecticides. Toxic hepatopathy occurred in cats[20] exposed to rotenone and requires therapeutic consideration.

Other Important Pesticides

ZINC PHOSPHIDE

Circumstantial and General Information. This rodenticide is used rather commonly and is stable for long periods under dry conditions.[21] Upon ingestion, acid catalysis of the metallophosphide causes production of phosphine gas, which is responsible for acute poisoning. The intact zinc phosphide is believed to produce hepatic and renal damage that results in more chronic effects. Secondary poisoning has been suggested as being more common with this rodenticide since the baits are objectionable due to their odor. In addition, ingestion of the bait commonly results in emesis, which lessens the opportunity for primary poisoning.

Clinical Signs. Following ingestion, the onset of clinical signs can vary greatly from 15 minutes to 18 hours. Generally, signs of poisoning are present within four hours. Emesis and depression are common initial presenting signs. Respiratory distress characterized by rapid, deep, stertorous motions may quickly follow, which can lead to death. Terminal seizures accompany this agonal course. Variations in degree of gastrointestinal manifestations and convulsive activity make clinical diagnosis extremely difficult. Dogs may display central nervous disorders that resemble strychnine, Compound 1080/1081, or metaldehyde poisoning. Death can occur peracutely or over a two-day time period related to hypoxia secondary to pulmonary damage, seizure activity, and/or cardiovascular collapse.

Clinical Laboratory Information. Hematological and biochemical data vary, depending on the course of the illness. Necropsy findings reveal lesions of gastroenteritis (often hemorrhagic), pulmonary edema, and hepatopathy and nephropathy in animals surviving for longer periods.

Toxicological Analysis. An odor from the stomach that resembles acetylene or rotten fish (garlic-like) is characteristic of zinc phosphide–poisoned animals. The stomach should be removed intact, frozen, and submitted for toxic analysis at a reputable veterinary diagnostic laboratory for confirmation of poisoning. Determination of zinc in the stomach, liver, and kidney is also recommended.

Differentiation. Differential considerations are those listed in Tables 55–2, 55–4, and 55–6.

Therapy. Gastric lavage with a five per cent sodium bicarbonate solution or 1:5000 potassium permanganate[14] is indicated. General detoxicants such as calcium gluconate, sodium thiosulfate, and dextrose aid in combating the absorbed poison. No specific antidote is available. Pentobarbital or diazepam to control central nervous excitation, corticosteroids and fluid therapy for cardiovascular support, antibiotics for coverage, and an oxygen-rich environment to aid respiratory distress are important measures to provide. Morphine, aminophylline, and/or Lasix are indicated if pulmonary edema is present. Lactulose and multiple vitamins, lipotropic agents (methionine, choline), and nutritional changes may be required to aid recovery in light of hepatic or renal damage.

PYRIDYLIUM HERBICIDES (PARAQUAT AND DIQUAT)

Circumstantial and General Information. These herbicides are hazardous if an animal has access to a concentrated product either as a mishap in application or storage, or by finding them in a dump site. Diquat is highly corrosive (see **Caustics and Disinfectants**). Both affect the lung, but paraquat is most dangerous. Other herbicidal toxicity is minimal with the exception of arsenical and phenolic herbicides. These are described elsewhere.[22]

Clinical Signs. Animals presented commonly have evidence of an oily substance on the body hair and may show skin irritation. Initial signs of nausea, ulcerations of oral mucous membranes, salivation, and respiratory distress are commonly seen within one to three days following exposure. Pulmonary edema is responsible for the early signs of respiratory distress. The respiratory component worsens despite treatment, as progressive fibrosis ensues. Damage to proximal renal tubules may lead to renal failure.

Clinical Laboratory Information. Gastrointestinal signs may lead to dehydration and electrolyte losses that should be monitored. Blood gases are important to examine and the PO_2 should be used as a measure of therapeutic response.

Toxicological Analysis. Urine and serum should be collected, as well as portions of oily hair or gastric contents if obtained early in the course of illness. A sample of a suspected source would be best if available. Few laboratories have the expertise to perform analysis in biological tissues, but samples should be frozen until a suitable laboratory is found.

Differentiation. The combination of gastrointestinal and pulmonary signs suggests ingestion of a hydrocarbon solvent. Neurological effects are common with hydrocarbon exposure but not with paraquat. The progression of respiratory signs is too slow for alphanaphthylthiourea

TABLE 55–7. EXTERNAL IRRITATION OR BURNS AND/OR ACUTE DISORDERS OF THE UPPER GASTROINTESTINAL TRACT WITH POSSIBLE SYSTEMIC EFFECTS

Toxic Agent	Other Associated Findings for Differentiation
Quaternary ammonium disinfectants	contact irritation, systemic
Caustics	same
Household cleaners	
Rust removers	
Fluxes	
Swimming pool pH agents	
Paraquat/diquat	ulcerations, pulmonary
Toads	salivation, cardiac
Caterpillar	contact irritation
Hymenoptera stings	swelling, dyspnea
Agents producing dermatologic abnormalities	
Thallium	alopecia, erythema
Arsenical products	external exposure
Organic mercurial compounds	neurologic effects
Petroleum solvents	contact irritation
Plants	contact irritation
Euphorbia species	irritant sap
Caper surge	
Tinsel tree, others	
Ornamental Azalea species	histamine release, oxalates
Dieffenbachia	
Philodendron, others	
Infectious respiratory viruses in cats	viral panel

(ANTU) poisoning, which is acute and fulminating. Other causes of pulmonary edema should be considered, as given in Tables 55–2, 55–6, 55–7.

Therapy. Supportive and symptomatic treatment comprise the only therapeutic route to follow; however, the prognosis is grave due to the progressive nature of this disorder. Since no antidote exists, intensive fluid therapy and the application of activated charcoal or adsorbent clays (bentonite or Fuller's earth) are important in order to remove the ingested poison. Oxygen therapy is contraindicated since free radical formation is enhanced by its presence, which causes further lung damage. Corticosteroids seem to offer the best therapeutic approach and long-term therapy should be followed for several weeks. Morphine, aminophylline, furosemide, and/or nebulization may be indicated. Administration of Desferal at 100 mg/kg as a 24-hour infusion has promise of antidotal action.

ANTU

Alphanaphthylthiourea (ANTU) poisoning is predominately a respiratory problem and produces a marked pulmonary edema more precipitously than paraquat. It is commonly used as a tracking powder rodenticide. Treatment of ANTU is symptomatic, including sedation with morphine, suction of pulmonary fluid, oxygen, furosemide, aminophylline, and nebulization to prevent foaming. Table 55–6 illustrates other conditions causing similar signs.

AVITROL (4-AMINOPYRIDINE)

Circumstantial and General Information. This product is used to control pest birds such as blackbirds, starlings, crows, feral pigeons, and gulls. Ingestion of blackbirds killed by avitrol did not produce secondary poisoning in dogs. Feedlots, urban areas, and airports are areas where baits are used and provide opportunity for dogs and cats to be exposed. Grains and bread are used as baits, both of which dogs will ingest.

Clinical Signs. Initial apprehension, salivation, tremors, hyperexcitability, incoordination, and disorientation may lead to noninducible seizures with terminal cardiopulmonary arrest.[23]

Clinical Laboratory Information. Stress response and metabolic acidosis are anticipated abnormalities. Cardiovascular changes are similar to those found in strychnine poisoning.

Toxicological Analysis. Detection of avitrol in the stomach contents, urine, liver, or blood confirms the diagnosis.

Differentiation. Clinical signs in dogs or cats are similar to metaldehyde, anticholinesterase insecticides, and the CNS-affecting rodenticides (see Table 55–4).

Therapy. Treatment is similar to that of metaldehyde, including such drugs as diazepam and xylazine with supportive care. In humans, diphenhydramine (Benadryl) and naloxone have also been recommended.[24] Propranolol has been suggested for use as a cardioprotectant in humans and dogs (0.05 to 0.5 mg/lb or 0.1 to 1.0 mg/kg).

PHOSPHORUS

Circumstantial and General Information. Elemental yellow phosphorus exposure via a rodenticidal paste (Stearns' Electric Paste), fireworks materials, flare contents, or police or military gas canisters may occur under unusual circumstances.

Clinical Signs. Three clinical phases have been described in acutely poisoned humans.[25] Initial signs include nausea, vomiting, diarrhea, and severe abdominal pain. Provided shock and death do not develop, these signs can linger eight hours to three days. A period of recovery lasting hours to weeks may follow. Then, clinical signs with a more serious systemic effect upon hepatic, renal, nervous, and cardiovascular systems develop. Clinical effects observed during the final phase include severe gastrointestinal upsets, coagulopathy, hepatic enlargement, icterus, seizures, oliguria to anuria, and death within days to weeks. External exposure to yellow phosphorus can cause second to third degree burns to the skin.

Clinical Laboratory Information. Evidence of injury to the systems mentioned should be found in animals that survive a peracute episode. Acidosis, hypoglycemia, and monocytosis are variable but anticipated changes accompanying the final phase. Hepatic injury is most pronounced and coagulopathy is associated with this possibly via disseminated intravascular coagulopathy and/or loss of hepatic coagulation factor synthesis. Abnormal electrocardiograms (e.g., T-wave and S-T segment alterations) may be found. Animals less than a year old that survive may have radiographic evidence of dense metaphyseal bands (present at three weeks) in long bones as described in humans.[26]

Toxicological Analysis. A case report of a peracute poisoning in a cat[27] was characterized by acute illness, showing severe dyspnea with tongue protruding and hypersalivation, progressive weakness, tonoclonic convulsions with periods of apnea, and death within ten minutes. The characteristic "smoking stool" syndrome was observed in the cat's stomach contents along with severe gastric and esophageal irritation. Typical of phosphorus poisoning, a garlic odor was also detected upon necropsy. Toxicological analysis of the stomach content, liver, and possibly serum would have provided confirmatory information.

Differentiation. Mushroom poisoning is very similar to phosphorus intoxication. Other considerations are listed in Tables 55–2 and 55–6.

Therapy. Treatment for this is directed toward the initial phase of poisoning. Removal of the toxic agent is best performed using a gastric lavage. Multiple administrations of activated charcoal q4h at 1.5 mg/lb (3 gm/kg) loading followed by 0.5 gm/lb (1 gm/kg) for 24 hours was believed more advantageous to give than the recommended lavage solutions of potassium permanganate (1:5000) or cupric sulfate (0.2 per cent).[26] Supportive drug and fluid therapy to prevent shock and symptomatic therapy should be implemented. No antidote is available. The final clinical phase may require plasma or whole blood transfusions in cases of severe coagulopathy.

PESTICIDES CAUSING COAGULOPATHY

Circumstantial and General Information. Rodenticidal anticoagulant poisonings are of high potential incidence due to their availability to household owners and their important role in urban and agricultural rodent control programs. There are two basic classes of clinical concern: the *short-acting* (warfarin and related anticoagulants) or *long-acting* (indandiones and second generation anticoagulants) clinical types that have been described.[28] The short-acting types have clinical effects lasting less than a week. Ingestion of anticoagulant baits is the major route of exposure, but secondary poisoning can occur in dogs and cats. This type of poisoning is more probable with second generation anticoagulants. From a clinical perspective, it is crucial to identify which class of anticoagulant one is dealing with for proper therapy. The anticoagulant and the amount ingested primarily determine the length of coagulopathy.

Clinical Signs. Since coagulopathy is the hallmark of anticoagulant rodenticide poisoning, presentation of an animal with subcutaneous hemorrhages and/or bleeding from any orifice or wound site is straightforward evidence of this poisoning. However, internal bleeding without external hemorrhage is a more serious diagnostic challenge. Depression and pallor are the two common clinical signs associated with cases of internal hemorrhage only. Evidence of weakness, nonlocalized pain, hypothermia to fever, cold extremities, and/or dyspnea may accompany the presentation. Less commonly, central nervous system signs may predominate, varying with site of hemorrhage, or the animal may be found dead following a peracute hemorrhagic episode. Bleeding into a specific region may display signs related to that area, such as acute dyspnea associated with retropharyngeal bleeding.

Clinical Laboratory Information. Coagulation tests are the most important ones to perform when anticoagulant rodenticide poisoning is suspected. Citrated blood samples should be obtained prior to administration of the antidote to best evaluate the condition. The coagulation screening tests (OSPT, APTT, ACT, clotting time tests) are prolonged. The one-stage prothrombin time (OSPT) is the most sensitive assay to perform for anticoagulant-poisoned animals due to the short half-life of Factor VII. A confirmatory diagnostic test to perform is to follow the OSPT every six to eight hours (ideally) after vitamin K_1 therapy is begun for 24 to 48 hours. A more sensitive assay exists, referred to as the PIVKA test, which can be as readily performed as the OSPT.[29]

Blood loss anemia characterizes the complete blood count. Biochemical profiles show no pattern due to anticoagulant poisoning. Organ dysfunction may occur secondary to hemorrhage and/or anemia.

Chest radiographs are indicated when patients are dyspneic. Pleural or pulmonary hemorrhage, or cardiac tamponade needs to be considered. Such conditions call for emergency measures. No radiographic evidence for any of the above supports serious loss of red cell mass requiring a whole blood transfusion.

Toxicological Analysis. Anticoagulant screening assays are limited to few veterinary diagnostic laboratories. Samples of choice are plasma/serum and liver. In addition, recent studies of vitamin K analysis and its diagnostic importance have shown great promise in confirming anticoagulant rodenticide poisoning.[30]

Differentiation. Tables 55–1, 55–6, and 55–8 list several conditions that must be considered in the event of a bleeding animal.

TABLE 55–8. PALLOR AND/OR HEMOLYTIC DISORDERS ASSOCIATED WITH DEPRESSION FOR DIFFERENTIAL CONSIDERATION

Toxic Agent	Other Associated Findings for Differentiation
Anticoagulant rodenticides	blood loss anemia
Acetaminophen (cat, especially)	Heinz-body anemia
Plant onions	Heinz-body anemia
Mothballs (naphthalene)	Heinz-body anemia
Zinc	AIHA
Aspirin (accumulative toxicity)	gastric ulceration
Iron	shock
Phenol disinfectants/products	massive exposure, hemolysis
Mushroom (Group 1)	hemorrhagic diarrhea
(Group 2)	hemolysis, methemoglobinemia
Arsine gas	hemolysis
Autoimmune hemolytic anemia (AIHA)	Coomb's positive
Autoimmune thrombocytopenia (AITP)	PF3 positive
Von Willebrand's disease	VW factor, breed
Other congenital conditions (hemophilia)	factors VIII, IX, X
Disseminated intravascular coagulopathy (DIC)	primary problem
GI neoplasia	blood loss anemia
Internal blood loss (injury, hemangiosarcoma)	same

Therapy. Whole blood or plasma transfusions, shock therapy, paracentesis for removal of blood from vital areas, oxygen therapy, and drugs for pulmonary edema are life-sustaining considerations.[28] Vitamin K_1 should be administered SQ as a loading dose (2.5 mg/lb or 5.0 mg/kg) in multiple sites followed in 6 to 12 hours with 0.75 to 1.25 mg/lb (1.25 to 2.5 mg/kg) q12h PO for seven days. In severely ill animals, the divided dose can be given SQ for 24 to 48 hours. Dogs known to have cholestatic, maldigestive, or malabsorptive disease conditions may require continued SQ administration. Animals known to have been poisoned with a long-acting anticoagulant should be treated for a minimum of 14 days. This dose is sufficient for cats but possibly excessive.

Instruct the client to return the animal for another OSPT in two to three days after the last vitamin K_1 dose. Elevation of OSPT provides a sound reason to continue vitamin K_1 therapy for an additional one to three weeks followed by checkups.

Heavy Metals

LEAD

Circumstantial and General Information. Recognition of lead poisoning is important in companion animals since the close association between humans and animals affords valuable insight into human exposure and the risk of lead-induced health problems in humans.[31] Many sources of lead are available to household pets, but the dog is predominately affected due to its compulsive eating habits and the accumulative nature of lead once ingested. Construction materials, hobby materials, and automotive materials contain lead. Ingestion of a leaded object such as a sinker provides a continual single source of lead as digestion occurs. A dog of any age can be affected but dogs less than one year old are more frequently affected. Several factors affect manifestation of toxicity, such as low dietary calcium.

Clinical Signs. A combination of gastrointestinal and neurological signs are commonly observed. Anorexia, vomiting, diarrhea, constipation, and/or abdominal pain within seven to ten days prior to presentation usually occurs. Development of neurological signs motivates a client to seek medical assistance. Neurological signs can vary from sudden epileptiform seizures to that of subtle behavior changes. Continual whining or barking possibly associated with abdominal pain or a neurological manifestation alerts a client to the problem. Running-like seizures followed by a short terminal course can occur. Periodic seizures consisting of opisthotonos, clonic-tonic motions, and vocalization, followed by extended intervals of normal behavior, are seen. Petit seizures such as chewing gum fits may be the extent of seizure activity. Puppy hysteria characterized by extreme nervousness and hyperexcitability may characterize the neurological signs. Dullness with apparent blindness may be observed in some cases. No obvious neurological manifestations may be seen except for abnormal behavior of the animal, such as hiding under objects, showing more or less aggressiveness, or poor athletic performance. These may occur in combination with the above manifestations.

Cats tend to show more dramatic neurological manifestations of the disease. Gastrointestinal disorders are not as prominent as in the dog.

Clinical Laboratory Information. Hematologic changes are quite characteristic of lead-poisoned animals in more chronically exposed subjects. The presence of nucleated red blood cells in the absence of anemia and of basophilic stippled red cells is the classic hemogram of lead-poisoned animals. Blood smears taken for examination of basophilic stippling are best prepared with unanticoagulated blood, dried slowly, and stained without prior alcohol fixation.[32] A microcytic hypochromic anemia may develop in prolonged clinical cases. Anisocytosis, poikilocytosis, polychromasia, echinocytosis, and target cells are other observed hematological changes due to increased red cell fragility. A left shifted leukocytosis or leukopenia may accompany the other signs. A bone marrow examination may reveal a low M/E ratio caused by an arrest at the polychromatic metarubricyte stage and the possible presence of sideroblasts.

Radiographs may reveal radiodense materials within the gastrointestinal tract. Leaded objects such as toys or sinkers are obvious. Even leaded paint chips can be visualized but must be differentiated from gravel or bone chips. Electroencephalograms may demonstrate slowing of wave activity with increased amplitude as continuous and present in all leads.

Toxicological Analysis. Whole blood is the preferred sample for confirmatory diagnosis in a living animal. Lead concentrations of 35 μg/dl (0.35 ppm) or above are highly supportive of lead poisoning, while concentrations of 60 μg/dl or above are considered diagnostic. The urinary CaEDTA post-chelation test should be performed in chronically poisoned animals if blood lead levels are inconclusive. The antidote should be administered as described in the therapeutic section, followed by collection of a 24-hour sample or total 24-hour urine volume. The postchelation lead concentrations in lead-poisoned dogs are usually greater than ten times the prechelation lead concentrations, while dogs not poisoned with lead have approximately tenfold or less prechelation urine value.

Hematologic parameters that are confirmatory of lead poisoning can also be measured. These include aminolevulinic acid (ALA) in urine, ALA-dehydratase enzyme activity, and free erythrocyte protoporphyrin concentrations (FEPs) in red blood cells. Normal values are not established in dogs or cats.

Differentiation. Tables 55–2 and 55–4 list other gastrointestinal and neurological diseases that must be differentiated from lead poisoning.

Therapy. In most cases, administration of the antidote of choice, calcium EDTA (calcium disodium ethylenediaminetetra-acetate), is sufficient to alleviate the clinical problems in dogs and cats. The antidote serves to chelate and enhance urinary excretion of lead. Life-threatening clinical signs must be controlled by symptomatic and supportive therapy. If indicated, oral administration of magnesium sulfate (Epsom salt) provides binding of ingested lead and evacuation of the gastrointestinal tract. Cats require thorough external washing. Surgical removal of a discrete leaded object in the gastrointestinal tract is indicated.

Commercial preparations of calcium EDTA are best diluted to one per cent (10 mg/ml) solutions in isotonic saline or five per cent dextrose to avoid irritation. The recommended treatment regimen is subcutaneous administration of 13 mg/lb (27.5 mg/kg) q6h for five days followed by a five-day rest and repetition if necessary. For convenience, subcutaneous administration of calcium EDTA at 25 mg/lb (50 mg/kg) q12h for five days has been recommended. Penicillamine can be given orally and is useful for continued therapy at home. Recommended dosage is 50 mg/lb/day (110 mg/kg/day) given divided q6–8h for one to two weeks. If adverse effects such as vomiting, depression, and anorexia occur, the daily dose should be changed to 15 to 25 mg/lb/day (33 to 55 mg/kg/day), which is better tolerated.

ARSENIC

Circumstantial and General Information. Different chemical forms of arsenic are found in various materials. Arsenical medications, insecticides, herbicides, defoliants, wood preservatives, industrial materials, enamels, and miscellaneous construction materials provide potential sources of arsenic.[33] The most common potential sources for dogs and cats are home arsenical herbicides and pesticidal preparations such as ant baits.

Clinical Signs. Both inorganic and organic alkyl arsenicals produce similar clinical effects. Acute exposure can produce onset of emesis, nausea, abdominal pain, and diarrhea within 30 minutes of ingestion. Progressive depression and weakness develop, leading to vascular collapse and death, which can occur within several hours. Diarrhea is very fluid and may be hemorrhagic if an arsenite source was ingested. Less acute exposures may lead to a longer course with secondary complications such as renal failure. A less typical presentation is that of a dermatitis associated with cutaneous exposure.[34]

Clinical Laboratory Information. Alteration of biochemical profiles (especially relating to the liver and kidney), electrolytes, and metabolic acidosis are expected with arsenic poisoning.

Toxicological Analysis. Early samples of urine and whole blood are good for arsenic determination in suspected cases. The liver and kidney should be frozen for arsenic measurement following acute death.

Differentiation. Table 55–2 lists other conditions that produce acute gastrointestinal signs. The quick demise of an animal with gastrointestinal signs is characteristic of arsenic poisoning.

Therapy. Intensive fluid and electrolyte therapy is essential in treatment of this condition. The antidote of choice is British antilewisite (BAL; dimercaprol) for inorganic arsenicals. The dose of BAL is loading with 2.5 mg/lb (5 mg/kg) (acute cases only) followed with 1.25 mg/lb (2.5 mg/kg) q3–4h for two days and then progressively lengthening the dosing interval (q12h) until recovery is evident. Penicillamine has also shown promise as an effective chelator in humans.[35] The general detoxicant sodium thiosulfate can be used if other chelating agents are unavailable. The dose is approximated at 30 mg/lb (60 mg/kg) orally and 15 mg/lb (30 mg/kg) IV as a ten per cent solution, both of which are to be administered q8–12h. Experimental use of selenium and superoxide dismutase (Palosein, Coopers) has provided lung protection. Protectants and drugs for control of pain and prevention of shock are additional therapeutic considerations.

ZINC

Circumstantial and General Information. Poisoning problems have resulted in dogs from ingestion of medication (Desitin) and of zinc-containing objects, including pennies. Inhalation of fumes of zinc oxide associated with welding has produced acute pulmonary disorders, which is conceivable in dogs and cats. The clinical problems that developed in these cases are commonly encountered in practice, at times with no etiologic explanation.

Clinical Signs. Animals are noticeably less active and anorectic.[36] Abdominal upsets such as vomiting, diarrhea, and pain may accompany depression and weakness. Icterus related to a hemolytic anemia is common. These signs may develop over several days or longer with progressive debilitation. Exposure of the skin can incite papulovesicular lesions with exfoliation.

Clinical Laboratory Information. Evidence of damage to the renal, erythroid, pancreatic, and hepatic tissues has been observed. Azotemia with other signs associated with acute renal failure is commonly observed. Hemolytic anemia presenting in a manner similar to autoimmunohemolytic anemia is also predominant. Blood samples are Coomb's negative. Enzymatic or ultrasound evidence of pancreatitis may be observed. Hepatic damage associated with interruption of function (prolonged BSP retention) and elevation of hepatic enzymes is common.

Toxicological Analysis. Diagnosis is aided by abdominal radiographs to identify metallic objects and involvement of one or more of the body systems discussed. Confirmation is obtained by measurement of zinc in serum and urine, or liver and kidney if obtained at necropsy. In collection of blood samples, a plastic, glass screw cap tube or special blood tubes (metal-free) should be used.

Differentiation. Since renal, erythroid, pancreatic, and hepatic damage occurs, diseases that affect one or more of these systems require consideration as given in Tables 55–2, 55–3, and 55–8. Pancreatitis and autoimmune hemolytic anemia are initial disease considerations.

Therapy. Confirmation is normally lacking on presentation and symptomatic and supportive therapy is generally initiated to treat the abnormalities. Fluid therapy, possibly a whole blood transfusion, fasting, and dietary monitoring with a bland ration, cimetidine (2 mg/lb or 4 mg/kg q8h), antibiotics, and possibly steroids, if indicated for control of hemolysis, are regimens commonly employed. Calcium EDTA should be administered as a chelation antidote similar to that for lead poisoning, following confirmation of zinc poisoning.[14]

THALLIUM

Circumstantial and General Information. This metal has been used historically as an insecticide and a rodenticide.[14] Old storage areas may contain thallium sulfate or acetate. Industrial usage of thallium is common and may provide a source. Thallium usage in Mexico provides avenues of exposure to animals in bordering states. It is tasteless, odorless, and stable, so toxic ingestion is probable if available. Absorption via the skin is also a potential route of exposure. Excretion from the body is very slow.

Clinical Signs. In the acute form, gastrointestinal signs predominate, with respiratory distress commonly leading to death within three to five days. Anorexia, nausea, abdominal pain, a fluid to hemorrhagic diarrhea, and occasionally oral ulcerations are observed. Intense congestion of oral and ocular mucous membranes may lead to development of the "brick red" color. Respiratory distress results from direct toxic effects on the lungs with development of pulmonary edema and possibly progressive cardiac effects. Shock, renal failure, and/or hepatic disease due to direct toxic effects and dehydration may accompany other symptoms. Neurologic signs such as muscular fasciculations, ataxia, depression to irritability, convulsions, hyperesthesia, and coma have been observed.

The chronic form of poisoning is more characteristic, extends several weeks, and can follow an acute episode. General presenting signs include emaciation, marked weakness and depression, dehydration, and emesis in association with an afebrile skin disorder, accompanied by elevated pulse and respiratory rate. The characteristic feature of the skin is erythema of varying degrees that can be brick red in color. In addition, bilateral, nonpruritic alopecia begins in 7 to 14 days following exposure. The hair can easily be epilated. Glossitis, stomatitis, rhinitis, and conjunctivitis with corneal ulcerations may occur. Additional clinical problems described include persistent respiratory distress, paraphimosis, vocal abnormalities, malabsorption, secondary seborrhea, metabolic acidosis, chronic inflammatory leukogram, and neurologic (dementia) and locomotor problems (pain, stiffness, lameness).[37]

Clinical Laboratory Information. A skin biopsy or postmortem histologic findings are very supportive of chronic thallium poisoning.[38]

Toxicological Analysis. Confirmation of thallium poisoning is best performed on urine samples using the Gabriel-Dubin method.[39] A test analogous to the pre/post urinary lead chelation test using potassium can be performed in chronic cases of thallium poisoning.[40] Quantitative methods require sophisticated instrumentation.

Differentiation. Differential considerations for acute intoxication are similar to other disorders listed in Tables 55–2, 55–3, 55–4, and 55–6. Development of hair loss with erythema in 7 to 14 days is highly supportive of thallium intoxication. The integumentary changes include diseases such as pyoderma, canine distemper, pemphigus, pemphigoid, lupus erythematosus necrolysis, cutaneous lymphosarcoma (especially mycosis fungoides), contact irritant dermatitis, drug eruptions, and other conditions listed in Table 55–7.

Therapy. Enhancement of thallium excretion and symptomatic and supportive care are the goals.[39] Oral administration of ferric-cyanoferrate (Prussian blue) in a glucose solution at 50 to 100 mg/lb (100 to 200 mg/kg) q8h for one to five weeks is the most practical therapeutic method to enhance excretion. Several days may be required before evidence of improvement is noted. Return of the animal's appetite is one of the first signs of recovery. Diphenylthiocarbazone (Dithizone) has also been recommended during acute poisoning. Activated charcoal has been effective in humans and is recommended for use with Prussian blue.[14]

Potassium chloride should also be given orally at 1 to 2 gm q8–12h until clinical weakness is corrected unless the animal has renal azotemia. Fluid and electrolyte therapy, protectants, antibiotics, steroids if indicated, glucose (PO, SQ), trihexyphenidyl or similar drugs, and oxygen therapy for respiratory distress are supplemental considerations during acute poisoning. The skin condition should be treated with antibiotic ointments, moisturizing creams, and supportive/nutritional care with soft, protective bedding. The skin is very susceptible to pressure-induced necrosis. Hard pads eventually slough off; most of the alopecic areas regrow hair in part with time. Symptomatic therapy is required for conditions such as paraphimosis, oral or ocular ulcerations, or neurologic deficits.

MERCURY

This metal affects renal function and leads to acute renal failure. Sources include ingestion of thermometer contents or access to liniments that contain mercury. Exposure to organic mercurials is very unlikely, but exposure affects the central nervous system, leading to a variety of neurologic problems. Tables 55–3, 55–4, and 55–7 list the more common diseases. Therapy is similar to that for arsenic with regard to the antidote for chelation. Tissues for mercury determination are similar to those for arsenic.

BIOTOXINS

Living organisms are capable of producing poisonous agents, which are referred to as biotoxins. Snakebite and insect stings are by far the most commonly encountered problems. Toad poisoning is common in geographic areas where toxic species live. Plant poisoning and most mycotoxicoses occur seldom but may be encountered depending upon location and accessibility. Garbage poisoning due to bacterial toxins is also a common problem in dogs.

Snake Venom Poisoning

Circumstantial and General Information. Three factors influence the seriousness of a poisonous snakebite: size of the animal, location of the bite, and the type of snake. A venomous bite in the thorax of a small dog is highly lethal. Pit vipers, which include rattlesnakes, copperheads, and water moccasins, have toxins that produce tissue and vascular damage, hemolysis, coagulopathy, and cardiac effects (Mojave green rattler). The only neurotoxic venomous snake native to the United States is the coral snake (*Micrurus fulvius* and *euryxanthus*). The bite of a Mojave green rattler (*Crotalus scutulatus*) may produce curare-like signs. In metropolitan areas, however, the bite from a "pet" of a reptile enthusiast (e.g., elapids) may deliver highly toxic neuro- and/or cardiotoxic venoms or venoms similar to those of the pit vipers.[41]

Three basic clinical conditions can be assigned to venomous snakebites of pit vipers: mild, moderate, and severe forms.[42] The mild cases have minimal local reaction at the site of the bite and minimal systemic signs. Moderate cases have intense local reaction with few systemic effects. Severe cases have both severe local and systemic clinical effects.

Clinical Signs. Clinical diagnosis of snakebite of pit vipers is usually straightforward since tissue swelling at the site of the bite is always present in a true envenomation. The bite area is painful to the touch. Point of entry of the fangs may be observed as two puncture sites roughly 0.25 cm or more apart. A bloody discharge from the puncture sites is common. Observation of fang marks with little tissue reaction is evidence of a bite where little or no venom was imparted.

Animals may be mildly depressed to fully obtunded. Lameness may be observed and is easily mistaken for an injury. Signs of impending or fully developed vascular collapse are common. Local swelling may impinge upon the major airways, causing a life-threatening situation. Animals presented several hours after the initial bite may develop signs associated with hemolytic anemia, coagulopathy, and/or sepsis. Exotic poisonous snakes that belong to the Crotalidae (e.g., fer-de-lance), Viperidae (e.g., puff adder), or Colubridae (e.g., boomslang) families contain highly potent venoms similar to those of the pit vipers.

Animals bitten by exotic poisonous snakes or the coral snake, which possess predominately neurotoxic venoms, commonly have little reaction at the bite site. Muscle fasciculations may be present at the bite site and licking or biting related to paresthesias may occur. A progressive, flaccid paralysis is the major clinical effect caused by a peripheral curare-like effect on motor nerve endings and/or centrally by way of brain stem effects. Animals become disoriented, fasciculations may develop, and hypersalivation is common due to dysphagia. Ptosis, facial and ocular paresis with pupillary variations, strabismus, swallowing difficulties, dyspnea, prostration, unconsciousness, and rarely, convulsions upon excitation are associated symptoms. Respiratory paralysis and/or cardiac arrest lead to death within minutes to eight hours if the bite is severe.

Clinical Laboratory Information. Alterations of hemograms or biochemical profiles anticipated with pit viper bites include hemoconcentration to anemia, thrombocytopenia, hemolysis, coagulopathy, hypoxia, and azotemia. A complete blood count, clotting panel, electrolytes and blood gases, hematocrit, platelet count, and urinalysis should be performed periodically to assess systemic effects and response to antivenin treatment. Determination of plasma fibrinogen and fibrin split

TABLE 55–9. CONDITIONS FOR CONSIDERATION IF A VENOMOUS ANIMAL IS SUSPECTED SOURCE

Toxic Agent	Other Associated Findings for Differentiation
Snakebite	
Pit viper type	marked local reaction, systemic
Neurotoxic type	little local, rapid debilitation
Hymenoptera	immediate intense pain, allergic
Spider bite	
Black widow	neurologic signs
Brown recluse	local necrotizing lesion
Caterpillars	local contact irritation
Centipede	local inflammation
Scorpion	highly painful, systemic effects
Lizards	severe bite wounds, systemic
Traumatic injury	swelling, pain
Abscess	gradual onset, cytology
Small mammalian bite (rat)	pattern of teeth marks, local
Puncture wound of trachea	subcutaneous emphysema
Angioneurotic edema	hypersensitivity reaction*
Cutaneous neoplasia	progressive onset, cytology
Anticoagulant swelling	

*Such as postvaccination.

products evaluates progression of anticoagulant effects. An electrocardiogram is recommended during the critical and intensive phases of poisoning.

Toxicological Analysis. No assays exist to identify snake venoms in a diagnostic laboratory. If the snake was killed, it should be brought in for identification. This information is helpful in assessing therapeutic requirements.

Differentiation. Injuries with associated fractures, Hymenoptera stings, small mammal bites, and abscesses may be confused with a snakebite. Table 55–9 lists differentiation for local lesions and Table 55–10 addresses cardiac dysrhythmias commonly associated with exotic snakes.

Therapy. Three phases following pit viper envenomation are described as the *critical* phase, requiring emergency care (two hours), the *intensive* phase (24 hours), where a prognosis is based on therapeutic response, and the *convalescent* phase, lasting approximately ten days.[43] Antibodies (antivenin and tetanus antitoxin), anti-inflammatories, and antibiotics are the basics of treatment.

TABLE 55–10. DISEASE CONSIDERATIONS WHEN CARDIAC ABNORMALITIES ARE ENCOUNTERED

Toxic Agent	Other Associated Signs for Differentiation
Plant	GI upset, 12- to 24-hr course
Oleander	
Lily-of-the-valley	
Foxglove	
Toad	rapid course, salivation
Snakebite	hypotension and arrhythmias
Petroleum solvents	respiratory, CNS, and/or GI
Iatrogenic digoxin	GI upset
Carbon monoxide	cherry-red blood
Primary cardiac diseases	cardiac exam, primary system
Secondary cardiac effects	evidence of other systems involved
Pancreatitis	
Gastric torsion	
Shock	
Anemia	
Acute tamponade (rupture of hemangiosarcoma)	
Others	

The administration of antivenin, the antidote, should be reserved for moderate and severe cases. It is a *must* in severe envenomations.

Upon presentation, corticosteroids such as prednisolone sodium succinate (20 mg/lb or 35 mg/kg) should be administered IV or IM. Administer one vial of polyvalent antivenin every 30 minutes to one hour IV, along with a broad-spectrum antibiotic such as trimethoprim-sulfa, chloramphenicol, ampicillin, amoxicillin, or a cephalosporin. Generally, administration of one to two vials is sufficient, but as many as 20 may be required before a positive response is observed, allowing for cessation of antivenin administration. Antibiotic therapy should be continued through the convalescent phase. Tetanus prophylaxis is indicated.

Administration of fluids and drugs to combat shock provides supportive care. Development of hypotension is characteristic of lethal pit viper bites. Lactated Ringers' solution should be administered while monitoring for pulmonary edema. Plasma expanders or whole blood may be used if indicated. Dexamethasone should be given at 2 to 4 mg/lb (4 to 8 mg/kg) IV during the intensive phase with tapering of oral dosing through the convalescent phase. Antihistamines are contraindicated in snakebite.[44]

Treatment of bites received from the coral snake or exotic poisonous snakes is similar to that for pit viper bites, except that a different antivenin must be used. The antivenin to be used depends on the type of snake responsible for the bite. Zoological parks and aquariums stock antivenin to all exotic snakes in their collections, and the closest facility should be contacted. Animals that are inflicted with neurotoxin snake envenomation commonly require tracheostomy, aspiration, and positive-pressure oxygen therapy to provide lifesaving support. Exotic species containing venoms similar to the pit vipers' must be handled in like manner but a related antivenin should be sought. Surgical management of tissue necrosis associated with the bite area is important with these highly poisonous snakes.

Anaphylactic reactions to the administration of antivenin are due to the horse antiserum. Epinephrine (0.05 ml/lb or 0.1 ml/kg IV or IM of 1:10,000 solution; repeat every 5 to 15 minutes) should be given immediately. Antihistamines are indicated in this situation. Antivenin should be continued only when a severe bite case is involved. Administer 0.5 to 1 mg/lb (1 to 2 mg/kg) diphenhydramine (Benadryl) IV followed by slow infusion of antivenin diluted 1:5 or 1:10 or more, if indicated, over a 15 to 20 minute period. Repeat antivenin administration in this manner hourly as needed. Benadryl should be repeated if indicated. Alternate administration of small amounts of epinephrine and antivenin has been effective in humans.[41]

Toad Poisoning

Circumstantial and General Information. Mouthing or ingestion of toads may cause mild to severe problems in dogs or cats. All toads contain glands in their skin that taste offensive to animals and may incite local effects (e.g., salivation). The Colorado river toad (*Bufo* *alvarius*) and the marine toad (*Bufo marinus*) are toxic species.[45] The parotid gland of these toads contains bufotoxins. Observation of animals "playing" with a toad allows for a rapid diagnosis. Flushing of the animal's mouth with water from a hose is the best preventative measure. Symptomatic and laboratory evidence are secondary means to support this diagnostic challenge if the history is unsupporting.

Clinical Signs. Onset of signs occurs within minutes of mouthing the toad.[46] Mouth irritation with hypersalivation is the most characteristic presenting clinical sign. Development of cardiac irregularities suggests exposure to the toxic species of toads. Associated cardiac signs include cyanosis, depression, weakness, collapse, pulmonary edema, and convulsions. Emesis and diarrhea may develop. Death is common within 30 minutes following contact with the toad.

Clinical Laboratory Information. When toad poisoning is suspected, monitoring with an ECG is desirable. A progression of dysrhythmias may occur that can lead to ventricular fibrillation.

Toxicological Analysis. No diagnostic methods exist to identify the bufotoxins. Presence of toad parts in stomach contents is confirmatory evidence.

Differentiation. Caustics, metaldehyde, anticholinesterase insecticides, and an oral or upper GI foreign body are conditions listed in Table 55–7 that may produce similar acute clinical signs. Pronounced cardiac arrhythmias suggest other conditions listed in Table 55–10.

Therapy. Emergency treatment for poisoning caused by toads containing the bufotoxins is essential. Immediate administration of propranolol (Inderal) (2.5 mg/lb or 5.0 mg/kg IV rapidly) with a repeat dose in 20 minutes if needed, has been recommended in dogs.[46] Others have recommended 0.75 to 2.5 mg/lb or 1.5 to 5.0 mg/kg for dogs and cats.[47] Induce anesthesia with pentobarbital, intubate, and flush the oral cavity with water. Establish an ECG monitor or obtain serial lead II ECG readings. If the arrhythmias persist, an IV drip of 0.01 to 0.1 mg/lb (0.02 to 0.2 mg/kg) propranolol can be administered. Potassium and phenytoin (Dilantin) administration may be given as described in the section on Poisonous Plants. If ventricular fibrillation is present upon presentation, the procedures described for cardiac glycoside intoxication should be followed, using defibrillation, epinephrine, or chemical defibrillation. Atropine (0.04 mg/kg) may be indicated to alleviate salivation and pulmonary secretions, and to provide cardioprotective actions against atrioventricular block (AV-block) and sinoatrial arrest.

Hypersalivation and anxiety associated with mouthing toads that do not contain bufotoxin require little emergency treatment, but acepromazine (IM, SQ 0.1 to 0.5 mg/lb or 0.2 to 1.0 mg/kg) and atropine (0.02 mg/lb or 0.04 mg/kg IV, SQ) may provide relief of the distressing signs.

Arthropod Bites or Stings

Circumstantial and General Information. This phylum contains four-fifths of the known animals in the world.[48] Venomous insects and arachnids are readily available to animals. Younger animals that learn to feed on insects are at high risk. Insects of Hymenoptera are the commonly encountered bees, bumblebees, wasps, hornets, yellow jackets, and fire (*Solenopsis* spp.) or harvester ants (*Pogonomyrmex* spp.).

Several species of caterpillars (Lepidoptera) equipped with simple, hollow, brittle spines associated with venom-secreting glands can produce nettling stings. The puss caterpillar (*Megalopyge opercularis*) is a commonly encountered species in human practice.

Spiders and scorpions are the arachnids that may produce a venomous bite or sting. The black widow (*Lactrodectus* spp.) and brown recluse or fiddleback (*Loxosceles* spp.) spiders may inflict a troublesome bite. The venom of the black widow is a neurotoxin, while that of the brown recluse causes local vascular thrombosis and necrosis. Few scorpions are toxic and are of limited geographic importance. The yellow, 2.0 to 7.5 cm *Centruroides sculpturatus* scorpion encountered in Arizona is capable of delivering a neurotoxic venom and is considered the scorpion of major importance. Centipedes bear a pair of curved hollow fangs equipped with venom glands in the first anterior segment, which can result in irritation to animals and humans. Millipedes eject secretions that produce contact irritation, but problems in humans occur primarily in tropical countries. Tick paralysis is covered in another section.

Clinical Signs. Hymenoptera stings are very common, especially in younger animals that indiscriminately investigate moving objects. External stings inflict immediate pain evidenced in dogs by yelping and running in a frenzied manner. Wheal and flare reaction occurs if the point of stinger entry can be located on the skin. Edema is variable but may extend well beyond the site and persist for up to four days. Stings in the orolingual and oropharyngeal regions are frequent, since ingestion of these insects is common in the novice animal. Stings in these locations produce excessive salivation and respiratory distress, which can be life-threatening due to swelling in addition to the pain and frenzy. This holds true for single, uncomplicated stings. However, in the event of multiple, uncomplicated stings, the degree of pain and vascular effects may lead to death in an acute manner. In humans, 40 to 50 hornet stings can be fatal.

Hypersensitive animals are in more serious trouble due to the complications superimposed by a single sting. Less severe reactions may result in hives, nausea, and wheezing. Severe reactions lead to marked dyspnea, cyanosis, and collapse commonly associated with a febrile reaction. Death occurs due to primary hypotension and/or hypoxia associated with pulmonary secretions, bronchial constriction, or tissue swelling. Systemic allergic reactions occur within 15 minutes to 6 hours. Delayed atypical reactions have been observed in humans 10 to 14 days after the event, and include the Arthus reaction, serum sickness, arthralgia, fever, nephrotic syndrome, acute glomerulonephritis, hepatorenal syndrome, necrotic angiitis, thrombocytopenic purpura, transverse myelitis, lymphadenopathy, birth defects, and others.

Stings from the fire ant produce immediate pain

followed by sterile vesicular development within two hours progressing to pustules within 24 hours. These are prone to secondary bacterial infections.

Animals that mouth a venomous caterpillar suddenly become distressed, accompanied by pawing at the mouth and headshaking. Signs associated with irritation and swelling ensue.

Bites from black widow spiders in humans are modestly painful with swelling of the local area or extremity. Severe muscle cramping develops within 30 minutes, spreading by continuity. Muscles of the limbs, abdomen, thorax, and lower back may become involved. Acute abdominal pain is quite characteristic. An ascending paralysis eventually develops. In addition, restlessness, depression, nausea with hypersalivation, ataxia, and weakness frequently accompany the neuromuscular signs. Seizures and coma may develop. Little information is available on the spider's comparative toxicity in humans and small animals. Dogs and cats may be more resistant since a paucity of cases have been reported, but diagnostic criteria are nonexistent.

The brown recluse bite is less likely to occur since this spider has weak fangs compared with the black widow. In humans, following a latent period of one to four hours, a painful reddish blister appears, surrounded by a blue-white halo. The site of the bite may become hemorrhagic and markedly erythemic in conjunction with more systemic signs of local lymphadenopathy and collapse. Necrosis occurs, leading to indurated ulcer formation at the bite site, which is slow in healing. Generalized signs of fever, arthralgia, and/or hemolytic anemia occasionally develop in humans early in the course of the disease; these are undoubtedly associated with immunologic mechanisms.

Animals stung by a venomous scorpion react in a manner similar to those affected by a Hymenoptera sting (immediate pain). However, a hyperesthesia develops that produces extreme response to any manipulation of the site. Neurologic signs follow, including hyperactivity, hypermotility, disorientation, hypertension, pulmonary edema, and convulsions. Stings of nonvenomous scorpions may produce pain and local edema to a limited extent.

Centipede bites result in pain and local swelling that may progress to regional lymphangitis and lymphadenopathy.

Clinical Laboratory Information. Clinical tests that evaluate renal and pulmonary function, hemograms, leukograms, Coomb's tests, and urinary analysis are useful to evaluate the degree of insult to the animal's body following envenomation.

Toxicological Analysis. Capturing the culprit responsible for envenomation is the only means of confirming the diagnosis. Examination of the suspected area where the animal was "stung" may prove useful, as a nest or hive may be found.

Differentiation. Considerations for bites or stings are listed in Table 55–9. Stings in the mouth result in signs that may be difficult to differentiate from conditions listed in Table 55–7.

Therapy. As a general rule, since puncture wounds are made by these creatures, prophylactic treatment for tetanus is indicated and possibly antibiotic therapy to cover against entry of other opportunistic organisms. Cleaning of the wound site should be considered. The use of bandages is not recommended for most of these conditions.

External uncomplicated stings of Hymenoptera require lotion application or administration of antihistamines (e.g., diphenhydramine). Multiple stings may require the administration of analgesics and corticosteroids in addition to antihistamine therapy. Stings in the mouth or pharynx require handling similar to that of multiple stings with the option of performing emergency procedures such as a tracheotomy. Alleviation of generalized symptoms can be aided with ten per cent calcium gluconate. Sting complications evidenced by hyperimmune reactions require the immediate administration of epinephrine every 20 to 30 minutes as needed along with corticosteroids.

The general therapeutic protocol for bites of spiders or stings of scorpions showing only local swelling and pain include a short-acting corticosteroid, a mild analgesic, and application of a cold pack. Animals showing or which develop systemic signs require additional therapy.[47]

Historically, calcium gluconate has been an effective treatment for black widow bites if given every two to four hours in humans. Methocarbamol given q6h is now the recommended drug in humans to alleviate muscle spasms, abdominal pain, and other neurologic disorders. Opioid analgesics (morphine, meperidine) are indicated if signs persist. Antivenin is available, and should be requested from a regional poison control center if deemed worthwhile.

Symptomatic and supportive therapy is required if the systemic signs occur with the bite of a brown recluse. Steroid therapy is highly recommended if initiated 72 hours following the bite. Following this time period, use of anti-inflammatories is not recommended; the condition should then be treated as a slow-healing ulcer.

Scorpion stings leading to systemic signs generally require an anesthetic agent. Diazepam or pentobarbital is effective in controlling excitability and seizures. Muscle spasms can be alleviated by use of methocarbamol or calcium gluconate. The use of antihypertensives is indicated in this disease complex in humans. Phentolamine or other sympatholytics are commonly used. Drugs for pulmonary edema may be indicated. Opiates should not be used since they potentiate toxicity in humans. In rare instances, antivenin may be desired and is available through the Poisonous Animals Research Laboratory of Arizona State University (Table 55–5).

Centipede bites can be handled in a manner similar to arachnid bites that show only local signs. Local infiltration with a local anesthetic alleviates any pain.

Poisonous Lizards

The Gila monster (*Heloderma suspectum*) and Mexican beaded lizard (*Heloderma horridum*) are the only two poisonous lizards in North America. Bites are extremely rare and very unlikely due the sluggish nature of captive specimens. Wild creatures travel in the evening and night and can move with alarming alacrity for defensive purposes. In the event of a bite, the animal will probably be presented with the lizard still attached. They bite "for keeps." The lizards do not have fangs like a snake, but the upper teeth are bathed in venom from eight venom glands located on the lower jaw. Removal of the lizard must be done most discreetly following decapitation. Treatment is similar to snakebite and antivenin can be requested from the Poisonous Animals Research Laboratory of Arizona State University. These bites are most painful even when no venom is produced. Therefore, wound care and relief of pain are in order.

Poisonous Plants

Cultivated plants outside the home and house plants provide opportunities for dogs and cats to contact toxic substances. Younger animals are more apt to chew on plants during destructive moods, but other situations may also cause an animal to do this. Plants have been classed by others for convenience to comprehend the vastness of possibilities and should be referred to if plant toxicity is suspected.[51–53] Treatment is based on the ABC's (airway, breathing, circulation) with symptomatic and supportive care. Activated charcoal and catharsis (if indicated) are appropriate detoxification measures to apply. Observation of plant material in stomach contents or vomitus is variable.

Plants containing cardiac glycosides are worthy of discussion. *Nerium oleander* is very common in some locations. Leaves or other parts of the plant deposited into a water dish can poison a dog or cat. Signs of poisoning develop within three hours, as vomiting and nausea progress to tenesmus and diarrhea. Varying conditions of the heart may be auscultated, including tachycardia, missed beats, blocks, and bradycardia. Bradycardia is the most characteristic sign of cardiac glycoside intoxication. However, the rate and pulse can vary from slow to fast, strong to weak. Weakness, depression, and collapse associated with cyanosis, respiratory distress, and terminal struggling may develop. The course of illness may persist for 24 hours or longer. Tables 55–2 and 55–10 list other conditions that have similar clinical signs.

Treatment for oleander poisoning requires careful evaluation of the heart and application of one or more drugs to alleviate associated dysrhythmias.[54] Infusion of potassium solutions IV at 0.25 to 0.5 mEq/mg/hr (0.5 to 1.0 mEq/kg/hr) with cardiac monitoring is recommended as supplementary treatment for hypokalemic animals, provided AV block is not present. Administration is still recommended in severely hypokalemic animals with cardiac glycoside-induced AV block.

Animals with pronounced sinus bradycardia and/or heart block should be initially treated with atropine SQ at 0.02 mg/lb (0.04 mg/kg), which should be repeated if little response is observed. Isoproterenol (Isuprel) can be used by IV administration of 0.002 to 0.025 μg/lb/min (0.005 to 0.05 μg/kg/min) PRN in dogs and cats to attempt to achieve a heart rate between 80 and 120 beats/min if little response to atropine is observed.

Ventricular tachyarrhythmias and premature contractions may be controlled by lidocaine, phenytoin, or propranolol. Lidocaine is the preferred drug, given slowly IV as a bolus over two to three minutes 1 to 2 mg/lb (2 to 4 mg/kg) followed by 12 to 50 μg/lb/min (25 to 100 μg/kg/min) constant infusion. If the effect of lidocaine is lost during infusion, administer a 1 mg/lb (2 mg/kg) bolus and increase the rate of infusion. Phenytoin should be administered in divided doses IV at 1 mg/lb (2 mg/kg) over two to three minutes and repeated four times if necessary (total dose of 5 mg/lb [10 mg/kg]). Overzealous administration of phenytoin can result in cardiovascular collapse. Propranolol (Inderal) is administered IV at 0.05 mg/lb (0.1 mg/kg) total dose divided five times (0.01 mg/lb or 0.02 mg/kg) or to effect in dogs, similar to phenytoin administration. Possibly higher doses for propranolol may be required as described under the section on Toad Poisoning. Oral administration once or as needed is recommended for cats at 2.5 to 5.0 mg/cat less than three lb (six kg) body weight and at 5.0 to 7.5 mg/cat more than three lb (six kg) body weight. Propranolol prevents reflex tachycardia caused by increased peripheral vascular resistance and desensitizes the myocardium to adrenergic agents. Readministration of the 0.01 mg/lb (0.02 mg/kg) multiple boluses may be required for maintenance.

In the event of ventricular fibrillation, the prognosis for therapeutic response is extremely poor. Defibrillation (3 watt-sec/kg external) should be attempted. Epinephrine (5 μg/lb or 10 μg/kg) administered IV may be useful in turning fine fibrillation into course fibrillation, which is more responsive to defibrillation. Chemical defibrillation (3 mg acetylcholine/lb [6 mg acetylcholine/kg] and 0.5 mEq potassium chloride/lb [1 mEq potassium chloride/kg] injected intracardially) followed by cardiopulmonary resuscitation, ventilation, and adrenergic drugs is an alternative approach.

Gastrointestinal upset should be controlled with fluid and electrolyte replacement, pain control, protectants, antidiarrheals, and/or antiemetics. Depression, weakness, delirium, and mental confusion may persist for some time following correction of the life-threatening cardiac effects. Administration of activated charcoal with a cathartic is recommended following stabilization of the animal.

Mushroom Poisoning

Fungi that form complex matrices in soil and other decaying matter reproduce via fruiting bodies that we refer to as mushrooms. These have historically and contemporarily caused severe illness in humans. Dogs and cats are not particularly fond of these growths, but ingestion, particularly by dogs, is always a possibility.

Ingestion of the mushroom is seldom observed; therefore, diagnosis can only be inferred from the clinical signs and circumstantial evidence. Questioning the owner as to the presence of mushrooms is important in solving the problem. If the fruiting bodies can be obtained, a mycologist must be sought to properly identify the specimen. The specimen should be obtained intact and in its entirety, the color noted, and placed in a paper bag followed by refrigeration. Stomach contents and/or vomitus can be saved for spore identification.

There are several classes of clinical signs associated with mushroom poisoning. The symptomatology presented is that described in humans and serves as a model.[55] Estimation of onset of signs following ingestion of the mushroom should be attempted since this is helpful in classification.

Delayed Gastrointestinal Onset Followed by Hepatic or Renal Effects (Group 1). *Amanita* spp. and *Galerina* spp. are responsible for these effects. Cyclopeptides referred to as amatoxins are the toxic agents. Following ingestion, 6 to 12 hours commonly pass before a sudden onset of abdominal pain, vomiting, nausea, diarrhea (occasionally hemorrhagic), and pyrexia with tachycardia and hypotension. These signs can subside, but in one to two days evidence of hepatic and renal damage via clinical laboratory testing or by clinical signs of depression and progressive distress may occur. Icterus, acute abdomen with adynamic ileus, coagulopathy, seizures, and coma develop as the course lengthens. Tables 55–2, 55–3, and 55–8 list other disease considerations.

Under most conditions, signs are treated symptomatically since no diagnosis has been made. In the event of known exposure, treatment of early signs is best provided by administration of activated charcoal every three to six hours for 24 to 36 hours, plus supportive therapy. In the event of hepatic and renal damage, lactulose (1 to 3 tablespoons PO q6 to 8h), dietary management, thiamine and multiple vitamins, parenteral fluids, diazepam for seizure control, non-nephrotoxic antibiotic coverage, plasma or whole blood transfusion, and peritoneal dialysis or hemodialysis are management options.

Delayed Gastrointestinal Onset Followed by Hepatic Effects (Group 2). *Gyromitra* spp., referred to as false morels, are responsible for this syndrome. Clinical signs are similar to the gastrointestinal phase of Group 1 but the onset is more variable (2 to 24 hours) and commonly resolves in several days with no further problems. However, the syndrome may progress with persistent abdominal pain, depression, anorexia, pyrexia, hepatomegaly, icterus, and rarely, seizures and/or coma. Spontaneous recovery is typical. Occasionally, methemoglobinemia and hemolysis occur. Tables 55–2 and 55–8 list the differentiation needed.

Therapy is similar to that for Group 1, but administration of pyridoxine hydrochloride (Vitamin B_6) at 12 mg/lb (25 mg/kg) IM, IV, or SQ provides antidotal supplementation, leading to quicker recovery.

Acute Clinical Signs Typical of Anticholinesterase Poisoning (Group 3). Two genera (*Clitocybe* and *Inocybe*) of the class Basidiomycetes are toxic. Onset of clinical signs occurs within 15 minutes to two hours following ingestion, typified by the SLUD syndrome (salivation, lacrimation, urination, and diarrhea). Respiratory distress related to bronchial secretions and muscular constriction is observed. Marked bradycardia with hypotension characterizes the cardiac effects. Abdominal pain, nausea, and miosis accompany these signs. Respiratory complications and/or vascular collapse may lead to death within ten hours. Table 55–4 lists other conditions for differentiation.

Atropine is the antidote of choice. The dose is similar to that for anticholinesterase insecticide therapy (0.2 mg/lb or 0.4 mg/kg IV, SQ, PRN) using cessation of salivation, bronchospasm, and return to normal sinus rhythm and blood pressure as endpoints for treatment. The central nervous effects commonly observed with anticholinesterase insecticides are minimal. Administration of activated charcoal is advisable. Cathartics or emetics are contraindicated.

Gastrointestinal Disorder Very Acute in Onset and Recovery (Group 4). *Chlorophyllum molybdites*, *Gomphus floccosus*, and *Lactarius* spp. are mushrooms that cause gastrointestinal irritation within two hours following ingestion. Abdominal pain, watery to hemorrhagic diarrhea, and dehydration with electrolyte losses are commonly observed. Hypersensitivity reactions may occur, resulting in urticaria, bronchial constriction and wheezing, vascular collapse, and even hemolysis. The acute gastrointestinal symptoms quickly resolve in three to four hours, leading to complete recovery in 24 hours. Symptomatic and supportive care are indicated in addition to activated charcoal administration. There is also a group of mushrooms (*Coprinus* spp.) that causes illness only following alcohol ingestion. Table 55–2 lists other differential considerations.

Psychoactive Effects Resulting in a "Spaced-out" Presentation (Group 5). The common mushroom species of *Amanita muscaria* (fly agaric) and *Amanita pantheria* represent one group responsible for these problems. Signs of disorientation, euphoria, and ataxia (as if "drunk") appear within 0.5 to 2 hours following ingestion. Mydriasis, myoclonus, and seizures and/or coma can occur. Recovery is usually complete within six to ten hours. Fatalities are rare. Urine provides a good sample for toxicologic analysis of isoxazole derivatives. Table 55–4 lists other conditions resulting in psychoactive effects.

A second group of mushrooms includes three genera that gained prominence during the counterculture movement of the 1960s. *Psilocybe* spp., *Paneolus* spp., and *Gymnopilus* spp. are the genera. Clinical signs are very similar to the *Amanita* spp. but the toxic psychoses are quite marked but short-lived (four-hour course).

The removal of the toxins is the basic goal of therapy, using activated charcoal orally along with lavage if indicated. The use of barbiturate or diazepam should be avoided unless seizure activity is present. Flaccid paralysis and apnea may result due to potentiation caused by the isoxazole derivatives. Therefore minimal doses should be used to effect only. Chlorpromazine or haloperidol is a recommended sedative. Other supportive care, such as fluids, may be indicated. Placement of the animal in a quiet, dark area is helpful in avoiding self-destructive reactions.

Mycotoxins

Aflatoxin is the most common mycotoxin that comes to mind when this category is mentioned. Historically, this biotoxin has caused major outbreaks. Clinical cases occur infrequently but are reported in dogs.[56] Acute exposure results in acute hepatic damage associated with depression, anorexia, vomiting, hemorrhagic diarrhea, icterus, and death. Chronic exposure is less definitive, but depression, anorexia, polyuria, polydipsia, and weakness predominate clinically and hepatic damage and failure are the most probable laboratory findings. A chronic outbreak of aflatoxicosis in Walker hounds was characterized by development of disseminated intravascular coagulation secondary to chronic-active hepatitis.[57] Diagnosis depends upon identification of aflatoxin in the feed or body tissues and/or fluids. Table 55–2 lists other disease considerations.

MOLDY WALNUT POISONING

This is a very common poisoning where walnuts are grown in the geographic regions with milder climates. A penicillium mold, *Penicillium crustosum*, grows upon the rich substrate provided by the meat of the nut when the fruit has fallen to the ground. Cooler temperatures above freezing allow mycotoxin production. The mycotoxin is penitrem A, which is a tremorigen. Ingestion of the walnut contents is common in dogs that have access to them. Any rich substrate maintained under cooler temperatures can serve as a growth medium and source for mycotoxin production. For example, moldy cream cheese that was refrigerated for a long period of time provided a source for poisoning in a dog.[58]

Clinical signs develop generally within one to three hours following ingestion and are basically identical to those of metaldehyde poisoning (see section on Pesticides Affecting the Central Nervous System). Table 55–4 lists other disease considerations. Ataxia, urination, defecation, polypnea, hyperthermia, mydriasis, and convulsive actions accompanying generalized tremors have been observed.[59] The metabolic acidosis that can develop rapidly with metaldehyde poisoning is not as marked with penitrem A. Diagnosis can be made by finding walnut pieces on examination of vomitus or gastric lavage contents. A mycotoxin screen of the stomach contents provides confirmation. Treatment is the same as for metaldehyde poisoning.

Garbage Poisoning

The term, as used in this chapter, refers in general to ingestion of an unknown substance, which encompasses actual garbage, rotten food sources (e.g., carrion), or contaminated water as reviewed.[60] Dogs frequently encounter such substances and readily consume the material. Cats are less prone to do so. Enterotoxins and endotoxins are commonly found in sources containing spoiled or putrefied organic material along with the bacteria that produce them. Ingestion of this material produces onset of emesis and diarrhea within a two-day period following ingestion. Acute abdominal signs may accompany the illness. Weakness, incoordination, and dyspnea leading to shock, with pupillary dilation and terminal seizures, may result. Changes in the leukogram from leukopenia to leukocytosis may be evident and decreased or elevated temperatures may occur. Adynamic ileus and/or gastroplegia can develop. Spontaneous recovery in as little as five to six hours may take place. Less acute forms[61] are typified by increased flatulence, halitosis, mucus-covered feces, and generalized lethargy and soreness. The haircoat may appear dull, with a rancid, seborrheic odor. Table 55–2 lists other disease considerations.

Treatment is similar to that of other poisonings. Removal of the ingested material is desirable since it serves as a reservoir for the organisms. The presenting signs help to perform this task, but a lavage or "through-and-through" enema may be indicated. Radiographs or ultrasound help to evaluate the presence of larger objects that often are unpalpable and may require surgical intervention. Supportive and symptomatic therapy recommended include antiemetic drugs such as diphenhydramine (0.25 to 1.0 mg/lb or 0.5 to 2.0 mg/kg IV,IM,SQ) or dimenhydrinate (0.5 to 0.75 mg/lb or 1 to 1.5 mg/kg); oral glucose (10 to 50 per cent) and electrolytes; kaopectate (1 to 3 ml/lb or 2 to 5 ml/kg PO q1 to 6h); broad-spectrum antibiotics (trimethoprim-sulfa); dietary management including *Lactobacillus acidophilus* sources; and maintenance fluids and electrolytes. Atropine (0.02 mg/lb or 0.04 mg/kg) may be required for parasympatholytic effects. Shock therapy should be instituted if pallor, tachycardia, and shallow respirations are present with prolonged capillary refill time and a weak, rapid pulse. Relapses of gastrointestinal signs can occur within approximately two days if therapy is insufficient.

Less frequent but more serious intoxications result from ingestion of putrefied substances containing botulism or from consumption of water containing blue-green algae. Neurologic effects are common with blue-green algae, including muscle fasciculations, seizures, weakness, and paralysis. Botulism is more commonly associated with neurologic deficits leading to respiratory paralysis. Emesis occurs with both disorders. Hepatic damage is common with blue-green algae poisoning. Table 55–4 lists other disease problems that cause similar signs. Therapy is basically symptomatic and supportive.

HOUSEHOLD MATERIALS

Home Medications

Many drugs are kept in homes. Three are very common and two are commonly administered to ill animals by a well-meaning owner only to make the animal's condition worse. Unexpected ingestion of the third could lead to serious problems, particularly if the owner is unaware of ingestion. Improper application of certain enema preparations can lead to serious problems in veterinary practices as well.

ASPIRIN

Circumstantial and General Information. A review of toxicity is available.[62] Acetylsalicylic acid or related derivatives may be given to a dog or cat suffering from some disorder by a sympathetic owner. Inadvertent ingestion by a dog or cat of candy-coated aspirin tablets or of spilled oil of wintergreen (methyl salicylate) also can lead to acute intoxication. Much information is available on aspirin poisoning in humans and is referred to below.[14]

Clinical Signs. Ingestion or owner dosing of several adult tablets results in acute poisoning with development of signs within four to six hours. Depression, vomiting, anorexia, hyperpnea, and pyrexia are early signs. The hyperpnea leads to respiratory alkalosis that is overridden by metabolic acidosis. Progressive depression and weakness result in loss of consciousness and death within a day or so. Disorders resulting from accumulative toxicity of aspirin therapy include hepatopathy, nephrosis, bone-marrow depression, tinnitus, and hearing loss. The classic disorder is the development of gastric ulcerations that cause occult to overt hemorrhage.

Clinical Laboratory Information. Hypoglycemia (occasionally hyperglycemia), ketonuria, and hyperchloridemic acidosis are common laboratory findings in humans. Hypokalemia may not be evident due to the acidosis, but potassium depletion is characteristic of salicylism. Renal and hepatic function are impaired in acute poisoning and may be reflected in the biochemical panels.

Toxicological Analysis. Inspection of stomach contents or vomitus for presence of pills followed by analysis is confirmatory evidence. Serum may also be tested chemically.

Differentiation. Diseases characterized by depression and increased respirations and acidosis should be considered. Ethylene glycol intoxication is one primary differentiation that is distinct due to the presence of oxalate crystalluria (see Tables 55–1 and 55–6 for other diseases listed).

Therapy. A significant metabolic imbalance is generated with salicylism. Therapy is directed toward removing unabsorbed poison and correcting hypokalemia, acidosis, dehydration, ketosis, and hyperthermia. Activated charcoal and a saline cathartic should be administered orally, especially in an acute intoxication. A large amount of potassium may be required in combination with bicarbonate and/or glucose to correct acidosis, ketosis, and oftentimes marked potassium depletion. Bicarbonate (1.5 mEq/lb or 3 mEq/kg IV) and potassium chloride (1 mEq/lb or 2 mEq/kg PO) are often required to alkalinize the urine because of paradoxical aciduria, which significantly increases salicylate excretion. Fluid replacement to restore the hypovolemia prevents development of shock and associated problems. A tepid bath may be required for control of hyperthermia. High environmental oxygen exposure is beneficial and renal dialysis is recommended.

ACETAMINOPHEN

Circumstantial and General Information. This drug has become a popular home analgesic.[62] Similar to aspirin, exposure is caused by accidental ingestion of pills or home treatments. Cats are more susceptible to poisoning. One adult tablet can produce illness in a cat and more tablets may result in death.[63]

Clinical Signs. Cats characteristically develop hemolytic anemia. Symptoms in the cat occur within one to two hours following ingestion. Depression, salivation, vomiting, and anorexia are characteristic. Mucous membranes are cyanotic due to methemoglobinemia. Dark-colored urine is observed due to hemolytic anemia and hemoglobinuria. As signs progress, icterus, facial edema, dependent edema of the extremities, and lethargy may develop. Respiratory distress may develop, leading to terminal seizures due to methemoglobinuria. Death can ensue following a 12- to 48-hour course. Less acute cases can recover spontaneously but full recovery may take as long as three weeks.

Dogs become depressed or anorectic, and may vomit within one or more hours after ingestion. This continues, progressively leading to development of abdominal pain, icterus, and death within two to five days. Dark-colored mucous membranes and urine may be observed, but to a lesser degree than in the cat. The liver is the primary target organ of toxicity.

Clinical Laboratory Information. Heinz-body anemia is characteristic in the cat and also the dog if large enough doses are ingested. Methemoglobinemia can reach fatal levels in the cat (above 70 per cent). Hemolysis is common and urine is strongly positive for hemoglobin. Hepatic damage occurs in cats but is not a predominant life-threatening event. Biochemical evidence of hepatic damage is anticipated within 12 to 48 hours in dogs. Renal and myocardial damage have been related to acetaminophen toxicity in humans.

Toxicological Analysis. Inspection of stomach contents or vomitus for presence of pills followed by analysis is confirmatory evidence. Serum and urine should be frozen for acetaminophen analysis.

Differentiation. Diseases that produce hemolytic anemia and/or methemoglobinemia are major considerations in the cat or dog. Conditions that cause acute abdominal distress are considerations in the dog. Tables 55–1, 55–2, and 55–7 illustrate these diseases.

Therapy. A gastric lavage is not indicated if vomiting has occurred. An osmotic cathartic can be administered orally but activated charcoal is contraindicated if the antidote is to be administered. N-acetylcysteine (Mucomyst) is the recommended antidote, given at 70 mg/lb or 140 mg/kg PO loading followed by three to five treatments with 35 mg/lb or 70 mg/kg PO q4h diluted to five per cent in water, an isotonic solution, or five to ten per cent glucose. Sodium sulfate has been used as an alternative antidote in cats by administering 25 mg/lb or 50 mg/kg IV as a 1.6 per cent solution in sterile water q4h for six treatments.

Additional therapy includes the administration of vitamin C in cats to reverse the methemoglobinemia. This can be given IV or SQ at 200 mg/cat q8h or 125 mg/cat PO q6h until corrected. Oxygen therapy, whole blood transfusions, renal diuresis, lactulose, medications to support hepatic function, and dietary management for hepatic and renal impairment are also considerations. Cats with methemoglobin concentrations high enough to produce respiratory distress must be handled with extreme care.

IRON

Circumstantial and General Information. Little has been reported about iron poisonings in dogs and cats, but iron-containing preparations in households are extremely available. These products are responsible for acute intoxications in children, and the following discussion is based on the extensive findings in humans.[14] A potentially fatal dose of elemental iron in a child is 400 mg. Containers of different chewable vitamin products have contained 0.4 to 3.0 gm of iron. Fatalities have been associated with as few as ten 0.3 gm tablets of ferrous sulfate. Candy-coated medications offer appetizing sources to dogs or cats if circumstances allow.

Clinical Signs. Acute poisoning is fundamentally characterized by gastroenteritis and vascular collapse. Sudden onset of vomiting, abdominal pain, and diarrhea associated with hemorrhagic gastroenteritis can occur half an hour or more following ingestion. Depression, pallor, cyanosis, ataxia, weak and/or rapid pulse with hypotension, and coma can ensue rapidly. Often, however, peripheral vascular collapse does not occur and an asymptomatic period develops in 6 to 24 hours following ingestion. A second crisis arises following this asymptomatic time period, characterized by cyanosis, pulmonary edema, vasomotor collapse, coma, and death, which may occur within 12 to 48 hours. Cases that develop hepatitis become icteric. Animals that survive may acquire gastric scarring and contraction, leading to chronic digestive problems that become evident three to four weeks later.

Clinical Laboratory Information. Considerable variation occurs with hemograms, blood gases, electrolytes, and biochemical measurements. Acidosis, hyperglycemia, and leukocytosis are common during the second crisis stage. Evidence of hepatic necrosis and failure may be observed in some cases as a predominant delayed phase of poisoning. Coagulopathy related to disseminated intravascular coagulopathy or hepatic dysfunction may be observed. Radiographs may show radiodense areas corresponding to the intact or partially chewed iron tablets.

Toxicological Analysis. The lethal range is reached when serum iron exceeds the TIBC. In humans, serum iron greater than 500 μg/dl is considered potentially lethal, while concentrations in excess of 300 μg/dl are associated with the development of clinical signs.[14]

Differentiation. Any disease that produces an acute gastroenteritis must be considered. Mushroom and phosphorus poisonings are two intoxications that are very similar in clinical course. Inorganic arsenical poisoning is likewise a strong candidate for consideration. Tables 55–1, 55–3, 55–5, and 55–7 list other disease considerations.

Therapy. Provided a tentative diagnosis is established, immediate oral administration of milk of magnesia should be performed since insoluble hydroxide salts are formed. Even if vomiting has occurred, apomorphine may be administered if appropriate, to dislodge any tablets. A gastric lavage slurry of 50 per cent sodium bicarbonate is recommended and a portion should be left in the stomach.

Deferoxamine mesylate (Desferal) is the antidote of choice. This drug chelates iron by forming ferrioxamine, which is eliminated primarily via the kidneys. Administrative schedules used in humans provide guidelines for application to animals. Intravenous infusion is used in severely affected patients with a dose of 20 mg/lb (40 mg/kg) at a rate not exceeding 7.5 mg/lb/hour (15 mg/kg/hour) in order to avoid hypotension. Repeat every 4 to 12 hours at 10 mg/lb (20 mg/kg) as determined by the animal's response. The intramuscular or subcutaneous route can be used in less acutely affected individuals at 10 mg/lb (20 mg/kg) every 3 to 12 hours. Length of treatment can extend to three days in severe poisonings.

Supportive care is required. Acidosis is relatively refractory but 1 to 3 mEq of sodium bicarbonate/lb (3 to 5 mEq/kg) may be beneficial. Prophylactic antibiotic coverage is recommended. Drugs and procedures (such as oxygen therapy) to treat pulmonary edema and manage shock are important considerations. Coagulation disorders or blood loss anemia may require whole blood or plasma transfusions, fluids, and/or heparin. Symptomatic care may be required if seizures or hyperthermia occur. Dietary management and follow-up evaluation of gastric damage are advocated.

FLEET-LIKE ENEMA INTOXICATION

Fleet-like enema preparations contain high amounts of sodium and phosphate. Administration of these products to cats or small dogs can produce illness within 30 to 60 minutes. Depression and ataxia are observed first, followed by tetany and/or seizures. Volume depletion followed by cardiovascular collapse may occur in severe cases. Hyperosmolality is responsible for the condition owing to hypernatremia and hyperphosphatemia. High-anion gap metabolic acidosis associated with lactate accumulation occurs along with hypokalemia. These changes occur rapidly within one hour after administration. Hyperglycemia is common in cats. The nervous system is quickly dehydrated by this hypertonic state, but this is not noted by physical examination. In addition, hypocalcemia and hypomagnesemia can occur, producing the excitatory neuromuscular signs. The course of illness generally resolves in 24 hours if death does not occur. Tables 55–1, 55–2, and 55–4 list other disease conditions that produce similar signs.

Treatment can vary from conservative to intensive. Basic fluid replacement should be done slowly. Oral administration of water with calcium gluconate and potassium chloride added is sufficient in mild cases. Animals more seriously affected should have serum sodium concentrations determined and the fluid deficit estimated by multiplying 60 per cent of the body weight (kg) by the ratio of the patient's sodium concentration to the normal sodium value. Intravenous administration of five per cent dextrose in water containing four to five mEq/l of potassium chloride and seven to ten mEq/l of calcium gluconate is recommended to replace the calculated deficit. Rapid administration of half the calculated deficit should be done for shock patients. Should brain edema occur (and oliguria), mannitol administration is indicated. If tetany is present, calcium gluconate (ten per cent) should be administered IV at 0.25 to 0.75 ml/lb (0.5 to 1.5 ml/kg) until bradycardia occurs. Further discussions of this condition and therapy are available.[64]

Household Hazards

MOTHBALLS

Although common to many homes, a paucity of case reports exists on naphthalene intoxication in dogs and cats. Ingestion of two gm is lethal in children. Acute ingestion can result in severe, rapidly progressive hemolytic anemia. Delayed signs of hemolysis can occur in three to seven days in humans.[14] Nausea, cyanosis, pallor, dark-colored urine, progressive depression, fever, and respiratory distress are observed. Heinz-body anemia and hemoglobinuria are anticipated laboratory findings. Hepatic and renal damage may also be manifested. If clinical signs are characterized by a neurological disorder (e.g., ataxia, tremors, seizures), moth crystals that contain paradichlorobenzene should be suspected.[2] Table 55–8 lists other causes of hemolytic anemias.

Diagnosis is best made by examination of the stomach contents. The smell of remaining mothballs is proof enough. Mothballs are not appreciably soluble in an aqueous solution such as the stomach; hence, they should not dissolve quickly. Gas from the stomach may also be sufficient evidence.

No specific antidote has been recommended. Therefore, supportive and symptomatic therapy are implied. Renal dialysis using mannitol and furosemide, whole blood transfusion, and oxygen therapy are indicated. A "through-and-through" enema following light anesthesia is appropriate, with subsequent administration of activated charcoal and saline cathartic in early cases of poisoning.

CAUSTICS AND DISINFECTANTS

Numerous products in the home contain toxic chemicals.[65] Substances containing strong acids or bases are very dangerous. Alkali burns are more penetrating than acid burns. Milder substances include soaps, detergents, and other cleaning products.[66] Heavy-duty detergents contain alkaline builders that can produce basic burns. The cationic disinfectants (quaternary ammonium compounds) commonly used in veterinary practices (Roccal) are very toxic in concentrated solutions.[67] Similarly, phenolic disinfectants are toxic to pets, especially cats.[68] Contact irritation that progresses to ulceration is common in most cases. Systemic effects such as depression, incoordination, a progressive coma leading to respiratory failure, or shock may occur. Esophagoscopy and gastroscopy using a flexible fiberoptic endoscope are recommended approximately 48 hours following ingestion of caustics. Emesis *should not be induced*. Milk or large quantities of water should be administered orally, followed by supportive care and NPO for two to five days. The basic principles of poison removal and supportive care may be implemented, depending on the agent as indicated in the review articles given. Table 55–7 lists various conditions that affect external surfaces or upper gastrointestinal areas.

PETROLEUM PRODUCTS

A review of exposure, chemical properties, clinical effects in dogs and cats, and therapy should be consulted.[69] A combination of neurological and respiratory signs accompanied by gastrointestinal irritation and cardiac abnormalities strongly suggests petroleum hydrocarbon exposure. Aspiration pneumonia is a usual finding, secondary to emesis that commonly is seen with ingestion of these materials. The broad array of clinical signs must include several differential lists found in Tables 55–2, 55–4, 55–6, 55–7, and 55–10.

CHOCOLATE AND SIMILAR SUBSTANCES

Theobromine is the major toxic component in chocolate. Ingestion of eight four-oz solid milk chocolate bars by a 30 lb dog may cause problems. Nervous excitation results in choreic movements, fasciculations, delirium, and seizures (see Table 55–4). Cardiac arrhythmias may cause death. Treatment is symptomatic. This subject has been reviewed.[70]

CIGARETTES

Ingestion of a package or more of cigarettes, cigars, or other tobacco products could lead to nicotine intoxication. Nervous excitation with parasympathomimetic effects followed by paralysis is observed. Other acute neurologic disorders must be considered (Tables 55–1 and 55–4). Stomach contents are most revealing. Treatment is symptomatic and requires ventilation support.

ETHYL ALCOHOL

Intake of large quantities of these beverages or yeast-containing food products[71] results in a drunk dog. Clinical signs of the obvious "drunk dog" are somewhat comical, but more serious presentations of a comatose animal with no history are diagnostically difficult. Acute intoxication results in vomiting, respiratory distress due to depression, agitation, and/or delirium, characterized by constant crying or depression that progresses to ataxia, incoordination, aimless wandering, and collapse. This condition can linger for one to two days. Animals may become unconscious and die.[72] Tables 55–1 and 55–4 list other conditions that could be confused with this condition. Hyperosmolality is characteristic. Differentiation from ethylene glycol reveals no oxalate crystalluria. The ketotic breath of the animal may be helpful in recognizing ethanol intoxication. Hypoglycemia is common with acute ethanol ingestion, but is variable. Blood alcohol levels can be readily determined. Diuresis, warmth, tracheal intubation, and ventilation support are major considerations.

References

1. Carson, TL: Toxic gases. *In* Kirk, RW (ed), Current Veterinary Therapy IX. Philadelphia, WB Saunders Co, p 203, 1986.
2. Beasley, VR: Prevalence of poisonings in small animals. *In* Kirk, RW (ed), Current Veterinary Therapy IX. Philadelphia, WB Saunders Co, p 120, 1986.
3. Oehme, FW: Information resources for toxicology. *In* Kirk, RW (ed), Current Veterinary Therapy IX. Philadelphia, WB Saunders Co, p 129, 1986.

4. Yeary, RA: Syrup of Ipecac as an emetic in the cat. JAVMA 161:1677, 1972.
5. Rumack, BH and Peterson RG: Poisoning: Prevention of absorption. Topic Emerg Med 1(3):13, 1979.
6. Bailey, EM, Jr: Emergency and general treatment of poisonings. *In* Kirk, RW (ed), Current Veterinary Therapy IX. Philadelphia, WB Saunders Co, p 135, 1986.
7. Frye, FL: Enterogastric lavage in small animal practice. Vet Med Sm An Clin 69:835, 1974.
8. Grauer, GF, et al.: Early clinicopathologic findings in dogs ingesting ethylene glycol. Am J Vet Res 45:2299, 1984.
9. Green RA, et al.: Hyperosmolemic changes following experimental ethylene glycol intoxication in dogs. Vet Clin Path 7:8, 1978.
10. Thrall, MA, et al.: Identification of calcium oxalate monohydrate crystals by x-ray diffraction in urine of ethylene glycol-intoxicated dogs. Vet Pathol 22:625, 1985.
11. Grauer, GF and Thrall, MAH: Ethylene glycol (antifreeze) poisoning. *In* Kirk, RW (ed): Current Veterinary Therapy IX. Philadelphia, WB Saunders Co, p 206, 1986.
12. Tarr, BD, et al.: Low-dose ethanol in the treatment of ethylene glycol poisoning. J Vet Pharmacol Ther 8:254, 1985.
13. Lloyd, WE: Sodium fluoroacetate (Compound 1080) poisoning. *In* Kirk, RW (ed): Current Veterinary Therapy VIII. Philadelphia, WB Saunders Co, p 112, 1983.
14. Arena, JM and Drew, RH (eds): *In* Poisoning, 5th. Springfield, IL, Charles C Thomas, 1986.
15. Taitelman, U, et al.: Fluoroacetamide poisoning in man: The role of ionized calcium. Arch Toxicol, Suppl 6:228, 1983.
16. Osweiler, GD: Strychnine poisoning. *In* Kirk, RW (ed): Current Veterinary Therapy VIII. Philadelphia, WB Saunders Co, p 98, 1983.
17. Sofola, O and Odusoste, K: Sympathetic cardiovascular effects of experimental strychnine poisoning in dogs. J Pharmacol Exper Ther 196:29, 1976.
18. Blaine, DR: Treatment of metaldehyde poisoning in dogs with megadoses of acepromazine maleate. VM/SAC 72:1009, 1977.
19. Booze, TF and Oehme, FW: Metaldehyde toxicity: A review. Vet Hum Toxicol 27:11, 1985.
20. Ramsay, FK, et al.: Diagnostic aspects of diseases produced by toxicants in small animals. Anim Hosp 3:221, 1967.
21. Casteel, SW and Bailey, EM: A review of zinc phosphide poisoning. Vet Hum Toxicol 28:151, 1986.
22. Yeary, RA: Herbicides. *In* Kirk, RW (ed), Current Veterinary Therapy IX. Philadelphia, WB Saunders Co, p 153, 1986.
23. Osweiler, GD: Toxicology of rodenticides and bird toxicants. *In* Kirk, RW (ed), Current Veterinary Therapy IX. Philadelphia, WB Saunders Co, p 165, 1986.
24. Spyker, DA, et al.: Poisoning with 4-aminopyridine: Report of three cases. Clin Toxicol 16:487, 1980.
25. Gleason, MN, et al.: Phosphorus. *In* Clinical Toxicology of Commercial Products, 3rd, Baltimore, Williams and Wilkins, p 192, 1969.
26. Snodgrass, WR and Doull, J: Early aggressive activated charcoal treatment of elemental yellow phosphorus poisoning. Vet Hum Toxicol 24(Suppl):96, 1982.
27. Frye, FL and Cucuel, JPE: Acute yellow phosphorus poisoning in a cat. VM/SAC 64:995, 1969.
28. Mount, ME, et al.: The anticoagulant rodenticides. *In* Kirk, RW (ed): Current Veterinary Therapy IX, Small Animal Practice. Philadelphia, WB Saunders Co, p 156, 1986.
29. Mount, ME: Proteins induced by vitamin K absence or antagonists (PIVKA). *In* Kirk, RW (ed): Current Veterinary Therapy IX, Small Animal Practice. Philadelphia, WB Saunders Co, p 513, 1986.
30. Mount, ME and Kass, PH: Diagnostic importance of vitamin K_1 and its epoxide measured in sera of dogs exposed to an anticoagulant rodenticide. Am J Vet Res, submitted, 1986.
31. Zook, BC: Lead intoxication in urban dogs. *In* Oehme, FW (ed), Toxicity of Heavy Metals in the Environment. New York, Marcel Dekker, p 179, 1978.
32. Zook, BC, et al.: Basophilic stippling of erythrocytes in dogs with special reference to lead poisoning. JAVMA 157:2092, 1970.
33. Fowler, BA, et al.: Arsenic. *In* Friberg, L, et al. (eds), Handbook on the Toxicology of Metals. New York, Elsevier/North-Holland Biomedical Press, p 295, 1979.
34. Evinger, JV and Blakemore, JC: Dermatitis in a dog associated with exposure to an arsenic compound. JAVMA 184:1281, 1984.
35. Watson, WA, et al.: Acute arsenic exposure treated with oral D-penicillamine. Vet Hum Toxicol 23:164, 1981.
36. Breitschwerdt, EB, et al.: Three cases of acute zinc toxicosis in dogs. Vet Hum Toxicol 28:109, 1986.
37. Crawford, MA and Jensen, RK: Thallium intoxication in the dog. Vet Hum Toxicol 28:533, 1986.
38. Muller, GH, et al.: Thallium toxicosis. *In* Small Animal Dermatology, 3rd ed, Philadelphia, WB Saunders Co, p 651, 1983.
39. Aronson, CE: Thallium intoxication. *In* Kirk, RW (ed), Current Veterinary Therapy, VI. Philadelphia, WB Saunders Co, p 124, 1977.
40. Coyle, V: Diagnosis and treatment of thallium toxicosis in a dog. J Sm An Pract 21:391, 1980.
41. Wingert, WA: Venomous snake bites. *In* Auerbach, PS and Geehr, EC (eds), Management of Wilderness and Environmental Emergencies. New York, Macmillan Publishing Co, p 352, 1983.
42. Parrish, HM, et al.: The clinical management of snake venom poisoning in domestic animals. JAVMA 130:548, 1957.
43. Clark, KA: Management of poisonous snakebites in dogs and cats. Mod Vet Pract 62:427, 1981.
44. Parrish, HM, et al.: The use of antihistamine (Phenergan) in experimental snake venom poisoning in dogs. JAVMA 129:522, 1956.
45. Fowler, ME: *In* Plant Poisoning and Biotoxins. Davis, University of California, p 196, 1981.
46. Palumbo, NE, et al.: Experimental induction and treatment of toad poisoning in the dog. JAVMA 167:1000, 1975.
47. O'Neill-Foil, CS and Waldron, DR: Bites and stings of venomous animals and toad poisoning. *In* Morgan, RV (ed), Manual of Small Animal Emergencies. New York, Churchill Livingstone, p 448, 1985.
48. Minton, SA: Arthropod envenomation. *In* Auerbach, PS and Geehr, EC (eds), Management of Wilderness and Environmental Emergencies. New York, Macmillan Publ Co, p 270, 1983.
49. Reszel, PA and Coventry, MB: Emergency treatment of bites and stings. *Proc Staff Meet Mayo Clin* 38:293, 1963.
50. Breen, JF: *In* Encyclopedia of Reptiles and Amphibians. Neptune City, TFH Publications Inc, p 194, 1974.
51. Fowler, ME: *In* Plant Poisoning in Small Companion Animals. Saint Louis, Ralston Purina Co, p 1, 1980.
52. Clay, BR: Poisoning and injury by plants. *In* Kirk, RW (ed), Current Veterinary Therapy VI. Philadelphia, WB Saunders Co, p 179, 1977.
53. Ruhr, LP: Ornamental toxic plants. *In* Kirk, RW (ed), Current Veterinary Therapy IX. Philadelphia, WB Saunders Co, p 216, 1986.
54. Wilcke, JR: Cardiac dysrhythmias. *In* Davis, LE (ed), Handbook of Small Animal Therapeutics. New York, Churchill Livingstone, p 267, 1985.
55. Geehr, EC: Toxic plant ingestions. *In* Auerbach, PS and Geehr, EC (eds), Management of Wilderness and Environmental Emergencies. New York, Macmillan Publishing Co, p 379, 1983.
56. Ketterer, PJ, et al.: Canine aflatoxicosis. Aust Vet J 51:355, 1975.
57. Greene, CE, et al.: Disseminated intravascular coagulation complicating aflatoxicosis in dogs. Cornell Vet 67:29, 1977.
58. Richard, JL and Arp, LH: Natural occurrence of the mycotoxin penitrem A in moldy cream cheese. Mycopathol 67:107, 1979.
59. Richard, JL, et al.: The mycotoxin, penitrem A, as a cause of moldy walnut toxicosis in a dog. Calif Vet 6:12, 1981.
60. Coppock, RW and Mostrom, MS: Intoxication due to contaminated garbage, food, and water. *In* Kirk, RW (ed), Current Veterinary Therapy IX. Philadelphia, WB Saunders Co, p 221, 1986.
61. Eberhart, GW: Garbage- and food-borne intoxications (enterotoxemias). *In* Kirk, RW (ed), Current Veterinary Therapy VI. Philadelphia, WB Saunders Co, p 176, 1977.
62. Oehme, FW: Aspirin and acetaminophen. *In* Kirk, RW (ed), Current Veterinary Therapy IX. Philadelphia, WB Saunders Co, p 188, 1986.
63. Finco, DR, et al.: Acetaminophen toxicosis in the cat. JAVMA 166:469, 1975.
64. Atkins, CE: Hypertonic sodium phosphate enema intoxication.

In Kirk, RW (ed), Current Veterinary Therapy IX. Philadelphia, WB Saunders Co, p 212, 1986.

65. Osweiler, GD: Household and commercial products. *In* Kirk, RW (ed), Current Veterinary Therapy IX. Philadelphia, WB Saunders Co, p 193, 1986.
66. Temple, AR and Veltri, JC: Outcome of accidental ingestions of soaps, detergents, and related household products. Vet Hum Toxicol, Supplement 21:31, 1979.
67. Oehme, FW: Poisonings from phenolic chemicals. *In* Kirk, RW (ed), Current Veterinary Therapy VI. Philadelphia, WB Saunders Co, p 145, 1977.
68. Oehme FW: Poisonings from phenolic chemicals. *In* Kirk, RW (ed), Current Veterinary Therapy VI. Philadelphia, WB Saunders Co, p 145, 1977.
69. Coppock, RW, et al.: Volatile hydrocarbons (solvents, fuels) and petrochemicals. *In* Kirk, RW (ed), Current Veterinary Therapy IX. Philadelphia, WB Saunders Co, p 197, 1986.
70. Hooser, SB and Beasley, VR: Methylxanthine poisoning (chocolate and caffeine toxicosis). *In* Kirk, RW (ed), Current Veterinary Therapy IX. Philadelphia, WB Saunders Co, p 191, 1986.
71. Thrall, MA, et al.: Ethanol toxicosis secondary to sourdough ingestion in a dog. JAVMA 184:1513, 1984.
72. Ratcliffe, RC and Zuber, RM: Acute ethyl alcohol poisoning in dogs. Aust Vet J 53:48, 1977.

56 ACUPUNCTURE THERAPY IN SMALL ANIMAL PRACTICE

SHELDON ALTMAN

Until recently, it was uncommon to treat chronic pain and chronic degenerative diseases in animals. Due to economic factors, inconvenience, and concern for suffering, the usual solution to these problems was euthanasia. Because of advances in nutrition and veterinary medicine, small animals are living longer and are experiencing debilitating geriatric conditions not commonly seen several decades ago. Even in young animals, trauma, disease, and congenital deformities can cause chronic pain, neurologic degeneration, or physiologic upsets that are not always successfully treated with current surgical or pharmacologic methods. Our clients are better informed about medical techniques available to treat human beings and have higher expectations of what veterinary medicine can do for their pets. Veterinarians have a renewed appreciation of the human-animal bond. Added to the strong desire to heal, which led most veterinarians into the profession, small animal practitioners have been seeking additional ways to help their patients. Some have explored new (in actuality old or even ancient) methods of healing. This environment has led to the use of acupuncture in modern veterinary practice.

Acupuncture is derived from the Latin, *acus*, meaning needle, and *punctura*, meaning puncture. In the narrowest sense, acupuncture is the insertion of very fine needles into specific predetermined points on the body to produce physiologic responses (Figure 56–1). Today many other means are used to stimulate acupuncture points in addition to needles. These will be discussed later.

Some of the most common applications of acupuncture are to relieve pain, to cause autonomic nerve responses, and occasionally, to induce surgical analgesia.

The specific points used, the depth to which the needles are inserted, the type of stimulation applied to the needles, and the duration of each treatment session vary according to the condition being treated. In humans, most acupuncture points are described as lying on "meridians" or "channels," which connect loci having functional relationships. According to traditional oriental philosophy, the acupoints communicate with the body organs and tissues through these meridians. There are 361 traditional meridian acupoints. Some of these occur bilaterally, bringing the total of meridian acupoints to 670. In addition, there are "extra" points that lie outside these channels and 133 acupuncture points in the ear,[1] bringing the total number of points to over 1000. To those veterinarians learning human acupuncture anatomy and transposing this knowledge to canine or feline anatomy, the task is a formidable one. A recent handbook published in Hong Kong,[2] describing acupuncture points in dogs and cats, lists 32 single points and 40 bilateral points, for a total 112 selection possibilities. Several other charts have been published with numbers of points varying between these two extremes (Figure 56–2).[3–8]

Traditionally, each acupuncture point has one or several actions when stimulated. When used in combination with other points, the results are modified. An analogy can be made to playing musical notes. If played as single notes, the tone is plain, direct, and easily recognized. As other notes are added, major, minor, or other chords are produced, giving a totally different quality of sound to the original note. Sometimes the wrong combinations of notes produce a dischord. Similarly, simultaneous stimulation of points in harmony can enhance specific actions beyond the capabilities of single point stimulation. In other cases, the effects can be obliterated or medical problems exacerbated by improperly combining acupoints.

HISTORICAL BACKGROUND

Most people have only recently heard of acupuncture, but it is actually one of the oldest forms of medical

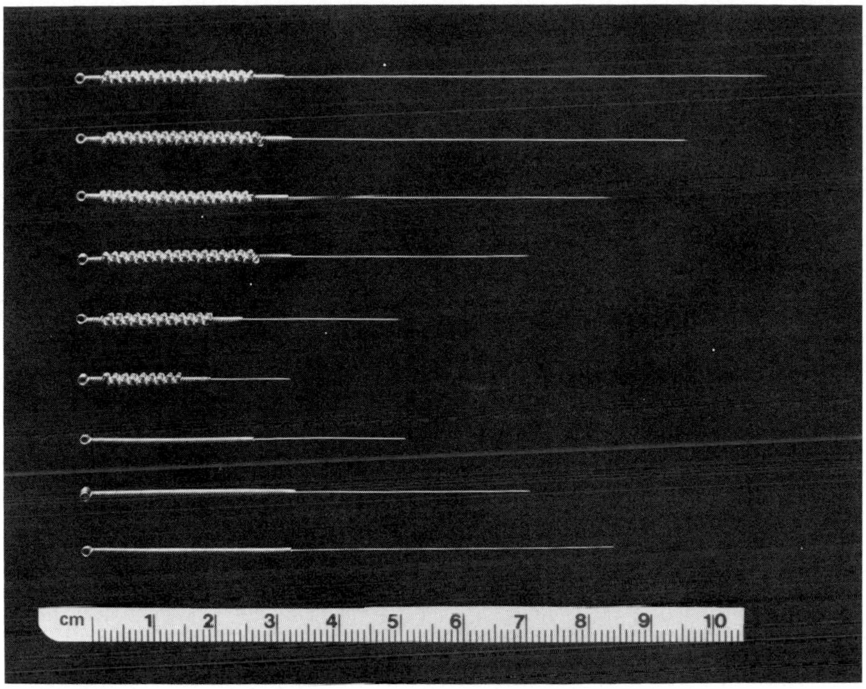

FIGURE 56–1. Typical needles used for acupuncture therapy.

treatment. Acupuncture-like therapy is thought to have existed in India as long as 7000 years ago. In the Orient, acupuncture has been used as a preventive and therapeutic modality for several thousand years. Stone and fish-bone needles were used in China during the Stone Age, an estimated 3000 years B.C. Bamboo, jade, copper, iron, gold, silver, and now stainless steel have been used as technology and the use of various metals and alloys developed. The *Huang Ti Nei Ching*, or "Yellow Emperor's Classic on Internal Medicine," is one of the oldest known documents on traditional Chinese medicine. It was published some time between 400 and 200 B.C. It is considered the bible of traditional Chinese medicine (TCM), describing the Oriental philosophy of anatomy, physiology, pathology, diagnosis, and treatment of maladies of that time. In fact, it even stated that blood flows continuously throughout the body, controlled by the heart. This was some 2000 years before William Harvey made the same discovery for western

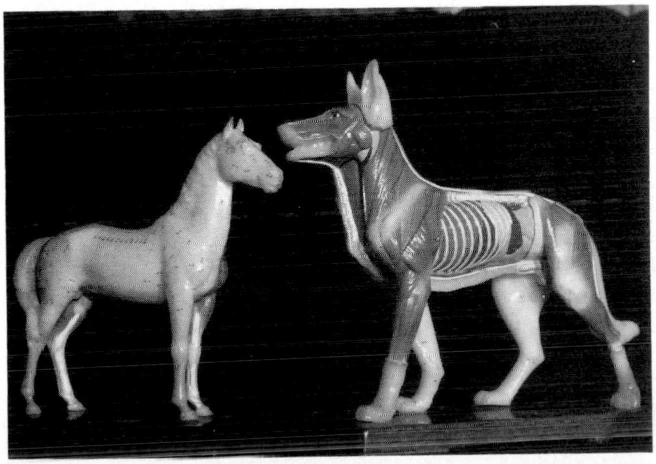

FIGURE 56–2. Chinese animal models with acupuncture points represented and numbered.

medicine in 1628. As far as acupuncture is concerned, 365 traditional points for the human being were detailed, nine basic types of needles were illustrated, indications for the use of acupuncture points to treat a variety of diseases were detailed, and "forbidden" or contraindicated points were described.

Further books and commentaries were published in China during the following centuries as the medical knowledge of the *Nei Ching* was passed from generation to generation and new knowledge and experience were added along the way. These books discussed more information on pain therapy and treatment of disease using acupuncture and moxibustion (the heating of acupuncture points by the burning of an herb, *Artemisia vulgaris*, on the points), yet the basic concepts of point and meridian anatomy and therapy have remained virtually the same as those described in the *Huang Ti Nei Ching*. TCM divided medical professionals into four distinct disciplines: physicians, surgeons, veterinarians, and dieticians.[9] Often their training and practice overlapped so that all or several of these disciplines were practiced by a single practitioner. Until occidental medical philosophies were introduced during the Ching Dynasty (1644 to 1911), TCM was the exclusive form of therapy practiced in China. Included in TCM are acupuncture, moxibustion, Tuei-Na (manipulative therapy or massage), Chi-Gung (breathing exercises), Shu-Shieh (nutrition and diet), and herbal medicine.[9]

In 1929, the growing popularity and influence of western medicine and surgery caused the Chinese government to ban the practice of traditional Chinese medicine. The ban, however, was widely ignored by much of the populace. The practice became somewhat clandestine, but TCM practitioners were readily available. During the days of the Red Revolutionary Army in China, Mao Tse-tung's troops were stricken severely with malaria. His medics had run out of atabrine and quinine and his troops were too ill to fight effectively due to the disease. Mao's plans for victory were in real jeopardy. According to modern legend, Mao was approached by TCM practitioners who offered conditionally to treat his troops. Their stipulation was that if the battle and revolution were won, TCM would occupy a place of honor in the new order. Acupuncturists then began to treat his soldiers and returned them to duty within three days. This demonstration apparently convinced Mao of the effectiveness of acupuncture. When he came to power, he insisted that traditional Chinese medicine (including acupuncture), along with modern western medicine, be studied by Chinese physicians. He ordered that the old and new medicines be given equal status in training, research, and practice under the new government. He stated emphatically that "Chinese Medicine and Pharmacology are a great treasure house and efforts should be made to explore them and raise them to a higher level."[10] Today, modern western medicine and acupuncture are practiced together in China and in other Oriental countries. An estimated 1,300,000 "barefoot doctors," 100,000 pharmacists, 200,000 nurses, 250,000 medical doctors, 150,000 veterinarians and 700,000 "barefoot veterinarians" have training in acupuncture. Research in acupuncture is being conducted in China, Taiwan, Russia, Belgium, Czechoslovakia, Italy, Romania, France, Germany, Japan, Korea, Portugal, Switzerland, the USA, and Canada.

Veterinary acupuncture is probably almost as old as acupuncture itself. A treatise on the use of acupuncture on Indian elephants estimated to have been written 3000 years ago was discovered recently in Sri Lanka.[11] Shun Yang (also called Pao Lo), who lived about 480 B.C., was the first recorded full-time practitioner of Chinese veterinary medicine. He is considered the father of the profession in China. A rock carving from the Han Dynasty (about 200 B.C.) shows soldiers acupuncturing their horses with arrows to stimulate them before battle. Government veterinarians and barefoot veterinarians (paraveterinary medical personnel) have treated cows, horses, pigs, and chickens from the Chou Dynasty until present times in China.[12] Japan had a history of veterinary acupuncture that seems to end at the middle 1800s when western medicine was introduced.[13] In France, veterinary acupuncture was used in the 1700s and early 1800s and was revived again in the past 20 to 30 years.[13–15] Today, most published reports on veterinary acupuncture come from France, Belgium, Taiwan, Austria, China, and the USA. The most complete reviews of the literature to date have been compiled by Phillip A. Rogers, M.R.C.V.S., who has become a liaison for veterinary acupuncturists around the world.[16–18]

EVIDENCE OF EFFICACY

CLINICAL EVIDENCE

Clinical studies and experimental reports encourage a closer look at acutherapy. In 1979, the World Health Organization (WHO) published its views on acupuncture after an interregional seminar held in Beijing (Peking). The WHO concluded that "acupuncture is clearly not a panacea for all ills; but sheer weight of evidence demands that acupuncture must be taken seriously as a clinical procedure of considerable value." A provisional list of 40 human diseases lending themselves to acupuncture treatment was compiled.[19] In veterinary medicine, a wide variety of reproductive disorders, musculoskeletal problems, pulmonary and gastrointestinal disorders, neurological disorders, and dermatological diseases have been treated with considerable success in many species.[13, 16, 17, 20–26]

In small animals, clinical reports on the successful treatment of reproductive disorders, intervertebral disk syndrome,[27–32] musculoskeletal problems,[33–36] dermatological conditions,[37] pain therapy,[38, 39] neurological disorders,[40, 41] and anesthetic emergencies[42, 43] in the canine have been published.[20, 21] In the feline, arthritis, nerve paralysis, and eczema have been treated.[18] Acupuncture analgesia has been used in small animal surgery, but it is not likely to gain popularity in view of more practical conventional anesthetic techniques.[44–48]

RESEARCH

Controlled studies under laboratory conditions have demonstrated that various physiologic changes can be elicited by the use of acupuncture. Some interesting effects reported are changes in uterine contraction,[17] gastrointestinal change[17, 49, 51, 53] cardiovascular changes,[17, 51–56] transient changes in hemograms and immune responses,[57, 58] and analgesic effects.

THEORIES OF MODES OF ACTION

The clinical and experimental results of acupoint stimulation leave little doubt that acupuncture does something. The fact that it has been used as an effective medical procedure on such a large portion of the world's population for over 4000 years makes it probably the most thoroughly field-tested technique known to medicine. But how are these effects mediated? What biophysical mechanisms are involved in the acupuncture process? We need to find the true basis for the action of acupuncture point stimulation in order to upgrade and better refine the procedures that have been used since the dawn of civilization.

Explanations of the mechanisms of acupuncture vary widely. The proposals include traditional oriental meridian theories, gate control and multiple gate control theories, reflex stimulation, neurophysiologic interference theories, holographic and dermatome theories, autonomic nervous system input theories, biochemical reactions, and many psychologic and hypnosis theories.[59] Research at the U.C.L.A. Acupuncture Research Project seems to indicate that a combination of at least three factors is necessary to obtain successful therapeutic results in humans: 1. immune-inflammatory reaction due to the physical act of traumatizing tissue as it is stimulated, causing a generalized response; 2. peripheral neural stimulation at the acupuncture points, modulating central neural regulation and causing more specific responses; and 3. psychologic support.[59] The effectiveness of acupuncture on animals and the lack of response to placebo acupuncture cast doubt on the validity of the psychologic and hypnosis theories and the need for psychologic support.

Modern Theories

NEUROLOGIC THEORIES

Probably the most popular theories of acupuncture are neurologic explanations.

Gate Theory. The gate theory has been proposed to explain analgesic effects of acupuncture.[60] When large myelinated A-beta or delta afferent nerve fibers that conduct touch and pressure sensations are stimulated, impulses from small unmyelinated C nerve fibers that carry pain sensations are blocked from passing a hypothetical "gate" located in the substantia gelatinosa of the spinal cord. As a result, the pain impulses cannot be transmitted higher in the central nervous system and no perception of pain takes place.[61] Acupuncture points may represent areas where greater numbers of large touch and pressure receptor fibers and small unmyelinated pain receptor fibers converge. Both sets of afferents synapse with neurons carrying impulses to the brain that are recognized as pain. Both afferents also synapse with interneurons, which can inhibit the input of these peripheral nerves to the neurons carrying the impulses higher in the CNS. In effect, an "accelerator and brake" effect is present. The pressure and touch afferents facilitate the interneurons, acting as an accelerator. The pain afferents inhibit the interneurons, acting as a brake. Increased stimulation of the touch and pressure afferents produces blockage of pain impulses coming to the synapse with the neurons that comprise the pain pathway to the brain. Stimulation of the acupuncture points increases input over the large afferents, thus producing an analgesic effect[62] (see Figure 56–3).

One of the shortcomings of this theory is the fact that cells of the substantia gelatinosa are believed to terminate in the medulla. This raises the following question: how can needles placed in the extremities produce analgesia to areas supplied by cranial nerves? Multiple gate theories have been proposed to solve this dilemma, with the second gates proposed to exist in either the thalamus or the brain stem. The thalamic gate theory[63] suggests that activation of large A-beta fibers by peripheral needling causes impulses to ascend to the thalamic level, causing the reticular and limbic system to shut the gate on pain sensations ascending through the spinothalamic and bulbothalamic tracts. The brain stem theory postulates that there is a brain stem central biasing mechanism, or reticular activating system, which controls transmission information being received through the integumental sensory afferents.[64] The central biasing mechanism theory has also been used to try to explain how stimulation of a point innervated by one nerve tract can provide pain relief at a site innervated by a completely different nerve complex.[61] Two questions not answered by the gate theory are why the analgesic effect lasts for 30 to 60 minutes after discontinuing stimulation when used for surgical analgesia and why chronic pain can be eliminated after multiple acupuncture treatments.

A theory of memory banks in pain-receiving cells has been proposed. Chronic pain is said to be the storage of the original pain sensation in these memory banks after a patient has been healed of an injury. Some illustrative examples cited are phantom limb pain and dental causalgia in people. Acupuncture is said to produce an amnesic effect in the memory banks of pain-receiving cells, thus diminishing or obliterating chronic pain. It has been proposed that these memory banks in pain-receiving cells can be activated or deactivated by weather or barometric pressure conditions, explaining why some chronic pain seems to be weather-affected.[11]

Inhibitory Surround. Another neurological theory used to explain acupuncture analgesia using points supplied by nerve complexes unrelated to the site of pathology is the cortical inhibitory surround hypothesis. According to this theory, a peripheral stimulus is mediated through afferent pathways and is projected onto the cerebral cortex. When a site of focal excitation is elicited in the cortex, the area immediately surrounding it is inhibited. Thus, if a point, or combination of points, whose cortical projection sites are adjacent to the cortical projection site of an area causing pain are stimulated, the resulting inhibition surrounding the stimulated cortical areas could obliterate or diminish the pain interpretation at the cortical level.[59]

Autonomic Theories. Another approach to explaining the mechanisms of acupuncture has been through the investigation of the autonomic nervous system.[51] In studies using rabbits, the ability to produce acupuncture analgesia in the nasal area is lost if the sympathetic chains are surgically interrupted.[65] In support of the autonomic nervous system approach, acupuncture points do, in many cases, correspond with Head's areas of referred pain.[66] According to Head's postulate, "the cutaneous pain felt in visceral disease is located in the areas where sensory nerves enter the spinal cord at the same segmental levels which supply nerves to the viscera concerned." It may be that cutaneous stimulation by needles is transmitted to the internal viscera through somatovisceral neuronal synapses in the spinal cord. During the process of such synapses, either the parasympathetic or sympathetic components of the visceral nerves seem to be selectively stimulated and the function of the autonomic nervous system is regulated[66] (Figure 56–4). If this is true, the ancient Chinese may have really been astute when they stated that external acupuncture points and meridians were connected to internal organs. Stimulation, in classical oriental terms, may have referred to activating the sympathetic nervous system, and sedation may have referred to parasympathetic activation.[67]

HUMORAL THEORIES

A humoral factor seems to be involved in acupuncture and has been demonstrated in cross-circulation experiments in rats.[68] When analgesia was achieved in 36 rats after 10 to 20 minutes of acupuncture stimulation, blood was allowed to circulate from the analgesic donor rats to paired recipients. Twenty-seven of the nonacupunctured recipient rats had significant increases in pain threshold, while the remaining nine did not. Both donors

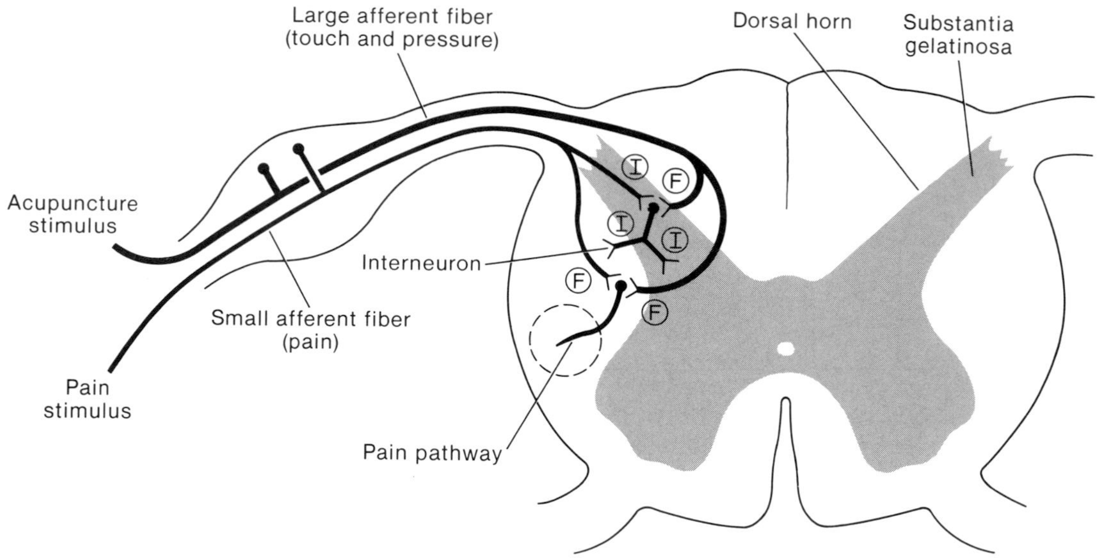

FIGURE 56–3. Gate theory. Acupuncture stimulus carries impulses to interneuron in substantia gelatinosa of spinal cord. Pain stimulus also sends impulses to same area. I = inhibition, F = facilitation. Acupuncture stimulus facilitates interneuron action, which causes inhibition of pain afferent synapse with pain pathway to brain. (Adapted from Latshaw, WK: Current theories of pain perception related to acupuncture. JAAHA 2:449, 1975.)

and recipients returned to normal control levels after acupuncture was discontinued. No such analgesic effects occurred in a control group of 19 pairs of rats. It has also been demonstrated that the effect of acupuncture can be reversed with naloxone,[69–71] leading one to suspect that acupuncture causes the release of a substance or substances that are neutralized by narcotic-antagonistic drugs. A series of methionine or leucine-linked molecules synthesized in the brain have been isolated. These compounds, enkephalins and endorphins, may be the humoral factors involved in acupuncture. They seem to fit the prerequisites necessary for a humoral explanation of acupuncture effects: they are produced endogenously, they seem to increase after acupuncture stimulation, they have physiological effects resembling morphine (e.g., they attach to opiate receptors, are analgesic in effect, and are antagonized by naloxone), and they are rapidly destroyed[72, 73] (Figure 56–4).

COMBINATION THEORY

Another theory ties the neurologic and humoral concepts together and describes acupuncture phenomena as follows: Nerve impulses caused by peripheral acupuncture stimuli are transmitted to the subcortical layer of the cerebrum by afferent A-delta myelinated nerve fibers. From the cerebrum, the impulses are transmitted to the thalamus and from the thalamus to the pituitary gland. Beta-lipotropin is stored in the anterior pituitary gland. When the acupuncture-activated stimulus arrives, the beta-lipotropin is acted upon by two enzymes: proenkephalinase to release enkephalins and proendorphinase to release endorphins. Enkephalin is then transmitted through A-delta myelinated nerve fibers to interneurons in the posterior horn of the spinal cord, in the substantia gelatinosa. There it acts as a neurotransmitter, or neuromodulator, to block release of substance P (a peptide neurotransmitter associated with the transmission of pain impulses) caused by afferent C-unmyelinated nociceptor messages coming from the site of pain stimulus. Since this release of substance P is blocked, no pain messages reach the pain-receiving cells in the dorsal horn of the spinal cord in the substantia gelatinosa. At the same time, endorphin is transmitted through efferent A-delta fibers to interneurons in the medulla oblongata, medial thalamus (nucleus centralis medialis, nucleus parafascicularis, and nucleus centralis lateralis), and the cerebral cortex. At these sites the endorphins block the release of substance P caused by impulses coming in from afferent C-unmyelinated nerve fibers arising at the site of noxious stimuli. Therefore, no pain messages reach the pain-receiving cells in the medulla oblongata, medial thalamus, and cerebral cortex. When acupuncture analgesia ends, enzyme enkephalinase destroys enkephalins and enzyme endorphinase destroys endorphins, returning the system to normal, so that new pain signals can be received if further injury should occur[11] (Figure 56–5).

BIOELECTRICAL THEORY

Another group of researchers, after 15 years of studying factors that initiate and control healing mechanisms, have described a complete control system, separate from the nervous system but working in conjunction with it.[74] It is, in essence, a primitive data transmission and control system whose prime function is sensing injury and starting the healing process, then stopping the process when healing is complete. The system works on DC electronic signals generated and distributed by the

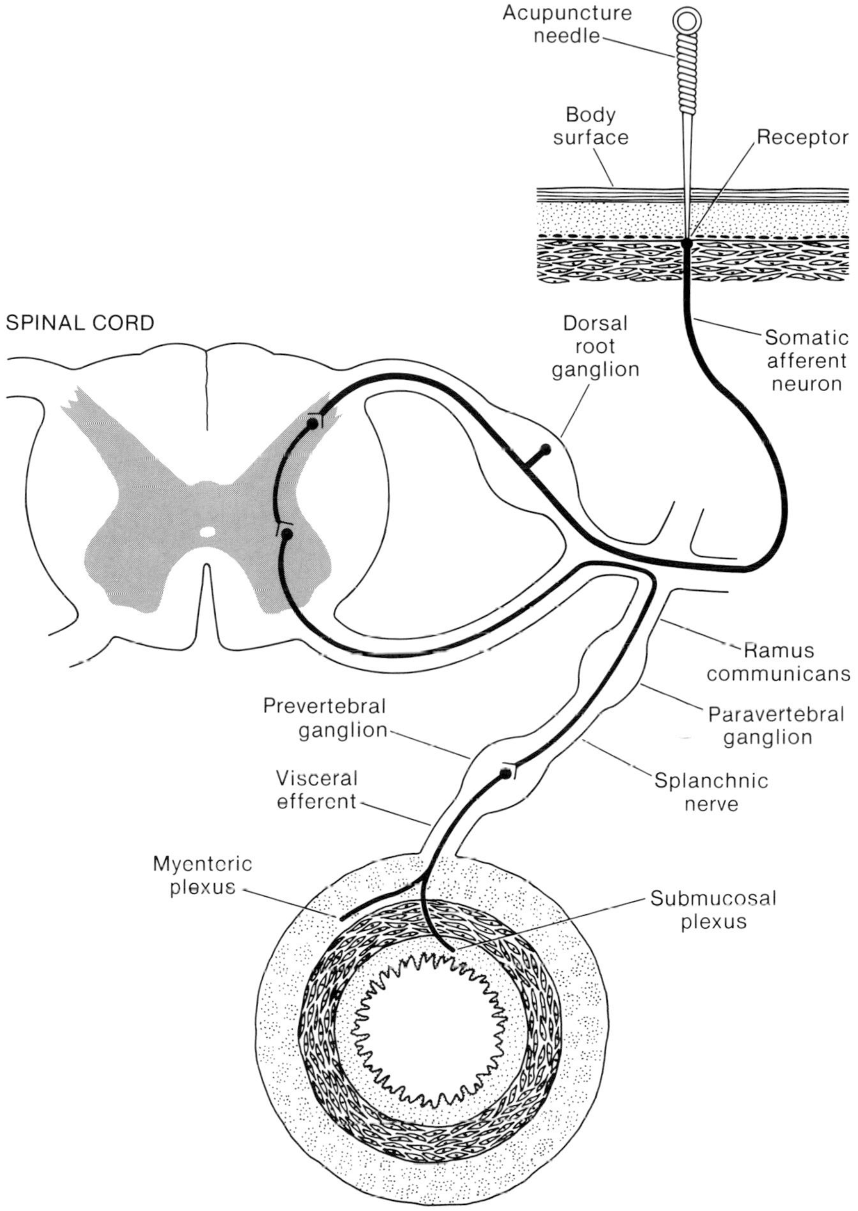

FIGURE 56–4. Acupuncture stimulation of somato-visceral reflex to affect organ function. (Adapted from Jenkins, TW: Functional Mammalian Neuronanatomy. 2nd ed. Philadelphia, Lea & Febiger, 1978, p. 150.)

perineural cells—Schwann cells peripherally and satellite and glial cells centrally. It could be compared to a computer system with peripheral transmission lines and central integrating areas. The output or control system has been studied for its effects on growth processes; the input portion of the system indicates damage or injury has been received.

In the transmission of DC signals, resistance, capacitance, and inductance reduce the magnitude of the signal as the transmission distance increases. Booster amplifiers in the system are needed to restore signal strength. It is considered that the acupuncture meridians are really DC communication channels and the acupuncture points are the booster amplifier locations. A metallic needle inserted into these amplifier points could alter the signal itself or the system's ability to transmit signals.[75] The theories of this group have been supported by their data on the electrical properties demonstrated at acupuncture points (higher conductance, lower resistance, organized field patterns, and differences in electrical potential).[74, 76–80]

Since no single theory seems to explain all of the effects of acupuncture, a combination of all of the above, or as yet undiscovered physiologic phenomena, may be responsible for the action of acupoint therapy. The author's personal opinion is that the mechanism involved depends on the particular point used, i.e., certain points or groups of points work through one set of mechanisms, other points are mediated by other physiologic reactions, depending on anatomic site, type of innervation, and the nature, magnitude, and duration of the stimulus. The fascinating fact is that the magnificent biological "machines" that we and our animal patients live in may have built-in reset buttons and adjustment controls that

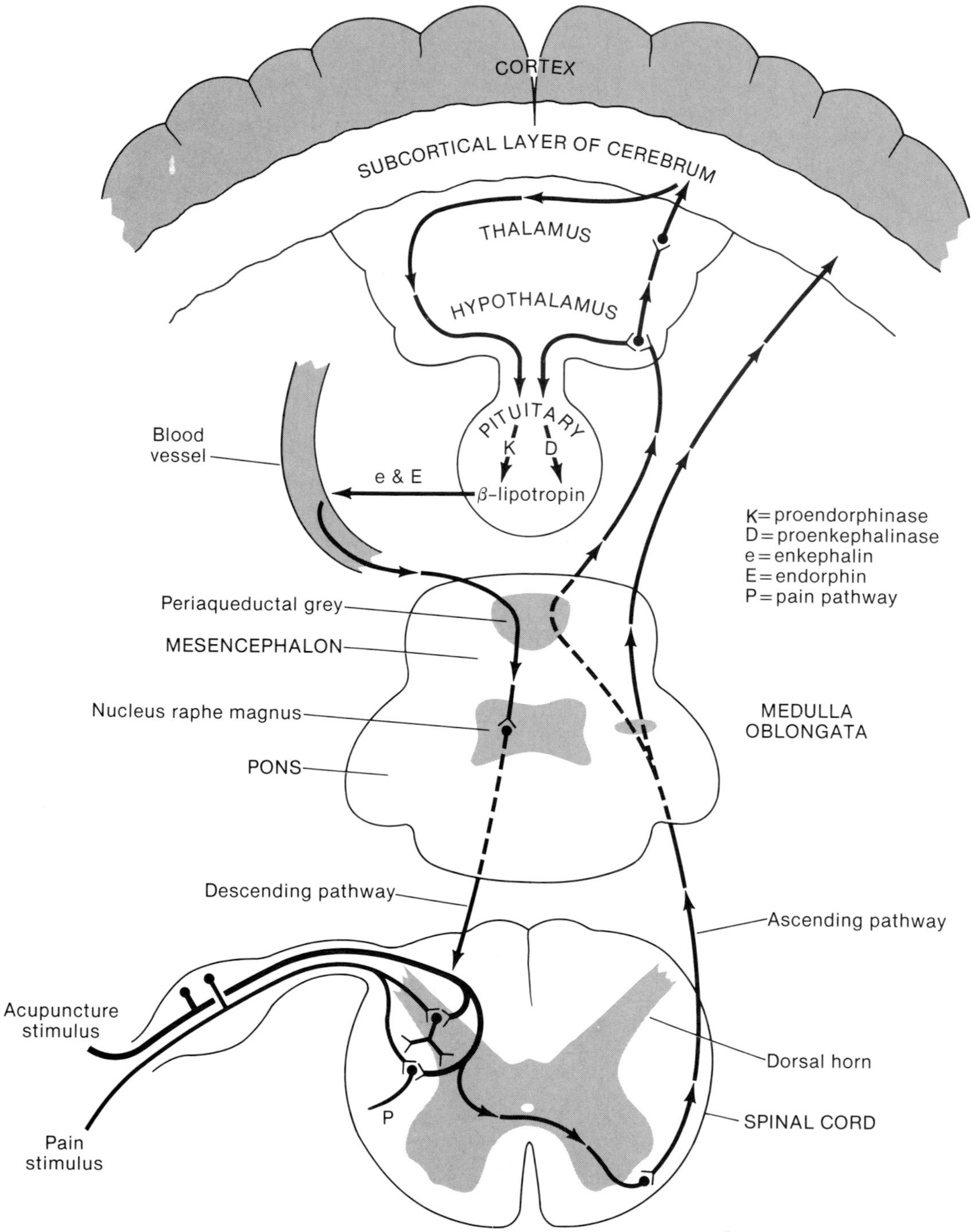

FIGURE 56–5. Combination of neurological and humoral factors to mediate acupuncture response. Acupuncture stimulus causes ascending impulses to reach centers in the subcortex, thalamus, and hypothalamus. These centers transmit impulses to the pituitary, initiating production of endorphins and enkephalins. These endogenous chemicals bind with receptors in the periaqueductal gray, causing a descending impulse to block pain reception in the substantia gelatinosa and other sites in the pain pathway. (Adapted from Yang, MP and Kok, SH: Endorphin in the Mechanism of Acupuncture Anesthesia. AJ Chin Med 7:147, 1979.)

are ours for the using, should we learn the secrets of how they work.

TRADITIONAL ORIENTAL MEDICINE

The basis for traditional Chinese medicine (TCM) is the theory that a life energy (Chi), consisting of positive (Yang) and negative (Yin) components, flows through the body in channels called meridians. These conduits are close to the surface at specific points on the body, the acupuncture points. Each meridian is supposed to correspond to a particular organ, from which energy is either generated or stored at a particular time of day. In contemporary thinking, Chi can be compared to electronic energy, the meridians to printed circuits, the internal organs to generators and storage batteries, the yin and yang energy polarities to the negative and positive electrical polarities, and the body itself to an electronically operated machine. Imbalances in the energy levels between the positive (Yang) and negative (Yin) polarities or impairment of flow through the meridians allows pathologic processes to begin and proceed. Imbalances or blockages can be produced by external factors (wind, cold, summer heat, excessive dampness, excessive dryness, or excessive heat), emotional factors (joy, anger, melancholy, pensiveness, grief, prolonged tension or stress, and fright), and miscellaneous pathogenic factors (irregular food intake, too much or too little physical stress and exertion, traumatic injuries, and impaired circulation).[81] By adjusting energy levels through stimulating specific acupuncture points or combinations of points, a homeostatic condition is reestablished and healing can take place. Various laws are used to explain pathology, selection of therapy, and prevention of recurrence. The study of traditional oriental medicine is intricate but fascinating, and gives one an appreciation of the powers of observation and astuteness of the early practitioners.

CURRENT USES OF ACUPUNCTURE IN SMALL ANIMAL MEDICINE

INDICATIONS

In two large-scale clinical studies on the West Coast, the most common causes for referral for acupuncture therapy in small animal practice were, in decreasing order of frequency: 1. paresis, paralysis, and pain in small dogs, usually resulting from intervertebral disc syndrome or trauma, 2. large dog paresis or paralysis syndromes resulting from neural compression caused by type II disc protrusions, spondylopathies and spinal instabilities, spondylolisthesis and cauda equina syndrome, and degenerative myelopathy, 3. pain due to hip dysplasia and resulting coxofemoral osteoarthritis, 4. other arthritic pain syndromes, 5. miscellaneous conditions not responding to conventional therapy, including allergy and dermatitis, lick granulomas, central nervous system disorders (ataxia, chorea, epilepsy), chronic respiratory diseases, gastrointestinal problems, osteochondritis dissecans, traumatic peripheral nerve injuries, and miscellaneous pain syndromes.[20, 21]

PRECAUTIONS

The most important contraindication for acupuncture is treating before an adequate diagnosis has been made or before at least an honest and diligent attempt has been made to determine the etiology of the condition being treated. This is contraindicated because acupuncture may mask or alter clinical signs so that later accurate diagnosis is more difficult (e.g., pain and neurologic syndromes). Or, it may cause a life-threatening condition (e.g., neoplasia) that should be dealt with by using another modality to have proper therapy delayed until it is too late to save the patient. Another factor to consider in acute cases is that elimination of pain may encourage the animal to be too active, thus hindering healing of the original condition.

Certain precautions should be taken in applying acupuncture therapy. If possible, acupuncture should be avoided under the following conditions: immediately after a heavy meal; after exertion or on a fatigued animal; on a subject that is extremely frightened, enraged, or emotional; on pregnant animals, especially if points below the umbilicus are to be used; if the subject has just been bathed or is going to be bathed within a short time after treatment; if injections of atropine, narcotics, narcotic antagonists, or corticosteroids have been used; or if the animal cannot be comfortably restrained and observed throughout the treatment period. The practitioner should always be aware of the anatomy of the area being punctured to avoid traumatizing underlying internal structures. Care must be exercised to avoid thermal burns with moxibustion and electrical shock or electrolytic burns with electroacupuncture.[82] In addition, it is inadvisable to insert needles in animals with severe blood dyscrasias or clotting deficiencies or into areas where local malignancies or skin infections are present.

SEQUELAE

Sequelae are seldom seen when acupuncture is employed by a knowledgeable practitioner. However, some can occur. The most common one seen is exacerbation of the problem being treated, especially in pain cases. The worsening is usually short-lived (less than 24 to 48 hours) and is frequently not a poor prognostic sign. The problem is commonly caused by "over-acupuncturing." Either too many points were used, wrong points selected, too much stimulation applied, or needles were left in place too long. Correcting these procedures in future sessions usually takes care of the problem. Some other sequelae that may be seen are: bent or broken needles; "needle-lock" or "frozen needles" when needles become caught in tissue, usually because of muscle spasms or becoming tangled in fascia, making them difficult to remove; injury to vital organs such as heart, liver, kidneys, and spleen; hematomas; pneumothorax; infections; nausea; vomiting; and in one instance, syncope.[83–85]

Techniques

As described previously, various physiologic events take place when acupuncture points are stimulated. The methods of applying the stimuli vary considerably, from a method as simple as applying finger pressure, to a method as complex as electronic stimulation, where such variables as waveform, amplitude, frequency, and patterns of stimuli can all be adjusted to achieve different results.

METHODS OF STIMULATION

Acupressure. Acupressure, or transdermal pressure therapy, was probably one of the earliest forms of point therapy. We unconsciously practice it on ourselves every time we rub or massage an area of pain or scratch a pruritic area. The early Chinese physicians described eight different forms of therapeutic massage:[86] thrusting, grasping, pressing, rubbing, rolling, pinching, rubbing between the palms, and tapping. Acupressure is probably best defined as finger pressure applied to the body surface in a general pattern or at designated points or locations.[87] Many styles of acupressure are in current use, among them Shiatsu, Do-In, Jun Shin Do Jitsu, and Tsubo therapy.

Shiatsu is thumb pressure massage, usually using double thumb pressure in an overall body pattern. Do-In is seldom used in animal treatment, as it is usually a human self-treatment technique to relieve headache, indigestion, cramping, and dizziness. In using Jun Shin Do Jitsu, the practitioner holds consecutive sets of two points simultaneously. Tsubo therapy is similar to Shiatsu in the use of thumb pressure, but attention is given to specific groups of points with interrelated therapeutic properties, and points are treated for a longer period of time. In veterinary medicine, acupressure is used rarely, mostly to relieve muscle spasm and relieve pain. It can be taught to owners to augment veterinarian-applied acupuncture.

Cupping, Vacuum Therapy. Negative pressure can be applied to points by the ancient technique of cupping. Three types of cups are described for use. One type is made of bamboo, with a small mouth and base and a slightly enlarged midsection. The other two types are globular, small-mouthed pots made of clay and glass.[88] A combustible solution, such as alcohol, is applied to the interior of the cup and ignited. The cup is then applied firmly over the point. As oxygen is consumed by the fire in the cup, a vacuum is created, and the skin is pulled up into the cup. The implications of applying a burning vessel to the skin of our patients can be imagined with alarm. Cupping is used in humans in China regularly and its use in large animals has been described. The author knows of no one using cupping in veterinary acupuncture in the United States.

Needles. The *Nei Ching* described nine traditional types of needles. Today, 25 to 34 gauge filiform stainless steel needles, one-half to two inches (1.25 to 5 cm) long, are most commonly used in small animal treatments (Figure 56–1). The length of the needles used is determined by the size of the animal and the location of the points being treated. Shorter needles (one-half inch or 1.25 cm) are used in small breeds and in points over bony areas such as the head, face, and distal limbs, and in areas where body cavities might be penetrated, such as the belly and lateral thorax. Medium needles (one inch or 2.5 cm) are used along the dorsal midline, paravertebrally, and in the upper thighs. Longer needles (one and a half to two inches or 3.75 to 5 cm) are used around the hip joints and popliteal fossae of large canine breeds. Cats can usually be treated using mostly one-half inch (1.25 cm) needles. The needles are solid, flexible, with a smooth shaft and, if examined under a microscope, the point appears rounded and pencil-like. Good quality needles should be flexible enough to bend to at least a 90° angle without breaking and then be straightened to its original shape without kinking. The best quality needles are manufactured in China, Korea, and Japan. Disposable presterilized needles are available, but the standard needles can be straightened, sharpened, honed, autoclaved, and reused many times, and are more economical. The proper techniques of inserting needles to the correct depth, at the proper angle, applying the appropriate manipulation to the needles while in situ, and proper removal of the needles are more difficult than one would imagine. Proper training and much practice are necessary before attempting to treat animal patients.

Temperature Variation. USE OF HEAT. Moxibustion is described in the *Nei Ching,* indicating it is probably almost as old as acupuncture itself. Moxa is the Chinese name for the powdered leaves of the mugwort, *Artemisia vulgaris.* The leaves of this medicinal herb are cured, dried, and ground in a mortar. The pale yellow fiber left is sifted to separate the moxa "wool" from the stems. For direct moxibustion, the moxa wool, or "punk," is rolled into the shape of a tiny cone and placed directly on the acupuncture point being treated. It is then ignited, and allowed to burn down toward the skin. It is removed with a forceps before it can cause a thermal burn. The procedure is repeated several times. A local area of intense erythema over the acupoint is produced. A base of bland ointment can be applied to the shaved skin before the moxa cones are applied. This adheres the cone to the skin and protects the skin from injury.

Indirect moxibustion is much more commonly used. The moxa can be obtained pre-rolled into a cigar-shaped stick and wrapped in a specially treated paper. In ancient times it was rolled and sealed in mulberry bark. The moxa stick is ignited and then moved back and forth slowly over an acupuncture point or over a needle inserted into an acupuncture point. The procedure is carried out until the skin becomes slightly erythematous. Care must be exercised in using both direct and indirect moxibustion in order not to burn the patient or singe the surrounding hair. These techniques are particularly effective in treating chronic pain problems.

Other methods of using heat to stimulate acupuncture loci are the employment of infrared lamps at a distance of 18 to 24 inches from the body surface to heat needles already in place and the use of electronic thermal devices developed specifically for that purpose. Irritant blister pastes to further stimulate these areas have been used in large animals, but their use in small animals is discouraged.

Use of cold. Cryotherapy is effective in many acute pain conditions. Ice cubes, Dry Ice, prepackaged chemical coolants, and ethyl chloride spray have been used. The stimulation of acupuncture points with cold is not advocated for chronic pain conditions.

Ultrasound. Sonapuncture, ultrasonic stimulation of acupuncture loci, has been advocated because it is noninvasive and shortens the treatment time. Only 10 to 30 seconds per point are required; small sound heads or probes as small as one-quarter inch (5 mm) in diameter are available.

Aquapuncture. Injection of solutions into acupuncture points is rapid, easily accomplished in most cases, and may be the only way to treat an animal that can only be restrained for a very short time. In small animals a 25-gauge one-half to one inch (1.25 to 2.5 cm) hypodermic needle can be used. Examples of substances advocated for injection include distilled water, electrolyte solutions (preferable hypotonic or hypertonic), vitamins (especially B_{12} and C), antibiotics, herbal extracts, local anesthetics, analgesics (e.g., phenylbutazone), and steroidal and nonsteroidal anti-inflammatory agents. Amounts injected range from 0.25 cc to 2 cc, depending on the site of injection and size of the animal. A dermojet can also be used for aquapuncture. It is held approximately one-half inch (1.25 cm) from the skin, and when activated, sprays a high pressure jet of solution into the top layers of skin, producing a wheal.

Electroacupuncture. Electronic devices have been developed to augment the stimulation given to acupuncture points (see Figure 56–6). They are either attached to inserted needles and deliver electronic stimulation percutaneously or an electroconductive medium and probes are used to pass the stimulus transcutaneously to underlying nerve structures. The electronic stimulation is more intense than manual manipulation of needles and usually causes more profound effects. Its use is almost essential to produce acupuncture analgesia for surgery. Most of the better machines are battery-powered to avoid the danger of electrocution, are AC rather than DC to avoid the danger of electrolysis burns, and are small enough to be easily portable. Many different types of electrostimulators are available. The better ones share these common characteristics: they are operated by transistor, cell, or rechargeable battery packs; they have a pulse generator that produces the frequency and pulse shape of the current; they possess frequency and pulse control knobs to regulate the pulse generator; and they have a current control to modulate the amplitude of the current going to the body.[89] Electroacupuncture is very commonly used in both human and animal acupuncture in Europe and the United States.

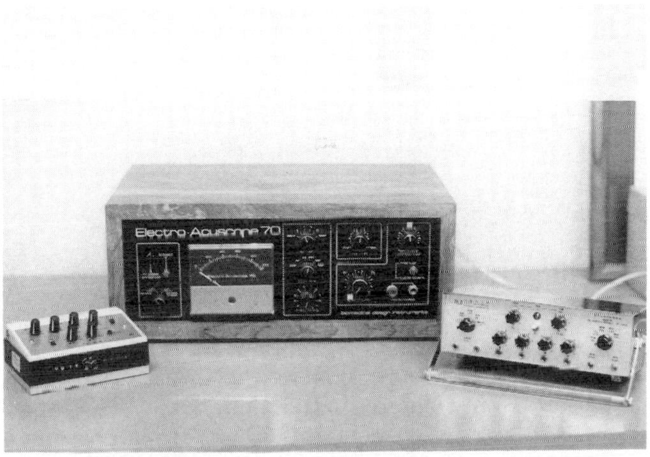

FIGURE 56–6. Electrical devices designed to stimulate acupuncture points transcutaneously without needles, or percutaneously in conjunction with needles.

Implantation. A more prolonged stimulation of acupuncture points can be achieved by implanting various materials into the loci. The most familiar examples are press needles or staples in the ears of humans to treat certain addictions, smoking, or obesity problems. These techniques are seldom used in small animals. Sutures can also be buried at acupoints to provide long-term therapy. Catgut or stainless steel has been used. The most common implantation technique in small animals is the use of metallic beads around the hip joints to treat chronic pain due to hip dysplasia-induced osteoarthritis. Under general anesthesia and aseptic conditions, a large-gauge hypodermic needle (14 gauge) is inserted into the proper acupuncture points. Several small gold beads are inserted through the lumen of the needle. A stylet is passed down the lumen of the needle to keep the beads in place as the needle is withdrawn. Then the hypodermic needle and stylet are withdrawn, in that order, leaving the beads permanently in the deeper tissues. In addition to treating chronic hip pain, the technique has been used to treat epilepsy in dogs.[90]

Laserpuncture. The use of low-intensity lasers to stimulate acupuncture points is very popular with many large animal practitioners, especially those engaged in equine practice. This practice was started in 1973, but as yet laser biostimulation has not been accepted wholeheartedly by all veterinary acupuncturists. The advocates of laser therapy cite good results in the treatment of pain, inflammatory conditions, and neurogenic disorders, and enhancement of healing in wounds, burns, ulcers, tendons, and bones.[91, 92] The term laser is derived by combining the first letters of Light Amplication by Simulated Emission of Radiation. Low-intensity laser therapy has been defined as "a form of intense light therapy using various frequencies and wave lengths which promote positive physiologic changes within cells that support the living organism in healing and reducing or eliminating pain."[91] The two types of lasers most commonly used in acupuncture are the red light emitters (wave length of 632 to 650 nm, generated by either a helium-neon gas tube or a laser-simulating diode device) and the infrared light emitters (wave length 902 nm, generated by a gallium-arsenite diode). The red light penetrates to a depth of 0.8 to 15 mm and the infrared light penetrates to a depth of 10 mm to 5 cm. The detractors claim that very little penetration of tissues takes place with the emissions from low intensity, or "cold" lasers—at least not enough to cause physiologic changes.

The advantages claimed for laser acupoint therapy are noninvasiveness, asepsis, freedom from pain, minimal restraint requirements, and short treatment time. The disadvantages are cost of laser units, limitations in treating large areas, and limitations on accurate data about the optimal parameters to use to achieve specific effects, e.g., wavelength, time of exposure, intensity of energy, frequency of light emissions, and frequency of treatment.[92] Claims of laser biostimulation effects made by clinical and research investigators include: increased phagocytosis, increased tissue granulation, increased collagen synthesis, increased vascularization, increased acetylcholine release, increased production of T and beta lymphocytes, increased synthesis of serotonin, inhibition of prostaglandin effects on tissues (e.g., pain, inflammation, and vasoconstriction), stimulation and release of beta-endorphins, and increased synthesis of ketosteroids and hydroxycorticosteroids.[91]

Acupuncture Points

DESCRIPTION

From the oriental point of view, there are two main groupings of acupuncture loci: those lying on the 14 meridians or channels and those not on these 14 meridians, designated "extra points." The points have traditional Chinese names, but are more commonly designated in the United States and Europe by an alphanumeric code showing the particular meridian upon which the point is located and the number of the point on the meridian (e.g., BL-60 would designate the sixtieth point on the bladder meridian). The points are further classified according to action as source, connecting, accumulating, association, alarm, master, action, trigger, terminal, tonification, and sedation points. It is beyond the scope of this chapter to explore these classifications more deeply.

Acupuncture points have been classified into four groupings based on their relationship to neural structures. Type I corresponds to known anatomic entities, e.g., the motor points of muscles, type II corresponds to the focal meeting of superficial nerves in the sagittal plane, type III points lie over the superficial nerves or nerve plexi, and type IV lie over the Golgi tendon organs at the muscle-tendon junction. Some of the physical attributes of acupoints are as follows: most have much lower electrical skin resistance than surrounding skin, thermographically, many are hotter than surrounding skin, and local tenderness on palpation is common. Most lie in anatomic depressions. They are located by using relationships with anatomic landmarks, proportional measurements using anatomic descriptions and maps, palpation (points usually feel like small indentations or nodules under the skin), and electronic point finders. The point finders are used to find the areas of lower electrical resistance or higher conductance on the skin. Unfortunately, interference by hair or skin moisture can give false readings in some cases.

SELECTION OF POINTS

The first task of an aspiring veterinary acupuncturist is to learn the anatomical locations of the acupuncture points. Then one must learn the physiological consequences of stimulating each point and the effects produced when they are used in combination with certain other points. Then, after a diagnosis is made and it is determined that acupuncture is indicated, the next task is the selection of points to be used (prescription) and the duration of the therapy session and type of stimulus (dosage). In traditional Chinese medicine, several laws[93] are used to determine these parameters. At the risk of sounding like a Chinese menu, the traditional laws are listed, but not dealt with in detail in this chapter.

Yi Pan Yun Yong Fa—local points used in combination with major distal points (e.g., mandibular pain can be treated with needles in the jaw plus needles in the toes on related meridians).

Tan Hseuh Tu Yung Fa—use of only a single point known to have a specific action for a specific malady (e.g., a point on the midline directly between the eyes is used for treating epilepsy).

Shuang Hsueh Ping Yong Fa—use of two symmetrical points (e.g., treating points bilaterally for a more intense effect).

Szu Chih Hsiang Ying Fa—use of points on all four extremities.

Lien Suo Ping Chen Fa—use of a chain of points on the same extremity for more profound effects.

Nei Wai Hu Ying Fa—use of two points at the same level on a body part, usually head or trunk, one point located anteriorly, the other posteriorly (e.g., one needle at the foramen magnum, the other in the nasal philtrum to treat brain disorders).

Lun Huan Chiao Ti Fa—encircling a point (e.g., using points surrounding a burn).

Hsun Ching Ch'u Hsueh Fa—use of points at the distal part of a meridian to treat disorders at the proximal end and vice versa (e.g., the use of a point on the hand to treat epistaxis, since the distal end of the meridian terminates next to the nares).

Piao Li Hsiang P'ei Fa—the relationship between an exterior point and an internal organ is employed, probably by stimulating a somato-visceral reflex.

Tui Cheng Ch'u Hsueh Fa—the application of known and well-proven formulas. This method is used by novice oriental practitioners and by most occidental practitioners.

Alarm Points and Associated Points—use of alarm points or associated points, which are specific points for diagnosis and treatment of disorders of internal organs or disorders along the related meridians (e.g., McBurney's Point for appendicitis in humans).

The Five Element Theory—use of traditional oriental laws of relationships between meridians, known as the Five Element Theory.

EXPECTED RESULTS

In acute problem cases, treating the animal every two to three days usually causes steady improvement until desired results are achieved. If treated only once weekly, the improvement seems to peak at the third or fourth day and then decreases, until at the next treatment the condition is only slightly better than when therapy was last given. At each treatment, however, improvement peaks a little higher and wanes more slowly, until progress becomes steady. In chronic cases, improvement is usually achieved more slowly and may vary in response at each treatment session until desired effects are seen. As mentioned earlier, exacerbation of signs may be seen after treatment, but usually is only temporary.

In two large-scale clinical evaluations, acceptable improvement was seen in 50 to 63.4 per cent of the cases treated.[20, 21] This does not seem to be an especially high response level until one considers that most of the cases were presented on a "nothing-to-lose" basis because they were refractory to more conventional therapies.

ATTITUDES TOWARD THE USE OF ACUPUNCTURE

REASONS FOR PAST NONACCEPTANCE

At the grass roots level, acupuncture has been received with attitudes ranging from apathy to antagonism, but seldom with soaring enthusiasm in the veterinary community. There are several understandable reasons for this lack of popularity. The use of foreign terms, such as "yang," "yin," "chi," and "meridian," sometimes casts a stigma on a new modality, simply due to unfamiliarity with the terms and concepts. The first impressions made by early investigators who claimed to be able to obtain fantastic results, with little clinical or research data and only doubtful anecdotal support, were unfavorable to and unforgivable by a community of professionals used to controlled studies, scientific investigation, and hard facts. A few advocates presented their findings with almost an aura of mysticism, which turned many veterinarians away. Many of the approaches to acupuncture have been presented in an unscientific manner, unpalatable to veterinarians with a sound scientific education. The lack of an all-inclusive physiologic explanation made still others hesitant to accept the validity of acupuncture. To those able to overcome these hurdles came the further problems of lack of easily accessible information and educational opportunities. The facts that many hours of study and a considerable commitment in class time, financial expense, and travel are required have discouraged other veterinarians. The misgivings of practitioners about how they will be perceived by their colleagues and clients if they practice acupuncture have also been factors in the hesitation to become involved.

PRESENT RESURGENCE OF INTEREST

Fortunately, in spite of these obstacles, a greater acceptance of veterinary acupuncture is gradually occurring. Media interest has led to client interest. Client interest has forced veterinarians to seek the help of veterinary acupuncturists. The favorable results obtained have stimulated the curiosity, as well as the misgivings of veterinary organizations. Articles and papers on veterinary acupuncture are now being accepted by more veterinary journals. Local, regional, state, and national meetings, seminars, and conventions have featured speakers on acupuncture. However, regard for the rights of the pet-owning public and concern for the image of the veterinary profession have prompted the American Veterinary Medical Association and several state associations to designate ad hoc committees to investigate the validity of acupuncture therapy and the credentials of those professing to know how to use the modality. In a policy statement approved by the A.V.M.A. House of Delegates in 1980, the following Guidelines on Acupuncture were approved:

> The A.V.M.A. has grave concern about acupuncture, regarding it as experimental. The public must be protected from those who make claims for acupuncture that are not based on adequate controlled experiments or documented research.
>
> Veterinarians must be aware of their legal responsibilities when acupuncture is used. The administration of an acupuncture needle should be regarded as a surgical procedure under the state veterinary practice acts.[94]

In January, 1986, the A.V.M.A.'s Alternate Therapies Study Committee began a two-year study on the safety and efficacy of procedures and regimens that differ from traditional forms of veterinary medicine and surgery. One of the modalities being studied is acupuncture. The committee is charged with reporting its findings to the Council on Veterinary Service. This body is faced with the task of determining if a given modality is appropriate as an alternative form of therapy in veterinary medicine, then proposing recommendations to certify or accredit practitioners in the approved modalities to be sure they are qualified.[95] The ad hoc committee recommended that the guidelines on acupuncture be changed to read:

> Veterinary acupuncture and acutherapy are considered valid modalities, but the potential for abuse exists. These techniques should be regarded as surgical and/or medical procedures under state veterinary practice acts. It is recommended that extensive educational programs be undertaken before a veterinarian is considered competent to practice acupuncture. There is a need to establish criteria for competency assessment.[96]

The concern of the A.V.M.A. has been shared by the veterinarians actually doing acupuncture. The International Veterinary Acupuncture Society (I.V.A.S.) was formed and chartered in 1974 to promote "excellence in the practice of veterinary acupuncture as an integral part of the total veterinary health delivery system. The Society endeavors to establish uniformly high standards of veterinary acupuncture through its educational programs and accreditation examination. I.V.A.S. seeks to integrate veterinary acupuncture and the practice of western veterinary science...."[97] The I.V.A.S. requires 120 hours of accredited class instruction, the passing of a comprehensive examination, and submission of five detailed case reports in order to receive Society Certification. The I.V.A.S. has drafted a code of ethics that details the duties of its member practitioners in general, the commitment of practitioners to the patient and to the profession, the ethics of the practitioner in commercial undertakings, and the relationship of the practitioner to the general public in making public statements, advertising, and professing education, training, and experience.

SOURCES OF INFORMATION AND EDUCATION

Veterinarians have been exposed to acupuncture largely through the efforts of three groups: the aforementioned International Veterinary Acupuncture Society (I.V.A.S.), the National Association for Veterinary Acupuncture (N.A.V.A.), and the Center for Chinese Medicine. I.V.A.S. courses are comprised of four intensive four-day sessions at monthly or longer intervals. The courses feature lectures by a faculty of American, European, and Oriental experts, literature reviews, broad support with hand-out materials, and live demonstrations with hands-on opportunities. The courses provide at least 120 hours of class time and are given every other year. Information regarding the courses and the organization can be obtained by writing to the current executive director. The address can be found in the A.V.M.A. annual directory under the heading "National, International, Allied, and Specialty Veterinary Organizations."

In 1973, the California Veterinary Medical Association (C.V.M.A.) appointed a committee to study the applications of acupuncture in veterinary medicine. Most literature available was in either Chinese, German, or French. The committee decided to have the information translated into English. The committee then undertook a clinical field trial with the help of the staff of the U.C.L.A. Pain Control Unit's Acupuncture Research Project. When encouraging results were obtained, the California Board of Examiners in Veterinary Medicine became concerned about the possibility of fraud or deceptive practices. They established stringent guidelines for the continuing acupuncture investigations. Included in these regulations were the requirements that cases should be treated in a facility set aside for acupuncture only and that the project had to be run by a nonprofit organization primarily under the control of veterinarians. To conform to the Board of Examiners' ruling, N.A.V.A. was formed by some of the original veterinary and nonveterinary acupuncture investigators.[98] For almost five years animals were treated at several locations in Southern California by a volunteer staff, with donations providing the sole funding for the clinics. Three in-depth courses were given in 1975 and 1976 and a compendium of veterinary acupuncture literature was published. Recently, the organization has been comparatively inactive and functions mainly in an advisory and information-disseminating capacity. Information can be obtained by writing to the current executive secretary, whose address appears under the heading of "National, International, Allied, and Specialty Veterinary Organizations" in the annual A.V.M.A. directory.

The Center for Chinese Medicine is a nonprofit educational organization providing continuing education courses in acupuncture in many fields of health care. The Center began offering two-day introductory seminars in veterinary acupuncture in 1977. The courses are held in various cities in the United States several times a year. With very few exceptions, the courses have been lecture only and introductory in nature. More information can be obtained directly from the Center.[99]

Through these three organizations and various local, regional, and national veterinary meetings, probably over 1000 veterinarians have been exposed to some form of acupuncture courses, varying from one day to more than 100 hours. There are an estimated 350 to 400 veterinarians using acupuncture on a daily basis in the United States.[100] I.V.A.S. reports 197 international members, most located in the United States, with 86 having been certified by examination after fulfilling educational and case report requirements. In many countries outside of the United States, acupuncture is taught and practiced by veterinarians associated with small national veterinary acupuncture associations.

LEGAL AND ETHICAL IMPLICATIONS OF ACUPUNCTURE

Legal briefs in Journals of the American Veterinary Medical Association[101, 102] indicate that the use of acupuncture constitutes the practice of veterinary medicine and/or surgery and that nonveterinarians practicing acupuncture on animals are probably in violation of local practice acts, unless special provisions exist for the treatment of an animal by a nonveterinary acupuncturist under the direction and control of a licensed veterinarian. No regulations exist, however, to insure the competence of a licensed veterinarian to practice acupuncture on animal patients. Eventually, to protect both the public and profession, provisions will have to be considered to assure that veterinarians or accredited nonveterinary acupuncturists under veterinary supervision are indeed educated and qualified in the practice of acupuncture on animals.[12] It is the author's hope that the profession will soon accept the certification of an organization such as the I.V.A.S. or that a College of Veterinary Acupuncturists can be formed to examine and accredit candidates as other specialty boards accredit diplomates.

References

1. Huang, HL: Ear Acupuncture, a complete text by the Nanking Army ear acupuncture team. Emmaus, PA, Rodale Press, Inc, 1974.
2. Lee-kin (translated by Tin-shen): A Handbook of Acupuncture Treatment for Dogs and Cats. Hong Kong Medicine and Health Publishing Co, 1985.
3. Klide, AM and Kung, SH: Veterinary Acupuncture. Philadelphia, University of Pennsylvania Press, 1977.
4. Young, HG: Atlas of Veterinary Acupuncture Charts, 2nd ed. Thomasville, GA, Oriental Veterinary Acupuncture Specialties, 1978.
5. Altman, S: An Introduction to Acupuncture for Animals. Monterey Park, CA, Chan's Corporation, 1981.
6. Weinstein, W (ed): Veterinary Acupuncture, Vol. 2—Dog. N Hollywood, CA, Eastwind Publishing Co, 1975.
7. Shores, A: Canine Acupuncture Chart, 1975.
8. Janssens, LAA: Acupuncture Points and Meridians in the Dog. Antwerp, Blondian Print, 1984.
9. Mok, M: Medicine—East meets West. Int J Chin Med 1:1, 1984.
10. Wei-Kang, F: The Story of Chinese Acupuncture and Moxibustion. Peking, Foreign Languages Press, 1975.

11. Concon, AA: Energetic concepts of classical Chinese acupuncture. A J Acup 7:41, 1979.
12. Altman, S: Acupuncture: a modern look at an ancient art. Calif Vet 31:6, 1977.
13. Joechle, W: Acupuncture in veterinary medicine: fact, fraud, or hoax? Pract Vet July/Aug, p 4, 1975.
14. Janssens, L: An overview: veterinary acupuncture in Europe. A J Acup 9:151, 1981.
15. Joechle, W: Veterinary acupuncture in Europe and America: past and present. A J Acup 6:149, 1978.
16. Rogers, PAM: Success claimed for acupuncture in domestic animals: a veterinary news item. Irish Vet J 28:182, 1974.
17. Rogers, PAM, et al.: Stimulation of the acupuncture points in relation to analgesia and therapy of clinical disorders in animals. Vet Ann, 17th Issue:258, 1977.
18. Rogers, PAM: 1 Esker Lawns, Co. Dublin, Ireland, Personal communication.
19. Bannerman RH: World Health Organization Viewpoint on Acupuncture, World Health, 1979, as reprinted in A J Acup 8:231. 1980.
20. Altman, S: Clinical use of veterinary acupuncture. VM/SAC, 76:1307, 1981.
21. Joechle, W: How effective is acupuncture: A report by the National Assoc for Vet Acup. Calif Vet 31:22, 1977.
22. Gideon, L: Acupuncture, clinical trials in the horse. JAVMA 170:220, 1977.
23. Feng, K (translated and edited by Hwang, YC): A method of electro-acupuncture treatment for equine intestinal impaction. A J Chin Med 9:174, 1981.
24. Kuussaari, J: Acupuncture treatment of aerophagia in horses. A J Acup 11:363, 1983.
25. Lakshmipathi,OR, et al.: Caesarean section in an ewe under acupuncture anesthesia. A J Acup 12:161, 1984.
26. White, SS and Christie, M: Traditional acupuncture and tetanus in the horse. A J Acup 12:359, 1974.
27. Buchli, R: Successful acupuncture treatment of a cervical disc syndrome in a dog. VM/SAC 70:1302, 1975.
28. Janssens, LA: Acupuncture treatment for canine thoracolumbar disk protrusions—a review of 78 cases. VM/SAC 78:1580, 1983.
29. Janssens, LA: The treatment of canine cervical disc disease by means of acupuncture; a review of 32 cases. JAAP 26:203.
30. Janssens, LA: The investigation and treatment of canine thoracolumbar disc disease: a personal view on the practical approach in a one person veterinary practice. Presented at 12th Ann Int Cong Vet Acup, PA, Sept, 1976.
31. Janssens, LA: Acupuncture treatment for thoracolumbar disc hernia in the dog—preview results. Presented at 12th Ann Int Cong Vet Acup, PA, Sept, 1976.
32. Still, J: Acupuncture treatment of thoracolumbar disc disease type I and II in the dog (back pain and hind limb paresis)—a study of 35 cases. Unpublished report, 1986. (author's address: 19, AV. Gustave Latinis, 1030 Bruxelles, Belgium.)
33. Buchli, R: Acupuncture treatment of post-myositis syndrome. VM/SAC 71:465, 1976.
34. Janssens, LA: Acupuncture therapy for the treatment of chronic osteoarthritis in dogs—a review of 61 cases. VM/SAC 71:465, 1976.
35. Schoen, AM: Critical evaluation of veterinary acupuncture therapy for chronic arthropathies. Proc of 9th Ann Int Conf on Vet Acup, IVAS, 73, 1983.
36. Schoen, AM: An introduction to veterinary acupuncture, mechanisms of action, indications, and clinical applications. Proc AAHA 53rd Ann Meet, 374, 1986.
37. Bullock, J: Acupuncture treatment of canine lick granuloma. Calif Vet 32:14, 1978.
38. Clifford, DH and Lee, MO: Trends in acupuncture research 1: Acupuncture in the control of pain. VM/SAC 73:1513, 1978.
39. Janssens, LA: Myofascial pain syndrome in dogs: the treatment of trigger points. A review of 41 cases. Presented at 12th Ann Int Cong Vet Acup, PA, Sept, 1976.
40. Stefanatos, J: Treatment to reduce radial nerve paralysis. VM/SAC 79:67, 1984.
41. Klide, A: Acupuncture therapy for the treatment of intractable idiopathic epilepsy in 5 dogs. Proc 10th Ann Int Conf on Vet Acup, IVAS, 55, 1984.
42. Altman, S: Acupuncture as an emergency treatment. Calif Vet 33:6, 1979.
43. Janssens, L, et al.: Respiratory and cardiac arrest under general anesthesia: treatment by acupuncture of the nasal philtrum. Vet Rec 105:273, 1979.
44. O'Boyle, MA and Vajda, GK: Acupuncture anesthesia for abdominal surgery. MVP 56:705, 1973.
45. Young, HG: Regional analgesia in dogs with electro-acupuncture. Calif Vet 33:11, 1979.
46. Janssens, L: Practical possibilities of acupuncture analgesia in small animal practice. Proc 8th Ann Int Vet Acup Conf Vet Acup, IVAS, 33, 1982.
47. Lee, GTC, et al.: Acupuncture anesthesia used in rabbit abdominal operations. A J Acup 4:149. 1976.
48. Wright, M and Mc Grath, CJ: Physiologic and analgesic effects of acupuncture in the dog. JAVMA 178:502, 1981.
49. Lee, GTC: A study of electrical stimulation of acupuncture locus *Tsusanli* (ST-36) on mesenteric microcirculation. A J Chin Med 2:53, 1975.
50. Clifford, DH: Acupuncture in veterinary medicine. In Kirk, RW (ed): Current Veterinary Therapy IX, Small Animal Practice. Philadelphia, WB Saunders Co, 1986, p 36.
51. Clifford, DH and Lee, MO: Trends in acupuncture research—2: acupuncture and the autonomic nervous system. VM/SAC 74:35, 1979.
52. Lee, DC and Lee, MO: Endorphins, naloxone, and acupuncture. Calif Vet 33:24, 1979.
53. O'Conner, J and Bensky, D: A summary of research concerning the effects of acupuncture. A J Chin Med 3:377, 1975.
54. Chin, DTJ and Ching, K: A study of the mechanisms of the hypotensive effect of acupuncture in the rat. A J Chin Med 2:413, 1974.
55. Lee, DC, et al.: Cardiovascular effects of acupuncture in anesthetized dogs. A J Chin Med 2:271, 1974.
56. Lee, MO, et al.: Cardiovascular effects of acupuncture at *Tsusanli* (ST-36) in dogs. J Surg Res, 18:51, 1975.
57. Brown, ML, et al.: The effects of acupuncture on white blood counts. A J Chin Med 2:383, 1974.
58. Rogers, PAM and Bossey, J: Activation of the defense systems of the body in animals and man by acupuncture and moxibustion. Acup Res Quart 5:47, 1981.
59. Bresler, DE and Kroening, RJ: Three essential factors in effective acupuncture therapy. A J Chin Med 4:81, 1976.
60. Melzack, R and Wall, P: Pain mechanisms: a new theory. Science 150:971, 1965.
61. Levin, N: Acupuncture in acute and chronic pain problems. Anesthesiol Rev, Jan, 1976, p 10.
62. Latshaw, WK: Current theories of pain perception related to acupuncture. JAAHA 2:449, 1975.
63. Man, PL and Chen, CH: Mechanism of acupunctural anesthesia. Diseases of the Nervous System 33:730, 1972, as quoted by Woods, W: Relief of localized pain by transcutaneous electrostimulation. A J Acup 3:137, 1973.
64. Bresler, DE, et al.: Traditional and contemporary theories of acupuncture, Part Two: contemporary theories of acupuncture. Acupuncture, Acupressure, and TENS for Pain Control. Pacific Palisades, CA, Center for Integral Medicine, 1980, p 88.
65. Loony, GL: Autonomic theory of acupuncture. Proc 2nd World Symposium on Acupuncture and Chinese Medicine. A J Chin Med 2:332, 1974.
66. Toyama, P and Nishizwa, M: The physiological basis of acupuncture therapy. J Nat Med Assn, Sept, 1972, p 397.
67. Altman, S: Acupuncture: taking a closer look. MVP 58:1003, 1977.
68. Lung, CH, et al.: An observation of the humoral factor in acupuncture analgesia in rats. A J Chin Med 2:203, 1974.
69. Mayer, DJ, et al.: Acupuncture and Central Control Pain. Proc of 1st World Congress on Study of Pain, 1975.
70. Ha, H, et al.: Naloxone reversal of acupuncture analgesia in the monkey. Exp Neurol 73:298, 1981.
71. Cheng, RS and Pomeranz, BH: Electroacupuncture is mediated by stereospecific opiate receptors and is reversed by antagonists of type 1 receptors. Life Sci 26:631, 1980.
72. Rogers, PAM: The primitive nervous systems and enkephalins. A J Chin Med 4:410, 1976.

73. Wong, J and Cheng, R: The Science of Acupuncture Therapy. Self-published, no date.
74. Reichmanis, M, et al.: Electrical correlates of acupuncture points. IEEE Transactions on Biomed Engineering, Nov, 1975, p 553.
75. Becker, RO and Selden, G: The Body Electric. NY, William Morrow and Co Inc., 1985, p 233.
76. Becker, RO, et al.: Electrophysiological correlates of acupuncture points and meridians. Psychoenergetic Systems, 1:105, 1976.
77. Brown, ML, et al.: Acupuncture loci: techniques for location. A J Chin Med 2:67, 1974.
78. Bergsmam, O and Woolley-Hart, A: Differences in electrical skin conductivity between acupuncture points and adjacent skin areas. A J Acup, 1:27, 1983.
79. Reichmanis, M, et al.: Laplace plane analysis of impedence on the H. Meridian. A J Chin Med 7:188, 1979.
80. Reichmanis, M, et al.: DC skin conductance variation at acupuncture loci. A J Chin Med 4:69, 1976.
81. Beijing College of Traditional Chinese Medicine: Essentials of Chinese Acupuncture. Beijing, Foreign Language Press, 1980, p 39.
82. Altman, S: An Introduction to Acupuncture for Animals. Los Angeles, Chan's Corp, 1984, p 142.
83. Rogers, PAM: Serious complications of acupuncture . . . or acupuncture abuses? A J Acup 9:347, 1981.
84. Chu, LSW, et al.: Acupuncture Manual, A Western Approach. NY, Marcel Dekker, Inc, 1979, p 27.
85. Altman, S: personal experience.
86. Bresler, DE, et al.: Acupuncture for Control and Management of Pain. Pacific Palisades, CA, The Center for Integral Medicine, 1976.
87. Siciliano, FR: Acupressure technique for pain control. Paper presented to Center for Integral Med, Jan, 1980.
88. Silverstein, ME, et al.: Acupuncture and moxibustion—a handbook for the barefoot doctors of China (a translation). NY, Schocken Books, 1975.
89. Chan P: Electroacupuncture, Its Clinical Applications in Therapy. Los Angeles, Chan's Books and Products, 1974.
90. Klide, AM, et al.: Acupuncture therapy for the treatment of intractable, idiopathic epilepsy in 5 dogs. Proceedings 10th Ann Int Conf on Vet Acup, IVAS, 1984, p 55.
91. Basko, IJ: A new frontier: Laser therapy. Calif Vet 37:17, 1983.
92. Jaggar, DH: A review of the low intensity laser and its application to acupuncture. Proc 8th Ann Int Vet Acup Conf, IVAS, 1982, p 99.
93. Wei-Ping, W: Chinese Acupuncture. Translation into English by Chancellor, PM, of the French edition by Lavier, J, Wellingsborough, England. 3rd impression, 1974, p 49.
94. AVMA 1987 Directory, p 460.
95. Anonymous: New committee studies alternative therapies. JAVMA 188:669, 1986.
96. Minutes of meeting of AVMA, Alternate Therapies Study Committee, Chicago, IL, Jan 20-21, 1987.
97. Anonymous: The International Veterinary Acupuncture Society. A brochure available by writing to ML Snader, VMD, RD 1, Chester Springs, PA 19425.
98. Anonymous: Guide to Acupuncture for Animals. A brochure prepared by NAVA and available by writing to R Glassberg, DVM, 1905 Sunnycrest Dr, Fullerton, CA 92635.
99. Center for Chinese Medicine: Courses in acupuncture for animals. 5266 E. Pomona Blvd, Suite 6, Los Angeles, CA, 90022.
100. Altman, S: Veterinary Acupuncture in California: a status report. Calif Vet 35:39, 1981.
101. Hannah, H: Legal Brief: Veterinary medicine and acupuncture. JAVMA 170:802, 1977.
102. Hannah, H: Legal Brief: More about acupuncture. JAVMA 171:44, 1977.

57 ADVERSE DRUG REACTIONS

LLOYD E. DAVIS

An adverse drug reaction is defined as any noxious and unintended response to a drug that occurs at appropriate doses of a given drug used for prophylaxis, diagnosis, or therapy and that occurs within a reasonable time frame of administration of the drug. The true incidence of drug-related disorders in veterinary practice is unknown, but it is obvious that such reactions occur and that many of them are fatal. The incidence of drug-related illness in animals is probably lower than that reported in human medicine. This may be related to shorter duration of therapy and the fact that fewer drugs are generally used in a given patient due to the economic constraints of veterinary medical practice. Nevertheless, our modern armamentarium of veterinary drugs is very effective in modifying physiologic processes and the risks have increased along with improved efficacy. The veterinarian can probably reduce the frequency of drug-induced disorders in animal patients by placing the same emphasis on the planning of therapy that the astute clinician normally places on diagnosis.

Most drugs employed in practice that have been evaluated in the target species are relatively safe for their intended use. Inordinate risk has been associated with some drugs that have been evaluated and approved for use in people but have not been studied in the animal species being treated. Some prominent examples are acetaminophen in cats, indomethacin and ibuprofen in dogs, and phenylbutazone in ponies. Use of such drugs has resulted in fatal drug reactions. It is generally advisable to employ drugs of a given class that have proven to be relatively safe in veterinary use. *The newest drug available is not always the best or safest choice for therapy*.

All pharmacologically active compounds present some risk to the patient. However, the therapeutic index varies considerably among different compounds. Generally, your willingness to accept this risk for your patient should vary in proportion to the severity or seriousness of the disease being treated. A drug with a narrow therapeutic index might be quite acceptable in a life-threatening situation (e.g., intravenous administration of lidocaine for ventricular tachycardia) or for treating a disease with high mortality (e.g., cytotoxic drugs for lymphosarcoma). There is no justification for administering such drugs to animals with self-limiting disease or for medically trivial purposes. Fatal drug reactions often result from inappropriate or trivial use of drugs (e.g., anaphylaxis from penicillin given for a viral infection, or pancytopenia from an overdose of estrogen administered to a bitch for mismating). The veterinarian should always keep in mind the possibility of adverse reactions occurring with any drug that he or she uses.

It is important when treating animals as outpatients to properly inform the client about the potential adverse reactions to a drug that has been dispensed. With proper information, the owner of the animal can seek help, and the drug can be withdrawn or the dosage modified at an early stage if a drug-induced disorder develops.

FACTORS RELATED TO THE DEVELOPMENT OF ADVERSE DRUG REACTIONS

As each patient is a unique being whose exact genome and particular circumstance is unlikely to be duplicated, it is not surprising that there are a number of factors to be considered in the individualization of therapy. These patient characteristics, the environment, and the nature of the dosage form need to be considered when dealing with adverse drug reactions.

Drug Factors

Adverse reactions in animals may occur in response to components of the dosage form other than the active drug. Considerable morbidity has been seen from propylene glycol used as a vehicle for injectables. When injected intravenously, propylene glycol causes hemolysis, heart block, and hypotension; when injected subcutaneously, it causes extensive edema by its osmotic effects. An allergic reaction following injection of vitamin B_{12} was confirmed to be associated with the benzyl alcohol employed as a preservative.[2]

Many adverse reactions observed in practice are dose-related and are associated with individual variation in pharmacokinetic behavior or individual sensitivity to action of the drug. These incidents can be corrected by modification of the dosage regimen and seldom require withdrawal of the drug. Variations in bioavailability, due to change from one product to another or to change in patient factors, could result in greater plasma concentrations of the drug. Incorrect route of administration is a frequent cause of adverse drug reactions. Barbiturates, chloral hydrate, levarterenol, and some other drugs administered subcutaneously cause sloughing of skin. Oral dosage forms given intravenously may cause sudden death. Particulate suspensions intended for intramuscular administration cause severe pulmonary embolism and death if administered in the vein.

Age

The incidence of adverse drug reactions is greater in the very young (less than 30 days old) and the very old animal. This is due to differences in body composition, rate of biotransformation of drugs, alteration in protein binding of drugs, and differential sensitivity of some tissues.

Habitus

The very obese as well as the asthenic animal may be more liable to develop adverse reactions to certain drugs. This is frequently caused by dosage errors introduced by calculating the dose on the basis of body weight. Drugs with low lipid solubility are not distributed into the excessive volume of adipose tissue. A common example is digoxin toxicity in obese dogs. Digoxin dosage should be predicated on the lean body mass. In contrast, digitoxin that is highly lipid-soluble is dosed on the basis of the total body weight, as its volume of distribution includes the body fat. Very lean animals such as greyhounds and whippets show prolonged effects to barbiturates and certain other drugs. Severe inanition from starvation or illness may modify the rate of biotransformation of drugs as well as drug distribution.

Sex

Adverse drug reactions occur more commonly in women than in men.[3] It is unknown whether there is a difference in incidence of drug reactions between the sexes of domesticated animals.

Pregnancy

Sensitivity to drugs and drug disposition may vary during pregnancy and parturition. Potential adverse effects on the embryo and fetus must be considered when treating animals after breeding and during pregnancy.[4]

Species

The more frequent occurrence of adverse drug reactions in some species than in others is related to drug disposition factors.

Disease

The presence of dysfunctions of various organ systems is an important factor in the occurrence of adverse drug reactions. Generally, the pharmacodynamic and pharmacokinetic properties of drugs have been determined in healthy animals. These properties can be greatly altered by intercurrent or associated disease conditions.[5] Renal diseases may greatly modify the elimination rate of a drug by delaying excretion or inhibiting biotransformation. Additionally, uremia may alter receptor sensitivity and change the extent of protein binding of a drug. Hepatic coma may be precipitated by certain drugs administered to animals with hepatitis or cirrhosis.

Immunologic Status

Patients with a past history of allergic reaction to a drug are more likely to suffer a reaction to the same or similar drug. Atopic individuals are at much greater risk than the general population of suffering adverse reactions to a variety of drugs.[6] Immunodeficient individuals may not respond normally to appropriate antibacterial therapy.

Breed Characteristics

A number of congenital disorders that may predispose affected individuals to adverse drug effects occur in various breeds of dogs and other species. For example, latent epilepsy in poodles, German shepherds, Belgian tervurens, beagles, Welsh corgis, and St. Bernards may be unmasked by corticosteroids. Von Willebrand's disease in Cairn terriers, Doberman pinschers, German shepherds, German shorthaired pointers, golden retrievers, miniature schnauzers, poodles, Scottish terriers, Shih Tzus, and Siberian huskies may predispose these animals to bleeding in response to anticoagulants and nonsteroidal anti-inflammatory drugs. The temperament of different breeds of animals varies considerably and will influence responses to drugs that affect behavior.

Presence of Other Drugs

The incidence of adverse drug reactions increases dramatically with the number of drugs given simultaneously to the patient.

Environmental Factors

Animals, as well as people, live in a much more complex environment now than they did a number of years ago. They are exposed to feed additives, agricultural chemicals, insecticides, atmospheric pollutants, and other chemicals that may modify their response to drugs. These may serve to increase or decrease the risk of developing inappropriate reactions to drugs given therapeutically. Crowding of animals in high-confinement situations may result in unusual responses. The lethal dose of amphetamine in rats was eight times smaller when animals were caged together than when they were isolated.[7] The significance of this to domesticated animals is unknown, but it may be wise to try to isolate animals that are undergoing drug therapy. Altitude is another environmental factor to consider, although little definitive information is available. Extremes of ambient temperature (either cold or hot environments) could provoke adverse effects to drugs that would not occur at neutral temperatures. An example is the effect of phenothiazine tranquilizers on temperature regulation in that normal control is lost and the patient may quickly develop pyrexia or hypothermia. The optimal environmental temperature for mammals is 75° F (24° C) as this requires no expenditure of energy for either heat production or heat loss. It has been observed that following severe trauma mortality increased 100 per cent at temperatures of 55° F (13° C) or 95° F (35° C) as compared to 75° F (24° C).[8]

Timing of Adverse Drug Reactions

Adverse drug reactions can occur at any time during therapy. Cardiac standstill may occur immediately following administration of quinidine to a patient with complete heart block. Anaphylactic reactions develop within minutes of administration of the allergen. Reactions to other drugs may require weeks to develop (e.g., reserpine-induced hypotension or exfoliative dermatitis from gold salts) and some may require months (e.g., calcinosis cutis or iatrogenic Cushing's disease from corticosteroids).

ALLERGIC DRUG REACTIONS

Allergic drug reactions (also called hypersensitivity reactions) are adverse effects of drugs based on immunologic mechanisms. They are dependent on a combination of antigen and antibody. Other types of adverse drug reactions due to direct toxicity, drug interactions, and modification of drug disposition by disease are not related to immunologic processes and can generally be anticipated and avoided by the clinician. Allergic reactions in a given patient generally cannot be anticipated by the veterinarian unless the animal has a prior history of allergy to some drug. The clinician should be particularly circumspect about using drugs to treat atopic individuals, since they have a greater tendency to develop an allergy to therapeutic agents. The true incidence of allergic reactions to drugs in veterinary practice is unknown. In humans, allergic reactions accounted for six to ten per cent of all drug reactions.[9] A comparatively small number of drugs account for most of the allergic drug reactions that occur in humans.

Characteristics of Allergic Response to a Drug

1. Generally allergic responses are not dose-related. Some individuals respond to exposure to minute quantities of the drug with severe allergic manifestations. Herein lies the risk of administering subtherapeutic doses of active drugs as placebos.[10]
2. The presence of circulating or cellular antibodies may be demonstrated in the patient.
3. The same reaction occurs when a test dose of the drug is given, although in some cases a more severe type of reaction occurs when the patient is challenged. For example, an animal might exhibit angioneurotic edema on initial exposure and develop anaphylaxis when given a test dose.
4. Eosinophilia is a common concomitant finding.
5. Mast cell degranulation may occur.
6. The clinical picture conforms to a known allergic pattern such as anaphylaxis, serum sickness, hemolytic anemia, thrombocytopenia, agranulocytosis, urticaria, allergic gastroenteritis, systemic lupus erythematosus, skin eruptions, or rashes.
7. The reaction does not resemble any known pharmacologic action of the drug.
8. There is a delay in the development of the allergic state following the initial exposure. Oftentimes this may not be apparent because of the lack of an adequate history of prior exposure to the drug. For example, animals may have been exposed to residues of antimicrobials in milk, meat, or other feedstuffs.

Immunologic Mechanisms

When foreign proteins are administered to animals, the incidence of allergic reactions approaches 100 per cent. This is not the case with most drugs, which are composed of small molecules. Some drugs almost never produce an immune response, whereas others induce antibody production in an appreciable number of individuals, with the serious consequences of an allergic drug reaction occurring in only a few subjects.

This is explained by the fact that in order for small drug molecules to become immunogenic, they must be able to form covalent bonds with macromolecules such as endogenous proteins, and to a lesser extent, polysaccharides or polynucleotides. Many, and probably most, drugs are not capable of forming covalent bonds with the functional groups of the amino acids comprising proteins.

The reactive moieties appear to be metabolites of the drug concerned rather than the parent compound. Some drug metabolites are chemically reactive and easily form covalent bonds with macromolecules. Such compounds have been implicated in the production of a number of serious toxic problems.[11] In the case of penicillin allergy in humans, it has been shown that several metabolites of penicillin conjugate with protein and induce antibody formation.[12] The principal reactive product seems to be the penicilloyl moiety resulting from the cleavage of the lactam ring of penicillin, although antibodies that are specific to other metabolic products have been demonstrated.[13] Most individuals that are treated with penicillin undergo an immune reaction to the penicilloyl group, but few of these develop allergic manifestations. In all probability, either the right types of antibody are not formed in the nonreactors or IgG may serve as a blocking antibody, protecting against the serious IgE-mediated allergic responses.[14] The problem of penicillin allergy is compounded by the fact that penicillin dosage forms may be contaminated with proteins introduced during their manufacture or by polymeric complexes that form spontaneously in the commercial preparation.[15] These are macromolecular substances that can act as complete antigens. Although drug allergy to penicillin has been characterized to the greatest extent, allergic mechanisms associated with metabolites have been documented for other drugs. Identification of the role of active metabolites in drug allergy also has been made for aminoglycoside antibiotics.[16]

A further problem that must be considered when confronted with a patient with a history of previous allergic reactions to a drug is the matter of cross-reactivity. If an animal has been sensitized to penicillin G, it is likely that it might develop an allergic drug reaction to a semi-synthetic penicillin such as ampicillin or carbenicillin.[17] All of these compounds have the basic penicillin nucleus, which can form the penicilloyl metabolite. Less apparent is the fact that a particular portion of the drug molecule might serve as the hapten in inducing the immune reaction. This structure can be common to pharmacologically disparate groups of drugs. For example, the sulfamyl group is found in the sulfonamide group of antimicrobials, furosemide, and the thiazide diuretics and sulfonylurea group of oral hypoglycemic drugs. An animal that had a previous reaction to a sulfonamide prescribed for treatment of an infection may at a later date react to a diuretic being used to relieve its edema.

Clinical Manifestations of Allergic Drug Reactions

Immediate Hypersensitivity. Anaphylaxis is an acute, systemic, life-threatening, allergic reaction characterized by hypotension, bronchospasm, angioedema, urticaria, erythema, pruritus, pharyngeal and/or laryngeal edema, cardiac dysrhythmias, vomiting, colic, and hyperperistalsis. Many of these clinical signs may be present in the patient or any one of them may appear as an isolated reaction. Anaphylactic manifestations most commonly follow parenteral administration of drugs but may occur upon inhalation or oral exposure. The appearance of signs develops within seconds to minutes following injection and is at its peak in 10 to 30 minutes. The onset may be delayed for an hour or two following administration of a relatively insoluble, repository dosage form such as benzathine penicillin. If the reaction is not fatal, the manifestations subside over a period of hours. Death generally is attributable to cardiac arrest, shock, or asphyxia. Approximately ten per cent of the cases of systemic anaphylaxis have a fatal outcome.[12] Penicillin seems to be the most common drug causing acute anaphylaxis in humans, and the incidence appears to be about four reactions per 10,000 injections.[18] The greatest risk seems to be in patients receiving a second course of therapy within two to eight weeks after an initial course. However, serious anaphylactic reactions can occur in patients with no previous history of having received the drug.

Mechanism of Reaction. Anaphylactic manifestations are associated with IgE antibodies to antigens with multiple-combining sites. Receptors on the surface of basophils and mast cells of the sensitized animal combine with the Fc portion of IgE during development of the immune response. Upon subsequent exposure, antigen forms cross-bridges between antibody molecules, which trigger the release of inflammatory mediators from the cells. This bridging of adjacent immunoglobulin molecules seems to be essential to the subsequent release of mediators of immediate hypersensitivity.[19] Univalent haptens such as parent drug or unconjugated metabolites fail to initiate a response and may inhibit the reaction. Subsequent to the antigen-antibody reaction, changes occur in the cell membrane that lead to fusion of cytoplasmic granules with the surface membrane, changes in concentration of intracellular cyclic-AMP, flux of calcium ion and release of prostaglandin D_2.[20] Canaliculi that communicate with extracellular fluid are formed and mediators are released into the surrounding environment.

An alternate mechanism for the production of anaphylaxis is the reaction among aggregates of antigen with specific IgG antibody that activates the complement system.[21] This leads to the release of anaphylatoxin, which can directly stimulate the degranulation of mast cells.

Treatment. The release of mediators of immediate hypersensitivity can be modified by physiologic modulation and by pharmacologic intervention. Secretion is inhibited by beta-adrenergic or PGE_1 stimulation and augmented by adenosine, cholinergic stimulation, and alpha-adrenergic stimulation.[20] The clinician can reduce the release of mediators by administering epinephrine, beta-adrenoceptor agonists, and phosphodiesterase (or adenosine) inhibitors such as theophylline. Corticosteroids modify the effects of the mediators on target tissues but do not modify the initial secretory response.

Typical Reactions. It is difficult to explain the variable occurrence of different manifestations of acute allergic drug reactions in different individuals or even in the same subject. One factor is the route of administration of the drug. Inhalation or airborne exposure may have a greater likelihood of producing asthma, conjunctivitis, and rhinitis. Topical application would be expected to induce urticaria with few systemic signs. Oral administration may stimulate vomiting, diarrhea, urticaria, angioedema, or anaphylaxis. Parenteral injection may cause peracute onset of anaphylactic shock, bronchospasm, angioedema, or urticaria. The type of reaction is likely to vary among species due to differences in the distribution of mast cells. Dogs have a high density of mast cells present in their liver. Anaphylaxis in dogs is generally manifested by vomiting and diarrhea followed by profound shock due to obstruction of the hepatic circulation, although cutaneous manifestations may appear in some cases. It is well known that guinea pigs respond to allergens by bronchoconstriction, resulting in asphyxia. Anaphylaxis in rabbits is associated with circulatory collapse due to acute pulmonary hypertension and right-sided heart failure. The "shock" organ in swine and rats appears to be the small intestine. Cats, ruminants, and primates seem to react most commonly with acute respiratory distress due to bronchospasm. Horses appear to manifest hypotension with collapse, urticaria, and angioedema.

Serum Sickness. Serum sickness is a systemic allergic reaction that occurs in response to some drugs and to biologics, and is manifested by lymphadenopathy, neuropathy, vasculitis, nephritis, arthritis, urticaria, and fever. The pathogenesis appears to be associated with the formation of immune complexes of antigen with IgG antibody, which are deposited in the affected tissues, activate complement, and initiate an inflammatory response. Serum sickness develops as specific antibodies appear while there is an excess of antigen in the blood. This is accompanied by a decline in serum complement titers.[22] IgE may be involved in the development of cutaneous manifestations.

Generally, the onset of serum sickness in response to a drug is delayed until 10 to 20 days after the beginning of therapy. This is the time usually required for sensitization to occur. An accelerated form of the reaction (onset in two to three days) may occur in individuals that have been previously sensitized to the drug. Clinical signs may persist for several days after withdrawal of the drug.

Antimicrobial drugs that have been incriminated most frequently in the production of serum sickness include the sulfonamides, penicillins, para-aminosalicyclic acid, and streptomycin.[12] Serum sickness in dogs treated for several weeks with sulfonamide-trimethoprim is relatively common and is associated with fever and polyarthropathy. The clinical signs abate during the week following withdrawal of the drug. Werner and Bright[23] have documented the immunologic basis for this adverse reaction and have attributed the reaction to sulfadiazine.

Hematologic Manifestations. The adverse drug reactions of hemolytic anemia, thrombocytopenia, and agranulocytosis may in some cases be immune-mediated. There are several mechanisms that have been demonstrated in human patients.[22] The hapten may react with a protein in the blood, anti-drug antibody is produced, and the antigen-antibody complex is then adsorbed to the cell membrane. This induces agglutination and when complement is activated, lysis occurs. Since the attachment of the antigen-antibody complex to erythrocytes is transitory, a negative reaction to the Coombs' test is usually observed. This mechanism seems to be responsible for some cases of hemolytic anemia and thrombocytopenia. A drug or reactive metabolite of the drug may covalently bind to components of the erythrocytic membrane.[24] Circulating antibody of the IgG, IgM, or IgA classes combines with the sensitized erythrocytes, resulting in hemolysis (IgG or IgM) or shortened life span of the erythrocyte (IgA). Clinical signs of anemia occur if the marrow does not compensate rapidly. Generally, a positive reaction to the Coombs' test is observed in such cases. A third mechanism is drug-induced damage to the blood-cell membrane, rendering it antigenic.[25] IgG antibodies are then formed against the cell membrane itself, resulting in autoimmune hemolytic anemia or thrombocytopenia. A fourth mechanism, which causes a positive Coombs' reaction but is not associated with an immunologic reaction with drug or cell wall antigens, is that of nonspecific, drug-induced binding of immunoglobulins to erythrocytic membranes. This reaction has been delineated in individuals receiving cephalothin.[22]

Drugs that have been associated with immune-mediated thrombocytopenia include stibophen, sulfonamides, isoniazid, and rifampin.[26] Drugs that most frequently cause immune-mediated hemolytic anemia in humans are penicillin, alpha-methyldopa, dipyrone, quinine, quinidine, stibophen, p-aminosalicylic acid, phenacetin, and rifampin.[12]

Agranulocytosis is a serious allergic drug reaction that appears to be much more severe (five to ten per cent mortality) in humans than in animals.[27] The reason for this species difference is not apparent at this time. Direct cytotoxic effects of drugs do produce severe leukopenia and pancytopenia in domesticated animals and will be discussed later. Immunologic mechanisms have not been well-elucidated for drug-induced agranulocytosis. In some cases, it has been possible to demonstrate serum antibodies. When blood from a patient with amidopyrine agranulocytosis was administered to normal recipients, they developed acute agranulocytosis.[28] An antineutrophil antibody was demonstrated in sera from neutropenic patients.[29] Immediate reactions are probably related to destruction of granulocytes in the blood, whereas agranulocytosis with or without pancytopenia may be related to immunologic effects on stem cells in the bone marrow. The drugs most frequently associated with agranulocytosis are phenylbutazone, amidopyrine, oxyphenbutazone, sulfonamides, cephalothin, semi-synthetic penicillins, chloramphenicol, p-aminosalicylic acid, phenothiazines, gold compounds, anticonvulsants, propylthiouracil, indomethacin, dipyrone, tolbutamide, barbiturates, antihistamines, and arsenicals.[26]

AUTOIMMUNE REACTIONS INDUCED BY DRUGS. Certain drugs may induce the formation of antibodies directed against the recipient's own tissues. In addition to hemolytic anemia and thrombocytopenia, which have already been discussed, drugs have been implicated in the development of systemic lupus erythematosus (SLE),[30] polymyositis,[31] hepatitis,[32] tubular nephropathy,[33] and inhibition of coagulation factor VIII.[34]

Parker[35] has discussed several possible mechanisms for drug-induced autoimmunity. These include (1) denaturation or exposure of a normal tissue constituent as a result of binding or cytotoxicity, (2) breaking immunologic tolerance, (3) interference with suppressor T-cell function, (4) blocking of reticuloendothelial system interfering with immune-complex disposal, (5) activation of latent viral infection, (6) drug acting as an immunologic adjuvant, and (7) cross-reaction between hapten and normal tissue antigen.

Drug-induced SLE has been observed in patients

treated with isoniazid, griseofulvin, tetracycline, and antimalarial drugs.[14]

CUTANEOUS MANIFESTATIONS. The immediate hypersensitivity reactions of angioedema and urticaria were discussed previously. A fairly common allergic drug reaction seen in animal patients as well as in veterinarians who handle drugs is contact dermatitis (which is a delayed hypersensitivity reaction). The drug or chemical acts as a hapten, which combines with proteins in the skin. The conjugate stimulates an immunologic response by lymphocytes in the regional lymph node.[57] Reactions can only occur upon exposure of the sensitized cells to the conjugate. If the antigen entered the blood, systemic reactions would occur or if injected, a delayed hypersensitivity reaction may develop at the injection site.[22]

Sensitized lymphocytes and monocytes are primarily involved in delayed hypersensitivity reactions. These cells are observed in affected areas during histopathologic studies and are responsible for the release of chemical mediators. When exposed to antigen, sensitized lymphocytes undergo blast transformation, release macrophage inhibitory factor, stimulate multiplication of monocytes, cause enzymatic changes in macrophages, and cause cell injury.

Diagnosis of Drug Allergy

Immunologic testing may be useful for investigating suspected therapy-related disorders or to assess whether a patient might be sensitive to a drug prior to initiation of therapy. Though this objective might be useful, it is difficult to achieve in most practice settings. Patch testing is useful for the diagnosis of contact sensitivity due to a delayed hypersensitivity reaction to a suspected drug or chemical. Erythema and induration of the patch-site becomes apparent at 24 to 48 hours, if the test is positive.

Intradermal tests for immediate hypersensitivity may be misleading. Erythematous reactions may occur due to nonspecific irritation caused by the product, yet the patient may not be hypersensitive. A frequent problem is lack of response in an allergic individual. Penicillin injected intradermally in a highly sensitive individual may produce no reaction but when a dose is given, the animal may develop anaphylaxis. The problem is that the parent drug probably is not antigenic. A reactive product, penicilloyl polylysine, was developed for cutaneous skin testing.[36] Reactivity to this compound occurred in 75 per cent of individuals with documented penicillin allergy, and testing with penicillin and penicilloic acid detected the remaining 25 per cent.[12] Serologic tests have limited value for the prediction of allergic drug reactions. As discussed earlier, many individuals develop antibodies during therapy with drugs or metabolites that bind covalently to cells but only a very few develop allergic drug reactions. Positive agglutination reactions merely indicate that the patient has received the drug and do not predict an allergic drug reaction.[37] Most of the tests *in vitro* require the services of a clinical immunology laboratory and the patient should probably be referred to a specialty clinic for diagnosis.

ACUTE ADVERSE DRUG REACTIONS RESEMBLING ALLERGY

Cardiovascular

Certain drugs may produce acute systemic reactions by mechanisms that are not immunologically mediated. These may be due to nonspecific release of mediators of hypersensitivity or due to direct effects of the drug on responding tissues. Injection of hypertonic solutions can stimulate the release of histamine.[38] This is probably an important mechanism, particularly in larger animals where relatively large volumes of concentrated solutions can be administered rapidly into a vein.

Acute collapse may occur as a result of the pharmacodynamic effects of certain vehicles and drugs. These incidents may be confused with systemic anaphylactic reactions. Cardiovascular effects of chloramphenicol, aminoglycosides, tetracyclines, polymyxins, propylene glycol, and several other drugs can produce sudden ataxia, shivering, dyspnea, and collapse following intravenous administration. These clinical signs are associated with various cardiac arrhythmias, hypotension, brief cardiac standstill, and decreased pulmonary and renal blood flow.[1] Tetracycline itself (in saline) produces a negative inotropic effect on the heart with a fall in blood pressure and severe conduction disturbances in the heart.[39] These effects were shown to be related to dose and rate of administration, and their intensity could be lessened by pretreatment with calcium borogluconate. The effects are probably related to the ability of tetracyclines to form chelates with calcium. This type of cardiovascular reaction has been reported in horses,[40] cattle,[1, 39] cats,[41] dogs, and humans. Propylene glycol alone has been shown to produce similar cardiovascular effects.[1] Rapid IV administration of a variety of drugs that are contained in propylene glycol vehicles (e.g., tetracyclines, chloramphenicol, and dexamethasone) may produce acute collapse through cardiovascular effects of the solvent.

Another cause of acute collapse following IV administration of water-insoluble drugs contained in an organic solvent is intravascular precipitation of the drug. When such solutions are introduced into an aqueous system, the drug may no longer remain in solution. The resultant precipitate or crystals are trapped in the pulmonary arterioles, producing embolism. I observed this while working with thalidomide during the 1960s. This was an extremely insoluble compound, which I wanted to study following intravenous injection. The powder was dissolved in dimethylsulfoxide and administered to two pigs. Immediately, the animals developed severe dyspnea, became cyanotic, and died. Following necropsy, frozen sections of lung were examined with polarized light. The vessels were loaded with refractile crystals of thalidomide. Acute pulmonary reactions resulting in death have been reported in patients being treated with amphotericin B, in combination with leukocyte transfusions.[42] These cases were characterized by acute development of dyspnea, hypoxemia, and interstitial infiltrates. The authors postulated that the amphotericin lysed aggregates of transfused leukocytes that were trapped in small pulmonary blood vessels, releasing neutrophil proteases which damaged the tissues.

Hematologic Reactions

Acute hemolytic reactions that are not immunologically mediated occur. Administration of drugs contained in hypotonic solutions or in some organic vehicles can cause rapid lysis of circulating erythrocytes with the development of hemoglobinemia and hemoglobinuria. The effects are generally transient and persistent anemia seldom develops. Species differences in resistance of erythrocytes to chlorpromazine-induced hemolysis have been reported.[43] Canine red cells were most resistant; human, murine, equine, and bovine cells were intermediate; and caprine and simian cells were least resistant.

Oxidant drugs and chemicals can cause hemolytic anemia accompanied by methemoglobinemia and Heinz body formation. The integrity of erythrocytic structure and function are maintained by close interrelationships among glucose metabolism, reduced glutathione and NADPH.[44] Normally, sulfhydryl groups in proteins of the cellular membrane and in globin are exposed to attack by oxidizing substances in blood and by oxygen. Oxidized SH groups are reduced in the presence of reduced glutathione and structural stability is maintained. NADPH is associated with the enzymes glutathione reductase and methemoglobin reductase, which catalyze the reduction of glutathione and the conversion of methemoglobin to hemoglobin. Oxidant drugs interfere with the functional activity of membrane sulfhydryl groups and stimulate lipid peroxidation within the membrane.[45] This damages the membrane and causes hemolysis. Highly reactive forms of oxygen are generated within the cell in the presence of oxidant drugs.[46] In the absence of sufficient reduced glutathione, peroxides persist and oxidize the sulfhydryl groups in the membrane and in globin. This results in hemolysis and the formation of Heinz bodies within the erythrocyte.[47] These doubly refractile bodies are formed from denatured globin molecules resulting from oxidation.

Heinz body anemia in response to oxidant drugs is encountered most frequently in cats and the neonates of most species. This may be explained by the fact that feline hemoglobin contains eight reactive sulfhydryl groups as compared to two in hemoglobin from other species.[44] This renders the feline hemoglobin more susceptible to oxidation and the formation of Heinz bodies. Furthermore, the spleen of the cat has been shown to play a minor role in the removal of cells containing Heinz bodies as compared to the horse or dog.[48] The neonatal animal is at risk because of reduced ability of the fetal erythrocyte to detoxify peroxides.[49] Several antimicrobial drugs cause hemolysis with Heinz body formation. Drugs that have been associated with this adverse reaction include sulfonamides, quinacrine, nitrofurans, neoarsphenamine, and nalidixic acid.[22]

Drug Fever

Drug fever may be produced as a result of drug allergy or by mechanisms that are not immune-mediated. In immune reactions, lymphokines from lymphocytes stimulate the release of endogenous pyrogen from neutrophils which, in turn, induces fever. Drugs may disrupt cell membranes, resulting in the direct elaboration of pyrogens into the circulation, e.g., amphotericin B. If drugs are prepared for injection with water that has not been properly distilled, bacterial pyrogens in the water may cause a febrile response. Excessive doses of certain drugs act to uncouple oxidative phosphorylation in tissues. Instead of energy produced by metabolism being trapped in high energy phosphate bonds, it is dissipated as heat. This mechanism is responsible for drug fever associated with salicylate and disophenol toxicity.

Drug fevers may result in body temperatures that exceed those commonly seen with infections. One may find rectal temperatures of 108 to 109° F (42° C) with disophenol intoxication. More commonly, one encounters sustained fever of 103 to 104° F (40° C) during the course of drug therapy. You should suspect this drug reaction in patients that have a sustained fever but in which the magnitude of the fever is out of proportion to the overall appearance of well-being of the animal. If the patient is bright, alert, eating, and active, it is likely that the fever is caused by the therapy rather than a disease. Defervescence generally occurs rapidly following withdrawal of the drug. Penicillins and cephalosporins are the most common cause of drug fever in cattle and dogs, and tetracycline the most common cause in cats.

TOXIC DRUG REACTIONS

Direct toxic effects of drugs on organs can occur as an exaggeration of the expected pharmacologic effect or may be related to actions that are unconnected with any desired therapeutic effect. Often the mechanisms for these effects are complex and obscure.

Nephrotoxicity

There are several reasons for the kidneys' vulnerability to toxic effects of drugs. Twenty to 25 per cent of the total cardiac output perfuses the kidneys each minute, thereby delivering appreciable amounts of drug over a given period of time. The blood vessels and glomeruli present a large endothelial surface area for contact with drugs and drugs are concentrated in the tubular fluid by the normal reabsorption of water. Some drugs are also concentrated in epithelial cells of the nephron by active transport from peritubular capillaries. Nephrotoxicity may be manifested as nephrotoxic renal failure, acute glomerulonephritis, interstitial nephritis, lower nephron nephrosis, and nephrotic syndrome. Drugs that are nephrotoxic are listed in Table 57–1.

Hepatotoxicity

The liver is vulnerable to toxic injury because of its strategic location and its central role in the biotransfor-

TABLE 57–1. DRUGS PRODUCING NEPHROTOXICITY

Antimicrobial Drugs	Analgesics
Ampicillin, I	Ibuprofen, I
Amphotericin B, T	Naproxen, I
Bacitracin, T	Phenacetin, T
Cephaloridine, T	Phenylbutazone, T, V
Colistin, T	Salicylates, T
Gentamicin, T	Antineoplastic Drugs
Kanamycin, T	Adriamycin, N
Methicillin, I	Cis-Platin, T
Neomycin, T	Cyclophosphamide, T, V
Oxacillin, I	Daunorubicin, N
Penicillin, I, V	Methotrexate, O
Polymyxin B, T	Mithramycin, T
Sulfonamides, O, I	Diuretics
Tetracyclines, T, V	Furosemide, I
Tobramycin, T	Mannitol, T
Heavy Metals	Thiazides, I, V
Arsenicals, T, N	Miscellaneous
Bismuth, T	Captopril, N
Cadmium, T	Dextrans, V
Copper, T	EDTA, T
Gold salts, T, N	Lithium, N
Mercurials, T, N	Penicillamine, N
Uranium, T	Phenazopyridine, T
	Phenindione, I
	Probenecid, N

Mechanisms are indicated by I = interstitial, N = nephrotic syndrome, O = obstructive, T = tubular and V = vasculitis.

From Davis, LE: Veterinary Clinical Pharmacology. Philadelphia, WB Saunders Company, *in preparation*.

mation of drugs. Drugs administered orally are absorbed into the portal vein and are presented to the liver in relatively high concentrations. If the drug is toxic to tissues or if it is converted to chemically reactive metabolites, hepatotoxicity may result. This toxic drug reaction may be classified as hepatocellular or cholestatic depending on the mechanism of injury. Icterus also can be caused by drugs through extrahepatic mechanisms, e.g., intravascular hemolysis or direct yellow discoloration of tissues (quinacrine). Hepatotoxic reactions are probably less common than nephrotoxicity and may be more difficult to recognize as drug-related. They should be suspected in any patient developing icterus, abnormal serum concentrations of transaminases or alkaline phosphatase, or hepatomegaly, while receiving a drug. The onset of clinical signs may be abrupt or insidious and severity may vary from asymptomatic changes in serum enzymes to fulminant hepatic necrosis. Hepatotoxicity is more commonly associated with chronic administration of medication or gross overdoses of certain drugs than with short courses of therapy.

Hepatocellular injury, degeneration, and necrosis result from the cytotoxic effects of the drug or its reactive metabolites on cellular components. Damage also can be mediated by immune mechanisms. This type of reaction is accompanied by marked increase in serum transaminase and bilirubin concentrations and prolonged prothrombin time when there has been extensive necrosis. In less severe injury, the transaminase concentrations are elevated with no evidence of jaundice. Affected animals have clinical signs associated with hepatic failure (see Chapters 88 and 89). Drugs that have caused hepatitis appear in Table 57–2. Probably the most significant causes of drug-related hepatotoxicity encountered in veterinary practice are the halogenated anesthetics, acetaminophen, isoniazid, corticosteroids, and anticonvulsants, although many of the drugs listed could potentially be a problem in animals being treated.

Acetaminophen toxicity generally is seen in animals that have accidentally ingested an overdose by eating tablets or capsules that were accessible to them or that the owner administered to them. This adverse reaction is seen more frequently as the drug becomes more popular as an over-the-counter drug. At lower doses, the primary reaction seen (particularly in cats) is Heinz body anemia. With increased amounts of the drug, hepatotoxicity of the hepatocellular type is seen. Affected animals develop icterus and facial edema, and are quite ill. Laboratory values for bilirubin, alanine aminotransferase, and BSP retention are elevated.[50]

The mechanism for the development of hepatotoxicity has been elucidated by Mitchell and coworkers in a series of elegant experiments.[51] Understanding of this mechanism is essential to the effective treatment of this adverse reaction. At usual doses, acetaminophen is conjugated with glucuronate and sulfate and a portion is oxidized to reactive intermediates. The intermediate is conjugated with glutathione and excreted as the mercapturic acid derivative, which is not biologically active. There is a limited reserve of glutathione available in the liver. As a consequence, with overdosage the supply of glutathione becomes exhausted, and the reactive metabolite combines covalently with cellular macromolecules, and the cell dies. The cat has an additional disadvantage in that it has only a limited ability to form glucuronides.[52] Following an overdose of acetaminophen, administration of N-acetylcysteine can provide sulfhydryl groups and act as a substitute for glutathione within the liver and erythrocyte. This has been shown to be effective in preventing hepatic necrosis and in

TABLE 57–2. DRUGS CAUSING HEPATOTOXICITY

Anesthetics	Cardiovascular Agents
Chloroform	Procainamide
Halothane	Quinidine
Methoxyflurane	Warfarin
Anticonvulsants	Antineoplastics
Carbamazepine	Busulfan
Phenobarbital	Cyclophosphamide
Primidone	L-Asparginase
Valproic acid	6-Mercaptopurine
Antimicrobials	Methotrexate
Ampicillin	Mithramycin
Carbenicillin	Urethane
Erythromycin estolate	Endocrine Agents
5-Fluorocytosine	Anabolic steroids (C-17 alkylated)
Griseofulvin	Corticosteroids
Isoniazid	Methimazole
Nitrofurantoin	Propylthiouracil
Quinacrine	Tranquilizers
Tetracyclines	Diazepam
Thiabendazole	Haloperidol
Analgesics	Phenothiazines
Acetaminophen	Other Drugs
Ibuprofen	Cimetidine
Indomethacin	Danthron
Naproxen	Dapsone
Phenylbutazone	Iodochlorhydroxyquin
Salicylates	Nicotinamide
	Stibophen
	Vitamin A

From Davis LE: Veterinary Clinical Pharmacology. Philadelphia, WB Saunders Company, *in preparation*.

improving methemoglobinemia and clinical signs of toxicity in the cat.[53] The recommended dosage regimen for N-acetylcysteine (Mucomyst) is 140 mg/kg as an initial dose, followed by 70 mg/kg orally every six to eight hours for four to five days. Acetophenetidin (phenacetin) is metabolized to acetaminophen and presents the same hazard. It may be encountered in a number of over-the-counter analgesic preparations, such as Anacin, Empirin Compound, and many sinus remedies.

TABLE 57–3. DRUGS THAT HAVE CAUSED APLASTIC ANEMIA

Antineoplastic	Endocrine Agents
Busulfan	Estrogens
Cyclophosphamide	Thiouracil
Cytosine arabinoside	Thiocyanate
Methotrexate	Methimazole
Mustargen	Tolbutamide
Vinblastine	Tranquilizers
Vincristine	Meprobamate
Antimicrobials	Phenothiazines
Amphotericin B	Antihistaminics
Chloramphenicol	Chlorpheniramine
Methicillin	Tripelennamine
Pyrimethamine	Miscellaneous
Quinacrine	Benzene
Sulfonamides	Carbamazepine
Tetracyclines	Carbon tetrachloride
Analgesics	Chlordane
Phenylbutazone	DDT
Phenacetin	Disophenol
Indomethacin	Gamma-Benzene hexachloride
Heavy Metals	
Organic arsenicals	
Gold salts	
Colloidal silver	

From Davis, LE: Veterinary Clinical Pharmacology. Philadelphia, WB Saunders Company, *in preparation*.

Aplastic Anemia

Aplastic pancytopenia is an uncommon adverse drug reaction in animal patients but when it occurs, its effects are devastating. True aplastic anemia is characterized by complete failure of hematopoiesis in which the red bone marrow has been replaced by fatty tissue. The affected animal shows signs of pallor of the mucous membranes, weakness, petechiation, hemorrhage, and increased susceptibility to infections. Diagnosis is confirmed by the presence of a hypocellular fatty bone marrow, determined by a bone marrow biopsy.

The mechanism by which drugs and certain chemicals produce their toxic effects on the bone marrow is not understood. There appears to be suppression of or damage to pluripotent stem cells in the marrow by either direct toxic or immune-mediated mechanisms.[54] There is also some evidence of individual susceptibility, perhaps a genetically determined predisposition, to the development of aplastic anemia in response to certain drugs. Some agents suppress the bone marrow in all individuals in a predictable, dose-related manner. Examples are the effects of ionizing radiation, cytotoxic drugs used in the treatment of cancer, and certain solvents and insecticides. Over 80 drugs have been incriminated as the cause of aplastic anemia in human patients. The reaction occurs infrequently despite widespread use of some of the drugs. In susceptible individuals, pancytopenia may occur with usual doses of the drugs administered for relatively short periods of time.

The drugs that have most frequently been implicated as causes of aplastic anemia in humans are chloramphenicol, phenylbutazone, mephenytoin, trimethadione, organic arsenicals, gold compounds, quinacrine, sulfamethoxypyridazine, and thiouracil.[55] There have been cases documented in the veterinary medical literature involving some of these same drugs (see Table 57–3). Chloramphenicol-induced aplastic anemia is probably very rare among animals. The more usual blood dyscrasia seen with chloramphenicol is dose-related leukopenia, which is reversible upon cessation of therapy. Watson et al.[56] described three cases of dyscrasias associated with phenylbutazone in the dog and four more in their discussion. Two of the cases had pancytopenia, the other had nonregenerative anemia and thrombocytopenia. Two of the patients died. These dogs had received usual therapeutic doses of phenylbutazone for periods ranging from four to eight weeks. A case of erythroid aplasia associated with thiacetarsamide treatment was described in which the dog survived for seven months before succumbing to the disorder.[57]

Probably the most commonly encountered cause of pancytopenia in the dog is estrogen toxicity. Dogs are known to be particularly sensitive to the myelotoxic effects of estrogens.[58] Following administration of a toxic dose of estrogen, there is an initial leukocytosis and left shift, followed by anemia, thrombocytopenia, and granulocytopenia. However, any combination of these findings could occur. Several clinical cases have been described.[59,60] Leukopenia and leukocytosis were seen among the cases; all had thrombocytopenia and anemia. Hemorrhages, petechiation, and presence of ecchymoses were common. Estradiol cyclopentylpropionate was the most common cause of marrow failure in these cases. This drug is intended for use in cattle for breeding purposes and should not be administered to dogs.

Drugs may exert direct toxic effects on other organs, which are regarded as adverse drug reactions, e.g., retinopathy, ototoxicity, and pulmonary infiltrates.

Medication Errors

Adverse drug reactions that are not related to patient characteristics or to unusual properties of the drug can occur. Relative safety and efficacy of drugs depends on an uninterrupted chain from the manufacturer through the distributor, the prescribing veterinarian, and the owner or the veterinary assistant, to the patient. In studies of human patients, it was found that from 25 to 59 per cent of the people committed errors in the self-administration of prescribed medication.[61] In hospitals, it was found that the average nurse made one error for every six medications given.[62] Errors encountered in a veterinary hospital may consist of omission of a dose, miscalculation of dosage, administration of a wrong drug, or improper administration of a drug. Clients may have difficulty in administering a drug to their animal. They may be handicapped, elderly, or have no assistance at home. A frequent cause of adverse reactions is the overly zealous owner. If such an owner is not sure that the animal swallowed the medication, he may repeat it to make certain, thereby giving an overdose.

It is important to show clients how to administer medication to an animal and to have them do it while you observe them. For complex management situations, such as control of the diabetic patient, it is useful to have detailed instructions printed that can be provided to the client at the animal's discharge. When dispensing medication, provide complete instructions for use on the package and advise the client about any possible side effects that might be associated with the drug. A small amount of time spent in education of the client can pay large dividends in terms of safe use of the drug you have prescribed.

MANAGEMENT OF ADVERSE DRUG REACTIONS

Generally, the adverse drug reactions encountered fall into one of two categories. Most are dose-related and the drugs produce their effects either by a direct extension of their expected pharmacologic effects or by organ toxicity. A smaller percentage are idiosyncratic and generally unpredictable. Hence, they constitute an inherent risk in drug therapy that is unavoidable. The main objectives to pursue in any animal that develops an adverse reaction to a drug are (1) provide life support; (2) stop administration of the drug; (3) enhance elimination of the drug; (4) if continued therapy is required, modify the dosage regimen or change to another drug; and (5) if available, administer drug antagonists or antidotes.

As has been discussed previously in this chapter, adverse drug reactions vary considerably in their time course. They may range from sudden death from cardiac standstill to a course of weeks to months with certain organ toxicities. Emphasis is placed on the emergency management of acute reactions, as most organ toxicity is managed in the same manner as diseases of those organs from other causes. For example, a patient with acute renal tubular necrosis produced by drugs is treated in much the same manner as an animal with severe renal disease (see Chapter 108). Similarly, drug-induced bronchoconstriction is managed as one would approach the patient with asthma.

In the case of sudden collapse following injection of a drug, cardiopulmonary resuscitation should be undertaken if there are signs of cardiac arrest present (see Chapter 35).

Resuscitation may be more difficult in patients with cardiac arrest attributable to certain drugs than in cases due to other etiologies. The drug causing arrest may pharmacologically antagonize efforts to establish autonomous activity of the heart. For example, if quinidine caused arrest of the heart in a patient with complete heart block by extinguishing ventricular pacemakers, the quinidine also exerts depressant effects on excitability and contractility of the myocardium. This may render the heart refractory to treatment.

Acute hypersensitivity reactions can have a rapid onset and must be treated immediately. These include anaphylaxis, angioedema, and urticaria. Anaphylaxis is life-threatening because of profound shock or bronchospasm (depending on species) leading to hypoxia of tissues and cardiac dysrhythmias. Angioedema involving the pharynx, glottis, and larynx may obstruct the airway and cause asphyxia. The immediate course of action is to administer epinephrine intravenously or intramuscularly (*not subcutaneously*). It is often very difficult to perform a venipuncture under these circumstances because of poor venous pressure. The adrenergic receptors in the arterioles of skeletal muscle are of the beta type. Consequently, epinephrine produces vasodilation at the injection site, providing for rapid absorption of the drug into the circulation.

The rationale for administering epinephrine is that it stimulates both alpha- and beta-adrenergic receptors, producing pharmacologic effects that are antagonistic to the effects of many of the mediators of immediate hypersensitivity. Stimulation of alpha receptors increases blood pressure and decreases blood flow in the skin and mucous membranes. The beta-adrenergic effects increase cardiac output, dilate constricted bronchioles, and inhibit further release of mediators from mast cells. This comprises definitive therapy for this emergency. Antihistaminics or corticosteroids are not effective in primary treatment of these acute allergic reactions. Antihistaminics block the H_1 histamine receptor, but histamine is only one among several mediators involved in the pathophysiology of immediate hypersensitivity. The onset of action of corticosteroids is too slow for these drugs to be of value in these circumstances. After initial control of clinical signs with epinephrine, an antihistaminic or glucocorticoid may be useful to prevent a relapse. Generally though, this is not necessary.

In less urgent situations, stop therapy and allow time for the processes of biotransformation and excretion to remove the drug from the body. Most dose-related effects abate as the drug is eliminated from the body. An example is a patient that is comatose from an excessive dose of a depressant. This should not be a cause for undue alarm, as veterinarians induce coma every time they anesthetize a patient. As long as vital functions are maintained, all that is required is supportive care. Fluids should be provided to maintain renal function, hydration, and blood pressure. The eyes should be protected from drying with methylcellulose drops as tear formation is likely to be inhibited. The patient should be turned regularly to prevent decubitus ulcers and congestion of dependent parts. If pulmonary and renal functions are adequate, the animal should be able to maintain homeostasis.

In some cases, active efforts should be made to enhance elimination of the drug following an overdose. In acute salicylism in the cat, the main problems are severe metabolic acidosis with increased anion gap, drug fever, prostration with coma, and gastrointestinal ulceration and bleeding. As the elimination rate of salicylate in the cat is slow ($T1/2 = 38$ hours) and dose-dependent, one cannot wait for resolution of the problem by normal elimination because the metabolic derangements are so profound that the animal would die before appreciable amounts of the drug had been eliminated. In this situation, increase the renal clearance of salicylate by maintaining a brisk alkaline diuresis with the intravenous infusion of mannitol and sodium bicarbonate solutions. Since salicylate is a weak acid with a pK_A of 3.0, it will be largely ionized in urine at a pH of 8.0. This prevents passive reabsorption of the salicylate from the distal tubules and enhances removal of the drug from the blood. Salicylate toxicity in the cat is a serious adverse reaction with high mortality. Successfully treated cases may require a week or more of intensive care before they fully recover.

Sometimes an overdose of a drug may cause nephrotoxicity along with other toxic effects. If acute renal failure has occurred, the only way of enhancing removal of the drug may be by peritoneal dialysis. Not all drugs are readily dialyzable; it depends on the extent of protein binding in plasma, their lipid solubility, and the extent of distribution in tissues.

In a small number of circumstances, antagonists may be available to prevent or mitigate the adverse effects. The administration of acetylcysteine to prevent hepatic necrosis and hemolytic anemia from acetaminophen was discussed earlier. Excessive muscarinic effects of cholinergic drugs can be controlled with atropine. Naloxone reverses the gastrointestinal and CNS effects of opiates and prazosin antagonizes acute hypertension produced by overdosage of decongestants or appetite suppressants, such as phenylpropanolamine.

The most discouraging adverse drug reaction to manage is aplastic anemia. A high percentage of these patients eventually succumb to hemorrhage or overwhelming sepsis. Severe aplastic anemia in humans has been defined by the International Aplastic Anemia Study Group as meeting the following criteria: (1) Neutrophil count less than $500/mm^3$, (2) platelet count less than $20,000/mm^3$, (3) less than one per cent reticulocytes, and (4) severe or moderate hypocellularity of bone marrow.[54] Ninety-one per cent of patients with severe aplastic anemia died within four months of diagnosis.

Blood transfusions may be necessary in animals with symptomatic anemia or bleeding due to thrombocytopenia, but sensitization to the donor cells eventually develops and renders the patient refractory to the benefits of transfusion. Prednisolone (1 mg/kg) may improve capillary integrity in thrombocytopenia but prolonged therapy was associated with a worse outcome in a large study of aplastic anemia.[63] Anabolic steroids stimulate production of erythrocytes, platelets, and leukocytes by normal bone marrow of animals,[64] but controlled clinical[54] and experimental[65] studies have failed to show efficacy in improving aplastic anemia. This has been the experience noted in case reports of bone marrow failure in animal patients. The most successful approach to the problem in human patients has been by allogeneic bone marrow transplantation following immunosuppression by cyclophosphamide or total-body irradiation combined with cyclophosphamide.[54] Nevertheless, long-term survival was still only 44 per cent.[66] Antimicrobial therapy should not be instituted routinely unless there is documented evidence of an infection. Patients with leukopenia are at increased risk to infection and indiscriminate exposure to antibiotics may lead to the production of resistant strains of organisms that would be more difficult to control should sepsis occur.

CONCLUSIONS

Adverse drug reactions are more easily prevented than treated once they occur. They constitute a major aspect of risk/benefit assessment by the veterinarian. Accordingly, rational use of a drug in practice requires a knowledge of its pharmacologic actions, side effects, and potential risk factors inherent in the patient. The clinician also must be able to recognize that an adverse reaction has occurred so that he can stop treatment to prevent further damage, and can plan a course of action for dealing with the reaction. Therapeutic enthusiasm is difficult to justify in the absence of a diagnosis or when a potent drug is used for trivial medical purposes, as the risks may far outweigh any potential benefits to be gained by therapy.

References

1. Gross, DR, et al.: Cardiovascular effects of intravenous administration of propylene glycol and of oxytetracycline in propylene glycol in calves. Am J Vet Res 40:783, 1979.
2. Grant, JA, et al.: Unsuspected benzyl alcohol sensitivity. N Engl J Med 306:108, 1982.
3. McQueen, EG: Pharmacological basis of adverse drug reactions. In Avery, GS (ed): Drug Treatment. Acton, MA, Publishing Sciences Group, 1976, p 169.
4. Davis, LE: Adverse effects of drugs on reproduction in dogs and cats. Mod Vet Pract 64:969, 1983.
5. Davis, LE: Interactions of disease and drugs. Proc 2nd Intl Cong Vet Anes Santa Barbara, Vet Pract Publ Co, 1985, p 32.
6. Smith, JW, et al.: Studies on the epidemiology of adverse drug reactions. II. An evaluation of penicillin allergy. N Engl J Med 274:998, 1966.
7. Lasagna, L and McCann, W: Effect of tranquilizing drugs on amphetamine toxicity in aggregated mice. Science 125:124, 1957.
8. Elman, R, et al.: Mortality in severe experimental burns as affected by environmental temperature. Proc Soc Exp Biol Med 51:350, 1942.
9. Borda, IT, et al: Assessment of adverse drug reactions within a drug surveillance program. JAMA 205:99, 1968.
10. Davis, LE, et al.: Monitoring drug concentrations in animal patients. JAVMA 176:1156, 1980.
11. Gillette, JR, et al.: Biochemical mechanisms of drug toxicity. Ann Rev Pharmacol 14:271, 1974.
12. Parker, CW: Allergic reactions in man. Pharmacol Rev 34:85, 1982.
13. Yamana, T, et al.: Kinetics and mechanism of penicillin aminolysis involved in penicillin allergy. J Pharm Pharmacol 27:56, 1975.
14. Parker, CW: Drug allergy. In Parker, CW (ed): Clinical Immunology. Philadelphia, WB Saunders, 1980, p 1219.
15. Stewart, GT: Allergic residues in penicillins. Lancet 1:1177, 1967.
16. Pirila, V and Pirila, L: Sensitization to the neomycin group of antibiotics. Acta Dermatol Venereol 46:489, 1966.
17. Adkinson, NF Jr, et al.: Routine use of penicillin skin testing on an inpatient service. N Engl J Med 285:22, 1971.
18. Idsoe, O, et al.: Nature and extent of penicillin side reactions, with particular reference to fatalities from anaphylactic shock. Bull WHO 38:159, 1968.
19. Sullivan, TJ and Parker, CW: Pharmacological modulation of the inflammatory mediator release by rat mast cells. Am J Pathol 85:437, 1976.

20. Sullivan, TJ and Kulczycki, A Jr: Immediate hypersensitivity responses. In Parker, CW (ed): Clinical Immunology. Philadelphia, WB Saunders, 1980, p 115.
21. Austen, K: Histamine and other mediators of allergic reactions. In Samter, M and Alexander, HL (eds): Immunological Diseases. Boston, Little, Brown and Co, 1971.
22. Cluff, LE, et al.: Clinical problems with drugs. In Major Problems in Internal Medicine Series, Vol 5. Philadelphia, WB Saunders, 1975, p 68.
23. Werner, LL, et al.: Drug-induced immune hypersensitivity disorders in two dogs treated with trimethoprim-sulfadiazine. Case reports and drug-challenge studies. JAAHA 19:783, 1983.
24. Thiel, JA, et al.: The specificity of hemagglutination reactions in human and experimental penicillin hypersensitivity. J Allergy 35:399, 1964.
25. Bakemeier, RF and Leddy, JP: Erythrocyte antibody associated with alphamethyldopa: Heterogeneity of structure and specificity. Blood 32:1, 1968.
26. Petz, LD and Fudenberg, HH: Immunological mechanisms in drug-induced cytopenias. In Brown, EG (ed): Progress in Hematology, Vol 9. New York, Grune and Stratton, 1976.
27. Hartl, PW: Drug allergic agranulocytosis (Schultz's disease). Semin Hematol 2:313, 1965.
28. Moeschlin, S and Wagner, K: Agranulocytosis due to the occurrence of leukocyte agglutinins. Acta Haematol 8:29, 1952.
29. Weitzman, SA, et al.: Drug-induced immunological neutropenia. Lancet 2:1068, 1978.
30. Tan, EM: Drug-induced autoimmune disease. Fed Proc 33:1894, 1974.
31. Cucher, BG and Goldman, AL: D-penicillamine-induced polymyositis in rheumatoid arthritis. Ann Intern Med 86:615, 1976.
32. Eddlestone, AL: Immunology and the liver. In Parker, CW (ed): Clinical Immunology. Philadelphia, WB Saunders, 1980, p 1009.
33. Border, WA, et al.: Antitubular basement-membrane antibodies in methicillin associated interstitial nephritis. N Engl J Med 291:381, 1974.
34. Klein, KG, et al.: Studies on an acquired inhibition of factor VIII induced by penicillin allergy. Clin Exp Immunol 26:155, 1976.
35. Parker, CW: Hapten immunology and allergic reactions in humans. Kroc Foundation conference on drug-related systemic lupus erythematosus. Arthritis Rheum 24:1024, 1981.
36. Parker, CW, et al.: Immunogenicity of haptenpolylysine conjugates. J Immunol 94:289, 1965.
37. deWeck, AL and Blum, G: Recent clinical and immunological aspects of penicillin allergy. Int Arch Allergy Appl Immunol 27:221, 1965.
38. Findlay, SR, et al.: Hyperosmolar triggering of histamine release from human basophils. J Clin Invest 67:1601, 1981.
39. Gyrd-Hansen, N, et al.: Cardiovascular effects of intravenous administration of tetracycline in cattle. J Vet Pharmacol Ther 4:15, 1981.
40. Potter, WL: Collapse following intravenous administration of oxytetracycline in two horses. Aust Vet J 49:547, 1973.
41. Tauberger, G, et al.: Comparative investigations of the circulatory actions of doxycycline and rolitetracycline after i.v. injections. Arzneimittel Forschung 21:1465, 1971.
42. Wright, DG, et al.: Lethal pulmonary reactions associated with the combined use of amphotericin B and leucocyte transfusions. N Engl J Med 304:1185, 1981.
43. Biery, EA, et al.: Rates of chlorpromazine-induced hemolysis in seven species of animals. J Vet Pharmacol Ther 1:149, 1978.
44. Kanecko, JJ: Porphyrin, heme and erythrocyte metabolism. In Kanecko, JJ (ed): Clinical Biochemistry of Domestic Animals, 3rd Ed. New York, Academic Press, 1980, p 119.
45. Jacob, HS and Jandl, JH: Effects of sulfhydryl inhibition on red blood cells. II. Studies *in vivo*. J Clin Invest 41:1514, 1962.
46. Carrell, RW, et al.: Activated oxygen and hemolysis. Br J Haematol 30:259, 1975.
47. Beutler, E: Drug-induced hemolytic anemia. Pharmacol Rev 21:73, 1969.
48. Jain, NC: Demonstration of Heinz bodies in erythrocytes of the cat. Bull Am Soc Vet Clin Pathol 2:13, 1973.
49. Gross, RT, et al.: Hydrogen peroxide toxicity and detoxication in the erythrocytes of newborn infants. Blood 29:481, 1967.
50. Finco, DR, et al: Acetaminophen toxicosis in the cat. JAVMA 166:469, 1975.
51. Mitchell, JR, et al.: Toxic drug reactions. Handb Exp Pharmacol 28:383, 1975.
52. Davis, LE and Westfall, BA: Species differences in the biotransformation of salicylate. Am J Vet Res 33:1253, 1972.
53. Gaunt, SD, et al.: Clinicopathologic evaluation of N-acetylcysteine therapy in acetaminophen toxicosis in the cat. Am J Vet Res 42:1982, 1981.
54. Camitta, BM, et al.: Aplastic anemia: Pathogenesis, diagnosis, treatment and prognosis. N Engl J Med 306:645, 712, 1982.
55. Weatherall, DJ, et al.: The blood and blood-forming organs. In Smith, LH and Their, SE (eds): Pathophysiology. The Biological Principles of Disease. Philadelphia, WB Saunders, 1981, p 383.
56. Watson, ADJ, et al.: Phenylbutazone-induced blood dyscrasias suspected in three dogs. Vet Rec 107:239, 1980.
57. Watson, ADJ: Bone marrow failure in a dog. J Sm Anim Pract 20:681, 1979.
58. Crafts, RC: The effect of endocrines on the formed elements of the blood. II. The effects of estrogens in the dog and monkey. Endocrinology 29:606, 1941.
59. Lorvenstine, LJ, et al.: Exogenous estrogen toxicity in the dog. Calif Vet 26:14, 1972.
60. Pyle, RL, et al.: Estrogen toxicity in a dog. Canine Pract 3:39, 1976.
61. Stewart, RB and Cluff, LE: A review of medication errors and compliance in ambulant patients. Clin Pharmacol Ther 13:463, 1972.
62. Barker, KN and McConnell, WE: How to detect medication errors. Mod Hosp 99:95, 1962.
63. Cooperative Group for the Study of Aplastic and Refractor Anemia: Androgen therapy of aplastic anemia—a projective study of 352 cases. Scand J Haematol 22:343, 1979.
64. Adamson, JW: Pharmacological stimulation of marrow function. Clin Haematol 32:533, 1976.
65. Morley, A, et al.: A controlled trial of androgen therapy in experimental chronic hypoplastic marrow failure. Br J Haematol 32:533, 1976.
66. Advisory Committee of the International Bone Marrow Transplant Registry: Allogeneic bone marrow transplantation for 144 patients with severe aplastic anemia. JAMA 245:1132, 1981.

SECTION V

CANCER—NEOPLASIA

58 TUMOR BIOLOGY

STEVEN E. CROW

In this chapter the processes that make neoplastic cells behave differently from normal cells are briefly reviewed. In addition, some of the diverse clinical syndromes caused by biochemical products of tumor cells are outlined. Lastly, the methods and usefulness of grading and staging clinical cancers are described. This introduction to the fascinating biology of neoplasia is intended to help the student or clinician to better understand the scientific basis for present and future clinical oncology applications. That knowledge can be very helpful in making appropriate choices regarding diagnostic and therapeutic procedures for animals with benign or malignant neoplasms.

Clinical management of cancer in small animal practice requires an understanding of the biologic behavior of neoplastic cells. The properties of cancer cells that are quantitatively or qualitatively different from those of normal cells represent potential sources of therapeutic exploitation. In addition, those differences are responsible for many of the seemingly inexplicable consequences of neoplasia.

The natural history of a neoplasm is the course that a particular type of tumor usually takes without treatment. It encompasses all of the effects of the tumor on function of the animal host. Knowledge of the natural behavior of a specific neoplasm or group of neoplasms is important in deriving both diagnostic and therapeutic plans. Specific questions about the nature of the neoplastic process include:

1. What are the earliest detectable changes associated with a neoplasm?
2. How long does it take for these early changes to progress to a clinically evident tumor?
3. Does the neoplasm spread to other organs or tissues? If so, what route of metastasis is most common?
4. What organs are most commonly involved with metastases?
5. What remote (paraneoplastic) effects are associated with the neoplasm?
6. How often does a specific type of neoplasm cause an observed constellation of clinical signs?
7. How does the tumor cause clinical signs and death?

Answers to these and other questions are important in making patient management decisions. Unfortunately, definitive answers to these clinical challenges are often lacking in veterinary medicine.

For example, a seven-year-old male golden retriever was examined following splenectomy for a ruptured hemangiosarcoma. Diagnosis was confirmed following a two-week history of episodic weakness. A regenerative anemia was present at the same time that the abdominal mass was identified radiographically. No metastatic nodules were observed in the lungs or in the liver. Should this dog receive adjuvant chemotherapy?

This simple question has no simple solution. Resolution of uncertainty depends on answers to more discrete questions such as the following: Is the dog otherwise healthy? How long has the neoplasm been present in this dog? Do hemangiosarcomas usually metastasize? How can metastases be detected? How long do dogs with this presentation usually survive following splenectomy? Do hemangiosarcomas respond to chemotherapy?

In this chapter, a basis for obtaining answers for some of these questions is established by examining some of the important biological processes that occur in neoplastic cells. Mechanisms for inhibition of tumor growth are reviewed and the pathogeneses of commonly observed paraneoplastic syndromes are described. Finally, clinical tools for predicting the biologic behavior of neoplasms (histopathologic grading and clinical staging) are discussed (see Figure 58–1).

DESCRIBING NEOPLASIA

Accurate description of neoplasms and measures of their clinical course are needed to facilitate communication among veterinary medical personnel. In this section, definitions of commonly used (and commonly misused) terms derived from clinical and reference sources 1–3 are given. In most cases, they describe characteristics of neoplasms from a clinician's viewpoint. Since some of the terms are often, though erroneously, used synonymously, careful attention was paid to their correct application to clinical circumstances.

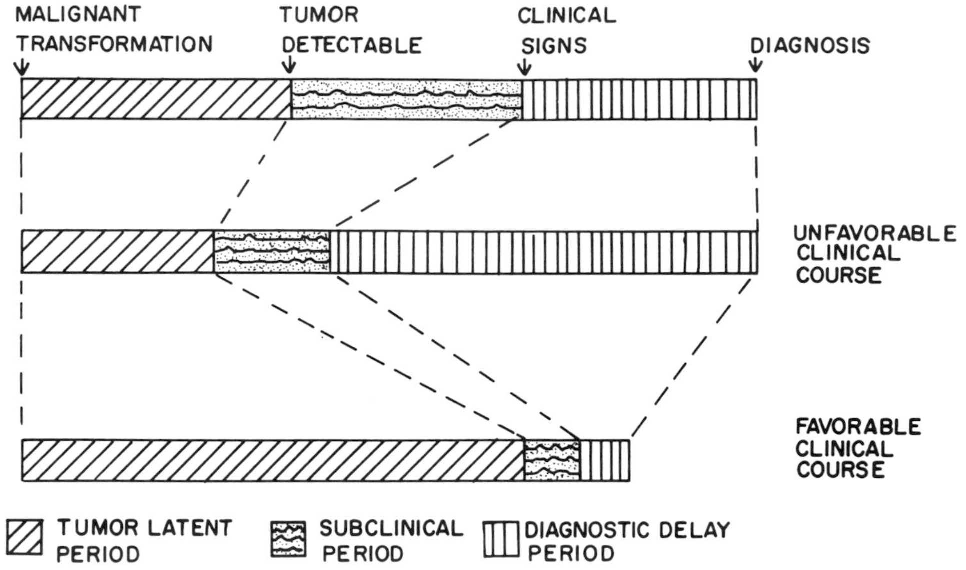

FIGURE 58–1. Graphic representation of two possible clinical courses for a neoplasm. In the unfavorable course, there is (1) rapid development of the neoplasm prior to the earliest time of detection (short latent period), (2) rapid progression to clinical illness (short subclinical period), and (3) slow recognition of the neoplasm (long diagnostic delay). A more favorable sequence features a long latency, very short subclinical period, and minimal diagnostic delay.

PHYSICAL CHARACTERISTICS OF NEOPLASMS

Papule, Nodule, Tumor. These terms indicate a growth of tissue of different texture or consistency surrounded by normal tissue(s). The maximum diameter of a papule is usually 3 mm, while nodules are less than 20 mm across. Tumor is used to describe larger growths; it is also frequently used as a synonym for neoplasm.

Sessile, Pedunculated. These terms describe the attachment of a nodule or tumor at its base. A sessile tumor has a base approximately equal to the largest diameter of the mass. A pedunculated tumor is connected to surrounding tissues by a narrow stalk. The clinical usefulness of these characteristics is questionable because the true extent of the neoplasm cannot always be determined by inspection or palpation.

Metastasis. This describes a pathologic process in which disease arising in one location spreads to another anatomic location by lymphatic, hematogenous, or transcoelomic extension. While this term can be correctly used to describe infectious processes, the term metastasis is usually reserved to describe one of the most important features of malignant neoplasms.

Invasiveness. This is the property a neoplasm or other disease process exhibits toward adjacent tissues. This attribute of malignant neoplasms is important to recognize because it limits the usefulness of some forms of therapy, e.g., surgery and cryosurgery.

Expansiveness. Expansiveness is the ability of neoplasms to expand within tissues, usually without destroying adjacent structure or function. However, large expansile masses can result in necrosis of surrounding tissues by exerting excessive pressure.

Mobility, Immobility. These terms describe a palpable characteristic of neoplasms. Immobile tumors are attached to immovable structures such as muscle, bone, or viscera. Mobile lesions may be invasive but usually involve relatively mobile organs or tissues such as skin or intestine.

SUBJECTIVE DESCRIPTIONS

Subjective descriptions of the clinical course of a neoplasm are difficult to quantitate but are nevertheless clinically useful.[1, 2]

Fulminant. This describes a disease progression that is sudden and intense. In neoplasms, it describes a rapid growth phase frequently associated with profound clinical signs, usually leading to death. Fulminant growth is most often seen as a late manifestation of leukemias, lymphomas, and metastatic tumors.

Progressive. This describes a continual worsening of disease with unremitting clinical signs, leading to debility and death.

Stable. A stable neoplasia shows persistent clinical signs without evidence of progression. Quality of life is relatively unchanged during this phase of disease.

Quiescent. During this stage, clinical signs are imperceptible or reduced in severity. No apparent growth of the tumor is observed during this clinical phase.

TEMPORAL MEASURES

The following terms are temporal measures of neoplasms. They are most often used by clinicians to describe periods in the natural or clinical history of an animal's neoplasm.[1, 2]

Latent Period. The latent period is the elapsed time between cellular transformation and the earliest possible clinical detection.

Pre-diagnosis Period. The pre-diagnosis period is the interval between earliest possible detection and definitive diagnosis. This delay, also known as lead time, may result from inattentiveness or inconclusive diagnostic studies or both.

Post-diagnosis Delay. The post-diagnosis delay is the elapsed time between definitive diagnosis and the initiation of appropriate anti-neoplastic treatment. This period is prolonged by indecisiveness, attention to conflicting intercurrent disorders, or intentional omission of therapy.

Doubling Time. Doubling time is the time in which a neoplasm doubles in volume (*not* in diameter). The doubling time of metastatic tumors has been used to predict future rate of growth.[4, 5]

A clinical course, i.e., natural history, that connotes a favorable prognosis for an animal with a neoplasm is characterized by a long latent period and long doubling time. Proper management requires early detection and prompt intervention (see Figure 58–1). At present, the only periods that can be changed by the veterinarian are the pre- and postdiagnosis delay periods. Every opportunity to shorten those intervals should be seized. Future advances in diagnosis may allow the clinician to detect neoplasms before clinical signs are evident, thereby reducing the subclinical period as well.

Additional terms that describe clinical events relevant to treatment and response to treatment are included in Chapter 59.

CELLULAR BIOLOGY OF CANCER

DIFFERENTIATION AND DE-DIFFERENTIATION

The concept that basic cellular mechanisms underlying the neoplastic state are related to mutational and hence, irreversible, changes in the genome has been challenged by many investigators.[6, 7] An epigenetic mechanism similar to that associated with normal cellular differentiation is a more plausible explanation for neoplastic transformation.[8] Nonmutational defects result in persistent alterations in the expression of genes, which are potentially reversible. This latter hypothesis is attractive because it introduces new possible avenues for both control and prevention of cancer.

The specific programming of the genetic information present in a cell's nucleus (i.e., gene expression) is largely governed by that cell's cytoplasm.[9, 10] It is now clear that all of the essential properties that characterize the malignant state (unrestrained growth, ability to metastasize) are present in normal cells. Further, the genome of a cancer cell is not irreversibly programmed.[11, 12] The oncogene theory postulates that all cells contain a viral oncogene; whether cancer develops is a function of either expression or repression of that portion of the host genome.[13, 14]

CELL SURFACE AND CYTOPLASMIC ALTERATIONS

Neoplastic cells exhibit physical and biochemical properties different from those of normal cells. These changes may be fundamentally important in causing altered behaviors observed in tumor cells.[15] Even though alterations in cellular processes are consistently found in a wide variety of tumor cell types, the changes differ markedly from one type of neoplasm to another. Thus, few generalities can be made about cellular changes associated with malignant transformation.[15]

One unique characteristic of cancer cells is defective growth control. Depending on which tumor is examined, that defect may be related to a variety of specific alterations, including decreased cyclic AMP and increased cyclic GMP levels, decreased fibronectin, decreased chalones, altered cytoskeleton, or increased levels of proteases on the cell surface.[15]

A second fundamental alteration of neoplastic cells is decreased adhesiveness. This defect may be partially responsible for separation and dissemination of metastatic cells. Proposed mechanisms for this change include diminished levels of surface glycosyl transferases and incomplete surface carbohydrate chains.

Increased proteases on the tumor cell membrane may contribute to the invasiveness of cells and may damage surface receptors involved in growth control.[16]

Another defect of tumor cells is abnormal contact inhibition (CI). CI is the restraint of directional locomotion of a cell after contact with another object, usually another cell. Normal cells show strong contact inhibition. The abnormality in tumor cell CI is not a lack of the property, but rather, subtle changes in migration patterns are observed.[17]

A fifth defect of tumor cells is disruption of the cytoskeleton. The microtubules and microfilaments of the cytoskeleton appear to play roles in arranging cells in distinct tissue patterns and in coordinating transport of intercellular signals.[15]

Finally, metabolic pathways and enzyme systems are deranged in cancer cells. For example, many tumor cells metabolize carbohydrates preferentially by anaerobic glycolysis, rather than by oxidative phosphorylation.[18, 19]

Many of the alterations seen in neoplastic cells are listed in Table 58–1. These biochemical alterations are possible points of vulnerability for cancer cells. Consequently, much research is being conducted into the basic workings of cancer cells. While much has been learned, it is obvious that mechanisms involved in the neoplastic process are numerous and complex. Unravelling their mysteries will undoubtedly lead to new, more effective means of controlling neoplastic growth.

TABLE 58–1. QUALITATIVE CHANGES IN TRANSFORMED CELLS

Altered Functions
Permeability
Transport
Phagocytosis
Adhesion and contact inhibition of movement (impaired)
Intercellular communication and contact inhibition of growth (impaired)
Mobility of surface components
Lectin agglutinability (increased)
Cell Surface Alterations
Charge density
Enzymes
Ion density
New antigens
Lost antigens
Lost or modified glycolipids
Lost or modified glycoproteins
Intracellular Alterations
Cytoplasmic transmitters
Cyclic nucleotide concentrations
Cytoskeletal control

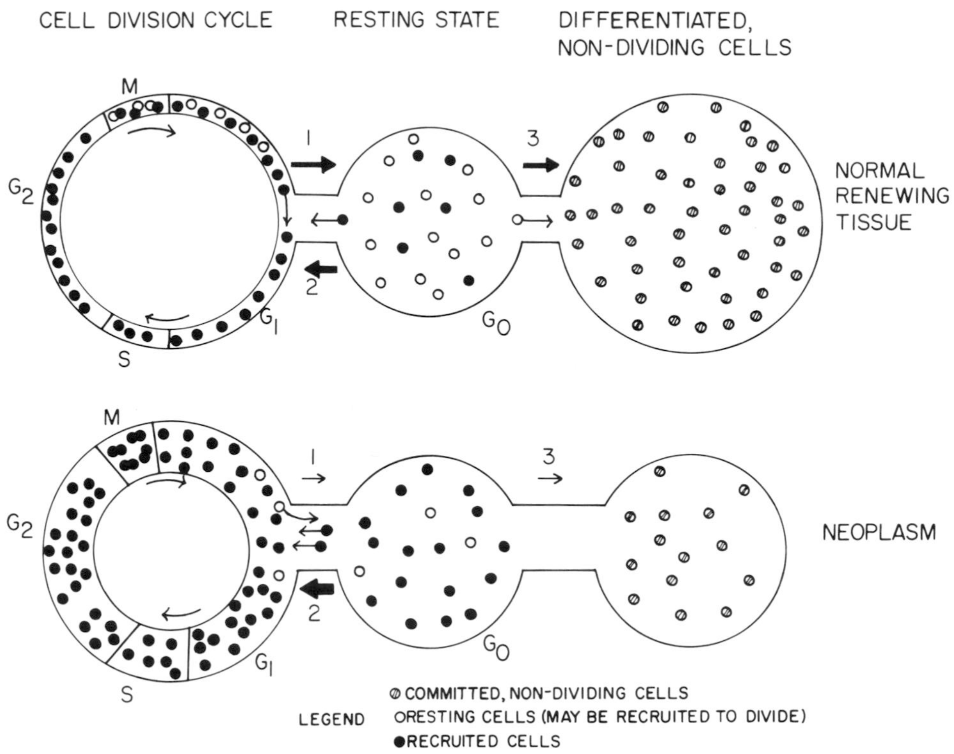

FIGURE 58–2. Comparison of the three populations of cells in a normal renewing tissue and in a neoplasm. Note that a greater percentage of tumor cells are dividing even though the cell cycle time is not significantly different. The normal tissue contains a larger proportion of nondividing cells.

THE CELL CYCLE

A tissue grows primarily by increasing its number of cells. Some tissues can grow by increasing the size of cells (hypertrophy) or by producing increased amounts of intercellular substance. Neoplasms, resembling embryonic tissues, grow primarily by increasing their cell numbers.[20] Some cancers, e.g., well-differentiated fibrosarcoma and inflammatory carcinoma, grow by both increasing their cell numbers and their intercellular substance.

All tissues, including neoplasms, contain a mixture of three different cell populations: cycling cells, resting cells, and nondividing cells. Cycling cells are continuously proceeding from one mitosis to another. Resting cells are normally dormant but may reenter the cell cycle if needed to replenish cell numbers. Nondividing cells leave the cell cycle after one or more divisions and differentiate. They are then unable to divide and eventually die.[21]

The growth rate of tissues (including tumors) can be determined using three measurements of the cell cycle: cell-cycle time, growth fraction, and rate of cell loss. Cell-cycle time is the interval between mitoses. Growth fraction refers to the percentage of cells in a neoplasm (or any tissue) that are cycling. Rate of cell loss refers to the fraction of cells that die or migrate out of the tissue. It was once thought that the major difference between tumors and normal tissues was that neoplasms have short cell-cycle times. Instead, it is now apparent that differences in growth fraction have the greatest effect on growth rate of tumors. The length of the cell cycle of a tumor is approximately the same as that of normal tissue; however, the percentage of cells in the temporary resting state and the percentage of cells traversing the cell cycle are markedly increased (Figure 58–2). Ultimately, whether a tumor (or other tissue) continues to grow depends on the difference between the rates of cell birth and cell loss.[20] It has been determined that 97 per cent of cells in some skin tumors will eventually die naturally.[22] However, as long as cell division replenishes the population faster than cells are lost, the tumor will continue to grow.[20]

The growth of transformed cells can be arrested by depriving them of nutrients, whereas normal cells need specific growth factors in order to reenter the cell cycle.[23, 24] These growth requirements are important because they may represent points for therapeutic intervention. They also bring into question the advisability of using hyperalimentation for support of animals with advanced malignancies.[25]

METASTASIS

A key feature of malignant tumors is that their cells are able to spread beyond the limits of the tissue of origin. Two mechanisms defined earlier in this chapter account for this mobility: invasiveness and metastasis.

Metastasis is responsible for a majority of therapeutic failures in human oncology practice.[3] In veterinary medicine, many failures are due to inadequate management of the primary neoplasm, but failure due to metastatic complications is also very important. Consequently, it is important to understand what is known about the prevention and/or interruption of this usually fatal process.

The development of a metastatic site involves a sequence of steps: (1) invasion of cells from the primary tumor into surrounding tissues, (2) penetration of lymph and/or blood vessels, (3) release of tumor emboli into the circulation, (4) lodgement of tumor emboli in capillaries or lymphatic vessels of distant organs, (5) penetration of the wall of the arresting vessel, (6) infiltration into the surrounding tissue, (7) proliferation in the new environment, and (8) vascularization of the new tumor.[26]

The most crucial step in this complex process appears to be the first step, invasion. Mechanisms for this process are unknown. Plausible explanations include mechanical expansion, loss of cell adhesiveness, excessive cellular motility, destruction of stroma by lytic enzymes, or damage to surrounding structures by host defense mechanisms. Whatever the mechanism(s), it is clear that the rate of division does not correlate well with invasiveness.[26] For example, well-differentiated fibrosarcomas may have only zero to one mitotic figures per high power field, but can be very invasive to surrounding structures, including bone. Conversely, perianal adenomas are rapidly growing neoplasms with numerous mitoses present, but they are not usually highly invasive neoplasms.

The inflammatory response, a normal host response to tissue damage, may actually assist the process of invasion in some malignant neoplasms.[27] Lysozymes from leukocytes enhance invasion by destroying growth-limiting structures such as the basement membrane.[26, 27]

Considerable controversy exists regarding the role of the regional lymph node (RLN) in control of cancer, both in the primary site and in the prevention of metastatic disease. Even though metastasis to lymph nodes is a common clinical finding, the RLN is immunologically involved in the host response to neoplasms.

The lymph node has long been regarded as a temporary barrier to neoplastic dissemination. Experimental evidence indicates that some tumor cells are trapped in the lymph node while others pass through into the efferent lymphatics.[28, 29] When tumor emboli localize in a lymph node, growth usually occurs in the subcapsular sinus.[28] The RLN contains immune cytotoxic mechanisms that may kill tumor cells, so that clinical or histologic absence of metastasis does not necessarily indicate that the animal is free of lymphatic metastases.[30] Also, removal or irradiation of the RLN during this period may inhibit tumor immunity.[31]

A widely accepted approach to management of lymph nodes associated with primary solid tumors is to leave them in place early in the course of disease, but to remove the RLN when there is obvious tumor infiltration.[32] This recommendation is based on the belief that removal early in the course of disease may promote metastasis. Late in the tumor's course the lymph node has lost its capacity for tumor immunity.[33]

Another limiting factor in forming metastatic foci is cell damage. Blood and lymph are hostile environments for many tumor cells. Cell loss is probably due to destruction by natural killer (NK) cells or mechanical disruption by turbulence, shearing, or reticuloendothelial (RE) cells.[34, 35] Tumor emboli are protected from attack by travelling in clusters or by becoming enveloped in fibrin.[36] Consequently, it has been suggested that anticoagulation of the blood could result in fewer surviving metastatic cells.[37]

The mere presence of tumor cells in the blood does not constitute metastasis because most circulating cells die quickly. Studies have indicated that as few as one-tenth of one per cent of cancer cells in the circulation survive to form secondary foci.[38]

The most frequent sites for metastases are the lung and liver (in human beings), perhaps because these two organs receive such a large proportion of the venous drainage.[39] Although reasons for cancer cells arresting at certain sites and not at others are not known, it is clear that some type of selectivity must occur during the development of secondary neoplasms. Why does prostatic carcinoma tend to metastasize to bones, especially the lumbar vertebrae? Similarly, why do primary lung cancers of human beings metastasize to the brain? In veterinary medicine, it has long been recognized that mast cell tumors tend to metastasize to skin. Primary bone tumors spread most commonly to lungs and/or other bones. Experimentally, certain clones of melanomas have been shown to "home in" on specific organs. The predominant "seed and soil" theory suggests that tumor cells set up housekeeping in sites that are biochemically and/or physically attractive to them.[40–42]

Multiplication of new tumor foci begins soon after blood vessels start to grow into the tumor. Initially, tumor cells exchange nutrients and catabolites with surrounding interstitial tissues by simple diffusion. Rapid growth starts with vascularization. Tumor cells are able to initiate and then maintain proliferation of blood vessels. A diffusible factor called tumor angiogenesis factor (TAF) has been isolated from several animal and human tumors.[43–46] TAF affects capillary endothelium in two ways: it causes mitosis and migration of endothelial cells. The discovery of this substance has potential clinical implications. If TAF is inhibited, thereby preventing capillaries from penetrating the tumor, growth ceases and the tumor enters a dormant phase. The term antiangiogenesis has been applied to therapeutic approaches based on this concept.[47]

In sum, to establish secondary foci, tumor cells must complete all of the steps in the metastatic process. Exceptional ability to complete one or more of the steps does not compensate for the inability to complete a preceding or subsequent step. Each of the steps in the metastatic process is a potential area for the control of metastasis. Destruction of tumor angiogenesis factor and the use of anticoagulants such as heparin to prevent tumor cell lodgement in capillaries are examples of clinical applications that have resulted from research on basic tumor biology.

TUMOR HETEROGENEITY

Although cells from a neoplasm frequently look monomorphic when examined by light microscopy, primary malignant neoplasms are not uniform in composition. Instead they differ in their biological characteristics, including invasiveness and ability to metastasize.[48] Development of variant cells is apparently due to selective forces, not random events, during progressive growth. This selection results in heterogeneity.[48] Numerous studies have shown that subpopulations of tumor cells from a single anatomic site may differ markedly with respect to hormone dependence, drug resistance, isoantigenic expression, and karyotype. Also, there is wide variation in their ability to form metastases.[49]

Neoplasms undergo phenotypic changes during their natural history. A tumor that originally appears to be benign may transform or progress over a period of months or years into a metastatic, lethal malignancy.[50, 51]

Within a primary neoplasm containing billions of cells, only a few cells are capable of metastasizing.[48] This phenotypic diversity has serious implications for the treatment of cancer. A pessimistic view of tumor heterogeneity sees chemotherapy as a relatively futile endeavor that may result in the selection of highly resistant clones of cells. Optimistically, selective forces may be identified, leading to new therapeutic options. If the process were a random event, there would be little cause for hope.

In contrast to the marked heterogeneity of primary tumors, metastatic foci usually contain a relatively homogeneous population of cells with similar metastatic potential.[35, 49] This difference supports the principle of using chemotherapy for metastatic disease, but avoiding its use for management of a primary solid tumor.

PARANEOPLASTIC SYNDROMES

Previous sections of this chapter have detailed some of the discernible differences of tumor cells that help to explain their capacity to cause morbidity and mortality in animals. Biochemical alterations in the cytoplasm or expression of previously repressed portions of the genome lead to many fascinating and sometimes puzzling clinical consequences. The changes observed are often profound and seem to have no direct association with the growth of neoplastic cells in either primary or secondary sites. In fact, these remote effects are often present before any physical evidence of a mass or growth is observed. These systemic complications of cancer are collectively known as paraneoplastic disorders. Because they often cause a constellation of recognizable clinical signs, they are more frequently referred to as paraneoplastic syndromes (PNS).

It has been estimated that up to 75 per cent of human cancer patients experience one or more remote effects of their neoplasm during the course of their disease.[52] Because many animals with cancer are euthanatized when clinical signs of illness become evident, the frequency of paraneoplastic disorders in dogs and cats is not known. Clinical experiences of several veterinary oncologists suggest that approximately one out of every four cancer-bearing dogs can be documented to have one or more remote effects of their neoplasm at the time of diagnosis.[53] Whatever the actual prevalence of PNS may be, there is no question that these disorders contribute significantly to the morbidity and mortality of neoplasia in dogs. The relative importance of PNS in cats is less clear. Very few of the disorders discussed here have been documented in domestic cats.

In addition to the reasons cited above, PNS are of interest to the veterinarian because investigation of their pathophysiology has provided important insights in the area of tumor biology. Also, PNS may provide important markers of the status of an animal's tumor, including evidence of relapse or response to therapy.

Common paraneoplastic syndromes of dogs and cats are listed in Table 58–2. A thorough discussion of all of the common paraneoplastic syndromes is beyond the scope of this chapter, but the mechanisms and importance of paraneoplastic disorders in small animal practice will be discussed. For a more detailed examination of each syndrome, the reader is referred to specific discussion of neoplastic disorders throughout this textbook.

ANEMIA

Anemia is the most commonly observed hematologic abnormality in animals with cancer.[54] A number of mechanisms for cancer-associated anemia have been described, some of which are related to treatment of the associated neoplasm.[55] The following discussion is limited to those anemias that are true paraneoplastic syndromes.

Anemia of chronic inflammatory disease (ACID) is a common complication of advanced cancer. Large masses with central necrosis and disseminated metastases are particularly likely to cause this nonregenerative type of anemia. This disorder is characterized by shortened erythrocyte life span, abnormal iron metabolism, depressed erythropoiesis, and excessive iron storage. Despite an adequate supply of iron in the bone marrow, insufficient iron is made available for hemoglobin synthesis due to an unexplained block in the release and use of iron from cells of the macrophage-phagocytic (MP) system. The anemia is usually mild to moderate in severity. In dogs, the packed cell volume (PCV) is usually 28 to 35 per cent. Morphologically, ACID is characterized as normocytic and normochromic. Biochemical analyses show decreased serum iron, decreased total iron-binding capacity, and decreased iron-binding saturation. Examination of the bone marrow reveals normal cellularity with excessive MP sequestration of iron.[55]

Microangiopathic hemolytic anemia is occasionally observed in animals with cancer, most commonly associated with disseminated intravascular coagulation. It results from damage to the RBC membrane by injured arteriolar endothelium and intravascular fibrin deposition. The anemia may be mild to severe; it is characterized by a strongly regenerative erythron. Presence of schistocytosis, intravascular hemolysis (elevated unconjugated bilirubin), and DIC establish the diagnosis.[56–58]

Immunohemolytic anemia may be a complication of neoplastic disease. Immune-mediated anemia is most frequently associated with lymphoproliferative malignancies in humans.[59] Diagnosis is based on demonstrating an autoantibody attached to red blood cells. Hemolytic anemia has been observed in cats with lymphosarcoma.[60] Positive direct Coombs' tests have been reported in dogs with lymphosarcoma.[61]

Hemorrhagic anemias associated with neoplasms are most frequently caused by invasion of primary or secondary tumors. Neoplasms that often cause significant blood loss include splenic hemangiosarcomas, nasal car-

TABLE 58–2. COMMON PARANEOPLASTIC SYNDROMES OF DOGS AND CATS

Category	Syndrome	Associated Neoplasm(s)
Ectopic or excessive hormonal effect	Hyperadrenocorticism	Pituitary adenoma Adrenal carcinoma
	Hyperinsulinism	Islet cell carcinoma
	Hyperestrinism	Sertoli cell tumor Seminoma Granulosa cell tumor
	Hyperthyroidism (thyrotoxicosis)	Thyroid adenomatous hyperplasia (or adenoma)
	Pseudohyperparathyroidism	Lymphosarcoma Apocrine gland carcinoma Circumanal gland carcinoma
Hematologic manifestations	Polycythemia	Renal carcinoma
	Anemia	
	—of inflammatory disease	Many neoplasms
	—microangiopathic	Angiosarcoma
	—aplastic	Sertoli cell tumor
	Disseminated intravascular coagulation	Angiosarcoma Prostatic carcinoma
Miscellaneous	Hyperviscosity	Plasma cell myeloma
	Hypertrophic osteopathy	Large thoracic tumors Carcinomas, sarcomas of urinary bladder
	Histaminosis, hemorrhagic gastroduodenitis	Mast cell tumors
	Fever of undetermined origin	Various neoplasms, especially lymphomas

cinomas, and intestinal adenocarcinomas. However, some types of cancer can result in bleeding or clotting disorders, which may in turn cause severe hemorrhage. Myeloproliferative disorders can lead to profound thrombocytopenia. Hepatocellular carcinomas or other liver neoplasms may affect coagulation factor synthesis, and many types of cancer may incite DIC.

Aplastic anemia associated with excessive production of estrogen by testicular neoplasms has recently been reported in dogs.[62–64] Diagnosis is established by demonstrating hypoplasia of all hematopoietic cell lines in the bone marrow and the presence of an estrogen-secreting neoplasm of the testis. Sertoli cell tumors and seminomas are potential causes of this syndrome.[62–64]

CACHEXIA

Cancer cachexia (CC) is a perplexing complication of cancer. Although it is most often associated with advanced malignancies, it may be an early clinical manifestation of disease. It is characterized clinically by anorexia, weight loss, and muscle weakness. Other commonly associated features include hepatomegaly, hypoalbuminemia, and nonregenerative anemia.[65] Cachexia is the most important cause of death of human beings with solid tumors.[66]

Although decreased food intake resulting from inappetence plays a major role in progressive weight loss, experimental evidence has implicated a variety of paraneoplastic processes in the pathogenesis of CC.[67, 68] Anorexia may be related to the production of peptides or nucleotides that affect the hunger and satiety centers of the hypothalamus.[69, 70] Human cancer patients have altered sensitivity to urea and sucrose;[71] it is likely that anorexia in cancer-bearing animals may also be related to altered taste.

Marked alterations in carbohydrate and lipid metabolism are known to occur in many types of cancer.[18, 19] Increased energy expenditure and increased basal metabolic rate are common findings in advanced cancer and are occasionally seen in early stages of neoplasia.[19] However, the contribution of these changes to the genesis of cachexia is not known.

Malabsorption occurs in a large percentage of neoplastic diseases, even though they are anatomically unrelated to the gastrointestinal tract. Villous atrophy, decreased D-xylose absorption, and increased fecal fat excretion occur in approximately 50 per cent of human cancer patients.[72] Maldigestion was found in a dog with pancreatic adenocarcinoma.[73]

FEVER

Persistent, low-grade fevers are commonly associated with some forms of cancer in animals, especially lymphoproliferative disorders.[74] Frequently, these fevers are undetected by the animal's owner. Occasionally they are the earliest clinical sign observed and may be a challenging diagnostic problem. Differential diagnoses include immune-mediated disorders such as systemic lupus erythematosus (SLE) and systemic fungal, bacterial, or viral infections. Malignancies produce fever in most instances by the interaction of lymphocytes with tumor-related antigens. The sensitized lymphocytes produce lymphokines, which stimulate the release of endogenous pyrogen by neutrophils and macrophages. Also, there is some evidence that tumors cells may be direct sources of endogenous pyrogen.[75, 76]

HYPERTROPHIC OSTEOPATHY

Hypertrophic osteopathy (HO) is an unusual PNS characterized by reluctance to move and progressive lameness of all four limbs. Onset of illness is usually gradual but may be acute. Physical examination reveals firm swelling of the long bones of the distal extremities. Early cases are hallmarked by diffuse pain of affected limbs, but this sign tends to subside as the disorder progresses. Radiographic findings include bilaterally symmetrical periosteal proliferation and obvious soft tissue swelling. Metacarpal and metatarsal bones are usually the first bones to be affected.[77, 78] Because the first descriptions of this syndrome involved either pleural effusion or primary lung tumors as the precipitating cause, HO was originally called hypertrophic pulmonary osteoarthropathy. However, recent reports indicate that the bony changes can occur as a complication of lesions in other viscera, especially the urinary bladder.[79–84] Because joints are not usually affected, the more accurate designation of osteopathy is preferred.[77, 78]

The etiology of HO is poorly understood. Several theories have been proposed for the pathogenesis of the aberrant periosteal activity. A hormonal cause for HO has been proposed. Growth hormone has been studied, and HO has been associated with increased urinary excretion of estrogens in human patients with bronchogenic carcinoma.[85, 86] No correlation was found between estrogens and liver-associated HO.[87–89] A second hypothesis is the neural reflex theory. There is considerable clinical and experimental evidence supporting the existence of a neural afferent component for HO. Transsection of the vagus nerve or intercostal nerves causes regression of HO in some animals.[90, 91] A third theory is that HO is caused by hypoxia associated with left-to-right cardiovascular shunting.[92] There is little clinical correlation or experimental evidence to support this hypothesis at present.

Management of HO entails removal of the inciting lesion, i.e., the neoplasm.[93]

ENDOCRINOPATHIES

One of the most interesting biological changes in cancer cells is the ability to secrete hormones or hormone-like substances. In some instances, neoplastic cells continue to function like cells of their native tissues but in other cases they may produce atypical humoral substances.[94] Regardless of the appropriateness of the cellular product, this aberrant or excessive secretion may result in profound clinical signs.

Tumors originating from endocrine glands can continue to produce hormone, even if the tumor is malignant.[94] For example, a majority of functional islet cell tumors (insulinomas) are malignant. Lymph node and hepatic metastases may be present at the time of diagnosis. Examples of paraneoplastic endocrinopathies associated with benign neoplasms include feline hyperthyroidism (thyroid adenoma), hyperadrenocorticism (pituitary adenoma), and hypergastrinemia (non-beta islet cell tumor of pancreas). Hyperestrinism (hyperestrogenism) has been reported to occur with both malignant and benign testicular tumors (seminoma, Sertoli cell tumor) and ovarian tumors (granulosa cell tumor).[95] The systemic effects of endocrine gland neoplasms are known as topic paraneoplastic syndromes. Hormone levels in these disorders are elevated but are not adequately controlled by counter-regulatory mechanisms.

Hyperhistaminemia causes severe morbidity and frequently causes death in patients with advanced mast cell tumors.[96] Histamine is released when mast cells degranulate or lyse. In large or rapidly growing mast cell tumors, serum and tissue histamine levels can become markedly elevated. Mast cell tumors have been associated with gastrointestinal ulceration in dogs and cats.[97–98] Ulcers are usually multiple and occur in the stomach and/or duodenum. In one study of dogs with mast cell tumors, 83 per cent had ulcers in the stomach or duodenum at necropsy.[97] A small percentage of these ulcers perforated the intestinal wall. The mechanism of ulceration is thought to be due to H_2 receptors that stimulate histamine production, which results in increased secretion of hydrochloric acid by parietal cells of the stomach. In addition, histamine may cause damage to submucosal arterioles and venules, leading to tissue necrosis.[99, 100]

Some nonendocrine tumors secrete biologically active substances such as enzymes, prostaglandins, and peptides.[101] In many cases, the active product has not been definitely identified. Nevertheless, the metabolic abnormalities closely mimic those of "normal" hormones. Signs caused by this type of tumor product are called ectopic paraneoplastic syndromes.[101]

The most commonly occurring ectopic PNS in small animal practice is hypercalcemia associated with lymphosarcoma and apocrine gland carcinoma in the dog.[102–104] Signs commonly observed in dogs with hypercalcemia are polyuria and polydipsia, weakness, anorexia, and muscle twitching. Hypercalcemia of malignancy, once thought to be caused by a parathormone-like substance, is apparently caused by release of an osteoclast-activating factor. It is associated with infiltration of the bone marrow by tumor cells.[105, 106] Because there is the potential of irreversible renal failure due to calcium deposition, many veterinary internists consider hypercalcemia associated with malignant tumors to be a medical emergency. Early and aggressive treatment of this complication is recommended.[107] Dogs with lymphosarcoma and hypercalcemia respond less favorably and survive for shorter periods than dogs with lymphosarcoma without elevated serum calcium levels.[108]

HYPERVISCOSITY

Monoclonal gammopathies are associated with lymphoproliferative disorders such as plasma cell myeloma, lymphosarcoma, and lymphocytic leukemia. Hyperviscosity results from accumulation of M component in serum. Because of their high molecular weights, macroglobulins (IgM) are most frequently associated with hyperviscosity. Polymerized IgA may also cause severe changes in serum viscosity. Most cases showing clinical signs have serum that is eight to ten times more viscous than normal serum. Although serum electrophoresis demonstrates the presence of excessive quantities of immunoglobulins, diagnosis of hyperviscosity syndrome (HVS) requires demonstration of increased serum viscosity and presence of clinical abnormalities. Signs of HVS include coagulation defects, visual impairment, retinal congestion or hemorrhages, renal function impairment, and central nervous system deficits (e.g., depression, stupor, coma). Nephrotoxicity may be the consequence of light chains being deposited as amyloid or the direct effect of immunoglobulins or Bence-Jones protein on renal tubular epithelial cells. Bleeding diatheses are due to the effect of M component on platelet function and coagulation factors.[55, 109–113]

DISSEMINATED INTRAVASCULAR COAGULATION

Bleeding and clotting disorders are extremely common complications of malignant diseases in human beings.[2] While clinical signs of coagulation disorders are relatively uncommon in animals with small, localized tumors, coagulation abnormalities were demonstrated in 83 per cent of untreated dogs with large tumor burdens.[57] Disseminated intravascular coagulation (DIC) is a nonspecific complication of many disease processes, characterized by concurrent activation of coagulation and fibrinolysis. DIC results in excessive consumption of both platelets and coagulation factors. Neoplasms apparently initiate DIC by releasing tissue thromboplastin or by causing vascular stasis.[56] DIC has been observed as a complication of several types of neoplasms in animals, including transitional cell carcinoma, hemangiosarcoma, and prostatic carcinoma.[53, 57]

MYASTHENIA GRAVIS

Thymoma is a relatively uncommon tumor of dogs, which is accompanied by a high prevalence of paraneoplastic disorders. The best documented of these complications is an autoimmune neuromuscular disease, myasthenia gravis.[114] The hallmark of this PNS is appendicular muscle weakness that is accentuated by exercise. Regurgitation may be observed if secondary megaesophagus is present. Dysphagia may occur and aspiration pneumonia is a common sequelae to this disorder. Diagnosis is confirmed by demonstration of a mediastinal mass (and subsequent biopsy) and dramatic, transient improvement in muscle function following a single intravenous injection of edrophonium chloride. Ninety per cent of dogs with acquired myasthenia gravis have a positive titer for serum antiacetylcholine receptor antibody.[114]

Many other paraneoplastic disorders have been documented in animals.[54, 95] Some PNS have been described only in human beings but are suspected in dogs and cats as well.[94, 101] Careful evaluation of animals with cancer will undoubtedly result in documentation of many PNS that are presently not well defined in veterinary medicine.

PATHOLOGIC DIAGNOSIS AND GRADING OF NEOPLASMS

Because inflammatory and hyperplastic processes can mimic neoplasms, a lesion suspected clinically of being a neoplasm must be definitely diagnosed by histopathologic examination. Surgical biopsy, exfoliative cytology, and core biopsy techniques are suitable methods for obtaining diagnostic samples in most neoplastic disorders of dogs and cats. However, the amount of information obtained from any of these sampling techniques depends not only on the expertise of the pathologist but on the skill of the clinician. The latter must supply pertinent information about the lesion and patient and must submit representative samples. Small nodules should be submitted whole, including surrounding excised tissues. When a lesion is too large for fixation without sectioning, a drawing of the entire lesion should be submitted with labelled sections of the tumor. When excision has been attempted, special attention should be given to identifying circumferential margins.

It is not always possible to definitely distinguish benign from malignant disease by histopathologic examination. Benign processes can mimic cancer. Canine cutaneous histiocytoma is an example of a benign neoplasm that has several histopathologic features of malignancy (anaplasia, high mitotic rate). Only when the animal's age and the gross appearance of the lesion are known can a pathologist make a definitive diagnosis. Conversely, malignant neoplasms may appear benign microscopically, e.g., thyroid carcinoma.

Clinical features that may affect the behavior of a neoplasm include the anatomic site of origin and the animal's age, species, or sex. For instance, squamous cell carcinomas arising on the eyelids, pinnae, or nasal planum of cats and dogs are invasive neoplasms that rarely metastasize to distant sites.[115] In contrast, squamous cell carcinomas arising in the oropharynx or nail bed epithelium of dogs frequently spread to regional lymph nodes and lungs.[116, 117] Similarly, osteosarcomas of flat bones are less likely to metastasize to lungs than are osteosarcomas of long bones.[118, 119] Circumanal gland tumors are usually benign in sexually intact male dogs but are frequently malignant in bitches.[120]

Although malignant neoplasms are much less common in young animals, cancers of dogs less than two years of age are frequently very aggressive.[121]

In many neoplasms, the histologic grade is the most important prognostic indicator. A grade is an evaluation of the degree of differentiation of the tumor. Both numeric and descriptive grading scales have been adopted for a variety of malignant tumors of dogs and cats. Low numeric grades or well-differentiated neoplasms are relatively normal morphologically, while high numeric grades or poorly differentiated neoplasms are anaplastic, bearing minimal resemblance to normal cellular and architectural features of the tissue of origin.[3]

Studies of the degree of differentiation of cutaneous mast cell tumors in dogs have shown excellent correlation between pathologic grade and post surgical survival (Table 58–3).[122, 123] Several investigators have attempted to correlate prognosis (measured by responsiveness to treatment and total survival) with subclassification of lymphosarcomas. Unfortunately, conclusions from these studies have been somewhat conflicting.[124–126] Occasionally, other pathologic criteria have been useful correlates

TABLE 58–3. CORRELATION BETWEEN PATHOLOGIC GRADE AND SURVIVAL IN DOGS WITH MAST CELL TUMORS

Histopathologic Description	1500-day Survival (%)
Well-differentiated	93
Intermediate differentiation	47
Poorly differentiated	6

for prognostication. Lymphocytic infiltration was associated with a better prognosis in canine mammary adenocarcinomas.[127] Other criteria that may be possible prognostic indicators include mitotic index, hormone receptors, and invasiveness.[127–129]

CLINICAL STAGING OF NEOPLASMS

With the advent of new and more effective means of treatment, clinical management of cancer in animals has become more complex. Only three decades ago most solid tumors were treated almost exclusively by surgery. Metastatic disease, if detected, was rarely treated. In veterinary medicine, pathologists chronicled the natural history of neoplasms by describing the progression of histopathologic changes that occurred in the various body organs. These studies were invaluable in providing the knowledge of what to expect from many types of malignant neoplasms of dogs and cats. However, subtle differences in clinical presentation were often not noted. Today, as a result of the collaborative efforts of the World Health Organization and representatives of the Veterinary Cancer Society, classification schemes have been designed for most neoplasms of domestic animals.[130] These clinical staging criteria are important in further defining the biologic consequences of animal neoplasms. By adding clinical measurements to pathologic descriptions of lesions, many of the unanswered questions about the clinical course of naturally occurring neoplasms can be more scientifically investigated. In the following paragraphs, the application of clinical staging schemes is addressed.

Useful cancer staging systems describe the origin and extent of a primary neoplasm, sites of metastases, and histologic type. Many schemes also include pathologic grading. Staging may help in delivering better patient management by providing prognostic information, assisting in selection of appropriate treatment modalities, giving the veterinarian greater insight into the tumor's biology in a particular animal, thereby helping to minimize morbidity, and facilitating the exchange of information in both clinical and research settings.

Because of the biologic diversity of neoplasms, no single clinical staging scheme is applicable to all types of tumors. Consequently, four different methods are used to classify the clinical presentation of neoplastic disorders.[2] The criteria examined include depth of invasion, tissue/organ involvement, TNM (tumor, regional lymph node, distant metastatic sites), and bone marrow morphology.

TABLE 58–4. ASTLER-COLLER MODIFICATION OF DUKES' CLASSIFICATION FOR COLORECTAL CANCER

Stage	Extent of Neoplasm	Five-Year Survival (%)
A	Limited to mucosa	75–100
B_1	Into muscularis mucosae	65
B_2	Beyond muscularis mucosae	50
C_1	Stage B_1 with positive lymph node(s)	40
C_2	Stage B_2 with positive lymph node(s)	15
D	Distant metastases	<5

TABLE 58–5. STAGING OF CUTANEOUS MELANOMAS IN HUMAN BEINGS (CLARK'S LEVELS OF INVASION)

Stage	Extent of Tumor	Five-Year Survival (%)
I	Confined to epidermis	100
II	Beyond basal lamina into papillary dermis	85
III	Into papillary dermis and abutting but not invading reticular dermis	65
IV	Into reticular dermis	50
V	Into subcutaneous fat	15

The depth of invasion criterion has been used successfully in human medicine to describe risk categories for patients with cutaneous melanomas and colorectal carcinomas. In 1932, Dukes described a clinical staging scheme that helped to predict survival and remission following resection of large bowel cancer.[131] Although based on pathologic evidence of invasion into the submucosa, muscularis, and serosa of the colon, as well as extension to mesenteric lymph nodes, this scheme featured clinically measurable parameters rather than morphologic grading criteria. Table 58–4 shows the usefulness of the scheme in predicting survival following surgery. Numerous modifications and refinements of Dukes' original classification scheme have helped to make this an even more useful clinical tool.[2]

Similarly, the biologic behavior of human cutaneous melanoma can be accurately predicted by careful examination of resected tissues. Table 58–5 provides convincing testimony to the clinical importance of assessing the level of invasion of all cutaneous melanomas in human beings.[132]

Unfortunately, neither of these schemes has proven useful in animals as yet, owing largely to late diagnosis of both melanoma and colorectal carcinoma in dogs and cats. Melanomas are common tumors in dogs but because they occur most frequently in the oral cavity,[133] diagnosis is usually not made until they have deeply invaded the mucous membranes. When melanomas occur on the skin, they are frequently hidden from view by hair until they are larger than 1 cm in diameter. Diagnosis of carcinoma of the large intestine is usually not made until overt hematochezia or tenesmus is noticed.[134] By that time, regional lymph node metastases are often present.[135]

Other neoplasms of dogs and cats that may be staged by depth of invasion criteria in the future include squamous cell carcinoma of the eyelids, pinnae, and nasal planum; mast cell tumors; and perianal gland tumors.

Lymphosarcoma and other lymphoproliferative disorders are most frequently staged using the tissue/organ involvement criterion. In addition to the pathologic classification discussed earlier in this chapter, the anatomic distribution of organs or tissues infiltrated with tumor cells is used. Prognosis for both Hodgkin's and non-Hodgkin's lymphomas is closely correlated with clinical stage in human patients.[136, 137] Most studies in dogs and cats indicate that responsiveness to therapy, length of remission, and survival may correlate with stage of disease.[138–141] The recommended scheme for clinical staging of canine lymphosarcoma (based on organ involvement) is shown in Table 58–6.

TABLE 58–6. VETERINARY CANCER SOCIETY/WORLD HEALTH ORGANIZATION STAGING SYSTEM FOR LYMPHOSARCOMA

Anatomic Distribution
A. Generalized (multicentric)
B. Alimentary
C. Thymic (anterior mediastinal)
D. Skin (cutaneous)
E. Leukemia*
F. Miscellaneous

Clinical Stages
I One lymph node or lymphoid structure involved
II Regional lymph nodes or lymphoid structures involved, limited to one side of diaphragm
III Lymph nodes or lymphoid structures or both sides of diaphragm involved
IV Hepatic and/or splenic involvement (with or without Stage III)
V Manifestation in the blood, bone marrow, or other organ

Each stage is subclassified into:
(a) without systemic signs
(b) with systemic signs

*Only blood and bone marrow involved.

The TNM classification scheme is the most widely applicable type of staging protocol. It can be applied to most solid tumors. In this system, tumors (T) are classified into three to five groups, usually using size and mobility characteristics to define groups (see Table 58–7). Involvement of ipsilateral and contralateral regional lymph nodes as well as "downstream" lymph nodes is noted in the three to five nodal (N) categories. Finally, two to four categories of distant metastatic expression are established. Simple computation shows that as many as 100 combinations of categories can be derived from such a simple scheme. Since so many groups would be extremely cumbersome, three to five numerical stages are usually derived (as shown at bottom of Table 58–7). The clinical usefulness of this process remains to be demonstrated in veterinary medicine. Neoplasms whose clinical course appears to correlate with a TNM classification scheme in veterinary medicine include mammary carcinoma, mast cell tumors, and oropharyngeal tumors.[142–145]

TABLE 58–7. PROPOSED TNM CLASSIFICATION SYSTEM FOR CUTANEOUS TUMORS

Primary Tumor
T_0 Primary neoplasm not evident
T_1 Less than 1 cm, mobile
T_2 1–3 cm in diameter, not deeply attached
T_3 3–5 cm in diameter, partially fixed to underlying structures
T_4 >5 cm in diameter, invading deeper structures

Regional Lymph Node
N_0 Palpable normal size, consistency
N_1 Enlarged, firm (ipsilateral)
N_2 Fixed to surrounding tissues
N_3 Involvement of lymph nodes beyond first station

Distant Metastasis
M_0 No evidence of metastasis
M_1 Single visceral metastasis
M_2 Multiple visceral metastases

Stage Assignment

I	T_1	N_0	M_0
	T_2	N_0	M_0
II	$T_{0,1}$ or $_2$	N_1	M_0
	T_3	N_0	M_0
III	T_3	N_1	M_0
	T_4	N_0	M_0
	any T	N_2	M_0
IV	any T	N_3	M_0
	any T	any N	M_1 or $_2$

TABLE 58–8. PERFORMANCE SCALE FOR DOGS AND CATS WITH CHRONIC DISEASES

Scale	Description
0	Normal activity; may have minor signs of disease that require no special care.
1	Slight limitation in normal activity; ambulatory; able to eat, drink, and eliminate normally.
2	Notable limitation in activity; has difficulty in eating, drinking, eliminating, or ambulating.
3	Disabled; requires assistance from humans in order to move; unable to do one of the following: eat, drink or eliminate.
4	Severely ill or moribund; requires immediate supportive care.

In addition to staging schemes that determine the extent of the neoplastic process, evaluation of the general health of the patient is advised. Use of scales such as that outlined in Table 58–8 are sometimes useful in helping both the clinician and the owner/client to keep the relative importance of the neoplastic disease in better focus.

Whenever possible, a routine set of standard tests should be obtained from animals with a particular kind of neoplasm. This is especially important when the animal is included in an experimental trial. However, staging procedures can be expensive and they are occasionally hazardous. Consequently, only studies that impact on management decisions should be performed in high-risk patients. For example, it is unwise to administer general anesthesia to obtain a bone marrow aspiration and core biopsy from a dog with hypercalcemic nephropathy secondary to multicentric lymphosarcoma. Even though the procedure may yield information about bone marrow infiltration, that knowledge may be relatively useless unless renal function is improved.

References

1. Dorland's Medical Dictionary, 26th edition. Philadelphia, WB Saunders, 1981.
2. Casciato, DA and Lowitz, BB: Manual of Bedside Oncology. Boston, Little, Brown and Company, 1983, p 3.
3. Bonfiglio, TA and Terry, R: The Pathology of Cancer. *In* Rubin P (ed): Clinical Oncology for Medical Students and Physicians—A Multidisciplinary Approach, 6th ed. Rochester, NY, American Cancer Society, 1983, p 20.
4. Bech-Nielsen, S, et al.: The use of tumor doubling time in veterinary clinical oncology. J Am Vet Radiol Soc 17:113, 1976.
5. Plesnicar, S, et al.: The significance of doubling time values in patients with pulmonary metastases of osteogenic sarcoma. Cancer Lett 1:351, 1976.
6. Markert, CL: Neoplasia: a disease of cell differentiation. Cancer Res 28:1908, 1968.
7. Braun, AC: The Cancer Problem: A Critical Analysis and Modern Synthesis. New York, Columbia University Press, 1969.

8. McKinnell, RG, et al.: Transplantation of pluripotential nuclei from triploid frog tumors. Science 165:394, 1969.
9. Braun, AC: On the origin of the cancer cell. Am Sci 58:307, 1970.
10. Davidson, EH: Gene Activity in Early Development. New York, Academic Press, 1968.
11. Friend, C, et al.: Hemoglobin synthesis in murine-induced leukemic cells in vitro: stimulation of erythroid differentiation by dimethylsulfoxide. Proc Natl Acad Sci USA 68:378, 1971.
12. Christman, JK, et al.: Correlated suppression by 5-bromodeoxyuridine of tumorigenicity and plasminogen activator in mouse melanoma cells. Proc Natl Acad Sci USA 72:47, 1975.
13. Huebner, RJ and Todaro, GJ: Oncogenes of RNA tumor viruses as determinants of cancer. Proc Natl Acad Sci USA 64:1087, 1969.
14. Todaro, GJ and Huebner, RJ: The viral oncogene hypothesis: new evidence. Proc Natl Acad Sci USA 69:1009, 1972.
15. Nicolson, GL and Poste, G: The cancer cell: dynamic aspects and modifications in cell-surface organization. N Engl J Med 295:197, 1976.
16. Dorsey, JK and Roth, S: Adhesive specificity of normal and transformed mouse fibroblasts. Dev Biol 33:249, 1973.
17. Ponten, J: Contact inhibition. *In* Becker FE(ed): Cancer—A Comprehensive Treatise, vol 4. New York, Plenum Press, 1975, p 55.
18. Gold, J: Cancer cachexia and gluconeogenesis. Ann NY Acad Sci 230:103, 1974.
19. Waterhouse, C: How tumors affect host metabolism. Ann NY Acad Sci 230:86, 1974.
20. Baserga, R: The cell cycle. N Engl J Med 304:453, 1981.
21. Baserga, R and Weibel, F: The cell cycle of mammalian cells. Int Rev Exp Pathol 7:1, 1969.
22. Tubiana, M: The kinetics of tumour cell proliferation and radiotherapy. Br J Radiol 44:325, 1971.
23. Schiaffonati, L and Baserga, R: Different survival of normal and transformed cells exposed to nutritional conditions nonpermissive for growth. Cancer Res 37:541, 1977.
24. Moses, HL, et al.: Mechanism of growth arrest of chemically transformed cells in culture. Cancer Res 38:2807, 1978.
25. Tannenbaum, A and Silverstone, H: Nutrition in relation to cancer. Adv Cancer Res 1:451, 1953.
26. Fidler, IJ: Mechanisms of cancer invasion and metastasis. *In* Baker, FE (ed): Cancer—A Comprehensive Treatise, vol. 4. New York, Plenum Press, 1975, p 1010.
27. Prehn, RT: The immune reaction as a stimulator of tumor growth. Science 176:170, 1972.
28. Fisher, B and Fisher, ER: Studies concerning the regional lymph node in cancer. I. Initiation of immunity. Cancer 27:1001, 1971.
29. Fisher, B and Fisher, ER: Studies concerning the regional lymph node in cancer. II. Maintenance of immunity. Cancer 29:1496, 1972.
30. Fisher, B, et al.: Studies concerning the regional lymph node in cancer. IV. Tumor inhibition in regional lymph nodes. Cancer 33:631, 1974.
31. Fisher, B, et al.: Studies concerning the regional lymph node in cancer. VIII. Effect of asynchronous tumor foci on lymph node cell cytotoxicity. Cancer 36:521, 1975.
32. Crile, G: Possible role of uninvolved regional nodes in preventing metastasis from breast cancer. Cancer 24:1283, 1969.
33. Jeglum, KA: Treatment of metastasis. Vet Clin N Am 15:659, 1985.
34. Sugarbaker, EV and Ketcham, AS: Mechanisms and prevention of cancer dissemination: an overview. Semin Oncol 4:19, 1979.
35. Poste, G and Fidler, IJ: The pathogenesis of tumor metastasis. Nature 283:139, 1979.
36. Warren, BA: Environment of the blood-borne tumor embolus adherent to vessel wall. J Med 4:150, 1973.
37. Hoover, HC, et al.: Osteosarcoma: improved survival with anticoagulation and amputation. Cancer 41:2475, 1975.
38. Liotta, LA, et al.: Stochastic model of metastases formation. Biometrics 32:535, 1976.
39. del Regato, JA: Physiopathology of metastasis. *In* Weiss L, Gilbert HA (eds): Pulmonary Metastasis. Boston, Hall, 1978, p 104.
40. Fidler, IJ, et al.: Relationship of host immune status to tumor cell arrest, distribution, and survival in experimental metastasis. Cancer 40:23, 1977.
41. Kinsey, DL: An experimental study of preferential metastasis. Cancer 13:674, 1960.
42. Hart, IR and Fidler, IJ: The role of organ selectivity in the determination of metastatic patterns of the B16 melanoma. Cancer Res 40:2281, 1980.
43. Folkman, J, et al.: Isolation of a tumor factor responsible for angiogenesis. J Exp Med 133:275, 1971.
44. Folkman, J: Tumor angiogenesis: therapeutic implications. N Engl J Med 285:1182, 1971.
45. Folkman, J: Tumor angiogenesis factor. Cancer Res 34:2109, 1974.
46. Folkman, J: Tumor angiogenesis: a possible control point in tumor growth. Ann Intern Med 82:96, 1975.
47. Folkman, J: Anti-angiogenesis: new concept for therapy of solid tumors. Ann Surg 175:409, 1972.
48. Fidler, IJ and Kripke, ML: Metastasis results from pre-existing variant cells with a malignant tumor. Science 197:893, 1977.
49. Fidler, IJ and Kripke, ML: Metastatic heterogeneity of cells from the K-1735 melanoma. *In* Grundman E (ed): Metastatic Tumor Growths. Stuttgart, Verlag, 1980.
50. Prehn, RT: Tumor progression and homeostasis. Adv Cancer Res 23:203, 1976.
51. Livingston, RB: Treatment of small cell carcinoma: evolution and future directions. Semin Oncol 5:299, 1979.
52. Payan, HM, et al.: Hematologic and biochemical paraneoplastic disorders. Arch Pathol Lab Med 102:19, 1978.
53. Crow, SE, et al.: Unpublished observations. Michigan State University, 1977-1985.
54. Weller, RE: Paraneoplastic disorders in companion animals. Comp Cont Ed Pract Vet 4:423, 1982.
55. Madewell, BR and Feldman, BF: Characterization of anemias associated with neoplasia in small animals. JAVMA 176:419, 1980.
56. Antman, KH, et al.: Microangiopathic hemolytic anemia and cancer: a review. Medicine 58:377, 1979.
57. Madewell, BR, et al.: Coagulation abnormalities in dogs with neoplastic disease. Thromb Diath Haemorr 44:35, 1980.
58. Feldman, BF, et al.: Disseminated intravascular coagulation: antithrombin, plasminogen, and coagulation abnormalities in 41 dogs. JAVMA 179:151, 1981.
59. Sacks, PV: Autoimmune hematologic complications in malignant lymphoproliferative disorders. Arch Intern Med 134:781, 1974.
60. Scott, DW, et al.: Autoimmune hemolytic anemia in the cat. JAAHA 9:530, 1973.
61. Dodds, WJ: Autoimmune hemolytic disease and other causes of immune-mediated anemia: an overview. JAAHA 13:437, 1977.
62. Morgan, RV: Blood dyscrasias associated with testicular tumors in the dog. JAAHA 18:970, 1982.
63. Edwards, DF: Bone marrow hypoplasia in a feminized dog with a Sertoli cell tumor. JAVMA 178:494, 1981.
64. Sherding, RG, et al.: Bone marrow hypoplasia in eight dogs with Sertoli cell tumor. JAVMA 178:497, 1981.
65. Crow, SE and Oliver, J: Cancer cachexia. Comp Cont Ed Pract Vet 3:681, 1981.
66. Nathanson, L: Effect of cancer on the host. *In* Horton J, Hill GJ (eds): Clinical Oncology. Philadelphia, WB Saunders, 1977, p 71.
67. Theologides, A: Weight loss in cancer patients. CA—A Cancer J Clin 27:205, 1977.
68. Maxwell, A: Cachexia of malignancy: some possible factors. New Phys 12:452, 1963.
69. Theologides, A: Anorexia-producing intermediary metabolites. Am J Clin Nutr 29:552, 1976.
70. Anand, B: Nervous regulation of food intake. Physiol Rev 41:667, 1961.
71. DeWys, W and Walters, K: Abnormalities of taste sensation in cancer patients. Cancer 36:1888, 1975.
72. Dymock, IW: Small intestinal function in neoplastic disease. Br J Cancer 21:505, 1967.
73. Bright, JM: Pancreatic adenocarcinoma in a dog with maldigestion syndrome. JAVMA 187:420, 1985.
74. Chiapella, AM: Fever of unknown origin in dogs and cats. *In* Kirk RW (ed): Current Veterinary Therapy VII. Philadelphia, WB Saunders, 1980, p 28.

75. Klastersky, J, et al.: Fever of unexplained origin in patients with cancer. Eur J Cancer 9:649, 1973.
76. Dinarello, CA and Wolff, SM: Pathogenesis of fever in man. N Engl J Med 298:607, 1978.
77. Thrasher, JP: Hypertrophic pulmonary osteoarthropathy in dogs. JAVMA 139:441, 1961.
78. Brodey, RS: Hypertrophic osteoarthropathy in the dog: a clinicopathologic survey of 60 cases. JAVMA 159:1242, 1971.
79. Halliwell, WH and Ackerman, P: Botryoid rhabdomyosarcoma of the urinary bladder and hypertrophic osteoarthropathy in a young dog. JAVMA 165:911, 1974.
80. Vulgamott, JC and Clark, RG: Atrial hypertension and hypertrophic pulmonary osteopathy associated with aortic valvular endocarditis in a dog. JAVMA 177:243, 1980.
81. Nafe, LA, et al.: Hypertrophic osteopathy in a cat associated with renal papillary adenoma. JAAHA 17:659, 1981.
82. Randolph, JA, et al.: Hypertrophic osteopathy associated with adenocarcinoma of the esophageal glands in a dog. JAVMA 184:98, 1984.
83. Rendano, VT and Slauson, DO: Hypertrophic osteopathy in a dog with prostatic adenocarcinoma and without pulmonary metastasis. JAAHA 18:905, 1982.
84. Caywood, DD, et al.: Hypertrophic osteoarthropathy associated with an atypical nephroblastoma in a dog. JAAHA 16:855, 1980.
85. Steiner, H, et al.: Ectopic growth-hormone production and osteoarthropathy in carcinoma of the bronchus. Lancet 1:768, 1968.
86. Dupont, B, et al.: Plasma growth hormone and hypertrophic osteoarthropathy in carcinoma of the bronchus. Arch Med Scand 188:25, 1970.
87. Ginsberg, J and Brown, J: Increased oestrogen excretion in hypertrophic pulmonary osteoarthropathy. Lancet 1:1274, 1961.
88. Jao, JY, et al.: Pulmonary hypertrophic osteoarthropathy, spider angiomata, and estrogen hyperexcretion in neoplasia. Ann Intern Med 70:581, 1969.
89. Epstein, O, et al.: Hypertrophic hepatic osteoarthropathy, clinical, roentgenologic, biochemical, hormonal and cardiorespiratory studies and review of literature. Am J Med 67:89, 1979.
90. Flavell, G: Reversal of pulmonary hypertrophic osteoarthropathy by vagotomy. Lancet 1:260, 1956.
91. Jolman, CW: Osteoarthropathy in lung cancer: disappearance after section of intercostal nerves. J Thorac Cardiovasc Surg 45:679, 1963.
92. Mendlowitz, M and Leslie, A: The experimental stimulation in the dog of the cyanosis and hypertrophic osteoarthropathy which are associated with congenital heart disease. Am Heart J 24:141, 1942.
93. Madewell, BR, et al.: Regression of hypertrophic osteopathy following pneumonectomy in a dog. JAVMA 172:818, 1978.
94. Bunn, PA and Minna, JD: Paraneoplastic syndromes. *In* DeVita VT, et al. (eds): Cancer—Principles and Practice of Oncology, 2nd ed. Philadelphia, JB Lippincott, 1985, p 1797.
95. Morrison, WB: Paraneoplastic syndromes of the dog. JAVMA 175:559, 1979.
96. Macy, DW: Canine and feline mast cell tumors: biologic behavior, diagnosis, and therapy. Semin Vet Med Surg 1:72, 1986.
97. Howard, EB, et al.: Mastocytoma and gastroduodenal ulceration. Vet Pathol 6:146, 1969.
98. Byers, JC and Fleischman, RW: Peptic ulcer associated with a mast cell tumor in a dog. Canine Pract 8:42, 1981.
99. Holeman, R and Langdell, RD: Histamine-induced increase in fibrinolytic activity. Proc Soc Exp Biol Med 115:584, 1964.
100. Kenyon, AJ, et al.: Histamine-induced suppressor macrophage inhibits fibroblast growth and wound healing. Am J Vet Res 44:2164, 1983.
101. Gomez-Uria, A and Pazianos, AG: Syndromes resulting from ectopic hormone-producing tumors. Med Clin N Amer 59:431, 1975.
102. Osborne, CA and Stevens, JB: Pseudohyperparathyroidism in the dog. JAVMA 162:125, 1973.
103. Drazner, FH: Hypercalcemia in the dog and cat. JAVMA 178:1252, 1981.
104. MacEwen, EG and Siegel, SD: Hypercalcemia: a paraneoplastic disease. Vet Clin N Am 7:187, 1977.
105. Meuten, DJ, et al.: Hypercalcemia in dogs with lymphosarcoma: biochemical, ultrastructural, and histomorphometric investigations. Lab Invest 49:553, 1983.
106. Mundy, GR, et al.: Evidence for secretion of an osteoclast stimulating factor in myeloma. N Engl J Med 291:1041, 1974.
107. Giger, U and Gorman, NT: Oncologic emergencies in small animals. Part II. Comp Cont Ed Pract Vet 6:805, 1984.
108. Weller, RE, et al.: Chemotherapeutic responses in dogs with lymphosarcoma and hypercalcemia. JAVMA 181:891, 1982.
109. MacEwen, EG and Hurvitz, AI: Diagnosis and management of monoclonal gammopathies. Vet Clin N Am 7:119, 1977.
110. Braund, KG, et al.: Neurologic complications of IgA multiple myeloma associated with cryoglobulinemia in a dog. JAVMA 174:1321, 1979.
111. MacEwen, EG, et al.: Hyperviscosity syndrome associated with lymphocytic leukemia in three dogs. JAVMA 170:1309, 1977.
112. Braund, KG, et al.: Neurologic manifestations of monoclonal IgM gammopathy associated with lymphocytic leukemia in a dog. JAVMA 172:1407, 1978.
113. Shull, RM, et al.: Serum hyperviscosity syndrome associated with IgA multiple myeloma in two dogs. JAAHA 14:58, 1977.
114. Aronsohn, M: Canine thymoma. Vet Clin N Am 15:755, 1985.
115. Theilen, GH and Madewell, BR: Tumors of the skin and subcutaneous tissues. *In* Theilen GH, Madewell BR (eds): Veterinary Cancer Medicine. Philadelphia, Lea and Febiger, 1979, p 129.
116. Todoroff, RJ and Brodey, RS: Oral and pharyngeal neoplasia in the dog: a retrospective survey of 361 cases. JAVMA 175:567, 1979.
117. Harvey, HJ: Oral tumors. Vet Clin N Am 15:493, 1985.
118. Ling, GV, et al.: Primary bone tumors in the dog: a combined clinical, radiographic, and histologic approach to early diagnosis. JAVMA 165:55, 1974.
119. Jongeward, SJ: Primary bone tumors. Vet Clin N Am 15:609, 1985.
120. Theilen, GH and Madewell, BR: Tumors of the Skin and Subcutaneous Tissues. *In* Theilen GH, Madewell BR (eds): Veterinary Cancer Medicine. Philadelphia, Lea and Febiger, 1979, p 146.
121. Severi, L (ed): Tumors of early life in man and animals. Proceedings of the Sixth Perugia Quadrennial International Conference on Cancer. Monteluce, Italy. 1978.
122. Bostock, DE: The prognosis following surgical removal of mastocytomas in dogs. J Sm Anim Pract 14:27, 1973.
123. Patnaik, AK, et al.: Canine cutaneous mast cell tumor: morphologic grading and survival time in 83 dogs. Vet Pathol 21:469, 1984.
124. Squire, RA, et al.: Clinical and pathologic study of canine lymphoma: clinical staging, cell classification and therapy. J Natl Cancer Inst 51:565, 1973.
125. Weller, RE, et al: Histologic classification as a prognostic criterion for canine lymphosarcoma. Am J Vet Res 41:1310, 1980.
126. Gray, KN, et al.: Histologic classification as an indication of therapeutic response in malignant lymphoma of dogs. JAVMA 184:814, 1984.
127. Kurzman, ID and Gilbertson, SR: Prognostic factors in canine mammary tumors. Semin Vet Med Surg 1:25, 1986.
128. Fowler, EH, et al.: Biologic behavior of canine mammary neoplasms based on a histogenetic classification. Vet Pathol 11:212, 1974.
129. MacEwen, EG, et al.: Estrogen receptors in canine mammary tumors. Cancer Res 42:2255, 1982.
130. TNM: Classification of tumours in domestic animals. Geneva, World Health Organization, 1980.
131. Dukes, CE: The classification of cancer of the rectum. J Pathol Bacteriol 35:323, 1932.
132. Clark, WH, et al.: The histogenesis and biologic behavior of primary human malignant melanomas of the skin. Cancer Res 29:705, 1969.
133. Priester, WA and McKay, FW: The occurrence of tumors in domestic animals. Natl Cancer Inst Monogr 54:159, 1980.
134. Crow, SE: Tumors of the alimentary tract. Vet Clin N Am 15:577, 1985.
135. Brodey, RS and Cohen, D: An epizootiological and clinicopathologic study of 95 cases of gastrointestinal neoplasms in the dog. *In* Proceedings of the 101st Annual Meeting of the AVMA, 1964.
136. Coltman, CA (ed): Hodgkin's disease. Semin Oncol 7:91, 1980.

137. Golomb, HM (ed): Non-Hodgkin's lymphoma. Semin Oncol 7:221, 1980.
138. Crow, SE, et al.: Chemoimmunotherapy for canine lymphosarcoma. Cancer 40:2102, 1977.
139. Weller, RE, et al.: Chemoimmunotherapy for canine lymphosarcoma: a prospective evaluation of specific and non-specific immunomodulation. Am J Vet Res 41:516, 1980.
140. Cotter, SM: Treatment of lymphoma and leukemia with cyclophosphamide, vincristine and prednisone: I. Treatment of dogs. JAAHA 19:159, 1983.
141. MacEwen, EG, et al.: Evaluation of some prognostic factors for advanced multicentric lymphosarcoma in the dog: 147 cases (1978–1981). JAVMA 190:564, 1987.
142. Bostock, DE: The prognosis following surgical excision of canine mammary neoplasms. Eur J Cancer 11:389, 1975.
143. MacEwen, EG, et al.: Canine mammary cancer: therapeutic studies (abstr). *In* Proceedings of the 12th Annual Scientific Program, ACVIM, 1984, p 41.
144. Macy, DW: Canine mast cell tumors. Vet Clin N Am 15:783, 1985.
145. White, RAS, et al.: Clinical staging for oropharyngeal malignancies in the dog. J Sm Anim Pract 26:581, 1985.

59 APPROACH TO TREATMENT OF CANCER PATIENTS

E. GREGORY MACEWEN and ROBERT C. ROSENTHAL

Prior to the initiation of any type of cancer therapy, the clinician must establish a diagnosis and the extent of disease (using clinical staging) and select the appropriate therapy to be used. The appropriate therapy is based on the type of tumor, the clinical stage, and proven responsiveness to the particular treatment.

DIAGNOSTIC CONSIDERATIONS

Before any therapeutic intervention can proceed, a thorough clinical examination is necessary to determine the presence of a tumor, determine the nature and extent of the neoplastic process, determine if any concurrent medical problems exist, and establish a prognosis based on the above information.

History. A complete history should be performed first and should include information about the duration and rate of tumor growth and/or the clinical signs associated with the tumor. In addition, any specific clinical manifestations associated with the neoplastic process should be identified and any history of any previous therapy should be recorded. Related to previous therapy, special attention should be given to the details of therapy, the extent of treatment, and an overall assessment of the success of that previous therapy. Additional information that may be important is the evaluation for any possible environmental factors associated with the development of the tumor. For example, when dealing with a cat with leukemia, it is important to know if any other cats in the household have died of any feline leukemia virus-related diseases. In a dog with a vaginal tumor, for example, it would be important to know if this dog roams free and could have been exposed to another dog carrying a transmissible venereal tumor. Clustering of disease is also an important factor to identify and evaluate. Clustering of disease may indicate either an infectious process or the possibility of some common environmental factor that could be associated with this neoplastic process. A history of the family lines, as it relates to the development of tumors, may indicate a possible genetic predisposition for certain neoplastic diseases. These are just a few examples of important information that needs to be gathered during the initial evaluation of the patient.

Physical Examination. The next important facet of patient evaluation includes a thorough physical examination. Particular attention must be directed toward regional lymph nodes and other possible metastatic sites. The tumor should be defined and information recorded such as tumor size, location, fixation, consistency, invasiveness, and inflammation or ulceration. This information is important to stage the disease adequately.

Diagnostic Tests. Hematologic and biochemical profiles give further information with regard to the extent of disease, as well as concurrent medical or paraneoplastic problems, and provide information important for future therapeutic decision making. The thoracic cavity and area of the tumor may need to be radiographed. Radiography of the thoracic cavity is primarily to determine if any pulmonary metastasis has developed, and radiography of the primary tumor may be necessary to further determine the extent of the disease and whether or not there appears to be any extensive invasion, such as bone involvement.

The history, physical, and radiographic findings and hematologic and biochemical profiles can provide important information regarding possible associated paraneoplastic conditions. Paraneoplastic disease syndromes are defined as disease conditions or clinical signs associated with products secreted or released from the tumor or conditions that result secondarily to the primary tumor (see Chapter 58, Table 58–2).

Clinical staging provides a description of the extent of the cancer in the affected animal at the time of diagnosis. Determining the clinical stage of a disease is important for the following reasons:

1. Prognosis is often associated with the clinical stage.
2. Clinical stage usually influences the type and extent of therapy to be given.
3. Using the system helps to maintain uniformity in reporting the results of cancer therapy.

A system for clinically staging both solid and hematopoietic tumors was adopted by the World Health Organization (WHO) and the Veterinary Cancer Society in 1978 and published in the World Health Organization TNM classification of tumors in domestic animals.[1] The system for solid tumors is based on the TNM system currently used in human oncology. "T" stands for tumor and describes the tumor by size (diameter in centimeters), number (single or multiple), and invasiveness. "N" represents the regional lymph nodes and describes them as of normal size, enlarged, or clinically or histologically metastatic. "M" designates metastasis beyond the regional lymph nodes to sites such as the lung.

In addition to hematology, clinical chemistry, and immunologic studies, veterinarians frequently collect samples for microscopic evaluation of cellular detail as part of the diagnostic process. Diagnostic cytology, exfoliative cytology, and cytopathology are similar terms used to describe the microscopic examination of cells that either exfoliate freely from epithelial surfaces or that are removed from tissues by mechanical means such as aspiration, scraping, or flushing. Cytologic evaluation remains one of the most useful techniques to arrive at a presumptive diagnosis, but histopathologic evaluation is required for definitive diagnosis. Nonetheless, cytology has considerable value as a diagnostic technique. The aims of cytologic examination can be summarized as follows: differentiation among normal, inflammatory, hyperplastic, dysplastic, and neoplastic processes; determination of the histogenesis of the neoplasm; detection of dissemination or recurrence of the neoplasms; monitoring the course and consequences of therapy; and monitoring the course of disease. It is beyond the scope of this chapter to provide the reader with all the methods of collection and preparation of specimens and their examination and interpretation. The reader is referred to a number of comprehensive review articles on cytology.

The definitive diagnosis is obtained by histopathologic evaluation of a representative tissue biopsy. Careful thought must be given to determining the most appropriate biopsy procedure. In order to optimize the chances of an accurate morphologic diagnosis, the largest amount of tissue possible, including both tumor and tumor margins, needs to be examined. The biopsy material should be representative of the tumor and the normal surrounding tissue. In addition to establishing a definitive diagnosis from the biopsy material, other information to obtain includes such important facts as the degree of invasiveness of the tumor, whether or not there is evidence of microscopic embolization of tumor cells into lymphatic vessels or blood vessels, and if it is a complete surgical excision, and whether or not the surgical borders are free of any tumor.

Tissue fixation is frequently disregarded when a surgical biopsy is performed. Chemical fixatives are the most common methods of tissue preservation for the surgical pathologist. Ten per cent buffered formaldehyde (formalin) fixation satisfies many of the essential criteria for an all-purpose fixative. For adequate fixation ten unit volumes of formalin are needed for each unit volume of tissue to be fixed. Formalin has excellent penetrating capabilities; however, the smaller the tumor size, the more rapid the fixation. When possible, the clinician should remove a small segment of tissue from an area likely to be representative of the neoplastic process and rapidly fix that segment. In addition, he or she should fix the remaining anatomically undisturbed tissue and submit both specimens to the pathologist for examination. When choosing tissues to be examined by a pathologist, one should include definable anatomic landmarks, and margins between normal and abnormal tissue should be clearly labeled for the pathologist.

The pathologist should be advised of the clinical features of the problem when reviewing biopsy material. Details such as the patient's signalment, as well as the size, color, growth rate, clinical signs, and the exact anatomic positioning of the biopsy material are essential. The radiographic appearance should be carefully described or copies of the radiographs may be sent for review when pertinent. When there are special considerations, such as a comparison to previous biopsy, these should be specifically requested.

Successful interpretation of biologic material obviously depends upon the experience and qualifications of the pathologist. Extensive experience in interpretation of biopsy material in domestic animals is essential if the morphologic findings are to be accurate and meaningful. Medical (MD) pathologists are often asked to make pathologic interpretations of animal tissues. Animal tumors, however, differ in many important respects from human tumors in regard to the significance of the morphologic features. Practitioners relying on MD pathologists to diagnose animal tumors will have problems due to inaccurate interpretation. Many veterinary schools and state diagnostic and private veterinary pathology laboratories around the country are available to provide excellent histopathologic services. Practitioners interested in clinical oncology are encouraged to choose one of these and learn to work and communicate closely with the veterinary pathologist.

Both radiography and ultrasonography are important diagnostic aids in the diagnosis and staging of neoplasms. Real time ultrasonography has made rapid gains in veterinary medicine and is an important method of diagnosing and staging neoplasms in selected locations.[2–6] Ultrasound-guided biopsy has improved the success and safety of obtaining the initial histologic diagnosis and may assist with the detection of possible recurrence.[7] Ultrasonography is also becoming important for planning radiotherapy treatment and for serially assessing treatment responses or complications following radiotherapy or chemotherapy.[2]

Ultrasound images display the cross-sectional anatomy and internal architecture of the cavity under study. Neoplasia is usually seen as a change in the internal architecture, with disruption of normal organ parenchymal pattern. These changes are not identified radiographically unless the size, shape, radiographic density, or position of organs is altered to a marked degree. Ultrasound and radiography are complementary procedures and are not mutually exclusive. However, the use of ultrasound as part of an initial screening procedure is becoming more commonly accepted in the veterinary profession. Ultrasound can be particularly beneficial in the evaluation of the liver for either primary or metastatic disease, the spleen, pancreas, kidney, bladder, prostate, ovary, adrenal gland, and the gastrointestinal tract.[2–7] Ultrasonography will become more important as a clinical aid to the diagnosis of neoplasia and determination of the extent of disease.

Another ancillary tool used in cancer diagnosis has been termed immunodiagnostics, including such tests as the ELISA or indirect fluorescent antibody tests for feline leukemia virus. Another area in which immunodiagnostics are beginning to play a role is in the use of monoclonal antibodies produced against one particular antigen, such as a tumor-associated antigen. Radiolabeled monoclonal antibodies are used now in human medicine to determine the extent of disease, but their use in veterinary medicine has only begun to be studied.

THERAPEUTIC CONSIDERATIONS

Surgery

The major role of surgery in the diagnosis of cancer lies in the acquisition of tissue for exact histologic diagnosis. A variety of techniques exists for obtaining tissues suspected of malignancy, including aspiration biopsy, needle biopsy, incisional biopsy, and excisional biopsy.[8]

Incisional biopsy refers to removal of a small wedge of tissue from a larger tumor mass. Incisional biopsies often are necessary for diagnosing large masses that would require major surgical procedures for local excision. Incisional biopsies are the preferred method of diagnosing soft tissue and bony sarcomas because of the magnitude of the surgical procedure necessary to extricate these lesions definitively. The veterinary surgeon must be aware of opening new tissue planes contaminated with tumor by performing incisional biopsies of large lesions.

In excisional biopsy, the entire suspected tumor is removed, including sufficient margins of surrounding normal tissue. Excisional biopsies are the procedure of choice for most tumors when they are performed without contaminating new tissue planes or further compromising the ultimate surgical procedure. When at all possible, the surgeon should perform an excisional biopsy rather than an incisional biopsy. However, an inappropriately performed excisional biopsy can compromise subsequent surgical excision. When this is a possibility, incisional biopsies should be performed.

Surgery remains the most important therapy for most solid tumors. Surgery can be a simple, safe method of curing patients with solid tumors when the tumor is confined to the anatomic site of origin. Unfortunately many animals with solid tumors have extension of the tumor either beyond the major anatomic site or they have overt or micrometastasis present. The extension of the surgical resection to include areas of regional spread can cure some of these animals, although regional spread often is an indication of undetectable distant micrometastases. Surgical procedures include scalpel excision, cryosurgery, and electrosurgery. Scalpel excision is used most often. Cryosurgery is useful in areas where scalpel excision is limited (i.e., the oral cavity and the extremities). Electrosurgery combines the advantage of hemostasis with controlled dissection. The surgeon treating cancer should be skilled in all of these methods.

Some basic principles regarding oncologic surgery are important.[9] The clinician should avoid manipulation of the tumor mass. It has been demonstrated in human beings that manipulation of the tumor may dislodge tumor cells and can potentially increase the incidence of metastases. All excisions should be made wide and deep. Ideally there should be at least a 1 cm margin around the tumor with histologically confirmed clear margins. If necessary, one can allow the defect to heal as an open wound or use reconstructive surgery. It is better to err on the side of being too aggressive than not being aggressive enough. Protect the skin margins to prevent tumor cell seeding. An en bloc resection of the primary tumor, including intervening lymphatics and lymph node, should be performed if the clinician suspects lymph node metastasis. Vessels should be ligated early in the surgical procedure to prevent dissemination of tumor emboli. Gloves, drapes, and instruments should be changed frequently to avoid contaminating the surgical field with tumor cells. All tissues excised should be submitted for complete histopathologic evaluation.

Surgery is not limited to the primary treatment of a malignancy. It can also be used to reduce the extent of tumor. The concept of cytoreductive surgery has received much attention in the recent years.[10] In some instances, the extensive local spread of cancer precludes the removal of all gross disease by surgery. Cytoreductive surgery is of benefit only when other effective treatment modalities are available to control unresectable residual disease. Except in rare palliative settings, there is no role for cytoreductive surgery in patients for whom little other effective therapy currently exists.

Surgical excision is sometimes required for the relief of pain or functional abnormalities. The appropriate use of surgery in these settings can improve the quality of life in animals affected with cancer. Palliative surgery may include the relief of mechanical problems such as intestinal obstruction or the removal of bleeding masses.

The value of surgery for the treatment of metastatic disease is often overlooked. As a general rule, patients with a single site of metastatic disease that can be resected without major morbidity should undergo resection of that metastatic cancer. In humans, many patients undergoing resection of their metastatic disease have benefited quite dramatically from this strategy. This approach is especially applicable for cancers that tend not to be highly responsive to systemic chemotherapy. In humans, the resection of pulmonary metastasis in patients with soft tissue and bony sarcomas can cure up to 30 per cent of patients.[11] In veterinary medicine few studies have been performed to evaluate the benefits of resecting metastatic disease, but certainly in human medicine this benefit has been realized.

Surgery can also be used to treat oncologic emergencies. These emergencies generally involve the treatment of exsanguinating tumors, perforation, drainage of abscess, or impending disruption of vital organs.

Chemotherapy

Chemotherapy is another major treatment modality. Unlike surgery, it is usually intended to have a systemic effect. Chemotherapy may be employed with a number of goals in mind. Ultimately, the goal of chemotherapy is to cure the disease, but whether this occurs in veterinary medicine is debatable. Nonetheless, there are other benefits from its use. Chemotherapy may help to control generalized, rapidly progressive disease not amenable to surgery or radiation therapy or help to increase the disease-free interval after such initial therapy. It may help to prevent spread of the neoplasm by controlling early metastases that are proliferating rapidly and have a relatively small likelihood of containing resistant cells. Chemotherapy may also benefit the patient by symptomatic relief of related problems and temporary restoration of deteriorated function.[13]

Of the three major types of therapy, surgery, chemotherapy, and radiation therapy, only chemotherapy is intended to deal with systemic or undetected metastatic disease. Metastatic disease is the primary cause of death in patients with neoplasia regardless of the mode of therapy. Clearly, the more effective the chemotherapy in controlling the distant spread of the disease, the longer the comfortable survival of the patient. An understanding of the basic principles of chemotherapy can help provide a basis for sensible, effective chemotherapy and prolonged survival.

BIOLOGIC BASIS

There are three aspects of cell kinetics that must be considered when discussing the biologic basis of chemotherapy: cell cycle, growth classes of tissues, and gompertzian growth of tumors.[12, 14–16]

Both normal and neoplastic cells proceed around the cell cycle in orderly progression from mitosis to mitosis. Mitosis M marks the beginning of the cell cycle. Cell division in mammalian cells takes an average of 30 to 90 minutes. The G_1 (gap 1) phase is the period of greatest temporal variability. Days to weeks may be involved in this period of RNA and protein synthesis, depending on the tissue type. From G_1, cells may enter a G_0 phase, which is a resting, nonproliferating state. Cells may remain in G_0 for long periods or return to G_1 and proceed in the cell cycle. The period of DNA synthesis (S phase) follows G_1 and generally lasts about two hours. This is followed by the G_2 (gap 2) phase, another period of RNA and protein synthesis, which generally lasts about six to eight hours. Various chemotherapeutic agents affect the cell cycle at different phases. A knowledge of the cell cycle is fundamental to the establishment of a sensible chemotherapeutic plan.

Not all tissues behave in the same manner regarding their growth and renewal characteristics. Tissues may be termed static, expanding, or renewing. This classification separates highly differentiated tissues (static tissues such as nerves or striated muscle) that do not undergo mitosis from those with the capacity for mitosis. Tissues in the expanding group (organs and glands) can undergo mitosis with the proper stimulus. The renewing tissues are those with mitotically active cell populations and include leukocytes, erythrocytes, mucosa, epidermis, and gametes. This group of tissues with short half-lives is precisely the group of tissues most susceptible to the drug effects intended to kill neoplastic cells.[12]

Just as tissues can be grouped, cells within tissues can also be categorized. A cell may have stem cell potential, may be maturing, or may be functional. A stem cell is an undifferentiated cell found in tissue undergoing renewal. Stem cells can synthesize DNA and divide. One daughter cell remains a stem cell, whereas the other differentiates more fully.[17] Stem cells respond to stimuli such as hormones or possibly to chemical feedback from mature cells, which may stimulate or inhibit division. The loss of mature cells may cause the stem cell compartment to become more active. Neoplastic cells may be dividing, temporarily nondividing, or permanently nondividing. In malignant neoplastic tissue, only a small proportion of the cells are differentiated. The remainder are dividing or retain the capacity to do so. In normal tissues, only a small proportion of the cells are dividing.[16]

In both normal and neoplastic cell populations, there are relatively more dividing cells in a small population and relatively fewer dividing cells in a large population. Gompertzian growth refers to a growth pattern exhibiting increased doubling time and decreased growth fraction as a function of time.[13] The increase in doubling time is related to both the decreased proportion of proliferating cells and the increased cell loss from exfoliation, metastasis, and cell death. It is evident that the cytoreductive effects of surgery or radiation therapy can induce a renewed level of proliferative activity within a tumor and render the tumor more susceptible to chemotherapeutic attack as its constituent cells proceed around the cell cycle.

The development of resistance is related to the mutation rate of the genetically unstable neoplastic cells. Therefore, the larger the number of tumor cells (tumor mass), the greater the number and proportion of resistant clones. Once such clones emerge, clinical resistance develops relatively rapidly; approximately 1.8 logs of growth (6 doublings) are required to go from a 95 per cent chance of no resistant cells to less than a five per cent chance of no resistant cells. Thus, there is a greater chance of success in treating a small mass or, theoretically, micrometastatic disease, than a large tumor burden.[18]

PHARMACOLOGIC FACTORS

To affect a tumor, the chemotherapeutic agent must reach the site of action. Its effectiveness is measured in terms of its concentration and exposure time at the site. The effective contact time, the product of drug concentration multiplied by drug exposure time, is affected by a number of important factors.[13] Route of administration and absorption may influence the efficacy of an administered drug. Chemotherapeutic agents may be administered orally, subcutaneously, intravenously, or intramuscularly for systemic effect. Local effect may be obtained by topical administration or introduction of the drug into the pleural cavity, peritoneal cavity, urinary bladder, or cerebrospinal fluid. Biotransformation of the drug also needs to be considered. Prednisone is frequently included in chemotherapeutic protocols but needs to be converted to prednisolone by the liver before it becomes an active drug.[19] Cyclophosphamide is likewise metabolized by the liver to an active form and is therefore effective orally or parenterally but not when locally instilled.

Distribution of a drug partially determines its effectiveness. If the drug does not reach the tumor, its exposure will be nil and the neoplastic cells will be unaffected. The blood-brain barrier represents such a problem in distribution. Most chemotherapeutic agents cannot gain access to the brain. The effect of tumors on the integrity of the blood-brain barrier is still open to question. Drugs normally excluded from the brain may enter the cancer-afflicted brain because of disruption of the blood-brain barrier.

Once a drug has been properly administered, adequately absorbed, and biologically transformed into an active form as necessary, there are other pharmacologic factors to be considered. Drug resistance, interactions, and toxicities all may affect the usefulness of a therapeutic agent. It is not unusual for the first trial of a drug to be beneficial and later trials to be much less so. Resistance to a drug may develop by several means. Acquired resistance by the tumor may occur owing to decreased activation or increased deactivation of the drug, reducing its effective contact time. Resistance may also be related to impermeability of the tumor cell to the drug, shifts in enzyme specificity, increased repair of cytologic lesions, or bypassing of inhibited reactions with alternate biochemical pathways.[13] Patients may be receiving multiple drug therapy, including therapies directed at problems other than the tumor. There are several ways interactions could occur between a chemotherapeutic agent and another drug. Direct chemical or physical interactions, interference with absorption or receptor binding, or altered metabolism or excretion each might have an impact on a drug's net effect. For example, antibiotics might alter gastrointestinal absorption by affecting microbial flora; aspirin may interfere with binding of drugs to serum albumin.[13] The chemotherapeutic protocol itself may call for multiple drugs given simultaneously or sequentially. The potential for drug interaction is great. Such possibly harmful interactions may either decrease the effectiveness of a drug to nonbeneficial levels or increase its toxicity. In addition, some factors of cell resistance mentioned earlier may alter drug concentrations and lead to interactions.[13]

Chemotherapy treads a narrow path between efficacy and toxicity. In fact, chemotherapeutic protocols are most often limited not by the degree of tumor cell killing but by toxicities to the patient. Recalling one of the biologic bases for chemotherapy, i.e., that the proliferating neoplastic cells can be attacked most effectively as they traverse the cell cycle, helps to explain some of the more commonly noted toxicities related to renewing tissue classes. The most commonly encountered problems relate to gastrointestinal toxicity, bone marrow suppression, and immunosuppression.[20, 21] Vomiting and anorexia may be noted as the gastrointestinal epithelium is affected. Although this problem is usually not life-threatening, it can be detrimental to the patient. Antiemetics may or may not be helpful. Other gastrointestinal toxicities seen less frequently include diarrhea, stomatitis, esophagitis, and gastrointestinal ulceration.[22]

Bone marrow toxicity leading to leukopenia and immune suppression affecting both humoral and cell-mediated immunity are two very serious problems associated with chemotherapy. Bone marrow toxicity may affect all the cellular components of the blood. Anemia and thrombocytopenia can be life-threatening, but leukopenia and the associated risk of infection are the primary and more common problems. Different chemotherapeutic agents cause different patterns of myelosuppression; some are more profound and persistent than others. Chemotherapy may need to be postponed until acceptable numbers of white blood cells return to the peripheral blood. Recommended leukocyte counts at which to postpone therapy have been published.[13, 23, 24] One such guideline is 4000 total white blood cells per microliter with at least 2500 granulocytes per microliter. As veterinary chemotherapists use more intensive protocols in the future, these guidelines will almost certainly be amended to reflect both the acceptance of more myelosuppression (to gain an increased likelihood of cure) and improved methods of dealing with myelosuppression. Generally, chemotherapy can be reinstituted in one to two weeks based on a return to normal white blood cell parameters. When resuming chemotherapy, it may be advisable to decrease the amount of the offending drug by 25 per cent, although it is always important to keep in mind the relationship of toxicity and efficacy.

The problems of immunosuppression relate closely to bone marrow toxicity and myelosuppression. There is great variation in the amount of immunosuppression encountered with chemotherapy, and the clinician must be constantly aware of its dangers. The combination of reduced nonspecific immunity (myelosuppression) and impaired humoral and cell-mediated immunity can render the patient prone to serious, life-threatening infection with little or no means of defense. Fortunately, immunosuppression associated with chemotherapy usually does not last long beyond the time of drug administration. Nonetheless, chemotherapeutic protocols should include as few immunosuppressive drugs as feasible without compromising the treatment.

Less common toxicities involve other body systems. Hemorrhagic cystitis associated with cyclophosphamide is a well-known complication that limits the prolonged use of that drug.[25] The bladder is not the only susceptible organ of the genitourinary system. The kidney is subject to damage from methotrexate, streptozotocin, and platinum compounds; doxorubicin is potentially nephrotoxic in cats.[26] Sterility in males and congenital malformations are also possible complications. Skin reactions and alopecia are less frequent in veterinary medicine than in human medicine, but they do occur.[27] Clipped hair may not regrow or may regrow in a different color. Wire-haired and curly-coated breeds seem more likely to develop alopecia. The lung, liver, heart, and central nervous system are all subject to toxicity from various chemotherapeutic agents although these manifestations are seen far less often than the others. Anti-cancer drugs themselves may be mutagenic. Their increased use may reveal this to be a more serious problem than is currently appreciated.

A final pharmacologic factor influencing chemotherapy is excretion. Most antineoplastic drugs are excreted by the kidneys or liver; if these organs are not functioning adequately to rid the body of the drug, rapid accumulation may result in severe, perhaps unmanageable, toxicity. The amount of drug given or the dosage interval may need to be adjusted to compensate for impaired excretion.[28]

The clinician must understand what can realistically be expected of a chemotherapeutic protocol. This understanding lays the groundwork for reasonable guidelines for chemotherapy.

Although patients may benefit from the use of a single chemotherapeutic drug, more often there are advantages in the use of multiple drugs in combination. Chemotherapeutic drugs kill a constant fraction of the tumor; the fraction killed by one drug is independent of that killed by another. Drugs can be used in combination to specifically attack different portions of the cell cycle. Drugs can be chosen that have different major toxicities, thus limiting toxicity of any one type and allowing each drug to be used in a full dose. It is toxicity and not the ability to kill cancer cells that limits the administration of chemotherapy. Combination chemotherapy also helps avoid the problems of both inherent drug resistance and the emergence of resistant subpopulations due to acquired resistance.[29] Intermittent treatment schedules allow intensive attack on the neoplasm and a rest period for recovery of normal cells before the next treatment. In theory, there should be added benefit from intensifying the chemotherapeutic attack when very small numbers of neoplastic cells remain. At the biochemical level, combinations may act by sequential, concurrent, or complementary inhibition, and it may be possible to design protocols based on these drug interactions. However, it appears that to date, the most successful combined regimens have been empirical in nature, employing drugs known to be individually active against the tumor.[30] There are many unanswered questions concerning not only the best combinations for any particular cancer but also how best to schedule chemotherapy in relation to surgery, radiotherapy, immunotherapy, and hyperthermia. Although the list of considerations governing the use of chemotherapy is long and seems to be growing, some basic principles are:[31, 32] use drugs known to be effective as single agents, use drugs with different mechanisms of action, use drugs with different toxicities, and use an intermittent treatment schedule.

GUIDELINES FOR CHEMOTHERAPY

To safely and effectively use the principles of chemotherapy previously discussed, the clinician must satisfy certain guidelines.[14, 21, 32] A thorough history and physical examination along with an appropriate data base are necessary for chemotherapy. In all cases, a histologic diagnosis of malignancy is imperative. An understanding of the biologic behavior of the tumor aids in both prognosis and the selection of drugs with a known effect against the tumor. The clinician must also understand the drugs and their toxicities. Toxic doses of drugs vary among species, and human dosages cannot always be adopted without modification. Safe dosage schedules for the species being treated should be used. Monitoring the toxicities associated with the treatment and evaluation of patient response follow hand in hand. Both are important to the proper management of chemotherapy. Monitoring toxicity to alter or limit treatment is needed for the well-being of the patient. The patient should be evaluated to judge the effect of the treatment on the disease as well as the recovery of the patient. No chemotherapy should be undertaken without the full understanding and cooperation of the owner concerning the goals of the therapy as well as the costs and the necessary commitment to a regular follow-up regimen. Certainly not all owners elect chemotherapy; some opt for no therapy and some for euthanasia. Chemotherapy can, however, help extend the patient's happy, comfortable life in many instances. This is the primary consideration in offering chemotherapy as a realistic alternative in the management of neoplasia.

DRUGS USED IN CHEMOTHERAPY

Chemotherapeutic agents can be placed into broad classifications that help make them more easily understood, yet each drug has its own characteristics and peculiarities. A brief classification with comments on the mechanisms, indications, and toxicities of selected drugs (Table 59–1) should help the clinician provide effective, rational chemotherapy. Note that doses are expressed as mg per meter squared (body surface area) rather than mg per kg. This has been considered a physiologically more accurate method of dosing chemotherapeutic drugs and allows more precise comparison of doses between species.[20, 33] See Table 59–2 for conversions from weight in kilograms to meters squared of body surface area for dogs. The table is also applicable to domestic cats, but is not appropriate for larger, nondomestic cats. Some recent work suggests that a dosing regimen based on body weight might, in fact, be preferred for anticancer drugs that have an elimination rate not primarily determined by organ function or for which the dose-limiting toxicity does not correlate with metabolic rate.[35, 36]

Alkylating Agents. Alkylating agents are compounds that substitute an alkyl radical ($R—CH_2—CH_2^+$) for a hydrogen atom on some organic compounds. Alkylation causes breaks in the DNA molecule and crosslinking of the twin strands of DNA and thereby interferes with the DNA replication and RNA transcription.[12, 37] Most contain more than one alkylating group and are considered polyfunctional alkylating agents. The alkylating agents are cell-cycle-phase nonspecific drugs.

Cyclophosphamide is the most widely used alkylating agent in veterinary medicine. It has been employed for lymphoreticular neoplasia, various sarcomas and carcinomas, mast cell tumors, and transmissible venereal tumors, both as a single agent and in combination with other drugs.[14] Cyclophosphamide requires hepatic activation and thus must be given by oral or intravenous routes. Its major dose-limiting toxicities are hematologic and gastrointestinal in nature. Leukopenia may be most severe within a week or two of administration, with recovery usually following within ten days. Anemia and thrombocytopenia are less common.[37, 38]

A unique and important toxicity associated with cyclophosphamide is sterile hemorrhagic cystitis. Active metabolites of cyclophosphamide cause mucosal ulceration, necrosis of smooth muscle and small arteries, and hemorrhage and edema in the urinary bladder. The renal pelves may also be affected. The patient may show signs of hematuria, pollakiuria, and stranguria.[25] Early recognition of signs, diuresis, and cessation of cyclophosphamide administration help limit the problem in most cases. Some cases may be persistent and require more aggressive therapy, such as the instillation of one per cent formalin solution into the bladder.[39] Measures helpful in avoiding cyclophosphamide-associated sterile hemorrhagic cystitis include not administering cyclophosphamide to a patient with concurrent cystitis or hematuria, administering the daily dose in the morning and providing free access to fresh water at all times, as well as ample opportunity to urinate, and being certain the patient urinates before the owners retire for the night.

Chlorambucil is often used in chemotherapy of canine lymphosarcoma as a replacement for cyclophosphamide, either in maintenance regimens or when myelosuppression or sterile hemorrhagic cystitis has been a problem. Although chlorambucil acts more slowly than cyclophosphamide and seems to have less myelosuppressive toxicity, regular monitoring of white blood cell parameters is warranted.[12, 14]

Antimetabolites. The antimetabolites are structural analogues of normal metabolites required for cell function and replication; they interfere with these processes by substitution for, or competition with, a metabolite. The antimetabolites are highly schedule-dependent, S-phase-specific drugs. Many questions remain unanswered regarding their best use.[37, 38]

Methotrexate inhibits dihydrofolate reductase competitively and interferes with both DNA and RNA synthesis. It has been used in the therapy of lymphoreticular neoplasms and myeloproliferative disorders as well as metastatic transitional cell tumor, transmissible venereal tumor, Sertoli cell tumor, and osteogenic sarcoma. Methotrexate toxicity to the bone marrow and gastrointestinal tract can be severe; with high-dose regimens, appropriately timed "rescue" may be achieved by administering citrovorum factor (folinic acid), the specific antidote. More commonly in veterinary medicine, methotrexate is given in a low-dose regimen that is far less toxic and does not require "rescue."[12, 14, 37, 38]

Plant Alkyloids. Vincristine and vinblastine are alkyloids extracted from the periwinkle plant, *Vinca rosea*. They act specifically in the M phase by binding with the microtubular protein tubulin and blocking mitosis by interfering with chromosomal separation in metaphase. Although vincristine and vinblastine share a common mechanism of action, resistance to one does not imply resistance to the other. They also have different major toxicities. Vincristine affects the nervous system. Paresthesia, loss of deep tendon reflexes, and sensory neuropathy are more easily assessed in human patients than animal patients. Lymphoid hypoplasia and constipation are more frequent veterinary complications. Vinblastine toxicity is primarily hematologic; myelosuppression may be a severe problem. Both drugs have been used in the treatment of lymphoreticular neoplasms. Vincristine is the treatment of choice for transmissible venereal tumor and has been used for various sarcomas and carcinomas.[40, 41] Vinblastine has been used in the treatment of carcinomas and mast cell tumors.[37, 38, 40]

Antibiotics. The antitumor antibiotics are natural products derived from various strains of the soil fungus *Streptomyces*. They are cytotoxic, cell-cycle-phase nonspecific drugs that damage DNA by binding (intercalating) DNA and inhibiting DNA or RNA synthesis.[37] Doxorubicin has been the most frequently used member of this class in veterinary medicine. It has important hematologic, gastrointestinal, and cardiac toxicities. Although signs of gastrointestinal upset, vomiting, and diarrhea can usually be managed symptomatically and supportively, myelosuppression may be a dose-limiting problem in the short term. Cumulative cardiac toxicity results in a dose-related cardiomyopathy. All patients receiving doxorubicin should be evaluated carefully for cardiac disorders before and during the course of treatment. The evaluation of serial endomyocardial biopsies would be an ideal approach but is not practical. The true role of ECGs and echocardiograms is not known, but these procedures might also be helpful. Dosages should be reduced if hepatic damage develops. Doxorubicin must be administered slowly through a free-flowing intravenous line. Patient restlessness, facial swelling, or head shaking may signal excessively rapid administration. If these signs are seen, administration should be stopped temporarily and started at a slower rate when signs abate. Pretreatment with antihistamines may help avoid some of these complications. Despite its apparently numerous drawbacks, doxorubicin has had wide application in the treatment of canine lymphosarcoma as both a first-line and a salvage drug. It has also been used for various carcinomas and sarcomas with limited success.[12, 14, 37, 38]

Hormones. Unlike other chemotherapeutic agents, hormones are not primarily cytotoxic drugs and are therefore less toxic to the patient. Hormonal agents are more selective than cytotoxic drugs in their actions.[42] Peptide hormones interact with cell membrane-bound nucleotide cyclase systems such as those that convert adenosine triphosphate (ATP) to cyclic adenosine monophosphate (cAMP) which acts as a "second messenger" to deliver and amplify regulatory signals to intracellular sites. Steroid hormones enter the cells and bind to a specific receptor protein. "Transformation" ("activation") of this newly formed complex allows it to pass the nuclear membranes, where it binds to DNA. This binding alters the transcription of the cell's messenger RNA, resulting in synthesis of new protein. Steroid-induced increases in free fatty acids may cause dissolution of the nuclear membrane, leading to cell death.[37]

TABLE 59–1. CHEMOTHERAPEUTIC AGENTS USED IN VETERINARY MEDICINE

Name	Brand Name (Manufacturer)	Cell Cycle Specificity*	Possible Indications	Suggested Dosages	Toxicity
Alkylating Agents					
Cyclophosphamide	Cytoxan (Mead Johnson)	CCNS	Lymphoreticular neoplasms, mammary and lung carcinomas, miscellaneous sarcomas	50 mg/m^2 PO or IV 4 days/week	Leukopenia, anemia, thrombocytopenia (less common), nausea, vomiting, sterile hemorrhagic cystitis
Chlorambucil	Leukeran (Burroughs Wellcome)	CCNS	Lymphoreticular neoplasms, chronic lymphocytic leukemia	2 mg/m^2 PO 2 to 4 days/week	Mild leukopenia, thrombocytopenia, anemia, nausea, vomiting (not common)
Nitrogen mustard	Mustragen (Merck Sharp & Dohme)	CCNS	Lymphoreticular neoplasms	5 mg/m^2 IV	Leukopenia, thrombocytopenia, nausea, vomiting, anorexia
Triethylene-thiophos-phoramide	Thio-TEPA (Lederle)	CCNS	Various carcinomas and sarcomas	9 mg/m^2 as a single dose or divided over 2 to 4 days (60 mg in 60 ml water for bladder instillation, 30 minutes/week)	Leukopenia, thrombocytopenia, anemia
Busulfan	Myleran (Burroughs Wellcome)	CCNS	Granulocytic leukemias, myeloproliferative disorders	3 to 4 mg/m^2 PO daily	Leukopenia thrombocytopenia, anemia
Melphalan	Alkeran (Burroughs Wellcome)	CCNS	Multiple myeloma, monoclonal gammopathies, lymphoreticular neoplasms	1.5 mg/m^2 PO for 7 to 10 days, repeat cycle	Leukopenia, thrombocytopenia, anemia, anorexia, nausea, vomiting
Dacarbazine	DTIC (Dome Laboratories)	CCNS	Malignant melanoma, various sarcomas	200 mg/m^2 IV for 5 days every 3 weeks	Leukopenia, thrombocytopenia, anemia, nausea, vomiting, diarrhea (often decreases with later cycles)
Lomustine	CeeNU (Bristol)	CCNS	Various carcinomas, lymphosarcoma	100 mg/m^2 PO every 6 weeks	Leukopenia, thrombocytopenia (both develop in 3 to 6 weeks), nausea, vomiting (transient)
Antimetabolites					
Methotrexate	Methotrexate (Lederle)	S	Lymphoreticular neoplasms, myeloproliferative disorders, various carcinomas and sarcomas	2.5 mg/m^2 PO daily	Leukopenia, thrombocytopenia, anemia, stomatitis, diarrhea, hepatopathy, renal tubular necrosis
6-Mercaptopurine	Purinethol (Burroughs Wellcome)	S	Lymphosarcoma, acute lymphocytic leukemia, granulocytic leukemia	50 mg/m^2 PO daily until response or toxicity	Leukopenia, nausea, vomiting, hepatopathy
5-Fluorouracil	Fluorouracil (Roche Laboratories)	S	Various carcinomas and sarcomas	200 mg/m^2 IV weekly	Leukopenia, thrombocytopenia, anemia, anorexia, nausea, vomiting, diarrhea, stomatitis
	Efudex Cream (Roche Laboratories)		Cutaneous tumors	Apply twice daily for 2 to 4 weeks	
Cytosine arabinoside	Cytosar-U (Upjohn)	S	Lymphosarcoma, myeloproliferative disorders	100 mg/m^2 SQ or IV drip for 4 days	Leukopenia, thrombocytopenia, anemia, nausea, vomiting, anorexia
Plant Alkyloids					
Vincristine	Oncovin (Eli Lilly)	M	Transmissible venereal tumor, lymphosarcoma	0.5 mg/m^2 IV weekly	Peripheral neuropathy, paresthesia, constipation
Vinblastine	Velban (Eli Lilly)	M	Lymphosarcoma, various carcinomas	2.5 mg/m^2 IV weekly	Leukopenia, nausea, vomiting

TABLE 59–1. CHEMOTHERAPEUTIC AGENTS USED IN VETERINARY MEDICINE *Continued*

Name	Brand Name (Manufacturer)	Cell Cycle Specificity*	Possible Indications	Suggested Dosages	Toxicity
Antibiotics					
Doxorubicin	Adriamycin (Adria Laboratories)	CCNS	Lymphosarcoma, osteogenic sarcoma, various carcinomas and sarcomas	30 mg/m² IV every 3 weeks (do not exceed 240 mg/m² total)	Leukopenia, thrombocytopenia, nausea, vomiting, cardiac toxicity, reactions during administration
Actinomycin D	Cosmegen (Merck Sharp & Dohme)	CCNS	Lymphosarcoma, various carcinomas and sarcomas	1.5 mg/m² IV or weekly	Thrombocytopenia, leukopenia, stomatitis, proctitis, nausea, vomiting
Bleomycin	Blenoxane (Bristol Laboratories)	CCNS (G_1, S, and M)	Squamous cell carcinomas, other carcinomas	10 mg/m² IV or SQ for 3 to 9 days, then 10 mg/m² IV weekly (do not exceed 200 mg/m² total)	Allergic reactions following administration, pulmonary fibrosis
Hormones					
Prednisolone		NA	Lymphoreticular neoplasms, mast cell tumors, CNS tumors	Vary widely depending on indication: 60 mg/m² PO daily to 20 mg/m² PO every 48 hours	Hyperadrenocorticism, secondary adrenocortical insufficiency
Diethylstilbestrol		NA	Perianal adenomas prostatic neoplasms (adjunctively)	1.1 mg/kg IM once (do not administer more than 25 mg) or 1 mg PO every 72 hours	Bone marrow toxicity, feminization
Miscellaneous					
L-asparaginase	Elspar (Merck Sharp & Dohme)	NA	Lymphoreticular neoplasms	20,000 units/m² IP or IM weekly	Anaphylaxis, leukopenia
o,p'-DDD	Lysodren (Calibiochem)	NA	Adrenocortical tumors	50 mg/kg PO daily to effect, then 50 mg/kg PO every 7 to 14 days PRN	Adrenocortical insufficiency
cis-Platinol	Platinol (Bristol)	CCNS	Various carcinomas and sarcomas	60–70 mg/m² IV drip q 3–5 weeks; saline diuresis before and after treatment required, do not use in cats	Nausea, vomiting, renal toxicity, bone marrow toxicity

*Notes: CCNS = cell-cycle-phase-nonspecific; S = S phase-specific; M = M phase-specific; NA = not applicable.

Adrenal corticosteroids may also alter the normal intracellular balance between endonucleases and reparative enzymes leading to cell death.[43]

Adrenal corticosteroids have important clinical uses in the therapy of lymphosarcoma and mast cell tumors and may be of benefit in the therapy of central nervous system neoplasms because of their ability to cross the blood-brain barrier. Their beneficial actions in other solid tumors probably relate more to anti-inflammatory effects than to direct antitumor effects.[19]

Sex hormones have been used in the treatment of hormone-dependent tumors of mammary, prostatic, or perianal gland origin. Hormonal therapy may be supplemental or ablative. With increasing availability of estrogen receptor analysis, rational hormonal therapy of mammary gland tumors will become likely. Currently, antiestrogenic therapy remains investigational. Hormones also have a valuable role as replacement therapy following ablative surgery, in the management of some metastatic problems, and in dealing with paraneoplastic syndromes such as hypercalcemia and anemia.[42]

Miscellaneous Agents. A number of other drugs that do not fall easily into any of the previously mentioned categories have also been used to treat animal cancers.

L-asparaginase is an enzyme preparation derived from a variety of bacteria. By hydrolyzing asparagine to aspartic acid and ammonia, L-asparaginase deprives neoplastic cells that lack the ability to synthesize L-asparagine out of extracellular sources, thereby rapidly inhibiting protein synthesis. L-asparaginase acts against cells in the G_1 phase. It has been used in the therapy of canine lymphoreticular neoplasms. Anaphylaxis has been the most dangerous side effect. Other toxicities include gastrointestinal disturbances, hepatotoxicity, hemorrhagic pancreatitis, and coagulation defects.[12, 37, 38] After conjugation with polyethylene glycol, L-asparaginase has a prolonged serum half-life and is less toxic. This form of L-asparaginase (PEG-asparaginase) has been used alone and in combination with other drugs in cases of canine lymphosarcoma.[44, 45]

The cell-cycle nonspecific drug o,p'-DDD directly suppresses both normal and neoplastic adrenocortical cells. With proper management, o,p'-DDD may be beneficial in patients with inoperable adrenocortical carcinoma as well as patients with adrenocortical hyperplasia secondary to a pituitary neoplasm. In addition to careful monitoring for impending hypoadrenocorticism, the clinician must be aware of toxic manifestations, including vomiting, diarrhea, and depression.[38]

Platinum complexes have been shown to have tumoricidal activity; cis-diaminedichloroplatinum (CDDP) is a cell-cycle-phase nonspecific drug that inhibits DNA

TABLE 59–2. CONVERSION TABLE OF WEIGHT IN KILOGRAMS TO BODY SURFACE AREA IN SQUARE METERS FOR DOGS

kg	m²	kg	m²
0.5	0.06	26.0	0.88
1.0	0.10	27.0	0.90
2.0	0.15	28.0	0.92
3.0	0.20	29.0	0.94
4.0	0.25	30.0	0.96
5.0	0.29	31.0	0.99
6.0	0.33	32.0	1.01
7.0	0.36	33.0	1.03
8.0	0.40	34.0	1.05
9.0	0.43	35.0	1.07
10.0	0.46	36.0	1.09
11.0	0.49	37.0	1.11
12.0	0.52	38.0	1.13
13.0	0.55	39.0	1.15
14.0	0.58	40.0	1.17
15.0	0.60	41.0	1.19
16.0	0.63	42.0	1.21
17.0	0.66	43.0	1.23
18.0	0.69	44.0	1.25
19.0	0.71	45.0	1.26
20.0	0.74	46.0	1.28
21.0	0.76	47.0	1.30
22.0	0.78	48.0	1.32
23.0	0.81	49.0	1.34
24.0	0.83	50.0	1.36
25.0	0.85		

synthesis and has some alkylating activity. It has been used in human medicine for testicular, ovarian, and bladder carcinoma; its true indications in veterinary medicine are still being evaluated, but CDDP may be helpful in the therapy of some lung tumors, squamous cell carcinomas, and osteosarcomas.[46–50] It causes nausea and vomiting, which may be severe and prolonged. Renal insufficiency is usually the dose-limiting toxicity, but myelosuppression may also be a problem. CDDP should not be used in cats because of its extreme pulmonary toxicity.[51] CDDP is rapidly finding its way into use in veterinary medicine.

Of the drugs available to treat cancer, it is not clear that the best use of any single drug—let alone the best drug combination or multimodality therapy—has been clearly established for any neoplasm. An understanding of the drugs available for use and their mechanisms, indications, and toxicities helps the clinician to provide rational chemotherapy. The clinician may be able to prognose with some accuracy on several bases. A histologic diagnosis provides a beginning. With that information in hand, knowledge of the biologic behavior of the tumor helps to predict response. The larger the tumor burden, the greater the number of residual tumor cells that will remain after first-order kinetic tumor cell kill along with resistant cells. Larger tumors are also more likely to have more profound metabolic effects on the host that are likely to limit its ability to tolerate chemotherapy. Note that these factors are consistent with the principles and guidelines for therapy previously discussed. The distribution of metastases may also affect response. However, rapidly growing tumors should theoretically be more amenable to chemotherapeutic intervention with S phase-specific drugs. To some extent, clinical parameters are quantitated by staging the tumor. The expanded use of clinical staging protocols undoubtedly contributes valuable information.

Chemotherapy has progressed tremendously in the past 40 years but is still in its infancy in veterinary medicine. An understanding of the biologic and pharmacologic principles underlying chemotherapy, the chemotherapeutic agents, and the potentials and limitations of drug therapy will enhance the delivery of appropriate therapy. The near future will present promising new therapeutic and prognostic options for a very challenging problem for the clinician.

Biologic Therapy

Biologic therapy must be viewed as a broader approach than simple stimulation of the immune system. Immunotherapy is a subcategory of biologic therapy that involves the use of cells or substances of the immune defense system to induce a positive antitumor effect. Biologic therapy can be categorized into the following approaches:[52–54] increase the host antitumor response through augmentation or restoration of effector mechanisms, increase the host defense mechanism by the administration of natural biologics, augment the host antitumor response using modified tumor cells or vac-

TABLE 59–3. CURRENT CLASSIFICATIONS OF BIOLOGIC RESPONSE MODIFIERS

Immunomodulator and/or Immunostimulating Agents
- BCG
- *Corynebacterium parvum*
- Cimetidine
- Levamisole
- Muramyl dipeptide (MDP)
- Muramyl tripeptide (MTP)
- Mixed bacterial vaccines (MBV)
- Picibanil (OK432)
- Prostaglandin inhibitors (aspirin, indomethacin)
- Thiabendazole
- Tilorones
- Tuftsin

Interferons and Interferon Inducers
- Interferons (alpha, beta, gamma)
- Poly ICLC
- Tilorones

Thymosins
- Thymosin alpha-I
- Thymosin fraction 5
- Other thymic fractions

Lymphokines and Cytokines
- Colony-stimulating factor (CSF)
- Interleukin-3 (IL-3)
- Granulocyte-Macrophage-CSF
- Lymphocyte activation factor (LAF–interleukin-1) (IL-1)
- Macrophage activation factor (MAF)
- Macrophage inhibition factor (MIF)
- T-cell growth factor (TCGF–interleukin-2) (IL-2)
- Tumor-necrosis factor (TNF)

Monoclonal Antibodies
- Anti-T cell
- Anti-T-suppressor cell
- Antitumor antibody conjugates (including antibody fragments and/or conjugates with drugs, toxins, and isotypes)

Effector Cells
- Macrophages
- NK cells
- T-cell clones
- T helper cells
- Lymphokine activated T cells (LAK-cells)

Miscellaneous Approaches
- Bone marrow transplantation and reconstitution
- Plasmapheresis and *ex vivo* treatments (activation columns and immunoabsorbents)
- Virus infection of cells (oncolysates)
- Blood constituent therapy (serum factors)

Antigens
- Tumor vaccines

cines, decrease the transformation and/or increase differentiation of tumor cells, and increase the ability of the host to tolerate damage by other cytotoxic modalities such as chemotherapy and radiation.

Table 59–3 lists the current biologic approaches used to treat cancer and has been edited to include those that are of primary importance in veterinary oncology.

TUMOR IMMUNOLOGY

Ample clinical evidence exists that the immune system plays a vital role in the development and progression of many neoplastic conditions. Three major areas of evidence exist to suggest that the host immune defenses against cancer do exist.

Evidence of tumor infiltration with lymphocytes and plasma cells resembling similar infiltrations of organ transplants suggests an antitumor immunologic mechanism. In some situations the presence of infiltrated mononuclear cells is associated with a better prognosis. A recent study of canine mammary carcinoma revealed that dogs with tumors with lymphoid cellular infiltrates had a lower recurrence rate and prolonged survival time after mastectomy.[55] In human beings, high incidences of cancer have been associated with primary and secondary immunodeficiencies. In most cases the immunodeficiencies are associated with an increase in epithelial and lymphoproliferative tumors.[56]

Spontaneous regression of established tumors is rare but well documented in human beings.[57] These observations have been made primarily in patients affected with malignant melanoma, choriocarcinoma, and adenocarcinoma of the kidney. The identification of spontaneous regressions of cancer in veterinary medicine is quite rare.

It is unrealistic to attribute the complex tumor immune system interactions to a function of one cell population. Antitumor activity is the result of interactions among various effector cell populations. Such interaction may be mediated through direct cell-to-cell contact or via biologic substances produced by the effector cells. The important cellular components associated with tumor immunity include killer cells, macrophages, and natural killer cells (NK). Killer cells are believed to be of monocyte-macrophage lineage and destroy target cells that have reacted with antibody. This is referred to as antibody-dependent cellular cytotoxicity (ADCC). Macrophages also play a major role as effectors against tumor cells, but macrophages generally express little cytotoxicity unless activated by lymphokines, bacterial substances, or interferon.[58] Activated macrophages are considered cytotoxic to most tumor cells regardless of their phenotypic expression. The tumor cell destruction by activated macrophages results predominantly from a nonphagocytic, contact-mediated secretion of cytotoxic substances. Tumor necrosis factor (TNF) or cachectin is one substance that may participate in the *in vivo* destruction of tumor cells.[59–60] Other important components associated with macrophage activation are the release of catalytic proteases, superoxide anions, and hydrogen peroxide, all of which are thought to play a role in macrophage-associated cytotoxicity. Another cell that is considered important in tumor cytotoxicity is the natural killer cell, also termed the large granular lymphocyte (LGL). The susceptibility of a target cell to lysis by NK cells depends on the degree of differentiation of the target and its capacity to repair membrane damage. NK activity can be regulated by interferon, stimulated by interleukin-2, and inhibited by PGE.[61] NK activity is probably more pronounced against lymphoreticular tumors than solid tumors.

B cells also play an important role in antitumor activity. An end-differentiated B lymphocyte is called a plasma cell. Plasma cells are very active in antibody production, synthesizing and secreting many thousands of antibody molecules per minute, but the cells live only three to six days. In the initial or primary response to an antigen, IgM is the predominant product; IgG usually predominates in the secondary response. Antibodies may be involved in the direct lysis of tumor cells or in the recruitment of cells carrying Fc receptors, such as NK cells and macrophages. In addition, antibodies may form soluble immune complexes, which may subvert the cellular immune responses.

T-cell immunity is probably most important in tumors expressing strong tumor-associated (specific) antigens. Even though T cells may be quite effective in mediating potent antitumor immunity, they do not appear to play a major role in immune surveillance against malignant cells. T cell activation includes the generation of helper T cells and suppressor T cells, as well as cytotoxic T lymphocytes. Amplification of their response requires interleukins and various lymphokines. The important lymphokines and cytokines are:[61]

1. migration inhibition factor (MIF), which functions to arrest macrophages at the antigenic tumor site,
2. macrophage activating factor (MAF), which is very similar to gamma interferon and will activate the macrophage,
3. lymphotoxins, which lyse tumor cells *in vitro*,
4. transfer factor (TF), which transfers the specific immune response to other lymphocytes,
5. interferons (IFN), which have immunoregulatory and anti-proliferative functions. They may suppress or enhance antibody production, express cell surface antigens, modulate T cell function, and regulate natural killer cell and macrophage function.
6. interleukin-1 (IL-1), which is a macrophage-derived cytokine that can enhance T cell proliferation. IL-1 may also augment the release of B cell growth factor. IL-1 causes fever and stimulates the liver to secrete acute phase proteins.
7. interleukin-2 (IL-2), which amplifies the proliferation of other T cells. IL-2 is produced by T helper cells and helps to generate the T cytotoxic cells. T cytotoxic proliferation is controlled by IL-2.
8. interleukin-3 (IL-3) or colony-stimulating factor, which can stimulate the production of granulocyte-macrophage progenitor cells that help to increase the overall effector cell population necessary for tumor cell control.

BACTERIAL PRODUCTS

Bacterial products exert their major effects on the activation of B and T lymphocytes, natural killer cells, and macrophages. The two most commonly studied biologic agents are *Corynebacterium parvum* and BCG. A recently completed study to evaluate *C. parvum* in dogs with canine oral melanoma evaluted 89 dogs with oral melanoma, all treated with surgery alone and/or *C. parvum*. It was reported that the median survival time was 228 days for those treated by surgery alone versus 370 days for those treated by surgery plus *C. parvum*. These differences in median survival times are only of borderline significance. When dogs with Stage 1 (primary tumor less then 2 cm in diameter) were excluded from the analysis, the median survival time for dogs that had surgery alone was 121 days versus 288 days for the dogs treated by the combined surgery and *C. parvum* therapy. These median survival times were highly significant ($p<0.001$). This study indicates that *C. parvum* had activity in retarding disease progression in dogs with malignant melanoma and further indicates that *C. parvum* may be more effective in the treatment of dogs with advanced oral melanoma.[62]

Studies using the attenuated mycobacterium BCG or BCG cell walls have resulted in some beneficial effects. The BCG cell wall preparations have been used successfully to treat bovine ocular squamous cell carcinoma and equine sarcoids.[63, 64] In a recent study, dogs with malignant mammary tumors were randomly selected to receive intertumoral injections of BCG cell walls four weeks before surgery. Twenty-four dogs were treated with BCG cell walls before surgery and 42 were treated with surgery alone. The mean time of tumor-free survival was significantly extended in the BCG cell wall-treated group.[65] Other studies using BCG components have failed to show any BCG activity in canine osteosarcoma or canine mammary tumors.[66, 67]

Another bacterial product that has been studied over the last few years is *Staphylococcus aureus*. *Staphylococcus aureus* (Staph A) of the Cowan 1 strain contains a cell wall protein called Protein A. Protein A binds to the Fc portion of certain immunoglobulins. Protein A has been used to absorb immunoglobulins and immune complexes extracorporeally from the plasma of tumor-bearing animals.[68] The removal of these immune complexes, or so-called blocking factors, has been associated with antitumor activity. Presumably the removal of the immune complexes allows for immunologic modulation, but the exact mechanism of action has not been totally determined. Recently, a study was reported using intravenous Protein A in cats with lymphoma and leukemia.[69] Fifteen FeLV infected cats, nine with lymphosarcoma and six with leukemia, were treated. Three of six with leukemia had a partial response, one of eight with lymphosarcoma had a partial response. None of the cats converted to FeLV-negative. Other studies of canine mammary adenocarcinoma have shown that the extracorporeal immunoabsorption of plasma over Staph A (with Protein A) has resulted in tumoricidal activity.[70, 71] The mechanism of this tumor activity may include removal of the immune complexes, but other effects could include activation of plasma factors such as complement or the release into the plasma of bacterial products that may have further immunomodulatory activity.[72]

A major drawback to the further study of these bacterial agents is the lack of chemical definition and the inability to produce a pure pharmacologic product. One peptide that has been purified and extracted from the BCG cell wall has been termed muramyl dipeptide (MDP). In experimental models MDP and its more lipophilic analogue (MTP) have been shown to increase the immune response against viruses, bacteria, parasites, and vaccines.[73] In addition, antitumor activity of MDP has been observed in a variety of experimental models.[74] Due to the small molecular weight of the muramyl peptides, a unique drug delivery system has been used to decrease drug excretion, increase half-life, and enhance delivery to the macrophages. The system used consists of microscopic phospholipids called liposomes. The MTP is encapsulated within the lipid bilayers of the vesicle and these microscopic vesicles can then be injected intravenously into a recipient animal. The liposomes are phagocytized by the monocytes and distributed to organs including the lung, liver, spleen, and lymph nodes. Once phagocytized, the liposome is digested and the active drug released into the cell. The rationale is to deliver MTP directly to the monocyte-macrophage lineage that results in their activation and enhanced cytotoxicity.[73, 75]

Another bacterial product which has been studied is a mixture of *Serratia marcescens* and *S. pyogenes*.[76] This combination has been termed a mixed bacterial vaccine (MBV). Antitumor activity in dogs and cats has been documented, although the responses are few in number. In addition significant effects in causing regression of eosinophilic granuloma in cats have been reported.[77] These studies reported on 42 cats with MBV therapy. Eight of these cats had a primary untreated eosinophilic granuloma and 34 of these were considered recurrent granulomas after failing corticosteroid therapy. Of the 42 cats treated, 16 had a complete regression of disease and 13 had a partial regression (at least a 50 per cent regression). The overall response rate, complete response plus partial response for the 33 evaluable cases, was 87 per cent. These results give further stimulus to the use of biologic bacterial agents for both neoplastic and non-neoplastic diseases.

CHEMICAL IMMUNOMODULATORS

Several chemically defined nonspecific immune stimulants are currently under study. The drug that has received the most attention is levamisole. Levamisole has been shown to modulate T-cell function and also to restore delayed cutaneous hypersensitivity reactions in immunosuppressed cancer patients.[78] Clinical trials in human patients using levamisole in combination with other therapies have yielded mixed results.[79–81] Positive effects have been seen in non-oat cell lung carcinoma and colon carcinoma in humans. The drug also stimulates increased phagocytic activity in macrophages.[82] Three prospective, randomized, double-blind clinical trials to evaluate levamisole in treating canine and feline mammary tumors and canine lymphosarcoma have recently been reported.[83–85] Using a total of 306 animals in these trials, these studies were unable to demonstrate any beneficial effect on disease-free interval or survival time when levamisole was combined with surgery (for mammary tumors) or combination chemotherapy (for lymphosarcoma).

Other chemical agents that have immunomodulatory activity are the H_2 blockers cimetidine and ranitidine. Human patients receiving cimetidine exhibit enhanced cell-mediated immunity, as evaluated by increased response to skin test antigens and restoration of sensitivity following development of acquired tolerance to haptens such as 1-chloro-2,4-dinitrobenzene (DNCB). Although the mechanisms of this enhancement have not clearly been defined, most studies suggest that cimetidine functions by inhibiting suppressor cell activity.[86] It has been suggested that suppressor cell activity may be mediated through the release of a soluble factor induced by histamine.[87] Knowledge of the potential of the H_2 antagonists as biologic response modifiers awaits further *in vitro* and *in vivo* study.

TUMOR CELL VACCINES

Tumor cell vaccines are used to enhance specific mechanisms associated with the antitumor response. Modified cancer vaccines potentially offer means whereby the immunogenicity of tumor cells may be artificially enhanced for use in active immunization protocols.

In veterinary oncology, tumor cell vaccines have been used in combination with chemotherapy to treat canine lymphosarcoma,[88] and more recently, the intralymphatic administration of tumor cell vaccines has been used to treat dogs with lymphosarcoma after they have been placed in remission by means of combination chemotherapy.[89]

A major limitation of vaccine therapy is the source, availability, and preparation of the tumor antigens. The present vaccines require viable but nontumorigenic cells prepared from individual donors.

The use of modified tumor cell vaccines in canine lymphosarcoma has been shown to correlate with the production of antibodies against supposed lymphosarcoma antigens. Researchers have found that some dogs undergoing intralymphatic vaccination develop high concentrations of antibodies and have the longest survival times.[90]

LYMPHOKINES AND CYTOKINES

Many of the specific biologics potentially available for therapy are cell products of lymphocytes (lymphokines) or of cells in general (cytokines). The lymphokines can modulate both T and B cell function, which can also alter tumor growth and metastasis. Several of these lymphokines, such as lymphotoxins, interleukin-1 and 2, macrophage-activating factor, and tumor necrosis factor, are under study for potential antitumor activity. As recombinant DNA technology becomes more available and these cytokines and lymphokines are manufactured in larger quantities, veterinary oncologists will have the opportunity to study these for potential therapeutic usefulness.

One group of substances that has received quite extensive study in human oncology, and to a very limited degree in veterinary oncology, is the interferons. The interferons are a family of proteins produced by a number of cells with different origins. Type 1 (alpha and beta) interferons are produced by leukocytes and fibroblasts, respectively. Type 2 (gamma) interferon is produced by lymphocytes and macrophages. Each interferon type has distinctive capabilities and alters a variety of immunologic and other biologic responses. Interferons can be directly cytotoxic or have secondary immunostimulatory effects. The critical mechanisms operative at the cellular level are unclear, but they may be mediated by the same inhibitors of DNA and RNA synthesis that occur in virus-infected cells. Cell cycle analysis has shown that interferon causes extension of all phases of cell cycle and prolongation of overall cell generation time.[91]

In vitro studies have shown that the immunomodulatory effects of interferon predominantly involve the potentiation of NK cells and increased cytotoxic activity of activated monocytes.[92] Macrophage-activating factor and gamma interferon appear to be identical. These substances act to increase the number and density of Fc receptors, which in turn are associated with an increase in antigen-presenting function. Enhancement of phagocytosis, as well as antiviral and bactericidal activity and antitumor cytotoxicity, occurs.

The antitumor activity of interferon has been demonstrated in human patients with hematologic, breast, renal, and head and neck cancers, but the best responses have been seen in a variety of lymphomas.[93] The future of interferon therapy in animals probably depends on the availability of genetically produced recombinant DNA interferon. Interferons tend to be species-specific; however, studies are under way using hybrid forms of alpha interferon produced from both human and bovine leukocytes to treat neoplasms in domestic animals.

MONOCLONAL ANTIBODIES

Antibody therapy for cancer in animal tumor models and in humans is considered one of the new approaches under the broad category of biologic response modifiers. Monoclonal antibody therapy may be effective when used alone for antibody-mediated, complement-dependent cytotoxicity or when conjugated with drugs, toxins, or radioisotopes.[94] A problem with monoclonal antibody therapy is the emergence of malignant clones that phenotypically lack the relevant antigen against which the monoclonal antibody has been produced.

Conjugation of immunoglobulin with drugs, toxins, or radioisotopes could circumvent requirements for host participation in antibody-mediated tumor cell killing. In theory, antibodies could serve as magic bullets to carry toxic moieties directly to the tumor and minimize systemic toxicity. In practice, a relatively small fraction of radionuclide or immunotoxin conjugates has localized to tumor transplants. Potential problems include stability of the conjugates, nonspecific uptake by the reticuloendothelial system, premature renal clearance, prolonged circulation in the peripheral vascular compartment, inaccessibility of antigenic determinants within tumor cells, and permeability of tumor vasculation. Monoclonal antibodies have been effective in ridding the bone marrow of malignant cells. This approach has been especially useful in patients undergoing autologous bone marrow transplantation. The selective monoclonal antibodies have been used outside the body to lyse marrow-contaminating malignant cells prior to the reinfusion of that marrow.[95]

SERUM FACTORS

Serum components have been shown to have antileukemic activity in mice, cats, and dogs.[96-99] Serum components studied have been normal serum, plasma, whole blood, and plasma cryoprecipitate. One dog with acute lymphoblastic leukemia remained in complete remission for 19 months after two months of plasma therapy.[99] The occasional, but well documented, remissions in human leukemia patients after transfusion of normal blood or plasma might represent the human counterpart of this phenomenon. A heparin precipitate from plasma that has antileukemic activity in mice bears resemblance to a fraction of plasma called cold-insoluble globulin (CIG) or fibronectin. Fibronectin is a major glycoprotein found in the blood and tissues and has been shown to enhance macrophage-mediated tumoricidal activity and stimulate T-cell blastogenesis.[100, 101] Fibronectin has also been shown to decrease metastasis in a murine melanoma model.[102]

The authors have been studying the effect of fibronectin in both canine and feline leukemia and lymphoma. Complete responses in a small number of cats undergoing infusions with freshly prepared fibronectin have been documented. The mechanism of antitumor activity is not understood. Further studies are warranted to evaluate the antitumor effects of purified fibronectin as a treatment for leukemia or lymphoma in cats.

FUTURE PERSPECTIVES

Biologic therapy has great potential in the area of cancer treatment. Extirpation by surgery, sterilization by radiation therapy, and cytotoxicity by chemotherapy are the major modalities of cancer treatment today. The manipulation or augmentation of the immune system offers new opportunities for cancer control. The availability of new, genetically engineered biologics and refined bacterial pharmaceuticals is increasing the clinician's armamentarium of possible approaches. Much of the success of biologic therapy has been documented in experimental animal models and *in vitro* immunologic assays. In general, many clinical trials in human and spontaneous animal tumors have yielded inconsistent results. Practically speaking, most approaches using biologic therapy must be considered to be investigational. Ongoing clinical trials in veterinary oncology will help to determine the efficacy of various biologics used to treat cancer. Until these results are published, caution must be exercised in using these agents in the clinical setting.

Radiation Therapy

Radiation therapy is another of the established treatment modalities. Because of the high cost of the equipment and the highly technical nature of its use, radiation therapy is largely restricted to the referral setting.

BIOLOGIC CONSIDERATIONS

Ionizing radiation used in radiation therapy comes from either x-rays or gamma rays. X-rays are produced in the electron shells surrounding an atomic nucleus; gamma rays are generated as unstable radioactive elements decay to a stable state. Otherwise, these energy sources are physically and biologically similar.[103] In tissue exposed to radiation, the energy from the source ionizes molecules in cytoplasmic and nuclear components. Although the physical, physiochemical, and chemical events occur within 10^{-6} seconds, the biologic consequences occur over, and last for, a period of years.[104] The most critical cellular component affected is DNA. The irradiated cell with damaged DNA dies because it is unable to complete mitosis successfully. Therefore, it is clear that tissues with a large fraction of rapidly cycling cells will be more likely to show an effect soon after radiation. However, this does not mean that slowly proliferating cells are spared, but rather that a longer time is necessary to appreciate the damage. These concepts have important implications for the evaluation of toxicity and treatment planning. Several terms require clarification. Radiosensitivity refers to the degree to which cells (normal or neoplastic) are damaged by ionizing radiation. It is influenced by the cells' mitotic rate, their potential for further mitoses, and their degree of differentiation. Other factors influencing the radiosensitivity of a tumor are its size and cell type, the presence of concurrent infection, and the patient's overall condition. The term radioresponsiveness has been used with much the same meaning but refers more correctly to the relative time until visible structural or functional changes occur. Radioresponsiveness is measured by clinical criteria. The term radiocurability refers to the ability of radiation to reduce the number of neoplastic cells to a critical mass that has no further clinical impact during the patient's life.[105] Just as chemotherapy is limited by toxicity, radiation therapy is limited by the response of normal tissue in the irradiated field.

Tissues that are undergoing constant renewal, such as gastrointestinal epithelium, the hair coat, and bone marrow, are likely sites of acute toxicity to the extent that they are included in the radiation field. Mucositis, alopecia, and myelosuppression are expected responses. Mucositis and myelosuppression are generally transient at the usual doses employed in radiation therapy; alopecia persists due to damaging effects of radiation on the more slowly proliferating elements of the skin, such as the microvasculature and connective tissue. These tissues and bone tissue are dose-limiting in that, unlike more rapidly proliferating tissues, they regenerate slowly and are likely to demonstrate necrosis rather than repair. Necrosis is an unacceptable consequence of therapy and is, therefore, dose-limiting.

In theory, the use of fractionated radiation therapy offers a differential advantage to normal cells over neoplastic cells. In veterinary practice, most protocols call for ten fractions delivered on a three-times-a-week basis for practical reasons. Four factors that determine the response of both normal and tumor tissues to repeated radiation exposure are reoxygenation, repopulation, redistribution, and repair. Hypoxic tissue is relatively radioresistant. Because the vasculature in tumors is sinusoidal, there are areas of the tumor that are too far from an adequate blood supply to be fully nourished but are not frankly necrotic. Such areas represent hypoxic sanctuaries from radiation. If as little as one per cent of a tumor is persistently hypoxic, the tumor will probably not be curable by radiation at or below doses tolerated by normal tissues.[103] Since well-oxygenated cells die following radiation, previously hypoxic cells may become better vascularized and better oxygenated. After reoxygenation, those cells are more susceptible to subsequent radiation. The improved nutritional status of some tumor cells may herald accelerated growth. This cellular regeneration or repopulation probably occurs to the same extent in normal and neoplastic tissues and does not offer any real advantage in planning fractionated radiation therapy. Similarly, exposed surviving cells may become synchronized in their phase of the cell cycle, probably due to the elimination of most of the cells in M phase and the blockade of other cells' normal progression. The synchrony (called redistribution) is transient, and as yet it has not been possible to take practical advantage of redistribution in planning fractionated radiation therapy. Repair mechanisms apply to both normal and neoplastic tissue and have not been employed to gain therapeutic advantage. Of these four theoretical responses, it appears that only reoxygenation provides any increase in the relative radiosensitivity of neoplastic cells.

In addition to external beam radiation, other means of delivery are available. Interstitial brachytherapy delivers radiation from a radioisotope (cobalt-60, cesium-137, gold-198, iridium-192, or iodine-125) sealed in a metallic container in the form of a seed, needle, or applicator. This approach allows the clinician to maximize the dose delivered to the tumor while limiting the dose to surrounding normal tissue. Negative aspects include potential exposure of both medical personnel and owners, as well as the need for isolation facilities in the hospital. Systemic radiotherapy with oral or injectable radionuclides is another means of delivering radiation. Iodine-131 has been used for the treatment of thyroid neoplasia in dogs and cats.[106, 107] These methods are used less frequently than external beam radiation.

Different organs and tissues have different inherent tolerances to radiation. Gonads, lymphoid tissue, and bone marrow are extremely radiosensitive and, in general, proliferating cells are more sensitive than end-differentiated tissues. Among normal tissues, there may be as much as a 20-fold difference in radiosensitivity. Neoplastic and normal tissues, however, overlap in many instances in their radiosensitivity, thus complicating the administration of radiation therapy and underlining the importance of the factors discussed above.[108]

PRACTICAL CONSIDERATIONS

As with chemotherapy, the success of radiation therapy is limited by its attendant toxicity. Side effects may be acceptable or unacceptable. Acceptable side effects are generally related to renewing tissues and are frequently seen during or shortly following therapy. Acceptable side effects include mucositis and moist desquamation. These problems resolve with time because some stem cells remain following therapy. Supportive measures such as gentle cleaning and the application of mild ointments may be helpful during the 10 to 14 days required for healing in most cases. Myelosuppression may occur if a large field including bone marrow is radiated. If these complications are anticipated, the hemogram should be monitored and treatment delayed if necessary. Hair loss will probably be permanent, but hair may regrow in a different color. Because they neither threaten life nor materially diminish the quality of life, these effects should be acceptable to most owners. However, they may be considered so objectionable by some that therapy is declined.

In tissues that are not undergoing constant renewal, side effects may not be noted for months to years after therapy is completed. Muscles, bones, and nerves are potentially affected with late necrosis, fibrosis, and nonhealing ulcerations, which are unacceptable side effects. The incidence of late complications is directly related to the dose per fraction; however, decreasing the dose per fraction and increasing the number of fractions is not always practical in veterinary medicine due to the usual requirement for hospitalization and repeated sedation or anesthesia. This dilemma may be resolved by the use of radioprotectors or radiosensitizers.[109]

Cancer therapy requires the understanding and cooperation of the owner in every instance. It is vital that there be a clear understanding of the expected and likely outcome. The histologic type of the tumor is not the only factor governing response. In addition, it is necessary to consider the site of the tumor as well as the extent of the disease, including the presence of metastases and the overall condition of the patient. Following radiation therapy, there may be marked or minimal response noted in the tumor size. A neoplasm may be responsive but change little in size if there is either slow proliferation or a large amount of stromal support. The primary goal of radiation therapy is to stop continued growth of the tumor while preserving normal tissue function. Failure should be defined on the basis of regrowth of a tumor that initially decreased in size or disappeared rather than on the fact that a tumor did not shrink at all or disappear.[110]

It is generally agreed that perianal adenomas, perianal adenocarcinomas, squamous cell carcinomas, acanthomatous epulis of periodontal origin, mast cell tumors, and transmissible tumors are radioresponsive, but quantitating that response precisely has been difficult. This is due in part to the various ways in which response data have been reported and in part to the variation in protocols used as well as the inherent variability of individual tumors within histologic types. See Table 59–4 for a summary of responses to radiation therapy. As suggested by the table, each tumor type may need to be considered different at each anatomic site.[103, 105, 110, 114] It is clear there is wide variation and that there are many factors to be considered with each tumor type. Consult the discussion of each type individually.

TABLE 59–4. RADIATION THERAPY RESPONSE

Tumor Type	Location	Response to Radiation Therapy	Reference
Acanthomatous	epulis	good	110
Epithelial tumors	nasal	<50%	112
		0–90%	111
	adenocarcinoma	12 months	113
	undifferentiated carcinoma	6 months	113
Fibrosarcoma	general	10–50%	112
		0–50%	111
	oral	<10%	112
		poor	110
	nasal	fair–good	110
Hemangiopericytoma		fair–good	114
Malignant melanoma	oral	fair–good	110
Mast cell tumors		40–60%	112
		50–90%	111
		variable	110
Perianal gland adenoma		70%	112
		70–100%	111
		good	110
Perianal gland adenocarcinoma		50%	112
		0–70%	111
Sarcomas	nasal	11 months	113
Squamous cell carcinoma	general	30–70%	112
		30–90%	111
	nasal plane	<10%	112
		poor	110
	nasal cavity	fair–good	110
		6 months	113
	tonsil	poor	110
	sublingual	fair	110
Tooth-germ neoplasms		>70%	112
		50–100%	111
Transmissible venereal tumor		>90%	112
		90–100%	111
		excellent	110

110: Thrall and Dewhirst, 1986.
111: Feeney and Johnston, 1983. Probability of cure.
112: Feeney, 1982. Two-year radiocurability rates.
113: Adams et al., 1987. Median survival time.
114: Evans, 1987.

Hyperthermia

Hyperthermia is the newest therapeutic option to find application in veterinary medicine, although it, like biologic response modification, must still be considered experimental when compared to the established modalities of surgery, radiation therapy, and chemotherapy. Despite its recent and relatively limited use in animal patients, hyperthermia has a long history. More than 90 years ago the observation of spontaneous regression of tumors in febrile patients stimulated the investigation of hyperthermia induced by the injection of infectious agents and bacterial toxins.

BIOLOGIC CONSIDERATIONS

Since those early observations were made, much has been learned about the delivery and effects of heat on normal and neoplastic tissues, but the exact mechanism of killing is still not known with certainty. At temperatures above 45°C, cells are destroyed nonselectively due to protein denaturation and coagulation. Heat has some selective lethal effect on tumor cells between 41° and 45°C. Proposed mechanisms of cell killing at 41° to 45°C include various effects on cell respiration, lysosomes, nucleic acid synthesis, and cell membranes. The effect of hypoxia on tumor cells is an important consideration in hyperthermia as well. Heating depresses oxidative metabolism without altering anaerobic pathways. This relative metabolic shift results in the accumulation of lactic acid and a subsequent lowering of cellular pH. At increased temperatures, lysosomes become more labile than normal. Lysosomal activity is further enhanced by low pH. Together, these effects may contribute to hyperthermic cell killing. Heat-induced depression of RNA and DNA synthesis is not directly lethal to tumor cells, but interference with these processes ultimately inhibits the proliferative capability and growth of the tumor. Finally, effects on the permeability, fluidity, and overall function of the plasma and nuclear membranes may result in cell death. The impact of these mechanisms is probably accentuated in tumor cells that are hypoxic and have a low pH compared to normal cells. Compounding these effects are other vascular factors. The sinusoidal nature of tumor vasculature provides a less efficient cooling mechanism than does the capillary network of normal tissues. Temperatures greater than 41°C further inhibit physiologic cooling by causing collapse and destruction of the tumor microcirculation. With the destruction of neoplastic cells, immunologic responses may come into play and further the process.[115, 116]

Temperature alone is not the only factor to be considered in the application of hyperthermia. The time of exposure to heat is also critical. In general, the higher the temperature, the shorter the time required to achieve a given effect, but there are limits imposed by the ability of normal tissues to withstand heating.[116] In addition, scheduling and protocol design must take into account the phenomenon of thermotolerance, and heat-induced increase in heat resistance. Since thermotolerance subsides within 72 hours after the application of heat, treatments should be scheduled at least three days apart.[118]

Heat can be applied in a systemic, regional, or localized manner. Systems for generating heat include ultrasound, microwaves, radiofrequency waves, hot water blankets, and radiant heat devices.[115, 118] There is also the potential for the application of heating techniques for marrow purging outside the body in conjunction with autologous bone marrow transplantation.[119] Each system has its proponents and advantages, but the means of application are complex and specific. Currently the clinical application of hyperthermic techniques is almost entirely limited to institutional practices, but practitioners should be aware of its availability and are advised to consult clinical oncologists regarding its availability and applicability in individual situations. It appears that hyperthermia is most effective when combined with other modalities, such as chemotherapy and/or radiation therapy. However, many questions remain to be resolved. There is a considerable body of work currently being generated at several veterinary schools in the area of whole body hyperthermia using radiant heat. This work should help answer many questions regarding the best application of hyperthermia in the adjunct setting.[118, 120–124]

Multimodality Therapy

Surgery was the first cancer therapy and cancer surgery is referred to in Egyptian documents over 3500 years old.[125] Radiation therapy and chemotherapy are much younger. Although some drugs have been used for almost two thousand years, modern chemotherapy began only after the toxic effects of nitrogen mustard gas on the bone marrow were noted in World War I. Since that time, scores of new chemotherapeutic agents have been developed and used. The use of radiation therapy has a much shorter history. The first report of a cure by radiation appeared in 1899.[126] It was also about this time that the first scientific considerations were given to the use of heat as a therapeutic modality, although the application of radiation has eclipsed hyperthermia until very recently. Biologic response modification has been an attractive concept since modern ideas about the immune system began to develop. Only very recently, however, have the techniques of molecular biology opened the door to specific interventions.[127] Most veterinarians will continue to be concerned primarily with questions regarding the best ways to use surgery and chemotherapy together and, to a lesser extent, radiation, hyperthermia, and biologic response modification. Surgery and radiation are considered local treatments; chemotherapy and biologic response modification are systemic. Hyperthermia may be either local or systemic. Surgical excision remains the most widely recommended therapy for most tumors in pets, but chemotherapy and other modalities are finding wider application in both the primary and adjunctive settings.

The classic approach has been to use only one local therapy, usually surgery but sometimes radiation, first. The patient was then observed until the disease recurred. At the time of relapse, chemotherapy might have been attempted. This approach, of course, lessened the likelihood of a good response to drug therapy because of the late and recurrent nature of the disease. Now it is common practice to plan adjuvant chemotherapy as part of the initial treatment. While local therapy is still very important in reducing the total tumor burden by removing or reducing the bulk of the primary tumor, the known biologic behavior of many of the commonly encountered tumors indicates that cure is not attained by these means. It is here that chemotherapy, planned and conducted in conjunction with other therapies, is likely to be most beneficial. When applied to the very much smaller tumor burdens left after surgery, this therapy may have a better chance of being effective. Whether adjunctive chemotherapy will bring about a cure seems to depend at least in part on the metastatic burden at the time of the primary therapy.[128]

Another means of combining modalities is neoadjuvant chemotherapy, the use of drugs before the definitive treatment (surgery or radiation) for the primary tumor. As with adjuvant chemotherapy, the prospects for "cure" seem to vary with the metastatic burden at the time therapy is undertaken, but there are some advantages to the neoadjuvant approach. By moving chemotherapy "up front," it may be possible to reduce the size of the surgical or radiation field even if the chemotherapy is not itself curative. Noncurative cytoreduction (by surgery or radiation) leads to increased proliferation, which in turn leads to increased resistance, increased shedding of tumor cells, and increased protection of tumor cells in sanctuaries. Neoadjuvant chemotherapy should help diminish these problems. Also, early chemotherapy may have an effect on undetected micrometastatic disease, which theoretically is kept somewhat in check by a suppressive effect from the primary tumor.[129, 130] Some implications for surgery are obvious; any significant decrease in the size of the primary will make the surgical procedure easier and less deforming. In addition, even if tumor cells are dislodged at the time of surgery, they may have been sterilized by chemotherapy and therefore be less likely to cause spread of the disease by direct implantation. The smaller the tumor burden at the time of surgery, the less the chance that disseminated intravascular coagulation will be a problem. Neoadjuvant chemotherapy is not without its potential disadvantages. There is always the possibility that the tumor will be totally unresponsive to the chosen drugs. In that case, the patient will have had suffered unwarranted toxicity, immunosuppression, and delay in other, more effective therapy.

The concepts of combined or multimodality therapy

are still relatively new to veterinary medicine. More thought should be given to planning the entire course of cancer treatment in order to present a client with a fully developed plan that includes whatever modalities might benefit the patient. It is worthwhile, then, to have in mind the indications for and problems with various combinations of surgery, radiation, and chemotherapy. In general, in combined modality treatments, chemotherapy and biologic therapy can be considered useful to combat micrometastatic disease, radiation to sterilize local or regional disease, and surgery to remove the gross tumor. The true role of either local or systemic hyperthermia is not known yet but most likely lies in an adjunct setting. Probably the most common combination considered presently is surgery followed by chemotherapy. Local treatment rids the patient of the primary tumor, and chemotherapy eliminates the micrometastatic burden. For diseases known not to be cured by surgery alone, the consideration of postoperative drugs is an attractive one but has not been fully evaluated. Tumors that might benefit from such therapy (but have not yet been proven to do so) include gastrointestinal tumors, hemangiosarcomas, malignant mammary tumors, some malignant melanomas, soft tissue sarcomas, squamous cell carcinomas, and thyroid carcinomas. In any case, adjuvant chemotherapy should not be undertaken unless there is some evidence that the tumor being treated is at least somewhat responsive to the drug or drugs used. A significant problem is evaluation of the efficacy of adjunctive treatment. If surgery were curative, unnecessary therapy would appear to have been beneficial, the owner would have assumed unwarranted expense, and the patient would have suffered unnecessary toxicity. In addition, there has been much concern about the effects of chemotherapy on wound healing. Although in experimental situations some chemotherapeutic drugs can affect some phases of healing, the clinical effects are minimal.[131, 132] Consultation with veterinary oncologists regarding complex multimodality treatment plans will help the practitioner provide the best care for animal cancer patients.

References

1. Owen, LN (ed), TNM: Classification of Tumors in Domestic Animals. WHO, Geneva, 1981.
2. Nyland, TG and Kantrowitz, BM: Ultrasound in diagnosis and staging of abdominal neoplasia. *In* Gorman, NT (ed): Oncology—Contemporary Issues in Small Animal Practice. New York, Churchill Livingstone, 1986, p 1.
3. Kantrowitz, BM, et al.: Adrenal ultrasonography in the dog: detection of tumors and hyperplasia in hyperadrenocorticism. Vet Radiol 27(2), 1987, in press.
4. Nyland, TG: Ultrasonic patterns of cancer hepatic lymphosarcoma. Vet Radiol 25:167, 1984.
5. Feeney, DA, et al.: Two-dimensional gray-scale ultrasonography for assessment of hepatic and splenic neoplasia in the dog and cat. JAVMA 184:68, 1984.
6. Konde, LJ, et al.: Sonographic appearance of renal neoplasia in the dog. Vet Radiol 26:74, 1985.
7. Hager, DA, et al.: Ultrasound-guided biopsy of the canine liver, kidney, and prostrate. Vet Radiol 26:82, 1985.
8. Withrow, SJ and Lowes, N: Biopsy techniques for use in small animal oncology. JAAHA 17:889, 1981.
9. Harvey, HJ: General principles of veterinary oncologic surgery. JAAHA 12:335, 1976.
10. Silberman, AW: Surgical debulking of tumors. Surg Gynecol Obstet 155:577, 1982.
11. Rosenberg, SA: Principles of surgical oncology. *In* Devita, VT Jr, et al. (eds): Cancer: Principles and Practice of Oncology, 2nd ed. Philadelphia, JB Lippincott, 1982, p 215.
12. Madewell, BR and Theilen, GH: Chemotherapy. *In* Theilen, GH, and Madewell, BR (eds): Veterinary Cancer Medicine. Philadelphia, Lea & Febiger, 1987.
13. Haskell, CM: Principles of cancer chemotherapy. *In* Haskell, CM (ed): Cancer Treatment. Philadelphia, WB Saunders, 1980.
14. Hess, PW, et al.: Chemotherapy of canine and feline tumors. JAAHA 12:350, 1976.
15. Schabel, FM: The use of tumor growth kinetics in planning "curative" chemotherapy of advanced solid tumors. Cancer Res 29:2384, 1969.
16. Yoxall, AT and Hind, JER (eds.): Veterinary applications of the pharmacology of neoplasia. *In* Pharmacological Basis of Small Animal Medicine. London, Blackwell Scientific Publications, 1975.
17. Pierce, GB and Fennell, RH, Jr: Pathology. *In* Holland, JF and Frei, E, III (eds): Cancer Medicine, 2nd ed. Philadelphia, Lea & Febiger, 1982.
18. Goldie, JN and Coldman, AJ: A mathematic model for relating the drug sensitivity of tumors to their spontaneous mutation rate. Can Trt Rep 63(11):1727, 1979.
19. Rosenthal, RC and Wilcke, JR: Glucocorticoid therapy. *In* Kirk, RW (ed): Current Veterinary Therapy VIII. Philadelphia, WB Saunders, 1983, p 854.
20. Couto, CG: Toxicity of anticancer chemotherapy. Proc Kal Kan Symposium 10:37, 1987.
21. MacEwen, EG: Cancer chemotherapy. *In* Kirk, RW (ed): Current Veterinary Therapy VII. Philadelphia, WB Saunders, 1980.
22. Harris, JB: Nausea, vomiting and cancer treatment. CA 28:194, 1977.
23. Giger, U and Gorman, NT: Acute complications of cancer and cancer therapy. *In* Gorman, NT (ed.): Oncology. New York, Churchill Livingstone, 1986, p 147.
24. Hess, PW: Principles of cancer chemotherapy. Vet Clin N Am 7:21, 1977.
25. Crow, SE, et al.: Cyclophosphamide-induced cystitis in the dog and cat. JAVMA 171:259, 1977.
26. Cotter, SM, et al.: Renal disease in five tumor-bearing cats treated with Adriamycin. JAAHA 21(3):405, 1985.
27. Conroy, JD: The etiology and pathogenesis of alopecia. Comp Cont Ed 1:806, 1979.
28. Bennett, WM, et al.: Guidelines for drug therapy in renal failure. Ann Intern Med 86:754, 1977.
29. Chabner, BA: The role of drugs in cancer treatment. *In* Chabner, BA (ed): Pharmacologic Principles of Cancer Treatment. Philadelphia, WB Saunders, 1982.
30. Carter, SK and Livingston, RB: Principles of cancer chemotherapy. *In* Carter, SK, et al. (eds): Principles of Cancer Treatment. New York, McGraw-Hill, 1981, p 95.
31. Rosenthal, RC: Chemotherapy. *In* Slatter, DH (ed): Textbook of Small Animal Surgery. Philadelphia, WB Saunders, 1985, p 2405.
32. Damon, LE and Cadman, EC: Advances in rational chemotherapy. Cancer Invest 4(5):421, 1986.
33. Freireich, EJ, et al.: Quantitative comparison of toxicity of anticancer agents in mouse, rat, hamster, dog monkey, and man. Can Chemo Rep 50(4):219, 1966.
34. Henness, AM, et al.: Use of drugs based on square meters of body surface area. JAVMA 171:1076, 1977.
35. Vriesendorp, HM: Optimal prescription method for cancer chemotherapy. Exp Hematol (suppl. 16) 13:57, 1985.
36. Page, RL, et al.: Unexpected toxicity associated with the use of body surface area for dosing melphalan in the log. Cancer Res 48:288, 1988.
37. Haskell, CM: Drugs used in cancer chemotherapy. *In* Haskell, CM (ed): Cancer Treatment. Philadelphia, WB Saunders, 1980.
38. Carter, SK and Livingston, RB: Drugs available to treat cancer. *In* Carter, SK, et al. (eds.): Principles of Cancer Treatment. New York, McGraw-Hill, 1981, p 111.
39. Weller, RE: Intravesical instillation of dilute formalin for treat-

ment of cyclophosphamide-induced hemorrhagic cystitis in two dogs. JAVMA 172:1206, 1978.
40. Calvert, CA, et al.: Vincristine for treatment of transmissible veneral tumor. JAVMA 181:163, 1982.
41. Rosenthal, RC: Clinical applications of vinca alkaloids. JAVMA 179:1084, 1981.
42. Rosenthal, RC: Hormones in cancer therapy. Vet Clin North Am 12:67, 1982.
43. Wielckens, K, et al.: Glucocorticoid-induced lymphoma cell death: The good and the evil. J Steroid Biochem 27:413, 1987.
44. MacEwen, EG, et al.: A preliminary study on the evaluation of asparaginase:polyethylene glycol conjugate against canine malignant lymphoma. Cancer 59:2011, 1987.
45. MacEwen, EG, et al.: PEG-asparaginase therapy of canine lymphosarcoma; preliminary results. Proc Vet Can Soc 7:40, 1987.
46. Himsel, CA, et al.: Cisplatin chemotherapy for metastatic squamous cell carcinoma in two dogs. JAVMA 189(12):1575, 1896.
47. Mehlaff, CJ, et al.: Surgical treatment of primary pulmonary neoplasia in 15 dogs. JAAHA 20(5):799, 1984.
48. Knapp, DW, et al.: Cisplatin therapy in 41 dogs with malignant tumors. J Vet Int Med 2:41, 1988.
49. Shapiro, W, et al.: Use of cisplatin for treatment of appendicular osteosarcoma in dogs. JAVMA 192:507, 1988.
50. Page, R: Cisplatin, new antineoplastic drug in veterinary medicine. JAVMA 186(3):288, 1985.
51. Knapp, DW, et al.: Cisplatin toxicity in cats. Proc VCS 6:4, 1986.
52. Oldham, RK: Biological response modifiers. J Natl Cancer Inst 70:789, 1983.
53. MacEwen, EG: Approaches to cancer therapy using biological response modifiers. Vet Clin N Am 15:667, 1985.
54. MacEwen, EG: Current concepts in cancer therapy: Biologic therapy and chemotherapy. Sem Vet Med Surg 1:5, 1986.
55. Kurzman, I and Gilbertson, SR: Prognostic factors in canine mammary tumors. Sem Vet Med Surg 1:25, 1986.
56. Kersey, JH, et al.: Immunodeficiency and cancer. Adv Cancer Res 18:211, 1973.
57. Everson, TC and Cole, WH: Spontaneous Regression of Cancer. Philadelphia, WB Saunders, 1966.
58. Fidler, IJ: Immunomodulation of macrophages for cancer and antiviral therapy. *In* Tomlinson, E and Davis, SS (eds): Site-Specific Drug Delivery. New York, John Wiley & Sons, 1986, p 111.
59. Helson, L, et al.: Effects of murine tumor necrosis factor on heterotransplanted human tumors. Exp Cell Biol 17:53, 1979.
60. Old, LJ: Tumor necrosis factor. Scientific American 258:59, 1988.
61. Johnton, WI: Basic concepts of immunity. *In* Torrence, PF (ed): Biological Response Modifiers. New York, Academic Press, 1985, p 21.
62. MacEwen, EG, et al.: Canine oral melanoma: Comparison of surgery versus surgery plus *Corynebacterium parvum*. Cancer Invest 45:397, 1985.
63. Kleinshuster, SJ, et al.: Efficacy of intratumorally administered mycobacterium cell walls in the treatment of cattle with ocular carcinoma. JNCI 17:1165, 1981.
64. Murphy, JM, et al.: Immunotherapy of ocular equine sarcoid. JAVMA 174:269, 1979.
65. Winters, WP and Harris, SC: Increased survival and interferon induction by BCG-CW immunotherapy in pet dogs with malignant mammary tumors. Proc Am Assoc Cancer Res 244:1982.
66. Meyer, JA, et al: Canine osteogenic sarcoma treated by amputation and MER. Cancer 49:1613, 1982.
67. Parodi, AL, et al.: Intratumoral BCG and *Corynebacterium parvum* therapy of canine mammary tumor before radical mastectomy. Cancer Immunol Immunother 15:172, 1983.
68. Forsgen, A and Sjoquist, J: Protein A from *S. aureus*: Pseudo-immune reaction with human gamma-globulin. J Immunol 97:822, 1966.
69. Harper, HD, et al.: Antitumor activity of Protein A administered intravenously to pet cats with leukemia and lymphosarcoma. Cancer 55:1863, 1985.
70. Terman, DS, et al.: Extensive necrosis of spontaneous canine mammary adenocarcinoma after extracorporeal perfusion over *Staph aureus*. J Immunol 124:795, 1980.
71. Messerschmidt, GL, et al.: Long-term follow-up of dogs with spontaneous mammary tumors treated with ex-vivo plasma perfusion over *Staph aureus*. Cowan I. J Natl Cancer Inst 71:535, 1983.
72. Gordon BR, Matus RE, Hurvitz, AI: Perfusion of plasma over *S. aureus*: Release of bacterial products is related to regression of tumor. J Biol Resp Modif 3:266, 1984.
73. Fidler, IJ: Macrophages and metastasis—A biological approach to cancer therapy. Cancer Res 45:4714, 1985.
74. Chedid, L, et al.: Potential use of muramyl peptides in cancer therapy and prevention. *In* Jeljaszewicz, J, et al. (eds): Bacteria and Cancer. New York, Academic Press, 1982, p 49.
75. Tanka, A, et al.: Stimulation of the reticuloendothelial system of mice by muramyl dipeptide. Infect Immunol 24:302, 1979.
76. MacEwen, EG: General concepts of immunotherapy of tumors. JAAHA 12:363, 1976.
77. MacEwen, EG and Hess, PW: Evaluation of effects of immunomodulation of feline eosinophilic granuloma complex. JAAHA 23:519, 1987.
78. Tripodi, D, et al.: Drug-induced restoration of cutaneous delayed hypersensitivity in anergic patients with cancer. N Engl J Med 289:354, 1973.
79. Rojas, AF, et al.: Levamisole in advanced breast cancer. Lancet 1:211, 1976.
80. Borden, EC, et al.: Interim analysis of a trial of levamisole and 5-fluorouracil in metastatic colorectal carcinoma. *In* Terry, WD and Rosenberg, SA (eds): Immunotherapy of Human Cancer. New York, Elsevier-North Holland, 1982, p 231.
81. Amery, WK, et al.: Four-year results from double-blind study of adjuvant levamisole treatment in resectable lung cancer. *In* Terry, WD and Rosenberg, SA (eds): Immunotherapy of Human Cancer. New York, Elsevier-North Holland, 1982, p 123.
82. Hoebeke, J and Franch, G: Influence of tetramisole and its optical isomers on the mononuclear phagocytic system: effect of carbon clearance in mice. J Reticuloendothelial Soc 14:317, 1973.
83. MacEwen, EG, et al.: Evaluation of effect of levamisole and surgery on canine mammary cancer. J Biol Resp Mod 4:418, 1985.
84. MacEwen, EG, et al.: Evaluation of effect of levamisole on feline mammary cancer. J Biol Resp Mod 5:541, 1984.
85. MacEwen, EG, et al.: Levamisole as adjuvant to chemotherapy for canine lymphosarcoma. J Biol Resp Mod 4:427, 1985.
86. Ershler, WB, et al.: Pharmacologic modulation of the immune response by cimetidine. Intern J Immunopharmacol 43:359, 1982.
87. Jin, Z, et al: Inhibition of suppressor cell function by cimetidine in an immune model. Clin Immunol Immunopathol 38:350, 1986.
88. Crow, SE, et al.: Chemoimmunotherapy for canine lymphosarcoma. Cancer 40:2101, 1977.
89. Jeglum, KA, et al.: Chemotherapy versus chemotherapy with intralymphatic tumor cell vaccine in canine lymphoma. Cancer 1987, in press.
90. Jeglum, KA and Winters, WO: Antibody response to lymphoma antigens in canine tumor patients following intralymphatic active specific immunotherapy. J Biol Resp Mod, 1987, in press.
91. Borden, EC and Bull, LA: Interferon: Biochemical cell growth inhibiting and immunological effects. *In* Brown ER (ed): Progress in Hematology, Vol 12. New York, Grune and Stratton, 1981, p 299.
92. Taylor-Papadimitriou, J: Effects of interferons on cell growth and function. *In* Gresser I (ed): Interferon 2. New York, Academic, 1980, p 13.
93. Goldstein, D and Laszb, J: Interferon therapy in cancer: From imaginon to interferon. Cancer Res 46:4315, 1986.
94. Oldham, RK: Monoclonal antibodies in cancer therapy. J Clin Oncol 9:582, 1983.
95. Foon, KA: Biological therapy of cancer. Breast Cancer Research and Treatment 7:5, 1985.
96. Kassel, RL, et al.: Serum-mediated leukemia cell destruction in AKR mice. J Exp Med 138:925, 1973.
97. Kassel, RL, et al.: Plasma-mediated leukemia cell destruction: current status. Blood Cells 3:605, 1977.

98. Hardy, WD, Jr, et al.: Treatment of feline lymphosarcoma with blood constituents. *In* Clemson, J and Yohn, DS (eds): Basel, Switzerland, Karger, 1976, p 518.
99. MacEwen, EG, et al.: Temporary plasma-induced remission of lymphoblastic leukemia in a dog. Am J Vet Res 42:1450, 1981.
100. Perri, RT, et al.: Fibronectin enhances in vitro monocyte-macrophage-mediated tumoricidal activity. Blood 60:430, 1982.
101. Lause, OB, et al.: Induction of lymphocyte blast transformation by purified fibronectin in vitro. J Immunol 132:1294, 1984.
102. Terranova, VP, et al.: Modulation of the metastatic activity of melanoma cells by laminin and fibronectin. Science 226:982, 1984.
103. Thrall, DE: Radiation therapy in the dog: principles, indications, and complications. Comp Cont Ed Pract Vet 4(8):652, 1982.
104. Sutherland, RT and Mulcahy, RT: Basic principles of radiation biology. *In* Rubin, P (ed): Clinical Oncology: A Multidisciplinary Approach. American Cancer Society, 1983, p 40.
105. Rubin, P and Siemann, D: Principles of radiation oncology and cancer radiotherapy. *In* Rubin, P (ed): Clinical Oncology: A Multidisciplinary Approach. American Cancer Society, 1983, p 58.
106. Mitchell, M, et al.: Canine thyroid carcinomas: clinical occurrence, staging by means of scintiscans, and therapy of 15 cases. Vet Surg 8:4(112), 1979.
107. Meric, SM, et al.: Serum thyroxine concentrations after radioactive iodine therapy in cats with hyperthyroidism. JAVMA 188(9):1038, 1986.
108. Denekamp, J: Cell kinetics and radiation biology. Int J Radiat Biol 49(2):357, 1986.
109. Walker, MA: A review of drugs that may be used in conjunction with radiotherapy. Vet Rad 23(5):220, 1982.
110. Thrall, DE and Dewhirst, ME: Application of radiotherapy in the control of neoplasia. *In* Gorman, NT (ed): Oncology. New York, Churchill Livingstone, 1986, p 71.
111. Feeney, DA and Johnston, GB: Radiation therapy: Applications and availability. *In* Kirk, RW (ed): Current Veterinary Therapy VIII. Philadelphia, WB Saunders, 1983, p 428.
112. Feeney, DA: Radiation therapy. Proc Am Col Vet Surg 10:10, 1982.
113. Adams, WM, et al.: Radiotherapy of malignant nasal tumors in 67 dogs. JAVMA 191:311, 1987.
114. Evans, SM: Canine hemangiopericytoma: a retrospective analysis of response to surgery and orthovoltage radiation. Vet Radiol, 1987, in press.
115. Dewhirst, MW and Connor, WG: Hyperthermia. *In* Slatter, DH (ed): Textbook of Small Animal Surgery. Philadelphia, WB Saunders, 1985, p 2427.
116. Richardson, RC: Hyperthermia—An old cancer therapy revisited. *In* Kirk, RW (ed): Current Veterinary Therapy VIII. Philadelphia, WB Saunders, 1983, p 423.
117. Thompson, JM: Advances in the use of hyperthermia. *In* Gorman, NT (ed): Oncology. New York, Churchill Livingstone, 1986, p 89.
118. Robins, HI: Role of whole-body hyperthermia in the treatment of neoplastic disease: its current status and future prospects. Cancer Res (Suppl) 44:4878, 1984.
119. Robins, HI, et al.: Potentiation of differential hyperthermic sensitivity of AKR leukemia and normal bone marrow cells by lidocaine or thiopental. Cancer 54:2831, 1984.
120. Hugander, A, et al.: Temperature distribution during radiant heat whole body hyperthermia: experimental studies in the dog. Cancer Res, 1987, accepted for publication.
121. Macy, DW, et al.: Physiological studies of whole-body hyperthermia in dogs. Cancer Res 45:2769, 1985.
122. Page, RL, et al.: Cardiovascular and metabolic response of tumor-bearing dogs to whole body hyperthermia. Cancer, 1987, accepted for publication.
123. Rosenthal, RC, et al.: Canine serum alkaline phosphatase following whole body hyperthermia. Proc Am Col Vet Int Med, 1987.
124. Thrall, DE, et al.: Temperature measurements in normal and tumor tissue in dogs undergoing whole body hyperthermia. Cancer Res 46:6229, 1986.
125. Hill, GJ: Historic milestones in cancer surgery. Semin Oncol 6(4):409, 1979.
126. Kaplan, HS: Historic milestones in radiobiology and radiation therapy. Semin Oncol 6(4):479, 1979.
127. MacEwen, EG: Current concepts in cancer therapy: biologic therapy and chemotherapy. Semin Vet Med Surg (Sm An) 1(1):5, 1986.
128. Griswold, OP: Body burden of cancer in relationship to therapeutic outcome: consideration of preclinical evidence. Can Trt Rep 70(1):81, 1986.
129. Sugarbaker, EV, et al.: Inhibitory effect of a primary tumor on metastasis. *In* Day, SB, et al. (eds): Cancer Invasion and Metastasis: Biologic Mechanisms and Therapy. New York, Raven Press, 1977, p 227.
130. Gorelik, E, et al.: Growth of a local tumor exerts a specific inhibitory effect on progression of lung metastases. Int G Cancer 21:617, 1978.
131. Ferguson, MK: The effect of antineoplastic agents on wound healing. Surg Gynecol Obstet 154:421, 1982.
132. Shamberger, R: Effect of chemotherapy and radiotherapy on wound healing: experimental studies. Rec Res Can Ther 98:17, 1985.

SECTION VI

THE NERVOUS SYSTEM

60 THE NEUROLOGIC EVALUATION OF PATIENTS

WILLIAM R. FENNER

The diagnosis of diseases of the nervous system should be no more difficult than the diagnosis of illness or injury to any other organ system. What distinguishes neurology is the absolute necessity of understanding functional neuroanatomy. To comprehend how anatomy is important in patients with nervous system disease, it is necessary to review the roles of the patient history, the neurologic examination, and diagnostic aids in evaluating patients with nervous system disease. In patients with neurologic disease, the location of the lesion determines what signs are seen. The cause of the lesion determines the order in which the signs appear and whether they persist, worsen, or regress. Put another way, anatomy determines the signs and etiology determines the course. The neurologic examination reveals where the problem is, but the history reveals the nature of the problem. Then, the clinician must choose and interpret appropriate diagnostic aids. For example, suppose a patient's history reveals a slowly progressive disease and the examination reveals that the disease is focal and confined to the cervical spinal cord. What could cause such a problem? An expanding mass is the logical answer. The next question is, "Based on a knowledge of which pathologic processes can affect that specific portion of the nervous system in that particular species, is the expanding mass a tumor, granuloma, abscess, or hypertrophic ligament from vertebral instability?" The clinician chooses diagnostic aids that distinguish between those various possibilities. The types of tissue reaction that occur in the nervous system are limited and include inflammation, degenerations, and neoplastic transformation among others. The etiology of the signs determines the type of tissue reaction in each patient, which in turn determines the changes seen in the diagnostic tests. These changes in spinal fluid composition, radiographic appearance, or electrophysiologic status, when placed in the context of the history and physical findings, allow the clinician to arrive at a diagnosis.

In short, clinical neurology starts with localizing a disorder. Then the history and localization are used to choose appropriate diagnostic tests. The results of the tests are combined with the history and localization to determine a set of deductions that best explains the clinical data. The thought processes used in doing this are outlined in Figure 60–1.

TAKING THE HISTORY

The neurologic evaluation of any patient should start with the taking of a careful and accurate history. The clinical signs seen in a patient with nervous system injury reflect where the injury has occurred. How those signs start (the onset) and how they change (the course) reflect what caused the injury. Because of this, the patient's history is essential to understanding a patient's disease. The history has two components, a general history of the animal and a specific history of the presenting illness. The information obtained from a history can be subdivided into three broad categories: anatomic information, etiologic information, and prognostic information.

Anatomically, the history can provide two types of information. First, the history may determine if neuro-

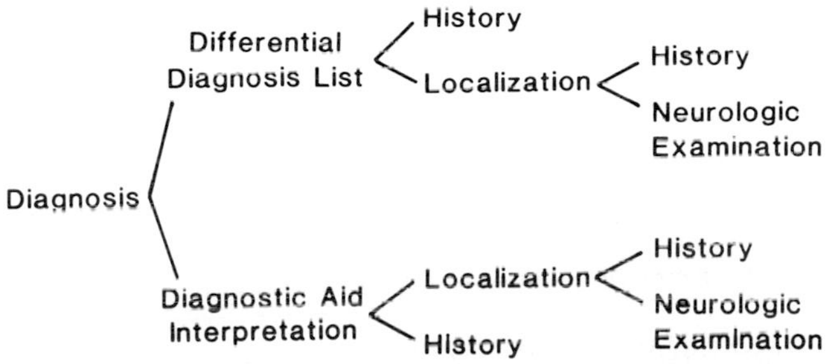

FIGURE 60–1. Diagnostic approach to patients with neurologic disease.

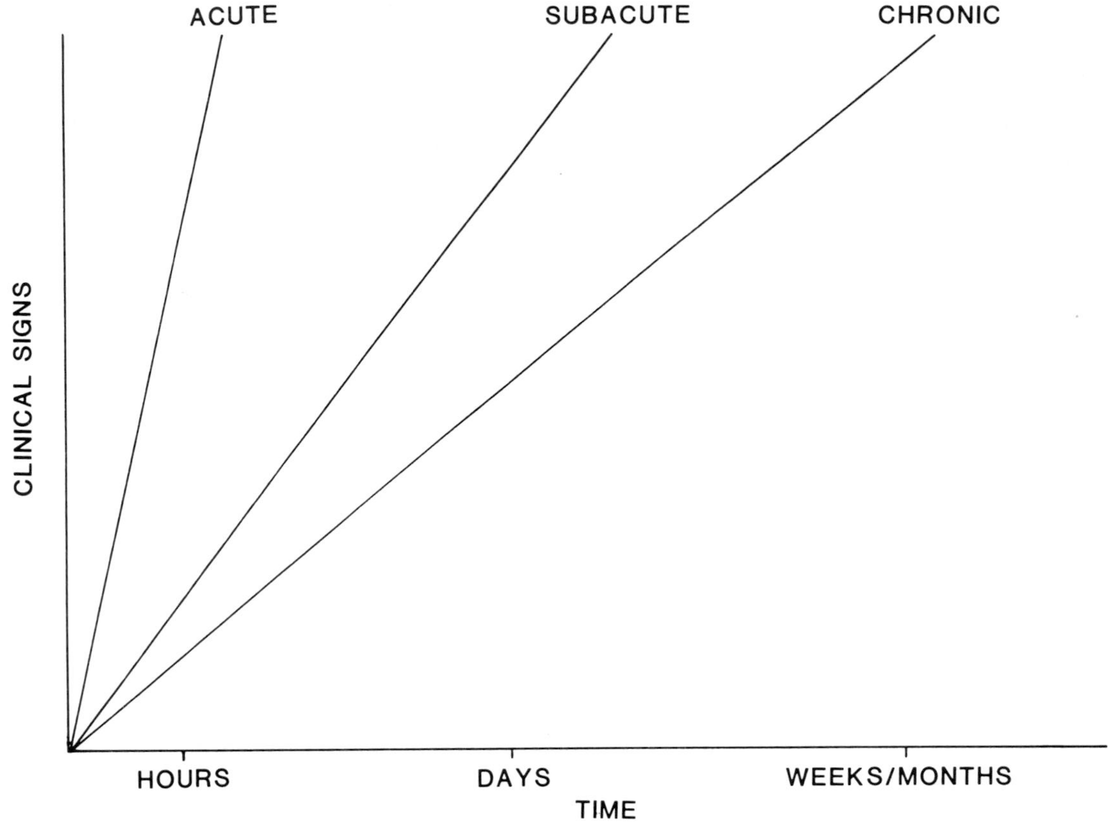

FIGURE 60–2. Time/sign graph demonstrating onset of neurologic signs.

logic dysfunction exists at all. Examples where the history may confirm the presence of neural dysfunction include epilepsy, narcolepsy, and myasthenia gravis. Second, the information obtained from the history may be essential in helping to localize the problem within the nervous system. Examples of this include a history of epilepsy or behavior disorders, which would localize a lesion to the cerebrum, or a history of neck or back pain, which would localize a problem along the spine.

The second category of information is etiologic, where the history allows you to arrive at a differential diagnosis. Each of the major classes of disease tends to follow a certain general historical pattern. For example, degenerations are slowly progressive, while trauma is acute and static. Knowing the history allows the clinician to place those pathologic processes that most resemble the historical course of the patient into the diagnostic list, while eliminating the others. This etiologic information is also helpful in choosing and interpreting diagnostic aids. For example, many disease processes, such as trauma, neoplasia, and infarcts, can cause an elevation of spinal fluid protein without elevating the white blood cell count of spinal fluid. With such a spinal fluid analysis, the clinician uses the history to find which one of them is most in keeping with the patient's clinical course. The etiologic portion of the history may also aid in choosing therapy. The history reveals whether or not certain therapies have already failed and allows treatment of secondary problems, such as pain, which may slow the patient's recovery.

The final category of information gained from the history is prognostic. The history allows a prognosis to be made because it is the history of response to the indicated therapy that will determine client satisfaction and patient outcome.

COLLECTING INFORMATION

First, obtain a general review of the animal's health. If this is a long-term patient, much of this information is already in the medical records. If it is a new patient, this general information may be critical to the success of the diagnosis. Review the patient's signalment and use. Age and breed are important because certain diseases, such as globoid cell leukodystrophy in Cairn terriers and spinal muscular atrophy in Brittany spaniels, are known to have age and breed predilections. Certain disorders are known to occur preferentially in one gender, such as prostatic neoplasia in males and mammary neoplasia in females. The use of the animal is important because it often determines the extent of diagnosis and therapy. For example, epilepsy may be acceptable in a pet but not in a guide dog.

Inquire about the animal's environment and diet for exposure to known toxins or nutritional deficiencies. Then obtain a general medical history, which should include the vaccination status of the animal, a general review of body symptoms, and a specific review of any previous illnesses that the patient has had. A previous illness or injury may have resulted in permanent neurologic damage that can confuse the current neurologic examination if it is not taken into consideration. Some prior medical or surgical problem could also result in an abnormal laboratory value or abnormal radiographs.

Knowing about the problem avoids chasing an unlikely diagnosis. Obtain a complete review of any current problems that the animal has, as they may provide clues to the nature of the neural dysfunction.

After the general review, proceed to the primary complaint. Ask when the signs started, as well as what the initial signs were. Inquire if additional signs appeared and if so, what they were and when they appeared. Ask if any previous therapy has been attempted, and if so, what effect it had on the patient. Remember that the average client is most concerned about one major problem, such as epilepsy. Concentration on that major problem may prevent the owner from mentioning more subtle abnormalities. The clinician can elicit these subtleties by asking screening questions about all areas of the nervous system. Too much questioning about normal areas can elicit meaningless information and tire the owner. As a clinician, try to find a balance between excess and inadequacy.

Try to get the client to describe what he or she sees, not what he or she thinks is causing the problem. For example, a client might say, "My dog is blind." If you let it go at that, the logical conclusion is that there is a visual deficit. However, if you ask, "Why do you think the dog is blind? What is it doing?" you may find that the owner suspects blindness because the pet loses its balance and bumps into objects while falling. In short, try to separate clinical fact from clinical fiction. Ask how, when, and where the disease started, then what happened next. Most diseases fall into one of three patterns of onset: acute, subacute, or chronic. With acute illnesses, the signs develop rapidly, usually reaching their maximal intensity within 24 hours. Peracute disorders usually reach maximal intensity within minutes of onset. Examples of acute or peracute illnesses include trauma, some toxic or metabolic injuries, and infarcts. Acute exacerbations may also develop in the course of a more chronic illness, such as brain herniation during the course of a brain tumor. Subacute illnesses usually have signs that develop progressively over a period of several days or a few weeks. Examples of subacute illnesses include most of the inflammatory diseases, many metabolic diseases, and some neoplastic disorders. Illnesses that are chronic in onset are those in which the signs continue to develop over a period of months or even years. Examples of chronic diseases include degenerations, nutritional disorders, some metabolic disorders (especially the intrinsic ones), and tumors (Figure 60–2).

Related to onset, but measuring a slightly different parameter, is clinical progression. Learn whether the signs have changed and if so, how they changed. If the signs are static, they do not change over the course of the disease. This is most characteristic of anomalies of the nervous system; however, some traumatic and vascular injuries may show a partial recovery followed by a static course. If the signs are progressive, there is an increase in the severity of signs over time, the number of signs over time, or both. Progression is characteristic of inflammations, degenerations, and neoplasia. In the case of improvement, there is a progressive decrease over time in the number of signs, the severity of signs, or both. An improving course is most characteristic of trauma, toxins, and vascular injury. Finally, the signs may wax and wane; i.e., they vary in intensity over time; at some times they may be severe and at others, improved. This waxing and waning pattern is especially characteristic of metabolic disorders; however, it may also be seen with spinal instabilities (Figure 60–3).

Learn the exact character of the signs, preferably through an actual description of the signs seen by the client. If the animal's clinical picture changes, is it

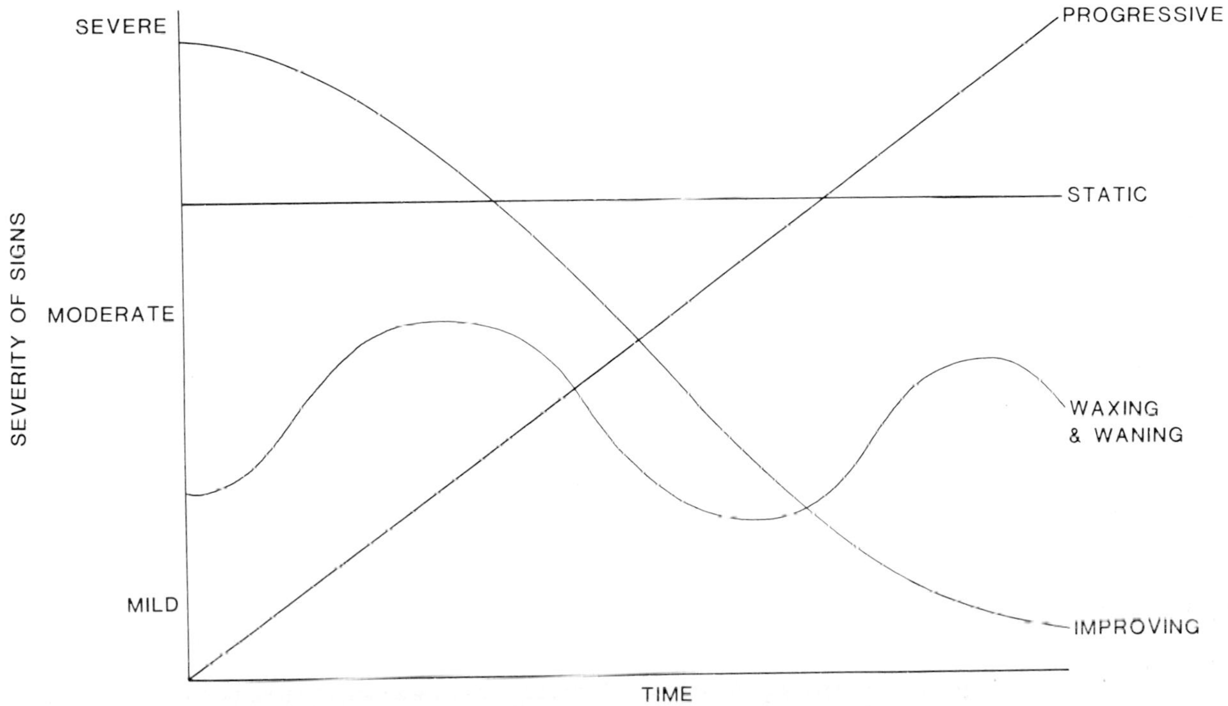

FIGURE 60–3. Time/sign graph demonstrating progression of neurologic signs.

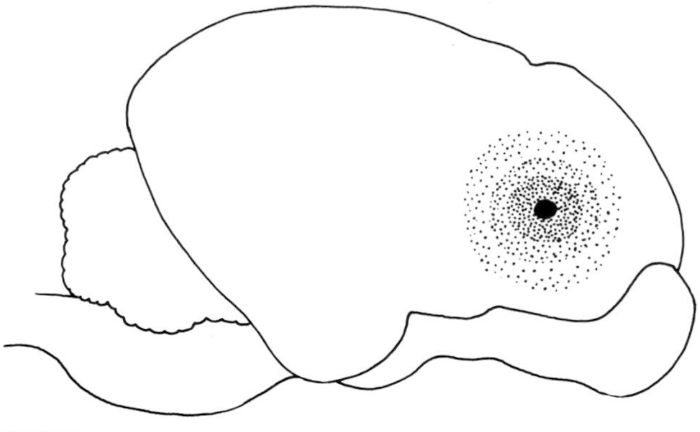

FIGURE 60–4. Anatomic representation of a logical progression/regression of neurologic disease.

because new signs developed as time progressed or was it simply a matter of the old signs worsening? An example of worsening of the same sign is a patient that starts out with pelvic limb weakness and over a period of a week becomes paralyzed in the pelvic limbs. An example of the development of new signs is a patient that starts out with pelvic limb weakness, but over a period of two weeks also develops a head tilt. These data give an idea of the anatomic progression of the disease.

The anatomic course of the disease is how the disease spreads to involve other portions of the nervous system. Try to decide whether the signs represent a logical progression or a random change. A logical progression is seen in those disorders where the signs change because of progressive involvement of the anatomic areas that are closest to the site of the initial problem. If the disorder is progressive, the next involvement will be that area immediately outside the area of initial involvement. If the disorder is regressive, the first area to improve should be the most peripheral area of the injury. Logically progressive disorders are usually expanding masses, which include neoplasia, abscesses, granulomas, and edema fluid around trauma. Logically regressive disorders are usually diminishing masses, which include hematomas, infarcts, and edema fluid (Figure 60–4). A special variant of logical progression accompanies the systems disorders. These are conditions where the problem affects functionally related areas of the nervous system, even though those areas may be widely separated physically. An example is spinal muscular atrophy of the Brittany spaniel, where the disease process involves one functional system, the ventral horn cell of the spinal cord (Figure 60–5). Most of these latter conditions are degenerations and thus chronic in nature.

In diseases where there is random progression, the signs do not appear in any related order; rather they appear in unrelated portions of the nervous system. This is most characteristic of inflammatory diseases, especially those caused by infectious agents. This pattern may also be seen with some toxic, nutritional, and metabolic disorders (Figure 60–6).

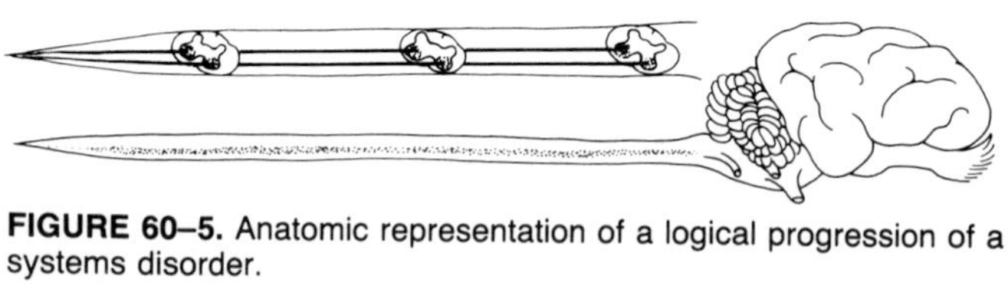

FIGURE 60–5. Anatomic representation of a logical progression of a systems disorder.

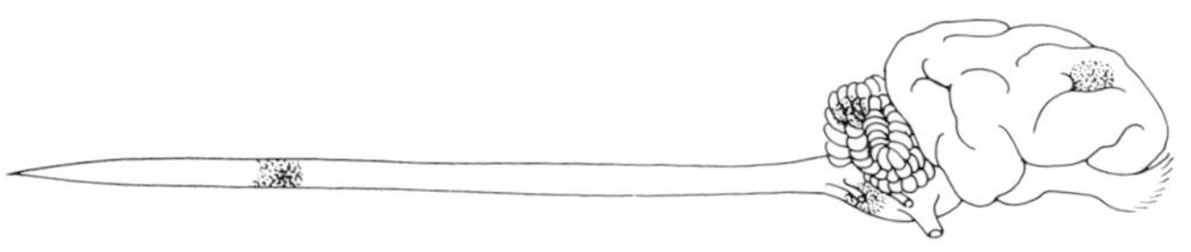

FIGURE 60–6. Anatomic representation of a random progression of a neurologic disorder.

In certain conditions, the signs are diffuse at the onset of the disease. In these disorders there is widespread, symmetrical involvement of the nervous system from the earliest stage of the illness. This pattern is very similar to systems disturbances, except that the process is not limited to a single functional system. Diffuse progression is characteristic of metabolic, toxic, nutritional, and degenerative disorders. It may also be seen in some inflammatory disorders (Figure 60–7).

Ask if there are any aggravating factors. Do the signs worsen with exercise, excitement, or stress, as would narcolepsy, myasthenia gravis, and cardiac syncope? Do convulsive episodes occur primarily during sleep, which is more characteristic of true epilepsy? Are the signs worsened by a meal, as is true of some metabolic disorders? In short, is there any portion of the history that shows that the signs depend on a specific event? If so, consider what type of disorder is most likely to be worsened by such an event. A final area to investigate is the effects of previous therapy. Have any therapies been tried already? If so, were they adequate in duration, dosage, and route of administration? If so, were they effective? If possible, have the client keep a record of the times that drugs were given and their effect on the illness.

ORGANIZING THE INFORMATION

After all the information is collected, reorganize it and repeat it to someone else so that he or she understands it the first time. If the history can be explained to someone else, it is probably clearly understood and can be used for diagnosis. This information allows the

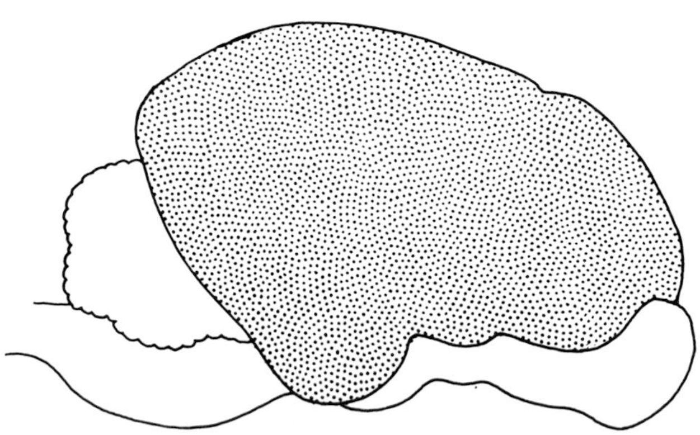

FIGURE 60–7. Anatomic representation of a diffuse neurologic disorder.

clinician to make a time sign graph, which can then be used to determine the major classes of disease processes that may be causing the patient's signs, i.e., degenerations, metabolic diseases, or nutritional diseases (Figure 60–8). Each of the major categories of disease tends to have a historical pattern that runs true for that pathologic process, across species and etiologic lines. These are summarized briefly here.

DISEASE CATEGORIES

Toxic Injuries. Toxic injuries to the nervous system result from exposure of the nervous system to an injurious chemical. The chemical is frequently environmental, i.e., lead, mercury, organophosphates, but may also be produced by microorganisms in the patient, as occurs in tetanus or botulism. The toxin may affect the nervous system by impairing neuronal respiration or axon transport, by impairing release of neurotransmitters, by enhancing the action of neurotransmitters, or by mimicking the action of neurotransmitters. The effects of the toxins that affect neurotransmitters are frequently reversible if exposure to the toxin is ended. The effects of the toxins that impair neuronal respiration or axon transport may be irreversible if they cause the death of the neuron or axon. Toxic injuries are usually acute in onset, with the signs being diffuse at onset. There is a widespread, symmetrical involvement of the nervous system from the earliest stage of the illness. This involvement may be confined to a functional system (tetanus – inhibitory interneurons) or to a morphologic region (lead poisoning = cerebrum). Patients with toxic injuries usually begin improving shortly after they are removed from the source of the toxin. In short, toxic illnesses are usually monophasic.

Metabolic and Nutritional Injuries. Metabolic and nutritional injuries include those conditions where the nervous system either is deprived of a factor essential for survival or is exposed to a toxin that is produced as a by-product of the failure of another organ system. The deficiency state may be due to the lack of a nutrient in the diet, as occurs in thiamine deficiency, to an inherited enzyme deficiency, as occurs in lysosomal storage disorders, or to an inability of the organism to maintain an adequate supply of the nutrient, as occurs in hypoglycemia due to an excess of insulin. The toxic states usually reflect damage to other organ systems, with resultant loss of the ability to remove toxic by-products from the systemic circulation, i.e., as occurs in renal failure. The onset of these conditions is quite variable. Acute onset is the rarest form and is usually seen with substrate deficiencies such as hypoglycemia. Subacute onset of signs is probably the most common in metabolic and nutritional disorders, with the chronic form being relatively uncommon. All metabolic and nutritional diseases tend to be diffuse at onset, with a widespread, symmetrical involvement of the nervous system from the earliest stage of the illness. Most of these conditions wax and wane, although some patients with enzyme deficiencies have chronically progressive signs.

Trauma. Traumatic injuries are generally acute in onset, producing local swelling, loss of blood supply, hypoxia, and necrosis. As soon as this process has stabilized, the nervous system begins to repair itself. The success of this repair is determined by the severity of the initial injury and whether or not there is any residual compression from the initiating process, e.g., a herniated intervertebral disc. The signs are generally focal and improving and have a logical pattern of regression. If there is instability associated with the injury, as

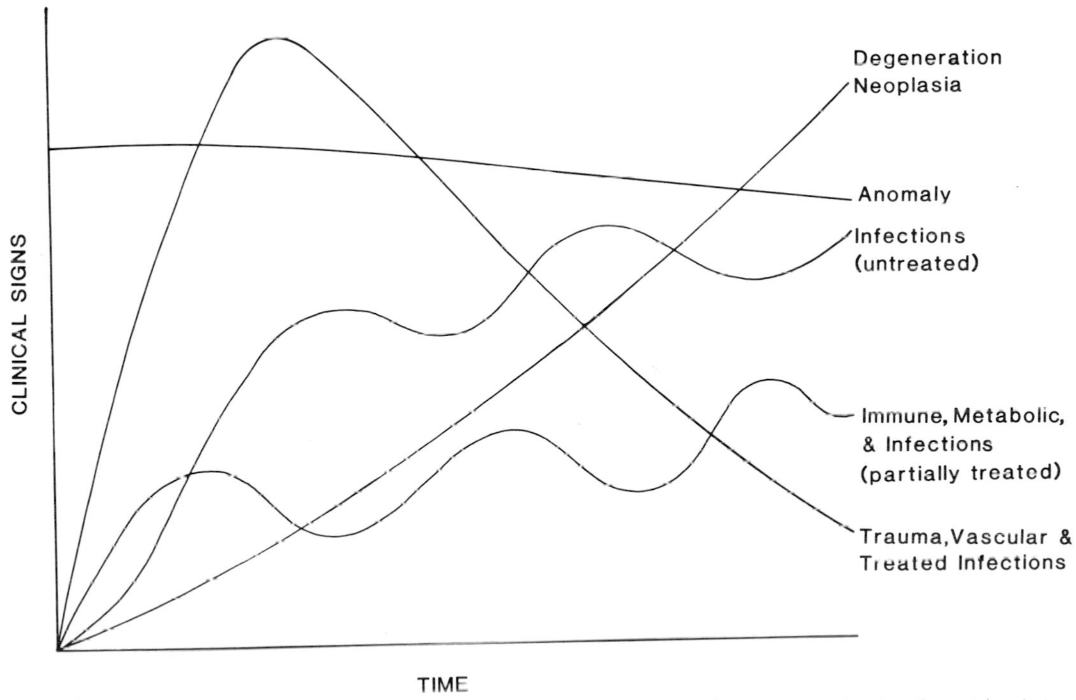

FIGURE 60–8. Time/sign graph demonstrating the onset and progression of common pathogenetic mechanisms of neurologic disease.

in spinal fractures, the signs may wax and wane or progress.

Vascular Injuries. Vascular injury to the nervous system may result from loss of blood supply (ischemia) or from hemorrhage into the nervous tissue. In most cases the initial process is focal, regardless of type. It is possible with systemic bleeding disorders to have multifocal or diffuse hemorrhage, with subsequent multifocal onset. The onset is almost always acute, with a logical progression of local signs. These conditions usually improve, resulting in a monophasic illness. Rarely, in the case of bleeding disorders, there may be progression of signs.

Malformations and Anomalies. Malformations and anomalies may cause nervous system dysfunction in one of two ways, each having a different clinical course. If the anomaly or malformation is in the substance of the nervous tissue itself, e.g., syringomyelia, the clinical signs are usually apparent at birth and do not progress. If, however, the malformation is in the tissues that support the nervous system, e.g., the skull or spine, the anomaly may not cause signs until late in the course of the animal's life. This occurs because in those cases, the signs usually reflect compression of the nervous system. This compression takes months or years to occur as a result of chronic instability, compounded by the body's attempts to correct that instability. Regardless of the type of onset, the signs are usually logical in their progression and represent a local injury.

Tumors. Tumors generally produce signs as a result of compression and replacement of the parenchyma of the nervous system by proliferating neoplastic tissue. The nervous system may also suffer vascular compromise (ischemia), bleeding, edema, and inflammation around the tumor site. These secondary changes often produce as many clinical signs as the primary tumor itself. Normally, the signs are subacute or chronic in onset, with a logical progression of local signs. Metastatic diseases may be random in their progression and more rapid in their onset.

Inflammations. Inflammations are considered in two categories, focal inflammations and disseminated inflammations. Focal inflammations may be abscesses, which are local regions of necrosis and suppuration that usually occur in response to bacterial infection. The clinical signs reflect a rapidly expanding mass lesion that is produced by the inflammatory process and its associated tissue edema. The signs are typically acute to subacute in onset, with a logical progression of local signs. If the patient has received inadequate therapy, the signs may wax and wane rather than progress. Focal inflammations also include granulomas, which represent an accumulation of inflammatory cells intermingled with a fibrotic reaction. This is the result of the body's attempts to remove or neutralize some chronic irritant, e.g., a fungal organism, a protozoal organism, a foreign body, or a parasite. The predominant cell type seen in the granuloma is a reflection of the chronicity of the process as well as the initiating agent. Depending on the etiology, granulomas may be focal (solitary), such as occurs with a foreign body, or multifocal (disseminated), such as occurs with an infection. Granulomas tend to be slower in onset and progression than abscesses; they are usually subacute to chronic. Focal granulomas are logically progressive in most cases, representing expansion of a local mass.

Disseminated inflammations may result from infectious causes or immune disorders or the cause may be unknown. In all cases there is a widespread infiltration of the nervous system with inflammatory cells, whose type is determined by its etiology. In addition, there is frequently edema of adjacent tissue, secondary reaction to inflammatory by-products, and vascular compromise. Disseminated inflammations cause a widespread failure of the nervous system. The onset of signs in an inflammation is generally subacute, although it may also begin acutely or chronically, depending on the cause of the inflammation. Typically, the course is one of random progression, although in some cases the signs may wax and wane.

THE NEUROLOGIC EXAMINATION

After reviewing the history, the clinician should proceed to the neurologic examination of the patient. This consists of observing an animal, watching its gait, carefully palpating it for abnormal muscle tone and mass, performing tests of reflexes and reactions in that animal, and finally, interpreting the information in order to answer a series of questions about that patient. Simply put, the questions are: Does the patient have a disease of the nervous system? If so, does it involve one or more parts of the nervous system? If only one part, which one? The goals of the neurologic examination are primarily to confirm the presence of a neurologic disease and to localize it within the nervous system. The neurologic examination cannot be understood without at least some knowledge of neuroanatomy. Morphologically, the nervous system may be subdivided two ways: into functional systems and into anatomic regions. The functional systems are composed of all the cells and their processes that are concerned with a specific function; examples are the motor system, the pain perception system, the consciousness system, and the balance system. These functional systems run through many different focal anatomic regions, but not all anatomic regions contain cells for all functional systems. The focal anatomic regions are small sections of the nervous system (such as the brain stem, cerebrum, and cerebellum in the brain) that are organized around certain functions or reflexes that are unique to that small area. Each focal anatomic region contains fibers or cells of one or more functional systems.

The major functional systems are consciousness, motor, nociception (pain perception), proprioception (joint perception, muscle stretch perception, and balance), and autonomic. The major anatomic regions are cerebrum, cerebellum, brain stem, and spinal cord. When the anatomic regions with their unique features and their functional systems are combined, they are distinguished as follows: cerebrum = consciousness, motor regulation, pain perception, joint perception, vision, learning, behavior, and some cranial nerve responses; cerebellum = muscle stretch perception, balance, and fine motor regulation; brain stem = consciousness, motor regulation, pain perception, joint perception, muscle stretch perception, balance, the autonomic systems, and cranial nerve reflexes and vegetative functions; the spinal cord = motor regulation, pain perception, joint perception, muscle stretch perception, balance, the autonomic systems, and spinal reflexes. These combinations yield a brief summary of the clinical signs expected with lesions in each local anatomic region (see Table 60–1). The neurologic examination allows the clinician to test the various functional systems and local reflexes. He or she can then use a knowledge of neuroanatomy to localize the disease process.

The examination should be conducted in a logical, methodical, and consistent manner. It is important to develop a particular order and follow it on all patients. Start with the general and advance to the specific, leaving the painful portions of the examination until the end. Remember that all reactions and responses require sensory input as well as motor output. Too often beginners assume that all abnormalities are reflections of lesions on the motor side of the reflex arc.

TABLE 60–1. SUMMARY OF CLINICAL SIGNS WITH LESIONS IN ANATOMIC REGIONS

Anatomic Region	Clinical Signs
Cerebrum	Mentational changes Visual deficits (normal pupils) Circling Weakness (hemitetraparesis) Seizures Abnormal postural reactions
Cerebellum	Ataxia Intentional tremor Normal strength Ataxic postural reactions Pathologic nystagmus Head tilt (variable) Rare menace deficit
Brain stem	Cranial nerve deficits Pathologic nystagmus Weakness Abnormal postural reactions Ataxia Depressed mental state Respiratory depression Cardiac arrhythmias Head tilts Circling
Vestibular injury	Pathologic nystagmus Ataxic postural reactions Ataxia Head tilts Circling Falling or rolling Positional strabismus
Spinal cord injury	Weakness Abnormal postural reactions Ataxia Respiratory distress (rarely) Bladder and bowel paralysis Pain Abnormal spinal reflexes Horner's syndrome (rarely)
Peripheral spinal nerve injury	Weakness Loss of spinal reflexes Depressed postural reactions Hypotonia Atrophy
Peripheral cranial nerve injury	Loss of cranial nerve function

It is a good idea to make a list of all of the findings as the examination progresses. When the examination is over, try to explain all of the findings with a lesion confined to a single focus within the nervous system (follow the flow chart in Figure 60–9). If all of the signs can be explained with a single lesion, the cause is probably a focal disease such as an infarct or neoplasm. If all the signs cannot be explained in this way, it is probably a disseminated disorder such as an inflammation or degeneration. In this sense, the neurologic examination also helps to determine the etiology of a problem. In addition, there are certain problems that only occur in specific regions of the nervous system. If a disorder is localized to that region, then by default that differential is included in the diagnostic considerations. An example is an extrusion of intervertebral disc material with spinal cord compression. If a problem is localized to the spinal cord, disc extrusion becomes one of the differentials, but if the problem is localized to the brain, it cannot be one of the differentials.

Normal findings on the neurologic examination may be as important as the abnormal in arriving at a localization. Take, for example, a tetraparetic dog whose sole findings on neurologic examination are exaggerated limb reflexes in all four limbs. A lesion involving both cerebral hemispheres, the brain stem, or the cranial cervical spine could result in such a weakness, but the cerebral and brain stem injury would each result in disorders of mental status and cranial nerve function. It is the lack of such deficits that allows a clinician to localize that patient's injury to the cervical spinal cord. Secondary objectives that are achieved by performing the neurologic examination include determining the extent of nervous system involvement, assistance in choosing diagnostic aids, and assistance in arriving at a prognosis.

The tools required to perform the neurologic examination on a patient are simple and inexpensive. They include an instrument for striking tendons, such as a reflex hammer or bandage scissors, a strong light source, a pair of hemostats, and a safety pin (Figure 60–10). With these tools a clinician should be able to perform a complete neurologic examination.

Technique of the Examination

The author divides the neurologic examination into six parts: general observations, gait and stance, tests of postural reactions, cranial nerve examination, spinal reflex examination, and evaluation of pain perception. Of these divisions, the general observations, gait and stance, and tests of postural reactions all evaluate general functional systems. The cranial nerve examination tests primarily local anatomic regions, while the spinal reflex examination and evaluation of pain perception test both functional systems and anatomic regions.

Reflexes are responses to a stimulus that are simple, practically invariable, inherited, and usually useful to the organism. They require a sensory nerve in the peripheral nervous system (PNS), a connection (synapse) in the CNS, and a motor nerve (PNS). Reactions,

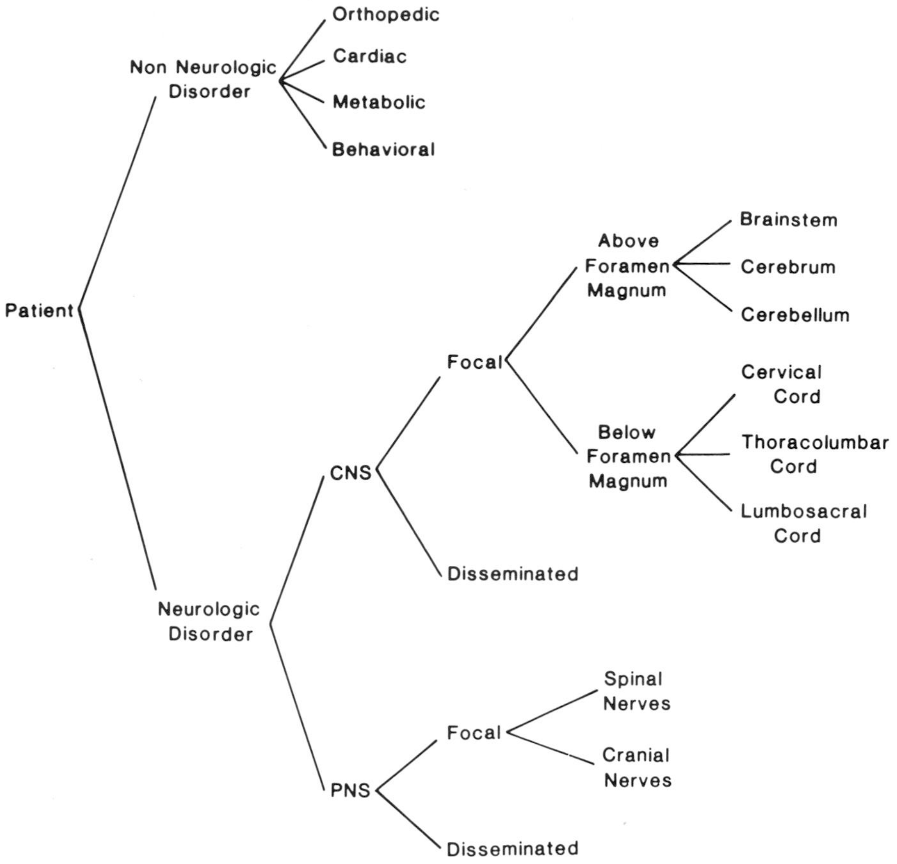

FIGURE 60–9. Localization flow chart for neurologic diagnosis.

on the other hand, are responses to stimuli that are complex and are integrated in the brain. Reactions require a sensory nerve (PNS), an ascending sensory pathway to the brain, integration in the brain, a descending motor pathway, and a motor nerve (PNS).[1, 2]

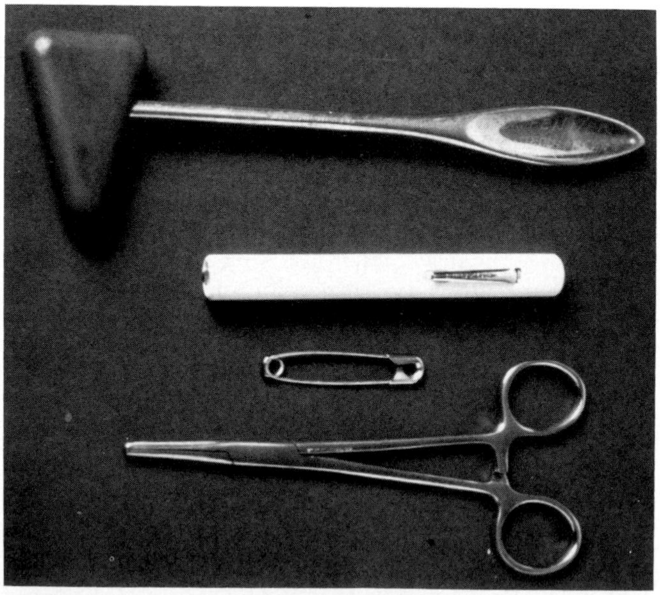

FIGURE 60–10. Tools needed to perform the neurologic examination.

General Observations

Mental Status Evaluation. Mental status is regulated by the brain stem and cerebrum, and its evaluation must be concerned with both the patient's level of consciousness and the content of that consciousness. The level of consciousness is regulated by the brain stem reticular activating system (RAS) and its interactions with the cerebrum. Abnormalities of the ascending reticular activating system (ARAS) or of the cerebrum may result in an abnormal level of consciousness that varies with the severity of the pathologic process as well as the rapidity of its onset.[3] A normal animal is described as being alert. Depression is an abnormal state in which the animal is excessively sleepy, but is easily aroused. As the injury increases in severity, the patient develops stupor. In this state, an animal can only be aroused by a painful stimulus. Finally, as the injury becomes very severe, the patient develops coma. Such a patient cannot be aroused, even with a painful stimulus. Any rostral brain stem injury, whether focal or diffuse, as well as many diffuse cerebral injuries, is capable of producing abnormalities in level of consciousness. Cerebral injuries that cause abnormal consciousness are generally rapid in onset.

The content of consciousness is concerned with mentational disorders. A normal animal is described as appropriate. A patient that is unaware and unconcerned with its surroundings may be described as demented. Such a patient may head press, walk off tables, and in other ways demonstrate a complete disregard for its own safety and well-being. If this disregard is superimposed on a state of agitation and over-responsiveness to the environment and to stimuli, the animal is called delirious or hysterical. A good example of delirium is the behavior displayed by many animals recovering from barbiturate anesthesia. Abnormal mentation is a reflection of a cerebral disorder, whether from a structural or metabolic cause. Often, changes in consciousness are only recognized by the owner, emphasizing the value of a careful history.

Head posture evaluates the special proprioceptive system. The normal animal holds its head on a plane parallel to the ground. If the animal holds one ear closer to the ground than the other ear, it is described as having a head tilt (Figure 60–11). Such a postural abnormality may be a reflection of pain about the head, but it is frequently a sign of vestibular dysfunction. An injury to the inner ear, peripheral portions of cranial nerve VIII, brain stem, and cerebellum may result in vestibular dysfunction. In general, the animal tilts its head towards the lesion, with the affected side held lower to the ground. In addition to head posture, look at neck position. In some animals the chin is tucked under or pulled tightly towards the sternum, in a form of excessive ventroflexion of the neck. This postural abnormality is usually a sign of severe weakness of the neck muscles. It has been reported in feline hypokalemic polymyopathies, occipital malformation in the dog, and cervical vertebral malformations. It is also seen in some cats with thiamine deficiency, suggesting that a vestibular abnormality may also cause such a postural deficit.

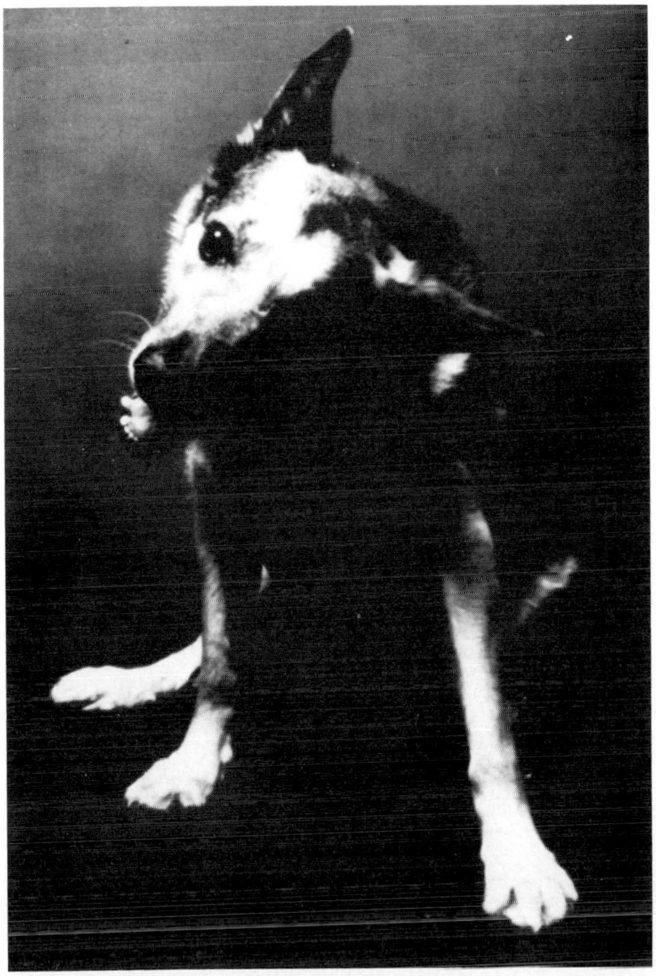

FIGURE 60–11. A patient demonstrating a head tilt.

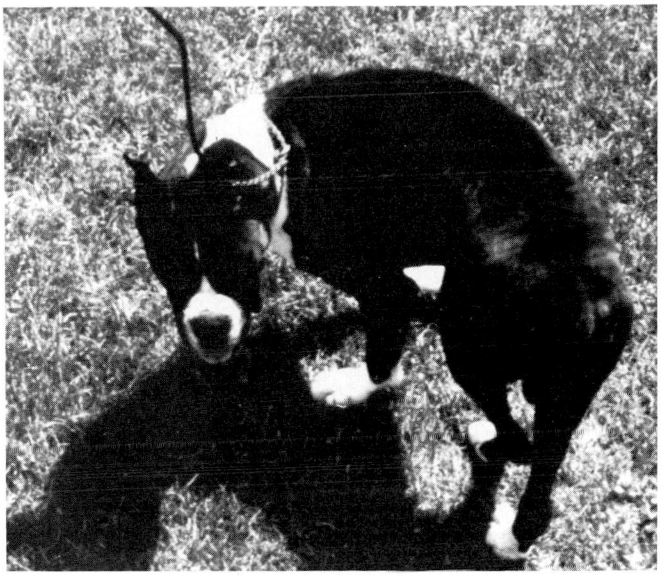

FIGURE 60–12. A patient circling as the result of a cerebral injury.

Coordination of the head is almost totally regulated by the cerebellum. Disturbances of head coordination appear as a head tremor and usually imply a lesion of the cerebellum or its connections in the brain stem. This tremor is often exaggerated by attempts to eat or drink (intention tremor).

Circling. Walking in circles tends to be seen in animals with brain diseases. A lesion in any part of the brain may cause circling, with the animal circling toward the diseased side. The circling seen with brain stem and cerebellar injuries is usually the result of a vestibular injury, so these animals usually have head tilts in addition to circling. It is not known why animals with cerebral injury circle, but they rarely have head tilts (Figure 60–12).

Evaluation of Limb Posture. A normal animal stands with its limbs at about shoulder or hip width, generally with the weight equally distributed on all four limbs (Figure 60–13). An abnormality of posture may be caused by abnormal position sense (proprioception), by weakness, or by pain. Many animals in pain have orthopedic disorders rather than neurologic disturbances. Often the specific type of abnormal stance may be helpful in further characterizing the functional system that is abnormal. A broad-based stance usually reflects a loss of balance and so is seen with cerebellar, brain stem, and peripheral vestibular disorders. High cervical cord lesions that involve the spinocerebellar pathways and diffuse PNS lesions may also cause a broad-based stance. Knuckling of limbs may be caused by either loss of conscious proprioception to a limb or paresis of a limb. Knuckling is seen with injury to the PNS, spinal cord, brain stem, and cerebrum. Holding up a limb is usually a sign of pain in the affected limb. This may be caused by injuries to peripheral nerves, nerve roots, or the meninges if the pain is neural in origin.

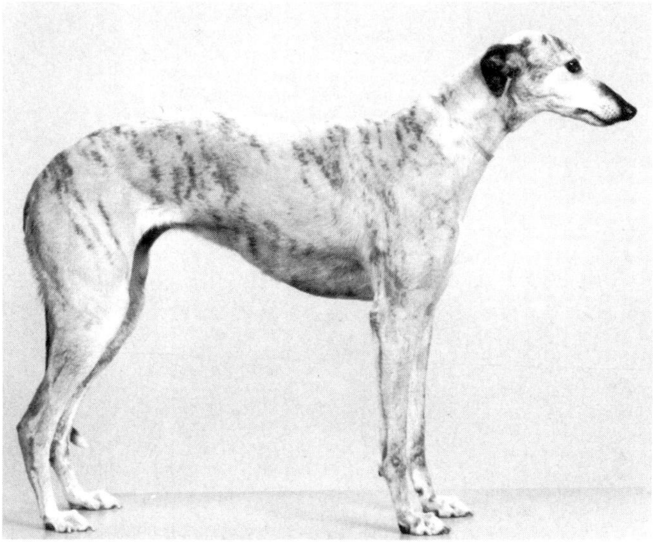

FIGURE 60–13. Normal stance in a dog.

Observation of Gait

A normal gait requires the use of almost the entire nervous system. A disturbance of gait may be caused by injury to almost any part of the nervous system. Sensory disturbances, i.e., loss of proprioception, tend to result in ataxia or loss of coordination of limb movements. Motor disturbances may cause either ataxia, as occurs with cerebellar lesions, or weakness, as occurs with lesions in all other parts of the motor system.[1, 4] While evaluating the gait, walk beside the animal and listen carefully for the scuffing of nails. The clinician can often hear an abnormal gait better than he or she can see one. Also, look carefully at an animal's toes for signs of abnormal wear, which may give a clue to a gait disturbance that is not observed during the examination. Try to observe the gait in an area with good footing, such as grass or carpeting. Avoid areas where there are a lot of distractions, such as high traffic areas of the hospital or the wards where other animals will distract the patient being examined. If there are steps or curbs available, make the patient go up and down; this increases the demands on the nervous system, allowing subtle abnormalities to be detected earlier.

Try to characterize all of the abnormalities present in the gait and the limbs that are affected. Ataxia or loss of coordination of the limbs is seen as swaying, veering, crossing over of the limbs, scuffing of the toes, and so on. Ataxia may be seen with cerebellar, brain stem, spinal cord, and PNS injuries of either the spinal nerves or cranial nerve VIII. A cerebral lesion very rarely causes ataxia. Weakness is characterized by stumbling, falling, tripping, or inability to initiate or sustain an activity. Weakness may be caused by injury to the cerebrum, brain stem, spinal cord, or peripheral spinal nerves. Spasticity is an increase in muscle tone resulting in decreased flexion of the limbs during movement. As a result, the gait is rigid and choppy. Spasticity implies a lesion of an upper motor neuron (UMN) and may be seen with injuries to the cerebrum, brain stem, and spinal cord. Dysmetria is an abnormal length of stride, with the limb movements either exaggerated in length (hypermetria) or foreshortened (hypometria). This gait disturbance may be seen with injury to the cerebellum, spinal cord, brain stem, peripheral spinal nerves, and cranial nerve VIII. While observing the gait, try to grade the severity of dysfunction in each limb, so that improvement or worsening of the condition can be quantitated.

Attitudinal and Postural Reactions

After evaluation of the gait, the clinician can further evaluate the integrity of the interconnecting pathways that regulate posture and movement with a series of reactions known as the attitudinal and postural reactions (A and P reactions). These tests evaluate the proprioceptive fibers of the peripheral nerves, spinal cord, brain stem, cerebrum, and cerebellum. Some of the tests evaluate special proprioception as well, which is determined by the inner ear. Finally, they test the long motor pathways of the upper motor neurons and their connections to the lower motor neurons (LMN). These tests are good screening tools for the detection of nervous system injury, but are not very helpful in specifically localizing the problem. These tests often pick up deficits that are not yet severe enough to have caused a gait deficit.

The technique involved in these procedures is either to place the limb in an abnormal position to see if the patient returns the limb to a normal position or to make the patient carry more weight on a limb than normal to see if it uses the limb normally.

Since these tests evaluate functional systems, they do

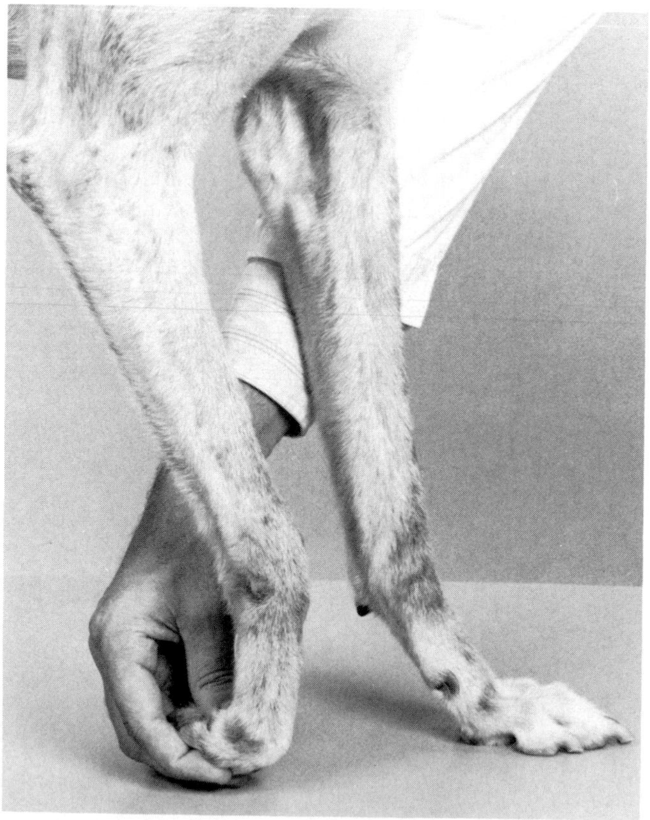

FIGURE 60–14. Testing for deficits in conscious proprioception.

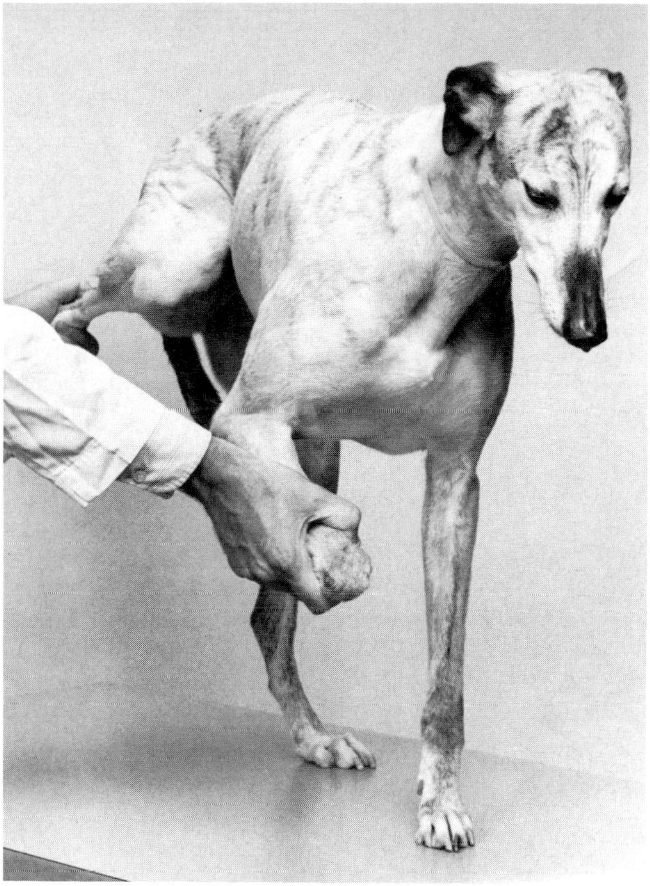

FIGURE 60–15. Hemistanding a patient to test strength.

not precisely localize lesions; however, knowing which limbs are abnormal along with the type of abnormality seen often gives clues to the location of the lesion. With lesions of the cerebrum, the clinical deficit is normally seen in both of the limbs on the opposite side of the body from the diseased hemisphere (contralateral). With brain stem lesions, the clinical signs are usually bilateral, but worse on the side of the brain stem injury. With lesions of cerebellum, spinal cord, and peripheral nerve, the clinical signs are almost always on the same side of the body as the nervous system injury (ipsilateral). With cerebellar injuries, the A and P reactions are usually still present, but ataxic. With peripheral vestibular injuries, the A and P reactions are preserved, but the animal tends to lean, fall, and roll to the diseased side when the maneuvers are performed. With lesions in all other locations in the nervous system, the A and P reactions are actually lost or absent.

Proprioceptive Positioning. In this test, a limb is abnormally abducted or adducted, or the paw is turned so that the animal's weight is borne on the dorsal surface of its paw (stands knuckled over) (Figure 60–14). If the A and P reactions are intact, the animal briskly brings the limb back to a normal resting position.

Hemihopping/Hemistanding/Hemiwalking. In this test, the patient's limbs on one side are held off the ground, while the patient is forced to walk sideways on its two remaining limbs (Figure 60–15). A normal animal has no trouble maintaining itself during this test. Weak animals sag and/or collapse on the abnormal side. This test is very good for determining asymmetries that were not detected during evaluation of the gait.

Wheelbarrowing. In this test, either the patient's thoracic or pelvic limbs are held off the ground, while the patient is hopped forwards and then backwards on its two remaining limbs (Figure 60–16). A normal animal has no trouble supporting itself during this test. Generally, the limbs move symmetrically. Animals tend to wheelbarrow forward better on the thoracic limbs, so differences between abilities going forward and abilities going backward are less significant than differences between the left and right limbs. This test is good for detecting subtle thoracic limb deficits that were not seen while evaluating the gait.

Hopping. In this test, the clinician supports all limbs except one, making the animal hop on that one limb. The animal should be made to bear as much of its weight as possible on the limb being tested (Figure 60–17). This test is very good for detecting subtle loss of strength, as well as left-to-right asymmetry between paired limbs.

Additional A and P reactions include the extensor postural thrust reaction, righting reaction, visual placing reactions, tactile placing reactions, and tonic neck reactions.[4] All of these tests evaluate the same basic pathways, although each individual test may evaluate one portion of the nervous system more completely than another. These tests are all well described in standard neurology texts.[1,4] In most animals, performing two or three of these tests is adequate; performing them all on one patient is overkill. Be certain to record which tests are performed and the abnormalities found, so that on future examinations the same tests can be repeated for comparison.

Cranial Nerve Examination

In the cranial nerve examination, evaluation of the function of each cranial nerve is attempted. Cranial

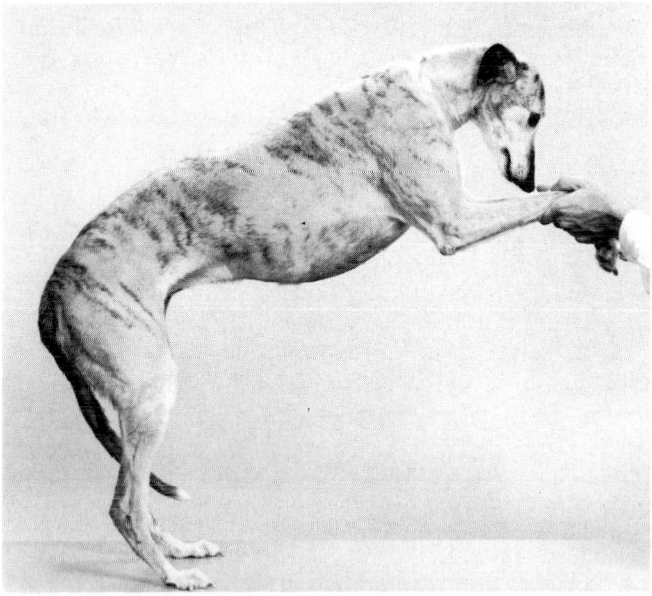

FIGURE 60–16. Wheelbarrowing an animal.

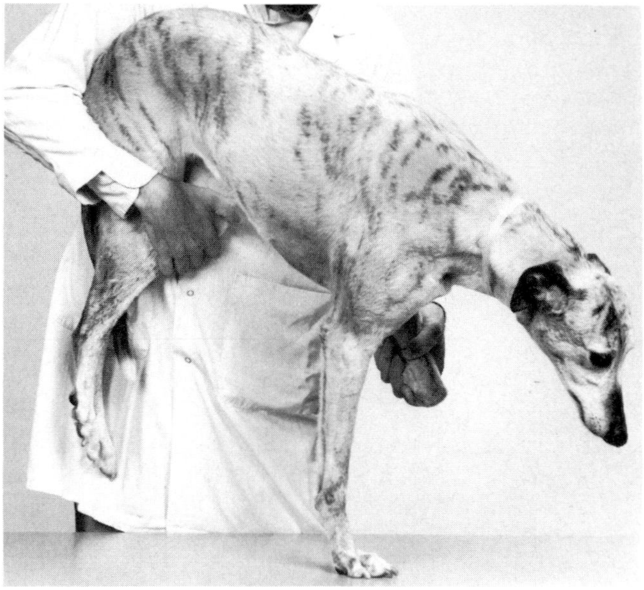

FIGURE 60–17. Hopping an animal, using the thoracic limbs.

nerves I and XI are the two that are the most difficult to test; these are not usually evaluated on a routine clinical neurologic examination. Except for Horner's syndrome, a cranial nerve deficit confirms the presence of a lesion above the foramen magnum. Cranial nerve abnormalities also provide fairly precise localization of neurologic problems in most cases.

Animals have 12 pairs of cranial nerves, two of which originate in the cerebrum, the rest of which are considered of brain stem origin. Since some cranial nerves are either motor or sensory, but not both, the testing of a cranial nerve reflex or response generally tests more than one nerve. In addition, many of the cranial nerve reflexes and responses are under higher control. As such, testing a cranial nerve response usually tests two peripheral cranial nerves, one motor and one sensory; a central connection, usually the brain stem; and a higher regulatory center, usually the cerebrum.[2, 5] This chapter describes the cranial nerve examination by test, not by nerve; it briefly reviews the cranial nerves and their functions before moving on to the actual tests themselves.

The olfactory nerve (CN I) originates in the cerebrum, is sensory in function, and provides the sense of smell. This nerve is difficult to test and clinical disorders of smell are rarely recognized in veterinary medicine.

The optic nerve (CN II) also originates in the cerebrum (diencephalon), is sensory, and provides vision and pupillary accommodation to light. This nerve is tested with the menace response, which tests vision by observation of pupil size and the pupillary light response, both of which test pupillary accommodation.

The oculomotor nerve (CN III) originates in the brain stem (mesencephalon) and provides motor innervation to the eyeball. It has a parasympathetic division, which constricts the pupil in response to light (pupillary accommodation) and a somatic division, which moves the eyeball by stimulation of extraocular muscles. This nerve is tested with the pupillary light response, by observation of pupil size and symmetry, by observation of ocular position, and by observation of ocular motility (the doll's eye maneuver and pathologic nystagmus).

The trochlear nerve (CN IV) originates in the brain stem (mesencephalon) and provides motor innervation to the eyeball. It moves the eyeball by stimulation of extraocular muscles. This nerve is tested by observation of ocular position and by observation of ocular motility (the doll's eye maneuver and pathologic nystagmus).

The trigeminal nerve (CN V) is both motor and sensory. It originates in the brain stem (mesencephalon) and provides pain and proprioceptive information from the head, as well as motor innervation to the muscles of mastication. This nerve is tested by corneal reflex, eye blink reflex, evaluation of jaw tone, and by painful stimuli to the face.

The abducens nerve (CN VI) originates in the brain stem (mesencephalon) and provides motor innervation to the eyeball. It moves the eyeball by stimulation of extraocular muscles and the retractor oculi muscle. This nerve is tested by observation of ocular position, by the retractor oculi reflex, and by observation of ocular motility (the doll's eye maneuver and pathologic nystagmus).

The facial nerve (CN VII) originates in the brain stem (myelencephalon). It provides motor innervation to the muscles of facial expression, is sensory to the tongue (taste), and innervates the lacrimal and salivary glands. This nerve is tested by observing facial symmetry, stimulating the eye to blink, and monitoring tear production.

The vestibulocochlear nerve (CN VIII) is a purely

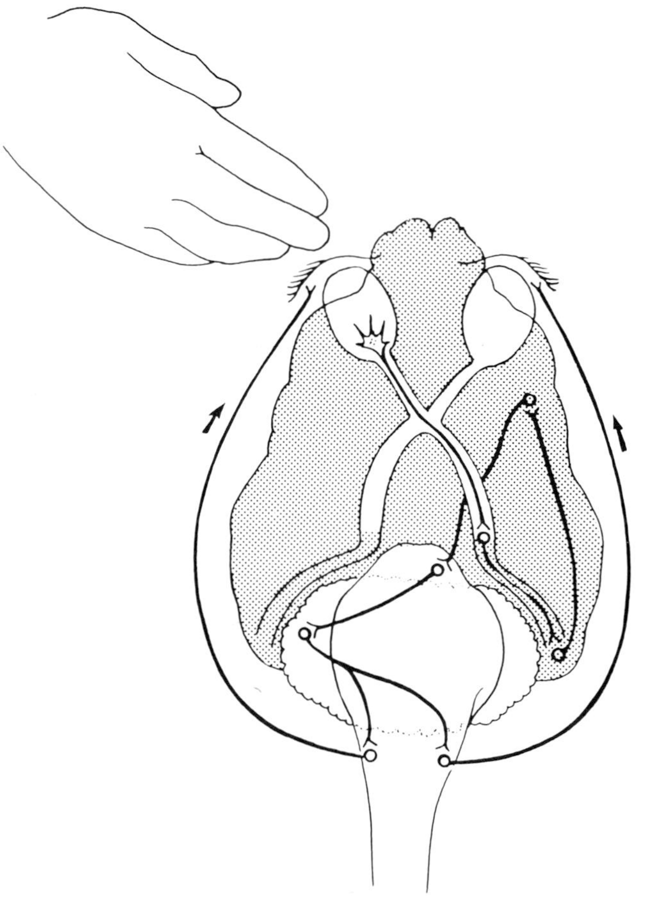

FIGURE 60–18. Anatomic representation of the menace pathways.

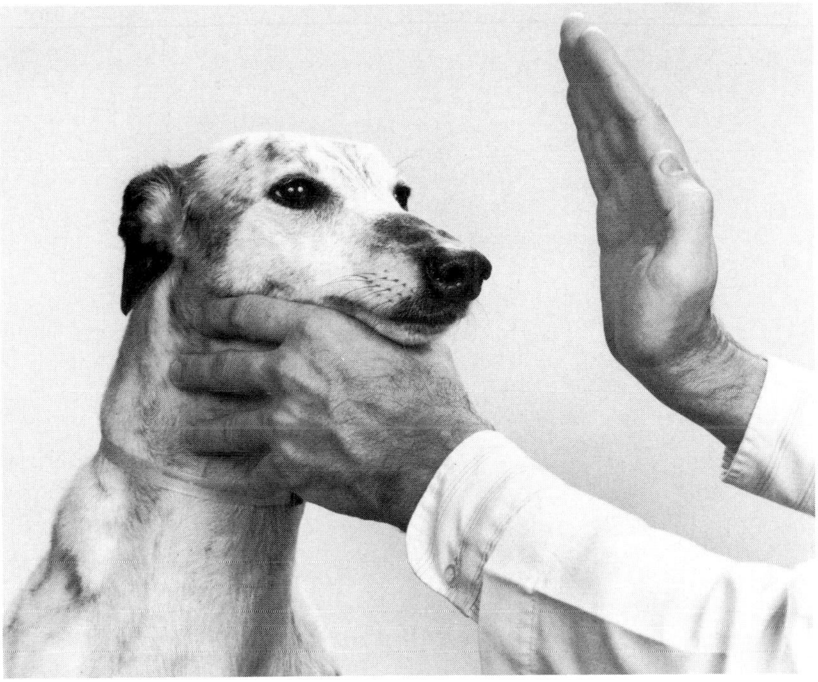

FIGURE 60–19. Testing the menace reactions in a patient.

sensory nerve, which originates in the brain stem (myelencephalon). It is responsible for detection of changes in posture relative to gravity, detection of spinning, regulation of extraocular muscle tone, and hearing. It is tested by observing extraocular motility, posture of the head, gait, and balance, and by electrical testing of hearing.

The glossopharyngeal nerve (CN IX) originates in the caudal brain stem, the myelencephalon. It is responsible for taste, sensation in the pharynx, and motor innervation of the pharynx, larynx, and some salivary glands. It is tested by observing the gag reflex and swallowing motions.

The vagus nerve (CN X) originates in the brain stem and is concerned with many autonomic functions. It regulates gastrointestinal motility, has regulatory functions over the heart, provides motor function for swallowing (along with CN IX), and regulates esophageal motility, among other functions. It is tested mainly by observing the gag reflex and swallowing behavior.

The spinal accessory nerve (CN XI) originates in the posterior brain stem and cranial cervical spinal cord. It is concerned with innervation of the muscles that elevate the shoulders and, to a lesser extent, with the elevators of the head. There is no reliable method of testing this nerve in veterinary neurology except using electrodiagnostics to test for denervation.

The hypoglossal nerve (CN XII) originates in the brain stem (myelencephalon) and is responsible for motor innervation of the tongue. This nerve may be tested indirectly by watching the animal use its tongue and directly by electrodiagnostic testing.

A more comprehensive review of the structure and function of the cranial nerves may be obtained by reading a neuroanatomy or clinical neurology textbook.[1, 4] For this discussion, the cranial nerve reflexes compose the more vital material.

Tests of Cranial Nerve Function

THE MENACE RESPONSE

The menace response is used to test cranial nerve II (sensory), cranial nerve VII (motor), and their central connections in the brain stem and cerebrum (Figure 60–18). The test is performed by making a menacing gesture toward an animal (Figure 60–19). The normal response is an avoidance response, for example, an eye blink or turning of the head. Loss of the menace response normally indicates a lesion in one of the following sites: retina (ipsilateral), optic nerve (ipsilateral), optic tract (contralateral), cerebrum (contralateral), brain stem (ipsilateral), or facial nerve (ipsilateral). Some animals with cerebellar disorders may have an ipsilateral loss of the menace response as well.[1] The mechanism of the menace deficit is not well understood. False-positive menace responses may also occur. The most common cause of this is the production of air currents by the movement of the hand that stimulates the corneal reflex. Sounds and other distractions may make the menace response hard to evaluate.

THE PUPILLARY LIGHT REFLEX (PLR)

This reflex tests the reflex portion of cranial nerve II and the visceral function of cranial nerve III (Figure 60–20). The test is performed by illuminating one eye with a bright light source (Figure 60 21). The normal response is rapid constriction of both pupils. The pupillary constriction in the eye being illuminated is called the direct pupillary response, while the constriction in the opposite pupil (the one being illuminated indirectly) is called the consensual response. An abnormal PLR is failure of one or both pupils to constrict. A lesion of the optic nerve produces loss of constriction in both

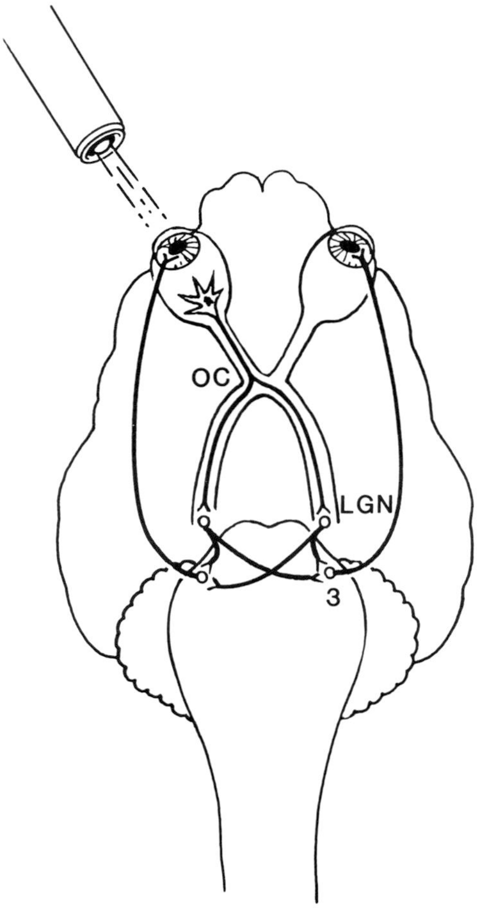

FIGURE 60–20. Anatomic representation of the pathways of the pupillary light reflex. OC = optic chiasm, LGN = lateral geniculate nucleus, and 3 = cranial nerve 3.

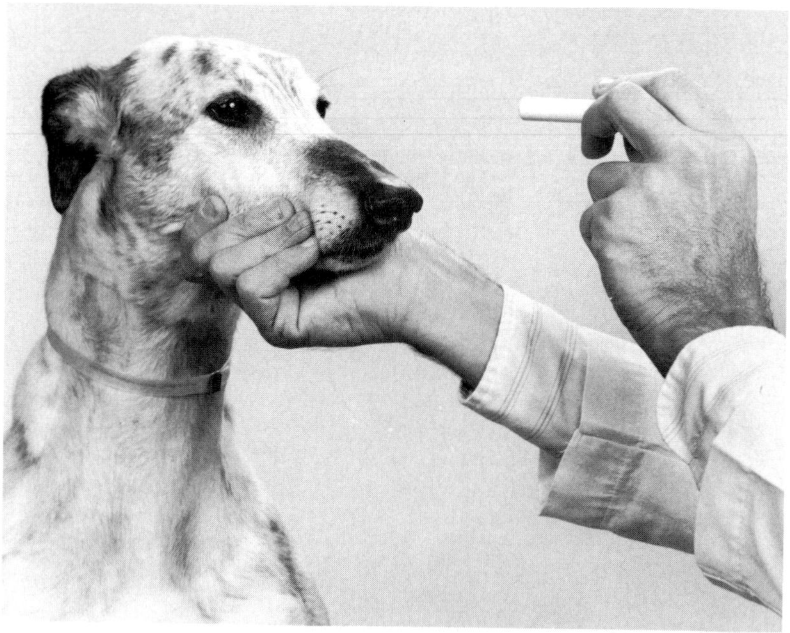

FIGURE 60–21. Testing the pupillary light reflex in a patient.

pupils when the affected eye is illuminated, but, when the normal eye is illuminated, both pupils constrict. If there is a lesion in the oculomotor nerve or brain stem, then the affected pupil fails to constrict regardless of which eye is illuminated. The unaffected eye constricts normally when each eye is illuminated. Ophthalmic diseases such as posterior synechia or severe iris atrophy may produce loss of pupillary responsiveness. Because of this, a thorough eye examination is essential in patients with abnormal pupils. Other causes of a misleading PLR are increases in sympathetic tone and a weak light source, which slows the PLR.

PUPILLARY SYMMETRY

In this test the clinician simply observes the eye to make certain that both pupils are equal to each other in size. If the oculomotor nerve and sympathetic nerve to the eye are both normal, the two pupils should always be equal in size. Unequal pupils, a condition called anisocoria, are an indication of possible damage to one of those two nerves. If the oculomotor nerve is abnormal, the large pupil is the denervated one and the PLR is absent in that eye. If the sympathetic nerve is abnormal, the small pupil is the abnormal one and the PLR is normal in both eyes. A number of ophthalmic disorders, including glaucoma, iritis, uveitis, and synechia, may produce anisocoria. Because of this, all patients with anisocoria should have a complete ophthalmic examination.

PUPIL SIZE

The size of the pupil is determined by the amount of ambient light (optic nerve) and the integrity of the pupillary muscles (oculomotor nerve and sympathetic nerve). Abnormally large pupils may be seen with excitement (sympathetic stimulation), bilateral optic nerve injury, cranial nerve III paralysis, and ophthalmic disease. Abnormally small pupils may be seen with loss of sympathetic tone, excess parasympathetic tone, and ophthalmic disease.

OCULAR POSITION

In a normal animal, both eyes should appear to be looking ahead in the same direction. This normal resting position is determined by the influence of the cerebrum and cranial nerve VIII on the extraocular muscles (cranial nerves III, IV, and VI) (Figure 60–22).[6] If one of these cranial nerves is not functioning, deviation of the eyeball (strabismus) may be observed. A medial strabismus is usually the result of an injury to the abducens nerve. A ventrolateral strabismus may result from an injury to either the oculomotor nerve or the vestibulocochlear nerve. A lesion to the trochlear nerve results in intorsion (a form of rotation) of the eye, which is only seen in animals with oval pupils or on retinal examination. If the cerebrum is not functioning, there may be a lateral gaze deviation, where both eyes are looking in the same direction but off to one side. This is uncommon in most veterinary patients. The author

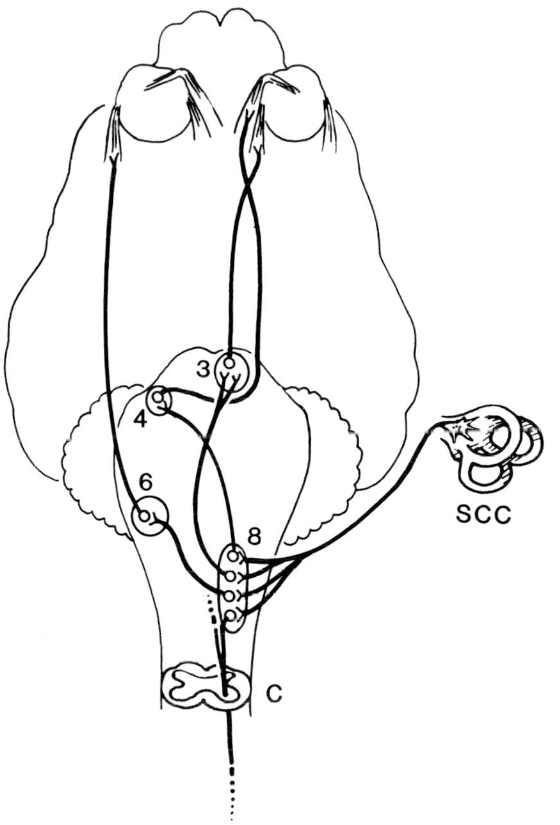

FIGURE 60–22. Anatomic representation of the pathways for ocular position. SCC = semicircular canal; C = cervical spinal cord; 3 = cranial nerve 3; 4 = cranial nerve 4; 6 = cranial nerve 6; and 8 = cranial nerve 8.

usually sees this phenomenon only in acute, severe injuries. Animals with retrobulbar masses may show a strabismus if the mass physically displaces the eyeball.

OCULAR MOTILITY (VOLUNTARY AND INVOLUNTARY)

Voluntary eye movement is initiated by cerebral stimulation of cranial nerves III, IV, and VI. Watch the animal as it looks around the examination room to see if it is able to move its eyes in all directions. With a cerebral lesion, both eyes are involved and there is a tendency for the eyes to look towards the side of the diseased cerebral hemisphere (conjugate gaze deviation). With a lesion of the cranial nerves, only one eye is involved. That eye tends to have a strabismus at rest and lack the ability to move.

Clinicians can initiate involuntary, rhythmic oscillations of the eye, known as nystagmus, by turning the head. This maneuver stimulates cranial nerve VIII, which in turn stimulates cranial nerves III, IV, and VI, which innervate the extraocular muscles. This involuntary eye movement is known as "physiologic nystagmus." It is manifested as a rhythmic oscillation of both eyes, first moving slowly away from the direction in which the head is turning, then rapidly in the same direction as the head is turning. This slow-rapid, slow-rapid oscillation continues as long as the head is being turned. A lesion of cranial nerve VIII or its central connections can result in loss of the ability to initiate this physiologic nystagmus; it will not be seen in either eye. A lesion of the cranial nerves that innervate the eyeball only paralyzes the one eye. In that case there will be loss of physiologic nystagmus in one eye, but not the other.

PATHOLOGIC NYSTAGMUS

A normal animal whose head is not being turned will not demonstrate spontaneous nystagmus. If nystagmus is present under such circumstances, it is a sign of pathology and is called "pathologic nystagmus." Pathologic nystagmus is usually the result of an imbalance in the special proprioceptive system, which includes the inner ear, cranial nerve VIII, the brain stem, and the cerebellum. A lesion of any of these four structures can cause pathologic nystagmus. By noting the direction(s) of the nystagmus, whether or not the direction changes, and what head positions the nystagmus occurs in, some conclusions may be drawn about the patient's problems. In horizontal nystagmus, the eyes move in a plane parallel to the animal's head (the eyes move from side to side). This type of nystagmus is most commonly seen in peripheral vestibular disease. The fast component of the nystagmus is away from the diseased side. In vertical nystagmus, the eyes move in a plane perpendicular to the animal's head (the eyes move up and down). This type of nystagmus is most commonly seen in central vestibular disease. With rotatory nystagmus, the eyes rotate in a clockwise or counterclockwise manner in the orbit. This type of nystagmus has components of both horizontal and vertical movement and is not localizing; it may be seen with a lesion anywhere in the special proprioceptive system.

Nystagmus is also classified by whether it is present at all times or not. Resting nystagmus is seen when the patient's head is at rest (not moving) and in a normal position. This type of nystagmus is most characteristic of peripheral vestibular disease. Positional nystagmus is present when the patient's head is still but the head is in an abnormal position, such as turned on its side or upside down. Positional nystagmus is most characteristic of central vestibular dysfunction, e.g., brain stem and cerebellar lesions. It is also seen during the compensation phase of peripheral vestibular diseases.

Finally, pathologic nystagmus is classified by whether or not it persists or can be reproduced for more than two weeks. Most pathologic nystagmus that is the result of an injury to the peripheral vestibular system spontaneously resolves over 10 to 14 days following the injury that initially caused it. After the nystagmus has resolved it can only be reproduced by new damage to the vestibular system. This appears to be a result of CNS compensation for the original injury. Nystagmus that results from injury to the CNS often cannot be compensated for. As a result, it persists over time. It may have any direction or method of induction, but whenever the animal is examined for it, it is present. This type of nystagmus is characteristic of all brain stem diseases and of progressive cerebellar diseases.

CRANIAL MUSCLE SYMMETRY

The superficial muscles of the head can be divided into·two major groups. The first is the muscles of facial expression. These muscles are innervated by the facial nerve (cranial nerve VII) and include the muscles of the eyelid and lip. The second group is the muscles of mastication, which are innervated by the trigeminal nerve (cranial nerve V). These muscles include the temporal and masseter muscles. Facial paralysis may result from injury to the contralateral cerebrum, ipsilateral brain stem, and ipsilateral peripheral nerve. Clinically, drooping of the lip, deviation of the nasal philtrum, increases in palpebral fissure (pseudoptosis), and in some animals, true ptosis (drooping of the eyelid) are seen. The diminished muscle function can be confirmed by testing the facial (palpebral and/or corneal) reflexes. Masticatory muscle paralysis may result from ipsilateral injury to the brain stem or peripheral nerve. The clinical appearance is loss of muscle mass and weakness of the jaw, often manifested as a dropped jaw and an inability to close the mouth.

FACIAL REFLEXES

Palpebral Reflex. This reflex tests the maxillary division of cranial nerve V and its brain stem connection to cranial nerve VII. The reflex is initiated by touching the palpebral margins, which produces an eye blink (Figure 60–23). Lack of the reflex is generally manifested as loss of eye blink. In some animals with incomplete paresis of cranial nerve V or VII, lagophthalmos, which is incomplete closure of the palpebral margins, may be seen.

Corneal Reflex. This reflex tests the ophthalmic portion of cranial nerve V and its brain stem connection to cranial nerve VII. The reflex is initiated by lightly touching the cornea, which produces an eye blink. Lack of this reflex is generally manifested as loss of eye blink. In some animals with incomplete paresis of cranial V or VII, lagophthalmos may be seen.

Retractor Oculi Reflex. This reflex tests the ophthalmic division of cranial nerve V and its brain stem connection to cranial nerve VI. The reflex is initiated by lightly touching the cornea, which produces retraction of the eye into the orbit. Lack of this reflex is usually a sign of neurologic dysfunction. In some animals with loss of the retrobulbar fat pad, the eye may be enophthalmic and incapable of retraction; in others, a retrobulbar mass may prevent retraction.

Facial Sensory Examination. This test examines cranial nerve V and its cerebral connections (Figure 60–24). It is performed by lightly stimulating the nasal mucosa, which should produce an avoidance response such as head turning. The nasal mucosa is a more reliable site for stimulation than the lips, which are fairly insensate in some animals.

THE ORAL CAVITY

Gag Reflex. This reflex tests cranial nerves IX and X and their brain stem connections. To initiate the test,

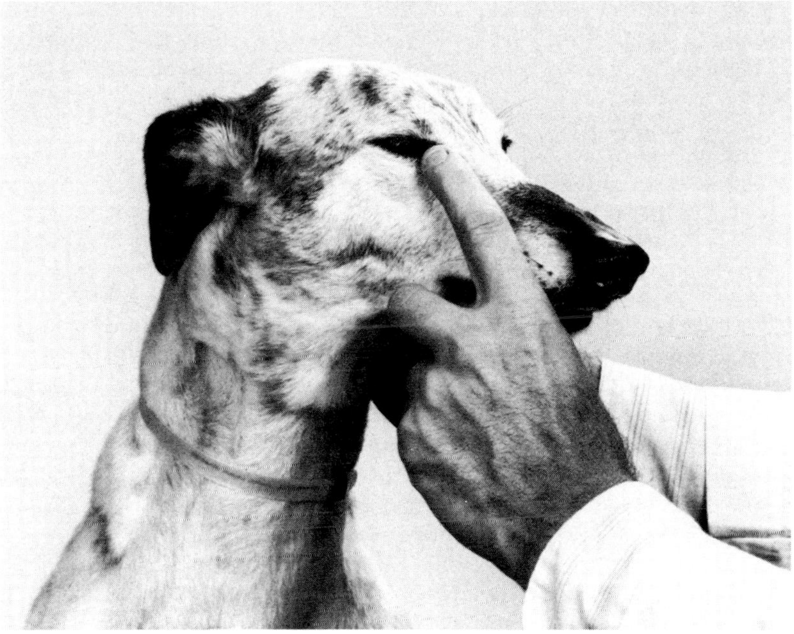

FIGURE 60–23. Testing the palpebral reflex in a patient.

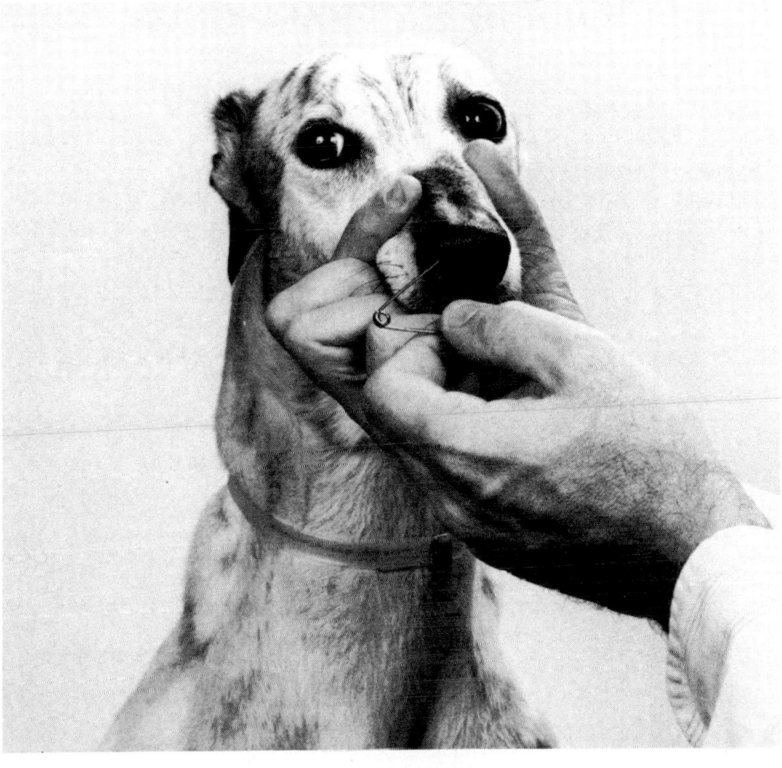

FIGURE 60–24. Testing the integrity of facial sensation.

lightly stimulate the oropharynx, which should produce a swallowing reflex. This reflex appears to be under a high degree of cerebral control in farm animals, but in the dog and the cat, loss of the reflex usually implies brain stem or peripheral nerve dysfunction.

Oral Examination. The oral examination evaluates the tongue (cranial nerve XII) and completes the evaluation of cranial nerves IX and X. Look for atrophy of the tongue, which can be produced by brain stem or peripheral nerve injury. Also look for deviation of the tongue, which can be caused by cerebral injuries as well as brain stem and peripheral nerve injuries. Examine the pharynx for evidence of paralysis of the soft palate, and look at the larynx for evidence of laryngeal paralysis. Either of these conditions may result from brain stem injuries or peripheral nerve injuries.

Conclusion. Most cranial nerve tests evaluate more than one nerve, as well as evaluating the central nervous system connections between two nerves. All of the tests can be abnormal as a result of peripheral nerve or brain stem injury, and many of them can be abnormal as a result of cerebral injury. Only a few may be abnormal as a result of cerebellar injury. Table 60–2 lists the cranial nerve tests discussed, with their sensory and motor nerves, normal response, and portions of CNS tested.

When evaluating the examination performed to this point, it may help to divide the brain into its local subdivisions and consider each one's major "functional" categories. The cerebrum is concerned with "brain" functions, so if it is abnormal, abnormalities of learning, behavior, and vision are seen. The brain stem is concerned with "head" function and is further subdivided into the midbrain, pons, and medulla. If the midbrain is abnormal, there is abnormality of eyeball function. If the pons is abnormal, the face does not function properly. If the medulla is abnormal, the mouth, tongue, and throat do not function as they should.[7] Finally, there is the cerebellum, which is concerned with coordination of movement of the whole body. If it is abnormal, disregulation of all voluntary motor coordination, with associated tremors and ataxia, occurs.

Spinal Segmental Reflexes

From the cranial nerve examination, the author proceeds to the spinal reflex examination. The spinal segmental reflexes directly test the reflex arcs of the spinal cord. They also indirectly test the higher centers in the brain that regulate the spinal reflexes. If an injury occurs within the reflex arc, it causes loss of the reflex. Loss of this reflex allows precise localization of the site of injury. Since such a change involves a lesion in the lower motor neuron, loss of reflexes is called a LMN sign or a LMN reflex change. If a lesion occurs cranial to a reflex arc, it disconnects the reflex from its higher (upper motor neuron) regulation. This regulation tends to be inhibitory, so loss of UMN regulation results in exaggeration of reflexes. This exaggeration reflects a lesion in the CNS involving UMN pathways, so such reflex changes are called UMN signs or UMN reflexes. UMN changes confirm the presence of a CNS lesion, but are not as precisely localizing as LMN reflexes. Spinal reflexes may be subdivided into three types. They are proprioceptive reflexes, nociceptive reflexes, and special (released) reflexes. This division is based on the type of sensory stimulation required to elicit the reflex for the first two categories and on the special conditions required to elicit the third.

PROPRIOCEPTIVE

These reflexes are initiated by the stretching of tendons or muscle spindles. They are strongly influenced by the UMN and so are very likely to be exaggerated with UMN lesions. Because increases in reflex activity need to be recognized as well as decreases in reflex activity, it is important to grade the strength of these reflexes. One standard grading scale is 0 = absent reflex, 1 = diminished reflex, 2 = normal reflex, 3 = increased reflex, 4 = increased reflexes with clonus. When interpreting proprioceptive reflexes, loss of the reflexes is the most important change, both indicating the presence of nervous system dysfunction and precisely localizing it. Exaggeration of proprioceptive reflexes is the next

TABLE 60–2. CRANIAL NERVE TESTS

Maneuver	Sensory Nerve	Motor Nerve	Normal Response	Portion of CNS Tested
Menace	II	VII	Blink	Cerebrum
Pupillary light reflex	II	III	Pupil constriction	Midbrain
Doll's eye	VIII	III/IV/VI	Nystagmus	Brain stem
Lid blink	V	VII	Lid closure	Pons/medulla
Retractor oculi	V	VI	Eye retraction	Pons/medulla
Gag reflex	IX/X	IX/X	Swallow	Medulla
Eye position at rest	VIII	III/IV/VI	Normal conjugate position	Vestibular brain stem
Temporal muscle palpation		V	Full, symmetrical muscles	Pons (brain stem)
Positional nystagmus	VIII	III, IV, VI	No eye movements	Cerebellum/vestibular
Tongue examination	V	XII	Normal movement, no atrophy	Caudal medulla

most important change, since it confirms the presence of nervous system dysfunction, but only localizes the injury to a region cranial to the reflex being tested. Normal reflexes are the least helpful, as both mild LMN and UMN injuries may fail to change the reflexes. Of course, normal reflexes are also seen in patients with normal nervous systems. As part of the evaluation of proprioceptive reflexes, evaluate the muscle tone of each limb. Injuries in the reflex arc (LMN injuries) produce hypotonia of the limb, while injuries of the UMN pathways produce a hypertonia or spasticity of the affected limbs. Proprioceptive reflexes and muscle tone are best evaluated in a relaxed animal in lateral recumbency. Since large dogs tend to have slightly more brisk reflexes than small dogs and cats, the clinician should practice eliciting the different reflexes in animals of various sizes to use as a normal data base.[1]

Thoracic Limb Reflexes. Thoracic limb reflexes are summarized in Figure 60–25.

TRICEPS REFLEX. This reflex tests the radial nerve, which arises from spinal cord segments C7-T1 or T2 (Figure 60–26). The reflex is elicited by striking the tendon of insertion of the triceps muscle. A normal response is a slight extension of the limb at the elbow. The reflex is often difficult to obtain in normal animals and when present, is hard to interpret.

EXTENSOR CARPI RADIALIS REFLEX. This reflex tests the radial nerve, and thus also tests spinal cord segments C7-T1 or T2. The reflex is elicited by striking the muscle belly of the extensor carpi radialis muscle, which results in extension of the carpus (Figure 60–27). This reflex is easier to elicit in many animals than the triceps reflex but is also difficult to interpret.

BICEPS REFLEX. This reflex evaluates the musculocutaneous nerve, which arises from spinal cord segments C6-C8. The reflex is initiated by striking a finger, which is placed on the tendon of insertion of the biceps muscle (Figure 60–28). A normal response is a slight flexion of

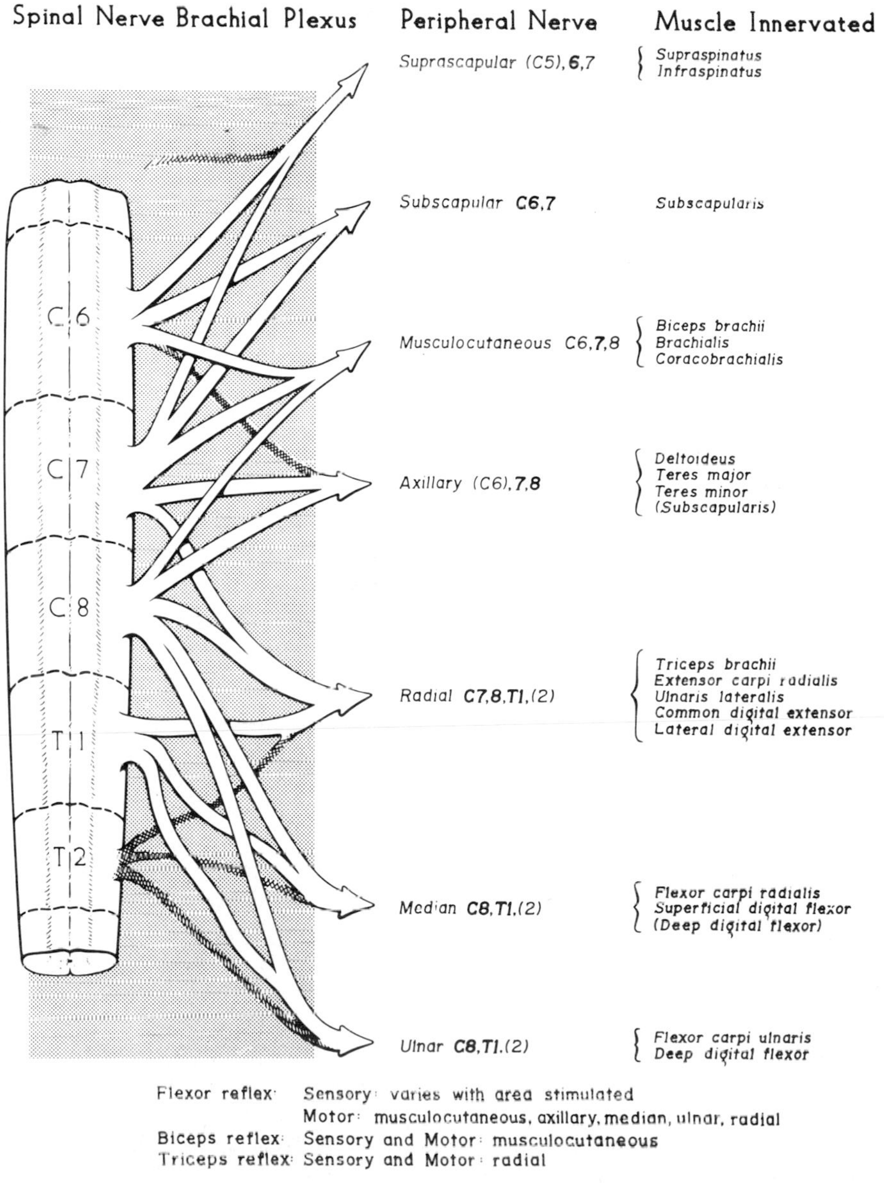

FIGURE 60–25. An anatomic representation of the thoracic limb reflexes. (From DeLahunta, A.: Veterinary Neuroanatomy and Clinical Neurology. Philadelphia, W.B. Saunders Co., 1983, p. 63.)

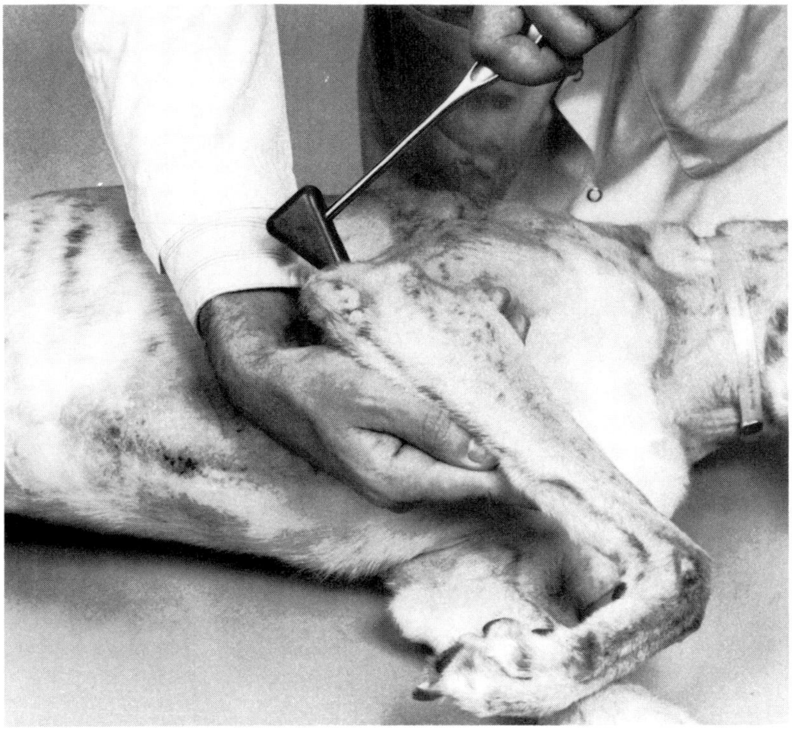

FIGURE 60–26. Testing the triceps reflex in a patient.

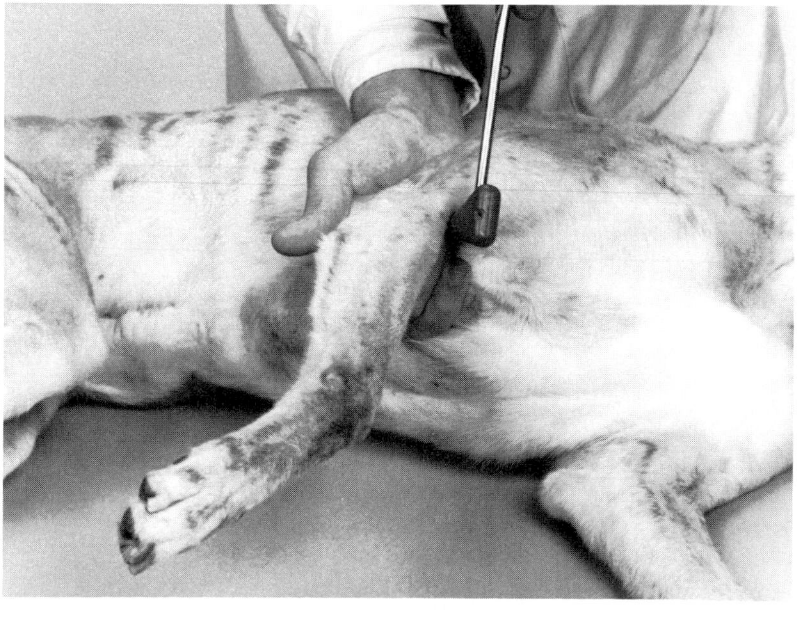

FIGURE 60–27. Testing the extensor carpi radialis reflex in a patient.

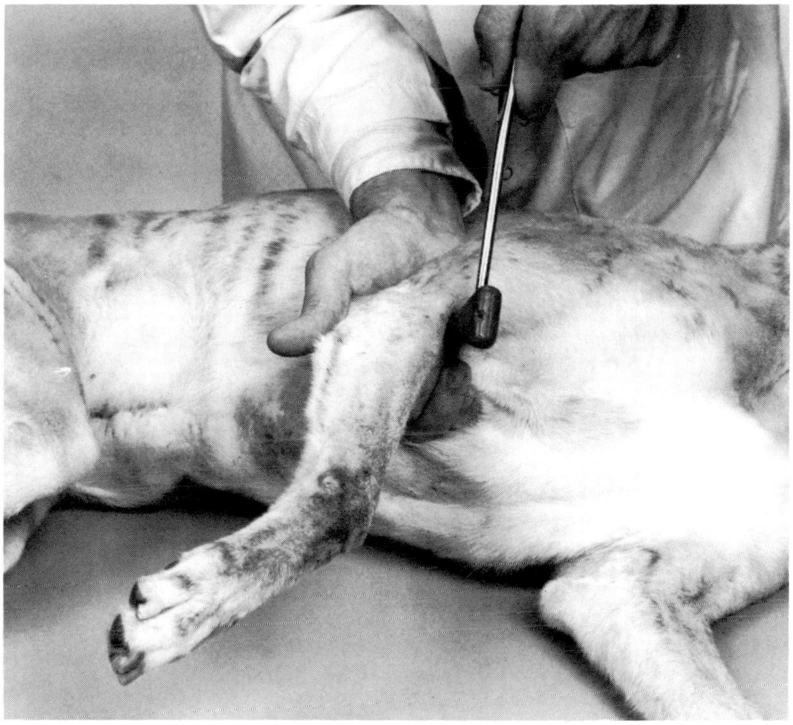

FIGURE 60–28. Testing the biceps reflex in a patient.

the elbow. This reflex is more difficult to obtain than the triceps reflex and is also difficult to interpret.

Pelvic Limb Reflexes. Pelvic limb reflexes are summarized in Figure 60–29.

Patellar reflex. This reflex tests the femoral nerve, which arises from spinal cord segments L4-L6. The reflex is elicited by striking the patellar tendon, which produces extension of the stifle (Figure 60–30). This reflex is probably the most reliable tendon reflex in veterinary medicine. With this reflex, a phenomenon known as a false localizing sign may occur. In this condition, paralysis of the sciatic nerve results in a hyperactive patellar reflex, possibly due to functional loss of the antagonist muscles that oppose the extensors of the stifle.

Anterior tibialis reflex. This reflex tests the peroneal branch of the sciatic nerve, which originates from spinal cord segment L6-S1 or S2. The reflex is initiated by striking the belly of the cranial tibial muscle (Figure 60–31). The normal response is flexion of the tarsus. The author does not consider this reflex to be very reliable, but it can usually be obtained.

Gastrocnemius reflex. This reflex tests the tibial branch of the sciatic nerve, which originates from spinal cord segment L6-S1 or S2. The reflex is initiated by striking either the belly of the gastrocnemius muscle or its tendon of insertion just proximal to the tuber calcaneous. The expected normal response is extension of the tarsus; however, in the author's experience, many patients have flexion of the tarsus. The author does not believe that this reflex is reliable, and it is also difficult to interpret.

Remember that all proprioceptive reflexes need to be evaluated for increases in reflex activity as well as decreases.

NOCICEPTIVE

These reflexes are initiated by nociceptive (painful) stimuli, such as pinching, compression, or pin pricks. In spite of the type of stimulus used, it is important to realize that these reflexes test only the integrity of a spinal reflex arc. The fact that a reflex is present tells nothing about the health of the nociceptive pathways traveling cranially to the brain. These reflexes do not have a large UMN influence; therefore, they do not normally become exaggerated with UMN lesions. The most significant change seen is loss of a nociceptive reflex, which indicates a LMN lesion.

Flexor Reflexes. These reflexes are initiated by compression of a digit, and the normal response is withdrawal of the limb from the source of the stimulus (Figure 60–32). The thoracic limb flexor response uses all of the peripheral nerves of the thoracic limb and tests spinal cord segments C6-T2. The loss of the reflex indicates a lesion in the reflex arc. The pelvic limb flexor reflex tests primarily the sciatic nerve and its branches. It tests L6-S2 nerve roots, as their fibers compose the sciatic nerve. The loss of the reflex indicates a lesion in the reflex arc.

Perineal Reflexes. These reflexes are normally initiated by lightly pricking the perianal region; they test the perineal and pudendal nerves, spinal cord segments S1-S3, and the cauda equina. The reflex is initiated by lightly stroking the perianal skin (Figure 60–33). The expected response is constriction of the anal sphincter and flexion of the tail. If a mild weakness is suspected, the best way to test the reflex is during a digital rectal examination, so that the examiner can feel the strength of contracture of the sphincter.

Panniculus Reflex (cutaneous reflex). This reflex is

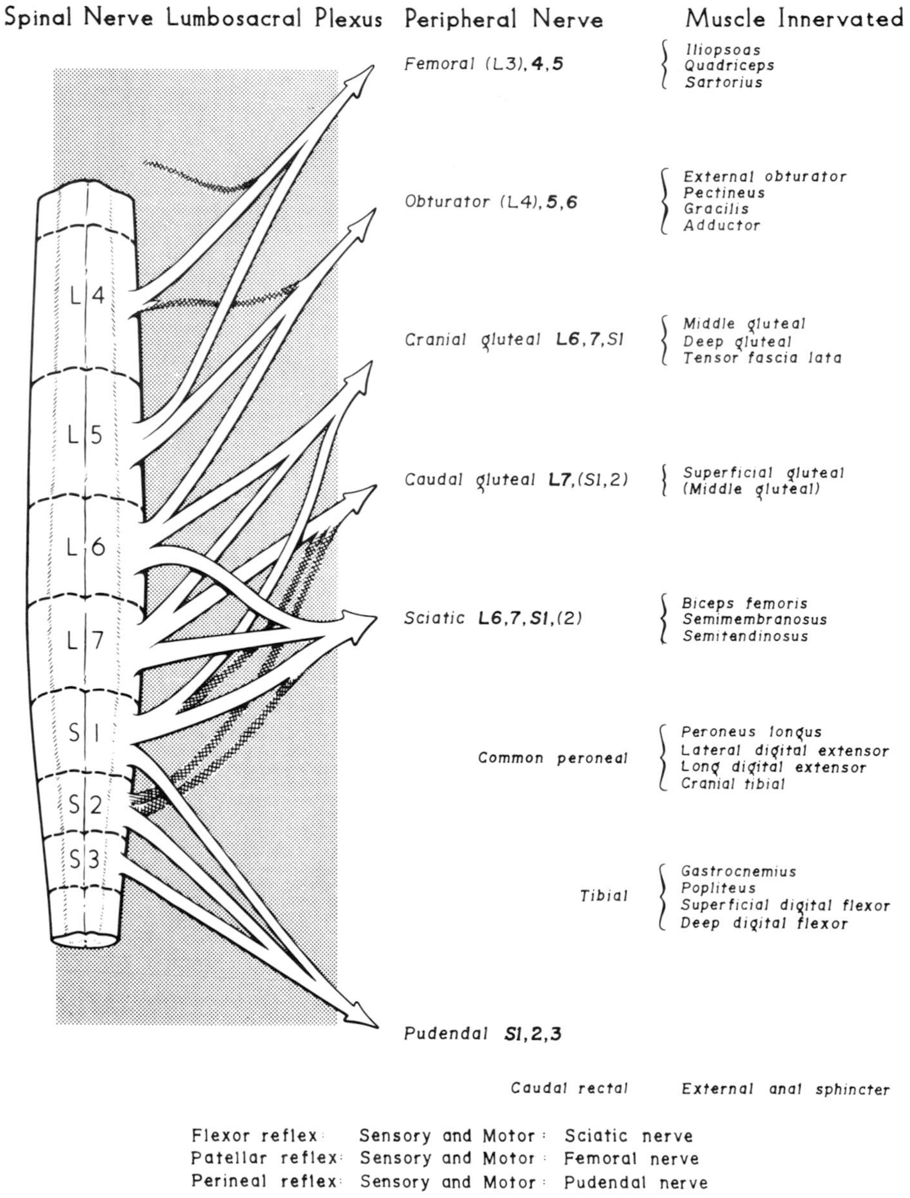

FIGURE 60–29. An anatomic representation of the pelvic limb reflexes. (From DeLahunta, A.: Veterinary Neuroanatomy and Clinical Neurology. Philadelphia, W.B. Saunders Co., 1983, p. 64.)

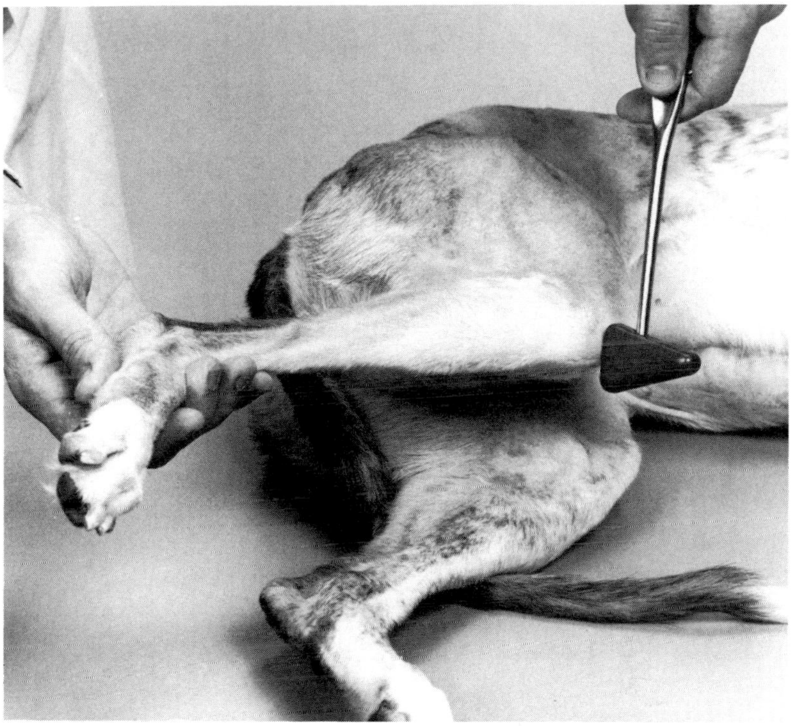

FIGURE 60–30. Testing the patellar reflexes in a patient.

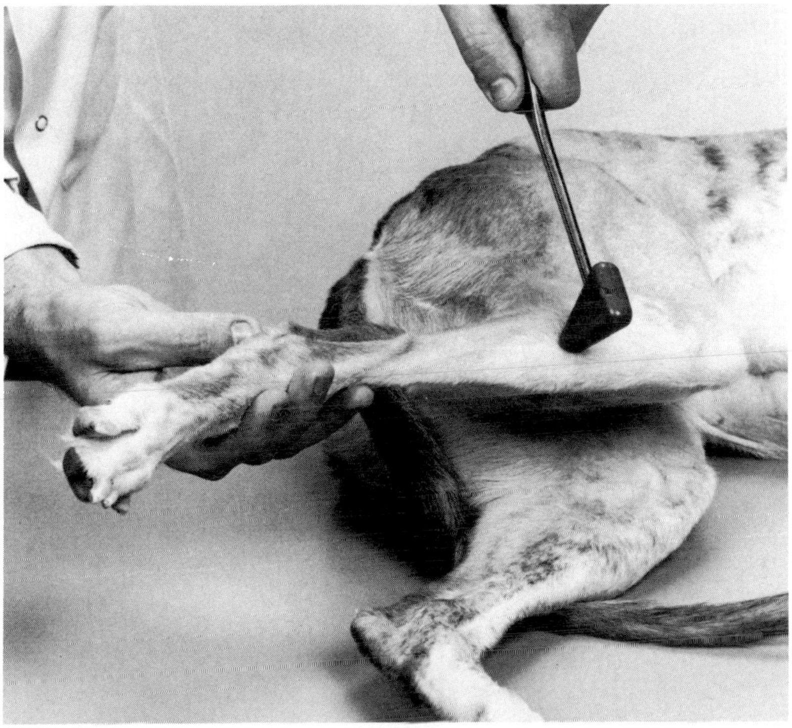

FIGURE 60–31. Testing the anterior tibial reflex in a patient.

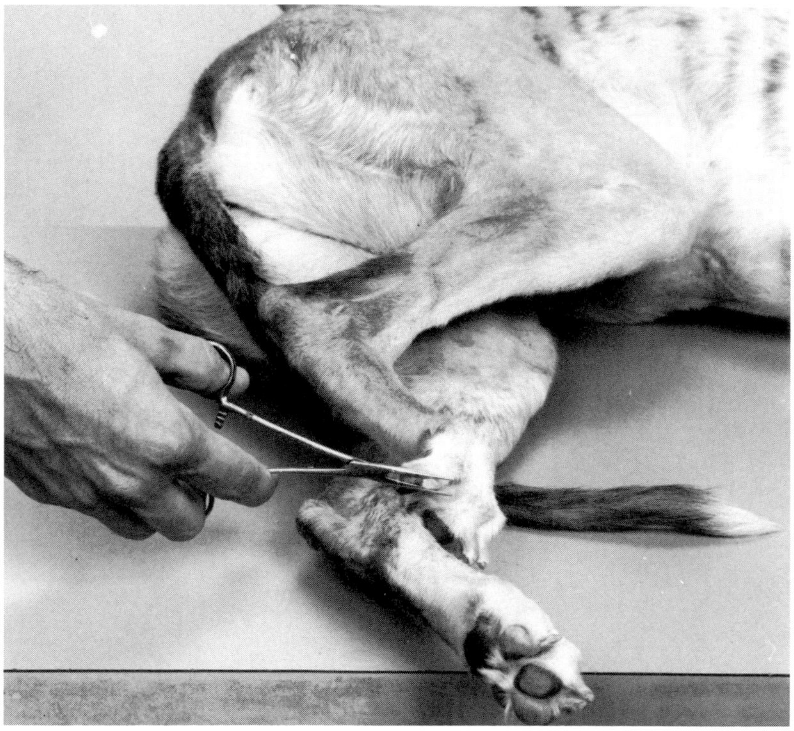

FIGURE 60–32. Testing the flexor reflexes in the pelvic limb.

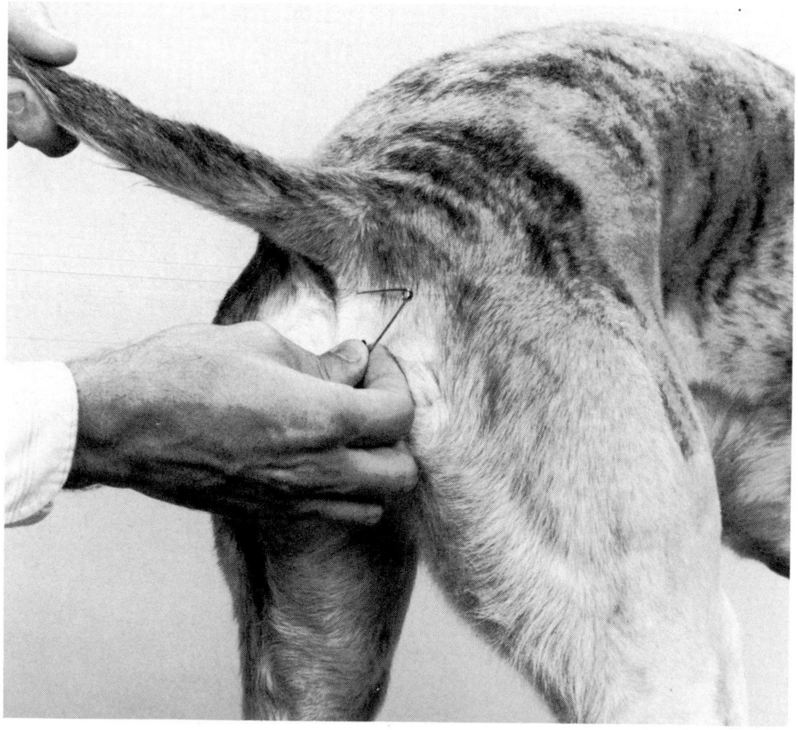

FIGURE 60–33. Testing the perineal reflex in a patient.

initiated by stimulating the skin of the trunk with a pin or hemostat. The clinician should be able to obtain it from the entire thoracic trunk, caudal to the posterior lumbar trunk. The stimulus is carried to the CNS by the dorsal root that supplies the dermatome being stimulated and travels cranially in the CNS to synapse on the LMN of the lateral thoracic nerve. This reflex may be useful in helping to localize transverse spinal cord lesions, if there is a clear demarcation from an area of absent reflex to a zone where the reflex is present. In some normal animals, this reflex may not be present, so it must be interpreted cautiously.

SPECIAL (RELEASED) REFLEXES

These are reflexes that are suppressed by the UMNs of normal animals. If there is a disconnection between the reflex arc and the UMNs, these reflexes become released or uninhibited. The presence of these reflexes is then an indicator of loss of UMN inhibition to a reflex arc.

Babinski Reflex. This reflex is only elicited in the pelvic limbs. It is elicited by lightly stroking the plantar aspect of the metatarsus. In normal animals the toes either do nothing or flex slightly. In the presence of UMN disease, the toes spread apart and elevate (dorsiflex), which is known as a positive Babinski. The presence of a positive Babinski reflex is considered an indication of damage to the UMN pathways to the pelvic limb.

Crossed Extensor Reflex. This reflex may be seen in any limb. It is produced by eliciting a flexor response. In a normal animal, the limb being stimulated flexes and the contralateral, paired limb does nothing. In the presence of UMN disease, when one limb is flexed, the contralateral paired limb involuntarily extends (Figure 60–34). This "crossed extension" is a consistent sign of loss of UMN control of the limb that extends. It is important that the patient be carefully observed during this test, so that voluntary extension and/or struggling is not confused with a crossed extension reflex. Table 60–3 reviews the spinal reflexes.

NOCICEPTIVE EVALUATION

Animals may have two types of sensory disturbances. The first of these is a decrease in the ability to perceive pain. If this decrease is mild, it is called hypalgesia or hypesthesia. If the loss is total it is referred to as analgesia or anesthesia. The second type of sensory disturbance is an increased sensitivity or exaggerated response to pain. Hyperesthesia refers to increased sensitivity; hyperpathia is an exaggerated response to pain. In veterinary patients it is impossible to distinguish between the two.

Loss of Pain Perception. This is tested by producing enough pain to initiate cerebral recognition and response. This is normally done by compressing the digits vigorously; the expected response is turning of the head and/or vocalization (Figure 60–35). This evaluation tests peripheral nerve, spinal cord, brain stem, and cerebrum. The cerebellum is not involved in the nociceptive pathways, so lesions of the cerebellum do not affect pain perception. Peripheral nerve lesions usually cause focal sensory loss, confined to the distribution of the involved nerve(s). Spinal cord lesions cause a bilateral, symmetrical sensory loss that is apparent caudal to the level of the injury. Brain stem lesions rarely produce detectable analgesia, since a lesion of that severity results in the death of the animal. Cerebral lesions produce only hypalgesia. The sensory deficit is unilateral and contralateral to the diseased hemisphere.

Exaggerated Responsiveness to Pain. This is tested by digital manipulation of the paraspinal muscles, stimulation of the paraspinal region with a hemostat or safety pin, or a similar maneuver. The objective is to produce a recognizable stimulus that does not normally bother the patient. This is repeated up and down the spine, searching for an area where the patient shows an unusually acute response to the stimulus. Such an exaggerated response is normally an indication of a nerve root or meningeal lesion, e.g., a herniated disc or meningitis. This test is most valuable in localizing spinal cord lesions.

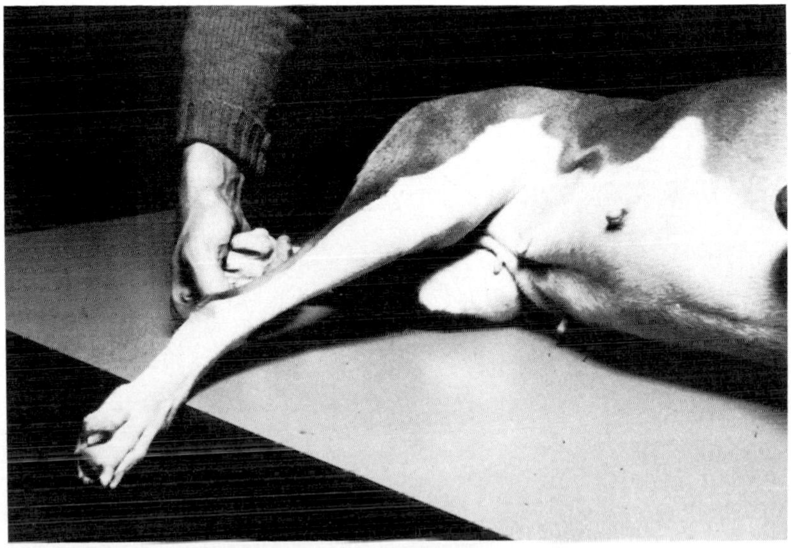

FIGURE 60–34. Demonstration of a crossed extensor reflex in a patient.

TABLE 60–3. TESTING SPINAL REFLEXES

Reflex Tested	PNS Tested	CNS Tested	Response	Interpretation
Triceps	Radial nerve	$\mathbf{C_7}$, $\mathbf{C_8}$, $\mathbf{T_1}$, (2)	Exaggerated Normal Diminished	UMN lesion ± No lesion LMN lesion
Biceps	Musculocutaneous nerve	C_6, $\mathbf{C_7}$, C_8	Exaggerated Normal Diminished	UMN lesion ± No lesion LMN lesion
Thoracic flexor	Musculocutaneous axillary, median ulnar, and radial nerves	C_6, $\mathbf{C_7}$, $\mathbf{C_8}$, $\mathbf{T_1}$, (2)	Normal Diminished	± No lesion LMN lesion
Patellar	Femoral nerve	L_4, $\mathbf{L_5}$, L_6	Exaggerated Normal Diminished	UMN lesion ± No lesion LMN lesion
Cranial tibial	Sciatic nerve	$\mathbf{L_6}$, $\mathbf{L_7}$, $\mathbf{S_1}$, (2)	Exaggerated Normal Diminished	UMN lesion ± No lesion LMN lesion
Pelvic flexor	Primarily sciatic nerve	$\mathbf{L_6}$, $\mathbf{L_7}$, $\mathbf{S_1}$, (2)	Normal	± No lesion
Perineal	Pudendal nerve	$\mathbf{S_1}$, $\mathbf{S_2}$, $\mathbf{S_3}$	Normal Diminished	± No lesion LMN lesion
Crossed extensor	—	**UMN** to Limb	Present	UMN lesion

Bold = Essential to reflex
Normal = Always supplies axons to nerve, not essential to reflex
( ) = Supplies axons to nerve in some animals, not essential to reflex

INTERPRETATION OF FINDINGS

It is usually helpful to begin by making a list of the abnormal findings, along with a list of the anatomic regions of the nervous system. Mark each anatomic region where a lesion could produce the listed sign (Figure 60–36). Then ask several questions. Does the patient have a neurologic disease? If there are plusses after any of the listed signs, this question is answered in the affirmative. Is the disease in the CNS or PNS? If the animal has cranial nerve deficits, the evaluation of the limbs and mental status can be used to answer this question. If there are only isolated cranial nerve deficits with no other signs, then the lesion is probably in the PNS. If there are CNN deficits and limb signs are present, the lesion is probably in the CNS. If the disease is below the foramen magnum and there are any UMN reflex changes present, then the lesion is in the CNS. If

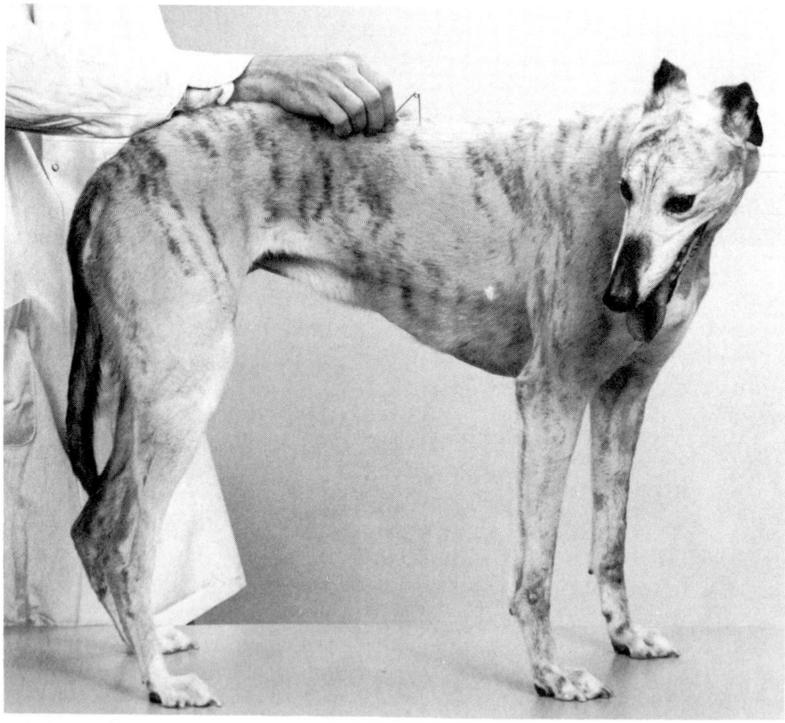

FIGURE 60–35. Testing for back pain in a patient.

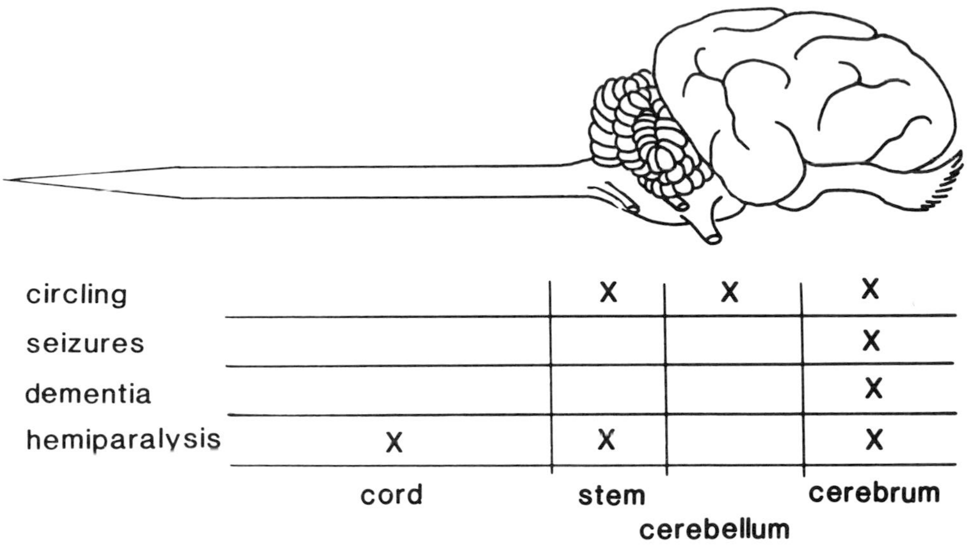

FIGURE 60–36. Demonstration of using signs to localize a lesion.

all spinal reflexes are LMN, then the lesion is probably in the PNS. Is the disease above or below the foramen magnum? If the animal has any abnormality of cranial nerves, historical seizures, abnormal head posture, abnormal head coordination, or an abnormal level of consciousness, then the lesion is above the foramen magnum. If the lesion involves the limbs alone, then the lesion is most likely below the foramen. Here negative findings are as important as positive findings. For example, an UMN tetraparetic patient could have a cerebral, brain stem, or cervical cord injury. If the patient has no head signs, then look for a cord lesion based on the negative head findings combined with the positive limb findings. After you have localized the pathologic process to above or below the foramen and to CNS or PNS, you can try to localize the lesion more precisely.

There are several benefits to be gained by localizing the disease. The clinician now knows whether the problem is a focal or disseminated disease. This is helpful because the probable etiologies are different for each class. Disseminated diseases tend to be caused by inflammations, metabolic diseases, and degenerations, among other causes. Focal diseases tend to be caused by masses, trauma, and vascular lesions. The localization also automatically eliminates some differentials from your diagnosis. A dog with signs suggesting a focal cerebral mass probably does not have an intervertebral disc extrusion. Finally, localization helps the clinician to choose diagnostic aids. Certain diagnostic tools are of value only with lesions in certain anatomic regions. An example is the electroencephalogram, which is only helpful in patients with cerebral injuries. Using this tool in patients with peripheral nerve disease is poor use of time and a waste of the client's money.

The next step in interpreting the findings is to return to the history, combine the information with the examination, and choose diagnostic aids. After interpreting the diagnostic aids, a diagnosis can be made (Figure 60–1).

Diagnostic Aids. Most of the diagnostic tests that are used to aid in the diagnosis of patients with nervous system disease are not covered here. The choice of diagnostic aid is largely based on where the disease process occurs and is more appropriately discussed in the following chapters. The major exception to this rule is cerebrospinal fluid (CSF) analysis, which is used in the evaluation of many parts of the CNS.

CSF taps are useful in the evaluation of many patients with CNS disease because they are safe and inexpensive, and very helpful when positive. They require only anesthetization and intubation. The only essential equipment is a needle with a stylet and an endotracheal tube. The clinician should have a laboratory capable of handling the sample rapidly, but with refrigeration and properly prepared slides, timing is not as crucial as it once was.

CSF COLLECTION. The technique is well explained in several textbooks of neurology.[1, 4] For fluid collection, the tap is generally performed in the neck with the fluid being obtained from the cerebellomedullary cistern. In larger dogs it is also possible to collect fluid from the lumbar subarachnoid space, but the technique is more time consuming and difficult. For cervical collection, the animal is placed under general anesthesia. Although the animal may be placed in either lateral or sternal recumbency, the author finds the technique easier in lateral recumbency. The animal should be intubated and preferably maintained on oxygen. The dorsal part of the cranial neck is clipped and prepared for an aseptic procedure using a surgical scrub. The head is held at a 90° angle to the spine, with the line of the nose and occipital crest parallel to the table. A stylet needle is used to collect the fluid. Generally a 20- or 22-gauge needle is adequate. From the occipital protuberance, draw a line to the cranial wings of the atlas. Using aseptic technique, insert the needle at the intersection of the two lines. Direct the bevel of the needle cranially. Slowly advance the needle toward the vertebra, angling slightly cranially. When entering the subarachnoid space, there will be a slight loss of resistance. The subarachnoid space is fairly shallow here, less than one-half inch in cats, so remove the stylet frequently to check for fluid. If bone is encountered, move the needle cranially or caudally until it enters the subarachnoid space. If blood-tinged spinal fluid comes out, replace the stylet and wait for 30 to 60 seconds, then remove the stylet again. Often the blood will have cleared, allowing a diagnostic collection to occur. If pure blood is obtained, the needle is probably off the midline and in a vertebral sinus. If this occurs, obtain a new needle, reposition the animal, and try again. In most cases, the patient's spinal fluid will not be contaminated and adequate fluid can still be collected.

When clear spinal fluid is obtained, attach a manometer if spinal fluid pressure is to be measured. If not, immediately collect the sample for analysis. This is best done by allowing the fluid to drip into a collection container. Aspiration of the sample is likely to result in blood contamination of the spinal fluid. Always hold the needle while you are collecting spinal fluid; do not allow the needle to enter the spinal cord. After collecting the fluid sample, replace the stylet and remove the spinal needle.

CSF INTERPRETATION. Evaluation should consist of both gross examination and laboratory examinations. First look at the color and clarity of the fluid. Normal spinal fluid should be clear and colorless. Cloudy fluid often indicates an increase in the number of white blood cells (WBC) (pleocytosis), with more than 200 WBC/μl needed to produce clouding. A yellow tint to the fluid is called xanthochromia. This may be the result of previous hemorrhage or protein elevations in excess of 150 mg/dl. Pink or red spinal fluid may be the result of either red blood cells (RBC) or hemoglobin in the spinal fluid. One way to tell if the pink color is from blood cells or hemoglobin is to examine the supernatant following spinning. If the supernatant remains pink, the color is from hemoglobin. This usually indicates the hemorrhage occurred many hours ago rather than as a result of the CSF tap. Following subarachnoid bleeding, the RBCs peak within 24 hours and disappear within 10 days. Hemoglobin appears within 4 hours, peaks within 48 hours, and then disappears within 14 days. Bilirubin appears within 9 hours, peaks within 72 hours, and disappears within 16 days.[8]

After looking at the color, evaluate the cells in the spinal fluid. A measurement of five cells/μl is the upper limit of normal for both RBC and WBC in spinal fluid. If RBC contamination is suspected, correct for the number of WBC either by attributing 1 WBC to each 700 RBC or by using the following formula: $W = WBCf - (WBCb \times RBCf)/RBCb$. Usually, the cell count is higher in cisternal CSF than in lumbar CSF, so this must be considered when looking at cell numbers. Generally, five to ten white cells/μl are suggestive of pathology and more than ten cells/μl are definite evidence of a pathologic process. A range of 5 to 50 WBC/μl is considered a mild elevation, while ranges of 50 to 200 WBC are considered a moderate elevation, and more than 200 WBC, a marked elevation in the white count. Normally, the WBC in CSF are derived from blood and consist predominantly of small lymphocytes. The presence of large lymphoid cells (stimulated lymphocytes) may occur following any nonspecific immune stimulus, such as infection, subarachnoid hemorrhage, infarction, or neoplasia. Mononuclear phagocytes may be present in some normal animals. Activated monocytes (histiocytes), which contain vacuoles in their cytoplasm and are larger than their parent cells, are found only in disease states. Macrophages are simply histiocytes containing phagocytized material. PMNs are rarely seen in normal CSF, unless there is a traumatic tap. A mild increase in the numbers of neutrophils may be the result of recent myelography, hemorrhage, or infarction, as well as the result of neoplasia (especially meningioma) and acute viral infections.[9] A marked increase in the number of neutrophils usually indicates a bacterial or immune disease of the nervous system. Eosinophils are rarely seen in CSF. If present, parasitic and fungal diseases are likely causes, although they may also be seen rarely following myelograms and hemorrhage, with tumors, and in idiopathic conditions.

Tumor cells are not shed in the CSF unless the tumor is contiguous with the subarachnoid space. This is most likely to occur with lymphomas and meningiomas.

Protein evaluations should be performed on all CSF samples. Normally, lumbar CSF has a greater protein content than cisternal CSF. The author feels this to be the most useful chemical change in spinal fluid. About 75 per cent of the protein in spinal fluid is albumin, with most of the remainder being globulin. Although total proteins alone are helpful, an electrophoresis to determine the pattern of protein elevation yields even more information. If the CSF is composed primarily of albumin, the electrophoretic pattern resembles that of plasma. This pattern indicates increased endothelial permeability and may result from a nonspecific disruption of the blood-brain barrier or from defective resorption of protein. If the primary protein is globulin, it indicates the intrathecal production of globulin. Any inflammatory disorder may produce such a change. If there is no associated elevation in the cell count, then the inflammatory disorder is not affecting the meninges; it is an encephalitis rather than meningoencephalitis. A mixed elevation suggests both intrathecal production and damage to the blood-brain barrier. If the total protein is elevated and it is a mixed elevation, calculation of the IgG-albumin index will, in theory, correct for the IgG that crosses a damaged blood-brain barrier, allowing the clinician to determine whether or not local production has occurred. The index is calculated as follows: $\text{INDEX} = [\text{IgG (CSF)} \times \text{albumin (serum)}] / [\text{IgG (serum)} \times \text{albumin (CSF)}]$. A normal index is approximately 0.85.[10]

A number of chemistry values are being examined for use as markers of CNS disease, including LDH, CPK, and lactate levels. There are problems with blood contamination in the samples affecting the values, as well as lack of specificity of the tests.[8]

Degenerations, anomalies, and metabolic, toxic, and nutritional diseases usually have no effect on CSF; they do not change cell type, cell number, or chemistry values. These are the conditions where advances in knowledge of CSF chemistry have the greatest chance of improving diagnostic abilities. With neoplasia, there is normally an increase in protein. There may be an increase in pressure if the mass is above the foramen magnum. Rarely, there is an increase in the cell count. Inflammations of the nervous system usually result in an increase in the number of cells in CSF, as well as an increase in the protein values. The WBC type reflects the type of inflammation present. In some cases, there may be mild elevations of spinal fluid pressure as well. In infarctions of the nervous system, there is usually an early elevation in protein, which resolves rapidly. If there is significant hemorrhage, there may be an elevation of RBC, while with necrosis, there may be an elevation in WBC. In cases of trauma, there is an elevation of the RBC and protein. If the trauma was to the brain, there may be elevations of pressure as well.

References

1. deLahunta, A: Veterinary Neuroanatomy and Clinical Neurology, 2nd ed. Philadelphia, WB Saunders Co, 1983.
2. House, EL and Pansky, B: A Functional Approach to Neuroanatomy, 2nd ed. New York, McGraw-Hill, 1967.
3. Plum, F and Posner, JB: The Diagnosis of Stupor and Coma, 3rd ed. Philadelphia, FA Davis, 1983.
4. Oliver, JE, et al.: Veterinary Neurology. Philadelphia, WB Saunders Co, 1987.
5. Brodal, A: Neurological Anatomy, 3rd ed. New York, Oxford University Press, 1981.
6. Baloh, RW and Honrubia, V: Clinical Neurophysiology of the Vestibular System. Philadelphia, FA Davis, 1979.
7. Daube, JR, et al.: Medical Neurosciences: An Approach to Anatomy, Pathology, and Physiology by Systems and Levels. Boston, Little, Brown and Co, 1978.
8. Fishman, RA: Cerebrospinal Fluid in Diseases of the Nervous System. Philadelphia, WB Saunders Co, 1980.
9. Carillo, JM, et al.: Intracranial neoplasm and associated inflammatory response from the central nervous system. JAAHA 22:397, 1986.
10. Sorjonen, DC: Total protein, albumin quota, and electrophoretic patterns in cerebrospinal fluid of dogs with central nervous system disorders. JAVMA 48:301, 1987.

61 DISEASES OF THE BRAIN

CRAIG E. GREENE and KYLE G. BRAUND

Clinical signs of diseases of the brain are listed in Table 61–1. The history, physical examination, and neurologic examination should provide information necessary to answer the following questions: Is it a neurologic disease? Is it a peripheral nerve, spinal cord, or brain disease? If the brain is involved, what part of the brain is affected? After a brief review of some diagnostic techniques used to detect intracranial disorders, a review of the various diseases of the brain is presented.

ANCILLARY DIAGNOSTIC TECHNIQUES

The signalment and history often indicate the type of disease process. Results of the neurologic examination, as summarized in Table 61–2, should localize the lesion to a portion of the brain (see Chapter 60). To confirm the diagnosis, one or more special diagnostic techniques may be indicated. Hematologic and serum biochemistry profiles are useful in evaluating systemic diseases that affect the brain secondarily and are covered in appropriate chapters. Cerebrospinal fluid (CSF), radiographic, and electrophysiologic examinations are specific adjuncts to diagnosis of brain disease and are briefly discussed here. See specific references for a more detailed discussion.

Cerebrospinal Fluid

CSF examination is an important diagnostic procedure for the dog or cat with suspected brain disease. Techniques for the collection, analysis, and interpretation of results of CSF analysis are presented in Chapter 60. The composition of the CSF reflects pathologic processes in the brain; however, a normal CSF does not eliminate the presence of organic disease. Alterations are primarily detected if the disease process is relatively acute and is in contact with the subarachnoid space or ventricular system. The primary contraindication to CSF analysis in brain disorders is increased intracranial pressure, cranial trauma, or poor anesthetic risk. Increased intracranial pressure can be suspected with rapid progression of neurologic signs within 24 hours, the sudden development of pupillary abnormalities, or the presence of papilledema on funduscopic examination. Despite its limitations, CSF analysis is probably the private practitioner's most definitive means of detecting the presence of intracranial inflammation.

Radiography of the Brain

Survey radiographs (noncontrast, "plain") of the head demonstrate abnormalities of the bony calvarium or alterations in the air-filled spaces of the skull (nasal passages, sinuses, and bulla ossea). Soft tissue changes in the brain cannot be seen because brain tissue, CSF, and blood all have similar radiographic density. Contrast procedures, such as arteriography, venography, ventriculography, or nuclear imaging must be used to detect changes within the brain. Most of the procedures are beyond the scope of veterinary practice; however, indications and contraindications of these techniques are reviewed.

SURVEY RADIOGRAPHY

Technique. Diagnostic radiographs of the skull require general anesthesia of the patient in order to achieve proper positioning. A basic series should include lateral, ventrodorsal, and frontal views (Figures 61–1, 61–2, and 61–3). An open mouth frontal view and lateral

TABLE 61–1. SIGNS OF DISEASE OF THE BRAIN

Seizures*
Altered mental status*
Behavioral abnormality
Lethargy, confusion, stupor, coma
Motor and proprioceptive dysfunction
Ataxia†
Abnormal position or movement of the head
Hemiparesis or tetraparesis†
Involuntary movement disorders
Abnormal vision, pupillary or eye movements
Other cranial nerve abnormalities

*May also be caused by extracranial abnormality.
†May also be caused by spinal cord or peripheral nerve disease (see Chapters 35 and 36).

TABLE 61–2. SIGNS OF LESIONS IN THE BRAIN

Anatomic Area	Mental Status	Posture	Movement	Postural Reactions	Cranial Nerves
Cerebral cortex	Behavior, depression, seizures	Normal	Gait normal to slight hemiparesis (contralateral)	Deficits (contralateral)	Normal (vision may be impaired–contralateral)
Diencephalon (thalamus & hypothalamus)	Behavior, depression (endocrine and autonomic)	Normal	Gait normal to hemiparesis or tetraparesis	Deficits (contralateral)	CN II
Brain stem (midbrain-medulla)	Depression, stupor, coma	Normal, turning, falling	Hemiparesis to tetraparesis, ataxia	Deficits (ipsi- or contralateral)	CN III–XII
Central vestibular (medulla)	Depression	Head tilt, falling	Hemiparesis, usually ipsilateral, ataxia	Deficits (ipsi- or contralateral)	CN VII; may also affect V & VII; nystagmus
Peripheral vestibular (labyrinth)	Normal	Head tilt	Normal to ataxia	Normal, although may be awkward	CN VIII, sometimes VII and/or Horner's syndrome, nystagmus
Cerebellum	Normal	Normal	Tremors, dysmetria, ataxia	Normal to dysmetric	Normal; may be menace deficit and/or nystagmus

From Oliver, J. E., Jr., and Lorenz, M. D.: Handbook of Neurologic Diagnosis. Philadelphia, W. B. Saunders Co., 1983.

oblique views are used for evaluating the bulla ossea (Figures 61–4 and 61–5).[1–3]

Indications. Fractures of the calvarium following cranial trauma are the primary indication for survey radiographs. Evaluation of the bulla ossea in vestibular disease is useful, although negative findings do not rule out middle ear disease. Any contrast procedure should be preceded by survey radiographs. Congenital hydrocephalus can be suspected on the basis of the calvarial changes seen on the survey radiographs.

Contraindications. The need for general anesthesia is the only contraindication for survey radiography.

CEREBRAL ARTERIOGRAPHY

Technique. Arteriograms are made by injection of contrast media into the internal carotid artery or the

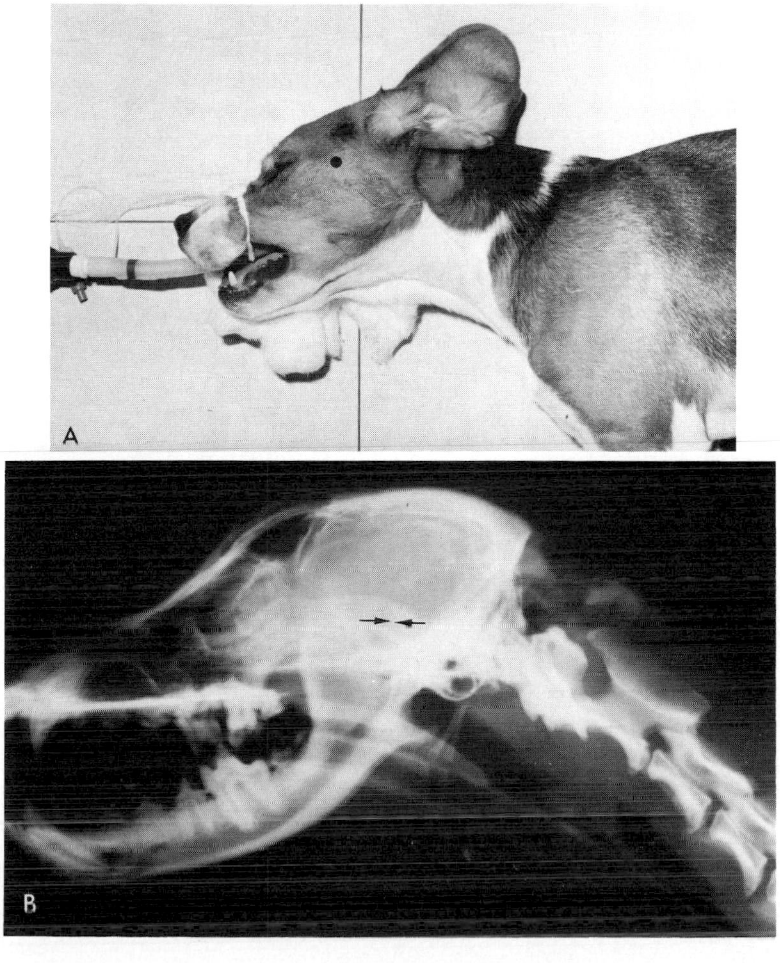

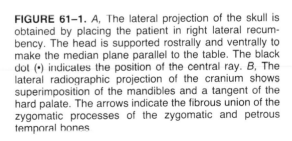

FIGURE 61–1. *A,* The lateral projection of the skull is obtained by placing the patient in right lateral recumbency. The head is supported rostrally and ventrally to make the median plane parallel to the table. The black dot (•) indicates the position of the central ray. *B,* The lateral radiographic projection of the cranium shows superimposition of the mandibles and a tangent of the hard palate. The arrows indicate the fibrous union of the zygomatic processes of the zygomatic and petrous temporal bones.

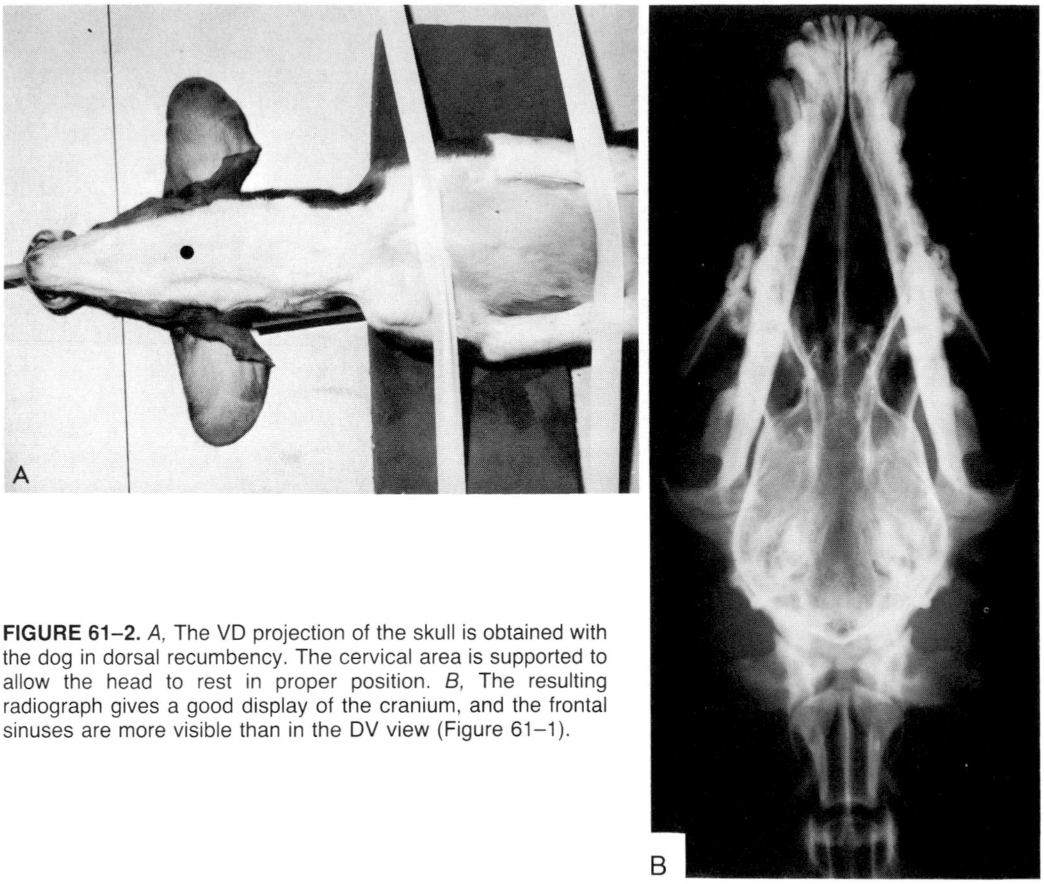

FIGURE 61–2. *A,* The VD projection of the skull is obtained with the dog in dorsal recumbency. The cervical area is supported to allow the head to rest in proper position. *B,* The resulting radiograph gives a good display of the cranium, and the frontal sinuses are more visible than in the DV view (Figure 61–1).

vertebral artery. Carotid arteriography outlines the arterial circle of the brain (circle of Willis) and the rostral and middle cerebral arteries. The caudal cerebral, rostral cerebellar, and basilar arteries are filled in some cases. Vertebral arteriography outlines the basilar, cerebellar, and caudal cerebral arteries, and at times the entire arterial circle and all of its branches (Figure 61–6). Vertebral arteriography requires catheterization of the femoral artery and is limited to medium to large dogs because of the greater size of the vessels.[2, 4]

A rapid film changer is necessary to make rapid, serial radiographs of the contrast medium as it progresses through the arterial, capillary, and venous circulation.

Indications. Arteriography is useful for identifying

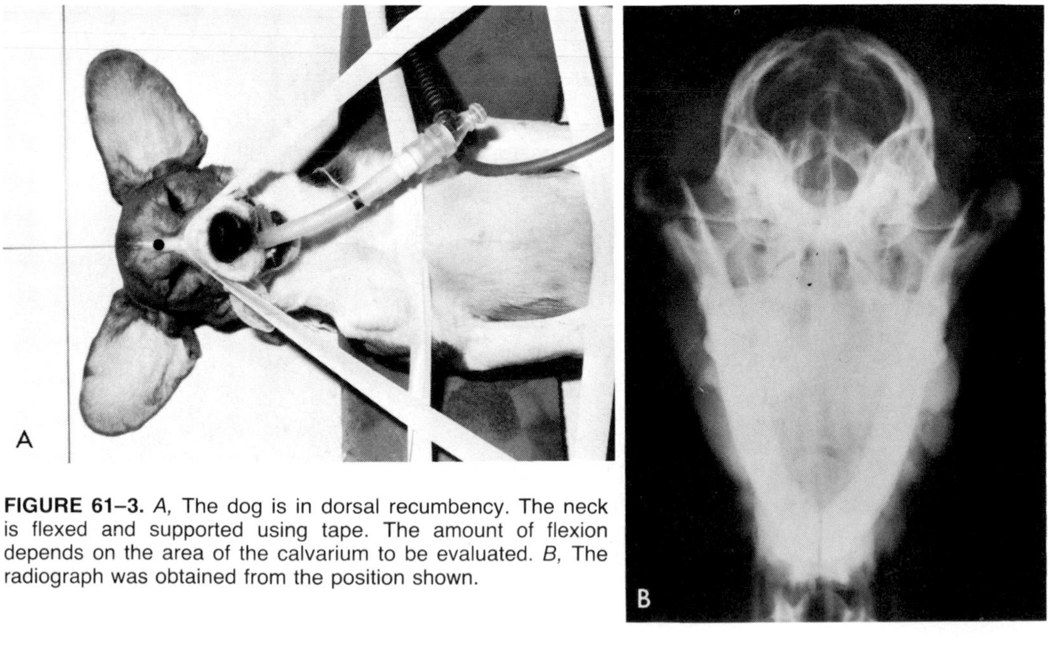

FIGURE 61–3. *A,* The dog is in dorsal recumbency. The neck is flexed and supported using tape. The amount of flexion depends on the area of the calvarium to be evaluated. *B,* The radiograph was obtained from the position shown.

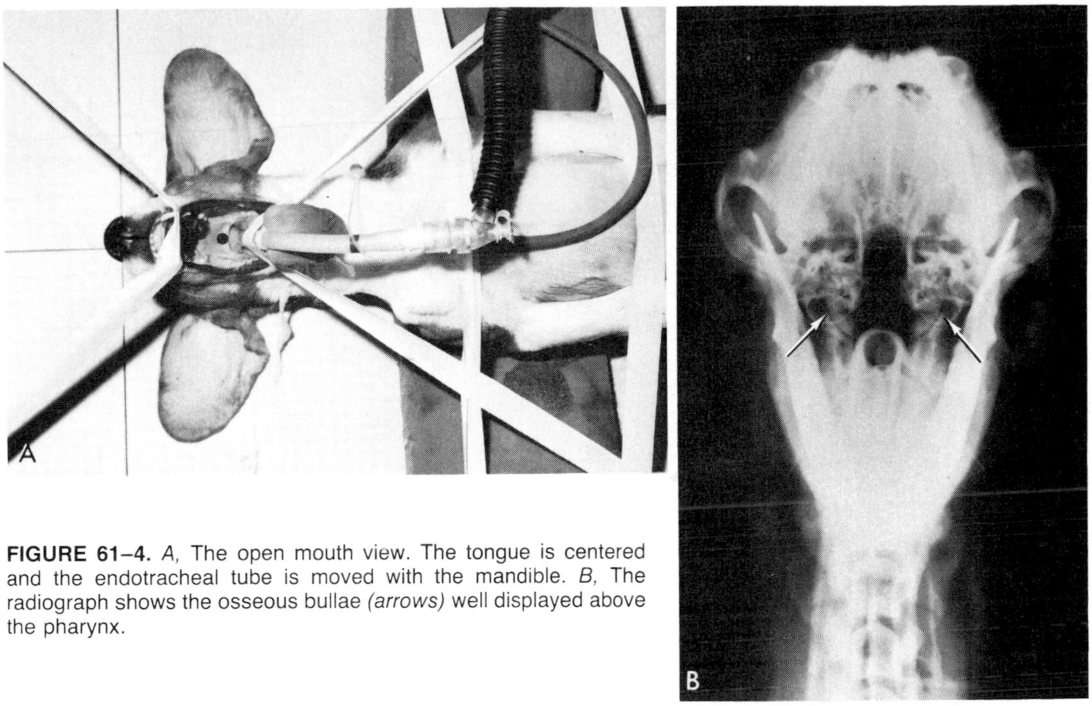

FIGURE 61–4. *A*, The open mouth view. The tongue is centered and the endotracheal tube is moved with the mandible. *B*, The radiograph shows the osseous bullae *(arrows)* well displayed above the pharynx.

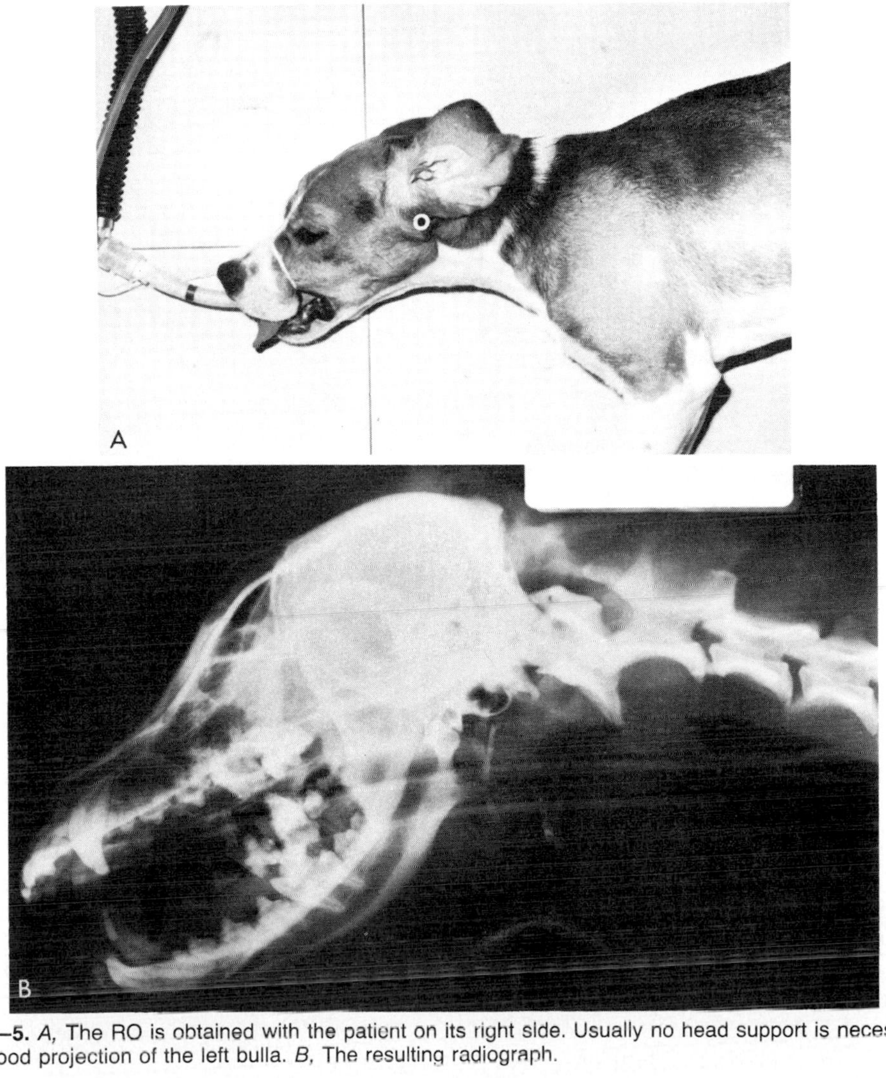

FIGURE 61–5. *A*, The RO is obtained with the patient on its right side. Usually no head support is necessary. This RO gives good projection of the left bulla. *B*, The resulting radiograph.

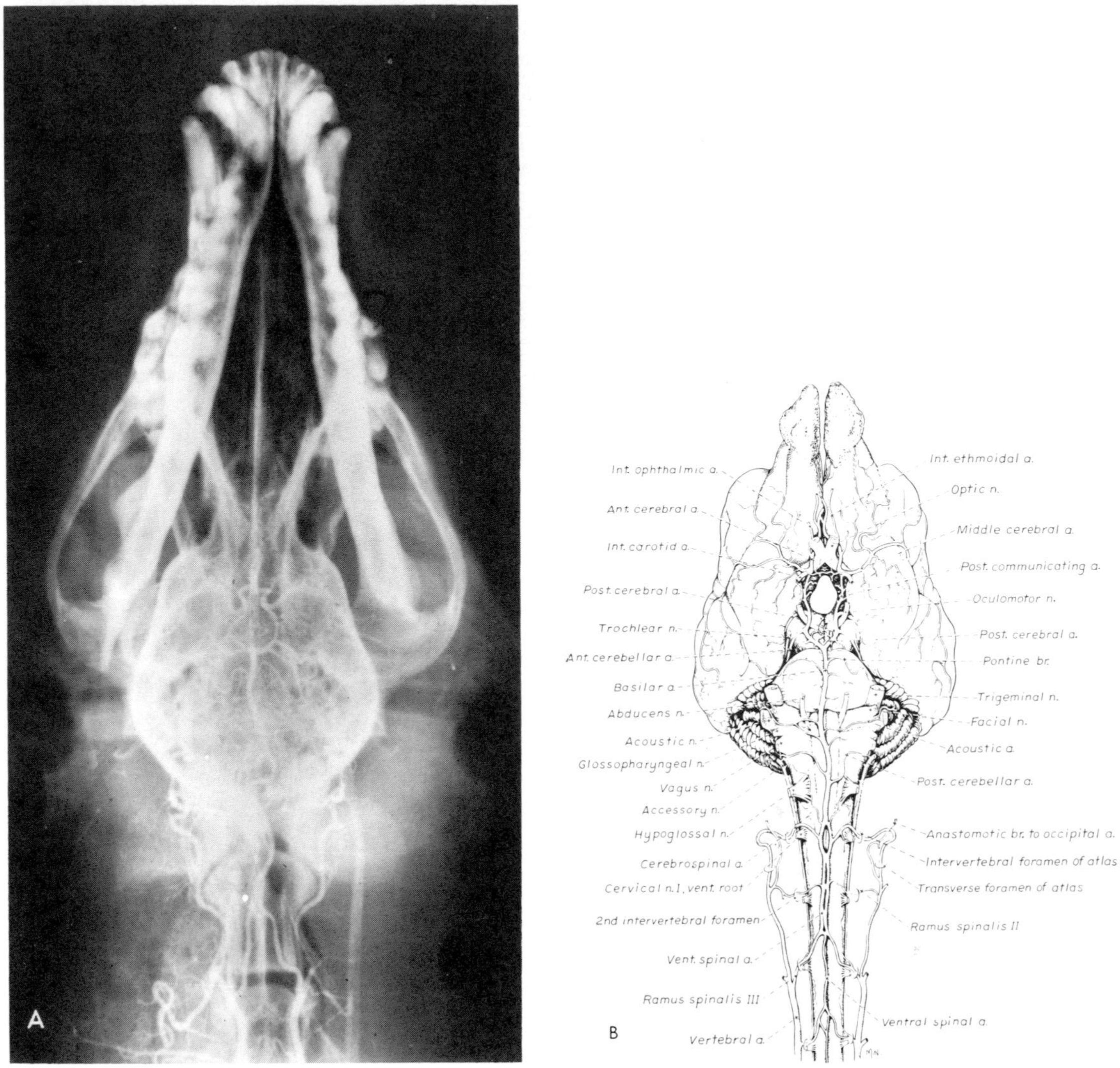

FIGURE 61–6. *A,* Cerebral arteriography. This normal arteriogram was taken 1.5 seconds after injection of contrast medium into the vertebral artery at the C4 level. *B,* The drawing is supplied for identification of specific arteries. (*B* is from Miller, ME, Christensen, GC, and Evans, HE: Anatomy of the Dog. Philadelphia, WB Saunders, 1964.)

mass lesions of the cerebrum. Masses may be identified by deviation of vessels, obstruction of vessels, or increased vascularity. Pooling of contrast material may occur if the blood-brain barrier has broken down (tumor blush). Intramedullary lesions of the brain stem and very small lesions are difficult to visualize with arteriography.

Contraindications. The procedure requires general anesthesia, surgical exposure, and catheterization of an artery. Sepsis and embolism are possible, although infrequent, complications. The equipment for rapid exposure of radiographs is usually available only at institutions.

CAVERNOUS SINUS VENOGRAPHY

Technique. Contrast media is injected, usually via a catheter, into the angularis oculi vein, while the jugular veins are compressed. A single dorsoventral radiograph is made as the injection is completed. The contrast media opacifies the ophthalmic plexus in the orbit and the cavernous sinus in the calvarium (Figure 61–7).[2, 5]

Indications. The cavernous sinuses on the floor of the cranial vault are closely related to the pituitary gland and cranial nerves II, III, IV, and VI. Mass lesions involving these structures may be detected. Bilateral injection is needed in some cases to be certain of abnormality. The technique does not require any special equipment.

Contraindications. Anesthesia is required.

VENTRICULOGRAPHY

Technique. Needles are placed in the lateral ventricles through small twist drill holes in the skull or through the open fontanelle in animals with congenital or neonatally acquired hydrocephalus. Air or a positive contrast medium is injected slowly. If air is used, radiographs are made with a horizontal beam with the head in varying positions to move the "bubble" to various parts of the ventricular systems[2, 4] (see Figure 61–8).

Indications. Ventriculography is used most frequently to confirm a diagnosis of hydrocephalus. Any mass

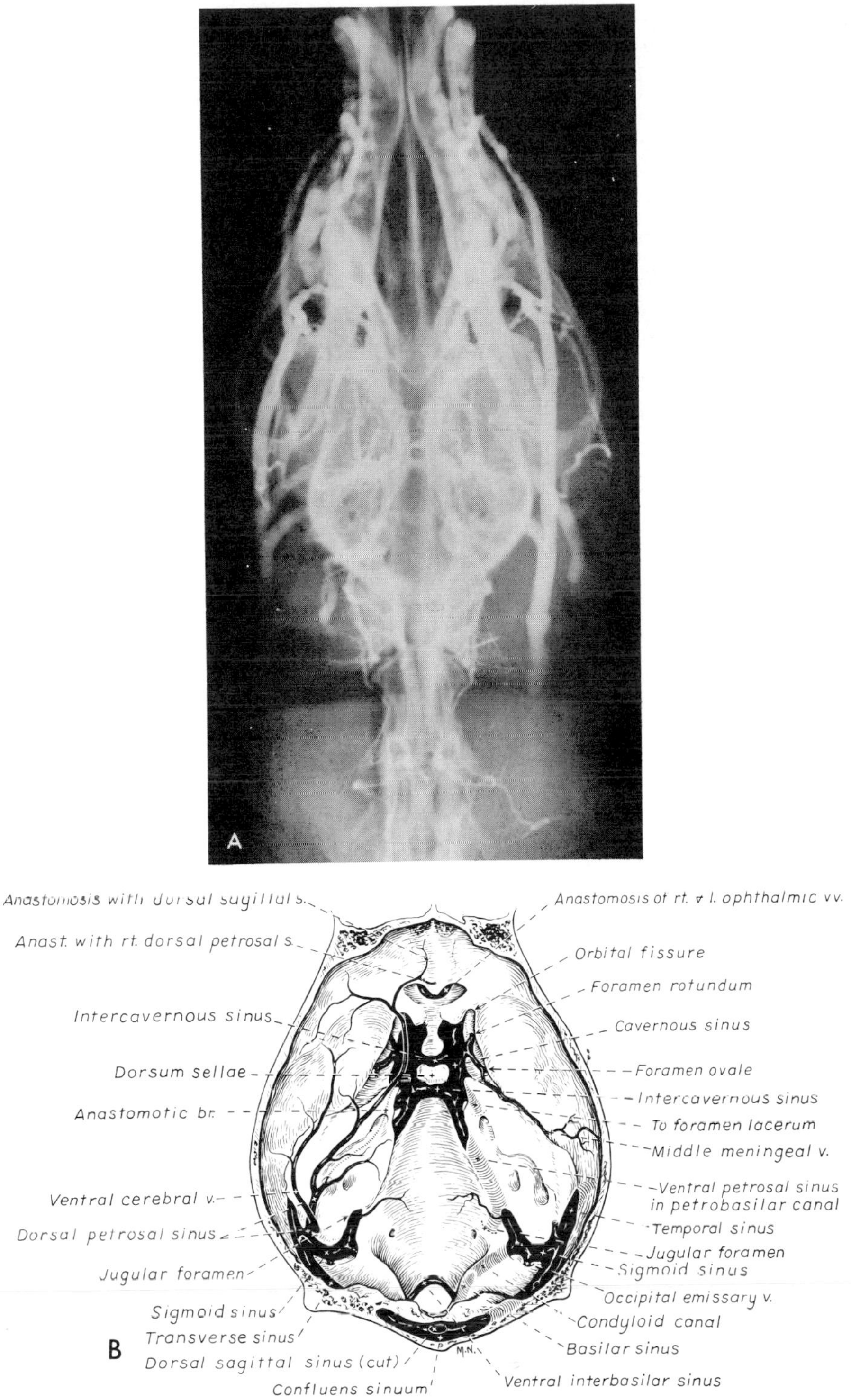

FIGURE 61–7. *A,* Cranial sinus venography. This DV projection of the skull is a normal venogram. *B,* The drawing illustrates the intracranial venous sinuses. (*B* is from Miller, ME, Christensen, GC, and Evans, HE: Anatomy of the Dog. Philadelphia, WB Saunders, 1964.)

lesion displacing the ventricles can be detected with ventriculography.

Contraindications. Anesthesia is required and the procedure is invasive. Increased intracranial pressure is not a contraindication, as removal of ventricular fluid can be beneficial. Positive contrast media can be toxic, causing seizures and an inflammatory response. Oil-based contrast materials may produce granulomatous changes and secondary hydrocephalus. Removal of too much fluid in hydrocephalic animals may cause collapse of the cerebral cortex and subdural hemorrhage. Air ventriculography has rarely caused problems.

NEW TECHNIQUES

A number of newer diagnostic techniques offer significant advantages over the methods described. Unfor-

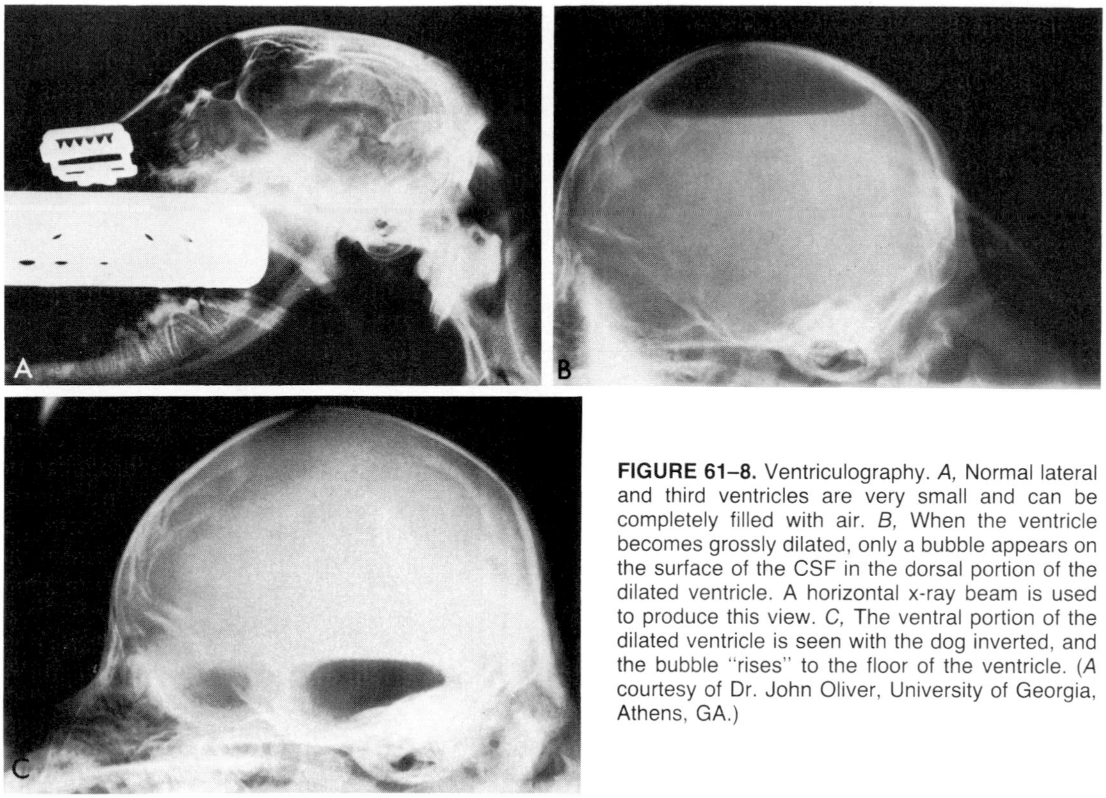

FIGURE 61–8. Ventriculography. *A,* Normal lateral and third ventricles are very small and can be completely filled with air. *B,* When the ventricle becomes grossly dilated, only a bubble appears on the surface of the CSF in the dorsal portion of the dilated ventricle. A horizontal x-ray beam is used to produce this view. *C,* The ventral portion of the dilated ventricle is seen with the dog inverted, and the bubble "rises" to the floor of the ventricle. (*A* courtesy of Dr. John Oliver, University of Georgia, Athens, GA.)

tunately, these techniques, which require very expensive equipment and considerable technical expertise, are available at few veterinary institutions.

Brain Scans. Brain scanning with radioactive isotopes can be used to identify a lesion in the brain if the blood-brain barrier has been breached. The primary indication is for brain tumors or other mass lesions. Older scanning equipment requires general anesthesia for restraint during the scan. New high-speed "cameras" may allow evaluation of the conscious patient. Facilities for handling radioactive isotopes must be available. Animals are usually radioactive for several days after the procedure, thus necessitating their hospitalization in isolation.

Computerized Axial Tomography. Computerized axial tomographic (CT) scans have revolutionized diagnosis of human cerebral disease. Computer enhancement of tomograms of the brain allows visualization of soft tissue densities in thin slices of the brain. When used in conjunction with CT scanning, isotope or contrast enhancement clearly outlines almost any lesion of the brain. The equipment is very expensive and only available at major veterinary referral centers at present.

Ultrasonography. Newer ultrasonographic techniques that may rival CT scans in their versatility are also becoming available.[6] The old echoencephalograms that could only detect a midline shift in the brain have never been very useful.[7] However, the newer technique can provide an image similar to the CT scan and at a much lower cost.

Nuclear Magnetic Resonance Imaging. Contrast-enhanced nuclear magnetic resonance imaging offers a potential new alternative to noninvasive localization of brain lesions. Studies in dogs have shown the procedure to be valuable in detecting focal experimental brain lesions.[8] Inert paramagnetic substances are injected intravenously and are leaked into the surrounding brain tissue in areas of a damaged blood-brain barrier, where they can be detected in the presence of a strong external magnetic field.

Electrophysiologic Diagnosis

ELECTROENCEPHALOGRAPHY

The electroencephalogram (EEG) is a graphic record of the electrical activity of the cerebral cortex. The activity is influenced by subcortical structures. The EEG cannot provide an etiologic diagnosis, but it can help determine whether brain disease is present or if the disease is focal or diffuse. Less reliable predictions include the time course or whether the disease is inflammatory or degenerative. Serial recordings may determine if the disease is progressing or improving.

Technique. Methods used to record EEGs vary widely, especially in the arrangement of the electrodes on the scalp (montage) and the method of restraint or depth of anesthesia. One or more of the references should be consulted for details.[9–11]

Indications. The EEG may be useful in any disease affecting the brain, but primarily those involving the cerebral cortex. Inflammatory diseases and hydrocephalus have the most characteristic changes.

Interpretation. EEGs from normal awake and anesthetized animals are depicted in Figure 61–9. Diseases may cause changes in amplitude, frequency, or both. Alteration in activity may be summarized as follows. Low-voltage fast activity (LVFA) and spikes indicate an

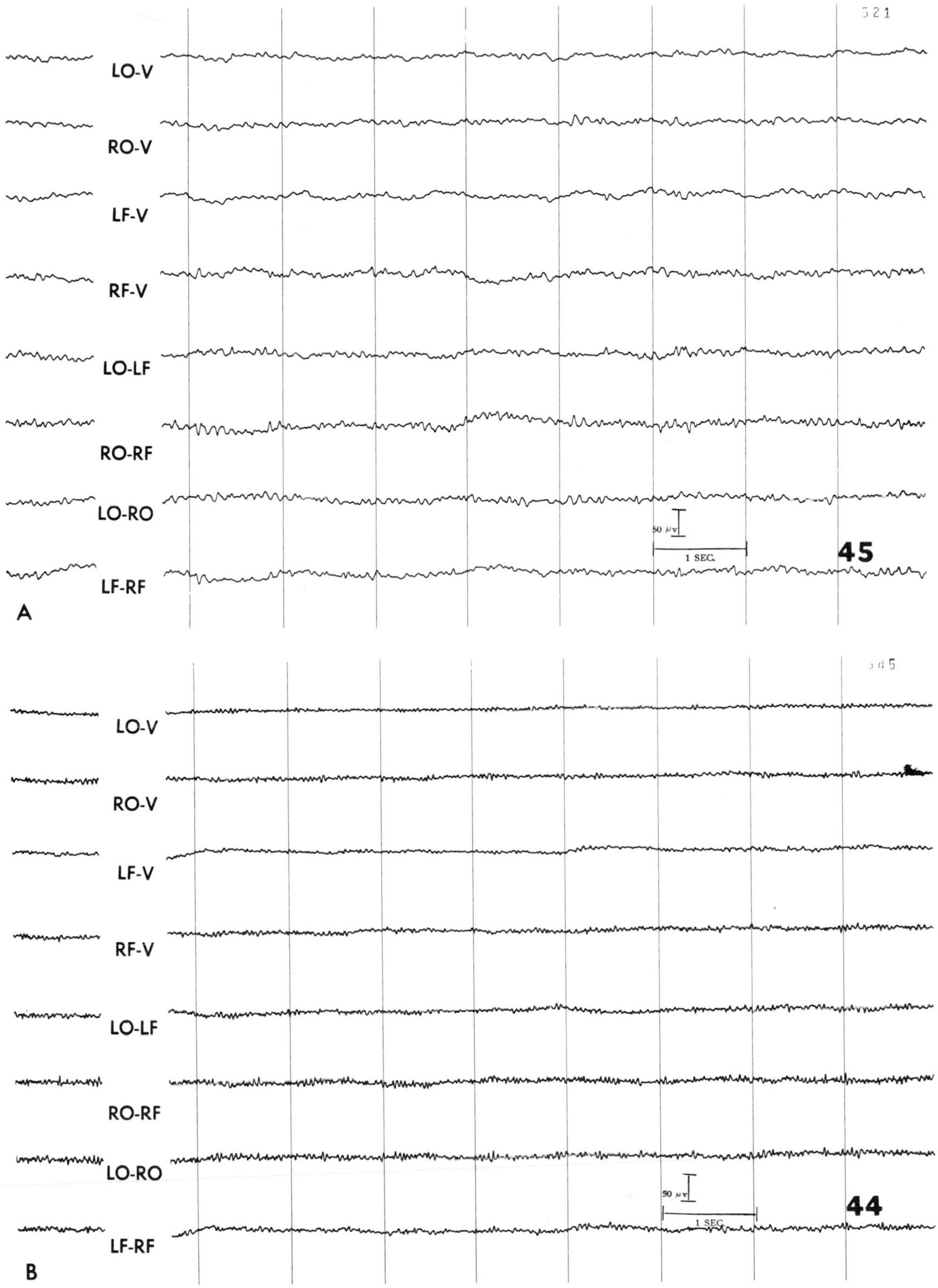

FIGURE 61–9. Normal electroencephalograms obtained without chemical restraint. *A*, Relaxed. *B*, Alert.

ongoing irritative process, such as inflammatory disease (Figure 61–10). Persistent high-voltage slow activity (HVSA) indicates death of neurons, such as degenerative disease (Figure 61–11). LVFA and HVSA are not pathognomonic of any given disease, but are suggestive of several diseases. Focal EEG abnormality indicates a cortical lesion (Figure 61–12). Generalized EEG abnormality indicates a generalized cortical disease or a disease in subcortical structures projecting diffusely to the cortex.[12] Increased intracranial pressure also causes HVSA.

EVOKED POTENTIALS

The development of equipment that can average electrical signals, extracting low amplitude, time-locked po-

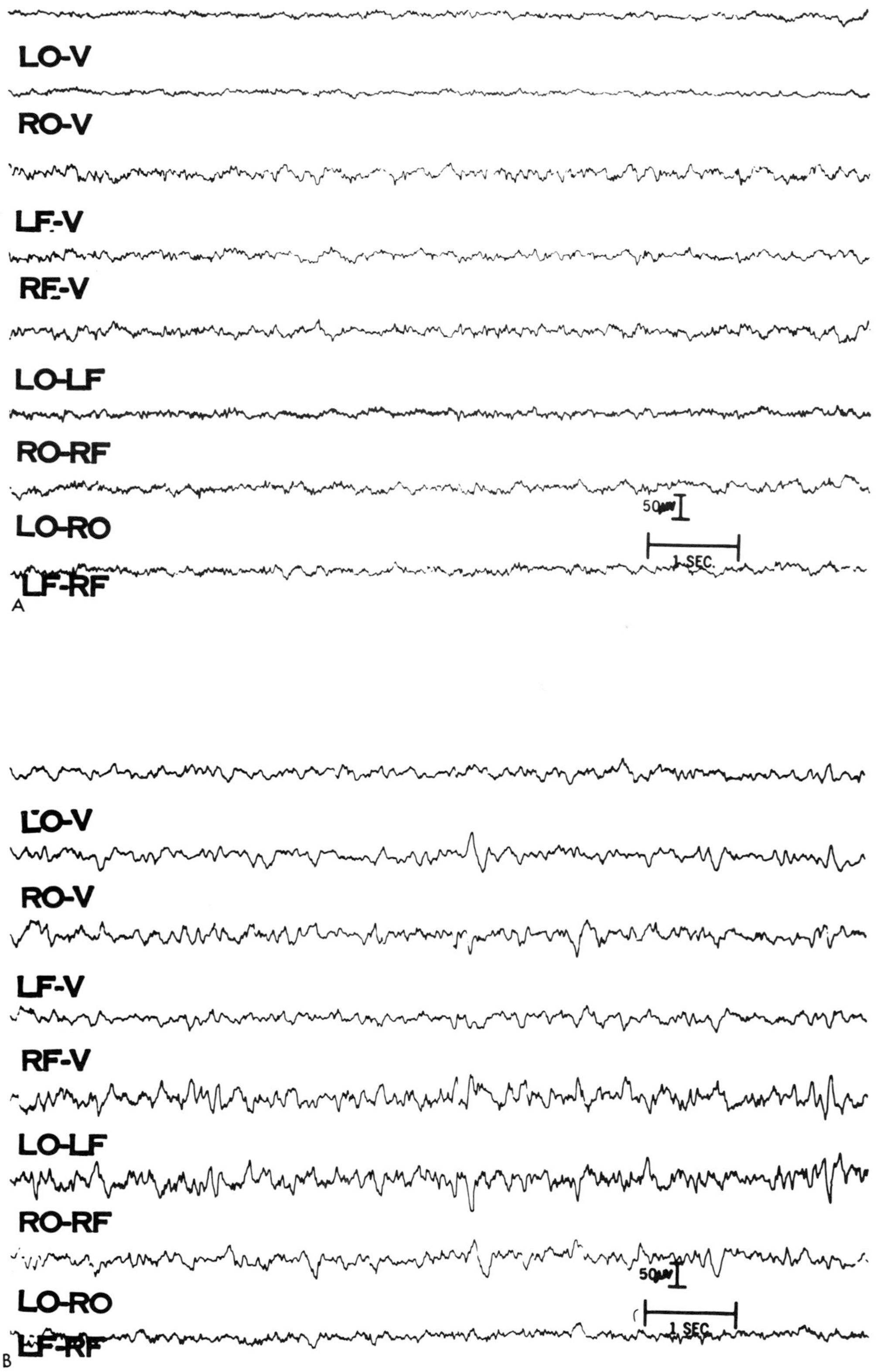

FIGURE 61–10. Sequential electroencephalograms from a patient with distemper encephalitis. *A*, Animal presented for examination; early encephalitis. *B*, Five days after first recording; transition from early to acute stage.

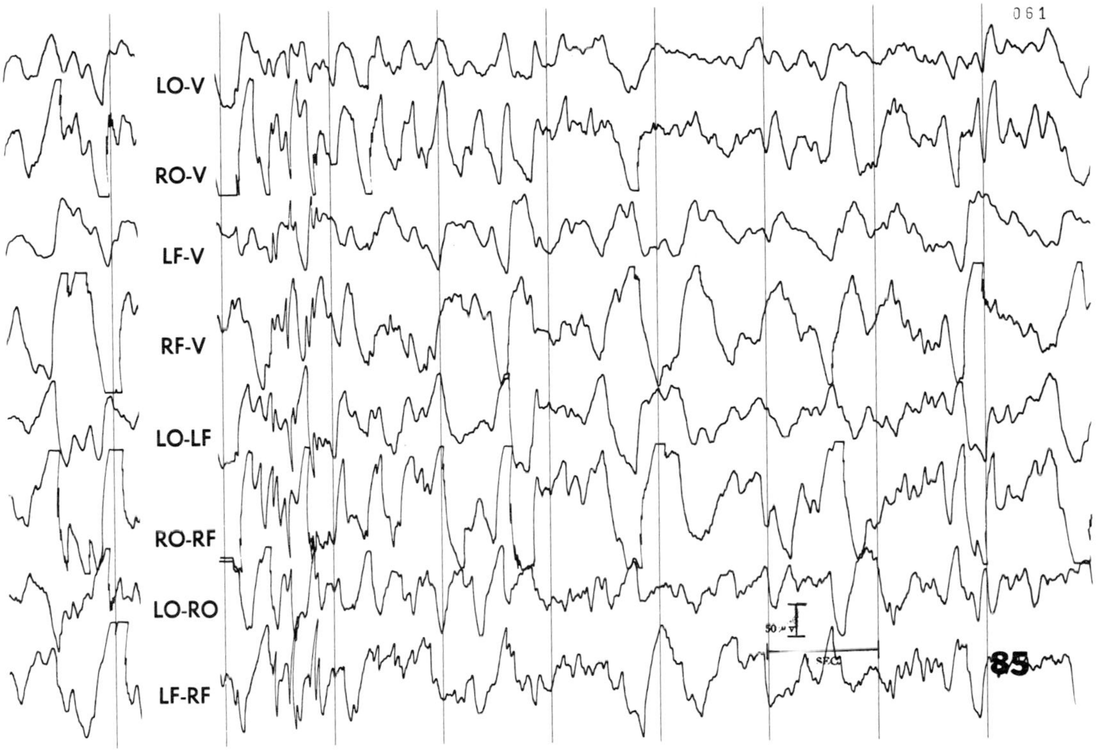

FIGURE 61–11. Electroencephalographic pattern typically seen in hydrocephalus.

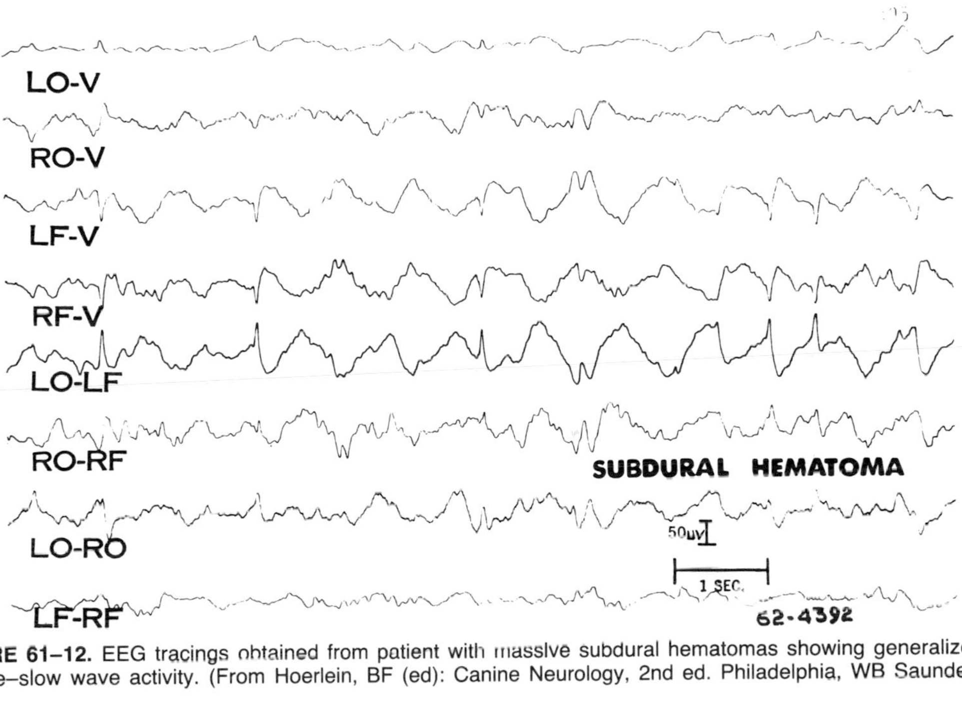

FIGURE 61–12. EEG tracings obtained from patient with massive subdural hematomas showing generalized high voltage–slow wave activity. (From Hoerlein, BF (ed): Canine Neurology, 2nd ed. Philadelphia, WB Saunders Co., 1971.)

tentials from the random background electrical activity, has provided a method for evaluation of sensory mechanisms. Visual, auditory, and somatosensory systems can be tested. Somatosensory evoked potentials are primarily used for evaluation of the spinal cord and peripheral nerves and are described in Chapters 62 and 64.

BRAIN STEM AUDITORY EVOKED RESPONSES (BAER)

Technique. All evoked potential measurements require a computerized signal averager to extract the response from the background EEG activity. Subcutaneous needle electrodes are placed on the vertex of the skull and near the petrous bone. A click stimulus is provided to the ear by an earphone. The response is a series of wave forms representing activity starting in the cochlea and relayed up the auditory pathway in the brain stem.[13]

Indications. The BAER is the best objective method for assessment of hearing in animals. Lesions of the brain stem caudal to the midbrain cause alterations in the wave forms that can aid in localization.

Interpretation. If there is no response at all, the cochlea is not functioning. Congenital deafness seen in some animals is an example. Lesions above the cochlear nucleus cause a decrement in the wave forms arising at the level of the lesion and all succeeding waves.

VISUAL EVOKED RESPONSES (VER)

Technique. The recording technique is similar to that of BAER except the recording electrodes are placed at the vertex and over the contralateral occipital cortex. The stimulus is a strobe light. The electroretinogram (ERG) may also be recorded by placing an electrode near the eye or using a contact lens electrode.

Indications. The VER is designed to provide an objective assessment of vision.

Interpretation. Unfortunately, recent research indicates that the VER is almost totally ERG. The potentials from the retina are so large that they obscure cortical potentials.[14] Redding has indicated that a later wave form consistent with a cortical potential can be demonstrated.[15] Development of a method using reversing grid pattern stimulation offers some hope for development of VER as a useful tool.

IMPEDANCE AUDIOMETRY

The compliance of the tympanic membrane, middle ear, and ossicles, the patency of the auditory tube, and the function of the facial nerve through the stapedius reflex can be evaluated. An impedence audiometer is required to perform the tests. Clinical trials are under way to define the capabilities of this test. Results are promising for diagnosis of middle ear and auditory system problems.[16]

ELECTROMYOGRAPHY (EMG)

Although primarily used for evaluation of peripheral nerves and muscle, EMG is equally useful for evaluating those muscles innervated by cranial nerves. Techniques and indications are discussed in Chapter 65.

DEVELOPMENTAL DISORDERS

Hydrocephalus

Hydrocephalus is the pathologic accumulation of CSF in the ventricular system or subarachnoid space of the brain. This can occur from increased production of fluid in the choroid plexus, decreased meningeal absorption of fluid, or obstruction of CSF flow. Clinically, the last two mechanisms are more common. Reduced absorption of CSF in the meninges may result from previous episodes of meningitis or subarachnoid hemorrhage. An open pathway from the ventricular system to the subarachnoid space with reduced absorption rate is called communicating hydrocephalus. Obstruction of flow from the ventricles to the subarachnoid space results in accumulation of CSF proximal to the point of obstruction. This form of hydrocephalus is called obstructive or noncommunicating hydrocephalus. The usual site of obstruction in most cases is the cerebral aqueduct or the lateral foramina of the fourth ventricle. Obstructive hydrocephalus can be either congenital or acquired later in life.

Certain breeds of dogs have a predisposition for hydrocephalus. The highest incidence is found in toy breeds and brachycephalic dogs. In these dogs the condition may be present at birth and may be associated with malformation of the mesencephalic aqueduct. Clinical signs are not always seen with mild hydrocephalus, which may be an incidental finding at necropsy of toy breed dogs. Furthermore, many clinically normal toy breed dogs may have open fontanelles without corresponding ventricular dilation.

Causes. The cause of congenital hydrocephalus may relate to the presence of toxins and infections prior to birth that close the mesencephalic aqueduct. Nutritional factors, vitamin deficiencies, and intraventricular injections have produced hydrocephalus experimentally. Congenital cases of hydrocephalus are not always associated with increased intracranial pressure at birth. The cranial vault increases in size to compensate for the increased volume of fluid so that there is no increase in intracranial pressure.

Development of neonatal hydrocephalus has been reported as a result of periventricular encephalitis and aqueduct obstruction in young dogs.[17] Several species of bacteria were isolated. Similar reports of hydrocephalus have been associated with feline infectious peritonitis virus infection and *Actinomyces* meningitis.[18, 19] Neonatally acquired hydrocephalus is associated with a rapid enlargement of the cranial vault and progression of neurologic signs beginning at six to eight weeks of age.

Clinical Signs. Clinical signs of hydrocephalus in neonatal animals are variable. Enlargement of the cranial vault with open fontanelles is present when the disease occurs in neonates (Figure 61–13). Neurologic signs may vary from mild depression to severe convulsive

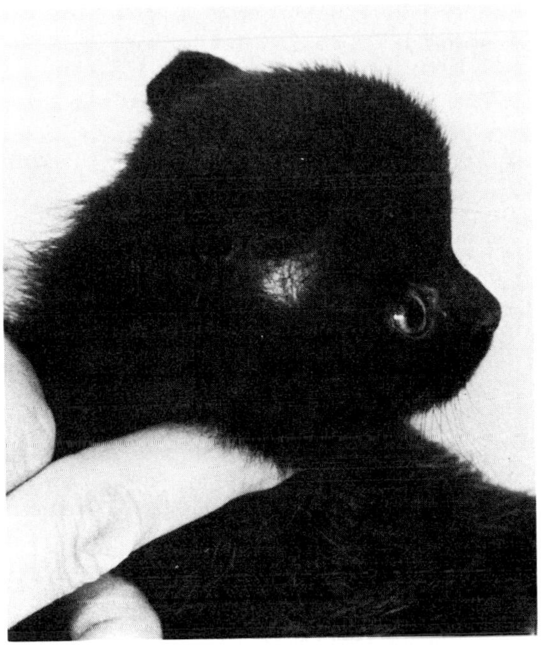

FIGURE 61–13. Kitten with hydrocephalus demonstrating the prominent, rounded calvarium that is especially apparent in the frontal area.

seizures. In most cases the earliest signs include altered mental status, visual deficits, and motor dysfunction.

On neurologic examination the animal with overt hydrocephalus is usually depressed. Animals have a normal gait, with slight hypermetric movements, and may circle continuously in one direction. Postural reactions, including proprioception, are usually depressed although the deficits can be subtle. Hopping movements are characterized by poor initiation and exaggerated follow-through. Follow-through on wheelbarrowing is usually hypermetric when the neck is extended. Severely affected animals drag their forelimbs. Reflexes in the limbs are normal to hyperactive, suggesting an upper motor neuron deficit. The normal gait with abnormal postural reaction and upper motor neuron dysfunction suggests forebrain disease. It is not uncommon for one side to be slightly more affected than the other.

Blindness can be detected in severely affected animals that bump into objects placed in their path. Menace deficits are also present and pupillary reflexes are normal. Papilledema can be found in cases having markedly increased intracranial pressure. Hydrocephalic animals with enlarged cranial vaults have a ventral strabismus, caused by the deformity of the orbit from the expanding skull. Ocular movements are normal. Facial sensory perception can be reduced, as evidenced by decreased avoidance of noxious stimulation to the inside of the nares. Auditory function is usually deficient in animals with severe motor deficits. Seizures may be an early manifestation of hydrocephalus. Some animals exhibit hyperesthesia to neck palpation or extension, presumably as a result of discomfort caused by increased intracranial pressure.

Radiographic examination of the skull in congenital cases reveals enlargement of the calvarium, with thinning of the dorsal wall and open sutures. The inner appearance of the skull may have a homogeneous density; however, this can be an unreliable criterion (Figure

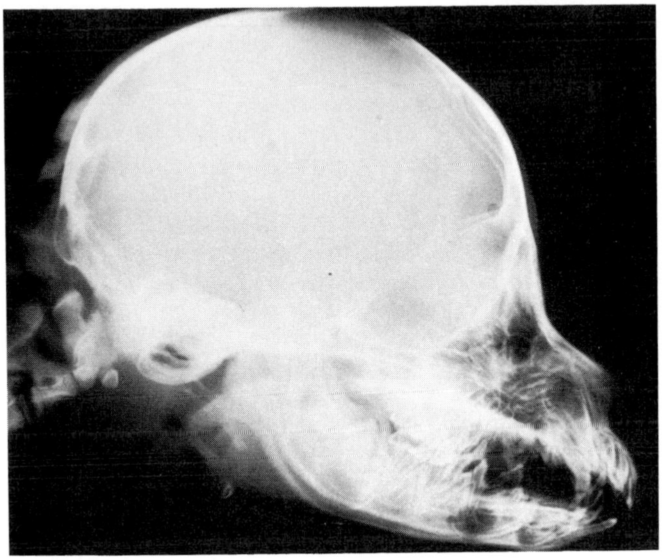

FIGURE 61–14. Lateral radiograph of a congenitally hydrocephalic dog with enlarged cranial vault, open fontanelle, and homogeneous density of calvarium.

61–14). Survey radiographs are normal in cases of hydrocephalus acquired later in life. The sizes and shapes of the ventricles are best assessed by pneumoventriculography or CT scans, although an estimate of size may be obtained by needle puncture (Figures 61–8, 61–15, and 61–16). Care must be taken not to remove too much fluid from the cerebellomedullary cistern in cases of hydrocephalus because of the danger of tentorial herniation. Excessive removal of fluid directly from the ventricles may produce subdural hematoma (Figure 61–17). The electroencephalographic changes in hydrocephalus are usually very characteristic and may be diagnostic (Figure 61–11).

The clinical course of the disease varies depending on the cause, the age of onset, and degree of neurologic deficits. Hydrocephalus is usually rapidly progressive

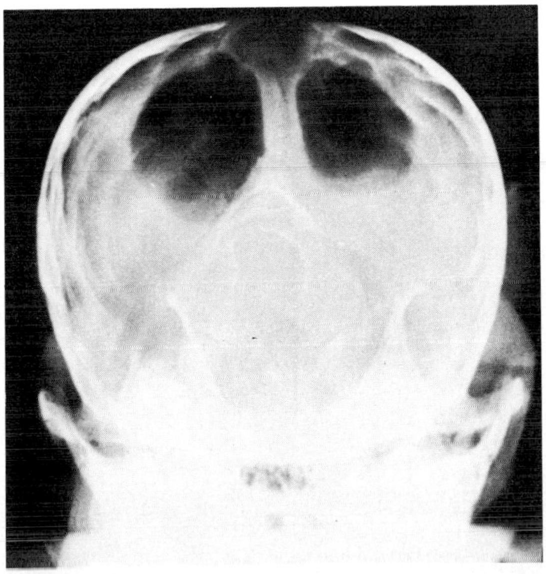

FIGURE 61–15. Radiograph of the skull of a Chihuahua after air has been injected into the lateral ventricles (pneumoventriculogram). The ventricles are grossly distended and the cerebral cortex is thin.

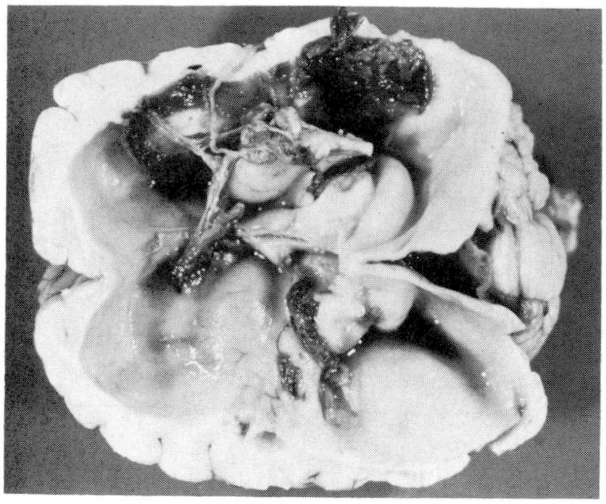

FIGURE 61–16. Horizontal section through brain of hydrocephalic dog with marked thinning of cerebral cortex. Basal nuclei and brain stem structures appear normal grossly. Hemorrhage in ventricles is secondary to a ventricular tap.

when an inflammatory process obstructs the mesencephalic aqueduct of neonatal or adult animals. Compensation may occur in congenitally affected animals so that neurologic signs remain static. Some dogs with mild hydrocephalus are clinically normal.

Treatment. Hydrocephalus results from some abnormality of CSF flow or absorption. If the precipitating cause can be defined, the treatment may be apparent. For example, removal of a choroid plexus papilloma that is secreting abnormal quantities of fluid or removal of a mass lesion obstructing the flow may result in recovery. However, such problems are rarely diagnosed in animals. Usually, the obstruction or impairment of absorption is the result of a permanent alteration in structure. In these cases, treatment must be directed at reduction of CSF production or drainage of the excess fluid.

Glucocorticoids, diuretics, and osmotic agents have been used in the medical management of hydrocephalus in animals that are not severely affected. Oral glucocorticoids have been successful in some cases. Dexamethasone is administered at an oral dose of 1 mg divided four times daily for 3 to 5 lb dogs.[20] This dose is gradually reduced during a two- to three-week course of therapy. Therapy is reinstituted and continued if the signs recur.

High-dose, long-term glucocorticoid therapy in young dogs or cats results in growth suppression, Cushingoid signs, and potential adrenal insufficiency. Some of these side effects may be minimized by intermittent dosage regimens.

Many cases of hydrocephalus eventually decompensate and require surgical correction. Fluid should be removed by ventricular or cisternal puncture prior to attempting surgical therapy to determine if surgical reduction of pressure will be rewarding. Hydrocephalus must be defined as communicating or obstructive to administer appropriate surgical therapy. Obstructive hydrocephalus in humans may be treated by direct drainage of fluid into the subarachnoid space, accomplished by a third ventricle stoma. An opening is made in the floor of the third ventricle. Fluid then drains into the interpeduncular cistern, from which it is distributed over the hemisphere where it can be absorbed.

Most surgical procedures devised to treat hydrocephalus have used tubing to shunt the fluid to another part of the body, such as the dorsal sagittal sinus, ureters, jugular vein, right atrium, peritoneal cavity, pleural cavity, or parotid duct.[21–26] The most frequently used methods are ventriculoatrial and ventriculoperitoneal shunts. Complications of shunts include obstruction to flow, infection, mechanical damage to nervous tissue, and disseminated intravascular coagulation (DIC).

Client education is of major importance in the treatment of hydrocephalus. The damage to the brain that has already occurred is permanent. In congenital hydrocephalus, especially in toy breeds, the surgical procedure is more difficult and complications are more frequent than in acquired hydrocephalus in older, larger dogs. Although many of these dogs can lead relatively normal lives, they are not totally normal animals.

Acquired hydrocephalus in an older dog is more likely to have a favorable prognosis. Signs are more severe because of the closed cranial vault, and the animal is

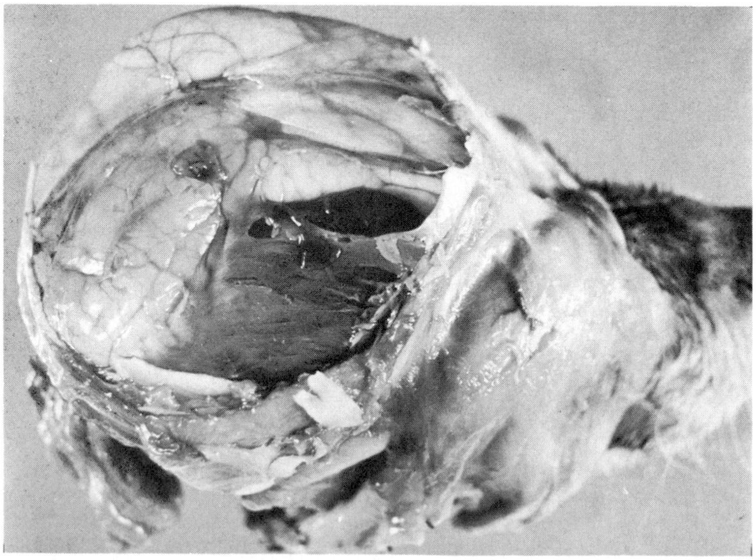

FIGURE 61–17. Large subdural hematoma in a dog with hydrocephalus. This resulted when too much fluid was aspirated from the lateral ventricle.

likely to be presented for treatment earlier in the course of the disease. The mature dog that is no longer growing does not require revision of the shunt because of increase in body length. Animals in this group are more likely to have complete recovery, and the fewer years of life expectancy reduces the likelihood of complications.

In spite of the many problems associated with the treatment of hydrocephalus, many owners want their animals treated. The surgical procedure is not difficult and the results can be very rewarding. The techniques of surgery are well described by others.[2, 22, 24, 25]

Congenital Syndromes

PORENCEPHALY AND HYDRANENCEPHALY

Porencephaly is a congenital defect extending from the surface of the cerebral hemisphere into the subadjacent ventricle. It may occur as a result of destructive processes or malformation during development. Hydranencephaly refers to cystic formation in the cerebral hemispheres as a result of prenatal destructive processes. Hydranencephalic, unlike porencephalic, defects are lined by an ependymal layer.

Causes of porencephaly and hydranencephaly in dogs and cats are prenatal traumatic or infectious processes. The clinical signs are similar to those of hydrocephalus in neonates. Neurologic deficits are variable because of the nonselective damage to the nervous system from teratogenic agents.

OTOCEPHALIC SYNDROME

The otocephalic syndrome, a complex group of abnormalities of the head, has been described as a hereditary phenomenon in the beagle.[27, 28] These animals have a variety of defects, ranging from complete distortion of all craniofacial structures anterior to the rostral occipital poles of the cerebral cortex, to minor defects in the brain, skull, and mandible. Many of these animals have some degree of hydrocephalus. A shortened lower jaw (partial agnathia) is a distinctive characteristic. Epileptic seizures are observed in mature dogs. Various degrees of neurologic signs are seen in surviving animals.

LISSENCEPHALY

Abnormalities in cerebrocortical convolutions occur from defects in neural migration during development. Intrinsic defects in the migration of neurons may be caused by metabolic or degenerative influences during pregnancy. Lissencephaly and pachygyria are developmental abnormalities that show an absence or limited number of cerebral convolutions (Figure 61–18). It is a rare anomaly that has been reported as a suspected inherited disorder in the Lhasa apso dog.[29] It has been reported in association with cerebellar hypoplasia in a cat and in wirehaired fox terriers and Irish setter dogs.[30, 31]

Neurologic abnormalities relating to lissencephaly include behavioral, visual, and convulsive disorders. These clinical signs have been noted within the first year of life. Neurologic abnormalities in these animals were mild or delayed in onset after birth, which indicates that dogs and cats are less dependent on the cerebral cortex for sensorimotor function than humans.

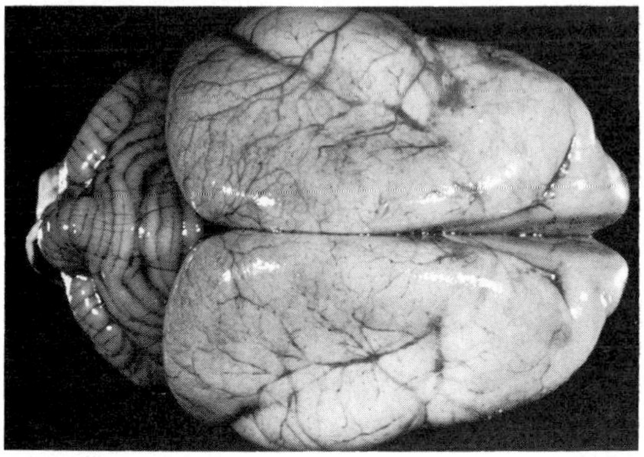

FIGURE 61–18. Brain of a Lhasa apso dog with lissencephaly. A few rudimentary sulci are present. (From Greene, CE, et al.: Lissencephaly in two Lhasa apso dogs. JAVMA 169:405, 1976.)

Subtle alterations are present in mental status. Affected dogs are intermittently depressed, confused, or hyperactive when stimulated by the presence of people or other dogs. The gait, as expected with a forebrain lesion, is normal. Postural reactions are mildly deficient or normal. Mild proprioceptive deficits are present in the hindlimbs, as evidenced by slow correction of knuckling of the digits. Bilateral menace deficits are present and animals collide with stationary objects when running.

Treatment for lissencephaly is not usually required because the neurologic deficits that are present are mild unless they are accompanied by cerebellar disease. Seizures may be controlled with anticonvulsant therapy.

CEREBELLAR MALFORMATION AND DEGENERATION

The cerebellum is responsible for the regulation of motor activity. Several congenital and neonatal infectious diseases result in maldevelopment of the cerebellum that produces cerebellar disease during the neonatal period. Dogs and cats have an incompletely developed cerebellum at birth, so diseased animals are not recognized as abnormal until they are several weeks of age.

In utero or perinatal infection with feline panleukopenia virus produces cerebellar malformations in young kittens (Figure 61–19). Cerebellar hypoplasia and cerebellar malformations have also been reported in dogs.[32–35] A familial association has been reported in Airedales and Boston terriers and in bull mastiffs affected with hydrocephalus.[28, 36] Although canine parvovirus is related to feline panleukopenia virus, cerebellar degeneration has not been associated with prenatal or neonatal infections in dogs. Herpesvirus has been associated with cerebellar damage in pups.

The diagnosis of cerebellar malformation should be entertained when cerebellar signs are present early in the neonatal period. Cerebellar signs are usually nonprogressive, unlike those seen with leukodystrophies, which also affect postnatal animals. Conditions causing dysmyelinogenesis, demyelination, and spongy degen-

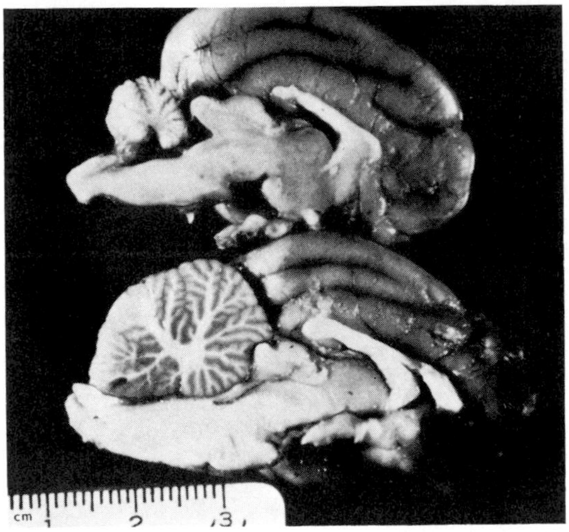

FIGURE 61–19. Brain of a normal cat *(bottom)* and kitten with cerebellar malformation *(top)* secondary to in utero panleukopenia virus infection. (From Oliver, JE, Jr, and Lorenz, MD: Handbook of Veterinary Neurologic Diagnosis. Philadelphia, WB Saunders, 1987.)

eration can also cause cerebellar signs (generalized body tremors) in neonatal animals. Unlike cerebellar malformation, the neurologic damage in these disorders is nonselective, so postural reaction initiation is deficient and upper motor neuron signs are present.

CONGENITAL MALFORMATION OF FORAMEN MAGNUM

Bardens has described a defect in the development of the occipital bone of toy breeds that was attributed to enlargement of the foramen magnum.[37] Clinical signs become apparent between two and six months and vary from cervical pain to seizures.

The clinical signs and course of disease are not characteristic and may reflect other intracranial disorders. The defect can be evaluated on frontal radiographs of the skull, preferably using the open mouth approach. At necropsy, these animals have a ligamentous structure that completes the foramen seen as a radiographic defect, but the clinical significance of this defect is questionable. Other disease, especially hydrocephalus, should be considered in any animal with such a skull defect.

HYPOMYELINOGENESIS

Congenital hypomyelinogenesis, an inadequate synthesis of myelin present at birth, has been reported in a wide variety of animals. Affected animals manifest tremors and oscillations of the head and body. These disorders may result from in utero infections or genetic and/or metabolic defects that result in failure of myelination of the central nervous system.

Cerebrospinal hypomyelinogenesis has been reported in pups of a number of dog breeds, including the Dalmatian, Weimaraner, lurcher, spaniel, and chow chow.[38–42] The genetic basis of inheritance in the spaniel dog was presumed to be a sex-linked recessive. The generalized body tremors are usually apparent when the pups begin to ambulate. They become more severe when they attempt to perform motor functions and disappear when they are resting or asleep. Postural reactions are slightly altered or absent, depending on the severity of the defect in limbs. Rear limbs are usually more severely affected. Segmental reflexes are normal. Cranial nerve examination usually is normal, although pendular nystagmus may be seen in those pups with head involvement. Affected dogs that survive and are mildly affected frequently improve and may be clinically normal at one year of age. Complete clinical improvement in some pups is attributed to partial involvement with delayed myelination of the nervous system. Gross and histologic examination of the brain at necropsy reveals an absence of myelinated white matter (Figure 61–20). Special staining must be used since myelin cannot be visualized using routine hematoxylin and eosin (H&E) staining.

Tremors have been associated with other congenital disorders affecting the white matter of the CNS.[43, 44] Hypomyelinogenesis and spongy degeneration was reported in a litter of three- to five-week-old puppies with rhythmic body tremors that disappeared with rest.[43] A litter of five kittens was born with hypomyelinogenesis and cerebellar hypoplasia.[45] The defective myelination was thought to be caused by an intrauterine effect on the fetuses.

DEGENERATIVE DISEASES

Metabolic Storage Diseases

Metabolic storage diseases are rare inherited diseases of humans and animals. As a result of partial or complete deficiency of a single lysosomal enzyme, there is an accumulation or storage of that enzyme's substrate and substrate by-products within lysosomes (organelles responsible for the intracellular digestion of polymeric material such as protein, polysaccharides, mucopolysaccharides, and complex lipids).[46–48] While lysosomal storage diseases are often widespread throughout the body,

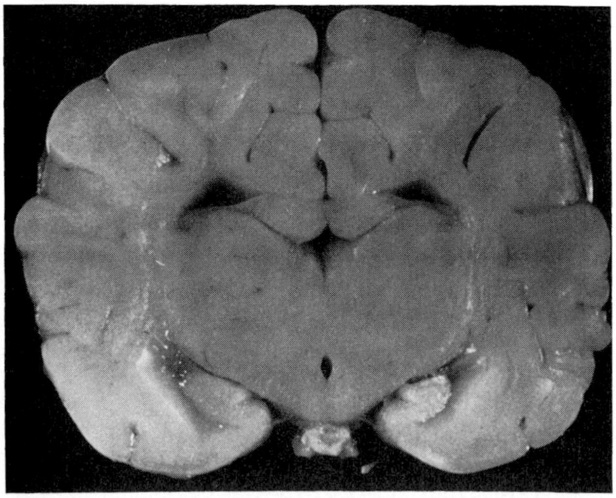

FIGURE 61–20. Frontal section of the brain of a puppy with hypomyelinogenesis. Lack of white matter is evident grossly. (From Greene, CE, et al.: Congenital cerebral hypomyelinogenesis in a pup. JAVMA 171:534, 1977.)

the majority affect the central nervous system (see Table 61–3).

Certain generalizations can be made about this group of diseases: (a) These diseases are rare and seen mainly in dogs and cats, (b) animals are usually normal at birth, (c) affected animals fail to grow as rapidly as their littermates, (d) as these conditions usually have a recessive mode of inheritance, only part of a litter is likely to be affected, (e) specific diseases are known to be present in certain breeds, (f) there is often a history of inbreeding, (g) many of the diseases manifest as neurologic disorders in young animals, usually at a few months of age, (h) the disease is always progressive and has a fatal outcome, (i) the age of onset and speed of progression are usually directly related, and (j) more than one system may be involved.

Diagnosis of metabolic storage diseases can be made by determining lysosomal enzyme activities from brain, viscera, or a preparation of white blood cells. The activity of the deficient enzyme is usually very low, while that of lysosomal enzymes tends to be increased. At present, no treatment is available.

GANGLIOSIDOSIS

Ganglioside storage diseases are inherited (autosomal recessive) defects of lysosomal hydrolase enzymes that result in accumulation of gangliosides and complex metabolites within lysosomes of most neurons throughout the nervous system. The storage material produces widespread neuronal degeneration.

In dogs and cats, several gangliosidoses have been identified and categorized according to the enzyme deficit and degree of visceral involvement. GM1 gangliosidosis, due to a deficiency of β-galactosidase, has been reported in the dog and cat. GM1 gangliosidosis with visceral involvement has been termed GM1 type 1 (the human eponym is Norman-Landing disease) and the form has occurred in a five-month-old beagle-cross dog and a three-month-old crossbred cat.[49, 50] GM1 gangliosidosis without visceral involvement is termed GM1 type 2 (the human eponym is Derry's disease). This is the more common form and has been reported in Siamese, Korat, and domestic cats.[51, 52] Signs first appear when cats are two to five months of age.

TABLE 61–3. STORAGE DISEASES IN DOGS AND CATS

Disease	Enzyme Deficit	Signalment	Clinical Signs	Key Reference*
Gangliosidosis				
GM1				
Type 1	β-galactosidase (ganglioside)	Beagle-cross dogs (5 mo)	Tremors, incoordination, spastic paraplegia, impaired vision	49
Type 2	β-galactosidase (ganglioside)	Siamese, Korat, and domestic cats (2–5 mo)	As above	52
GM2				
Type 1	Hexosaminidase A (ganglioside)	German shorthaired pointer (6–12 mo) Japanese spaniel (18 mo)	Ataxia, impaired vision, dementia Dementia	53, 54
Type 2	Hexosaminidase A and B (ganglioside)	Domestic cats (3 mo)	Same as cats with GM1 gangliosidosis	55
Sphingomyelinosis	Sphingomyelinase (sphingomyelin)	Siamese, domestic cats; poodle (3–4 mo)	Ataxia, tremors, hypermetria	56, 57
Glucocerebrosidosis	β-glucosidase	Sydney silky dog (6–8 mo)	As for sphingomyelinosis	59
Ceroid lipofuscinosis	Unknown defect (lipopigments accumulate)	English setter, dachshund, cocker spaniel, Chihuahua, saluki, etc.; cats (usually >1 yr)	Personality change, impaired vision, ataxia, seizures	62, 70
Fucosidosis	α-L-fucosidase (α-L-fucose?)	Springer spaniel (usually >1.5 yr)	Ataxia, personality change, dysphonia, dysphagia, seizures	68, 71
Mannosidosis	α-mannosidase (mannoside)	Domestic cat, Persian cats (2–7 mo)	Ataxia, tremors, hypermetria	73, 75
Glycogenosis				
Type II	α-glucosidase (glycogen)	Lapland dog (6 mo)	Weakness, exercise intolerance, seizures	81
Type III	Amylo-1,6-glucosidase (glycogen)	German shepherd dog (2–6 mo)	Muscle weakness, hepatomegaly	84
Mucopolysaccharidosis				
Type I	α-L-Iduronidase (mucopolysaccharide)	Domestic cat (10 mo)	Progressive lameness, facial deformities, skeletal malformations	85
Type VI	Arylsulfatase B (mucopolysaccharide)	Siamese cat (2–3 mo)	As for Type I, plus paraparesis, seizures	86, 88, 89
Globoid leukodystrophy	β-galactosidase (galactocerebrosidase)	Cairn terrier, West Highland terrier, beagle, bluetick hound (2–4 mo), mixed, poodle, Pomeranian, bassett hound (>1 yr); domestic cat (5–6 wk)	Ataxia, tremors, paraparesis, hypermetria, impaired vision	93
Metachromatic leukodystrophy	Arylsulfatase (sulfatide)	Domestic cat (2 wk)	Progressive motor dysfunction, seizures, opisthotonos	106

*For additional references, see text.

GM2 gangliosidosis also has been reported in dogs and cats. GM2 type I (the human eponym is Tay-Sachs disease) is caused by a deficiency of hexosaminidase A and has been reported in German shorthaired pointer dogs and in Japanese spaniels.[53, 54] There is no visceral involvement. Clinical signs are first observed in animals six to nine months of age. A second form of the disease, termed GM2 type 2 (the human eponym is Sandoff's disease), has been reported in domestic cats. Storage material occurs in visceral organs as well as in neurons and results from a deficiency of both A and B isoenzymes of hexosaminidase.[55] Clinical signs are observed in kittens approximately three months of age.

Clinical signs of gangliosidosis are very similar in dogs and cats and are highlighted by their relentlessly progressive nature. Ataxia, discrete head tremor, and dysmetria typically are the first signs observed, followed by spastic paraplegia or tetraplegia, visual impairment, depression, sometimes dementia, seizures, and death. Corneal clouding has been seen in feline gangliosidosis.

SPHINGOMYELINOSIS

Sphingomyelinosis (the human eponym is Niemann-Pick disease) is a rare and presumably heritable lysosomal storage disease that has been reported in a five-month-old miniature poodle dog and in three- to four-month-old Siamese cats.[56, 57] The disease results from a profound deficiency of lysosomal sphingomyelinase activity, with resultant accumulations of sphingomyelin, cholesterol, and gangliosides in neurons and visceral cells of the mononuclear-phagocyte system. Pathologic lesions are characterized by widespread cytoplasmic swelling and vacuolation of neurons in central and peripheral nervous systems, and foamy macrophages in the lung, spleen, lymph nodes, liver, adrenal glands, and intestine. Changes are most marked in the Purkinje cells of the cerebellum and neurons of the cerebellar roof nuclei and hippocampus and in dorsal root and peripheral ganglion cells. Most lymphocytes and monocytes in blood smears contain cytoplasmic vacuoles.

Clinical signs include ataxia, hypermetria, continuous head tremors, and loss of equilibrium. Signs can progress to visual impairment, total paresis, and death. A neurogenic syndrome, without central nervous system signs, has recently been observed.[58]

GLUCOCEREBROSIDOSIS

Glucocerebrosidosis (the human eponym is Gaucher's disease) is a rare lysosomal storage disease caused by a deficiency of glucocerebrosidase (β-glucosidase). The disorder has been reported in Australian silky terriers.[59, 60] Glucocerebroside accumulates in neurons throughout the brain. The cytoplasm of these cells is foamy, is finely vacuolated, and often contains weakly eosinophilic granules. Severe degenerative changes can occur in the cerebellum. Glucocerebroside storage occurs also in visceral cells of the mononuclear-phagocytic system.

Clinical signs reportedly occur around six months of age and are characterized by severe incoordination, wide-based stance, stiff gait, generalized tremors, and hypermetria.

CEROID LIPOFUSCINOSIS

Ceroid lipofuscinosis is believed to be a lysosomal storage disease associated with accumulation of lipofuscin and its related pigment ceroid, particularly in neurons and glial cells of the CNS. The pathogenesis of this disease is unknown; however, in English setters, a deficiency of p-phenylenediamine-mediated peroxidase, an enzyme that presumably prevents accumulation of peroxidized lipids, may be involved.[61] The presence of the pigment alone is unlikely to be the cause of the CNS disorder, since the pigment is present in normal aged dogs.

Neuronal ceroid lipofuscinosis occurs as an autosomal recessive trait in English setters.[62] There have been sporadic case reports in Chihuahuas, dachshunds, terrier-crosses, saluki dogs, corgis, and border collies.[63–68] A generalized form has been reported in cocker spaniels.[69] Neuronal ceroid lipofuscinosis also has been reported in cats.[70]

Neuronal ceroid lipofuscinosis is characterized pathologically by distention of large and small neurons with fine granular storage material that stains pinkish with H&E, black with Sudan black and Luxol fast blue, orange with Sudan III, are periodic acid–Schiff-positive, and show autofluorescence with ultraviolet light. Affected neurons are distributed throughout the brain and spinal cord.

Clinical signs usually occur in mature animals between one and nine years of age, although most reports are of animals under two years of age. Signs are extremely variable and include personality changes, visual impairment, generalized ataxia, head tremors, seizures, and tetraparesis. Hematology, serum biochemistries, urinalysis, CSF analysis, and skull and spinal radiographs are normal.

FUCOSIDOSIS

Fucosidosis is a lysosomal storage disease resulting from a deficiency of the enzyme α-L-fucosidase in various tissues, including central and peripheral nervous systems, kidney, pancreas, lymph nodes, and lung. As a consequence of this enzyme deficiency, there is an intralysosomal accumulation of a substrate, probably α-L-fucose. This disease, reported in English springer spaniels, is believed to be inherited as an autosomal recessive trait.[68, 71, 72]

The lesions in the CNS are characterized by extensive cytoplasmic vacuolations and swelling of many neurons and supporting glia throughout the brain and spinal cord. Occasional axonal spheroids are present in the cerebellar white matter. Many phagocyte-like cells with a foamy, vacuolated, PAS-positive cytoplasm are present either free in the parenchyma or as pronounced cuffs about larger vessels. Peripheral nerves are infiltrated by foamy macrophages and fibers are separated by edematous, finely fibrillar ground substance. There is minimal degenerative change in peripheral nerves.

Clinical signs develop in English springer spaniels one

and a half to three years of age. Signs are characterized by progressive change in temperament, loss of learned behavior, seizures, visual deficits, loss of balance, and apparent deafness. Additional signs can include head tremor, nystagmus, dysphonia, dysphagia, anisocoria, circling, head pressing, and spasms of jaw chomping. Hematologic studies indicate that 3 to 40 per cent of lymphocytes have marked cytoplasmic vacuolation. CSF analysis can reveal low glucose levels and elevated nucleated cell count, up to 500/mm^3, comprising macrophages and lymphocytes.

MANNOSIDOSIS

Mannosidosis is a lysosomal storage disease resulting from a deficiency of the enzyme acidic α-D-mannosidase in various organs, including brain, kidney, and liver. As a consequence of this enzyme deficiency, there is accumulation of mannose-rich material in the tissues and excretion in the urine of mannose-rich oligosaccharides. This rare disease has been reported in a seven-month-old domestic shorthaired cat presented with multiple skeletal anomalies, diminutive size, and neurologic disturbances characterized by progressive generalized ataxia and intention tremors.[73, 74] An hereditary form of mannosidosis has also been reported in Persian kittens in which similar neurologic signs, but no skeletal abnormalities, appeared at two months of age.[75] Microscopic lesions are characterized by extensive vacuolation of lymphocytes, visceral organs, and neurons and glial cells of the nervous system. Poor myelination of the cerebral white matter and axonal spheroid formation in cerebral and cerebellar white matter have been observed in two- and three-month-old Persian kittens.

GLYCOPROTEINOSIS

It has been suggested that glycoprotein-containing neuronal inclusion bodies found in beagles with epilepsy and rarely in other breeds are similar to Lafora bodies in human myoclonic epilepsy.[76, 77] These basophilic inclusions contain polysaccharide, are PAS-positive, and occur also in peripheral nerve, liver, spleen, and lymph nodes. However, the relationship between seizures and these inclusion bodies remains to be proven, since similar inclusions have been observed in older dogs of various breeds with no signs of clinical disease.[78, 79] Furthermore, in a recent study of epilepsy-prone beagles, only six of 68 dogs (8.8 per cent) had Lafora-like inclusion bodies.[80]

GLYCOGENOSIS

Glycogen storage diseases are rare disorders in dogs and cats. These diseases represent inborn errors of metabolism that lead to accumulations of glycogen due to the deficient activity of one of the enzymes involved in glycogen degradation or synthesis. The enzyme defects result in inadequate use of glycogen, glycogen accumulation within muscle cells, and often fasting hypoglycemia. Clinical signs of weakness, exercise intolerance, vomiting, collapse, and seizures may be observed.

A glycogen storage disease (glycogenosis type II) due to acid α-glucosidase enzyme deficiency, has been reported recently in related Lapland dogs.[81] Clinical signs develop in animals after six months of age and are characterized by progressive muscle weakness, frequent vomiting and regurgitation, megaesophagus, dysphonia, persistent panting, and cardiac abnormalities. Death occurred before the age of two years. The main lesions consisted of massive glycogen accumulation in most organs and tissues, especially in skeletal muscle. An autosomal recessive mode of inheritance is suggested. Attempts are being made to identify heterozygous animals by their partial deficiency of acid α-glucosidase.[82]

A glycogenosis similar to Cori's disease (glycogenosis type III) of humans, associated with a deficiency of the debranching enzyme amylo-1,6-glucosidase, has been reported in German shepherd dogs.[83, 84] Muscular weakness has been noted as early as two months of age. Other clinical signs included progressive abdominal distention as a result of hepatomegaly. Glycogen-like material occurred in liver, smooth and skeletal muscle, and nerve and glial cells of the CNS.

MUCOPOLYSACCHARIDOSIS

Mucopolysaccharidoses comprise a group of generic lysosomal diseases that result from deficits in the metabolism of glycosaminoglycans that accumulate in various connective tissues and/or are excessively excreted in urine. There are two mucopolysaccharidoses described in cats, both considered to be recessively inherited. Mucopolysaccharidosis I (the human eponym is Hurler's syndrome), caused by a deficiency of α-L-iduronidase, has been reported in a ten-month-old domestic shorthaired cat.[85] This cat was presented because of progressive lameness, a broad face with depressed nasal bridge, small ears, corneal clouding, and multiple bone dysplasia, including fusion of vertebrae over the cervicothoracic junction, pectus excavatum, and bilateral coxofemoral subluxation. The cat excreted excessive amounts of glycosaminoglycans in its urine and glycosaminoglycan storage was evident in fibroblasts and neurons. Gross postmortem findings included hepatosplenomegaly. Swollen, vacuolated neurons were seen in the central nervous system.

Mucopolysaccharidosis VI (the human eponym is Maroteaux-Lamy syndrome) has been reported in two- to three-month-old Siamese cats.[86, 87] This disorder is caused by a deficiency of the enzyme arylsulfatase B. The clinical features of affected animals are almost identical to those of cats with mucopolysaccharidosis I; however, Siamese cats have toluidine blue-positive granules in circulating neutrophils. It has been estimated that approximately 25 per cent of cats four to seven months of age with mucopolysaccharidosis VI develop clinical signs of thoracolumbar spinal cord dysfunction secondary to cord compression from focal bony protrusions into the vertebral canal.[88] Clinical signs are characterized by varying degrees of pelvic limb paresis that may progress to paraplegia, incontinence, and decreased pain sensation caudal to the level of the thoracolumbar lesion. Seizures have been reported in an affected two-year-old Siamese cat.[89]

Prognosis can be favorable with surgical decompression of the spinal cord early in the course of the disease; however, the long-term prognosis for cats with mucopolysaccharidosis I or VI remains to be determined.

GLOBOID CELL LEUKODYSTROPHY

Globoid cell leukodystrophy (the human eponym is Krabbe's disease) is a rare lysosomal storage disease that results in progressive degeneration of white matter of the central, and sometimes peripheral, nervous systems. The disease is caused by an accumulation of galactocerebroside, possibly within oligodendrocytes and Schwann cells, as a result of a deficiency of the enzyme β-galactosidase.

Significant lesions are confined to the nervous system, where any level of the brain and spinal cord may be affected. The disease is characterized by destruction of white matter and replacement by aggregates (often in a perivascular fashion) of nonsudanophilic, nonmetachromatic, PAS-positive macrophages called globoid cells.

Globoid cell leukodystrophy is inherited as an autosomal recessive trait in young (three- to six-month-old) Cairn and West Highland white terriers.[90–98] The disease also has been reported in a four-month-old beagle, a two-year-old poodle, a four-year-old basset hound, four-month-old bluetick hounds, two Pomeranians ranging in age from 5 1/2 months to 14 years, and in domestic shorthaired kittens.[99–104]

The clinical signs associated with this disease are variable. Animals often present with either signs of an ascending posterior paralysis or signs of a cerebellar syndrome, or both.

Results of ancillary aids usually are nonspecific. Hematology, serum biochemistry, ophthalmology, and spinal/skull radiography are normal. Analysis of CSF can reveal an elevated protein level, but cell counts usually fall within normal limits (albuminocytologic dissociation). PAS-positive cells are rarely identified in CSF.[105]

METACHROMATIC LEUKODYSTROPHY

Metachromatic leukodystrophy has been reported in a domestic cat, with progressive motor dysfunction, seizures, and terminal opisthotonos.[106] The neurologic signs are first noted at two weeks of age. Histologic findings of demyelination and gliosis are accompanied by sulfatide accumulation within neurons that stain metachromatically. It is believed to be due to a deficiency in arylsulfatase.

Other Degenerative Disorders

DALMATIAN LEUKODYSTROPHY

A progressive neurologic disorder, possibly transmitted by an autosomal recessive gene, has been described in Dalmatian dogs.[107] Gross pathologic changes include brain atrophy, dilatation of lateral ventricles, and cavitation of the central white matter of the cerebral hemispheres. Within affected areas of white matter, there is a diffuse loss of myelin, widespread vacuolation, edema, and presence of numerous lipid-filled macrophages.

Clinical signs are noted between three and six months of age and are characterized by visual deficiency and progressive ataxia and weakness in all limbs. Results of routine hematology, urinalysis, and CSF are within normal limits.

FIBRINOID LEUKODYSTROPHY

A rare fibrinoid leukodystrophy (a synonym is Alexander's disease) characterized by diffuse pallor and rarefaction of CNS white matter and pressure of irregularly shaped eosinophilic structures designated "Rosenthal fibers" has been reported in two Labrador retriever dogs and in a Scottish terrier.[108, 109] The fibers are arranged most densely around blood vessels, and subependymal and subpial areas. Affected white matter can be characterized by increased vascularity. Astrocytic proliferation is commonly seen. Neuronal loss may be evident in the cerebral cortex and subcortical grey structures. The cause of this disease is not known; however, an astrocytic dysfunction is suspected. Clinical signs are noted at about six months of age and include pelvic and limb paresis, progressive ataxia, generalized weakness, and personality changes.

DEMYELINATING MYELOPATHY OF MINIATURE POODLES

A rare, suspected hereditary disorder in miniature poodles has been reported.[110–112] Pathologically, diffuse demyelination can occur throughout all columns of the spinal cord; however, spinal cord grey matter and dorsal and ventral nerve roots are preserved. There may be loss and degeneration of axons. In some dogs, the most severe lesions occur in dorsal and ventral white columns of cervical and thoracic spinal cord segments. Focal areas of malacia also have been observed in cerebral and cerebellar peduncles, cerebellar root nuclei, and tegmentum of the midbrain. Lesions can be characterized by the presence of lipid-laden macrophages. Clinical signs first appear between two and four months of age. Initial signs of pelvic limb paresis progress to spastic paraplegia and tetraplegia. Analysis of CSF is within normal limits. Prognosis is poor; there is no treatment. There have been no additional reports of this disease during the past 20 years.

SPONGIFORM DEGENERATION

Rare, variable spongiform degenerative conditions, possibly hereditary in nature, have been recognized in young dogs and cats. A suspected genetic disorder occurs in the Egyptian Mau breed of cat (a small breed derived from the Siamese cat).[113] There is widespread vacuolation of white and grey matter of brain and spinal cord. There is no evidence of myelin breakdown. Clinical signs are first noticed in kittens at seven weeks of age and are characterized by pelvic limb ataxia and hypermetria. Subsequent signs include intermittent periods of severe depression and reduced activity, with frequent flicking movements of distal pelvic limbs when at full flexion. The condition may improve with age.

Spongiform degeneration, described in a Samoyed puppy, was characterized by a generalized vacuolation of white matter throughout brain and spinal cord, with most severe changes being found in the cerebellum.[114] Pelvic limb tremors were observed at 12 days of age, progressing to generalized tremors over the next five days. A similar spongiform change has been described in the cerebral and cerebellar white matter, but not in spinal cord, of silky terrier puppies.[43] A large number of Alzheimer type II protoplasmic astrocytes were found in severely affected areas. Clinical signs were noted at birth and consist of uncontrolled intermittent contractures of the vertebral column, especially muscles of the thoracolumbar region at intervals of approximately two per second. Occasionally, the pelvic limbs were lifted off the ground during these contractures. The episodes were intensified with excitement. Low-intensity contractions continued during sleep. Signs did not appear to be progressive.

Spongiform degeneration of the white matter of the CNS and peripheral nervous system, with most prominent lesions in cerebellar peduncle, deep cerebellar white matter to cerebral white matter, has been observed in two young female Labrador retriever littermates, between four and six months of age.[115] Clinical signs were characterized by progressive ataxia and dysmetria of head, trunk, and limbs, hyporeflexia with clonus, and extensor rigidity with episodes of exaggerated rigidity and opisthotonos and muscle atrophy. Routine hematology, serum biochemistries, urinalysis, and CSF tests have been within normal limits. Prognosis of dogs with this disorder appears to be guarded to poor. Treatment with acepromazine (0.25 mg/kg IM) may reduce the episodes of extensor rigidity. Phenobarbital, 2 mg/lb/day (5 mg/kg/day), PO may produce temporary improvement of signs.

LEUKOENCEPHALOMYELOPATHY OF ROTTWEILERS

A degenerative disorder of the spinal cord and lower brain stem recently has been reported in rottweiler dogs.[116, 117] All dogs had a history of progressive gait abnormalities, which began insidiously at ages varying from 1.5 years to 3.5 years. Demyelinating lesions are found in the brain stem, deep cerebellar white matter, and spinal cord. Axons are preserved. Lesions tended to be bilaterally symmetrical. The cause and pathogenesis are unknown. Clinical signs included ataxia, tetraparesis, dysmetria, delayed proprioceptive positioning, and exaggerated spinal reflexes. All diagnostic studies, including CSF analysis, EMG, plain radiography, and myelography, were normal. One dog was treated with glucocorticoids for two months without improvement. The clinical and pathologic course and treatment remain to be evaluated. Pedigree data suggest that the disease is transmitted genetically.

HEREDITARY QUADRIPLEGIA AND AMBLYOPIA IN THE IRISH SETTER

This is an autosomal recessive, lethal disease of Irish setters. All animals are affected at birth. Although they make coordinated walking or paddling movements, they are unable to stand or walk unaided, and propel themselves on their bellies with a swimming type of action.[118] Signs progress to visual impairment, nystagmus, head tremor, and seizures. No convincing neuropathologic changes have been found to account for the clinical signs.[119]

Results of routine hematologic, radiographic, urine, and CSF tests are within normal limits. Prognosis is poor; there is no treatment.

CEREBELLAR DEGENERATION

There are many degenerative disorders affecting the nervous system of domestic animals. The majority of these disorders are hereditary or are suspected of being hereditary in nature and are characterized by premature aging and degeneration and death of various neuronal cell populations. The cause and pathogenesis are not known. The mechanism of premature degeneration of cells, termed "abiotrophy," implies an inherent lack of trophic or nutritive factor. Degenerative diseases tend to be breed-related. Unlike congenital syndromes, these animals are normal at birth. Clinical signs frequently begin within a few months after birth. Progressive neurologic deficits generally develop with degenerative disorders.

Antemortem diagnosis is based on clinical signs, age, breed, and by ruling out acquired diseases. Examination of biopsy material from selected sites, such as the cerebellum, may confirm a diagnosis in some instances. In general, electrodiagnostic aids, clinical biochemistry, CSF analysis, and radiology are of limited value in the diagnosis of degenerative disease. Prognosis is guarded to poor; there is no treatment. Cerebellar degeneration has been reported in several breeds of dogs.

Inherited Cerebellar Degeneration in the Kerry Blue Terrier. This is an autosomal recessive disease that affects Kerry blue terriers. Degenerative lesions initially are observed in the Purkinje cell (+/− granule cell) layers and are followed by symmetrical, bilateral neuronal degeneration in the olivary nuclei three to four months after the onset of clinical signs. Several months later, neurons of the substantia nigra and caudate nuclei degenerate in a symmetrical fashion.[120]

Clinical signs of stiffness of pelvic limbs and head tremors reflect cerebellar disease and are seen between eight and 16 weeks of age. Subsequent signs include dysmetria-hypermetria and, often, inability to stand by one year of age. The condition is progressive and prognosis, poor. There is no treatment.

Inherited Cerebellar Degeneration in the Gordon Setter. This is believed to be an autosomal recessive, late-onset cerebellar disease affecting mature Gordon setters between six and 30 months.[121, 122] Lesions are restricted to the cerebellum and characterized by profound loss of Purkinje cells throughout most of the cerebellar cortex. The molecular layer is moderately thinned and the granule cell layer varies in thickness. It has been suggested that the degenerative process begins in Purkinje cells and that granule cells may be secondarily affected.[123] Dogs appear normal during the first six months of life, but between nine and 18 months they may develop a mild thoracic limb stiffness, hypermetria, broad-based stance, and occasional stumbling. Nystagmus can occur late in the condition. These signs progress very slowly or remain static after a short period of progression. There is no treatment; prognosis is guarded. The disease is usually slowly and insidiously progressive over several years.

Inherited Cerebellar Degeneration in the Rough Coated Collie. This is an autosomal recessive disease reported in rough coated collie dogs in Australia in which there is early and rapid degeneration of Purkinje cells and granule cells of the cerebellum.[124] Other changes include neuron depletion in cerebellar root nuclei, lateral vestibular nuclei, inferior olivary nuclei, and the ventral horns of the spinal cord. Posterior incoordination occurs between one and two months of age. Subsequently, animals develop a broad-based stance, hypermetria, and head tremors and, occasionally, a "bunny-hopping" gait. Affected animals frequently fall sideways or forward, with their legs in extension. Severely affected dogs typically spend most of their time lying down. Clinical signs may stabilize after 12 months of age. There is no treatment.

Cerebellar Degeneration in the Border Collie. This condition appears to be very similar to that described in the rough coated collie.[125] There is a reported loss of granule and Purkinje cells from the anterior folia of the cerebellar vermis, which is flattened grossly. The disease is believed to be familial. Clinical signs are first noted at six to eight weeks of age and are characterized by ataxia, hypermetria, and head tremor. Prognosis is guarded to poor, since clinical signs reportedly deteriorate with time.

Cerebellar Degeneration in Bull Mastiffs. This is believed to be an autosomal recessive cerebellar disease affecting bull mastiff puppies usually between four and nine weeks of age (in one affected dog, initial signs were noted at seven months of age).[36] Pathologic findings are characterized by moderate to severe communicating hydrocephalus, with dilatation of all ventricles and the cerebral aqueduct. Symmetrical lesions occur in the cerebellar nuclei, lateral vestibular nuclei, and inferior colliculi. The cerebellar lesions consist of vacuolation, gliosis, and frequent axonal spheroids. The Purkinje cells appear normal. There is no cerebellar atrophy, although occasional "torpedos" have been seen in the granule cell layer. A specific deficit or abiotrophy within the Purkinje system could account for degenerating axons in cerebellar and lateral vestibular nuclei but would not explain the lesions in the inferior colliculus. The concentrations of spheroids in and adjacent to nerve cell nuclei and the paucity of degenerative changes in their nerve cell bodies may suggest that this disease is another form of neuroaxonal dystrophy.

Clinical signs include ataxia, most obvious in pelvic limbs, hypermetria, proprioceptive deficits, and head tremor, which is accentuated as animals attempt to eat. All affected animals to date have had visual deficits and slowed menace reflexes. Less constant signs include hysterical behavior, compulsive movements, circling, depression, and nystagmus.

Ancillary aids such as hematology, serum biochemistry, and CSF analysis are within normal limits. Ventriculography may reveal enlarged lateral ventricles. The contrast passes from lateral ventricles to fourth ventricles without hindrance and into the spinal subarachnoid space, suggesting there is no blockage and that this is a communicating form of hydrocephalus. Prognosis is guarded; there is no treatment.

Cerebellar Degeneration in Other Breeds. Cerebellar degeneration, usually involving Purkinje cells, has been reported in families of Samoyeds (with swollen axons of Purkinje neurons in the granule cell layer), Airedale terriers, Finnish harriers, and Bern running dogs. A genetic basis has been suggested. A similar disorder has been observed in single litters of Labrador retrievers, golden retrievers, beagles, cocker spaniels, Cairn terriers, and Great Danes.[126] The authors have observed isolated cases of Purkinje cell degeneration and loss in German shepherd, springer spaniel, pit bull and poodle puppies between the ages of six and 16 weeks. Clinical signs are characterized by the typical cerebellar syndrome.

NEUROAXONAL DYSTROPHY

Neuroaxonal dystrophy (NAD) is a degenerative neurologic disease that has been reported in cats and dogs. NAD is transmitted as an autosomal recessive trait in cats and is suspected of being inherited in dogs. The disease is characterized by membrane-filled swellings ("spheroids") of distal or preterminal axons within the central nervous system. The pathogenic mechanisms underlying the development of this type of axonal abnormality are not well understood. In general, clinical signs of cerebellar-like disease develop in young animals and are typically progressive. Ancillary laboratory tests such as CSF analysis, skull/spinal radiography, and electrodiagnostics are normal. There is no treatment. Prognosis is guarded due to the progressive nature of the disease.

Feline Hereditary Neuroaxonal Dystrophy. Domestic tricolor cats have been found to have an autosomal recessive condition that is characterized pathologically by gross atrophy of the cerebellar vermis and microscopically by marked ballooning of cell processes (spheroids) in nuclear groups extending from the medulla to the thalamus and cerebellar vermis.[127] These changes are accompanied by loss of neurons, including Purkinje and granule cells of the cerebellar vermis. Inner ear lesions have been reported.

Clinical signs occur in kittens around five to six weeks of age, at which time head tremors and head shaking are observed. Signs progress to marked incoordination of gait and hypermetria. Affected kittens have a lilac color, which darkens with age. Unaffected littermates are black.

Neuroaxonal Dystrophy in Rottweilers. A recessive mode of inheritance is suspected in rottweilers with NAD.[128, 129] The cerebellum is mildly atrophic and appears to be small. Massive numbers of axonal spheroids are present in many regions of the neuraxis, especially in the dorsal horn of the spinal cord, nuclei gracilis and cuneatis, granular layer of the cerebellum, and vestibular nucleus. In some dogs, a marked loss of cerebellar Purkinje cells has been reported. Clinical signs are characterized by slowly progressive ataxia, hypermetria, and wide-based stance, beginning in the first year of life. As the neurologic deficit progresses, head intention tremors, postural and spontaneous nystagmus, and menace deficit may be noted. Some rottweilers have been observed up to six years of age.

Neuroaxonal Dystrophy in Collie Sheep Dogs. A cerebellar neuroaxonal dystrophy in Collie sheep dogs has been reported in New Zealand and Australia.[130] The history of several affected pups in litters from successive matings of the same sire and dam is suggestive of an autosomal recessive mode of inheritance. Numerous spheroids, associated with mild wallerian degeneration, are present in the central cerebellar, adjacent peduncular and folia white matter, and associated cerebellar roof and lateral vestibular nuclei. Clinical signs develop from two to four months of age, and include hypermetria, wide-based stance, difficulty in maintaining balance, intention tremor, and ataxia. Body growth, learning ability, and social behavior with other dogs appears to be normal.

Neuroaxonal Dystrophy in Other Breeds. Neuroaxonal dystrophy recently has been reported in two female Chihuahua puppies.[131] Clinical signs began at seven months of age and were characterized by sudden onset of tremors and exaggerated gait. Spheroids were numerous throughout the white matter of the brain.

It is possible that a degenerative cerebellar disease of bull mastiff dogs may be another form of NAD.[36]

HEREDITARY ATAXIA IN TERRIERS

Hereditary ataxia is an autosomal recessive disorder in smooth-haired fox terriers in Sweden that has been reported as a clinical entity since 1941.[132, 133] A similar condition has been described in Britain in Jack Russell terriers, a type of short-legged, smooth-haired terrier developed within the smooth-haired fox terrier breed.[134] Pathologically, a focal, wallerian degeneration is found in the dorsolateral and ventromedial white matter of the cervical and thoracic spinal cord. In Jack Russell terriers, degenerative changes also are found in central auditory pathways and peripheral nerves.

Clinical signs in both breeds occur between two and six months of age, when weakness and pelvic limb incoordination are observed. The incoordination progresses to involve all limbs and a prancing or dancing type of gait is observed. Animals appear to be unable to gauge the extent of a movement, which is unpredictable in direction. Severely affected animals frequently fall and are unable to rise to their feet.

Clinical signs may stabilize after several months and some affected animals are able to live a relatively normal life in spite of the abnormal movements. In no case has the disease, per se, proved to be fatal. Routine hematologic, radiographic, urine and CSF tests are within normal limits.

Acquired Tremors

A syndrome associated with a sudden onset has been described that affects young mature dogs of small breeds.[135] The shaking is exacerbated by excitement and activity but postural reactions remain normal. Thus, the neurologic examination closely resembles that for dogs with congenital cerebrospinal hypomyelinogenesis and those that the authors have observed resulting from CNS intoxication. Although a diffuse disruptive process of the CNS is suspected, the pathologic findings in a few dogs have consisted of a mild, diffuse nonsuppurative encephalitis.[135] CSF examination is usually normal.

Treatment early in the course of the disease with immunosuppressive doses of glucocorticoids is thought to reduce the course and severity of the illness, and some dogs may recover from the disease spontaneously within several weeks.

CEREBROVASCULAR DISEASES

Cerebral Anoxia and Hypoxia

Cerebral hypoxia and anoxia can result from cardiac failure, anemia, or other defects in the oxygen-carrying capacity of the blood. Iatrogenic hypoxia results from improper anesthesia or intoxication with cyanide, carbon monoxide, or oxidative compounds that produce methemoglobinemia. Focal hypoxia of the brain can result from neoplasia, infections, subarachnoid hemorrhage, parasitic or degenerative processes that damage the cerebrovascular network or cause vasoconstriction. The results of oxygen deprivation to the brain depend upon the severity and duration of the insult. The response of individual neurons is variable with regard to metabolic rate and oxygen need. Oxygen demands are highest in the cerebral cortex and decrease progressively toward the caudal medulla.

Diffuse cerebral ischemia in the dog or cat produces significant irreversible neuronal injury in as few as 15 minutes of severe ischemia.[136] Tolerance of anoxia was longer than previous established times for cardiac arrest. The areas of greatest injury included the neocortex, hippocampus, basal ganglia, thalamus, rostral brain stem, and cerebellum. Polioencephalomalacia was the histologic lesion produced by cerebral anoxia.

Cerebral anoxia may occur in any breed of dog associated with stress, seizures, and respiratory arrest. Abnormalities in the respiratory system of the brachycephalic breeds make them more susceptible to oxygen deficiencies with induction of anesthesia.

Clinical signs that occur following cerebral hypoxia include ataxia, tetraparesis, collapse, convulsions, and coma. Pupils may be mydriatic or miotic depending on the extent of neuronal damage. Diffuse cerebrocortical hypoxia alone produces symmetrically small pinpoint pupils. Rostral brain stem injury is associated with fixed pupils that are either midpoint or dilated.

Edema of the brain is concurrent with cerebral oxygen deficiency. In the closed cranial vault, edema of the brain results in compression of the cerebrum and associated cranial nerves. Cardiac arrest or fibrillation in which resuscitation or spontaneous conversion is successful may still result in permanent brain damage if the blood supply to the brain has been removed for more than five to ten minutes. Intracranial pressures have been reduced in cats following resuscitation from cerebral hypoxia by hyperventilation to reduce arterial carbon dioxide concentration.[137]

Neely and Youmans experimentally increased the intracranial pressure in dogs, effectively reducing cerebral circulation.[138] Death occurred in 9 to 12 minutes when intracranial pressures of 100 mmHg were applied. Artificial respiration was given to resuscitate dogs with similar intracranial pressures; the intracranial pressures were exerted for 5, 10, 15, 20, and 25 minutes. All dogs survived for 48 hours and could stand, see, and hear the following day. When pressures of 100 mmHg of mercury were applied for longer than 25 minutes, survival was never longer than 24 hours. The severity and extent of neuronal necrosis following cerebral hypoxia in cats was shown to be associated with blood glucose concentration.[139] Presumably this results from anaerobic glycolysis and the production of increased brain lactate concentrations. Therefore, attempts should be made to reduce serum glucose concentrations using insulin, and the use of hypertonic glucose to reduce brain edema might be avoided when cerebral edema is the result of hypoxia.

Hoerlein reported two dogs that were resuscitated after more than ten minutes of cardiac massage following cardiac arrest.[140] Both dogs had signs of severe brain damage and remained comatose for several days after resuscitation, but became relatively normal within two months. Sight and hearing were severely impaired, as was retention of learned responses. It was speculated that extreme cerebrocortical damage from anoxia is not as incapacitating in the dog or cat with regard to life and locomotion, as it is in humans.

Hypertonic mannitol commonly has been recommended to treat compromised cerebral circulation, since it is known to reduce brain edema and intracranial hypertension and increase cerebral blood flow. However, when given at a dose of 1 gm (2 gm/kg) IV, it did not appear to improve cerebral blood flow in dogs following cerebral ischemia.[141]

Polioencephalomalacia

Polioencephalomalacia refers to variable degrees of diffuse necrosis of cerebral grey matter. Other nuclear grey matter areas can be affected. This lesion is commonly found with various intoxicants such as lead and cyanide, and with thiamine deficiency and hypoglycemia. It frequently results from cardiac arrest, cranial trauma, or cerebrovascular hypoxia from any cause. Persistent seizures of any cause can lead to polioencephalomalacia because of respiratory arrest and cerebral hypoxia. Focal polioencephalomalacia can follow selective insults to the nervous system, such as occur with microfilaria or vasculitis. Distemper infections in the nervous system can result in selective malacia of the paleocortex.[142] Focal polioencephalomalacia can result from disturbances in cerebral blood flow from any cause.

Once polioencephalomalacia develops, it results in a persistent seizure focus. Dogs with extensive cerebrocortical necrosis are usually comatose or depressed with tetraparesis. They may present in status epilepticus. Menace deficits are usually present with normal pupillary reflexes.

Hemorrhage

In contrast to the high incidence in humans, massive intracerebral hemorrhage resulting from spontaneous rupture of vessels and/or saccular aneurysms rarely occurs in animals.[143] Intracranial and intraspinal hemorrhages occasionally have been reported in dogs in association with arteriovenous vascular malformations, e.g., telangiectatic hemartomas and angiomas.[144, 145] Small, ring-like hemorrhages reportedly increase in frequency in dogs over 11 years of age.[143] The hemorrhages are associated with an amyloid angiopathy and occur mainly in the upper layers of the cerebral cortex. Cerebellar cortex, white matter, and subcortical and brain stem grey matter are rarely involved. Clinical signs compatible with a cerebral syndrome are observed.

Hemorrhage can often be present in the CNS of animals with migrating parasitic disorders (cuterebriasis in dogs), protozoan infections (toxoplasmosis in dogs), bacterial meningitis, viral diseases (canine hepatitis), degenerative disorders (thiamine deficiency in cats), toxins (warfarin poisoning), systemic metabolic disorders (disseminated intravascular coagulopathies, platelet dysfunction [thrombocytopenia], and coagulation factor deficiencies), and cranial or spinal trauma.

Hemorrhage into primary and secondary brain tumors also is observed frequently in dogs, especially oligodendrogliomas, glioblastomas, ependymomas, and hemangioendotheliomas.

Onset of clinical signs in animals with sudden hemorrhage is usually acute. Presence of macrophages in CSF containing red blood cells or hemosiderin ("siderophages") may suggest a recent hemorrhagic episode. Prognosis of animals with hemorrhage is guarded.

Infarction

Infarction or necrosis (a synonym is malacia) of CNS parenchyma results from cerebrospinal vascular occlusion. Vascular occlusion of cerebral blood vessels can result from many causes, including diseases of the blood vessel itself, such as vasculitis, atherosclerosis, or fibrosis.[146] Atherosclerotic deposits in cerebral vessels have been a complication of chronic hyperlipidemic disorders in dogs and cats.[147, 148] Seizures have been noted with increased frequency in dogs with persistent hyperlipemia.[149] Emboli to the nervous system can occur from bacteria, parasites, fibrocartilaginous material, neoplastic cells, and fibrin clots. Diffuse cerebral infarction is a sequela to disseminated intravascular coagulation.

Feline Ischemic Encephalopathy

There is an ischemic necrosis of cerebral tissue that occurs sporadically in adult male and female cats of all ages, especially in summer months.[150, 151] Lesions may be unilateral or bilateral and may involve up to 75 per cent of one cerebral hemisphere. The major area of infarction is frequently in the distribution of the middle cerebral artery. Vascular occlusive lesions, including thrombosis and vasculitis, have been found only occasionally. Affected animals do not have cardiomyopathy.

Clinical signs are nonprogressive and variable but acute in onset. Clinical signs include depression, circling to seizures, and change in attitude, often to the point of aggression. Mydriasis and visual impairment may be present. Clinical signs may be modified or disappear with time (several days to weeks). Hematology, skull radiographs, and CSF analysis usually are normal. Abnormal brain trace pattern may be detected with electroencephalography. Prognosis is usually favorable since many of the signs seen initially do ameliorate; however, behavioral changes and uncontrollable seizures may persist.

INFLAMMATORY DISEASES

Infectious agents that affect the CNS of dogs and cats generally produce signs of both a neurologic and a systemic nature. (The reader is referred to Chapters 46 to 49 for discussions of each disease.) This review concentrates on central nervous system lesions produced by each agent.

Viral Diseases

RABIES

Rabies is a fatal nervous disorder caused by a neurotropic virus. The disease usually is transmitted by bites from infected animals, and all warm blooded animals appear to be susceptible to the disease. Rabies infection has been reported following vaccination with modified live virus vaccines.[152–155]

The incubation period is more prolonged and variable than other CNS infections, depending on the site of the bite and amount of inoculum. This is because rabies virus gains access to the central nervous system by centripetal migration up nerves. Postvaccinal cases generally have an incubation period of one to two weeks, while natural cases vary from two weeks to one year.

The clinical signs of rabies include progressive lower motor neuron dysfunction and ascending paralysis from the site of inoculation. Complete paralysis usually does not occur until after behavioral signs are seen. The classic clinical spectrum of behavioral changes, lasting 24 to 36 hours, begins with a prodromal syndrome manifest by dullness and depression. The animal may scratch or chew at the site of inoculation.

In the furious stage of rabies, which lasts five to ten days, the animal may run aimlessly and bite at anything in its path. Salivation is profuse and conjunctivitis and prolapse of the third eyelid occur. When confined, the animal may attack its cage and bedding. Cats are notorious for showing erratic or unusual behavior during this interval.

Dumb rabies is associated with the signs of progressive lower motor neuron paralysis. Neurons in the cranial nerve nuclei become affected. Facial and masseter muscle paralysis prevents adequate food and water intake and changes in facial expression. The eyelids may squint and anisocoria may be present. Vocalization may stop at the time of complete paralysis and the condition progresses to coma when medullary neurons become affected.

The classic description of the stages of rabies is somewhat artificial and not all animals progress through or show these three phases of infection. Neurologic signs of any type can occur. Rabid dogs may display any form of rabies and frequently changes in behavior occur. The topographic localization of rabies infection of the brain explains the specific neurologic deficits seen at various stages of the clinical illness.[156]

Vaccine-induced rabies in dogs and cats begins with paralysis in the inoculated limb within seven to 21 days of inoculation.[153, 154] Progressive paralysis begins in an ascending fashion. Progressive lower motor neuron signs and muscular rigidity develop. Pain sensation and reflex function usually are depressed caudal to the point of ascending paralysis. Partial paresis of the forelimbs occurs. Two dogs with postvaccinal rabies recovered within one to two months following the onset of clinical signs.[154]

Increased CSF protein and leukocyte count are mild and similar to that of other viral encephalitides, such as canine distemper. Virus identification in nervous tissue is done on fresh or refrigerated tissues using immunofluorescent (FA) methods. Unlike the older test for Negri bodies, it is not necessary that animals show neurologic signs because the FA method detects virus in the brain as soon as, or prior to, its occurrence in saliva. The FA methods have been used to detect virus in cutaneous nerves, such as those in the sensory vibrissae of the maxillae, theoretically allowing an antemortem diagnosis.[157] Measurement of CSF antibody to rabies virus is an accurate means of diagnosing rabies in cases when infection has been present for at least several weeks; however, a negative titer does not eliminate the possibility of infection.

Because of potential public health complications, suspected rabid animals should be euthanatized. Animals with vaccine-induced rabies do not represent a health hazard because of attenuation of the virus and the fact that it is not shed in the saliva. Animals with vaccine-induced rabies may improve with time. Experts should be consulted because of the difficulty in distinguishing vaccine virus from virulent virus without monoclonal antibody or genetic analysis techniques.

Prevention of rabies infection requires adequate vaccination. Killed vaccines are being used with more frequency because of the lack of side effects and the ability to use one vaccine in many species. The Compendium of Animal Rabies Vaccines published by the Association of State Public Health Veterinarians should be consulted for available products.

CANINE DISTEMPER

The spread of distemper virus to the CNS depends on the immunocompetence of the dog at the time of infection.[158] In most cases of distemper, the virus enters the nervous system regardless of whether nervous signs are noted. Distemper virus may directly injure neuronal elements or secondarily alter the cell membrane so that it is destroyed by host immune responses. Distemper virus may also damage myelin-producing cells or elicit an immune-mediated myelinolysis. Specific antimyelin antibody has been found in the sera of dogs with distemper encephalitis.[159] The role of antimyelin antibodies in the pathogenesis of CNS lesions is controversial, since the antibodies may increase as a result of the release of myelin products in the systemic circulation.

Usual sites of acute distemper encephalitis are periventricular and subependymal nervous tissue. Antiviral antibody in the CSF appears to suppress the release of intracellular virus and may induce formation of an incomplete virus and latent or chronic CSF infection.[160, 161]

Clinical signs of distemper vary, depending on the virulence of the virus, environmental conditions, and host age and immune status. Neurologic signs of distemper frequently begin one to three weeks after recovery from systemic illness. Mature, partially immune dogs may develop neurologic signs without prior history of systemic disease.

Neurologic complications of canine distemper indicate a poor prognosis. Neurologic signs are variable and correlate to the area of involvement. Seizures, cerebellar and vestibular signs, sensory ataxia, and myoclonus are common.

Myoclonus, a forceful involuntary twitching of muscles, reflects irritation or loss of inhibition to the particular lower motor neuron segment innervating the muscle group. There may be paresis of the affected limb or muscle group. The neural mechanism for myoclonus originates in the area of spinal cord or brain stem motor neurons and is modified by higher centers.[162]

Young puppies may be infected from transplacental transmission of distemper virus. They usually develop neurologic signs during the first four to six weeks of life. Depending on the state of gestation, abortions, stillbirths, and birth of weak puppies are noted. Prenatally or neonatally infected dogs that survive usually show persistent immunodeficiencies.[158]

Clinical diagnosis of canine distemper is primarily based on clinical suspicion. Hematologic and biochemical changes are nonspecific. Electroencephalography can indicate the presence of inflammatory disease, but it does not provide a specific diagnosis. CSF abnormalities can be found in dogs with neurologic distemper. Increased cell and protein contents are characteristic, with most of the cells being lymphocytes. Increased protein levels in CSF have been globulin (IgG and IgM) with specific anticanine distemper virus activity.[163]

Specific neutralizing antibody in CSF is the most definitive evidence for CNS distemper without CNS disease. CSF antibody may be artificially increased during traumatic tapping because of whole blood contamination or from other causes of CNS inflammation. Specialized CSF electrophoresis is needed to identify whether the CSF globulin is locally produced or due to nonspecific leakage of all blood proteins. This test can only be performed by specially equipped diagnostic or research laboratories.

Immunofluorescent techniques can be used for the specific diagnosis of canine distemper. However, they can be unreliable in detecting distemper antigen in all cases with nervous system involvement. Neutralizing antibody either clears the virus from the tissues other than the nervous system or binds to the virus, producing false-negative results. Examination of cells in CSF in these cases usually is only rewarding in very acute cases because antibody neutralizes viral antigen. Fluorescent antibody testing can be performed on frozen sections of nervous tissue at necropsy.

Pathologic findings in the nervous system of dogs with canine distemper are variable. Young puppies dying of acute fatal encephalitis can have acute noninflammatory neuronal and myelin degeneration or demyelination. Older, and in most cases more immunocompetent, animals develop widespread perivascular lymphocytic infiltrates, which may progress to sclerosis in more chronically affected animals. Multifocal demyelinating lesions are commonly found in the cerebellopontine angle, the cerebral peduncles, optic tracts, and the spinal cord. Intranuclear and intracytoplasmic inclusions can be detected in most cases.

Atypical chronic forms of distemper infection have been recognized in the CNS. The clinical signs are usually gradually progressive and localizing. Multifocal perivascular infiltration with demyelination and necrosis is a common pathologic finding. This may progress to sclerosing panencephalitis.[164]

Therapy for neurologic disturbances in canine distemper is unrewarding, as progressive encephalitis often leads to tetraplegia, semicoma, and incapacitation such that euthanasia is recommended. Dogs should not be euthanatized unless their neurologic disturbances are progressive or incompatible with life.

Seizures, myoclonus, and optic neuritis are three neurologic manifestations that can be tolerated if the signs are nonprogressive. No drug has been shown to control myoclonus. Recommendations have been made to administer anticonvulsants after the systemic disease but prior to the development of seizures. There is no evidence to show that anticonvulsants prevent entry of the virus into the nervous system, but they may suppress foci from causing seizures.

FELINE INFECTIOUS PERITONITIS

Feline infectious peritonitis (FIP) has been recognized as a cause of CNS disease in the cat for a decade. Sporadic reports prior to this time describe a nonsuppurative meningoencephalitis of unknown origin.[165]

The CNS form of FIP occurs in cats of various ages. Cats that develop the neurologic or ophthalmologic signs of FIP rarely have abdominal or pleural effusion. Ocular signs that may precede or accompany the neurologic disease are characterized by a granulomatous anterior uveitis. Other nonspecific signs of systemic illness include anorexia, pale mucous membranes, dehydration, and pyrexia.[166] Noneffusive pyogranulomatous lesions, which most commonly occur in the kidney, may be detected by abdominal palpation.

Neurologic deficits with CNS involvement are variable, depending on the duration and site of the infection in the nervous system. The disease tends to localize and spread along CNS vasculature, resulting in meningitis and ependymitis. Signs of meningitis in very early cases are muscular twitching and hyperesthesia. Seizures are common when the process involves the surface of the cerebral hemispheres. Cerebellar and vestibular systems are involved because of their superficial location. Cranial nerve dysfunction is common for a similar reason. Spinal cord involvement is manifested by pelvic limb paresis or tetraparesis. Paraspinal hyperesthesia is often detectable in these cases. Multifocal and diffuse neurologic signs are frequently apparent because of the spread of infection in the subarachnoid and ventricular spaces. Hydrocephalus has been reported in young kittens as a result of obstruction of the cerebral aqueduct.[18]

Hypergammaglobulinemia is a common finding on the biochemical profile. CSF abnormalities include increases in protein and predominantly neutrophilic pleocytosis. CSF changes are present in most cases because of meningeal localization. The direct immunofluorescent test for FIP antibody in serum can be performed as an aid in confirming the diagnosis, although the results can be ambiguous. When clinical signs are compatible with those of active FIP, sequential titers should be performed to detect a rise in antibody titer of sufficient magnitude. Single high titers (greater than 1:1600, but dependent upon the laboratory used) only indicate previous or recent exposure to FIP virus. Exposure to feline enteric coronavirus produces lower titers.

Pathologic lesions in the nervous system are confined to microscopic examination. A pyogranulomatous meningitis and ependymitis are characteristic findings. Adjacent parenchymal inflammation includes neutrophilic, histiocytic, and plasma cell infiltration.

Treatment for the neurologic signs in FIP is unrewarding. High doses of immunosuppressive or anti-inflammatory medications temporarily halt or reverse many of the clinical signs.

AUJESZKY'S DISEASE

Aujeszky's disease (pseudorabies) is a neurotropic viral disease of cattle, sheep, dogs, cats, rats, and swine. The latter is adapted to the virus and serves as inapparent carrier of infection.

Animals with clinical signs show intense pruritus and may scratch or bite themselves to the point of self mutilation. Like rabies virus, this herpesvirus migrates up peripheral nerves to the central nervous system where it causes polioencephalomyelitis. Clinical signs relate to ascending lower motor neuron paralysis. Anorexia and depression are followed by paresis, convulsions, and coma in three days. Ingestion of infected swine, cattle, or rat offal is a common source of infection in dogs and cats. This results in the development of cranial muscle paralysis and death within 48 hours.[167, 168] The pruritus, lack of aggression, and rapid death distinguish this disease from rabies.

Lesions in the brain are those of an acute polioencephalomyelitis in the caudal medulla.[167] Perivascular mononuclear infiltrations with microabscess formation and intranuclear eosinophilic viral inclusion bodies (Cowdry type A) are characteristic.[169]

A vaccine for treating affected animals is not available in the United States. Active and passive immunizations have been reported to allow recovery.[170] Care should be taken in disposal of carcasses of dead animals. Rodent control and isolation of infected animals helps to limit the spread of infection.

HERPESVIRUS INFECTION

Newborn puppies can develop systemic infections with canine herpesvirus as a result of in utero exposure or by contact with their dam during the first week of life. The virus is temperature-sensitive and primarily infects neonates with subnormal body temperatures, although older immunosuppressed dogs have been systemically infected.

Some pups that survive the systemic illness show neurologic signs from viral encephalomyelitis. The virus is thought to enter the CNS by hematogenous means, although ganglioneuritis of the trigeminal nerve has been found in puppies infected by oronasal exposure.[171] The virus has a predilection for cerebellar and vestibular portions of the nervous system. The neurologic disease is usually nonprogressive and mild deficits may be compatible with survival in infected puppies.

CANINE PARVOVIRUS INFECTION

As with feline panleukopenia virus infection in cats, canine parvovirus infection can cause degeneration and necrosis of CNS tissue when infection occurs prenatally or perinatally.[172, 173] Because the parvoviruses show an affinity for replicating cells, they affect only the CNS in the developing nervous system. Affected puppies show neurologic abnormalities within the first few weeks of life, in addition to other systemic signs. Widespread, rather than selective, cerebellar degeneration and necrosis has been a feature of the CNS lesions.

POSTVACCINAL ENCEPHALITIS

Neurologic complications have been documented following vaccination in dogs and cats. Historically, complications following rabies vaccination have received the most attention. Allergic encephalomyelitis was a common complication of the use of the first rabies vaccines of nervous tissue origin. Encephalomyelitis following the use of modified live rabies vaccines has been discussed previously.

Encephalomyelitis with inclusion body formation was reported after combined distemper/infectious canine hepatitis vaccination in the dog.[174] Fatzer and Fankhauser and Bestetti made similar observations.[175, 176] The latter authors demonstrated pseudomyxovirus nucleocapsids of canine distemper by electron microscopy. Postvaccinal distemper has also been reported following immunosuppression in dogs and in association with parvovirus infection in three-week-old puppies.[177, 178]

Fankhauser et al. reported atrophy of the Purkinje cells in three of six pups given modified live measles vaccine at six weeks of age.[179] Cerebellar signs were noted beginning five days after vaccination.

A modified live canine coronavirus vaccine has been

found to cause systemic vasculitis and meningoencephalitis similar to lesions produced by FIP.[180]

Modified live feline panleukopenia vaccines should not be used in kittens younger than two to four weeks. Cerebellar degeneration can occur from vaccine virus infection.

Modified live vaccines should never be used in pregnant animals because of the risk of inducing resorption, abortion, or malformations.

Rickettsial Diseases

Rocky Mountain spotted fever (RMSF) and ehrlichiosis are tick-borne rickettsial diseases that produce meningoencephalitis in dogs. In the acute phase, both diseases produce an immune-mediated vasculitis that results in inflammation and necrosis of a variety of tissues, including the meninges and CNS.

Both syndromes are accompanied by multisystemic signs, which often accompany the neurologic features, including lethargy, confusion, stupor, convulsive seizures, and coma. These forebrain signs have been noted less commonly with ehrlichiosis. Central or peripheral vestibular dysfunction has been one of the most common signs of either disease. Signs of spinal cord involvement, including paraparesis, ataxia, and paraspinal hyperesthesia, have been found with both diseases.

Hematologic and biochemical alterations are nonspecific but thrombocytopenia is one of the more consistent (but not absolute) laboratory findings, making platelet count a suitable screening procedure. Serologic confirmation is still needed, and there appears to be no cross reaction between these parasites.

Rickettsiae appear to be extremely sensitive to the effect of tetracycline (10 mg/lb or 22 mg/kg given q8h), with the polysystemic signs of RMSF and acute ehrlichiosis disappearing within 24 to 48 hours. Delays in recovery of neurologic deficits are noted, presumably because of the persistent and irreversible neurologic lesions that are produced.

Bacterial Diseases

Bacteria can enter the nervous system by the vascular system or direct extension. Signs of bacterial meningitis include pyrexia, hyperesthesia, stiffness, and cervical rigidity. Neurologic deficits indicate parenchymal involvement, and the term meningoencephalitis is used. Bacterial infections spread to the central nervous system via the blood, following infection and/or abscess formation elsewhere in the body. Persistent or intermittent bacteremia is a common source for infection. Bacteria commonly isolated from CSF in the dog and cat include *Pasteurella* sp. and *Staphylococcus* sp. *Actinomyces*, *Cryptococcus*, *Blastomyces*, and *Histoplasma* can cause clinical signs of meningoencephalitis indistinguishable from that caused by bacteria. Bacterial meningitis can be associated with ependymitis, aqueductal obstruction, and hydrocephalus.[19] Cerebrospinal fluid examination with bacterial and fungal culture allows an appropriate diagnosis. Bacterial or fungal meningoencephalitis results in a marked increase in protein and cell count in the cerebrospinal fluid. Leukocyte counts are usually greater than 500 cells/mm^3, with a preponderance of polymorphonuclear cells. CSF findings are similar with fungal infections but organisms can often be demonstrated. CSF fluid with this composition should be cultured.

Antibiotic therapy should be instituted when CSF results suggest bacterial meningitis. The antibiotic may be changed when the culture results are returned. Antibiotic effectiveness in the nervous system depends on adequate penetration of the intact blood-brain and blood-cerebrospinal fluid barriers.[181] Certain antibiotics that are otherwise ineffective penetrate these barriers in the presence of inflammation. Chloramphenicol, a highly lipid-soluble antibiotic, has the highest penetrability of the central nervous system and its concentration exceeds that in serum. Trimethoprim/sulfonamide combinations also penetrate well. Ampicillin and penicillin enter the nervous system with meningeal inflammation but their effectiveness wanes as the inflammatory process resolves. When given parenterally, aminoglycosides, which are highly polar, do not give adequate CSF concentrations under any circumstances. Intrathecal therapy with aminoglycosides and other antibiotics should only be used in refractory cases.

Glucocorticoids have been recommended for treating meningoencephalitis because of their anti-inflammatory effects. Glucocorticoid therapy should never be used in the treatment of bacterial or fungal meningitis. It allows the spread of infection and reportedly produces a worsening of neurologic status. Osmotic diuretics may be used instead of glucocorticoids to control cerebral edema. Treatment of systemic mycosis is discussed in Chapter 49.

INTRACRANIAL ABSCESS

Abscesses in the brain can be considered a variant of bacterial meningoencephalitis. The localization of pus and infection may result in focal or lateralizing signs on neurologic examination similar to a mass lesion (Figure 61–21).

Diagnostic and therapeutic findings are the same as those for bacterial meningoencephalitis except that mass lesions can be detected with specialized radiographic

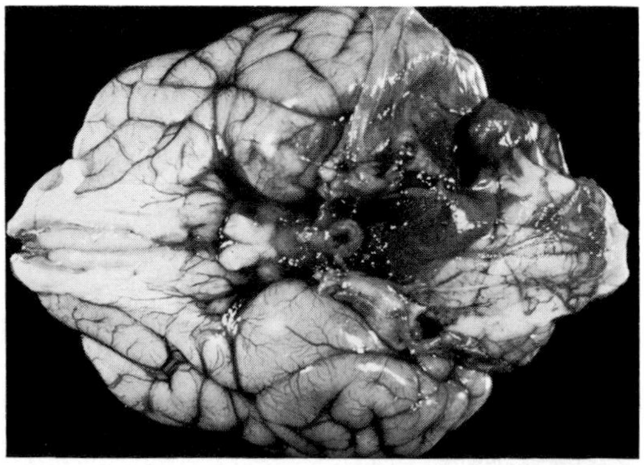

FIGURE 61–21. Intracranial abscess in the cerebellopontine angle of a mixed breed dog, resulting from extension of infection from otitis media.

techniques. Surgical drainage of abscesses in the central nervous system is impractical in most cases.

TETANUS

Tetanus can occur in the dog and cat as a result of soil contamination of necrotic wounds with *Clostridium tetani*. The incubation period is five to eight days.

The anaerobic organism produces an exotoxin at the site of infection. This toxin is released in the systemic circulation and affects the nervous system. Tetanus toxin blocks the activity of inhibitory interneurons within the central nervous system. This results in release from inhibition and subsequent hyperexcitability of lower motor neurons.

Clinical signs reflect tonic spasms of skeletal muscles with intermittent clonus and can be exacerbated by external stimuli. The third eyelid often prolapses, the lids retract, and the facial muscles in dogs have a characteristic expression (Figure 61–22). Tonus of the masseter, digastric, and facial muscles causes retraction of the lips and difficulty in opening the mouth and swallowing. Dyspnea and opisthotonos are common. Hypersensitivity to external stimuli increases as the disease progresses. The animal may die of respiratory paralysis, although recovery is frequent with supportive care.

Treatment of tetanus should begin with a thorough examination for the site of infection. If discovered, the wound should be adequately debrided and drainage provided. Massive doses of penicillin (25,000 to 50,000 IU/lb) are used. Intravenous administration of antitoxin is the most effective route of parenteral therapy. Intrathecal antitoxin has been more effective than parenteral administration in humans. Most canine and feline cases are mild and respond to supportive care, so antitoxin may not be necessary. Respiratory support must be provided by means of ventilatory assistance in severely affected cases. Tracheal intubation and oxygen administration may be required.

Mycotic Diseases

SYSTEMIC MYCOSES

Specific fungi that spread multisystemically are contracted from infected soil in particular geographic regions. The organisms usually enter the body and cause infection in the upper or lower respiratory systems. Dissemination throughout the body to other organs, including the nervous system, occurs in certain cases. Immunosuppression and debilitation are thought to contribute to their dissemination. Of fungi producing systemic mycoses, *Cryptococcus* is most likely to spread to the CNS.

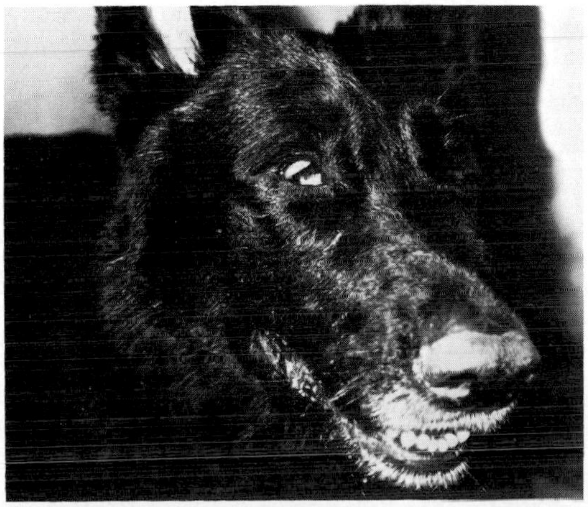

FIGURE 61–22. Bilateral protrusion of the third eyelids in a dog with tetanus. Note the hypertonus of the facial muscles.

Fungal organisms may enter the nervous system by the blood vascular route or by extension from the upper respiratory tract through the cribriform plate of the ethmoid bone. They spread through the CSF and cause disseminated meningoencephalitis. Neurologic signs are usually multiple and may be associated with other signs of systemic illness in the animal.

CSF cytology and culture are the most definitive means of establishing infection within the CNS. Serologic testing is less reliable and serially paired samples are required for more accurate diagnosis.

Treatment requires specific chemotherapy, which is discussed in Chapter 49, although neurologic deficits may not improve following therapy. The infection may be difficult to control within the CNS because of poor penetration of parenterally or orally administered antifungal agents. Even combination chemotherapy with multiple antifungal drugs has not been rewarding in treating CNS infections in dogs and cats.[158] Intrathecal administration has been employed in human cases.

PROTOTHECOSIS

Prototheca is an achlorophyllous alga that can cause disseminated and CNS infections in immunosuppressed dogs and cats. The organism is ubiquitous in the environment and may gain access to the body through normal body orifices or by wound penetration. Soil and stagnant water seem to be common sources of the organism. Establishment of localized or systemic infection probably results from failure of the host's defense mechanisms.

Disseminated protothecosis has been reported in animals, including the dog and cat, but CNS involvement has only recently been described.[182, 183]

Clinical findings in animals are diverse and reflect the variable localization of the organism following dissemination. Persistent bloody diarrhea is a common feature. Blindness is common and results from the extensive retinal lesions that are often produced. Central nervous signs in dogs have included ataxia, circling, incoordination, and paresis or paralysis. Central nervous signs have not been seen in cats; only the cutaneous form has been observed.

Diagnosis of the disease is made by culture, and histologic and immunofluorescent detection of the organism in any tissue or body fluid. The CSF analysis often exhibits increases in neutrophils, or eosinophils and organisms may be seen. Gram staining of yeast or fungal isolates allow rapid identification of the organism. Rectal scrapings should be performed in any animal showing CNS signs regardless of whether bloody diarrhea is seen.

Surgical removal is the therapy of choice for localized superficial infections with *Prototheca* that occur in humans. There is no known effective treatment for disseminated protothecosis. Unfortunately, most of the cases reported in dogs and cats have been disseminated. Limited success with the combined use of amphotericin B and tetracycline has been found in the treatment of cutaneous protothecosis in humans.

PHAEOHYPHOMYCOSIS

Phaeohyphomycosis refers to infections of the skin and subcutaneous tissue with brown pigmented fungi. When the infection disseminates in dogs and cats, it can affect the central nervous system.[184–186] Disseminated infection is most common in the immunocompromised host. The most frequent genus of fungi known to spread to the CNS of dogs and cats is *Cladosporium*. Extraneural lesions have not been observed in animals with CNS infections.

Animals with CNS dissemination show a rapid progression of neurologic signs characterized by forebrain dysfunction, nuchal rigidity, ataxia, altered behavior, depression, seizures, and coma. CSF abnormalities have included increased protein and a neutrophilic pleocytosis. The organism has not been cultured antemortem in any case.

Necropsy findings on coronal sections of the brain include grossly discolored to cavitated lesions. Histologically, lesions are pyogranulomatous foci surrounded by septate branching hyphae. Therapy has not been tried and may prove unrewarding because of the rapid progression of neurologic signs once they develop.

Protozoal Diseases

TOXOPLASMOSIS

Toxoplasma is a ubiquitous protozoan parasite that causes multisystem dysfunction in all mammalian species. As the only definitive host, the cat appears to be well adapted to the parasite, since clinical *Toxoplasma* infection is rarer in the cat than other species.[187] *Toxoplasma* encephalitis in dogs and cats is rare unless concurrent immunosuppression is present. *Toxoplasma* encephalitis in dogs commonly complicates infection with canine distemper virus. Young puppies frequently develop encephalomyelitis, radiculoneuritis, and myositis with concurrent infections. Previously infected dogs and cats may develop *Toxoplasma* encephalitis and myositis when given large doses of immunosuppressive drugs such as glucocorticoids. Seizures, pelvic limb paresis, and ataxia have been the most common neurologic signs in postnatally infected dogs and cats. Neurologic signs can vary, however, with the area of the CNS that is affected. Polymyositis is characterized by generalized lower motor neuron signs, hyperesthesia, and muscle atrophy and these signs may mask CNS involvement. Ophthalmoscopic examination should be performed because retinochoroiditis and anterior uveitis are frequent findings. Consult Chapter 46 for diagnosis and therapy.

CANINE ENCEPHALITOZOONOSIS

Encephalitozoonosis, a disease of several mammalian species, including humans, has been reported in dogs.[188] It is caused by an obligate intracellular protozoan parasite, *Encephalitozoon cuniculi*. The etiologic agent of this disease in humans may be closely related, but not identical, to this parasite.

Clinical signs are seen in puppies in the first few months of life. Nervous signs predominate despite the multisystemic involvement by the parasite. Disorientation, circling, behavioral changes, convulsions, fatigue, weight loss, and death have been reported.[188] The majority of puppies in a litter are affected.

Hydrocephalus is found on gross examination of the nervous system. Microscopically, there is a granulomatous encephalitis characterized by perivascular mononuclear cell infiltration and necrosis. Extensive inflammatory foci are found in the brain and meninges. Protozoa can be demonstrated with a modified Gram stain on nervous tissue and can be cultivated in tissue culture. A serologic test is available that can be used to aid in the diagnosis of the disease.

ACANTHAMOEBIASIS

Acanthamoeba is a free-living protozoon that causes disease in people and animals. Previous literature refers to these organisms as *Hartmanella* sp. Affected dogs are thought to have been infected neonatally or as adults that are immunocompromised by other concurrent illnesses.[189–193] The mode of transmission in dogs is unknown, but systemic hematogenous spread following ingestion or inhalation is suspected.

Clinical findings resemble those of canine distemper. Affected animals develop lethargy, increased rectal temperatures, and dyspnea, followed by neurologic signs such as seizures and progressive ataxia, incoordination, and eventual death.

Premortem diagnosis has been limited in established cases. A fluorescent antibody method has been used to measure circulating serum antibody, although its significance is unknown. Direct FA procedures have been used to identify the organism in tissue samples. FA staining is often needed to identify the organisms in tissues because they resemble tissue macrophages.

Metazoal Parasitic Diseases

Most CNS signs related to parasitic infection are associated with direct invasion of the CNS by some form of the parasite. The signs relate more to the site of invasion than to the type of parasite involved. Localization within the brain and spinal cord is possible by means of neurologic testing. The determination of cause usually depends upon examination at necropsy. The presence of large numbers of eosinophils in cerebrospinal fluid may make the clinician suspicious of parasitic infection.

DIROFILARIASIS

Although reported in dogs, cats are especially prone to develop neurologic signs such as dementia, ataxia, circling, mydriasis, and seizures as a result of aberrant worm migration (see Chapter 80).[194]

CUTEREBRIASIS

Cuterebrae have been discovered in the brain of dogs and cats with neurologic signs.[195–198] In these abnormal hosts, the infection is a larval migrans. The fly normally deposits its eggs near the burrows of rodents. Dogs and cats become infected accidentally by investigating these areas or by ingesting infected rodents. The larvae normally mature in subcutaneous tissue but may make an ectopic migration into the brain. CSF fluid in one dog had increased WBC and protein, with an eosinophilic pleocytosis.

LARVAL MIGRANS

Cases of visceral larval migrans were studied by Barrons and Saunders.[199] Granulomas caused by migrating *Toxocara* larvae were observed microscopically in the brain and other tissues of animals. Similarly, abnormal migration of visceral larvae were reported by Richards and Sloper.[200] Cerebrospinal nematodiasis caused by *Ancylostoma caninum* was reported in a dog.[201] A 12-week-old cocker spaniel had signs of imbalance, torticollis, and pain on flexion of its neck that progressed to tetraparesis and death. *Angiostrongylus cantonensis* is a lungworm of rodents that causes larval migrans and eosinophilic meningoencephalitis in humans. The life cycle in the rat normally consists of a migration to the brain prior to localizing in the pulmonary arteries. *A. cantonensis* was reported to cause progressive posterior paresis and ataxia in a litter of puppies in Australia.[202] Histologic findings in the puppies were randomly distributed, consisting of granulomatous inflammation at all levels in the brain and spinal cord.

COENUROSIS

Cerebral coenurosis has been reported in the cat and the dog.[203–205] The brain is a common site of cyst development in unusual intermediate hosts of *Taenia* species. The neurologic signs were obvious in all cases. Preventative measures should be taken to avoid animal contact with feces of definitive hosts of these tapeworms.

Inflammatory Diseases of Unknown Cause

GRANULOMATOUS MENINGOENCEPHALOMYELITIS

Granulomatous meningoencephalomyelitis (GME) is a worldwide sporadic, nonsuppurative inflammatory disease of the central nervous system of dogs and, rarely, of cats.[164, 206–218] Lesions of GME may be disseminated or focal. The disseminated form has been previously described as "inflammatory reticulosis" and "histiocytic encephalitis." The focal form of GME has been described as "neoplastic reticulosis."

The cause of GME is unknown. The lesions resemble experimental allergic encephalomyelitis, suggesting a possible immunologic basis for the disease. Immunohistologic studies indicate that many of the lymphocyte cells present in GME are immunoglobulin-bearing cells.[219] It is possible that GME represents an altered host response to an infectious agent; distemper and rabies-like inclusion bodies and *Toxoplasma*-like organisms have been reported in some dogs.[216, 220, 221]

Lesions are confined to the central nervous system and are characterized by dense aggregations of mesenchymal cells arranged in a whorling, perivascular pattern. Perivascular cuffs are usually composed of histiocytes (macrophages) and varying numbers of lymphocytes, monocytes, and plasma cells set in nests of reticular fibers. Neutrophils and multinucleate giant cells are sometimes present in small numbers.

In the disseminated form of GME, lesions usually are distributed widely throughout the central nervous system, especially in the white matter of the cerebrum, lower brain stem, cerebellum, and cervical spinal cord. Comparable lesions can occur in grey matter and in leptomeningeal and choroid plexus vasculature. Coalescence of granulomatous lesions from many adjacent blood vessels can produce a true space-occupying mass, which represents the focal form of GME. The cells of this mass may or may not have neoplastic features such as variable mitotic index and varying degrees of pleomorphism. Focal lesions usually are single and most commonly occur in the brain stem (especially in the pontomedullary region) and cerebral white matter. Animals with focal GME usually have accompanying disseminated lesions. In some dogs, an ocular form occurs with granulomatous cuffs initially involving the optic nerves, optic disc, or the retina. In these dogs, disseminated or focal lesions of GME can develop subsequently.

Disseminated and focal forms of GME are more common than the ocular form. GME appears to occur more commonly in small (toy) breed dogs, particularly in poodles and terriers. The majority of confirmed cases occur in young to middle-aged dogs (eight months to eight years of age). The disease occurs in both sexes; however, there may be a higher prevalence in females.

Disseminated GME is usually acute in onset, with a progressive course over a one- to eight-week period. In approximately 25 per cent of affected dogs, there is rapid deterioration of clinical signs, leading to death within one week. In more than 50 per cent of the cases, the clinical course lasts from two to six weeks. The ocular form also tends to have a sudden onset and may remain static or may be progressive, especially if disseminated lesions coexist. The focal form of GME has a more insidious onset and can progress slowly over a three- to six-month period.

Clinical signs are variable and reflect lesion localization. The ocular form of GME is characterized by acute onset of blindness and dilated pupils that are unresponsive to light stimulation as a result of unilateral or bilateral optic neuritis. Ophthalmic examination may reveal a hyperemic and edematous disc. Vessels may be dilated and focal hemorrhage may be present.[222–225]

Focal GME usually produces clinical signs suggestive of a single, space-occupying lesion, e.g., cerebral, midbrain, pontomedullary, vestibular, cerebellar, or cervical syndrome. In animals with disseminated GME, clinical signs usually reflect a multifocal syndrome. Common signs include incoordination, ataxia and falling, cervical pain, head tilt, nystagmus, facial and/or trigeminal nerve paralysis, circling, seizures, and depression. Occasionally, fever accompanies the clinical signs.

Hematologic, serum biochemical, and radiographic studies are usually normal, while electroencephalographic tracings are frequently nonspecific. The most useful diagnostic aid is cerebrospinal fluid analysis. In most dogs, CSF is abnormal, with mild to pronounced pleocytosis ranging from 50 to 700+ WBC/mm^3, and consisting of lymphocytes, monocytes, and numbers of large anaplastic mononuclear cells with abundant lacy cytoplasm. Computerized tomography may detect a mass lesion in dogs with the focal form of GME. Glucocorticoid therapy reportedly decreases CSF cellularity; however, a statistically significant steroid effect was not noted in a recent study.[217, 226] Protein in CSF is variably elevated, ranging from 60 to 250 mg/dl. Occasionally, protein can be elevated without pleocytosis. An increased concentration of IgG in CSF has been reported.[215]

Prognosis for permanent recovery is poor. The shortest survival periods, ranging from several days to weeks, are seen with the disseminated and ocular forms. Dogs with the focal form can survive for three to six months or longer. Long-term therapy is generally unsatisfactory, although temporary remission is often achieved with corticosteroid medication (e.g., oral prednisolone, 0.5 to 1 mg/lb/day [1 to 2 mg/kg/day] initially, before reducing the dose to 2.5 to 5 mg, given on alternate days). Most dogs require continued therapy to prevent recurrences of clinical signs. Improvement may last for several months in some dogs, although nearly all eventually succumb to the disease. Cessation of corticosteroid therapy is invariably associated with rapid and dramatic clinical deterioration. The ocular form of GME can be treated initially with repositol retrobulbar corticosteroids (e.g., 2.5 mg of betamethasone) in conjunction with oral prednisolone therapy.

IDIOPATHIC FELINE POLIOENCEPHALOMYELITIS

This is a chronic, slowly progressive neurologic disease that has been described in cats of various ages.[227] In this report five of six cats were female and of different breeds. The cause of feline polioencephalomyelitis is unknown. Pathologic changes suggest a viral infection; however, viral isolation attempts have been unsuccessful. The pathogenesis of this disease may be associated with panleukopenia or feline leukemia virus.

Pathologic changes consist of severe neuronal degeneration and loss, especially in segments of the thoracic spinal cord and, to a lesser extent, in the cerebral cortex, basal and diencephalic nuclei, midbrain, periaqueductal grey matter, and oculomotor and pontomedullary nuclei. Diffuse degeneration of white matter (demyelination and axonal necrosis) is usually present in the ventral and lateral columns of the spinal cord.

Clinical signs include incoordination, paresis, and hypermetria. Intention tremors involving the head may be seen. Affected cats are usually mentally alert. Cranial nerve function is normal except for depressed direct and consensual pupillary reflexes in some animals. Postural reactions and segmental reflexes of the spine may be noticeably depressed in affected limbs. Occasionally, a localized area of apparent hyperesthesia is evident. In some cases, a psychomotor-like pattern of seizures that is characterized by hallucinations, wild stares, clawing, and hissing and biting at imaginary objects has been noted in sleeping animals. Some cats have leukopenia, myeloid hypoplasia, and nonregenerative anemia. EEG traces may be abnormal. The prognosis is guarded and data on treatment are lacking.

PYOGRANULOMATOUS MENINGOENCEPHALOMYELITIS

Pyogranulomatous meningoencephalomyelitis is an acute, rapidly progressive disease lasting two to three weeks that, to date, has been recognized in mature pointers.[228]

The cause of the meningoencephalomyelitis is unknown. Special histologic stains for microorganisms, cultures of blood and cerebrospinal fluid, and studies of animal inoculations have all been negative. Clinical and pathologic data suggest a bacterial etiology.

Pathologic changes are found throughout the brain and spinal cord, but are most severe in the upper segments of the cervical spinal cord and in the lower brain stem. These changes are characterized by extensive mononuclear (plasma and lymphocytic cells) and polymorphonuclear inflammatory infiltrations in the leptomeninges and parenchyma. Large perivascular cuffs are seen. In some cases, central necrosis of grey matter and edema are found in segments of the cervical cord along with infiltration of macrophages, monocytes, neutrophils, and plasma cells. These changes are probably secondary to impaired spinal circulation from the meningeal reaction. An increased population of reticuloendothelial cells is occasionally observed among the perivascular cells. Focal ependymitis may be present along ventricular pathways.

Clinical signs include cervical rigidity, kyphosis, nose held close to the ground, reluctance to move, incoordination, head tilt, falling/rolling, spontaneous and positional nystagmus, and seizures. Occasionally, bradycardia, vomiting, and atrophy of the cervical muscles are seen. Signs of parenchymal involvement include paralysis of the trigeminal and facial nerves, and Horner's syndrome.

Marked, predominantly neutrophilic pleocytosis (500 to 1000 WBC/mm^3) and an increased concentration of protein (sometimes over 700 mg/dl) are found on examination of the cerebrospinal fluid of affected animals. In the small series of cases observed thus far, prognosis has been poor. Antibiotic therapy has resulted in temporary remission of signs.

PUG ENCEPHALITIS

A syndrome of chronic granulomatous meningoencephalitis has been described in pugs.[135] The usual onset of the disease is between nine months and four years of age and is generally progressive. The pathologic process consists of meningeal inflammation within the cranium affecting the forebrain, peripheral cranial nerves, and, occasionally, the cerebellum. Generalized seizures may be the first presenting complaint, although partial motor seizures, signs of forebrain defects (circling with a normal gait and contralateral postural reaction defects), and vestibular or other cranial neuropathies may be noted.

Cerebrospinal fluid examination usually shows an inflammatory process with increased lymphocytes, mononuclear cells, and protein. Diffuse white matter degeneration with perivascular mononuclear infiltrates is found primarily in the cerebral cortex, often with an associated lymphocytic meningitis.

The cause of this disorder is unknown although a familial predisposition suggests an immune pathogenesis or immunodeficiency with secondary infectious process. Antimicrobial and glucocorticoid therapy has been unrewarding, as has been the control of seizures using anticonvulsants.

CORTICOSTEROID-RESPONSIVE MENINGITIS

A meningeal syndrome characterized by anorexia, vomiting, muscular rigidity, cervical pain, hyperesthesia, and fever has been described primarily in large (greater than 30 lbs) young dogs (4 to 16 months).[229, 230] Signs of parenchymal involvement, including incoordination and postural deficits, are less common.

Peripheral neutrophilia and monocytosis are the main hematologic abnormalities. CSF findings include increased protein and neutrophilic pleocytosis, with no organisms being identified or cultured. A few of the dogs have had positive lupus erythematosus cell tests, although antinuclear antibody test results have been negative.

Antimicrobial therapy has little effect on the course or outcome of the disease. Glucocorticoid therapy has been given beginning with antiedema (1.0 mg/lb/day [2.2 mg/kg/day] dexamethasone) or immunosuppressive (1.0 mg/lb/day [2.2 mg/kg/day] prednisolone) therapy, with gradual tapering to anti-inflammatory and intermittent dosage schedules. Eventually the glucocorticoids have been discontinued in some of the dogs with no signs of relapse.

NEOPLASIA

It is now well established that central nervous system neoplasia in dogs and cats is common. Indeed, nervous system tumors occur in dogs with a frequency and variety similar to that in humans.[231] Primary nervous system tumors originate from neuroectodermal, ectodermal, or mesodermal cells normally present in or associated with the brain, spinal cord, or peripheral nerves. Secondary tumors affecting the nervous system may originate from surrounding structures, such as bone and muscle, or from hematogenous metastasis of primary tumors in other organs. Tumor emboli can lodge and grow anywhere in the brain, meninges, choroid plexus, or spinal cord. In animals, primary tumors rarely metastasize outside the cranial cavity or the vertebral canal.[232] Neoplastic angioendotheliomatosis, which violates these generalizations, is a rare, distinct neoplastic syndrome in which proliferations of tumor cells populate the lumina of arteries, capillaries, and venules with resultant thrombosis without extravascular invasion. Cerebral angioendotheliomatosis has been described in a Doberman that developed progressive weight loss, posterior paresis, and profound depression.[233] Presumably these neoplastic cells originate from endothelial sources, but immunocytochemistry did not confirm it in this case.

Classification of nervous system tumors in animals has followed the criteria used for human tumors (see Table 61–4).[231, 232, 234, 235] Classification is primarily based upon the characteristics of the constituent cell type, its pathologic behavior, topographic pattern, and secondary changes seen within and surrounding the tumor. To a much lesser extent, classification is based on the biological behavior of the tumor. Although many animal neoplasms have characteristics analogous to corresponding tumors in humans, 15 to 20 per cent of neuroectodermal tumors (especially gliomas) remain unclassified. Unlike the factors of age and breed, no gender predisposition for the various types of nervous system tumors has been detected.[232, 236]

Pathogenesis

With intracranial tumors, accurate clinicopathologic correlations are frequently impossible.[237] The actual location of a tumor may be masked by secondary effects. Except in brain tissue actually infiltrated by a tumor, a mass lesion within the nonexpansible cranial cavity often leads to local necrosis, edema, subtentorial herniation of the cingulate gyrus, compression of the hypothalamus, and coning of the cerebellum, as a result of herniation of the cerebellar vermis through the foramen magnum. Two other forms of brain herniation reported in dogs with brain tumors are: herniation of portions of the temporal cortex ventral to the tentorium cerebelli ("caudal transtentorial" herniation) and herniation of the rostral cerebellar vermis ventral to the tentorium cerebelli ("rostral transtentorial" herniation).[238] Herniation, combined with attenuation of the ventricular system, especially at the level of the mesencephalic aqueduct, can lead to hydrocephalus and elevated intracranial pressure; ischemic necrosis of herniated tissue can ensue.[237–240] Immunoproliferative diseases such as macroglobulinemia-associated lymphocytic leukemia can also produce a spectrum of neurologic abnormalities as a result of serum hyperviscosity.[241] The transient signs and changing patterns have been attributed to increased intravascular erythrocyte aggregation and associated impaired blood flow in the vascular beds of affected areas. Primary tumors usually have a slowly progressive growth pattern; bone tumors and secondary, highly malignant, metastatic tumors frequently demonstrate a more acute progression.

Incidence

The incidence of neoplasia of the nervous system in domestic animals appears to vary according to the vet-

TABLE 61–4. CLASSIFICATION OF TUMORS OF THE NERVOUS SYSTEM

Tumor Type	Predilection Sites	Species/Breed	Incidence
Primary Tumors			
1. *Tumors of nerve cells*			
Ganglioneuroma	Variable, e.g., cerebellum, cranial nerve roots, eye, cervical ganglion	Dogs	Rare
2. *Tumors of neuroepithelium*			
Ependymoma	Third and lateral ventricles	Dogs, cats	Rare
Neuroepithelioma	Meninges, thoracolumbar spinal cord	Dogs (German shepherd)	Uncommon
Choroid plexus papilloma	Fourth ventricle	Dogs	Common
3. *Tumors of neuroglia*			
Astrocytoma	Piriform area, convexity of cerebral hemispheres, thalamus, hypothalamus	Dogs (brachycephalic), cats	Common
Oligodendroglioma	Cerebral hemispheres	Dogs (brachycephalic)	Common
Glioblastoma	As for astrocytoma	Dogs (brachycephalic)	Uncommon
Spongioblastoma	Variable, e.g., ependymal surfaces, cerebellum, optic nerve/tracts	Dogs (brachycephalic)	Rare
Medulloblastoma	Cerebellum	Dogs, cats	Uncommon
Gliomas (unclassified)	Periventricular areas, especially in cerebral hemispheres	Dogs	Common
4. *Tumors of peripheral nerves and nerve sheaths*			
Nerve sheath tumors (schwannoma, neurofibroma, neurinoma)	Peripheral nerves	Dogs, cats	Common
5. *Tumors of meninges, vessels, and other mesenchymal structures*			
Meningiomas	Convexities of cerebral hemispheres and floor of the vault	Dogs (dolichocephalic), cats	Common
Angioblastoma	Variable	Dogs, cats	Common
Sarcoma	Variable	Dogs, cats	Common
Focal granulomatous meningoencephalomyelitis (reticulosis)	Cerebral hemispheres and brain stem	Dogs, cats	Common (dogs)
6. *Tumors of the pineal gland, pituitary gland, and craniopharyngeal duct*			
Pinealoma	Pineal body	Dogs	Rare
Pituitary adenoma	Pituitary gland	Dogs (brachycephalic), cats	Common
Craniopharyngioma	Hypophyseal-infundibular areas	Dogs	Rare
7. *Tumors of heterotopic tissues (malformation tumors)*			
Epidermoid, dermoid, teratoma	Variable (fourth ventricle and cerebellopontine angle for epidermoid)	Dogs	Rare
Secondary Tumors			
1. *Metastatic tumors*			
Mammary gland adenocarcinoma, pulmonary carcinoma, prostatic carcinoma, chemodectoma, malignant melanoma, lymphosarcoma salivary gland adenocarcinoma, etc.	Variable	Dogs, cats	Relatively common
2. *Primary tumors from surrounding tissues*			
Osteosarcoma, lipoma, chondrosarcoma, fibrosarcoma, nasal adenocarcinoma, hemangiosarcoma, multiple myeloma, calcifying aponeurotic fibromatosis, epidermoid cyst, etc.	Variable	Dogs, cats	Relatively common

From Braund KG: Clinical Syndromes in Veterinary Neurology. Baltimore, Williams & Wilkins, 1986, pp. 142–143 (with permission).

erinary institution. Neoplasms of the nervous system occur more frequently in dogs than in any other domestic species.[242] In one survey, intracranial neoplasms were discovered in 2.83 per cent of 6175 dogs at postmortem examination.[243]

Primary tumors of the nervous system in animals occur more often in the brain than in the spinal cord or the peripheral nerves.[231, 232, 234, 244] Brain tumors in dogs and cats tend to occur in mature adults, usually over five years of age. The most frequent canine brain tumors are meningiomas, gliomas (astrocytomas, oligodendrogliomas) (Figure 61–23), and undifferentiated sarcomas.[245, 246] Primary reticulosis (the focal form of granulomatous meningoencephalomyelitis), pituitary adenomas, and plexus papillomas also are commonly reported.[234, 247–249] Metastatic brain tumors are relatively uncommon. Dogs of brachycephalic breeds with common ancestry (e.g., boxers, English bulldogs, and Boston terriers) over two years old have the highest incidence of brain tumors among domestic animals (Table 61–5). Of these tumors, the gliomas (including those that are unclassified) are the most numerous. The common locations of

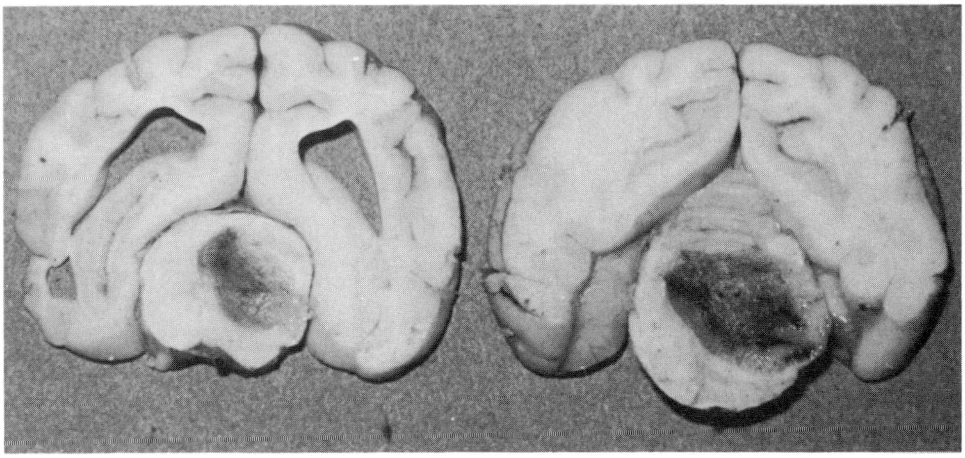

FIGURE 61–23. Oligodendroglioma in the brain stem of a seven-year-old boxer. The neoplasm extended from the caudal mesencephalon to the rostral medulla. Clinical signs included a left facial palsy and right hemiparesis.

glial tumors (and other neoplasms of the nervous system) are outlined in Table 61–4. Pituitary adenomas also are frequently reported in brachycephalic breeds.

Meningiomas are the most commonly reported feline primary brain tumors.[246, 250, 251] Usual locations include the tela choroidea of the third ventricle and the supratentorial meninges. In contrast, one study reported that 58 per cent of meningiomas in dogs occurred on the ventral aspect of the brain.[252] There is a high incidence of multiple meningiomas in cats.[253]

TABLE 61–5. ESTIMATED RELATIVE RISK[1] *(R)* OF CANINE NERVOUS-TISSUE TUMORS FOR ALL BREEDS WITH ≥4 TUMORS OBSERVED, BY BREED AND BY SEX WITHIN TUMOR CATEGORY

Tumor Category	Risk Category	Cases Observed	R
Glial (96)	Breed		
	Boxer	33	23.3[2]
	Boston terrier	6	5.2[2]
	All breeds combined	96	1
	Poodle, miniature or toy	6	0.7
	All other purebred	38	0.7[2]
	Mixed breed	13	0.5[3]
	Sex		
	Male	42	0.8
	Female	54	1
Meningeal (50)	Breed		
	German shepherd dog	6	1.4
	Poodle, miniature or toy	5	1.1
	All breeds combined	50	1
	All other purebred	32	0.9
	Mixed breed	7	0.6
	Sex		
	Female	26	1
	Male	24	1
Peripheral nerve (53)	Breed		
	Beagle hound	4	2.4
	German shepherd	5	1.1
	Mixed breed	14	1
	All breeds combined	53	1
	All other purebred	30	0.9
	Sex		
	Female	31	1.3
	Male	22	1

[1]Adjustment made for age and sex in determining breed *R* and for age and breed determining sex *R*.
[2]Significantly different ($p<0.05$) from $R = 1$.
[3]Significantly different ($p<0.01$) from $R = 1$.
From Hayes, H. M., Jr., Priester, W. A., and Pendergrass, T. W.: Occurrence of nervous tissue tumors in cattle, horses, cats and dogs. Int. J. Cancer 15:39–47, 1975.

Clinical Signs

Clinical signs of nervous system neoplasia vary according to the location of the tumor and secondary effects.[110, 238, 254, 255] Onset of clinical signs can be acute or insidious, and the clinical course can progress rapidly or slowly. Accurate description of the temporal clinical course for the various brain tumors in animals, seemingly feasible from a retrospective study, is presently unknown. The inaccurate representation probably results from a variety of factors, including the relatively low incidence of brain tumors in animals when compared with tumors of other organs or systems, the historical inaccuracies as to onset of clinical signs and subsequent clinical course, and finally, incomplete clinicopathologic correlations.

Diagnosis

Diagnosis of a tumor of the nervous system is based on the animal's age and breed and on diagnostic aids that include plain-film radiography, contrast radiography, or specialized radiographic techniques such as radionuclide imaging (scintigraphy) and computerized axial tomography.[256] Plain-film radiography detects evidence of bone neoplasia. At present, computerized axial tomography is the method of choice for localizing brain tumors.[257–261] Computerized axial tomography currently is being used to define characteristics of various brain tumors in animals.[262] Furthermore, differentiation of neoplastic from non-neoplastic brain lesions in dogs is being facilitated by the use of computerized tomography.[263] Examination of CSF can indicate an elevation in protein content, but this is a variable finding; tumor cells are rarely found in the CSF.[264, 265]

Prognosis and Treatment

Prognosis of animals with nervous system tumors is guarded to poor. Inability to accurately localize a tumor mass in the brain usually precludes surgical intervention; however, this situation should change with the advent of computerized axial tomography.[266] In veterinary medicine, the roles of radiotherapy and chemotherapy in nervous system tumor management have been limited, primarily because of the expensive equipment required (e.g., cobalt 60 teletherapy and the use of clinical linear accelerators). Results of one study demonstrated that canine brain tumors may be treated effectively by use of megavoltage radiation.[267] The success rate of chemotherapy on solid tumors in animals generally has been poor compared with that in humans. Glucocorticoids may ameliorate clinical signs by reducing edema around the tumor and may produce temporary regression of lymphoid and reticulohistiocytic tumors.

CRANIAL TRAUMA

Cranial trauma is a relatively common entity in dogs and cats, usually resulting from a fall or an automobile accident. Head injury frequently causes severe neurologic dysfunction. It can produce shear stresses that induce transient loss of consciousness with minimal parenchymal damage, or more severe cerebral contusion, brain degeneration with or without laceration and hemorrhage, and sometimes cranial fractures, which, if they involve the floor of the cranial vault, may damage cranial nerves.

An important consequence of head injury is cerebral edema. Edema of the brain can be produced by vascular leakage ("vasogenic" edema) and by cellular hypoxia that leads to accumulation of fluid within cells, especially neurons and astrocytes ("cytotoxic" edema). Vasogenic edema is prominent in white matter, whereas cytotoxic edema affects grey and white matter.[268] Cerebral edema can increase intracranial pressure, which reduces cerebral perfusion and further exacerbates cellular hypoxia. The size of the brain may increase dramatically as a result of cerebral edema, leading to possible brain herniation. The brain can herniate in several ways. The three most common herniations are when the cingulate gyrus herniates under the falx cerebri, the occipital or temporal lobe herniates under the tentorium cerebelli (transtentorial herniation) (Figure 61–24), and the cerebellum herniates through the foramen magnum.[269]

Hemorrhage can be an important factor in cranial trauma (Table 61–6). Contusions may lead to subdural hemorrhage, which in animals is often diffusely distributed over the cerebral cortex.[270] Hemorrhage into the brain substance from damaged vessels is commonly observed (Figure 61–25). This form of bleeding may be short-lived due to vessel spasm and microthrombi formation.[271] Disruption of arachnoid vessels can lead to bleeding into the subarachnoid space. Bleeding into the inner ear is not infrequent.[272]

Pathologic alteration may include subdural or subarachnoid hemorrhage, bone fragments embedded within brain parenchyma, ischemic laminar necrosis of the cerebral cortex, profound hemorrhage into the substance of the brain (especially the midbrain, with associated focal or multifocal necrosis of midline structures), and edema. Midbrain compression as a result of transtentorial herniation may cause closure of the mesencephalic aqueduct and obstruct CSF flow and further increase intracranial pressure. Obstructive hydrocephalus may ensue.

Lesions may be dispersed at multiple levels of the brain. This results in a wide variation of clinical signs commensurate with a multifocal syndrome. Some animals may be completely normal after a brief period of unconsciousness lasting a few seconds. Other animals may be comatose, confused, delirious, or depressed. Pupil size may be normal, pinpoint (suggestive of mild or moderate midbrain compression), or dilated and unresponsive to light (suggestive of severe midbrain compression, e.g., from transtentorial herniation). Normal conjugate eye movements may be depressed or absent when the head is rotated (this is suggestive of severe brain stem pathology). Other signs can include blindness that may be transient (up to 24 hours) or permanent, various cranial nerve deficits, vestibular and/or cerebellar signs, and abnormal respiration. Limbs of recumbent animals may be rigidly extended.

TABLE 61–6. SIGNS CHARACTERISTIC OF FOCAL BRAIN STEM HEMORRHAGE AT ONE LEVEL*

Level	Consciousness	Pupils	Eye Movement	Motor Function	Autonomic Responses
Diencephalic	Apathy to stupor	Small but reactive	Normal	Hemiparesis to tetraparesis	Normal to Cheyne-Stokes respiration
Midbrain	Stupor to coma	Bilateral dilated or midposition, unresponsive	Ventrolateral strabismus, bilateral	Decerebrate rigidity	Hyperventilation (variable)
Pons	Coma	Midposition, unresponsive	Oculocephalic reflexes absent	Decerebrate rigidity to flaccid paralysis	Rapid shallow respiration, loss of micturition reflex
Medulla	Coma	Midposition, dilated terminally	Absent	Flaccid paralysis	Irregular to apnea

*Assuming a large intramedullary hemorrhage confined primarily to one level. The most frequent is in the caudal midbrain and pons following acute head injury. Asymmetric or smaller lesions will produce less severe signs.

From Oliver, J. E., Jr.: Intracranial injury. *In* Kirk, R. W. (ed.): Current Veterinary Therapy VII. Philadelphia, W. B. Saunders Company, 1980.

Diagnosis typically is based on historical information relating to the accident, clinical evidence of cranial injury, such as abrasions or penetrating wounds, and/or clinical signs. Skull fractures may be demonstrated using radiography.

Treatment of animals with cranial trauma can be medical, surgical, or both. Medical management is aimed at treating cerebral edema and tissue hypoxia by establishing an oxygen-rich environment, maintaining central venous blood pressure using isotonic lactated Ringer's solution, and administration of high levels of glucocorticoids and hypertonic agents such as mannitol. Comatose patients should be intubated and given oxygen. Conscious animals that are depressed or delirious can be placed in an oxygen cage or supplied oxygen via a tracheostomy tube. Dexamethasone can be given using a dose of 1 to 2 mg/lb (2 to 4 mg/kg), IV, which is repeated at six- to eight-hour intervals for 24 to 36 hours, and then at decreased doses at the same interval for another 36 to 48 hours. Glucocorticoids are considered to be effective in treating vasogenic edema.[269] Mannitol can be administered at a dose of 1 gm/lb (2 gm/kg) IV, given over a ten-minute period and repeated two to three times at three- to four-hour intervals. Hypertonic solutions such as mannitol are believed to be effective in reducing cytotoxic edema.[269]

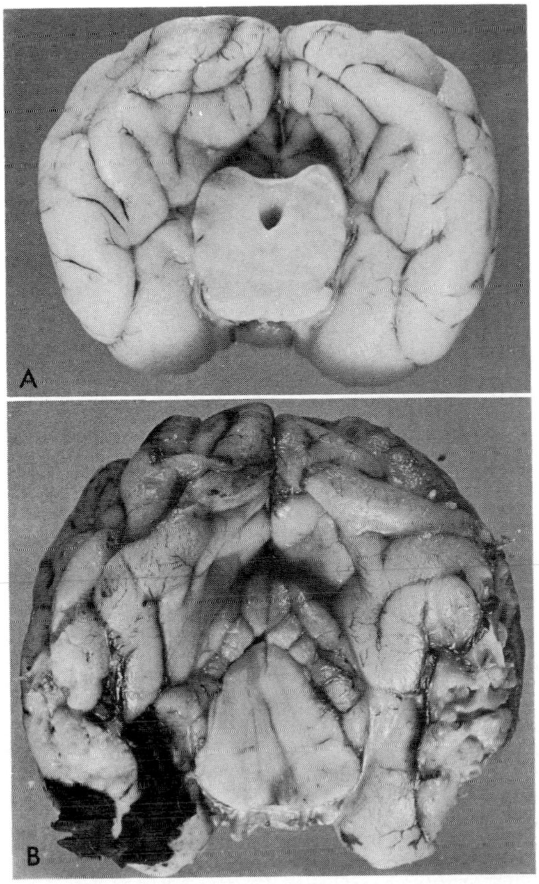

FIGURE 61–24. *A*, Caudal view of brain transected at midbrain. Normal brain with open cerebral aqueduct. *B*, Severe cerebral edema has caused herniation of the cerebrum under the tentorium cerebelli, compressing and distorting the brain stem. The cerebral aqueduct is closed, causing further increase in intracranial pressure. (From Oliver, JE, Jr: Neurologic examinations II. VM SAC 67:658, 1972.)

Animals presented with seizures or status epilepticus can be treated with valium, using a dose of 5 to 10 mg IV or IM repeated as needed every 30 minutes. Alternatively, barbiturates can be used if seizures persist. General supportive treatment includes maintaining normal body temperature, prevention of decubital ulcers by placing animals on a padded surface with frequent turning, and bladder emptying.

Surgical management can be considered under the following circumstances: animals with skull fractures and penetrating wounds, comatose animals with miotic pupils whose condition has not improved after 24 to 36 hours of medical therapy, and animals whose signs are deteriorating despite medical treatment. Various surgical techniques are available for cerebral decompression.[2] A bilateral/lateral craniotomy approach affords excellent exposure for removal of bone fragments and blood clots, for vessel ligation, and for decompression (Figure 61–26).

Prognosis is guarded. Some animals are normal after a brief period of unconsciousness. Others may remain in stable condition for several days before showing signs of deterioration. Stuporous or comatose animals with dilated unresponsive pupils have a poor prognosis. A period of coma lasting 48 hours or longer is a grave prognostic sign. Deteriorating clinical signs such as depression progressing to coma or normal or miotic pupils becoming dilated and unresponsive are ominous and indicative of progressive brain swelling or transtentorial herniation. Long-term sequelae of head trauma include seizures and/or focal, persistent neurologic deficits.

TOXICOLOGIC DISORDERS

Many toxic agents cause CNS signs, either as the primary effect or secondarily, in the later stages of the

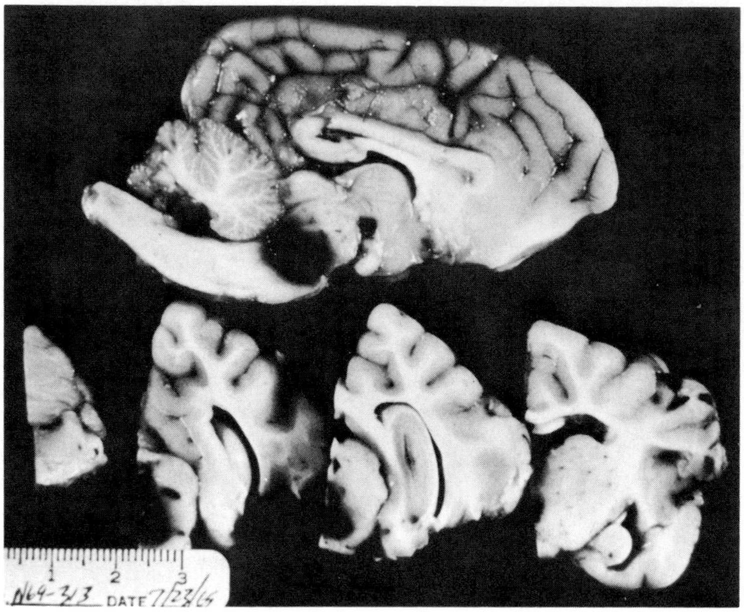

FIGURE 61–25. The brain of a boxer that was hit by a car. Hemorrhage in the brain stem extends from the caudal aspect of the mesencephalon into the rostral pons. This dog was comatose and exhibited decerebrate rigidity. (From Oliver, JE, Jr: Neurologic examinations II. VM SAC 67:658, 1972.)

syndrome. Toxicologic problems are reviewed in detail in Chapter 55.

CNS Signs of Toxicity

Most common toxic agents that affect the nervous system produce one or more of the following signs: seizures; depression or coma; tremors, ataxia, and paresis; and generalized lower motor neuron signs.[273, 274] Toxicities causing lower motor neuron signs are discussed in Chapter 55. Toxic agents that are commonly associated with the other signs are listed in Table 61–7.

SEIZURES

An acute onset of seizures that do not spontaneously stop (status epilepticus) should always suggest toxicity. Status epilepticus may result from other causes, but poisoning with insecticides or rodenticides is the most common cause. Strychnine poisoning causes tetany, which is exacerbated by noise or stimulation of the animal. The animal usually does not lose consciousness because the primary effect is a loss of inhibition in the spinal cord. Chlorinated hydrocarbon insecticides usually produce tonic/clonic seizures with muscle fasciculation that often persists between seizures. The autonomic nervous system is minimally affected when compared with the effects of organophosphate toxicity. Organophosphates also produce tonic/clonic seizures, but there is also marked autonomic activity, including miosis, salivation, and sometimes vomiting, diarrhea, and urination. Carbamates are very similar to organophosphates.

Lead poisoning is usually chronic and the seizures

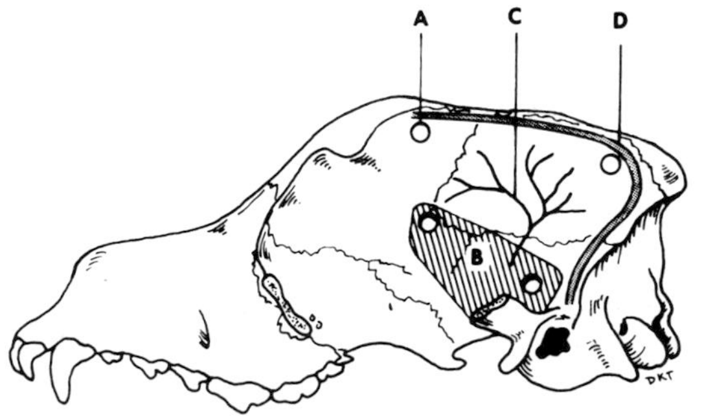

FIGURE 61–26. Important landmarks for placement of bur holes *(A)* include venous sinuses *(D)* and middle meningeal artery *(C)*. The hatched area *(B)* can be removed for exploration of the cranial vault or for decompression. (From Oliver, JE, Jr: Neurologic emergencies in small animals. Vet Clin N Am 2:341, 1972.)

TABLE 61–7. SIGNS OF TOXICITY OF THE NERVOUS SYSTEM

Signs	Common Toxic Agents
Seizures	Chlorinated hydrocarbons
	Organophosphates
	Carbamates
	Strychnine
	Sodium fluoroacetate (1080)
	Thallium
	Lead
	Staphylococcus toxin
	Toad *(Bufo sp.)*
	Amphetamines
	Zinc phosphide
Depression or coma	Drugs
	Narcotics
	Barbiturates
	Tranquilizers
	Marijuana
	ANTU
	Ethylene glycol
Tremor, ataxia, or paresis	Hexachlorophene
	Metaldehyde
	Lead
	Organophosphates
	Chlorinated hydrocarbons
	Tranquilizers
	Marijuana

From Oliver, J. E., Jr., and Lorenz, M. D.: Handbook of Veterinary Neurologic Diagnosis. Philadelphia, W. B. Saunders Company, 1983.

may be episodic. Other toxicities causing seizures are less common.

DEPRESSION OR COMA

An increasing number of animals present with signs of overdoses of prescription or "street" drugs.[275–277] Clinical signs are dose-dependent, ranging from depression and ataxia to coma. Diagnosis is complicated by the reluctance of the owner to admit availability.

Coma may be the terminal phase of many intoxications. It is important to differentiate coma resulting from overdose of a sedative type of drug, such as a barbiturate, from terminal coma from other causes. Terminal coma usually produces some loss of brain stem reflexes, such as dilated pupils, fixed midposition eyes, and irregular respiration. Drug-induced coma usually does not abolish all brain stem reflexes so that the pupils are usually miotic, the eyes may move with changing head positions, and respiration is regular, although it may be shallow.

TREMORS, ATAXIA, AND PARESIS

Hexachlorophene poisoning may cause signs of cerebellar dysfunction, especially in cats and very young dogs (fewer than eight weeks of age).[278–280] Although acute death may follow ingestion of large amounts, induced vomiting usually prevents retention of the toxic substance.[278] Chronic exposure usually causes tremors and ataxia. Washing the bitch's mammary glands with a hexachlorophene soap has produced the syndrome in nursing puppies. Bathing puppies and cats in hexachlorophene soap has also caused toxicity.[280] Vacuolation of the white matter, presumably edema, is the primary histopathologic finding. Animals that are not severely affected recover when the source is removed, although residual tremors have been seen in some cases.

Chronic organophosphate toxicity can cause tremors, ataxia, and paresis. It has been associated with the use of flea collars and topical insecticides.[281] A similar syndrome may be seen with chronic lead poisoning.[282–284]

DIAGNOSIS

The history is the most important factor in establishing a diagnosis of toxicity. If the source is to be ascertained, the clinician may have to ask the owner more leading and specific questions than are needed for most medical problems. Insecticides and rodenticides are commonly recognized poisons, but the source of lead or the availability of drugs may be more difficult to identify.

The clinical signs as outlined will suggest the most likely causes. Specific diagnostic tests and treatment for each toxic agent are discussed in Chapter 55.

METABOLIC DISORDERS

Nutritional Disorders

Nutritional disorders in the dog and cat may occur with either deficiencies or excesses. Vitamin and mineral deficiencies are the result of deficient diet or malabsorption. The former is becoming increasingly rare because of widespread commercially available balanced diets. Cats generally have greater requirements for many soluble vitamins and nutrients than dogs. This, coupled with their finicky dietary habits, makes them more susceptible to nutritional disturbances. Neurologic disturbances have been observed as a complication of many of the vitaminoses.

HYPOVITAMINOSIS A

In the growing dog, vitamin A deficiency may result in abnormally thick cranial bones. This thickening may cause compression and delayed growth of associated nervous tissue.[285] Deficiencies of vitamin A in growing animals may also cause an increase in CSF pressure, resulting in hydrocephalus.[286] Morris has recommended daily dietary levels of 50 IU per lb (100 IU per kg) of body weight of vitamin A for normal maintenance and twice that for growth.[287] The signs of vitamin A deficiency include poor growth, xerophthalmia (conjunctivitis that produces abnormally dry, lusterless eyes), suppurative skin disease, and impaired bone growth. Bones in the axial skeleton are usually shortened and thickened. Neurologic signs are essentially related to constrictive effects of nervous tissue.

HYPOVITAMINOSIS B

Deficiencies of thiamine, riboflavin, niacin, pantothenic acid, and biotin have all been observed to cause weakness or convulsions in animals.[287, 288]

Thiamine Deficiency. Thiamine deficiency has been observed to cause lesions in the periventricular grey matter of the brain stem, archicerebellum, and cerebral cortex of dogs and cats. Although thiamine deficiency may occur following nutritional deficiencies, it is presently uncommon in animals fed commercial diets.[289] It may also occur following extensive diuresis or anorexia without adequate supplementation. This is especially true of cats because they have greater thiamine requirements than dogs.[290] Thiamine deficiency has also occurred in cats fed all-fish diets containing thiaminase and in dogs fed cooked meat, where the cooking destroyed the thiamine.[291, 292]

Initial clinical signs of thiamine deficiency are inappetence, weight loss, and coprophagia, progressing to a sudden onset of mild ataxia, followed by convulsions. The convulsions in cats and dogs are characterized by ventroflexion of the head, hyperesthesia, and dilated, unresponsive pupils. Dogs develop upper motor neuron paraparesis that progresses to tetraparesis and convulsions. Terminally, the animals are semicomatose. Opisthotonos and persistent extensor tonus of the limbs may be present. Electrocardiographic abnormalities have also been described, in addition to neurologic abnormalities.[292]

Symmetrical polioencephalomalacia is the characteristic lesion of thiamine deficiency. Lesions can vary in severity from bilateral, spongy change to frank necrosis. Lesions in the dog and cat are generally located in the brain stem, which is not the case with hypoxia and intoxicants that affect the cerebral cortex. Lesions in thiamine deficiency are found in the nuclei of the caudal colliculi, vestibular nuclei, cerebellar folia near the fourth ventricle, and oculomotor nuclei.

Treatment for thiamine deficiency should be instituted in any animal when it is suspected by history and clinical observation. Therapy early in the disease, with 1 to 2 mg of thiamine hydrochloride IM, results in clinical improvement.[135] Thiamine should be administered as an adjunctive measure in dogs or cats with prolonged anorexia or undergoing chronic diuresis.

Riboflavin Deficiency. Deficiencies of riboflavin result in dry, scaly skin, erythema of the pelvic limbs and chest, anemia, and muscular weakness, particularly of the hind quarters. Degeneration of neurons in the brain and spinal cord occurs in riboflavin-deficient dogs. Clinical signs of cramping, ataxia, and convulsions have been reported.

Niacin Deficiency. Niacin deficiency is characterized by anorexia, weight loss, diarrhea, oral ulceration, and neurologic signs. Weakness, convulsions, and coma have been reported. Widespread degeneration of nervous tissue has been found in spinal cord neurons and dorsal and ventral spinal nerve roots.[2]

Pantothenic Acid Deficiency. Pantothenic acid deficiencies were observed to cause anorexia, hypoglycemia, hypochloremia, and azotemia. Nervous signs included convulsions, coma, and death. The daily maintenance dose of pantothenic acid is 25 mg/lb (50 mg/kg) body weight.

Biotin Deficiency. Biotin deficiency is uncommon with most diets but it can occur with ingestion of raw eggs. The clinical signs are tension, aimless wandering, spasticity of the hindlimbs, and progressive paralysis. A return to a normal diet is usually curative.

Vitamin B_{12} Deficiency. Although vitamin B_{12} deficiency usually causes only anemia in dogs and cats, Newberne and O'Dell reported indications that vitamin B_{12} deficiency promoted the development of hydrocephalus in rat puppies.[293] A purified diet, low in cobalt and vitamin B_{12}, resulted in a high incidence of hydrocephalus.

HYPERVITAMINOSIS A

Hypervitaminosis A has been associated with cervical spondylopathy in the cat.[294–297] The condition is most common in younger cats fed diets rich in liver. The clinical signs are anorexia, dullness, and musculoskeletal and neurologic deficits.

Inability to move the head and neck and forelimb lameness result from proliferation of bone around the cervical spinal vertebrae. More severe neurologic deficiencies and tetraparesis or paralysis may result as bone is deposited around the spinal nerves and cord.

Mineral, Electrolyte, and Acid-Base Disturbances

HYPOCALCEMIA AND HYPERCALCEMIA

The pathophysiology and treatment of calcium disorders is discussed in Chapter 94. Clinical signs of hypocalcemia include neuromuscular excitability and grand mal convulsions. Seizures may be intermittent and only temporarily controlled with anticonvulsant therapy. Intravenous organic calcium preparations are initially used to control convulsions. Hypercalcemia is usually associated with CNS depression, muscular weakness, and fine muscle fasciculations. Blood calcium can be reduced as a lifesaving measure by administering glucocorticoids and diuretics.

HYPOKALEMIA

Potassium deficiencies can result from decreased intake of potassium or increased loss of potassium in gastrointestinal fluid or urine. A drop in extracellular potassium partially explains the loss of neuromuscular function, manifested by weakness, depression, ileus, reduced renal concentrating abilities, and abnormal cardiac conduction. Diuresis is a commonly incriminated factor. Lower motor neuron paralysis is characteristic. Medical management of hypokalemia involves the reduction of ongoing loss and replacement therapy. Supplementation is easiest and safest by the oral route. Vomiting and gastrointestinal irritation can be minimized with commercially available wax matrix products. Intravenous therapy with a diluted potassium salt solution requires cautious monitoring over a lengthy time period. Subcutaneous therapy is relatively safe, but also requires dilution of potassium chloride prior to use. It is the preferred method of parenteral administration when anorexia, ileus, and gastrointestinal complications preclude oral therapy.

HYPERKALEMIA

Hyperkalemia is a life-threatening phenomenon. It occurs most commonly when the kidney is unable to excrete sufficient potassium, as occurs with oliguric renal failure. Adrenal insufficiency also results in reduced renal ability to excrete potassium. Clinical signs are bradycardia, depression, and neuromuscular weakness.

Treatment is directed toward shifting potassium into cells, by administration of alkali or glucose plus insulin therapy and by diuresis with fluids or diuretics. Adverse effects of hyperkalemia can be antagonized by the administration of calcium and/or glucose and insulin solutions.

HYPONATREMIA

Severe sodium depletion can cause mental derangement and CNS depression. Hyponatremia with *hypovolemia* can be caused by loss of an excess of sodium that may occur with diuretic therapy, with adrenal insufficiency, or with gastrointestinal diseases. CNS signs in severe cases usually result from dehydration. In contrast, hyponatremia with *hypervolemia* occurs with water retention in the syndrome of inappropriate secretion of antidiuretic hormone (SIADH). A metabolic encephalopathy results whenever the brain becomes overhydrated and cerebral edema occurs. SIADH has been reported in a dog with heartworm disease that had nervous signs of anorexia, depression, weakness, and incoordination.[298]

Treatment of hyponatremic-hypovolemia consists of replacement of lost sodium by oral or parenteral fluid therapy. Oral sodium therapy with simultaneous water restriction can be used to correct inappropriate secretion of ADH with hyponatremic-hypervolemia.

HYPERNATREMIA

Hypernatremia may also be associated with hyper- or hypovolemic states. *Hypovolemic*-hypernatremia can occur with water deprivation and diabetes insipidus. Primary adipsia and hypodipsia have been found to cause hypovolemic-hypernatremic syndromes in dogs.[39, 299, 300] Hypernatremia and *hypervolemia* are associated with renal sodium retention, such as occurs with hyperaldosteronism. Results of urine specific gravity or osmolality can help distinguish these two syndromes. Hyperaldosteronism may occur rarely in the dog or cat as primary hypersecretion. More commonly, it is secondary to congestive heart failure, nephrotic syndrome, and cirrhosis, when the kidneys retain sodium in an attempt to maintain effective plasma volume.

Hypernatremia with hypovolemia is associated with increased serum osmolality. The brain responds to serum hyperosmolality by increasing brain osmolality to prevent intracellular dehydration. Nervous tissue forms "idiogenic osmoles" through various biochemical pathways. These intracellular substances move slowly across the blood-brain barrier relative to water. Clinical signs of hypernatremic syndromes include irritability, confusion, seizures, or coma. A rapid decrease in serum osmolality during oral or parenteral fluid replacement results in brain edema and may trigger the neurologic signs. Hypovolemic-hypernatremic syndromes should be corrected slowly over 24 to 48 hours. The use of hypotonic rather than isotonic fluids is controversial, although isotonic fluids would seem to offer less of a gradient to water moving into the CNS during rehydration. In hypervolemic states associated with sodium retention, the use of diuretics such as furosemide is essential.

ACID-BASE DISTURBANCES

A complex relationship exists between the pH of the brain, CSF, and serum. The pH of CSF usually is similar to the pH of the brain. Changes in pH of CSF occur more readily with shifts in P_{CO_2}, such as occur with respiratory acidosis or alkalosis. Only slight changes in pH of CSF occur in metabolic acidosis or alkalosis because of the low permeability of the blood-CSF barrier to bicarbonate.

For similar reasons, caution must be used when rapidly correcting metabolic acidosis with bicarbonate infusions. Following bicarbonate infusions, CO_2 readily forms and diffuses into the CSF, causing paradoxical CSF acidosis. A deterioration in CNS signs occurs in these patients.

Respiratory alkalosis may be associated with signs of CNS hyperexcitability and vasoconstriction, with reduced cerebral blood flow.[301] Hyperventilation can cause respiratory alkalosis, which may trigger the seizure focus in a predisposed pet.

Endocrine Disturbances

HYPOGLYCEMIA

Glucose is an essential substance for neuronal function. A deficiency of glucose results in a variety of neurologic signs, including depression, posterior paresis, and grand mal convulsions. These signs can frequently be reversed with the administration of hypertonic glucose solutions.

Hypoglycemia can be caused by decreased production or increased use or catabolism of glucose. Decreased production of glucose is associated with decreased intake or malabsorption, hepatic insufficiency, or glycogen storage disorders.

Increased catabolism of blood glucose occurs with hyperinsulinism and excessive renal loss. Increased exercise may lead to overuse of blood glucose. Not all of these mechanisms have been well documented as causing hypoglycemia or nervous disorders in dogs and cats.

OTHER ENDOCRINE DISORDERS

Hypothyroidism can cause CNS signs of severe sluggishness, mental depression, and collapse in some dogs. Cranial nerve deficits and peripheral neuropathies have also been noted. These are usually corrected within two to three days of administration of thyroid hormone. Hypothyroidism, hyperlipemia, and resultant atherosclerosis with arteriovascular occlusion have been reported to cause seizures, disorientation, and progressive semicoma in a dog.[148] Hyperthyroidism, documented in older cats and dogs with thyroid neoplasia, can be associated with nervousness, restlessness, polydipsia, polyuria, and cardiac enlargement. Hyperadrenocorticism and diabetes insipidus usually are not associated with primary neurologic disturbances unless they are caused by pituitary tumors that are expanding in the cranial vault.

Polysystemic Disorders

UREMIA

Uremia is associated with a wide variety of neurologic complications involving the central and peripheral nervous systems. Signs of central nervous dysfunction can include behavioral alterations, incoordination, tetany, and convulsions. Tetanic movements of the facial muscles have been observed in chronically uremic dogs.[39]

Numerous theories exist to explain the neurologic signs accompanying uremia. A number of suspected "uremic toxins" that accumulate in renal failure have been identified. "Middle molecules" with intermediate molecular weights, 500 to 5000, have been evaluated for potential neurotoxicity without success. The enteric flora may act on dietary or endogenous proteins to produce toxic amines that affect the central nervous system.

TABLE 61–8. DRUG APPENDIX

Generic	Trade	Dosage	Route	Frequency	Description
Dexamethazone	Azium (V)	1 mg/3–5 lbs	PO	q6, 8, or 12h	Hydrocephalus
		2.2 mg/2.2 lbs	IV or PO	q24h	Glucocorticoid responsive meningitis antiedema CNS dosage
		2–4 mg/2.2 lbs	IV	q6–8h	Cranial trauma
Prednisolone	Many and generic (V)	1–2 mg/2.2 lbs	PO	q24h	Granulomatous meningoencephalomyelitis
		2.2 mg/2.2 lbs	PO	q24h	Glucocorticoid responsive meningitis immunosuppressive CNS dosage
Betamethasone (repositol)	Celestone Soluspan (H)	2.5 mg	Retrobulbar	q2–4wk	Ocular granulomatous meningoencephalomyelitis (with prednisolone)
Mannitol	Many and generic (V)	2 g/2.2 lbs	IV		Brain edema, cranial trauma
Tetracycline	Many and generic (V)	22 mg/2.2 lbs	PO, IV	q8h	Rickettsiae
Penicillin	Many and generic (V)	50,000–100,000 IU/2.2 lbs	IM, IV	q12h	Tetanus
Diazepam	Valium (H)	5–10 mg	IV, IM	prn	Seizures
Vitamin A	Aquasol A (V)	100 IU/kg	PO	q24h	Deficiency state
Thiamine HCl	Many and generic (V)	1–2 mg	IM	q24h	Deficiency state
Pantothenic Acid	Injacom 100 + B complex (V)	50 mg/kg	PO	q24h	Deficiency state

V = Veterinary drug; H = Human drug

Efforts have centered around the role of parathormone as a potential neurotoxin. Dogs with renal failure have marked increases in circulating parathormone and increased brain calcium, which was thought to be associated with neurologic complications.[302] Although decreased energy metabolism in the uremic brain has been suspected of being caused by interference with brain metabolism, decreased brain energy consumption in uremia has been shown to result from reduced energy demands rather than an ability to generate sufficient energy.[303]

HEPATIC INSUFFICIENCY

Acute or chronic hepatic parenchymal failure or portacaval shunts are associated with central nervous system dysfunction in the dog and cat. Research with experimental animals has shown that hepatic encephalopathy results from a variety of complex metabolic derangements in the CNS from the extracellular accumulation of toxic products that are not removed by the failing liver. In addition to the accumulation of cerebrotoxic compounds, there is evidence to suggest that the permeability of the blood-brain barrier is altered, resulting in increased uptake of these substances. Elevated plasma ammonia occurs from ineffective conversion of ammonia to urea. Excess ammonia enters the nervous system directly, producing cytotoxic edema.[304] In the CNS, ammonia is detoxified by astrocytes, where it combines with alpha ketoglutarate, eventually forming glutamine.[305] The degree of neurologic dysfunction in hepatic insufficiency has been directly correlated with glutamine concentrations in CSF. Elevated plasma concentrations of aromatic amino acids such as tryptophan are thought to contribute to the neurotoxicity of hepatic failure. The toxicity of tryptophan may relate to its metabolite, serotonin, an important, centrally acting neurotransmitter. Decreased hepatic removal of mercaptans, the metabolites of methionine, and of short-chain fatty acids compound the toxic encephalopathy. Increased plasma and CSF concentrations of various false neurotransmitter substances that alter normal neural transmission have been found in hepatic insufficiency. False neurotransmitters include gamma-aminobutyric acid, octopamine, serotonin, histamine, phenylethanolamine, and catecholamines. See Chapter 89 for a full discussion of the diagnosis and therapy of this syndrome.

Neurologic signs are variable, depending on the onset and severity of the disease. There may be depression, stupor, blindness, behavioral changes, aggression, head pressing, and signs of forebrain motor dysfunction. Grand mal seizures are seen in many cases. Animals with acute or severe hepatic dysfunction may be tetraplegic, with little voluntary motor activity. Pinpoint pupils may be present in the most severely affected cases. Cranial neuropathies rarely have been observed. Neurologic signs of hepatic encephalopathy may vary with time and be noticeably exacerbated by high-protein diets and administration of exogenous ammonia for diagnostic purposes.

HYPOTHERMIA

Exposure to cold can cause seizures, coma, and death. Hypothermia of less than 53.5° F (12° C) causes consistent brain damage.[306] Clinically, hypothermia can be encountered in the neonate during the first week of life. It is a common postoperative complication and may delay anesthetic recovery. Hypothermia can also result from hypothalamic lesions in dogs and cats.

Supportive and corrective measures should be taken to assure regulation of a normal body temperature. Blankets, warm water immersion, heating pads, and hot water bottles can provide adequate warmth in these circumstances.

HYPERTHERMIA

Heat stroke is a polysystemic disorder that results from forced confinement of animals in a hot environment. Experimentally, heat stroke does not occur in dogs until their rectal temperature exceeds 109.4° F (43° C). Malignant hyperthermia, a syndrome that occurs following anesthetic procedures, results in extreme pyrexia. Both lead to elevated body temperatures and deleterious effects on body function and the central nervous system.

Although the cause of these two disorders is different, the pathophysiologic alterations and treatment of these conditions are similar. Pathophysiologic alterations, including cell necrosis, electrolyte disturbances, vascular collapse, and hypotensive shock, compromise function of the central nervous system. Disseminated intravascular coagulation, which usually complicates hyperthermic conditions, can result in cerebral hypoperfusion and cerebrocortical necrosis.

The nervous signs associated with hyperthermia range from depression to stupor, convulsions, and coma. Cerebral edema and polioencephalomalacia may develop, which explain some of these nervous signs.

Therapy for this condition involves reducing body temperature by supportive means. Seizures should be controlled with anticonvulsants. Muscular rigidity should be controlled with muscle relaxants and sedation. Cerebral edema should be treated with glucocorticoids and diuretics such as mannitol. The latter also promotes increased cerebral circulation.

References

1. Conrad, CR: Radiographic examination of the central nervous system. *In* Ettinger SJ (ed): Textbook of Veterinary Internal Medicine, 1st ed. Philadelphia, WB Saunders, 1975, p 333.
2. Hoerlein, BF: Canine Neurology, Diagnosis, and Treatment, 3rd ed. Philadelphia, WB Saunders, 1978.
3. Ticer, JW: Radiographic Technique in Small Animal Practice. Philadelphia, WB Saunders, 1975.
4. Conrad, DR and Oliver, JE Jr: Cerebral arteriography. *In* Ticer JW (ed): Radiograph Techniques in Small Animal Practice. Philadelphia, WB Saunders, 1975, p 278.
5. Oliver, JE, Jr: Cranial sinus venography. JAVRS 10:66, 1969.
6. Brown, JA, et al.: Ultrasound evaluation of experimental hydrocephalus in dogs. Surg Neurol 22:273, 1984.
7. Redding, RW and Knecht, CD: Neurologic examination. *In* Ettinger SJ (ed): Textbook of Veterinary Internal Medicine. Philadelphia, WB Saunders, 1975, p 283.
8. Brasch, RC, et al.: Contrast enhanced NMR imaging: animal studies using gadolinium-DTPA complex. Roentgenology 142:625, 1984.
9. Klemm, WR and Hall, CL: Electroencephalograms on anesthetized dogs with hydrocephalus. Am J Vet Res 32:1859, 1971.
10. Redding, RW: Canine electroencephalography. *In* Hoerlein BF (ed): Canine Neurology, Diagnosis and Treatment, 3rd ed. Philadelphia, WB Saunders, 1978, p 150.
11. Klemm, WR: Animal electroencephalography. New York, Academic Press, 1969.
12. Klemm, WR and Hall, CL: Current status and trends in veterinary electroencephalography. JAVMA 164:529, 1974.
13. Marshall, AE, et al.: Brainstem auditory evoked response in the diagnosis of inner ear injury in the horse. JAVMA 178:282, 1981.
14. Malnati, GA, et al.: Electroretinographic components of the canine visual evoked response. Am J Vet Res 42:159, 1981.
15. Redding, RW and Ingram, JT: The visual evoked response of the dog. Proc AVNA, Washington, DC, July 1980.
16. Penrod, JP and Coulter, DB: The diagnostic uses of impedance audiometry in the dog. JAAHA 16:941, 1980.
17. Higgins, RJ, et al.: Internal hydrocephalus and associated periventricular encephalitis in young dogs. Vet Pathol 14:236, 1977.
18. Krum, S, et al.: Hydrocephalus associated with the noneffusive form of feline infectious peritonitis. JAVMA 167:745, 1975.
19. Anvik, JO and Lewis, R: Actinomyces associated with hydrocephalus in a dog. Can Vet J 17:42, 1976.
20. Swaim, SF: Personal communication, 1975.
21. Parkinson, D and Jain, KK: Hydrocephalus: A shunt between the ventricle and Stensen's duct. Can J Surg 4:183, 1961.
22. Few, AB: The diagnosis and surgical treatment of canine hydrocephalus. JAVMA 179:286, 1966.
23. Nulsen, FE and Becker, DP: Control of hydrocephalus by valve-regulated shunt. J Neurosurg 26:361, 1967.
24. Gage, ED and Hoerlein, BF: Surgical treatment of canine hydrocephalus by ventriculoatrial shunting. JAVMA 153:1418, 1968.
25. Gage, ED: Surgical treatment of canine hydrocephalus. JAVMA 157:1729, 1970.
26. Little, JR, et al.: Comparison of ventriculoperitoneal and ventriculoatrial shunts for hydrocephalus in children. Mayo Clin Proc 47:396, 1972.
27. Fox, MW: The otocephalic syndrome in the dog. Cornell Vet 54:250, 1964.
28. Fox, MW: Diseases of possible hereditary origin in the dog. J Hered 56:169, 1965.
29. Greene, CE, et al.: Lissencephaly in two Lhasa apso dogs. JAVMA 169:405, 1976.
30. Frauchiger, E and Fankhauser, R: Vergleichende Neuropathologic des Menschen and der Tiere. Berlin, Springer-Verlag, 1957.
31. deLahunta, A: Comparative cerebellar disease in domestic animals. Comp Cont Ed Pract Vet 2:8, 1980.
32. Dow, RW: Partial agenesis of the cerebellum in dogs. J Comp Neurol 72:549, 1940.
33. Cordy, DR and Snelbaker, HA. Cerebellar hypoplasia and degeneration in a family of Airedale dogs. J Neuropathol Exp Neurol 11:324, 1952.
34. Carpenter, MB: A study of congenital feline cerebellar malformation. J Comp Neurol 105:51, 1956.
35. Oliver, JE, Jr and Geary, JC: Cerebellar anomalies–Two cases. VM SAC 60:697, 1965.
36. Carmichael, S, et al.: Familial cerebellar ataxia with hydrocephalus in bull mastiffs. Vet Rec 112:354, 1983.
37. Bardens, JW: Congenital malformation of the foramen magnum in dogs. Southwest Vet 18:1965.
38. Greene, CE, et al.: Congenital cerebrospinal hypomyelinogenesis in a pup. JAVMA 171:534, 1977.
39. Greene, CE: Personal observations. University of Georgia, Athens, GA 1986.
40. Mayhew, IG, et al.: Tremor syndrome and hypomyelination in Lurcher pups. J Sm Anim Pract 25:551, 1984.
41. Griffiths, IR, et al.: Shaking pups: a disorder of central myelination in the spaniel dog. Clinical genetic and light microscopical observations. J Neurol Sci 50:423, 1981.
42. Vandevelde, M, et al.: Dysmyelination of the central nervous system in the Chow-Chow dog. Acta Neuropathol 42:221, 1978.
43. Richards, RB and Kakulas, BA: Spongiform leukoencephalopathy associated with congenital myoclonia syndrome in the dog. J Comp Pathol 88:317, 1978.
44. van den Akker, S: A case of leukodystrophia in a dog. Folia Psychiat Neurol Neurochis 5:536, 1958.
45. Fatzer, R: Leukodeptrophische Erkrankungen im Gehirn junger Katzen. Schweiz Arch Tierheilkd 117:641, 1975.
46. Blakemore, WF and Palmer, AC: Cerebral lipidoses and leucodystrophies in animals. Vet Ann 12:129, 1971.
47. Jolly, R: Lysosomal storage diseases. Neuropathol Appl Neurobiol 4:419, 1978.
48. Jolly, RD and Blakemore, WF: Inherited lysosomal storage diseases: an essay in comparative medicine. Vet Rec 92:391, 1973.
49. Read, DH, et al.: Neuronal-visceral GM1 gangliosidosis in a dog with β-galactosidase deficiency. Science 194:442, 1976.
50. Blakemore, WF: GM1 Gangliosidosis in a cat. J Comp Pathol 82:179, 1972.
51. Baker, HJ and Lindsey, JR: Animal model of human disease: human GM1 gangliosidosis animal model: Feline GMI gangliosidosis. Am J Pathol 74:649, 1974.

52. Baker, HJ, et al.: Neuronal GM1 gangliosidosis in a Siamese cat with β-galactosidase deficiency. Science 174:838, 1971.
53. Karbe, E: Animal model of human disease: GM2 gangliosidosis (Amaurotic idiocies) types I II and III. Animal model: canine GM2 gangliosidosis. Am J Pathol 71:151, 1973.
54. Cummings, JF, et al.: GM2 gangliosidosis in a Japanese spaniel. Acta Neuropathol 67:247, 1985.
55. Cork, LC, et al.: GM2 ganglioside lysosomal storage disease in cats with β-hexosaminidase deficiency. Science 196:1014, 1977.
56. Bundza, A, et al.: Niemann-Pick disease in a poodle dog. Vet Pathol 16:530, 1979.
57. Crisp, CE, et al.: Lipid storage disease in a Siamese cat. JAVMA 156:616, 1970.
58. Steiss, JE and Cuddon, PA: Personal observations. University of Saskatchewan, Saskatoon, Canada; University of California, Davis, CA, 1985.
59. Hartley, WJ and Blakemore, WF: Neurovisceral glucocerebroside storage (Gaucher's disease) in a dog. Vet Pathol 10:191, 1973.
60. Van De Water, NS, et al.: Canine Gaucher disease—the enzymatic defect. Aust J Exp Biol Med Sci 57:551, 1979.
61. Patel, V, et al.: Phenylene diamine-mediated peroxidase deficiency in English setters with neuronal ceroid-lipofuscinosis. Lab Invest 30:366, 1974.
62. Koppang, N: Neuronal ceroid-lipofuscinosis in English setters. J Sm Anim Pract 10:639, 1970.
63. Rac, R and Giesecke, PR: Lysosomal storage disease in Chihuahuas. Aust Vet J 51:403, 1975.
64. Cummings, JF and deLahunta, A: An adult case of canine neuronal ceroid-lipofuscinosis. Acta Neuropathol 39:43, 1977.
65. Vandevelde, M and Fatzer, R: Neuronal ceroid-lipofuscinosis in older dachshunds. Vet Pathol 17:686, 1980.
66. Hoover, DM, et al.: Neuronal ceroid-lipofuscinosis in a mature dog. Vet Pathol 21:359, 1984.
67. Appleby, EC, et al.: Ceroid-lipofuscinosis in two Saluki dogs. J Comp Pathol 92:375, 1982.
68. Hartley, WJ, et al.: A suspected new canine storage disease. Acta Neuropathol 56:225, 1982.
69. Nimmo-Wilkie, JS and Hudson, EB: Neuronal and generalized ceroid-lipofuscinosis in a Cocker spaniel. Vet Pathol 19:623, 1982.
70. Green, PD and Little, PB: Neuronal ceroid-lipofuscin storage in Siamese cats. Can J Comp Med 38:207, 1974.
71. Kelly, WR, et al.: Canine α-L-fucosidosis: A storage disease of Springer Spaniels. Acta Neuropathol 60:9, 1983.
72. Littlewood, JD, et al.: Neuronal storage disease in English Springer spaniels. Vet Rec 112:86, 1983.
73. Burditt, LJ, et al.: Biochemical studies on a case of feline mannosidosis. Biochem J 189:467, 1980.
74. Blakemore, WF: A case of mannosidosis in the cat: clinical and histopathological findings. J Sm Anim Pract 27:446, 1986.
75. Vandevelde, M, et al.: Hereditary neurovisceral mannosidosis associated with α-mannosidase deficiency in a family of Persian cats. Acta Neuropathol 58:64, 1982.
76. MacKenzie, CD and Johnson, RP: Lafora's disease in a dog. Aust Vet J 52:144, 1976.
77. Tomchick, TL: Familial Lafora's disease in the beagle dog. Fed Proc 32:8, 1973.
78. Holland, JM, et al.: Lafora's disease in the dog. Am J Pathol 58:509, 1970.
79. Cusick, PK, et al.: Canine neuronal glycoproteinosis—Lafora's disease in the dog. JAAHA 12:518, 1976.
80. Montgomery, DL and Lee, AC: Brain damage in the epileptic beagle dog. Vet Pathol 20:160, 1983.
81. Walvoort, HC, et al.: Canine glycogen storage disease type II: a clinical study of four affected Lapland dogs. JAAHA 20:279, 1984.
82. Walvoort, HC, et al.: Heterozygote detection in a family of Lapland dogs with a recessively inherited metabolic disease: canine glycogen storage disease type II. Res Vet Sci 38:174, 1985.
83. Rafiquzzaman, M, et al.: Glycogenosis in the dog. Acta Vet Scand 17:196, 1976.
84. Ceh, L, et al.: Glycogenesis type III in the dog. Acta Vet Scand 17:210, 1976.
85. Haskins, ME, et al.: Mucopolysaccharidosis in a domestic shorthaired cat—a disease distinct from that seen in the Siamese cat. JAVMA 175:384, 1979.
86. Cowell, KR, et al.: Mucopolysaccharidosis in a cat. JAVMA 169:334, 1967.
87. Langweiler, M, et al.: Mucopolysaccharidosis in a litter of cats. JAAHA 14:748, 1978.
88. Haskins, ME, et al.: Spinal cord compression and hindlimb paresis in cats with mucopolysaccharidosis VI. JAVMA 182:983, 1983.
89. Breton, L, et al.: A case of mucopolysaccharidosis VI in a cat. JAAHA 19:891, 1983.
90. Howell, J McC and Palmer, AC: Globoid leukodystrophy in two dogs. J Sm Anim Pract 12:633, 1971.
91. Fankhauser, R, et al.: Leukodystrophie von Typus Krabbe beim Hund. Schweiz Arch Tierheilkd 105:198, 1965.
92. McGrath, JT, et al.: A morphologic and biochemical study of canine globoid cell leukodystrophy. J Neuropathol Exp Neurol 28:171, 1969.
93. Fletcher, TF, et al.: Globoid cell leukodystrophy (Krabbe type) in the dog. JAVMA 149:165, 1966.
94. Fletcher, TF, et al.: Experimental Wallerian degeneration in peripheral nerves of dogs with globoid cell leukodystrophy. J Neuropathol Exp Neurol 30:593, 1971.
95. Fletcher, TF, et al.: Ultrastructural features of globoid-cell leukodystrophy in the dog. Am J Vet Res 32:177, 1971.
96. Fletcher, TF and Kurtz, HJ: Animal model for human disease: Globoid cell leukodystrophy, Krabbe's disease. Am J Pathol 66:375, 1972.
97. Suzuki, Y, et al.: Studies in globoid leukodystrophy: enzymatic and lipid findings in the canine form. Exp Neurol 29:65, 1970.
98. Hirth, RS and Nielsen, SW: A familial canine globoid cell leukodystrophy ("Krabbe type"). J Sm Anim Pract 8:569, 1967.
99. Johnson, GR, et al.: Globoid cell leukodystrophy in a beagle. JAVMA 167:380, 1975.
100. Zaki, F and Kay, WJ: Globoid cell leukodystrophy in a miniature poodle. JAVMA 163:248, 1973.
101. Luttgen, PJ, et al.: Globoid cell leukodystrophy in a basset hound. J Sm Animal Pract 24:153, 1983.
102. Boysen, BG, et al.: Globoid cell leukodystrophy in the bluetick hound dog. Clinical manifestations. Can Vet J 15:303, 1974.
103. Selcer, EA and Selcer, RR: Globoid cell leukodystrophy in two West Highland white terriers and one Pomeranian. Comp Cont Ed Pract Vet 6:621, 1984.
104. Johnson, KH: Globoid leukodystrophy in the cat. JAVMA 157:2057, 1970.
105. Roszel, JF, et al.: Periodic acid Schiff-positive cells in cerebrospinal fluid of dogs with globoid cell leukodystrophy. Neurology 22:738, 1972.
106. Baker, HJ: Inherited metabolic disorders of the nervous system in dogs and cats. *In* Kirk RW (ed): Current Veterinary Therapy V. Philadelphia, WB Saunders, 1974, p 700.
107. Bjerkas, I: Hereditary "cavitating" leukodystrophy in Dalmatian dogs. Acta Neuropathol 40:163, 1977.
108. McGrath, JT and Batt, R: A leukodystrophy in the dog. J Neuropathol Exp Neurol 37:78, 1975.
109. Cox, NR, et al.: Myeloencephalopathy resembling Alexander's disease in a Scottish terrier dog. Acta Neuropathol (in press).
110. McGrath, JT: Neurologic Examination of the Dog, 2nd ed. Philadelphia, Lea and Febiger, 1960, p 207.
111. Douglas, SW and Palmer, AC: Idiopathic demyelination of brainstem and cord in a miniature poodle puppy. J Pathol Bacteriol 82:67, 1961.
112. Steinberg, SA, et al.: Clinico-pathologic conference. JAVMA 143:404, 1963.
113. Kelly, DF and Gaskell, CJ: Spongy degeneration of the central nervous system in kittens. Acta Neuropathol 35:151, 1976.
114. Mason, RW, et al.: Spongiform degeneration of the white matter in a Samoyed pup. Aust Vet Pract 9:11, 1979.
115. O'Brien, DP and Zachary, JF: Clinical features of spongy degeneration of the central nervous system in two Labrador retriever littermates. JAVMA 186:1207, 1985.
116. Gamble, DA and Chrisman, CL: A leukoencephalomyelopathy of Rottweiler dogs. Vet Pathol 21:174, 1984.
117. Wouda, W and van Nes, JJ: Progressive ataxia due to central demyelination in rottweiler dogs. Vet Quart 8:89, 1986.
118. Palmer, AC, et al.: Hereditary quadriplegia and amblyopia in the Irish setter. J Sm Anim Pract 14:343, 1973.

119. Palmer, AC: Introduction to Animal Neurology, 2nd ed. Oxford, Blackwell Scientific, 1976, p 202.
120. deLahunta, A and Averill, DR: Hereditary cerebellar cortical and extrapyramidal nuclear abiotrophy in Kerry blue terriers. JAVMA 168:1119, 1976.
121. Cork, LC, et al.: Canine inherited ataxia. Ann Neurol 9:492, 1981.
122. deLahunta, A, et al.: Hereditary cerebellar cortical abiotrophy in the Gordon setter. JAVMA 177:538, 1980.
123. Troncoso, JC, et al.: Canine inherited ataxia: ultrastructural observations. J Neuropathol Exp Neurol 44:165, 1985.
124. Hartley, WJ, et al.: Inherited cerebellar degeneration in the rough coated collie. Aust Vet Pract 8:79, 1978.
125. Gill, JM and Hewland, ML: Cerebellar degeneration in the border collie. N Z Vet J 8:170, 1980.
126. deLahunta, A: Diseases of the cerebellum. Vet Clin N Am 10:91, 1980.
127. Woodard, JC, et al.: Feline hereditary neuroaxonal dystrophy. Am J Pathol 74:551, 1974.
128. Cork, LC, et al.: Canine neuroaxonal dystrophy. J Neuropathol Exp Neurol 42:286, 1983.
129. Chrisman, CL, et al.: Neuroaxonal dystrophy of rottweiler dogs. JAVMA 184:464, 1984.
130. Clark, RG, et al.: Suspected neuroaxonal dystrophy in collie sheep dogs. N Z Vet J 30:102, 1982.
131. Blakemore, WF and Palmer, AC: Nervous disease in the Chihuahua characterized by axonal swellings. Vet Rec 117:498, 1985.
132. Bjorck, G, et al.: Hereditary ataxia in smooth-haired fox terriers. Vet Rec 69:87, 1957.
133. Bjorck, G, et al.: Hereditary ataxia in fox terriers. Acta Neuropathol (Suppl) 1:45, 1962.
134. Hartley, WJ and Palmer, AC: Ataxia in Jack Russell terriers. Acta Neuropathol 26:71, 1973.
135. deLahunta, A: Veterinary Neuroanatomy and Clinical Neurology, 2nd ed. Philadelphia, WB Saunders, 1983.
136. Ginsberg, MD, et al.: Diffuse cerebral ischemia in the cat. III. Neuropathological sequelae of severe ischemia. Ann Neurol 5:350, 1979.
137. Todd, MM, et al.: Cerebrovascular effects of prolonged hypocarbia and hypercarbia after experimental global ischemia in cats. Crit Care Med 13:720, 1985.
138. Neely, WA and Youmans, JR: Anoxia of the canine brain without damage. JAVMA 183:1085, 1963.
139. Courten-Myers, GM, et al.: Brain injury from marked hypoxia in cats: role of hypotension and hyperglycemia. Stroke 16:1016, 1985.
140. Hoerlein, BF: Heat stroke. *In* Kirk RW (ed): Current Veterinary Therapy III. Philadelphia, WB Saunders, 1968, p 103.
141. Arai, T, et al.: Effects of mannitol on cerebral circulation after transient complete cerebral ischemia in dogs. Crit Care Med 14:634, 1986.
142. Braund, KG and Vandevelde, M: Polioencephalomalacia in the dog. Vet Pathol 10:661, 1979.
143. Dahme, E and Schroder, B: Kongophile Angiopathie cerebrovascular Mikroaneurysmen und cerebrale Blutungen beim alten Hund. Zentralbl Veterinarmed A 26:601, 1979.
144. Fankhauser, R and Luginbuhl, H: Pathologische Anatomie des Zentralen und Peripheren Nervensystems der Haustiere. Berlin, Paul Parey, 1968.
145. Fankhauser, R, et al.: Cerebrovascular disease in various animal species. Ann N Y Acad Sci 127:817, 1965.
146. Detweiler, DK, et al.: The significance of naturally occurring coronary and cerebral arterial disease in animals. Ann N Y Acad Sci 149:868, 1968.
147. Manley, LW, et al.: Canine hyperlipoproteinemia and atherosclerosis. Am J Pathol 87:205, 1977.
148. Patterson, JS, et al.: Neurologic manifestations of cerebrovascular atherosclerosis associated with primary hypothyroidism in a dog. JAVMA 186:499, 1985.
149. Rogers, WA, et al.: Lipids and lipoproteins in normal dogs and dogs with secondary hyperlipoproteinemia. JAVMA 166:1092, 1975.
150. deLahunta, A: Feline neurology. Vet Clin N Am 6:433, 1976.
151. Zaki, FA and Nafe, LA: Ischemic encephalopathy and focal granulomatous meningoencephalitis in the cat. J Sm Anim Pract 21:429, 1980.
152. Anon: Postvaccinal rabies in the cat. US Dept HEW, CDC, Morbid Mortal Weekly Rep 29(Feb 29):86, 1980.
153. Barnard, BJH, et al.: Neurological symptoms in a cat following vaccination with high egg passage flurry rabies vaccine of chicken embryo origin. Ondersterpoort J Vet Res 44:195, 1977.
154. Pedersen, NC, et al.: Rabies vaccine virus infection in three dogs. JAVMA 172:1092, 1978.
155. Vandevelde, M and Fatzer, R: Neurologische komplikaties bij drie Londen na vaccinatic met een rabies weefsel kultuurvaccin. Vlamms Diergneesk T 43:253, 1974.
156. Murphy, FA: Rabies pathogenesis. Arch Virol 54:279, 1977.
157. Howard, DR: Skin biopsy provides accurate rabies diagnosis. Norden News 56:32, 1981.
158. Greene, CE (ed): Clinical Microbiology and Infectious Diseases of the Dog and Cat. Philadelphia, WB Saunders, 1984.
159. Krakowka, S, et al.: Myelin-specific autoantibodies associated with central nervous system demyelination in canine distemper virus infection. Infect Immunol 8:819, 1973.
160. Lincoln, SD, et al.: Etiologic studies of old dog encephalitis. I. Demonstration of canine distemper viral antigen in the brain of two cases. Vet Pathol 8:1, 1971.
161. Higgins, RJ, et al.: Primary demyelination in experimental canine distemper virus-induced encephalomyelitis in gnotobiotic dogs. Sequential immunologic and morphologic findings. Acta Neuropathol 58:1, 1982.
162. Breazile, JE, et al.: Experimental study of canine distemper myoclonus. Am J Vet Res 27:1375, 1976.
163. Cutler, RW and Averill, DR: Cerebrospinal fluid gammaglobulins in canine distemper encephalitis. Neurology 19:1111, 1969.
164. Vandevelde, M: Primary reticulosis of the central nervous system. Vet Clin N Am 10:57, 1980.
165. Kronevi, T, et al.: Feline ataxia due to nonsuppurative meningoencephalomyelitis of unknown etiology. Nord Vet Med 26:720, 1974.
166. Kornegay, JN: Feline infectious peritonitis. The central nervous system form. JAAHA 14:580, 1978.
167. Hagemoser, WA, et al.: Studies on the pathogenesis of pseudorabies in domestic cats following oral inoculation. Can J Comp Med 44:192, 1980.
168. Hoerlein, BF and Vandevelde, M: Primary disorders of the central nervous system. *In* Hoerlein BF (ed): Canine Neurology, 3rd ed. Philadelphia, WB Saunders, 1978, p 321.
169. Fankhauser, R, et al.: Morbus Aujesky bei Hund and Katze in der Schweiz. Schweiz Arch Tierheilkd 117:623, 1975.
170. Stepenko, MLF: Outbreak of Aujezky's disease in dogs. Veterinarian 3:61, 1962.
171. Percy, DH, et al.: Pathogenesis of canine herpesvirus encephalitis. Am J Vet Res 31:145, 1970.
172. Johnson, BJ and Castro, AE: Isolation of canine parvovirus from a dog brain with severe necrotizing vasculitis and encephalomalacia. JAVMA 184:1398, 1984.
173. Lenghaus, C and Studdert, MJ: Generalized parvovirus disease in neonatal pups. JAVMA 181:41, 1982.
174. Hartley, WJ: A postvaccinal inclusion body encephalitis in dogs. Vet Pathol 11:301, 1974.
175. Fatzer, R and Fankhauser, R: Enzephalomyelitis bei jungen Hunden nach Staupe. HCC Impfung Prakt Tierarztl 57:280, 1976.
176. Bestetti, G, et al.: Encephalitis following vaccination against distemper and infectious hepatitis in the dog. Acta Neuropathol 43:68, 1978.
177. Appel, MJG and Gillespie, JH: Canine distemper virus. Virol Monogr 11:1, 1972.
178. Krakowka, S, et al.: Canine parvovirus potentiates canine distemper encephalitis attributable to modified live-virus vaccine. JAVMA 180:137, 1982.
179. Fankhauser, R, et al.: Purkinjezellatrophie nach Masernivins—Vakzinierung beim Hund. Schweiz Arch Neurol Neurochir Psychiatr 112:353, 1973.
180. Wilson, RB, et al.: A neurologic syndrome associated with the use of a canine coronavirus-parvovirus vaccine in dogs. Comp Cont Ed Pract Vet 8:117, 1986.
181. Fenner, WR: Treatment of central nervous system infections in small animals. JAVMA 185:1176, 1984.
182. Tyler, DE, et al.: Disseminated protothecosis with central nervous system involvement in a dog. JAVMA 176:987, 1980.
183. Imes, GD, et al.: Disseminated protothecosis in a dog. Onderstepoort J Vet Res 44:1, 1977.

184. Jang, SS, et al.: Feline brain abscesses due to *Cladosporium trichoides*. Sabouraudia 15:115, 1977.
185. Reed, C, et al.: Leukemia in a cat with concurrent *Cladosporium* infection. J Sm Anim Pract 15:55, 1974.
186. Ribas, JL, et al.: Cerebral phaeohyphomycosis: an unusual mycosis of dogs and cats. Proc 3rd Annu Med Forum, ACVIM, San Diego, June, 1985, p 151.
187. Kyle, RJ: *Toxoplasma* encephalitis in a cat. N Z Vet J 23:13, 1975.
188. Shadduck, JA, et al.: Isolation of the causative organism of canine encephalitozoonosis. Vet Pathol 15:449, 1978.
189. Bauer, RW, et al.: Acanthamebiasis infection in a greyhound dog. Case report. 13th Annu Southeast Vet Pathol Conf, Tifton, GA, May 17, 1986.
190. Culbertson, CG, et al.: *Acanthamoeba* observations on pathogenicity. Science 127:1506, 1958.
191. Ayers, KM, et al.: *Acanthamoeba* in a dog. Vet Pathol 9:221, 1972.
192. Pearce, JR, et al.: Amebic meningoencephalitis caused by *Acanthamoeba castellani* in a dog. JAVMA 187:951, 1985.
193. Griffin, JL: Pathogenic free-living amoeba. *In* Krier, JP (ed): Parasitic Protozoa, vol 2. New York, Academic Press, 1978, p 507.
194. Fukushima, K, et al.: Aberrant dirofilariasis in a cat. JAVMA 184:199, 1984.
195. Hatziolos, BC: *Cuterebra* larva causing paralysis in a dog. Cornell Vet 57:129, 1967.
196. MacDonald, JN, et al.: *Cuterebra* encephalitis in a dog. Cornell Vet 66:372, 1976.
197. Hatziolos, BC: *Cuterebra* larva in the brain of a cat. JAVMA 148:787, 1966.
198. McKenzie, BE, et al.: Intracerebral migration of *Cuterebra* larva in a kitten. JAVMA 172:173, 1978.
199. Barrons, CN and Saunders, LZ: Visceral larva migrans. Pathol Vet 3:315, 1966.
200. Richards, MA and Sloper, JC: Hypothalamic involvement in visceral larva migrans in a dog suffering from diabetes insipidus. Vet Rec 76:449, 1964.
201. Buick, TD, et al.: Spinal nematodiasis of the dog associated with *Ancylostoma caninum*. Aust Vet J 53:602, 1977.
202. Mason, KV, et al.: Granulomatous encephalomyelitis of puppies due to *Angiostrongylus cantonensis*. Aust Vet J 52:295, 1976.
203. Georgi, JR, et al.: Cerebral coenurosis in a cat. Report of a case. Cornell Vet 59:27, 1969.
204. Hayes, MA and Creighton, SR: Coenurosis in the brain of a cat. Can Vet J 19:341, 1978.
205. Jauregui, PH and Marquez-Monter, H: Cysticercosis of the brain in dogs in Mexico City. Am J Vet Res 38:1641, 1977.
206. Braund, KG: Granulomatous meningoencephalomyelitis. JAVMA 186:138, 1985.
207. Braund, KG, et al.: Granulomatous meningoencephalomyelitis. JAVMA 172:1195, 1978.
208. Cordy, DR: Canine granulomatous meningoencephalomyelitis. Vet Pathol 16:325, 1979.
209. Palmer, AC: Pathogenesis and pathology of the cerebello-vestibular syndrome. J Sm Anim Pract 11:167, 1970.
210. Koestner, A: Primary lymphoreticuloses of the nervous system in animals. Acta Neuropathol Suppl VI:85, 1975.
211. Koestner, A and Zeman, W: Primary reticuloses of the central nervous system in dogs. Am J Vet Res 23:381, 1962.
212. Cuddon, PA and Smith-Maxie, L: Reticulosis of the central nervous system in the dog. Comp Cont Ed Pract Vet 6:23, 1984.
213. Glastonbury, JRW and Frauenfelder, AR: Granulomatous meningoencephalomyelitis in a dog. Aust Vet J 57:186, 1981.
214. Sarfaty, D, et al.: Differential diagnosis of granulomatous meningoencephalomyelitis, distemper, and suppurative meningoencephalitis in the dog. JAVMA 188:387, 1986.
215. Murtaugh, RJ, et al.: Focal granulomatous meningoencephalomyelitis in a pup. JAVMA 187:835, 1985.
216. Alley, MR, et al.: Granulomatous meningoencephalomyelitis of dogs in New Zealand. N Z Vet J 31:117, 1983.
217. Russo, ME: Primary reticulosis of the central nervous system in dogs. JAVMA 174:482, 1979.
218. Fankhauser, R, et al.: Reticulosis of the central nervous system (CNS) in dogs. Adv Vet Sci Comp Med 16:35, 1972.
219. Vandevelde, M, et al.: Immunohistologic studies in primary reticulosis of the canine brain. Vet Pathol 18:577, 1981.
220. Cameron, AM and Conroy, JD: Rabies-like neuronal inclusions associated with a neoplastic reticulosis in a dog. Vet Pathol 11:29, 1974.
221. Vandevelde, M, et al.: Primary reticulosis of the central nervous system in the dog. Vet Pathol 15:673, 1978.
222. Fischer, CA and Jones, GT: Optic neuritis in dogs. JAVMA 160:68, 1972.
223. Fischer, CA and Liu S-K: Neuro-ophthalmic manifestations of primary reticulosis of the central nervous system in a dog. JAVMA 158:1240, 1971.
224. Garmer, NL, et al.: Reticulosis of the eyes and the central nervous system in a dog. J Sm Anim Pract 22:39, 1981.
225. Smith, JS, et al.: Reticulosis of the visual system in a dog. J Sm Anim Pract 18:643, 1977.
226. Bailey, CS and Higgins, RJ: Characteristics of cerebrospinal fluid associated with canine granulomatous meningoencephalomyelitis: a retrospective study. JAVMA 188:418, 1986.
227. Vandevelde, M and Braund, KG: Polioencephalomyelitis in cats. Vet Pathol 16:420, 1979.
228. Braund, KG: Encephalitis and meningitis. Vet Clin N Am 10:31, 1980.
229. Russo, EA, et al.: Corticosteroid responsive aseptic suppurative meningitis in three dogs. Southwest Vet 35:197, 1983.
230. Meric, SM, et al.: Corticosteroid-responsive meningitis in ten dogs. JAAHA 21:677, 1985.
231. Luginbuhl, H: A comparative study of neoplasms of the central nervous system in animals. Acta Neurochirurg (Suppl) 10:30, 1964.
232. Luginbuhl, H, et al.: Spontaneous neoplasms of the nervous system in animals. Prog Neurol Surg 2:85, 1968.
233. Summers, BA and de Lahunta, A: Cerebral angioendotheliomatosis in a dog. Acta Neuropathol 68:10, 1985.
234. Fankhauser, R, et al.: Tumors of the nervous system. Bull WHO 50:53, 1974.
235. Braund, KG: Neoplasia of the nervous system. Comp Cont Ed Pract Vet 6:717, 1984.
236. Hayes, KC and Schiefer, B: Primary tumors in the CNS of carnivores. Pathol Vet 6:94, 1969.
237. Palmer, AC: Tumors of the central nervous system. Proc Royal Coll Med 69:49, 1976.
238. Kornegay, JN, et al.: Clinicopathologic features of brain herniation in animals. JAVMA 182:1111, 1983.
239. Palmer, AC: Clinical and pathological features of some tumors of the central nervous system in dogs. Res Vet Sci 1:36, 1960.
240. Palmer, AC: Clinical signs associated with intracranial tumours in dogs. Res Vet Sci 2:326, 1961.
241. Braund, KG, et al.: Neurologic manifestations of monoclonal IgM gammopathy associated with lymphocytic leukemia in a dog. JAVMA 172:1407, 1978.
242. Hayes, HM, et al.: Occurrence of nervous-tissue tumors in cattle, horses, cats and dogs. Int J Cancer 15:39, 1975.
243. McGrath, JT: Intracranial pathology of the dog. Acta Neuropathol (Suppl) 1:3, 1962.
244. Zaki, FA: Spontaneous central nervous system tumors in the dog. Vet Clin N Am 7:153, 1977.
245. McGrath, JT: Morphology and classification of brain tumors in domestic animals. *In* Proceedings, Brain Tumors in Brain and Animals, National Institute of Environmental Health Sciences, Research Triangle Park, NC, Sept, 1984.
246. Braund, KG and Ribas, JL: Central nervous system meningiomas. Comp Cont Ed Pract Vet 8:241, 1986.
247. Fankhauser, R and Vandevelde, M: Zur klinik der Tumoren des Nervensystems beim Hund und Katze. Schweiz Arch Tierheilkd 123:553, 1981.
248. Zake, FA and Nafe, LA: Choroid plexus tumors in the dog. JAVMA 176:328, 1980.
249. Braund, KG and Ribas, JL: Brain ventricular tumors. Proc 3rd Annu Med Forum, ACVIM, San Diego, June, 1985, p 157.
250. Zaki, FA and Hurvitz, AI: Spontaneous neoplasms of the central nervous system of the cat. J Sm Anim Pract 17:773, 1976.
251. Nafe, LA: Meningiomas in cats: a retrospective clinical study of 36 cases. JAVMA 174:1224, 1979.
252. Andrews, EJ: Clinicopathologic characteristics of meningiomas in dogs. JAVMA 163:151, 1973.
253. Luginguhl, H: Studies on meningiomas in cats. Am J Vet Res 22:1030, 1961.
254. Kay, WJ: Diagnosis of intracranial neoplasms. Vet Clin N Am 7:145, 1977.

255. Palmer, AC, et al.: Clinical signs including papilloedema associated with brain tumors in twenty-one dogs. J Sm Anim Pract 15:359, 1974.
256. Kallfelz, FA, et al.: Scintiographic diagnosis of brain lesions in the dog and cat. JAVMA 172:589, 1978.
257. Fike, JR, et al.: Computerized tomography of brain tumors of the rostral and middle fossas in the dog. Am J Vet Res 42:275, 1981.
258. Fike, JR, et al.: Anatomy of the canine brain using high resolution computed tomography. Vet Radiol 22:236, 1981.
259. LeCouteur, RA, et al.: Computed tomography of brain tumors in the caudal fossa of the dog. Vet Radiol 22:244, 1981.
260. LeCouteur, RA, et al.: X-ray computed tomography of brain tumors in cats. JAVMA 183:301, 1983.
261. Schunk, KL: Computed tomography of brain tumors in small animals. Proc 3rd Annu Med Forum, Am Coll Vet Intern Med, San Diego, June 1-4, 1985, p 159.
262. Turrel, JM, et al.: Computered tomographic characteristics of primary brain tumors in 50 dogs. JAVMA 188:851, 1986.
263. Fike, JR, et al.: Differentiation of neoplastic from non-neoplastic lesions in dog brain using quantitative CT. Vet Radiol 27:121, 1986.
264. Roszel, JF: Membrane filtration of canine and feline cerebrospinal fluid for cytologic evaluation. JAVMA 160:720, 1972.
265. Vandevelde, M and Spano, JS: Cerebrospinal fluid cytology in canine neurologic disease. Am J Vet Res 38:1827, 1977.
266. Shell, L, et al.: Surgical removal of a meningioma in a cat after detection by computerized axial tomography. JAAHA 21:439, 1985.
267. Turrel, JM, et al.: Radiotherapy of brain tumors in dogs. JAVMA 184:82, 1984.
268. Klatzo, I: Neuropathological aspects of brain edema. J Neuropathol Exp Neurol 26:1, 1967.
269. Fishman, RA: Brain edema. N Engl J Med 293:706, 1975.
270. Palmer, AC: Concussion: the result of impact injury to the brain. Vet Rec 111:575, 1982.
271. Smith, DR, et al.: Experimental in vivo microcirculatory dynamics in brain trauma. J Neurosurg 30:664, 1969.
272. Palmer, AC: The accident case. IV. The significance and estimation of damage to the central nervous system. J Sm Anim Pract 5:25, 1964.
273. Oliver, JE and Lorenz, MD: Handbook of Neurologic Diagnosis. Philadelphia, WB Saunders, 1983.
274. Osweiler, GD: Incidence and diagnostic considerations of major small animal toxicoses. JAVMA 155:2011, 1969.
275. Meriwether, WF: Acute marijuana toxicity in a dog. VM/SAC 64:577, 1969.
276. Stowe, CM, et al.: Amphetamine poisoning in dogs. JAVMA 168:504, 1976.
277. Godbold, JC, et al.: Acute oral marijuana poisoning in the dog. JAVMA 175:1101, 1979.
278. Scott, DW, et al.: Hexachlorophene toxicosis in dogs. JAVMA 162:947, 1973.
279. Ward, BC, et al.: Hexachlorophene toxicity in dogs. JAAHA 9:167, 1973.
280. Bath, ML: Hexachlorophene toxicity in dogs. J Sm Anim Pract 19:241, 1978.
281. Bell, TG, et al.: Ataxia, depression, and dermatitis associated with the use of dichlorovos-impregnated collars in the laboratory cat. JAVMA 167:579, 1976.
282. Kowalazyk, DF: Lead poisoning in dogs at the University of Pennsylvania Hospital. JAVMA 168:428, 1976.
283. Knecht, CD, et al.: Clinical clinicopathologic and electroencephalographic features of lead poisoning in dogs. JAVMA 175:196, 1979.
284. Zook, BC, et al.: Lead poisoning in dogs. JAVMA 155:1329, 1969.
285. Editorial: Bone overgrowth and nerve regeneration in vitamin A deficiency. Nut Rev 1:419, 1943.
286. Dublin, WB: Fundamentals of Neuropathology. Springfield, IL, Charles C. Thomas, 1954.
287. Morris, ML: Nutrition. *In* Catcott EJ (ed): Canine Medicine. Santa Barbara, American Veterinary Publications, Inc, 1968, p 89.
288. Eddy, D: The Avitaminoses, 2nd ed. Philadelphia, Williams and Wilkins, 1941.
289. Bagga, RB, et al.: Thiamine deficiency encephalopathy in a specific pathogen-free cat colony. Lab Anim Sci 18:323, 1978.
290. Morris, ML: Veterinary Dietetics. Topeka, Kansas, Mark Morris Associates, 1981.
291. Read, DH, et al.: Polioencephalomalacia of dogs with thiamine deficiency. Vet Pathol 14:103, 1977.
292. Read, DH, et al.: Experimentally induced thiamine deficiency in dogs: clinical observations. Am J Vet Res 42:984, 1981.
293. Newberne, PM and O'Dell, BL: Histopathology of hydrocephalus resulting from a deficiency of vitamin B_{12}. Proc Soc Exp Biol Med 97:62, 1958.
294. English, PB and Seawright, AA: Deforming cervical spondylosis. Aust Vet J 49:376, 1964.
295. Lucke, VM, et al.: Deforming cervical spondylosis in the cat associated with hypervitaminosis A. Vet Rec 82:141, 1968.
296. Fry, PD: Cervical spondylosis in the cat. J Sm Anim Pract 7:711, 1968.
297. Baker, JR and Huges, IB: A case of deforming cervical spondylosis in a cat associated with a diet rich in liver. Vet Rec 83:44, 1968.
298. Breitschwerdt, EB and Root, CR: Inappropriate secretion of antidiuretic hormone in a dog. JAVMA 175:181, 1979.
299. Crawford, MA, et al.: Hypernatremia and adipsia in a dog. JAVMA 184:818, 1984.
300. Hall, EJ: Hypernatremia and adipsia in a dog (letter). JAVMA 185:4, 1984.
301. Young, RKS and Yagel, SK: Cerebral physiological and metabolic effects of hyperventilation in the neonatal dog. Ann Neurol 16:33, 1984.
302. Arieff, AI and Massry, S: Calcium metabolism of brain in acute renal failure. J Clin Invest 53:397, 1974.
303. Mahoney, CA, et al.: Uremic encephalopathy: role of brain energy metabolism. Am J Physiol 247:F527, 1984.
304. Fujiwara, M, et al.: Hyperammonemia-induced cytotoxic brain edema under osmotic opening of blood-brain barrier in dogs. Res Exp Med 185:425, 1985.
305. Fraser, CL and Arieff, AI: Hepatic encephalopathy. N Engl J Med 313:865, 1985.
306. Egerton, N, et al.: Neurologic changes following profound hypothermia. Ann Surg 157:366, 1963.

62 DISEASES OF THE SPINAL CORD

RICHARD A. LECOUTEUR and GEORGINA CHILD*

Spinal cord disorders of cats or dogs are the most frequently encountered neurologic diseases in small animal practice. Neurologic deficits resulting from such diseases commonly affect locomotion, and therefore are easily recognized by dog and cat owners. Early diagnosis and accurate prognosis are essential for all spinal cord disorders, including those that are not amenable to treatment. Fortunately, many spinal cord diseases respond to appropriate medical and/or surgical treatment. Management of spinal cord disorders of small animals demands the ability to complete and interpret results of a neurologic examination, the ability to compile a list of diagnostic possibilities, and a knowledge of available diagnostic procedures and current treatment recommendations.

The objectives of this chapter are to outline a diagnostic approach to diseases of the spinal cord; to review aspects of the neurologic examination that pertain to localization of diseases that affect the spinal cord; to introduce and discuss regional localization of disorders that affect the spinal cord; and to provide a comprehensive alphabetical listing of disorders that affect the canine and/or feline spinal cord, with emphasis on etiology and pathogenesis, clinical findings, diagnosis, and treatment. The alphabetical listing of diseases can be used in association with Tables 62–1 through 62–4 to formulate a plan for diagnosis and treatment of a dog or cat with spinal cord disease.

MECHANISMS OF DISEASE

Diseases that affect the spinal cord may be divided into two groups.[1, 2] The first group comprises disease processes that affect both the nervous system and other organ systems. The second group includes diseases that are unique to the nervous system, such as disorders of myelin, neurons, or supporting cells (glial cells and the like). Categories of disease that may be included in either of these two groups include congenital and familial disorders, infections, immunologic and metabolic disorders, toxicities, nutritional disorders, trauma, vascular disorders, degenerations, neoplasia, and idiopathic disorders.

The localization of specific functions in the nervous system has important effects on the clinical presentation and nature of progression of diseases affecting the spinal cord. Localization of function in the spinal cord causes a similar pathologic process to result in many different clinical presentations, depending on what part(s) of the spinal cord it affects.[1] For example, a spinal cord neoplasm located at the level of C3 vertebra may result in tetraparesis whereas the identical neoplasm located at the level of T13 vertebra may result in paraparesis with the thoracic limbs unaffected. Furthermore, localization of function in the spinal cord renders it inherently vulnerable to focal lesions that in other organs where function is more uniformly distributed might not result in detectable clinical signs.[2] For example, a small infarction of the cervical spinal cord may result in tetraplegia, whereas a similar lesion occurring in hepatic parenchyma likely would not compromise liver function.

The unique susceptibility of the nervous system to a localized lesion is compounded by its strictly limited capacity to restore function in damaged tissue.[2] The pathologic reactions of the spinal cord to disease are to a degree nonspecific so that various disorders may induce a somewhat similar histologic appearance. With the exception of neoplasia and congenital malformations, most disorders of the spinal cord are characterized morphologically by the combination of a number of lesions that are not diagnostic when viewed in isolation.[3] Certain of these lesions may be recognizable grossly, while others are seen only by means of microscopic examination and involve the cellular elements of the

*The authors would like to acknowledge the use of class notes of Dr. Terrell A. Holliday, University of California, Davis, California, in the preparation of sections of this manuscript that describe clinical signs of spinal cord disease, and the Berkeley Veterinary Research Foundation for financial support in the production of manuscript photographs.

TABLE 62–1. DISEASES AFFECTING THE CERVICAL REGION (SPINAL CORD SEGMENTS C1–C5)

Category of Disease	Disease
Anomalous (Hereditary/ congenital)	*Atlantoaxial subluxation
	*Congenital vertebral anomalies
	Spina bifida
	Myelodysplasia
	Syringomyelia/hydromyelia
	Globoid cell leukodystrophy
	Hereditary ataxia
	Pilonidal sinus/epidermoid cyst
	Calcium phosphate deposition disease in Great Dane dogs
Degenerative	*Intervertebral disk disease
	*Cervical spondylomyelopathy
	Demyelinating myelopathy of miniature poodles
	Leukoencephalomyelopathy of rottweilers
	Neuroaxonal dystrophy of rottweilers
	Spondylosis deformans
	Dural ossification
Inflammatory/ infectious	*Diskospondylitis
	*Corticosteroid-responsive meningitis
	*Granulomatous meningoencephalomyelitis/reticulosis
	*Distemper myelitis
	*FIP meningitis/myelitis
	Bacterial/fungal/rickettsial/protothecal meningitis/myelitis
	Protozoal myelitis
	Pyogranulomatous meningoencephalomyelitis
	Feline polioencephalomyelitis
	Spinal nematodiasis
Neoplastic	*Neoplasia
Traumatic	*Spinal cord trauma
Vascular	*Ischemic myelopathy
	Necrotizing vasculitis
	Progressive hemorrhagic myelomalacia
	Hemorrhage
	Vascular malformations and benign vascular tumors
Nutritional	Hypervitaminosis A in cats
Idiopathic	Spinal arachnoid cysts
	Multiple cartilaginous exostoses

*Common causes of spinal cord disease.

spinal cord.[3] A topographic study of the lesions observed must therefore be combined with morphologic studies in order to arrive at an etiologic diagnosis.

Clinical syndromes affecting the spinal cord may be characterized by a single focal lesion (transverse myelopathy) or by several focal lesions (multifocal disorders). Certain diseases may have a diffuse (or disseminated) distribution. Clinical differentiation of diffuse and multifocal disorders may be difficult. Myelopathies may be extrinsic, in which spinal cord dysfunction is secondary to diseases of the vertebrae, meninges, or epidural space, or may be intrinsic, in which the disease begins as an intramedullary lesion. Extrinsic myelopathies are almost always transverse myelopathies.

As the nervous system can respond in only a limited number of ways to the numerous causes of myelopathies, it is necessary to follow a systematic diagnostic approach in an animal with a spinal cord disorder. Such an approach ensures that less frequently encountered causes of myelopathy are not misdiagnosed and consequently treated inappropriately.

Diagnostic Approach to a Spinal Cord Problem

SIGNALMENT

Accurate diagnosis of a spinal cord disorder must include consideration of an animal's age, breed, and sex. Diseases may be specific to certain species and breeds. Such diseases have been summarized by several authors.[4–11]

HISTORY

An accurate and complete history constitutes the initial step in the diagnosis of all neurologic problems. Important aspects of history include rapidity of onset of the problem and the nature of its progression.[9, 10] This information may be helpful in determining the cause of a problem. For example, neoplastic diseases affecting the spinal cord most often result in focal signs that have an insidious onset and a gradual progression. In contrast, vascular disorders such as infarction or hemorrhage may produce an acute onset of focal signs without evidence of progression. Inflammatory, degenerative, or metabolic disorders generally cause a diffuse distribution of

TABLE 62–2. DISEASES AFFECTING THE CERVICAL ENLARGEMENT (SPINAL CORD SEGMENTS C6–T2)

Category of Disease	Disease
Anomalous	*Congenital vertebral anomalies
	Spina bifida
	Myelodysplasia
	Syringomyelia/hydromyelia
	Hereditary myelopathy of Afghan hounds
	Calcium phosphate deposition disease of Great Dane dogs
	Globoid cell leukodystrophy
	Pilonidal sinus/epidermoid cyst
Degenerative	*Intervertebral disk disease
	*Cervical spondylomyelopathy
	Spondylosis deformans
	Dural ossification
Inflammatory/ infectious	*Diskospondylitis
	Distemper myelitis
	FIP meningitis/myelitis
	Protozoal myelitis
	Bacterial/fungal/rickettsial/protothecal meningitis/myelitis
	Feline polioencephalomyelitis
	Spinal nematodiasis
	Granulomatous meningoencephalomyelitis/reticulosis
Neoplastic	*Neoplasia
Traumatic	*Spinal cord trauma
Vascular	*Ischemic myelopathy
	*Progressive hemorrhagic myelomalacia
	Necrotizing vasculitis
	Hemorrhage
	Vascular malformation and benign vascular tumors
Nutritional	Hypervitaminosis A of cats
Idiopathic	Multiple cartilaginous exostoses
	Spinal arachnoid cysts

*Common causes of spinal cord disease.

TABLE 62–3. DISEASES AFFECTING THE THORACOLUMBAR REGION (SPINAL CORD SEGMENTS T3–L3)

Category of Disease	Disease
Anomalous	*Congenital vertebral anomalies
	Spina bifida
	Myelodysplasia
	Syringomyelia/hydromyelia
	Mucopolysaccharidosis
	Globoid cell leukodystrophy
	Hereditary myelopathy of Afghan hounds
	Pilonidal sinus/epidermoid cyst
Degenerative	*Intervertebral disk disease
	*Degenerative myelopathy
	Hound ataxia
	Spondylosis deformans
	Dural ossification
Inflammatory/ infectious	*Diskospondylitis
	*Distemper myelitis
	*FIP meningitis/myelitis
	Bacterial/fungal/rickettsial/protothecal meningitis/myelitis
	Protozoal myelitis
	Feline polioencephalomyelitis
	Spinal nematodiasis
	Granulomatous meningoencephalomyelitis/reticulosis
Neoplastic	*Neoplasia
Traumatic	*Spinal cord trauma
Vascular	*Ischemic myelopathy
	Progressive hemorrhagic myelomalacia
	Hemorrhage
	Necrotizing vasculitis
	Vascular malformations and benign vascular tumors
Idiopathic	Multiple cartilaginous exostoses
	Spinal arachnoid cysts

*Common causes of spinal cord disease.

signs that have an insidious onset and gradual progression. Traumatic and congenital diseases may result in either a focal or multifocal distribution of signs, most often with an acute onset and without progression, although such diseases may have a progressive course.[9, 10]

While careful consideration of these factors is helpful in determining the cause of a spinal cord problem, there is a sufficient number of exceptions to the general statements listed above that such information must be used with caution and should not be the sole basis for excluding a disorder from a list of differential diagnoses. For example, an acute onset of signs does not rule out neoplasia as a potential cause of myelopathy, as a neoplasm may be associated with rapid decompensation of neural tissue, particularly if vascular factors such as infarction or hemorrhage are involved.

PHYSICAL EXAMINATION

A physical examination consists of a series of observations that provide information regarding the general health of all body systems. Results of this examination are used to supplement information collected in the history and may implicate involvement of body systems other than the nervous system. For example, an animal presented with a primary complaint of back pain may in fact have abdominal pain related to an underlying gastrointestinal or urinary system disorder.

A thorough orthopedic examination should be completed in any dog suspected of having a spinal cord disorder. Particular attention should be paid to the examination of joints for signs of effusion or abnormal motion. Disorders such as rupture of anterior cruciate ligaments bilaterally or bilateral patellar luxations may mimic paraparesis due to a neural disorder.

NEUROLOGIC EXAMINATION

A neurologic examination is an extension of a physical examination. The technique of the neurologic examination is described in depth in Chapter 60. When spinal cord disease is suspected, it is essential to complete a thorough, comprehensive, and unbiased examination of the nervous system. Errors in diagnosis commonly occur when only the region of an obvious neurologic deficit is examined and more subtle alterations in other parts of the nervous system are overlooked.

The objectives of the neurologic examination are to detect the presence of and to determine the location and extent of a disorder of the nervous system.[9]

PROBLEM LIST

A complete list of problems should be compiled following completion of physical and neurologic examinations. All identified problems should be included, despite the fact that certain of the problems listed may not appear to be directly related to the presenting

TABLE 62–4. DISEASES AFFECTING THE LUMBAR ENLARGEMENT (SPINAL CORD SEGMENTS L4–Cd5 AND CAUDA EQUINA)

Category of Disease	Disease
Anomalous	*Spinal bifida
	*Sacrocaudal dysgenesis
	Congenital vertebral anomalies
	Myelodysplasia
	Syringomyelia/hydromyelia
	Globoid cell leukodystrophy
	Pilonidal sinus/epidermoid cyst
Degenerative	*Intervertebral disk disease
	*Lumbosacral vertebral canal stenosis
	Spondylosis deformans
	Dural ossification
Inflammatory/ infectious	*Diskospondylitis
	*Protozoal myelitis
	Distemper myelitis
	FIP meningitis/myelitis
	Bacterial/fungal/rickettsial/protothecal meningitis/myelitis
	Feline polioencephalomyelitis
	Spinal nematodiasis
	Granulomatous meningoencephalomyelitis/reticulosis
Neoplastic	*Neoplasia
Traumatic	*Spinal cord trauma
Vascular	*Ischemic myelopathy
	*Progressive hemorrhagic myelomalacia
	Hemorrhage
	Necrotizing vasculitis
	Vascular malformations and benign vascular tumors
Idiopathic	Multiple cartilaginous exostoses
	Spinal arachnoid cysts

*Common causes of spinal cord disease.

complaint of an animal. Problems should be listed at the most current level of understanding and should be updated, redefined, or combined as more information is collected. Careful attention to maintenance of a problem list ensures that all aspects of an animal's complaint are addressed during a work-up. This is essential, as often there is a tendency for a clinician to focus a work-up on an obvious neurologic deficit while ignoring a related problem. For example, a dog or cat with signs consistent with spinal cord infarction may have signs that reflect an underlying cardiovascular or endocrine problem.

DIFFERENTIAL DIAGNOSIS LIST

A list should be compiled of possible causes for each problem included on the problem list. Such a list should be exhaustive and the most probable causes should be listed first. Ranking of differential diagnoses is based on information collected in the history regarding signalment, nature of onset and progression of signs, and on results of the physical and neurologic examinations.

MINIMUM DATA BASE

The minimum data base for a dog or cat with signs of spinal cord disease includes factors considered above (signalment, history). Initial clinicopathologic tests include a complete blood count, blood chemistry profile, and urinalysis. Results of these tests may result in addition of further problems to a problem list or may permit redefinition or combination of existing problems.

Results of initial blood and urine tests may support a diagnosis of a metabolic, toxic, or infectious disorder that is either producing or complicating signs of spinal cord dysfunction. Additional diagnostic tests may be required to investigate disorders suspected on the basis of results of initial screening tests. For example, hyperglobulinemia detected in a cat with signs of myelopathy may support completion of a serum feline infectious peritonitis (FIP) titer.

Thoracic or abdominal radiographs may be obtained as part of the minimum data base in dogs or cats with a spinal cord disorder. This is especially necessary in older animals, in animals in which abnormalities of cardiovascular or respiratory function are suspected, or in animals in which neoplasia is included on a list of differential diagnoses.

ANCILLARY DIAGNOSTIC INVESTIGATIONS

Several diagnostic procedures aid in the differentiation of causes of a myelopathy. Certain of these procedures further aid in defining the exact location and extent of a disorder affecting the spinal cord. The selection of an appropriate technique or techniques depends on results of physical and neurologic examinations and on the ranking of causes on a differential diagnosis list. As a general rule, techniques are selected to first investigate the most likely causes of a spinal cord disorder. The least invasive diagnostic tests and those with the lowest morbidity should be completed first.

The recommended essential procedures for diagnosis of a myelopathy in advised order of completion are noncontrast vertebral radiography, cerebrospinal fluid (CSF) analysis, and myelography. Additional procedures may be added to this list, depending on the nature of the problem being investigated.

Noncontrast Vertebral Radiography. Noncontrast vertebral radiography is essential in the accurate diagnosis of a disorder affecting the spinal cord.[4, 6, 12–14] A minimum requirement is that radiographs include the entire region of the vertebral column that may produce the observed clinical signs. Due to the limitations of a neurologic examination in outlining multiple lesions of the spinal cord, and for the purpose of comparison if problems related to other regions of the vertebral column occur in the future, the entire vertebral column should be radiographed whenever possible. Correct technique, exact positioning, and use of appropriate projections are essential considerations for the production of noncontrast vertebral radiographs that are of diagnostic quality. This subject has been extensively reviewed by several authors.[4, 6, 12, 13]

Further diagnostic investigations may be indicated on the basis of results of noncontrast vertebral radiography. For example, a finding of diskospondylitis may be followed by culture and sensitivity testing of blood, urine, or an aspirate from an infected disk or by serologic testing for *Brucella canis*. Differentiation of an infectious lesion from a vertebral neoplasm may be difficult on the basis of results of noncontrast vertebral radiography. In such cases, a biopsy by means of needle aspiration or surgical excision may be indicated.

Cerebrospinal Fluid Analysis. Cerebrospinal fluid collection and analysis are essential in cases where noncontrast vertebral radiographs do not fully define location, nature, and extent of a disorder affecting the spinal cord. Collection of CSF may be done by means of a cisternal or a lumbar subarachnoid puncture. It has been recommended that CSF be collected from a cisternal site if cervical spinal cord disease is suspected and from a lumbar location if a thoracolumbar disorder is involved. However, a lumbar collection site (most often between L5 and L6 vertebrae) may be used for most dogs or cats with a spinal cord disorder regardless of the suspected location of the problem. Precautions must be used in the collection of CSF from animals in which an increased intracranial pressure is suspected. Techniques for CSF collection and analysis have been discussed by other authors.[4, 6, 8, 14–17]

Analysis of CSF collected from a dog or cat with a spinal cord disorder should always include a total and differential white blood cell count and a quantitative estimation of protein content. Results for CSF from normal dogs have been published.[18] It should be noted that normal values differ in CSF collected from lumbar and cisternal collection sites.[18] Similar data for feline CSF do not exist, although it is anticipated that results for this species would be similar to those of dogs.

Results of CSF analysis may support further examination of CSF. For example, CSF may be submitted for bacterial or fungal culture and sensitivity testing, or for completion of viral titers.[15]

Myelography. Contrast radiography should be done in those animals where results of noncontrast vertebral radiography and CSF analysis do not fully define a disorder affecting the spinal cord.[4, 6, 12–14] Myelography is the radiographic examination of the spinal cord and emerging nerve roots following injection of contrast material into the subarachnoid space. Patterns of myelographic change can be used to differentiate intramedullary, intradural-extramedullary, and extradural space-occupying lesions (Figure 62–1).[4]

This technique is difficult to perform, and myelography is not without undesirable consequences in all cases.[4] Therefore, myelography should only be considered if positive findings are essential for diagnosis and prognosis, or to determine a precise site for surgery. Although myelography may be completed by means of either a cisternal or lumbar injection site, a lumbar injection site is preferred for dogs or cats with spinal cord disease at any level of the vertebral column. Use of dynamic radiographic techniques and completion of oblique projections may augment diagnostic information gained from a myelographic study.[4]

Electrophysiology. There are several electrophysiologic techniques that may be applied to diseases affecting the spinal cord.[6] Electromyographic (EMG) examination of paraspinal and limb musculature may be used to further define the extent of a spinal cord lesion.[19] This technique is ideally done prior to completion of noncontrast vertebral radiographs as results may help determine the exact region or regions of the spinal cord that are affected, thus facilitating concentration of noncontrast radiographic studies to such an affected area. The role of EMG examination in the diagnosis of spinal cord disease is, however, somewhat limited.[20] Abnormal EMG results associated with spinal cord disease are seen only when the lower motor neurons (LMNs) in the ventral horn of the spinal cord or their axons in the ventral root are affected by a pathologic process.[19] The EMG often is normal in association with disorders that primarily affect the spinal cord white matter. Furthermore, specific information regarding the cause of a myelopathy is not available by means of EMG examination.

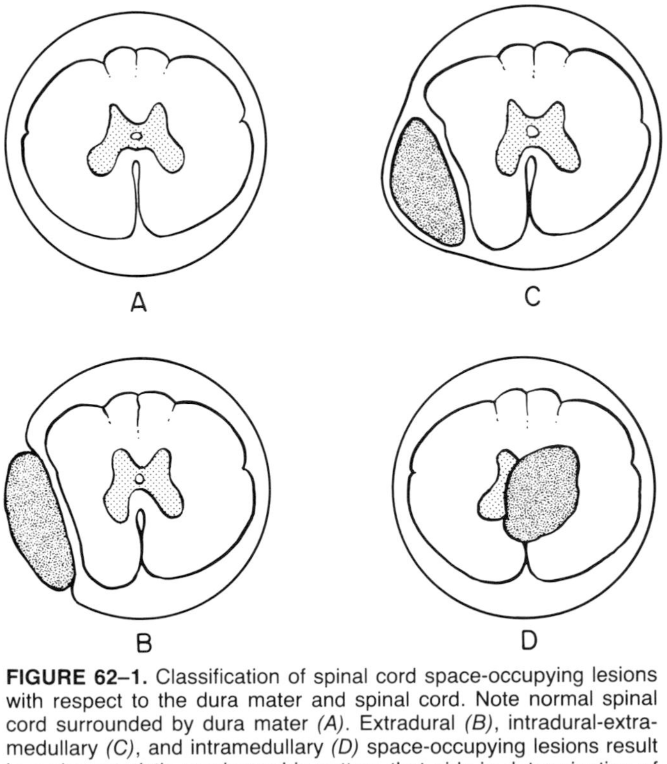

FIGURE 62–1. Classification of spinal cord space-occupying lesions with respect to the dura mater and spinal cord. Note normal spinal cord surrounded by dura mater *(A)*. Extradural *(B)*, intradural-extramedullary *(C)*, and intramedullary *(D)* space-occupying lesions result in a characteristic myelographic pattern that aids in determination of exact location of a lesion.

Electromyographic examination may be used to define the extent of a lesion affecting the brachial or lumbar enlargement of the spinal cord.[21, 22] This may be accomplished by mapping the distribution of EMG abnormalities caused by denervation in muscles of a thoracic or pelvic limb, and by correlating this information with the spinal nerve root origins of the nerves that supply the affected muscles of a limb.[21] As it is possible by means of EMG to distinguish between disuse atrophy and atrophy that occurs secondary to denervation, such electrophysiologic findings may be valuable in precisely defining location and extent of a spinal cord lesion.[23]

Sensory or motor nerve conduction velocities may be measured in either a thoracic or pelvic limb of dogs or cats.[24] The results of such studies may also aid in identification of nerve roots affected by a spinal cord disorder. Spinal cord potentials (cord dorsum potentials) evoked by stimulation of a peripheral sensory nerve may be used in combination with sensory nerve conduction velocity determinations to determine involvement of sensory nerve roots proximal to the dorsal root ganglia.[25]

Percutaneously recorded evoked spinal cord potentials may provide a method for the localization of spinal cord lesions in dogs or cats, as is the case in humans.[25, 26] Furthermore, such studies may provide a noninvasive method for ascertaining the severity of a lesion, determining an accurate prognosis, and evaluating the response to therapy.

A variety of pressure, flow, and electrophysiologic techniques have been developed to assess the function of the lower urinary tract.[6] Cystometry, urethral closure pressure profile recording, electromyography of urethral sphincter, uroflowmetry, and evoked spinal cord potential measurements following pudendal nerve stimulation have all been investigated in dogs or cats.[6] Combinations of these electrophysiologic tests may provide information regarding the functional status of spinal cord segments involved in micturition.

Additional Diagnostic Techniques. There are several additional diagnostic techniques that may be used for the accurate localization of a spinal cord disorder.[6]

Linear tomography is a radiographic technique that may be used to cause selective blurring of images of superimposed objects, while maintaining some degree of image sharpness relative to a structure of concern.[27, 28] This is accomplished by coordinating tube-film movement about a central pivot point and thus requires specialized radiographic equipment. Since tomography is used to eliminate distracting shadows of superimposed structures, it is of value in assessment of complex objects such as the vertebral column. The lumbosacral junction, with overlying bodies of the ileum, and the thoracic vertebral column, with overlying ribs, are regions of the spine in which linear tomography has particular application in vertebral radiography.

Other diagnostic techniques currently in use for the diagnosis of disorders affecting the vertebral column include epidurography, transosseous vertebral sinus venography, and diskography.[6] These techniques are discussed further under the section entitled lumbosacral vertebral canal stenosis.

X-ray computed tomography (CT) and magnetic resonance imaging (MRI) are being used with increasing frequency in the diagnosis of spinal cord disorders of dogs and cats.[9] These techniques will aid in the accurate determination of location and extent of spinal cord diseases in the future.

CLINICAL SIGNS OF SPINAL CORD DISEASES

A complete neurologic examination is described in Chapter 60. Complete assessment of an animal's gait and posture, postural reactions, spinal reflexes, cranial nerve function, and state of consciousness is essential in determining the presence or absence of spinal cord disease, the most likely location(s) of a spinal cord lesion, and whether a focal, multifocal, or disseminated disease process is present involving the spinal cord and/or other parts of the nervous system.[8]

Bailey and Morgan describe five groups of clinical signs that are seen to a varying degree in all animals that have a disease affecting the spinal cord.[4] These clinical signs are depression or loss of voluntary movement, alteration of spinal reflexes, changes of muscle tone, muscle atrophy, and sensory dysfunction. Careful assessment of each of these groups of clinical signs in an animal suspected to have a disease affecting the spinal cord facilitates lesion localization and diagnosis. Neurologic disorders that result in either loss of voluntary movement alone or sensory dysfunction alone are unlikely to be spinal cord disorders, as the majority of spinal cord diseases do not affect selected tracts while sparing anatomically adjacent pathways.

Diseases of the spinal cord may also result in dysfunction of bladder, urethral sphincter and anal sphincter, and in loss of voluntary control of urination and defecation.[5] This may be due to interruption of spinal cord pathways connecting brain stem and cerebrum to bladder and rectum that are important in normal detrusor reflex function and voluntary control of micturition and defecation, or may be due to interruption of the parasympathetic nerve supply to the bladder and urinary and anal sphincters (L7 to S3 spinal cord segments and spinal nerves). Spinal cord diseases also indirectly interfere with excretory functions by impairing the ability of an animal to assume the posture necessary for normal defecation or urination.

Voluntary Movement. Loss of voluntary movements due to interruption of motor pathways at any point from cerebrum to muscle fibers is referred to as paralysis (plegia). Lesser degrees of motor loss are referred to as paresis (or weakness). The terms tetraplegia (or quadriplegia) and tetraparesis (or quadriparesis) refer to absence of voluntary movements in thoracic and pelvic limbs and weakness of movements in thoracic and pelvic limbs, respectively. The terms paraplegia and paraparesis describe absence of voluntary movements and depression of voluntary movements in only the pelvic limbs. Hemiplegia and hemiparesis refer to paralysis or motor dysfunction, respectively, of a pelvic limb and a thoracic limb on the same side.[1, 4]

Voluntary movements must be differentiated from reflex movements on the basis of neurologic examination findings and general observations.

Ataxia (incoordination) is seen in association with paresis, and probably occurs due to interference with both ascending and descending spinal cord pathways. Many ascending spinal cord tracts contribute to the transmission of sensory information to the cerebrum for coordination of voluntary movements; however, interference with the spinocerebellar tracts probably causes a large part of the ataxia seen in association with spinal cord disease in animals. It must be remembered that observation of gait is the only means available for clinical testing of these pathways.

Spinal Reflexes. Spinal reflexes are stereotyped involuntary responses that occur independently of the brain, and can be elicited regularly by specific stimuli.[29] The central nervous system (CNS) components of spinal reflex arcs are located entirely within the spinal cord. Disturbance of spinal reflexes occurs in almost all animals with spinal cord disease. A spinal reflex may be normal, depressed (hyporeflexia) or absent (areflexia), or exaggerated (hyperreflexia).[9] Classification of spinal reflexes into one of these three categories is essential for localization of a spinal cord lesion.

Depression of a spinal reflex in association with spinal cord disease most frequently occurs as a result of involvement by a pathologic process of spinal cord segments mediating the reflex.[4] It must be remembered that involvement of motor nerves arising from, or sensory nerves traveling to, such spinal cord segments, or abnormalities of the effector organ (muscle), may also result in depression of spinal reflexes.

Exaggeration of a spinal reflex in association with spinal cord disease occurs when a lesion affects the spinal cord cranial to segments that mediate a reflex. Neural mechanisms that result in spinal reflex exaggeration are not completely understood.[4] The concept that reflex exaggeration simply results from interruption of descending inhibitory pathways is useful in the exercise of lesion localization; however, other factors are likely to be involved, such as collateral axonal sprouting or the development of denervation supersensitivity.[30, 31] It is important to remember that reflex exaggeration may result from a brain lesion as well as from a spinal cord lesion.

Spinal cord lesions that affect both gray and white matter may result in depression of spinal reflexes mediated by spinal cord segments involved in a pathologic process, and in exaggeration of spinal cord reflexes mediated by spinal cord segments caudal to a lesion.[9] This is useful in lesion localization, particularly for a lesion that affects the cervical enlargement (C6 to T2 spinal cord segments), where thoracic limb hyporeflexia and pelvic limb hyperreflexia may be present.

Interpretation of reflex abnormalities must be approached with the knowledge that two (or more) lesions located within the same anatomic division of the spinal cord may result in reflex changes identical to those produced by a single lesion.[9] For example, two lesions between T3 and L3 spinal cord segments cause hyperreflexia in the pelvic limbs that is indistinguishable from that resulting from a solitary lesion in this location. Further, hyporeflexia produced by one spinal cord lesion may mask hyperreflexia that would otherwise result from a second lesion in a more cranial location.[9] For example, a lesion in the lumbar enlargement (L4 to S3 spinal cord segments) causes hyporeflexia in the pelvic limbs that masks the hyperreflexia that otherwise results from a second lesion cranial to the L4 spinal cord segment.

Depression of spinal reflexes caudal to a lesion may be seen for several days following spinal cord injury in humans or primates. This phenomenon is called spinal shock. Sudden withdrawal of suprasegmental facilitation has been stated to be the likely cause.[32] It is apparent that spinal shock occurs in quadrupeds; however, it is too brief in duration to be of clinical significance.[33] Hyporeflexia observed immediately following spinal cord injury should be attributed to damage to spinal cord segments mediating the reflexes, or to other systemic complications, such as hypovolemic shock, that frequently accompany spinal cord trauma.

Muscle Tone. Maintenance of normal muscle tone is a function of spinal reflexes (tonic muscle stretch reflexes).[4] Alterations of muscle tone are therefore interpreted in a similar fashion to that for alterations in spinal reflexes described above. Abnormal muscle tone may be depressed (hypotonia), absent (atonia), or exaggerated (hypertonia), depending on the location of a spinal cord lesion.

Muscle Atrophy. Two types of muscle atrophy may occur in association with a spinal cord disease. Denervation atrophy is seen when α motor neurons (LMNs) that innervate a muscle are damaged by a lesion affecting their spinal cord segment(s) of origin.[4] Denervation atrophy is evident within a week of injury, usually is severe, and is associated with EMG abnormalities. Disuse atrophy may be seen in muscles innervated by LMNs caudal to a spinal cord lesion. Disuse atrophy usually is slower in onset and progression than denervation atrophy, most often is less severe in character, and is not associated with EMG alterations.

Sensory Dysfunction. Abnormalities of sensory (ascending) pathways of the spinal cord contribute to the ataxia of spinal cord disease; however, specific clinical tests of their function do not exist. Perception in animals must be inferred from certain behavioral responses that indicate ascending sensory signals have reached the cerebral cortex (e.g., aversive response to a noxious stimulus). Interruption of sensory signals at any point between (and including) sensory receptors in the periphery and cerebral cortex may depress or obliterate normal sensory function. Therefore, results of clinical examination for signs of sensory dysfunction alone may not be of value in localizing a lesion to the spinal cord. However, when combined with results of other parts of a neurologic examination, signs of sensory dysfunction can provide important diagnostic and prognostic information.[4]

Conscious proprioception (perception of body position or movement) and pain perception are tested during a neurologic examination. Conscious proprioception is a sensitive indicator of spinal cord function, and depression or loss of conscious proprioception frequently is the sign first produced by a myelopathy.

Pain perception may be normal, depressed (hypesthesia) or absent (anesthesia), or exaggerated (hyperesthesia). Two types of pain perception are sometimes distinguished in animals. Cutaneous ("superficial") pain perception is manifested by a response to pricking or pinching of the skin, and deep pain perception is manifested by reaction to pinching the toes or tail across bone with hemostatic forceps. Areas of decreased or absent cutaneous pain perception may aid in identification of specific nerves, nerve roots, and spinal cord segments involved in a pathologic process. This technique of cutaneous mapping is especially useful in lesions that affect the cervical or lumbar enlargements.[23]

Deep pain perception appears to be the sensory function that is most resistant to a spinal cord disease, and is the last spinal cord function to disappear in myelopathies of any type. An animal with a complete bilateral loss of deep pain perception due to a transverse myelopathy is necessarily paralyzed caudal to the lesion. Therefore, loss of deep pain perception is a very grave prognostic sign.[4]

Hyperesthesia in association with a spinal cord disease may indicate nerve root or spinal nerve involvement, or may be consistent with meningeal irritation.[4] A focal area of hyperesthesia over the vertebral column may indicate the location of a spinal cord lesion.

LOCALIZATION OF SPINAL CORD DISEASES

Motor, sensory, reflex, and sphincter abnormalities may be used to determine the location of a lesion within one of four major longitudinal divisions of the spinal cord. The divisions are cervical (C1 to C5 spinal cord segments), cervical enlargement (C6 to T2), thoracolumbar (T3 to L3), and lumbar enlargement (L4 to Cd5) (Figure 62–2).[10] It is essential to remember that these divisions refer to spinal cord segments, not vertebrae, and that spinal cord segments do not correspond exactly with vertebrae of the same number (Figure 62–3).[34] Some variations may be encountered due to slight differences between animals in segments that form cervical and lumbar enlargements. The diseases most commonly associated with neurologic signs referable to each of these four regions are listed in Tables 62–1 through 62–4.

A disorder of each of the four regions of the spinal cord results in a combination of neurologic signs that is specific for the region involved. Recognition of a characteristic group of clinical signs therefore allows accurate localization of a spinal cord lesion.[10] This concept of neurologic syndromes as a basis for lesion localization has been recommended by several authors.[5, 6, 10] The presence of neurologic deficits indicative of involvement of more than one region of the spinal cord is highly

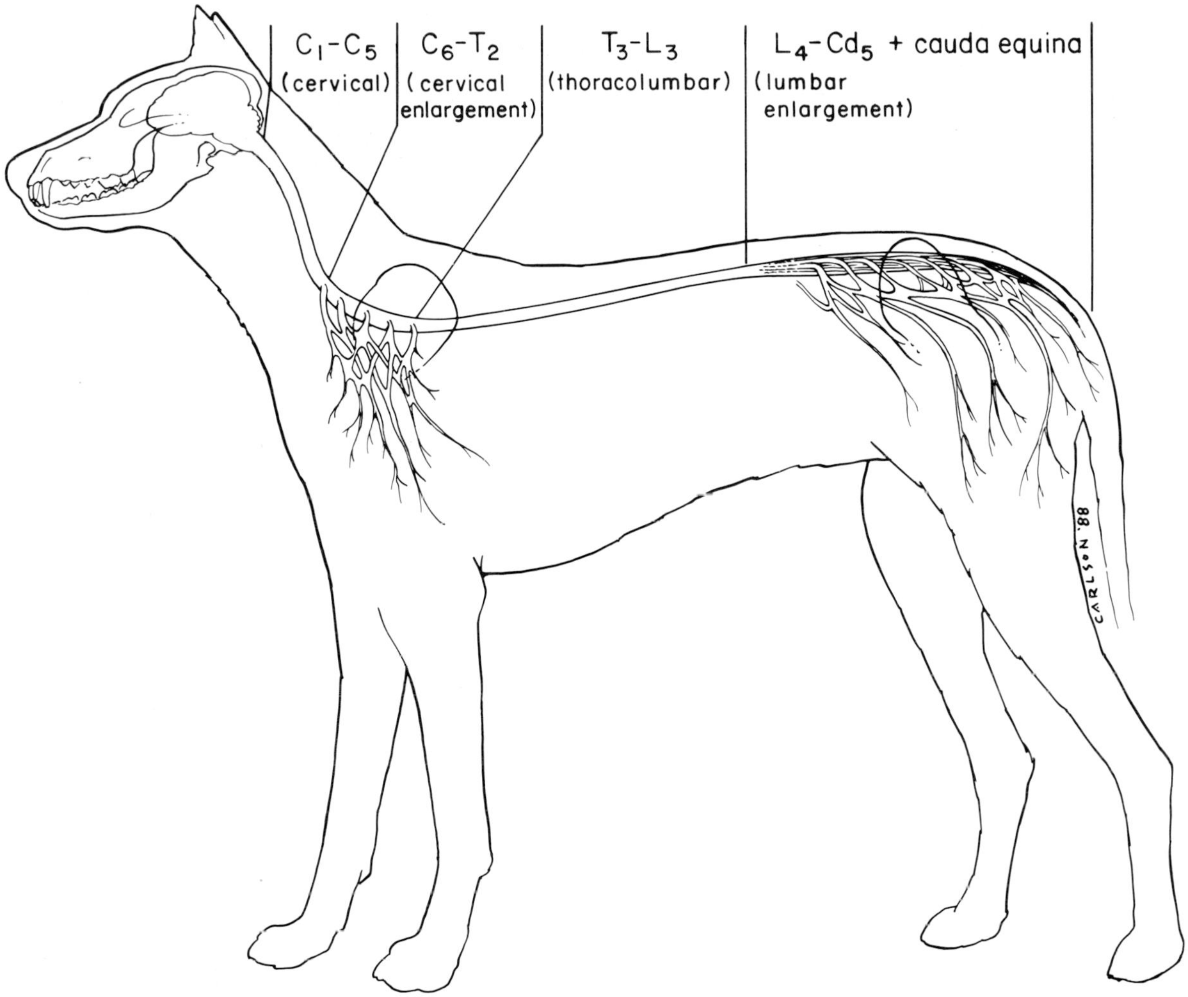

FIGURE 62–2. Regional divisions of the spinal cord.

suggestive of multifocal or disseminated spinal cord disease.

The functional differences between upper motor neurons (UMNs) and LMNs may be used to localize lesions to one of the functional regions of the spinal cord (Table 62–5).[1, 4]

Cell bodies of spinal cord LMNs are located in the spinal cord gray matter. Their axons leave the spinal cord via the ventral nerve roots to become part of a peripheral nerve, and to terminate on a muscle. The LMNs of the thoracic limb have their cell bodies in C6 to T2 spinal cord segments that form the cervical enlargement, while LMNs of the pelvic limb arise from the L4 through S1 spinal cord segments of the lumbar enlargement. Anal and urethral sphincter LMNs originate from S1 through S3 spinal cord segments. Signs of

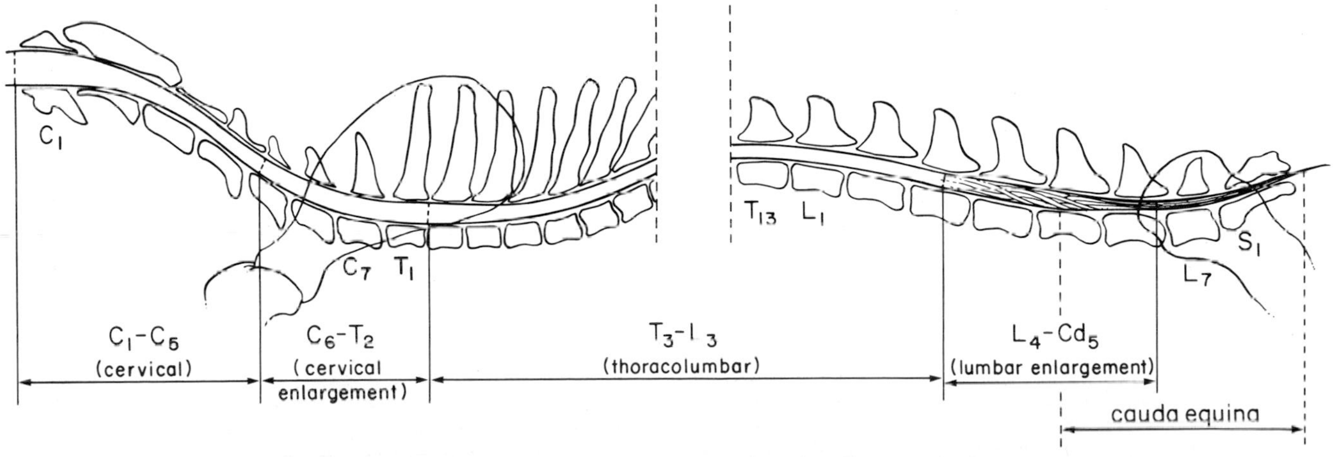

FIGURE 62–3. Anatomic relationship of spinal cord segments and vertebral segments.

TABLE 62–5. SUMMARY OF NEUROLOGIC DEFICITS EXPECTED WITH A LESION IN EACH OF THE FOUR REGIONAL DIVISIONS OF THE SPINAL CORD

	Cervical (C1–C5 Spinal Cord Segments)	Cervical Enlargement (C6–T2 Spinal Cord Segments)	Thoracolumbar (T3–L3 Spinal Cord Segments)	Lumbar Enlargement (L4–Cd5 Spinal Cord Segments + Cauda Equina)
Upper motor neuron (UMN) or Lower motor neuron (LMN) signs	Pelvic limbs: UMN Thoracic limbs: UMN	Pelvic limbs: UMN Thoracic limbs: LMN	Pelvic limbs: UMN Thoracic limbs: normal	Pelvic limbs: LMN Thoracic limbs: normal
Meningeal/nerve root signs	Apparent cervical pain, rigidity, spasms in cervical muscles.	Apparent cervical pain, rigidity, thoracic limb lameness, "root signature."	Apparent back pain, may be focal area of hyperesthesia.	Apparent lumbar or lumbosacral pain; may be focal area of hyperesthesia, pelvic limb lameness, pain on sitting or rising.
Voluntary movement	Tetraparesis or hemiparesis Tetraplegia or hemiplegia	Tetraparesis or hemiparesis. May be primarily paraparesis. Tetraplegia or hemiplegia.	Paraparesis or paraplegia. Normal voluntary movement in thoracic limbs.	Paraparesis or paraplegia. Paralysis of the tail. Normal voluntary movement in thoracic limbs.
Muscle tone/atrophy	Normal or increased muscle tone in all 4 limbs. Disuse atrophy of muscles of all 4 limbs in chronic conditions.	Normal or increased muscle tone in pelvic limbs. Decreased, normal, or increased tone in thoracic limbs. Denervation atrophy may be present in thoracic limb(s). Disuse atrophy of all 4 limbs in chronic conditions.	Normal or increased muscle tone in pelvic limbs. Normal tone in thoracic limbs (except when Schiff-Sherrington sign present). Disuse atrophy of the pelvic limbs in chronic conditions.	Normal or decreased muscle tone in pelvic limbs and tail. Normal tone in thoracic limbs (except when Schiff-Sherrington sign present). Denervation atrophy may be present in pelvic limb(s).
Spinal reflexes	Normal or exaggerated spinal reflexes in all 4 limbs. Normal panniculus reflex. Normal anal reflexes.	Normal or exaggerated spinal reflexes in pelvic limbs. Normal, decreased, or absent spinal reflexes in thoracic limbs. Normal, decreased, or absent panniculus reflex. Normal anal reflexes.	Normal or exaggerated spinal reflexes in pelvic limbs. Normal spinal reflexes in thoracic limbs. Panniculus reflex may be decreased or absent caudal to lesion (for lesions cranial to L2-L3). Normal or exaggerated anal reflexes.	Normal, decreased, or absent spinal reflexes in the pelvic limbs. May be pseudoexaggeration of patellar reflexes with lesions caudal to L5. Normal spinal reflexes in thoracic limbs. Normal panniculus reflex. Normal, decreased, or absent anal reflexes.
Sensory dysfunction	Ataxia of all 4 limbs. Conscious proprioception and postural reactions depressed or absent in all 4 limbs or ipsilateral thoracic and pelvic limbs. Cutaneous sensation and deep pain perception usually normal.	Ataxia of all 4 limbs or pelvic limbs only. Conscious proprioception and postural reactions decreased or absent in all 4 limbs, ipsilateral thoracic and pelvic limbs, *or* pelvic limbs only. Cutaneous sensation and deep pain perception may be normal, decreased, or absent in thoracic and pelvic limb(s).	Ataxia of pelvic limbs. Conscious proprioception and postural reactions decreased or absent in pelvic limb(s). Cutaneous sensation and deep pain perception may be normal, decreased, or absent in pelvic limb(s) and tail. Sensory function normal in thoracic limbs.	Ataxia of pelvic limbs. Conscious proprioception and postural reactions decreased or absent in pelvic limb(s). Cutaneous sensation and deep pain perception may be normal, decreased, or absent in pelvic limb(s) ± perineum and tail. Sensory function normal in thoracic limbs.
Urination/defecation	May be loss of voluntary control of urination and defecation, detrusor areflexia, and urinary sphincter hypertonus or reflex dyssynergia.	Similar to C1–C5.	Similar to C1–C5.	May be urinary and/or fecal incontinence, flaccid anus and/or large, distended, and easily expressed bladder.
Other signs	Severe lesions result in respiratory paralysis. May be unilateral Horner's syndrome (unusual). Cranial cervical lesions may result in positional strabismus, facial hyperesthesia, or caudal brainstem dysfunction.	Unilateral Horner's syndrome. May be paralysis of diaphragm.	Schiff-Sherrington sign.	Schiff-Sherrington sign.

LMN dysfunction, which in diseases affecting the spinal cord reflect damage to the spinal cord segment(s) from which LMNs originate, are depression or loss of voluntary motor activity, depression or loss of muscle tone, and rapid, severe atrophy of an affected muscle due to denervation.[1, 4]

Upper motor neurons arise from cell bodies located in the brain. Their axons form descending pathways of the spinal cord, and terminate on interneurons that in turn synapse with LMNs. Lesions affecting UMNs result in UMN signs. These UMN signs result from an increase in the excitatory state of LMNs. Upper motor neuron signs include depression or loss of voluntary motor activity, normal or exaggerated segmental spinal reflexes, appearance of abnormal spinal reflexes (e.g., crossed extensor reflex), increased muscle tone, and muscle atrophy due to disuse.[1, 4]

Unilateral signs resulting from spinal cord disease are unusual; however, signs frequently are asymmetric. In the majority of cases, a lesion resulting in asymmetric signs is located on the side of greater motor and sensory deficit. Signs most commonly recognized in association with a lesion of each of the major spinal cord regions are summarized in Table 62–5.

Cervical (C1 to C5). Fatal respiratory paralysis resulting from interruption of descending respiratory motor pathways or damage to motor neurons of the phrenic nerve (C5 to C7 spinal cord segments) occurs in a complete transverse myelopathy. Lesions that are less than complete may not affect respiration, and in such cases other signs may be detectable.

Ataxia and paresis of all four limbs usually are seen. Tetraplegia rarely is seen, as lesions of sufficient severity to cause tetraplegia also produce respiratory paralysis. Hemiparesis occasionally may be present in association with a cervical lesion. Lesions of the cervical spinal cord may result in paraparesis with minimal neurologic deficits in thoracic limbs. The reasons for this are poorly understood.

Spinal reflexes and muscle tone are intact in all limbs, and may be normal or exaggerated. Muscle atrophy generally is not present; however, disuse atrophy may develop in cases that have a chronic course. Anal reflexes are intact and anal tone usually is normal. Bladder dysfunction may occur due to detrusor muscle areflexia, with normal or increased urinary sphincter tone, and loss of voluntary control of micturition. Reflex dyssynergia may also be seen. Although voluntary control of defecation may be lost, reflex defecation occurs when feces are present in the rectum.

Horner's syndrome (ptosis, miosis, and enophthalmos) rarely may be present in an animal with a severe destructive cervical lesion.

Conscious proprioception and other postural reactions usually are depressed or absent in all limbs. Complete loss of conscious proprioception may be present without detectable loss of pain perception.

Cervical hyperesthesia ("spasms," apparent pain on palpation, cervical rigidity, and abnormal neck posture) may be seen in some animals with cervical myelopathy. Occasionally an animal may hold a thoracic limb in a partially flexed position, a posture that may be consistent with C1 to C5 nerve root or spinal nerve entrapment ("root signature"), although this posture is seen more commonly with a disorder of the cervical enlargement.

Disorders that affect the cervical region of the spinal cord must be differentiated from brain lesions that result in tetraparesis. This can be accomplished by doing a complete neurologic examination; however, occasionally this distinction can be difficult. In most circumstances a cervical lesion does not result in neurologic deficits attributable to involvement of the medulla oblongata; however, there are several notable exceptions to this rule.[4] Positional strabismus, resulting from loss of the vertebral joint proprioceptive input to the attitudinal reflexes, may be seen in association with a cranial cervical lesion (C1 to C3 spinal cord segments). A cranial cervical lesion may also cause facial hypesthesia as a result of involvement of the spinal nucleus and tract of the trigeminal nerve. Cranial cervical trauma often results in clinical signs referable to injury to the caudal brain stem (head tilt, pharyngeal paresis, facial paresis) or cerebellum.

The Schiff-Sherrington sign (syndrome or phenomenon) consists of hypertonicity of thoracic limb muscles and hyperextension of the neck, and is seen in association with spinal cord lesions caudal to the cervical enlargement. It is essential to differentiate this sign from thoracic limb hypertonicity caused by a cervical lesion.

Cervical Enlargement (C6 to T2). Ataxia and paresis of all four limbs usually are present. Occasionally paresis of thoracic limbs and paralysis of pelvic limbs may be seen.

Spinal reflexes and muscle tone may be normal or depressed in thoracic limbs, and normal or exaggerated in pelvic limbs. The nature of thoracic limb reflex alterations depends on the exact craniocaudal location of a lesion within this region. Muscle atrophy often is severe in thoracic limbs. Panniculus reflex may be depressed or absent unilaterally or bilaterally due to interruption of the LMNs involved in this reflex (C8 and T1 spinal cord segments).

If bladder dysfunction occurs, it is similar to that observed with a lesion in the cervical region, with loss of voluntary control of urination. Anal reflexes and anal tone most often are normal although voluntary control of defecation may be absent.

Unilateral Horner's syndrome is commonly observed with a spinal cord lesion of the cervical enlargement, particularly a lesion involving T1 to T3 spinal cord segments or nerve roots.

Conscious proprioception and other postural reactions usually are depressed in all four limbs. Alterations in these functions may be more pronounced in the pelvic limbs than in thoracic limbs. Occasionally, conscious proprioception is absent only in a thoracic and pelvic limb on the same side.

Severe depression or loss of pain perception rarely is seen in association with a lesion of the cervical enlargement, except in intrinsic myelopathies (e.g., ischemic myelopathy). There may be hyperesthesia at the level of a lesion of the cervical enlargement, thoracic limb lameness, or apparent neck pain.

Thoracolumbar (T3 to L3). The majority of spinal cord lesions of dogs or cats occur in this region. Typically thoracic limb gait is normal, and paresis and ataxia, or paralysis, are seen in pelvic limbs.

Thoracic limb spinal reflexes are normal. Pelvic limb spinal reflexes and muscle tone are normal to exaggerated, depending on the severity of the lesion. Muscle atrophy is not seen in thoracic limbs. Pelvic limb muscle atrophy, if present, is the result of disuse and is seen in animals with a severe, chronic lesion.

Anal reflexes and anal tone usually are normal or exaggerated. Voluntary control of defecation may be lost. Reflex defecation occurs when the rectum is filled with feces; however, it may not be at an appropriate time or place. Degree of bladder dysfunction varies depending on the severity of a spinal cord lesion. There may be loss of voluntary control of urination, detrusor muscle areflexia with normal or increased urinary sphincter tone, or reflex dyssynergia in which initiation of voiding occurs and is stopped by involuntary contraction of the urethral sphincter. The bladder can be manually expressed in some animals, but not in others due to increased tone of the urinary bladder sphincter. This is often referred to as a "UMN bladder." Although "overflow" incontinence may occur with lesions of the spinal cord in this region secondary to overfilling of the bladder, detrusor muscle tone and urinary sphincter tone are present, distinguishing this type of incontinence from that due to lesions of the lumbar enlargement and cauda equina ("LMN bladder").[5]

Conscious proprioception and other postural reactions are normal in the thoracic limbs, and depressed or absent in the pelvic limbs.

Pain perception is normal in the thoracic limbs and may be normal, depressed, or absent in the pelvic limbs. Panniculus reflex may be reduced or absent caudal to a lesion. In the lumbar region the panniculus reflex may be present in lesions caudal to L3 due to the pattern of cutaneous innervation of lumbar spinal nerves.[35] There may be an area of hyperesthesia at the level of a lesion.

The Schiff-Sherrington sign may be seen with a lesion in this region. Usually it is an indication of an acute and severe spinal cord lesion, although such a lesion may be reversible.

Lumbar Enlargement (L4 to Cd5) and Cauda Equina. Involvement of this region by a pathologic process results in varying degrees of pelvic limb paresis and ataxia, or paralysis, and is often accompanied by dysfunction of bladder and by paresis or paralysis of anal sphincter and tail. Thoracic limb function is normal.

Pelvic limb reflexes and muscle tone are reduced or absent. Muscle atrophy often is present in pelvic limbs. Conscious proprioception and other postural reactions are reduced or absent in pelvic limbs.

Anal tone and anal reflexes are reduced or absent. The rectum and colon may become distended with feces, and fecal incontinence, with continual leakage of feces, is often seen. Constipation may result from the inability to void feces. Paresis or paralysis of the urethral sphincters and detrusor muscle result in overfilling of the bladder and "overflow" incontinence. Affected animals have a large residual volume of urine in the bladder, and the bladder is easily expressed manually.

The Schiff-Sherrington sign occasionally may be seen with an acute lesion affecting this region of the spinal cord.

The term cauda equina is used to describe the lumbar, sacral, and caudal nerve roots and spinal nerves as they extend caudally from the caudal tip (conus medullaris) of the spinal cord within the vertebral canal. Lesions that affect cauda equina result in clinical signs that are indistinguishable from lesions that affect the spinal cord segments from which the nerves of the cauda equina arise (L6 to Cd5).

ALPHABETICAL LISTING OF DISEASES

Atlantoaxial Subluxation (Atlantoaxial Instability) and Malformations of the Odontoid Process

Etiology and Pathogenesis. Subluxation, instability, or malformation of the atlantoaxial joint that permits excessive flexion of the joint may result in compression of the spinal cord due to dorsal displacement of the cranial portion of the body of the axis into the vertebral canal. These conditions may result from congenital or developmental abnormalities, trauma, or a combination.[36, 37]

The axis arises from six or seven centers of ossification.[38] The cranial epiphysis develops between the body of the axis and the odontoid process (dens). An accessory center for the apex of the dens is present in many dogs. Ossification centers of the dens and cranial epiphysis of the axis normally do not unite until a dog is between seven and nine months of age.[38] The pathogenesis of malformation of the odontoid process is unknown; however, it may result from a degenerative process similar to that occurring in necrosis of the femoral head in small breeds of dog.[8]

Agenesis or hypoplasia of the dens, non-union of the dens with the axis (odontoid process dysplasia), and dorsal angulation of the odontoid process with compression of the spinal cord have been associated with atlantoaxial instability in dogs.[39–43]

Normally, the dens is attached to the atlas by two ligaments, the transverse ligament of the atlas and the dorsal atlantoaxial ligament. The transverse ligament is structurally more important, and extends from one side of the body of the atlas to the other. The transverse ligament crosses the dorsal aspect of the dens, and helps to maintain the dorsoventral alignment of atlas and axis. The dens is normally attached to the occipital bone by an apical and two lateral (alar) ligaments. Lack of ligamentous support for the atlantoaxial joint, with progressive stretching and weakening of the dorsal atlantoaxial ligament, may occur in combination with normal development of the dens. Insufficient ligamentous support of the atlantoaxial joint resulting in atlantoaxial instability may occur in any breed of dog.

Traumatic atlantoaxial luxation occurs in all breeds of dog or cat[44] and usually results from rupture of the atlantoaxial ligaments or fracture of the dens at its junction with the axis. Onset of signs is usually acute, and coincides with the trauma; however, occasionally the onset of signs is delayed. Traumatic atlanto-occipital luxation and instability have been described in dogs.[45, 46]

Hyperextension of the head may be the cause of this injury.[45] Of the three dogs described, mild neurologic deficits and cervical pain were present in two, and vestibular abnormalities and tetraparesis were seen in one.

Clinical Findings. Congenital or developmental malformations occur most frequently in toy or miniature breeds of dog; however, they may rarely occur in any breed. Animals with congenital or developmental abnormalities of the atlantoaxial joint usually develop clinical signs during the first year of life, although clinical signs may occur at any age (Figure 62–4). Occasionally a dog with a congenital atlantoaxial abnormality may be normal until slight trauma occurs at an older age, at which time clinical signs may occur. These animals are often presented with a history of minor trauma.

Clinical signs associated with congenital atlantoaxial instability may have an acute onset, may be slowly progressive or may be intermittent. Signs are indicative of a transverse myelopathy between C1 and C5. Traumatic atlantoaxial luxation may occur in animals of any age. Clinical signs associated with traumatic atlantoaxial instability are usually acute in onset. Signs vary from reluctance to be patted on the head and cervical pain to tetraparesis or tetraplegia.[8] Severe spinal cord trauma as a result of atlantoaxial luxation may result in death due to respiratory paralysis. Rarely following atlantoaxial subluxation, hemorrhage and edema may ascend the medulla and result in dysphagia, facial paralysis, vestibular deficits, opisthotonos, or death.[47] Abnormalities in alignment of the atlas and axis may be palpable.

Atlanto-occipital luxation results in trauma to the medulla oblongata and clinical signs indicative of a caudal brain stem or cranial cervical spinal cord injury. Severe injuries may result in respiratory paralysis and death.

Diagnosis. As the clinical appearance of an animal with atlantoaxial subluxation may resemble that in other cervical myelopathies, diagnosis is made on the basis of radiographic findings. Atlantoaxial instability is best demonstrated by means of a lateral radiographic projection of the cervical spine with the neck in slight ventroflexion. Radiographically the body of the axis is displaced dorsally and cranially into the vertebral canal and the distance between the dorsal arch of the atlas and spinous process of the axis is increased (Figure 62–5). If preliminary views are not diagnostic of atlantoaxial instability, slight flexion of the head may be necessary. As muscle tone in the neck helps support atlantoaxial alignment, radiographs may be completed without anesthesia in a cooperative animal. Extreme care must be taken when manipulating an animal suspected of having atlantoaxial instability under anesthesia or during radiography, as flexion of the animal's neck may result in further spinal cord compression. Splinting the animal's neck and head in extension prior to anesthesia helps in preventing excessive flexion of the head during induction of anesthesia, intubation, and positioning for radiography. Abnormalities of the dens may be seen on ventrodorsal views or slightly oblique lateral views (such that the wings of the atlas are not superimposed on the dens). An open-mouth view may show agenesis, nonunion, or fracture of the dens[48]; however, the degree of cervical flexion required for completion of this view may result in further spinal cord compression. Therefore obtaining an open-mouth view usually is not recommended.

Animals with congenital or developmental abnormal-

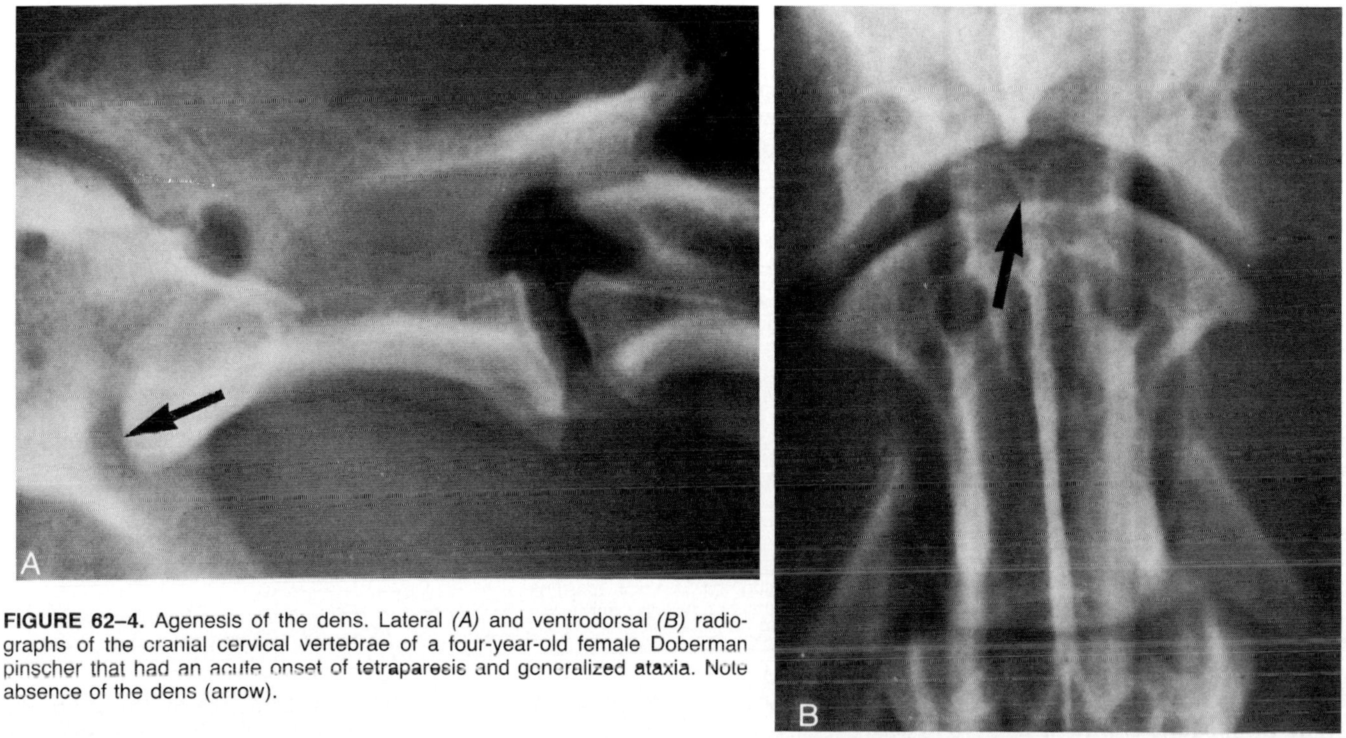

FIGURE 62–4. Agenesis of the dens. Lateral *(A)* and ventrodorsal *(B)* radiographs of the cranial cervical vertebrae of a four-year-old female Doberman pinscher that had an acute onset of tetraparesis and generalized ataxia. Note absence of the dens (arrow).

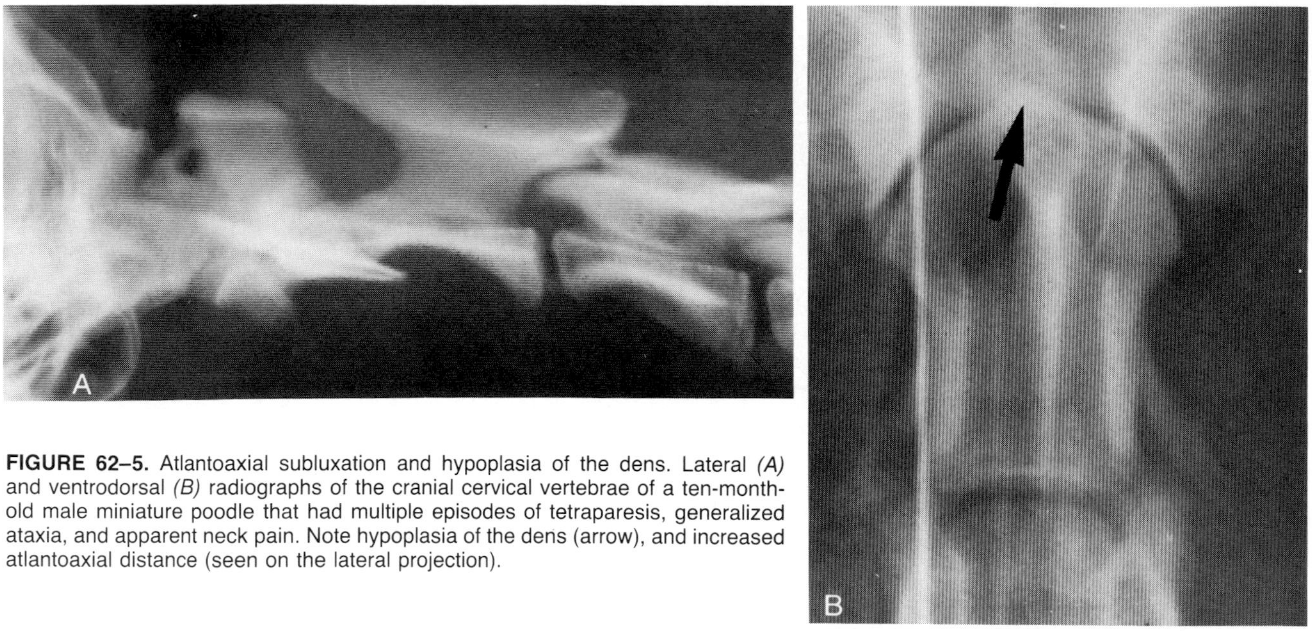

FIGURE 62–5. Atlantoaxial subluxation and hypoplasia of the dens. Lateral *(A)* and ventrodorsal *(B)* radiographs of the cranial cervical vertebrae of a ten-month-old male miniature poodle that had multiple episodes of tetraparesis, generalized ataxia, and apparent neck pain. Note hypoplasia of the dens (arrow), and increased atlantoaxial distance (seen on the lateral projection).

ities of C2 may have additional vertebral abnormalities such as shortening of C1 or abnormal atlanto-occipital articulation. Agenesis or malformation of the dens may be an incidental finding and is probably not of clinical significance unless associated with radiographic findings of atlantoaxial instability. However, spinal cord compression associated with hypoplasia of the dens without radiographic evidence of atlantoaxial instability has been reported in a dog.[41] Similarly, abnormal angulation of the dens may cause spinal cord compression. In these cases, myelography is necessary to demonstrate spinal cord compression.

Treatment. Animals with an acute onset of neurologic deficits resulting from atlantoaxial instability or traumatic atlanto-occipital luxation should be treated medically, as described for other forms of spinal cord trauma. In addition, the head and neck should be splinted in extension. Animals with mild luxations and cervical pain only or with minimal neurologic deficits, or animals with multiple vertebral abnormalities such as atlantoaxial instability and shortening of the body of C1, may respond to splinting of the head and neck in extension and strict cage rest for at least six weeks.[49] Casting material or a metal metacarpal splint may be used for this purpose. Care must be taken to ensure that respiration is not compromised. Splinting the head and neck allows formation of fibrous tissue to stabilize the atlantoaxial joint, and is most successful in small dogs. However, clinical signs may recur. A toy poodle with multiple anomalies of C1 and C2 was successfully managed by one of the authors for several years by means of a removable, firm, foam cervical collar that prevented excessive flexion of the neck. Manual reduction of atlanto-occipital dislocation and casting of the head in flexion for eight weeks has been used to treat affected dogs.[45]

Surgical stabilization and/or decompression is indicated in animals with moderate to severe neurologic deficits or recurrent episodes of neck pain unresponsive to medical therapy or splinting, and in animals in which angulation of the dens results in spinal cord compression. Various surgical techniques have been described, utilizing either a dorsal or a ventral approach.[50–58]

Dorsal stabilization may be achieved by use of stainless steel wire, nonabsorbable suture material, or nuchal ligament to attach the spinous process of the axis to the dorsal arch of the atlas. Hemilaminectomy may also be done by means of a dorsal approach if spinal cord decompression proves necessary. Dorsal stabilization is not without risk, as additional spinal cord trauma and respiratory arrest may result from passing stainless steel or nonabsorbable suture under the arch of C1, or from excessive flexion of the neck during surgery. Other problems encountered include breakage of the suture material or tearing of the suture material through the dorsal arch of C1 prior to adequate fibrous tissue formation and stabilization of the atlantoaxial joint. Modifications of the dorsal wiring technique have been reported.[39, 54]

A ventral approach to the atlantoaxial joint that utilizes a cancellous bone graft and a cross-pinning technique for stabilization has been described.[56] This technique provides a permanent fusion of the axis and atlas and therefore has advantages when compared to the dorsal technique. Fixation of the atlantoaxial joint via a ventral approach is especially indicated in animals in which the dorsal structures (such as the dorsal arch of the atlas, or the dorsal spinous process of the axis) cannot support fixation devices, or in cases in which odontoidectomy is necessary to achieve spinal cord decompression, such as angulation or malformation of the dens.[43] A neck brace is recommended for two to four weeks postoperatively. Complications encountered with the ventral approach include improper pin placement and pin migration. Pin migration may be prevented by molding polymethyl methacrylate around exposed portions of pins following placement. A modification of the ventral fixation technique using lag screw fixation in place of pins has been described.[59]

The prognosis for animals with atlantoaxial instability varies depending on the severity of spinal cord injury that occurs. Prognosis is fair to good for those with mild to moderate neurologic deficits and guarded for those with an acute onset of tetraplegia.

Bacterial, Fungal, Rickettsial, or Protothecal Meningomyelitis

Etiology and Pathogenesis. Bacterial or fungal meningitis and/or myelitis occur infrequently in dogs and cats. Several routes of infection exist. Direct implantation of organisms may occur following a bite wound, spinal puncture, or surgery, or may accompany migration of a foreign body such as a grass awn. Extension may occur from a focus of infection such as a paravertebral infection, diskospondylitis, or dermoid sinus, or from infection following tail docking. Infection may also result from hematogenous spread of systemic infection such as endocarditis. As clinical signs produced by bacterial or fungal agents depend more on the neural structures affected than on the agent responsible, these agents are discussed together.

Meningitis may be accompanied by infection of the underlying parenchyma of the spinal cord (myelitis). Meningitis and/or myelitis may be focal, multifocal, or disseminated in distribution and are frequently accompanied by meningoencephalitis. Pathologically, meningitis is characterized by infiltration of inflammatory cells into the leptomeninges. Inflammation may occur throughout the entire subarachnoid space of the brain and spinal cord. Myelitis is characterized by necrosis and infiltration of inflammatory cells within spinal cord parenchyma.

Bacteria that have been isolated from cats or dogs with meningitis and myelitis include *Staphylococcus aureus, S. epidermidis, S. albus, Pasteurella* sp, *Actinomyces,* and *Nocardia.*[60–65] Fungal infections have been caused by *Cryptococcus neoformans, Blastomyces dermatitidis, Histoplasma capsulatum,* and *Coccidioides immitis. Cryptococcus neoformans* is found ubiquitously and frequently causes infection in immunosuppressed animals.[66–69] Cryptococcosis is more common in cats than dogs and infection may result from extension of nasal infection through the cribriform plate. *Blastomyces, Histoplasma,* and *Coccidioides* infections are found in certain geographic areas in the United States and in such cases the CNS is infected by hematogenous spread.

Focal epidural infections have been reported to occur, generally as a result of migrating grass awns or penetrating wounds. Proliferation of inflammatory tissue may result in an extradural space-occupying lesion causing spinal cord compression and clinical signs of a transverse myelopathy.[63] Abscessation may occur within the spinal cord and may have the radiographic appearance of an intramedullary mass.

Rickettsial or protothecal infections may cause meningomyelitis similar in clinical presentation to that resulting from bacterial or fungal infection of the CNS. Ehrlichiosis *(Ehrlichia canis* infection) and Rocky Mountain spotted fever (RMSF, caused by *Rickettsia rickettsii)* may cause meningoencephalitis or meningomyelitis in dogs. Rocky Mountain spotted fever is transmitted primarily by two outdoor ticks *(Dermacentor variabilis* and *D. andersoni)*, while ehrlichiosis is transmitted by a tick that is frequently found inside houses *(Rhipicephalus sanguineus)*.[70] Acutely, both diseases may induce immune-mediated vasculitis in a variety of tissues including the CNS.[70] Borreliosis caused by *Borrelia burgdorferi* has been reported to occur in dogs, and may be expected to cause meningomyelitis as it does in humans.[71–73]

Prototheca wickerhamii and *Prototheca zopfii,* species of ubiquitous, colorless unicellular algae, have been isolated from pyogranulomatous lesions of the spinal cord and other organs.[74, 75] Protothecosis rarely occurs, and infection may depend on inadequate host immune response.

Clinical Findings

Bacterial or fungal infections. Clinical signs of meningitis include apparent spinal pain, hyperesthesia, and cervical or thoracolumbar rigidity, occasionally manifest as a "sawhorse" posture. Irritation of the numerous nerve endings in the meninges results in reflex muscle spasms when affected animals are stimulated. Fever is intermittent and is more likely to occur in association with concurrent bacteremia or disseminated fungal infection. Fever may occur in association with primary CNS infections due to presence of leukocytic pyrogens in the CSF or in the hypothalamic circulation.

Neurologic deficits are indicative of associated myelitis or radiculitis, and abnormalities depend on the location and extent of infection. Focal myelitis may result in signs of transverse myelopathy. Disseminated bacterial meningomyelitis often is associated with meningoencephalitis, and clinical signs usually are acute and rapidly progressive. Focal bacterial meningitis and/or myelitis and fungal meningomyelitis may be associated with development of more slowly progressive clinical signs.

Paraparesis and pelvic limb ataxia are common presenting signs in animals with cryptococcal meningitis and/or myelitis. Progressive paralysis of a single pelvic limb has been reported in two cats with cryptococcal infection of the lumbar spinal cord.[66] Cats with CNS cryptococcal infections may show an acute onset of clinical signs despite chronic destruction of nervous tissue.[66]

Clinical signs of bacterial or fungal meningitis and myelitis are indistinguishable from other causes of meningitis and myelitis in animals. Causes include granulomatous meningoencephalitis (GME), corticosteroid-responsive meningitis and necrotizing vasculitis of the meningeal arteries, canine distemper virus myelitis of dogs, and CNS toxoplasmosis and FIP meningomyelitis in cats. The differential diagnosis of meningitis also includes intervertebral disk protrusion (especially in the cervical spine), spinal fracture, diskospondylitis, polymyositis, and polyarthritis.

Rickettsial infections. Central depression is the most consistent clinical finding in dogs with rickettsial infection.[76] Other abnormalities indicative of spinal cord and/or meningeal involvement include paraparesis, tetraparesis, ataxia, and generalized or localized hyperesthesia.[76, 77] Cervical rigidity may occur in animals with RMSF.[76] Intermittent neck pain was the predominant clinical sign in two dogs with positive *E. canis* titers seen by these authors. Neurologic abnormalities indicative of cerebral involvement include vestibular disturbances, seizures, cerebellar abnormalities, and coma.[76] Other clinical signs that occur in dogs with rickettsial infections include listlessness, depression, fever, anorexia, lymphadenopathy, dyspnea, diarrhea, vomiting, hemorrhagic diathesis, and joint pain.[76, 78] Dogs of all ages may be infected and clinical signs are often indistinguishable from those of systemic viral infections (especially canine distemper), septicemia, and immune-mediated disorders.[78]

Protothecal infections. Clinical signs reported in dogs with CNS protothecosis have included ataxia, circling, and paresis or paralysis.[70] Only the cutaneous form of this disease has been reported in cats.[70]

Diagnosis of Bacterial and Fungal Infections. A diagnosis of bacterial or fungal meningitis and/or myelitis is made on the basis of results of CSF analysis, and isolation of a causative organism by culture of CSF. Clinical signs may reflect meningeal irritation or myelopathy that may be indistinguishable from signs caused by other noninfectious myelopathies such as intervertebral disk disease. Presence of fever or abnormal hemogram cannot be relied upon for diagnosis of meningitis/myelitis, as neither may be present in affected animals.

Bacterial or fungal meningitis has been reported to result in moderate to severe CSF pleocytosis. More than 5000 white blood cells/μl may be present in some cases. Polymorphonuclear (PMN) cells predominate. Mixed mononuclear and PMN pleocytosis occurs with fungal meningitis, and eosinophils may be present, especially in cases of cryptococcal meningitis (Figure 62–6).[68] The CSF appears turbid if the cell count is greater than 500 white blood cells/μl. In the experience of the authors, disseminated bacterial meningomyelitis is rarely recognized ante mortem in dogs or cats. Focal bacterial epidural, meningeal, or parenchymal infections more commonly occur. Cerebrospinal fluid findings in affected animals reflect the degree of leptomeningeal or ependymal involvement, and the CSF white blood cell count may be normal or only slightly elevated (less than 50 white blood cells/μl).

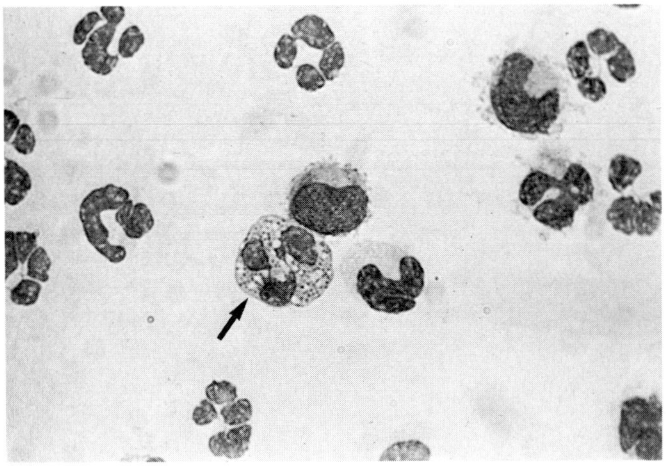

FIGURE 62–6. Meningomyelitis. White blood cells in cerebrospinal fluid (prepared by cytocentrifugation and stained with a modified Wright's stain) from an eight-year-old greyhound with a history of apparent lumbar spinal pain that was progressive in severity. Total CSF white blood cell count was 2300/μl, with the predominant cell type being polymorphonuclear leukocyte. Four per cent of white blood cells were eosinophils (arrow). A causative organism was neither seen in, nor isolated from, CSF. A diagnosis of granulomatous meningomyelitis was confirmed at necropsy.

Cerebrospinal fluid protein is usually moderately to markedly elevated due to increased capillary permeability and leakage of serum proteins into the CSF, and probably also due to local production of immunoglobulins. If CSF protein content is high, fibrin clots may develop. Cerebrospinal fluid pressure is usually normal but occasionally is elevated,[65] especially in animals with cryptococcal meningitis. Hemorrhage into the CSF may occur; a red or pink supernatant is indicative of recent hemorrhage. Xanthochromia develops if more than 48 hours have elapsed following hemorrhage. Cerebrospinal fluid glucose content may be decreased (CSF glucose is normally 60 to 80 per cent of a simultaneously determined plasma glucose concentration) as a result of glucose utilization by microorganisms and possibly by PMN leukocytes. However, low CSF glucose concentration is not a consistent finding in animals with bacterial meningitis.

Bacteria or fungal organisms may be identified by Gram's stain or acridine orange stain of sedimented or centrifuged CSF. Cryptococcal organisms often are observed in cell preparations of CSF and can be identified by staining with Wright's stain or Gram's stain, or using a wet mount preparation with India ink.

Cerebrospinal fluid from all animals with CSF abnormalities consistent with meningitis should be submitted for both aerobic and anaerobic bacterial culture,[79, 80] and antibiotic sensitivity testing of any cultured bacterial isolates. Cerebrospinal fluid fungal culture may also be done. Negative CSF cultures are common, even in those animals in which bacteria or fungal organisms can be identified in CSF. Culturing the sediment of centrifuged CSF, or filtering CSF and culturing the filter, may increase the likelihood of obtaining a positive CSF culture. Causative organisms may be isolated from blood cultures of animals that are bacteremic or have systemic fungal infection. *Histoplasma* organisms may be found in buffy coat or bone marrow neutrophils or monocytes. It is recommended that a large volume of CSF, preferably two or three milliliters, be collected for bacterial and/or fungal culture. If a delay in processing of a CSF sample is anticipated, CSF can be aseptically inoculated into a blood culture bottle for submission to a diagnostic laboratory.

Serology may also be useful in diagnosis of CNS fungal infections. The titer of antibody-coated latex agglutination to cryptococcal (capsular) antigen may be useful in the diagnosis of cryptococcal meningitis and in assessing the response to therapy. The latex cryptococcal agglutination titer (LCAT) is more sensitive than the indirect fluorescent antibody test and can be used on CSF. However, animals with localized CNS infection may have a negative titer.[81]

Focal epidural inflammatory lesions may appear as an

extradural mass on myelography. Chronic focal meningitis may result in obstruction of CSF flow and blockage of contrast material on myelography due to arachnoid adhesions.

Diagnosis of Rickettsial Infections. The characteristic histopathologic lesion of RMSF is necrotizing vasculitis, perivascular accumulation of PMN cells, and lymphoreticular cell infiltration in most tissues of the body including the meninges and CNS.[82] The histopathologic lesion occurring in canine ehrlichiosis is generalized lymphoid and plasma cell accumulation in bone marrow, meninges, kidney, and other organs.[83] Dogs with RMSF commonly have leukocytosis, thrombocytopenia, and hypoalbuminemia. Dogs with ehrlichiosis commonly have anemia, leukopenia, thrombocytopenia, and hypoalbuminemia, although hypergammaglobulinemia may occur.[76] Platelet counts may be normal in dogs with either disease. Biochemical abnormalities are not specific for either disease.[76]

Results of CSF analysis of dogs with RMSF may be normal or may show a mild increase in protein (less than 60 mg/dl) and nucleated cells (less than 80 cells/dl) with lymphocytes being the predominant cell type.[78] Currently, there is little information on the expected CSF findings in animals with ehrlichiosis. In one reported case, CSF protein and nucleated cells were increased, with lymphocytes being the predominant cell type.[76]

Diagnosis of both diseases is based on serology. A single positive serum titer for *E. canis* using an indirect immunofluorescent antibody technique is considered diagnostic for ehrlichiosis.[76] In acute phases of the disease morulae may be seen in circulating mononuclear cells. A four-fold increase in serum antibody titer in samples collected two to three weeks apart is considered diagnostic for RMSF.[76] Treatment with chloramphenicol may depress a rise in antibody titer.[78]

Direct fluorescent specific antibody staining of skin biopsies provides rapid diagnosis of RMSF. Positive staining may occur in skin from areas with or without hemorrhagic lesions.[76, 84]

Diagnosis of Protothecal Infection. Neutrophilic or eosinophilic leukocytes often are increased in CSF of animals with protothecosis.[70] Culture of CSF on fungal media may result in isolation of the organism.[70] Rectal scrapings should also be done. Fluorescent antibody examination may demonstrate the organism in tissue sections.[70]

Treatment of Bacterial Infections. In treating bacterial meningitis and/or myelitis it is desirable to use an antimicrobial that is specific for the causative organism, and that crosses the blood-brain barrier (or blood–spinal cord barrier) in therapeutic concentrations, in order that drug concentrations may be maintained after the acute phase of inflammation has subsided. The blood-brain, blood–spinal cord, and blood-CSF barriers are most permeable to antimicrobials with high lipid solubility, low ionization potential, and low protein binding affinity.

Antibiotics may be administered to animals with suspected bacterial meningitis prior to obtaining results of culture and sensitivity testing. Selection should be based on tentative organism identification (by Gram's stain or acridine orange stain) from CSF, the suspected source of infection, and the ability of an antibiotic to reach effective tissue concentrations in CNS.

High-dose intravenous therapy with a bactericidal drug should be used where possible, although many bactericidal drugs penetrate poorly into the CSF. Penicillin and penicillin derivatives in high doses have been recommended for the treatment of CNS infections caused by gram-positive cocci (e.g., penicillin G 5000–10,000 U/lb IV every six hours for at least seven days).[84a] Oxacillin may be used for the treatment of meningitis caused by penicillin-resistant strains of *Staphylococcus*.

Most cephalosporins penetrate poorly into the CNS.[84a] Several third generation cephalosporins (e.g., cefotaxime) reach effective CNS concentrations, and are considered the drugs best suited for treatment of gram-negative meningitis.[73, 84a, 85] First and second generation cephalosporins do not reach effective CSF concentrations, and should not be used in treatment of CNS infections.[84a] The cephalosporins largely have replaced the aminoglycosides, which penetrate poorly into the CNS.

Metronidazole is useful for treatment of most anaerobic infections, is bactericidal, and diffuses well into all tissues including the CNS.[73] Metronidazole has had an increasing role in the therapy of brain abscesses of humans.[85a] Metronidazole is used in combination with high doses of penicillin when aerobes are present.[85a] Toxicity (central vestibular signs and cerebellar dysfunction) has been reported in dogs treated with metronidazole.[86]

Chloramphenicol reaches higher CSF concentrations than most other antibiotics; however, it is bacteriostatic, and many strains of *Staphylococcus* have been shown to be resistant to this drug.[86a] Chloramphenicol may be given at a dosage of 20 mg/lb IV QID or 25 mg/lb orally TID in dogs, and 5 to 10 mg/lb/day divided BID in cats. Adverse effects of chloramphenicol include gastroenteritis in dogs and cats, and bone marrow depression in cats. Because of the high frequency of adverse effects, and as bactericidal drugs are preferred for treatment of CNS infections, use of chloramphenicol is restricted to infections caused by susceptible organisms that are resistant to other agents.[86a]

Most sulfonamides penetrate effectively into the CSF. Sulfadiazine (which is less protein bound than other sulfonamides) penetrates into the CSF and nervous tissue better than sulfamethoxazole and is effective if given orally. Data are not available regarding the concentration of trimethoprim in CSF of dogs; however, CSF concentrations may be as high as 35 per cent of serum concentrations in other species.[87] Trimethoprim-sulfadiazine combinations usually are bactericidal in action, and are effective for treatment of some bacterial CNS infections.

In general, tetracycline, a broad-spectrum bacteriostatic drug, only reaches effective CNS concentrations when meninges are inflamed. However, newer tetracyclines (minocycline, doxycycline) penetrate the CNS better than tetracycline and have better activity against anaerobes and some aerobic organisms.[86a]

Intrathecal administration of antibiotics has been used in humans. Although possible for use in dogs, multiple

CSF punctures, each requiring anesthesia, are needed. Some drugs are toxic when directly introduced into the CNS (e.g., penicillin may cause seizures), and drugs may not diffuse freely through CSF especially if there is a blockage of CSF flow.

Treatment with antibiotics should be started as soon as possible after submission of CSF for culture. After results of culture and sensitivity are known, therapy may be altered. Treatment is continued for two to four weeks; however, treatment for longer periods is often necessary and relapses are possible. It is also important to identify possible sources of infection outside the CNS (endocarditis, diskospondylitis, paravertebral abscess). Localized spinal cord or meningeal infections that are well encapsulated may be resistant to antibiotic therapy. Surgical exploration is indicated if focal meningeal or epidural infection refractory to medical therapy is suspected.

Use of corticosteroids in cases of bacterial meningitis and myelitis is controversial.[73] Corticosteroids may decrease inflammation and thereby decrease the resulting spinal cord and nerve root damage; however, such treatment may also decrease host defense mechanisms, and in turn may result in worsening of clinical signs and in a higher incidence of relapse.

Prognosis in cases of bacterial meningitis and myelitis depends both on the ability to eliminate the causative organism, and on the extent of neurologic deficits. Neurologic deficits occurring as a result of spinal cord or nerve root inflammation may be permanent.

Treatment of Fungal Infection. Fungal infection of the CNS of dogs or cats is extremely difficult to eliminate. The disease is often multisystemic, and is seldom recognized in the early stages of CNS involvement.[73]

Amphotericin B is frequently used to treat systemic fungal infections, although it is poorly absorbed into the CSF and nervous tissue. Intrathecal administration of amphotericin B has been recommended,[88] especially in animals with *Coccidioides immitis* meningitis, but may result in arachnoiditis and cranial nerve toxicity.

Combinations of drugs have been recommended.[73] Amphotericin B, ketoconazole (poor CNS penetration), and flucytosine (good CNS penetration) are the main agents used. Rifampin has been used to enhance amphotericin B activity.[73] Combined treatment with amphotericin B and 5-fluorocytosine (5FU) has been recommended for use in cases of cryptococcosis.[89] Long-term, high dose ketoconazole therapy is reported to be effective for treatment of cryptococcosis in cats.[89a]

Because of the difficulty in obtaining therapeutic concentrations of antifungal agents within nervous tissue, the prognosis for CNS mycotic infections is poor. In the future, newer generation imidazoles (e.g., fluconazole) that are currently under investigation may be efficacious for treatment of fungal infections of the CNS.[73]

Treatment of Rickettsial Infections. Rickettsial organisms appear to be extremely sensitive to tetracyclines (10 mg/lb orally TID for 14 days).[84, 90] Tetracyclines are bacteriostatic, and elimination of the organisms from the body depends on the immunocompetence of an affected animal. Doxycycline has better CNS penetration than that seen with oxytetracycline or tetracycline, and is used in animals with meningitis or myelitis resulting from RMSF or ehrlichiosis.[73] Chloramphenicol is used in place of tetracycline to treat young dogs prior to the eruption of permanent teeth. Severely affected dogs, especially those with neurologic involvement, may die despite therapy. Supportive therapy should be given as necessary; however, caution should be used in giving IV fluids to dogs with RMSF, as increased vascular permeability increases the risk of cerebral and pulmonary edema associated with overhydration. Neurologic deficits may be permanent in affected dogs.[76] Recovery may be prolonged, and pancytopenia persistent, in dogs with chronic ehrlichiosis.[78]

Treatment of Protothecal Infection. Effective therapy for disseminated protothecosis has not been described.[70]

Calcium Phosphate Deposition Disease in Great Dane Dogs

Etiology and Pathogenesis. A disease characterized by progressive incoordination and paralysis has been described in Great Dane puppies.[91] Pathologically, periarticular calcium phosphate mineralization and bone deformity are found in the axial and appendicular skeleton. Bones are shorter than normal and have a thin cortex and increased medullary trabeculae and curvature. Caudal cervical vertebral canal stenosis results from dorsal displacement of C7, and deformation of the vertebral articular processes results in spinal cord compression.

The pathogenesis of this disease is unknown. It may be familial, as related animals have been found to be affected. Serum calcium and phosphate concentrations of affected dogs are similar to those of normal age-matched Great Dane dogs; however, blood pH is lower in affected dogs. The mineralization of soft tissues and the bone deformity are thought to be a primary alteration rather than secondary to another major underlying disease process. This disease does not appear to be related to cervical spondylomyelopathy that is also seen in Great Dane dogs.

Clinical Signs. Clinical signs in one- to two-month-old Great Dane puppies are indicative of a progressive caudal cervical myelopathy.

Diagnosis. Radiographs show dorsal displacement of C7 and focal radiographic densities between the spinous processes of the caudal cervical vertebrae. The lesions of the spinous processes correspond to mineral deposits in the vertebral diarthrodial joints seen on histopathologic examination.

Treatment. Treatment for this condition has not been described.

Cervical Spondylomyelopathy

Etiology and Pathogenesis. Several terms have been used to describe a disease of the cervical vertebral column of Great Dane dogs, Doberman pinscher dogs, and other large breeds of dog. These terms include "wobbler" syndrome, caudal cervical malformation-malarticulation, cervical spondylopathy, cervical vertebral instability, and cervical vertebral stenosis.[92] The term "wobbler" describes a dog with generalized ataxia and tetraparesis that may be seen with a variety of cervical myelopathies, and its use is therefore to be discouraged.[4] The number of different terms that have been used reflects the many unanswered questions that remain regarding etiology and pathogenesis of this condition. The term cervical spondylomyelopathy accurately reflects the complexity of the syndrome, and has therefore become widely accepted.

While etiology remains undetermined, the high incidence of this syndrome in certain breeds of dog suggests that heredity is a contributing factor.[92] Osteochondrosis resulting from overnutrition and rapid growth in Great Dane dogs may also be a factor.[92] It is likely that these and other as yet undefined factors contribute to the development of the syndrome.

Congenital, developmental, and degenerative forms of stenosis of the vertebral canal of humans have long been known; however, the clinical significance of these problems has only recently been recognized.[93] Stenosis of the vertebral canal of humans may be clinically "silent" as long as it is not complicated by other factors such as instability or intervertebral disk protrusion.[93] In other words, the addition of a dynamic factor may be necessary for the manifestation of clinical signs in cases of vertebral canal stenosis.[93] The role of a dynamic factor has been noted in dogs.[94–96]

Cervical vertebral canal stenosis in association with spinal cord compression in dogs was first described in 1967.[97] Deformity of C3 that resulted in spinal cord compression in young male basset hounds was reported.[97] Malformation of vertebral bodies in association with spinal canal stenosis has since been reported by numerous authors to occur in the cervical spine of other breeds of dog.[92, 98–105] In addition, malformation of vertebral arches, including articular processes and intervertebral joints, has been reported to contribute to stenosis of the vertebral canal.[96, 99, 100, 102, 105–108]

Stenosis of the vertebral canal or intervertebral foramina may also be seen in association with encroachment of soft tissue structures into the vertebral canal. Hypertrophy of the interarcuate ligament (ligamentum flavum),[99–106] dorsal longitudinal ligament or dorsal anulus fibrosus,[106] and joint capsule of vertebral joints[99] has been reported. It has been suggested that soft tissue stenosis may result from hypertrophy or hyperplasia of ligamentous structures that occur secondary to instability or stress.[100–102, 104, 106, 109, 110] Type II disk protrusion also is a component of soft tissue stenosis in many affected dogs;[92] however, it has been speculated that the dorsal anulus fibrosus is a "redundant" structure, and that spinal cord compression results from collapse of the underlying disk that causes passive dorsal "buckling" of the anulus fibrosus.[109] The dorsal longitudinal ligament was reported not to contribute to stenosis in one study.[109]

Vertebral instability, either alone or in combination with vertebral malformation and/or soft tissue stenosis, has been suggested as an initiating cause of spinal cord compression and associated neurologic abnormalities.[92] Chronic progressive compression of the spinal cord results from stenosis of the vertebral canal that is caused by a combination of the above factors. Histopathologic alterations seen in the spinal cord are characteristic of chronic compression. Focal involvement of both gray and white matter may be present at the level of the stenosis, although occasionally only white matter is affected. In gray matter, hypertrophied astrocytes may be present, and loss of neurons may be noted. It is speculated that extradural compression results in microvascular stasis, which in turn causes neuronal edema, hypoxia, and cell death. White matter degeneration is noted in tracts cranial and caudal to the level of focal compression. Myelin degeneration appears to predominate over axonal degeneration. Infiltration of spinal cord parenchyma by inflammatory cells is seldom seen. On the basis of these pathologic alterations, it is possible that remyelination of remaining axons could result in neurologic improvement following resolution of the stenosis by means of surgery.[92]

Cervical spondylomyelopathy occurs most frequently in young (less than two years of age) Great Dane dogs, and middle aged or older (three to nine years of age) Doberman pinscher dogs. Other breeds of dog that have been reported to be affected include Saint Bernard, Weimaraner, Labrador retriever, German shepherd, boxer, basset hound, Rhodesian ridgeback, Dalmatian, Samoyed, Old English sheepdog, and bull mastiff.[92, 111] Males appear to be affected more frequently than females.[92, 102]

The C5-6 and C6-7 interspaces appear to be affected most commonly, although alterations consistent with a diagnosis of cervical spondylomyelopathy may be seen at the level of C4-5, and less frequently at C3-4. Reported incidence of sites affected varies. A review of 111 dogs revealed 76 per cent had spinal cord compression at C6-7, and 32 per cent had compression at C5-6. Spinal cord compression may be present at more than one site in the cervical spine. Stenosis of the vertebral canal of basset hounds has been reported to occur at C2-3.[97, 107]

Although the lesions seen in all breeds of dog of all age groups are similar, certain pathologic changes are more characteristic of each particular group. Younger Great Dane dogs frequently have dorsal spinal cord compression as a result of elongation of the cranial aspect of the dorsal arch of affected vertebrae. Older Doberman pinscher dogs frequently have severe ventral spinal cord compression centered over the anulus fibrosus of the affected interspace.[92]

Clinical Findings. The clinical signs that occur in dogs with cervical spondylomyelopathy reflect chronic compression of the cervical spinal cord. Clinical signs are most often insidious in onset and are gradually progressive over several months or years; however, less frequently clinical signs may develop acutely, perhaps following an apparently insignificant traumatic episode. Gait deficits are frequently noted initially in the pelvic limbs. A mild pelvic limb ataxia progresses in severity until a wide-based, crouching stance and dragging or knuckling of the toes of the pelvic limbs may be seen. Abnormalities may be more easily observed when an affected dog rises from a lying position, turns, or negotiates stairs or a curb.

Neurologic abnormalities that may be noted in the

pelvic limbs include depression or loss of conscious proprioception and exaggerated spinal reflexes. Thoracic limb abnormalities most often occur after the development of neurologic deficits in pelvic limbs, and thoracic limb deficits seldom progress to the level of severity of pelvic limb abnormalities. Thoracic limb deficits usually are of mild severity, and only may be evident during intensive evaluation of postural reactions, particularly thoracic limb hopping reactions. Neurogenic atrophy of supraspinatus or infraspinatus muscles may be detected; however, widespread lower motor neuron involvement in thoracic limbs rarely is seen. In dogs with a chronic course, a stiff, spastic, "choppy" thoracic limb gait may be seen, often in combination with a rigid flexion of the neck. Although affected dogs may resist extension of the neck, apparent neck pain, as seen frequently with an acute cervical disk protrusion, is seldom elicitable.

Diagnosis. In addition to a complete physical and neurologic examination, a complete blood count, serum biochemistry profile and urinalysis are done in affected dogs. Dogs with a history, clinical findings, or serum biochemical findings consistent with a systemic or metabolic disease should be assessed by means of appropriate testing. Disorders such as congestive cardiomyopathy or hypothyroidism frequently are diagnosed in Great Dane dogs or Doberman pinscher dogs. Thyrotropin stimulation testing is recommended in any Doberman pinscher dog with clinical signs consistent with cervical spondylomyelopathy.

Radiography is the most accurate method for delineating the pathologic alterations of cervical spondylomyelopathy. Diagnosis of cervical vertebral canal stenosis has been made on the basis of noncontrast lateral radiographs of the cervical spine; however, numerous studies have emphasized that noncontrast radiographs of the cervical spine may be normal in affected dogs.[92] Abnormalities that may be present on noncontrast radiographs include malalignment or "slipping" of vertebrae, remodeling of vertebrae with cranial stenosis of the vertebral canal, new bone formation (spondylosis deformans), narrowing or collapse of one or more intervertebral disk spaces, calcification of the nucleus pulposus of one or more intervertebral disks, sclerosis of vertebral endplates, and degenerative changes of vertebral articular facets (Figures 62–7 and 62–8). It is important to note that features such as vertebral remodeling with spondylosis deformans, narrowing of intervertebral disk spaces, and asymmetry of articular facets may not be associated with clinically significant vertebral canal stenosis. "Tilting" between adjacent vertebrae that may be apparent on plain spinal radiographs may, in fact, be within normal limits.[112]

Myelography is essential to determine the location or locations, and nature and extent, of spinal cord compression present. Myelography findings are essential in considering treatment options and any surgical repair that is to be attempted. The importance of ventrodorsal projections in defining lateral spinal cord compression,[108] and dynamic or "stressed" radiographs in outlining dorsal spinal cord compression,[92] in combination with myelography, has been emphasized by several authors. "Traction" radiographs have been recommended as a method of showing the dynamic nature of a lesion.[92, 109]

The abnormality most frequently recognized in Doberman pinscher dogs following myelography is ventral spinal cord compression resulting from an hypertrophied, hyperplastic, or "redundant" dorsal anulus fibrosus (Figure 62–7). Other findings include dorsal spinal cord compression resulting from hypertrophied or hyperplastic ligamentum flavum, dorsolateral spinal cord compression resulting from malformed articular processes, or spinal cord compression resulting from malformed or malaligned vertebrae.

Dynamic or "stress" radiography, following myelography, is of particular value in demonstration of instability, ventral spinal cord compression as a result of dorsally protruding intervertebral disks, or dorsal spinal cord compression as a result of ventrally protruding interarcuate ligament or joint capsule. A dorsal extended view is most appropriate for demonstration of dorsal spinal cord compression due to interarcuate ligament hypertrophy/hyperplasia.[113] It has been reported, however, that routine use of "stressed" views is not warranted because of the possibility of misinterpretation of alterations, and the risk of further injury to a spinal cord that may already be severely compromised.[100] "Stress" radiography may be useful in selected cases but should be performed with caution. "Traction" radiography, where firm traction is placed on the cervical spine during exposure of a lateral radiograph, may further delineate the dynamic nature of a lesion (Figure 62–8).[92] By means of this technique, spinal cord compression resulting from "redundant" or protruding anulus fibrosus may be relieved by the procedure. Failure to relieve the compression by means of "traction" may indicate a static lesion such as a disk protrusion. "Traction" views are recommended following myelography, as they do not appear to increase spinal cord compression, and provide information that is useful in the selection of an appropriate surgical technique.

Advanced imaging modalities such as CT or MRI may provide further information regarding this syndrome in the future.[114]

Treatment. Numerous treatment regimens have been recommended for the management of dogs with cervical spondylomyelopathy.[92, 98] The large number of recommended treatments reflects the variety of lesions demonstrated by various diagnostic techniques, the variable results that have been achieved by investigators, and the personal bias of individual surgeons. It is likely that this trend will continue until controlled prospective studies are done to further investigate the etiology and pathogenesis of this disease.

The course of the disease without therapy is difficult to predict. In most dogs the disease course is chronic and progressive. Prognosis in the absence of treatment is considered guarded to poor in most affected dogs. Therapy is directed either toward the relief of clinical signs by means of medical treatment and management practices or toward surgical relief of spinal cord compression.

Medical therapy consists of use of anti-inflammatory medications and management procedures that reduce neck movement, such as close confinement or use of a neck brace.[92, 115] Some affected dogs may be maintained at an acceptable level of neurologic function for months

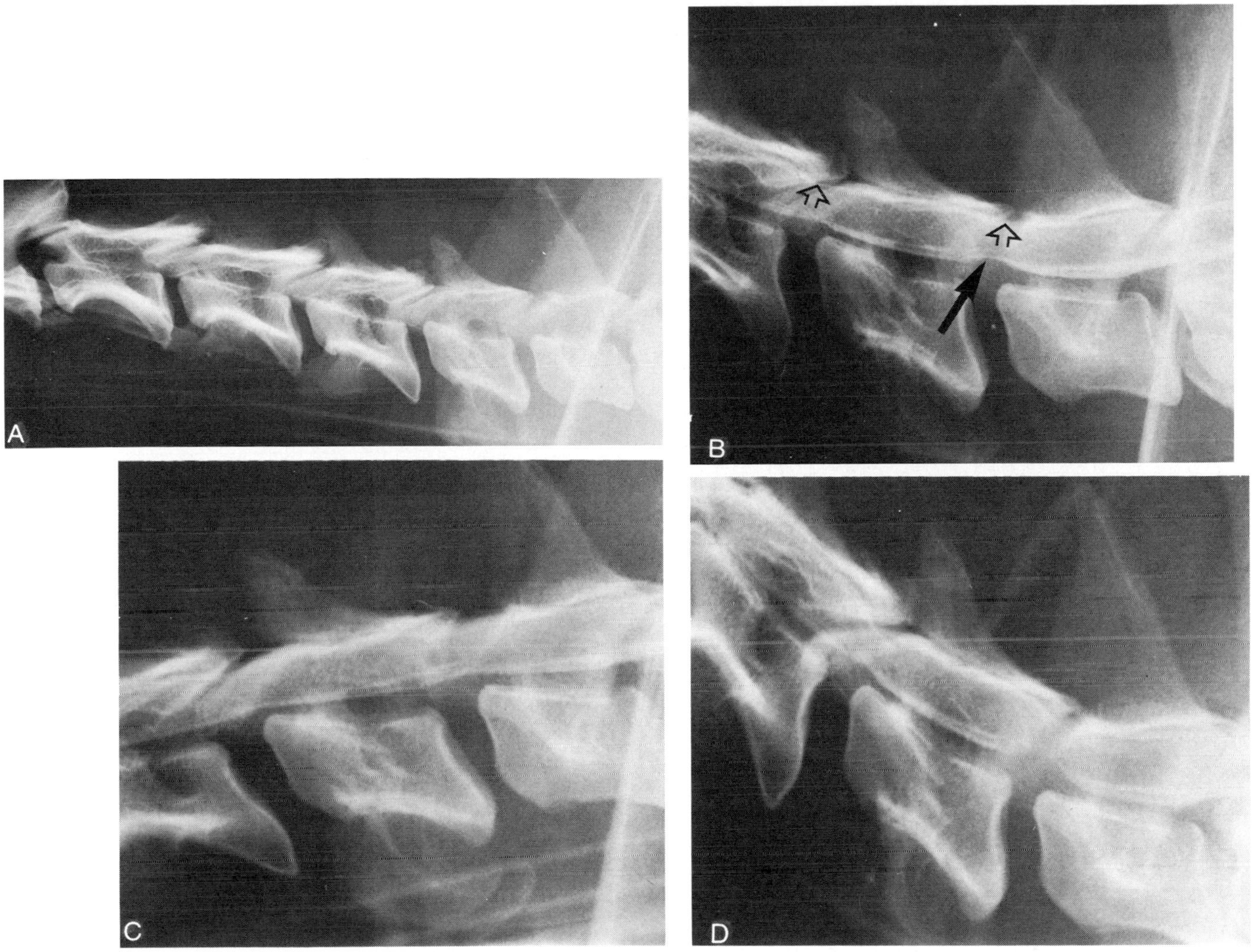

FIGURE 62–7. Cervical spondylomyelopathy. Radiographs of the cervical vertebrae of an 11-year-old male Doberman pinscher with a history of tetraparesis and generalized ataxia that had been gradually worsening for the previous two months. Slight narrowing of the C6-C7 disk is seen on a noncontrast lateral projection *(A)* completed with the cervical spine in a nonstressed position. A C6-C7 extradural mass causing ventral spinal cord compression (solid arrow) is seen on a lateral projection of a myelogram *(B)* of the caudal cervical spine (in a non-stressed position). There is also an extradural mass causing dorsal spinal cord compression at C5-C6 and C6-C7 (open arrows). "Stressed" lateral projections of a myelogram completed with the neck in a flexed *(C)* and extended *(D)* position demonstrate that the extradural spinal cord compressions are reduced following neck flexion and are worsened following neck extension.

to years by means of corticosteroid administration. In some dogs, corticosteroid therapy may be discontinued during periods of improved neurologic function, and reestablished during periods of relapse of neurologic abnormalities. Adverse effects of long-term corticosteroid therapy must be considered, and it must be remembered that this approach does not address the underlying sustained spinal cord compression in most cases. Use of a neck brace or cage confinement is recommended in association with corticosteroid administration; however, these techniques are likely only to be useful in those dogs in which there is a dynamic component to the spinal cord compression. Supplementation of hypothyroid dogs with synthetic levothyroxine (T4) products is recommended, and in some dogs may result in dramatic clinical improvement.

Techniques for surgical management have been developed in order to address the problem of underlying spinal cord compression that is present in dogs with cervical spondylomyelopathy.[92, 98] The high potential for morbidity and postoperative complications associated with surgical management of cervical spondylomyelopathy must be considered prior to recommending surgery.[92, 116] These considerations must be balanced with the present knowledge of the natural progression of the disease.

Surgical procedures may use either a dorsal or ventral approach to the vertebral column. The primary objectives of all surgical procedures are decompression of the spinal cord, stabilization of the vertebral column, or both. Decompressive procedures involve removal of the source of compression, whether it be ligamentum flavum, dorsal anulus fibrosus, or another structure. Although instability may not be apparent on "stressed" radiographs, surgical stabilization procedures have been recommended by many authors. Atrophy of ligamentous

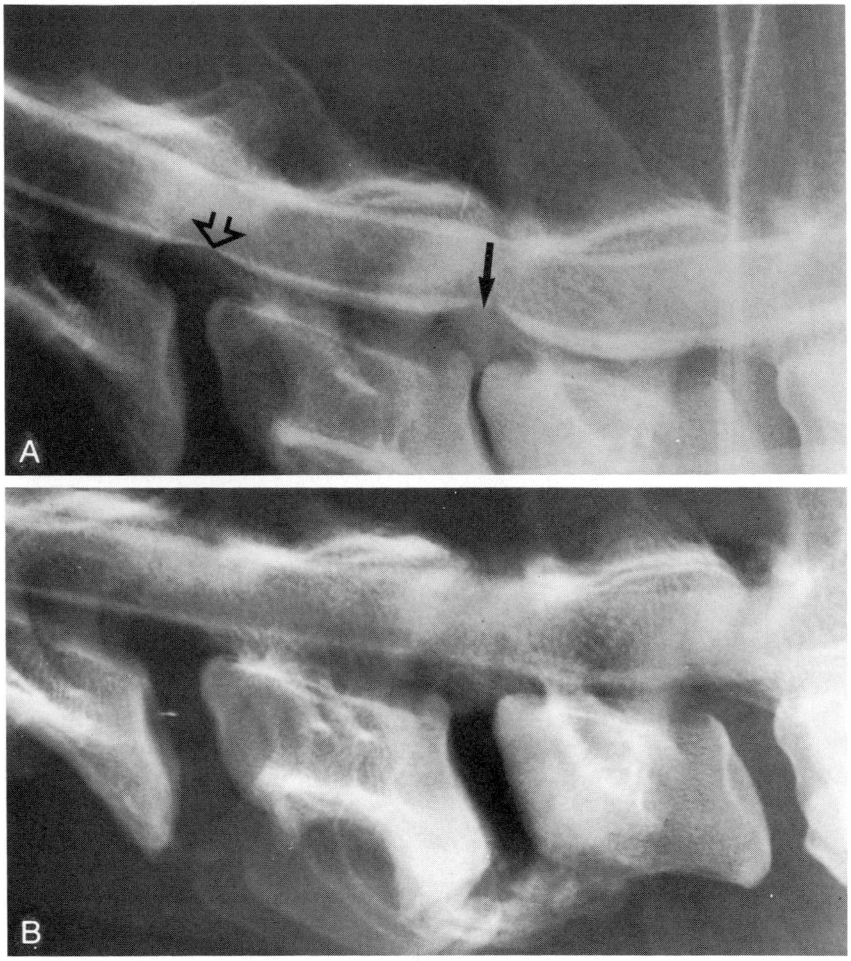

FIGURE 62–8. Cervical spondylomyelopathy. Caudal cervical myelogram of an 11-year-old male German shepherd mixed breed dog with a history of progressively worsening tetraparesis and generalized ataxia. Slight narrowing of the C5-C6 disk and collapse of the C6-C7 disk are seen on a lateral projection *(A)* completed with the cervical spine in a nonstressed position. There is an extradural mass causing ventral spinal cord compression at both C5-C6 (open arrow) and C6-C7 (solid arrow). The extradural compressions are relieved following "traction" of the cervical vertebrae *(B)*. Note that the C5-C6 and C6-C7 disks are restored to a normal width following traction.

structures that are causing compression has been suggested to occur following immobilization.[92] Further, stabilization has been reported to remove the dynamic exacerbation of dorsal anulus fibrosus compression that may occur with extension of the neck. The selection of an appropriate surgical technique must be based on results of a myelogram that includes both "stressed" and "traction" radiographs.

A dorsal approach for decompression of the spinal cord by means of a dorsal laminectomy may be used in dogs where only ligamentum flavum compression of the spinal cord is present, or where ligamentum flavum compression is more severe than concurrent dorsal anulus compression.[98, 113] Dorsal laminectomy is unlikely to effectively relieve ventral spinal cord compression resulting from dorsal anulus fibrosus compression.[117]

Dogs with multiple levels of spinal cord compression have been difficult to treat successfully. Medical therapy, with surgical decompression of the most severely affected site, has been recommended. Recently, a continuous dorsal laminectomy extending from the caudal aspect of C4 to the cranial aspect of T1 was recommended for use in Doberman pinscher dogs with multiple-level, dynamic, dorsal and ventral extradural compressive lesions of the caudal cervical vertebral column.[118]

Dorsal stabilization procedures utilizing either wire or lag screw fixation of articular facets have been used in association with dorsal laminectomy.[119] Effectiveness of such stabilization techniques for management of caudal cervical spondylomyelopathy has not been adequately investigated.

Advantages of dorsal techniques include excellent exposure of ligamentous structures located dorsal to the spinal cord and avoidance of ventral vertebral sinuses. Disadvantages include the inability to decompress dorsal anulus fibrosus compression of the spinal cord, and worsening of neurologic function that may be seen postoperatively despite gentle handling of neural tissues.[92] Further, dorsal stabilization and fusion techniques that utilize articular processes and facets are not as effective biomechanically as techniques that utilize vertebral bodies.

A ventral approach to the cervical vertebral column permits completion of a ventral "slot" that provides adequate relief of spinal cord compression that results from dorsal anulus fibrosus hypertrophy or hyperplasia.[92] This approach is superior to a dorsal laminectomy in dogs that have a significant dorsal anulus fibrosus compression of the spinal cord. The ventral "slot" procedure may be done at adjacent interspaces; however, this may be associated with an increased incidence of postoperative complications. It has been reported that two thirds of dogs with cervical spondylomyelopathy demonstrate clinical improvement following only ventral decompression.[113, 120] Inadequate or incomplete removal of abnormal tissue from the vertebral canal is likely to be responsible for the majority of failures.[92]

Fenestration may be completed by means of a ventral approach. Clinical results of surgical fenestration in large breeds of dog have been poor, with neurologic improvement occurring in only 7 of 34 dogs reported in two studies.[92] It is likely that surgical fenestration does not diminish spinal cord compression resulting from soft tissue stenosis of the vertebral canal. Recently, chemonucleolysis has been investigated as an alternative to ventral decompression for the treatment of type II cervical disk protrusion in large breeds of dog.[121] Initial results suggest that this technique may be useful in selected cases with dorsal anulus fibrosus compression of the spinal cord.[121]

Ventral stabilization of the cervical vertebral column by means of either vertebral body lag screw fixation or a transverse "slot" procedure has been investigated.[92, 113] Neither technique provides adequate decompression of spinal cord, and these procedures are of undetermined efficacy in the management of caudal cervical spondylomyelopathy at this time.

A recently developed ventral technique that combines vertebral distraction and fusion has been recommended by several investigators.[92] The technique involves completion of a ventral "slot." The "slot" provides a means to effect a ventral decompression in those dogs in which dorsal anulus fibrosus spinal cord compression is not relieved with "traction" myelography. The "slot" penetrates to a depth of three quarters of the depth of the affected disk space in those dogs in which ventral spinal cord compression is relieved by "traction." The majority of anulus fibrosus–associated spinal cord compressions appear to be relieved by traction. The affected vertebrae are distracted, and are rigidly stabilized with an orthopedic implant that maintains distraction. The "slot" is packed with a bone graft to accelerate bony fusion. Techniques used for stabilization include an allogenic cortical bone graft alone or combined with a plastic plate applied to the ventral aspect of the vertebral bodies, a Harrington rod combined with a cancellous bone graft, and fixation with Steinmann pins and polymethyl methacrylate combined with a cancellous bone graft.[92] A maximum of two adjacent interspaces may be fused using these techniques. These techniques have the disadvantages that an orthopedic implant is required, and fusion at one level may lead to disk degeneration at adjacent levels.[92]

Prognosis for dogs with cervical spondylomyelopathy is difficult to determine. In general, medical therapy may be expected to provide clinical improvement for a variable period of time (weeks to years). It must be remembered that medical therapy does not alter sustained and often progressive spinal cord compression. Surgical therapy that relieves spinal cord compression is often associated with postoperative complications;[92] however, the following statements may be made. The prognosis for dogs with a chronic history of worsening signs is not as favorable as for dogs with acute onset of signs. Mildly affected dogs have a fair prognosis for recovery.[92] Dogs with a single level of compression appear to have a better prognosis after surgery than those with multiple-level compressions.[113] One report of long-term follow-up of dogs treated by fusion revealed that up to 19 per cent of dogs developed spinal cord compression at an adjacent interspace an average of 20 months after surgery.[92] Overall, prognosis must be considered guarded, regardless of the type of therapy.

Congenital Vertebral Anomalies

Etiology and Pathogenesis. Congenital anomalies frequently occur in the vertebral column of cats or dogs; however, the majority of such anomalies are not clinically significant. If a vertebral anomaly causes instability or deformity of the vertebral canal, then spinal cord compression and associated clinical signs may result.

Vertebral anomalies develop due to disturbances in embryonic development. Vertebrae develop from the embryonic mesoderm. The mesodermal layer differentiates into the central notochord and lateral serially arranged somites, separated by transverse clefts in the mesoderm. Each of these somites forms a dermatome (laterally), myotome (intermedially), and sclerotome (medially). The vertebrae are formed from sclerotomes. Each sclerotome separates into cranial and caudal halves and the sclerotomes then recombine, such that the caudal half of one joins the cranial half of the adjacent sclerotome, surrounding the intersegmental blood vessels, which in turn penetrate and supply each vertebral body. The recombined sclerotomic masses migrate to surround the neural tube (developing spinal cord) and notochord to form the primordial vertebrae. The notochord is obliterated except at each intervertebral disk where it becomes the nucleus pulposus of a disk. Chondrification of each primitive vertebra then occurs from four centers that merge to form a solid cartilaginous vertebra. Ossification occurs subsequently from four centers (two in the vertebral body that merge to become one, and one in each side of the vertebral arch). At birth, ossification of the vertebrae is only partial and three centers of ossification are identifiable. Secondary ossification centers develop and join the vertebral processes and endplates.

The most frequently recognized vertebral anomalies are alteration in location of the anticlinal vertebra, anomalies of articular processes, variations in numbers of vertebrae, transitional vertebrae, butterfly vertebrae, block vertebrae, nonfusion of sacral vertebrae, or hemivertebrae.[122] Of these anomalies, hemivertebrae are the most significant as a cause of neurologic abnormalities.

HEMIVERTEBRAE. Hemivertebrae result from hemimetameric displacement of somites during recombination of sclerotomes to form the primordial vertebrae, resulting in unilateral hemivertebrae.[123] Lack of vascularization, resulting in failure of ossification of one half of the vertebral body, may be the cause of unilateral hemivertebrae and of dorsal and ventral hemivertebrae. Hemivertebrae are wedge-shaped, and the apex may be directed dorsally, ventrally, or medially across the midline. Hemivertebrae may be associated with moderate to severe angulation of the spine (kyphosis, scoliosis, or lordosis), and may be displaced dorsally during growth by pressure from adjacent vertebrae. Hemivertebrae occur most commonly in the thoracic spine of "screw-tailed" brachycephalic breeds (French and English bulldogs, pugs, and Boston terriers) but may occur at any location in any breed of dog.[124] A familial incidence has been reported in English bulldogs and Yorkshire terriers.[125] Thoracic hemivertebrae are inherited (autosomal recessive) in German short-haired pointer dogs.[125] Kinked tails result from development of caudal hemivertebrae. Abnormal vertebral development has been associated with neonatal mortality of bulldogs.[127]

Block vertebrae. Block vertebrae result when the segmentation of somites is disturbed, and may occur at any level of the vertebral column.[123] Block vertebrae involve the vertebral bodies, vertebral arches, dorsal spinous processes, or entire vertebrae. Partial "blockage" of vertebral bodies may occur allowing partial development of an intervertebral disk. The sacrum is considered a "normal" block vertebra, with remnants of disk material or intervertebral disk spaces frequently seen radiographically.[122] Block vertebrae may be the same length as the number of involved vertebrae, or may be shorter, and can result in abnormal angulation of the spine.

Butterfly vertebrae. Butterfly vertebrae result from persistence of the notochord. In some instances, sagittal cleavage of the notochord may result in a sagittal cleft dorsoventrally through the vertebral body.[123] On a dorsoventral radiograph of the vertebral column, such vertebrae resemble a butterfly with wings spread. Compensatory growth of the adjacent normal vertebrae often fills in the funnel-shaped depression of the vertebral endplates. Butterfly vertebrae are most common in brachycephalic "screwtailed" breeds (French and English bulldogs, pugs, Boston terriers).

Transitional vertebrae. Dogs may have variations in the number of cervical, thoracic, lumbar, or sacral vertebrae.[122] Furthermore, congenital absence or alteration in the shape of vertebral articular processes and variation in the location of the anticlinal (usually T11) and diaphragmatic (usually T10) vertebrae may occur. Vertebrae that have the characteristics of two major divisions of the vertebral column are referred to as transitional vertebrae. Alterations may be unilateral or bilateral, and most commonly involve vertebral arches and transverse processes and less frequently the vertebral bodies.

Transitional vertebrae may occur at the cervicothoracic, thoracolumbar, or lumbosacral junctions. Observed alterations include transverse processes of C7 resembling a rib, a transverse process on the most caudal thoracic vertebra in place of a rib (lumbarization of the last thoracic vertebra), the first sacral vertebra having a transverse process (lumbarization), or the last lumbar vertebra having a transverse process that has fused with the ilium (sacralization). These alterations may be accompanied by alteration in size and shape of the vertebral body, or the plane of the vertebral body or intervertebral disk. The total number of presacral vertebrae must be known in order to determine accurately those vertebrae that are abnormal. The pelvis may be attached to the sacrum in an oblique manner due to unilateral sacralization or lumbarization. The first caudal vertebra may be partially or completely fused with the sacrum.

Stenosis of the thoracic spinal canal has been reported in English bulldogs.[128] This disorder apparently results from a vertebral anomaly in this breed of dog.

Multiple spinal anomalies may occur in a single dog. Kyphosis, scoliosis, and lordosis are most commonly associated with hemivertebrae;[129] however, cervical kyphosis, scoliosis, and vertebral rotation have been described as the sole cause of spinal cord compression in an Afghan hound.[130]

Clinical Findings. Congenital vertebral anomalies frequently occur. Forty-seven per cent of 145 dogs surveyed were affected in one study.[122] Clinical signs related to anomalous vertebrae are not present in the majority of affected animals. In most animals in which clinical signs develop, trauma to the spinal cord has occurred secondary to vertebral instability or progressive deformity with growth. Block vertebrae and butterfly vertebrae most often are stable and rarely are associated with clinical signs of spinal cord dysfunction.

Hemivertebrae are more often associated with neurologic dysfunction than are other vertebral anomalies. Hemivertebrae may result in vertebral instability and/or narrowing of the spinal canal, especially in the dorsoventral plane, due to moderate to severe angulation of the spine, which can result in spinal cord compression or intermittent trauma to the spinal cord. Clinical signs produced depend on the location of the anomaly and usually reflect a progressive or intermittent transverse myelopathy. Most frequently, clinical signs of a transverse myelopathy in the T3-L3 spinal segments are evident. Abnormal spinal conformation may be visible or palpable. Acute onset of neurologic deficits may occur following trauma to an already unstable spine, or clinical signs may become evident as a dog grows, due to spinal cord compression that results from progressive spinal deformity. Clinical signs usually occur in dogs less than one year of age.

Severely altered transitional vertebrae at the lumbosacral junction may cause instability and predispose the region to secondary changes such as arthritis due to abnormally positioned synovial joints, nerve root pressure from osteophyte formation, or intervertebral disk changes. Evidence of severe secondary changes was not found in one study and the clinical significance of these anomalies remains unknown.[122]

Stenosis of the thoracic spinal canal in English bulldogs may result in spinal cord compression and clinical signs referable to a transverse myelopathy between T3 and L3.

Diagnosis. Diagnosis of a vertebral anomaly is made by means of radiographs of the vertebral column (Figure 62–9).[122, 131] Radiographically, hemivertebrae and adjacent vertebrae appear to be formed of normal bone, and disk spaces are usually well-formed or widened.[4] Vertebral bodies appear to have a portion absent, and do not appear to be compressed. Adjacent vertebrae frequently have an altered shape that conforms to the defect found in the congenitally affected segment. Vertebral endplates are smooth and of normal thickness.

Hemivertebrae should be differentiated from vertebral compression due to a traumatic fracture, pathologic fracture due to vertebral neoplasia, or osteomyelitis. Most often these other problems result in disruption of

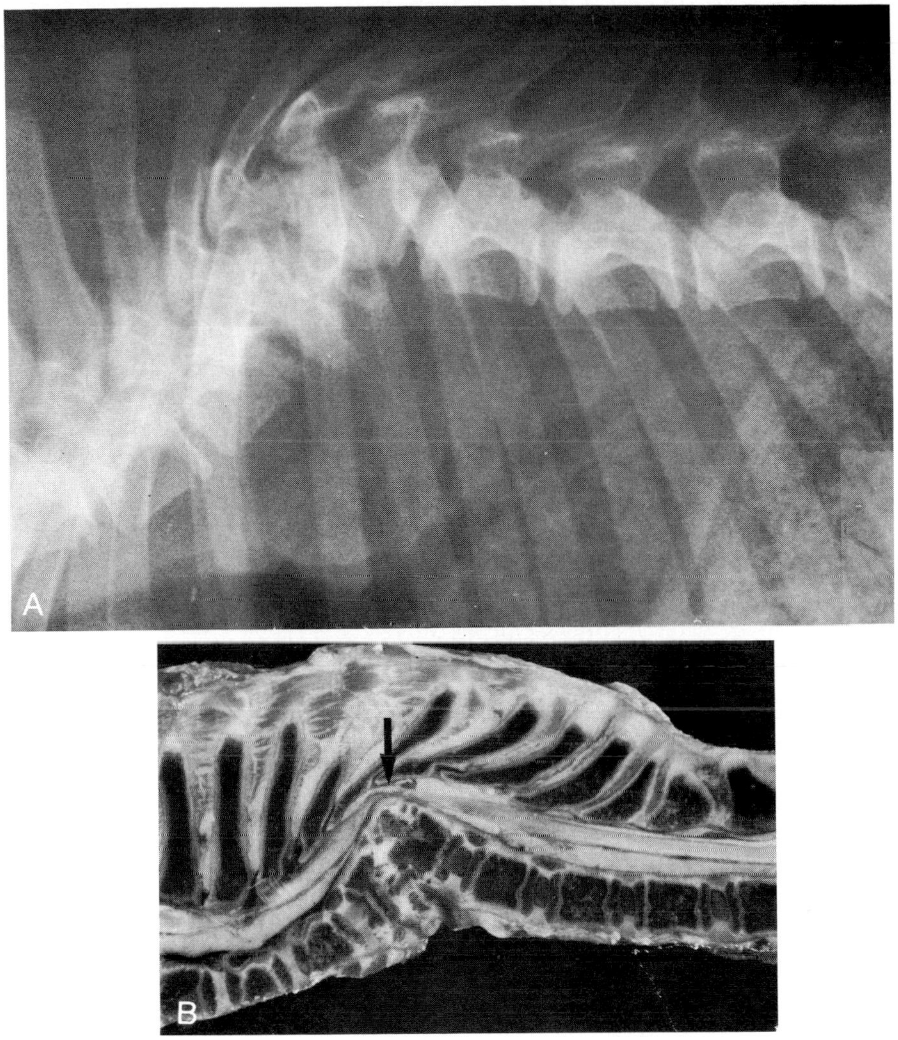

FIGURE 62–9. Hemivertebrae. Lateral radiograph *(A)* of the midthoracic region of the vertebral column of a three-month-old male malamute that had a history of inability to use the pelvic limbs since birth. Pain perception was absent in the pelvic limbs. Note the kyphosis associated with hemivertebrae affecting three midthoracic vertebrae. Severe spinal cord compression (arrow) is seen in a gross necropsy specimen *(B)* of the vertebral column sectioned in the midsagittal plane.

the trabecular pattern or ventral and lateral cortical shadows of vertebrae. Vertebral osteophytes may be seen in association with either unstable hemivertebrae or acquired vertebral lesions. In most cases, myelography is necessary to determine the presence of spinal cord compression resulting from a congenital anomaly.

Treatment. Vertebral anomalies resulting in spinal cord compression and instability of the vertebral column may be treated by means of surgical decompression and stabilization. It is important to determine that a congenital anomaly is the cause of an animal's myelopathy by ensuring that the clinical signs are consistent with the observed abnormality. Further, it is essential that radiographs and a myelogram of the entire vertebral column have been obtained. Caution must be exercised in completing surgery on an animal with a vertebral anomaly, and prognosis must be guarded. Animals may have more than one spinal abnormality, and vertebral anomalies may be associated with congenital spinal cord anomalies that are not amenable to surgical treatment.[132]

Corticosteroid-Responsive Meningitis (Aseptic Meningitis)

Etiology and Pathogenesis. Corticosteroid-responsive meningitis occurs in young, medium to large breeds of dog, and may be the most frequently occurring form of meningitis in dogs.[5, 8, 86, 133, 134] The etiology is unknown; however, immune-mediated mechanisms seem likely, as a causative agent has not been identified and affected animals improve when treated with corticosteroids. A positive LE clot test that may be an indicator of an immune-mediated disease process has been detected in several animals.[133, 134] Dogs in one study did not have detectable antinuclear antibody.[134] It has been suggested that repeated vaccinations with multivalent modified live vaccines may be a cause of immune-mediated disease by sensitizing the host to viral antigens. This may account for the presence of the disease in young dogs, which generally receive several vaccinations within the first year of life.[135]

One affected dog was examined pathologically.[133] Histologic changes indicated chronic active suppurative leptomeningitis.

The clinical and clinical pathologic findings associated with this disease are very similar to those seen in dogs with necrotizing vasculitis of the spinal meningeal arteries. Both diseases appear to have a similar pathogenesis.

Clinical Findings. Affected dogs generally are between seven and 16 months of age. There is not an apparent sex predilection. Clinical signs include reluctance to move, arched back, stiff gait, apparent cervical and/or thoracolumbar pain, fever, muscle rigidity or spasms, apparent pain on opening the mouth, and less commonly, neurologic deficits such as decreased conscious proprioception, paraparesis, or tetraparesis. Optic neuritis has been reported in an affected animal.[134] Clinical signs are indistinguishable from those of meningitis and myelitis due to other causes (bacterial, fungal, viral) and necrotizing vasculitis of spinal meningeal arteries. Clinical signs may be acute in onset and progressive, or may have a waxing and waning course over a period of weeks or months.

Diagnosis. Diagnosis is made on the basis of increased white blood cells in CSF, failure to isolate an infectious agent from CSF, and response to therapy with corticosteroids. Ninety per cent of affected dogs may have a mature neutrophilia in peripheral blood.[136] The CSF white blood cell count may be normal, or may range from 50 to more than 3000 cells/μl, with predominantly mature neutrophils. Bacteria or fungi are not seen within white blood cells. Occasionally a single CSF sample may be normal.[134] Protein concentration in the CSF most often is increased (40 to 350 mg/dl). Bacterial (aerobic and anaerobic) and fungal cultures of the CSF, urine, and blood are negative. It may be difficult to distinguish this disease from granulomatous meningoencephalomyelitis (GME) on the basis of CSF analysis, although GME is usually seen in older dogs, has a higher percentage of mononuclear cells in the CSF, and is often progressive despite transient improvement with corticosteroid therapy.

Treatment. Initially, a corticosteroid is given at a dose sufficient to produce a remission of clinical signs (prednisone 1–2 mg/lb/day). Corticosteroids are reduced slowly over several months to the lowest dose necessary to maintain a remission of clinical signs. Maintenance treatment using every other day dosage is preferred. Approximately 50 per cent of affected animals have recurrence of clinical signs following discontinuation of corticosteroid therapy.[136] Increasing the corticosteroid dose may be necessary if clinical signs recur.[134] Therapy for up to six months may be necessary to prevent recurrence of clinical signs. Ideally, a CSF puncture should be repeated, and results of analysis should prove to be within normal limits, prior to cessation of therapy. Prognosis for eventual resolution of clinical signs is good. Treatment with antibiotics may be indicated initially if the diagnosis is uncertain and bacterial meningitis is suspected.

Degenerative Myelopathy of Dogs

Etiology and Pathogenesis. Degenerative myelopathy (also called chronic degenerative radiculomyelopathy) is characterized by slowly progressive ataxia and paresis of the pelvic limbs. Degenerative myelopathy is characterized histologically by demyelination, axonal degeneration, and astrocytosis in the white matter of the spinal cord.[137, 138] These changes are found throughout the spinal cord and are most severe in thoracic spinal cord segments, especially in dorsolateral and ventromedial funiculi.[137–139] Spinal cord lesions are not restricted to particular fiber tracts, are not continuous throughout the length of the spinal cord, and in most cases are not bilaterally symmetrical.[139] In some dogs, severe degeneration of the lumbar dorsal nerve roots (with sparing of the ventral nerve roots) and lesions in the dorsal and intermediate gray matter of the spinal cord have been found.[137] Similar lesions have not been found in all studies,[138, 139] which may be due to examination at different stages of the disease process.

Etiology of degenerative myelopathy is unknown. A primary demyelinating disease or a primary axonal degeneration with secondary demyelination is possible.[139] Dural ossification (osseous metaplasia or "ossifying pachymeningitis"), spondylosis deformans, chronic intervertebral disk protrusion, or infectious or vascular disorders may occur concurrently with degenerative myelopathy.[137, 138]

There are clinical and pathologic similarities between degenerative myelopathy and a myelopathy associated with vitamin B_{12} deficiency in humans.[40] An enteropathy characterized by abnormalities in the specific activity of small intestinal brush border lysosomal enzymes has been described in dogs with degenerative myelopathy; however, hypovitaminosis B_{12} was not a consistent feature.[140] The relationship between this enteropathy and degenerative myelopathy is not known.

Impairment in the proliferative response to thymus-dependent mitogens by peripheral blood leukocytes, which correlates with the clinical status of affected dogs, has been found in dogs with degenerative myelopathy.[141] Lymph node and spleen cell populations are normal in these dogs. Myelin basic protein (MBP) specific hypersensitivity was not detected in dogs with degenerative myelopathy by leukocyte proliferation in the presence of MBP *in vitro*.[141] The depressed response to thymus-dependent mitogens by peripheral blood leukocytes was associated with the presence of peripheral blood suppressor cells.[142] The relationship between this impaired response to thymus-dependent mitogens, the presence of peripheral blood suppressor cells, and the development of degenerative myelopathy has not been established.

It has been suggested that degenerative myelopathy may result from an autoimmune response to a neural antigen (distinct from MBP), and the abnormal immunologic findings from an attempt by the host to control an autoimmune event.[141] Suggestions that the disease is due to a "dying back" process[137] have not been supported by morphologic and morphometric studies.[139] "Dying back" of neurons is seen in toxic neuropathies and is characterized by degeneration of long fiber tract systems in the spinal cord with the location of the most severe lesions in the terminal, or near terminal, regions of affected pathways. Lesions are bilaterally symmetric and predominantly involve large-diameter fibers, a pattern that is not found in degenerative myelopathy.

The occurrence of degenerative myelopathy predominantly in German shepherd dogs and German shepherd mixed breed dogs suggests a genetic basis for the disease, although evidence indicating a hereditary susceptibility in the German shepherd breed does not exist. Analysis of the pedigrees of affected dogs is needed. Degenerative myelopathy has been described in three closely related Siberian huskies, suggesting a hereditary basis for the disease in this breed.[143]

Clinical Findings. Degenerative myelopathy generally occurs in dogs six years of age or older. Males are affected more often than females. It has been reported most commonly in German shepherd dogs and German shepherd mixed breed dogs although it does occur in other large and medium breeds of dog including collie and collie crosses, Labrador retrievers, Siberian huskies, Chesapeake Bay retrievers, and Kerry blue terriers.[137–139, 143]

Affected dogs usually are presented with a slowly progressive paraparesis and pelvic limb ataxia. Onset of clinical signs is gradual with the abnormal pelvic limb gait often attributed to hip dysplasia or a traumatic incident. Neurologic deficits often are more noticeable when the dog walks on smooth surfaces. Affected dogs may have worn pelvic limb toenails. Although neurologic deficits are most often present bilaterally they may be asymmetric.[137, 138] Paraparesis and ataxia progressively worsen such that most affected dogs become nonambulatory within several months to one year after neurologic deficits are first detected. Paralysis of the pelvic limbs rarely occurs, probably because most large dogs are euthanatized if they become nonambulatory.

Apparent pain or discomfort is not evident in affected dogs. Voluntary control of urination and defecation is retained, although affected dogs may not be able to urinate or defecate in an appropriate place due to severe paraparesis or inability to assume a voiding posture. This is important, as some dogs are presented for apparent incontinence in the house, which may suggest a lesion of the cauda equina or sacral spinal cord segments.

Muscle atrophy is not severe in the initial stages of the disease, but may become noticeable in later stages; it is due to disuse rather than denervation. Cutaneous and deep pain perception remains intact throughout the course of the disease.

Neurologic examination findings usually are indicative of a transverse myelopathy between T3 and L3. Abnormalities include decreased or absent conscious proprioception and placing reactions in the pelvic limbs, normal to exaggerated patellar reflexes, normal to exaggerated withdrawal reflexes in the pelvic limbs, normal anal sphincter tone and anal reflex, normal muscle tone in the tail, and in some cases crossed extensor reflexes in the pelvic limbs. The panniculus reflex usually is normal bilaterally. It is important to note that patellar reflexes may be decreased or absent unilaterally or bilaterally in some cases, possibly as a result of degeneration of the dorsal root ganglia or dorsal gray matter of the lumbar spinal cord (i.e., an afferent rather than a LMN lesion).[137] Pathologic changes in dorsal root ganglia may be part of the disease process or may be an age-related change.[144]

Diagnosis. Diagnosis of degenerative myelopathy is based on clinical findings and age and breed of dog and by ruling out all other causes of a transverse myelopathy in the T3 to L3 region of the spinal cord. Diseases to be considered in the differential diagnosis include diskospondylitis, myelitis, spinal cord compression due to type II intervertebral disk protrusion, or spinal neoplasia. Radiographs of the vertebral column may be normal, or may demonstrate degenerative changes such as dural ossification, spondylosis deformans, or narrowed intervertebral disk spaces.

An increased protein content (40–100 mg/dl) is often found in CSF collected from the lumbar subarachnoid space. Cerebrospinal fluid protein level is usually normal in samples collected from the cisternal subarachnoid space. The white blood cell count is normal in both lumbar and cisternal CSF.

Significant myelographic abnormalities are not found. Occasionally dogs may have more than one spinal cord lesion, for example, spinal cord compression due to a type II disk protrusion and degenerative myelopathy, making degenerative myelopathy very difficult to identify. Degenerative myelopathy may be suspected if a dog fails to improve after two weeks of treatment with corticosteroids.

Treatment. Effective treatment has not been reported, and affected dogs usually progress to a state of severe nonambulatory paraparesis within a year of initial diagnosis. Occasionally, depending on animal and owner compliance, a dog may be managed with intensive nursing care, and may be supported in a cart for many months.

Degenerative Myelopathy of Cats

Etiology and Pathogenesis. Degenerative myelopathy has been described in a six-year-old cat.[145] Histologic examination of spinal cord confirmed diffuse demyelination and marked astrocytosis in white matter. Lesions were most severe in the midthoracic to midlumbar spinal cord segments. Axonal degeneration was relatively uncommon; however, findings were morphologically similar to those of degenerative myelopathy of dogs. The etiology of the myelopathy was not determined; however, the cat was FeLV positive, and the possibility of virus-induced myelopathy was considered. Recently retroviruses have been associated with the development of chronic progressive myelopathy in humans.[146, 147] In light of this information, all cats with progressive myelopathy should be tested for both FeLV and FTLV.

Clinical Findings. In the single report of degenerative myelopathy, the affected cat showed progressive symmetric paraparesis over a period of several months. Neurologic deficits were consistent with a transverse myelopathy between T3 and L3 spinal cord segments. Clinical improvement was not apparent after treatment with corticosteroids.

Diagnosis. The diagnosis of this condition is similar to that described for degenerative myelopathy of dogs.

Treatment. As for degenerative myelopathy of dogs, effective treatment has not been described.

Demyelinating Myelopathy of Miniature Poodles

Etiology and Pathogenesis. Demyelination of the brain stem and spinal cord has been reported in young miniature poodles.[148–150] Extensive symmetrical demyelination within all funiculi and segments of the spinal cord is seen on histologic examination. The demyelination is most severe in cervical segments and in tegmentum. Lesions also are found in white matter in other areas of the midbrain, medulla, cerebellar peduncles, cerebellum, and corpus callosum. The majority of axons are spared. The etiology and pathogenesis of the disease are unknown; however, a hereditary basis for the disorder is suspected.[8, 148]

Clinical Findings. Affected dogs are between two and five months of age. Clinical signs are indicative of a progressive, diffuse myelopathy. Initially, progressive paraparesis is seen, followed by tetraparesis, paraplegia, and tetraplegia over a period of two weeks. Withdrawal reflexes are normal, and extensor thrust reflexes are present. Muscle tone in all limbs is increased, and tetraplegic dogs may lie in lateral recumbency with forelimbs held in extension. Pain perception remains normal. Cranial nerve deficits are not present, and affected animals are alert and responsive. Affected animals are not in apparent pain.

Diagnosis. Diagnosis is made on basis of breed, age, and clinical signs, and by ruling out other causes of diffuse myelopathy, including canine distemper myelitis. In one dog for which CSF results were reported, the white blood cell count was normal.[148]

Treatment. Effective treatment for this disorder has not been described and prognosis is hopeless.

Diskospondylitis (Spondylitis, Vertebral Osteomyelitis)

Etiology and Pathogenesis. Bacterial or fungal infection of the intervertebral disks and adjacent vertebral bodies (diskospondylitis), or of only the vertebral bodies (spondylitis), may result in extradural spinal cord or cauda equina compression due to extension of granulation tissue and bony proliferation within the vertebral canal, or due to pathologic fracture or luxation of an infected vertebra or vertebrae. Less commonly, diskospondylitis may lead to diffuse or focal meningitis and myelitis.

Diskospondylitis and spondylitis result from implantation of bacteria or fungi introduced by migrating plant awns (grass seeds, foxtails), hematogenous spread, extension of a paravertebral infection, a penetrating wound, or previous disk or vertebral surgery.

Diskospondylitis and spondylitis occur more commonly in dogs in areas where grass awn infections are a problem. Several theories exist to explain migration of grass awns to the vertebral column. Awns may be swallowed and migrate through the bowel wall (possibly at the caudal duodenal flexure), through the mesentery to the attachment to ventral epaxial muscles, and to the vertebral column.[151] Evidence of scarring, however, has not been found in the gut or abdomen of dogs with diskospondylitis. As dogs with diskospondylitis thought to be due to plant awn migration have lesions most commonly in the cranial lumbar spine (L2-L4) it has been suggested that awns may be inhaled and migrate through the lungs to the diaphragm, and lodge at the crural insertion on the lumbar vertebrae.[4] Plant awns may also migrate through skin and paravertebral or abdominal muscles to the vertebral column. Grass seeds are able to travel long distances due to the direction of the barbs. Forward progress may be aided by muscle movements.[151]

Hematogenous spread of bacteria or fungi is probably the most common cause of diskospondylitis. Sources of infection include bacterial endocarditis and sites of dental extraction. Urinary tract infections have been implicated as a primary focus of infection. Retrograde flow in the vertebral veins has been suggested as a possible route of infection to the vertebral column. Whether diskospondylitis associated with urinary tract infection is due to venous or arterial dissemination of bacteria, or whether there is a direct causal relationship between urinary tract infection and diskospondylitis, has not been established. Many dogs with diskospondylitis have concurrent urinary tract infection. Diskospondylitis due to *Brucella canis* infection most likely results from bacteremic spread from a genital infection.[152]

Affected intervertebral disks may have evidence of degeneration (collapsed disk space, spondylosis deformans) or trauma (traumatic disk protrusion, vertebral luxation). Prior disease or injury to the disk has been suggested as a factor in the pathogenesis of diskospondylitis.[4, 153]

Diskospondylitis has been found in a number of dogs in a single kennel.[154] Immunologic studies completed in affected dogs showed evidence of immunosuppression, which may play a role in the pathogenesis of diskospondylitis. Diskospondylitis and vertebral osteomyelitis also have been reported associated with *Mycobacterium avium* infection in basset hounds.[155] An inherited immunodeficiency was suggested as a predisposing factor in these dogs.[155]

Organisms most commonly isolated from blood, affected vertebrae, and urine of dogs with diskospondylitis are coagulase-positive *Staphylococcus* spp *(aureus, intermedius)*. Other organisms that have been isolated include *Bacteroides capillosus, Brucella canis, Nocardia* sp, *Streptococcus canis, Corynebacterium* sp, *Escherichia coli, Proteus* sp, *Pasteurella* sp, *Paecilomyces* sp, *Aspergillus* sp, and *Mycobacterium* sp.[155–170] *Coccidioides immitis* may cause vertebral body osteomyelitis.[171] *Hepatozoon canis* infection has been associated with periosteal bone proliferation of the vertebrae as well as other bones of the body.[172] *Spirocerca lupi* infection may cause productive bony changes on the ventral aspect of thoracic vertebrae where the aorta and the esophagus run in parallel course.[165]

Clinical Findings. Diskospondylitis may occur in dogs of any age and is most commonly seen in giant and large breeds of dog. Diskospondylitis has been reported in a cat.[173] Diskospondylitis may occur at any level of the vertebral column, and multiple lesions may be seen, in either adjacent vertebrae (particularly in the cranial thoracic spine)[174] or nonadjacent vertebrae (especially in cases where hematogenous spread of an infecting organism occurs). Diskospondylitis occurs more commonly in thoracic and lumbar spine than in cervical spine. The lumbosacral disk space frequently is involved.

Clinical findings depend on the location of the affected vertebra or vertebrae. The most common clinical signs are weight loss, anorexia, depression, fever, reluctance to run or jump, and apparent spinal pain (which may be severe). Hyperesthesia may be present only over the site of the lesion or may be poorly localized, especially with involvement of multiple sites.

Diagnosis. Diagnosis may be difficult, as clinical signs often are nonspecific. Diskospondylitis should always be considered in an animal with fever of unknown origin. If the lumbosacral intervertebral disk is involved, dogs often show a stilted, short-strided pelvic limb gait and shifting pelvic limb lameness. Clinical signs commonly are present for several weeks or months before a diagnosis of diskospondylitis is made.

Neurologic deficits associated with spinal cord or cauda equina compression may be present, and may reflect either a transverse or a multifocal myelopathy. Neurologic deficits associated with a transverse myelopathy (T3-L3) occur most commonly and include paraparesis, decreased conscious proprioception, exaggerated spinal reflexes, and much less commonly, paraplegia. Cervical lesions most commonly cause only apparent cervical pain, and lumbosacral lesions may cause neurologic deficits due to compression of nerves of the cauda equina. Rarely animals may demonstrate clinical signs of diffuse suppurative meningitis associated with extension of infection to involve the spinal meninges. Dogs may have a history of draining tracts in the paravertebral area associated with grass seed migration. Diskospondylitis has been described in dogs with osteomyelitis in other sites (femur and sternum).[155a]

Affected animals may have a normal or elevated peripheral white blood cell count. Typical radiographic findings are destruction of the bony endplates adjacent to an infected disk, collapse of the intervertebral disk, and varying degrees of new bone production. Early lesions may consist only of lytic areas in affected vertebral endplates. More advanced lesions show a mixture of bone lysis and extensive new bone production, with osteophytes bridging adjacent vertebrae containing a central destructive focus (Figure 62–10). Affected vertebral bodies may be shortened and bony proliferation may result in fusion of one or more vertebrae. Dogs with paravertebral grass seed migration may have radiographic abnormalities suggestive of paravertebral abscess formation and periosteal bone formation on the ventral aspect of vertebral bodies. This occurs most frequently in the cranial lumbar region.

Diskospondylitis may be superimposed on other vertebral abnormalities including fracture and associated callus formation, spondylosis deformans, or a surgical site. Infection may be difficult to distinguish from a healing fracture, unstable fracture or congenital malformation, or postoperative changes. Diskospondylitis usually can be distinguished from a neoplastic lesion, as neoplasms rarely cross intervertebral disk spaces. Lesions of spondylosis deformans have intact (and more sclerotic) vertebral endplates compared with the roughened and lytic vertebral endplates present in diskospondylitis. However, older dogs may have a pattern of bony destruction of endplates that is due to a noninflammatory process associated with degeneration of the disk. In such cases, destruction of endplates occurs secondary to instability of the disk. This degenerative problem may be difficult to distinguish from diskospondylitis.[4]

Diskospondylitis may be present in more than one site in the vertebral column, especially following hematogenous route of infection. Therefore, it is important to radiograph the entire spine in animals known or suspected to have diskospondylitis. Occasionally, clinical signs may occur before characteristic radiographic changes are evident. If diskospondylitis is suspected, and characteristic lesions cannot be found, a dog should be radiographed again in two to four weeks. Well-positioned, good quality radiographs, usually with the animal under general anesthesia, are required for diagnosis of early cases of diskospondylitis. Tomography may also be a useful method for radiographic diagnosis of diskospondylitis, particularly at the lumbosacral junction (Figure 62–11). Nuclear bone scans, which are available in some institutions, may be useful either for detection of early lesions prior to development of radiographically evident lesions, or in animals in which it is uncertain whether lesions are due to infection or to other causes (e.g., severe spondylosis deformans).

Collection of CSF is indicated in animals with neurologic deficits. Cerebrospinal fluid may be normal, or may have an increased protein content in cases where diskospondylitis lesions cause extradural compression of spinal cord or result in meningitis and/or myelitis. The CSF white blood cell count may be normal, or may be elevated, with an increase in PMN neutrophils in CSF from animals with meningitis or myelitis.

Myelography is indicated in animals with neurologic deficits indicative of spinal cord compression and is mandatory in cases in which decompressive surgery is considered. Myelographic findings usually indicate extradural compression, which results from extension of granulation tissue and bony proliferation within the spinal canal. Clinical signs do not always correlate well with the degree of compression seen on myelography, and depend on factors such as rate and duration of compression as well as degree of compression.

Aerobic, anaerobic, and fungal cultures of blood and urine should be done prior to treatment in an attempt to isolate causative organisms. Some authors consider any organism other than *S. aureus* cultured from the urine unlikely to be the causative organism unless it is also cultured from blood or a vertebral lesion.[160] Cultures of CSF are indicated if the WBC count is elevated. Cultures of fluid from draining sinuses may also be done.

Efforts should be made to diagnose *B. canis* infection in all dogs with diskospondylitis. The serologic diagnosis of canine brucellosis is difficult as surface antigens of *B. canis* cross-react with antibodies to other nonpathogenic organisms seen in dogs. The rapid slide agglutination test may be used as a screening test. This test has a high negative predictive value; that is, over 99 per cent of dogs negative by the slide test are truly free of disease. A tube agglutination test and agar gel immunodiffusion test are also available, and each provides somewhat greater diagnostic specificity.[88] As dogs with *B. canis* infection remain bacteremic for months to years, blood culture is an effective method for diagnosis.

Surgical biopsy may be indicated in affected dogs in which a causative organism is not isolated from blood or urine, and/or animals that are unresponsive to treat-

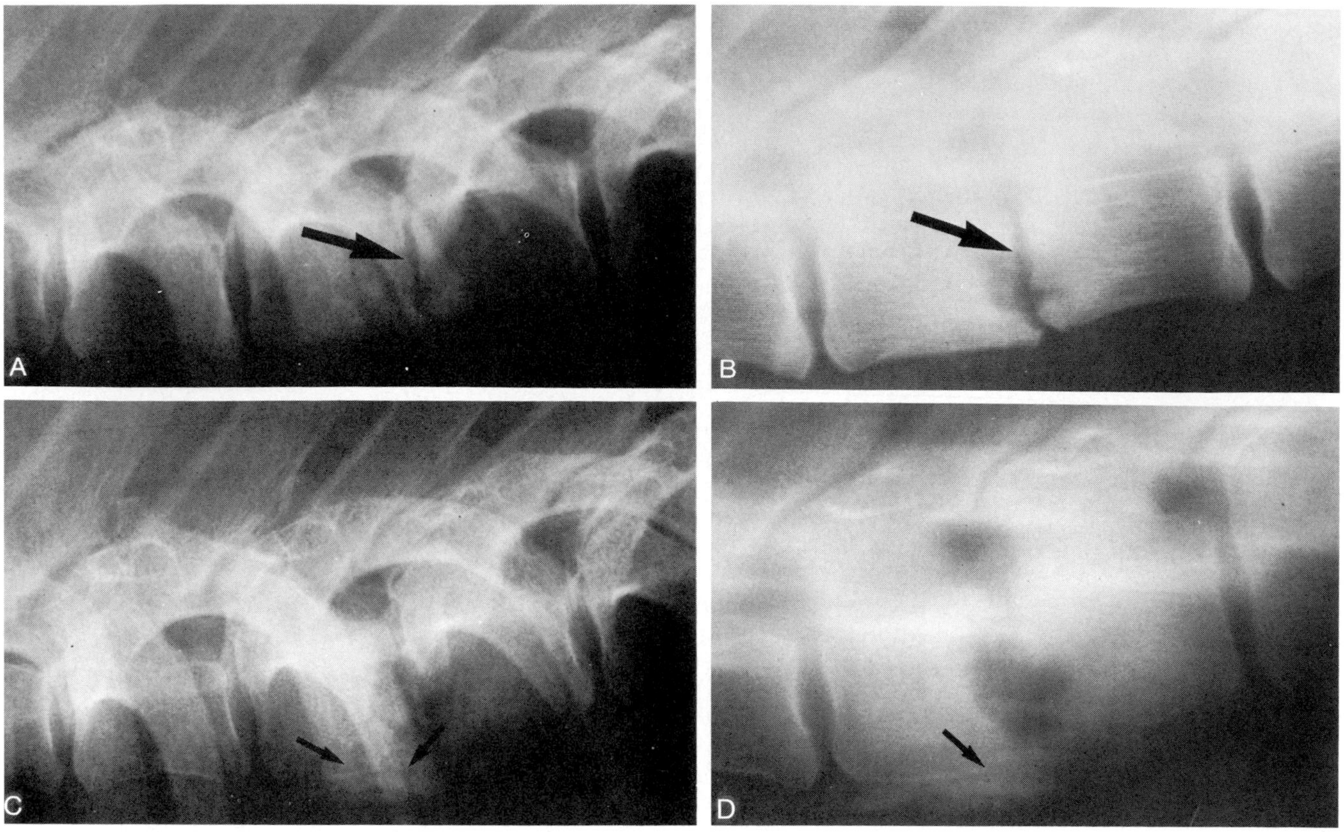

FIGURE 62–10. Diskospondylitis. Lateral radiograph *(A)* and linear tomogram *(B)* of the midthoracic vertebral column of a one-year-old female Doberman pinscher eight weeks following the onset of apparent back pain. Note the collapse of the T6-T7 disk (arrow), destruction of vertebral endplates, and well-delineated lysis of the T6 and T7 vertebral bodies. These changes are easily observed on the tomogram, where superimposed ribs are not a factor. Lateral radiograph *(C)* and linear tomogram *(D)* of the midthoracic vertebrae completed three months following *A* and *B*. The dog had received a four-week course of a broad-spectrum antibiotic that resulted in clinical improvement following the initial radiographic examination; however, signs of spinal pain had returned. Note progression of the radiographic changes seen three months earlier, and the presence of bony proliferation (arrows) at T6-T7. Following surgical biopsy and culture of the T6-T7 disk, therapy with an appropriate antibiotic drug was commenced. Complete radiographic resolution of the diskospondylitis and fusion of the T6-T7 vertebrae was apparent after six months of continued antibiotic therapy.

ment with broad-spectrum antibiotics. Fluoroscopy guided needle aspiration of lesions is possible in some animals. However, cultures of samples collected in this way are often negative, especially if animals have been treated with antibiotics prior to completion of a biopsy.

Treatment. Treatment of diskospondylitis in animals without neurologic deficits, or with mild neurologic deficits, consists of long-term use of an antimicrobial that is effective against the causative organism(s) determined by results of blood and/or urine cultures. If an organism is not cultured, dogs without severe neurologic deficits may be treated empirically, assuming infection with the most common organism isolated from animals with diskospondylitis (coagulase-positive *Staphylococcus* sp). Antibiotics that are most effective for this purpose are cephalosporins, or penicillinase-resistant penicillins such as oxacillin and cloxacillin. A trimethoprim/sulfonamide combination or chloramphenicol is less effective but is less expensive, and may be effective in some cases.

Clinical signs may recur if the infection is not completely eliminated prior to cessation of antibiotic therapy, and repeated cultures of blood and urine and ongoing treatment with an appropriate antibiotic may be necessary. Treatment is continued for at least six weeks, and vertebral radiographs are done every two to three weeks to monitor progression/regression of a lesion. Antibiotic administration may be necessary for up to six months before radiographic evidence of resolution of lesions is seen. Obtaining radiographs to monitor response to therapy is important also to monitor for development of new lesions.

Lesions resulting from *B. canis* infection appear to be less severe and more slowly progressive than those caused by other bacterial diskospondylitides.[175] A combination of minocycline or tetracycline and streptomycin is recommended for treatment of *B. canis* infections.[84a, 88, 176, 177] Treatment is expensive and often is ineffective, probably due to intracellular location of bacteria. A decreasing antibody titer is considered an indication of resolving infection. Recrudescence of infection after cessation of antibiotic therapy occurs commonly although periodic antibiotic therapy may keep affected dogs free of clinical signs.[175] Infected dogs should be

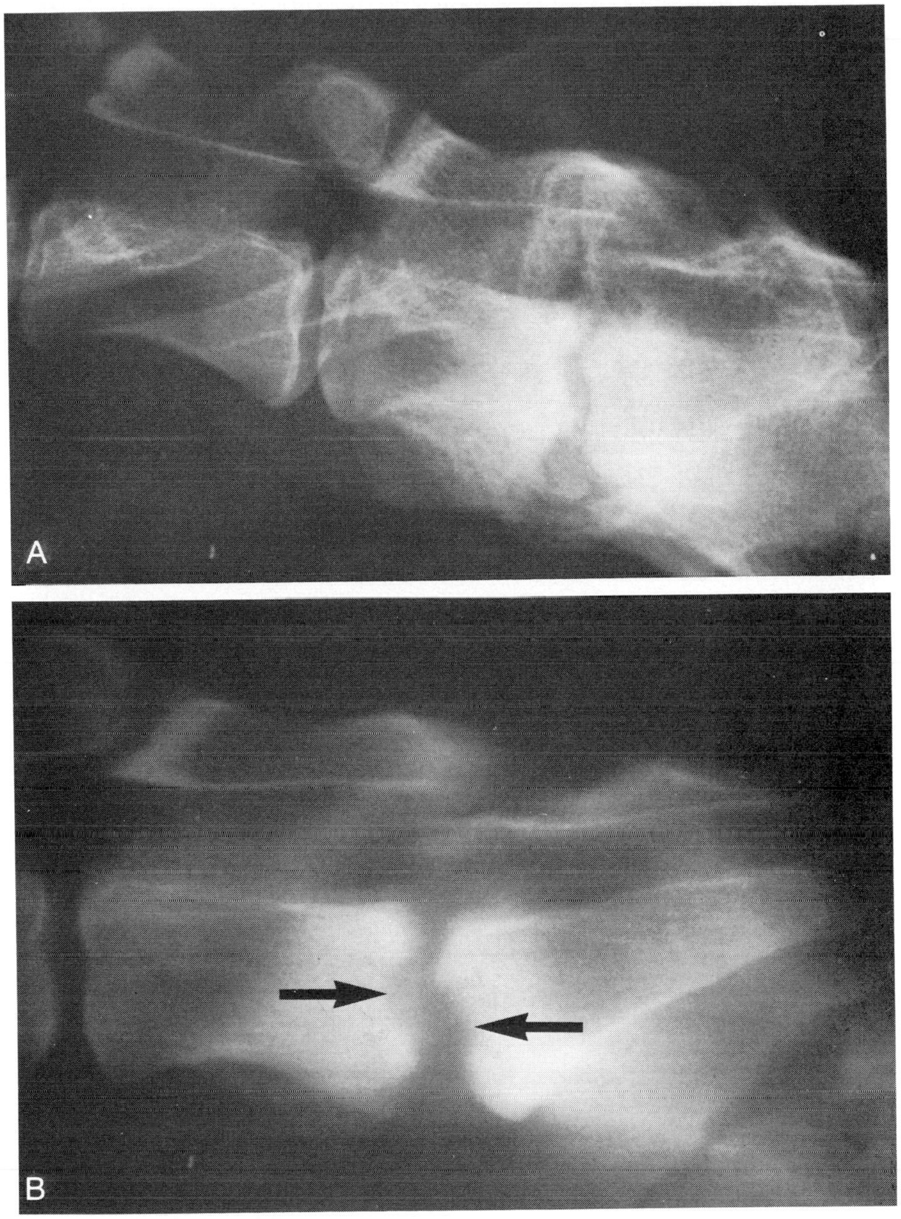

FIGURE 62–11. Diskospondylitis. Lateral radiograph *(A)* and linear tomogram *(B)* of the lumbosacral region of the vertebral column of a four-year-old German shepherd that had a one-month history of apparent lumbar pain and pelvic limb weakness. Note sclerosis of vertebral endplates, spondylosis deformans, new bone formation, and collapsed disk seen on the radiograph of L7-S1. A tomogram of this region confirms the presence of bone lysis (arrows) consistent with a diagnosis of diskospondylitis. *Staphylococcus aureus* was cultured from urine, blood, and material obtained from the L7-S1 disk by means of needle aspiration.

neutered to eliminate risk of transmission. *B. canis* infections have public health significance, as people may become infected. Symptoms in people are usually mild and nonspecific, and the infection can be treated successfully with tetracycline.[178] The overall risk of human infection from dogs with diskospondylitis due to *B. canis* infection is low unless the animal is aborting or excreting organisms in the urine.[88]

Clinical improvement in animals with diskospondylitis (resolution of fever, improved appetite, reduction of apparent spinal pain) should be seen within two weeks of starting antibiotic therapy. If clinical improvement is not seen, treatment should be reevaluated. Antibiotic therapy should be reviewed, and surgical biopsy of a lesion may be considered. Use of analgesics and restriction of exercise during the first weeks of treatment may be helpful.[159]

Surgical exploration of a lesion should be considered in animals that are unresponsive to treatment or have persistent draining tracts suggestive of grass seed migration. Objectives of surgery are curettage of lesions and harvesting of material for bacterial and fungal culture. A cancellous bone graft has been recommended following curettage of a disk space. Decompressive surgery is indicated if evidence of spinal cord compression is found on myelography, and in animals showing severe or progressive neurologic deficits. Diskospondylitis lesions may be stable due to extensive osteophyte production; however, surgical stabilization of the vertebrae may be necessary if decompression is necessary over more than one intervertebral disk space or there is radiographic evidence of vertebral instability prior to surgery.

Prognosis for animals with diskospondylitis depends on the ability to eliminate the causative organism(s) and on the degree of neurologic dysfunction. Animals with severe neurologic deficits have a guarded to poor prognosis.

Distemper Myelitis and Myoclonus

Etiology and Pathogenesis. Infection with canine distemper (CD) virus may result in a progressive, diffuse, multifocal, or focal myelopathy. Affected animals may or may not have a history of systemic illness. Dogs of any age may be affected but those with myelitis due to CD infection are usually less than three years of age. Dogs that have been vaccinated according to recommended schedules may be affected.

Canine distemper virus is a neurotropic virus. Infection with CD virus may result in both gray and white matter changes. The white matter of the cerebellum, cerebellar peduncles, optic nerves, optic tracts, and spinal cord is most severely affected. Focal or diffuse demyelination may occur in the white matter of the spinal cord. The mechanism by which demyelination occurs is not known but it may be due to a primary effect of the virus on glial cells,[178, 179] or immunologic mechanisms may be the primary cause.[180, 181] Both mechanisms may be involved with the direct viral effects occurring acutely, and local immune responses may result in chronic progressive demyelination.[182–184]

Further histopathologic changes seen in the spinal cord and throughout the CNS include perivascular cuffing by mononuclear cells, gliosis, microglial proliferation, inflammatory cell infiltration of the pia-arachnoid, and neuronal changes (nuclear pyknosis, chromatolysis, shrunken cells, and neuronophagia). Intranuclear and intracyloplasmic inclusions may or may not be present. The presence of inclusions is not an indication of the severity of the disease.

Clinical Findings. Canine distemper myelitis may occur as a focal or a diffuse disease at any location in the spinal cord. Clinical signs reflect the location of the lesion(s). The T3-L3 spinal cord segments are affected most often, and clinical signs indicative of a transverse myelopathy in this region are seen. Neurologic abnormalities include paraparesis or paraplegia and normal to exaggerated reflexes in the pelvic limbs. Neurologic deficits are progressive and are bilateral; however, they may be asymmetrical.

Affected dogs may have clinical signs indicative of current or previous systemic CD infection, including naso-ocular discharge, gastroenteritis, pneumonia, and hyperkeratosis of the nose or foot pads. Neurologic deficits indicative of multifocal or disseminated CNS infection may be present. Neurologic deficits commonly seen in dogs with CD infection are vestibular and/or cerebellar abnormalities and visual deficits. Chorioretinitis with retinal hyperreflectivity and "medallion" lesions may be present on ophthalmoscopic examination.

Self-mutilation occasionally is seen in dogs with CD infection. The limbs and tail are the common sites of mutilation. Paresis or paralysis of the limbs may also be present. The location of the lesion in the peripheral or central neural pathways resulting in self-mutilation is unknown.[11]

Diagnosis. Antemortem diagnosis often is difficult. Clinical signs of multifocal CNS disease, particularly neurologic deficits indicative of spinal cord and cerebellovestibular disease, are highly suggestive of CD infection.

Hematologic findings in dogs with CD infection are nonspecific. Abnormalities of CSF may be useful in diagnosis of CD infection; however, CSF may be normal. The CSF white blood cell count and protein content are usually mildly to moderately elevated in CD infection. Cells seen in CSF are predominantly lymphocytes (10–60 cells/μl). The presence of interferon in CSF appears to be a reliable indicator of virus persistence.[185]

Increased CD virus–specific antibody titers in CSF may be useful in the diagnosis of CD infection. Increased anti–CD virus antibody in CSF may offer evidence for chronic CD infection, as antibody is produced locally in the CNS, and significant levels of increased titers have rarely been present in vaccinated dogs or in dogs with systemic CD infection without CNS involvement. Cerebrospinal CD antibody may be artifactually increased if the blood-brain/spinal cord barrier is disrupted during CSF collection, causing whole blood contamination of CSF. Negative CD antibody results do not rule out a diagnosis of CD.[88, 185]

Serologic demonstration of levels of neutralizing, precipitating, or cytotoxic antibody is not sufficient for a diagnosis of CD. Antibody may be induced by vaccination, and although a persistently elevated or rising serum antibody titer may be suggestive of CD infection, titers may not increase after onset of clinical disease. The only specific serologic test available would be demonstration of virus-specific IgM in dogs that have not been vaccinated within three weeks prior to sampling.[185] Specific antibody may not be present in dogs with acute distemper infection.[186]

Immunofluorescence may be used to demonstrate viral antigen in conjunctival or vaginal imprints, in cells from tracheal washings, in lymphocytes in CSF, or in buffy-coat preparations. Unfortunately in subacute and chronic forms of CD, viral antigen has disappeared from buffy coat and surface epithelium, and therefore negative test results do not rule out a diagnosis of CD.

Other techniques available for the antemortem diagnosis of CD include demonstration of inclusion bodies in cells of the buffy coat and use of advanced immunologic techniques.[88]

Treatment. Clinical signs of CD myelitis may be either rapidly or more slowly progressive. Periods of apparent improvement may be seen followed by progression of clinical signs. A specific antiviral drug having an effect on CD in dogs is not presently available. Favorable results have been reported by some investigators with short-duration (one to three days) corticosteroid therapy.[88] Intravenous administration of modified live vaccine in dogs with CD is only effective if given before clinical signs appear. Treatment of CD myelitis is almost always unrewarding. Symptomatic and supportive therapies are indicated in certain cases. The prognosis is poor for recovery. In dogs that recover from CD infection, residual signs such as myoclonus or optic neuritis may improve with time. Immunization by vaccination is the only effective approach to CD prevention at the present time.

DISTEMPER MYOCLONUS

Myoclonus is the rhythmic twitching of a muscle or muscle group and is most often associated with CD infection. This condition has been incorrectly named "chorea" by some investigators; however, this term applies to a movement disorder of humans produced by a basal ganglia disorder. Any muscles may be involved including the facial and masticatory muscles or limb muscles. The pathogenesis of myoclonus is unknown. It is thought to result from an abnormality in the motor neuron and interneuron pools of the medulla and spinal cord. Myoclonus is not dependent on descending pathways from the brain, but is abolished following transection of ventral spinal roots of nerves innervating affected muscles. Animals may recover from systemic CD infection, and occasionally from CNS infection; however, myoclonus may persist. Myoclonus is generally permanent and may persist during sleep. Myoclonus may be alleviated by continuous oral therapy with procainamide.[8] Other drugs used to treat myoclonus in humans, such as clonazepam, may be useful in the control of myoclonus but have not yet been used extensively in dogs.[8]

Dural Ossification

Etiology and Pathogenesis. Dural ossification (osseous metaplasia of the dura mater; "ossifying pachymeningitis") is the formation of bony plaques on the inner surface of the dura mater. Bony plaques are found most commonly in the cervical and lumbar spine and may occur laterally, ventrally, or dorsally. Dural ossification is found in over 40 per cent of large and small breeds of dog over two years of age, and in over 60 per cent of dogs five years of age or older.[187, 188] Although many dogs with dural ossification also have spondylosis deformans, a direct correlation between the two conditions does not exist. The etiology of dural ossification is unknown.

Clinical Findings. Dural ossification rarely results in neurologic deficits or apparent spinal pain in dogs. Other causes of spinal cord disease should be ruled out before attributing clinical significance to dural ossification.

Diagnosis. Radiographically, bony plaques appear as thin radiopaque lines (linear shadows), which are most easily viewed at the site of intervertebral foramina (Figure 62–12).[4] These linear shadows need to be distinguished from calcified herniated disk material within the spinal canal, vertebral osteophytes, and the accessory processes of the lumbar vertebrae.[188]

Treatment. There is not a specific treatment for dural ossification; however, surgical removal of a bony plaque from the vicinity of a nerve root rarely may be necessary to alleviate apparent pain due to nerve root compression.

Feline Infectious Peritonitis, Meningitis, and Myelitis

Etiology and Pathogenesis. Pyogranulomatous meningitis and myelitis may occur in cats with FIP. Feline infectious peritonitis results from a coronavirus infection and is most commonly seen in younger cats between six months and five years of age. Infected cats may also have concurrent FeLV infection.[189, 190] Meningeal and spinal cord lesions are probably the result of immune complex–mediated vasculitis. Involvement of the CNS is more frequently observed in the noneffusive (dry) form than in the effusive (wet) form of FIP. Multifocal and diffuse involvement of the CNS is common and a consistent clinical course is not associated with FIP.[191]

Clinical Findings. Feline infectious peritonitis may result in focal, multifocal, or diffuse involvement of the spinal cord, brain, and meninges, and clinical signs reflect the location of these lesions. Leptomeningitis with infiltration of spinal nerve roots has also been reported.[192] The most commonly recognized neurologic signs are pelvic limb ataxia, hyperesthesia (especially over the back), and generalized ataxia.[189, 191]

Affected animals usually manifest other clinical signs indicative of disseminated disease such as persistent fever (frequently greater than 105° F), weight loss, enlarged kidneys, chorioretinitis, panophthalmitis, or anterior uveitis.

Diagnosis. Diagnosis is made on the basis of clinical signs, clinical pathology (blood, CSF), and serology. Hematologic changes include neutrophilia, lymphopenia, and elevated serum fibrinogen and gamma globulins. Cerebrospinal fluid usually is abnormal with an elevated white blood cell count and protein level. The differential CSF white blood cell count is variable but PMN cells, lymphocytes, and monocytes usually are present. Polymorphonuclear cells may be the predominant cell type in CSF. Protein concentration may be very high (greater than 2000 mg/dl),[189] and CSF may be viscous and may clot. This should be taken into consideration when performing a CSF puncture, as fluid may flow into the needle very slowly.

Results of cytologic examination of CSF, however, depend on the degree of meningeal involvement. Meningeal inflammation may be extensive and CSF in these cases is generally very abnormal. In the presence of focal or parenchymal inflammation, CSF may be normal.

Cats with FIP generally have a high antibody titer. Presence of a positive antibody titer is not diagnostic of FIP, but in the presence of clinical signs, hypergammaglobulinemia, and abnormal CSF findings consistent with FIP is highly suggestive of FIP infection.[190] Similarly, a low antibody titer does not rule out FIP. The differential diagnosis list for CNS FIP includes toxoplasmosis, cryptococcosis, and lymphosarcoma.

Treatment. Prognosis for cats with FIP of the CNS is poor. The FeLV status of cats suspected to have FIP should be determined prior to commencing treatment, as the prognosis for cats with both viruses is hopeless.[190] The most effective treatment protocols combine high levels of corticosteroids (prednisolone 1 to 2 mg/lb orally once daily in the evening), cytotoxic drugs (either cyclophosphamide 1 mg/lb orally once daily for four consecutive days of each week, or melphalan 1 mg orally every third day) and broad-spectrum antibiotics (ampicillin 10 mg/lb orally q8h), together with maintenance of nutrient intake and electrolyte balance.[190] Cats receiving cytotoxic drugs should be routinely monitored for evidence

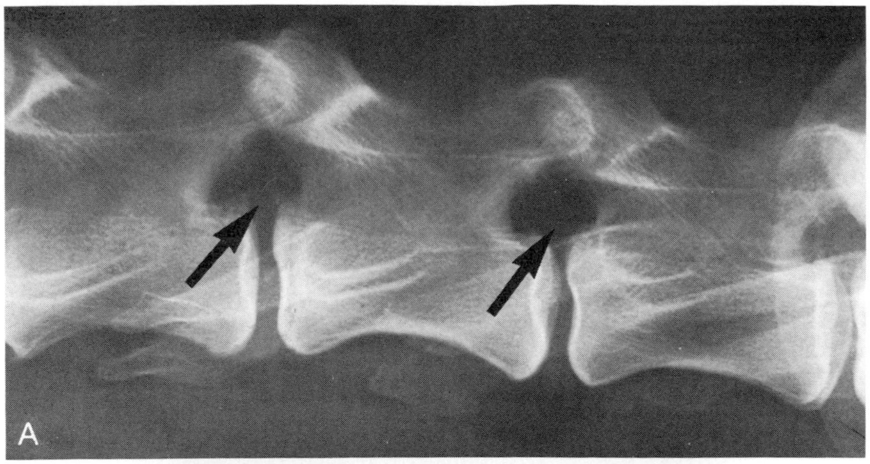

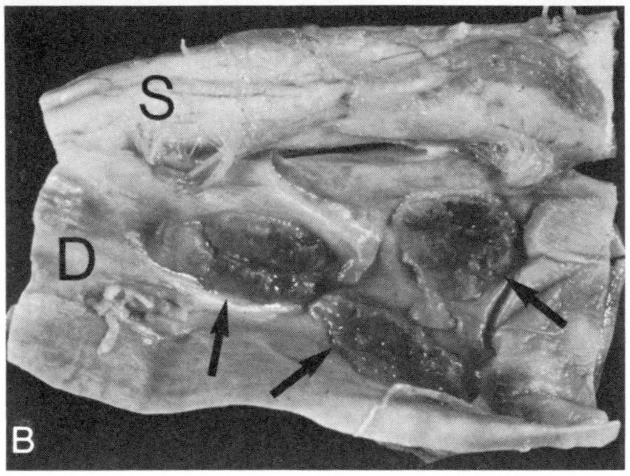

FIGURE 62–12. Dural ossification. *A*, Lateral projection of the midlumbar region of a 12-year-old male German shepherd. Note the bone plaques (arrows) in the dura mater that are seen as sharply defined linear densities. Dural ossification often is present at the level of an intervertebral foramen and should not be confused radiographically with extruded disk material. This dog did not have clinical signs of spinal cord disease. *B*, Gross necropsy specimen of the spinal cord (S) of a nine-year-old female German shepherd with dural ossification. The dura mater (D) has been longitudinally incised and reflected exposing nodular-appearing plaques of ossification of the dura mater (arrows). This dog did not have clinical signs of spinal cord disease.

of kidney dysfunction or bone marrow suppression. If a positive response to therapy is seen, treatment should be continued for at least three months.[190] Cats with neurologic disease associated with FIP usually respond poorly to treatment.[189]

Feline Polioencephalomyelitis

Etiology and Pathogenesis. Feline polioencephalomyelitis is a chronic, slowly progressive encephalomyelitis of unknown etiology described in immature and mature cats.[88] Histopathologically, the disease is characterized by neuronal degeneration and perivascular cuffing by mononuclear cells. Demyelination and axonal loss is most conspicuous in the ventral and lateral columns of the spinal cord and most severe in the thoracic spinal cord segments.[193, 194] Lymphocytic meningitis, neuronophagia, and glial nodules also have been described, and lesions may be found in the cerebral cortex, diencephalon, midbrain, and medullary nuclei.[88]

The pathogenesis of the disease is unknown. A viral etiology is suspected on the basis of the histopathologic changes although a specific viral agent has not been isolated. The chronic clinical course, distribution of lesions, and lack of inclusions distinguish this disease from rabies, pseudorabies, and FIP. Feline panleukopenia virus, FeLV, and arboviruses have been suggested as possible agents in the pathogenesis of lesions. Further virologic and serologic tests are needed to determine the role of viral infection in the pathogenesis of this disorder.

Clinical Findings. Clinical signs include ataxia, paraparesis, tetraparesis, hypermetria, head tremors, and localized hyperesthesia. Spinal reflexes, pupillary light reflexes, and postural reactions may be normal or depressed. Two animals have been described as having episodes of hallucinations, clawing, hissing, and biting at imaginary objects during sleep. These "seizures" preceded other clinical signs by more than two years in one cat. Clinical signs usually are indicative of multifocal CNS disease but may be suggestive of focal transverse myelopathy in the thoracolumbar region or lumbar enlargement. Clinical signs are slowly progressive over several months.

Diagnosis. Antemortem diagnosis is difficult and is made by ruling out other multifocal CNS diseases. Two affected cats have been reported to be leukopenic, and one affected cat had an elevated CSF protein concentration (40 mg/ml).[193]

Treatment. Treatment of affected cats has not been reported.

Globoid Cell Leukodystrophy (Krabbe Type Leukodystrophy)

Etiology and Pathogenesis. Globoid cell leukodystrophy is an inherited lysosomal storage disease that results from a deficiency in beta-galactosidase (galactocerebrosidase). Globoid cell leukodystrophy is characterized by bilaterally symmetric demyelination of the white matter of the brain, spinal cord, spinal nerve roots, and peripheral nerves, and by accumulation, especially perivascularly, of large phagocytic cells with foamy-appearing cystoplasm (globoid cells) containing nonmetachromatic, nonsudanophilic, and PAS-positive material. Ultrastructurally, this material consists of degenerated myelin sheaths and various types of inclusions thought to represent galactocerebroside accumulation.[195] Globoid cell leukodystrophy appears to be inherited as an autosomal recessive trait in Cairn terriers[196] and West Highland white terriers,[197] and findings in other breeds of dog suggest a recessive factor.[195] The condition may not be inherited as a simple autosomal recessive trait in cats.[198]

The disease is seen in young animals and is progressive. In some affected animals, neurologic deficits occur predominantly in pelvic limbs, and in others cerebellar signs predominate. The reasons for the predominant pelvic limb abnormalities in some dogs are not known.

Clinical Findings. Globoid cell leukodystrophy has been reported to occur in several breeds of dogs including Cairn terriers and West Highland white terriers and in domestic cats.[195, 196, 198-203] Clinical signs generally are first seen between two and six months of age. However, neurologic abnormalities were not evident in an affected basset hound until four years of age.[200] Affected cats usually show abnormalities by six weeks of age.

Progressive paraparesis and paraplegia predominate in some affected animals. Spinal reflexes in the pelvic limbs may be normal or exaggerated, indicative of T3-L3 transverse myelopathy. Neurologic signs in affected animals usually progress to quadriparesis, dysmetria, head tremor, behavioral changes, and/or blindness. Spinal reflexes may be decreased or absent and muscle atrophy may be evident in some animals, indicative of LMN disease. Clinical signs usually progress over a period of two to six months, although clinical signs were observed to progress for two years in one dog.[201] Clinical signs in cats with globoid cell leukodystrophy are generally more indicative of cerebellar disease and are more rapidly progressive than in dogs.[198]

Diagnosis. Diagnosis is made on the basis of age, breed, and presence of progressive neurologic deficits and by ruling out other causes of progressive myelopathy such as canine distemper myelitis.

Cerebrospinal fluid may contain phagocytic cells containing PAS-positive material (globoid cells) and CSF protein content may be increased.[204] In some animals CSF may be normal. Brain and/or peripheral nerve biopsy may show characteristic demyelination and globoid cell accumulation and may be done to confirm a diagnosis of globoid cell leukodystrophy.

Treatment. Treatment for globoid cell leukodystrophy has not been described.

Granulomatous Meningoencephalomyelitis (GME, Reticulosis)

Etiology and Pathogenesis. Granulomatous meningoencephalomyelitis is a nonsuppurative meningoencephalomyelitis of unknown etiology in dogs. It is characterized histopathologically by large perivascular accumulations of mononuclear cells throughout the brain, spinal cord, and meninges (Figure 62–13). Controversy exists as to the naming of this disease and origin of the primary cell types involved in these perivascular accumulations. The terms granulomatous meningoencephalomyelitis and inflammatory reticulosis have been used when perivascular accumulations are predominantly macrophages, lymphocytes, plasma cells, and neutrophils, with a low mitotic index.[205] The term neoplastic reticulosis has been used in those cases in which accumulated cells are predominantly reticulohistiocytic cells, with a high mitotic index. Histiocytic cells may arise either from the mesenchymal elements of the CNS or from blood monocytes.[206, 207] One author has suggested epithelioid cells in GME result from differentiation of macrophages that originate from the migration and maturation of blood monocytes.[208] Others suggest that histiocytic cells result from the proliferation of undifferentiated mesenchymal elements of the adventitia of blood vessels, leptomeninges, and microglia of the spinal cord and brain.[209, 209a]

A resident mononuclear phagocyte cell population has been identified in the normal brain of normal dogs.[209, 209a] Recent immunologic studies in dogs have shown that some inflammatory and neoplastic reticuloses of the CNS are immunoglobulin-bearing lymphosarcomas (B-cell tumors).[209, 209a] Other immunoglobulin-lacking neoplastic reticuloses may be true reticulosarcomas. Many inflammatory reticuloses with a polyclonal immunoglobulin-bearing cell population are true inflammatory processes (granulomatous meningoencephalomyelitis). The pathogenesis of these inflammatory lesions is unknown.[88, 209, 209a] This discussion is limited for the most part to GME. Microorganisms have not been demonstrated in lesions, nor have any been isolated following culture of affected tissue. However, GME has features suggestive of a cell-mediated immunologic response, possibly to the sustained presence of an infectious organism.[210]

The lesions of GME vary in location but generally are disseminated randomly throughout the nervous sys-

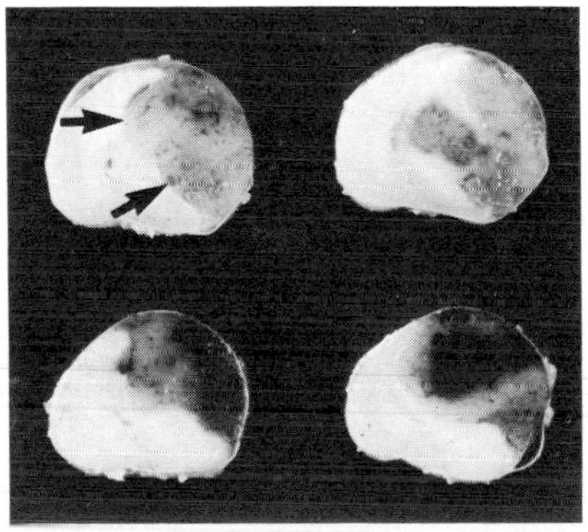

FIGURE 62–13. Granulomatous meningoencephalomeylitis. Gross necropsy specimens of the cervical spinal cord from a four-year-old female miniature poodle with a history of apparent neck pain and progressive tetraparesis and generalized ataxia. An intramedullary space-occupying lesion is seen in adjacent transverse sections of the midcervical spinal cord (arrows). The histopathological diagnosis was granulomatous meningomyelitis.

tem and can be found in the cerebral hemispheres, cerebellum, spinal cord, brain stem, diencephalon, and midbrain. Optic nerves also may be affected. White matter generally is more severely affected than gray matter. Perivascular accumulation of cells may be massive and lesions may coalesce to form large granulomas that cause clinical signs indicative of a focal, space-occupying lesion. Edema and necrosis of parenchyma between lesions may be seen. Lesions in the leptomeningeal vasculature result in clinical signs of meningitis. Neoplastic reticuloses identified as lymphosarcomas are focal mass lesions rather than disseminated disease processes.[209, 209a] The distribution of meningeal lesions is not related to that of parenchymal lesions.[205]

Clinical Findings. Granulomatous meningoencephalomyelitis has been reported frequently in purebred and mixed breeds of dog. A higher incidence has been found in female dogs, small breed dogs, and poodle, poodle-mixed breed dogs, and Airedale terriers.[205, 206, 208, 210, 211] Affected dogs usually are between one and nine years of age, although dogs may be affected at any age.

Clinical signs are variable and may indicate focal or multifocal cerebral, brain stem, cerebellar, and/or spinal cord involvement. Granulomatous meningoencephalomyelitis may involve the spinal cord at any level; however, lesions appear to be most severe in the cervical spinal cord and clinical findings are often indicative of cervical spinal cord disease. Findings include apparent cervical pain, rigidity, reluctance to move, hyperesthesia, cervical paraspinal muscle spasms, exaggerated spinal reflexes, decreased conscious proprioception, paraparesis, tetraparesis, or paraplegia.[210–212] Affected animals usually have an acute onset of clinical signs that are progressive over several days to months.

Diagnosis. Antemortem diagnosis is difficult and usually is made on the basis of clinical findings and results of CSF analysis. Clinical signs may be indistinguishable from other causes of cervical pain and cervical myelopathy. This is an important consideration in assessing animals suspected to have cervical intervertebral disk disease. Cerebrospinal fluid collection and analysis are indicated in such cases, especially if surgical decompression or fenestration is being considered.

Dogs with GME may have intermittent fever.[212] Complete blood count and appearance on spinal and skull radiographs frequently are within normal limits. The CSF is abnormal in most affected dogs. The CSF white blood cell count generally is elevated (may be greater than 1000 WBC/μl). Mononuclear cells predominate.[211, 212] The percentage of lymphocytes and monocytes varies considerably. Polymorphonuclear cells may also be present and constituted 0 to 62 per cent of the differential white blood cell count in one study.[211] In the same study, less than one per cent of the differential white blood cell count consisted of macrophages with ingested debris, plasma cells, and cells undergoing mitosis.[211] The total and differential CSF white blood cell counts do not reflect the severity of meningeal involvement or the degree of necrosis.[211] Protein concentration in CSF is usually elevated, while CSF pressure may be normal or increased. Alterations in CSF were similar in untreated and corticosteroid-treated dogs in one study.[211] Meningeal lesions may render CSF collection from cisternal puncture difficult. Although CSF collected from the lumbar subarachnoid space of affected dogs may have fewer white blood cells than cisternal CSF, it is of use in diagnosis. The difference in white blood cell counts probably reflects a greater distance of the lumbar subarachnoid space from the site of the majority of lesions.[211] Bacterial and fungal cultures are negative and organisms are not identified in CSF cell preparations. Noncontrast radiography and myelography may confirm an intramedullary space-occupying lesion of the spinal cord (Figure 62–14).

Treatment. Granulomatous meningoencephalomyelitis is either continuously or episodically progressive, and the prognosis is very poor for recovery of affected animals. Treatment with corticosteroids may result in improvement of clinical signs for several days to several months or years. Immunosuppressive doses of corticosteroids should be given, and therapy must be sustained for long periods. The corticosteroid regimen used for treatment of corticosteroid-responsive meningitis should be used for therapy of dogs with GME. Clinical remissions of greater than one year occur in some cases; however, clinical signs usually recur with discontinuation of treatment with corticosteroids. Radiation therapy may be useful in treatment of GME of the spinal cord in the future.

Hemorrhage

Etiology and Pathogenesis. Intramedullary, intrameningeal, or epidural hemorrhage may occur due to coagulopathies including thrombocytopenia, clotting factor deficiencies, disseminated intravascular coagulation, and anticoagulant poisonings (warfarin and the like). Acute hemorrhage may also occur in association with tumors, vascular malformations, acute intervertebral disk protrusion, trauma, parasitic migration, or meningitis. Spontaneous intramedullary hemorrhage with hematoma formation has been reported in the cervical spinal cord of a dog.[213] Spontaneous subperiosteal vertebral hemorrhage and hematoma formation associated with spinal cord compression and transverse myelopathy have been reported in dogs.[214]

Clinical Findings. Observed neurologic deficits depend on the location of the hemorrhage and usually indicate a focal or multifocal myelopathy. Clinical signs most often are acute in onset and neurologic deficits may be severe. Extensive gray matter necrosis may occur with intramedullary hemorrhage, resulting in LMN signs over a relatively large area of the spinal cord, especially if the cervical or lumbosacral spinal cord is involved. Epidural hemorrhage may result in spinal cord compression and clinical signs indicative of a transverse (focal) myelopathy. Subarachnoid hemorrhage may result in clinical signs suggestive of meningitis, including cervical rigidity, hyperesthesia, and increased body temperature.

Diagnosis. Animals with coagulopathies may have evidence of hemorrhage elsewhere in the body (skin, mucous membranes, retina, or sclera). Diagnostic tests for coagulopathy include determination of prothrombin time, partial thromboplastin time, platelet count, activated clotting time, fibrinogen levels, and evaluation of

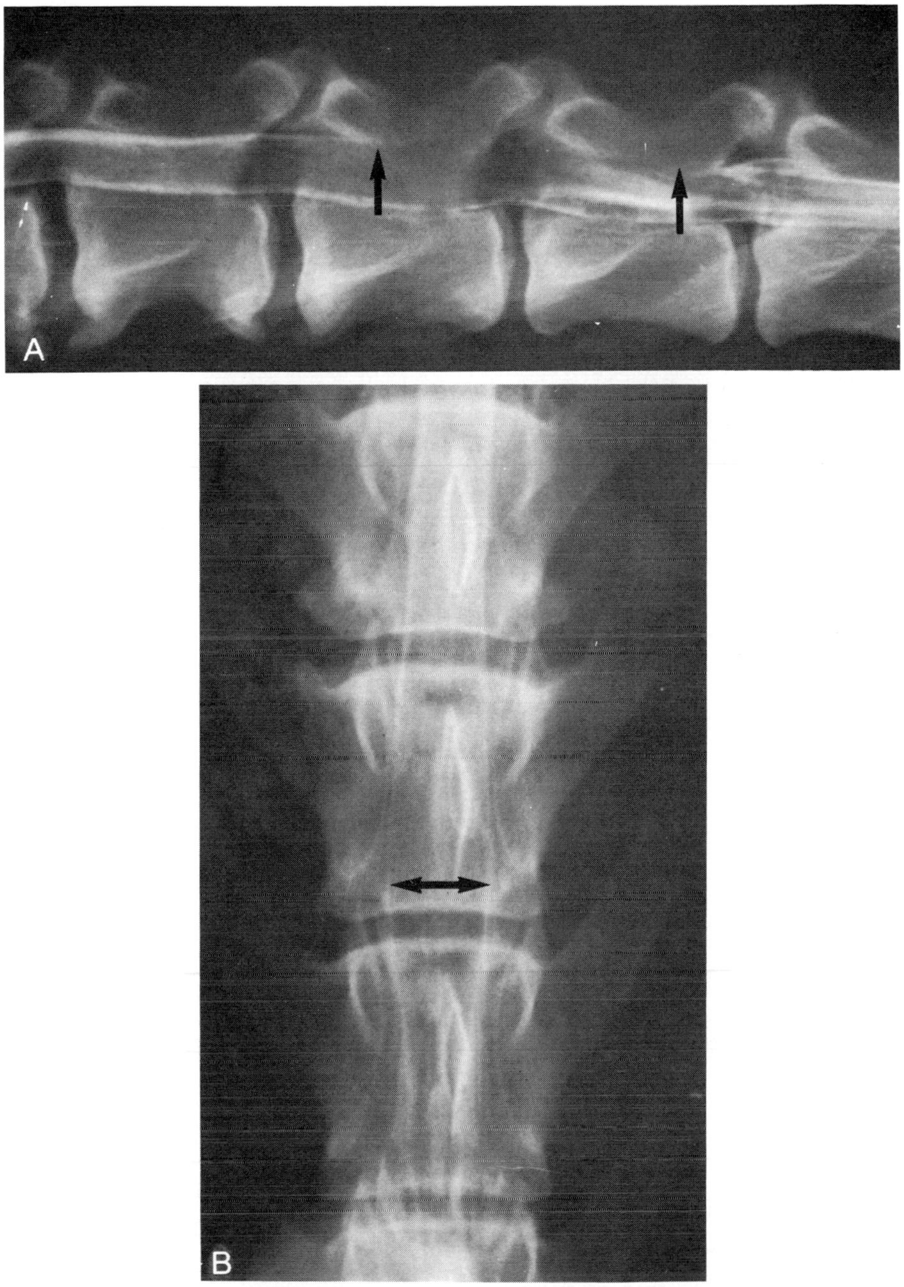

FIGURE 62–14. Granulomatous meningoencephalomyelitis. Lateral *(A)* and ventrodorsal *(B)* projections of a midlumbar myelogram of a 10-year-old male golden retriever. On the lateral projection there is loss of the dorsal contrast column at the level of the L4 and L5 vertebrae (between arrows). Intramedullary expansion of the spinal cord (double-headed arrow) is present at the level of L4-L5 vertebrae on the ventrodorsal projection. The histopathologic diagnosis was granulomatous meningomyelitis within spinal cord parenchyma.

specific clotting factor activity. Subarachnoid CSF puncture may be contraindicated in animals with a coagulopathy because of the high probability of inducing further hemorrhage. Red blood cells may be present in CSF for a short time following subarachnoid hemorrhage, and CSF supernatant may be red or pink in color. Xanthochromia may be present in CSF 48 hours or more after the hemorrhage has occurred. Cerebrospinal fluid white blood cell count and protein may also be elevated.

Myelography is indicated in cases in which epidural hemorrhage is suspected to be the cause of spinal cord compression and in which noncontrast radiographs and results of CSF analysis are normal and evidence of coagulopathy is not found. Epidural hemorrhage is not distinguishable from other extradural space-occupying lesions on myelography. Hemorrhage may be secondary to other abnormalities such as intervertebral disk extrusion, as a result of laceration of a vertebral venous sinus.

Treatment. Treatment is directed at the underlying cause in animals with coagulopathies. Epidural and intramedullary hematomas not associated with coagulopathy may be removed surgically.[213] Prognosis depends on the severity of neurologic deficits present at the time of diagnosis.

Hereditary Ataxia (Ataxia in Smooth-Haired Fox Terriers and Jack Russell Terriers)

Etiology and Pathogenesis. An inherited, progressive, generalized ataxia has been reported to occur in young smooth-haired fox terriers in Sweden and Jack Russell terriers in England.[215–217] This disease is characterized pathologically by demyelination bilaterally throughout the dorsolateral and ventromedial white matter of the spinal cord.[216] In Jack Russell terriers, widespread Wallerian-type degeneration in the white matter of the brain and degenerative changes in the central auditory pathways and peripheral nerves may be seen.[217] Hereditary ataxia is inherited as an autosomal recessive trait in smooth-haired fox terriers.[216] Etiology of ataxia in Jack Russell terriers is not known; however, clinical and pathologic findings suggest it may be congenital.[217]

Progressive ataxia also has been described in a five-month-old Pyrenean mountain dog.[218] Clinical signs were most obvious in the pelvic limbs and deficits included absent conscious proprioception and decreased patellar and withdrawal reflexes. Diffuse axonal degeneration of the dorsolateral, lateral, and ventral white matter of the medulla and spinal cord segments cranial to L5 was present at necropsy. Spinocerebellar tracts, caudal and middle cerebellar peduncles, and cerebellar folia were also involved. Axonal degeneration was also present in tibial nerve. Etiology and pathogenesis of this condition were not determined.

Clinical Findings. Both males and females are affected. Neurologic abnormalities are first seen between two and six months of age and include pelvic limb ataxia and "swinging" of the hindquarters. Ataxia becomes progressively worse over six months to two years and involves all four limbs. Affected animals often have a "prancing" pelvic limb gait.[217] Dysmetria may be severe and affected dogs fall to the ground with slight change in position.[216]

Diagnosis. Diagnosis is made on the basis of age, breed, and clinical findings.

Treatment. Treatment is not effective. Affected animals are eventually unable to walk.

Hereditary Myelopathy of Afghan Hounds (Necrotizing Myelopathy or Myelomalacia of Afghan Hounds)

Etiology and Pathogenesis. Hereditary myelopathy is a disease characterized by extensive spongiform degeneration of myelin with micro- and macrocavitation within the spinal cord white matter of young Afghan hounds.[219–221] Typically, paresis and ataxia in pelvic limbs that progress to paraplegia within 10 to 14 days occur in affected dogs.

Histopathologically, lesions are found in all funiculi of the white matter of midthoracic spinal cord segments. Ventral funicular alterations may extend to the mid- and caudal lumbar spinal cord segments. Lesions are also found in the caudal cervical spinal segments and in neurons surrounding the dorsal nucleus of the trapezoid body and ventral gray columns of the medulla.[219] Many axons are spared despite extensive myelin degeneration. Lesions are not typical of other demyelinating or leukodystrophic diseases. Pathogenesis of this disease is unknown. The cause of the myelin defect is believed to be genetic and an autosomal recessive mode of inheritance has been suggested.[219]

Clinical Findings. Clinical signs most commonly occur between three and eight months of age, although dogs as old as 13 months have been affected. The disease is seen in both males and females. Initially, affected dogs may have a "bunny-hopping" gait, followed by progressive paresis and ataxia in the pelvic limbs. Patellar reflexes usually are exaggerated and muscle tone is increased in the pelvic limbs. Thoracic limb gait is initially stiff and awkward, and progresses to become paretic. Swaying of the trunk often is evident when animals walk with pelvic limbs supported. Pain perception initially is normal, but with progression of the disease becomes impaired caudal to the cranial thoracic region. Neurologic deficits are indicative of a caudal cervical or cranial thoracic myelopathy. Late in the course of the disease affected dogs may become recumbent, and hypotonia and decreased spinal reflexes may occur. Paresis or paralysis of the intercostal muscles may result in abdominal breathing. The clinical course of the disease is rapid with severe neurologic deficits evident within two weeks of onset of clinical signs.

Diagnosis. Diagnosis of hereditary myelopathy is made on the basis of age, breed of dog, and clinical signs and by ruling out other causes of rapidly progressive caudal cervical or cranial thoracic myelopathy in young dogs, including canine distemper myelitis and necrotizing vasculitis of the spinal meningeal arteries. Cerebrospinal fluid may be normal or may have an elevated protein concentration. Significant abnormalities are not present on spinal radiographs or myelography.[219]

Treatment. Treatment for hereditary myelopathy has not been described, and prognosis for affected animals is hopeless.

Hound Ataxia

Etiology and Pathogenesis. Hound ataxia is a term used to describe a myelopathy of hunting foxhounds, harrier hounds, and beagles in the United Kingdom.[222, 223] Progressive paresis and ataxia of the pelvic limbs occur in affected dogs. Histologically, bilaterally symmetric Wallerian degeneration is present in all funiculi of spinal cord white matter. Lesions are more severe in cervical and thoracic spinal cord segments. Dorsolateral columns are relatively spared by the disease. Degeneration of ascending tracts in the brain stem, cerebellar peduncles, and Wallerian degeneration of the sciatic nerves have also been reported. The severity of histologic lesions does not appear to be related to the severity of neurologic deficits.

Etiology and pathogenesis of this condition are unknown. It is unlikely to be genetic as dogs of different breeding develop the disease when introduced to an affected pack. A nutritional or toxic etiology seems most likely as all animals were kenneled (hunt conditions) and fed a restricted diet ("paunch" and "knacker's meat").

Clinical Findings. Affected animals (male and female) were between two and seven years of age. The clinical findings are indicative of a transverse myelopathy between T3 and L3 spinal cord segments. A gradual onset of ataxia in the pelvic limbs, paraparesis, and a "stilted" gait in the pelvic limbs (without evidence of pain) characterize this disease. At a fast gait exaggerated retraction of the pelvic limbs may occur. Some affected dogs may drag their hind feet. Conscious proprioception in the pelvic limbs is decreased in some animals; however, spinal reflexes in the pelvic limbs and pain perception are normal. Muscle atrophy is not seen. In most affected animals the panniculus reflex is absent bilaterally caudal to the midthoracic or cranial lumbar spinal cord segments. Affected hounds are usually severely debilitated within 6 to 18 months of the onset of clinical signs.

Diagnosis. Diagnosis is made on the basis of age, breed of dog, and clinical findings and by ruling out other causes of progressive T3 to L3 myelopathy, including compressive lesions of the spinal cord (type II intervertebral disk protrusion, diskospondylitis, neoplasia) and intramedullary lesions such as neoplasia. Cerebrospinal fluid has been reported to be normal in affected dogs.

Treatment. Therapy for hound ataxia has not been described.

Hypervitaminosis A of Cats

Etiology and Pathogenesis. Hypervitaminosis A in cats is characterized by extensive confluent exostosis that is most prominent in the cervical and thoracic spine.[224, 225] It is caused by a chronic excess of dietary vitamin A and is usually a result of feeding a diet consisting largely of liver. Exostosis may extend to involve the entire spine, ribs, and pelvic and thoracic limbs with complete fusion of the spine and joints. Compression of spinal nerve roots or nerves may occur if new bone formation extends into intervertebral foramina.

Clinical Findings. Clinical signs in affected cats include apparent cervical pain and rigidity, thoracic limb lameness, ataxia, reluctance to move, paralysis, and hyperesthesia or anesthesia of the skin of the neck and forelimbs. The three most proximal diarthrodial joints of the cervical spine are almost always first affected. Osseous lesions develop insidiously and clinical disease usually is advanced in cats older than two years of age before significant clinical features are recognized.

Diagnosis. Radiographic evidence of extensive exostosis of the cervical vertebral column and a history of excessive dietary intake of vitamin A or liver are necessary for diagnosis.

Treatment. Reduction of dietary intake of vitamin A prevents the development of further exostosis; however, it may be difficult to persuade affected cats to eat anything other than liver.

Intervertebral Disk Disease

Etiology and Pathogenesis. Degeneration of intervertebral disks may result in protrusion or extrusion of disk material into the spinal canal resulting in spinal cord compression and clinical signs ranging from apparent pain to complete transverse myelopathy. Degenerative changes may occur in any of the intervertebral disks (C2-3 to L7-S1); however, disk protrusion or extrusion occurs most commonly in the cervical, caudal thoracic, and lumbar spine. The intervertebral disks between T1 and T11 are stabilized dorsally by the intercapital ligaments that join opposite rib heads across the floor of the spinal canal over the dorsal anulus fibrosus of the intervertebral disk.[34] These ligaments are closely associated with the dorsal longitudinal ligament located on the floor of the spinal canal and the dorsal anulus fibrosus of each disk. As a result, disk protrusion or extrusion is less likely in this region.

Two types of disk herniation (type I and type II) have been reported to occur in dogs by Hansen.[226] Type I disk herniation occurs with degeneration and rupture of the dorsal anulus fibrosus and extrusion of nucleus pulposus into the spinal canal. Type I disk extrusion is most commonly associated with chondroid disk degeneration (Figure 62–15). Type II disk protrusion is characterized by bulging of the intervertebral disk without complete rupture of the anulus fibrosus. Type II disk protrusion is most commonly associated with fibroid disk degeneration (Figure 62–16).

Chondroid metaplasia of the nucleus pulposus and Type I disk extrusion occur most commonly in chondrodystrophoid breeds including dachshund, beagle, Pekingese, Lhasa apso, Shih Tzu, and breeds with chondrodystrophoid tendencies including miniature poodle and cocker spaniel.[227, 228] Chondroid disk degeneration and type I disk extrusion may occur in any breed,

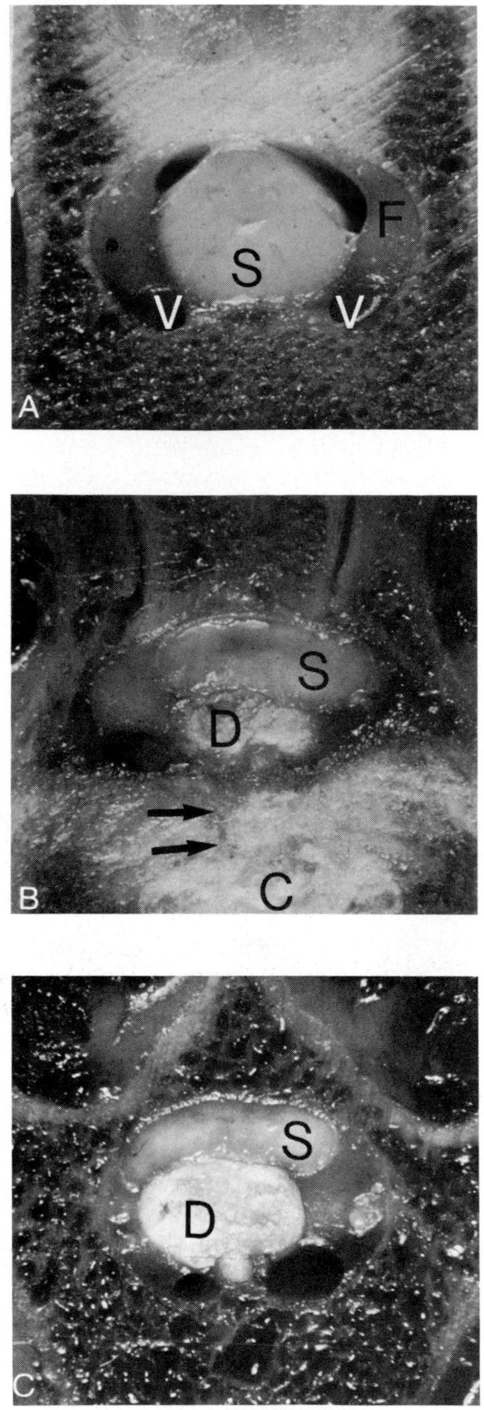

FIGURE 62–15. Type I disk extrusion. Gross necropsy specimens from a four-year-old male dachshund that had an acute onset of pelvic limb paralysis. Pain perception was absent in the pelvic limbs. Myelography confirmed acute disk extrusion at T11-T12 that had caused severe spinal cord compression. *A,* Transverse section of the T12 vertebral canal 1 cm caudal to the extruded T11-T12 disk. Note the normal appearance of the spinal cord (S) within the spinal canal. Epidural fat (F) and internal vertebral venous plexuses or vertebral sinuses (V) are also present within the spinal canal. *B,* Transverse section of the vertebral canal at the level of the T11-T12 disk. Calcified disk material (C) is present within the nucleus pulposus. A fissure (arrows) is present within the dorsal anulus fibrosus, and calcified material from the nucleus pulposus (D) has extruded through the fissure into the spinal canal. Dorsal displacement and compression of the spinal cord (S) have occurred. *C,* Transverse section of the vertebral canal 5 mm cranial to B. Extruded calcified material (D) from the nucleus pulposus is compressing the spinal cord (S) at this level.

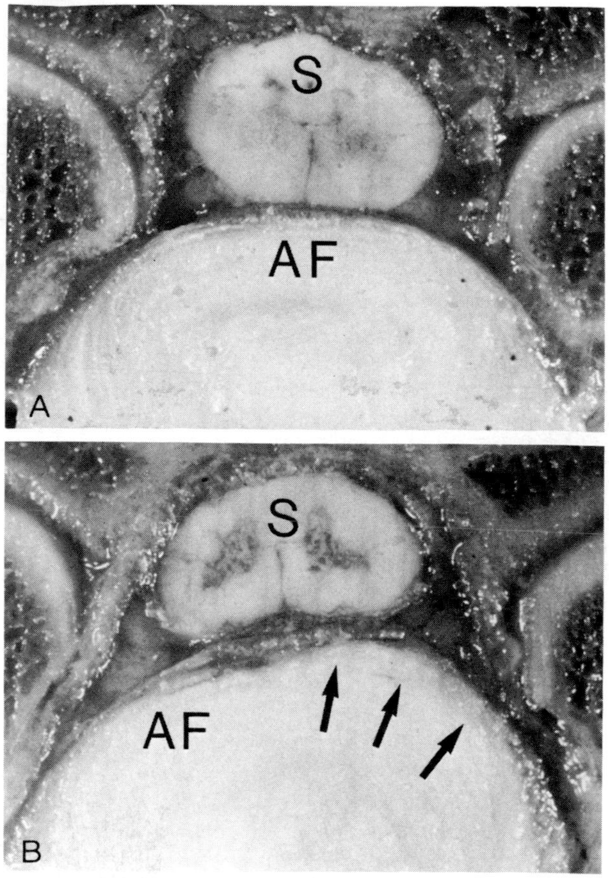

FIGURE 62–16. Type II disk protrusion. Gross necropsy specimens from a seven-year-old female Doberman pinscher that had a history of progressively worsening tetraparesis and generalized ataxia. Myelography confirmed Type II disk protrusion at C6-C7. The disk protrusion appeared to be predominantly on the left. *A,* Transverse section of the vertebral canal at the level of the C5-C6 disk. Note the normal appearance of the spinal cord (S) within the spinal canal, and the close anatomic relationship of the dorsal anulus fibrosus (AF) to the spinal cord. *B,* Transverse section of the vertebral canal at the level of the C6-C7 disk. Note the compression of the left spinal cord (S) that is resulting from dorsal bulging (arrows) of the anulus fibrosus (AF) at this level.

including large breeds of dog. These authors have noted an unusually high incidence of type I disk extrusion in Doberman pinscher dogs.[229]

Recent studies have demonstrated differences between the vertebral canal and spinal cord mensuration in dachshunds and German shepherd dogs.[229a] The spinal cord of dachshunds was found to terminate further caudally than that of German shepherd dogs. Further, the ratio of spinal cord to vertebral canal heights in the lumbar region was notably greater in dachshunds than in German shepherd dogs. The smaller lumbar epidural space in dachshunds may explain the occurrence of severe clinical signs seen in this breed in association with apparently small amounts of extruded disk material. It is also possible that the larger epidural space present in large breeds of dog may account for the fact that small amounts of extruded disk material within the spinal canal in these breeds may not cause spinal cord compression and associated clinical signs.

Chondroid degeneration of disks is characterized by an increase in collagen content of the disk, alteration of specific glycosaminoglycan concentration of the nucleus pulposus, and a decrease in water content of the disk.[230, 231] The normally gelatinous nucleus pulposus becomes progressively more cartilaginous and granular and eventually may mineralize (calcify). Extrusion of degenerative nucleus pulposus occurs through fissures in, or rupture of, the anulus fibrosus.[232] Hansen has reported that in chondrodystrophoid breeds of dog 75 to 100 per cent of all disks undergo chondroid metaplasia by one year of age.[226] Recently, the radiographic pattern of degenerative changes that occur with aging in the vertebral column and intervertebral disks of beagles has been described.[232a] This study aids in the differentiation of clinically insignificant degenerative changes and pathologic changes that may produce clinical signs.

Fibroid disk degeneration occurs in older dogs of all breeds but is most often recognized as a clinical problem in older, large-breed, nonchondrodystrophoid dogs and is characterized by fibrous metaplasia of the nucleus pulposus. An increase in the noncollagenous glycoprotein content of intervertebral disks occurs in nonchondrodystrophoid breeds of dog with aging.[230] Calcification of the disk may occur, but is rare. Protrusion of the disk occurs with a bulging of the anulus fibrosus due to partial rupture of the anular bands. Rupture of the anulus fibrosus and extrusion of nucleus pulposus (characteristic of type I disk extrusion) uncommonly is seen in association with type II disk protrusion. Intervertebral disk protrusion or extrusion may occur in a ventral, dorsal, or lateral direction. In most instances, only dorsal protrusions or extrusions are of clinical significance as meningeal irritation and nerve root and/or spinal cord compression may occur. Occasionally a lateral disk protrusion or extrusion may result in nerve root or spinal nerve compression with associated clinical signs.

The cause of intervertebral disk degeneration is unknown. Trauma does not appear to play a major role in chondroid degeneration but may be a factor in acute disk extrusion. Mechanical and anatomic factors are probably important, as disk extrusions are most common in the cervical and T11 to L3 regions of the vertebral column. Genetic factors probably have a role in the accelerated degeneration of disks in chondrodystrophoid breeds but the exact influence of these factors is not known.[233, 234] Hypothyroidism and autoimmune disease have also been proposed as contributing factors.[235–237]

Type I disk extrusion often results in more severe clinical signs than type II protrusion although the mechanical distortion and compression of the spinal cord caused by type II protrusion may be greater. Nucleus pulposus is most often extruded into the spinal canal acutely (minutes to hours) or subacutely (days) from disks undergoing chondroid degeneration, whereas slowly progressive spinal cord compression most often accompanies protrusion of disks undergoing fibroid degeneration as the bulging fibrous mass increasingly enlarges within the spinal canal. The spinal cord changes seen in acute versus chronic spinal cord compression differ, and are reflected in the difference in clinical signs and response to treatment seen in these different types of intervertebral disk disease (see Spinal Cord Trauma). The severity of spinal cord injury depends on the velocity at which the compressive force is applied, the degree of compression, and the duration of the compression.[238] Vascular factors, as well as mechanical distortion of the spinal cord as a result of herniated disk material, are important in the pathogenesis of resulting spinal cord lesions.[239] Severe spinal cord lesions may be found in spinal cord that does not have evidence of compression, presumably as a result of vascular changes.[239]

Hemorrhage, edema, and necrosis of both spinal cord gray and white matter are characteristic of acute spinal cord injury associated with acute type I disk extrusion. Hemorrhage and edema are not a major feature of chronic spinal cord compression in which white matter changes such as demyelination, focal malacia, vacuolization, and loss of axons are seen.[4, 240] Type I disk extrusions often are associated with rupture of vertebral venous sinuses, and hemorrhage into the epidural space may increase the degree of spinal cord compression. Pulmonary emboli arising from the nucleus pulposus have been described in three chondrodystrophoid dogs with acute thoracolumbar transverse myelopathies as a result of type I disk extrusions, presumably as a result of disk material entering the vertebral venous sinuses.[241] Nucleus pulposus may also penetrate the dura mater. Traumatic rupture of the anulus fibrosus and extrusion of normal nucleus pulposus may occur, resulting in spinal cord compression and an acute onset of clinical signs indicative of a transverse myelopathy.

Degenerative disk disease also occurs in cats,[242–244] although the incidence of clinical signs associated with disk protrusion is low. Degenerative changes and distribution of disk protrusions are similar to type II disk protrusions in nonchondrodystrophoid dogs. Clinical signs seen usually are indicative of a slowly progressive transverse cervical[245] or thoracolumbar myelopathy. Type I disk extrusion associated with calcification of intervertebral disks and an acute onset of neurologic deficits rarely have been reported in cats.[246] Diagnosis and treatment are similar to that described for dogs.

Clinical Findings. Chondroid degeneration and type I disk extrusion most commonly occur in dogs three years of age and older, but may occur in younger animals. Fibroid degeneration and type II disk protrusion most commonly occur in dogs older than five years of age. There does not seem to be a sex predilection for intervertebral disk disease.

Clinical signs seen with intervertebral disk disease vary depending on whether type I or type II disk herniation is present, the location of the lesion, and severity of the spinal cord lesion. Clinical signs seen in association with type I disk extrusion include apparent pain and/or motor and/or sensory deficits. These clinical signs usually develop rapidly, within minutes or hours of disk extrusion. However, clinical signs may progress slowly over several days or manifest periods of improvement and subsequent worsening over weeks or months. These findings are probably associated with extrusion of small amounts of disk material into the spinal canal over a period of time.[1]

Clinical signs associated with type I disk extrusion in the cervical spine usually are less severe than those associated with extrusions in the thoracolumbar region. Although large amounts of disk material may be extruded in the cervical region, the vertebral canal in this region is larger in diameter in relation to the spinal cord than is the case in the thoracolumbar region. Apparent neck pain is the most common clinical finding in dogs with cervical disk extrusion. Affected dogs often hold the head and neck rigidly and cry out when moved, and may show spasms of cervical musculature. Neurologic deficits indicative of a cervical myelopathy such as proprioceptive deficits, tetraparesis, or tetraplegia are seen less commonly.

Ipsilateral Horner's syndrome and hyperthermia have been described in cases of acute, severe, dorsolateral cervical disk extrusions.[247] Lower motor neuron deficits in the thoracic limbs may be seen in caudal cervical disk extrusions. Thoracic limb lameness may also be seen in caudal cervical disk extrusions as a result of nerve root compression, particularly from lateral disk extrusions where disk material enters an intervertebral foramen.

Clinical findings in animals with thoracolumbar type I disk extrusion depend on the severity of spinal cord injury, and range from apparent back or abdominal pain to complete paraplegia and loss of deep pain perception. Neurologic deficits usually are indicative of a transverse myelopathy between T3 and L3, as most disk extrusions in this region occur between T11 and L3.[248, 249] Lower motor neuron signs may be seen in the pelvic limbs if disk extrusion occurs caudal to L3 as a result of compression of the lumbosacral spinal cord or nerves of the cauda equina. Lower motor neuron signs also may be seen in paraplegic animals with progressive hemorrhagic myelomalacia (PHM). The clinical signs and diagnosis of PHM are discussed later.

The panniculus reflex may be depressed or absent caudal to the site of disk extrusion. The site of a lesion is usually one or two vertebral spaces cranial to the loss or depression of panniculus reflex.[35] The Schiff-Sherrington sign may be seen in animals with acute type I disk extrusion caudal to T2.

Clinical signs seen in both cervical and thoracolumbar type I disk extrusion may be asymmetrical, especially if extrusion occurs dorsolaterally within the spinal canal. Apparent pain associated with disk extrusions results from inflammation and/or ischemia caused by compression of meninges and/or spinal nerve roots. Extruded disk material initiates an extradural inflammatory reaction that results in fibrous adhesions between the dura mater and extruded disk material.[250, 251] Pain may also arise from stimulation of sensory nerve endings in the anulus fibrosus and dorsal longitudinal ligament.[252, 253] The nucleus pulposus of each disk does not contain nerve fiber endings.[252]

Clinical signs associated with type II disk protrusion generally are slowly progressive over a period of months. Clinical signs, however, may develop acutely over days in some animals. Neurologic deficits usually are indicative of a cervical or thoracolumbar myelopathy. Paraparesis or tetraparesis, depending on the site of the lesion, is the most common clinical finding, and deficits may be asymmetrical. In the cervical spine type II protrusions most commonly occur in caudal cervical disks. In some cases, caudal cervical type II disk protrusion may be part of the spectrum of abnormalities associated with cervical spondylomyelopathy. Apparent neck or back pain may or may not be a feature of type II disk protrusion.

Diagnosis. A tentative diagnosis of type I disk protrusion or extrusion may be made on the basis of age, breed, history, and clinical signs; however, other causes of transverse myelopathy or apparent pain should be considered in the differential diagnosis. It must be remembered that apparent spinal pain is seen in animals with meningitis. Dogs with thoracolumbar disk extrusions may show apparent abdominal pain, and in such animals causes of abdominal pain such as pancreatitis and peritonitis must be considered in the differential diagnosis.

The differential diagnosis in animals with type II disk protrusion includes all other causes of progressive transverse myelopathy, the most likely being neoplasia or degenerative myelopathy.

Spinal radiographs and, in almost all cases, CSF analysis and myelography are necessary to confirm a diagnosis of disk extrusion or protrusion. General anesthesia is required to achieve the precise positioning needed to obtain radiographs of diagnostic value. Foam wedges or sandbags are usually needed to align the vertebral column parallel to the table top for lateral projections. Care must be taken, however, in anesthetizing and positioning animals that have acute type I disk extrusions, as further extrusion of disk material and further spinal cord compression may occur with manipulation and movement of the spine.

Calcification of the nucleus pulposus is best seen on lateral radiographic views and usually is seen in one or more disks of most chondrodystrophoid dogs greater than one year of age.[232a] Calcified disks also may be seen in older nonchondrodystrophoid breeds of dog. The radiographic density of such disks varies from a slight haziness to that equal to the density of the vertebral body.[4] Calcified material within the nucleus pulposus is indicative of disk degeneration, but alone is not of clinical significance (Figure 62–17).

The disk space of an extruded disk may be narrower than adjacent disk spaces and may be wedge-shaped with a decrease in the width of the disk space dorsally. However, positioning is important as some disk spaces (C7-T1, T9-10 or T10-11, and L7-S1) are normally narrower than adjacent spaces and cervical and lumbosacral disks are normally wedge-shaped on hyperextension and flexion of the spine.[4] "Spikes" of calcified material suggestive of disk extrusion may extend dorsally from a disk. Calcified material may be present within the vertebral canal but often is difficult to visualize due to overlying vertebral articular processes or ribs. Intervertebral foramina are larger in the lumbar spine and calcified material often is easily visualized in the spinal canal in this region. Disk material within the spinal canal may appear as a hazy, indistinct shadow or as a dense mass with distinct margins.[4] The former pattern often is seen associated with explosive disk extrusion and dissemination of disk material along the spinal canal whereas the latter pattern usually is associated with a slower extrusion of disk material over a longer time with desiccation, fibrosis, and possibly further mineralization of the disk material within the spinal canal (Figure 62–18).[4] In many cases of disk extrusion calcified material is not visualized within the spinal canal, as disk material is probably not sufficiently mineralized to be visible on

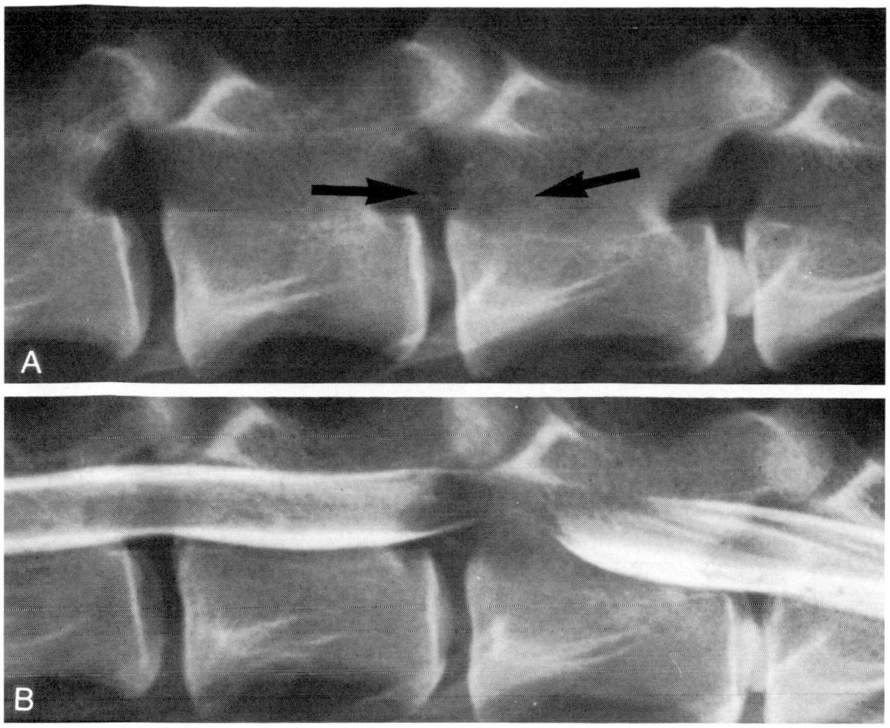

FIGURE 62–17. Type I disk extrusion. Lateral radiograph *(A)* and myelogram *(B)* of the mid-lumbar vertebrae of a ten-year-old female Doberman pinscher with an acute onset of pelvic limb paresis. A slightly narrowed L3-L4 disk is present on plain radiographs, and calcified nucleus pulposus is seen within the vertebral canal at this level (arrows). The nucleus pulposus of the L4-L5 disk is calcified; however, it remains *in situ* and is not of clinical significance at this time. A myelogram confirms the presence of ventral spinal cord compression at the level of the L3-L4 disk, and demonstrates that the calcified L4-L5 disk is not associated with spinal cord compression.

radiographs. Ventrodorsal views, and in some cases oblique views (Figure 62–19), are important in determining laterality of any visible mineralized material within the spinal canal. Vertebral osteophytes and vertebral endplate sclerosis may be seen associated with chronic disk degeneration and extrusion or in cases of chronic disk degeneration without disk extrusion or protrusion.[232a]

Type II disk protrusion may be associated with narrowing of the disk space, osteophyte production, and endplate sclerosis. Calcification of disk material rarely is seen in association with type II disk protrusion. In some animals with type I or type II disk herniation obvious abnormalities are not seen on noncontrast vertebral radiographs (Figure 62–20).

Myelography is almost always necessary to confirm that disk material has herniated into the spinal canal resulting in spinal cord compression. Myelography is most important in determining the site (or sites) of disk herniation and in lateralization of disk material within the spinal canal prior to surgical decompression. Myelography should not be done solely as a means of confirming a diagnosis of likely type I disk herniation in animals with signalment, history, clinical signs, and radiographs that are highly suggestive of disk extrusion in which surgical decompression is not anticipated. Myelography, however, is necessary for diagnosis in most cases of type II disk protrusion as a means of distinguishing disk protrusion from other causes of slowly progressive transverse myelopathy such as spinal neoplasia and degenerative myelopathy.

Cerebrospinal fluid should be collected and analyzed prior to myelography to rule out inflammatory or infectious disease of the spinal cord and/or meninges. Clinical

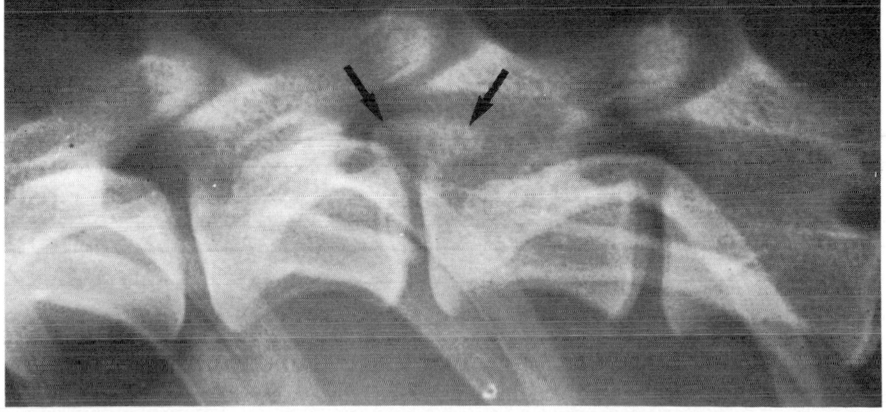

FIGURE 62–18. Type I disk extrusion. Lateral radiograph of the thoracolumbar region of the vertebral column of a four-year-old spayed female Dachshund with a history of acute onset of pelvic limb paresis. Note the narrowed intervertebral T12-T13 disk, and the calcified disk material within the vertebral canal at this level.

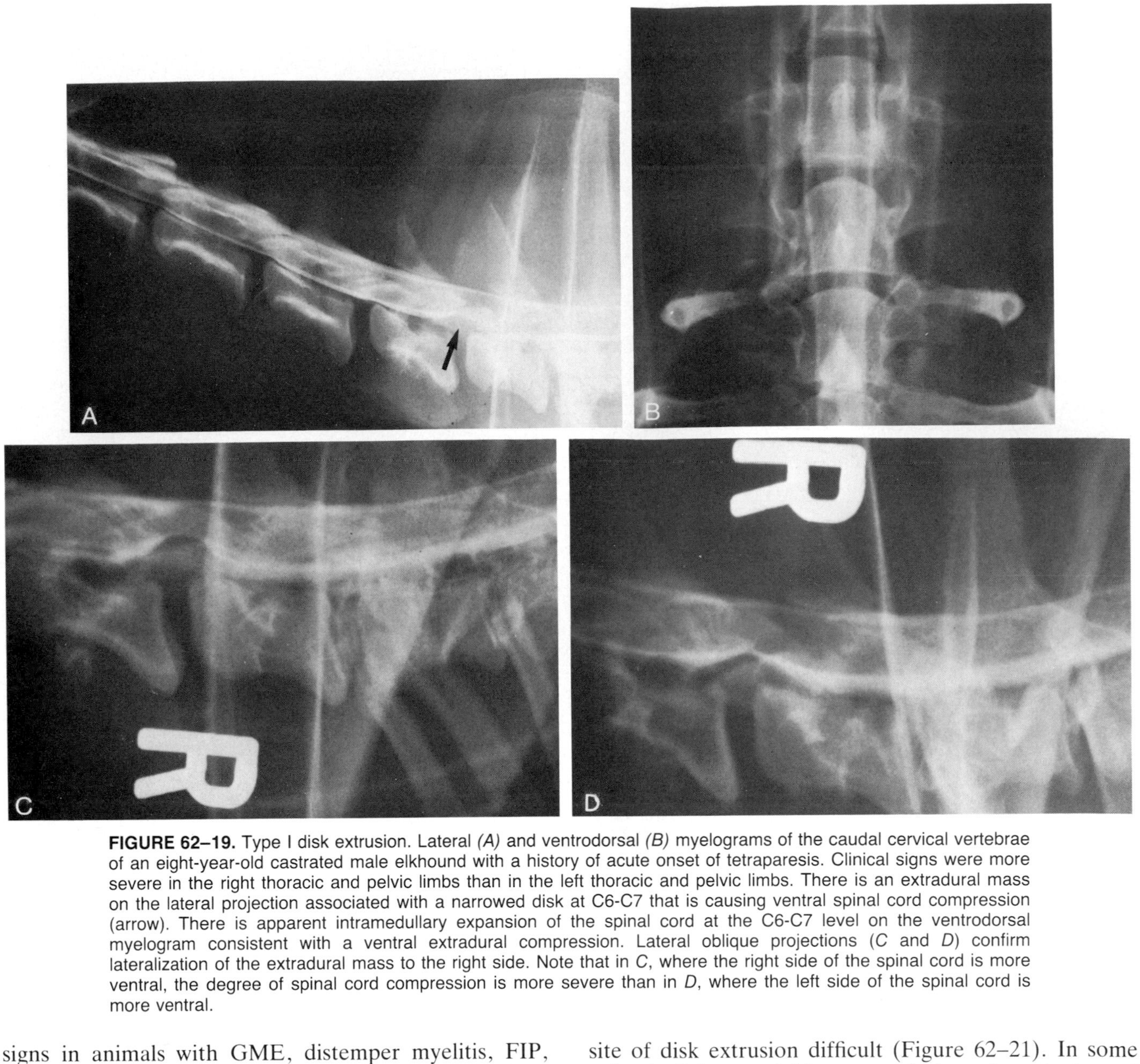

FIGURE 62–19. Type I disk extrusion. Lateral *(A)* and ventrodorsal *(B)* myelograms of the caudal cervical vertebrae of an eight-year-old castrated male elkhound with a history of acute onset of tetraparesis. Clinical signs were more severe in the right thoracic and pelvic limbs than in the left thoracic and pelvic limbs. There is an extradural mass on the lateral projection associated with a narrowed disk at C6-C7 that is causing ventral spinal cord compression (arrow). There is apparent intramedullary expansion of the spinal cord at the C6-C7 level on the ventrodorsal myelogram consistent with a ventral extradural compression. Lateral oblique projections (*C* and *D*) confirm lateralization of the extradural mass to the right side. Note that in *C*, where the right side of the spinal cord is more ventral, the degree of spinal cord compression is more severe than in *D*, where the left side of the spinal cord is more ventral.

signs in animals with GME, distemper myelitis, FIP, spinal lymphoma, and other disorders may mimic those of cervical or thoracolumbar disk disease.

The characteristic myelographic findings in both type I and type II disk herniation into the spinal canal are extradural compression of the spinal cord with displacement of the spinal cord and narrowing of the subarachnoid space on lateral and/or ventrodorsal views, depending on the location of the compressive mass. Type II, and most type I, disk herniations result in a ventral or ventrolateral epidural mass that causes dorsal displacement of the spinal cord. Disk material may extend over more than one vertebral segment in type I extrusions and may result in deviation or narrowing of contrast columns over more than one vertebral length. Disk material may completely encircle the spinal cord. Acute type I disk extrusions often are accompanied by spinal cord edema and swelling. The spinal cord may be widened over several spinal cord segments and the myelographic appearance is similar to that of an intramedullary mass, making precise determination of the site of disk extrusion difficult (Figure 62–21). In some animals disk material is scattered along the spinal canal without obvious mechanical distortion of the spinal cord.

Rarely, in the cervical region, type I disk extrusion may occur laterally (Figure 62–22) or intraforaminally resulting in neck pain or thoracic limb pain due to nerve root compression. In such cases myelograms may be normal; however, increased density associated with calcified disk material may be visualized intraforaminally on ventral oblique radiographs of the cervical spine.[254]

Traumatic disk protrusion is usually associated with narrowing of the intervertebral disk space on radiographs. Other abnormalities such as vertebral fracture, luxation, or instability also may be seen. Myelography is useful in determining the presence or absence of spinal cord compression in such cases, and therefore whether surgical decompression is indicated.

Treatment

TYPE I DISK EXTRUSION. The appropriate treatment for animals with type I disk extrusion depends on the

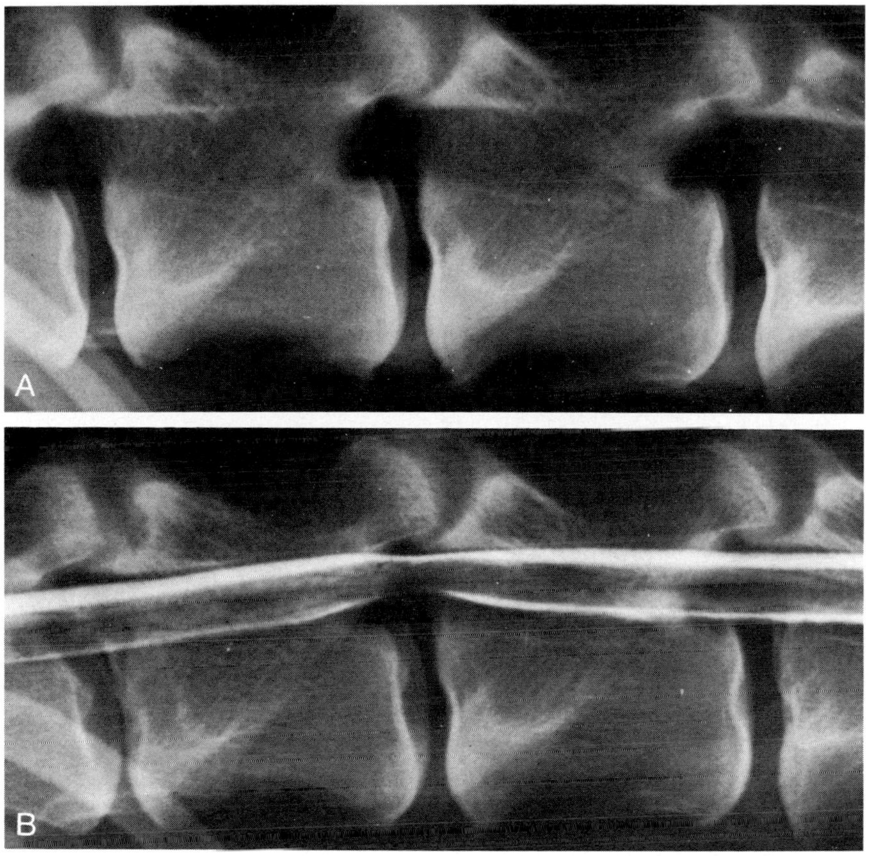

FIGURE 62–20. Type II disk protrusion. Lateral radiograph *(A)* and myelogram *(B)* of the mid-lumbar vertebral column of a seven-year-old castrated male Great Dane with a three-month history of corticosteroid-responsive back pain. The dog was neurologically normal at the time of this study. Slight narrowing of the L2-L3 disk and mild ventral spondylosis deformans are seen on the lateral radiograph. The myelogram confirms severe ventral spinal cord compression at the level of L2-L3 associated with a type II disk protrusion.

animal's neurologic status. Each animal should be evaluated individually. Medical treatment directed at decreasing spinal cord edema by means of corticosteroids is indicated in all animals with an acute onset of neurologic deficits. The recommended dose is as for spinal cord trauma. The use of corticosteroids in dogs with type I disk extrusion has been associated with pancreatitis, gastrointestinal bleeding, or colonic perforations.[255–257] The incidence of these complications may be reduced by using lower doses of corticosteroids and administering potent injectable corticosteroids for as short a time as possible (maximum of one to two days).

Nonsurgical (medical or conservative) treatment is recommended for animals with apparent pain only or animals that have mild neurologic deficits but are ambulatory and have not had previous clinical signs associated with disk disease (Table 62–6). These animals should be strictly confined to a small area such as a hospital cage or a quiet place away from other pets for at least two weeks and walked (on a leash or harness) only to urinate and defecate. The objective of confinement is to allow fissures in the anulus fibrosus to heal, thus preventing further extrusion of disk material, and allowing resolution of the inflammatory reaction caused by small amounts of extruded disk material. Confinement cannot be accomplished effectively by the majority of dog owners.

Use of analgesics, muscle relaxants, and anti-inflammatory drugs such as corticosteroids is not recommended in most cases as it is believed their use encourages animals to exercise and risk further disk extrusion. Very cautious use of analgesics or anti-inflammatory agents occasionally may be indicated; however, strict confinement followed by a period of restricted exercise

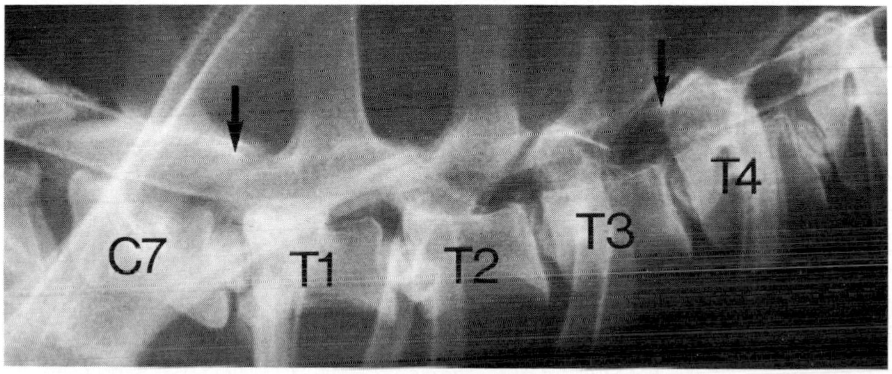

FIGURE 62–21. Type I disk extrusion. Lateral myelogram of the cervicothoracic region of the vertebral column of a nine-year-old male long-haired dachshund with an acute onset of tetraparesis. The dog had lower motor neuron signs in thoracic limbs, upper motor neuron signs in pelvic limbs, and a left Horner's syndrome. Multiple calcified disks are seen caudal to C7-T1. Contrast material is not visible between the caudal aspect of C7 and the cranial aspect of T4 (between arrows). Spinal cord swelling over the length of three vertebrae makes precise localization of a disk extrusion difficult.

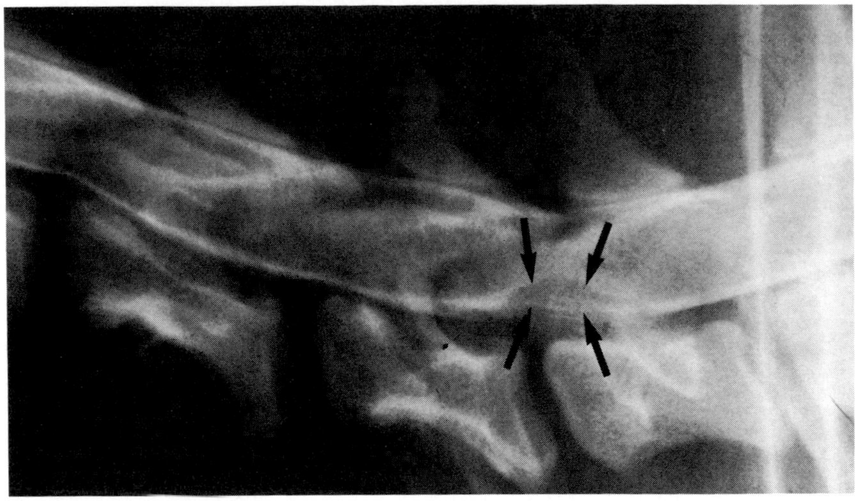

FIGURE 62–22. Type I disk extrusion. Lateral myelogram of the caudal cervical vertebral column of an eight-year-old male beagle with a one-week history of apparent neck pain and left thoracic limb lameness. There is a narrowed intervertebral disk at C6-C7 with an associated extradural mass causing ventral spinal cord compression. Note the "double" contrast columns at this level (arrows). This myelographic appearance is characteristic of a lateralizing extradural mass. In this dog the mass is a calcified disk that has extruded laterally toward the left C6-C7 intervertebral foramen.

is imperative. Owners should also be warned that an animal's neurologic status may deteriorate due to extrusion of further disk material despite this treatment and to observe the animal very carefully. If the neurologic status worsens, an animal's treatment should be reevaluated. Owners should also be warned that a recurrence of clinical signs is very common due to further disk extrusion at the same or a different site[248, 249, 258] and subsequent episodes may be more severe, especially in the thoracolumbar spine.

Animals with severe cervical pain frequently do not respond to cage rest. These dogs often have large amounts of disk material within the spinal canal and dogs that do not show improvement after seven to ten days of confinement should be evaluated further by means of radiographs and possibly myelography, and ventral cervical decompression should be considered.

TABLE 62–6. SUMMARY OF INDICATIONS FOR THERAPY FOR TYPE I INTERVERTEBRAL DISK EXTRUSION OF DOGS

Type of Therapy	Indications
1. Medical	Apparent back pain only–1st episode or *Mild* ataxia and paresis–1st episode or Paralysis with absent pain perception for more than 24 hours
2. Surgical	
a. Fenestration only	Apparent back pain only–2nd or multiple episodes
b. Decompression (and fenestration)	*Mild* ataxia and paresis–2nd or multiple episodes or Moderate/severe ataxia and paresis, or paralysis–1st episode or Deterioration of neurologic status despite adequate medical therapy or Paralysis with absent deep pain perception for less than 24 hours

Surgical disk fenestration has been recommended as a prophylactic measure to prevent further extrusion of disk material into the spinal canal. Fenestration of the disks most likely to herniate (C2-3 through C6-7 in the cervical spine and T11-12 through L3-4 in the thoracolumbar spine) is recommended in animals that have had one or more episodes of apparent neck or back pain and have evidence of intervertebral disk disease on radiographs (Table 62–6). Various surgical techniques have been described.[6, 249, 259, 260] Fenestration of disks does not remove disk material from the spinal canal and therefore is not recommended as the sole surgical procedure in dogs that have evidence of disk material within the spinal canal and spinal cord compression on radiographs and myelography. Disk fenestration should be done with care in animals showing evidence of pain, as disk material may be forced into the spinal canal resulting in a worsening of neurologic status.

The role of disk fenestration in the management of intervertebral disk disease is controversial. Most authors feel fenestration of cervical disks is of value in preventing further disk extrusion and recurrence of apparent neck pain.[249, 258, 261] In the thoracolumbar region some investigators report that disk fenestration does prevent recurrence of disk extrusion at the same or different sites, while others report that only spinal cord decompression at the site of initial disk extrusion is indicated, as the low incidence of recurrence at other sites makes disk fenestration unnecessary.[248, 249, 262–266]

Disk fenestration in the thoracolumbar region is not easily done and complications such as scoliosis, pneumothorax, and hemorrhage may occur.[267] Disk fenestration in the cervical region is achieved more easily and rarely is associated with such complications. Fenestration does not prevent recurrence of disk extrusion in all animals.[248] The effectiveness of fenestration depends largely on the amount of nucleus pulposus removed.[268] Completion of disk fenestration is recommended at the time of spinal cord decompression. The authors recommend fenestration in either the cervical or thoracolumbar region of the vertebral column for dogs that have recurrent bouts of apparent pain resulting from type I intervertebral disk disease.

Animals with neurologic deficits such as paresis or paralysis with deep pain perception intact, animals with recurrent bouts of apparent back or neck pain, or animals with apparent back or neck pain (or mild neurologic deficits) that are unresponsive to strict confinement should be evaluated by means of spinal radiographs, CSF analysis, and myelography (Table 62–6). Surgical decompression of the spinal cord and removal of disk material from the spinal canal should be considered. Although many dogs with moderate or severe paresis improve neurologically if treated with corticosteroids and cage rest,[269] neurologic recovery is often more rapid and more complete in animals following surgical decompression of the spinal cord. In addition the neurologic status of some dogs with type I disk extrusion, especially in the thoracolumbar spine, suddenly worsens over a period of hours or days despite medical treatment. Such deterioration usually results from further disk extrusion that may result in irreversible spinal cord damage and permanent paralysis. This progression of signs always is a risk with medical treatment of animals with thoracolumbar disk disease. Progression is impossible to predict on the basis of history, clinical signs, or radiography. Owners should be made aware of treatment options and offered the opportunity of referral to an appropriate surgical facility when animals are initially presented. Surgical decompression should be done as soon as possible to prevent further spinal cord damage incurred as a result of sustained compression or further extrusion of disk material. In addition, if surgery is delayed two to three weeks, disk material hardens and becomes adherent to dura mater, and becomes difficult or impossible to remove from the spinal canal.

Prognosis for neurologic recovery in animals that retain deep pain perception postsurgically is fair to very good. The major factors that correlate with the degree of neurologic improvement seen postsurgically are the animal's neurologic status prior to surgery, the rapidity of onset of clinical signs, and the time interval between onset of clinical signs and surgical decompression. Animals that have severe neurologic signs, a rapid onset of clinical signs (hours), and a long period of time before surgery generally have a prolonged recovery period and may have varying degrees of permanent neurologic deficit.

The incidence of recurrence of clinical signs due to disk extrusion is greater in nonsurgically than surgically treated dogs. One author found that one third of dogs with type I disk herniation that were treated nonsurgically had a recurrence of clinical signs, and generally showed greater severity of neurologic deficits at the time of recurrence.[249] Another author reported a recurrence rate of 40 per cent in nonsurgically treated dogs.[248]

The advantages and disadvantages of various techniques for spinal cord decompression have been discussed.[6, 248, 254, 259, 260] Surgical treatment is not without risks. Anesthesia is necessary, and surgery occasionally results in further spinal cord damage due to surgical manipulation. Nonsurgical treatment should be attempted in animals that are poor anesthesia or surgical candidates or if surgical treatment is not possible financially.

In animals with clinical signs of a complete transverse myelopathy, without deep pain perception for a period of greater than 24 hours, the prognosis for return of spinal cord function is very poor despite medical or surgical treatment.[4, 249] A small percentage of these animals may improve neurologically if given sufficient time; however, surgical treatment does not appear to increase the probability of improvement and usually is not recommended. In cases in which deep pain perception has been absent for less than 24 hours, the prognosis for return of spinal cord function is guarded to poor; however, surgical treatment may increase the likelihood of neurologic improvement in this group. Use of evoked spinal cord potential monitoring may aid in deciding whether or not spinal cord function remains and whether improvement is likely.

Regardless of whether medical or surgical treatment is instituted, animals that are paretic or paralyzed require intensive nursing care. Neurologic improvement may take weeks or months and this requires owner cooperation and enthusiasm regarding care and physical therapy. Manual expression, intermittent catheterization, and/or indwelling catheterization of the bladder are often required to ensure emptying of the bladder. Weekly urinalysis, especially in animals that do not have voluntary control of micturition, is important in monitoring for urinary tract infection. It is also important to keep animals well padded, clean, and dry to prevent formation of pressure sores, and to ensure caloric and water intake is adequate. Physical therapy does not result in neurologic improvement but helps prevent disuse muscle atrophy associated with paraplegia or tetraplegia. Physical therapy should not be attempted in animals treated medically for at least the first two weeks following onset of signs, as further extrusion of disk material may occur.

TYPE II DISK PROTRUSION. Treatment with corticosteroids may result in neurologic improvement for variable periods of time in animals with type II disk protrusion. However, corticosteroid therapy is not curative. The reason for this improvement is not clear as intramedullary hemorrhage and edema seen in cases of acute spinal cord injury are not a feature of chronic spinal cord compression. In the thoracolumbar spine surgical removal of protruded disk material is generally impossible without causing further spinal cord damage. Surgical decompression without removal of protruded disk material may result in improvement; however, the neurologic status of some dogs is worsened permanently despite very careful surgical technique.[4] The reasons for this are not known but increased vascular permeability has been described in the spinal cord associated with release of chronic spinal cord compression[270] and this probably plays a role in this phenomenon. Ventral decompression in the cervical spine allows removal of protruded type II disk material and neurologic improvement may occur; however, some dogs, especially those with moderate to severe neurologic deficits prior to surgery, may manifest temporary or permanent worsening of clinical signs postoperatively. Neurologic improvement may take several months and is believed to be primarily due to remyelination of axons in the white matter of the spinal cord.

Chemonucleolysis. Injection of the proteolytic enzyme chymopapain into the nucleus pulposus of intervertebral disks to cause diskolysis has been used infrequently in veterinary medicine.[271–274] The precise mechanism by which chymopapain causes dissolution of the nucleus pulposus is unknown. In one study in dogs, dissolution of the nucleus pulposus was demonstrated histologically in all cervical intervertebral disks injected with chymopapain via a ventral surgical approach.[274] Similar pathologic findings were found in lumbar disks of dogs injected with chymopapain transcutaneously under fluoroscopic guidance via a lateral approach.[275] Significant postoperative clinical complications were not seen. Radiographic narrowing of the intervertebral disk spaces was found in both the cervical and lumbar chymopapain-injected spaces. Cervical injection resulted in a more noticeable narrowing than lumbar injection.[275] However, successful injection as determined histologically was not always detected radiographically.[274] These studies have described only the acute response to chymopapain. However, another study has shown chymopapain injection results in progressive dissolution of nucleus pulposus and eventual regeneration of nuclear ground material.[276]

Chemonucleolysis may be of benefit in animals with intervertebral disk disease when the nucleus pulposus is still contained within an intact or partially ruptured anulus fibrosus. Dissolution of nucleus pulposus in these cases may relieve pressure of the protruding disk on the spinal cord and nerve roots.[274] Chemonucleolysis may also be useful as a prophylactic measure in animals with evidence of intervertebral disk degeneration to prevent acute type I disk extrusion.

Chemonucleolysis is not indicated in cases of type I disk extrusion, as the enzyme is unable to reach sequestered nucleus pulposus within the spinal canal.[277] Chemonucleolysis has been used in the treatment of type II disk protrusion in the cervical spine of large breeds of dog. The majority of dogs in one study improved clinically despite persistence, or only slight decrease, in the degree of spinal cord compression on myelography.[121] Injection of chymopapain via a surgical approach to the intervertebral disks is recommended to prevent inadvertent intrathecal injection or accidental penetration of the vertebral arteries, spinal arteries, or spinal nerve roots.[274] Further evaluation of the effect of chemonucleolysis in dogs with intervertebral disk disease is needed; however, it seems likely that this technique may have advantages over the presently used methods for surgical disk fenestration.

Ischemic Myelopathy Due to Fibrocartilaginous Embolism

Etiology and Pathogenesis. Ischemic myelopathy results from ischemic necrosis of spinal cord gray and white matter associated with fibrocartilaginous emboli that occlude arteries and/or veins of the leptomeninges and spinal cord parenchyma. This disease is characterized by an acute onset of neurologic deficits and is generally nonprogressive after several hours.

The substance occluding spinal cord arteries and veins has histologic and histochemical properties similar to fibrocartilage of intervertebral disks and is presumed to originate from the nucleus pulposus of an intervertebral disk. Pathogenesis of the fibrocartilaginous embolism is not known.

In humans, it has been postulated that cartilaginous disk material extrudes into the cancellous bone of the adjacent vertebra (Schmorl's nodes) and enters the sinusoidal venous channels of the bone marrow from which the material may subsequently drain into the venous plexuses in the vertebral canal. Increased venous pressure (e.g., during coughing, straining) may result in reversal of blood flow in these veins, forcing fibrocartilage back into the veins of the leptomeninges and spinal cord.[278]

Dogs, however, are anatomically different from humans in that the vertebral endplates consist of compact bone adjacent to the fibrocartilaginous disk material. Schmorl's nodes rarely occur in dogs and have not been observed in dogs with ischemic myelopathy. Valves may also prevent the reversal of blood flow in some vertebral veins. Fibrocartilage has been observed in the longitudinal venous sinuses in several dogs with ischemic myelopathy, and herniation of nucleus pulposus directly into the overlying venous sinuses has been suggested as a cause.[279] These theories do not explain the fact that occlusion commonly occurs in arteries as well as veins and in some animals only arterial embolism can be demonstrated.

Arteriovenous anastomosis in the spinal cord vasculature may account for arterial occlusion with emboli arising from the venous system of vertebral bodies or venous sinuses.[8, 280] Direct penetration of disk material into the arterial circulation seems unlikely, as evidence of hemorrhage (expected with extrusion into thick muscular arterial walls) has not been demonstrated in dogs with ischemic myelopathy. Fibrocartilage has been demonstrated in a large peridiskal artery in one dog.[281]

The variable distribution of infarction and hemorrhage does not match the pattern expected from the occlusion of any one major leptomeningeal artery,[8, 280] and numerous vessels in the leptomeninges and spinal cord parenchyma must be occluded simultaneously to cause necrosis of the spinal cord in the dog.[282] A direct relationship has not been noted between intervertebral disk disease and ischemic myelopathy. However, fibrocartilaginous embolism has been described in several dogs with degenerative intervertebral disk disease that on histopathologic examination had both macroscopic and microscopic extrusion of nucleus pulposus and fibrocartilage material into the blood vessels around the extruding disk.[281, 283] The majority of affected animals, however, do not have evidence of degenerative intervertebral disk disease, and the disease is most common in relatively young (one to five years of age) large and giant breeds of dog that have a low incidence of degenerative disk disease and type I disk extrusion.

The relationship of exercise or minor trauma to the occurrence of fibrocartilaginous embolism also is not known. Many affected dogs have a history of mild to moderate exercise prior to the onset of clinical signs.

Fibrocartilaginous embolism and ischemic myelopathy have been reported in a cat.[284]

Clinical Findings. Ischemic myelopathy most commonly occurs in large and giant breeds of dog, generally between one and nine years of age. The disease has been described in many breeds including smaller dogs such as miniature schnauzers and Shetland sheepdogs.[280] Both males and females may be affected and ischemic myelopathy has been described in several females during estrus.[285]

Ischemic myelopathy is characterized by an acute onset of neurologic deficits that may be severe. Clinical signs may progress over several hours but are generally not progressive after 12 hours. Affected animals usually do not have a history or evidence of trauma but may have a history of exercise prior to the onset of clinical signs. Apparent pain usually is not present at the time of examination or during the course of the disease, although dogs are often reported to "cry out" at the onset of clinical signs.

Neurologic deficits usually are bilateral and are often (but not always) asymmetrical. Clinical signs seen depend on the location and extent of the spinal cord lesion. Many spinal cord segments may be involved and neurologic deficits present may indicate extensive gray and white matter necrosis. If fibrocartilaginous embolism occurs in the cervical enlargement, unilateral or bilateral LMN signs in the thoracic limbs and UMN signs in the pelvic limbs are seen. The absence of a panniculus reflex unilaterally or bilaterally often is noted in lesions involving the T1 spinal cord segment. An ipsilateral Horner's syndrome commonly is seen in dogs with fibrocartilaginous embolism of the cervical enlargement as a result of damage to preganglionic sympathetic cell bodies in the spinal cord segments T1 and T2. A Horner's syndrome may also be seen in severe lesions in the cervical spinal cord, due to interruption of the tecto-tegmental spinal tract. Other lesions of sufficient severity to damage neurons of the tecto-tegmental spinal tract are rare, as most disease processes result in bilateral damage to the spinal cord and bilateral severe lesions in the cervical cord usually result in respiratory paralysis and death. Horner's syndrome has, however, been reported in association with cervical disk protrusion and a cervical spinal tumor.[247, 285]

Fibrocartilaginous embolism in the lumbosacral spinal cord causes unilateral or bilateral LMN signs in the pelvic limbs, anal and urinary sphincters, and tail. Lesions may also occur in the C1 to C5 and T3 to L3 spinal cord segments and result in symmetric or asymmetric UMN signs to all four limbs or pelvic limbs, respectively. Neurologic deficits may range from decreased conscious proprioception and mild paresis to complete paralysis and analgesia in affected limbs.

Diagnosis. Ischemic myelopathy should be suspected in any dog (especially large and giant breeds of dog) with an acute onset of nonprogressive neurologic deficits that are not associated with apparent spinal pain, especially if deficits are asymmetrical or indicate that at least several spinal cord segments are involved. A diagnosis is made by ruling out other causes of myelopathy. Spinal radiographs are normal. Cerebrospinal fluid may be normal or may have an elevated protein concentration as a result of leakage of protein through damaged vascular endothelium. The white blood cell count of CSF may be normal or may be mildly increased in the early stages, probably as a result of an inflammatory response triggered by spinal cord ischemia. Xanthochromia may be present 48 hours or more after a subarachnoid hemorrhage. Appearance on a myelogram usually is normal, although mild intramedullary swelling as a result of spinal cord edema may be seen for up to 24 hours after the onset of clinical signs.

Treatment. Corticosteroids (as recommended for spinal trauma) may be given initially to reduce any secondary spinal cord edema; however, after several days, edema usually is resolved. Good nursing care is essential in recumbent animals to prevent pressure sores, urinary tract infections, and contracture of denervated muscles. Prognosis depends on the severity of an animal's neurologic deficits. Animals that retain pain perception in affected limbs and tail usually regain neurologic function although recovery may take several weeks to months and LMN signs may persist (muscle atrophy and/or paresis). Animals with absent pain perception for 24 hours are likely to have irreversible spinal cord damage and have a poor prognosis for return of function in affected limb or limbs. Many animals show improvement within two weeks of onset of signs, unless extensive gray matter destruction has occurred.

Clinical improvement seen in the first two weeks may be accounted for by resolution of edema and hemorrhage, and establishment of collateral circulation to areas that were ischemic but not necrotic. Later clinical improvement is probably due to compensation by remaining spinal cord neurons.[8]

Leukoencephalomyelopathy of Rottweiler Dogs

Etiology and Pathogenesis. Leukoencephalomyelopathy is a demyelinating disorder of the brain and spinal cord that has been reported to occur in rottweiler dogs. It is characterized by progressive tetraparesis and hypermetria, especially of the thoracic limbs. Leukoencephalomyelopathy has been reported in two dogs in the United States.[286] A similar disorder recently has been reported in 16 rottweiler dogs in the Netherlands.[287]

Histopathologic examination demonstrated demyelination in white matter of the spinal cord, brain stem, and cerebellum, with intact naked axons and thinly myelinated axons accompanied by reactive astrogliosis. The spinal cord lesions were found in the lateral funiculi and occasionally the dorsal funiculi, predominantly in the cervical and thoracic spinal cord, and tended to be bilaterally symmetric. The lack of neuronal fiber degeneration makes primary demyelination more likely than secondary demyelination.

Etiology of this disease is unknown. It may be the result of an acquired primary demyelinating disease but whether the lesions seen are due to a single demyelinating event or due to repeated demyelination and remyelination is not known. As the lesions are bilaterally symmetric, toxic, metabolic, and nutritional mechanisms may be involved. Infectious causes, such as CD virus, may also result in demyelination. Vascular mechanisms may also be involved, as lesions had a segmental distribution; however, axon degeneration would be expected. An inherited condition in which myelin formation is defective and cannot be maintained (leukodystrophy) is also possible. The two dogs in the United States report were related, as were the 16 dogs reported in the Netherlands.

Other leukodystrophies have been reported in young animals, although an adult-onset leukodystrophy has not been described in dogs. The relationship of this disease to neuroaxonal dystrophy of rottweiler dogs is not known. Histopathologic lesions and clinical findings differ from those described in dogs with neuroaxonal dystrophy; however, a dog related to a dog with leukoencephalomyelopathy was diagnosed as having neuroaxonal dystrophy.

Clinical Findings. Both males and females have been reported to be affected. Clinical findings reported were tetraparesis, hypermetria (especially of the forelimbs), decreased conscious proprioception (especially of the pelvic limbs), and exaggerated spinal reflexes. Clinical signs became apparent between 18 months and three and a half years of age, and abnormalities were slowly progressive over several months to one year. Neurologic abnormalities were consistent with a transverse myelopathy of the cervical spinal cord. Neurologic deficits referable to structures rostral to the foramen magnum wer not detected.

Diagnosis. Diagnosis may be made on the basis of age and breed of an affected dog, and by ruling out other causes of cervical myelopathy such as CD myelitis, granulomatous meningoencephalomyelitis, cervical spondylomyelopathy, or spinal neoplasia. Results of radiography, CSF analysis, and myelography were normal in dogs reported.

Treatment. Treatment has not been effective. Improvement was not seen in one dog treated with corticosteroids.

Lumbosacral Vertebral Canal Stenosis

Etiology and Pathogenesis. Lumbosacral vertebral canal stenosis is a term that encompasses a spectrum of disorders that result in narrowing of the lumbosacral vertebral canal with resulting compression of the cauda equina.[288] The term *cauda equina syndrome* describes a group of neurologic signs that results from compression, destruction, or displacement of those nerve roots and spinal nerves that form the cauda equina.[4, 289–291] Disorders of the cauda equina that result in cauda equina syndrome may be either congenital or acquired, or may be a combination of both these categories (Table 62–7).[289, 290] The majority of disorders included in Table 62–7 are discussed in separate sections (e.g., intervertebral disk disease or diskospondylitis).

The term lumbosacral vertebral canal stenosis is used by these authors to describe an acquired disorder of large breeds of dog that results from several or all of the following: type II disk protrusion (dorsal bulging of the anulus fibrosus), hypertrophy/hyperplasia of the interarcuate ligament, thickening of vertebral arches or articular facets, and (infrequently) subluxation/instability of the lumbosacral junction.[4, 292] It is likely that several separate disorders presently are included within this single syndrome.

TABLE 62–7. DISORDERS THAT RESULT IN SIGNS OF CAUDA EQUINA DYSFUNCTION IN DOGS

1. Congenital disorders
   a. Vertebral and/or nerve root anomalies (e.g., spina bifida)
   b. Idiopathic lumbar stenosis
2. Acquired disorders
   a. Infections (e.g., diskospondylitis)
   b. Neoplasia (e.g., malignant nerve sheath neoplasia)
   c. Intervertebral disk disease
   d. Iatrogenic stenosis (e.g., postsurgical scarring)
   e. Lumbosacral vertebral canal stenosis (with/without "retrolisthesis")
3. Combined disorders
   a. Combination of congenital and acquired disorders (e.g., disk degeneration and lumbosacral vertebral canal stenosis)

Other terms that have been used to describe this disorder are lumbosacral instability, lumbosacral malformation/malarticulation,[293] lumbar spinal stenosis, lumbosacral spondylolisthesis, and cauda equina syndrome. As stated above, cauda equina syndrome may result from numerous causes other than lumbosacral vertebral canal stenosis; therefore, use of this term to describe this condition is inappropriate. In humans, the term spondylolisthesis refers specifically to a forward (anterior) movement of a lower lumbar vertebra relative to a lumbar vertebra or sacrum directly below it. This problem rarely occurs in dogs, in which the most frequently encountered problem is a ventral "slippage" of the sacrum relative to the body of the L7 vertebra.[294] The term retrolisthesis has been proposed to describe this "reverse spondylolisthesis" of dogs.[289] Lumbar spinal stenosis is a term that perhaps is best used to describe a congenital ("idiopathic") syndrome reported to occur in young dogs by Tarvin and Prata.[295] Lumbosacral instability is a misleading term, as instability is not demonstrated consistently in association with lumbosacral vertebral canal stenosis.

Certain similarities between vertebral and soft tissue alterations seen in dogs with lumbosacral vertebral canal stenosis and Doberman pinscher dogs with caudal cervical spondylomyelopathy have been noted. As the etiology and pathogenesis for either condition are incompletely understood, such comparisons are of little significance at the present time.[293]

Clinical Findings. Acquired degenerative lumbosacral vertebral canal stenosis occurs most commonly in large-breed dogs. Males appear to be affected more frequently than females. German shepherd dogs appear to be affected more often than dogs of other breeds.[293] Dogs with the congenital ("idiopathic") form appear to be of the smaller breeds.[295] Affected dogs in both categories are between three and seven years of age, although the problem may be noted to occur at any age.[4, 293] Degenerative lumbosacral vertebral canal stenosis rarely is recognized in cats.[296]

Signs of cauda equina compression seen frequently in affected dogs include the following: apparent pain on palpation of the lumbosacral region, on caudal extension of the pelvic limbs, or on elevation of the tail;[293] difficulty rising; pelvic limb lameness (often unilateral); pelvic limb muscle atrophy; paresis of the tail; scuffing of the toes; urinary and/or fecal incontinence, or "inappropriate" voiding due to an inability to assume a voiding posture; self-mutilation of the perineum, tail, or pelvic limbs; and rarely, paraphimosis.[289] These signs most often are insidious in onset and progress gradually over months, and are easily confused with those of hip dysplasia or degenerative myelopathy.

Abnormalities detected on neurologic examination include gait deficits related to sciatic nerve paresis (e.g., dragging of toes). In addition, depression or loss of conscious proprioception, normal or slightly exaggerated patellar reflexes ("pseudoexaggeration" related to loss of antagonism to femoral nerve–innervated muscles by sciatic nerve–innervated muscles), depressed or absent flexion reflexes in pelvic limbs, decreased anal tone and anal sphincter reflexes, atonic bladder, hypesthesia of the perineum and tail, and muscle atrophy may be seen. These abnormalities relate to deficits of the sciatic, pudendal, caudal, and pelvic nerves, whose nerve roots comprise the cauda equina.[291]

Diagnosis. Characteristic clinical findings may be consistent with a diagnosis of degenerative lumbosacral vertebral canal stenosis. Careful mapping of areas of loss of cutaneous sensation may assist in determining involved nerve roots.[23] However, presence of this syndrome must be confirmed by means of plain radiographs and special radiographic techniques. Diagnosis of this condition requires completion of several specialized radiographic procedures in sequence. Rarely can this condition be diagnosed on the basis of plain radiographic findings alone.

Plain radiographic findings include spondylosis deformans ventral and lateral to the lumbosacral articulation,[297] sclerosis of vertebral endplates, "wedging" or narrowing of the L7-S1 disk space, and secondary degenerative joint disease in the region of L7-S1 articular facets (Figure 62–23).[292, 293] Ventral displacement of the sacrum with respect to L7 ("retrolisthesis") and diminished dorsoventral dimensions of the lumbosacral spinal canal may be seen; however, such findings must be interpreted with caution, as they may be seen in normal dogs in association with slight rotation of the vertebral column on lateral radiographs.[294] Every effort must be made to ensure that such rotation does not occur during exposures for lateral radiographic projections. General anesthesia is mandatory for obtaining radiographs of the lumbosacral vertebral column. A ventrodorsal projection also is recommended.

"Stressed" plain radiographic projections (flexed and extended views), completed with careful attention to avoid rotation, often assist in determining the presence of instability or "retrolisthesis." Several attempts to separate normal dogs from dogs with lumbosacral vertebral canal stenosis by means of objective measurements made from radiographs have not been successful.[294] Appearance on plain radiographs helps to eliminate other causes of cauda equina syndrome (e.g., diskospondylitis or vertebral neoplasia). Linear tomography, when available, may provide specific information regarding the diameter of the lumbosacral vertebral canal that cannot be obtained from plain radiographs.[289, 293]

Electromyography may complement information available from a neurologic examination and from plain spinal radiographs by confirming denervation in muscles innervated by the nerves of the cauda equina. Motor nerve conduction velocity determinations in sciatic and tibial nerves and measurement of evoked spinal cord potentials may also provide indirect evidence of cauda equina dysfunction.

Several contrast radiographic techniques exist for examination of the lumbosacral vertebral canal. Use of such techniques is necessary for demonstration of soft tissue vertebral canal stenosis.

Myelography most often is not of use in the diagnosis of lumbosacral problems, as it has been reported that the terminal portion of the subarachnoid space of dogs fills unreliably with contrast material at this level, resulting in misinterpretation of findings.[289] Some investigators maintain, however, that myelography is reliable when an animal is tilted for sufficient time (up to 15 minutes) to ensure adequate filling of the caudal subarachnoid space.

Transosseous vertebral sinus venography (filling of vertebral sinuses with contrast material) and epidurography (filling of the lumbosacral epidural space with contrast material) have been used by many investigators in an attempt to outline soft tissue stenosis of the lumbosacral vertebral canal.[298–300] Results obtained with either of these techniques must be interpreted cautiously, as falsely positive studies occur with both.[289] A recent study comparing venography, epidurography, and myelography in normal dogs and dogs with an experimentally induced mass lesion at the lumbosacral junction demonstrated that in the lateral projections epidurography was sensitive in demonstrating a lesion in 41.7 per cent of dogs, compared to 22.2 per cent with venography and 0 per cent with myelography.[301]

A technique that may have use in the future for confirmation of lumbosacral soft tissue stenosis is diskography.[302] Diskography consists of radiography completed following the injection of contrast material into the nucleus pulposus of an intervertebral disk (Figure 62–24). Results of diskography in the lumbar and cervical region of dogs have been reported.[302, 303] This technique would appear to have special application to the lumbosacral disk space.

In the future, CT and MRI, either alone or combined with the contrast techniques listed above, will provide further information regarding soft tissue stenosis of the lumbosacral vertebral canal. Surgical exploration may be indicated in dogs in which results of ancillary diagnostic tests do not provide a definite diagnosis of soft tissue stenosis.

Treatment. Some affected dogs in which clinical signs are mild or in which apparent lumbosacral pain is the sole problem improve temporarily after strict confinement and restricted leash exercise for a period of four to six weeks. Use of analgesic drugs or corticosteroids has been recommended; however, their use must be accompanied by strict confinement.

Clinical signs commonly recur in affected dogs treated only by means of medical therapy.[293] Dogs with recurrence of signs, or dogs that are moderately to severely affected at the time of initial presentation (especially those with urinary/fecal incontinence), should be consid-

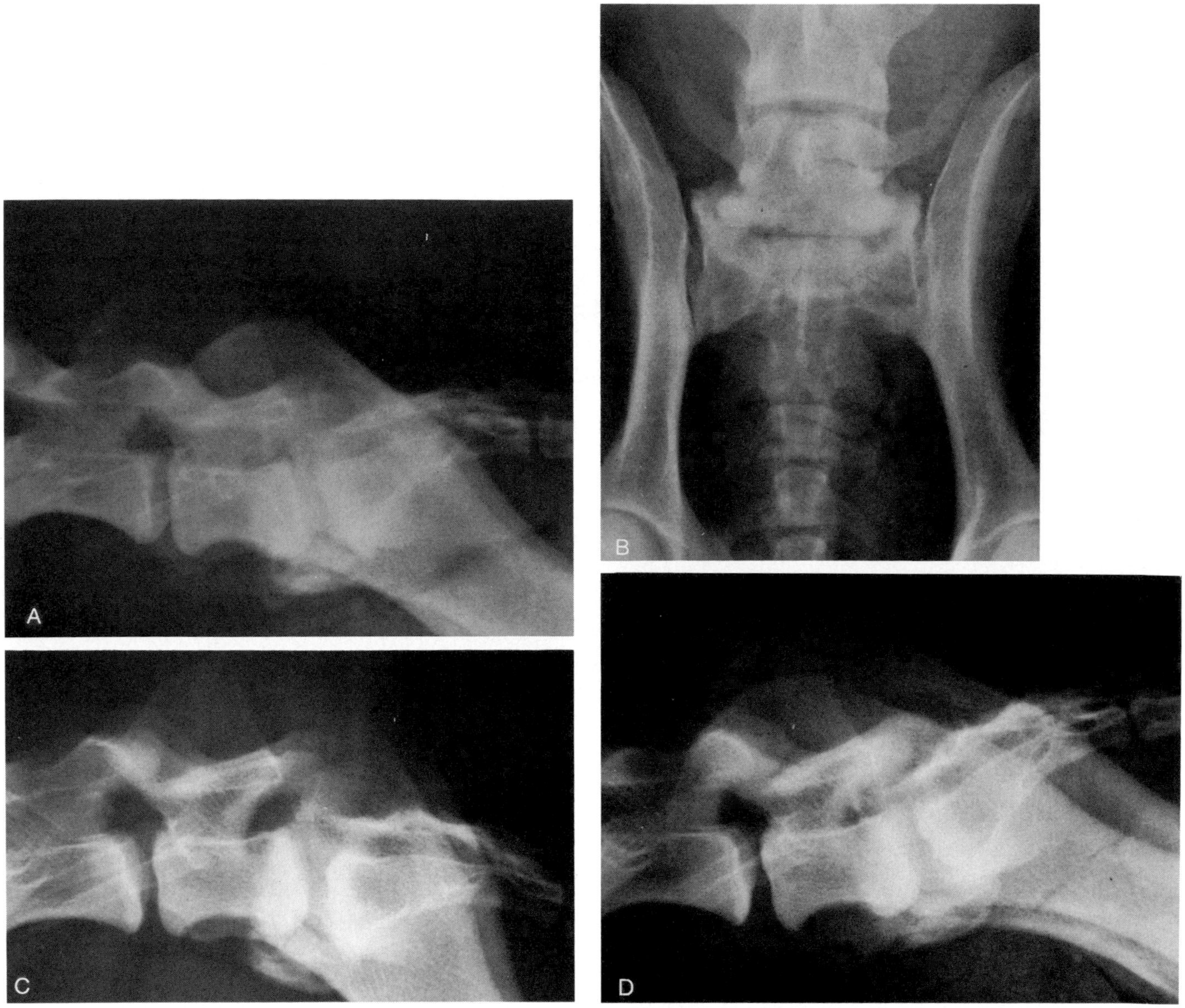

FIGURE 62–23. Lumbosacral vertebral canal stenosis. Lateral *(A)* and ventrodorsal *(B)* radiographs of the lumbosacral region of the vertebral column of a seven-year-old female Vizsla. The dog had a history of apparent spinal pain, hypotonic tail, urinary incontinence, and pelvic limb paresis. Sclerosis of vertebral endplates of L7 and S1, L7-S1 spondylosis deformans, "wedging" of the L7-S1 disk, and malalignment of L7-S1 are evident on the nonstressed lateral projection. Spondylosis deformans is seen lateral to the L7-S1 vertebral articulation on the ventrodorsal projection. A flexed lateral projection *(C)* confirms the presence of "retrolisthesis," with excessive ventral movement of the sacrum with respect to the body of L7. Instability of the lumbosacral articulation is further suggested by the extended projection *(D)*, where "wedging" of the L7-S1 disk is seen. Use of these stressed projections is essential for confirmation of instability in association with lumbosacral vertebral canal stenosis.

ered candidates for surgical therapy. Dorsal decompressive laminectomy of L7 and S1 vertebrae is recommended.[293] This procedure may be combined with foraminotomy or facetectomy in dogs in which compression of spinal nerves at the level of the intervertebral foramina is suspected.[293] In animals with radiographically confirmed instability or significant "retrolisthesis," fusion of the lumbosacral articulation may be necessary. A dorsal approach for fusion has been recommended,[304] and successful ventral lumbosacral fusion by means of a lag screw fixation has been reported.[305] These authors prefer a ventral approach that utilizes an autologous ileal graft placed in a "slot" made in the caudal body of L7 and the cranial body of S1.

Dogs should be confined for two to four weeks postoperatively. Postoperative complications include seroma formation at the surgical site and formation of a laminectomy scar at the site of the laminectomy.[293] Both can be avoided by use of appropriate surgical technique.

Attention to bladder emptying may be necessary in dogs with bladder atony prior to surgery.[293] The bladder should be manually expressed three times daily in such

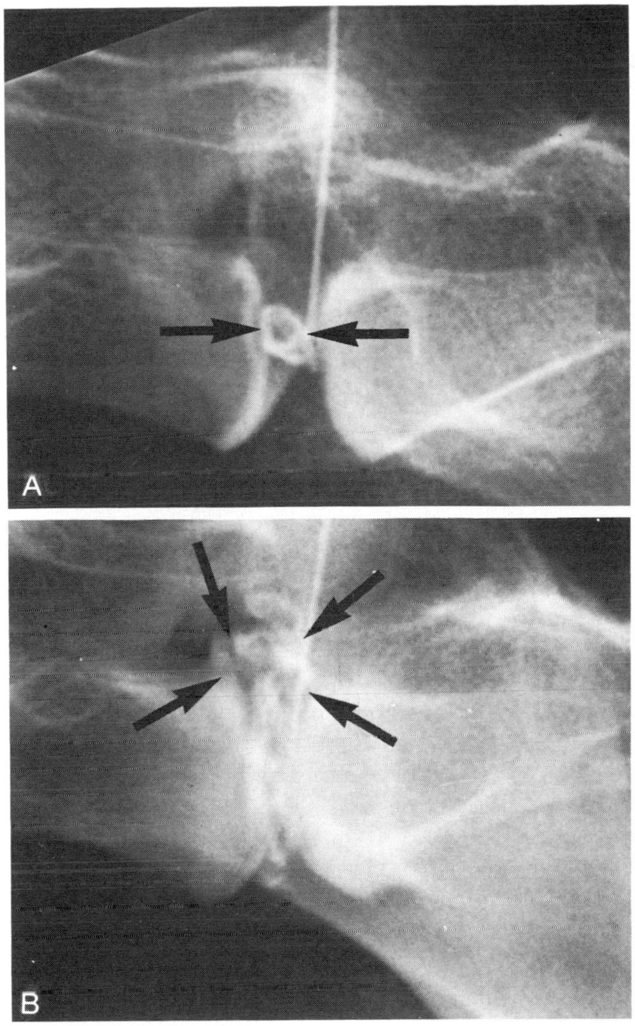

FIGURE 62–24. Lumbosacral vertebral canal stenosis. *A*, Diskogram at L7-S1 in a normal five-year-old male St. Bernard. Note the placement of a spinal needle in the nucleus pulposus of the L7-S1 disk. Contrast material is confined to the region of the nucleus pulposus (arrows). *B*, Diskogram at L7-S1 in a six-year-old male Great Dane with a history of apparent spinal pain and self-mutilation of the right side of the tail. Note the irregular pattern of contrast filling of the disk and the "dome-shaped" region of contrast material that has accumulated within the vertebral canal (arrows). This abnormal diskogram is consistent with a diagnosis of L7-S1 disk degeneration with bulging of the dorsal anulus fibrosus into the vertebral canal. This diagnosis was confirmed following a dorsal laminectomy completed over this site.

dogs. Urine should be submitted for culture and sensitivity testing prior to and two weeks after completion of surgery, and appropriate antibiotic therapy instituted as indicated by results.

Prognosis for affected dogs is dependent on the severity of signs prior to surgery. Return to normal function may be expected in dogs that are mildly affected prior to surgery. Dogs with bladder atony or a flaccid anal sphincter prior to surgery have the poorest prognosis.

Mucopolysaccharidosis

Etiology and Pathogenesis. The mucopolysaccharidoses are a group of genetic diseases that result from defects in the metabolism of glycosaminoglycans. Two subclasses have been recognized in cats, and paraparesis associated with spinal cord compression has been reported in Siamese cats with mucopolysaccharidosis VI (MPS VI).[306] Mucopolysaccharidosis VI is the result of a deficiency of the lysosomal enzyme arylsulfatase B and, in addition to causing characteristic physical deformities, can result in skeletal changes, including fusion of the cervical vertebrae, variable fusion of thoracic and lumbar vertebrae, bony proliferation and bony protrusion into the vertebral canal in the thoracic and lumbar spine causing compression of the spinal cord, and bony proliferation in the intervertebral foramina, causing nerve root compression.[307] Bony proliferative changes and associated spinal cord compression occur prior to, or at the time of, epiphyseal closure (about nine months of age) and are probably nonprogressive after this time. Mucopolysaccharidosis VI is an inherited abnormality and has an autosomal recessive mode of inheritance.

Mucopolysaccharidosis I due to a deficiency in α-L-iduronidase has been reported in a domestic short-haired cat.[308] The clinical features were similar to MPS VI but bony proliferative changes and associated spinal cord compression were not found. Although vacuolar changes were observed in neurons of brain and cervical spinal cord, presumably as a result of storage of glycosaminoglycans, neurologic deficits were not found clinically. Mucopolysaccharidosis I probably has an autosomal recessive mode of inheritance.

Clinical Findings. The characteristic physical findings in cases of MPS VI are small head, flat, broad face, widely spaced eyes, corneal clouding, small ears, depressed bridge of the nose, large forepaws, and concave deformity of the sternum. Affected kittens are smaller than normal littermates with physical deformities noticeable by eight weeks of age. Neurologic deficits due to skeletal changes and spinal cord compression are seen between four and seven months of age and progress over two to four weeks. Neurologic findings are indicative of a transverse myelopathy between T3 and L3, and include absent conscious proprioception, normal to exaggerated pelvic limb reflexes, and decreased pain perception in the pelvic limbs. The thoracic limb gait may be normal or affected cats may have a crouching posture. Spinal reflexes in the thoracic limbs are normal.

Diagnosis. Radiographs of the spine show vertebral fusion and bony protrusions into the spinal canal and intervertebral foramina of the thoracolumbar spine. However, bony proliferation is not an indication of neurologic dysfunction. Myelography is necessary to demonstrate spinal cord compression. Subarachnoid CSF puncture may be difficult due to proliferative changes around the vertebrae. MPS VI can be confirmed by measurement of arylsulfatase B activity in leukocytes.[309]

Treatment. As skeletal changes are nonprogressive after about nine months of age, decompressive surgery may result in improvement in neurologic signs. However, spinal cord compression may be present at more than one site. The underlying lysosomal enzyme deficit is not amenable to treatment at present. Bone marrow transplantation is being investigated as a possible therapy for MPS VI.[310]

Multiple Cartilaginous Exostoses (Osteochondromatosis)

Etiology and Pathogenesis. Cartilaginous exostoses are benign proliferative lesions of cartilage and bone associated with epiphyseal regions.[8] Any bone formed by endochondral ossification may be affected and multiple lesions develop in most cases. The vertebrae, ribs, and long bones are frequently involved, and clinical signs of spinal cord disease may be seen as a result of spinal cord compression caused by extension of exostoses into the spinal canal. The formation of exostoses is related to abnormal differentiation of cartilage cells. Histologically, lesions consist of a thin cortex covered by hyaline cartilage, with a center of cancellous bone containing nodules of cartilage undergoing endochondral ossification. Multiple cartilaginous exostoses have been reported in both dogs and cats.[311–318] Neither breed nor sex predilection has been established. Lesions usually are recognized in animals less than one year of age but may remain undetected until later in life if not associated with clinical signs. Growth of exostoses stops spontaneously when normal bone growth at the epiphyseal plates ceases.[8] Continued growth or reactivation of growth of exostoses is suggestive of neoplasia. Subsequent development of a neoplasm has been reported at the site of cartilaginous exostoses.[319, 320]

The etiology of multiple cartilaginous exostoses is unknown. The disease may be familial.[312–314] In one report of a cat, electron microscopy showed C-type particles resembling those of feline leukemia virus associated with the plasma membrane of chondroblastic elements of the exostoses.[317]

Solitary cartilaginous exostosis has been described in the cervical spine of three large-breed dogs three to five months of age.[321] These lesions comprised a partially calcified mass consisting of cartilage, strands of connective tissue, and foci of dystrophic calcification, located between the dorsal aspect of C1 and C2, that resulted in spinal cord compression and clinical signs of a cervical myelopathy and apparent cervical pain. These lesions were considered to be different from those of multiple cartilaginous exostoses, as pathologically bone formation was not seen. These masses were attached to the vertebral periosteum and dorsal atlantoaxial ligament. Abnormal embryonic development leading to the formation of abnormal masses of mesenchymal tissue along the midline was suggested as a possible cause of these lesions.

Clinical Signs. Multiple cartilaginous exostoses may occur anywhere in the vertebral column but most commonly are found in the thoracic and lumbar spine. They may result in spinal cord compression and clinical signs indicative of a progressive transverse myelopathy between T3 and L3. Neurologic deficits are often asymmetric. Torticollis and neurologic deficits consistent with a cervical myelopathy were reported in a dog with exostoses of the cervical spine.[315]

Diagnosis. Radiographically, lesions tend to be circular and smooth, with sclerotic borders.[314] Lesions are usually multiple and may be cystic or proliferative, with an increased radiodensity. Myelography is necessary to demonstrate associated spinal cord compression. Extension of exostoses into the spinal canal results in extradural compression of the spinal cord. Surgical biopsy is necessary to differentiate cartilaginous exostoses from neoplastic lesions. Vertebral osteomas may also occur in young dogs and result in similar clinical signs.[8]

Treatment. Surgical excision of cartilaginous exostoses with spinal cord decompression is the recommended treatment for lesions causing spinal cord compression and neurologic deficits. Treatment is not necessary for animals with multiple cartilaginous exostoses of the vertebral column that do not result in neurologic deficits. The prognosis for animals that have stopped growing is good; however, the prognosis for animals that are still growing is guarded, as lesions may continue to expand and subsequently result in spinal cord compression.

Myelodysplasia

Etiology and Pathogenesis. The term myelodysplasia describes a number of malformations of the spinal cord believed to result from incomplete closure or development of the neural tube. Malformations found histopathologically include the following: anomalies of the central canal (hydromyelia, duplication of the central canal, or absence of the central canal); anomalies of the central gray matter, ventral median fissure, and dorsal median septum; gray matter ectopias, chromatolysis, and loss of nerve cell bodies; and syringomyelia, usually in the dorsal columns.[322] Lesions are found throughout the spinal cord but are more severe in the lumbar region.

Myelodysplasia is considered to be an inherited condition in the Weimaraner dog, transmitted by a mutant gene with some degree of dominance but reduced penetrance and variable expressivity.[323] Both males and females are affected. Embryos (24 to 28 days) from matings of severely dysraphic Weimaraner dogs show aberrantly positioned mantle cells ventral to the central canal in the neural tube floorplate area.[324] The neural tube was closed in all of the dysraphic embryos studied. Dysraphic fetuses show structural abnormalities thought to be an exacerbation of the abnormal migration of mantle cells, such as absence of the ventral median fissure and concomitant fusion of the ventral horns, flattening of the ventral horns, and disruption of the spinal nuclei.[325] Syringomyelia is seen pathologically in older dysraphic Weimaraner dogs and may be indicative of progressive disease, although clinical signs in affected dogs remain static.[322] Evidence of syringomyelia was not found in dysraphic embryos or fetuses.[324, 325] Myelodysplasia has been described in other breeds of dogs or cats, including a Dalmatian, a rottweiler, mixed-breed dogs, and Manx cats.[8, 132, 326–328] Etiology and pathogenesis of the condition in these animals are unknown.

Clinical Findings. Clinical signs vary in severity and usually are referable to a transverse myelopathy between T3 and L3. Clinical abnormalities usually are evident at four to six weeks of age, when puppies become ambulatory,[322] although abnormal reflexes have been reported in affected newborn puppies.[323, 329] The major clinical finding in affected dogs is a symmetric "bunny-hopping" pelvic limb gait, which has been speculated to be due to altered neural mechanisms in the lumbar spinal cord.[330] Other clinical findings are crouching stance, abduction or overextension of one or both pelvic limbs, decreased conscious proprioception in the pelvic limbs, scoliosis, and in one case, torticollis.[327] Spinal reflexes and pain perception usually are normal. In Weimaraner dogs, other findings include abnormal hair "streams" in the dorsal neck region, koilosternia (gutter-like depression in the chest), and occasionally, a head tilt.[322]

Myelodysplasia of Weimaraner dogs is a nonprogressive condition. The sudden onset and progression of clinical signs reported in a one-and-a-half-year-old, mixed-breed dog may have been associated with progressive syringomyelia and hydromyelia.[327]

Treatment. There is not an effective treatment. In Weimaraner dogs and probably in other dogs or cats, clinical signs are not progressive and affected animals may be acceptable pets.

Necrotizing Vasculitis

Etiology and Pathogenesis. Necrotizing vasculitis of the extradural and intradural spinal meningeal arteries has been reported to occur in young dogs of several breeds.[136, 331–333] Pathologic changes that have been described include fibrinoid degeneration, intimal and medial necrosis, inflammatory cell infiltration, periadventitial accumulation of inflammatory cells, meningeal fibrosis, and hyalinization and mineralization of meningeal arterial walls. Neurologic deficits may result from the rupture of structurally weakened blood vessels causing extensive meningeal hemorrhage, and compression of the spinal cord. Thrombosis of vessels and infarction of the spinal cord may also be contributing factors.[333] Subsequent meningeal fibrosis around nerve roots and spinal cord also may result in axonal degeneration. Pathologic changes are seen throughout the spinal cord. Similar lesions also have been found in the cardiac arteries of several dogs.[332, 333] Etiology of this disease has not been determined.

The occurrence of this disease in three Bernese Mountain dog littermates suggests a genetic predisposition to the disease.[331] This disease has also been recognized in an inbred colony of beagle dogs.[332] Immune-mediated mechanisms are suspected in the pathogenesis of the disease. Lymphocytic thyroiditis and renal amyloidosis, which are also thought to have an immunologic basis, were found in several dogs.[332] Infectious agents have not been isolated, although a viral-induced immune-mediated reaction is a possible cause. Antinuclear antibody was not present in three dogs tested.[331] Vasculitis of spinal arteries has also been reported as part of polysystemic necrotizing vasculitis in an older dog.[334]

Clinical Findings. Affected dogs usually are four to 12 months of age. Clinical signs include fever, anorexia, cervical rigidity, hunched posture, apparent spinal pain, shifting lameness, apparent pain on opening the mouth and in some animals, neurologic deficits, including paraparesis, tetraparesis, and paraplegia. Clinical findings usually are indicative of meningitis and, in some animals, of multifocal or diffuse myelopathy.

Diagnosis. Affected animals may have a peripheral mature neutrophilic leukocytosis. Cerebrospinal fluid generally has a marked pleocytosis (may be greater than 10,000 WBC/μl) with predominantly mature nontoxic neutrophils present. Bacterial or fungal organisms have not been identified in white blood cells of CSF. Cerebrospinal fluid protein concentration also is elevated. Blood and CSF bacterial (aerobic and anaerobic) cultures are negative. This disease often cannot be distinguished from other meningitides (including viral, bacterial, or fungal meningitis, GME or aseptic suppurative meningitis) on the basis of clinical and CSF findings.

Treatment. Treatment with corticosteroids usually results in a rapid improvement in clinical signs. However, relapses commonly occur when treatment is discontinued. Neurologic deficits may persist despite treatment in dogs with severe neurologic abnormalities. Treatment for longer than six months may result in permanent resolution of clinical signs.[331] A dose of corticosteroids sufficient to produce a remission of clinical signs (1–2 mg/lb prednisone) is given initially, followed by maintenance oral therapy at a dose tapered slowly to be the lowest dose possible that controls clinical signs (preferably every other day dosage).[136] It has been suggested that corticosteroid therapy should be continued until clinical signs have resolved and results of CSF analysis are normal. If signs recur, the dose should again be increased. Antibiotic therapy does not result in improvement in clinical signs. As this condition is often indistinguishable from septic meningitis, treatment with a broad-spectrum antibiotic that reaches satisfactory concentrations in the CSF (e.g., trimethoprim-sulfadiazine or chloramphenicol) is suggested initially in animals in which the diagnosis is uncertain.

Neoplasia

Etiology and Pathogenesis. The spinal cord may be a site of primary or metastatic neoplasia, or may be compressed or invaded by primary or metastatic tumors arising from the vertebrae and surrounding tissues.[335–374] Primary neoplasms may arise from the neuroectodermal, ectodermal, or mesodermal cells of the spinal cord, spinal nerve roots, spinal nerves, or meninges.

Primary neural tumors include astrocytoma, glioma, ependymoma, neuroepithelioma, malignant nerve sheath neoplasm (schwannoma, neurofibroma, neurofibrosarcoma), meningioma, meningeal sarcoma, and reticulum cell sarcoma. Primary lymphosarcoma of the spinal cord also has been reported in a dog.[337]

Tumors of spinal nerves that extend into the spinal canal or spinal nerve roots may cause extradural or intradural compression of the spinal cord. These tumors may also invade the spinal cord parenchyma. The distinction between schwannoma, Schwann cell sarcoma, neurofibroma, and neurofibrosarcoma is difficult to make histologically but all have similar features clinically and on gross pathology.[336] The term malignant nerve sheath neoplasm has been proposed for this tumor.[336] These tumors may involve any cranial or spinal nerve or dorsal or ventral nerve root and commonly spread to involve adjacent nerves and nerve roots. Malignant nerve sheath tumors commonly arise from nerve roots or spinal nerves contributing to the brachial plexus. These tumors may arise from more than one site.[338]

Lymphosarcoma may also involve peripheral nerves and extend along spinal nerves and nerve roots into the spinal canal, resulting in clinical signs of spinal cord disease.[336]

Meningeal sarcomatosis is a rare condition characterized by diffuse infiltration of the leptomeninges by neoplastic mesenchymal cells. In one reported case in a dog, clinical signs were lameness, reluctance to sit, apparent spinal pain, seizures, and urinary incontinence.[339]

The spinal cord may also be compressed by tumors originating from surrounding structures. Most commonly these tumors arise from bone, cartilage, fibrous tissue, and blood vessels of vertebrae, and less commonly from the hemopoietic elements of bone and tissue outside the vertebral column, including muscle, fat, and paraganglia.[340, 341] Primary vertebral tumors, which may cause compression of the spinal cord due to either extension of tumor mass into the spinal canal or pathologic fracture of the vertebra, include osteosarcoma, chondrosarcoma, fibrosarcoma, hemangioma, hemangiosarcoma, plasma cell myeloma, and giant cell sarcoma (arising from primitive stromal elements of bone marrow) and undifferentiated sarcomas.[336] Tumor metastases from sites elsewhere in the body may also be found in vertebrae, epidural space, meninges, and rarely the parenchyma of the spinal cord. Secondary tumors occur due to hematogenous or lymphatic spread of tumor emboli and include hemangiosarcoma, lymphosarcoma, mammary adenocarcinoma, pulmonary carcinoma, prostatic carcinoma, and malignant melanoma. Clinical signs associated with secondary spinal tumors may comprise the initial presenting complaint for affected animals, or may occur late in the course of the disease or during or after treatment for a primary tumor. With the prolonged survival times that accompany recent therapeutic regimes for osteosarcoma of long bones, an increased frequency of vertebral metastases can be expected, particularly in cranial thoracic vertebrae. Embolic tumor cells may pass directly to the lumbar vertebrae from tumors in the pelvic area by reversal of blood flow in the vertebral veins with increases in central venous pressure.

Retrospective studies have shown the most commonly occurring spinal tumors in dogs to be primary and secondary bone tumors, and tumors of spinal nerves and nerve roots.[335, 342, 343] Primary intramedullary tumors occur less commonly than extradural or intradural-extramedullary tumors. Spinal tumors of all types occur more frequently in large breeds of dog. Epidural lymphosarcoma is the most commonly occurring spinal tumor in cats.[344, 345] Primary intramedullary tumors rarely occur in cats. Etiology of vertebral and spinal cord tumors is unknown. Lymphosarcoma in cats may be associated with FeLV infection; however, not all cats with spinal lymphosarcoma test positive for FeLV.

Spinal tumors may occur in animals of any age. Although tumors more commonly occur in animals more than five years of age, spinal cord neuroepithelioma in dogs[351] and lymphosarcoma in cats are found most commonly in young animals.[336] Neuroepithelioma has also been classified as medulloepithelioma and ependymoma.[346–348] One report classified a similar spinal tumor as nephroblastoma.[349] These tumors have been reported in large breeds of dog aged six months to three years. German shepherd dogs have a higher incidence of this tumor than other breeds.[8] A similar tumor has been described in an older dog.[350] Neuroepitheliomas are generally located in an intradural and extramedullary location, closely associated with the pia mater of the spinal cord and separated from the spinal cord by a thin band of connective tissue. The tumor may replace most of the spinal cord and may also have an intramedullary component. Neuroepitheliomas often appear as an intramedullary mass on myelography. These tumors occur in T10-L2 spinal cord segments and may be the result of neoplastic transformation of remnants of embryonic medullary (neuro)epithelium in this region of the spinal cord.[346] However, immunocytochemical studies do not support a neuroectodermal origin for these tumors. The mixed epithelial and mesenchymal patterns seen in these tumors are similar to nephroblastomas.[351]

Metastatic spinal tumors have also been reported to occur in young dogs.[352] Primary spinal cord, meningeal, and nerve root tumors rarely metastasize outside the spinal canal; however, tumors may arise from multiple sites or may metastasize along CSF pathways (meningioma, ependymoma). Primary vertebral tumors commonly metastasize to other organ systems.

Clinical Findings. Clinical signs depend on the location of the tumor. Tumors may involve more than one spinal cord segment and more than one spinal tumor may be present, resulting in multifocal signs. However, most animals present with clinical signs referable to a transverse myelopathy. Tumors may occur anywhere within the spinal cord or spinal canal and usually result in progressive neurologic deficits. The duration of clinical signs may vary considerably (from one week to one year in one study).[335] Animals may present with the following signs: an acute onset of severe neurologic deficits associated with pathologic fracture of a vertebra, resulting in spinal cord compression; epidural, subarachnoid, or intramedullary hemorrhage; or spinal cord ischemia associated with tumor expansion. Neurologic deficits are usually bilateral but may be asymmetrical.

Tumors of nerves of the brachial plexus initially cause progressive LMN signs in the ipsilateral thoracic limb, including muscle atrophy and paresis. The affected limb is often painful on palpation or movement; cutaneous sensation generally remains intact.[336] If the tumor extends into the spinal canal, UMN signs to the pelvic limbs may become apparent. Tumors of the nerves of the cauda equina or lumbosacral plexus, with extension into the spinal canal, may cause unilateral or bilateral LMN signs in the pelvic limbs, tail, perineum, urinary bladder, and anal sphincter.

Apparent pain is a common finding associated with extradural and intradural tumors,[353, 374] and was the predominant clinical sign in a study of dogs with vertebral tumors.[354] Apparent pain may be intractable, especially in animals with a tumor affecting spinal nerve roots. This may be due to stretching or inflammation of the meninges surrounding the expanding tumor. Intramedullary tumors are reported to cause a more rapid progression of clinical signs and are much less likely to be painful than extradural or intradural-extramedullary tumors.[335] In general, however, extradural, intradural-extramedullary, and intramedullary tumors cannot be distinguished on the basis of clinical findings.

Diagnosis. A tentative diagnosis of spinal tumor can be made on the basis of radiographic, CSF, and myelographic findings. Definitive diagnosis can only be made after biopsy of a suspected lesion.

Radiography. Bone lysis with a cortical "break" is the most common radiographic finding in animals with vertebral tumors (Figure 62–25).[354] Other radiographic findings include destruction of vertebral endplates, collapse of an adjacent disk space, collapse and shortening of a vertebral body, pathologic fracture, bone sclerosis and bony production, cyst-like expansile lesions, or adjacent soft tissue masses.[354] Bone tumors most commonly occur in the vertebral body but may also be found in the dorsal spinous processes, transverse processes, and articular facets. Primary and secondary bone tumors or specific tumor types cannot be distinguished radiographically. Primary bone tumors usually involve one vertebra but may involve multiple vertebrae. More than half of the secondary bone tumors in one study involved more than one vertebra.[354] Rarely metastatic tumors (e.g., carcinoma) may arise within a disk space. Such tumors may have a radiographic appearance that resembles that of diskospondylitis. Metastases from intrapelvic soft tissue tumors often produce periosteal new bone on the ventral aspect of multiple lumbar vertebral bodies in association with paravertebral soft tissue mass formation. Vertebral lesions of multiple myeloma are characterized by "punched out" lytic lesions.

Vertebral lesions may also occur with spread of tumors from surrounding soft tissues into the vertebrae. Bone tumors are not always easily detected by means of radiography, due to inconsistent vertebral shape, overlying rib and soft tissue shadows, and improper patient positioning.[354] Other diseases, such as bacterial or fungal diskospondylitis, spondylitis, or vertebral osteomyelitis, must be considered in the differential diagnosis of vertebral tumors.

Expanding tumors within the spinal canal may result in widening of the vertebral canal and loss of bone density due to ischemia and necrosis of overlying bone. Similarly, tumors of spinal nerves extending into the spinal canal may cause widening of intervertebral foramina (Figure 62–26).

Cerebrospinal fluid analysis. Cerebrospinal fluid may be normal or may have an increased protein concentration and/or white blood cell count. A mild to moderate increase in CSF white blood cell count may occur in animals with tumors arising from or invading the leptomeninges. Polymorphonuclear cells may predominate, probably as a result of meningeal inflammation and necrosis. Tumor cells rarely are found in CSF,[355] except in CSF from animals with lymphosarcoma, in which abnormal lymphocytes are often present in association with meningeal infiltration.[356, 357] Abnormal cells have also been found in the CSF of a dog with myeloblastic leukemia and leukemic meningitis.[358] Collection of CSF from the lumbar subarachnoid space may yield more cells than cisternal collection, due to probable caudal flow of CSF in animals.[8] Inability to demonstrate tumor cells in CSF may be the result of the methods used to analyze CSF. The use of cell concentrating techniques that yield a greater percentage of cells present in CSF may result in the preservation of more neoplastic cells. Xanthochromia, suggesting previous subarachnoid hemorrhage, occasionally is present.[359] Cerebrospinal fluid protein concentration may be increased due to abnormal permeability of blood–spinal cord or blood-meningeal barrier, as a result of extradural compression or meningeal or parenchymal tumor infiltration.

Myelography. Myelography may be helpful in differentiating intramedullary, intradural-extramedullary, and extradural tumors (Figure 62–27). Cisternal and lumbar injection of contrast material may be necessary to outline both the cranial and caudal extent of a tumor. It is important to obtain survey radiographs of the entire vertebral column prior to and after injection of contrast, as more than one tumor may be present and the neurologic deficits of one tumor may "mask" those produced by another. Several radiographic views (at least lateral and ventrodorsal) are necessary to determine whether a tumor is intramedullary, intradural-extramedullary, or extradural. Tumors may have a

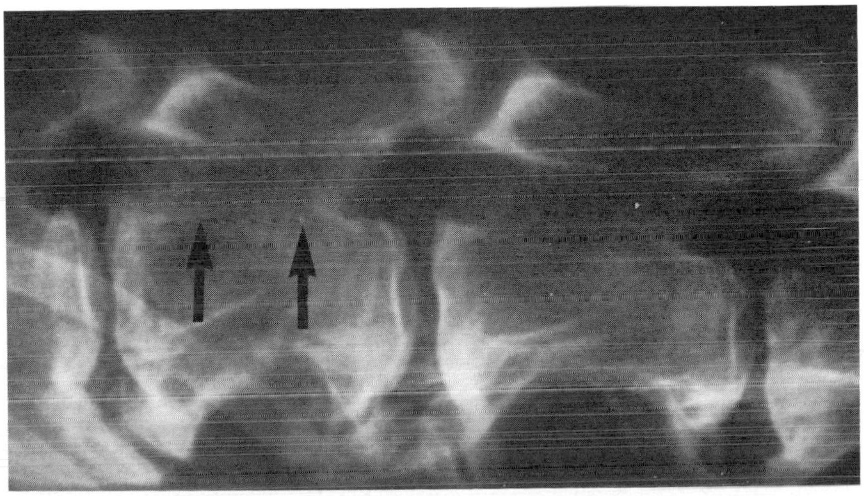

FIGURE 62–25. Vertebral neoplasia. Lateral radiograph of the cranial lumbar vertebral column of an 11-year-old spayed female German shepherd with a history of progressively worsening pelvic limb paresis and ataxia. Note the extensive spondylosis deformans ventral to the L1-L2, L2-L3, and L3-L4 disks. There appears to be slight narrowing of the L1-L2 disk. Patchy lysis of the L2 vertebral body associated with loss of the dorsal cortex (cortical "break") of the body (arrows) is consistent with neoplasia. The histopathologic diagnosis was metastatic adenocarcinoma.

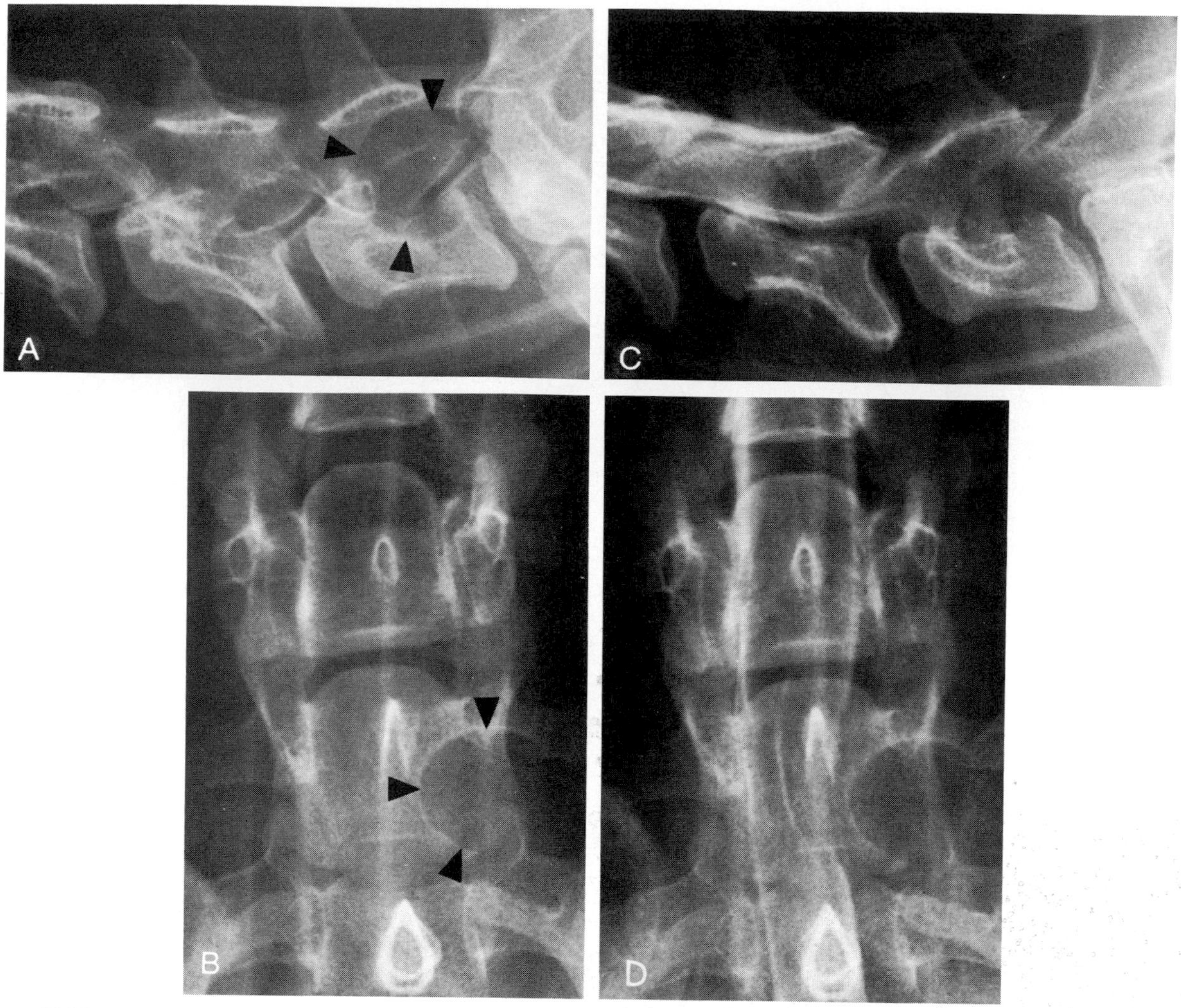

FIGURE 62–26. Malignant nerve sheath tumor. Lateral *(A)* and ventrodorsal *(B)* radiographs of the caudal cervical vertebral column of a ten-year-old spayed female long-haired dachshund. The dog had a one-year history of progressively worsening left thoracic limb lameness. Enlargement of the left C7-T1 intervertebral foramen is seen on both lateral and ventrodorsal projections (arrowheads). There is absence of contrast material over the length of the C7 vertebra on the lateral myelogram *(C)*. The ventrodorsal myelogram *(D)* confirms the presence of a left-sided extradural mass adjacent to the enlarged intervertebral foramen. Histologic diagnosis was malignant nerve sheath neoplasm.

mixed myelographic appearance, with extradural, intradural, and/or intramedullary components (e.g., nerve root tumors, meningioma, and neuroepithelioma). Myelographic findings may also be misleading, as extradural tumors may appear intramedullary on some views, or spinal cord edema associated with acute extradural compression may appear the same as an intramedullary mass. Other mass lesions resulting in spinal cord compression, intramedullary swelling, and intradural lesions must be considered in the differential diagnosis of spinal tumors. Such mass lesions include intervertebral disk protrusion, epidural abscess or granuloma formation, spinal cord edema associated with spinal cord trauma, vascular malformation, or subarachnoid cyst. The authors have seen two dogs with progressive myelopathy associated with intramedullary astrocytoma in which myelographic findings were normal.

Other diagnostic tests. As many spinal tumors are secondary tumors and primary vertebral tumors commonly metastasize, careful attention should be directed toward eliminating the presence of other tumors by performing a thorough physical examination, survey thoracic and abdominal radiographic examinations, rectal examination, complete blood count and other diagnostic tests as necessary. For example, animals with lymphosarcoma may show abnormal circulating lymphocytes and/or hypercalcemia, and animals with plasma cell myeloma may show aplastic anemia, myelophthisis, hypercalcemia, elevated serum protein, monoclonal gammopathy on serum electrophoresis, and/or Bence Jones proteinuria.

In the future, both CT and MRI will aid in exact determination of location and extent of spinal tumors. Use of these advanced imaging modalities will aid in precise surgical planning and radiation therapy planning (Figure 62–28).

Biopsy. Biopsy of suspected lesions is necessary to differentiate neoplasms from other vertebral and spinal cord abnormalities and to determine histologic type. An open surgical technique is most often used to obtain an

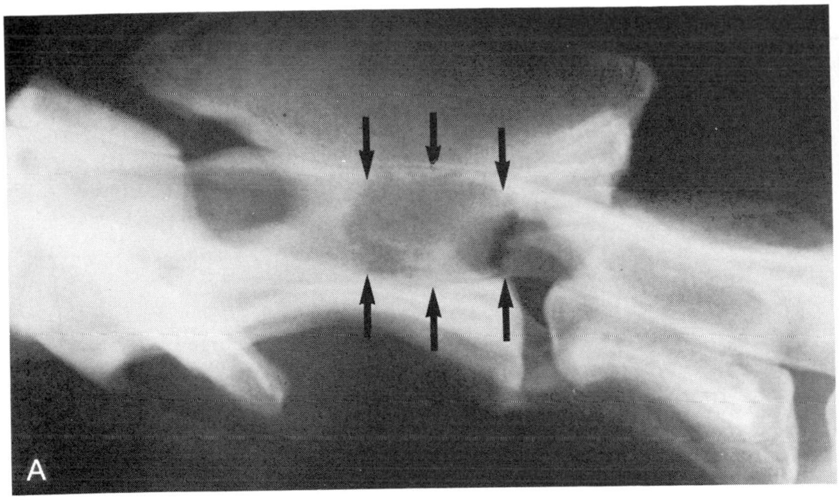

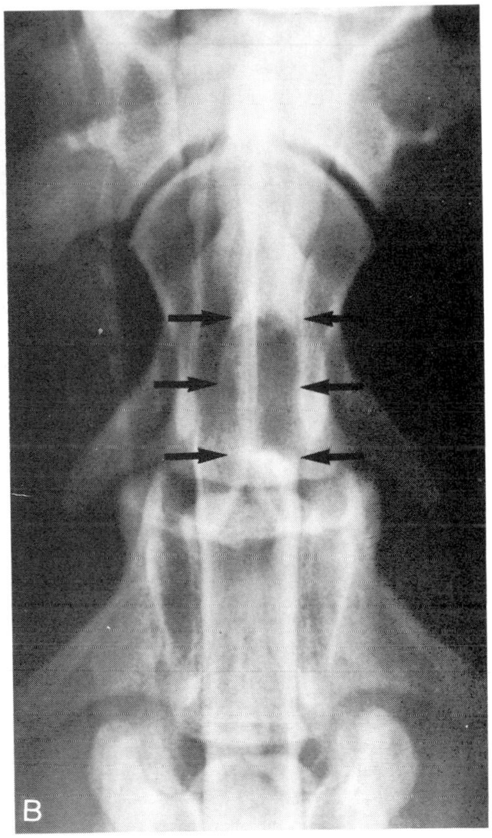

FIGURE 62–27. Intradural-extramedullary space-occupying lesion. Lateral *(A)* and ventrodorsal *(B)* projections of a myelogram of the cranial cervical vertebral column of a 12-year-old male golden retriever. Note the filling defect in the subarachnoid space within C1 (arrows). This pattern is typical of an intradural-extramedullary mass. The histopathologic diagnosis was meningioma.

adequate specimen of most spinal tumors; however, in the future fluoroscopy- or CT-guided needle biopsy techniques will become available for use in dogs and cats.[375]

Treatment. The majority of vertebral tumors are not surgically resectable, due to the malignant characteristics of the tumor and the decreased stability of the vertebral column that may result from extensive surgery. Surgical decompression of the spinal cord and debulking of tumor mass may be palliative in some cases. Surgical resection of solitary plasma cell myeloma may be possible.[4] Some tumors within the spinal canal are surgically resectable,

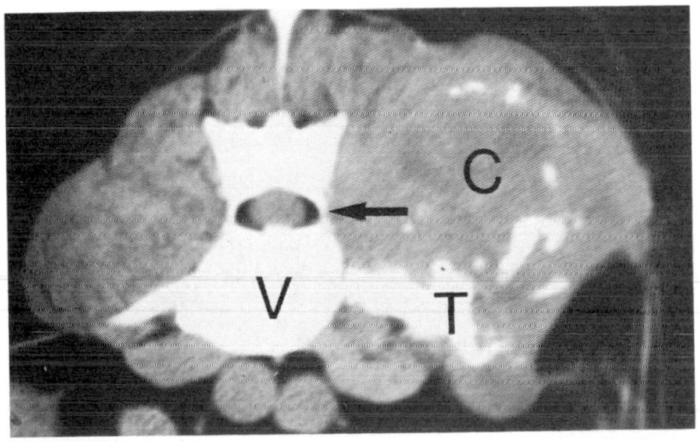

FIGURE 62–28. Computed tomography. Transverse CT image of the vertebral column of a 13-year-old spayed female Old English sheepdog at the level of the L4 vertebral body (V). Note the chondrosarcoma (C) arising from the transverse process (T) of L4. There are areas of calcification within the neoplasm. The tumor involves the lateral lamina (arrow) of L4. Exact determination of location and extent of a neoplasm is possible by means of CT.

including some tumors that appear intramedullary on myelography, such as neuroepithelioma. Surgical exploration of solitary tumors within the spinal canal is recommended in animals in which clinical signs are indicative of an incomplete transverse myelopathy, even in animals in which myelographic findings are consistent with an intramedullary mass. Intradural nerve root tumors are rarely completely surgically resectable, and the recurrence rate is high due to intramedullary spread of tumor cells. Resection of ventral nerve roots contributing to the brachial or lumbosacral plexus may necessitate amputation of the affected limb.[336]

There is not a direct relationship between tumor size and rate of progression or severity of clinical signs. The spinal cord is able to compensate for pressure applied gradually, and animals with spinal tumors may remain ambulatory despite having little normal spinal cord tissue remaining. Compression applied to the spinal cord rapidly, such as may occur with a pathologic fracture, may cause severe and irreversible spinal cord damage.

Corticosteroids may decrease spinal cord edema associated with spinal cord tumors and result in clinical improvement for a variable period of time. Radiation therapy and chemotherapy may be helpful in animals with spinal lymphosarcoma. Most chemotherapeutic agents do not cross the blood–spinal cord or blood-CSF barrier in sufficient concentrations to eliminate tumor cells in the meninges or spinal cord. Several chemotherapeutic agents, including methotrexate and cytosine arabinoside, may be given intrathecally and have been used in the treatment of meningeal lymphosarcoma and leukemic meningitis.[357] Complications of intrathecal use of chemotherapeutic agents include arachnoiditis and seizures. Chemotherapy may be helpful in treatment of plasma cell myeloma.

Chemotherapy and radiotherapy have not been used in the treatment of a sufficient number of primary spinal cord, nerve root, and meningeal tumors to assess results; however, initial experience suggests that further use of radiation therapy is warranted. Various chemotherapeutic regimens have been used in the treatment of various bone tumors and tumors that metastasize to bone, generally with poor results. Chemotherapy regimens in the future may offer more hope in the treatment of vertebral tumors. In general, the prognosis for animals with nonresectable spinal tumors is poor.

Neuroaxonal Dystrophy of Rottweiler Dogs

Neuroaxonal dystrophy is a disease of rottweiler dogs characterized by the accumulation of axonal spheroids throughout the neuraxis.[376–379] Clinically, affected animals have progressive ataxia in all limbs and severe hypermetria, especially of the thoracic limbs. Histologically, axonal spheroids are found in massive numbers throughout the brain and spinal cord, especially in the dorsal horns of the spinal cord and nucleus gracilis and nucleus cuneatus. The cerebellum is mildly atrophic in some dogs. Afferent fibers entering the sensory nuclei in the spinal cord, brain stem, and diencephalon are primarily affected. Electron microscopy has shown axonal spheroids to be enlarged distal portions of axons and synaptic terminals, containing accumulations of smooth membrane-bound vesicles, membranous lamellae, dense bodies, and other organelles.[376] Histologic lesions may be mild in young dogs.

A recessive mode of inheritance with variable penetrance in rottweiler dogs is suspected from preliminary breeding studies.[376] Etiology and pathogenesis of distal membranous axonopathies are not understood, but location of lesions suggests a derangement in the presynaptic portion of neurons or abnormalities in axonal transport.[376] Axonal dystrophies have been associated with toxins, nutritional deficiency, aging, and genetic disorders in other species and humans.

Clinical Findings. Affected dogs may be clumsy as puppies, or clinical signs may not be seen until dogs are more than 12 months of age. Both male and female dogs are affected. Clinical signs may progress slowly over several years. The initial clinical finding is progressive ataxia of all limbs. Paresis or abnormalities in conscious proprioception have not been found in affected dogs. Patellar reflexes may be exaggerated; however, other reflexes are normal. These findings are consistent with a transverse myelopathy of the cervical spinal cord or multifocal spinal cord disease. As the disease progresses other signs become apparent, including hypermetria (especially of the thoracic limbs), incoordination, tremors of the head, positional nystagmus, decreased menace response, and crossed extensor reflexes. Thoracic limb hypermetria may be severe in older dogs, especially when climbing stairs. The neurologic deficits seen in older dogs are predominantly referable to abnormalities in the cerebellum or input to the cerebellum.

Diagnosis. Diagnosis is made on the basis of age, breed, and neurologic findings and by ruling out other causes of cervical spinal cord and cerebellar disease. This disease is unusual in that it is slowly progressive over several years, but in the initial stages may appear clinically similar to other causes of a cervical myelopathy, including CD myelitis and cervical spondylomyelopathy. Cerebrospinal fluid may have an elevated protein concentration (40 mg/dl was reported in one dog[378]). Spinal radiographs and myelograms are normal.

Treatment. Currently, treatment is not effective. Clinical improvement has not been detected during treatment with corticosteroids. Due to the slow progression of the disease, affected dogs may be acceptable pets for several years. Affected dogs should not be used for breeding, although a diagnosis of neuroaxonal dystrophy may not be made until after these dogs have produced litters.

Pilonidal Sinus and Epidermoid Cyst (Dermoid Sinus, Pilonidal Cyst)

Etiology and Pathogenesis. A pilonidal sinus is an invagination of the skin dorsal to the spine, extending below the skin to variable depths and in some cases as far as the dura mater, where it may communicate with the subarachnoid space.[380] The formation of pilonidal sinuses is related to failure of complete separation of the neural groove from the epidermis during embryonic development.[381] Pilonidal sinuses may occur anywhere along the dorsal midline from cervical to sacrocaudal regions and may be single or multiple. Purebred and crossbred Rhodesian ridgeback dogs are most commonly affected, although other breeds of dogs may be affected.[382] There have not been reports of sinuses occurring along the ridge of hair of Rhodesian ridgeback dogs.[383] Histologically, sinuses are lined with stratified squamous epithelium and sweat glands; sebaceous glands and hair follicles are found. The sinuses contain inspissated sebum, hair, and exfoliated cells, and commonly become inflamed or infected.[384] If sinuses communicate with the subarachnoid space, extension of infection results in meningitis or myelitis. Pilonidal sinuses are likely to occur as a hereditary defect in Rhodesian ridgeback dogs, but the mode of inheritance is not definitely known.[383]

Epidermoid cysts have been reported to occur in the brain and spinal cord of dogs.[385, 386] Such cysts are thought to arise from entrapment and subsequent growth of primordial epithelial cells during closure of the neural tube. Morphologically similar cysts have developed in humans following injury or after repeated lumbar subarachnoid punctures for CSF collection, presumably from mechanical implantation of epidermal cells.[386] An intramedullary spinal epidermoid cyst reported in a dog was thought to have a congenital cause.[386] Apparently spinal epidermoid cysts rarely occur in dogs.

Clinical Signs. Clinical signs of meningitis and myelitis may be seen in animals as a result of extension of infection from a pilonidal sinus to the subarachnoid space. Localized or generalized spinal pain and rigidity may be seen associated with meningitis. Neurologic deficits indicative of a transverse or diffuse myelopathy may be seen as a result of myelitis.

Neurologic signs resulting from a spinal epidermoid cyst depend upon its location. In the only reported case in a dog, signs were consistent with a progressive transverse myelopathy between T3 and L3 spinal cord segments.[386]

Diagnosis. A pilonidal sinus may be palpable as a cord of fibrous tissue under the skin of the dorsal midline. Palpation may be painful if the sinus is infected. An opening in the skin on the dorsal midline is usually found and hair may or may not be seen protruding from this opening. Cerebrospinal fluid in animals with meningitis or myelitis is generally abnormal and indicative of bacterial infection. Fistulography performed by injecting a radiographic contrast material such as metrizamide, which is not an irritant to nervous tissue, into the sinus demonstrates whether pilonidal sinuses are continuous with the subarachnoid space. Myelography may also demonstrate communication.

Diagnosis of a spinal epidermoid cyst is based on clinical signs and results of plain spinal radiography, CSF analysis, and myelography. Typically an epidermoid cyst should be suspected in the presence of an intramedullary, expansile lesion on myelography in a young dog with progressive neurologic deficits.[386] Diagnosis is confirmed by means of an open surgical biopsy, which may provide the only means to rule out spinal neoplasia (e.g., neuroepithelioma).

Treatment. Animals with meningitis and/or myelitis associated with a pilonidal sinus should be treated in the same way as an animal with meningitis and myelitis due to another cause. Antibiotic therapy should be selected on the basis of CSF culture, culture of the contents of the pilonidal sinus, and sensitivity testing. Complete surgical excision of the pilonidal sinus is essential. Laminectomy may be necessary to remove portions of a pilonidal sinus from within the spinal canal. Recurrence of infection is likely in dogs in which a pilonidal sinus is incompletely removed. Prognosis depends on the severity of neurologic deficits prior to surgery, the response to antibiotic therapy, and whether or not the pilonidal sinus is removed completely. Complications of surgical removal include wound dehiscence and seroma formation. Affected animals should not be used for breeding.

Treatment of spinal epidermoid cysts of dogs has not been reported. Surgical excision may be possible in some animals.

Progressive Hemorrhagic Myelomalacia

Etiology and Pathogenesis. Acute, severe spinal cord injury may result in progressive ascending and descending infarction and hemorrhagic necrosis of the spinal cord parenchyma. Progressive hemorrhagic myelomalacia (PHM) occurs infrequently and usually follows peracute explosive extrusion of a thoracolumbar disk, but may also be seen in animals after spinal cord trauma. This condition previously has been termed "hematomyelia."

The majority of dogs with thoracolumbar disk protrusions have evidence of a localized myelopathy affecting up to four spinal cord segments.[239] In animals with PHM, hemorrhagic necrosis of the entire spinal cord may occur over a period of one to two days (Figure 62–29). Etiology of this syndrome is not known; however, spinal cord pathology indicates severe ischemia. The characteristic histologic findings include necrosis of neural and mesenchymal elements, hemorrhage, necrosis of intramedullary and meningeal blood vessels, and perivascular deposits of fibrin.[387] Marked subarachnoid hemorrhage and thrombosis of spinal cord vasculature are also present. The cause of the spinal cord ischemia is unknown.

Clinical Signs. Clinical signs depend on the location of the lesion; however, most affected animals initially have clinical signs indicative of a transverse myelopathy between T3 and L3, with UMN signs in the pelvic limbs. Neurologic deficits usually are severe (paraplegia and absent deep pain perception in pelvic limbs) and peracute in onset (hours). Clinical signs indicating a diffuse myelopathy progress over a period of hours to one to two days. As infarction and hemorrhagic necrosis of the spinal cord progress cranially and caudally, LMN signs may be seen in the pelvic limbs, anus, and thoracic limbs, and the level of cutaneous anesthesia extends cranially. The Schiff-Scherrington sign may be present prior to involvement of the spinal cord cranial to T3. Diaphragmatic paralysis and bilateral Horner's syndrome may be seen,[6] with involvement of the cervical spinal cord. Affected animals often are in extreme pain and are anxious and show an increased body temperature.

Diagnosis. A diagnosis is made on the basis of progressive clinical signs indicative of a diffuse myelopathy. Any animal with an acute onset of paraplegia due to a lesion between T3 and L3 that shows LMN signs in the pelvic or thoracic limbs should be suspected of having more than one lesion, or PHM.

Treatment. Progressive hemorrhagic myelomalacia is in most cases fatal within 24 to 48 hours due to respiratory paralysis. Effective medical or surgical treatments do not exist, and euthanasia is recommended. Difficulty often arises when treating animals that are presented with an acute onset of paraplegia with or without deep pain perception within hours of the onset of clinical

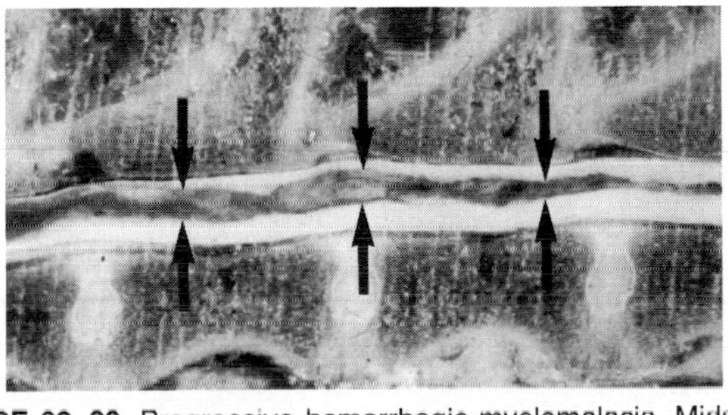

FIGURE 62–29. Progressive hemorrhagic myelomalacia. Midsagittal view of a gross necropsy specimen of the vertebral column of a four-year-old female dachshund that had an acute T11-T12 disk extrusion. Note the hemorrhagic myelomalacia within the L2 and L3 spinal cord segments (arrows).

signs. Ideally, if decompressive surgery is indicated, it should be performed as soon as possible; however, a small percentage of these cases may show clinical signs of PHM after surgery. Hemorrhagic myelomalacia in some cases may not progress to involve the cervical cord[4, 387] and affected animals may survive; however, the spinal cord damage incurred and associated severe neurologic deficits are permanent.

Protozoal Myelitis

Etiology and Pathogenesis. *Toxoplasma gondii* infection may cause a focal or disseminated myelopathy in dogs and cats. Animals are infected after ingesting meat containing toxoplasma bradyzoites and/or tachyzoites, after ingesting cat feces containing sporulated oocysts, or by transplacental or congenital infection.[388] The infective organism is spread hematogenously to most organs of the body, including the CNS. The incidence of disease associated with *Toxoplasma gondii* is thought to be low; however, opportunistic infection in immunosuppressed animals may be more widespread than previously reported. Immaturity and concurrent CD virus infection may result in an increased susceptibility of dogs to toxoplasmosis.[389, 390] In dogs with systemic toxoplasmosis, the incidence of CNS involvement is high.[391] In cats, concurrent infection with FeLV or FTLV or administration of corticosteroids may predispose to the development of clinical signs of toxoplasmosis through immunosuppression and reactivation of latent infection.[392]

Pathologically, CNS toxoplasmosis lesions are characterized by diffuse perivascular cuffing, infiltration of tissues by inflammatory cells (predominantly mononuclear cells), hemorrhage, necrosis, edema, and neuronal degeneration.[391] Granulomatous reactions may be seen. Encysted or free forms of *Toxoplasma gondii* may be present. Observed tissue reactions may occur as a result of cell rupture, immune-complex deposition, delayed hypersensitivity reaction, or degeneration of toxoplasma cysts.

A protozoan parasite, *Neospora caninum*, structurally distinct from *Toxoplasma gondii*, has been identified.[393] The newly discovered organism, belonging to a new genus and new species, formed meronts in many tissues of dogs, especially brain and spinal cord, resulting in meningoencephalomyelitis. *Neospora caninum* organisms do not react to toxoplasma immunoperoxidase staining techniques, and the life cycle is unknown. Clinically the new protozoal disease appears similar to toxoplasmosis; however, CNS signs and myositis were seen more commonly than in toxoplasmosis.[393]

Clinical Findings. Affected animals usually have clinical signs of progressive multifocal or disseminated CNS disease. Clinical signs indicating a focal transverse or diffuse myelopathy only may be seen initially. Neurologic deficits depend on site of involvement and may be UMN or LMN. If lower motor neurons are involved, denervation may result in severe muscle atrophy.

In dogs less than one year of age, a syndrome of progressive paralysis and rigid extension of one or both pelvic limbs may be seen in association with *Toxoplasma gondii* infection. Muscle atrophy and contracture of affected limbs is seen and limbs cannot be flexed. Muscle changes may be the result of myositis and myonecrosis and/or denervation due to myelitis or radiculitis in the caudal lumbar and sacral spinal cord segments.[394–397]

Animals with CNS toxoplasmosis may or may not have other clinical signs indicative of systemic infection (fever, lymphadenopathy, pneumonia, apparent muscle pain, gastrointestinal tract disease, iritis, or chorioretinitis).

Diagnosis. Antemortem confirmation of CNS toxoplasmosis in dogs or cats is extremely difficult.[88] Results of routine hematologic and biochemical tests may be abnormal in cats or dogs with acute systemic toxoplasmosis; however, such results reflect only the organ systems involved and are not specific for toxoplasmosis. Cerebrospinal fluid may be normal, or may have an elevated white blood cell count with a mixed mononuclear pleocytosis, and an elevated protein concentration. Xanthochromia may be present if subarachnoid hemorrhage has occurred. Radiography of the thorax or abdomen of animals with acute disease may demonstrate effusion, pneumonia, or abdominal masses.[88]

Toxoplasma organisms may be identified in cytologic preparations of thoracic or peritoneal effusions, or in biopsies of lymph node or muscle examined by conventional histopathologic techniques, or by other methods such as immunoperoxidase staining. It is difficult, however, to be certain of the association between clinical disease and demonstration of organisms.[88]

Numerous serologic tests have been used in the diagnosis of toxoplasmosis.[88] This subject has been reviewed in detail by Greene (1984).[88] Serologic testing for antibody (immunoglobulin G or IgG) is of limited use for determining active infection, unless paired titers done two to three weeks apart demonstrate a four-fold increase. Certainly, a negative titer does not rule out a diagnosis of toxoplasmosis. Currently it is recommended that for serologic diagnosis of toxoplasmosis in dogs or cats a single serum sample should be submitted for immunoglobulins G and M (IgG and IgM) determinations, and for calculation of levels of circulating antigen to *Toxoplasma gondii*.[398, 399] Further, in cats suspected of having toxoplasmosis, both FeLV and FTLV (FIV) titers should be determined.[392]

Fecal examination for oocysts is the most practical method for determining the public health risk of a cat suspected to have toxoplasmosis. Oocysts are shed in feces of infected cats for only a short time (five days to two weeks postinfection).[88]

Treatment. Several antibacterial agents have been recommended for treatment of toxoplasmosis in dogs and cats. Available drugs are effective in CNS tissues only against actively proliferating forms of the organism, and are not active against encysted forms, which are dependent on host humoral and cell-mediated immune responses for eradication.[88] Clindamycin is presently recommended for treatment of systemic infection of dogs or cats.[88, 392] Oral therapy at a total daily dosage of 12 mg/lb (25 mg/kg) divided q12h appears effective in cats, while a daily dose of 5 to 18 mg/lb (10 to 40 mg/kg) divided q6h or q8h should be effective in dogs. Therapy should be continued for two to four weeks.

The effectiveness of clindamycin in penetrating CNS tissues of dogs or cats has not been determined, and it is therefore recommended that sulfadiazine or triple-sulfas be given orally at a daily dosage of 50 mg/lb divided q12h for CNS toxoplasmosis. Addition of pyrimethamine at a daily dosage of 0.25–0.5 mg/lb permits reduction of the sulfadiazine dosage by half. Hematologic monitoring for bone marrow suppression is essential for cats placed on this therapeutic regimen.

The public health risk posed by a cat with active *Toxoplasma gondii* infection must be considered prior to and during treatment for toxoplasmosis.[88]

Pyogranulomatous Meningoencephalomyelitis

Etiology and Pathogenesis. Pyogranulomatous meningoencephalomyelitis is an acute, rapidly progressive disease that has been described in mature pointers.[400] Pathologic changes are most severe in the cranial cervical spinal cord and caudal brain stem. Lesions are characterized by extensive mononuclear and polymorphonuclear infiltration of the leptomeninges and spinal cord parenchyma and formation of large perivascular cuffs. Central gray matter necrosis and edema in the cervical spinal cord may occur in association with impaired spinal cord circulation secondary to meningitis. A causative agent has not been identified, although a bacterial etiology is suggested by clinical and pathologic data.

Clinical Findings. Clinical signs are indicative of meningitis and cervical myelopathy, and include cervical rigidity, kyphosis, nose held to the ground, reluctance to move, incoordinated hypermetric gait, and atrophy of cervical muscles. Other reported abnormalities are bradycardia, vomiting, trigeminal and facial nerve paralysis, and Horner's syndrome. Clinical signs are rapidly progressive over two to three weeks.

Diagnosis. Diagnosis is made on the basis of clinical signs and results of CSF analysis. There is an increased CSF white blood cell count (500–1000 cells/μl) with predominance of polymorphonuclear cells. Protein concentration is also increased in CSF, and may be greater than 700 mg/ml. Organisms have not been identified on cell preparations or culture of CSF.

Treatment. Temporary remission of clinical signs may occur with antibiotic therapy; however, prognosis for recovery is very poor.

Sacrocaudal Dysgenesis in Manx Cats

Etiology and Pathogenesis. Manx cats have varying degrees of taillessness associated with sacral and/or caudal vertebral deformities. Some tailless cats have a normal sacrum, spinal cord, and cauda equina. Others show varying dysgenesis or agenesis of the sacral and/or caudal vertebrae that may be associated with spina bifida and/or malformations of the terminal spinal cord and/or cauda equina. Spinal cord malformations include absence or partial development of sacral and caudal spinal cord segments or cauda equina, myelodysplasia, meningocele, meningomyelocele, diastematomyelia of sacral segments (duplication), myeloschisis (cleft within the spinal cord), syringomyelia in the lumbar and sacral spinal cord segments, shortening of the spinal cord, and subcutaneous cyst formation.[328, 401–405] These spinal cord and cauda equina malformations are associated with variable neurologic deficits.

Sacrocaudal dysgenesis is inherited as an autosomal dominant trait and may be lethal in some homozygote cats.[406] Sacrocaudal dysgenesis and associated malformations have been recognized in most breeds of cats, many not of true Manx breeding. Sacrocaudal agenesis in a Maltese kitten has been reported.[407]

Clinical Findings. Clinical signs are variable depending on the degree of spinal cord and cauda equina malformation and include paraparesis, paraplegia, megacolon, atonic bladder, absent anal and urinary bladder sphincter tone, absent anal reflex, urinary and fecal incontinence, and perineal analgesia. Affected cats often walk plantigrade in the pelvic limbs with a "bunny hopping" gait. Vertebral abnormalities may be palpable in the lumbosacral region and in some cats a meningocele, congenital or the result of necrosis of the overlying skin, may exit through the skin and drain CSF.

Clinical signs usually are evident soon after birth and may remain static or may be progressive. Worsening of neurologic deficits may be due to progressive syringomyelia in the lumbar and sacral spinal cord.

Diagnosis. Diagnosis is made on the basis of clinical findings and radiographic findings indicative of dysgenesis or agenesis of the sacral and caudal vertebrae. Myelography may demonstrate meningocele or attachment of spinal cord to subcutaneous tissues in the lumbosacral region. The degree of spinal deformity does not always correspond with the degree of neurologic impairment. Clinical findings are the most important factors to consider in determining prognosis.

Treatment. Prognosis for severely affected cats is hopeless and treatment is not available. Cats with urinary and fecal incontinence may be managed with manual bladder expression and fecal softening agents; however, recurrent urinary tract infection, megacolon, and chronic constipation are common problems. Meningocele in cats with minimal neurologic deficits may be surgically correctable. Many tailless cats do not have neurologic deficits, and sacral and caudal deformities often are an incidental radiographic finding.

Spina Bifida

Etiology and Pathogenesis. Spina bifida is a term used to describe a group of developmental defects characterized by failure of fusion of the vertebral arches with or without protrusion or dysplasia of the spinal cord, meninges, or both. It has been described in both dogs and cats.[408–414] Malformations have been variously named spina bifida occulta, cystica, manifesta and operta, depending on whether vertebral arch only, vertebral arch and spinal cord, and/or meningeal abnormalities are present.

Anomalies of the vertebral arch and spinal cord are influenced by the development of the neural tube.

Normally an area of embryonic ectoderm thickens along the dorsal midline to form the neural plate. The neural plate subsequently folds (forming the neural groove and then the neural tube that separates from the ectoderm and develops into the spinal cord) and is surrounded by the sclerotomic masses that form the vertebrae.

Spina bifida is a midline cleft in one or more vertebral arches. The cleft may consist of only nonfusion of the dorsal spinous processes, or most of the vertebral arch of one or several adjacent vertebrae may be absent. The spinal cord and meninges may be normal (spina bifida occulta) or may be abnormal and there may be protrusion of the meninges and/or spinal cord through the vertebral defect. Spina bifida may be caused by nonfusion of the two halves of the primordial vertebral arch due to failure of the neural tube to close as the result of overgrowth of the cells of the neural tube,[415] or may be due to cleft formation in the neural tube after closure. It has been suggested that after formation of the neural tube, clefts split its dorsal wall and a neuroschistic bleb encroaches on the somites and prevents fusion of the vertebral arches.[416] If the neuroschistic bleb is retained, defects of the spinal cord occur. Healing of the bleb may also occur and result in spina bifida occulta (vertebral arch defect without concomitant spinal cord abnormalities).

Myelodysplasia consisting of hydromyelia, syringomyelia, anomalies of the dorsal septum, anomalies of the central gray matter, abnormal position of the central gray matter, anomalies of the dorsal and ventral horns, and myeloschisis (cleft in the dorsal part of the spinal cord) may occur in association with spina bifida. The most severe defects involve myelorachischisis, with superficial location of the neuroectoderm that is continuous with the skin. Myelorachischisis may be due to failure of the formation of the neural tube or rupture of the neuroschistic bleb after neural tube closure.[416] Spina bifida with myelorachischisis has been reported to occur in dogs and cats.[417, 418]

Etiology of spina bifida is unknown and probably multifactorial[419] with genetic and environmental components. Nutritional factors may have a role in the neural tube defects. Spina bifida can be induced in the offspring of laboratory animals by exposing pregnant females to a variety of chemical or environmental toxins.

Clinical Findings. Spina bifida is usually an incidental radiographic finding; however, if associated with spinal cord malformations, it may result in clinical signs of spinal cord or cauda equina dysfunction. Large dorsal arch defects are most often associated with spinal cord abnormalities. There is a high incidence of spina bifida in English bulldogs. Spina bifida may occur anywhere in the spinal column but occurs most commonly in the caudal lumbar spine where clinical signs are indicative of a transverse myelopathy from L4 to S3 spinal cord segments (pelvic limb ataxia or paresis, complete paraplegia, fecal and urinary incontinence, decreased or absent anal and urinary bladder sphincter tone, perineal analgesia, and decreased spinal reflexes in the pelvic limbs). Clinical signs usually become evident when affected animals start to walk.

Spina bifida also has been reported in the thoracic spine of a dog[408] and may be associated with other spinal deformities such as scoliosis. Other associated anomalies include dimpling of the skin or "streaming" (abnormal direction) of the hair coat over the affected region or a palpable abnormality in the spinal column. Meningoceles may cause necrosis of the overlying skin and drainage of CSF. Meningoceles may be present in the absence of clinical signs associated with spinal cord malformation.

Diagnosis. Absence of the vertebral arch or failure of fusion of the dorsal spinous processes in one or more vertebrae may be evident on plain radiographs (Figure 62–30). Myelography may demonstrate meningocele.

Treatment. Treatment is not effective for affected animals with clinical signs of spinal cord malformation. Meningocele may be amenable to surgery if neurologic abnormalities are not evident. Treatment is not necessary for animals with vertebral defects in the absence of spinal cord dysfunction (spina bifida occulta).

Spinal Arachnoid Cysts (Meningeal, Leptomeningeal Cysts)

Etiology and Pathogenesis. Spinal arachnoid cysts rarely have been reported in dogs or cats.[420–422] The pia and arachnoid membranes form the walls of these cysts and accumulation of CSF results in expansion of the overlying dura and compression of the spinal cord.

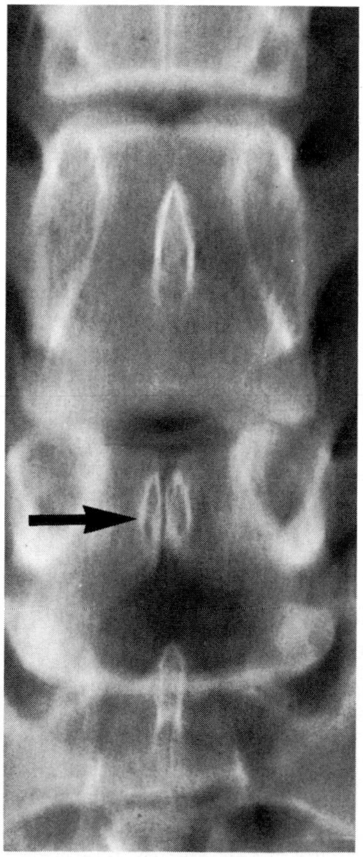

FIGURE 62–30. Spina bifida. Ventrodorsal radiograph of the caudal lumbar vertebral column of an eight-year-old spayed female chow. A deficit in fusion of the embryologic neural tube has resulted in nonfusion of the spinous process of L7 (arrow). This congenital defect was an incidental finding in this dog.

Arachnoid cysts are separated from the underlying spinal cord by an intact pia mater. Pathogenesis of arachnoid cysts is unknown. Evidence of inflammation or neoplasia has not been reported. Trauma resulting in arachnoid tears may be a factor in the formation of arachnoid cysts. Spinal arachnoid cyst formation was associated with a congenital vertebral anomaly (hemivertebrae) in one dog and vertebral instability causing increased stress on spinal cord and meninges was suggested as a possible cause.[420] Repeated trauma or chronic arachnoiditis was postulated as a cause in another dog that repeatedly pushed through heavy doors with its head.[422] A spinal arachnoid cyst was diagnosed in a dog less than one year of age by one of the authors. A congenital abnormality was considered to be the most likely cause in this dog.

Clinical Findings. In reported cases a single arachnoid cyst was found in either the cranial cervical or caudal thoracic spinal canal and neurologic deficits were indicative of a progressive transverse myelopathy in either the C1-C5 or T3-L3 spinal cord region. Apparent cervical pain and spasms of the cervical muscles were a feature of cervical lesions; however, apparent pain was not evident in dogs with thoracic lesions. Neurologic deficits may be asymmetrical.

Diagnosis. Diagnosis is made on the basis of myelographic, surgical, and histopathologic findings. Plain radiographs of the spine may be normal or may show enlargement of the vertebral canal with smooth cortical margins presumably as a result of pressure atrophy of bone overlying the cyst.[420] Abnormalities in CSF analysis have not been reported. Care should be taken in attempting a cisternal subarachnoid puncture in an animal suspected of having a cervical arachnoid cyst, as lesions usually are located on the dorsal midline. One reported dog was injured inadvertently during attempted cisternal puncture.[421]

Pooling of contrast material within the subarachnoid space, resulting in widening of the subarachnoid space and spinal cord compression, is seen on myelography (Figure 62–31). In all reported cases, lesions have been intradural-extramedullary and located on the dorsal midline. Lesions may extend over more than one spinal cord segment.

Treatment. Surgical exploration is necessary to confirm a diagnosis of subarachnoid cyst and to decompress the spinal cord. Complete surgical excision is not usually possible, as cysts are closely associated with the pia mater of the spinal cord. However, partial excision of a subarachnoid cyst has resulted in decompression of the spinal cord and clinical improvement without recurrence reported.[421, 422]

Spinal Nematodiasis

Etiology and Pathogenesis. Aberrant migration and growth of parasites within the spinal canal rarely occurs in dogs or cats. The route of migration of most parasites that enter the spinal canal is unknown. Parasites may cause extensive damage to neural parenchyma due to infarction, spinal cord compression, or granuloma formation. Parasites reported to occur in CNS of dogs include *Dirofilaria immitis, Toxocara canis* larvae, *Angiostrongylus cantonensis* (rat lungworm of Australia), and *Ancylostoma caninum* (Australia).[423–428]

Clinical Findings. Clinical signs depend on location of the lesions. Lesions may be focal or multifocal. Spinal nematodiasis usually is seen in immature animals, with the exception of *Dirofilaria immitis*. Clinical signs often have an acute onset and usually are progressive. Clinical signs rarely occur with aberrant *Toxocara* migration in dogs; however, a single *Toxocara* larva has been found in the cauda equina of a dog.[425] Clinical signs reported associated with *Angiostrongylus cantonensis* in the dog include paraparesis, paraplegia, urinary and fecal incontinence, paralysis of the tail, and apparent pain.[427] *Ancylostoma caninum* migration in the spinal cord has been reported to result in paraparesis, apparent neck pain, and tetraplegia.[426] Adult *Dirofilaria immitis* have been found in the spinal epidural space and subarachnoid space in dogs.[423, 424] Acute onset of paraplegia has been described in two dogs associated with *Dirofilaria immitis* migration in the thoracolumbar spinal cord.[423, 424] Acute onset of clinical signs was seen in one animal despite a chronic granulomatous reaction in the spinal cord. Whether aberrant migration of an adult worm or migration of a larval form with subsequent maturation occurs is not known.

Diagnosis. Definite diagnosis is difficult ante mortem as it requires isolation or demonstration of the parasite within the CNS.

An increase in white blood cell count, especially eosinophils, and/or protein may be present in the CSF. Affected animals usually have a large parasite burden and nematode eggs or larvae may be found in the feces. Dogs with *Dirofilaria immitis* infestation may have circulating microfilaria. Lesions may be located by means of myelography.

Treatment. Prognosis for animals with spinal nematodiasis depends on the severity of neurologic deficits that result and usually is poor. Medical therapy often is ineffective in eliminating parasites in the CNS. Surgical removal of *Dirofilaria immitis* adults from the spinal epidural space has been reported.[424]

Spinal Cord Trauma

Etiology and Pathogenesis. Acute spinal cord injuries of dogs or cats result most commonly from direct physical trauma such as missile injury or vertebral fracture or luxation. Also, spinal cord trauma is the underlying cause of neurologic signs in numerous myelopathies (e.g., intervertebral disk protrusion or extrusion). Chronic spinal cord compression usually is seen in association with chronic progressive diseases such as neoplasia or type II disk protrusion.[429]

Following injury, the spinal cord may undergo sustained compression, distraction, or both.[238] The severity of a spinal cord injury, as determined by the eventual degree and quality of recovery, is related to three factors: the velocity with which the compressive force is applied, the degree of compression (transverse deformation), and the duration of the compression.[238] The

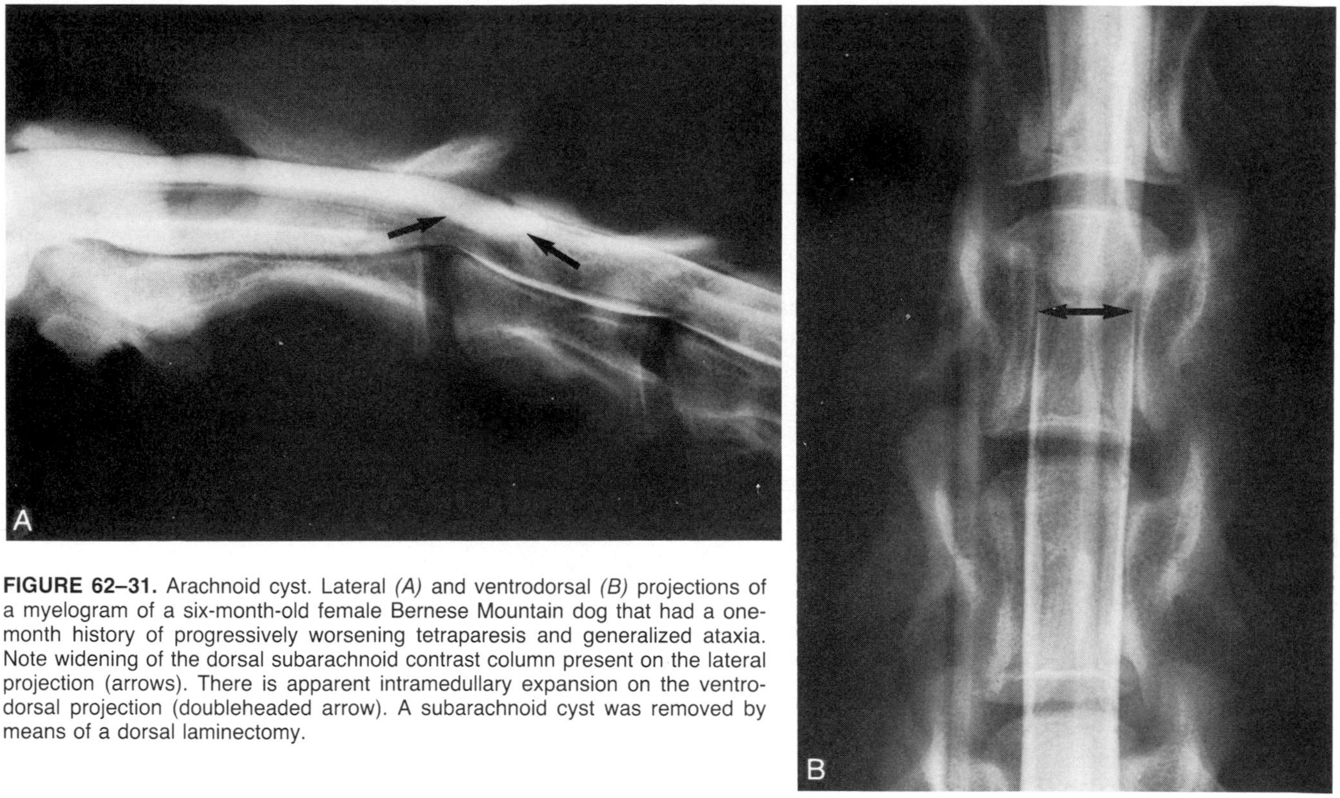

FIGURE 62–31. Arachnoid cyst. Lateral *(A)* and ventrodorsal *(B)* projections of a myelogram of a six-month-old female Bernese Mountain dog that had a one-month history of progressively worsening tetraparesis and generalized ataxia. Note widening of the dorsal subarachnoid contrast column present on the lateral projection (arrows). There is apparent intramedullary expansion on the ventrodorsal projection (doubleheaded arrow). A subarachnoid cyst was removed by means of a dorsal laminectomy.

relative roles of these factors in determining the severity of a spinal cord injury have yet to be determined.

An understanding of differences between acute and chronic spinal cord injury is essential for effective management and determination of prognosis in cats or dogs with spinal trauma. Extensive experimental work has been done in order to elucidate the mechanisms involved in the production of lesions following spinal cord trauma, and results of such research provide information that is essential for effective therapy of spinal injuries.[430]

ACUTE SPINAL CORD INJURY. It has long been recognized that blunt traumatic injury to the spinal cord causes neurologic deficits through both direct and indirect mechanisms.[431, 432] The direct effects are due to immediate disruption of neural pathways in spinal gray or white matter produced by the trauma. These effects have also been termed "immediate" effects and have been considered by most investigators not to be amenable to therapy.[431] Indirect effects develop during the first few hours following injury, and result in delayed secondary injury to the spinal cord. The mechanisms of this secondary process remain largely undetermined; however, it is likely that they result in part from release of endogenous pathophysiologic "factors" in response to the initial trauma. It has been hypothesized that such "factors" produce injury by reducing spinal cord blood flow or by altering the local metabolic environment within injured spinal cord tissue.[431] The secondary damage has been considered potentially reversible through the use of either physical (e.g., hypothermia) or pharmacologic interventions.[431, 432]

Trauma to the spinal cord triggers a progressive series of autodestructive events that lead to varying degrees of tissue necrosis depending on the severity of the injury.[432] Pathologic changes that occur in traumatized spinal cord tissue include petechial hemorrhages that progress to hemorrhagic necrosis, lipid peroxidation, lipid hydroxylation with subsequent prostaglandin and leukotriene (eicosanoid) formation, loss of calcium ions from the extracellular space and loss of potassium ions from the intracellular space, ischemia with consequent decline in tissue oxygen tension and energy metabolites and development of lactic acidosis, and inflammation and neuronophagia by PMN leukocytes.

In spite of extensive investigation, the mechanisms responsible for the initiation and propagation of these pathophysiologic and biochemical events remain undetected. Recent evidence suggests, however, that the overall initiator of this autodestructive cascade of events is mechanical deformation of any type (i.e., impact or compression injury), and that the primary sites of injury are the cellular and subcellular membranes of glia, neurons, and vascular endothelial cells. Lipid peroxidation and activation of membrane lipases, with release of fatty acids leading to production of eicosanoids, are the earliest mechanically stimulated biochemical events described at the present time.[433]

The sequence of pathologic alterations that occurs following spinal cord injury has been reviewed by several authors.[434–436] Within five minutes of injury postcapillary venules become congested. This is followed by opening of endothelial gap junctions here and at the capillary level, resulting in diapedesis of red blood cells and extravasation of fluid proteins and electrolytes through the "leaky" vasculature. Within 30 minutes of injury, microscopic hemorrhages appear in the central gray matter, and coalesce over the following several hours (central hemorrhagic necrosis) (Figure 62–32). Vacuolization develops within endothelial cells, indicating a profound ischemic or hypoxic insult, that subsequently leads to coagulative necrosis of the neuronal population. Adjacent white matter is relatively less severely affected; however, periaxonal swelling and retraction balls may be observed. These events may lead to autodissolution of the spinal cord within 24 hours, even in the absence of ongoing mechanical compression.

A special feature of spinal cord injury is progressive hemorrhagic myelomalacia. This condition occurs following spinal cord trauma and appears to be a progression of central hemorrhagic necrosis and edema to areas of the spinal cord not directly involved in the initiating injury.

Chronic spinal cord compression. It has been shown experimentally that when slow compression of the spinal cord is compared to dynamic (or rapid) compression of an equal amount, the extent of spinal cord dysfunction is determined by the contact velocity of compression.[437] The major pathologic substrate for neural dysfunction after slow balloon compression is thought to be physical injury to the neural membranes, irrespective of blood flow changes, and the ability of that membrane to recover appears to be related to rapidity and duration of compression.[437, 438] Clinical observations support the conclusion that spinal cord conduction is resistant to slow compression. Further, it has been demonstrated that levels of compression that do not have an effect when applied slowly cause an immediate loss of conduction through the injured site when applied rapidly.[437, 438]

Chronic spinal cord compression results either from a slowly developing lesion (e.g., neoplasia), or from an acute compression that is sustained.[439] In contrast to acute spinal cord injury, chronic compression affects white matter more severely than it affects gray matter. Hemorrhage and edema, the major findings of acute trauma, are not significant in chronic compression.[439] Characteristic lesions are degeneration of myelin, focal areas of malacia, vacuolization, and loss of white matter axons. Mechanical deformation is likely to be the major factor in pathogenesis of these lesions; however, ischemia and venous obstruction also may be important considerations.[439]

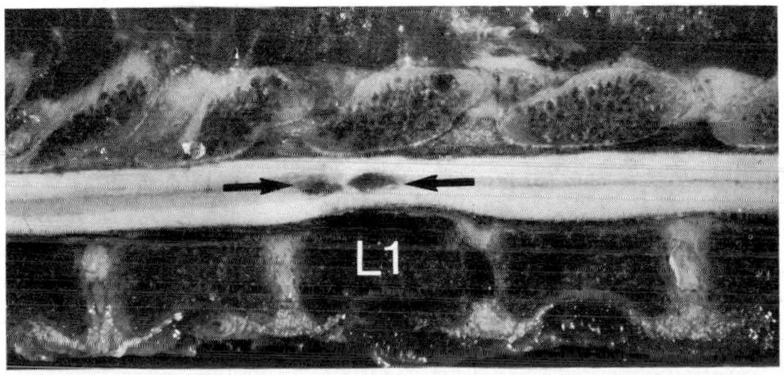

FIGURE 62–32. Central hemorrhagic necrosis. Midsagittal view of a gross necropsy specimen of the vertebral column of a one-year-old male Shih Tzu dog that sustained a compression fracture of L1 vertebra. Note the central hemorrhagic necrosis within the spinal cord gray matter (arrows).

Clinical Findings

Acute spinal cord injury. Dogs or cats with a spinal injury frequently have serious injuries to other organ systems. A primary concern is to balance the relative urgency of non-neurologic injuries (hemorrhage, shock, airway obstruction, or limb fractures) and the need for early treatment of spinal cord injury.[429]

A complete neurologic examination is done to localize the site(s) of injury, and to determine severity. Careful palpation of the vertebral column may aid in identification of a vertebral fracture or luxation. Administration of tranquilizers or analgesic drugs should be delayed until completion of the neurologic examination, as such medications may alter an animal's responses. A neurologic examination should be done with care to prevent further injury resulting from excessive movement of a vertebral instability.

Several aspects of the neurologic examination are of special importance in assessment of a dog or cat with a spinal cord injury. Recognition of the Schiff-Sherrington sign is important. Following trauma, this sign must be differentiated from other postures associated with cranial injury (e.g., decerebrate rigidity or decerebellate posture). Both deep and cutaneous pain perception should be assessed, as results of these tests are important in determining prognosis. It should be remembered that vertebral column injuries may be multiple, and that a neurologic examination may not indicate presence of a second lesion.[429]

Chronic spinal cord compression. Clinical signs of chronic spinal cord compression may progress over weeks or months, or may be seen to occur acutely. Acute onset of neurologic signs with chronic spinal cord compression frequently is seen in association with such disorders as spinal neoplasia or type II disk protrusion. Sudden onset of signs may accompany pathologic fracture of a vertebra, and spinal cord hemorrhage or infarction. In some cases sudden decompensation of chronically compressed spinal cord may occur in the absence of pathologic changes. In these cases it is assumed that compensatory mechanisms within the spinal cord are exhausted, and that sudden decompensation has occurred.[439]

Diagnosis

Acute spinal cord injury. Results of a neurologic examination are used to determine the site and severity of a spinal injury. Radiographs of the entire spinal column should be done. Two radiographic views are essential. Ventrodorsal views may be accomplished by means of a horizontal beam. Evoked spinal cord potential testing may be of use in determining location and severity of a spinal cord lesion in animals following trauma.

The objectives of radiographic examination of an animal following acute spinal trauma are the following: precise determination of location and extent of a lesion, demonstration of multiple lesions that may not be apparent on the basis of a neurologic examination, and assessment of the need for surgical therapy and determination of the most appropriate surgical procedure to be used.[238, 429] Accurate interpretation of radiographs depends on a knowledge of results of a neurologic examination.

It is recommended by these authors that a myelogram be completed in animals that have sustained spinal trauma. Results of a myelogram may determine the extent of spinal cord swelling resulting from concussion in animals without evidence of a spinal fracture or luxation, and may confirm that surgical decompression by means of laminectomy is not necessary in animals with a fracture that is evident on plain radiographs. In the diagnosis of intervertebral disk disease a myelogram is considered essential prior to surgery.

Chronic spinal cord compression. Methods for diagnosis of chronic spinal cord compression are the same as for acute spinal cord injury. A myelogram is considered essential in all such cases.[429]

Treatment. Management of an animal with spinal trauma follows a list of priorities, with the focus of treatment being prevention of secondary spinal cord damage that occurs after the initial injury.[429] Immediate treatment of non-neural injuries is limited to those problems that are life-threatening, such as shock or hemorrhage.

Acute spinal cord injury. Treatment of acute spinal cord trauma should always be instituted as soon as possible following injury. The specific objectives of therapy are the following: relief of edema, control of intra- or extramedullary hemorrhage, relief of spinal cord compression, and, in cases of vertebral fracture/luxation, removal of bone fragments from the spinal canal and stabilization of the vertebral column.[429] Treatment of acute spinal cord trauma may be medical, surgical, or a combination of both.

Based on experimental findings in a large number of experimental models in animals, a variety of medical treatments have been advocated for the treatment of acute spinal cord injury. Such treatments have been reviewed by several authors.[430, 432, 433, 435] Recently, interest has focused on the use of antioxidants and free radical scavengers. Unfortunately, the role of these numerous therapies in the management of a dog or cat with a spinal injury remains to be determined. The large number of suggested therapies underlines the fact that the mechanisms responsible for delayed secondary effects in the injured spinal cord are incompletely understood.

Corticosteroids are routinely and widely used in the treatment of acute spinal cord injury. Despite a positive clinical impression that corticosteroids have beneficial effects, their use is controversial.[432, 440, 441] Some studies have failed to demonstrate significant improvement of neurologic recovery in association with corticosteroid administration. The use of low or high doses of corticosteroids in the treatment of spinal trauma also has yielded conflicting results.

Use of high doses of corticosteroids may result in complications leading to increased morbidity and mortality (e.g., gastrointestinal bleeding, pancreatitis, colonic perforation); therefore, low dose regimens are recommended. Dexamethasone sodium phosphate should be given at an initial dosage of 0.25 to 1 mg/lb IV, and may be repeated at a dose of 0.1 mg/lb q6h or q8h. Immediate post-trauma administration of methylprednisolone sodium succinate (60 mg/lb divided q8h) has been demonstrated to be effective in preserving feline spinal cord tissue following injury.[440, 441]

A decision regarding surgical therapy must be made as soon as non-neural injuries have been treated and medical management has been instituted.[429] Ideally, this is within two hours of injury. Indications for surgery following spinal cord injury are the following: moderate to severe paresis, or paralysis, associated with myelographic evidence of spinal cord compression; progressive worsening of neurologic signs despite adequate medical therapy; and luxation or fracture of the vertebral column, in association with distraction, malalignment, instability, or myelographic evidence of spinal cord compression. Any animal with sustained compression of the spinal cord following injury, regardless of the cause, must be considered a candidate for surgical decompression of the spinal cord. In general, it is best to initiate surgical therapy in any animal in which there is uncertainty regarding the indications for surgical versus medical therapy. Neurosurgical procedures require specialized knowledge and equipment, and prompt referral to a qualified surgeon may be indicated.

The major objectives of surgical management of spinal trauma are decompression of sustained spinal cord compression and realignment and stabilization of vertebrae if necessary.[429] Surgical decompression by means of laminectomy is beneficial when there is myelographic evidence of extradural spinal cord compression. Laminectomy alone is not sufficient for decompression in most cases, and the compressing mass (e.g., disk material, hematoma, bone fragments) should be removed where possible. In cases where spinal cord swelling is the major source of compression, or where there is discoloration of the spinal cord, durotomy or myelotomy may be combined with laminectomy.

The most effective methods for alignment and stabilization of the vertebral column require surgical exposure, and can therefore be done at the time of decompression. Satisfactory methods of external fixation of spinal fractures do not exist. Methods of surgical fixation have been reviewed by several authors.[6, 442] Use of polymethyl methacrylate and Steinmann pin fixation for the majority of spinal fractures or luxations is favored by these authors.[443] Surgical management of spinal cord injury of animals provides the best opportunity for rapid and complete recovery in animals with sustained compression or instability, and facilitates postinjury care, as the risk of further injury resulting from movement of an unstable vertebral column is minimized. However, conservative management, including strict confinement for four to six weeks, may be efficacious in animals with minimal neurologic deficits and without myelographic evidence of sustained spinal cord compression or vertebral displacement or instability.

Regardless of the type of stabilization used, strict confinement is recommended for two weeks after surgery. Potential complications encountered in dogs or cats with a spinal injury include development of a urinary tract infection or pressure sores. Careful attention to nursing care is essential regardless of the type of therapy.

Prognosis for an animal with an acute spinal cord

injury depends on numerous factors; however, results of a neurologic examination should be the main determinant. Assessment of pain perception is essential for accurate prognosis. Perception of a painful stimulus must be differentiated from reflex activity that is mediated at the level of the spinal cord. Owners of affected animals should be made aware at the outset of therapy of factors such as prognosis, expense involved, expected time from treatment to recovery, and the need for prolonged physical therapy in most cases. Following a severe spinal injury, an animal may require many months to recover, and residual neurologic deficits may persist.

Chronic spinal cord compression. The approach to treatment of chronic spinal cord compression is different from that for acute spinal cord injury. As previously stated, hemorrhage and edema usually are not prominent factors in chronic compression. Therefore medical management by means of corticosteroids would not be expected to be efficacious; however, many animals with chronic spinal cord compression improve clinically following corticosteroid administration. The reason for such a response is undetermined; however, it may be due to effects of corticosteroids at the membrane level resulting in improved conduction in remaining axons.[4] Occasionally, animals may be maintained for months or years by means of corticosteroid therapy alone.

Surgical decompression of the spinal cord should be approached with caution in animals with chronic spinal cord compression. Pathologic alterations within the spinal cord may be irreversible, in which case the most that may be achieved is to arrest progression of neurologic deficits. In some cases compensation for the irreplaceable loss of neural tissue may occur.[439] Neurologic status may be worsened by surgical decompression, even with meticulous surgical technique.[4] Such deterioration may be the result of reactive hyperemia that follows decompression, which in turn results in vascular protein leakage in the affected spinal cord segment.[270] However, surgical decompression should be considered in most animals that have neurologic deficits associated with chronic spinal cord compression.

Spondylosis Deformans

Etiology and Pathogenesis. Spondylosis deformans is characterized by the formation of osteophytes (bony spurs) around the margins of vertebral endplates. Osteophytes may form at one or multiple intervertebral disk spaces and may appear to bridge or almost bridge intervertebral disk spaces. Bony ankylosis between adjacent osteophytes was not a frequent finding in one study.[444] The radiographic appearance of solid bony bridges may represent only an interdigitation of the adjacent osteophytes.[444] Changes in the intervertebral disks have been found to be important in the pathogenesis of spondylosis deformans. Osteophyte production in spondylosis deformans is the noninflammatory bony response to degenerative changes in the intervertebral disks. These degenerative changes involve the anulus fibrosus and lead to the formation of intradiskal fissures.[444]

The incidence and size of vertebral osteophytes increases with age. All breeds of dog are affected, although large canine breeds may have a higher incidence of spondylosis deformans. The caudal thoracic, lumbar, and lumbosacral spinal segments are affected most frequently. As these segments are areas of greatest spinal mobility, dynamic and mechanical factors may play a role in osteophyte formation.[6, 444] Spondylosis deformans is uncommon in the cervical and cranial thoracic segments in dogs. In cats, the incidence of spondylosis deformans forms a bell-shaped curve with the highest incidence at the level of T7-T8.[445]

Spondylosis deformans has also been called ankylosing spondylosis or ankylosing spondylitis, although it is not an inflammatory condition and ankylosis is uncommon.

Clinical Findings. In most affected animals, spondylosis deformans is not of clinical significance. Rarely, bony spurs may project into the spinal canal or intervertebral foramina, resulting in compression of spinal cord or spinal nerves. In such affected animals clinical signs depend on the location of the lesion, and include apparent spinal pain, lameness, and signs of transverse myelopathy or peripheral neuropathy. Other causes of spinal cord disease, peripheral nerve disease, and apparent spinal pain should be investigated and ruled out before attributing an animal's clinical signs to spondylosis deformans. Localized pain or lameness is reported to occur in animals with fracture of vertebral osteophytes.[6]

Diagnosis. A diagnosis of spondylosis deformans is based on results of radiographs of the spine (Figure 62–33). Bony osteophytes associated with spondylosis deformans may be seen at one or multiple intervertebral disk spaces ventral to the vertebral bodies on lateral projections and lateral to the vertebral bodies on dorsoventral views. These osteophytes have a curved, "beak-like" appearance with smooth ventral and lateral borders. Osteophytes range in size from small bony spurs to those that equal the dorsoventral dimensions of the vertebral body. Spurs from adjacent vertebrae may interdigitate.[4] Osteophytes form predominantly around the ventral and lateral margins of the vertebral endplates and those apparent on lateral radiographs appear to be projecting dorsally into the spinal canal. Such osteophytes generally are located lateral to the spinal canal.[4] Extensive osteophyte production dorsolateral to the vertebral body may compress spinal nerves at the level of the intervertebral foramina.

Bone may form in the mass of connective tissue formed between developing osteophytes and remain unattached to the vertebral bodies. These apparently free bone fragments are usually seen ventral to the intervertebral disk and may eventually become incorporated into developing osteophytes. These bone fragments may appear radiographically to be fractured osteophytes, but in fact they are not formed as a result of trauma.[446]

Vertebral osteophytes may occur at disk spaces that are of normal or narrowed width. Dorsally or dorsolaterally projecting osteophytes need to be distinguished

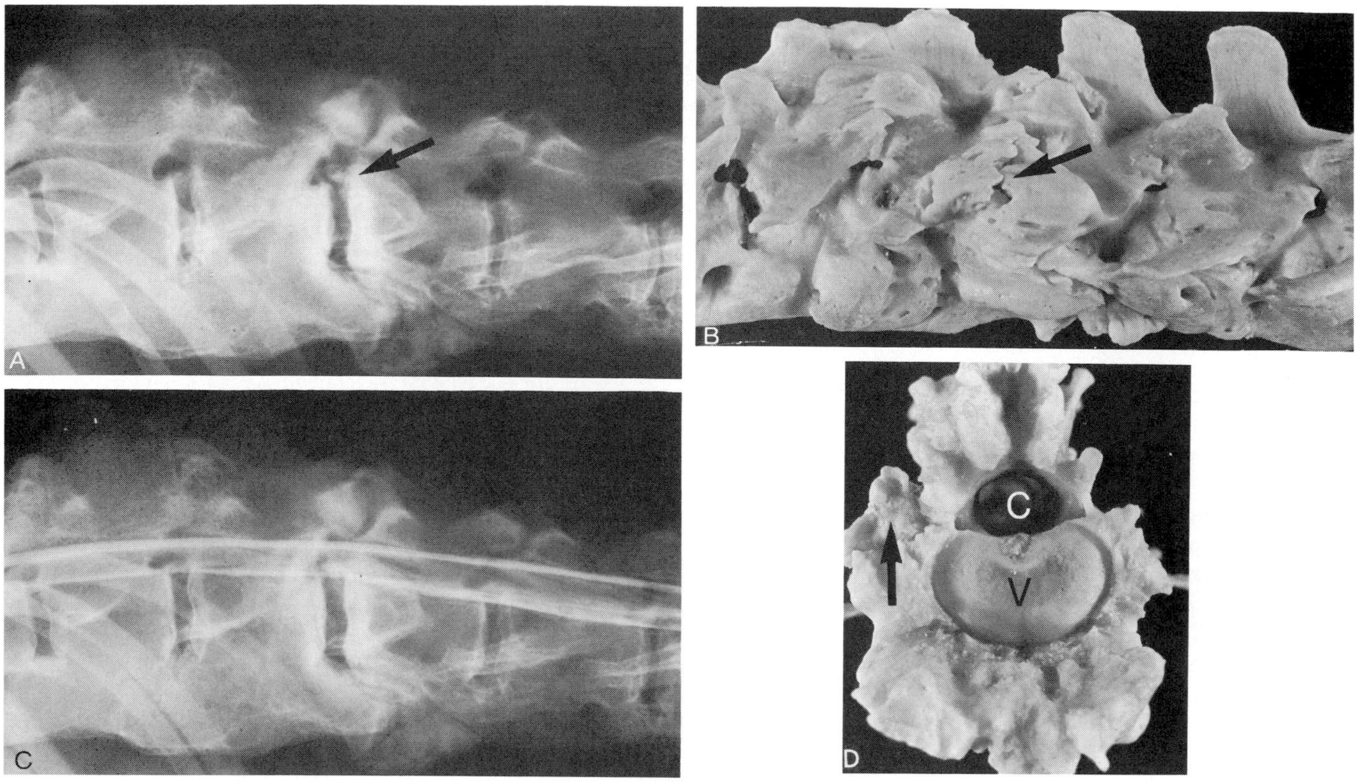

FIGURE 62–33. Spondylosis deformans. Lateral radiograph *(A)*, lateral myelogram *(B)*, and gross pathologic specimen *(C)* of the cranial lumbar vertebral column of a 12-year-old male golden retriever dog. Note the extensive spondylosis deformans that is present in the absence of disk narrowing or myelographic abnormalities. Osteophytes (arrow) may appear to project into the spinal canal on the lateral view; however, these are actually dorsolateral and do not result in spinal cord compression. The typical location of osteophytes is seen in *D*, where the spinal canal (C) of the L2 vertebra (V) is not encroached upon by the ventrally and laterally located osteophytes. The arrow in *D* indicates osteophytes located in close proximity to the intervertebral foramen. This dog was neurologically normal.

from calcified disk material on lateral radiographs.[4] Vertebral osteophytes may also form as a result of instability between adjacent vertebrae due to vertebral fracture or luxation, diskospondylitis, congenital vertebral malformations, and surgery such as disk fenestration. However, the term spondylosis deformans is used specifically to define the formation of vertebral osteophytes secondary to disk degeneration.[4] Disk protrusion may occur at the same site as spondylosis deformans resulting in spinal cord compression. Myelography is necessary to determine whether disk protrusion or dorsal vertebral osteophyte formation is causing spinal cord compression.

Treatment. Spondylosis deformans rarely results in spinal cord compression. However, if spinal cord compression or nerve root entrapment is indicated on a myelogram of an animal with neurologic deficits, surgical decompression may result in clinical improvement. Removal of dorsally projecting osteophytes should not be attempted. As in animals with chronic type II disk protrusion, worsening of neurologic signs may occur after spinal cord decompression despite very careful surgical technique. Analgesics may be of benefit in animals with evidence of pain suspected to be the result of spinal nerve compression by vertebral osteophyte production. In most animals, spondylosis deformans is not of clinical significance and treatment is not necessary.

Syringomyelia and Hydromyelia

Etiology and Pathogenesis. A distinction cannot be made clinically between syringomyelia (cavitation of the spinal cord) and hydromyelia (dilation of the central canal). Syringomyelia may occur secondary to hydromyelia (communicating syringomyelia) or may not communicate with the central canal (noncommunicating syringomyelia). Syringomyelia may be associated with spinal cord tumors, myelitis, meningitis, and spinal cord trauma.[322] The cause of syringomyelia is not known but the condition may result from venous obstruction or distention, or may be due to mechanical disruption or shearing of spinal cord tissue planes.

Hydromyelia with or without syringomyelia may be associated with congenital malformations such as myelodysplasia; meningomyelocele or hydrocephalus; or lesions resulting in obstruction of CSF flow into the spinal subarachnoid space at the foramen magnum such as chronic arachnoiditis, trauma, congenital malformations, and vascular malformations; or it may be idiopathic.[8, 322, 408, 447, 448] Hydromyelia and syringomyelia in these animals probably results from intracranial and spinal cord venous[449] or arterial[450] pressure changes and associated CSF pressure changes.

Syringomyelia in Weimaraner dogs with myelodysplasia may be the result of progressive hydromyelia, abnormalities in the central canal, or abnormal vascular patterns in local areas of the spinal cord leading to low-grade ischemia, degeneration, rarefaction, and cavitation in the spinal cord.[322]

Regardless of the cause, cavitation can be progressive, probably along planes of structural weakness such as the gray matter of the dorsal horns, and subsequent necrosis and edema of spinal cord parenchyma around such a cavitation (or dilated central canal) can result in the onset and progression of clinical signs.

Clinical Findings. Clinical signs depend on the location of the lesion and whether or not other spinal cord lesions are present. Clinical findings include progressive spinal deformity (scoliosis, torticollis) (Figure 62–34) LMN or UMN signs, depending on location, and apparent spinal pain. Clinical signs may be acute or may be progressive over weeks to several years.[448] In Weimaraner dogs with myelodysplasia, clinical signs do not appear to be progressive.[322]

Diagnosis. Myelography may show obstruction of the flow of CSF at the foramen magnum if hydromyelia or syringomyelia is due to chronic arachnoiditis or arachnoid adhesions. Cisternal puncture for the collection of CSF is contraindicated in these animals due to likely inadvertent puncture of the spinal cord. Lumbar CSF may show evidence of chronic inflammation. Myelography in other cases may be normal or may show intramedullary swelling of the spinal cord. Computed tomography of the spinal cord may be useful in the diagnosis of cavitary lesions of the spinal cord.

Treatment. Treatment in dogs has not been reported. Surgical drainage of cavitary lesions in humans has resulted in improvement in some cases.

Vascular Malformations and Benign Vascular Tumors

Etiology and Pathogenesis. Spinal arteriovenous malformations and benign vascular tumors (hemangioma, cavernous angioma) have been reported to occur in dogs.[451, 452] Arteriovenous malformations consist of one or more anomalous arteries arising from radicular arteries that drain without a capillary bed into one or more veins communicating with veins on the surface of the spinal cord, resulting in the formation of tangles of tortuous distended vessels on or within the spinal cord. These malformations may be extramedullary, intramedullary, or both. Hemangioma is regarded as a benign neoplasm of endothelium that consists of discrete masses of tangled capillaries with or without cavernous or solid areas.[451] Multiple hemangiomas may occur and are predominantly extramedullary, but may be intramedullary. These tumors may arise from the meninges.

Clinical Findings. An arteriovenous malformation has been reported in a dog less than one year of age.[451] Hemangioma has been reported in two dogs (six and seven years of age)[451] and a cavernous angioma has been reported in a four-month-old dog.[452] Arteriovenous malformations and vascular tumors may occur anywhere in the spinal canal and clinical signs usually reflect a progressive transverse myelopathy. An acute onset or sudden worsening of clinical signs may occur due to hemorrhage or thrombosis associated with abnormal vasculature of the malformation or tumor. Clinical signs may be the result of spinal cord compression or ischemia.

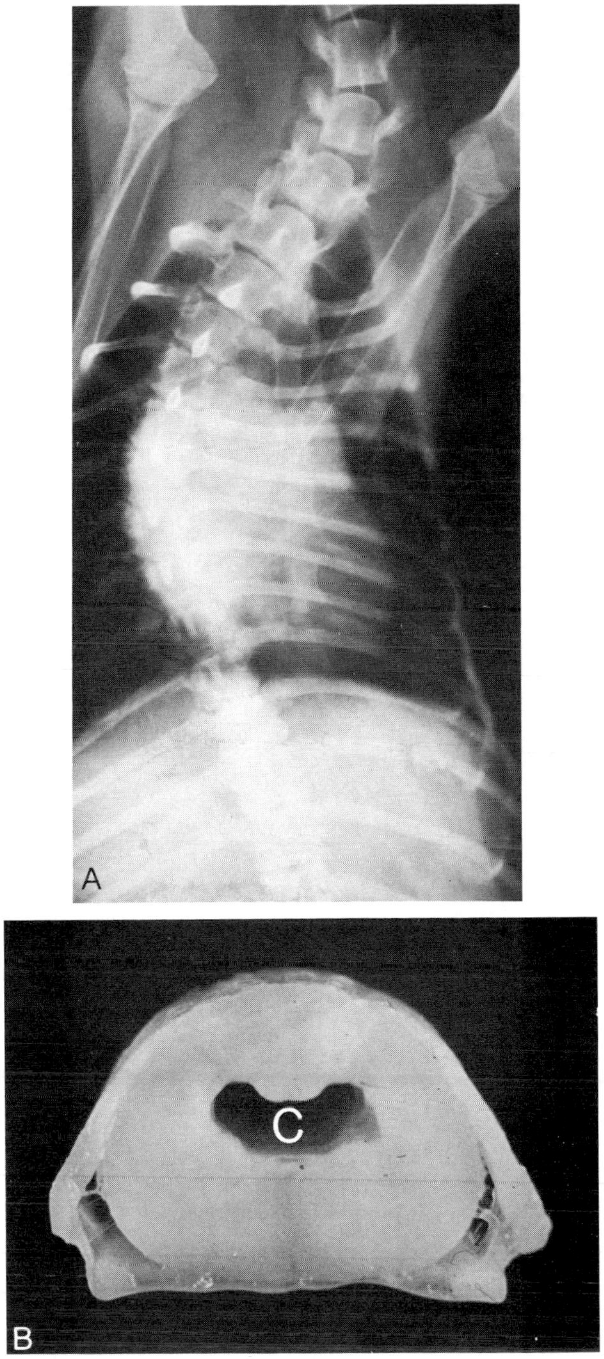

FIGURE 62–34. Scoliosis and hydromyelia. Ventrodorsal radiograph *(A)* of the caudal cervical and thoracic vertebral column of a one-year-old female beagle. Note the scoliosis of the vertebral column. The spinal cord throughout the region of scoliosis *(B)* had an enlarged central canal (C) consistent with a diagnosis of hydromyelia.

Diagnosis. Cerebrospinal fluid may be normal or may have an elevated protein concentration. Cerebrospinal fluid may be xanthochromic and the white blood cell count may be mildly elevated if subarachnoid hemorrhage has occurred or a meningeal inflammatory response is associated with tumor growth.

Myelography may show evidence of an intradural or intramedullary mass. Surgical biopsy is necessary to distinguish these lesions from other neoplasms, subarachnoid cysts, and other intradural and intramedullary lesions.

Treatment. Surgical removal of a vascular malformation or vascular tumor may be possible.

References

1. LeCouteur, RA: Tetraparesis. *In* Ford, RB (ed): Clinical Signs and Diagnosis in Small Animal Practice. New York, Churchill Livingstone, 1988, p 316.
2. Morris, JH and Schoene, WC: The nervous system. *In* Robbins, SL, et al. (eds): Pathologic Basis of Disease. Philadelphia, WB Saunders, 1984, p 1370.
3. Kornegay, JN: Pathogenesis of diseases of the central nervous system. *In* Slatter, DH (ed): Textbook of Small Animal Surgery. Philadelphia, WB Saunders, 1985, p 1266.
4. Bailey, CS and Morgan, JP: Diseases of the spinal cord. *In* Ettinger, SJ (ed): Textbook of Veterinary Internal Medicine, 2nd ed. Philadelphia, WB Saunders, 1983.
5. Oliver, JE Jr and Lorenz, MD: Handbook of Veterinary Neurologic Diagnosis. Philadelphia, WB Saunders, 1983.
6. Oliver, JE Jr, et al.: Veterinary Neurology. Philadelphia, WB Saunders, 1987.
7. Luttgen, PJ: Paraplegia. *In* Ford, RB (ed): Clinical Signs and Diagnosis in Small Animal Practice. New York, Churchill Livingstone, 1988, p 295.
8. deLahunta, A: Veterinary Neuroanatomy and Clinical Neurology, 2nd ed. Philadelphia, WB Saunders, 1983.
9. Kornegay, JN: Management of animals with neurologic disease. *In* Kornegay, JN (ed): Neurologic Disorders, Contemporary Issues in Small Animal Practice, vol 5. New York, Churchill Livingstone, 1986, p 1.
10. Braund, KG: Clinical Syndromes in Veterinary Neurology. Baltimore, Williams and Wilkins, 1986.
11. Chrisman, CL: Problems in Small Animal Neurology. Philadelphia, Lea and Febiger, 1982.
12. Walker, MA: The vertebrae. *In* Thrall, DE (ed): Textbook of Veterinary Diagnostic Radiology. Philadelphia, WB Saunders, 1986, p 41.
13. Bartels, JE: Intervertebral disk disease. *In* Thrall, DE (ed): Textbook of Veterinary Diagnostic Radiology. Philadelphia, WB Saunders, 1986, p 51.
14. Vandevelde, M and Fankhauser, R: Ein Fuhrung in die veterinarmedizinische Neurologie. Berlin, Verlag Paul Parey, 1987.
15. Cook, JR and DeNicola, DB: Cerebrospinal Fluid. Vet Clin North Am 18:475, 1988.
16. Mayhew, IG and Beal, CR: Techniques of analysis of cerebrospinal fluid. Vet Clin North Am 10:155, 1980.
17. Roszel, JF: Membrane filtration of canine and feline cerebrospinal fluid for cytologic evaluation. JAVMA 160:720, 1972.
18. Bailey, CS and Higgins, RJ: Comparison of total white blood cell count and total protein content of lumbar and cisternal cerebrospinal fluid of healthy dogs. Am J Vet Res 46:1162, 1985.
19. Farnbach, GC: Clinical electrophysiology in veterinary medicine. Part I: Electromyography. Comp Cont Ed 11:791, 1980.
20. Chrisman, CL: Electromyography in the localization of spinal cord and nerve root neoplasia in dogs and cats. JAVMA 166:1074, 1975.
21. Bailey, CS: Clinical evaluation of the cutaneous innervation of the canine thoracic limb. JAAHA 20:939, 1984.
22. Bailey, CS, et al.: Spinal nerve root origins of the cutaneous nerves of the canine pelvic limb. Am J Vet Res 49:115, 1988.
23. Bailey, CS and Kitchell, RL: Cutaneous sensory testing in the dog. J Vet Int Med 1:128, 1987.
24. Farnbach, GC: Clinical electrophysiology in veterinary neurology. Part II: Peripheral nerve testing. Comp Cont Ed 11:843, 1980.
25. Holliday, TA, et al.: Percutaneous recording of evoked spinal cord potentials of dogs. Am J Vet Res 40:326, 1979.
26. Shores, A, et al.: Spinal-evoked potentials in dogs with acute compressive thoracolumbar spinal cord disease. Am J Vet Res 48:1525, 1987.
27. Geary, JC: Veterinary tomography. J Am Vet Radiol Soc 8:32, 1967.
28. Barber, DL: Imaging: radiography—II. Vet Radiol 22:149, 1981.
29. Roberts, TDM: Neurophysiology of Postural Mechanisms. New York, Plenum Press, 1967.
30. McCouch, GP, et al.: Sprouting as a cause of spasticity. J Neurophysiol 21:205, 1958.
31. Cannon, WB and Rosenbleuth, A: The Supersensitivity of Denervated Structures. New York, Macmillan, 1949.
32. Denny-Brown, D: The cerebral control of movement. The Sherrington Lectures VIII. Springfield, Charles C Thomas, 1966.
33. Sherrington, CS: The integrative action of the nervous system, 2nd ed. New Haven, Yale University Press, 1947.
34. Evans, HE and Christensen, GC: Miller's Anatomy of the Dog, 2nd ed. Philadelphia, WB Saunders, 1979.
35. Bailey, CS, et al.: Cutaneous innervation of the thorax and abdomen of the dog. Am J Vet Res 45:1689, 1984.
36. Oliver, JE and Lewis, RE: Lesions of the atlas and axis in dogs. JAAHA 9:304, 1973.
37. Geary, JC, et al.: Atlanto-axial subluxation in the canine. J Small Anim Pract 8:577, 1967.
38. Hare, WCD: Radiographic anatomy of the cervical region of the canine vertebral column. Part II. Developing vertebrae. JAVMA 139:217, 1961.
39. Cook, JR and Oliver, JE: Atlantoaxial luxation in the dog. Comp Cont Ed 3:242, 1981.
40. Ladds, P, et al.: Congenital odontoid process separation in two dogs. J Small Anim Pract 12:463, 1970.
41. Zaki, FA: Odontoid process dysplasia in a dog. J Small Anim Pract 21:277, 1980.
42. Parker, AJ, et al.: Abnormal odontoid process angulation in a dog. Vet Rec 93:559, 1973.
43. Swaim, SF and Greene, CE: Odontoidectomy in a dog. JAAHA 11:663, 1975.
44. Richter, K, et al.: Traumatic displacement of the dens in a cat: Case report. JAAHA 19:751, 1983.
45. Greenwood, KM and Oliver, JE: Traumatic atlanto-occipital dislocation in two dogs. JAVMA 173:1324, 1978.
46. Crane, SW: Surgical management of traumatic atlanto-occipital instability in a dog. Vet Surg 7:39, 1978.
47. Bailey, CS and Holliday, TA: Diseases of the spinal cord. *In* Ettinger, SJ (ed): Textbook of Veterinary Internal Medicine. Philadelphia, WB Saunders, 1975.
48. Morgan, JP: Radiology in Veterinary Orthopedics. Philadelphia, Lea and Febiger, 1972.
49. Gilmore, DR: Nonsurgical management of four cases of atlantoaxial subluxation in the dog. JAAHA 20:93, 1984.
50. Gage, ED and Smallwood, JE: Surgical repair of atlanto-axial subluxation in a dog. Vet Med 65:583, 1970.
51. Gage, ED: Atlantoaxial subluxation. *In* Bojrab, MJ (ed): Current Techniques in Small Animal Surgery, Philadelphia, Lea and Febiger, 1975, p 376.
52. Shires, P: Atlantoaxial instability. *In* Bojrab, MJ (ed): Current Techniques in Small Animal Surgery, 2nd ed. Philadelphia, Lea and Febiger, 1983, p 549.
53. Chambers, JN, et al.: The use of nonmetallic suture material for stabilization of atlantoaxial subluxation. JAAHA 13:602, 1977.
54. Renegar, WR and Stoll, SG: Thus use of methylmethacrylate bone cement in the repair of atlantoaxial subluxation stabilization failures—case report and discussion. JAAHA 15:313, 1979.
55. LeCouteur, RA, et al.: Stabilization of atlantoaxial subluxation in the dog using the nuchal ligament. JAVMA 177:1011, 1980.
56. Sorjonen, DC and Shires, PK: Atlantoaxial instability: A ventral surgical technique for decompression, fixation, and fusion. Vet Surg 10:22, 1981.
57. Kishigami, M: Application of an atlantoaxial retractor for atlantoaxial subluxation in the cat and dog. JAAHA 20:413, 1984.
58. Hurov, L: Congenital atlantoaxial malformation and acute subluxation in a mature basset hound—surgical treatment by wire stabilization. JAAHA 15:177, 1979.
59. Denny, HR, et al.: Atlanto-axial subluxation in the dog: A review of thirty cases and an evaluation of treatment by lag screw fixation. J Small Anim Pract 29:37, 1988.
60. Bestetti, G, et al.: Paraplegia due to *Actinomyces viscosus* infection in a cat. Acta Neuropathol 39:231, 1977.

61. Braund, KG: Encephalitis and meningitis. Vet Clin North Am 10:31, 1980.
62. Rhoades, HE, et al.: Nocardiosis in a dog with multiple lesions of the central nervous system. JAVMA 142:278, 1963.
63. Stowater, JL, et al.: Actinomycosis in the spinal canal of a cat. Fel Pract 8:26, 1978.
64. Kornegay, JN, et al.: Bacterial meningoencephalitis in two dogs. JAVMA 173:1334, 1978.
65. Bullmore, CC and Sevedge, JP: Canine meningoencephalitis. JAAHA 14:387, 1978.
66. Wilkinson, GT: Feline cryptococcosis: a review and seven case reports. J Small Anim Pract 20:749, 1979.
67. Palmer, AC, et al.: Cryptococcal infection of the central nervous system of a dog in the United Kingdom. J Small Anim Pract 22:579, 1981.
68. Sutton, RH: Cryptococcosis in dogs: A report on six cases. Aust Vet J 57:558, 1981.
69. Wagner, JL, et al.: *Cryptococcus neoformans* infection in a dog. JAVMA 153:945, 1968.
70. Greene, CE: Infectious diseases affecting the central nervous system. *In* Kornegay, JN (ed): Neurologic Disorders, Contemporary Issues in Small Animal Practice, vol 5. New York, Churchill Livingstone, 1986, p 57.
71. Kornblatt, AN, et al.: Arthritis caused by *Borrelia burgdorferi* in dogs. JAVMA 186:960, 1985.
72. Magnarelli, LA, et al.: Borreliosis in dogs from southern Connecticut. JAVMA 186:955, 1985.
73. Luttgen, PJ: Inflammatory disease of the central nervous system. Vet Clin North Am 18:623, 1988.
74. Tyler, DE, et al.: Disseminated protothecosis with central nervous system involvement in a dog. JAVMA 176:987, 1980.
75. Imes, GD, et al.: Disseminated protothecosis in a dog. Onderstepoort J Vet Res 44:1, 1977.
76. Greene, CE, et al.: Rocky Mountain spotted fever in dogs and its differentiation from canine erhlichiosis. JAVMA 186:465, 1985.
77. Hibler, SC: Rickettsial infections in dogs. Part I. Rocky Mountain spotted fever and coxiella infections. Comp Cont Ed 7:856, 1985.
78. Greene, CE: Update on neurologic and serologic findings on RMSF in dogs. Proceedings, 5th Ann Vet Med Forum, ACVIM, San Diego, CA, 1987, p 691.
79. Dow, SW and Jones, RL: Anaerobic infections. Part II. Diagnosis and treatment. Comp Cont Ed 9:827, 1987.
80. Dow, SW, et al.: Central nervous system infection associated with anaerobic bacteria in two dogs and two cats. J Vet Int Med 2:171, 1988.
81. Prevost, E, et al.: Successful medical management of severe feline cryptococcosis. JAAHA 18:111, 1982.
82. Keenan, KP, et al.: Studies on the pathogenesis of *Rickettsia rickettsii* in the dog: Clinical and clinicopathologic changes of experimental infection. Am J Vet Res 38:851, 1977.
83. Hildebrandt, PK, et al.: Pathology of canine ehrlichiosis (tropical canine pancytopenia). Am J Vet Res 34:1309, 1973.
84. Breitschwerdt, E: Rocky Mountain spotted fever. Proceedings, 4th Ann Vet Med Forum, ACVIM, Washington, DC, 1986, p 5.
84a. The choice of antimicrobial drugs. Med Lett Drugs Ther 30:33, 1988.
85. Meric, SM: Canine meningitis—a changing emphasis. J Vet Int Med 2:26, 1988.
85a. Scully, BE: Metronidazole. Med Clin North Am 72:613, 1988.
86. Dow, SW, et al.: Central nervous system toxicity associated with metronidazole in dogs. JAVMA 1988. In press.
86a. Francke, EL and Neu, HC: Chloramphenicol and tetracyclines. Med Clin North Am 71:1155, 1987.
87. Hird, JFR: Clinical use of antibiotics in small animal practice. *In* Yoxall, AT and Hird, JFR (eds): Pharmacological Basis of Small Animal Medicine. Melbourne, Blackwell Scientific Publications, 1979, p 63.
88. Greene, CE: Clinical Microbiology and Infectious Diseases of the Dog and Cat. Philadelphia, WB Saunders, 1984.
89. Weir, EC, et al.: Short-term combination chemotherapy for treatment of feline cryptococcosis. JAVMA 174:507, 1979.
89a. Hansen, BL: Successful treatment of severe feline cryptococcosis with long-term high doses of ketoconazole. JAAHA 23:193, 1987.
90. Hribernik, T: Canine ehrlichiosis. Comp Cont Ed 3:997, 1981.
91. Woodard, JC, et al.: Calcium phosphate deposition disease in Great Danes. Vet Pathol 19:464, 1982.
92. VanGundy, T.E.: Disc-associated wobbler syndrome in the Doberman pinscher. Vet Clin North Am 18:667, 1988.
93. Naylor, A: Factors in the development of the spinal stenosis syndrome. J Bone Joint Surg 61-B:306, 1979.
94. Olsson, SE: The dynamic factor in spinal cord compression. J Neurosurg 15:308, 1958.
95. Olsson, SE: Dynamic and static compression of the canine spinal cord. Proceedings, Gaines Symp Sm Anim Dis, Ohio State Univ, Columbus, OH, 1980, p 24.
96. Olsson, SE, et al.: Dynamic compression of the cervical spinal cord. A myelographic and pathologic investigation in Great Dane dogs. Acta Vet Scand 23:65, 1982.
97. Palmer, AC and Wallace, ME: Deformation of cervical vertebrae in basset hounds. Vet Rec 80:430, 1967.
98. Trotter, EJ: Canine wobbler syndrome. *In* Newton, CD, Nunamaker, DM (eds): Textbook of Small Animal Orthopaedics. Philadelphia, JB Lippincott, 1985, p 765.
99. Trotter, EJ, et al.: Caudal cervical vertebral malformation-malarticulation in Great Danes and Doberman pinschers. JAVMA 168:917, 1976.
100. Chambers, JN and Betts, CW: Caudal cervical spondylopathy in the dog: A review of 20 clinical cases and the literature. JAAHA 13:571, 1977.
101. Mason, TA: Cervical vertebral instability (wobbler syndrome) in the dog. Vet Rec 104:142, 1979.
102. Denny, HR, et al.: Cervical spondylopathy in the dog—a review of thirty-five cases. J Small Anim Pract 18:117, 1977.
103. Wolvekamp, WT and Wentink, GH: Vertebral body deformation causing wobbler syndrome in a Great Dane. Tijdschr Diergeneesk 100:775, 1975.
104. Geary, JC: Canine spinal lesions not involving discs. JAVMA 155:2038, 1969.
105. Wright, F, et al.: Ataxia of the Great Dane caused by stenosis of the cervical vertebral canal: Comparison with similar conditions in the basset hound, Doberman pinscher, ridgeback, and the thoroughbred horse. Vet Rec 82:1, 1973.
106. Selcer, RR and Oliver, JE, Jr: Cervical spondylopathy—wobbler syndrome in dogs. JAAHA 11:175, 1975.
107. Wright, JA: The use of sagittal diameter measurements in the diagnosis of cervical spinal stenosis. J Small Anim Pract 20:331, 1979.
108. Rendano, VT and Smith, LL: Cervical vertebral malformation malarticulation (wobbler syndrome)—the value of the ventrodorsal view in defining lateral spinal cord compression in the dog. JAAHA 17:627, 1981.
109. Seim, HB III and Withrow, SJ: Pathophysiology and diagnosis of caudal cervical spondylomyelopathy with emphasis on the Doberman pinscher. JAAHA 18:241, 1982.
110. Raffe, MR and Knecht, CD: Cervical vertebral malformation—a review of 36 cases. JAAHA 16:881, 1980.
111. Raffe, MR and Knecht, CD: Cervical vertebral malformation in bull mastiffs. JAAHA 14:593, 1978.
112. Wright, JA: A study of the radiographic anatomy of the cervical spine in the dog. J Small Anim Pract 18:341, 1977.
113. Read, RA, et al.: Caudal cervical spondylomyelopathy (wobbler syndrome) in the dog: a review of thirty cases. J Small Anim Pract 24:605, 1983.
114. Sharp, NJH, et al.: Evaluation of ventral decompression in cervical vertebral instability of the Doberman using conventional and computed tomography enhanced myelography. Abstract, Am Coll Vet Surg 22nd Annual Meeting. Vet Surg 16:102, 1987.
115. Shores, A: Canine cervical vertebral malformation/malarticulation syndrome. Comp Cont Ed 6:326, 1984.
116. Clark, DM: An analysis of intraoperative and early postoperative mortality associated with cervical spinal decompressive surgery in the dog. JAAHA 22:739, 1986.
117. Allen, BL, et al.: The biomechanics of decompression laminectomy. Spine 12:803, 1987.
118. Lyman, R: Continuous dorsal laminectomy for treatment of Doberman pinschers with caudal cervical vertebral instability and malformation. Proceedings, 5th Ann Vet Med Forum, ACVIM, San Diego, CA, 1987, p 303.
119. Swaim, SF: Evaluation of four techniques of cervical spinal fixation in dogs. JAVMA 166:1080, 1975.

120. Chambers, JN, et al.: Update on ventral decompression for caudal cervical disk herniation in Doberman pinschers. JAAHA 22:775, 1986.
121. Bailey, CS, et al.: Chemonucleolysis in Type II disk disease. Proceedings, 6th Ann Vet Med Forum, ACVIM, Washington, DC, 1988, p 763.
122. Morgan, JP: Congenital anomalies of the vertebral column of the dog: A study of the incidence and significance based on a radio-graphic and morphologic study. J Am Vet Radiol Soc 9:21, 1968.
123. Bailey, CS: An embryological approach to the clinical significance of congenital vertebral and spinal cord abnormalities. JAAHA 11:426, 1975.
124. Leyland, A: Ataxia in a Doberman pinscher. Vet Rec 116:414, 1985.
125. Kramer, JW: Characterization of heritable thoracic hemivertebra of the German shorthaired pointer. JAVMA 181:814, 1982.
126. Done, SH, et al.: Hemivertebra in the dog: clinical and pathological observations. Vet Rec 96:313, 1975.
127. Drew, RA: Possible association between abnormal vertebral development and neonatal mortality in bulldogs. Vet Rec 94:480, 1974.
128. Knecht, CD, et al.: Stenosis of the thoracic spinal canal in English bulldogs. JAAHA 15:181, 1979.
129. Grenn, HH and Lindo, DE: Hemivertebrae with severe kyphoscoliosis and accompanying deformities in a dog. Can Vet J 10:214, 1969.
130. Parker, AJ, et al.: Cervical kyphosis in an Afghan hound. JAVMA 162:953, 1973.
131. Wright, JA: Congenital and developmental abnormalities of the vertebrae. J Small Anim Pract 20:625, 1979.
132. Shell, LG, et al.: Spinal dysraphism, hemivertebra, and stenosis of the spinal canal in a rottweiler puppy. JAAHA 24:341, 1988.
133. Russo, EA, et al.: Corticosteroid-responsive aseptic suppurative meningitis in three dogs. Southwestern Vet 35:197, 1983.
134. Meric, SM, et al.: Corticosteroid-responsive meningitis in ten dogs. JAAHA 21:677, 1985.
135. Dodds, WJ: Immune-mediated diseases of the blood. Adv Vet Sci Compar Med 27:163, 1983.
136. Meric, SM: Steroid-responsive suppurative meningitis of dogs. Proceedings, 6th Ann Vet Med Forum, ACVIM, Washington, DC, 1988, p 237.
137. Griffiths, IR and Duncan, ID: Chronic degenerative radiculomyelopathy in the dog. J Small Anim Pract 16:461, 1975.
138. Averill, DR: Degenerative myelopathy in the aging German shepherd dog: Clinical and pathologic findings. JAVMA 162:1045, 1973.
139. Braund, KG and Vandevelde, M: German shepherd dog myelopathy—a morphologic and morphometric study. Am J Vet Res 39:1309, 1978.
140. Williams, DA, et al.: Enteropathy associated with degenerative myelopathy in German shepherd dogs. Scientific Proceedings, ACVIM Annual Mtg, New York, 1983, p 40.
141. Waxman, FJ, et al.: Progressive myelopathy in older German shepherd dogs. I. Depressed response to thymus-dependent mitogens. J Immunol 124:1209, 1980.
142. Waxman, FJ, et al.: Progressive myelopathy in older German shepherd dogs. II. Presence of circulating suppressor cells. J Immunol 124:1216, 1980.
143. Bichsel, P and Vandevelde, M: Degenerative myelopathy in a family of Siberian husky dogs. JAVMA 183:998, 1983.
144. Griffiths, IR and Duncan, ID: Age changes in the dorsal and ventral lumbar nerve roots of dogs. Acta Neuropathol 32:75, 1975.
145. Mesfin, GM, et al.: Degenerative myelopathy in a cat. JAVMA 176:62, 1980.
146. Bhagavati, S, et al.: Detection of human T cell lymphoma/leukemia virus type I DNA and antigen in spinal fluid and blood of patients with chronic progressive myelopathy. N Engl J Med 318:1141, 1988.
147. Brew, BJ: Another retroviral disease of the nervous system. Chronic progressive myelopathy due to HTLV-I. N Engl J Med 318:1195, 1988.
148. Douglas, SW and Palmer, AC: Idiopathic demyelination of brainstem and cord in a miniature poodle puppy. J Path Bact 82:67, 1961.
149. McGrath, JT: Neurologic Examination of the Dog with Clinicopathologic Observations, 2nd ed. Philadelphia, Lea and Febiger, 1960.
150. Steinberg, SA: Clinicopathologic conference. JAVMA 143:404, 1963.
151. Johnston, DE and Summers, BA: Osteomyelitis of the lumbar vertebrae in dogs caused by grass-seed foreign bodies. Aust Vet J 47:289, 1971.
152. Henderson, RA, et al.: Discospondylitis in three dogs infected with *Brucella canis*. JAVMA 165:451, 1974.
153. Gage, DE: Treatment of discospondylitis in the dog. JAVMA 166:1164, 1975.
154. Turnwald, GH, et al.: Diskospondylitis in a kennel of dogs: Clinicopathologic findings. JAVMA 188:178, 1986.
155. Carpenter, JL, et al.: Tuberculosis in five basset hounds. JAVMA 192:1563, 1988.
155a. Gilmore, DR: Diskospondylitis and multifocal osteomyelitis in two dogs. JAVMA 182:64, 1983.
156. Gilmore, DR: Lumbosacral diskospondylitis in 21 dogs. JAAHA 23:57, 1987.
157. Betts, CW: Osteomyelitis of the vertebral body and the intervertebral disk: Diskospondylitis. *In* Newton, CD and Nunamaker, DM (eds): Textbook of Small Animal Orthopaedics. Philadelphia, JB Lippincott, 1985, p 725.
158. Kornegay, JN: Canine diskospondylitis. Comp Cont Ed 1:930, 1979.
159. Johnson, RG and Prata, RG: Intradiskal osteomyelitis: A conservative approach. JAAHA 19:743, 1983.
160. Kornegay, JN and Barber, DL: Diskospondylitis in dogs. JAVMA 177:337, 1980.
161. Berg, JN, et al.: Identification of the major coagulase-positive *Staphylococcus* sp. of dogs as *Staphylococcus intermedius*. Am J Vet Res 45:1307, 1984.
162. Bennett, D, et al.: Discospondylitis in the dog. J Small Anim Pract 22:539, 1981.
163. Hirsh, DC and Smith, TM: Osteomyelitis in the dog: Microorganisms isolated and susceptibility to antimicrobial agents. J Small Anim Pract 19:679, 1978.
164. Bradney, IW: Vertebral osteomyelitis due to *Nocardia* in a dog. Aust Vet J 62:315, 1985.
165. LaCroix, JA: Vertebral body osteomyelitis: A case report. J Am Vet Radiol Soc 14:17, 1973.
166. Hurov, L, et al.: Diskospondylitis in the dog: 27 cases. JAVMA 173:275, 1978.
167. Patnaik, AK, et al.: Paecilomycosis in a dog. JAVMA 161:806, 1972.
168. Day, MJ, et al.: Disseminated aspergillosis in dogs. Aust Vet J 63:55, 1986.
169. Wood, GL, et al.: Disseminated aspergillosis in a dog. JAVMA 172:704, 1978.
170. Nestel, BL and Nestel, HM: Spinal tuberculosis in the dog. JAVMA 131:234, 1957.
171. Millman, TM, et al.: Coccidioidomycosis in the dog: Its radiographic diagnosis. J Am Vet Radiol Soc 20:50, 1979.
172. Craig, TM, et al.: *Hepatozoon canis* infection in dogs: Clinical, radiographic, and hematologic findings. JAVMA 173:967, 1978.
173. Norsworthy, GD: Diskospondylitis as a cause of posterior paresis. Fel Pract 9:39, 1979.
174. Kornegay, JN, et al.: Cranial thoracic diskospondylitis in two dogs. JAVMA 174:192, 1979.
175. Kornegay, JN: Diskospondylitis. *In* Kirk, RW (ed): Current Veterinary Therapy VIII. Philadelphia, WB Saunders, 1983, p 718.
176. Flores-Castro, R and Carmichael, LE: Canine brucellosis: Current status of methods for diagnosis and treatment. Proceedings, 27th Gaines Vet Symp, College Station, Texas, 1977, p 17.
177. Meyer, ME: Canine brucellosis. Labrador Retriever Magazine 1:10, 1976.
178. Higgins, RJ, et al.: Primary demyelination in experimental canine distemper virus induced encephalomyelitis in gnotobiotic dogs. Acta Neuropathol 58:1, 1982.
179. Summers, BA, et al.: Early events in canine distemper demyelinating encephalomyelitis. Acta Neuropathol 46:1, 1979.
180. Koestner, A, et al.: Canine distemper: A virus-induced demyelinating encephalomyelitis. *In* Zeman, W, and Lenette, EH

(eds): Slow Virus Diseases. Baltimore, Williams and Wilkins, 1974, p 86.
181. Krakowka, S, et al.: Myelin-specific autoantibodies associated with central nervous system demyelination in canine distemper virus infection. Infect Immun 8:819, 1973.
182. Vandevelde, M, et al.: Immunological and pathological findings in demyelinating encephalitis associated with canine distemper virus infection. Acta Neuropathol 56:1, 1982.
183. Vandevelde, M, et al.: Demyelination in experimental canine distemper virus infection: Immunological, pathologic, and immunohistological studies. Acta Neuropathol 56:285, 1982.
184. Raine, CS: On the development of CNS lesions in natural canine distemper encephalomyelitis. J Neurol Sci 30:13, 1976.
185. Appel, MJG: Canine distemper. *In* Barlough, JE (ed): Manual of Small Animal Infectious Diseases. New York, Churchill Livingstone, 1988, p 49.
186. Appel, MJG: Pathogenesis of canine distemper. Am J Vet Res 30:1167, 1969.
187. Sandersleben, J von and Sergany, MAM: Ein Bietrag zur sogenannten Pachymeningitis spinalis ossificans des Hundes unter Beruch-sichtigung pathogenetischer and atiologischer Gesischtspunkte. Zentralbl Veterinaermed 13A:526, 1966.
188. Morgan, JP: Spinal dural ossification in the dog: Incidence and distribution based on a radiographic study. J Am Vet Radiol Soc 10:43, 1969.
189. Pedersen, NC: Feline infectious peritonitis: Something old, something new. Fel Pract 6:42, 1976.
190. Barlough, JE and Scott, FW: Feline infectious peritonitis. *In* Barlough, JE (ed): Manual of Small Animal Infectious Diseases. New York, Churchill Livingstone, 1988, p 63.
191. Kornegay, JN: Feline infectious peritonitis: The central nervous system form. JAAHA 14:580, 1978.
192. Legendre, AM and Whitenack, DL: Feline infectious peritonitis with spinal cord involvement in two cats. JAVMA 167:931, 1975.
193. Vandevelde, M and Braund, KG. Polioencephalomyelitis in cats. Vet Pathol 16:420, 1979.
194. Hoff, EJ and Vandevelde, M: Non-suppurative encephalomyelitis in cats suggestive of a viral origin. Vet Pathol 18:170, 1981.
195. Johnson, GR, et al.: Globoid cell leukodystrophy in a beagle. JAVMA 167:380, 1975.
196. Hirth, RS and Nielsen, SW: A familial canine globoid cell leucodystrophy ("Krabbe type"). J Small Anim Pract 8:569, 1967.
197. Suzuki, Y, et al.: Studies in globoid leukodystrophy: Enzymatic and lipid findings in the canine form. Exp Neurol 29:65, 1970.
198. Johnson, KH: Globoid leukodystrophy in the cat. JAVMA 157:2057, 1970.
199. Fletcher, TF, et al.: Globoid cell leukodystrophy (Krabbe type) in the dog. JAVMA 149:165, 1966.
200. Luttgen, PJ, et al.: Globoid cell leucodystrophy in a basset hound. J Small Anim Pract 24:153, 1983.
201. Zaki, FA and Kay, WJ: Globoid cell leukodystrophy in a miniature poodle. JAVMA 163:248, 1973.
202. Boysen, BG, et al.: Globoid cell leukodystrophy in the bluetick hound dog. I. Clinical manifestations. Can Vet J 15:303, 1974.
203. McGrath, JT, et al.: A morphologic and biochemical study of canine globoid leukodystrophy. J Neuropathol Exp Neurol 28:171, 1969.
204. Roszel, JF, et al.: Periodic acid-Schiff-positive cells in cerebrospinal fluid of dogs with globoid cell leukodystrophy. Neurology 22:738, 1972.
205. Cordy, DR: Canine granulomatous meningoencephalomyelitis. Vet Pathol 16:325, 1979.
206. Russe, ME: Primary reticulosis of the central nervous system in dogs. JAVMA 174:492, 1979.
207. Vandevelde, M: Primary reticulosis of the central nervous system. Vet Clin North Am 10:57, 1980.
208. Fankhauser, R, et al.: Reticulosis of the central nervous system (CNS) in dogs. Adv Vet Sci Compar Med 16:35, 1972.
209. Vandevelde, M: Morphological and histochemical characteristics of GME and reticulosis: One disease or two? The Bern perspective. Proceedings, 4th Ann Vet Med Forum, ACVIM, Washington, DC, 1986, p 11.
209a. Vandevelde, M, et al.: Immunohistological studies on primary reticulosis of the canine brain. Vet Pathol 18:577, 1981.
210. Alley, MR, et al.: Granulomatous meningoencephalomyelitis of dogs in New Zealand. NZ Vet J 31:117, 1983.
211. Bailey, CS and Higgins, RJ: Characteristics of cerebrospinal fluid associated with canine granulomatous meningoencephalomyelitis: A retrospective study. JAVMA 188:418, 1986.
212. Braund, KG, et al.: Granulomatous meningoencephalomyelitis in six dogs. JAVMA 172:1195, 1978.
213. Martin, RA, et al.: Focal intramedullary spinal cord hematoma in a dog. JAAHA 22:545, 1986.
214. Withrow, SJ and Doige, CE: Subperiosteal vertebral hematoma as a cause of acute paraplegia in two dogs. JAAHA 15:295, 1979.
215. Bjorck, G, et al.: Hereditary ataxia in smooth-haired fox terriers. Vet Rec 69:871, 1957.
216. Bjorck, G, et al.: Hereditary ataxia in fox terriers. Acta Neuropathol Suppl I:45, 1962.
217. Hartley, WJ and Palmer, AC: Ataxia in Jack Russell terriers. Acta Neuropathol 26:71, 1973.
218. Wright, JA and Brownlie, S: Progressive ataxia in a Pyrenean Mountain dog. Vet Rec 116:410, 1985.
219. Averill, DR and Bronson, RT: Inherited necrotizing myelopathy of Afghan hounds. J Neuropathol Exp Neurol 36:734, 1977.
220. Cummings, JF and deLahunta, A: Hereditary myelopathy of Afghan hounds, a myelinolytic disease. Acta Neuropathol 42:173, 1978.
221. Cockrell, BY, et al.: Myelomalacia in Afghan hounds. JAVMA 162:362, 1973.
222. Palmer, AC and Medd, RK: Hound ataxia. Vet Rec 109:43, 1981.
223. Palmer, AC, et al.: Spinal cord degeneration in hound ataxia. J Small Anim Pract 25:139, 1984.
224. Clark, L: Hypervitaminosis A: A review. Aust Vet J 47:568, 1971.
225. Seawright, AA, et al.: Hypervitaminosis A and deforming cervical spondylosis of the cat. J Compar Pathol 77:29, 1967.
226. Hansen, HJ: A pathologic-anatomical study on disc degeneration in dog. Acta Orthop Scand Suppl II, 1952.
227. Priester, WA: Canine intervertebral disc disease—occurrence by age, breed, and sex among 8,117 cases. Theriogenology 6:293, 1976.
228. Braund, KG, et al.: Morphological studies of the canine intervertebral disc. The assignment of the beagle to the achondroplastic classification. Res Vet Sci 19:167, 1975.
229. Parker, AJ, et al.: Cervical disc prolapse in a Doberman pinscher. JAVMA 163:75, 1973.
229a. Morgan, JP, et al.: Vertebral canal and spinal cord mensuration: A comparative study of its effect on lumbosacral myelography in the Dachshund and German shepherd dog. JAVMA 191:951, 1987.
230. Ghosh, P, et al.: The variation of the glycosaminoglycans of the canine intervertebral disk with aging. Gerontology 23:87, 1977.
231. Ghosh, P, et al.: A comparative chemical and histological study of the chondrodystrophoid and nonchondrodystrophoid canine intervertebral disc. Vet Pathol 13:414, 1976.
232. Olsson, SE: On disc protrusion in dog (enchondrosis intervertebralis). Acta Orthop Scand Suppl VIII: 1951.
232a. Morgan, JP and Miyabayashi, T: Degenerative changes in the vertebral column of the dog: A review of radiographic findings. Vet Radiol 29:72, 1988.
233. Ghosh, P, et al.: Genetic factors in the maturation of the canine intervertebral disc. Res Vet Sci 19:304, 1975.
234. Ball, MU, et al.: Patterns of occurrence of disc disease among registered Dachshunds. JAVMA 180.519, 1982.
235. Greene, JA, et al.: Hypothyroidism as a possible cause of canine intervertebral disc disease. JAAHA 15:199, 1979.
236. Paatsama, S, et al.: Effect of estradiol testosterone, cortisone acetate, somatotropin, thyrotropin and parathyroid hormone on the lumbar intervertebral disc in growing dog. J Small Anim Pract 10:351, 1969.
237. Naylor, A: The biophysical and biochemical aspect of intervertebral disc herniation and degeneration. Ann Roy Coll Surg Engl 31:91, 1962.
238. Holliday, TA: Spinal cord trauma. *In* Proceedings, 49th Ann Mtg, AAHA, Las Vegas, NV, 1982, p 229.
239. Griffiths, IR: Some aspects of the pathology and pathogenesis of the myelopathy caused by disc protrusions in the dog. J Neurol Neurosurg Psychiatry 35:403, 1972.

240. Gooding, MR, et al.: Experimental cervical myelopathy: Effect of ischaemia and compression of the canine cervical spinal cord. J Neurosurg 43:9, 1975.
241. Riser, WH and Rinehard, MK: Canine intervertebral disc disease: Its development and its association with pulmonary and spinal cord embolism. Abstract, 35th Ann Mtg Am Coll Vet Pathol, Toronto, Ontario, 1984, p 100.
242. King, AS, et al.: Protrusion of the intervertebral disc in the cat. Vet Rec 70:509, 1958.
243. King, AS and Smith, RN: Disc protrusions in the cat: Distribution of dorsal protrusions along the vertebral column. Vet Rec 72:335, 1960.
244. King, AS and Smith, RN: Disc protrusion in the cat: Age incidence of dorsal protrusions. Vet Rec 72:381, 1960.
245. Littlewood, JD, et al.: Intervertebral disc protrusion in a cat. J Small Anim Pract 25:119, 1984.
246. Seim, HB III and Nafe, LA: Spontaneous intervertebral disk extrusion with associated myelopathy in a cat. JAAHA 17:201, 1981.
247. Griffiths, IR: A syndrome produced by dorsolateral "explosions" of the cervical intervertebral discs. Vet Rec 87:737, 1970.
248. Levine, SH and Caywood, DD: Recurrence of neurological deficits in dogs treated for thoracolumbar disk disease. JAAHA 20:889, 1984.
249. Hoerlein, BF: Canine Neurology: Diagnosis and Treatment, 3rd ed. Philadelphia, WB Saunders, 1978.
250. Hoerlein, BF: Intervertebral disc protrusions in the dog. I. Incidence and pathological lesions. Am J Vet Res 14:260, 1953.
251. McCarron, RF, et al.: The inflammatory effect of nucleus pulposus. Spine 12:760, 1987.
252. Forsythe, WB and Ghoshal, NG: Innervation of the canine thoracolumbar vertebral column. Anat Rec 208:57, 1984.
253. Bogduk, N, et al.: The innervation of the cervical intervertebral discs. Spine 13:2, 1988.
254. Felts, JF and Prata, RG: Cervical disk disease in the dog: Intraforaminal and lateral extrusions. JAAHA 19:755, 1983.
255. Moore, RW and Withrow, SJ: Gastrointestinal hemorrhage and pancreatitis associated with intervertebral disk disease in the dog. JAVMA 180:1443, 1982.
256. Crawford, LM and Wilson, RC: Melaena associated with dexamethasone therapy in the dog. J Small Anim Pract 23:91, 1982.
257. Toombs, JP, et al.: Colonic perforation following neurosurgical procedures and corticosteroid therapy in four dogs. JAVMA 177:68, 1980.
258. Russell, SW and Griffiths, RC: Recurrence of cervical disc syndrome in surgically and conservatively treated dogs. JAVMA 153:1412, 1968.
259. Shores, A: Intervertebral disc disease. *In* Newton, CD and Nunamaker, DM (eds): Textbook of Small Animal Orthopaedics. Philadelphia, JB Lippincott, 1985, p 739.
260. Walker, TL and Betts, CW: Intervertebral disc disease. *In* Slatter, DH (ed): Textbook of Small Animal Surgery. Philadelphia, WB Saunders, 1985, p 1396.
261. Denny, HR: The surgical treatment of cervical disc protrusions in the dog: A review of 40 cases. J Small Anim Pract 19:251, 1978.
262. Davies, JV and Sharp, NJH: A comparison of conservative treatment and fenestration for thoracolumbar intervertebral disc disease in the dog. J Small Anim Pract 24:721, 1983.
263. Funkquist, B: Investigations of the therapeutic and prophylactic effects of disc evacuation in cases of thoraco-lumbar herniated discs in dogs. Acta Vet Scand 19:441, 1978.
264. Hoerlein, BF: The status of the various intervertebral disc surgeries for the dog in 1978. JAAHA 14:563, 1978.
265. Prata, RG: Neurosurgical treatment of thoracolumbar disks: The rationale and value of laminectomy with concomitant disk removal. JAAHA 17:17, 1981.
266. Brown, NO, et al.: Thoracolumbar disk disease in the dog: A retrospective analysis of 187 cases. JAAHA 13:665, 1977.
267. Bartels, KE, et al.: Complications associated with the dorsolateral muscle separating approach for thoracolumbar disk fenestration in the dog. JAVMA 183:1081, 1983.
268. Shores, A, et al.: Structural changes in thoracolumbar disks following lateral fenestration. A study of the radiographic, histologic and histochemical changes in the chondrodystrophoid dog. Vet Surg 14:117, 1985.
269. Wilcox, KR: Conservative treatment of thoracolumbar intervertebral disc disease in the dog. JAVMA 147:1458, 1965.
270. Griffiths, IR: Vasogenic edema following acute and chronic spinal cord compression in the dog. J Neurosurg 42:155, 1975.
271. Saunders, EC: Treatment of the canine intervertebral disc syndrome with chymopapain. JAVMA 145:893, 1964.
272. Widdowson, WL: Effects of chymopapain in the intervertebral disc of the dog. JAVMA 150:608, 1967.
273. Biggart, JF: Discolysis: An introduction. Calif Vet 10:10, 1984.
274. Atilola, MAO, et al.: Cervical chemonucleolysis in the dog: A surgical technique. Vet Surg 17:135, 1988.
275. Atilola, MAO, et al.: Canine chemonucleolysis: An experimental radiographic study. Vet Radiol 29:168, 1988.
276. Garvin, PJ, et al.: Long term effects of chymopapain on intervertebral discs of dogs. Clin Orthop 92:281, 1973.
277. McCuloch, JA: Chemonucleolysis. J Bone Joint Surg 59B:45, 1977.
278. Feigin, I, et al.: Fibrocartilaginous venous emboli to the spinal cord with necrotic myelopathy. J Neuropathol Exp Neurol 24:63, 1975.
279. Zaki, FA and Prata, RG: Necrotizing myelopathy secondary to embolization of herniated intervertebral disk material in the dog. JAVMA 169:222, 1976.
280. deLahunta, A and Alexander, JW: Ischemic myelopathy secondary to presumed fibrocartilaginous embolism in nine dogs. JAAHA 12:37, 1976.
281. Griffiths, IR: Spinal cord infarction due to emboli arising from the intervertebral discs in the dog. J Compar Pathol 83:225, 1973.
282. Norrell, HA, et al.: Ischaemic myelopathy in dogs. Surgical Forum 18:429, 1967.
283. Hayes, MA, et al.: Acute necrotizing myelopathy from nucleus pulposus embolism in dogs with intervertebral disk degeneration. JAVMA 173:289, 1978.
284. Zaki, FA, et al.: Necrotizing myelopathy in a cat. JAVMA 169:228, 1976.
285. Zaki, FA, et al.: Necrotizing myelopathy in five Great Danes. JAVMA 165:1080, 1974.
286. Gamble, DA and Chrisman, CL: A leukoencephalomyelopathy of rottweiler dogs. Vet Pathol 21:274, 1984.
287. Wouda, W and van Nes, JJ: Progressive ataxia due to central demyelination in rottweiler dogs. Vet Quarterly 8:89, 1986.
288. Kornegay, JN: Vertebral diseases of large breed dogs. *In* Kornegay, JN (ed): Neurologic Disorders. New York, Churchill Livingstone, 1986, p 197.
289. Lenehan, TM: Canine cauda equina syndrome. Comp Cont Ed 5:941, 1983.
290. Denny, HR, et al.: The diagnosis and treatment of cauda equina lesions in the dog. J Small Anim Pract 23:425, 1982.
291. Berzon, JL and Dueland, R: Cauda equina syndrome: Pathophysiology and report of seven cases. JAAHA 15:635, 1979.
292. Walla, VL Jr: Die kompression der cauda equina beim hund. Kleintierpraxis 31:313, 1986.
293. Oliver, JE Jr, et al.: Cauda equina compression from lumbosacral malarticulation and malformation in the dog. JAVMA 173:207, 1978.
294. Wright, JA: Spondylosis deformans of the lumbo-sacral joint in dogs. J Small Anim Pract 21:45, 1980.
295. Tarvin, G and Prata, RG: Lumbosacral stenosis in dogs. JAVMA 177:154, 1980.
296. Hurov, L: Laminectomy for treatment of cauda equina syndrome in a cat. JAVMA 186:504, 1985.
297. Larsen, JS and Selby, LA: Spondylosis deformans in large dogs —relative risk by breed, age and sex. JAAHA 17:623, 1981.
298. McNeel, SV and Morgan, JP: Intraosseous vertebral venography: A technic for examination of the canine lumbosacral junction. J Vet Radiol Soc 19:168, 1978.
299. Feeney, DA and Wise, M: Epidurography in the normal dog: Technic and radiographic findings. Vet Radiol 22:35, 1981.
300. Kido, DK, et al.: Metrizamide epidurography in dogs. Radiol 128:119, 1978.
301. Hathcock, JT, et al.: Comparison of three radiographic contrast procedures in the evaluation of the canine lumbosacral spinal canal. Vet Radiol 29:4, 1988.
302. Garrick, JG and Sullivan, CR: A technic of performing diskography in dogs. Mayo Clinic Proc 39:270, 1964.
303. Wrigley, RH, Reuter, RE: Canine cervical diskography. Vet Radiol 25:274, 1984.

304. Slocum, B, and Devine, T: L7-Sl fixation-fusion for treatment of cauda equina compression in the dog. JAVMA 188:31, 1986.
305. Betts, CW, et al.: An unusual case of traumatic spondylolisthesis in a red bone hound: Diagnosis and therapy. JAAHA 12:470, 1976.
306. Haskins, ME, et al.: Spinal cord compression and hindlimb paresis in cats with mucopolysaccharidosis VI. JAVMA 182:883, 1983.
307. Konde, LJ, et al.: Radiographically visualized skeletal changes associated with mucopolysaccharidosis VI in cats. Vet Radiol 28:223, 1987.
308. Haskins, ME, et al.: Mucopolysaccharidosis in a domestic short-haired cat—a disease distinct from that seen in the Siamese cat. JAVMA 175:384, 1979.
309. Haskins, ME, et al.: Mucopolysaccharide storage disease in three families of cats with arylsulfatase B deficiency: Leukocyte studies and carrier identification. Pediatr Res 13:1203, 1979.
310. Wenger, DA, et al.: Bone marrow transplantation in the feline model of arylsulfatase B deficiency. *In* Krivit, W and Paul, NW (eds): Bone Marrow Transplantation for Treatment of Lysosomal Storage Diseases. March of Dimes Birth Defects Foundation, Birth Defects Original Article Series. New York, AR Liss, 22:177, 1986.
311. Alexander, JE and Pettit, GD: Spinal osteochondrosis in a dog. Can Vet J 8:47, 1967.
312. Gee, BR and Doige, CE: Multiple cartilaginous exostoses in a litter of dogs. JAVMA 156:53, 1970.
313. Chester, DK: Multiple cartilaginous exostoses in two generations of dogs. JAVMA 159:895, 1971.
314. Gambardella, PC, et al.: Multiple cartilaginous exostoses in the dog. JAVMA 166:761, 1975.
315. Alden, CL and Dickerson, TV: Osteochondromatosis of the cervical vertebrae in a dog. JAVMA 168:142, 1976.
316. Prata, RG, et al.: Spinal cord compression caused by osteocartilaginous exostoses of the spine in two dogs. JAVMA 166:371, 1975.
317. Pool, RR and Carrig, CB: Multiple cartilaginous exostoses in a cat. Vet Pathol 9:350, 1972.
318. Riddle, WE and Leighton, RL: Osteochondromatosis in a cat. JAVMA 156:1428, 1970.
319. Owen, LN and Bostock, DE: Multiple cartilaginous exostoses with development of a metastasizing osteosarcoma in a Shetland sheepdog. J Small Anim Pract 12:507, 1971.
320. Banks, WC and Bridges, CH: Multiple cartilaginous exostoses in a dog. JAVMA 129:131, 1956.
321. Bichsel, P, et al.: Solitary cartilaginous exostoses associated with spinal cord compression in three large-breed dogs. JAAHA 21:619, 1985.
322. McGrath, JT: Spinal dysraphism in the dog. Pathologia Veterinaria (Suppl) 2:1, 1965.
323. Shelton, ME: A possible mode of inheritance for spinal dysraphism in the dog with a more complete description of the clinical syndrome. MS Thesis, Iowa State University, Ames, Iowa, 1977.
324. Engel, HN and Draper, DD: Comparative prenatal development of the spinal cord in normal and dysraphic dogs: Embryonic stage. Am J Vet Res 43:1729, 1982.
325. Engel, HN: Comparative prenatal development of the spinal cord in normal and dysraphic dogs: Fetal stage. Am J Vet Res 43:1735, 1982.
326. Neufeld, JL and Little, PB: Spinal dysraphism in a Dalmatian dog. Can Vet J 15:335, 1974.
327. Geib, LW and Bistner, SI: Spinal cord dysraphism in a dog. JAVMA 150:618, 1967.
328. Martin, AH: A congenital defect in the spinal cord of the Manx cat. Vet Pathol 8:232, 1971.
329. Draper, DD, et al.: Neurologic, pathologic and genetic aspects of spinal dysraphism in dogs. (Abstr.) Anat Histol Embryol 4:369, 1975.
330. Confer, AW and Ward, BC: Spinal dysraphism: A congenital myelodysplasia in the weimaraner. JAVMA 160:1423, 1972.
331. Meric, SM, et al.: Necrotizing vasculitis of the spinal pachyleptomeningeal arteries in three Bernese Mountain dog littermates. JAAHA 22:459, 1986.
332. Harcourt, RA: Polyarteritis in a colony of beagles. Vet Record 102:519, 1978.
333. Hoff, EJ and Vandevelde, M: Case report: Necrotizing vasculitis in the central nervous systems of two dogs. Vet Pathol 18:219, 1981.
334. Kelly, DF, et al.: Polyarteritis in the dog: A case report. Vet Record 92:363, 1973.
335. Luttgen, PJ, et al.: A retrospective study of twenty-nine spinal tumours in the dog and cat. J Small Anim Pract 21:213, 1980.
336. LeCouteur, RA: Nervous system neoplasia. *In* Withrow, SJ and MacEwen, EG (eds): Clinical Veterinary Oncology. Philadelphia, JB Lippincott, 1988. In press.
337. Dallman, MJ and Saunders, GK: Primary spinal cord lymphosarcoma in a dog. JAVMA 189:1348, 1986.
338. Vanvelde, M, et al.: Neoplasms of mesenchymal origin in the spinal cord and nerve roots of three dogs. Vet Pathol 13:47, 1976.
339. Kusewitt, DF, et al.: Meningeal sarcomatosis in a dog. Vet Pathol 17:646, 1980.
340. Funkquist, B: Hourglass extradural lipoma in a dog. JAVMA 138:302, 1961.
341. Lewis, JC, et al. Paraganglioma involving the spinal cord of a dog. JAVMA 168:864, 1976.
342. Wright, JA: The pathological features associated with spinal tumours in 29 dogs. J Compar Path 95:549, 1985.
343. Prata, RG: Diagnosis of spinal cord tumors in the dog. Vet Clin North Am 7:165, 1977.
344. Northington, JW and Juliana, MM: Extradural lymphosarcoma in six cats. J Small Anim Pract 19:409, 1978.
345. Haynes, JS and Leininger, JR: A glioma in the spinal cord of a cat. Vet Pathol 19:713, 1982.
346. Kennedy, FA, et al.: Spinal cord medulloepithelioma in a dog. JAVMA 185:902, 1984.
347. Luttgen, PJ and Bratton, GR: Spinal cord ependymoma: A case report. JAAHA 12:788, 1976.
348. Zachary, JF, et al.: Intramedullary spinal ependymoma in a dog. Vet Pathol 18:697, 1981.
349. Bridges, CH, et al.: Spinal cord nephroblastoma in a dog. Proceedings, 35th Ann Mtg Am Coll Vet Pathol, Toronto, 1984, p 97.
350. Clark, DM and Picut, CA: Neuroepithelioma in a middle-aged dog. JAVMA 189:1330, 1986.
351. Summers, BA, et al.: A novel intradural extramedullary spinal cord tumor in young dogs. Acta Neuropathol 75:402, 1988.
352. MacCoy, DM, et al.: Pelvic limb paralysis in a young miniature pinscher due to metastatic bronchogenic adenocarcinoma. JAAHA 12:774, 1976.
353. Wright, JA, et al.: The clinical and radiological features associated with spinal tumours in thirty dogs. J Sm Anim Pract 20:461, 1979.
354. Morgan, JP, et al.: Vertebral tumors in the dog: A clinical, radiologic, and pathologic study of 61 primary and secondary lesions. Vet Radiol 21:197, 1980.
355. Vandevelde, M and Spano, JS: Cerebrospinal fluid cytology in canine neurologic disease. Am J Vet Res 38:1827, 1977.
356. Rosin, A: Neurologic disease associated with lymphosarcoma in ten dogs. JAVMA 181:50, 1982.
357. Couto, CG, et al.: Central nervous system lymphosarcoma in the dog. JAVMA 184:809, 1984.
358. Weller, RE, et al.: Myeloblastic leukemia and leukemic meningitis in a dog. Mod Vet Pract 61:42, 1980.
359. Zaki, FA, et al.: Primary tumors of the spinal cord and meninges in six dogs. JAVMA 166:511, 1975.
360. Suter, PF, et al.: Myelography in the dog: Diagnosis of tumors of the spinal cord and vertebrae. J Vet Radiol 12:29, 1971.
361. Raskin, RE: An atypical spinal meningioma in a dog. Vet Pathol 21:538, 1984.
362. Nafe, LA, et al.: An enlarged intervertebral foramen associated with an anaplastic sarcoma in a dog. JAAHA 19:299, 1983.
363. Jones, BR: Spinal meningioma in a cat. Aust Vet J 50:229, 1974.
364. Clemmons, RM, et al.: Lumbar epidural chondrosarcoma in a dog treated by excision and chemotherapy. JAVMA 183:1006, 1983.
365. Shores, A, et al.: Meningeal sarcoma mimicking a sciatic neuropathy in a dog. J Small Anim Pract 25:719, 1984.
366. Ferrell, JF, et al.: Cervical ganglioneuroma in a dog. JAVMA 144:508, 1964.
367. Jones, BR, et al.: Malignant glioma of the spinal cord in a dog. J Small Anim Pract 15:763, 1974.

368. Goedegebuure, SA: A case of neurofibromatosis in the dog. J Small Anim Pract 16:329, 1975.
369. Wright, JA: An undifferentiated sarcoma affecting the first three cervical vertebrae of a puppy. J Small Anim Pract 19:267, 1978.
370. Gilmore, DR: Neoplasia of the cervical spinal cord and vertebrae in the dog. JAAHA 19:1009, 1983.
371. Wise, DT, et al.: Posterior paresis caused by extension of hemangiosarcoma from lungs to thoracic vertebrae of a dog. JAVMA 171:544, 1977.
372. van Bree, H, et al.: Cervical cord compression as a neurologic complication in an IgG multiple myeloma in a dog. JAAHA 19:317, 1983.
373. Parker, AJ, et al.: Vertebral chondrosarcoma with extensive pulmonary metastases in a dog. J Small Anim Pract 12:673, 1971.
374. Prata, RG and Carillo, JM: Nervous system. *In* Slatter, DM (ed): Textbook of Small Animal Surgery. Philadelphia, WB Saunders, 1985, p 2499.
375. Destouet, JM and Monsees, B: Percutaneous bone biopsy: Techniques and results. Applied Radiol Mar/Apr:19, 1985.
376. Cork, LC, et al.: Canine neuroaxonal dystrophy. J Neuropathol Exp Neurol 42:286, 1983.
377. Troncoso, JC, et al.: Canine neuroaxonal dystrophy. J Neuropathol Exp Neurol 41:363, 1982.
378. Chrisman, CL, et al.: Neuroaxonal dystrophy of rottweiler dogs. JAVMA 184:464, 1984.
379. Evans, MG, et al.: Neuroaxonal dystrophy in a rottweiler pup. JAVMA 192:1560, 1988.
380. Leyh, R and Carithers, RW: Dermoid sinus in a Rhodesian ridgeback. Iowa State Vet 1:36, 1979.
381. Gerlach, J: Dermal sinuses and dermoids. *In* Vinken, PJ and Bruyn, GW (eds): Handbook of Clinical Neurology. Amsterdam, North Holland Publishing, 32:449, 1978.
382. Selcer, EA, et al.: Dermoid sinus in a Shih Tzu and a boxer. JAAHA 20:634, 1984.
383. Mann, GE and Stratton, J: Dermoid sinus in the Rhodesian ridgeback. J Small Anim Pract 7:631, 1966.
384. Cord, LH, et al.: Mid-dorsal dermoid sinuses in Rhodesian ridgeback dogs—a case report. JAVMA 131:515, 1957.
385. Kornegay, JN and Gorgacz, EJ: Intracranial epidermoid cysts in three dogs. Vet Pathol 16:646, 1982.
386. Tomlinson, J, et al.: Intraspinal epidermoid cyst in a dog. JAVMA 193:1435, 1988.
387. Griffiths, IR: The extensive myelopathy of intervertebral disc protrusions in dogs ("the ascending syndrome"). J Small Anim Pract 13:425, 1972.
388. Jones, SR: Toxoplasmosis: A review. JAVMA 163:1038, 1973.
389. Hartley, WJ, et al.: Toxoplasma meningoencephalomyelitis and myositis in a dog. NZ Vet J 6:124, 1958.
390. Moller, T and Neilsen, SW: Toxoplasmosis in distemper-susceptible carnivora. Pathol Vet 1:189, 1964.
391. Koestner, A and Cole, CR: Neuropathology of canine toxoplasmosis. Am J Vet Res 21:831, 1960.
392. Lappin, MR, et al.: Diagnosis and management of clinical feline toxoplasmosis. J Vet Int Med 1988. In press.
393. Dubey, JP, et al.: Newly recognized fatal protozoan disease of dogs. JAVMA 192:1269, 1988.
394. Averill, DR and deLahunta, A: Toxoplasmosis of the canine nervous system: Clinicopathologic findings in four cases. JAVMA 159:1134, 1971.
395. Drake, JC and Hime, JM: Two syndromes in young dogs caused by *Toxoplasma gondii*. J Small Anim Pract 8:621, 1967.
396. Holliday, TA, et al.: Skeletal muscle atrophy associated wth canine toxoplasmosis. A case report. Cornell Vet 53:288, 1963.
397. Core, DM, et al.: Hindlimb hyperextension as a result of *Toxoplasma gondii* polyradiculitis. JAAHA 19:713, 1983.
398. Lappin, MR, et al.: Diagnosis of recent *Toxoplasma gondii* infection in cats utilizing an enzyme-linked immunosorbent assay for immunoglobulin M. Am J Vet Res 1988. In press.
399. Lappin, MR, et al.: Enzyme-linked immunosorbent assay for the detection of circulating antigens of *Toxoplasma gondii* in the serum of cats. Am J Vet Res 1988. In press.
400. Braund, KG: Encephalitis and meningitis. Vet Clin North Am 10:31, 1980.
401. DeForest, ME and Basrur, PK: Malformations and the Manx syndrome in cats. Can Vet J 20:304, 1979.
402. James, CCM, et al.: Congenital anomalies of the lower spine and spinal cord in Manx cats. J Pathol 97:269, 1969.
403. Segedy, AK, et al.: Sacral spinal cord agenesis in a kitten. JAVMA 174:510, 1979.
404. Tomlinson, BE: Abnormalities of the lower spine and spinal cord in Manx cats. J Clin Pathol 24:480, 1971.
405. Leipold, HW, et al.: Congenital defects of the caudal vertebral column and spinal cord in Manx cats. JAVMA 164:520, 1974.
406. Todd, NB: The inheritance of taillessness in Manx cats. J Heredity 52:228, 1961.
407. Frye, FL: Spina bifida occulta with sacrococcygeal agenesis in a cat. Anim Hosp 3:328, 1967.
408. Furneaux, RW, et al.: Syringomyelia and spina bifida occulta in a samoyed dog. Can Vet J 14:317, 1973.
409. Wilson, JW: Spina bifida in the dog and cat. Comp Cont Ed 4:626, 1982.
410. Wilson, JW, et al.: Spina bifida in the dog. Vet Pathol 16:165, 1979.
411. Parker, AJ, et al.: Spina bifida with protrusion of spinal cord tissue in a dog. JAVMA 163:158, 1973.
412. Parker, AJ and Byerly, CS: Meningomyelocoele in a dog. Vet Pathol 10:266, 1973.
413. Clark, L and Carlisle, CH: Spina bifida with syringomyelia and meningocoele in a short-tailed cat. Aust Vet J 51:392, 1975.
414. Done, JT: Developmental disorders of the nervous system in animals. Adv Vet Sci Comp Med 20:69, 1976.
415. Patten, BM: Overgrowth of the neural tube in young human embryos. Anat Rec 113:381, 1952.
416. Padget, DH: Neuroschisis and human embryonic maldevelopment: new evidence on anencephaly, spina bifida and diverse mammalian defects. J Neuropathol Exp Neurol 29:192, 1970.
417. Chesney, CJ: A case of spina bifida in a chihuahua. Vet Rec 93:120, 1973.
418. Frye, FL and McFarland, LZ: Spina bifida with rachischisis in a kitten. JAVMA 146:481, 1965.
419. Kalter, H and Warkany, J: Congenital malformations, etiologic factors and their role in prevention. New Engl J Med 308:424, 1983.
420. Parker, AJ and Smith, CW: Meningeal cyst in a dog. JAAHA 10:595, 1974.
421. Parker, AJ, et al.: Spinal arachnoid cysts in the dog. JAAHA 19:1001, 1983.
422. Gage, ED, et al.: Spinal cord compression resulting from a leptomeningeal cyst in the dog. JAVMA 152:1664, 1968.
423. Luttgen, PJ and Crawley, RR: Posterior paralysis caused by epidural dirofilariasis in a dog. JAAHA 17:57, 1981.
424. Shires, PK, et al.: Epidural dirofilariasis causing paraparesis in a dog. JAVMA 180:1340, 1982.
425. Barron, CN and Saunders, LZ: Visceral larva migrans in the dog. Pathol Vet 3:315, 1966.
426. Buick, TD, et al.: Spinal nematodiasis of the dog associated with *Ancylostoma caninum*. Aust Vet J 53:602, 1977.
427. Mason, KV, et al.: Granulomatous encephalomyelitis of puppies due to *Angiostrongylus cantonensis*. Aust Vet J 52:295, 1976.
428. Sprent, JFA: On the invasion of the central nervous system by nematodes. I. The incidence and pathological significance of nematodes in the central nervous system. Parasitol 45:50, 1950.
429. LeCouteur, RA: Central nervous system trauma. *In* Kornegay, JN (ed): Neurologic Disorders. Contemporary Issues in Small Animal Practice, vol 5. New York, Churchill Livingstone, 1986, p 147.
430. de la Torre, JC: Spinal cord injury, review of basic and applied research. Spine 6:315, 1981.
431. Collins, WF and Kauer, JS: The past and future of animal models used for spinal cord trauma. *In* Popp, AJ, et al. (eds): Neural Trauma. New York, Raven Press, 1979, p 273.
432. Faden, AI: Recent pharmacological advances in experimental spinal injury. Theoretical and methodological considerations. Trends Neurosci 6:375, 1983.
433. Anderson, DK, et al.: Spinal cord injury and protection. Ann Emerg Med 14:816, 1985.
434. Eidelberg, E: The pathophysiology of spinal cord injury. Radiologic Clin North Am 15:241, 1977.
435. Braund, KG: Acute spinal cord traumatic compression. *In* Bojrab, MJ (ed): Pathophysiology in Small Animal Surgery. Philadelphia, Lea and Febiger, 1981, p 220.
436. Berg, RJ and Rucker, NC: Pathophysiology and medical man-

agement of acute spinal cord injury. Comp Cont Ed 7:646, 1985.
437. Anderson, TE: Spinal cord contusion injury: Experimental dissociation of hemorrhagic necrosis and subacute loss of axonal conduction. J Neurosurg 62:115, 1985.
438. Kobrine, AI, et al.: Experimental acute balloon compression of the spinal cord. Factors affecting disappearance and return of the spinal evoked response. J Neurosurg 51:841, 1979.
439. Vandevelde, M: Spinal cord compression. *In* Bojrab, MJ (ed): Pathophysiology in Small Animal Surgery. Philadelphia, Lea and Febiger, 1981, p 228.
440. Faden, AI, et al.: Megadose corticosteroid therapy following experimental traumatic spinal injury. J Neurosurg 60:712, 1984.
441. Means, ED, et al.: Effect of methylprednisolone in compression trauma to the feline spinal cord. J Neurosurg 55:200, 1981.
442. Walker, TL, et al.: Diseases of the spinal column. *In* Slatter, DH (ed): Textbook of Small Animal Surgery. Philadelphia, WB Saunders, 1985, p 1367.
443. Blass, CE, et al.: Cervical stabilization in three dogs using Steinmann pins and methylmethacrylate. JAAHA 24:61, 1988.
444. Morgan, JP: Spondylosis deformans in the dog. Acta Orthop Scand suppl 96, 1967.
445. Beadman, R, et al.: Vertebral osteophytes in the cat. Vet Record 76:1005, 1964.
446. Morgan, JP and Biery, DN: Spondylosis deformans. *In* Newton, CD, Nunamaker, DH (eds): Textbook of Small Animal Orthopaedics. Philadelphia, JB Lippincott, 1985, p 733.
447. Schmahl, W and Kaiser, E: Hydrocephalus, syringomyelia, and spinal cord angiodysgenesis in a Lhasa-apso dog. Vet Pathol 21:252, 1984.
448. Child, G, et al.: Acquired scoliosis associated with hydromyelia and syringomyelia in two dogs. JAVMA 189:909, 1986.
449. Gardner, WJ: Hydrodynamic mechanism of syringomyelia: Its relationship to myelocele. J Neurol Neurosurg Psychiatry 28:247, 1965.
450. Williams, B: Current concepts of syringomyelia. Brit J Hosp Med 4:331, 1970.
451. Cordy, DR: Vascular malformations and hemangioma of the canine spinal cord. Vet Pathol 16:275, 1979.
452. Zaki, FA: Vascular malformation (cavernous angioma) of the spinal cord in a dog. J Small Anim Pract 20:417, 1979.

63 NEURO-OPHTHALMOLOGY

ALEXANDER de LAHUNTA

Examination of the eye and its adnexa is a major component of the neurologic examination of a patient. Many cranial nerves are involved in the innervation of these structures and the central visual pathway comprises a significant portion of the prosencephalon. One of the most reliable indicators of a cerebral lesion is a loss of vision with preservation of pupillary light responses. This discussion of neuro-ophthalmology is organized in the manner that the author performs the examination of the eye in the neurologic examination of a patient.[1] Features of the examination are summarized in Table 63–1.

The order in which one performs the neurologic examination varies from individual to individual and often depends on the nature of the patient's disability. If the patient is ambulatory, the author usually examines the gait and postural reactions first. While watching the dog walk through the corridors of the hospital and around objects, a visual deficit may be apparent only if it is severe. Even almost completely blind animals often avoid objects amazingly well, especially in a familiar environment. Owners rarely recognize a visual deficit until it is a total bilateral deficit. This often results in a complaint of the sudden onset of blindness.

TABLE 63–1. SUMMARY OF FEATURES OF OCULAR PART OF NEUROLOGIC EXAMINATION

Test or Observation	Neurologic Components
Menace response	II–central visual pathway–VII (cerebellum)
Size of pupils	II, III, sympathetics, prosencephalon ocular disease (cerebellum)
Pupillary light reflex	II–pretectal nuclei–III
Eyelids	
Size of fissure	III, sympathetics, VII Masticatory muscle atrophy (cerebellum)
Third eyelid	Sympathetics Masticatory muscle atrophy (cerebellum)
Position of eyeballs	III, IV, VI, vestibular system, orbit
Normal nystagmus	VIII–brain stem–III, VI
Abnormal nystagmus	Vestibular system, congenital–visual system
Palpebral reflex	V–VII

MENACE RESPONSE

The clinician may begin the cranial nerve examination with the eye and the animal's response to a menacing gesture. It is convenient to examine most dogs by standing over them and gently extending their head and neck so that both eyes can be observed. Cats and toy breed dogs are better examined while sitting on the floor with one's back against a wall, legs held together and flexed, and the patient lying with its back between the clinician's thighs. This allows good control of the patient's head for the cranial nerve examination.

The menace response is elicited by making a threatening gesture with the hand at each eye while the other hand covers the opposite eye. If the other eye is not covered, an alert animal may be blind in the eye being tested but pick up the threat with its normal eye and respond by blinking bilaterally. It is crucial to the validity of this test that the threatening hand not touch the patient or create enough air currents to be felt by the patient.

The normal response to this threat is a rapid blink (closure of the palpebral fissure). The motor component is mediated through the facial nerve and its nucleus in the medulla. The afferent side of this response is extensive and involves a cerebral pathway, which implicates this as a learned response. Therefore, this response may not become fully developed until 10 to 12 weeks of age in some small animals. The following structures must be normal for the impulses to be generated by the threat and ultimately reach the facial motor neurons in the medulla: cornea, aqueous, lens, vitreous, retina, optic nerve, optic chiasm (65 per cent of optic nerve axons cross in the cat, 75 per cent in the dog), optic tract, lateral geniculate nucleus, and optic radiation, and visual cortex of occipital lobe (Figure 63–1). It is assumed that the visual cortex projects to the motor cortex, which in turn projects via the internal capsule and crus cerebri to the medulla. Alternate pathways from the visual cortex to the brain stem may exist.

Because the majority of optic nerve axons cross in the optic chiasm, the impulses generated in the retina of the threatened eye primarily project to the opposite

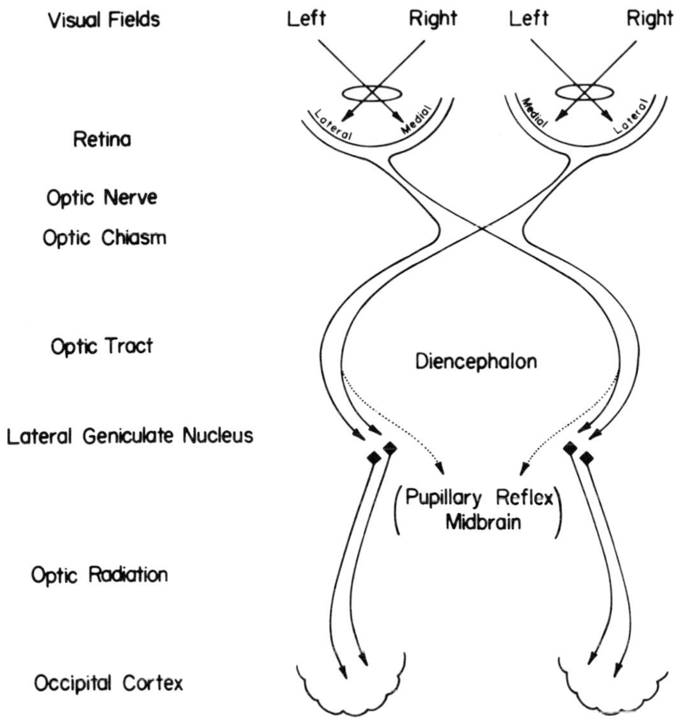

FIGURE 63–1. Schematic drawing of central visual pathway for visual perception.

optic tract, lateral geniculate nucleus, optic radiation and visual cortex. Therefore, a loss of menace response on one side is a reliable indicator of a lesion in the opposite central visual pathway even though there are still intact optic nerve axons projecting ipsilaterally. Most of the optic nerve axons that cross in the chiasm arise from the ganglion cell layer of the medial two-thirds of the retina and those that project ipsilaterally come from the lateral retina. Ideally, these could be tested separately by a threat from the lateral and medial visual fields, respectively. However, this is not reliable in the small animal patient and clinical experience has established a close relationship between a unilateral menace defect and a contralateral central lesion. Because of the close interaction between the cerebrum and the cerebellum, serious cerebellar lesions prevent the menace response but do not interfere with visual perception. Animals with such lesions always have significant signs of cerebellar ataxia. A unilateral cerebellar lesion causes an ipsilateral menace deficit.

If the menace response does not occur, the clinician should first check the facial nerve innervation of the orbicularis oculi by touching the eyelids to see that they close the fissure normally. If a facial paralysis exists, then observe for head or eyeball retraction when that eye is threatened. With slight retraction of the eyeball, the third eyelid passively protrudes. A dog or cat with "flashing third eyelids" often has a facial paralysis; this is an indication that vision is intact.

If there is no facial paralysis and no menace response occurs, lightly strike the animal two to three times with the threatening hand and then repeat the threat without touching the patient. This often arouses and directs the attention of the patient to what you are doing and is followed by a normal response.

With all young animals who may not yet have learned this response and occasionally with stoic, older animals, the clinician can assess their vision by rolling a roll of tape by them on the floor from different directions. A normal, alert, young animal that may not respond to the menace readily follows the roll of tape. The same effect can be accomplished by dropping cotton balls in front of the animal. The visual placing postural reaction test also tests their vision. The animal is held off the ground and brought to the edge of a table. If it sees the table, it elevates its limbs to place them on the table's surface before the limbs touch the table. A blind animal does not elevate its limbs until they touch the table's edge. As a rule, total blindness can be suspected when the patient does not direct its eyes at you during the examination.

PUPILLARY LIGHT REFLEX

The size and response of pupils to light should be assessed following the menace test. If there is a visual deficit, further location of the lesion depends on a careful examination of the eyeballs and the pupils. It is very important to evaluate the size of the pupils in normal room light before stimulating the retina with a strong accessory light source. If the pupils cannot be seen without extra light, hold a penlight parallel with the median plane of the patient and at a distance that just allows you to see the pupillary margins. Assess the size of the pupils and compare them with each other. The pupillary light reflex appears to be remarkably resistant to serious ocular diseases. Animals with extensive retinal or optic nerve disease (optic neuritis, progressive retinal degeneration) can be functionally blind and yet the pupils may still respond to a bright light. The clinician who is unaware of this fact may direct a strong light source into the fundus of a blind dog, observe a pupillary response, and erroneously diagnose a lesion in the central visual pathway in the brain. Although blind with pupils that respond to a bright light source, these animals have pupils that are dilated more than normal in room light. This can be verified by comparison with other animals in the same room light who have normal vision.

The pupillary light reflex only involves a pathway through the brain stem (Figure 63–2). The motor component of the reflex is the parasympathetic lower motor neuron located in the oculomotor nerve (cranial nerve III). The preganglionic cell bodies are in the rostral part of the oculomotor nucleus in the rostral midbrain. The axons of these cell bodies course ventrally and leave the midbrain in the oculomotor nerve on the medial side of the crus cerebri. This nerve courses through the cavernous sinus lateral to the pituitary gland and leaves the cranial cavity through the orbital fissure. It lies on the ventrolateral aspect of the optic nerve and, at about two-thirds the distance to the eyeball, it terminates in a number of branches to extraocular muscles. At this termination there is a small ganglion, the ciliary ganglion, that contains the cell bodies of the postganglionic axons in this parasympathetic pathway. These axons

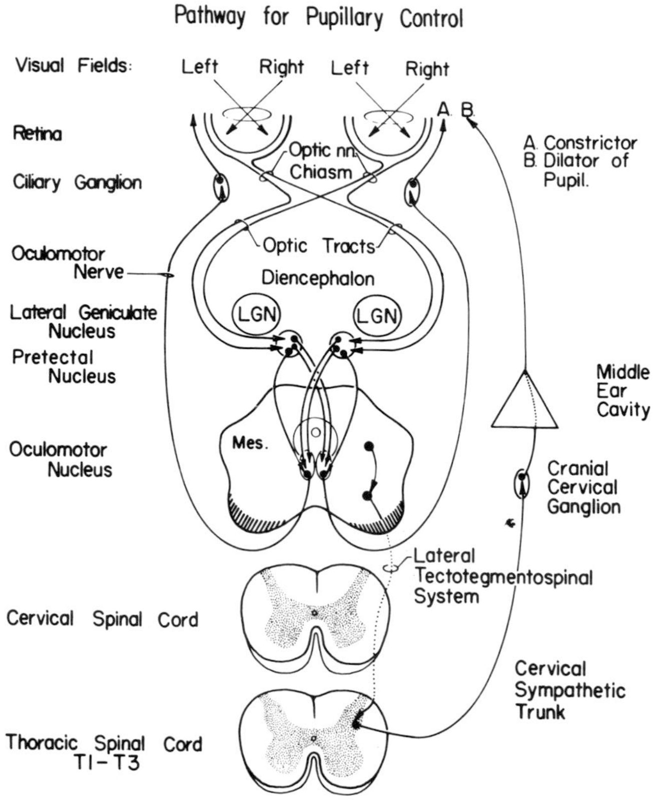

FIGURE 63–2. Schematic drawing of neuroanatomic pathway for control of pupil size.

course to the eyeball in ciliary nerves, penetrate the sclera, and follow the choroid to the iris and the constrictor muscle of the pupil.

The afferent pathway follows that for visual perception (menace response) to the level of the lateral geniculate nucleus in the caudal thalamus. There the retinal neurons in the optic tract that are concerned with the pupillary light reflex pass over the lateral geniculate nucleus and terminate near the midline of the caudal thalamus in the pretectal nucleus. Most of the axons of these pretectal neurons cross through the caudal commissure to terminate in the contralateral oculomotor parasympathetic nucleus. Because a significant number of optic nerve axons do not cross at the optic chiasm and some pretectal neurons project ipsilaterally, the impulses generated by light directed into one eye reach both oculomotor nuclei, and a bilateral response occurs. The response in the stimulated eye is called the direct response. That in the opposite eye is the indirect or consensual response. As a rule, these responses are equal in small animals. Occasionally the indirect response is smaller, which can be explained by the double crossing of the majority of these axons. This first occurs at the optic chiasm and then again at the caudal commissure.

Remember that it takes a serious lesion of the afferent side of this reflex to cause an abnormality. It would be rare for this reflex to be abnormal in an animal with an afferent lesion that was not blind in that eye. As a rule, afferent lesions that interrupt this reflex occur in the eyeball, optic nerve, or optic chiasm. Rarely, both optic tracts are affected sufficiently to cause pupillary abnormalities. A single optic tract lesion is rare and may cause no pupillary light reflex abnormality or cause a depressed response when the eye opposite to the lesion is stimulated.

Animals with unilateral lesions in the retina or optic nerve have no menace response in that eye. Frequently there is no asymmetry of pupil size or the pupil in that eye is slightly larger. Light directed into the affected eye causes no response in either eye. Light directed into the unaffected eye elicits a bilateral response. In order to assess direct and indirect responses, the clinician should direct the light back and forth between the eyes. In animals with a unilateral lesion, as the light is directed from the unaffected to the affected eye, the pupil in the affected eye will dilate back to the resting state created by the room light. This occurs because the strong light source was taken away from the unaffected eye and the lesion in the affected eye has interrupted the afferent pathway for this reflex. This phenomenon is readily apparent as the light is repeatedly moved between the eyes. Further confirmation of a unilateral lesion is made by covering the normal eye and observing further dilation of the pupil in the affected eye. This proves that its normal size at rest or with only slight dilation is due to the room light entering the normal eye.

A lesion of the efferent pathway in the parasympathetic component of the oculomotor nerve causes a widely dilated pupil in the ipsilateral eye at rest. The menace response is normal in each eye. Light directed into either eye only causes constriction of the pupil in the eye on the side opposite from the lesion.

The optic chiasm and the oculomotor nerves are accessible for compression by extramedullary, space-occupying lesions in the region of the hypophyseal fossa. A retrobulbar or intracranial lesion that affects both the optic nerve and parasympathetic part of the oculomotor nerve on the same side causes a widely dilated pupil in the ipsilateral eye at rest. There is no menace response from this affected eye. Light directed into the affected eye elicits no response in either eye. Light directed into the unaffected eye causes pupillary constriction only in that eye.

PUPIL SIZE

From this discussion it should be apparent that it is important to evaluate and compare the size of the pupils in room light or under an equal amount of light from an accessory source. The influence of lesions in the eyeball, optic nerve, and oculomotor nerve has been considered. The one remaining neurologic component that can influence the size of the pupil is the sympathetic innervation of the iris smooth muscle that dilates the pupil. The size of the pupil at rest represents a balance between the amount of light stimulating the retina and influencing the oculomotor neurons to constrict the pupil and the emotional status of the patient that influences the sympathetic system, resulting in pupillary dilation.

A defect in the sympathetic innervation of the structures of the head is referred to as Horner's syndrome; all the signs observed relate to the eye. Anisocoria results from the loss of innervation of the dilator of the pupil, producing miosis on the affected side. This is apparent at rest and when either eye is stimulated with light. In darkness this pupil dilates due to the inactivity of oculomotor neurons. Due to loss of tone in smooth muscle normally maintained by sympathetic innervation, there is also a protrusion of the third eyelid and slight narrowing of the palpebral fissure (ptosis). Enophthalmos results from loss of tone in the periorbital smooth muscle, but distinguishing this feature from the other eyelid changes is both difficult and unimportant.

Sympathetic innervation of these structures is maintained by both upper and lower motor neuron systems (Figure 63–2). Lesions involving the latter are the most common causes of Horner's syndrome. The upper motor neuron system involves a pathway arising in the hypothalamus and midbrain that courses through the remaining brain stem and the lateral funiculus of the cervical spinal cord to terminate on preganglionic cell bodies of the lower motor neuron system. These cell bodies are located in the intermediate gray column from T1 to L4 or L5. Those that project to the head are located predominately from T1 to T3. Their axons leave the spinal cord in the segmental ventral roots and branch off the spinal nerve just beyond the intervertebral foramen in the communicating ramus to the thoracic sympathetic trunk. As a rule these preganglionic axons do not synapse here but pass through the cervicothoracic and middle cervical ganglia and course cranially in the cervical sympathetic trunk where it is associated with the vagus nerve in the carotid sheath. At the base of the skull ventral to the tympano-occipital fissure these preganglionic axons terminate on cell bodies of second neurons in the cranial cervical ganglion. Postganglionic axons course through the middle ear and enter the cranial cavity to join the ophthalmic nerve (branch of cranial nerve V). The ophthalmic nerve traverses the orbital fissure and branches in the periorbita to supply sympathetic innervation to the smooth muscle of the periorbita, eyelids, and the iris dilator muscle of the pupil.

Severe cervical spinal cord lesions that interrupt this upper motor neuron can cause Horner's syndrome. Such a bilateral lesion is life-threatening due to its simultaneous interference with the upper motor neuron that controls respiration. Acute unilateral lesions such as an intervertebral disk extrusion on one side or infarction from fibrocartilaginous emboli cause hemiplegia and an ipsilateral Horner's syndrome. There are many lesions that can interfere with the lower motor neuron sympathetic innervation of the head. The specific location of the lesion is usually determined by the nature of the other clinical signs that are present. Examples are given in Table 63–2.

A rare observation is a mildly dilated, slowly responsive pupil that occurs in animals with severe cerebellar disease that affects the cerebellar nuclei.

Evaluation of the size of the pupils is important in assessing the location and extent of brain damage from intracranial injury and following the response to therapy. Brain stem contusion with hemorrhage and laceration of the midbrain and pons are common results of serious injury. This lesion interrupts the parenchymal components of the oculomotor neurons, causing bilateral, widely dilated, unresponsive pupils, which is a grave sign. Injuries that predominately involve the prosencephalon often result in very miotic pupils, which is assumed to represent a release of the parasympathetic oculomotor neurons from upper motor neuron inhibition. These can change rapidly to dilated, unresponsive pupils if there is progressive brain stem edema or hemorrhage. They can just as readily return to normal size if the cerebral edema resolves. Frequently there is remarkable anisocoria with one mydriatic and one miotic pupil. Usually each shows a slight response to light. These should be watched carefully as an indication of whether to treat the patient more vigorously or not. Severe caudal brain stem lesions that are life-threatening often result in partly dilated, fixed, unresponsive pupils.

TABLE 63–2. LESION LOCATION AND ASSOCIATED NEUROLOGIC SIGNS

Location	Lesion	Associated Neurologic Signs
T1–T3 spinal cord	Injury Neoplasia Embolic myelopathy	Tetraparesis to tetraplegia with LMN forelimb signs and UMN hindlimb signs
T1–T3 ventral roots proximal spinal nerves	Avulsion	Diffuse LMN paralysis of ipsilateral thoracic limb
Cranial thoracic sympathetic trunk	Lymphosarcoma, other neoplasms	None
Cervical sympathetic trunk	Neoplasia Injury–surgical; drug injections; dog bites	None or laryngeal hemiplegia
Postganglionic axons in middle ear	Otitis media	Peripheral vestibular ataxia, facial paralysis
Retrobulbar	Injury Neoplasia	Optic and oculomotor nerve defects

Anisocoria can also result from specific diseases of the eye. Keratitis or uveitis may cause miosis in the affected eye and glaucoma causes mydriasis. Iris atrophy is a common cause of dilated, unresponsive pupils in older animals and usually is bilateral. This can be confirmed in the absence of synechia by the inability of the iris to respond to a few drops of a two per cent solution of pilocarpine, which acts directly on the muscle, causing constriction in the normal eye. In teaching hospitals, a common cause of dilated, unresponsive pupils is the prior administration of a mydriatic drug for fundic examination. The same effect can occur in animals that consume drugs containing atropine or plants with belladonna alkaloids.

PHARMACOLOGIC TESTING

It is possible to use direct- and indirect-acting autonomic nervous system drugs to help determine whether the lesion in the parasympathetic or sympathetic innervation of the eye is in the first or second neuron of the lower motor neuron system.[2, 3] This is based on the phenomenon of denervation hypersensitivity that occurs with second neuron lesions and uses very low concentrations of the drug.

In the parasympathetic system, lesions of the second neuron that denervate the pupil constrictor make it hypersensitive to low concentrations of the direct-acting drug pilocarpine. A 0.1 per cent solution causes constriction of the pupil of the denervated iris but not a normal iris or an iris in which the lesion involves the first neuron. With first neuron lesions, indirect-acting drugs cause pupil constriction by way of the intact second neuron. These drugs include physostigmine (0.5 per cent solution) and phospholine iodine (0.06 per cent solution). These do not produce pupillary constriction with second neuron lesions.

The same concept applies to the sympathetic system innervation of the dilator of the pupil. For the direct-acting drug, a 1/10,000 dilution of epinephrine can be used. This should only cause dilation of a denervated pupil. Alternatively, 0.1 ml of a 0.001 per cent epinephrine solution causes dilation in 20 minutes if the pupil is denervated and 30 to 40 minutes if the lesion is in the preganglionic neurons. Cocaine (ten per cent solution) or hydroxyamphetamine (one per cent solution) can be used as the indirect-acting drugs. These do not cause normal mydriasis if the lesion is in the second neurons that directly innervate the pupil dilator muscle.

These tests have been used to confirm the involvement of both components of the autonomic nervous system lower motor neuron in the ocular signs of the ganglionopathy referred to as feline dysautonomia or the Key-Gaskell syndrome.[4, 5] Ciliary ganglia lesions cause the dilated pupils and lesions of the cranial cervical ganglia cause the protruded third eyelids.

PALPEBRAL FISSURE

The size of the palpebral fissure depends primarily on the normal tone in the levator palpebrae superioris muscle innervated by the oculomotor nerve and the smooth muscle innervated by the sympathetic neurons. The orbicularis oculi innervated by the facial nerve is responsible for closure of the fissure. Its function is observed when the menace response is tested. In facial paralysis in small animals, the size of the palpebral fissure is usually unchanged or slightly enlarged due to loss of tone in the orbicularis oculi. There is insufficient striated muscle innervated by the facial nerve that terminates in the eyelids to help keep the fissure open. Therefore its paralysis does not result in ptosis.

A small palpebral fissure or ptosis results from a lesion in the oculomotor or sympathetic neurons that supply the eye. With a complete oculomotor paralysis, the ipsilateral pupil is dilated and unresponsive to light directed into either eye. There is also a lateral and slightly ventral strabismus, with decreased ability to adduct the eye normally. A lesion in the sympathetic innervation also produces an elevated third eyelid and miosis.

A small palpebral fissure occurs indirectly when extensive atrophy of the muscles of mastication occurs and the eyeball retracts into the orbit. This atrophy can result from an extensive myositis of these muscles or from their denervation when lesions affect the mandibular nerve component of the trigeminal nerve.

A narrowed palpebral fissure occurs with spasm of the facial muscles on one side. Hemifacial spasm is thought to result from a unilateral lesion affecting the facial nerve. As a rule this lesion is an otitis media affecting the facial nerve in its canal through the temporal bone. The fissure is narrowed due to overactivity of the orbicularis oculi. Similarly, the ear on the affected side is elevated slightly and the lips are retracted. This disease rarely occurs bilaterally. Tetanus regularly produces a bilateral narrowing of the palpebral fissures due to the uninhibited facial neuron activity.

Occasionally animals with serious cerebellar disease that involves the cerebellar nuclei have one palpebral fissure that is slightly wider or a mildly elevated third eyelid. This has also been produced experimentally with lesions in the nuclei of the cerebellum.

THIRD EYELID

Normally, the third eyelid is maintained in its position ventromedial to the eyeball by the tone in its smooth muscle, which keeps it retracted. This is a function of its sympathetic innervation. The normally protruded position of the eyeball in the orbit also contributes to the normal position of the third eyelid.

Lesions of the sympathetic neurons cause a constant protrusion of the third eyelid that is a feature of Horner's syndrome. The third eyelid also passively protrudes if the eyeball is actively retracted (as in tetanus) or the eyeball sinks in the orbit from atrophy of the muscles of mastication (trigeminal nerve paralysis).

STRABISMUS

Strabismus is an abnormal position of the eyeball. It results from lesions of the cranial nerves that innervate the striated extraocular muscles (cranial nerves III, IV, and VI) or occurs in some head positions with lesions in the vestibular system. Oculomotor nerve lesions cause a lateral and slightly ventral strabismus due primarily to loss of innervation of the medial rectus and secondarily to the denervation of the dorsal and ventral rectus muscles and the ventral oblique muscle. Eyeball adduction is deficient. This is observed on testing normal vestibular nystagmus. As the head is moved in a dorsal plane, side to side, the eyeballs normally develop a jerk nystagmus with the quick phase in the direction of the head movement. The jerk-like movement toward the nose is adduction from the action of the medial rectus innervated by the oculomotor nerve (III). The same abrupt movement away from the nose, abduction, is a function of the lateral rectus innervated by the abducent nerve (VI). The latter is deficient in lesions of the abducent neurons and a medial strabismus is observed. Ptosis and a dilated unresponsive pupil accompany a complete loss of oculomotor nerve function.

Trochlear nerve (IV) lesions are rare or unrecognized.

Denervation of the dorsal oblique muscle results in a strabismus that is difficult to recognize in the dog because of the round pupil and because the dog may recover rapidly due to the compensatory activity of the other extraocular muscles. In the cat with its vertical pupil, the dorsal aspect of the pupil deviates laterally with a lesion of the trochlear neurons. In the dog a fundic examination may reveal a similar lateral displacement of the superior retinal vein.

Strabismus is often seen in hydrocephalic animals that have an enlarged cranial cavity. Both eyes often deviate ventrolaterally. This is thought to result from a malformation of the orbit that occurs when the cranial cavity is distorted by the early development of the brain abnormality. These eyes adduct and abduct normally on testing normal vestibular nystagmus and no ptosis or pupillary abnormality is present.

Strabismus can also be observed in some positions of the head when animals have lesions in the vestibular system. This can occur peripherally with lesions in the inner ear and vestibulocochlear nerve (VIII) or centrally with lesions in the vestibular nuclei of the medulla or vestibular pathways in the cerebellum. This involves the eye on the same side as the vestibular abnormality, is usually a ventrolateral strabismus, and is only present in some positions of the head. It is most evident when the head and neck are extended and the eye on the affected side fails to elevate normally in the palpebral fissure. Sclera is evident dorsally in the "dropped" eye. Normally both eyes elevate and remain in the center of the fissure so that no sclera is visible. This ventrolateral strabismus can be differentiated from the strabismus of an oculomotor nerve lesion by the presence of signs of vestibular system disturbance and the ability to adduct the eye normally on testing normal nystagmus.

NYSTAGMUS

Nystagmus is an involuntary movement of the eyes that is most commonly a jerk movement with quick and slow phases. The direction refers to the quick phase, which normally occurs when the head is moved from side to side or up and down. The quick phase is in the direction of the head movement. Abnormal nystagmus most commonly occurs with disturbances of the vestibular system. In acute or progressive lesions, it may be spontaneous or resting, which means it is constant regardless of the position of the head. In more prolonged, less progressive lesions, it may only be present when the head is held flexed to either side or extended. This is called positional nystagmus. With all disturbances of the peripheral components of the vestibular system, the quick phase of the abnormal nystagmus is opposite to the side of the head tilt and balance loss, which are on the same side as the lesion. This nystagmus can be horizontal or rotatory. In determining the direction of rotatory nystagmus, follow the position of 12 o'clock at the pupillary aperture. With lesions of the central components of the vestibular system, the quick phase can be away from the lesion, be toward the lesion, change directions with different positions of the head, or be vertical.

Congenital nystagmus is rare and usually is rapid and pendular (the speed is equal in both directions of the movement). This occasionally occurs transiently over a few weeks in litters of young puppies. It often accompanies other congenital abnormalities in the visual system. This is probably the reason that it is seen more often in Siamese cats, who have increased numbers of optic nerve axons that cross in the chiasm and have alterations of the architecture of their central visual pathway. There is no evidence of visual deficit. These cats may also show a medial strabismus. A remarkable, rapid, constant, pendular nystagmus has been observed in Belgian sheep dogs that are lacking in the development of the optic chiasm. Each optic nerve is directly continuous with the ipsilateral optic tract. This is presumed to be inherited. Congenital nystagmus is occasionally observed in puppies with retinal and optic nerve anomalies (collie eye syndrome), retinal detachment, or intraocular hemorrhage.

PALPEBRAL REFLEX

The palpebral reflex is used to test the ability of the animal to close its eyelids. This tests both the sensory (V) and motor (VII) innervation of the eyelids. The sensory innervation occurs through branches of the ophthalmic and maxillary nerves from the trigeminal nerve (cranial nerve V). Although the ophthalmic nerve branches are predominately medial and the maxillary are lateral, there is extensive overlap, so that the only autonomous zone of the ophthalmic nerve is a small area of skin dorsomedially. For the maxillary nerve branches this zone is ventrolateral to the lateral angle of the eyelids. Sensory deficits are uncommon compared to facial paralysis and can be mistaken for the latter. Animals with only a trigeminal nerve lesion blink spontaneously and when the eye is menaced, providing they are visual. Loss of ophthalmic nerve innervation to the cornea via ciliary nerves may result in a neurotrophic keratitis.

References

1. de Lahunta, A: Veterinary Neuroanatomy and Clinical Neurology, 2nd ed. Philadelphia, WB Saunders, 1983.
2. Scagliotti, RH: Neuro-ophthalmology. *In* RW Kirk (ed): Current Veterinary Therapy Small Animal Practice VII. Philadelphia, WB Saunders, 1980, p 510.
3. Slatter, DH: Fundamentals of Veterinary Ophthalmology. Philadelphia, WB Saunders, 1981.
4. Canton, DD, et al.: Dysautonomia in a cat. JAVMA 192:1293, 1988.
5. Sharp, NJH, et al.: Feline dysautonomia (the Key-Gaskell syndrome): A clinical and pathological study of forty cases. J Sm Anim Pract 25:539, 1984.

64 PERIPHERAL NERVE DISORDERS

CHERYL L. CHRISMAN

Peripheral nerves are the communication pathway between the central nervous system and the rest of the body. There are 12 pairs of cranial nerves and 36 pairs of spinal nerves that enter and exit from the brain stem and spinal cord, respectively.[1]

Sensory peripheral nerves carry the modalities touch, temperature, pain, proprioception, olfaction, vision, audition, and equilibrium into the central nervous system. The most common clinical manifestations of sensory peripheral neuropathies are anesthesia, self-mutilation or hyperesthesia if touch and pain modalities are affected and ataxia of the limbs and knuckling of the toes if proprioception is affected. Anosmia, blindness, deafness, and dysequilibrium are signs of specific cranial nerve sensory dysfunctions.

Motor peripheral nerves have cell bodies in the ventral horn gray matter of the spinal cord, and the axons exit through the ventral root to innervate skeletal muscle, smooth muscle, or glands. Disorders of motor nerves to skeletal muscles are considered in this chapter. The primary sign is paresis or paralysis of affected muscles with depressed spinal reflexes. Muscle atrophy is present if the disorder is chronic. Most peripheral nerves are mixtures of sensory and motor fibers (Figure 64–1), and both sensory and motor dysfunctions are seen in most peripheral nerve disorders.[2]

PHYSIOLOGY AND PATHOPHYSIOLOGY

Peripheral nerves are capable of transmitting an electrical signal along their membranes. In the resting state potassium and protein ions are contained within the nerve cell and sodium ions are actively extruded (Figure 64–2). The result is that the interior of the nerve cell is negative compared to a positive exterior. If the nerve is stimulated to a specific threshold level by a chemical or electrical stimulus, an action potential is created as sodium rushes into the cell, making the interior positive compared to the exterior, a state referred to as depolarization (Figure 64–2). The action potential travels along the neuronal membrane as an electrical impulse to the nerve terminal, which contains packets of a neurotransmitter chemical. When the nerve terminal depolarizes neurotransmitter is released and stimulates either another nerve cell (in the case of sensory nerves) or a skeletal muscle receptor (in the case of motor nerves). The sensory and motor nerves are covered with lipid insulation called a myelin sheath, which is interrupted periodically at areas called nodes of Ranvier. Saltatory conduction occurs when the electrical impulses jump from node to node rather than being propagated along the entire nerve; this greatly shortens conduction time. The myelin is produced by Schwann cells, which wrap around the nerve fiber (Figure 64–1). Once the nerves depolarize, repolarization to their original state occurs so the nerve can again be stimulated (Figure 64–2).

In the motor nerve terminal are vesicles containing the neurotransmitter acetylcholine. When the electrical impulse reaches the nerve terminal, acetylcholine is released. The acetylcholine reacts with the endplate receptor site on the muscle to produce depolarization and an endplate potential (EPP). The enzyme acetylcholinesterase, present at the neuromuscular junction, removes acetylcholine from the receptor site on the muscle and repolarization occurs. The acetylcholine is then reabsorbed into the nerve terminal so it can be used again. Microelectrode recordings at the neuromuscular junction show a constant leakage of acetylcholine from the nerve terminal, and the resultant subthreshold changes are referred to as miniature endplate potentials (MEPPs). The myotrophic effect of the motor nerve is well known and has been attributed in part to the production of MEPP. If MEPPs are decreased or absent, owing to motor nerve injury, the muscle undergoes severe atrophy.

The mechanisms of disease affecting peripheral nerves and the specific diseases discussed in this chapter are listed in Table 64–1. Congenital, traumatic, vascular, neoplastic, infectious, inflammatory, and some idiopathic mechanisms affect one or a small group of nerves and produce focal cranial or spinal nerve deficits. The

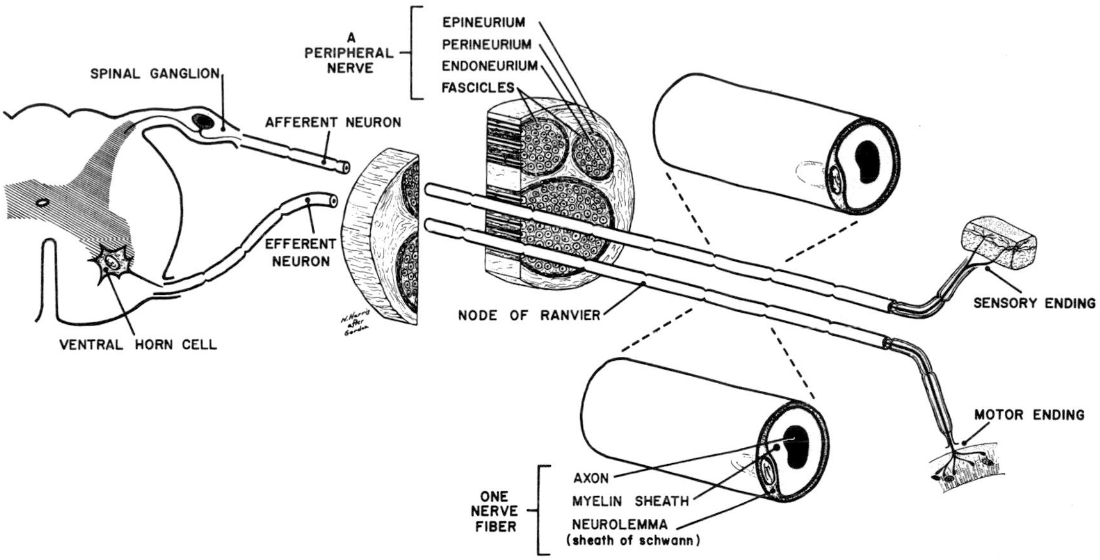

FIGURE 64–1. Diagram showing the various parts of a peripheral nerve. (From Miller, M., Christensen, G., and Evans, H.: Anatomy of the Dog. Philadelphia, W. B. Saunders Company, 1964.)

immunologic mechanisms may produce focal or diffuse signs. Metabolic, endocrine, toxic, and other idiopathic mechanisms most commonly produce multifocal or diffuse cranial and/or spinal nerve deficits, which may be asymmetrical or symmetrical.

Dysfunction of peripheral nerves is due to a disease affecting the nerve itself or its myelin sheath. Congenital and familial mechanisms of disease may result in a lack of development of a nerve or a metabolic defect within the nerve or Schwann cell, which results in the eventual death of either. If the Schwann cell metabolism is altered by a metabolic, endocrine, toxic, or idiopathic disorder,

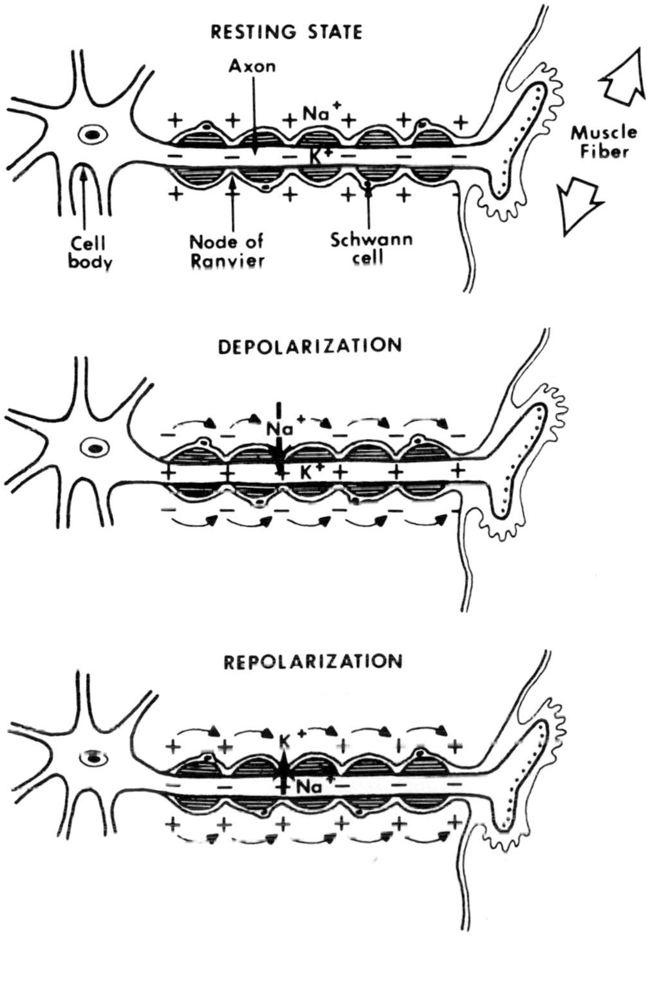

FIGURE 64–2. Anatomy and physiology of a motor peripheral nerve. (From Chrisman, C: Problems in Small Animal Neurology. Philadelphia, Lea and Febiger, 1982.)

TABLE 64–1. MECHANISMS OF DISEASE AND SPECIFIC PERIPHERAL NERVE DISORDERS

Congenital and Familial Disorders
Focal Neuropathies
Optic nerve hypoplasia
Congenital vestibulopathy (Doberman pinschers)
Laryngeal paralysis (Bouvier des Flandres)
Megaesophagus
Polyneuropathies
Progressive spinal muscular atrophy (Brittany spaniels)
Globoid cell leukodystrophy
Boxer neuropathy
Dachshund sensory neuropathy
Sensory neuropathy (English pointers)
Dancing Doberman disease
Giant axonal neuropathy (German shepherds)
Hypertrophic neuropathy (Tibetan mastiffs)
Polyneuropathy with inherited primary hyperchylomicronemia (cats)
Traumatic and Vascular Disorders
Focal Neuropathies
Brachial plexus avulsion
Other cranial and spinal nerve injury
Ischemic neuromyopathy
Neoplasia
Focal Neuropathies
Neurinoma (schwannoma, neurilemmoma)
Neurofibroma, neurofibrosarcoma
Lymphosarcoma
Polyneuropathies
Paraneoplastic polyneuropathy
Metabolic and Endocrine Disorders
Polyneuropathies
Diabetic polyneuropathy
Hyperinsulinism polyneuropathy
Hypothyroid polyneuropathy
Paraneoplastic polyneuropathy
Miscellaneous metabolic polyneuropathies
Toxic Disorders
Polyneuropathies
Chemical agents
Heavy metals
Drugs
Clostridium botulinum toxin
Tick neurotoxin
Snake venom neurotoxin
Infectious Disorders
Focal Neuropathies
Toxoplasma gondii meningoradiculitis
Other miscellaneous viral, bacterial, or fungal meningitides that affect nerve roots as well
Inflammatory/Suspected Immune-Mediated Disorders
Focal Neuropathies
Optic neuritis
Trigeminal neuritis
Brachial plexus neuritis
Polyneuropathies
Ganglioradiculitis or cranial polyneuropathy
Acute polyradiculoneuritis
Chronic progressive and relapsing polyradiculoneuritis and polyneuritis
Feline polyneuritis
Idiopathic Disorders
Focal Neuropathies
Idiopathic trigeminal neuropathy
Idiopathic facial nerve paralysis
Feline idiopathic vestibular syndrome
Canine geriatric vestibular syndrome
Cricopharyngeal achalasia
Megaesophagus
Spontaneous laryngeal paralysis
Polyneuropathies
Distal denervating disease
Distal symmetrical polyneuropathy
Sensory neuronopathy
Feline and canine hyperesthesia syndromes

segmental demyelination of the peripheral axon results.[3] Nerve transmission is greatly slowed (Figure 64–3). If the normal flow of axoplasm from the cell body to the nerve terminal and back to the cell body is interrupted, as seen in some metabolic, toxic, and idiopathic disorders, nerve terminal degeneration results. This terminal degeneration is referred to as a "dying back neuropathy"

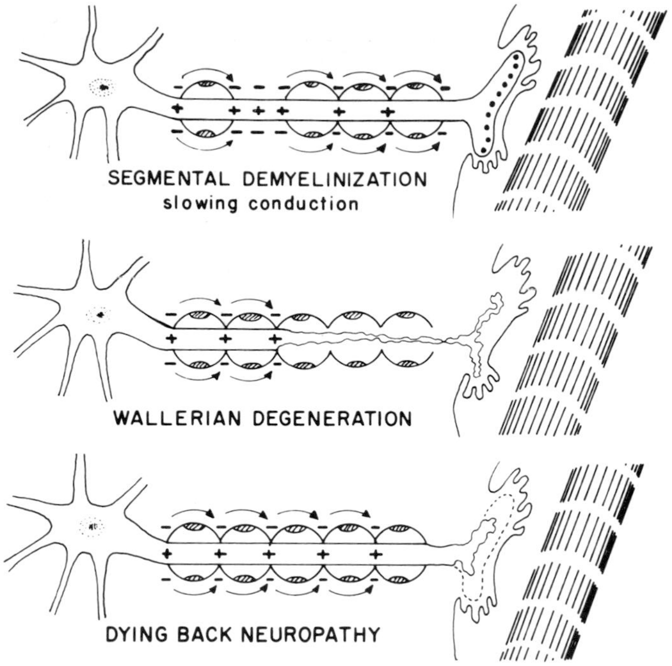

FIGURE 64–3. Pathology and pathophysiology of a motor peripheral nerve. (From Chrisman, C: Electromyography in animals. *In* Bojrab, J (ed): Pathophysiology in Small Animal Surgery. Philadelphia, Lea and Febiger, 1981.)

or distal axonopathy (Figure 64–3). Certain drugs and toxins like botulism toxin or tick toxin may block the release of neurotransmitter substance from nerve terminals. Other substances affect acetylcholinesterase and alter normal neuromuscular transmission.

If the nerve is severely damaged or disrupted, the portion disconnected from the cell body degenerates. This process is referred to as wallerian degeneration (Figure 64–3). Degeneration may occur on the proximal stump back to the next node of Ranvier or farther. If degeneration involves the cell body, the entire nerve may die. If the cell body is spared, the nerve may be capable of regeneration, so long as the nerve sheath (Schwann cell or neurilemmal sheath) remains intact and is not severely damaged from the insult. Regeneration occurs at an average rate of one mm per day or one inch per month.

CLINICAL EVALUATION

HISTORY

The purpose of the history is to establish the signs and course of the suspected peripheral nerve disorder so an accurate differential diagnosis can be made. The signalment (breed, age, and sex) of the dog or cat and clinical signs should initially be considered to determine the likelihood of one of the known congenital or familial peripheral nerve disorders. If the signs were acute in onset, stable, and focal, the possibility of a traumatic or vascular insult should be ascertained. Exposure to ticks, dead carrion potentially causing botulism, snakes, and all drugs and chemicals ingested or contacted should be

TABLE 64–2. CRANIAL PERIPHERAL NERVES

Nerve	Function	Tests of Function	Signs of Dysfunction
1. Olfactory	1. Smell	1. Blindfold animal and see if it can find food to eat	1. Inability to find food
2. Optic	2. Vision	2. Pupillary light reflex (sensory portion) Menace response; walk through a maze; throw cotton balls	2. Blind, with loss of pupil response to light
3. Oculomotor	3. Constrict pupil; extraocular muscles—dorsal, medial and ventral rectus, and ventral oblique—move eyeball Levator muscle of the upper lid—open eyelids	3. Pupillary light reflex (motor portion) Oculocephalic response or vestibular nystagmus; eyeball movement	3. Dilated pupil; paralyzed eyeball deviated downward and outward Ptosis
4. Trochlear	4. Extraocular muscles—superior oblique	4. Eyeball movement	4. Slight upward and inward rotation of eyeball seen on ophthalmoscopic exam
5. Trigeminal	5. Motor to muscles of mastication—chew, close mouth Sensation to the face	5. Palpate muscles of head; feel jaw tone Eye blink, ear twitch, and lip retraction response to touching or pinching (sensory)	5. Atrophied temporalis or masseter muscles Bilateral—dropped jaw, loss of sensation to the head
6. Abducens	6. Extraocular muscles—lateral rectus—move eyeball laterally	6. Eyeball movement	6. Paralyzed eyeball deviated medially
7. Facial	7. Muscles of facial expression; elevate ears, close eyes, curl lips Lacrimal and salivary glands	7. Eye blink, ear twitch and lip retraction response to touching or pinching (motor); Schirmer tear test	7. Inability to close the eyelid, move the ear, or curl the lips Dry eyes and mucous membranes
8. Vestibulo-cochlear	8. Vestibular equilibrium—changes in eyeball position and limb tone with changes in head position Cochlear—hearing	8. Observe head posture, balance and gait; observe for nystagmus and positional strabismus and nystagmus When sleeping try to arouse	8. Unilateral—head tilt, circling, rolling, or leaning to one side; rotary or horizontal nystagmus; positional nystagmus and strabismus Bilateral—fall to either side; wide lateral head movements Bilateral—deafness
9. Glosso-pharyngeal	9. Sensory to the pharynx	9. Swallow reflex (sensory)	9. Dysphagia—difficulty swallowing
10. Vagus	10. Motor to the pharynx, larynx Parasympathetic to viscera of thorax and abdomen	10. Swallow reflex; auscultate and examine larynx	10. Dysphagia—difficulty swallowing Laryngeal paralysis—unilateral and bilateral Bilateral—megaesophagus
11. Spinal accessory	11. Motor to muscles of neck	11. Palpate neck musculature	11. Atrophy of musculature Unilateral—slight deviation of the neck away from the lesion
12. Hypoglossal	12. Motor to the tongue	12. Observe drinking and ability to pull tongue into mouth; palpate tongue	12. Unilateral—atrophy and contracture of one side; Bilateral—inability to retract tongue

explored to determine if toxicity is a likely cause. Metabolic, endocrine, or paraneoplastic dysfunctions that might have an associated polyneuropathy should also be considered. Primary neoplastic processes of peripheral nerves are generally focal, chronic, and progressive. A previous knowledge of immune-mediated and idiopathic peripheral nerve disorders is important to determine if these fit the signalment, clinical course, and signs of the animal.

NEUROLOGIC EXAMINATION

The purpose of the neurologic examination is to determine if a peripheral cranial or spinal motor and/or sensory nerve disorder is present, if it is focal, diffuse or multifocal, symmetrical or asymmetrical, and how severe the dysfunction is (see Chapter 60). A summary of cranial nerve functions, tests of function, and signs of dysfunction can be found in Table 64–2.

Peripheral spinal nerves are evaluated by testing motor ability, spinal reflexes, superficial skin sensation, deep pain response, limb coordination, and proprioception and observing muscle atrophy. Tables 64–3 and 64–4 summarize neurologic abnormalities found with lesions of the peripheral nerves to the thoracic limb and pelvic limb, respectively.

DIAGNOSTIC AIDS

Diagnostic aids that specifically evaluate peripheral nerves include electromyography and nerve biopsy.

Electromyography. Electromyography (EMG) is performed to evaluate the electrical function of the peripheral nerve and skeletal muscle it innervates, together called the motor unit.[4–6] There are two types of studies

TABLE 64–3. LESIONS OF NERVES OF THE THORACIC LIMB AND NEUROLOGIC EXAMINATION FINDINGS

Roots	Nerve	Muscle Atrophy	Gait and Posture Deficit	Spinal Reflex Alterations	Distribution of Sensory Loss
C6–C7	Suprascapular	1. Supraspinatus 2. Infraspinatus	1. None	1. None	1. None
C7–C8	Axillary	1. Deltoid	1. None	1. None	1. Small area of sensory loss of dorsolateral aspect of brachium
C6–C8	Musculocutaneous	1. Biceps brachii	1. No flexion of elbow	1. Decreased or absent flexion of elbow during flexor reflex 2. Decreased or absent biceps tendon reflex	1. Some sensory loss of medial aspect of forearm
C7–T2	Radial	1. Triceps brachii 2. Extensor carpi radialis 3. Ulnaris lateralis 4. Common and lateral digital extensors	1. No extension of elbow 2. No extension of carpus and digits 3. Unable to support weight on limb	1. Decreased or absent triceps tendon reflex 2. Decreased or absent extensor carpi radialis muscle response	1. Decreased or absent sensation on the cranial aspect of the limb from the toes to elbow
C8–T1	Median and Ulnar	1. Flexor carpi radialis 2. Superficial digital flexor 3. Flexor carpi ulnaris 4. Deep digital flexor	1. No flexion of carpus 2. No flexion of digits	1. Decreased or absent flexion of carpus and digits during flexor reflex	1. Decreased or absent sensation on the caudal aspect of the limb from toes to elbow 2. Ulnar nerve—loss of sensation from 5th

TABLE 64–4. LESIONS OF NERVES OF THE PELVIC LIMB AND NEUROLOGIC EXAMINATION FINDINGS

Roots	Nerve	Muscle Atrophy	Gait and Posture Deficit	Spinal Reflex Alterations	Distribution of Sensory Loss
L5–L6	Obturator	1. Pectineus 2. Gracilus	1. Slight abduction of hip	1. None	1. None
L4–L5	Femoral	1. Quadriceps femoris	1. Unable to extend stifle 2. Limb collapses with weight	1. Decreased or absent patellar tendon reflex	1. Decreased or absent sensation on medial surface of thigh, stifle, leg, and paw
L6–S1	Sciatic	1. Semimembranosus 2. Semitendinosus 3. All muscles of peroneal and tibial nerves	1. Unable to actively flex stifle 2. Hock flexes and extends passively 3. Hock dropped 4. Knuckled onto digits 5. Caudal gluteal muscle involvement will produce adduction of hip	1. Decreased or absent flexor reflex 2. Decreased or absent cranial tibial muscle response 3. Decreased or absent gastrocnemius tendon reflex	1. Decreased or absent sensation below the stifle to the toes except medial surface
L6–S1	Tibial	1. Gastrocnemius 2. Superficial and deep digital flexors	1. Dropped hock and tarsus 2. Overflexion of hock and overextension of digits	1. Decreased or absent gastrocnemius tendon reflex	1. Decreased or absent sensation on caudal and plantar surface of limb from stifle to paw
L6–S1	Peroneal (fibular)	1. Peroneus longus 2. Cranial tibial 3. Lateral and long digital extensor	1. Stand knuckled onto digits 2. Overextension of hock and overflexion of digits	1. Decreased or absent cranial tibial muscle response	1. Decreased or absent sensation on cranial and dorsal surface of limb from stifle to paw

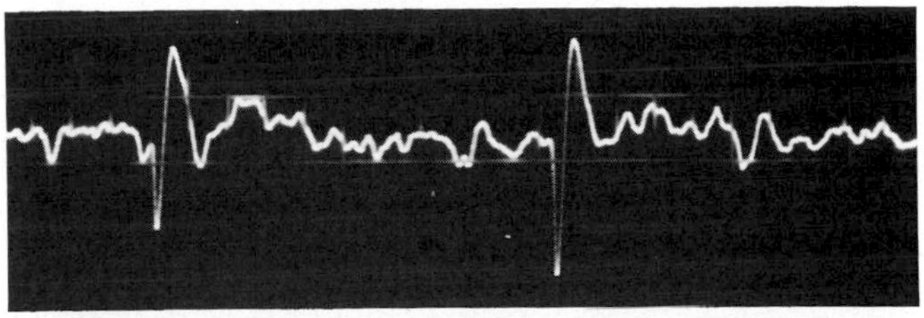

FIGURE 64–4. Positive waves may be seen after insertional activity in neuromuscular disease: 100 microvolts per centimeter, 30 milliseconds per major division.

often performed during the EMG examination, needle EMG and nerve stimulation.

Needle EMG. The needle EMG is performed by inserting a needle recording electrode into a muscle and observing its response during contraction, at rest, and during the induced mechanical irritation caused by insertion of the electrode. The responses can be visualized on an oscilloscope and heard with the aid of an audio amplifier and speaker. Since the health and the electrical activity of the muscle are directly affected by the peripheral nerve that innervates it, the muscle's response is a reflection of the health of the nerve as well. All cranial and spinal nerve skeletal muscle can be examined. Paravertebral muscle examination can be used to localize ventral nerve root disease. Limb muscles can be examined to determine if nerves of the brachial and lumbosacral plexus might be diseased. The needle EMG is therefore used to determine if the disease process is focal, diffuse, or multifocal and may detect abnormalities not seen on the neurologic examination.

When the recording needle electrode is held still and the normal patient has complete muscle relaxation, little activity is seen. If the recording electrode is held still in the muscle but the muscle is not relaxed, motor unit action potentials (MUAPs) are seen. These action potentials represent muscle fiber contraction due to reflex or voluntary stimulation by the nerve. MUAPs may vary in amplitude but are generally biphasic or triphasic. The number of action potentials depends on the strength of the contraction. In a struggling animal, these potentials may obliterate all other electrical activity, so generally the animal must be anesthetized for the rest of the examination. Many of the MUAPs may be polyphasic, with four or more phases in motor-unit disease.

A sharp burst of electrical activity appears in the normal relaxed muscle when the recording electrode is inserted and stops when the electrode is stationary. This electrical activity is called the insertional activity and represents potentials produced by the mechanical irritation of the muscle cell membrane with the tip of the recording electrode. The sound associated with insertional activity is sharp and crisp, stopping abruptly upon cessation of electrode movement.

After a nerve is injured, it generally takes a minimum of five days for the muscle to demonstrate abnormal insertional activity. It may take three weeks for maximal changes to be seen. In either neuropathy or myopathy, as the needle electrode is moved in the muscle, a burst of electrical activity with a characteristic wave form appears and continues after the electrode stops moving. Positive sharp waves with an initial primary deflection downward or in the positive direction on the oscilloscope, followed by a smaller upward or negative phase may be seen following insertion (Figure 64–4). Only a few positive sharp waves may appear after insertion or there may be trains of 50 or 100 per second. The trains of positive sharp waves may sound like a racing car speeding by.

Bizarre high-frequency discharges are another electrical disturbance that may be seen after insertional activity. These are trains of polyphasic discharges that reach a frequency of 200 per second (Figure 64–5). It is thought that these discharges originate from the muscle spindles within the muscle. These have been referred to as pseudomyotonic discharges, but this term is confusing, as bizarre high-frequency discharges are seen in both nerve and muscle disease. Myotonic discharges are trains of positive sharp waves and bizarre high-frequency discharges that wax and wane visually and audibly following insertion of the electrode and are found only in animals with the muscle membrane defect myotonia (see Chapter 65).

Spontaneous electrical discharges called fasciculation and fibrillation potentials occur if a muscle is denervated or diseased. When the electrode is still within the belly of the muscle and the muscle is relaxed, the potentials spontaneously appear on the oscilloscope. Fasciculation potentials are visible through the skin or mucous membranes. Amplitude, duration, and shape of these potentials may vary. They are identified by an irregular firing rate and rhythm, usually less than three or four per second. Fibrillation potentials have an amplitude of 5 to 30 microvolts, a duration of 0.5 to 2 milliseconds, and frequency of 2 to 10 per second (Figure 64–6). Their sound resembles that of eggs frying. The fasciculations are thought to be spontaneous discharges from part or all of the motor unit, whereas fibrillation potentials are thought to be discharges from single muscle fibers.

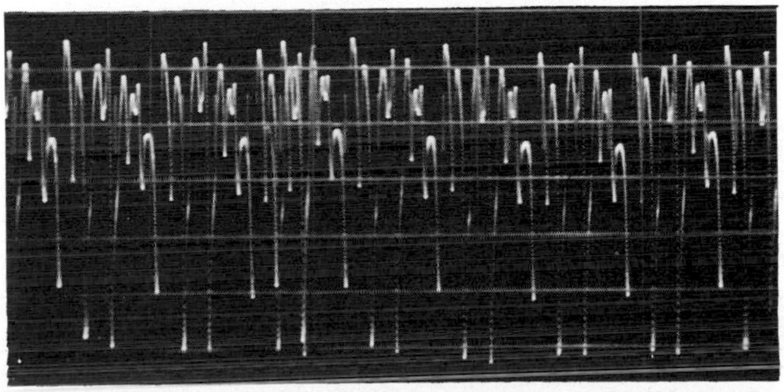

FIGURE 64–5. Bizarre high-frequency discharges may be seen after insertional activity in neuromuscular disease: 100 microvolts per centimeter, 30 milliseconds per major division.

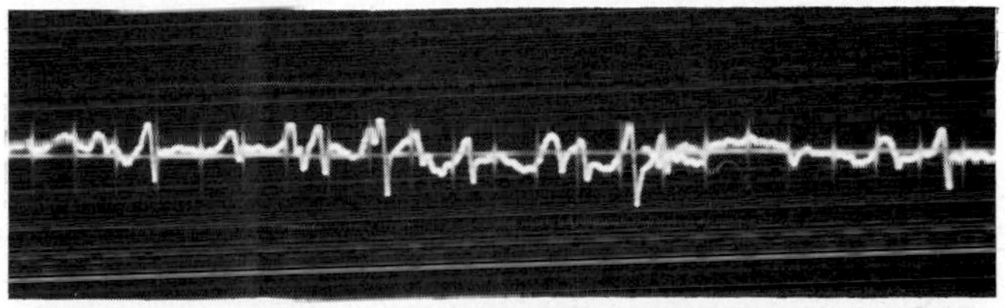

FIGURE 64–6. Fibrillation potentials are spontaneously occurring electrical discharges seen in neuromuscular disease: 100 microvolts per centimeter, 30 milliseconds per major division.

Fibrillation potentials may be seen with positive sharp waves during electrode insertion in many neuropathies and myopathies.

Nerve stimulation. Nerve stimulation studies are used to help localize the lesion within the motor unit to nerve root, peripheral axon, neuromuscular junction, or muscle. Nerve stimulation can help determine the integrity of a traumatized nerve 72 hours after the injury. The distal segment of a severed nerve may still respond prior to that time. The motor nerve is evaluated by placing stimulating electrodes in an area of the nerve to be tested and a recording electrode in the corresponding muscle it innervates (Figure 64–7). The nerve is given a supramaximal electrical stimulus and, after a brief delay, an action potential is recorded from the muscle and displayed on the oscilloscope. The time delay measured on the oscilloscope, from the time of the stimulus artifact to the onset of the action potential, is called the nerve latency and is measured in milliseconds. This time includes the conduction along the myelinated axons, the slowing through the nonmyelinated terminal branches, the delay of transmission across the neuromuscular junction, and the contraction of the muscle. In order to determine the conduction along the axon alone, a second site on the nerve must be stimulated and its latency determined (Figure 64–8). The conduction velocity for that nerve is then calculated by subtracting the two latencies and dividing this value into the distance between the two stimulation sites. The velocity is expressed in meters per second. Conduction velocities for peripheral nerves of the limbs are usually 50 meters per second or greater in most laboratories. The conduction velocity depends on the temperature of the limb and is slower in a cool limb. During nerve-stimulation studies, not only the latency but also the amplitude and the shape of the evoked response should be examined. If the response has a low amplitude, neuromuscular junction disease may be present. Repetitive nerve stimulation at five stimulations per second is used to evaluate the neuromuscular junction, and in a disease such as myasthenia gravis, the action potential amplitude decreases on the first three stimulations (see Chapter 65).

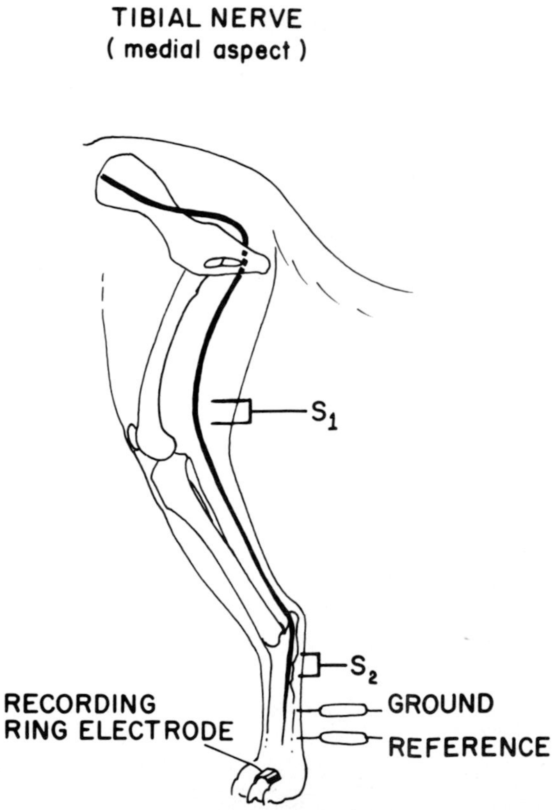

FIGURE 64–7. The electrode placement for tibial nerve stimulation. S1, the proximal stimulation site; S2, the distal stimulation site. The time from S1 to the recording ring electrode is conduction latency 1. The time from S2 to the recording ring electrode is conduction latency 2. (From Chrisman, C: Electromyography in Animals. *In* Bojrab, J (ed): Pathophysiology in Small Animal Surgery. Philadelphia, Lea and Febiger, 1981.)

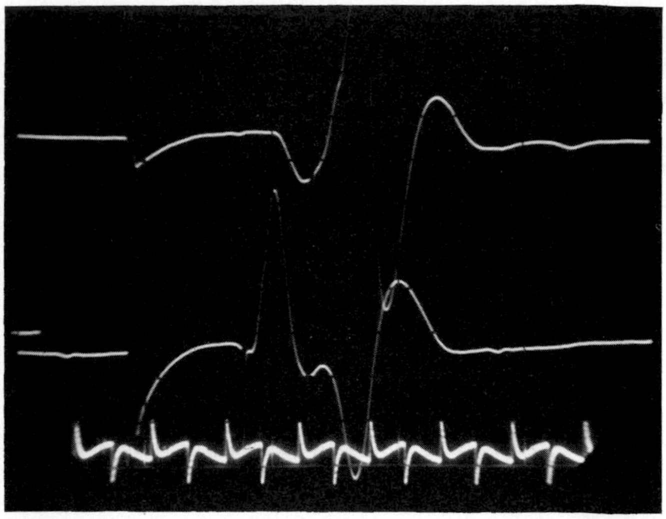

FIGURE 64–8. Nerve conduction. Conduction latency = time between the stimulus artifact on the left and the onset of the action potential to the right. Top tracing is stimulated proximally on the nerve; middle tracing is stimulated distally on the nerve: 2000 microvolts per centimeter, 5 milliseconds per major division.

Nerve conduction velocity = distance between stimulated points (meters) ÷ (conduction latency$_1$ − conduction latency$_2$)

Sensory nerve conduction studies of the peripheral nerves of the limbs may also be performed by stimulating the sensory nerves of the toe and recording the evoked action potential over the nerve itself.[7–9] The nerve action potential is a low-amplitude negative response. The latency is measured from the stimulation artifact to the onset of the response. The conduction velocity is calculated by dividing the latency into the distance between the stimulating and recording sites. Fifty meters per second and above is considered normal for peripheral sensory nerves.

Table 64–5 outlines EMG changes with disease at various sites within the neuromuscular system.

Biopsy and Pathology of Peripheral Nerves. If a polyneuropathy is suspected, a nerve biopsy may be examined microscopically. A biopsy may be obtained by removing only a fascicle of the nerve a few centimeters in length and leaving the rest intact. The nerves may be embedded in Epon and one-micron transverse and longitudinal sections cut and stained with toluidine blue for light microscopy. Transverse and longitudinal nerve sections are evaluated for number, size, and density of nerve fibers as well as for the presence of

TABLE 64–5. NEEDLE EMG AND NERVE STIMULATION STUDIES IN NEUROMUSCULAR DISORDERS

Disorder	Needle EMG Findings	Nerve Stimulation	Nerve Conduction Velocity
Polyradiculopathy	Trains of positive waves and fibrillation potentials; bizarre high-frequency discharges; decreased number MUAPs; polyphasic MUAPs	Evoked response normal or polyphasic, amplitude may be reduced	Normal
Polyradiculoneuropathy or polyneuropathy	Trains of positive waves and fibrillation potentials; bizarre high-frequency discharges; decreased MUAPs; polyphasic MUAPs	Evoked response normal or polyphasic, amplitude may be reduced	Decreased
Neuromuscular junction (NMJ)	Normal insertion; decreased or no MUAPs (NMJ blockade)	Decreased or no evoked response (NMJ blockade); decremental response on repetitive stimulation (myasthenia gravis)	Normal (if can record), unless concurrent polyneuropathy
Polymyopathy	May be normal insertion or trains of positive waves and fibrillation potentials; increased number but decreased amplitude of MUAPs	Evoked response normal or low amplitude and polyphasic	Normal

inflammatory cells. Another part of the fascicle biopsied may be specially prepared and the individual fibers teased apart for longitudinal examination. Segmental demyelination and axonal degeneration are readily seen on examination of teased fiber preparations.

If nerve terminal disease in suspected, then a biopsy of the muscle at the motor point, the area where the nerve enters the muscle, is obtained and a methylene blue stain can be applied. Nerve terminal degeneration and regeneration may be seen, supporting the diagnosis of a distal axonopathy.

FOCAL DISEASES OF CRANIAL PERIPHERAL NERVES

Anosmia, blindness, strabismus, pupillary dilatation, dropped jaw, atrophy of the head muscles, increased or decreased facial sensation, facial paralysis, deafness, head tilt, equilibrium loss, dysphagia, megaesophagus, laryngeal paralysis, and tongue paralysis are all signs associated with cranial nerve dysfunction.[10, 11] These signs may be associated with disease of the peripheral cranial nerves or their respective nuclei in the brain stem, from the diencephalon through the myelencephalon or medulla oblongata (see Chapter 60).

If a focal disease process is affecting one or more peripheral cranial nerves without brain stem involvement, then no abnormalities should be detected on evaluation of the strength, coordination, and proprioception of the limbs or spinal reflexes. If other abnormalities are found along with the cranial nerve deficits on the neurologic examination, then a focal or multifocal brain stem lesion or multifocal or diffuse neuromuscular disorder is more likely. Only focal disease processes affecting one or more peripheral cranial nerves are discussed in this section.

The most common mechanisms for focal cranial nerve disease, in order of decreasing frequency, are traumatic, idiopathic, neoplastic, and inflammatory or infectious disorders.

OLFACTORY NERVES (CRANIAL NERVE I)

Hyposmia or anosmia is a decreased ability or inability to smell and may be caused by blockage of the nasal passages or primary disease of the olfactory nervous system. The owner may complain that the animal is unable to find its food but readily eats if food is placed in its mouth.

Rhinitis that produces mucosal swelling, collection of exudates, and blockage of nasal passages is the most common cause of hyposmia or anosmia. The olfactory impairment generally returns to normal once the rhinitis clears.

Nasal neoplasms, such as mucoid epidermoid carcinomas, may block nasal passages, erode through the cribriform plate, and directly affect olfactory nerves and bulbs to produce alterations in olfaction. The initial primary complaint is usually a chronic nasal discharge and not olfactory disturbances. By the time olfactory disturbances develop, the prefrontal cerebral cortex is also involved and personality disorders are often apparent. Other neoplasms of the prefrontal cerebral cortex also may affect olfaction.

Cranial trauma, a common cause of permanent and transient hyposmia and anosmia in humans, is rare in animals owing to the protective effect of the large frontal sinuses.

OPTIC NERVES (CRANIAL NERVE II)

Disorders of the optic nerves producing blindness and dilated pupils are discussed in Chapter 63 and include optic nerve hypoplasia, optic neuritis, optic nerve trauma, or neoplastic processes affecting the optic nerves.

OCULOMOTOR (CRANIAL NERVE III), TROCHLEAR (CRANIAL NERVE IV), AND ABDUCENS (CRANIAL NERVE VI) NERVES

The oculomotor, trochlear, and abducens nerves innervate the extraocular muscles and produce eyeball movement. If these cranial nerves are diseased, strabismus, an uncontrollable deviation from the normal axis of one or both eyeballs, is seen.

Bacterial or viral infections of individual cranial nerves unassociated with brain stem involvement are rare. Traumatic injury to these cranial nerves may occur with skull fractures in the area of the orbital fissure where all three nerves exit the skull. The result is a fixed, immobile eyeball.

Neurofibroma, neurofibrosarcoma, neurinoma, and lymphosarcoma are tumors of peripheral nerves that might affect cranial nerves III, IV, and VI and produce strabismus. Meningiomas may also compress these nerves where they exit the brain stem. Eventually limb proprioceptive deficit and weakness, evidence of brain stem compression, can be detected on the neurologic examination.

Diagnosis and prognosis of strabismus may be aided by serial neurologic examinations to differentiate a static or improving disease process such as trauma from a progressive disorder such as infection or neoplasia (see Chapter 63).

TRIGEMINAL NERVES (CRANIAL NERVE V)

If the motor portions of the trigeminal nerves are affected by a disorder bilaterally, the animal is unable to close its mouth and the jaw hangs open. Occasionally trauma to the nerves bilaterally at the temporomandibular joint produces this syndrome.[12]

Idiopathic Trigeminal Neuropathy. An acute onset of inability to close the mouth with no associated trauma is seen in dogs.[13, 14] Occasionally, affected dogs have bilateral ptosis, miosis, and enophthalmus of the eyes (Horner's syndrome) as the sympathetic nerves travel for a short distance with the trigeminal nerves and are simultaneously affected (Figure 64–9). There is no masseter and temporalis muscle atrophy and sensation of the head is usually normal. Positive waves and fibrillation potentials are found in the temporalis and masseter muscles on needle EMG examination. Stimulation of the trigeminal nerves at the base of the ear evokes a contraction of masseter and temporalis muscles. Affected animals recover in one to two weeks. During that period, nutrition should be maintained by feeding a gruel that the animal can lap with the tongue. The cause of the trigeminal neuropathy is unknown. Necropsy of one case was performed and a bilateral nonsuppurative neuritis of the trigeminal nerves was found.[15] It is unknown if idiopathic trigeminal neuropathy is always a trigeminal neuritis, such as might be associated with an immune-mediated process. The prognosis appears to be excellent for recovery of trigeminal nerve function without medication. Horner's syndrome may be a permanent change in some cases. No recurrence of the signs in the same dog have been reported.

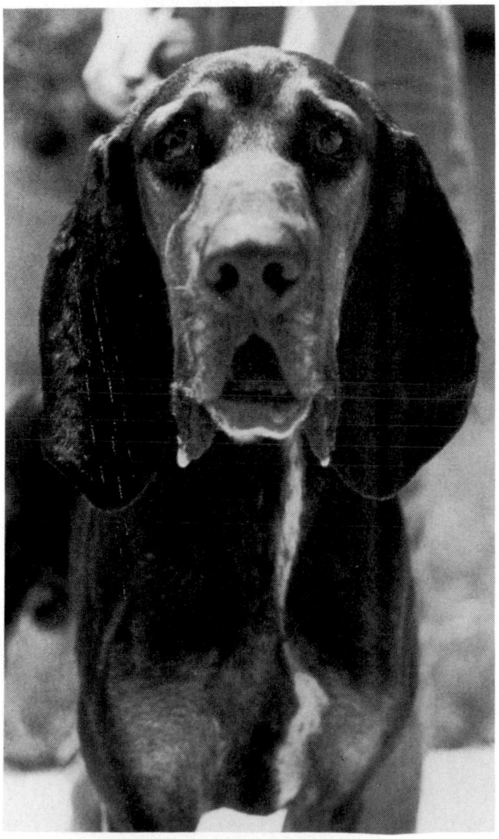

FIGURE 64–9. Idiopathic trigeminal neuropathy in a dog with a bilateral Horner's syndrome and an inability to close the mouth.

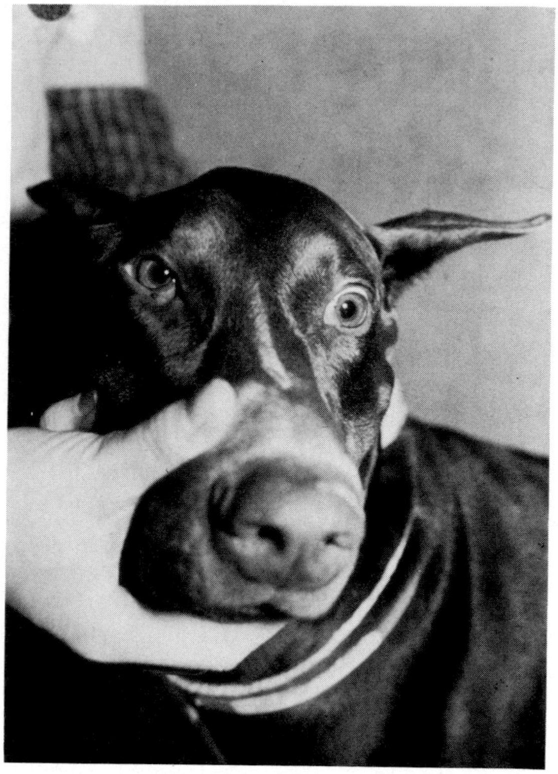

FIGURE 64–10. Atrophy of the right temporalis and masseter muscles from unilateral trigeminal nerve disease.

Trigeminal Nerve Trauma and Neoplasia. The most common cause of unilateral trigeminal nerve disease is trauma or neoplasia.[16] A weakness in jaw tone may be detected but often goes unnoticed owing to the remaining strength of the opposite side. A unilateral temporalis and masseter muscle atrophy is the most consistent abnormality (Figure 64–10). Bilateral temporalis and masseter muscle atrophy may be seen in chronic bilateral trigeminal nerve disease, but is more commonly due to a myositis (see Chapter 65). Traumatic lesions either remain the same or improve and produce a cosmetic defect due to the asymmetry of the head musculature. Peripheral nerve and meningeal tumors continue to grow and affect brain stem structures and produce signs of conscious proprioceptive deficits and paresis or paralysis of the limbs. Peripheral nerve tumors can be unrewarding to remove, since the tumor has often spread up the nerve root into the brain stem.

Sensory Trigeminal Neuropathy. Decreased facial sensation may accompany trigeminal nerve trauma or neoplasia but is rarely a complaint. Increased facial sensation is commonly seen in humans and rarely seen in animals. The author evaluated one dog with chronic face pain and inflammation associated with a foreign body found at the base of the ear involving the trigeminal nerve. Some peripheral nerve tumors may also be painful. For other cases of episodic or continual face pain or hypersensitivity, no underlying cause can be discovered. Some of these animals rub and mutilate their faces and chins. Various therapeutic trials with anticonvulsants, tranquilizers, corticosteroids, large doses of vitamin B, and hormones have given varying results in different animals. For some animals no relief can be found and the owner may prefer euthanasia.

There is one report of a two-year-old collie with an acute onset of excessive salivation, coughing, and dysphagia associated with the loss of touch and pain sensation from the face, tongue, and oral mucosa.[17] There was no change over 18 months and lesions were found at necropsy only in the gasserian ganglion and major branches of the trigeminal nerve bilaterally. The cause was unknown.

FACIAL NERVES (CRANIAL NERVE VII)

Loss of facial expression because of lack of ear and lip movement and inability to close the eyelid is the primary sign associated with facial nerve paralysis (Figure 64–11). In unilateral facial nerve paralysis an asymmetry of the face is readily apparent. Chronic, complete denervation of facial muscles may lead to muscle fibrosis and contracture of the lips and ears on the affected side (Figure 64–12). If parasympathetic fibers to the lacrimal and salivary glands are affected, the cornea and mucous membranes on that side may be dry.

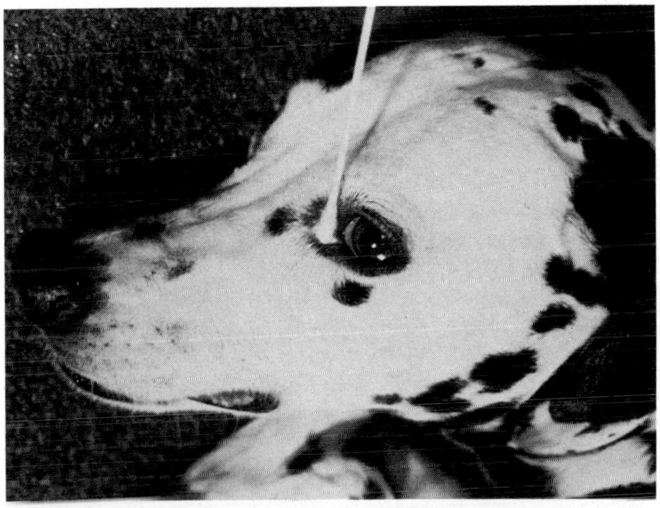

FIGURE 64–11. Facial nerve paralysis in a dog showing deviation of the nose to the normal side and inability to close the eyelid when the medial canthus is touched with a cotton swab. (From Chrisman, CL: Disorders of the vestibular system. Comp Cont Ed 10:747, 1979.)

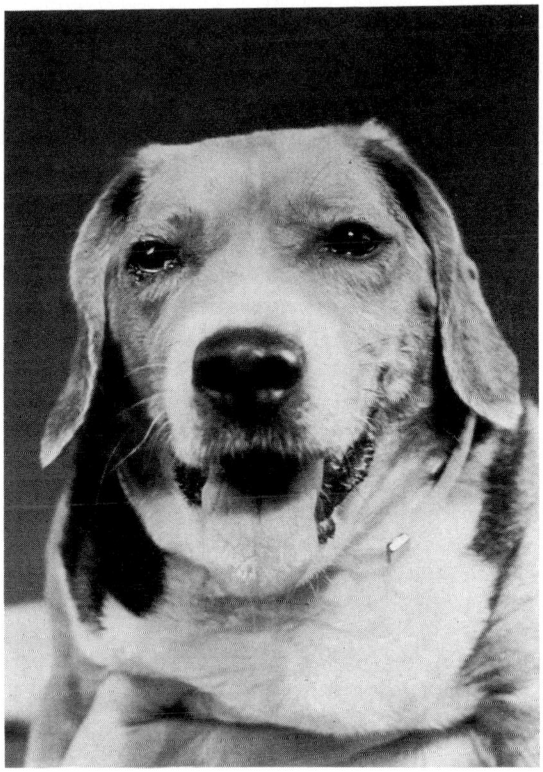

FIGURE 64–12. Chronic bilateral facial nerve paralysis with contracture of all facial muscles. (From Chrisman, CL: Disorders of the vestibular system. Comp Cont Ed 10:747, 1979.)

Middle Ear Infections. Otitis media from otitis externa or pharyngitis or of hematogenous origin may affect the facial nerve and produce paralysis. If severe inflammation of the nerve occurs, the prognosis for recovery is poor. A head tilt and other signs of vestibular nerve involvement are seen if the inner ear becomes affected. Long-term antibiotics are the therapy of choice (see drugs listed under Inner Ear Infections in the drug index).

Trauma to the Facial Nerve. A traumatic insult to the facial nerve may occur on the side of the face or base of the ear and produce paralysis of the lip or eye.[18] As a guide to prognosis, the facial nerve can be stimulated electrically at the base of the ear to determine if the distal segments are intact. If there is no response to electrical stimulation, the prognosis is poor. Traumatic lesions of the petrous temporal bone of the skull often produce facial and vestibular nerve deficits at the same time.

Neoplasia of the Facial Nerve. Facial nerve neoplasia may produce signs of facial paralysis alone if the tumor affects the nerve at the level of the middle ear or more peripherally. Concomitant vestibular deficits are seen with tumors from the inner ear to the brain stem. Meningiomas of the pontine-medullary junction may initially produce facial and vestibular nerve deficits, but as they grow and enlarge, ipsilateral hemiparesis of the limbs and other signs associated with brain stem compression are seen.

Idiopathic Unilateral and Bilateral Facial Nerve Paralysis. Idiopathic facial nerve paralysis has been reported in dogs, especially cocker spaniels.[19] The signs may be unilateral or bilateral. The underlying cause is unknown, but some cases may be due to a hypothyroid-induced peripheral neuropathy.[15] Some affected animals are hypothyroid, but others are not. Hypothyroid dogs may improve on thyroid replacement therapy. Some dogs spontaneously recover and others have permanent paresis or paralysis.

The main complication of facial nerve paralysis, other than the cosmetic defect, is the possibility of exposure keratitis if the tear glands are denervated. A Schirmer tear test should be performed; if moisture is low, artificial tears should be administered daily.

VESTIBULOCOCHLEAR NERVES (CRANIAL NERVE VIII)

Head tilt, circling, leaning, rolling to the affected side, and horizontal and rotary nystagmus are all signs associated with unilateral peripheral vestibular nerve disease.[20–22] Falling to either side, wide head excursions, and generalized equilibrium loss are associated with bilateral peripheral vestibular nerve disease. Deafness is most commonly produced by bilateral receptor and cochlear nerve disease.

Congenital and Familial Vestibulocochlear Nerve Disease. Equilibrium disturbances and deafness from birth may be associated with lack of development of either or both the vestibular or auditory receptors of the inner ears. Congenital deafness with normal equilibrum is common in Dalmatians, English setters, and blue-eyed white cats. The deafness is permanent. A congenital vestibulopathy is seen in Doberman pinschers between 4 to 16 weeks of age and a head tilt and circling are the most obvious signs. Many affected puppies improve with age; others retain the head tilt or circle when excited.

Ototoxic Drugs. The aminoglycoside antibiotics, particularly streptomycin, dihydrostreptomycin, gentamicin, and kanamycin, may produce equilibrium disturbances and deafness.[23] The toxic damage produced by these drugs is often permanent.

Inner Ear Infections. A common cause of unilateral and bilateral vestibular disorders is an inner ear infection (Figure 64–13). The animal should be anesthetized so that the external ear canals, tympanic membranes, and pharynx can be carefully examined and radiographs of the skull obtained. In chronic infections, thickening or lysis of the osseous bullae and petrous temporal bone may be seen. Skull radiographs are often normal with acute infections. Bacterial cultures and antibiotic sensitivity tests aid in selecting an appropriate antibiotic. If no cultures are available, chloramphenicol, trimethoprim sulfa, or cephalexin is recommended (see drug index). The signs may improve after a few days on the therapy, but the antibiotic should be continued for four to six weeks unless contraindicated for other reasons. In most cases the signs may quickly return if only one to two weeks of antibiotic therapy are given. If the tympanic membrane is ruptured, irritating or oil-based external ear medications should not be used, as they may damage or accumulate in the middle ear. If the infection is diagnosed early and treated aggressively, the prognosis is good, but a residual head tilt and facial nerve paralysis may occur. Some cases develop chronic bilateral infections that lead to osteomyelitis of the osseous bullae and petrous temporal bone. Radical surgical drainage procedures may be needed to clear or control the infection. On occasion, especially in cats, the infection may ascend the vestibulocochlear and facial nerves to the brain stem and produce a brain stem abscess or meningitis.

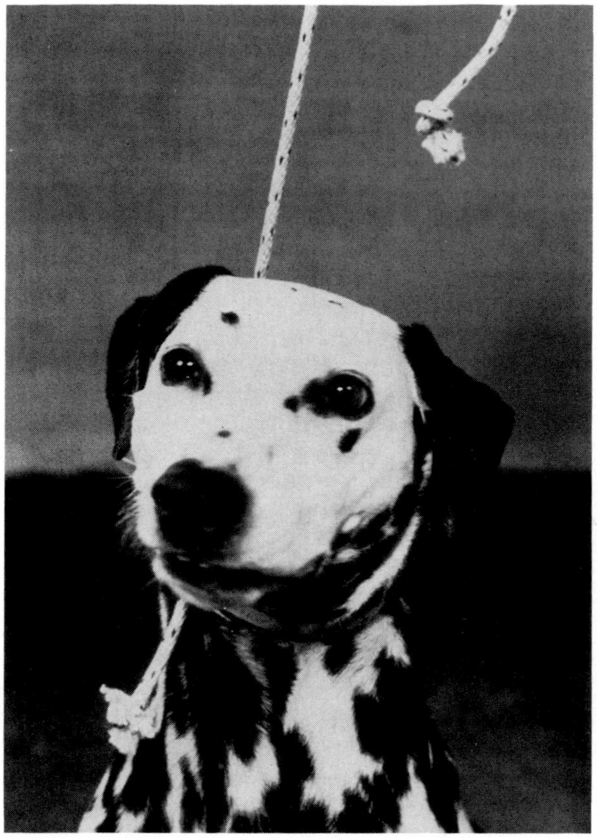

FIGURE 64–13. A dog with a left middle and inner ear infection and an associated left head tilt and facial nerve paralysis. (From Chrisman, CL: Disorders of the vestibular system. Comp Cont Ed 10:747, 1979.)

Vestibular Nerve Tumors. Neurofibromas, neurofibrosarcomas, neurinomas, and squamous cell carcinomas produce a slow, progressive head tilt and usually an associated facial nerve paralysis on the same side.[16, 24] Meningiomas of the pontine-medullary region may initially produce a head tilt and facial paralysis on one side, but evidence of brain stem compression, such as ipsilateral hemiparesis and conscious proprioceptive deficits, as well as trigeminal and abducens nerve paralysis, will eventually be seen.

Idiopathic Vestibular Neuropathies. In cats and aged dogs, an idiopathic, acute vestibulopathy is commonly seen.[20, 22, 25] Equilibrium may be so severely altered that the animal may initially be unable to stand, will roll or continually fall to one side, and have a severe head tilt. Spontaneous horizontal or rotary nystagmus is also common. The condition has been incorrectly referred to as "stroke" in geriatric dogs, as it is a peracute neurologic dysfunction. Many dogs may be mistakenly euthanatized because the condition initially appears so severe. Skull radiographs and cerebrospinal fluid are normal. Within 72 hours, both dogs and cats improve and are often able to stand. Equilibrium is often still abnormal, but the nystagmus decreases and then disappears. Regardless of therapy, most dogs and cats are normal within two weeks. Improvement of the signs on serial neurologic examinations is the best guide to prognosis. Sometimes a permanent head tilt remains, but the animals can function well and are acceptable pets. The underlying cause is presently unknown. The author has seen bilateral idiopathic vestibulopathies in cats. Most of these animals have dysequilibrium, fall to either side, and are deaf. Affected animals may slowly improve equillibrium and hearing over many months but usually retain some residual deficit.

GLOSSOPHARYNGEAL AND VAGUS NERVES (CRANIAL NERVES IX AND X)

Dysphagia. Bilateral glossopharyngeal or vagus nerve lesions may produce dysphagia or difficulty in swallowing. Focal bilateral disease of these nerves is rare. Dysphagia is most commonly associated with multifocal and diffuse neuromuscular diseases, such as polyneuropathies, myasthenia gravis, neuromuscular junction blockade, and polymyopathies. Dysphagia can result in aspiration of fluids and pneumonia and be a complication of many of these diseases. Cricopharyngeal achalasia produces dysphagia, but the cause of the disorder is currently unknown (see Chapter 67).

Megaesophagus. Cervical vagus nerve lesions produce megaesophagus and laryngeal paralysis, while bilateral thoracic vagus nerve lesions located distal to the recurrent laryngeal nerve produce megaesophagus alone. Megaesophagus is often associated with polymyositis and myasthenia gravis (see Chapter 65). The underlying neuromuscular disturbance in congenital and idiopathic megaesophagus and esophageal achalasia is currently unknown (see Chapter 83).

Laryngeal Paresis or Paralysis. Diseases of the cranial and recurrent laryngeal branches of the vagus nerve produce laryngeal paresis or paralysis.[26–28] A change in the voice, increased upper airway noise, and dyspnea are the main signs of disease. Bilateral lesions produce bilateral laryngeal paresis or paralysis and the animal may have severe cyanosis. Unilateral vagus nerve lesions produce ipsilateral laryngeal hemiplegia and little noticeable dysphagia or megaesophagus. As with dysphagia and megaesophagus, laryngeal paresis or paralysis may be associated with diffuse or multifocal neuromuscular disease.

Bouvier des Flandres and Siberian huskies may have a congenital laryngeal paralysis by four to six months of age.[29] A loss of endurance, laryngeal stridor, dyspnea, and cyanosis are prominent clinical signs. Partial laryngectomy is the therapy of choice. An idiopathic, spontaneous laryngeal paralysis with no other neurologic deficits has been reported in adult large breed dogs and cats.[30] Surgical correction is often necessary to restore a patent airway.[31]

Trauma and neoplasia of the recurrent laryngeal nerve may be a cause of laryngeal hemiplegia.[32] The prognosis for neoplasia is generally poor.

SPINAL ACCESSORY NERVES (CRANIAL NERVE XI)

Primary disease of the spinal accessory nerve is rare and is manifested by atrophy of its muscle supply in the neck. Fractures of the base of the skull may injure the nerve and produce atrophy.

HYPOGLOSSAL NERVE (CRANIAL NERVE XII)

Symmetrical tongue weakness or atrophy is usually associated with a diffuse or multifocal neuromuscular or central nervous system disease.

Hypoglossal Nerve Trauma and Neoplasia. Difficulty in lapping water and in eating and unilateral muscle atrophy with no other signs may be due to injury or neoplasia of the hypoglossal nerve. The prognosis for neoplasia is generally poor.

FOCAL DISEASES OF SPINAL NERVES

SPINAL NERVE ROOT DISORDERS

Most of the common spinal root disorders are discussed in Chapter 62. Intervertebral disc herniation, congenital vertebral abnormalities, spondylosis deformans, inflammation, and tumors may directly affect the nerve roots. If nerve roots of the brachial plexus or lumbosacral plexus are involved, there may be decreased or absent spinal reflexes and muscle atrophy in the affected limb. Electromyographic examination of the paravertebral muscles aids in detecting and localizing motor nerve root disease. *Toxoplasma gondii* infection of the spinal cord and meninges may also produce a radiculitis. Other bacterial, viral, and fungal agents may produce a radiculitis in association with meningitis.

TRAUMATIC PERIPHERAL NEUROPATHIES

General Diagnosis, Therapy, and Prognosis. The most common cause of focal spinal nerve disease is trauma.[33] A recent automobile accident, fall, or some other incident producing injury may be ascertained from the history. Physical examination may show lacerations, bruising, or fractures. In many cases, there may be no signs of trauma. Neurologic evaluation includes examining for voluntary movement, limb reflexes, muscle atrophy, and superficial and deep sensations. This examination localizes the nerves injured and determines the severity of the injury.

Neurapraxia is a loss of nerve function caused by a physiologic dysfunction, not degeneration of the nerve. Neurapraxia lasts 3 to 12 weeks in humans, but its duration in animals is unknown. Neurotmesis is a complete severance of a nerve, and no function will return unless the nerve is repaired by surgery. Axonotmesis is a rupture or severance of axons within a nerve with the supporting structures and the neurilemmal sheath of the nerve still intact. The axons undergo wallerian degeneration, then sprout and regrow along the intact neurilemmal sheath to reinnervate the muscle. The rate of growth averages about one millimeter per day or one inch per month. Most nerve injuries are the result of stretching, direct blows, excessive pressure, or injections, and are often a combination of neurapraxia and axonotmesis. Local edema and hemorrhage at the site of injury also contribute to the loss of nerve function.

The EMG examination may be used to evaluate nerve integrity and to differentiate between neurapraxia, neurotmesis, and axonotmesis. Nerve stimulation studies should be delayed for 72 hours after the injury. An outline of serial EMG changes associated with peripheral nerve injuries can be found in Table 64–6.

When an injury can be localized to a certain portion of the nerve, the distance from the injury site to the muscle to be reinnervated may be measured and a time for regeneration estimated using one inch per month as a guide. The closer the nerve injury is to the muscle it must reinnervate, the better the prognosis. As time goes on, the neurilemmal sheath tube shrinks and denervated muscle fibers become fibrotic. Any injury over 12 inches long will probably not even make anatomic contact with the muscle, because the neurilemmal tube will be closed. Serial improvement of signs and MNCV returning to normal on neurologic and EMG examinations, respectively, are the most accurate indications of an improving prognosis.[34]

During the period when the nerve is regenerating, the denervated muscle undergoes severe atrophy. Because of disuse, the denervated muscle has a decreased blood supply, which further contributes to muscle atrophy. Physical therapy can assist in overcoming circulation problems and delaying muscle atrophy. It is the primary treatment for all nerve injuries. Physical therapy may include the use of heat, ultrasound, and exercises. In veterinary medicine, the most practical source of heat and the most effective form of massage is the whirlpool. Animals should receive whirlpool therapy two or three times daily for 15 to 20 minutes on affected areas. The water should not be too hot, in order to avoid damaging the desensitized skin. If a whirlpool is not available, warm water baths or hot towels and simultaneous massage may be substituted.

Denervated muscles must be protected from overstretching by gravity or strong antagonist muscles. A spoon splint leg brace supporting the carpus or tarsus may be used to facilitate walking but should be removed often to insure good circulation to the foot. Passive manipulation of all joints and stretching of the tendons should be performed several times daily to prevent contractures. The desensitized limb must be protected from lacerations and abrasions, which commonly occur on the dorsal surface of the paw. Even with the best regimen of physical therapy, muscles that remain denervated atrophy and fibrose and permanent contracture of muscles and tendons results.

During certain stages of the regeneration period, the animal may begin to mutilate the paw because of tingling or itching sensations produced by the regeneration of sensory nerves. This period is usually transient but can be very frustrating for the owner and veterinarian. The animal may produce severe lesions by self-mutilation, regardless of attempts to bandage and protect the foot. Elizabethan collars, muzzles, wire mesh foot guards, and leather boots are among the many things that have been tried in individual cases. Corticosteroid therapy often has little effect.

The overall prognosis for most nerve injuries depends on the severity of the injury, how much of the dysfunction is due to neurapraxia and how much to axonotmesis, how far the injury occurs from the muscles denervated, and the owner's commitment to provide months of physical therapy.

If there is no response to electrical stimulation, surgical exploration of the nerve may be performed to repair the nerve. Peripheral nerve surgery techniques are well described elsewhere.[35]

If electromyography is not available, serial neurologic

TABLE 64–6. SERIAL ELECTROMYOGRAPHIC CHANGES ASSOCIATED WITH PERIPHERAL NERVE INJURIES

Phase	Needle EMG Findings	Nerve Stimulation Studies
Acute (1–7 days)	May be normal insertional activity Axonotmesis or neurotmesis after 5–7 days may get positive sharp waves and fibrillation potentials May get MUAPs if some intact axons In neurapraxia, EMG may be normal	No response on proximal stump May be a response on distal stump for 72 hours after injury A response after 72 hours indicates some nerve integrity Low amplitude of evoked response indicates axonotmesis Slowed conduction velocity in severe injury In neurapraxia, distal segment will stimulate normally
Subacute (10–21 days)	In neurapraxia, EMG will be normal In axonotmesis or neurotmesis—many positive sharp waves and fibrillation potentials Appearance of MUAP is a good sign	It is a good sign if amplitude of evoked response increases It is a good sign if conduction velocity increases more toward normal
Chronic (longer than 3 months)	Fibrosis of the muscle may be felt during insertion of the electrode Fibrillation potentials will still be present in denervated muscle fibers MUAPs may be decreased in number, polyphasic, and increased in amplitude	Amplitude of evoked response should be increasing with regeneration but may be polyphasic The nearer the conduction velocity is to normal the better the prognosis

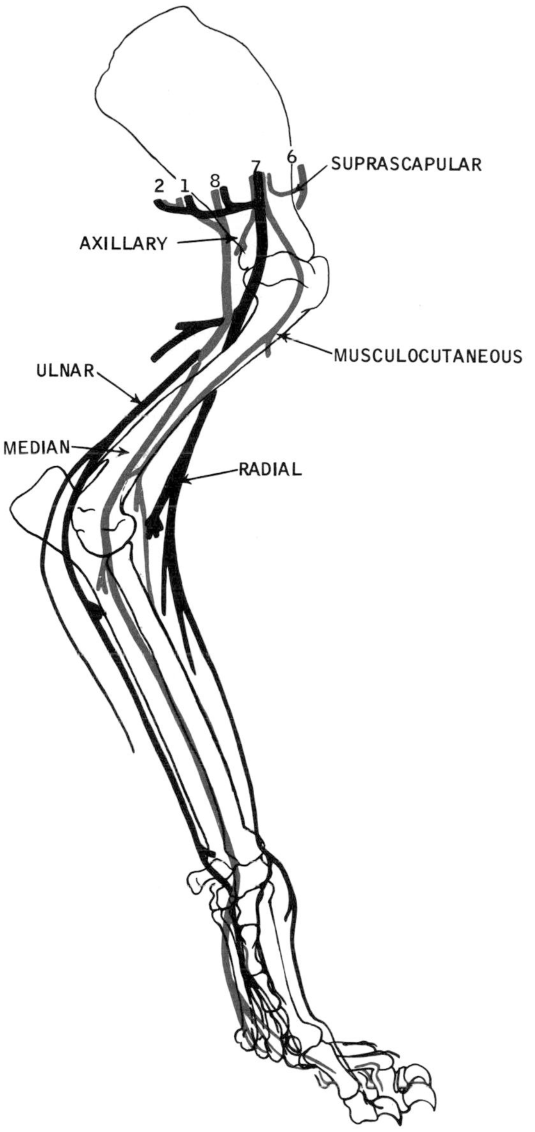

FIGURE 64–14. Diagram of the major nerves of the forelimb from a medial view. (From Hoerlein, B. F. [ed] Canine Neurology, 3rd ed. Philadelphia, W. B. Saunders Company, 1978.)

examinations should be performed over several months. If there has been no change in the neurologic status for several months and surgical repair is impossible, then surgery for joint fusion or tendon transplant of the carpus or tarsus may be considered.[36] Amputation of the limb is a last resort and is considered only when no improvement occurs after several months of critical evaluation.

Brachial Plexus Avulsion or Stretch. Brachial plexus nerve root avulsion is one of the most common traumatic nerve disorders in the dog and cat.[37–40] The nerve roots and brachial plexus are shown in Figure 64–14. During severe abduction of the forelimb, nerve roots of the brachial plexus are stretched or torn from the spinal cord. In extreme abduction the dorsal edge of the scapula moves medioventrally, temporarily inverting to produce severe tension on the nerve roots of the brachial plexus. The physical examination may show no evidence of fractures or bruising, but the animal is unable to bear any weight on the limb, which is dragged when gaiting (Figure 64–15).

Neurologic examination of the forelimb in complete avulsion shows no flexor reflex, extensor thrust reflex, triceps and biceps tendon reflexes, sensation over the limb below the elbow, or deep sensation from the digits (Table 64–3).[41] Atrophy may become apparent in all the muscles of the forelimb. Diagnosis is further supported by thoracic fluoroscopy, which dynamically demonstrates a flaccid diaphragm on the side of the lesion. Sympathetic innervation to the pupils and eyelids arises from spinal cord segments C7 to T2 and courses rostrally to innervate these structures. If the avulsion includes these nerve roots close to the spinal cord, ptosis, miosis, and enophthalmus (Horner's syndrome) result on the affected side.

Positive waves, fibrillation potentials, bizarre high-frequency discharges, and lack of voluntary motor units in the forelimb muscles (and often C6-T2 paravertebral muscles on the same side) are found on needle EMG examination if the avulsion is complete. Nerve stimulation three to seven days after the injury shows no response of the nerves of the limb. If the nerve roots are torn from the spinal cord in complete avulsion, surgical repair is usually unsuccessful and limb amputation may be necessary. If the brachial plexus is neurapraxic or partially damaged, as previously discussed, repeated neurologic and EMG examinations enable the reinnervation process to be followed as a guide to prognosis. If conscientious physical therapy is instituted,

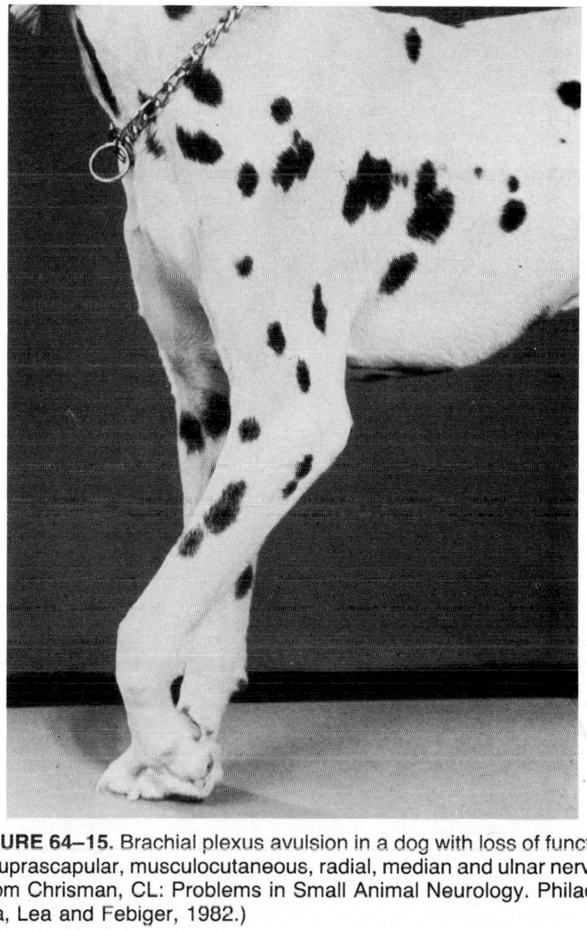

FIGURE 64–15. Brachial plexus avulsion in a dog with loss of function of suprascapular, musculocutaneous, radial, median and ulnar nerves. (From Chrisman, CL: Problems in Small Animal Neurology. Philadelphia, Lea and Febiger, 1982.)

muscle atrophy and tendon contraction may be minimal, and the limb may be functional again.

Suprascapular Nerve Injury. The suprascapular nerve may be injured as it crosses the cranial border of the distal scapula and may produce atrophy of the supraspinatus and infraspinatus muscles (Figure 64–14). There is little motor deficit in the affected limb during gaiting (Table 64–3). Electromyographic examination may show positive waves, fibrillation potentials, and bizarre high-frequency discharges in muscles innervated by the suprascapular nerve. If MUAPs are seen, some axons within the nerve remain intact. Nerve stimulation studies may be performed by stimulation of the suprascapular nerve at the cranial border of the distal scapula. If there is no indication that the nerve is intact, the nerve may be surgically explored. Although loss of this nerve causes little functional loss to the limb when gaiting, the associated muscular atrophy produces a cosmetic defect that becomes very apparent in shorthaired dogs and cats.

Radial Nerve Injury. Radial nerve injury is most frequently associated with brachial plexus injury but may occur alone with fractures of the humerus (Figure 64–14). On neurologic evaluation there is a loss of extensor thrust reflex and the leg can bear no weight and knuckles onto the dorsum of the paw (Table 64–3). Sensation may be diminished or lost over the dorsal and lateral aspects of the foreleg and the dorsal aspect of the paw. Atrophy of the triceps and the extensors of the carpus and digits occurs. When injury occurs without damage to the innervation of the triceps, extension of the elbow is possible and the animal will bear weight but will knuckle onto the dorsum of the paw. In time, the animal may compensate and knuckle less. However, lack of physical therapy may lead to contracture of the flexor tendons of the carpus, which can cause the animal to knuckle continually and injure the dorsum of the paw. Needle EMG examination may show positive waves, fibrillation potentials, and bizarre high-frequency discharges. MUAPs may be seen if the nerve is intact. The radial nerve may be stimulated on the lateral humerus and the response recorded in one of the extensor muscles of the carpus. If there is a lack of response to electrical stimulation, the nerve should be surgically explored and repaired.

Median and Ulnar Nerve Injury. Injury of the median and ulnar nerves may occur with distal humeral fractures, fractures of the radius and ulna, or a blow to the nerves in these regions (Figure 64–14). A loss of flexion of the carpus and digits occurs. Owing to the inability to flex, there is overextension or sinking of the carpus with weight bearing. In ulnar nerve damage, there is decreased or absent sensation to the caudal forearm, the dorsolateral aspect of the fifth digit, and the lateral volar side of the paw. In median nerve damage, there is decreased or absent sensation to the medial volar paw (Table 64–3).

Positive waves, fibrillation potentials, and bizarre high-frequency discharges in the specific muscles innervated by each nerve are seen on needle EMG examination. MUAPs are seen only if the nerves are intact. Stimulation of the ulnar nerve may be performed at the caudal medial elbow and again at the medial carpus, with the recording electrode in the volar interosseous muscles of the digits. If there is no response to electrical stimulation, the nerve should be surgically explored and repaired.

Sciatic Nerve Injury. Sciatic nerve injury is commonly caused by fractures of the ilium, fractures and surgical trauma at the proximal femur, and improper intramuscular injections (Figure 64–16).[42–47] The extensor muscles of the stifle joint are intact and enable the animal to support weight. As the animal is gaited, the hock flexes and extends passively, and knuckling of the paw is seen. There is a loss of the flexor reflex of the stifle and hock (Table 64–4). Injury to the sciatic nerve within the pelvic canal produces loss of hip extension, the hip flexes, and the limb is deviated toward the midline. Sciatic nerve injury results in decreased or absent sensation on the lateral surface of the limb below the stifle and on the rostral and caudal surfaces of the tarsus and paw. Sensation of a narrow strip of skin down the medial side of the limb to the dorsal surface of the

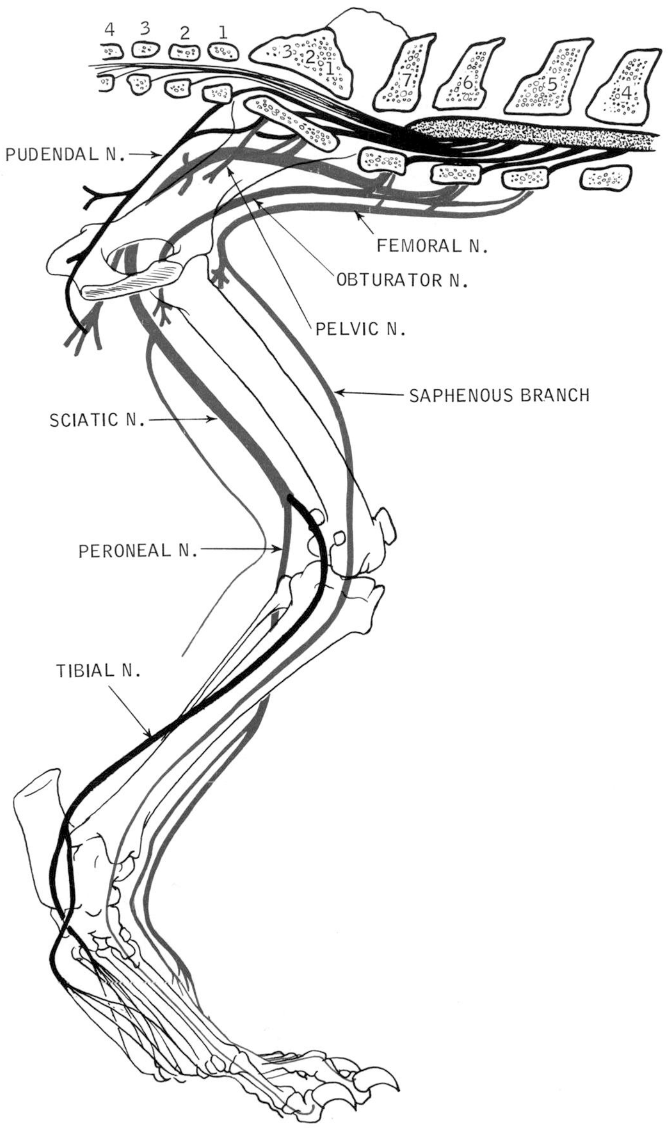

FIGURE 64–16. Diagram of the major nerves of the hindlimb from a medial view. (From Hoerlein, B. F. [ed]: Canine Neurology, 3rd ed. Philadelphia, W. B. Saunders Company, 1978.)

second digit is supplied by the saphenous nerve, a branch of the femoral nerve, so it is normal. Distribution of EMG abnormalities may aid in localizing the level of sciatic nerve injury. The sciatic nerve may be stimulated at the caudal aspect of the hip joint. If the nerve is unresponsive to electrical stimulation, exploration and repair of the nerve should be performed.

Peroneal or Fibular Nerve Injury. The peroneal nerve is a terminal branch of the sciatic nerve and is especially vulnerable to trauma on the lateral aspect of the stifle joint (Figure 64–16).[48] A lack of flexor reflex of the hock occurs and the animal knuckles during gaiting (Table 64–4). There is also a lack of sensation on the dorsal surface of the limb below the stifle and on the dorsal surface of the paw. Needle EMG abnormalities of positive waves, fibrillation potentials, and bizarre high-frequency discharges may be found in the flexor muscles of the hock and the extensors of the digits. The peroneal nerve may be stimulated on the lateral aspect of the stifle to determine whether it is intact and how severe the injury is. Exploration and repair of the nerve should be performed if it is unresponsive to electrical stimulation. In time, the animal may compensate and knuckle less, even though innervation is still deficient. Lack of physical therapy results in contracture of the digital flexor tendons and the animal continually knuckles, which produces severe abrasions on the dorsal surface of the paw. Surgical fusion of the tarsus may be necessary as a last resort.

Tibial Nerve Injury. The tibial nerve is also a terminal branch of the sciatic nerve (Figure 64–16). The animal is unable to extend the hock and stands with the hock flexed. Sensation is diminished or absent on the caudal aspect of the limb and on the plantar surface of the paw (Table 64–4). Needle EMG abnormalities of positive waves, fibrillation potentials, and bizarre high-frequency discharges may be seen in the extensors of the hock and flexors of the digits. The tibial nerve may be stimulated on the medial aspect of the rear limb at the stifle joint and again at the medial surface of the tarsus, with the recording electrode in the interosseous muscles of the plantar surface of the paw.

Femoral Nerve Injury. Injury to the femoral nerve is manifested by an inability to extend the stifle, which results in an inability to bear weight on the affected limb. The patellar reflex is absent and there is a loss of extensor thrust of the stifle. Sensation is decreased or absent on the medial surface of the thigh, stifle, leg, and paw (Table 64–4). Needle EMG abnormalities are localized in those muscles innervated by the femoral nerve. The nerve may be stimulated on the medial surface of the thigh (Figure 64–16). If the nerve is unresponsive to electrical stimulation, surgical exploration and repair of the nerve should be performed, if possible. In time, however, the animal may compensate for the inability to support weight by taking quick steps before the leg collapses.

Obturator Nerve Injury. The obturator nerve may be injured where it passes down the shaft of the ilium, resulting in an inability to adduct the thigh (Figure 64–16, Table 64–4). During parturition, neurapraxia may occur and produce a transient loss of function. If the nerve is severely damaged, the EMG abnormalities of positive waves and fibrillation potentials are seen in the external obturator, pectineus, adductor, and gracilis muscles.

Pudendal Nerve Injury. The pudendal nerve, with motor innervation to the skeletal muscles of the penis, vulva, urethra, and anal sphincter, may occasionally be injured during surgical intervention in the area of the anus. The nerve roots composing this nerve (S1, S2, and S3) may be injured as a result of a herniated intervertebral disc or a vertebral fracture. Neurologic manifestations of injury include a unilateral or bilateral loss of anal sphincter tone and anesthesia of the penis or clitoris, the vulva, part of the scrotum, and the perianal skin. There is often a loss of the anal reflex. Decreased numbers or absence of MUAPs and positive waves and fibrillation potentials may be found on needle EMG examination of the denervated external anal sphincter. The cauda equina may be stimulated with an epidural needle electrode placed between vertebrae L7 and S1 and an action potential recorded from the external anal sphincter to determine pudendal nerve integrity.

Lumbosacral Plexus Injury. Lumbosacral plexus or nerve root injuries are much less common than brachial plexus injuries but do occur occasionally, associated with severe pelvic and proximal rear limb trauma (Figure 64–16). Combined femoral and sciatic nerve deficits of the rear limb are seen. The neurologic and EMG examinations can be used to outline the nerves affected and to determine the severity of involvement for the formulation of an accurate prognosis.

ISCHEMIC NEUROPATHIES

In cats with cardiomyopathy (Chapter 77), an ischemic reaction of blood vessels to hind limb nerves and muscles may cause an acute paraplegia with depressed or absent spinal reflexes.[49] Depending on the degree of ischemia, motor nerve conduction velocity is slow or absent. The prognosis in most cases is poor. Dogs with heartworms or traumatic insults occluding blood vessels may have ischemic neuropathies.[50–52]

PERIPHERAL NERVE NEOPLASIA

Primary neoplasia of peripheral nerves in dogs and cats is produced from Schwann cells and supporting structures.[53] Schwann cells produce neurinomas, also called schwannomas or neurilemmomas.[54] Neurofibromas and neurofibrosarcomas form from connective tissue around the nerve bundles and occur as single tumors involving only one nerve or as multiple tumors involving several nerves, a plexus, or multiple nerve roots (Figure 64–17).

Primary peripheral nerve tumors grow very slowly and most commonly affect adult dogs. The initial presenting complaint is lameness of a limb. The brachial plexus or nerve roots C6 to T2 are common sites of neoplasia; an affected animal often begins limping on one forelimb.[55] As the tumor enlarges over the next several months, atrophy of affected muscles becomes apparent as paresis of the limb develops. There is often pain associated with limb movement. Ultimately the limb may be paralyzed, with decreased or no sensation

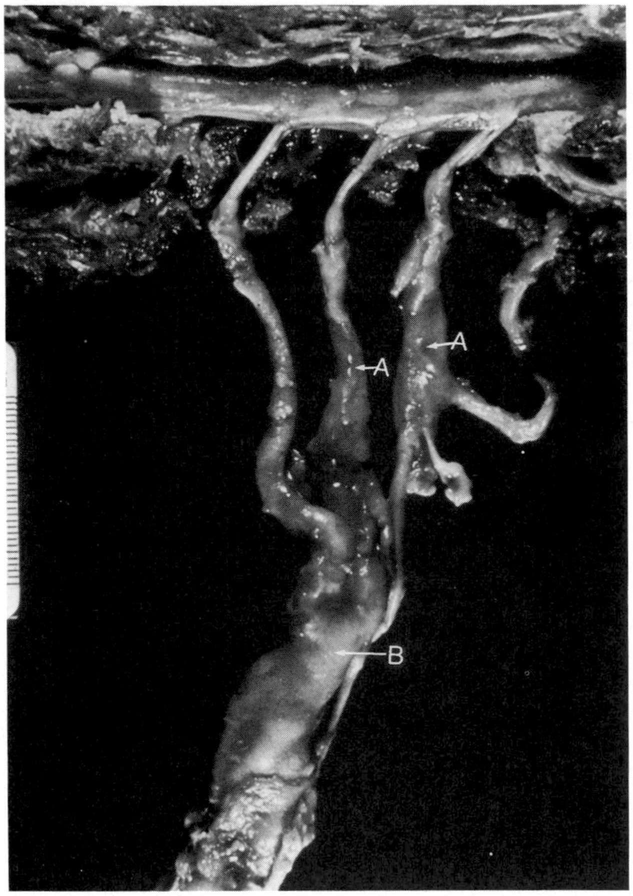

FIGURE 64–17. Neurofibrosarcoma producing thickening of the nerve roots *(A)* and brachial plexus *(B)* in a dog.

below the tumor site but extreme pain at the tumor site. Sometimes a palpable enlargement along the nerve or plexus may be found in the later stages of tumor development.

The diagnosis of neoplasia is suspected from the gradual progression of paresis, atrophy, and pain. Surgical exploration and removal of the tumor is the therapy. The portion of the nerve containing the tumor must be removed and the ends anastomosed. In the case of the brachial plexus tumor, the limb may have to be amputated, because the tumor is so large that too much nervous tissue must be removed for anastomosis to be possible. The prognosis for brachial plexus neurofibromas and neurofibrosarcomas is poor. There are usually multiple tumors, which grow along nerve roots into the spinal canal. They ultimately produce severe pain and hemiplegia or quadriplegia.

Neurofibromas and neurofibrosarcomas may affect any peripheral nerve or nerve roots and therefore can produce cranial nerve deficits, quadriparesis, quadriplegia, or ataxia of all four limbs, or paraparesis and paraplegia.

Lymphosarcoma is the most common metastatic neoplasia of nerve roots.[56, 57] In cats and dogs, the limb paresis and muscle atrophy due to lymphosarcoma often occurs more rapidly than that caused by neurinomas, neurofibromas, and neurofibrosarcomas, and severe neurologic deficit may be seen within a few weeks after the onset of signs. The prognosis is poor because the nerve roots are diffusely infiltrated with abnormal lymphocytes and surgical removal is usually impossible.

Other tumors of bone and muscle may not directly invade but may entrap peripheral nerves and produce signs of deficit in a limb. Prognosis varies with the tumor type and ability to remove or treat and relieve the pressure on the nerve.

MULTIFOCAL DISEASES OF PERIPHERAL NERVES

FAMILIAL POLYNEUROPATHIES

Progressive Spinal Muscular Atrophy. An autosomal recessive inherited abiotrophy of ventral horn cells, as well as other neurons, occurs in Swedish Lapland dogs and Brittany spaniels.[58, 59] A generalized weakness beginning at five to seven weeks of age, which rapidly progresses to a flaccid quadriplegia with severe muscle atrophy in a few weeks, is the course of the disorder in Swedish Lapland dogs. In affected Brittany spaniels, paravertebral muscle atrophy slowly progresses over the first year of life to produce a flaccid quadriplegia with severe muscle atrophy and tendon contractures. There is no therapy for either breed.

Globoid Cell Leukodystrophy. An autosomal recessive disorder that has been described in several breeds of dogs and cats is most common in West Highland White and Cairn terriers.[60] Widespread demyelination occurs throughout the central and peripheral nervous system owing to a deficiency of the enzyme beta-galactocerebrosidase. Generalized weakness begins in affected animals from four to six months of age and progresses to complete quadriplegia in a few weeks. Severe degenerative changes in the axons and myelin sheath may be seen on histologic examination of a peripheral nerve biopsy. Leukocytes may be assayed for the enzyme β-galactocerebrosidase. Carrier animals have enzyme levels that fall in between those of normal and affected animals.

Boxer Neuropathy. An autosomal recessive disorder of peripheral and central neuronal axons has been described in three families of boxer dogs in the United Kingdom.[61, 62] Clinical signs of pelvic limb ataxia begin in dogs under six months of age. Patellar reflexes are depressed bilaterally. There is no treatment, but clinical signs progress so slowly that affected dogs may be acceptable pets for months or years. A similar disorder has been described in a Pyrenean mountain dog.[63]

Dachshund Sensory Neuropathy. Affected long-haired dachshund puppies have decreased superficial and deep sensation over the entire body, urinary incontinence, and proprioceptive deficits in the pelvic limbs.[64, 65] Patellar reflexes are normal but flexor reflexes are absent due to the lack of pain sensation; no paresis or muscle atrophy is present. Needle EMG and motor nerve conduction velocity are normal. Sensory nerve conduction is reduced or absent. The prognosis is poor but the progression of the disease may be slow. A genetic basis is suspected. There is degeneration in distal sensory peripheral nerves.

Sensory Neuropathy of English Pointers and Short Hair Pointers. An autosomal recessive sensory neuropathy has been described in English pointers in the United States and a similar condition has been described in short hair pointers in Germany.[66, 67] At three months of age affected puppies begin to mutilate their paws and digits. There is a complete loss of sensation to the digits in the hind limbs but gait and spinal reflexes are normal. The needle EMG is also normal. A developmental hypoplasia and progressive degeneration of sensory nerves is suspected. The prognosis is poor.

Dancing Doberman Disease. Adult Doberman pinschers are presented for holding up one pelvic limb while standing; no underlying bone or joint disease can be detected (Figure 64–18). The clinical signs may remain the same for years, with only one limb affected. In other dogs the signs may progress to affect the other limb as well, so while standing the animal alternately flexes and extends each pelvic limb in a dancing motion, then sits down. Over several months to years the gastrocnemius, semitendinosus, and semimembranosus muscles atrophy and mild pelvic limb weakness and conscious proprioceptive deficits develop.[68] Positive sharp waves and fibrillation potentials are found initially in gastrocnemius and then the semitendinosus and semimembranosus muscles on needle EMG examination. A distal neuropathy of the tibial nerve is suspected but there may be a myopathic component to the disease as well. One dog studied over five years developed a generalized polyneuropathy and at necropsy a generalized distal axonopathy was found. Other dogs studied over several years have remained static or progressed only slightly. A simultaneous degeneration and regeneration process of the distal nerves is suspected. The genetic basis of this disorder is not known, but there appears to be a breed predisposition.

Giant Axonal Neuropathy. A central and peripheral distal axonopathy has been described in 14- to 16-month-old German shepherds.[69–71] The clinical signs include paresis and proprioceptive deficits of the pelvic limbs in particular and depressed patellar reflexes bilaterally.

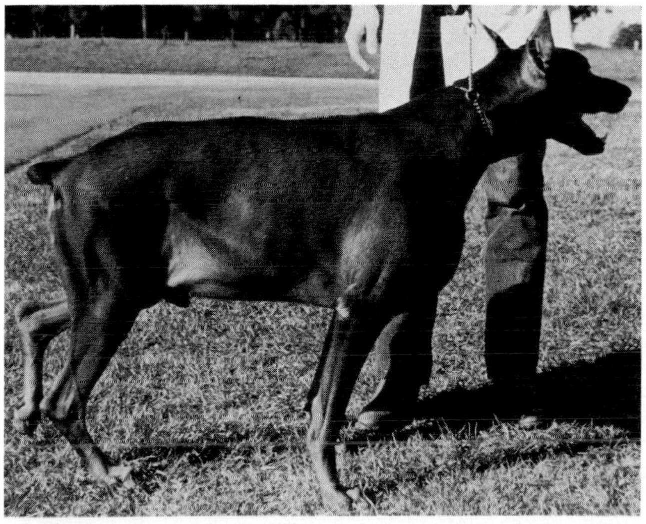

FIGURE 64–18. A nine-year-old Doberman pinscher with a characteristic stance and an associated suspected tibial distal neuropathy of the left hind leg.

There is atrophy of pelvic limb musculature below the stifles, as well as megaesophagus and a diminished bark. An autosomal recessive inheritance is suspected. Slow axoplasmic transport is altered and swollen axons contain masses of neurofilaments, thus the name giant axonal neuropathy. There is no therapy and the prognosis is poor.

Hypertrophic Neuropathy. An autosomal recessive polyneuropathy has been reported in Tibetan mastiff puppies with clinical signs of quadriparesis and hyporeflexia beginning at 7 to 12 weeks of age.[72, 73] Some puppies are severely affected within three weeks; other puppies are only mildly affected. An inherited metabolic defect of the Schwann cell is suspected as widespread demyelination is found throughout the peripheral nerves and roots. There is no therapy.

Polyneuropathy with Inherited Hyperchylomicronemia in Cats. Cats with inherited hyperchylomicronemia may develop a mutifocal polyneuropathy due to nerve compression by lipid granulomata.[74] In one study, 9 out of 20 cats with an inherited hyperchylomicronemia developed multifocal neuropathies and had a combination of signs of Horner's syndrome, facial, trigeminal, recurrent laryngeal, peroneal, femoral, radial, and tibial nerve paralysis. Cats with the peripheral neuropathy improved two to three months after the initiation of a low-fat diet.

The sites of nerve lesions in affected cats were at spinal foramina and bony prominences. It is suspected that minimal trauma at these sites produces lipid granulomata in cats with high blood lipid levels and a multifocal compression neuropathy occurs.

METABOLIC AND ENDOCRINE POLYNEUROPATHIES

Diabetic Polyneuropathy. Dogs and cats with diabetes mellitus may develop pelvic limb weakness, conscious proprioceptive deficits, depressed patellar reflexes, and muscle atrophy, as well as generalized weakness.[75–78] Fibrillation potentials and positive waves are found on needle EMG examination. Motor nerve conduction velocity is decreased.[79] All dogs and cats diagnosed as having a peripheral neuropathy should be evaluated for diabetes mellitus (Chapter 96). Neuronal degeneration (especially in distal nerves) and segmental demyelination are the primary pathological changes (Figure 64–19). If mild, the clinical signs may improve after insulin therapy is regulated.

Hyperinsulinism Polyneuropathy. A polyneuropathy may occur concurrently in dogs with hypoglycemia and and hyperinsulinism from an islet cell adenocarcinoma.[80, 81] Affected dogs have paraparesis or quadriparesis with depressed patellar reflexes only or generalized depression of all spinal reflexes (Figure 64–20). Fibrillation potentials and positive waves are found on needle EMG examination. Motor nerve conduction velocity is decreased. All dogs diagnosed with a polyneuropathy should be evaluated for hyperinsulinism hypoglycemia. Clinical signs may improve once the tumor is removed and insulin levels return to normal.

Hypothyroid Polyneuropathy. Dogs with hypothyroidism and lymphocytic thyroiditis may have concurrent

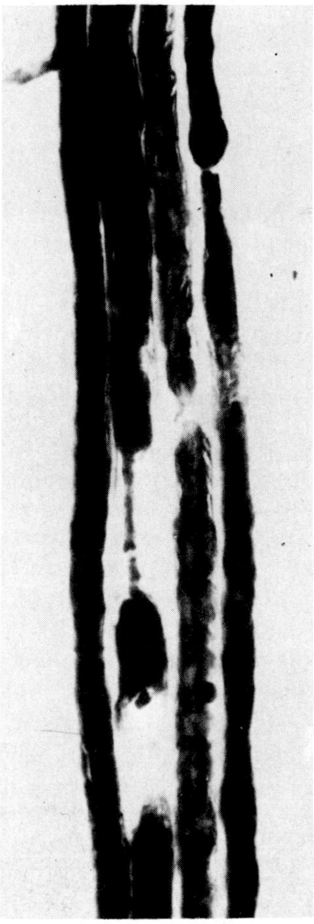

FIGURE 64–19. Nineteen-year-old male tabby cat, diabetic for three years. Four teased nerve fibers with the second from the left demonstrating paranodal (segmental) demyelination typical of diabetic neuropathy. Sciatic nerve, osmium tetroxide stain × 250. (Courtesy of D. R. Averill, Jr., and Departments of Pathology, Angell Memorial Animal Hospital and Harvard Medical School.)

paraparesis or quadriparesis with depressed spinal reflexes.[82, 83] Positive waves, fibrillation potentials, and bizarre high-frequency discharges may be present in distal limb musculature on needle EMG examination. Motor and sensory nerve conduction velocities are slower than normal, as is characteristic of peripheral nerve disease. Sural nerve biopsy may demonstrate segmental demyelination on examination of a teased fiber specimen. A polymyopathy has also been described with hypothyroidism (Chapter 95). Any dog presented with a polyneuropathy should be evaluated for hypothyroidism (Chapter 95). Affected dogs often improve when thyroid replacement therapy is instituted.

Paraneoplastic Polyneuropathy. Some neoplastic processes may release a substance that alters the function of peripheral nerves and produces polyneuropathy in dogs.[84, 85] Affected dogs may have paraparesis and quadriparesis with depressed spinal reflexes. Positive waves, fibrillation potentials, and bizarre high-frequency discharges may be found on needle EMG examination. Motor nerve conduction velocities are slow. Segmental demyelination and axonal degeneration are found on histologic examination of peripheral nerves. Any dog presented with a chronic polyneuropathy should be examined for a concurrent neoplastic process. Thoracic radiographs may be useful in detecting pulmonary tumors, which may cause a paraneoplastic polyneuropathy in dogs. The overall prognosis is often poor.

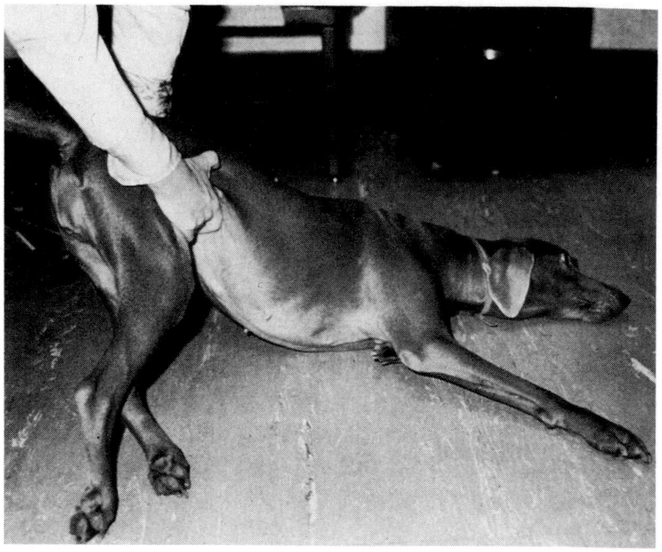

FIGURE 64–20. A dog with an insulinoma and a concurrent polyneuropathy characterized by a flaccid quadriparesis. (Courtesy of Dr. Julia Blackmore, Ft. Pierce, Florida.)

Miscellaneous Metabolic Polyneuropathies. In humans, chronic uremia and hepatopathies may produce polyneuropathy. More studies need be performed in animals with these conditions to determine if their generalized weakness is in part due to a polyneuropathy.

TOXIC POLYNEUROPATHIES

Chemical Agents, Heavy Metals, and Drugs. Many agents are known to produce polyneuropathy in humans and animals.[86] For any quadriparetic animal with a chronic polyneuropathy of unknown cause, the possibility of toxicity should be considered. Any chronic medications the animal has been receiving, as well as environmental exposure to chemicals, should be reviewed for their potential ability to produce a polyneuropathy. Table 64–7 lists some chemicals, heavy metals, and drug therapies that are known to produce polyneuropathy in humans and animals. Once the offending drug is removed, regeneration of peripheral nerves occurs and the animal often returns to normal.

Neomycin may inhibit the release of acetylcholine from the nerve terminal. Used in conjunction with muscle relaxants, it may block the neuromuscular transmission and produce quadriparesis. Streptomycin, kanamycin, gentamicin, polymyxin B, tetracyclines, and sulfonamides may also block neuromuscular junction activity and produce generalized weakness and depressed spinal reflexes in some animals.

Organophosphates cause one of the most common toxicities affecting the normal transmission of acetylcholine.[87] These drugs cause a phosphorylation of acetylcholinesterase, which renders it inactive. This leads to an initial overstimulation of the postsynaptic membrane by acetylcholine, followed by depression. Synapses of

TABLE 64–7. CHEMICAL AGENTS THAT MAY PRODUCE POLYNEUROPATHY

Industrial and Cosmetic Chemicals	Heavy Metals
Acrylamide	Arsenic
Tri-ortho-cresyl phosphate	Lead
Di-isopropyl fluorophosphate (DFP)	Mercury
Parathion	Thallium
Malathion	Gold
Other organophosphorus compounds	**Drugs**
Carbon disulfide	Chloramphenicol
Trichloroethylene	Clioquinol
N-hexane	Diphenylhydantoin
Carbon monoxide	Disulfiram
Methyl bromide	Isoniazid
Chlorophenothane (DDT)	Nitrofurantoin
Lindane	Thalidomide
Polychlorinated biphenyls	Vincristine
Carbon tetrachloride (CCl_4)	Vinblastine
Dichlorophenoxyacetic acid (2,4-D)	Ampicillin
Pentachlorophenolate	Erythromycin
Gasoline	Tetracycline
Methylbutylketone (MBK)	
Zinc pyridinethione (ZPT)	

the autonomic and central nervous systems are affected, as well as the neuromuscular junction. Signs of toxicity include miosis, excessive salivation, muscle tremors, convulsions, and quadriparesis. Serum and red blood cell acetylcholinesterase levels can be measured and are markedly decreased in organophosphate toxicity. Atropine sulfate is used therapeutically to block autonomic and central nervous system effects but has little effect on the neuromuscular junction. If neuromuscular involvement is severe and generalized weakness is the primary sign, diphenhydramine therapy may improve the neurologic deficit a few hours after administration.[87] Treatment of organophosphate toxicity is described further in Chapter 55. Chronic organophosphate exposure may produce a polyneuropathy as well, with quadriparesis and depressed spinal reflexes. Recovery is slow once the exposure is discontinued, as nerves must regenerate.

***Clostridium botulinum* Toxin.** The organism *Clostridium botulinum* produces a neurotoxin that may be ingested from spoiled food or carrion. Type C botulism intoxication is reported in dogs.[88–90] The neurotoxin inhibits the release of acetylcholine from neuromuscular junctions as well as autonomic synapses and decreases conduction of the peripheral nerves. The onset of signs often occurs within 24 to 48 hours after ingestion of the carrion and the severity of signs may vary greatly with each individual. Signs may range from mild generalized weakness, with more involvement of rear limbs than of forelimbs, to a flaccid quadriplegia with absent spinal reflexes. Evidence of cranial nerve disturbances such as mydriasis, weak jaw tone, facial muscle weakness, dysphagia, and megaesophagus may also be seen. Bradycardia, hypothermia, and decreased respirations are often present. In severe cases affected dogs are dead within 24 hours from respiratory paralysis and aspiration of fluids.

Needle EMG studies are initially normal but may show fibrillation potentials after five to seven days in cases that survive for that period of time. Motor nerve conduction velocity may be normal or decreased. The amplitude of the evoked response is reduced. Serum from affected dogs may be injected into healthy mice, which usually become similarly affected in 24 to 48 hours.

Mildly affected dogs may recover in three to four weeks with polyvalent antitoxin (if available), penicillin, and general supportive care.

Tick Neurotoxin. The females of the eastern wood tick (*Dermacentor variabilis*), the western mountain tick (*Dermacentor andersoni*), and the Australian tick (*Ioxodes holocyclus*) can attach to dogs and cats, engorge with blood, and secrete a toxin that blocks proper neuromuscular junction activity and produces flaccid quadriplegia.[91, 92] Clinical signs may vary in severity from mild paraparesis with depressed patellar reflexes to an acute ascending quadriplegia with no spinal reflexes, facial nerve paresis, and respiratory distress, which may appear identical to that caused by botulism or acute polyradiculoneuritis (discussed later in this section). The animal should be thoroughly examined for an engorged female tick, which may be found anywhere on the body, but often appears on the face, behind the ears, or on some other region of the head or neck. If the animal is bathed or dipped to remove ticks, care should be taken when applying organophosphates, as these may further depress neuromuscular junction function.

The EMG examination may be used to differentiate tick paralysis and acute polyradiculoneuritis.[91, 93] No abnormalities of insertional activity are seen on needle EMG, and there are few if any MUAPs in severe tick paralysis. When a motor nerve is directly stimulated there is little or no response to electrical stimulation, indicating that the neuromuscular junction is blocked.[94] The evoked response is normal or only slightly reduced in acute idiopathic polyradiculoneuritis. The EMG associated with botulism is similar to tick paralysis, but botulism is very rare compared to tick intoxication.

Therapy consists of removal of the tick and, in severe cases, the administration of hyperimmune canine serum, if available.[92]

Once the tick is removed, recovery often occurs rapidly and the animal may be completely normal in 24 to 72 hours. Occasionally animals worsen slightly for 48 hours but then improve; the overall prognosis for recovery is excellent.

Snake Venom Neurotoxin. Dogs bitten by a coral snake may develop generalized weakness and depressed spinal reflexes produced by a venom-induced neuromuscular junction blockade.[95] The author studied one affected dog that had no needle EMG abnormalities but had reduced evoked potentials upon nerve stimulation. The dog recovered with supportive nursing care and no other specific therapy.

INFLAMMATORY AND SUSPECTED IMMUNE-MEDIATED POLYNEUROPATHIES

Brachial Plexus Neuritis. Acute paralysis of the thoracic limbs bilaterally may be produced by an immune stimulus in dogs and cats.[96–98] Flexor reflexes of the thoracic limbs are depressed or absent and severe muscle atrophy may develop rapidly. Positive waves and fibrillation potentials may appear in denervated muscles on needle EMG. If there is no response to direct nerve stimulation, the prognosis is poor. Nerve biopsy on one dog showed severe wallerian degeneration. The prognosis for recovery varies with the severity of clinical signs. In some cases the neuritis may be due to vaccination with a modified live rabies vaccine.

Ganglioradiculitis or Cranial Polyneuropathy. Adult dogs may develop a combination of multiple cranial nerve deficits, such as blindness with a dilated pupil, facial paresis, facial hypalgesia, temporalis and masseter muscle atrophy, a head tilt, megaesophagus and dysphagia with or without mild ataxia, and paresis of the limbs. If limb paresis is present, then patellar reflexes are often depressed. Positive waves and fibrillation potentials are found on needle EMG of affected skeletal muscles. Cerebrospinal fluid analysis is normal. No inciting cause is known, but a nonsuppurative cranial and spinal ganglioradiculitis has been found in a few dogs studied.[99] The author has treated suspected cases with corticosteroid therapy; some dogs exhibited slow improvement after one month on therapy.

Acute Polyradiculoneuritis. Acute polyradiculoneuritis is the most common polyneuropathy of dogs and is widely known as coonhound paralysis because it was first described in raccoon-hunting dogs.[100–103] Adult dogs of any breed, age, or sex are affected. The history may indicate that the clinical signs develop 7 to 14 days after a raccoon bite or scratch or a recent vaccination with a modified live rabies vaccine. In other cases no inciting immunologic stimulus can be determined. Pelvic limb weakness develops and progresses over a period of two to ten days to become a symmetric hyporeflexic or areflexic quadriparesis or quadriplegia. In some patients progression is more rapid, so that little difference is seen between the pelvic and thoracic limbs, and a few begin with thoracic limb weakness. Some animals develop cranial nerve signs, most commonly a flaccid unilateral or bilateral facial paralysis, a hoarse voice, or difficulty in swallowing. Although most patients become too weak to rise, in mild cases affected dogs are able to stand and walk with assistance throughout the course of the disease and have only depressed patellar reflexes.

Affected quadriparetic or quadriplegic dogs may or may not have generalized hyperesthesia. They are afebrile, bright, and alert, and are mentally appropriate. They are usually able to eat if supported but should be monitored for swallowing difficulties. Occasionally dogs may lose control of bowel or bladder function but often they can still wag their tails.

The cisterna magna cerebrospinal fluid analysis, complete blood count, and serum enzymes are within normal limits. Positive sharp waves and fibrillation potentials beginning seven to ten days after the onset of the signs are seen on needle EMG. Peripheral nerve conduction times may be within normal limits, if the lesion resides primarily in ventral spinal roots proximal to the site of conduction time determination. Weeks after the onset, conduction time may be slow, owing to secondary degeneration of peripheral nerve fibers.

Rapid, symmetric loss of skeletal muscle bulk ensues once dogs become recumbent. The atrophic muscles may show spontaneous fasciculations, or fasciculation may be produced by direct percussion of the muscles. Multifocal, grouped muscle fiber atrophy without inflammatory changes characteristic of denervation atrophy is seen on histologic examination of the muscle. On peripheral nerve biopsy examination, only secondary degeneration shows, since the inflammatory lesions are in the nerve roots.

Some animals that develop severe signs rapidly over a few days sustain breathing difficulties; this impaired respiration is due to involvement of the intercostal and phrenic nerves and may be fatal. Under such circumstances respiratory assistance may be required. An oxygen chamber, nasal intubation and oxygen therapy or tracheostomy, endotracheal intubation, and positive pressure ventilation are alternative methods of support. Fortunately, this is a rare phenomenon, and respiratory assistance is usually only required for three to five days before spontaneous respiration returns. Patients that recover slowly suffer the difficulties of recumbency. Pressure sores may be prevented by using an air mattress, a water bed, or thick straw bedding and turning the patient over regularly. If decubital ulcers develop, these should be debrided and treated with topical antibiotics daily. Daily bathing may be necessary to keep the skin free of excreta. Systemic antibiotics should be used if skin ulceration becomes serious. There is no other specific treatment. Corticosteroid therapy may shorten the progression of the disease if given within 48 hours of the onset of signs.

The recovery period is extremely variable, from a few days in mild cases to one and a half to two months in others. Most affected dogs do not get any worse after ten days but should be monitored for pharyngeal and respiratory paralysis during that period. Most dogs recover completely, but a small proportion are left with mild weakness and muscle atrophy. Recurrence of signs may occur three weeks to two years after recovery.

The cause of acute polyradiculoneuritis is unknown. The lesion is lymphocytic radiculitis, with demyelination almost exclusively limited to the ventral spinal roots, but affecting the dorsal spinal roots in some cases (Figure 64–21). No agent has been isolated from affected tissues or materials collected from raccoons known to

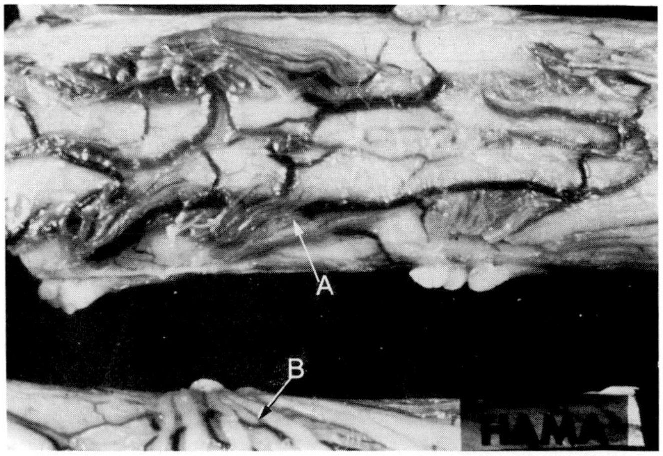

FIGURE 64–21. Ventral nerve roots *(A)* shrunken and discolored in a dog with acute polyradiculoneuritis compared to normal dorsal roots *(B)*. (From Chrisman, CL: Clinical manifestations of multifocal peripheral nerve and muscle disorders of dogs. Comp Cont Ed 7:355, 1985. Courtesy of D. R. Averill, Jr., Maybee, MIchigan.)

have precipitated the disorder and a cell-mediated autoimmune disorder is suspected. The antibodies against known canine viral diseases do not rise during the course of the disease. Only approximately half of the cases have a definite history of an encounter with a raccoon, suggesting that there may be multiple etiologies or that the raccoon is a carrier of a common agent.

Chronic Progressive and Relapsing Polyradiculoneuritis and Polyneuritis. The clinical manifestations of chronic polyradiculoneuritis and polyneuritis are similar in character to acute polyradiculoneuritis, but the course and localization of signs are different.[104–106] Weakness affects adult dogs and cats and may be of such a slow onset that the signs in one limb may be mistaken for the lameness of musculoskeletal disease. Typically, such signs may wax and wane for weeks. A continued progression may result in flaccid paraparesis or quadriparesis over a period of months, with asymmetry of the weakness often prevalent. Spinal reflexes may be absent and muscles atrophic in the affected limbs. There may be unilateral or bilateral facial weakness or other cranial neuropathies. Some cases have elevated spinal fluid protein and, on rare occasions, increased cells. CSF analysis in most cases is normal. Needle EMG studies indicate involvement of many peripheral nerves, and nerve conduction velocity is slow if peripheral axons are affected or normal if the lesion is restricted to nerve roots or terminals. There may be a mild to moderate lymphocytic and plasma cell inflammation in the sensory branches of the radial nerve taken for biopsy. Inflammatory lesions may be disseminated in peripheral nerves and nerve roots and there may be varying degrees of axonal necrosis and myelin loss found on necropsy.[104]

All animals should be evaluated for concurrent metabolic, endocrine, paraneoplastic, or toxic disturbances, since the polyneuropathy associated with these is clinically similar and the prognosis may be better. Administration of corticosteroids or cytotoxic agents has had no effect on the course of many cases of chronic polyneuritis of unknown origin. The prognosis is often grave; most animals become progressively worse and are eventually euthanatized. The diagnosis of polyradiculoneuritis is confirmed on necropsy.

Feline Polyneuritis. Two cases of feline polyneuritis have been described.[107] One cat had an acute onset of quadriparesis with absent tendon reflexes and a depression of other reflexes similar to acute polyradiculoneuritis in dogs. The second cat had a chronic course with some remissions of muscle twitching, hypermetria, and biting at the hind paws. In both cases no underlying cause was found, but on necropsy examination there was a generalized peripheral nerve mononuclear cell infiltration and destruction of myelin and axons.

OTHER IDIOPATHIC POLYNEUROPATHIES

Some dogs and cats are presented with polyneuropathies that do not fit into the classification of previously described polyneuropathies. Although the clinical syndrome may appear to be similar, no toxic, endocrine, metabolic, or other systemic disturbance can be elucidated and no inflammation is found upon histologic examination of the nerves.

Distal Denervating Disease. In Great Britain a group of dogs have been described that developed quadriparesis or quadriplegia over a few days to three weeks.[108] Spinal reflexes were absent and muscle atrophy became severe. Needle EMG abnormalities confirmed diffuse denervation. In a few dogs very distal motor peripheral nerves showed axonal degeneration. Most dogs recovered with no therapy in four to six weeks. No cause for this disorder was found. Whether this syndrome is different from other causes of distal axonopathy remains to be seen.

Distal Symmetrical Polyneuropathy. Another distal polyneuropathy producing flaccid paraparesis and quadriparesis has been described in dogs.[109, 110] One of the cases developed the signs following treatment with arsenicals for heartworms and the development of disseminated intravascular coagulation.[110, 111] The distal axonopathy involved motor and sensory nerves, unlike the distal denervating disease described previously. There is no treatment and the prognosis was reported as poor.[110] Where these cases fit in the overall classification of peripheral neuropathies remains to be seen. Concurrent toxicities, metabolic or endocrine disturbances, and paraneoplastic disorders should be eliminated as causes of the signs, since all of these have been reported to produce distal axonopathies in dogs.

Sensory Neuropathy. Progressive ataxia and loss of proprioception may occur in adult dogs over several months to years.[112, 113] There is no associated weakness, but tendon reflexes are depressed. Sensation of the head and body may be increased or decreased. Affected animals may have difficulty chewing and swallowing and develop an abnormal extension in the pelvic limbs. Needle EMG is normal. There is no treatment and the prognosis for recovery is poor. Upon necropsy, a pronounced degeneration and loss of dorsal root ganglion cells and large diameter fibers in the dorsal root and dorsal columns of the spinal cord is found.

Feline and Canine Hyperesthesia Syndromes. A clinical syndrome of periodic, hysterical, intense chewing or licking of the back, tail, and rear limbs has been observed in cats (especially the Siamese) and in dogs. It has been referred to as the idiopathic hyperesthesia syndrome.[114, 115] Sensory polyneuropathies in animals may have associated hyperesthesia and may lead to self-mutilation. Initially there is no dermatitis, but in chronic cases, dermatitis develops as a result of the constant mutilation. Presently, little is known concerning an etiology of these conditions. Diagnostic tests, including needle EMG, CSF, and radiography, are often normal. Corticosteroids, phenobarbital, diazepam, and hormones have all been tried individually on a two-week trial basis each (see drug index) with mixed success in alleviating the signs. Acupuncture and cobra venom have also been tried on a few occasions with response in some cases. The sensory peripheral nervous system has not been completely evaluated in these cases to rule out a sensory polyneuropathy. Some mild abnormalities have been found on sensory nerve EMG studies associated with lick granulomas in dogs, another idiopathic self-mutilation syndrome.[116]

References

1. Hoerlein, BF: Peripheral nervous system. *In* Hoerlein, BF (ed): Canine Neurology, 3rd ed. Philadelphia, WB Saunders, 1978, p 233.
2. Chrisman, CL: Clinical manifestations of multifocal peripheral nerve and muscle disorders of dogs. Comp Cont Ed 7:355, 1985.
3. Duncan, ID and Griffiths, IR: Neuromuscular disease. *In* Kornegay, JN (ed): Contemporary Issues in Small Animal Practice: Neurologic Disorders. New York, Churchill Livingstone, 1986, p 169.
4. Steinberg, SH: A review of electromyographic and motor nerve conduction velocity techniques. JAAHA 15:621, 1979.
5. Farnbach, G: Clinical electrophysiology in veterinary neurology, Part I. Electromyography. Comp Cont Ed 10:791, 1980.
6. Chrisman, CL: Electromyography in animals. *In* Bojrab, MJ (ed): Pathophysiology in Small Animal Surgery. Philadelphia, Lea and Febiger, 1981, p 831.
7. Holliday, TA, et al.: Sensory nerve conduction velocity. Technical requirements and normal values for branches of the radial and ulnar nerves of the dog. Am J Vet Res 38:1543, 1977.
8. Redding, RW, et al.: Sensory nerve conduction velocity of cutaneous afferents of the radial, ulnar, peroneal and tibial nerves of the dog: Reference values. Am J Vet Res 43:517, 1982.
9. Redding, RW and Ingram, JT: Sensory nerve conduction velocity of cutaneous afferents of the radial, ulnar, peroneal and tibial nerves of the cat: Reference values. Am J Vet Res 45:1042, 1984.
10. Chrisman, CL: Signs related to autonomic and somatic cranial nerve dysfunction. *In* Chrisman, CL (ed): Problems in Small Animal Neurology. Philadelphia, Lea and Febiger, 1982, p 215.
11. Shell, L: Cranial nerve disorders in dogs and cats. Comp Cont Ed 4:458, 1982.
12. Robins, G: Dropped jaw—mandibular neurapraxia in the dog. J Sm Anim Pract 17:753, 1976.
13. Srivastava, HN: A case of trigeminal paralysis in the dog. Indian Vet J 47:270, 1970.
14. Hoelzle, RJ: Idiopathic trigeminal neuropathy in a dog. Vet Med Sm Anim Clin 78:345, 1983.
15. deLahunta, A: General Somatic Efferent System, Special visceral efferent system. *In* deLahunta A (ed): Veterinary Neuroanatomy and Clinical Neurology. Philadelphia, WB Saunders, 1983, p 110.
16. Zachary, JF, et al.: Multicentric nerve sheath fibrosarcomas of multiple cranial nerve roots in two dogs. JAVMA 188:723, 1986.
17. Carmichael, S and Griffith, IR: Case of isolated sensory trigeminal neuropathy in a dog. Vet Rec 109:280, 1981.
18. Renegar, WR: Auriculopalpebral nerve paralysis following prolonged anesthesia in a dog. JAVMA 174:1007, 1979.
19. Braund, KG: Idiopathic facial paralysis in the dog. Vet Rec 105:296, 1979.
20. Chrisman, CL: Vestibular Diseases. *In* Chrisman, CL (ed): The Veterinary Clinics of North America. Advances in Neurology. Philadelphia, WB Saunders, 1980, p 103.
21. Schunk, KL and Averill, DR: Peripheral vestibular syndrome in the dog. A review of 83 cases. JAVMA 182:1354, 1983.
22. Schunk, KL: Peripheral vestibular disease in small animals. *In* Kirk RW (ed): Current Veterinary Therapy IX. Philadelphia, WB Saunders, 1986, p 794.
23. Fowler, NC: The ototoxicity of neomycin in the dog. Vet Rec 82:267, 1968.
24. Indrieri, RJ and Taylor, RF: Vestibular dysfunction caused by squamous cell carcinoma involving the middle ear and inner ear in two cats. JAVMA 184:471, 1984.
25. Burke, EE, et al.: Review of idiopathic feline vestibular syndrome in 75 cats. JAVMA 187:94, 1985.
26. Harvey, HJ, et al.: Laryngeal paralysis in hypothyroid dogs. *In* Kirk, RW (ed): Current Veterinary Therapy VIII. Philadelphia, WB Saunders, 1983, p 694.
27. Gaber, CE, et al.: Laryngeal paralysis in dogs: a review of 23 cases. JAVMA 186:377, 1985.
28. O'brien, JA: Laryngeal paralysis in dogs. *In* Kirk RW (ed): Current Veterinary Therapy IX. Philadelphia, WB Saunders, 1986, p 789.
29. Venker-van Haagen, AJ, et al.: Spontaneous laryngeal paralysis in young Bouviers. JAAHA 14:714, 1978.
30. Hardie, EM, et al.: Laryngeal paralysis in three cats. JAVMA 179:879, 1981.
31. Harvey, CE and Venker-van Haagen, AJ: Surgical management of pharyngeal and laryngeal airway obstruction in the dog. Vet Clin North Am 5:515, 1975.
32. Schaer, M, et al.: Laryngeal hemiplegia due to neoplasia of the vagus nerve in a cat. JAVMA 174:513, 1979.
33. Raffe, MR: Peripheral Nerve Injuries in the Dog. (Parts I and II). Comp Cont Ed 1:269, 1979.
34. Steinberg, SH: The use of electrodiagnostic techniques in evaluating traumatic brachial plexus root injuries. JAAHA 15:621, 1979.
35. Swaim, S: Peripheral nerve surgery. *In* Hoerlein, BF (ed): Surgery Canine Neurology. Philadelphia, WB Saunders, 1978, p 296.
36. Bennett, D and Vaughan, LC: The use of muscle relocation techniques in the treatment of peripheral nerve injuries in dogs and cats. J Sm Anim Pract 17:99, 1976.
37. Griffiths, IR: Avulsion of the brachial plexus. Part I. Neuropathology of the spinal cord and peripheral nerves. J Sm Anim Pract 15:165, 1974.
38. Griffiths, IR, et al.: Avulsion of the brachial plexus, Part 2. Clinical aspects. J Sm Anim Pract 15:177, 1974.
39. Van Nes, JJ: Evaluation of traumatic forelimb paralysis of dogs. Res Vet Sci 40:144, 1986.
40. Wheeler, SJ, et al.: The diagnosis of brachial plexus disorders in dogs: a review of twenty two cases. J Sm Anim Pract 27:147, 1986.
41. Bailey, CS: Patterns of cutaneous anesthesia associated with brachial plexus avulsions in the dog. JAVMA 185:889, 1984.
42. Bennett, D: An anatomical and histological study of the sciatic nerve, relating to peripheral nerve injuries in the dog and cat. J Sm Anim Pract 17:379, 1976.
43. Withrow, SJ and Amis, TC: Sciatic nerve injury associated with intramedullary fixation of femoral fractures. JAAHA 13:562, 1977.
44. Gilmore, DR: Sciatic nerve injury in twenty-nine dogs. JAAHA 20:403, 1984.
45. Walker, TL: Ischiatic nerve entrapment. JAVMA 178:1284, 1981.
46. Fanton, JW, et al.: Sciatic nerve injury as a complication of intramedullary pin fixation of femoral fractures. JAAHA 19:687, 1983.
47. Chambers, JN and Hardie, EM: Localization and management of sciatic nerve injury due to ischial or acetabular fracture. JAAHA 22:539, 1986.
48. Bennett, D and Vaughan, LC: Peroneal nerve paralysis in the cat and dog: An experimental study. J Sm Anim Pract 17:499, 1976.
49. Griffiths, IR and Duncan, ID: Ischemic neuromyopathy in cats. Vet Rec 104:518, 1979.
50. MacCoy, DM and Trotter, EJ: Brachial paralysis subsequent to traumatic partial occlusion of the right subclavian artery. JAAHA 13:625, 1977.
51. Burt, JK, et al.: Femoral artery occlusion by *Dirofilaria immitis* in a dog. J Am Vet Rad Soc 18:166, 1977.
52. Slonka, GF, et al.: Adult heartworms in arteries and veins of a dog. JAVMA 170:717, 1977.
53. Goedegebuure, SA: A case of neurofibromatosis in the dog. J Sm Anim Pract 16:329, 1975.
54. Patnaik, AK, et al.: Canine malignant melanotic schwannomas: a light and electronmicroscopic study of two cases. Vet Rec 21:483, 1984.
55. Carmichael, S and Griffiths, IR: Brachial plexus tumors in seven dogs. Vet Rec 108:437, 1981.
56. Fox, JG and Gutnick, MJ: Horner's syndrome and brachial paralysis due to lymphosarcoma in a cat. JAVMA 160:977, 1972.
57. Presthus, J and Teige, J: Peripheral neuropathy associated with lymphosarcoma in a dog. J Sm Anim Pract 27:463, 1986.
58. Sandefeldt, E, et al.: Hereditary neuronal abiotrophy in the Swedish Lapland dog. Cornell Vet 63:71, 1973.

59. Lorenz, MD, et al.: Hereditary canine spinal muscular atrophy in Brittany spaniels: Clinical manifestations. JAVMA 175:833, 1979.
60. Kurtz, HJ and Fletcher, TF: The peripheral neuropathy of canine globoid-cell leukodystrophy (Krabbe-Type). Acta Neuropathol 16:226, 1970.
61. Griffiths, IR, et al.: A progressive axonopathy of boxer dogs affecting the central and peripheral nervous system. J Sm Anim Pract 21:29, 1980.
62. Griffiths, IR: Progressive axonopathy: an inherited neuropathy of Boxer dogs. 1. Further studies of the clinical and electrophysiological features. J Sm Anim Pract 26:381, 1985.
63. Wright, JA and Brownlie, S: Progressive ataxia in a Pyrenean Mountain Dog. Vet Rec 116:410, 1985.
64. Duncan, ID, et al.: The pathology of a sensory neuropathy affecting long haired dachshund dogs. Acta Neuropath 58:141, 1982.
65. Duncan, ID and Griffiths, IR: A sensory neuropathy affecting long-haired dachshund dogs. J Sm Anim Pract 23:831, 1982.
66. Cummings, JC, et al.: Acral mutilation and nociceptive loss in English pointer dogs. Acta Neuropath 53:119, 1981.
67. Cummings, JF, et al.: Hereditary sensory neuropathy. Amer J Path 112:136, 1983.
68. Chrisman, CL: Distal polyneuropathy of Doberman pinschers. *In* Proceedings of the 3rd Annual Medical Forum, ACVIM, San Diego, June, 1985, p 164.
69. Duncan, ID and Griffiths, IR: Canine giant axonal neuropathy. Vet Rec 101:438, 1977.
70. Duncan, ID and Griffiths, IR: Peripheral nervous system in a case of canine giant axonal neuropathy. Neuropathol Appl Neurobiol 5:25, 1979.
71. Duncan, ID, et al.: Inherited canine giant axonal neuropathy. Muscle Nerve 4:223, 1981.
72. Cummings, JF, et al.: Canine inherited hypertrophic neuropathy. Acta Neuropath 53:137, 1981.
73. Cooper, BJ, et al.: Canine inherited hypertrophic neuropathy: clinical and electrodiagnostic studies. Am J Vet Res 45:1172, 1984.
74. Jones, BR, et al.: Peripheral neuropathy in cats with inherited primary hyperchylomicronaemia. Vet Rec 119:268, 1986.
75. Braund, KG and Steiss, JE: Distal neuropathy in spontaneous diabetes mellitus in the dog. Acta Neuropath 57:263, 1982.
76. Katherman, AE and Braund, KG: Polyneuropathy associated with diabetes mellitus in a dog. JAVMA 182:522, 1983.
77. Johnson, CA, et al.: Peripheral neuropathy and hypotension in a diabetic dog. JAVMA 183:1007, 1983.
78. Kramek, BA, et al.: Neuropathy associated with diabetes mellitus in the cat. JAVMA 186:42, 1984.
79. Steiss, JE, et al.: Electrodiagnostic analysis of peripheral neuropathy in dogs with diabetes mellitus. Am J Vet Res 42:2061, 1981.
80. Chrisman, CL: Postoperative results and complications of insulinomas in dogs. JAAHA 16:677, 1980.
81. Shahar, R, et al.: Peripheral polyneuropathy in a dog with functional islet B-cell tumor and widespread metastasis. JAVMA 187:175, 1985.
82. Sims, MH, et al.: Depressed thyroid function in two tetraplegic dogs. JAVMA 171:178, 1977.
83. Indrieri, RJ, et al.: Neuromuscular abnormalities associated with hypothyroidism and lymphocytic thyroiditis in three dogs. JAVMA 190:544, 1987.
84. Sorjoren, DC, et al.: Paraplegia and subclinical neuromyopathy associated with a primary lung tumor in a dog. JAVMA 180:1209, 1982.
85. Braund, KG, et al.: Peripheral neuropathy associated with malignant neoplasms in dogs. Vet Path 24:16, 1987.
86. Krinta, G, et al.: Clioquinol and 25 hexanedione induce different types of distal axonopathy in the dog. Acta Neuropathol 47:213, 1979.
87. Clemmons, RM, et al.: Correction of organophosphate-induced neuromuscular blockade by diphenhydramine. Am J Vet Res 45:2167, 1984.
88. Barsanti, JA, et al.: Type C botulism in American fox hounds. JAVMA 172:809, 1978.
89. Cornelissen, JM, et al.: Type C botulism in five dogs. JAVMA 21:401, 1985.
90. Van Nes, JJ, et al.: Electrophysiologic evidence of peripheral nerve dysfunction in 6 dogs with botulism type C. Res Vet Sci 40:372, 1986.
91. Barsanti, JA: Botulism, tick paralysis and acute polyradiculoneuritis. *In* Kirk RW (ed): Current Veterinary Therapy VII. Philadelphia, WB Saunders, 1980, p 773.
92. Ilkiw, JE: Tick paralysis in Australia. *In* Kirk, RW (ed): Current Veterinary Therapy VII. WB Saunders, Philadelphia, 1980, p 777.
93. Chrisman, CL: Differentiation of tick paralysis and acute polyradiculoneuritis in the dog using electromyography. JAAHA 11:455, 1975.
94. McLennan, H and Oikawa, I: Changes in function of the neuromuscular junction occurring in tick paralysis. Can J Physiol Pharmacol 50:53, 1972.
95. Meerdink, GL: Bites and stings of venomous animals. *In* Kirk, RW (ed): Current Veterinary Therapy VIII. Philadelphia, WB Saunders, 1983, p 156.
96. Cummings, JF, et al.: Canine brachial plexus neuritis: A syndrome resembling serum neuritis in man. Cornell Vet 63:59, 1973.
97. Alexander, JW, et al.: A case of brachial plexus neuropathy in a dog. JAAHA 10:515, 1974.
98. Bright, RM, et al.: Brachial plexus neuropathy in the cat: a case report. JAAHA 14:612, 1978.
99. Cummings, JF, et al.: Ganglioradiculitis in the dog: a clinical, light and electron-microscopic study. Acta Neuropathol 60:29, 1983.
100. Cummings, JF: Idiopathic polyneuritis, Guillain-Barre syndrome. Am J Pathol 66:189, 1972.
101. Northington, JW, et al.: Acute idiopathic polyneuropathy in the dog. JAVMA 179:375, 1981.
102. Northington, JW and Brown, MJ: Acute canine idiopathic polyneuropathy. A Guillain-Barre like syndrome in dogs. J Neurol Sci 56:259, 1982.
103. Cummings, JF, et al.: Coonhound paralysis; further clinical studies and electron microscopic observations. Acta Neuropath 56:167, 1982.
104. Cummings, JF and deLahunta, A: Chronic relapsing polyradiculoneuritis in a dog. A clinical, light and electron microscope study. Acta Neuropathol 28:191, 1974.
105. Cummings, JF and deLahunta, A: Canine Polyneuritis. *In* Kirk, RW (ed): Current Veterinary Therapy VI. Philadelphia, WB Saunders, 1977, p 825.
106. Flecknell, PA and Lucke, VM: Chronic relapsing polyradiculoneuritis in a cat. Acta Neuropathol 41:81, 1978.
107. Lane, JR and deLahunta, A: Polyneuritis in a cat. JAAHA 20:1006, 1984.
108. Griffiths, IR and Duncan, ID: Distal denervating disease: A degenerative neuropathy of the distal motor axon in dogs. J Sm Anim Pract 20:579, 1979.
109. Braund, KG, et al.: Distal symmetrical polyneuropathy in a dog. Vet Path 17:422, 1980.
110. Braund, KG: Clinical syndromes in veterinary neurology. Baltimore, Williams and Wilkins, 1986, p 92.
111. Dillon, AR and Braund, KG: Distal polyneuropathy after canine heartworm disease therapy complicated by disseminated intra vascular coagulation. JAVMA 181:239, 1982.
112. Wouda, W, et al.: Sensory neuronopathy in dogs: A study of four cases. J Comp Path 93:437, 1983.
113. Steiss, JE, et al.: Sensory neuronopathy in a dog. JAVMA 190:205, 1987.
114. Tuttle, J: Feline hyperesthesia syndrome. Vet Professional Topics, University of Illinois 2:2, 1979.
115. Chrisman, CL: Self mutilation. *In* Chrisman, CL (ed): Problems in Small Animal Neurology. Philadelphia, Lea and Febiger, 1982, p 437.
116. Van Nes, JJ: Electrophysiologic evidence of sensory nerve dysfunction in 10 dogs with acral lick dermatitis. JAAHA 22:157, 1986.

DRUG INDEX

Middle and Inner Ear Infections

1. Chloramphenicol (Chloromycetin) 25 mg/lb (50 mg/kg) orally q8 hours for 4 to 6 weeks.
2. Trimethoprim and sulfadiazine (Tribrissen) 7 mg/lb (15 mg/kg) orally q12 hours for 4 to 6 weeks.
3. Cephalexin (Keflex) 15 mg/lb (30 mg/kg) orally q12 hours for 4 to 6 weeks.

Organophosphate Toxicity

1. Atropine sulfate 0.1 mg/lb (0.2 mg/kg) initial dose divided 1/4 intravenously and 3/4 subcutaneously or intramuscularly for acute autonomic signs.
2. Diphenhydramine (Benadryl) 2 mg/lb (4 mg/kg) orally q8 hours daily until neuromuscular weakness resolves.

Inflammatory and Suspected Immune-Mediated Polyneuropathies

1. Prednisone 1 mg/lb (2.5 mg/kg) daily for 5 to 7 days, then reduce to 0.6 mg/lb (1.25 mg/kg) for 5 to 7 days, then reduce to 0.3 mg/lb (0.62 mg/kg) for 5 to 7 days, then reduce to 0.3 mg/lb (0.62 mg/kg) every other day for 5 times. If signs improve and then worsen as the dose decreases, increase back to previous dose. If signs resolve in 1 to 2 weeks, taper drug dosage to alternate day therapy over 1 week and discontinue. If signs return within a few weeks after recovery, maintain on alternate day therapy to prevent future recurrences.

Hyperesthesia Syndromes (Trial with 1 Drug at a Time)

1. Prednisone for 1 month as given above in inflammatory and suspected immune-mediated polyneuropathies.
2. Phenobarbital 0.5 mg/lb (1 mg/kg) orally q12 hours for 2 weeks to see if signs are controlled. If not, taper and discontinue.
3. Diazepam (Valium) 1 to 2 mg orally q6 to 8 hours for cats and 5 to 10 mg orally q 6 to 8 hours for dogs for 2 weeks to see if signs are controlled. If not, taper and discontinue.
4. Megestrol acetate (cats—hyperesthesia syndrome) 5 to 10 mg orally every 3 or 4 days to control signs. Must get a written release from owner giving permission to use, as not approved for use in cats. Can produce diabetes mellitus in cats. Use only when trials of prednisone, phenobarbital, or diazepam have been unsuccessful.

65 DISORDERS OF THE SKELETAL MUSCLES

VINCE PEDROIA

HISTORICAL PERSPECTIVE

In 1961 Ormrod described a dog with weakness resembling human myasthenia gravis.[1] By 1981, Pflugfelder et al. had reported on the immunocytochemical localization of immune complexes at the neuromuscular junction of myasthenic dogs, suggesting the autoimmune nature of the disease.[2]

In 1961 Bardens et al. suggested that puppies with hypoglycemia had Von Gierke's glycogen storage disease.[3] In 1985 Vora et al. demonstrated with enzymology and glycogen analyses a familial phosphofructokinase deficiency (glycogen storage disease type VII) in springer spaniels.[4]

Winter and Stephenson described one of the first cases of eosinophilic masticatory myositis in 1952 and in 1985 Shelton et al. demonstrated autoantibodies directed against specific myofiber types in eosinophilic masticatory myositis.[5, 6]

These examples illustrate the wide array of disorders responsible for muscle dysfunction and the sophisticated investigations being conducted into the myopathies of animals.

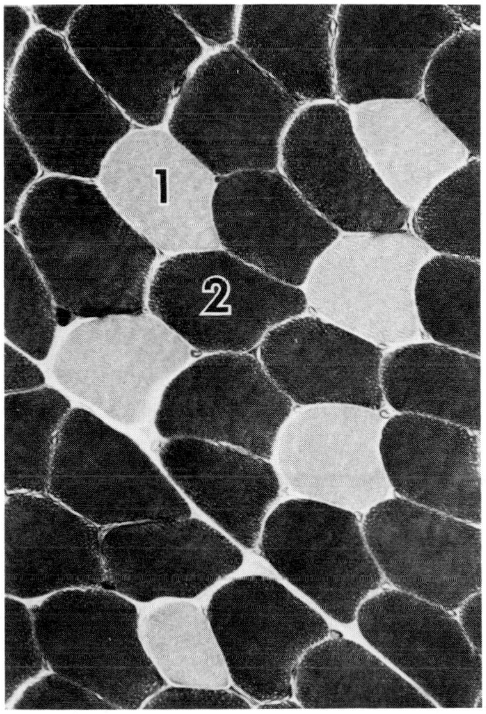

FIGURE 65–1. Transverse section of canine muscle fibers stained for myofibrillar ATPase. Type 1, slow-twitch muscle fibers, are lightly stained, while type 2, fast-twitch muscle fibers, are darkly stained. × 450. (Courtesy of G. H. Cardinet, III.)

STRUCTURE

The skeletal muscles are composed of fusiform cells called myofibers. In transverse sections the cells are polygonal, with multiple peripheral nuclei (Figure 65–1). In longitudinal sections there are characteristic light and dark bands, which are the basis for the term "striated muscle." The myofiber is bound by a complex outer membrane called the sarcolemma, which includes a plasma membrane that maintains the resting membrane potential and propagates the action potential. T tubules are invaginations of the sarcolemma into the cell, which convey the action potential to the interior. Each myofiber receives a single branch of a motor neuron at a deep primary cleft in the sarcolemma. At the bottom of the primary cleft are tiny secondary clefts. The acetylcholine receptors (ACHR) are on the ridges between these secondary clefts. Between the terminal membrane of the nerve fiber and the plasma membrane of the sarcolemma is a basal lamina, which binds acetylcholinesterase.

A motor neuron may innervate a few or several hundred myofibers to form motor units. Stimulation of the motor neuron activates all elements of the motor unit. Injury to the motor neuron above its point of branching denervates the entire unit, whereas injury to individual branches denervates only single myofibers. The myofibers of a motor unit are not packed closely

TABLE 65–1. PROPERTIES OF MOTOR UNIT MYOFIBER TYPES

	Histochemical Myofiber Type				
Masticatory	*Type I*	*Masticatory Variant Type I*	*Type 2A*	*Type 2B*	*Type 2C*
Physiologic properties					
Twitch	Slow	—	Fast	Fast	—
Fatigability	Resistant	—	Resistant	Fatigable	—
Histochemical properties					
Myofibrillar ATPase					
pH 9.8	Light	Light	Dark	Dark	Dark
Preincubation					
pH 4.5	Dark	Intermediate	Light	Dark	Dark
pH 4.3	Dark	Light	Light	Light	Dark
Other nomenclature	I	—	II	II	—
	Beta red	—	Alpha red	Alpha white	—
	S (Slow twitch, oxidative)	—	FOG (Fast twitch, oxidative, glycolytic)	FG (Fast twitch, glycolytic)	—

together but are widely scattered with fibers from other units interspersed between them.

The motor nerve fibers in a muscle nerve are heterogeneous. There are large fibers that arise from large cell bodies, have rapid conduction velocities, and discharge in a phasic pattern with brief bursts of action potentials of high frequency. Conversely, there are smaller fibers, which arise from smaller cell bodies, have slower conduction velocities, and have a tonic pattern of discharge with prolonged bursts of action potentials of lower frequency.

The myofibers of a muscle are also heterogeneous. When stained for myofibrillar adenosine triphosphatase (ATPase), a checkerboard array appears (Figure 65–1). The light fibers are type 1 and the dark ones, type 2. Most muscles have both types with several subgroups (Table 65–1).[7] The large phasic motor nerve fibers innervate the type 2 myofibers and the smaller tonic motor nerve fibers innervate the type 1 fibers. Hence, all myofibers of a given motor unit are of the same type. It appears that there is a neurotropism such that the physiologic and biochemical properties of the myofibers are determined by the nature of their innervation. This neurotropism is dramatically demonstrated during reinnervation.

After nerve injury, branches of surviving nerve fibers produce sprouts that contact and reinnervate the denervated myofibers. The reinnervated fibers acquire characteristics consistent with their new nerve supply. Hence, type one fibers can become type twos and twos can become ones. This results in a pathologic condition called "type grouping," where the normal checkerboard array disappears and clusters of fibers of the same type appear (Figure 65–2). This is the hallmark of denervation with reinnervation as occurs with many neuropathies[8] (see Chapter 64).

PHYSIOLOGY

Spontaneous release of single quantum of acetylcholine into the synaptic space results in binding of sufficient acetylcholine to the ACHR to produce a feeble muscle membrane depolarization called a miniature end plate potential (MEPP). Arrival of a nerve impulse produces synchronous release of sufficient quanta to produce a larger depolarization, the end plate potential (EPP), which prompts the generation of the muscle fiber action potential. The binding of acetylcholine to the receptors causes a conformational change in the receptors that results in the opening of ion channels. The resulting ion flux leads to the EPP. Diffusion from the receptors and hydrolysis by acetylcholinesterase removes the acetylcholine and terminates the depolarization.

The action potential generated at the neuromuscular junction (NMJ) spreads along the plasma membrane and into the cell via the T tubule system. Within the cell the T tubules encounter cisterns of the intracellular sarcoplasmic reticulum, where the electrical events on the surface promote calcium release from the sarcoplasmic reticulum into the intracellular space, which initiates the contractile process. This interaction of electrical and contractile events is called "excitation-contraction coupling."

Within the myofibers there are myofibrils that are composed of series of contractile elements, the sarcomeres. Sarcomeres are made of interdigitating myofilaments of actin and myosin, with the regulatory proteins troponin and tropomyosin. The interaction of calcium with troponin initiates a chain of events leading to binding of actin to myosin, hydrolysis of ATP by myosin ATPase, and a change in conformation of the myosin globular heads such that the filaments slide past each other and the sarcomere shortens. Resorption of calcium by the sarcoplasmic reticulum arrests the process. A review of muscle structure and function is available elsewhere.[9]

MYOPATHY

Normal muscle tone and concerted movement require interaction of the central nervous system with the motor units. In addition, information from receptors in the periphery, such as the muscle spindle apparatus (which monitors muscle length) and the Golgi tendon organs (which respond to muscle tension), influences the motor units by input to the lower motor neurons. Motor units must be recruited in appropriate numbers and at appropriate rates to achieve the desired movement.

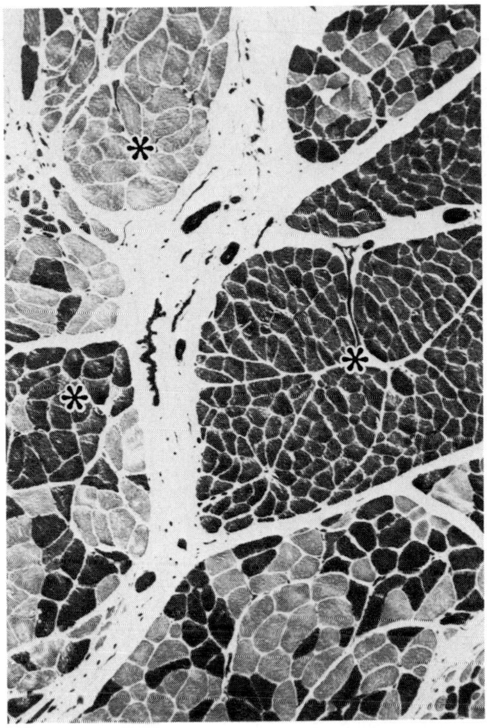

FIGURE 65–2. Transverse section of a muscle biopsy obtained from a dog with a chronic neuropathic disorder. The distribution pattern of fiber types becomes clustered (*) to form "type grouping" of type 1 and type 2 muscle fibers. × 60. (Courtesy of G. H. Cardinet, III.)

Loss of function of some or all of the myofibers of a unit reduces the effectiveness of that unit and if the disorder is widespread enough clinical disability appears. The diseases that affect the muscle fibers are called myopathies. Any part of the myofibers may be affected, from the motor endplates of the neuromuscular junctions to the bioenergetic system within the cells. In addition, the disease may affect only one type of myofiber. These diseases may be focal, multifocal, or generalized.

The general features of patients with myopathies are contrasted with the signs of other nervous system disorders in Table 65–2. Details of specific myopathies are given in subsequent sections.

TABLE 65–2. GENERAL FEATURES OF MYOPATHIES, NEUROPATHIES, AND MYELOPATHIES

	Myopathy	Neuropathy	Myelopathy
Weakness	+	+	+
Exercise-related	+	−	−
Altered sensation	−	+	+
Reflexes	Not affected	Depressed	Exaggerated or Depressed
Tone	Not affected	Reduced	Increased or reduced
Atrophy	±	+	If LMN or Disuse
EMG abnormal	+	+	If LMN
NCV	Normal	Slow	Normal
Muscle biopsy changes	Specific pathology	Denervation; type grouping	Denervation if LMN

Myasthenia Gravis

Myasthenia gravis (MG) occurs as both an acquired, autoimmune disorder and a congenital, familial one. It has been described in humans, dogs, and cats, but not in other species. However, experimental MG has been described in several species.

All of these patients manifest premature fatigue that is relieved with rest and anticholinesterase therapy. Decrementing of the amplitude of compound muscle action potentials with repetitive nerve stimulation and reduced endplate potentials are consistent electrophysiologic features. The basis of these abnormalities is a paucity of ACHR on the postsynaptic sarcolemma.[10–13]

PATHOPHYSIOLOGY

The paucity of ACHR in acquired MG is associated with autoimmunity. IgG has been demonstrated to be associated with the neuromuscular junctions (NMJ) of these patients, using *Staphylococcus* Protein A-horseradish peroxidase conjugates, which bind to the immunoglobulin.[2] It has been determined that up to 100 per cent of the remaining ACHR in the muscle of myasthenic patients has IgG bound to it.[10] In addition, circulating IgG, which reacts with ACHR, has been demonstrated in 90 per cent of dogs with acquired MG.[10, 11, 14, 15] The significance of the levels of titers of anti-ACHR antibodies with regard to the clinical course of the disease remains unclear. Additional evidence of an immune process is the appearance in the serum of antistriational antibody with affinity for the A bands of the myofibrils.[10, 11, 14–16] The mechanism whereby this autoimmunity leads to destruction of the ACHR is not proven but demonstration of elements of the complement system at the NMJ suggests a complement-mediated process.[17]

The stimulus for this immune disturbance is unknown. The role of the thymus has received considerable attention. For example, 87 per cent of humans with myasthenia gravis have pathology of the thymus.[18] Of these, 75 per cent have hyperplasia with germinal centers and 25 per cent have thymomas. There are only four reports of thymomas in myasthenic dogs, but it appears the thymus has not received thorough inspection in most cases.[10, 19–21] Thymectomy is not an effective treatment for human myasthenia gravis when associated with thymoma but it is moderately effective when associated with hyperplasia. Thymectomy failed to resolve the need for anticholinesterase therapy in one case in which it was reported in the dog.[21]

In congenital myasthenia gravis there is no evidence of autoimmunity. There is a reduced density of ACHR but no circulating antibodies to ACHR nor IgG deposited on the postsynaptic sarcolemma.[10–13] The pathogenesis involves neither an increased destruction of ACHR nor a failure of the sarcolemma to synthesize the ACHR, but instead a failure of insertion of the ACHR into the postsynaptic membrane.[22] In the Jack Russell terrier, smooth fox terrier, and springer spaniel, a familial basis is apparent and in the smooth fox terriers an autosomal recessive mode of inheritance has been established.[23–27]

ACQUIRED MYASTHENIA GRAVIS

The incidence and prevalence of acquired MG are unknown. Fifty-nine cases of acquired MG in dogs have been described.[1, 11, 14, 15, 19–21, 28–37] The incidence appears to warrant consideration of this diagnosis during the evaluation of dysphagia, megaesophagus, and premature fatigue. The ages of the patients that have been reported ranged from 8 weeks to 11 years. There was only one case younger than 8 months and one case older than 8 years. Among the 59 cases there were 34 females and 25 males. Breed predisposition was not evident. However, large breeds predominated and one report of 23 cases included 11 German shepherd dogs.[37]

The hallmark of myasthenia gravis is premature fatigue that is relieved by rest. These patients rise to walk readily but promptly develop a spastic pelvic limb gait, then tetraparesis, and finally collapse. Tachypnea and dyspnea are common signs during these episodes. Some patients have manifested drooping of the eyelids and the ears. Most patients demonstrate sialosis associated with dysphagia and regurgitation associated with megaesophagus. Some patients are presented for signs of dysphagia or megaesophagus or their sequela, aspiration pneumonia. Prehension and mastication may be affected. Laryngeal dysfunction has not been described.

Neurologic examination after rest is normal, except for pharyngeal function. During collapse muscle tone may be reduced, spinal reflexes depressed, and placing functions such as proprioception absent. Administration of an anticholinesterase drug enhances recovery and restores exercise tolerance. A positive test is restoration of strength that lasts for two to three minutes. This is reason enough for a presumptive diagnosis and institution of therapy. Edrophonium (Tensilon) is the drug of choice, as its duration of action is a few minutes only and therefore, if a cholinergic crisis occurs, the patient is at minimal risk. The response to anticholinesterase drugs is highly variable and precise dose recommendations cannot be given. The recommended dose of edrophonium is 0.5 to 5.0 mg intravenously. The dose can be raised and repeated within a few minutes if restoration of exercise tolerance does not ensue. The hallmarks of cholinergic crisis are exacerbation of weakness and signs of muscarinic stimulation: salivation, miosis, vomiting, and diarrhea. If muscarinic signs appear and the test has failed, it should be abandoned. Failure of the test would presumptively exclude MG from consideration but other means of diagnosis should be pursued if the clinical presentation is consistent with MG.

Laboratory evaluations are not expected to contribute to establishing the diagnosis except as they reflect complications such as aspiration pneumonia. Two patients with acquired MG had depressed serum T_4 levels but its relationship to the MG remains obscure.[11] Serum creatine kinase has been elevated in some cases but is not predictable.

Megaesophagus can be confirmed with thoracic radiographs. Cranial mediastinal masses may be thymomas. Dysphagia can be confirmed with contrast radiography, but extreme caution is advised as the risk of aspiration is high.

Electromyography reveals normal insertional activity

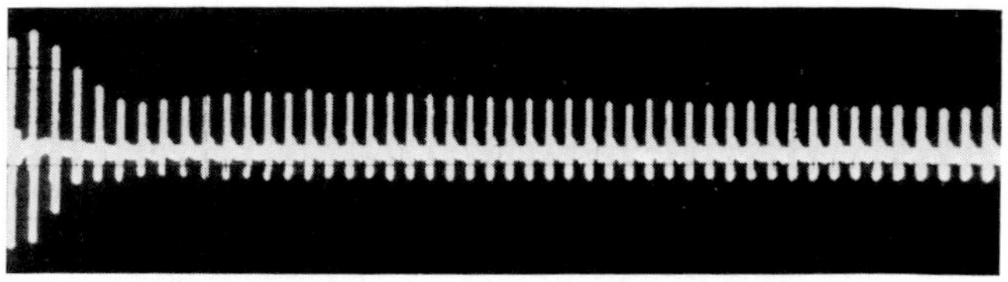

FIGURE 65–3. Compound muscle action potentials evoked by repetitive stimulation of a peripheral nerve. There is decrementing of their amplitude, which is an indication of myasthenia gravis.

without spontaneous myofiber discharges. Motor and sensory nerve conduction velocities are normal. Repetitive stimulation of a peripheral nerve at rates of 1 to 30 per second may result in a decrement in the amplitude of the compound muscle action potential (Figure 65–3). This is relieved by administration of edrophonium.

Muscle biopsy is normal in most cases. There have been sporadic reports of myositis associated with MG.[20, 36] Sections of muscle can be examined for IgG bound to the NMJ using the staphylococcal Protein A-horseradish peroxidase method (Figure 65–4).[2] In addition, a qualitative test for serum IgG with affinity for ACHR involves application of patient serum to normal muscle sections, followed by staphylococcal Protein A-horseradish peroxidase methods.[16] Quantitative methods for determination of serum anti-ACHR antibodies involve measuring the abilities of patient serum to inhibit the binding of I^{125} alpha-bungerotoxin to solubilized ACHR.[10, 11, 14, 15]

Management of Acquired Myasthenia Gravis. Management of acquired MG is a significant challenge due

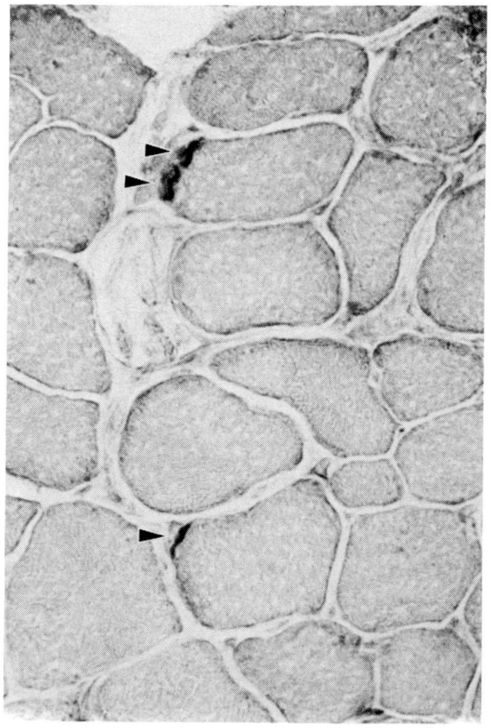

FIGURE 65–4. Transverse section of a muscle biopsy obtained from a dog with acquired myasthenia gravis. Detection and localization of IgG at neuromuscular junctions (arrowheads) is accomplished following incubation of the sections with staphylococcal Protein A conjugated to horseradish peroxidase. × 450. (Courtesy of G. H. Cardinet, III.)

to the severity of dysphagia and megaesophagus and the variability of the response to anticholinesterase drugs. Treatment fails in most cases. Most patients have life-threatening pneumonia or develop it soon after hospitalization.

Prompt treatment with anticholinesterase drugs is indicated. Neostigmine (Prostigmin) is the treatment of choice until exercise tolerance is established and regurgitation abolished. The recommended dose is 0.5 to 2.5 mg IM three times per day. Again, the dose is variable and cholinergic crises must be differentiated from episodes of MG. Food is withheld until a dose of neostigmine is found that restores exercise tolerance but does not induce muscarinic signs. Then the feeding of a liquid diet from an elevation is begun. Once regurgitation is abolished, oral pyridostigmine (Mestinon) can be given; the dose recommended is 7.5 to 30 mg PO two times per day. Again, the precautions given for neostigmine apply. Treatment of aspiration pneumonia is discussed in Chapter 69. When follow-up radiographs have been taken of successful cases, megaesophagus has persisted, although clinical signs have abated.

Corticosteroids are the treatment of choice once the patient is stable and infections have resolved. These should be given concurrently with the anticholinesterase medications for two weeks. Then the anticholinesterase drugs should be gradually reduced. An anti-inflammatory dose of prednisone is recommended. If the patient remains in remission, the steroids can be tapered slowly. Many patients that survive the early phases resolve the disease and tolerate a withdrawal of therapy. Other immunosuppressive drugs have been discussed for use in humans and azathioprine (Imuran) has been used in one group of dogs with some success.[37]

CONGENITAL MYASTHENIA GRAVIS

Congenital myasthenia gravis has been observed in the springer spaniel, the Jack Russell terrier, and the smooth fox terrier. Clinical signs appear in these puppies at six to eight weeks of age. The signs are similar to those of acquired MG, including regurgitation due to megaesophagus. There is a positive Tensilon test and benefit from maintenance anticholinesterase therapy, but long-term survival does not occur. Definitive diagnosis requires demonstration of a reduced density of AChR without evidence of autoimmunity. A presumptive diagnosis can be made from clinical presentation, response to anticholinesterase therapy, and repetitive nerve stimulations.

FELINE MYASTHENIA GRAVIS

Within the descriptions of four cases of feline myasthenia gravis is evidence to suggest that acquired, immune-mediated, and congenital forms occur.[38–40] The disorder appears to be rare. The clinical features are similar to those of the dog. Megaesophagus has been reported. The clinical signs of MG in the cat are similar to those of toxicity due to organophosphorous compounds. Therefore OP toxicity should be excluded before administration of anticholinesterase compounds for testing or treatment. Information is sparse regarding treatment and prognosis of MG in cats.

Myotonia

Myotonia implies a condition in which contraction persists after stimulation. The hallmark of myotonic disorders is stiffness that is exacerbated after rest and improves with exercise. Myotonia occurs with a variety of neuromuscular disorders. It seems appropriate at this time to reserve the term myotonia for describing a clinical sign rather than a diagnosis. Electromyography often reveals a typical high-frequency myofiber activity called a myotonic discharge, characterized by varying frequency and amplitude, resulting in a sound resembling a dive-bomber airplane. Hence the term "dive-bomber potentials" has been applied. Frequencies vary from approximately 100 to 200 per second, with amplitudes from approximately 150 to 400 μV. These potentials persist after neuromuscular blockade, confirming their origin within the myofibers. Myotonic discharges are a hallmark of human myotonia congenita.

Another type of high-frequency myofiber activity has been detected with electromyography in some neuromuscular diseases. This is called bizarre high-frequency discharge or pseudomyotonic discharge (Figure 65–5). It has an abrupt onset and termination without the waxing and waning of frequency and amplitude of the myotonic dive-bomber activity. Bizarre high-frequency discharge appears in some neuromuscular diseases characterized by myotonia and also in patients with neuromuscular disorders without myotonia, such as neuropathies and myositis.

PATHOPHYSIOLOGY

Myotonia seems to arise from an abnormality of the plasma membrane. In human myotonia congenita, familial myotonia of goats, and experimental myotonia produced by carboxylic acids, the muscle plasma membrane resistance is increased.[41] This resistance is attributed to an attenuated chloride conductance due to a reduction in chloride channels. Normally, chloride leak-

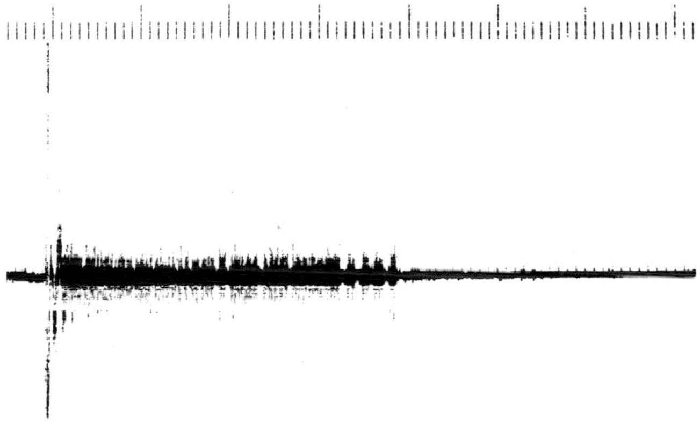

FIGURE 65–5. Bizarre high-frequency discharge. The brief high-amplitude burst at the left is the normal insertion activity associated with penetration by the EMG needle. About four seconds of BHFD ensues and terminates abruptly. (Courtesy of T. A. Holliday.)

age prevents a depolarizing afterpotential due to an accumulation of extracellular potassium in the T tubules. Without this efflux of chloride, the afterpotential persists and generates additional action potentials. Thus, a sustained series of action potentials follows the original nerve-mediated potentials and contraction persists. The pathophysiology of bizarre high-frequency discharge has not been explored.

HUMAN MYOTONIA

There are three familial myotonias in humans: myotonia congenita, dystrophic myotonia, and paramyotonia congenita.[42] Attempts have been made to compare these to conditions in animals and to assign these terms to animal diseases, but although similarities exist, precise comparisons cannot be made.

MYOTONIA OF CHOW CHOW DOGS

A familial myotonia with an unknown mode of inheritance has been described in chow chow dogs.[43–48] An autosomal recessive mode has been suggested but not proven. Clinical signs usually appear at approximately eight to 12 weeks of age. Some patients have been five to nine months old. These puppies have stiffness that is most severe in the muscles of the pelvic limbs. This often results in a bunny-hopping gait. Stiffness can be so severe that ambulation is impossible. Exercise tends to alleviate the signs. There can be muscle hypertrophy, including the tongue, and percussion of affected muscles results in a persistent myotonic dimple.

Serum creatine kinase is elevated consistently. Electromyography reveals myotonic discharges with normal conduction velocities and few to no spontaneous discharges, such as fibrillations and positive sharp waves. There are no changes in compound muscle action potential amplitude with repetitive nerve stimulation. Muscle biopsies usually reveal several changes: variation of fiber sizes, central nuclei, increased subsarcolemmal nuclei, fiber necrosis, and fiber splitting. Both types of fibers are affected. These changes have been regarded as "dystrophic." However, their relationship to human conditions is equivocal.

The clinical signs of these dogs usually stabilize and they can survive. Treatment with membrane-stabilizing drugs such as phenytoin, quinidine, and procainamide has produced variable results.

TYPE 2 MYOFIBER DEFICIENCY OF LABRADOR RETRIEVER DOGS

A rare neuromuscular disorder of the Labrador characterized by myotonia has been described and determined to be familial with an autosomal recessive mode of inheritance.[49–52] The clinical signs appear between three and six months of age and as the dogs mature, the signs stabilize. The signs include difficulty in holding the head erect, stiffness and extension of the limbs, shortened gait, hopping with the pelvic limbs, and collapse. The problem abates with rest. Activity, excitement, cold, and administration of edrophonium exacerbate the signs.

The only significant clinicopathologic abnormalities are creatinuria and a lower than normal serum creatine kinase level. Electromyography reveals spontaneous myofiber discharges, including fibrillations and bizarre high-frequency discharges. Nerve conduction velocities are normal and repetitive nerve stimulations do not reveal changes in the amplitude of compound muscle action potentials. The predominant pathologic change is a paucity of type 2 myofibers.

Studies of urinary electrolyte excretion reveal that these dogs excrete larger than normal quantities of sodium, potassium, and calcium and that their urinary volumes are increased. In addition, plasma aldosterone levels are elevated. The significance of these findings remains to be seen.

The pathogenesis of this condition is obscure. The evidence suggests a myopathy but the possibility of neuropathy has not been excluded. Successful therapy has not been achieved.

OTHER MYOTONIC CONDITIONS

A myopathy of juvenile golden retrievers has been described.[53] The clinical signs were similar to those of the chow chow dogs but electromyography revealed bizarre high-frequency discharge rather than myotonic discharge. Muscle biopsies were characterized by variable fiber sizes, hyaline fibers, central nuclei, proliferation of endomysium, necrotic fibers with phagocytosis, and regeneration. Both types of fibers were affected.

There have been additional reports of myopathies characterized by myotonia in Irish terriers, a Staffordshire terrier, and a Rhodesian ridgeback.[54–56] Myotonia has been recognized as a feature of hyperadrenocorticism and is discussed in another section.

Disorders of Glycogen Metabolism

It appears that there are several types of glycogen storage disorders in dogs and these affect the muscles as well as other organs. Generalized glycogen storage disease associated with hypoglycemia has been described in six- to eight-week-old toy breeds. These dogs exhibited stupor, weakness, and coma. The first report regarded these as similar to Von Gierke's syndrome.[3] Later the same authors assigned these cases to three categories: Von Gierke syndrome (deficiency of glucose-6-phosphatase or type I), generalized glycogen storage, and Cori's disease (amylo-1,6-glucosidase deficiency, limited dextrinosis, debrancher enzyme deficiency, or glycogen storage disease type III).[58] Enzymatic investigations were not performed. Since then a generalized glycogenesis presumed to be α-glucosidase deficiency has been described.[59]

Amylo-1,6-glucosidase deficiency has subsequently been confirmed with enzymatic and glycogen structure studies.[60–61] This disorder occurred in nine- to 15-month-old female German shepherd dogs. These dogs exhibited poor growth and weakness. Blood glucose was measured in one case and found to be lower than normal.

Mammalian phosphofructokinase (PFK) exists in multimolecular forms that result from random combinations of three subunits: M (muscle), P (platelet), and L (liver). Humans homozygous for deficiency of the M subunit (glycogen storage disease type VII) experience exertional weakness and compensated hemolysis. PKF deficiency has been identified in springer spaniel dogs.[4, 62, 63] Nuclear magnetic resonance spectroscopy was used to investigate the bioenergetics of these dogs and a glycolytic block was confirmed. The dogs suffered from chronic hemolytic anemia and sporadic hemolytic crises. Weakness was not a problem. Enzymatic investigations demonstrated that the dogs lacked the M subunit. Apparently weakness does not occur because the muscle fibers contain an anomalous PFK composed of L subunits and also because canine muscle has a higher oxidative potential due to a predominance of type 1 and type 2A fibers.

These reports confirm that disorders of carbohydrate metabolism occur in the dog. Their role in clinical myopathies remains to be further elucidated.

Nemaline Myopathy

Myopathies associated with nemaline rods have been described in dogs and cats.[64, 65] Several rare syndromes occur in humans.[42] Nemaline rods are intramyofiber structures aligned along the long axis of the fibers. They are up to 6 μm in length and are associated with the Z bands of the sarcomeres. With trichrome stains they have a characteristic red color and in cross-sections they appear in clusters within the myofibers. Their significance and specificity remain unclear.

A familial syndrome in young cats characterized by large numbers of nemaline rods has been reported.[65] These cats had the following characteristic signs: apprehension, reluctance to move, and abrupt exaggerated movements when prompted that produced a rapid, hopping, hypermetric gait. The signs involved all limbs without loss of strength or balance. Patellar reflexes were consistently depressed. Atrophy was an inconsistent feature. Creatine kinase levels in serum were modestly elevated. EMG and CSF were normal.

Pathologic findings in the muscles included type 1 myofiber paucity, atrophy of type 1 and type 2A fibers, fiber splitting, and central nuclei. Nemaline rods were most prevalent in atrophied type 1 and type 2A fibers.

The pathogenesis of this disorder and the significance of the nemaline rods remain unclear. It appears at this point that nemaline rods are a nonspecific neuromuscular disease change.

Muscular Dystrophy

Muscular dystrophy in humans refers to a group of familial degenerative myopathies. Vascular and neurogenic hypotheses regarding pathogenesis prevailed at one time. Now the most convincing evidence suggests that defects of the plasma membrane resulting in inappropriate calcium flux may be the cause of at least Duchenne dystrophy.[42]

There have been several reports suggesting that canine myopathies were "dystrophic."[66, 67] The myopathies of Irish terriers and golden retrievers mentioned earlier and some of the cases of myotonia manifested pathologic changes suggesting disorders resembling human dystrophies. At this time correlation of canine disorders to those of humans seems unwarranted, pending further investigation regarding pathogenesis, heritability, and pathology.

Hypothyroid Myopathy

Neuropathy and myopathy have been reported to be associated with hypothyroidism in humans.[68] There are few reports of this association in animals (see Chapter 95).[64, 69, 70] Type 2 myofiber atrophy has been a consistent feature of muscle biopsies of hypothyroid humans and dogs with neuromuscular disorders (Figure 65–6). Whether this change is neurogenic or myopathic remains to be demonstrated. At this time the role of hypothyroidism in neuromuscular disorders remains unclear. It appears to be warranted to examine thyroid functions in patients with neuromuscular disorders and to treat accordingly if hypothyroidism is confirmed.

Hyperadrenocorticism

Dogs with hyperadrenocorticism manifest a variety of clinical signs of muscular dysfunction. Many cases present with generalized atrophy presumed to be related to an enhanced catabolic state due to impaired protein synthesis and, perhaps, an impairment of the anabolic effects of insulin.[16] However, several cases have been described where weakness was associated with hypertro-

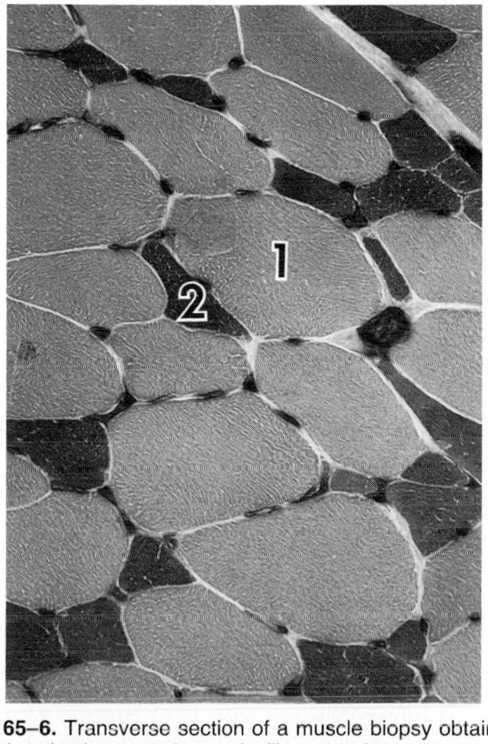

FIGURE 65–6. Transverse section of a muscle biopsy obtained from a dog with selective type 2 muscle fiber atrophy. 1 = type 1; 2 = type 2. × 450. (Courtesy of G. H. Cardinet, III.)

phy and stiffness or myotonia (see the section on myotonia). Some cases have had no clinical evidence of myopathy.[71–74]

Regardless of the clinical features, electromyography has consistently revealed high-frequency discharges. Some were myotonic and others were bizarre high-frequency discharges. Biopsies of these cases yielded highly variable results but type 2 myofiber atrophy was a consistent feature. Whether this change was neuropathic or myopathic was not proven. Some cases revealed myofiber necrosis and phagocytosis, others had patterns suggesting denervation and nerve fiber pathology. These findings suggest a disorder both of peripheral nerves and myofibers or a "neuromyopathy."

Although there is a confusing array of information available it seems clear that there are profound neuromuscular effects of hyperadrenocorticism and these are highly variable. Their significance remains to be resolved.

Polymyositis

Generalized inflammatory myopathy of dogs has been associated with toxoplasmosis, SLE, and leptospirosis.[75–79] Atrophic and eosinophilic forms have been described.[80, 81] Most cases of polymyositis have necrosis and phagocytosis of myofibers with a mononuclear infiltrate.[82–84] Direct immunofluorescence has revealed immune complexes on the sarcolemma of these cases.[83] In addition, autoantibodies directed toward the sarcolemma have been identified.[16] Hence, these cases are presumed to be autoimmune in nature.

Dogs with polymyositis are usually adults; there is no apparent male or female predisposition. The predominant clinical signs are weakness, pain, fever, atrophy, and stiffness. Regurgitation associated with megaesophagus is a common feature and these patients often have aspiration pneumonia. Differentiation of these patients from cases of neuropathy or myelopathy may be difficult (Table 65–2).

Levels of serum enzymes such as aspartate aminotransferase, lactic dehydrogenase, and creatine kinase may be elevated but inconsistently; they do not reflect the severity of the disease. When elevated they cannot be regarded as diagnostic. For example, creatine kinase is elevated in polyneuropathies. ANA tests are usually negative.

Electromyography reveals spontaneous myofiber discharges, including fibrillations, positive sharp waves, prolonged insertional activity, and bizarre high-frequency discharges. Motor unit potentials may be polyphasic. Nerve conduction velocities and repetitive stimulation studies are normal.

Muscle biopsies reveal myofiber necrosis with phagocytosis and a mononuclear infiltrate. There is evidence of regeneration and fibrosis. A fiber type predisposition is not apparent in these cases.

Dogs with polymyositis should be treated with immunosuppressive corticosteroids. An infectious cause or aspiration pneumonia are contraindications. The goal is prompt remission with large doses, followed by long-term, low-dose, alternate-day therapy. Relapses are to be expected. Other immune-mediated disorders and other problems associated with immune disturbances, such as neoplasia, should be sought.

Toxoplasmosis

Myositis due to toxoplasmosis occurs in juvenile and adult forms.[75–77] It appears that concurrent CNS infection always occurs. It is mentioned here because serologic confirmation is very unreliable and muscle biopsy is regarded as the best means of antemortem diagnosis (Figure 65–7). If a diagnosis is confirmed, trimethoprim/sulfonamide therapy is recommended.

Dermatomyositis

A disease of juvenile collies characterized by concurrent dermatitis and myositis has been described and called dermatomyositis (DM).[85–88] The disease is familial and it appears to be inherited as an autosomal dominant with variable expressivity. Dermatitis appears at seven to 11 weeks of age with a fluctuating course for several years. Some cases have had temporary remissions, whereas others have had complete resolutions. The intensity of dermatitis is highly variable and myositis may not be clinically apparent. It has been suggested that this condition is the same as epidermolysis bullosa,

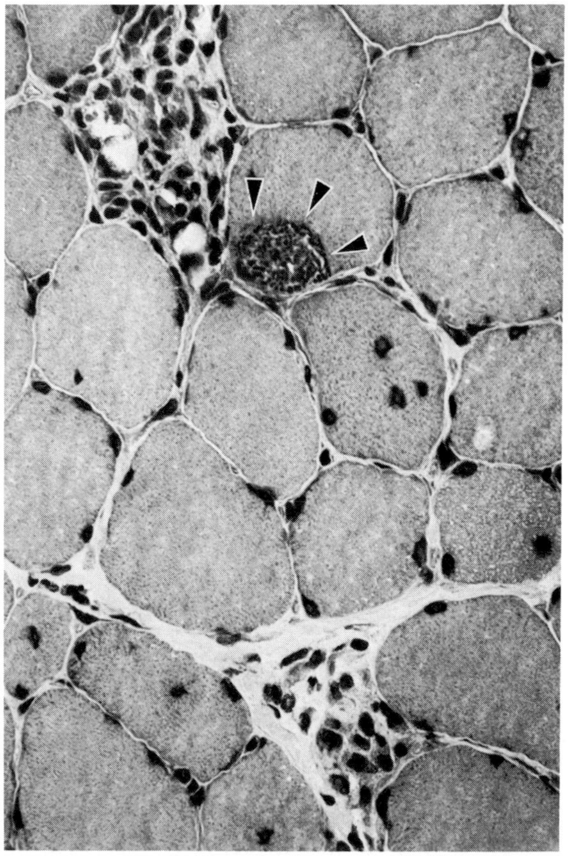

FIGURE 65–7. Transverse section of a muscle biopsy obtained from a dog with myositis associated with toxoplasmosis. One fiber contains an intrafiber cyst of the *Toxoplasma* spp. organisms *(arrowheads)*. × 450. (Courtesy of G. H. Cardinet, III.)

which has been described in collies and Shetland sheepdogs.

The predominant dermatologic signs are erythema, alopecia, ulceration, and crusts of the face, lips, pinnae, tail, and the skin over the prominent bones. Secondary pyoderma occurs and vesicles appear occasionally.

Resolving lesions exhibit alopecia and hypo- or hyperpigmentation. Histologic abnormalities include acanthosis, vacuolation of basal cells, and separation of the dermoepidermal junction. The dermis may have no lesions early in the course of the disease, but later a prominent inflammation with a perivascular mononuclear infiltrate usually appears. There may be concurrent pyoderma or demodecosis. Serum and cutaneous immunologic investigations are not remarkable except for circulating immune complexes, whose role is not defined.

The myositis in DM also has a variable expression. Most cases show few or no clinical signs. The patients with signs of myositis are those with severe dermatitis. Masticatory muscle myositis predominates. Some cases manifest poor growth, difficulty in prehending or masticating, dysphagia, generalized paresis, or exercise intolerance. Creatine kinase, CSF, and other clinicopathologic signs are not consistently abnormal.

Electromyography reveals spontaneous myofiber discharges, such as positive sharp waves, fibrillation potentials, and bizarre high-frequency discharges. These changes appear to have limited distribution and the masticatory muscles may be the only muscles involved in some cases. Nerve conduction velocities are normal. Muscle biopsies reveal myofiber necrosis with mononuclear infiltrate, atrophy, regeneration, and fibrosis. Both fiber types appear to be affected. There has been no documentation of immunoglobulin associated with these lesions nor circulating autoantibodies to myofibrillar proteins.[16]

The fluctuating course of this disease makes prognostication difficult. Likewise, the efficacy of therapy has been difficult to judge. Corticosteroids have been tried but response has been equivocal. Affected animals must not be used for breeding.

A similar condition has been described in the Shetland sheepdog, where it appeared to be familial.[89] Additional reports will be required to clarify the condition in this breed. The evidence of myositis is meager.

Masticatory Muscle Myositis

Masticatory muscle myositis (MMM) is a common disorder of the dog. It occurs as a component of polymyositis, but in most cases the inflammation is limited to the masticatory muscles. In some cases eosinophilia or an eosinophilic infiltrate led to the use of the term eosinophilic myositis.[90–93] Atrophic myositis was the term used to describe other cases.[94–96] The nature of these conditions and possible relationships between them have been debated extensively. Recent investigations have suggested an autoimmune basis for MMM and have revealed that eosinophilic myositis and eosinophilia are unusual. Most cases of MMM have necrosis and phagocytosis of myofibers, with mononuclear accumulations.[97]

PATHOGENESIS

Histochemical investigations using the myofibrillar adenosine triphosphatase staining properties of myofibers have revealed that the myofibers of the masticatory muscles are distinct from those of the limbs.[98] This probably relates to their origin from the first branchial arch rather than the somites and may be related to the nature of their innervation by the mandibular branch of the trigeminal nerve. Two types of fibers of the masticatory muscles have been described: a variant of type 1 and type 2M (Table 65–2). Additional investigations have demonstrated that these myofibers also contain a unique group of myosin components.[99]

These findings led the way to further studies that have revealed details regarding the pathogenesis of MMM. It appears that the type 2M myofibers are the target of an autoimmune disturbance (Figure 65–8).[6, 97] Necrosis and phagocytosis are limited to these fibers and the density of the variant type 1 fibers increases, whereas the density of the type 2M fibers decreases.[97] Immunocytochemical methods using the staphylococcal Protein A-horseradish peroxidase method reveal IgG bound to affected myofibers and IgG with affinity for type 2M fibers in the serum of affected patients. In addition, ELISA and immunoblot methods confirm that the serum of these patients contains antibodies directed toward the unique myosin components of these fibers. The stimulus for this autoimmunity remains obscure. These autoantibodies are directed against proteins usually sequestered from the immune system. The means whereby the immune system encounters these myofibrillar components and the role of the antibodies in the pathogenesis of the myositis is unknown. Nevertheless, the information gathered so far supports the autoimmune nature of the disorder. Further work will elucidate the mechanisms involved.

CLINICAL FEATURES

Masticatory muscle myositis occurs in adult dogs of the large breeds. A male or female predisposition is not apparent. The expression of the disorder is variable. Most patients are presented for bilateral atrophy of temporalis and masseter muscles with trismus. Some cases manifest swelling of those muscles and unilateral cases occur occasionally. Recurrent cases occur. Concurrent MMM and optic neuritis has been reported. The outcome of most cases is severe atrophy with preservation of function that is presumed to be related to sparing of the variant type 1 fibers from the immune attack. Some cases develop permanent trismus, presumed to be due to fibrosis.[99] Laboratory investigations do not reveal consistent abnormalities. Eosinophilia occurs occasionally but is not always associated with an eosinophilic myositis. Serum creatine kinase may be modestly elevated, but often the value is normal. Electromyography reveals spontaneous myofiber discharges limited to the masticatory muscles. Abnormalities beyond the masticatory muscles suggest an alternate neuromuscular disorder. Bizarre high-frequency discharges have been observed. Biopsy of affected muscles reveals necrosis and phagocytosis of type 2M myofibers with a mononuclear

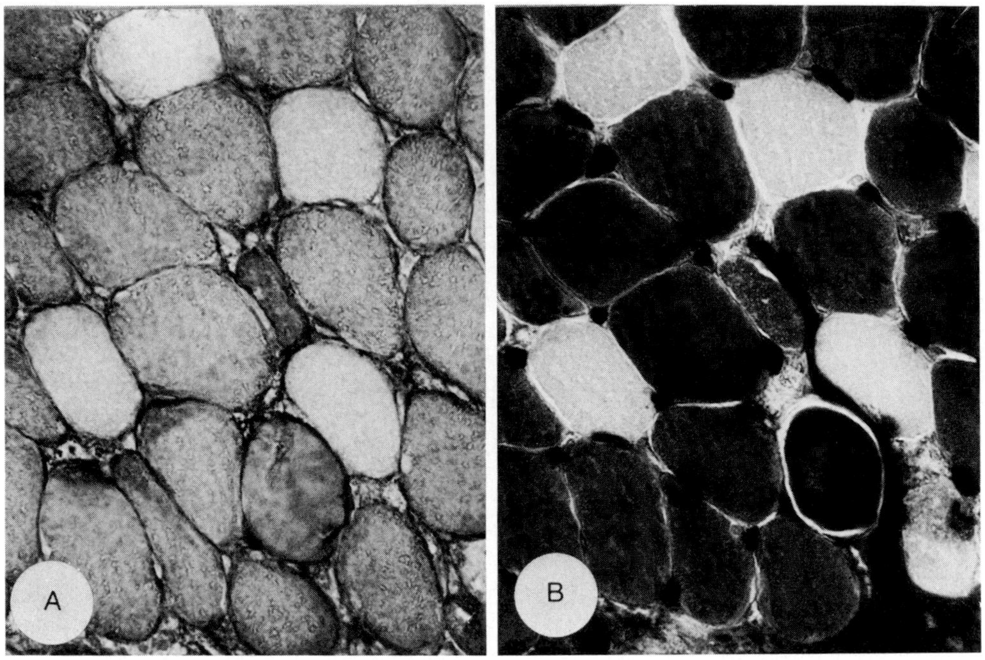

FIGURE 65–8. Adjacent transverse sections of a temporalis muscle biopsy obtained from a dog with masticatory muscle myositis. The sections were stained for IgG localization *(A)* and myofibrillar ATPase *(B)*. Fibers that are positively stained for IgG *(A)* are darkly stained type 2M fibers *(B)*, while fibers unstained for IgG *(A)* are lightly stained type 1 fibers *(B)*. × 450. (From Shelton GD, Cardinet GH, and Bandman E: Canine masticatory muscle disorders: A study of 29 cases. Muscle and Nerve 10:753–766, 1987.)

infiltrate. Infrequently, eosinophils are a major feature. Immunologic investigations can be conducted; the findings have been discussed in an earlier section.

MANAGEMENT

Immunosuppressive doses of corticosteroids are indicated for the treatment of MMM with trismus, whether associated with swelling or atrophy. Chronic cases with severe atrophy and without interference with mastication are probably the result of previous episodes of inflammation and may not require therapy. Patients with severe trismus and atrophy may fail to respond due to fibrosis and the prognosis is poor. Attempts to force the jaws open are not indicated. The goal is to achieve normal function. There is little hope of preventing or alleviating atrophy. Once function has been restored, long-term, low-dose, alternate-day therapy can be instituted.

References

1. Ormrod, AN: Myasthenia in a cocker spaniel. Vet Rec 73:489, 1961.
2. Pflugfelder, CM, et al.: Acquired canine myasthenia gravis: immunocytochemical localization of immune complexes at neuromuscular junctions. Muscle and Nerve 4:289, 1981.
3. Bardens, JW, et al.: Clinical observations on a Von Gierke-like syndrome in puppies. Allied Vet Jan-Feb, 1961.
4. Vora, S, et al.: Characterization of the enzymatic lesion in inherited phosphofructokinase deficiency in dog: an animal analogue of human glycogen storage disease type VII. Proc Natl Acad Sci USA 82:8109, 1985.
5. Winter, H and Stephenson, HC: A case of eosinophilic myositis in a dog. Cornell Vet 42:531, 1952.
6. Shelton, GD, et al.: Fiber type-specific autoantibodies in a dog with eosinophilic myositis. Muscle and Nerve 8:783, 1985.
7. Braund, KG, et al.: Observations on normal skeletal muscle of mature dogs: A cytochemical, histochemical, and morphometric study. Vet Pathol 19:577, 1982.
8. Dubowitz, V and Brooke, MH (eds): Muscle Biopsy, a Modern Approach. Saunders, London, 1974.
9. Cardinet, GH and Stephens-Orvis, J: Skeletal muscle function. *In* Kaneko JJ (ed): Clinical Biochemistry of Domestic Animals, 3rd ed. New York, Academic Press, 1980, p 545.
10. Lennon, VA, et al.: Myasthenia gravis in dogs: acetylcholine receptor deficiency with and without anti-receptor autoantibodies. *In* Rose NR, et al. (eds): Genetic Control of Autoimmune Disease. Amsterdam, Elsevier North Holland, 1978, p 295.
11. Lennon, VA, et al.: Acquired and congenital myasthenia gravis in dogs: a study of 20 cases. *In* Satoyoshi E (ed): Myasthenia Gravis: Pathogenesis and Treatment. Univ Tokyo Press, 1981, p 41.
12. Miller, LM, et al.: Congenital myasthenia gravis in 13 smooth fox terriers. JAVMA 182:694, 1983.
13. Oda, K, et al.: Congenital canine myasthenia gravis: 1. deficient junctional acetylcholine receptors. Muscle and Nerve 7:705, 1984.
14. Garlepp, M, et al.: Antibodies to the acetylcholine receptor in myasthenic dogs. Immunology 37:807, 1979.
15. Garlepp, MJ, et al.: Autoimmunity in spontaneous myasthenia gravis in dogs. Clin Immunol Immunopathol 31:3401, 1984.
16. Shelton, GD and Cardinet, GH: Pathophysiologic basis of canine muscle disorders. J Vet Int Med 1:36, 1987.
17. Engel, AG: Morphologic and immunologic findings in myasthenia gravis and in congenital myasthenic syndromes. J Neur Neurosurg Psychiatr 43:577, 1980.
18. Drachman, DB: Myasthenia gravis. N Engl J Med 298:136, 1978.
19. Hall, GA, et al.: Thymoma with myasthenia gravis in a dog. J Pathol 188:177, 1972.
20. Darke, PGG, et al.: Myasthenia gravis, thymoma and myositis in a dog. Vet Rec 97:392, 1975.
21. Poffenbergar, E, et al.: Acquired myasthenia gravis in a dog with thymoma: a case report. JAAHA 21:119, 1985.
22. Oda, K, et al.: Congenital canine myasthenia gravis: II. Acetylcholine receptor metabolism. Muscle and Nerve 7:717, 1984.
23. Johnson, RP, et al.: Myasthenia in springer spaniel littermates. J Sm Anim Pract 16:641, 1975.
24. Jenkins, WL, et al.: Myasthenia gravis in a fox terrier litter. J S Afr Vet Assn 47:59, 1976.
25. Palmer, AC and Goodyear, JV: Congenital myasthenia in the Jack Russell terrier. Vet Rec 103:433, 1978.

26. Miller, LM, et al.: Inheritance of congenital myasthenia gravis in smooth fox terrier dogs. J Hered 75:163, 1984.
27. Wallace, ME and Palmer, AC: Recessive mode of inheritance in myasthenia gravis in the Jack Russell terrier. Vet Rec 114:350, 1984.
28. Palmer, AC and Barker, J: Myasthenia in the dog. Vet Rec 95:452, 1974.
29. Palmer, AC, et al.: Autoimmune form of myasthenia gravis in a juvenile Yorkshire terrier x Jack Russell terrier hybrid contrasted with congenital (non-autoimmune) myasthenia gravis of the Jack Russell. J Sm Anim Pract 21:359, 1980.
30. Witt, WM and Ludwig, RD: Anticholinesterase-responsive weakness in the canine similar to myasthenia gravis of man. JAAHA 14:138, 1978.
31. Johnson, NW and McDonald, IF: Myasthenia gravis in a dog. Vet Rec 101:216, 1977.
32. Marlow, CA: Myasthenia gravis in a dog. Vet Rec 101:123, 1977.
33. Fraser, DC, et al.: Myasthenia gravis in the dog. J Neurol Neurosurg Psychiat 33:431, 1970.
34. Zacks, SI, et al.: A myasthenic syndrome in the dog: A case report with electron microscopic observations on motor end plates and comparisons with the fine structure of end plates in myasthenia gravis. Ann NY Acad Sci 135:79, 1966.
35. Lorenz, MD, et al.: Neostigmine-responsive weakness in the dog, similar to myasthenia gravis. JAVMA 161:795, 1972.
36. Cain, GR, et al.: Myasthenia gravis and polymyositis in a dog following fetal hematopoctic cell transplantation. Transplantation 41:21, 1986.
37. Schutt, VI and Kersten, U: Myasthenia gravis - eine ubersicht uber den krankheitsverlauf bei 23 Hunden. Kleintierpraxis 31:121, 1986.
38. Dawson, JRB: Myasthenia gravis in a cat. Vet Rec 86:562, 1970.
39. Mason, KV: A case of myasthenia in a cat. J Sm Anim Pract 17:467, 1976.
40. Indrieri, RJ, et al.: Myasthenia gravis in two cats. JAVMA 182:57, 1983.
41. Rowland, LP: Diseases of the motor unit: The motor neuron, peripheral nerve, and muscle. *In* Schwartz JH (ed): Principles of Neural Science. Amsterdam, Elsevier, 1985, p 196.
42. Walton, Sir John (ed): Brain's Diseases of the Nervous System. Oxford Univ Press, 1985.
43. Griffiths, IR and Duncan, ID: Myotonia in the dog: a report of four cases. Vet Rec 93:184, 1973.
44. Duncan, ID and Griffiths, IR: A myopathy associated with myotonia in the dog. Acta Neuropathol (Berl) 341:297, 1975.
45. Wentink, GH, et al.: Three cases of myotonia in a family of chows. Tijdschr Diergeneesk 99:729, 1974.
46. Farrow, BRH and Malik, R: Hereditary myotonia in the chow chow. J Sm Anim Pract 22:451, 1981.
47. Jones, BR, et al.: Myotonia in related chow chow dogs. N Z Vet J 25:217, 1976.
48. Shores, A, et al.: Myotonia congenita in a chow chow pup. JAVMA 188:532, 1986.
49. Kramer, JW, et al.: A muscle disorder of labrador retrievers characterized by deficiency of Type II muscle fibers. JAVMA 169:817, 1976.
50. Kramer, JW, et al.: Inheritance of a neuromuscular disorder of labrador retriever dogs. JAVMA 179:380, 1981.
51. Moore, MP, et al.: Electromyographic characterization of labrador retriever dogs with inherited Type II muscle fiber deficiency. Fed Proc 43:708, 1984.
52. Hegreberg, GA, et al.: Electrolyte loss associated with an inherited Type II muscle fiber deficiency in dogs. Fed Proc 43:708, 1984.
53. Kornegay, JN: Golden retriever myopathy. *In* Kirk RW (ed): Current Veterinary Therapy IX. Philadelphia, WB Saunders Co, 1986, p 792.
54. Wentink, GH, et al.: Myopathy with a possible recessive X-linked inheritance in a litter of Irish terriers. Vet Pathol 9:328, 1972.
55. Shires, PK, et al.: Myotonia in a Staffordshire terrier. JAVMA 183:229, 1983.
56. Simpson, ST and Braund, KG: Mytonic dystrophy-like disease in a dog. JAVMA 186:495, 1985.
58. Bardens, JW: Glycogen storage disease in puppies. VMSAC 61:1174, 1966.
59. Mostafa, IE: A case of glycogenic cardiomegaly in a dog. Acta Vet Scand 11:197, 1970.
60. Rafiquzzaman, M, et al.: Glycogenosis in the dog. Acta Vet Scand 17:196, 1976.
61. Ceh, L, et al.: Glycogenosis Type III in the dog. Acta Vet Scand 17:210, 1976.
62. Giger, U, et al.: Inherited phosphofructokinase deficiency in dogs with hyperventilation-induced hemolysis: increased in vitro and in vivo alkaline fragility of erythrocytes. Blood 65:345, 1985.
63. Giger, U, et al.: Myopathy in phosphofructokinase deficient dogs studied by in vivo ^{31}p-NMR. Muscle and Nerve 9(5S):187, 1986.
64. Cardinet, GH and Holliday, TA: Neuromuscular diseases of domestic animals: a summary of muscle biopsies from 159 cases. Ann NY Acad Sci 317:290, 1979.
65. Cooper, BJ, et al.: Nemaline myopathy of cats. Muscle and Nerve 9:618, 1986.
66. Innes, JRM: Myopathies in animals. Br Vet J 107:131, 1951.
67. Whitney, JC: Progressive muscular dystrophy in the dog. Vet Rec 70:611, 1958.
68. Layzer, RB (ed): Neuromuscular Manifestations of Systemic Disease. Philadelphia, FA Davis Co, 1985, p 79.
69. Sims, MH, et al.: Depressed thyroid function in two tetraplegic dogs. JAVMA 171:178, 1977.
70. Indrieri, RJ, et al.: Neuromuscular abnormalities associated with hypothyroidism and lymphocytic thyroiditis in three dogs. JAVMA 190:544, 1987.
71. Duncan, ID, et al.: Myotonia in canine Cushing's disease. Vet Rec 100:30, 1977.
72. Greene, CE, et al.: Myopathy associated with hyperadrenocorticism in the dog. JAVMA 174:1310, 1979.
73. Braund, KG, et al.: Subclinical myopathy associated with hyperadrenocorticism in the dog. Vet Pathol 17:134, 1980.
74. Braund, KG, et al.: Experimental investigation of glucocorticoid-induced myopathy in the dog. Exp Neurol 68:50, 1980.
75. Suter, MM, et al.: Polymyositis-polyradiculitis due to toxoplasmosis in the dog: serology and tissue biopsy as diagnostic aids. Zbl Vet Med A 31:792, 1984.
76. Hartley, WJ, et al.: *Toxoplasma* meningoencephalomyelitis and myositis in a dog. N Z Vet J 6:124, 1958.
77. Drake, JC and Hime, JM: Two syndromes in young dogs caused by *Toxoplasma gondii*. J Sm Anim Pract 8:621, 1967.
78. Krum, SH, et al.: Polymyositis and polyarthritis associated with systemic lupus erythematosus in a dog. JAVMA 170:61, 1977.
79. Lavrain, AR: Lesions of skeletal muscle in leptospirosis. Am J Pathol 31:501, 1955.
80. Oghiso, Y, et al.: Clinical and pathological studies on a spontaneous case of canine systemic atrophic myositis. Jap J Vet Sci 38:553, 1976.
81. Scott, DW and deLahunta, A: Eosinophilic polymyositis in a dog. Cornell Vet 64:47, 1974.
82. Meier, H: Myopathies in the dog. Cornell Vet 48:313, 1958.
83. Kornegay, JN, et al.: Polymyositis in dogs. JAVMA 176:431, 1980.
84. Farnbach, GL: Myositis in the dog. Comp Cont Ed Pract Vet 1:183, 1979.
85. Hargis, AM, et al.: Familial canine dermatomyositis. Am J Pathol 116:234, 1984.
86. Kunkle, GA, et al.: Dermatomyositis in collie dogs. Comp Cont Ed Pract Vet 7:185, 1985.
87. Haupt, KH, et al.: Familial canine dermatomyositis: clinical, electrodiagnostic, and genetic studies. Am J Vet Res 46:1861, 1985.
88. Haupt, KH, et al.: Familial canine dermatomyositis: clinicopathologic, immunologic, and serologic studies. Am J Vet Res 46:1870, 1985.
89. Hargis, AM, et al.: A skin disorder in three shetland sheepdogs: comparison with familial canine dermatomyositis of collies. Comp Cont Ed Pract Vet 7:306, 1985.
90. Whitney, JC: Eosinophilic myositis in dogs. Vet Rec 67:1140, 1955.
91. Harding, HP and Owen, LN: Eosinophilic myositis in the dog. J Comp Pathol 66:109, 1956.
92. Head, KW, et al.: A case of eosinophilic myositis in a dog. Br Vet J 114:22, 1958.
93. Lescure, F: Myosite des masticateurs et cecite chez le chien. Revue Med Vet 136:761, 1985.

94. Whitney, JC: Atrophic myositis in a dog: the differentiation of this disease from eosinophilic myositis. Vet Rec 69:130, 1957.
95. Martin, WP and Thompson, R: An unusual case of masticatory muscular atrophy in a dog. Can Vet J 1:371, 1960.
96. Whitney, JC: A case of cranial myodegeneration (atrophic myositis) in a dog. J Sm Anim Pract 11:735, 1970.
97. Shelton, GD, et al.: Canine masticatory muscle disorders: a study of 29 cases. Muscle and Nerve 10:753, 1987.
98. Orvis, JS and Cardinet, GH: Canine muscle fiber types and susceptibility of masticatory muscles to myositis. Muscle and Nerve 4:354, 1981.
99. Shelton, GD, et al.: Electrophoretic comparison of myosins from masticatory muscles and selected limb muscles in the dog. Am J Vet Res 46:493, 1985.

DRUG INDEX

1. Edrophonium (Tensilon), Roche Laboratories, Nutley, NJ
   10 mg/ml
   Recommended dosage: 0.05 to 0.1 mg/lb (0.1 to 0.2 mg/kg) IV for testing for myasthenia gravis
2. Neostigmine (Prostigmin), Roche Laboratories, Nutley, NJ
   0.25, 0.50, and 1.0 mg/ml
   Recommended dosage: 0.02 mg/lb (0.04 mg/kg) IM q.i.d. for initial control of myasthenia. The dose and frequency are highly variable. Slow increases recommended. Atropine can be used concurrently to control muscarinic effects.
3. Pyridostigmine (Mestinon), Roche Laboratories, Nutley, NJ
   Tablets, 60 mg; syrup, 60 mg/5 ml
   Recommended dosage: 0.22 mg/lb (0.5 mg/kg) b.i.d. for maintenance in myasthenia. Doses and frequency are highly variable. Slow increases recommended. Atropine can be used concurrently. Corticosteroids recommended concurrently.

SECTION VII

THE RESPIRATORY SYSTEM

66 CLINICAL APPROACH TO THE PATIENT WITH RESPIRATORY DISEASE

MICHAEL SCHAER, NORMAN ACKERMAN, and
ROBERT R. KING

Animals with various types of respiratory diseases are commonly encountered by small animal practitioners. Many respiratory diseases of the dog and cat may be diagnosed based on the history and physical findings; others, not so routine, present the clinician with a formidable diagnostic challenge. The correct approach to respiratory diseases requires a meticulous history and a complete physical examination in order to prescribe appropriate therapy and to justify further diagnostic procedures. The first section of this chapter discusses the general approach to the patient with respiratory disease and provides the clinician with the general diagnostic methodology concerning respiratory disorders. The second and third sections describe the principles of thoracic radiographic techniques and interpretation and the diagnostic procedures for the lower respiratory tract, respectively. Prior to proceeding with the detailed discussion regarding the history and physical examination, please note the selected definitions pertinent to abnormalities of the respiratory system provided in Table 66–1.

TABLE 66–1. DEFINITIONS RELATING TO DISEASES OF THE RESPIRATORY SYSTEM

Cough	A sudden explosive forcing of air through the glottis, excited by an effort to expel mucus or other matter from the bronchial tubes or larynx.
Hemoptysis	The spitting of blood derived from the lungs or bronchial tubes.
Dyspnea	Subjective difficulty or distress in breathing; frequently, but not necessarily, rapid breathing, usually associated with serious disease of the heart, lungs, or pleural space.
Tachypnea	Very rapid breathing; polypnea.
Hyperpnea	A condition in which the respiration is deeper and more rapid than normal.
Stridor	A high-pitched, noisy respiration, usually associated with upper airway obstruction.
Rale	An adventitious sound of varied character heard on auscultation of the thorax in many cases of pulmonary and bronchial disease.
Rhonchus	A loud rale; especially a whistling or sonorous rale produced in the larger bronchi or the trachea.

GENERAL APPROACH

HISTORY

The written history should contain all medical facts concerning the patient's life, as well as a complete description of the presenting complaint. The clinician must allow sufficient time for the owner to provide this information, which is vital for reaching a correct diagnosis. The examiner must be able to distinguish subjective information from objective information in order to proceed down the correct diagnostic pathway and to avoid an unnecessary expenditure of time and money. Table 66–2 provides a list of the important historical subjects essential for a complete anamnesis.

Signalment. The animal's age and breed must be noted because of the increased incidence of certain diseases in specific breeds and in various age groups. For instance, many of the viral respiratory diseases of the dog and cat commonly occur in the young animal because of the owner's failure to have the pet vaccinated against diseases such as feline rhinotracheitis, feline calicivirus, canine parainfluenza, and canine distemper.

TABLE 66–2. ESSENTIALS FOR THE COMPLETE ANAMNESIS

Age, breed, and sex of the animal
Origin of the animal; previous locales where animal has been
Present environment, exposure to other animals, health status of any other animals and humans at home
Prior medical problems
Vaccination and heartworm status
The current complaint
 a. Last known period of normalcy
 b. Disease onset–acute or gradual
 c. Progression and duration
 d. Intervening signs
 e. Previous treatments for current illness and animal's response; previous medication for problems unrelated to present illness
 f. Present status, i.e., weight loss, attitude, level of activity, appetite status, exercise tolerance

On the other hand, pulmonary neoplasia occurs more frequently in the middle and older age groups.

Certain breeds are predisposed to specific respiratory tract disorders. The brachycephalic breeds commonly have disorders involving the upper respiratory tract, such as stenotic nares, elongated soft palate, and eversion of the lateral laryngeal ventricles. The small toy breeds of dogs have a high incidence of collapsed trachea. Although nasal neoplasia can affect most breeds of dogs, the dolichocephalic and mesocephalic breeds have a higher incidence of this disorder. The Chapters in Section VIII describe the various congenital and acquired forms of heart disease in the dog and cat that can eventually lead to respiratory distress.

The intact male and female pets that have the opportunity to stray are predisposed to trauma. Examples of the associated pathology include gunshot wounds, pneumothorax, hemothorax, and diaphragmatic hernia.

Origin. The animal's geographic origin should be noted while taking the history, as an aid to diagnosis. Histoplasmosis is most commonly found in the states bordering on the Mississippi River Valley and coccidioidomycosis is common in the southwestern parts of the United States. Heartworm disease was confined to the southeastern United States and states bordering on the Gulf of Mexico; however, today dirofilariasis is prevalent throughout most of the USA and many other areas of the world. With today's ease of rapid travel, certain infectious diseases are no longer geographically restricted as they were in the past.

Present Environment. The animal's current environment should be described by the owner. The indoor dog and cat that are under close owner scrutiny are less likely to acquire chest trauma without the owner's knowledge; the outdoor pet is more likely to acquire trauma unobserved by the owner. Unvaccinated animals that are boarded in kennels are more likely to contract infectious respiratory diseases than the pet without environmental exposure to such infectious pathogens. Occupational respiratory diseases are commonly reported in humans. Animals exposed to similar air pollutants are certainly also at risk for pneumoconioses.

Prior Medical Problems. A careful inquiry into the animal's past medical history should be made. A previous history of malignant neoplasia can suggest respiratory disease due to thoracic metastasis. Examples of malignant tumors that have a high predilection for pulmonary metastasis include malignant melanoma, osteosarcoma, hemangiosarcoma, mammary adenocarcinoma, and cutaneous adnexal carcinoma. Dogs and cats that are afflicted with infectious respiratory diseases can become victims of secondary complications such as bacterial pneumonia, chronic sinusitis, and chronic bronchitis. A history of trauma may contribute to the diagnosis of a dyspneic animal as in pneumothorax, hemothorax, chylothorax, and diaphragmatic hernias. Animals with prior histories of bacterial pneumonia, smoke inhalation, or allergic pneumonia are predisposed to chronic lung diseases such as chronic bronchitis, bronchiectasis, and pulmonary fibrosis. These complications are usually associated with protracted patient morbidity.

Current Complaint. After obtaining the historical data, the clinician should focus on the current complaint. This is best begun by inquiring when the animal was last normal and when the problem began. Oftentimes the owner is unaware of the pet's respiratory disease and presents the animal with the complaints of decreased appetite and exercise intolerance. This is frequently true of dogs and cats that have pleural effusions. Pet owners are more aware of respiratory disease when their pets show more obvious signs, such as nasal discharge, sneezing, coughing, and gagging. It is important to determine whether the signs of disease are acute or chronic. A dog that begins coughing a few days following kennel boarding is quite likely to have acquired infectious tracheobronchitis. On the other hand, an eight-year-old poodle with the same type of harsh resonant cough that is unchanged for several years is more likely to have a disorder such as collapsed trachea. A young indoor dog or cat that becomes acutely dyspneic with diffuse moist pulmonary rales is certainly a candidate for noncardiogenic pulmonary edema from electrocution.

Progression and Duration. The nature of disease progression and duration should be accurately described. Animals showing respiratory abnormalities when placed in specific environments should be suspected of having hypersensitivity-related disease. However, with repeated exposure to the sensitizing antigen, the patient's respiratory signs can change from intermittent to continuous. Progressive respiratory disease frequently shows systemic manifestations such as weight loss, mental depression, dull hair coat, decreased appetite, and exercise intolerance.

The history should also contain a description of other intervening signs. The onset of vomiting, diarrhea, or seizures in an unvaccinated dog that first presented with respiratory illness should lead the clinician to suspect an infectious disease such as canine distemper. A cat that is examined for a chronic cough, fever, and focal lung consolidation several weeks after having been treated for pyothorax is a good candidate for a diagnosis of lung abscess.

Previous Treatments. A complete history of previous medications can reveal important information. Animals with allergic lung disease typically respond to symptomatic treatments containing glucocorticoids. This response frequently lasts as long as the effects of glucocorticoids continue, and the patient soon suffers a relapse when the drug is no longer available. Chronic bacterial bronchitis frequently responds to antibiotic treatment, but patients with this ailment periodically suffer relapses. Some drugs and chemicals are known to be a direct cause of pulmonary disease, especially in humans. Such drugs include busulfan, bleomycin, methotrexate, nitrofurantoin, and the sulfonamides. The pulmonary changes are fairly specific for each type of drug but generally include infiltrates and pulmonary fibrosis associated with pulmonary hypersensitivity.

Present Status. The present status of the patient should be evaluated. Signs indicating chronic progressive disease were mentioned earlier. These signs can occur in various combinations and should signal the clinician that hospitalization for a diagnostic work-up and therapeutic support measures are warranted. In contrast, the patient with a nasal and ocular discharge associated with a recent onset of coughing is often treated symptomatically as an outpatient if the animal is alert, active, and eating well.

In summary, the history is a source of many important diagnostic clues. Allow enough time to obtain this vital diagnostic information, which should be correlated with the physical examination findings in order to deduce the most likely diagnosis as soon as possible.

THE PHYSICAL EXAMINATION

A thorough physical examination is essential for all patients with respiratory disease. It should be performed as methodically as possible. When the animal does not present with an acute respiratory emergency requiring an abbreviated initial physical examination and immediate therapy, the clinician should direct his undivided attention to the entire animal before examining the respiratory system specifically. Much can be gained by simply observing the animal from a distance, taking careful note of its body condition, mentation, posture, locomotion, and respiratory pattern. An animal with respiratory disease that looks dull and emaciated usually has a serious illness. The typical features of a dyspneic animal include anxious behavior, posturing with elbows abducted and neck extended, rapid respiratory rate with an increased abdominal breathing component, and sometimes open-mouth breathing. This patient requires immediate supportive therapy and an expedient, nonstressful, diagnostic examination.

The temperature and the pulse and respiratory rates should be taken and recorded after an initial general observation of the patient. Fever is usually associated with inflammatory diseases such as bacterial and viral infections. However, the examiner should be aware that not all patients with infections have fever. Furthermore, it is common for a normal dog or cat to spike body temperatures as high as 104° F (40° C) from pure excitement.

Although most dogs and cats with respiratory disease have increased pulse and respiratory rates, there are rare occasions where exceptions occur. As seen with pyrexia, the excited normal patient can also have increased pulse and respiratory rates.

Hydration. The patient's hydration status should be noted. Febrile inappetent cats with upper respiratory virus infections of only a few days' duration are commonly dehydrated at the time of the physical examination. Any animal with signs of dyspnea and anorexia is prone to dehydration, which warrants fluid replacement during the initial phase of therapy. Dehydrated animals with bacterial pneumonia commonly have tenacious mucous plugs obstructing the lower airways. Establishing euhydration helps mobilize and remove these mucous obstructions from the bronchi and bronchioles.

The patient's complete health status should be thoroughly assessed prior to commencing parenteral rehydration. Those without underlying cardiac disease or hypoalbuminemia can be safely rehydrated with isotonic polyionic parenteral fluids (such as lactated Ringer's solution). Animals with cardiac disease are predisposed to pulmonary edema during parenteral fluid therapy. These patients should, therefore, receive either 0.45 per cent saline or half-strength lactated Ringer's solution and the rate of infusion usually should not exceed 1 ml/pound/hour. Ideally, cardiac patients receiving parenteral fluid therapy should have central venous pressure (CVP) monitoring in an intensive care setting. The intravenous fluids should be temporarily discontinued when the CVP reaches 8 to 10 cm H_2O and reinstituted when it reduces to safer levels, such as 2 to 5 cm H_2O. Animals with hypoalbuminemia are predisposed to pulmonary edema and pleural effusions because they lack sufficient plasma oncotic pressure. Therefore, parenteral fluids administered to such patients should be given very cautiously and be accompanied by close monitoring.

Abdomen and Lymph Nodes. Thorough palpation of the abdomen and the peripheral lymph nodes is very important. Any detectable hepatomegaly, splenomegaly, lymphadenopathy, or other mass lesions might indicate a multicentric neoplastic process in the dyspneic animal. Gastric tympany associated with an acute onset of dyspnea in a puppy or kitten is a clue to the diagnosis of aerophagia associated with acute chest trauma or pulmonary edema due to electrocution. The detection of ascites in a patient with respiratory disease suggests abnormalities such as hypoproteinemia, neoplasia, heart failure, systemic inflammatory disease, or diffuse hemorrhage (see Chapter 28).

Skin and Musculoskeletal Systems. The skin and musculoskeletal systems should be evaluated for any localized swellings or inflammatory foci. The digits and pads of an unpigmented cat or dog should be assessed for peripheral cyanosis. Animals affected with cardiomyopathy or bacterial endocarditis can present with any combination of dyspnea, intermittent claudication, or an inability to use a particular limb. This limb dysfunction might be due to an arterial thromboembolus or vasospasm, causing regional tissue ischemia or anoxia. Dogs showing signs of painful, warm, firm, symmetrical swelling that involves their distal appendages might have hypertrophic osteopathy and associated severe underlying pulmonary disease.

Head. The animal's head should be inspected thoroughly. Dyspneic animals frequently splay their nostrils during both inspiration and expiration. Evaluation of the nasal area should note the presence and character of any nasal discharge and abnormal nasal sounds. A lack of movement of a wisp of cotton held directly in front of a nasal opening usually indicates ipsilateral nasal obstruction. Visualization and palpation of the nasal bones can detect asymmetrical swellings typical of neoplastic or granulomatous diseases. Cyanosis is particularly noticeable when examining the nonpigmented, oral mucous membranes. Dyspneic hypoxemic dogs and cats often have pale mucous membranes, which can easily be mistaken for anemia. Since anemia and hypoxemia can coexist in a patient, certain diagnostic laboratory tests and thoracic radiographs are required in order to make the correct assessment. This latter problem is well illustrated in the animal suffering from anticoagulant rodenticide intoxication, in which thoracic hemorrhage results in anemia and dyspnea. The remainder of the oral examination should assess the pharyngeal area for presence of neoplasms, foreign bodies, or structural and functional abnormalities.

Eyes. A superficial eye examination can detect conjunctivitis and abnormal ocular discharges that vary from serous or mucoid to purulent in character. Funduscopy is important for the detection of characteristic chorioretinopathies that accompany various diseases such as canine distemper, toxoplasmosis, systemic mycoses, feline leukemia, and infectious feline peritonitis.

Thorax. Finally, the thorax should be evaluated. Before proceeding with auscultation, the clinician should observe the character and rate of breathing. Dyspneic animals display a thumping type of breathing pattern associated with an exaggerated abdominal component and increased respiratory rate. Visualization and palpation of the thorax can reveal abnormal rib and sternal conformation that may be associated with pectus excavatum, tumors, granulomas, and trauma. Cervical palpation can oftentimes detect paratracheal mass lesions or specific tracheal structural abnormalities. Inspection of the thoracic skin might reveal fistulous tracts that connect to deep thoracic wall tissues, reflecting the possibility of intrathoracic involvement as well.

Accurate thoracic auscultation requires the examiner's concentration, a good quality stethoscope, and a quiet examination room. Before evaluating the heart sounds, each side of the chest should be palpated for the detection of a cardiac thrill or a deflection of the apical heart beat. With auscultation, the intensity of the heart sounds should be noted. Any unilateral dullness of cardiac sounds can reflect pathology involving the lungs or pleural cavity ipsilaterally. Muffled heart sounds do not always reflect chest pathology; this may be a normal finding in the deep-chested dog or the extremely obese patient. The heart rate and rhythm should be noted with simultaneous evaluation of the femoral artery pulse quality. The detection of a pulse deficit is a sign of cardiac arrhythmia. Auscultation over the heart valves can detect murmurs or splitting of the systolic or diastolic component. The clinician must realize that the detection of a heart murmur in a coughing or dyspneic animal does not always mean that a definitive diagnosis of congestive heart failure is in order. For example, a ten-year-old toy poodle that has a mitral insufficiency and a collapsed trachea may be coughing primarily because of the collapsed trachea. A meticulous history, thorough physical examination, thoracic radiographs, and an electrocardiogram are in order to correctly define this dog's problem.

Pulmonary auscultation is a definite clinical skill. Accurate listening is often hampered by the friction sounds resulting from the animal's hair rubbing against the stethoscope diaphragm and the tremulous movements of the excited patient. The examiner should auscultate all areas of the chest cavity and take particular note of audible asymmetry. An effort should be made to distinguish cardiac from respiratory sounds in order to avoid mistaking breathing sounds for heart murmurs.

Normal breathing in the dog and cat produces vesicular sounds that are equated to the sound of a "mild wind blowing through the trees." Bronchovesicular sounds merely reflect the flow of air through the bronchial passageways. They are often accentuated in the hyperventilating animal. Normally the bronchovesicular sounds are heard equally bilaterally. Asymmetrical sounds are associated with chest pathology such as pleural effusions, diaphragmatic hernias, pneumothorax, large pulmonary and pleural masses, and pulmonary consolidation.

Coughing animals frequently have harsh bronchovesicular sounds. These sounds are most often associated with disorders of the trachea and bronchi. Tracheal palpation in these animals usually easily elicits a cough reflex. In comparison to normal vesicular sounds, these sounds are characterized as harsh with an exaggerated intensity.

Rales are abnormal breathing sounds produced by the movement of air through bronchi with a luminal diameter compromised as a result of fluid accumulation or bronchial wall thickening. Rales vary in intensity, pitch, and quality, depending on the cause and the area of localization along the bronchopulmonary tree. Medical textbooks clearly describe many different types of rales that are unfortunately not readily apparent during auscultation of the actual patient. Table 66–3 provides descriptions of the various types of breath sounds. More important than the classification of the rales is the clinician's ability to detect the mere presence of abnormal lung sounds and to pursue the problem diagnostically in a logical and expedient manner.

Pleural friction sounds result from rubbing of the apposing pleural surfaces. In the normal animal these sounds are never auscultated. When they are heard, they signify alteration of the pleural surfaces by inflammatory or neoplastic disease.

Percussion of the thorax should not be neglected during the examination of dogs and cats. With practice, percussion is useful in detecting areas of dullness in the chest cavity resulting from abnormal fluid accumulations, mass effect, or lung consolidation. Areas of hyperresonance suggest the presence of pneumothorax.

DIAGNOSTIC APPROACH TO THE NONDYSPNEIC PATIENT WITH RESPIRATORY DISEASE

Before commencing with a diagnostic work-up for respiratory disease, the clinician must first recognize that a respiratory disorder is present and, based on the history and physical examination findings, be able to localize the area of involvement. Often the pet owner misinterprets the frequent gagging and retching move-

TABLE 66–3. CLASSIFICATION OF BREATH SOUNDS

Normal Breath Sounds	
Vesicular	Quiet, rustling sounds heard over peripheral lung regions; inspiration (I) and early expiration (E) normally audible; I louder and longer than E
Bronchial	Harsher blowing or tubular sounds heard over the trachea and anterior thorax; E usually louder and longer than I; presence in an abnormal location usually indicates consolidation
Bronchovesicular	A combination of the above sounds heard when these areas overlap or in early disease
Adventitious (Abnormal) Breath Sounds	
Discontinuous sounds—crackles—distinct, intermittent snapping sound of very short duration; may indicate fluid accumulation or fibrosis; more frequent during I	
Fine crackles Medium crackles Coarse crackles	Depending upon loudness and duration
Continuous sounds—rhonchi and wheezes—slightly longer duration, yet still only a fraction of the respiratory cycle; may have a musical quality; indicate airway narrowing; more frequent during E	
Wheeze—high pitch	
Rhonchus—low pitch	
Stridor—an inspiratory, high-pitched wheeze; originates in laryngeal area	
Pleural friction rub—a combination of continuous and discontinuous sounds; described as a creaky leather sound; produced when inflamed pleural surfaces rub together; may occur on I or E	

Modified from Murphy, RLH Jr: A Simplified Introduction to Lung Sounds. Wellesley Hills, MA, Stethophonics, 1977.

ments following a coughing episode and presents the animal with a mistaken primary complaint of vomiting. In order to avoid wasting time and money on unnecessary tests, the owner's subjective descriptions should be brought into the proper clinical perspective by the examining clinician. Table 66–4 describes the historical signs most often seen with pathology associated with certain anatomic locations along the respiratory tract. The following sections pertaining to the diagnostic workup of specific anatomic areas are very general because of the more detailed discussions found elsewhere in the text.

TABLE 66–4. CLINICAL SIGNS ASSOCIATED WITH SPECIFIC ANATOMIC INVOLVEMENT OF THE RESPIRATORY SYSTEM

Anatomic Area	Usual Signs
Nasal cavity	Nasal discharge, snorting, sneezing, nasal rubbing
Pharynx	Hypersalivation, gagging, retching; occasionally dysphagia, stridor in occlusive disorders
Larynx	Gagging, dyspnea, stridor, occasionally cough
Trachea	Harsh, resonant cough followed by gag; stridor often accompanies occlusion
Bronchi or bronchioles	Cough often followed by gagging or retching
Alveoli	Cough when associated with bronchial pathology; occasionally tachypnea only without cough; dyspnea
Pleural effusions	Tachypnea; coughing is absent unless bronchial pathology is associated with the effusion; dyspnea

NASAL CAVITY AND SINUSES

The diagnostic approach to disorders of the nasal cavity and sinuses varies according to the suspected underlying disorder. The cat or dog with transient viral, irritant, or hypersensitivity rhinitis is usually diagnosed on the basis of the history and physical examination only. However, signs indicative of a chronic or progressive nasal disorder usually require some or all of the following diagnostic procedures: preanesthetic hematologic and serum biochemical evaluations, thoracic radiographs, oral examination during anesthesia, high quality radiographs of the nasal cavity and sinuses, nasal cultures for bacteria and fungi isolation, serology for fungal titer determinations, rhinoscopy, nasal flush and cytology, and biopsy. A blood coagulation evaluation and a serum *Ehrlichia* titer should be done whenever epistaxis is the primary complaint. The selection of these tests depends on the specific problem of each patient, after taking the age and other physical problems into consideration.

THE PHARYNX AND LARYNX

A complete evaluation of the pharynx and larynx is best performed on a sedated or anesthetized animal. Before inducing a deep plane of anesthesia, a neurologic examination is imperative to rule out disorders of the ninth and tenth cranial nerves, which are characterized by soft palate asymmetry, loss of the gag reflex, and abnormal laryngeal movements. Radiography, pharyngoscopy, laryngoscopy, culture, and biopsy are the diagnostic tests indicated for a complete evaluation of pharyngeal and laryngeal disorders. In the normal animal, examination of the oropharynx should reveal an absence of inflammation, mass lesions, and strictures. The posterior aspect of the soft palate should normally have minimal contact with the epiglottis and the laryngeal opening should symmetrically abduct and adduct during breathing.

TRACHEA AND BRONCHI

The preliminary medical evaluation of the coughing dog with a serious or protracted tracheal and/or bronchial disorder should include a complete blood count, serum biochemical profile, urinalysis, fecal parasite evaluation, microfilaria test, thoracic radiography, and electrocardiography. Depending on the history and physical examination findings and the results of preliminary diagnostic tests, serologic tests for the detection of occult dirofilariasis or mycotic diseases may also be required. Usually the correct diagnosis is made with the history, physical examination, and the preceding diagnostic tests. If the problem remains enigmatic after these procedures, the subsequent evaluation of the tracheal-bronchial structures should include tracheal wash for culture and cytology, tracheoscopy, bronchoscopy, and bronchial brush biopsy. These procedures are discussed later in this chapter. Before anesthetizing the animal with serious tracheal and bronchial disease, the clinician must carefully consider the risk-to-benefit ratio for these diagnostic procedures and thoroughly discuss them with the pet owner. An arterial blood gas and pH analysis should also be done on this type of patient.

ALVEOLI

Often the exact diagnosis of alveolar disease is easily achieved by correlating the history, physical examination, aforementioned blood tests, and thoracic radiographs. Potentially stressful procedures such as bronchoscopy and the tracheal wash are very risky when the diagnosis is obvious, as in congestive heart failure or the noncardiogenic pulmonary edema associated with an electric cord bite. However, when the diagnosis is not so readily apparent and the patient is deteriorating from undiagnosed progressive lung disease, use of the special diagnostic tests is certainly justified. Bronchoscopy and bronchial brush biopsy do not always provide the clinician with the specific diagnosis of pulmonary alveolar disorders. Therefore, more invasive diagnostic procedures such as transthoracic fine needle aspirate, lung biopsy, or a surgical thoracotomy with lung biopsy are required.

PLEURAL EFFUSIONS

The diagnostic approach to pleural effusions should be preceded by the clinician's understanding that pleural effusion is merely a sign of a more specific underlying problem such as hypoalbuminemia, thoracic neoplasia, lung torsion, or pleuritis. Therefore, the diagnostic work-up should include a complete blood count and serum biochemical profile, urinalysis, thoracic radiographs, and a needle thoracentesis to obtain pleural fluid for cytology and culture. Specific blood tests such as prothrombin and partial thromboplastin times are indicated when a hemorrhagic pleural effusion resulting from a systemic bleeding disorder is suspected. Frequently, the thoracic pathology causing pleural effusions is obscured by pleural fluid on the initial radiographs. Removing this fluid via chest drainage and repeating the chest radiographs frequently reveals a clearer view of the underlying abnormality.

DIAGNOSTIC APPROACH TO THE DYSPNEIC PATIENT WITH RESPIRATORY DISEASE

The dyspneic patient is a definite diagnostic challenge to the clinician, requiring the utmost skill and clinical prudence. The risk-to-benefit ratio of various diagnostic tests should be carefully evaluated prior to their selection. For example, there is seldom enough time or need to await the results of blood tests and to perform various radiographic procedures on a patient that presents with an acute onset of stridorous breathing due to an obvious obstructing pharyngeal foreign body. Similarly, the cat with acute pulmonary edema from hypertrophic obstructive cardiomyopathy seldom has the initial fortitude to withstand the stress of positioning for chest radiographs and electrocardiography. These situations call for sound clinical judgment to determine if immediate emergency treatment should precede any form of diagnostic work-up. The exact type of emergency treatment depends on the initial history and physical examination findings. Following relief of the patient's respiratory distress, the clinician should then pursue a methodical diagnostic work-up.

Radiography

Thoracic radiographs may confirm or deny a clinical impression or suspicion, provide information that adds support to a diagnosis already suggested by the history or physical examination, produce information not otherwise detectable, and allow evaluation of disease progression or regression. A thoracic radiograph is not a substitute for a complete physical examination. It is most useful when specific information is needed following formulation of a tentative diagnosis or list of differential diagnoses. To ensure that previously unsuspected conditions are not overlooked, the radiograph should be evaluated completely without considering the history or physical abnormalities and then reevaluated while looking for answers to those questions raised by the historical or physical findings.

Since air within the lung contrasts with the normal intrapulmonary tissue dense structures (pulmonary vessels, larger bronchi, and pulmonary interstitium), radiography is more suitable for gross morphologic evaluation of the lung; however, functional pulmonary abnormalities may also be evaluated.[1] Fluoroscopy, serial radiography, and cine or videoradiography are generally required for evaluation of functional pulmonary abnormalities such as restrictive, obstructive, or vascular diseases. Limited functional information can be inferred by comparison of arterial size to venous size and comparison of expiratory and inspiratory radiographs.

EFFECT OF TECHNICAL QUALITY ON RADIOGRAPHIC APPEARANCE

Respiratory Phase. Optimum pulmonary contrast and detail are achieved in thoracic radiographs obtained at the peak of inspiration (Figure 66–1). The pulmonary vessels are shorter, wider, and less sharply defined and the lung is denser when radiographs obtained at expiration are compared to those obtained at peak inspiration.[2] This loss of vascular definition and increased density can easily be misinterpreted as evidence of pulmonary disease. Most resting animals will not inspire fully; interference with respiration by closing the animal's mouth and obstructing the nares may be necessary.

At full inspiration the lung lobes cranial to the cardiac silhouette and the accessory lung lobe are large and lucent. There is slight separation of the heart from the sternum, the pulmonary cupula extends cranial to the first rib, the ventral tracheal angulation is marked, and the diaphragm is flat, separated from the heart, and contacts the heart close to the apex. The lumbodiaphragmatic angle is wide, and the caudal vena cava is almost parallel to the vertebral column, distinct, thin, and elongated.[2]

Exposure Time. Respiratory motion can result in poor vascular and bronchial detail and mimic pulmonary disease. Short exposure times of 1/60 to 1/120 second

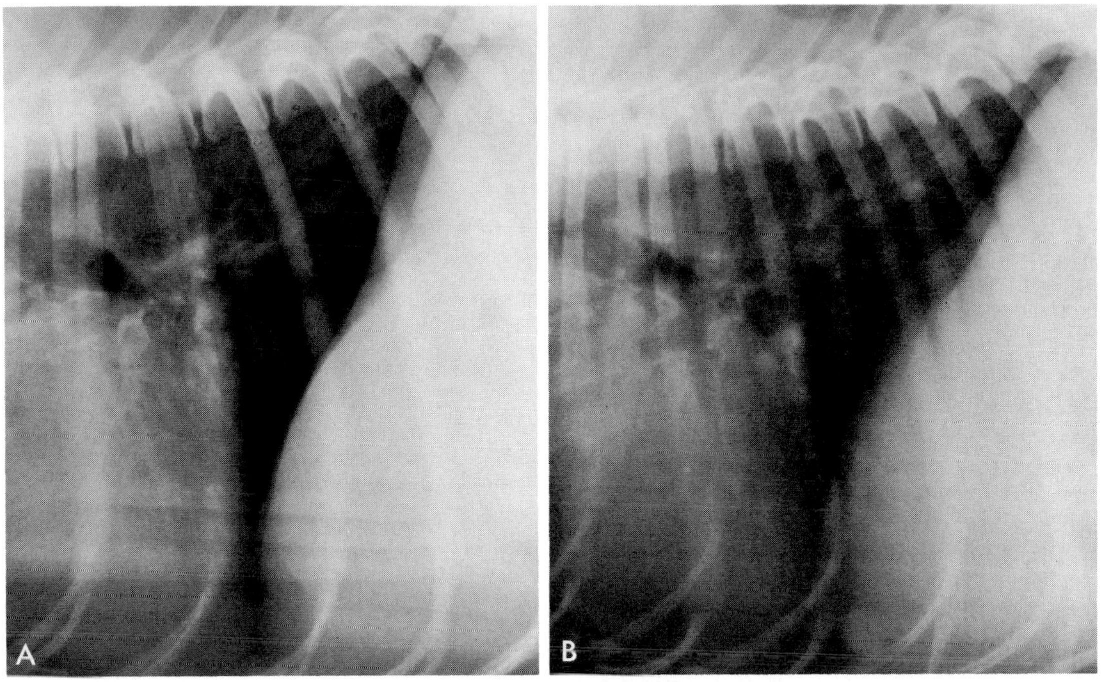

FIGURE 66–1. Lateral thoracic radiograph obtained at peak inspiration *A* and expiration *B*. The pulmonary vessels are shorter, wider, and less sharply defined and the lung is denser at expiration *B* when compared with inspiration *A*.

are therefore necessary. Blurring of ribs or other bony structures indicates that motion artifact is present.

Grids and Collimators. Scatter radiation that diminishes pulmonary detail and radiographic contrast can be reduced by using a stationary fine line or a Potter-Bucky (moving) grid and proper x-ray beam collimation. Scatter radiation becomes significant when radiographing obese animals or those with thoracic diameters 12 to 14 cm or greater.

Technique Charts. A technique chart is essential for producing consistent thoracic radiographs. Radiographic underexposure or overexposure can dramatically alter the lung's appearance, diminish contrast and detail, and obscure significant abnormalities (Figure 66–2). Underexposure creates an illusion of increased pulmonary density. Overexposure makes the lungs black and may obliterate subtle intrapulmonary infiltrates. Technique standardization is important for comparison of radiographs taken at different times during the disease course and during the animal's life. It also makes comparison with other animals of similar age, breed, or physical condition more meaningful.

Darkroom Procedure. Standardization of radiographic technique includes standardization of darkroom procedures. Many excellent radiographs are ruined in the darkroom. Strict attention to time and temperature in radiographic processing and proper mixing and replenishing of chemicals prevents most processing artifacts. Underdeveloping is more often a problem than overdeveloping. It results in increased pulmonary density. Careful handling of the film before and after processing is important, as emulsion defects, scratches, chemical stains, and undeveloped areas on the film may mimic or obliterate pulmonary abnormalities.

Positioning. At least two radiographs are needed for proper thoracic evaluation. A right or left lateral recumbent radiograph and a dorsoventral (sternal recumbent) or ventrodorsal (dorsal recumbent) radiograph are generally obtained. The lung's appearance differs when right and left lateral recumbent and dorsoventral and ventrodorsal radiographs are compared (Figure 66–3).[3–5] The dependent lung lobes collapse even in the conscious animal. This alters the lung's radiographic appearance and may obscure pulmonary lesions in the dependent lung and enhance those in the nondependent lobe.

In lateral recumbency the diaphragmatic crus on the dependent side is usually anterior to the opposite crus and the cranial lung lobe bronchus on the dependent side is dorsal to the opposite bronchus. The cardiac silhouette usually contacts the sternum when the animal is in right lateral recumbency and is separated slightly from the sternum in left lateral recumbency. The cranial lobe vessels in the dependent lung lobe are less frequently identified than those in the opposite lung lobe.[5]

The accessory lung lobe inflates more completely when the dog is in dorsal recumbency than when the dog is sternal. This increases the distance from the cardiac silhouette to the diaphragm when the ventrodorsal radiograph is compared to the dorsoventral.[4]

Obtaining both right and left lateral recumbent radiographs may be a satisfactory substitute for obtaining a lateral and a ventrodorsal (or dorsoventral) radiograph in patients who resist sternal or dorsal recumbency.[5] The right lateral recumbent radiograph demonstrates most lesions in the left lung lobes and the left lateral recumbent radiograph demonstrates most right lung lobe lesions. The combination of lateral and ventrodorsal (or dorsoventral) radiographs is still preferred, since lesion localization is more accurate. Improved detection of intrapulmonary neoplasia has been demonstrated when three views (both right and left lateral and dorsal recum-

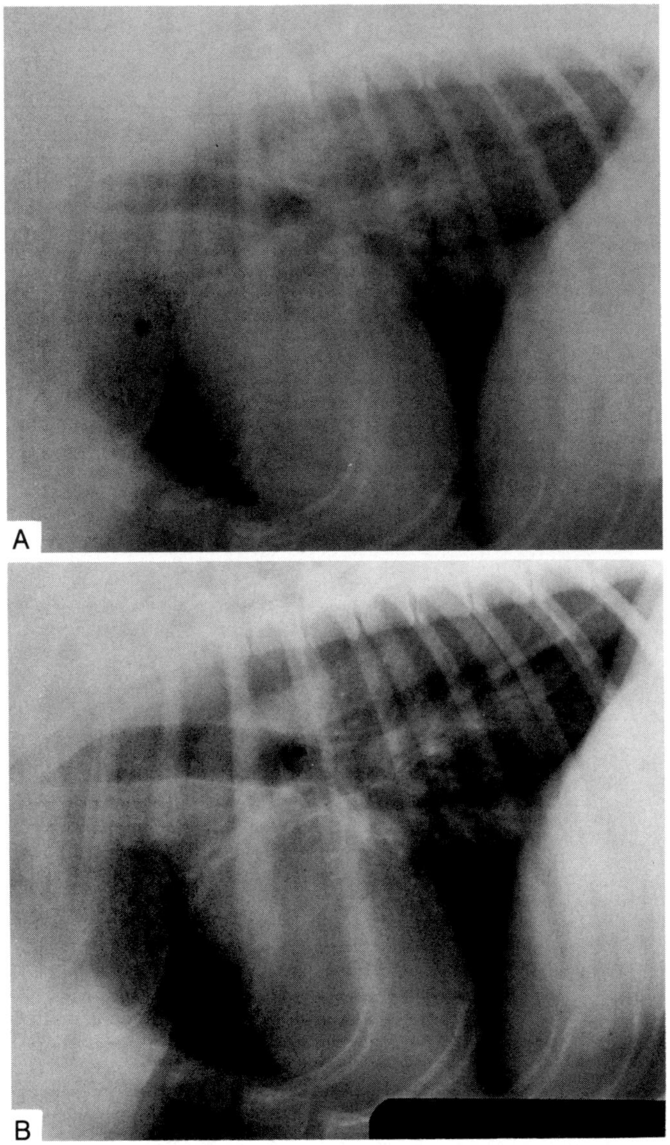

FIGURE 66–2. Lateral thoracic radiograph underexposed *A* and properly exposed *B*. The apparent increased density *A* has been corrected *B* by increasing the radiographic exposure. Proper exposure also permits more complete evaluation of the cranial lung lobes, which are obscured by the overlying tissues of the forelimbs.

bent) are obtained.[6] Consistency in patient positioning and x-ray technique is much more important than the position in which the patient is placed (i.e., right or left lateral; dorsal or sternal recumbent).

INTERPRETATION OF RADIOGRAPHS

Once a technically satisfactory radiograph is obtained, a systematic examination of the film reduces the possibility of overlooking an abnormality. The system used is a matter of personal preference; however, once adopted, it should be used every time. Placing the radiograph on the view box in a standard manner facilitates radiographic interpretation. Lateral radiographs are usually placed with the animal's head toward the viewer's left and ventrodorsal or dorsoventral radiographs are placed with the animal's right side on the viewer's left. When this is done consistently certain anatomic structures are seen in specific regions on the radiograph and both normal structures and abnormalities are recognized more quickly. A systematic approach familiarizes the viewer with normal anatomic variations and common technical artifacts.[1]

Normal Radiographic Features. The radiographic features of the lung of the normal dog and cat are illustrated in Figures 66–4 and 66–5. The trachea can be identified and traced to its bifurcation at about the fifth intercostal space. Beyond this point only the larger bronchi may be identified. The smaller peripheral bronchi are generally not visible except in older dogs and in larger dogs with bronchial wall calcification. The bronchial walls produce thin, nontapering tissue-dense lines, which are found in parallel pairs or may be viewed on end as a tissue-dense circle with a lucent center. Pulmonary vessels produce tissue-dense lines that branch and taper toward the lung periphery. When seen on end, vessels appear as round, solid, tissue-dense shadows. Pulmonary arteries are dorsal to the bronchus in the lateral radiograph and lateral to the bronchus in the dorsoventral radiograph. Pulmonary veins are located ventral to the bronchus in the lateral radiograph and medial to it in the dorsoventral. Pulmonary arteries follow the bronchial tree and may be traced back to their origin just cranial to and to the left of the tracheal bifurcation. Pulmonary veins may be recognized converging on the left atrial area. Bronchial arteries cannot be identified.

Pulmonary Density. Once radiographic technical quality has been evaluated and judged acceptable, the second step in thoracic radiographic interpretation is to evaluate the overall pulmonary density. Determine whether the lung is increased (whiter) or decreased (blacker) in density when compared to other radiographs of the same or similar animals. Reevaluate the lung density in relation to all technical factors (exposure, phase of respiration, animal's age, physical condition). If the density is not a technical artifact, consider whether it is focal or diffuse. Focal pulmonary densities are those involving a portion of a lung lobe or single lobe. A difference in radiographic density is evident when comparing the affected right lung lobe to the unaffected left. A diffuse pulmonary density affects the lung lobes equally and is a manifestation of a generalized disease. The density in the right lung lobes is similar to that in the left lobes.

Pulmonary Density Distribution. The next step is to look at the distribution of the lung density and determine which area of the lung is involved. For this purpose the lung may be divided into hilar, middle, and peripheral; dorsal and ventral; cranial, middle, or caudal segments. Certain pulmonary abnormalities have predilected sites; however, a great deal of variation is noted.

Pulmonary Pattern Recognition. Pulmonary pattern recognition is important in order to determine what structures are responsible for the increased or decreased pulmonary density. Three patterns of pulmonary density (vascular, interstitial, and alveolar) may be noted.[1, 7]

Vascular pattern. The vascular pattern presents radiographically as an increase in the size, number, and/or prominence of the pulmonary vessels and an alteration in vessel shape (contour), branching, or course (Figure 66–6). It may result when the large pulmonary

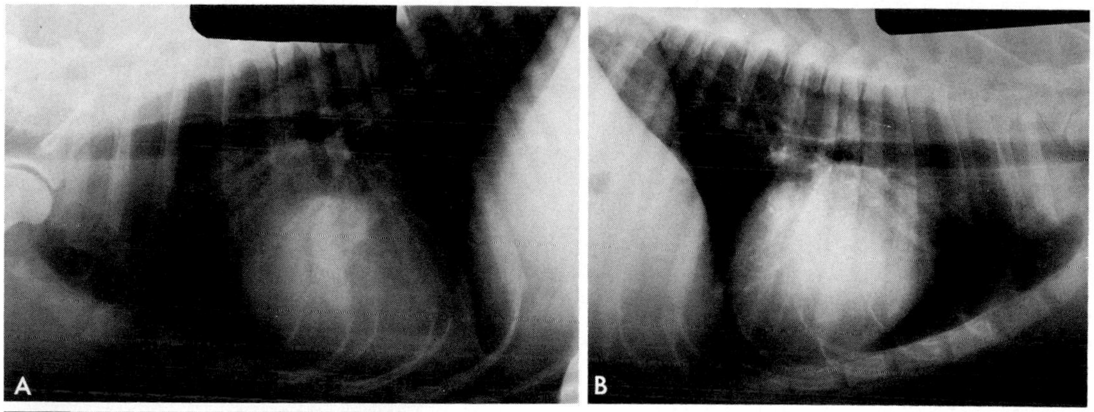
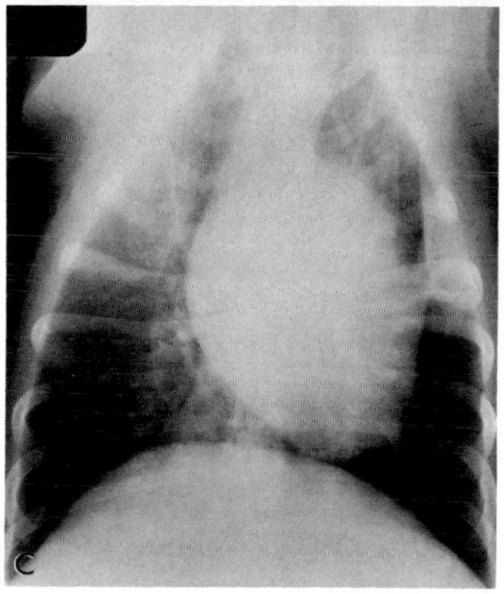

FIGURE 66–3. Right lateral recumbent *A,* left lateral recumbent *B,* and ventrodorsal *C* radiographs of a three-year-old pointer with a cough of one week's duration. The alveolar density is easily identified in the right lateral recumbent radiograph *A* but not readily seen in the left lateral recumbent radiograph *B.* In the ventrodorsal radiograph the alveolar infiltrate is evident in the caudal segment of the left cranial lung lobe. The difficulty in identification of the lung lesion is due to collapse of the dependent lung and contact of the lesion with the heart, obliterating the lesion's margins.

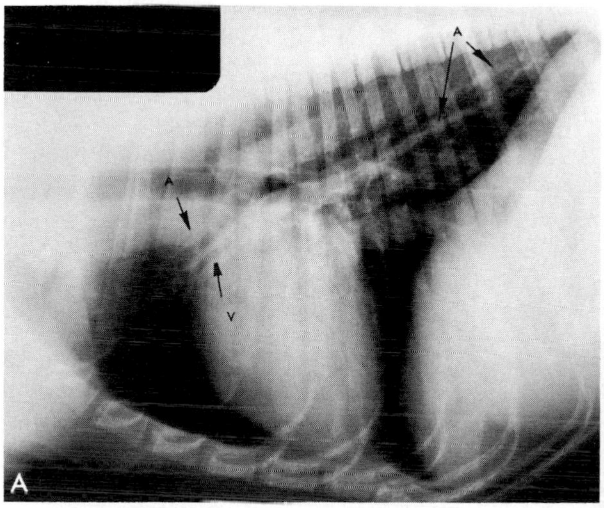

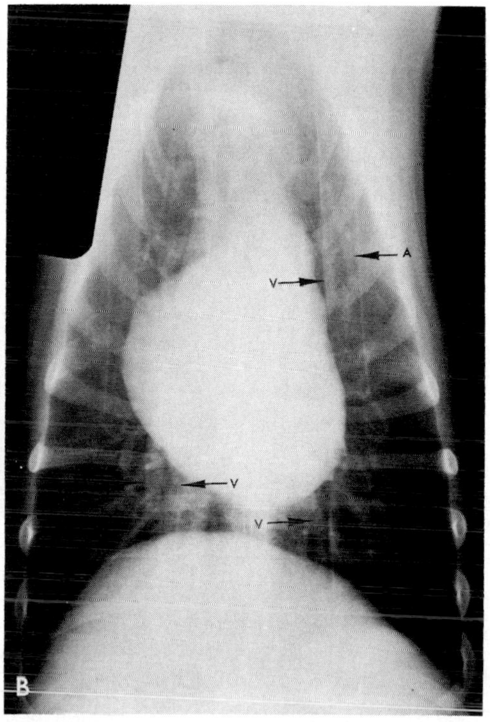

FIGURE 66–4. Lateral *A* and ventrodorsal *B* radiographs of a normal one-year-old Doberman. The pulmonary arteries (A) in the cranial lung lobe are visible dorsal and the pulmonary veins (v) ventral to the adjacent bronchus. The dog was in right lateral recumbency and therefore the right crus is anterior to the left and the left cranial lobe bronchus is ventral to the right. In the ventrodorsal radiograph the pulmonary arteries (A) are lateral and the pulmonary veins (V) are medial to the adjacent bronchus.

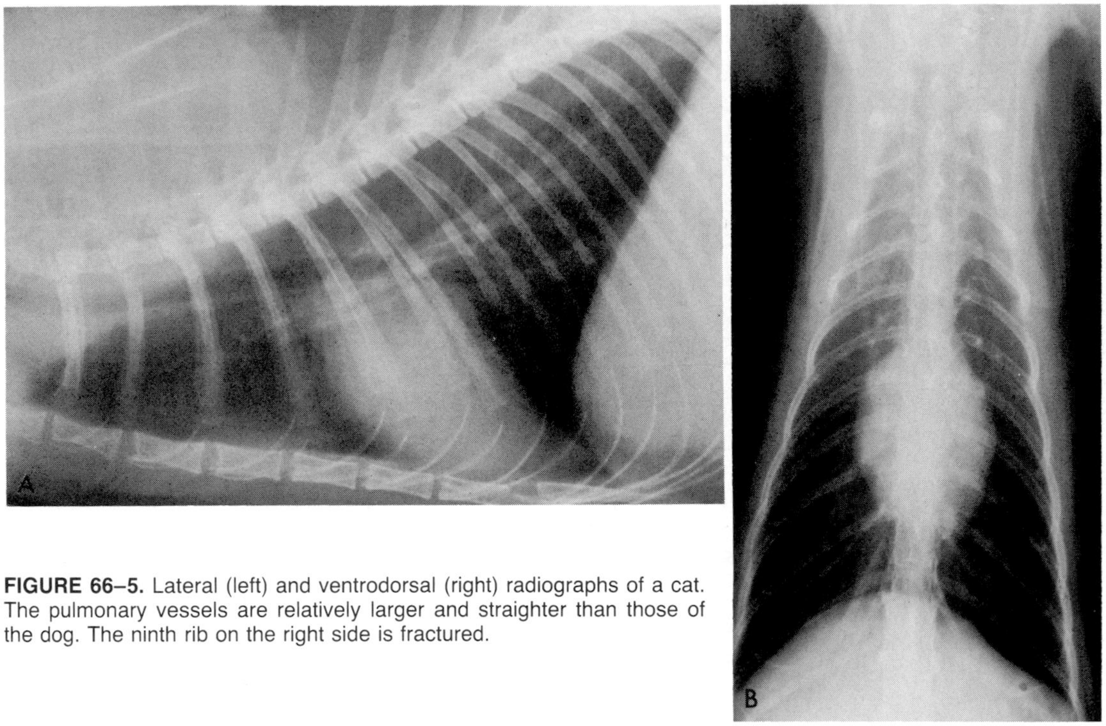

FIGURE 66–5. Lateral (left) and ventrodorsal (right) radiographs of a cat. The pulmonary vessels are relatively larger and straighter than those of the dog. The ninth rib on the right side is fractured.

vessels become bigger or when a greater number of the smaller, more peripheral pulmonary vessels are visible. Pulmonary vascular congestion (increased pulmonary vascularity) is a nonspecific radiographic change. It may occur during the course of an infectious pulmonary disease, in response to an inhaled irritant, from left-to-right cardiac shunts, or from pulmonary venous congestion. Standardized systems for measuring pulmonary arterial size and comparison with rib diameters have been proposed. Quantitation is difficult and the size of the pulmonary artery is usually compared to (and should be the same as) the size of the adjacent pulmonary vein.[1] Pulmonary vascular size and number evaluation is subjective, based on past experience.

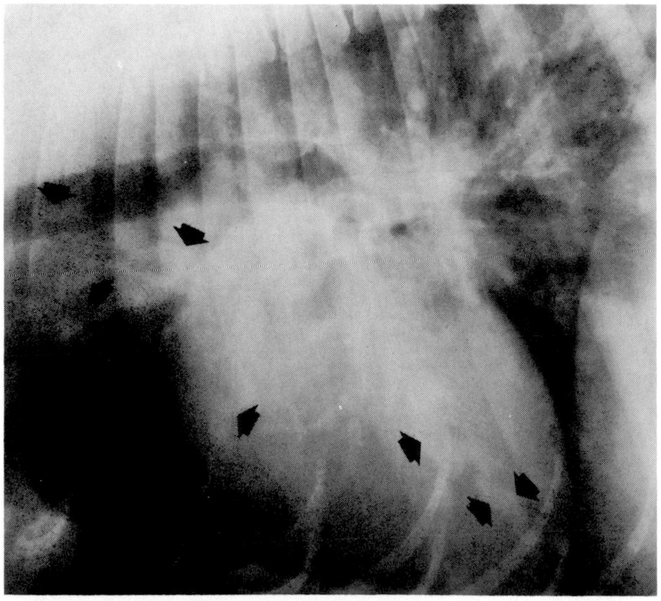

FIGURE 66–6. Lateral thoracic radiograph of a dog with dirofilariasis. The enlarged and irregular pulmonary arteries are visible (arrows).

Decreased pulmonary vascularity produces a radiolucent lung with a few small pulmonary vessels identified. This may be due to hypovolemia, thrombosis, or right-to-left vascular shunts. Overexposure of the radiograph mimics decreased vascularity; however, careful examination of the radiograph using a high intensity lamp prevents this misinterpretation. When due to hypovolemia, decreased pulmonary arterial and venous size is frequently accompanied by microcardia and decreased caudal vena cava size.

Interstitial pattern. Conditions that affect the pulmonary connective tissue (interalveolar septa, perivascular tissue, and peribronchial tissue) produce an increased pulmonary interstitial density. Its radiographic appearance has been described as a fine, indistinct, linear, reticulated, or honeycomb pattern, with or without small, round, and/or irregular nodular densities.[1, 7] Nodular interstitial densities are often larger than and separate from the adjacent vessels and can be distinguished from the round, end-on vascular densities. An increase in pulmonary interstitial density blurs normal vascular shadows. Well-defined, thin, linear densities that do not completely obscure the vascular shadows indicate a chronic or inactive disease (Figure 66–7). Poorly defined, thick lines that coalesce and become patchy are indicative of an active process (Figure 66–8).

Pulmonary interstitial density increases as an animal ages as a result of chronic inhalation of an irritant such as dust or smoke, or as a scar following resolution of a previous, active disease.[8] This produces pulmonary interstitial fibrosis. Mycotic pneumonia, metastatic neo-

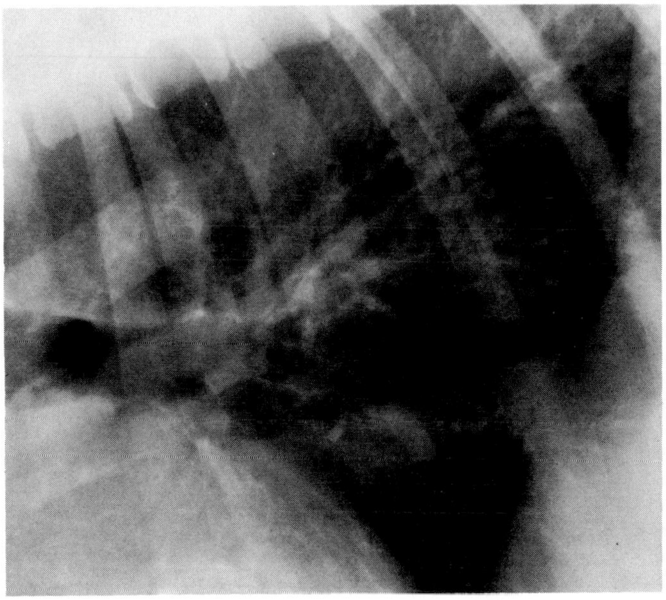

FIGURE 66–7. Close-up of a lateral thoracic radiograph of a six-year-old dog. The well-defined, thin linear densities that incompletely obscure the vascular shadows are indicative of chronic or inactive pulmonary disease.

plasia, smoke inhalation, allergic pneumonia, and pulmonary contusion produce radiographic patterns indicating an active pulmonary interstitial disease.

ALVEOLAR PATTERN. The alveolar pattern has been described as patchy or fluffy, poorly defined densities that tend to coalesce.[7] The most prominent feature of the alveolar pattern, the air bronchogram, is a radiolucent branching structure representing the bronchial lumen surrounded by fluid (Figure 66–9). The bronchial wall and adjacent pulmonary vessel are not visible.

Recognition of the air bronchogram is important for several reasons. It indicates that the tissue density is in the lung rather than being pleural, mediastinal, or extrathoracic. It also indicates the fluid nature of the pulmonary density (i.e., pus, blood, edema), since solid masses such as tumors or organizing granulomas compress and obliterate bronchial structures and do not

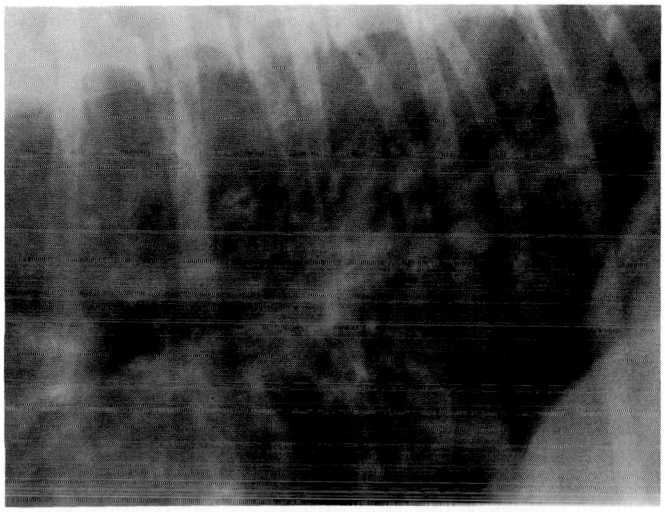

FIGURE 66–8. Close-up of a three-year-old dog with an allergic pneumonia. The poorly defined, thickened interstitial densities are indicative of an active process. (Compare with Figure 66–7.)

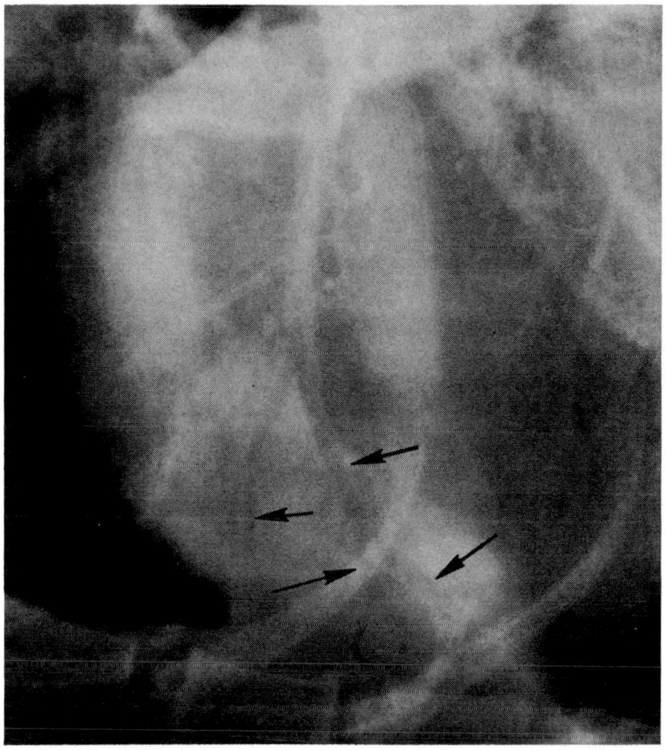

FIGURE 66–9. Close-up of lateral thoracic radiograph of a dog with an alveolar infiltrate in the right middle lung lobe. The air bronchogram is visible (arrows). This infiltrate was due to a bacterial pneumonia.

produce air bronchograms. The alveolar pattern may be seen in association with left heart failure, electric shock, central nervous system trauma, pulmonary hemorrhage, bacterial pneumonia, and some toxins (ANTU).

Most pulmonary diseases produce a mixed density pattern due to their active nature. A prominent vascular pattern may progress to an interstitial pattern with loss of vascular outlines. This may progress to an alveolar pattern with air bronchograms. After treatment, the pulmonary density may disappear in the reverse sequence. Fortunately, most diseases have a predominant pattern and typical distribution when the animal first becomes symptomatic and this provides the basis for the radiographic diagnosis (Table 66–5). Treatment or duration of the disease alters the specificity of the radiographic changes.

Location. The location of the pulmonary abnormality should be considered. Aspiration pneumonia is most often ventral or cranioventral in position. Thromboembolism, when occurring secondary to dirofilariasis, is usually located caudal and dorsal. Primary lung tumors are often found in the pulmonary hilus (most commonly in the right caudal lobe).

Density. Pulmonary abscesses and some necrotic pulmonary neoplasms may communicate with a bronchus and produce a radiolucent area (cavitary lesion) within the otherwise solid tissue density. The inner margins of these lesions are irregular. Pulmonary cysts or bullae are round or oval air-filled structures with thin, smooth walls. Calcification may be seen within a tissue-dense neoplasm, abscess, or organized hematoma. Small, calcified nodular densities are most likely pleural calcification or calcified granulomas.

TABLE 66–5. RADIOGRAPHIC PATTERNS OF PULMONARY DISEASE

Vascular
- *Increased*
  - Left-to-right intracardiac shunts (patent ductus arteriosus, ventricular and atrial septal defect)
  - Venous congestion (left heart failure)
  - Arteriovenous fistula
  - Dirofilariasis
  - Pulmonary arterial hypertension
- *Decreased*
  - Right-to-left intracardiac shunts (tetralogy of Fallot)
  - Pulmonic stenosis
  - Hypovolemia (shock, dehydration, Addison's disease)
  - Emphysema
  - Thromboembolism
  - Right heart failure
  - Pericardial fluid
  - Constrictive pericarditis

Interstitial
- *Disseminated*

Chronic
- Age
- Scarring
- Mild, chronic irritant (smoke, dust)
- Bronchitis
- Bronchiectasis

Acute
- Mycotic
- Metastatic
- Lymphosarcoma
- Left heart failure
- Parasitic
- Dirofilariasis
- Disseminated intravascular coagulation, coagulopathies (warfarin, von Willebrand's disease)
- Feline infectious peritonitis
- Uremia
- Viral
- Bacterial
- Bronchiectasis

Focal or Multifocal
- *Chronic*
  - Old infarct
  - Recurrent aspiration
  - Recurrent bacterial infection
  - Foreign body
  - Granuloma
- *Acute*
  - Embolism
  - Bacterial
  - Aspiration
  - Foreign body
  - Contusion
  - Uremia

Alveolar
- *Disseminated*
  - Cardiogenic (left heart failure)
  - Noncardiogenic
    - Allergic
    - Central nervous trauma
    - Electric shock
    - Toxin (ANTU)
    - Postexpansion
    - Neoplasia (rare) (carcinomatosis, lymphosarcoma)
- *Focal or Multifocal*
  - Bacterial
  - Aspiration
  - Hemorrhage
  - Embolism
  - Parasitic
  - Mycotic
  - Lung lobe torsion

Pulmonary density may increase secondary to decreased lung volume in conjunction with pleural air or fluid (pneumothorax, hydrothorax). Under these circumstances identification of the diseased lung lobe may be difficult. In most instances of hydrothorax or pneumothorax, lung lobe collapse is uniform. If a single lobe is more collapsed (more dense) than the others, pulmonary disease is probably present in that lobe. This can be confirmed by repeating the radiographs after the fluid or air is removed.

Bronchial Distribution. The bronchial distribution and lung lobe arrangement should also be evaluated. Abnormal position may occur with lung lobe torsion, displacement by a pulmonary or pleural mass, diaphragmatic hernia, left atrial enlargement, or esophageal diseases.

Heart. The heart should be critically evaluated when pulmonary density is abnormal. Left heart enlargement accompanies cardiogenic pulmonary edema (Figure 66–10). Right heart enlargement may be present in noncardiogenic pulmonary edema (cardiac enlargement secondary to the pulmonary disease).

Other Thoracic Structures. The position of the diaphragm and mediastinum and width of the intercostal spaces should be evaluated. Lung lobe atelectasis results in a small, tissue-dense lung lobe with decreased thoracic volume on the affected side. This volume loss may be compensated for by overinflation of the remaining normal lung lobes, cranial displacement of a diaphragmatic crus, shifting of the mediastinum or heart toward the affected side, or failure to expand the intercostal spaces. Inflammation, edema, or neoplastic infiltration of a lung lobe produces a tissue-dense lobe of normal or increased size and these compensatory changes are not seen.

Nodular Density. Most nodular densities are interstitial solid masses or fluid-filled cavities; they compress the adjacent lung or bronchi as they enlarge. Nodular densities may be solitary or multiple and well or poorly circumscribed. They may form large masses. A definitive diagnosis based solely on the nodule's radiographic appearance is impossible. Enlargement of a solitary nodule after an interval of three to four weeks is an indication for lung biopsy.[1]

Decreased Pulmonary Density. Considerable pathology must be present before focal or diffuse decreases in pulmonary density can be detected. Focal decreases are more easily recognized than generalized changes because they contrast with the normal lung density. An expiratory radiograph may accentuate the density difference between normal and affected lung. Bullae or blebs may be intrapulmonary or subpleural and are the most frequent focal radiolucencies. Emphysema and oligemia may be focal or diffuse.

The radiographic changes that accompany pulmonary disease do not always permit a specific radiographic diagnosis. Identification and recognition of patterns and

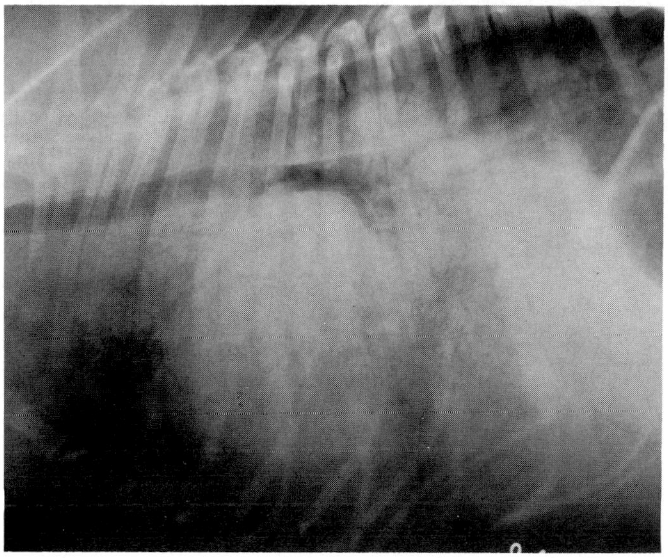

FIGURE 66–10. Lateral thoracic radiograph of a dog. A hilar alveolar infiltrate is present. The enlarged cardiac silhouette can be identified because of the tracheal elevation. This indicates that the alveolar density is the result of left heart failure.

consideration of density distribution aids in determining a differential diagnosis; however, all aspects of the radiograph should be examined before a radiographic diagnosis is made. When all radiographic features are combined, the radiographic diagnosis can be quite specific. In most cases a final diagnosis is based on the physical, historical, and clinical data as well as the radiographic changes.

PULMONARY DIAGNOSTIC PROCEDURES

The past 15 years have witnessed the development of numerous diagnostic procedures in veterinary medicine for determining the etiologies of pulmonary infiltrates, solitary masses, and diffuse lung diseases. This section discusses the clinical indications, efficacy, and safety of four such procedures: transtracheal aspiration, bronchoscopy, percutaneous fine needle aspiration, and open lung biopsy.

TRANSTRACHEAL ASPIRATION

Transtracheal aspiration was originally proposed for use in humans as a method for obtaining representative airway secretions from the lower respiratory tract.[9] Theoretically, oropharyngeal flora do not extend beyond the larynx and the airways below this level are normally sterile. Thus, specimens collected for microbiologic or cytologic examination are expected to be uncontaminated by oral flora. The indications for transtracheal aspiration (washing) include chronic coughing, evidence of pulmonary parenchymal disease, and the presence of radiographic patterns compatible with bronchopulmonary infiltration.

Preparation. The items needed for transtracheal aspiration are inexpensive and readily available. Sterile gloves, local anesthetic agent, sterile (nonbacteriostatic) saline, 6-ml and 12-ml syringes, 16- to 18-gauge intravenous needle catheter devices, and material for sterile preparation of the skin are needed. For large dogs, a 14-gauge needle and a #3 French polypropylene catheter can be used. Large and medium-sized dogs can be restrained by backing them into a corner in a sitting position. A second person straddles the dog and raises the head for catheter placement. Small dogs and cats are best restrained on a table with the head elevated. Most small animals require some form of chemical restraint, such as acetylpromazine, diazepam, ketamine hydrochloride, or oxymorphone to facilitate accurate needle placement into the larynx (see Table 66–6).[10] Some movement of the animal during the procedure is common.

Method. With the animal restrained, the ventral area of the neck over the larynx and proximal cervical trachea is shaved and surgically scrubbed with a germicidal preparation. The cricothyroid ligament is located by moving the index finger cranially along the trachea until the ridge of the cricoid cartilage is located. A triangular depression (cricothyroid ligament) is found just cranial to the ridge on the cricoid cartilage. In large dogs, the catheter can be introduced between the cervical tracheal rings, but cartilage fracture or chondritis may result. Once the site for percutaneous transtracheal aspiration is located, the skin and subcutaneous tissues are infiltrated with a local anesthetic. The landmarks should again be identified and the catheter needle inserted, with the beveled part of the needle kept in a ventral position, through the skin into the tracheal lumen. Care should be taken to ensure that the catheter is threaded distally into the trachea and not directed toward or coughed into the larynx or pharynx. Catheter passage through the needle should be easy and usually induces coughing. The catheter tip should not extend beyond the carina (see Figure 66–11). Inability to pass the catheter indicates failure to enter the tracheal lumen or passage of the needle through both the ventral and dorsal tracheal walls. Paratracheal catheter placement can occur and that possibility should be considered if saline can be easily injected through the catheter but a negative pressure is present on aspiration. If the catheter has been improperly placed, it should be removed and the procedure repeated. Following proper catheter placement, the metal needle is withdrawn (to prevent laceration of the catheter), leaving the catheter within the trachea. If secretions are very viscid, they may be aspirated directly into a sterile syringe. If no material is obtained, several milliliters of sterile nonbacteriostatic saline are injected through the catheter and aspirated as soon as the animal coughs. When material is in the catheter, some resistance to suction is noted. If air alone is obtained, it must be expelled and the procedure repeated. An adequate sample (1 to 2 ml), with flecks of mucoid or purulent debris, is usually obtained after two or three washes, but instillation of 30 to 50 ml of saline may be required in a large dog. Respiratory distress following tracheal washing is rare because the large surface area of the bronchial mucosa rapidly absorbs the saline. Specific guidelines for the maximum total volume of instilled fluid have not been determined,

TABLE 66–6. RECOMMENDED DOSAGE OF SELECTED DRUGS FOR PULMONARY DIAGNOSTIC TECHNIQUES

Drug	Dose	Comments
Acetylpromazine	0.025–0.5 mg/lb IM or IV up to 3.0 mg (dog and cat)	Use very low doses in boxers (syncope); far better sedation if combined with meperidine. To avoid overdosage, patients seldom need more than 1.0 mg when drug is given as IV push
Acetylpromazine + Meperidine	0.02 mg/lb IM (dog and cat) 1–3 mg/lb IM (dog), 1 mg/lb IM (cat)	Good sedation
Ketamine Hydrochloride + Acetylpromazine	2–10 mg/lb IM (cat) 0.02–0.5 mg/lb IM (cat)	Give glycopyrolate (0.05 mg/lb IM) or atropine (0.02 mg/lb IM) to prevent hypersalivation
Ketamine Hydrochloride + Diazepam	2–5 mg/lb IM (cat) 0.12–0.25 mg/lb IM (cat)	Use glycopyrolate or atropine; very good cardiovascular stability
Acetylpromazine + Oxymorphone	0.02–0.5 mg/lb IV (dog) 0.02–0.5 mg/lb IV (dog)	Good restraint; reversible narcotic
Diazepam + Oxymorphone	0.1 mg/lb IV (dog) 0.005–0.05 mg/lb IV (dog)	Good for debilitated animals; reversible narcotic

but 0.75 ml/pound (1.5 ml/kg) body weight can be used as a clinical guideline. After a sample has been obtained, the syringe is capped with a sterile needle with rubber plug to prevent contamination and the catheter is removed from the trachea. Gentle pressure with a gauze sponge should be applied to the puncture site for several minutes following the procedure.

A tracheobronchial washing technique has been recently described in intubated, lightly anesthetized animals.[11] The animal is positioned with the affected lung down and a sterile 14-gauge needle catheter device is passed through the endotracheal tube. Catheter placement should be in the lower main stem bronchus (Figure 66–12). Viscid airway secretions can be aspirated directly; however, instillation of 2 to 3 ml of sterile nonbacteriostatic saline into the airway, followed by immediate aspiration, is usually required. After an adequate sample is obtained, the catheter is removed.

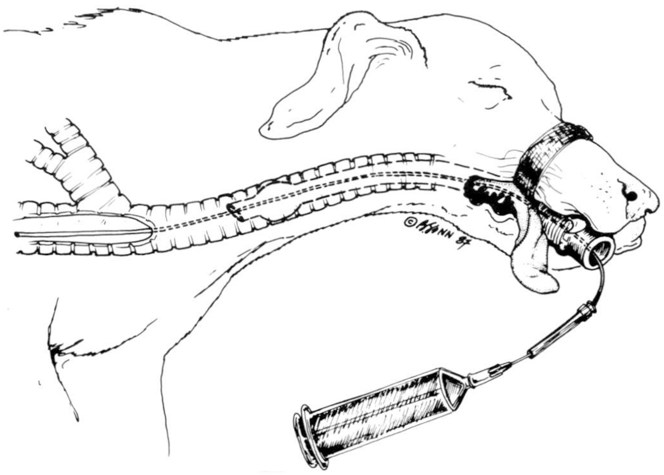

FIGURE 66–12. Schematic representation of the proper anatomic placement of a catheter in the main stem bronchial lumen during tracheobronchial washing.

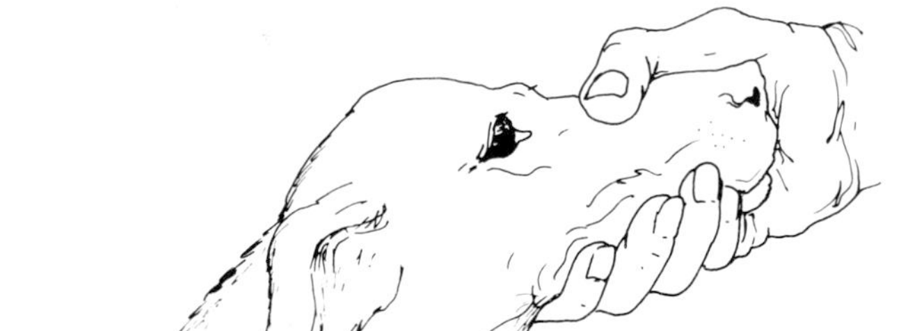

FIGURE 66–11. Conceptual drawing of the correct anatomic placement of a catheter in the tracheal lumen during transtracheal aspiration. Note that the needle has been withdrawn from the neck and has been covered by the plastic needle guard to prevent accidental laceration of the catheter during the procedure.

Supplemental oxygen may be needed for hypoxemic patients.

Specimens. Specimens of airway secretions recovered by either tracheal or bronchial aspiration should be rapidly processed for culture and cytologic examinations.[12, 13] Delay may result in false-negative culture results. Material can be cultured for aerobic and anaerobic bacteria, mycoplasma, and fungus organisms. Aerobic bacteria predominate, probably because oropharyngeal anaerobes are killed by ambient oxygen tension. Anaerobes are infrequently present unless aspiration pneumonia or pulmonary abscessation is present. The role of mycoplasma in respiratory infections of dogs and cats is incompletely understood. Fungal species are uncommonly found unless the patient is immunosuppressed, is receiving chronic antibiotic therapy, or has systemic mycosis.

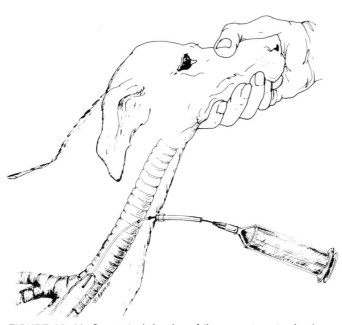

Respiratory tract specimens also should be submitted for cytologic examination (Figure 66–13). Information gained from examination of new methylene blue wet mounts and Wright-Giemsa or Gram stains of air-dried smears of aspirated material is often as useful as culture results.[14] Aspirated airway secretions normally contain cellular elements and mucus. Large mononuclear cells predominate; neutrophils, eosinophils, small mononu-

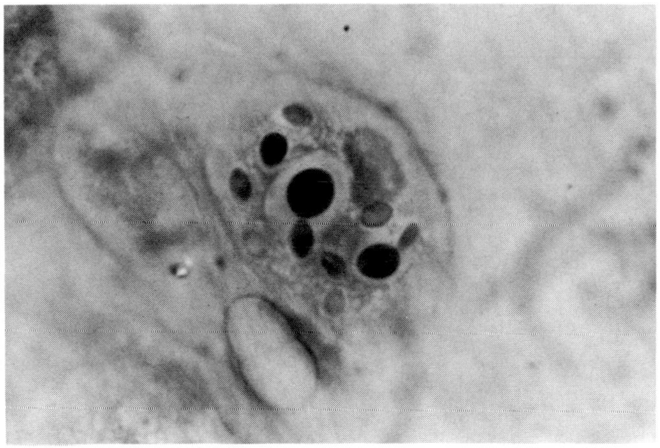

FIGURE 66–13. Transtracheal aspiration from a cat with cryptococcosis. Typical budding yeast form of *Cryptococcus* sp. is present within a macrophage. (Periodic acid-Schiff stain, × 250. Slide courtesy of Dr. D. J. Meyer.)

clear cells, and ciliated epithelial cells account for 10 to 15 per cent of the remaining cell types. An increase in neutrophil numbers suggests inflammatory or infectious conditions, while eosinophil counts are elevated in allergic (hypersensitivity) and parasitic lung diseases. Lymphocyte counts may be increased or decreased in acute and chronic pulmonary diseases. Mucus hypersecretion and Curschmann spirals suggest chronic inflammatory disease. Organisms contained within phagocytic cells are generally pathogenic, with one species usually predominating. Rational medical management can be made based on cytologic findings, pending culture results. Variable types of bacteria suggest oropharyngeal contamination and the presence of squamous epithelial cells, often with *Caryophanon* sp. on their surface, substantiates the suspicion. Other elements such as parasite larvae, ova, or neoplastic cells are uncommon findings but, when present, establish a diagnosis.

Results. The sensitivity (recovery of organisms responsible for disease) and specificity (lack of contaminant organisms) of transtracheal aspiration in the diagnosis of bronchopneumonia has been addressed in several human but only one experimental canine study.[12, 13, 15] Probable pathogens were recovered from 335 of the 383 human patients (87 per cent).[12] Forty-four of the remaining 48 individuals had received antibiotic treatment prior to transtracheal aspiration, perhaps eliminating or inactivating the infecting pathogen(s). Approximately one per cent of the patients had false-negative results, probably related to faulty catheter placement, infection location, or airway occlusion between the trachea and the nidus of infection. In dogs, organisms responsible for infection were recovered in 50 to 90 per cent, but specificity was poor.[13] Pure cultures were obtained in only 10 to 20 per cent of the animals. Further clinical studies are needed to more completely assess the reliability of tracheobronchial aspiration in dogs and cats. Although some controversy exists regarding sensitivity and specificity of the procedure, it is easy to perform, inexpensive, and helpful in many cases of infectious and inflammatory tracheobronchial disease. Transtracheal aspiration should be the initial procedure, but alternative methods with greater sensitivity and specificity, such as percutaneous fine needle aspiration lung biopsy or catheter sheathed brush systems, should be used when transtracheal aspiration is not diagnostic, when complicated respiratory problems are encountered, or following unsuccessful resolution of a previously diagnosed pulmonary disease.

Complications. Complications associated with the transtracheal washing technique in humans include localized subcutaneous emphysema, mediastinal emphysema, paratracheal infection, transient hemoptysis, aspiration pneumonia, cardiac arrhythmias associated with severe hypoxemia or acidosis, acute respiratory failure, and sudden death without significant hemorrhage.[12, 16] One author (RRK) has encountered mild transient hemoptysis and subcutaneous emphysema. Complications can be minimized if the procedure is done by experienced clinicians on cooperative animals in whom the anatomic landmarks are easily identified. Before the procedure, abnormalities posing excess risk such as hypoxemia and coagulation defects should be assessed and corrected. Not unexpectedly, the patients that are most susceptible to complications are also most likely to benefit from the procedure.

BRONCHOSCOPY

Bronchoscopes. The rigid bronchoscope was first introduced into human medicine in 1904, with the smaller, flexible bronchofiberscopes being introduced as a clinical diagnostic tool in 1967.[17, 18] The rigid bronchoscope consists of a hollow tube with a blunted, beveled tip. A fiberoptic light bundle or electric light bulb provides distal illumination. Rigid scopes are available as small as 3 mm in diameter and 20 cm in length. A variety of larger diameters and lengths are available. Some bronchoscopes have a sidearm at the proximal end for supplemental oxygen administration, which is a distinct advantage in hypoxemic patients. The fiberoptic bronchoscope consists of a control section connected to a flexible insertion tube that contains a number of optical fibers bundled together with both ends tightly bound, steering cables, and usually one or more suction channels. An accurate optical image is obtained if the arrangement of fibers at one end of the bundle is identical to the other end. An external light source is needed and one or more fiber bundles serve to transmit the light to the end of the scope, where the illuminated optical image is transmitted back through the viewing fiber bundles to the observer. Insertion tube diameters range from 2.5 mm (with suction channel) in the specialized ultra-thin scopes, to 6.0 mm, with working tube lengths from 60 to 145 cm. Suction channels may be 1.2, 1.8, 2.0, or 2.2 mm in diameter, with a larger, 2.6 mm channel available on special scopes. Suction channels of 1.8 or 2.0 are generally satisfactory but the 2.6 mm channel is superior for suctioning tenacious secretions and for bronchial biopsies. A variety of forceps (grasping and biopsy) and brushes (cytology and culture) are available.

Indications. Bronchoscopy permits visualization of the tracheobronchial tree and specimen collection. Remote areas of the bronchial tree can be brought within sight and manipulative reach with the flexible fiberoptic scopes. Rigid scopes provide better visualization of the upper airways and main stem bifurcation. Indications for bronchoscopy include the need to remove foreign bodies, chronic coughing of undetermined origin, prior abnormal cytologic findings, unresolved pneumonia, hemoptysis, the need to suction obstructing secretions, a need for airway examination with culture, biopsy, lavage, or cytology, and the need for a conduit for selective bronchography.[18, 19] It is also useful in the preoperative assessment of tentatively and definitively diagnosed conditions such as neoplasia, bronchiectasis, lung lobe torsion, and lung abscessation, where inspection of the entire respiratory tract for evidence of metastasis or progression of the disease may offer important information concerning the successful resolution of the problem. The choice of scope, rigid or flexible fiberoptic, depends on the patient, the type and severity of the disorder, and the purpose of the procedure.

A major limitation in the use of these instruments has been their expense. Rigid fiberoptic bronchoscopes are relatively inexpensive but the cost of flexible bronchofiberscopes is often prohibitive unless one specializes in pulmonary medicine. Catheter brushes (for cytology and culture) and biopsy forceps are reasonably inexpensive and can often be used with both rigid and flexible fiberoptic scopes.

Examination. Bronchoscopic examination can be done with the patient sedated or anesthetized. A narcotic sedative (oxymorphone) combined with a muscle relaxant (diazepam) works well in dogs (Table 66–6). In cats, a dissociative anesthetic (ketamine hydrochloride) and a muscle relaxant (diazepam) are frequently used (Table 66–6). One author (RRK) prefers general anesthesia with the patient in sternal recumbency because the lungs are in a normal anatomic orientation and are easily expanded. The flexible fiberoptic bronchoscope is passed through an endotracheal tube. This method permits removal and reinsertion of the instrument atraumatically, lessens the possibility of scope damage, and guarantees airway patency should cardiopulmonary complications occur. Supplemental oxygen can be administered through a nasal cannula when an endotracheal tube is not used, but this is less reliable.

Introduction of a rigid bronchoscope should always be performed with the patient anesthetized. Prior to introducing the bronchoscope, areas for selective evaluation should be determined and appropriate instruments and materials should be available. The rigid scope is introduced through the larynx with the patient in dorsal recumbency with its head extended. Ventilation and oxygen supplementation can be maintained through the sidearm attachment. The smaller-diameter flexible instrument is best introduced through a T-tube into the endotracheal tube. To reduce friction, lubricating jelly should be applied to the distal end of the instrument. The bronchoscope is guided through the endotracheal tube and into the major airways. The tracheobronchial tree should be systematically examined, with initial inspection beginning with the trachea and carina. Each lobe and first through fourth or fifth order bronchi should be identified and inspected.[18, 20] With experience, bronchoscopy can be completed in five to ten minutes. Sampling procedures such as lavage, culture, brushing, and transbronchial biopsy require additional time.

Bronchopulmonary lavage is performed following placement of a flexible fiberoptic bronchoscope (or catheter) into the distal airways.[21–23] Wedging the instrument or catheter limits the region of lavage and results in better fluid recovery. Several instillations and subsequent withdrawals of 5 to 10 ml of sterile 0.9 per cent saline are made (Figure 66–14). The total volume instilled varies with the animal's size (50 to 100 ml in medium to large dogs and 25 to 50 ml in small dogs and cats). A recovery of 80 to 90 per cent can be expected in normal animals, but fluid volume and color is reduced or changed with smaller airway collapse secondary to inflammation, infection, and neoplasia. Total and differential nucleated cell counts can be determined in the recovered fluid and may be helpful in defining the etiology of alveolar and interstitial infiltrates, such as allergic pneumonitis, infection, and chronic bronchitis (Figure 66–15).[21–23] Furthermore, the supernatant fluid may be analyzed for immunologic and biochemical mediators of disease.[21, 23] This technique is least valuable in the diagnosis of infection because the bronchoscopic channel may be contaminated by oropharyngeal organisms during introduction.

The plugged telescoping catheter brush system has much greater sensitivity and specificity for the diagnosis of infection than bronchopulmonary lavage fluid.[13, 24] Brush contamination is prevented by a disposable, biodegradable plug that is not ejected until the catheter reaches the sampling area. The inner cannula is advanced, followed by the brush, and the sample is taken (Figure 66–16). The brush is retracted into the cannula and the entire device is withdrawn. Recovery of viable organisms is enhanced if cultures are made at the time of sample collection.[13] Contamination rates from double-sheathed catheter brush samples are low (less than 20 per cent) and the likelihood of obtaining a culture of resident organisms in the distal airways is high (80 per cent).[13]

Mucosal abnormalities that are too distant or do not protrude sufficiently into the bronchial lumen to be

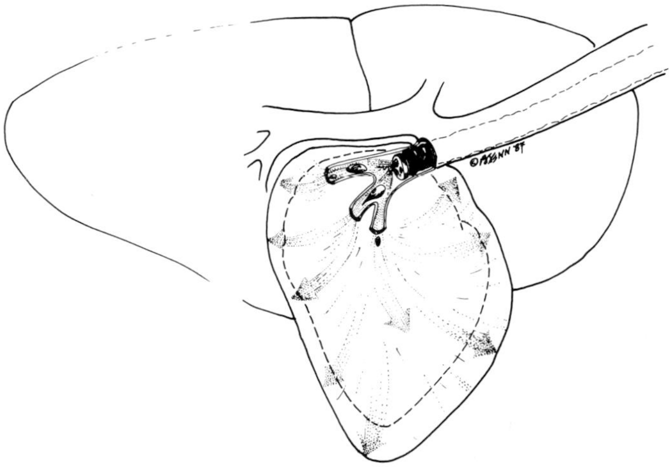

FIGURE 66–14. Conceptual drawing of the bronchoalveolar lavage procedure. The bronchoscope's tip is wedged into a bronchus to improve fluid recovery. A volume of sterile saline at room temperature is introduced through the suction channel in 5- to 10-ml increments. Aspiration by syringe is performed immediately after the instillation of each 5- to 10-ml increment.

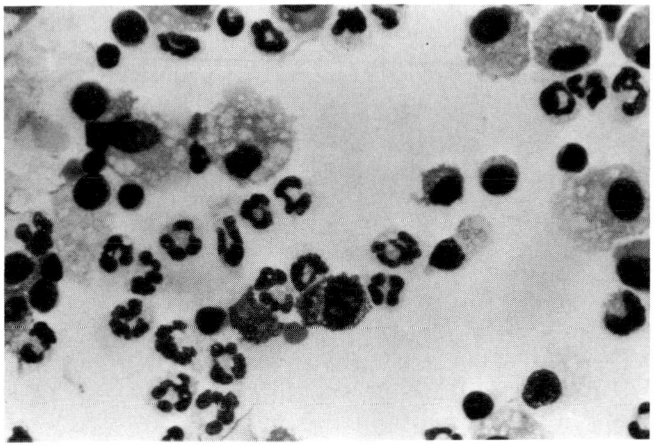

FIGURE 66–15. Bronchoalveolar lavage cytocentrifuge preparation from a dog with chronic bronchitis. Neutrophils predominate; differentiated alveolar macrophages are large cells with abundant pale foamy cytoplasm; undifferentiated alveolar macrophages are smaller, and the cytoplasm contains no or few vacuoles. Several plasma cells and lymphocytes (small, dark mononuclear cells) are present. (Wright-Giemsa stain, × 250.)

caught by biopsy forceps can be evaluated by brushing the bronchial mucosa.[13, 18, 25] A rigid bronchoscope is unsatisfactory if areas distal to second-order bronchi are involved. Flexible fiberscopes allow brush positioning parallel to the bronchus to be brushed. Bronchofiberscopes with inner channels greater than 1.6 mm in diameter permit passage of a catheter-sheathed cytology brush, which eliminates contamination when the brush is inserted into and removed from the suction channel. Several brushings are done, using a separate brush for each area. The amount of cellular material desquamated varies with the degree of abrasion and brush composition and construction. Newer brushes are made with matted nylon instead of wire bristles. Although stiff wire brushes result in better rubbing action, they are more likely to bend and injure normal bronchial mucosa. Small tissue fragments are swept into the interstices of the brush and after streaking slides, the brush can be placed in a petri dish with saline to obtain more cellular fragments. This is especially useful in evaluating pulmonary neoplasms. In humans, positive diagnoses have been reported in 80 to 90 per cent of the cases with tumor grossly visible by bronchoscopy and approximately 50 per cent with invisible tumors.[26]

Specimens. Cytologic specimens should be processed immediately.[13, 25] Wright-Giemsa and Gram stains are used routinely. The Papanicolaou stain may be used if neoplasia is suspected and improved nuclear detail is desired. Management of the cytologic specimen is discussed elsewhere.[27]

Transbronchial Biopsy. Transbronchial biopsy is an important alternative to open lung biopsy.[18, 28] In diffuse pulmonary disease, peripheral biopsies are recommended and either the rigid or flexible scopes can be used; however, if infiltrates are localized in the cranial lobes, the flexible instrument is superior for positioning. The flexible instrument is preferred and either forceps or needle aspiration biopsy can be employed.[28, 29]

For forceps biopsy the scope is positioned in the chosen bronchus and a 1 to 2 ml bolus of lidocaine with epinephrine, 1:20,000 strength, is instilled into the airway to promote vasoconstriction and bronchodilation.[28] The forceps (alligator jaw type) is passed through the bronchoscope and into a peripheral airway (Figure 66–17). The forceps is retracted 1 to 2 cm and positive pressure ventilation is used to expand the lungs. The forceps is advanced and opened and the animal is allowed to exhale. While maintaining expiration, the forceps is gently advanced 1 cm and the jaws are closed, trapping a small portion of the bronchial wall. The forceps is completely withdrawn from the bronchoscope, leaving the tip of the instrument wedged into the bronchial segment to tamponade any bleeding. Four or five specimens are obtained and placed in a sterile bottle or petri dish containing saline solution. Lung tissue is fluffy and floats, while bronchial tissue is dense and sinks. Biopsy specimens (Figure 66–18) are placed into ten per cent formalin solution after touch impressions are made for cytologic examination. If bleeding occurs, a red mirror of blood is seen at the tip of the bronchoscope. The instrument should be kept in a wedged position for several minutes until a clot forms.

The second transbronchial biopsy technique uses an 18- to 22-gauge, 13 to 20 mm aspiration biopsy needle.[29] Lidocaine and epinephrine are not usually needed. The aspiration needle is passed through the bronchoscope with the needle tip retracted. The needle is advanced beyond the protective sheath and inserted into the lesion

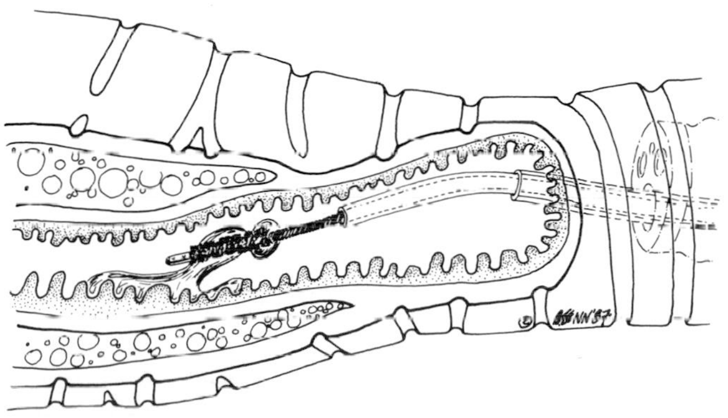

FIGURE 66–16. Schematic representation of airway secretion collection using the telescoping catheter brush system. As demonstrated here, the sample is obtained by moving the brush back and forth across the mucosa and airway secretions.

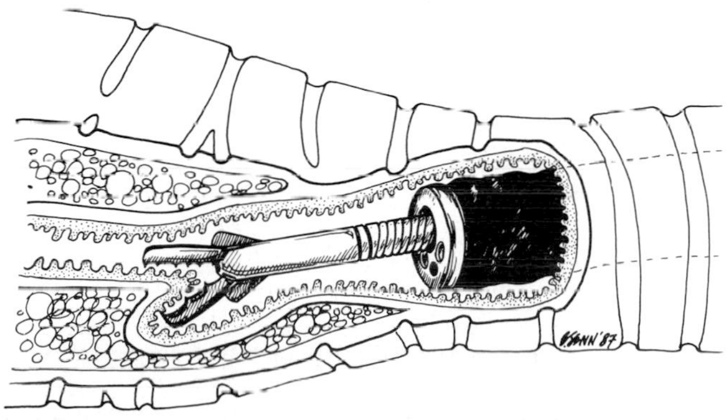

FIGURE 66–17. Conceptual drawing of a transbronchial lung biopsy. Invagination of the bronchial wall into the alligator forceps occurs during expiration.

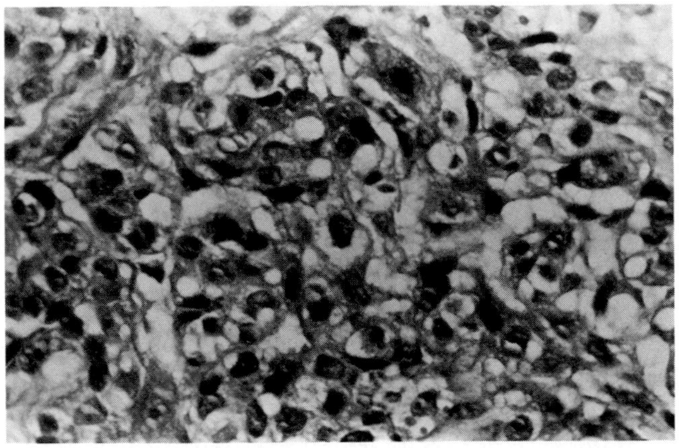

FIGURE 66–18. Transbronchial lung biopsy showing polymorphic neoplastic nests of cells with vacuolated cytoplasm that stained positive for mucin; characteristic of adenocarcinoma. (Hematoxylin and eosin, × 250.)

(Figure 66–19). Suction is applied at the proximal end of the biopsy catheter with a 20-ml syringe, and the needle is moved in and out, taking care to leave the needle tip in the bronchial mucosa. Suction is gradually released, the needle is withdrawn from the bronchial wall and retracted into the sheath; both the aspiration catheter and bronchoscope are then removed as a unit. After withdrawal of the sheath from the scope, the needle is advanced, a saline- or air-filled syringe is attached, and the aspirated material is ejected onto a glass slide or into formalin. Pinpoint-size hemorrhages in the bronchial wall make identification of the biopsy site easy. Multiple aspiration biopsies should be performed.

The diagnostic accuracy of transbronchial biopsy for noninfectious pulmonary disease in humans is 60 to 80 per cent, with transbronchial aspiration biopsy the more sensitive technique (80 per cent).[28, 29] False-negative and false-positive results are reported in fewer than two per cent of the cases. The forceps biopsy method (sensitivity 50 to 90 per cent, specificity 70 to 90 per cent)[13] seems to be superior to the needle aspiration technique (sensitivity 30 per cent, specificity 30 per cent) for the diagnosis of infections.[30]

In general, bronchoscopy is considered safe, with fewer complications occurring when the flexible bronchofiberscope is used.[18] In humans, the most frequently reported problems (pneumothorax, hemorrhage, bronchospasm, and respiratory compromise) occur in fewer than 0.1 per cent of all bronchoscopic procedures. Deaths are even less common (0.01 per cent). Pneumothorax (5.9 per cent) and hemorrhage (5.5 per cent, often associated with the use of anticoagulant drugs) are reported as frequent complications of transbronchial forceps biopsy.[28] Arterial hypoxemia with 10 to 20 mm Hg drop in oxygen tension is common during bronchoscopy and supplemental oxygen during the procedure is recommended for patients with arterial oxygen tensions less than 60 mm Hg while breathing room air.[31] Insertion of the flexible bronchofiberscope through an endotracheal tube can result in air flow resistance and it is recommended that endotracheal tube diameter be 3 mm greater than the fiberoptic bronchoscope insertion tube to minimize this potential problem. Despite reported complications, bronchoscopy is safe even in severely compromised patients, provided that proper precautions are taken.[18]

PERCUTANEOUS FINE NEEDLE ASPIRATION LUNG BIOPSY

Percutaneous lung biopsy has been used in humans since the latter part of the nineteenth century, but its popularity declined because of frequent complications.[32] In recent years percutaneous aspiration biopsy, percutaneous cutting (core) biopsy, suction-excision biopsy, and trephine biopsy have been enhanced by fluoroscopy and ultrasonography, which is used to visualize and localize discrete lung lesions.[32, 33] Patchy or diffuse lung disease is less clearly outlined and nonspecific or misleading specimens are frequently obtained. Fine needle aspiration biopsy is preferred since the other techniques are far more hazardous and more likely to cause a pneumothorax and marked pulmonary hemorrhage.[34]

Indications for percutaneous fine needle aspiration biopsy include identification of discrete lesions, confirmation of lung metastasis, obtaining material for microbiologic examination and culture, and evaluation of solitary pulmonary lesions. Percutaneous fine needle aspiration biopsy should also be used for patients considered poor surgical risks for open lung biopsy.

The technique of percutaneous fine needle aspiration

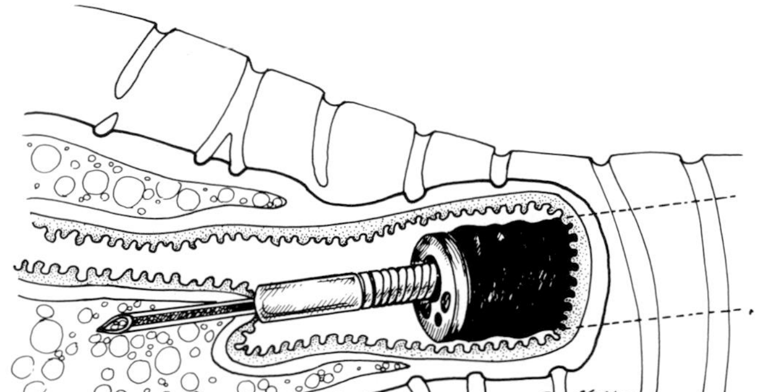

FIGURE 66–19. Schematic drawing of a transbronchial needle aspiration biopsy. The specimen is obtained by applying suction at this proximal end of the biopsy catheter.

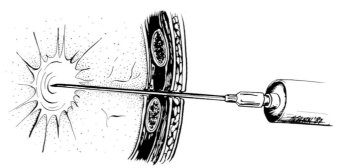

FIGURE 66–20. Conceptual drawing of a percutaneous fine needle aspiration biopsy. The specimen is obtained by applying suction and moving the needle back and forth within the lesion.

biopsy is a rapidly and easily learned. When possible, routine prebiopsy laboratory studies should include arterial blood gas tension and bleeding time determinations. Platelet count, prothrombin time, partial thromboplastin time, or activated coagulation time tests are determined if a bleeding disorder is suspected. Hypoxemia and coagulation abnormalities should be corrected prior to biopsy to reduce the risk of complications.

The patient should remain relaxed and quiet throughout the procedure. Atropine and diazepam or a reversible narcotic-analgesic can be used to suppress coughing, secretions, and vasovagal reflex. When required, oxygen may be administered by nasal cannula. The risks of the procedure are increased in uncooperative or coughing animals. Although it is a relative contraindication because of the patient's inability to clear endobronchial hemorrhage, anesthesia may be necessary.

The patient should be positioned in lateral or sternal recumbency. The biopsy area is localized using lateral and ventrodorsal or dorsoventral thoracic radiographs. Fluoroscopic or ultrasonic guidance is extremely helpful but is not always necessary. The biopsy site is clipped, prepared with an appropriate germicidal solution, and surgically draped. The skin, subcutaneous tissue, muscle, and parietal pleura are infiltrated with 1 to 2 per cent lidocaine solution. A small skin and subcutaneous tissue stab incision is made with a scalpel blade before the needle is introduced. A disposable spinal needle of 19- to 23-gauge with stylet is advanced through the chest wall to an appropriate depth, which is estimated from previous chest radiographs, fluoroscopy, or ultrasonography, or by detecting a change in lung consistency (Figure 66–20). For microbial cultures and with diffuse lesions, the needle is advanced into the pulmonary parenchyma approximately 1 to 3 cm. Once the tip is positioned within the lesion, the stylet is removed and a 10- to 20-ml syringe is quickly attached to the needle hub. The lesion is sampled by moving the needle back and forth over a 0.5 to 1.0 cm distance while exerting continuous suction on the syringe. An alternative method, particularly useful for obtaining fluid for microbial culture, is to use a 10-ml syringe containing 2 to 3 ml of nonbacteriostatic saline solution. The saline solution is expelled once the area of interest is localized, and a firm negative pressure is applied and maintained as the needle is advanced and rotated. Suction is maintained while the needle is withdrawn to prevent pulmonary venous air embolism. Many large tumors have necrotic centers and it is important to obtain a sample from the lesion periphery if possible. Insertion and withdrawal are performed rapidly to minimize pleural tearing. Following needle removal, the skin and subcutaneous tissues are gently massaged to prevent air leaking into the pleural space from the incision site.

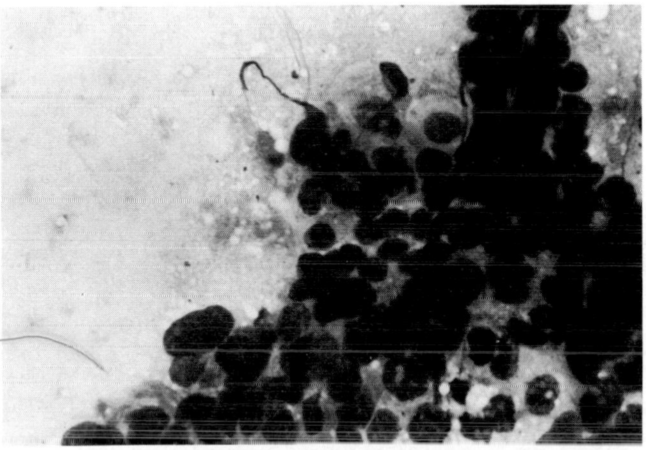

FIGURE 66–21. Percutaneous fine needle aspiration cytology specimen showing anisokaryosis and granular chromatin. Most cells have indistinct cytoplasm but an occasional oval cell can be observed. This specimen was suggestive of carcinoma. (Wright-Giemsa, × 100.)

Material obtained can be smeared onto glass slides and stained for cytologic examination (Figure 66–21) or inoculated into broth or onto solid media for culture. If a small core of tissue is obtained, it should be transferred to ten per cent buffered formalin solution for histologic examination. To obtain a representative sample, one to five lung aspirates can be taken from different depths in a centrifugal fashion. Obtaining a biopsy from a large peripheral mass is relatively easy, but more centrally located 0.5 to 1.0 cm lesions require considerable skill and fluoroscopic or ultrasonographic guidance.[32, 33]

After the biopsy, expiratory chest radiographs are obtained and evaluated for pneumothorax. All animals should be observed frequently for 24 hours after biopsy for evidence of respiratory distress. If pneumothorax occurs following the first or second aspiration, placement of a chest tube should be considered before the procedure is repeated.

For identification of nontreated pulmonary infections, aspiration consistently yields the highest specificity (80 to 100 per cent) and sensitivity (90 to 100 per cent) of all available procedures, except for open lung biopsy.[13, 32] The diagnostic accuracy for lung neoplasms is approximately 80 to 95 per cent.[32, 33, 35] Missed diagnoses are usually due to needle placement away from the lesion, the sampling of peripheral inflammatory processes not representative of the entire lesion, poorly differentiated tumor types, and poorly exfoliative tumors.

Complications of percutaneous fine needle aspiration biopsy of the lung are common and potentially serious.[13, 32, 33] Pneumothorax is most common (20 to 50 per cent), with up to 50 per cent of the affected patients requiring chest tube drainage. Less frequently encountered problems include hemoptysis (three to eight per cent), localized interstitial infiltrate adjacent to the puncture site (one to four per cent), and hemorrhagic pleural effusion (less than one per cent). Deaths are rare (less than 0.1 per cent) and usually occur subsequent to air embolism or endobronchial hemorrhage. Needle tract implant metastases and infections have been reported several times, but are considered rare and are not an absolute contraindication. A new procedure, employing ultrathin (24- to 25-gauge) needle aspiration reportedly produces fewer complications (pneumothorax eight per cent, hemoptysis four per cent) while maintaining similar diagnostic yields.[36]

Patient selection is very important, and screening for abnormalities of platelet count, clotting function, and arterial oxygen tension is essential. The value of this technique should always be weighed against the patient's ability to withstand transient pneumothorax or hemoptysis.

OPEN LUNG BIOPSY

Bronchoscopic and percutaneous fine needle aspiration biopsy techniques have decreased the need for open lung biopsy. However, open lung biopsy remains the standard to which all other techniques are compared. Indications for lung biopsy via thoracotomy include undiagnosed pulmonary infiltrates, presence of a resectable solitary mass, persistent pleural effusion, and hilar lymphadenopathy (when associated with undiagnosed parenchymal disease).

The various surgical approaches are well described in standard texts.[37, 38] Definitive diagnosis is made in 70 to 100 per cent of the cases.[39, 40] In up to one-half of the patients, the results of biopsy-proven diagnosis effect a change in therapy. Pneumothorax is the most common complication, occurring in approximately eight per cent of cases. Bleeding problems (hemothorax and hemoptysis) are rare (less than one per cent). Mortality has been reported up to three per cent, although selection of cases influences mortality rate.

SUMMARY AND CONCLUSIONS

A variety of diagnostic modalities are available to the clinician seeking the cause of a pulmonary disease. The four procedures discussed should be regarded as complementary. For example, transtracheal aspiration and bronchoscopy are indicated for central and endobronchial lesions, fine needle aspiration biopsy for more peripheral lesions or focal pulmonary infiltrates, and bronchoscopy or open lung biopsy for more diffuse processes. Complications are a major concern because many animals requiring these procedures have limited respiratory reserves and the diagnostic value may not outweigh the complication rate.

The sensitivity and specificity are also important factors when considering the best approach. In most instances, except for transtracheal washing, the differences may be insignificant; however, the theoretical advantages of a procedure should not be interpreted as sufficient to substantiate its use before a less invasive technique is tried.

References

1. Suter, PF: Thoracic radiography: a text atlas of thoracic diseases in the dog and cat. Wettswil, Switzerland, Peter F Suter, 1984.
2. Silverman, S and Suter, PF: Influence of inspiration and expiration on canine thoracic radiographs. JAVMA 166:502, 1975.
3. Carlisle, CH and Thrall, DE: A comparison of normal feline thoracic radiographs made in dorsal versus ventral recumbency. Vet Radiol 23:3, 1982.
4. Ruehl, WW and Thrall, DE: The effect of dorsal versus ventral recumbency on the radiographic appearance of the canine thorax. Vet Radiol 22:10, 1981.
5. Spencer, CP, et al.: The canine lateral thoracic radiograph. Vet Radiol 22:262, 1981.
6. Lang, J, et al: Sensitivity of radiographic detection of lung metastasis in the dog. Vet Radiol 27:74, 1986.
7. Suter, PF and Chan, KF: Disseminated pulmonary diseases in small animals; a radiographic approach to diagnosis. JAVRS 9:67, 1968.
8. Reif, JS and Rhodes, WH: The lung of aged dogs: Radiographic-morphologic correlation. Vet Radiol 7:5, 1966.
9. Pecora, DV: A comparison of transtracheal aspiration with other methods of determining the bacterial flora of the lower respiratory tract. N Engl J Med 269:664, 1963.
10. Creighton, SR and Wilkins, RJ: Transtracheal aspiration biopsy: Technique and cytological evaluation. JAAHA 10:219, 1974.
11. Moise, NS and Blue, J: Bronchial washings in the cat: Procedure and cytologic evaluation. Comp Cont Ed Pract Vet 5:621, 1983.
12. Bartlett, JG: Diagnostic accuracy of transtracheal aspiration bacteriologic studies. Am Rev Resp Dis 115:777, 1977.
13. Moser, KM, et al.: Sensitivity, specificity, and risk of diagnostic procedures in a canine model of *Streptococcus pneumoniae* pneumonia. Am Rev Resp Dis 125:436, 1982.
14. Greenlee, PG and Roszel, JF: Feline bronchial cytology: Histologic/cytologic correlation in 22 cats. Vet Pathol 21:308, 1984.
15. Bartlett, JG, et al.: Percutaneous transtracheal aspiration in the diagnosis of anaerobic pulmonary infection. Ann Intern Med 79:535, 1973.
16. Pratter, MR and Irwin, RS: Transtracheal aspiration guidelines for safety. Chest 76:518, 1979.
17. Ikeda, S: Atlas of Flexible Bronchofiberscopy. Baltimore, University Park Press, 1974.
18. Sackner, MA: Bronchofiberscopy: State of the art. Am Rev Resp Dis 111:62, 1975.
19. Landa, JF: Indications for bronchoscopy. Chest 73:686, 1978.
20. Amis, TC and McKiernan, BC: Systematic identification of endobronchial anatomy during bronchoscopy in the dog. Am J Vet Res 47:2649, 1986.
21. Crystal, RG, et al.: Bronchoalveolar lavage. Chest 90:122, 1986.
22. Rebar, AH, et al.: Bronchopulmonary lavage cytology in the dog: Normal findings. Vet Pathol 17:294, 1980.
23. Reynolds, HY: Bronchoalveolar lavage. Am Rev Resp Dis 135:250, 1987.
24. Wimberley, NW, et al.: Use of a bronchoscopic protected catheter brush for the diagnosis of pulmonary infections. Chest 81:556, 1982.
25. Shroff, CP: Abrasive bronchial brushing cytology. Acta Cytol 29:101, 1985.
26. Zavala, DC, et al.: Use of the bronchofiberscope for bronchial brush biopsy. Chest 63:889, 1973.
27. Meyer, DJ: Management of the cytology specimen. Comp Cont Ed Pract Vet 9:10, 1987.
28. Zavala, DC: Transbronchial biopsy in diffuse lung disease. Chest 73:727, 1978.
29. Horsley, JR, et al.: Bronchial submucosal needle aspiration performed through the fiberoptic bronchoscope. Acta Cytol 28:211, 1983.
30. Shure D, et al.: Transbronchial needle aspiration in the diagnosis of pneumonia in a canine model. Am Rev Resp Dis 131:290, 1985.
31. Dubrawsky, C, et al.: The effect of bronchofiberscopic examination on oxygen status. Chest 67:137, 1975.
32. Sagel, SS, et al.: Percutaneous transthoracic aspiration needle biopsy. Ann Thorac Surg 26:399, 1978.
33. Yang, PC, et al.: Peripheral pulmonary lesions: Ultrasonography and ultrasonically guided aspiration biopsy. Radiology 155:451, 1985.
34. Roudebush, P, et al.: Percutaneous fine-needle aspiration biopsy of the lung in disseminated pulmonary disease. JAAHA 17:109, 1981.
35. Johnston, WW: Percutaneous fine needle aspiration biopsy of the lung. Acta Cytol 28:218, 1984.
36. Zavala, DC and Schoell, JE: Ultrathin needle aspiration of the lung in infectious and malignant disease. Am Rev Resp Dis 123:125, 1981.
37. Nelson, AW: Lower respiratory system. *In* Slatter DH (ed): Textbook of Small Animal Surgery. Philadelphia, WB Saunders, 1985, p 1016.
38. Archibald, J and Harvey, CE: Thorax. *In* Archibald J (ed): Canine Surgery. Santa Barbara, American Veterinary Publications, 1974, p 424.
39. Aaron, BL, et al.: Open lung biopsy, a strong stand. Chest 59:18, 1971.

40. Stillwell, PC, et al.: Limited thoracotomy in the pediatric patient. Mayo Clin Proc 56:673, 1981.

Selected References for Approach to Respiratory Diseases

American Board of Internal Medicine: Clinical competence in internal medicine. Ann Intern Med 90:402, 1979.
Bordow, RA and Moser, KM (eds.): Manual of Clinical Problems in Pulmonary Medicine with Annotated Key References. 2nd ed. Boston. Little, Brown and Company, 1985.
Brodey, RS: Hypertrophic osteoarthropathy in the dog: a clinicopathologic survey of 60 cases. JAVMA 159:1242, 1971.
Cantwell, HD, et al.: Pleural effusion in the dog: principles for diagnosis. JAAHA 19:227, 1983.
Kaplan, W: Epidemiology of the principal systemic mycoses of man and lower animals and the ecology of their etiologic agents. JAVMA 163:1043, 1973.
Kolata, RJ and Burrows, CF: The clinical features of injury by chewing electrical cords in dogs and cats. JAAHA 17:219, 1981.
Legendre, AM, et al.: Canine nasal and parasinus tumors. JAAHA 19:115, 1983.
Moise, NS and Blue, J: Bronchial washings in the cat: procedure and cytologic evaluation. Comp Cont Ed Pract Vet 5:621, 1983.
Reif, JS: Physical examination of the canine respiratory system. Vet Clin N Am 1:71, 1971.
Reigelman, RK: The hidden holes in the history. Postgrad Med 70:40, 1981.
Thayer, GW and Robinson, SK: Bacterial bronchopneumonia in the dog: a review of 42 cases. JAAHA 20:731, 1984.

67 DISEASES OF THE NOSE AND THROAT

PETER G. C. BEDFORD

THE NOSE

STRUCTURE AND FUNCTION

The nose consists of a bony nasal cavity, the nasal conchae or turbinate bones within this cavity, the paranasal sinuses, and the paired, distally situated nasal cartilages that form the framework of the mobile rhinarium (Figure 67–1). The roof of the nasal cavity is formed by the paired nasal bones, the lateral walls by the premaxillae and maxillae, and the floor (or hard palate) by the vomer, the paired palatine bones, the palatine processes of the maxillae, and the premaxillae. The posterior limit is the ethmoid bone and anteriorly the rhinarium opens to the exterior via two external nares or nostrils. The nasal cavity is divided in the midline by a bony and cartilaginous septum into two separate nasal chambers or fossae. Each chamber is subdivided into a number of longitudinal air-conducting channels, or meati, by the presence of the nasal conchae, scroll-like cartilaginous or ossified structures covered with ciliated pseudocolumnar epithelium. The conchae are divided into three parts, the anteriorly situated dorsal and ventral conchae and the posteriorly situated ethmoidal concha. Alternative terminology can be used for these structures: the dorsal nasal concha is also called the dorsal nasoturbinate, the ventral nasal concha is also called the maxilloturbinate, and the ethmoidal concha is also called the ethmoturbinate. The dorsal nasal concha is an elongated scroll attached to the ethmoid and nasal bones, and the dorsal nasal meatus passes above it. The ventral nasal concha, a number of tightly folded scrolls, extends from the first to the third premolar teeth. The middle nasal meatus passes between it and the dorsal nasal concha while the ventral nasal meatus lies between it and the hard palate. The brittle bony ethmoidal conchae are outgrowths of the ethmoid bone that fill the caudal part of the nasal cavity and extend dorsally into the frontal sinuses. Olfactory nerve endings are found primarily within the mucosa covering the ethmoidal conchae, and additional sensory nerves supplied to the mucosa lining each nasal chamber also contribute to olfaction. In addition, the paired tubular structures known collectively as the vomeronasal or Jacobson's organ are also lined with olfactory neuroepithelium. They are found in the anterior ventral part of the nasal septum, and the incisive duct provides a common connection between them and the nasal and oral cavities. The vomeronasal organ probably functions in identification and sexual behavior[1, 2] and lip curling may help in its function by aiding the aspiration of smells.[3]

The paranasal sinuses are extensions of the nasal cavity; only the frontal sinuses are of any clinical significance in the dog and cat. Their involvement in nasal disease is usually due to their impaired drainage through diseased ethmoidal conchae, or the extension of neoplasia from the nasal cavity. The cavities of the sphenoidal sinus of the dog and the presphenoidal sinus of the cat are within the presphenoid bone and are filled with turbinate scrolls. The maxillary sinus of the dog is simply a shallow recess in the lateral wall of the nasal cavity, opposite the carnassial tooth.

The anterior part of the nose, the rhinarium, is formed from three paired cartilages. The external naris opens into the nasal vestibule between the ventrolateral nasal cartilage and the dorsolateral and accessory cartilages. These latter are jointly referred to as the wing of the nostril. This is the most mobile part of the rhinarium, its movement being controlled by the insertion of fibers from the levator labii maxillaris and the nasolabialis muscles. The nasal vestibule, just posterior to the nostril, is almost obliterated in both the dog and the cat by the presence of the distended termination of the ventral nasal concha, the alar fold. As this structure is fused to the wing of the nostril, most of the incoming air is diverted ventrally into the common and ventral nasal meati. During sniffing there is forced inspiration and the nostrils are dilated. An increased volume of air enters the vestibule, some passing dorsally to the ethmoidal conchae and their olfactory neuroepithelium.

Olfaction is obviously a major function of the nose in the dog and cat, both of which have a highly developed sense of smell. The nasal mucosa is well vascularized,

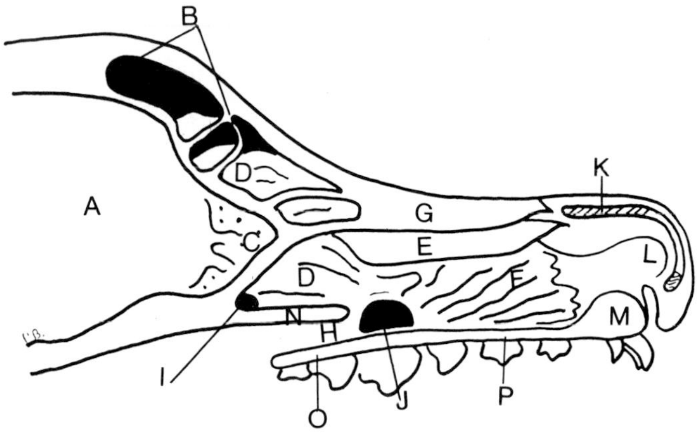

FIGURE 67–1. Diagram of left rhinarium, nasal chamber, and paranasal sinuses of the dog. *A,* Cranial cavity, *B,* frontal sinus, *C,* cribriform plate, *D,* ethmoidal concha, *E,* dorsal nasal concha, *F,* ventral nasal concha, *G,* nasal bone, *H,* internal naris (choana), *I,* position of sphenoidal sinus, *J,* maxillary sinus or recess, *K,* dorsolateral nasal cartilage, *L,* alar fold, *M,* premaxilla, *N,* vomer, *O,* palatine bone, *P,* palatine process of maxilla.

and inspired air is warmed and humidified to the point of saturation as it passes through the conchae. In addition the mucus layer that lines the conchal air passages serves as a filter medium to trap bacteria and particulate material.

Diagnosis

The history and the clinical signs seen in patients with nasal disease are relatively specific, the problems experienced in treatment being related to the differential diagnosis of a clinical picture characterized by discharge and sneeze, and to the very nature of the diseases themselves. While the diagnosis and treatment of foreign body rhinitis or a nasal polyp is uncomplicated and attended routinely by a good prognosis, the diagnosis of cause and methodology of treatment of hyperplastic rhinitis remain uncertain and the prognosis is often unsatisfactory. In most patients the initial response of the nasal mucosa to disease is the production of a serous discharge, usually accompanied by sporadic or persistent sneezing. With chronicity, the discharge usually becomes much thicker and more mucoid; in the presence of bacterial infection and necrosis, it is often purulent; and where tissue breakdown and erosion have occurred or the mucosa is severely congested, the discharge may be bloodstained or even accompanied by hemorrhage. Sneezing is commonplace in the acute situation but tends to occur less frequently in long-standing disease. When it does occur in this latter situation it can be paroxysmal, and epistaxis may result. Sneezing and snorting are prompted by irritation and are reflex actions designed to clear the airway. Gagging and retching in the presence of nasal disease reflect the nasopharyngeal drainage of discharge and are possibly more common in chronic disease situations.

Diagnosis involves careful consideration of the history; age and breed are particularly relevant when considering rhinomycosis or neoplasia. Physical examination of the conscious patient has its limitations, but may be of value where palatine defects or long-standing neoplasia are present. The type of discharge may indicate cause, and hematology and serology can be useful on occasion. Endoscopy is of limited value, but radiography often proves to be the linchpin in diagnosis while rhinotomy is occasionally necessary.

THE HISTORY

The presence of nasal discharge is the commonest clinical feature, but one which can be missed or reported inaccurately if the patient is a nostril licker. This is an important consideration, for most cats and many dogs fall into this category. Fortunately, sneezing is also common and is not as easily masked, although the amount of sneezing can be markedly reduced in chronic disease. Noisy breathing results from obstruction of one or both nasal chambers, due to congestion of the conchal mucosa and the presence of discharge or neoplasia. When obstruction is severe, the patient mouth breathes, a feature that is particularly noticeable during excitement or exercise. Occasionally an owner may notice the patient pawing or rubbing its nose, while other patients seem to experience pain and resent having their faces touched. Facial deformity over the nasal chambers or frontal sinuses may be present, but this feature usually indicates long-standing disease. Anorexia or depressed appetite is associated with loss of olfaction, but may also reflect pain.

PHYSICAL EXAMINATION

A complete physical examination of the patient must include evaluation of the whole respiratory tract, with particular reference to laryngeal, tracheal, and pulmonary function. Auscultation should be attempted both during open-mouth and closed-mouth breathing; occluding one nostril at a time during the latter can be helpful in determining the extent of any blockage. Visual or palpable asymmetry of the nasal cavity or frontal sinuses is of obvious significance, and softness of bone in these areas indicates invasion by endonasal neoplasia. In the presence of normal facial contour, pain elicited by palpation may indicate a destructive rhinomycosis. Proptosis or deviation of the eye suggests an extension of a turbinate-based tumor into the orbit. Epiphora and the presence of discharge in the medial canthus are suggestive of blockage or erosion of the nasolacrimal duct, while hemorrhage from the lacrimal puncta may occasionally accompany long-standing neoplasia. Where possible in the conscious animal, the oral cavity and oropharynx should be examined; palatine defects and oronasal fistulae are of obvious etiological significance, and with time endonasal neoplasia can invade the hard palate and gingival areas.

The external nares should be examined for movement during inspiration, patency, the presence of discharge, ulceration, and tumor formation. Collapse of the external naris can follow trauma or necrosis of the nasal cartilages, but inspiratory bilateral collapse with complete loss of patency is a congenital feature of the brachycephalic breeds. The physical nature of any discharge may indicate cause or dictate features of secondary pathogenic significance.[4] Swabs should be taken for culture to identify fungal and bacterial organisms, and antibiotic sensitivity should be assessed, for although most of the bacteria isolated are contaminants, they may be of pathogenic significance. However, microbiological results are not always meaningful and should be read in the general context of the clinical picture. Patency of the rhinarial and nasal cavity airways can be assessed quite simply using a strand of cotton wool held in front of each external naris in turn, but percussion of the frontal sinuses is a valueless exercise. Hematologic examination may be helpful, while the serologic confirmation of aspergillosis is an essential diagnostic procedure, particularly in the young dolichocephalic dog.

Further evaluation necessitates the use of general anesthesia, with endotracheal intubation required to prevent any possible inhalation of discharge and to render irrigation of the nasal chambers safe. The teeth, hard and soft palates, and the tonsils should be reexamined, and the nasopharynx checked for discharge and neoplasia by using a dental mirror and illumination (Figure 67–2) or a small, flexible endoscope.[5] Where size of the external naris permits, anterior rhinoscopy is easily achieved in the dog using a long auriscope cone or a small endoscope. Evaluation of the vestibule; the common, dorsal, and ventral nasal meati; and the dorsal and ventral conchae is possible, but of limited value

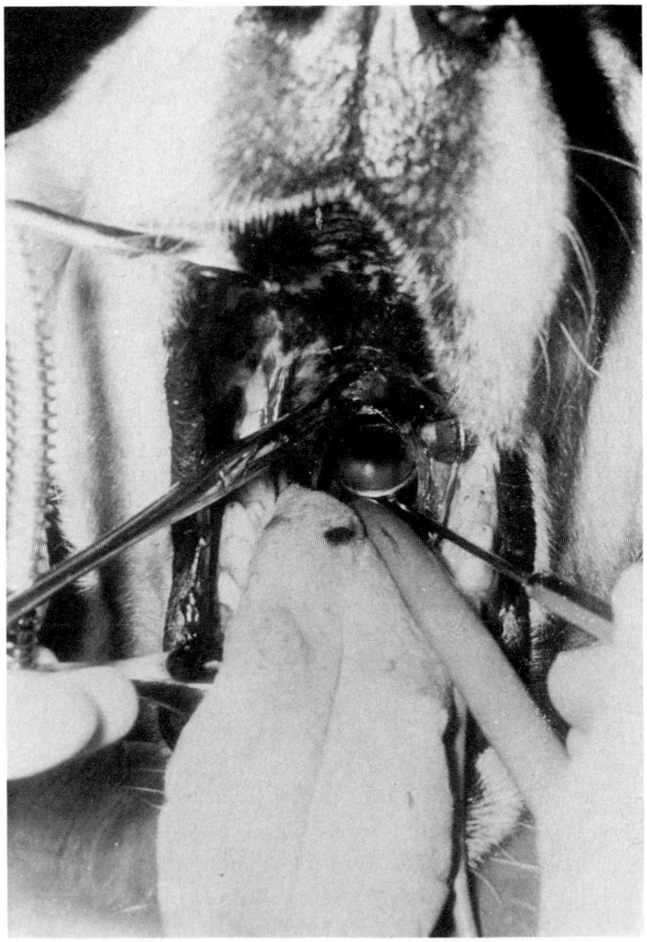

FIGURE 67–2. Posterior rhinoscopy. A warmed dental mirror is used to examine the nasopharynx and choanae.

unless a foreign body or established neoplasia is present. Copious discharge and induced hemorrhage from congested mucosa can complicate the procedure, but foreign bodies can be removed without resorting to rhinotomy and the presence of nasal polyps can be confirmed. The identification of neoplasms involving the ethmoidal concha is difficult when tumor formation is in its early stages. Occasionally fungal colonies, particularly those involving the ventral nasal conchae, may be identified.

Irrigation of the nasal cavity can dislodge the occasional foreign body, but this technique is perhaps of more value in aiding the interpretation of any radiographic findings by removing discharge obscuring the smaller air passages. It is also of some value in obtaining material for culture or cytologic investigation.[6] The nasopharynx should be packed off, and warm sterile water or physiological saline flushed through each nasal chamber using lubricated tubing, with the patient in lateral recumbency.

RADIOGRAPHIC EXAMINATION

Given the limitations of anterior and posterior rhinoscopy, radiography remains the one important noninvasive diagnostic procedure for routine application. Several projections of the nasal cavity and frontal sinuses are possible,[7] but in all interpretation relies upon contrast between bone (Figure 67–3), soft tissue, and air. Nasal discharge, blood, hyperplastic tissue change, and neoplasia mask the negative contrast of the air-filled spaces and cavities, while areas of increased negative contrast are due to tissue destruction. The dorsoventral (occlusal) projection using nonscreen film placed inside the mouth is the most useful, for the nasal conchae are easily demonstrated and the nasal chambers can be compared with each other (Figures 67–3*B* and 67–4). Using nonscreen film means that the dorsoventral view does not suffer from a complicating superimposition of the mandible over the nasal cavity. Similarly, the lateral projection suffers from superimposition of one-half of the skull over the other (Figure 67–5). This can be confusing where bilateral disease is present but helpful in the three-dimensional location of lesions. The ventrodorsal open-mouth projection foreshortens the nasal cavity but allows additional examination of the ethmoidal conchae (Figures 67–2*A* and 67–6), while the anteroposterior projection allows assessment of the frontal sinuses only (Figures 67–2*C* and 67–7).

There are occasions when diagnosis is not possible without exploratory surgery. Early tumor formation may be confused with hyperplastic rhinitis, and the etiology of chronic inflammation may not be apparent. The noninvasive collection of specimens for cytologic and histopathological examination is not always rewarding in either the dog or the cat, and rhinotomy can thus prove necessary. It also permits direct examination of the intranasal structures. If the evidence gathered by rhinotomy indicates that radical turbinectomy offers an enhanced chance of cure, then this exploratory procedure is easily converted into a therapeutic one. There is something of a species difference between the dog and cat in terms of rhinotomy and radical turbinectomy, for the procedure is well tolerated in the former but of possible serious consequence in the latter.

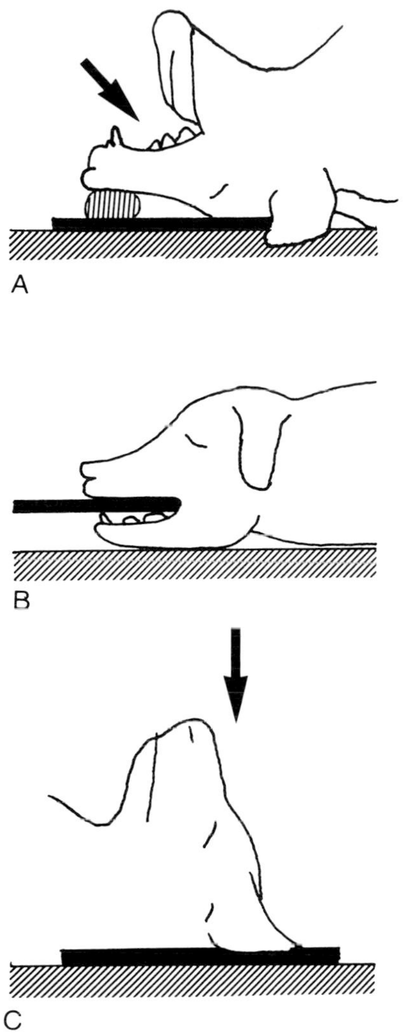

FIGURE 67–3. Positions for radiography of the nasal cavity. *A*, The ventrodorsal projection; *B*, the dorsoventral projection; *C*, the anteroposterior projection.

The nasal chamber is opened by removing a large flap incorporating nasal, maxillary, and frontal bone from the posterior edge of the rhinarium to the posterior one-third of the ipsilateral frontal sinus. The section does not cross the midline and does not involve the bony dorsal nasal septum (Figure 67–8). As such, the bone flap need not be replaced since postoperative facial distortion does not occur. The flap needs to be wide enough to allow adequate examination of the dorsal nasal and ethmoidal conchae and to permit the use of biopsy or other surgical instruments. Hemorrhage is not severe even when tissue is biopsied, but heavy bleeding accompanies radical turbinectomy and fluid therapy is necessary. Turbinectomy involves the removal of all conchal tissues and, where necessary, the contralateral conchae can be excised through the cartilaginous part of the nasal septum. Should the contralateral frontal sinus require curettage and postoperative irrigation, then it must be trephined separately. Hemorrhage is controlled by packing the nasal chamber with a sterile gauze bandage, which is removed some five days later. Occasionally subcutaneous emphysema may accompany rhinotomy, but this is of no clinical consequence. Routine antibiotic therapy during the postoperative phase is dictated on the basis of swabbing every five days, and complete healing may take up to six weeks.

Conditions of the Rhinarium

CLEFT OF THE PRIMARY PALATE

The primary palate consists of the lip and premaxillae, and the term "harelip" is used to describe the unilateral or bilateral congenital clefts that are occasionally seen in the dog, but rarely in the cat (Figure 67–9*A*). Such clefts may or may not accompany defects of the hard and soft palates (the secondary palate). Suckling is almost impossible because any communication with the rhinarial airway interferes with the creation of negative pressure within the mouth, but such animals can be nursed for the first two or three months of life, after which time corrective surgery is generally possible. The wing of the nostril can be repositioned, and full depth closure of the cleft is easily accomplished even when the tissue deficiency is considerable (Figure 67–9*B*).

CONGENITAL STENOSIS OF THE EXTERNAL NARES

Bilateral stenosis and inspiratory collapse of the external nares are parts of the brachycephalic airway obstruction syndrome.[10, 11] The dyspnea seen commonly

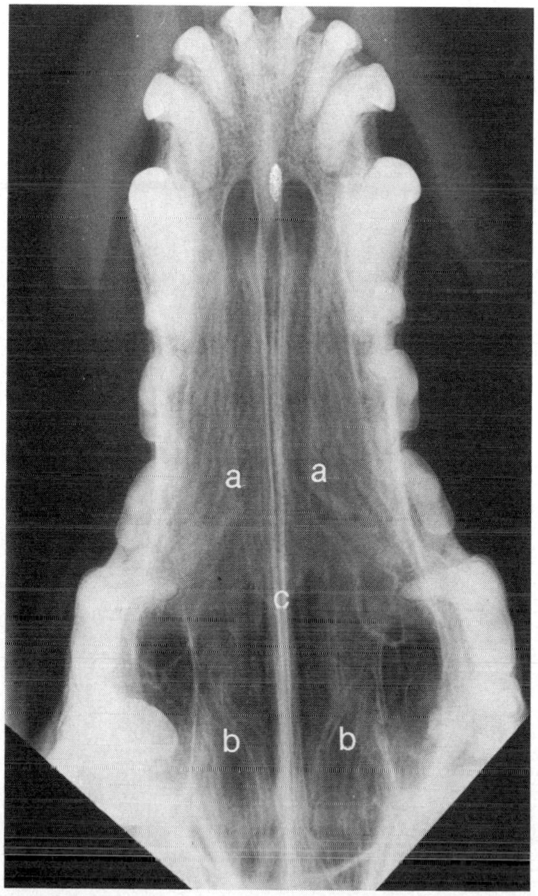

FIGURE 67–4. Radiography of the nasal cavity: dorsoventral or occlusal projection of a standard poodle, ten years old. *a*, nasal conchae; *b*, ethmoidal conchae; *c*, nasal septum.

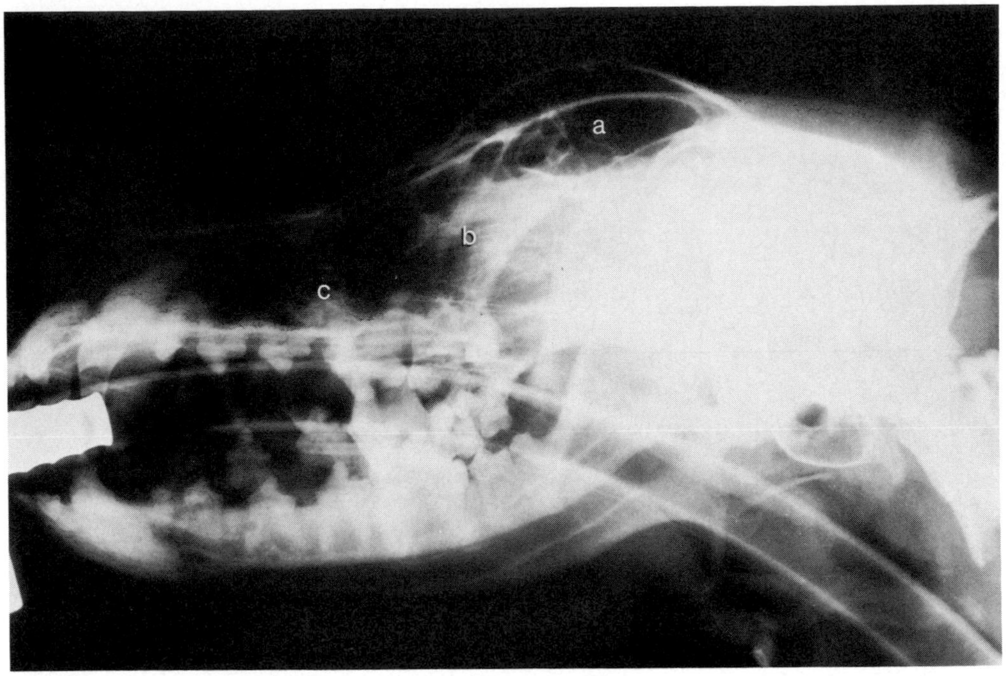

FIGURE 67–5. Radiography of the nasal cavity: lateral projection of a standard poodlle, ten years old. *a*, frontal sinus; *b*, ethmoidal concha; *c*, ventral nasal concha.

in these breeds is due to the combined effect of the abnormal nares, reduced nasal and pharyngeal air space, an excess of soft palate, and possible distortion and collapse of the larynx. At rest the airway through the external naris is extremely narrow but patent. During inspiration the naris does not dilate, but the wing of the nostril is sucked medially against the philtrum, thus closing down the air space. Total closure means that the dog must mouth breathe, but in the presence of partial occlusion, nasal breathing is possible if the inspiratory effort is increased to overcome the obstruction. This increased effort exerts a collapsing force on the soft tissues within the upper respiratory tract, and the dyspnea experienced is complicated by any resulting pharyngeal edema and may be further compounded by soft palate occlusion of the laryngeal aditus.

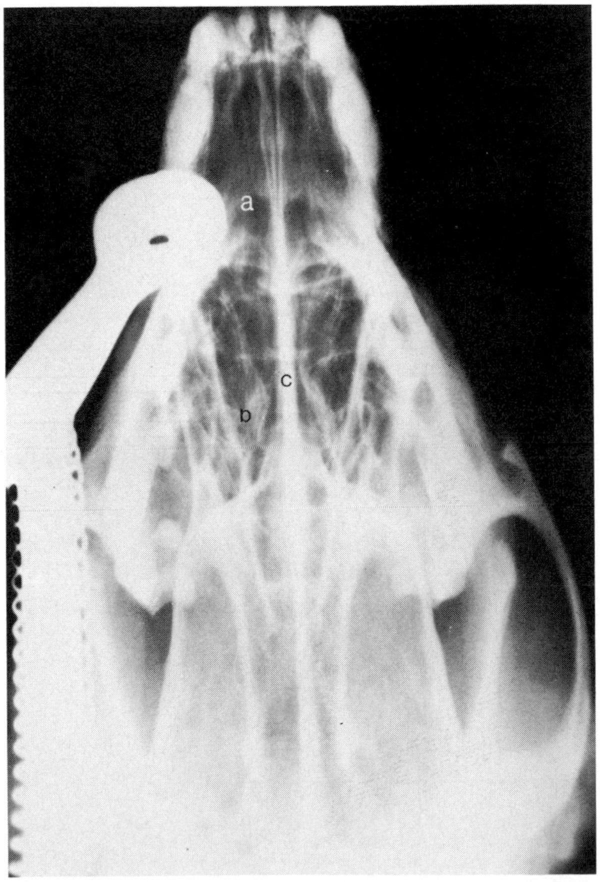

FIGURE 67–6. Radiography of the nasal cavity: ventrodorsal projection of a standard poodle, ten years old. *a*, nasal conchae; *b*, ethmoidal conchae; *c*, nasal septum.

The relief of dyspnea caused by stenotic nares is simply obtained by abducting the wing of the nostril surgically or removing part of its structure.[12] Ellipsoidal resection of skin and integument from the dorsolateral aspect of the rhinarium creates the necessary abduction, or, alternatively, the occluding distal portion of the wing of the nostril can be removed by scalpel or diathermy to expose the entrance to the nasal vestibule.

TRAUMA AND FOREIGN BODIES

Wounds of the rhinarium usually heal without complication, but where there is damage to the dorsolateral

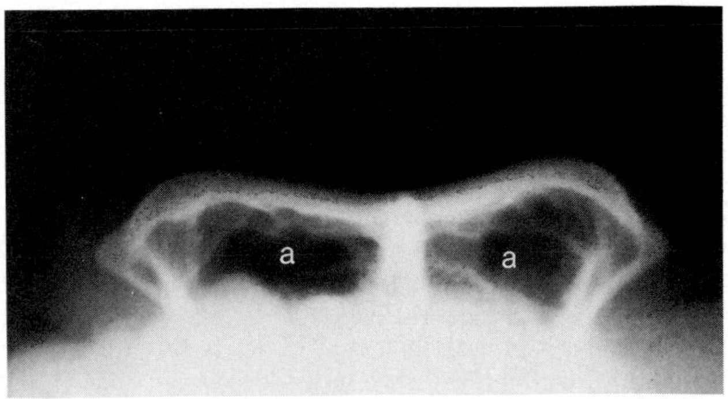

FIGURE 67–7. Radiography of the nasal cavity: anteroposterior projection of a standard poodle, ten years old. *a*, frontal sinuses.

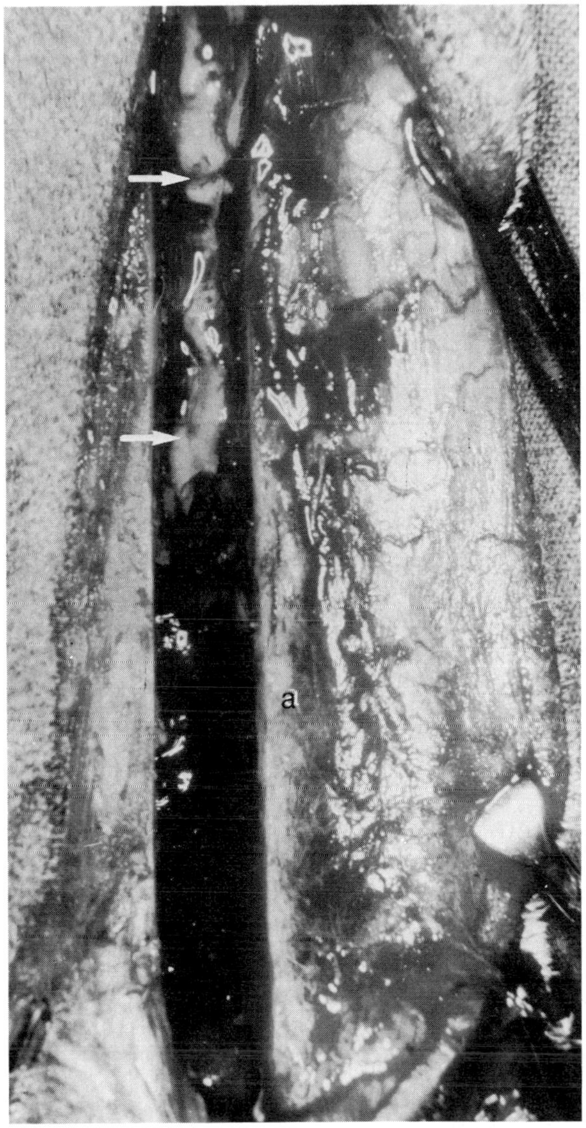

FIGURE 67–8. Exploratory rhinotomy, demonstrating the presence of *Aspergillus* colonies (arrows) on the right dorsal nasal and ethmoidal conchae. *a*, right maxilla.

nasal cartilages, stenosis and collapse of the nares may occur. Foreign bodies seldom lodge within the nostril, despite the presence of the alar fold. Most objects find their way into the ventral nasal concha and meatus.

PEMPHIGUS VULGARIS

Persistent licking of nasal discharge may occasionally cause excoriation of the rhinarium, but this should not be confused with the intractable ulceration caused by pemphigoid mucocutaneous disease, particularly seen in the German shepherd dog (Figure 67–10). The condition can occur at any age, and lesions affecting other mucocutaneous junctions may be present. Both nostrils may be involved, and crusting, rhinorrhea, hemorrhage, and persistent sneezing may all accompany the ulceration. The condition is progressive and erosion of the nasal cartilages can lead to distortion or even collapse of the nostrils. The picture is often complicated by bacterial contamination, and diagnosis may necessitate biopsy and the demonstration of autoantibodies by immunofluorescence. Treatment is always difficult and both cryotherapy and radiotherapy are claimed to be effective in chronic disease. Steroid therapy can often offer effective control, and prednisolone given at a dose rate of 5 to 10 mg/lb q 24h is used in early disease.

NEOPLASIA

Squamous cell carcinoma of the rhinarium is seen with equal frequency in the dog and cat (Figures 67–11 and 67–12). In the dog, the tumor usually originates within the medial wall of the nasal vestibule, but can extend laterally into the wing of the nostril and may infiltrate through the philtrum to demonstrate bilateral involvement. Although the tumor is slow to metastasize, excision is followed by rapid recurrence, and early radiotherapy or cryotherapy is the treatment of choice. The tumor is seen in white-nosed cats and usually presents as a bleeding "ulcer" involving the dorsal rhinarium and the external naris. Tumor growth may be triggered by ultraviolet light, and carcinoma of the pinna may occur in the same patient. As with the dog, metastasis is slow and cryosurgery offers effective treatment.

Fibrosarcomas can involve the rhinarium and although metastasis is uncommon, recurrence usually follows excision. The malignant melanoma is also seen in both species; recurrence and metastasis are common.

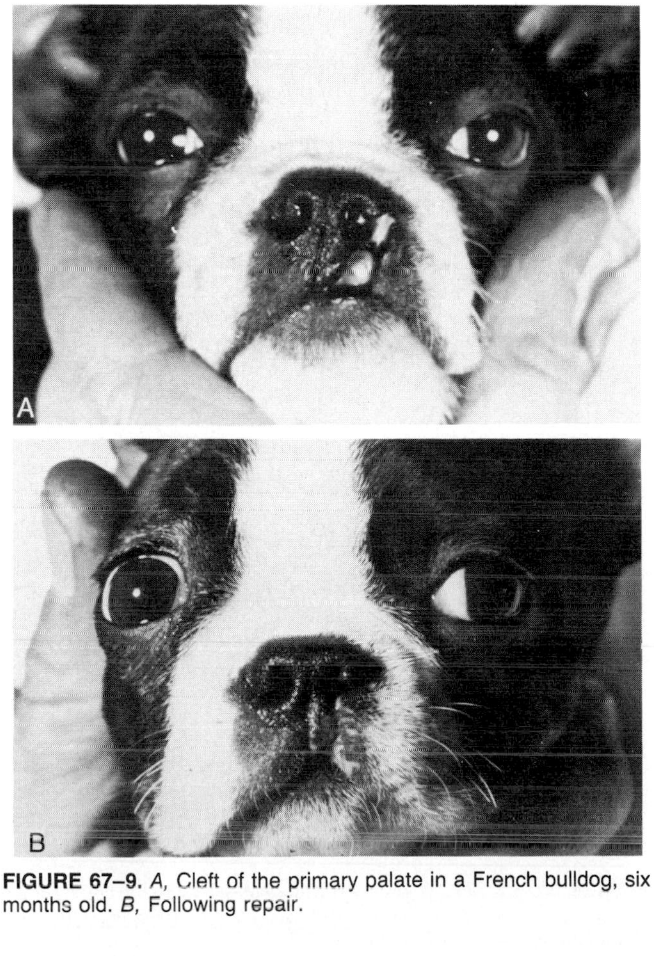

FIGURE 67–9. *A*, Cleft of the primary palate in a French bulldog, six months old. *B*, Following repair.

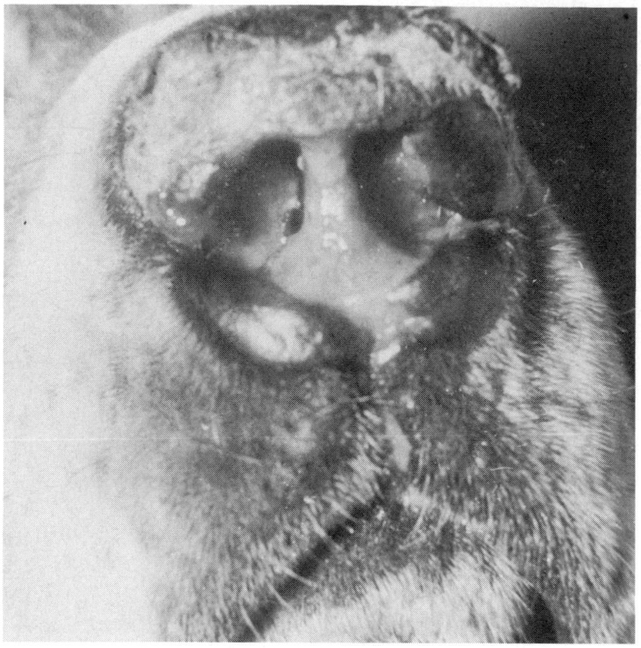

FIGURE 67–10. Extensive erosion of the rhinarium due to pemphigus vulgaris in a German shepherd dog, six years old.

Conditions of the Nasal Cavity

TRAUMA

Epistaxis invariably accompanies nasal trauma, but the extent can vary considerably. The simple measures, which are cage rest and ice packs, are often sufficient to control minor hemorrhage, but the pressure packing of both the rhinarial airway and the internal nares with gauze sponges under general anesthesia can be essential when severe epistaxis is present. Mucous membrane color, capillary refill time, and the rate and strength of the pulse are simple pointers to clinical status, and the necessity for replacement therapy is based upon these features and hematocrit values.

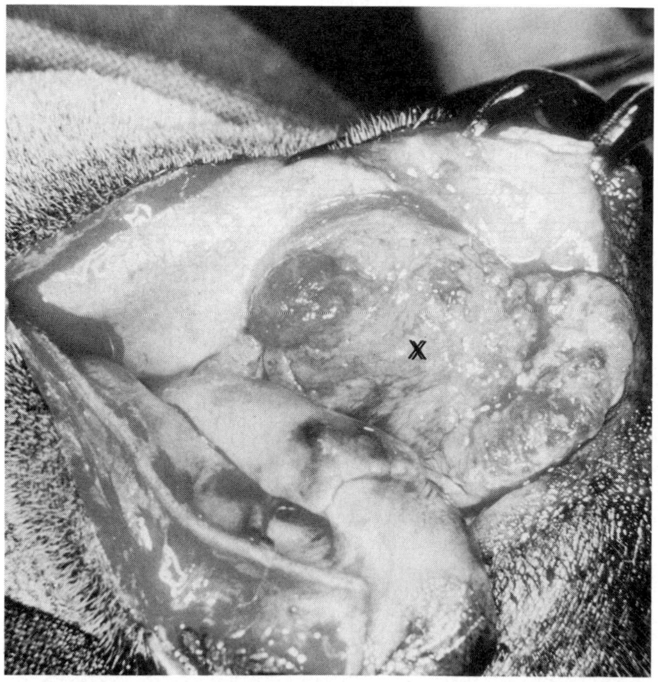

FIGURE 67–11. Lateral rhinotomy to expose squamous cell carcinoma (X) involving the medial wall of the right external naris of a German shepherd dog, nine years old.

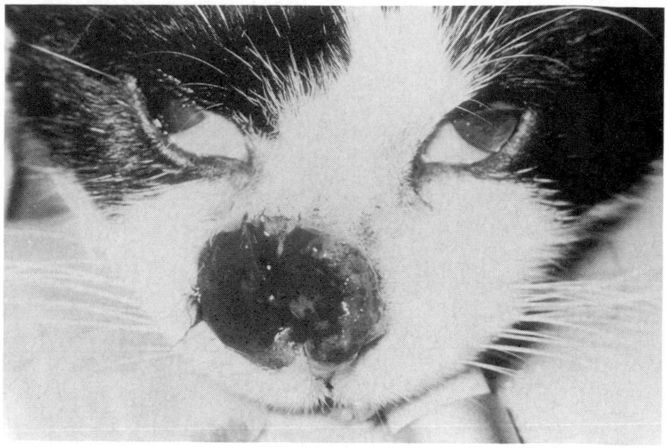

FIGURE 67–12. Extensive squamous cell carcinoma of the rhinarium in a domestic short-haired cat, five years old.

Obstruction of the nasal cavity following trauma is due to the presence of blood clots and edema, and mouth breathing may persist for several days. The displacement of fractured maxillary and nasal bone can reduce the patency of the nasal cavity, and either such fractures should be repaired or the bone fragments removed. Secondary infection can complicate the picture, and necrosis of the conchae may be seen in the long term. Splitting the hard palate along the maxillary and palatine symphyses can occur during the jumping cat's five-point landing as the result of the mandibular teeth being forced upwards between the maxillary dental arcades. The palatine mucosa swells with edema and possible hemorrhage, but the cleft is not seen until tissue necrosis has taken place several days after the event.

FOREIGN BODY RHINITIS

Most intranasal foreign bodies are of vegetable origin, and are simply inhaled through the external nares into the anterior nasal cavity. Others enter through palatine defects, and occasionally bone or wood may enter the posterior nasal cavity from the nasopharynx (Figure 67–13). Shotgun or airgun pellets, other "missile type" foreign bodies,[13] and the results of bizarre human behavior complete the list.

The entry of foreign body material into the nasal cavity is invariably of sudden onset and accompanied by violent and persistent sneezing, together with head-shaking and nose-pawing. The foreign body may be dislodged and leave a mild inflammatory response of two or three days' duration. Sneezing and discharge persist when the foreign body is retained, and occasionally hemorrhage may result from the violence of the sneezing episodes. With time, though, these initial features give way to a clinical picture characterized by chronic nasal discharge with secondary bacterial and possible fungal infections complicating the situation. Gagging and retching due to the nasopharyngeal drainage of discharge may be a feature of rhinitis due to foreign body material in the posterior nasal cavity.

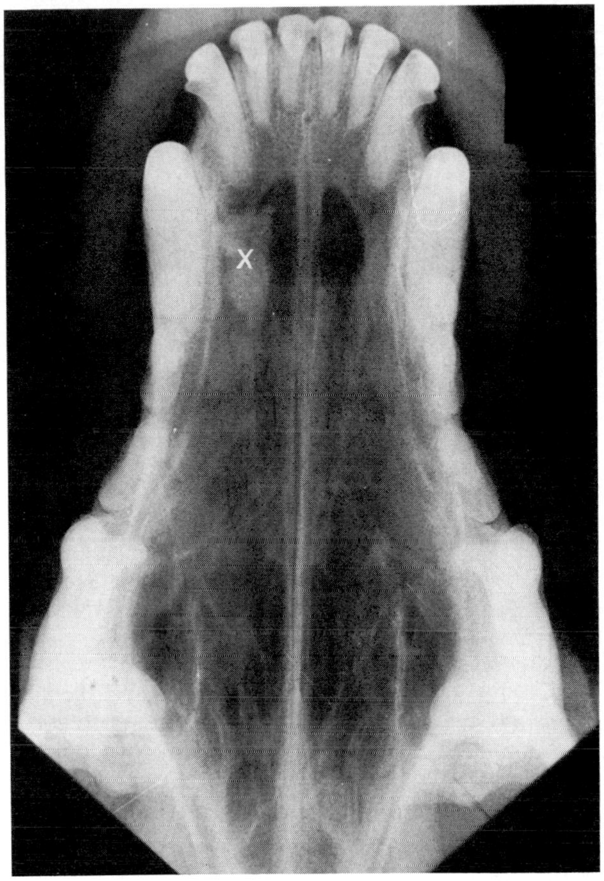

FIGURE 67–13. Radiograph of the nasal cavity demonstrating the presence of a piece of bone (X) in the anterior left nasal chamber of a Doberman pinscher, two years old.

Radiography does not reveal the presence of vegetable foreign bodies, but anterior rhinoscopy under general anesthesia may allow identification and removal of foreign body material from the dorsal and ventral nasal conchal regions. Rhinotomy may prove necessary in the treatment of foreign body rhinitis from other causes.

RHINITIS DUE TO PALATINE DEFECTS

Congenital and traumatic defects of both the hard and soft palates permit the passage of food material into the nasal cavity (Figures 67–14 and 67–15). The initial inflammatory response is complicated by secondary bacterial and possibly fungal infections, and a purulent discharge may be present. The additional problem in the neonate is an inability to suckle adequately because the defect does not allow creation of a negative pressure within the buccal cavity. Congenital hypoplasia and traumatic defects of the soft palate prevent adequate closure of the nasopharynx during swallowing, and food and fluid are expelled into the nasal cavity. Feeding and drinking at head level may prevent severe involvement in the presence of a minor lesion, but palatoplasty is essential when the defect is extensive. Traumatic defects such as those caused by the dog running onto a piece of wood should be repaired as quickly as possible, and several techniques covered elsewhere in this chapter are used in the repair of the hypoplastic soft palate.

Small traumatic defects through the hard palate may be repaired by pedicle flaps lifted from adjacent palatine material (Figure 67–16), but larger defects and congenital clefts require more complicated surgery. The traditional Langenbeck technique involves the use of two bipedicle mucoperiosteal flaps lifted from the palate adjacent to the cleft (Figures 67–17 and 67–18). These are sutured in the midline to bridge the defect; the donor sites are left to granulate. The viability of the flaps depends primarily on the maintenance of blood supply from the straight palatine arteries, and an alternative technique[14] is preferred mainly because there is less dependence on these major blood vessels (Figure 67–19). In addition this alternative technique allows closure of the cleft at the incisive foramen, something that is difficult to achieve with the Langenbeck approach.

A mucoperiosteal flap that is the length of the cleft and is based on the nasal mucosa is lifted on one side of the cleft (Figure 67–20*A*). It is then rotated through 180° and sutured into elevated mucoperiosteal tissue on the contralateral edge of the cleft (Figure 67–20*B*). The flap's blood supply from the palatine artery is destroyed during surgery, but adequate vascularity is maintained via the nasal mucosa. The donor site is left to granulate, the whole repair process taking some four to six weeks to complete (Figure 67–20*C*). Antibiotic coverage is

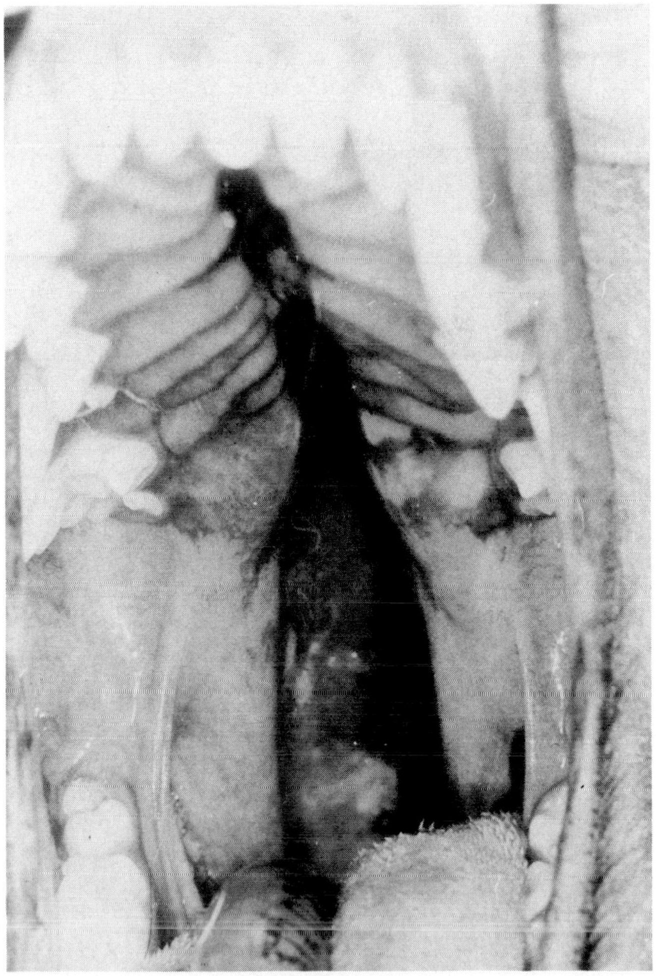

FIGURE 67–14. Congenital midline cleft hard and soft palates in a Jack Russell terrier, seven months old.

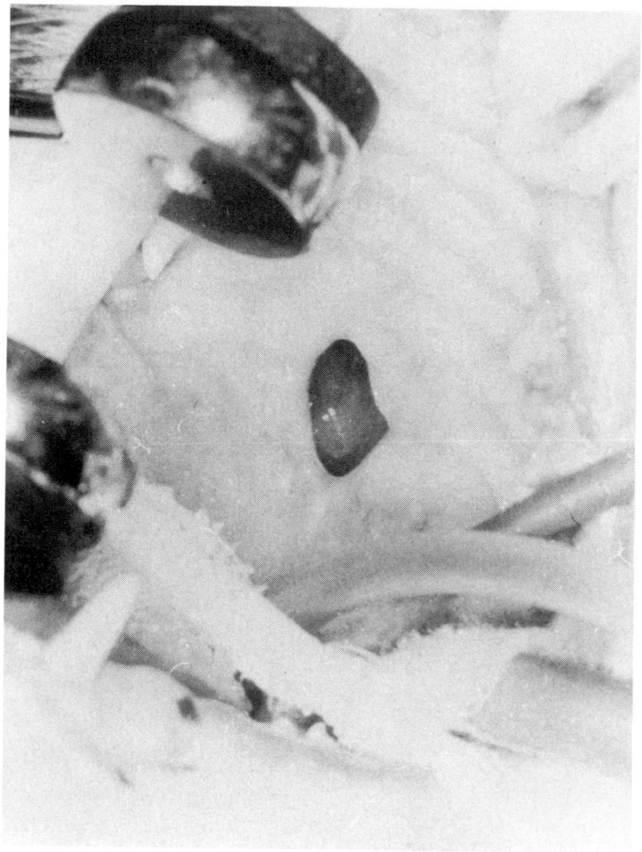

FIGURE 67–15. Traumatic midline defect of the hard palate in a domestic short-haired cat, four years old.

maintained for ten days, but may be extended as continuation treatment for the rhinitis.

RHINITIS DUE TO DENTAL DISEASE

Periodontal disease is commonplace in the dog and cat, but periapical abscess associated with this problem together with caries and dental fractures is seldom involved in rhinitis. Treatment consists of removal of the diseased tooth and curettage of the alveolus. Oronasal fistula formation following this surgery and the loss of canine teeth in older animals may result in low-grade nasal discharge. Such defects can be sealed by using pedicle flaps of buccal mucosa.

VIRAL RHINITIS

Several viruses are involved in upper respiratory tract disease in the dog and cat.[15] Most viral-induced rhinitis in the dog is seen as acute, but transient, relatively low-grade disease that may predispose the patient to secondary, often chronic, bacterial infection. The effects of infection with canine distemper are well recognized, but adenovirus, herpes virus, reovirus, and a parainfluenza virus similar to simian SV5 can be involved. A specific rhinitis syndrome attributed to primary herpes virus infection with secondary *Bordetella bronchiseptica* and *Pasteurella multocida* involvement has been described in the Irish wolfhound.[16] Hereditary immunodeficiency may be associated, with puppies inhaling dormant herpes virus in uterine and vaginal fluids during whelping. A rhinitis characterized by the presence of a watery, bilateral discharge, noisy respiration, and bouts of sneezing is seen in the neonate, the discharge becoming catarrhal, purulent, and even blood-tinged with the passage of time. Puppies may eventually recover, but many are left with hyperplastic rhinitis (Figure 67–21) and pulmonary disease. Growth retardation may occur. Medical treatment is ineffective and although radical turbinectomy may relieve the nasal disease, the overall

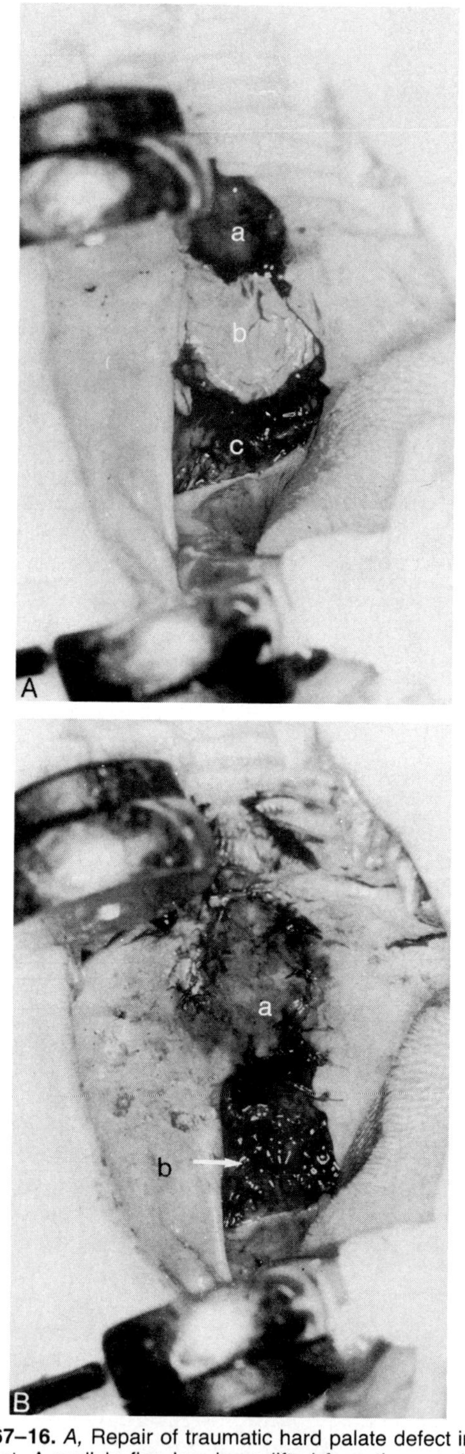

FIGURE 67–16. *A,* Repair of traumatic hard palate defect in a three-year-old cat. A pedicle flap has been lifted from the anterior part of the soft palate. *a,* The defect; *b,* the pedicle flap; *c,* the donor site. *B,* The pedicle flap has been sutured into the prepared edges of the defect. *a,* The pedicle flap; and arrow, the donor site.

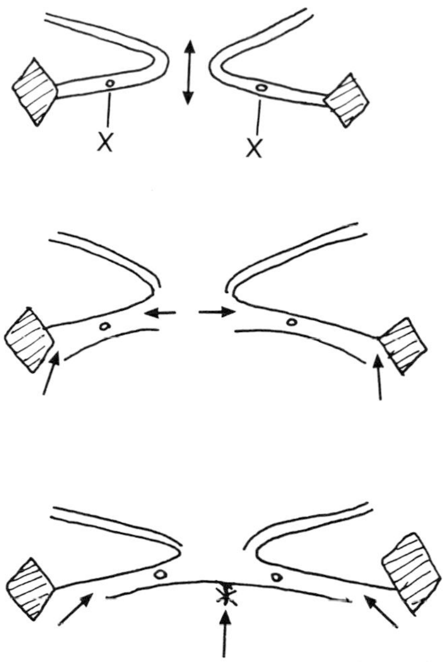

FIGURE 67–17. The Langenbeck technique for cleft hard palate repair. Top, The cleft in vertical section; x = palatine arteries. Center, Incisions at the edges of the cleft and along the gingival margins allow the two mucoperiosteal flaps to be moved into the midline. Bottom, The cleft is closed in the midline, and the donor sites are left to granulate.

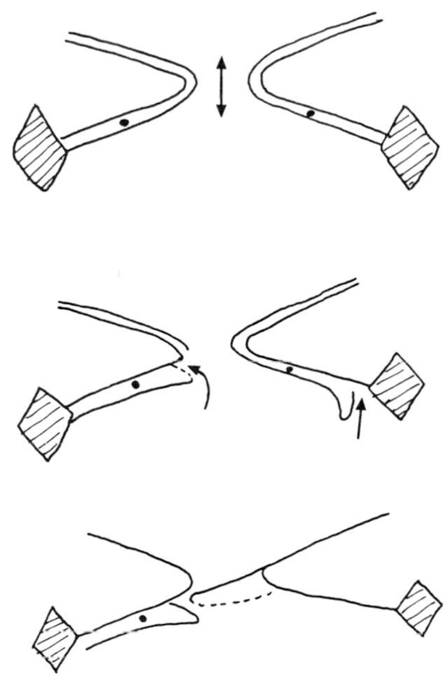

FIGURE 67–19. Repair of the cleft hard palate using a single pedicle of mucoperiosteal tissue. Top, The cleft in vertical section; shows palatine arteries. Center, The mucoperiosteal flap is lifted by incision along the gingival margin, and the contralateral edge of the cleft is elevated. Bottom, The flap is sutured into the prepared contralateral edge of the cleft.

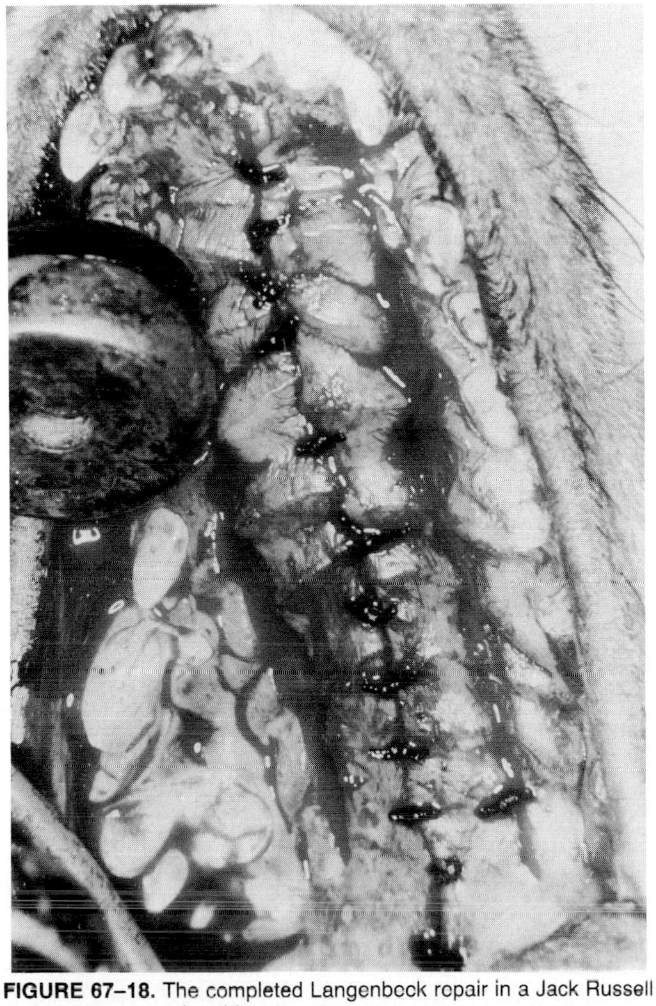

FIGURE 67–18. The completed Langenbeck repair in a Jack Russell terrier, seven months old.

prognosis is related to the extent of the pulmonary involvement.

The two main agents in feline upper respiratory tract disease are feline rhinotracheitis virus (FVR) and feline calicivirus (FCD). FVR, a herpes virus, is extremely contagious and the disease produced is more severe than that caused by FCD. Mild to severe rhinitis occurs, and although the picture can be complicated by bacterial and mycoplasmal infections, turbinate osteolysis can be produced by the virus acting alone. FCD, a group of RNA viruses, is also highly contagious and severe rhinitis may be part of the general picture. Carrier states exist for both organisms, with the intermittent shedding of virus being induced by stress. Differential diagnosis of the two viruses is almost impossible, but unnecessary in terms of treatment. Broad-spectrum antibiotics are essential background therapy and several regimens have been advocated.[17] A two- to three-week course of ampicillin (15 mg/lb q12h) or a potentiated sulfonamide (10 mg/lb q12h) can be accompanied by multivitamin therapy. Any dehydration must be corrected, and both subcutaneous and intravenous glucose/saline solutions are preferred. Feeding by pharyngostomy tube can overcome anorexia and provide an alternative route for fluid and antibiotic medication. The nasal passages should be kept as free as possible by simple cleansing and the use of nebulized decongestants and steam inhalations. Failure of the rhinitis to respond to systemic antibiotics may be corrected by administering antibiotic through the frontal sinuses.[18] Under general anesthesia the sinuses are entered using a 2 mm drill, and warm physiological saline is used to flush the nasal chambers clear of discharge before the antibiotic is administered. This technique can be repeated every two or three days until the rhinitis has been alleviated.

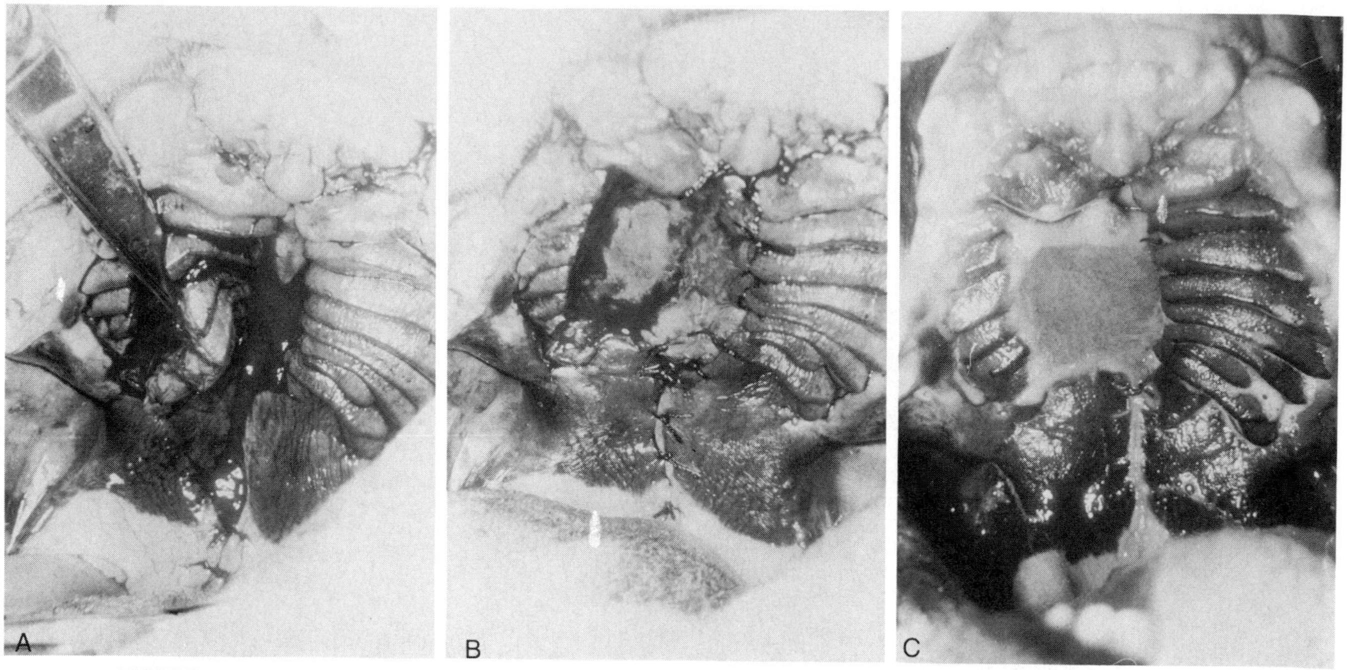

FIGURE 67–20. *A,* A mucoperiosteal pedicle flap based on the left edge of the cleft is raised (the soft palate cleft has been repaired prior to incision) in a bulldog, four months old. *B,* The flap has been sutured into the contralateral edge of the cleft. *C,* The appearance of the mucoperiosteal pedicle flap repair three weeks after surgery.

Unfortunately, the acute disease situation often gives way to a chronic rhinitis. Hyperplastic change involving the mucous gland elements and the epithelial stroma is responsible for constant copious discharge, sneezing, and snuffling. Long-term combined antibiotic and vitamin therapy and frontal sinus antibiotic infusion can prove unrewarding. Decongestants may bring some relief, but the effect is temporary. The frontal sinuses can be involved, not so much by an extension of inflammation and infection, but by mucus retention and mucocoele formation as the result of impaired drainage through the diseased ethmoidal conchae. As such the term "sinusitis" is a misnomer, and exploration and drainage of the frontal sinuses is therefore of limited value. Many patients and owners can cope with the situation, but for others turbinectomy is a logical step. This surgery should not be undertaken lightly, for the cat is a poor rhinotomy patient, and the postoperative period is complicated by possible bacterial infection. The procedure is the same as that already outlined as a diagnostic technique, and fluid and supportive therapy is vital during and following the surgery. All the conchae should be removed, and care is particularly necessary when removing the ethmoidal components from the cribriform plate in this species. Packing the nose with gauze bandage may not be necessary, and should be avoided if possible because the cat is a poor mouth breather. Any packing should be removed on the fifth postoperative day, and at this stage the nasal cavity can be irrigated free of blood clots and debris. Feeding by pharyngostomy tube is usually necessary for ten days postoperatively.

BACTERIAL RHINITIS

A number of bacteria can be isolated from rhinitis patients, and while some are of contaminant significance only, others exert a pathogenic effect (Figure 67–22). It is likely that most require predisposing inflammation or damage to create an environment in which they can multiply in order to exert their pathogenic effect as secondary invaders. This may not be the case with *Bordetella bronchiseptica* and *Pasteurella multocida*, since there is some evidence to show that they may cause acute rhinitis in the dog.[19] Antibiotic therapy can be more effective if selected on the basis of sensitivity tests, but treatment should consider both cause and effect.[20] Hyperplastic changes within the mucosa can result from uncontrolled infection and render that infection difficult to treat. Antibiotics will have some effect, but dyspnea, inadequate drainage, and recurrence of infection will only be prevented by turbinectomy. Unlike cats, dogs tolerate this procedure well, and complications other than postoperative infection are rare. *Staphylococcus aureus* and gram-negative bacteria such as *Pseudomonas* or *E. coli* can be encountered during the six-week healing phase; they present additional problems in the overall treatment of the condition.

FUNGAL RHINITIS

Nasal mycosis is much more common in the dog than the cat. *Aspergillus fumigatus*[21] is the commonest fungus found in canine rhinomycosis, but *Penicillium* species and *Cryptococcus neoformans* may cause disease on occasion. Nasal rhinosporidiosis attributed to *Rhinosporidium seeberi* has been recorded as an occasional condition in North America, the disease being due to the growth of granulomatous masses within the anterior nasal cavity.[22–24] In the cat it is *Cryptococcosus neoformans* that is the commonest fungal pathogen, with *Aspergillus*[26] and *Penicillium* species being isolated rarely.

Aspergillosis is primarily a disease of the young to

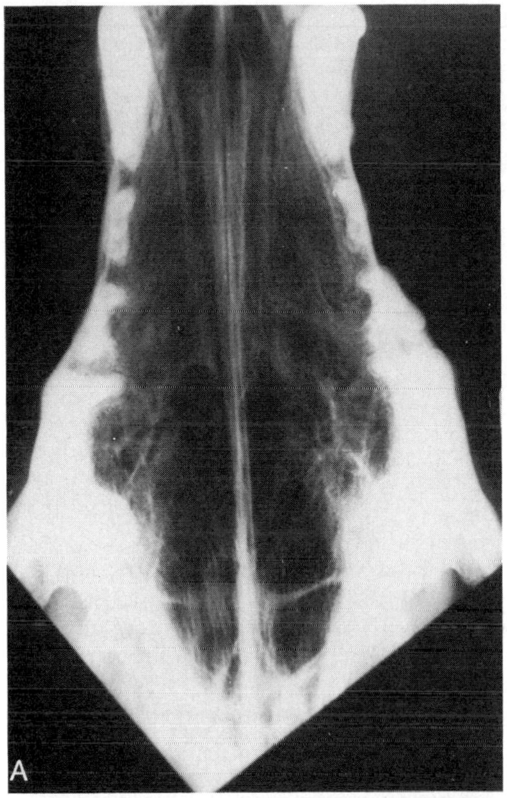

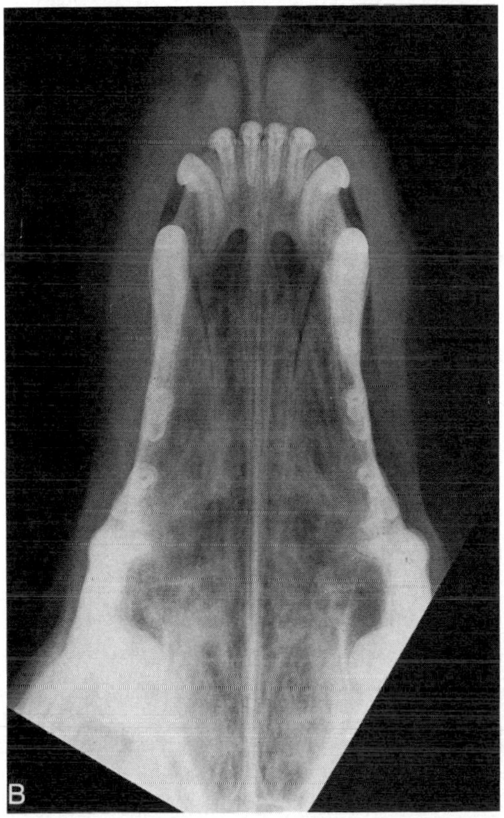

FIGURE 67–21. *A,* The normal nasal cavity in a four-year-old Irish wolfhound. *B,* Hyperplastic rhinitis in a 14-month-old Irish wolfhound.

middle-aged dolichocephalic dog. Infection is first seen in the caudal region of the ventral nasal conchae, but with time it spreads forward and can extend posteriorly to involve the ethmoidal conchae and the frontal sinuses.

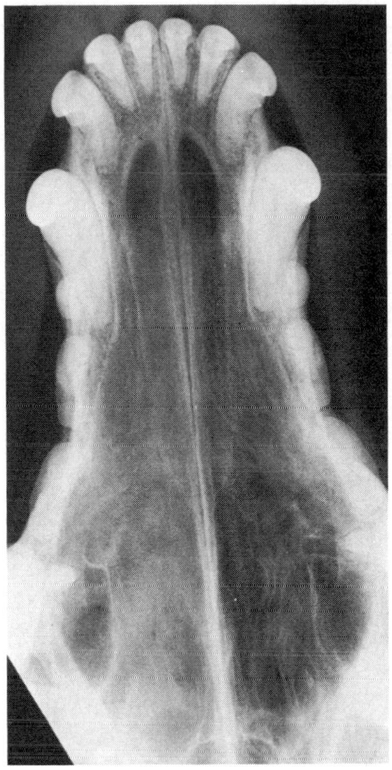

FIGURE 67–22. Acute unilateral rhinitis (left half of x-ray) with heavy *Pasteurella multocida* infection in a Weimaraner, nine months old.

There may be infiltration of the maxillae and nasal bones, and this may account for the pain elicited by palpation in some patients. Facial distortion and fistula formation do not occur. A unilateral or bilateral mucopurulent nasal discharge is present, with blood-staining or rank hemorrhage indicating the destructive nature of the infection. Diagnosis is confirmed by demonstrating the branching septate hyphae of the fungus or the "sunburst" appearance of its conidiophores in smears or cultures of the discharge, but a negative result at this stage should not rule out the presence of the organism. An agar gel double-diffusion test reliably confirms the presence of antibodies in serum,[27–29] and radiography may reveal the areas of localized tissue destruction caused by the fungus[30] (Figure 67–23). Exploratory rhinotomy demonstrates the whitish "jam mold" colonies on the conchal mucosa or biopsy material can be harvested to culture the organism.

Aspergillus spores are commonplace, and it is possible that disease is seen in some patients as the result of a specific immune deficiency. This may partially explain the variation in response that occurs with medical therapy. It is likely, though, that most rhinomycoses follow predisposing tissue damage caused by trauma, bacterial infection, and neoplasia, and these latter two factors should be borne in mind when therapy is instituted. Treatment involves some discussion of the possible zoonotic hazard, and a guarded prognosis must always be given. In early disease, systemic and local antifungal therapy may be employed, and in some cases may best be treated by rhinotomy and curettage of the diseased tissues. A six-week course of oral thiabendazole[31] at 50 mg/lb q24h should be completed before surgery to reduce the amount of curettage necessary. On occasion,

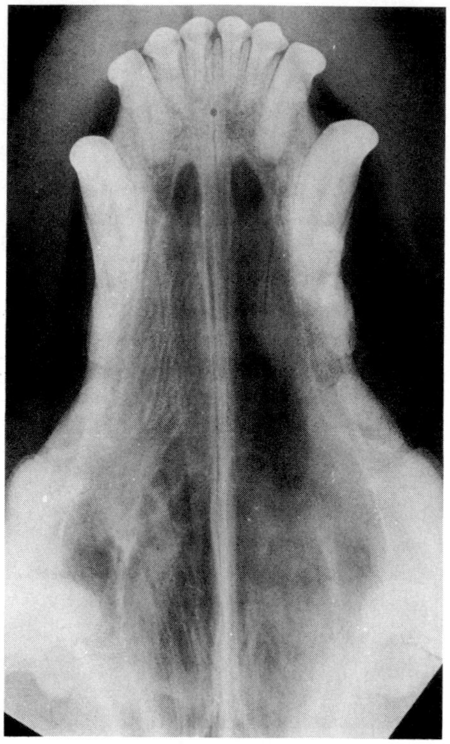

FIGURE 67–23. *Aspergillus fumigatus* infection of the right nasal chamber in a German shepherd dog, three years old.

the degree and severity of hemorrhage accompanying the disease necessitates turbinectomy before the completion of this course. Following surgery, the nasal cavity is flushed for five days with Lugol's iodine, and broad-spectrum antibiotics are used for approximately two weeks. The oral thiabendazole treatment is continued for at least two weeks and as long as six weeks. Thiabendazole appears to be nontoxic in this species, but an occasional patient may exhibit lethargy and intermittent vomiting on long-term therapy. In the author's case series, approximately 50 per cent of patients respond to this therapeutic approach. A more effective way of treating nasal aspergillosis is required and other treatment regimens are possible. The use of systemic ketoconazole alone or combined with topical enilconazole offers an acceptable alternative[32–34] and recent experience using topical enilconazole alone has been most encouraging. Frontal sinus trephination permits twice daily sinus and nasal chamber irrigation over a ten-day period, the enilconazole being used at 20 mg/lb body weight made up to a 10 ml dose with sterile water.

A noninvasive type of aspergillosis occurs infrequently in the dog,[35] characterized by compact masses of mycelia ("fungal balls") filling the larger conchal air spaces without damaging the surrounding tissue. Secondary bacterial contamination influences the nature of the discharge seen. Diagnosis can be difficult because patients may be serologically negative and the radiographic features of tissue destruction are not present. Anterior rhinoscopy or rhinotomy is necessary, and treatment calls for turbinate dissection with routine postoperative antibiotics. Fungal balls may follow local trauma and impaired local immunity, but the difference between this type of aspergillosis and the invasive form is not completely understood.

Cryptococcal rhinitis in the cat usually occurs in the older patient and other body systems may be involved. A severe chronic rhinitis with persistent sneezing and discharge is accompanied by the destruction of facial bone, and radiographs demonstrate osteolysis of the maxillae and nasal and frontal bones. Treatment is possible using long-term doses of amphotericin B, but is not advocated because of the nature of the disease and possible drug-induced renal failure. See Chapter 49 for a more complete discussion of the diagnosis and treatment of this condition.

PARASITIC RHINITIS

Intranasal parasite infection is uncommon in the dog and does not occur in the cat. The presence of the nasal mite *Pneumonyssus caninum* is of little clinical significance, for the associated rhinitis is both mild and transient. Disease due to the tongue worm, *Linguatula serrata*,[36] may be characterized by a severe rhinitis in which coughing and violent sneezing occur and a blood-stained discharge is seen. The host can be severely affected, and the identification of the cause of rhinitis can be difficult. Eggs may be present in the nasal discharge, but the parasite's long life cycle does not guarantee that all swabs will be diagnostic. Rhinotomy may thus prove necessary, and the parasite's physical removal is the only certain method of treatment.

NEOPLASIA

Benign fibrous polyps that originate within the anterior nasal cavity are an occasional finding in both the dog and cat (Figure 67–24). Enlargement causes airway obstruction, and pressure-induced destruction of the anterior ethmoidal conchae can cause hemorrhage and a blood-stained nasal discharge. Secondary bacterial and possibly fungal infections may complicate the clinical picture. The presence of a polyp is confirmed by anterior rhinoscopy and radiography, and anterior rhinotomy is necessary to effect removal. Recurrence, although possible, is rare.

Malignant endonasal neoplasia is the commonest cause of nasal discharge in the older dolichocephalic canine patient, but such tumors are uncommon in the cat.[37] The adenocarcinoma is the most common neoplasm in the dog's nasal cavity, but fibrosarcoma, chon-

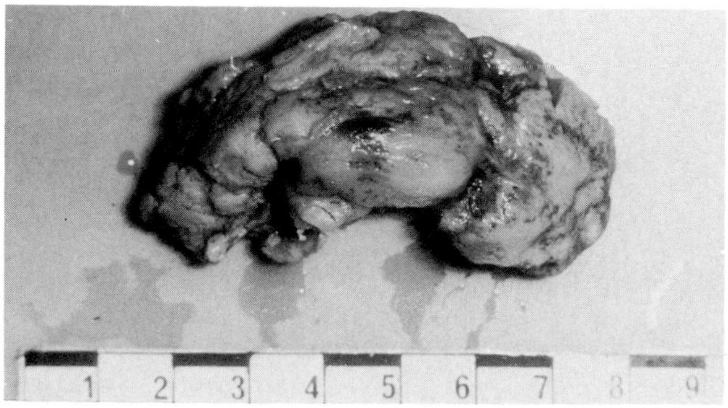

FIGURE 67–24. A fibrous polyp removed from the left nasal conchal region. The point of attachment was the nasal septum of a Great Dane, two years.

drosarcoma, osteosarcoma, and squamous cell carcinoma have all been recorded. All originate within the ethmoidal concha,[38] but invasion of the maxilla, palatine bone, and the frontal sinus occur with time. A unilateral mucopurulent discharge becomes bilateral when there is transseptal spread to the contralateral chamber. The discharge may be blood-stained, and bouts of epistaxis can occur spontaneously or during violent sneezing. Erosion of the nasolacrimal duct produces an "ocular" discharge, and posterior drainage of discharge with coughing and retching can occur when the tumor mass occludes the nasal chamber. Distortion of the facial contour denotes local invasion, but metastasis other than to regional lymph nodes appears to be rare. The radiographic features[39, 40] are those of bone destruction or proliferation and the replacement of air space with soft tissue shadow (Figure 67–25). Occasionally the differential radiographic diagnosis of early tumor and chronic hyperplastic rhinitis can be difficult, and exploratory rhinotomy can be necessary.

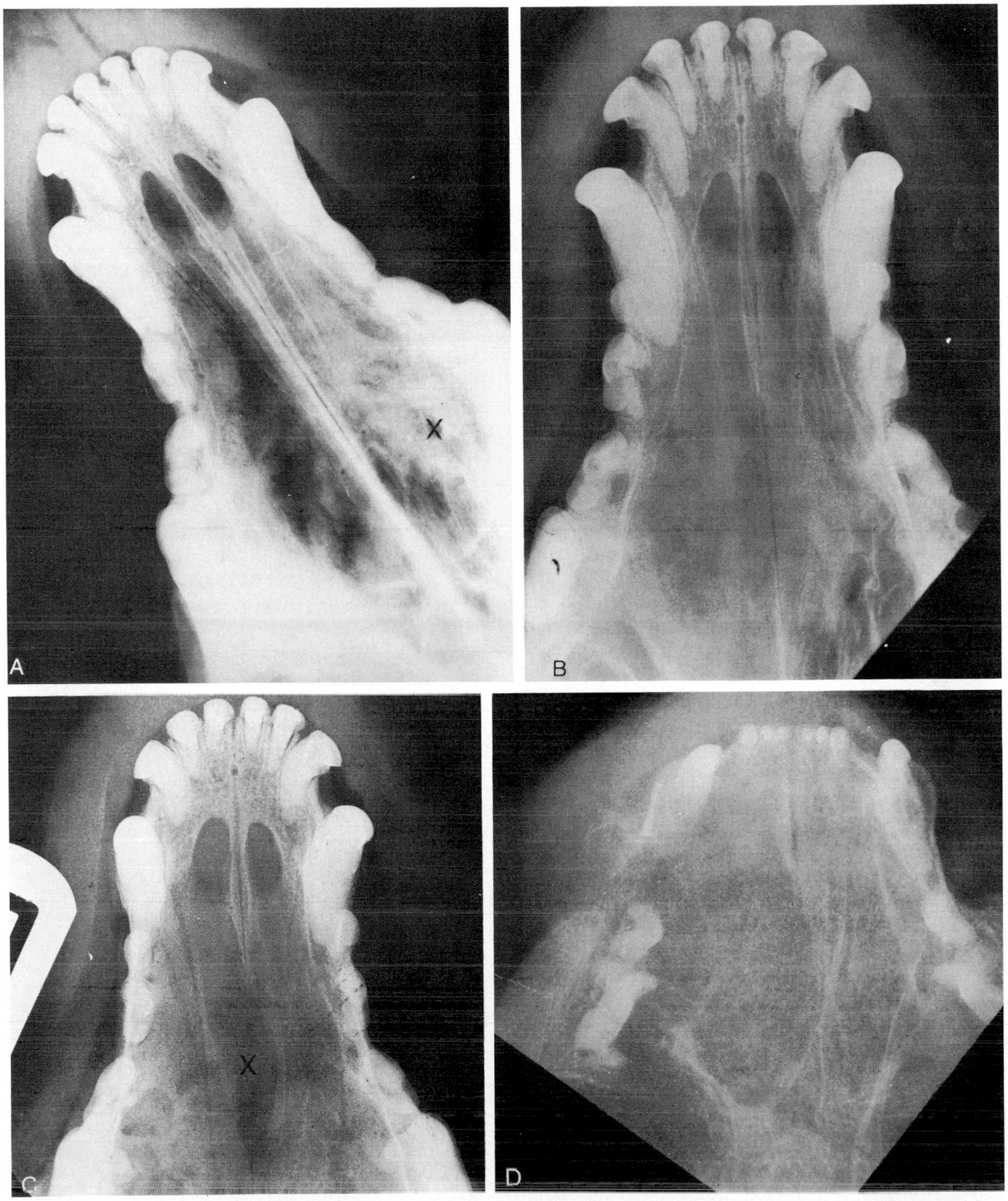

FIGURE 67–25. *A,* Endonasal neoplasia (X) predominantly within the right ethmoid concha in a crossbred, eight years old. *B,* Bilateral endonasal neoplasia with breakdown of the nasal septum in a collie-cross, ten years old. *C,* Bilateral endonasal neoplasia with invasion of the hard palate (X) in the midline in a standard poodle, six years old. *D,* Bilateral endonasal neoplasia with breakdown of the nasal septum in a British short-haired cat, nine years old.

Curettage is not an effective treatment for endonasal neoplasia, and no matter how complete the turbinectomy, recurrence should be expected, usually within three months. The prognosis is therefore grave because the ineffectiveness of cytotoxic therapy and the problems of radiotherapy mean that treatment may not be a practical possibility.[41, 42]

Transmissible venereal tumor has been recorded, but it remains an unusual diagnosis.[43]

Lymphosarcoma as part of a multicentric tumor problem is the most common endonasal neoplasm in the cat, but other carcinomas are seen occasionally. Dyspnea, purulent nasal discharge, epistaxis, and facial distortion are the expected clinical features, and treatment is not advisable, given the nature of these two tumor types.

Conditions of the Paranasal Sinuses

Primary conditions of the paranasal sinuses in both the dog and cat are rare occurrences (Figure 67–26). The dolichocephalic and mesocephalic canine frontal sinus is a relatively large structure, but in the brachycephalic and small breeds and in the cat the frontal sinus is reduced in size and may be virtually absent. The dorsal extension of the ethmoidal conchae into the sinuses allows their involvement in inflammatory and neoplastic disease as an extension of nasal cavity disease. Sinusitis, when it occurs, is thus an extension of a rhinitis, and both bacterial and fungal infections may be present. Malignancy of the ethmoidal conchae can fill the sinus cavity and even break out through the frontal bones (Figure 67–27). These potential complications should be considered during the diagnosis and treatment of nasal disease, and radiographic evaluation of the frontal sinuses, together with their trephination or exposure during rhinotomy to facilitate therapy, can be of value. Acute and chronic hyperplastic rhinitis in the cat can respond to lavage through the frontal sinuses, while sinus irrigation following rhinotomy is often an essential part of therapy for aspergillosis. Disease based within the ethmoidal conchae can interfere with the normal drainage of the frontal sinus, and resultant retention mucocoele formation may eventually disrupt the continuity of the frontal bones. True primary frontal sinusitis in both the dog and the cat can be treated by trephination and lavage, but the therapeutic approach to primary neoplasia is restricted by the same limitations that apply to endonasal neoplasia.

The other paranasal sinuses are of little anatomical or clinical significance. The canine maxillary sinus or recess, an outpouching of the nasal cavity at the level of the carnassial tooth, which is in open communication with the middle and ventral nasal meati, can be involved occasionally in cyst formation and periapical carnassial tooth abscessation. Congenital cyst formation in which there may be distortion of the lateral maxilla above the carnassial tooth, is extremely rare; most malar abscesses break out externally on the face with a discharging sinus just below the ventral orbital rim.

THE PHARYNX

Structure and Function

The pharynx is that area common to the respiratory and digestive tracts that lies between the oral and nasal cavities anteriorly and the esophagus and larynx posteriorly. It extends from the posterior limit of the orbit to the second cervical vertebra. The presence of a long soft palate divides the pharynx into a dorsal nasopharynx and a ventral oropharynx, while that portion that lies above the epiglottis is known as the laryngopharynx. The nasopharynx conducts air from the internal nares or choanae to the intrapharyngeal opening at the distal border of the soft palate. Its lateral walls bear the single slit-like internal openings of the eustachian tubes; the lymphoid tissue in its dorsal wall is referred to as the pharyngeal tonsils or adenoids. During deglutition, the posterior nasopharynx is closed by the upward displacement of the soft palate. Palatine movement is achieved by both muscle action and passive displacement resulting

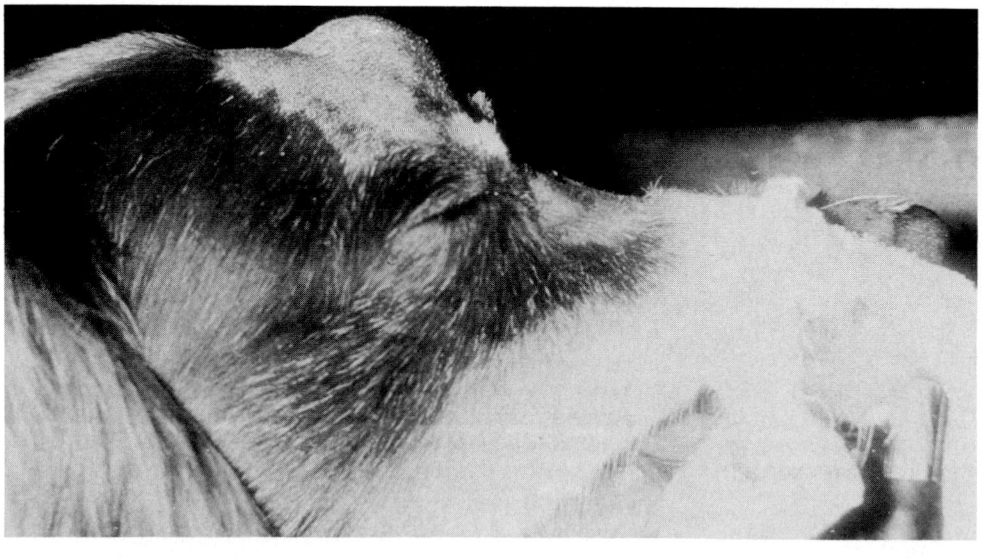

FIGURE 67–26. Fibrosarcoma of the left frontal sinus in a springer spaniel, ten years old.

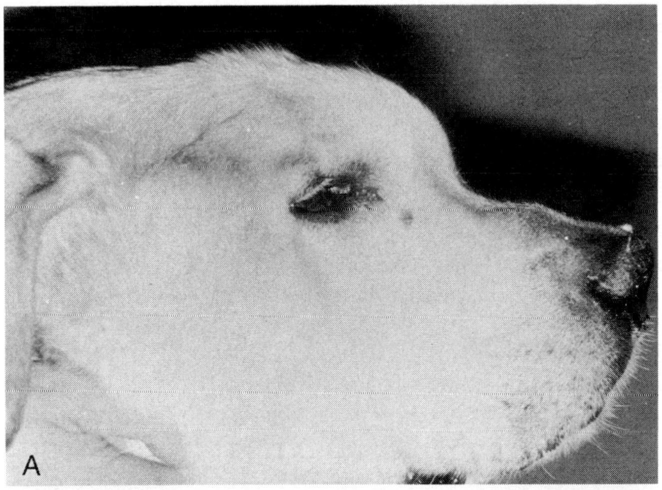

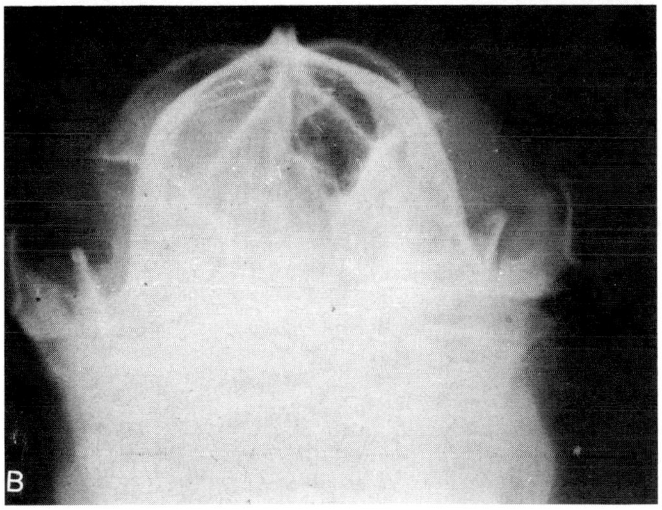

FIGURE 67–27. *A,* Disruption of the frontal bones caused by the invasion of a turbinate-based tumor into the frontal sinuses of a Labrador, twelve years old. *B,* Invasion of the left frontal sinus. Anteroposterior projection of a Labrador cross, ten years old.

from the movement of a food bolus and the presence of the root of the tongue. The oropharynx extends from the isthmus of the fauces to the interpharyngeal opening and the epiglottis, and is involved in both deglutition and mouth breathing. During deglutition its dimensions constantly change due to movements of the root of the tongue, the soft palate, and the epiglottis. Its lateral walls, the fauces, bear the paired palatine tonsils. Each tonsil is contained within a tonsillar fossa, crypt, or sinus situated just caudal to the palatoglossal arch. There is no tonsillar afferent lymphatic supply, but efferent vessels drain into the medial retropharyngeal lymph nodes. The diffuse lymphoid material in the root of the tongue is referred to as the lingual tonsil. The laryngopharynx extends from the intrapharyngeal opening to the esophagus. A plicated ridge of tissue, called the limen pharyngoesophageum, marks its junction with the esophagus. During swallowing, the root of the tongue pushes a bolus of food into the posterior oropharynx, and the three pairs of constrictor muscles plus two pairs of shortener muscles squeeze the bolus into the esophagus. The epiglottis guards the laryngeal aditus with the rima glottidis closed.

The soft palate is a long and substantial muscular structure in both the dog and cat. Its thickest portion, some 5 mm in the average dog, is at the level of the junction between its middle and posterior thirds. Paired palatine muscles and components of the paired tensor and levator veli palatini muscles, the pterygopharyngeal muscles, and the palatopharyngeal muscles contribute to its structure. It extends posteriorly from the hard palate, the junction of these two structures in the dolichocephalic and mesocephalic dog breeds and the cat being just caudal to the last upper molar teeth. In the brachycephalic dog this junction is approximately one centimeter further into the pharynx, and, as such, the intrapharyngeal opening does not exist and the distal soft palate lies within the anterior laryngeal aditus.

During nose breathing the soft palate lies beneath the epiglottis, with the nasopharynx in direct communication with the laryngeal aditus. Minimal resistance to increased respiratory effort during exercise is obtained by mouth breathing, and here the epiglottis is depressed by the action of the hypoepiglotticus muscle and the soft palate is tensed and elevated. Thus the oropharynx and laryngeal aditus simply become a direct extension of the buccal cavity.

Diagnosis

The clinical features of pharyngeal disease are usually dramatic but often nonspecific. Inappetence, anorexia, pain, dysphagia, retching, gagging, dyspnea, and coughing may all implicate the pharynx as the focus of disease, and a complete physical examination of the area involving general anesthesia is essential. Microbiological investigation is of limited value because a plethora of bacteria are always cultured. Radiography may demonstrate foreign body presence or tumor formation, and fluoroscopy and barium swallow studies are essential in the differential diagnosis of dysphagia of no apparent cause.

Disease Conditions of the Pharynx

TRAUMA AND FOREIGN BODIES

The history is usually quite specific, with the patient demonstrating a combination of dyspnea, retching, gulping, and dysphagia. The severity of these signs varies with the amount of damage, the size of foreign body, and the duration of the problem. Large foreign bodies wedged in the pharynx usually cause marked distress and dyspnea, with tracheotomy a necessary emergency treatment on occasion. Sticks that are run onto can lacerate the soft palate and the pharyngeal walls, and though these are usually removed immediately by owners, splinters can remain within the wounds to cause subsequent abscess formation. Foreign bodies that have penetrated the lateral fauces may produce retrobulbar or submandibular abscesses, those that pass through the dorsal wall of the nasopharynx or laryngopharynx may result in deep-seated retropharyngeal abscessation, while those due to penetration beneath, or lateral to, the larynx can drain ventrally or into the mouth. The surgical exploration of foreign body wounds and abscess sites may not always reveal the cause; the success of treatment often relies on drainage and antibiotic therapy. The first indication of grass seed penetration is often an abscess or the discharging sinus it produces. Pins and needles are the easiest buried foreign bodies to identify and remove; radiography greatly facilitates their location.

Choke chain damage and other severe compression trauma can fracture the hyoid apparatus, can induce critical pharyngeal and laryngeal edema, and can cause pharyngeal and laryngeal paralysis. Damage to the hypoepiglotticus muscle impairs epiglottic depression during mouth breathing, and patients that breathe normally at rest may show distress during exercise.[44]

INFECTION

Pharyngitis is not a common primary entity in either the dog or the cat. Infection here is usually associated with concurrent respiratory or systemic disease. Tonsillar hypertrophy as the result of lymphoid activity is a secondary feature in upper respiratory tract infection, but accompanies mouth breathing, alimentary tract disease, and even chronic anal disease attended by licking. Primary tonsillitis does occur, but is seldom seen except as a syndrome common to young dogs, usually within the smaller breeds. Such dogs can be very ill, with pyrexia, coughing, retching, and general malaise completing the clinical picture. The response to broad-spectrum antibiotic therapy is usually rapid, and tonsillectomy is seldom considered. Tonsillectomy is indicated where tonsillar bulk is compromising the oropharyngeal airway, and is therefore of possible value in the treatment of the brachycephalic airway obstruction syndrome.

THE NASOPHARYNGEAL POLYP

Dyspnea with possible rhinorrhea in young cats may be due to the presence of fibrous polypoid masses within the nasopharynx.[45, 46] The polyp represents a most important differential diagnosis in feline upper respiratory tract disease. Such masses appear to originate within the eustachian tube, and either may emerge into the tympanic bulla and external auditory canal or may enlarge to fill the nasopharynx. Recent observations have shown that some polyps may possibly be congenital in origin.[47] With growth, the obstructive dyspnea becomes marked but deglutition remains normal. Examination under general anesthesia may demonstrate ventral bowing and tautness of the soft palate, and the lesion itself is easily located by examining the nasopharynx (Figure 67–28). Radiography demonstrates the presence of the polyp (Figure 67–29), and removal is effected by locating its pedicle attachment and firmly twisting it out of the eustachian tube. It is not necessary to split the soft palate to facilitate surgery, and recovery is uneventful, with little indication of recurrence.

SOFT PALATE DEFECTS

Wounding and hypoplasia of the soft palate can result in ineffective sealing of the posterior nasopharynx during deglutition, and food and fluid can pass forward into the nasal chambers. Foreign body rhinitis results, and feeding is attended by sneezing, gagging, and retching. Occasionally, feeding at head level ameliorates the problem, but repair of all but the slightest defect is essential. The foreshortened maxillae of brachycephalic dogs means that there is a relative excess of soft palate length in these breeds. At rest, the soft palate lies above the epiglottis within the laryngeal aditus and is responsible for the commonplace classical snoring inspiratory noise that is accepted as normal for such dogs. During increased inspiratory effort due to exercise, excitement, obstruction elsewhere within the upper respiratory tract, or pulmonary disease, the soft palate is sucked into the aditus and vestibule and severely reduces the laryngeal airway. The palate is often swollen and thickened with edema, and the resulting obstructive dyspnea can be considerable, even life-threatening. Excess soft palate is

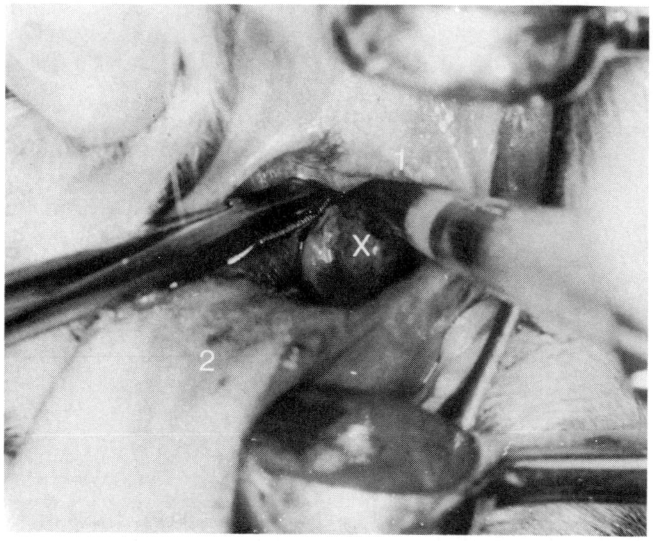

FIGURE 67–28. Nasopharyngeal polyp in a crossbred male cat, ten months old. The soft palate has been elevated to reveal the lesion (X). 1, soft palate; 2, tongue.

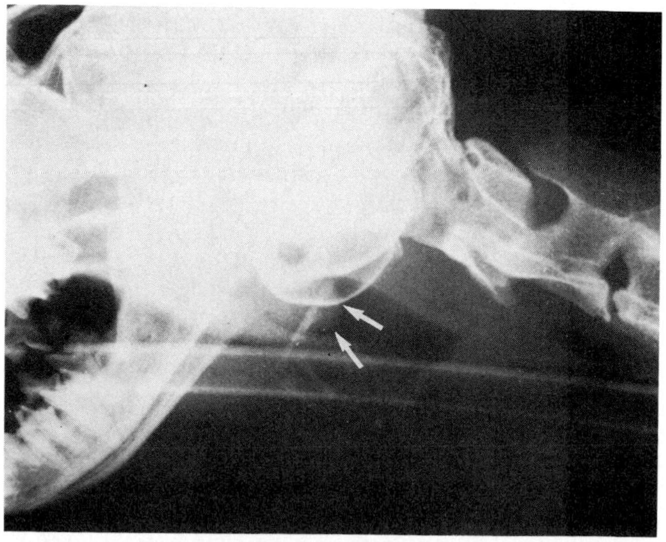

FIGURE 67–29. Nasopharyngeal polyp in an Abyssinian cat, six months old. The radiograph demonstrates the presence of the polyp (arrows) within the nasopharynx.

the single most important factor in the brachycephalic airway obstruction syndrome, and partial palatectomy is essential in almost all but the slightest defects.

Traumatic defects are repaired as accurately as possible, with effective repair often being completed even when tissue has been lost (Figure 67–30). Repair of full thickness tears should involve two layers of suturing, and tonsillar sinus material can be mobilized to close lesions in which tissue has been lost, or is too badly damaged to effect repair. Tracheotomy helps to maintain an airway during and following surgery, and is particularly useful in the smaller patient in terms of managing pharyngeal edema and removing the restriction to access that the presence of an endotracheal tube creates. (In general this comment relates to any surgery involving the soft palate.) A ventral midline skin incision and the separation of the sternohyoid muscle midline raphe exposes the ventral trachea. The trachea is opened by a transverse, 180° scalpel incision through the membranous tissue linking two adjacent cartilaginous rings, and the tracheotomy tube inserted through the incision into the lumen. The tube is secured to the skin, and left in situ for four or five days following surgery. Constant supervision is necessary to ensure that it remains patent, and hourly checks can be essential during the first 48 hours. The use of a metal-sleeved tube renders inspection and cleaning a simple procedure. Corticosteroid therapy is helpful in managing the pharyngeal edema, and routine antibiotic coverage is required. The use of a humidified air supply helps to prevent drying of the lower pulmonary membranes.

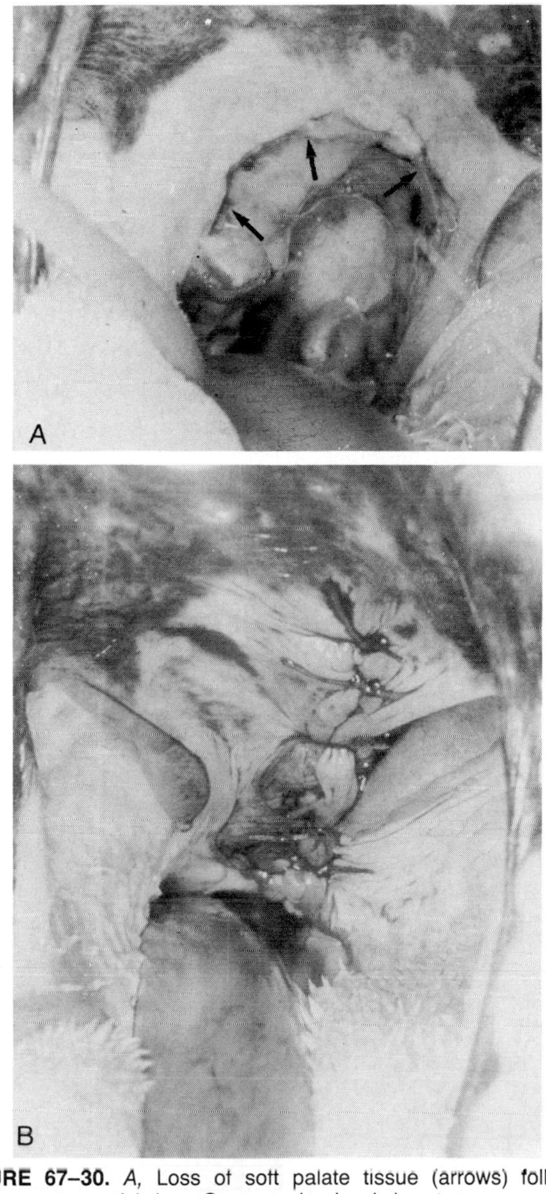

FIGURE 67–30. *A*, Loss of soft palate tissue (arrows) following running onto a stick in a German shepherd dog, two years old. *B*, Two-layer repair of the defect.

Congenital soft palate hypoplasia is seen with or without hard palate defects, and midline clefts (Figure 67–14), unilateral defects (Figure 67–31), and gross hypoplasia (Figure 67–32) are seen infrequently in the dog, and are rare in the cat. Despite the common belief, there is no evidence to suggest that such defects are inherited, and repair is possible in many patients if the neonatal stage can be successfully managed. Puppies cannot adequately suckle, and the nasal return of milk is often the first feature noticed by the owner. As with hard palate defects, surgery is best attempted at two to three months of age. Midline clefts are repaired by splitting each edge of the cleft into a posterior nasopharyngeal flap and an anterior oropharyngeal flap. The two pairs of flaps are sutured separately in the midline, with nonabsorbable suture material being preferred for the anterior flaps. There is usually sufficient tissue cranially, but the caudal cleft repair can be under tension. Unilateral hypoplasia requires a different approach and although in theory a mucous membrane flap can be lifted from the lateral nasopharyngeal wall to close the defect, a repair technique involving tonsillar sinus tissue is preferred (Figure 67–33). The lateral edge of the hypoplastic soft palate is split into posterior and anterior flaps, the tonsil is excised, the debrided edge of the posterior sinus wall is sutured to the posterior palatine flap, and the debrided edge of the anterior sinus wall is sutured to the anterior palatine flap. This double-layered technique gives strength to the repair and sufficiency of tonsillar sinus wall tissue counters tension on the suture lines. The use of a pharyngostomy tube can help ensure success with the more complicated repair techniques. Where there is bilateral hypoplasia, repair is impossible and survival depends upon the feeding regimen.

Obstructive dyspnea caused by a relative excess of soft palate is treated by partial palatectomy. The palate material beyond the distal one-third of the tonsils is removed by simple scissor excision. The epiglottis should not be used as a landmark because both it and the larynx itself are movable. The palate is grasped at the midpoint of its free border, and long-handled, slightly curved dissection scissors are used to remove first one half and then the other. Any hemorrhage usually occurs towards the tonsillar sinuses, not centrally. It must be remembered that the soft palate is quite a substantial structure and the scissor cut must be full thickness. Diathermy and crushing techniques are not advocated because of ensuing pharyngeal edema, and any hemor-

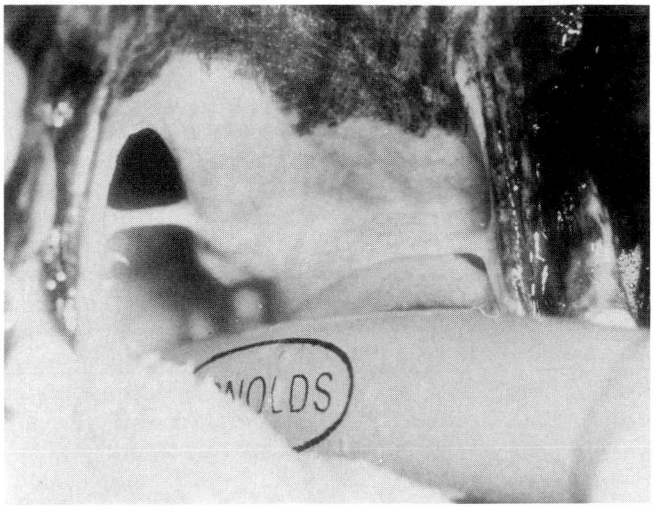

FIGURE 67–31. Unilateral soft palate hypoplasia in a German shepherd dog, eight months old.

rhage is controlled by subsequent closure of the wound using several simple interrupted sutures of nonabsorbable material.

A condition of dramatic presentation but of no apparent clinical consequence is that of the "reverse sneeze," in which the soft palate is made to vibrate for several seconds while there is accompanying expiratory flapping of the upper lips. It is seen occasionally in all breeds, perhaps more commonly in the smaller breeds. Owners are often alarmed, but collapse does not occur and the dog returns to normal immediately. The cause remains unknown but it has been speculated that nasopharyngeal spasm or glottic entrapment of the soft palate might be responsible. Treatment is not necessary, but pulling the tongue forward, compressing the thorax, massaging the pharynx, and even clapping of the hands all can produce the desired relief.

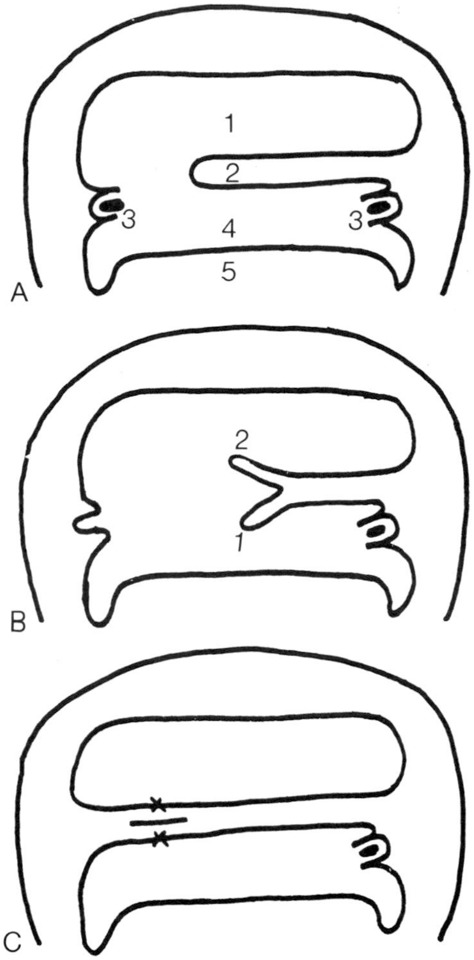

FIGURE 67–33. Repair technique for unilateral soft palate hypoplasia: dorsoventral section of the pharynx. *A,* Diagram of the cleft. 1, nasopharynx; 2, soft palate; 3, tonsillar sinus; 4, oropharynx; 5, tongue. *B,* The right tonsil has been excised and the soft palate split into anterior (1) and posterior (2) flaps. *C,* The posterior palatine flap has been sutured to the posterior tonsillar sinus wall and the anterior palatine flap to the anterior tonsillar sinus wall.

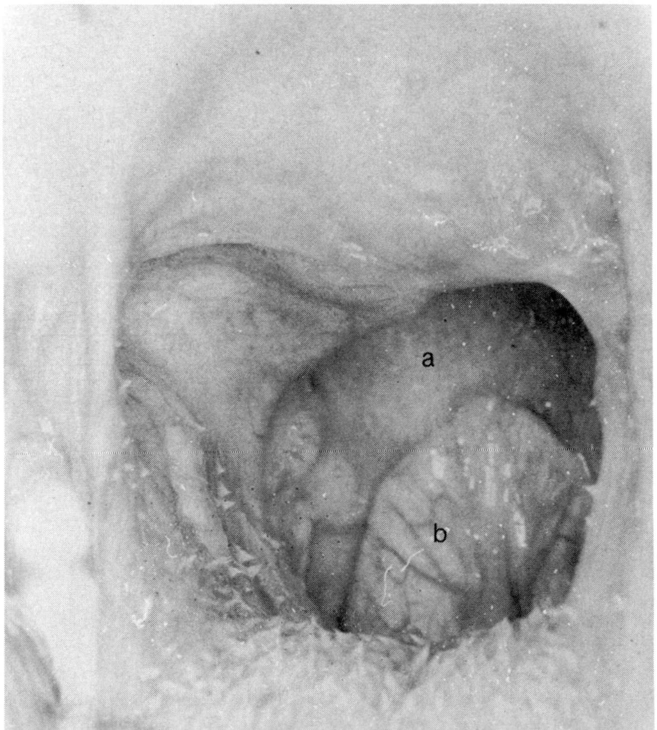

FIGURE 67–32. Gross soft palate hypoplasia in a springer spaniel, five months old. *a,* dorsal wall of nasopharynx; *b,* ventral surface of epiglottis; *c,* dorsum of tongue.

PHARYNGEAL PARALYSIS

During deglutition, a bolus of food is squeezed through the oropharynx and laryngopharynx by a "stripping" wave of constriction within the pharyngeal muscles. Liquids and semi-solids tend to pass through the piriform recesses, whereas solid food moves in the midline. Dysphagia due to myopathy or lesions of the glossopharyngeal, vagus, and trigeminal nerves is rare, and often the etiology remains unknown. Trauma is an obvious cause, but in other patients although the failure of muscle action can be demonstrated using barium swallows and fluoroscopy, identification of the cause and related treatment remain impossible. Quidding, spluttering, coughing, and sneezing attend attempted swallowing, and inhalation pneumonia may accompany the problem. Fortunately, most dysphagia is due to discomfort or pain, and trauma, infection, tonsillitis, and neoplasia are obvious local factors. Cricopharyngeal achalasia or malfunction in which there is failure of the proximal esophageal sphincter to relax is an important, nonpainful differential diagnosis. Patients with temporary pharyngeal paralysis can be supported by pharyngostomy intubation, but those with permanent paralysis carry a grave prognosis. An unusual complication that may follow feline dysautonomia is sneezing and gagging during deglutition. The mechanism remains unknown, but food and fluid can only pass into the nasopharynx in the presence of soft palate dysfunction.

CRICOPHARYNGEAL ACHALASIA

The cricopharyngeus muscle forms a sphincter around the proximal esophagus and relaxation in sequence with pharyngeal muscle constriction permits food and fluid to pass into the esophagus. Inability to relax this sphincter is seen as a congenital lesion in cocker and springer spaniels or may be acquired unusually as the result of presumed fibrosis in canine or feline patients of any age.[48] It is an uncommon condition in which the patient attempts to swallow food, and the food is returned into the mouth or nasal chambers. Fluids may be swallowed, and the congenital lesion usually becomes apparent when the puppy starts to take solid food. Quidding, coughing, spluttering, and sneezing are all features of the problem, and the diagnosis is confirmed using fluoroscopy and barium swallows in the conscious patient. An inhalation pulmonary involvement may be present.

Treatment can be reasonably successful and is achieved by resecting the dorsal part of the cricopharyngeus muscle. A ventral midline skin incision from the hyoid bone to the distal one-third of the trachea with midline dissection of the sternohyoid muscle straps allows exposure of the trachea and ventral larynx. Section of the left sternothyroid muscle allows a clockwise rotation of the larynx to expose the dorsal aspect of the proximal esophagus. A wide strip of cricopharyngeus muscle is dissected out, down to the level of the esophageal mucosa. The wound is not sutured, the hope being that any subsequent fibrosis will be unable to close the sphincter. A bulky diet should be fed during the immediate postoperative phase to help reduce the chances of stricture.

PHARYNGOSTOMY INTUBATION

This technique is of value in supporting the anorectic patient, those in which prehension, mastication, and deglutition are not possible and where swallowing might interfere with the results of pharyngeal surgery.[49] An 8 mm diameter rubber or polyethylene tube is passed through the lateral wall of the pharynx at the level of the piriform fossa, down the esophagus and into the stomach so that some 4 cm of tubing passes through the cardia. The piriform fossa is located by placing a finger tip or the end of a hemostat against the lateral wall of the pharynx behind the soft palate and immediately posterior to the stylohyoid/epihyoid articulation. Incision here avoids the hypoglossal nerve and the carotid and maxillary blood vessels. The tubing is sutured to the skin, and a cap is used to prevent any leakage of food. Patients are fed up to 100 ml of liquid food four to eight times per day, and the tube can be used for several weeks without complication. Regurgitation of the tube occurs if it is too long or too short, and radiography can be used to check that the end is correctly positioned in the stomach. Occasionally interference with the movement of the epiglottis during swallowing may predispose the patient to the inhalation of food particles and fluids. Aspiration pneumonia and obstruction of the laryngeal aditus are thus potential complications.[50]

NEOPLASIA

In the dog and cat squamous cell carcinoma of the tonsil is the commonest pharyngeal tumor (Figure 67–34), but malignant melanoma and lymphosarcoma may also involve this site in the canine patient.[51] The presenting clinical features of tonsillar squamous cell carcinoma are pain, anorexia, the drooling of saliva, which might be blood-stained, halitosis, and possible palpable submandibular lymphadenopathy. Bilateral involvement is not uncommon, and the diseased tonsil may be enlarged and hard or soft, and bleeds readily when touched. In some patients the tonsil may look quite

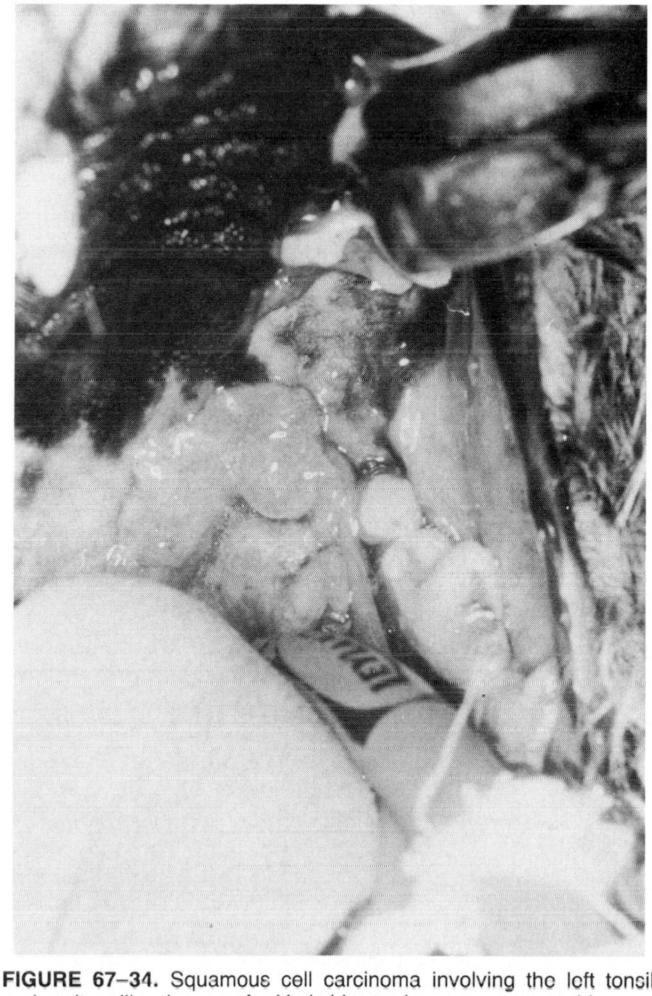

FIGURE 67–34. Squamous cell carcinoma involving the left tonsil and peritonsillar tissues of a Yorkshire terrier, seven years old.

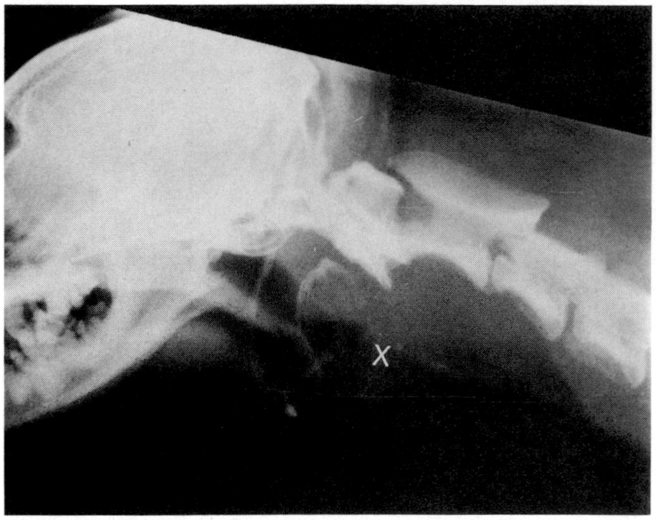

FIGURE 67–35. Squamous cell carcinoma of the tonsil in a Chihuahua, nine years old. The radiograph demonstrates retropharyngeal lymph node metastasis (x). Some calcification has occurred.

normal in size and color, and it is the metastatic lesions in the retropharyngeal lymph nodes that are the main cause of the clinical signs seen (Figure 67–35). The metastases can enlarge considerably to distort the dorsal pharyngeal wall and even displace the larynx. Severe cervical pain can even render the lesion an important differential diagnosis in assumed disc protrusion. Tonsillectomy is of no value, due to the presence of retropharyngeal and possible pulmonary metastases.

Occasionally, enlargement of the tonsil can be caused by non-neoplastic cystic swelling, and dysphagia is relieved by surgical excision. Swelling due to retropharyngeal abscessation can cause pain and dysphagia, and treatment involves drainage and antibiotic therapy.

THE LARYNX

Structure and Function

The larynx is a complex tubular valve constructed of cartilage, ligament, and muscle, which guards the entrance to the trachea. It is supported by the hyoid apparatus, and bordered dorsally by the laryngopharynx and anteriorly by the intrapharyngeal opening, the distal soft palate, and the oropharynx. Its framework consists of a leaf-shaped epiglottis cranially, a shield-shaped thyroid cartilage, a ring-shaped cricoid cartilage, and the paired arytenoid cartilages. Several muscles and ligaments unite these cartilages, and the luminal surface is lined with a ciliated pseudocolumnar epithelium. The roof of the larynx is formed by the cricoid and arytenoid cartilages, and the walls and floor by the cricoid and thyroid cartilages. Ventrally these two cartilages are linked by the cricothyroid membrane, and dorsolaterally they are joined via the cricothyroid articulations. The true vocal cords or ligaments are straps of elastic tissue contained within the vocal folds or labiae vocale, each fold being suspended from the vocal process of the arytenoid cartilage and attached ventrally to the thyroid cartilage. Together the arytenoid cartilages and the vocal folds are referred to as the glottis, and the gap between the folds is called the rima glottidis; this gap is the narrowest part of the intralaryngeal airway. Closure of the glottis prevents food and fluid from entering the trachea during swallowing. The arytenoid cartilages and vocal folds meet in the midline to seal off the airway, and probable posterior displacement of the epiglottis over the laryngeal vestibule may close off the aditus. Pharyngeal contents pass to the esophagus mainly within the piriform recesses. During inspiration at rest and throughout respiration during exertion the glottis is actively open. This is achieved by the action of one pair of abductor muscles of the larynx, the cricoarytenoideus dorsalis muscles, upon the arytenoid cartilages. The vocalis muscle attached to the caudal part of each vocal cord is partially responsible for regulating the sounds made during phonation. The false vocal cords, or vestibular folds, are mucosal plicae that run between the cranial thyroid cartilage and the cuneiform processes of the arytenoid cartilages, anterior to the true vocal cords. The laryngeal ventricles are mucosal pockets that end blindly and are located between the two sets of vocal cords. The aryepiglottic membrane runs from the corniculate process of the arytenoid cartilage over the cuneiform process of the cartilage to insert into the lateral edge of the epiglottis. Its continuation onto the ventral surface of the epiglottis is referred to as the glosso-epiglottic or subepiglottic mucosa and in turn this membrane is continuous with the papillae-bearing cornified mucosa on the dorsum of the tongue. Innervation of the larynx is derived entirely from the vagus; the motor nerve supply to all the musculature except the cricothyroid muscle is provided by the paired recurrent laryngeal nerves, and the sensory nerve supply is provided by the cranial and recurrent laryngeal nerves.

The larynx functions in two basic ways, acting as a valve in deglutition and inspiration, and being responsible for the production of voice. Closure of the rima glottidis by the vocal folds during swallowing is probably supported by movement of both the aryepiglottic and vestibular folds,[52] the passive caudal displacement of the epiglottis to cover the laryngeal aditus, and limited reorientation of the larynx as a whole at the level of the cricotracheal junction. Variation in the size of the rima glottidis helps regulate air flow to the lungs, with maximum abduction of the larynx occurring during deep inspiration. Tension within the vocal cords is responsible for the sounds produced in phonation.

Diagnosis

Laryngeal disease is indicated by coughing, altered phonation, and varying degrees of obstructive dyspnea. The covering and lining mucous membrane is rich in sensory nerve endings, and reflex coughing is prompted by the presence of inflammatory products or foreign body material. Coughing also occurs when there is failure of vocal cord activity in laryngeal adduction, and as such it may be a feature of laryngeal paralysis. Attention may be drawn initially to paralysis by change in the tone or volume of the bark. Stridor and reduced exercise tolerance are also features of laryngeal paralysis, but both accompany any obstructive dyspnea, cyanosis, and asphyxiation, further complicating the obstruction in some patients. The laryngeal collapse that occurs as a long-term extension of the brachycephalic airway obstruction syndrome, chronic proliferative laryngitis, and laryngeal neoplasia are all associated with chronic stridor, whereas the asphyxiation that is due to laryngeal spasm is transient and spontaneous in otherwise normal patients.

Observation of the patient at rest is helpful, but exercise may be necessary to induce dyspnea. The presence of mouth breathing indicates severe laryngeal obstruction, but both the nasal chambers and the oropharynx can be checked for patency at this stage of the examination. Palpation of the larynx may produce a cough or reveal neoplastic distortion and local lymphadenopathy, other soft tissue swellings due to abscess formation or neoplasia, and subcutaneous emphysema, which may accompany pharyngeal trauma. Tracheal collapse is an important differential diagnosis and palpation of this structure provokes the characteristic "honking" cough and reveals the flattened conformation of the trachea. Auscultation is valueless in the diagnosis of laryngeal disease; upper respiratory tract noise masks any accompanying pulmonary disease.

Satisfactory examination of the larynx requires general anesthesia. Gross abnormality of the anterior larynx, arytenoid displacement, and distortion of the epiglottis are easily discernible, and the glottis itself may be examined adequately by depressing the epiglottis with the blade of the laryngoscope (Figure 67–36). Cricoarytenoideus dorsalis muscle activity in abduction is checked by observing movement of the arytenoid cartilages under very light anesthesia. Reduced movement, fibrillation, and no movement at all of one or both the arytenoids and the vocal cords during inspiration dictate a diagnosis of laryngeal paralysis, but this assessment can only be made when a strong jaw reflex is present. With deeper anesthesia the infraglottic cavity and trachea can be examined using a small caliber endoscope. Radiography is not an essential diagnostic procedure but displacement of the larynx by space-occupying lesions, hyoid fractures, foreign bodies, and neoplasia may all be identified. The demonstration of anterior mediastinal neoplasia may explain relatively sudden onset laryngeal paralysis.

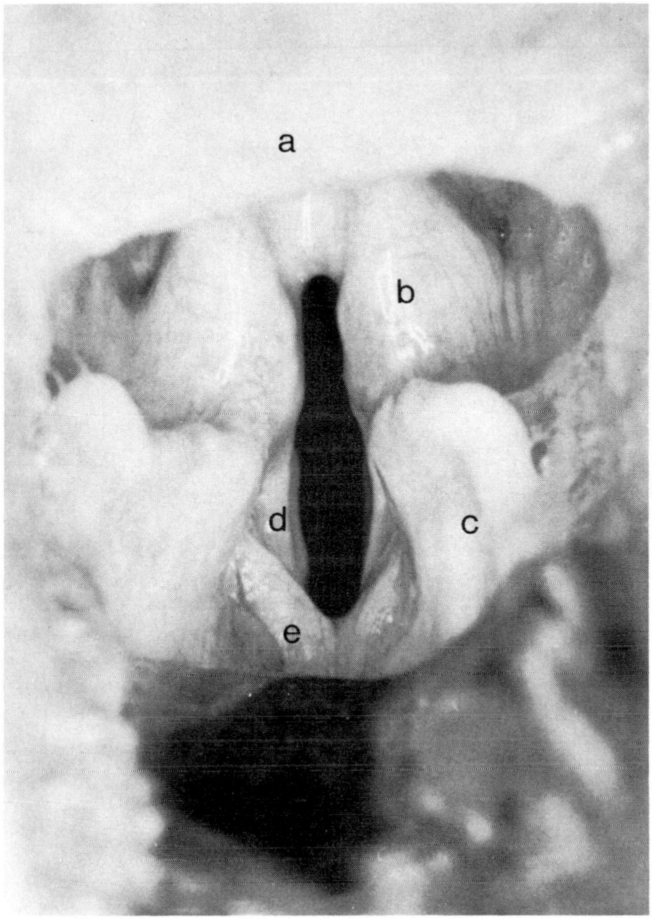

FIGURE 67–36. The anterior aspect of the canine larynx: the epiglottis has been depressed using a laryngoscope blade (X). *a,* Soft palate; *b,* left arytenoid cartilage; *c,* left lateral edge of epiglottis; *d,* right vocal cord; *e,* right ventricular fold.

Disease Conditions of the Larynx

TRAUMA

The larynx is seldom subjected to traumatic damage because its position in the neck is a relatively well-protected one in both the dog and the cat. However, compression injuries and puncture wounds are possible in both species, and choke chain damage in the dog may cause fracture of the hyoid apparatus and even the laryngeal cartilages. Severe trauma may result in critical airway obstruction as the result of dislocation of the arytenoid cartilages from their articulation with the cricoid or separation of the laryngo-tracheal junction. Treatment involves the maintenance of an airway and tracheotomy can be necessary until surgical repair has been completed and the associated edema and swelling have regressed. Infection is the specific complication of bite wounds, and both antibiotics and corticosteroids have their place in any treatment regimen. Hyoid fractures result in possible dyspnea, but local perilaryngeal swelling due to hemorrhage and edema is more likely. Repair is not necessary except where accompanying fracture displacement of the laryngeal cartilages has occurred. The possibility of damage to the laryngeal nerves should be considered in the prognosis given, with laryngeal paralysis being a potential complication.

Attempted intubation during anesthesia when the glottic reflex is still present or the tube used is too large and non-lubricated can damage the laryngeal mucosa, particularly at the level of the rima glottidis. Hyperemia, edema, possible spasm, and even erosion of the mucosa can accompany such poor practice, and persistent "tube cough" may require corticosteroid and antibiotic therapies. Panting in obese animals and brachycephalics can induce severe laryngeal edema; this situation is critical in those patients with existing obstructive dyspnea. Cage rest in a cool, moist environment, sedation, and corticosteroid therapy may have to be supported by tracheotomy in the severely affected patient.

FOREIGN BODIES

Intralaryngeal foreign bodies are rare in dogs and cats, since their presence in the vestibule and glottis stimulates reflex closure of the rima glottidis, which prompts their removal by coughing. Spiky objects such as chicken bones and needles can become lodged within the glottis during the initial laryngeal spasm, and grass seeds and barley awns that have passed through the rima glottidis lodge in the distal trachea, bronchi, and bronchioles. The presence of foreign body material within the infraglottic cavity appears to be an unusual occurrence.[53]

INFECTION

Acute inflammation of the larynx following endotracheal intubation or accompanying the presence of a glottic foreign body may be complicated by bacterial infection. Several viruses and bacteria may cause laryngitis in the dog and cat but this is usually part of a generalized respiratory tract infection, as occurs with rhinitis. A chronic proliferative laryngitis of unknown etiology occurs as an unusual cause of obstructive disease in the dog and cat. It is characterized by granulomatous tissue change, principally involving the arytenoid mucosa and the aryepiglottic folds. Systemic and intralesional corticosteroid therapy can be helpful in producing transient relief, but the severe dyspnea caused by long-term airway stenosis may best be treated by partial laryngectomy or even tracheostomy.

LARYNGEAL SPASM

Spasm in which the rima glottidis is closed and the glottis is further obstructed by the aryepiglottic folds is a life-threatening condition. Primary laryngospasm in which there is a spontaneous, seemingly unprovoked closure of the glottis is an unusual and little understood occurrence in both the dog and cat, but laryngospasm associated with endotracheal intubation in the cat is well recognized. Its occurrence has led to the essential use of local analgesic sprays prior to intubation and in support of general nongaseous anesthesia when pharyngeal surgery is undertaken in this species. There is no treatment for primary laryngospasm, although cordectomy or tracheostomy offers a possible solution.

LARYNGEAL PARALYSIS

Failure of the larynx to abduct during inspiration due to recurrent laryngeal nerve damage or disease is a significant clinical entity in the dog. While the unilateral paralysis due to accidental and surgical trauma or following neuropraxia related to the presence of space-occupying lesions is seldom of importance, except perhaps in performance dogs, bilateral paralysis causes stridor, cough, reduced exercise tolerance, and even cyanosis and collapse. Congenital unilateral and bilateral paralysis is uncommon but has been recorded in the Siberian husky and the Bouvier des Flandres breeds.[54] Bilateral paralysis is most commonly encountered in elderly dogs of the larger breeds, as the result of a neurogenic atrophy of the laryngeal musculature.[55] The Labrador retriever, the Afghan hound, the setter, the springer spaniel, and the greyhound are the breeds most commonly cited. A muted bark and the presence of a soft, moist cough are often early additional features, but given time, the roaring sound of inspiratory dyspnea becomes the dominant sign. Exercise and excitement increase the level of stridor, and the reduced exercise tolerance may give way to collapse on exertion.

Rest and corticosteroid therapy to reduce the associated laryngeal and pharyngeal edema can be helpful in the early stages of the disease, but the maintenance of an adequate laryngeal airway becomes essential for the well-being of these patients. Various surgical techniques employing cordectomy have been used to relieve the dyspnea. Good results cannot be guaranteed following such surgery. The initial immediate improvement often

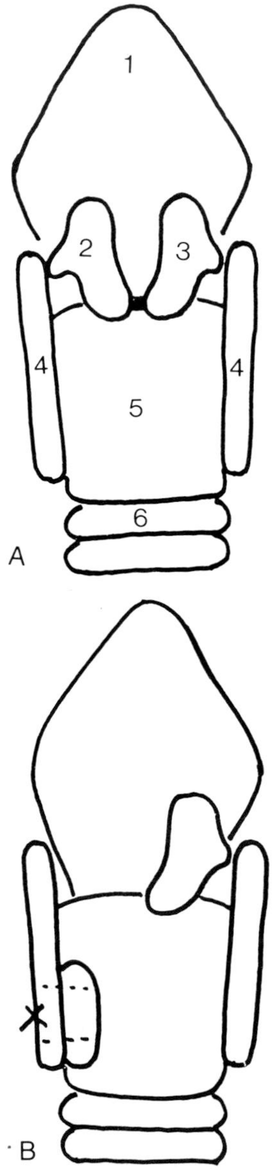

FIGURE 67–37. Arytenoid lateralization. *A*, Diagrammatic dorsal view of the larynx. 1, Epiglottis; 2, left arytenoid cartilage; 3, right arytenoid cartilage; 4, thyroid wings; 5, cricoid cartilage; 6, trachea. *B*, The left arytenoid cartilage has been mobilized and sutured to the posterior thyroid wing.

gives way to airway obstruction associated with fibrous tissue webbing and cicatrization.[56, 57] Fortunately, alternative techniques based on arytenoid tie-back or lateralization make a good prognosis possible in most patients thus treated.[58] Laryngeal tie-back surgery in which the left arytenoid cartilage is abducted by fixation to the cricoid cartilage has proved successful in the horse, and the extension of the same principle to canine disease was a natural one. Either arytenoid cartilage is dissected free from the anterior rim of the cricoid cartilage and sutured firmly to the caudal wing of the ipsilateral thyroid cartilage (Figure 67–37). This results in permanent unilateral abduction of the larynx and produces a rima glottidis that offers reduced obstruction to inspiration. A unilateral tie-back has been shown to be as effective as a bilateral one,[59] and is a simpler technique that produces no postoperative cough. The dorsolateral aspect of the larynx is exposed by incising skin and panniculus muscle above the level of the external maxillary artery. The thyropharyngeus muscle is cut along the cornual length of the thyroid cartilage, and the caudal articulation between this cartilage and the cricoid cartilage is broken down. The muscular process of the arytenoid cartilage is then identified on the anterior dorsal aspect of the cricoid cartilage, and the cricoarytenoid articulation is disrupted using blunt dissection. The sesamoid band that joins the two arytenoids medially is cut, leaving the dissected arytenoid cartilage attached to the larynx only by the vocal cord and laryngeal mucosa. The articular facet of this cartilage is then attached to the posterior medial surface of the caudal thyroid wing using a 0 silk mattress suture (Figure 67–38). Postoperative laryngoscopy confirms and demonstrates the degree of abduction obtained (Figure 67–39). Hematoma formation, edema, and disruption of the surgical anastomosis are potential complications, but all three may be managed successfully.

A castellated laryngofissure combined with vocal cord resection has been advocated for the treatment of laryngeal paralysis in the dog,[60] and may offer a useful alternative to lateralization. All surgery involving this area may be complicated after recovery by inhalation pneumonia.

LARYNGEAL COLLAPSE

The obstructive dyspnea of the brachycephalic patient can be further complicated by severe restriction of the anterior laryngeal airway caused by the displacement of the glosso-epiglottic mucosa, the eversion of the mucosal lining of the lateral ventricles, a subsequent inward and downward rotational distortion of parts of the arytenoid cartilages, and a dorsal scrolling of the epiglottis (Figure 67–40).

The glosso-epiglottic mucosa is loosely attached to the ventral surface of the epiglottis and the dorsum of the tongue. Increased inspiratory effort can suck the mucosa into the laryngeal aditus to complicate the obstruction already caused by the presence of the soft palate[61] (Figure 67–41). Displacement is temporary, since the mucosa is returned to its normal position on expiration. Treatment is by simple scissor excision of the mucosa. The lateral ventricles are well-developed structures in the dog. The combination of the soft palate blockage of the laryngeal aditus and the increased inspiratory effort needed to overcome the effects of this block subjects the walls of the laryngeal airway to a considerable collapsing force. It is not surprising therefore that the

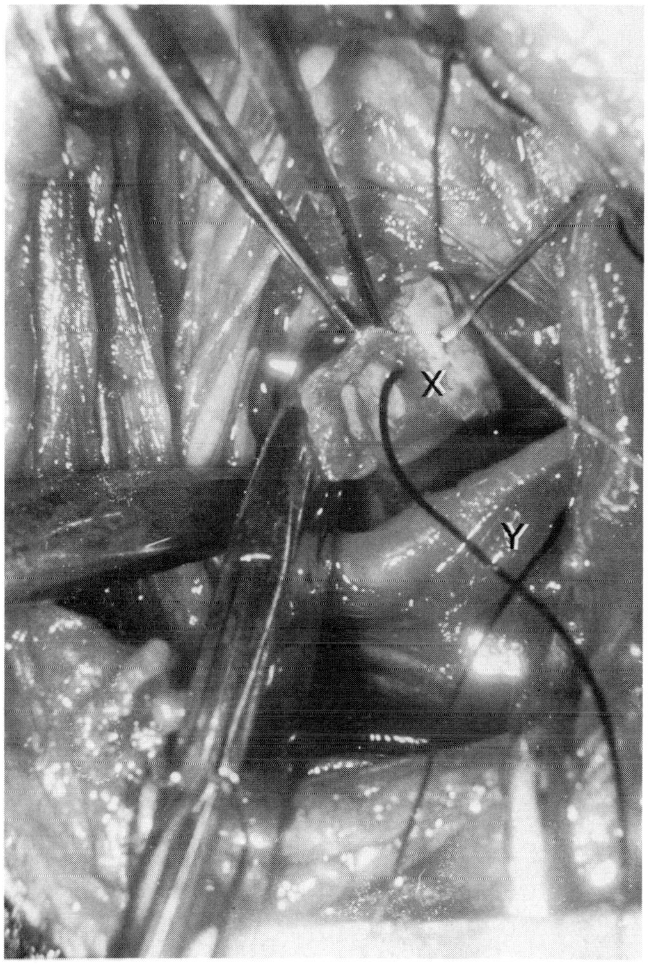

FIGURE 67–38. Arytenoid lateralization in an Irish setter, seven years old. The left arytenoid cartilage (x) is being sutured to the posterior wing of the thyroid cartilage (y).

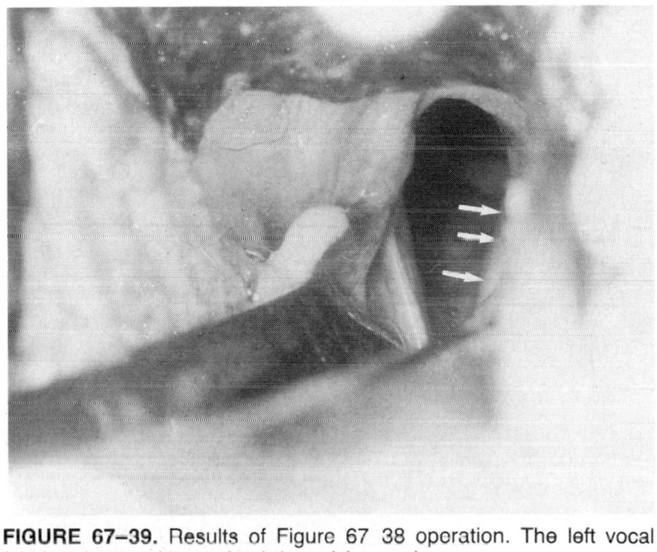

FIGURE 67–39. Results of Figure 67 38 operation. The left vocal fold has been adequately abducted (arrows).

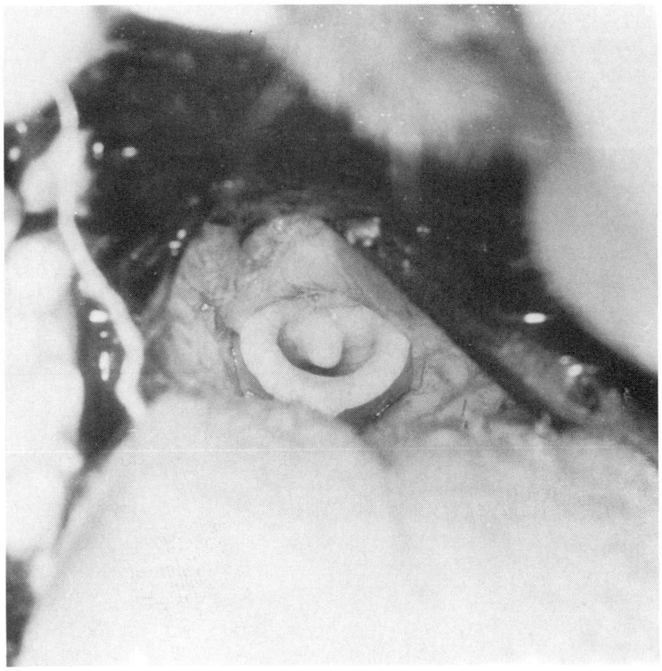

FIGURE 67–40. Laryngeal collapse in a pug, seven years old. Displacement of the arytenoid cartilages and scrolling of the epiglottis produces severe airway obstruction.

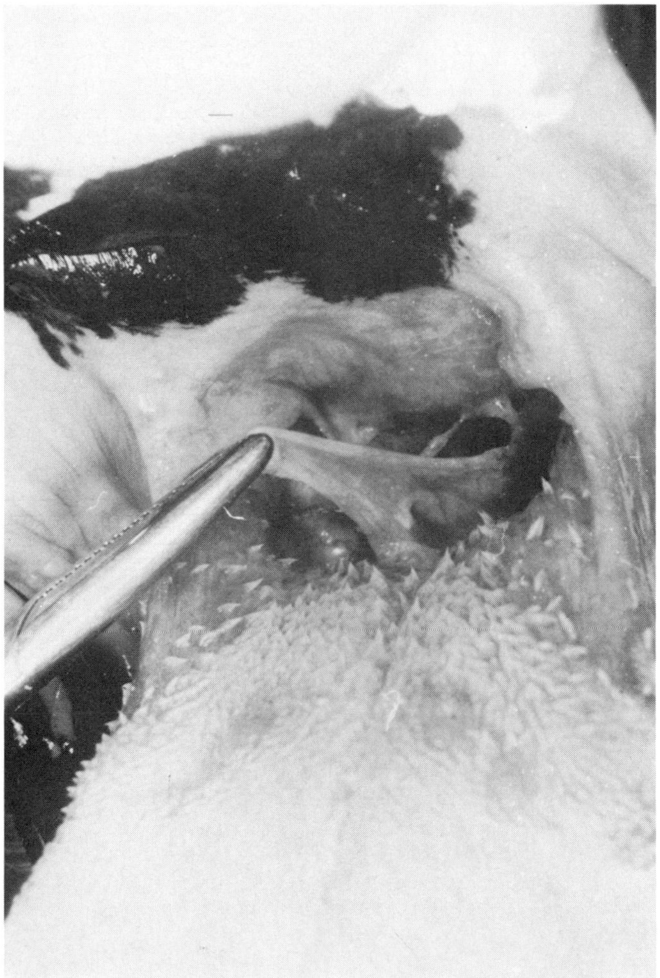

FIGURE 67–41. Displacement of the glosso-epiglottic mucosa during laryngeal collapse in a bulldog, two years old. The loose mucosa is being demonstrated using forceps.

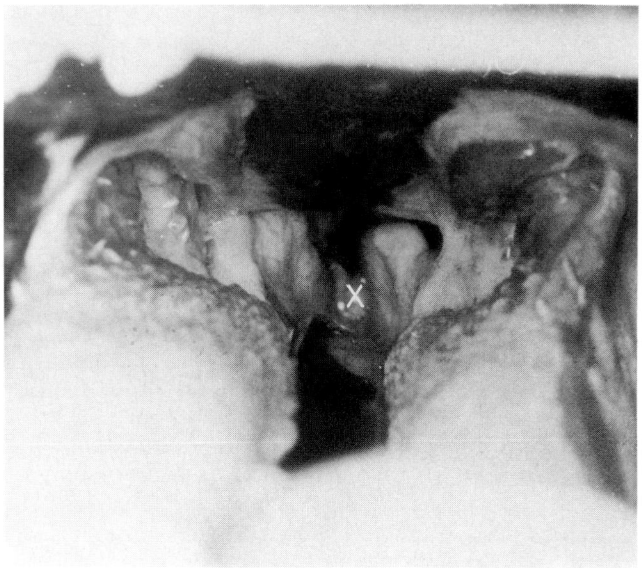

FIGURE 67–42. Eversion of the laryngeal ventricle linings (X) during laryngeal collapse.

lining mucosa of the ventricles can be everted into the airway, where they are seen as balls of tissue lying anterior to the vocal cords (Figure 67–42). Early in the process of laryngeal collapse the linings may be returned into the ventricles during expiration, but subsequent fibrosis results in their permanent presence in the airway. Their excision is as vital as partial soft palatectomy and the removal of any displacing glosso-epiglottic mucosa in preventing further distortion of the larynx. It is achieved by simple excision, long-handled dissection scissors being used to effect their removal. Hemorrhage is usually minimal, but tracheotomy will safeguard the airway during the surgery and recovery periods.

The same collapsing force that lifts the glosso-epiglottic mucosa and everts the ventricle linings also pulls the aryepiglottic folds medially into the aditus. This in turn leads to the collapse of the corniculate and cuneiform processes, pulling them medially and ventrally into the laryngeal aditus. At the same time the lateral edges of the epiglottis into which the aryepiglottic folds insert are pulled dorsally and medially, and scrolling occurs. Distortion of the arytenoid cartilages and epiglottis results in severe, potentially fatal, glottic airway obstruction, and partial laryngectomy is only partially successful in the management of these patients. The postoperative distortion of the glottis caused by granulation-type repair and webbing can be as severe as that caused by the collapse[62] (Figure 67–43); tracheostomy may offer a more acceptable alternative solution.

NEOPLASIA

Inflammatory polyps arising from vocal cord tissue are an uncommon cause of mild obstructive dyspnea in the dog. An altered bark may be noticed and a cough may be present. Simple excision using laryngeal cup forceps is not accompanied by complication or recurrence. Chondroma and granuloma formation may follow accidental and surgical trauma and can cause severe obstructive dyspnea. Dissection may prove impossible

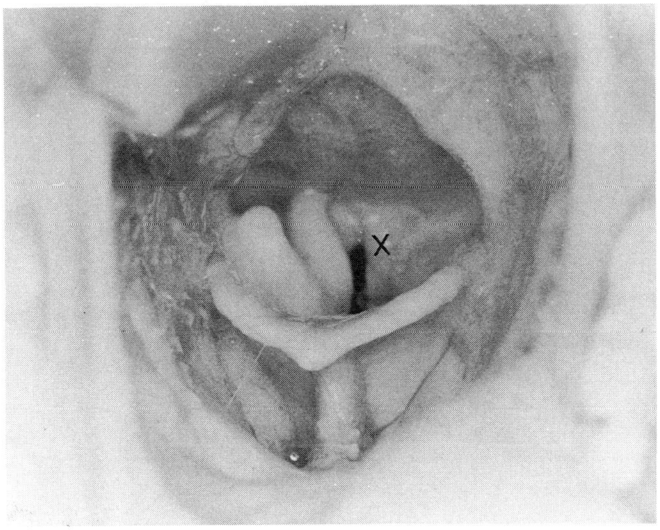

FIGURE 67–43. Postoperative webbing (X) following partial left laryngectomy in a bulldog, four years old.

and tracheostomy may be necessary. Primary neoplasia is rare, but adenocarcinomas, osteosarcomas, mast cell tumors, oncocytomas, chondrosarcomas, and leiomyomas can promote obstructive dyspnea,[63–66] while thyroid adenocarcinomas, lymphosarcomas, and heart-base and anterior mediastinal tumors may cause recurrent and cranial laryngeal neuropraxia.

References

1. Ramser, R: Zur Anatomie des Jacobsonschen Organs beim Hunde. Dissertation, Friedrick Wilhelms University, Berlin, 1935.
2. Eisenberg, JF and Kleinman, DG: Olfactory communication in mammals. Ann Rev Ecol Systemat 3:1, 1972.
3. Schneider, KM: Das Flehmen. Zeit. f. Gesamte Tiergartnerei, Leipzig 3:183, 1930.
4. Bedford, PGC: The differential diagnosis of nasal discharge in the dog. Veterinary Annual, 18th ed, Bristol, John Wright, 1978, p 232.
5. Venker van Haagen, AJ: Otoscopy, rhinoscopy and bronchoscopy in small animal clinics. Veterinary Quarterly 7:222, 1985.
6. Withrow, SJ, et al.: Aspiration and punch biopsy techniques for nasal tumors. JAAHA 21:551, 1985
7. Webbon, PM and France, C: Radiography. Atlas of canine surgical techniques. In Bedford, PGC (ed.): Oxford, Blackwell Scientific Publications, 1984, p 33.
8. Spreull, JSA: Surgery of the nasal cavity of the dog and cat. Vet Rec 75:105, 1963.
9. Bedford, PGC: Surgery of the head and neck region. In Bedford, PGC (ed.): Atlas of Canine Surgical Techniques. Oxford, Blackwell Scientific Publications, 1984, p 66.
10. O'Brien, JA and Harvey, CE: Diseases of the upper airway. In Ettinger, SJ (ed.): Textbook of Veterinary Internal Medicine, Philadelphia, WB Saunders, Vol 1 p 565.
11. Harvey, CE: Upper airway obstruction syndromes in dogs. In Kirk, RW (ed.): Current Veterinary Therapy. Vol. VI, WB Saunders, Philadelphia, p 233.
12. Harvey, CE and O'Brien, JA: Upper airway obstruction surgery: stenotic nares surgery in brachycephalic dogs. JAAHA 18:535, 1982.
13. Fallon RK, et al.: Unusual nasal foreign body (metal arrowhead) in a dog. JAVMA 186:710, 1985.
14. Howard, PR, et al.: Mucoperiosteal flap technique for cleft palate repair in dogs. JAVMA 165:352, 1974.
15. Wright, NG, et al.: Canine respiratory virus infection. J Sm Anim Pract 15:27, 1974.
16. Wilkinson, GT: Some observations on the Irish wolfhound rhinitis syndrome. J Sm Anim Pract 10:5, 1969.
17. Lane, JG: Feline nasal disorders. In Wright, PSG (ed.): ENT and Oral Surgery of the Dog and Cat. Bristol, John Wright, 1982, p 74.
18. Winstanley, EW: Trephining frontal sinuses in the treatment of rhinitis and sinusitis in the cat. Vet Rec 95:289, 1974.
19. Thompson, H, et al.: Experimental respiratory disease in dogs due to *Bordetella bronchiseptica*. Res Vet Sci 20:16, 1976
20. Harvey, CE: Therapeutic strategies involving antimicrobial treatment of the upper respiratory tract in small animals. JAVMA 185:1159, 1984.
21. Lane, JG, et al.: The diagnosis and successful treatment of *Aspergillus fumigatus* infection of the frontal sinuses and nasal chambers of the dog. J Small Anim Pract 15:79, 1974.
22. Allison, N, et al.: Nasal rhinosporidiosis in two dogs. JAVMA 188:869, 1986.
23. Easley, JR, et al.: Nasal rhinosporidiosis in the dog. Vet Pathol 23:50, 1986.
24. Hoff, B and Hall, DA: Rhinosporidiosis in a dog. Can Vet J 27:231, 1986.
25. Barrett, RE and Scott, DW: Treatment of feline cryptococcosis. JAAHA 11:511, 1975.
26. Goodall, SA, et al.: The diagnosis and treatment of a case of nasal aspergillosis in a cat. J Sm Anim Pract 25:627, 1984.
27. Lane, JG and Warnock, DW: The diagnosis of *Aspergillus fumigatus* infection of the nasal chambers of the dog with particular reference to the double diffusion test. J Sm Anim Pract 18:169, 1977.
28. Richardson, MD, et al.: Rapid serological diagnosis of *Aspergillus fumigatus* infection of the frontal sinuses and nasal chambers of the dog. Res Vet Sci 33:167, 1982.
29. Richardson, MD and Warnock, DW: Antigen selection for optimal serological diagnosis of *Aspergillus fumigatus* infection of the nasal chambers of the dog. Vet Rec 114:354, 1984.
30. Sullivan, M, et al.: The radiological features of aspergillosis of the nasal cavity. J Sm Anim Pract 27:167, 1985.
31. Harvey, CE: Nasal aspergillosis and penicillinosis in dogs. Results of treatment with thiabendazole. JAVMA 184:48, 1984.
32. Bauck LB: Treatment of canine nasal aspergillosis with ketoconazole. Vet Med Small Anim Clin 78:1713, 1983.
33. Sharp, NJH, et al.: Canine nasal aspergillosis: Serology and treatment with ketoconazole. J Sm Anim Pract 25:149, 1984.
34. Sharp, NJH and Sullivan, M: Treatment of canine nasal aspergillosis with systemic ketoconazole and topical enilconazole. Vet Rec 118:560, 1986.
35. Hargis, AM, et al.: Noninvasive nasal aspergillosis (fungal ball) in a six year old standard poodle. JAAHA 22:504, 1986.
36. Blagburn, BL, et al.: Canine linguatulosis. Canine Pract 10:54, 1983.
37. Beck, ER and Withrow, SJ: Tumors of the canine nasal cavity. Vet Clin N Am 15:521, 1985.
38. Sande, RD and Alexander, JE: Turbinate bone neoplasms in dogs. Mod Vet Pract 51:23, 1976.
39. Morgan, JP, et al.: Tumors in the nasal cavity of the dog: a radiographic study. J Am Vet Radiol Soc 13:18, 1972.
40. Gibbs, C, et al.: Radiological features of intranasal lesions in the dog: a review of 100 cases. J Sm Anim Pract 20:515, 1979.
41. Bradley, PA and Harvey, CE: Intranasal tumors in the dog: an evaluation of prognosis. J Sm Anim Pract 14:459, 1973.
42. Thrall, DE and Harvey, CE: Radiotherapy of malignant nasal tumors in 21 dogs. JAVMA 183:663, 1983.
43. Parrent, R: Presence of canine transmissible venereal tumor in the nasal cavity of dogs in the area of Dakar (Senegal). Can Vet J 24:287, 1983.
44. Lane, JG: Obstructions of the upper respiratory tract. In Wright, PGC (ed.): ENT and Oral Surgery of the Dog and Cat. Bristol, John Wright, 1982, p 90.
45. Bedford, PGC, et al.: Nasopharyngeal polyps in the cat. Vet Rec 109:551, 1981.
46. Lane, JG, et al.: Nasopharyngeal polyps arising in the middle ear of the cat. J Sm Anim Pract 22:511, 1981.

47. Bedford, PGC and Brownlie, SE: Early occurring nasopharyngeal polyp in a kitten. Vet Rec 117:668, 1985.
48. Rosin, E and Hanlon, GF: Canine crico-pharyngeal achalasia. JAVMA 160:1496, 1972.
49. Bohning, RH, et al.: Pharyngostomy for the maintenance of the anorectic animal. JAVMA 186:611, 1970.
50. Crowe, DT and Downs, MO: Pharyngostomy complications in dogs and recommended technical modifications: Experimental and clinical investigations. JAAHA 22:493, 1986.
51. Todoroff, RJ and Brodey RS: Oral and pharyngeal neoplasia in the dog: A retrospective survey of 361 cases. JAVMA 175:567, 1979.
52. Pressmen, JL and Keleman, G: Physiology of the larynx. Physiol Rev 35:506, 1955.
53. Bedford, PGC and Grey B: Intralaryngeal foreign body as an unusual cause of dyspnea in a dog. J Sm Anim Pract, in press.
54. Venker-van Haagen, AJ: Investigations on the pathogenesis of hereditary laryngeal paralysis in the Bouvier. Thesis. Utrecht University. 1980.
55. O'Brien, JA, et al.: Neurogenic atrophy of the laryngeal muscles of the dog. J Sm Anim Pract 14:521, 1973.
56. Harvey, CE and O'Brien, JA: Upper airway obstruction surgery. Treatment of laryngeal paralysis in dogs by partial laryngectomy. JAAHA 18:551, 1982.
57. Harvey, CE: Partial laryngectomy in the dog. Healing and swallowing function in normal dogs. Vet Surg 12:192, 1983.
58. Harvey, CE and Venker-van Haagen, AJ: Surgical management of pharyngeal and laryngeal airway obstruction in the dog. Vet Clin N Am 5:515, 1985.
59. Lane, JG: Surgery of the conducting airways. In Wright, PSG (ed.): ENT and Oral Surgery of the Dog and Cat. Bristol, John Wright, 1982, p 113.
60. Smith, MM, et al.: Evaluation of a modified castellated laryngofissure for alleviation of upper airway obstruction in dogs with laryngeal paralysis. JAVMA 188:1279, 1986.
61. Bedford, PGC: Displacement of the glosso-epiglottic mucosa in canine asphyxiate disease. J Sm Anim Pract 24:199, 1983.
62. Harvey, CE: Upper airway obstruction surgery. Partial laryngectomy in brachycephalic dogs. JAAHA 18:548, 1982.
63. Wheeldon EB, et al.: Neoplasia of the larynx of the dog. JAVMA 180:642, 1982.
64. Lightfoot, RM, et al.: Laryngeal leiomyoma in a dog. J Sm Anim Pract 24:753, 1983.
65. Mays, MBC: Laryngeal oncocytoma in two dogs. JAVMA 185:677, 1984.
66. Saik JE, et al.: Canine and feline laryngeal neoplasia: a 10 year study. JAAHA 22:359, 1986.

68 DISEASES OF THE TRACHEA

STEPHEN J. ETTINGER and JAMES W. TICER

HISTORY AND COMMON ASSOCIATIONS

In pathologic conditions affecting the trachea, the most commonly recognized clinical signs are coughing; stertorous, noisy inspiratory sounds; stridulent or wheezing expiratory sounds; pulmonary edema; and occasionally, cyanosis. The type as well as the specific nature of the cough may help in elucidating the specific disease entity present. The clinical differentiation of the coughing state requires the clinician to evaluate the type of cough, to examine the patient, and to ask specific questions of the owner with respect to the nature of the cough. Chapter 18 identifies the most commonly encountered general causes of coughing in small animals. The structural, histologic, and functional considerations of the trachea have been reviewed in normal[1] dogs and in eight dogs with tracheal pathology.[2]

PHYSICAL EXAMINATION

Diseases of the trachea may present with degrees of severity varying from a normal-appearing patient to one with severe respiratory distress and secondary cyanosis. Respiratory sounds may be normal in a well-compensated patient or may be stertorous, raspy, or noisy with moist, dry, or sibilant rales. Evaluation of the coughing animal has been described in Chapter 18.

Palpation of the trachea, from the larynx to the thoracic inlet, is an important aspect of the evaluation of the respiratory system of the patient. Lesions obstructing the airway, such as lymphadenopathy, goiter, cysts, or neoplasia, may be palpated. A description of laryngeal palpation can be found in Chapter 67. The thyroid gland may be palpated caudal and slightly dorsal to the cricoid cartilage. In most dogs, these glands are palpable on the trachea at the caudal angle of the mandible. The thyroid gland is difficult to palpate in the normal cat. In cats with thyroid hyperplasia or neoplasia, a hidden enlargement may be readily palpated after the animal has been sedated or anesthetized, although in some cases it may be recognized without sedation. The trachea is usually a relatively noncollapsible, elliptically C-shaped structure that is somewhat compliant upon compression. Obvious borders or angles usually cannot be felt; however, the tracheal cartilages with their fibroelastic annular ligaments can usually be palpated. It is difficult to palpate the trachea in heavy or obese dogs and cats. When disease of the trachea is being considered, one must first complete a thorough oral, laryngeal, and pharyngeal examination. Tracheal disease can often complicate or be confused with other upper respiratory lesions.

SPECIAL DIAGNOSTIC EXAMINATIONS

Usually, examination of the oral and pharyngeal cavities and trachea under anesthesia is performed after routine radiographs or the physical examination (or both) have suggested the presence of a pathologic condition in that area. In some cases, oral examination without anesthesia may reveal abnormalities that may warrant further evaluation of the patient under anesthesia. A description of the oral and pharyngeal cavities under anesthesia may be found in Chapter 67. Anesthesia provides an opportunity for careful digital palpation of the entire cervical trachea, from the larynx to the thoracic inlet. The size and shape of the trachea, including deviations in the cartilaginous rings, dorsoventral or lateral compression of the trachea with dorsolateral angulations, stenotic regions, and large space-occupying lesions may be evaluated by palpation.

After the oral and pharyngeal examination has been completed, one may examine the trachea and the bronchi by endoscopy. When culture and antibiotic sensitivity testing of tracheal exudates are being considered, it is usually advisable to perform this procedure prior to further endoscopic examination. Culture of the trachea in cats and in most toy and medium-sized breeds of dogs may be satisfactorily performed using commercially available, laboratory culturette swabs. These six- to eight-inch-long swabs are inserted into the trachea under general anesthesia while sterility is maintained by holding the epiglottis down with a laryngoscope or forceps and the tube is allowed to pass into the trachea. Cultures may be taken from most levels of the trachea by using this technique. A preferable method of obtaining specimens from the lower respiratory tract is that of transtracheal aspiration. This technique requires only local anesthesia. This method uses puncture of the cricothyroid membrane and threading of a sterile catheter into the trachea.[3] Although it is an excellent method of obtaining aspirates from the mid-respiratory tract, it may be of limited value for tracheal culture. Another technique that works well is to insert a sterile endotracheal tube into the trachea after the animal has been anesthetized and flush sterile saline through a small sterile catheter placed in the tracheal tube. The animal is then held upside down and the fluid is collected in a sterile vial as it runs out of the front of the tube. While perhaps not as precise as other methods, it is practical and easy to perform with equipment usually found in the small animal practice setting. Following culture of the trachea, endoscopic examination of the trachea may be performed. Culture material may also be obtained through the accessory channel of most endoscopes. The endoscope is passed slowly from cranial area to the caudal. Pertinent information, such as color and appearance of the mucous membranes of the trachea, is noted. Production of mucus, pus, or other exudative material on these membranes or the presence of submucosal nodules secondary to *Filaroides osleri* near the tracheal bifurcation may also be seen. Dorsoventral compression of the trachea with draping of the dorsal membrane and such obvious lesions as ulcers or space-occupying masses may also be observed. Following routine endoscopic examination of the trachea, selective bronchoscopy may be performed as indicated. The authors recommend endoscopy using either rigid or flexible fiberoptic sterile endoscopic equipment. This equipment may not be readily available to most practicing veterinarians. Normal and pathologic conditions of the canine trachea, as visualized through rigid endoscopic equipment, have been reported.[4]

CLINICOPATHOLOGY

Diseases of the trachea only occasionally have definitive, demonstrative, clinicopathological findings. A complete blood count may indicate an eosinophilic leukocytosis in the presence of an allergic response. These findings are not specific for tracheal pathology and should be considered in that light when positive findings are present. Culture and antibiotic sensitivity testing of exudates from the tracheal mucosa may be helpful if an infectious tracheitis is present. Often, cases of chronic tracheitis, tracheobronchitis, and collapsed trachea do not produce significant pathologic bacterial cultures. Nevertheless, culture and antibiotic sensitivity testing are of value when a growth develops. The commonly encountered species of *Staphylococcus* and *Streptococcus* and *Escherichia coli* are usually found. Cultures of bronchial washings are more likely to be positive. Cytologic examination of tracheal smears and exudates may reveal bacteria, red and white cells, worm larvae, neoplastic cells, or cells reflecting a chronic response. Occasionally the larvae of respiratory system parasites such as *Filaroides osleri, Crenosoma vulpis,* or *Capillaria aerophila* are recognized. Bronchiolar and alveolar parasites such as *Filaroides milksi* or *Aelurostrongylus abstrusus* (in cats) may also be found. The first-stage larvae of *Aelurostrongylus* may be recognized on routine fecal examination.

RADIOGRAPHIC EXAMINATION

Ventrodorsal (VD) and lateral views of the cervical and thoracic trachea are necessary for routine radiographic examination. Generally, the reduced exposure technique used to evaluate the thorax is inadequate for the tracheal examination, especially in the region of the thoracic inlet, since visualization of adjacent soft tissue structures is needed to evaluate peritracheal tissues that may be an integral part of tracheal disease syndromes. The use of a single examination with a large film that is designed to produce diagnostic information about both the pulmonary parenchyma and cervical region is therefore not recommended. The lateral radiographic examination must be performed with careful positioning of the patient to avoid artifactual deviations of the trachea, especially in the caudal cervical and cranial mediastinal regions. Excessive flexion of the occipitoatlantal articulation may cause deviations of the trachea, which may artifactually suggest extratracheal masses, particularly in the cranial mediastinal region. The forelimbs should remain in their natural position during the initial examination. Subsequent radiographs, with the limbs pulled caudally or cranially, may be needed if a suggested lesion is noted in the area covered by the shoulders. VD views are necessary to evaluate the course of the trachea. VD oblique views are needed at times to evaluate the thoracic tracheal lumen when superimposition of the sternum prevents sufficient radiographic detail for diagnostic quality. These views are usually not necessary, however, since the trachea usually courses to the right of the cranial mediastinum and reaches the midline only at the tracheal bifurcation (carina). Uniform x-ray beam penetration of the patient may be enhanced by placing the patient's head toward the anode (positive) side of the x-ray tube, thus taking advantage of the so-called heal effect. This results in a more uniform exposure of the resulting radiographs, since the relatively more intense x-ray beam of the cathode (negative) side of the tube is placed over the thickest part of the patient. If the thoracic trachea is of primary interest and the initial thoracic radiographs exhibit insufficient exposure of the region, the kV of the machine setting should be increased by 15 per cent and the studies repeated. Additional radiographic detail may be obtained by closing the collimator further so that only the trachea and adjacent peritracheal tissues are exposed. This reduces the amount of scatter radiation and thereby improves detail. Tracheal radiographs should be surveyed for continuity of mucosal lining, diameter, and placement within the cervical and thoracic regions. The normal tracheal diameter generally decreases slightly from the cranial to the caudal end. The normal ventrodorsal diameter of the trachea at the third rib should be approximately three times the width of the third rib at the level of the trachea.[5]

Another method of determining normal tracheal diameter uses the ratio of the inner diameter of the trachea at the thoracic inlet to the distance between the ventral edge of the first thoracic vertebra and the dorsal edge of the manubrium. The normal ratio is 0.16 or greater.[6] Abrupt changes in the luminal diameter should not occur. Occasionally, the caudal cervical esophagus is superimposed over the dorsal aspect of the trachea and is seen on lateral radiographic projection. This overlying density may be confused with a dorsal tracheal collapse caused by an inverting dorsal tracheal membrane.[7] If a sufficient exposure has been used, the continuity of the tracheal lumen may be traced through this overlying shadow. If, after careful examination, the cause of this shadow remains obscure, a repeat lateral radiograph produced on maximum expiration usually shows increased cervical tracheal diameter when the cause is tracheal collapse. When tracheal collapse due to dorsal membrane inversion is suggested by the clinical examination, a pair of lateral radiographs of the entire trachea should be produced at the maximum inspiratory phase and at the maximum expiratory phase of the respiratory cycle. Normal aging processes may result in the dystrophic mineralization of tracheal rings, and these should not be considered pathologic.

Contrast studies of the tracheal lumen are indicated in cases showing signs of tracheal rupture or fracture, when suspected radiolucent foreign bodies may not be evident on noncontrast survey radiographs, and when a more detailed examination of the luminal surface is required. Partial or complete obstruction due to a neoplasm or stenosis may also be evaluated with positive contrast studies of the trachea. Contrast materials should not be introduced into the respiratory system when acute pulmonary disease is accompanied by fever or recent hemoptysis,[8] when there is hypersensitivity to the contrast material, in chronic nephritis when iodine materials are being used, when vital lung capacity is depressed, in acute bronchitis, or with severe emphysema.[9] General anesthesia is necessary to permit introduction of contrast material and to suppress coughing.[10] Short-acting anesthesia is recommended, since rapid recovery enhances the reappearance of the cough reflex. Atropine sulfate should not be used when preparing the patient for anesthesia, since it interferes with mucociliary action that helps to remove contrast material.[11] An endotracheal tube is passed to assure adequate ventilation. The contrast medium may then be introduced through the endotracheal tube with the catheter attached to a syringe. The contrast material of choice is 50 to 60 per cent weight per volume suspension of barium sulfate in a carboxymethylcellulose base.[10] Dilution should be made with sterile saline. In a 20- to 30-lb dog, 2 to 3 cc are instilled into the cervical trachea and the patient is allowed to respire normally for approximately one minute; then VD and lateral radiographs are made. The degree of tracheal lumen opacification is evaluated. More contrast material may be added safely if the tracheal bifurcation is not outlined adequately. Fluoroscopic control of this procedure is desirable and preferred.

Motion studies of the diseased trachea are highly desirable for evaluating pathodynamics. Image-intensification equipment is necessary to obtain adequate radiographic detail safely. These studies are extremely valuable, if not indispensible, for the study of the collapsed trachea and other coughing syndromes. Patients should be placed in lateral recumbency and the entire trachea visualized. A cough may usually be stimulated by digital pressure applied at the thoracic inlet. Videotape recordings of these dynamic studies add to their usefulness. Playback observations in slow motion frequently result in the detection of functional features that may have been missed during the initial examination.

TRACHEAL DISEASES

TRACHEITIS

Tracheitis refers to an inflammation of the epithelial lining of the trachea. The inflammatory response may result from noninfectious diseases.

Features. Tracheitis is usually associated with a nonproductive or slightly productive cough that is characterized as resonant and harsh, occurring in paroxysms, and often terminated by gagging. In some cases, especially in collapsed trachea, the sound of the tracheitis cough is of a higher frequency. Since tracheitis may be primary or secondary, the history varies with the etiology. In tracheobronchitis (kennel cough) of an infectious nature, the patient has had some exposure to other animals in a kennel or hospital situation. Exposure to animals at dog shows may also result in this disease. Usually, coughing with tracheobronchitis develops three to five days after the initial exposure to the virus. In tracheitis associated with respiratory tract infections, there are the auscultable rales of pulmonary interstitial and alveolar disease. When pneumonia has occurred previously, tracheitis may be a residual lesion that is responsible for the coughing. When a collapsed trachea is the cause of the coughing, the onset may occur at any time; often the owner cannot recall any situation that was responsible for the syndrome.

Most patients with tracheitis are asymptomatic with the exception of a cough. The physical examination is often normal, and no fever is present. Palpation of the trachea near the thoracic inlet elicits the typical tracheal cough. Examination of the oral cavity and oropharynx is unlikely to reveal abnormalities. When chronic coughing has been present, the tonsils may be enlarged and may extend further out of the crypts than normal. There may be an increased amount of phlegm in the caudal region of the pharynx. Since tracheitis may occur secondary to disease of the oropharynx, there may be evidence of pharyngeal or laryngeal disease upon careful examination of these regions. Auscultation of the heart is usually within normal limits unless chronic mitral valvular fibrosis is responsible for a systolic murmur. Since tracheitis may also develop secondary to chronic cardiac coughing, one must also eliminate this syndrome from the list of differential diagnoses. Snapping of the second heart sound as a result of increased pulmonary resistance may be present over the pulmonic area. Auscultation of the lungs is normal unless the tracheitis is secondary to pulmonary disease. When tracheobronchitis is present, coarse bronchial lung sounds may be auscultated over the entire lung field. Since chronic tracheitis may be associated with cor pulmonale, pulmonary fibrosis, and pulmonary emphysema, a patient with a history of chronic coughing may demonstrate increased vesicular rales, inspiratory and expiratory sibilant sounds, and crackling rales.

Etiology. Most of the common bacterial agents responsible for upper and lower respiratory tract infection also produce inflammation of the trachea. Bacterial tracheitis may develop secondary to viral infection of the respiratory system in conditions such as canine distemper, tracheobronchitis, and the feline pneumonitis complex. (Viral pulmonary disease in the dog and cat is described in Chapters 47 and 48.) The noninfectious causes of chronic tracheitis are probably more common. Prolonged barking can irritate the trachea, and tracheitis may develop. Coughing as a result of a collapsed trachea or cardiac disease may produce a secondary tracheitis. Control of the primary disease may relieve the secondary tracheitis; however, recognition of the secondary syndrome is important, since it may also require therapy. Inhalation of smoke and noxious gases may irritate the tracheal lining, producing a tracheitis. Superimposition of a bacterial infection may occur secondary to the chronic cough caused by irritation. Tracheitis caused by infestation of parasites such as *Filaroides osleri, Crenosoma vulpis,* or *Capillaria aerophile* may also occur.

Other Diagnostic Aids. Tracheitis as a primary disease does not have any specific radiographic features. The radiographic features that occur when tracheitis is secondary to other diseases are discussed under those conditions. Irregularity of the tracheal contour may result when nodules are present owing to parasitic granuloma[12] or nodular hyperplastic tracheitis.[13] These may be outlined with a small amount of positive contrast medium. In cases of chronic tracheitis, the electrocardiogram is essentially normal. Spiking of the P wave (P pulmonale) suggests right-sided heart strain. Hematology and other blood chemical studies are usually within normal limits unless secondary, allergic, or associated diseases are present. Similarly, cultures of the tracheal lining for pathogenic bacteria are often negative. Occasionally, when a pus-like exudative material is found on the tracheal lining, bacterial culture may be positive and specific antibiotic sensitivity testing is then beneficial. Aspiration and examination of the exudate may reveal parasitic ova. Bronchoscopic examination may reveal parasitic nodules typical of lungworms.

Differential Diagnosis. Probably of greatest importance in the differential diagnosis is the recognition of the disease as a primary or secondary problem. In addition, diseases of the oral cavity, pharynx, and respiratory system may cause coughing similar to that of the tracheal cough.

Therapy. Tracheal coughing is usually treated with antitussive and bronchodilating preparations. Many of these preparations also contain expectorants. In most cases, a five- to seven-day course with bronchodilators and broad-spectrum antibiotics is justified for outpatient treatment of the cough. If it becomes apparent that the patient is not responding satisfactorily to medication after a brief trial course, then a more complete examination is indicated. As a minimum, radiographs of the thoracic/cervical trachea and screening laboratory data are then necessary. Table 68–1 lists some of the useful bronchodilator-antitussive combination medications used by the authors. Tracheitis, when caused by bacterial infection, is best treated with antibiotics. When possible, determine the drug of choice by culture and sensitivity testing of the tracheal mucosa. Occasionally, short-term therapy with corticosteroids may be warranted; however, it is important to stress that this provides symptomatic relief only and it may be detrimental to the primary condition (i.e., heart failure or infectious disease). When chronic coughing has been part of the history, nebulization four to six times daily may help to liquefy mucoid material collecting in the trachea. When nebulization is not possible, the dog or cat can be placed in a bathroom with steam produced from a hot shower. This procedure should last 15 to 20 minutes, three times daily. Following either method, gentle coupage of the thoracic wall helps to loosen secretions and stimulate expectoration.

DISEASE DUE TO *FILAROIDES OSLERI* (LUNGWORM)

Filaroides osleri is a worldwide parasitic organism causing a disease seen most often in young dogs under two years of age. It occurs in individual situations but is often seen as a kennel-related problem (especially in Greyhounds).[14] Although most often described in young dogs, it does persist in older animals, often without significant pathophysiologic effects.

Although described as a lungworm, this parasite most commonly affects the region proximal to the tracheal carina. Occasionally it affects the lumen and lining of the larger bronchi, but only very rarely does it extend deeper into the pulmonary system.

Reports of direct transmission through stool and saliva suggest that this metastrongyle may not require an intermediate host to complete its life cycle. Experimental and natural direct transmissions have been demonstrated.[15]

Dogs usually present with chronic, mild to severe (at times) inspiratory wheezing-dyspneic sounds, coughing, and/or debilitation. Panting is usually not prominent except in very advanced cases.

The severity of the clinical signs may be overplayed in the literature. Most dogs seen by the authors experience definite but mild, often nonprogressive respiratory signs. Exercise intolerance does occasionally occur, and coughing is typically characterized as a harsh tracheobronchial sound associated with attempts at terminal retching. A small amount of white to blood-tinged mucus is common, but at times larger amounts of exudate are brought up.

Tracheal sensitivity occurs but physical palpation is not abnormal. Heart sounds are most often normal but may be less apparent when obvious respiratory embarrassment with wheezing, rhonchi, or pulmonary edema is present.

TABLE 68–1. DRUGS USED FOR TRACHEAL DISEASES

Generic Name and Preparation	Trade Name	Dosage
Aminophylline 1½ gr 100 mg tablets	—	5 mg/lb q6–12h as needed
Theophylline elixir 80 mg/tbls capsules 100 and 200 mg	Elixophyllin, Theolixir	5 mg/lb q6–12h as needed
Oxtriphylline 400 and 600 mg SA tablets	Choledyl SA	Similar to aminophylline; reported to cause fewer GI problems
Theophylline with glyceryl guaiacolate 150 mg theophylline 90 mg glyceryl guaiacolate per capsule or tbls	Quibron	1 capsule q8–12h for larger dogs; ¼ to 1 tbls elixir q8–12h for smaller dogs and cats
Aminophylline 1½ gr with ¼ or ½ gr phenobarbital	—	½ to 1 tablet q6–12h
Theophylline 130 mg Ephedrine HCl 24 mg Phenobarbital 8 mg	Tedral tablets	¼ to 1 tablet q8–12h
Hydrocodone bitartrate 5 mg Homatropine methylbromide 1.5 mg per tablet or per tsp	Hycodan	½ to 1 tablet (or teaspoon) q6–24h as needed; may increase dosage if sedative effect does not occur
Hydrocodone 5 mg Phenyltoloxamine 10 mg per tablet or per tsp	Tussionex	½ to 1 tablet (or teaspoon) q6–24h as needed; may increase dosage if sedative effect does not occur
Butorphanol tartrate 5, 10, 25 mg tablets	Torbutrol	0.25 mg/lb q6–12h; may cause sedation
Prednisone 2 mg Trimeprazine 5 mg per tablet or spansule	Temaril-P	1 tablet/20 lb q12h; good for allergic and noninfectious inflammatory coughing (i.e., tracheal collapse)
Guaifenesin 100 mg Dextromethorphan 15 mg per 5 cc	Robitussin-DM	Nonnarcotic; OTC preparation; for temporary antitussive effect. Dosage similar to that for adults and children
Thiabendazole	Mintezol	35 mg/lb/day for 2 days 70 mg/lb/day for 21 days
Levamisole	—	3.5 mg/lb/day for 10–30 days
Ivermectin	Ivomec	1000 μg/lb once a week for 8 weeks

The radiographic examination is helpful if the disease process is extensive and the nodules are very large. The tracheal lining may be diffusely thickened, be interrupted with indistinct solid masses, or show ill-defined, two- to ten-mm semicircular lesions protruding into the lumen (Figure 68–1*A*).[16] This gives the appearance of nodules or growths within the lumen. Radiographic contrast studies are occasionally helpful, but due to the dog's precarious clinical status, direct bronchoscopic examination is safer, more specific, and not as likely to injure the pet. Rigid or flexible fiberoptic scopes that extend into the region of the carina work well. Nodules (one to five mm wide and high and cream colored) are diagnostic and larvae are often seen peeking into the luminal edge of the growth. Brushings and biopsies of the nodules provide a definitive diagnosis (see Figure 68–1*B*). There are multiple nodules involving the caudal one third of the trachea and the initial lumen beyond the carina.[13, 16, 17] Despite reports of surgical removal this is usually not feasible due to the large number of nodules. Removal of a large obstructing nodule potentially may be therapeutic in rare situations.

Larvae are occasionally detected in the feces. Usual flotation methods dehydrate the larvae. The Baermann technique is preferred. Eggs, when seen, are 50 × 80 μ, thin-shelled, colorless, and larvated. The larvae are 230 μ long with a distinct, kinked tail. Both larvae and eggs may be visualized in the sputum and washings from affected dogs' tracheas.

Many drugs have been reported to be effective in treating lungworms, but each has a distinct disadvantage, such as thiacetarsamide sodium, which must be given intravenously twice daily for three weeks.[18] Some clinicians have successfully used thiabendazole therapy.[19] Vomiting is reduced by first administering an antiemetic, and the drug is given as a divided dose twice daily in the food at 30 mg/lb for two days and then 65 mg/lb for 21 days. There are some reports indicating moderate success with diethylcarbamazine therapy. Levamisole therapy orally was successful in a series of young dogs using 3.5 mg/lb daily for 10 to 30 days.[20] Side effects of salivation, vomiting, diarrhea, and restlessness are known to occur with this drug. These may be reduced in intensity with atropine, but the clinician should stop therapy if excessive side effects are present. Because of the lack of success with the previously mentioned drugs, the authors have treated several dogs with oral ivermectin at 1000 mcg/lb once weekly for two months. The nodules were reduced in size but did not resolve entirely. All of these dogs became asymptomatic and continue to thrive. Hearsay reports of success with fenbendazole and albendazole exist, but the authors are not aware of any published confirming reports.

COLLAPSED TRACHEA

There are two types of collapsed trachea, the dorsoventral and the lateral forms. The lateral form is unusual and occurs most commonly after central chondrotomy has been used as a method of treating the dorsoventral form of collapse. Lateral collapse rarely occurs sponta-

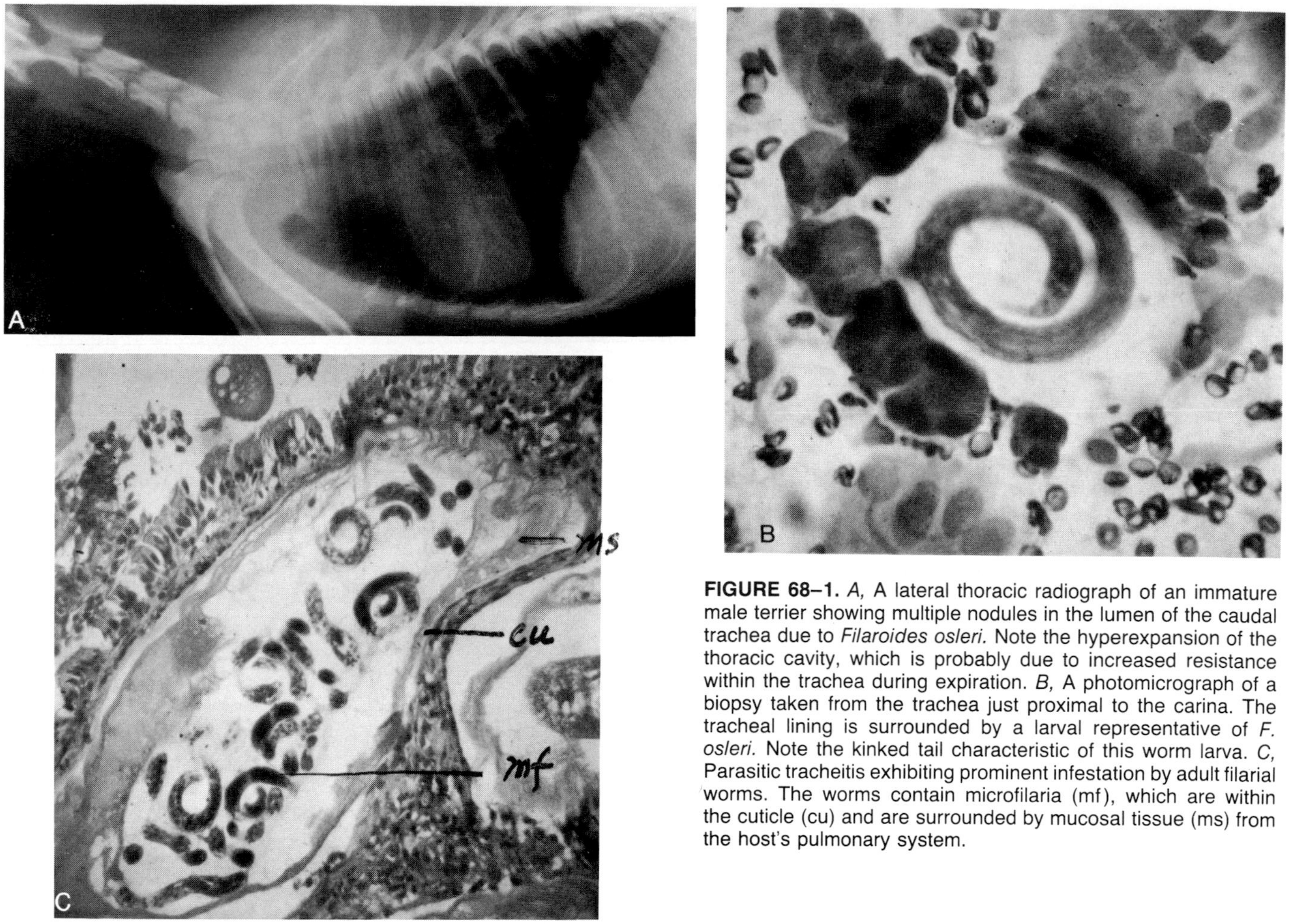

FIGURE 68–1. *A,* A lateral thoracic radiograph of an immature male terrier showing multiple nodules in the lumen of the caudal trachea due to *Filaroides osleri.* Note the hyperexpansion of the thoracic cavity, which is probably due to increased resistance within the trachea during expiration. *B,* A photomicrograph of a biopsy taken from the trachea just proximal to the carina. The tracheal lining is surrounded by a larval representative of *F. osleri.* Note the kinked tail characteristic of this worm larva. *C,* Parasitic tracheitis exhibiting prominent infestation by adult filarial worms. The worms contain microfilaria (mf), which are within the cuticle (cu) and are surrounded by mucosal tissue (ms) from the host's pulmonary system.

neously, although one case was described in a large dog.[21] Dorsoventral flattening (narrowing of the trachea) is a commonly described lesion that is often associated with a pendulous dorsal membrane. In many cases, secondary tracheitis makes treatment of the syndrome difficult. The collapsed trachea may involve the cervical region only, but more commonly both the cervical and thoracic areas of the trachea are involved. Occasionally, only the thoracic trachea is involved and the collapse extends into the bronchi not infrequently. Extension of the tracheal collapse to the bronchi is what is sometimes described as collapsing of the trachea at the carina. This condition has not been reported in cats.

Etiology. The etiology of the collapsed trachea is unknown. The condition, as described, is an acquired disease that usually occurs in middle-aged to aged animals. It has been described in young dogs as a congenital lesion.[22–25] The clinical syndrome and findings in congenital cases are essentially similar to those described in the acquired disease. Congenital collapsed tracheas have been described as malformations of the rings with compression at the thoracic inlet. There may be a dorsoventral flattening of the trachea, with a shallow arc-like formation occurring in the congenital type in the dog.[26] In dogs with acquired collapsed trachea, there is no loss of potential tracheal ring size, but the rings do lose their ability to remain firm and thus subsequently collapse. They become hypocellular and the matrix varies. Glycoprotein and glycosaminoglycan are deficient or totally lacking in dogs with collapsed tracheas.[2] There is a report that the ratio of the width of the trachea to its height was significantly increased in dogs with collapsed trachea as compared with normal dogs.[27] The essential lesion was due to removal of the organic matrix from the tracheal cartilage.

Features. Tracheal collapse produces a syndrome aptly described as a "respiratory distress syndrome."[28] The disease is usually paroxysmal in nature, often with a long history of chronic coughing, occasionally beginning in puppyhood. The cough may be described as chronic, harsh, or dry; if the owner is asked specifically, however, the cough often is described as a "goose honk" sound, occurring initially during the day and occasionally extending into the evening hours.[29] With rare exception, the disease is recognized in toy and miniature breeds, most often Chihuahuas, Pomeranians, toy poodles, Shih Tzus, Lhasa apsos, and Yorkshire terriers. Originally described as occurring most commonly in fat dogs, the authors and others[30] have seen the problem in both fat and thin animals. The condition is observed most commonly in middle-aged to aged animals, developing any time from three years of age onward. It is occasionally associated with chronic mitral valvular fibrosis and must frequently be differentiated from heart failure due to this condition. Often patients in a compensated cardiac state are presented with a cough due to a collapsed trachea. The pressure of the enlarged left atrium on the left main stem bronchus may aggravate or precipitate the tracheal cough, even in the absence of heart failure. The characteristic cough is elicited by excitement, tracheal pressure (such as that caused by pulling on a leash), and drinking water or eating food. Often, the owner indicates that the patient begins to cough when it is picked up or held and when excessive pressure is placed on the thoracic inlet.

One cannot discount a psychological component to this problem. Many dogs have learned that coughing attracts love and attention and use the cough to this end. These animals do not cough while in the hospital, but begin a paroxysm of coughing that is quite dramatic immediately upon seeing the owner.

Physical examination usually reveals a normal dog. Depending upon the state of anxiety and the respiratory distress of the moment, the patient's color varies from normal to cyanotic. The patient is afebrile but may develop a fever with extreme respiratory distress and agitation. Hyperthermia may result if the distress is not relieved. Perhaps the most significant finding during the physical examination is the elicitation of a "goose honk" cough when the trachea is palpated in the region of the thoracic inlet. Occasionally, in moderately thin patients, the dorsoventral compression of the trachea and an angle at the lateral edges of the trachea can be palpated. This is rarely possible in obese dogs. The cardiac sounds vary from normal to those with systolic murmurs associated with either compensated or decompensated cardiac disease. In the normal dog's heart, the second heart sound is less pronounced than the snapping second heart sound that is often auscultated in dogs with collapsed tracheas. The lung sounds vary from normal vesicular sounds to rattling, stridulous sounds associated with sibilant rales and wheezing. In dogs with varying degrees of respiratory distress, inspiratory noises during breathing and an expiratory grunt with an abdominal effort are recognized.

A significant feature of the physical examination is the frequent association of hepatomegaly with collapsed trachea. It has been the authors' continued experience that hepatomegaly occurs in a large percentage of patients with this syndrome. Marked hepatomegaly can result in decreased ventilatory capacity, thus compromising respiratory exchange. Often therapeutic reduction in the size of the liver is associated with a reduction in the degree of respiratory distress and coughing. Although liver biopsies have been made in patients with this collapsed trachea-hepatomegaly syndrome, no specific abnormalities other than hepatic fatty metamorphosis have been recognized.

Additional Examinations. In most uncomplicated cases, there are usually no electrocardiographic abnormalities other than P pulmonale resulting from right-sided heart strain. With the possible exception of dental tartar and enlarged, hyperemic tonsils, examination of the oral cavity is usually normal. Culture of the tracheal lining occasionally produces a common bacterial growth; however, a larger percentage of the dogs cultured for bacteria have no growth. Tracheoscopy reveals a decreased dorsoventral diameter of the trachea with a pendulous dorsal membrane. The lumen, when viewed end on, is described as a flattened ellipse.[28] When passing a tracheal tube from the oropharynx, one is acutely aware that the tracheal diameter and tidal volume increase as the tube is passed beyond the thoracic inlet. In most cases, the tracheal mucous membranes are hyperemic but usually show no exudate. On occasion, a copious, frothy catarrhal exudate is present.[28] In a study of 20 surgically managed cases,[31] 30 per cent of the dogs were observed to have laryngeal paresis or paralysis. This high figure does not correlate with the large number of dogs that the authors have seen who cough intermittently with this disease for many years. It may, however, represent an important specific subset of patients.

Radiography. Radiographic examination of patients with collapsed tracheas requires both still and motion studies. The trachea and liver should be examined on DV and lateral radiographs of the thorax and cranial abdomen. Separate VD and lateral radiographs of the cervical and cranial thoracic regions should be obtained

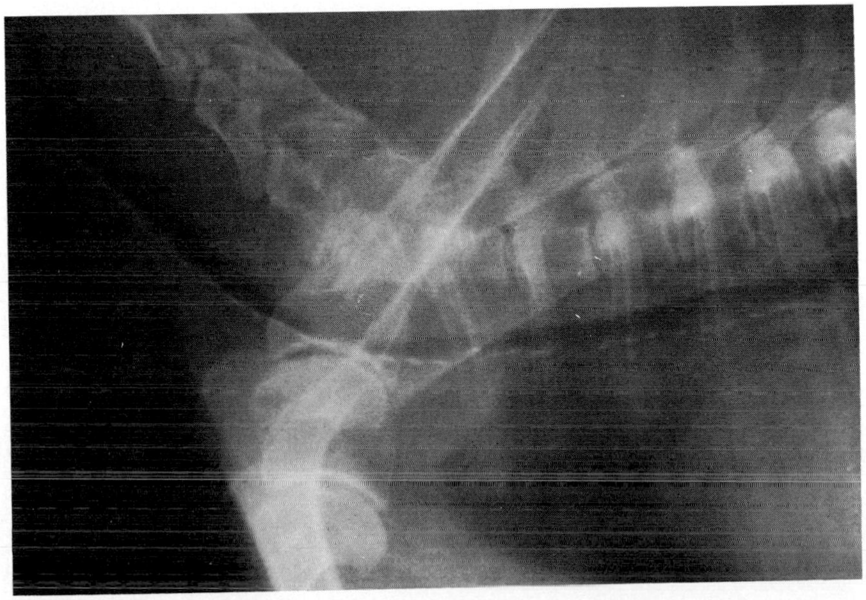

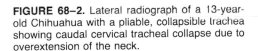

FIGURE 68–2. Lateral radiograph of a 13-year-old Chihuahua with a pliable, collapsible trachea showing caudal cervical tracheal collapse due to overextension of the neck.

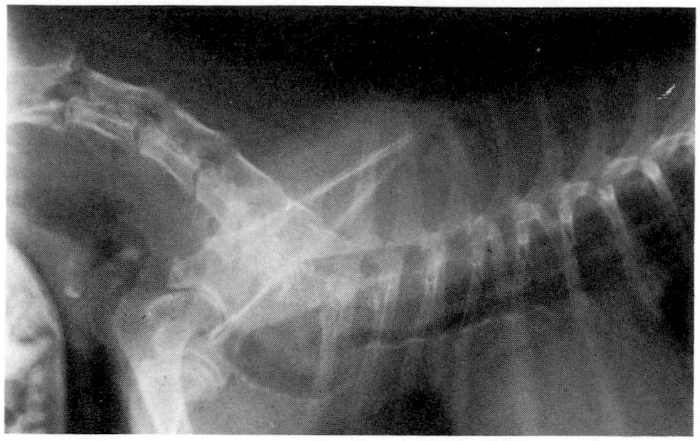

FIGURE 68–3. The "kinking" of the trachea that may occur with excessive flexion of the neck. These undesirable causes of narrowing of the trachea must be avoided while the dog is being x-rayed and, more importantly, during recovery from an anesthetic.

to assess the contour of the trachea. At times, lateral radiographs made during both the maximum inspiratory phase and expiratory phase of the respiratory cycle are needed to demonstrate a collapsed trachea. If both the cervical and thoracic trachea are collapsible, the inspiratory study usually shows collapse of the cervical segment and dilation of the thoracic segment. Conversely, the study made on expiration usually shows a collapse of the thoracic segment (and occasionally stem bronchi) and an unchanged or dilated cervical segment. Occasionally, a "sky line" view of the trachea at the thoracic inlet is helpful in diagnosing the disease. Care should be taken not to overflex or overextend the occipito-atlantal articulation when obtaining the lateral views, since this may produce pressure on the trachea that can cause narrowing of the lumen (Figure 68–2) or an abnormal tracheal course in the caudal cervical or thoracic region (Figure 68–3). There is also a subtle loss of

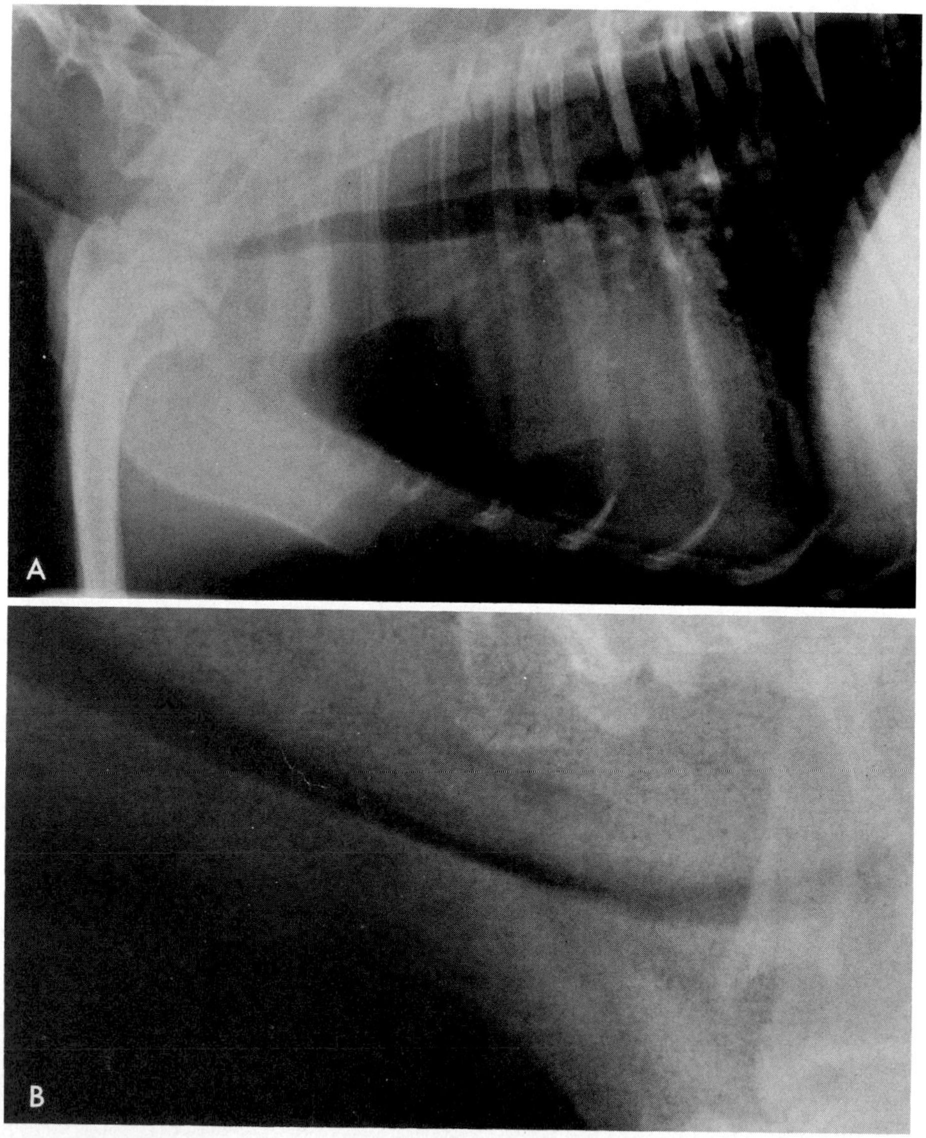

FIGURE 68–4. *A,* Lateral radiograph of an eight-year-old male Yorkshire terrier with collapsed cervical trachea. *B,* 100-mm spot film of the cervical trachea showing generalized narrowing. Dynamic studies showed that the thoracic trachea remained unchanged during the respiratory cycle.

radiographic detail at the dorsal lumen margin, which is produced by inversion of dorsal tracheal membrane. The ventral margin of the tracheal lumen remains well demarcated and is unaffected by the collapsing process. The collapsed region usually involves approximately one-third of the tracheal length, and the extremities of the collapse blend into the normal lumen size over a distance of 2 to 3 cm (Figure 68–4). The course of the trachea is usually unaffected in uncomplicated cases. DV or VD views of the thorax usually show no demon-

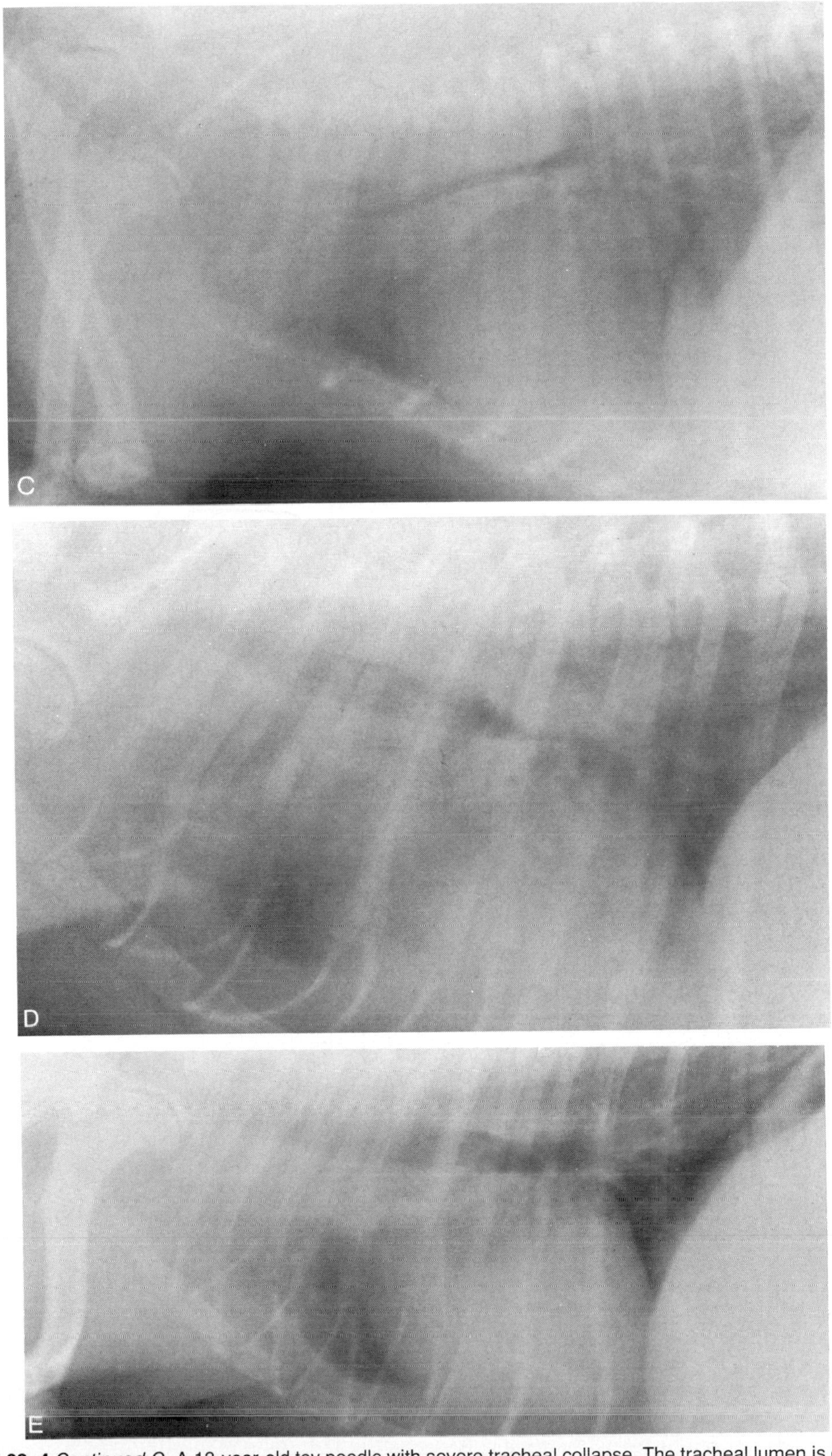

FIGURE 68–4 *Continued C,* A 13-year-old toy poodle with severe tracheal collapse. The tracheal lumen is completely collapsed at the thoracic inlet during portions of the respiratory cycle. *D,* A ten-year-old Shih Tzu with collapsed stem bronchi on expiration. *E,* Same dog as in *D,* with open bronchi during inspiration.

strable changes in the trachea; however, concomitant lung disease may be seen, especially when bronchitis is present. Patients with a collapsing trachea may show radiographic evidence of severe obesity or hepatomegaly, which adds to the complexity of the syndrome. Motion studies of normal respiratory function and cough, using image intensification fluoroscopy, should be made in order to assess the severity of the lesion. Severe cases may show collapse only during the forced expiration due to coughing. Slow-motion studies of videotape recordings are often helpful in delineating the magnitude of the collapse, especially when produced by coughing.

Differential Diagnosis. The differential diagnosis of collapsed trachea requires consideration of such common conditions as tonsillitis, laryngeal collapse, stenosis of the nares, eversion of the lateral ventricles, elongation of the soft palate, bronchitis or primary tracheitis, foreign body tracheitis, and decompensated chronic mitral valvular disease. The list of causes of coughing that could be confused with collapsed trachea is extensive (see Chapter 18).

Treatment. The majority of cases can be successfully treated symptomatically. Bronchodilator preparations containing expectorants and sedatives usually suffice to control this disease (see Table 68–1). Nebulization or vaporization provides additional relief. In some cases hospitalization with sedation for a period of several days, associated with corticosteroid therapy and nebulization, helps to reduce the degree of tracheitis. Occasionally, when other therapy fails, the authors have found that digitalization, for some unexplained reason, can be of assistance in controlling this cough. It is important to recognize that other disease states, specifically chronic lung disease and hepatomegaly, may be present. The authors have noted that the treatment of patients with special diets for lipoprotein abnormalities associated with fatty infiltration of the liver helps in the medical management of the collapsed trachea syndrome in selected cases. In obese patients, weight loss is a primary objective. Several authors have reported on the surgical correction of this condition.[1, 30, 32, 33, 64] In the authors' experience, the use of central chondrotomy has been ineffective in controlling this disease. Plication of the dorsal tracheal ligament has been used to shorten the gap between the free ends of the tracheal cartilage.[34] The authors wish to reemphasize the need for effective and intensive medical therapy in this condition. Although there are a few favorable reports on the surgical correction of this disease, the surgeons with whom the authors have been associated have suggested that this may be due to individual surgical technique and/or experience with these procedures. It seems that if surgical intervention is necessary, it should be performed by a surgeon who has obtained good results with prior cases. Other surgical methods have been described and include tracheal ring prostheses[1] and intraluminal Silastic devices.[1, 35, 36] These efforts do not resolve the problem of main stem bronchial collapse and usually do not effectively resolve even isolated thoracic inlet disease. Tracheal resection and anastomosis has been reviewed.[1, 37] It may be that the favorable results reported by others reflect the fact that these patients were treated medically postsurgically with the drug therapy, hospitalization, sedation, and enforced cage rest that the authors often find to be effective without surgery.

SEGMENTAL TRACHEAL STENOSIS

Segmental tracheal stenosis is an unusual condition affecting small animals. It may occur as a congenital lesion or it may result from trauma to the trachea.[38] The syndrome produces respiratory distress with stridorous respiratory sounds and the subsequent development of cyanosis. Secondary upper respiratory tract infections result and develop into overwhelming pulmonary disease. This complicates the primary condition and is likely to be responsible for the death of the patient. Stenosis of the trachea has occurred at the site of a tracheotomy performed when the affected animal was young.[39] In that patient, the area about the tracheotomy site failed to grow and developed to only one-third the size of the adult trachea. Necrosis of the cartilage and thickening of the tracheal wall developed in a 12-year-old dog, possibly as a result of excessive endotracheal cuff pressures during a prior surgical procedure.[40] The condition was surgically corrected by removal of a 2 cm segment of fibronecrotic trachea. A four-ring segment of trachea that was stenosed to a three-mm diameter following experimental thoracic surgery in a German shepherd has been excised.[41] The authors have observed tracheal stenosis following recovery from bite wounds of the cervical trachea (Figure 68–5).

In a six-month-old Siberian husky an intrathoracic tracheal stricture of unknown cause was surgically corrected. This dog later required a second surgery to correct progressive, multifocal, fibrotic strictures of the respiratory tree. A specially designed harness (martingale-type) using adhesive separately around the thorax and muzzle was recommended for use during treatment to limit extension of the neck during tracheal healing.[42] The adhesive was attached over the muzzle and head on the midline and along the right and left sides by gauze. Tracheal resection in the dog was recently reviewed, describing both the split cartilage and the annular ligament techniques.[1, 38]

An eight-month-old cat presented for dyspnea was reported to have an area of web-like granulation tissue that caused a tracheal stenosis at the level of the fourth intercostal space. The cause of the lesion was unknown.[43] Two young cats with constricted lumens of the trachea cranial to the thoracic inlet were described. One author identified these as tracheal collapse but they fit best into the segmental classification. In one case, histopathology was normal, but in the second, squamous metaplasia was observed. Both cats were middle-aged males.[44]

HYPOPLASTIC TRACHEA

The hypoplastic trachea syndrome is a congenital defect resulting in inadequate growth of the tracheal rings. The condition varies from mild to severe, the severity determining the prognosis for long-term survival of the patient. The condition was first described in 1972, although the congenital tracheal collapses previously reported by others may have actually been hypoplastic tracheas.[5]

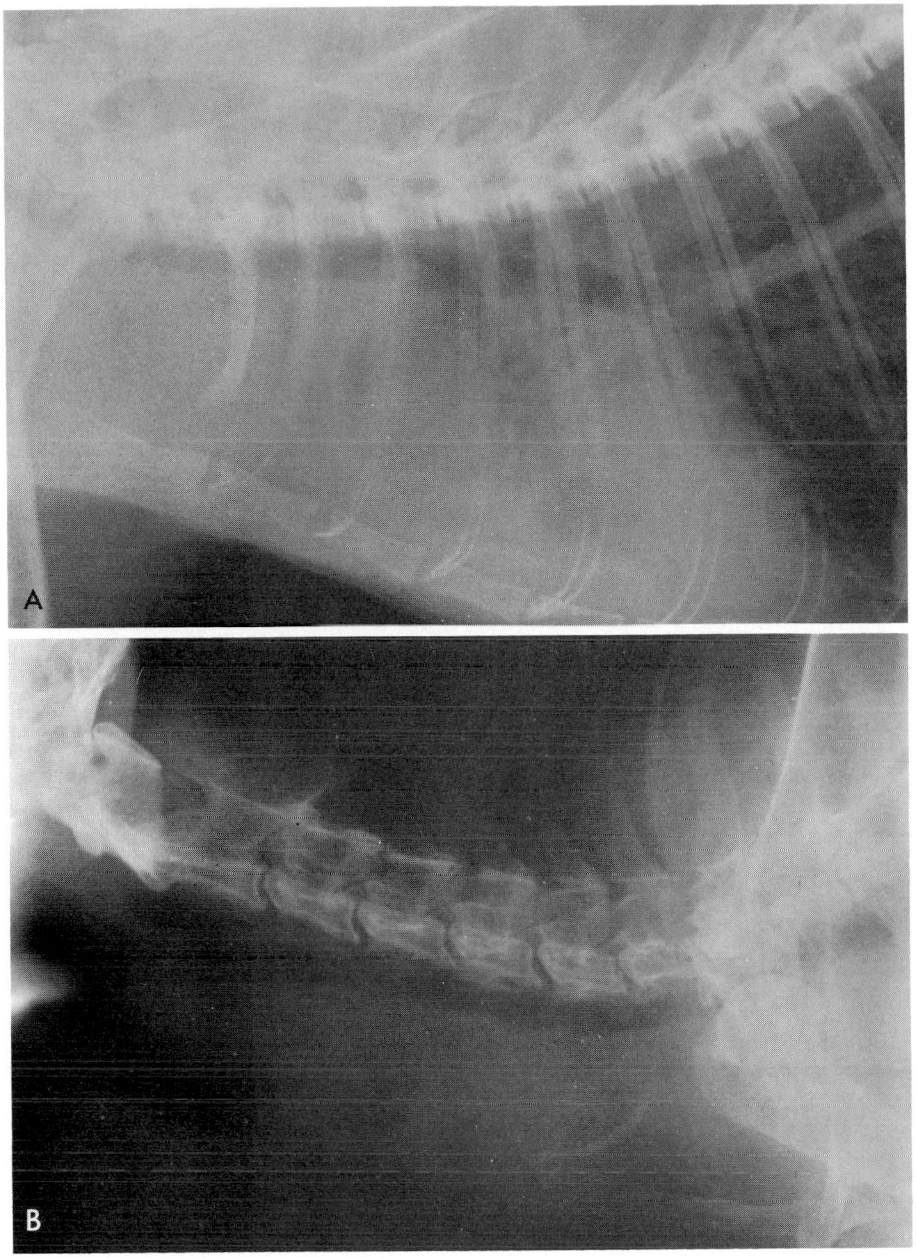

FIGURE 68–5. *A*, Lateral thoracic radiograph of a seven-year-old male poodle that had acquired a tracheal tear in a dog fight six weeks earlier. There was an open, contaminated wound that healed by secondary intention and resulted in a partial stenosis at the level of C3–C4. *B*, Same patient five weeks after resection and anastomosis.

Features. This congenital disease state is recognized primarily in young, brachycephalic animals. The first complete report involved a series of dogs, most of which were English bulldogs.[5] The condition is associated with secondary respiratory tract infections. Other congenital abnormalities may be associated with this problem. The clinical features of a hypoplastic trachea are those of bronchopneumonia associated with a moist, productive cough, auscultable moist rales, and a fever. Although acute bronchopneumonia is intermittent and relapsing, chronic respiratory distress and coughing are likely to occur continuously. Physical examination reveals a sensitive trachea that, when palpated, evokes coughing. Excitement increases or exacerbates the episodes of coughing. Except during periods of acute bronchopneumonia, coughing is usually more severe and serious during the day. Most cases of hypoplastic trachea are treated initially as an upper respiratory tract infection, usually with an adequate response to antibiotic and bronchodilator therapy. However, frequent relapses are common, especially as the animal grows in size while the trachea remains abnormally small. Except for the history and the frequent, recurrent episodes of upper respiratory tract infection, there are no other obvious clinical features. The heart sounds, unless associated with congenital cardiac defects, are normal. Clinical pathology reveals a leukocytosis with a left shift during acute exacerbations of the bronchopneumonia. The radiographic features are the most important and usually provide the definitive diagnosis for this syndrome (Figure 68–6). DV and lateral radiographs of the thorax and VD and lateral views of the cervical region should be obtained to assess the tracheal diameter and the pulmonary changes that are often associated with hypoplastic trachea at the time the patient is presented for examination. Pneumonic signs are often responsible for the owner's concern. The diameter of the trachea at the third rib as seen on the lateral view should be approximately three times the width of the third rib at the level of the trachea.[5] Another method of determining normal tracheal diameter uses the ratio of the inner diameter of the trachea at the thoracic inlet to the distance between the ventral edge of the first thoracic vertebra and the dorsal edge of the manubrium. The normal ratio is 0.16 or greater.[6] Precise measurement of tracheal lumen diameter may be difficult, owing to decreased radiographic detail in the cranial mediastinal region, especially in the brachycephalic breeds and particularly in young animals. Detail may be increased by the addition of a positive contrast medium such as a barium sulfate suspension or an organic iodine solution. Contrast studies are particularly useful in differentiating

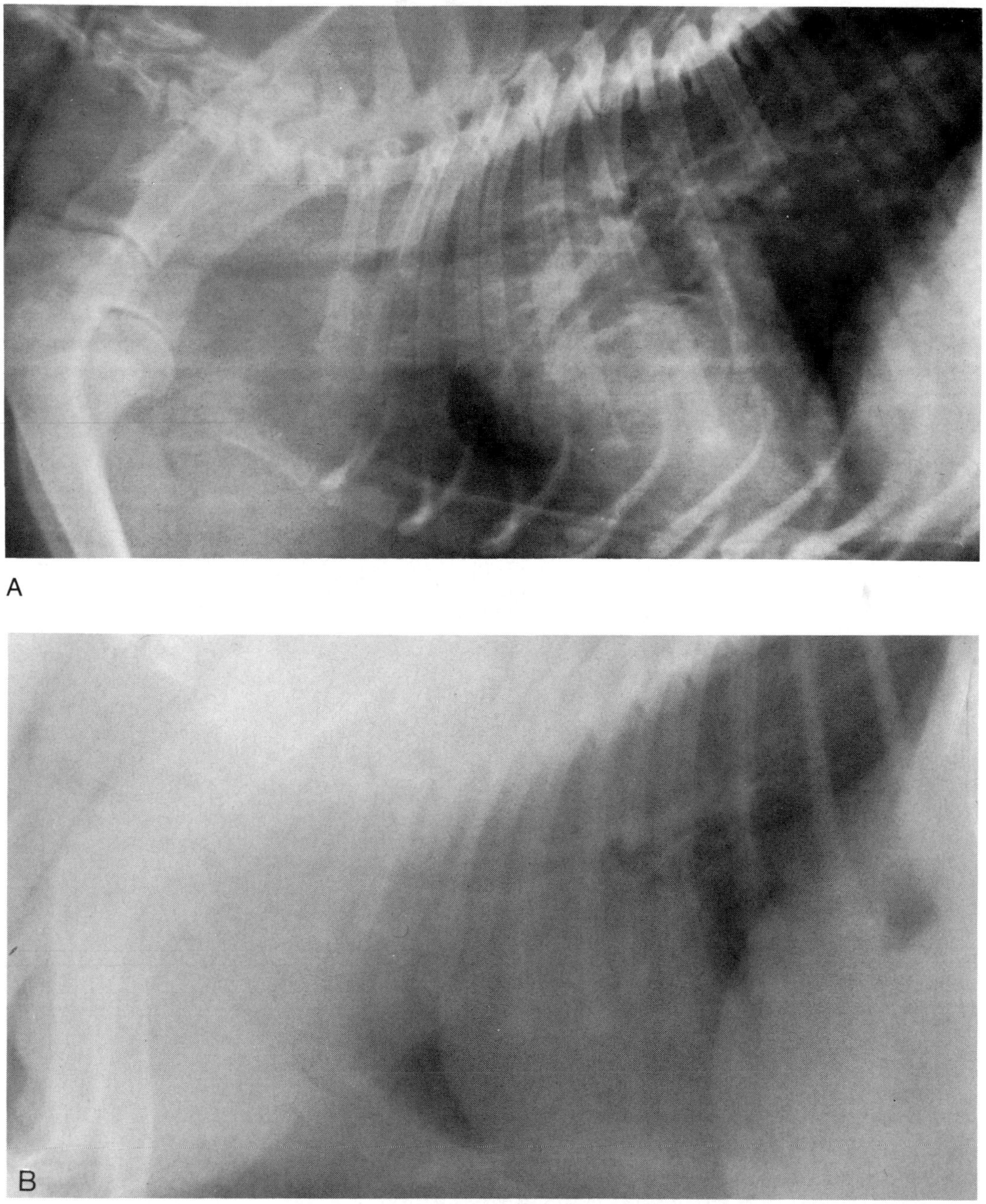

FIGURE 68–6. *A,* Lateral cervical and thoracic radiograph of a one-year-old female bulldog. The radiograph of the thorax clearly demonstrates a markedly hypoplastic trachea, in addition to pulmonary changes suggesting bronchitis. The ratio of the tracheal diameter to the height of the thoracic inlet was 0.07. The normal ratio is 0.16 or greater. The indistinct outline of the trachea is due to the accumulation of large amounts of mucus in the trachea. *B,* Hypoplasia of the trachea in a four-month-old female boxer presented with a productive gagging cough and moderate respiratory distress. Lateral thoracic radiographs show a severely hypoplastic trachea. The ratio of the tracheal diameter to the height of the thoracic inlet was 0.05. *C,* Same dog as in *B* at 11 months of age, when the ratio had increased to 0.06; there was a marked improvement in the clinical condition. *D,* Same dog as in *B* and *C* at two years of age. The ratio had increased to 0.12 and the patient was clinically normal for the breed. (Courtesy of Dr. Lawrence E. Stickles, Santa Cruz, California.) *E,* A four-month-old female Great Dane. A lateral radiograph of the cervical region demonstrates severe hypoplasia of the trachea. Presumably the trachea was injured during the previous anesthetic episode.

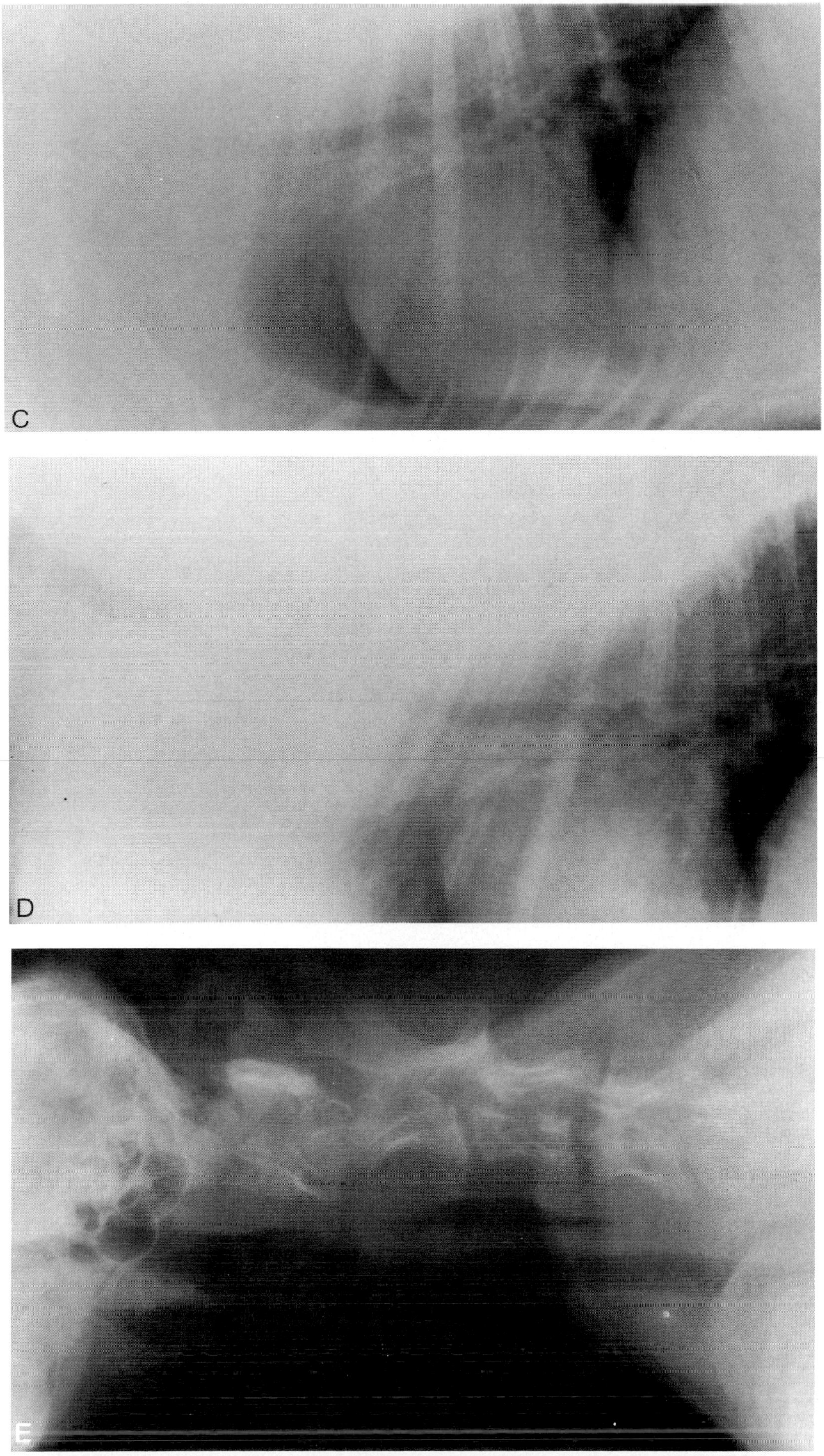

FIGURE 68–6 *Continued*

hypoplastic trachea from segmental tracheal collapse or stenosis. Fluoroscopic control of contrast media administration is desirable in patients with hypoplastic trachea, since overfilling and alveolarization of media may decrease the respiratory exchange of the compromised patient. Motion studies are helpful in differentiating hypoplastic trachea from segmental collapse, since variation of lumen size does not occur during the respiratory cycle in patients with severe hypoplastic trachea.

Prognosis and Therapy. The prognosis for dogs with a hypoplastic trachea depends on the degree of hypoplasia. Many patients with slightly hypoplastic to even moderately hypoplastic tracheas can live normal, satisfactory lives with only an occasional need for bronchodilator therapy and antibiotics. It is important to prevent bronchopneumonia from developing by keeping the affected animal in a draft-free environment and preventing excessive exposure to moisture and cold. Prevention of excessive weight gain helps the animal by limiting the strain placed on the respiratory system by obesity. When recurrent upper respiratory tract infections occur, the use of antibiotics is in order, preferably determined by culture and sensitivity testing. Antibiotics should be used only when indicated rather than on a continual prophylactic basis. In some dogs, regular intermittent therapy with antibiotics (three to five days every three weeks) has proved successful. Since the syndrome affects primarily the brachycephalic breeds, it is advisable to discourage breeding animals with this condition. There is no evidence at this time indicating that the lesion is hereditary, however. There are no known surgical corrective procedures for the treatment of hypoplastic trachea.

OBSTRUCTIVE TRACHEAL DISEASE AND FOREIGN BODIES

Tracheal foreign bodies are not common in clinical situations. When they do occur, foreign bodies are usually small enough to pass beyond the tracheal bifurcation, causing the subsequent development of inhalation pneumonia. When foreign bodies are reasonably large, they are likely to come to rest at the carina (tracheal bifurcation). Dogs and cats may inhale pebbles, nails, marbles, pins, and grass awns into the trachea and bronchi. There are numerous case reports in the literature that describe other, similar inhaled objects. Tracheal obstructions are also uncommon, although they occur more frequently than tracheal foreign bodies. Pathologic conditions responsible for tracheal obstruction include laryngeal paralysis (see Chapter 82); cancer of the larynx; thyroid and parathyroid tumors; enlargement of the mandibular, retropharyngeal, or prescapular lymph nodes due to infection, neoplasia, or granuloma, such as histoplasmosis[45] or coccidiomycosis;[46] peritracheal abscesses and cysts; and tracheal ring neoplasia (see Tracheal Neoplasia), cranial mediastinal masses, thymomas, esophageal tumors, or esophageal granulomas secondary to *Spirocerca lupi*. Nodular amyloidosis in the trachea of a dog has been reported.[47]

Features. Stridor and loud rhonchi (rattling in the throat) are indicative of obstruction of a large air passage and indicate the need for laryngoscopy and bronchoscopy.[48] Chronic coughing may occur as frequently as stertorous breathing. Respiratory distress and dyspnea are usually obvious to the owner. Pulmonary edema develops in more advanced states. In most instances, these conditions do not respond to symptomatic therapy, and the animal's condition continues to deteriorate despite continued intensive symptomatic treatment. Coughing is the most common complaint associated with *Histoplasma*-induced tracheobronchial lymphadenopathy in dogs.[45] Continued signs of coughing, dyspnea, and stridor in the absence of a known cause are a definite indication for radiography of the thorax. Bronchoscopy is another tool that may reveal information relevant to the etiology of the signs of upper airway obstruction. Another sign that occurs in association with tracheal obstruction is vomiting or regurgitation. Animals with cranial mediastinal masses are often presented for regurgitation or dysphagia. Frequently this is associated with severe retching. At times, the spasms are so severe that cyanosis, syncope, and seizures may develop. The latter are of brief duration and are precipitated by attempts at swallowing food. Thyroid hyperplasia and neoplasia in the dog are commonly associated with coughing and dysphagia. In the cat, these signs are uncommon, as the mass apparently does not restrict the tracheal lumen.

Radiographic Examination. Tracheal foreign bodies have varying degrees of radiopacity, but since the air in the tracheal lumen provides a ready-made contrast medium, radiographic detection of radiodense objects is seldom difficult. Inhaled foreign bodies that allow respiratory function that is compatible with life are generally small enough to pass caudally through the entire length of the trachea to become lodged at the carina or in one of the main stem bronchi. A valve-like action develops at the obstruction site so that inhalation of air is prevented, but exhalation occurs, resulting in atelectasis of the obstructed lung lobes. Transudation of serous fluid into the bronchi distal to the obstruction occurs with consequent loss of the outline of the foreign body owing to the displacement of the surrounding air contrast. Relatively radiolucent foreign bodies are thereby rendered invisible to radiographic examination. Dorsoventral and both left and right lateral radiographic views are necessary to evaluate the changes caused by obstructive foreign bodies. Atelectatic lung lobes appear as consolidated masses with lobar distribution. These are better visualized when the lesion is on the nondependent side in lateral projection. Air bronchograms are not seen. The subsequent lobar volume loss results in a mediastinal shift toward the collapsed side owing to overexpansion of the normal lobes. The cardiac silhouette also shifts. Pleural effusion may occur in chronic cases. Extraluminal masses causing obstructive tracheal disease are generally recognized radiographically as linear decreases in lumen diameter over a length determined by the size of the mass (Figure 68–7). These masses usually occur dorsal or lateral to the trachea but may also be found ventrally or circumferentially (Figure 68–8). Esophageal barium-contrast studies may be helpful in delineating the extent of the lesion (Figure 68–9). Motion studies of barium swallows may also be desira-

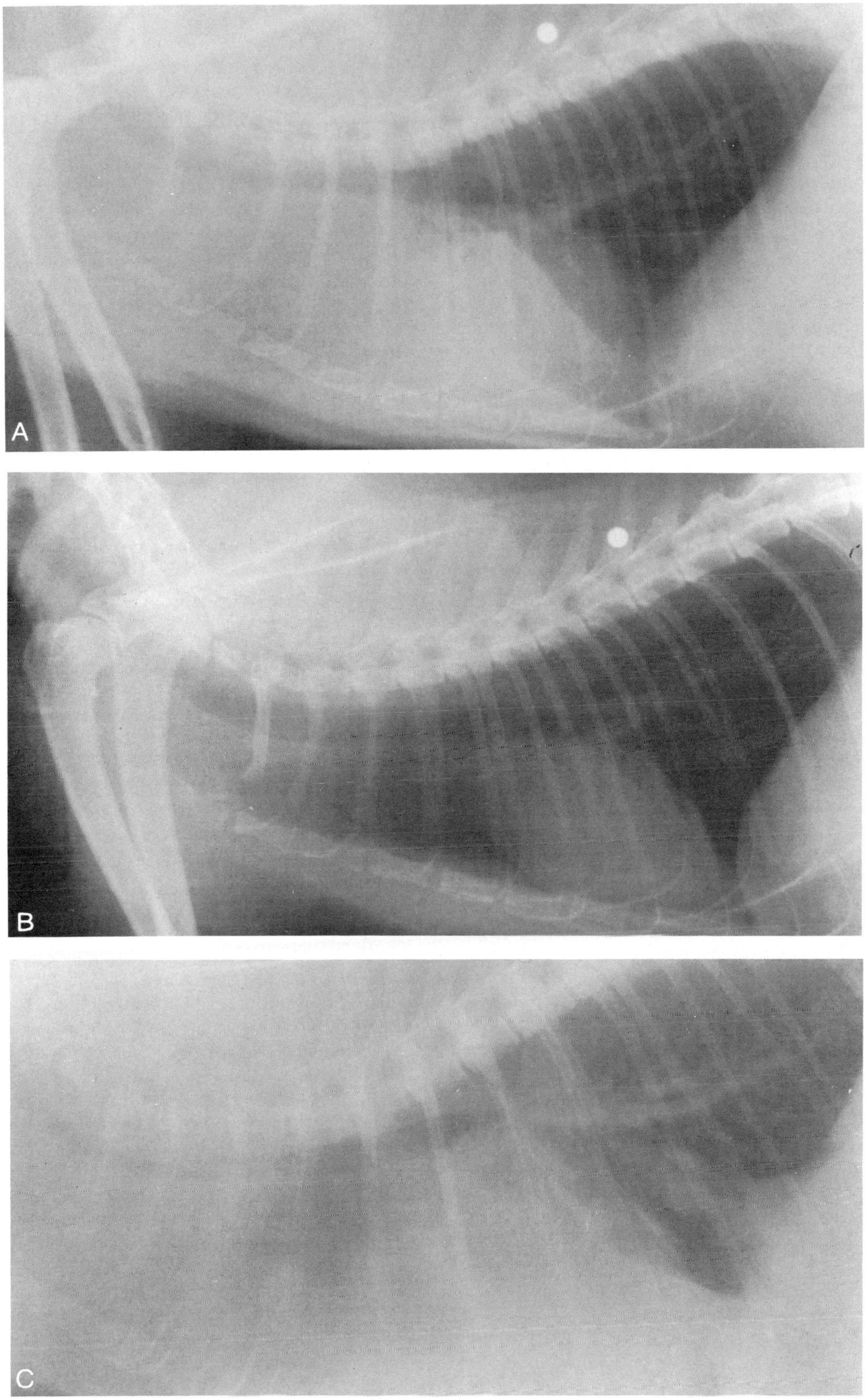

FIGURE 68–7. *A,* A lateral thoracic radiograph of a five-year-old domestic shorthaired cat, presented for dyspnea and emesis, shows an elevation and compression of the trachea at the thoracic inlet along with pleural fluid. The cranial lung lobes are displaced caudally. These signs were secondary to a lymphosarcoma of the cranial mediastinum. *B,* Same cat as in *A,* five weeks after chemotherapy. Notice the reexpansion of the previously compressed trachea. *C,* A lateral thoracic radiograph of an eight-year-old female Burmese cat with pleural fluid secondary to cardiomyopathy. Note that the tracheal elevation is not accompanied by tracheal compression as in the previous case of a mediastinal mass.

ble. Esophageal studies are often needed to differentiate the etiology of tracheal narrowing or displacement in the cranial mediastinal region, particularly in brachycephalic breeds, in which cranial mediastinal masses are often difficult to delineate. Concomitant narrowing of the trachea and esophagus in the cranial mediastinum is highly suggestive of an extraluminal mass.

Treatment. Treatment for upper-airway obstructive disease requires restoration of a normal flow of oxygen to the lung tissue and removal of the obstructive lesion. When a foreign body is recognized, the patient should be held upside down and shaken vigorously to dislodge it. This procedure may be performed using a short-acting anesthetic. Should this method be unsuccessful, the patient is intubated with an endotracheal tube or a tracheotomy is performed. Then, using bronchoscopy and snares, the foreign body is carefully removed from the tracheal lumen, if reactive tissue has not embedded the foreign body. This may also be monitored using fluoroscopic visualization of the procedure. Extreme caution is required to prevent penetration of the tracheal lining. When endoscopic equipment is unavailable or in certain cases in which the equipment is mechanically too large to remove foreign objects, surgical removal through thoracotomy and either an open tracheotomy or a lobar excision is required. A procedure using apical lobectomy may be considered to reach a pin or other object embedded at the tracheal bifurcation.[49] This uses a dissection-extraction technique that permits removal of the foreign object while maintaining normal thoracic surgical ventilation.

In the treatment of obstructive tracheal disease, the use of endotracheal intubation or tracheotomy or both is paramount. If the obstructive site is known to be above the thoracic inlet, an endotracheal tube may be passed below the obstruction, temporarily relieving the clinical signs. When obstructive disease is present, surgical extirpation of the offending mass should be considered. If the obstructing lesion is high in the cervical region, tracheotomy may provide temporary relief for the patient until palliative therapy can be provided. Heart-base tumors may obstruct the trachea (Figure 68–9) and can, in advanced cases, be responsible for chronic coughing, dyspnea, and vomiting. Thymomas or other cranial mediastinal masses are causes of tracheal obstruction that do not benefit from tracheal intubation.

TRACHEAL NEOPLASIA

In the dog, neoplastic disease of the upper airway usually occurs in the nasal passages, whereas laryngeal and tracheal involvement is less common. In cats, laryngeal involvement is quite infrequent and tracheal tumors are very unusual. A squamous cell carcinoma in the trachea was found in a ten-year-old cat presented for dyspnea of a short duration. A middle-aged Siamese cat with progressive dyspnea had a histiocytic lymphosarcoma removed from the midcervical trachea. There was a good response to medical therapy after surgery. Osteosarcoma, adenocarcinoma, squamous cell carcinoma, osteoma, and chondroma have been reported as tracheal tumors.[20, 23, 48, 50–53, 63] A tracheal adenocarcinoma in a seven-year-old cat was aspirated and treated successfully for 17 months. Aspiration was performed via suction during bronchoscopy.[54]

Osteochondroma in the dog was first reported in 1970.[55] Since that report, there have been a number of similar descriptions of tracheal masses with much the same histopathology.[56] All but one case occurred in dogs under one year of age; the other patient was two years old. All cases involved large breed dogs; there was no sex prevalence. On careful evaluation of the histopathology, the authors proposed that these lesions are not osteochondromas or ecchondromas but rather are proliferations that are better described as tracheal osteochondral dysplasias.[56] A primary tracheal chondrosarcoma was reported in a six-year-old German shepherd dog.[57] A tracheal leiomyoma arising from the smooth muscle bands connecting the tracheal cartilages was removed from an aged poodle mix dog.[58] In a tracheal mass obstructing the laryngeal inlet region, the pathology indicated nodular amyloidosis, although the authors were unable to rule out metastatic medullary carcinoma of the thyroid glands.[47]

Features. Most patients with tracheal tumors show signs of upper airway obstruction, i.e., coughing, stridorous breathing, and dyspnea. Occasionally, cyanosis of the mucous membranes or gagging or both may occur. Loud rhonchi are auscultable over the entire cervical region and are transmitted to both the right and left lung fields. In some cases, the tumors are palpable and recognized during the physical examination. In other cases, endoscopy and radiography are required to demonstrate the lesion. In such cases, confirmation of the lesion is made by cytologic examination of the tracheal washings or biopsy of the pathologic tissue.

Radiographic Examination. Tracheal neoplasms decrease luminal size in a nonlinear manner, resulting in a mass protruding into the lumen. These masses are outlined by the tracheal air, which provides a natural contrast medium. Disruption of the mucosal continuity is seen at the base of the neoplasm. This is in contradistinction to the silhouette produced by masses that may be extraluminal, such as enlarged mediastinal or hilar lymph nodes, in which the line produced by the luminal air-mucosa interface is seen to pass uninterrupted through the mass. Positive contrast studies can be performed to increase the specificity of the sign.

Treatment. Surgical correction of artificially induced tracheal abnormalities has been performed with fascia lata, fibrin film, rigid tubes of Pyrex or tallium, polyethylene tubes, and by suturing connective tissue over the defect.[59] The first reported successful surgical correction of a tracheal tumor in small animals took place in 1970.[55] In that case, an osteochondroma involving three tracheal rings and appearing as an intraluminal mass was removed from a one-year-old dog. Teflon mesh anchored with stainless steel sutures to the annular ligament of the cartilages was used in the correction. Muscle tissue was then sewed around the Teflon mesh. A full-blown, endotracheal cuff must be maintained below the surgical site during tracheal repair, to prevent aspiration of blood.[40, 48] Stenosis of the trachea and subsequent res-

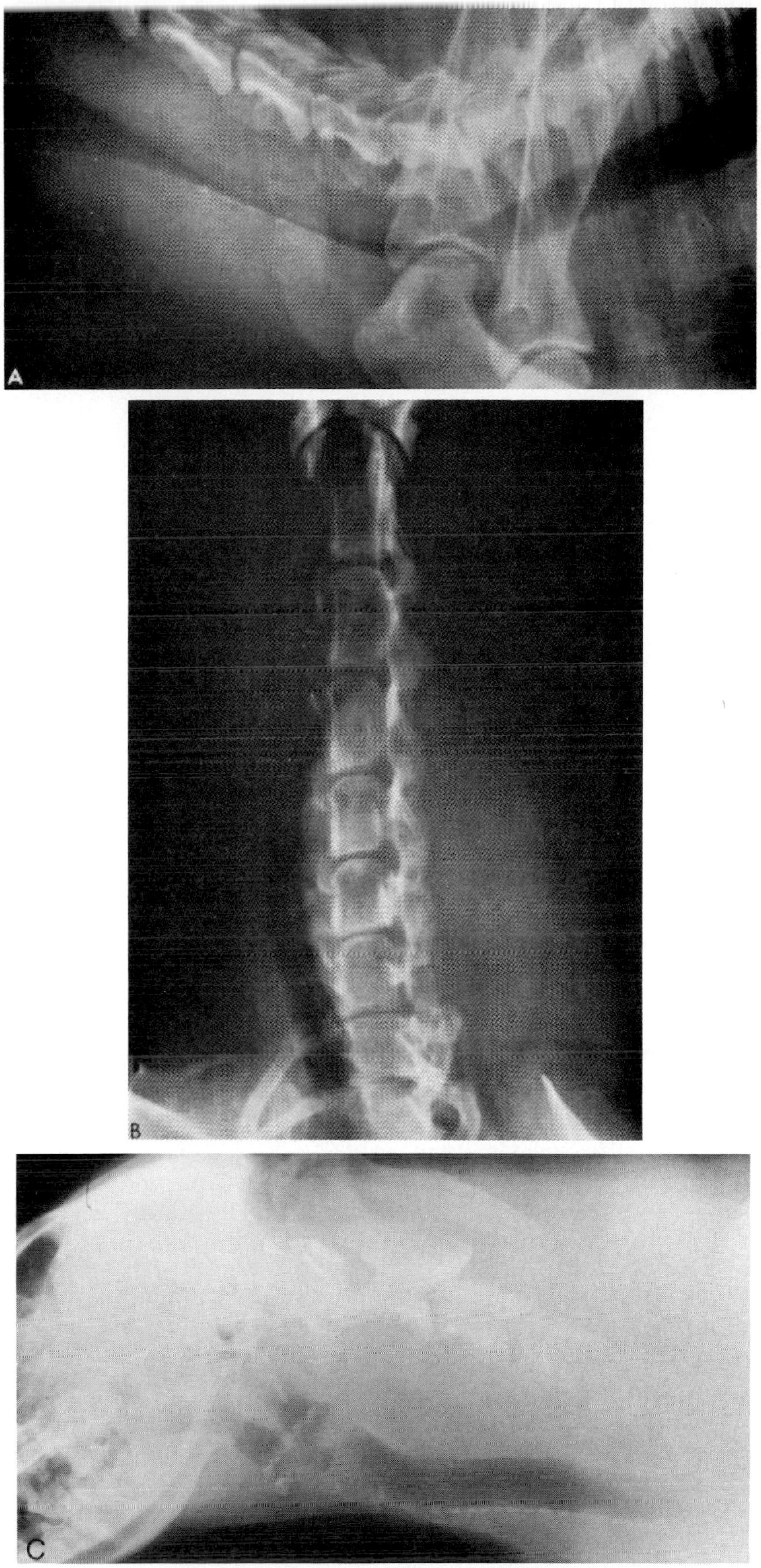

FIGURE 68–8. A middle-aged poodle presented for respiratory distress with coughing and stridor. *A* and *B*, Lateral and dorsoventral radiographs of the cervical region demonstrate the trachea pushed to the right and the collapsing of the trachea. *C*, A lateral cervical radiograph of an eleven-year-old male cockapoo showing ventral displacement of the larynx and trachea due to a thyroid carcinoma.

piratory distress are the major hazards of tracheal surgery. Various techniques have been described in the cases of successful removal of tracheal osteochondral dysplasias (osteochondromas).[56] Tracheal resection and anastomosis with good results, leaving a lumen size of at least 80 per cent of the normal trachea, have been described.[1, 60] These reports stress the importance of not tying knots within the tracheal lumen.

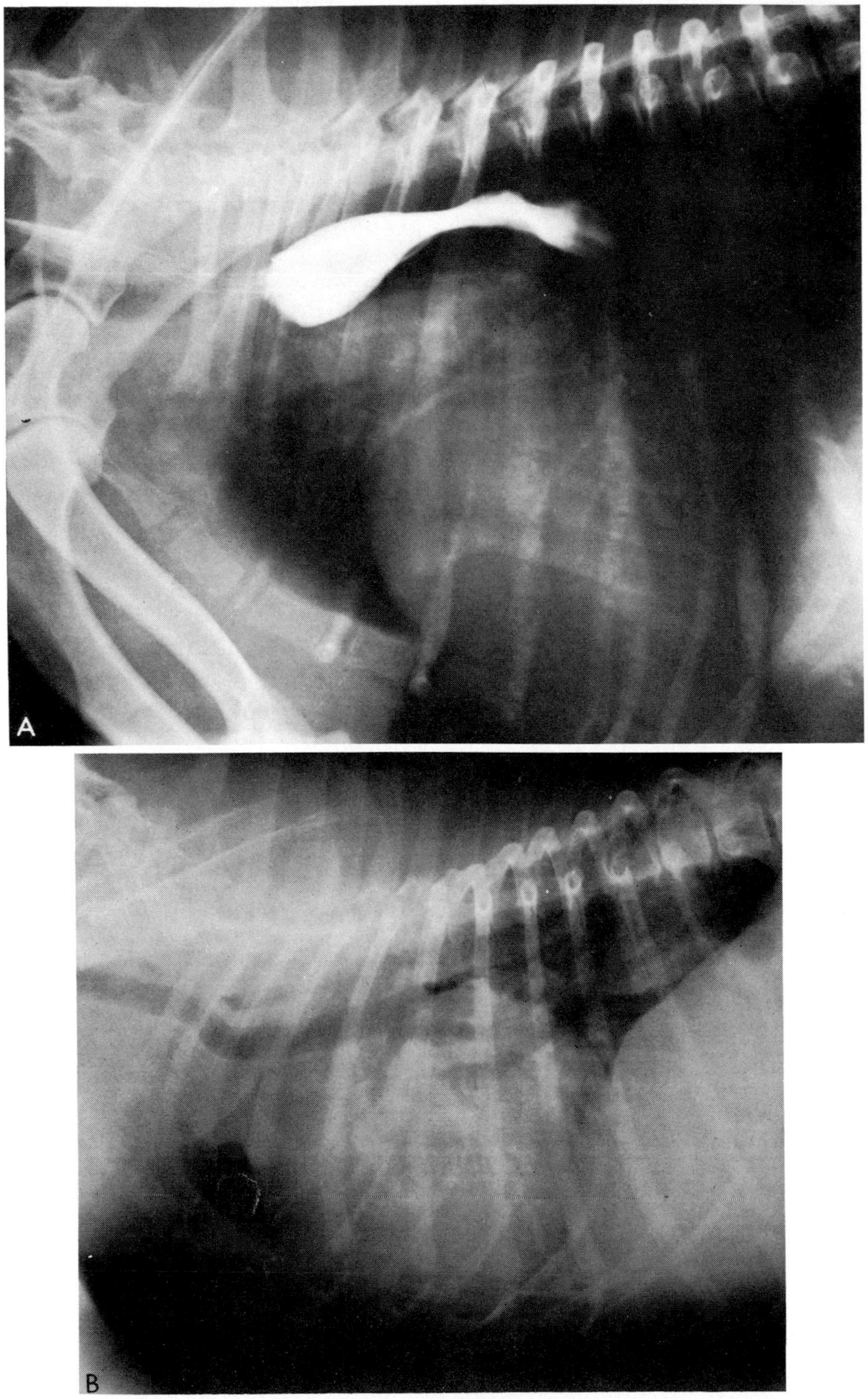

FIGURE 68–9. A 12-year-old male boxer presented for emesis and a rapid, irregular heart rate. *A,* The lateral view of the thorax. Following the administration of oral barium, normal passage of the barium to the level of the base of the heart is revealed. At the base of the heart, the barium courses abnormally in a dorsal direction but continues to flow beyond the heart. Elevation of the esophagus just cranial to and at the base of the heart is suggestive of cardiomegaly or a heart-base tumor or both. *B,* A grossly enlarged and rounded cardiac silhouette and deviation of the thoracic trachea. This film, highly suggestive of pericardial effusion, was taken three months after *A.* After pericardial effusion was confirmed by pericardiocentesis, all of the pericardial fluid was removed. The tracheal bifurcation is outlined owing to a slightly oblique projection.

TRACHEAL TRAUMA

With the exception of lacerations of the tracheal wall resulting in secondary subcutaneous emphysema, traumatic injury to the trachea is an unusual condition in small animals. A ventrolateral tear of the annular ligament produces secondary subcutaneous emphysema over the entire body.[61] This latter condition develops frequently in dogs or cats involved in fights during which a tooth punctures or lacerates the tracheal wall. Air escapes from the tracheal opening and enters the subcutaneous tissue of the neck. In some cases, the subcutaneous emphysema involves only the peritracheal region, although it may become considerably more extensive and involve the entire subcutaneous area of the body. Such tears may also be responsible for the development of pneumomediastinum in both the dog and cat. Subcutaneous emphysema is generally recognized by the crackling sensation of the animal's skin. The tissue beneath the skin appears swollen. The presence of such a lesion should immediately indicate the possibility of a tracheal tear.

Other reports of tracheal trauma are infrequent. A case of tracheal stenosis was described in a dog that had previously undergone surgery for a minor unrelated procedure. Endotracheal intubation was performed, and following this procedure, a cough, dyspnea, and cyanosis developed. Radiographs indicated stenosis of the trachea cranial to the thoracic inlet. During subsequent surgical correction of the stenotic lesion, it was noted that the tracheal epithelium was replaced by fibrous connective tissue. The authors suggested that trauma from endotracheal intubation and excessive pressure on the endotracheal cuff may have been responsible for this lesion.[40] Reconstruction of a short segment of necrotic window of the cervical tracheal tissue with polypropylene mesh was reported.[31] The authors have seen a three-month-old female Great Dane with hypoplastic trachea that was presented in severe respiratory distress two days after being anesthetized and intubated for an ear crop. A large mucosal tear in the cranial aspect of the cervical trachea had created a flap-like obstruction that was dislodged during the placement of an endotracheal tube to relieve the distress. Tracheal hypoplasia should always be considered when intubation is difficult (see Figure 68–6*E*). Damage as a result of blunt trauma to the tracheal rings is a condition that is expected to occur. However, despite the seeming likelihood, the authors have not encountered this lesion. Esophagotracheal fistula is a significant side effect of tracheal trauma in humans, but it is uncommon in small animals.[62]

Radiographic Examination. Fractures of the trachea produce radiographic signs of peritracheal, intermuscular, and subcutaneous emphysema when the lesion is located in the cervical region. Pneumomediastinum may also be present with cervical lesions and when the lesion is intrathoracic. Fractures or lacerations of the trachea or tracheobronchial tree should always be considered in cases of persistent, increasing subcutaneous emphysema when no cutaneous lacerations can be located (see Figure 68–10). Positive-contrast studies, using a water-soluble organic iodide solution instead of a barium suspension, are indicated when the location of the lesion is not obvious from the noncontrast radiographic examination. Post-traumatic tracheal stenosis may usually be located with a noncontrast radiographic examination

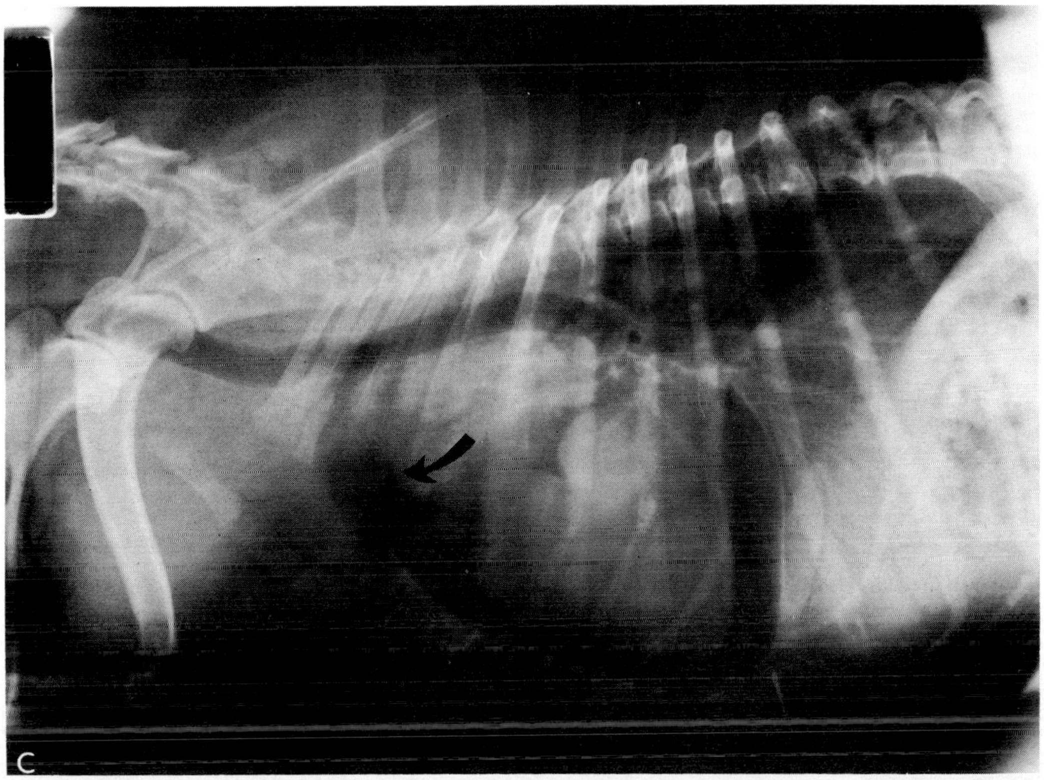

FIGURE 68–9 *Continued C,* A pneumopericardium demonstrates the heart-base tumor (arrow).

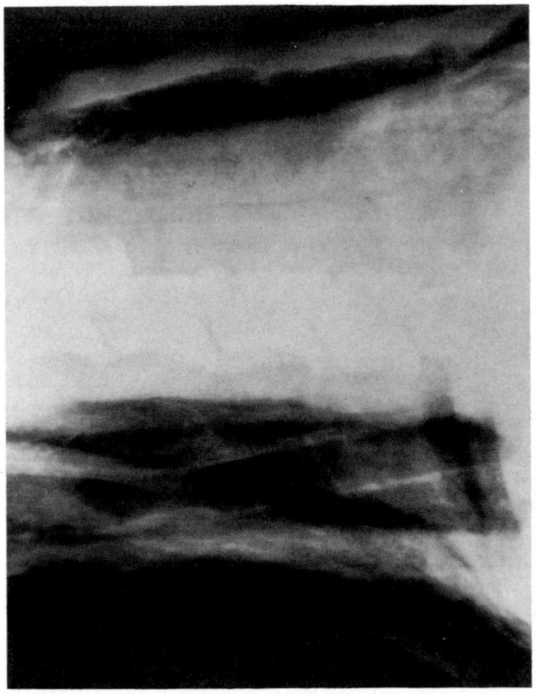

FIGURE 68–10. Lateral cervical radiograph of a ten-year-old male cocker spaniel with tracheal narrowing and rupture at the level of C3 resulting from a dog fight. There is extensive cervical and subcutaneous emphysema with concomitant pneumomediastinum. Note that the outer tracheal wall is visible throughout its length owing to the free extraluminal air providing contrast.

(see Figure 68–5). These lesions produce a segmental narrowing of the lumen with rather abrupt margins.[40]

Treatment. If the subcutaneous air collection is regressing and there are no signs of pulmonary distress, it is usually recommended that the patient be cage rested, allowing the emphysema to regress by slow absorption. If the condition is becoming further aggravated by continued air leakage, then closure of the laceration site is essential. The severity of subcutaneous emphysema may be reduced by aspiration through a large bore needle and wrapping the body with elastic bandages. In most cases, however, this procedure is not necessary. Perhaps of greater importance is the determination of the presence of other pathologic conditions such as pneumothorax or hemothorax. If such a condition is present, the clinician should consider immediate thoracocentesis.

References

1. Hedlund, DS: Surgical diseases of the trachea. Vet Clin N Am 17:301, 1987.
2. Dallman, MJ: Normal and Collapsed Canine Tracheas: A Histochemical, Scanning Electron Microscope and Statistical Study. Dissertation, University of Missouri-Columbia, 1981.
3. Creighton, SR and Wilkins, RJ: Transtracheal aspiration biopsy: Technique and cytologic evaluation. JAAHA 10:219, 1974.
4. VenKer-Van Haagen, AJ: Bronchoscopy of the normal and abnormal canine. JAAHA 15:397, 1979.
5. Suter, P, et al.: Congenital hypoplasia of the canine trachea. JAAHA 8:120, 1972.
6. Harvey, CE and Fink, EA: Tracheal diameter. JAAHA 18:570, 1982.
7. O'Brien, TR: Radiographic Diagnosis of Abdominal Disorders in the Dog and Cat: Radiographic Interpretation. Clinical Signs—Pathophysiology. Philadelphia, WB Saunders Co, 1978.
8. Whitehouse, WM: Bronchography. *In* Potchen, EJ, et al. (eds): Principles of Diagnostic Radiology. New York, McGraw-Hill, 1971.
9. Nelson, SW, et al.: Barium sulfate and bismuth subcarbonate suspension as bronchographic media. Radiology 72:829, 1959.
10. Zontine, W: Bronchography. *In* Ticer, JW (ed): Radiographic Technique in Small Animal Practice. Philadelphia, WB Saunders Co, 1975.
11. Herman, R, et al.: A clinical evaluation of propyliodone bronchography. J Am Vet Rad Soc 13:27, 1972.
12. Carrig, CB: *Filaroides osleri*. JAVMA 166:1007, 1975.
13. DeRick, A, et al.: Tracheal obstruction due to a nodular hyperplastic tracheitis in a dog. J Sm Anim Pract 18:473, 1977.
14. Bogan, JA and Duncan, JL: Anthelmintics for dogs, cats, and horses. Br Vet J 140:361, 1984.
15. Polley, L and Creighton, SR: Experimental direct transmission of the lungworm *Filaroides osleri* in dogs. Vet Rec 100:136, 1977.
16. Suter, PF: Thoracic Radiography: A Textbook. Zurich, 1984.
17. Burrows, D, et al.: Pneumothorax due to *Filaroides osleri* infestation in the dog. J Sm Anim Pract 3:613, 1972.
18. Dorrington, JE: *Filaroides osleri*: The success of thiacetarsamide sodium therapy. J S Afr Vet Med Assoc 34:435, 1963.
19. Hill, BL and McChesney, AE: Thiabendazole treatment of a dog with *Filaroides osleri*. JAAHA 12:487, 1976.
20. Darke, PGG: Use of levamisole in the treatment of parasitic tracheobronchitis in the dog. Vet Rec 99:293, 1976.
21. Binnington, AG and Kreplin, CMA: An unusual lateral tracheal collapse in a dog. Can Vet J 18:190, 1977.
22. Davies, R and Mason, R: Abnormality of the trachea in a dog. Vet Rec 82:191, 1968.
23. Maksic, D and Small, E: Diagnostic radiography of the canine thorax. Vet Med 60:41, 1965.
24. Schiller, A, et al.: Treatment of tracheal collapse in the dog. JAVMA 145:669, 1964.
25. Zook, B and Hathaway, J: Tracheal stenosis and congenital cardiac anomalies in a dog. JAVMA 149:298, 1966.
26. Jubb, K and Kennedy, P: Pathology of Domestic Animals. New York, Academic Press, 1963, p 124.
27. Done, SA and Drew, RA: Observations on the pathology of tracheal collapse in dogs. J Sm Anim Pract 17:783, 1976.
28. O'Brien, J, et al.: Tracheal collapse in the dog. J Am Vet Rad Soc 7:12, 1966.
29. Ettinger, S and Suter, P: Canine Cardiology. Philadelphia, WB Saunders Co, 1970.
30. Done, S, et al.: Tracheal collapse in the dog: A review of the literature and report of two new cases. J Sm Anim Pract 11:743, 1970.
31. Furneaux, RW: Tracheal reconstruction with knitted polyprolene mesh in a dachshund dog. J Sm Anim Pract 14:619, 1973.
32. Leonard, H: Collapse of the larynx and adjacent structures in the dog. JAVMA 136:360, 1960.
33. Leonard, H: Surgical correction of collapsed trachea in dogs. JAVMA 158:598, 1971.
34. Rubin, GJ, et al.: Surgical reconstruction for collapsed tracheal rings. J Sm Anim Pract 14:607, 1973.
35. Hobson, HP: Total ring prosthesis for surgical correction of collapsed trachea. JAAHA 12:822, 1976.
36. Slatter, DH and Pettit, GD: A surgical method of correction of collapsed trachea in the dog. Aust Vet J 50:41, 1974.
37. Lau, RE, et al.: Tracheal resection and anastomosis in dogs. JAVMA 176:134, 1980.
38. Bradley, RL, et al.: Tracheal resection and anastomosis for traumatic tracheal collapse in a dog. Comp Sm Anim Med 9:234, 1987.
39. Potter, B, et al.: Tracheal stenosis as a sequel to tracheotomy. Vet Rec 76:485, 1964.
40. Knecht, C, et al.: Iatrogenic tracheostenosis in a dog. JAVMA 160:1427, 1972.
41. Gordon, W: Surgical correction of tracheal stenosis in a dog. JAVMA 162:479, 1973.
42. Hauptman, J, et al.: Intrathoracic tracheal stricture management in a dog. JAAHA 21:505, 1985.

43. Leonpacher, RJ: Tracheal stenosis in a cat. Mod Vet Pract 57:287, 1976.
44. Hendricks, JC and O'Briend, JA: Tracheal collapse in two cats. JAVMA 187:418, 1985.
45. Ackerman, N, et al.: Respiratory distress associated with histoplasma-induced tracheobronchial lymphadenopathy in dogs. JAVMA 163:963, 1973.
46. Cramlet, SH, et al.: Radiodense mass over the base of the heart compressing the trachea. JAVMA 167:1097, 1975.
47. Dill, GS, et al.: Nodular amyloidosis in the trachea of a dog. Vet Path 9:238, 1972.
48. Brodey, R, et al.: Osteosarcoma of the upper airway in a dog. JAVMA 155:1460, 1969.
49. Eyster, et al.: Surgical removal of a foreign body from the tracheal bifurcation of a cat. JAAHA 12:481, 1976.
50. Cain, JR and Manley, P: Tracheal adenocarcinoma in a cat. JAVMA 182:614, 1983.
51. Moulton, J: Tumors in Domestic Animals. Berkeley, University of California Press, 1961.
52. Veith, LA: Squamous cell carcinoma of the trachea in a cat. Feline Pract 4:30, 1974.
53. Beaumont, PR: Intratracheal neoplasia in two cats. J Sm Anim Pract 23:29, 1982.
54. Neer, TM and Zeman, D: Tracheal adenocarcinoma in a cat and review of the literature. JAAHA 23:377, 1987.
55. Gourley, I, et al.: Tracheal osteochondroma in a dog: A case report. J Sm Anim Pract 11:327, 1970.
56. Carb, A and Halliwell, WH: Osteochondral dysplasias of the canine trachea. JAAHA 17:193, 1981.
57. Aron, DN, et al.: Primary tracheal chondrosarcoma in a dog. JAAHA 16:31, 1980.
58. Bryan, RD, et al.: Tracheal leiomyoma in a dog. JAVMA 178:1070, 1981.
59. Markowitz, J, et al.: Experimental Surgery Including Surgical Physiology, 5th ed. Baltimore, Williams & Wilkins, 1964.
60. Bojrab, MJ and Dallman, MJ: Tracheal resection and anastomosis. Canine Pract 7:69, 1980.
61. Chalifoux, A, et al.: Generalized subcutaneous emphysema in a dog. Mod Vet Pract 53:50, 1972.
62. Stogdale, L, et al.: A congenital oesophagotracheal fistula in a two-year-old dog. J South Afr Vet Assoc 48:212, 1977.
63. Schneider, PR, et al.: Histiocytic lymphosarcoma of the trachea in a cat. JAAHA 14:485, 1979.
64. Anderson, G: Surgical correction of tracheal collapse using Teflon rings. Oklahoma Vet 23:6, 1971.

69 DISEASES OF THE LOWER RESPIRATORY TRACT (LUNG) AND PULMONARY EDEMA*

ELEANOR C. HAWKINS, STEPHEN J. ETTINGER, and PETER F. SUTER

For the purposes of this chapter, lower respiratory tract disease refers to disease of the bronchial tree and pulmonary parenchyma. The presentation, diagnosis, treatment, and prognosis of specific lower respiratory tract diseases will be discussed in categories of bronchial diseases, non-neoplastic pulmonary diseases, and neoplastic pulmonary diseases (Table 69–1). General therapeutic principles which can be applied to the management of most patients with lower respiratory disease will be described initially (Table 69–2).

GENERAL THERAPEUTIC MANAGEMENT OF LOWER RESPIRATORY TRACT DISEASE

Treatment of patients with respiratory disease should be based on the specific disease process and the severity of clinical signs. It is much preferable to alleviate clinical signs by removing the underlying disease process rather than to attempt to counter the body's responses with palliative therapy. A definitive diagnosis should be aggressively sought to allow for specific therapy. However, certain general principles should be considered for all patients showing signs of respiratory disease. These general considerations include oxygenation and ventilation, airway humidification, physiotherapy, and acid-base balance. Bronchodilation, cough suppression, use of expectorants, and nebulization of medications have selected applications for patients with respiratory disease.

OXYGENATION AND VENTILATION

Oxygenation of blood is readily assessed clinically by measurement of the partial pressure of oxygen in arterial blood (P_aO_2). If a blood gas analyzer is not present on site, the heparinized specimen can be transported on ice to a nearby human hospital. Normal P_aO_2 values range from 80 to 100 mm Hg for patients breathing room air. Hemoglobin saturation with oxygen, and thus whole blood oxygen content, does not begin to decrease greatly until the P_aO_2 falls below 60 mm Hg.

Lower respiratory tract diseases can result in inadequate oxygenation due to decreased ventilation, improper matching of ventilation and perfusion within the lungs (V/Q mismatching), and interference with the diffusion of gases across the alveolar membrane. Disease in small animals primarily results in one or both of the first two problems.

Differentiation between hypoventilation and V/Q mismatching can be helpful in managing the hypoxemic patient. Measurement of arterial blood gases and calculation of the gradient of alveolar and arterial oxygen concentrations (A-a gradient) will allow the distinction to be made (Table 69–3).[1,2] Hypoventilation, in general, causes the carbon dioxide tension (P_aCO_2) to become relatively high and the A-a gradient to remain normal. Causes of hypoventilation include: upper airway obstruction; diseases affecting pulmonary or thoracic wall compliance, such as pleural effusion, pneumothorax and extreme abdominal distention; and decreased function of respiratory muscles, as may be seen with lower motor neuron paralysis, coma, or drug-induced suppression

*In this chapter, the section on the lower respiratory tract was written by Eleanor C. Hawkins and the section on pulmonary edema by Stephen J. Ettinger and Peter F. Suter.

TABLE 69–1. LOWER RESPIRATORY TRACT ABNORMALITIES

Bronchial Diseases
- Canine infectious tracheobronchitis
- Feline allergic bronchitis (feline asthma)
- Canine allergic bronchitis
- Chronic bronchitis
- Primary ciliary dyskinesia
- Bronchiectasis
- Bronchial foreign bodies
- Bronchial parasites
- Bronchial compression
- Bronchoesophageal fistulas
- Bronchial mineralization
- Bronchial neoplasia

Non-Neoplastic Pulmonary Diseases
- Infectious diseases
- Viral diseases
- Rickettsial diseases
- Bacterial diseases
- Protozoal diseases
- Fungal diseases
- Parasitic diseases
- Hypersensitivity and immune-mediated diseases
- Eosinophilic diseases
- Mononuclear (granulomatous) diseases
- Traumatic lung diseases
- External trauma (pulmonary contusions)
- Internal trauma (aspiration, near-drowning, smoke inhalation)
- Cystic-bullous disease
- Miscellaneous conditions
- Pulmonary thromboembolic disease
- Obesity
- Congenital abnormalities
- Pulmonary mineralization
- Acute respiratory distress syndrome
- Lung lobe torsions
- Sequelae to pulmonary disease
- Chronic obstructive pulmonary disease
- Emphysema
- Abscessation
- Lobar consolidation
- Atelectasis
- Cor pulmonale

Neoplastic Pulmonary Disease
- Primary pulmonary neoplasia
- Metastatic pulmonary neoplasia
- Lymphosarcoma

Pulmonary Edema

of respiration. Ventilation-perfusion abnormalities are identified by a low P_aCO_2 relative to the degree of hypoxemia, as predicted by a large A-a gradient. Causes of V/Q mismatching include most pulmonary parenchymal diseases.

Therapeutic intervention is recommended when the P_aO_2 declines below 60 mm Hg or the P_aCO_2 rises above 60 to 75 mm Hg.[3, 4] More severe hypoxemia can result in tissue hypoxia, cardiac arrhythmias, mental depression, and eventual loss of consciousness. Carbon dioxide tensions greater than 60 mm Hg can be associated with

TABLE 69–2. THERAPEUTIC CONSIDERATIONS FOR ALL PATIENTS WITH LOWER RESPIRATORY TRACT DISEASE

Oxygenation	Physical therapy
Ventilation	Acid-base status
Airway hydration	

TABLE 69–3. CALCULATION OF ALVEOLAR-ARTERIAL OXYGEN GRADIENT[a, b]

The alveolar-arterial oxygen gradient (A-a gradient) is an estimate of the difference between the concentration of oxygen in the alveoli (P_AO_2) and the actual measured arterial oxygen tension (P_aO_2). Normal values for the A-a gradient are 0–15 mm Hg. Hypoventilation causing hypoxemia will result in a normal gradient. A larger A-a gradient implies ventilation-perfusion abnormalities.

$$\text{A-a gradient} = P_AO_2 - P_aO_2$$

The P_AO_2 is calculated by the following formula, and for an individual patient on room air the variable factor is arterial carbon dioxide tension (P_aCO_2).

$$P_AO_2 = P_IO_2 - P_aCO_2/R$$

P_IO_2 is the oxygen tension of the inspired gas, which for room air at body temperature at sea level is about 150 mm Hg. The value can be calculated more exactly by the equation:

$$P_IO_2 = (P_B - P_{H_2O}) \times F_IO_2$$

PB is barometric pressure (mm Hg)
P_{H_2O} is the partial pressure of water in the air at body temperature (mm Hg)
F_IO_2 is the fractional concentration of oxygen in the air (generally 21 per cent)
R is the respiratory exchange ratio, which varies with diet but is generally assumed to be approximately 0.8.

[a]Amis, TC: Clinical respiratory physiology. *In* Kirk, RW (ed): Current Veterinary Therapy VIII. Philadelphia, WB Saunders, 1983, p 191.
[b]Haskins, SC: Blood gases and acid-base balance: Clinical interpretation and therapeutic implications. *In* Kirk, RW (ed): Current Veterinary Therapy VIII. Philadelphia, WB Saunders, 1983, p 201.

significant hypoxemia, and eventual respiratory depression and narcosis.[3] In the absence of blood gas analysis the presence of cyanosis, muddy mucous membranes, deterioration in mental status, or cardiac arrhythmias in conjunction with increased respiratory efforts are indications for treatment of hypoxemia. Though other factors are involved, such as the red cell mass, cyanosis is generally observed at oxygen tensions less than 50 mm Hg.[1]

Hypoventilation can be corrected with ventilatory support and room air. Increasing the inspired concentration of oxygen may improve oxygenation, but will not correct the hypercapnia and resultant alkalosis.

Hypoxemia resulting from V/Q abnormalities should respond readily to increased alveolar oxygen concentrations achieved by increasing the concentration of inspired oxygen. An exception is with complete shunts, in which case blood flows directly from artery to vein without passing alveoli, and altering alveolar oxygen concentrations will not affect blood oxygenation.

Some pulmonary parenchymal diseases are severe enough that blood oxygen tensions cannot be adequately maintained without prolonged administration of 100 per cent oxygen, which is toxic to the patient, or are associated with collapse of alveoli and decreased compliance. In these situations, positive pressure ventilatory support as well as oxygen supplementation may be necessary.

Oxygen Supplementation. The fractional concentration of inspired oxygen can be increased over that in room air (about 21 per cent) by supplementation, though potential side effects must be addressed. Administration of 50 per cent oxygen for longer than 24 hours, or 100 per cent oxygen for over 12 hours should be avoided due to potentially fatal effects on the lungs. Patients which cannot be maintained on lower concentrations of oxygen should be provided with positive pressure ventilatory support. Humidification is essential if oxygen administration is necessary for more than a few hours to avoid severe airway drying. Ventilation and humidification are discussed later.

Oxygen supplementation can be provided through masks, transtracheal catheters, nasal catheters, oxygen cages, and tracheal tubes. Masks are used for the emergency stabilization of patients requiring oxygen support. They should fit snugly over the muzzle to minimize dead space, and ophthalmic ointment should be applied to protect against corneal drying. Fractional concentrations of 50 to 60 per cent oxygen can be achieved with a properly fitting mask and flow rates of 8 to 12 L/min.[4] Long-term supplementation requires other methods.

Oxygen can also be administered for short periods through an intravenous catheter positioned transtracheally. The catheters are placed using the same technique as for tracheal washings. These systems cannot be maintained for prolonged periods and may result in tracheitis. Fractional concentrations of 30 to 40 per cent can be achieved with flow rates of only 1 to 2 L/min.[4]

Nasal catheters can be used for oxygen supplementation for longer periods of time and allow free movement of the patient's head. The technique has been described for use in dogs.[5] One ml of lidocaine is dripped into the nostril with the nose slightly elevated. A polyurethane or rubber catheter is lubricated with lidocaine jelly and placed in the ventral meatus by aiming the tip dorsomedially and inserting to the level of the carnassial tooth. The external end of the catheter is sutured to the muzzle within one cm of its exit from the nostril. An intravenous administration set is used to connect the catheter to the oxygen source. Fractional concentrations of oxygen of 40 per cent or more can be achieved with flow rates of 25 to 50 ml/lb (50 to 100 ml/kg) body weight using the described method.[5] Potential complications include epistaxis and gastric distension.

Oxygen cages can be used to provide increased oxygen concentrations with minimal stress to the patient. The animal is in a completely isolated environment, and careful attention must be paid to temperature, humidity, and concentrations of oxygen and carbon dioxide within the cage. If these parameters are not controlled, considerable stress can be placed on these fragile patients and death can result. Oxygen cages can usually provide fractional concentrations of 35 to 50 per cent oxygen.[6]

Tracheal tubes can be used to bypass upper airway obstructions and can be cuffed to allow for positive pressure ventilatory support. These tubes can be placed orally, in which case the patient must be unconscious or chemically restrained, or transtracheally (tracheostomy tube). Patients can be restrained for oral intubation with narcotic agents. The addition of diazepam or nondepolarizing muscle relaxants, such as pancuronium bromide, may be needed for additional relaxation or if ventilation is required. Placement of tracheostomy tubes is described in many surgery textbooks and emergency manuals.

Patients maintained with tracheal tubes require careful monitoring and frequent nursing care to prevent obstruction of the tube with secretions since patients generally cannot breathe around their tracheal tubes. Tracheostomy tubes, which have an inner tube that can be removed for cleaning, are preferred over single-lumen tubes that must be suctioned. The frequency of cleaning or suctioning required is dependent on the individual patient, the size of the tube, and the amount of secretions produced. Immediately following placement the tubes should be monitored at least every 30 minutes, but the interval can often be increased to several hours. Sterile saline should be injected through the tube at a rate of 0.1 to 0.2 ml/lb/hr (0.2 to 0.4 ml/kg/hr) every few hours to moisten the mucosa and secretions.[4]

Additional nursing care is required to minimize mucosal damage and infection. The cuff should be deflated and the tube repositioned slightly every few hours to minimize pressure damage to the mucosa. The use of a high volume, low pressure cuff is recommended. The cuff need not be inflated at all if ventilation is not required. To minimize the likelihood of infection, tubes should be replaced at least every 48 hours. All manipulations should be performed using sterile technique, and the tube should be removed as soon as it is no longer required. Nevertheless, infection is common and the tip of the tube should be cultured following removal. Prophylactic antibiotic therapy is not recommended.

If an anesthetic machine is used to deliver oxygen through a tracheal tube, adequate flow rates should be maintained to avoid rebreathing. Minimum oxygen flow should be 2.5 times the minute volume (100 ml/lb/min or 200 ml/kg/min).[4] Fractional concentrations of up to 100 per cent can be delivered.

Ventilation. Ventilatory support can be provided on an emergency basis with an anesthetic machine or ambu bag. The prolonged maintenance of a patient requires a ventilator and the patient must be closely monitored for appearance of deleterious side effects of positive-pressure ventilation, such as decreased venous return resulting in decreased cardiac output and hypotension; ischemia of abdominal organs, sometimes resulting in renal failure; pulmonary damage; pneumothorax; and impaired airway clearance, and obstruction of the tracheal tube.[7] Small disruptions to the system can result in the death of the patient.

Four types of ventilatory support are intermittent positive pressure ventilation (IPPV), positive end expiratory pressure (PEEP), continuous positive airway pressure (CPAP), and high frequency ventilation (HF). Patients are generally started with IPPV, which is comparable to bagging the patient by hand. This method can overcome inadequate respiratory efforts by the patient and can counter decreased compliance and alveolar collapse. Pressures of 15 to 20 cm of water are generally adequate for the inflation of normal lungs, though higher pressures may be necessary to overcome decreased compliance of diseased lungs.

Success of ventilation is judged by blood gas analysis. If there is inadequate response, PEEP can be initiated. The patient must exhale against the mild positive expiratory pressure (usually 5 to 10 cm of water) and early airway closure is countered. However, the increased pressure can severely compromise venous return and cause deterioration of the patient.[6,8] Continuous positive airway pressure is similar to PEEP except that increased pressure is maintained within the airways throughout expiration and inspiration.[6,9] All of these methods of ventilation can cause changes to the pulmonary parenchyma.

High frequency ventilation has not gained widespread use in clinical veterinary medicine, though some reports have been published.[10,11] The technique allows for ventilation without creating positive intrathoracic pressure and the resulting cardiovascular compromise. Oxygen can be administered through an intravenous catheter, avoiding the problems associated with tracheal tube maintenance. There are several variations of the technique, but all utilize small tidal volumes administered at frequencies of 60 to 2500 cycles/minute.

Patients who have been maintained with ventilatory support must be gradually weaned from the ventilator since the maintenance of normal or low P_aCO_2 will interfere with the normal respiratory drive. Support is discontinued slowly to allow the P_aCO_2 to increase. If the patient does not begin normal spontaneous ventilation the support is resumed and discontinuation is attempted later.

A review of ventilatory techniques in veterinary patients has been published.[7]

AIRWAY HUMIDIFICATION

Normal airway clearance mechanisms are dependent on the maintenance of adequate airway hydration. Drying of airways results in increased viscosity of secretions and decreased ciliary function, interfering with the clearance of secretions from the lungs. Additional effects of airway drying include inflammation and degeneration of the mucosa, vascular shunting, decreased compliance, atelectasis, and increased risk of infection.[4]

Maintaining airway hydration should be a consideration in all patients with lower respiratory disease. Special attention is necessary where the nasal cavity is bypassed, such as with the use of tracheal tubes, and where oxygen supplementation is required, since canister gas does not contain water vapor.

The most important method of maintaining airway hydration is maintaining the systemic hydration of the patient. Strict attention to fluid balance is essential. The importance of systemic hydration cannot be overemphasized and should deter the clinician from arbitrarily treating a coughing patient with diuretics.

The addition of water to inspired gases is indicated in patients receiving oxygen supplementation. The simplest system incorporates a canister of water into the oxygen line such that the gas is bubbled through the water. Complete water saturation within the airways cannot be achieved by bubbling through water at room temperature because the air becomes heated to body temperature within the airways and can carry more moisture. Humidifiers are available using the same principle which also heat the gas to body temperature. They should be placed in close proximity to the patient to minimize cooling and condensation within the tubing of the system.

Disposable filters can be incorporated into the ventilation system which retain the heat and moisture from expired air to be returned with the inspired gases. These filters can interfere with the flow of air as they become plugged with secretions and can provide a site for bacterial growth. They must be changed daily to minimize these problems.[4]

The addition of water to inspired air also can be used for patients with heavy respiratory secretions in an attempt to facilitate clearance. The efficacy of such techniques is not well established but subjectively results in improvement in some cases.[6] The addition of water can be attempted with nebulizers or vaporizers.

Nebulizers add water droplets to the system. Saline is recommended for use as a non-irritating, mucolytic agent. It can be added to the air in drops ranging in size from 0.8 to 6.0 μ or more through a variety of nebulizers, including jet, ultrasonic and Babington nebulizers.[6] The resultant aerosols are administered by mask or into an enclosed space such as an oxygen cage or a cage with plastic over the door. The treatment is administered for 30 to 45 minutes every 4 to 12 hours and should be followed by physiotherapy to facilitate clearance of rehydrated secretions.[6]

Nebulizers also can be used to provide moisture to the airways of patients with tracheal tubes. The use of nebulizers for the local administration of drugs is described later.

Potential problems associated with nebulization include overhydration, overheating, electrolyte imbalances, bronchospasms, and the transmission of infection from patient to patient. Detrimental changes in pulmonary function can also occur. Patients should be carefully monitored before and after therapy. If nebulization appears to worsen their status, it should not be continued. Bronchodilators are definitely indicated when medicants are aerosolized. They may be useful with saline nebulization.

Chronic therapy in the home can potentially be performed through nebulization. Usually, home therapy is carried out with vaporizers available in local pharmacies or by placing the patient in a steamy bathroom during showers. While this moisture is not likely to reach distal airways, subjective improvement in patient attitude is frequently reported in cases with upper airway, tracheal, or bronchial disease. The patient should not be allowed to become overheated, and treatment should be followed by physiotherapy.

PHYSIOTHERAPY

Physiotherapy is indicated to help prevent the pooling of secretions in the dependent portions of the lung of patients with limited mobility, heavy secretions, or a depressed cough reflex. It is especially important following nebulization or vaporization therapy. Ideally, material trapped in dependent portions of the lung is loosened and coughed out of the lungs.

Exercise may be beneficial for a variety of reasons, including change in position and deep breathing efforts. Frequent, mild exercise is less likely to be detrimental than vigorous exercise, and efforts should cease if the patient exhibits signs of respiratory distress. Patients which are sedated, unconscious, or otherwise limited in mobility should be turned every two hours so that the same areas of lung are not always dependent.

Percussion is a technique for the mechanical jarring of secretions and stimulation of cough. The palm of the hand is used to strike the rib cage in a clapping motion over the area of the lungs. The force approaches that used in enthusiastic applause, but should not be uncomfortable to the patient. The technique is performed for 5 to 10 minutes, by the clock, several times daily. When teaching the technique to owners, the exact location of the lung fields should be demonstrated since a large portion of the rib cage protects abdominal organs.

ACID-BASE BALANCE

The respiratory system has a major influence on systemic pH. Lower respiratory disease of sufficient magnitude to cause tissue hypoxia leads to the development of metabolic acidosis. The lungs may compensate for the acidosis through hyperventilation and compensatory respiratory alkalosis. Extremely severe pulmonary disease and hypoventilation can result in retention of carbon dioxide and primary respiratory alkalosis.

Blood gas values should be critically evaluated to ensure that the primary process (metabolic or pulmonary) is identified and treated, rather than the compensatory response. Therapeutic intervention for hypoxemia and hypercapnia is described in oxygenation and ventilation. Chapter 53, on fluid therapy, addresses the management of acid-base disorders of metabolic origin.

BRONCHODILATION

Bronchodilators can be useful in the management of a variety of lower respiratory diseases. They are widely used in the treatment of allergic bronchitis, where bronchoconstriction is felt to contribute to clinical signs. They also have been used to manage chronic bronchitis, pulmonary edema, tracheal collapse and a variety of parenchymal diseases. In addition to effects on airway lumen size, the methylxanthine bronchodilators may improve respiratory function by increasing the contractility of respiratory muscles and decreasing fatigue.[12]

Methylxanthines, sympathomimetic drugs, and anticholinergic drugs can be used for their bronchodilatory properties. The methylxanthines, particularly theophyllines, are widely used and are well tolerated for chronic use. In addition to the properties described above, theophyllines improve myocardial contractility and act as mild diuretics. Arrhythmias can occur at toxic concentrations or in the presence of hypoxemia or preexisting cardiac disease. Other signs of toxicity include restlessness, tachycardia and nausea.[13] These problems are occasionally observed.

Theophyllines are available in a wide variety of formulations for intravenous, intramuscular and oral administration. Oral absorption is rapid and is the preferred method of administration. Intramuscular injection is painful, and intravenous administration must be performed slowly over several minutes.[13] Sustained-release oral preparations are particularly convenient for owners.

Serum theophylline concentrations can be measured at human hospitals, and therapeutic concentrations are considered to be 5 to 20 μg/ml.[14, 15] These levels are achieved by administering theophylline itself or a drug with theophylline activity, such as aminophylline or oxtriphylline. Theophylline is administered at an initial dosage of 4 mg/lb (9 mg/kg) q6h to q8h in the dog and 2 mg/lb (4 mg/kg) q8h to q12h in the cat.[13, 14] Certain sustained-release products may require administration only every 12 to 24 hours. Two products, Theo-Dur Tablets and Slo-Bid Gyrocaps, appear to require only daily administration to cats at a dosage of approximately 50 mg/cat[16] and twice daily administration to dogs at dosages of 9 mg/lb (20 mg/kg) and 11 to 14 mg/lb (25 to 30 mg/kg), respectively.[17] Aminophylline is administered at 5 mg/lb (11 mg/kg) q6h to q8h in the dog and 2.5 mg/lb (5 mg/kg) q8h to q12h in the cat.[14, 15] Oxtriphylline is available in a pediatric syrup that is well accepted by dogs and is administered at a dosage of 6 mg/lb (14 mg/kg) q6h to q8h.[13]

In critical cases or chronic cases that do not respond to therapy, the dosage should be assessed by the measurement of serum concentrations.[13, 15] The drug should be given at a consistent dosage for at least one day in dogs and two days in cats. Samples are obtained two hours after oral administration to measure peak concentrations and prior to dosing to determine persistence of the drug. The dosage should be modified to maintain values within the therapeutic range. Slow release products require longer to reach steady state and peak concentrations.

Sympathomimetic drugs cause bronchodilation through β_2 adrenergic effects. The two most clinically useful sympathomimetic drugs are epinephrine and terbutaline. Epinephrine is used primarily for the emergency management of cats with severe allergic bronchitis. A rapid response can be seen. However, epinephrine has profound β_1 effects in addition to β_2 effects. The stimulation of cardiac sympathetic receptors in the presence of hypoxemia can induce fatal arrhythmias. Epinephrine should not be used if a response can be attained with rapid-acting corticosteroids and oxygen therapy.

Terbutaline is selective for β_2 receptors. Subjectively, it has been successful in some cases where theophylline products were not. Its advantage has not been proven objectively. Recommended dosages for terbutaline are 1.25 to 5.0 mg/dog q8h and 1.25 mg/cat q8h.

Anticholinergic drugs counter parasympathetically induced bronchoconstriction. They are not recommended for routine clinical use due to the potential for increasing viscosity of bronchial secretions and undesirable systemic effects.[13]

COUGH SUPPRESSION

Coughing is an extremely important defense mechanism assisting the clearance of secretions and debris from the airways. Cough suppressants are indicated only for patients that have fatiguing or persistent, non-productive coughs. These patients are usually suffering from bronchial inflammation. Even in these cases elimination of the underlying cause, such as bacterial infection, is the preferred treatment. Cats rarely, if ever, require cough suppressant therapy. When intervention is necessary, cough suppressants should be used at the lowest dosage required to allow the patient to rest and to break the irritating coughing cycle.

A variety of cough suppressants are available for use in dogs. Dextromethorphan hydrobromide is a mild suppressant and can be administered at a dosage of 1 mg/lb (2 mg/kg) q6h to q8h.[6] Hydrocodone bitartrate is an effective narcotic cough suppressant, administered at a dosage of 0.125 mg/lb (0.25 mg/kg) q8h to q24h. Butorphanol tartrate is administered at 0.25 mg/lb (0.55 mg/kg) q6h to q12h PO or 0.025 mg/lb (0.055 mg/kg) q6h to q12h SQ. The latter two drugs should not be administered to cats.

EXPECTORANTS

The desired effect of expectorant therapy is to increase the volume and decrease the viscosity of bronchial secretions. The ability of expectorants to achieve this effect is questionable.[6, 18] Rather than over-medicate patients, methods known to facilitate the clearance of secretions should be used until evidence is produced for the inclusion of expectorants in the management of pulmonary patients. The importance of airway hydration has been previously addressed.

NEBULIZATION OF MEDICATIONS

The delivery of medications locally through nebulization has been accepted for use in humans. Unpleasant and toxic systemic effects can be avoided, and medication can be provided at the source of the problem. Some examples of aerosolized drugs include N-acetylcysteine, antibiotics and corticosteroids.

The potential benefits of nebulized medications in veterinary medicine must be balanced by the potential complications and the lack of patient cooperation. Mucolytic agents, such as N-acetylcysteine, can be irritating and induce bronchospasms, while saline alone is felt to have substantial benefits for improved mucus clearance. Antibiotics administered by aerosol can predispose the patient to opportunistic infections.[3] The local administration of poorly absorbed corticosteroids has not been investigated in clinical veterinary medicine.

The distribution of inhaled medications in the lung is affected by the cooperation of the patient. Deep, sustained inhalations greatly enhance the distribution of droplets. Such cooperation cannot be achieved in veterinary medicine and droplets may not pass beyond the nasal cavity.

The technology for aerosolizing medications for the local delivery to the pulmonary tree is available. The actual application in veterinary clinical medicine is limited.

BRONCHIAL DISEASES

Patients with bronchial disease commonly are presented with coughing as the major complaint. Other signs of pulmonary disease, such as exercise intolerance, increased respiratory efforts, and cyanosis; and systemic signs, such as weight loss, anorexia, and depression, can occur as well. The trachea can be concurrently affected, and pneumonia can occur secondary to diseased airways and decreased clearance mechanisms.

Physical examination may reveal pharyngitis and increased tracheal sensitivity. Auscultation can reveal normal lung sounds, increased bronchovesicular sounds, crackles, or wheezes.

Thoracic radiographs inconsistently demonstrate a bronchial pattern when inflammatory disease is present. Inflammation is more effectively confirmed by analysis of tracheal or bronchial wash fluid. Septic inflammation is diagnostic for primary or secondary infection. Eosinophilic inflammation occurs with allergic (hypersensitivity) responses or parasitic diseases. Nonseptic, chronic inflammation is suggestive of chronic bronchitis. Neoplasia uncommonly involves the bronchial tree, but can secondarily result in virtually any type of inflammatory response.

Thoracic radiographs may show evidence of other bronchial diseases, such as bronchial masses (foreign bodies, granulomas, abscesses, or neoplasia), bronchiectasis, or bronchial compression. Further diagnostic evaluation of these cases may include bronchoscopy, bronchography, or exploratory thoracotomy.

CANINE INFECTIOUS TRACHEOBRONCHITIS

Several viruses and bacteria, alone or in combination, can result in acute, self-limiting signs of bronchitis known as canine infectious tracheobronchitis, or kennel cough. The organisms commonly associated with the disease are canine adenovirus 2 (CAV2), canine parainfluenza virus (CPV), and *Bordetella bronchiseptica*. Other organisms which may contribute to signs include canine adenovirus 1, reovirus, herpesvirus, and mycoplasma. Invasive infectious agents, such as distemper virus or systemic mycoses, may cause signs indistinguishable from infectious tracheobronchitis during transient infections or early in the course of severe infections. The agents involved in infectious tracheobronchitis are readily spread from dog to dog.

Presentation. Dogs with infectious tracheobronchitis are presented with an acute onset of a honking cough that is often worse with exercise and may be productive or nonproductive. A careful history will frequently reveal recent exposure to a new puppy or to dogs during kenneling, hospitalization, or showing. Lack of current vaccinations may be discovered, though current vaccinations do not eliminate the possibility of disease.

Coughing can be induced by tracheal palpation. Increased bronchovesicular sounds may be auscultatable. Debilitation, persistent fever, chorioretinitis, or other signs of systemic disease should alert the clinician to a more serious problem.

Diagnostic Evaluation. Diagnostic tests are primarily performed for the early identification of more serious disease, rather than to definitively diagnose infectious tracheobronchitis. The CBC is typically unremarkable. Thoracic radiographs are normal, though a mild bronchial pattern could occur. Tracheal wash fluid analysis reveals acute inflammation characterized by increased neutrophils. Bacteria may be apparent, and culture and sensitivity testing may be useful in the selection of antibiotics. Viral isolation can be performed, but the information obtained is useful only for epidemiologic purposes.

Treatment. Most cases of infectious tracheobronchitis resolve without treatment within seven to ten days.[19] The patient should be rested and exciting stimuli should be avoided until signs have resolved. Cough suppressants are indicated only if the cough is nonproductive and is persistent or interferes with sleep (see General Therapeutic Management).

Antibiotics are indicated only when there are complications or signs of systemic involvement, and they should be initiated after culturing of tracheal wash fluid. Although the potential involvement of *Bordetella* makes arbitrary antibiotic therapy tempting, the beneficial response anecdotally attributed to antibiotics would often occur without them. Chloramphenicol, amoxicillin/clavulanate, tetracycline, and gentamicin have been found to be effective against *Bordetella* isolates *in vitro*.[20, 21] Therapeutic concentrations of systemically administered antibiotics may not always be achieved at the bronchial epithelium where the *Bordetella* reside, and the high end of the recommended dosage range generally should be used to treat these infections.[19] Clinical improvement should be noted within three to five days of antibiotic therapy, but the drug should be continued for a minimum of 14 days.[19] Unresponsive infections may benefit from nebulized antibiotics.[22, 23]

Corticosteroids often decrease the severity of signs through their anti-inflammatory effects. The self-limiting nature of the disease and the disadvantage of interfering with the protective mechanisms of the respiratory tract make their use undesirable.

Prognosis. The prognosis for recovery is excellent.

Prevention and Control. Prevention of infectious tracheobronchitis in pet animals is best achieved through avoidance of exposure and vaccination. Parenteral vaccines against CAV2 and CPV are readily available in combination with canine distemper virus vaccines. These vaccines are effective in decreasing the severity of clinical signs resulting from these agents but the CPV vaccine does not completely prevent infection.[23] The vaccines are given every three weeks to puppies under 14 weeks of age to overcome the interference of maternal antibodies. Yearly booster vaccines are recommended.

Vaccines against *Bordetella* are available for parenteral and intranasal administration. Vaccination against Bordetella is recommended only for high risk patients or kennel situations in which case intranasal vaccines are preferred. The intranasal route of administration produces a localized immune response. After three weeks of age, only one vaccination is necessary followed by yearly booster vaccines.

In kennels experiencing frequent outbreaks of infectious tracheobronchitis, control should be aimed at sanitation and ventilation. Cages should be kept clean and dry using routine disinfectants. Animal to animal contact should be avoided, both within the kennel area and during exercise, and routine sanitation procedures reviewed with animal caretakers. Ventilation should provide 12 to 15 air changes per hour.[19]

FELINE ALLERGIC BRONCHITIS (FELINE ASTHMA)

Feline allergic bronchitis refers to a syndrome in cats with similarities to asthma in humans. It is commonly referred to as feline asthma. Signs of feline allergic bronchitis are due to inflammation and reversible airway obstruction. Signs due to permanent airway changes, such as fibrosis, are generally referred to as chronic bronchitis though these changes may be the result of chronic allergic disease. The reversible airway obstruction in feline asthma is a result of bronchoconstriction, bronchial smooth muscle hypertrophy, inflammatory cell infiltrates, increased mucus production and decreased mucus clearance.[24, 25] Exhalation of air becomes difficult as the narrowed airways collapse with increased intrathoracic pressure during expiration. Air is trapped in the peripheral lung as a result of the above and from obstruction of airways with mucus plugs. Abnormalities in the distribution of ventilation and perfusion occur.

The specific mechanisms for the syndrome in cats have not been thoroughly investigated, and most of the explanations of pathogenesis in cats are taken from experiments in humans and dogs. A Type I hypersensitivity response is postulated, with contributions from histamine, slow-reacting substance of anaphylaxis, prostaglandins, major basic protein, other mediators of inflammation, and possibly the autonomic nervous system.[25, 26, 27]

A source of antigenic stimulation causing the exaggerated bronchial response is rarely found, but inhaled allergens and infectious agents have been incriminated. Suspected allergens include litter dust, perfumes, cigarette smoke, fireplace smoke, and insulation materials. Seasonal associations in some cats suggest plant source allergens. Bacterial infections are associated with exacerbations of signs in humans, and pathogenic bacteria have been cultured from tracheal wash fluid of 25 per cent of cats with bronchial disease.[28] Parasitic infections, especially with *Aleurostrongylus* or *Dirofilaria,* can result in similar signs. Mycotic infections occasionally result in an eosinophilic response.

Presentation. Allergic bronchitis can occur in any age cat, but many cats begin showing signs at one to three years of age.[27] Siamese and Himalayan cats may be more frequently affected.[27] Presenting signs range from occasional or frequent coughing episodes to bouts of severe respiratory distress. The cats are usually asymptomatic between episodes and rarely show systemic signs of disease. Careful history taking may reveal association of signs with seasons or antigenic stimuli in the environment.

Physical examination findings vary with the severity of disease. A cat presented between episodes may show no obvious abnormalities. Expiratory wheezes and crackles may be auscultated with more advanced disease. With severe involvement, the cat may be presented in severe respiratory distress with open mouth breathing, cyanosis, and a pronounced abdominal component to expiration. In the distressed patient, wheezes and crackles may be marked, though occasionally decreased vesicular sounds are auscultated due to air trapping and decreased ventilation.

Diagnostic Evaluation. Thoracic radiographs classically reveal a bronchial pattern, and interstitial patterns and patchy alveolar densities can occur (Figures 69–1 and 69–3). Early cases may exhibit no obvious radiographic changes. During severe attacks or with chronic disease, hyperinflation of the lungs may result in increased radiolucency and flattening of the diaphragm.

A complete blood count (CBC) reveals eosinophilia in up to 75 per cent of cases,[24] though other causes of eosinophilia, such as parasitism, also should be considered. The absence of a peripheral eosinophilia should not eliminate this diagnosis.

Tracheal wash fluid analysis is indicated in these patients. A marked inflammatory response is expected and is characterized by eosinophilia. In some cases the predominant cell type is nondegenerative neutrophils with few eosinophils (Figure 69–2). Whether these latter cases represent a separate etiology and pathogenesis is unknown, but their clinical presentation and response to therapy are similar to cases with eosinophilia. The tracheal wash fluid should be carefully examined for infectious agents. Bacterial culture should be performed routinely.

Special fecal concentration techniques should be performed to investigate for underlying parasitic disease (see Parasitic Diseases). Heartworm testing should also be performed, especially in areas with high incidence of the disease.

Treatment. Cats presenting in severe respiratory distress should be stabilized based on classic presenting signs prior to specific diagnostic evaluation. A rapid acting corticosteroid, such as prednisone sodium succinate (50 to 100 mg/cat), should be administered intravenously. If the administration route results in too much stress, intramuscular injection can be used. Oxygen should be administered, preferably in a cage to minimize stress. The combination of glucocorticoids, oxygen, and rest nearly always results in stabilization. Rarely, more aggressive therapy with epinephrine (0.1 ml of 1:1000 given SQ) is necessary. Epinephrine can potentially induce fatal arrhythmias, especially in the hypoxic heart.

Chronic management of feline allergic bronchitis consists of elimination of potential antigenic stimuli, anti-inflammatory therapy and bronchodilators. Environmental sources of antigen are rarely discovered, but they usually are not pursued aggressively by careful history taking and elimination trials. This lack of interest is unfortunate since elimination of offending allergens can result in a cure, while other treatments are only successful in controlling signs. The possible role of litter can be tested by switching to sandbox sand or newspaper for several weeks. Indoor cats may show improvement following replacement of furnace filters and use of air cleaners. Possible infectious sources of hypersensitivity are discovered through a thorough initial diagnostic evaluation with repeated evaluation if treatment failure occurs.

Anti-inflammatory therapy with corticosteroids is rapidly effective in controlling signs in the majority of cases. A short acting oral preparation, such as prednisone or prednisolone, is preferred to allow the most control of treatment. A dosage of 0.25 to 0.5 mg/lb (0.5 to 1.0 mg/kg) q8h to q12h is used initially. Higher dosages can be prescribed if necessary to control signs. Once signs are controlled, the drug is rapidly tapered to alternate evening therapy at the lowest effective dosage. Where oral medication cannot be reliably administered, repositol steroids such as methylprednisolone acetate can be

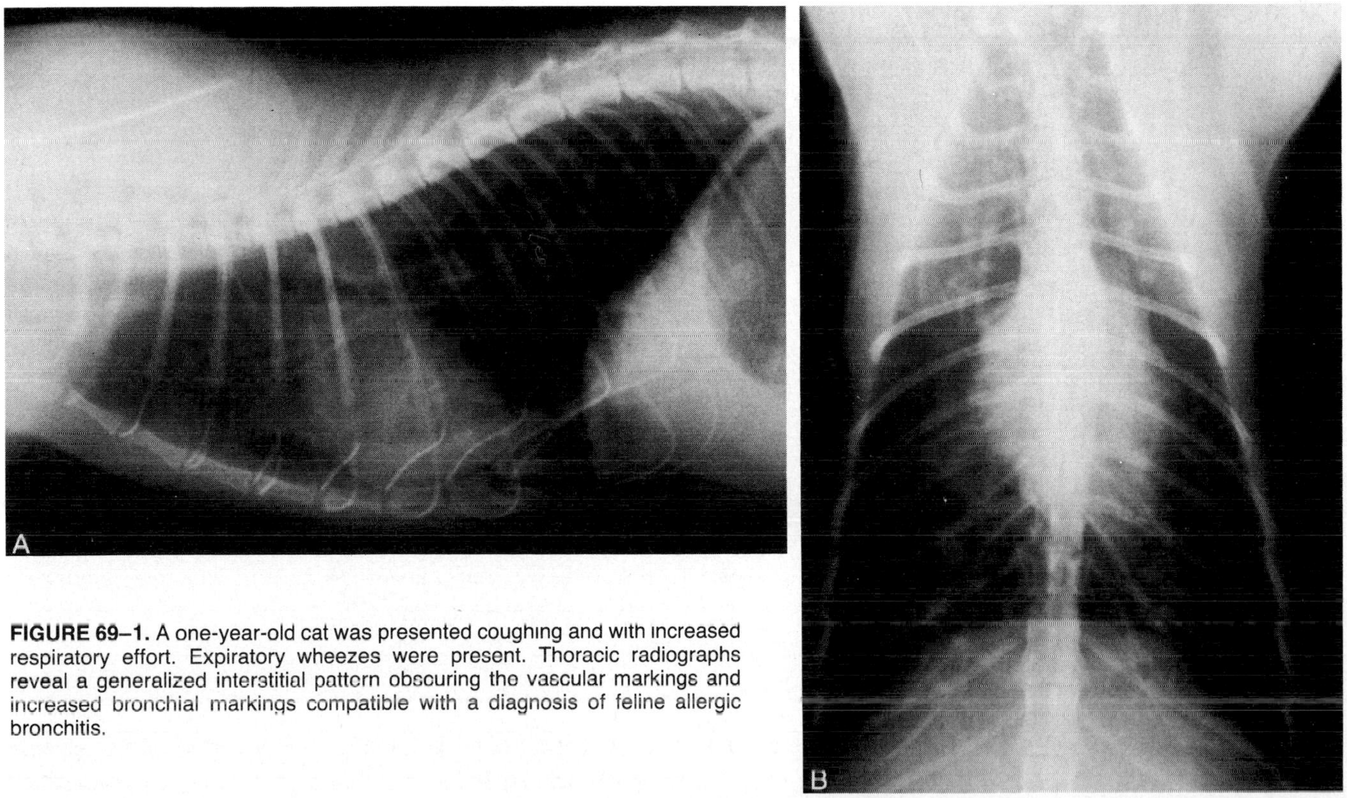

FIGURE 69–1. A one-year-old cat was presented coughing and with increased respiratory effort. Expiratory wheezes were present. Thoracic radiographs reveal a generalized interstitial pattern obscuring the vascular markings and increased bronchial markings compatible with a diagnosis of feline allergic bronchitis.

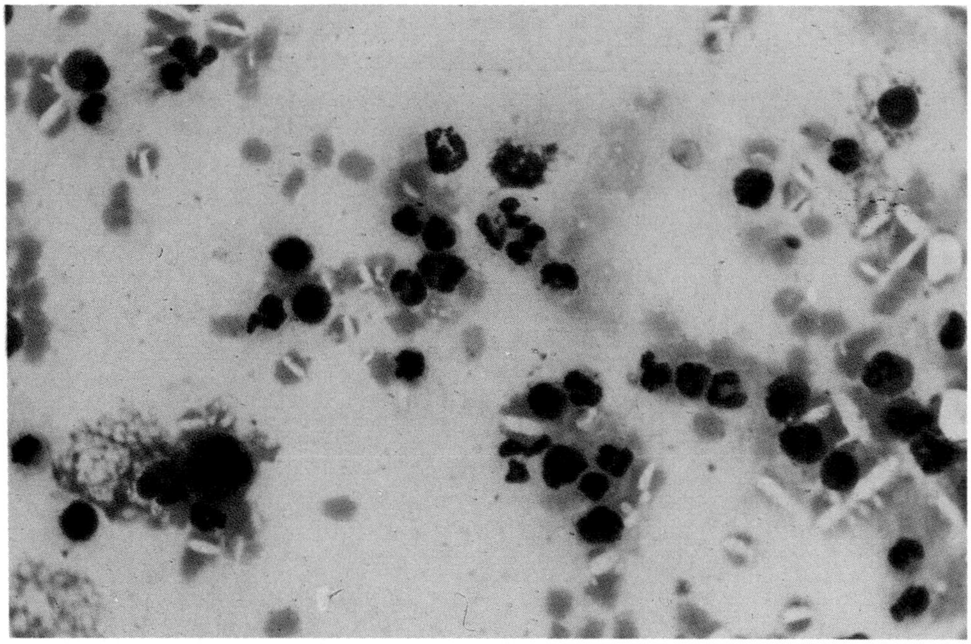

FIGURE 69–2. Tracheal wash fluid cytology from the cat in Figure 69–1 demonstrating moderate numbers of mature, nondegenerate neutrophils and low to moderate numbers of eosinophils. A few macrophages are present. The major differential diagnoses of lungworms and dirofilariasis were pursued with fecal examinations and heartworm tests. No evidence for parasitic disease was found. Bacterial culture was negative.

used at a rate of 1 to 2 mg/lb (2 to 4 mg/kg) IM as often as needed to control signs (usually 10 to 30 days).

The response to corticosteroids is generally marked, but the amount of steroids required to control signs is extremely variable. Some cats require as little as 1.25 mg of prednisone every third day while others experience recurrence when any tapering is attempted.

The duration of therapy necessary is also variable, with some cats requiring life-long treatment and some cats requiring only occasional courses of drug. In humans, therapy may be continued beyond cessation of signs since occult small airway disease usually persists, and allowing such inflammation to persist may contribute to permanent bronchial changes.[25, 29] Radiographic

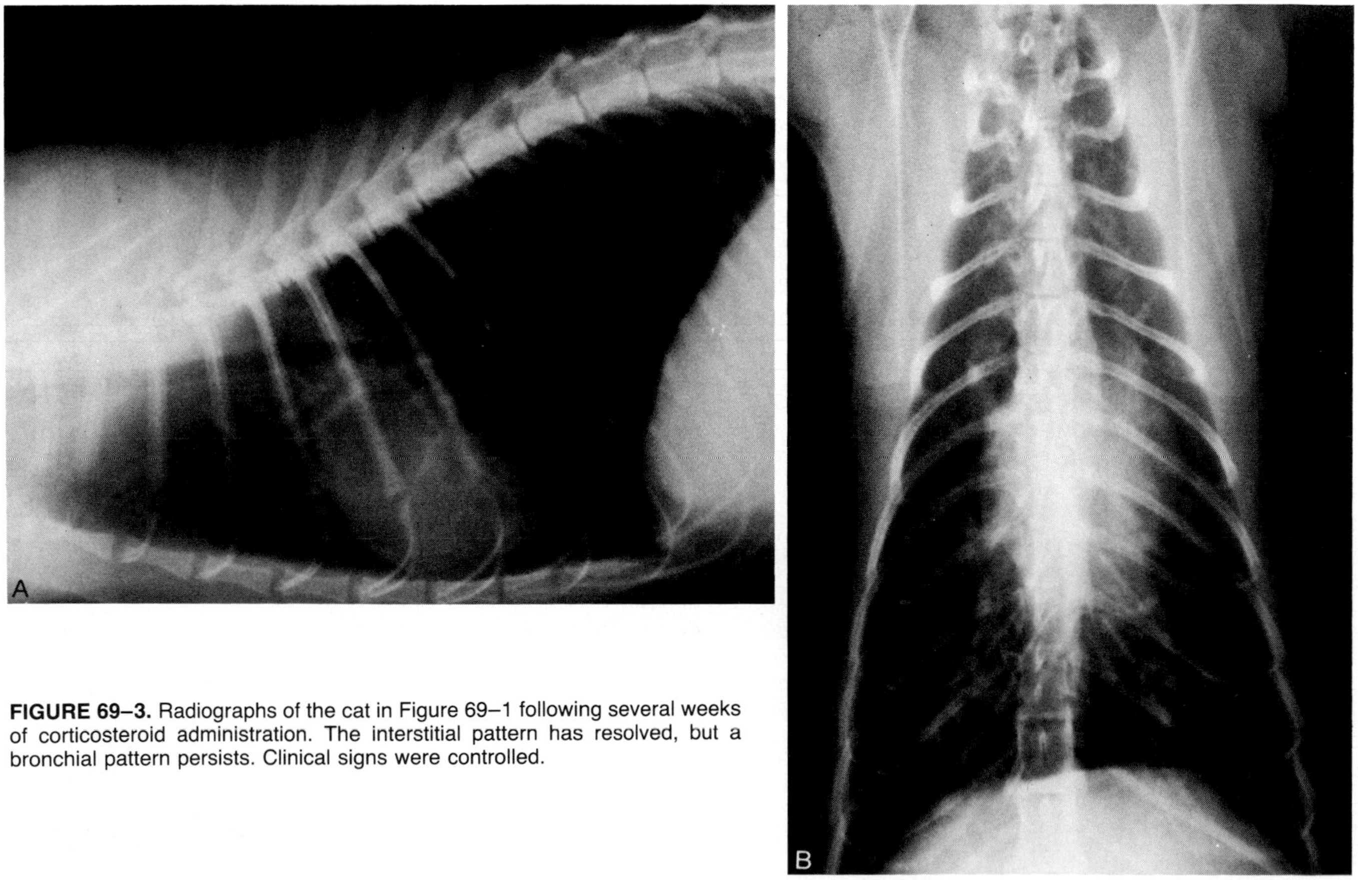

FIGURE 69–3. Radiographs of the cat in Figure 69–1 following several weeks of corticosteroid administration. The interstitial pattern has resolved, but a bronchial pattern persists. Clinical signs were controlled.

and tracheal wash evaluations may be useful prior to and after discontinuation of therapy to detect continued inflammatory disease. The benefits of such evaluation have not been proven in cats.

Bronchodilators can be helpful in controlling signs and may decrease the dosage of corticosteroids required. Although reduction in signs may occur with bronchodilators alone, they are recommended in conjunction with corticosteroids because of the potential for permanent airway damage resulting from persistent inflammation. The use of bronchodilators is discussed under General Therapeutic Management.

Cats that do not respond to therapy or that experience sudden worsening of signs during constant levels of therapy should be re-evaluated for inciting or complicating disease. As in the initial evaluation, infectious agents or environmental stimuli should be considered.

Prognosis. The prognosis for cats with allergic bronchitis is good for control, though death can occur from a severe exacerbation of signs. Cure is achieved through the identification and elimination of an inciting antigen or spontaneous remission. When medication is discontinued, over half of patients will show recurrence of signs.[28]

Complications, such as chronic bronchitis and emphysema, result in a lesser prognosis though the rate of complications in cats has not been documented. These problems are discussed under Chronic Bronchitis and Cystic-Bullous Disease.

Canine Allergic Bronchitis

Allergic bronchitis in the dog is not a well defined clinical entity. The term is used to describe a syndrome of coughing, bronchitis, and eosinophilic inflammation that responds to steroid therapy. A positive association with offending antigens has not been well documented. Many clinicians have seen occasional cases that respond to environmental manipulations, such as eliminating smoking in the house, though chronic bronchitis may improve with decreased exposure to irritants without implying a specific hypersensitivity reaction.

The dog has been used as an experimental model for allergic bronchitis with hypersensitivity responses created with ragweed and ascarid antigens.[30–32] Extremely high levels of exposure have been necessary.[30]

Dogs with signs of allergic bronchitis frequently have co-existing problems, such as chronic bronchitis, bacterial infection, and tracheal collapse. These problems may be primary, secondary, or concurrent to the hypersensitivity response. In any case, they complicate the clinical diagnosis and management of allergic bronchitis.

Presentation. Dogs with allergic bronchitis are presented with typical signs of bronchial disease. A careful history should be taken to discover any relationship to potential allergens.

Diagnostic Evaluation. Radiographs typically show a bronchial pattern. A diffuse interstitial pattern and patchy alveolar densities can occur, though cases demonstrating these patterns may have eosinophilic pulmonary disease (see Hypersensitivity and Immune-Mediated Disease). A peripheral eosinophilia may be present.

Tracheal wash fluid analysis reveals eosinophilic inflammation. A careful examination of all slides should be made for infectious agents that may be acting as antigen sources for the hypersensitivity response. Lungworms, fungal agents, and bacteria should all be considered. Fluid should be submitted for bacterial culture.

Ancillary tests should be performed to further investigate for underlying antigenic sources, such as fecal examinations for lungworms and heartworm testing. The clinical usefulness of skin testing in these cases has not been established.

Treatment. The treatment of choice is the elimination of offending antigens. Infections should be treated with appropriate antibiotics. Possible environmental sources should be eliminated as a diagnostic and therapeutic trial.

Corticosteroids are administered for their anti-inflammatory effects. Prednisone or prednisolone at a dosage of 0.25 to 0.5 mg/lb (0.5 to 1.0 mg/kg) q12h will usually control signs. The drug should be tapered as quickly as possible to the lowest, alternate morning dosage that will control signs.

Prognosis. The prognosis for controlling clinical signs is good; however, long-term continuous or intermittent therapy is often required. As previously mentioned, co-existing conditions, such as chronic bronchitis, bacterial infection, and tracheal collapse, may complicate management. The reader is encouraged to review these sections for additional management techniques.

Chronic Bronchitis

The clinical definition of chronic bronchitis in dogs was adapted by Wheeldon in 1974 from the definition in humans. Chronic bronchitis is defined as a persistent cough occurring for at least two consecutive months in the past year in the absence of a specific pulmonary disease.[33] The latter requirement has important implications to the clinician, as chronic bronchitis cannot be appropriately diagnosed without careful elimination of other active pulmonary disease. The term chronic bronchitis in cats is less well defined, but is generally distinguished from allergic bronchitis by the presence of irreversible changes.

Chronic bronchitis has been well characterized in dogs histologically from both spontaneous and experimentally induced cases.[33, 34] Bronchial gland hyperplasia and hypertrophy and increased goblet cells are present with increased mucus or a mucopurulent exudate within the airways. Hyperplasia, loss of cilia, and sometimes ulceration of the bronchial epithelium are seen. Increased mixed inflammatory cells are present in the lamina propria.

Grossly, these alterations result in hyperemic, thickened bronchial walls, increased mucus with obstruction of small airways, and sometimes polypoid proliferations of the epithelial surface.[33] Airway walls are often weakened.

The factors initiating these changes are not known. In humans, smoking, atmospheric pollution, and infection are important components, and allergic and genetic factors may be involved.[18, 33, 35] In affected animals inhaled irritants subjectively appear to contribute to clinical signs, and experimental exposure of dogs to pollutants such as sulfur dioxide is used to create models for bronchitis. Infectious agents are associated with acute tracheobronchitis in the dog, but their role as initiating factors of chronic bronchitis is not established. *Bordetella* has been isolated from many dogs with chronic bronchitis,[33, 35] but these infections may be secondary to alterations in normal pulmonary defense mechanisms rather than inciting causes. Allergic bronchitis was discussed previously, and can result in chronic alterations. Genetic factors in humans include deficiency of α-1-antitrypsin, though this problem has not been documented in animals. Chronic bronchitis can be a component of ciliary dyskinesia in the dog, and this condition is discussed separately.

Signs occur as a result of inflammation, increased secretions, and chronic obstructive pulmonary disease. Inflammation and increased secretions result in chronic cough. Obstructive pulmonary disease is the result of the histologic changes described above, bronchoconstriction, airway collapse or early airway closure, and secondary fibrosis. The obstructive disease causes air trapping and an abnormal distribution of ventilation and perfusion within the lung.[35] As the chronic bronchitis progresses, bullous emphysema and bronchiectasis may further aggravate signs and management. The reader is referred to Bronchiectasis and Cystic-Bullous Diseases.

Concurrent diseases also may complicate the management of chronic bronchitis. Infection may be a result of reduced airway defenses. Tracheal collapse and mitral regurgitation commonly occur in the breeds with high incidence of chronic bronchitis and may cause similar signs. Careful evaluation is necessary to determine the contribution of these conditions to the clinical signs.

Presentation. Small breed adult dogs are most commonly affected with chronic bronchitis. By definition, signs of bronchial disease must be of at least two months duration. The signs often demonstrate gradual progression of disease, but the animals are usually presented following an acute exacerbation of signs. The cough may or may not be productive and may be worse with exercise or excitement. The attitude and appetite are normal unless the cough has become continuous. Severe exacerbations may be accompanied by cyanosis and exhaustion. Careful history may reveal an association with smoke, dust, or other environmental irritants.

On physical examination the patients are often overweight. Auscultation may reveal normal airway sounds, increased bronchial sounds, crackles from excessive mucus or exudate, or expiratory wheezes from airway obstruction. A respiratory sinus arrhythmia may be detected.[36] Tracheal collapse, tracheitis, or mitral insufficiency may be detected as concurrent problems. Remember that dogs presenting with cough and a cardiac murmur often are not in heart failure, and treating them as such can be harmful.

Thoracic radiography classically reveals a bronchial pattern. A concurrent mild interstitial pattern is common. Patchy peripheral alveolar densities can occur due to decreased clearance of mucus or secondary bronchopneumonia. Air trapping can sometimes be appreciated radiographically as hyperinflated lungs with increased radiolucency of lung fields and flattening of the diaphragm. Radiographic changes are not always apparent in spite of marked clinical signs.[33] Expiratory radiographs or fluoroscopy can be useful in detecting collapse of large airways. Collapse may be apparent in the intrathoracic trachea or mainstem bronchi.

Complete blood counts are generally unremarkable. Possible abnormalities include mature neutrophilia as a result of stress, polycythemia as a result of chronic hypoxemia, and anemia as a result of chronic inflammatory disease. A neutrophilic leukocytosis and left shift can occur with secondary bronchopneumonia. Eosinophilia should raise suspicions for allergic or parasitic disease.

Tracheal wash fluid should be collected for cytologic and microbiologic analysis. Cytologic findings are variable. A proteinaceous background is common from the increased mucus. Epithelial cells may demonstrate hyperplastic changes. Inflammatory cell infiltrates may be minimal, show mild chronic inflammation, or show severe, septic inflammation. Eosinophilia suggests a hypersensitivity response and was discussed under Allergic Bronchitis. Bacteria are frequently isolated by culture, and sensitivity testing can be valuable in the selection of antibiotics.

Bronchoscopic examination reveals increased mucus or mucopurulent exudate, and hyperemic, swollen, irregular bronchial walls. Large airway collapse is often marked (Figure 69–4).

Treatment. There is no single treatment that will effectively control signs in all patients. Each patient should be treated individually with frequent reassessment until the most effective regimen is found. Frequently, intense management is required to control the presenting exacerbation, and then therapy can be decreased to maintenance levels once severe signs are controlled.

Initial treatment should be aimed at eliminating factors contributing to the sudden worsening of signs. Such factors may include inhalation of irritants, excitement, and infection. The patient should be kept away from smoke, dust, and pollutants to the best of the owner's

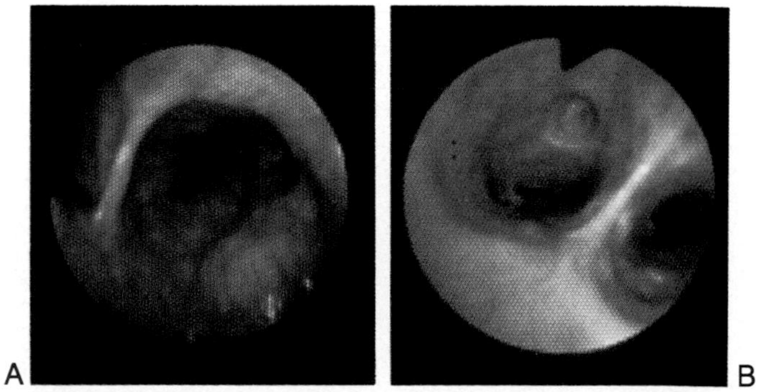

FIGURE 69–4. Two dogs with chronic bronchitis as visualized bronchoscopically. The narrowing of mainstem bronchi is apparent due to inflammation, swelling, and hyperplasia (A) and airway collapse (B). These changes interfere with normal airway clearance mechanisms and contribute to signs of chronic obstructive pulmonary disease. Hyperemia and increased mucus were present in both, but are not demonstrated photographically.

ability. Excitement and stress should be minimized, and some dogs may require mild tranquilization if severe, fatiguing coughing is present. Acepromazine or phenobarbital may be useful for this purpose. Potential bacterial invaders should be treated with an antibiotic with a broad spectrum including *Bordetella* pending culture and sensitivity results (see Canine Infectious Tracheobronchitis).

A trial with bronchodilator therapy is instituted to combat bronchoconstriction and to decrease respiratory muscle fatigue. Bronchodilators are discussed under General Therapeutic Management.

Maintenance of the water content of respiratory secretions is extremely important in assisting bronchial clearance mechanisms. Systemic dehydration should be avoided and diuretics are contraindicated. Airway humidification should be followed by physiotherapy. These techniques are also described.

Weight loss should be aggressively pursued in all overweight patients. The clinical response to weight loss can be dramatic, but direct involvement of the veterinarian is usually required for a successful weight loss program. Sending the dog home with a controlled diet is rarely as effective as also having the owners exercise the dog, keep records of exercise and weights, and periodically recheck with the veterinarian for weight measurements and progress reports.

Other therapy is prescribed on an individual basis. Cough suppressants are indicated only to control continuous or fatiguing, nonproductive coughing. Expectorants have questionable effectiveness and in general are not useful. Corticosteroids will often improve clinical signs and may slow the airway changes associated with chronic inflammation, but the added insult to pulmonary defenses in an already severely compromised patient makes such therapy potentially harmful.

Prognosis. Though the prognosis for recovery from chronic bronchitis is extremely poor due to irreversible changes, control of signs is generally achievable. Both the veterinarian and the owner must be willing to persevere through exacerbations, tailor therapy over time, and accept the chronic nature of the disease. Many patients live good-quality lives for many years.

Primary Ciliary Dyskinesia (Immotile Cilia Syndrome)

Cilia carry out important functions in multiple organs of the body. The respiratory system is extremely dependent on functioning cilia for effective clearance of respiratory secretions, inhaled particles, and infectious agents. Congenital abnormalities of ciliary structure and function have been identified in humans and dogs. The term immotile cilia syndrome has been used to refer to functionally immotile cilia.[37] However, affected cilia are rarely immotile but rather have ineffective motion. Primary ciliary dyskinesia has been suggested as a more accurate term.[38]

Ciliary dyskinesia is a result of one or more defects of ciliary microtubules identifiable by electron microscopy. Many different clinical features are possible. The triad of situs inversus (the transposition of abdominal and thoracic organs from left to right), chronic rhinitis and sinusitis, and bronchiectasis is referred to as Kartagener's syndrome in humans, and similar signs have been reported in dogs.[37, 38] Situs inversus does not always occur with ciliary dyskinesia. Bronchiectasis is a result of chronic airway obstruction with mucus and chronic inflammation.[38] Additionally, ciliary dysfunction can result in otitis media, hearing loss, hydrocephalus, dilated renal tubules, and male infertility.[37, 38]

In a report of English springer spaniels with the syndrome, the disease was produced in offspring of affected parents. Results of several matings suggested that genetic transmission was not dominant, sex-linked, or chance mutation.[37]

Presentation. Reported cases of ciliary dyskinesia have been identified in dogs less than one and a half years old.[38] Littermates with the syndrome have been reported in English pointers and English springer spaniels.[37, 38] Persistent bilateral nasal discharge is a frequent presenting sign. The disease should be considered in any young patient with chronic, recurring signs of respiratory infection or infertility. Other organs can be affected as described above.

Diagnostic Evaluation. Routine diagnostic evaluation often reveals evidence of respiratory infection. Radiographs may reveal bronchitis, bronchiectasis, or bronchopneumonia. Situs inversus, characterized by dextrocardia, in conjunction with respiratory infection or infertility is an extremely suggestive finding. A leukocytosis may be present on CBC. Septic inflammation is often apparent on tracheal fluid analysis and bacterial culture is generally positive.

Definitive diagnosis is by electron microscopy. Nasal mucosa or tracheal mucosa biopsies, or spermatozoa in the intact male, can be submitted for examination.

Treatment. Ciliary dyskinesia cannot be directly treated. The majority of clinical signs are the result of bacterial infections. These infections can be treated with appropriate antibiotics as they occur. General principles of therapy for respiratory disease can also be applied.

Prognosis. The long-term prognosis in canine cases is guarded, though some animals have been maintained for over five years with intermittent therapy.

Prevention. Though infertility is a problem in many affected animals, the disease can be produced by breeding phenotypically normal animals.[37] Breeders should give careful consideration to using dogs for breeding when an immediate relative has been diagnosed with ciliary dyskinesia.

Bronchiectasis

Bronchiectasis is the permanent dilation of bronchi. The dilation may be localized (saccular), or extend down the airways (cylindrical). The dilation greatly interferes with normal airway clearance, and mucus and exudate can accumulate distal to the abnormality.

The disease is seen clinically most often as a complication of chronic pulmonary disease, especially chronic bronchitis or allergic bronchitis. It may be a component of primary ciliary dyskinesia.

Presentation. Clinical cases of bronchiectasis are usually discovered in dogs as a complication of chronic airway disease. The author is unaware of reports in cats.

Diagnostic Evaluation. The diagnosis is generally made from thoracic radiographs obtained during the evaluation of patients with chronic bronchial disease, though changes are likely to be present prior to their appearance radiographically. The airway walls do not appear parallel and lose their normal gentle taper.[39] The diameter of the airway lumens is greater than expected away from the central lung. Consolidation may be present distal to the bronchus (Figure 69–5).[39] In dogs, multiple lobes are usually involved.[40] Further characterization can be obtained through bronchoscopy or bronchography, but these studies are rarely indicated solely to document bronchiectasis.

Treatment. Therapeutic recommendations are generally the same as for chronic bronchitis. These cases are especially prone to recurrent infections and corticosteroid therapy should be avoided. Decreased clearance can be improved with attention to airway humidification, physiotherapy, and minimal use of cough suppressants. If changes are localized to a few bronchi, surgical resection can be considered.[36, 40]

Prognosis. Bronchiectasis may not be a permanent change in dogs. Clinical signs of chronic bronchitis are generally more difficult to control when bronchiectasis is present.

Bronchial Foreign Bodies

Bronchial foreign bodies occur as a result of aspiration of small objects. The normal protective reflexes are quite effective in the prevention of foreign body aspiration, but occasional cases are seen. Objects that may be found include grass awns, marbles, and teeth.

Presentation. Hunting breeds are prone to grass foreign bodies due to repeated exposure during exercise. Puppies may aspirate foreign bodies during play. Patients are often presented with an acute onset of severe, paroxysmal coughing or respiratory distress. If the object is lodged in a distal airway, signs may not be so dramatic and cases may present with chronic recurrent pneumonia.

Diagnostic Evaluation. When patients are presented with sudden, acute signs, radiographs are taken of the thorax and neck. A soft tissue or mineral density may be apparent in the airways. The definitive diagnosis is generally made with bronchoscopy. The foreign body is identified by systematic evaluation of all airways, assuming it has not travelled into the peripheral lung beyond the functional length or diameter of the scope. If a foreign body is not visible, each airway should be examined for localized exudate or hemorrhage. Bronchography may be useful for localization of disease where bronchoscopy is not available.

For animals with recurring bronchopneumonia, thoracic radiographs should be evaluated soon after initiation of antibiotics and within one week of discontinuation of antibiotics in an attempt to identify a focal source of persistent infection or inflammation. Such a focus may represent a foreign body, and bronchoscopy or surgical exploration is indicated.

The surgical approach to foreign bodies is pursued after the disease has been localized bronchoscopically or radiographically. The affected lobe may not be grossly apparent externally.

Treatment. Treatment consists of removal of the foreign body, generally through bronchoscopy or lobectomy. Bronchoscopic removal is preferred. Secondary bacterial infections are treated with appropriate antibiotic therapy (see Bacterial Pneumonia).

Prognosis. When a foreign body is identified and can be removed, the prognosis is excellent. Some foreign bodies, especially grass awns, may escape detection and result in chronic pulmonary disease. They may also migrate through the pleural space resulting in pneumothorax, discospondylitis, or signs from invasion of other

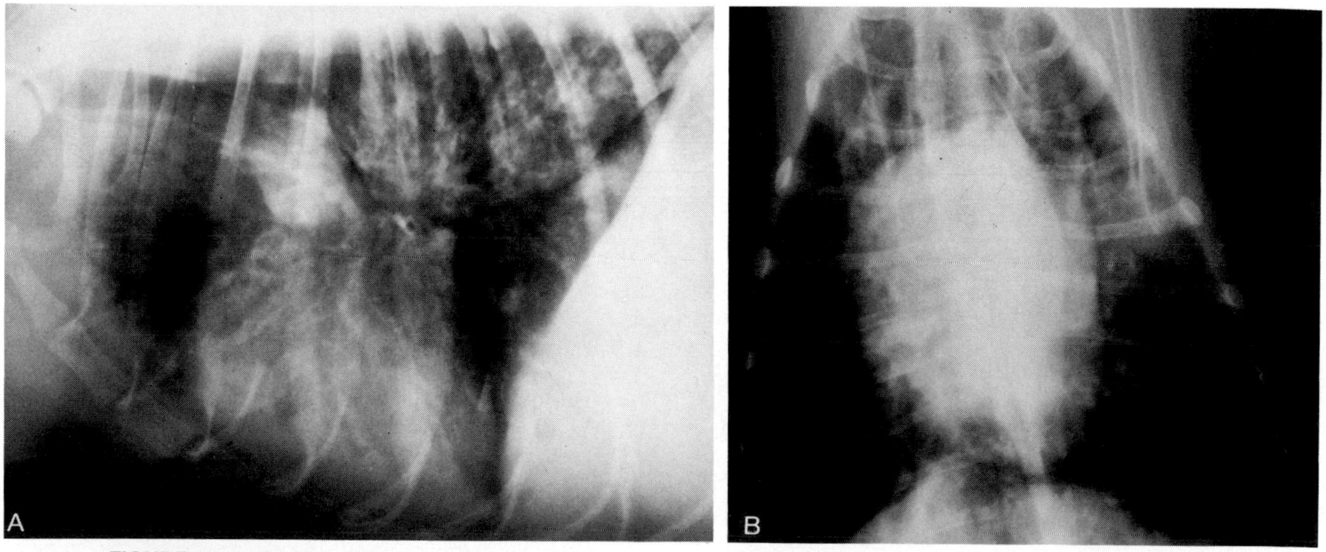

FIGURE 69–5. Bronchiectasis is suggested in this dog by the presence of prominent, wide airways extending beyond the hilar region. Peribronchial and interstitial densities are present throughout the lung fields, and ventral consolidation is visible in the lateral projection. Hilar lymphadenopathy is apparent. Cytologic analysis of tracheal wash fluid revealed marked eosinophilic inflammation. No etiologic agents were found. Decreased airway clearance probably contributed to the consolidation of the peripheral lung.

organs, though the origin of grass awns found in distant parts of the body can almost never be determined.

Bronchial Parasites

Several lungworms result primarily in signs of bronchial disease. These parasites include: *Capillaria aerophila* in the dog and cat, and *Crenosoma vulpis* and *Oslerus osleri* in the dog (see Chapter 68).

Bronchial Compression

Bronchial compression from structures outside of the airways can cause coughing. Compression can be the result of hilar lymphadenopathy, pulmonary neoplasia, or left atrial enlargement. The diagnosis is made on thoracic radiography.

Hilar lymphadenopathy occurs as a result of inflammatory pulmonary disease due to infection, neoplasia, or immune disease. The reader is referred to those sections of this chapter. Left atrial enlargement as a result of mitral insufficiency occurs commonly in the same small breeds where tracheal collapse and chronic bronchitis are seen and can contribute to clinical signs through the compression of mainstem bronchi. The problem of atrial enlargement and bronchial compression is distinct from heart failure.

Bronchoesophageal Fistulas

Bronchoesophageal fistulas occur most frequently as a result of esophageal foreign bodies which penetrate the wall of the esophagus and involve an adjacent airway.[41] Congenital fistulas or fistulas resulting from trauma or neoplasia can occur, and congenital lesions may not become clinically apparent for years.[41] The connection created between the esophagus and airways can allow saliva and ingested material to enter into the lungs. The result is recurrent aspiration pneumonia. Pleuritis also can occur.

The diagnosis of bronchoesophageal fistula is made through contrast radiography. An esophagram is performed using a thin solution of barium sulfate.[41]

Animals are initially managed as described under Aspiration Pneumonia. The problem is corrected surgically.

Bronchial Mineralization

Bronchial mineralization can be seen radiographically as an incidental finding in aged dogs. Chondrodystrophic breeds are more commonly affected and calcification may be evident at an early age. No correlation to disease has been made.[42]

Bronchial Neoplasia

Bronchial neoplasia is discussed under Pulmonary Neoplastic Diseases.

NON-NEOPLASTIC PULMONARY DISEASE

Patients with pulmonary disease frequently are presented with signs of coughing, increased respiratory effort, or exercise intolerance. Cats are less apt to cough than dogs, except with allergic or parasitic disease. General systemic signs, such as weight loss, anorexia, and depression, may occur concurrently or as the only complaint. In general, the history and physical examination will localize the disease to within the thoracic cavity.

Thoracic radiographs are used to further localize and characterize the disease process. Any radiographic pattern or combination of patterns may result from non-neoplastic pulmonary diseases, but certain patterns are suggestive of particular diseases.

Cytologic or histologic evaluation is required to obtain a definitive diagnosis for most pulmonary diseases. Cytologic specimens often are obtained by tracheal wash. More invasive methods, such as bronchoscopic collection, lung aspirates, or lung biopsies, may be necessary. Less invasive tests, such as antibody titers for certain infectious diseases or fecal examinations for parasites, may be helpful in confirming a specific diagnosis.

Non-neoplastic pulmonary diseases include infectious disease (viral, bacterial, protozoal, fungal, and parasitic), hypersensitivity and immune-mediated disease, traumatic lung disease, cystic-bullous disease, miscellaneous conditions, and sequelae to active disease. These diseases will be discussed with consideration for pathogenesis, presenting signs, diagnostic evaluation, treatment, prognosis, and, where applicable, control and zoonotic potential.

INFECTIOUS PULMONARY DISEASES

Viral Diseases

CANINE DISTEMPER

Canine distemper virus can infect epithelial tissues throughout the body, resulting in signs due to respiratory, gastrointestinal, neurologic, or ophthalmologic involvement. Respiratory system involvement is usually identified with severe disease, and bacterial pneumonia is a common complication. Mild, transient signs could be mistaken for infectious tracheobronchitis.[43]

Presentation. Canine distemper can occur in puppies and adult dogs. Puppies are particularly susceptible in the absence of colostral antibody protection and prior to completion of the distemper vaccination series. A history of exposure may be discovered, with an expected incubation period of three to six days.[44]

Client complaints may include anorexia, depression, conjunctivitis, nasal discharge or cough. These signs are often followed at some time by vomiting and diarrhea.

Physical examination during the respiratory phase may reveal bilateral serous or mucopurulent nasal discharge and conjunctivitis. A fever may be present. Crackles may be auscultated throughout the lungs. It is essential to perform a funduscopic examination as chorioretinitis is an important supportive sign.

Diagnostic Evaluation. The viral infection is characterized by a generalized, interstitial pattern on thoracic radiographs and a lymphopenia. Tracheal wash cytology may reveal acute, nonseptic inflammation. The occurrence of secondary bacterial pneumonia causes a mixed bronchial and alveolar pattern to develop radiographically. The septic inflammation can result in a neutrophilia and degenerative neutrophiles and bacteria may be demonstrated on tracheal wash analysis.

The diagnosis of canine distemper is usually based on age, history, and the classic involvement of multiple organ systems. The clinical application of specific diagnostic tests are discussed in Chapter 47.

Treatment. There is no antiviral treatment available for canine distemper virus infection. Some dogs will recover with appropriate supportive care. Specific treatment should be directed against secondary bacterial involvement.

Prognosis. The prognosis for dogs with severe clinical signs is poor. About 50 per cent of dogs that do survive may develop neurologic signs of distemper[44] but may not appear until one to three weeks following resolution of initial signs.[43]

Control. Excellent vaccines are available to aid in the prevention of distemper. Proper vaccination protocols combined with isolation of puppies until the initial vaccination series has been completed can greatly reduce the likelihood of disease.

OTHER CANINE VIRAL PNEUMONIAS

Viral agents other than canine distemper virus have been associated with respiratory diseases in the dog. Two of the more common of these viruses are canine adenovirus two and canine parainfluenza virus, which are associated with canine infectious tracheobronchitis. Mild interstitial pneumonia can be caused by viruses, but clinically apparent disease generally occurs as a result of concurrent or secondary bacterial infection. There is no specific treatment for these viruses. The reader is directed to a discussion of these problems in this chapter.

FELINE CALICIVIRUS

Feline calicivirus is a major cause of feline upper respiratory infections, but the virus can infect other tissues in the body and can result in an interstitial pneumonia in cats.[45] Fluorescent antibody and virus isolation testing can be performed to definitively diagnose the agent, but the clinical usefulness of these tests is limited due to the time involved until results are available and the lack of specific therapy once the agent is identified. Care should be taken to identify any secondary or concurrent infections that can be specifically treated, otherwise treatment is supportive only.

FELINE INFECTIOUS PERITONITIS

A common clinical presentation of feline infectious peritonitis (FIP) is pleural effusion. However, FIP can involve the pulmonary parenchyma in the noneffusive form of the disease, resulting in peribronchiolar pyogranulomatous inflammation. This dry form of the disease is rarely apparent clinically.[46]

FELINE LEUKEMIA VIRUS INFECTION

Feline leukemia virus does not directly cause lower respiratory tract disease. The virus may contribute to other diseases with pulmonary involvement, such as lymphosarcoma, toxoplasmosis, and FIP. Treatment and prognosis for such patients is based upon these latter diagnoses.

RICKETTSIAL DISEASES

The two major rickettsial agents in dogs, *Rickettsia rickettsii* and *Ehrlichia canis*, generally result in vague, multi-systemic signs of disease. Pulmonary signs occur more commonly with Rocky Mountain spotted fever (RMSF) than with ehrlichiosis. In one review, 46 of 63 cases of RMSF showed signs of pneumonitis, dyspnea, or cough.[47] Thoracic radiographs may demonstrate a diffuse interstitial pattern (see Chapter 46).

Bacterial Diseases

BACTERIAL PNEUMONIA

Bacterial pneumonia is a common cause of respiratory disease in dogs, but is an unusual finding in cats. Primary bacterial infection in dogs can occur as a result of *Bordetella bronchiseptica*[48] and possibly *Streptococcus zooepidemicus*.[49] A wide variety of other bacteria can result in pneumonia, often as secondary invaders.[50]

The possibility of an underlying problem should not be overlooked in animals with bacterial pneumonia. In fact, bacterial infection may complicate any other pulmonary disease process. Possible primary etiologies include aspiration due to megaesophagus or bronchoesophageal fistulas, foreign bodies, neoplasia, lung parasites, mycotic infections, viral infections, bronchial disease, and trauma.

Pneumonia resulting from infection with *Mycobacterium* will be discussed separately.

Presentation. Animals with bacterial pneumonia are presented with signs typical of lower respiratory disease. Localizing signs, such as cough, exercise intolerance, respiratory distress, and nasal discharge are common. However, subtle, nonspecific signs, such as depression, anorexia, and weight loss, may be the only complaints.

Physical findings also are typical of lower respiratory disease. Mucopurulent nasal discharge and an increased respiratory effort may be apparent. Mucous membranes may be cyanotic with severe disease or following exertion. Lung sounds are usually increased with moist crackles audible over all or part of the lung fields. A fever may be present. Animals with mild or localized disease may not have obvious signs, and radiographs may be necessary to support clinical intuition.

Diagnostic Evaluation. Thoracic radiographs may show only an interstitial pattern early in the disease. An alveolar pattern develops as the disease progresses. Distribution of lesions may be helpful in identifying underlying problems. Focal lesions may be associated with foreign bodies. Involvement of primarily the dependent lung lobes is supportive of aspiration pneumonia. A marked bronchial pattern suggests primary airway disease. Abnormalities characteristic of other diseases, such as hilar lymphadenopathy, pulmonary artery enlargement, or mass lesions, should be examined carefully since an alveolar pattern can mask these lesions. Repeated radiographic evaluations following resolution of pneumonia are indicated to avoid overlooking these patterns.

The CBC may reveal a neutrophilic leukocytosis and left shift with a monocytosis. It is fairly common to find only a stress response or a normal leukogram.

Tracheal wash fluid analysis is valuable for the diagnosis and treatment of bacterial infections. Cytologic evaluation typically reveals septic inflammation with a predominance of degenerate neutrophils. Bacteria are typically present both intra- and extra-cellularly. The specimen should be cultured for identification of bacteria and sensitivity testing. Culturing for anaerobes and mycoplasma should be considered in difficult cases. Mycoplasma are not likely to be a major cause of pneumonia in cats.[51]

More invasive diagnostic techniques, such as bronchoscopy or lung aspiration, may be necessary if the tracheal wash specimen is nondiagnostic. This situation may occur with localized disease. In one study, 19 per cent of tracheal wash preparations from dogs with bacterial bronchopneumonia did not show inflammation.[52]

Treatment. Antibiotics are the primary treatment for bacterial infections. Antibiotics should be selected based upon the results of sensitivity testing from tracheal wash or similar specimens obtained during bronchoscopy. There appears to be much variability with *in vitro* sensitivity of common pulmonary isolates in different parts of the country and over time,[53] emphasizing the importance of culture and sensitivity testing for individual patients. In a report of 42 dogs with bronchopneumonia, significantly more dogs responded to treatment based upon sensitivity testing than on empirical treatment.[52]

Reasonable initial antibiotic selection can be made based upon microscopic examination of the specimen and tentative organism identification pending results of sensitivity testing. Gram-negative rods, which include most rod shaped organisms, are frequently sensitive to trimethoprim/sulfonamides, chloramphenicol, or gentamicin.[52, 54] Gram-positive cocci are often sensitive to trimethoprim/sulfonamides or cephalosporins.[54] *Bordetella bronchiseptica* isolates are often sensitive to chloramphenicol, gentamicin, and tetracycline.[20] Little data are available concerning some of the newer antibiotics such as amikacin and amoxicillin/clavulanate, though one study showed 93 per cent sensitivity of *Bordetella bronchiseptica* isolates to amoxicillin/clavulanate potassium in 14 canine isolates.[21] Growth of more than one organism has been reported in over 40 per cent of dogs with bacterial pneumonia.[54, 55] Multiple organisms with different antibiotic resistance patterns may complicate the selection of effective antibiotics. Table 69–4 shows a compilation of bacterial isolates from several reports.

Another consideration in the selection of antibiotics, in addition to the organism(s) involved, is the antibiotic concentration achieved within the pulmonary parenchyma and airways. Concentrations within the parenchyma are likely to correlate well with serum concentrations.[56] There appears to be poorer antibiotic penetration into bronchial secretions, with serum concentrations exceeding bronchial concentrations.[56] Inflammation may improve penetration early in the treatment of bacterial infections.

In most infections, routine administration of appropriate antibiotics is adequate to achieve a therapeutic response. Several options can be considered in more complicated infections. Dosages at the high end of the recommended range can be administered to increase local drug concentrations.[50] Antibiotics can be selected that in humans have been shown to reach relative high concentrations in the sputum, such as clindamycin and tobramycin.[56] For all severe cases parenteral, bactericidal antibiotics are recommended for initial therapy.

In cases of persistent bronchial infections due to *Bordetella*, aerosol administration of antibiotics can be used.[22, 57] This route of therapy is not indicated in cases of bronchopneumonia and should not replace systemic therapy.[57]

General therapeutic measures should always be applied in addition to antibiotic therapy. Adequate oxygenation should be maintained with supplementation as needed. The importance of maintaining airway hydration cannot be overemphasized. Physiotherapy and bronchodilators may also be useful. Corticosteroids and cough suppressants should be avoided since they further impair the patient's defense mechanisms.

Once a plan of therapy has been established, the patient should be monitored for 48 to 72 hours. If no improvement in signs is observed in that time, therapy should be re-evaluated.[50] If improvement is observed, treatment should continue a minimum of one week beyond the total resolution of signs (including active radiographic changes). Radiographs should be re-eval-

TABLE 69–4. AEROBIC BACTERIA ISOLATED FROM TRACHEAL WASHINGS FROM 177 DOGS WITH BACTERIAL PNEUMONIA[a, b, c]

Bacteria	Number Isolated
Streptococcus (hemolytic and non-hemolytic)	49
E. coli	44
Pasteurella	38
Klebsiella	28
Staphylococcus	25
Pseudomonas	22
Bordetella	20
Others	30

[a]Thayer, GW and Robinson, SK: Bacterial bronchopneumonia in the dog: A review of 42 cases. JAAHA 20:731, 1984.

[b]Hirsch, DC: Bacteriology of the lower respiratory tract. *In* Kirk, RW (ed): Current Veterinary Therapy IX. Philadelphia, WB Saunders, 1986, p 247.

[c]Harpster, NK: The effectiveness of the cephalosporins in the treatment of bacterial pneumonias in the dog. JAAHA 17:766, 1981.

uated approximately one week after discontinuation of therapy to detect early evidence of recurrence, to note any persistent changes which suggest an underlying disease process, and to detect complications, such as consolidation, atelectasis, or abscessation.

Prognosis. Bacterial pneumonias are generally responsive to appropriate antibiotic therapy and supportive care. The severity and chronicity of the infection, the presence of underlying disease, and the development of complications can affect the long-term prognosis.

MYCOBACTERIAL INFECTIONS

Dogs and cats are susceptible to infections caused by *Mycobacterium tuberculosis* and *M. bovis* (true tuberculosis), but are relatively resistant to infections by *M. avium*.[58] A variety of opportunistic saprophytic Mycobacteria can also cause clinical disease in the dog and cat.

Presentation. True tuberculosis in the dog and cat is often clinically inapparent. When clinical infection occurs, mycobacteria may involve only regional lymph nodes, or may disseminate throughout the body, causing severe signs. Localizing signs of disseminated tuberculosis in cats classically represent involvement of the intestinal tract, while signs in dogs are the result of pulmonary involvement. Saprophytic Mycobacteria generally cause cutaneous lesions, although *M. fortuitum* has been reported to cause pneumonia in the dog.[59, 60] In one series of cases the major clinical signs in dogs with tuberculosis were vague and nonspecific, such as anorexia, weight loss, and lethargy.[61] Discussion in this chapter will be limited to patients with pulmonary signs.

Historic and physical findings in dogs with pulmonary involvement reflect severe lower respiratory disease and may mimic neoplasia, severe bacterial pneumonia, or mycotic disease. A prior lack of response to antibiotics may be reported.

Diagnostic Evaluation. Radiographs may show hilar lymphadenopathy and a nodular interstitial pattern. Granulomas, mineralization of pulmonary lesions, and pleural or pericardial effusions may be apparent.[58] Pulmonary hypertrophic osteopathy can occur.[58] The abnormalities on CBC are generally nonspecific.[61]

Tracheal wash fluid analysis could potentially reveal chronic inflammatory changes and perhaps intracellular organisms. Unfortunately, these specimens may be noninflammatory.[60]

The diagnosis depends on the identification of organisms. Pleural fluid, lung aspirates, or lung biopsies may be required. Specimens should be cultured for Mycobacterium so that the organisms can be identified as saprophytic or nonsaprophytic, though Mycobacteria are slow growing, and primary identification of organisms should be based on cytologic or histologic evaluation. Fecal and urine cultures may be useful even when pulmonary signs predominate.[36] Acid-fast staining will enhance the appearance of the organisms.

Treatment. Treatment for true tuberculosis based on human data should consist of at least 2 drugs for a period of 18 months or more. Such drugs include isoniazid (4.5 to 9 mg/lb or 10 to 20 mg/kg, up to 300 mg, q24h, PO), rifampin (4.5 to 9 mg/lb or 10 to 20 mg/kg, q12h, PO), streptomycin (4.5 to 7 mg/lb or 10 to 15 mg/kg, q12h, IM or SQ) and ethambutol (7 mg/lb or 15 mg/kg, q24h, PO).[58] Gastrointestinal signs, neuropathies and allergic reactions have been noted with the orally administered drugs.[62] More toxic drugs have been used for resistant infections in humans, such as para-aminosalicylic acid, pyrazinamide, ethionamide, cycloserine, kanamycin, or viomycin.[58]

Saprophytic Mycobacterium infections do not respond to anti-tuberculosis therapy. Organisms may be sensitive to streptomycin, kanamycin, amikacin, minocycline, doxycycline, sulfamethoxazole, sulfamethoxazole-trimethoprim, or amoxicillin/clavulanate.[59, 60, 63, 64] Sensitivity testing should be performed. The presence of large granulomas or consolidated lung tissue may require surgical removal since antibiotic penetration is likely to be poor. Duration of therapy is dependent upon clinical response, but several months may be required.

Prognosis. Animals with true tuberculosis have a grave prognosis. Euthanasia has been recommended for these patients due to the expense and duration of therapy combined with the potential human health threat.[36, 65, 66]

The prognosis for saprophytic Mycobacterium infections is guarded. Extensive treatment may be required.

Zoonotic Potential. There have not been reports of dogs or cats as a source of Mycobacterium in human infections. The potential for transmission exists and owners should be made aware of the risk. General sanitation measures should be reviewed if treatment is elected. The source of infection should be identified if possible, in cases of *M. tuberculosis* or *M. bovis,* to avoid further spread to humans or other animals.

Protozoal Diseases

TOXOPLASMOSIS

Toxoplasmosis is caused by the protozoal organism *Toxoplasma gondii*. It can occur in the dog and the cat, though cats are the definitive host for the organism. Healthy animals exposed to the organisms rarely develop clinical signs. Immunodeficiency syndromes or concurrent diseases, such as feline leukemia virus infections or canine distemper, predispose the animals to clinical disease.

Clinical disease can occur in an acute or chronic form. Acute disease can result in signs from multiple organ involvement, including the lung, liver, lymph nodes, muscles, uterus and fetuses, central nervous system, and eye. Chronic disease generally affects the nervous system, muscles, or eyes. Pulmonary signs were present in 9 of 12 cats with acute toxoplasmosis and in 4 of 17 cats with chronic toxoplasmosis.[67] Pulmonary involvement only is addressed below.

Presentation. Historic and physical findings are typical of severe lower respiratory disease.[68, 69] Anorexia, weight loss, cough, exercise intolerance, and respiratory distress may be reported. A mucopurulent ocular and nasal discharge may be present, and the patient may be febrile. Auscultation reveals increased bronchovesicular sounds or crackles. Generalized lymphadenopathy can occur as well as signs of involvement of other organ systems. Funduscopic examination should be performed for evidence of chorioretinitis. In dogs, the disease can present similarly to canine distemper and, in fact, the two diseases may occur together.

Diagnostic Evaluation. Radiographs of the thorax reveal fluffy interstitial and alveolar densities throughout the lung fields. Nodular patterns, diffuse interstitial patterns, consolidation, and effusions can occur.[70]

The CBC may reveal a leukopenia in infected cats due to a neutropenia with a degenerative left shift and lymphopenia.[67] Eosinopenia and monocytopenia may also be present. Leukocytosis may occur during recovery.[68]

Tracheal wash fluid analysis can show non-specific inflammation. In one report organisms were not identified in tracheal exudate obtained agonally,[70] but careful examination of the fluid for oocysts is warranted and could provide a definitive diagnosis.

Biopsy of infected tissues and histologic evaluation may allow for the identification of organisms, but such evaluation is rarely feasible in an animal with acute, severe pulmonary disease. Organisms have been found on fluid analysis of pleural effusions.[68]

The diagnostic application of fecal examinations and serum titers is discussed in Chapter 46 as is the treatment, prognosis, and zoonotic potential of toxoplasmosis.

PNEUMOCYSTOSIS

Pneumocystis carinii is a protozoal organism, which causes pulmonary disease in immunocompromised patients. Increased awareness of this disease has occurred as a result of human immunodeficiency virus infections (AIDS) and immunosuppressive anti-cancer therapies. Latent or subclinical infections can occur in several species, including humans and cats.[71] Clinical disease can also occur in several species, including humans and dogs.

Clinical infections in the dog are generally limited to the lung, though systemic spread has been reported.[72] The organisms adhere to the epithelial cells lining the alveoli without invading into deeper tissues. Signs appear when the organisms multiply to a sufficient extent to interfere with alveolar ventilation.[71] Signs also can occur as a result of a severe inflammatory response. This response may be successful in eliminating the infection.[71]

Presentation. Dogs with clinical pneumocystosis present with signs reflective of chronic pneumonia, such as weight loss, exercise intolerance, respiratory distress, and sometimes a non-productive cough.[71, 73, 74] Careful questioning for evidence of immunosuppressive disease or therapy is indicated. Increased bronchovesicular sounds may be audible, but moist sounds are not expected.[71] Pyrexia is uncommon.[71, 73, 74]

Diagnostic Evaluation. Radiographs typically show a diffuse alveolar pattern. Depending upon the inflammatory reaction, interstitial or localized disease may be present.

A CBC generally reflects an inflammatory response. An eosinophilia or monocytosis can be seen.[71]

The diagnosis is made through the identification of organisms. Tracheal wash analysis can reveal organisms, but other specimens may be necessary. Bronchoalveolar lavage fluid analysis has been valuable in the diagnosis of the disease in humans and can be performed in dogs.[75, 76] Lung aspirates or lung biopsies can be examined. The identification of organisms can be enhanced with the application of methenamine silver or Giemsa stains, as the organisms are not obvious with routine hematoxylin and eosin stain.[71]

Serum antibody testing and direct fluorescent antibody testing to detect pneumocystis antigen are available for humans. Their application to the dog has not been investigated.

Treatment. Specific protocols for therapy have not been established for the dog. Pentamidine isethionate can be administered at a dosage of 2 mg/lb (4 mg/kg) q24h SQ for 2 weeks.[71] Toxic effects include vasodilation and hypotension, hyperglycemia, hypocalcemia, hypokalemia, renal and liver dysfunction, swelling at the injection site, and systemic anaphylaxis.[62, 71] Obviously, careful monitoring of patients is essential. The drug may continue to be effective at lower dosages when combined with sulfonamides.[71]

Trimethoprim and sulfamethoxazole combinations have also been used to treat infections in humans. A very high dosage is used in humans (14 mg/lb or 30 mg/kg, q6h PO for 2 weeks), and half this dosage administered PO or IV has been proposed for use in the dog.[71]

General therapy should include elimination of immunosuppressive factors whenever possible.

Prognosis. Few cases have been described in the dog. Because the disease occurs in immunosuppressed animals, the prognosis is poor unless the immunosuppression can be reversed.

Zoonosis. Experimental transmission of pneumocystosis between species is difficult.[71] No data are available to link disease in humans with a canine or feline source.

Fungal Diseases

The historic, physical, clinical, pathologic, and radiographic signs of pulmonary mycotic infections can be extremely similar to those signs produced by neoplasia, immune disease, or other infections. Patients showing respiratory signs in conjunction with weight loss, lymphadenopathy or chorioretinitis should be considered potential candidates for mycotic disease. A definitive diagnosis is essential since treatment is prolonged, costly, and potentially toxic. Systemic mycoses are discussed in Chapter 49.

HISTOPLASMOSIS

Histoplasmosis is caused by *Histoplasma capsulatum*. Exposure occurs primarily through inhalation of organisms. Following exposure, most animals develop a localized, asymptomatic infection of the lungs that is resolved by cell-mediated immunity. Depending on the amount of organisms inhaled and the immune status of the animal, systemic dissemination may occur and clinical signs develop. Reactivation of a previous infection may also occur. The majority of patients presented to the veterinarian have signs of disseminated disease.[77–79]

Presentation. Lung involvement with histoplasmosis is common, and signs are typical of lower respiratory tract disease.

Diagnostic Evaluation. Thoracic radiographs classically exhibit a diffuse, miliary interstitial pattern when pulmonary disease is present, though alveolar patterns or areas of consolidation may occur with severe inflammation. Hilar lymphadenopathy may be present and can be sufficiently severe to cause signs from bronchial compression. Calcification of pulmonary lesions can occur.

Tracheal wash fluid analysis may be normal or reveal chronic inflammation. Macrophages should be critically examined for the presence of organisms.

Cytologic identification of organisms is the preferred method of diagnosis. Organisms frequently cannot be identified in tracheal wash fluid, and collection of other specimens may be required. Pulmonary tissue can be sampled more deeply through needle aspiration or biopsy, or bronchoalveolar lavage. Other potential sites for specimen collection, and the application of fungal cultures and serum tests, are described in Chapter 49.

Treatment. Dogs presenting with only mild respiratory signs may overcome the infection without therapeutic intervention, and these cases are rarely diagnosed. Whether or not treatment of these transient infections decrease the likelihood of persistent latent infections is not known.

The majority of cases are diagnosed following systemic dissemination of disease. These patients require aggressive therapy as described in Chapter 49.

Acute exacerbation of respiratory signs and cyanosis may be observed in severe cases following initial treatment. Short-acting corticosteroids at low doses and oxygen supplementation are indicated until the patient is stable. Though steroids are useful in the stabilization of these acutely deteriorating patients, they should not be continued beyond stabilization.

Prognosis. Histoplasmosis may range in severity from mild localized disease to severe systemic disease. The prognosis for patients with mild, localized signs is good. Cases that are presented with severe pulmonary involvement have a guarded prognosis.

Zoonotic Potential. See Chapters 37 and 49.

BLASTOMYCOSIS

Blastomycosis is caused by *Blastomyces dermatitidis*. The route of exposure is probably through inhalation, with the lungs as the primary site of infection.[77, 79, 80, 81] Dissemination may occur to a variety of organs. Animals may be exposed to the organism without developing clinical signs,[82] but once clinical signs develop the animals are generally considered to have progressive disease.[77, 81]

Presentation. Client complaints relate to the organ systems involved. Typical respiratory signs were present in 43 per cent of dogs in a review of 47 cases.[83]

Diagnostic Evaluation. Radiographic changes of the thorax were noted in 85 per cent of cases.[83] A diffuse, miliary interstitial pattern, as is seen with histoplasmosis, is typical (Figure 69–6). An alveolar or bronchial pattern can also occur. Hilar lymphadenopathy occurs, but perhaps less frequently than with other mycotic diseases.[79] Pleural effusion may be apparent and one case has been reported in association with chylothorax.[84]

Tracheal wash fluid analysis can be unremarkable or reveal chronic inflammation. Careful examination of slides should be performed to identify any organisms that might be present.

As is the case with histoplasmosis, cytologic identification of organisms is the preferred method of diagnosis. In addition to tracheal wash fluid, cytologic evaluation can be performed on lung aspirates or biopsies, or bronchoalveolar lavage fluid (Figure 69–7). Other potential sites for specimen collection, and the use of fungal cultures and serum tests, are discussed in Chapter 49.

Treatment. Treatment of blastomycosis is discussed in Chapter 49. Acute exacerbation of respiratory signs can occur following initial treatment, as described for histoplasmosis, and can be managed similarly.

Prognosis and zoonotic potential are discussed in Chapters 37 and 49.

COCCIDIOIDOMYCOSIS

Coccidioidomycosis is caused by *Coccidioides immitis*. Infection can occur through the respiratory tract as with the other systemic mycoses. Localized, asymptomatic pulmonary infections occur, but are rarely diagnosed. Severe pulmonary infection and systemic dissemination are responsible for clinically recognized infection.[85]

Presentation. Patients with pulmonary disease are presented with typical lower respiratory signs.

Diagnostic Evaluation. Thoracic radiographs are abnormal in the majority of cases,[86] with changes similar to those seen with the other mycoses. A diffuse interstitial pattern occurs, and bronchial or alveolar components are possible. Hilar lymphadenopathy was present in 74 per cent of reviewed cases, and pleural effusion or thickening was noted in 47 per cent.[86]

Tracheal wash fluid analysis may be unremarkable or reveal chronic inflammation. The slide should be carefully examined for any organisms that might be present.

Cytologic identification of organisms provides a definitive diagnosis, and if tracheal wash preparations are non-diagnostic other specimens should be examined from organs suspected of being infected. Such specimens include lung aspirates or biopsies, bronchoalveolar lavage fluid, and pleural fluid.

Further diagnostic procedures, treatment, prognosis and zoonotic potential are discussed in Chapter 49.

CRYPTOCOCCOSIS

Cryptococcosis generally affects the nasal cavity, nasal sinuses, eyes, skin, or brain of cats, and the central nervous system or eyes of dogs. Pulmonary lesions have been reported in 50 per cent of feline cases, though clinical signs relative to the lower respiratory tract are rare and an antemortem diagnosis of pulmonary involvement is uncommon.[79, 87] Thoracic radiographs are normal in most cases in spite of pulmonary involvement discov-

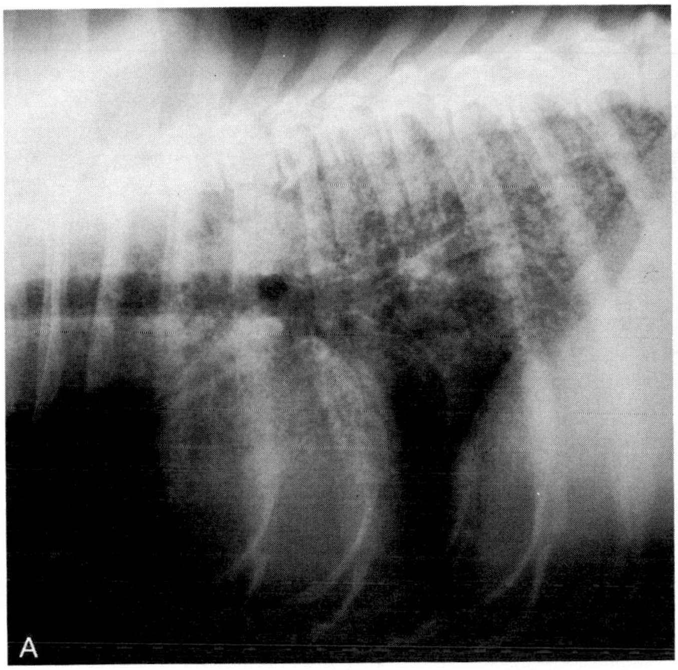

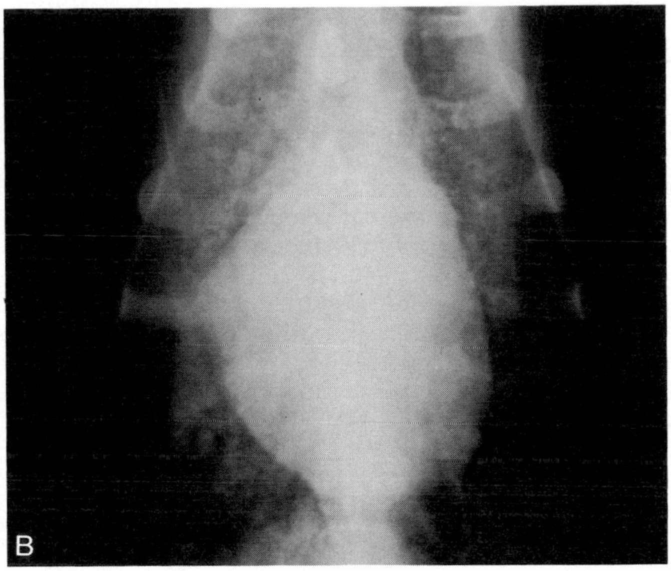

FIGURE 69–6. Radiographs demonstrating the typical diffuse, miliary interstitial pattern of pulmonary mycotic disease.

ered on necropsy, but can show a bronchoalveolar pattern, consolidation, or nodules.[87, 88] The reader is referred to Chapter 49 for a complete discussion of the disease.

ASPERGILLOSIS

Aspergillosis is a disease that predominantly involves the nasal cavity and sinuses of dogs. Severe pulmonary infections occur occasionally in cats. They are generally associated with immune compromise and are often diagnosed post-mortem.[77, 79, 88] A case of bronchopulmonary aspergillosis has been reported in the dog.[89]

Parasitic Diseases

Lungworms can result in a variety of clinical signs in dogs and cats as a result of the parasites themselves and of the inflammatory reaction they induce, though frequently the infections are asymptomatic. The inflammatory response is typically eosinophilic, but nonspecific chronic inflammatory changes can predominate. Secondary bacterial infections can occur and may obscure the diagnosis of parasitic disease.

A definitive diagnosis is based on the identification of organisms. The diagnosis may be hampered by intermittent shedding of characteristic eggs or larvae.

The prognosis for most lungworm infections is good since severe disease is rarely present. However, the clinical effectiveness of specific antiparasitic therapy is not always well established.

PARAGONIMUS KELLICOTTI

Paragonimus kellicotti, lung flukes, cause pulmonary disease in dogs and cats in the states surrounding the Great Lakes, and in the midwest and southern United States. Adult flukes reside in cysts within the parenchyma of the lung. Eggs are passed into the airways, are coughed up, swallowed, and passed in the feces. Aquatic snails and crayfish are required intermediate hosts. The crayfish are ingested, and the flukes migrate to the lungs through the diaphragm. The adult worms, as well as eggs trapped in alveoli and airways, result in pulmonary pathology.

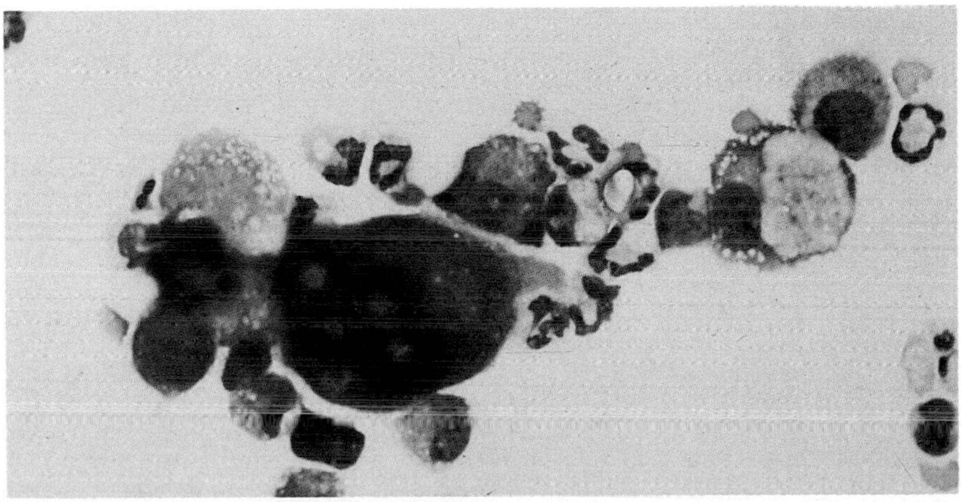

FIGURE 69–7. Bronchoalveolar lavage fluid cytology from the dog in Figure 69–6 demonstrates macrophages and mature nondegenerate neutrophils. A single extracellular budding yeast form of *Blastomyces dermatitidis* and a giant cell with four phagocytized yeast forms are present. The fungal forms are 10–20 μ in size, are deeply basophilic, and have a thick cell wall.

Presentation. Animals may not exhibit signs as a result of Paragonimus infection. When they occur, clinical signs result from an inflammatory reaction to the parasite, from secondary bacterial infection, or from cyst rupture and pneumothorax. The major sign of the inflammatory disease is coughing.[90, 91] Occasionally hemoptysis occurs.[92] In cats, wheezing can occur and be confused with feline allergic bronchitis. Respiratory distress is uncommon except when cysts result in pneumothorax. Lung sounds may be increased with inflammatory disease, or decreased with pneumothorax.

Diagnostic Evaluation. Thoracic radiographs demonstrate air-filled cysts or tissue density masses averaging 1 cm in diameter.[39] The masses most commonly involve the caudal lung lobes, and may be well-defined or not, depending on the inflammatory reaction.[39, 91] Pneumothorax may be present. Diffuse inflammatory signs may be apparent, resulting in bronchial, interstitial, or patchy alveolar patterns.[92]

A CBC and tracheal wash fluid analysis may reveal eosinophilic inflammation.[90] The disease is definitively diagnosed by the identification of eggs. These may be found in tracheal wash fluid or in feces. The eggs are single operculated, ovoid eggs approximately 90 μ in length (Figure 69–8).[93] Concentration techniques should be performed on fecal specimens to increase the likelihood of identifying the eggs. Routine flotation will concentrate the eggs, but can distort their appearance. Sedimentation is the preferred technique and can be performed without expensive equipment.[91, 92] Eggs may be shed intermittently and multiple fecal examinations may be necessary for their detection.

Treatment. No treatment for Paragonimus infection has been well established in the clinical setting. Fenbendazole (11 to 23 mg/lb or 25 to 50 mg/kg, q12h for 10 to 14 days) has been effective in experimental infections in dogs, and has been used in cats.[94] Albendazole (11 mg/lb or 25 mg/kg, q12h for 10 to 21 days) has been effective experimentally in cats.[92] One dog was treated successfully with praziquantel at a dosage of 11 mg/lb (25 mg/kg) q8h PO for 3 days.[95] Treatment with praziquantel at a dosage of 2 mg/lb/day (5 mg/kg/day) for 2 days was not effective.

AELUROSTRONGYLUS ABSTRUSUS

Aelurostrongylus abstrusus is a small (less than 1 cm) lungworm of cats. Adult worms reside primarily within the bronchioles. First stage larvae are coughed out of the airways, swallowed and passed in the feces. A mollusk (snail or slug) intermediate host is required, and transport hosts such as small mammals or birds play a role in infecting cats. An inflammatory response to the parasites can result in clinical signs.

Presentation. Aelurostrongylus infections may be asymptomatic. Clinical signs can range from mild coughing to severe wheezing and respiratory distress. Increased lung sounds may be heard. The clinical presentation mimics feline allergic bronchitis. Secondary bacterial infections can occur.

Diagnostic Evaluation. Thoracic radiographs can show small, poorly defined, nodular densities throughout the lung fields, similar to metastatic neoplasia or mycotic disease. The caudal lung fields are most heavily involved.[39, 92] Inflammatory reactions can also result in bronchial, interstitial, and alveolar patterns. These patterns can be confused with allergic bronchitis.

Tracheal wash fluid analysis may reveal eosinophilic inflammation, which can be reflected in the CBC. The disease is definitively diagnosed by the identification of first stage larvae in tracheal wash fluid or feces. Larvae are characterized by dorsal and ventral cuticular spines on their tails (Figure 69–8).[92] Feces should be examined following concentration of larvae using the Baermann technique. The technique can be performed with inexpensive equipment.[92]

Treatment. Infection with Aelurostrongylus is usually self-limiting, and asymptomatic infections do not necessarily warrant treatment.[92] Experimental infections have resolved spontaneously within six months.[96] The presence of inflammation may be an indication for treatment since the inflammatory cells themselves can potentially induce changes to the airways.

Specific anti-parasitic therapy can be attempted with fenbendazole. Dosage regimens vary from as little as 11 mg/lb /day (25 mg/kg/day) for 5 days to 25 mg/lb/day (55 mg/kg/day) for 21 days.[97, 98] The author uses 11 to 23 mg/lb (25 to 50 mg/kg) q12h for 10 to 14 days as described for Paragonimus. Levamisole has been suggested for treatment, but is associated with potential toxic effects in cats. Ivermectin has been used successfully to treat at least one case of Aelurostrongylus using a dose of 180 μg/lb (400 μg/kg) SQ.[99] A dose of 90 μg/lb (200 μg/kg) was unsuccessful. Toxic effects were not seen when ivermectin was used in 23 cats in doses of 180 μg/lb (400 μg/kg), but toxicity trials have not been performed in the cat.[100]

Non-specific treatment with corticosteroids may be helpful in decreasing the severity of clinical signs. The potential side effects and potential for decreased anti-parasitic action of drugs should be considered. Bronchodilator therapy may also provide symptomatic relief.

CAPILLARIA AEROPHILA

Capillaria aerophila is a 2 to 4 cm lungworm that resides in the nasal cavity, trachea, and bronchi of dogs and cats. Eggs are coughed up, swallowed, and passed in the feces. Infection is direct or through earthworm intermediate hosts.[92, 101]

Presentation. The majority of cases are asymptomatic. Occasionally a chronic cough is reported.

Diagnostic Evaluation. Thoracic radiographs in symptomatic patients may reveal a bronchial or interstitial pattern. Tracheal wash fluid typically shows eosinophilic inflammation. The diagnosis is made by the identification of eggs in tracheal wash or fecal specimens examined by flotation. The eggs are double operculated like Trichuris ova, but are smaller (< 70 μ), less pigmented, and have asymmetrical terminal plugs (Figure 69–8).[93] Intermittent shedding of ova may occur.[101]

Treatment. Treatment is probably not necessary when clinical signs are absent. Specific treatment protocols have not been evaluated, but levamisole (3.5 mg/lb/day or 8 mg/kg/day, PO for several treatments in dogs), fenbendazole (11 to 23 mg/lb or 25 to 50 mg/kg, q12h

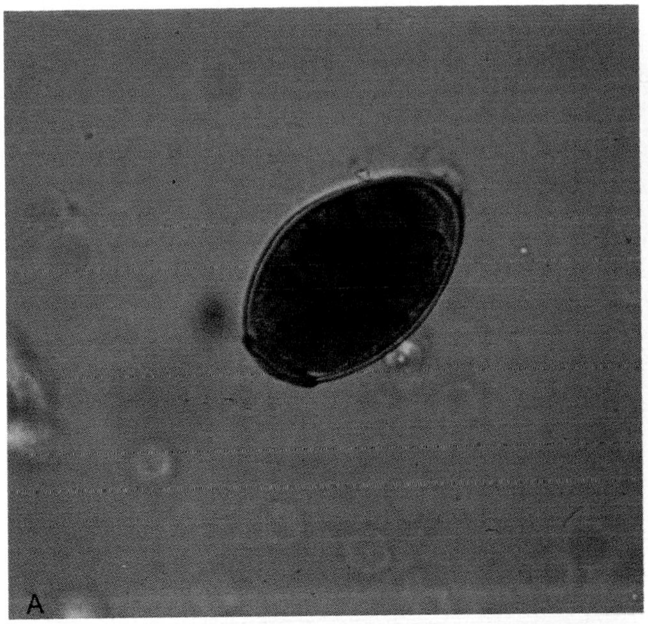
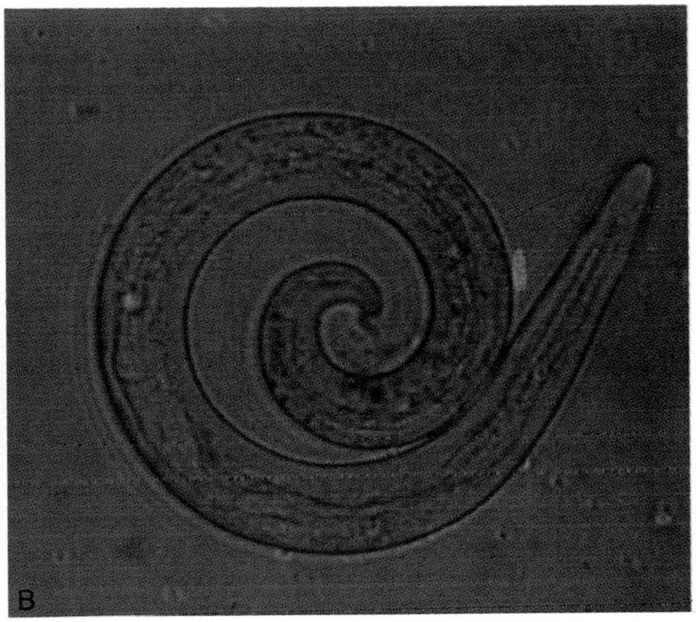
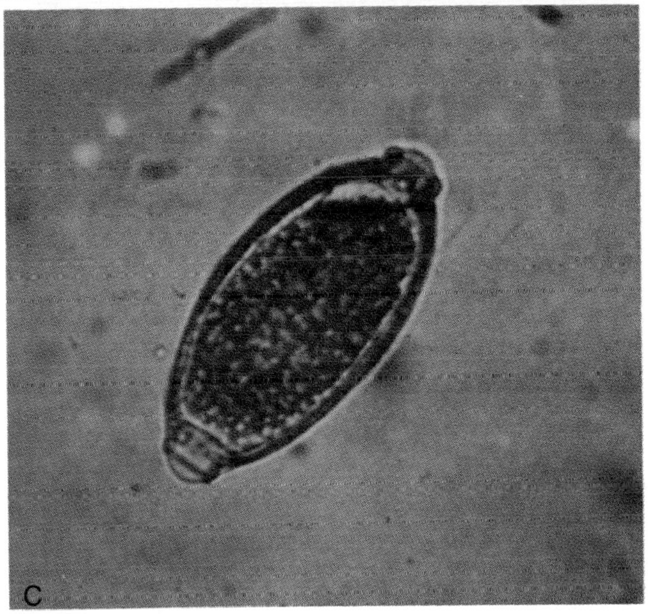

FIGURE 69–8. Diagnostic specimens of common lung parasites. *Paragonimus kellicotti* ova (A) are found in feces examined by sedimentation or flotation, or in tracheal wash fluid. They have a single operculum and are approximately 90 μ in length. *Aelurostrongylus abstrusus* larvae (B) are found in feces examined by the Baermann technique, or in tracheal wash fluid. They are characterized by ventral and prominent dorsal cuticular spines on their tails. *Capillaria aerophila* ova (C) are found in feces examined by flotation, and tracheal wash fluid. They have two opercula but are smaller (<70 μ) and less pigmented than *Trichuris* ova. (Courtesy of Dr. K. Kazacos.)

for 10 to 14 days), and ivermectin have been proposed.[92, 101] Ivermectin was effective in eliminating infection in one cat at an oral dose of 140 μg/lb (300 μg/kg), but was not effective in another cat at an oral dose of 45 μg/lb (100 μg/kg).[102]

OSLERUS OSLERI

Oslerus (Filaroides) osleri is a lungworm that resides at the carina and in the major bronchi of dogs. This parasite is discussed in Chapter 68.

FILAROIDES HIRTHI

Filaroides hirthi is a small lungworm (less than 2 mm) that resides in the terminal bronchioles and alveoli of dogs.[92] Larvae are coughed up, swallowed, and passed in the feces. No development of larvae outside of the dog is required, and autoinfection can worsen the worm burden within the patient. The worms often induce a granulomatous inflammatory reaction. The parasite can be endemic in research colonies of dogs and interfere with interpretation of pathologic findings following experiments.

Presentation. The majority of cases do not demonstrate clinical signs. Severe respiratory tract signs, including tachypnea and respiratory distress, have been reported in three cases.[103–105] Two of these cases occurred in potentially immunocompromised patients and were fatal.[104, 105]

Diagnostic Evaluation. Thoracic radiographs may reveal a diffuse, miliary interstitial pattern or focal nodules.[92, 103] A definitive diagnosis may be difficult. Tracheal wash specimens should be evaluated for larvae or larvated eggs. Fecal specimens are best examined using zinc sulfate flotation,[106] though the Baermann technique can be used. Larvae demonstrate a kinked tail characteristic of *Filaroides* spp.[93]

Treatment. Albendazole (23 mg/lb or 50 mg/kg, q12h for 5 days, repeated in 21 days)[92] and fenbendazole (23 mg/lb/day or 50 mg/kg/day for 14 days)[103] have been used to treat infections. Signs may suddenly worsen during treatment, perhaps due to a reaction to worm death.[103]

ANDERSONSTRONGYLUS (FILAROIDES) MILKSI

Andersonstrongylus milksi reside in the bronchioles and alveoli of dogs and can result in a mild inflammatory response. Clinical signs rarely occur. Embryonated eggs or larvae may be found in tracheal wash specimens, and larvae may be present in fecal specimens examined by the Baermann technique.[92, 107]

CRENOSOMA VULPIS

Crenosoma vulpis is a worm that resides in the trachea, bronchi, and bronchioles of dogs. Larvae are coughed up, swallowed, and passed in the feces. Mollusks serve as intermediate hosts.[92, 108] Spines on the worms cause mucosal abrasions and can result in occlusion of smaller airways.[96] Infection is uncommon.

Presentation. Dogs are presented with signs of tracheobronchitis. Bronchopneumonia, sneezing, and nasal discharge can occur.[96] Radiographs may reveal bronchial, alveolar, interstitial, or mixed patterns.[108]

The diagnosis is made by identification of larvae in tracheal wash fluid or in fecal specimens examined by the Baermann technique. Larvae have a straight tail, unlike those of Filaroides and Oslerus.[96]

Treatment. Two drugs have been used successfully in eliminating infection: diethylcarbamazine (35 mg/lb or 80 mg/kg, q12h for three days), and levamisole (3.5 mg/lb or 8 mg/kg, PO once).[108]

ANGIOSTRONGYLUS VASORUM

Angiostrongylus is rarely diagnosed in the United States. The 2.5 cm worm resides in the pulmonary artery and right ventricle of dogs.[96] The larvae are coughed up, swallowed, and passed in the feces. Mollusks serve as intermediate hosts. Pulmonary artery obstruction, endarteritis, and thrombosis occur, as well as parenchymal damage due to larval migration.[96, 109] Hemorrhages due to anticoagulant factors have been reported.[96, 109]

Presentation. Dogs may be presented with congestive heart failure, lower respiratory signs, including hemoptysis, and subcutaneous hemorrhages.

Diagnostic Evaluation. Radiographs show changes similar to heartworm disease. Larvae may be found in feces or tracheal washings and are identified by a small cephalic button and wavy tail.[96]

Treatment. Levamisole (4.5 mg/lb/day or 10 mg/kg/day, for 2 days) has been recommended for treatment.[109]

Intestinal Parasite Migration

Toxocara canis undergoes migration through the lung of dogs following infection. There are generally no clinical signs from this stage, but in heavy infections pulmonary signs may result from damage and the inflammatory reaction to the migrating larvae.[96] Coughing and tachypnea are usually noted in puppies less than six weeks of age. Fecal examination may reveal no ova, since larvae begin migrating prior to the shedding of eggs. A peripheral eosinophilia may be present.

Signs are usually mild and resolve without treatment. Glucocorticoids can be administered in low dosages to control severe signs but are rarely necessary. Routine anthelmintic therapy is not effective against the larval stage.

Other intestinal parasites with lung migration as part of their life cycle include *Ancylostoma caninum* and *Strongyloides stercoralis*. Transient signs, such as coughing, might be noted.[96] No specific treatment for pulmonary involvement is recommended.

DIROFILARIA IMMITIS

Heartworm disease in the dog and cat (see Chapter 80) can result in marked pulmonary pathology and respiratory signs.

Hypersensitivity and Immune-Mediated Diseases

The immune system, systemic and local, plays a major role in the pathogenesis, clinical signs, progression and recovery of virtually all pulmonary diseases. In some instances the resultant inflammatory response dominates the clinical disease. These diseases can be arbitrarily characterized by their inflammatory response as primarily eosinophilic (or hypersensitivity) and primarily mononuclear (granulomatous). In some instances an antigenic source is discovered, and treatment can be directed toward eliminating the cause. In most instances no offending agent can be found, and immunosuppressant therapy is necessary to control the response.

EOSINOPHILIC (HYPERSENSITIVITY) DISEASES

Eosinophilic pulmonary diseases can be further characterized as primarily bronchial or parenchymal. Bronchial hypersensitivity diseases include feline allergic bronchitis, canine allergic bronchitis, and bronchial parasitic diseases. These conditions were discussed under Bronchial Diseases.

Pulmonary parenchymal hypersensitivity diseases are also known as pulmonary infiltrates with eosinophils, or PIE. The syndrome is characterized by interstitial or alveolar pulmonary infiltration, radiographically, and the presence of eosinophilic inflammation. Although these conditions are seen in dogs and cats, they have not been well defined.[27, 110] Dirofilariasis has been found in some of the reported cases.[111]

Presentation. Signs of PIE are extremely variable, depending upon the severity of disease. Coughing is often the primary complaint and is nonresponsive to antibiotic therapy. Other signs of pulmonary disease can occur, as well as weight loss, depression, and anorexia.

The owner should be questioned about potential exposure to drugs and inhaled allergens.

Physical examination may reveal a fever, though animals are usually normothermic. Lung sounds may be increased due to increased exudation and airway narrowing, or decreased with areas of consolidation.

The CBC classically reflects the eosinophilic response. However, peripheral eosinophilia may be absent in spite of marked pulmonary involvement.

Radiographs can show a mild interstitial pattern, alveolar densities, and even large masses which can be confused as neoplasia or fungal granulomas. Hilar lymphadenopathy may be severe. Dilated, tortuous pulmonary arteries may be present as a result of pulmonary hypertension and should increase the index of suspicion for heartworm disease. A bronchial component also may be present (Figure 69–5).

Cytologic evaluation is necessary for diagnosis. Tracheal wash fluid can be obtained readily and may be adequate for diagnosis. Deeper specimens may be required with localized or interstitial disease obtained through bronchoalveolar lavage, thoracic aspirates, or lung biopsy. Eosinophilic inflammation predominates, though other types of inflammatory cells are also present. Specimens should be critically evaluated for any source of antigen. Antigenic sources include parasites, but also bacteria, fungi, and neoplasia.

Further evaluation for an antigenic source should be pursued with examination of feces for lungworms and microfilarial examination of blood. In dogs with radiographic evidence of heartworm disease and in cats, occult adult antigen heartworm tests should be performed. Animals residing in or having visited areas of the country with endemic mycotic diseases also should be tested for those diseases. Fundoscopic examination should be performed to identify lesions suggestive of infectious diseases.

Treatment. When possible, an etiology should be identified and removed. Medications should be discontinued. Exposure to inhaled allergens should be eliminated by changing the animal's environment. Infectious agents should be treated appropriately.

If no allergen can be found, immunosuppression is required. Corticosteroids are frequently successful in controlling the inflammatory process. An initial dosage of 0.5 mg/lb (1 mg/kg) q12h of prednisone is suggested. The patient should be re-evaluated after 5 to 7 days. Radiographs should be evaluated at that time to assess response, but also to identify any change that might suggest deterioration due to an undiagnosed primary disease.

If signs have resolved, the steroid dosage can be gradually tapered to alternate day therapy at 0.25 mg/lb (0.5 mg/kg). Discontinuation of drug can be attempted after 4 to 6 weeks of therapy, but in many cases long-term therapy is required.

If the process is not controlled, the initial steroid dosage can be doubled. Cases with markedly asymmetric lesions or mass lesions apparent radiographically may exhibit clinical behavior similar to the mononuclear diseases described below, and cytotoxic drugs may be required.

Prognosis. If a primary allergen is identified, the prognosis is dependent on the ability to eliminate the antigen. If no source is identified, the prognosis for control is good, though many animals require long-term, low-dose steroid therapy to manage the clinical signs. As previously mentioned, a few cases may behave similarly to the mononuclear diseases described next.

Mononuclear (Granulomatous) Diseases

Several conditions in humans have been identified in which the pulmonary parenchyma is infiltrated with mononuclear inflammatory cells. These diseases include Wegener's granulomatosis, lymphomatoid granulomatosis, Goodpasture's syndrome, and systemic lupus erythematosus. Wegener's granulomatosis and lymphomatoid granulomatosis are characterized by necrotizing vasculitis and granulomatous inflammation.[112, 113] Some cases of lymphomatoid granulomatosis progress to lymphoma.[113] Goodpasture's syndrome is a result of anti-basement membrane antibodies, which attack the glomerular basement membranes and the basement membranes of pulmonary alveoli and capillaries.[114] Systemic lupus erythematosus (SLE) is a multisystemic autoimmune disease, and lung vasculature occasionally may be involved.[114]

Reported cases in dogs have included lymphomatoid granulomatosis, granulomatosis associated with a positive LE cell test, and pneumonitis as a component of SLE.[115–118] Other cases of inflammatory pneumonitis have been diagnosed in dogs and cats and resolution was achieved with immunosuppressant therapy. These diseases have not been well characterized pathologically.

Inciting causes for these syndromes are rarely identified. They may represent immune-mediated, allergic, or pre-neoplastic conditions.[115] Some infectious agents that can cause similar responses include feline infectious peritonitis virus, rickettsia, atypical bacteria, protozoa, fungi, parasites (including *Dirofilaria*), and bacteria secondary to foreign bodies. The diseases produced by these agents are discussed in Infectious Pulmonary Diseases. Another differential diagnosis is pulmonary neoplasia, either of mononuclear cell origin or inciting a granulomatous inflammatory response. Neoplastic pulmonary disease is discussed in a separate section.

Goodpasture's syndrome has not been reported in dogs, and SLE is discussed in Chapter 119. The remainder of this section will address granulomatosis.

Presentation. Animals are presented with any combination of respiratory signs. Signs of other organ involvement may be present.

Diagnostic Evaluation. Thoracic radiographs reveal an interstitial pattern with multiple, ill-defined nodules of varying size. Hilar lymphadenopathy is frequently present.[115]

Cytologic evaluation of tracheal wash fluid, bronchoalveolar lavage fluid, or lung aspirates reveals granulomatous inflammation without evidence of an etiologic agent. Histopathologic evaluation of a biopsy is required for a definitive diagnosis. Other more accessible organs can be biopsied if they are involved, such as the skin or kidneys.

Treatment. Treatment consists of immunosuppression and should be withheld pending the elimination of infectious differential diagnoses. High dosages of prednisone (1 to 2 mg/lb/day or 2 to 4 mg/kg/day) are administered. Cyclophosphamide also may be necessary to control signs based on response in humans. Cyclophosphamide and vincristine have been used to treat canine lymphomatoid granulomatosis.[115] Since these diseases are poorly defined in animals, it is prudent to begin with steroids alone and add cytotoxic drugs if a beneficial response is not seen.

Re-evaluation with radiographs is recommended within one week of initiating therapy, both to evaluate response to drugs and to identify previously undiagnosed infectious disease (Figures 69–9 and 69–10). Tapering of therapy to a maintenance level, and continuation of therapy for several months before attempting total discontinuation is suggested as for other immune-mediated diseases.

Prognosis. Prognosis is difficult to address because of the lack of clinical reports. Response has been seen in some cases to corticosteroids alone and to corticosteroids and cytotoxic drugs. Of five reported cases treated for lymphomatoid granulomatosis, three were still in complete remission 7, 12, and 32 months from the time of treatment.[115]

Traumatic Lung Disease

Injury to the lung can occur as a result of external or internal trauma. External trauma refers to injury sustained to the lung from outside of the body, such as being hit by a car, being kicked, or falling. Also included in this category are penetrating wounds, such as from gunshots, stabbings, or bites. The subject of management of pulmonary trauma is too broad for this chapter, but the isolated component of pulmonary contusions will be addressed. Internal trauma refers to lung injury sustained from inhalation or aspiration of damaging material. Aspiration pneumonia, near-drowning, and smoke inhalation are discussed.

PULMONARY CONTUSIONS

Pulmonary contusions refer to hemorrhage and edema within the lung and occur as a result of traumatic injury. Respiratory signs develop from ventilation/perfusion abnormalities as alveoli become filled with fluid or collapse. Secondary pneumonia, pain, pneumothorax, hemothorax, rib fractures, diaphragmatic hernias, traumatic myocarditis, and circulatory shock can add to the clinical signs.

Presentation. The patient is presented with historic or physical examination findings confirming a traumatic incident. The lungs should be carefully auscultated. Recent hemorrhage and edema results in moist lung sounds, while consolidated lobes cause an absence of sounds. In both instances the changes are often localized. Diffusely decreased lung sounds are suggestive of pleural involvement.

Ribs should be carefully palpated for fractures. The skin overlying the thorax should be examined thor-

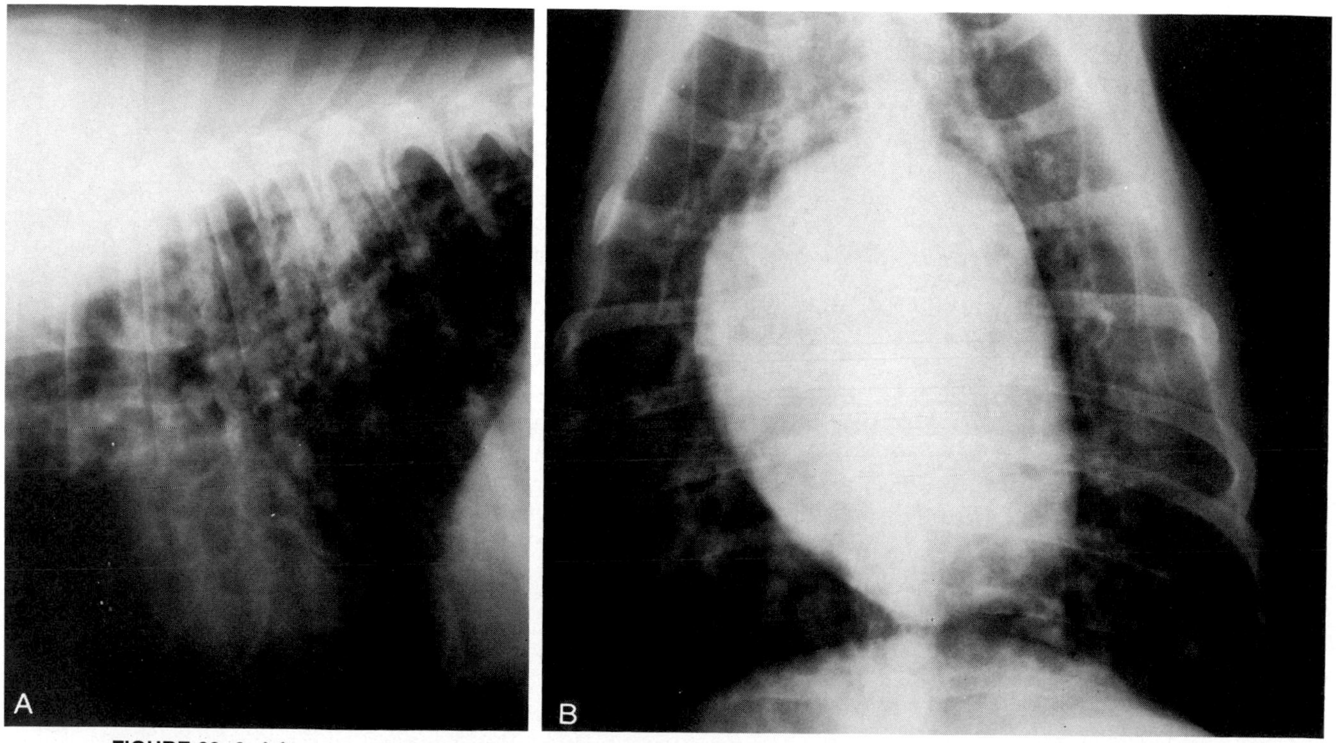

FIGURE 69–9. A four-year-old dog was presented for chronic coughing and weight loss. Radiographs show a diffuse interstitial pattern with fluffy nodular densities. A tracheal wash was nondiagnostic. Granulomatous inflammation was present on bronchoalveolar lavage fluid analysis. There was no evidence of neoplasia and no etiologic agents were seen or cultured. Fungal and toxoplasma titers and heartworm tests were negative. A thrombocytopenia was present also and was assumed to be immune-mediated. Neoplastic or infectious pulmonary disease could not be completely eliminated from the differential diagnoses, but further diagnostic measures were declined and a presumptive diagnosis of immune-mediated disease was made. An immunosuppressive dosage of prednisone was prescribed.

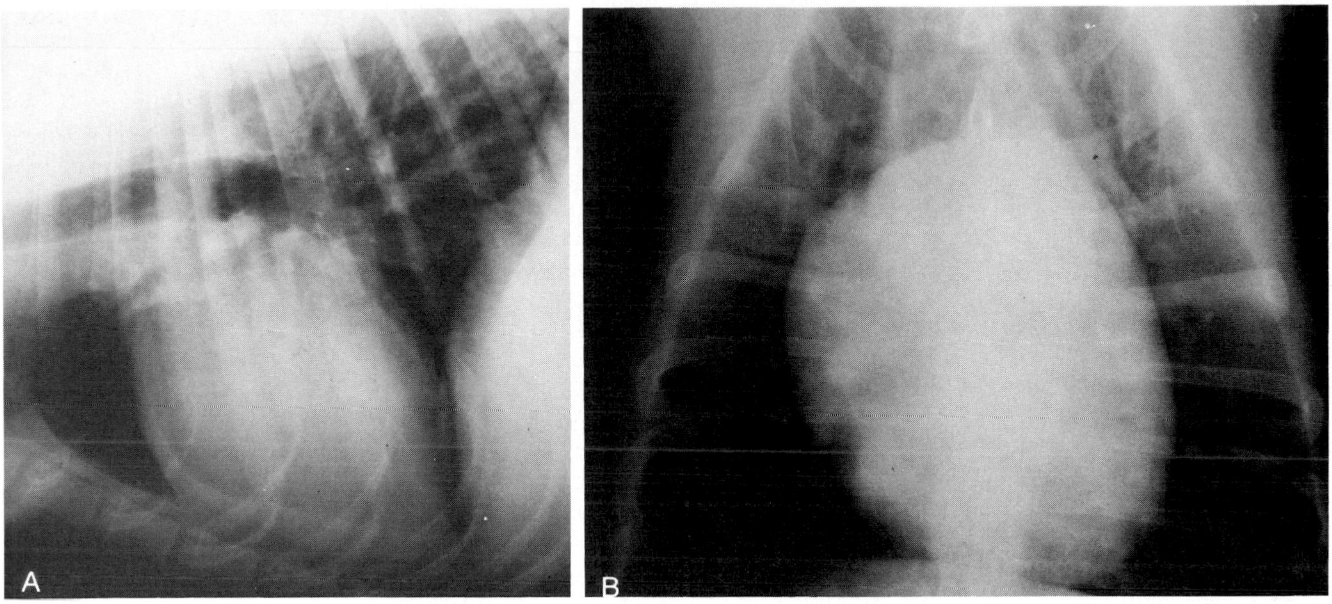

FIGURE 69–10. Radiographs from the dog in Figure 69–9 show marked resolution of disease after 1 week of corticosteroids. The thrombocytopenia also had resolved.

oughly, visually and by palpation, for penetrating wounds or subcutaneous emphysema that may be obscured by coat. Penetrating wounds should be examined critically to determine the full extent of involvement. The examination is especially important in bite wounds, where the degree of external trauma may be far less than the deeper injury.[119] Surgical exploration may be required.[119]

The patient should be carefully monitored, even though apparently stable. Deterioration may occur rapidly for up to 24 hours after the traumatic incident.[120]

Diagnostic Evaluation. Pulmonary contusions are evidenced radiographically by localized areas of an interstitial pattern, alveolar pattern, or consolidation. These changes become apparent 2 to 12 hours following the trauma.[121] Other trauma-induced changes may be apparent.

Bite wounds are often contaminated with one or more of a variety of organisms.[119] Material should be submitted for bacterial culture and sensitivity testing.

Treatment. The critical patient should be stabilized following principles of shock-trauma management. Animals showing clinical signs of hypoxemia should be provided oxygen supplementation. Short-acting corticosteroids may be indicated during stabilization.[120] Diuretics have been suggested to decrease pulmonary edema, but animals with pulmonary lesions severe enough to warrant the treatment are rarely stable enough to be administered volume-depleting drugs. Certainly, overhydration should be avoided. A beneficial response may be seen to bronchodilator therapy.[120]

Once the animal is stabilized, little therapy is generally required beyond cage rest. Antibiotics are indicated for puncture wounds. The effectiveness of prophylactic antibiotics in blunt thoracic trauma is debatable. Careful patient monitoring, in most cases, will result in the early detection of infection and allow appropriate antibiotics to be administered.

Prognosis. Improvement is usually seen within 24 to 48 hours of injury with complete resolution of signs in 3 to 10 days.[121] Complications occasionally develop, and re-evaluation of patients radiographically is indicated following trauma for the early detection of pneumonia, collapsed lung lobes, traumatic lung cysts, lung lobe torsions, or other related injuries. Hemoptysis is uncommon and is considered a poor prognostic sign.[120]

ASPIRATION PNEUMONIA

Aspiration pneumonia occurs when foreign material is inspired into the lungs. Aspiration may occur from the loss of normal protective mechanisms or iatrogenically. Normal protective mechanisms can be circumvented with megaesophagus or other esophageal disorders, pharyngostomy or nasogastric tubes, cleft palate, some laryngoplasties, and abnormal consciousness due to neurologic disease, anesthesia, or severe debilitation. Iatrogenic aspiration can occur by administering food, medication or diagnostic compounds (such as barium) through stomach tubes, pharyngostomy tubes or nasogastric tubes that have been incorrectly positioned in the trachea. The oral administration of mineral oil to cats to treat hair balls can result in aspiration due to a lack of stimulation of protective reflexes by the flavorless, nonirritating oil.

Aspiration can result in respiratory signs due to many mechanisms, including physical obstruction of airways by debris; severe inflammation in response to gastric acid, food particles, mineral oil, antacids or other reactive materials, bacterial infection, physical damage to the alveolar surfaces, decreased pulmonary compliance, and bronchoconstriction.[122] The severity of signs is dependent on the characteristics of the aspirated material and the respiratory and systemic status of the patient prior to aspiration.[122]

Presentation. Owners may present patients with acute aspiration following vomition or regurgitation, loss of-consciousness, or forced oral administration of mineral oil, food, or drugs. Some patients experience aspiration during hospitalization for an underlying problem. The clinician should be aware of patients at risk for aspiration and monitor them for early clinical signs.

Most cases demonstrate acute, severe respiratory distress, with signs apparent within two hours of aspiration.[122] The owners may report acute coughing prior to the development of respiratory distress. Other cases present with a history of chronic recurrent pneumonia.

Physical examination reveals harsh or moist lung sounds, especially in the ventral lung fields. A fever may be present. A thorough oral examination should be performed to identify vomitus or foreign material, cleft palate, or an abnormal gag reflex. The thoracic inlet should be observed to detect ballooning of the esophagus during expiration characteristic of megaesophagus.

Diagnostic Evaluation. Thoracic radiographs often support a diagnosis of aspiration pneumonia. The characteristic change is a bronchoalveolar pattern involving primarily the dependent lung lobes (Figure 69–11). Consolidation may be present. Radiographic changes may be inapparent initially, then gradually progress for one to two days following aspiration. Radiographs should be critically examined for evidence of megaesophagus. A barium swallow may be necessary to confirm this diagnosis, but should be delayed until the patient is stabilized.

Mineral oil aspiration in cats can cause a diffuse, nodular interstitial pattern. The pattern mimics those seen with neoplastic, fungal, and parasitic diseases. A careful history and cytologic analysis should be performed before making a diagnosis of one of these more serious diseases.

Tracheal wash fluid analysis shows acute or chronic inflammation, depending on the duration of injury. Tracheal wash fluid is especially valuable for the identification of bacteria since the marked inflammatory response created by aspiration can result in fever and a peripheral leukocytosis with or without septic involvement.

Once the patient is stabilized, further diagnostic evaluation can be performed to identify underlying diseases. The search for such a problem should be aggressive since aspiration is a secondary problem and will likely recur without elimination of the underlying cause.

Treatment. The severely distressed patient needs immediate oxygen supplementation. If material is still present in the upper airways based on radiographs or auscultation, airway suctioning or bronchoscopy and foreign body removal should be performed. These procedures may require sedation, and ventilatory support should be available. Positive pressure ventilation may also be necessary to overcome decreased lung compliance. Bronchodilator therapy should be administered, and food should be withheld. General Therapeutic Management should be reviewed for details on oxygenation, ventilation, and bronchodilator therapy. Airway humidification and physiotherapy are also discussed and should be included in the management of these cases. Cardiovascular collapse should be treated aggressively with intravenous fluids.

The use of corticosteroids for treatment of acute aspiration is controversial. Though the drugs decrease inflammation and stabilize membranes, they can also inhibit helpful protective responses of the lung. In acute cases where the patient is deteriorating, administration of short-acting corticosteroids is justified.

Some clinicians recommend the use of antibiotics in all cases, while others prefer to monitor clinical progress until evidence of bacterial pneumonia develops. Even if antibiotics are used routinely, monitoring is essential since a population of resistant bacteria can easily develop.

Patients with minimal signs due to aspiration of barium or mineral oil often require no specific therapy. They should be monitored for the development of further signs or sequelae.

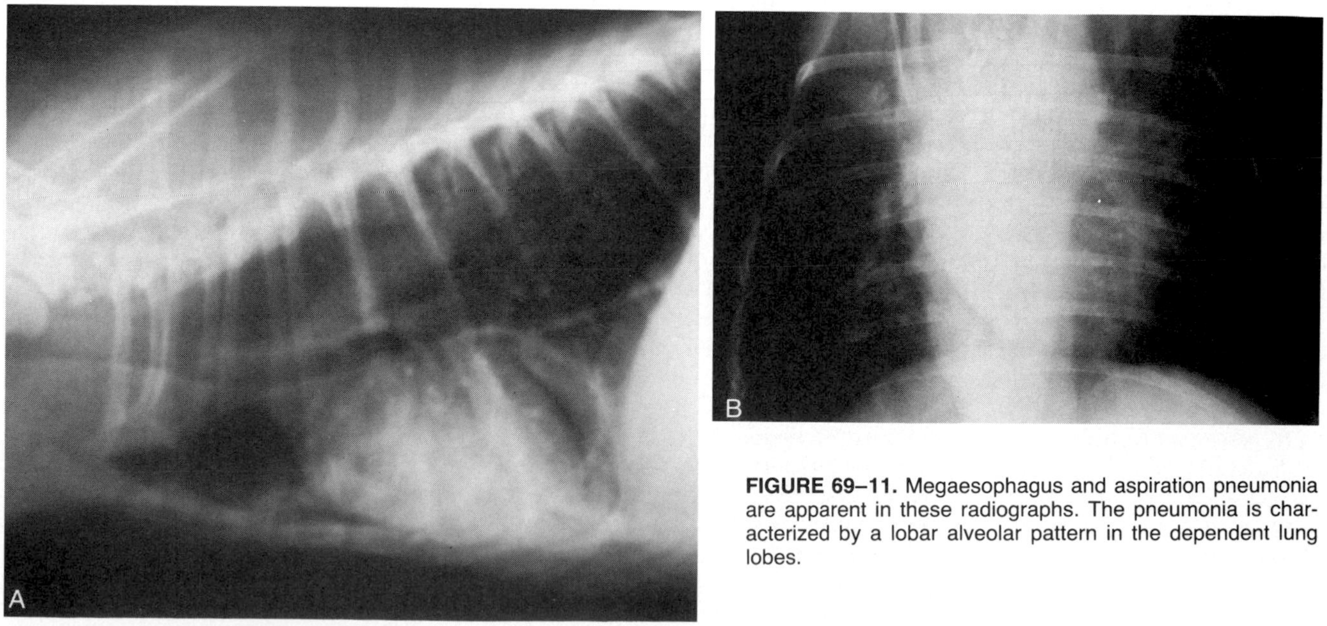

FIGURE 69–11. Megaesophagus and aspiration pneumonia are apparent in these radiographs. The pneumonia is characterized by a lobar alveolar pattern in the dependent lung lobes.

Prognosis. Prognosis is dependent on the amount and character of the material aspirated, the condition of the animal prior to aspiration, and the inciting cause of aspiration. The prognosis can be excellent, as with mild aspiration of barium or mineral oil, or grave. Long-term complications can occur and radiographs should be evaluated following recovery to identify such problems. Possible sequelae include abscesses, granulomas, and consolidated lobes.

Prevention. Guidelines for prevention of aspiration generally pertain to the management of animals with full stomachs prior to the induction of anesthesia and are discussed in surgery and anesthesia texts.

NEAR-DROWNING

Near-drowning occurs as a result of submersion in water. Carbon dioxide concentrations in the bloodstream rise, stimulating breathing efforts. Aspiration occurs in most cases and results in severe pulmonary damage. In ten per cent of cases, laryngospasm prevents the aspiration of water.[123] Dry-drowning results, and pulmonary disease is absent.

Pulmonary damage occurs through a variety of mechanisms. The consequences of the aspiration pneumonia are discussed in the previous section and result from inhalation of vomitus, and debris or chemicals within the water. Bacteria are often present in the water, causing complicating infections. The water itself is harmful. Fresh water dilutes the effects of surfactant, resulting in alveolar collapse and decreased compliance. It may result in hyponatremia as a result of the diffusion of the hypotonic water out of the alveolar space. Hypertonic salt water causes the diffusion of water from within the tissues into the alveoli, creating pulmonary edema (secondary drowning) and potentially hypernatremia.[123]

The changes in the lungs cause severe ventilation/perfusion abnormalities and profound hypoxemia. Hypoxemia quickly leads to metabolic acidosis. The combination of hypoxemia and acidosis is responsible for neuronal death, cerebral edema and herniation, and ultimately death of the patient.[123]

Presentation. Patients are presented following a rescue. Physical examination generally reveals loss of consciousness and either severe respiratory distress or respiratory arrest. The cardiovascular status may be markedly abnormal due to shock, hypoxemia, and acidosis. Hypothermia may be present. Auscultation of the lungs reveals severe moist crackles or an absence of lung sounds. Near-drowning that occurs in waters shared by boaters may be complicated by traumatic injury due to propellers.

Diagnostic Evaluation. Initial evaluation centers on the monitoring of vital functions. General status, neurologic status, blood gases, serum electrolytes, hematocrit and protein concentration, electrocardiogram, and urine output should be frequently monitored.

Once the patient is stabilized, thoracic radiographs are useful to determine the extent of involvement. Radiographic changes may lag behind clinical signs during the initial 24 to 48 hours.[123] A mixed bronchial, alveolar and interstitial pattern is likely. The presence of radiodense material filling airways (sand bronchograms) is a rare, potentially fatal complication.[124] Radiographic evaluation should be continued during and following recovery for the detection of progressive bronchopneumonia, consolidation, or abscessation. Recovering cases should show marked radiographic improvement within ten days.[123]

Tracheal wash evaluation may be indicated if secondary bacterial pneumonia is suspected. Bacterial culture and sensitivity testing should be performed in addition to cytologic analysis.

Treatment. During initial stabilization, alterations in monitored parameters should be treated aggressively as they occur. Hypoxemia is treated with oxygen supplementation. Ventilatory support may be necessary to overcome the decreased compliance. Bronchodilators may be useful. Acidosis is treated with correction of hypoxemia, routine shock therapy, and bicarbonate supplementation. Electrolyte and serum protein abnormalities can be countered with the intravenous administration of appropriate fluids or plasma. Arrhythmias first should be treated through correction of hypoxemia, acidosis and electrolyte imbalances. Anti-arrhythmic therapy should be attempted only if arrhythmias persist. Decreasing urine output may be an indication of cardiovascular failure and signal the need for more aggressive therapy. Comatose or severely dyspneic patients may benefit from mild bicarbonate supplementation (0.5 to 1 mg/lb or 1 to 2 mg/kg IV) prior to the availability of blood gas results.[123]

Animals with abnormal consciousness should be treated with corticosteroids to decrease cerebral edema. Mannitol may also be indicated (see Chapter 61).

Following stabilization, patients are treated with general supportive care. The management of bacterial complications has been discussed.

Prognosis. Prognosis is dependent upon the patient's condition on presentation. Poor prognostic indicators are coma, pH less than seven, and the need for resuscitation or mechanical ventilation.[123] If metabolic stabilization has been achieved, the neurologic status should be closely monitored. As long as the neurologic status shows continued improvement, time should be allowed for functional recovery to occur.

Prevention. Client education is necessary for prevention. In one survey, half of the dogs in immersion accidents were four months old or less.[123] Cold water and rapid currents are particularly exhausting even for the experienced swimmer. Pools, ditches and some rivers provide no avenues for exit. Pool accidents can be extremely upsetting when the front paws are raw and bleeding from frantic attempts to escape. Boating accidents occur when dogs leap from boats, often unobserved, for no apparent reason. In areas of the country where water recreation is popular, client information posters, newsletters, or periodic newspaper articles may be a useful way to avoid accidents.

SMOKE INHALATION

Pulmonary damage due to the inhalation of chemicals can occur during exposure to pollutants, poorly ventilated housing, exhaust from gasoline or diesel engines, improperly functioning heaters, and a variety of other sources.[125] The most commonly identified source of inhalation damage is smoke inhalation as a result of fire.

Smoke inhalation results in respiratory signs through several mechanisms. Carbon dioxide inhalation results in the formation of carboxyhemoglobin with the displacement of oxygen from hemoglobin. Tissue hypoxia results. Heat from inhaled hot air can injure the upper airways to the level of the larynx, and the resultant inflammation and edema can cause upper airway obstruction. Thermal injury can occur to deeper airways through the inhalation of heated particles.[122] These particles can cause injury themselves and can carry chemicals that are caustic to the epithelial cells of the lungs.[122] Chemicals resulting from the combustion of plastic and other materials can be directly toxic to lung tissue. Pulmonary macrophage function and the mucociliary apparatus are adversely affected by smoke inhalation, predisposing the lungs to secondary bronchopneumonia.[122, 126] Concurrent burns to the skin can worsen the pulmonary status, perhaps due to the release of depressant factors, inhibition of immune mechanisms, or development of disseminated intravascular coagulation.[127]

Presentation. Animals presented with smoke inhalation are generally brought from the scene of a fire. The presence of burns around the face, singed vibrissae, oral inflammation, and soot-stained nasal discharge or saliva are supportive of inhalation exposure. The absence of these signs does not eliminate the possibility that significant exposure occurred.

Mucous membranes may be bright red, due to carboxyhemoglobin, or cyanotic. Cyanosis may not be apparent if high concentrations of carboxyhemoglobin are present even with extremely low blood oxygen content.[122] Furthermore, carbon monoxide intoxication may be significant in the absence of the characteristic reddening of mucous membranes.[125] Therefore, animals with suspected carbon monoxide exposure should be treated as such pending confirmatory laboratory results.

Respiratory signs often progress with time. Cough, increased respiratory efforts, and upper airway signs may be present initially. Severe pulmonary edema, epithelial sloughing, secondary infections, and acute respiratory distress syndrome may occur days after exposure.[122, 126] Hypoxemia may result in arrhythmias and abnormal mentation.[125]

Diagnostic Evaluation. Thoracic radiographs are particularly valuable in following progression and resolution of injury.[126] Common pulmonary patterns have been described, in order of frequency, as diffuse bronchial patterns, diffuse patchy consolidation, hyperinflation, and massive consolidation especially of dorsal lung fields.[126] As with other traumatic disease, radiographic signs may lag behind clinical signs.[126]

Blood gas analyses must be evaluated with caution. The $P_{A_{O_2}}$ is a reflection of dissolved oxygen and generally reflects whole blood oxygen content. With carbon monoxide poisoning, the $P_{A_{O_2}}$ may be normal in spite of decreased oxygen content since the carbon monoxide interferes with the oxygen saturation of hemoglobin. The $P_{A_{O_2}}$ can be used as an indication of pulmonary function.

Carboxyhemoglobin concentrations in venous blood can be measured by human hospitals. Specimens must be transported on ice.[127] Treatment should not pend results, but recovery can be monitored by such evaluation.

The patient's cardiac and neurologic status should be carefully monitored with electrocardiograms and serial neurologic examinations. Serum electrolyte and plasma protein concentrations also should be regularly assessed.

Deterioration in status or complications following initial stabilization may require further evaluation with radiographs, tracheal wash analyses, or bronchoscopy. Cytologic evaluation and culture and sensitivity testing of collected specimens may provide useful information.

Treatment. A patent airway is essential, and animals with laryngeal obstruction may require tracheostomies (see Chapter 67). In compromised patients, oxygen supplementation should begin as soon as an airway is established. Supplementation can be initiated at the scene of the fire by face mask when rescue personnel are in attendance.

Carbon monoxide is eliminated by the lungs, and removal is greatly facilitated by the administration of 100 per cent oxygen. The half-life of carboxyhemoglobin is four hours with room air and one-half hour with 100 per cent oxygen.[127] Oxygen therapy should be continued until carboxyhemoglobin concentrations are less than ten per cent.[125] If oxygen therapy is required for an extended period, lower concentrations should be administered.

Pulmonary injury should be managed using general principles of therapy, including oxygenation, airway humidification, and physiotherapy. Bronchodilators may be useful. Antibiotic therapy, as in other traumatic injuries, generally should be withheld until infection occurs. Careful monitoring for evidence of infection is essential. Corticosteroids may be necessary for acute stabilization, but continued use should be avoided due to potential interference with already damaged protective mechanisms.

Other systems also should be attended. Cardiovascular abnormalities will often respond to correction of hypoxemia and fluid and electrolyte management. While dehydration would be detrimental, overhydration should also be avoided. Deterioration in neurologic signs may suggest cerebral edema. Corticosteroid therapy, and perhaps mannitol, are indicated. Skin burns require meticulous management.

Treatment of pulmonary sequelae, such as bronchitis, bronchopneumonia, abscesses, and consolidation or atelectasis are discussed in other sections. The patient should be evaluated following apparent recovery to detect persisting disease.

Prognosis. Patients presented with minimal signs of smoke inhalation on physical and radiographic examination have a good prognosis for recovery, assuming marked deterioration does not occur within the first 24 to 48 hours.[126] The prognosis is progressively more guarded with increasingly severe respiratory signs, neurologic signs, and cutaneous burns. The development of bronchopneumonia is more likely when factors beside inhalation injury are involved, such as the use of a tracheostomy tube or cutaneous burns.[127]

Cystic-Bullous Disease

Circumscribed regions of air and fluid (cavitary lesions) can occur within the lung parenchyma due to cysts, bullae, blebs, and pneumatoceles. Similar lesions result from parasitic cysts and abscesses, and the reader is referred to other sections for discussion of these conditions.

Cysts are fluid-filled or air-filled lesions surrounded by a thin wall of respiratory epithelium.[128] They may be congenital, but are often associated with thoracic trauma.[129]

Bullae are air accumulations formed by the loss of alveolar walls. They often occur as a progression of emphysema due to chronic obstructive pulmonary disease, as may be seen with chronic bronchitis. Alveoli are able to fill with air, but expiration is impeded by airway closure. Pre-existing collagen defects may predispose some animals to the formation of these cavities.[130] In dogs with chronic bronchitis, the changes are usually confined to the edges of lung lobes.[36] Bullae that occur at the pleural surface are called blebs.[128]

Pneumatoceles result from the entry of air into necrotic lesions. They may occur as a result of abscesses, granulomas, or neoplasia.[128] The term has been used to describe a variety of other cavitary lesions.

Respiratory signs reflect the primary disease process (such as pulmonary contusions or chronic obstructive disease), ventilation-perfusion abnormalities, interference with function of adjacent normal structures, and pneumothorax due to dissection of air or rupture of cysts. Secondary infections can occur.

Presentation. Patients generally are presented either with signs of a primary pulmonary disease process or with signs of pneumothorax.

Diagnostic Evaluation. Patients with associated primary processes, such as traumatic contusions, severe bronchopneumonia, aspiration pneumonia, and granulomas, should be radiographed periodically to detect the presence of cystic change or other complications. Patients with pneumothorax should have thoracic radiographs evaluated following removal of air from the pleural space to allow full lung expansion for the evaluation of the pulmonary parenchyma.

Initially cavitary lesions may be totally obscured by overlying densities. They may appear as fluid lines without obvious walls on horizontal beam radiographs. As silhouetting densities resolve, the margins of the lesions can often be identified. Bullous emphysema is rarely apparent radiographically. It is usually observed at exploratory thoracotomy or on post-mortem examination of patients with chronic pulmonary disease.

A definitive diagnosis of cavitary lesions is obtained with thoracotomy, excision, and histopathologic examination. This aggressive approach is not always necessary or indicated.

Treatment. The treatment and monitoring of various primary processes are discussed in other sections of this chapter. Pneumothorax is managed medically as discussed in Chapter 70. Cavitary lesions may resolve with supportive care and treatment of primary disease, but total resolution may require many weeks. In humans, surgical exploration is suggested if the lesions do not decrease in size within six weeks post-trauma in adults and three to four months in children.[129]

Surgical exploration and removal of cavitary lesions by partial or total lobectomy may become necessary more quickly in the presence of continued pneumothorax or unresolving localized infection.[128, 130] Dry-gauze pleurodesis is suggested following removal of bleb lesions.[128] Bullous emphysema is difficult to correct surgically. Pleurodesis can be considered.[130]

Incidental cystic lesions or nonprogressive lesions can be approached conservatively or surgically. If observation is elected, the owners should be warned of the potentials for pneumothorax and infection. Surgical intervention may eliminate those risks, but carries anesthetic and postoperative risks of its own.

Prognosis. Patients whose cavitary lesions result in overt clinical signs have variable prognoses dependent on the primary disease process and the extent of involvement. Resolution of the primary disease decreases the likelihood of further cavitary lesions. Localized lesions can be successfully removed surgically, if indicated. Multiple, diffuse lesions may not be surgically resectable and may be associated with conditions where recurrence is probable, such as bullae due to chronic airway disease. Prognosis in such cases is guarded, though in one report three of six patients with recurrent pneumothorax due to bullous emphysema survived at least two years after surgery.[130]

Miscellaneous Conditions

PULMONARY THROMBOEMBOLIC DISEASE

Pulmonary thromboembolic disease is the result of the obstruction of pulmonary arteries and arterioles. Circulating particles or emboli, such as bacteria, foreign bodies (intravenous catheters), air, fat, parasites, and fragments of thrombi from elsewhere in the body, can be trapped by the extensive pulmonary vascular system. Thrombi can develop within vessels as a result of stasis of blood, damage to the endothelial lining of blood vessels, and systemic hypercoagulability. Blood clots are normally eliminated shortly after they form by the fibrinolytic system. In disease states, the balance between clot formation and dissolution is disturbed.

The interference in pulmonary blood flow results in abnormal ventilation/perfusion relationships within the lung. This change initially results in hypoxemia and hypocapnia, though hypercapnia can occur in severe conditions.[131] Pulmonary hypertension may occur due to massive obstruction or reflex vasoconstriction, and may lead to cor pulmonale.[131] Pulmonary infarction is relatively uncommon.[131, 132] Sudden respiratory distress can occur due to hypoxemia and as a reflex initiated by receptors in the pulmonary artery.[132] Other complications may include decreased cardiac blood flow and mild pleural effusion.[132]

The most commonly recognized cause of pulmonary thromboembolism in small animal medicine is dirofilariasis. Other diseases associated with the condition include nephrotic syndrome, bacterial endocarditis, hyperadrenocorticism, and immune-mediated hemolytic anemia.[133] Thrombus formation can occur postoperatively. Thromboembolic disease resulting from cardiomyopathy is usually associated with systemic embolization.

Presentation. Patients generally experience a peracute onset of extremely severe respiratory distress and tachypnea that is poorly responsive to routine supportive measures. A split second heart sound may occur as a result of pulmonary hypertension. Occasionally cough, hemoptysis, or crackles may be present.[131] Signs may be present related to a predisposing disease process.

Diagnostic Evaluation. Thoracic radiographs are often surprisingly normal. A patient with profound respiratory distress and minimal radiographic changes should be an immediate suspect for thromboembolism. Severe cases may demonstrate decreased size of peripheral vessels with normal or slightly increased central pulmonary artery size, mild right heart enlargement, and mild pleural effusion.[134] Atelectasis can occur with localized disease.[134] Unique features associated with dirofilariasis are discussed in Chapter 80.

Blood gas analysis reveals hypoxemia. Carbon dioxide tensions may be decreased, but with severe disease become elevated. Metabolic acidosis is commonly present as a result of hypoxemia.

A definitive diagnosis of pulmonary thromboembolic disease is obtained with contrast radiography. The study should be performed early in the course of disease prior to the partial dissolution of clots.[131] Ideally, contrast material is injected through a catheter placed in the pulmonary artery; however, nonselective angiography can be used and is a more practical technique.[134] A catheter is advanced to the level of the right atrium, and 0.5 to 1.0 ml/lb (1 to 2 ml/kg) of contrast material is injected. Optimum visualization occurs about three seconds after beginning the injection.[131] A positive angiogram reveals filling defects or sudden interruptions in blood flow. Unaffected regions of the lung may show vessel dilation and rapid contrast transit.[131]

Ventilation and perfusion scanning with radioisotopes are noninvasive safe procedures that can confirm a diagnosis of thromboembolism. The facilities for such testing in animals are limited.

Ancillary tests are essential for the diagnosis of underlying disease processes.

Treatment. Therapeutic recommendations are based largely on experiences in humans.[131, 135] Prevention of continued thrombosis is achieved with anticoagulant therapy using heparin. Coumarin products are required for long-term interference with coagulation. Aspirin, in very low doses, may be useful for its ability to decrease platelet function. Thrombolytic drugs have not gained widespread acceptance in veterinary medicine due to lack of selectivity and expense. The reader is referred to Chapter 116 for a discussion of anticoagulant therapy.

Prognosis. The prognosis is variable, depending upon the severity of disease and the ability to correct predisposing problems. In most cases, the prognosis is guarded to poor.

OBESITY (PICKWICKIAN SYNDROME)

Obesity can affect the lungs in a variety of ways. Intra-thoracic and intra-abdominal fat may interfere with expansion of the thoracic cavity and lungs during inspiration resulting in hypoventilation. Work of breathing, oxygen consumption, and cardiac output during activity are increased in people with excess body mass.[136] Obesity may reflect relatively low levels of exercise and conditioning.

The term pickwickian syndrome refers to a specific condition in humans characterized by obesity, somnolence, hypoventilation, and erythrocytosis.[137] A central neurologic abnormality may be involved.[137] It should be defined by extreme obesity, elevated $PaCO_2$, and an absence of pulmonary disease.[137] It should not be used indiscriminately to describe all obese patients with respiratory disease.

The specific contribution of obesity to clinical pulmonary disease in small animal medicine has not been measured. The clinician should not use obesity as an excuse to avoid pursuing specific disease entities, such as tracheal collapse. However, the beneficial effects of weight reduction in patients with chronic bronchial or pulmonary disease can be dramatic.

CONGENITAL ABNORMALITIES

Congenital abnormalities are rare. The most frequently reported congenital abnormality involving the lower respiratory tract is ciliary dyskinesia and was discussed with bronchial diseases. Other reported abnormalities include anomalous tracheobronchial tree, bronchial cartilage hypoplasia and congenital emphysema, congenital bronchoesophageal fistulas, and pulmonary vascular anomalies.[41, 134, 138, 139] Severe pectus excavatum also can interfere with normal pulmonary function.

The presence of respiratory signs in very young animals or related animals should raise the index of suspicion for congenital disease, though young animals are quite susceptible to infectious diseases, which occur more commonly. With some anomalies, animals may reach several years of age prior to the development of signs or may never develop signs at all.

PULMONARY MINERALIZATION

Mineralized thoracic densities in the airways, pleura, parenchyma, or lymph nodes may be incidental radiographic findings. Chondrodystrophoid dogs may demonstrate airway mineralization at an early age. Mineralization of the airways or the pleura can occur in aged dogs, although the increased pleural density is usually a result of fibrosis.[42] Diffuse nodular mineralization of unknown etiology involving the pulmonary parenchyma can be a non-progressive lesion and can be misinterpreted as metastatic neoplasia.[42] Mineral densities in the local lymph nodes can result from the prior aspiration of barium.

Mineralization can also occur in areas of inflammation or necrosis, such as in the center of masses resulting from fungal infections, tuberculosis, parasites, or neoplasia. The mineralized densities often persist following resolution of active disease.

Systemic diseases resulting in soft tissue mineralization, such as renal secondary hyperparathyroidism and hyperadrenocorticism, can result in mineral deposition in the bronchial walls and other organs.[134] The presenting signs generally reflect the primary disease process or dysfunction of other organs.

ACUTE RESPIRATORY DISTRESS SYNDROME (SEE PULMONARY EDEMA)

LUNG LOBE TORSIONS (SEE CHAPTER 70)

Sequelae to Pulmonary Disease

CHRONIC OBSTRUCTIVE PULMONARY DISEASE

In humans the term chronic obstructive pulmonary disease (COPD) is used clinically to describe chronic lung disease with components of bronchitis and emphysema resulting in obstruction to air flow.[132] Specific documentation of obstructive disease generally is not possible without pulmonary function tests. In small animal medicine, function testing is not readily available and the term is generally applied to patients with clinically apparent respiratory compromise due to chronic bronchitis and its complications.

EMPHYSEMA

Pulmonary emphysema in dogs and cats is generally associated with chronic bronchial disease. It can occur congenitally. The reader is referred to Chronic Bronchitis and Cystic-Bullous Disease.

PULMONARY ABSCESSATION

Pulmonary abscesses, though rare, can occur as a complication of bacterial pneumonia, foreign bodies, trauma (including aspiration), parasitic or fungal infections, and neoplasia. They are identified radiographically as nodular or cavitary lesions. The walls may be thick or thin and are often ill-defined. If air is present within the cavity, a fluid line may be apparent on horizontal beam radiographs.

The diagnosis is suspected from radiographic appearance, especially when found during or following an episode of an associated disease. Surgery is indicated if the diagnosis must be confirmed through excision and histologic evaluation, or if the lesion does not resolve after several months of aggressive antibiotic therapy.

LOBAR CONSOLIDATION

Consolidation refers to the filling of airways with cells or fluid and can occur with inflammatory, neoplastic, or hemorrhagic disease. An entire lung lobe becomes involved when localized lesions coalesce, when processes spread through channels of collateral ventilation throughout the lung lobe, and when there is complete bronchial obstruction.[134] Lobar consolidations are recognized radiographically as soft tissue densities with apparent lung lobe borders (Figure 69–12).

Consolidation can be a result of any severe inflammatory disease process. Primary pulmonary neoplasia will result in a consolidated pattern in a small percentage of cases,[140] and pulmonary hemorrhage (contusion) and lung lobe torsions can also cause lobar consolidation. If treatment of the primary disease does not result in resolution of the consolidation, surgical excision may be necessary.

ATELECTASIS

Atelectasis refers to the collapse of lung due to the loss of air from the alveoli. Compression atelectasis commonly results from pneumothorax and pleural effusion. Obstructive atelectasis occurs as a complication of total airway obstruction and the absorption of alveolar gases into the blood. The obstruction may be a result of foreign bodies, but is more often due to mucus, inflammation, airway collapse, or airway compression. Inhalation anesthesia, prolonged recumbency, or decreased ciliary clearance can potentiate the tendency for atelectasis to occur. Atelectasis also can occur as a result of alveolar collapse from the loss of surfactant. Decreased surfactant is a common problem in premature infants, but can occur in acquired diseases such as acute respiratory distress syndrome and drowning.

The primary differential diagnosis for atelectasis is pulmonary consolidation resulting from the replacement of alveolar air with fluid or cells. Atelectatic lobes have concave margins, are reduced in size, and result in rearrangement of the unaffected lung lobes as is evident by changes in location of the interlobar fissures and diaphragm and shifting of the mediastinum.[134] The lobes are not always noticeably shrunken since edema and inflammatory infiltration can be present within the parenchyma.[134]

Treatment is directed at the inciting cause. Physiotherapy may be beneficial. Prolonged atelectasis can result in abscessation or fibrosis, and surgical intervention may be necessary in obstructive atelectasis if signs are persistent.

COR PULMONALE

Cor pulmonale refers to hypertrophy of the right ventricle as a result of pulmonary hypertension. Pulmonary hypertension is most often associated with chronic pulmonary diseases such as chronic bronchitis in which alveolar hypoxia results in persistent pulmonary vasoconstriction.[132] Pulmonary hypertension can also occur due to thromboembolic disease.

In veterinary medicine cor pulmonale is recognized by the presence of right heart enlargement on thoracic radiography in conjunction with chronic pulmonary disease. Cardiac ultrasonography can be performed to further characterize chamber enlargement and to identify any primary heart diseases. Pressure measurements are rarely performed. Eventually right heart failure can occur.

Aggressive treatment should be directed at the pulmonary disease since the condition is a secondary event. If such an approach fails, hydralazine theoretically may be beneficial as a vasodilator.[141] The clinical application

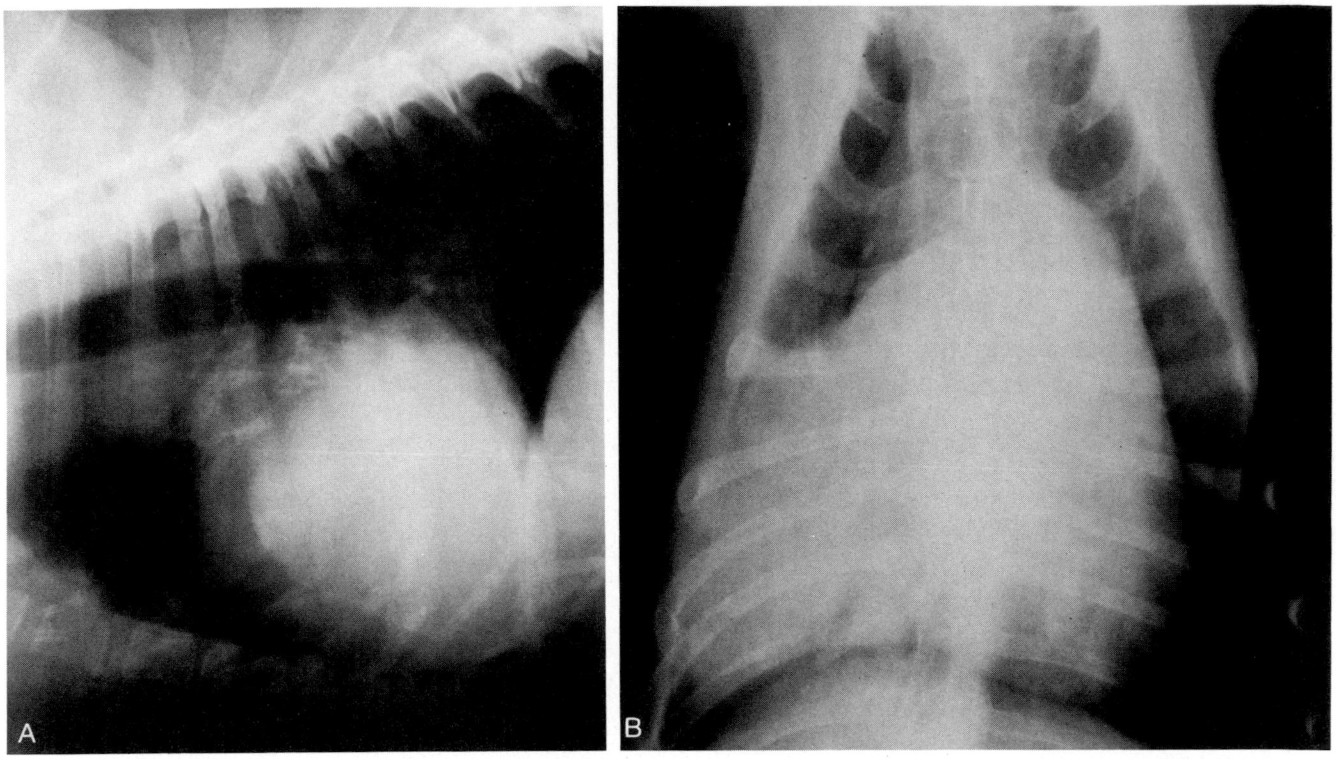

FIGURE 69–12. A 12-year-old dog was presented for coughing and shortness of breath of a two-week duration. Radiographs show consolidation of the right middle lung lobe. The bronchus was compressed and could not be entered bronchoscopically. Bronchoalveolar lavage fluid revealed mild, chronic inflammation. A lobectomy was performed and torsion of the lobe was found. On microscopic examination, infarction and fibrosis were identified. There was no evidence of an active inflammatory process or neoplasia.

of such therapy in veterinary medicine has not been established.

Neoplastic Pulmonary Disease

Lung tissue can be affected by primary pulmonary neoplasia, metastatic neoplasia, lymphosarcoma, and neoplasia invading from adjacent tissues. Neoplasia of adjacent tissues, such as the pleura, mediastinum, thoracic wall, esophagus, and heart, are discussed in other sections.

Primary Pulmonary Neoplasia

Neoplasia arising primarily from the lungs is uncommon in the dog and cat, especially when compared to the incidence in man or the incidence of metastatic pulmonary neoplasia. The number of cases diagnosed appears to be increasing with time and, assuming that the trends of longer life-spans and improved diagnostic and therapeutic methods continue, the clinician will be faced with more and more of these cases.[142–144]

Classification of primary pulmonary neoplasia has been standardized utilizing the World Health Organization classification scheme. Some authors find the system incompatible with clinical findings.[145] The great majority of primary pulmonary tumors in dogs and cats are carcinomas. Adenocarcinomas are most frequently found, accounting for 70 to 80 per cent of pulmonary carcinomas,[145] followed by squamous cell and anaplastic carcinomas.[142, 143, 146–151] Fibrosarcomas, osteosarcomas, chondrosarcomas, hemangiosarcomas, and benign adenomas occur infrequently.[142, 143, 146, 149–151]

Metastatic disease resulting from the spread of primary lung tumors is common due to the malignant nature of most of these tumors. Neoplastic cells frequently metastasize to other areas of the lung through blood vessels, lymphatics, or airways. In one series of canine cases 18 of 26 dogs had metastases, of which 17 involved the lungs.[146] The pulmonary metastatic lesions may be smaller than the original tumor, or multiple uniform nodules can occur. Uniform nodules may represent multicentric disease rather than metastases. Another common site of metastasis is the bronchial lymph nodes. The pleura can be involved. Extrathoracic metastatic lesions can involve the long bones, liver, spleen, pancreas, kidneys, adrenal glands, heart, brain, esophagus, abdominal or mediastinal lymph nodes, and eyes.[143, 146–148, 152, 153] Involvement of multiple digits has been seen in several cats.[151, 154]

Clinical signs can result from the primary pulmonary tumors and intrathoracic metastases, from extrathoracic metastases, and from paraneoplastic conditions. Primary tumors and intrathoracic metastases can cause respiratory signs from compression or obstruction of airways, regional ventilation/perfusion abnormalities, or pleural effusion. Inflammatory reactions to the tumors, secondary infections, intrapulmonary hemorrhage, cavitary lesions, pneumothorax, and hemothorax also can contribute to respiratory signs. Nonrespiratory signs from the primary tumor, such as weight loss, anorexia, and depression, can occur with or without concurrent respiratory signs. Occasionally pulmonary tumors compress the major thoracic veins resulting in ascites, jugular distention, or edema of the head and neck. Esophageal compression can lead to dysphagia or regurgitation.

Extrathoracic metastatic disease results in signs associated with the systems involved. Cases may present for those signs alone without historic evidence of respiratory disease.

A variety of paraneoplastic syndromes have been associated with primary pulmonary tumors in humans, but few have been reported in small animals.[155] Hypertrophic pulmonary osteopathy (HPO) is the most frequently reported syndrome in dogs, with less frequent occurrence in cats.[134, 155] One review of 29 primary canine lung tumors reported 5 cases of HPO, although another review of 29 cases reported none.[143, 146] Paraplegia and a neuromyopathy was reported in one dog with an anaplastic pulmonary carcinoma.[156]

Presentation. Dogs and cats presented with primary pulmonary tumors are usually middle-aged or older animals. The mean age at presentation is 9 to 12 years, with patients as young as two years reported.[142, 143, 146, 148] No particular sex or breed predisposition is obvious, although one review revealed a high incidence in boxers relative to the hospital population.[142, 146]

Client complaints can reflect respiratory signs, signs of metastasis or HPO, or nonlocalizing signs, all of which are usually chronic.[142, 143, 146, 148] Respiratory system involvement is suggested by cough, exercise intolerance, respiratory distress, and rarely hemoptysis. The cough is generally nonproductive. Lameness or signs of dissemination to other organs occur from metastases or HPO. Nonlocalizing signs include weight loss, anorexia, and depression. Dysphagia, vomiting, and rarely ascites or edema of the head and neck also can occur.

Physical examination can reflect signs of respiratory disease, other organ involvement, or general debilitation. The lungs should be carefully auscultated for localized areas of increased or absent lung sounds. Pleural effusion may result in a generalized decrease in lung sounds. Lameness may be noted due to bone metastases or HPO, and the involved limb may be swollen and painful. The patient may exhibit poor condition and weight loss.

Abnormalities may be discovered on physical examination that are unrelated to the pulmonary neoplasia, and the tumor may be an incidental finding. A number of animals are presented with other primary tumors elsewhere in the body.[142, 157]

Diagnostic Evaluation. Radiographs are the most valuable diagnostic aid in the evaluation of patients with pulmonary neoplasia. Lung patterns are quite varied and include diffuse involvement, single circumscribed mass lesions, lobar consolidations, and multiple circumscribed masses (Figures 69–12 and 69–13).[140, 143, 148] Diffuse involvement is a common occurrence and can result in reticulonodular, alveolar, or peribronchial densities.[140, 143] These patterns can occur alone or in combination. Cavitation of mass lesions, hilar lymphadenopathy, and calcification of lesions can be seen.[140, 143, 148]

Radiographs of the lungs do have important limitations that must be considered. Radiographs are insensitive to masses less than 1 cm in diameter.[155] Improving the sensitivity of thoracic radiographs is discussed with metastatic pulmonary neoplasia. More important to the client and the patient, a definitive diagnosis of neoplasia cannot be made based upon radiographs alone. The signalment, history, physical findings, and radiographs may strongly suggest a neoplastic process, but the definitive diagnosis is obtained through cytologic or histologic evaluation of tissue. Conditions that can mimic pulmonary neoplasia to a surprising degree include infections (especially parasitic, fungal, and atypical bacteria), foreign body reactions, hypersensitivity and immune-mediated diseases, and lung lobe torsions. Diffuse lung tumors can be indistinguishable radiographically from pneumonia, hemorrhage, and edema in addition to the above diseases. All of these conditions offer a significantly better prognosis than primary neoplasia and should be aggressively pursued whenever the condition of the patient and the client's desires will allow.

Pleural effusion or pneumothorax can be observed radiographically in patients with pulmonary neoplasia.[140, 143, 148] Neoplasia of the chest is a common cause of pleural effusion in small animals.[158] Pneumothorax is much less common. Patients should be re-evaluated radiographically following the removal of fluid or air from the pleural space to allow the lungs to expand fully for accurate radiographic evaluation.

Radiographs of the bones should be evaluated in animals presenting with lameness, limb pain, or swelling for evidence of HPO or bone metastases. Signs involving other organ systems also should be pursued.

A definitive diagnosis of pulmonary neoplasia requires the cytologic or histologic evaluation of specimens. Pleural fluid, tracheal washings, bronchial brushings, and bronchoalveolar lavage fluid can be evaluated cytologically. These specimens can be collected relatively noninvasively, but they are frequently nondiagnostic. Interpretation of such specimens must be carefully performed, since inflammatory processes can result in some cytologic criteria of malignancy in cells such as the pleural mesothelium or respiratory epithelium. The presence of non-neoplastic abnormalities, such as bacterial infection, nonseptic inflammation, or hypersensitivity responses, does not totally eliminate the possibility of underlying neoplasia.

Transthoracic or transbronchial biopsies can be obtained from lesions near the thoracic wall or involving the major airways respectively. Transthoracic needle biopsies are best performed with fluoroscopic or ultrasonographic guidance. Peripheral lesions can be biopsied using two radiographic views to provide anatomical guidance. Transbronchial biopsies can be guided by visualization of lesions during bronchoscopy or fluoroscopically. A relatively small specimen is obtained and must be representative of the primary disease for an accurate diagnosis to be made. Potential complications of biopsy include hemothorax, pneumothorax, and abscess rupture.

Thoracotomy is the most invasive method of obtaining lung tissue, but there are major advantages to this approach. Excellent specimens can be provided to the pathologist for analysis. The other lung lobes and re-

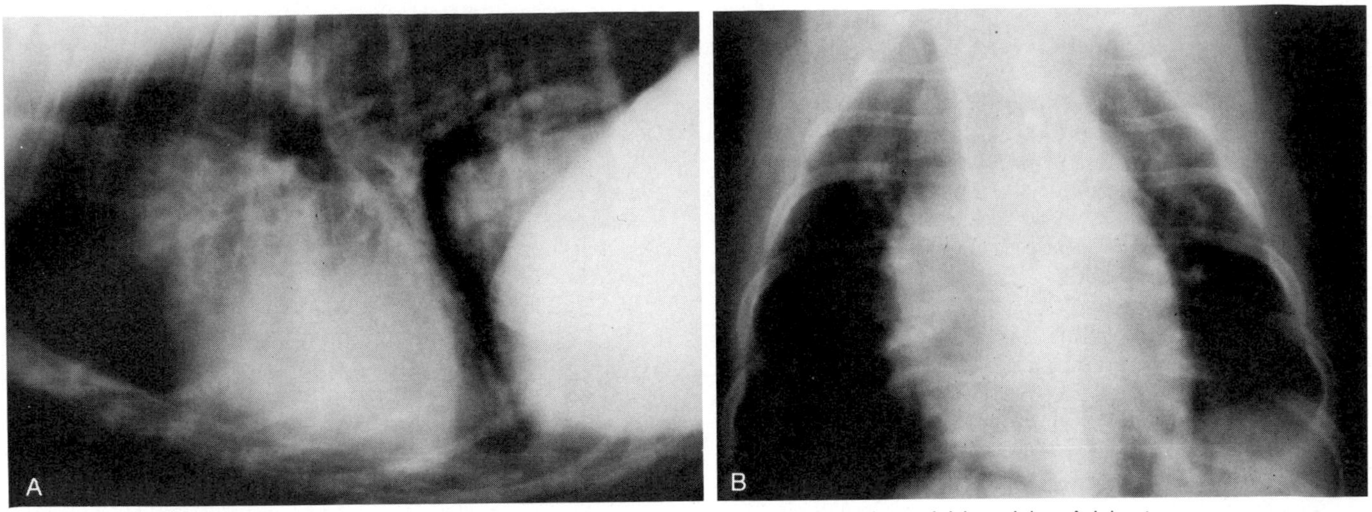

FIGURE 69–13. Radiographs showing a well-circumscribed mass in the left caudal lung lobe. A lobectomy was performed. The histologic diagnosis was pulmonary adenocarcinoma.

gional lymph nodes can be examined and biopsied, and the treatment of choice, lobectomy, can be performed (Figure 69–14).

In situations where aggressive diagnostic evaluation is not desirable, further information can be obtained non-invasively by the repeated evaluation of thoracic radiographs over time. Radiographs taken every four to six weeks, depending upon the rate of progression of clinical signs, can be evaluated to determine the course of the disease. If no change is seen radiographically after several months, the lesions may be non-neoplastic or extremely slow growing. If changes typical of malignant neoplasia occur rapidly, the clinical diagnosis of primary pulmonary neoplasia is more likely correct. This approach is not recommended for potentially resectable lesions because the tumor may become nonresectable during the delay.

Computerized tomography and nuclear imaging are being used in the evaluation of pulmonary neoplasia in humans. Their use in dogs and cats is limited due to availability and expense.

Therapy. Excision of tumor with wide surgical margins is the treatment of choice for primary pulmonary neoplasia. Lobectomy is usually required. If the disease is determined to be non-resectable at surgery, signs may be temporarily palliated with the excision of areas of major involvement. This improvement may be a result of relief of compression on adjacent tissues, elimination of sites of necrosis and inflammation, or improvement of ventilation/perfusion relationships.

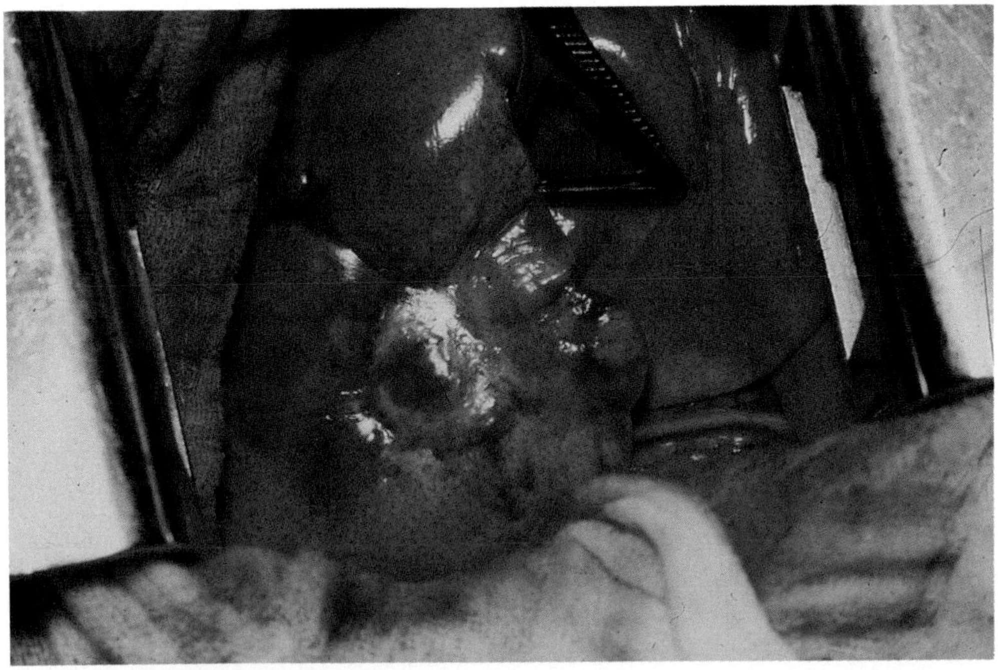

FIGURE 69–14. Papillary adenocarcinoma involving the left cranial lung lobe of a dog.

Tumors that cannot be excised can be treated with systemic chemotherapeutic drugs, though promising results have not been published. Cyclophosphamide, doxorubicin hydrochloride, methotrexate, and nitrogen mustard have been used in humans.[159] Cisplatin and vindesine (a vinca alkaloid) in combination were successful in achieving greater than 50 per cent reduction of measurable lesions in two dogs with advanced, recurrent pulmonary carcinoma.[160]

Prognosis. The long-term prognosis for most primary pulmonary tumors is guarded to poor, though the course may be slow. The majority of tumors are malignant, and many are nonresectable at the time of diagnosis. Some cases will respond to surgical excision. In one report, three dogs with single masses were treated by lobectomy. One dog was euthanatized upon recurrence of dyspnea 16 months later, one dog showed recurrence of tumor radiographically at 19 months, and the third dog had a benign tumor and remained well.[143] Another report of 15 dogs that were treated by lobectomy based on single lung lobe involvement without identifiable metastases or extrathoracic disease on preoperative evaluation demonstrated a mean survival of ten months (range 7 to 19 months) in 9 dogs that had died, and a mean survival of 20 months (range 8 to 46 months) in 6 dogs that were alive and asymptomatic at the time of publication.[160] Though statistical significance was not present, dogs with adenocarcinoma had longer mean survival times than dogs with squamous cell carcinoma, and dogs without lymph node metastasis had longer survival times than those with lymph node involvement.[160]

Metastatic Pulmonary Neoplasia

The lungs are a common site of metastases, second only to lymph nodes draining the organ with the primary tumor.[140] Malignant cells must successfully complete many steps in order to establish tumors in distant sites. The primary tumor must be vascularized, the local tissues must be invaded, neoplastic cells must exfoliate from the primary mass, cells must be carried to other organs, and cells must leave the circulation at the new site, invade local tissues, and proliferate.[161] Only a few cells ever successfully complete this process, and the longer a cell is in circulation the less likely it is to develop into a metastatic lesion.[161] The lungs contain the first capillary system through which most circulating neoplastic cells pass.[140, 155]

Any malignant tumor potentially can result in metastatic disease. Tumor types with high incidences of pulmonary metastatic lesions include thyroid carcinomas and mammary carcinomas.[140] Pulmonary metastases from osteosarcoma, hemangiosarcoma, transitional cell carcinoma, oral and digital melanoma, and squamous cell carcinoma also occur commonly.[162] Metastatic disease is often the limiting factor in the treatment of primary malignancies, and in humans 50 per cent or more of malignant tumors have metastasized prior to diagnosis.[163]

Detection of metastases is routinely attempted through the evaluation of thoracic radiographs because of the high incidence of metastases to the lung and the ability to detect metastases in the lung because of contrast with air. Unfortunately, the discovery of metastases on thoracic radiographs represents a late finding in the course of disease.[144, 155] Limitations of thoracic radiography are discussed under Diagnostic Evaluation.

Pulmonary metastases, themselves, can result in clinical signs and may be responsible for the presentation of a patient. Signs result from similar mechanisms as discussed for Primary Pulmonary Neoplasia.

Presentation. Animals with pulmonary metastatic disease can be presented for signs caused by the primary tumor or for signs caused by the pulmonary involvement. The presenting signs with advanced pulmonary metastases are similar to those described for primary pulmonary neoplasia.

Diagnostic Evaluation. A presumptive diagnosis of pulmonary metastatic disease frequently is made on the basis of a histopathologically diagnosed primary malignant tumor and suggestive thoracic radiographs. Radiographic patterns associated with metastatic tumors are the same as those described in the discussion of primary pulmonary neoplasia (Figures 69–15 and 69–16). Clinical evidence may be sufficiently convincing to discontinue the diagnostic evaluation at this point, but the clinician should be aware that occasionally erroneous conclusions will be made. To further obscure an accurate diagnosis, radiographic evaluation is relatively insensitive and may fail to detect metastatic lesions.

A diagnosis of pulmonary metastases may be incorrectly made as a result of two primary tumors in the

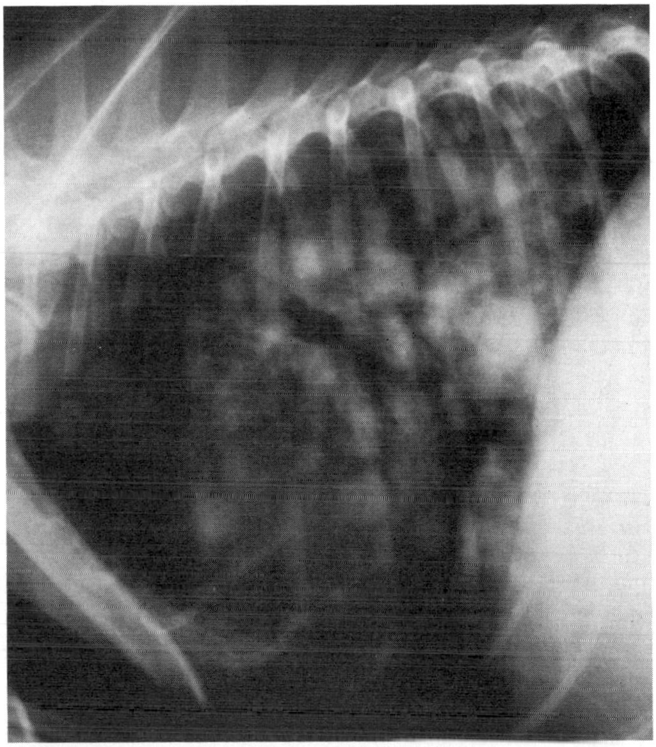

FIGURE 69–15. A reticular interstitial pattern with multiple nodules throughout the lung fields is suggestive of metastatic neoplasia. Fungal infection, immune-mediated disease, or other inflammatory processes must be included in the differential diagnoses and are supported by the ill-defined borders of many of the nodules. This patient had had a malignant melanoma removed from a distal limb previously, and the tumor had metastasized to the lung.

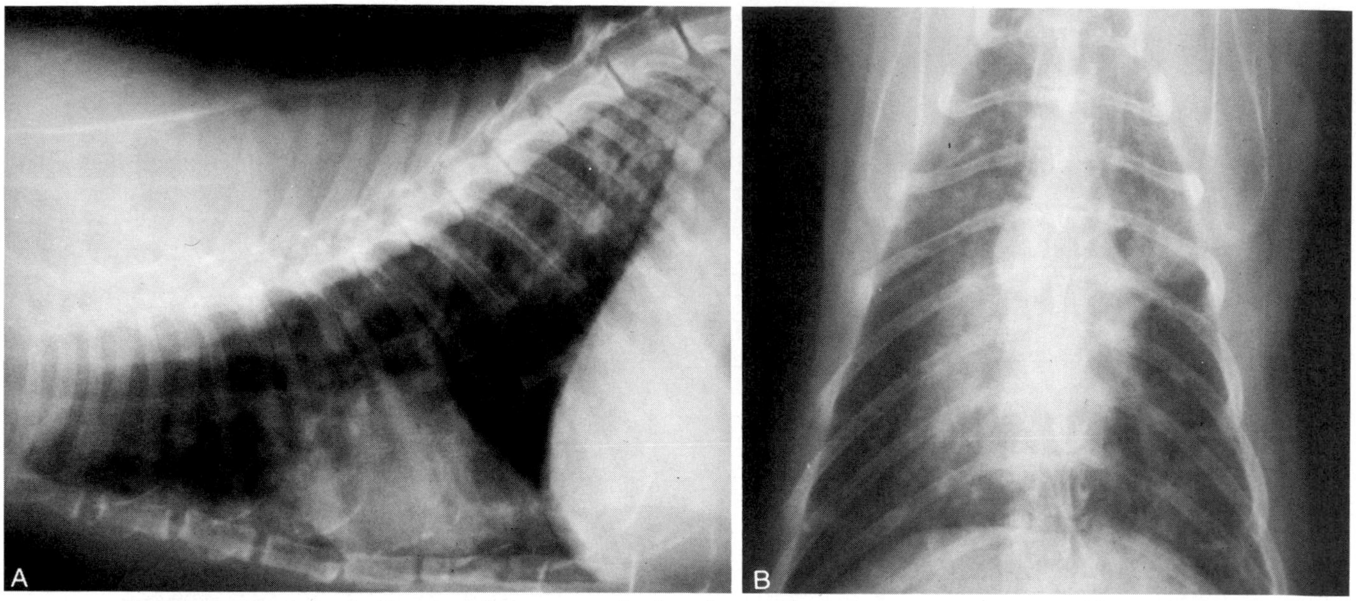

FIGURE 69–16. *A,* A cat with metastatic mammary gland carcinoma. The metastases are represented by a marked, diffuse interstitial pattern. *B,* A bronchial component also is visible.

same patient or due to the misinterpretation of benign radiographic lesions. Fifteen of 29 dogs with primary pulmonary neoplasia were found to have coincidental tumors at other sites in the body.[146] In another report, two cats with mammary tumors had pulmonary masses; one was an abscess and one was a primary lung tumor.[157] In these cases the pulmonary lesions were not the result of metastasis from the extrapulmonary tumors. Radiographic patterns that can be misinterpreted as metastatic disease can occur as a result of atypical bacterial infections, immune-mediated or hypersensitivity diseases, parasitic infections, fungal infections, and other non-neoplastic diseases. A definitive diagnosis of metastatic neoplasia can be obtained through the cytologic or histologic evaluation of specimens as described for primary pulmonary tumors. Re-evaluation of the patient radiographically at one to two month intervals is especially useful for these cases.

The relative insensitivity of thoracic radiographs is well established. Under the best circumstances, thoracic radiographs can only detect lesions greater than 3 to 5 mm diameter.[140] One study showed that conventional radiographs failed to detect 25 per cent of canine pulmonary metastases that were found at necropsy.[164] Three of eight dogs with pulmonary metastases from transitional cell carcinoma of the bladder were not diagnosed radiographically because the unstructured interstitial densities apparent were interpreted as compatible with age.[165] Sensitivity can be improved by performing both right and left lateral recumbent views and by having multiple readers interpret the radiographs.[166] Improved sensitivity from two lateral views can be attributed to increased contrast in the well-aerated, nondependent lung lobes and magnification of the lung furthest from the film (Figure 69–17).[166, 167] Radiographs should be exposed during inspiration. If pleural effusion is present, it should be removed and radiographs taken again with the lungs fully expanded.

Treatment. Surgical excision of single or small numbers of metastatic lesions could potentially contribute to cure of disease and may palliate clinical signs. Unfortunately, metastatic disease is rarely identified prior to the development of diffuse, nonresectable, pulmonary lesions.

Chemotherapeutic agents are recommended based on the sensitivity of the primary tumor, though tumor heterogeneity may result in a different sensitivity pattern in the metastatic cells.[161] The advanced stage at which

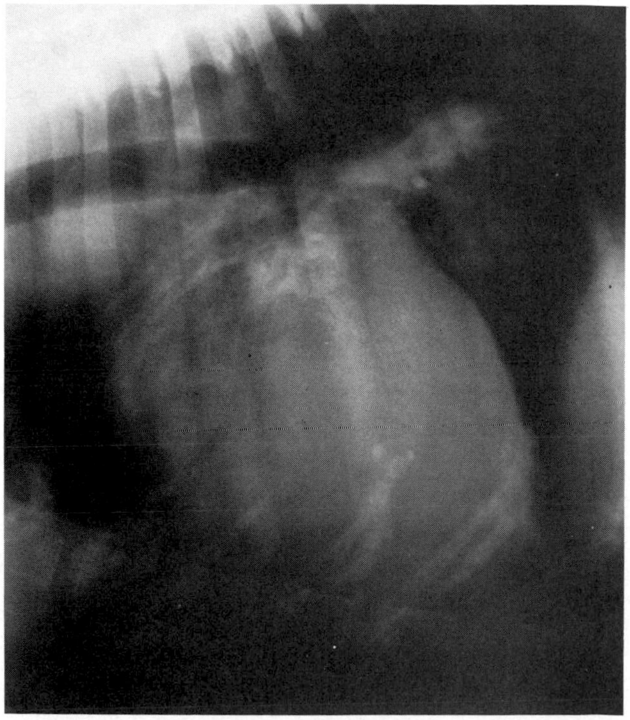

FIGURE 69–17. This radiograph is from the same dog as Figure 69–14 but was exposed with the patient in left lateral recumbency rather than right. The absence of air contrast in the poorly ventilated dependent lobes obscures the presence of the infiltrated lobe. Because of this effect, both lateral views should be taken to improve the sensitivity of radiographs used to screen for neoplastic disease.

metastases are detected may account for a generally poor long-term response.[155]

Other potential treatment modalities include immunotherapy and antimetastatic drugs. No recommendations for specific immune modulating agents can be made at this time. Anti-metastatic drugs are being evaluated for the prevention of metastases. These drugs interfere with one or more of the steps required for successful seeding of neoplastic cells in distant organs.

Prognosis. The long-term prognosis for patients with pulmonary metastatic disease is grave. Therefore, the clinician should be extremely careful in making the diagnosis.

Lymphosarcoma

Lymphosarcoma can involve the pulmonary parenchyma in the multicentric form of the disease. Thoracic radiographs reveal an irregular reticular pattern, often with ill-defined nodular densities.[140] Hilar, mediastinal, or sternal lymphadenopathy may be apparent (Figure 69–18). Rarely a single mass lesion or a peribronchial pattern occurs.[140] Radiographic changes are similar to changes caused by severe inflammatory pulmonary diseases.

Neoplastic cells may be identifiable on respiratory cytologic or histologic specimens (Figure 69–19), but the disease is generally diagnosed through other more accessible systems, such as the peripheral lymph nodes. The disease is discussed thoroughly in Chapter 115.

PULMONARY EDEMA

Pulmonary edema can be defined as an abnormal accumulation of liquid and solute in the interstitial tissues, airways, and alveoli of the lung.[168] Pulmonary edema is the result of a disease process rather than the disease itself.

Normal fluid content of extravascular pulmonary tissue is maintained by a delicate balance between outward transcapillary fluid transport and pulmonary lymphatic drainage. In pulmonary edema, movement of liquid and blood from the interstitial space and occasionally the alveoli is not as great as the return of liquid to the blood through the lymphatic drainage.[169]

The barrier that exists between the pulmonary capillaries and alveolar gas consists of three layers, each structurally distinct. These include the capillary endothelial cells, the alveolar-capillary interstitial space, and the lining of the alveolar wall. Clefts in the capillary endothelium are referred to as the loose junctions and the alveolar cell unions are called the tight junctions. Alveolar flooding, the final stage of pulmonary edema occurs where the tight junctions break down. A further protective barrier to alveolar flooding is the hydrophobic lipoprotein, surfactant, that lines the alveoli.[170]

For clinical purposes, it suffices to distinguish between accumulation of fluid in the pulmonary connective tissue framework, consisting of the peribronchial, perivascular tissue sheaths and the alveolar walls, and the accumulation of fluid within the alveolar airspaces, including the terminal and respiratory bronchioli. Fluid can accumulate in the interstitial spaces either acutely or chronically. This is referred to as interstitial pulmonary edema in contrast to alveolar edema, in which the airspaces are filled with fluid. Independent of the cause, interstitial edema usually precedes alveolar edema, resulting in considerable overlap between the two events. The clinical differentiation of the two types of pulmonary edema can thus be difficult or impossible. The fluid first appears in the perivascular and peribronchial tissue spaces. After the limits of the loose interstitial spaces

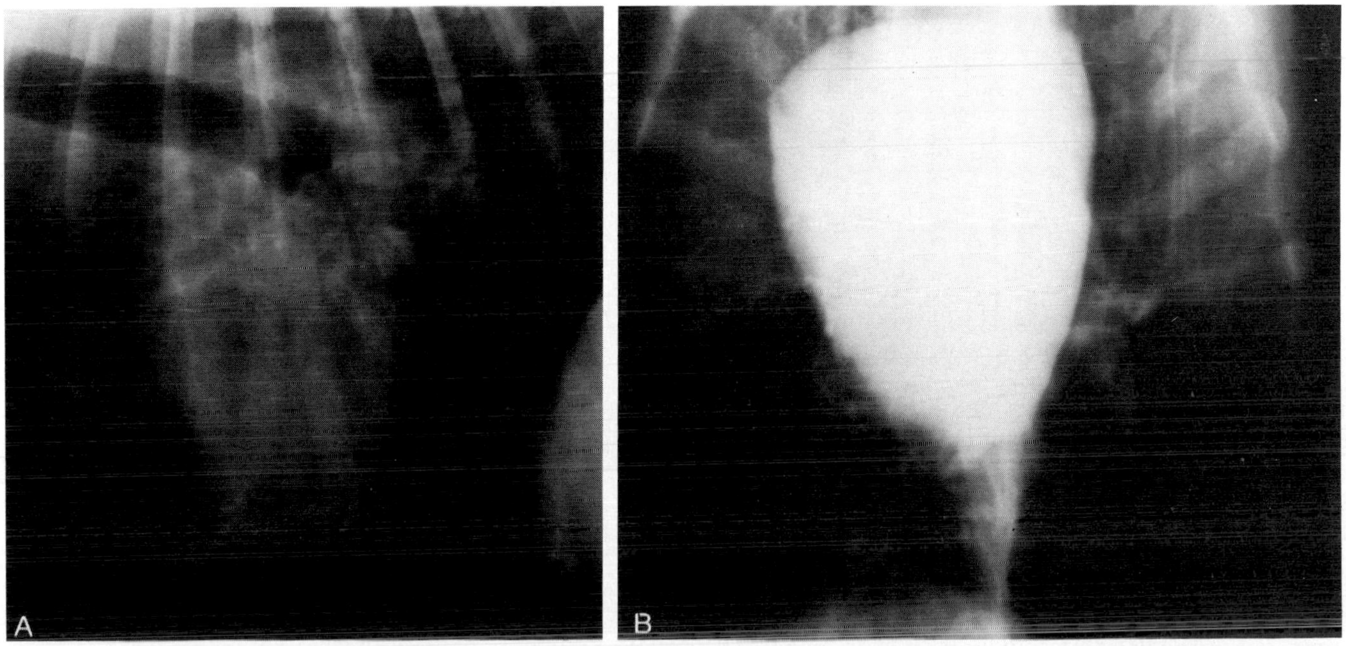

FIGURE 69–18. These radiographs demonstrate an increased interstitial pattern and hilar lymphadenopathy compatible with pulmonary involvement with multicentric lymphosarcoma. Inflammatory diseases or other neoplasia could result in a similar pattern.

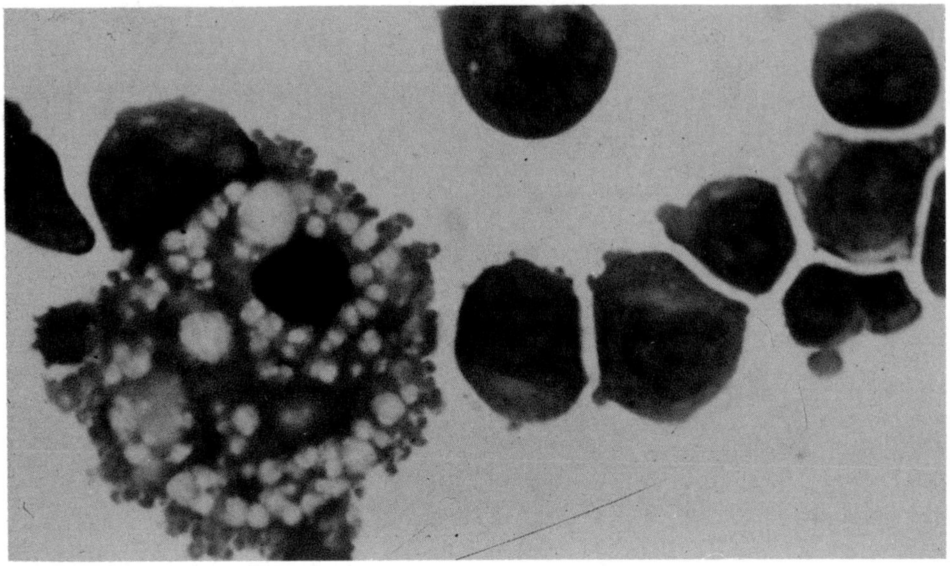

FIGURE 69–19. Cytologic evaluation of bronchoalveolar lavage fluid from the patient in Figure 69–18 confirmed the presence of lymphosarcoma in the lung. The malignant lymphoblasts exhibit mild anisocytosis, anisokaryosis, and variation in nuclear/cytoplasmic ratios. A single prominent, and often irregular, nucleolus is present in most cells. A large, active, vacuolated macrophage is present.

are exceeded and pressures continue to rise, the tight junctions of the alveolar membranes break down and alveolar edema occurs.[171] The accumulation of fluid, particularly in the airspaces of the lung, interferes with the pulmonary gas exchange and leads to respiratory embarrassment and eventually death by suffocation.

ETIOLOGY AND PATHOPHYSIOLOGY

A number of physiologic mechanisms protect the integrity of the interstitial spaces and prevent the accumulation of fluid in the pulmonary airspaces. Pulmonary edema develops when one or more of the following homeostatic mechanisms are interfered with. These mechanisms include such disturbances as: (1) an increase in the capillary hydrostatic pressures, (2) a loss of negative interstitial hydrostatic pressure, (3) increased capillary permeability to proteins, (4) insufficient interstitial lymphatic drainage, (5) decreased colloid osmotic pressure in the capillaries and/or the interstitium, (6) an abnormally high alveolar surface tension, and (7) an enlarged capillary surface area. Under clinical circumstances, a single factor or several of these factors combined can be responsible for the formation of pulmonary edema. The clinical importance of the various etiologic factors differs. An abnormally high alveolar surface tension is probably only rarely involved in edema formation. An elevated capillary hydrostatic pressure forcing fluid into the interstitium and a reduced colloid osmotic pressure of the plasma failing to hold fluid within the capillaries are among the most important factors.

It has been shown that a net vectorial sum of the Starling forces across the pulmonary capillaries is essential for the presence of a liquid layer coating the alveolar walls in a normal state. Therefore, even minor modifications of the permeability of the capillary wall and alveolar epithelium are important. Within limits, an increased rate of net capillary filtration into the interstitium can be compensated for by raising pulmonary lymphatic flow. The expanded pulmonary lymph system has a protective action against pulmonary edema.[172] Interstitial pulmonary edema forms only when the leakage of liquid into the interstitium exceeds the transport capacity of the lymphatics. High cardiac output markedly increasing pulmonary blood flow in large left-to-right shunts (patent ductus arteriosus [PDA], ventricular septal defect [VSD], or arteriovenous fistulas) can lead to pulmonary edema without elevation of pulmonary wedge pressure. The importance of an increased capillary flow for edema formation is supported by a temporary increase in pulmonary extravascular water during heavy exercise.[173]

For practical clinical purposes, the etiologies of lung edema can be subdivided into two major types: cardiogenic edema with increased left atrial and pulmonary venous pressure (25 to 35 mm Hg),[174] and noncardiogenic edema with a normal pulmonary venous pressure.[175–177] Staub has proposed a more precise classification of edemas into high pressure edema and permeability edema.[178] Instead of the expression high pressure edema, the term hemodynamic edema or imbalance of Starling forces is sometimes encountered.[179, 180] A summary of the various etiologies of pulmonary edemas is given in Table 69–5. In many types of pulmonary edema, both pressure and permeability are increased. Most pulmonary edemas in dogs and cats are cardiogenic in origin.

Left heart failure remains the most common cause of pulmonary edema in the dog and cat. It is associated with increased filling pressures of the heart. These are the result of either an increase in the diastolic volume or a decrease in the compliance of the left atrium and ventricle, or both. The increase in the filling pressure results in increased pressures transmitted backwards into the pulmonary veins and capillaries. Pulmonary capillary wedge pressures may already have returned to normal when there is still marked pulmonary edema, since the rate of removal of both interstitial and alveolar edema is relatively slow.

With increasing knowledge of pulmonary pathophysiology, Ingram and Braunwald have added two classifications of lymphatic insufficiency and unknown etiologies as additional categories for the etiology of pulmonary edema (Table 69–5).[180] This demonstrates the fact that although the clinical features of pulmonary edema are well recognized, some aspects of the etiopathophysiology still remain unclear.

High pressure edema in the absence of heart failure occurs with the overexpansion of extracellular volume by crystalloid fluid infusions and decreased protein osmotic pressure. Fluid overload is well tolerated in normal dogs; however, an equal amount of fluid infused into an animal with hypoproteinemia, renal disease, or left-sided heart failure may cause pulmonary edema. Cats made experimentally hypovolemic by bleeding and then infused with lactated Ringer's solution experienced a significant rise in the CVP and some died of pulmonary and/or cerebral edema.[181] Although classic high pressure pulmonary edema is associated with left-sided heart failure, there is experimentally supported evidence that systemic venous hypertension may occasionally contribute to pulmonary edema formation.[182]

TABLE 69–5. CLASSIFICATION OF PULMONARY EDEMA BASED UPON INITIATING MECHANISM

I. Imbalance of Starling Forces
   A. Increased pulmonary capillary pressure
      1. Increased pulmonary venous pressure without left ventricular failure (e.g., mitral stenosis)
      2. Increased pulmonary venous pressure secondary to left ventricular failure
      3. Increased pulmonary capillary pressure secondary to increased pulmonary arterial pressure (so-called overperfusion pulmonary edema)*
   B. Decreased plasma oncotic pressure
      1. Hypoalbuminemia secondary to renal, hepatic, protein-losing enteropathic, or dermatological disease or nutritional causes**
   C. Increased negativity of interstitial pressure
      1. Rapid removal of pneumothorax with large applied negative pressures (unilateral)
      2. Large negative pleural pressures due to acute airway obstruction along with increased end-expiratory volumes (asthma)*
   D. Increased interstitial oncotic pressure
      1. No known clinical or experimental example
II. Altered Alveolar-Capillary Membrane Permeability (Adult Respiratory Distress Syndrome)
   A. Infectious pneumonia—bacterial, viral, parasitic
   B. Inhaled toxins (e.g., phosgene, ozone, chlorine, Teflon fumes, nitrogen dioxide, smoke)
   C. Circulating foreign substances (e.g., snake venom, bacterial endotoxins, alloxan†, alpha-naphthyl thiourea†)
   D. Aspiration of acidic gastric contents
   E. Acute radiation pneumonitis
   F. Endogenous vasoactive substances (e.g., histamine, kinins*)
   G. Disseminated intravascular coagulation
   H. Immunological—hypersensitivity pneumonitis, drugs (nitrofurantoin), leukoagglutinins
   I. Shock lung in association with nonthoracic trauma
   J. Acute hemorrhagic pancreatitis
III. Lymphatic Insufficiency
   A. Post lung transplant
   B. Lymphangitic carcinomatosis
   C. Fibrosing lymphangitis (e.g., silicosis)
IV. Unknown or Incompletely Understood
   A. High altitude pulmonary edema
   B. Neurogenic pulmonary edema
   C. Narcotic overdose
   D. Pulmonary embolism
   E. Eclampsia
   F. Post cardioversion
   G. Post anesthesia
   H. Post cardiopulmonary bypass

*Not certain to exist as a clinical entity.
**Not certain that this, as a single factor, leads to clinical pulmonary edema.
†Predominantly an experimental technique.
From Ingram, RH Jr, and Braunwald, E: Pulmonary edema: Cardiogenic and noncardiogenic. *In* Braunwald, E (ed): Heart Disease: A Textbook of Cardiovascular Medicine, 3rd ed. Philadelphia, WB Saunders, 1988, p 349.

Occasionally, pulmonary edema occurs when large amounts of pleural fluid or gas are aspirated rapidly. It has been postulated that the increased negative interstitial pulmonary pressure could be responsible for this type of lung edema.[183] Extrathoracic airway obstruction, namely severe obstructive laryngeal diseases of any cause, can result in pulmonary edema in dogs and cats.

Acute respiratory failure with massive pulmonary edema is well known as the adult respiratory distress syndrome (ARDS), or shock lung syndrome.[184] Adult respiratory distress syndrome is the common response of the lung to a great variety of injuries. These injuries alter the permeability of the pulmonary vascular endothelium by such mechanisms as circulating humoral agents, intrapulmonary release of noxious substances, microembolization, and pulmonary intravascular clot formation. These mechanisms are amplified by interacting factors such as massive fluid therapy, prolonged O_2 application, pulmonary infection, and myocardial depression.[185] ARDS occurs with pulmonary or extrathoracic trauma, shock, septicemia, endogenous toxemias, and a wide variety of noxious substances reaching the lungs via the airways.

Epithelial disruption appears to be responsible for the excessive alveolar flooding in experimentally induced oleic acid low pressure permeability edema in dogs. This results in greater impairment of gas exchange than when compared to high pressure-induced edema.[186]

Pulmonary edema following pancreatitis in the dog is one of the many forms of ARDS.[187] Disseminated intra vascular coagulation triggered by alterations in the clotting mechanisms can result in pulmonary edema.[185]

Aspiration of liquids, particularly gastric content, during anesthesia or unconsciousness can lead to pulmonary edema. The damage to the alveolar lining of the lung and the severity of the pulmonary edema depend on the amount, the pH, the osmolarity, and the inherent toxic constituents of the aspirate.

Permeability edema signifies that an increase has occurred in the transendothelial conductance for water and that the microvascular barrier restriction to the flow of plasma proteins has decreased.[178] Permeability pulmonary edema is associated with protein-rich exudate, which easily forms hyaline membranes. A significant number of the etiologies that chemically or physically alter the permeability of the alveolar linings or the pulmonary capillary epithelium also damage the myocardium. Toxic inhalants such as ozone damage the alveolar lining. Other inhalants such as smoke can contain noxious fumes freed by the burning process, which will cause both pulmonary and myocardial damage. In smoke inhalation, chemical injury can lead to delayed onset of pulmonary edema. Furthermore, insults caused by smoke may be combined with the effects of intense heat, which in themselves may damage the respiratory epithelium and cause edema. Histologically, toxic inhalants are often found to cause hyaline membranes within the airspaces.[185] Spontaneous cases of smoke inhalation in the dog show an almost identical response as the disease in humans.[188] The number of toxic inhalants capable of damaging the alveolar wall and pulmonary capillaries is almost unlimited. Even exposure to 100 per cent oxygen for several days may damage the alveolar lining and capillary membranes and lead to pulmonary edema. A variety of toxic substances such as organophosphates, herbicides, ANTU (α-naphthylthiourea), venoms of snakes or bees, and bacterial endotoxins can reach the lung via the systemic circulation. Pulmonary edema formation in dogs and cats with terminal uremia is common.[189] The edema formation is usually confined to the interstitium.

Infectious diseases, including viral, bacterial, and parasitic pneumonia, damage the capillaries and the alveolar walls and result in inflammatory lung edema. The rapid development of an infectious pulmonary edema can be favored by preexisting congestive heart disease or an increased amount of lung liquid from other causes.

In anaphylactic, idiosyncratic, or other immunogenic reactions, and also in some of the other types of pulmonary edemas, arachidonic acid metabolites and the liberation of vasoactive substances (such as histamine, serotonin, kinins, prostaglandins, and proteolytic enzymes) increase microvascular pressures and thus increase the transvascular fluid filtration rate. This intensifies the damage to the underlying tissue.[185, 190] Hypersensitivity or idiosyncrasy reactions to therapeutic agents, radiographic contrast media, vaccines, or other biological products are uncommon when one considers their extensive use. Allergies to inhaled plant materials such as pollen, or to food can result in pulmonary edema. It may be difficult, however, to identify the allergen in a particular case.

Drowning or near-drowning, which fills the alveoli with water, must be considered a form of pulmonary edema.[185] Fresh water may be rapidly reabsorbed into the vascular compartment. This results in sudden hypervolemia and hemolysis.[191] Sea water, however, produces osmotic injury to the pulmonary capillaries. The result is hemoconcentration and fulminant pulmonary edema. "Secondary drowning" refers to pulmonary edema formation hours or days after the initial drowning and may be due to surfactant washout or pulmonary distress syndrome.[192]

Neurogenic pulmonary edema has been produced experimentally in dogs by increasing the intracranial pressure.[193] The increased intracranial pressure, which can be due to any type of brain or head injury, stimulates a massive sympathetic discharge. The resulting liberation of catecholamines may be a consequence of a hypothalamic injury.[194] The sympathetic discharge raises peripheral resistance and blood pressure, and blood volume is shifted from the systemic to the pulmonary circulation. Pulmonary venous pressure and capillary permeability rise dramatically and allow fluid to leak or even hemorrhage to occur. Central venous pressure and pulmonary wedge pressure drops back to normal within 5 to 15 minutes, thus averting heart failure, but pulmonary capillary permeability stays high for several hours or days owing to volume-mediated capillary damage.[185]

Alpha-adrenergic and β-adrenergic overactivity, inducing neurogenic lung edema, can be counteracted by sympatholytic, antiepinephrine, or general anesthetic agents, and the development of neurogenic pulmonary edema can be prevented. Pulmonary edema in dogs and cats with heat stroke or electrocution due to biting into electric cords may be associated with neurogenic factors.[195, 196] The presence of supraventricular tachycardia in electrocuted animals and the favorable response to intravenous digitalis therapy suggests that cardiac factors are involved. Neurogenic pulmonary edema may occur following seizures due to a wide variety of causes such as intoxication with chlorinated hydrocarbons, infections, or degenerative changes. Hypoglycemia in severely stressed hunting dogs was suspected as the inciting factor for pulmonary edema.[196] Paroxysmal pulmonary edema may occur secondary to sympathoadrenal stimulation that affects both the peripheral vasculature and the left ventricle.[197] It results in a sudden shift of large amounts of blood from the periphery to the heart and lungs. This causes a systolic overload of the left ventricle because of a large venous return. The formation of a paroxysmal pulmonary edema may or may not be associated with left ventricular failure.

Földi experimentally produced pulmonary edema in dogs with hemodynamically inconsequential mitral insufficiency by partially ligating the pulmonary lymphatics.[198] Lymphatic obstruction also contributes to the formation of lung edema in disseminated pulmonary lymphosarcoma and widespread metastatic lung disease in which the lymphatics are blocked by neoplastic cells (lymphangitis carcinomatosis) and in severe hilar lymphadenopathy.

HISTORY AND CLINICAL SIGNS

The history and clinical signs may reveal a gradual or sudden onset of pulmonary edema, depending on the cause and severity of the process. Some forms of edema are recognizable if a careful medical history is obtained. The common clinical signs of pulmonary edema are tachypnea, dyspnea, and moist rales. The degree of respiratory distress varies from mild, when the signs may only be noticeable during exercise, to fulminant and most severe, when the animal is unable to lie down because of air hunger. The physical signs may also differ with the location of the pulmonary fluid. When the fluid is confined to the interstitial spaces, no contact of the fluid with respiratory air occurs, and therefore the auscultatory sounds will be unassuming. The confirmation of the interstitial pulmonary edema essentially depends on the radiographic diagnosis.[199, 200]

Owing to the accumulation of interstitial fluid, the lungs lose their normal elasticity and compliance, and vital capacity is reduced. These functional alterations are reflected to a varying degree in the depth and frequency of the respiratory rate. By shallow and more rapid breathing, the increased work of breathing can be reduced. Initially, tachypnea and dyspnea will be noticed only after exercise or excitement; later, they will also be present at rest. The increased pulmonary circulation during exercise may precipitate the entry of fluid into the alveolar spaces, where it may interfere with the pulmonary surfactant and further reduce compliance and vital capacity of the lung.[185] One sign reported in dogs with interstitial pulmonary edema is restlessness at night and an inability to breathe in a recumbent position (orthopnea). It can be associated with a nonproductive cough. The alteration in pulse quality depends on the presence and type of heart disease.

With interstitial fluid accumulation, flow resistance in the pulmonary arteries will increase, resulting in an increased mean pulmonary artery pressure. Hypoxia, which develops with pulmonary edema, will further increase the pulmonary arteriolar constriction, leading to local pulmonary hypertension and increased right ventricular load, which in turn jeopardizes its normal function (cor pulmonale). The easily collapsible small terminal airways may narrow in lung edema, and the walls of the large conducting airways can become edematous, thereby promoting bronchial constriction, which is recognized as wheezing (asthma).

Acute alveolar edema is associated with respiratory distress that is much more severe than that due to interstitial pulmonary edema. The signs consist of shallow, very rapid, open-mouth breathing, wheezing, and bubbling noises. The noises, originating in the trachea and the large airways, may be of sufficient intensity to be heard without auscultation. Varying amounts of pale or pinkish frothy fluid may be seen passing from the mouth or nose. Affected animals are usually reluctant to lie down; instead they remain in sternal recumbency or assume a sitting position with the forelimbs abducted to allow for wider thoracic excursion. The associated open-mouth breathing in cats can be very dramatic. The wide-eyed appearance expresses marked anxiety. Air hunger may be indicated by the animal's desire to seek a place with cool, moving air. The mucous membranes appear pale or muddy. The pulse progresses to rapid and weak and may further deteriorate as the severity of the condition deteriorates. On auscultation, the intensity of the moist crepitant rales makes it frequently impossible to hear the normal cardiac sounds or cardiac murmurs.

With increasing severity of the pulmonary edema, animals will become cyanotic. The filling of the alveolar airspaces produces an intrapulmonary venoarterial shunt. The fluid-filled alveoli are unable to contribute to gas exchange, and inhalation of 100 per cent oxygen will not lead to the expected increase in arterial oxygen tension because of the perfusion of nonventilated alveoli. Due to the severe stress and increased respiratory efforts, the body temperature may become elevated, mimicking an infectious disease. This is often seen during the warm summer season or in humid climates as a result of the disturbed heat-exchange mechanism via airways and circulation.

It may be difficult or impossible to differentiate clinically between high pressure cardiogenic and permeability pulmonary edema because of the difficulty in properly hearing cardiac sounds. Left-sided heart failure does occur in the absence of tachyarrhythmias or valvular heart murmurs. A gallop rhythm heralding heart failure can be difficult to hear in the presence of lung edema. Often the history may provide some clues suggesting cardiac origin, such as a nocturnal cough, exertional dyspnea, or syncopal episodes. A cardiac origin of pulmonary edema is often indicated by a symmetric perihilar pulmonary density and cardiomegaly seen radiographically. Measuring the pulmonary artery wedge pressure might assist the clinician in separating cardiogenic high pressure edema from high permeability, normal pressure edema. Permeability pulmonary edema can have a wide variety of etiologies and, accordingly, the history may be specific (such as smoke inhalation or accident) or ambiguous. It can be difficult to differentiate between the true cause and precipitating factors such as exercise, excitement, or changes in climate. In the absence of a complete history or signs of an associated disease, the cause of the pulmonary edema often cannot be determined. Chronic or subacute pulmonary edema may go unnoticed by the owner and may be detected incidentally when an animal is radiographed for a coincidental problem. In retrospect, the owner may report that the animal had coughed occasionally or had shown a reduced exercise tolerance. The presence of protein-rich transudate in the interstitial spaces will provoke the formation of collagen, reticulum, and elastic fibers. As a result of these interstitial changes, pulmonary fibrosis and stiffness of the lung will occur.[185]

CLINICOPATHOLOGY

Arterial hypoxemia is the major abnormality seen in lung edema. Parallel with hypoxemia, acid-base imbalance, initially respiratory alkalosis or acidosis and later combined respiratory and metabolic acidosis, will occur.[185] The arterial level of carbon dioxide may or may not be elevated in pulmonary edema, depending on the balance between relatively unaffected regions of the lung and affected, nonventilated regions and on whether the dog or cat will be able to markedly increase the ventilatory rate. Clinicopathology examinations may have to be delayed in animals with fulminant pulmonary edema. Once the emergency has been brought under control, however, laboratory data may be helpful. A complete blood count and blood chemistry provide information on the specifics of the disease. Hematocrit and plasma protein determination assist in diagnosing hemodilution, hypoproteinemia, or hemoconcentration. Comparison of the protein concentrations of edema fluid and that of the plasma aids in the diagnostic separation of increased permeability from high pressure pulmonary edema.[201] Protein content of normal canine pulmonary interstitial fluid is between 0.5 and 0.8 of the serum protein values. The average protein concentration in canine alveolar fluid was equal to the plasma protein concentration in dogs with permeability edema.[202] In dogs with cardiogenic edema, the protein concentration of alveolar fluid was less than half that of plasma. The differential blood count helps in differentiating infectious from noninfectious pulmonary edema. Blood gas analysis of PO_2, PCO_2, and arterial pH is among the most valuable laboratory data. Unfortunately, the availability of these measurements is often limited to institutions.

Electrocardiography

Electrocardiography (ECG) provides the clinician with a rapid assessment of cardiac size and electrical conductivity. Cardiomegaly observed radiographically may be confirmed by ECG; arrhythmias auscultated are defined more precisely. Diagnosis of feline cardiomegaly, often not identified radiographically, is supported from the ECG tracing. Ultrasonography further identifies cardiac function, hypertrophy, dilation, and pathology.

Radiographic Examination

Radiographic examination of the thorax is the most frequently utilized method for detecting pulmonary edema. Unfortunately, it lacks the sensitivity for assessing early interstitial edema, especially in high permeability edema prior to the development of clinical signs. Radiography usually fails to identify the cause of the edema in non-cardiac states.[203] Yet, it remains the single most effective clinical tool to identify and differentiate the clinical state of pulmonary edema.

Radiographic examination is rarely needed for the initial diagnosis of acute pulmonary alveolar edema. Clinically stressful procedures and valuable time need not be wasted taking radiographs in emergency situations. The life-threatening condition must be brought under control by treating the patient symptomatically. After emergency measures have been instituted and the patient is more comfortable, the radiographic examination is indicated for a detailed evaluation of the dog's or cat's thorax and for refined information about the anatomic distribution, location, and extent of the edema fluid. Radiography is important in reassessing the tentative clinical diagnosis in animals in which the origin of the edema remains obscure, or when other conditions besides edema must be considered. Additional information such as pleural effusion, pulmonary metastases, cardiomegaly, hilar lymphadenopathy, dilation of pulmonary veins, or signs of a previous trauma can be gained from the radiograph. These changes are of particular importance in differentiating cardiogenic from noncardiogenic pulmonary edema. Radiography serves to document the response to therapy and is of particular importance for the assessment of residual interstitial edema after the acute signs of alveolar edema have subsided.

Radiographically, one can differentiate between interstitial and alveolar edema.[176] On most radiographs, the two types of edema coexist, but the alveolar edema effectively blocks the interstitial edema from being seen except in areas where interstitial edema alone is present. Alveolar edema is characterized by an alveolar pattern consisting of mottled or blotchy, soft tissue disseminated pulmonary densities (Figures 69–20 and 69–21). Interstitial pulmonary edema is recognized radiographically as a diminished pulmonary radiolucency and loss of contrast of the pulmonary vessels, which is often referred to as hilar or general pulmonary haze (Figure 69–22). The central portion of the pulmonary veins can be dilated, bronchial cuff formation may occur, and the interlobar fissures of the lung may become visible because of subpleural interstitial edema.

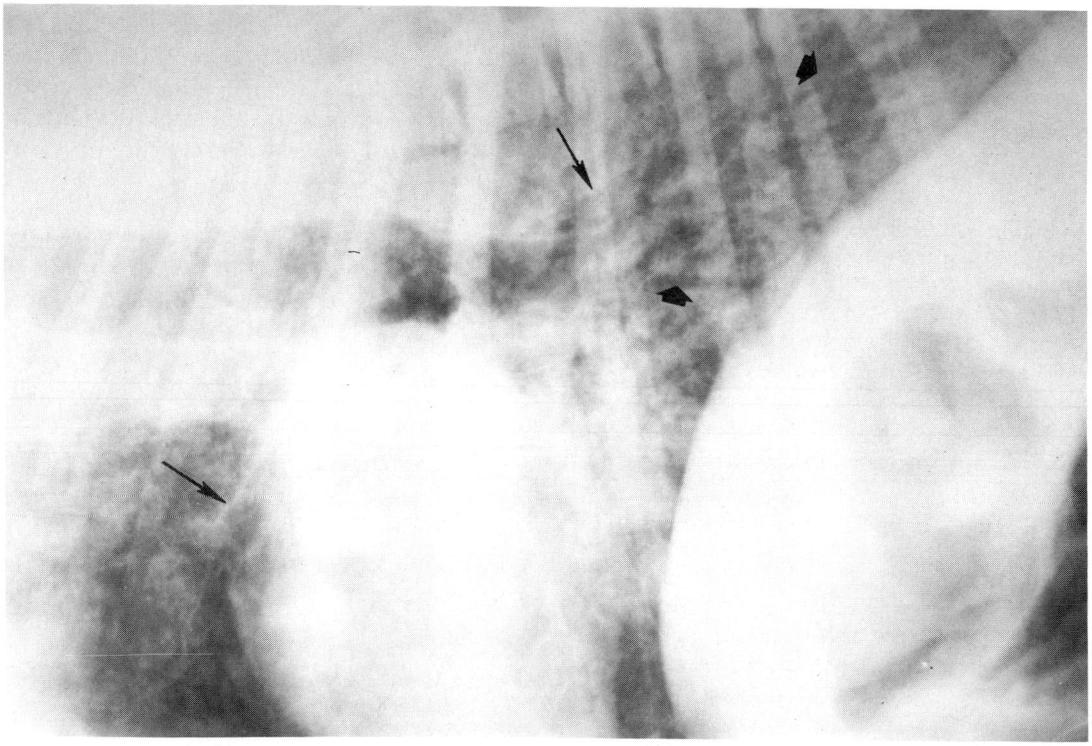

FIGURE 69–20. Lateral radiograph, four-month-old Great Dane with severe noncardiogenic pulmonary edema caused by smoke inhalation. The lung field appears mottled and blotchy, or grainy confluent densities are present. Airbronchograms (wide arrows) are seen, supporting a radiographic diagnosis of a disseminated alveolar pulmonary pattern. A number of ill-defined lines are seen in the dense lung field (small arrows). They represent an increased density of the bronchial walls and are due to edema of the bronchial walls and peribronchial tissue. The cardiac silhouette is partially obscured by the increased pulmonary density; nonetheless, one can assume that no significant cardiomegaly is present. The involvement of all lung lobes and the normal-appearing peripheries of the cranial and middle lobes are compatible with a diagnosis of lung edema rather than pneumonia.

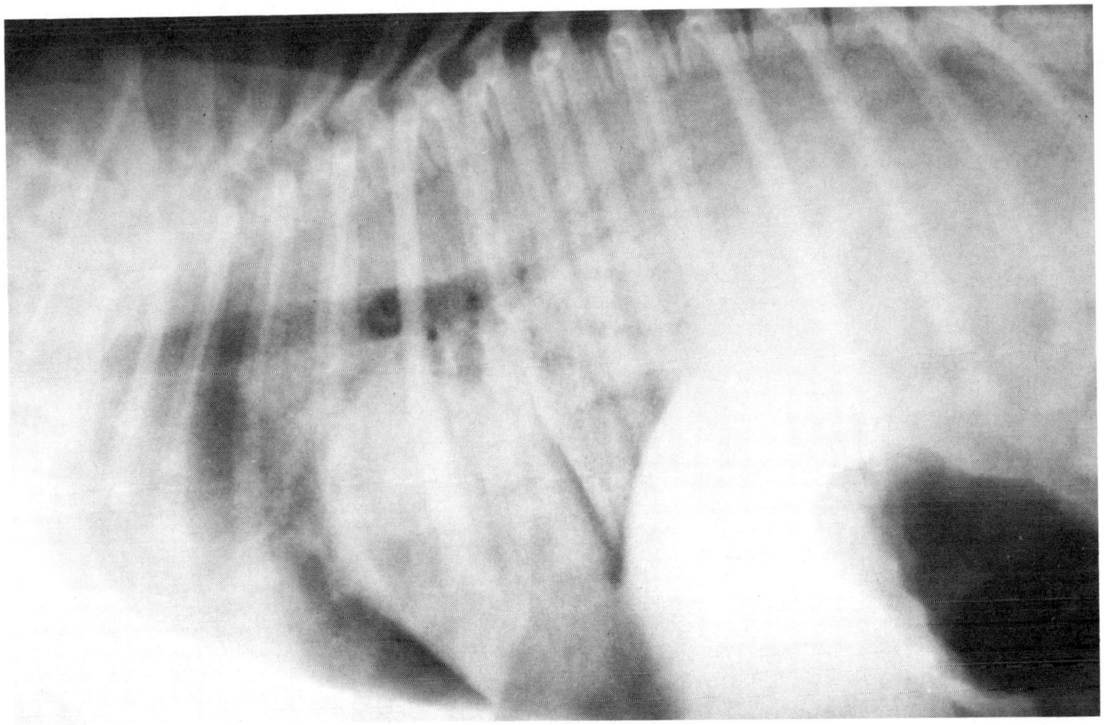

FIGURE 69–21. Lateral radiograph, two-month-old, male basenji pup with severe pulmonary edema predominantly involving the caudal lobes. The pup was in severe respiratory distress and was bleeding slightly from the mouth. The cardiac silhouette appears normal in size, which is supported by the normal position of the trachea. The cranial and middle lung lobes seem only slightly affected by the disease process. Airbronchograms can be seen within the markedly increased density of the caudal lobes, supporting the diagnosis of an alveolar pattern. Confinement of the density to the caudal lobes and a normal-appearing cardiac silhouette are commonly seen with accidents of electrocution. Inspection of the pup's mouth revealed burn marks on the gum and lips, confirming the suspicion that the pup had bitten into an electric cord.

Both alveolar and interstitial pulmonary edema patterns are seen with a variety of etiologies. By evaluating the anatomic location of the edema and determining cardiac size, a specific diagnosis can often be made. In the majority of dogs, but less often in cats, cardiogenic pulmonary edema is associated with cardiomegaly, in particular enlargement of the left atrium and left ventricle. In a small number of dogs with acute heart failure, cardiomegaly may not be noticeable radiographically.

In dogs, the alveolar and interstitial pulmonary edema is usually diffuse and symmetric or may favor the right caudal lung lobe. In cats, pulmonary edema may be multifocal and asymmetric. In dogs, cardiogenic pulmonary edema may begin in the right caudal lobe. A unilateral distribution of the edema is found secondary to hypostasis or atelectasis in animals that have been lying on the same side for a prolonged period of time. In dogs with experimental high pressure edema, there were significantly greater increases in density in the more central and dependent zones of the lung than in the nondependent dorsal peripheral zones as shown by computed tomography.[204]

In most cases of cardiogenic pulmonary edema, the most frequent location of the radiographic density is perihilar, with the periphery of the lungs seemingly uninvolved.[205] This hilar distribution of pulmonary edema may be due to differences in ventilation, length of pulmonary microvasculature, and lymphatic drainage of the hilar versus the peripheral portions of the lung.[206] A so-called reversed butterfly effect, with the hilar regions of the lung apparently uninvolved and alveolar consolidations taking up the pulmonary periphery, has been seen rarely in permeability edemas. A unifocal or multifocal asymmetric distribution of alveolar or interstitial densities in the middle or peripheral portions of the lungs of dogs is unusual and should be associated with pneumonia, infarcts, or hemorrhage, rather than with pulmonary edema. Focal or peripheral lobar location of an alveolar pattern, in particular an involvement of the cranial and middle lobes, is more typical of bronchopneumonia than of noninflammatory pulmonary edema. Occasionally, alveolar edema can be atypical in location and appearance. In the early phases of acute edema, when only small groups of alveoli are filled with fluid, the radiographic density may appear as a finely granular opacity composed of large numbers of miliary-sized nodules. As the edema progresses, multiple, ill-defined nodules four to six mm in diameter, which tend to coalesce into blotchy alveolar densities, are seen.

Alveolar consolidations confined to the caudal lobes suggest neurogenic or electric cord bite as the etiology. Permeability edemas due to blood-borne toxic factors result in symmetric involvement of the entire lung.[203] Inhalations of toxic fumes produces the earliest and most severe edema in the caudal lobes, allergic conditions peripherally, while neurogenic storms affect the peripheral or middle portions of the caudal lobes.[203]

Atypical location of pulmonary edema can be the result of a preexisting or associated disease such as pneumonia, emphysema, pleural effusion, or pleural

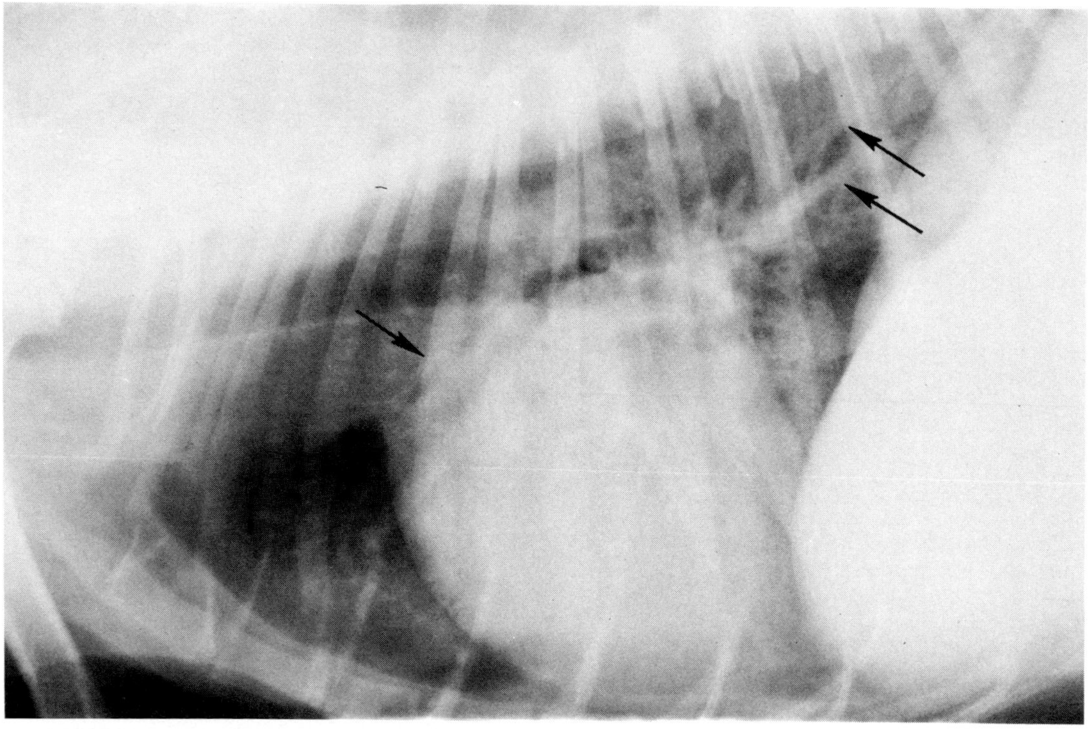

FIGURE 69–22. Lateral radiograph, 14-year-old female cocker spaniel with interstitial pulmonary edema. A slight dyspnea had been noticed by the owner for two weeks prior to the onset of a sudden severe tachypnea and dyspnea and a short loss of consciousness. An acute alveolar pulmonary edema was diagnosed on a prior radiograph. After treatment with furosemide, the dog showed a marked clinical improvement. Radiographically the presence of an interstitial pulmonary edema is supported by the increased disseminated density of the lung field and the lack of contrast with the vascular structures of the lung. The vascular structures (arrows) are blurred, but they can still be seen against the increased background density. Notice that alveolar density (Fig. 69–21) effectively blocks the arteries from being perceived. The visibility of the vascular structures in interstitial edema can be explained by the confined fluid within the interstitial tissue rather than in the alveoli as in an alveolar pattern. This pattern needs to be differentiated from increased densities and loss of contrast of the lungs in radiographs made at expiration or from an interstitial pattern caused by pulmonary fibrosis due to old age or preceding diseases.

adhesions. Infection associated with edema may modify or aggravate its course. Unilateral pulmonary edema, which is readily confused with other alveolar or interstitial diseases, can be due to unilateral emphysema in the unaffected side, lobectomy and subsequent overexpansion of the remaining lobes on the ipsilateral side, unilateral damage to the lung on the affected side by aspiration or a unilateral venous or lymphatic occlusion caused by hilar masses or pleural effusion, and unilateral thromboembolism.

The interstitial and alveolar patterns can change rapidly in distribution and location. Pulmonary edema in cases of allergy can develop within minutes. Therapy may rapidly take effect and change an edema from alveolar to interstitial within a few hours. A marked, rapid change in type, extent, and location of pulmonary densities on sequential radiographs provides support for a tentative diagnosis of pulmonary edema. Technical effects, such as those resulting from obesity, underexposure, and expiratory phase radiographs, diminish the contrast of the lung field giving it a denser appearance, which can be misdiagnosed as pulmonary edema. It is possible to make a radiograph of an animal with pulmonary edema look "normal" by a forceful inflation of the lungs by positive pressure ventilation. According to Staub,[173] this can be explained by the spreading of the interalveolar fluid over the alveolar walls and by counteracting the tendency of half-filled alveoli to collapse.

DIFFERENTIAL DIAGNOSIS

Since pulmonary edema is a complication of a pathological process rather than a disease in itself, the specific cause may be obscure. A carefully gathered history, a systemic physical examination, a complete multiphasic blood chemistry screening, and a radiographic examination of the thorax will usually be sufficient to arrive at a tentative diagnosis. It is essential to consider carefully all possible differential diagnoses (Table 69–5). The differentiation of pulmonary edema of cardiogenic origin from noncardiogenic edemas is usually based on the presence of cardiac murmurs, a characteristic history, and cardiomegaly seen on the radiographs. It may be possible to separate inflammatory from noninflammatory pulmonary edema by the presence of fever and leukocytosis. In permeability edema due to allergy, gaseous inhalation, or chemical intoxication, it may often be impossible to identify the cause. Traumatic pulmonary edema (pulmonary contusion) and pulmonary hemorrhage can often be verified by associated bruises or contusions and rib fractures on the radiographs. Disseminated intravascular coagulation, which can be associated with pulmonary edema, may be recognized by poor blood clotting and petechial hemorrhages into mucous membranes. The differentiation of interstitial pulmonary edema, which may not cause overt clinical signs from other conditions, such as pneumonia, granulomatous conditions, pulmonary fibrosis, or disseminated neoplasms, strongly depends on serial radiographic and laboratory examinations.

TREATMENT OF PULMONARY EDEMA

A rational approach to the treatment of pulmonary edema requires a series of rapid decisions based on firm clinical findings. The first decision to be made requires a clinical evaluation of the severity of the edema. Acute fulminating alveolar pulmonary edema demands immediate intensive treatment directed at the life-threatening signs. In subacute and chronic pulmonary edema, efforts to identify the primary cause should come first. Then, treatment may be directed specifically at the underlying problem. Mild pulmonary edema may vanish spontaneously with rest. The objectives in treating pulmonary edema are improvement of respiratory gas exchange, removal of abnormal fluid accumulations, and correction of acid-base imbalances. A discussion of general pulmonary therapy is at the beginning of this chapter. Specific details relevant to pulmonary edema will be further discussed here.

When acute pulmonary edema is present, the clinician should attempt to answer the following questions in order to choose the most appropriate therapy: Is the edema cardiogenic or noncardiogenic? Is there an arrhythmia, a gallop rhythm, or a murmur? Is the body temperature markedly elevated (suggesting severe anxiety and distress, heat stroke, central nervous system disturbance, or acute pneumonia)? Is there any indication of an upper airway obstruction? Have drugs, vaccines, or any other foreign substances been introduced into the body during the past 24 hours? Could an electric shock or toxic substance be responsible? Is there a history of recent thoracic trauma? Is the patient receiving large volumes of intravenous fluids?

In acute severe edema, further diagnostic tests are deferred until therapeutic measures are applied. Nevertheless, a lateral or dorsoventral radiograph and single-lead electrocardiogram done with minimal restraint are advisable if the diagnosis is in doubt.

Permeability pulmonary edema of the acute fulminating type is treated by oxygen supplementation, corticosteroids, parenteral diuretics, bronchodilators, and sedation. Depending on etiology, additional procedures may include heparin in some clotting abnormalities, antibiotics in infections, mannitol in brain trauma, or positive pressure ventilation in severe hypoxia. Edema caused by congestive heart failure is treated similarly. In addition, digitalis therapy and peripheral vasodilators, if not already being administered, are instituted.

Peripheral vasodilation in noncardiogenic permeability edemas may have an adverse effect on the edema due to an increase in cardiac output and a decrease in peripheral vascular resistance.[207] Antisympathetic interventions, such as phenoxybenzamine, may prevent increases in pulmonary venous pressures. Such an effect may significantly reduce lung injury edema and microvascular pressure of noncardiogenic origin.[208]

Diuretics. In small-animal medicine, the diuretic of choice for acute pulmonary edema is furosemide. In addition to its diuretic effect, furosemide reduces afterload and improves left ventricular emptying. It also brings about peripheral vascular response of venodilation. Used intravenously at the rate of 0.5 to 2 mg/lb (1.1 to 4.4 mg/kg) of body weight, its effect commences within minutes, and reaches a peak diuresis within 30 minutes. Furosemide may be safely used at least once in the presence of decreased glomerular filtration. It should not be repeated if no urine is produced. If urine production is maintained, furosemide may be repeated after two hours and thereafter may be given three times per day if necessary until a satisfactory response is evident. The patient can be given oral furosemide at 1 to 2 mg/lb (2.2 to 4.4 mg/kg) of body weight.

Any product capable of inducing a rapid intensive diuresis may alter electrolyte levels. It is advisable to regularly determine serum electrolyte levels in patients receiving multiple doses of any diuretic. When used in combination with the digitalis glycosides, furosemide appears to contribute to the development of digitalis intoxication, probably because of its profound effects on electrolyte depletion. Oral supplementation of potassium chloride may be beneficial with prolonged use of diuretics, but preferably when deficiencies are recognized by serum electrolyte determination.

For subacute and chronic pulmonary edema, thiazide or xanthine derivatives may be chosen. Mannitol diuresis may be preferred with neurogenic edema due to trauma.

Furosemide has nondiuretic venodilating effects that reduce pulmonary shunts and lung water in the early phases of permeability edema. However, once the injury is well established, only the diuretic effect is significant.[209, 210] The combined effect of furosemide and dobutamine significantly reduced permeability-induced lung water in short-term studies on dogs.[211]

Bronchodilating Agents. Injectable aminophylline has inherent diuretic, mild positive inotropic, and venodilation properties, in addition to a salutary bronchodilating effect. It may enhance the diuresis induced by furosemide. Aminophylline also provides a desirable stimulating effect on the central nervous system. Aminophylline is given intravenously, by deep intramuscular injection, subcutaneously, or orally. The usual dosage range is 4.5 mg/lb (10 mg/kg) of body weight, repeated every six to eight hours. The side effects of vomiting (i.e., agitation, hypotension, and tachycardia) must be avoided.

Sedation. Sedation is important for both medical and humane purposes. Hyperexcitable and frightened animals further aggravate the vicious cycle of detrimental effects of restlessness. Morphine depression of the respiratory center changes the rapid violent movements to a slower deeper rhythm. Morphine also diminishes the acute sympathoadrenal barrage aggravating the pulmonary edema.

Administered simultaneously, morphine sulfate and chlorpromazine reduce the venous cardiac return. Morphine dilates the splanchnic vasculature and chlorpromazine produces peripheral vasodilation as a result of α-adrenergic blockade. Morphine sulfate is reported to have some beneficial cardiac effects as well.[212] Morphine may raise the intracranial pressure and is contraindicated in neurogenic pulmonary edema.

Morphine sulfate is preferable to meperidine and

codeine. Inactivity helps to reduce the secondary effects of emesis. Therefore, morphine sulfate is best given to patients that will remain quietly recumbent, rather than to those that will be moved about. Low doses, 0.02–0.05 mg/lb, are given subcutaneously, intramuscularly, or intravenously and may be repeated as indicated, since very large doses may be needed in the dog to be effective. Morphine sulfate must not be administered with atropine. Atropine is contraindicated because it increases the cardiac rate and also makes secretions more viscid, thereby impairing expectoration. New morphine-like derivatives with less respiratory depressing effects may be useful in treating pulmonary edema. Morphine is often contraindicated in cats because of CNS stimulation but has been used with good results in many cases.

Chlorpromazine is administered subcutaneously, intramuscularly, or intravenously in very low doses. When used in association with morphine, chlorpromazine is given at the rate of 0.25 mg/lb (0.55 mg/kg) of body weight. With neurogenic edema due to trauma, seizures, or eclampsia, pentobarbital titrated to deep sedation may be used. A mild hypothermia may be of benefit with anesthesia. Assisted positive pressure ventilation helps to remobilize the edema fluid in anesthetized animals.

Digitalis. When pulmonary edema is secondary to heart failure, rapid digitalization is indicated if cardiac glycosides have not been administered within the past week. When glycosides are being administered, it is imperative to identify the likelihood of digitalis intoxication by a history of vomiting and electrocardiographic abnormalities. Cardiogenic pulmonary edema not resulting from digitalis intoxication may require modifications of the daily maintenance dose of glycoside. Such increased doses can be administered orally, with rapid beneficial effects.

Oxygen. Supplementary oxygen is necessary in severe pulmonary edema. When cages with proper temperature (maximum 65° F) and humidity control systems are available, oxygen may be administered at a flow of six to ten liters per minute, depending upon the animal's size. Nebulization of alcohol has been advocated as a method to reduce surface tension and prevent foam formation. Oxygen administered either into a chamber or through a nasal or an endotracheal tube, should be humidified to prevent drying of the mucous membranes. Depending on the severity of hypoxemia, oxygen concentration should be from 50 to 100 per cent. Maximum gas flows are usually required when cages are used because of initial dead space and the leaks regularly found in such systems.

When well-controlled oxygen chambers are not available, the patient is most likely to find comfort in a quiet area near an open window or an air conditioner providing a flow of cool air. Beneficial effects of oxygen administration can only be expected when the oxygen can reach the alveoli and the gas exchange across the alveolar capillary membrane is functional. Oxygen therapy is of questionable value in the treatment of acute pulmonary alveolar disease as long as the airways and alveoli are blocked by frothy fluid. Fluid accumulation obstructing the airways needs to be resolved by tracheobronchial suction and by the therapeutic measures referred to above before oxygen therapy can reduce hypoxemia.

Severe pulmonary edema of various etiologies and the concomitant hypoxia in dogs and cats can be treated successfully with continuous positive airway pressure (CPAP) or positive end-expiratory pressure (PEEP) breathing.[213] Mechanical ventilation requires tracheal intubation or a cervical tracheostomy. PEEP can be created by using a respirator or by letting the animal breathe spontaneously and exhale against a 5- to 20-cm water pressure. PEEP improves gas exchange in edema, not by altering lung water accumulation, but rather by increasing lung volume and redistributing the excess alveolar water into the compliant perivascular space.[214, 215] CPAP keeps a sufficient number of airways and alveolar units open in cases that have failed to respond adequately to conventional measures. The use of PEEP ventilation is only advocated for clinics that have proper equipment as well as a staff of sufficient size to continuously monitor the patient and equipment.

Acid-Base Balance. Combined respiratory and metabolic acidosis may develop and is aggravated by a reduction in cardiac output and subsequent impairment of liver function. Hypochloremic, hyponatremic, hypokalemic alkalosis is a potential side effect of vigorous diuretic therapy. Acid-base imbalances need to be defined and then treated accordingly. Most clinical veterinary situations do not have the benefits of immediate blood gas analysis. The clinician is obligated to treat the patient based on an assessment of clinical findings.

Preload Reduction. Other techniques used in the management of acute pulmonary edema include rotating tourniquets and phlebotomy. Rotating tourniquets applied every 15 minutes to the limbs are less likely to be helpful in animals than they are in humans because of the comparatively smaller muscle mass of animal limbs. Phlebotomy is advocated up to a maximum of 25 per cent of the total blood volume to help reduce venous return. Phlebotomy should never be performed by restraining the patient. The authors use the saphenous or jugular vein, whichever is readily available for venipuncture. Nitroglycerin ointment applied transcutaneously to a hairless area induces a rapid reduction in preload. When applying the ointment, the doctor or technician should wear gloves because of the transcutaneous absorption route.

Other Measures. Soluble corticosteroids are indicated in high dosages in shock, allergy, and endotoxin-induced pulmonary edema. Other therapeutic agents that have been advocated in specific pulmonary edema states include antihistamines in allergic conditions. Isoproterenol may be useful in certain noncardiac pulmonary edema and shock states. Atropine sulfate is indicated exclusively in organophosphate-induced pulmonary edema. Pulmonary edema resulting from hyperactive clotting mechanisms may require heparin and low molecular-weight-dextran therapy. Alpha-adrenergic blockade may be in order in neurogenic pulmonary edema when a sympathoadrenal storm has occurred.

The need for antibiotics is questionable if the pulmonary edema can be resolved promptly. Broad-spectrum antibiotics are indicated in infectious pulmonary edema and in chronic edema.

Fluid therapy may improve tissue oxygenation but may also increase pulmonary edema. Colloids and albumin therapy are without benefit and may increase the pulmonary alveolar liquid.

References

1. Amis, TC: Clinical respiratory physiology. *In* Kirk, RW (ed): Current Veterinary Therapy VIII. Philadelphia, WB Saunders, 1983, p 191.
2. Haskins, SC: Blood gases and acid-base balance: clinical interpretation and therapeutic implications. *In* Kirk, RW (ed): Current Veterinary Therapy VIII. Philadelphia, WB Saunders, 1983, p 201.
3. Haskins, SC: Management of pulmonary disease in the critical patient. *In* Zaslow, IM (ed): Veterinary Trauma and Critical Care. Philadelphia, Lea & Febiger, 1984, p 339.
4. Court, MH, et al.: Inhalation therapy. Vet Clin North Am 15:1041, 1985.
5. Fitzpatrick, RK and Crowe, DT: Nasal oxygen administration in dogs and cats: experimental and clinical investigations. JAAHA 22:293, 1986.
6. McKiernan, BC: Principles of respiratory therapy. *In* Kirk, RW (ed): Current Veterinary Therapy VIII. Philadelphia, WB Saunders, 1983, p 216.
7. Pascoe, PJ: Short-term ventilatory support. *In* Kirk, RW (ed): Current Veterinary Therapy IX. Philadelphia, WB Saunders, 1986, p 269.
8. Luce, JM: The cardiovascular effects of mechanical ventilation and positive end-expiratory pressure. JAMA 252:807, 1984.
9. Orton, CE and Wheeler, SL: Continuous positive airway pressure therapy for aspiration pneumonia in a dog. JAVMA 188:1437, 1986.
10. Bjorling, DE and Whitfield, JB: High-frequency jet ventilation during pneumothorax in dogs. Am J Vet Res 47:1984, 1986.
11. Bjorling, DE, et al.: High-frequency jet ventilation during bronchoscopy in a dog. JAVMA 187:1373, 1985.
12. Murciano, D, et al.: Effects of theophylline on diaphragmatic strength and fatigue in patients with chronic obstructive pulmonary disease. N Engl J Med 311:349, 1984.
13. Papich, MG: Bronchodilator therapy. In Kirk, RW (ed): Current Veterinary Therapy IX. Philadelphia, WB Saunders, 1986, p 278.
14. McKiernan, BC, et al.: Pharmacokinetic studies of theophylline in cats. J Vet Pharm Ther 6:99, 1983.
15. McKiernan, BC, et al.: Pharmacokinetic studies of theophylline in dogs. J Vet Pharm Ther 4:103, 1981.
16. Dye, JA, et al.: Sustained release theophylline pharmacokinetics in the cat. Proceedings of the Sixth Veterinary Respiratory Symposium. Chicago, The Comparative Respiratory Society, 1986, p 8.
17. McKiernan, BC: Respiratory therapeutics. Proceed Fifth Vet Med Forum, San Diego, ACVIM, 1987, p 165.
18. Preuter, JC and Sherding, RG: Canine chronic bronchitis. Vet Clin North Am 15:1085, 1985.
19. Thayer, GW: Canine infectious tracheobronchitis. *In* Greene, CE: Microbiology and Infectious Diseases of the Dog and Cat. Philadelphia, WB Saunders, 1984, p 430.
20. Roudebush, P and Fales, WH: Antibacterial susceptibility of Bordetella bronchiseptica isolates from small companion animals with respiratory disease. JAAHA 17:793, 1981.
21. Kilgore, WR, et al.: β-Lactamase inhibition: a new approach in overcoming bacterial resistance. Comp Cont Ed Pract Vet 8:325, 1986.
22. Bemis, DA and Appel, MJ: Aerosol, parenteral, and oral antibiotic treatment of Bordetella bronchiseptica in dogs. JAVMA 170:1082, 1977.
23. Appel, MJ: Canine infectious tracheobronchitis (kennel cough): a status report. Comp Cont Ed Pract Vet 3:70, 1981.
24. Carpenter, JL: Bronchial asthma in cats. *In* Kirk, RW (ed): Current Veterinary Therapy V. Philadelphia, WB Saunders, 1974, p 208.
25. Moise, NS and Spaulding, GL: Feline bronchial asthma: pathogenesis, pathophysiology, diagnostics and therapeutic considerations. Comp Cont Ed Pract Vet 3:1091, 1981.
26. Moses, BL and Spaulding, GL: Chronic bronchial disease of the cat. Vet Clin North Am 15:929, 1985.
27. Noone, KE: Pulmonary hypersensitivities. *In* Kirk RW (ed): Current Veterinary Therapy IX. Philadelphia, WB Saunders, 1986, p 285.
28. Dietze, AE and Moise, NS: Feline bronchial disease. Proceed 4th Ann Eastern States Vet Conf, Orlando, 1987, p 2.
29. Frigas, E and Gleich, GJ: The eosinophil and the pathophysiology of asthma. J Allergy Clin Immunol 77:527, 1986.
30. Wilkie, BN: Allergic respiratory disease. *In* Cornelius, CE, et al. (eds): Advances in Veterinary Science and Comparative Medicine, Vol 26: The Respiratory System. New York, Academic Press, 1982, p 233.
31. Chung, KF, et al.: Antigen-induced airway hyperresponsiveness and pulmonary inflammation in allergic dogs. J Appl Physiol 58:1347, 1985.
32. Booth, BH, et al.: Immediate-type hypersensitivity in dogs: cutaneous, anaphylactic, and respiratory responses to Ascaris. J Lab Clin Med 76:181, 1970.
33. Wheeldon, EB, et al.: Chronic bronchitis in the dog. Vet Rec 94:466, 1974.
34. Chakrin, LW and Saunders, LZ: Experimental chronic bronchitis: pathology in the dog. Lab Invest 30:145, 1974.
35. Amis, TC: Chronic bronchitis in dogs. *In* Kirk, RW (ed): Current Veterinary Therapy IX. Philadelphia, WB Saunders, 1986, p 306.
36. Wheeldon, EB, et al.: Chronic respiratory disease in the dog. J Sm Anim Pract 18:229, 1977.
37. Edwards, DF, et al.: Immotile cilia syndrome in three dogs from a litter. JAVMA 183:667, 1983.
38. Morrison, WB, et al.: Primary ciliary dyskinesia in the dog. J Vet Int Med 1:67, 1987.
39. Kneller, SK: Thoracic radiography. *In* Kirk, RW (ed): Current Veterinary Therapy IX. Philadelphia, WB Saunders, 1986, p 250.
40. Meyer, W and Burt, JK: Bronchiectasis in the dog: its radiographic appearance. J Am Vet Radiol Soc 14:3, 1973.
41. Park, RD: Bronchoesophageal fistula in the dog: literature survey, case presentations, and radiographic manifestations. Comp Cont Ed Pract Vet 6:669, 1984.
42. Reif, JS and Rhodes, WH: The lungs of aged dogs: a radiographic-morphologic correlation. J Am Vet Radiol Soc 7:5, 1966.
43. Greene, CE: Canine distemper. *In* Greene, CE (ed): Clinical Microbiology and Infectious Diseases of the Dog and Cat. Philadelphia, WB Saunders, 1984, p 386.
44. Moise, NS: Viral respiratory diseases. Vet Clin North Am 15:919, 1985.
45. Hoover, EA and Kahn, DE: Experimentally induced feline calicivirus infections: clinical signs and lesions. JAVMA 166:463, 1975.
46. Pedersen, NC: Feline infectious peritonitis and feline enteric coronavirus infections: feline infectious peritonitis. Fel Pract 13(5):5, 1983.
47. Greene, CE: Rocky Mountain spotted fever. JAVMA 191:666, 1987.
48. Batey, RG and Smits, AF: The isolation of Bordetella bronchiseptica from an outbreak of canine pneumonia. Aust Vet J 52:184, 1976.
49. Garnett, NL, et al.: Hemorrhagic streptococcal pneumonia in newly procured research dogs. JAVMA 181:1371, 1982.
50. Thayer, GW: Infections of the respiratory system. *In* Greene, CE (ed): Clinical Microbiology and Infectious Diseases of the Dog and Cat. Philadelphia, WB Saunders, 1984, p 238.
51. Pedersen, NC: Mycoplasmal infections. *In* Holzworth, J (ed): Disease of the Cat: Medicine and Surgery. Philadelphia, WB Saunders Co, 1987, p 308.
52. Thayer, GW and Robinson, SK: Bacterial bronchopneumonia in the dog: a review of 42 cases. JAAHA 20:731, 1984.
53. Jones, SD and McKiernan, BC: Lower respiratory tract disease in the dog: bacterial cultures and sensitivities. *In* Proceed 6th Vet Respir Symp, Chicago, The Compar Respir Soc, 1986, p 16.
54. Hirsch, DC: Bacteriology of the lower respiratory tract. *In* Kirk, RW (ed): Current Veterinary Therapy IX. Philadelphia, WB Saunders, 1986, p 247.

55. Harpster, NK: The effectiveness of the cephalosporins in the treatment of bacterial pneumonias in the dog. JAAHA 17:766, 1981.
56. Pennington, JE: Penetration of antibiotics into respiratory secretions. Rev Infect Dis 3:67, 1981.
57. McKiernan, BC: Therapeutic strategies involving antimicrobial treatment of the lower respiratory tract in small animals. JAVMA 185:1155, 1984.
58. Greene, CE: Mycobacterial infections. *In* Greene, CE (ed): Clinical Microbiology and Infectious Diseases of the Dog and Cat. Philadelphia, WB Saunders, 1984, p 633.
59. Jang, SS, et al.: Pulmonary Mycobacterium fortuitum infection in a dog. JAVMA 184:96, 1984.
60. Turnwald, GH, et al.: Survival of a dog with pneumonia caused by Mycobacterium fortuitum. JAVMA 192:64, 1988.
61. Liu, S, et al.: Canine tuberculosis. JAVMA 177:164, 1980.
62. Greene, CE, et al.: Antimicrobial chemotherapy. *In* Greene, CE (ed): Clinical Microbiology and Infectious Diseases of the Dog and Cat. Philadelphia, WB Saunders, 1984, p 144.
63. Dalovisio, JR, et al.: Clinical usefulness of amikacin and doxycycline in the treatment of infection due to Mycobacterium fortuitum and Mycobacterium chelonei. Rev Infect Dis 3:1068, 1981.
64. Swenson, JM, et al.: Rapidly growing mycobacteria: testing of susceptibility to 34 antimicrobial agents by broth microdilution. Antimicrob Agents Chemother 22:186, 1982.
65. Farrow, BR and Love, DN: Bacterial, viral, and other infectious problems. *In* Ettinger, SJ (ed): Textbook of Veterinary Internal Medicine, 2nd ed. Philadelphia, WB Saunders, 1982, p 269.
66. Bekaert, DA: Handbook of Diseases Transmittéd from Dogs and Cats to Man. Calif Vet Handbook Suppl 9:14, 1982.
67. Petrak, M and Carpenter, JD: Feline toxoplasmosis. JAVMA 146:728, 1965.
68. Greene, CE and Prestwood, AK: Coccidial infections. *In* Greene, CE (ed): Clinical Microbiology and Infectious Diseases of the Dog and Cat. Philadelphia, WB Saunders, 1984, p 824.
69. Dubey, JP: Toxoplasmosis in cats. Feline Pract 16(4):12, 1986.
70. Feeney, DA, et al.: An unusual case of acute disseminated toxoplasmosis in a cat. JAAHA 17:311, 1981.
71. Greene, CE and Chandler, FW: Pneumocystosis. *In* Greene, CE (ed): Clinical Microbiology and Infectious Diseases of the Dog and Cat. Philadelphia, WB Saunders, 1984, p 859.
72. Tvedten, HW, et al.: Systemic Pneumocystis carinii infection in a dog. JAAHA 10:592, 1974.
73. Copland, JW: Canine pneumonia caused by Pneumocystis carinii. Aust Vet J 50:515, 1974.
74. McCully, RM, et al.: Canine pneumocystis pneumonia. J S Afr Vet Assoc 50:207, 1979.
75. Orenstein, M, et al.: Value of bronchoalveolar lavage in the diagnosis of pulmonary infection in acquired immune deficiency syndrome. Thorax 41:345, 1986.
76. Mann, JM, et al.: Nonbronchoscopic lung lavage for diagnosis of opportunistic infection in AIDS. Chest 91:319, 1987.
77. Legendre, AM: Systemic mycotic infections of dogs and cats. *In* Scott, FW (ed): Contemporary Issues in Small Animal Practice, Infectious Diseases. New York, Churchill Livingstone, 1986, p 29.
78. Barsanti, JA: Histoplasmosis. *In* Greene, CE (ed): Clinical Microbiology and Infectious Diseases of the Dog and Cat. Philadelphia, WB Saunders, 1984, p 687.
79. Roudebush, P: Mycotic pneumonias. Vet Clin North Am 15:949, 1985.
80. Barsanti, JA: Blastomycosis. *In* Greene, CE (ed): Clinical Microbiology and Infectious Diseases of the Dog and Cat. Philadelphia, WB Saunders, 1984, p 675.
81. Pyle, RL, et al.: Canine blastomycosis. Comp Cont Ed Pract Vet 3:963, 1981.
82. Smith, CD, et al.: Distribution of Blastomyces dermatitidis in dogs with skin test and serologic results following airborne infections. Sabouraudia 13:192, 1975.
83. Legendre, AL, et al.: Canine blastomycosis: a review of 47 clinical cases. JAVMA 178:1163, 1981.
84. Willard, ME, et al.: Chylothorax associated with blastomycosis in a dog. JAVMA 186:72, 1985.
85. Barsanti, JA and Jeffery, KL: Coccidioidomycosis. *In* Greene, CE (ed): Clinical Microbiology and Infectious Diseases of the Dog and Cat. Philadelphia, WB Saunders, 1984, p 710.
86. Millman, TM, et al.: Coccidioidomycosis in the dog: its radiographic diagnosis. J Am Vet Radiol Soc 20:50, 1979.
87. Barsanti, JA: Cryptococcosis. *In* Greene, CE (ed): Clinical Microbiology and Infectious Diseases of the Dog and Cat. Philadelphia, WB Saunders, 1984, p 700.
88. Holzworth, J, et al.: Mycotic diseases. *In* Holzworth, J (ed): Diseases of the Cat: Medicine and Surgery. Philadelphia, WB Saunders, 1987, p 320.
89. Southard, C: Bronchopulmonary aspergillosis in a dog. JAVMA 190:875, 1987.
90. Dubey, JP, et al.: Experimental Paragonimus kellicotti infection in dogs. Vet Parasitol 5:325, 1979.
91. Dubey, JP, et al.: Induced paragonimiasis in cats: clinical signs and diagnosis. JAVMA 173:735, 1978.
92. Barsanti, JA and Prestwood, AK: Parasitic diseases of the respiratory tract. *In* Kirk, RW (ed): Current Veterinary Therapy VIII. Philadelphia, WB Saunders, 1983, p 241.
93. Williams, JF and Zajac, A: Diagnosis of gastrointestinal parasitism in dogs and cats. St Louis, Ralston Purina Company, 1980.
94. Dubey, JP, et al.: Fenbendazole for treatment of Paragonimus kellicotti infection in dogs. JAVMA 174:835, 1979.
95. Kirkpatrick, CE and Shelly, EA: Paragonimiasis in a dog: treatment with praziquantel. JAVMA 187:75, 1985.
96. Urquhart, GM, et al.: Veterinary Parasitology. Essex, England, Longman Scientific and Technical, 1987.
97. Miller, BH, et al.: Pleural effusion as a sequelae to aleurostrongylus in a cat. JAVMA 185:556, 1984.
98. Vig, MM and Murray, PA: Successful treatment of Aelurostrongylus abstrusus with fenbendazole. Comp Cont Ed Pract Vet 8:214, 1986.
99. Kirkpatrick, CE and Megella, C: Use of ivermectin in treatment of Aelurostrongylus abstrusus and Toxocara cati infections in a cat. JAVMA 190:1309, 1987.
100. Franc, M, et al.: Essai de traitement de l'otacariase du chat par les ivermectines (Trial on treatment of otacariasis of cat by ivermectins). Revue Med Vet 136:693, 1985.
101. Greenlee, PG and Noone, KE: Pulmonary capillariasis in a dog. JAAHA 20:983, 1984.
102. Blagburn, BL, et al.: Anthelmintic efficacy of ivermectin in naturally parasitized cats. Am J Vet Res 48:670, 1987.
103. Rubash, JM: Filaroides hirthi infection in a dog. JAVMA 189:213, 1986.
104. August, JR, et al.: Filaroides hirthi in a dog: fatal hyperinfection suggestive of autoinfection. JAVMA 176:331, 1980.
105. Craig, TM, et al.: Fatal Filaroides hirthi infection in a dog. JAVMA 172:1096, 1978.
106. Georgi, JR, et al.: Patency and transmission of Filaroides hirthi infection. Parasitol 75:251, 1977.
107. Corwin, RM, et al.: Lungworm (Filaroides milksi) infection in a dog. JAVMA 165:180, 1974.
108. Stockdale, PH and Smart, ME: Treatment of crenosomiasis in dogs. Res Vet Sci 18:178, 1975.
109. Williams, JF: Parasitic diseases of the respiratory tract. *In* Kirk, RW (ed): Current Veterinary Therapy VII. Philadelphia, WB Saunders, 1980, p 262.
110. Neer, TM, et al.: Eosinophilic pulmonary granulomatosis in two dogs and literature review. JAAHA 22:593, 1986.
111. Confer, AW, et al.: Four cases of pulmonary nodular eosinophilic granulomatosis in dogs. Cornell Vet 73:41, 1983.
112. Israel, HL, et al.: Wegener's granulomatosis, lymphomatoid granulomatosis, and benign lymphocytic angiitis and granulomatosis of lung. Ann Intern Med 87:691, 1977.
113. Fauci, AS, et al.: Lymphomatoid granulomatosis: prospective clinical and therapeutic experience over 10 years. N Engl J Med 306:68, 1982.
114. Tizard, I: Veterinary Immunology: An Introduction. Philadelphia, WB Saunders, 1987, p 337.
115. Posterino, NC, et al.: Canine pulmonary lymphomatoid granulomatosis: 8 cases (1981-1986). Vet Can Soc News 11(1):1, 1987.
116. Lucke, VM, et al.: A lymphomatoid granulomatosis of the lungs in young dogs. Vet Pathol 16:405, 1979.
117. Berkwitt, L, et al.: Pulmonary granulomatosis associated with immune phenomena in a dog. JAAHA 14:111, 1978.
118. Drazner, FH: Systemic lupus erythematosus in the dog. Comp Cont Ed Pract Vet 2:243, 1980.

119. McKiernan, BC, et al.: Thoracic bite wounds and associated internal injury in 11 dogs and 1 cat. JAVMA 184:959, 1984.
120. Morgan, RV: Respiratory emergencies: Part I. Comp Cont Ed Pract Vet 5:228, 1983.
121. Krahwinkel, DJ: Thoracic trauma. *In* Kirk, RW (ed): Current Veterinary Therapy VII. Philadelphia, WB Saunders, 1980, p 268.
122. Tams, TR: Aspiration pneumonia and complications of inhalation of smoke and toxic gases. Vet Clin North Am 15:971, 1985.
123. Farrow, CS: Near-Drowning. *In* Kirk, RW (ed): Current Veterinary Therapy VIII. Philadelphia, WB Saunders, 1983, p 167.
124. Bonilla-Santiago, J and Fill, WL: Sand aspiration in drowning and near-drowning. Radiol 128:301, 1978.
125. Carson, TL: Toxic gases. *In* Kirks, RW (ed): Current Veterinary Therapy IX. Philadelphia, WB Saunders, 1986, p 203.
126. Farrow, CS: Inhalation injury. *In* Kirk, RW (ed): Current Veterinary Therapy VIII. Philadelphia, WB Saunders, 1983, p 173.
127. Tams, TR and Sherding, RG: Smoke inhalation injury. Comp Cont Ed Pract Vet 3:986, 1981.
128. Anderson, GI: Pulmonary cavitary lesions in the dog: a review of seven cases. JAAHA 23:89, 1987.
129. Aron, DN and Kornegay, JN: The clinical significance of traumatic lung cysts and associated pulmonary abnormalities in the dog and cat. JAAHA 19:903, 1983.
130. Kramek, BA, et al.: Bullous emphysema and recurrent pneumothorax in the dog. JAVMA 186:971, 1985.
131. Burns, MG: Pulmonary thromboembolism. *In* Kirk, RW (ed): Current Veterinary Therapy VIII. Philadelphia, WB Saunders, 1983, p 257.
132. Center, D and McFadden, R: Pulmonary defense mechanisms. *In* Sodeman, WA and Sodeman, TM (eds): Sodeman's Pathologic Physiology: Mechanisms of Disease. Philadelphia, WB Saunders, 1985, p 460.
133. Klein, MK, et al.: Pulmonary thromboembolism associated with immune-mediated hemolytic anemia in dogs: 10 cases. Proceed 6th Ann Vet Med Forum. Washington, DC, ACVIM, 1988, p 757.
134. Suter, PF: Lower airway and pulmonary parenchymal disease. *In* Suter, PF: Thoracic Radiography. Wettsweil, Switzerland, PF Suter, 1984, p 517.
135. Feldman, BF: Thrombosis—diagnosis and treatment. *In* Kirk, RW (ed): Current Veterinary Therapy IX. Philadelphia, WB Saunders, 1986, p 505.
136. Cherniack, RM, et al.: Obesity. Amer Rev Respir Dis 134:827, 1986.
137. West, JB: Disorders of ventilation. *In* Braunwald, E, et al. (eds): Harrison's Principles of Internal Medicine, 11th ed. New York, McGraw-Hill, 1987, p 1129.
138. Sartin, EA and Dubielzig, RR: Congenital anomalies in the respiratory tree of a dog. JAAHA 20:775, 1984.
139. Amis, TC, et al.: Congenital bronchial cartilage hypoplasia with lobar hyperinflation (congenital lobar emphysema) in an adult Pekingese. JAAHA 23:321, 1987.
140. Suter, PF, et al.: Radiographic recognition of primary and metastatic pulmonary neoplasms of dogs and cats. J Am Vet Radiol Soc 15:3, 1974.
141. McFadden, ER and Braunwald, E: Cor pulmonale. *In* Braunwald, E (ed): Heart Disease, 3rd ed. Philadelphia, WB Saunders, 1988, p 1597.
142. Mehlhaff, CJ and Mooney, S: Primary pulmonary neoplasia in the dog and cat. Vet Clin North Am 15:1061, 1985.
143. Barr, FJ, et al.: The radiological features of primary lung tumours in the dog: a review of 36 cases. J Small Anim Pract 27:493, 1986.
144. Stann, SE and Bauer, TG: Respiratory tract tumors. Vet Clin North Am 15:535, 1985.
145. Moulton, JE et al.: Classification of lung carcinomas in the dog and cat. Vet Pathol 18:513, 1981.
146. Brodey, RS and Craig, PH: Primary pulmonary neoplasms in the dog: a review of 29 cases. JAVMA 147:1628, 1965.
147. Taylor, GN, et al.: Primary pulmonic tumors in beagles. Am J Vet Res 40:1316, 1979.
148. Koblik, PD: Radiographic appearance of primary lung tumors in cats: a review of 41 cases. Vet Radiol 27:66, 1986.
149. Seiler, RJ: Primary pulmonary osteosarcoma in a dog with associated hypertrophic osteopathy. Vet Pathol 16:369, 1979.
150. Stephens, LC, et al.: Primary pulmonary fibrosarcoma associated with Spirocerca lupi infection in a dog with hypertrophic pulmonary osteoarthropathy. JAVMA 182:496, 1983.
151. Carpenter, JL, et al.: Tumors and tumor-like lesions. *In* Holzworth, J (ed): Diseases of the Cat: Medicine and Surgery. Philadelphia, WB Saunders, 1987, p 406.
152. Moore, JA and Taylor, HW: Primary pulmonary adenocarcinoma in a dog. JAVMA 192:219, 1988.
153. Hamilton, HB, et al.: Pulmonary squamous cell carcinoma with intraocular metastasis. JAVMA 185:307, 1984.
154. Jensen, HE and Arnbjerg, J: Bone metastasis of undifferentiated pulmonary adenocarcinoma in a cat. Nord Vet Med 38:288, 1986.
155. Madewell, BR and Theilen, GH: Tumors of the respiratory tract. *In* Theilen, GH and Madewell, BR (eds): Vet Canc Med. Philadelphia, Lea & Febiger, 1987, p 535.
156. Sorjonen, DC, et al.: Paraplegia and subclinical neuromyopathy associated with a primary lung tumor in a dog. JAVMA 180:1209, 1982.
157. Nafe, LA, et al.: Mammary tumors and unassociated pulmonary masses in two cats. JAVMA 175:1194, 1979.
158. Noone, KE: Pleural effusions and diseases of the pleura. Vet Clin North Am 15:1069, 1985.
159. Crow, SE: Clinical diagnosis and management of carcinomas. *In* Gorman, NT (ed): Contemporary Issues in Small Animal Practice, Oncology. New York, Churchill Livingstone, 1986, p 213.
160. Mehlhaff, CJ, et al.: Surgical treatment of primary pulmonary neoplasia in 15 dogs. JAAHA 20:799, 1984.
161. Rosenthal, RC: Tumor metastasis: biology and treatment. Comp Cont Ed Pract Vet 6:767, 1984.
162. Crow, SE: Neoplasms of the respiratory tract. *In* Kirk, RW (ed): Current Veterinary Therapy VII. Philadelphia, WB Saunders, 1980, p 249.
163. Schabel, FM. Concepts for systemic treatment of micrometastases. Cancer 35:15, 1975.
164. Reif, JS, et al.: Canine pulmonary disease and the urban environment I: the validity of radiographic examination for estimating the prevalence of pulmonary disease. Arch Environ Health 20:676, 1970.
165. Walter, PA, et al.: Radiographic appearance of pulmonary metastases from transitional cell carcinoma of the bladder and urethra of the dog. JAVMA 185:411, 1984.
166. Lang, J, et al.: Sensitivity of radiographic detection of lung metastases in the dog. Vet Radiol 27:74, 1986.
167. Biller, DS and Meyer, CW: Case examples demonstrating the clinical utility of obtaining both right and left lateral thoracic radiographs in small animals. JAAHA 23:381, 1987.
168. Spencer, H: Pathology of the Lung. Pergamon Press, Oxford, 1968.
169. Harris, P and Heath, D: Pulmonary Edema. *In* The Human Pulmonary Circulation, 3rd ed. New York, Churchill Livingstone, 1986, p 373.
170. Ingram, RH, and Braunwald, E: Pulmonary edema: Cardiogenic and noncardiogenic. *In* Braunwald, E (ed): Heart Disease, 3rd ed. Philadelphia, WB Saunders, 1988, p 545.
171. Greene, DG: Newer Concepts of Pulmonary Edema. *In* Frontiers of Pulmonary Radiology. New York, Grune and Stratton, 1969.
172. Ortega, P, et al.: Electron and Eight Microscopy Studies of Progressive Pulmonary Edema in Experimental Heart Failure in the Dog. *In* Viamonte, M. (ed.). Progress in Lymphology II. Stuttgart, Germany, Georg Thieme, 1970, p 32.
173. Staub, NC: The pathophysiology of pulmonary edema. Human Pathol I:419, 1970.
174. Meszaros, WT: Lung changes in left heart failure. Circulation 48:859, 1973.
175. Luisada, AA: Paroxysmal pulmonary edema and the acute cardiac lung. Am J Cardiol 20:69, 1967.
176. Rigler, LG, and Suprenant, EL: Pulmonary edema. Semin Roentgenol 2:33, 1967.
177. Harle, TS, et al.: Pulmonary edema without cardiomegaly. Am J Roentgenol 103:555, 1970.
178. Staub, N.C: Pulmonary edema due to increased microvascular permeability to fluid and protein. Circ Res 43:143, 1978.

179. Fishman, AP, and Pietra, GG: Hemodynamic Pulmonary Edema. *In* Fishman, AP, and Renkin, EM (eds.): American Physiological Society. Bethesda, MD, 1979, p 79.
180. Ingram, RH and Braunwald, E: Pulmonary Edema: Cardiogenic and Non-Cardiogenic. *In* Braunwald, E (ed): Heart Disease, 3rd ed. Philadelphia, WB Saunders, 1988, p 544.
181. Boothe, HW, Jr, et al.: Cardiovascular effects of rapid infusion of crystalloid in the hypovolaemic cat. J Sm Anim Prac 26:8, 1985.
182. Miller, WC, et al.: Contribution of systemic venous hypertension to the development of pulmonary edema in dogs. Circ Res 43:598, 1978.
183. Trapnell, DH, and Thurston, JGB: Unilateral pulmonary edema after pleural aspiration. Lancet 1:1367, 1970.
184. Interiano, B, et al.: Acute respiratory distress syndrome in pancreatitis. Ann Intern Med 77:923, 1972.
185. Robin, ED,: Permeability Pulmonary Edema. *In* Fishman, AP and Renkin, EM (eds.): Pulmonary Am Physiol Society. Bethesda, MD, 1979, p 217.
186. Montaner, JS, et al.: Alveolar epithelial damage. A critical difference between high pressure and oleic acid-induced low pressure pulmonary edema. J Clin Invest 77:1786, 1986.
187. Lees, GE, et al.: Pulmonary edema in a dog with acute pancreatitis and cardiac disease. JAVMA 172:690, 1978.
188. Farrow, CS: Smoke inhalation in the dog: Current concepts of pathophysiology and management. VM/SAC 70:404, 1975.
189. Jubb, KVF, and Kennedy, PC: Pathology of Domestic Animals, Vol 2. New York, Academic Press, 1971.
190. Malik, AB, et al.: Pulmonary microvascular effects of arachidonic acid metabolites and their role in lung vascular injury. Fed Proc 44:36, 1985.
191. Swann, HG: Mechanism of circulatory failure in fresh and sea water drowning. Circ Res 4:241, 1956.
192. Hunter, TB, and Whitehouse, W: Fresh-water near-drowning: Radiological aspects. Radiology 112:51, 1974.
193. Ducker, TB, and Simmons, RL: Increased intracranial pressure and pulmonary edema. The hemodynamic response of dogs and monkeys to increased intracranial pressure. J Neurosurg 28:118, 1968.
194. Bean, JW, and Beckman, DL: Centrogenic pulmonary pathology in mechanical head injury. J Appl Physiol 27:807, 1969.
195. Kolata, RJ: The Clinical Features of Electric Cord Bite Injury in Dogs. Proceed 41st Ann Meet AAHA, 1974, p 460.
196. Lord, PF, et al.: Acute pulmonary edema and seizures in hunting dogs. Nord Vet Med 27:112, 1975.
197. Luisada, AA: Pulmonary Edema in Man and Animals. St. Louis, Warren H Green, 1970.
198. Földi, M: Diseases of Lymphatics and Lymph Circulation. Springfield, Ill, Charles C Thomas, 1969.
199. Grainerger, RG: Interstitial pulmonary edema and its radiological diagnosis. A sign of pulmonary venous and capillary hypertension. Br J Radiol 31:201, 1958.
200. Logue, RB, et al.: Subtle roentgenographic signs of left heart failure. Am Heart J 65:464, 1963.
201. Fein, A, et al.: The value of edema fluid examination in patients with pulmonary edema. Am J Med 67:32, 1979.
202. Vreim, CE, et al.: Protein composition of lung fluids in anesthetized dogs with acute cardiogenic edema. Am J Physiol 231:1466, 1976.
203. Suter, PF and Lord, PF: Thoracic Radiography, 1st ed. Weitsweil, Switzerland, PF Suter, 1984.
204. Hedlund, LW, et al.: Hydrostatic pulmonary edema. An analysis of lung density changes by computed tomography. Invest Radiol 19:254, 1984.
205. Suter, PF, and Chan, KF: Disseminated pulmonary diseases in small animals: A radiographic approach to diagnosis. J Am Vet Rad Soc 9:67, 1968.
206. Fleischner, FG: The butterfly pattern of acute pulmonary edema. Am J Cardiol 20:39, 1967.
207. Bishop, MJ and Cheney, FW: Vasodilators worsen gas exchange in dog oleic-acid lung injury. Anesthesiology 64:435, 1986.
208. Dauber, IM and Weil, JV: Lung injury edema in dogs. Influence of sympathetic ablation. J Clin Invest 72:1977, 1983.
209. Ali, J and Wood, LD: Pulmonary vascular effects of furosemide on gas exchange in pulmonary edema. J Appl Physiol 57:160, 1984.
210. Rusch, VW, et al.: Effect of furosemide on fully established low pressure pulmonary edema. J Surg Res 41:141, 1986.
211. Molloy, WD, et al.: Treatment of canine permeability pulmonary edema: short-term effects of dobutamine, furosemide, and hydralazine. Circulation 72:1365, 1985.
212. Vassalle, M: Role of catecholamine release in morphine hyperglycemia. Am J Physiol 200:530, 1961.
213. Haskins, SC: Standards and Techniques of Equipment Utilization. *In* Sattler, FP, et al. (eds.): Veterinary Critical Care. Philadelphia, Lea and Febiger, 1981.
214. Saul, GM, et al.: Effect of graded administration of PEEP on lung water in noncardiogenic pulmonary edema. Crit Care Med 10:667, 1982.
215. Malo, J, et al.: How does positive end-expiratory pressure reduce intrapulmonary shunt in canine pulmonary edema? J Appl Physiol 57:1002, 1984.

70 MEDIASTINAL, PLEURAL, AND EXTRAPLEURAL DISEASES

TIM BAUER

DISORDERS OF THE DIAPHRAGM

As the principal muscle of respiration, the diaphragm is responsible for the majority of inspiration during normal respiration.[1,2] The most common clinical problems involving the diaphragm are paralysis and hernia. While there are relatively few primary disorders of the diaphragm, it is frequently affected by disorders above and below it.

Diaphragmatic Displacement

The right hemidiaphragm is normally more cranial than the left.[3] One or both hemidiaphragms can be moved cranially or caudally by a variety of abdominal and thoracic conditions.

BILATERAL DISPLACEMENT

Bilateral caudal displacement of the diaphragm is a characteristic of obstructive airway disorders. It is more profound in chronic disorders, causing air trapping and hyperinflation.[4] The diaphragms are flattened; this may be more pronounced in the lateral radiograph. While large pleural effusions have the same effect, diaphragmatic displacement is difficult to recognize because the effusion obliterates the diaphragmatic contour. Pneumothorax, either simple or under tension, displaces the diaphragm caudally. Cranial displacement may occur normally with obesity or pregnancy. Intra-abdominal disorders producing displacement include ascites, hepatomegaly, intra-abdominal masses, obstructive ileus, and acute gastric dilatation.

UNILATERAL DIAPHRAGMATIC DISPLACEMENT

Unilateral caudal displacement of a hemidiaphragm may occur with unilateral pneumothorax, pulmonary cysts, or bullae. Pleural effusion or mass may produce displacement but may be hard to discern radiographically. Unilateral cranial displacement, unlike bilateral displacement, is most commonly a result of intrathoracic disease.[5] Processes causing loss of lung volume, such as atelectasis or pulmonary resection, move a hemidiaphragm cranially. Pulmonary restriction due to adhesions or fibrothorax may likewise cause displacement. Pulmonary embolism or thrombosis often affects lung volumes and as such, provokes small changes in the diaphragm.[6,7]

EVENTRATION

Diaphragmatic eventration is a condition in which a hemidiaphragm is thinned and frequently is moved cranially. The diaphragm is atrophic or may be devoid of muscle fibers.[7] The etiology is unknown but the condition is assumed to be either acquired or congenital. While there have been sporadic reports of incidents, the importance of this process is unknown in veterinary patients.

PARALYSIS OF THE DIAPHRAGM

Diaphragmatic paralysis is the most clinically important disorder of diaphragmatic function. It may be unilateral or bilateral and may be a permanent or transient phenomenon.[8] Innervation is by the phrenic nerves arising from the cervical roots of C4-C7.[9,10] Dysfunction arises from disruption of the phrenic pathway anywhere between its origin and the diaphragm. Unilateral paralysis may be caused by traumatic or surgical transection, infiltrative or mass lesions, and neuropathic disorders. Bilateral paralysis is most commonly a result of cervical spinal trauma but may be caused by the disorders previously mentioned.

Patients with unilateral paralysis are rarely symptomatic and the diagnosis may be an incidental finding.

Bilateral paralysis may cause significant dyspnea and anxiety. Dyspnea may be accentuated by eating, ileus, or recumbency, as all these may further reduce lung volumes.

The diagnosis of diaphragmatic paralysis may be suspected by the clinical setting and radiographic findings of cranial displacement of the diaphragm. The diagnosis is made by fluoroscopic demonstration of diminished or absent diaphragmatic motion during normal inspiration.[11]

DIAPHRAGMATIC HERNIA

The term "diaphragmatic hernia" loosely refers to all disorders in which abdominal viscera traverse the diaphragm and enter the thoracic cavity. The abdominal viscera may be contained within a hernial sac or may be free in the pleural space. Herniation of abdominal contents through the diaphragm may occur at any level and may be congenital or acquired.[12, 13] Traumatic rupture is usually the result of severe trauma, most frequently nonpenetrating to the abdomen and caudal chest. Intra-abdominal pressures rise rapidly during insult. This is accentuated if it occurs against a closed glottis. The diaphragm ruptures, allowing various abdominal organs to gain access to the pleural space.[14]

The veterinary literature is full of clinical reports of diaphragmatic hernia, but few report similar distributions of herniation sites or organs involved.[15–19] It appears that there is a predilection for the lateral aspects of the diaphragm. Pleural effusion seems to occur in only 40 to 50 per cent of the cases reported.[20] This seemingly low incidence may reflect the stage at which the case is diagnosed as well as the anatomic nature of the hernia and incarcerated organs.

Despite the frequency of this disorder, it often remains a difficult diagnosis to make definitively. Radiographic evaluation remains the most important single method of confirming the diagnosis. Multiple contrast studies may be helpful in documenting the lesion; barium swallow, contrast pleurography, contrast peritonography, and even mesenteric angiography have been employed (Figure 70–1*A* and *B*). Ultrasonography or nuclear liver/spleen scans may be of assistance in complicated cases. Negative contrasts such as diagnostic pneumothorax or pneumoperitoneum may outline the diaphragm or demonstrate abdominothoracic communication.

History. Diaphragmatic hernia may present as an acute, subacute, or chronic disorder; the history may be the same. Frequently there is no history of trauma, either recent or past; inquiry referable to past traumatic events may prove fruitful. There may be a vague history of gastrointestinal distress that is episodic; low-grade respiratory signs may be observed, possibly provoked by exercise or recumbency. Signs may be progressive and escalate over a period of time.

Acute presentation following trauma may be referable to factors other than herniation. Animals in acute distress may have all their signs secondary to pulmonary compression and atelectasis but more frequently the signs are associated with hypotension, lung contusion, and other intra-abdominal injuries.

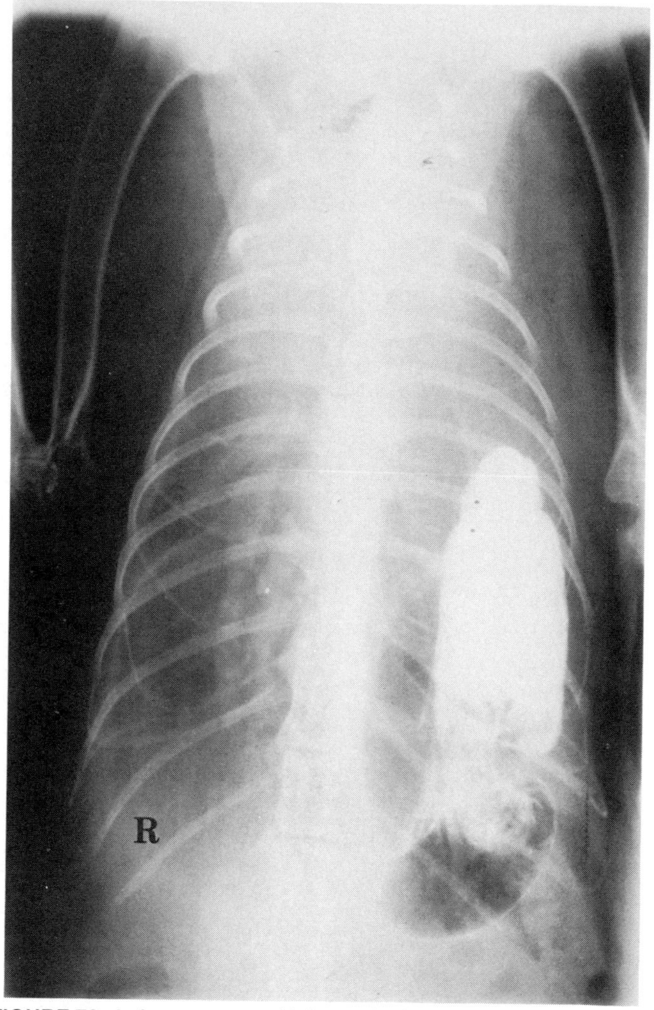

FIGURE 70–1. A seven-year-old domestic shorthaired cat with pleural effusion secondary to a diaphragmatic hernia. The gastrogram demonstrates abdominal viscera in the left hemithorax. While not visible on this view, healed rib fractures were evident on survey films.

As hernias may have been present for weeks to years, the patient with chronic herniation may be presented for longstanding signs or acute signs referable to pleural effusion, sudden incarceration of a viscus, or lung torsion.

Management. Diaphragmatic hernia is a surgical disorder; however, not all acutely ill patients require immediate surgical intervention. Primary care in the acute patient is directed toward the management of concurrent injury. While the apparent presence of diaphragmatic hernia may by the only tangible finding, treatment of hypotension, anemia, and acute ventilatory failure may be necessary prior to elective correction. An acute intra-abdominal injury such as splenic or hepatic rupture, avulsion of the kidney, or retroperitoneal or omental bleeding frequently accompanies trauma significant enough to produce herniation. Persistent hypotension despite transfusion and the finding of hemoperitoneum or hemothorax may be a more important indication for laparotomy than the finding of a hernia.

Patients with longstanding herniation may present with pleural effusion of unknown etiology. While thoracocentesis is always indicated in such cases, any index of suspicion should prompt extra care during such procedures to avoid puncture of a viscus or solid organ. Likewise, tube thoracostomy may be necessary, but placement is dictated by the radiographic findings. Whenever possible, contrast studies should be performed before drainage.

PERITONEAL PERICARDIAL DIAPHRAGMATIC HERNIA

This congenital condition is frequently an incidental finding in older patients who have been examined radiographically for other reasons. It is not known as an acquired anomaly; this should be kept in mind when debating the causal relationship of signs in older individuals.[21, 22]

Radiographically the cardiac silhouette may appear to be a centrally located globular structure. There may be gas shadows present if bowel is involved or there may be granular densities representing ingesta (Figure 70–2). Uncommonly, calcification of entrapped tissue occurs.[3] Sternal deformity may be a concurrent finding with either a bifid appearance or absence or fusion of sternebral segments.

Clinical signs may not be present and there may be no historical recognition of thoracic or abdominal signs. For unknown reasons these hernias may become symptomatic late in life. Strangulation of incarcerated viscera may occur, causing acute signs of bowel obstruction or increases in intrapericardial fat, or hepatic and splenic strangulation, which may prompt formation of pericardial effusions and signs of heart failure.

The diagnosis may be strongly suspected by the appearance of the routine thoracic radiographs. The diagnosis may be confirmed by numerous studies. This is done prior to any contemplated surgical intervention. Upper gastrointestinal contrast studies, echocardiography, liver/spleen scans, angiography, or peritonography may demonstrate the lesion.

There may be valid clinical debate about the necessity of correcting these lesions. It may be unnecessary and indeed unwise to correct such lesions in older asymptomatic patients in which these findings are incidental. Likewise, symptomatic presentation may not be due to this striking finding and as such, a search should be made for other potential causes of vague intra-abdominal signs. This may obviate the surgical exploration. In young symptomatic patients, surgical correction should be attempted as quickly as possible. Response is usually excellent with a total resolution of all signs.

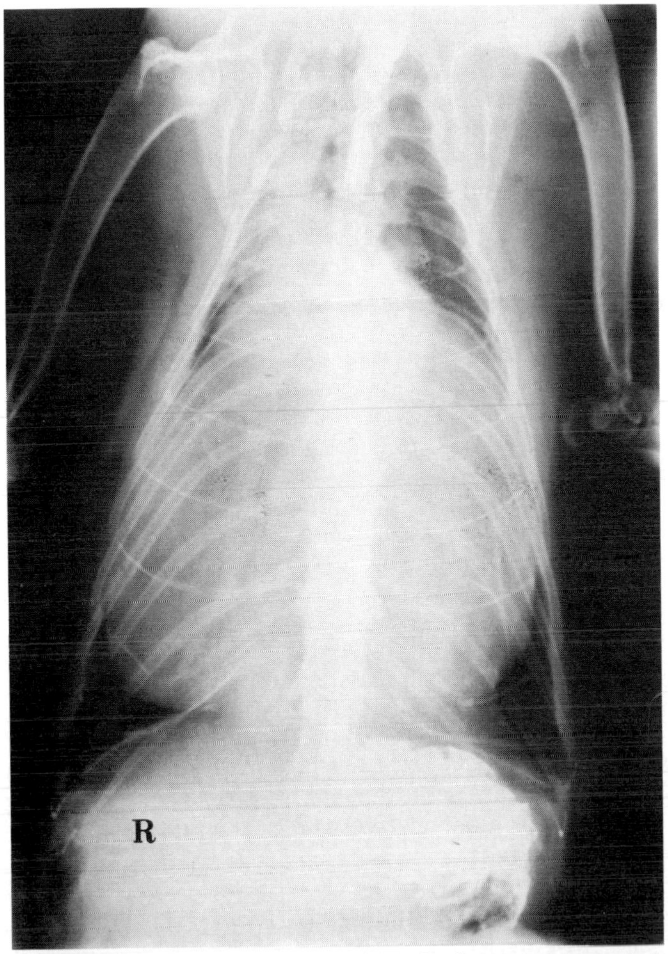

FIGURE 70–2. Peritoneal pericardial hernia discovered as an incidental finding on survey radiographs obtained for unrelated reasons. A barium swallow has been performed to delineate esophageal and gastric borders.

DISORDERS OF THE CHEST WALL

BLUNT CHEST TRAUMA

Nonpenetrating chest trauma is a major cause of serious and fatal thoracic dysfunction in animals. Although a preponderance of these injuries results from motor vehicle trauma, other causes such as falls from heights, being kicked, and sports-related injuries such as those caused by Frisbees, may be responsible for many cases. Blunt chest trauma may be responsible for a number of injuries that occur alone or in combination: pulmonary injuries such as contusion, laceration or hematoma; chest wall disruption; fracture of the tracheobronchial tree; rupture of the diaphragm; and hemothorax, pneumothorax, or pneumomediastinum.

The term "flail chest" refers to chest wall disruption with multiple linear rib fractures and associated paradoxical segmental motion of the fractured section. The multiple rib or sternal fractures in essence isolate the wound from the rest of the thoracic wall, enabling it to move independently during respiration (Figure 70–3). This phenomenon effectively reduces transpulmonary pressure and leads to hypoventilation.[23, 24] This is further compounded by any process that reduces pulmonary compliance, such as hemorrhage, contusion, or edema.[25]

Clinical recognition may be hampered by a multiplicity of thoracic injuries. When the flail segment is dorsal, the overlying muscles may splint the lesion, decreasing visibility. As transpulmonary pressure rises, the paradoxical motion is increasingly evident. Radiographically, multiple rib fractures are evident; this may be accompanied by elevation of the affected hemidiaphragm and associated loss of lung volume.

Management of flail chest is determined by the patient's respiratory status and concomitant chest injuries. A variety of measures have been recommended to

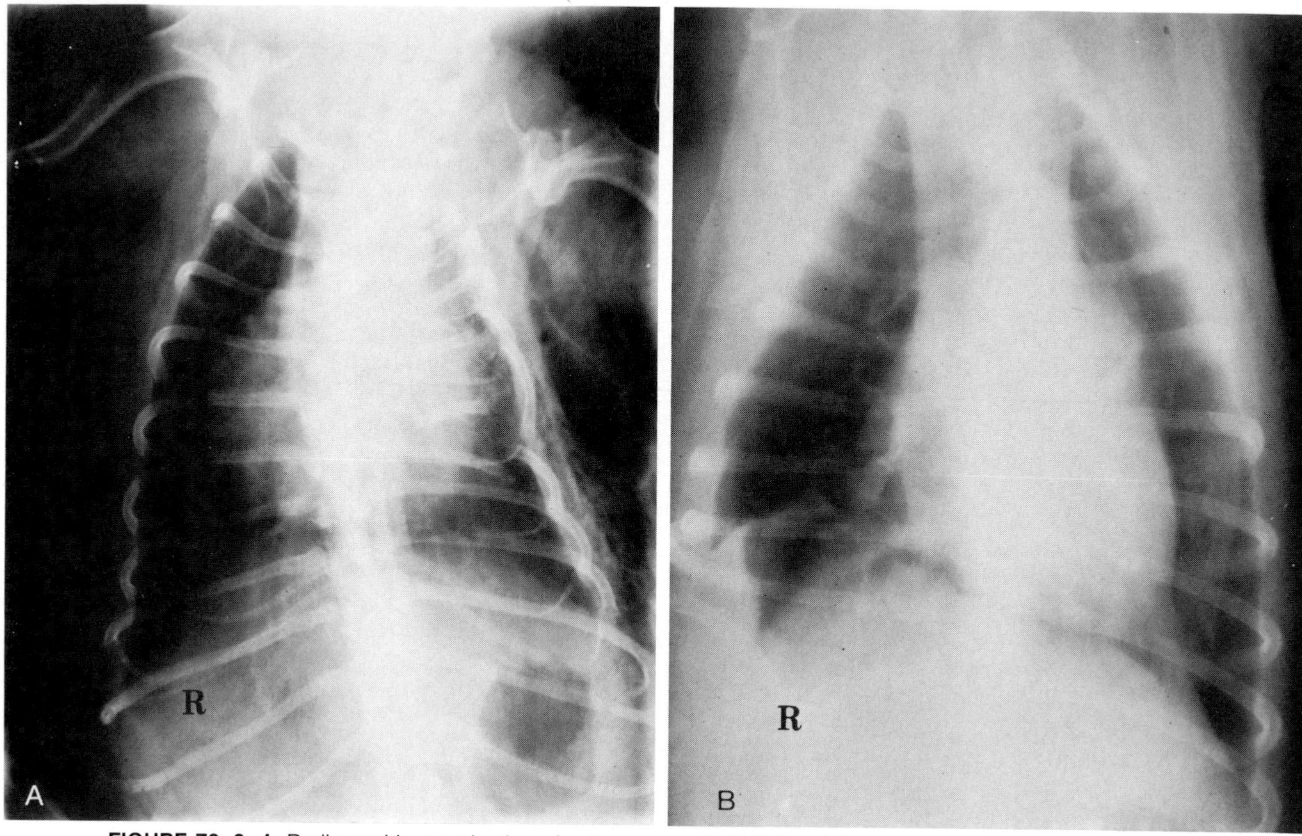

FIGURE 70–3. *A*, Radiographic examination of a three-year-old Shih Tzu following a motor vehicle accident. Note the multiple free rib segments in the left hemithorax and a large volume of free subcuticular air. *B*, Radiographic examination of a golden retriever following a motor vehicle accident. This patient has loss of lung volume secondary to a large flail segment. Note the elevated right hemidiaphragm and pleural effusion.

externally stabilize the flail segment, including splints and thoracic bandages.[26–28] These appear to be of little use and with thoracic compression may provoke further hypoventilation. These measures have been supplanted by mechanical ventilation, which reverses the underlying pathophysiology.[23, 29, 30] Those patients without respiratory failure do not usually require such intervention. Narcotic analgesia coupled with intercostal nerve blocks frequently reduces dyspnea and promotes patient cooperation in dealing with the injury. Flail segments usually heal without surgical repair. Internal fixation of the rib fractures with K-wires or pins may be helpful in stabilizing the hemiflail segments.

Pneumothoraces, both simple and tension types, are discussed elsewhere (in this chapter). Hemothorax or hemorrhage into the pleural space may be of intercostal or pulmonary origin. Signs and findings of pleural effusion, hypotension, and shock may be concurrent findings. Management is dictated by the size of the hemothorax. Small hemothoraces that provide radiographic evidence of costophrenic blunting or visible pleural fissure lines may be treated conservatively and should resorb in one to two weeks. With large, trauma-related hemothoraces, tube thoracostomy is indicated to reduce hemothorax, monitor further bleeding, and tamponade the bleeding site by lung reexpansion. Significant fibrothorax rarely occurs secondary to hemothorax.[31–33] Thoracotomy may rarely be required with persistent bleeding from systemic vessels. Every attempt should be made to avoid surgery, using the above measures and transfusion.

Patients with large nontraumatic or postsurgical hemothoraces should be managed without chest tube insertion whenever possible. Chest wall bleeding in patients with coagulopathies should resolve with the appropriate therapy for the underlying disorder. While ill-advised if fresh whole blood and plasma are available, autotransfusion of pleural blood may be life-saving with large hemothoraces associated with warfarin-related diatheses.

THORACIC WALL DEFORMITY

There are numerous congenital and acquired thoracic cage deformities that variably affect the contour and volume of the thorax. Deformities of the sternum, ribs, and thoracic spine are frequently encountered, both clinically and radiographically, and are frequent incidental findings. Unlike humans, in whom these deformities may provoke progressive symptomatic respiratory disorders, animals rarely experience respiratory failure as a result of thoracic deformity, if it is unaccompanied by primary cardiac or pulmonary defects. Frequently animals that are mildly symptomatic as infants are asymptomatic as adults.

THORACIC WALL MASSES AND INFILTRATIVE DISORDERS

This group of disorders includes primary neoplasia that arises from the skeletal portion of the thorax, metastatic tumors, tumors that directly invade the chest wall from without or within, and granulomatous or purulent infectious disorders.

Primary Chest Wall Malignancy. Chondrosarcoma is the most frequently encountered primary neoplasm of the chest wall and accounts for approximately one-third of this tumor's distribution.[3, 34] The tumors typically arise from the costochondral junction or the sternum. It may be found in the midportion of the first two ribs on rare occasions.

These tumors are typically slow-growing and may be advanced at the time of diagnosis. They tend to be locally invasive and frequently invade the pleura and mediastinum, causing effusion (Figure 70–4). Chondrosarcomas rarely metastasize to distant sites.[35] These tumors may be characterized as benign by pathologists only to return later and invade adjacent structures following resection.

Osteosarcomas of the chest wall are typically nonpainful, rapidly growing tumors that most frequently arise at the costochondral junction.[36] This tumor has a predilection for the appendicular skeleton rather than the ribs.[35] When they occur in the thoracic wall, they may be large and directly invade the underlying pleura and lung. As with peripheral osteosarcoma, this tumor has a propensity for pulmonary metastasis. Complete surgical resection may prove difficult, as with chondrosarcoma.

Soft tissue sarcomas, such as fibrosarcoma and hemangiosarcoma, may occur anywhere in the chest wall. These are often large infiltrative masses that may produce bone destruction. Frequently these invade the pleura, causing effusion. Hemangiosarcoma of the skin and thoracic soft tissues may not be as aggressive as the visceral forms and may not metastasize as rapidly.

Multiple Myeloma. Multiple myeloma or plasmacytoma is a systemic disease that occasionally presents as a rib lesion. Multiple "punch-out" lytic lesions may be present in the ribs and less frequently in the sternum. Systemic disease is usually present at the time bone lesions are discovered; fever, weakness, and abnormal serum protein are often clinical features of this disease.

Osteochondromatosis. Osteochondromatoses or cartilaginous exostoses are uncommon tumors. They are cartilage-covered bone tumors and are considered benign. They appear on ribs or vertebral segments and are frequently found in younger animals. Most frequently single lesions grow to various magnitudes until skeletal maturation is complete. These tumors are solitary or multiple and may grow large enough to restrict intrathoracic and chest wall structures. Some tumors take on malignant characteristics and continue to grow like other bone malignancies. Causes of these tumors in dogs and cats are somewhat speculative. It has been postulated that some of these tumors in dogs may be heritable, while C-type viral particles have been seen in feline tumors.[37, 38]

Metastatic Chest Wall Tumors. Tumor metastasis to the chest wall, ribs, and thoracic spine appears less frequently in veterinary patients than humans, in whom it occurs frequently with such tumors as bronchogenic carcinoma and breast carcinoma.[39, 40] Osteosarcoma in dogs may metastasize to ribs, involving the rib shaft rather than the costochondral junction. When such findings are present, survey films of the appendicular skeleton are in order if no primary tumor is clinically evident.

Mammary carcinoma has been reported to metastasize to bone; however, only a small number of these were rib lesions.[41, 42] It must be kept in mind that these diagnoses are made on the basis of survey radiographs. Routine use of bone scans might increase the observed incidence.

Treatment. The treatment of primary as well as metastatic chest wall tumors is surgical; this, in turn, may be followed by chemotherapy or radiation. The goals of chest-wall resection are complete removal of the tumor,

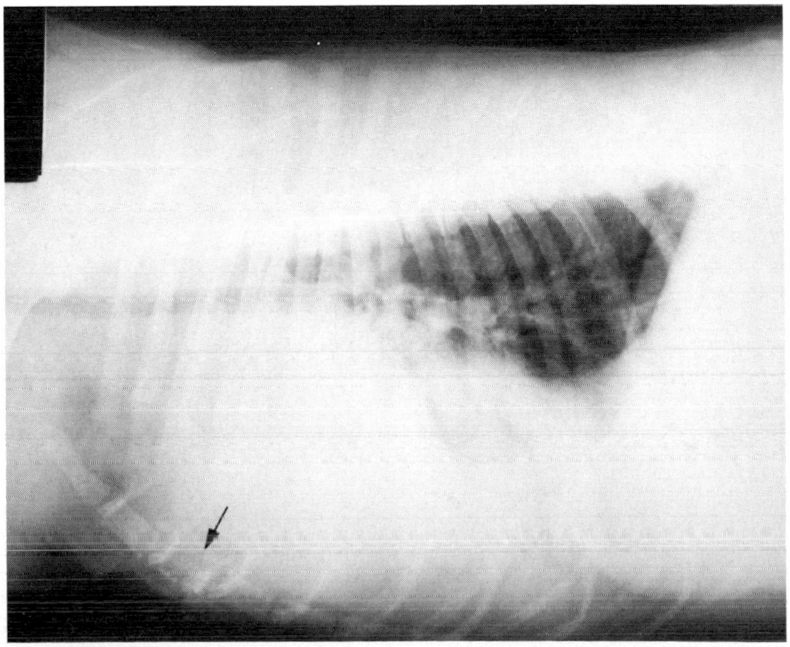

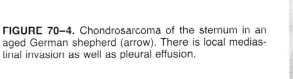

FIGURE 70–4. Chondrosarcoma of the sternum in an aged German shepherd (arrow). There is local mediastinal invasion as well as pleural effusion.

leaving disease-free tissue margins and reconstruction of the chest wall to close the defect and to provide cosmetically acceptable coverage with integument.

Resection of benign tumors can be done locally without wide margins. As with other malignancy, wide resection is indicated. This means that at least 1.5 cm of normal rib, cartilage, or sternum should be resected in all directions around the tumor. As malignant tumors may extend distances within the medullary space, or extend along the periosteum and pleura, the longest possible segment of ribs should be resected.

Infectious Chest Wall Disorders. Numerous non-neoplastic conditions may present as chest wall masses or chest wall thickening and must be considered in the differential diagnosis of chest wall masses. Since the treatment of these non-neoplastic conditions is different from that of neoplasia, it is imperative that they be recognized prior to radical surgical resection.

Cellulitis, abscesses, or granuloma formation may be seen with infections with *Actinomyces* species, *Nocardia* species, anaerobic organisms, aerobic organisms, and fungi, such as *Blastomyces*, *Aspergillus*, *Coccidioides*, and *Cryptococcus*. Some of these may be associated with migration of foreign bodies or bite wounds, others with systemic dissemination or local invasion.

While many of these may be grossly and radiologically extrapleural, others have associated intrathoracic radiographic findings. Pleural effusion, sternal or tracheobronchial adenopathy, or pulmonary infiltrates may be concurrent findings. Frank empyema may accompany any of the previously mentioned causes.

When bacterial chest wall abscesses are unaccompanied by a history of known trauma, the possibility of a foreign body-related cause should be sought. Likewise, empyema associated with chest wall or sternal abscesses should prompt similar exploration. It is the author's opinion that primary pleural infection rarely extends through the parietal pleura and infects the thoracic wall integument. Rather, the converse situation is generally found, with extrapleural infection fistulating into the pleural space. Many foreign bodies are situated in the extrapleural tissues and are removable without thoracotomy.

DISORDERS OF THE PLEURA AND PLEURAL SPACE

Anatomy and Physiology

The pleura is a microscopic membrane of mesothelial origin.[43] Anatomically, it covers the surfaces of the rib cage, mediastinum, and lung. The mediastinum, chest wall, and diaphragm are covered by parietal pleura. The lung and its associated fissures are covered by visceral pleura. This extends to the hilum, where it is met by the reflections of mediastinal parietal pleura.[10]

The potential space between visceral and parietal pleura is referred to as the pleural space or cavity; it contains a few milliliters of fluid that lubricate the surface during respiratory motion.[44, 45] The fluid grossly resembles serum and has a protein content of approximately 1.5 grams per deciliter. Unlike humans, the majority of companion animals have a single contiguous pleural space that exists due to fenestrations of the mediastinum; thus pleural fluid freely communicates between right and left hemithoraces. Visceral and parietal pleura have a separate vascular supply. The visceral supply is mainly via the pulmonary artery; however, the bronchial arterial circulation plays a major role.[46] Pleural veins anastomose with bronchial veins at the hilum.

The parietal pleural blood supply is regional and courses from branches of intercostal circulation on the chest wall, from intercostal and pericardial origin in the mediastinum, and from the diaphragmatic vasculature along its surface. Venous drainage is mainly into the azygous and internal mammary venous complexes.

As with vascular supply, visceral and parietal pleura have separate lymphatics. In addition, there are trans-diaphragmatic lymphatics that directly connect the peritoneal and pleural spaces.[47, 48] The lymphatics of parietal pleura have stoma, which are apparently essential for the removal of particulate matter from the pleural space. These are not found in the visceral pleural lymphatics.

There exists a precarious balance between hydrostatic and oncotic forces within the pleura (Starling forces). Hydrostatic and oncotic pressures within the systemic circulation, pulmonary circulation, and the intrapleural space collectively produce a water gradient of approximately nine centimeters, which favors transudation of pleural fluid from parietal pleura into the pleural space. These same forces provide a gradient of approximately ten centimeters of water, favoring absorption of the fluid into the visceral pleura's vasculature.[49] The result of this is the continual net flow of fluid through the pleural space. This delicate balance can be interrupted by any disorder that alters oncotic pressure, systemic or pulmonary capillary pressure, lymphatic compliance, capillary permeability, or effective surface area.

History and Physical Findings

There are relatively few clinical signs exhibited by animals with thoracic disorders. These signs, which may occur acutely or develop insidiously over several days or weeks, are often alarming to the client and cause variable degrees of discomfort for the patient. In addition to the complete review of systems, it is important to obtain from the client a detailed description of the signs and their progression.

Clinical Manifestations of Pleural Effusion

The most common sign associated with pleural effusion is shortness of breath. Depending on the cause, some patients may have cough, fever, or the subjective finding of pleural pain (elicited by firm palpation of the intercostal spaces).

Frequently the degree of dyspnea does not directly correlate with the volume of pleural fluid. Concurrent pulmonary parenchymal disease, anemia, or congestive heart failure may play a major role in the clinical picture. Patients with even extremely large volumes of fluid may tolerate them with little dyspnea if they have accumulated chronically.

Cough is a variable finding. Cats infrequently have a

cough unless the condition is accompanied by small airway disease. Dogs may frequently cough due to bronchial compression by large effusions.

Fever is a finding not limited to patients with effusions of infectious etiology. Immunologic disorders, neoplasia, and trauma may be associated with episodic fever. Fever may be associated with large pleural effusions in dogs due to ineffective ventilation and heat exchange.

Patients with very large pleural effusions may have perceptible changes in thoracic cage conformation.[50] In the presence of unilateral effusions, the affected hemithorax may bulge palpably and produce an asymmetric appearance in the thorax. Intercostal muscles may be flat or convex on palpation, and there may be an absence of a palpable cardiac impulse.

Pleural effusions of any significant magnitude may be detected by thoracic percussion. Percussion of the chest has two major functions: to identify the normal anatomic boundaries of the thoracic and extrathoracic structures and to determine if there is aerated lung at appropriate sites. Because interpretation of percussed sound, as with breath sounds, is subjective, considerable practice is required to develop reliable percussion technique.

Percussion over a normal lung produces a low frequency vibration responsible for the resonant note obtained.[51] When underlying structures are dense, such as over the cardiac region, consolidated lung, pleural fluid, or other thoracic masses, a characteristic dulling of the vibration is noted. The character of the note obtained varies with the area of the chest examined, amount of subcuticular tissue, and depth of breathing or body posture. It is sufficient to characterize the sound as normal or dull. Hyperresonance has been reported with emphysema or pneumothorax, but this may be difficult to recognize.

Diagnosis

In pulmonary medicine, as in every medical discipline, the establishment of a precise diagnosis is of paramount importance. While this is not always possible in every patient, recommendations regarding treatment and prognosis should be based on the most precise morphologic and etiologic diagnosis obtained by reasonable diagnostic methods. Just as retrieval and identification of an infectious agent from the lung provides important diagnostic and therapeutic information, recognition of a degenerative, neoplastic, or immunologic process has prognostic and therapeutic implications.

DIAGNOSTIC APPROACH

Clinicians dealing with thoracic disorders have a variety of diagnostic techniques at their disposal. How and when each is employed depends on the clinician's knowledge of, and skill with, each technique, as well as his or her understanding of the patient and the disease process.

Diagnostic techniques can be divided into categories based upon their invasiveness and diagnostic yield; it is clearly preferable to use procedures with minimal invasiveness and high diagnostic yield. Unfortunately, in the field of thoracic medicine, few procedures possess both of these characteristics.

The first category consists of procedures that require minimal invasiveness, but usually do not produce a definitive diagnosis. While these may suggest a disease process, reliance on them as the only diagnostic studies may lead to serious misdiagnoses. These procedures include the history, physical examination, thoracic radiography, electrocardiography, hematologic evaluation, and biochemical and blood gas analysis.

The second category may be called procedures that require minimal invasiveness and may yield a definitive diagnosis when combined with procedures from the first group. Among these procedures are serologic tests, urine culture, blood culture, Gram stain, peripheral lymph node aspiration, and cytology.

The last category consists of procedures that are invasive and may place some patients at significant risk, but have the highest diagnostic yields. These procedures provide the most valuable information and in most instances carry fewer risks than thoracotomy. They are listed in increasing order of invasiveness: pulmonary scintigraphy (ventilation/perfusion scanning), transtracheal aspiration, thoracocentesis, laryngoscopy, bronchoscopy, bronchography, percutaneous pleural biopsy, fine needle aspiration of the lung, transbronchial lung biopsy, cardiac catheterization and angiography, cutting needle biopsy, mediastinoscopy, thoracoscopy, and open lung biopsy (Table 70–1).

The rate at which one proceeds from noninvasive procedures depends on the clinical situation. In the seriously ill patient, a definitive diagnosis should be obtained as rapidly as possible, and the early use of invasive procedures may be justified. The patient's clinical progress should dictate the techniques used; changes in the clinical condition should prompt appropriate changes in the diagnostic approach.

THORACIC RADIOGRAPHY

Thoracic radiography remains a major tool in the investigation of chest disease.[3] While there are a limited number of ways in which the lung, mediastinum, and pleura can react to injury (and produce radiographic patterns), the chest radiograph is invaluable when interpreted in light of other clinical information. Whenever possible, previous studies should be evaluated, as they may document the progression of the disorder and, in some cases, provide a normal study for comparison. While the attending clinician is usually best qualified to interpret these studies, it is useful to obtain the second opinion of a colleague or radiologist. Impartial objectivity and unfamiliarity with the patient and client may result in useful observations overlooked on initial evaluations.

IDENTIFICATION OF PLEURAL EFFUSION

The most important methods of recognizing a pleural effusion are physical examination and thoracic radiography. When a significant effusion is present within the pleural space, the separation of visceral pleura and air-filled lung from the parietal pleural surface causes diminished conduction of sound, resulting in a characteristic loss or muffling of auscultable breath sounds and dullness on percussion.[51] Careful examination with the patient in a standing position may allow definition of a

TABLE 70–1. ORGANISMS CULTURED FROM PLEURAL FLUID (LISTED IN ORDER OF APPARENT FREQUENCY)

Cats	Dogs
Bacteroides	Fusobacterium
Actinomyces	Actinomyces
Peptostreptococcus	Corynebacterium
Streptococcus	Streptococcus
Pasteurella	Bacteroides
Fusobacterium	Pasteurella
Mycoplasma	*E. coli*
	Klebsiella
	Peptostreptococcus
	Fungal agents

Order and organisms may vary by geographic location.

fluid level on the chest wall. The chest radiograph is the definitive study used to confirm the clinical diagnosis of pleural effusion and usually demonstrates small effusions not detectable on physical examination. The radiographic appearance of a pleural effusion is determined by the elastic recoil of the lung, volume of effusion, gravity, patient position, and patency of the mediastinum (unilateral or bilateral effusion).[52] Loculation of fluid may occur in empyema or chronic hemothorax due to pleural fibrosis and adhesions. Positional variations and horizontal beam radiographs can be useful in confirming such cases.[3] Both diagnostic ultrasound and fluoroscopy can also be used to locate loculated pockets of pleural fluid, although fluoroscopy is limited by its inability to differentiate between fluid, masses, and thickened pleura.

PLEURAL BIOPSY

Biopsy of the pleura can be accomplished either as an open procedure at thoracotomy or less invasively with closed techniques using a biopsy needle. Pleural biopsy is a particularly useful means of diagnosing pleural neoplasia and granulomatous disorders resulting in pleural effusion.[53] As the technique yields tissue samples, the histopathologic anatomy is preserved, often yielding a diagnosis where cytopathologic examination has been negative or equivocal. As such, biopsy is most frequently performed on pleural effusions of unknown etiology when thoracocentesis and cytopathologic studies have been negative. Contraindications for closed needle pleural biopsy are few: bleeding disorders, significant pulmonary insufficiency, pyoderma or cellulitis over biopsy site, and empyema.

While many biopsy needles have been used in the past, the two most frequently used instruments are the Abrams and Cope pleural biopsy needles.[54–59] While selection of either instrument largely depends on personal preference, the four-part Cope needle has the added benefit of allowing thoracocentesis and procurement of several biopsy samples without withdrawing the instrument from the patient between samples (Figure 70–5).

Regardless of the technique or needle used, the approach is similar. The chosen site is surgically prepared and cutaneous and pleural anesthesia achieved with two per cent lidocaine. A small stab wound is made along the caudal rib margin to avoid the intercostal vessel. Pleural fluid should not be removed in any volume prior to the biopsy unless the patient is sufficiently dyspneic to warrant such. Removal of pleural fluid precludes the use of pleural biopsy, as the fluid serves to separate visceral and parietal surfaces. Pleural drainage should be undertaken after a number of biopsies are taken. As pleural changes may be diffuse, multiple biopsy sites are frequently used; this should increase the yield of the procedure. If these multiple samples are not diagnostic, rebiopsy does not have a significantly higher yield unless new radiographic findings suggest a new localized lesion in a previously unbiopsied site.[60] When pleural neoplasia is suspected, the ventral one-third of the chest appears to be of the highest yield, as metastatic lesions are more frequently located ventrally and spread dorsally. As would be anticipated, the more diffuse the process, the greater the biopsy yield.

The complications of closed pleural needle biopsy requiring therapy are infrequently encountered when patient selection is proper and the procedure is accomplished by a trained individual.[61] Possible complications include hemothorax, pneumothorax or subcuticular emphysema, empyema, and needle track implantation of neoplasms. Significant iatrogenic pneumothorax or hemothorax that are symptomatic require prompt tube thoracostomy and water seal drainage. Subcutaneous air

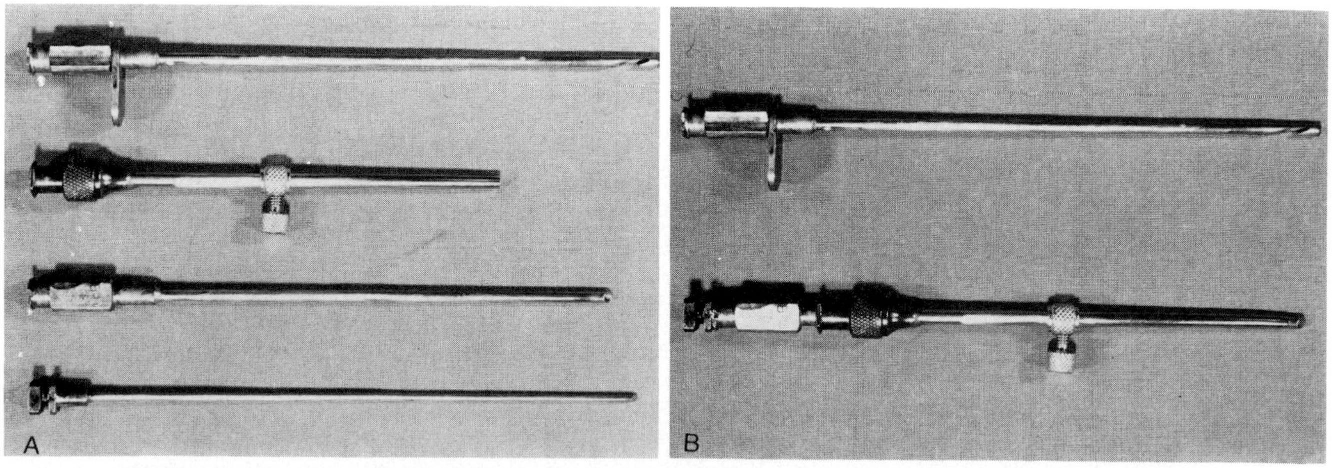

FIGURE 70–5. *A*, Cope pleural biopsy needle separated into component parts. *B*, Cope needle assembled with internal trocar. Once inserted in the pleural space, the trocar is removed and the hooked biopsy needle is inserted.

or fluid accumulation may require pressure dressings for a short period following biopsy.

OPEN BIOPSY

Diagnostic thoracotomy and biopsy under direct visualization should be used as a last resort. Open biopsy obviously carries the risks of general anesthesia and surgery. When needle biopsy and less invasive means have not suggested a diagnosis, open biopsy and exploration may not always identify the cause of the pleural effusion. Those patients that are seen for open biopsy are those with the most elusive disorders.

THORACOSCOPY

Direct examination of the pleural space by thoracoscopy and biopsy of the pleura or other lesions may be advisable when laboratory analysis of pleural fluid and percutaneous pleural biopsy have failed to provide a diagnosis.[53] Surgical exploration and postmortem examination in such cases often show discrete metastases or granulomas that were missed by percutaneous random biopsy. In addition, some primary pleural tumors and metastatic sarcomas can produce effusion without exfoliating large numbers of neoplastic cells, resulting in false-negative findings on cytologic examination of pleural fluid. The primary indication for thoracoscopy over thoracotomy is the debilitated or elderly patient in which thoracotomy poses an unacceptable risk and less invasive procedures have failed to provide a diagnosis.

Several fiberoptic instruments designed specifically for thoracoscopy, and others designed for arthroscopy or bronchoscopy, work satisfactorily.[62, 61] The author has used both the Storz arthroscopic and Olympus bronchoscope with acceptable results. The most appropriate instruments are the rigid thoracoscopes (Storz, Dyonics, Wolf) that provide a fiberoptic tube in biopsy channel (Figure 70–6).

The procedure is performed using general anesthesia or deep narcotic sedation and local anesthesia. If a large effusion is present, it should be drained prior to this examination. With the patient in lateral recumbency, a cannula is inserted into the pleural space and a partial pneumothorax is induced to cause retraction of lung lobes so that pleural surfaces can be examined. Most patients tolerate partial pneumothorax well, and the author has not experienced significant hypoxemia in patients receiving supplemental oxygen. The thoracoscope is introduced through a small intercostal stab incision after blunt separation of the intercostal muscles with a small forceps. The pleural space is examined with the aid of suction and limited rotation of the thorax. Biopsy of lesions on the parietal pleural surface poses little risk other than hemorrhage. Biopsy of visceral pleural lesions risks pleural laceration and further pneumothorax. Visualization of the mediastinum is difficult, and the author's attempts at hilar or heart base examination have been disappointing.

DIAGNOSTIC THORACOCENTESIS

Thoracocentesis should be performed on all patients with a pleural effusion not previously examined. Since all pleural fluids (blood, exudates, and transudates) are radiographically indistinguishable, thoracocentesis is essential for establishing a definitive diagnosis. In addition, removal of fluid improves radiographic visualization of lung and pleura, as well as providing relief from associated dyspnea. A relative contraindication for thoracocentesis is the presence of a bleeding disorder caused by anticoagulation, severe thrombocytopenia, or a heritable coagulopathy. As with all diagnostic procedures, the risks of thoracocentesis versus its benefits must be evaluated for each patient's condition.

In all but the most uncooperative patients, the procedure is accomplished without sedation. There are several methods of thoracocentesis, all of which are acceptable, depending on the clinician's preference and experience with each technique. The required equipment is very simple and is summarized in Figure 70–7. In most cases, the patient is placed in standing or comfortable sitting positions. Lateral recumbency is usually unsatisfactory for retrieval of samples in patients with small or moderate effusions unless a chest tube is being inserted. Occasionally samples are difficult to obtain in the upright position in patients with a small effusion. In such cases, a sample can often be obtained by using a ventral approach with the patient positioned in lateral recumbency and the thorax exposed in a space between two tables; this technique is rarely necessary.

Two per cent lidocaine is used for regional anesthesia prior to the procedure. The skin and subcuticular tissues over the seventh or eighth intercostal space at or just

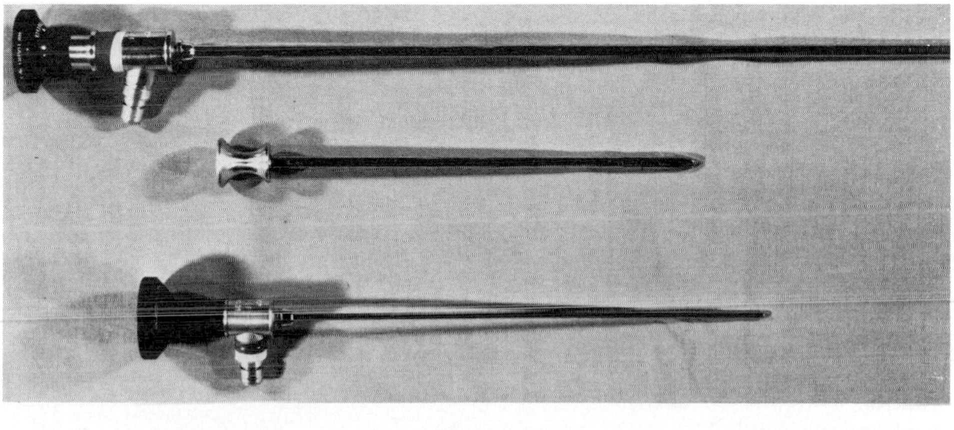

FIGURE 70–6. Rigid fiberoptic instruments used for thoracoscopy. The larger of the two is 5 mm × 30 cm, and the smaller, 2.5 mm × 18 cm. The insertion trocar is pictured in the middle.

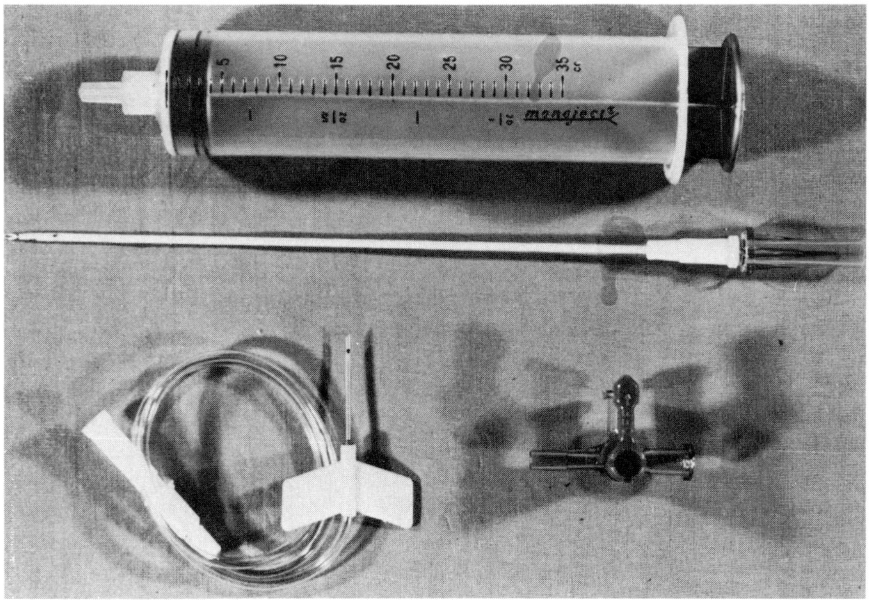

FIGURE 70–7. Equipment for thoracocentesis. Commercially available presterilized thoracocentesis trays containing catheters, stopcock, sampling vials, and skin preparation materials are available (not shown). The components most frequently used for thoracocentesis are pictured.

above the costochondral junction is infiltrated with a 25-gauge needle to the depth of one-half to one centimeter. A 22-gauge needle is then inserted and small injections are made as the needle is advanced through the intercostal muscles toward the pleural space. This technique provides adequate anesthesia of the parietal pleura, which is often quite sensitive when penetrated by even small-bore needles. The chosen device with syringe attached is inserted through the surgically prepared and anesthetized intercostal space, taking care to avoid the intercostal artery located just caudal to each rib. Slight suction is applied as the tip penetrates the parietal pleura, and samples are withdrawn for bacterial culture, cytologic evaluation, and biochemical or serologic analysis, when indicated. If fluid is not readily aspirated, the needle or catheter should be withdrawn and repositioned. There is no benefit to increased negative syringe pressure, which tends to suck lung or pleura over the needle, causing unnecessary trauma and obstruction of flow. Following sampling or complete drainage, the device is withdrawn and pressure is applied over the puncture site for a few moments. A dressing or pressure bandage is usually not required. It is important to obtain both aerobic and anaerobic cultures in cytologically infected fluids. Many empyemas in the dog and cat have an anaerobic component. Minimal fluid analysis should include determination of pH, specific gravity, protein concentration, packed cell volume, total white count, differential white cell count, and as previously mentioned, culture and cytologic evaluation.

THERAPEUTIC THORACOCENTESIS

Thoracocentesis as a therapeutic procedure is frequently necessary when a large pleural effusion causes lung compression and hypoventilation. Following removal of large pleural effusions, dyspnea is usually markedly reduced. This is accomplished by two means: the lungs reexpand and the thoracic musculature subsequently operates on a more effective point on its length tension curve.[65] Even modest effusions may need to be removed when accompanied by underlying pulmonary or pulmonary vascular disease. Prior to any attempt at needle aspiration or tube thoracostomy, chest radiographs should be obtained to confirm the diagnosis of effusion and evaluate its location and potential loculation.

Whenever infected fluids are present (e.g., empyema) tube thoracostomy is mandatory and should be performed as the primary means of drainage.[66] Likewise, when large sterile effusions are present in canine patients, a chest tube rather than needle aspiration should be used. The most effective chest tubes are those thoracic catheters manufactured for this purpose. Most Foley and nonballoon-type urinary catheters are inappropriate due to their small lumen and predilection to collapse or obstruct. Most chest tubes have depth markers that are radiopaque and have both end and side ports to facilitate drainage. The size catheter selected is governed by the width of the patient's intercostal space and viscosity of pleural fluid (approximately 10 to 16 French in cats and 16 to 32 French in dogs). Insertion of large-bore chest tubes appears to be best facilitated by trocarization. Many manufacturers provide presterilized chest tubes with their own internal trocars. While the incidence of iatrogenic laceration of lung, mediastinum, or heart appears negligible with these instruments, care must always be taken when using this method of tube thoracostomy.

At the insertion site, a one-half to one cm skin incision is made and the trocar catheter advanced subcutaneously one to three intercostal spaces with a rotary motion. To avoid overzealous insertion, the trocar is gripped with the right hand, and the left hand grasps the tip one to two cm above the skin to act as a guard and prevent deep insertion. Again with a twisting motion, the tube is inserted through the intercostal muscles; when resistance abruptly decreases, the trocar tip is withdrawn and the tube inserted to the desired position.

The tube is secured to the chest wall by means of a

series of butterfly bandages to prevent inadvertent dislodgement. A single purse-string suture is placed at the site of entry. Following insertion, the tube is attached to an underwater drainage unit; water seal drainage creates a constant negative intrapleural pressure in favor of drainage at 10 to 20 cm of water. Higher pressures do not provide greater drainage, but rather serve to obstruct the chest tube ports.

While chest drainage can be satisfactorily accomplished with a three-chamber bottle system, the newer disposable plastic systems are safer and offer more monitoring features. They are helpful in providing early patient ambulation, as they are easily portable and maintain negative pleural pressures.

The possible complications of needle drainage or tube thoracostomy include hemorrhage, pneumothorax, pulmonary edema, bradycardia, and laceration of abdominal or thoracic viscera. Pneumothorax may result from puncture or laceration of visceral pleura and lung or leakage of air into the chest through the aspirating device. Significant pneumothorax is rare if the centesis is performed carefully with appropriate equipment; thoracic radiographs are not routinely obtained following thoracocentesis for evaluation of pneumothorax if clinical signs are not observed.

Bleeding is also an uncommon complication in patients with normal hemostasis. Bleeding from the puncture wound usually indicates puncture of an intercostal vessel and is easily controlled with slight digital pressure. Pleural bleeding is usually the result of a vascularized neoplasm, pulmonary laceration, or penetration of inflamed and hypervascular pleural surfaces. Such bleeding is self-limiting in most cases.

Air embolism may theoretically be induced. This presumably occurs if the visceral pleura is punctured, thus lacerating superficial vessels, allowing alveolar air to enter the systemic circulation. Pleural shock, i.e., bradycardia and hypotension, may occur with pleural puncture, but occurs more frequently when large volumes of pleural fluid are rapidly withdrawn. This is presumably an exaggerated vagal response and can be immediately reversed with atropine and volume expansion if necessary.[67] This phenomenon would appear to occur most frequently in feline patients with a cardiogenic cause for their effusion.

Reexpansion pulmonary edema may occur after rapid removal of large volumes of pleural fluid.[68] In contrast to the same phenomenon in humans, the edema appears rapidly following the expansion and appears to provoke only mild clinical signs.[69] The etiology is speculative and includes rapid shifts in pulmonary circulation, derangement of surfactant function, and increases in lung permeability. Animal models have been used to study this phenomenon and suggest that large volumes of pleural fluid are required over several days to provoke reexpansion edema.[70, 71]

MEDIASTINOSCOPY

Mediastinoscopy is a surgical procedure used for the diagnosis of cranial mediastinal disorders when mass lesions have been detected by physical examination and thoracic radiography. The procedure allows mediastinal access and visualization without thoracotomy. It can provide valuable information in the diagnosis of disorders of the mediastinal lymphatic chain, such as lymphoma, infectious or granulomatous disorders, and other primary or metastatic neoplasms. Before mediastinoscopy is considered, the peripheral lymph nodes should be carefully examined in case a simple superficial lymph node aspirate or biopsy may provide a diagnosis.

The procedure is performed using general anesthesia with the patient positioned in dorsal recumbency. A midline incision is made at the thoracic inlet between the manubrium and the ventral surface of the trachea. Blunt dissection is carried along fascial planes caudally into the mediastinum. A Carlens or similar mediastinoscope is introduced and direct visualization accomplished. The cranial lymph nodes can be visualized by this procedure, whereas hilar mass lesions can only be seen if they bulge forward into the cranial mediastinum. Care must be taken to avoid injury to the major vascular structures in this region; prior to manipulation or biopsy, fine-needle aspiration should be performed to prevent accidental biopsy of the great vessels.

The author has had limited experience with mediastinoscopy. He has been successful in obtaining tissue and avoiding thoracotomy in several patients where other techniques failed to yield a precise anatomic diagnosis. For those considering this procedure, it is advisable to enlist the aid of an interested surgeon who can learn the technique and gain the necessary experience and proficiency to perform it safely and reliably.

The contraindications for mediastinoscopy include previous mediastinal surgery that has obliterated fascial planes, bleeding disorders, and vena caval syndrome with venous congestion and edema. Potential complications include pneumothorax, bleeding, and infection.

Disorders Associated with Pleural Effusion

PLEURAL EFFUSION DUE TO CONGESTIVE HEART FAILURE

While pure right-sided heart failure or biventricular failure represents a major cause of pleural effusion, the clinician should remain vigilant for concurrent disorders masquerading as heart failure. Malignancy, parapneumonic effusion, and pulmonary embolism or thrombosis may all coexist with known heart disease, particularly in older patients.

In both canine and feline patients, biventricular failure may produce pleural effusion of significant magnitude. While left ventricular failure is capable of producing effusions, they tend not to be large in volume. In the experimental canine model, it has been shown that systemic venous hypertension produces more pleural fluid than does pulmonary venous hypertension.[72]

Patients with heart failure almost invariably have significant physical findings: distended neck veins, gallop rhythms, splitting of heart sounds, and pathologic murmurs. The heart is almost invariably enlarged on routine radiographs and echocardiographic evaluation reveals significant anatomic or functional abnormalities.

The pleural effusion of congestive heart failure is a

transudate and typically is straw-colored, although occasionally bloody or pseudochylous. The specific gravity usually is 1.013 or less with a protein below 3 gm/dl.[73] Under the majority of circumstances, diagnostic thoracocentesis is unnecessary unless concurrent illness is questioned. Therapeutic pleural drainage is not unusual in that it allows the most rapid resolution of severe dyspnea associated with large effusions.

Appropriate therapy for the underlying heart disease should result in medical management of the effusion. In those patients with recurrent effusions unresponsive to management, pleurodesis may be considered, but only as a last resort and after reevaluation and consultation.

NEOPLASTIC PLEURAL EFFUSION

The majority of pleural tumors are metastatic in origin; primary pleural tumors are uncommon.[35] While pleural spread of neoplasia is frequently accompanied by effusion, this is not always the case.

It appears in humans that the mechanism most frequently evoked in the production of malignant effusion is the obstruction of pleural lymphatics.[74, 75] Obstruction of major mediastinal nodes may also play a major role, or less frequently, obstruction of the thoracic duct. There are numerous secondary mechanisms that may produce effusions of various magnitudes: increase in oncotic pleural pressure if the malignancy deposits proteinaceous debris in the pleural space; exudation due to mechanical pleural irritation; increase in vascular permeability due to local release of prostaglandins or complement; parapneumonic effusion secondary to atelectasis due to airway obstruction or infection; pericarditis with hemodynamic sequelae; and obstruction of major veins by compression, such as superior vena caval syndrome.[76] The volume of pleural fluid present is dependent upon several factors: the stage at which diagnosis is made, type of neoplasia, and the patency of the mediastinum. The latter is particularly important, as neoplastic mediastinitis may limit the effusion to one hemithorax. Characteristically, the effusion rapidly returns after evacuation no matter what the mechanism of production, unless some intervention is instituted to augment pleural dynamics, i.e., chemotherapy, radiation, or pleurodesis.

Cytopathologic examination of sediment from suspected malignant effusions is a necessity but is by no means invariably positive. While there are no statistics available to confirm or deny the author's impression, it appears that only 40 to 50 per cent of confirmed neoplasia yields positive pleural fluid cytology. There are patients in which serial examination of samples are additive; however, as a rule, unless the method of collection is changed, e.g., needle drainage of loculated pockets or tube drainage with concentration of large volumes of pleural fluid, the yield will not increase. Yield is often highest with initial thoracocentesis when multiple techniques are used, such as the combination of pleural biopsy, cell filtration, and cell block preparations. Cytologic examination rarely identifies the primary anatomic origin of the tumor, but may be suggestive.

Frequently, pleural fluids are not positive when infiltrative tumors have obstructed lymphatic flow (except for lymphoma). Definitive diagnosis is frequently not possible even for the most talented cytopathologists, in that normal or stimulated mesothelial cells, with light microscopy, may be difficult to evaluate. Atypia, nuclear variation, high mitotic index, and acinar formation may be frequent findings with any process that irritates the pleura.

The presence of pleural involvement and neoplastic cells in any patient with neoplasia other than lymphoma represents metastasis, and hence a poor prognosis and a short mean survival time. This appears to be true even for those patients that are thought to be asymptomatic for their thoracic spread. Again, the presence of pleural effusion cannot be directly equated to pleural spread of a tumor; while this is frequently the case, there are those patients with localized neoplasia whose effusion is secondary to lymphatic obstruction, pulmonary vascular disease, or secondary sequelae such as lung torsion. As such, the presence of effusion is not an absolute indication of inoperability.

The treatment of neoplastic pleural effusion depends on multiple factors, i.e., type of neoplasia, anatomic involvement, anticipated prognosis, and clinical signs present. In a patient with advanced disease and a poor short-term prognosis, therapeutic thoracocentesis may be the only reasonable means of providing palliative care. Systemic chemotherapy is suggested in patients with potentially responsive neoplasia. With lymphoma or mammary carcinoma, chemotherapy alone may resolve the effusion without invasive therapy.[77] Pleurodesis is the most frequently used treatment for neoplastic effusions, the objective being to obliterate the pleural space and thus eliminate a potential space in which the fluid can accumulate.[78, 79] The indication for pleurodesis is a patient whose signs of dyspnea are related solely to the presence of effusion and recur following thoracocentesis and re-accumulation. Several drugs have been effective, including bleomycin talc, tetracycline, quinacrine, and nitrogen mustard.[79–83] The long-term relief provided by pleurodesis is variable.

As quantification of effectiveness is impossible, the subjective clinical impression of improved pulmonary function and decrease in dyspnea is considered evidence of a successful procedure. The successful management of these effusions is at best palliative as the underlying malignancy is virtually never curable. The goal of therapy is to improve the length and quality of life.

It would appear that all the previously mentioned drugs are effective to one degree or another. There is a distinct lack of evidence to suggest that one is more appropriate than another in veterinary patients. At this time, the author's experience is largely limited to the use of tetracycline as a sclerosing agent.

Pleurodesis with tetracycline is accomplished by closed-tube thoracostomy and water seal drainage of the pleural space. Complete drainage appears to be necessary for optimal effect; to assess effectiveness of drainage, a chest film is obtained 12 to 24 hours following chest tube placement. If complete drainage has been accomplished, tetracycline (100 to 250 mg in cats and 500 mg to 1 gm in dogs) is injected into the chest tube in 20 to 60 ml of saline. The chest tube is clamped and drainage interrupted for 6 hours, during which time the patient is turned every 30 minutes to allow the fluid to contact all pleural surfaces. The tube is unclamped and water seal suction resumed for 24 to 72 hours, or until drainage diminishes to 15 to 20 ml per day in cats or 100 to 150 ml per day in dogs. Many patients appear anxious or in overt pain while tetracycline is being instilled. It is recommended that patients be medicated with narcotics prior to administration. While there have been few experienced acute reactions to the use of intrapleural tetracycline, the most common side effects are apparent pain, fever, vomition, and rarely, hypotension.

In the moribund patient that is in the terminal stages of an advanced cancer, closed drainage is the most reasonable means of reducing dyspnea. While simple thoracocentesis is useful, more complete drainage and better lung re-expansion is possible by closed-tube thoracostomy and short-term water seal drainage. Repeated attempts at needle aspiration frequently cause more patient discomfort and increase the risk of pneumothorax.

PLEURAL EFFUSIONS ASSOCIATED WITH PULMONARY INFECTION/PARAPNEUMONIC EFFUSION

Patients with pneumonia may experience pleural effusions secondary to their infection in the absence of overt empyema.[3] Parapneumonic effusions, while sterile inflammatory exudates, are grossly serous or hemorrhagic rather than purulent. The effusion resolves spontaneously with appropriate treatment of the pulmonary infection.

The frequency of associated effusion depends on the associated causative microorganism. While all bacterial pneumonias are capable of producing parapneumonic effusion, the author has observed that *Klebsiella* and streptococcal infections appear to have the highest incidence.

EMPYEMA

Pyothorax, or empyema, is the accumulation of infected material and fluid within the pleural space. Causative agents may reach the pleural space by three routes: as a result of systemic sepsis, infection reaches the pleura by either lymphatics or blood; as a result of spread from an adjacent structure (pneumonia with bronchopleural communication and parapneumonic spread, rupture of the esophagus, mediastinitis, or subphrenic infection); by direct introduction of organisms as a result of penetrating trauma, foreign bodies, thoracocentesis, or surgery. Aberrations of all the normal forces that keep the pleural space free of fluid probably play a role in the accumulation of large effusions encountered in this disorder.[84] Inflammation produces an increase in regional blood flow, resulting in capillary hypertension. Increased capillary permeability results in colloid flux toward the pleural space, causing a rise in pleural oncotic pressure. With loss of favorable oncotic gradient, fluid removal must be maintained by regional lymphatics, the effectiveness of which may be compromised by fibrosis or obstruction with cellular and infectious debris. The clinical recognition of empyema begins with the detection of physical findings compatible with loss of lung volume and is confirmed by observation of pleural effusion on chest radiographs. Laboratory examination of the effusion is the only definitive means of making the diagnosis; thus, thoracocentesis is required. Presence of organisms on gram or acid-fast stains, and their subsequent growth in culture media, are an absolute requirement for both diagnosis and definitive therapy.

Clinical Presentation. Fever, anorexia, weight loss, and shortness of breath are the chief signs associated with empyema. An infectious prodrome may have been noted days to weeks prior to the owner seeking medical attention. The subacute or acute nature of the process may be marked by a prior history of surgery, hospitalization for a seemingly unrelated illness, or having been away from home for several days.

Radiographic Findings. In most cases, a moderate-to-large pleural effusion is present, obscuring the cardiac silhouette and a large portion of the pulmonary and pleural detail.

In most cases, the effusions are bilateral; however, in a significant number the exudate is unilateral because of pleural and mediastinal involvement. Although large amounts of free pleural gas are rarely present, pneumohydrothorax may be a finding when standing or horizontal beam lateral views are obtained in patients with anaerobic infections or necrotizing pneumonia. Gas may be retrieved following tube thoracostomy. On immediate post-drainage films, many patients have pulmonary infiltrates or identifiable consolidation, most frequently involving the left cranial lobes in both feline and canine patients.[66] Most of these findings are absent on subsequent evaluations.

Microbiology. The gram stain is the most important tool for rapid assessment of microorganisms in pleural fluid. Specimens collected by transtracheal aspiration may also be of value in early assessment.

Both dogs and cats with empyema have a high incidence of anaerobic infection, either as a sole pathogen or in combination with aerobic organisms. For this reason, it is of extreme importance to submit both aerobic and anaerobic cultures.[85] Anaerobes are capable of creating a fetid odor; this is mainly due to the volatile amines, short-chain fatty acids, and organic acids they produce. The absence of a fetid smell, however, does not rule out the presence of anaerobes. The morphology of anaerobes as seen on gram stains may set them apart from aerobic organisms.

The lists of causative organisms overlap in the two species. In general, feline patients tend to have a higher incidence of pure anaerobic infection and fewer enteric infections.

Therapy. Tube thoracostomy should be performed as soon as the diagnosis is made.[84] Chest tube drainage is best accomplished by continuous water seal suction at approximately 20 cm. Only a small number of patients require bilateral chest tube placement as a result of persistent loculation of fluid or a complete mediastinum, which prevents adequate evacuation of both hemithoraces with a single chest tube. The use of continuous water seal suction is ideal. It is the key to complete and rapid removal of infected pleural exudate. Tube thoracostomy without continuous water seal drainage is a less than ideal means of pleural drainage. Continuous removal facilitates a more complete and rapid resolution of the empyema pocket. As is true of treatment of any abscessed cavity, medical resolution cannot take place without complete drainage of the infected material. Patients will not improve clinically until effective drainage is established.

After volume restoration, tube thoracostomy is performed without general anesthesia. In those patients that appear anxious or uncooperative, low-dose narcotic sedation prior to the procedure may be used. Extreme caution must be used in sedating these patients; respiratory reserve is usually minimal, and any decrease in respiratory effort or drive as the result of sedation may prove fatal.

Cytologic examination of pleural fluid should be undertaken frequently to assess the effectiveness of antimicrobial therapy. Gram stains may be evaluated every 48 hours throughout the course of drainage. Gram stains frequently fail to reveal any bacteria after two to three days. Serial cultures are obtained when patients continue to produce an infected effusion despite antimicrobial therapy, and when a change is noted in organism morphology on gram stain. In a few cases, an organism may be obtained on subsequent culture that was not isolated at the time of primary bacteriologic workup.

In most patients, therapy should be instituted with moderately high doses of parenteral synthetic penicillin. An oral agent may be substituted as the clinical condition improves. Duration of treatment depends chiefly on clinical impression and response to therapy. The author arbitrarily uses three months of oral therapy after complete tube drainage.

Penicillin remains the drug of choice for most forms of anaerobic pleural pulmonary infection.[86] *Bacteroides fragilis* is present in approximately 15 per cent of the feline isolates and in a smaller percentage of canine patients. *Bacteroides fragilis* has generally been shown to be penicillin-resistant *in vitro*; for this reason, either chloramphenicol or clindamycin is employed when it is isolated.[86]

In community-acquired infection, there is a high probability that the causative organisms will be sensitive to ampicillin. As such, unless hospital-acquired infection is known to exist or the gram stain suggests otherwise, patients should be started on a synthetic penicillin. For canine patients, the author has employed ampicillin, 1 gm every 4 hours for the first 48 hours, then every 6 hours for the remainder of the first week. At discharge, the dosage is decreased to every 8 hours. Feline patients are treated with an average dose of 250 mg on the same schedule.

Hospital-acquired infection is less predictable and, under most circumstances, should be treated with a single agent. While cultures are pending, treatment with a combination of a cephalosporin and aminoglycoside is suggested.

Discussion. The established diagnosis of empyema constitutes a medical emergency and should be treated without delay. Tube thoracostomy should be performed to achieve effective drainage of infected material. Chest tube size should be governed by the size of the intercostal space; large-bore chest tubes are more effective in draining viscous exudates. This procedure is associated with a low rate of complications, none of which has proven fatal in the author's experience.

Neither proteolytic enzymes nor pleural space lavage need be used, as excellent results in both drainage and pleural space sterilization have been obtained without their use. There is no convincing evidence that enzymes adequately lyse established fibrin plaque. They may be of use in maintaining patency of small chest tubes; however, this problem is alleviated by the use of the largest possible tube and frequent "stripping" of the water seal tubing.

Empyema in the immunologically competent patient, regardless of the cause, appears to be a readily treatable disease if treated early and vigorously, as described above. Previous case reviews show a mortality rate of 40 to 80 per cent when therapy consists of thoracocentesis and antibiotic therapy alone. If allowed to persist untreated or if treated only with antibiotic therapy, the disorder may progress to the chronic stage. The consequences of improper or late management are costly and often result in pulmonary dysfunction and limitation if the patient survives. It is the author's belief that thoracocentesis or tube thoracostomy without continuous water seal drainage seldom, if ever, should be employed as the sole means of pleural space evacuation. Successful treatment requires prompt and thorough removal of infected material from the pleural space, the most satisfactory means being tube thoracostomy with continuous water seal drainage and long-term antibiotic therapy. Such intervention should yield a good to excellent prognosis.

AUTOIMMUNE DISORDERS ASSOCIATED WITH PLEURAL EFFUSION

Many autoimmune disorders may be associated with the presence of a pleural effusion. In veterinary patients the volumes tend to be small, often just large enough to be radiographically observable (Figure 70–8). Among the disorders producing effusion are systemic lupus erythematosus, rheumatoid arthritis, idiopathic thrombocytopenia, and autoimmune hemolytic anemia. There are those disorders with an immunologic basis in which effusions are not clearly caused directly by the disorder. Among these disorders are angiitis and granulomatosis, and often such poorly defined entities as Wegener's granulomatosis. Unlike systemic lupus erythematosus and rheumatoid arthritis, the effusions of these patients may be large and responsible for significant clinical signs.

It is unknown how many patients with systemic lupus erythematosus have effusion as a manifestation of their disease. The volume of the effusion is usually small and there is often some question as to the etiology of the effusion, as this patient population may have other systemic complications of their immunologic disorder. Only a small number of canine patients have undergone thoracocentesis. The effusion is usually an inflammatory exudate, although it may occasionally be a transudate, particularly in those patients that are volume overloaded, either iatrogenically or due to concurrent renal

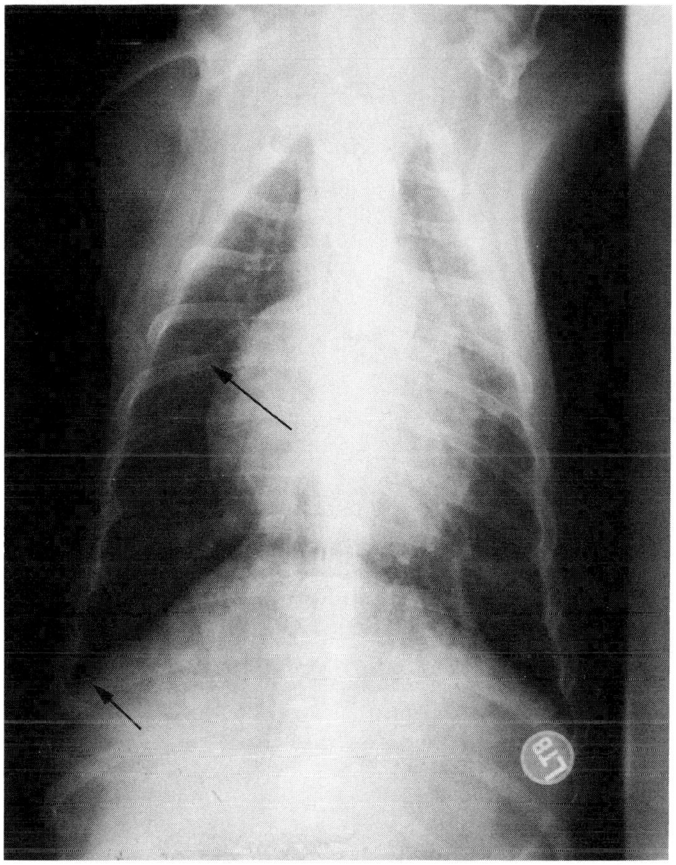

FIGURE 70–8. A six-year-old Labrador retriever with systemic lupus erythematosus. The arrows point out the small pleural effusion, a pleural fissure line is present, and there is blunting of the costophrenic angle. Thoracocentesis yielded a sterile exudate. Treatment of this patient's immunopathy with a corticosteroid resolved the effusion.

failure. The cell population is variable, but usually contains both lymphocytes and polymorphonuclear cells. One of the potential benefits of cytopathologic examination of these fluids may be the early detection of lupus erythematosus cells, which may be absent in the blood. Likewise, some patients serologically negative for antinuclear antibody in serum may have strongly positive titers in pleural fluid.

Pleural effusion may be present in patients with both rheumatoid arthritis and serologically negative, immunologically based polyarthritis. Unlike systemic lupus erythematosus, when pleural effusion is present there is almost invariably significant interstitial pulmonary disease present. As with systemic lupus erythematosus, these disorders typically yield small accumulations of pleural fluid and are probably systemic manifestations of the joint disease.

PLEURAL EFFUSIONS ASSOCIATED WITH HEPATIC DISORDERS

Pleural effusion may be seen in patients with hepatic cirrhosis; almost invariably there is associated ascites.[87] The effusions are transudates and may be hemorrhagic. Several factors probably play a role in the production of these effusions: systemic venous hypertension, hypoproteinemia, and an increase in lymphatic pressure and volume. Direct lymphatic or anatomic communication between the diaphragm and pleural space may play a role in some patients' effusions.[88–90]

The volume of effusion may be large and cause significant dyspnea. The fluid is a transudate with less than 3 gm/dl protein. Thoracocentesis is frequently necessary to palliate dyspnea; however, if possible, only enough fluid should be removed to make the patient comfortable. Chronic therapy revolves around proper alimentation to increase plasma protein concentrations, low sodium diets, and the use of diuretics. In the patient with large volumes of fluid that actually reaccumulate, tube thoracostomy may be advisable; in such patients it is important to frequently monitor central venous pressure, as hypovolemia may be induced by evacuation of large volumes of pleural and/or peritoneal fluid.

PLEURAL EFFUSION ASSOCIATED WITH PANCREATITIS

Pleural effusion may be associated with acute fulminant pancreatitis. It usually is small and self-limiting, with no specific treatment necessary.[91] Patients with pronounced dyspnea usually have pulmonary edema as the cause rather than a large volume of pleural effusion.

The pathogenesis of the effusion associated with pancreatitis is not specifically known and may represent multiple etiologies.[97] It is known that the subpleural and subperitoneal lymphatics communicate and are capable of transporting both particulate matter and fluids from the abdomen to the pleural space. It has been shown that pancreatic enzymes can likewise be transported in peritoneal fluid to the pleural space via the same lymphatics.[93, 94] In addition, lipase is capable of producing chemical inflammation, which may increase the lymphatics' permeability and hence increase the net flux of fluid from the peritoneum toward the pleural space.

The pleural fluid is typically an exudate that frequently has a high white cell count. Rarely, the fluid is a transudate or chylous. While not invariably the case, a high pleural fluid lipase is frequently present and exceeds that of the serum. This may be markedly exaggerated in patients with acute pancreatitis. This is not a pathognomonic finding, as patients with parapneumonic effusion, chylothorax, and effusion secondary to abdominal carcinomas may increase lipase activity over that of the serum, particularly with impairment of renal function.

INFREQUENT CAUSES OF PLEURAL EFFUSION

Abdominal Surgery. Major abdominal procedures may be followed by pleural effusions of various magnitudes, usually small. Subphrenic inflammation associated with gastric, hepatic, or duodenal procedures may increase transdiaphragmatic lymphatic flow. The acute appearance of small postoperative pleural effusion usually is not clinically relevant, and is self-limiting; however, it should be examined to rule out infection or concomitant pleural or pulmonary illness.

Esophageal Rupture. While frank empyema may be the end result of esophageal perforation, the acute consequences may be a sterile pleural effusion.[95, 96] If the effusion is secondary to mediastinitis (associated with initial stages of rupture), esophageal secretions and bacteria are contained within the mediastinal pleura. The encapsulated abscess may be responsible for a modest volume of effusion. Frank esophageal secretions with saliva may be present with esophageal-pleural fistulas (see Figure 70–9).

Diagnostic Procedures. Small pleural effusions may be recognized following a number of invasive diagnostic procedures. Transthoracic liver biopsy, pleural needle biopsy (in the absence of pleural effusion), mediastinoscopy, thoracoscopy, and rarely, percutaneous kidney biopsy may be associated with pleural irritation via trauma or extravasation of iodinated contrast, resulting in pleural effusion. Frank hemorrhage may occasionally be the cause of effusion.

Glomerulonephritis. Patients with glomerulonephritis may develop effusions for numerous reasons, among them hypoproteinemia and decreased oncotic pressure, pulmonary embolus or thrombosis, or hypertension and congestive heart failure.[97] The effusion is a transudate; patients with hypoproteinemia usually have accompanying ascites. In these patients, the pleural effusion may be very large.

Pyometra and Postpartum Status. These effusions are small and the etiology is unknown. They are usually recognized on routine radiographs taken to evaluate the underlying event. They resolve spontaneously and require no intervention.

Pulmonary Thrombosis or Embolism. The pleural effusions associated with pulmonary vascular obstruction are usually small, and their magnitude appears to be related to the size of the associated pulmonary infiltrates.[91] The effusions may be exudative or transudative. The white cell counts are typically low, but the fluid may be hemorrhagic. Direct treatment of these effusions is unnecessary. Patients with pulmonary vascular disease are typically dyspneic, tachycardic, and anxious; these signs are not related to the effusions or pulmonary infiltrate, but rather to alterations in pulmonary perfusion.

Hyperthyroidism. Feline patients with hyperthyroidism may develop effusion with or without documented cardiac failure, although the latter is by far more prevalent. The effusion is transudative and may be pseudochylous. While medical management of the hyperthyroid state appears to resolve the small effusions of patients without apparent congestive heart failure, patients with overt congestive heart failure appear to be best managed with appropriate cardiac medication and surgical thyroidectomy. Despite medical management and marked depression of T_4, patients in heart failure may continue to develop large effusions requiring thoracocentesis. Surgical intervention appears to markedly reduce or abolish such effusions.

Lung Torsion. In some cases, it is questionable whether the pleural fluid was present prior to lung lobe torsion or caused by the event. The effusion is typically an exudate and frankly hemorrhagic.[98] The effusion arises from strangulation of the bronchus, lymphatics, and the bronchus' vascular pedicle. Rotation along the lung's long axis obstructs lymphatic and venous drainage, while the artery remains patent. Progressive lobar

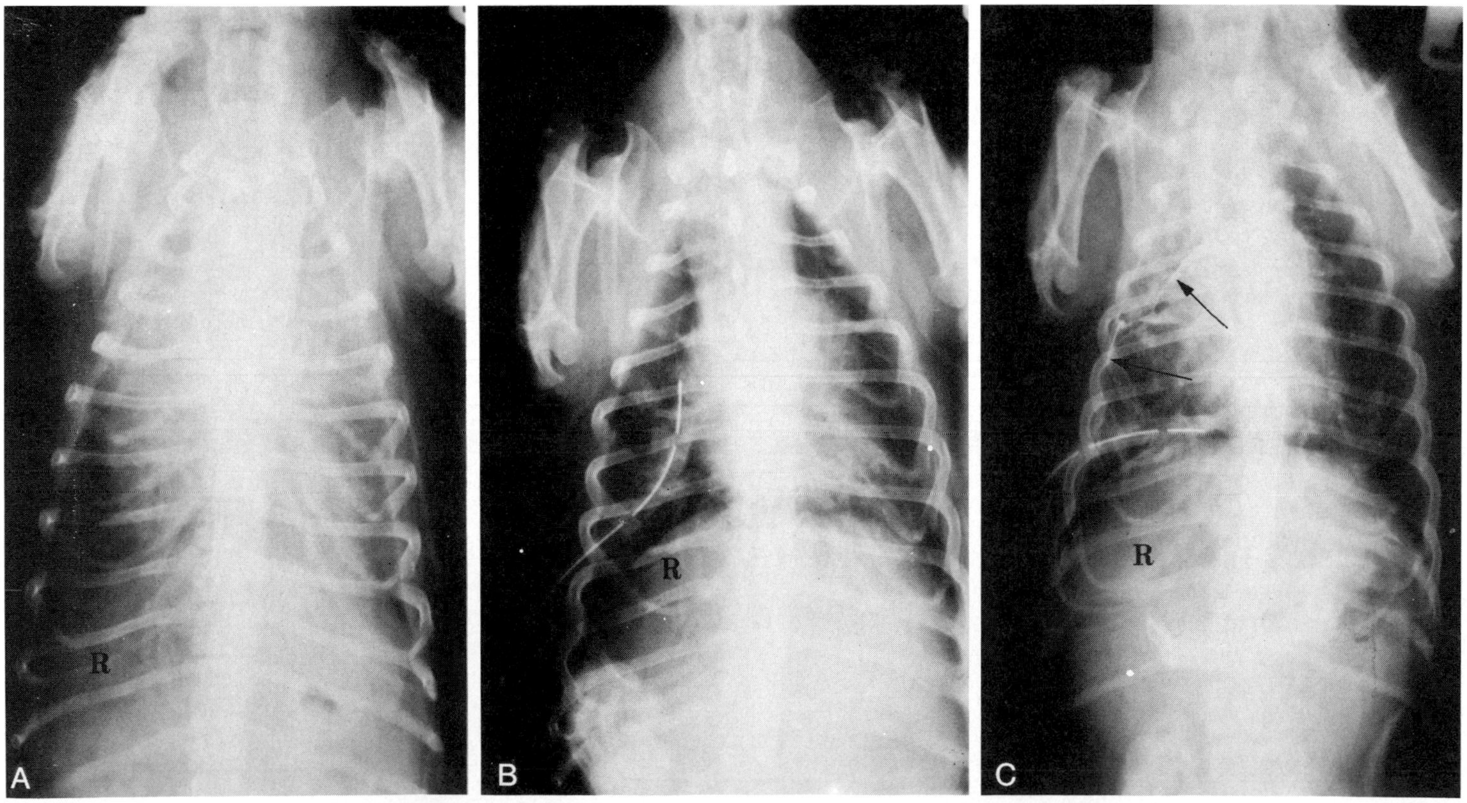

FIGURE 70–9. *A*, A four-year-old Dachshund with pleural effusion and fever. *B*, Tube thoracostomy yielded an infected exudate with strands of mucoid viscous material, which grossly appeared to represent esophageal material. *C*, Following a Renovist II and water swallow, free contrast is seen in the pleural space (arrows). Subsequent thoracotomy revealed esophageal rupture and mediastinal abscessation, but the patient made an uneventful recovery following surgical closure of the esophagus and medical management of the associated empyema.

engorgement with blood ensues, producing an expansile mass. Patients are frequently acutely ill, dyspneic, and in extremis. Tube thoracostomy rather than simple thoracocentesis is advisable to remove the large volume of effusion and prevent recurrence prior to surgical intervention. Extreme caution must be exercised during thoracostomy to avoid laceration of the torsed lung lobe. When effusions are bilateral, the tube should be introduced first into the contralateral hemithorax.

Trauma. Most pleural effusions appearing immediately following both major abdominal and thoracic trauma are hemothoraces. Most frequently, the effusions are self-limiting; however, tube thoracostomy may be necessary in nonresolving effusions to prevent pleural peel formation and fibrothorax. Thoracic surgery and decortication may rarely be required if spontaneous resolution or tube drainage does not clear the pleural blood; this complication appears to be rare.

Traumatic Diaphragmatic Hernia. Traumatic diaphragmatic hernia with incarceration of abdominal viscera is a cause of post-traumatic pleural effusion. The effusion may be transudative or exudative and mildly hemorrhagic. While most effusions appear early, some patients do not develop large effusions until several weeks or months following the traumatic event.

Central Venous Catheters. Both large- and small-bore venous catheters may cause pleural effusion by thrombosis and venous obstruction. Experimental ligation produced chylothorax in both dogs and cats.[99] Perforation and frank hemorrhage may also be a result of such central venous monitoring devices. For unknown reasons, these patients may appear in acute pain and exhibit signs similar to those of cervical vertebral disk prolapse. These effusions may be transudative and chylous or frank hemothoraces. If perforation or thrombosis is suspected, venacavagrams should be obtained prior to removing the offending intravascular cannula.

PLEURAL EFFUSION OF UNDETERMINED ETIOLOGY

Despite exhaustive evaluation and even thoracic surgery, the causes of some pleural effusions will remain undetermined. While some patients' diseases will eventually be diagnosed, a significant number will remain undiagnosed even after years of follow-up.

Pleural Effusion with Eosinophilia. Pleural effusions with eosinophil counts higher than that of the peripheral blood appear to be encountered frequently. The significance of these mildly eosinophilic effusions and their relationships to the etiologic cause of the effusion is unknown; hence their diagnostic significance is questionable. It would appear that small accumulations of eosinophils are a common reaction to various pleural insults.[100, 101] There is no consensus on what constitutes pleural fluid eosinophilia; arbitrarily, the author refers to eosinophilic effusions as those with ten per cent or more of the total cells being eosinophils.

While almost any disorder causing pleural effusion is capable of episodically being eosinophilic in veterinary patients, parasitic, immunologic, and hypersensitivity disorders appear to be the most frequent causes. The pathogenesis of pleural fluid eosinophilia in these disorders is not clearly evident. In the setting of experimentally induced eosinophilic pleural effusion in dogs, both the pleura itself and the associated fluid contain increased numbers of eosinophils.[102] In animals, blood cells contain eosinophilic chemotactic factor.[103] This may explain why any effusion that is hemorrhagic or one where there is significant diapedesis of red cells may become eosinophilic. Other substances contained in white blood cells, such as histamine, kinins, and immune complexes, may attract eosinophils. Neoplasia-related chemotaxis may occur with mast cell sarcoma, various forms of lymphosarcoma, or leukemia, and even with some carcinomas.[104] Rarely, eosinophilic pleural effusion and fever may be observed after pacemaker insertion or introduction of vascular catheters that have recently been sterilized with ethylene oxide.

The disorders that most frequently produce effusions with profound eosinophilia are those pulmonary disorders associated with angiitis and granulomatosis. These effusions may have 50 to 75 per cent of the white cells present as eosinophils. When this occurs, it frequently is associated with peripheral eosinophilia of a similar magnitude. Other disorders with pulmonary eosinophilia, such as heartworm disease, chronic eosinophilic pneumonia, and hypereosinophilic syndrome, may produce pleural effusions with significant eosinophilia. The degree of the eosinophilia produced by these and other hypersensitivity disorders is variable and should not be used as a standard for their diagnosis. Likewise, mild pleural fluid eosinophilia is of little use in the differential diagnosis of underlying effusions.

Chylothorax and Pseudochylothorax

Chylothorax is the accumulation of chylous fluid in the pleural space. This fluid has a high triglyceride concentration and demonstrates a chylomicron band in lipoprotein electrophoresis.[105, 106] The fluid has the gross appearance of skim milk. In patients not ingesting lipids or fats, the fluid may become more opaque. These effusions may become pink or blood-tinged following trauma or traumatic thoracocentesis. When centrifuged, both true chyle and pseudochyle do not clear as do milky fluids of other etiologies. Not all milky effusions are true chyle; the differentiation between chyle and pseudochyle may be difficult and require the use of biochemical or dye tests. True chyle contains fat, the amount of which varies depending upon the amount of dietary fat ingested, and as such it stains with Sudan III (although this is not a pathognomonic test).[107] The demonstration of chylomicrons in pleural fluid confirms the diagnosis of true chylothorax; such demonstration requires the use of lipoprotein electrophoresis. The diagnosis of chyle and pseudochyle may be made by adding diethylether and alkali to a sample of pleural fluid. When mixed, the milky nature of the fluid dissipates if it is due to cholesterol rather than chylomicrons.[108] If there is continued doubt as to the diagnosis, the patient may be fed a fatty meal mixed with a lipotrophic dye; butter may be mixed with coal tar dye or green dye.[109] The dye appears in pleural fluid one to two hours after ingestion, if the fluid is true chyle. Table 70–2 identifies the major characteristics of chyle and pseudochyle.

TABLE 70–2. MAJOR CHARACTERISTICS OF CHYLE AND PSEUDOCHYLE

Findings	Chyle	Pseudochyle
Appearance	Milky	Milky
Stain with Sudan III	Positive	Negative
Clearing with ether	Positive	Negative
Cytology	Lymphocytes and fat globules	Few cells typically, but may have PMN's and lymphs in some cases

The etiology of chylothorax includes a malignancy, trauma, and congenital, pancreatic, parasitic, infectious, and idiopathic causes. Chylothorax may be associated with chylous ascites in patients with systemic lymphatic disorders, such as lymphangiectasis.[111]

The treatment of chylothorax has changed in the last 20 years, and what once carried a poor to grave prognosis currently has a fair to good prognosis. Early treatment of chylothorax centered on frequent thoracocentesis and attempts at thoracic duct ligation.[110] Attempts at readministration of chyle via pleural venous shunts have resulted in vena cava thrombosis and occasional anaphylactic reactions.

Conservative management should be considered for patients not having a neoplastic or infectious cause for their effusions. Such means include thoracocentesis and attempts to reduce lymphatic flow and hence pleural accumulation. This is achieved by decreasing fluid intake and feeding carbohydrate-rich diets that are free of fats.[105] Medium-chain triglycerides are substituted because they are taken up directly by the portal circulation. It is important to avoid long-chain fatty acids, as they greatly increase lymphatic flow. A commercially prepared diet, MCT oil, Mead Johnson Laboratories, is available. Hills Pet Products produces a relatively low fat diet, R/D, which may alternatively be used.

A conservative approach is warranted in patients with traumatic, postoperative, or congenital chylothorax. The duration of therapy depends upon the patient's status and ability to tolerate the diet and thoracocentesis.

Chylothorax secondary to malignancy commonly does not resolve in the face of systemic chemotherapy other than with lymphomas. A combination of chemotherapy and pleurodesis is advocated; however, multiple attempts at creating pleural synthesis may be necessary. In patients with lymphoma, mediastinal radiation may aid in resolution of chylothorax.

For those patients in which conservative therapy fails, tube thoracostomy and water seal drainage is suggested. This is followed by pleurodesis (previously described).[113] Attempts at thoracic duct ligation followed by pleurodesis do not appear to yield a higher rate of resolution then pleurodesis alone. It is unclear whether successful surgery results from discrete ligation or the creation of postoperative pleural symphysis. The use of pleurodesis yields a variable outcome. In an unpublished series, four of nine cats treated by pleurodesis alone experienced complete resolution. Three were asymptomatic but continued to have radiographic evidence of pleural fluid, one was not helped, and one patient developed constrictive pericarditis secondary to pleurodesis, with additional signs of congestive heart failure.

Pneumothorax

Pneumothorax may occur through any one of four pathways. Air enters the pleural space via puncture of the pulmonary visceral pleura, chest wall disruption, entry of mediastinal air, and diaphragmatic rupture.[114] The pathogenesis of the pneumothorax plays a role in its management and associated clinical signs. Small lesions of the visceral pleura frequently close as lung volumes decrease; however, the volume of intrapleural air increases until the leak seals. Large air leaks persist and the lung collapses radiographically, appearing as a small hilar mass.

Pneumothorax may occur under tension if the lung or pleura acts as a one-way valve, i.e.,allowing air to pump into the pleural space by respiratory motions, but preventing its flow back toward the airway (Figure 70–10). In this case, the intrapleural pressures rise drastically and become supratmospheric.[115] This phenomenon may occur as a unilateral process with the involved lung pressed against the mediastinum, sealing its normal anatomic fenestrations. When this occurs, significant mediastinal shift toward the contralateral hemithorax is seen radiographically.[3]

TRAUMATIC PNEUMOTHORAX

Blunt or penetrating trauma to the thorax or abdomen may be the most frequent cause of pneumothorax in

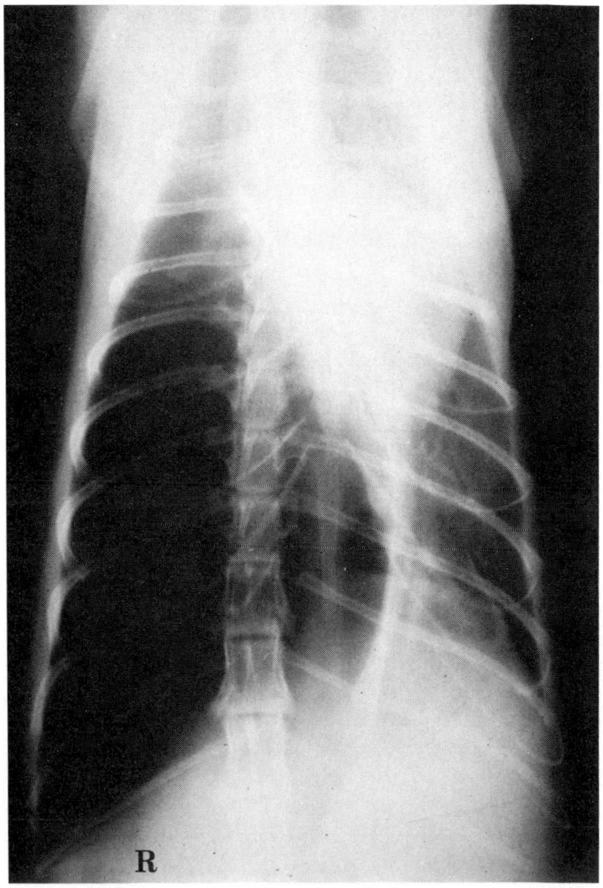

FIGURE 70–10. Tension pneumothorax. The right hemithorax is lucent without visible vascular or bronchial markings. There is a marked mediastinal shift to the left.

TABLE 70–3. CAUSES OF PNEUMOTHORAX

Traumatic–blunt or penetrating
Pulmonary cysts
Pulmonary cavitations–infectious or neoplastic
Pulmonary emphysema–bullae or blebs
Iatrogenic–thoracocentesis, lung biopsy, needle aspiration, mechanical ventilation, placement of large or central venous catheters, surgical
Spontaneous
Parasitic lung disease

veterinary patients. Radiographs should be obtained in any patient that has sustained chest trauma and has even slight dyspnea.

Findings other than pneumothorax may include rib fractures, subcuticular emphysema, pneumomediastinum, pulmonary contusions, and in rare cases, rupture of the trachea or major bronchus. Pneumothorax occurs by a number of mechanisms: direct laceration by rib fractures, chest wall disruption, or thoracic compression against a closed glottis, resulting in greatly increased transpleural pressures, rupturing lung or bronchus.[30, 116]

SPONTANEOUS PNEUMOTHORAX

The author uses this term to describe pneumothorax not associated with a known iatrogenic or traumatic cause, and when no apparent pulmonary pathology is present on radiographs following lung reinflation. Spontaneous pneumothorax rarely occurs in cats, and is seen most frequently in large, deep-chested dogs, particularly hounds.[117] These animals have typically been well without past pleural or pulmonary history. In some cases, recent exertion may have taken place; however, one case review had no such findings. It is assumed that these cases represent rupture of a small subpleural bleb, the etiology of which appears to be unknown.

PULMONARY CYSTS

The rupture of large pulmonary cysts or pneumatoceles may produce pneumothoraces with large volumes (Figure 70–11). This is due to resultant bronchopleural communication. Frequently, even with the lung collapsed, multiple or single large bullae are visible radiographically. Due to the magnitude of the bronchopleural fistula, the lung may not reexpand because of persistent air leakage; this may persist despite tube thoracostomy and water seal drainage. Surgical resection is frequently necessary.

LUNG ABSCESSES OR NECROSIS OF PULMONARY NEOPLASIA PRODUCING PNEUMOTHORAX

The formation of either infectious or sterile abscess cavities secondary to tumor necrosis may produce acute pneumothorax.[3, 118] The subpleural cavity may rupture and produce pneumothorax with empyema; frequently, these are under tension and are life-threatening when superimposed on the underlying illness.

Lung abscess may occur secondary to foreign body aspiration or primary pneumonia. It appears that *E. coli*, *Pseudomonas*, and *Klebsiella* are most frequently involved in these necrotizing infections. Acute necrotizing pneumonia without overt abscesses may cause pneumothorax. Patients with aspiration-related infections may be more prone to these complications, possibly due to the added chemical injury.

IATROGENIC PNEUMOTHORAX

Inadvertent production of a pneumothorax may occur as a complication of a wide variety of both diagnostic and therapeutic maneuvers. Thoracocentesis, Cope needle biopsy, fine needle aspiration, transtracheal aspiration, bronchoscopy and transbronchoscopic lung biopsy, mechanical ventilation, transthoracic liver biopsy, intercostal nerve block, tracheostomy, placement of central venous cannulas, and pacemaker implantation may all be associated with pneumothorax.[119] Probably the most important diagnostic aid is the awareness on the part of the veterinarian that pneumothorax may

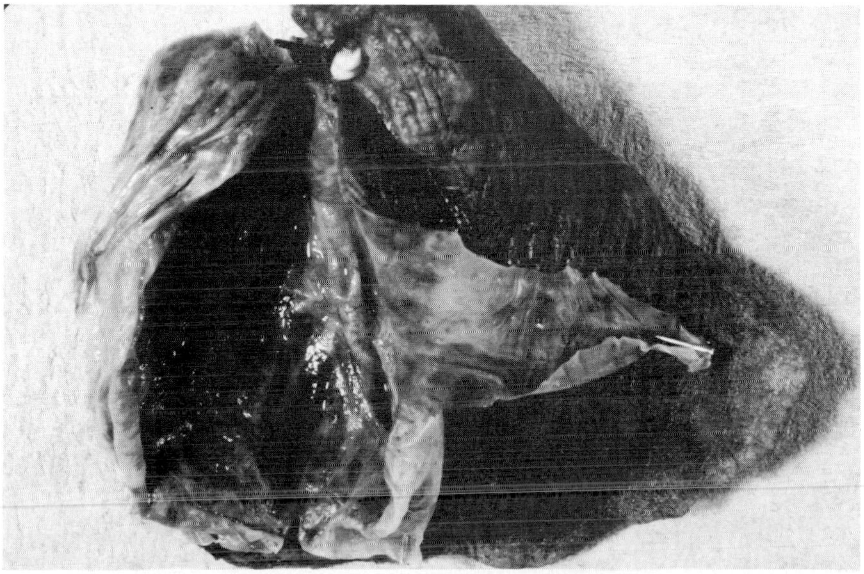

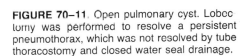

FIGURE 70–11. Open pulmonary cyst. Lobectomy was performed to resolve a persistent pneumothorax, which was not resolved by tube thoracostomy and closed water seal drainage.

occur under these circumstances and that the development of dyspnea, tachycardia, hypotension, or cyanosis should suggest this possibility.

DIAGNOSIS AND TREATMENT OF PNEUMOTHORAX

The presence of any significant pneumothorax is readily recognizable on both DV and lateral radiographs. The dorsal ventral projection is of the most importance, as it helps identify both unilateral and tension pneumothoraces.[3] Lateral decubitus views may be of assistance in identifying small volumes of intrapleural air. Likewise, end expiratory exposures accentuate the findings of pneumothorax. The hallmark of pneumothorax is a lucent hemithorax with absence of vascular markings. This finding depends on the volume of intrapleural air.

Physical findings associated with a large pneumothorax are relatively distinctive. The chest is resonant on percussion, but breath sounds are diminished or absent on auscultation. When unilateral tension pneumothorax occurs, the affected side may appear to bulge.

Management of pneumothorax is dictated by the context in which it occurs and the presence or absence of complications. In the patient with spontaneous pneumothorax, there are three therapeutic options: observation if the patient is relatively asymptomatic (in the absence of fever or hydropneumothorax, not every patient requires thoracocentesis), thoracocentesis to remove pleural air and reexpand lungs, or if there is recurrence, tube thoracostomy and water seal drainage. Of these options, a single-needle aspiration is the least effective and usually will not resolve the problem; however, the course will probably not be complicated by such therapy. Tube thoracostomy and water seal drainage for three to four days allows prompt and complete reexpansion of the lung. In addition, this may produce adhesions and help prevent recurrence. Should recurrence be a problem in a patient without radiographic evidence of the cause, either pleurodesis or thoracotomy may be curative. At thoracotomy, gauze sponge abrasion of the pleural surfaces is undertaken to produce pleural synthesis. The author has found neither of these options to be necessary following tube thoracostomy and resolution by this method of drainage.

Unlike spontaneous pneumothorax, traumatic or iatrogenic pneumothorax may reasonably respond to a single-needle aspiration. Following reduction of pneumothorax, the patient's clinical and radiographic progress should be followed. If dyspnea and radiographic evidence of pneumothorax return, tube thoracostomy and drainage should be instituted. The use of chest tubes attached to Heimlich valves rather than water seal drainage units is discouraged, as they are unreliable and will no longer function when moistened by condensation or pleural fluids. The small lung volumes of most companion animals further preclude the use of these valves.

The radiographic presence of a pulmonary cyst, lung abscess, or lung torsion or evidence of esophageal perforation is an indication for surgical intervention. While initial tube thoracostomy may be required to reduce the pneumohydrothorax and stabilize the patient preoperatively, the complications of these lesions do not frequently resolve without pulmonary resection or surgical closure.

Unlike the above conditions, pneumothorax associated with necrotizing pneumonia in the absence of overt abscesses is not a surgical emergency. However, it necessitates chest tube insertion in all cases. By definition, such cases represent both pneumonia and empyema, as there is direct pleural communication with the infected lung. Failure to treat these patients aggressively frequently results in lung abscess formation and the formation of frank empyema.

In other categories of pneumothorax, prompt tube insertion with closed drainage should be instituted. The more significant the underlying pulmonary or cardiac disease and associated clinical dysfunction, the more urgent the indication for tube drainage.

Mediastinal Disorders

The mediastinum is the central portion of the thoracic cavity, covered by the reflections of parietal pleura. It physically separates the two hemithoraces.[10] In most dogs and cats, the mediastinum is incomplete; thus, a unilateral process causing effusion or pneumothorax affects the contralateral hemithorax.[112] Inflammatory disorders may seal the mediastinal fenestrations, keeping a process unilateral.[120, 121] The anatomic boundaries of the mediastinum are the thoracic inlet cranially, the diaphragm caudally, the thoracic spine dorsally, and the sternum ventrally.

The mediastinum has been bisected into various anatomic subdivisions by various authors.[112, 121a] The main purpose of any subdivision is to aid in radiographic localization of the mediastinal pathology. To simplify anatomic description, this section refers to the ventral, central, and dorsal mediastinal compartments (Figure 70–12).

The ventral mediastinal boundaries are the thoracic inlet cranially, the sternum ventrally, and the dorsal pericardial surfaces caudally to the cardiophrenic ligament. It contains the heart, ascending segments of the great vessels, cranial vena cava, and sternal lymphatics.

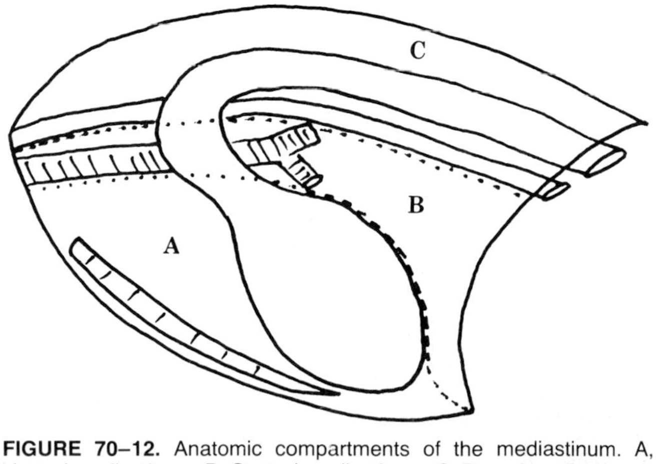

FIGURE 70–12. Anatomic compartments of the mediastinum. A, Ventral mediastinum; B, Central mediastinum; C, Dorsal mediastinum.

The central mediastinum extends from the dorsal surface of the ventral compartment to the dorsal surface of the esophagus. It contains the trachea, esophagus, aortic arch, main pulmonary arteries, caudal vena cava, and the tracheobronchial and hilar lymphatics.

The dorsal compartment continues from the dorsal esophageal margins to the ventral surface of the thoracic spine. It contains the descending aorta.

While it is logical to classify mediastinal lesions on the basis of their anatomic location, it should be apparent that there is overlap from one compartment to another. Some lesions indeed may extend into all three subdivisions, while others are discrete. Nevertheless, consideration of anatomic placement will allow exclusion of numerous processes and will allow formulation of a complete differential diagnosis.

HISTORY

A history of recent trauma or diagnostic or surgical procedures is critical to the diagnosis of hemomediastinum, pneumothorax, or pneumomediastinum. A history of recent visits to other emergency or primary care clinics may be omitted by clients who are unreasonably fearful that they have betrayed their loyalty to their regular veterinarian.

A history of previous procedures or malignancy should be sought in the presence of mediastinal enlargement. Previous tumors may have been removed but not submitted for histopathologic evaluation; confirmation should be obtained that tumors were called histopathologically benign, rather than grossly benign. When the clinical picture warrants, another histopathologic opinion should be obtained on biopsy material.

Geographic location needs to be ascertained when contemplating exposure to specific fungal or parasitic disorders. Many animals are obtained later in life, and inability to provide a full history may be an important feature.

PHYSICAL FINDINGS

Once mediastinal disease is recognized, a complete physical examination should always be repeated. Extrathoracic abnormalities are frequently present in cases of lymphosarcoma, metastatic carcinoma, and systemic fungal dissemination. These findings lead to alternative diagnostic options. Signs of mediastinal disease are frequently vague and associated with lesion size, location, pathologic consequences, and peripheral vascular signs. Large infiltrative masses of the anterior segments of the ventral and central mediastinum may produce obstruction of the vena cava. Vena cava syndrome is characterized by edema and symmetric swelling of the head, neck, and frequently, the front limbs (Figure 70–13). This phenomenon is related to both peripheral venous hypertension and lymphatic stasis. Veins of the front limbs and neck are distended. Frequently, thin-skinned animals may have a paucity of visible scalp or cutaneous veins. Obstruction must be at the level of the

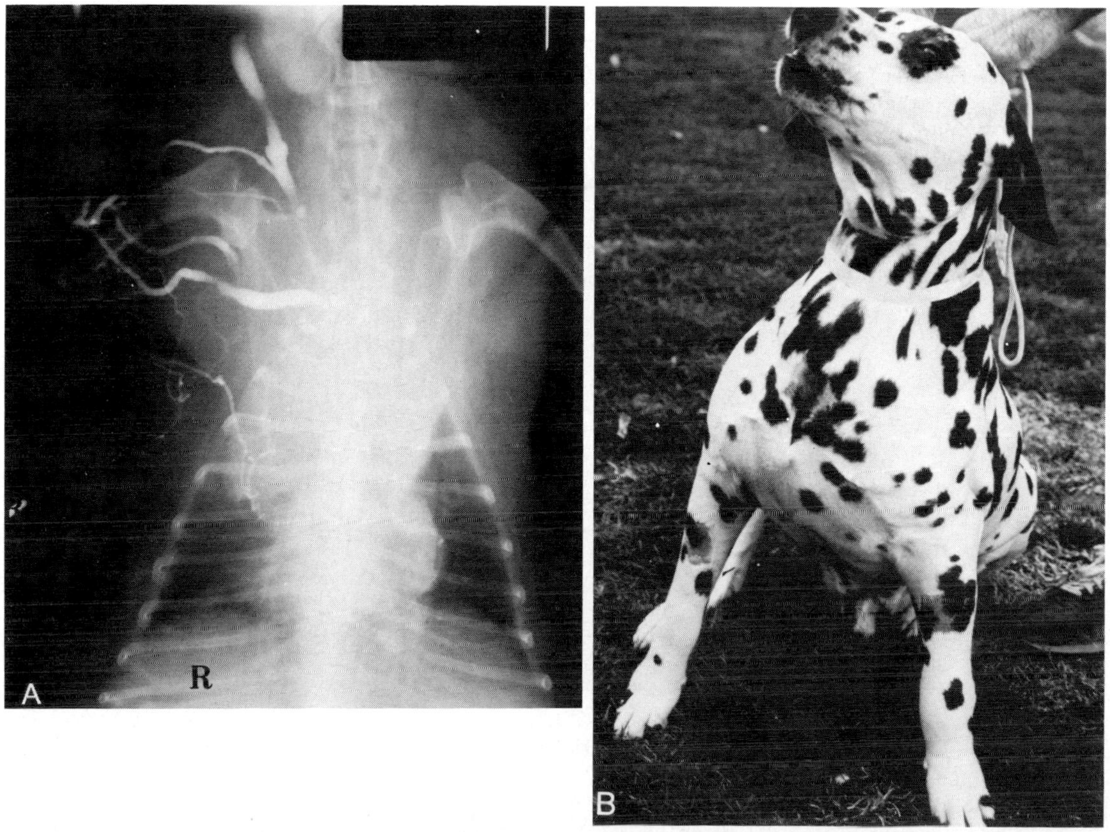

FIGURE 70–13. *A*, Aged beagle with a mediastinal mass and superior vena cava syndrome. Contrast medium has been injected into the right cephalic vein. Contrast medium is seen to reflex retrograde into the external jugular vein and into dilated cutaneous vessels. *B*, Dalmation with mediastinal lymphosarcoma causing vena cava obstruction. Note the symmetrical swelling of the face, neck, and front feet.

vena cava; unilateral obstruction of neck veins without arterial venous fistulization does not produce these signs. The diagnosis is made by venography. Contrast is injected into the saphenous vein and serial flat films are obtained. Frequently, not only compression of the vena cava but also redirection of venous flow towards dilated superficial cutaneous veins of the neck and thorax are seen.

Respiratory Signs. Signs are largely related to airway or pulmonary parenchymal compression. Mass lesions may compress the trachea or segmental bronchi, producing airway obstruction. Infiltrative processes may entrap peripheral nerves, causing laryngeal paralysis. Upper airway obstruction, changes in vocalization, and stridor may predominate as clinical signs.

Dysphagia. Surprisingly, even very large masses that markedly displace and compress the esophagus do not typically produce dysphagia. Segmental esophageal dysfunction, megaesophagus, esophageal foreign bodies, tumors, or mediastinitis most frequently cause signs of dysphagia or regurgitation.

Ophthalmologic Changes. Infiltrative processes or mass lesions may produce Horner's syndrome. Hyphema may be present in patients with occult lymphosarcoma. Rarely, this can be observed with metastasis of hemangiosarcoma.

DIAGNOSTIC STUDIES IN MEDIASTINAL DISEASE

Depending upon the results of these examinations, patients are placed into four diagnostic groups: patients diagnosable by noninvasive and minimally invasive procedures, such as serology, extrathoracic needle aspiration or biopsy, thoracocentesis, bronchoscopy, and endobronchial secretion evaluation; patients requiring angiography to define vascular lesions; patients requiring intrathoracic lymph node or mass aspiration or biopsy, accomplished percutaneously or via mediastinoscopy; patients requiring open diagnosis by a thoracotomy.

Radiography. The cornerstone of recognition is the presence of a mediastinal abnormality on standard thoracic radiographs. The exact location of the lesion within the mediastinum is determined both to help select further diagnostic tests and to aid in establishing a differential diagnosis. As with other thoracic radiographs, it is of prime importance to review past thoracic radiographs, if such exist.

Other More Invasive Procedures. Venocavography is employed to substantiate the diagnosis of vena cava compression or obstruction. Angiography is used to define aortic or pulmonary trunk dilation or obstruction. Chemoreceptor tumors or periaortic carcinomas and sarcomas may "blush" during aortography.

Bronchoscopy is of limited use in defining mediastinal disorders unless pulmonary parenchymal pathology coexists. Extrinsic compression of the trachea or hilum may be visually demonstrated.

Lymphangiography may be useful in documenting mediastinal lymphatic disorders. It typically is not helpful in the presence of adenopathy.

Esophograms or contrast gastrograms may demonstrate esophageal pathology and extrinsic displacement or compression. In the case of perforation, barium or Gastrografin may be seen to escape into the mediastinum or pleural space. Diaphragmatic hernia may be likewise visualized with small-bowel studies.

Radioisotope studies may aid in the diagnosis of ectopic thyroid tissue. Venograms may alternatively be performed with radioactive isotope techniques.

Echocardiography is useful in detecting pericardial effusions, cysts, and masses.[122] Other cystic masses may be visualized in the cranial mediastinum. Neoplasia of the heart may be well visualized.

Thoracocentesis and pleural biopsy are important studies when pleural effusion accompanies mediastinal disease. Cytologic examination is mandatory with any undiagnosed effusion.

Mediastinoscopy may provide a means of obtaining biopsy tissue without thoracotomy.[123] Masses in the cranial mediastinal compartment are accessible via this technique.[53] Mediastinoscopy is technically difficult if not impossible in patients with superior vena cava syndrome, infiltrative cancers of the head and neck, or mediastinal hemangiosarcoma.

Needle aspiration of the cranial mediastinal compartment is a useful means of establishing a diagnosis. Closed cutting needle biopsy of the ventral and central mediastinal compartments is ill-advised due to the superimposition of major vascular and visceral structures. When attempting to introduce a needle into the mediastinum, the anatomic planes should be kept in mind. Needles are placed parallel to the sternum rather than the lateral aspect of the thoracic wall. This approach allows the needle to course longitudinally through the mediastinum, avoiding the lung.

Diagnostic thoracotomy is contemplated only when the previously discussed techniques have failed to provide a diagnosis. In those cases in which a mediastinal mass remains etiologically undiagnosed, exploratory thoracotomy without undue delay appears to best serve the patient.

DISORDERS CAUSING ACUTE WIDENING OF THE CRANIAL SEGMENTS OF THE VENTRAL AND CENTRAL MEDIASTINUM

There is considerable variability in the normal radiographic appearance of the canine mediastinum.[112] Factors such as obesity, variation in thymic size and rib cage conformation, and specific breed conformities make it difficult if not impossible to evaluate small or moderate degrees of mediastinal widening. Previously obtained radiographs are of immeasurable value in judging small amounts of mediastinal change.

In comparison, cats rarely have accumulations of mediastinal fat that mimic mediastinal widening. Their thoracic conformation is similar in all breeds, and their normal mediastinal width rarely exceeds that of the sternum.

MEDIASTINAL HEMORRHAGE

Both dogs and cats may experience mediastinal hemorrhage secondary to trauma, thoracic surgery, or coagulopathies (Figure 70–14). It has been reported that

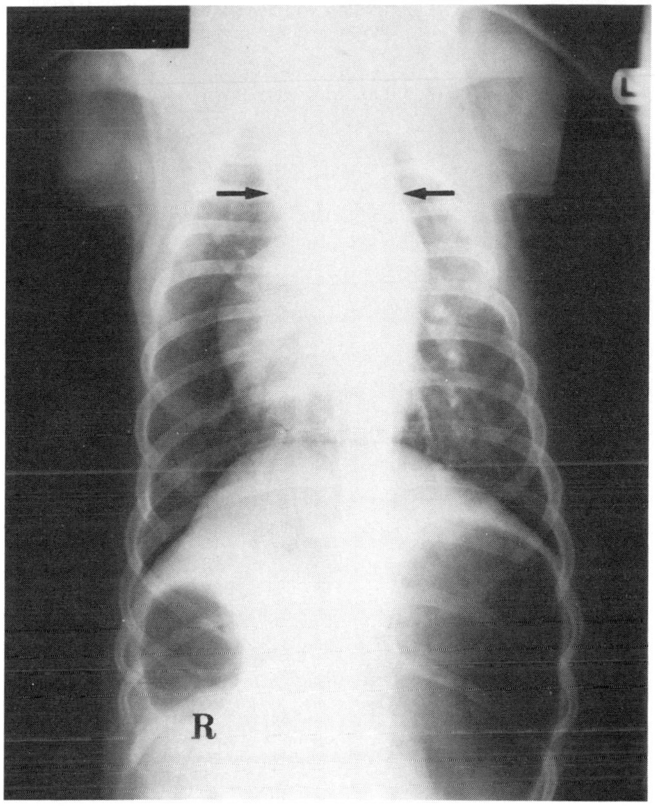

FIGURE 70–14. Golden retriever with mediastinal hemorrhage, secondary to warfarin-induced hemorrhagic diasthesis. Arrows show extent of mediastinal widening. This patient's clinical signs were related to airway compression and obstruction.

young dogs may experience spontaneous and fatal hemorrhage related to thymic vascular disruption.[124] Non-traumatic dissection of the aorta or vena cava is a rare event in both dogs and cats. As such, hemomediastinum virtually always represents a medical disorder, and surgical exploration is not warranted.

MEDIASTINAL EDEMA

Edema may appear in the mediastinum secondary to both infection and traumatic causes. While patients in heart failure and with lymphangiectasis may grossly have edema present at surgical exploration or necropsy, the magnitude of these changes is not radiographically apparent.

MEDIASTINITIS

Mediastinitis may represent an acute, subacute, or chronic disorder. Many patients have obvious findings on their survey radiographs, while others may have no concrete radiographic findings on initial evaluation. By definition, mediastinitis includes any process producing inflammation within the mediastinal space; the working definition, however, appears only to include infectious causes in veterinary patients.

Acute Mediastinitis. Acute mediastinitis most frequently arises from perforation or rupture of the trachea or esophagus. These patients may have persistent radiographic findings suggesting the etiology, such as tracheal fracture or esophageal foreign body. Head and neck infection may extend via fascial planes and thoracic inlet into the mediastinum. Acute mediastinitis infrequently stems from sepsis, pneumonia, pericarditis, or empyema. When not treated promptly, mediastinitis may progress to abscesses, such cases frequently progressing to frank empyema. Mediastinitis may be recognized following tube thoracostomy and closed drainage of an empyema pocket (Figure 70–15).

Chronic Mediastinitis. Granulomatous mediastinitis may result from infection by a number of agents. *Histoplasma*, *Cryptococcus*, *Coccidioides*, *Actinomyces*, and *Nocardia* species are the most frequently encountered organisms. *Actinomyces* species and *Corynebacterium* species have been reported as causes for mediastinal granulomas in dogs. Unlike the same disorders in humans, these lesions tend to present themselves as discrete mediastinal masses. Both mediastinal abscesses and granulomas may masquerade as neoplasia.

Treatment of Mediastinitis. Acute mediastinitis associated with esophageal perforation is a surgical emergency. These patients frequently are presented in extremis with dysphagia, dyspnea, and fever. Pneumothorax and frank empyema may be present at the time of admission. In such cases, tube thoracostomy and pleural drainage should be instituted preoperatively and pleural fluid cultured both aerobically and anaerobically. Patients with esophageal perforation almost invariably have anaerobic organisms as a portion of their infection; *Bacteroides fragilis* infection may complicate such cases. Until culture results are available, antimicrobial therapy is started with both an aminoglycoside and penicillin in patients with normal renal function. Azotemic patients should either be dosed according to their creatinine clearance, or a second- or third-generation cephalosporin substituted. Whenever possible, chronic mediastinitis is treated surgically. Abscess drainage or granuloma removal may prove a formidable challenge and may necessitate segmental pulmonary resection. Antifungal or antimicrobial therapy depends on the etiologic agent.

PNEUMOMEDIASTINUM

Pneumomediastinum, or the presence of air within the mediastinum, may occur seemingly spontaneously, secondary to trauma, as a result of mechanical ventilation, or related to both diagnostic and therapeutic maneuvers.[119, 123] Air may enter the mediastinum by several routes. Penetrating wounds of the head, neck, and cranial thorax may allow air to dissect into the mediastinum via the thoracic inlet. Air may move cranially from the abdomen and retroperitoneum; this may appear spontaneously following abdominal surgery or rupture of a gas-filled viscus, or on rare occasions may be associated with bowel obstruction without rupture. Most frequently, pneumomediastinum results from airway or alveolar rupture; air is transmitted from the air space or airway to the interstitium, where it tracks toward the hilum, ultimately filling the mediastinum. Pneumomediastinum may occur as a sole event or in combination with pneumothorax. Pneumothorax can result from a primary pulmonary leak or as a result of rupture of the mediastinal pleura. Radiographically, pneumomediastinum is characterized by ability to visualize mediastinal structures usually not seen, i.e., aorta, vena cava, azygous vein, and esophagus.[112] In addition, there may be subcuticular emphysema present and fascial planes of the neck and front limbs may be radiographically recognizable (Figure 70–16). On rare occasions, pneumocardium may be present.

Clinical Manifestations

Clinical signs depend on the underlying cause, volume and pressure of mediastinal air, presence or absence of concurrent pneumothorax, and presence or absence of concurrent infection.[95, 96, 125]

TABLE 70–4. CAUSES OF PNEUMOMEDIASTINUM

1. Spontaneous pneumomediastinum
   Cough, exertion, profound dyspnea, emphysema, cysts or cavitary lesions, idiopathic
2. Mechanical ventilation
   C-PAP, high inspiratory pressures due to poor lung compliance, overzealous bagging
3. Bronchial or tracheal rupture
   Traumatic intubation, endotracheal tube cup perforation, rupture secondary to blunt trauma, penetrating wound laceration
4. Esophageal rupture
   Foreign body, blunt or penetrating trauma, endoscopy
5. Mediastinoscopy
   Occurs as a routine with this procedure
6. Percutaneous insertion of a large-bore central venous or pulmonary artery catheter
   Appears more frequently in large, deep-chested dogs
7. Tracheostomy
8. Transtracheal aspiration

Many patients are relatively asymptomatic. Pneumomediastinum may only be recognized after routine thoracic radiographs. As previously mentioned, the only physical findings may be subcuticular emphysema; this may take on enormous proportions, with the patient appearing balloon-like. Even such massive subcutaneous emphysema is not dangerous, but admittedly probably uncomfortable.

Markedly increased pressures within the mediastinum can produce acute catastrophic hypotension and ventilatory failure.[126] Decreased venous return results from compression of the great veins. Acute pneumothorax, which may be under tension, may produce profound dyspnea. Patients with esophageal rupture and mediastinitis may appear to be in pain and in extremis. Frequently, there are radiographically evident foreign bodies present within the esophagus and cranial to the cardiac silhouette; in these patients, there may be evidence of pleural effusion as well as pneumomediastinum and/or pneumothorax.

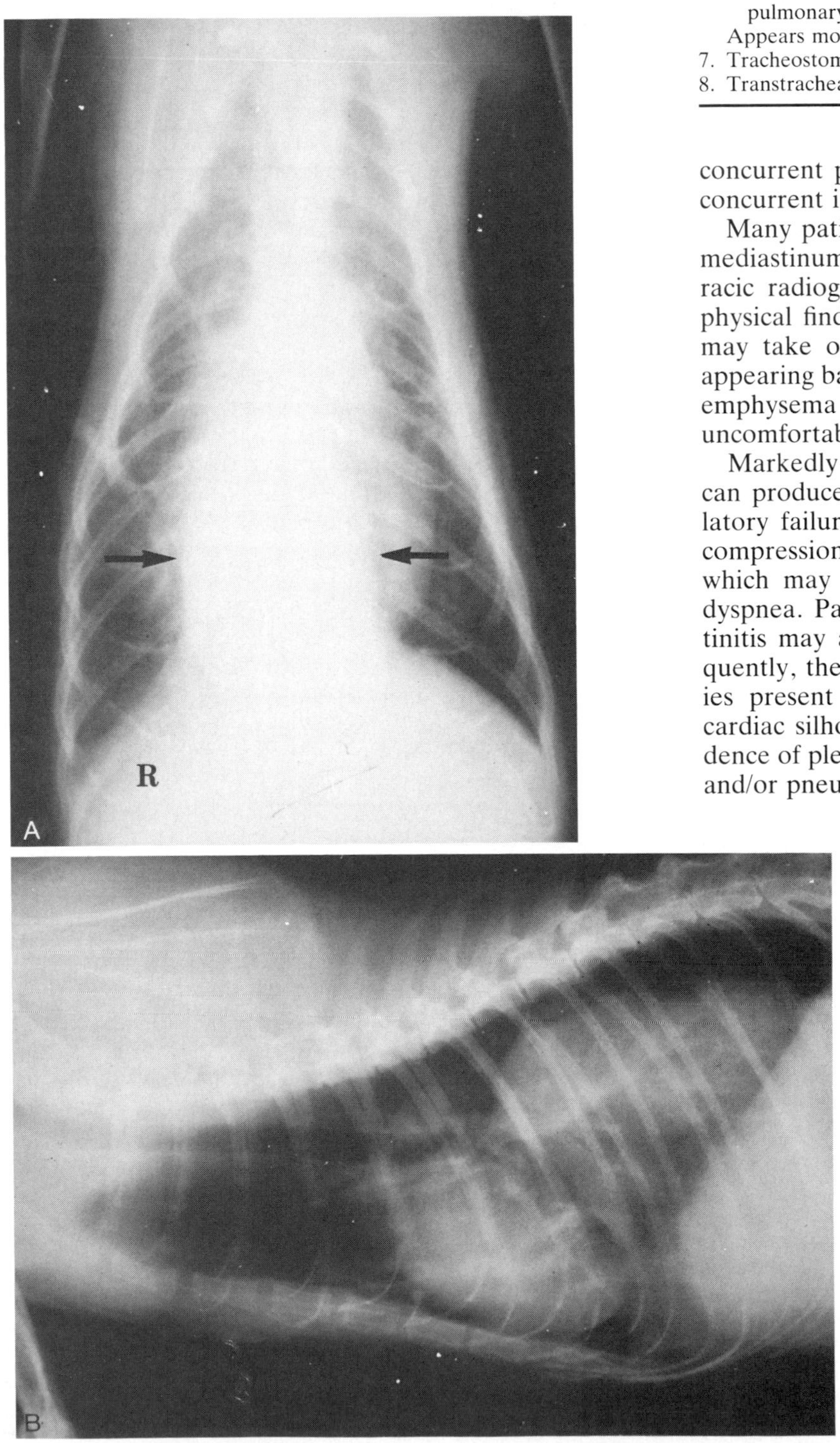

FIGURE 70–15. *A*, Mediastinal granuloma or abscess outlined by arrows. These radiographic findings were observed following a tube thoracostomy and treatment of an anaerobic empyema. *B*, Lateral projection of the same patient.

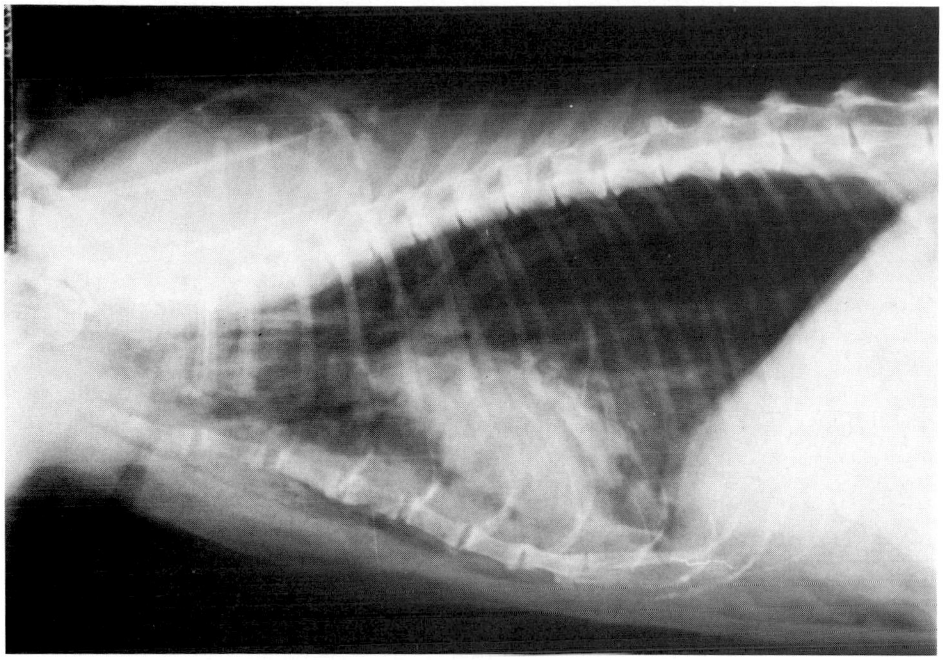

FIGURE 70–16. Pneumomediastinum in an aged Siamese cat following anesthesia for an elective dental procedure. Note visualization of mediastinal structure not normally recognizable.

Treatment

Most uncomplicated cases of pneumomediastinum require no treatment at all. It may, however, take 10 to 20 days for all mediastinal and subcutaneous air to spontaneously resolve. In those patients with large volumes of subcutaneous air, needle aspiration of the subcutis may be performed to reduce the volume.

Most patients who are significantly dyspneic have associated pneumothorax. Simple thoracocentesis may reduce dyspnea temporarily, but recurrence is frequent, requiring tube thoracostomy and water seal drainage. Patients in circulatory collapse should be volume-expanded to restore blood pressure; the use of pressors is rarely necessary. Attempts to cannulate the mediastinum are ill advised; such attempts may result in laceration of the mediastinal viscera.

BENIGN LYMPHADENOPATHY

Numerous infectious disorders produce thoracic lymph node enlargement. Typically, thoracic lymph node enlargement produced by viral infections, sepsis, pneumonia, and immunologic disorders tends to be only mild to moderate, so that nodes are radiographically inapparent.[112] To this degree the differential diagnosis of hilar, parahilar, and sternal lesions associated with adenopathy is limited.

Bacterial infection causing empyema or mediastinitis produces adenopathy that may be radiographically recognizable.[112] Frequently the primary process prevents recognition of node enlargement until pleural or mediastinal fluid is resorbed. Sternal node enlargement is the most frequently visualized, and radiographic en-

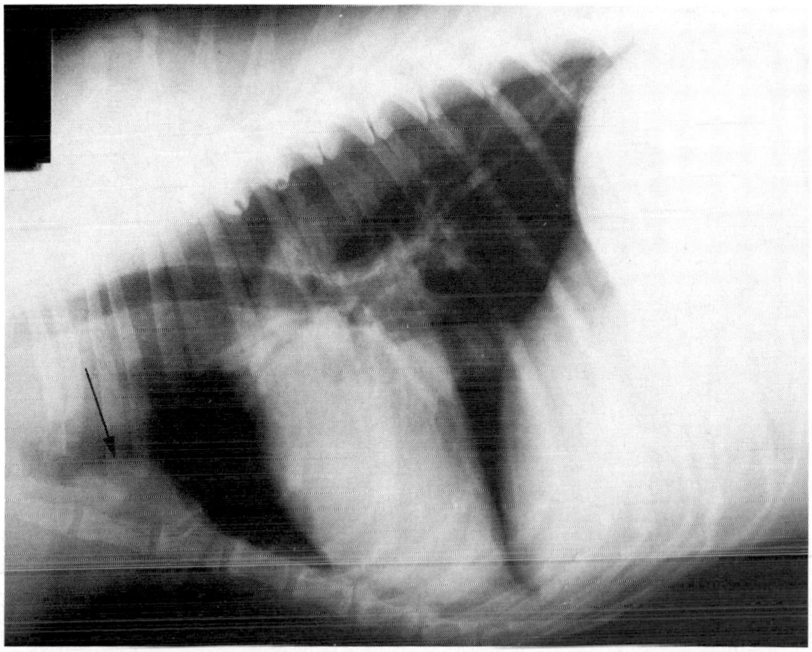

FIGURE 70–17. Sternal adenopathy following resolution of an *E. coli* empyema in an aged Afghan hound. Arrows identify enlarged sternal lymph node.

largement may persist weeks after resolution in infected pleural effusions or widespread pulmonary infections (Figure 70–17). While obviously a subjective evaluation, the magnitude of enlargement produced by these processes is much less than that of other agents discussed in this section.

FUNGAL DISORDERS

Mediastinal adenopathy may be the major radiographic finding in patients with systemic fungal disorders (Figure 70–18). Coccidioidomycosis, histoplasmosis, blastomycosis, and cryptococcosis may all produce mediastinal adenopathy in severe cases.[112, 127–129] The diagnosis is suggested by the infectious presentation and geographic location; the diagnosis is confirmed by the appropriate serology or biopsy of extrathoracic sites. Each of these disorders has sequelae that aid in the clinical differentiation; the appropriate portions of this text should be consulted.

MYCOBACTERIAL DISORDERS

Primary tuberculosis in dogs and cats may produce mediastinal node enlargement as a component of their complex.[130] Suffice it to say that the reported incidence of canine and feline tuberculosis is negligible in the U.S.A. and this diagnosis need only be contemplated with exclusion of the more frequently encountered infections and neoplastic causes.

BACTERIAL INFECTION ASSOCIATED WITH GRANULOMATOSIS

Mediastinal granulomas of identifiable or unknown etiology may cause mediastinal enlargement. These disorders may be fulminant, acute and suppurative, or be responsible for chronic granulomatous mediastinitis. *Actinomyces* and *Nocardia* species are the most frequently involved agents and may be responsible for both thoracic and extrathoracic spread. Adenopathy with pleural effusion is a frequent finding; pulmonary infiltrates may be present, but less frequently. In the absence of pleural effusion or extrathoracic sites that are accessible, definitive diagnosis may be a challenge. Cultures of respiratory secretions in the absence of overt pulmonary infection are infrequently positive. Blood and urine cultures rarely yield the causative organism. Open lymph node biopsy may be necessary to confirm the diagnosis. The author is unaware of any such cases successfully diagnosed by a mediastinoscopy. These lesions may mimic neoplasia both clinically and radiographically. While uncommon, they are an example of a potentially curable disorder that at first glance may be written off as incurable cancer.

NONINFECTIOUS GRANULOMATOUS DISORDERS WITH EOSINOPHILIA

These poorly understood disorders akin to lymphomatoid or allergic granulomatosis in humans are associated with hilar adenopathy, pleural masses and eosinophilia. The hilar adenopathy is striking and appears to be a consistent finding (Figure 70–19). It is unclear whether these syndromes are benign or malignant; suffice it to say the clinical course is far from benign. Hilar adenopathy persists despite pulmonary resection, steroid therapy, or treatment with soft tissue sarcoma protocols. Many patients have systemic involvement; pulmonary vascular disease with thrombosis and obstruction is a consistent complication.

The diagnosis is suspected in the presence of the salient clinical features. Peripheral eosinophilia is frequently striking. If pleural effusion is present, it too is frequently eosinophilic. The diagnosis is made by lung and lymph node biopsy, which is frequently undertaken at the time of pulmonary mass resection.

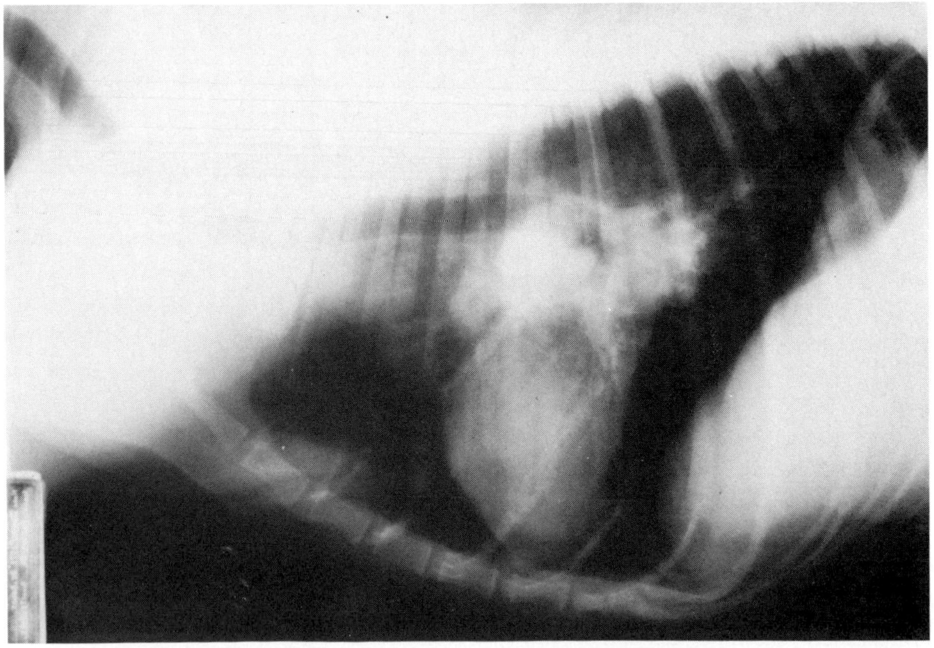

FIGURE 70–18. Hylar adenopathy in a dog with coccidioidomycosis.

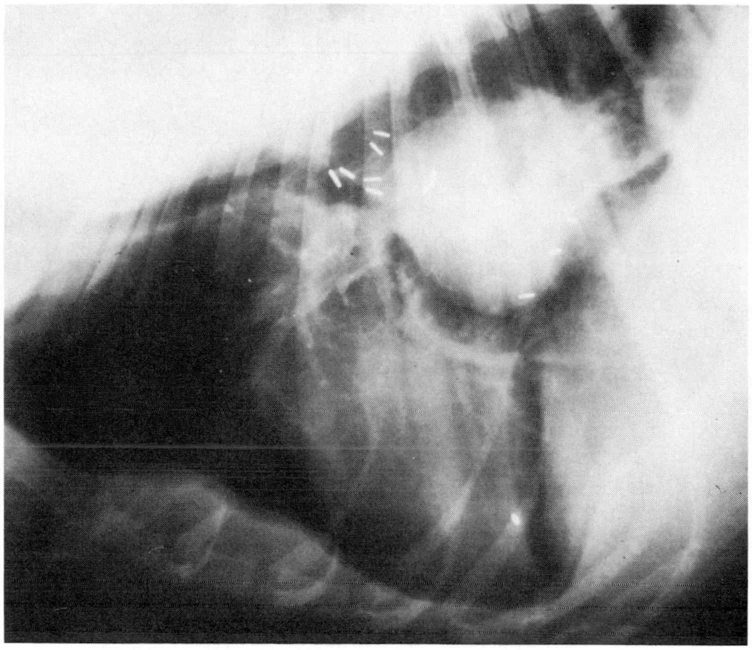

FIGURE 70–19. Persistent hylar adenopathy following pulmonary resection in a Boxer with pulmonary eosinophilia associated with angiitis and granulomatosis.

NEOPLASTIC LYMPHADENOPATHY

Lymphoma and lymphosarcoma frequently manifest their major clinical signs as those of mediastinal and pleural disease (Figure 70–20). These are often present even with the alimentary and multicentric forms. Feline patients experience approximately 70 per cent of their tumor distribution in the mediastinum and alimentary tract; canine patients experience the majority of their disease as the multicentric form.[35, 131] The distribution of thoracic lesions differs in canine and feline patients. Cats, with their propensity for the thymic form, may have perihilar or sternal node involvement. In comparison, dogs infrequently have thymic lymphosarcoma; they normally exhibit sternal, perihilar, or mediastinal involvement.[112, 131] Both dogs and cats may infrequently develop pulmonary thoracic lymphosarcoma. When this occurs it may mimic pulmonary carcinoma with hilar spread. This form may be difficult to diagnose without lung biopsy.

TABLE 70–5. LOCATIONS OF MEDIASTINAL LESIONS

- Ventral mediastinum
  - Dilated superior vena cava, thyroid and parathyroid tumors
  - Thymic tumors
  - Lymphoma
  - Mediastinal cysts
  - Fat pads
  - Lymphadenopathy
  - Cardiomegaly
- Central mediastinum
  - Mediastinitis
  - Aortic dilatation
  - Esophageal disorders
  - Lymphadenopathy
  - Thyroid and parathyroid tumors
  - Neurogenic tumors
  - Pulmonary artery dilatation
  - Lymphoma
- Dorsal mediastinum
  - Descending aortic dilatation, paravertebral infiltrative or mass disorders

Unlike thymoma, thoracic lymphosarcoma is frequently accompanied by pleural effusion.[112] The volume of effusion does not appear to correlate well with tumor mass. Cats subjectively appear to develop proportionately larger volumes than dogs. Dyspnea may be related to airway compression by large tumor masses or to pleural effusion. For this reason, it is imperative to evaluate the dorsoventral radiograph, which helps to distinguish effusion from mass.

Diagnosis

Whenever possible, the diagnosis of lymphosarcoma is made from extrathoracic evaluation. Bone marrow or hematologic evaluation may provide a diagnosis in some patients. Histopathologic rather than cytopathologic confirmation is preferable, as such a careful search for peripheral node involvement may yield diagnostic options. The presence of neoplastic cells in pleural fluid is variable. Needless to say, any patient with pleural effusion should undergo diagnostic, if not therapeutic, thoracocentesis. Needle aspiration of most lymphomas is diagnostically rewarding, although histiocytic lymphoma may not exfoliate cells and have negative pleural fluid cytology and a variable yield from needle aspiration. Closed cutting needle biopsy is ill-advised, due to the proximity of vascular and visceral structures. Infrequently, thoracotomy is necessary to confirm the diagnosis; this is most frequent when lymphomas are present in the caudal segments of the central mediastinum.

METASTATIC INVASION OF MEDIASTINAL LYMPH NODES

Mediastinal lymphadenopathy may be due to metastatic carcinoma; pulmonary carcinomas appear the most common cause. In such cases there is usually a pulmonary mass or infiltrate that is a diagnostic aid. Pulmonary lymphosarcoma mimics this pattern.

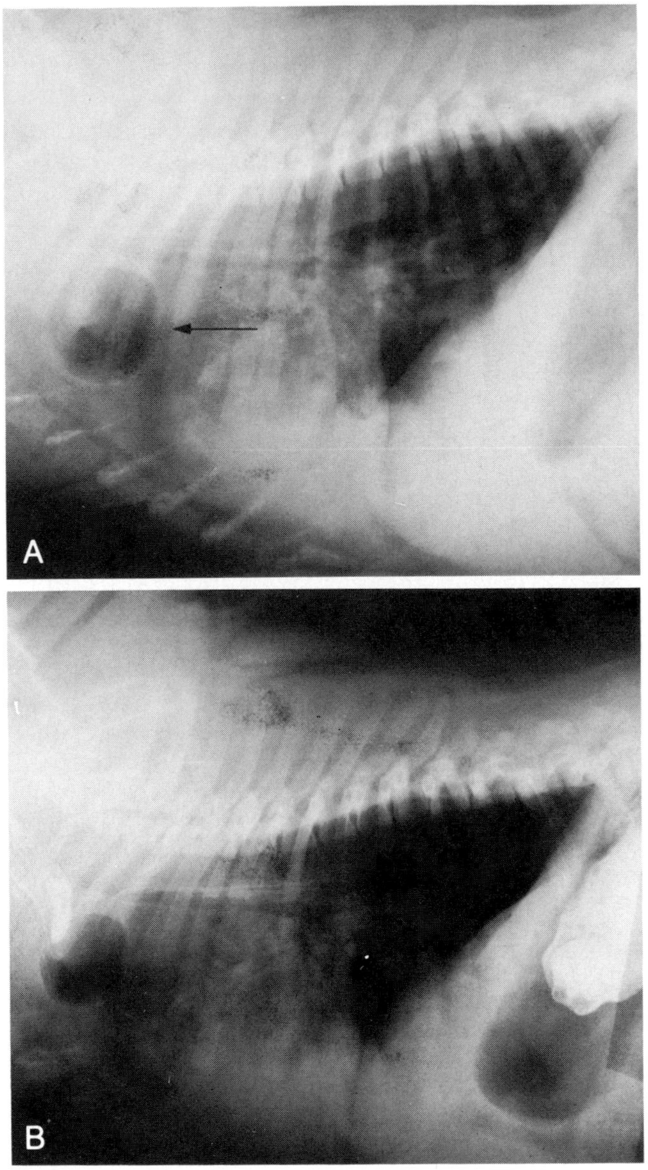

FIGURE 70–20. *A*, A young English bulldog with clinical signs referable to recurrent aspiration pneumonia. Arrow points to lucent mediastinal lesion. *B*, Same patient following barium swallow. Lucency is observed to represent esophageal diverticulum.

Anaplastic or undifferentiated carcinoma of the head and neck may appear to be entirely mediastinal in its spread. It may appear as small sternal or tracheobronchial masses, with or without pleural effusion. While the frequency of these tumors is similar, cats appear to experience more frequent mediastinal spread. Cervical or mediastinal tumor infiltration may provoke Horner's syndrome, laryngeal paralysis, or megaesophagus.

Mediastinal lymph node metastases may arise from tumors of the gastrointestinal tract, urogenital organs, and mammary glands. As with other tumors, extrathoracic sites should be explored whenever possible.

THYROID CARCINOMA

Extension of thyroid carcinoma into the cranial ventral mediastinum is more frequent in dogs than cats but uncommon in both species.[132] In patients with mediastinal spread, there may be palpable physical findings of a discrete or infiltrative process in the neck and thoracic inlet. While overt vena cava syndrome may not be present, there may be venous engorgement due to tumor infiltration of neck veins. Similar involvement of peripheral nerves may lead to laryngeal paralysis and signs of airway obstruction.

CYSTS

Benign cysts of the ventral mediastinum are uncommon and arise from diverse cell lines, including pleural, lymphatic, bronchogenic, and thymic origins.[133] They typically are inadvertent findings on thoracic radiographs obtained for other reasons. Patients are typically asymptomatic and these masses are not known to be pathologic. When they are present, they may mimic solid neoplasia and as such their identification is important. This is accomplished by needle aspiration of the mass. It should be noted that many solid neoplasias have a cystic component; benign cysts should be radiographically absent or diminished in size following aspiration.

CHEMODECTOMA

Chemodectomas or heart-base, aortic body, or nonchromaffin paragangliomas are neoplasms of chemoreceptor cells of the aortic and carotid bodies.[35] They may appear as discrete, well-encapsulated masses or infiltrative masses, intertwining themselves around the great vessels and mediastinal structures. Less commonly, there is direct cardiac extension.

The recognition of such tumors often is related to intrapericardial invasion, with production of pericardial effusion and signs of right heart failure. Survey radiographs may reveal the presence of a mediastinal widening or less frequently a discrete mass. Since there is a predilection for this tumor in brachycephalic breeds, mediastinal widening may be difficult to assess because their normal anatomy has considerable variability.[35, 112] Diagnosis ultimately requires surgical biopsy; however, presumptive diagnosis may be established by aortography or echocardiographic evaluation.

SCIRRHOUS CARCINOMA

Carcinomas of the mediastinum are not frequently encountered and may pose a diagnostic challenge. The radiographic and clinical signs of pleural effusions may predominate. Following thoracocentesis, mild mediastinal widening or small mass lesions may be present in the ventral or central mediastinum early in the course of the disease. The natural history of this neoplasm involves spreading to and involving the entire mediastinum, producing symmetrically thickened surfaces that are difficult to perceive radiographically. This tumor does not typically exfoliate cells, and pleural fluid cytology yields an extremely inflammatory exudate without neoplastic cells. Diagnostic needle aspirates even with fluoroscopic guidance may be unsuccessful, thus necessitating an open biopsy for confirmation. Cats appear to have a higher incidence of this tumor. It is unclear whether these are primary or metastatic tumors. Meticulous necropsy dissection and histopathologic review has failed to find tumor other than thoracic carcinoma in four cats. While it could easily be argued that these represent metastasis of a microscopic mammary or abdominal carcinoma, it can be argued with equal validity that these arise from epithelial tissues of the mediastinum.

MISCELLANEOUS TUMORS

Numerous tumors occur with relatively low frequency as primary masses of the central and ventral mediastinal compartments. They include hemangiosarcoma, fibrosarcoma, myxoma, and mesothelioma.[35] Both hemangiosarcoma and myxoma may have cardiac invasion with signs of tamponade or venous obstruction. Associated thoracic findings are variable, ranging from pulmonary spread to pleural effusion.

DIGESTIVE TRACT LESIONS

For purposes of this section, esophageal lesions are subdivided into those of dilation, foreign bodies, and neoplasia. Primary tumors of the esophagus are rare.[35, 133] Even more uncommon are tumors large enough to appear as discrete masses that displace other structures. Tumors include leiomyoma, leiomyosarcoma, *Spirocerca lupi*-related sarcoma, osteosarcoma, fibrosarcoma, and squamous carcinoma. These masses, with the exception of osteosarcoma, are rarely calcified; they are recognized via esophagrams or esophagoscopy.[112]

Disorders of dilation as a result of megaesophagus, vascular ring lesions, and diverticula primarily present as areas of lucency, either discrete or linear, comprising the length of the mediastinum. These gas-filled structures may have fluid levels or granular densities representing ingesta. Frequently densities that suggest pulmonary infections secondary to aspiration are present.

Foreign bodies are more frequently cranial to the heart. Associated radiographic findings are dependent upon duration and degree of obstruction and the presence or absence of perforation (see mediastinitis). Diaphragmatic hernia may simulate mediastinal mass lesions. Infrequently, viscera may be incarcerated within the mediastinum, appearing radiographically as a discrete mass. More frequently the presentation is that of pleural disease or pleural masses with effusion. Pericardial diaphragmatic hernia may mimic simple pericardial effusion, pericardial masses, or cardiomegaly.

VASCULAR LESIONS

The incidence of aneurysm in dogs and cats is very low and is not a major consideration in a differential diagnosis. The most frequently observed enlarged structures are those produced by congenital or acquired cardiac or vascular disorders, i.e., aortic stenosis, pulmonic stenosis, pulmonary vascular diseases such as heartworm or pulmonary thrombosis, patent ductus arteriosus, and arteriovenous valve insufficiency.[134] Infrequent right atrial obstruction or large arteriovenous fistulas may produce radiologically recognizable vena cava or azygos vein dilation.

In most cases, the characteristic physical, radiographic, and echocardiographic findings preclude the necessity for angiocardiographic evaluation or aortography.

THYMOMA

While there are numerous neoplasms of the thymus gland, true thymomas are uncommon in both the dog and cat.[133, 135] These tumors are solid and discrete when observed early in their course. Later they are expansile, often extending both cranially, caudally, and laterally, making surgical removal impossible. Local invasion is common but the metastatic potential of thymomas is apparently very low.[35, 136] Despite this tendency, it is often difficult to classify individual cases as malignant or benign. As previously mentioned, with this tumor's potential for local invasiveness, perhaps it is more reliable to consider this tumor's physical characteristics rather than histopathology in defining malignancy. Tumors that are fully encapsulated and noninvasive appear to carry a better prognosis for surgical resection.

The clinical signs associated with thymoma are related to both tumor size and the presence or absence of paraneoplastic syndromes.[35] Dyspnea, malaise, weight loss, and anorexia predominate in the clinical picture. Large pleural effusions are not typically present, unlike other thymic tumors. If vomition is present, it is usually related to megaesophagus rather than obstruction. As with any mass lesion of the cranial mediastinum, superior vena cava syndrome may be present.

A number of associated disorders have been recognized; these include Cushing's syndrome, myasthenia gravis, hypogammaglobulinemia, and aplastic anemia.[137] Thymoma is often recognized in the course of the workup of these disorders. As in humans, it has been reported that surgical removal of the thymoma may palliate or resolve the signs of myasthenia gravis.[112]

References

1. Proceedings of the International Symposium on the Diaphragm. Am Rev Respir Dis 119:1, 1979.
2. Campbell, EJM, et al.: The Respiratory Muscles: Mechanics and Neural Control. WB Saunders, Philadelphia, 1970.
3. Suter, PF and Lord, PF: *In* Thoracic Radiography: A Text Atlas of Thoracic Diseases of the Dog and Cat. Switzerland, PF Suter CH 8907 Wettswil, S, 1984
4. Sharp JT: Thoracoabdominal motion in chronic obstructive pulmonary disease. Am Rev Respir Dis 115:47, 1977.
5. Lillington, GA and Jamplis, RW: A Diagnostic Approach to Chest Diseases: Differential Diagnosis Based on Roentgenographic Patterns. 2nd ed. Williams & Wilkins, Baltimore, 1977.
6. Moser, K: Pulmonary embolism: State of the art. Am Rev Respir Dis 115:829, 1977.
7. Fraser, RG and Pare, JAP: Diagnosis of Diseases of the Chest. WB Saunders, Philadelphia, 1979.
8. Spitzer, SA, et al.: Transient bilateral diaphragmatic paralysis. Chest 64:355, 1973.
9. Chrisman, CL: Problems in Small Animal Neurology. Lea & Febiger, Philadelphia, 1982.
10. Miller, ME, et al.: Anatomy of the Dog. WB Saunders, Philadelphia, 1964.
11. Loh, L, et al.: The assessment of diaphragmatic function. Medicine 56:165, 1977.

12. Feldman, DB, et al.: Congenital diaphragmatic hernia in neonatal dogs. JAVMA 153:942, 1968.
13. Stevenson, DE: Congenital diaphragmatic hernia in beagle pups. J Sm Anim Pract 4:339, 1963.
14. Bernatz, PE, et al.: Problem of the ruptured diaphragm. JAMA 168:877, 1958.
15. Brasmer, TH and Witter, RE: Diaphragmatic hernia: A series of cases. No Am Vet 33:108, 1952.
16. Kent, GL: Feline diaphragmatic hernia. JAVMA 116:348, 1950.
17. Carb, A: Diaphragmatic hernia in the dog. JAVMA 136:559, 1960.
18. Toomey, A and Bograb, MJ: Traumatic diaphragmatic hernias. Comp Cont Educ 11:866, 1980.
19. Wilson, GP, et al.: A review of 116 diaphragmatic hernias in dogs and cats. JAVMA 159:1142, 1971.
20. Walker, RG and Hall, LW: Rupture of the diaphragm: Report of 32 cases in dogs and cats. Vet Rec 77:830, 1965.
21. Barrett, RB and Kittrell, JE: Congenital peritoneopericardial diaphragmatic hernia in a cat. J Am Vet Rad Soc 7:21, 1966.
22. Bolton, GR, et al.: Congenital peritoneopericardial diaphragmatic hernia in a dog. JAVMA 155:723, 1969.
23. Avery, EE, et al.: Critically crushed chests. J Thorac Surg 32:291, 1956.
24. Blair, E: Pulmonary barriers to oxygen transport in chest trauma. Am J Surg 42:55, 1976.
25. Fulton, RL and Peter, ET: Physiologic effects of fluid therapy after pulmonary contusion. Am J Surg 126:773, 1973.
26. LeRoux, BT and Stemmler, P: Maintenance of chest wall stability: A further report. Thorax 26:424, 1971
27. Moore, BP: Operative stabilization of non-penetrative chest injuries. J Thorac Cardiovasc Surg 70:619, 1974.
28. Paris, F: Surgical stabilization of traumatic flail chest. Thorax 30:521, 1975.
29. Davidson, IA: Crush injuries of the chest. Thorax 24:563, 1969.
30. Jette, NT and Barash, PG: Treatment of flail injury of the chest. Anaesthesia 32:475, 1977.
31. Read, RA: Successful treatment of organizing hemothorax by decortication in a dog–a case report. JAAHA 17:167, 1981.
32. Griffith, GL: Acute traumatic hemothorax. Ann Thorac Surg 26:204, 1978.
33. Wilson, SM: Traumatic hemothorax: Is decortication necessary? J Thorac Cardiovasc Surg 77:489, 1979.
34. Brody, RS, et al.: Canine skeletal chondrosarcoma: A clinicopathologic study of 35 cases. JAVMA 165:68, 1974.
35. Theilen, GH and Madewell, BR: Tumors of the respiratory tract and thorax. *In* Veterinary Cancer Medicine. Lea & Febiger, Philadelphia, 1987.
36. Wolke, RE and Nielsen, SW: Site incidence of canine osteosarcoma. J Sm Anim Pract 7:489, 1966.
37. Chester, DK: Multiple cartilaginous exostoses in two generations of dogs. JAVMA 15:895, 1971.
38. Pool, RR and Carrig, CB: Multiple cartilaginous exostoses in a cat. Vet Path 9:350, 1972.
39. Brody, RS, et al.: Metastatic bone neoplasms in the dog. JAVMA 148:29, 1966.
40. Stelzer, P and Gay, WA: Tumors of the chest wall. Surg Clin North Am 60:779, 1980.
41. Krook, L: A statistical investigation of carcinoma in the dog. Acta Pathol Microbiol Scand 35:407, 1954.
42. Misdorp, W: Malignant mammary tumors in the dog and cat compared with the same in the woman. Dissertation, Univ. of Utrecht, 1964.
43. Wang, NS: The regional difference of pleural mesothelial cells in rabbits. Ann Rev Respir Dis 110:623, 1974.
44. Miserocchi, G and Agostoni, E: Pleural liquid and surface pressures at various lung volumes. Respir Physiol 39:315, 1980.
45. Stewart, PB and Burgen, ASV: The turnover of fluid in the dog's pleural cavity. J Lab Clin Med 52:212, 1958.
46. McLaughlin, RF, et al.: A study of the subgross pulmonary anatomy in various mammals. JAMA 175:149, 1961.
47. Higgins, GM and Graham, AS: Lymphatic drainage from the peritoneal cavity in the dog. Arch Surg 19:453, 1929.
48. Lemon, WS and Higgins, GM: Lymphatic absorbtion of particulate matter through the normal and the paralyzed diaphragm: An experimental study. Am J Med Sci 178:536, 1929.
49. Kinasewitz, GT and Fishman, AP: Influence of alterations in Starling forces on visceral pleural fluid movement. J Appl Physiol 51:671, 1981.
50. Rabinov, K, et al.: Tension hydrothorax—an unrecognized danger. Thorax 21:465, 1966.
51. Davis, S, et al.: The shape of a pleural effusion. Br Med J 1:437, 1963.
52. Fleischner, FG: Atypical arrangement of free pleural effusion. Radiol Clin N Am 1:347, 1963.
53. Bauer, TG and Thomas, WP: Pulmonary edema. *In* Kirk, RW (ed): Current Veterinary Therapy VIII. WB Saunders, Philadelphia, 1983.
54. DeFrancis, N, et al.: Needle biopsy of parietal pleura: Preliminary report. N Engl J Med 252:948, 1955.
55. Moghissi, K: A new type of pleural biopsy instrument. Br Med J 1:1534, 1961.
56. Carpenter, RL and Lowell, JR: Pleural biopsy and thoracocentesis by new instrument. Dis Chest 40:182, 1961.
57. Harvey, C and Harvey, HP: Subclavian lymph node, pleural and pulmonary biopsy in diagnosis of intrathoracic disease. Postgrad Med J 34:204, 1958.
58. Abrams, LD: A pleural biopsy punch. Lancet 1:30, 1958.
59. Cope, C: New pleural biopsy needle. JAMA 167:1107, 1958.
60. Mungall, IPF, et al.: Multiple pleural biopsy with the Abrams needle. Thorax 35:600, 1980.
61. Schools, GS: Needle biopsy of parietal pleura: A current status. Texas State J Med 59:1056, 1963.
62. Ash, SR and Manfredi, F: Directed biopsy using small endoscope. N Engl J Med 291:1398, 1974.
63. Boushy, SF, et al.: Thoracoscopy: Technique and results in eighteen patients with pleural effusion. Chest 74:386, 1978.
64. Oldenburg, FA and Newhouse, MT: Thoracoscopy: A safe, accurate diagnostic procedure using the rigid thoracoscope and local anesthesia. Chest 75:45, 1979.
65. Estenne, M, et al.: Mechanism of relief of dyspnea after thoracocentesis in patients with large pleural effusions. Am J Med 74:813, 1983.
66. Bauer, TG: Pyothorax. Current Veterinary Therapy IX. WB Saunders, Philadelphia, 1986.
67. Simpson, K: Death from vagal inhibition. Lancet 1:551, 1949.
68. Bernstein, A: Re-expansion pulmonary edema. Chest 77:708, 1980.
69. Bauer, T and Thomas, WP: Pulmonary diagnostic techniques. Vet Clin N Am 13:273, 1983.
70. Miller, WC, et al.: Experimental pulmonary edema following re-expansion of pneumothorax. Am Rev Respir Dis 108:664, 1973.
71. Paolin, J and Cheney, FW: Unilateral pulmonary edema in rabbits after re-expansion of collapsed lung. J Appl Physiol 46:31, 1979.
72. Mellins, RB, et al.: Effect of systemic and pulmonary venous hypertension on pleural and pericardial fluid accumulation. J Appl Physiol 29:564, 1970.
73. Creighton, SR and Wilkins, RS: Pleural effusion. *In* Kirk, RW (ed): Current Veterinary Therapy. WB Saunders, Philadelphia, 1977.
74. Meyer, PC: Metatastic carcinoma of the pleura. Thorax 21:437, 1966.
75. Wang, NS: The preformed stomas connecting the pleural cavity with the lymphatics in the parietal pleura. Ann Rev Respir Dis 111:12, 1975.
76. Leckie, WJH and Tothill, P: Albumen turnover in pleural effusions. Clin Sci 29:339, 1965.
77. Stann, SE and Bauer, TG: Respiratory tract tumors. Vet Clin N Am 3:535, 1985.
78. Austin, EH and Flye, MW: The treatment of recurrent malignant pleural effusion. Ann Thorac Surg 28:190, 1979.
79. Good, JT and Sahn, SA: Intrapleural therapy with tetracycline in malignant pleural effusions. The importance of proper technique. Chest 74:602, 1978.
80. Desser, RK, et al.: The management of malignant pleural effusions (monograph). Materia Medica Division, Creative Annex, Inc, New York, 1984.
81. Pearson, FG and MacGregor, DC: Talc poudrage for malignant pleural effusion. J Thorac Cardiovasc Surg 51:732, 1966.
82. Taylor, SA, et al.: Quinacrine in the management of malignant pleural effusion. Br J Surg 64:52, 1977.
83. Karnofsky, DA, et al.: Use of nitrogen mustards in palliative treatment of carcinoma with particular reference to bronchogenic carcinoma. Cancer 1:634, 1948.

84. Thomas, DF, et al.: Management of streptococcal empyema. Ann Thorac Surg 2:658, 1966.
85. Bartlett, JG and Gorbach, SL: Bacteriology of empyema. Lancet 1:338, 1974.
86. Sanford, JP: Guide to antimicrobial therapy. Antimicrobial Therapy Inc, West Bethesda, MD, 1987.
87. Hardy, RM: Disorders of the liver. *In* Ettinger, SJ (ed): Textbook of Internal Medicine: Veterinary Diseases of the Dog and Cat. WB Saunders, Philadelphia, 1983.
88. Sulavik, S and Katz, S: Pleural Effusion: Some Infrequently Emphasized Causes. Charles C Thomas, Springfield, IL, 1963.
89. Islam, N, et al.: Hepatic hydrothorax. Br J Dis Chest 59:222, 1965.
90. Johnston, RF and Loo, RV: Hepatic hydrothorax: Studies to determine the source of the fluid and report of thirteen cases. Ann Int Med 61:385, 1964.
91. Suter, PF and Lord, PF: Lower airway and pulmonary parenchymal diseases. *In* Suter, PF: Thoracic Radiography: A Text Atlas of Thoracic Diseases of the Dog and Cat. Wettsweil, Switzerland, 1984.
92. Kay, MD: Pleuropulmonary complications of pancreatitis. Thorax 23:397, 1968.
93. Egdahl, RH: Mechanism of blood enzyme changes following the production of experimental pancreatitis. Ann Surg 148:389, 1958.
94. Perry, TT: Role of lymphatic vessels in the transmission of lipase in disseminated pancreatic fat necrosis. Arch Pathol 43:456, 1947.
95. Finley, BS, et al.: The management of non-malignant intrathoracic esophageal perforations. Ann Thorac Surg 30:575, 1980.
96. Michel, L, et al.: Operative and nonoperative management of esophageal perforations. Ann Surg 194:57, 1981.
97. DiBartola, SP and Chew, DS: Glomerular disease in the dog and cat. *In* Kirk, RW (ed): Current Veterinary Therapy IX. WB Saunders, Philadelphia, 1986.
98. Lord, PF, et al.: Lung lobe torsion in the dog. JAAHA 9:473, 1973.
99. Blalock, A, et al.: Experimental production of chylothorax by occlusion of the superior vena cava. Ann Surg 104:359, 1936.
100. Chapman, JS: The reaction of serous cavities to blood. J Lab Clin Med 46:48, 1955.
101. Cohen, S and Ward, P: In vitro and in vivo activity of a lymphocyte and immune complex dependent chemotactic factor for eosinophils. J Exp Med 133:133, 1971.
102. Kabaker, I: Contribution a l'etude experimentale des pleuresies a eosinophiles au cours du pneumothorax artificiel (English abstract). Stassbouro Med 95:277, 1935.
103. Chapman, JS: Effects of solvents on eosinophilic stimulating substance of erythrocyte stroma. Proc Soc Exp Biol Med 51:516, 1961.
104. Wasserman, SI, et al.: Tumor associated eosinophilotactic factor. N Engl J Med 290:420, 1974.
105. Harpster, NK: Chylothorax. *In* Kirk, RW (ed): Current Veterinary Therapy IX. WB Saunders, Philadelphia, 1986.
106. Seriff, NS, et al.: Chylothorax: Diagnosis by lipoprotein electrophoresis of serum and pleural fluid. Thorax 32:98, 1977.
107. Denborough, MA and Nestel, PJ: Milky effusions. Med J Aust 2:874, 1964.
108. Hughs, RL, et al.: The management of chylothorax. Chest 76:212, 1979.
109. Williams, KR and Burford, TH: The management of chylothorax. Ann Surg 160:131, 1964.
110. Patterson, DF and Munson, TO: Traumatic chylothorax in small animals treated by ligation of the thoracic duct. JAVMA 133:452, 1958.
111. Bradley, R and DeYoung, DW: Chylothorax with concurrent chyloabdomen in a dog. VM/SAC 72:1024, 1977.
112. Suter, PF and Lord, PF: Mediastinal abnormalities. *In* Suter, PF: Thoracic Radiography: A Text Atlas of Thoracic Diseases of the Dog and Cat. Wettsweil, Switzerland, 1984.
113. Strausser, JL and Flye, MW: Management of non-traumatic chylothorax. Ann Thorac Surg 31:520, 1981.
114. Dines, DE, et al.: Pneumothorax (monograph). Mayo Clinic & Mayo Foundation, Rochester, 1983.
115. Simmons, DH and Hemingway, A: Acute respiratory effects of pneumothorax in normal and vagotomized dogs. Am Rev Tuberc 76:195, 1957.
116. Walker, RG: Traumatic pneumothorax in small animals. Vet Rec 71:859, 1959.
117. Yoshioka, MM: Management of spontaneous pneumothorax in twelve dogs. JAAHA 18:57, 1982.
118. Schaer, M, et al.: Spontaneous pneumothorax associated with bacterial pneumonia in the dog: Two case reports. JAAHA 17:783, 1981.
119. Antoni, RO and Ponka, JL: The hazards of iatrogenic pneumothorax in certain diagnostic and therapeutic procedures. Surg Gynecol Obstet 113:24, 1961.
120. Park, RD and Parker, AJ: Radiographic manifestations of exudative pleuritis in the cat. Feline Pract 4:40, 1974.
121. Robertson, SA, et al.: Thoracic empyema in the dog; a report of twenty-two cases. J Sm Anim Pract 24:103, 1983.
121a. Myer, W: Radiography review: The mediastinum. J Am Vet Rad Soc 19:197, 1978.
122. Thomas, WP, et al.: Detection of cardiac masses by two dimensional echocardiography. J Vet Radiol 25:65, 1984.
123. Carlens, E: Mediastinoscopy. A method for inspection and tissue biopsy in the superior mediastinum. Dis Chest 36:343, 1959.
124. Kohler, H: Spontaneous fatal hemorrhage in the thymus gland of dogs. Wiener Tieraztl Mschr 62:341, 1975.
125. Bernard, WF: A study of the pathogenesis and management of spontaneous pneumothorax. Dis Chest 42:403, 1962.
126. Macklin, CC: Pneumothorax with massive collapse from experimental local over-inflation of lung substance. Can Med Assoc 36:414, 1937.
127. Ackerman, N, et al.: Respiratory distress associated with histoplasma-induced tracheobronchial lymphadenopathy in dogs. JAVMA 163:963, 1973.
128. Maddy, KT: Disseminated coccidioidomycosis of the dog. JAVMA 132:483, 1958.
129. Menges, RW: Blastomycosis in animals. Vet Med 55:45, 1960.
130. Olsson, SE: On tuberculosis in the dog. A study with special reference to x-ray diagnosis. Cornell Vet 47:193, 1957.
131. Ackerman, N and Madewell, BR: Thoracic and abdominal radiographic abnormalities in the multicentric form of lymphosarcoma in dogs. JAVMA 176:36, 1980.
132. Eigenmann, EJ: Endocrine Tumors. *In* Theilen, GH and Madewell, BR (eds): Veterinary Cancer Medicine, 2nd ed. Lea & Febiger, Philadelphia, 1987.
133. Jubb, K and Kennedy, P: Pathology of Domestic Animals, 2nd ed. Academic Press, New York and London, 1970.
134. Ettinger, SJ and Suter, PF: Canine Cardiology. WB Saunders, Philadelphia, 1970.
135. Parker, GA and Casey, HW: Thymomas in domestic animals. Vet Pathology 13:353, 1976.
136. Mitcham, SA, et al.: Malignant thymoma with widespread metastases in a dog: Case report and brief literature review. Can Vet J 25:280, 1984.
137. Batata, MA: Thymomas: Clinicopathologic features, therapy and prognosis. Cancer 34:389, 1974.

SECTION VIII

THE CARDIOVASCULAR SYSTEM

71 PATHOPHYSIOLOGY OF HEART FAILURE

DAVID H. KNIGHT

Heart failure occurs when blood returning to the heart cannot be pumped out at a rate commensurate with the metabolic demands of the body. The syndrome represents a complex interaction of compensatory responses that attempt to preserve nominal cardiac function and regional blood flow. This is achieved with variable success, depending on the severity of the underlying cardiac disease and the extent to which overuse of compensatory mechanisms produces deleterious side effects. It should be understood that in addition to a complex pathogenesis, heart failure has many etiologies (Table 71–1). Therefore, it cannot be defined in simple, universally applicable terms. Conditions that impose volume or pressure systolic mechanical overloads on the heart, depress myocardial contractility, interfere with ventricular filling, or increase systemic metabolic requirements compromise cardiac function and elicit some combination of compensatory responses. Consequently, the clinical presentation of heart failure is neither uniform nor necessarily obvious. Before rational decisions can be made regarding therapeutic options, it is essential that each patient be individually evaluated to determine what is causing the heart to fail and which compensatory responses are in greatest need of modification in order to alleviate the clinical manifestations of heart failure.

A distinction has been made between *myocardial*, *heart*, and *circulatory failures*.[1] If myocardial contractility is sufficiently depressed, heart (pump) failure will ensue and perfusion will be inadequate. This cascade of complications with increasingly wide ramifications illustrates the fundamental importance of ventricular contractility to the integrity of the circulatory system. However, depressed contractility (myocardial failure) is not an a priori prerequisite for heart failure. The heart may fail acutely without loss of contractility if it is suddenly subjected to an unmanageable load. For example, acute mitral regurgitation resulting from rupture of primary chordae tendineae could produce hemodynamic instability and a severe decline in useful cardiac work due entirely to mechanical inefficiency of the pump. In this instance, normal myocardial function is only a transient state, since heart failure caused by chronic hemodynamic overloading eventually depresses contractility.[2] Also, interference with venous return due to cardiac tamponade or restrictive pericarditis unloads the ventricles during diastole despite high filling pressure and severely compromises cardiac output without any direct adverse effect on contractility. The peripheral circulatory responses to either a hemodynamic overload or inhibition of ventricular filling are similar and signs of congestion and edema develop.

Although circulatory failure is usually attributable to

TABLE 71–1. POTENTIAL CAUSES OF HEART FAILURE IN DOGS AND CATS

Myocardial Dysfunction	Systolic Mechanical Overload		Diastolic Mechanical Inhibition	Hyperkinetic Circulation
	PRESSURE	VOLUME		
Idiopathic dilated cardiomyopathies*	Subaortic stenosis*	Aortic regurgitation*	Hemopericardium with cardiac tamponade	Thyrotoxicosis
Myocarditis*	Pulmonic stenosis*	Mitral regurgitation*	Neoplasia*	Pregnancy
Abnormal rhythm	Pulmonary hypertension (heartworm disease)*	Tricuspid regurgitation*	Pericarditis*	Pyrexia
Taurine deficiency (cats only)*			Left atrial tear*	Anemia
	Systemic hypertension	Left to right shunts Patent ductus arteriosus* Ventricular septal defect* Peripheral arteriovenous fistula Overtransfusion	Restrictive pericarditis Feline hypertrophic cardiomyopathy*	

*Major, primary causes of heart failure. Other causes are either infrequent or contribute secondarily to the onset of failure in already compromised hearts.

heart failure, it may also occur in the absence of primary cardiac dysfunction. Hypovolemia can lower blood pressure and produce circulatory collapse (shock) by underloading a normal heart. Conversely, profound anemia and high metabolic states may create a mismatch in circulatory supply and demand that exceeds the capacity of the normal heart. Eventually, if circulatory failure is not corrected, cardiac function will deteriorate. Therefore, when either heart or circulatory failure develops, the clinician must be concerned about the preservation of myocardial function regardless of whether it was depressed initially.

Heart failure is a complicated topic that is often made more confusing by the vague and interchangeable use of terms that are intended to emphasize certain aspects of the syndrome. The following are brief definitions of clinically relevant and frequently used terms.

Congestive Heart Failure. This term is inclusive for the spectrum of clinical manifestations resulting from circulatory congestion and edema due to heart failure. The cardinal feature of congestive heart failure is elevated filling pressure of one or both ventricles. Regardless of etiology, the neurohumoral responses are similar. The terms congestive heart failure and heart failure may be used interchangeably.

Right- and Left-sided Heart Failure. Signs of congestion and edema may be limited to the venous circulation, organs, and body cavities draining into either the right or left sides of the heart. The terms right and left are used to designate which ventricle is failing and is responsible for the clinical manifestations. Failure of the right ventricle is associated with ascites, pleural effusion, and peripheral edema, while pulmonary edema is the hallmark of left ventricular failure. No distinction is implied by the substitution of ventricular failure for heart failure.

Generalized Heart Failure. As performance of the entire heart declines in chronic heart failure, the distinction between failure of the right and left sides is lost. Because the right and left ventricles are aligned in series and share a common septum, malfunction of one side eventually has a negative impact on the other. Signs of congestion involving both the systemic and pulmonary venous circulations are designated generalized heart failure. However, in generalized heart failure the overt signs of congestion and edema may occur predominantly behind one or the other side of the heart.

Forward and Backward Failure. These terms originated from conceptually oversimplified theories about the mechanisms of heart failure. Forward failure attributes the clinical manifestations to low cardiac output, while backward failure relates to the pooling of blood behind the ventricles, causing clinical signs of congestion and edema. Based on the current understanding of the pathogenesis of heart failure, these terms are used infrequently.

Acute and Chronic Heart Failure. The pulmonary venous circulation has a lower pressure and blood volume capacity than the systemic venous circulation, and therefore it is less able to accommodate hemodynamic imbalances. Consequently, pulmonary edema may develop very rapidly. Because of its critical effect on respiration, the clinical manifestations tend to become evident sooner and have more serious implications. Under these circumstances, the onset of left heart failure may be described as being "acute." If it persists or the patient is marginally in and out of failure over an extended period of time, the term "chronic" is more applicable. On the other hand, edema accumulates more slowly in the larger systemic venous circulation. Because it causes less functional impairment, it can be tolerated for a relatively long time. Since the clinical signs of right heart failure have an insidious onset and are not immediately evident, the term "chronic" is ordinarily more appropriate in that context.

High Output Heart Failure. High output failure designates a state in which cardiac output is substantially elevated before the onset of clinical signs and remains elevated until late in the clinical course of failure. Conditions causing a reduction in peripheral vascular resistance due to increased metabolism or a peripheral arteriovenous fistula necessitate a compensatory increase in cardiac output, leading to a hyperkinetic circulation. Since this is only possible when blood volume is expanded, the signs of high output failure are largely indistinguishable from other causes of heart failure if the hyperkinetic features are not put into proper perspective. As ventricular function declines late in the course of severe high output failure, cardiac output may return to the normal range.

Compensated Heart Failure. Compensated heart failure implies that cardiac output can be maintained in the normal range at rest or increased to a limited extent during exertion at the expense of deleterious side effects resulting from an interplay of compensatory mechanisms. Signs of congestion and edema are usually prominent features.

Decompensated Heart Failure. A decompensated failing heart is unable to maintain normal cardiac output even at rest despite full use of compensatory mechanisms. Thus, low output heart failure is a late development characterized by cachexia, renal insufficiency, and mental dullness, in addition to signs of congestion and edema.

Refractory Heart Failure. When heart failure persists despite all attempts to control heart rate, increase contractility, or favorably modify filling pressure and outflow impedance, it is considered to be intractable. These patients usually display signs of both low cardiac output and congestion. Some cases that have been classified as intractable in the past may be responsive to the more vigorous treatments currently being practiced.

DETRIMENTS OF CARDIAC OUTPUT

The product of heart rate and ventricular stroke volume is the simplest expression of cardiac output.[3, 4] The ability of the ventricle to perform work by ejecting a volume of blood (stroke volume) can be analyzed in terms of myocardial contractility and the forces stretching the relaxed myocardium or opposing shortening during contraction, i.e., the preload and afterload. The following construct illustrates the effect of these variables on cardiac output:

$$\text{Heart Rate} \times \frac{\text{Contractility} \times \text{Preload}}{\text{Afterload}}$$

Under normal circumstances, heart rate is the major determinant of transient changes in cardiac output, as long as stroke volume remains relatively stable. At any level of contractility, stroke volume varies directly with preload and inversely with afterload. Factors that have a major effect on preload, afterload, and contractility are listed in Table 71–2. The relationships of these three variables to the pressure/volume events of the cardiac cycle are explained in Figure 71–1.

HEART RATE

Heart rate is normally determined by how rapidly diastolic depolarization (phase 4 of the action potential) of the sinoatrial pacemaker cells reaches the threshold potential. The frequency of discharge is under autonomic control. Acetylcholine released from parasympathetic nerves slows the heart, and norepinephrine released from sympathetic nerves and the adrenal medulla has a positive chronotropic effect. An increase or decrease in the activity of one component of the autonomic nervous system is usually accompanied by a reciprocal change in the other. In heart failure, adrenergic control is defective. The normal heart rate increase in response to exercise or a fall in blood pressure may be attenuated due to the high level of circulating catecholamines and an abnormally elevated heart rate at rest.[5] Also, the parasympathetically mediated baroreceptor reflex that slows heart rate in response to elevated blood pressure may be blunted.[6] Abnormalities in the arterial baroreflex control of heart rate are at least partially reversible if heart failure is successfully treated.[7]

A modest increase in contractility occurs at accelerated heart rates (Bowditch effect). This is less apparent in normal conscious dogs than in anesthetized dogs with depressed hearts or in isolated cardiac muscle.[8] The positive inotropic effect associated with increases in heart rate appears to be largest when the rate change occurs over the low end of the physiologic range of heart rates.[9] Merely pacing the heart of a normal, conscious dog does not produce a sustained increase in cardiac output because peripheral blood flow is reflexively adjusted to systemic metabolic requirements.[10] Pacing raises output only if ventricular volume is maintained during diastole by expanding the blood volume. Normally, during exercise (or other circumstances increasing oxygen consumption) a reduction in peripheral arteriolar vascular resistance facilitates venous return to the heart and maintains ventricular diastolic volume. The increase in cardiac output is usually directly proportional to heart rate under these conditions. However, at very high heart rates, diastole becomes sufficiently short to compromise ventricular filling and limit further increases in cardiac output. Conversely, stroke volume reaches a maximum at slow heart rates. When heart rate is also fixed, as in complete heart block, the ability to adjust cardiac output is seriously impaired even if myocardial function is normal.

The relationship between stroke volume (cardiac output) and heart rate is complex. Some coherence to the cardiac output/heart rate relationship has recently been provided.[11] Ventricular filling pressure (preload), myocardial contractility, and state of the arterial vasculature (afterload) influence stroke volume independently and in combination. The change in stroke volume with heart rate depends on the effect heart rate has on these variables. The heart rate at which maximal cardiac output is achieved differs with the circumstances.

An inverse relationship exists between heart rate and stroke volume. The rate at which stroke volume declines tends toward zero as heart rate increases (Figure 71–2 *A*). On the other hand, stroke volume remains relatively constant at very low heart rates. The rate at which stroke volume declines as heart rate accelerates is greatest when stroke volume is small to begin with (Figure 71–2*B*). Under these conditions, cardiac output actually may fall as heart rate increases (Figure 71–2*C*). However, if stroke volume is large initially, a rise in cardiac output accompanies an increase in heart rate despite a decrease in stroke volume. Somewhere in between these extremes, an increase in heart rate may produce no change in cardiac output. Since heart rate is a major determinant of myocardial oxygen consumption, cardiac efficiency depends on the preservation of stroke volume relative to heart rate so that the energy expended by cardiac acceleration will produce an increase in cardiac output.

PRELOAD

The tension generated by contracting striated muscle (cardiac or skeletal), and therefore the velocity and extent of shortening against the same afterload, is a function of sarcomere length. The length to which myocardial fibers are stretched in the intact heart is determined by the effective (transmural) filling pressure

TABLE 71–2. FACTORS INFLUENCING THE THREE MAJOR DETERMINANTS OF VENTRICULAR PERFORMANCE

Preload	Afterload	Contractility
Blood volume	Arterial pressure	Sympathetic nerve stimulation
Body position	Vasomotion	Circulating catecholamine
Skeletal muscle venous pump	Vascular stiffness	Intrinsic myocardial depression
Venous tone (neurogenic)	Ventricular chamber radius	Loss of myocardium
Intrathoracic pressure	Ventricular wall thickness	Pharmacologic agents
Intrapericardial pressure	Preload	Metabolic factors
Atrial contraction		Hypoxia
Ejection fraction		Hypercapnia
		Acidosis
		Postextrasystolic potentiation

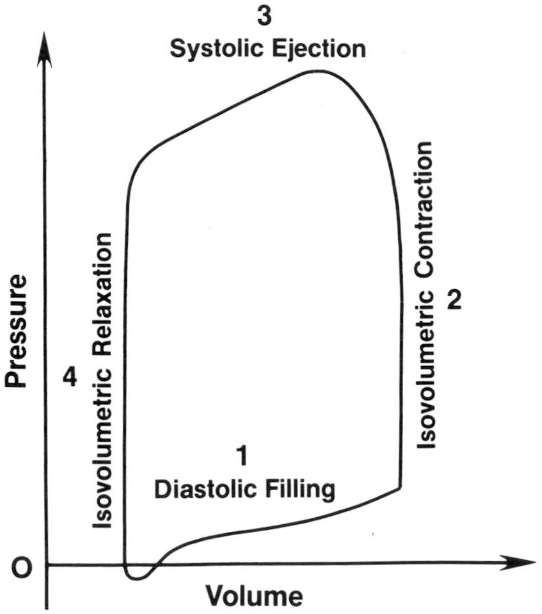

FIGURE 71–1. Simultaneous changes in intraventricular pressure (P) and volume (V) during the normal cardiac cycle are depicted in a loop diagram. Phase I is the filling period between the opening and closing of the atrioventricular (AV) valve. The extent of filling determines the preload (myocardial fiber length) at the onset of systole (Phase 2). During this second phase, an isovolumetric contraction takes place while the AV and semilunar (SL) valves are both closed. Normally, ejection begins with the opening of the SL valve at the onset of Phase 3. The load opposing muscle fiber shortening (afterload) varies during the systolic period. Afterload incorporates the intraventricular pressure and ventricular geometry (chamber radius and wall thickness) as expressed by wall tension in the LaPlace relationship. Systole continues until the active contractile process reaches a maximum.[26] This condition is achieved when the elastance (stiffness) of the muscle fibers is maximal (E max). E max can be approximated by the upper left corner of the loop diagram where the P/V ratio also reaches a maximum. Since E max is essentially unaffected by loading conditions, it can be used as an index of myocardial contractility. Ejection ceases shortly after completion of the active contractile process. At that time, the SL valve closes and the ventricle begins to relax isovolumetrically until the AV valve reopens and the cycle repeats.

The area within the P/V loop represents the net work performed by the ventricle. Early in diastole, ventricular filling may be an active process in which elastic recoil in the ventricular wall sucks blood into the chamber.[15] Once the equilibrium volume is restored, the hydrostatic pressure of blood returning to the heart performs work on the ventricle during the remainder of Phase I.

or preload. This relationship between resting length of the contractile units (sarcomeres) and active tension has an anatomic basis in the degree of overlapping between the actin and myosin filaments (Figure 71–3).[12] As the sarcomere is progressively stretched toward an optimal length (2.2 μ), the number of Ca^{++}-activated cross bridges between filaments increases, resulting in a progressively more forceful contraction (Figure 71–4).

This fundamental property of cardiac muscle is the basis for the Frank-Starling phenomenon, also known as Starling's law of the heart. By this mechanism of heterometric autoregulation, the right and left ventricles are able to adjust their respective outputs to beat-to-beat differences in venous return. In this way a balance is achieved over several beats between the outputs from both sides of the heart. In cats and dogs, the upper limit of normal left ventricular filling pressure stretches the sarcomeres to the length producing peak tension during contraction (Figure 71–5).[13] This means that contraction normally begins somewhere on the ascending limb of the sarcomere length–active tension curve. At physiologic end-diastolic pressures, sarcomeres are stretched to their optimal length in the midwall of the left ventricle and to a lesser extent on both sides of this zone.[13] Since sarcomere length increases across the full thickness of the wall as filling pressure rises, it has been hypothesized that lengthening of sarcomeres in the inner and outer regions of the wall enables the Frank-Starling mechanism to also operate in the range of pathologically high preloads.[14]

In the normal mammalian ventricle, an equilibrium volume exists at which filling pressure is zero. During systole, the ventricle becomes smaller than the equilibrium volume and some of the energy of contraction is stored, to be expended as an elastic recoil at the onset

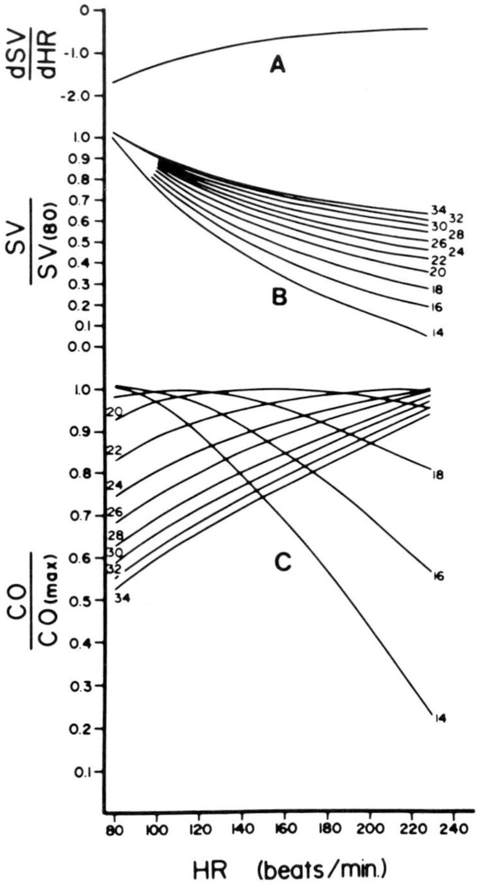

FIGURE 71–2. *A*, Quadratic regression function representing the stroke volume-heart rate (dSV/dHR) relationship in dogs. The dSV/dHR function is HR-dependent and tends toward zero at high heart rates. *B*, Family of curves representing the SV-HR function normalized with respect to the SV at a HR of 80 beats per minute (SV_{80}) plotted as the ratio of actual SV to SV_{80}. The value of the SV used for normalization is shown to the right of each curve. SVs were largest at 80 beats per minute and the smaller this value, the more rapidly it declined with increasing HR. *C*, Family of curves resulting from multiplication of SV by HR to yield cardiac output (CO), each normalized to its respective maximum CO value. Parameters identify output curves with associated SV ratio curves (B). Depending on the value of SV80 and the range of HRs, CO may increase, decrease, or remain essentially unchanged. (From Melbin, J, et al.: Coherence of cardiac output with rate changes. Am J Physiol 243:H499, 1982, by permission of the American Physiologic Society.)

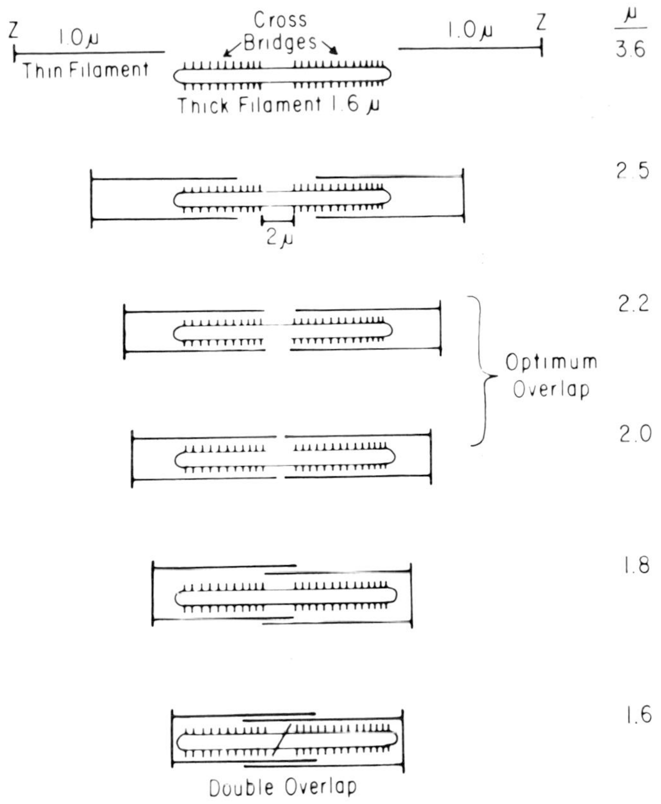

FIGURE 71–3. Schematic representation of the relative positions of the thick myosin filaments and the thin actin filaments in vertebrate striated muscle at six selected sarcomere lengths ranging from 1.6 μ to 3.6 μ. The area of overlap between actin filaments and portions of the myosin filaments containing force-generating cross-bridges remains constant between 2.0 μ and 2.2 μ and decreases linearly at lengths beyond 2.2 μ. (From Sonnenblick, EH and Skelton, CL: Reconsideration of the ultrastructural basis of cardiac length-tension relations. Circ Res 35:517, 1974, by permission of the American Heart Association.)

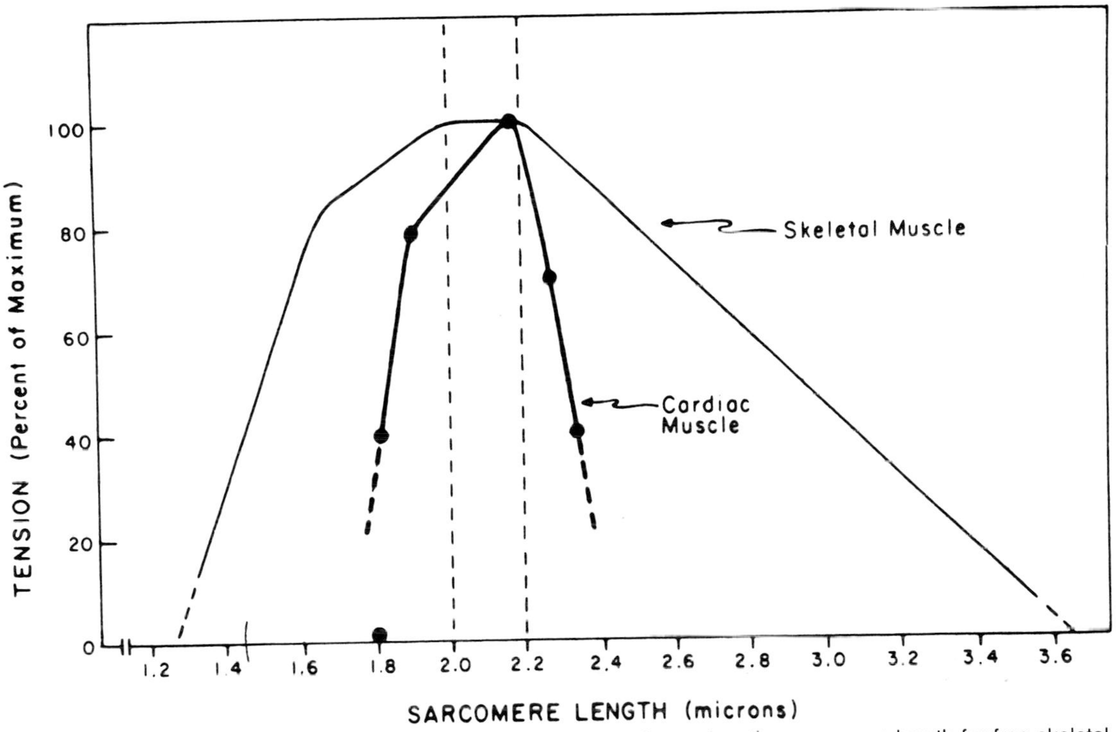

FIGURE 71–4. Relation between actively developed isometric tension and resting sarcomere length for frog skeletal muscle fibers and cat right ventricular papillary muscles. The curve for skeletal muscle fibers is derived from the data of Gordon et al.[77] In both tissues, peak developed tension is attained at a sarcomere length of 2.2 μ. At a sarcomere length of 2.0 μ, tension development is substantially decreased in cardiac muscle but remains maximal in skeletal muscle. At sarcomere lengths less than 2.0 μ, developed force falls in both types of muscle, but it falls more precipitously in cardiac tissue. At sarcomere lengths longer than 2.0 μ, cardiac muscle is resistant to further extension and its developed force declines precipitously compared with the linear fall determined for skeletal muscle. In cardiac muscle, this decrease in force cannot be entirely explained by sarcomere elongation and a decrease in myofilament overlap. (From Sonnenblick, EH and Skelton, CL: Reconsideration of the ultrastructural basis of cardiac length-tension relations. Circ Res 35:517, 1974, by permission of the American Heart Association.)

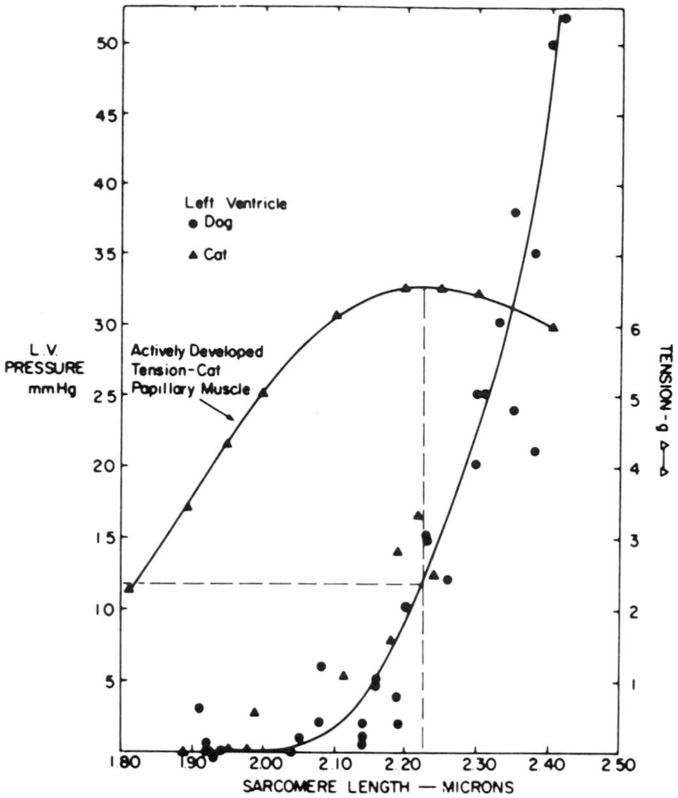

FIGURE 71–5. Relation between left ventricular pressure and average sarcomere length in the midwall of a canine left ventricle. The upper curve represents the relation between tension development and sarcomere length, as obtained from studies of cat papillary muscle. The lower curve relates left ventricular filling pressure to midwall sarcomere length for both dog and cat. At a left ventricular filling pressure of 12 mmHg, which approximates the upper limit of normal filling pressure in the intact animal, average midwall sarcomere length is about 2.2 μ. This sarcomere length is also associated with the upper limits of the length–active tension curve, as shown by the vertical dashed line. Further increments in filling pressure yield only minor further increments in sarcomere length for very large increments in filling pressure. (From Spotnitz, JH, et al.: Relation of ultrastructure to function in the intact heart: Sarcomere structure relative to pressure-volume curves of the intact left ventricles of dog and cat. Circ Res 18:49, 1966, by permission of the American Heart Association.)

of diastole. This produces a negative filling pressure at the beginning of diastole and blood may actually be sucked into the ventricle.[15] The elastic recoil is strongest in vigorously contracting ventricles that achieve a small end-systolic volume. It is not ordinarily apparent in the failing heart that empties poorly and must operate at a higher filling pressure and larger end-diastolic volume in order to achieve a more favorable length–active tension relationship. Under these conditions, it appears that the response of the depressed myocardium is better characterized by the Frank-Starling mechanism.

The ventricular diastolic pressure-volume relationship is curvilinear (Figure 71–5). In the normal ventricle, the early phase of diastole proceeds rapidly at a low filling pressure. However, as the chamber dilates, it becomes progressively less distensible or compliant (dV/dP) and an exponential increase in filling pressure is required if blood is to continue flowing into the ventricle. Consequently, in dilated ventricles, particularly at large chamber volumes, acute increases in end-diastolic volume may require filling pressures that exceed the physiologic range. This increase in hydrostatic pressure is a major contributing factor in the pathogenesis of edema. Over time, chronic high filling pressure can shift the diastolic pressure-volume relationship so that larger end-diastolic volumes can be achieved without further increases in pressure.[16] This is made possible by lengthening myocardial cells through the addition of sarcomeres and slippage between adjacent cells rather than progressive stretching of sarcomeres.

Ischemia, fibrosis, and incomplete relaxation during tachycardia decrease ventricular compliance by making the myocardium less distensible.[4] Also, an increase in wall thickness independent of the mechanical properties of the myocardium impedes ventricular filling. This accounts for the lower filling pressure of the normal right ventricle compared to the left and the reduction in ventricular diastolic function often associated with concentric hypertrophy (see later).[17] Decreased ventricular compliance impairs diastolic function and, by necessitating abnormally high preloads, seriously limits the extent to which the Frank-Starling mechanism can be used to advantage.

A properly timed atrial systole augments stroke volume by forcibly injecting blood into the ventricular chamber and increasing the preload immediately before ventricular contraction. This is particularly important during tachycardia, when the filling cycle is abbreviated or in the presence of any condition that impedes filling by decreasing ventricular compliance.[18] Atrial fibrillation deprives the ventricles of this late diastolic boost and stroke volume declines, particularly when the heart rate is rapid. Atrial fibrillation increases the mean ventricular filling pressure and may exacerbate signs of congestion.[19]

Blood volume expansion is an important determinant of preload and the adequacy of ventricular filling. Neurohumoral regulation of venous tone is responsible for major changes in the volume and distribution of blood in the venous compartments. Venoconstriction increases the effective blood volume by reducing venous pooling, thereby promoting the return of blood to the heart and producing an increase in preload.

On the other hand, preload may be decreased in several clinical circumstances. Orthostatic pooling of blood in the limbs is not a significant problem in animals as it is in humans. Elevated intrathoracic pressure caused by pneumothorax or intermittent positive pressure respiration can have a major adverse effect on cardiac performance by impeding systemic venous return. Also by increasing ventricular extramural pressure, cardiac tamponade reduces the effective preload despite compensatory increases in filling pressure and can seriously compromise cardiac output (see Diastolic Mechanical Inhibition).

Preload reserve is an important adaptive mechanism, particularly for making immediate adjustments in ventricular function. However, its importance to chronic cardiac compensation is superseded by the development of cardiac hypertrophy, adrenergic support of the inotropic state of the myocardium, conservation of cardiac output by regional adjustments in flow distribution, and increases in heart rate.

AFTERLOAD

The time-varying tension that develops in the wall of a contracting ventricle is designated the afterload.[20] Afterload, which is expressed in units of pressure (mmHg) or stress (mmHg/cm²), is affected primarily by intraventricular pressure and chamber size. The load borne by each muscle fiber depends on the wall thickness. The relationships between wall tension (T), chamber pressure (P), radius (r), and wall thickness (h) can be represented by the LaPlace equation for thick-walled spheres ($T = Pr/2h$). As the radius of a sphere increases, the wall tension required to maintain that volume for a given distending pressure also increases. Systolic pressure reflects the product of the force-generating capability of the myocardium and the impedance to blood ejected from the ventricle. The latter is affected by the physical properties of the vascular bed downstream from the ejecting ventricle and any neurohumoral modifications imposed upon the dynamic state of the vessels.

When the afterload on a normal heart is increased abruptly, there is a brief, modest increase in contractile force that occurs after a few beats and subsequently, stroke volume is restored if the change in afterload is not large. This is known as the Anrep effect. It has little influence on the new equilibrium and is probably caused by reactive hyperemia of the myocardium as it recovers from a transient period of subendocardial ischemia.[21] More importantly, ventricular end-diastolic volume increases. The increase in preload (myocardial fiber length) is compensatory to the extent that it enables the ventricle to contract more forcefully and preserve stroke volume.

This adjustment obscures the important negative effect afterload has on stroke output. If contractility and preload remain unchanged, muscle fiber shortening decreases as afterload increases.[22] This reciprocal relationship becomes evident in normal hearts when venous return is impeded so that preload cannot rise. The negative effect of afterload is particularly evident in depressed hearts, operating at a high preload, far to the right on the diastolic function curve (Figure 71–6*B*). These hearts have already reached or possibly exceeded the optimal sarcomere length and therefore have no preload reserve remaining. If an increase in afterload is not appropriately matched by an increase in preload, stroke output declines.[23]

There is a cost associated with increased use of preload. Each increase in preload enlarges the ventricle, and as predicted by the LaPlace relationship, this further increases the afterload. However, due to geometric considerations, a net positive effect on stroke volume is preserved because at the larger chamber volume, the same stroke volume can be achieved with a smaller reduction in chamber radius.

The tension developed in muscle fibers is a powerful stimulus for hypertrophy. Myocardial hypertrophy compensates for chronic increases in afterload by distributing the force over a larger cross-sectional area, thereby returning wall stress toward normal.[24] However, if myocardial contractility is severely depressed and continues to deteriorate, neither additional increases in preload nor cardiac hypertrophy may be able to preserve cardiac function.[2]

CONTRACTILITY

Contractility is the property of muscle that determines the peak tension that can be developed starting from a specific resting fiber length. The relationship between resting length and peak isometric tension within the physiologic range is linear, and its slope is a measure of the inotropic state of the muscle.[25, 26] A more accessible measure of contractility in the intact ventricle can be derived from the end-systolic pressure-volume relationship (Figure 71–6). Although performance as it relates to muscle shortening in both excised and *in situ* hearts is sensitive to preload and afterload, contractility is, by definition, independent of both (Figure 71–6*B*,*C*).[27, 28] Preloading increases the total force of contraction by stretching the muscle (Frank-Starling mechanism) but does not affect the intrinsic length–active tension relationship. Similarly, afterload determines the extent of fiber shortening in an isotonic contraction (Figure 71–6*B*) that is possible at any inotropic state but does not affect the peak tension that would be generated by an isometric contraction at a designated preload (Figure 71–6*A*).

Chronic systolic mechanical overloading of any etiology requires the heart to perform more work at a given cardiac output. However, the myocardium possesses little reserve capacity for expending more energy.[29] Unlike skeletal muscles, the heart is a functional syncytium and is therefore unable to recruit more motor units by neuronal stimulation. Instead, the heart must respond by regulating the intensity of activity within individual myocardial cells. The adjustment involves a combination of responses that enhances the ability of the heart to pump blood and at the same time decreases its rate of energy consumption.

Sustained systolic overloading of the heart usually leads to a decline in myocardial contractility.[2] An explanation for this depressed function and its role in the pathogenesis of heart failure has been sought by examining myocardial energy supply, production, storage, and use, in addition to the structure and function of the contractile proteins. Much of the information gathered so far is conflicting and no unifying biochemical defect has been identified.[1, 30]

Heart failure can occur despite adequate coronary perfusion and delivery of oxygen to the myocardium. Furthermore, in some instances, oxidative phosphorylation remains at normal levels until late in the course of heart failure, suggesting that decreased mitochondrial energy production is not a cause of heart failure though it may play a role in perpetuating it.[1] Neither does it appear that decreased contractility is caused by a reduction of total high-energy phosphate stores, since normal concentrations of creatinine phosphate and ATP have been measured in papillary muscles removed from failing hearts.[17] In myocardial failure, chemical energy is converted into mechanical work at a reduced rate. A reduction in ATPase activity appears to be responsible.[31] Although this slows the velocity of contraction, it allows the moderately depressed myocardium to achieve normal peak tension more gradually with less oxygen consumption and thus more efficiency.[32] However, pumping efficiency is decreased by structural changes in the heart

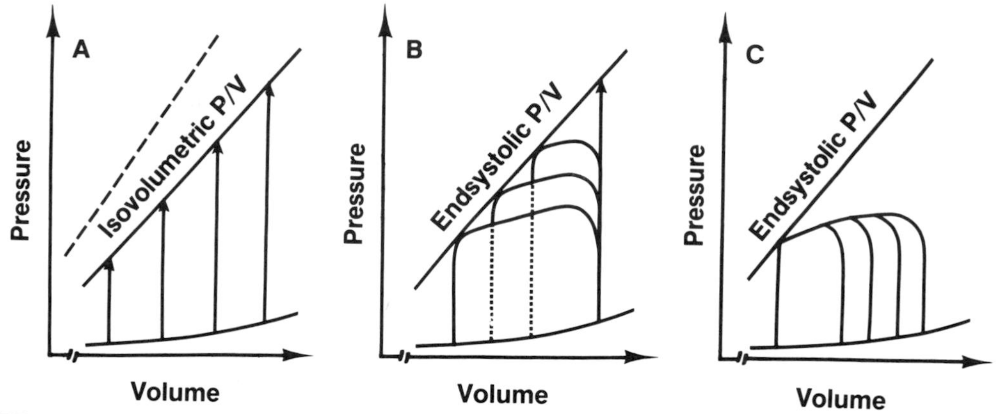

FIGURE 71–6. A schematic representation of the pressure-volume relationship in an isovolumetric *(A)* and ejecting ventricle *(B* and *C)*. *A*, If ejection is prevented by cross-clamping the aorta, an isovolumetric contraction is produced. At progressively larger volumes (preloads), the peak intraventricular pressure rises in accordance with the Frank-Starling mechanism. A straight line relationship exists between the peak pressure developed and each increment in volume. The slope of this P/V relationship reflects the inotropic state of the myocardium. Because the P/V relation line does not extrapolate to the origin, the volume axis has been shortened. If contractility increases (dashed line), as for example with adrenergic stimulation, a nonparallel, upward shift of the isovolumetric P/V line occurs. As a result, greater peak pressure is developed at each preload (fiber length). *B*, The inotropic state and ventricular filling curve are the same as in *A*. Four contractions against successively higher afterloads occur at the same preload. The first three produce ejections in which stroke volume declines as afterload increases. In each case, the end-systolic P/V relationship falls along the previously determined isovolumetric P/V line. The pressure developed in the isovolumetric fourth beat confirms the identity of this line. Both in the isovolumetric contraction and at end-systole in the ejecting ventricle, the contractile force is at a maximum for the corresponding fiber length and the muscle has reached its maximum elastance (stiffness). Consequently, the slope of the end-systolic P/V relationship can be substituted for the isovolumetric P/V relationship as an index of contractility. *C*, With contractility and end-systolic pressure held constant, four contractions at progressively higher preloads produce successively larger stroke volumes. The end-systolic P/V relationship is the same for each contraction because preload, like afterload, does not affect contractility.

(dilatation, valve dysfunction, loss of myocardial cells, fibrosis) and poor coordination of cardiac contraction caused by rhythm disturbances.

Cardiac contraction is initiated when Ca^{++} enters the myocardial cytosol from the sarcoplasmic reticulum and interacts with the regulatory proteins (tropomyosin and troponin). Ca^{++} catalyzes a complex physiochemical reaction between the contractile proteins (actin and myosin), producing a conversion of chemical energy into mechanical work.[29] The process responsible for delivering Ca^{++} to the contractile proteins is called excitation-contraction coupling. Excitatory impulses produce membrane changes that affect Ca^{++} entry into the cell and modify the phasic (beat-to-beat) control of myocardial contractility.[29] The total intracellular Ca^{++} available for contraction is normal in the depressed myocardium. However, the reuptake and binding of Ca^{++} in the sarcoplasmic reticulum at the completion of contraction is reduced. This interferes with relaxation as well as restoration of Ca^{++} in the sarcoplasmic reticulum for subsequent release during the next contraction. A redistribution occurs in which more Ca^{++} is stored in mitochondria, where it is less readily available to activate the myofilaments. High concentrations of mitochondrial Ca^{++} may also interfere with oxidative phosphorylation. Since reduction in the uptake of Ca^{++} by the sarcoplasmic reticulum occurs early in the course of myocardial failure, it may be an initiating event.[33] Abnormalities in excitation-contraction coupling may play an important role in the pathogenesis of some primary cardiomyopathies as well as severely depressing contractility secondary to chronic hemodynamic overloading. Ca^{++} interaction with contractile proteins is also critical to adrenergic stimulation of the myocardium and the action of positive and negative inotropic drugs.[1]

In the normal heart, stimulation of cardiac sympathetic nerves is the most important factor regulating the inotropic state and it is capable of producing rapid changes in contractility. Adrenal medullary release of epinephrine into the circulation is a slower, less volatile mechanism for adrenergic stimulation of the heart. In the failing heart, adrenergic neural control is defective and extracardiac adrenergic humoral stimulation plays an increasingly important role.[34] However, abnormal responsiveness to sympathetic stimulation is not a fundamental cause of intrinsic myocardial depression in heart failure.[35]

The failing heart is under progressively intense adrenergic stimulation. However, the positive chronotropic and inotropic responses to sympathetic nerve stimulation are blunted due to reductions in the synthesis, storage, and release of myocardial norepinephrine.[35, 36] The response to circulating catecholamines is also blunted by a decrease in the density of myocardial β-adrenergic receptors late in the course of the heart failure.[37] This is partially offset by an increase in plasma catecholamine concentration in patients with severe heart failure. Despite intensification of adrenergic stimulation, there is a net decrease in responsiveness of the failing heart and this may contribute to the decline in cardiac performance. Nevertheless, adrenergic stimulation remains an important support mechanism, as evidenced by the further deterioration of cardiac function that frequently follows the administration of β-adrenergic blockers to heart failure patients.

COMPENSATORY MECHANISMS

The same physiologic mechanisms that enable the normal heart to perform extraordinary amounts of work also assist the failing heart in preserving a nominal level of performance when there is a loss of contractility, abnormal loading conditions are imposed, or a combination of these occur. A continuum of cardiac function curves represents the spectrum of performance between normal hyperfunction and decompensated heart failure (Figure 71–7). Each function curve describes the net effect of homeostatic mechanisms on useful cardiac work performed over a range of ventricular filling pressures. Cardiac reserve reflects the extent to which compensatory mechanisms are still able to adjust cardiac output upward to meet the metabolic demand. Conceptually, the ability to respond depends on the shape of the function curve and the point along the curve at which the heart is operating. As cardiac function declines, an increase in ventricular filling pressure produces smaller increments of useful work (stroke or cardiac output). This causes the function curve to flatten out and the point at which the ventricle is operating shifts progressively to the right. Once cardiac output falls below normal at rest despite full use of preload reserve, the heart has decompensated and signs of poor perfusion coexist with signs of congestion. The integrity of cardiac function depends on three major compensatory mechanisms: (1) catecholamine release from cardiac adrenergic nerves and the adrenal medulla, (2) Frank-Starling mechanism, implemented by blood volume expansion through the complex interplay of the renal-adrenal-pituitary axis, and (3) cardiac hypertrophy with or without chamber enlargement.

SYMPATHETIC NERVOUS SYSTEM

In both the exercise-stressed normal individual and the patient in heart failure, increased cardiac output and conservation of blood flow by a redistribution to organs with metabolic priority are necessary. Reflex sympathoadrenal stimulation of the cardiovascular system is the most rapidly responsive mechanism for achieving these goals and preserving homeostasis. Although the response to local myocardial and circulating adrenomedullary norepinephrine is qualitatively similar in normal

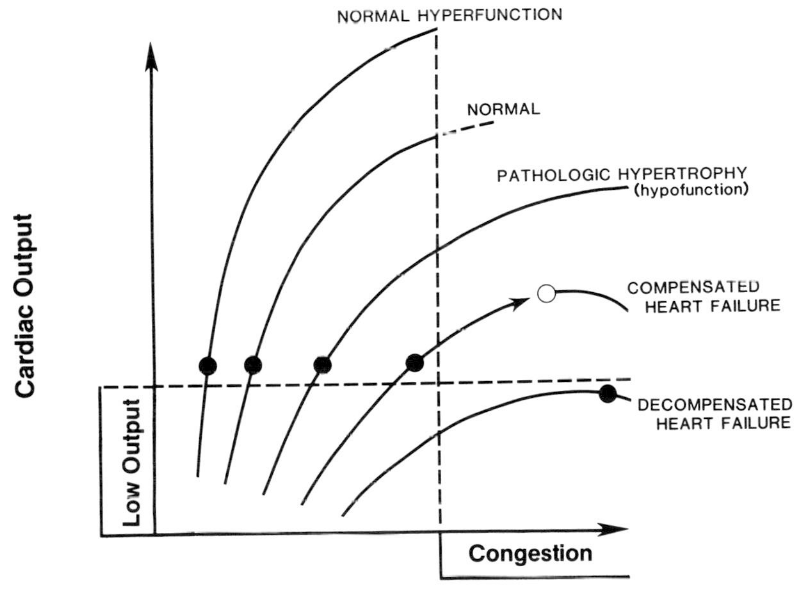

FIGURE 71–7. The continuous spectrum of cardiac performance attainable during different clinical states is illustrated by a family of ventricular function curves. A progressive downward displacement of the function curve to the right occurs as contractility declines and preload has incrementally less effect on cardiac performance. The operating points for hypothetical individuals at rest are indicated by the solid circles and the open circle represents a response to exercise. The normal ventricle, under the influence of catecholamine stimulation and volume loading (training effect), is able to improve its performance over the physiologic range of preloads by shifting to a steeper function curve (normal hyperfunction). Pathologic hypertrophy helps to maintain cardiac output in the presence of systolic overloading but at the expense of some increase in filling pressure and decrease in contractility. As a mismatch between afterload and ventricular contractility develops, there is greater reliance on preload reserve, and ventricular filling pressure and chamber volume increase. Ventricles that are marginally able to maintain normal resting cardiac output at high normal filling pressure (functional Class III, compensated heart failure) may be unable to respond to an increased workload without developing clinical signs of congestion. Decompensation (functional Class IV) is present when despite maximal use of all compensatory responses, including preload reserve, cardiac output cannot be maintained in the normal range at rest. Physical activity is significantly compromised in Class III and Class IV heart failure.

and failing hearts, important quantitative differences exist. If an abnormally intense pattern of vasoconstriction is not present at rest in heart failure, then it invariably occurs during exercise.[38]

The entire myocardium and peripheral vascular system are supplied with sympathetic nerve terminals. When cardiac output or blood pressure falls, the sympathetic nervous system coordinates increases in heart rate, strength of cardiac contraction (β-adrenergic effects), and selective peripheral vascular vasoconstriction (α-adrenergic effects) that attempt to restore hemodynamic equilibrium. At first the heart is very sensitive to direct β-adrenergic nerve stimulation, but as cardiac performance deteriorates, there is a significant decrease in maximum chronotropic and inotropic responsiveness due to depletion of cardiac norepinephrine stores.[7, 36] Depletion of myocardial norepinephrine is not responsible for the depressed contractility of failing hearts but it does partially deprive the heart of potentially useful support from sympathetic nerve stimulation. However, relative to cardiac nerve stimulation, sensitivity to circulating norepinephrine is enhanced and the heart becomes increasingly dependent on adrenomedullary-mediated catecholamines for inotropic support.[36]

Vasoconstriction of regional peripheral vascular beds by α-adrenergic stimulation is a reflex response to falling cardiac output and blood pressure. In heart failure, hypotension is prevented by constricting some vascular beds in favor of preserving blood flow to others. As with the normal exercise response, blood flow to the kidney, gastrointestinal tract, skin, and inactive skeletal muscles is restricted so that the brain, heart, and exercising muscle can be adequately perfused. As heart failure worsens and the background level of systemic adrenergic stimulation by circulating catecholamines intensifies, even minimal stress causes exaggerated changes in the regional circulations, resulting in detrimental side effects. Arteriolar vasoconstriction increases afterload and further impedes ventricular ejection. Although in the early adaptive stage venoconstriction is useful for increasing venous return and preload, it may exacerbate edema formation in later stages of heart failure, especially if blood volume is greatly expanded. Also, underperfusion of the kidneys perpetuates a vicious cycle of progressive blood volume expansion and peripheral vasoconstriction mediated by the renin-angiotensin-aldosterone system (Figure 71–8).

The increase in peripheral vascular resistance mediated by sympathetic vasoconstriction is compounded in the advanced stages of heart failure by an increase in vascular stiffness that is completely independent of catecholamine stimulation (Figure 71–9).[38, 39] The alterations in the mechanical properties of the vessels are caused by an increase in mural vascular sodium content and edema secondary to the renal retention of sodium and water that occurs with heart failure. Sodium-induced vascular stiffness probably occurs in all vessels. Functionally, it is particularly significant in skeletal muscle, where exercise produces large amounts of metabolic vasodilators that override adrenergically mediated vasoconstriction but not the effects of increased sodium content in the vessel wall. Consequently, autoregulation of resistance vessels and nutritive flow to skeletal muscle in heart failure patients is impaired during exercise.[40] Metabolic vasodilation normally provides for blood flow in excess of that required by exercising muscle. However, in heart failure there is less skeletal muscle blood flow relative to the work performed. This is partially compensated for by an increased extraction of oxygen from the blood perfusing the exercising muscles, and consequently, the arteriovenous oxygen difference widens.[39] The exercise intolerance displayed by heart failure patients is largely due to poor muscle perfusion.[40, 41] Failure to adequately dilate cutaneous vessels so that heat generated during exercise can be dissipated is another consequence of peripheral vasoconstriction and increased vascular stiffness.

RENAL-ADRENAL-PITUITARY INTERACTIONS

In the normal heart, sympathoadrenal stimulation is the primary mechanism for adjusting to transient increases in workload. However, cardiovascular disease imposes chronic, sustained changes in hemodynamics that require more stable, long-term adaptations. In this regard, the kidneys play a pivotal role in expanding blood volume and facilitating ventricular filling, thereby enabling the length–active tension relationship of the Frank-Starling mechanism to operate.

Blood volume expansion is the result of renal conservation of sodium and water brought about by a combination of intrarenal hemodynamic autoregulation and neurohumoral stimulation.[42] The sequence of events begins with a fall in cardiac output and blood pressure, which the kidney perceives as a decline in effective arterial blood volume (Figure 71–8). Systemic blood pressure is restored by reflex peripheral arteriolar vasoconstriction, which includes the afferent renal glomerular arterioles. The preglomerular arterioles are very sensitive to adrenergic stimulation and a disproportionate amount of blood is diverted from the kidneys. Renal plasma flow and filtration rate decrease, but this is partially compensated for by an increase in the filtration fraction, which enables the kidneys to maintain nominal excretory function. Normally, most of the sodium and water in the glomerular filtrate is reabsorbed during passage through the proximal tubules. The capacity of the proximal tubules to recover sodium and isotonic volumes of water is maintained, if not enhanced, as renal perfusion and the volume of filtrate decline. Consequently, a greater percentage of filtered sodium and water is absorbed in the proximal tubule and the total body content of both increases. If the effective blood volume is restored and increased ventricular filling improves cardiac performance and thus renal perfusion, then a new equilibrium is established at the expense of an elevation in ventricular filling pressure and expansion of the intravascular and interstitial fluid spaces.[43]

The hemodynamic effects of renal autoregulation are amplified by the renin-angiotensin-aldosterone humoral axis (Figure 71–8). Triggered by underperfusion, pressure-volume stretch receptors in the renal afferent arterioles stimulate release of *renin*, a proteolytic enzyme derived from the adjacent juxtaglomerular cells.[44, 45]

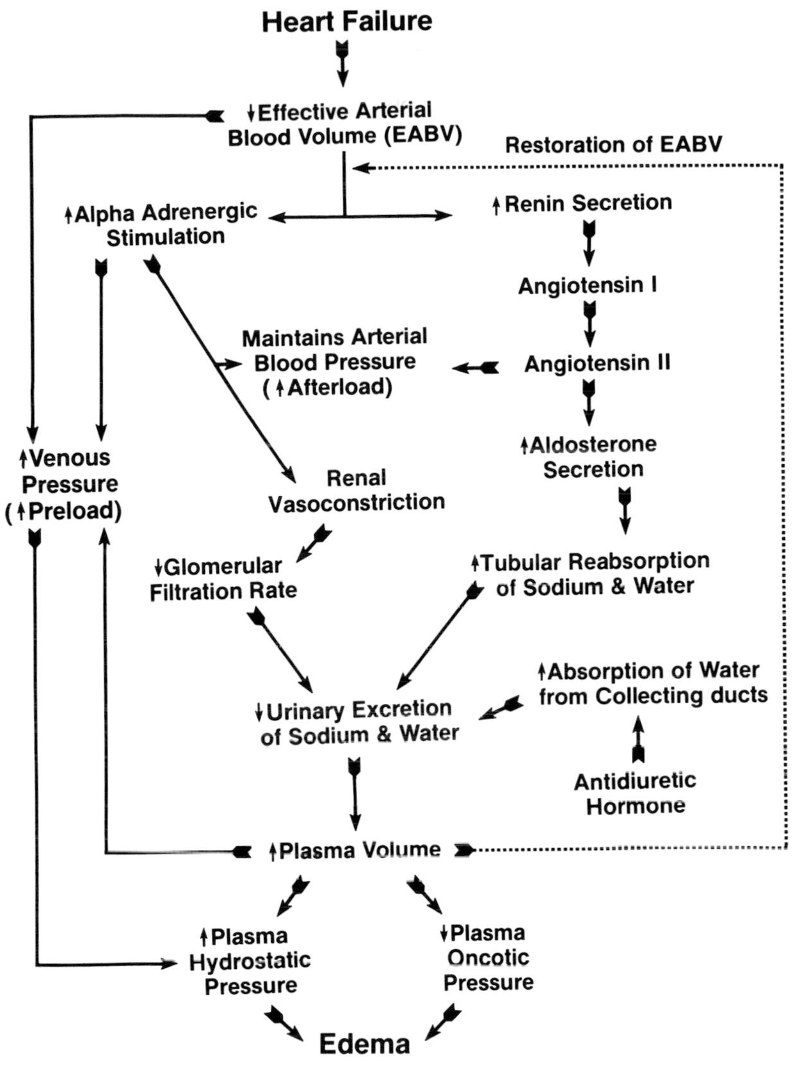

FIGURE 71–8. Mechanisms contributing to the development of edema in heart failure. (Modified from Cannon, PJ: The kidney in heart failure. N Engl J Med 296:26, 1977.)

Renin release is also stimulated by a decrease in the amount of sodium delivered to the distal tubules due to augmented proximal tubular reabsorption and by direct adrenergic stimulation of the juxtaglomerular cells. Renin acts on a serum globulin substrate, *angiotensinogen*, to produce *angiotensin I*. Primarily during circulation through the lung, the pharmacologically inactive peptide, angiotensin I, is converted into *angiotensin II* by an *angiotensin-converting enzyme*.[45]

Angiotensin II counters a decline in effective arterial blood volume by performing synergistic roles as a potent vasoconstrictor and a regulator of sodium-potassium homeostasis. Systemic blood pressure is supported by the widespread arteriolar vasoconstriction. As a consequence, renal perfusion is reduced further and the renal autoregulatory retention of sodium and water is enhanced, leading to expansion of blood volume. Because angiotensin II also constricts efferent glomerular arterioles, glomerular capillary pressure is maintained despite a reduction in renal perfusion and intrarenal hemodynamics are disturbed less than would otherwise be the case. When renal blood flow is low, the role of efferent arteriolar constriction in preserving the volume of glomerular filtrate is particularly important.[46]

In addition to its direct vasoconstrictor and renally mediated hemodynamic effects on blood pressure and volume, angiotensin II is a major stimulus for secretion of the adrenal mineralocorticoid *aldosterone*. Aldosterone promotes reabsorption of sodium from the distal renal tubules and collecting ducts, partially in exchange for potassium and hydrogen ions. Blood levels of aldosterone parallel those of renin and angiotensin II. If effective blood volume is restored, a positive feedback response withdraws the stimulus for renin-angiotensin-aldosterone secretion and blood levels return to normal, despite the expanded interstitial fluid volume (edema) at the new steady state. Thus aldosterone secretion is increased during periods when sodium is being actively retained to expand blood volume and establish a new hemodynamic equilibrium. If cardiac compensation is achieved, aldosterone blood levels decline. When the damaged heart is unable to improve its performance adequately, the kidney continues to be stimulated by these hormones and edema worsens. Rarely does protracted secretion of aldosterone by itself cause hypokalemia or alkalosis in heart failure patients, because the amount of sodium reaching the distal tubules and available for exchange with potassium is relatively small.[45]

Expansion of blood and interstitial fluid volumes is also facilitated by an increase in thirst, stimulated by

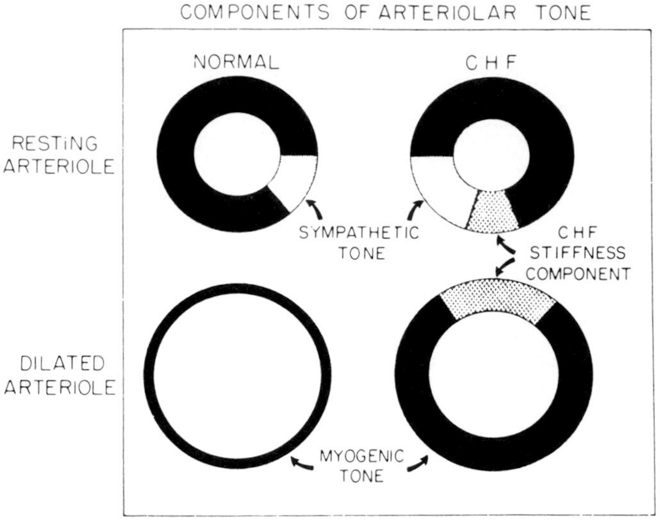

FIGURE 71–9. Diagrammatic representation of the components determining arteriolar tone at rest and with metabolic vasodilatation (horizontal rows) in normal subjects and patients with congestive heart failure (CHF) (vertical columns). The internal cross-sectional areas have been drawn to scale based on blood flow data obtained from humans. There are increased sympathetic arteriolar tone at rest and a vascular stiffness component secondary to increased vascular sodium content, which alters the mechanical properties of the arterioles. Vasoactive metabolites produced by exercising skeletal muscles counter the sympathetically mediated vasoconstriction in those vascular beds but not the vascular stiffness component that limits regional blood flow in CHF. (Reproduced by permission from Zelis, R and Mason, DT: Compensatory mechanisms in congestive heart failure—the role of the peripheral resistance vessels. N Engl J Med 282:962, 1970.)

angiotensin II.[45] Thus an increased water load complements the sodium retention promoted by renal vasoconstriction and aldosterone secretion. The epithelium of the renal collecting ducts is made more permeable to water by *antidiuretic hormone* (ADH), which is secreted by the posterior lobe of the pituitary gland. Although ADH secretion may be increased in heart failure patients, it does not play a major role in blood volume expansion or the pathogenesis of edema.[45] However, inappropriate ADH secretion occasionally may cause dilutional hyponatremia in some patients with severe heart failure or after heavy diuresis in those with milder degrees of failure.

Blood volume expansion due to renal retention of sodium and water can also cause dilutional hypoproteinemia. This creates an imbalance between vascular hydrostatic and oncotic pressures that favors the movement of fluid into the interstitial space. In progressive heart failure, the accumulation of edema fluid is limited only to the extent that the body can continue to perform vital functions. If a new hemodynamic equilibrium is not achieved collectively by the compensatory mechanisms invoked to preserve circulatory competence, then the feedback loops of these servosystems remain open. Consequently, the renin-angiotensin-aldosterone system continues to facilitate the conservation of sodium and water, thereby worsening the volume imbalance, to the eventual detriment of the body. If the hydrostatic imbalances that are the essence of the backward failure theory were the primary mechanism, the formation of edema would be self-limiting and body weight would stabilize.

The renin-angiotensin-aldosterone humoral axis and renal autoregulation serve primarily to preserve a positive sodium balance and arterial blood pressure. However, the rise and fall of these hormones does not completely explain the long-term homeostatic response to changes in sodium load or blood pressure. Increasing attention is being focused on a peptide of atrial tissue origin called the *atrial natriuretic hormone*.[47] What role atrial natriuretic hormone may play in the pathophysiology of heart failure has yet to be determined. However, some modulating effect is anticipated, since it opposes the renin-angiotensin-aldosterone activity at four operational levels: renin secretion, aldosterone secretion, angiotensin-mediated vasoconstriction, and aldosterone-mediated sodium retention. Thus, atrial natriuretic hormone may be a counterforce in heart failure that prevents edema from becoming worse than would otherwise be the case.

CARDIAC HYPERTROPHY

Hypertrophy is an adaptation to chronically increased tension on myocardial fibers caused by systolic mechanical overloading or impaired contractility.[48] Fiber tension is affected by the pressure, volume, and wall thickness of a cardiac chamber as expressed by the LaPlace relationship. An increase in either pressure or volume creates additional wall stress (force/unit cross-sectional area). Hypertrophy addresses this imbalance by increasing muscle mass, in part through the generation of additional contractile units (myofilaments), thereby distributing the wall force over a larger cross section. If the hypertrophic response is fully compensatory, cardiac pump (but not myocardial) hyperfunction is achieved at normal sarcomere length and wall stress by the addition of contractile units.[23]

One of two patterns of ventricular hypertrophy develops, depending on the nature of the stress.[49] Pressure-overloaded ventricles adapt to increases in systolic wall tension by increasing wall thickness relative to the chamber volume, which remains essentially unchanged so long as cardiac function is successfully preserved. This increase in wall thickness and muscle mass relative to chamber volume is called *concentric hypertrophy*. Volume-overloaded ventricles adapt to chronic, obligatory increases in stroke volume by undergoing extensive end-diastolic enlargement. A similar change occurs in ventricles with primary contractile deficits. Under these circumstances, wall thickness relative to chamber volume is normal at best and is usually reduced despite an increase in muscle mass. This pattern is referred to as *eccentric hypertrophy*.[48, 49]

In nonfailing, pressure-overloaded ventricles, wall stress is normalized by the addition of contractile units arranged in parallel.[49] This increases total wall force and thus mechanical advantage, allowing total stroke volume to remain essentially unchanged. Since sarcomeres are difficult to stretch beyond their optimal length, the chamber dilatation that results from chronic volume overloading cannot be accounted for simply on the basis of sarcomere elongation.[13] Under severe, acute volume loading, slippage between the myofibrils in individual cells permits some elongation by pulling the sarcomeres out of register. However, it takes a combination of slippage between myocardial cells and myocardial cell elongation to produce the large increases in chamber size caused by chronic volume loading.[49] Cell lengthening is accomplished in part by the addition of sarcomeres in series at the intercalated discs and slippage between fibrils.[50, 51] As new filaments are added at the periphery of the fibrils, the fibrils widen and the diameter of the myocardial fibers increases. Dilatation, unlike wall thickening, produces no intrinsic mechanical advantage since at the larger volume, wall stress is increased. In eccentric hypertrophy, the requirement for increased contractile force is partially offset by the fact that less fiber shortening is required when comparable stroke volumes are achieved from a larger end-diastolic volume. Thus, stroke volume can be maintained in the chronically dilated heart despite a decline in ejection fraction.

By adding contractile units, hypertrophy effectively increases the total contractile force in the ventricular wall, but not the force per unit. Intrinsic depression of the myocardial inotropic state may not be immediately evident in a ventricle that has successfully adapted to a pressure overload.[24] However, decreased contractility of hypertrophied myocardium has been demonstrated even before there is evidence of cardiac failure (Figure 71–10).[36] Eventually, a decline in contractility becomes a critical factor in the pathogenesis of decompensated cardiac failure.[2]

CAUSES OF HEART FAILURE

A list of potential causes of heart failure is presented in Table 71–1. Some of these are best classified as secondary causes because their impact is insufficient to produce heart failure unless cardiac performance is already compromised. However, their contribution may be significant under these circumstances and should not be neglected. Overtransfusion, severe anemia, pyrexia, or cardiac arrhythmias producing drastic increases or decreases in heart rate may destabilize a patient in a precarious state of hemodynamic balance and either precipitate heart failure or make it impossible to control. Systemic hypertension in dogs and hyperthyroidism in cats are also of secondary importance even though they have the potential to cause heart failure. Both conditions are relatively uncommon and usually too mild to cause overt signs of heart failure in the absence of concomitant cardiac disease. The remaining causes listed in Table 71–1 represent major clinical entities that can be classified pathophysiologically into three functional types.

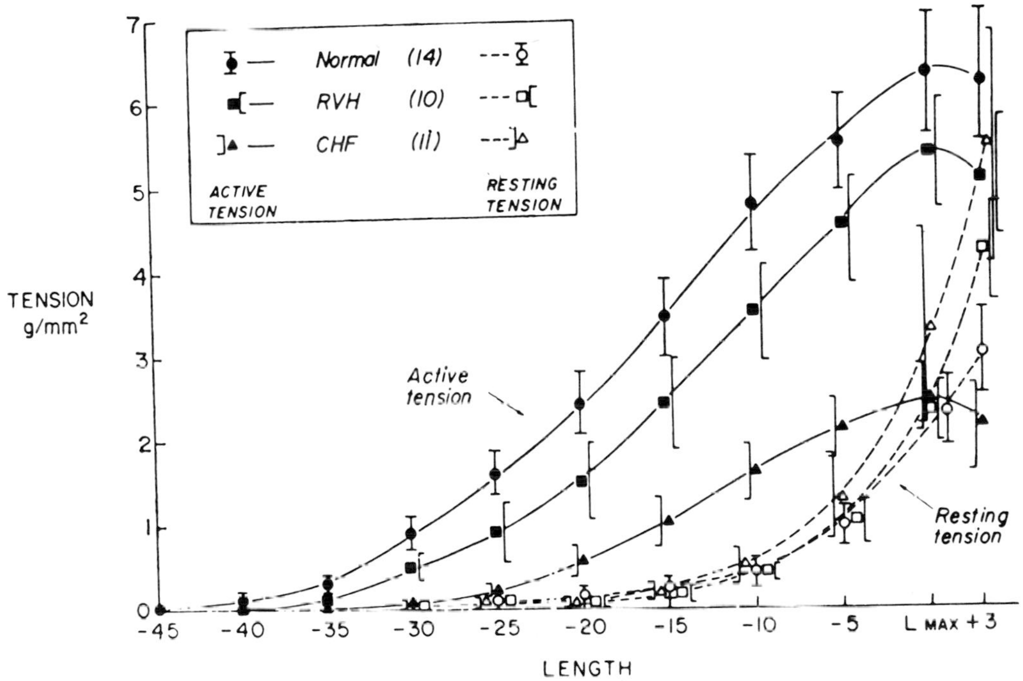

FIGURE 71–10. Relation between muscle length and tension of right ventricular papillary muscles from normal cats (circles) and cats with experimentally produced ventricular hypertrophy (squares) and heart failure (triangles). Open symbols = resting tension; solid symbols = actively developed tension. Each value is the average of the group; vertical lines with cross bars = ±1 SEM. Tension is corrected for cross-sectional area (g/mm²). Numbers in parentheses = number of animals. (From Spann, JF, et al: Contractile state of cardiac muscle obtained from cats with experimentally produced ventricular hypertrophy and heart failure. Circ Res 21:341, 1967, by permission of the American Heart Association.)

PRIMARY REDUCTION OF VENTRICULAR CONTRACTILITY

Dilated cardiomyopathy and chronic myocarditis, whatever their etiologies, produce profound depression of ventricular contractility, usually leading to intractable heart failure within a relatively short period of time. Heart failure in dilated cardiomyopathy is associated with low ejection fraction and stroke volume, tachycardia, and low cardiac output (Figure 71–11).[52] Hemodynamic performance is supported temporarily by using preload reserve (Frank-Starling mechanism) and eccentric ventricular hypertrophy.[2] A new equilibrium is attempted by shifting the diastolic pressure-volume relationship further to the right, forcing the ventricle to operate at a larger end-diastolic chamber volume and filling pressure (Figure 71–12). Dogs (and presumably cats) with dilated cardiomyopathy not only have poor systolic function but also have a very stiff ventricular myocardium that compromises diastolic function and necessitates inordinate increases in filling pressure.[53] Due to the spherical ventricular chamber dilation that characterizes ventricular geometry in this condition, orthogonal wall stresses are particularly high.[54] Furthermore, as these patients reach the intractable stage of heart failure, this mismatch between afterload and the inotropic state of the myocardium caused by the primary depression in contractility and loss of preload reserve is exacerbated by an inadequate degree of hypertrophy to normalize wall stress.[55] Progressive loss of contractility, expended preload reserve, and inadequate ventricular hypertrophy lead to deterioration of hemodynamic performance and a state of low output heart failure.

Cardiac performance in dilated cardiomyopathy is not as dependent on preload as previously thought. Both the congestive signs and stroke output can improve after normal filling pressure is restored with vasodilator and diuretic therapy.[56] This improvement does not appear to be completely explained by a simultaneous reduction in afterload due to a decrease in peripheral vascular resistance. At this late stage of the syndrome, the ventricle may be operating so far to the right on a very depressed (flattened) function curve that it no longer benefits from the elevated preload. At this time, high filling pressure not only contributes to signs of congestion but, having reached the point of diminishing re-

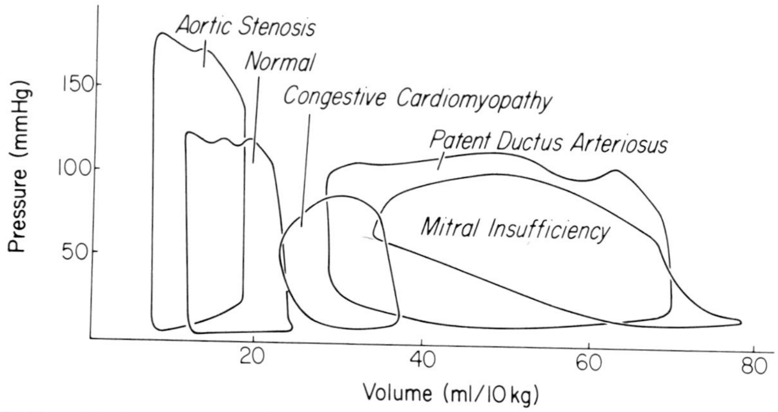

FIGURE 71–11. Left ventricular pressure-volume loops from dogs with different heart diseases compared with a normal loop. Aortic stenosis: In compensated aortic stenosis, there is increased stroke work because of the increased pressure the myocardium must work against to maintain output. In this example, a state of ventricular hyperfunction has been achieved by normalizing systolic wall stress through development of concentric hypertrophy. An increase in ejection fraction has enabled the left ventricle to maintain stroke volume from a slightly smaller end-diastolic volume. The increased slope of the diastolic filling curve reflects the reduction in ventricular compliance resulting from the compensatory increase in ventricular wall thickness. Dilated cardiomyopathy: In dilated cardiomyopathy, both the end-diastolic and end-systolic volumes are increased. Although a normal stroke volume has been maintained, ejection fraction is abnormally low (0.33) because of the disproportionate increase in end-systolic volume. However, the effective stroke volume is reduced due to regurgitation through a mitral valve made incompetent by ventricular dilatation.[52] This secondary effect is illustrated by the decreased slope of the ascending limb of the loop, which normally represents the isovolumetric contraction phase. The isovolumetric relaxation phase is abbreviated due to the combination of low end-systolic pressure related to a weak contraction and the high filling pressure, which hastens the reopening of the mitral valve. This dog was in heart failure. Patent ductus arteriosus: In the example of patent ductus arteriosus (PDA) with a left-to-right shunt, the pressure-volume loop is greatly elongated, indicating an increase in the ventricular volume and work parameters. The ejection fraction is normal. The isovolumetric contraction period ends and ejection begins at a lower pressure than in the normal loop because ductal flow reduces aortic diastolic pressure. In PDA with larger shunts and greater increases in end-diastolic volume, the isovolumetric contraction may disappear.[52] This can be explained by further lowering of aortic diastolic pressure or development of mitral regurgitation secondary to ventricular dilatation. Mitral regurgitation: In chronic, severe primary mitral regurgitation, end-diastolic, end-systolic, and stroke volumes are greatly increased. Because of immediate unloading into the atrium, there is no isovolumetric contraction. Isovolumetric relaxation is also lost. After the peak end-systolic pressure is reached, there is a small, additional decrease in ventricular volume due to a brief continuation of regurgitant flow. The high filling pressure and normal early diastolic ventricular compliance then allow a rapid inflow of blood and premature ventricular distension.[53] As volume loading increases, end-diastolic pressure rises. However, when mitral regurgitation has progressed gradually for a long time, the left atrium and ventricle are able to reach very large volumes with only modest increases in filling pressures. (Reprinted from Lord, PF: Quantitative left ventricular cineangiocardiography in the dog: Measurement and usefulness of left ventricular volume. Vet Rad 18:51, 1977, with permission of the publisher.)

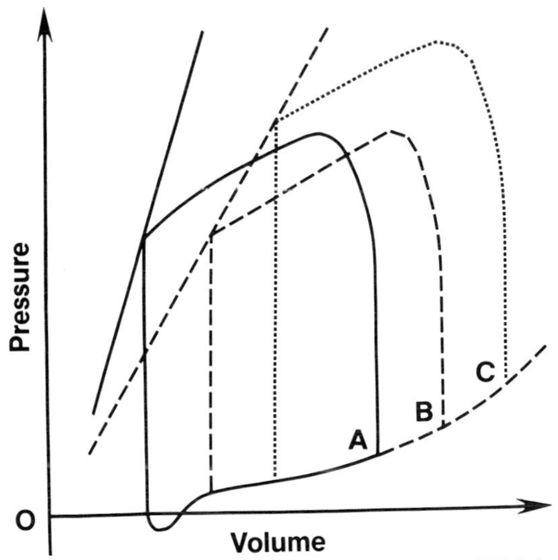

FIGURE 71–12. The hypothetical pressure/volume (P/V) loop of a normal ventricle *(A)* is compared with two P/V cycles under different loading conditions in a ventricle with decreased contractility *(B* and *C)*. The end-systolic P/V relationship over a range of end-systolic volumes is represented by a diagonal line for each ventricle. Loops B and C represent the response to acute changes in contractility *(B)* and afterloading *(C)* preceding chronic adaptation through normalization of ventricular wall stress (force/cross-sectional area) by the development of myocardial hypertrophy. In loop B, the arterial pressure is unchanged but in this depressed inotropic state, the ventricle is unable to reach the end-systolic volume of the normal ventricle and a compensatory increase in end-diastolic volume is needed to maintain a normal stroke volume. If afterload is increased by a rise in arterial pressure *(C)* or increased wall stresses related to chamber enlargement without adequate compensatory hypertrophy, preservation of stroke volume necessitates a further increase in preload and end-diastolic volume. As the ventricle becomes increasingly distended, there is an accelerated reduction in chamber compliance (dV/dP) and the filling pressure at end-diastole begins to rise rapidly. Preload reserve is expended as dilatation progresses. Eventually, end-diastolic filling pressure becomes pathologically elevated, contributing to the development of edema, which limits the usefulness of the Frank-Starling mechanism. In this setting of limited preload reserve, an afterload mismatch develops, such that further increases in afterload result in a decrease in stroke volume.[23]

turns, may actually be detrimental to cardiac performance as well. The functional improvement accompanying restoration of normal filling pressure in extremely dilated hearts may be attributable to lower wall stress throughout the cardiac cycle, which diminishes the afterload mismatch, reduces myocardial oxygen consumption during contraction, and improves coronary blood flow in diastole. In addition, even a small reduction in chamber volume may increase cardiac efficiency by improving AV valve competence in those patients with regurgitation secondary to ventricular dilatation.

SYSTOLIC MECHANICAL OVERLOAD

Cardiac work may be pathologically increased by imposing either an obligatory pressure or volume overload. Eventually, depressed contractility also becomes an important variable in the pathogenesis of heart failure caused by any disease that produces chronic systolic mechanical overloading of the heart.[2]

PRESSURE OVERLOADING

Subaortic stenosis and pulmonary hypertension are two classic examples of pressure overloading. Without compensatory adjustments, ventricular stroke volume would decline, since the high afterload opposes the velocity and extent of myocardial fiber shortening. Chronic pressure-overloaded ventricles rely primarily on concentric hypertrophy rather than the Frank-Starling mechanism (preload reserve) to preserve stroke output. Although a transient increase in preload initially assists the ventricle in making this adjustment, increased ventricular wall tension stimulates myocardial hypertrophy, which augments the total contractile force, enabling the muscle fibers to shorten against the elevated pressure load. Through the development of concentric hypertrophy, a new equilibrium is established between the force of contraction and the imposed load. So long as normal systolic wall stress (force/cm^2) is restored in the hypertrophied ventricle, stroke volume can be maintained without a chronic increase in end-diastolic volume or reduced ejection fraction.[24]

When ventricular performance is examined by analysis of pressure-volume relationships, the concentrically hypertrophied ventricle that has successfully adapted to a pressure overload displays hemodynamic hyperfunction (Figure 71–11).[57] However, after normalizing the total contractile force to the thickness of the hypertrophied ventricular wall, the systolic wall stress is only restored to normal.[58] Even though the balance between afterload and total contractile force may be reestablished without an increase in end-diastolic volume, the increase in wall mass decreases ventricular compliance, necessitating higher filling pressure.

Demand for higher cardiac output (in response to exercise, for example) would necessitate a further increase in intraventricular systolic pressure and wall stress due to the elevated and relatively fixed resistance to the ejection of blood. This can be accomplished initially by using preload reserve (Figure 71–12). However, if increased afterload, perhaps due to worsening of the underlying abnormality, is to be sustained, normal wall stress must be restored by additional hypertrophy. As hypertrophy becomes a less effective response, the pressure-loaded ventricle becomes increasingly dependent on preload.[58] Progressive ventricular dilatation is indicative of a decline in myocardial contractility and displaces the diastolic function curve further to the right.[59] This puts patients increasingly at risk of developing edema as the steep portion of the diastolic function curve is reached and filling pressure becomes critically elevated. Once myocardial preload reserve is expended and contractility is sufficiently depressed, cardiac output begins to fall below demand. Due to the particularly large mechanical restraints imposed by a high afterload, pressure-overloaded hearts decompensate, while the myocardium is less severely depressed than in volume-overloaded hearts at a comparable stage of heart failure.[2]

Volume Overloading. In conditions such as atrioventricular and semilunar valve regurgitation and left-to-right shunts due to patent ductus arteriosus and ventricular septal defect, the hydraulic efficiency of the heart is reduced because a substantial portion of the output is ejected in a retrograde direction or is short-circuited without reaching its intended destination. In the volume-loaded ventricle, total stroke output exceeds the effective (forward) stroke volume. In chronic cases, total stroke output is increased by extensive use of preload reserve and structurally remodeling the affected cardiac chambers to make them larger. As the ventricle increases in size, systolic wall stress is normalized by eccentric hypertrophy. Ventricular compliance remains high in dogs with mitral regurgitation and this is probably also true to a variable extent with other volume-overloading conditions.[53] The relatively flat diastolic function curve in such cases permits a large volume of blood to enter the ventricle before wall stress begins to rise and filling pressure becomes critically elevated (Figure 71–11).[52]

Aortic Versus Mitral Regurgitation. At equivalent total and effective stroke volumes, left ventricular function is more seriously compromised by aortic regurgitation.[60] The difference exists because in aortic regurgitation the entire stroke volume must be ejected into the relatively high impedance aorta, whereas in mitral regurgitation a large portion of the stroke volume (regurgitant fraction) is able to flow into the more compliant left atrium where pressure is low. Consequently, at comparable volume loads, afterload and total ventricular work are substantially higher with aortic regurgitation. In humans, chronic aortic regurgitation causes greater end-diastolic distension of the left ventricle than any other disease. This is less likely to occur in animals, where most cases of aortic regurgitation are caused by acute bacterial valvulitis and are usually fatal before the left ventricle has had time to reach the limits of adaptation.

In mitral regurgitation, on the other hand, the left ventricle is able to begin emptying immediately at a low afterload, which, even at its peak, does not exceed normal. Emptying continues briefly after closure of the aortic valves because mitral regurgitation continues until pressures in the atrium and ventricle equilibrate (Figure 71–11). Though the end-systolic volume of the afterload-reduced ventricle is normal at first, it eventually increases as contractility declines and the ventricle is forced to dilate in order to have the capacity to generate a large stroke volume. Despite the hemodynamic burden of major chronic mitral regurgitation, myocardial contractility is sustained well in the compensated state and the condition can be tolerated for a long time.[61] However, once decompensation occurs, the degree of myocardial depression in both mitral and aortic regurgitation is greater than that occurring at a comparable stage of pressure overloading.[2]

Ventricular Septal Defect Versus Patent Ductus Arteriosus. The comparison between left-to-right shunts due to ventricular septal defect and patent ductus arteriosus is analogous to that between mitral and aortic regurgitation.[62] At the same volume of left-to-right shunt, the left ventricular systolic mechanical overload is greater with a patent ductus because of higher afterload. In an uncomplicated ventricular septal defect, blood is shunted immediately into the low pressure right ventricle and pulmonary artery, whereas with a patent ductus, the entire left ventricular stroke volume must be ejected into the aorta at a substantially higher pressure. Because of the extra pressure load, it is more difficult for the left ventricle to empty as completely, i.e., to reach an equivalent end-systolic volume, and the ventricle tends to operate at a higher end-diastolic volume in order to maintain an effective stroke output (total stroke output less ductal flow). This accounts for the larger left atrial and ventricular volumes and lower ejection fraction in cases of patent ductus arteriosus compared to a ventricular septal defect at equivalent shunt volumes. Due to the greater pressure loading with aortic regurgitation and patent ductus arteriosus, myocardial oxygen consumption is higher in those conditions than with pure volume overloading (mitral regurgitation and uncomplicated ventricular septal defect).[2] In actual practice, ventricular septal defects in dogs are usually small and cause little hemodynamic disturbance in contrast to the typically large ductal flow, which, if not interrupted, usually leads eventually to left heart failure.

Acute Versus Chronic Overloading. The effects of pure pressure and volume overloads on ventricular contractility differ considerably over time. Severe, short-term pressure loading produces extensive hypertrophy and depresses contractility more than a comparable period of volume loading, which produces marked dilatation but substantially less hypertrophy. Eventually, however, chronic volume loading adversely affects contractility to a greater extent.[2] Structural changes in the myocardium of ventricles subjected to different loading conditions may provide a partial explanation. In the concentric hypertrophy of pressure loading, there is a decrease in the density of contractile elements and this may be responsible for depressing contractility.[63] Long-term overdistension of volume-loaded ventricles is associated with progressive slippage between muscle fibers and loss of register between myofibrils.[14] These changes could account for the profound depression of contractility in the late stages of volume overloading. Disengagement of actin-myosin filaments does not appear to be a factor. However, the marked decline in myocardial distensibility as sarcomeres are stretched to their optimal length can significantly compromise diastolic function (Figure 71–10). Although it takes a long time before contractility is seriously depressed by volume loading, the degree of impairment ultimately exceeds that occurring with a pressure overload and is more likely to be irreversible.[64]

Decompensation occurs when contractility is depressed to a level that cannot be compensated for by further increments in preload or hypertrophy. At that point, cardiac output falls below normal because of the mismatch between afterload and the inotropic state of the ventricle. Afterload mismatch is reached after less depression of contractility in chronic pressure-overloaded ventricles. Volume loading is generally tolerated better because of the lower afterload opposing myocardial shortening. When loss of contractility is a primary disorder, e.g., dilated cardiomyopathy, decompensation does not take place until an even lower level of inotropy has been reached. The degree of myocardial depression at the onset of decompensation in these three types of cardiac disease is inversely proportional to the systolic load; i.e., depression is least in pressure overloading and greatest in the myopathies.[2] This relationship has important prognostic implications, since there is greater potential for responding to therapy when contractility is least depressed.

DIASTOLIC MECHANICAL INHIBITION

Conditions causing a decrease in ventricular diastolic function impede venous return and initiate the compensatory adjustments that increase filling pressure. Cardiac causes of diastolic mechanical inhibition can be broadly categorized into pericardial and ventricular wall abnormalities. In dogs and cats, pericardial disorders are the most common and significant causes. Elevated intrapericardial pressure opposes cardiac filling by decreasing the transmural pressure gradient responsible for chamber distension during diastole. Right ventricular filling pressure normally is less than that of the left ventricle. Therefore, the right ventricle is particularly adversely affected by an increase in intrapericardial pressure and cardiac output is limited by a decrease in systemic venous return. As the intrapericardial pressure approaches the filling pressure in the right side of the heart and the transmural pressure declines toward zero, cardiac tamponade develops.[65] Cardiac compression reduces ventricular diastolic volume and the effective preload of both ventricles. Stroke volume and cardiac output decline, but a reflex increase in adrenergic stimulation increases systemic vascular resistance and temporarily prevents the blood pressure from falling. During the compensatory stage, signs of right heart failure (generalized systemic venous engorgement and abdominal and pleural effusions) predominate. However, if tamponade worsens, hypotension and circulatory collapse develop terminally.

Right heart failure with cardiac tamponade is most commonly caused by hemopericardium produced by benign sanguineous pericarditis or intrapericardial neoplasms. Both clinical entities may be complicated to some degree by restrictive pericardial disease.

Filling can also be impeded by conditions that stiffen the ventricular wall. Feline hypertrophic and restrictive cardiomyopathies primarily affect the left ventricle and therefore typically produce high left ventricular filling pressure and pulmonary edema. It appears that the type of hypertrophic cardiomyopathy usually encountered in the cat does not obstruct left ventricular outflow but the thick ventricular walls make the chamber less compliant and interfere with diastolic function. The subendocardial fibrosis of the left ventricular wall in the restrictive type produces a similar effect. Tachycardia also decreases ventricular compliance by preventing complete relaxation of the myocardium.[66] This relatively mild reduction in ventricular compliance, when coupled with a shortened filling cycle, may contribute to the development of a significant decline in diastolic function under circumstances where filling is already compromised. Although systolic dysfunction is the primary abnormality in subaortic stenosis, left ventricular chamber stiffness due to severe concentric hypertrophy and myocardial fibrosis are probably important contributing factors when left heart failure occurs with this anomaly.

CLINICAL MANIFESTATIONS OF HEART FAILURE

Except in those infrequent catastrophic instances when the heart is subjected to an acute loss of contractility or mechanical efficiency, heart failure and its clinical manifestations have a slow, insidious onset. If given time to make compensatory adjustments, the heart has a remarkable ability to maintain a normal cardiac output at rest and increase blood flow to levels permitting modest amounts of physical activity until late in the natural history of the underlying disease. Each compensatory mechanism eventually produces deleterious side effects. It is important to realize that these side effects are responsible for the clinical signs of heart failure. As the underlying disease progressively worsens and evokes stronger compensatory responses, a point of diminishing returns is reached after which continued reliance on these mechanisms is precluded by the intensification of their side effects.

With the exception of generalized venous engorgement, the other physical signs associated with heart failure (Table 71–3) may have a noncardiac pathogenesis. Therefore, provocative signs should not be attributed to heart failure unless there is also evidence of heart disease of sufficient severity to adequately explain them. To aid clinical recognition and etiologic classification of heart failure, the manifestations may be grouped to characterize failure of the right or left side of the heart or a combination of both (generalized failure). The number of signs occurring in an individual case is variable. Generally, the more severe the state of heart failure, the more obvious and numerous the signs become.

The classic signs of congestion and edema related to heart failure are manifestations of the blood-volume expansion, evoked to restore an effective blood volume and implement the Frank-Starling mechanism. The increase in systolic wall tension and stroke volume made possible by actively stretching the myocardium requires progressively higher filling pressures as the diastolic function curve is extended to the right (Figures 71–11 and 71–12). When chamber distension is allowed to proceed gradually, large volumes can be attained at modest elevations in filling pressure (Figure 71–11). This is accomplished by myofibrillar and intermyocardial cell slippage. However, as myocardial failure worsens,

TABLE 71–3. PHYSICAL SIGNS ASSOCIATED WITH HEART FAILURE

Pulmonary Signs (left heart)	Systemic Signs (right heart)
Rales (alveolar edema)	Generalized venous engorgement
Frothy, pink expectorant	Hepatomegaly
Shortness of breath, tachypnea	Serous effusions in body cavities
Nocturnal dyspnea (orthopnea)	Ascites
Cough	Pleural effusion
	Pericardial effusion
	Dependent peripheral edema
	Weight gain (retained fluid)
Signs Attributable to Either Left or Right Heart Failure	
Weakness and fatigue (general exercise intolerance)	
Exertional dyspnea	
Gallop rhythm (accentuated third heart sound)	
Poor peripheral perfusion	
Pale membranes	
Slow capillary refill time	
Mild cyanosis	
Cool extremities	
Tachycardia	
Weight loss (cachexia)	

progressively higher filling pressure is required as the operating point on the ventricular function curve is displaced further to the right (Figure 71–7). Since the stretched myocardium is relatively stiff, an acute compensatory increase in end-diastolic volume in response to the stress of exercise, for example, requires a rapid rise in filling pressure and exacerbates the signs of congestion and edema.

An abrupt increase in left ventricular filling pressure can be critical because pulmonary edema can form precipitously and rapidly become fatal. Pulmonary interstitial and peribronchial edema is associated with decreased pulmonary compliance and some increase in respiratory effort (dyspnea). This may progress to alveolar edema, which is functionally more significant since it interferes with gas exchange. Alveolar edema causes inspiratory, crackling lung sounds (rales). Similar lung sounds may occur with pneumonia or other pulmonary parenchymal diseases. In fulminating cases of left heart failure, edema fluid accumulates in the bronchi and trachea, where it mixes with air and may appear in the nose and mouth as a slightly blood-tinged froth.

After reclining for variable periods of time, some marginally compensated dogs may experience mild respiratory distress and resume a sitting position or move about restlessly. This is caused by a redistribution of edema, with fluid accumulating in the lung due to an increase in pulmonary capillary pressure related to the hydrostatic effects of assuming lateral recumbency. Since this is more likely to occur at night during the normal sleep period, this pattern of respiratory distress is called *paroxysmal nocturnal dyspnea*.

A cough is commonly attributed to left-sided heart failure in dogs. Actually, dogs in left heart failure cough weakly if at all, particularly when suffering from severe pulmonary edema, and cats seldom cough for any reason. The so-called "heart failure" cough is usually caused by severe left heart enlargement with compression of the left bronchus between the left atrium and aorta, as frequently happens with chronic mitral regurgitation. The vigorous, often strident, and usually nonproductive cough related to this complication is generally easily induced by tracheal manipulation. Its characteristics are similar to the cough of the collapsed trachea syndrome, which frequently is also present in small dogs. Paroxysmal cycles of coughing are common, particularly in conjunction with physical activity. Consequently, a cough may draw attention to left-sided heart disease, but is not necessarily indicative of heart failure in these cases.

Serous effusions accumulate more gradually in body cavities than in the lung and are not immediately compromising. However, pleural effusion may become life threatening. When pericardial effusion secondary to heart failure occurs, it is usually mild and does not significantly interfere with cardiac function.

Dogs have a predilection for developing ascites, but in cats pleural effusion is more common. Hepatomegaly due to chronic passive congestion is a prominent and consistent finding in all cases of pure right-sided and generalized heart failure. Since the accumulation of ascitic fluid is nearly limitless, it may cause severe abdominal distension and a large increase in gross body weight. Daily monitoring of body weight is an objective means of evaluating the efficacy of heart failure treatment when large effusions are present. Following successful diuresis, such patients frequently look emaciated and it becomes apparent in retrospect that considerable tissue edema had been present. Overt pitting edema in limbs and the body wall is relatively uncommon and usually a late manifestation of severe right and generalized heart failure.

High filling pressure in an enlarged, usually dilated ventricle that often has decreased diastolic compliance may produce an audible third heart sound in the dog and cat. This is associated with the rapid deceleration of blood as it enters the ventricle. A physiologic third heart sound is not audible in these species. Therefore, this diastolic sound has pathologic significance. The extra heart sound creates a triple rhythm reminiscent of the cadence of galloping hoof beats, hence the clinical expression *gallop rhythm* is given to this phenomenon. Since a tachycardia usually accompanies a gallop, summation of the normally inaudible third and fourth heart sounds may help to make ventricular filling an audible event. A faint, often intermittent gallop rhythm is sometimes audible in cats with heart rates in the 200 to 220 range but without evidence of heart failure. A physiologic summation gallop may explain this observation.

The sympathetic nervous system provides a means for rapidly fine tuning cardiac contractility, heart rate, and peripheral arterial and venous tone. Although the failing myocardium is partially depleted of norepinephrine and less responsive to cardiac nerve stimulation, it continues to be driven by high levels of circulating catecholamines.[35] As cardiac performance declines, the intensity of sympathetic stimulation increases,[67] raising the basal heart rate and causing widespread peripheral vasoconstriction. Consequently, tachycardia, blanched mucous membranes, and cool extremities are common signs of sympathetic overstimulation in heart failure.

By increasing contractility of the failing myocardium, sympathetic stimulation would be expected to increase myocardial oxygen consumption. However, if, as a result of an increase in contractility, the heart is able to operate at a smaller end-diastolic volume and pressure, systolic intramyocardial tension, which is also a major determinant of myocardial oxygen consumption, will decrease. The net effect may be an increase in cardiac performance without additional myocardial oxygen consumption.[68] However, sustained tachycardia and inappropriately elevated afterload are counterproductive, in part because each decreases cardiac efficiency by increasing myocardial oxygen consumption relative to the amount of useful work performed. In addition, tachycardia also compromises delivery of oxygen to the myocardium by shortening diastole and thus encroaching on the period during which most of the coronary flow is occurring. Theoretically, these complications could contribute to myocytolysis and further deterioration of myocardial function, eventually leading to decompensation.

Concentric hypertrophy is the primary compensatory response to a systolic pressure overload. Although the contractility of hypertrophied myocardium is depressed to some degree, a net increase in total contractile force and normalization of systolic wall stress is achieved if there is a compensatory increase in total myocardial mass. As myocardial cells hypertrophy, the increased diffusion distance and reduction in capillary density interfere with the ability of the coronary circulation to adequately perfuse the ventricle. This may be accentuated by excessive adrenergic stimulation that, as mentioned previously, can increase myocardial oxygen consumption. Thus myocardial ischemia can develop, particularly when heart rate and wall stress are transiently increased during exercise. In humans, the discomfort of angina pectoris under these circumstances is a major factor limiting the effectiveness of cardiac hypertrophy, particularly concentric hypertrophy. It is not apparent whether animals experience similar sensations. However, subaortic stenosis in dogs is associated with myocardial necrosis and fibrosis, ventricular dysrhythmias, and sudden death, all of which are attributed to myocardial injury related to ischemia in the severely pressure-overloaded left ventricle.

Myocardial hypertrophy, ischemia, and fibrosis decrease ventricular compliance and may contribute significantly to the increased filling pressure related to blood-volume expansion and venoconstriction.[69, 70] The passive length-tension relationship of hypertrophied myocardium is not altered on a unit basis. However, filling pressure must increase due to the increased thickness of the ventricular wall. Therefore, by normalizing wall stress in systole, hypertrophy (particularly the concentric type) can decrease diastolic compliance of the intact ventricle. Even higher filling pressure will be necessary if the myocardium also becomes stiffer due to ischemia or fibrosis. Each of these complications decreases preload reserve and enhances the likelihood of congestion and edema by making inordinately high filling pressure necessary to ensure adequate venous return.

When the compensatory mechanisms are no longer able to overcome the deterioration in ventricular systolic function, then cardiac output and regional blood flow become inadequate even at rest, and the function of other organs becomes seriously impaired. Signs of decompensating heart failure include cachexia, weakness, reduced urine flow, and hypotension, in addition to the side effects associated with congestion. Cerebral dysfunction is more apparent in humans but probably occurs to some extent in animals. Since most animals that reach this end stage of heart failure are forced out of necessity to be more active than their cardiac status justifies, few of them are maintained for long in this condition.

FUNCTIONAL CLASSIFICATION OF HEART FAILURE

In addition to the etiologic and pathophysiologic classifications of heart failure (Table 71–1), it is useful to categorize patients clinically by the degree of functional disability (Table 71–4). Since a parallel usually exists between the intensity of therapy and the severity of heart failure, a functional classification can help guide treatment decisions. More importantly, functional grouping makes comparison of clinical responses among different patients more meaningful, and as individual patients shift from one class to another, it provides a basis for assessing treatment efficacy and documenting the natural progression of disease. Increases in cardiac output by the normal heart depend on the same compensatory mechanisms that support the failing heart. Therefore, the reserve capacity for exercise is limited to the extent that these mechanisms are already being used at rest.

TABLE 71–4. FUNCTIONAL CLASSIFICATION OF HEART FAILURE

Class	Clinical Signs
I	Exercise capacity limited only during strenuous, athletic activity.
II	Fatigue, shortness of breath, coughing, etc., become evident when ordinary exercise is exceeded. Ascites may appear at this stage.
III	Comfortable at rest, but exercise capacity is minimal.
IV	No capacity for exercise. Disabling clinical signs are present even at rest.

The New York Heart Association Functional Classification is based on the development of clinical signs during exertion and the degree to which exercise capacity is impaired. This system can be modified for use in dogs (Table 71–4). The major limitation of this method is its subjectivity. The amount of physical activity that is considered normal depends upon lifestyle and the purpose for which the animal is kept. A lap dog may give little indication of the severity of its cardiac dysfunction, while a sporting dog may perform poorly despite being able to exercise at a relatively high intensity. Since signs of respiratory distress developing during transient periods of increased activity are heavily weighted in this system, dogs with left heart dysfunction are likely to be overclassified. On the other hand, dogs in right heart failure with grossly evident ascites, for example, may exercise at a rate that belies the severity of their cardiac dysfunction. In humans, a surprisingly poor correlation has been found between pump function at rest and exercise capacity.[67]

Exercise capacity can be objectively evaluated by comparing the work performed to oxygen consumption and blood lactate levels.[41] Unfortunately, these methods are impractical for routine clinical use in animals. Consequently, veterinary clinicians must continue to rely upon their subjective assessment, but must also be aware of its limitations. Clinical judgment improves if information obtained from physical findings and radiographic, echocardiographic, and other appropriate means of assessment is taken into consideration.

THERAPEUTIC CONSIDERATIONS

As the heart inexorably fails and there is progressively greater dependence on compensatory mechanisms, the deleterious side effects that are a consequence of these adjustments become increasingly troublesome. The first priority of heart failure therapy is to correct those side effects that may be life threatening. This objective is critically important when dealing with acute pulmonary edema. The extent to which each compensatory mechanism may be operative varies among patients and at different stages of heart failure. Therefore, an effort must be made to determine the individual's particular needs if the goals of therapy are to be achieved and counterproductive measures are to be avoided. Ordinarily, these decisions are based on limited amounts of objective information and a large measure of clinical judgment.

BLOOD VOLUME DEPLETION AND VENODILATION

Diuretics, salt-restricted diets, and venodilators primarily reduce preload. They may be very effective in relieving signs of congestion and edema, but they do not immediately improve cardiac function. As heart failure worsens and preload reserve is used up, the ventricular function curve flattens out (Figure 71–7). Consequently, further increases in preload produce little or no improvement in cardiac output and intensify the congestive signs. Conversely, as high filling pressure is reduced and the operating point on a severely depressed function curve begins to move back toward the left, only a small decline in cardiac output occurs (Figure 71–13). If ventricular chamber volume becomes smaller following a decrease in filling pressure, systolic wall tension (afterload) also declines (LaPlace relationship). Thus, without necessarily causing a fall in systemic blood pressure, preload-reducing maneuvers may also lower afterload. This has a small positive effect on ventricular performance and partially offsets any decline in cardiac output that might otherwise result from a decrease in preload. Therefore, when contractility is severely depressed and ventricular filling pressure is high, diuretics and venodilators are able to relieve congestion and edema without having a major adverse effect on cardiac output. However, the failing heart becomes more preload-dependent as the operating point is shifted further to the left and the slope of the ventricular function curve becomes steeper. In this critical range, decreases in filling pressure diminish venous return and cardiac output. When this begins to happen, additional diuretic or venodilator administration is contraindicated by the decline in cardiac output, renal blood flow, and glomerular filtration rate. The less ventricular function is depressed, the more sensitive cardiac performance becomes to a decrease in preload (Figure 71–13).

A second way that diuretics may also decrease afterload is by improving vascular compliance (Figure 71–9). Some of the salt and water retained by heart failure patients is accumulated in the vessel walls. This can significantly increase their stiffness and diminish their responsiveness to vasodilatory stimuli. By relieving vascular edema, diuretics improve vasomotor responsiveness to endogenous metabolic vasodilators and vasodilating drugs.

ARTERIOLAR VASODILATATION

Perfusion pressure is maintained by widespread and often intense arteriolar vasoconstriction in heart failure patients. Since the vessels of the heart and brain lack α-adrenergic receptors, they do not participate in the sympathetically mediated general increase in systemic vascular resistance, and a larger than normal proportion of the cardiac output is diverted to these vital organs. Although regional peripheral vasoconstriction facilitates a potentially useful redistribution of cardiac output, the increase in total vascular resistance eventually becomes a self-defeating process. By exacerbating the mismatch between afterload and contractility, arteriolar vasoconstriction makes it more difficult for the ventricle to eject blood, and both the stroke volume and ejection fraction decrease. In heavily preloaded, dilated ventricles that have not developed a compensatory degree of hypertrophy, systolic wall tension is high. These ventricles are particularly adversely affected by inappropriately ele-

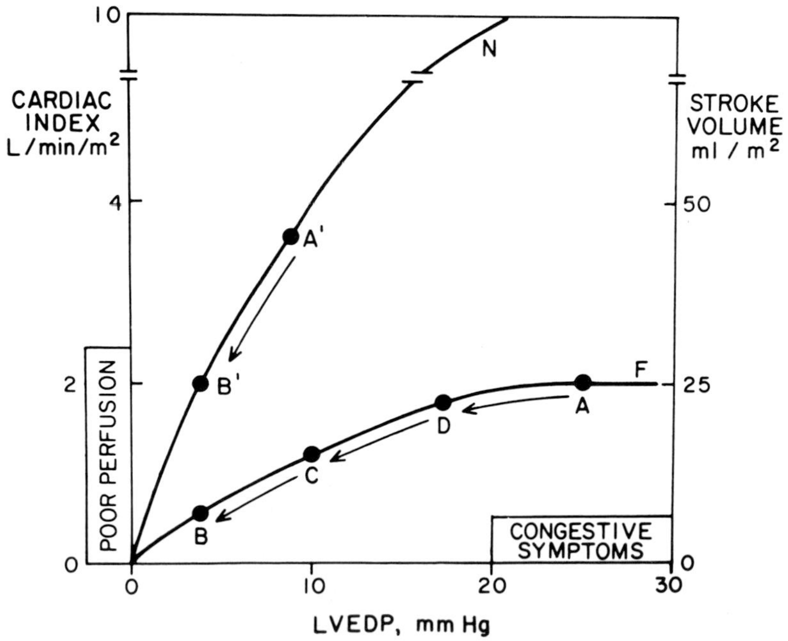

FIGURE 71–13. Effect of venodilator or diuretic therapy in a normal (N) subject (A′—B′) and in patients with heart failure (F) and markedly elevated left ventricular filling pressure (A—D), moderately elevated filling pressure (D—C), and normal filling pressure (C—B). In all instances venodilator or diuretic therapy results in a decline in filling pressure; except in the patient with marked elevation of filling pressure, cardiac output declines. (From Smith, FW and Braunwald, E: The management of heart failure. *In* Braunwald, E (ed): Heart Disease: A Textbook of Cardiovascular Medicine, 2nd ed. Philadelphia, WB Saunders, 1984.)

vated afterloads. The extent to which a given afterload limits shortening and thus reduces stroke output is directly proportional to the degree of myocardial depression (Figure 71–14). Accordingly, afterload reduction achieved with arteriolar vasodilators produces the greatest increase in stroke volume when myocardial contractility is severely depressed and a high preload ensures adequate venous return.[71] For this reason, their use is usually reserved for patients in the late stages of heart failure.

Figure 71–14 illustrates the effect of afterload reduction on muscle length (stroke volume). As preload reserve is used up in the late stages of heart failure, the ability of the myocardium to cope with increases in afterload is seriously limited. In this situation, even modest decreases in afterload produce sizable increases in fiber shortening. So long as vascular impedance is not drastically reduced, systemic blood pressure is maintained by a compensatory increase in cardiac output that is made possible by a combination of increased stroke volume and heart rate. To the extent that the augmented flow is distributed to underperfused, metabolically active tissues, such as exercising skeletal muscles, both hemodynamic and functional improvement is achieved. In humans, pure arteriolar vasodilatation invariably increases cardiac output, but not necessarily exercise capacity.[72]

The normal myocardium is much less sensitive to afterloading. An equivalent decrease in end-systolic wall tension produces a much smaller increase in fiber shortening than would occur in severely depressed myocardium (Figure 71–14). Therefore, a substantial increase in heart rate is necessary if the normal heart or one in which contractility is only modestly reduced is to be able to increase cardiac output sufficiently to prevent weakness or syncope due to hypotension. Tachycardia at rest is a frequent side effect of arteriolar vasodilatation at this stage in dogs. However, hypotension is more likely to become a troublesome side effect in patients with severely depressed myocardial contractility. Because their sympathetically mediated baroreceptor responses are attenuated, dogs in the late stages of heart failure experience less reflex tachycardia at equivalent degrees of hypotension.[6] Although there may be a substantial increase in stroke volume, the limited heart rate response may prevent cardiac output from rising sufficiently to prevent hypotension. For this reason, the dosage of afterload-reducing drugs must be carefully titrated, especially in advanced heart failure patients. With the possible exception of some cases of mitral regurgitation, arteriolar vasodilator therapy is likely to be of little or no benefit in the early stages of heart failure when preload is adequately controlled by diuretics and systolic function is only marginally compromised.

COMBINED EFFECT OF INCREASED CONTRACTILITY AND AFTERLOAD REDUCTION

A positive inotrope increases both the peak and incremental change in the force of myocardial contraction as the muscle is stretched. This shift moves the cardiac function curve toward normal and complements the action of arteriolar vasodilators (Figure 71–15) while counteracting the potential decline in performance resulting from a diuretic- or venodilator-induced reduction

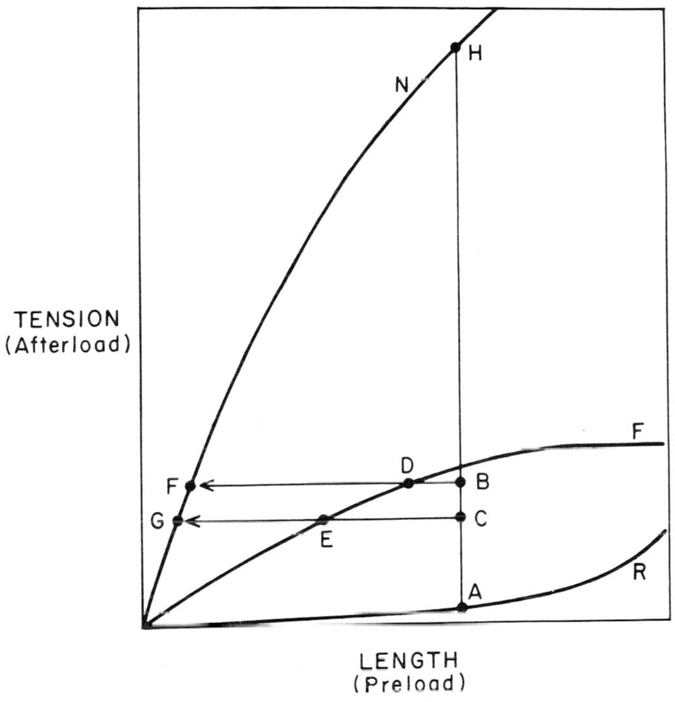

FIGURE 71–14. Length-tension relations in normal (N) and failing (F) heart muscle. R = length–resting tension curve for both normal and failing heart muscle. The effects of reducing afterloads from B to C on shortening are contrasted. In the normal muscle, shortening increases only slightly (from B—F to C—G). In failing muscle, there is substantial enhancement of shortening (B—D to C—E). H represents isometric tension development by normal muscle. (From Smith, FW and Braunwald, E: The management of heart failure. *In* Braunwald, E (ed): Heart Disease: A Textbook of Cardiovascular Medicine, 2nd ed. Philadelphia, WB Saunders, 1984.)

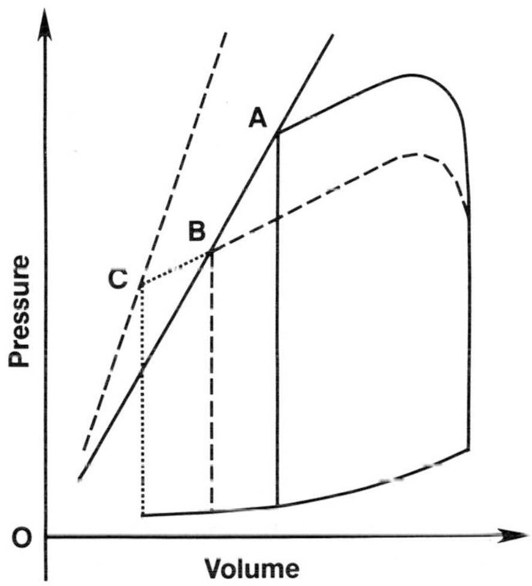

FIGURE 71–15. Schematic representation of the acute changes in the ventricular pressure/volume (P/V) relationship after decreasing the afterload and increasing myocardial contractility. The increase in stroke volume achieved by reducing afterload from *A* to *B* with an arteriolar dilating drug is further augmented by a positive inotrope, which shifts the end-systolic P/V relationship (represented by the diagonal lines) to point *C*. If there is an effective response to this drug combination, end-diastolic pressure and volume should subsequently decline.

in preload. For these reasons, positive inotropes are frequently used to advantage in combination with drugs that exert their effect entirely by modifying loading conditions.

Greater increases in cardiac output can be achieved with the combined use of arteriolar vasodilators and positive inotropes than with the use of either therapy alone (Figure 71–15).[72, 73] For reasons discussed in the preceding section on arteriolar vasodilators, this combined therapy has the greatest potential for improving cardiac performance when contractility is depressed and preload is high. The extent to which an increase in cardiac output and subsequent fall in ventricular filling pressure can be attributed to an increase in inotropy depends on how much contractile reserve remains. Severely depressed contractility and a large afterload mismatch characterize patients in low output heart failure due to the dilated forms of cardiomyopathy. In some of these patients, myocardial depression may be so profound that stimulating the heart produces little or no response. In effect, such cases have exhausted their contractile reserve.[74] Once it has been used up, the only way to improve cardiac performance is by reducing afterload.

In patients with severe chronic mitral regurgitation, there is already a large reduction in left ventricular afterload due to incompetence of the mitral valve. Contractility in these hearts is usually significantly depressed, although to a lesser degree than in the primary myopathic hearts. Because of the large regurgitant fraction, a smaller end-systolic volume is reached than would otherwise be possible. However, since the end-systolic volume still is frequently larger than normal, the benefit from cardiotonic therapy may be considerable.[52] Total stroke volume may not increase much following arteriolar vasodilatation, but a decrease in peripheral vascular resistance facilitates ejection of blood into the aorta, thereby decreasing the regurgitant fraction and increasing the effective (forward) stroke output.[75] Neither positive inotropes nor afterload-reducing drugs have an immediate effect on preload and therefore, they are not relied upon in the initial stages of combating life-threatening pulmonary edema. However, if they are successful in improving ventricular function, a further decline in filling pressure will gradually ensue.

Although some patients experience considerable clinical improvement following the administration of arteriolar vasodilating drugs, both with and without concomitant positive inotrope therapy, others fail to respond or become refractory to their long-term use.[76] It is important to realize that the clinical response to afterload-reducing drugs represents the net effect of drug-induced vasodilatation and counteractive mechanisms that attempt to preserve the existing hemodynamic state. By lowering blood pressure, vasodilators activate the sympathetic nervous system and the renin-angiotensin system, thereby triggering a reactive vasoconstrictor response. The existence of this equilibrium can be documented by the rebound and overshoot in blood pressure that frequently follows the abrupt withdrawal of direct-acting arteriolar vasodilators. This phenomenon is most likely to occur in heart failure patients with only mild ventricular impairment, in which circulating catecholamine levels had not risen substantially before vasodilatation, and circulatory reflexes remained largely intact. In addition to reactive vasoconstriction, patients that continue on chronic vasodilator therapy experience considerable salt and water retention due to neurohumoral responses and altered renal hemodynamics. Besides exacerbating the congestive signs, this also opposes vasodilatation by increasing arterial vascular stiffness. Independent of these counteractive mechanisms, certain classes of vasodilators become ineffective due to the development of true drug tolerance.[76]

Both short- and long-term hemodynamic benefit from vasodilator therapy is uncertain at the outset. It is frequently impossible to adequately assess those variables (contractility, loading conditions, state of neurohumoral activation) that are important determinants of successful vasodilator therapy. Therefore, the clinical status of these patients must be continuously reevaluated since these drugs will be ineffectual if certain hemodynamic prerequisites are not present. Eventually, progressive worsening of the underlying disease overwhelms all forms of therapy. Distinguishing this terminal state of clinical deterioration from an inappropriate choice of drugs and ineffective dosage can be a dilemma.

SUMMARY

The syndrome of heart failure is a complex, multisystem interaction of positive feedback mechanisms that attempt to restore cardiac performance. These mechanisms involve the heart, peripheral circulation, kidneys, and neuroendocrine system consisting of the sympathetic nervous system and the adrenal and pituitary glands. Pump function may be compromised by the failure of any of its constituent parts to perform adequately. Although myocardial failure is not always the primary cause of heart failure, it is a common denominator at the end stage of all long-standing pathologic increases in cardiac workload.

The cardiovascular system has considerable, though limited, capacity to maintain hemodynamic homeostasis. As the capacity to pump blood in response to metabolic requirements declines, reflex sympathoadrenal activation drives the heart faster and more forcefully. Also, autonomically induced regional peripheral vasoconstriction conserves cardiac output by diverting blood to organs with obligatory needs, maintains perfusion pressure, and assists venous return to the heart. If cardiac performance continues to deteriorate, the renal-adrenal-pituitary axis triggers blood volume expansion and permits further use of the Frank-Starling mechanism. Myocardial hypertrophy is a major cardiac adaptation to a sustained hemodynamic burden. The extent to which cardiac function is compromised depends on the duration and severity of underlying cardiac disease, effectiveness of compensatory mechanisms, and success of therapeutic maneuvers. Once cardiac reserve becomes severely limited, the same compensatory mechanisms that had a beneficial effect at an earlier stage become overused and produce deleterious side effects. Controlling the compensatory mechanisms is the major goal of therapy since only a few causes of heart failure are curable. The clinical manifestations of heart failure reflect the relative contributions of the cardiac and peripheral vascular compensatory mechanisms. Consequently, the clinical presentation of heart failure is variable and the approach to therapy needs to be individualized.

References

1. Braunwald, E: Pathophysiology of heart failure. *In* Braunwald, E (ed): Heart Disease: A Textbook of Cardiovascular Medicine. 2nd ed. Philadelphia, WB Saunders, 1984, p 447.
2. Mason, DT: Regulation of cardiac performance in clinical heart disease: Interactions between contractile state, mechanical abnormalities and ventricular compensatory mechanisms. *In* Mason, DT (ed): Congestive Heart Failure: Mechanisms, Evaluation, and Treatment. New York, York Medical Books, Dun-Donnelley Pub, 1976, p 111.
3. Braunwald, E: Regulation of the circulation. N Engl J Med 290:1124–1420, 1974.
4. Braunwald, E et al.: Contraction of the normal heart. *In* Braunwald, E (ed): Heart Disease: A Textbook of Cardiovascular Medicine. 2nd ed. Philadelphia, WB Saunders, 1984, p 409.
5. Higgins, CB, et al.: Alterations in the baroreceptor reflex in conscious dogs with heart failure. J Clin Invest 51:715, 1972.
6. White, CW: Reversibility of abnormal arterial baroreflex control of heart rate in heart failure. Am J Physiol 24:H778, 1981.
7. Covell, JW, et al.: Reduction of the cardiac response to postganglionic sympathetic nerve stimulation in experimental heart failure. Circ Res 19:51, 1966.
8. Higgins, CB et al.: Extent of regulation of the heart's contractile state in the conscious dog by alteration in the frequency of contraction. J Clin Invest 52:1187, 1973.
9. Maughan, WL, et al.: Effect of heart rate on the canine end systolic pressure-volume relationship. Circ 72:654, 1985.
10. Narahara, KA and Blettel, L: Effect of rate on left ventricular volumes and ejection fraction during chronic ventricular pacing. Circ 67:323, 1983.
11. Melbin, J et al.: Coherence of cardiac output with rate changes. Am J Physiol 234:H499, 1982.
12. Sonnenblick, EH and Skelton, CL: Reconsideration of the ultrastructural basis of cardiac length-tension relations. Circ Res 35:517, 1974.
13. Spotnitz, HM, et al.: Relation of ultrastructure to function in the intact heart: Sarcomere structure relative to pressure volume curves of the intact left ventricles of dog and cat. Circ Res 18:49, 1966.
14. Yoran, C et al.: Structural basis for ascending limb of left ventricular function. Circ Res 32:297, 1973.
15. Robinson, TF, et al.: The heart as a suction pump. Scientific Am 256(6):84, 1986.
16. LeWinter, MM, et al.: Time-dependent shifts of the left ventricular diastolic filling relationship in conscious dogs. Circ Res 45:641, 1979.
17. Leyton, RA, et al.: Cardiac ultrastructure and function: Sarcomeres in the right ventricle. Am J Physiol 221:902, 1971.
18. Linderer, T, et al.: Influence of atrial systole on the Frank-Starling relation and end-diastolic pressure-diameter relation of the left ventricle. Circ 67:1045, 1983.
19. Braunwald, E and Frahm, CJ: Studies on Starling's law of the heart. IV. Observations on hemodynamic functions of left atrium in man. Circ 24:633, 1961.
20. Noordergraaf, A and Melbin, J: Ventricular afterload: a succinct yet comprehensive definition. Am Heart J 95:545, 1978.
21. Vatner, SF, et al.: Effects of anesthesia, tachycardia, and autonomic blockade on the Anrep effect in intact dogs. Am J Physiol 226:1450, 1974.
22. Piene, H and Covell, JW: A force-length-time relationship describes the mechanics of canine left ventricular wall segments during auxotonic contractions. Circ Res 49:70, 1981.
23. Ross, JJ: Afterload mismatch and preload reserve: A conceptual framework for the analysis of ventricular function. Prog Cardiovasc Dis 18:255, 1976.
24. Sasayama, S, et al.: Adaptations of the left ventricle to chronic pressure overload. Circ Res 38:172, 1976.
25. Weber, KT and Janicki, JS: Instantaneous force-velocity-length relations: Experimental findings and clinical correlates. Am J Cardiol 40:740, 1977.
26. Sagawa, K: The end-systolic pressure-volume relation of the ventricle: Definition, modifications, and clinical use. Circ 63:1223, 1981.
27. Suga, H and Sagawa, K: Instantaneous pressure-volume relationship and their ratio in the excised, supported canine left ventricle. Circ Res 35:117, 1974.
28. Sodums, MT, et al.: Evaluation of left ventricular contractile performance utilizing end-systolic pressure-volume relationships in conscious dogs. Circ Res 54:731, 1984.
29. Katz, AM: Congestive heart failure: Role of altered myocardial cellular control. N Engl J Med 293:1184, 1975.
30. Pool, PE and Braunwald, E: Fundamental mechanisms in congestive heart failure. Am J Cardiol 22:7, 1968.
31. Luchi, RJ: Reduced cardiac myosin-adenosine triphosphate activity in dogs with spontaneously occurring heart failure. Circ Res 24:513, 1969.
32. Swynghedauw, E, et al.: Decreased contractility after myocardial hypertrophy: Cardiac failure or successful adaptation? Am J Cardiol 54:437, 1984.
33. Ito, Y and Chidsey, CA: Intracellular calcium and myocardial contractility. V. Calcium uptake of the sarcoplasmic reticulum fractions in hypertrophied and failing rabbit hearts. J Molec Cell Cardiol 6:237, 1974.
34. Rutenberg, HL and Spann, JF: Alterations of cardiac sympathetic neurotransmitter activity in congestive heart failure. *In* Mason DT (ed): Congestive Heart Failure: Mechanisms, Evaluation, and Treatment. New York, York Medical Books, Dun-Donnelley Pub, 1976, p 85.
35. Spann, JF, et al.: Cardiac norepinephrine stores and the contractile state of heart muscle. Circ Res 19:317, 1966.
36. Spann, JF, et al.: Contractile state of cardiac muscle obtained from cats with experimentally produced ventricular hypertrophy and heart failure. Circ Res 21:341, 1967.
37. Bristow, MR, et al.: Decreased catecholamine sensitivity and β-adrenergic receptor density in failing human hearts. N Engl J Med 307:205, 1982.
38. Zelis, R and Flaim, SF: Alterations in vasomotor tone in congestive heart failure. Progr Cardiovasc Dis 24:437, 1982.
39. Zelis, R and Mason, DT: Compensatory mechanisms in congestive heart failure—the role of peripheral resistance vessels. N Engl J Med 282:962, 1970.
40. Wilson, JR, et al.: Impaired skeletal muscle nutritive flow during exercise in patients with congestive heart failure. Role of cardiac pump dysfunction as determined by the effect of dobutamine. Am J Cardiol 53:1308, 1984.
41. Weber, KT, et al.: Oxygen utilization and ventilation during exercise in patients with chronic cardiac failure. Circ 65:1213, 1982.
42. Mason, DT, et al.: Alterations of hemodynamics and myocardial mechanics in patients with congestive heart failure: Pathophysiologic mechanisms and assessment of cardiac function and ventricular contractility. Prog Cardiovasc Dis 12:507, 1970.
43. Tonkon, MJ, et al.: Renal function and edema formation in congestive heart failure. *In* Mason DT (ed): Congestive Heart Failure: Mechanisms, Evaluation and Treatment. New York, York Medical Books, Dun-Donnelley Pub, 1976, p 169.
44. Peart, WS: Renin-angiotensin system. N Engl J Med 292:302, 1975.
45. Cannon, PJ: The kidney in heart failure. N Engl J Med 296:26, 1977.
46. Hall, JE, et al.: Control of glomerular filtration rate by renin-angiotensin system. Am J Physiol 233:F366, 1977.
47. Laragh, JH: Atrial natriuretic hormone, the renin-aldosterone axis, and blood pressure-electrolyte homeostasis. N Engl J Med 313:1330, 1985.
48. Grossman, W, et al.: Wall stress and patterns of hypertrophy in the human left ventricle. J Clin Invest 56:56, 1975.
49. Spotnitz, HM and Sonnenblick, EH: Structural conditions in the hypertrophied and failing heart. *In* Mason, DT (ed): Congestive Heart Failure: Mechanisms, Evaluation, and Treatment. New

York, York Medical Books, Dun-Donnelley Pub, New York, 1976, p 159.
50. Bishop, SP and Cole, CR: Ultrastructural changes in the canine myocardium with right ventricular hypertrophy and congestive failure. Lab Invest 20:219, 1969.
51. Laks, MM, et al.: Canine right and left ventricular cell and sarcomere lengths after banding the pulmonary artery. Circ Res 24:705, 1969.
52. Lord, PF: Left ventricular volumes of diseased canine heart: Congestive cardiomyopathy and volume overload (patent ductus arteriosus and primary mitral valvular insufficiency). Am J Vet Res 35:493, 1974.
53. Lord, PF: Left ventricular diastolic stiffness in dogs with congestive cardiomyopathy and volume overload. Am J Vet Res 37:953, 1976.
54. Laskey, WK, et al.: Left ventricular mechanics in dilated cardiomyopathy. Am J Cardiol 54:620, 1984.
55. Hirota, Y, et al.: Mechanisms of compensation and decompensation in dilated cardiomyopathy. Am J Cardiol 54:1033, 1984.
56. Stevenson, LW and Tillisch, JH: Maintenance of cardiac output with normal filling pressures in patients with dilated heart failure. Circ 74:1303, 1986.
57. Sasayama, S, et al.: Hyperfunction with normal inotropic state of the hypertrophied left ventricle. Am J Physiol 232:H418, 1977.
58. Ross, J: Afterload mismatch in aortic and mitral valve disease: Implications for surgical therapy. J Am Coll Cardiol 5:811, 1985.
59. Spann, JF, et al.: Ventricular performance, pump function and compensatory mechanisms in patients with aortic stenosis. Circ 62:576, 1980.
60. Wisenbaugh, T, et al.: Differences in myocardial performance and load between patients with similar amounts of chronic aortic versus chronic mitral regurgitation. J Am Coll Cardiol 3:916, 1984.
61. Eckberg, DL, et al.: Mechanics of left ventricular contraction in chronic severe mitral regurgitation. Circ 47:1252, 1973.
62. Mason, DT, et al.: Alterations of left ventricular performance and myocardial mechanics in patent ductus arteriosus and ventricular septal defect. Clin Res 16:240, 1968.
63. Wallenberger, A, et al.: Some metabolic characteristics of mitochondria from clinically overloaded hypertrophied hearts. Exp Molec Pathol 2:251, 1963.
64. Pinsky, WW, et al.: Permanent changes of ventricular contractility and compliance in chronic volume overload. Am J Physiol 237:H575, 1979.
65. Fowler, NO: Physiology of cardiac tamponade and pulsus paradoxus. Physiological, circulatory and pharmacologic responses in cardiac tamponade. Mod Concepts Cardiovasc Dis 47:115, 1978.
66. Braunwald, E, et al.: Studies on Starling's law of the heart: Determinates of the relationship between end-diastolic pressure and circumference. Circ Res 8:1254, 1960.
67. Francis, GS, et al.: Relationship of exercise capacity to resting left ventricular performance and basal plasma norepinephrine levels in patients with congestive heart failure. Am Heart J 104:725, 1982.
68. Sonnenblick, EH and Skelton, CL: Oxygen consumption of the heart: Physiological principles and clinical implications. Mod Concepts Cardiovasc Dis 40:9, 1971.
69. Kunis, R, et al.: Coronary revascularization for recurrent pulmonary edema in elderly patients with ischemic heart disease and preserved ventricular function. N Engl J Med 313:1207, 1985.
70. Dougherty, AH, et al.: Congestive heart failure with normal systolic function. Am J Cardiol 54:778, 1984.
71. Packer, M, et al.: Importance of left ventricular chamber size in determining the response to hydralazine in severe chronic heart failure. N Engl J Med 303:250, 1980.
72. Weber, KT, et al.: Vasodilator and inotropic agents in treatment of chronic cardiac failure: Clinical experience and response in exercise performance. Am Heart J 102:569, 1981.
73. Miller, RR, et al.: Combined vasodilator and inotropic therapy of heart failure: Experimental and clinical concepts. Am Heart J 102:500, 1981.
74. Sonnenblick, EH, et al.: New positive inotropic drugs for the treatment of congestive heart failure. Am J Cardiol 55:41A, 1985.
75. Greenberg, BH, et al.: Beneficial effects of hydralazine in severe mitral regurgitation. Circ 58:273, 1978.
76. Packer, M and LeJemtel, TH: Physiologic and pharmacologic determinants of vasodilator response: A conceptual framework for rational drug therapy for chronic heart failure. Prog Cardiovasc Dis 24:275, 1982.
77. Gordon, AM, et al.: Variation in isometric tension with sarcomere length in vertebrate muscle fibers. J Physiol (Lond) 184:170, 1966.

72 THE CLINICAL EVALUATION OF CARDIAC FUNCTION

DAVID SISSON

EVOLUTION OF THE CARDIAC EVALUATION

A carefully taken history and conscientiously performed physical examination usually suffice to establish the existence of heart disease. Together, they provide the basis for the selection of those diagnostic procedures required to determine the cause of cardiac dysfunction and to establish a causal relationship between the observed clinical signs and disease of the heart. Most veterinarians have been impressed with the importance of making an accurate anatomic and etiologic diagnosis, and they have been trained to recognize the various forms of congenital and acquired heart disease in animals. Most veterinarians are able to integrate the information made available from the history, the physical examination, the electrocardiogram, and thoracic radiographs to arrive at a provisional diagnosis. However, it is apparent that in many instances the information obtained from these procedures is inadequate or misleading. The interpretations of these studies are often extremely subjective, difficult to quantify, and therefore, difficult to interpret or communicate. Considerable clinical experience must be acquired before the value and limitations of these methods of evaluation are realized.

The diagnosis of some heart ailments is exceptionally difficult when the examination is limited to routine methods of evaluation. For example, it is extremely hard, if not impossible, to distinguish hypertrophic cardiomyopathy from dilated cardiomyopathy in cats unless some technique is used that allows visualization of the heart's internal anatomy.[1] The accurate assessment of cardiac function has been an equally elusive goal of the veterinary practitioner. Methods of evaluation currently employed do not permit any but the most crude assessments of cardiac function. With the exception of mitral regurgitation, the early stages of developing heart disease are rarely detected in animals. Prime examples include dilated cardiomyopathy, hypertensive heart disease, and cor pulmonale. It is also extremely hard to assess the severity of the common congenital and acquired cardiac disorders, to recognize the onset of heart failure, or to anticipate the requirement for therapeutic intervention. Until recently, the information needed to assess cardiac function could only be obtained by selective cardiac catheterization and quantitative angiocardiography.

New techniques and methodologies have emerged in recent years that have dramatically improved the accuracy of the cardiac evaluation. Most of these methods share a common attribute—they provide, in addition to invaluable qualitative diagnostic information, more objective, quantitative measures of cardiac performance than traditional methods of evaluation. Percutaneous right heart catheterization, radionuclide angiography, M-mode, two-dimensional, and Doppler echocardiography are now commonly used techniques that are available in most veterinary medical teaching hospitals. The development of these sophisticated technologies has greatly improved the diagnostic capabilities of the practicing cardiologist. Unfortunately, the veterinary profession is less aware of the opportunities presented to more accurately assess cardiac function in a minimally invasive fashion. These methods are being used with increasing frequency to assess basal cardiac function in patients with heart disease and, in serially performed studies, to objectively quantify patient responses to new and traditional therapies. The ability to assess cardiac function noninvasively promises to improve the management of individual patients with heart disease and to permit the formulation of more accurate prognoses. It is becoming increasingly important for the practicing veterinarian to understand the derivation of the common measures of cardiac function, to recognize the clinical relevance of the various indices of cardiac function, and to appreciate the attributes and limitations of the techniques used to make these evaluations.

EVALUATION OF THE LEFT HEART

SIZE AND MORPHOLOGY OF THE LEFT HEART

The size of the left atrium and left ventricle reflects the severity of underlying heart disease in most of the common cardiac disorders of the dog and cat. It can be accurately stated that for a given cardiac disease, a larger heart is usually more severely compromised than a smaller heart. Myocardial function is likely to become worse and the longevity of the patient is likely to be shorter as the heart becomes progressively enlarged. In humans with left heart failure due to cardiomyopathy or ischemic heart disease, the severity of the disease, as measured by patient survival, has been shown to correlate with the volume of the left ventricle both at end-systole and at end-diastole.[2] Similar observations have not yet been reported in dogs or cats with dilated cardiomyopathy, but similar results can be anticipated. In dogs and humans with mitral regurgitation, the severity of myocardial failure also correlates well with the size of the left ventricle at end-systole and end-diastole.[3–5] There are some notable exceptions to these generalizations, including those instances where valvular regurgitation develops suddenly due to bacterial endocarditis or rupture of a chorda tendineae.[6, 7] When heart failure develops acutely, there is insufficient time for the heart to hypertrophy and for these compensatory changes to become fully manifest. When the heart is presented with a sudden overwhelming volume or pressure overload, chamber size cannot be relied on to reflect the severity of disease or the functional state of the myocardium.

Functional evaluation of the heart often requires accurate measures of chamber size (volume) and wall thickness. When the cause of heart disease is known, a crude estimation of left ventricular size can be made inexpensively with routine thoracic radiographs. However, the information provided by routine thoracic radiography is extremely meager because of the inherent limitations of the method. These limitations result from many factors, including ambiguity resulting from conformational differences between the thoraces of the various breeds, the inability to identify the borders of the left and right ventricles, the inability to distinguish systolic from diastolic films, and most importantly, the inability to distinguish soft tissue (heart wall) from blood (chamber size). Thus, plain thoracic radiographs are unable to distinguish cardiac enlargement due to dilatation from that due to eccentric or concentric hypertrophy.

Selective biplane cineangiography surmounts these obstacles, providing the most accurate available measure of left ventricular volume.[8] Ventricular volume is calculated using the formula for an ellipsoid of revolution as described by Dodge.[9] Left ventricular volume calculated in this fashion overestimates the true volume of the left ventricle. Thus, these measurements must be adjusted using a regression equation derived from prior studies, which describe the relationship between the calculated volumes and actual volumes of excised, barium-filled canine hearts.[10, 11] While angiographic measures are considered the standard against which all other techniques are compared, the method is invasive, time-consuming, and expensive to perform. The requirement for general anesthesia places animals with severe heart failure at risk and compromises the data sought from the evaluation. For these reasons, selective catheterization and angiocardiography are used uncommonly for

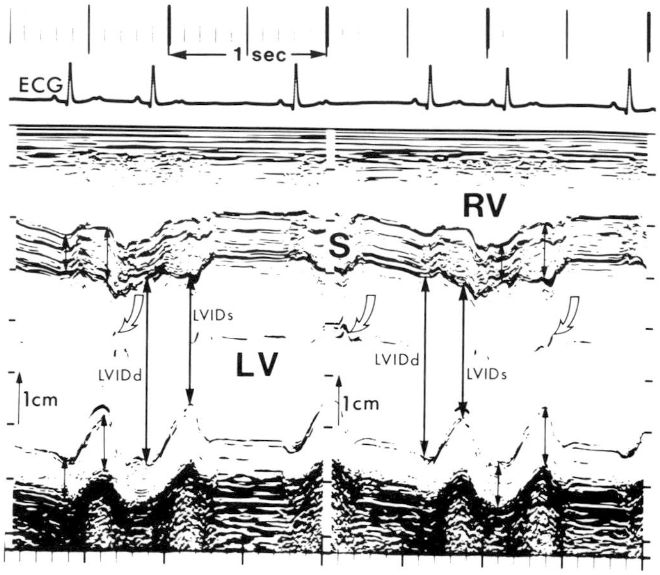

FIGURE 72–1. The short-axis internal dimensions of the left ventricle can be obtained at end-diastole (LVIDd) and at end-systole (LVIDs) from the M-mode echocardiogram at a point just below the tips of the mitral valve (open arrows). From these measures fractional shortening can be calculated and left ventricular volume, stroke volume, and ejection fraction can be estimated (see Table 72–1). RV = right ventricle; LV = left ventricle; S = interventricular septum.

functional evaluations of the heart even in well equipped and well staffed veterinary teaching hospitals. Single plane cineangiography provides a simpler and only slightly less accurate measure of left ventricular volume, but also is infrequently used for the evaluation of cardiac function in animals. Using this method, Lord reported end-diastolic volume in the normal dog as 25.4 ± 2.2 ml/10 kg, and end-systolic volume as 12.5 ± 1.2 ml/10 kg.[10]

Echocardiography has become the procedure of choice for the noninvasive evaluation of the left heart. With M-mode echocardiography, left ventricular volume can be estimated in normal dogs from measurements of the short axis diameter of the left ventricle (Figure 72–1). The necessary calculations require a number of geometric assumptions, none of which are entirely valid. Nonetheless, formulas for calculating left ventricular volume proposed by Pombo, Mashiro, Teichholz, and others have been applied with some success to the study of normal dogs.[12–15] These formulas are provided in Table 72–1. Studies in anesthetized dogs and of casts made of canine hearts fixed at end-systole and end-diastole have shown that the short axis of the left ventricle shortens more than the long axis.[16, 17] These observations appear to be best accommodated by

TABLE 72–1. LEFT VENTRICULAR VOLUME ESTIMATES FROM M-MODE ECHOCARDIOGRAMS

Author	Reference	Systolic Volume	Diastolic Volume
Fortuin	15	47 (ESD)–120	59 (EDD)–153
Mashiro	14	0.85 (ESD^3)	1.20 (EDD^3)
Pombo	12	ESD^3	EDD^3
Teichholz	13	$\frac{7\,(ESD^3)}{2.4 + ESD}$	$\frac{7\,(EDD^3)}{2.4 + EDD}$

ESD = end-systolic diameter, EDD = end-diastolic diameter.

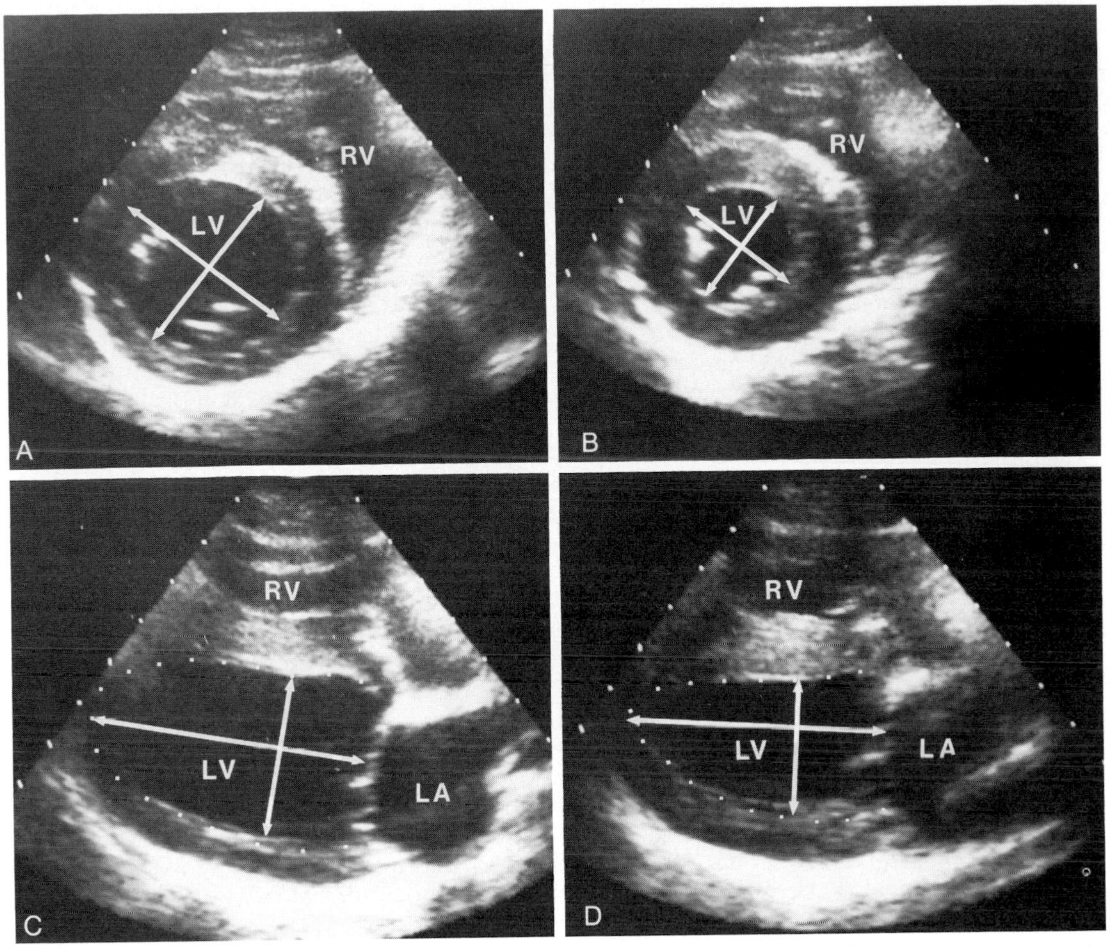

FIGURE 72–2. Two-dimensional echocardiography allows more accurate estimation of left ventricular volume, stroke volume, and ejection fraction than M-mode echocardiography. Short-axis orientation of the sector scanner (*A,* diastole; *B,* systole) permits measurement of both short-axis dimensions (arrows) and cross-sectional area. Long-axis orientation of the sector scanner (*C,* diastole; *D,* systole) permits measurement of long-axis dimensions and area allowing more accurate calculations of left ventricular volume using a variety of previously validated formulas.[28–31]

Teichholz's formula. In the author's laboratory, the Teichholz's equation most accurately predicts cardiac output and ejection fraction in normal dogs.

None of these formulas has been critically evaluated for the calculation of ventricular volume in dogs or cats with heart disease. These formulas are not likely to provide reliable estimates of ventricular volume in patients with dilated or eccentrically hypertrophied hearts, inasmuch as the geometric assumptions made are no longer valid. It has been shown that the short axis of the dog's ventricle enlarges more than the long axis when the heart hypertrophies eccentrically, i.e., the heart becomes more globoid.[18] When the left ventricle dilates acutely, the cross-section of the left ventricle changes from a circular configuration to an elliptical one.[18] Disease of the right heart often distorts the shape of the left ventricle because the configuration of the interventricular septum is altered.[19, 20] When these limitations are combined with technical errors of measurement, it soon becomes apparent that M-mode echocardiographic measurements of the left ventricle cannot be used to accurately estimate ventricular volume.[21, 22] Nonetheless, M-mode echocardiography can provide a useful estimate of relative ventricular size when it is simply reported as a cross-sectional dimension. Normal values for these measurements, indexed for body weight or body surface area, have been reported by a number of investigators.[23–27]

Theoretically, two-dimensional echocardiography should provide more accurate estimates of left ventricular volume than M-mode studies. Two-dimensional echocardiography permits measurement of the short and long axis of the heart from several different imaging planes and allows the examiner to identify global and regional changes in cardiac structure or function (Figure 72–2).[28] Fewer assumptions of ventricular shape are required, and the calculations of left ventricular volume resemble those described for biplane angiocardiography.[29] In the author's experience, it is impossible to obtain a satisfactory long axis view of the left ventricle in many dogs in order to make the necessary calculations. Volume may be underestimated because the long axis is foreshortened by improper angulation of the transducer.[30] The application of Simpson's rule for measuring left ventricular volume avoids the requirement of making any of these geometric assumptions.[31] With this method, the left ventricle is divided into a number of parallel slices and LV volume is obtained by adding together the volumes of all the slices. Unfortunately, the measurements and calculations required to obtain accurate estimates of left ventricular volume by this method are cumbersome to perform and generally require sophisticated and expensive image- and data-processing equipment. Unless such equipment becomes more readily available, such measurements will not be made routinely. Further research, coupled with improvements in equipment and software, can be expected to remedy many of these problems.

Left ventricular wall thickness can also be measured and used to assess cardiac function and the adequacy of compensation by the heart to an imposed hemodynamic burden. Measurements of wall thickness can be made from echocardiographic or angiographic studies. These measurements, as well as the derived estimates of ventricular mass, correlate well with measurements obtained at necropsy.[14, 32–34] When combined with measurements of chamber dimensions, extremely useful ratios of wall thickness to radius (or diameter or volume) can be calculated. In response to chronic volume overload, the heart hypertrophies eccentrically, and wall thickness increases modestly to normalize wall stress. The ratio of wall thickness to radius remains essentially normal in the compensated, volume-overloaded heart.[35, 36] As heart failure develops, the radius of the heart increases disproportionately to wall thickness, and this ratio diminishes.[37] In response to chronic pressure overload, the heart concentrically hypertrophies. The ratio of wall thickness to radius increases in proportion to the severity of the pressure overload (Laplace's law).[36] In fact, in the absence of heart failure, the severity of aortic stenosis can be crudely estimated from measures of wall thickness.[38] When heart failure ensues, the expected ratio of LV wall thickness to LV radius diminishes.[39] Such assessments require measurement of left ventricular pressure, cardiac output and calculation of the expected wall thickness. It has been suggested that poor cardiac performance in patients with aortic stenosis may result from inadequate hypertrophy rather than intrinsic depression of myocardial contractility.[40] In humans with heart failure due to ischemia or dilated cardiomyopathy, the ratio of left ventricular diastolic diameter to diastolic wall thickness appears to provide one of the best echocardiographic measures of the severity of disease, as judged by patient survival.[2] Such findings underscore the significance of the mismatching of wall stress to contractility in these disorders.

MEASUREMENT OF CARDIAC OUTPUT

Measurement of cardiac output is a very insensitive method of detecting cardiac dysfunction or myocardial failure. Even in the presence of overt heart failure, cardiac output can be maintained by the operation of a variety of compensatory mechanisms. Increases in heart rate, elevations of preload mediated by neurohumoral mechanisms, and cardiac hypertrophy act in concert to maintain cardiac output until late in the course of many cardiac diseases. The value of measuring cardiac output is increased when left ventricular filling pressure (LV end-diastolic pressure) is simultaneously determined.[40] In most instances, the measurement of pulmonary artery wedge pressure or pulmonary artery diastolic pressure can be used to estimate left ventricular end-diastolic pressure (preload). Cardiac output may be reduced in patients with a normal heart due to sudden elevations in afterload or, more commonly, due to reductions in preload caused by dehydration or hemorrhage. When filling pressure is decreased, a subnormal cardiac output may be due to inadequate preload rather than pump failure (Frank-Starling mechanism). When cardiac output is low and left ventricular filling pressures are high, myocardial contractility is probably depressed. It should be apparent that this statement presupposes that an elevated filling pressure indicates adequate preload. This is not always true, particularly when left ventricular compliance is abnormal.

In patients with severe heart failure, stroke volume and cardiac output are often depressed. In these patients, the sequential measurement of cardiac output is one of the most sensitive methods available to detect a hemodynamic response to afterload reduction or positive inotropic therapy. Cardiac output can be accurately measured by the Fick and indicator dilution techniques. The Fick method requires the measurement of oxygen consumption for several minutes under steady state conditions.[42] Cardiac output is then calculated by dividing oxygen consumption by the arterial-venous oxygen difference. The Fick method is most accurate when cardiac output is low and the arterial-venous oxygen difference is high.[43] When cardiac output is high, small errors in the measurement of oxygen content may cause large errors in the calculation of cardiac output. This is a laborious procedure to perform in anesthetized dogs and an impractical one to perform in most conscious dogs.

In most clinical circumstances, cardiac output is measured by the thermodilution technique due to its accuracy, safety, and relative simplicity.[44] Like all indicator dilution techniques, cardiac output is calculated based on the principle that the rate of blood flow can be accurately measured if the amount of indicator injected is known, if the concentration of the indicator can be continuously measured at some point downstream, and if the time for all of the mixture to pass the sampling site once can be determined. With the thermodilution technique, a known quantity of cold saline or 5 per cent dextrose in water is injected into the cranial vena cava or right atrium. The resultant temperature change in the circulating blood is continuously detected by a thermistor mounted on the tip of a Swan-Ganz catheter positioned in the pulmonary artery. A dedicated cardiac output computer is commonly used to calculate cardiac output (liters/minute). To facilitate comparisons between individuals, cardiac output is usually indexed for body surface area (liters/minute/meter^2). Stroke volume and stroke volume index can be easily calculated if the heart rate is simultaneously recorded. Normal values for cardiac output in the awake dog are given in Table 72–2.[45–53]

Cardiac output can also be measured by methods that permit the calculation of ventricular volume at end-systole and end-diastole (cardiac output = stroke volume × heart rate). Pertinent examples include echocardiographically and angiographically derived measure-

TABLE 72–2. CARDIAC OUTPUT AND CARDIAC INDEX IN NORMAL AWAKE DOGS

Author	Reference	CO (ml/min)	CI (ml/min/m² or /kg)	No. dogs
Manders	45	2200	89 (/kg)	14
Grimditch	46	1900	88 (/kg)	8
Bagshaw	47	—	3900 (/m²)	9
Bishop	48	2554	—	15
Sundet	49	2140	113 (/kg)	5
Yeo	50	3240	135 (/kg)	7
Liard	51	2448	125 (/kg)	19
Lin	52	3170	127 (/kg)	5
McKenzie	53	4200	187 (/kg)	9

CO = cardiac output, CI = cardiac index.

ments of cardiac output. Inasmuch as these methods require certain geometric assumptions for the calculation of left ventricular volume, they are less reliable than more direct measurements of cardiac output obtained using the Fick method or indicator dilution techniques.[54] In normal dogs and humans, M-mode derived measures of cardiac output have been reported to correlate well with more direct measures of cardiac output.[14, 55, 56] Unfortunately, this correlation is poor in cats.[57, 58] When the heart is enlarged, irregularly shaped, or is contracting asymmetrically, M-mode estimates of cardiac output are completely unrealistic. As previously mentioned, two-dimensional echocardiography provides a remedy for some of the errors induced by making erroneous assumptions about cardiac structure and function in disease states. In the presence of valvular regurgitation, an accurate geometric method of calculating cardiac output provides an estimate of total ventricular output rather than forward blood flow. By simultaneously measuring forward output (using indicator dilution techniques) and total ventricular output (using angiographic or echocardiographic derived measures) estimates of regurgitant flow and regurgitant fraction can be obtained.[59] Such calculations are useful for the evaluation of patients with chronic mitral regurgitation.

The equipment for measuring cardiac output is unavailable in most veterinary practices. An alternative to the measurement of cardiac output is provided by the calculation of the arterial-mixed venous oxygen (A-V O_2) difference. Arterial blood normally contains about 19 ml oxygen/dl, PaO_2 = 95 mm Hg, 95 per cent saturation, Hb = 15 g/dl. Mixed venous blood at rest contains about 15 ml oxygen/dl, PvO_2 = 40 mm Hg, 75 per cent saturation, Hb = 15 g/dl. The average extraction of oxygen is seen to equal 4 ml/dl at rest. As metabolic activity increases, e.g., with exercise, or when cardiac output is decreased, as in heart failure, the tissues extract up to three times more oxygen, up to a theoretical maximum of 11 ml/dl. This leaves a lesser amount of oxygen in the venous blood. In normal dogs at rest, PvO_2 levels usually exceed 35 mm Hg.[60] PvO_2 values lower than 35 mm Hg have been reported in dogs with heart failure due to chronic mitral regurgitation and in dogs with dilated cardiomyopathy.[60, 61]

The clinical value of these measures is uncertain at this time. PvO_2 levels depend on arterial oxygen saturation, cardiac output, and the rate of extraction of oxygen by the metabolizing tissues.[62, 63] The constancy of this latter value is difficult to ensure in animals in a hospital setting. The calculation of the arterial-mixed venous oxygen difference is of limited value in patients with hyperdynamic circulatory states, as observed in patients with chronic liver disease, hyperthyroidism, or peripheral A-V fistulas.[64] In patients with high output heart failure, the arterial-mixed venous oxygen difference is often normal or low due to arteriolar dilatation and the physiologic shunting of arterial blood to the venous circulation. In addition, systemic vascular resistance is usually substantially lower than normal in these disorders. The author has not observed a consistent correlation between cardiac output measured by thermodilution and PvO_2 in dogs with cardiomyopathy when both were measured simultaneously before and after therapy. This and all other measurements of cardiac output are inaccurate reflections of cardiac function unless the loading conditions of the heart are known.

The long-awaited ability to noninvasively measure cardiac output in clinical patients is rapidly becoming a reality. Doppler ultrasound provides the means to estimate cardiac output based on measurements of the velocity of blood flow in the aorta or in other locations, such as the pulmonary artery and mitral and tricuspid orifices.[65, 66] Sound waves with frequencies similar to those used to produce diagnostic ultrasound images are also used to measure blood velocity. Doppler studies are based on the principle that an emitted ultrasound pulse undergoes a change in frequency when it is reflected by moving targets. The Doppler equation describes the calculation of blood velocity (V) as a function of the Doppler frequency shift (f_s), the velocity of sound in soft tissue (c = 1540 m/sec), the frequency of the emitted ultrasound pulse (f_o), and the angle (r) between the emitted ultrasound pulse and the long axis of blood flow.

$$V = \frac{f_s \times c}{2\ f_o \cos r}$$

Stroke volume is calculated as the product of the Doppler flow velocity integral obtained from the aorta and the cross-sectional area of the aorta at its orifice. Cardiac output is then calculated as stroke volume multiplied by heart rate. Most studies report good correlation of cardiac output measured by Doppler techniques with measurements obtained by thermodilution or the Fick method.[67–71] The technique requires meticulous attention to detail and a skilled examiner. The most significant cause of error appears to be the noninvasive measurement of the diameter of the aorta.[65] Small errors in this measure result in large errors in calculations of cardiac output. While the equipment needed is not yet generally available to most veterinarians, the method is sufficiently developed that reports of its use in animals will probably appear with increasing frequency over the next few years.

PULMONARY VENOUS PRESSURE

Left heart failure is usually evidenced by dyspnea, pulmonary rales, and exercise intolerance. In most patients with left heart failure, the presence of pulmonary congestion can be ascertained by thoracic radiography.[72] The nature and distribution of lesions on chest x-rays and the concurrent presence of cardiomegaly (and a systolic murmur or gallop rhythm) usually correctly implicate the failing heart as the cause of pulmonary congestion. When pulmonary infiltrates of uncertain etiology are identified in patients with heart disease, other methods must be used to confirm the existence of heart failure. When equivocal evidence of left heart failure is present in these patients, left atrial pressure can be estimated by measurement of pulmonary artery wedge pressure using a Swan-Ganz catheter[73] (Figure 72–3). With this technique, a catheter with an inflatable balloon near the tip is introduced percutaneously through the external jugular vein and is advanced through the right heart to a branch of the pulmonary artery. The balloon not only aids the passage of the catheter, but also provides a means of occluding the vessel posterior to the catheter's terminal orifice. In this fashion, the pressure of the left atrium, as reflected retrograde through a continuous column of blood, is measured. Diastolic pulmonary artery pressure also provides an indirect estimate of mean left atrial pressure. In the absence of mitral valve disease, these measures provide useful estimates of the filling pressure of the left ventricle (LVEDP). There is no reliable, noninvasive method available for the measurement of pulmonary venous or left atrial pressure. Clinical investigations of the hemodynamic effects of vasodilators and positive inotropes should include measures of left atrial pressure obtained by the methods described.

Mean left atrial pressure in awake, normal dogs is less than 12 mm Hg in this author's laboratory. Interstitial pulmonary edema begins to develop when mean left atrial pressure exceeds 20 mm Hg.[74] Alveolar flooding begins to occur when mean left atrial pressure exceeds 25 mm Hg. When plasma oncotic pressure is abnormally low due to hypoproteinemia, pulmonary congestion may develop at lower pressures. The severity of pulmonary congestion does not always correlate with venous pressure, inasmuch as the capacity of the pulmonary lymphatics increases with longstanding elevations of left atrial pressure.[75] In dogs with chronic left heart failure, it is not uncommon to record mean left atrial pressures exceeding 35 mm Hg.[60] It should be realized that left atrial pressure may be extremely labile in the patient with mitral regurgitation. Sudden increases in afterload and fluid shifts from the systemic capacitance vessels can cause sudden and dramatic increases in left atrial and pulmonary venous pressures.

In patients with less severe disease, pulmonary congestion may be absent or may develop only following exercise. In these patients, resting cardiac output and left atrial pressure may be in the normal range at rest. The evaluation of cardiac function in these circumstances may require the application of a hemodynamic stress to unmask latent dysfunction. In normal animals, exercise elicits an increased stroke volume and cardiac output with no elevation in or only slightly elevated, filling pressures.[76] Patients with heart failure evidence reduced increases in cardiac output with exercise, and filling pressures increase markedly.[76] Other stresses, such as the administration of arterial vasoconstrictors, can be used in a similar fashion. The normal heart responds to this stress with little change in stroke volume and a small rise in end-diastolic pressure. In the failing ventricle, stroke volume falls and end-diastolic pressure rises markedly.[77]

The need to monitor left atrial pressure is perhaps greatest in patients with severe left heart failure and low cardiac output. It is desirable in these circumstances to maximize cardiac output by maintaining ample, yet not excessive, left ventricular filling pressures. These considerations are extremely important when vasodilation is accomplished with potent intravenous agents such as nitroprusside. The measurement of pulmonary artery wedge pressure is also extremely important in patients with coexisting heart and renal disease, which require vigorous fluid therapy. In these patients, the rate of fluid administration is moderated when wedge pressures increase to unacceptable levels. With less advanced disease and less vigorous therapy, reliance on thoracic radiographs to demonstrate resolution of pulmonary congestion, together with evaluation of the clinical response of the patient, is usually sufficient to ensure the welfare of the patient.

LEFT VENTRICULAR PRESSURES

The isovolumetric phase indices are measures of myocardial contractility made from recordings of the rate of rise of left ventricular pressure prior to the opening of the aortic valve. Peak dP/dt, $dP/dt/DP_{40}$ (dP/dt measured at a developed pressure [DP] of 40), and similar measures have been used to assess myocardial contractility in a variety of circumstances.[78–81] The accurate measurement of these parameters requires expensive, high-fidelity micro-tip pressure transducers. The isovolumetric phase indices are not used to measure basal contractility in the clinical setting but can be used to measure directional changes in myocardial contractility with an acute intervention. They have not been used for the study of clinical heart disease in animals.

The assessment of dogs with congenital subvalvular aortic stenosis requires quantitation of the translesional pressure gradient, the simultaneous measurement of cardiac output, and calculation of the size of the stenotic orifice. This is most accurately accomplished by cardiac catheterization. Gorlin's hydraulic equation is used to calculate the severity of stenosis.[82] Unfortunately, no studies have been performed to determine the clinical significance of making these measurements in the dog. The natural history of the disease is essentially unknown, although sudden death is thought to occur commonly. The relationship between sudden death and the severity of the stenosis has not been defined. Since there is no practical remedy for this disorder and selective cardiac catheterization is expensive, extensive evaluations of affected dogs are not commonly performed. Two-dimensional echocardiography is usually employed to make an anatomic diagnosis. This method also permits a crude estimation of the severity of stenosis based on measurements of left ventricular and septal wall thicknesses.[37]

Doppler ultrasound evaluation appears to offer an accurate, noninvasive means for estimating the severity of obstruction in dogs with aortic stenosis.[83, 84] The Bernoulli equation is used to predict the trans-stenotic pressure gradient (P), where $P = 4V^2$ and V is the peak flow velocity of the obstructive flow jets as measured by the Doppler examination.[85] In dogs with subvalvular aortic stenosis, pressure gradients estimated by Doppler evaluation correlate well with those measured at the time of cardiac catheterization. The onset of heart failure in dogs with subvalvular aortic stenosis is usually evidenced by increasing end-systolic and end-diastolic dimensions of the left ventricle and decreased ejection phase indices.

CONTRACTILE INDICES OF THE LEFT VENTRICLE

The ejection phase indices are the most common clinically used measures of cardiac contractility.[86] Despite objections that they are sensitive to acute changes in preload and altered afterload, they are of great use in the evaluation of basal contractility.[87, 88] All of these measures accurately distinguish normal patients from patients with myocardial dysfunction. Common measures of the ejection phase include the ejection fraction, the ejection rate, fractional shortening, and the mean and peak velocities of circumferential fiber shortening (VCF) (Table 72–3). The ejection fraction is simply a measure of the percentage of the end-diastolic volume that is ejected with each heart beat, i.e., the ratio of stroke volume to the end-diastolic volume of the left ventricle expressed as a percentage. Calculations of mean and peak VCF provide estimates of the rate of change of the left ventricular dimensions. These calculations require the additional measurement of ejection time. The ejection phase indices can be calculated using angiographically or echocardiographically derived measurements of left ventricular size. As previously discussed, all methods requiring estimation of volume are plagued by errors that result from the required geometric assumptions. Of these methods, the angiocardiographically derived measurements of the ejection phase indices serve as the standard.[8] Lord reported the average ejection fraction of normal halothane anesthetized dogs to be 61 per cent using single plane cineangiography.[10] He also reported the ejection fractions of several dogs with mitral regurgitation, patent ductus arteriosus, and dilated cardiomyopathy.[11] M-mode and two-dimensional echocardiographic studies provide less accurate measures of ejection fraction, particularly when the heart is irregularly shaped or when regional wall motion abnormalities are present. To avoid the errors inherent in making any geometric assumptions, most echocardiographers simply calculate fractional shortening and mean VCF as measures of the ejection phase.[89, 90] Boon et al. and Lombard reported fractional shortening in normal unsedated dogs to be 26.9 to 48.3 per cent (mean = 36.26 per cent) and 30 to 53 per cent (mean = 39 per cent), respectively.[23, 24] Boon also reported VCF in dogs as 1.58 to 2.79 cir/sec (mean = 2.07).[23] Pipers et al. reported the fractional shortening in the awake cat as 23 to 56 per cent (mean = 41 per cent), while Jacobs and Knight reported it as 49.8 per cent ± 5.27.[25, 26] Pipers et al. reported VCF in cats as 1.27 to 4.55 cir/sec (mean = 2.86), while Jacobs and Knight reported it as 3.65 cir/sec ± 0.63.[25, 26] Similar values have been obtained by others.[23–27]

TABLE 72–3. CALCULATION OF THE EJECTION PHASE INDICES

Ejection Fraction:	$\frac{EDV - ESV}{EDV} \times 100$
Ejection Rate (mean):	$\frac{EDV - ESV}{EDV \times ET}$
Fractional Shortening:	$\frac{EDD - ESD}{EDD} \times 100$
Mean Velocity of Circumferential Fiber Shortening:	$\frac{EDD - ESD}{EDD \times ET}$

EDV = end-diastolic volume, ESV = end-systolic volume, EDD = end-diastolic diameter, ESD = end-systolic diameter, ET = ejection time.

Radionuclide angiography is also being used with increasing frequency to measure cardiac performance during the ejection phase.[91–95] With this method, red blood cells or albumin tagged with technetium 99m is injected into a peripheral vein and the number of counts in the left ventricle at end-systole (ESC) and at end-diastole (EDC) is determined using a multicrystal gamma camera. Left ventricular ejection fraction is then calculated as (EDC − ESC)/EDC (Figure 72–4). Either first pass or gated equilibrium studies can be performed. Unlike any of the other methods discussed, no geometric assumptions regarding left ventricular shape are required in the calculations. Other technical problems have been identified, such as the necessity for background correction, the problem of accurate edge detection, and problems caused by superimposition of counts from the left ventricle and adjacent cardiac chambers. Ejection fractions calculated from gated radionuclide studies in normal dogs have been shown to correlate closely with those obtained by echocardiographic methods.[96]

Calculations of the ejection phase indices are most commonly made for the evaluation of dogs and cats with primary myocardial disease, e.g., dilated cardiomyopathy.[61, 97–101] A number of studies have demonstrated the reliability of the echocardiographic ejection phase indices in identifying dogs and cats with dilated cardiomyopathy. But, it must be recognized that the ejection phase indices do not provide a very sensitive method for the detection of hemodynamic changes in individual patients treated for heart failure. This is particularly obvious in dogs and cats with dilated cardiomyopathy and with very dilated hearts and low ejection fractions. For example, when cardiac output is increased by 20 per cent in a patient with an initial ejection fraction of 18 per cent, one would expect only a 3.6 per cent change in the ejection fraction, assuming that heart rate is constant. This magnitude of change lies well within the error of the techniques used to calculate ejection fraction.[102] Many animals with dilated cardiomyopathy have some degree of mitral regurgitation. This also complicates the interpretation of small changes in the ejection phase indices.

Significant hemodynamic and clinical improvement may occur without a change in the measured ejection phase indices. Small changes in the ejection phase

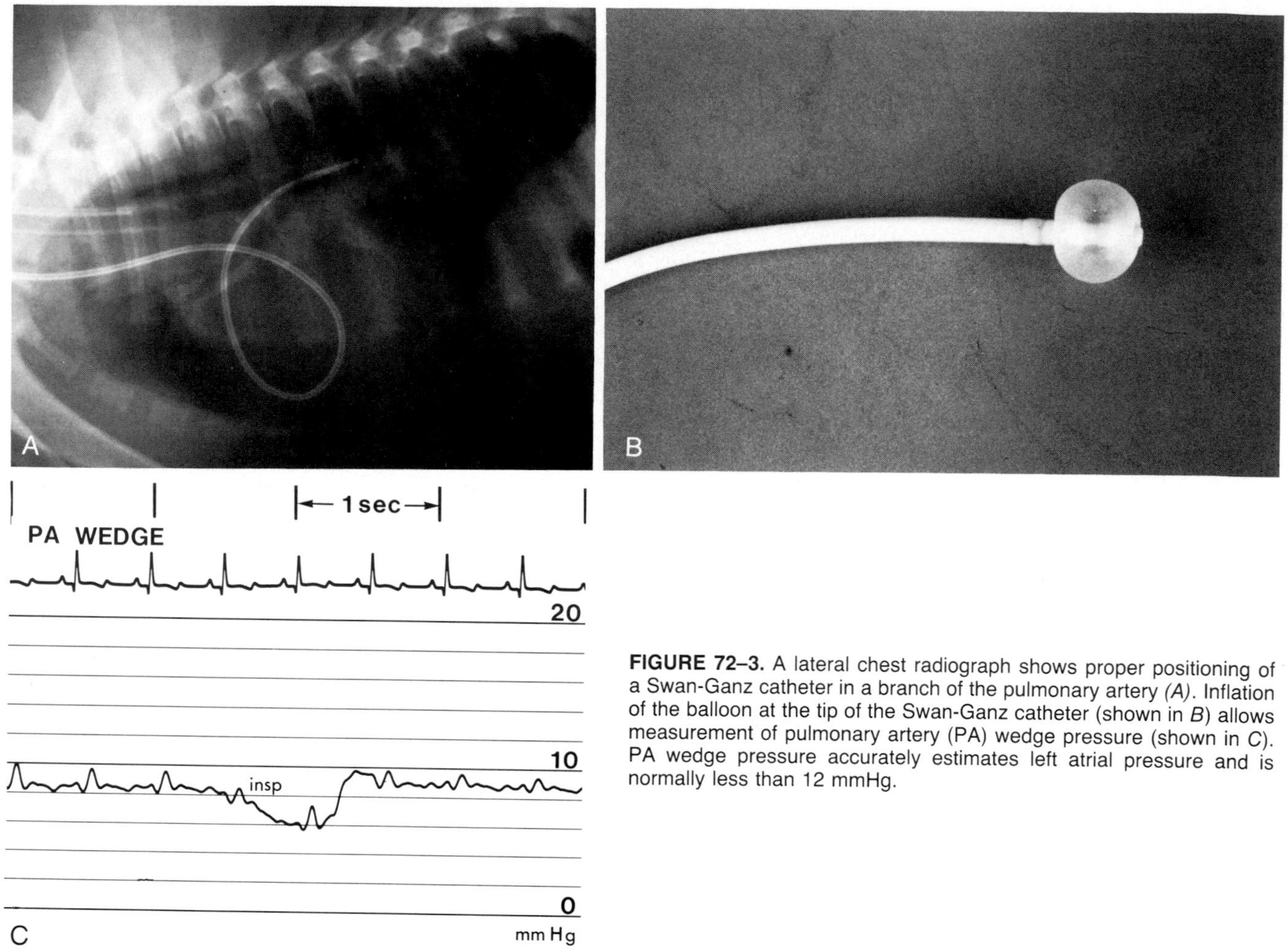

FIGURE 72–3. A lateral chest radiograph shows proper positioning of a Swan-Ganz catheter in a branch of the pulmonary artery *(A)*. Inflation of the balloon at the tip of the Swan-Ganz catheter (shown in *B*) allows measurement of pulmonary artery (PA) wedge pressure (shown in *C*). PA wedge pressure accurately estimates left atrial pressure and is normally less than 12 mmHg.

indices of individual patients cannot be relied on to judge the effectiveness of therapy. The significance of such measures must not be overinterpreted. Large changes in the ejection phase indices are required before they achieve significance in the individual patient. At this time, the application of the ejection phase indices as measures of hemodynamic improvement is more appropriately confined to the study of populations of patients in which statistical methods can be used to determine the significance of any measured differences.

Left ventricular function can also be assessed by more novel measures of the ejection phase using Doppler methods. Patients with cardiomyopathy can be distinguished from normal patients by measures of the peak flow velocity in the aorta or by calculation of the mean aortic flow velocity integral.[103,104] In addition, sequential measures of peak aortic flow velocity can be used to evaluate the response of individual patients to therapy. Knight has used this method to evaluate the response of dogs with myocardial failure to the experimental drug milrinone.[105]

Relative to the level of myocardial contractility, the ejection phase indices are falsely increased in dogs with mitral regurgitation (Figure 72–5).[3] This results from the unique loading conditions present in mitral regurgitation. Increased preload augments fiber shortening by the Frank-Starling mechanism and the impedance to ventricular ejection is markedly altered as large volumes of blood are ejected into the low-pressure left atrium. In patients with mitral regurgitation, myocardial contractility can only be measured accurately by methods that take into account these abnormal loading conditions.[106,107] Functional indices that are based on the end-systolic pressure-to-volume relationship are more appropriate measures of myocardial contractility in patients with mitral regurgitation. In spite of the inherent limitations of the method, measures of the ejection fraction continue to be used for the assessment of human patients with mitral regurgitation. It is simply recognized that a normal ejection fraction in these patients signifies a significant decline in myocardial contractility. In this circumstance, an ejection fraction less than 60 per cent is considered to represent significantly depressed myocardial function.[108,109] Using Teichholz's equation to estimate ventricular volume, Kittleson reported that an ejection fraction less than 80 per cent signifies moderate to severe myocardial failure in dogs with mitral regurgitation.[60]

When the loading conditions of the heart are abnormal or variable, the evaluation of myocardial contractility is best accomplished by determination of the end-systolic wall stress-to-volume relationship. A number of

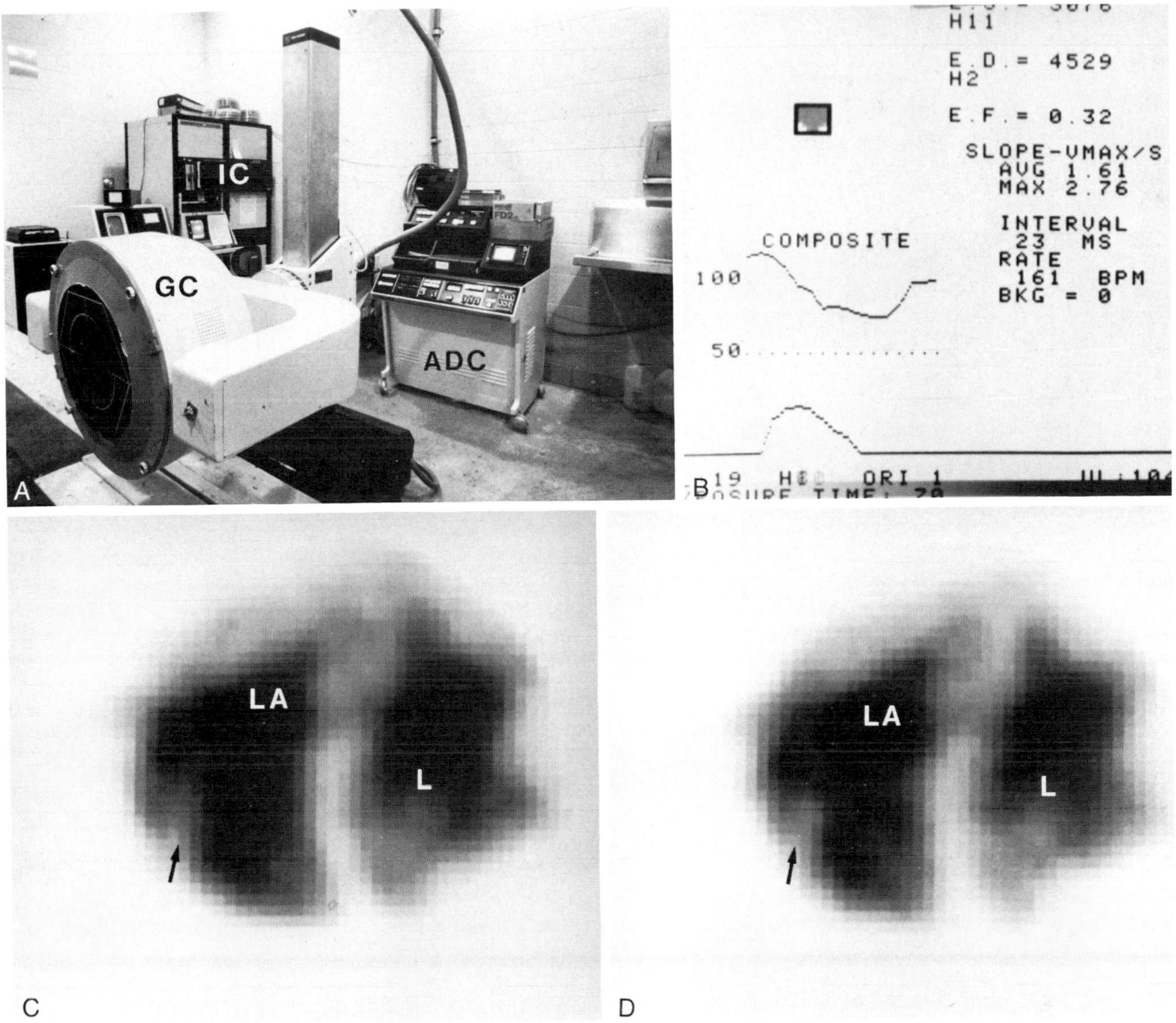

FIGURE 72–4. A multicrystal gamma camera (GC), an analog to digital converter (ADC), and dedicated imaging computer (IC) used to noninvasively measure left ventricular volumes and ejection fraction are shown in *A*. Ejection fraction is calculated from a time activity curve of the left ventricle following injection of red cells or albumin tagged with technetium 99m *(B)*. The ejection fraction (E.F. = 32 per cent) of a dog with cardiomyopathy is calculated as end-diastolic counts (E.D. = 4529)—end-systolic counts (E.S. = 3076)/end-diastolic counts. Computer generated images of the heart from a gaited equilibrium study are shown during at end-diastolic *(C)* and at end-systole *(D)*. The arrow indicates the interventricular septum which separates the right ventricle (anterior) from the left ventricle (posterior). LA = left atrium; L = liver.

"end-systolic" indices have been derived from studies that have demonstrated that there is a linear relationship between end-systolic pressure or wall stress and end-systolic volume over a wide range of loading conditions.[110–112] The slope of this line, as well as the intercepts, separate patients with and without left ventricular failure (Figure 72–6).[113] This relationship is most accurately established from angiographic measurements of left ventricular volume and wall thickness at end-systole combined with invasive pressure measurements made during a variety of loading conditions. This procedure requires meticulous measurements and is cumbersome to perform. However, a number of useful clinical indices of myocardial function have been derived from this relationship. It is possible to calculate useful estimates of myocardial contractility from measures of arterial pressure and ventricular dimensions at end-systole (using echocardiographic techniques).[114] The end-systolic pressure volume ratio and end-systolic volume index are less accurate approximations of left ventricular function that have been employed to assess function when cardiac loading conditions are abnormal.[6, 60, 115] The most common application of these measures in veterinary medicine is for the evaluation of myocardial contractility in dogs with mitral regurgitation. It has been suggested that myocardial contractility is normal or nearly normal if the size of the left ventricle at end-systole is normal when indexed for body surface area. In human patients with mitral regurgitation, preoperative myocardial contractility has been shown to be an

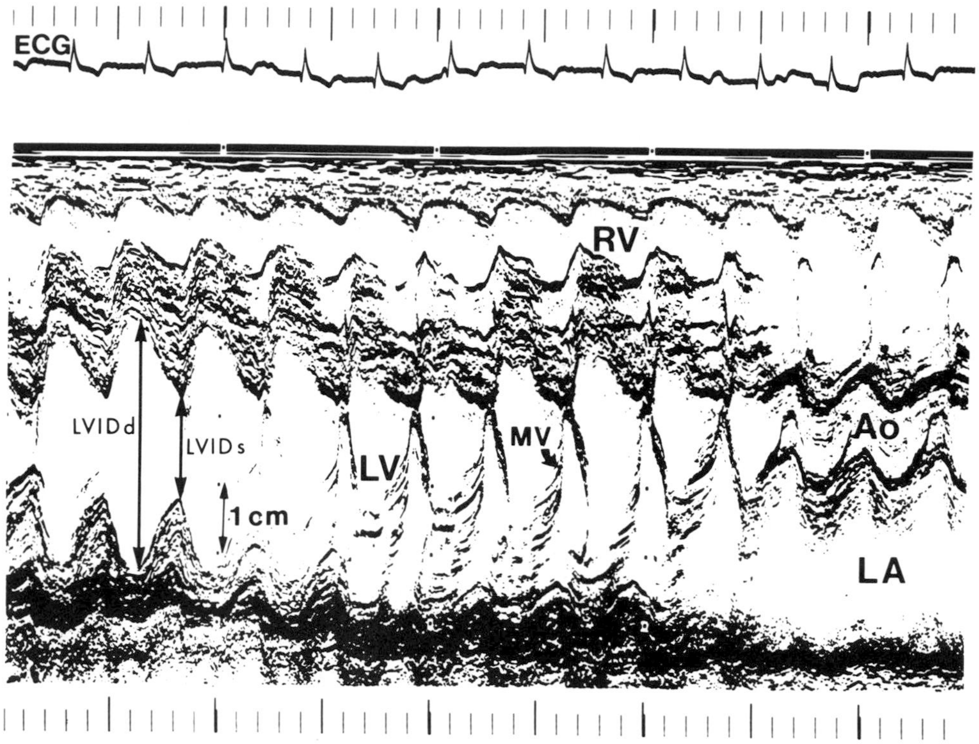

FIGURE 72–5. In the M-mode echocardiogram of a dog with mitral and tricuspid regurgitation, fractional shortening (LVIDd-LVIDs/LVIDd) is above normal (57 per cent). However, this measure and all other measures of the ejection phase cannot be used to accurately assess myocardial function when mitral regurgitation exists. One of the end-systolic indices would be more appropriate in these circumstances (see text). RV = right ventricle; LV = left ventricle; MV = mitral valve; AO = aorta; LA = left atrium.

important determinant of left heart function postoperatively and has prognostic value in predicting the surgical outcome.[6, 103–105] The evaluation of myocardial contractility in humans is performed primarily to determine the advisability of mitral valve replacement.

It must be emphasized that it is inappropriate to direct therapy solely toward any one measure of cardiac function, regardless of the method used to detect that abnormality. The manifestations of heart failure are caused by a complex cascade of initiating factors and compensatory mechanisms, all of which must be considered when planning or revising therapeutic plans. In recent years, therapy of patients with mitral regurgitation has focused on the reduction of systemic vascular resistance (SVR). Reports of improved cardiac output, reduced filling pressures, and decreased SVR with vasodilators and angiotensin converting enzyme inhibitors have influenced many to employ these therapies on a routine basis. It has been argued that inotropic therapy, namely digitalization, is inappropriate in most dogs with mitral regurgitation.[60] This argument was based on the observation of normal or nearly normal contractility in most affected dogs, as assessed by M-mode-derived measures of end-systolic volume. The accuracy of the method has never been validated in dogs. More sophisticated methods of evaluating myocardial contractility in dogs with experimental chronic mitral regurgitation have demonstrated significant myocardial impairment.[116] The potential beneficial effects of positive inotropes for the reduction of mitral regurgitant orifice size has apparently not been considered in recent studies.[3, 60] In experimental models of mitral regurgitation in dogs, positive inotropic therapy has been shown to markedly reduce mitral regurgitant flow by this mechanism, in the absence of myocardial failure.[117] It is quite possible that the most effective therapy for mitral regurgitation will include a positive inotrope together with an arterial or mixed vasodilator. Primary consideration in the evaluation of any medical evaluation must be given to the clinical response of the patient. To assume any practical value, every measure of cardiac performance must serve this goal.

ALTERNATE METHODS OF EVALUATION

Most veterinarians are unfamiliar with the use of systolic time intervals (STI) as a measure of left ventricular performance. Two time periods must be determined to use this method, the pre-ejection period (PEP) and the left ventricular ejection time (LVET).[118] The PEP is the interval of time from the beginning of ventricular depolarization to the beginning of ventricular ejection. The LVET is self-explanatory. These intervals can be determined by the simultaneous recording of the electrocardiogram, phonocardiogram, and carotid pulse tracing. They can also be obtained by a variety of other methods, such as M-mode echocardiography or Doppler interrogation. In the absence of conduction disturbances, the primary determinant of the PEP is the rate of pressure development during the isovolumetric phase of systole. The primary determinants of the LVET are the rate and extent of shortening of the left ventricle. The PEP lengthens during heart failure, while the LVET shortens. It is apparent that the ratio of PEP to LVET would be higher than normal in patients with left ventricular failure. The interested reader is referred to the references for a more complete discussion of these indices.[118–124]

EVALUATION OF THE RIGHT HEART

SIZE AND MORPHOLOGY OF THE RIGHT HEART

The assessment of right atrial and ventricular size using routine thoracic radiographs suffers from the same limitations described for the left heart. One of the most common mistakes made by veterinary practitioners is the overinterpretation of thoracic radiographs. Right heart enlargement is often perceived when, in fact, none exists. A significant problem in the interpretation of thoracic radiographs is the difficulty experienced in assessing the size of the right ventricle when the left ventricle is enlarged. For this reason, many veterinarians "see" biventricular enlargement when only the left heart is enlarged. Relevant examples include dogs with a patent ductus arteriosus or mitral regurgitation. It is equally difficult to recognize biventricular enlargement when it is present, e.g., in dogs with combined mitral and tricuspid regurgitation.

Echocardiographic evaluation offers a partial solution to the problems of assessing right ventricular and right atrial size and morphology. Echocardiographic studies offer more accurate assessments of chamber size and wall thickness than thoracic radiographs.[125, 126] Nonetheless, the lack of spatial orientation and complex geometry of the right ventricle limits the value of the M-mode echocardiogram for this purpose. Slight changes in the positioning of the transducer can markedly alter the apparent size of the right ventricle.[127] This represents a problem only when enlargement of the right heart is marginal. The right atrium cannot be adequately imaged in most animals using the standard imaging planes required for M-mode studies. Two-dimensional echocardiography is better able to assess the size of the right atrium and allows more accurate appraisal of right ventricular volume. The echocardiographic examination of the right heart is best accomplished by two-dimensional studies using multiple imaging planes, including the right parasternal long and short axis views, the left cranial views, and the left caudal parasternal four-chamber view.[128] Enlargement of the right heart is usually easily detected by these methods. However, the complex geometry of the right ventricle makes quantitative evaluation of this chamber difficult regardless of the method used.

Current methods for angiocardiographic or echocardiographic estimation of right ventricular volume are either too cumbersome to routinely employ or are simply too crude to be of much value.[129–132] These limitations do not diminish the value of echocardiography for imaging anatomic changes in the right heart resulting from congenital or acquired disorders. Pulmonic stenosis, tricuspid dysplasia, and septal defects can often be imaged by two-dimensional echocardiography.[133–135] Right heart enlargement due to pulmonary hypertension or tricuspid regurgitation can usually be appreciated even if it cannot be quantitated.[136]

RIGHT ATRIAL PRESSURE

Right heart failure in dogs and cats is usually manifested on physical examination by jugular distention, exaggerated jugular venous pulses, and ascites. Generalized venous distention and peripheral edema are less commonly observed in small animals than in humans, but may occur with severe heart failure. Pleural effusion may also develop in dogs and cats with severe, isolated right heart failure. More commonly, the presence of pleural effusion signifies the existence of biventricular heart disease, pericardial disease, obstruction of the cranial vena cava, or disease of the lung, pleura, or mediastinum.[137]

When right heart failure or pericardial disease is suspected, the measurement of right atrial pressure can be used to confirm the presence of cardiovascular disease and to serve as an unbiased reference point to gauge the effect of therapy. Right atrial pressure may be estimated by the determination of central venous pressure or may be directly recorded to allow inspection of the right atrial waveform. Central venous pressure (CVP) is measured in dogs and cats by inserting an intravenous catheter into the external jugular vein and positioning the tip in the right atrium or cranial vena cava. The catheter is attached via a three-way stopcock to a manometer and an intravenous infusion line (Figure 72–7). Normal CVP ranges from 3 to 10 cm H_2O, which equals 2 to 8 mm Hg (1.36 cm H_2O = 1 mm Hg). Central venous pressure may be elevated as a result of tricuspid valve incompetence, pump failure, or impaired ability of the right ventricle to fill. Impaired right ventricular filling can result from abnormal compliance of the right ventricle due to fibrosis or hypertrophy, the constraining effect of the pericardial sac due to effusion or fibrosis, and obstruction to the flow of blood by a mass or other lesion.

Dogs with overt right heart failure often have filling pressures in excess of 20 cm H_2O. Moderate elevations of CVP are sometimes measured in animals with expanded blood volume and/or high cardiac output. Some relevant examples include animals with severe hepatic

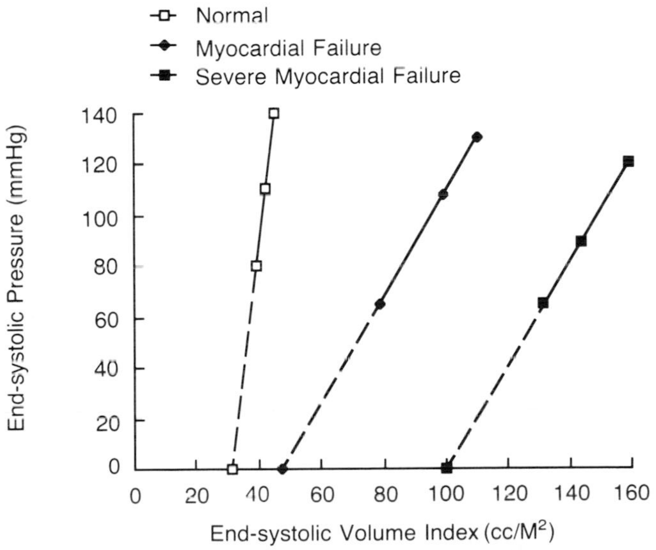

FIGURE 72–6. The end-systolic pressure volume relationship can be used to distinguish patients with normal myocardial function from those with moderate or severe myocardial failure. (Modified from Grossman W, et al.: Contractile state of the left ventricle in man as evaluated from end-systolic pressure-volume relations. Circulation 56:845, 1977, by permission of the American Heart Association, Inc.)

disease, pregnant animals, hyperthyroid cats, and patients that are inadvertently overhydrated by overzealous fluid administration. In some animals with acute right heart failure or less advanced disease, venous pressures at rest may be normal or only slightly elevated. In these patients, the application of a stress designed to increase venous return, such as exercise or abdominal compression, may result in a dramatic and sustained rise in CVP.[138] The combined measurement of CVP and cardiac output prior to, and following, a challenge with an intravenous fluid load is also helpful for the assessment of these patients. When cranial or caudal vena caval obstruction is suspected, the measurement of venous pressure in each of these locations often provides corroborating evidence as to the location of the lesion.

The direct recording of the jugular venous pulse or of right atrial pressure allows inspection of the pressure waveform and often permits recognition of the cause of systemic congestion or jugular pulsations.[139, 140] The normal atrial pressure tracing consists of an "a" wave due to atrial systole, an "x" descent during ventricular systole, a "v" wave due to atrial filling, and a "y" descent as the atrium empties into the right ventricle. The normal "x" descent may be interrupted by a small "c" wave caused by tricuspid valve closure. Regurgitant or "c-v" waves typify the right atrial pressure tracing of patients with tricuspid regurgitation. The prominent "c-v" waves of massive tricuspid regurgitation have been referred to as "ventricularization" of the atrial waveform.[141] Canon "a" waves are observed in patients with atrioventricular dissociation when the right atrium intermittently contracts against a closed tricuspid valve, e.g., as occurs in third degree heart block.[142] Giant "a" waves are common in diseases causing right ventricular hypertension.[143, 144] Abnormally steep "x" or "y" descents are frequently observed in human patients with pericardial disease.[145, 146]

PERFORMANCE OF THE RIGHT VENTRICLE

Functional evaluation of the right ventricle has been largely neglected in domestic animals and in humans with heart disease.[147] In part, this is the result of the predominance of left heart disease in these species. Early studies suggested that the contractile performance of the right heart was hemodynamically unimportant. Early experiments in normal dogs demonstrated that complete destruction of the right ventricular wall fails to alter right ventricular pressure development or cardiac performance.[148] From this work it was incorrectly concluded that the right ventricle was little more than a passive conduit for blood. Subsequent studies have demonstrated the functional importance of the right ventricle, particularly when pulmonary vascular resistance is increased and in patients with left heart disease.[147, 149, 150] It has become apparent that the contractile performance of the right heart is extremely important in determining the exercise capacity of patients with left heart disease.

Quantitative evaluation of right ventricular performance is difficult because the complex geometry of the right ventricle hampers precise measurement of right ventricular volume. The accuracy of the right ventricular ejection phase indices, which are based on end-systolic and end-diastolic volume estimates, suffers as a result. These problems severely limit the utility of angiography and echocardiography for assessing right ventricular function. Compared with that of the left ventricle, assessment of performance of the right ventricle is more difficult to assess because it is more sensitive to changes in preload and afterload.[147, 151] Regardless of the method used, the interpretation of functional studies of the right ventricle requires meticulous evaluation for tricuspid regurgitation and estimates of right ventricular end-diastolic volume and pulmonary artery pressure to define

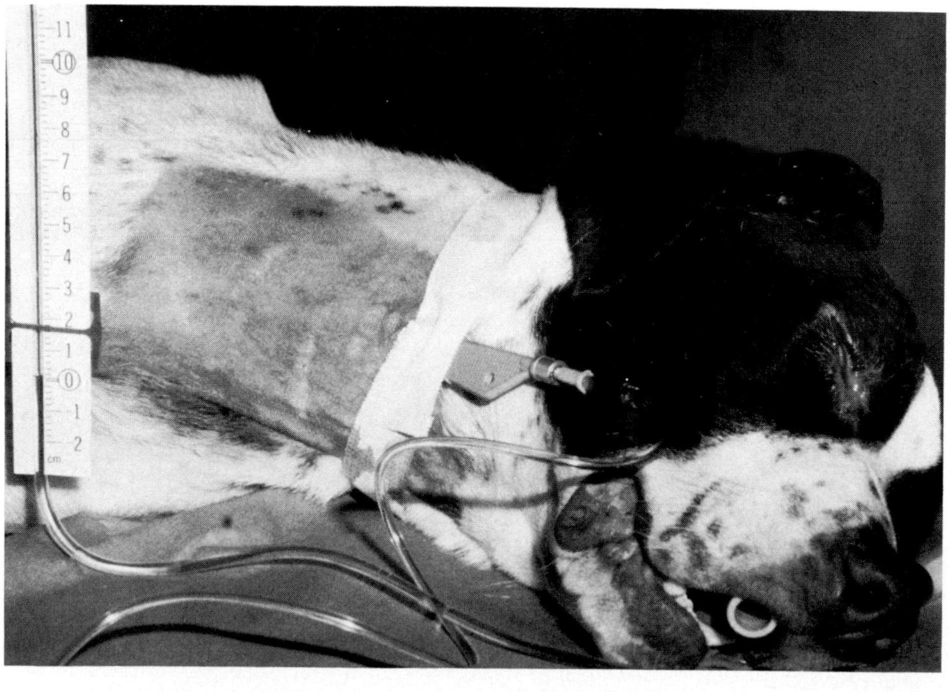

FIGURE 72–7. When pericardial disease or right heart failure is suspected, right atrial pressure can be estimated by measurement of central venous pressure using an intravenous catheter and a saline manometer. Central venous pressure is less than 10 cm H_2O in the normal dog. This measurement allows objective evaluation of response to therapy in dogs with right heart failure due to tricuspid regurgitation, heartworm disease, or cardiomyopathy.

the loading conditions present at the time of the evaluation.

In humans, radionuclide angiography is being used increasingly to obtain accurate measurements of the right ventricular ejection fraction.[152–154] The shape of the right ventricle need not receive consideration using this method. In most humans, technically satisfactory first-pass and gated equilibrium studies of the right heart can be obtained. Both methods appear to yield accurate and repeatable results. With first pass studies, isolation of the right ventricle (from the left) is obtained at the expense of counting density. With gated studies, counting density is much higher but there are technical problems with the identification of cardiac borders and the subtraction of background activity. In the author's experience, accurate gated radionuclide studies are more difficult to perform and are less accurate in dogs than in humans. The shape of the chest and anatomy and the orientation of the heart precludes sufficient isolation of the right from the left ventricle. For these reasons, first-pass studies are more appropriately performed in dogs. Unfortunately, the technique has not been used in clinical studies of the dog or cat.

INVASIVE HEMODYNAMIC EVALUATION

Invasive evaluation of the right heart can be quickly and easily accomplished by introduction of a Swan-Ganz catheter.[155] This catheter can be introduced by an experienced operator in conscious dogs using a valved catheter introducer. Inflation of the balloon at the tip of the catheter allows placement of the catheter in the pulmonary artery without the requirement for fluoroscopy. Pressure monitoring to determine the location of the catheter tip during introduction is essential to avoid complications.[155] By this technique, cardiac output can be measured and right atrial, right ventricular, pulmonary artery, and pulmonary artery wedge pressures can be obtained. With these measurements, stroke volume, stroke work, and pulmonary vascular resistance can be calculated. The simultaneous measurement of arterial blood pressure allows the calculation of systemic vascular resistance as well.

These measures do not provide a method for assessing the contractile performance of the right ventricle. However, they are essential to detect and assess the severity of pulmonary hypertension and overall cardiac performance. Such information is invaluable for the formulation of an accurate prognosis in dogs with advanced heartworm disease or cor pulmonale from other causes. These measures can also be used to clarify the cause of tricuspid regurgitation and to assess the relative contribution of left heart failure to dysfunction of the right heart.[156, 157] Right ventricular and pulmonary artery pressures are normal or only slightly elevated with isolated, structural tricuspid valve disease. Functional tricuspid regurgitation, resulting from pulmonary hypertension, develops most often when the mean pulmonary artery pressure exceeds 60 mm Hg.[158] Evaluation of the right side of the circulation is also important when assessing patients with left heart disease. Recent observations in humans with chronic left heart failure suggest that exercise capacity is more closely related to the level of pulmonary vascular resistance (PVR) and right heart performance than to the functional indices of the left ventricle.[159, 160] It has also been reported that the mortality rate is higher in patients with left heart failure and high PVR than in patients with left heart failure and normal or only modestly elevated PVR.[161]

As the use of Doppler becomes more widespread, the necessity of measuring intracardiac pressures invasively will diminish. Pressures in the right heart can be easily estimated by Doppler methods when only minor regurgitant lesions are present.[162] While there are certain technical problems, the severity of pulmonic stenosis can often be estimated in dogs by a careful Doppler evaluation.[163] The presence and severity of pulmonary hypertension can also be determined noninvasively using this methodology.[164, 165] The presence of small ventricular septal defects can be established even when the defect is not visible on the two-dimensional echocardiogram.[166, 167] Novel applications of this technology are evolving almost daily in what amounts to a forecast of the time when the invasive evaluation of cardiac function will become a rare event.

References

1. Harpster NK: Feline myocardial diseases. *In* Kirk RW (ed): Current Veterinary Therapy IX. Philadelphia, WB Saunders, 1986, p 380.
2. Archibald D, et al.: Prognostic value of echocardiographic parameters in chronic congestive heart failure: the VHEFT study. JACC 9:202A, 1987 (abstract).
3. Kittleson MD, et al.: Myocardial function in small dogs with chronic mitral regurgitation and severe congestive heart failure. JAVMA 184:455, 1984.
4. Zile MR, et al.: Chronic mitral regurgitation: predictive value of preoperative echocardiographic indexes of left ventricular function and wall stress. J Am Coll Cardiol 3:235, 1984.
5. Borow KM, et al.: End-systolic volume as a predictor of postoperative left ventricular regurgitation. Am J Med 68:655, 1980.
6. Kotler MN, et al.: M-mode and two-dimensional echocardiography in mitral and aortic regurgitation: pre- and postoperative evaluation of volume overload of the left ventricle. Am J Cardiol 46:1144, 1980.
7. Morganroth J, et al.: Acute severe aortic regurgitation. Pathophysiology, clinical recognition, and management. Ann Int Med 87:223, 1977.
8. Braunwald E: Assessment of Cardiac Function. *In* Braunwald E (ed): Heart Disease, A Textbook of Cardiovascular Medicine. Philadelphia, WB Saunders, 1984, p 467.
9. Dodge HT, et al: An angiocardiographic method for directly determining left ventricular stroke volume in man. Circ Res 11:739, 1962.
10. Lord PF, et al: Left ventricular volume measurements by single-plane cineangiocardiography: hemodynamic study of normal canine left ventricle. Am J Vet Res 31:2031, 1970.
11. Lord, PF: Left ventricular volumes of diseased canine heart: congestive cardiomyopathy and volume overload (patent ductus arteriosus and primary mitral valvular insufficiency). Am J Vet Res 35:493, 1974.
12. Pombo, JF, et al.: Left ventricular volumes and ejection function by echocardiography. Circulation 43:480, 1971.
13. Teichholz, LE, et al.: Problems in echocardiographic volume determinations: echoangiographic correlations. Circulation 46(Suppl II):75, 1972.
14. Mashiro, I, et al.: Ventricular dimensions measured noninvasively by echocardiography in the awake dog. J Appl Physiol 41:953, 1976.

15. Fortuin, NJ, et al.: Evaluation of left ventricular function by echocardiography. Circulation 46:26, 1972.
16. Ross, J, Jr. et al.: The architecture of the heart in systole and diastole: technique of rapid fixation and the analysis of left ventricular geometry. Circ Res 21:409, 1967.
17. Bishop, VS, et al.: Left ventricular internal diameter and cardiac function in conscious dogs. J Appl Physiol 27:619, 1969.
18. Ross, J, Jr, et al.: Diastolic geometry and sarcomere length in the chronically dilated canine left ventricle. Circ Res 28:49, 1971.
19. Kabashwa, T, et al.: Study of volume and/or pressure overload by real-time, two-dimensional echocardiography: motion of the interventricular septum and motion and shape of the left ventricular cavity. J Cardiogr 8:55, 1978.
20. Weyman, AE, et al.: Mechanism of abnormal septal motion in patients with right ventricular volume overload: a cross-sectional echocardiographic study. Circulation 54:179, 1976.
21. Rasmussen, S, et al.: Unreliability of M-mode left ventricular dimensions for calculating stroke volume and cardiac output in patients without heart disease. Chest 81:614, 1982.
22. Felner, JM, et al.: Sources of variability in echocardiographic measurements. Am J Cardiol 45:995, 1980.
23. Boon, J, et al.: Echocardiographic indices in the normal dog. Vet Radiol 24:214, 1983.
24. Lombard, CW: Normal values of the canine M-mode echocardiogram. Am J Vet Res 45:2015, 1984.
25. Pipers, FS, et al.: Echocardiography in the domestic cat. Am J Vet Res 40:882, 1979.
26. Jacobs, G and Knight, DH: M-mode echocardiographic measurements in nonanesthetized, healthy cats: effects of body weight, heart rate, and other variables. Am J Vet Res 46:1705, 1985.
27. Soderberg, SF, et al.: M-mode echocardiography as a diagnostic aid for feline cardiomyopathy. Am Vet Rad Soc J 24:66, 1983.
28. Haendchen, RV, et al.: Quantitation of regional cardiac function by two-dimensional echocardiography. Circulation 67:1234, 1983.
29. Folland, ED, et al.: Assessment of left ventricular ejection fraction and volumes by real-time two-dimensional echocardiography. Circulation 60:760, 1979.
30. Schnittger, I, et al.: Limitations of comparing left ventricular volumes by two-dimensional echocardiography, myocardial markers, and cineangiography. Am J Cardiol 50:512, 1982.
31. Rogers, EW, et al.: Echocardiography for quantitation of cardiac chambers. *In* Yu PN and Goodwin JF (eds): Progress in Cardiology. Volume 8. Philadelphia, Lea and Febiger, 1979.
32. Wyatt, HL, et al.: Cross-sectional echocardiography. I. Analysis of mathematic models for quantifying mass of the left ventricle in dogs. Circulation 60:1104, 1979.
33. Devereux, RB and Reichek, N: Echocardiographic determination of left ventricular mass in man. Anatomic validation of the method. Circulation 55:613, 1977.
34. Troy, BL, et al.: Measurement of left ventricular wall thickness and mass by echocardiography. Circulation 45:602, 1972.
35. Ross, J, Jr: Adaptations of the left ventricle to chronic volume overload. Circ Res 35(Suppl II):64, 1974.
36. Grossman, W, et al.: Wall stress and patterns of hypertrophy in the human left ventricle. J Clin Invest 56:56, 1975.
37. Gaasch, WH, et al.: The effect of aortic valve replacement on left ventricular volume, mass, and function. Circulation 58:825, 1978.
38. Mokotoff, DM, et al.: Noninvasive quantification of severity of aortic stenosis by echocardiographic wall thickness-radius ratio. Am J Cardiol 43:406, 1979 (abstract).
39. Gunther, S and Grossman, W: Determinants of ventricular function in pressure overload hypertrophy in man. Circulation 59:679, 1979.
40. Spann, JF, et al.: Ventricular performance, pump function, and compensatory mechanisms in patients with aortic stenosis. Circulation 62:578, 1980.
41. Ross, J, Jr: Assessment of cardiac function and myocardial contractility. *In* Hurst JW (ed): The Heart, 5th ed. New York, McGraw-Hill, 1986, p 310.
42. Yang, SS, et al.: From Cardiac Catheterization Data to Hemodynamic Parameters. Philadelphia, FA Davis, 1978.
43. Franch, RH: Cardiac catheterization. *In* Hurst JW (ed): The Heart, 4th ed. New York, McGraw-Hill, 1978, p 479.
44. Ganz, W and Swan, HJC: Measurement of blood flow by thermodilution. Am J Cardiol 29:241, 1972.
45. Manders, WT and Vatner, SF: Effects of sodium pentobarbital anesthesia on left ventricular function and distribution of cardiac output in dogs with particular reference to the mechanism for tachycardia. Circ Res 39:512, 1976.
46. Grimditch, GK, et al.: Effect of exhaustive exercise on myocardial performance. J Appl Physiol 51:1098, 1981.
47. Bagshaw, RJ and Cox, RH: Pulmonary vascular response to carotid sinus hypotension in the awake and anesthetized dog. Acta Anesethesiol Scand 27:323, 1983.
48. Bishop, VS and Peterson, DF: Pathways regulating cardiovascular changes during volume loading in awake dogs. Am J Physiol 231:854, 1976.
49. Sundet, WD, et al.: Cardiovascular and renin responses to vanadate in the conscious dog: Attenuation after calcium channel blockade. Proc Soc Exp Biol Med 175:185, 1984.
50. Yeo, CJ, et al.: The effects of intravenous substance P infusion on hemodynamics and regional flow in conscious dogs. Surgery 95:175, 1984.
51. Liard, JF, et al.: Cardiac output distribution during vasopression infusion or dehydration in conscious dogs. Am J Physiol 243:H663, 1982.
52. Lin, YC, et al.: Cardiovascular function during voluntary apnea in dogs. Am J. Physiol 245:R143, 1983.
53. McKenzie, JE, et al.: Relationships between adenosine and coronary resistance in conscious exercising dogs. Am J Physiol 242:H24, 1982.
54. Devereux, RB: Echocardiography: state of the art – 1984. Cardiology 71:118, 1984.
55. Kronik, G, et al.: Comparative value of eight M-mode echocardiographic formulas for determining left ventricular stroke volume. Circulation 60:1308, 1979.
56. Murray, JA, et al.: Echocardiographic determination of left ventricular dimensions, volumes, and performance. Am J Cardiol 30:252, 1972.
57. Teichholz, LE, et al.: Problems in echocardiographic-angiographic correlations in the presence or absence of asynergy. Am J Cardiol 37:7, 1976.
58. Dyson, DH, et al.: Comparison of 3 methods for cardiac output determination in cats. Am J Vet Res 46:2546, 1985.
59. Ajisaka, R, et al.: Echocardiographic assessment of left ventricular volume overloading in aortic insufficiency and mitral insufficiency. J Cardiogr 8:209, 1978.
60. Kittleson, MD, et al.: Acute hemodynamic effects of hydralazine in dogs with chronic mitral regurgitation. JAVMA 187:258, 1985.
61. Kittleson, MD, et al.: Efficacy of digoxin administration in dogs with idiopathic congestive cardiomyopathy. JAVMA 186:162, 1985.
62. Clemmer, TP: Oxygen transport. Int Anesthesiol Clin 19:21, 1981.
63. Means, BA and Taplett, LC: Quick Reference to Critical Care Nursing. Rockville, Maryland, Aspen Publishers, 1986.
64. Grossman, W and Braunwald, E: High cardiac output states. *In* Braunwald E (ed): Heart Disease, A Textbook of Cardiovascular Medicine. Philadelphia, WB Saunders, 1984, p 807.
65. Skjaerpe, T, et al.: Cardiac output. *In* Hatle L and Anglesen B (eds): Doppler Ultrasound in Cardiology, 2nd ed. Philadelphia, Lea and Febiger, 1985.
66. Valdes-Cruz, LM, et al.: A simplified mitral value method for 2-D echo Doppler cardiac output. Circulation 6B(Suppl III):230, 1983.
67. Valdes-Cruz, LM, et al.: Accuracy of two-dimensional echo Doppler for measuring low systemic and pulmonary blood flows: canine study. Paper presented 51st Annual Meeting, American Academy of Pediatrics.
68. Goldberg, SJ, et al.: Evaluation of pulmonary and systemic blood flow by 2-dimensional Doppler echocardiography using Fast Fourier Transform Spectral Analysis. Am J Cardiol 50:1394, 1982.
69. Freidman, MJ, et al.: 2-D echo-range gated Doppler measurements of cardiac output and stroke volume in open chest dogs. Circulation 62(Suppl III):101 (abstract).
70. Nishimura, RA, et al.: Noninvasive measurement of cardiac output by continuous-wave Doppler echocardiography: initial experience and review of the literature. Mayo Clin Proc 59:484, 1984.

71. Lewis, JF, et al.: Pulsed Doppler echocardiographic determination of stroke volume and cardiac output: clinical validation of 2 new methods using the apical window. Circulation 70:425, 1984.
72. Ingram, RH and Braunwald, E: Pulmonary edema: cardiogenic and noncardiogenic. *In* Braunwald, E (ed): Heart Disease, A Textbook of Cardiovascular Medicine. Philadelphia, WB Saunders, 1984.
73. Connoly, DC, et al.: Pulmonary artery wedge pressures in mitral valve diseases: relationship to left atrial pressure. Fed Proc 12:28, 1953.
74. Milne, ENC: Physiologic interpretation of the plain radiograph in mitral stenosis, including a review of criteria for the radiological estimation of pulmonary arterial and venous pressures. Br J Radiol 36:902, 1963.
75. Cross, CE, et al.: Mitral stenosis and pulmonary fibrosis: special reference to pulmonary edema and lung lymphatic function. Arch Inter Med 125:248, 1970.
76. Ross, J, Jr, et al.: Left ventricular performance during muscular exercise in patients with and without cardiac dysfunction. Circulation 34:597, 1966.
77. Ross, J, Jr and Braunwald, E: The study of left ventricular function in man by increasing resistance to ventricular ejection with angiotension. Circulation 29:739, 1964.
78. Quinones, MA, et al.: Influence of acute changes in preload, afterload, contractile state, and heart rate on ejection and isovolumic indices of myocardial contractility in man. Circulation 53:293, 1976.
79. Nejad, NS, et al.: Assessment of myocardial contractility from ventricular pressure recordings. Cardiovasc Res 5:15, 1971.
80. Wallace, AG, et al.: Hemodynamic determinants of the maximal rate of left ventricular pressure. Am J Physiol 205:30, 1963.
81. Burns, JW, et al.: Mechanics of isotonic left ventricular contractions. Am J Physiol 224:725, 1973.
82. Gorlin, R and Gorlin, SO: Hydraulic formula for calculation of the area of the stenotic mitral valve, other cardiac values, and central circulatory shunts. Am Heart J 41:1, 1951.
83. Gaber, C: Paper presented at the 5th Annual Veterinary Medical Forum, ACVIM, 1987.
84. Valdes Cruz, LM, et al.: Prediction of the gradient in fibromuscular subaortic stenosis by continuous wave 2-D Doppler echocardiography: animal studies. Circulation 68(Suppl III):366, 1983.
85. Holen, J, et al.: Determination of pressure gradient in mitral stenosis with a noninvasive ultrasound Doppler technique. Acta Med Scand 199:455, 1976.
86. Karliner, JS, et al.: Left ventricular myocardial mechanics: systolic and diastolic function. *In* Grossman, W (ed): Cardiac Catheterization and Angiography. 2nd ed. Philadelphia, Lea and Febiger, 1980, p 245.
87. Benzing, G, et al.: Evaluation of canine left ventricular contractility. Card Res 8:313, 1974.
88. Dodge, HT: Hemodynamic aspects of cardiac failure. *In* Braunwald E (ed): The Myocardium Failure and Infarction. New York, HP Publishing, 1974, p 70.
89. Quinones, MA, et al.: Percentage of shortening of the echocardiographic left ventricular dimension. Its use in determining ejection fraction and stroke volume. Chest 74:59, 1978.
90. Sahn, DJ, et al.: Recommendations regarding quantitation in M-mode echocardiography: results of a survey of echocardiographic methods. Circulation 58:1072, 1978.
91. Bacharach, SL, et al.: Left ventricular peak ejection rate, filling rate, and ejection fraction-frame rate requirement at rest and exercise. J Nucl Med 20:189, 1979.
92. Pavel, D, et al.: Ventricular phase analysis of radionuclide-gated studies. Am J Cardiol 45:398, 1980 (abstract).
93. Marshall, R, et al.: Assessment of cardiac performance with quantitative radionuclide angiography. Sequential left ventricular ejection fraction, normalized left ventricular ejection rate, and regional wall motion. Circulation 6:820, 1977.
94. Gould, KL: Quantitative imaging in nuclear cardiology. Circulation 66:1141, 1982.
95. Lippert, AC, et al.: Nuclear angiography in a dog with congestive cardiomyopathy. JAVMA 188:525, 1986.
96. Sisson, D: Paper presented at the 5th Annual Veterinary Medical Forum, ACVIM, 1987.
97. Lombard, CW: Echocardiographic and clinical signs of canine dilated cardiomyopathy. J Small Anim Pract 25:59, 1984.
98. Calvert, CA, et al.: Congestive cardiomyopathy in Doberman Pinscher dogs. JAVMA 181:598, 1982.
99. Wingfield, WE, et al.: Echocardiographic assessment of mitral valve motion, cardiac structures, and ventricular function in dogs with atrial fibrillation. JAVMA 181:46, 1980.
100. Moise, NS, et al.: Echocardiography, electrocardiography, and radiography of cats with dilation cardiomyopathy, hypertrophic cardiomyopathy, and hyperthyroidism. Am J Vet Res 147:1477, 1986.
101. Kittleson, MD, et al.: Echocardiographic and clinical effects of milrinone in dogs with myocardial failure. Am J Vet Res 46:1659, 1985.
102. Clark, RD, et al.: Serial echocardiographic evaluation of left ventricular function in valvular disease, including reproducibility guidelines for serial studies. Circulation 62:5621, 1980.
103. Gardin, JM, et al.: Evaluation of dilated cardiomyopathy by pulsed Doppler echocardiography. Am Heart J 106:1057, 1983.
104. Gardin, JM: Advances in the Doppler evaluation of left ventricular function. *In* Pohost GM, et al. (eds): New Concepts in Cardiac Imaging. Chicago, Year Book Medical Publishers, 1986, p 21.
105. Knight, D: Paper presented at the 5th Annual Veterinary Medical Forum, ACVIM, 1987.
106. Schuler, G, et al.: Temporal response of left ventricular performance to mitral valve surgery. Circulation 59:1218, 1979.
107. Carabello, BA, et al.: Assessment of preoperative left ventricular function in patients with mitral regurgitation: value of the end-systolic wall stress/end-systolic volume ratio. Circulation 64:1212, 1981.
108. Kay, JH, et al.: Surgical treatment of mitral insuffiency secondary to coronary artery disease. J Thorac Cardiovasc Surgery 79:12, 1980.
109. Corin, WJ, et al.: Inability of the end-systolic stress/end-systolic volume index ratio to predict postoperative outcome in chronic mitral regurgitation. J Am Coll Cardiol 9:85A, 1987 (abstract).
110. Suga, H, et al.: Load independence of the instantaneous pressure-volume ratio of the canine left ventricle and effects of epinephrine and heart rate on the ratio. Circ Res 32:314, 1973.
111. Mahler, F, et al.: Systolic pressure-diameter relations in the normal conscious dog. Cardiovasc Res 9:447, 1975.
112. Sagawa, K: The ventricular pressure-volume diagram revisited. Circ Res 43:677. 1978.
113. Grossman, W, et al.: Contractile state of the left ventricle in man as evaluated from end-systolic pressure-volume relations. Circulation 56:845, 1977.
114. Reichek, N, et al.: Noninvasive determination of left ventricular end-systolic stress: validation of the method and initial application. Circulation 65:99, 1982.
115. Slutsky, R, et al.: Peak systolic blood pressure/end-systolic volume ratio: assessment at rest and during exercise in normal subjects and patients with coronary artery disease. Am J Cardiol 46:813, 1980.
116. Kleaveland, JP, et al.: Depressed ventricular function in experimental mitral regurgitation. J Am Coll Cardiol 9:40A, 1987 (abstract).
117. Yoran, C, et al.: Dynamic aspects of acute mitral regurgitation: effects of ventricular volume, pressure, and contractility on the effective regurgitant orifice area. Circulation 60:170, 1979.
118. Lewis, RP: A critical review of the systolic time intervals. Circulation 56:146, 1977.
119. Lewis, RP: The use of systolic time intervals for evaluation of left ventricular function. *In* Noble O and Fowler NO (eds): Noninvasive Diagnostic Methods in Cardiology. Philadelphia, FA Davis, 1983.
120. Pipers, FS, et al.: A totally noninvasive method for obtaining systolic time intervals in the dog. Am J Vet Res 39:1822, 1978.
121. Weissler, AM: Current concepts in cardiology. Systolic time intervals. N Engl J Med 296:321, 1977.
122. Weissler, AM, et al.: Systolic time intervals in heart failure in man. Circulation 37:149, 1968.
123. Hirschfield, S, et al.: Measurement of right and left ventricular systolic time intervals by echocardiography. Circulation 51:304, 1975.
124. Ahmed, SS, et al.: Systolic time intervals as measures of the contractile state of the left ventricular myocardium in man. Circulation 46:559, 1972.
125. Baker, BJ, et al.: Echocardiographic detection of right ventricular hypertrophy. Am Heart J 105:611, 1983.

126. Lombard, CW: Right heart enlargement in heartworm-infected dogs. A radiographic, electrocardiographic, and echocardiographic correlation. Vet Radiol 25:210, 1984.
127. Felner, JM, et al.: Sources of variability in echocardiographic measurements. Am J Cardiol 45:995, 1980.
128. Thomas, WP: Two-dimensional, real-time echocardiography in the dog. Technique and anatomic validation. Vet Radiol 25:50, 1984.
129. Silverman, NH and Hudson, S: Evaluation of right ventricular volume and ejection fraction in children by two-dimensional echocardiography. Pediatr Cardiol 4:197, 1983.
130. Krebs, W, et al.: Right ventricular volume determination by two-dimensional echocardiography and radiography of model hearts using a subtraction method. Z Kardiol 71:413, 1982.
131. Saito, A, et al.: Right ventricular volume determination by two-dimensional echocardiography. J Cardiogr 11:1159, 1981.
132. Bommer, W, et al.: Determination of right atrial and right ventricular size by two-dimensional echocardiography. Circulation 60:91, 1979.
133. Bonagura, JD and Herring, DS: Echocardiography II: Congenital heart disease. Vet Clin North Am 15:1195, 1985.
134. Bonagura, JD and Pipers, FS: Diagnosis of cardiac lesions by contrast echocardiography. JAVMA IB2:396, 1983.
135. Sisson, D: The echocardiographic diagnosis of congenital heart disease. Proceedings of the 3rd Annual Medical Forum, 1985, p 171.
136. Sisson, D: Valvular heart disease. *In* Bonagura JD (ed): Contemporary Issues in Small Animal Practice—Cardiology. New York, Churchill-Livingstone, 1987.
137. Ross, JN: Heart failure. *In* Ettinger SJ (ed): Textbook of Veterinary Internal Medicine, 2nd ed. Philadelphia, WB Saunders, 1983.
138. Swartz, MH: Jugular venous pressure pulse: its value in cardiac diagnosis. Primary Cardiol 8:197, 1982, p 901.
139. Hartman, H: The jugular venous tracing. Am Heart J 59:698, 1960.
140. Benchimol, A and Tippit, HC: The clinical value of the jugular and hepatic pulses. Prog Cardiovasc Dis. 10:159, 1967.
141. Hurst, JW and Schlant, RC: Examination of the veins and their pulsation. *In* Hurst JW (ed): The Heart. New York, McGraw-Hill, 1978, p 193.
142. Wood, P: Diseases of the Heart and Circulation, 2nd ed. Philadelphia, JB Lippincott, 1957, p 47.
143. Perloff, JK: The Clinical Recognition of Congenital Heart Disease, 3rd ed. Philadelphia, WB Saunders, 1987, p 197.
144. Constant, J: Arterial and venous pulsations in cardiovascular diagnosis. J Cardiovasc Med 5:973, 1980.
145. Hancock, EW: Constrictive pericarditis: clinical clues to diagnosis. JAMA 232:176, 1975.
146. Shabetai, R, et al.: The hemodynamics of cardiac tamponade and constrictive pericarditis. Am J Cardiol 26:480, 1970.
147. Morris, JJ and Wechsler, AS: Right ventricular function: the assessment of contractile performance. *In* Fisk RL (ed): The Right Heart. Philadelphia, FA Davis, 1987, p 3.
148. Starr, I, et al.: The absence of conspicuous increment of venous pressure after severe damage to the right ventricle of the dog, with a discussion of the relation between clinical congestive failure and heart disease. Am Heart J 26:291, 1943.
149. Guiha, NH, et al.: Predominant right ventricular dysfunction after right ventricular destruction in the dog. Am J Cardiol 33:254, 1974.
150. Vlahakes, GJ, et al.: The pathophysiology of failure in acute right ventricular hypertension: hemodynamic and biochemical correlations. Circulation 63:87, 1981.
151. Weber, KT, et al.: Contractile mechanics and interaction of the right and left ventricles. Am J Cardiol 47:686, 1981.
152. Morrison, DA, et al.: Right ventricular ejection fraction measurement: contrast ventriculography versus gated blood pool and gated first pass radionuclide methods. Am J Cardiol 54:651, 1984.
153. Steele, P, et al.: Measurement of right and left ventricular ejection fractions by radionuclide angiography in coronary artery disease. Chest 70:51, 1976.
154. Parish, MD, et al.: Radionuclide evaluation of right and left ventricular function in children: validation of methodology. Am J Cardiol 49:1241, 1982.
155. Rackley, CE: The use of the Swan-Ganz catheters. *In* Hurst JE (ed): The Heart. New York, McGraw-Hill, 1978, p 511.
156. Sepulveda, G and Lukas, DA: The diagnosis of tricuspid insufficiency: clinical features in 60 cases with associated mitral valve disease. Circulation 11:552, 1955.
157. Wallace, CR and Hamilton, WF: Study of spontaneous congestive heart failure in the dog. Circ Res 11:301, 1962.
158. Hansing, CE and Rowe, GG: Tricuspid insufficiency: a study of hemodynamics and pathogenesis. Circulation 45:793, 1972.
159. Baker, BJ, et al.: Relation of right ventricular ejection fraction to exercise capacity in chronic left ventricular failure. Am J Cardiol 54:596, 1984.
160. Costanzo-Nordin, MR, et al.: Dilated cardiomyopathy: correlation between right ventricular function and exercise performance. The Right Heart, An International Multidisciplinary Symposium. Phoenix, AZ, 1985.
161. Baker, BJ and Franciosa, JA: Effect of the left ventricle on the right ventricle. *In* Fisk RL (ed): The Right Heart. Philadelphia, FA Davis, 1987, p 145.
162. Yock, PG and Popp, RL: Noninvasive estimation of ventricular pressures by Doppler ultrasound in patients with tricuspid or aortic regurgitation. Circulation 68(Suppl III):230, 1983 (abstract).
163. Gaber, C: Paper presented at the 5th Annual Veterinary Medical Forum, ACVIM, 1987.
164. Hatle, L, et al.: Noninvasive estimation of pulmonary artery systolic pressure with Doppler ultrasound. Br Heart J 45:157, 1981.
165. Kitabataka, A, et al.: Noninvasive estimation of pulmonary hypertension by a pulsed Doppler technique. Circulation 68:302, 1983.
166. Stevenson, JG, et al.: Diagnosis of ventricular septal defect by pulsed Doppler echocardiography—sensitivity, specificity, and limitation. Circulation 58:322, 1978.
167. Hatle, L and Rokseth, R: Noninvasive diagnosis and assessment of ventricular septal defect by Doppler ultrasound. Acta Med Scand 645:47, 1981.

73 THERAPY OF HEART FAILURE

BRUCE W. KEENE and JOHN E. RUSH

Heart failure is a well recognized clinical syndrome in veterinary medicine. The relative ease with which the syndrome is recognized, however, often belies the complex disease processes that ultimately lead to the clinical presentation. Heart failure can be simply defined as any situation where the heart's pumping ability is impaired to such a degree that adequate blood flow to the body can no longer be supplied while maintaining normal cardiac filling pressures. Cardiac filling pressures refer to ventricular end-diastolic pressure; which in the absence of stenotic valvular disease or pulmonary vascular disease is reflected in the diastolic atrial pressure. The mean pulmonary capillary wedge pressure reflects left ventricular end-diastolic pressure, the central venous pressure reflects the right ventricular end-diastolic pressure. Either exaggerated increases in cardiac filling pressures or attenuation of the normal rise in cardiac output that accompanies exercise (or both) may limit exercise capacity, resulting in shortness of breath and/or fatigue. Heart failure can develop as a result of any disorder that produces damage directly to the myocardium or places the heart under a chronically increased pressure or volume load. Until many important questions regarding the etiology and pathophysiology of the diseases that produce heart failure in dogs and cats are resolved, definitive therapy for the syndrome will remain unavailable. The veterinary clinician must apply the currently available knowledge of cardiac physiology, pathophysiology, and pharmacodynamics to the formulation of a rational therapeutic plan for the management of heart failure in each affected individual. Chapter 71 details the pathophysiology of heart failure in a variety of clinical settings. The purpose of this chapter is to review the currently available therapeutic strategies and drugs used to manipulate the properties of the heart and peripheral circulation to alleviate the clinical signs of heart failure.

The most obvious and effective strategy in the treatment of any clinical disorder is to identify and remove or prevent its cause. In dealing with heart failure, implementation of this strategy is often impossible because of inadequate knowledge, technical skill, financial resources, or a combination of these factors. A broad spectrum of clinically recognizable diseases result in heart failure in dogs and cats. Only a few of these diseases are caused by correctable defects, however, and the underlying etiology of the diseases that most commonly cause heart failure (chronic valvular disease and the cardiomyopathies) remains largely unknown. Examples of heart diseases in which a specific cause can be identified and sometimes surgically corrected include several congenital malformations (see Chapter 74). In addition to congenital heart diseases, some pericardial diseases are medically or surgically correctable (see Chapter 78), and most cases of heartworm disease can be managed by this straightforward approach of identification and removal or prevention of the cause of disease (see Chapter 80).

In the case of chronic valvular disease, a surgical "cure" might be possible even though the underlying cause of valvular degeneration is not well understood. At the present time, however, the cost and technical difficulty of valve replacement have prevented veterinary application of this procedure. Recently, research efforts directed toward the discovery of the underlying cause(s) of primary myocardial diseases have met with some success, and there is reason to believe that some heart diseases that are now managed primarily by palliating the signs of heart failure may soon be "curable" by correcting their underlying cause, or may at least be preventable if the initiating factor can be eliminated prior to the onset of heart failure and end stage disease.[1, 1a]

In most cases of heart failure, however, the clinician must make as refined a clinical diagnosis as possible, and, based on a thorough knowledge of the physiologic state of the patient and the pathophysiologic consequences of the disease, institute appropriate therapy. The therapeutic arsenal available for the management of heart failure has expanded rapidly in recent years, and this expansion has enhanced not only the therapeutic possibilities but also the responsibilities of the veterinarian. New and powerful positive inotropic and vasodilator drugs may be life-saving when used appropriately under well-monitored conditions, but these same drugs used inappropriately can be life-threatening. The decision to use any drug should be based on the need for the specific pharmacologic action(s) of the drug, the safety of the drug in a given setting, and the efficacy of the drug in that setting. Current knowledge of a particular drug's safety and efficacy can usually be obtained by consulting various texts or original manuscripts. The perceived need for a particular drug or intervention, however, depends upon a variety of factors, including the experience of the clinician and the information available about the condition of the patient and the pathophysiology of the disease. It must be recognized that despite a rich historical tradition of heart failure therapy in veterinary medicine, intensive study of the pharmacodynamics of cardioactive drugs, as well as of the pathophysiology and natural history of many heart diseases, has only recently been undertaken. Many of our therapeutic concepts, therefore, are based on anecdotal experience and may of necessity change as new data become available from prospectively monitored patients in placebo-controlled trials. The therapeutic recommendations contained in this chapter represent a synthesis of the available data from monitored drug trials in both human and veterinary patients with heart failure as well as the authors' clinical experience.

BASIC CONSIDERATIONS IN HEART FAILURE THERAPY

Many drugs are currently available that modify properties of the heart and circulation in heart failure. These drugs may act by affecting the heart or blood vessels directly, by stimulating or inhibiting the function of the autonomic nervous system, or by altering the patient's neurohumoral or endocrine responses to heart failure. Drugs that alter the heart rate and rhythm, contractility, preload, and afterload all play a role in the medical management of heart failure arising from a variety of causes. In the successful management of heart failure from causes not currently amenable to primary therapy, drugs must be carefully chosen to manipulate the heart and circulation to achieve the following therapeutic goals: (1) Relieve fluid accumulations due to excessive cardiac filling pressures as needed to improve tissue oxygenation and patient comfort. (2) Maintain or increase cardiac output to levels capable of supplying the oxygen and nutrients needed to support normal daily activity, mentation, and renal function. (3) Minimize myocardial oxygen demand (MVO_2) whenever possible, while accomplishing goals 1 and 2. (4) Control rhythm disturbances that might predispose the patient to sudden hemodynamic decompensation or death.

These general objectives are designed to return the patient to a comfortable (if relatively sedentary) existence, compensate for whatever physiologic defect resulted in heart failure, and whenever possible, to alter the stimulus for hypertrophy and the tendency toward arrhythmia. Clearly, these goals cannot be accomplished in the same way when dealing with patients that are suffering from pathophysiologically diverse diseases. For example, patients with diseases that cause heart failure due to diastolic dysfunction (e.g., hypertrophic cardiomyopathy) have different therapeutic needs from those whose disease causes failure because of systolic dysfunction (e.g., dilated cardiomyopathy). Even within the broad category of systolic dysfunction, diseases that cause failure secondary to chronic volume loads (e.g., mitral insufficiency) require different therapy than those that cause failure secondary to chronic pressure loads (e.g., aortic stenosis) or primary muscle failure (e.g., dilated cardiomyopathy). It is important that the veterinary clinician establish not only an accurate diagnosis, but that he or she also have methods available to assess the status of the heart and peripheral circulation before deciding on appropriate therapy. Failure to accomplish either of these critical steps often results in suboptimal therapy and can have catastrophic consequences for the patient.

Methods useful in the clinical assessment of the physiologic status of the heart and peripheral circulation have been reviewed extensively elsewhere.[2–4] The following brief summaries are offered to provide some basic background information necessary before contemplating the specific pharmacologic actions of individual drugs and other interventions used to alter these properties.

CONTRACTILITY

Contractility is an intrinsic property of the heart muscle that can change the force and velocity of contraction independently of the cardiac loading conditions. The cellular mechanisms of changes in contractility are based on load-independent factors that determine both the rate at which the actin-myosin binding sites responsible for contraction are activated and the rate at which these sites interact once activation has occurred.[5] It is widely believed that despite important differences in their pharmacologic mechanisms of action, all of the drugs used to increase contractility (positive inotropes) share the common final intracellular action of increasing the amount of calcium available at the site of regulation of the actin-myosin interaction, thereby enhancing ventricular contraction.[6]

Because the heart's performance as a pump is intimately linked to loading conditions during life, contractility is among the most difficult properties of the cardiovascular system to assess.[7] At any given level of cardiac contractility, the stroke volume (and thus the cardiac output if the heart rate is constant) varies directly with the preload and inversely with the afterload.[8] Quantitation of contractility would be useful in determining the diagnosis and prognosis, as well as in judging the need for positive inotropic therapy in patients with heart failure. Because drugs that increase contractility often have potentially adverse effects as well (for example, increasing MVO_2, arrhythmogenesis, central nervous system effects, or other toxic effects), it is advantageous to determine the baseline level of myocardial contractility before therapeutic decisions are made. Unfortunately, the indices available for the estimation of contractility are imperfect, and patients with heart disease often have intercurrent abnormalities of preload, afterload, contractility, and rhythm variables that cannot always be controlled, held constant, or easily isolated.

In general, the most clinically useful and widely applied of these indices in veterinary practice involve noninvasive procedures such as echocardiography. These techniques can be useful in therapeutic decision making, and appropriate application of these indices are reviewed elsewhere in this text (see Chapter 71). The clinician must be aware of the limitations of these techniques, however, and evidence exists that drugs may produce marked hemodynamic and clinical improvement in heart failure patients without causing a significant change in noninvasive ventricular function indices. This is true because the changes seen with effective treatment are often small, and the range of error for many noninvasive measurements is relatively large.[9, 10] As a result of these problems, changes in noninvasive parameters of ventricular function seen during the course of beneficial drug therapy have not always been shown to correlate closely with observed changes in the hemodynamic, clinical, or functional status of heart failure patients.[11, 12]

Several drugs are used primarily to manipulate contractility, and many others number contractile alterations among their most important side effects. Digitalis glycosides, catecholamines, and bipyridine derivatives are the most important and widely used positive inotropes in the therapy of heart failure, and their clinical pharmacology and practical use are discussed in this chapter.

PRELOAD

Preload is defined as the initial length of the cardiac muscle fiber prior to contraction.[13] Preload is thus closely related to the end-diastolic pressure and volume of the ventricle, factors that determine the degree of stretch on the cardiac myofibrils just before contraction occurs. The Frank-Starling relationship[14] states that cardiac output or stroke volume generally increases as the ventricular end-diastolic pressure increases, up to the point where optimal stretch of the muscle occurs. After that point, further increases in end-diastolic pressure do not result in improvement in cardiac output. Movement along a single curve by increasing or decreasing the preload with subsequent increases or decreases in stroke volume thus demonstrates the Frank-Starling relationship (see Chapter 71). Upward or downward displacement of the entire curve, such that a given level of ventricular end-diastolic pressure results in a greater or lesser stroke volume than the initial function curve dictated, represents a change in myocardial contractility.

With these definitions and relationships in mind, it is obvious that the clinical assessment of preload is important in the therapy of heart failure. Ideally, the clinician strives to optimize preload, that is, to maintain it at as high a level as possible without allowing excessive fluid buildup to occur in the lungs or body cavities. Plasma protein concentrations, lymphatic drainage capacity, capillary permeability, and other factors account for individual variations in the amount of preload tolerated to maximize cardiac function without allowing excessive fluid transudation to occur secondary to increases in capillary hydrostatic pressure. Just as excessive preload may result in clinical signs arising from fluid accumulation, inadequate preload can reduce cardiac output to levels incapable of supporting normal organ function, resulting in azotemia, hypothermia, fatigue, and other signs of forward heart failure.

Clinically, preload can be thought of as depending on the blood volume and the "tightness" with which that volume is held by the capacitance vessels, primarily the veins. Preload can be estimated clinically in a variety of ways. Direct measurement of the left ventricular end-diastolic pressure via catheterization of the left ventricle is generally considered too invasive for routine clinical use, and often the pulmonary capillary wedge pressure is substituted as a reasonable reflection of preload that does not require left heart catheterization. In routine practice settings, pulmonary venous distention evaluated radiographically is often a useful indicator of left ventricular preload. A more detailed discussion of the clinical assessment of preload can be found in Chapter 71.

Many drugs, as well as several nonpharmacologic maneuvers, are used to adjust the preload in the management of heart failure. Among these, diuretics, vasodilators (specifically venodilators), and salt restriction are the most important and widely used. These are discussed in detail in this chapter.

AFTERLOAD

Afterload is the sum of all the external factors that oppose ventricular ejection.[13] When the afterload is progressively raised, as often occurs secondary to the activation of a variety of neurohumoral and other mechanisms in heart failure,[15] an increasing portion of the heart's contractile energy must be expended in order to generate tension, and a correspondingly smaller amount is then available for myocardial fiber shortening and ejection of blood. The peripheral vascular resistance, arterial wall stiffness, physical properties of the blood (e.g., viscosity), and the preload all affect the amount of myocardial wall tension necessary for ventricular ejection, and therefore determine the afterload.[16] Since the amount of afterload is inversely related to the cardiac output or stroke volume at any given level of contractility and preload, afterload is clearly an important factor to consider in the therapy of heart failure. In addition to increasing cardiac output and possibly reducing mitral regurgitation, if present, reduction of excessive afterload also serves to reduce MVO_2, of which myocardial wall tension is a prime determinant.

Inappropriate or excessive reduction of afterload is counterproductive, however, because of the loss of perfusion pressure needed to maintain cerebral, cardiac, and renal blood flow. Reasonably accurate regulation of afterload is thus important to the successful management of heart failure, and monitoring some index of afterload provides significant clinical benefit, especially in the initial phases of therapy. Because myocardial wall tension is currently impossible to measure clinically, the mean arterial pressure or diastolic arterial pressure is often used as an index of afterload, although it provides an incomplete estimation. A variety of invasive and noninvasive methods are available in veterinary medicine for the measurement of arterial blood pressure.[17]

The drugs used to regulate afterload in the management of heart failure are primarily vasodilators, a broad category of compounds having a variety of mechanisms of action and uses, which are discussed in detail in this chapter.

HEART RATE

The heart rate is the only primary determinant of cardiac function that is easy to measure accurately. Over a wide range, the heart rate is directly related to cardiac output. At extremely high rates, however, such as might be seen with atrial fibrillation or other supraventricular or ventricular tachyarrhythmias, cardiac output and perfusion may actually diminish because of inadequate diastolic filling time and/or ventricular dyssynergy. Experimental evidence shows that paced rates of 260 can produce severe myocardial dysfunction and failure.[18] Heart rate is best measured electrocardiographically, especially in cases of supraventricular tachyarrhythmia, where pulse deficits occur and the heart rate by cardiac auscultation may be either difficult to obtain or misleading. The heart rate is an important determinant of both the cardiac output and MVO_2, and pharmacologic regulation of heart rate in heart failure complicated by supraventricular tachycardia is discussed in the following sections covering specific drugs (digitalis, β-blockers, and calcium antagonists). A detailed discussion of the therapy of specific cardiac arrhythmias and antiarrhythmic drugs can be found in Chapter 76.

MYOCARDIAL OXYGEN DEMAND

Myocardial oxygen demand (MVO_2) is determined by a combination of factors, including the intramyocardial wall tension, contractility, heart rate, and myocardial mass.[19, 20] The clinical importance of MVO_2 is twofold: MVO_2 is thought to be a potent mediator of myocardial hypertrophy, and excessive MVO_2 may, under some circumstances, outstrip the supply of oxygen, resulting in myocardial hypoxia that can predispose to arrhythmia and/or contractile dysfunction. Although veterinary patients do not routinely suffer from diseases that primarily restrict myocardial blood flow (e.g., atherosclerotic coronary artery disease), MVO_2 is still an important parameter to be considered in the management of heart failure in animals. Tachyarrhythmias may, for example, increase the MVO_2 while simultaneously decreasing the blood flow and thus the oxygen supply to the myocardium. Drugs used to increase contractility may also increase MVO_2, potentially predisposing the heart to hypoxia, ischemia, arrhythmia, and further hypertrophy.

Myocardial oxygen consumption is not generally measured in clinical settings, but by careful consideration of its determinants the clinician can attempt to minimize MVO_2 whenever possible, thus minimizing the risk of complicating whatever heart disease is present by the superimposition of myocardial hypoxia or ischemia during the management of heart failure.

CLASSIFICATION AND STAGING OF HEART FAILURE

In addition to understanding the pathophysiologic basis for heart failure arising in any particular patient, some judgment regarding the severity of the patient's disease is also necessary if appropriate therapy is to be initiated. To facilitate this clinical judgment in humans with coronary artery disease, three classification systems have been developed.[21-23] Of these, the New York Heart Association (NYHA) Functional Classification,[21] based largely on the degree of activity restriction resulting from the signs of heart failure, is probably the most widely used in human medicine. It has been adapted to veterinary use. The NYHA Functional Classification can be summarized as follows:

Class I—No limitation. Physical activity, including normal exercise, does not cause symptoms.

Class II—Slight limitation of physical activity. Ordinary physical activity results in symptoms.

Class III—Marked limitation of physical activity. Less than ordinary activity leads to symptoms.

Class IV—Inability to carry on any activity without symptoms. Symptoms present at rest.

Many clinicians and investigators find this classification to be inadequate, since it is based primarily on historical findings, and the true degree of exercise impairment may correlate poorly with that reported by the client. This may be particularly important in cats, as they commonly restrict their activity voluntarily, effectively masking their disease until it becomes so advanced that compensation is no longer possible. Also, such classification systems appear to be most useful in making therapeutic decisions with regard to a relatively homogeneous population of patients, such as a subset of humans with coronary artery disease. The classification is not truly quantifiable and may therefore be subject to considerable interobserver variability. Such classifications may be of little benefit or may even be harmful if used to make therapeutic decisions for individuals that, although symptomatically similar in terms of the severity of their heart failure, have acquired their symptoms as a result of etiologically and/or pathogenetically diverse diseases.

Because of the drawbacks of using clinical signs alone as a yardstick for decision making in the therapy of heart failure, other approaches have been developed to evaluate the status of patients. Various methods of quantifying the clinical signs, degree of fluid retention, ventricular function, hemodynamics, and exercise capacity of patients in heart failure have found advocates in both human and veterinary medicine.[24] While many of these techniques are potentially useful to the veterinary clinician, care must be exercised to avoid the myriad pitfalls associated with the use of any single method to evaluate this complex syndrome and every effort must be made to synthesize all of the information available about a patient in constructing an appropriate therapeutic plan.

DRUGS THAT IMPROVE CONTRACTILITY (POSITIVE INOTROPES)

The use of positive inotropic drugs to treat heart failure is based on the principle that the heart possesses contractile reserves that, even in the failing heart, can be activated to enhance cardiac performance and output. Experimental studies in animals support the existence of such reserves, even though their magnitude and therapeutic utility in the setting of severe myocardial failure has been questioned.[25, 26] Concern exists, for example, that activation of contractile reserves in severe heart failure may damage the myocardium, potentially shortening life expectancy.[27, 28] Other recent evidence suggests the existence of a "training effect" associated with some of the catecholamine positive inotropic agents, and suggests long-term benefits in cardiac performance following their short-term use.[29–31] The ongoing controversy surrounding the use of various positive inotropic agents generally revolves around one of the following factors: (1) All positive inotropes can potentially increase the myocardial oxygen demand, and all are potentially arrhythmogenic. (2) All result in increased intracellular calcium levels, or at least in increased sensitivity of the contractile proteins to intracellular calcium, situations that can potentially damage the contractile apparatus. (3) Despite some preliminary evidence of long-term improvement following dobutamine infusion,[30, 31] none of these agents has been shown to significantly alter the underlying pathology that caused the heart to fail, and they should be thought of as palliative, not curative agents. (4) The efficacy of most of these drugs is uncertain in many clinical settings.[32–39] (5) With the possible exception of some of the new phosphodiesterase inhibitors, all of the currently available positive inotropic drugs have a narrow therapeutic index, requiring meticulous patient monitoring. In addition, all of these drugs have potentially serious side effects even at therapeutic concentrations. (6) Despite seemingly major questions regarding their need, safety, and efficacy, these drugs have the potential to cause symptomatic improvement, thus enhancing the quality of the heart failure patient's life, at least temporarily. This clinical observation provides the strongest argument for their use.

Digitalis

The digitalis glycosides have been employed for over 200 years to treat heart failure, since William Withering recorded the "power of the foxglove over the motion of the heart" in the treatment of dropsy in 1785.[40] Digitalis, including both digoxin and digitoxin, is obtained from the leaves of the foxglove plants, *Digitalis lanata* and *Digitalis purpurea*. All of the digitalis glycosides share a chemical structure consisting of a steroid nucleus bound to an unsaturated lactone ring. This combination is called an aglycone, and, with specific ring fusions and additions, forms the basis for their pharmacologic activity.[41] Variations in the number of sugar molecules attached to the aglycone account for major pharmacokinetic differences, altering protein binding, metabolism, and excretion of these compounds. However, when administered at comparable dosages, few, if any, differences can be demonstrated between the glycosides in terms of their electrophysiologic, hemodynamic, or toxic effects, and administration of digoxin and digitoxin appear to result in similar inotropic responses.[42]

ACTIONS

Digitalis is used for both its positive inotropic and supraventricular antiarrhythmic actions. Though some controversy remains regarding the precise mechanism of its positive inotropic action, digitalis specifically binds to and inhibits Na^+-K^+-ATPase at the myocardial cell membrane and has been shown to increase contractility in both the normal and failing heart.[43–49] Inhibition of the Na^+-K^+-ATPase enzyme causes a reduction in sodium transport out of the cell, transiently raising the intracellular sodium concentration. This increase in intracellular sodium enhances calcium influx via the sodium-calcium exchange mechanism, and these phasic increases in intracellular calcium are directly responsible for the increased inotropic state.[50] The extent and importance of this inotropic effect appears to depend on a number of factors, including the heart rate, intracellular and extracellular electrolyte concentrations, and possibly, the initial degree of myocardial dysfunction.[48, 49] Speculation exists that in severe myocardial failure, increases in intracellular myocardial calcium concentrations caused by digitalis may be ineffective in increasing contractility and could even damage the myocardial cell.[51]

The antiarrhythmic effects of digitalis are caused by a combination of direct as well as neurally mediated (primarily parasympathomimetic) effects on the heart. Most of the antiarrhythmic effects are exerted on the specialized conduction tissues, increasing the refractory period while decreasing the conduction velocity in these tissues.[52] In the SA node, these effects result in a decreased slope of phase 4 (diastolic) depolarization and thus slow the heart rate. Investigations performed in conscious dogs, both intact and denervated, demonstrate that the neurally mediated parasympathomimetic effects of the drug are responsible for most of its ability to slow AV nodal conduction and increase AV nodal refractoriness.[53] These properties form the basis for the use of digitalis in slowing the ventricular response to atrial fibrillation and breaking or preventing atrial or AV nodal re-entrant tachycardias. They also account for the frequently observed prolongation of the P-R interval accompanying digitalis usage in the setting of sinus rhythm. Experimental evidence suggests that older animals are more sensitive to these effects than younger animals.[54] The neurally mediated effects of digitalis appear to originate primarily in the area postrema of the medulla.[55] This is the region of the chemoreceptor trigger zone that lacks a normal blood-brain barrier, facilitating penetration of the drug into the brain.[50]

The direct effects of digitalis on the myocardium shorten the refractory period of both atrial and ventricular muscle, tending to increase the incidence of spontaneous or ectopic activity.[56] In concert with the autonomically mediated changes induced by the effects of the drug on the central nervous system, this property accounts for the frequent appearance of cardiac arrhythmias seen in patients intoxicated with digitalis. ECG manifestations of digitalis action reported in animals with therapeutic serum concentrations of digoxin include a reduction in heart rate, prolongation of the P-R interval, nonspecific T wave changes, and mild ST segment depression or ST segment coving.[57–60]

The net hemodynamic effect of digitalis is often difficult to define because of the drug's broad spectrum of actions on a variety of tissues, as well as the complex reflex changes that accompany any therapeutic manipulation in the setting of heart failure. Digoxin causes mild venous and arteriolar constriction, an action that is most pronounced after IV injection.[61, 62] This acute effect of arteriolar constriction and increased systemic vascular resistance may sometimes precede the positive inotropic effects of digitalis, leading to increased left ventricular end diastolic pressure and potentially exacerbating signs of heart failure.[63] Alternatively, when heart failure is improved by digitalis administration, increased cardiac output may improve renal perfusion, and the resulting deactivation of the renin-angiotensin-aldosterone system is accompanied by a diuresis and reduction in α-adrenergic tone, with subsequent reductions in venous pressure and systemic vascular resistance.[64] Although all positive inotropic drugs have the potential to increase MVO_2, it has been proposed that digitalis might actually be capable of reducing MVO_2 when administered under the appropriate circumstances.[65] One obvious mechanism of MVO_2 reduction involves the effective treatment of tachycardia, prolonging diastole, and increasing coronary perfusion time and the potential oxygen supply to the myocardium. A second potential mechanism of MVO_2 reduction invokes a significant positive inotropic effect, which in and of itself would be expected to increase MVO_2. If the inotropic effect significantly increases ejection fraction, stroke volume, and cardiac output, however, the resulting neurohumorally mediated reductions in preload and afterload might permit the heart to operate at a smaller ventricular volume, thus generating less wall tension and requiring less oxygen.

PHARMACOKINETICS

Digoxin and digitoxin are the most commonly used digitalis preparations in veterinary medicine. Both compounds are available for intravenous and oral (PO) administration. Intramuscular injections are painful, potentially resulting in muscle necrosis in addition to erratic absorption; they should therefore be avoided.[41] The oral absorption of digitoxin (95 per cent) is more predictable and complete than that of digoxin, resulting in better bioavailability of digitoxin in the dog.[65] The elixir formulation of digoxin (available both as a liquid and in capsule form) is better absorbed (75 to 90 per cent) than the tablet (50 to 70 per cent), and dosage reductions of approximately 25 per cent have been recommended if the elixir is chosen for therapy.[67, 68] Oral absorption of both compounds can be reduced by food, antacids, kaolin-pectin preparations, neomycin, metoclopramide, and gastrointestinal malabsorption syndromes.

Elimination kinetics and routes of metabolism are different for digoxin and digitoxin. Digoxin elimination is heavily dependent on glomerular filtration. Animals with decreased glomerular filtration rates, whether or not they are azotemic, are thus at increased risk of toxicity.[69] Dosage reductions for animals with compromised glomerular filtration are necessary if digoxin therapy is chosen under these circumstances. Although nomograms relating dosage reductions to BUN or creatinine have been proposed, in the authors' experience digitalization of azotemic animals with digoxin must be approached with great caution and on an individual basis to avoid toxicity. Digitoxin is used in this situation whenever possible.[70] If digoxin must be used to digitalize an azotemic patient, the authors recommend reducing the dosage of digoxin by 50 per cent for every 50 per cent rise in the BUN and monitoring serum digoxin levels beginning 8 to 12 hours after the morning dose on the third, fifth, and seventh day of maintenance digitalization (sooner if signs of toxicity appear). Hypothyroidism is known to raise serum digoxin levels in humans, and may affect digitalis kinetics in the dog as well.[71, 72]

The half-life of digoxin in the dog is 20 to 40 hours, with a large amount of individual variation.[57, 66, 67] Since 90 per cent of steady-state blood levels of any drug are achieved after three half-lives, 2.5 to 5 days may be necessary to reach steady state levels after initiation of maintenance therapy. Alternatively, even a normal animal intoxicated with digoxin has 50 per cent of the drug remaining 20 to 40 hours after termination of therapy. Depending on the drug's half-life in the animal and the initial drug concentration, toxicity may persist for three to five days after cessation of therapy (longer in severe azotemia).

In contrast to digoxin, the half-life of digitoxin in the dog is only 8 to 12 hours.[57, 73, 74] Because of its shorter half-life, digitoxin is usually given three times a day in the dog compared to twice daily dosing for digoxin. Digitoxin is eliminated primarily by the liver, and the drug's disposition does not appear to be altered by most hepatic diseases.[74] Elevations of liver enzymes, therefore, may not contraindicate digitoxin therapy. Phenobarbital, primidone, phenytoin, phenylbutazone, and other hepatic microsomal enzyme inducers may increase the metabolism and excretion of digitoxin, whereas it has been suggested that hepatic microsomal inhibitors such as chloramphenicol or tetracyclines may decrease elimination.[75] In contrast to digoxin, digitoxin is highly protein-bound in plasma.[66] Protein binding necessitates that more total drug be present in the plasma in order to reach the concentration of free drug needed to interact with receptors and produce a therapeutic effect. While this means that both higher dosages and higher blood levels of digitoxin are necessary to reach therapeutic concentrations, it does not imply that toxicity is more likely. Actually, digitalis toxicity may well be less likely with digitoxin because of its more uniform absorption and excretion, and the prevalence of occult renal dysfunction in elderly animals, which predisposes them to digoxin intoxication. When it occurs, digitoxin toxicity is generally shorter lived and easier to manage because of the much shorter half-life of digitoxin as compared with digoxin.

Having briefly examined the pharmacokinetic profiles of digoxin and digitoxin in the dog, it may be somewhat surprising that digitoxin, with its superior bioavailability, hepatic metabolism, and shorter half life has not found widespread acceptance in veterinary practice. While there are no doubt many reasons for this fact, foremost among them is the lack of a concentrated dosage form for digitoxin. Without a means to deliver a reasonable amount of the drug in a reasonably small package, the use of digitoxin becomes inconvenient in patients weighing more than 10 to 15 kilograms. In practice, digoxin is almost always prescribed for large breed patients requiring digitalization. Small breed patients may be treated with either digoxin or digitoxin, and digitoxin is preferred when renal function is questionable. Digoxin and digitoxin should not be used simultaneously because of their pharmacokinetic differences and because digitoxin is metabolized in part to digoxin.[41]

The pharmacokinetics of digitoxin are not well studied in cats, with the two available investigations reporting a half-life of 2.5 days.[76, 77] Because of this long half-life, digitoxin is not generally used in this species. While several studies have examined the pharmacokinetics of digoxin in the normal cat, little documented information is available concerning the pharmacokinetics or efficacy of the drug in cats with heart failure.[76, 78–82] Digoxin half-life in normal cats has been reported to be between 10.4 and 58 hours.[80, 81] The most convincing data used both single IV and chronic oral dosing at clinically relevant concentrations of digoxin, with the resulting average half-life of 33 hours, with a trend toward prolongation with chronic oral dosing.[80, 82]

INDICATIONS AND CURRENT USE

Although the list of clear-cut indications for digitalis is shrinking, digoxin still forms the backbone of chronic therapy in animals with myocardial failure and/or symptomatic supraventricular arrhythmias. The advent of more potent positive inotropic drugs for the emergency support of contractility in acute heart failure or cardiogenic shock, coupled with evidence that myocardial contractility appears rarely to be severely compromised in dogs with chronic valvular disease, have placed two of the previous indications for digitalization in doubt.[83]

One of the current controversies in veterinary cardiology revolves around the clinical utility of digitalis in the therapy of chronic valvular disease in the dog. Based on M-mode echocardiographic indices of ventricular function, some authors have questioned the need for digitalization of most patients with chronic severe mitral insufficiency and normal sinus rhythm, assuming that digitalis is useful in this situation primarily as a positive inotrope. In their study of 16 dogs with severe heart failure secondary to chronic mitral regurgitation, only 3 (19 per cent) had calculated ejection fractions of less than 80 per cent, shortening fractions of less than 50 per cent, end-diastolic volume indices greater than 200 ml/M^2, and end-systolic volume indices greater than 30 ml/M^2; these are all criteria considered to indicate depressed myocardial function.[83] The finding of echocardiographically normal myocardial function in these patients raised the general question of whether inotropic support is indicated in most cases of heart failure secondary to chronic mitral regurgitation and specifically, whether digitalis should be more selectively prescribed in this setting.

Other investigators have also questioned the use of digitalis for the routine therapy of heart failure and found that dogs receiving neither digoxin or digitoxin lived longer than dogs receiving either drug, except in the presence of atrial fibrillation.[84] In addition, the owners surveyed in that study believed that their animals felt better when digitalis was not included in the therapeutic regimen, and animals not receiving digitalis had less depression, anorexia, vomiting, or diarrhea than animals receiving the drug. Although the anecdotal methodology and statistical analysis of this study have been criticized, it nevertheless raises the question of the need for, and efficacy of, digitalis in the therapy of heart failure.[85]

On the other side of the controversy, some experimental evidence in dogs with surgically induced mitral insufficiency and subsequent heart failure suggests not only hemodynamic but also myocardial energetic improvement after digitalis, returning intracellular calcium and sarcolemmal Na^+-K^+-ATPase values to normal.[86] Interestingly, and possibly germane to the controversy surrounding digitalis usage, is a clinical investigation of 21 children with signs of early heart failure secondary to a ventricular septal defect. Myocardial failure was not present under these circumstances, which hemodynamically mimics mitral regurgitation to some extent, but 57 per cent (12) of the subjects experienced clinical improvement on digoxin, despite the fact that echocardiographic measurements were improved in only 28 per cent (6 of the 12 with clinical improvement).[87]

Two explanations for the conflicting scientific and clinical body of information surrounding the efficacy of digoxin in the therapy of heart failure seem plausible. First, noninotropic mechanisms may be partly responsible for the clinical improvement of patients receiving digitalis.[88] Second, the historical tradition favoring the use of digitalis in the therapy of heart failure may bias studies using subjective endpoints, and powerful placebo effects have been shown to occur in veterinary medicine as well as human medicine in the evaluation of heart failure therapy.[89–91] This controversy may not subside until prospective, large-scale, blind, placebo-controlled studies are performed in veterinary medicine. In the interim, some recommendations can be made based upon current knowledge of the pathophysiology of chronic valvular disease and the pharmacodynamic properties of digitalis. At this time, no clinical evidence exists to suggest that digitalis has a sparing effect on the myocardium, and it is inappropriate to digitalize any patient based on finding a murmur. Considering currently available information regarding the risk-to-benefit ratio of digitalization, the authors prefer to use digitalis in the management of heart failure secondary to chronic valvular disease when one of the following criteria are met: (1) Concurrent presence of a persistent supraventricular tachyarrhythmia, including sinus tachycardia (heart rate greater 160 at home). (2) Echocardiographic evidence of left ventricular myocardial failure. (3) Persistent clinical evidence of right heart failure (ascites, pleural effusion).

In the therapy of cardiac diseases where the primary pathophysiologic defect is myocardial dysfunction (e.g., dilated cardiomyopathy) and in the absence of serious contraindications (e.g., ventricular arrhythmias that increase in frequency or severity with therapy), digitalization is indicated in both the dog and cat. This is not to imply, however, that digitalis is effective in improving myocardial function in all cases of cardiomyopathy.

An investigation of the effects of digoxin in giant breed dogs with dilated cardiomyopathy demonstrated echocardiographic evidence of functional improvement in only four of ten dogs studied, despite serum digoxin concentrations within the reported therapeutic range.[36] Dogs that improved significantly following digoxin administration also had significantly higher central venous oxygen tensions (a correlate of cardiac output) and lower heart rates after therapy, as well as significantly prolonged survival when compared to dogs that did not respond. Several clinical investigations performed in humans have questioned the efficacy of digitalis in the management of heart failure, especially in the presence of sinus rhythm.[32, 34, 35, 92, 93] Although the controversy surrounding the efficacy of digitalis is unresolved, at the time of this writing digitalis remains the only orally active positive inotrope approved for the long-term treatment of heart failure in the United States. Chapters 71 and 72 describe pathophysiologic studies that outline the beneficial effects and reasons for digitalization in heart failure conditions.

Digitalis is generally contraindicated in animals with sinus node dysfunction, unless their symptoms can be shown to arise from episodes of supraventricular tachycardia (e.g., tachycardia-bradycardia syndrome). Atrioventricular nodal dysfunction more serious than first degree AV block also represents an important contraindication to digitalis. Other conditions in which digoxin is relatively contraindicated include pericardial disease, hypertrophic cardiomyopathy, and aortic stenosis—in general conditions where diastolic dysfunction is the underlying pathophysiologic mechanism of disease and inotropic support is unnecessary or potentially harmful.

Although the actions of digitalis can potentiate ventricular arrhythmias present prior to digitalization, such arrhythmias do not constitute an absolute contraindication to therapy. One author has shown in human patients that digitalis exacerbates ventricular arrhythmias in approximately one-third of the cases, has no effect in one-third, and actually reduces the severity of arrhythmia in another third.[94] As there is currently no reliable way to determine which category a patient will fall in, digitalis is relatively contraindicated in the presence of severe ventricular arrhythmias.

Once the decision is made to digitalize a patient, oral digitalization using maintenance dosing from the beginning is usually the preferred method of reaching therapeutic levels. This method is thought to minimize the chances of toxicity, and steady state serum concentrations are generally reached within two to five days after initiating therapy.[95] Although once-daily digoxin dosing might appear to be adequate considering its 20 to 40 hour half-life, the dosage is usually divided and administered twice daily in an attempt to reduce the serum peaks and nadirs, while retaining the same mean serum concentration. Experimental evidence exists in the dog that twice daily dosing of digoxin actually results in a slightly lower mean serum concentration of digoxin, as well as decreased peak serum levels during the day, when compared with once daily administration.[96]

The dosage of digoxin should be based on lean body weight, since the drug is not distributed to adipose tissue or ascitic fluid. Based on a pharmacokinetic study in dogs with surgically induced heart failure, compensatory dosage reductions of 10, 20, 30, or 40 per cent of the standard dosage have been recommended for animals with mild, moderate, severe, or extreme ascites, respectively.[97] Because of individual variations in body composition, drug disposition, severity of disease, and owner compliance, digitalization remains as much an art as a science, despite the available pharmacokinetic knowledge. It is not too surprising, then, that a variety of published dosage recommendations can be found. In the dog, these include 0.010 mg/lb/day (0.022 mg/kg/day), 0.010 mg/lb (0.022 mg/kg) divided twice daily, the above dosages multiplied by 0.75 for the elixir and by 0.85 for the tablet, and 0.22 mg per square meter twice daily. The surface area-based dosage best reflects the fact that giant breed dogs require less digoxin than medium-sized or small dogs.[58] Clinically, it is the authors' experience that Doberman pinschers with dilated cardiomyopathy are particularly sensitive to digitalis and prone to toxicity even at seemingly minimal dosages (usually less than 0.25 mg q12h in the authors' clinic). Fasting may result in small but significant increases in serum digoxin concentration.[97] It has been recommended that the maximum dose of digoxin for any dog regardless of size not exceed 0.75 mg/day, which seems prudent unless proven inadequate by serum levels and lack of therapeutic response.[98] Recommended dosages for digitoxin also vary somewhat in the dog (0.01 to 0.03 mg/lb or 0.02 to 0.06 mg/kg two to three times daily), although estimation of lean body weight appears to be unnecessary for accurate dosing. (Editor's Note: In the clinical experience of the editor, dosages of digoxin exceeding 0.25 mg q12h are rarely if ever exceeded in the treatment of heart failure, even in the largest of dogs.)

In the authors' experience, digitalis dosage can best be adjusted by evaluating the serum drug concentration approximately one week after the initiation of therapy. Serum digoxin samples are obtained 8 to 12 hours after the previous dose; digitoxin levels are drawn 6 to 8 hours after drug administration. The therapeutic range for digoxin is 0.8 to 2.4 ng/ml; the range for digitoxin is 15 to 35 ng/ml.[57, 99] In patients with inadequate blood levels or those within the low end of the therapeutic range experiencing clinical signs suggestive of inadequate digitalization, the dose is cautiously increased (not more than 30 per cent), and repeat serum levels are obtained one week later.

When emergency digitalization is indicated in the dog (almost always because of hemodynamically significant, persistent supraventricular tachycardia accompanying severe heart failure), intravenous administration of digoxin can be accomplished safely and is preferred by the authors over rapid oral digitalization protocols. The recommended intravenous dosage of digoxin in the dog is 0.01 to 0.02 mg/lb (0.02 to 0.04 mg/kg), with 25 per cent given each hour for four hours.[100]

Cats display enormous individual variability in both their pharmacokinetic and clinical response to chronic oral administration of digoxin. Much of what is known about the use of digoxin in cats with heart failure is anecdotal, acquired through empirical and often uncontrolled therapeutic trials. In general, cats are easily intoxicated with digitalis, and this seems especially true of cats suffering from dilated cardiomyopathy. A variety of dosage regimens have been published, including 0.004 mg/lb (0.008 mg/kg) divided twice daily[101] and 0.001 to 0.01 mg/lb (0.004 to 0.02 mg/kg) divided twice daily.[102] Two authors have recommended the following dosages in cats: cats weighing 4 to 7 lb (1.9 to 3.2 kg) receive ¼ of a 0.125 mg tab every second to third day, cats weighing 7 to 13 lb (3.2 to 6.0 kg) receive ¼ tablet daily, and cats weighing more than 13 lb (6.0 kg) receive ¼ tablet twice a day.[103] In the authors' clinic, adult cats undergoing digitalization for dilated cardiomyopathy (by far the most common indication) are started directly on a maintenance schedule of ¼ of a 0.125 mg tablet every other day, and digoxin serum levels are evaluated on the seventh day of dosing. Digoxin elixir may be poorly tolerated by cats, apparently because of unpalatability. In emergency situations (e.g., persistent, hemodynamically significant supraventricular tachycardia or cardiogenic shock in settings where more potent inotropes are unavailable), rapid intravenous digitalization can be accomplished in cats by initial injection of 0.0011 mg/lb (0.0025 mg/kg) lean body weight, followed by 0.0005 mg/lb (0.00125 mg/kg) each hour for up to two hours or a total dosage of 0.002 mg/lb (0.005 mg/kg).

TOXICITY AND DRUG INTERACTIONS

The digitalis glycosides have a narrow therapeutic index, and digitalis intoxication is a common clinical problem in both human and veterinary medicine. Intoxication is reported to occur in between 5 and 35 per cent of digitalized humans, and its occurrence is often associated with high mortality rates.[104, 105] The one available clinical investigation in dogs receiving digoxin found that 25 per cent of 79 dogs studied had serum levels above the reported therapeutic range.[74]

Many clinical situations are known to affect digitalis pharmacokinetics and predispose the patient to digitalis intoxication. As previously mentioned, primary renal failure, or any cause of reduced glomerular filtration (e.g., heart failure) may lead to intoxication by decreasing the renal clearance of digoxin. Hypothyroid dogs may require lower doses of digoxin to avoid toxicity.[72] Hyperthyroid individuals may require increased amounts of digoxin because of enhanced drug clearance, although cellular sensitivity to digitalis may be heightened by the hyperthyroid state.[106] Hypoalbuminemia can result in digitoxin intoxication as diminished protein binding results in more unbound or free digitoxin in the serum.[74] Similarly, since digoxin is normally bound to skeletal muscle, geriatric animals with reduced muscle mass may have a decreased volume of distribution in addition to their often lower glomerular filtration rate, thus predisposing them to toxicity if compensatory dosage reductions are not made.[107] Body weight should be monitored regularly and frequently in patients with heart failure, and digitalis (as well as other drug) dosages adjusted accordingly.

Electrolyte abnormalities also significantly influence both the occurrence and severity of digitalis intoxication. Although hyperkalemia may be observed in severe digitalis intoxication, hypokalemia is the electrolyte abnormality that most frequently predisposes to digitalis intoxication. Hypokalemia tends to increase myocardial concentrations of digitalis and may also contribute to the development of cardiac arrhythmias during intoxication.[108] Anorexia, concurrent use of diuretics, and hyperaldosteronism are the most common contributors to the development of hypokalemia associated with heart failure or its therapy. Hypercalcemia can also complicate digitalis intoxication, potentiating cellular calcium loading and increasing ventricular automaticity.[109] Hypercalcemic patients or those receiving calcium supplementation may thus be inordinately predisposed to cardiac arrhythmias while receiving digitalis.

Many drugs interact with digitalis, often resulting in alterations of metabolism, excretion, volume of distribution, or absorption of one or both drugs. The digoxin-quinidine interaction is perhaps the best known example, in which quinidine has been demonstrated to displace digoxin from binding sites on the myocardium and skeletal muscle, as well as decreasing the total body clearance of digoxin. These actions (primarily reductions in clearance) can elevate the serum digoxin concentrations up to three times their original values.[110, 111] The quinidine-induced increase in serum digoxin level, however, is associated with a decreased inotropic response to digoxin.[112] The use of quinidine in patients receiving digoxin should be avoided when possible, and a reduced dosage of digoxin should be used if the combination is necessary. Digitoxin and quinidine have been shown to be free of this interaction in the dog.[113] Increased digoxin serum concentrations have also been reported to attend the concurrent administration of digoxin with verapamil, amiodarone, captopril, spironolactone, triamterene, and possibly cimetidine.[114–117] Additionally, propranolol, diltiazem, and parasympathomimetic drugs may exacerbate the vagal effects of digitalis.

In dogs, acute withdrawal of phenobarbital, as well as chronic phenobarbital therapy, has been associated with digoxin intoxication but the mechanism of these interactions is unclear and apparently unrelated to hepatic microsomal enzyme induction.[118, 119] These interactions are not observed with digitoxin. In normal dogs, furosemide, phenytoin, or hydrochlorothiazide administered concurrently with digoxin failed to produce any significant interactions, but clinical digitalis toxicity associated with reduced digoxin clearance was observed in a pharmacokinetic study evaluating digoxin administered together with furosemide, aspirin, and a low-salt diet in cats.[120, 121] Aspirin has also been shown to increase serum digoxin concentrations in the dog.[122]

The clinical manifestations of digitalis intoxication are caused by both direct and neurally mediated actions. Signs of intoxication vary among individuals, but anorexia, depression, and/or borborygmus are frequent early complaints, followed by nausea, vomiting, and diarrhea if therapeutic intervention is not prompt. In severe cases, vomiting may be persistent and protracted, resulting in volume contraction, electrolyte disturbances, and pre-renal azotemia—all of which tend to elevate serum digoxin concentrations and potentiate the drug's toxic effects.

Cardiac arrhythmias commonly attend digitalis intoxication and may contribute to both morbidity and mortality. Sinus bradycardia with varying degrees of AV block, ventricular bigeminy or tachycardia, junctional or supraventricular arrhythmias, and unusually slow ventricular response rates to atrial fibrillation are all signs of digitalis intoxication.[58, 60, 99] While electrocardiography provides a reasonably reliable indicator of moderate digoxin toxicity (2.5 to 6.0 ng/ml) in dogs, ECG evidence of toxicity should always be interpreted in light of the animal's clinical condition and cardiac rhythm prior to digitalis administration.[99] Electrocardiographic signs of effective digitalization and digitalis intoxication may overlap.[57, 58]

The availability of serum digitalis levels on a same-day basis at most local human hospitals has facilitated therapeutic digitalization and simplified the diagnosis of digitalis intoxication. Though the dose of digoxin required to produce intoxication is variable, signs of digoxin intoxication are consistently observed when serum digoxin concentrations rise above 2.5 ng/ml in normal dogs.[99] Serum concentrations greater than 6.0 ng/ml have been shown to cause life-threatening toxicity, manifested by vomiting, dehydration, hypothermia, azotemia, electrolyte disturbances, and elevations of CPK and LDH.[99] While elevated serum digitalis levels are not completely specific or sensitive for intoxication (i.e., some animals above the toxic range may not be sick and other animals that are within the therapeutic range may actually be toxic), they are clinically useful in identifying intoxicated animals and in guiding therapy.

In animals showing clinical or electrocardiographic signs of intoxication, digitalis should be discontinued pending evaluation of the serum drug concentration. The patient should receive appropriate supportive care until the clinical signs resolve. Serum levels and the patient in general should both be re-evaluated, and if digitalis is indicated, therapy can be reinstituted at appropriately reduced (usually 50 per cent) dosages.

If digitalis assays are not readily available, mild signs of digitalis intoxication can be managed by withdrawal of the drug for one to two days and restarting therapy with a 50 per cent dose reduction. Successful treatment of severe digitalis intoxication requires intensive care monitoring. Careful evaluation and management of the patient's hydration, renal function, and electrolyte status are essential. Signs of heart failure coexisting with digitalis intoxication further complicate the management of fluid and electrolyte balance and worsen the prognosis. Ventricular arrhythmias are usually managed with lidocaine or phenytoin (see Chapter 76). Cholestyramine binds to digitalis in the intestinal tract and may be useful in digitoxin intoxication by absorbing drug that is undergoing enterohepatic circulation, or in digoxin intoxication if a large dose of drug was recently administered.[123, 124]

Fab portions of anti-digoxin and anti-digitoxin antibodies are now available for the treatment of life-threatening digitalis toxicity in people. These antibodies offer fast, effective therapy and have been tested successfully in dogs, but their high cost is often prohibitive.[125–130]

Catecholamines

GENERAL PROPERTIES

The sympathetic nervous system performs a variety of homeostatic functions, in addition to mediating "fight or flight" reactions. Receptors for the sympathetic nervous system (adrenergic receptors), are classified as α-1, α-2, β-1, β-2, and dopaminergic by most investigators at this time. β-1 receptors predominate in the heart, and stimulation of those receptors results in positive inotropic and chronotropic (heart rate) responses. β-2 receptors are mostly located in vascular and bronchial smooth muscle, and stimulation of these receptors causes relaxation, with subsequent vasodilation and bronchodilation. α-1 receptors are located primarily at postsynaptic sites in both vascular smooth muscle and myocardium; their stimulation results mainly in vasoconstriction and a positive inotropic response.

Sympathomimetic drugs share a basic chemical structure consisting of a benzene ring with an ethylamine side chain. Sympathomimetic compounds with hydroxyl (—OH) groups substituted on the aromatic benzene ring are called catecholamines.[131] Variations on this structure account for the pharmacologic diversity and receptor specificity of these compounds, but they all share certain basic properties. All of the catecholamines have short serum half-lives, usually less than two minutes, and all undergo extensive first-pass hepatic metabolism following oral administration. This is due to the presence of two enzymes (catechol-O-methyltransferase [COMT] and monoamine oxidase [MAO]) that rapidly metabolize these compounds.[131] Because of these properties, these drugs are usually administered intravenously and are generally useful only for the short-term management of severe heart failure. Some evidence suggests, in fact, that long-term therapy with these agents or their orally active congeners may not be feasible because of "down-regulation" of β-adrenergic receptor density, which renders them ineffective during chronic use.[132] All of the catecholamines are potentially arrhythmogenic, and all can cause severe subendocardial hemorrhage, ischemia, and necrosis if administered in toxic doses.[133]

Catecholamines increase contractility primarily by stimulating the β-1 receptors on cardiac myocytes, thus stimulating adenylate cyclase and increasing cyclic 3′, 5′-AMP concentration within the cytosol. Cyclic-AMP-dependent protein kinases activated by the increased 3′, 5′-cAMP concentration then catalyze the phosphorylation of membrane proteins in the sarcolemma and sarcoplasmic reticulum. Phosphorylation of these membrane proteins is believed to regulate the calcium flux across the sarcolemma and sarcoplasmic reticulum and may also alter calcium binding to the regulatory proteins that control the contractile apparatus.[6] The end result of this receptor stimulation is increased intracellular calcium availability and/or sensitivity, the final common pathway by which most positive inotropic drugs enhance myocardial contractility.

Epinephrine

INDICATIONS AND CURRENT USE

Epinephrine is often the drug of choice for positive inotropic and circulatory support following cardiac arrest. Epinephrine is a potent α, β-1, and β-2 agonist that increases contractility, heart rate, blood pressure, and cardiac output.[35] While these actions are highly desirable in some situations, they result in a dramatic increase in cardiac work and oxygen demand, which, together with the drug's electrophysiologic effects, can be highly arrhythmogenic.[134] Epinephrine is therefore not recommended for the therapy of heart failure.

Epinephrine is available in 1 ml ampules containing 1 mg of epinephrine (1:1,000 dilution) or as prefilled syringes (1 mg/10 cc or 1:10,000 dilution). To reduce the likelihood of accidental overdosage, 1:1,000 solutions should be diluted to 1:10,000 solutions before use. The usual dosage used during resuscitation is 2 mcg/lb (5 mcg/kg) or 0.25 cc/10 lb (0.5 cc/10 kg) of a 1:10,000 solution administered intravenously or intratracheally. Intracardiac epinephrine should be avoided whenever possible, but can be dosed at 0.2 cc/10 kg of the 1:10,000 solution.

Isoproterenol

INDICATIONS AND CURRENT USE

Isoproterenol is the prototype β agonist. Intravenous administration increases contractility, heart rate, and cardiac output, but reduces arterial blood pressure.[135] Because of its arrhythmogenicity and hypotensive effects, isoproterenol is rarely used therapeutically except in the emergency treatment of high grade or complete AV block that has proven unresponsive to anticholinergics, where it may decrease AV node refractoriness and/or increase the spontaneous rate of the ventricular escape focus. Isoproterenol infusion is also used as a provocative test for mild subaortic stenosis during diagnostic left ventricular catheterization.[136] This drug currently has no place in the management of cardiac arrest or myocardial failure.

Isoproterenol is supplied in 0.2 mg vials that must be diluted for continuous intravenous infusion. Infusion rates vary from 0.02 to 0.04 mcg/lb/min (0.045 to 0.09 mcg/kg/min). Electrocardiographic monitoring should be employed, and the lowest effective infusion rate should be used to avoid ventricular arrhythmias and subendocardial myocardial damage.

Dopamine

ACTIONS

Dopamine is the biosynthetic precursor to norepinephrine in the catecholamine metabolic pathway. Specific dopaminergic receptors are located in renal, mesenteric, coronary, and cerebral vascular beds. Stimulation of these receptors with low dosages of dopamine (0.5 to 3.5 mcg/lb/min or 1 to 7.5 mcg/kg/min) results in vasodilation, accounting for the use of this drug in the treatment of acute oliguric renal failure, since improved renal blood flow may facilitate the return of renal function.[137, 138] Dopamine also stimulates α- and β-adrenergic receptors, causes release of norepinephrine from nerve endings in the heart, and at high infusion rates (5 to 10 μg/lb/min or 10 to 20 μg/kg/min) increases heart rate, inotropy, and blood pressure.[138, 139] The specific dopaminergic vasodilatory effects on the renal artery are overdriven and lost at higher infusion rates. High doses tend to be arrhythmogenic, increasing the myocardial workload and oxygen demand drastically, and potentially increasing the pulmonary capillary wedge pressure (thus worsening heart failure).[140, 141] Lower infusion rates (1 to 5 mcg/lb/min or 3 to 10 mcg/kg/min) result in increased cardiac output with little change or a slight decrease in total peripheral resistance and minimal change in heart rate – a desirable spectrum of effects for the acute management of myocardial failure.[142–144]

INDICATIONS AND CURRENT USE

Dopamine thus has three clinical uses, depending on the dosage range administered. Low doses are useful in the management of acute oliguric renal failure. Higher doses can be used for circulatory support in patients with cardiovascular depression, with the degree of chronotropy and pressor response, as well as arrhythmogenicity, being dose-dependent up to a dose of approximately 23 mcg/lb/min (50 mcg/kg/min). Dopamine may be useful at midrange dosages for the management of primary myocardial disease that has resulted in heart failure, and at higher dose ranges can be used for inotropic and circulatory support during resuscitation efforts. Because of the drug's propensity to cause a marked chronotropic and pressor response; however, it must be used under closely monitored circumstances regardless of the indication.

In the authors' clinic, dopamine is rarely used as a primary drug in the management of heart failure except in cases of cardiogenic shock related to anesthesia or in the setting of post-cardiac resuscitation, where arterial blood pressure support becomes critical. In this setting, dopamine infusion is initiated at 0.5 mcg/lb/min (1 mcg/kg/min), and the patient is closely monitored for increases in heart rate, the development of ventricular or supraventricular arrhythmias, and arterial blood pressure response. Infusion rates are then judiciously increased in 1 to 3 mcg/lb/min (3 to 5 mcg/kg/min) increments approximately every 8 to 10 minutes until the desired effects are achieved or signs of toxicity occur. Usual dosages for cardiocirculatory support are between 2.2 and 10 mcg/lb/min (5 and 20 mcg/kg/min); however, in rare cases up to 23 mcg/lb/min (50 mcg/kg/min) may be necessary and tolerated. Dopamine is available in 5 ml ampules that contain 40 mg/ml dopamine hydrochloride for dilution and subsequent continuous infusion.

TOXICITY AND DRUG INTERACTIONS

Side effects are dose-dependent and can include tachycardia, supraventricular and/or ventricular arrhythmias, vomiting, hypotension, or vasoconstriction. Toxicity can usually be effectively managed by slowing or discontinuing the infusion, as the half-life of the drug is less than two minutes.

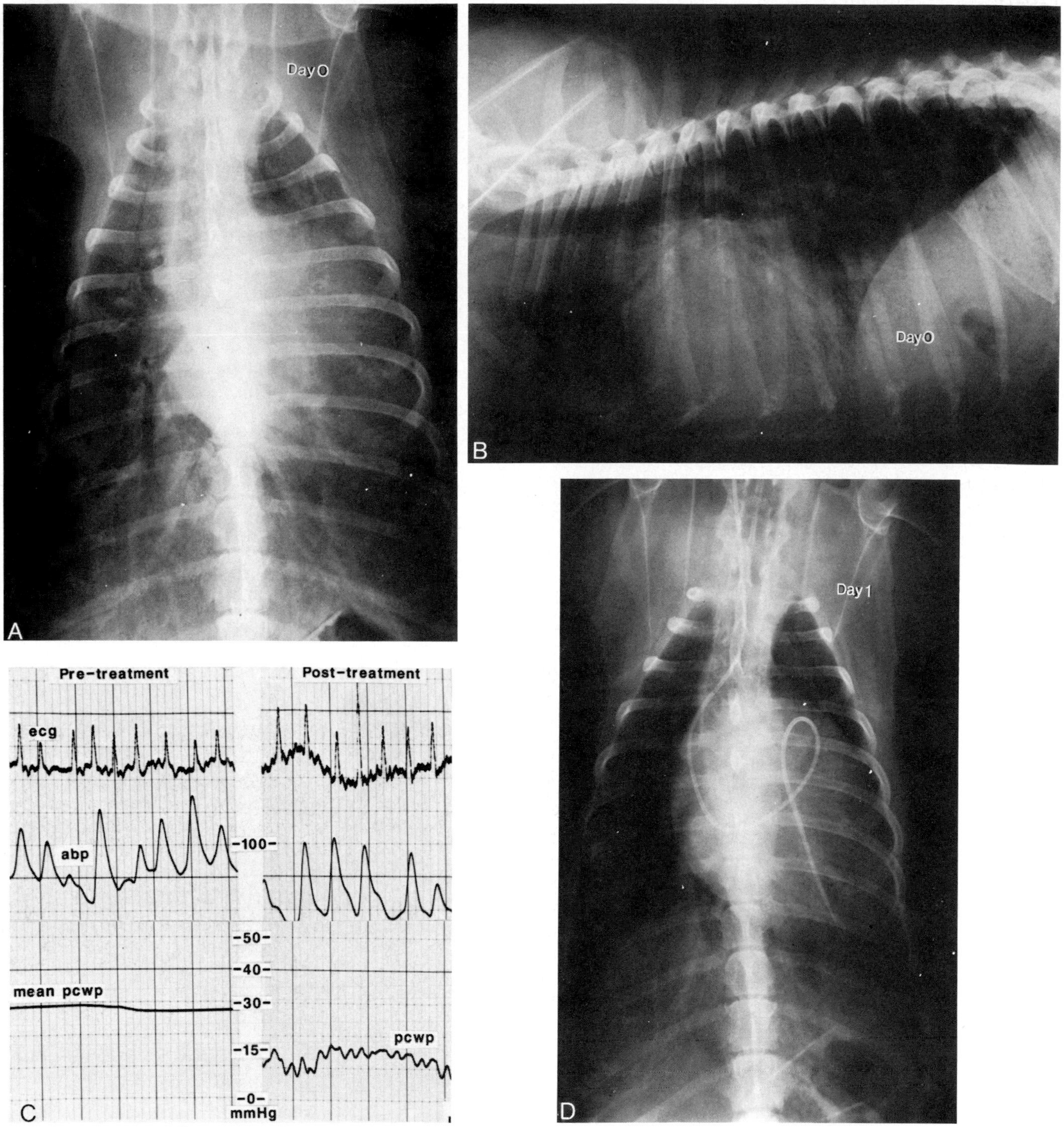

FIGURE 73–1. *A* and *B,* Thoracic radiographs (Day 0) taken at admission of a seven-year-old male standard poodle show generalized cardiomegaly, pulmonary venous distention, and pulmonary edema. *C,* An electrocardiogram (ECG) showed atrial fibrillation and echocardiography revealed a hypocontractile left ventricle and confirmed the diagnosis of dilated cardiomyopathy. Mean pulmonary capillary wedge pressure (pcwp) measured immediately following percutaneous placement of a Swan-Ganz thermistor-tipped catheter in the pulmonary artery was 28 mm Hg. An arterial line placed at the same time showed the arterial blood pressure (abp) to be approximately 108/90 mm Hg. The cardiac output measured in triplicate by thermodilution was 1.8 liters/min. *D* and *E,* Intravenous infusion of dobutamine (5 μg/kg/min) and nitroprusside (7 μg/kg/min) resulted in dramatic clinical, radiographic (Day 1), and hemodynamic improvement. Pcwp fell to 12 mm Hg, heart rate and abp decreased slightly (100/80 mm Hg), and cardiac output rose to 3.4 liters/min within two hours of beginning treatment. *F* and *G,* The animal was gradually weaned off of dobutamine and nitroprusside and onto digoxin, Lasix, and captopril, with sustained improvement in clinical signs and radiographic status (Day 2). A β-blocker (Atenolol) has since been added to the treatment regimen to further decrease the ventricular response to atrial fibrillation.

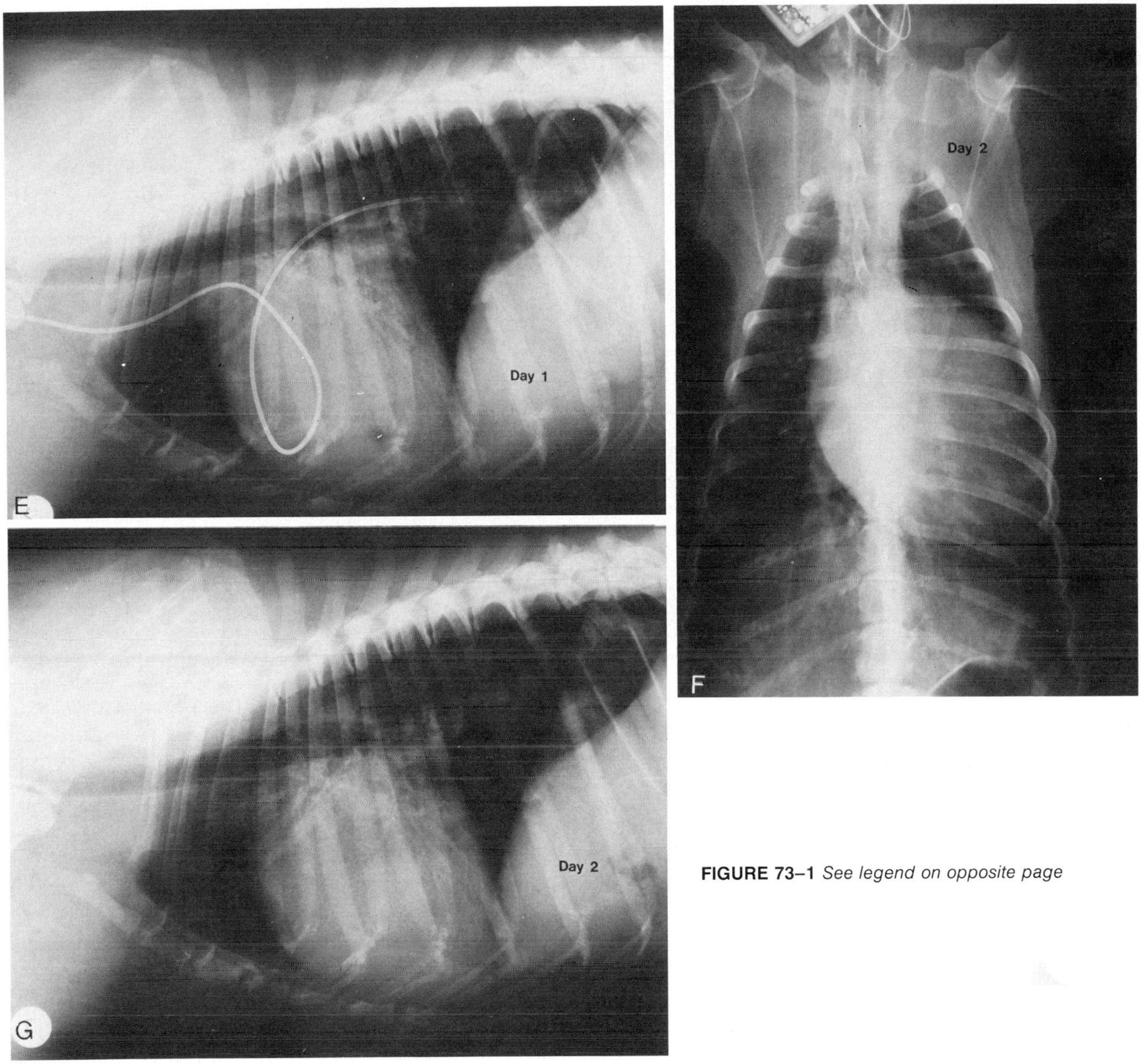

FIGURE 73–1 *See legend on opposite page*

Dobutamine

ACTIONS

Dobutamine, a synthetic analog of dopamine, is presently the most useful sympathomimetic amine used in the therapy of heart failure. Dobutamine provides the positive inotropic effects of dopamine, but lacks its vasodilatory effects on the renal, coronary, cerebral, and mesenteric vascular beds. Dobutamine is a β-1 agonist, with lesser degrees of α-1 and β-2 stimulatory properties. Dobutamine infusion increases cardiac contractility, cardiac output, coronary, and skeletal muscle blood flow. At appropriate doses, peripheral vascular resistance decreases such that little or no change in mean arterial blood pressure occurs.[145–147] At equipotent inotropic dosages, dobutamine is less likely to increase heart rate or arterial blood pressure than dopamine. The relative lack of α stimulation by dobutamine at low but inotropically effective dosages (1.5 to 3 mcg/lb/min or 3 to 7 mcg/kg/min) represents a significant advantage over dopamine in the therapy of heart failure.[147] Dobutamine has been shown to be superior to dopamine with respect to increasing cardiac output and decreasing left ventricular filling pressures in humans with low output heart failure.[148] One recent report in the human medical literature actually suggests a synergistic effect of dopamine and dobutamine in combination, but no such experience exists at the time of this writing in veterinary patients.[149]

Even though dobutamine increases myocardial oxygen demand in the normal heart, judicious use does not increase, and may even decrease, MVO_2 in heart failure. As with all catecholamines, tachycardia and supraventricular or ventricular ectopia may be observed at higher infusion rates (5 to 10 mg/lb/min or 10 to 20 mcg/kg/min).[150] Although α stimulation by dobutamine is minimal at infusion rates less than 10 mcg/lb/min (20 mcg/kg/min), these (pressor) effects may predominate if the patient is concurrently receiving a β-blocking drug. β blockers can effectively abolish the inotropic effects of dobutamine.[145]

Experimental evidence in dogs suggests that chronic dobutamine infusion may have a "conditioning" effect on the heart, and some clinical investigations in humans with heart failure secondary to primary myocardial disease have claimed that long-term hemodynamic benefits may accrue from dobutamine infusion.[29–31, 151] The first such study actually involved dopamine and found that 68 per cent of dilated cardiomyopathy patients given a three-day intravenous infusion reported symptomatic improvement for at least one week thereafter.[151] In a follow-up study using dobutamine infusions, some patients reported symptomatic improvement for up to six months.[30] A more recent study aimed at obtaining objective hemodynamic and metabolic evidence of improvement after dobutamine infusion demonstrated normalization of serum sodium and urea nitrogen concentrations during therapy, with some patients receiving long-term subjective benefits as well as objective improvement in echocardiographic indices and systolic time intervals. Analysis of endomyocardial biopsies performed before and after dobutamine infusion revealed improved ratios of ATP to creatine, probably indicating improved myocardial energetics after dobutamine infusion.[31] Based on these studies, intermittent outpatient therapy with dobutamine has been suggested as a method of long-term inotropic support in the management of heart failure.[152] Not all evidence concerning dobutamine is favorable, however. In one recent study, 13 human patients with severe congestive heart failure received 48 hours of intravenous dobutamine weekly, without evidence for prolonged survival and only partial symptomatic improvement of their heart failure between infusions.[153] Seventy-seven per cent of these patients died during the six month study, and while these patients represent a high-risk subset of heart failure patients with a known high mortality rate, these results are nevertheless disappointing. Prospective, controlled veterinary studies will be necessary to evaluate the therapeutic utility of intermittent dobutamine infusion in the long-term management of myocardial failure in animals.

INDICATIONS AND CURRENT USE

Currently, the routine clinical use of dobutamine is generally limited to veterinary patients with severe, intractable heart failure caused or complicated by myocardial failure or depression. Patients with atrial fibrillation or supraventricular tachycardia that depend on functional AV block to maintain a reasonable ventricular rate may experience enhanced AV nodal conduction with dobutamine, and these patients should be pretreated with digitalis prior to dobutamine therapy. Like all catecholamines, dobutamine may exacerbate ventricular or supraventricular ectopia and should be used with extreme caution in the presence of any tachyarrhythmia. Dobutamine is contraindicated in patients with hypertrophic subaortic stenosis or any heart disease characterized by ventricular hypertrophy that might result in outflow tract obstruction under catecholamine stimulation (e.g., hypertrophic cardiomyopathy).

Dobutamine must be administered by continuous intravenous infusion in a controlled environment. Therapy should be initiated at low dosages (0.5 to 1 mcg/lb/min or 1 to 2 mcg/kg/min in the dog, 0.25 mcg/lb/min or 0.5 mcg/kg/min in the cat) with continuous electrocardiographic monitoring, if possible. Central hemodynamic monitoring (arterial blood pressure, pulmonary capillary wedge pressure, and cardiac output) is extremely helpful in determining the response to therapy (see Figure 73–1), but is not essential for the successful use of the drug. If hemodynamic monitoring is unavailable, meticulous and frequent evaluation of the heart rate and rhythm, arterial pulse quality, mucous membrane color, capillary refill time, respiratory rate, and breath sounds usually permit sound therapeutic decisions to be made as treatment progresses. In the absence of hemodynamic monitoring capabilities, dosage must be titrated more slowly.

Clinical improvement usually occurs at infusion rates of 1 to 5 mcg/lb/min (2.5 to 10 mcg/kg/min) in the dog. Following initiation of therapy, the infusion rate is gradually increased over a period of hours, depending on the response to therapy. Sustained increases in heart rate or the appearance or exacerbation of supraventricular or ventricular ectopy should prompt immediate dosage reduction (usually by 50 per cent) or discontinuation of therapy, depending on the nature of the arrhythmia and the patient's general condition. In the authors' experience, effective dosages in the dog usually range from 1.0 to 5 mcg/lb/min (2.5 to 10 mcg/kg/min), with extra caution being necessary when using rates above 5 mcg/lb/min (10 mcg/kg/min). Infusion rates of 10 to 20 mcg/lb/min (20 to 40 mcg/kg/min) frequently result in tachycardia and vasoconstriction.

In patients that respond to therapy, dobutamine infusion is usually maintained for one to three days, because tachyphylaxis (tolerance) has been shown to occur in humans after 72 hours of continuous infusion.[154, 155] Cats appear to be exquisitely sensitive to dobutamine and may manifest toxic signs of seizures and/or vomiting. The authors' empirical experience in cats suggests that the infusion rate should not exceed 2 to 2.5 mcg/lb/min (4 to 5 mcg/kg/min). Dobutamine is available in 250 mg vials for reconstitution usually with 5 per cent dextrose in water.

TOXICITY AND DRUG INTERACTION

Once reconstituted, dobutamine is stable for approximately 6 hours at room temperature and should be used within 24 hours even if refrigerated. Alkaline solutions may inactivate the drug and should be avoided during reconstitution or administration.

Side effects observed with dobutamine are similar to those with dopamine, and include tachyarrhythmias, vomition, nervousness, and seizures (cats). Discontinuation of the drug is usually effective in alleviating arrhythmias or other toxic manifestations within 20 minutes, unless massive overdosage has resulted in permanent catecholamine-induced myocardial damage.

Orally Active Sympathomimetic Amines

The previously described sympathomimetic amines all share the property of requiring constant intravenous infusion to sustain their effects because of short half-lives and low oral bioavailability, due to extensive first-pass hepatic inactivation. Several orally active sympathomimetic amines are under investigation for potential use in the therapy of heart failure, including salbutamol, a drug that is currently available. Salbutamol, predominantly a β-2 agonist, is currently used in human medicine as a bronchodilator. While intravenous infusion of salbutamol has been shown to acutely improve systolic and diastolic cardiac function in human patients with dilated cardiomyopathy, its potential for long-term oral use will remain unknown in veterinary medicine until questions of efficacy and tachyphylaxis can be answered.[156] Levodopa has been used in human medicine to treat patients with Parkinson's disease. Levodopa is metabolized to dopamine at a slow rate after oral administration, and beneficial cardiovascular effects have been demonstrated in humans with congestive heart failure, as well as in dogs.[143, 157] Some other related compounds are under investigation, including pirbuterol, prenalterol, and butopamine. None of these drugs has been proven to be effective in the therapy of heart failure in veterinary patients and they are limited to investigational use.

BIPYRIDINE DERIVATIVES AND OTHER NEW INOTROPIC AGENTS

This new class of drugs has generated both excitement and controversy with regard to their potential for treating heart failure. These compounds are structurally dissimilar to both the catecholamines and digitalis glycosides. The two drugs that have been evaluated most extensively in both human and veterinary medicine are amrinone and milrinone, both bipyridine derivatives. Although the precise mechanism(s) of action of these agents is still uncertain, their positive inotropic effects are due at least in part to selective inhibition of the cyclic-AMP-specific cardiac phosphodiesterase F-III.[158, 159] Phosphodiesterase enzymes are responsible for the inactivation of cyclic-AMP, thereby reversing a cascade of events that leads to increased intracellular calcium concentrations. In the heart, increased calcium concentrations stimulate contractility. By inhibiting phosphodiesterase (cardiac phosphodiesterase III) and thus cAMP inactivation, these drugs increase contractility much more effectively than the older xanthine-derived drugs.

In addition to the positive inotropic and vasodilatory effects of these drugs, increased cAMP concentrations may also lead to undesirable stimulation of chronotropy or arrhythmogenesis.[160] The potential of these drugs to cause arrhythmia and raise MVO_2 is of obvious concern when dealing with a population of heart failure patients already at significantly increased risk of sudden death. Primarily because of their vasodilating effects, however, it appears that the bipyridine derivatives tend to reduce or cause no change in MVO_2 in the setting of heart failure.[161]

Amrinone

ACTIONS

Amrinone appears to increase cardiac contractility and cause vasodilation, decreasing preload and afterload. Amrinone is currently available for use in the United States. The *in vivo* positive inotropic properties of amrinone are somewhat difficult to measure because the effects of vasodilation also improve cardiac output and interfere with most clinically attainable indices of contractility.[162] In dogs with experimentally induced heart failure, amrinone infusion resulted in improved cardiac output, reduced left ventricular filling pressures, diminished myocardial oxygen demand, and improved contractility (dP/dt).[161] Another study demonstrated similar findings, with the additional benefit of decreased systemic vascular resistance.[163] A study in cats with experimentally induced right ventricular failure was unable to demonstrate a positive inotropic effect *in vitro*, but did demonstrate improved ventricular relaxation, indicating that amrinone may also enhance cyclic AMP dependent relaxation processes.[164] In addition, amrinone may improve coronary flow reserve by both dilating coronary arteries and decreasing the left ventricular end-diastolic pressure, allowing for better coronary flow in diastole.[165] The use of amrinone in dogs with naturally acquired heart disease has not been reported, and the initial enthusiasm for amrinone therapy of heart failure has been dulled by recent reports of extensive side effects and limited efficacy.[166, 171]

INDICATIONS AND CURRENT USE

Pending further investigation in dogs and cats with naturally occurring heart failure, the use of amrinone should be limited to the short-term therapy of patients with severe heart failure that is refractory to more conventional treatment. Published dosage recommendations for the dog and cat suggest an initial bolus of 0.5 to 1.5 mg/lb (1 to 3 mg/kg), followed immediately by a constant rate infusion of 5 to 50 μg/lb/min (10 to 100 μg/kg/min).[172] Monitoring recommendations (electrocardiographic and central hemodynamic) are the same as for dobutamine or dopamine. Amrinone has a short half-life (4.6 minutes in humans), but according to one author, peak effects are not seen until 60 minutes after intravenous infusion is started in the dog (90 minutes in cats).[172] The drug is eliminated both unchanged and in the form of several metabolites by the kidney. Amrinone is supplied in 20 ml vials of a 5 mg/ml solution.

TOXICITY AND DRUG INTERACTIONS

Hypotension, arrhythmia, or GI distress may indicate overdosage, and the infusion rate should be promptly decreased or the drug discontinued, depending on the nature and severity of signs. Amrinone has also been associated with thrombocytopenia, liver function abnormalities, and a syndrome of fever and lethargy in humans. Oral amrinone is associated with a high incidence of side effects in humans, with 83 per cent of patients reporting some disturbance, and 34 per cent requiring withdrawal from therapy in one multicenter placebo-controlled trial.[171]

Amrinone must be diluted in nondextrose-containing solutions and should not be injected together with furosemide in the same intravenous line, to avoid precipitation.

Milrinone

ACTIONS

Milrinone is another bipyridine derivative phosphodiesterase inhibitor, differing from amrinone primarily in its potency and intended route of administration. Milrinone is a carbonitrile derivative of amrinone that is thought to possess between 20 and 50 times the potency of amrinone. Milrinone appears to have a wide therapeutic index (about 100) and may prove to be useful in the long-term management of heart failure.[173] Though more potent, the hemodynamic effects of milrinone appear qualitatively similar to amrinone.[158]

In addition to its contractile effects, milrinone has also been shown to improve several indices of left ventricular diastolic function.[174] Milrinone has not been associated with the side effects of thrombocytopenia and gastrointestinal disturbance that have been reported with amrinone, and clinical trials in humans with severe heart failure have demonstrated milrinone's vasodilating and positive inotropic effects.[158, 175] In a clinical trial of human patients with severe heart failure, milrinone compared favorably as a single agent to either dobutamine or sodium nitroprusside with respect to their acute hemodynamic effects.[176] Milrinone caused a greater fall in pulmonary capillary wedge pressure and maintained a lower myocardial oxygen consumption than dobutamine, and although nitroprusside caused equal improvement in cardiac output and wedge pressure, milrinone caused significantly less hypotension than nitroprusside.

Unfortunately, other recent clinical investigations in humans have obtained mixed results, with findings suggesting no benefit in survival or even decreased long-term survival with milrinone.[177–179]

INDICATIONS AND CURRENT USE

The available published reports on the effects of milrinone in dogs with myocardial failure are promising.[173, 173a] At oral dosages of 0.2 to 0.44 mg/lb (0.5 to 1.0 mg/kg) q12h, all dogs showed echocardiographic evidence of improved ventricular function that was generally maintained throughout the four weeks of the study.[173] Six of the 14 dogs studied improved clinically during the study, and pulmonary edema was reported to be improved in the seven dogs so affected at the outset of the trial. Two dogs experienced increased ventricular ectopia that was chronologically correlated with milrinone administration, but did not require specific antiarrhythmic therapy. No evidence for drug tolerance was seen over the course of the investigation. At this time, milrinone is approved only for intravenous use; the oral form is unavailable except for investigational use. Further studies to demonstrate its long-term efficacy are needed before broad recommendations can be made concerning the use of milrinone in the dog, and to date, no studies have been published in cats. Imidazolone derivatives that possess cardiotonic and vasodilatory effects are being evaluated for use in the treatment of heart failure.[180–185]

DIURETICS

Diuretics are and will probably continue to be a pharmacologic mainstay of heart failure therapy. Along with salt restriction and venodilating drugs, they represent one of the three available methods of preload reduction. Diuretics act by a variety of mechanisms to reduce the plasma volume, thereby reducing venous, and ultimately, ventricular filling pressures. To understand why diuretics are often effective in relieving the clinical signs of congestive heart failure, a basic understanding of the kidney's response to reductions in cardiac output is necessary.

Reductions in cardiac output from any cause (heart failure, blood loss) may divert part of the large renal blood flow (normally about 20 per cent of the cardiac output or 3 to 5 ml/g/min) to organs with smaller "perfusion reserves" and a lower tolerance for blood flow reductions (e.g., the brain).[186] Such reductions in blood flow to the kidney result primarily in reduced pressure delivery to the glomerular capillaries, with cell damage or death occurring only in cases of severe renal hypoperfusion. The compensatory events that follow a reduction of renal blood flow are designed to restore blood volume (e.g., following hemorrhage), but are also responsible for the retention of salt and water that contributes to the congestive signs of heart failure.

In heart failure, decreased cardiac output and renal blood flow are accompanied by increased postglomerular vascular resistance and filtration fraction.[186] The increased filtration fraction results in increased peritubular capillary oncotic pressure, and this in turn enhances sodium resorption and ultimately, fluid retention. The excess salt and water retained by this mechanism, in addition to the activation of the renin-angiotensin-aldosterone axis, contributes to the elevated venous pressures that characterize congestive heart failure and form the basis for diuretic therapy.

Most diuretics inhibit the resorption of sodium or chloride in the renal tubules, resulting in the loss of more solute and water into the urine and the subsequent reduction of preload. Some diuretics (high-ceiling or loop diuretics) may also promote salt loss by shifting intrarenal blood flow in favor of the renal cortex. When used appropriately, diuretics can result in marked symptomatic improvement (e.g., resolution of pulmonary edema, pleural effusion, or ascites) with little change in cardiac output. This is possible because beyond a certain point, increases in preload that occur as a "compensatory" mechanism in heart failure are ineffective in raising the cardiac output, a situation that results in the flat portion of the ventricular function curve. In this situation, diuresis can reduce preload without causing a commensurate reduction in the force of cardiac contraction or cardiac output. If diuretics are used in an animal not operating on the flat portion of the ventricular function curve, however, significant reductions in cardiac output can and do occur. None of the diuretics has been shown to have any direct effect on the heart itself, and they should not be expected to increase cardiac output unless some afterload reduction also occurs as a result of their use.

High Ceiling or Loop Diuretics

GENERAL PROPERTIES

The family of high-ceiling or loop diuretics includes furosemide, ethacrynic acid, and bumetanide. These are all potent diuretics that act at the thick ascending limb of the loop of Henle to inhibit active chloride transport.[187–189] These drugs can increase the fractional clearance of sodium by more than 20 per cent, producing brisk diuresis and subsequent reduction of preload. Furosemide and bumetanide also have minor effects on the proximal renal tubule, causing mild bicarbonaturia and phosphaturia during peak diuresis.[190] Although the loop diuretics decrease renal vascular resistance and increase renal blood flow acutely, they can eventually decrease plasma volume and renal blood flow with chronic use.[191] Furosemide and ethacrynic acid tend to redistribute intrarenal blood flow away from the juxtamedullary regions to outer cortical nephrons.

In general, these drugs are effective in the face of hypoalbuminemia, acid-base or electrolyte imbalances, and low glomerular filtration rates, making refractoriness to therapy unusual in the absence of severe renal failure.[191] The action of the loop diuretics may be blunted if nonsteroidal anti-inflammatory drugs are used concurrently.[192] The loop diuretics have a steep dose-response curve and are therefore useful in patients with mild to severe congestive heart failure.

FUROSEMIDE

Actions. Furosemide is the most commonly used diuretic in veterinary medicine. In addition to the previously described diuretic actions, some studies suggest that intravenously administered furosemide may induce beneficial hemodynamic effects prior to the onset of diuresis. These effects are thought to increase systemic venous capacitance, thereby decreasing ventricular filling pressures and mean pulmonary artery pressure.[193] Although these acute hemodynamic effects have been invoked to explain the apparent immediate relief that sometimes appears to precede the onset of diuresis when furosemide is employed in the treatment of pulmonary edema, a recent study in humans with chronic congestive heart failure found that intravenously administered furosemide caused a transient reduction in cardiac performance secondary to activation of neurohumoral factors (e.g., norepinephrine, renin-angiotensin system).[194] The exact nature of the acute hemodynamic effects of intravenously administered furosemide in animals requires further study.

Indications and Current Use. Furosemide can be administered by intravenous, subcutaneous, intramuscular, and oral routes. It is widely considered to be "first line" therapy in the management of inappropriate fluid retention secondary to heart failure from any cause. The onset of action of intravenously administered furosemide is rapid, with diuresis beginning 5 minutes after injection and peaking approximately 30 minutes later. Administered orally, the onset of diuresis occurs within one hour and peak action occurs one to two hours after dosing. Furosemide is highly protein-bound, and has a half-life of approximately 15 minutes. The drug is cleared largely by secretion into the proximal renal tubules.

Furosemide is supplied as 12.5, 20, 40, and 50 mg tablets, as a 10 mg/ml elixir for oral use, and as a 50 mg/ml solution for injection. The recommended dosage of furosemide is variable, depending on the severity of clinical signs. The routine maintenance oral dosage for dogs with chronic congestive heart failure is approximately 0.5 to 1 mg/lb (1 to 2 mg/kg) q12h, increasing to 2 mg/lb (4 mg/kg) q8h in refractory cases. In dogs with acute, severe congestive heart failure, furosemide is usually administered parenterally at a dosage of 1 to 2 mg/lb (2 to 4 mg/kg), and that dose is often repeated in two to six hours until they are stable. Although some published doses of furosemide for cats are the same as for dogs, the authors' experience suggests that most cats respond well to lower dosages (0.5 to 1 mg/lb or 1 to 2 mg/kg q12h to q24h). Chronic therapy in the cat and some dogs can often be accomplished with intermittent administration every second or third day. The lowest effective dosage and frequency of administration are often best determined in conjunction with the owner's judgment and observation of clinical signs.[101]

Toxicity and Drug Interactions. Toxicity and adverse responses to furosemide are usually related to electrolyte and fluid loss, although furosemide is a sulfonamide derivative and can cause reactions in patients sensitive to sulfonamides. Overzealous therapy with furosemide (or any diuretic) can result in volume contraction, with subsequently diminished cardiac output and organ perfusion (e.g., pre-renal azotemia). Volume contraction associated with excessive diuretic use can serve to decrease the clearance and increase the serum concentrations of a variety of concurrently administered drugs, an effect that can precipitate intoxication from these other agents (e.g., digoxin).

Hypokalemia is the most common electrolyte imbalance accompanying furosemide therapy, although this complication is uncommon as long as the patient continues to eat normally. Anorexia predisposes to hypokalemia, especially if furosemide administration is continued. A common cause of anorexia in the management of heart failure is digitalis toxicity, a setting where hypokalemia may be especially troublesome in light of the exacerbation of digitalis toxicity caused by hypokalemia. Even in the absence of digitalis, some studies have suggested that diuretic-induced hypokalemia may be associated with an increased incidence of sudden death, presumably from ventricular arrhythmias.[195] Although a recent review of this evidence has questioned the validity of the association between hypokalemia and ventricular arrhythmia or sudden death in humans, hypokalemia should certainly be avoided where possible and managed judiciously when encountered (see Chapter 53).[196] At the authors' hospital, serum electrolyte levels are checked routinely in all hospitalized animals receiving diuretic therapy and at three- to six-month intervals in outpatients on chronic therapy, depending on their appetite, diuretic dosage, species, and disease.

Hyponatremia can also be a potentially serious complication of both advanced congestive heart failure and furosemide therapy.[197] Hyponatremia results from an imbalance between water intake and renal diluting capacity. In this situation, the kidneys are unable to produce maximally dilute urine to remove free water from the body, resulting in reduced serum sodium concentrations and hypotonicity.[198] The renin-angiotensin system influences the development of this syndrome primarily through the effects of angiotensin II in directly stimulating thirst while enhancing the release of antidiuretic hormone and reducing renal blood flow. These actions combine to increase water intake while decreasing the ability of the distal nephron to dilute the urine. Hypokalemia may predispose animals to hyponatremia by enhancing antidiuretic hormone secretion and by causing sodium ions to move into cells to replace lost potassium.

Despite low serum sodium levels in these heart failure patients, total body sodium levels are usually normal or increased. This condition has been termed dilutional hyponatremia and represents a serious (though fortunately infrequent) complication of advanced congestive heart failure and/or diuretic therapy. Dilutional hyponatremia is one of the few clinical situations where water restriction is indicated, and the prognosis for this infrequently seen condition is guarded to grave. In addition to water restriction, intensive therapy of the underlying cause of heart failure may improve cardiac output and renal perfusion in patients with dilutional hyponatremia. Further diuretic therapy is inappropriate. In consideration of the proposed pathogenesis of the condition, therapy with angiotensin-converting enzyme inhibitors has been advocated. Hypotension has been found to be a significant complication of the use of angiotensin-converting enzyme inhibitors in hyponatremic human patients, however, and caution is indicated pending further study.[197]

In addition to the potential problems associated with volume contraction and electrolyte disturbances, hearing loss has been reported to occur in some human patients following administration of furosemide and ethacrynic acid, especially after rapid intravenous injection.[199] The occurrence of this complication is difficult to evaluate in veterinary medicine, but excessively rapid intravenous administration of these drugs should probably be avoided.

Depletion of water soluble vitamins has been reported as a complication of diuretic therapy.[199a] Because these vitamins are important in the metabolic pathways that are responsible for the production of ATP, supplementation of B-complex vitamins has been recommended for patients on continuous diuretic therapy.

ETHACRYNIC ACID

Ethacrynic acid is rarely prescribed by veterinarians. The drug is similar to furosemide in most respects, including its mechanism of action, quality and quantity of the induced diuresis, and dose-response curve. Reported side effects of ethacrynic acid in humans include gastrointestinal disturbances and upper abdominal pain, and it is recommended that the drug be taken with food. Leukopenia, thrombocytopenia, and reversible deafness have also been reported.[191] Although the incidence of side effects in animals is unknown, considering the extensive experience accumulated by most veterinarians with furosemide and the similarity of furosemide and ethacrynic acid, the routine use of ethacrynic acid cannot be recommended at this time.

BUMETANIDE

Bumetanide is the most recent of the high-ceiling or loop diuretics to gain approval for use in animals. The drug is similar to furosemide in most respects, but is much more potent on a milligram basis. For this reason, it is expected that bumetanide will be used most frequently for large animals, where the advantage of smaller injection volumes may be significant. At the present time, the authors are unaware of any significant pharmacodynamic advantage of the drug in small animals.

THIAZIDE DIURETICS

Actions. The thiazide diuretics act on the proximal portion of the distal convoluted tubule to inhibit resorption of sodium and cause secretion of potassium. Some thiazides may have a secondary site of action in the proximal tubule.[200] These drugs produce a moderate diuresis, less dramatic than that observed with the loop diuretics. The diuretic effects are not strictly dose-dependent, in that a dose-response plateau is observed whereby dosage increases do not result in increased diuresis. All of the thiazide diuretics produce a similar diuresis, both quantitatively and qualitatively, permitting drug selection based primarily on pharmocokinetic properties and ease of administration. In general, the newer, more lipid-soluble thiazides (cyclothiazide, methychlothiazide) have longer durations of action than the older, water-soluble drugs (chlorothiazide and hydrochlorothiazide). The thiazide diuretics are not effective in patients with compromised renal function.[201] They are contraindicated in azotemic animals because they tend to decrease renal blood flow and may cause deterioration of renal function. Blood urea nitrogen and/or serum creatinine determinations should be made before therapy is begun.

Indications and Current Use. The thiazides are most

commonly used to produce a moderate diuresis in the early stages of heart failure, although their use in veterinary medicine has declined in recent years. Because the thiazide diuretics act at a different site on the renal tubule than either the loop diuretics or potassium-sparing diuretics, combinations of thiazides with other diuretics may be beneficial in relieving refractory fluid retention. Chlorothiazide and hydrochlorothiazide are the most commonly used thiazides in veterinary medicine. Chlorothiazide has its onset of action within one hour, and the peak action is reached approximately four hours after administration. The effects of chlorothiazide persist for 6 to 12 hours. Chlorothiazide is supplied in 250 and 500 mg tablets. The usual oral dosage in the dog and the cat is 10 to 20 mg/lb (20 to 40 mg/kg) q12h. Hydrochlorothiazide has an onset of action of approximately two hours, and peak activity occurs about four hours after administration. The duration of hydrochlorothiazide action is 12 hours, and the drug is available as 25 and 50 mg tablets. The recommended dosage in dogs and cats is 1 to 2 mg/lb (2 to 4 mg/kg) q12h.

Toxicity and Drug Interactions. In animals with normal renal function, the thiazide diuretics have little potential for toxicity. As with the loop diuretics, adverse effects are most commonly attributed to overuse, resulting in disturbances of electrolyte or fluid balance. Because of thiazide-induced secretion of potassium into the renal tubule, hypokalemia is the most commonly observed electrolyte disturbance. The frequency of this complication can be minimized by ensuring that diuretic use is restricted to patients who are eating normally or are under close supervision (including serum potassium monitoring).

POTASSIUM-SPARING DIURETICS

Actions. Spironolactone and triamterene are the potassium-sparing diuretics currently used in veterinary medicine. As previously discussed, potassium loss and hypokalemia represent potential complications of diuretic therapy. In patients receiving diuretic therapy, a potassium-sparing agent may be added to allow dosage reduction of the other diuretic, increase the serum potassium on a long-term basis, and/or provide an additional degree of diuresis. These diuretics produce only mild diuresis in normal individuals, however, heart failure patients with elevated plasma aldosterone concentrations may have a significantly greater diuretic response.

Spironolactone is a competitive antagonist of aldosterone, therefore serum aldosterone levels must be elevated if spironolactone is to be effective. Aldosterone secretion increases with activation of the renin-angiotensin system in response to reductions in serum sodium, elevations of serum potassium, or reductions in effective blood volume or cardiac output. Aldosterone acts on the renal tubule to increase the resorption of sodium and chloride while increasing the excretion of potassium. Spironolactone competes with aldosterone for occupation of its receptor site, causing a mild diuresis with the added beneficial effect of potassium retention. The onset of action after initiation of therapy is slow, and peak diuresis does not occur for 48 to 72 hours. The diuretic effect persists for two to three days after discontinuation of therapy.

Triamterene also causes a reduction in potassium secretion in the distal nephron. While triamterene was originally thought to be a nonsteroidal competitive antagonist of aldosterone, experimental studies have demonstrated that the diuretic effect of triamterene is maintained in adrenalectomized animals. While the exact mechanism of action is still undetermined, the drug is thought to act independently of aldosterone, probably through direct effects on electrolyte transport in the renal tubules.[202] The peak onset of action of triamterene occurs 6 to 8 hours after oral administration, and the diuretic effects persist for 12 to 16 hours.

Indications and Current Use. Because they work at a different site in the nephron than either the thiazides or the loop diuretics, the addition of a potassium-sparing agent to a diuretic regimen can provide an additional degree of diuresis sometimes required to keep patients with severe chronic fluid retention comfortable.[203] In the authors' practice, these agents are used mostly in management of refractory ascites or pulmonary edema secondary to heart failure that has become unresponsive to conventional management with furosemide as well as appropriate vasodilators and/or inotropic agents. Spironolactone is supplied in 25 mg tablets; the recommended dosage in the dog is 1 to 2 mg/lb/day (2 to 4 mg/kg/day). Triamterene is supplied in 100 mg capsules, and the usual dosage in the dog is 1 to 2 mg/lb/day (2 to 4 mg/kg/day), administered with meals to avoid gastrointestinal side effects.

Toxicity and Drug Interactions. Because of the potential for hyperkalemia, potassium-sparing diuretics should not be administered concurrently with potassium supplements or angiotensin converting enzyme inhibitors. While spironolactone or triamterene may be useful when added to existing diuretic regimens, neither drug is recommended as the sole diuretic agent in the therapy of heart failure.

VASODILATORS

Vasodilators have been used for many years in the therapy of heart failure in humans, and have gained increasing acceptance in veterinary medicine for the therapy of heart failure in dogs and cats. The rationale for the use of vasodilators in the management of heart failure is straightforward and is briefly summarized before discussing the clinical use of specific drugs.

Regardless of the underlying cause, reductions in cardiac output associated with heart failure initiate a variety of compensatory changes directed at restoring circulatory function.[204] Activation of the renin-angiotensin-aldosterone system, expansion of the intravascular fluid volume, and increases in sympathetic tone are compensatory changes that occur in response to reductions in cardiac output. These compensatory mechanisms act in concert to increase cardiac preload and afterload. Although these mechanisms serve to maintain the circulatory volume and perfusion pressure acutely, in the setting of chronic heart failure, excessively elevated preload may result in fluid accumulations without significant improvements in cardiac output, and excessive afterload requires increased amounts of the heart's contractile energy to be expended in generating tension. Increased ventricular wall tension increases the heart's oxygen demand and makes less energy available for myofiber shortening and actual ejection of blood.[205]

Venous dilating drugs, like diuretics, are employed as preload reducers. They increase venous capacitance, reduce venous pressures, and relieve abnormal fluid accumulations without seriously compromising cardiac output if they are used appropriately in patients operating on the flat portion of the ventricular function (Frank-Starling) curve. An additional benefit of preload reduction may accrue if ventricular size is also reduced by decreasing venous return, thus lowering ventricular wall tension and afterload. Arterial vasodilators are employed to reduce the impedance to left ventricular ejection, thereby reducing the tension generated in the myocardium, increasing the amount of contractile energy devoted to myofiber shortening (increasing the stroke volume and cardiac output), and reducing the MVO_2. In the setting of mitral regurgitation, afterload reduction has the additional advantage of reducing the amount of blood regurgitated into the left atrium, as it becomes easier for the left ventricle to eject blood into the aorta.[206–208] Successful afterload reduction may also reduce ventricular filling pressures, thus reducing preload as well as ventricular size.

Significant mechanical, hemodynamic, and metabolic advantages are found in keeping the dilated heart as small as possible, and such advantages could theoretically alter or delay the natural progression of myocardial failure and/or valvular heart disease.[209] These arguments, along with demonstrated hemodynamic efficacy in controlled clinical experiments and recent evidence of increased length of survival, form the basis for advocating the use of vasodilators in the therapy of heart failure.

Even though vasodilators have made a tremendous impact on the treatment of heart failure in both human and veterinary medicine in the past ten years, until recently no controlled trials had demonstrated that these drugs prolonged survival in addition to improving the patient's hemodynamic profile, clinical signs, and quality of life. In a controlled experiment on human patients with chronic heart failure published in 1986, patients receiving vasodilators (hydralazine and isosorbide dinitrate) lived significantly longer than patients managed with conventional therapy.[210] Other human studies have suggested that therapy with angiotensin-converting enzyme inhibitors may also prolong survival.[211] Several studies in veterinary patients have demonstrated beneficial effects of vasodilator therapy on the hemodynamic and clinical consequences of chronic heart failure in dogs.[212–217]

Although vasodilators promise attractive potential benefits in the management of heart failure, serious drawbacks are associated with their inappropriate or overzealous use. Venodilators, like diuretics, have the potential to reduce cardiac output if used inappropriately in patients not operating on the flat portion of their ventricular function curve. Inappropriate use of arterial dilators may cause serious hypotension and reflex tachycardia. All of these drugs have the potential to induce profound weakness and lethargy with injudicious use. It is important to remember that the hemodynamic effects of all of the vasodilators are very different in patients in heart failure than in normal animals. The beneficial actions of these drugs and avoidance of their potential adverse effects depend upon the presence of the increased sympathetic tone, activation of the renin-angiotensin-aldosterone system, vasopressin release, increased vascular stiffness, and blunted baroreceptor responses that characterize heart failure.[218, 219]

Vasodilators are generally classified by their site of action on the peripheral circulation and may selectively dilate arteries, veins, or both. Selection of a vasodilator depends on the pathophysiology of a particular patient's heart failure and the clinical signs present, as well as the clinician's past experience, availability of hemodynamic monitoring, and potential interactions with other therapeutic agents to be used. In consideration of the adverse effects associated with their inappropriate use, every effort to obtain a definitive diagnosis along with as much hemodynamic information as possible should be made prior to initiating vasodilator therapy.

Abrupt discontinuation of vasodilator therapy can be associated with a "rebound" phenomenon (increased systemic vascular resistance, ventricular filling pressures, and decreased cardiac output).[220] With this in mind, vasodilator therapy that is to be discontinued is generally tapered over a period of days, rather than stopped suddenly. Although a large number of vasodilators with a variety of different mechanisms of action have been tested in animals, this section discusses only those that are currently being used in the clinical management of heart failure in veterinary medicine.

HYDRALAZINE

Actions. Of the vasodilators available for use in veterinary patients, hydralazine has been the most extensively studied in clinical veterinary use.[213–216] Hydralazine is a direct-acting arteriolar dilator that appears to act either via elevation of local concentrations of PGI_2 or possibly by inhibiting calcium influx into smooth muscle cells.[221, 222] The direct actions of hydralazine are limited to arteriolar smooth muscle, and the drug has little effect on the venous capacitance vessels.

Initial clinical studies using hydralazine in dogs found that it improved the clinical status of dogs with mitral insufficiency and cough that had been previously unresponsive to therapy with digitalis, diuretics, bronchodilators, and antitussives.[214] More recent hemodynamic studies of dogs with heart failure secondary to naturally acquired mitral insufficiency demonstrated that hydralazine decreased blood pressure, pulmonary capillary wedge pressure, and total systemic vascular resistance; and increased cardiac index and venous oxygen tension, a correlate of cardiac output.[216] The authors of this study concluded that hydralazine administration produced significant hemodynamic improvement in dogs with severe mitral valve insufficiency.

Indications and Current Use. Hydralazine is rapidly absorbed from the intestinal tract and the onset of action occurs within one hour of oral administration. Hydralazine undergoes significant first-pass hepatic metabolism, primarily via acetylation.[223] Although not excreted by renal mechanisms, uremia has been reported to affect the biotransformation of hydralazine, increasing serum levels.[223] Pharmacodynamic studies in dogs with experimentally induced heart failure demonstrated that peak improvement in cardiac performance occurred 3 to 5 hours after oral hydralazine administration, with effects lasting an average of 11 to 13 hours.[217] Clinical studies using a combination of noninvasive blood pressure determinations and free-flowing jugular venous oxygen tensions to titrate the dosage of hydralazine to an objectively measured physiologic response have recommended an initial oral dosage of 0.5 mg/lb (1 mg/kg), to be increased by 0.5 mg/lb (1 mg/kg) to a maximum of 1.5 mg/lb (3 mg/kg), depending on the therapeutic response.[215] Where arterial blood pressure and venous oxygen tension measurements are available, the recommended therapeutic endpoints of hydralazine titration are a mean arterial blood pressure of 70 to 80 mm Hg and central venous oxygen tensions of greater than 30 mm Hg, provided these values are achieved prior to reaching the maximum dose of 1.5 mg/lb (3 mg/kg). The dosage of hydralazine required to reach these endpoints is then administered twice daily in most patients. If arterial blood pressure and/or blood gas monitoring are unavailable, an initial hydralazine dosage of 0.25 to 0.5 mg/lb (0.5 to 1 mg/kg) q12h is recommended, and this dosage is slowly increased to a maximum of 1.5 mg/lb (3 mg/kg) over several days. In this situation, the maintenance dose is determined by the patient's clinical response to therapy and radiographic evidence of resolution of pulmonary edema and/or decreased left atrial size. The dose of hydralazine in the cat has been reported to be 2.5 mg to 10 mg q12h, again starting with the lower dosage and slowly increasing the dose as needed, based upon the response to therapy.[224] Hydralazine is available in 1 ml vials of a 20 mg/ml solution for parenteral use, as well as 10 and 25 mg tablets for oral administration. In general, because of the rapid and predictable onset of action following oral administration, this route is preferred.

Hydralazine is used most frequently in the setting of chronic symptomatic mitral regurgitation, where the drug may result in decreased mitral regurgitant volume, with subsequently increased forward cardiac output and reduced left atrial size. In the authors' experience, hydralazine is often beneficial in patients with chronic cough secondary to left atrial enlargement that has caused compression or collapse of the left main stem bronchus. Hydralazine may be useful in any situation where arteriolar dilation is likely to be beneficial (e.g., low-output heart failure from any cause other than aortic stenosis or hypertrophic cardiomyopathy). Because of hydralazine's potential to cause hypotension, tachycardia, and other side effects, therapy should be initiated under careful supervision.

Toxicity and Drug Interactions. Hypotension is the most commonly reported complication of therapy with hydralazine. If hypotension is encountered, the drug should be discontinued for 24 hours and restarted at 50 per cent of the initial dose. Persistent hypotension may necessitate discontinuation of therapy, or in life-threatening situations, dopamine can be administered intravenously to increase cardiac output while supporting the arterial blood pressure. Another potentially significant side effect of hydralazine is reflex tachycardia. Although baroreceptor reflexes are diminished in heart failure, significant reduction in arterial blood pressure attending hydralazine therapy may still cause an increase in heart rate. Experimental evidence also suggests that hydralazine-induced histamine release may indirectly contribute to the increases in heart rate observed under some conditions.[225] The presence of persistent sinus tachycardia accompanying hydralazine therapy may require either dosage adjustment or the addition of digitalis or a β-adrenergic blocking agent to control the heart rate.

Decreases in arterial blood pressure also activate the renin-angiotensin-aldosterone system, which may lead to increased fluid retention and possibly the development of refractory fluid accumulations. Increases in serum aldosterone concentrations have been shown to accompany chronic hydralazine therapy in dogs with heart failure, and diuretics (primarily furosemide) should almost always be prescribed in conjunction with hydralazine to prevent excess fluid retention.[226, 227] Spironolactone, triamterene, or angiotensin-converting enzyme inhibitors may be useful adjuncts in managing refractory edema or ascites occurring during hydralazine therapy.

Gastrointestinal disturbances (most commonly anorexia and vomiting) sometimes occur during hydralazine therapy and may persist despite dosage reductions. These side effects represent a relatively frequent cause for discontinuation of hydralazine therapy and/or lack of owner compliance. A systemic lupus erythematosus–like syndrome, including positive ANA titers, reported in humans taking high doses of hydralazine (greater than 400 mg/day) appears to be more common in those who are genetically slow acetylators and has not been reported in veterinary patients.[228] (Editor's Note: In a recent clinical evaluation of vasodilating agents in dogs and cats with heart failure, drug therapy had to be discontinued or dosages significantly reduced due to side effects in nearly one-half of the animals treated.)

NITROGLYCERIN AND OTHER NITRATES

Actions. Nitroglycerin and the nitrates cause direct relaxation of venous smooth muscle. This action results in increased venous capacitance, subsequently reducing cardiac preload. When used in high dosages, these drugs also cause a minor amount of dilatation of the large arteries.[229] These actions consistently decrease right atrial and pulmonary capillary wedge pressures and result in smaller and more variable changes in cardiac output, arterial pressure, and systemic vascular resistance.[230]

Indications and Current Use. The nitrates are used primarily for the acute treatment of cardiogenic pulmonary edema in veterinary medicine. They are well absorbed orally, but are subject to extensive first-pass metabolism by the liver, necessitating high dosages if this route of administration is chosen. Nitroglycerin is also rapidly absorbed by sublingual and transcutaneous routes, and transcutaneously applied two per cent nitroglycerin ointment is the most frequently used nitrate in veterinary patients. Nitroglycerin ointment is applied to the inside of the pinna of the ear or other shaved or hairless region every four to six hours. This route of application appears to have a rapid onset of action, with decreases in central venous pressure measurable within 15 to 30 minutes of application.

The effective dose is variable, but in the authors' experience one-quarter to one inch of ointment usually results in measurable reductions in central venous or pulmonary capillary wedge pressure within 30 minutes. Ideally, the dosage should be titrated based on either central hemodynamic measurements and/or clinical signs. The lower end of the dosage range is appropriate for the initial therapy of cats and small dogs. Because nitroglycerin ointment can also be absorbed through the skin of the individual applying it, care must be taken to avoid excessive contact. Old ointment must be removed before the next dose is applied to the skin to prevent buildup. Newer self-adhesive transdermal therapeutic delivery systems providing sustained (24-hour) nitroglycerin levels are commonly used in humans, and have significant advantages in ease of application and consistency of dosage.[231] While these same advantages would seem to apply to veterinary patients, studies on the use of sustained transdermal nitroglycerin delivery systems in veterinary patients have not been reported. In the authors' hospital, 2.5 and 5 mg transdermal nitroglycerin patches are being used with safety and hemodynamic efficacy in the acute management of cardiogenic pulmonary edema in large breed dogs. These patches can be cut in quarters for use in small dogs and cats.

Although no controlled clinical veterinary studies have examined the efficacy of the nitrates in the management of heart failure, the results of some human studies suggest that their long-term usefulness is restricted by the development of tolerance.[232, 233] One recent investigation found that the hemodynamic response to nitroglycerin could be restored through intermittent (removing the patches overnight) rather than continuous usage in humans with heart failure, and these issues need to be addressed in veterinary patients.[234] At the present time, the use of nitroglycerin is most often restricted to emergency or acute-care settings in veterinary medicine. In cases where both preload and afterload reduction are indicated, nitroglycerin may be combined with an arterial vasodilator such as hydralazine to achieve those effects.

Toxicity and Drug Interactions. Overdosage with nitroglycerin can result in severely compromised cardiac output because of large reductions in preload. Hypotension, depression, lethargy, nausea, and pre-renal azotemia may follow. Some degree of lethargy and/or somnolence is often seen with nitroglycerin therapy in animals, and people frequently report nausea and headache with initial use. These side effects rarely preclude the drug's use in the acute management of life-threatening cardiogenic pulmonary edema, where its venodilating and preload-reducing actions may be life saving. They may, however, limit the drug's long-term usefulness and affect owner compliance if administration is perceived to be associated with decreased activity levels or quality of life.

SODIUM NITROPRUSSIDE

Actions. Sodium nitroprusside is a balanced vasodilator that acts directly on arterial and venous vascular smooth muscle. Intravenous administration of sodium nitroprusside increases cardiac output and lowers systemic vascular resistance, arterial blood pressure, and pulmonary capillary wedge pressure.[208] Nitroprusside may also reduce diastolic intraventricular pressures by enhancing ventricular compliance.[235] As with hydralazine, nitroprusside also reduces regurgitant fraction in human patients with mitral insufficiency.[208] Sodium nitroprusside has both an extremely rapid onset and an extremely short duration of action in the dog. Because of its short duration of action, it must be administered by constant intravenous infusion.

Indications and Current Use. Nitroprusside's potent hypotensive effect makes it the agent of choice when immediate (emergency) reduction of blood pressure and/or afterload is required. In veterinary critical care settings, the drug is most often used to improve cardiac output and reduce ventricular filling pressures (and thus pulmonary edema) in patients with severe heart failure. Because of its potent hypotensive effect, nitroprusside should ideally be used only in settings where arterial blood pressure can be monitored either continuously or at least frequently.

In canine patients with severe heart failure or cardiogenic shock secondary to dilated cardiomyopathy, nitroprusside therapy is often administered concurrently with dobutamine (Figure 73–1). The positive inotropic support of dobutamine appears to mitigate the hypotensive effects of nitroprusside, and in the authors' experience usually results in greater improvement in cardiac output and pulmonary capillary wedge pressure than either drug used as a single agent in this setting.

Sodium nitroprusside is supplied in 50 mg vials for dilution prior to intravenous use; the resulting solution should be protected from the light to avoid degradation. In the dog, the initial infusion rate used at the authors' hospital is 0.5 mcg/lb/min (1 mcg/kg/min), and the rate of infusion is increased by 0.5 mcg/lb/min (1 mcg/kg/min) every 5 minutes until the mean arterial pressure reaches the target level of approximately 70 mmHg. Clinical and hemodynamic response must be carefully monitored. Infusion rates greater than 2.0 to 3.5 mcg/lb/min (5.0 to 7.0 mcg/kg/min) are usually unnecessary.

Toxicity and Drug Interactions. Hypotension may develop rapidly and can be managed by simply reducing the infusion rate. Although the arterial blood pressure can be decreased to virtually any desired level by adjusting the infusion rate of nitroprusside, maximum clinical and hemodynamic benefit are usually obtained when the drug is used in combination with dobutamine as previously discussed. No clinical experience with nitroprusside has been reported in cats.

The ferrous ion of nitroprusside is metabolized to cyanide by the red blood cells and other tissues. Cyanide thus formed is further metabolized to thiocyanate in the liver, but high doses or protracted therapy (days) with nitroprusside can theoretically result in cyanide poisoning.[236] The earliest and most reliable indicators of intoxication are the development of metabolic acidosis and increased tolerance to the drug. If toxicity is encountered, the drug should be discontinued at once, and therapy with sodium nitrate and sodium thiosulfate should be initiated. Intoxication may be prevented by concurrent use of hydroxocobalamin, which results in the formation of a nontoxic compound, cyanocobalamin. In the authors' experience, such measures appear to be unwarranted if the drug is used as directed in the dog.

PRAZOSIN

Actions. Prazosin is a selective α-1 (postsynaptic) receptor blocker and thus causes dilation of both arteries and veins.[237] In people with heart failure, a number of clinical investigations have shown that the balanced vasodilation that results from the administration of prazosin increases cardiac output while reducing cardiac filling pressures and improving signs of heart failure. Although some studies have demonstrated sustained hemodynamic benefits either at rest or with exercise from chronic prazosin therapy, only one of several randomized double-blind, placebo-controlled trials performed on humans in heart failure has shown significant improvement in symptoms and exercise capacity after 1 to 12 months of treatment with prazosin compared to that with placebo.[238–244] Most investigations demonstrate that tolerance to the drug's actions develops with time, attenuating the beneficial hemodynamic effects.[245, 246] The exact mechanism of this tolerance to α-blockade is not known; however, it does not appear to be mediated by the renin-angiotensin system.[247] Other clinical investigations performed on humans with heart failure have shown that the regional distribution of the increased cardiac output resulting from prazosin therapy may not be as satisfactory as with other vasodilators, with renal, limb, and liver blood flow being relatively lower than that achieved with hydralazine therapy.[248] At the time of this writing, no controlled clinical studies of either the short- or long-term effects of prazosin have been performed on dogs or cats with heart failure, although reports of therapeutic success do exist.[212]

In addition to reports of prazosin's hemodynamic effects, one experimental study in dogs with surgically induced mitral insufficiency and subsequent heart (and myocardial) failure found that three months of prazosin therapy prevented the deterioration of myocardial function observed in control animals during the six-month study period.[249] The applicability of these investigations to the therapy of naturally occurring diseases in veterinary patients is uncertain, and the role of prazosin in the therapy of heart failure awaits further clarification.

Indications and Current Use. Prazosin is supplied in 1, 2, and 5 mg capsules. The dosage of prazosin in dogs is not well established and should be titrated to the clinical and/or hemodynamic response. General recommendations for initial therapy in small dogs are that 1 mg of prazosin be administered twice daily, whereas large dogs can be given up to 2 mg 3 times daily. Because the capsules cannot be divided, prazosin therapy in very small dogs and cats is inconvenient and may be hazardous if some accommodation for dosage reduction is not made. Capsules may be partially emptied, permitting more gradual titration from 0.5 mg per dose.

Toxicity and Drug Interactions. Hypotension is the most frequent side effect of prazosin, and this may result in syncope, lethargy, or general malaise. Because prazosin selectively blocks postsynaptic (α-1) receptors, presynaptic (α-2) receptors remain capable of providing normal feedback inhibition from norepinephrine, diminishing further neurotransmitter release and usually preventing the development of reflex tachycardia.

Because of the difficulty in dosing small patients and the questions of efficacy surrounding chronic administration, prazosin is infrequently employed as a "first choice" vasodilator in the authors' practice. While prazosin offers some advantage in that it supplies orally available balanced vasodilation, more definitive studies of the safety and efficacy of this drug are needed in veterinary patients. At the time of this writing, it seems prudent to reserve prazosin therapy for patients who are either refractory to, or intolerant of, the effects of other vasodilators.

Angiotensin-Converting Enzyme Inhibitors

Inhibition of the angiotensin-converting enzyme is currently an accepted approach to the management of human patients with severe chronic heart failure from a variety of causes.[250, 250a] Several angiotensin-converting enzyme inhibitors have been developed and studied for use in heart failure therapy. At this time, two of these drugs (captopril and enalapril) are available in the United States, although only one (captopril) is currently approved for the therapy of heart failure.

Excessive activation of the renin-angiotensin-aldosterone system appears to be an important mediator of the increased afterload and preload that eventually contribute to the clinical syndrome of heart failure.[251–253] In heart failure, renal renin is released through many mechanisms, including sympathetic stimulation and reductions in renal perfusion and perfusion pressure.[254] Renin acts on angiotensinogen, producing inactive angiotensin I. Angiotensin-converting enzyme (dipeptidyl carboxypeptidase) in the lungs and vascular endothelial cells then cleaves circulating angiotensin I to active angiotensin II. Angiotensin II is a potent vasoconstrictor that also functions to stimulate the release of aldosterone from the adrenal cortex. Angiotensin-converting enzyme inhibitors (ACE inhibitors) therefore perform two potentially useful functions in the management of heart failure, preventing both the direct vasoconstricting effects of angiotensin II on both arteries and veins, as well as reducing the retention of sodium and water by secondarily inhibiting aldosterone release. Angiotensin-converting inhibitors thus act as balanced vasodilators, reducing both afterload and preload.

CAPTOPRIL

Actions. Captopril was the first angiotensin-converting enzyme inhibitor to be developed and approved, and its effects in human patients with heart failure are well documented.[250, 255–258] The drug significantly increases cardiac output, while reducing systemic vascular resistance, pulmonary capillary wedge pressure, and right atrial pressure. The heart rate is usually unaffected or may be reduced by approximately ten per cent. Clinical trials of captopril in human patients with heart failure show that up to 85 per cent of patients refractory to digitalis and diuretics experience significant improvement in cardiac function, symptoms, and exercise tolerance and that these benefits persist in many patients for more than one year.[250, 258] Captopril therapy has been shown to result in significantly more clinical improvement in humans with heart failure than prazosin.[259] Captopril therapy also improved survival of hyponatremic patients compared to those treated with non-ACE inhibitor vasodilators.[260]

Decreasing circulating levels of angiotensin II may not be the only mechanism by which captopril diminishes systemic vascular resistance. Captopril has also been shown to inhibit the degradation of bradykinin, reduce the release of antidiuretic hormone (arginine vasopressin), lower the concentration of circulating catecholamines, and possibly increase the levels of some vasodilating prostaglandins.[250, 256, 261] Additionally, captopril therapy decreases diuretic-induced potassium loss in human heart failure patients.[262]

Indications and Current Use. In the dog, preliminary (unpublished) clinical studies of captopril have been encouraging. Most canine patients with NYHA class III or class IV heart failure have been shown to have elevated plasma aldosterone concentrations, which decreased following captopril therapy.[226] In the authors' practice, captopril is currently being used as part of the therapeutic regimen for dogs with heart failure secondary to chronic valvular disease, as well as dilated cardiomyopathy, and it appears to be an especially valuable adjunct in the management of refractory ascites or pleural effusion secondary to chronic heart failure. Hemodynamic effects of captopril are usually observed within 30 minutes of administration, with peak effects occurring 60 to 90 minutes later. The hemodynamic benefits of captopril in the dog seem to last for about eight hours after a single dose. Recent studies of humans have indicated that there may be a complex relationship between the short- and long-term effects of captopril, in that some patients who fail to show an initial hemodynamic response to the drug may have gradual improvement with prolonged exposure.[263, 264] The relevance of these findings to veterinary medicine is unknown at this time, but they may suggest that captopril should be continued despite initial lack of efficacy in the hope of obtaining a beneficial late response following prolonged administration. In healthy humans, 70 per cent of an orally administered dose is absorbed, 30 per cent is protein bound, and 35 per cent is eliminated by the kidney as unchanged drug. Renal elimination correlates with creatinine clearance and dosage reduction is required if severe renal dysfunction is present.[250]

Captopril is available in 12.5, 25, 50, and 100 mg tablets. The initial dosage in the dog is usually 0.10 to 0.22 mg/lb (0.25 to 0.5 mg/kg) q8h; this dosage may be titrated upward based on clinical response. (Editor's Note: Frequent toxic reactions often necessitate reduction of dosage rates to once or twice daily.)

Toxicity and Drug Interactions. As with the other vasodilators, hypotension is a potential complication of captopril therapy, and low initial doses with gradual dose titration are recommended to minimize this problem. Gastrointestinal disturbances, including anorexia, vomition, and diarrhea (sometimes severe and bloody), are the most frequently observed side effects of captopril therapy in the dog. These signs are at best difficult to distinguish from those of digitalis toxicity (if the drugs are being used concurrently) and can pose a diagnostic dilemma if digitalis serum levels are not readily available. In the authors' experience, discontinuation of captopril therapy has usually resulted in prompt resolution of GI disturbances, and therapy can often be resumed at reduced dosages.

Hyperkalemia may occur, especially if captopril is used concomitantly with potassium-sparing diuretics or potassium supplements.[255] Captopril therapy in human patients has also been reported to cause skin rashes, neutropenia, and a stable elevation of BUN and creatinine in some patients.[258] Renal insufficiency has been observed in veterinary patients receiving captopril and is the most serious reported side effect of captopril in the dog, apparently occurring infrequently and at dosages greater than 1 mg/lb (2 mg/kg) administered 3 times per day.[172] In humans, a recent investigation of renal insufficiency during long-term captopril and enalapril therapy for severe heart failure concluded that the deterioration of renal function after converting enzyme inhibition was not a toxic or immunologic reaction, but rather a hemodynamic consequence of therapy that could be remedied by sodium repletion.[265] Elucidation of the mechanism of renal dysfunction accompanying converting enzyme inhibition in dogs will require further study; however, based on human studies and empirical observations, some practical recommendations can be made.

In general, captopril dosage should not exceed 1 mg/lb (2 mg/kg) administered 3 times daily, and the drug should be used cautiously (with frequent monitoring of serum urea nitrogen and creatinine levels) in patients with demonstrated renal dysfunction. Diuretic dosages (especially furosemide) should be adjusted to the lowest levels compatible with patient comfort to avoid sodium depletion. The clinically useful dosage of captopril in the cat has been reported to range from 0.5 to 1 mg/lb (1 to 2 mg/kg) administered 3 times daily.[103] The combination of captopril and hydralazine was reported to dramatically improve cardiac output in a small group of human heart failure patients, but controlled studies in veterinary patients on the efficacy of captopril alone and in combination with other vasodilators are needed to test the applicability of these findings to clinical veterinary situations.[266]

ENALAPRIL

Actions. Enalapril is the other angiotensin-converting enzyme inhibitor currently available in the United States, and most of its actions appear to be qualitatively similar to captopril. The major advantage of enalapril in humans is its longer pharmacodynamic half-life, enabling more convenient once a day to twice daily administration.[256] Enalapril is a prodrug, requiring de-esterification in the liver to its active form, enalaprilate. This conversion may be delayed in human patients with compromised hepatic function.[268] Enalaprilate is eliminated primarily via renal mechanisms.

Recent placebo-controlled studies using enalapril in humans with heart failure have demonstrated improved oxygen uptake, hemodynamic parameters, and exercise tolerance both initially and after 12 weeks of therapy.[269] Clinical investigations in veterinary patients are needed before specific recommendations can be made regarding the usefulness of enalapril in veterinary medicine.

β-ADRENERGIC RECEPTOR BLOCKERS

GENERAL PROPERTIES

Sympathetic stimulation of cardiac (primarily β-1) β-adrenergic receptors increases the heart rate, the force of cardiac contraction, and myocardial oxygen consumption. In the peripheral circulation, β receptor stimulation (primarily β-2) results in vasodilation. Nonselective β receptor blockade, then, is generally associated with reductions of heart rate and contractility, slowing of electrical conduction, reduced myocardial oxygen consumption, and increased peripheral vascular resistance.

These effects may be desirable in the management of heart diseases characterized by concentric hypertrophy, as well as in the treatment of cardiac arrhythmias. In patients with pathologic hypertrophy (e.g., hypertrophic cardiomyopathy, semilunar valve stenosis, and tetralogy of Fallot), significant reductions in cardiac output can occur during periods of excitement, stress, exercise, or administration of positive inotropic drugs, as a result of tachycardia and ventricular outflow obstruction by a hyperdynamic or hypertrophied interventricular septum. Clinical signs precipitated by these events can often be mitigated by judicious β blockade. In cats with hypertrophic cardiomyopathy, for example, elevated end-diastolic left ventricular pressures and decreased ventricular compliance are exacerbated by β receptor stimulation (isoproterenol infusion), and this exacerbation can be prevented with β blockade.[101] The effectiveness of β blockade in treating diseases complicated or caused by myocardial hypertrophy depends on the contribution of sympathetic tone to the disease process. Blocking the effects of catecholamine release during periods of stress may decrease myocardial oxygen consumption and prevent tachyarrhythmias and increases in left ventricular end-diastolic pressure, thus helping to prevent the development of heart failure.[270] β blockade usually improves myocardial perfusion, but results in either no change or a decrease in cardiac output.[271] Drugs with β-2 blocking activity generally increase peripheral vascular resistance by blocking β-2–mediated vasodilation, but they may also antagonize the sympathetically mediated release of renin, potentially causing a decrease in peripheral vascular tone as well as a reduction in sodium and water retention.[272]

The primary use of β-adrenergic blocking drugs in veterinary medicine has been for their antiarrhythmic effects, often as a means of further slowing the ventricular response to atrial fibrillation when digitalis alone is inadequate. β blockade in the setting of heart failure requires caution, since the failing ventricle may be dependent on adrenergic tone to maintain systolic ventricular function, and the β blockers all have negative inotropic effects. While the management of chronic atrial fibrillation remains the primary indication for the use of β blockers in heart failure in veterinary patients, recent research has stimulated interest in other potential benefits of β blockade.

Endogenous catecholamine levels have been shown to be elevated in human patients with chronic heart failure, and elevated levels of plasma norepinephrine have been associated with a poor prognosis in human patients with heart failure.[273, 274] β blockers are known to improve human survival rates after myocardial infarction, and these drugs have also been shown to prevent the development or progression of some models of dilated cardiomyopathy in experimental animal models of the disease.[275, 276] Catecholamine-induced calcium-mediated mitochondrial and other subcellular damage has been implicated in the progression of many kinds of myocardial degeneration.[277] These studies and a large body of related research provides support for the idea that β blockade may be of benefit to patients in heart failure from a variety of causes and points out the need for controlled prospective veterinary studies to determine whether β blockade will prolong survival in heart failure patients, as well as whether plasma catecholamine levels might be of value in selecting patients that might benefit from β blockade.

PROPRANOLOL

Indications and Current Use. Propranolol is the prototype nonselective β blocker, most commonly used in the therapy of heart failure to slow the ventricular response to atrial fibrillation. Most patients are initially digitalized and receive propranolol only if the ventricular rate is not adequately reduced (80 to 130 beats per minute at the authors' clinic) by digoxin alone. Care must be exercised in patients with myocardial failure since the negative inotropic effects of β blockade can exacerbate signs of heart failure.

Propranolol is supplied in 10, 20, 40, and 80 mg tablets for oral use and in 1 mg/ml ampules for intravenous use. Oral bioavailability is low as a result of extensive first-pass hepatic metabolism. Chronic oral therapy increases bioavailability, presumably due to saturation of hepatic enzyme systems or reduction of hepatic blood flow. Although the plasma half-life of propranolol is only 1.5 hr in the dog, the pharmacodynamic effects of propranolol appear to last much longer.[278] This phenomenon is attributed to the presence of active metabolites, and oral dosing every eight hours is generally adequate to control the heart rate in both dogs and cats. Because the effects of propranolol depend on the baseline level of sympathetic tone, no universal dosage recommendations can be made.

Initial doses of propranolol should be low to avoid excessive depression of contractility and vaso- or bronchoconstriction; the dose is then gradually increased as dictated by the response to therapy. In the dog, propranolol is usually started at an oral dosage of 0.05 to 0.1 mg/lb (0.1 to 0.2 mg/kg) q8h, or about 10 mg q8h in a large breed dog. This dose is gradually increased over several days until the desired heart rate response is attained. Cats with hypertrophic cardiomyopathy but without overt signs of pulmonary edema or acute thromboembolism are generally started on one-quarter of a 10 mg tablet q8h, to be increased over a period of weeks up to a maximum dose of 10 mg q8h, if required, to control the heart rate and development of clinical signs with excitement or stress. The intravenous dose is much lower in both species, 0.01 mg/lb (0.02 mg/kg) as a slow bolus with increases up to 0.5 mg/lb (0.1 mg/kg) to reach the desired therapeutic effect. Intravenous propranolol is rarely indicated in the therapy of heart failure. (See Chapter 76 for further discussion of the antiarrhythmic indications and use of propranolol.)

Toxicity and Drug Interactions. Toxic effects of propranolol are almost always related to excessive β blockade. Propranolol should not be used in animals with asthma, bradycardia or heart block, or in patients with overt heart failure and poor myocardial function. Other potential side effects include gastrointestinal upsets, weakness, visual disturbances, and thrombocytopenia.[101] β blockers may reduce the sympathetic compensation for hypoglycemia and may necessitate changes in insulin dosage in the diabetic patient to prevent hypoglycemia. Propranolol significantly prolongs the half-life of lidocaine due to reductions in hepatic blood flow, and may thereby predispose to lidocaine toxicity if the two drugs are used together. Sudden withdrawal of β blocking drugs can cause enhanced sensitivity to β agonists, and may result in tachyarrhythmias and/or hypertension. β receptor blockers should therefore be tapered over several days if therapy is to be discontinued.

OTHER β BLOCKING DRUGS

Several newer β blocking drugs have received some attention for their potential use in veterinary patients. These drugs differ from propranolol in that they offer one or more novel properties that may confer an advantage in the setting of heart failure. These properties include intrinsic sympathomimetic activity, relative β-1 receptor specificity, and lipophilicity. Pindolol is a nonspecific β blocker that has significant intrinsic sympathomimetic activity, which means that it is capable of both stimulating and blocking β receptors, theoretically reducing the side effects of bronchoconstriction, increased peripheral vascular resistance, cardiac failure, depressed atrioventricular conduction, and bradycardia. Pindolol and other β blockers with intrinsic sympathomimetic activity may prove to be useful in the therapy of heart failure to prevent excessive β blockade.[279, 280] When the body has low sympathetic tone, these drugs exert mild positive inotropic effects, and when sympathetic tone is high, they act as β blockers.

β-1 receptor specificity, or so-called cardioselectivity, is also an important factor in analyzing the newer β blockers. Both atenolol and metoprolol exhibit β-1 receptor specificity at least at low dosages, and therefore minimize bronchoconstriction and possibly changes in peripheral vascular resistance. Lipophilicity is another consideration in choosing a β blocker, since lipophilic drugs cross biological membranes more easily than hydrophilic ones, and are subject to renal tubular resorption, thus requiring metabolism (usually by the liver) before elimination can occur. Propranolol is highly lipophilic, and is subject to extensive hepatic metabolism and a first pass effect that limits the oral bioavailability (2 to 17 per cent). Atenolol and nadolol have low lipophilicity and good bioavailability and are eliminated primarily by renal mechanisms. Lipophilicity may play an important role in the decision of which β blocking drug to use in an animal with compromised hepatic or renal function.

Atenolol is a hydrophilic, relatively specific β-1 blocker with a long pharmacodynamic half-life that allows twice daily dosing in the dog. The authors have successfully used atenolol as an adjunct to digitalization in controlling the ventricular response to atrial fibrillation in large breed dogs. Empirically, an initial oral dose of 12.5 mg (one-quarter of a 50 mg tablet) administered twice daily to dogs larger than 50 pounds has been a satisfactory starting point, although an occasional patient cannot tolerate this dosage because of increased lethargy and depression. Further studies on the pharmacodynamic properties of the new β-adrenergic blocking drugs are required before concrete recommendations can be made.

CALCIUM ANTAGONISTS

Calcium antagonists have a wide spectrum of therapeutic indications in human medicine, including some suggested uses in the therapy of heart failure. Three of these drugs, verapamil, diltiazem, and nifedipine, are approved for use in the United States. Although chemically diverse, these drugs share the ability to impede the flow of calcium entering cells. Differences in their chemical structures, mechanisms of action, and reflex changes induced by their actions account for their differing effects. While all are potent coronary arterial dilators, verapamil is a potent negative inotrope, useful as a supraventricular antiarrhythmic because of its effect of slowing conduction in the AV node. Nifedipine has insignificant negative inotropic and antiarrhythmic properties in the intact animal but is a potent arterial vasodilator, and diltiazem is intermediate in antiarrhythmic, inotropic, and vasodilating effects. Interest in these drugs in veterinary medicine centers on their antiarrhythmic properties (see Chapter 76), as well as their potential use in the therapy of heart failure.

There is evidence that myocardial damage from calcium overload occurs in human as well as animal models of cardiomyopathy, and abnormalities in diastolic function that accompany hypertrophic cardiomyopathy may be related to excess calcium.[277] Additionally, calcium antagonists have been shown to prevent or arrest the development of certain animal models of cardiomyopathy.[276, 281] The molecular pathogenesis of mitochondrial and myocyte calcium overload is currently unknown and may, in fact, result from a variety of insults. Experimental catecholamine-induced, calcium-mediated damage to the myocardium can also be prevented with calcium channel blocking drugs.[277]

Reports in the human medical literature have suggested the use of verapamil in treating hypertrophic obstructive cardiomyopathy in cases where propranolol is contraindicated.[282, 283] Although similarities exist between human and feline patients with hypertrophic cardiomyopathy, and some authors have suggested that calcium antagonists may be valuable in the therapy of hypertrophic cardiomyopathy in cats, clinical, hemodynamic and pharmacodynamic studies need to be performed before these drugs can be routinely recommended.[284, 284a]

One uncontrolled case study reports the use of verapamil in the conversion of atrial fibrillation to sinus rhythm in dogs.[285] While both verapamil and diltiazem may prove useful in the therapy of atrial fibrillation and other supraventricular arrhythmias, their potentially potent negative inotropic effects in the setting of heart failure dictate the need for extreme caution.[286–288] The calcium antagonists (especially verapamil) cannot be recommended at this time for the treatment of animals in heart failure except under investigational circumstances.

DIETARY MANAGEMENT OF HEART FAILURE

GENERAL CONSIDERATIONS

Dietary management of the patient with heart failure is an important component of successful medical therapy. Anorexia, weight loss, and eventual cachexia are an all too common and disheartening set of complications that accompany heart failure and its drug therapy. The dietary management of the heart failure patient may vary with the patient's original condition and diagnosis. However, two broad objectives are constant: sodium restriction, as an adjunct to regulating preload, and prevention, or reversal if possible, of the general debilitation and weight loss (cardiac cachexia) that attends nearly all cases of chronic heart failure in dogs and many cases in cats.

SODIUM RESTRICTION

Dogs with heart disease have a reduced capacity to excrete sodium loads, a finding that is exaggerated in the presence of clinical signs of congestive heart failure.[289–291] Such experimental findings form the basis for dietary sodium restriction in the management of heart failure, as decreased sodium intake translates into decreased sodium (and consequently fluid) retention. Dietary sodium restriction, along with diuretics and venodilators, is a method of preload restriction.

Like diuretics or venodilators, the level of sodium restriction can be titrated to fit the clinical needs of the patient. Mild, moderate, and severe sodium restriction have been defined by the American Heart Association as 15 mg/lb (30 mg/kg), 6 mg/lb (13 mg/kg), and 3 mg/lb (7 mg/kg) body weight per day, respectively.[292] Although these levels of sodium intake are much lower than the National Research Council's recommended minimum daily intake of sodium for dogs (45 mg/lb/day or 95 mg/kg/day), dogs have been found to be efficient sodium conservers, resulting in these lower recommended dietary levels.[292, 293] A general recommendation for total daily dietary intake of sodium in dogs with heart failure is less than 6.5 mg/lb/day (15 mg/kg/day).[59]

Commercial low-sodium diets are widely available and provide sodium restriction adequate for the management of most cases of heart failure.[294] Unfortunately, whether due to sodium restriction or simply dietary change, some animals find these diets unpalatable. Although reports of feeding studies indicate that more than 95 per cent of dogs accept a severely sodium restricted diet in a hospital environment if fed nothing else for three days, sodium restriction is usually more "painlessly" accomplished by the gradual introduction of the new diet.[295] Minor modifications such as warming, frying, sprinkling with a salt substitute or garlic powder (not garlic salt), or mixing with other low-sodium foods may improve patient acceptance, and a positive attitude on the part of the veterinarian also seems helpful.

Owners must learn to avoid salty treats and realize that even small, seemingly insignificant morsels may contain a large amount of sodium in relation to the size of their pet. Processed meats and foods are usually high in sodium and should be avoided unless they are specifically labeled as "low sodium" and the amount of sodium in each serving is known. Prepared snacks (both human and animal) are notoriously high in sodium, and potato chips, pretzels, and almost anything pre-prepared at fast-food restaurants should be avoided. Even the sodium content of the water in some geographic locations cannot be ignored, and distilled water should be used if the water supply contains more than about 150 ppm sodium.

Effective dietary restriction of sodium can potentially reduce the need for diuretics and/or venodilators in controlling signs of fluid accumulation. Recommendations have been made that dietary sodium restriction should begin as soon as the diagnosis of heart disease is established (e.g., cardiac murmur auscultated) and before clinical signs of heart failure are evident.[295] While this recommendation is theoretically attractive, the long lag time between the discovery of cardiac pathology and the onset of heart failure in many dogs brings the potential clinical significance of this intervention into question, and controlled clinical studies are needed to definitively answer the question of the optimal time to begin dietary sodium restriction. More detailed information regarding the sodium content of popular pet foods and human foods, as well as recipes for appropriate home-made low-sodium diets, can be found elsewhere.[296]

CARDIAC CACHEXIA

Cardiac cachexia is the term used to describe the dramatic weight loss, especially the loss of muscle mass, that accompanies cardiac failure. This finding is so consistent in the dog that in the authors' clinical experience, the presence of obesity should cause the clinician to seriously question the validity of the diagnosis of heart failure as a cause of respiratory signs. While the pathogenesis of this phenomenon is not completely understood, application of basic nutritional and metabolic principles to the management of heart failure has allowed some progress to be made in both the current understanding and the management of this condition.

Anorexia appears to be a major contributor to the pathogenesis of cardiac cachexia. Anorexia in heart failure has been related to a number of factors, including the activation of neurohumoral and endocrine compensatory mechanisms, a generalized feeling of malaise and lethargy that accompanies reduced cardiac output, and drug-induced effects on the central nervous system (chemoreceptor trigger zone) or other organ systems that may combine to produce nausea.[297] The loss of appetite may be compounded by dietary alterations, exercise restriction, and emotional reactions to a worried owner or the hospital environment. Despite enforced rest, the muscles of respiration as well as the myocardium often have increased metabolic needs and energy requirements that can contribute to catabolism and weight loss at a time when reduced cardiac output fails to deliver nutrients to and remove wastes from the cells. Elevated plasma catecholamine levels may also contribute to the increased metabolic demands of heart failure.

Serum levels of albumin, hemoglobin, folate, thiamine, potassium, calcium, magnesium, and iron are often decreased, and increased fecal fat, nitrogen, and energy excretion related to malabsorption have been reported.[298] In humans, cachexic heart failure patients have been shown to have a higher incidence of postoperative complications and death, and nutritional support prior to surgery improves not only survival rates but also indices of immune function.[299]

In light of these findings, it is clear that nutritional support of the cardiac patient is important. One important factor that the authors have found frequently overlooked in the hospital environment is some assurance that the normal calorie requirement of the patient is being met, assuming the patient will eat what is offered. This is especially important in giant breed dogs, who may lose weight in the hospital simply because they are not being fed adequate quantities of food. In general, a high quality commercial or home-made diet for dogs in heart failure should include 14 to 18 per cent of the dry matter as high quality protein in the dog, and higher levels in the cat (40 per cent).[295]

ANCILLARY THERAPY

MORPHINE

Morphine is useful in the treatment of acute cardiogenic pulmonary edema. Morphine has potent analgesic and anti-anxiety effects that help calm distressed and dyspneic animals, promoting deeper and slower respirations via mild depression of the respiratory centers.[139] Morphine reduces the heart rate and has venodilator properties that help to reduce preload.

Morphine is not generally used in cats because of the possibility of "morphine rage," an aggressive, agitated state sometimes produced by the drug. The recommended dosage of morphine in dogs is 0.05 to 0.10 mg/lb (0.1 to 0.25 mg/kg) subcutaneously, repeated as necessary to achieve the desired effect.[300] Small doses of morphine (0.02 to 0.4 mg/lb or 0.05 to 0.1 mg/kg) can be slowly administered intravenously at five-minute intervals if required, but rapid IV injection often causes severe agitation and vocalization and therefore is best avoided.

Overdosing may result in marked centrally mediated respiratory depression. Emesis and/or defecation shortly after injection are relatively common undesirable side effects.

REST AND STRESS MANAGEMENT

Animals with acute heart failure or an exacerbation of chronic heart failure should have cage rest or its equivalent at home until the signs of failure have improved. Strict rest is used to reduce the animal's oxygen and energy requirements and thus the strain on an already overtaxed, diseased heart. Cage rest has been demonstrated to improve survival in at least one clinical veterinary investigation, in which dogs with heart failure secondary to heartworm disease were shown to be significantly more likely to survive if they were cage rested before and after adulticide therapy.[301] In some heart failure patients (especially cats), the need for stress reduction may be incompatible with frequent office checks or hospitalization except in a dire emergency. These patients should be managed as much as possible at home and handled as little and as gently as possible if hospitalized. Subcutaneous injection of low dosages of morphine is extremely useful in managing anxiety related to acute pulmonary edema in dogs, and supplemental oxygen may be of benefit in both dogs and cats.

Patients with acute cardiogenic pulmonary edema should be considered extremely fragile and both stress and exercise kept to an absolute minimum. This rule translates into such patients being transported on a cart or carried, as necessary. In heart failure, essentially no effective cardiac reserves remain to handle the demand for increased cardiac output imposed by exercise, hence signs of heart failure often worsen dramatically (and sometimes with catastrophic results) if stress and excessive movement are not avoided.

Long-term therapeutic goals of increased exercise tolerance should never be confused with the rest and exercise restriction essential to survival in animals with acute heart failure. In the majority of cases, permanent, moderate-to-severe exercise restriction will be necessary (if not self-imposed by the animal) for animals with heart disease severe enough to cause signs of failure. Careful client education is needed to ensure that the owner is aware of the potential damage that excess exercise can do, and that the athletic expectations of the owner for their pet are realistic. Patient explanation of these facts can prevent some stress-induced exacerbations of heart failure and avoid disappointment and discouragement with therapy.

OXYGEN THERAPY

Oxygen therapy can be lifesaving in the patient with acute, severe pulmonary edema. Forty to 50 per cent oxygen should be administered in a temperature controlled, humidified environment, with minimal stress or discomfort for the patient. Nebulization through 20 per cent ethanol may reduce airway foaming.[139] Masks and other temporary devices are generally not recommended for use in heart failure patients.

BRONCHODILATORS

The use of bronchodilators, specifically the methylxanthine derivative theophylline (or one of its salts, e.g., aminophylline) has been advocated for the management of coughing or dyspnea associated with cardiogenic pulmonary edema.[302, 303] These drugs may be useful (though not essential) adjuncts in the acute management of pulmonary edema, as well as in the chronic therapy of patients that suffer from chronic bronchial diseases concurrently with heart disease.

Theophylline and theophylline salts are available in a variety of formulations from many sources, but all should be dosed based on the theophylline content. Based on pharmacokinetic data in dogs and cats, the dosage of theophylline in dogs should be 4 mg/lb (9 mg/kg) three to four times daily, and cats should receive 2 mg/lb (4 mg/kg) two to three times daily.[304, 305] Dosages for aminophylline should be 10 to 20 per cent higher. The usual route of administration is oral, as these drugs are rapidly and completely absorbed. However, slow IV injection is also possible in emergency situations where oral administration is not possible. Chronic bronchodilator therapy is not routinely employed by the authors in the management of heart failure uncomplicated by significant primary bronchial pathology.

A more detailed review of bronchodilator therapy is available for readers seeking specific information regarding the use of these drugs in settings other than heart failure (Chapters 18, 68, and 69).

THORACOCENTESIS AND ABDOMINOCENTESIS

Thoracocentesis (and more rarely abdominocentesis) can be a lifesaving procedure for the cardiac patient with severe pleural or peritoneal effusion. Both procedures should be performed aseptically following surgical skin preparation whenever possible. The effusions should be evaluated cytologically and biochemically, and bacterial culture performed if indicated.

The clinician should attempt to remove as much intrathoracic fluid as possible to correct the reduced lung volume associated with atelectasis. The physical removal of ascitic fluid is less commonly required, and only enough should be removed to facilitate more normal respiratory movements by relieving pressure on the diaphragm. Repeated fluid removal from the abdomen or thorax can lead to significant loss of total body protein and subsequent hypoproteinemia, predisposing to further fluid transudation. For this reason, mobilization of fluid through the use of diuretics, dietary sodium restriction, and vasodilators is preferred to centesis as a method of controlling fluid accumulations if they do not represent an immediately life-threatening problem. In all cases, however, diagnostic centesis to provide a small fluid sample for cytologic examination is indicated for any new effusion.

Thoracocentesis in cats with dilated cardiomyopathy may reveal the presence of a chylous effusion.[306] These cats may present a diagnostic challenge, and the presence of dilated cardiomyopathy as the underlying cause of effusion should be echocardiographically or angiographically confirmed. Therapy for dilated cardiomyopathy is then administered and the effusion reevaluated as needed, depending on the clinical progress of the patient.

FLUID THERAPY

Parenteral administration of fluids (either subcutaneously or intravenously) may be needed in managing animals in heart failure, especially if they are anorexic. Aggressive use of diuretics may also precipitate a need for fluid therapy. The clinician must objectively assess the need for and efficacy of fluid therapy, monitoring body weight, radiographic changes, serum creatinine, electrolytes, hematocrit, and plasma protein. In addition, the respiratory rate, pattern, and sounds, as well as the mucous membrane color and capillary refill time, may provide useful clinical information to guide fluid therapy. Central hemodynamic monitoring (central venous pressure, pulmonary capillary wedge pressure, arterial blood pressure, and cardiac output) is extremely useful in adjusting the fluid dosage to optimize the preload under emergency, life-threatening circumstances.

As a general recommendation, the authors prefer low-sodium solutions, and 0.45 per cent sodium chloride with 2.5 per cent dextrose appropriately supplemented with potassium chloride is often used. Both the type of fluid and the dosage must be tailored to individual needs, but conservative therapy, usually at maintenance levels or slightly below, is usually indicated.[307]

COUGH SUPPRESSANTS

Occasional patients (usually miniature or toy dogs) with a combination of chronic bronchial disease and heart disease (often mitral insufficiency with subsequent bronchial compression secondary to left atrial enlargement) require antitussives to quiet a persistent nonproductive cough. Hydrocodenone or butorphenol are the most commonly employed narcotic cough suppressants, although nonprescription strength cough syrup is effective in some animals. The dosage and frequency of administration of both hydrocodenone and butorphenol should be individualized in an attempt to control the cough while minimizing sedation.

INTEGRATED THERAPEUTIC STRATEGIES

The previous sections reviewed the actions, indications, and current usage of the therapeutic interventions commonly employed in the management of heart failure in veterinary medicine. Based upon this knowledge, the clinician must decide which drugs to use in a given clinical setting—an often difficult and highly individual decision. Because of the diverse pathophysiologic origins of heart failure, construction of a general algorithm for heart failure therapy is a complex task. The principles of therapy are clear, however, and the clinician should approach the patient by defining the properties of the heart and circulation that are responsible for the syndrome of heart failure in that individual, identifying the cause of these derangements if possible, and either correcting the underlying cause or modifying the properties of the heart and circulation to relieve the clinical signs. A complete data base and a definitive diagnosis are almost always prerequisites for the successful long-term management of heart failure.

For the common acquired heart diseases of dogs and cats (e.g., chronic valvular heart disease and the cardiomyopathies), appropriate therapy depends on the pathophysiology as well as the clinical stage of the disease. General therapeutic guidelines for veterinary patients with heart failure can be adapted to the modified New York Heart Association classification of heart failure discussed previously, and summarized as follows:

Class I—Client education, usually no medical therapy is indicated. Every effort should be made to make a definitive diagnosis and determine (and correct) the underlying cause of disease. Baseline functional data (ECG, chest radiographs, echocardiogram if indicated) should be obtained.

Class II—Specific therapy depends on the nature and pathogenesis of signs. For example, a vasodilator in combination with a diuretic may be used to reduce left atrial size and subsequent bronchus compression causing cough secondary to chronic mitral regurgitation. Often sodium restriction and/or a diuretic are adequate to relieve mild, intermittent signs due to fluid retention. Antiarrhythmic therapy is administered as indicated.

Class III—Conventional therapy (see below) is often indicated, usually accompanied by an appropriate vasodilator. Inotropic support (digitalis or other positive inotrope) is indicated for patients with myocardial failure (e.g., dilated cardiomyopathy), but probably not for others.

Class IV—Emergency measures, including strict cage rest, supplemental oxygen, morphine, vasodilators, intravenous positive inotropes, bronchodilators, and antifoaming agents are employed as needed in addition to conventional therapy. In some patients (especially cats and small dogs), acquisition of a complete data base (radiographs, and so on) must be delayed because of their fragile condition and susceptibility to stress. In these cases, emergency therapy must be based on a presumptive diagnosis obtained from the signalment, history, and physical examination.

Conventional medical therapy of heart failure consisted for many years of digitalis, diuretics, low-salt diet, rest, and antiarrhythmic drugs when indicated. In fact, with a few exceptions, current therapeutic recommendations for advanced heart failure usually encompass these conventional treatments, although as previously discussed, controversy surrounds the use of digitalis in some circumstances. Although guidelines for therapy based on the clinical stage of the patient with heart failure may be helpful in managing pathophysiologically homogeneous groups of patients, the thoughtful clinician is better served by constructing a treatment regimen based on careful evaluation of the preload, afterload, heart rate, rhythm, and myocardial oxygen demand. Pharmacologic or other therapeutic measures, used only when specifically indicated by meticulous evaluation of the patient's cardiovascular status, minimize the number of therapeutic interventions and reduce not only the complexity of therapy but the potential for drug-related side effects, toxicity, and interactions as well. This essentially "conservative" approach should increase therapeutic efficacy and owner compliance. The need for effective and objective monitoring of the patient's clinical status and response to therapy cannot be overemphasized. In the authors' practice, invasive central hemodynamic monitoring has proven extremely useful in the management of acute life-threatening heart failure, especially in large breed dogs. The use of a percutaneous catheter introduction system allows relatively atraumatic right heart and pulmonary artery catheterization, with subsequent monitoring of pulmonary capillary wedge pressure and cardiac output. When used in conjunction with a continuous ECG and either a peripheral arterial line or a noninvasive arterial blood pressure monitor, the clinician can objectively evaluate hemodynamic correlates of cardiac preload and afterload, as well as the cardiac output, heart rate, and rhythm. While this monitoring system is expensive and requires intensive nursing care, it allows the repeated measurement of essential hemodynamic parameters in response to potent inotropic and/or vasodilating agents (see Figure 73–1). Such monitoring facilitates therapy, allowing for rapid adjustments or changes in the treatment regimen, while providing objective evidence of therapeutic effects.

In circumstances where invasive monitoring is either not indicated (less severe failure) or not feasible because of either technical or financial constraints, effective decisions can be made based on the clinical, radiographic, and laboratory parameters previously noted. In the follow-up management of outpatients with chronic heart failure, appropriate monitoring depends on the therapeutic regimen and disease. Generally, body weight, renal function, electrolyte status, heart rate, rhythm, and serum digoxin concentration (if applicable) are obtained at varying intervals, depending on the diagnosis and volatility of the patient's disease and clinical status.

In nearly all cases of heart disease severe enough to cause clinical signs of heart failure, the long-term prognosis despite extraordinary therapeutic efforts must be guarded. Lack of owner compliance is a common cause of therapeutic failure, and inadequately explained, overly complex, and poorly tolerated or labeled medication regimens are a common cause of owner noncompliance. If the complexity, cost, or time restrictions imposed by a treatment plan engender client confusion, anger, or dissatisfaction despite the clinician's conscientious efforts to explain the drugs and disease, then even the best of plans must be changed. Following the initial hospitalization, the dosages of vasodilators, diuretics, and inotropic agents often require adjustment based on the client's clinical observations at home. The owner must understand at the outset that such adjustments will probably be needed and that they do not necessarily signal therapeutic failure. The owner must also understand, however, that therapeutic failure in most cases is eventually inevitable and that their veterinarian is also available for support and understanding at this time. As with any chronic illness in which significant amounts of time, effort, and money are invested, it is crucial that the veterinarian and client "stay on the same side" in the treatment of the pet and that an adversarial relationship never be allowed to develop.

It is the authors' experience that thorough client education and the availability of high quality, compassionate emergency services (or the primary clinician's home phone number) will serve to avoid most client relations problems regardless of the outcome of therapy. The owner (and the clinician) must be aware of the financial and emotional investment involved in managing a pet in heart failure. The protracted treatment of such a pet can be an exceptionally rewarding experience for both the client and the veterinarian or an exceptionally frustrating one. It requires a large measure of mutual respect, trust, cooperation, and caring if therapy is to succeed.

References

1. Keene, BW, et al.: Carnitine-linked defects of myocardial metabolism in canine dilated cardiomyopathy. ACVIM Research Reports Scientific Session, Proc 4th Ann Vet Med Forum, 2:14, 1986.

1a. Pion, PD, et al.: Myocardial failure in cats associated with low plasma taurine: A reversible cardiomyopathy. Science 237:764, 1987.

2. Sonnenblick, EH and Skelton, CL: Derived indices of ventricular and myocardial function. N Engl J Med 296:978, 1977.

3. Swan, HJC and Ganz W: Hemodynamic measurements in clinical practice: A decade in review. J Am Coll Cardiol 1:103, 1983.

4. Packer, M and LeJemtel, TH: Physiologic and pharmacologic determinants of vasodilator response: A conceptual framework for rational drug therapy for chronic heart failure. Prog Cardiovasc Dis 24:275, 1982.

5. Katz, AM and Bradly, AJ: Mechanical and biochemical correlates of cardiac contraction. Mod Conc Cardiovasc Dis 40:39, 1971.

6. LeJemtel, TH and Sonnenblick, EH: Nondigitalis cardiac inotropic agents. *In* Hurst, JW (ed): The Heart. 6th ed. New York, McGraw-Hill, 1986, p 1652.

7. Myhre, ESP, et al.: The effect of contractility and preload on matching between the canine left ventricle and afterload. Circulation 73:161, 1986.

8. Ross, J, Jr.: Cardiac function and myocardial contractility: A perspective. J Am Coll Cardiol 1:53, 1983.

9. DeMaria, AN, et al.: Effects of nitroglycerin on left ventricular cavitary size and cardiac performance determined by ultrasound in man. Am J Med 57:754, 1974.

10. Firth, BH, et al.: Assessment of vasodilator therapy in patients with severe congestive heart failure: Limitations of measurements of left ventricular ejection fraction and volumes. Am J Cardiol 50:954, 1982.

11. Engler, et al.: Clinical assessment and follow up of functional capacity in patients with chronic congestive cardiomyopathy. Am J Cardiol 49:1832, 1982.

12. Franciosa, JA, et al.: Lack of correlation between exercise capacity and indexes of resting left ventricular performance in heart failure. Am J Cardiol 47:33, 1981.

13. Schlant, RL and Sonnenblick, EH: Normal physiology of the cardiovascular system. *In* Hurst, JW (ed): The Heart. 6th ed. New York, McGraw-Hill, 1986, p 37.

14. Starling, EH: The Linacre Lecture on the Law of the Heart. London, Longmans, Green and Co, 1918.

15. Cohn, JN, et al.: Role of vasoconstrictor mechanisms in the control of left ventricular performance of the normal and damaged heart. Am J Cardiol 44:1019, 1979.

16. Braunwald, E, et al.: Contraction of the normal heart. *In* Braunwald, E (ed): Heart Disease—A Textbook of Cardiovascular Medicine, 2nd ed. Philadelphia, WB Saunders, 1984, p 409.

17. Hamlin, RL, et al.: Noninvasive measurement of systemic arterial pressure in dogs by automatic sphygmomanometry. Am J Vet Res 43:1271, 1982.

18. Wilson, JR, et al.: Experimental congestive heart failure induced by rapid ventricular pacing in the dog: Cardiac effects. Circulation 75:857, 1987.

19. Sarnoff, et al.: Hemodynamic determinants of oxygen consumption of the heart with special reference to the tension-time index. Am J Physiol 192:148, 1958.

20. Sonnenblick, et al.: Velocity of contraction as a determinant of myocardial oxygen consumption. Am J Physiol 209:919, 1965.

21. The Criteria Committee of the New York Heart Association. Diseases of the Heart and Blood Vessels: Nomenclature and Criteria for Diagnosis. 7th ed. Boston, Little, Brown, 286, 1973.

22. Campeau, L: Letter to the editor: Grading of angina effect by the Canadian Cardiovascular Society. Circulation 54:522, 1976.

23. Goldman, L, et al.: Comparative reproducibility and validity of symptoms for assessing cardiovascular functional class. Advantages of a new specific activity scale. Circulation 64:1227, 1981.

24. Packer, M: How should we judge the efficacy of drug therapy in patients with chronic congestive heart failure? The insights of six blind men. J Am Coll Cardiol 9:433, 1987.

25. Dyke, SH, et al.: Detection of latent function in acutely ischemic myocardium in dogs: comparison of pharmacologic inotropic stimulation and postextrasystolic potentiation (PESP). Circ Res 36:490, 1975.

26. Spann, JF, et al.: Contractile performance of the hypertrophied and chronically failing cat ventricle. Am J Physiol 223:1150, 1972.

27. Katz, AM: A new inotropic drug: Its promise and a caution. N Engl J Med 299:1409, 1978.

28. LeJemetel, TH and Sonnenblick, EH: Should the failing heart be stimulated? N Engl J Med 310:1384, 1984.

29. Liang, C, et al.: Conditioning effects of chronic infusions of dobutamine. Comparison with exercise training. J Clin Invest 64:613, 1979.

30. Unverferth, DV, et al.: Long-term benefit of dobutamine in patients with congestive cardiomyopathy. Am Heart J 100:622, 1980.

31. Unverferth, DV, et al.: The hemodynamic and metabolic advantages gained by a three-day infusion of dobutamine in patients with congestive cardiomyopathy. Am Heart J 105:29, 1983.

32. Mulrow, CD, et al.: Reevaluation of digitalis efficacy. Ann Int Med 101:113, 1984.

33. Fleg, JL, et al.: Is digoxin really important in treatment of compensated heart failure? A placebo-controlled crossover trial in patients with sinus rhythm. Am J Med 73:244, 1982.

34. Lee, D, et al.: Heart failure in outpatients: a randomized trial of digoxin versus placebo. N Engl J Med 306:699, 1982.

35. Taggart, et al.: Digoxin withdrawal after cardiac failure in patients with sinus rhythm. J Cardiovasc Pharmacol 5:229, 1983.

36. Kittleson, MD, et al.: Efficacy of digoxin administration in dogs with idiopathic congestive cardiomyopathy. JAVMA 186:162, 1985.

37. Bright, JM: Controversies in veterinary medicine: Is the long-term use of digitalis for treatment of low output failure unwarranted? JAAHA 19:233, 1983.

38. Baim DS, et al.: Survival of patients with severe congestive heart failure with oral milrinone. J Am Col Cardiol 7:661, 1986.

39. Packer M, et al.: Hemodynamic and clinical limitations of long-term inotropic therapy with amrinone in patients with severe chronic heart failure. Circulation 70:1038, 1984.

40. Withering, W: An Account of the Foxglove, CGJ and J Robinson, Paternoster-Row, London, 1785.

41. Hoffman, BF and Bigger, JT: Digitalis and allied cardiac glycosides. *In* Gilman AG, Goodman LS (eds): The Pharmacologic Basis for Therapeutics. 7th ed. New York, Macmillan Publishing, 1985, p 716.
42. Hamlin RL, et al.: Effects of digoxin and digitoxin on ventricular function in normal dogs and dogs with heart failure. Am J Vet Res 32:1391, 1971.
43. Matsui, H and Schwartz, A: Mechanism of cardiac glycoside inhibition of the (Na^+-K^+)-dependent ATPase from cardiac tissue. Biochim Biophys Acta 151:655, 1968.
44. Besch, HR, et al.: Correlation between the inotropic action of ouabain and its effects on subcellular enzyme systems from canine myocardium. J Pharmacol Exp Ther 171:1, 1970.
45. Lee, KS and Klaus, W: The subcellular basis for the mechanism of inotropic action of cardiac glycosides. Pharmacol Rev 23:193, 1971.
46. Hougen, TJ, et al.: Effects of inotropic and arrhythmogenic digoxin doses and of digoxin-specific antibody on myocardial monovalent cation transport in the dog. Circ Res 44:23, 1979.
47. Smith, TW: Discussion Paper: Use of antibodies in the study of the mechanism of action of digitalis. Annals NY Acad Sci 242:731, 1974.
48. Cotten, M deV and Stopp, PE: Action of digitalis on the nonfailing heart of the dog. Am J Physiol 192:114, 1958.
49. Smith, TW: The future of inotropic drugs in clinical practice. Eur Heart J 3:149, 1982.
50. Smith, TW and Braunwald, E: The management of heart failure. *In* Braunwald E (ed): Heart Disease: A Textbook of Cardiovascular Medicine. Philadelphia, WB Saunders, 1984, p 503.
51. Kittleson, MD: Drugs used in the management of heart failure. *In* Kirk, RW (ed): Current Veterinary Therapy VIII. Philadelphia, WB Saunders, 1983, p 285.
52. Rosen, MR, et al.: Electrophysiology and pharmacology of cardiac arrhythmias. IV. Cardiac arrhythmias and toxic effects of digitalis. Am Heart J 89:391, 1975.
53. Kim, YI, et al.: Dissociation of the inotropic effect of digitalis from its effect on AV conduction. Am J Cardiol 36:459, 1975.
54. Rosen MR, et al.: Ouabain-induced changes in electrophysiologic properties of neonatal, young, and adult canine cardiac purkinje fibers. J Pharmacol Exp Ther 194:255, 1975.
55. Somberg, JC and Smith, TW: Localization of the neurally mediated arrhythmogenic properties of digitalis. Science 204:321, 1979.
56. Kassebaum, DG: Electrophysiological effects of strophanthin in the heart. J Pharmacol Exp Ther 140:329, 1963.
57. DeRick, A, et al.: Plasma concentrations of digoxin and digitoxin during digitalization of healthy dogs and dogs with cardiac failure. Am J Vet Res 39:811, 1978.
58. Ettinger, S: Therapeutic digitalization of the dog in congestive heart failure. JAVMA 148:525, 1966.
59. Ettinger, S and Suter, PF: Canine Cardiology. Philadelphia, WB Saunders, 1970.
60. Tilley, LP: Essentials of Canine and Feline Cardiology. 2nd ed. Philadelphia, Lea and Febiger, 1985, p 190.
61. Stark, JJ, et al.: Neurally mediated and direct effects of acetylstophanthidin on canine skeletal muscle vascular resistance. Circ Res 30:274, 1972.
62. DeMots, H, et al.: Effects of ouabain on coronary and systemic vascular resistance and myocardial oxygen consumption in patients without heart failure. Am J Cardiol 41:88, 1978.
63. Smith, TW and Haber, E: Medical progress: Digitalis (second of four parts). N Engl J Med 289:1010, 1973.
64. Detweiler, DK and Knight, DH: Congestive heart failure in dogs: Therapeutic concepts. JAVMA 171:106, 1977.
65. Hamlin, RL: New ideas in the management of heart failure in dogs. JAVMA 171:114, 1977.
66. Breznock, EM: Application of canine plasma kinetics of digoxin and digitoxin to therapeutic digitalization in the dog. Am J Vet Res 36:993, 1973.
67. Button, C, et al.: Pharmacokinetics, bioavailability, and dosage regimens of digoxin in dogs. Am J Vet Res 41(8):1230, 1980.
68. Ghirardi, P, et al.: Bioavailability of digoxin in a new soluble pharmaceutical formulation in capsules. J Pharm Sci 66:267, 1977.
69. Gierke, KD, et al.: Digoxin disposition kinetics in dogs before and during azotemia. J Pharmacol Exp Ther 205:459, 1978.
70. Scialli, VT and Tilley, LP: Digitalis. Its clinical indication and practical usage. Burroughs Wellcome Co, Research Triangle Park, NC, 1979, p 1.
71. Doherty, JE and Perkins, WH: Digoxin metabolism in hypo- and hyperthyroidism. Ann Int Med 64:489, 1966.
72. Harris, SG: Digitalis glycosides. *In* Kirk, RW (ed): Current Veterinary Therapy V. Philadelphia, WB Saunders, 1974, p 320.
73. Katzung, BG and Meyers, H: Excretion of radioactive digitoxin by the dog. J Pharmacol Exp Ther 149:257, 1965.
74. Hamlin, RL: Basis for selection of a cardiac glycoside for dogs. Proc First Symp Vet Pharmacol Ther, 1978.
75. Davis, LE: Pharmacodynamics of digitalis, diuretics, and antiarrhythmic drugs. *In* Kirk RW (ed): Current Veterinary Therapy VI. Philadelphia, WB Saunders, 1980, p 352.
76. Okita, GT: Species difference in duration of action of cardiac glycosides. Fed Proc 26:1125, 1967.
77. Fischer, CS, et al.: The tissue distribution and excretion of radioactive digitoxin, studies on normal rats and cats, and rats with dietary-induced myocardial lesions. Circulation 5:496, 1952.
78. White, WS and Gisvold, O: Absorption rate studies of orally administered cardiac glycosides in cats. J Am Pharmacol Assoc Sci Ed 41:42, 1952.
79. Erichsen, DF, et al.: Therapeutic and toxic plasma concentrations of digoxin in the cat. Am J Vet Res 41:2049, 1980.
80. Weidler, DH, et al.: Pharmacokinetics of digoxin in the cat and comparisons with man and dog. Res Commun Chem Pathol Pharmacol 19:57, 1978.
81. Heinz, N and Flasch, H: Comparison of pharmacokinetics of digoxin and dihydrodigoxin in cats in single-dose studies. Naunyn Schmiedebergs Arch Pharmacol 303:181, 1978.
82. Bolton, GR and Powell, W: Plasma kinetics of digoxin in the cat. Am J Vet Res 43:1994, 1982.
83. Kittleson, MD, et al.: Myocardial function in small dogs with chronic mitral regurgitation and severe congestive heart failure. JAVMA 184:455, 1984.
84. Hamlin, RL, et al.: Treatment of heart failure in dogs without use of digitalis glycosides. VM/SAC 68:349, 1973.
85. Patterson, et al.: Veterinary Letterhead—On digitalis glycosides in treatment of heart failure: Criticism and reply. VM/SAC 68:708, 1973.
86. Prassad, K, et al.: Effects of chronic digoxin treatment on cardiac function, electrolytes, and sarcolemmal ATPase in the canine failing heart due to chronic mitral regurgitation. Am Heart J 108:1487, 1984.
87. Berman, W, et al.: Effects of digoxin in infants with a congested circulatory state due to a ventricular septal defect. N Engl J Med 308:363, 1983.
88. Aubier, M, et al.: Effects of digoxin on diaphragmatic strength generation in patients with chronic obstructive pulmonary disease during acute respiratory failure. Ann Rev Resour Dusm 135:544, 1987.
89. Hamlin, R and Smith, C: Placebo effects in veterinary medicine. Fed Proc 24:329, 1965.
90. Captopril Multicenter Research Group: A placebo-controlled trial of captopril in refractory chronic congestive heart failure. J Am Coll Cardiol 2:755, 1983.
91. Leier, CV, et al.: Chronic indoramin therapy in congestive heart failure: a double-blind, randomized, parallel placebo-controlled trial. J Am Coll Cardiol 9:426, 1987.
92. Gheorghiade, M and Beller, GA: Effects of discontinuing maintenance digoxin therapy in patients with ischemic heart disease and congestive heart failure in sinus rhythm. Am J Cardiol 51(8):1243, 1983.
93. Cohn, et al.: Variability of hemodynamic responses to acute digitalization in chronic cardiac failure due to cardiomyopathy and coronary artery disease. Am J Cardiol 35:461, 1975.
94. Lown, B, et al.: Effect of a digitalis drug on ventricular premature beats. N Engl J Med 67:1084, 1977.
95. Pedersoli, WM: Serum digoxin concentrations in healthy dogs treated without a loading dose. J Vet Pharmacol Ther 1:229, 1978.
96. Hamlin, RL and Hobson, JL: Digoxin in dogs: Once a day or twice a day? JAVMA 184:953, 1984.
97. Button, C, et al.: Application of individualized digoxin dosage regimens to canine therapeutic digitalization. Am J Vet Res 41(8):1238, 1980.

98. Darke, PG: Myocardial disease in small animals. Br Vet J 141:342, 1985.
99. Teske, RH, et al.: Subacute digoxin toxicosis in the beagle dog. Toxicol Appl Pharmacol 35:283, 1976.
100. Bonagura, JD: The clinical pharmacology of the cardiovascular drugs. Small Animal Medicine Veterinary Update Series, 1980.
101. Tilley, LP and Weitz, J: Pharmacologic and other forms of medical therapy in feline cardiac disease. Vet Clin North Am 7:415, 1977.
102. Harris, SG and Ogburn, PN: The cardiovascular system. *In* Catcott EJ (ed): Feline Medicine and Surgery, 2nd ed. Santa Barbara, American Veterinary Publications, 1975.
103. Bond, BR and Fox, PR: Advances in feline cardiomyopathy. Vet Clin North Am 14:1021, 1984.
104. Beller, GA, et al.: Digitalis intoxication—A prospective clinical study. N Engl J Med 284:989, 1971.
105. Sodeman, WA: Diagnosis and treatment of digitalis toxicity. N Engl J Med 273:35, 1965.
106. Hahn, AW: Digitalis glycosides in canine medicine. *In* Kirk, RW (ed): Current Veterinary Therapy VI. Philadelphia, WB Saunders, 1977, p 329.
107. Marcus, FI, et al.: Digitalis and sympathomimetic stimulants. *In* Opie, LH (ed): Drugs for the Heart, 1st ed. Orlando, Grune and Stratton, 1984, p 99.
108. Shapiro, W: Correlative studies of serum digitalis levels and the arrhythmias of digitalis intoxication. Am J Cardiol 41:852, 1978.
109. Gold, H and Edwards, DJ: The effects of ouabain on the heart in the presence of hypercalcemia. Am Heart J 3:45, 1927.
110. Warner, NJ, et al.: Tissue digoxin concentrations during the quinidine-digoxin interaction. Am J Cardiol 51:1717, 1983.
111. Bigger, JT: The quinidine-digoxin interaction: what do we know about it? N Engl J Med 301:779, 1981.
112. Goldman, S, et al.: Effect of the ouabain-quinidine interaction on left ventricular and left atrial function in conscious dogs. Circulation 67:1054, 1983.
113. Peters, DN, et al.: Absence of pharmacokinetic interaction between digitoxin and quinidine in the dog. J Vet Pharmacol Ther 4:271, 1981.
114. Schwartz, JB, et al.: Acute and chronic pharmacodynamic interaction of verapamil and digoxin in atrial fibrillation. Circulation 65:1163, 1982.
115. Fenster, PE and Whute, NW, Jr.: Pharmacokinetic evaluation of the digoxin-amiodarone interaction. J Am Coll Cardiol 5:108, 1985.
116. Cleland, JGF, et al.: The effects of captopril on serum digoxin and urinary urea and digoxin clearances in patients with congestive heart failure. Am Heart J 112:130, 1986.
117. Galimarini, D, et al.: Effect of alkalosis on ouabain toxicity in the dog. J Pharmacol Exp Ther 186:199, 1973.
118. Breznock, EM: Effects of phenobarbital on digitoxin and digoxin elimination in the dog. Am J Vet Res 36:371, 1975.
119. Pedersoli, WM, et al.: Serum digoxin concentrations in dogs before, during, and after concomitant treatment with phenobarbital. Am J Vet Res 41(10):1639, 1980.
120. Pedersoli, WM, et al.: Serum digoxin concentrations in healthy dogs before, during, and after concomitant treatment with furosemide, hydrochlorthiazide, and phenytoin. JAAHA 19:1031, 1983.
121. Snyder, PS, et al.: The effects of aspirin, furosemide, and commercial low salt diet on digoxin kinetics in normal cats. ACVIM Research Reports Scientific Session, Proc 5th Ann Vet Med Forum. 1987, in press.
122. Wilkerson, RH and Mockridge, PB: Effect of selected drugs on serum digoxin concentration in the dog. Am J Cardiol 45:1201, 1980.
123. Caldwell, JH, et al.: Interruption of the enterohepatic circulation of digitoxin by cholestyramine II. Effect of metabolic disposition of tritrium-labeled digitoxin and cardiac systolic time intervals in man. J Clin Invest 50:2638, 1971.
124. Bazzano, G and Bazzano, GS: Digitalis intoxication treatment with a new steroid-binding resin. JAMA 220:824, 1972.
125. Butler, VP, et al.: Effects of sheep digoxin-specific antibodies and their Fab fragments on digoxin pharmacokinetics in dogs. J Clin Invest 59:345, 1977.
126. Hess, T, et al.: Suicidal digoxin poisoning: Conventional treatment and antibody therapy. Klin Wochenschr 60:401, 1982.
127. Lloyd, BL and Smith, TW: Contrasting rates of reversal of digoxin toxicity by digoxin-specific IgG and Fab fragments. Circulation 58:280, 1978.
128. Ochs, HR, et al.: Reversal of inotropic effects of digoxin by specific antibodies and their Fab fragments in the conscious dog. J Pharmacol Exp Ther 207:64, 1978.
129. Schmidt, DH and Butler, VP: Reversal of digoxin toxicity with specific antibodies. J Clin Invest 50:1738, 1971.
130. Smith, TW, et al.: Cardiac glycoside-specific antibodies in the treatment of digitalis intoxication. *In* Haber and Krause (eds): Antibodies in Human Diagnosis and Therapy. New York, Raven Press, 1977.
131. Weiner, N: Norepinephrine, epinephrine, and the sypathomimetic amines. *In* Gilman AG and Goodman LS (eds): The Pharmacological Basis of Therapeutics, 7th ed. New York, Macmillan Publishing, 1985, p 145.
132. Colucci, WS, et al.: Decreased lymphocyte β-adrenergic receptor density in patients with heart failure and tolerance to the β-adrenergic agonist piubuterol. N Engl J Med 305:185, 1981.
133. Lockett, M: Dangerous effects of isoprenaline in myocardial failure. Lancet 2:104, 1965.
134. Shepherd, JT and Vanhoutte, PM: Neurohumoral regulation. *In* Shepherd JT, Vanhoutte PM: The Human Cardiovascular System. New York, Raven Press, 1979, p 107.
135. Shepherd, JT and Vanhoutte, PM: Pharmacodynamics. *In* Shepherd JT, Vanhoutte PM: The Human Cardiovascular System. New York, Raven Press, 1979, p 180.
136. Wynne, J and Braunwald, E: The cardiomyopathies and myocarditides. *In* Braunwald E (ed): Heart Disease: A Textbook of Cardiovascular Medicine, 2nd ed. Philadelphia, WB Saunders, 1984, p 1399.
137. Graziani, G, et al.: Dopamine and furosemide in oliguric renal failure. Nephron 37:39, 1984.
138. Marcus, FI, et al.: Digitalis and sympathomimetic stimulants. *In* Opie LH (ed): Drugs for the Heart, 1st ed. Orlando, Grune and Stratton, 1983, p 99.
139. Adams, HR: Cardiovascular emergencies: Drugs and resuscitative principles. Vet Clin North Am 11:77, 1981.
140. Harrison, DC, et al.: The pulmonary and systemic circulatory response to dopamine infusion. Br J Pharmacol 37:618, 1969.
141. Leir, CV, et al.: Comparative systemic and regional hemodynamic effects of dopamine and dobutamine in patients with cardiomyopathic heart failure. Circulation 58:466, 1978.
142. Goldberg, LI: Cardiovascular and renal actions of dopamine: Potential clinical applications. Pharmacol Rev 24:1, 1972.
143. Goldberg, LI and Raifer, SI: Sympathomimetic amines: Potential clinical applications in ischemic heart disease. Am Heart J 103:724, 1982.
144. Goldberg, LI, et al.: Sodium diuresis produced by dopamine in patients with congestive heart failure. N Engl J Med 268:1060, 1963.
145. Vatner, SF, et al.: Effects of dobutamine on left ventricular performance, coronary dynamics and distribution of cardiac output in conscious dogs. J Clin Invest 53:1265, 1974.
146. Beregovich, J, et al.: Hemodynamic effects of a new inotropic agent (dobutamine) in chronic cardiac failure. Br Heart J 37:629, 1975.
147. Akhtar, N, et al.: Hemodynamic effects of dobutamine in patients with severe heart failure. Am J Cardiol 36:202, 1975.
148. Loeb, HS, et al.: Superiority of dobutamine over dopamine for augmentation of cardiac output in patients with chronic low output cardiac failure. Circulation 55:375, 1977.
149. Kleinschmidt, R, et al.: Die Kombination von Dopamin und Dobutamin in der Differentialtherapie der akuen und chronischen Myokardinsuffizienz. Dtsch Med Wochenschr 15:598, 1985.
150. Bednarsky, RM and Muir, WW: Arrhythmogenicity of dopamine, dobutamine, and epinephrine on thiamylal-halothane anesthetized dogs. Am J Vet Res 44(12):2341, 1983.
151. Leier, CV, et al.: The cardiovascular effects of the continuous infusion of dobutamine in patients with severe heart failure. Circulation 56:468, 1977.
152. Applefeld, MA, et al.: Intermittent, continuous outpatient dobutamine infusion in the management of congestive heart failure. Am J Cardiol 51:455, 1983.
153. Krell, MJ, et al.: Intermittent, ambulatory dobutamine infusions in patients with severe congestive heart failure. Am Heart J 112:787, 1986.

154. Unverferth, DV, et al.: Tolerance to dobutamine after a 72 hour continuous infusion. Am J Med 69:262, 1980.
155. MacCannell, KL, et al.: Hemodynamic responses to dopamine and dobutamine infusions as a function of duration of infusion. Pharmacology 26:29, 1983.
156. Sharma, B and Goodwin, JF: Beneficial effect of salbutamol on cardiac function in severe congestive cardiomyopathy: Effect on systolic and diastolic function of the left ventricle. Circulation 58:449, 1978.
157. Rajfer SI, et al.: Beneficial hemodynamic effects of oral levodopa in heart failure. N Engl J Med 310:1357, 1984.
158. Alousi, AA, et al.: Cardiotonic activity of milrinone, a new and potent cardiac bipyridine, on the normal and failing heart of experimental animals. J Cardiol Pharmacol 5:792, 1983.
159. Colucci, WS, et al.: New positive inotropic agents in the treatment of congestive heart failure. N Engl J Med 314:290, 1986.
160. Scholz, H and Meyer, W: Phosphodiesterase-inhibiting properties of newer inotropic agents. Circulation 73:99, 1986.
161. Jentzer, JH, et al.: Beneficial effect of amrinone on myocardial oxygen consumption during acute left ventricular failure in dogs. Am J Cardiol 48:75, 1981.
162. Hermiller, JB, et al.: Amrinone in severe congestive heart failure: Another look at an intriguing new cardioactive drug. J Pharmacol Exp Ther 22:319, 1984.
163. Alousi, AA, et al.: The beneficial effect of amrinone on acute drug-induced heart failure in the anesthetized dog. Cardiov Res 19:483, 1985.
164. Bassett, AL, et al.: Enhanced relaxation and reduced positive inotropic effects of amrinone in ventricular muscle from cats with subacute heart failure. Adv Myocardiol 6:629, 1983.
165. Baim, DS: Effects of amrinone on myocardial energetics in severe congestive heart failure. Am J Cardiol 56:16b, 1985.
166. Packer, M, et al.: Failure of low doses of amrinone to produce sustained hemodynamic improvement in patients with severe chronic congestive heart failure. Am J Cardiol 54:1025, 1984.
167. Franciosa, JA: Intravenous amrinone: An advance or a wrong step? Ann Intern Med 102:399, 1985.
168. Wilsmhurst, PT and Webb-Peploe, MM: Side effects of amrinone therapy. Br Heart J 49:447, 1983.
169. Dunkman, WB, et al.: Adverse effects of long-term amrinone administration in congestive heart failure. Am Heart J 105:861, 1983.
170. Johnston, DL, et al.: Amrinone therapy in patients with heart failure: Lack of improvement in functional capacity and left ventricular function at rest and during exercise. Chest 86:394, 1984.
171. Massie, B, et al.: Long-term oral administration of amrinone for congestive heart failure: Lack of efficacy in a multicenter controlled trial. Circulation 71:963, 1985.
172. Kittleson, MD: Drug therapy of heart disease: Positive inotropic agents and captopril. Proc 9th Ann Kal Kan Symposium, October, 1985, p 19.
173. Kittleson, MD, et al.: Echocardiographic and clinical effects of milrinone in dogs with myocardial failure. Am J Vet Res 46:1659, 1985.
173a. Kittleson, MD, et al.: The acute hemodynamic effects of milrinone in dogs with severe idiopathic myocardial failure. J Vet Int Med 1:121, 1987.
174. Monrad, ES, et al.: Improvement in indexes of diastolic performance in patients with congestive heart failure treated with milrinone. Circulation 70:1030, 1984.
175. Sonnenblick, EH, et al.: Effects of milrinone on left ventricular performance and myocardial contractility in patients with severe heart failure. Circulation 73(suppl III):111, 1986.
176. Monrad, ES, et al.: Milrinone, dobutamine, and nitroprusside: Comparative effects on hemodynamics and myocardial energetics in patients with severe congestive heart failure. Circulation 73:168, 1986.
177. Gilbert, EM, et al.: Adverse outcome during long-term milrinone for advanced heart failure: A controlled pilot study. Circulation 72:111, 1985.
178. Rettig, G, et al.: Acute hemodynamic and long term clinical efficacy of milrinone in congestive heart failure. Circulation 72:111, 1985.
179. Baim, DS, et al.: Survival of patients with severe congestive heart failure treated with oral milrinone. J Am Coll Cardiol 7:661, 1986.
180. Ohyagi, A, et al.: Effect of ICI 118,587 on left ventricular function during graded treadmill exercise in conscious dogs. Am J Cardiol 54:1108, 1984.
181. Kariya, T, et al.: Studies on mechanism of cardiotonic activity of MDL 19205: Effects on several biochemical systems. J Cardio Pharmacol 4:509, 1982.
182. Amin, DK, et al.: Comparative hemodynamic effects of intravenous dobutamine and MDL-17,043, a new cardioactive drug, in severe congestive heart failure. Am Heart J 109:91, 1985.
183. Uretsky, BF, et al.: The acute hemodynamic effects of a new agent, MDL 17,043 in the treatment of congestive heart failure. Circulation 67:823, 1983.
184. Crawford, MH, et al.: Positive inotropic and vasodilator effects of MDL 17,043 in patients with reduced left ventricular performance. Am J Cardiol 53:1051, 1984.
185. Dage, RC, et al.: Cardiovascular properties of a new cardiotonic agent, MDL 19205. J Cardiovasc Pharmacol 6:35, 1984.
186. Hollenberg, NR: Pathophysiology of congestive heart failure: The role of the kidney. *In* Cohn JN (ed): Drug Treatment of Heart Failure. New York, Yorke Medical Books, 1983, p 53.
187. Imai, M: Effect of bumetanide and furosemide on the thick ascending limbs of Henle's loop of rabbits and rats perfused in vitro. Eur J Pharmacol 41:409, 1977.
188. Burg, MB and Green, N: Function of the thick ascending limb of Henle. J Clin Invest 52:612, 1973.
189. Rocca, AS and Kokko, JP: Sodium chloride and water transport in the medullary thick ascending limb of Henle: Evidence for active chloride transport. J Clin Invest 52:612, 1973.
190. Delaney, V and Bourke, E: Diuretics. *In* Hurst JW (ed): The Heart. 6th ed. New York, McGraw-Hill, 1985, p 1657.
191. Kim, KE, et al.: Ethacrynic acid and furosemide: Diuretic and hemodynamic effects and clinical uses. Am J Cardiol 27:407, 1971.
192. Laiwah, AC, et al.: Antagonistic effect of non-steroidal antiinflammatory drugs on furosemide-induced diuresis in cardiac failure. Br J Cardiol 283:714, 1981.
193. Dikshit, K, et al.: Renal and extrarenal hemodynamic effects of furosemide in congestive heart failure after myocardial infarction. N Engl J Med 288:1087, 1973.
194. Francis, GS, et al.: Acute vasoconstrictor response to intravenous furosemide in patients with congestive heart failure. Ann Int Med 103:1, 1985.
195. Multiple Risk Factor Intervention Trial: Risk factor changes and mortality results. JAMA 248:1465, 1982.
196. Papademetriou, V: Diuretics, hypokalemia, and cardiac arrhythmias: A critical analysis. Am Heart J 111:1217, 1986.
197. Lilly, LS: The clinical significance of hyponatremia in congestive heart failure. Pract Cardiol 12:53, 1986.
198. Bonagura, JD: Fluid and electrolyte management of the cardiac patient. Vet Clin North Am 12:501, 1982.
199. Bourke, E: Furosemide, bumetanide, and ototoxicity. Lancet 1:917, 1976.
199a. Gertler, MM and Rusk, HA: Rehabilitation principles in congestive heart failure. American Heart Association Monograph No 1, 2nd ed, 1966.
200. Materson, BJ: Insights into intrarenal sites and mechanisms of action of diuretic agents. Am Heart J 106:188, 1983.
201. Reubi, FC: The action and use of diuretics in renal disease. *In* Freidberg, C (ed): Heart, Kidney, and Electroytes. New York, Grune & Stratton, 1962, p 169.
202. Mudge, GH: Diuretics and other agents employed in the mobilization of edema fluid. *In* Gilman, AG, Goodman, LS (eds): The Pharmacologic Basis of Therapeutics. 6th ed. New York, Macmillan, 1980, p 908.
203. Frazier, HS and Yager, H: Drug therapy: The clinical use of diuretics. Med Intell 288:455, 1973.
204. Zelis, R, et al.: Abnormalities in the regional circulation accompanying congestive heart failure. Prog Cardiovasc Dis 18:181, 1977.
205. Braunwald, E: Vasodilator therapy—A physiological approach to the treatment of heart failure. N Engl J Med 297:331, 1977.
206. Harshaw, CW, et al.: Reduced systemic vascular resistance as therapy for severe mitral regurgitation of valvular origin. Ann Intern Med 83:312, 1975.
207. Yoran, C, et al.: Mechanism of reduction of mitral regurgitation with vasodilator therapy. Am J Cardiol 43:773, 1979.
208. Chatterjee, K, et al.: Beneficial effects of vasodilator agents in

severe mitral regurgitation due to dysfunction of subvalvar apparatus. Circulation, October, 1973, p 684.
209. Mason, DT, et al.: Panel Discussion. Am J Med 65:208, 1978.
210. Cohn, JN, et al.: Effect of vasodilator therapy on mortality in chronic congestive heart failure: Results of a veterans administration cooperative study. New Engl J Med 314:1547, 1986.
211. Furberg, CD and Yusuf, S: Effect of vasodilators on survival in chronic congestive heart failure. Am J Cardiol 55:1110, 1985.
212. Atwell, RB: The use of α blockade in the treatment of congestive heart failure associated with dirofilariasis and mitral valvular incompetence. Vet Rec, February 10, 1979, p 114.
213. Kittleson, MD and Hamlin, RL: Hydralazine therapy for severe mitral regurgitation in a dog. JAVMA 179:903, 1981.
214. Hamlin, RL and Kittleson, MD: Clinical experience with hydralazine for treatment of otherwise intractable cough in dogs with apparent left-side heart failure. JAVMA 180:1327, 1982.
215. Kittleson, MD, et al.: Oral hydralazine therapy for chronic mitral regurgitation in the dog. JAVMA 182:1205, 1983.
216. Kittleson, MD, et al.: Acute hemodynamic effects of hydralazine in dogs with chronic mitral regurgitation. JAVMA 187:258, 1985.
217. Kittleson, MD and Hamlin, RL: Hydralazine pharmacodynamics in the dog. Am J Vet Res 44:1501, 1983.
218. Zelis, R, et al.: A comparison of the effects of vasodilator stimuli on peripheral resistance vessels in normal subjects and in patients with congestive heart failure. J Clin Invest 47:960, 1968.
219. Zelis, R and Flaim, SF: Alterations of vasomotor tone in congestive heart failure. Prog Cardiovasc Dis 25:437, 1982.
220. Aronow, WS: Treatment of congestive heart failure II. Vasodilators and angiotensin-converting enzyme inhibitors. Rational Drug Therapy 16:1, 1982.
221. Greenwald, JE: Modulation of prostaglandin biosynthesis: Proposed mechanism of action of hydralazine. PhD dissertation, The Ohio State University, 1981.
222. Mclean, AJ, et al.: Interaction of hydralazine with tension development and mechanisms of calcium accumulation in K^+ stimulated rabbit aortic strips. J Pharmacol Exp Ther 207:40, 1978.
223. Rudd, P and Blaschke, TF: Antihypertensive agents and the drug therapy of hypertension. *In* Gilman, AG, Goodman, LS (eds): The Pharmacological Basis of Therapeutics. 7th ed. New York, Macmillan Publishing Co, 1985, p 795.
224. Keene, BW: Cardiovascular drugs. *In* Bonagura, JD (ed): Contemporary Issues in Small Animal Practice, Vol 7—Cardiology. New York, Churchill Livingstone, 1987, p 21.
225. Gershwin, ME and Smith, NT: Mode of action of hydralazine on guinea pig atria. Arch Int Pharmacodyn 170:108, 1967.
226. Knowlen, GG, et al.: Comparison of plasma aldosterone concentration among clinical status groups of dogs with chronic heart failure. JAVMA 183:991, 1983.
227. Koch-Weser, J: Drug therapy: Hydralazine. N Engl J Med 295:320, 1976.
228. Perry, H: Late toxicity to hydralazine resembling systemic lupus erythematosus or rheumatoid arthritis. Am J Med 54:56, 1973.
229. Mason, DJ and Braunwald, E: The effects of nitroglycerin and amylnitrate on arteriolar and venous tone in the human forearm. Circulation 32:755, 1965.
230. Vatner, SF, et al.: Effects of nitroglycerin on cardiac function and regional blood flow distribution in conscious dogs. Am J Physiol 234:H-244, 1978.
231. Chien, YW: Pharmaceutical considerations of transdermal nitroglycerin delivery: Various approaches. Am Heart J 108:207, 1984.
232. Sharpe, DN and Coxon, R: Nitroglycerin in a transdermal therapeutic system in chronic heart failure. J Cardiovasc Pharmacol 6:76, 1984.
233. Packer, M, et al.: Hemodynamic factors limiting the response to transdermal nitroglycerin in severe chronic congestive heart failure. Am J Cardiol 57:260, 1986.
234. Sharpe, DN, et al.: Hemodynamic effects of intermittent transdermal nitroglycerin in chronic congestive heart failure. Am J Cardiol 59:895, 1987.
235. Carroll, JD, et al.: The differential effects of positive inotropic and vasodilator therapy on diastolic properties in patients with congestive cardiomyopathy. Circulation 74:815, 1986.
236. Palmer, RF: Drug therapy: Sodium nitroprusside. N Engl J Med 292:294, 1975.
237. Brogden, RN, et al.: Prazosin: A review of its pharmacological properties and therapeutic efficacy in hypertension. Drugs 14:163, 1977.
238. Awan, NA, et al.: Efficacy of ambulatory vasodilator therapy with oral prazosin in chronic refractory heart failure. Circulation 56:346, 1977.
239. Bertel, O, et al.: Sustained effect of chronic prazosin treatment in severe congestive heart failure. Am Heart J 101:529, 1981.
240. Colucci, WS, et al.: Long-term therapy of heart failure with prazosin: A randomized double-blind trial. Am J Cardiol 45:337, 1980.
241. Parmley, WW, et al.: Hemodynamic effects of prazosin in chronic heart failure. Am Heart J 102:622, 1981.
242. Harper, RW, et al.: The acute and chronic haemodynamic effects of prazosin in severe congestive cardiac failure. Med J Aust 2 (suppl):36, 1980.
243. Markham, RV, et al.: Efficacy of prazosin in the management of chronic congestive heart failure: A six month randomized, double-blind, placebo-controlled study. Am J Cardiol 51:1346, 1983.
244. Reifart, N, et al.: Symptomatic and hemodynamic effects of prazosin in chronic congestive heart failure in a randomized double-blind trial over one year (abstr). J Am Coll Cardiol 5:461, 1985.
245. Arnold, S, et al.: Attenuation of prazosin effect on cardiac output in chronic heart failure. Ann Intern Med 91:345, 1979.
246. Packer, M, et al.: Hemodynamic and clinical tachyphylaxis to prazosin-mediated afterload reduction in severe chronic congestive heart failure. Circulation 59:531, 1979.
247. Packer, M, et al.: Role of the renin-angiotensin system in the development of hemodynamic and clinical tolerance to long-term prazosin therapy in patients with severe chronic heart failure. J Am Coll Cardiol 7:671, 1986.
248. Magorien, RD, et al.: Prazosin and hydralazine in congestive heart failure. Regional hemodynamic effects in relation to dose. Ann Int Med 95:5, 1981.
249. Prasad, K, et al.: Effect of prazosin treatment on the cardiac sarcolemmal ATPase in failing heart due to mitral insufficiency in dogs. Cardiovasc Res 19:406, 1985.
250. Romankiewicz, JN, et al.: Captopril: An update review of its pharmacologic properties and therapeutic efficacy in congestive heart failure. Drugs 25:6, 1983.
250a. Kramer, BL, et al.: Controlled trial of captopril in chronic heart failure: A rest and exercise hemodynamic study. Circulation 67:807, 1983.
251. Davis, JL: Adrenocortical and renal hormonal function in experimental cardiac failure. Circulation 25:1002, 1968.
252. Curtiss, C, et al.: Role of the renin-angiotensin system in the systemic vasoconstriction of chronic congestive heart failure. Circulation 58:763, 1978.
253. Laragh, JH: Hormones and the pathogenesis of congestive heart failure: Vasopressin, aldosterone, and angiotensin II. Circulation 25:1015, 1962.
254. Merril, AJ, et al.: Concentration of renin in renal venous blood in patients with chronic heart failure. Am J Med 1:468, 1946.
255. Dzau, VJ, et al.: Sustained effectiveness of converting-enzyme inhibition in patients with severe congestive heart failure. N Engl J Med 302:1373, 1980.
256. Ader, R, et al.: Immediate and sustained hemodynamic and clinical improvement in chronic heart failure by an oral angiotensin-converting enzyme inhibitor. Circulation 61:931, 1980.
257. Romankiewicz, JA, et al.: Captopril: An updated review of its pharmacological properties and therapeutic efficacy in congestive heart failure. Drugs 25:6, 1983.
258. Cody, RJ: Angiotensin-converting enzyme inhibitors in treatment of heart failure. Pract Cardiol 12:108, 1986.
259. Bayliss, J, et al.: Vasodilation with captopril and prazosin in chronic heart failure: Double blind study at rest and on exercise. Br Heart J 55:265, 1985.
260. Lee, WH and Packer, M: Prognostic importance of serum sodium concentration and its modification by converting enzyme inhibition in patients with severe chronic heart failure. Circulation 73:257, 1986.
261. Mettauer, B, et al.: Differential long-term intrarenal and neurohormonal effects of captopril and prazosin in patients with chronic congestive heart failure: Importance of initial plasma renin activity. Circulation 73:492, 1986.

262. Cleland, JGF, et al.: Total body and serum electrolyte composition in heart failure: The effects of captopril. Eur Heart J 6:681, 1985.
263. Packer, M, et al.: Hemodynamic patterns of response during long-term captopril therapy for severe chronic heart failure. Circulation 68:803, 1983.
264. Massie, BM, et al.: Lack of relationship between short-term hemodynamic effects of captopril and subsequent clinical responses. Circulation 69:1135, 1984.
265. Packer, M, et al.: Functional renal insufficiency during long-term therapy with captopril and enalapril in severe chronic heart failure. Ann Int Med 106:346, 1987.
266. Massie, B, et al.: Hemodynamic and clinical responses to combined captopril-hydralazine therapy. Circulation 66:11, 1982.
267. Gross, DM, et al.: Effect of N-[(s)-1-carboxy-3-phenylpropyl]-L-Ala-L-Pro and its ethyl ester (MK 421) on angiotensin converting enzyme in vitro and angiotensin I pressor responses in vivo. J Pharmacol Exp Ther 216:552, 1981.
268. Kubo, SH and Cody, RJ: Clinical pharmacokinetics of the angiotensin converting enzyme inhibitors—A review. Clin Pharmacokinet 10:377, 1985.
269. Kromer, EP, et al.: Effectiveness of converting enzyme inhibition (enalapril) for mild congestive heart failure. Am J Cardiol 57:459, 1986.
270. Fuster, VF, et al.: The natural history of idiopathic dilated cardiomyopathy. Am J Cardiol 47:525, 1981.
271. Muir, WW and Sams, R: Clinical pharmacodynamics and pharmacokinetics of β-adrenoceptor blocking drugs in veterinary medicine. Comp Cont Ed 156:155, 1984.
272. Conolly, ME, et al.: The clinical pharmacology of β-adrenoceptor-blocking drugs. Prog Cardiovasc Dis 19:203, 1976.
273. Viquerat, CE, et al.: Endogenous catecholamine levels in chronic heart failure. Am J Med 78:455, 1985.
274. Cohn, JN, et al.: Plasma norepinephrine as a guide to prognosis in patients with chronic congestive heart failure. N Engl J Med 311:819, 1984.
275. Hjalmarson, A, et al.: The Goteborg metoprolol trial-effects of mortality and morbidity in acute myocardial infarction. Circulation 67 (suppl 1):26, 1983.
276. Gwathmey, JK and Hamlin, RL: Protection of turkeys against furazolidone-induced cardiomyopathy. Am J Cardiol 52:626, 1983.
277. Opie, LH, et al.: Calcium and catecholamines: Relevance to cardiomyopathies and significance in therapeutic strategies. J Mol Cell Cardiol 17:21, 1985.
278. Kates, RE, et al.: Pharmacokinetics of propranolol in the dog. J Vet Pharmacol Ther 2:21, 1979.
279. Adams, HR: New perspectives in cardiopulmonary therapeutics: Receptor-selective adrenergic drugs. JAVMA 185:966, 1984.
280. Frishman, WH: Pindolol: A new β-adrenoceptor antagonist with partial agonist activity. N Engl J Med 308:940, 1983
281. Rouleau, JL, et al.: Verapamil preserves myocardial contractility in the hereditary cardiomyopathy of the Syrian hamster. Circ Res 50:405, 1982.
282. Roth, SJ, et al.: Intravenous verapamil for hypertrophic obstructive cardiomyopathy. Texas Heart Inst J 10:177, 1983.
283. Bonow, RO, et al.: Verapamil-induced improvement in left ventricular diastolic filling and increased exercise tolerance in patients with hypertrophic cardiomyopathy: short- and long-term effects. Circulation 72:853, 1985.
284. Allert, JA and Adams, HR: New perspectives in cardiovascular medicine: The calcium channel blocking drugs. JAVMA 190:573, 1987.
284a. Bright, JM, and Golden, AL: The use of calcium channel blockers in cats with hypertrophic cardiomyopathy. Proc of the 6th Ann Vet Med Forum, 184, 1988.
285. Johnson, JT: Conversion of atrial fibrillation in two dogs using verapamil and supportive therapy. JAAHA 21:429, 1985.
286. Lang R, et al.: Verapamil or digitalis for atrial fibrillation? Chest 83:491, 1983.
287. McGoon, et al.: Verapamil as a valuable cardiovascular therapeutic agent. Mayo Clinic Proc 57:495, 1983.
288. Theisen, K, et al.: Effect of the calcium antagonist diltiazem on atrioventricular conduction in chronic atrial fibrillation. Am J Cardiol 55:98, 1985.
289. Hamlin, RL, et al.: Detection and quantitation of subclinical heart failure in dogs. JAVMA 150:1513, 1966.
290. Pensinger, RR: Dietary control of sodium intake in spontaneous congestive heart failure in dogs. VM/SAC, July, 1964.
291. Wallace, CR and Hamilton, WF: Study of spontaneous congestive heart failure in the dog. Circ Res 11:301, 1962.
292. Morris, ML, et al.: Low sodium diet in heart disease: How low is low? VM/SAC, September 1976, p 1225.
293. Anonymous: Nutrient requirements of domestic animals, No 8. Nutrient requirements of dogs. National Academy of Sciences, Washington DC, 1974.
294. Thomas, WP: Low sodium diets. *In* Kirk, RW (ed): Current Veterinary Therapy VI. Philadelphia, WB Saunders, 1977.
295. Ross, JN, Jr: Heart failure. *In* Lewis, LD, et al. (eds): Small Animal Clinical Nutrition III. Topeka, Mark Morris Associates, 1987, p 11.
296. Lewis, et al.: Small Animal Clinical Nutrition III. Topeka, Mark Morris Associates, 1987.
297. Pittman, JG and Cohen, P: The pathogenesis of cardiac cachexia. New Engl J Med, 1964.
298. Heymsfield, SB, et al.: Nutritional support in cardiac failure. Symp on Surg Nutr 61:635, 1981.
299. Blackburn, GL, et al.: Nutritional support in cardiac cachexia. J Thorac Cardiov Surg 73:489, 1977.
300. Baggot JD: Pharmacodynamics. *In* Booth NH, McDonald LE (eds): Veterinary Pharmacology and Therapeutics. Ames, Iowa State University Press, 1982, p 23.
301. Calvert, CA and Thrall, DE: Treatment of canine heartworm disease coexisting with right-side heart failure. JAVMA 180:1201, 1982.
302. Bolton, GR: The role of bronchodilators in the treatment of congestive heart failure. *In* Kirk, RW (ed): Current Veterinary Therapy VI. Philadelphia, WB Saunders, 1977.
303. Ware, WA and Bonagura, JD: Canine myocardial diseases. *In* Kirk, RW (ed): Current Veterinary Therapy IX. Philadelphia. WB Saunders, 1986, p 370.
304. McKiernan, BC, et al.: Pharmacokinetic studies of theophylline in dogs. J Vet Pharmacol Ther 4:103, 1981.
305. McKiernan, BC, et al.: Pharmacokinetic studies of theophylline in cats. J Vet Pharmacol Ther 6:99, 1983.
306. Birchard, SJ, et al.: Chylothorax associated with congestive cardiomyopathy in a cat. JAVMA 189:1462, 1986.
307. Bonagura, JD: Fluid and electrolyte management of the cardiac patient. Vet Clin North Am 12:501, 1982.

DRUG INDEX

Generic	Trade	Dosage	Route	Frequency	Description
Digoxin	Lanoxin Lanoxicaps Cardoxin	Dog—0.05 mg/lb 0.01 to 0.02 mg/lb over 4 hrs Cat—¼ of a 0.125 mg tab 0.005 mg/kg over 4 hr	Orally IV Orally IV	q12h qod	Positive inotrope, supraventricular antiarrhythmic
Digitoxin	Crystodigin	Dog—0.01 to 0.03 mg/kg	Orally	q8–12h	Positive inotrope
Dopamine	Inotropin Dopastat	2 to 10 mcg/kg/min	IV	CRI*	Catecholamine resuscitation
Dobutamine	Dobutrex	Dog—1.2 to 20 mcg/lb/min Cat—0.2 to 2.2 mcg/kg/min	IV	CRI	Catecholamine—heart failure
Amrinone	Inocor	0.4 to 1.4 mg/kg, then 4.5 to 45 mcg/kg/min	IV IV	Bolus CRI	Positive inotrope—vasodilator
Milrinone	Unapproved	Dog—0.2 to 0.45 mg/kg	Orally	q12h	Positive inotrope—vasodilator
Furosemide	Lasix	Dog—0.45 to 2 mg/kg Cat—0.2 to 0.45 mg/kg	Orally, IV, IM, SQ	qd–q8h qod–qd	Loop diuretic
Chlorothiazide	Diuril	9 to 18 mg/lb	Orally	q12h	Thiazide diuretic
Hydrochlorothiazide	HydroDIURIL	1 to 2 mg/kg	Orally	q12h	Thiazide diuretic
Spironolactone	Aldactone	1 to 2 mg/kg	Orally	qd	Potassium-sparing diuretic
Triamterene	Dyrenium	1 to 2 mg/kg	Orally	gd	Potassium-sparing diuretic
Hydralazine	Apresoline	Dog—0.2 to 1.4 mg/kg Cat—1.2 to 4.5 mg	Orally	q12h q12h	Arterial vasodilator afterload reducer
Nitroglycerin	Nitrol Nitrodisc	¼ to 1″ 2.5 or 5 mg patch	Transcutaneous	q6h qd	Venous vasodilator preload reducer
Sodium nitroprusside	Nipride	Dog—2 to 10 mcg/kg/min	IV	CRI	Balanced vasodilator preload + afterload reducer
Prazosin	Minipress	Dog—0.5 to 2 mg initially	Orally	q8h–q12h	Balanced vasodilator preload + afterload reducer
Captopril	Capoten	0.2 to 0.9 mg/kg	Orally	q8h	ACE† inhibitor
Propranolol	Inderal	Dog—0.1 to 1 mg/kg Cat—1.2 to 4.5 mg 0.001 to 0.045 mg/kg	Orally IV	q8h–q12h q12h	Beta blocker, non-selective
Atenolol	Tenormin	0.12 to 0.45 mg/kg	Orally	q12h	B1 selective Beta blocker
Morphine	Morphine	Dog—0.04 to 0.12 mg/kg 0.02 to 0.45 mg/kg	SQ IV		Narcotic, sedative

*CRI = Constant rate infusion
†ACE = Angiotensin converting enzyme

74 CONGENITAL HEART DISEASE

JOHN D. BONAGURA

CLINICAL APPROACH TO CONGENITAL HEART DISEASE

Malformations of the heart and great vessels represent a small, but clinically significant, cause of cardiovascular disease in small animal patients.[1–14] The etiopathogenesis and resultant circulatory abnormalities of congenital heart diseases in animals parallel those of humans.[15, 16] There are marked similarities of clinical findings between small animals and humans with cardiac malformations. For this reason, many of the diagnostic and therapeutic principles employed in veterinary cardiology are identical to those used in the management of children with congenital heart disease.

The identification of congenital heart disease is critical to the evaluation of newly acquired pets and the assessment of purebred dogs and cats raised for future breeding. While the accurate assessment of congenital heart disease may require referral for echocardiography and cardiac catheterization, the practicing veterinarian should be cognizant of various cardiac malformations and must distinguish murmurs caused by significant defects from the innocent murmurs so often auscultated in neonates. Furthermore, the clinician must have a general appreciation of the genetic and etiologic basis of congenital heart disease in order to properly counsel breeders.[17–21] The purpose of this chapter is to review clinically relevant aspects of congenital heart disease including pathogenesis, pathology, pathophysiology of clinical signs, heritability, and clinical management.

Clinical Evaluation

HISTORY AND PHYSICAL EXAMINATION

The general diagnostic approach to the pet with congenital heart disease is similar to that used in the evaluation of acquired cardiac disorders.[1, 9, 15, 22–36] The breed and sex are particularly important because many cardiac malformations have a genetic basis. The noninvasive clinical evaluation includes the patient history, physical examination, thoracic radiography, electrocardiography, routine hematologic tests, and echocardiography (Table 74–1). Based on these evaluations, a tentative anatomical diagnosis can be rendered. Definitive diagnosis generally requires echocardiography and may necessitate cardiac catheterization and angiocardiography. The extent of a cardiac workup is influenced by client expectations, clinical signs, and surgical considerations.

History. The age, breed, and sex should be considered when evaluating animals with congenital heart disease. Maturity is a factor when assessing the effect of pulmonary vascular resistance on the magnitude of systemic to pulmonary shunts. Although the pulmonary vascular resistance falls immediately at birth, it continues to decline during the first one to two months of life,[31] and left to right shunting may be not be fully manifested until a number of weeks after birth. It has been shown that congenital subaortic stenosis may actually develop during the first two months of life,[2, 9] and the associated cardiac murmur can actually increase in intensity during the four months after birth. Breed associations with canine cardiac defects, summarized in Table 74–2, emphasize the genetic basis of some malformations. While human males are predisposed to congenital heart disease, both male and female pups develop cardiac malformations. A sex predisposition is not well established in dogs except for the higher prevalence of patent ductus arteriosus in female dogs.[1, 4, 8] The Siamese and Burmese breeds may be predisposed to some congenital heart defects, and male kittens seem to be at higher risk for cardiac malformation.[36]

TABLE 74–1. CLINICAL EVALUATION OF CONGENITAL HEART DISEASE

Signalment (breed predisposition)
History of clinical signs
Jugular pulses
Arterial pulse
Mucous membranes
Precordium
Cardiac auscultation
Electrocardiography
Thoracic radiography
Packed cell volume
Echocardiography
Doppler echocardiography
Contrast echocardiography
Cardiac catheterization
Angiocardiography

TABLE 74–2. BREED PREDILECTIONS IN CONGENITAL HEART DISEASE

Beagle	Pulmonic stenosis
Boxer	Subaortic stenosis, ?pulmonic stenosis, ?atrial septal defect
Bull terrier	Mitral dysplasia
Chihuahua	Patent ductus arteriosus (PDA), pulmonic stenosis
Collie	Patent ductus arteriosus
Doberman pinscher	Atrial septal defect
English bulldog	Tetralogy of Fallot, ventricular septal defect, pulmonic stenosis
German shepherd	Subaortic stenosis, mitral and tricuspid valve dysplasia, PDA
German shorthair pointer	Subaortic stenosis
Golden retriever	Subaortic stenosis, tricuspid valve dysplasia
Great Dane	Mitral and tricuspid valve dysplasia
Keeshond	Tetralogy of Fallot
Labrador retriever	Tricuspid valve dysplasia
Maltese	Patent ductus arteriosus
Newfoundland	Subaortic stenosis
Poodles	Patent ductus arteriosus
Pomeranian	Patent ductus arteriosus
Rottweiler	Subaortic stenosis
Samoyed	Pulmonic stenosis, ?atrial septal defect
Schnauzer	Pulmonic stenosis
Shetland sheepdog	Patent ductus arteriosus
Terrier breeds	Pulmonic stenosis
Weimaraner	Tricuspid dysplasia, peritoneopericardial hernia

Clinical signs of congenital heart disease include failure to grow, shortness of breath, abdominal swelling, cyanosis, weakness, syncope, seizures, and sudden death. However, many animals with congenital heart disease are relatively asymptomatic and the client may be unaware that the pet is afflicted with a serious cardiac malformation. The pup with severe aortic stenosis may appear almost normal during a cursory evaluation, yet may die suddenly after a brief period of exercise. Similarly, neonates with patent ductus arteriosus and incipient cardiac failure often seem to feel well until pulmonary edema becomes life-threatening.

Physical Examination. While some pets with congenital heart disease are examined for typical signs of congestive heart failure, most cases of congenital heart disease are identified at the time of immunization following auscultation of a cardiac murmur (Table 74–3). The veterinarian may face a dilemma, however, since normal pups and kittens can exhibit soft innocent systolic cardiac murmurs, which must be distinguished from murmurs caused by a cardiac malformation. While variable, the typical innocent murmur is soft (grade 1 to 3/6), is loudest at the pulmonic or aortic valve area, is protomesosystolic (or ejection) in timing, and varies with heart rate and changing body position. Some innocent murmurs are musical in quality. Innocent murmurs generally, but not invariably, diminish in intensity or resolve by the time the animal is 14 to 16 weeks of age.

Cardiac murmurs of congenital heart disease often are loud and accompanied by a precordial thrill. However, this association represents an oversimplification, since a murmur may not be audible even in the presence of severe cyanotic heart disease. Moreover, mild stenosis of a semilunar valve or ventricular outflow tract may generate only a soft systolic murmur that can be easily confused with an innocent flow murmur. Thus, any grade cardiac murmur is compatible with congenital heart disease. Additional auscultatory abnormalities, such as a loud or split second heart sound, may offer further evidence of congenital heart disease.

Abnormalities of the arterial pulse, mucous membranes, jugular venous pulse, or precordium may substantiate a clinical suspicion of congenital disease. Hyperkinetic arterial pulsations are characteristic of lesions causing diastolic run-off of aortic blood as occurs with patent ductus arteriosus or aortic regurgitation. Hypokinetic pulses are typical of subaortic stenosis or conditions like tricuspid dysplasia, which are characterized by diminished ventricular output. Cyanosis often indicates systemic to pulmonary shunting, but can develop in animals with severe congestive failure and secondary pulmonary dysfunction. Prominent jugular pulsations may suggest an abnormality of the right side of the heart such as pulmonic stenosis or tricuspid regurgitation. A precordial heave often indicates hypertrophy or enlargement of the underlying ventricle and provides insight into the underlying cardiac malformation. As a general rule, a precordial thrill accompanies loud cardiac murmurs and the location of this vibration is the point of maximal murmur intensity. The location of the precordial thrill often is characteristic of the associated defect (see specific cardiac defects for details).

Laboratory Tests. As a general principle, hematologic tests are not an important part of the congenital heart disease workup. While serum biochemical tests may be abnormal when there is congestive heart failure or intercurrent organ disease (e.g., portosystemic shunting), the CBC, biochemical profile, and urinalysis are typically normal. Of note is the presence of a higher than normal PCV in a neonate with right to left shunting. Polycythemia is often noted with tetralogy of Fallot, reversed patent ductus arteriosus, and complex cyanotic heart disease. Arterial hypoxemia, hypocarbia, and metabolic acidosis may be detected in severe cases of right to left shunting.

Despite a strong clinical suspicion of congenital heart disease based on history and physical examination, definitive evaluation of the neonate with a cardiac murmur generally requires more detailed studies. In this regard, the electrocardiogram (ECG) and thoracic imaging using radiography and Doppler echocardiography are required.

CARDIAC IMAGING

Radiography. Survey radiographs of the thorax are important for the identification of cardiomegaly, size of the great vessels, pulmonary circulatory dynamics, and congestive heart failure.[5, 22–24] Angiocardiography,[5, 24–26] useful for determining anatomical defects, delineating abnormal blood flow, and estimating ventricular function, is discussed later. The use of radionuclide studies to detect cardiac shunting has not been adequately evaluated in veterinary medicine. While specific radiographic features are discussed with the individual de-

TABLE 74–3. AUSCULTATORY FINDINGS IN CONGENITAL HEART DISEASE (CARDIAC MURMUR)

Lesion	Timing	Quality (PCG Configuration)	Point Maximal Intensity	Comments
Aortic regurgitation	Diastolic	Blowing (Decrescendo)	Left cardiac base	Usually associated with aortic stenosis, aortic endocarditis, or VSD
Aortic stenosis*	Systolic†	Ejection (Crescendo-decrescendo)	Left third to fourth ICS	Often equally loud at the right cardiac base
Atrial septal defect	Systolic; diastolic	Ejection; diastolic rumble	Pulmonic valve area Tricuspid valve area	Splitting of S_2 (Murmurs of relative pulmonic and tricuspid stenosis)
Mitral dysplasia‡	Systolic	Regurgitant (Holosystolic)	Fifth-sixth ICS (Left apex)	Radiates widely
Patent ductus arteriosus	Continuous	Machinery	Left base, dorsal	Loudest at S_2, radiates to right base
Pulmonary hypertension	Usually systolic; rarely diastolic	Decrescendo or ejection	Left cardiac base	Associated ejection sound, loud P_2, or split S_2
Pulmonic insufficiency	Diastolic	Blowing (Decrescendo)	Left cardiac base	May be heard at right hemithorax; may occur with pulmonic stenosis or pulmonary hypertension
Pulmonic stenosis	Systolic	Ejection (Crescendo-decrescendo)	Left second ICS (Pulmonic valve area)	Radiates to left, dorsal cardiac base; softer on right; possible ejection sound
Tetralogy of Fallot	Systolic	Ejection (Crescendo-decrescendo)	Left second ICS (Pulmonic valve area)	Murmur of VSD may be evident at the RSB; murmurs may be soft or absent
Tricuspid dysplasia‡	Systolic	Regurgitant (Holosystolic)	Right third-fourth ICS (Tricuspid valve area)	Radiates dorsally and to the left
Ventricular septal defect (VSD)	Systolic†	Regurgitant (Holosystolic)	Right sternal border (Second-fourth ICS)	May be loudest over pulmonic valve area (Relative pulmonic stenosis), S_2 may be split

PCG = phonocardiogram
ICS = intercostal space
RSB = right sternal border
S_2 = second heart sound
P_2 = pulmonic component of S_2
*Typically a subaortic obstruction
†At times, a diastolic murmur of aortic regurgitation may also be present
‡Mitral stenosis and tricuspid stenosis are rare but may generate diastolic murmurs over the affected valve area and adjacent ventricle

fects, some general comments about interpretation of survey radiographs can be made at this time.

Detection of cardiomegaly is relatively easy; however, the distinction between right and left ventricular enlargement may be difficult without echocardiography. The frequent occurrence of apex shifting may confuse the clinician, resulting in an erroneous diagnosis. Thus, the radiographic assessment should be done in conjunction with the ECG and preferably the echocardiogram. Moreover, there is a tendency to overinterpret the right ventricle in neonates, in which some right ventricular dominance is normal. This may lead to a presumptive diagnosis of pulmonic stenosis in a pup with a functional cardiac murmur.

Dilation of the great vessels can be a clue to the underlying cardiac malformation. Aortic widening in the cranial mediastinum is typical of the post-stenotic dilatation of subaortic stenosis or the aortic anomaly sometimes noted with tetralogy of Fallot. Aneurysmal dilation of the descending aorta is common with patent ductus arteriosus. Enlargement of the main pulmonary artery may accompany post-stenotic turbulent flow from pulmonic stenosis, increased flow caused by any left to right shunt, or pulmonary hypertension.

Pulmonary vascularity must be assessed with caution,[24] but is a useful guideline in determining pulmonary overcirculation, undercirculation, and venous congestion. Cranial lobar arteries and veins as well as peripheral pulmonary vascular markings should be assessed. Right to left shunts, like tetralogy of Fallot, are characterized by diminished peripheral perfusion and normal to small lobar vessels. Reversed or bidirectional shunts caused by pulmonary hypertension cause diminished peripheral perfusion with dilated lobar arteries and dilatation of the main pulmonary trunk. Vascularity can also be decreased in other conditions, such as pulmonic stenosis and severe tricuspid dysplasia. Conversely, left to right shunts, like atrioventricular septal defects and patent ductus arteriosus, have increased dimension of lobar arteries and veins with prominent peripheral vascular markings that may be misinterpreted as interstitial lung densities. Right or left ventricular failure may be heralded by widened diameter of the caudal vena cava or pulmonary veins, respectively.

Echocardiography. In recent years, the need for cardiac catheterization and angiocardiography for definitive diagnosis of congenital heart disease has been somewhat diminished owing to the development of echocardiography, a study that permits detailed imaging of cardiac anatomy.[27, 28] The addition of Doppler echocardiography, which can detect normal and abnormal blood flow and estimate intravascular pressures, promises to augment the usefulness of ultrasound studies.[29a–d] Contrast echocardiography, whereby intravascular echo targets are created by the rapid injection of saline or indocyanine-green dye,[27, 28, 30] is another method that can reliably detect some intracardiac shunts in situations where Doppler technology is unavailable.

Doppler echocardiography, which uses ultrasound to measure the velocity of moving red blood cell targets, permits noninvasive assessment of normal and abnormal flow and the detection of high-velocity jets in the heart and blood vessels, and allows the cardiologist to noninvasively estimate intracardiac and vascular blood pressures.[29b–d] A careful "echodoppler" study can replace the invasive cardiac catheterization and angiocardiogram in many instances. The velocities of the RBC can be displayed on a spectral tracing that also uses a [+] and [−] coding relative to a zero baseline to determine relative direction of blood flow (Figure 74–1*A*). When the transducer used contains two crystals (a constant transmitter and constant receiver), very high velocities can be recorded along the directed line of ultrasound. The velocities of all RBCs in the line are recorded at once and displayed. This is called *continuous-wave Doppler* and is used to measure the high velocities that are encountered as RBCs traverse a stenotic valve (Figure 74–1*B* and *C*) or a ventricular septal defect. If a method called pulsed or range-gated Doppler is used, the exact point of the velocity measurement can be determined. This is done by having the operator direct a depth-range "gate" that is superimposed over a cross-sectional image. This method, called pulsed Doppler, can be used to provide accurate information about the anatomic site of the RBC velocity and relative direction of flow (Figure 74–1*A*). If a method called color-flow mapping is used, hundreds of pulsed Doppler sample volumes can be overlayed on the cross-sectional anatomic image. The Doppler shift is then coded in color (red, toward; blue, away from the transducer origin), and the intensity of color is used to indicate the relative velocities of the RBCs at that exact point in the image. Turbulent blood flow can be detected using special "turbulence" or "variance" maps. This complex imaging method, which combines cross-sectional imaging, pulsed Doppler, and color designation of RBC direction and velocity, is called *color-flow imaging;* this technique is the noninvasive equivalent of the angiogram. Blood can be followed through the heart during phases of the cardiac cycle and abnormal flow assessed.

The modern "echodoppler" study proceeds as follows: (1) anatomic detail, cardiac function, and cardiac dimensions are determined by two-dimensional and M-mode echocardiography; (2) color-flow imaging (when available) or contrast echocardiography is used to detect abnormal blood flow; (3) pulsed Doppler is used to detect anatomic areas of high-velocity blood flow in the heart and great vessels; (4) high velocity flow is quantitated using continuous-wave Doppler. While the methods and calculations employed in these studies are beyond the scope of this chapter, one important calculation that is often used in evaluation of congenital heart disease is the modified Bernoulli equation, whereby the pressure drop across a stenosis or ventricular septal defect is estimated as Pressure Gradient = 4 (peak V)^2. When high velocity flow is detected, as in Figure

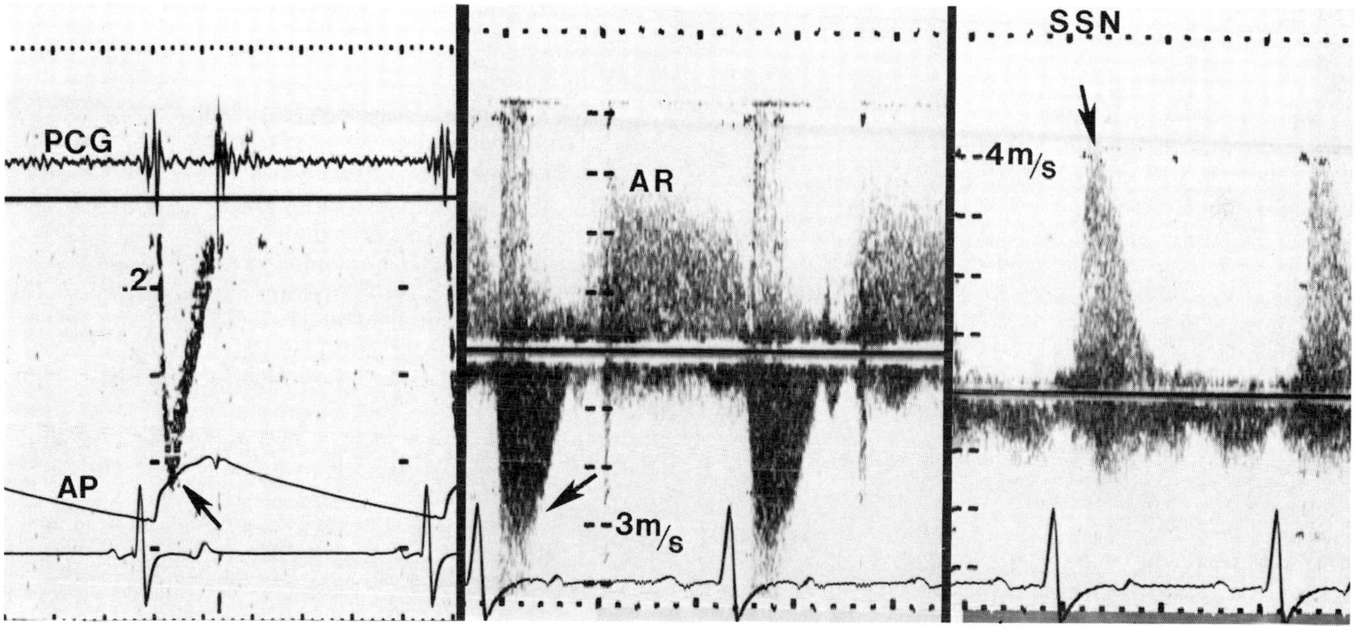

FIGURE 74–1. Pulsed and continuous-wave Doppler recordings obtained from a normal anesthesized dog (left) and a Newfoundland dog with discrete subaortic stenosis. The left panel demonstrates a normal velocity profile obtained across the aortic valve. A simultaneous phonocardiogram (PCG), arterial pressure (AP) tracing, and ECG are included to demonstrate the timing of the velocity waveform. The transducer was located at the left apex; therefore, the signal is negative or below the zero baseline (the calibration is 0.2 m/s per division). The center panel demonstrates high-velocity systolic flow across the region of the aortic valve (arrow) in a dog with left ventricular outflow obstruction. There is aortic regurgitation (AR) as well, indicated by the positive, high velocity diastolic signal. Another continuous-wave study (right panel) was obtained in this dog with the transducer located at the suprasternal notch and the echo beam directed into the ascending aorta and ventricular outflow tract. A high-velocity flow of approximately 4 m/s was recorded. The pressure gradient is estimated to be at least 64 mm Hg. (The calibration is 1.0 m/s per division.)

74–1*C*, the peak velocity can be used to estimate the pressure gradient across the obstruction and can be used to assess the severity of the defect and the need for surgical intervention. The interested reader is referred to the work of Hatle and Angelsen for greater detail.

The following are examples of questions that can be answered by echocardiography: Are there two ventricles and two atria? Are the ventricular walls hypertrophied? Are the atria or ventricular dimensions increased? Is there dilation of the aorta or pulmonary artery? Can the atrioventricular and semilunar valves be identified and do they appear normal? Are there obvious defects in the cardiac septa? Are the ventricular outflow tracts patent or stenotic?

ELECTROCARDIOGRAPHY

The electrocardiogram (ECG) is quite helpful in cases of congenital heart disease. While a normal ECG does not rule out a cardiac malformation, an abnormal ECG helps to rule out certain defects and increase the likelihood of others (see Figures 74–2 to 74–4).[5, 9, 15] For example, a normal ECG axis with increased QRS voltages is typical of patent ductus arteriosus but unlikely in pulmonic stenosis or tricuspid dysplasia. Left axis deviation may indicate left ventricular hypertrophy or congenital left anterior fascicular block. Persistence of a right ventricular hypertrophy pattern after the first few weeks of age in the dog is abnormal[31] and highly suggestive of pulmonic stenosis, tetralogy of Fallot, tricuspid dysplasia, atrial septal defect, large ventricular septal defect, or pulmonary hypertension. Right ventricular hypertrophy can also lead to conduction delay in the ECG with right axis deviation and widening of the QRS complex.[5, 32] Occasionally, the presence of congenital right bundle branch block may suggest an erroneous diagnosis of right ventricular hypertrophy in an animal with a left heart lesion, but as a general rule this finding is very suggestive of the aforementioned right-sided defects.

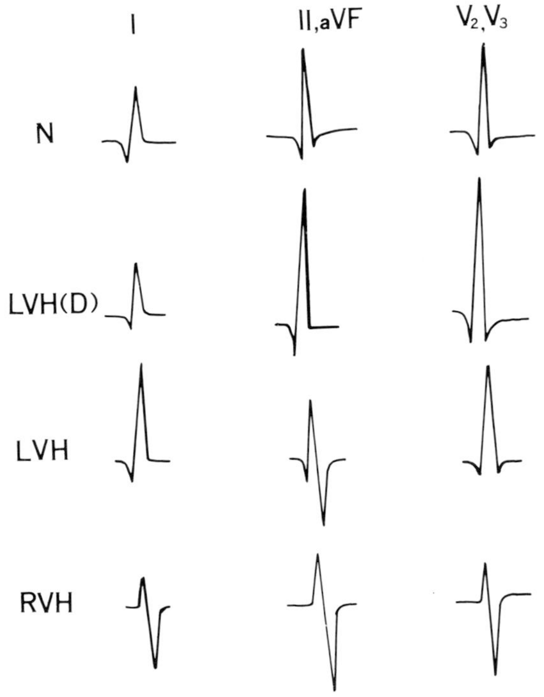

FIGURE 74–2. Electrocardiographic patterns of ventricular enlargement. Typical QRS complexes are shown for normal dogs (N), left ventricular hypertrophy and dilation (LVH (D)), left ventricular concentric hypertrophy (LVH), and right ventricular hypertrophy (RVH). Typical patterns for leads I, II, aV_F, and left precordial leads V_2, V_3 are shown.

ANGIOCARDIOGRAPHY AND CARDIAC CATHETERIZATION

Cardiac catheterization is an invasive procedure useful for the diagnosis of structural malformation of the heart and assessment of physiological derangements caused by these anatomical lesions.[5, 15, 24–26, 33–35] To many cardiologists, selective angiocardiograms plus catheterization data represent the "gold standard" by which to identify and assess congenital heart disease. While Doppler echocardiography is often superior to angiocardiography in the identification of anatomical defects (endocardial cushion defects exemplify this point), determination of intravascular pressures, cardiac output, and oximetry may profoundly affect the treatment of the patient.

Angiocardiography. Selective angiocardiography identifies most of the common congenital heart defects. The author's general approach is to perform both right and left ventriculograms and to record the movement of blood (contrast material) during the next 10 to 20 seconds. A supravalvular aortic injection is also performed and the movement of blood followed for 8 to 10 seconds. The right ventriculogram can generally identify the following lesions: tricuspid regurgitation, double-chambered right ventricle, pulmonic stenosis or atresia, right to left shunting ventricular septal defect, tetralogy of Fallot (and pseudotruncus arteriosus), transposition of the great vessels, truncus arteriosus, aorticopulmonary communication (with pulmonary hypertension), reversed patent ductus arteriosus, and abnormal pulmonary vascularity owing to pulmonary hypertension or vascular disease.

Following return of contrast to the left side of the heart from the right ventricular (or pulmonary artery) injection, the following lesions can generally be identified: anomalous pulmonary venous return (to the right atrium), atrial septal defect (left to right shunting), mitral stenosis, and subaortic and aortic valve stenosis. The left ventriculogram can usually identify mitral regurgitation, ventricular septal defect (left to right shunting), subaortic and aortic valve stenosis, truncus arteriosus (and pseudotruncus arteriosus), and supravalvular lesions listed below under the aortogram.

The aortogram generally delineates aortic regurgitation; subaortic, subpulmonic ventricular septal defect with prolapse of an aortic valve leaflet into the defect; abnormal coronary arteries; aorticopulmonary communication (left to right shunting); coarctation of the aorta; patent ductus arteriosus (left to right shunting); and abnormal pulmonary collateral circulation (bronchoesophageal circulation).

Additional injections of contrast media are indicated for identification of specific lesions. For example, injec-

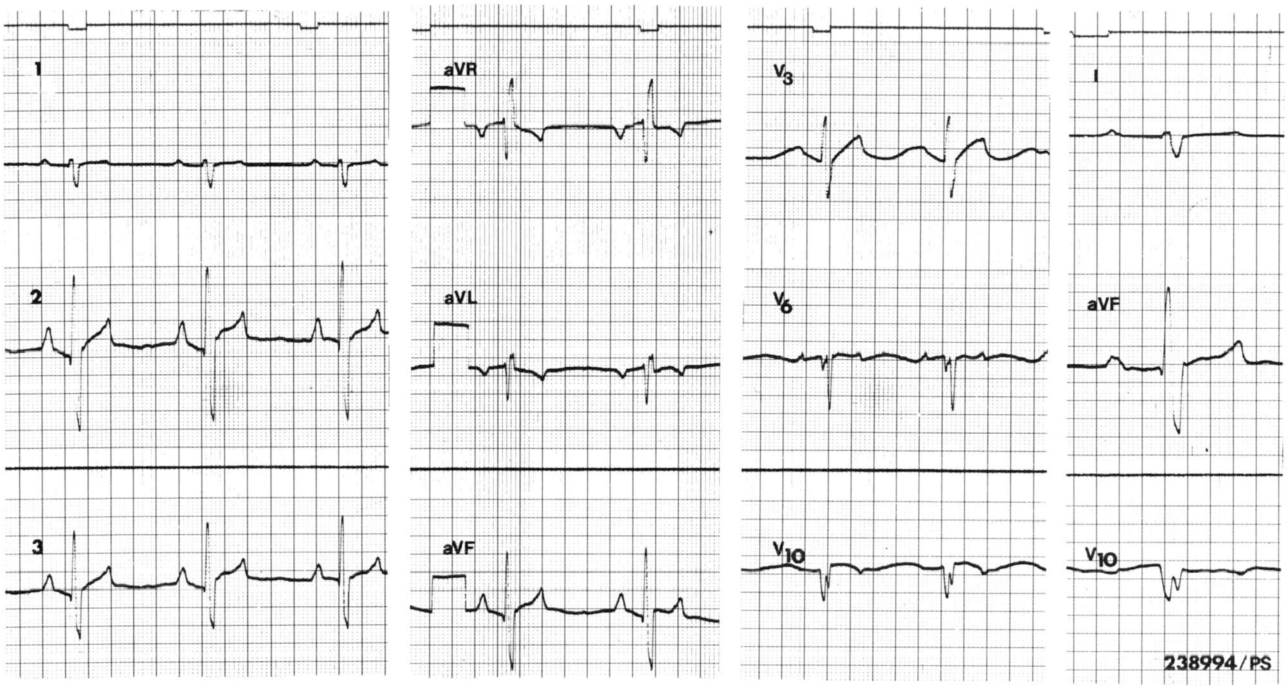

FIGURE 74–3A. Atrial enlargement and right ventricular hypertrophy in a dog with pulmonic stenosis. A right axis deviation in the frontal plane, with prominent S waves in leads 1, 2, 3, aVF, V_3, and V_6, is typical of right ventricular hypertrophy. P waves in lead 2 are quite prominent, which may also indicate atrial enlargement. 1 mV calibration is shown; paper speed = 50 mm/sec except for the right panel, which is 100 mm/sec.

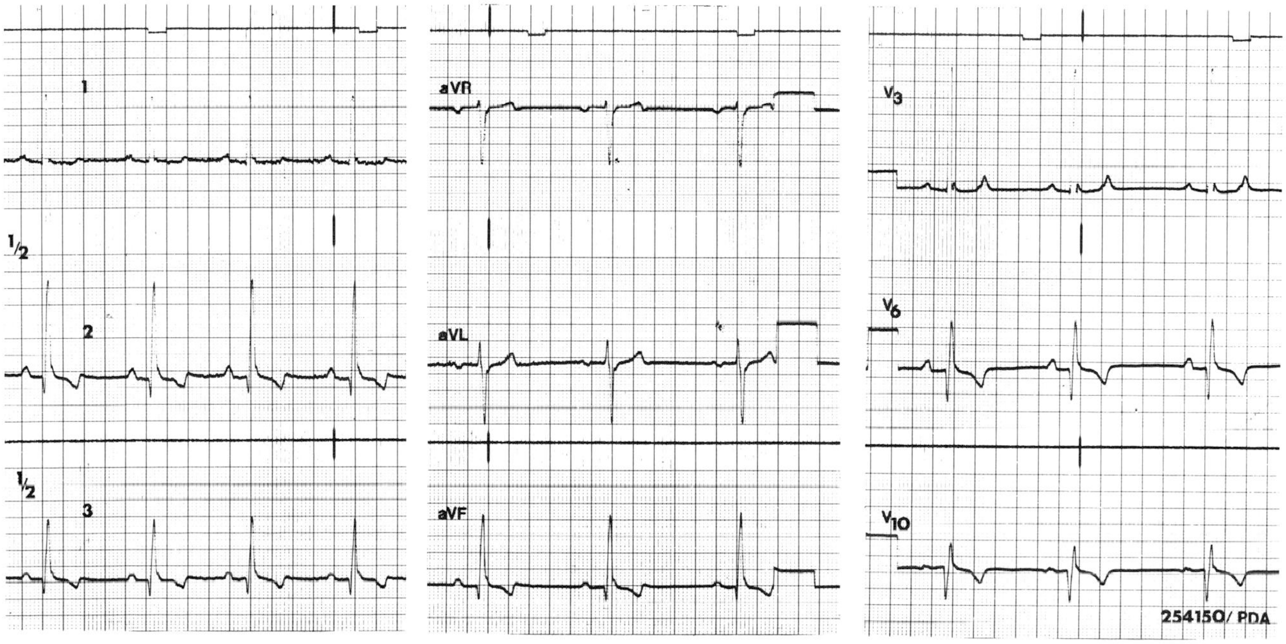

FIGURE 74–3B. Electrocardiogram from a dog with patent ductus arteriosus. The frontal axis is normal but there are increased voltages in leads 2, aVF, and 3. R-wave amplitude in V_3 is also large, exceeding 5 mvolts. Leads 2, 3, aVR, aVL, and V_3 are recorded at 5 mm = 1 mV; all other leads are at standard sensitivity; paper speed = 50 mm/sec.

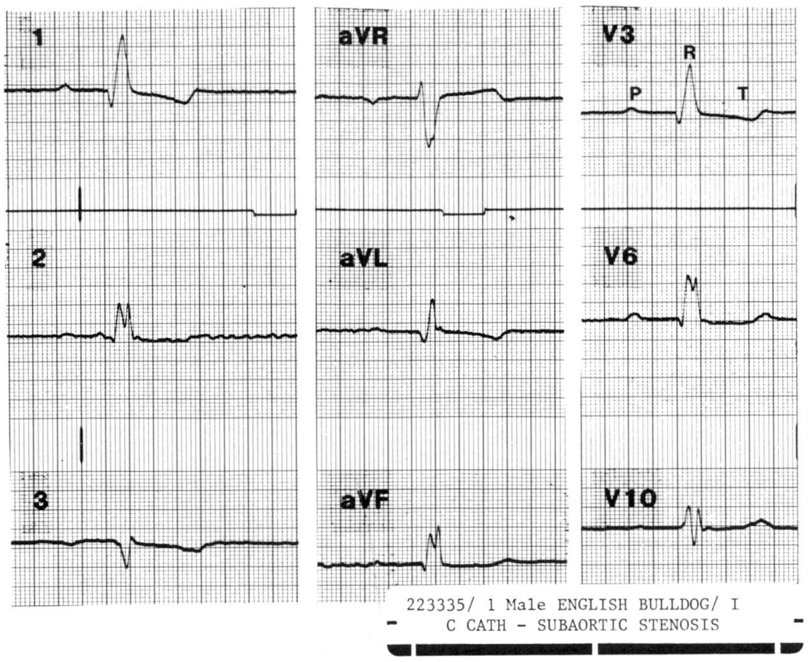

FIGURE 74–4. Electrocardiogram from a dog with congenital subaortic stenosis. The frontal axis is deviated to the left as evidenced by the prominent R-waves in leads 1 and aVL. The QRS duration is slightly prolonged and there is a minor ventricular conduction disturbance noted in lead 2 and lead aVF. The absence of S waves in leads 1 and V_3 militates against right ventricular enlargement.

tion of contrast into the left jugular vein identifies persistent left cranial vena cava. A right atrial injection is needed to document right to left shunting atrial septal defect or hypoplasia/atresia of the tricuspid valve and right ventricle. Abnormal position of the angiocardiographic catheter may also delineate a lesion as when an atrioventricular septal defect is crossed.

Cardiac Catheterization. Cardiac catheterization allows the clinician to sample blood for hemoglobin oxygen saturation (oximetry), measure cardiac output and stroke volume, perform qualitative indicator dilution studies, and record intravascular pressure abnormalities. While the reader is directed to the references for a more complete description of catheterization data,[5, 15, 33] some principles of interpretation are germane to this chapter (Figure 74–5).

Pressures should be equal across an opened cardiac valve. Thus, with valve stenosis there is a pressure gradient (an increase in pressure behind the stenosis, relative to the pressure distal to the valve), which is a crude indicator of the severity of obstruction (Figures 74–6 and 74–7). A diastolic gradient across an atrioventricular valve is indicative of mitral or tricuspid stenosis, while a systolic gradient across a semilunar valve denotes pulmonic or aortic stenosis. Such gradients are dependent on transvalvular flow and may be artificially diminished by heart failure, anesthetic agents, hypovolemia (from diuretics), or combinations of lesions that reduce transvalvular flow across the narrowed region (examples include mitral stenosis with aortic stenosis and tricuspid regurgitation with pulmonic stenosis). It should be mentioned that a gradient does not necessarily indicate valvular stenosis when there is a large left to right shunt as with atrioventricular septal defects. A systolic gradient of between 5 and 25 mm Hg is quite common in these cases and can be attributed to "relative" pulmonic stenosis, the physiologic obstruction caused by a tremendous volume of blood traversing a normal valve.

Normally there is a marked disparity between the systolic pressures of the systemic and pulmonary circulations. Systolic pressure within the left ventricle and aorta is approximately 120 mm Hg, while systolic pressures in the right ventricle and pulmonary artery are typically 25 to 30 mm Hg.[5] Since right and left ventricular outputs are virtually identical, the pulmonary vascular resistance must be markedly lower (approximately 12 per cent of the systemic resistance). Thus, if a communication exists between systemic and pulmonary circulations, blood will shunt from a higher pressure to a lower pressure system; i.e., left to right. Largely patent ductus arteriosus and (nonrestrictive) atrioventricular septal defects commonly lead to significant left to right shunting with marked pulmonary overperfusion. Catheterization will document the disparity in pressures in most cases; however, it is emphasized that measurement of peak systolic pressures may not necessarily indicate the tendency towards shunting because resistance is the key factor. For example, with a large ventricular septal defect, the ventricles will behave as a common chamber, and will equilibrate systolic pressures, and blood will preferentially flow out the path of least resistance. If the pulmonary resistance is normal, a tremendous left to right shunt will develop. If there is pulmonic stenosis or elevated pulmonary vascular resistance, then shunting will either be minimal, bidirectional, or right to left.

It is emphasized that measurement of pulmonary artery pressure alone does not accurately reflect the state of pulmonary vascular resistance. Pulmonary hypertension may result from either increases in flow through the lung, increased pulmonary vascular resistance, or both (pressure is proportional to flow × resistance). Unless cardiac output is measured by thermodilution or indicator dilution techniques, the clinician may be uncertain if pulmonary hypertension represents high flow (an indication for pulmonary artery banding or surgery) or high resistance (a contraindication for

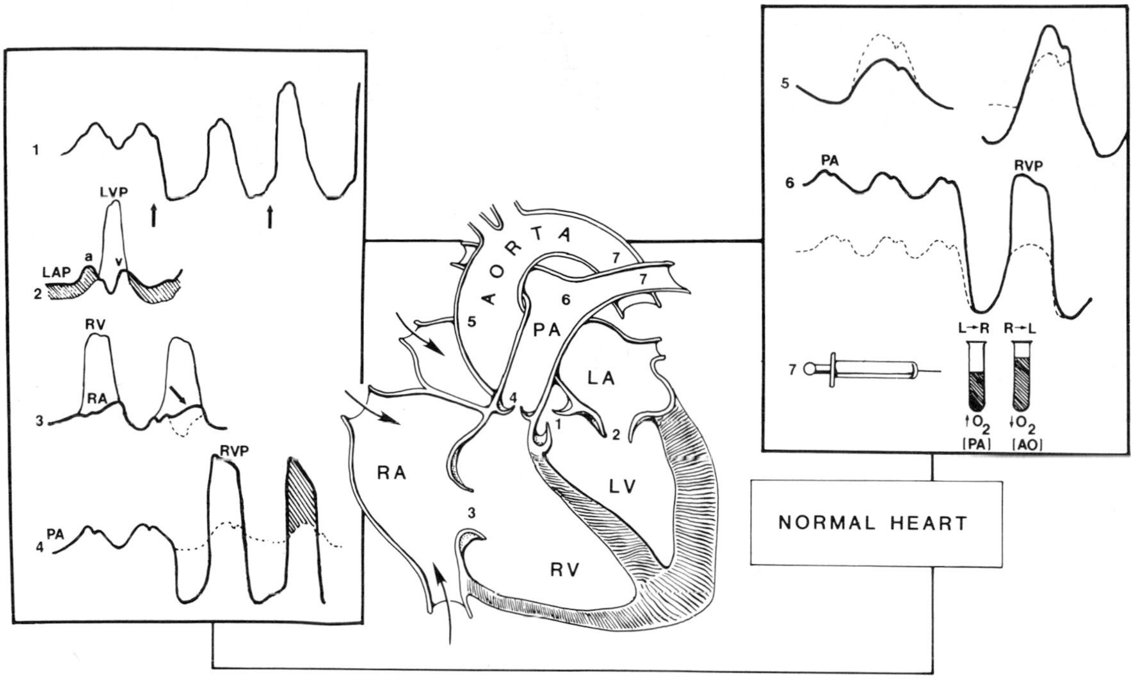

FIGURE 74–5. Illustration of a normal heart with potential hemodynamic abnormalities associated with congenital heart disease. Each curve corresponds to the numbered anatomic area. 1 = example of a pressure profile obtained by pushing the catheter from the aorta into the left ventricle (first arrow). If there is subaortic stenosis, the initial ventricular systole pressure will be identical to that of the aorta; however, as the catheter is advanced behind the obstruction (second arrow), the left ventricular systolic pressure increases and there is an obvious pressure gradient. Left ventricular end diastolic pressure (second arrow) may be high if there is left ventricular hypertrophy with increased stiffness or if there is left ventricular failure. 2 = superimposed left atrial and left ventricular pressures in a case of mitral dysplasia leading to mitral stenosis. The left atrial pressure exceeds the left ventricular pressure during diastole, which is not normal. The difference in pressure (crosshatched area) is the diastolic gradient and is an index of the severity of obstruction. 3 = changes in the right atrial pressure curve as a result of tricuspid regurgitation due to tricuspid valve dysplasia. Normally the right atrial pressure curve dips and is negative during ventricular systole (dotted line); however, with tricuspid regurgitation, increases in atrial pressure during systole may be recorded (arrow). With severe tricuspid regurgitation, the right atrial pressure curve may resemble that of the right ventricle, a situation termed ventricularization of the right atrial pressure curve. 4 = ventricular systolic pressure increases as a result of pulmonic stenosis. The dotted line shows the anticipated right ventricular systolic (but *not* the diastolic) pressure in the normal situation; however, as a result of stenosis there is an increase in systolic pressure (crosshatched area). 5 = alterations in the arterial pressure profile as a result of aortic stenosis *(left)* or patent ductus arteriosus *(right)*. Obstruction to left ventricular outflow causes a late rising pulse, while abnormal diastolic runoff leads to a low diastolic pressure and hyperkinetic pulse. The dotted lines indicate the approximate normal pressure profile. 6 = pulmonary hypertension with resultant increases in right ventricular systolic pressure. The dotted lines indicate the normal situation. Note that the right ventricular systolic pressure increase is not accompanied by a pressure gradient. 7 = oxygen saturation is altered when there is cardiac shunting. In left to right shunts, the pulmonary arterial oxygen saturation is increased, whereas with right to left shunts the aortic oxygen saturation is decreased and polycythemia may result from secondary increases in erythropoietin.

FIGURE 74–6. Left ventricular pressures obtained from an anesthetized dog with aortic stenosis. In the right panel the left ventricular pressure is superimposed on the aortic pressure curve. The crosshatched area indicates the pressure gradient in this dog. The panel on the left is taken at two different sensitivities. The last four ventricular pressure curves are recorded at the same sensitivity as the right panel. Notice the prominent atrial contribution to ventricular pressure (arrows), which probably indicates ventricular hypertrophy and stiffness. The elevated left ventricular end diastolic pressure is due, in large part, to this vigorous atrial contraction. The transducer was open to air and then closed to record pressure (lower arrow).

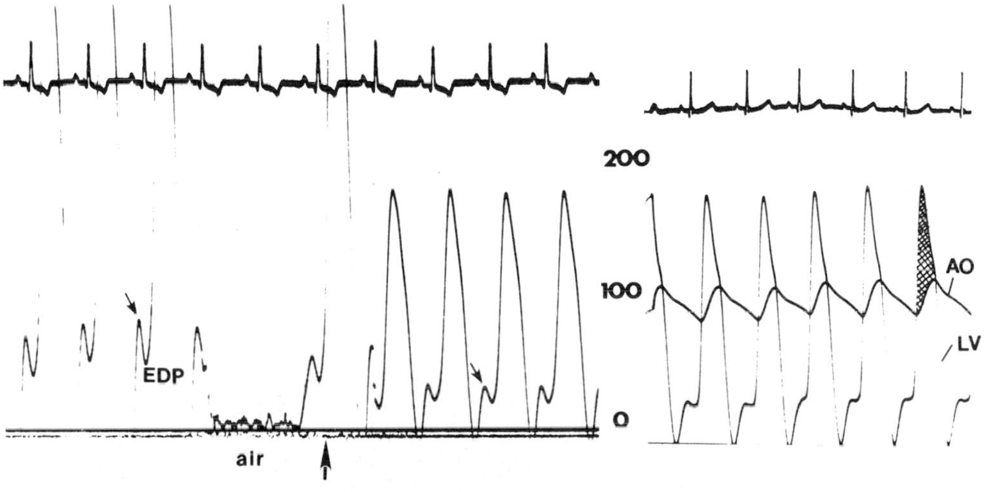

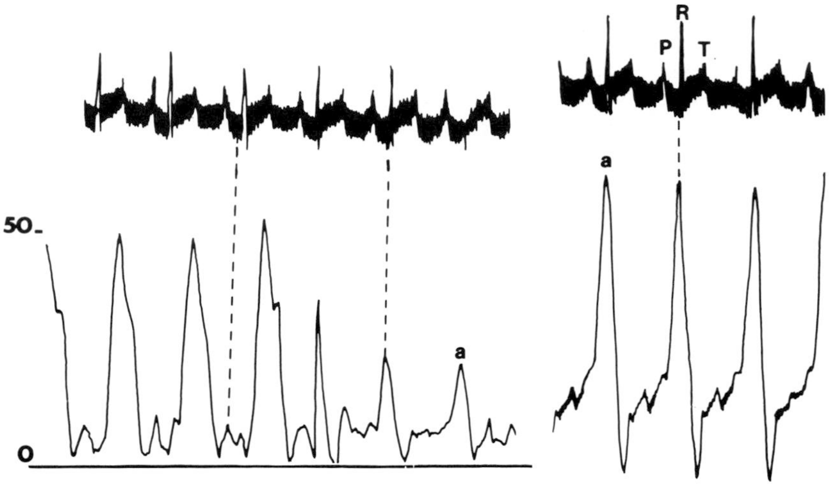

FIGURE 74–7. Right ventricular and right atrial pressure recordings showing a diastolic gradient in a dog with tricuspid dysplasia and tricuspid stenosis. The panel at the left shows the pull back from the right ventricle into the right atrium. Notice that the diastolic pressure (dashed lines) is relatively low in the right ventricle but is markedly higher in the right atrium. A vigorous atrial contraction (a) is obvious, particularly in the higher sensitivity recording at the right. This clearly shows that the increase in atrial pressure develops following atrial activation but before ventricular contraction. (Curves were retraced.)

most surgeries). Fortunately, other features such as oximetry and the peripheral perfusion of the lung on the thoracic x-ray film can provide insight about vascular resistance in these cases.

When cardiac catheterization reveals elevation of ventricular end-diastolic pressure, a number of hemodynamic abnormalities must be considered: ventricular hypertrophy or endocardial fibrosis with increased diastolic ventricular stiffness, volume overloading as with cardiac shunting or incompetent valves, ventricular failure, semilunar valve regurgitation, pericardial disease, or a combination of these problems (Figure 74–8).

Aortic and arterial pulse pressure characteristics can be altered in congenital disease by obstruction to left ventricular outflow, decreased cardiac output, hypovolemia, and abnormal aortic run-off. The arterial pulse of aortic stenosis is typically late-rising or hypokinetic. In situations of abnormal diastolic run-off, as with patent ductus arteriosus or aortic regurgitation, the pulse is bounding (hyperkinetic), characterized by a large left ventricular stroke volume and systolic hypertension and a decreased diastolic pressure. The arterial pulse pressure (systolic minus diastolic) may be diminished with ventricular failure or decreased stroke volume.

Hemoglobin oxygen saturation (per cent) and blood oxygen content (ml O_2/dl blood) depend on the partial pressure of oxygen, characteristics of the hemoglobin-oxygen dissociation curve, and the hemoglobin concentration.[15, 33] When oxygen saturations are recorded from the right and left circulations, oxygen step-ups or step-downs may be detected. For example, a marked increase in oxygen saturation (or content) in the right ventricular outflow tract suggests left to right shunting ventricular septal defect. Right to left shunting leads to desaturation of arterial blood beginning at the level of the shunt. Formulae have been devised to estimate the degree of cardiac shunting using oxygen content and indicator dilution techniques.[33, 35]

A word of caution is appropriate relative to oxygen saturation values on the right side of the heart. While the oxygen saturation values from mitral valve to left ventricle to ascending aorta to descending aorta normally are within one to two per cent of each other, the right atrium receives blood from a variety of sources, each with a different oxygen saturation, and there is incomplete mixing of blood in this chamber. Our experience has been to consistently measure the lowest oxygen saturation at the coronary sinus, and to find the cranial vena cava to be higher than the azygous vein or caudal vena cava in samples from anesthetized dogs breathing 33 per cent oxygen. Thus, caution must be exercised in attempting to diagnose atrial septal defects using single "high right atrial" samples compared with those within the right ventricle. While differences of greater than five per cent saturation are suspicious for shunting, even these differences can be encountered within the right atrium of some dogs who do not have intracardiac shunting.

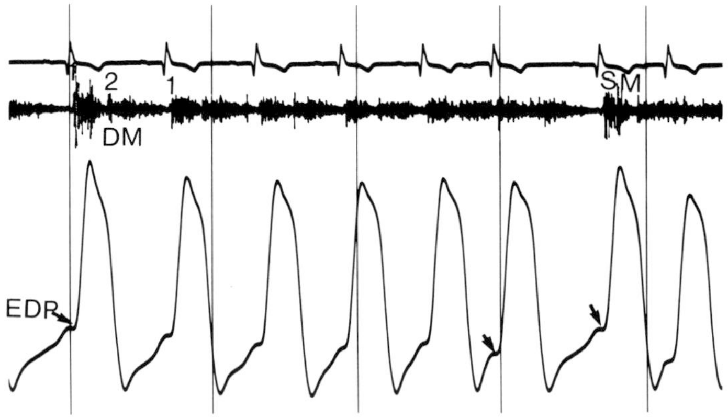

FIGURE 74–8. Left ventricular pressure curves obtained from a dog with congenital subaortic stenosis, aortic regurgitation, and heart failure. The ECG, phonocardiogram, and left ventricular pressure trace are shown. The first and second heart sounds, the diastolic murmur (DM) and the systolic murmur (SM) are indicated. The left ventricular end-diastolic pressure is quite high, but the development of maximum end-diastolic pressure (EDP) is more gradual than occurred in the animal in Figure 74–6. This is explained by the aortic regurgitation. Longer cardiac cycles permit increased regurgitation and more dramatic increases in left ventricular end-diastolic pressure (arrows).

CAUSES, PREVALENCE, AND CLASSIFICATION OF CONGENITAL HEART DISEASE

Causes of Cardiac Malformation

Congenital cardiac defects may develop as a result of genetic, environmental, chromosomal, infectious, toxicologic, nutritional, and drug-related factors.[17-21] Little is known about nongenetic factors as they pertain to spontaneous congenital heart disease in the dog and cat. Surveys of cats suggest that some breeds are predisposed to certain malformations. More is known about genetically transmitted defects in specific canine breeds (Table 74–2).

The elegant studies of Patterson and associates have clearly demonstrated a genetic basis for congenital heart disease in the dog. As discussed in the section on singular cardiac lesions, most studies suggest a polygenic basis for transmission. As stated by Patterson, "these genetic factors have specific effects on cardiac morphogenesis, resulting in specific types of cardiovascular malformations."[20] Multiple genes have an additive effect and produce a discrete phenotypic trait once a threshold has been attained. Such patterns of inheritance explain the spectrum of subclinical to severe malformations found in families of dogs with conotruncal septal defects and tetralogy of Fallot.[2] Unfortunately, the absence of a simple (Mendelian) mode of genetic transmission makes counseling of breeders difficult. Without careful attention to pedigree and results of future breeding trials, it may be difficult to eliminate or reduce the prevalence of cardiac defects in certain breeds. The interested reader is referred to Patterson's studies for more detail.[1-4]

Prevalence of Congenital Heart Disease. The exact prevalence of congenital heart disease in the dog and cat cannot be stated with certainty. Clearly, there are some regional differences in the recognition of specific malformations within certain breeds. The largest surveys suggest that patent ductus arteriosus is the most common malformation in the dog, and either atrioventricular septal defect or atrioventricular valve dysplasia most common among cats. A compilation of congenital heart defects has been reported by Patterson and Detweiler in dogs and by Liu and by Harpster in cats.[2, 12, 14, 36] In the largest survey of dogs, 325 malformations were detected in 290 dogs, and the overall prevalence in a university hospital canine population was 6.8 per 1,000 dogs.[1, 2, 14] The frequency of diagnoses in these 290 dogs was approximately 28 per cent for patent ductus arteriosus, 20 per cent for pulmonic stenosis, 14 per cent for aortic stenosis, 8 per cent for persistent right aortic arch, 7 per cent for ventricular septal defect, and less than 5 per cent for tetralogy of Fallot, persistent left cranial vena cava, and atrial septal defects.

Harpster's review of congenital heart disease in cats summarizes data from the literature, Angell Memorial Animal Hospital, and the Animal Medical Center. The prevalence of congenital heart disease was between 2 and 10 cats per 1,000 admissions and included a total of 287 reported anomalies. Atrioventricular septal defects (including ventricular septal defect, atrial septal defect, and endocardial cushion defect) accounted for approximately 24 per cent, atrioventricular valve dysplasia 17 per cent, endocardial fibroelastosis 11.5 per cent, patent ductus arteriosus 11 per cent, aortic stenosis 6 per cent, and tetralogy of Fallot 6 per cent of the reported diagnoses. Males were affected nearly twice as often as females in the series reported by Harpster.[36]

Table 74–4 is a compilation of the more frequently recognized congenital cardiac defects in the dog and the

TABLE 74–4. CARDIOVASCULAR MALFORMATIONS IN THE DOG AND CAT

Canine
Most common defects
Patent ductus arteriosus
Pulmonic stenosis
Subaortic stenosis
Atrioventricular valve dysplasia
Persistent right aortic arch
Ventricular septal defect
Tetralogy of Fallot
Peritoneopericardial diaphragmatic hernia
Persistent left cranial vena cava
Uncommon
Aortic interruption/hypoplasia
Aortic stenosis (valvular)
Aorticopulmonary window
Anomalous pulmonary venous return
Arteriovenous fistula
Coarctation of the aorta
Cor triatriatum
Double aortic arch
Double-chambered right ventricle
Double-outlet right ventricle
Ebstein's anomaly of the tricuspid valve
Endocardial cushion defect
Endocardial fibroelastosis
Ostium secundum atrial septal defect
Pulmonic valve insufficiency
Retroesophageal subclavian artery
Situs inversus
Vascular anomalies
Electrocardiographic disturbance
Right bundle branch block
Ventricular pre-excitation
Feline
Most common defects
Atrioventricular septal defects
Atrial septal defect
Endocardial cushion defect
Ventricular septal defect
Atrioventricular valve dysplasia
Mitral valve dysplasia
Tricuspid valve dysplasia
Patent ductus arteriosus
Endocardial fibroelastosis
Aortic stenosis
Tetralogy of Fallot
Peritoneopericardial hernia
Persistent right aortic arch
Pulmonic stenosis
Uncommon defects
Atrial malformation
Cor triatriatum
Anomalous right atrium
Double outlet right ventricle
Truncus arteriosus
Taussig-Bing complex
Vascular malformation
Anomaly of the vena cava
Stenosis of pulmonary vein

cat while Table 74–2 summarizes some of the breed predispositions recognized in dogs with congenital heart disease.

Classification of Congenital Heart Disease. While a number of classification systems can be used to classify congenital heart defects, the author has chosen to discuss clinically important malformations as follows:

Systemic to pulmonary shunting
- Patent ductus arteriosus
- Aorticopulmonary window (see vascular anomalies)
- Atrioventricular septal defects
  - Atrial septal defects
  - Ventricular septal defects
  - Endocardial cushion defects
- Anomalous pulmonary venous return

Malformations of cardiac valves
- Obstruction to right ventricular outflow
  - Pulmonic stenosis
  - Tetralogy of Fallot (see cyanotic heart disease)
  - Double-chambered right ventricle
- Obstruction to left ventricular outflow
  - Subaortic stenosis
  - Aortic stenosis
  - Supravalvular aortic stenosis
  - Coarctation of the aorta (see vascular lesions)
- Dysplasia of the mitral valve
- Dysplasia of the tricuspid valve

Cyanotic heart disease
- Eisenmenger physiology (reversed shunting—see systemic to pulmonary shunting)
- Tricuspid atresia/right ventricular hypoplasia
- Tetralogy of Fallot
- Transposition of the great vessels
- Double outlet right ventricle

Miscellaneous cardiac defects
- Endocardial fibroelastosis
- Anomalous development of the atria
- Multiple cardiac anomalies
- Pericardial defects
- Peritoneopericardial hernia

Vascular anomalies
- Vascular ring anomalies
  - Persistent right aortic arch
- Anomalies of the aorta
  - Aorticopulmonary communication
  - Coarctation
  - Interruption of the aortic arch
- Venous anomalies
- Persistent left cranial vena cava

While this system is somewhat arbitrary and may not be representative of the embryologic basis for maldevelopment, the pathophysiologic basis of clinical signs can be explained using this classification. Obviously, some lesions can be placed in more than one pathophysiologic class while others are quite rare or have been reported only in combination with other defects. Since most defects lead to measurable hemodynamic abnormalities, the reader is urged to review the previous section on cardiac catheterization before considering these individual malformations.

CARDIAC MALFORMATIONS CAUSING SYSTEMIC TO PULMONARY SHUNTING

Patent Ductus Arteriosus

The ductus arteriosus is derived from the left sixth aortic arch and acts to shunt fetal blood from the pulmonary artery to the systemic circulation.[37–42] This function diverts blood away from the unoxygenated fetal lung into the descending aorta, which is the anatomic site of systemic vascular entry for the ductus. Following parturition, the increase in oxygen tension leads to inhibition of local prostaglandins causing functional closure of the ductus, followed by anatomic obliteration during the ensuing weeks of life. Initial closure, probably accomplished by contraction of smooth muscle within the ductus, decreases ductal flow dramatically within the first 12 to 14 hours of life. While the ductus may be probe-patent in pups less than four days of age, it generally closes by seven or eight days post-whelping with histologic studies suggesting even earlier closure.[4, 41, 42] Abnormal patency of the ductus (Figures 74–9 and 74–10) is the most common congenital cardiac defect in the dog, is well recognized in the cat, and has been extensively studied and described.[37–61]

PATHOGENESIS

The failure of ductal closure probably results from histological differences within the wall of the ductus. Whereas the ductal wall contains a loose branching pattern of circumferential smooth muscle in normal pups, with PDA the wall more closely resembles that of the aorta. According to the work of Patterson, Buchanan, and colleagues[4] the increasing genetic liability to patent ductus arteriosus (PDA) represents "extension of the noncontractile wall structure of the aorta to an increasing segment of the ductus arteriosus, progressively impairing its capacity to undergo physiologic closure." The simplest form of this malformation is the ductus diverticulum, a blind funnel-shaped outpouching of the ventral aspect of the aorta. While this lesion can be recognized only by angiography or at the necropsy table, it represents the *forme fruste* of PDA and indicates that the dog possesses genes for this defect.[4, 8, 39–40] Increasing genetic liability results in PDA with left to right shunting or the less common, but more severe, reversed PDA wherein pulmonary hypertension develops, causing bidirectional or right to left flow through the ductus. Mode of transmission is polygenic.

PATHOPHYSIOLOGY

The pathophysiology of PDA with respect to genesis of clinical signs is summarized in Figure 74–11. Owing to the higher aortic than pulmonary blood pressure,

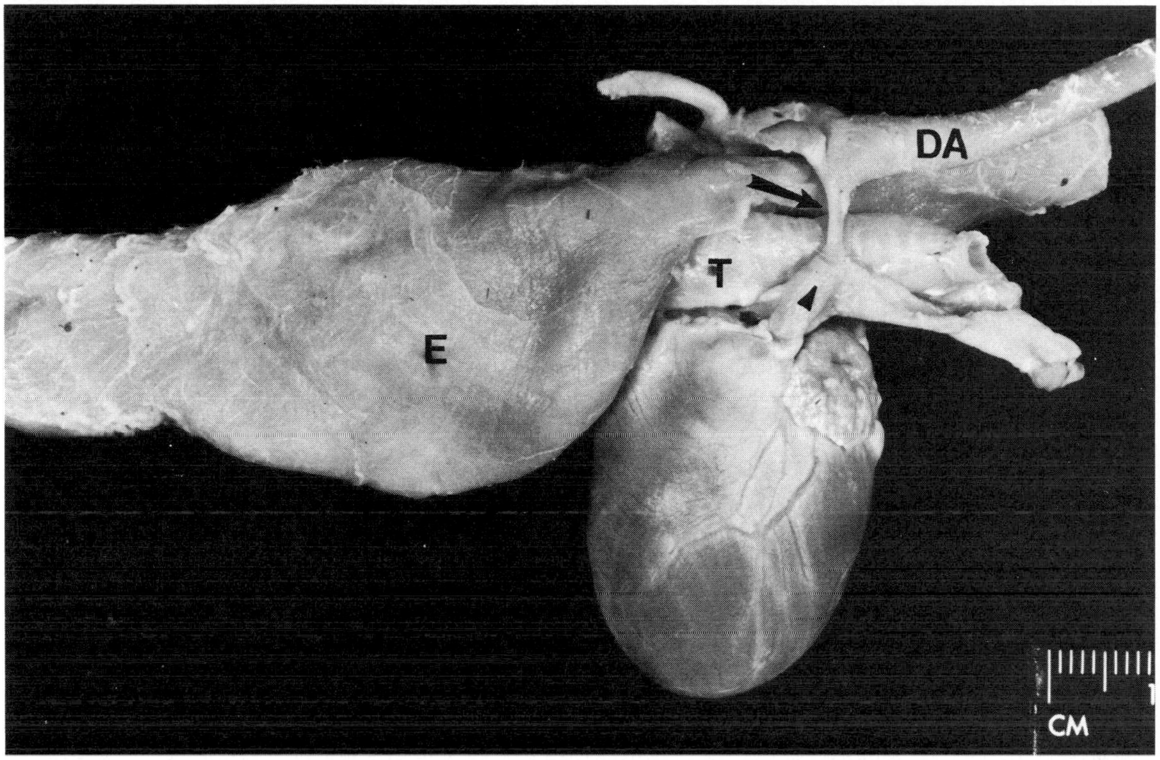

FIGURE 74–9. Left lateral view of the heart, the esophagus, and trachea of a cat with patent ductus arteriosus, right aortic arch, and vascular ring anomaly. The esophagus (E) is dilated proximal to the vascular ring. The trachea (T), ductus arteriosus (large arrow), and the aorta form the vascular ring. In the normal situation, the aortic arch would have formed to the left of the trachea and esophagus and there would not have been entrapment. DA = descending aorta; the junction of the pulmonary artery and the ductus is indicated by the arrowhead.

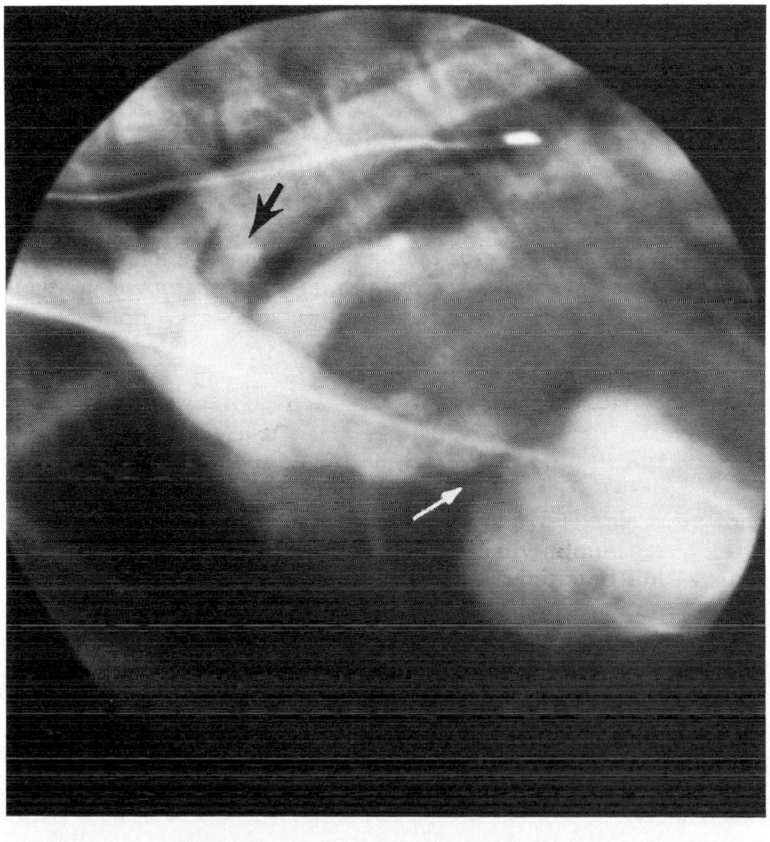

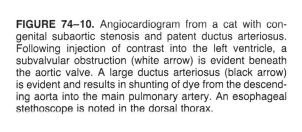

FIGURE 74–10. Angiocardiogram from a cat with congenital subaortic stenosis and patent ductus arteriosus. Following injection of contrast into the left ventricle, a subvalvular obstruction (white arrow) is evident beneath the aortic valve. A large ductus arteriosus (black arrow) is evident and results in shunting of dye from the descending aorta into the main pulmonary artery. An esophageal stethoscope is noted in the dorsal thorax.

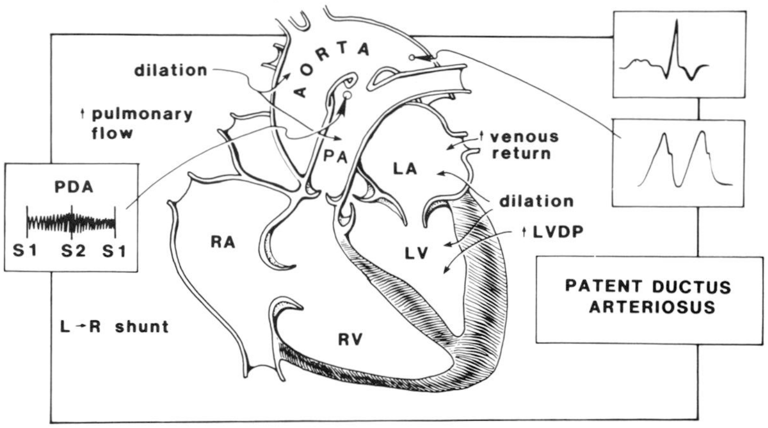

FIGURE 74–11. Schematic illustration of pathophysiologic changes that develop in patent ductus arteriosus. See text for details. (By permission from Bonagura, JD: Congenital heart disease. *In* Bonagura, JD (ed): Cardiology. New York, Churchill Livingstone, 1987.)

blood shunts continuously into the main pulmonary artery. This results in a continuous cardiac murmur, increased pulmonary flow, and increased venous return to the left atrium and left ventricle. Volume overloading of the left side of the heart causes atrial dilatation, ventricular dilatation, and hypertrophy and increases left ventricular diastolic pressure (LVDP). If the luminal defect is large and the pulmonary vascular resistance relatively normal, left ventricular failure with pulmonary edema develops from volume overload. The left ventricular stroke volume increases as a result of increased filling (Frank-Starling principle); however, aortic diastolic pressure is low owing to run-off of blood through the ductus. This causes a hyperkinetic, or waterhammer, arterial pulse. Increased volume flow in the aorta and pulmonary artery, combined with turbulence about the ductus, causes dilation of the aorta and main pulmonary artery. The right ventricle is spared unless there is pulmonary hypertension, in which case ventricular hypertrophy develops.

In a small percentage of cases, the lumen of the PDA is so large that pulmonary vascular pressure and resistance markedly increase. In Patterson's colony, this type of ductus was the most severe and reversal of the shunt developed within the first months of life.[39] This appears to fit the clinical picture in the dog wherein, unlike human patients, documentation of shunt reversal after six months of age is lacking.

Dogs and cats with reversed PDA exhibit high pulmonary vascular resistance, systemic systolic pressures in the right ventricle and pulmonary artery, decreased pulmonary flow, a small left ventricle, and marked hypertrophy of the right ventricle. The exact mechanism by which the pulmonary vascular resistance increases is not completely understood, but anatomic descriptions of the pulmonary vasculature have been described for both humans and animals. Histologic changes within small pulmonary vessels include hypertrophy of the media, thickening of the intima, and plexiform lesions of the vessel wall.[60, 61]

CLINICAL FINDINGS

The clinical features of PDA have been defined in both breeding colonies and in clinic populations.[1–4, 37–53] Female dogs of certain breeds are at greatest risk for development of PDA (Table 74–2). The Chihuahua, collie, Maltese, poodle, pomeranian, and Shetland sheepdog are frequently affected. Females developed PDA at a rate of 2.49 per 1000 versus 1.45 per 1000 for males.[2] Pups may be clinically healthy or thin, may be tachypneic, and may demonstrate signs of left-sided congestive heart failure. Clinical signs are unlikely to occur until the pulmonary vascular resistance declines.

Left to Right Shunting PDA. Arterial pulses are hyperkinetic, a continuous thrill may be palpated at the craniodorsal cardiac base, and a continuous murmur is audible (Figure 74–12). The point of maximal intensity is over the main pulmonary artery, high on the left base, and radiates cranial to the manubrium and to the right base.[5, 39, 47] Frequently, only the systolic murmur is evident over the mitral area, and this murmur has not been proven to be due to concurrent mitral regurgitation, though mitral incompetency can develop with severe left ventricular dilatation. In the cat, the murmur may be heard best more caudoventrally than in the dog and may be systolic in timing when there is progressive pulmonary hypertension. The left ventricular apical impulse is often displaced caudoventrally. Mucous membranes are pink unless there is left ventricular failure and pulmonary edema.

Electrocardiography indicates left atrial enlargement with widening of the P-waves and left ventricular dilatation characterized by a normal frontal axis and increased voltage Q-waves and R-waves in cranio-caudal leads II, III, and aVF (Figure 74–3*B*). Radiography documents pulmonary overcirculation, dilation of the main pulmonary artery and descending aorta, and left atrial and left ventricular enlargement (Figure 74–13). It is not uncommon in the cat for the left apex to be displaced into the right hemithorax (see Figure 74–14). Echocardiography substantiates cardiac and great vessel enlargement, and spectral and color-flow Doppler echocardiography indicates continuous and abnormal retrograde flow in the pulmonary artery.

Cardiac catheterization and angiocardiography (Figures 74–10 and 74–15) are unnecessary unless intercurrent malformations are strongly suspected. In dogs with PDA, associated cardiac defects are uncommon,[4, 44] and catheterization cannot be justified if noninvasive data support the diagnosis of uncomplicated PDA. Catheterization data may show elevated pulmonary capillary

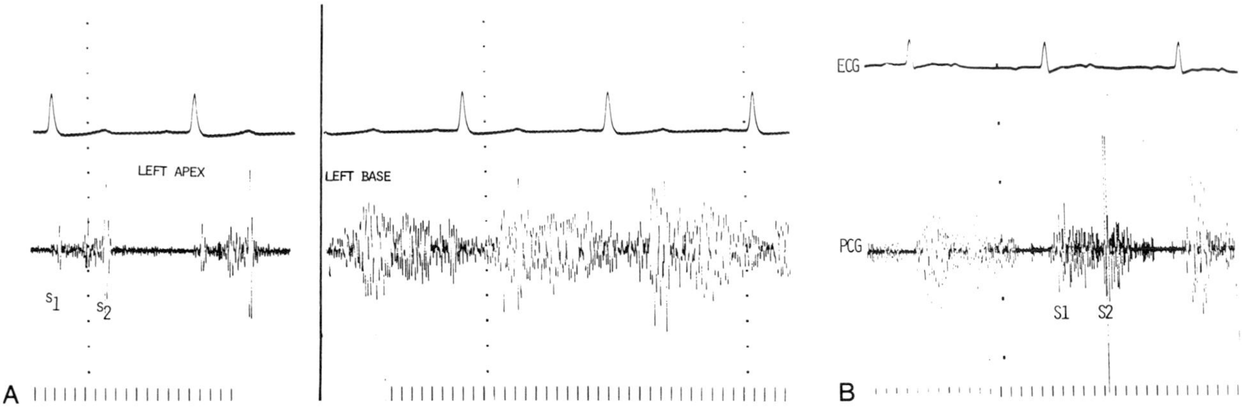

FIGURE 74–12. Phonocardiograms from two dogs with congenital heart disease. Panel A is from a dog with patent ductus arteriosus. The phonocardiogram at the left apex records a predominantly systolic murmur. At the left base the continuous murmur is readily evident. The murmur is quite loud at the time of the second heart sound. B = phonocardiogram from a dog with ventricular septal defect and aortic regurgitation. Both systolic and diastolic murmurs are evident. The second heart sound is prominent.

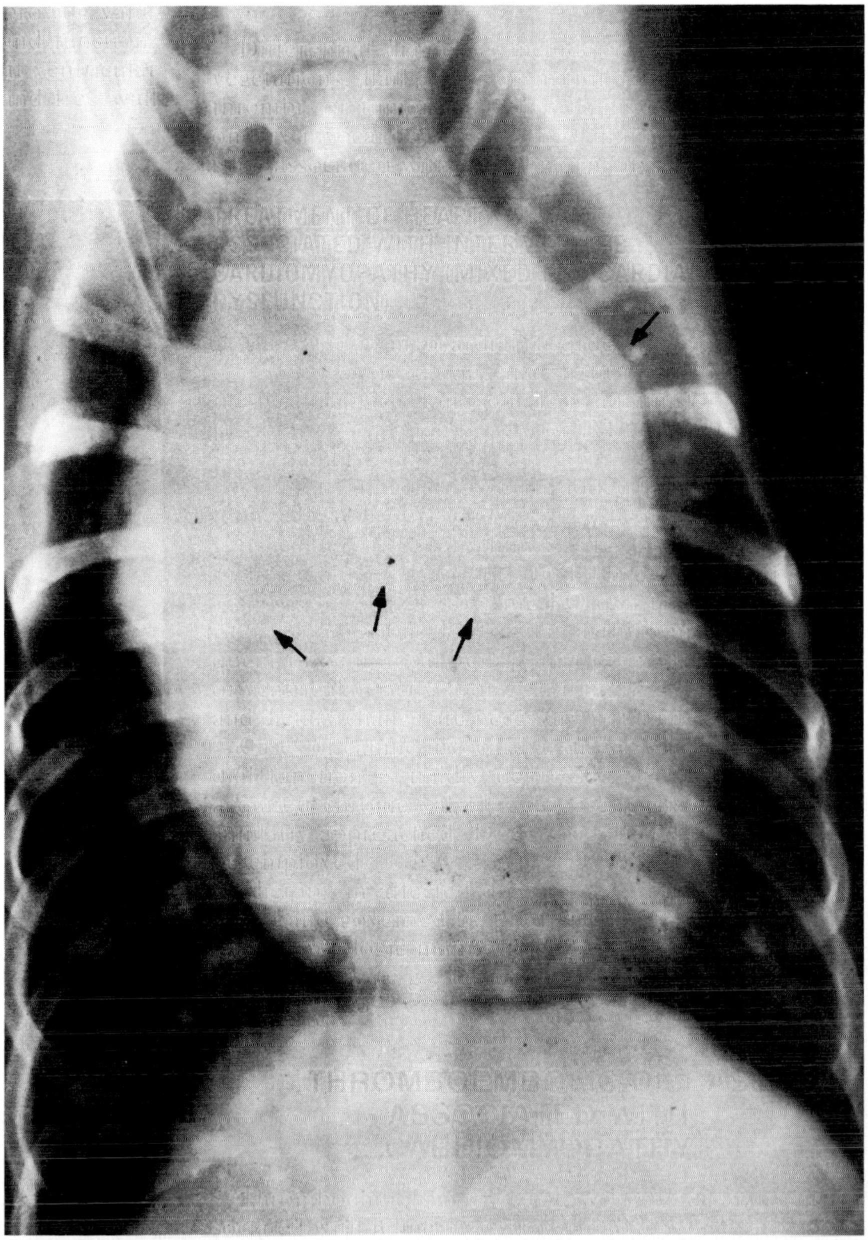

FIGURE 74–13. Ventrodorsal radiograph from a dog with patent ductus arteriosus. The heart is markedly elongated compatible with left ventricular dilation. The left auricle (single arrow) and the left atrium are markedly enlarged. The mainstem bronchi are deviated laterally about the enlarged left atrium (arrows). Pulmonary vascular markings are prominent.

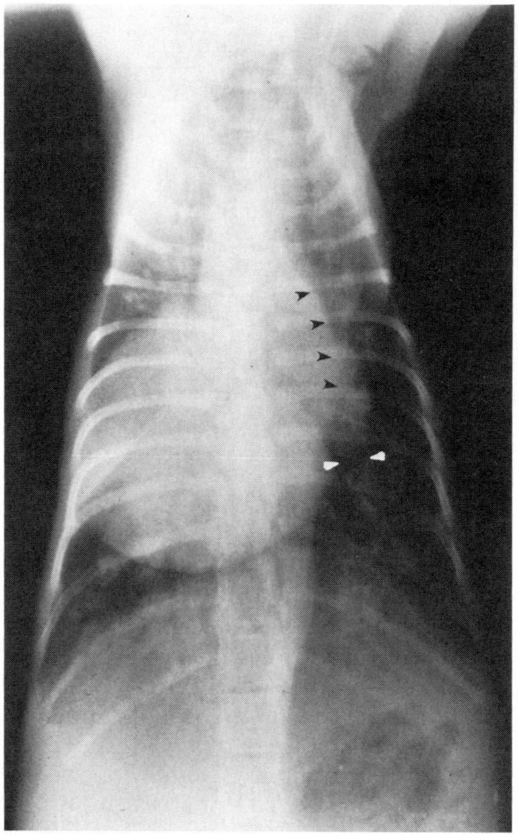

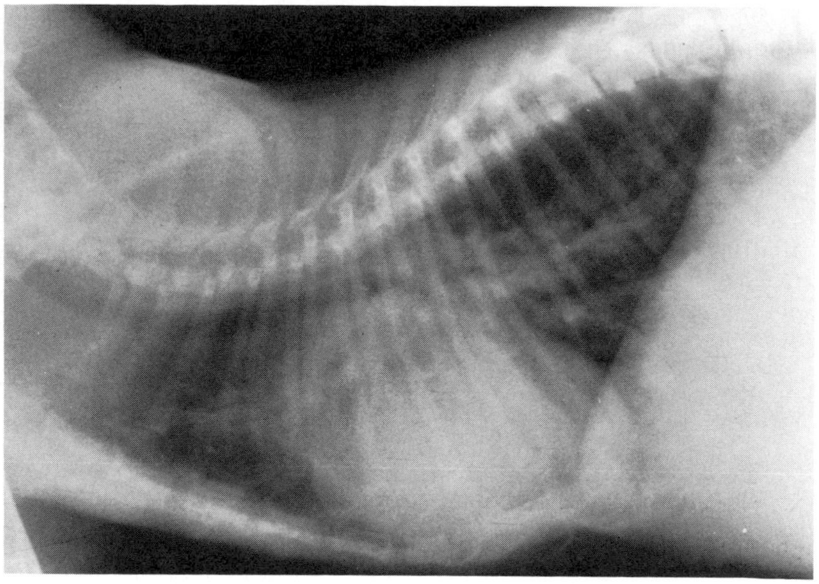

FIGURE 74–14. Radiographs from a kitten with patent ductus arteriosus. The left ventricle is markedly enlarged and the apex has shifted into the right hemithorax. The descending aorta bulges slightly (arrowheads) and the lobar pulmonary arteries are markedly enlarged (white arrowheads) compatible with pulmonary overcirculation. The lateral view shows significant elongation of the heart with tracheal elevation and marked increases in pulmonary vascularity in both the cranial and caudal lung lobes.

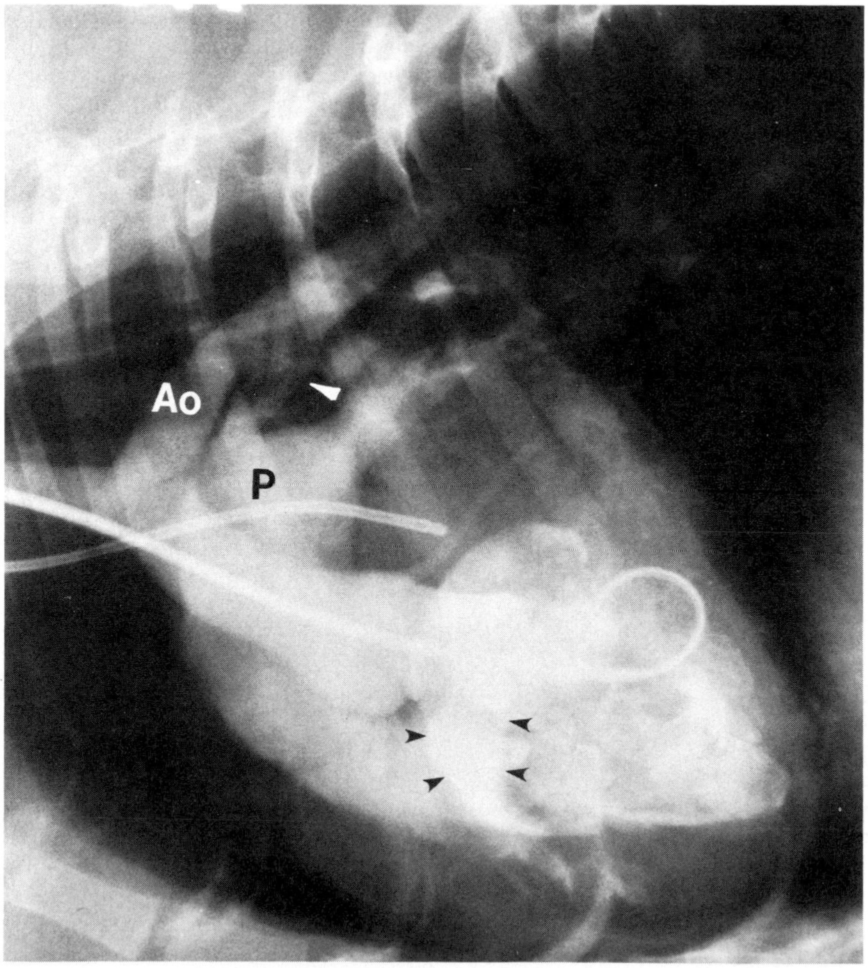

FIGURE 74–15. Left ventriculogram obtained from a dog with pulmonary hypertension caused by a ventricular septal defect and patent ductus arteriosus. A pigtail catheter is present within the left ventricle, with another catheter evident within the right atrium. Following injection of contrast into the left ventricle, a stream of dye crosses the ventricular septal defect (arrowheads), opacifies the hypertrophied right ventricular outflow tract and main pulmonary artery (P) and fills the distal pulmonary circulation. Contrast that exits into the aorta (Ao) outlines this vessel as well as the ductus arteriosus (white arrowhead), which connects the descending aorta with the dilated main pulmonary artery.

wedge, pulmonary artery, and left ventricular diastolic pressures.[39, 58] Pulmonary and right ventricular pressures are usually near normal in cases uncomplicated by heart failure or pulmonary vascular disease. An oxygen step-up is recorded in the descending aorta. When contrast material is injected into the left ventricle, or preferably the aorta, the ductus is evident and both aorta and pulmonary artery are opacified. Mitral regurgitation may be present if there is severe left ventricular dilatation, and pulmonic insufficiency may be noted owing to dilation of the pulmonary annulus.

PDA with Pulmonary Hypertension. When right to left shunting develops as a result of increased pulmonary vascular resistance (Figure 74–16), "reversed PDA" is present.[5, 8, 9, 39, 46, 59–61] The symptomatic patient exhibits shortness of breath, pelvic limb weakness or collapse, seizures, and differential cyanosis (cyanosis of the caudal mucous membranes with pink cranial membranes). Differential cyanosis is readily explained by the location of the right to left shunt from the pulmonary artery into the descending aorta (Figure 74–17). Perfusion of the kidneys with hypoxemic blood leads to secondary polycythemia and hyperviscosity, with the PCV often exceeding 65 per cent. Metabolic acidosis can develop.[59]

Clinical examination indicates that the continuous cardiac murmur is no longer present. An ejection sound, protosystolic murmur, and a loud or split second heart sound may be evident over the pulmonary area or left cardiac base. Right ventricular hypertrophy is evident as a right ventricular precordial heave, and by electrocardiography, radiography, and echocardiography. The thoracic x-ray film also indicates dilatation of the main pulmonary artery and proximal lobar arteries, peripheral hypoperfusion, and a "ductus bump" of the descending aorta (Figure 74–16). Echocardiography may permit imaging of the large pulmonary artery to aortic ductal communication.

Pulmonary hypertension with elevation of right ventricular systolic pressure is recorded at cardiac catheterization. Bidirectional shunting is commonly observed during angiography (Figure 74–17); however, the importance of the right to left shunt is emphasized by the thickening of the right ventricular walls, relatively small size of the left atrium and left ventricle, and the oxygen step-down in the descending aorta. Right ventriculograms outline a large ductus that appears to continue distally as the descending aorta.

Variable amounts of contrast flow cranial to the ductus. An erroneous diagnosis of pulmonic stenosis can be made since marked hypertrophy in the right ventricular outflow tract can lead to a mild systolic muscular obstruction that declines during diastole. Dilated lobar arteries showing increased distal tortuosity are commonly visualized, and bronchoesophageal collateral vessels may be prominent.

Natural History. Eyster has indicated that approximately 64 per cent of dogs diagnosed with left to right shunting PDA will be dead within one year of diagnosis without surgical treatment of the condition.[53] Complications of left to right PDA include pulmonary edema

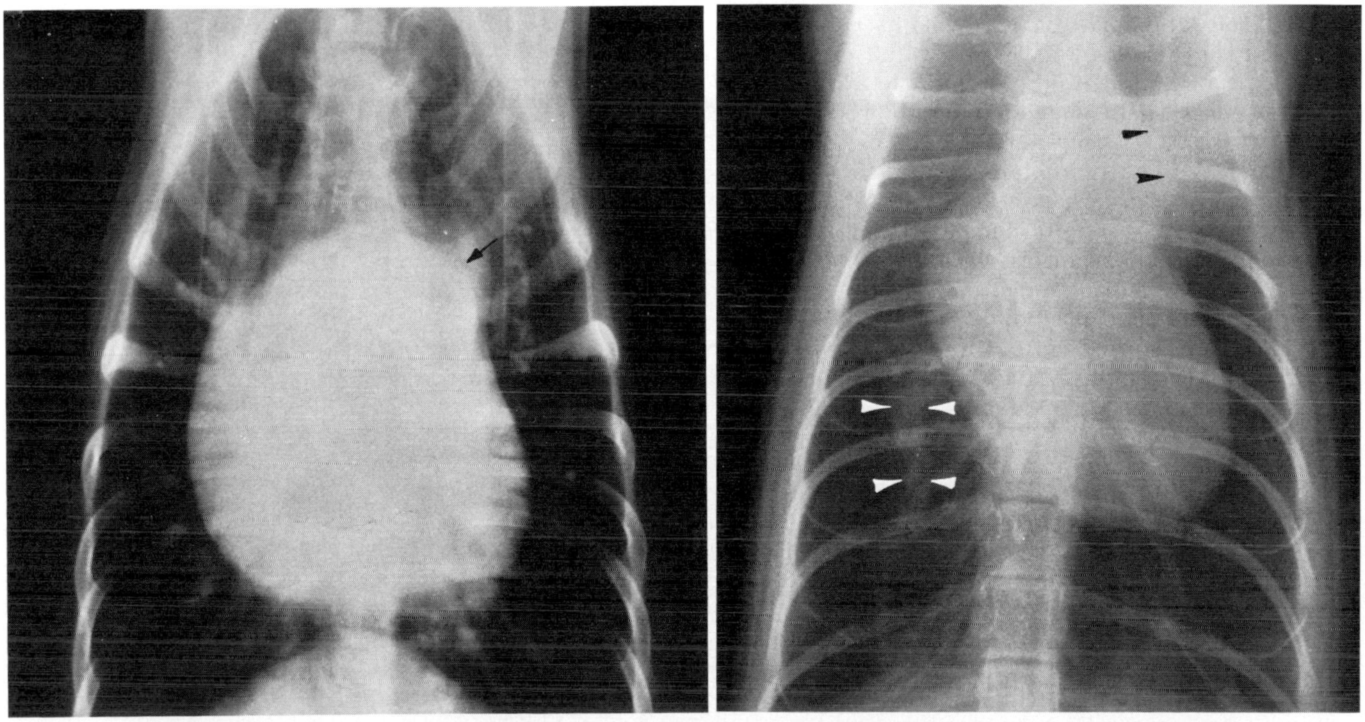

FIGURE 74–16. Dorsoventral radiographs from a dog *(left)* and a cat *(right)* with patent ductus arteriosus and pulmonary hypertension. Noted the marked dissimilarity between the appearance of the heart in this dog and the previous case (Figure 74–13). The right ventricle is rounded and there is significant bulging of the main pulmonary artery (arrow) compatible with pulmonary hypertension. The radiograph from the cat shows aneurysmal dilation (ductus bump) of the descending aorta (upper arrowheads) and dilation and tortuosity of a lobar pulmonary artery (lower arrowheads) compatible with pulmonary hypertension. A focal area of pneumonia is evident in the left cranial lung lobe.

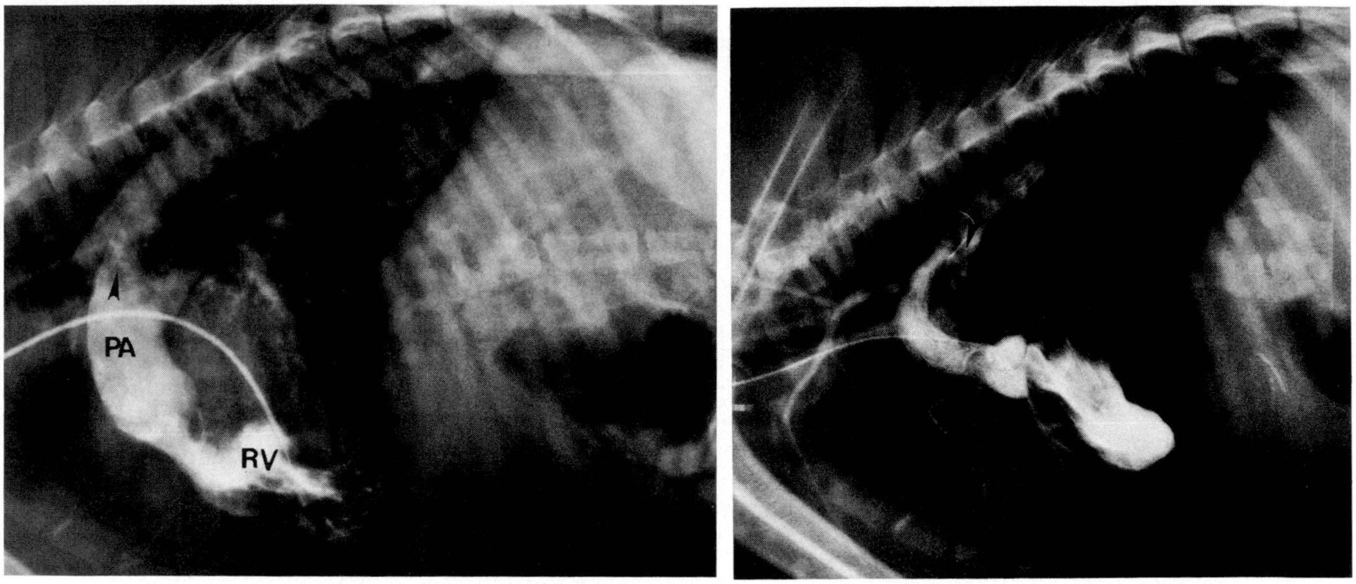

FIGURE 74–17. Right and left ventricular angiograms obtained from a dog with patent ductus arteriosus, pulmonary hypertension, and bidirectional shunting. The right ventriculogram opacifies the right ventricle (RV), the main pulmonary artery (PA), and the large ductus (arrowhead), which subsequently fills the descending aorta and opacifies the kidney. Note that the right ventricular wall is markedly hypertrophied, that there is secondary muscular hypertrophy of the infundibulum, which narrows the right ventricular outflow tract, and that the main pulmonary artery is dilated. The genesis of polycythemia is obvious. Desaturated blood perfuses the caudal portion of the body including the kidneys, which results in an increase in plasma erythropoietin. The left ventriculogram shows a small left ventricle that has been displaced dorsocaudally, prominence of the right coronary circulation, and some degree of left to right shunting (arrowhead) into the ductus. Note that the contrast in the descending and distal aorta has been diluted by the right to left shunt.

from left ventricular failure, atrial fibrillation from left atrial enlargement, pulmonary hypertension secondary to left ventricular failure (but *not* vascular disease), and development of mitral regurgitation presumably from left ventricular dilatation.[53, 58] Obviously some dogs with PDA survive to maturity and an occasional dog with PDA survives to more than ten years of age. While it is popular to extrapolate from humans and predict that pulmonary hypertension and shunt reversal may develop in mature dogs with PDA, the author is unaware of a documented case of shunt reversal that has occurred after a dog has attained six months of age.

When pulmonary hypertension in the neonate leads to reversed shunting, congestive heart failure is unlikely to develop. However, hypoxemia, polycythemia, and hyperviscosity can incapacitate the dog, and cardiac arrhythmias and sudden death may result. Dogs with reversed PDA often live for 2 to 5 years if they are not stressed and the PCV is controlled below 65 to 68 per cent.

Clinical Management. Surgery is recommended in all cases of left to right shunting PDA diagnosed in dogs less than two years of age. When this is diagnosed in older pets, a cardiologist should be consulted. Recommended preoperative studies include a PCV, fecal flotation, chest radiograph, and ECG. The latter tests help to stage the extent of the patient's disease. Doppler echocardiography can be used to verify the diagnosis or to rule out concurrent defects. The optimal time for surgery has not been determined but ductus ligation is often done between 8 and 16 weeks of age, or sooner if cardiac failure is imminent. Surgical techniques have been described in detail.[48–54] When congestive heart failure has developed, the patient is stabilized medically (see Table 74–5) prior to surgery. Treatment with prostaglandin inhibitors, often used in premature infants to encourage closure of the PDA, is unlikely to be successful in full-term pups or kittens and is not advocated. Transcatheter occlusion has not been described in the dog.[43, 45]

Prognosis with surgery is excellent, though it is inadvisable to use the dog for breeding. Surgical mortality of greater than five per cent should be considered excessive in uncomplicated cases.[53] Ductal recanalization has been reported but is quite uncommon, occurring in two per cent of the cases.[57] While detailed follow-up studies have not been reported, most pets act clinically normal following surgery and overall cardiac size normalizes, though the heart and great vessels continue to be misshapen in outline.[44] Soft left- or right-sided systolic murmurs are common following ductus ligation but are generally absent at the time of suture removal.[47] Persistent systolic murmurs are likely to indicate mitral regurgitation, ventricular septal defect, or subaortic stenosis. When atrial fibrillation or advanced congestive heart failure is present in PDA, the prognosis is guarded to poor. These patients are poor anesthetic risks.

Treatment of *reversed PDA* with secondary polycythemia consists of enforced rest, limitation of exercise, avoidance of stress, and maintenance of the PCV between 62 and 68 per cent. Excessive bleeding is discouraged since oxygen content of arterial blood may be diminished, leading to tissue hypoxia. Fluid volume should be maintained during phlebotomy by infusing crystalloid solutions.

Atrioventricular Septal Defects

During cardiac development the atria and ventricles are joined as a common chamber. The common atrioventricular canal is partitioned by growth of cardiac septa causing the four-chambered heart.[15] The atria are partitioned by two septa: septum I (primum), which forms first, and septum II (secundum), which develops to the right of septum I. The foramen ovale, a slit-like passageway for blood between these septa, permits right to left atrial shunting in the fetus, but functionally and anatomically closes in the neonate once left atrial pressure increases. The ventricular septum is formed by a variety of primordia. Eventually, the lower atrial septum is connected to the upper ventricular septum by growth and differentiation of the endocardial cushions. Defects in the ventricular septum or atrial septa I and II, and maldevelopment of the endocardial cushions, cause patencies of the atrioventricular septum. This form of congenital heart disease is relatively common in the cat, and is encountered in dogs as an isolated lesion and as a component of the tetralogy of Fallot.[4–13, 62–79]

PATHOGENESIS

The cause of most atrioventricular septal defects is unknown, and aside from its genetic basis in Keeshonden with conotruncal malformation, there are no consistent data about etiopathogenesis of spontaneous defects in dogs or cats.[4] Atrial septal defects (ASD) can be classified based on the region of malformation.[15, 16] Defects of the septum in or near the fossa ovale are ostium (or septum) secundum defects, patency of the lower atrial septum represents an ostium primum defect, and the rare sinus venosus atrial septal defects are found dorsocranial to the fossa ovale (Figure 74–18).[13, 62–67] Since the endocardial cushions are also responsible for partitioning the lowermost atrial septum, defects here are sometimes called endocardial cushion defects. This is particularly so when there is a high ventricular septal defect and anomalous development of the atrioventricular valves (e.g., clefts or common septal leaflet). Complete endocardial cushion defects are sometimes termed "common atrioventricular canal" or "canal" defects, since the primitive atrioventricular canal never partitions and there is communication between all four cardiac chambers.

Patent foramen ovale is not a true ASD inasmuch as the septa are present but can be pushed into an open position.[62] The clinical significance of patent foramen ovale pertains to right to left shunting that may develop in animals with elevated right atrial pressures, as may accompany severe pulmonic stenosis or dysplasia of the tricuspid valve.

Most ventricular septal defects (VSD) are located high on the ventricular septum.[68] Muscular or multiple ("swiss-cheese") defects are uncommon in small animals. The typical location of the single-orifice VSD is below the aortic valve. The right ventricular location of a VSD varies and is often described relative to the crista supraventricularis.[15] Subcristal VSD are often located just under the septal leaflet of the tricuspid valve, and may be partially occluded by this structure (Figure 74–

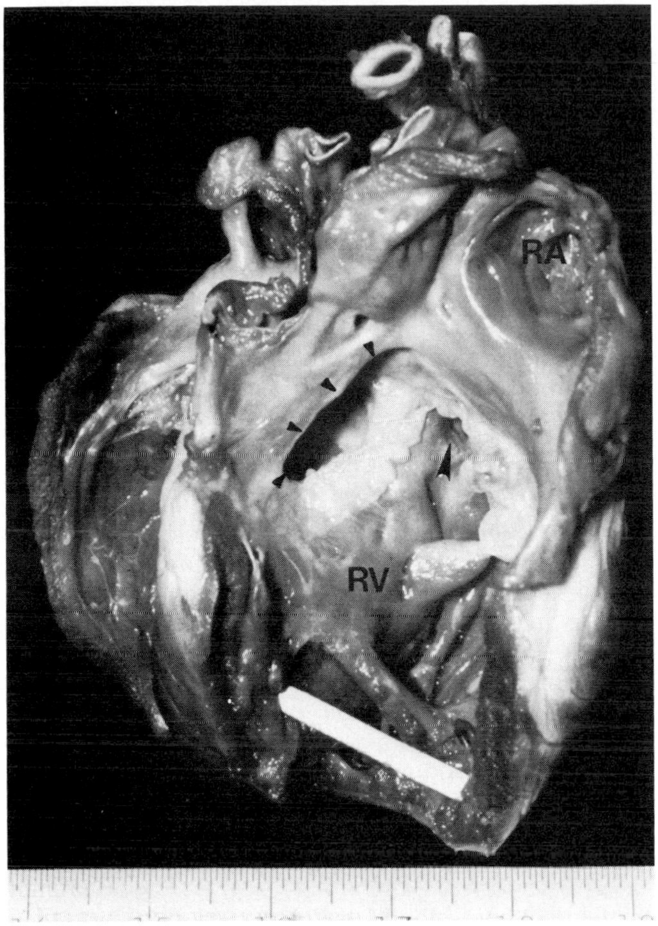

FIGURE 74–18. Endocardial cushion defect in a cat. The heart is viewed from the caudal aspect, and the right atrium (RA) and right ventricle (RV) are dilated. The left atrium and left ventricle are to the viewer's left. A large ostium primum atrial septal defect is evident in the lower portion of the atrial septum (arrowheads) just above the septal leaflet of the tricuspid valve. A smaller ventricular septal defect was also present (larger arrow) beneath a slightly cleft tricuspid valve cusp.

19). Large defects that literally obliterate the crista are not uncommon, particularly with tetralogy of Fallot.[2, 4] Some subaortic, supracristal (subpulmonic) defects cause the right aortic valve to prolapse into the defect, partially occluding the hole, but also causing aortic valve incompetency.

PATHOPHYSIOLOGY

The pathophysiology of isolated ASD and VSD is summarized in Figures 74–20 and 74–21. A principle applicable to any atrioventricular septal defect is that shunting will depend on the caliber of the orifice (i.e., restrictive or not) and the relative resistances in the systemic and pulmonary circulations.[15, 62, 68, 72, 73] Typically, blood shunts from left to right. However, conditions that increase right atrial or ventricular pressures will retard left to right shunting and may lead to reversed shunting. Thus, when atrioventricular septal defects are complicated by tricuspid or pulmonic stenosis, pulmonary atresia, or pulmonary hypertension, right to left shunting may develop.

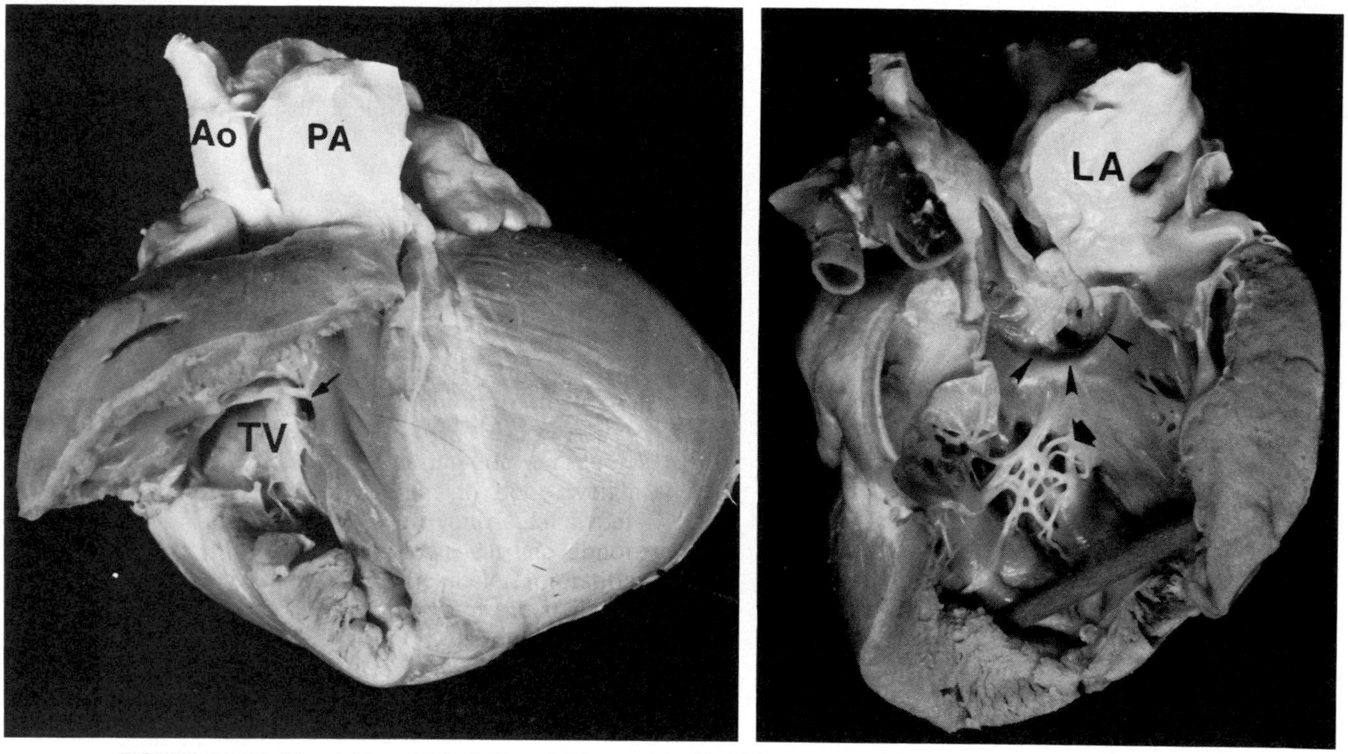

FIGURE 74–19. The right ventricle *(left)* and left ventricle *(right)* from a cat with a ventricular septal defect. The septal defect (arrow) has been partially covered by the tricuspid valve (TV) septal leaflet. The left ventricular aspect of the septal defect is evident as a large depression (arrrowheads) that has been markedly diminished in size by the overlying tricuspid valve leaflet. Only a small hole is left for shunting of blood. This cat lived for a number of years with this defect. Prominence of the left ventricular moderator bands is also noted (lower arrow). (Ao = Aorta, PA = pulmonary artery, LA = Left atrium.)

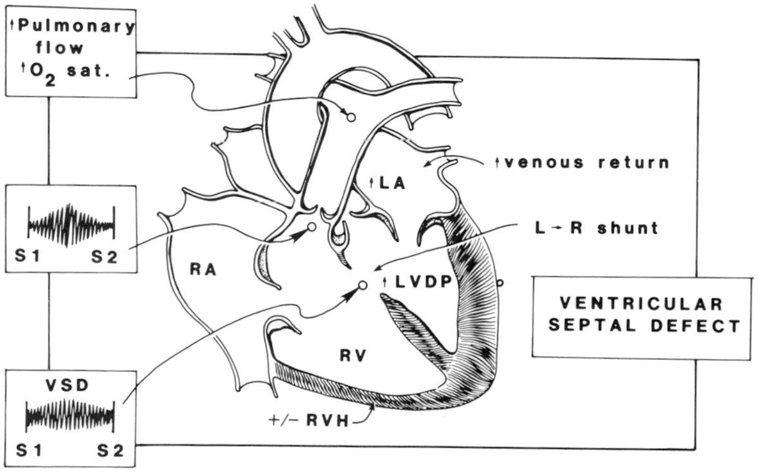

FIGURE 74–20. Schematic illustration demonstrating the pathophysiology of ventricular septal defect. See text for details. (By permission from Bonagura, JD: Congenital heart disease. *In* Bonagura, JD (ed): Cardiology. New York, Churchill Livingstone, 1987.)

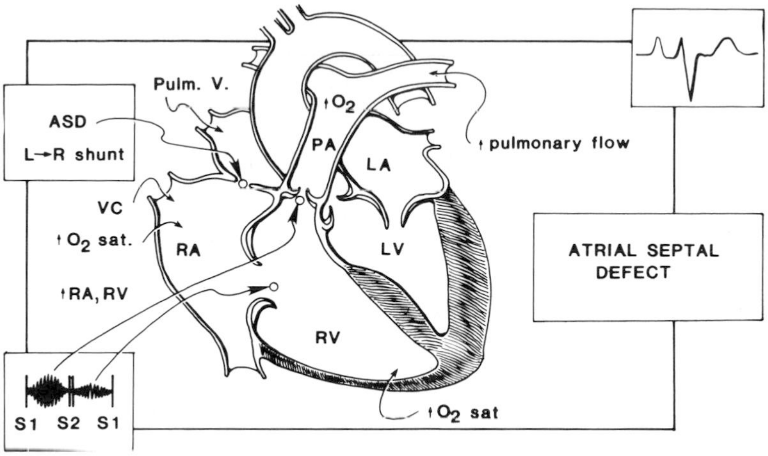

FIGURE 74–21. Schematic illustration demonstrating the pathophysiology of atrial septal defect. See text for details. (By permission from Bonagura, JD: Congenital heart disease. *In* Bonagura, JD (ed): Cardiology. New York, Churchill Livingstone, 1987.)

Atrial Septal Defect. It is convenient to think of a heart with a large atrial septal defect as having a common atrium.[15, 65] Accordingly, blood will flow along the atrioventricular path of least diastolic resistance. Since the right ventricular walls are thinner and more compliant, blood preferentially shunts into the right ventricle (Figure 74–21). The resultant volume overload of the right atrium (RA), right ventricle (RV), pulmonary artery (PA), and pulmonary veins leads to enlargement of these structures (Figures 74–22 to 74–24). Since the left atrium now receives more blood, one might suspect that this chamber would enlarge, but the increased return is shunted immediately into the lower pressure right atrium. When significant left atrial enlargement does occur, an endocardial cushion defect should be suspected with concurrent mitral regurgitation.

Left to right shunting increases hemoglobin oxygen saturation in the RA, RV, and PA. While the shunting of blood per se does not generate a cardiac murmur, excessive transvalvular flow velocity, which can be measured by Doppler echocardiography, can cause murmurs of relative valve stenosis. Delayed closure of the pulmonic valve (and early closure of the aortic valve) causes splitting of the second heart sound.[62, 63] Since the right side of the heart is volume overloaded, right ventricular failure is most likely to develop in advanced cases. Complete endocardial cushion defects, with mitral regurgitation, may cause bilateral congestive heart failure.

Ventricular Septal Defect. The pathophysiology of the isolated ventricular septal defect is influenced by many factors. Owing to the higher left than right ventricular pressures, left to right shunting develops and oxygen saturation in the right ventricular outflow tract

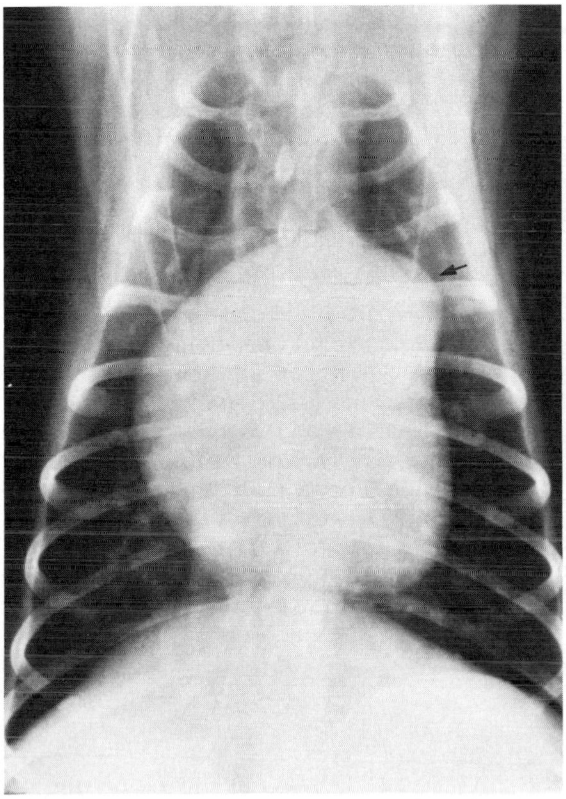

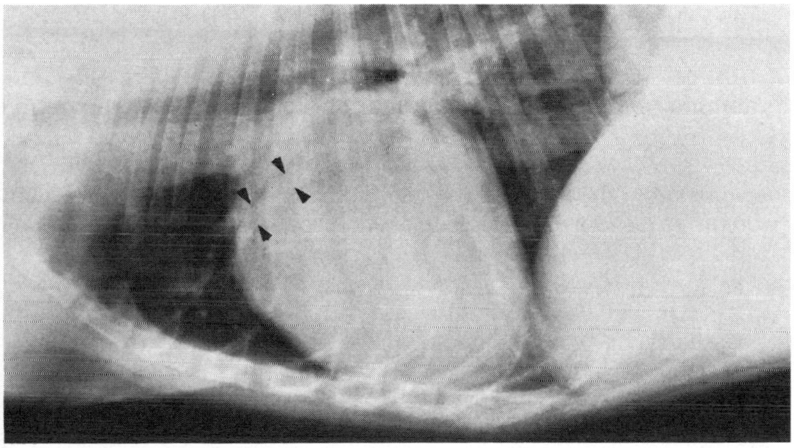

FIGURE 74–22. Ventrodorsal and lateral radiographs obtained from a dog with an endocardial cushion defect, mitral regurgitation, and significant left to right shunting at the atrial level. The right ventricle is somewhat rounded, and there is marked dilation of the main pulmonary artery (arrow) compatible with increased right ventricular and pulmonary flow. The lateral radiograph shows increased pulmonary vascularity with marked increases in the caliber of lobar pulmonary vessels. A dilated pulmonary vein (arrowheads) is indicated. This dog developed congestive heart failure.

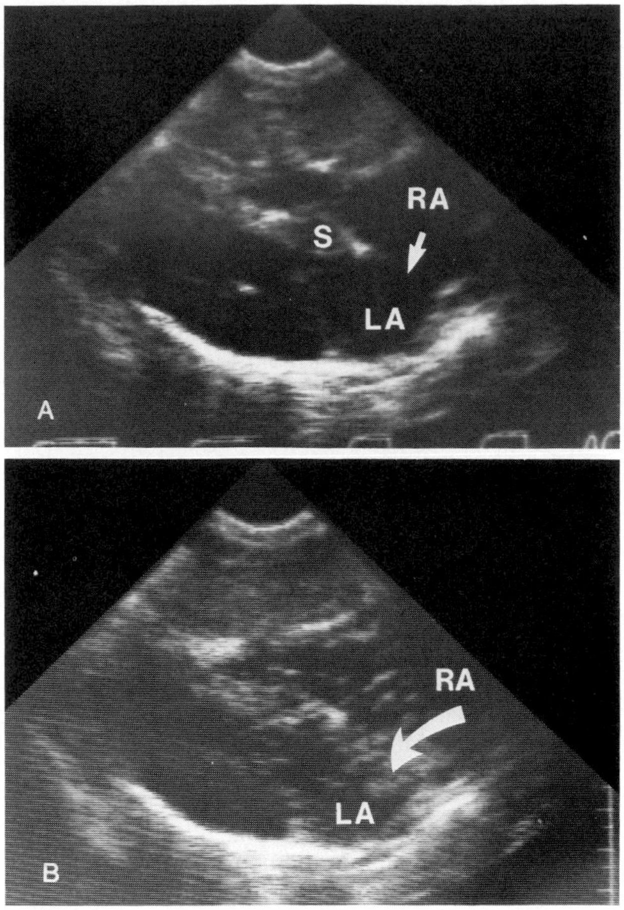

FIGURE 74–23. Cross sectional echocardiograms from a dog with right to left shunting ostium secundum atrial septal defect. *A* shows a large echo-free space between the right atrium (RA) and the left atrium (LA). The ventricular septum (S) is indicated. Following injection of saline into the cephalic vein, echo contrast is observed to traverse the atrial septal defect (large arrow) indicating right to left communication.

and the pulmonary artery is higher when compared to that in the right atrium (Figure 74–20). The peak RBC velocity across the defect can be quantitated by Doppler echocardiography and is directly proportional to the pressure difference across the defect ($\Delta P = 4V^2$). It has been demonstrated that with high ventricular septal defects, much of the shunt flow is pumped immediately into the pulmonary artery, with variable volumes ejected into the right ventricular chamber.[72, 73] Thus, the left ventricle does most of the volume work. Additionally, as pulmonary flow increases, there is increased venous return to the left atrium and left ventricle, and the left ventricular diastolic pressures (LVDP) can increase. Left ventricular failure can develop in situations of marked left to right shunt (e.g., greater than 2.5:1, pulmonary to systemic flow).

The degree of right ventricular hypertrophy (RVH) and enlargement depends on a variety of factors: size of the septal defect, pulmonary vascular resistance, and pulmonic valve function. Very large, nonrestrictive defects cause the two ventricles to behave as a common chamber, so that ventricular pressures equilibrate and RVH will be evident. Blood then goes to the path of least resistance. If the pulmonary valve and the vascular resistance are normal, tremendous left to right shunting is likely to occur. If pulmonary vascular resistance increases, then left to right shunting will be diminished and bidirectional shunting may be observed. In the animal with tetralogy of Fallot, the stenotic pulmonic valve offers such great resistance that right to left shunting predominates.

Eisenmenger's Physiology. As with PDA, the patient with a large atrioventricular septal defect and left to right shunt may develop high pulmonary vascular resistance leading to pulmonary hypertension. Consequently, resistance to right ventricular outflow increases and right ventricular systolic and diastolic pressures increase to systemic levels. Reversed shunting (right to left) then can develop, leading to a situation known as "Eisenmenger's physiology" (Figure 74–23). Anatomic changes in the pulmonary arteries have been observed in dogs and cats with reversed shunting and are described in the section on Cyanotic Heart Disease. As with PDA, shunt reversal often develops within six months after birth; however, it is unknown if some animals with ASD require the relatively long time for development of pulmonary hypertension noted in human patients with secundum ASD. Eisenmenger's physiology represents an irreversible condition. Afflicted animals become hypoxemic and cyanotic, and develop polycythemia and hyperviscosity.

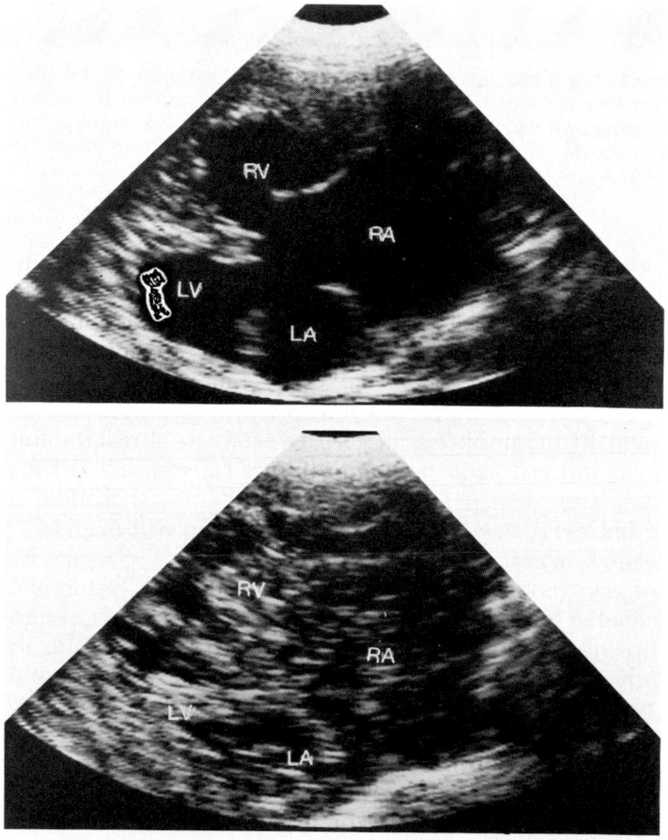

FIGURE 74–24. Cross sectional echocardiogram obtained from a cat with an endocardial cushion defect. A major area of echo dropout is observed at the junction of the right atrium (RA), left atrium (LA), right ventricle (RV), and left ventricle (LV). This cat had bidirectional shunting as is illustrated in the next panel. When saline is injected into the cephalic vein, all cardiac chambers become opacified with echo targets.

CLINICAL FINDINGS

Atrial Septal Defect. A left to right ASD is recognized through auscultation of soft systolic cardiac murmurs over the pulmonic and tricuspid valves and by identifying splitting of the second heart sound. The systolic murmur of relative pulmonic stenosis is easiest to identify and is heard best at the left cardiac base. A diastolic rumble of relative tricuspid stenosis may be audible at the right hemithorax. When a systolic murmur of mitral regurgitation is identified at the left apex, an endocardial cushion defect should be considered. Cyanosis is unexpected, unless there is stenosis of a right-sided heart valve or pulmonary hypertension, in which case S_2 should be loud. Cardiac failure may be evident in advanced cases. Differential diagnosis includes anomalous pulmonary venous return.[80]

Volume overloading of the right side of the heart is evident on thoracic radiography (Figure 74–22) and by echocardiography (Figures 74–23 and 74–24). The main pulmonary artery may be dilated. Pulmonary vascularity is increased unless there is pulmonary hypertension. The left atrium is normal to slightly enlarged. Marked left atrial enlargement suggests mitral insufficiency from a cleft mitral valve. The defect may be imaged as an area of abnormal sonolucency. Echocontrast (saline) may traverse the defect when there is bidirectional shunting (Figures 74–23 and 74–24). Doppler studies can identify abnormal blood flow adjacent to the defect, increased transpulmonic valve velocity, or associated mitral insufficiency. The electrocardiogram indicates right ventricular and possibly atrial enlargement with ASD, and either left or right ventricular enlargement with VSD. Intraventricular conduction disturbances (Figure 74–25) are not uncommon with atrioventricular septal defects, and a cranial axis deviation may suggest an ostium primum ASD.[4, 64, 66]

Cardiac catheterization is useful for evaluating the magnitude of shunting. By measuring oxygen content in the venae cavae and cardiac chambers, the magnitude of systemic to pulmonary shunting can be estimated; however, the shunt estimation will be affected by the variability of venous oxygen saturation found in the dog (see section on Cardiac Catheterization). If congestive heart failure has developed, central venous and right ventricular diastolic pressures are increased. Right ventricular systolic pressure is elevated if there is pulmonary hypertension or a large left to right shunt. High flow across the pulmonic valve causes "relative" pulmonic stenosis, identified in most cases by a pressure gradient of between 5 and 25 mm Hg and a coincident increase in ejection velocity recorded by Doppler techniques.[63] Angiocardiography is inferior to echocardiography, though it can be used to image an ASD. An injection of contrast material made in the right ventricle or pulmonary artery will outline left to right shunting defects during the left-sided phase of the study. Following pulmonary venous return, the atrial septum usually can be seen between the left atrium and aorta on the lateral projection (Figure 74–26).

Viewing this area for a jet of contrast, or more commonly a "spilling-over" of dye across this wall into the right atrium and auricle and venae cavae, permits identification of the shunt. The cardiac catheter often is advanced across large septal defects. With endocardial cushion defects, a left ventriculogram may outline a

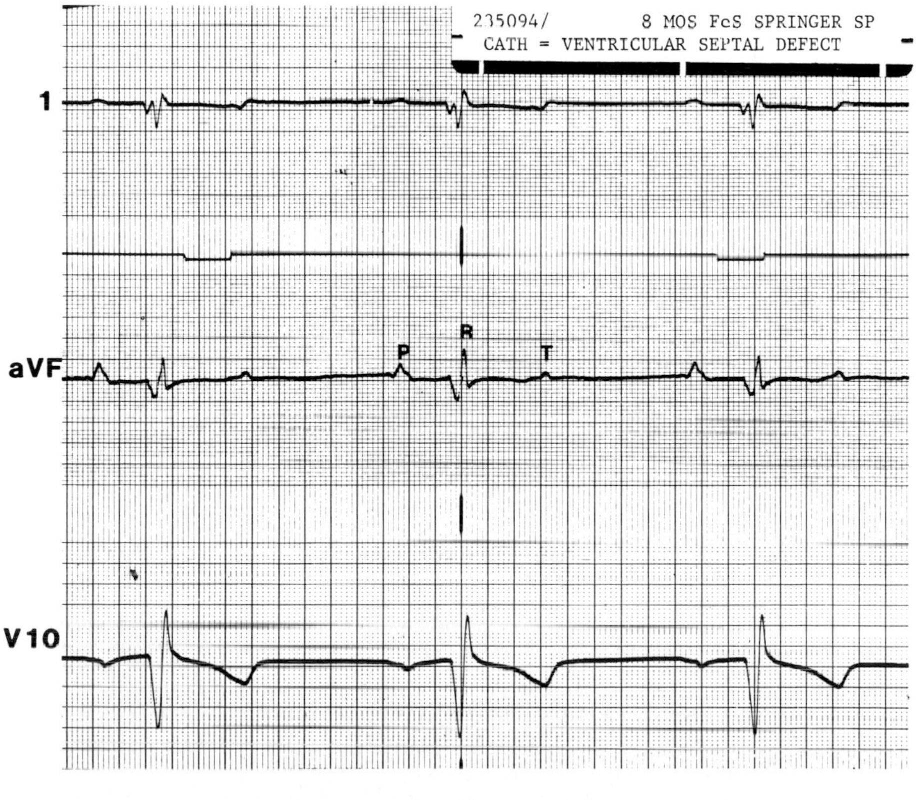

FIGURE 74–25. Electrocardiogram from a dog with a ventricular septal defect. An intraventricular conduction disturbance is present, characterized by a wide and abnormal Q wave in the aV_F and abnormal initial activation of the septum and ventricles in lead 1. Standard calibration: paper speed = 50 mm per second.

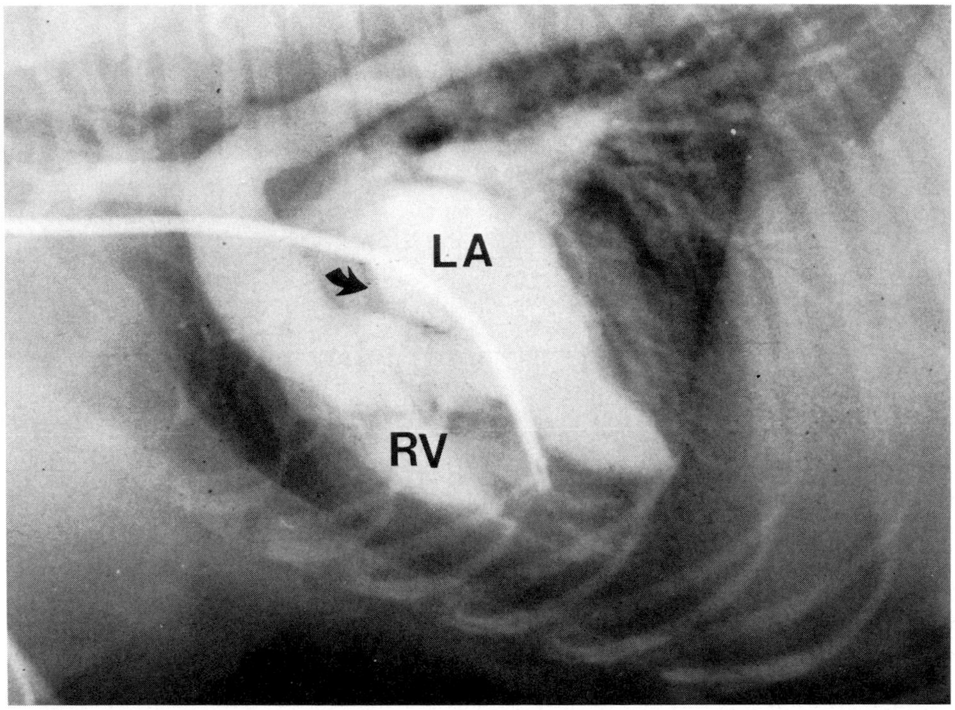

FIGURE 74–26. Angiocardiogram from a dog with an intact atrial septum and a small ventricular septal defect. Contrast was injected into the right ventricle and dye was allowed to return to the left atrium and left ventricle. Note that the atrial septum appears intact (arrow), and that there is no obvious opacification of the right auricle or caudal vena cava. Opacification of the right ventricle is evident as a result of a small left to right shunting ventricular septal defect. This is a suboptimal method for identifying ventricular septal defects since a selective left ventricular injection would rule out the possibility of residual contrast in the right ventricle.

VSD, mitral regurgitation, and possibly left ventricular to right atrial shunting.

Ventricular Septal Defect. The clinical features of VSD are variable. Most commonly, a harsh, holosystolic murmur heard best at the right sternal border will be present.[5–10, 68] A murmur of relative pulmonic stenosis, and possibly splitting of the second heart sound, may be evident at the left base and may be very prominent when the septal defect is subpulmonic. When a diastolic murmur of aortic regurgitation is present, prolapse of an aortic cusp should be suspected and the defect is likely to be supracristal (Figure 74–12). Mitral regurgitation is likely with an endocardial cushion defect.

Thoracic radiography demonstrates pulmonary overcirculation, left atrial and ventricular dilation, and variable degrees of right ventricular enlargement.[22–24] The main and lobar pulmonary arteries often are dilated. If the shunt is left to right, then peripheral pulmonary vascularity is increased. With cases of VSD and pulmonary hypertension, the main and proximal lobar vessels are distended, but the peripheral vascular markings are scant. Electrocardiography is also variable, indicating left atrial enlargement, left ventricular dilation, and/or right ventricular hypertrophy. Early ventricular activation can be a subtle abnormality (Figure 74–25).[69] The presence of a right axis deviation in a dog with VSD usually indicates either a large defect, with equilibration of ventricular pressures and concurrent pulmonic stenosis, or pulmonary hypertension. Echocardiography successfully delineates the VSD in most cases. Doppler studies can identify the high velocity jet of a restrictive VSD. Pressure drop across the defect (providing insight to right ventricular systolic pressure) can be estimated from the peak shunt velocity using the formula $\Delta P = 4V^2$. Echocontrast studies also can be utilized to demonstrate shunting.

Cardiac catheterization and angiocardiography document the anatomic lesions and estimate the degree of shunting.[68] An oxygen step-up is recorded in the right ventricle. Ventricular diastolic pressures are elevated with ventricular failure or severe diastolic overload. Pulmonary hypertension and elevated right ventricular systolic pressure may be detected in some cases. A systolic pressure gradient of 5 to 25 mm Hg, indicating relative pulmonic stenosis, is evident with some cases of left to right shunting VSD. The angiocardiogram (Figures 74–15 and 74–27) outlines the defect, shunt flow, and geometric alterations of the ventricles and great vessels. Aortic regurgitation may be observed following a supravalvular aortic injection.

NATURAL HISTORY

Potential outcomes of atrioventricular septal defects include (1) patient tolerance of the lesion, (2) partial or complete closure of a VSD by adherence of the septal tricuspid leaflet, right ventricular hypertrophy, or aortic valve prolapse, (3) progressive aortic regurgitation due to valve prolapse, (4) development of congestive heart failure, (5) development of pulmonary hypertension, and (6) reversal of the shunt with development of arterial hypoxemia and cyanosis. It is difficult to predict the survival of a patient without detailed Doppler echocardiographic studies and/or catheterization data, and even with this information there are inadequate data to allow accurate subsetting of patients. Cats with endocardial cushion defects not uncommonly develop biventricular congestive heart failure.

CLINICAL MANAGEMENT

Methods used in the management of atrioventricular septal defects are summarized in Table 74–5. Definitive treatment of these problems requires surgery using car-

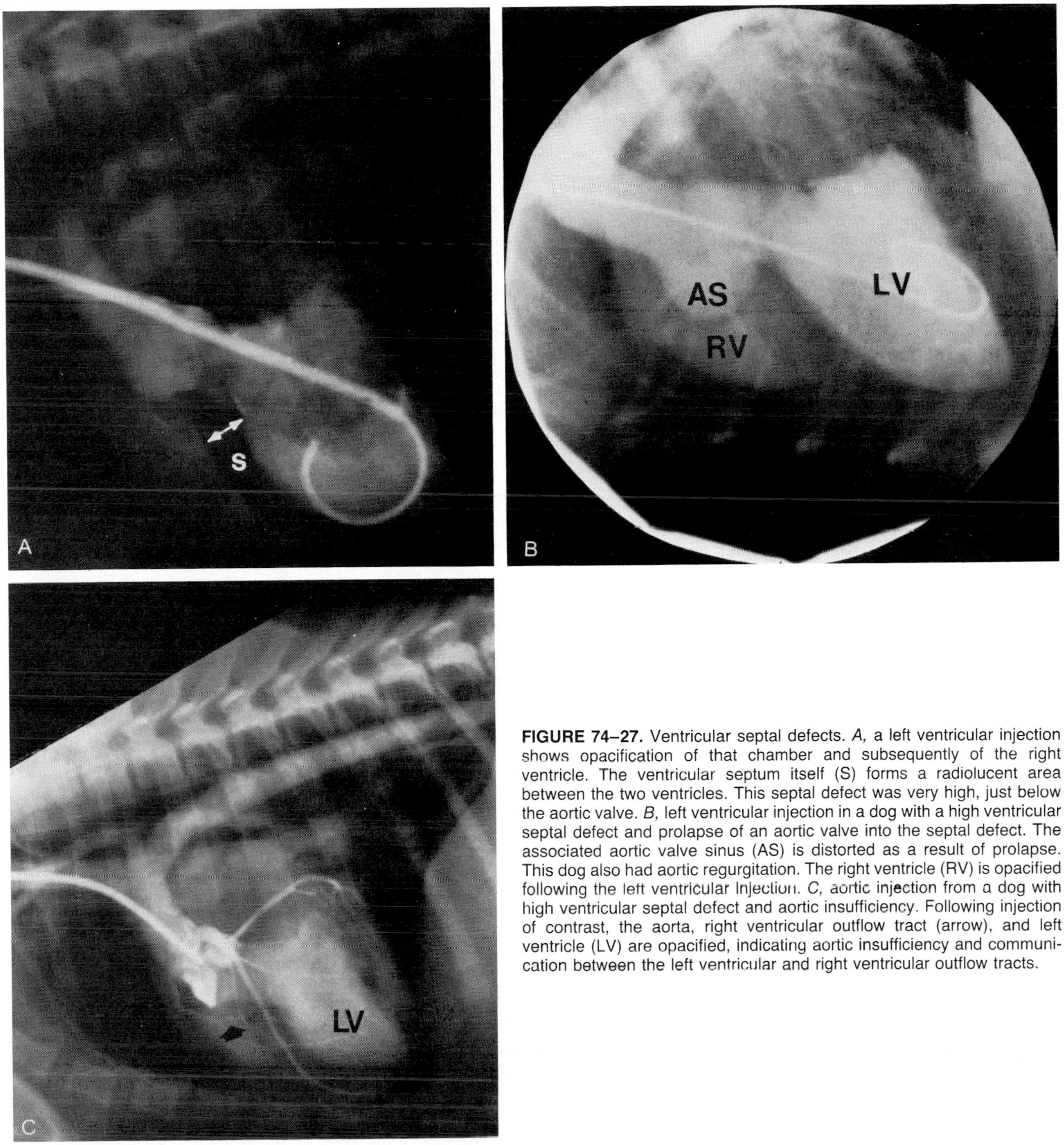

FIGURE 74–27. Ventricular septal defects. *A,* a left ventricular injection shows opacification of that chamber and subsequently of the right ventricle. The ventricular septum itself (S) forms a radiolucent area between the two ventricles. This septal defect was very high, just below the aortic valve. *B,* left ventricular injection in a dog with a high ventricular septal defect and prolapse of an aortic valve into the septal defect. The associated aortic valve sinus (AS) is distorted as a result of prolapse. This dog also had aortic regurgitation. The right ventricle (RV) is opacified following the left ventricular injection. *C,* aortic injection from a dog with high ventricular septal defect and aortic insufficiency. Following injection of contrast, the aorta, right ventricular outflow tract (arrow), and left ventricle (LV) are opacified, indicating aortic insufficiency and communication between the left ventricular and right ventricular outflow tracts.

diopulmonary bypass.[76, 77] This is rarely accomplished. Pulmonary artery banding can be used to create supravalvular pulmonary stenosis and decrease the magnitude of left to right shunting.[74, 75] This procedure is recommended for dogs and cats showing signs of left-sided congestive heart failure. Anemia should be avoided, since a low hematocrit leads to decreased pulmonary vascular resistance and increased shunting.[78] When left-sided congestive heart failure is severe, arterial vasodilators may be beneficial since they decrease systemic resistance and decrease left to right shunting.[79]

Treatment of Eisenmenger's physiology is discouraging and is similar to that discussed for reversed PDA. Maintenance of the PCV between 62 and 68 per cent is recommended. Excessive bleeding may promote tissue hypoxia, while hematocrits higher than 68 per cent are more likely to cause signs of hyperviscosity.

MALFORMATION OF CARDIAC VALVES

PULMONIC STENOSIS

Pulmonic stenosis (PS) is a common congenital heart defect in the dog and is occasionally recognized in the cat.[81–89] While obstruction to right ventricular outflow can develop in the infundibulum, subvalvular region, and above the pulmonic valve, dysplasia of the pulmonary valve is the most frequently observed defect in dogs. Subvalvular and/or valvular stenosis is recognized in animals with tetralogy of Fallot. Right ventricular outflow obstruction in the extreme form is represented as pulmonary artery atresia (see Figure 74–52).

Pathogenesis. Pulmonic stenosis has a genetic basis in certain breeds (Table 74–2), although the cause of this malformation in the cat is unknown. Abnormal development of pulmonary valve anlagen causes dysplasia of the valve. A polygenic mode of transmission was suggested by Patterson and associates.[86] They studied the heritability and pathology of isolated PS in the beagle. A spectrum of abnormalities was observed and graded as follows: grade 1: "slight thickening of pulmonary valve leaflets with little or no fusion or hypoplasia, producing minimal or no demonstrable pulmonary outflow obstruction" and grade 2: "moderate to severe thickening of pulmonary valve leaflets, usually with fusion or hypoplasia, or both, producing moderate to severe pulmonary outflow obstruction."

Clinical cases of PS usually represent a grade 2 lesion. Histologic abnormalities include thickening of the valve spongiosa and the presence of bands of fusiform cells in a dense collagen network. These changes may represent overproduction of normal valve elements or a failure of conversion of the cushion-like embryonic valve primordia. Blood-filled spaces and endothelium-lined spaces also are found in one or more cusps of affected dogs.[86]

We have observed similar findings in other breeds (Figure 74–28).[88] Many of these dogs have fibrous thickening at the immediate base of the valves; however, the valve leaflets are also abnormal. Such thickenings may account for the preponderance of "subvalvular" PS in some surveys. Pulmonic stenosis of the dog more closely resembles atypical PS in children.[15, 86]

Pathophysiology. The pathophysiology[15] of PS is summarized in Figure 74–29. Obstruction to right ventricular outflow causes an increase in ventricular systolic pressure (RVSP), leading to right ventricular hypertrophy (RVH), leftward septal deviation or flattening, and a systolic pressure gradient across the pulmonary valve (Figure 74–5). High-velocity and turbulent flow about the stenosis is associated with a systolic ejection murmur and post-stenotic dilation of the main pulmonary artery (PA). Increasing stiffness of the right ventricle is responsible for the vigorous atrial contraction ("a" wave) that may be evident in the jugular venous furrow. Progressive right atrial enlargement probably develops from various factors: (1) outflow obstruction, (2) elevated ventricular diastolic pressure, (3) secondary tricuspid regurgitation (TR) caused by high RV pressure and geometric changes within the ventricle, and (4) decreased cardiac output with compensatory retention of sodium and water. Diminished right ventricular coronary blood flow has been documented in dogs with PS.[85] Critical stenosis limits cardiac output with exercise. If right atrial pressures become markedly elevated, right-sided congestive heart failure develops.

Clinical Findings. Pulmonic stenosis is more common in certain breeds including the beagle, Samoyed, Chihuahua, English bulldog, schnauzer and other terrier breeds.[8, 9] Dogs with PS may be asymptomatic, develop signs related to low cardiac output, such as syncope and tiring, may manifest right-sided congestive heart failure,[88] or develop hypoxemia from right to left shunting across an atrioventricular septal defect. Clinical signs are more likely in dogs greater than one year of age. Typical physical examination findings include: prominent jugular pulse, left basilar ejection murmur over the pulmonic valve that radiates dorsally on the left cardiac base (Figure 74–30), and palpable right ventricular hypertrophy (right-sided heave). It is not uncommon in advanced cases to auscultate a holosystolic murmur of tricuspid regurgitation over the right hemithorax.

Right ventricular enlargement is almost always evident on the ECG [31, 32, 90] (Figure 74–2), echocardiogram (Figures 74–30 and 74–31), and thoracic radiograph (Figure 74–32).[8, 22–24, 88] Additional radiographic features of PS include post-stenotic dilation of the main pulmonary artery, variable dilation of the proximal left pulmonary artery, and pulmonary underperfusion. Echocardiography demonstrates hypertrophy and enlargement of the right ventricle with increased prominence of the papillary muscle, secondary muscular narrowing of the right ventricular outflow tract (most cases), increased echogenicity of the pulmonary valve, and dilation of the main pulmonary artery. Doppler studies reveal increased blood velocity across the stenosis and turbulence in the pulmonary artery. These noninvasive studies can be used to estimate the pressure gradient.

Cardiac catheterization permits subsetting of patients based on right ventricular systolic pressure.[87, 88, 93] The degree of stenosis is graded as mild (gradient up to 49 mm Hg), moderate (gradient of 50–99 mm Hg), or severe (gradient greater than 100 mm Hg). Futhermore,

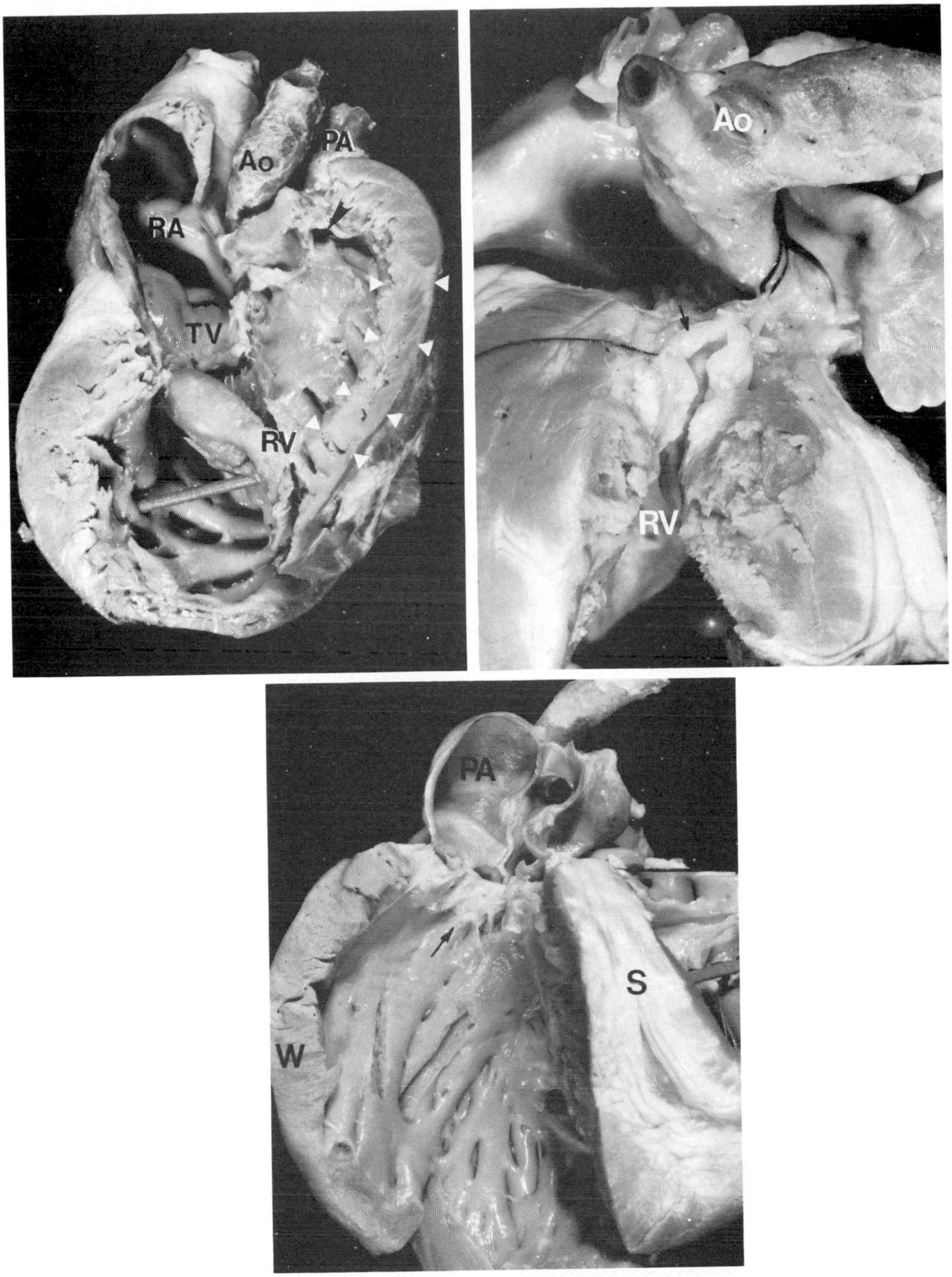

FIGURE 74–28. Pathology of pulmonic stenosis. Hearts obtained from three dogs with pulmonic valve dysplasia show some of the variable features. Upper right—dysplastic pulmonary valve viewed from above. The main pulmonary artery has been cut away to illustrate the thickened, partially fused pulmonary valve leaflets (arrow). The right ventricle (RV) and the aorta (Ao) are indicated. Lower center—right ventricular enlargement with hypertrophy of the right ventricular wall (W) is evident in this dog with pulmonic valve dysplasia (arrow). The pulmonic valve leaflets are thickened and malformed, and the thickening extends to the base of each valve. The main pulmonary artery (PA) is dilated as a result of poststenotic dilation. The ventricular septum is noted (S). Upper left—hypoplasia of the pulmonary valve (arrow) is evident in this specimen viewed from ventral surface. There is marked hypertrophy of the right ventricle, papillary muscles, infundibulum (white arrowheads), and supraventricular crest between the tricuspid valve (TV) and the pulmonary valve (upper arrow). The right atrium (RA), aorta (Ao), and the main pulmonary artery (PA) are indicated.

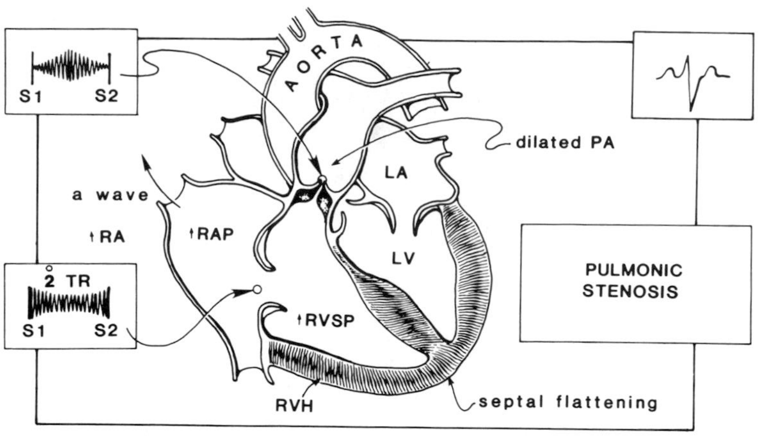

FIGURE 74–29. Schematic illustration of the pathophysiology of pulmonic stenosis. See text for details. (By permission from Bonagura, JD: Congenital heart disease. *In* Bonagura, JD (ed): Cardiology. New York, Churchill Livingstone, 1987.)

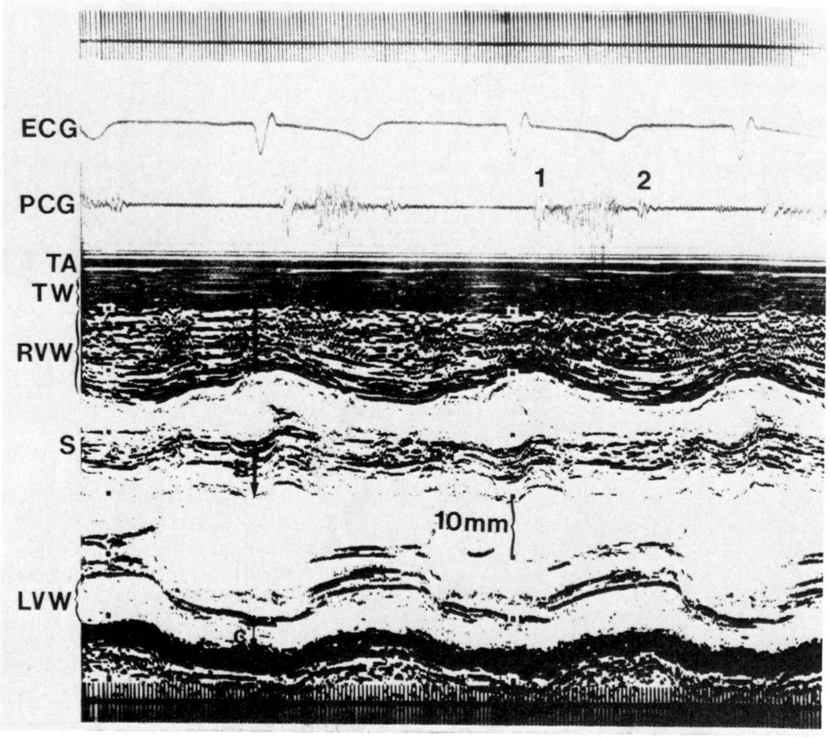

FIGURE 74–30. Echophonocardiogram from a dog with pulmonic stenosis. A systolic murmur is evident in the phonocardiogram (PCG) and there is marked right ventricular hypertrophy in this M-mode echocardiogram. TA = transducer artifact, TW = thoracic wall, RVW = right ventricular wall, S = septum, LVW = left ventricular wall.

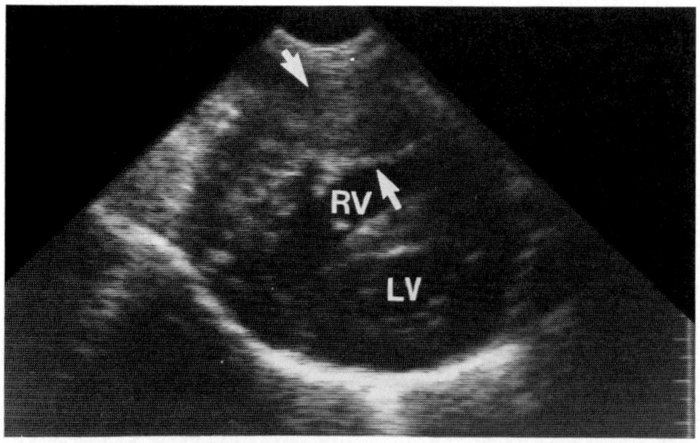

FIGURE 74–31. Cross sectional echocardiogram from a dog with pulmonic stenosis showing marked right ventricular hypertrophy in this short axis view. Compare this to the ventricular septum and left ventricular wall. The right ventricular (RV) and left ventricular (LV) lumina are evident as echo free spaces. The thickness of the right ventricular wall is delineated by the arrows.

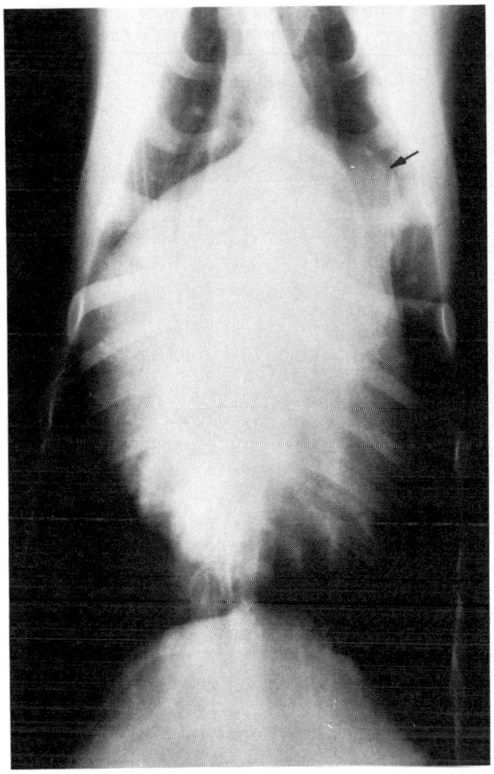

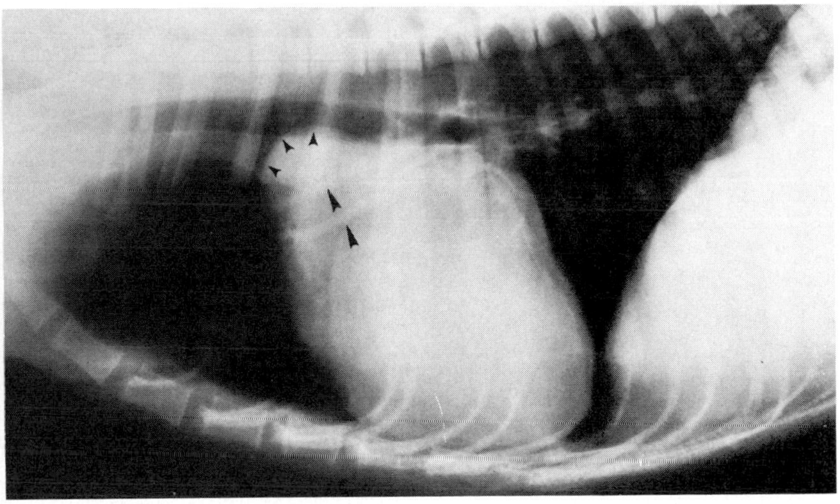

FIGURE 74–32. Ventrodorsal and lateral radiographs from a dog with pulmonic stenosis. In the ventrodorsal view, there is marked enlargement of the right side of the heart, shifting of the apex to the left, and dilation of the main pulmonary artery (arrow). The lateral view shows proximal but not distal tracheal elevation, post-stenotic dilation of the main pulmonary artery (arrowheads), and reduction of pulmonary circulation with relatively small lobar pulmonary arteries and veins (larger arrowheads).

elevated right ventricular end-diastolic pressure and a prominent atrial *a* wave are frequent findings.

Angiocardiography delineates the valvular obstruction and secondary changes in the ventricle and pulmonary artery. Angiocardiographic abnormalities include: dysplastic pulmonary valves, right ventricular hypertrophy, secondary dynamic muscular obstruction of the right ventricular infundibulum, enlargement of the right coronary artery, and post-stenotic dilation of the pulmonary artery. The angiographic features of pulmonic valve dysplasia consist of any combination of the following:[86, 88] narrowing at the immediate base of the valve sinuses, asymmetrical valve sinuses, hypoplasia of the annulus or a valve sinus, thickening of individual valve leaflets producing a lucent filling defect, narrowing of the dye column with a central or asymmetric jet of contrast observed within a narrowed valve orifice, or systolic doming of the valve (indicating fusion of the commissures). Many of these features are illustrated in Figures 74–33 to 74–36.

Natural History. Dogs with mild and even moderate PS can live normally. Animals with moderate to severe stenosis may develop complications including exertional syncope, cardiac arrhythmias, secondary tricuspid regurgitation, atrial fibrillation, congestive heart failure, and sudden death. When an ASD, patent foramen ovale, or VSD coexists with PS, the potential for right to left shunting, hypoxemia, and polycythemia must be appreciated (see section on Cyanotic Heart Disease). While systolic pressure gradients are not always predictive of clinical outcome, we have found a general correlation between pressure gradient and survival.

Clinical Management. Following noninvasive studies, the clinician generally can determine if the stenosis is likely to be mild or moderate to severe. Affected dogs should not be bred. If significant radiographic, ECG, and echocardiographic changes are evident, or if the patient has clinical signs of disease, the pressure gradient should be determined by cardiac catheterization or Doppler echocardiography. It cannot be stated with certainty at what pressure gradient an operation should be recommended; however, the dog with a gradient of greater than 50 mm Hg should be considered as a surgical or balloon valvuloplasty candidate. If the clinician elects to delay surgery in a dog with moderate to severe stenosis (gradient 50 to 99 mm Hg), then the patient should be reevaluated in 6 to 12 months. Over time, progressive infundibular hypertrophy can produce additional obstruction.

A number of surgical procedures have been advocated for the treatment of moderate to severe PS.[87, 91–94] Valvulotomy, partial valvulectomy, and patch-grafting over the outflow tract are most popular. Of critical concern is the nature of subvalvular muscular hypertrophy (Figure 74–34). If this is severe, simple valvulotomy may not be adequate to relieve obstruction. Moreover, valve dilation (Brock dilation) can be initially successful but subsequently fail as a result of scarring. Thus, until more data are available concerning postoperative regression of muscular hypertrophy, it is the author's recommendation that a patch graft technique be employed in cases of valve dysplasia with significant subvalvular muscular hypertrophy. The introduction of balloon valvuloplasty techniques[94b, c] to veterinary cardiology may be promising for cases of isolated stenosis with mobile valves; however, since most cases of PS in the dog resemble atypical PS in children, the ultimate benefit of valvuloplasty in dogs remains to be seen (Figure 74–34*C* and *D*).

When CHF or atrial fibrillation develops, the prog-

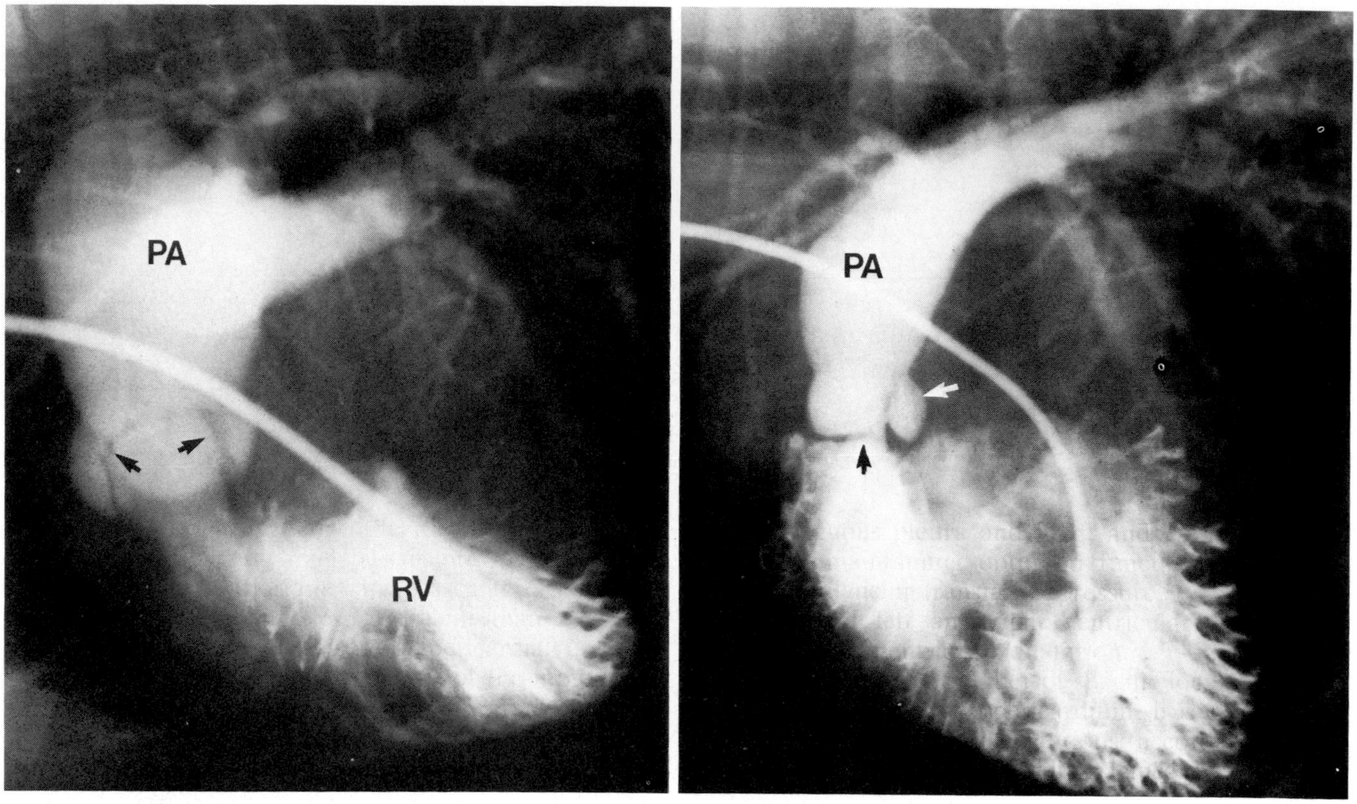

FIGURE 74–33. Angiocardiograms from two dogs with pulmonary valve dysplasia. Right—following injection of contrast into the right ventricle, dye is funneled into a relatively small area in the region of the pulmonary valves (lower arrow) before it fills the main pulmonary artery (PA). Slight distortion of the pulmonary valve sinuses is evident (upper arrow), and there is marked thickening at the base of the valve sinuses. Left—thickening of the pulmonary valve cusp (arrows) in a dog with pulmonic valve dysplasia. Following the right ventricular injection, contrast funneled in a relatively narrow area of the pulmonary valve, surrounded the valve by filling the sinuses, and opacified the post-stenotic dilation in the main pulmonary artery (PA). RV = right ventricle.

nosis is poor and medical treatment (Table 74–5), balloon valvuloplasty, and initial stabilization should be accomplished prior to any surgical intervention.

PULMONIC INSUFFICIENCY

Pulmonic insufficiency (PI) is an uncommon abnormality that has been observed in basset hounds and other breeds.[95, 96] Abnormal development of valve leaflets or dilation of the pulmonary artery annulus has been observed in pups with congenital PI. The resultant insufficiency leads to right ventricular dilation. Heart failure can develop in severe PI induced experimentally in dogs. Pulmonic insufficiency also can develop secondary to pulmonary hypertension or pulmonic valve dysplasia (and surgery) and is associated with dilation of the main pulmonary artery in dogs with PDA.

Clinical features include variable systolic and diastolic murmurs. Enlargement of the main pulmonary artery and right ventricle may be evident on thoracic radiography. The ECG shows right ventricular hypertrophy. Angiography (Figure 74–36) documents regurgitation in excess of that expected from the catheter and slow clearance of contrast from the dilated right ventricle. Echocardiography may show diastolic fluttering of the tricuspid valve if the regurgitant jets strike the atrioventricular valve. Doppler studies document PI and the regurgitant jet will be of high velocity (>2 m/s) when there is pulmonary hypertension.

The principal significance of this defect is that it not be confused with PDA, in which the supporting electrocardiographic and radiographic findings are quite dissimilar from those of congenital pulmonic insufficiency.[95] Treatment has not been described; however, some dogs tolerate the lesion well. Medical therapy of heart failure is indicated in dogs with signs of systemic venous congestion.

AORTIC STENOSIS

Aortic stenosis (more correctly termed subaortic stenosis [SAS] in the dog) is one of the most important congenital malformations of the canine heart and continues to confound breeders of large breed dogs.[97–109] Supravalvular stenosis is rare in dogs, although it has been described more often in the cat,[101] and pure valvular aortic stenosis per se is very uncommon, although the author has seen two cases in the dog and others report its occurrence. The lesions and clinical consequences of left ventricular outflow obstruction are summarized below.

Pathogenesis. Aside from sporadic case reports and the necropsy studies of Liu and associates[12, 13, 101] and Harpster,[36] little is known about aortic stenosis in the

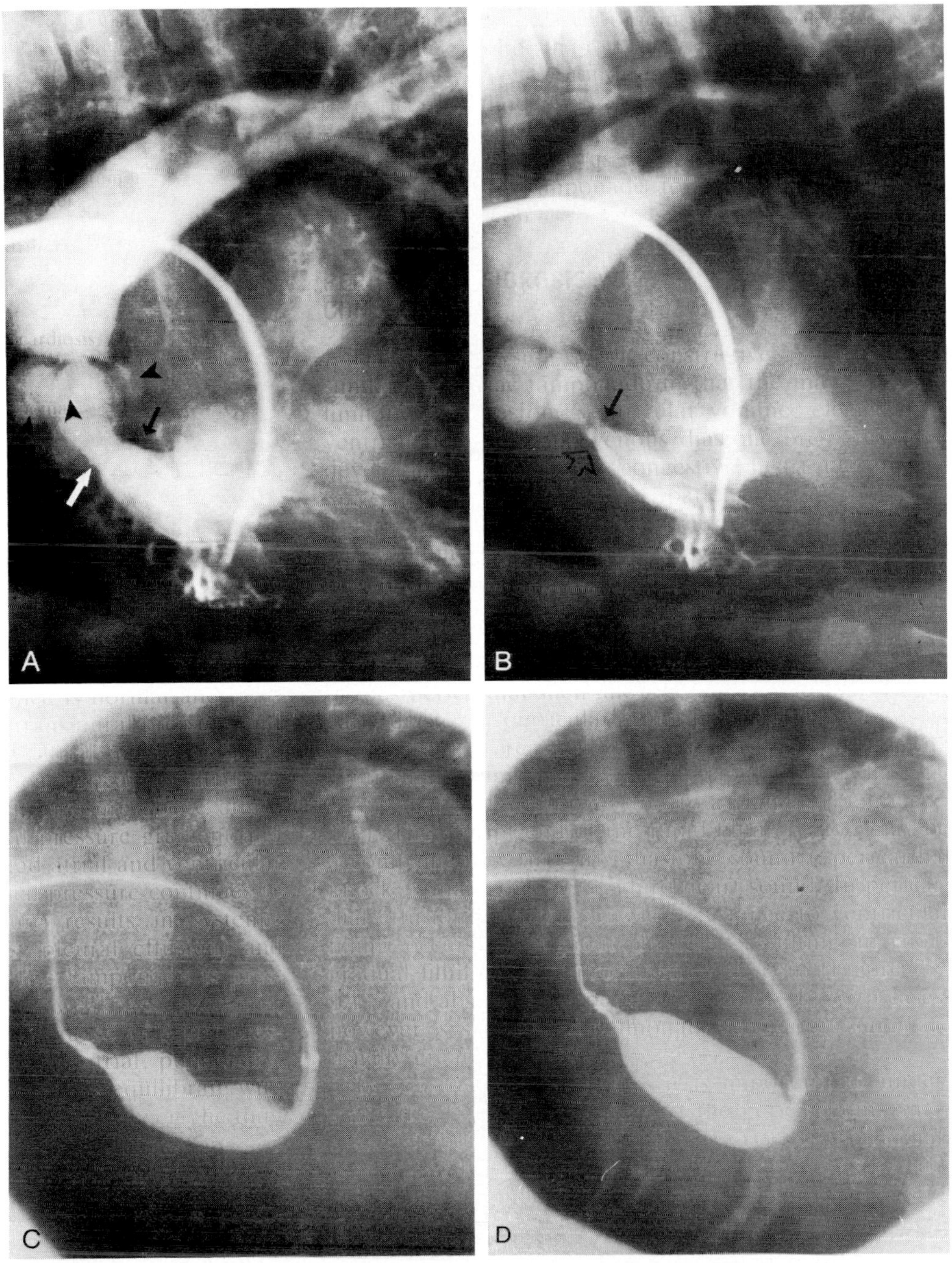

FIGURE 74–34. Pulmonic stenosis in the dog. A and B—Secondary muscular obstruction due to pulmonic valve dysplasia. *A,* Following injection of contrast into the right ventricle, narrowing is evident just below the pulmonary valves due to hypertrophy of the ventricular infundibulum (white arrow) and the supraventricular crest (black arrow). The pulmonary valve is dysplastic and the valve sinuses unequal in size (arrowheads). Note that in the later systolic frame *(B)* there has been marked attenuation of the subvalvular region as a result of dynamic muscular obstruction (arrows). *C* and *D*—Radiographs obtained from a different dog with congenital pulmonic stenosis during catheter balloon valvuloplasty. In *C,* a radiopaque guide wire has been passed across the pulmonary valve and into the main pulmonary artery. The balloon catheter has been advanced along the guide wire to straddle the obstruction (the extent of the balloon is noted by opaque markers). Following partial inflation of the balloon, the valve and annulus begin to distend. The dorsal aspect of the stenosis is evident as an indentation in the balloon. Following full inflation *(D)*, the stenosis has apparently been relieved; however, in this particular case, repeated dilations were unsuccessful in significantly reducing the systolic pressure gradient. Balloon dilation is less likely to be successful if the annulus is hypoplastic or the valves markedly thickened and dysplastic.

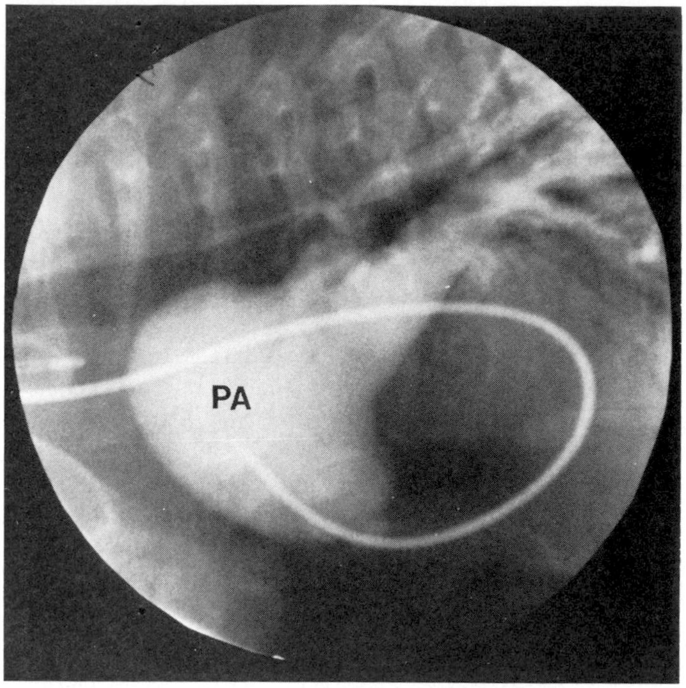

FIGURE 74–35. Subvalvular pulmonic stenosis or double-chambered right ventricle. Contrast was injected into the right ventricle, which resulted in opacification of this chamber and the main pulmonary artery (PA). The pulmonary valve area is wide and normal; however, there is marked narrowing of the dye column at the junction of the right ventricular inflow and outflow tracts. There is a focal area of filling within the ventral right ventricular wall. The obstruction was a consistent finding on repeated films, and the location is most compatible with a so-called double chambered right ventricle.

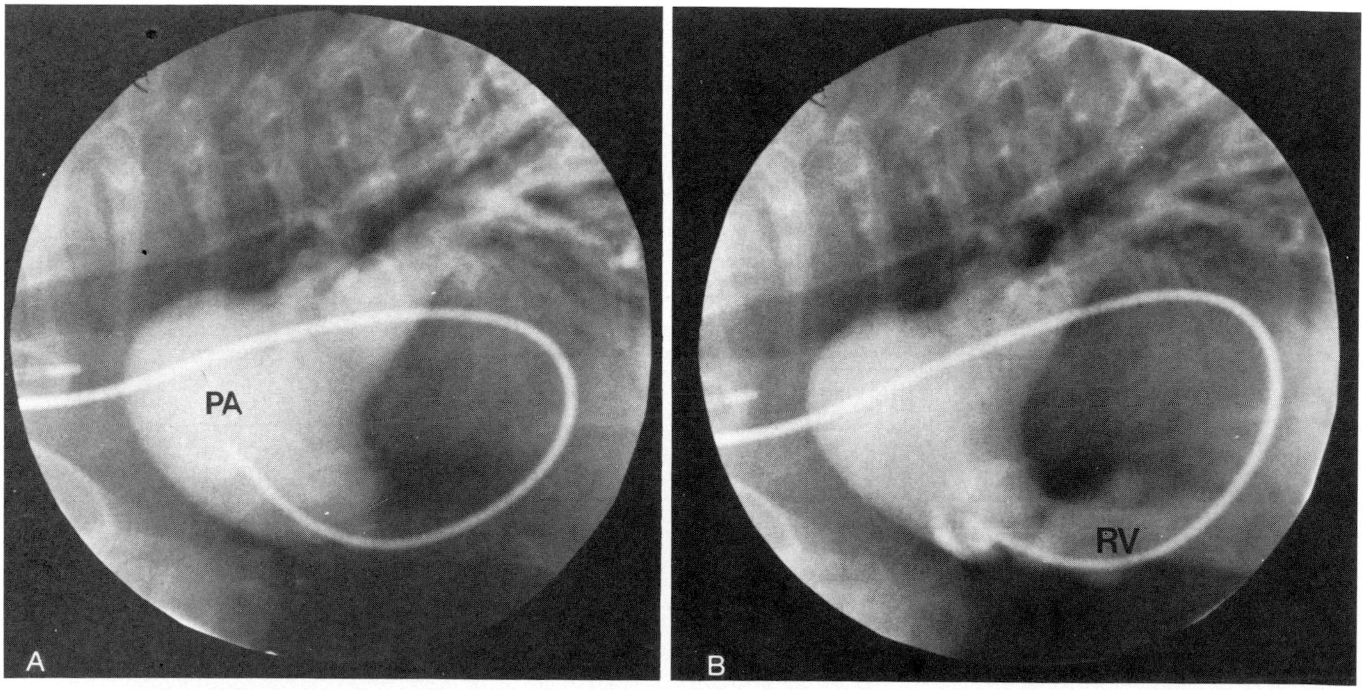

FIGURE 74–36. Pulmonic insufficiency in a bassett hound. *A*, The catheter has been advanced into the main pulmonary artery (PA) and contrast was injected. In the subsequent film *(B)*, contrast is noted to regurgitate back across the pulmonary valve into the right ventricle (RV). This dog also had an obvious diastolic murmur, diastolic fluttering of the tricuspid valve on echocardiography, and significant dilation of the right ventricle. A mild pulmonic stenosis was also present, but the predominant abnormality appeared to be pulmonic insufficiency. The cause of the marked dilation of the main pulmonary artery is unknown.

TABLE 74–5. THERAPY OF CONGENITAL HEART DISEASE

Lesion Treatment	Palliative Treatment	Definitive
Aortic stenosis	Medical therapy CHF,* beta-blockade, exercise restriction, ?balloon dilation	Ventricular to aortic valved conduit; surgical resection of subvalvular ring†
Atrial septal defect	Pulmonary artery banding, medical therapy CHF*	Suture or patch closures
Mitral dysplasia	Medical therapy CHF,* treat arrhythmias	? Valve replacement† Commissurotomy‡
Patent ductus arteriosus	Medical therapy CHF	Surgical ligation of PDA
Persistent right fourth aortic arch	Treatment of aspiration pneumonia; feeding liquids, gruel in upright position	Ligation and division of PDA or ligamentum arteriosum
Pulmonary hypertension (Eisenmenger's physiology)	Rest, phlebotomy (control PCV), oxygen	None
Pulmonic stenosis	Medical therapy CHF	Surgical treatment:§ valvulotomy, partial valvulectomy, Brock dilation, patch graft technique, ventricular-arterial conduit, balloon valvuloplasty
Tetralogy of Fallot	Systemic pulmonary shunt, phlebotomy (control PCV), ?propranolol, rest, oxygen	Surgical repair of VSD and PS†
Tricuspid dysplasia	Medical therapy CHF,* treat arrhythmias	?Valve replacement† or annuloplasty Commissurotomy‡
Ventricular septal defect	Medical therapy CHF,* pulmonary artery banding	Surgical closure‡

*Control of congestive heart failure: rest, sodium-restricted diet, furosemide, digitalis; hydralazine may decrease the magnitude of left to right shunting with septal defects or PDA. Antiarrhythmic treatment if required.

†Generally requires cardiopulmonary bypass, hypothermia, or both.

‡Commissurotomy for dysplasia causing valve stenosis; can be done as intracardiac operation or by balloon valvuloplasty.

§Procedure depends on type of valve malformation, degree of secondary muscular ventricular outflow obstruction, and surgical experience; temporary systemic venous occlusion may be required.

cat; however, SAS in dogs has been studied extensively in the Newfoundland dog. Data derived from colony studies of Pyle and Patterson[4, 99, 100, 103, 104] in this breed are identical to the clinical features observed in other breeds with SAS. Breeding studies in the Newfoundland established a genetic basis for the perpetuation of SAS.[4, 100] The mode of transmission is most compatible with a polygenic mechanism, or possibly an autosomal dominant with modifying genes. Pathology studies suggest that the subvalvular obstruction may not necessarily be present at birth, but instead develops postnatally, during the first four to eight weeks of life. This time sequence may have clinical significance relative to the identification of cardiac murmurs in pups of breeds known to be at risk for SAS.

Subaortic stenosis in Newfoundland dogs has been graded based on postmortem studies as follows:[4, 100] grade 1: the mildest form, consisting of "small, whitish, slightly raised nodules on the endocardial surface of the ventricular septum immediately below the aortic valve"; grade 2: a "narrow ridge of whitish, thickened endocardium" extending partially about the left ventricular outflow tract; grade 3: the most severe form, "a fibrous band, ridge, or collar completely encircling the left ventricular outflow tract just below the aortic valve" (Figure 74–37). This ring is raised above the endocardium, extends to, and may involve the cranioventral leaflet of the mitral valve and the base of the aortic valves.

The stenotic ring consists of loosely arranged reticular fibers, mucopolysaccharide ground substance, and elastic fibers. Discrete bundles of collagen and even cartilage are found in advanced lesions.[100]

Associated necropsy findings include concentric left ventricular hypertrophy, left atrial hypertrophy, and poststenotic dilation of the ascending aorta and aortic arch. Auscultation and cardiac catheterization of dogs with grade 1 lesions failed to reliably detect the postmortem lesion, whereas grade 2 lesions often were associated with soft cardiac murmurs and only minimal systolic pressure gradients. The clinical implication of these findings is clear; while genes coding for SAS may be carried by a dog, clinical detection may be quite difficult in mild cases, and genetic counseling may be fraught with error.

Flickinger and Patterson[103] and Pyle[104] also have shown that coronary circulation in dogs with SAS is abnormal. Lesions characterized by extensive changes of the intramural coronary arteries were found. Histologic changes include intimal proliferation of connective tissue and smooth muscle, and medial degeneration. These changes are presumably secondary to the high wall tension found in this condition. Focal areas of myocardial infarction and fibrosis have been observed in conjunction with these vascular changes. Pyle demonstrated abnormal coronary flow with diminished baseline diastolic flow and actual reversal of coronary flow during systole.[8, 104]

Pathophysiology. Figure 74–38 summarizes the clinical pathophysiology of SAS in the dog. Owing to ventricular outflow obstruction, left ventricular systolic pressure increases, and a pressure gradient is detected across the outflow tract (Figure 74–5). Obstruction to ejection causes a late rising arterial pulse. High velocity and turbulent flow across this area are associated with a systolic cardiac murmur and poststenotic dilation of the ascending aorta, aortic arch, and brachycephalic trunk. Left atrial hypertrophy develops as a consequence of the elevated left atrial pressure needed to fill the stiff, hypertrophied left ventricle (LVH).

In some cases a to-and-fro murmur of aortic stenosis/aortic regurgitation is evident. It is caused by involvement of the valve leaflets with the fibrous ring, dilation

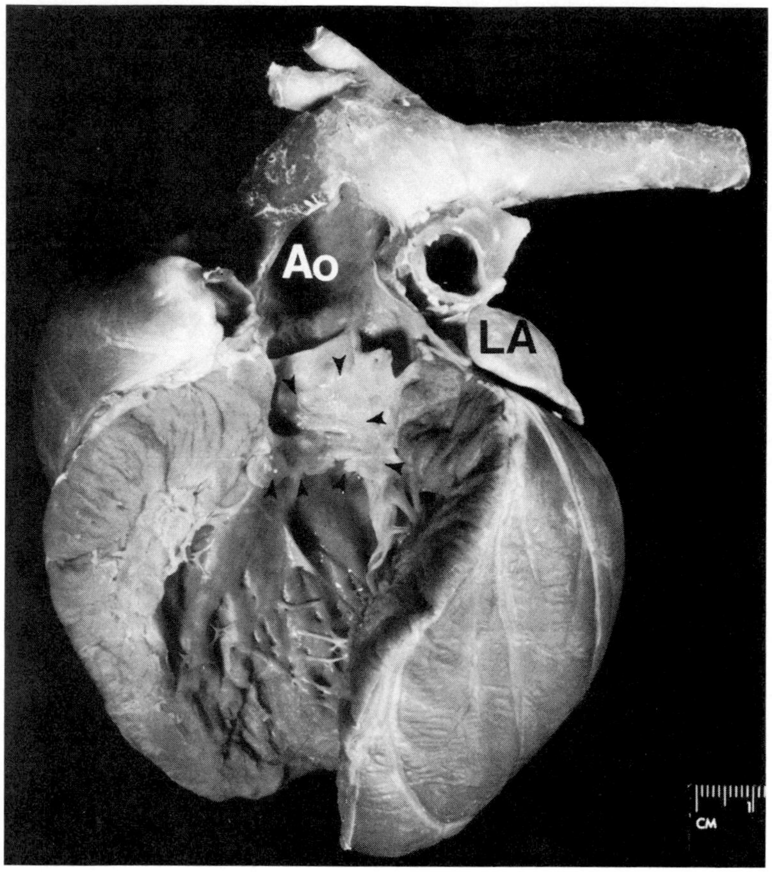

FIGURE 74–37. Specimen from a dog with congenital subaortic stenosis. An extensive subaortic valvular fibrous ring (arrowheads) extends from the cranioventral mitral leaflet to the base of the aortic valve cusps. There is post-stenotic dilation of the ascending aorta (Ao). The left auricle (LA) is indicated. There is marked left ventricular hypertrophy.

of the aortic annulus, and bacterial endocarditis. Left ventricular hypertrophy and myocardial ischemia are probably responsible for changes in the QRS complex and ST-T segment.

Critical SAS can lead to left-sided congestive heart failure. More often, exertional syncope or sudden death is reported, caused by undetermined mechanisms. Certainly, the development of myocardial ischemia and malignant ventricular arrhythmias must be considered a potential cause of hypotension.[8] In addition, severe hypotension might result from exercise-induced increases in left ventricular pressure, activation of ventricular mechanoreceptors, and inappropriate bradycardia or vasodilation.

Clinical Findings. Clinical findings[5–9, 98–100] in pups with mild SAS are minimal. Affected dogs are asymptomatic and have a soft to moderately intense ejection murmur that can easily be confused with a functional murmur. More severely affected dogs may be presented with exertional tiring, syncope, or left-sided congestive heart failure. Sudden death, without premonitory signs, is common.

Congenital SAS is most common among larger breeds including the Newfoundland, boxer, German shepherd,

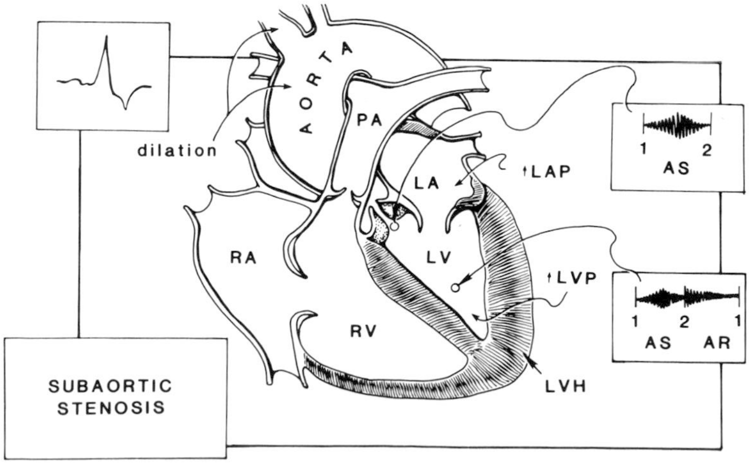

FIGURE 74–38. Schematic illustration demonstrating the pathophysiology of congenital subaortic stenosis. See text for details. (By permission from Bonagura, JD: Congenital heart disease. *In* Bonagura JD (ed): Cardiology. New York, Churchill Livingstone, 1987.)

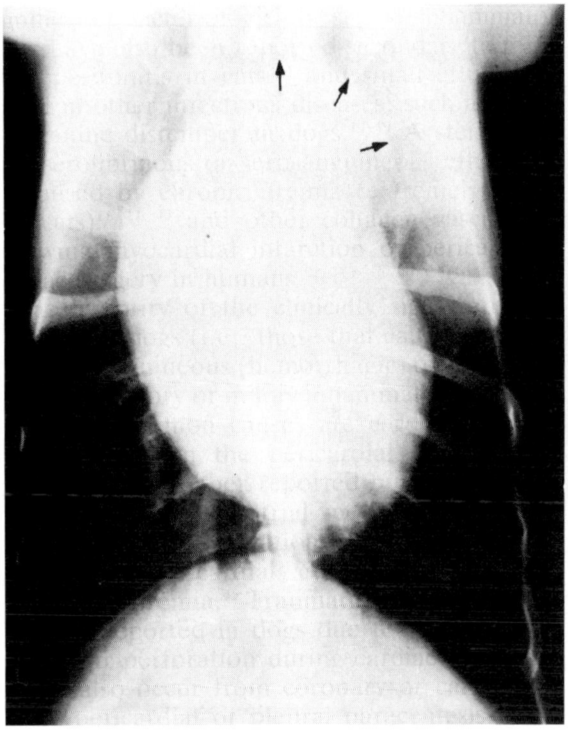

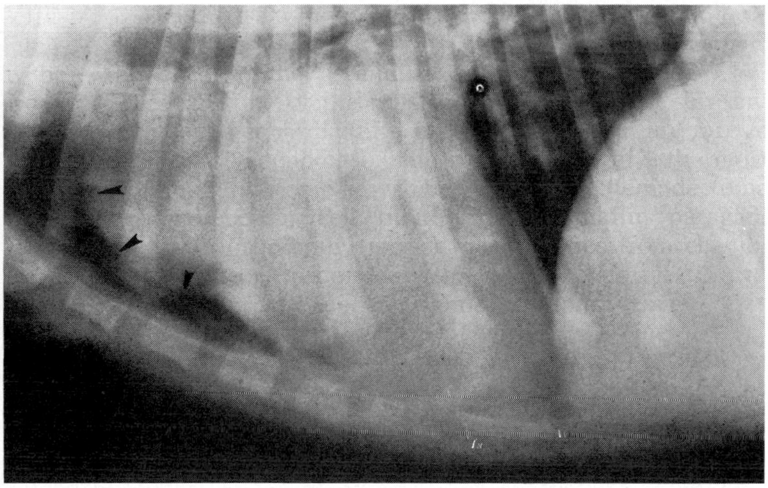

FIGURE 74–39. Thoracic radiographs from two dogs with congenital subaortic stenosis. The dorsoventral panel *(left)* shows minimal enlargement of the heart but significant dilation of the aorta within the mediastinum and in the area of the aortic arch (arrows). This is compatible with poststenotic dilation. Lateral view from a different dog *(right panel)* shows left atrial enlargement and dramatic poststenotic dilation of the aorta causing a cranioventral widening in the mediastinum (arrowheads). This dog also had aortic regurgitation.

and golden retriever.[8] Other large breeds, such as the Rottweiler and German short-haired pointer, also may be overrepresented in some parts of the United States.

Recognition of severe SAS is not difficult, as the ventricular outflow obstruction generates an ejection murmur of variable intensity, and in some cases, there is a soft diastolic murmur secondary to incompetency of the aortic valve. The murmur is most intense in the subaortic region (about the fourth intercostal space) and tends to radiate down the apex, up the carotid arteries, and even to the calvarium. Frequently, the systolic murmur is equally loud at the right cardiac base, presumably from radiation into the ascending aorta. As previously mentioned, SAS probably develops in the postnatal period; thus, the murmur may become more prominent during the first few months of life. We have noted an increasing number of dogs with both SAS and mitral regurgitation, but these murmurs are somewhat similar in timing and point of maximal intensity and therefore can be difficult to distinguish. Other physical examination abnormalities include an arterial pulse that is hypokinetic and tardy and a left ventricular apical impulse that is prominent from ventricular hypertrophy.

Thoracic radiography can be normal or indicate left ventricular hypertrophy (Figure 74–39).[8, 22–24] The mediastinum may be widened as a result of poststenotic dilation of the aorta. Pulmonary circulation is normal unless there is pulmonary edema and venous congestion. When marked left atrial enlargement is present, intercurrent mitral regurgitation should be suspected. Echocardiography demonstrates left ventricular hypertrophy, a subvalvular fibrous ring that can involve the mitral valve, and poststenotic dilation of the aorta (Figure 74–40).[27, 106] Doppler studies can be used to quantitate increased velocity flow and turbulence about the stenosis, and may also detect aortic regurgitation which is often inaudible during clinical examination. The systolic gradient can be estimated from the peak velocity using the relationship $\Delta P = 4V^2$ (Figure 74–1*C*).

The ECG may be normal, but in advanced cases indicates left ventricular hypertrophy. Either left axis deviation (Figure 74–4) or increased R-wave amplitude with a normal frontal axis can be observed. Widening of the QRS is not uncommon. ST-T segment depression is compatible with myocardial ischemia (or left ventricular hypertrophy). Ischemia should be strongly suspected when exercise precipitates even greater ST-T change or ventricular arrhythmias (Figure 74–41).

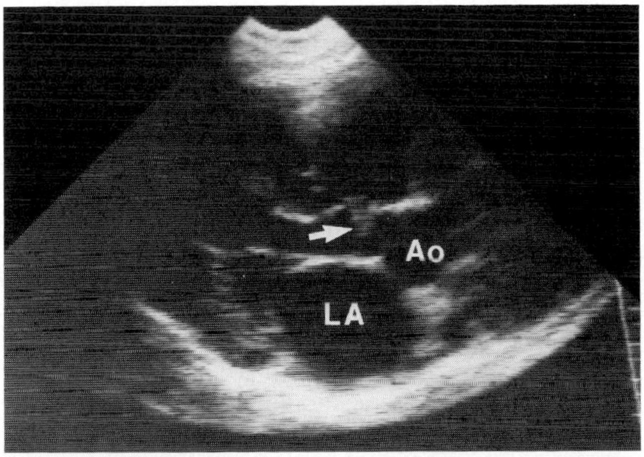

FIGURE 74–40. Cross sectional echocardiogram obtained from a dog with congenital subaortic stenosis. The view is obtained from the right hemithorax and shows the left atrium (LA), aorta (Ao), and the region of the left ventricular outflow tract. The left ventricular apex (not seen) is to the viewer's left. A significant fibrous obstruction is evident (arrow) just below the aortic sinuses of Valsalva.

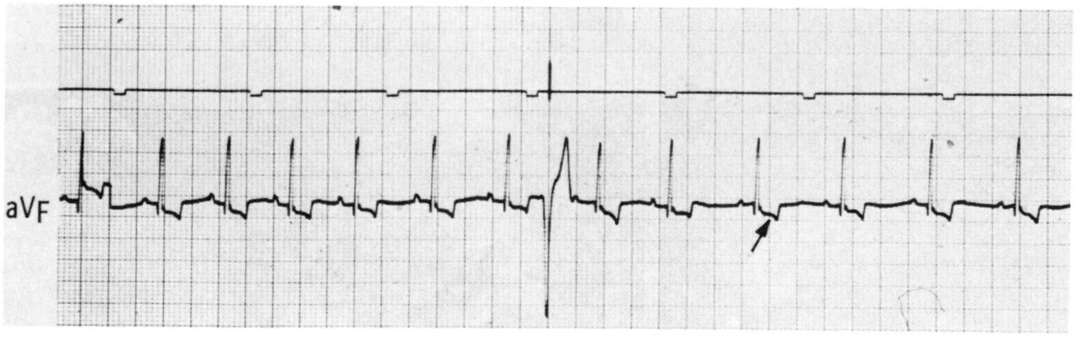

FIGURE 74–41. Electrocardiogram from a dog with congenital subaortic stenosis. There is a single interpolated ventricular premature complex and significant ST segment depression (arrow). This may indicate myocardial ischemia in this dog. Paper speed = 50 mm per second; calibration: 5 mm = 1 mV.

Cardiac catheterization demonstrates a gradient across the obstruction and generally records an elevation of ventricular diastolic pressure (Figures 74–5, 74–6, and 74–8) (see section on Cardiac Catheterization).[8, 105] Gradients of less than 50 mm Hg are compatible with mild SAS. The gradient during a post-extrasystolic potentiation, recorded after an induced ventricular premature beat, may be considerably higher than that recorded during sinus rhythm. One might suspect that such potentiation is suggestive of what develops in the unanesthetized dog during stress or exercise.

The left ventriculogram outlines a relatively small ventricular cavity and illustrates the subvalvular obstruction, poststenotic dilation, and intercurrent problems like mitral regurgitation (Figures 74–10 and 74–42). The lesion is most evident in the ventral aspect of the outflow tract when viewed on the lateral projection. A supravalvular aortic injection should be done to rule out aortic insufficiency. The left extramural coronary artery and its major branches are often noted to be prominent.

Natural History. Severe SAS is a discouraging condition, since most dogs either die suddenly or develop

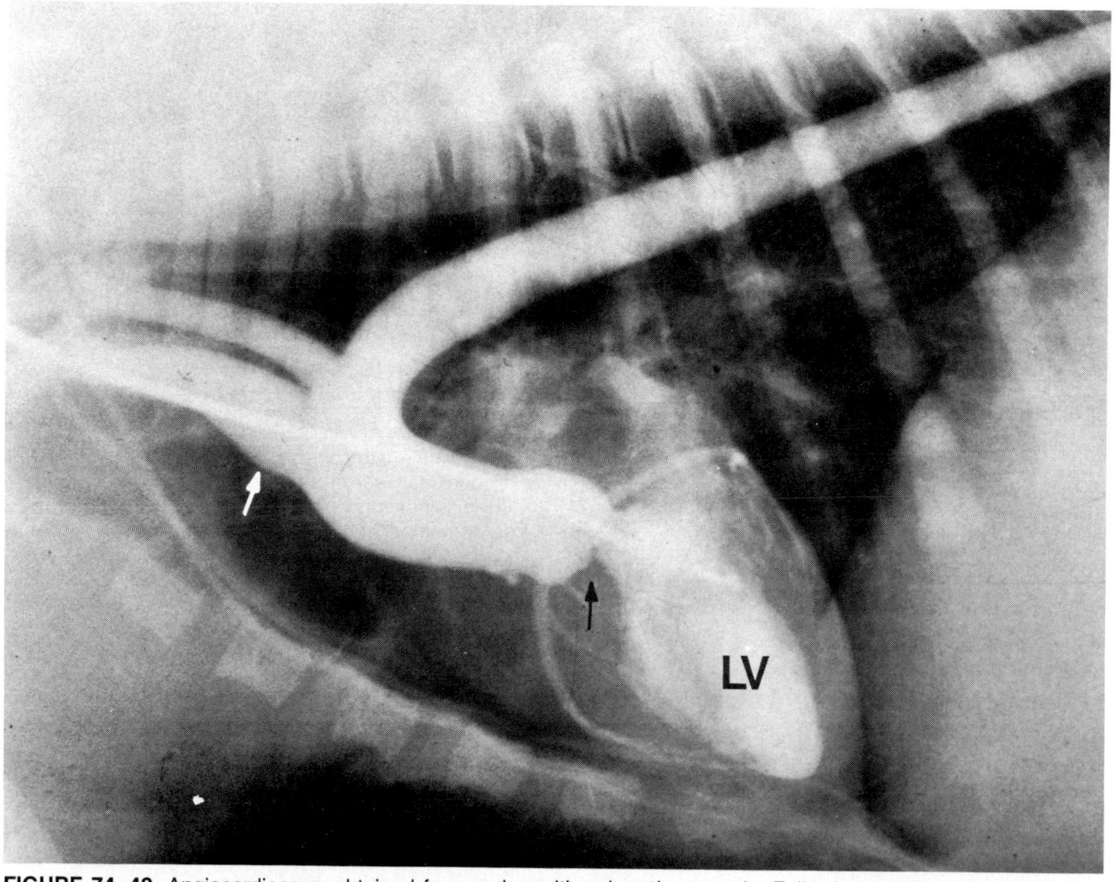

FIGURE 74–42. Angiocardiogram obtained from a dog with subaortic stenosis. Following injection of contrast into the left ventricle (LV) the subvalvular aortic obstruction (lower arrow) is obvious. There is poststenotic dilation of the ascending aorta and of the brachiocephalic trunk (upper arrow). The left ventricular wall appears thickened. The valve region is at the level of origin of the coronary arteries.

congestive heart failure. Mitral regurgitation, aortic regurgitation, aortic valve endocarditis, and atrial fibrillation are complicating factors that generally lead to the pet's demise. It is axiomatic that a clinical examination in an asymptomatic dog cannot reliably predict the severity of the stenosis. While a long and loud ejection murmur, markedly attenuated pulses, and abnormalities of the ECG and chest x-ray film suggest significant SAS, echocardiography (with Doppler) and/or cardiac catheterization are usually required to confirm the severity of the condition.

Dogs with minimal ventricular hypertrophy, only mild ventricular outflow obstruction, and a pressure gradient of less than 50 mm Hg are likely to be near-normal pets. Dogs with gradients of 75 mm Hg or more usually develop complications or sudden death.

Clinical Management. Dogs with mild SAS documented by detailed studies are treated normally, and are not used for breeding. Prophylaxis for bacterial endocarditis is prudent. Dogs with moderate to severe SAS should have restricted exercise. While surgical procedures have been employed to either remove the obstruction or bypass it with a left apical to aortic conduit, such surgery is rarely performed.[107] The author prescribes β-blocking drugs such as propranolol or nadolol (Table 74–5) empirically to dogs with a history of syncope (without CHF), gradients of greater than 100 torr, or with significant ST-T changes or premature ventricular complexes noted on a postexercise ECG. β-blockade is used in an attempt to decrease myocardial oxygen demand. The value of such treatment is unproven.

AORTIC REGURGITATION

With an increasing awareness of this condition, and the application of angiography and Doppler echocardiography to the study of congenital heart disease, aortic regurgitation (AR) is being recognized with increasing frequency as a complication of cardiac malformation.[108, 109] While isolated congenital AR appears to be rare, this condition can complicate high ventricular septal defects, aortic stenosis, and possibly tetralogy of Fallot. The potential mechanisms for AR with these conditions have been reviewed by Eyster et al.[108]

A diastolic murmur, heard best over the left hemithorax, is typical of AR (Figure 74–12), and the diagnosis is supported by palpation of a hyperkinetic arterial pulse. Left ventricular dilatation and hypertrophy develop. The pathophysiology and additional responses to AR are similar to those described for the acquired condition on page 1048. Significant AR can lead to left ventricular failure. Documentation of AR requires either angiocardiography (Figure 74–27) or Doppler echocardiography.

DYSPLASIA OF THE ATRIOVENTRICULAR VALVES

Malformations of the mitral and tricuspid valves are observed in both cats and dogs.[12, 113, 110–121] Mitral dysplasia in cats represents one of the most important types of cardiac malformation in this species. Malformed atrioventricular valves, as a general rule, are incompetent; yet, careful echocardiographic and catheterization studies may demonstrate valve stenosis as well. In many ways, congenital atrioventricular valve dysplasia is similar to acquired degenerative valvular disease in the dog. For this reason, only the salient features of these conditions will be reviewed, and the reader is directed to Chapter 75 on Valvular Heart Disease for greater detail.

Pathogenesis. The cause of mitral and tricuspid valve dysplasia is unknown. Undoubtedly, a genetic basis exists in certain breeds; however, detailed breeding trials have not been reported. The pathology of this condition has been described by Liu and Tilley and in the necropsy reports of others. A spectrum of lesions has been identified, including shortening, rolling, notching, and thickening of the valve leaflets, fusion and thickening of chordae tendineae or elongation of the chordae, direct insertion of the valve cusp into a papillary muscle, atrophy or hypertrophy of the papillary muscles, and upward malpositioning of the papillary muscles leading to a horizontal alignment of the cords (Figures 74–43 and 74–44).[113–120] These features are common to both left and right atrioventricular valves. Additionally, dogs and cats with tricuspid dysplasia can have fusion of papillary muscles, patency of the foramen ovale or concurrent ASD, and fibrinous epicarditis over the dilated right atrium.[116, 119]

Whether or not some cases of tricuspid dysplasia represent Ebstein's anomaly is unresolved.[120, 121] In the latter condition, the anomalous tricuspid valve is displaced down into the ventricle. Simultaneous intracardiac pressure and electrode studies are needed to document a ventricular electrogram in the lowermost portion of the downwardly displaced right atrium.[15]

Pathophysiology. The essential pathophysiologic abnormalities can be summarized as follows: 1) valve regurgitation with resultant volume overloading and diminished cardiac output, 2) dilation with hypertrophy of the ventricle and atrium on the affected side, 3) predisposition to cardiac arrhythmias, particularly atrial fibrillation, 4) potential for valve stenosis with obstruction to ventricular filling, and 5) potential for right to left shunting through the foramen ovale or an ASD in cases of tricuspid dysplasia.

While atrioventricular valve insufficiency is more common than stenosis, the possibility of valve obstruction should be considered if the ventricle is normal in size but the atrium is dilated, or if right to left atrial shunting is documented by echocardiography. In cases of dysplasia causing valve stenosis, a diastolic gradient will be recorded across the affected valve (Figures 74–5 and 74–7) and transmitral (or transtricuspid) flow velocity will be increased above normal values as measured by Doppler echocardiography. Valvular regurgitation leads to prominent cv waves in the atrial pressure curve (Figure 74–5). Cardiac output is limited even in the setting of elevated ventricular diastolic pressures.

Clinical Findings. The Great Dane, German shepherd, and possibly the Afghan hound are predisposed to mitral dysplasia.[111–114] Tricuspid dysplasia seems to be most common in large male dogs,[9] and the Old English sheepdog and Labrador retriever may be at increased risk. Presenting symptoms include signs referable to

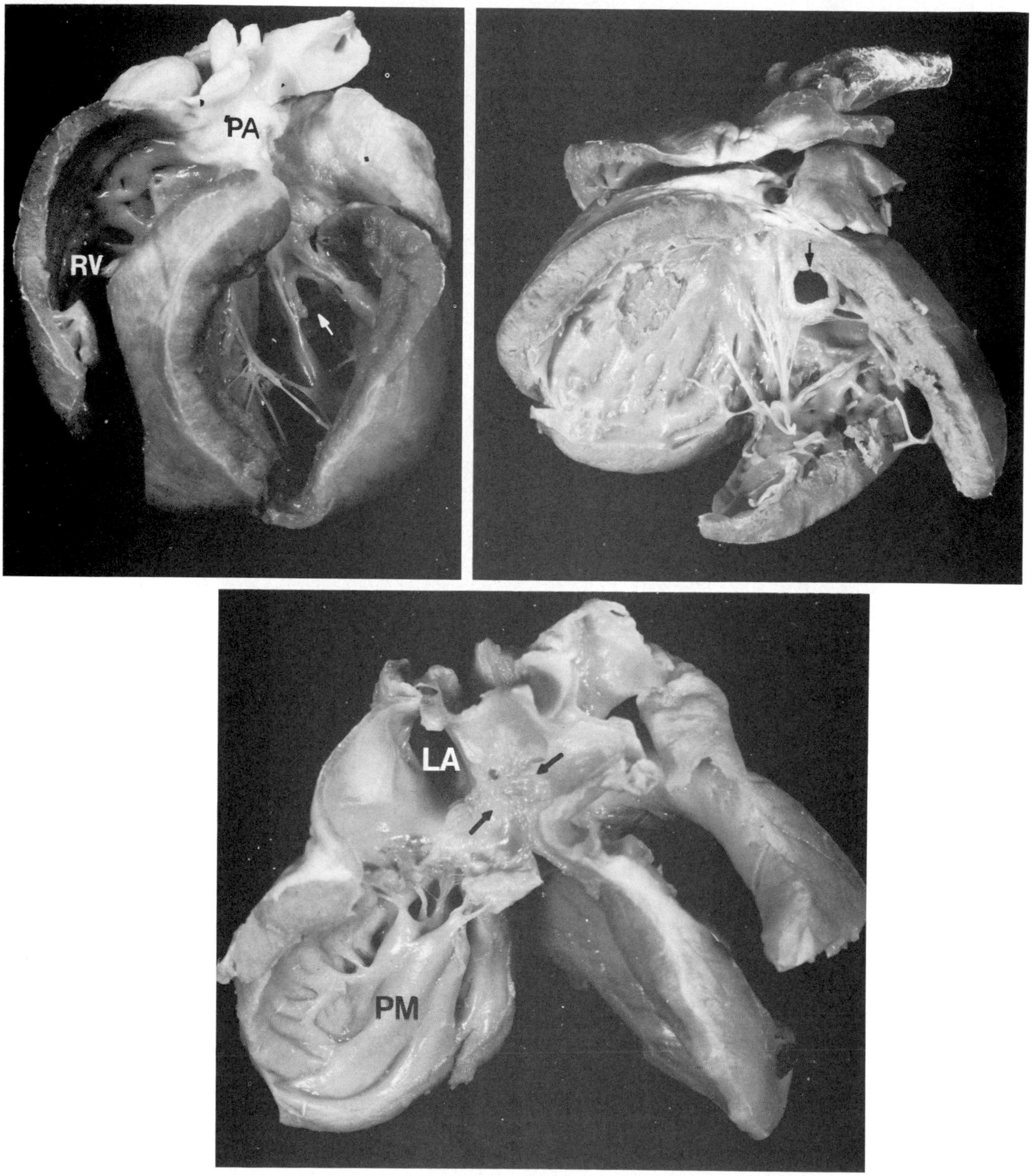

FIGURE 74–43. Mitral valve dysplasia. Three specimens are shown. Left—dysplastic mitral valve from a cat. The valve cusp is thickened and the leaflet is C-shaped (arrow). Both cranioventral and caudodorsal cusps were similar and resulted in an oval opening of mitral incompetency in this cat. The left auricle is markedly dilated. The right ventricle (RV) and pulmonary artery (PA) are marked. Ventricular moderator bands adjacent to the papillary muscles of the left ventricular seem prominent. Lower panel—heart of a mature cat with diabetes and congestive heart failure. The open left ventricle shows a singular papillary muscle (PM) with relatively short chordae tendineae attaching to an abnormal mitral valve. Jet lesions (arrows) are evident in the opened left atrium (LA). Right panel—a ring-type mitral valve dysplasia in a dog (arrow). This dog also had a patent ductus arteriosus (not shown).

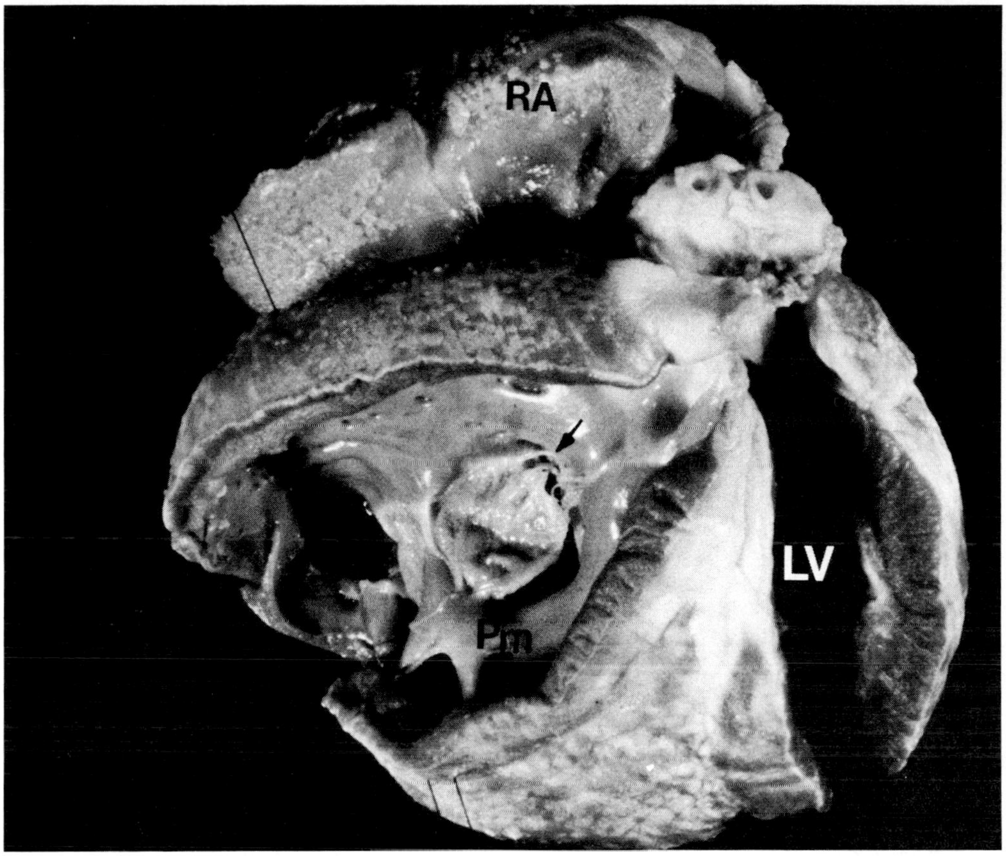

FIGURE 74–44. Post mortem specimen from a dog with tricuspid valve dysplasia. The right atrium (RA) is markedly dilated as a result of tricuspid regurgitation. The tricuspid valve itself is grossly malformed with short chordae tendineae (arrow), malformation of the valve leaflets and cusps, and abnormalities of the papillary muscles (Pm) characterized by a single large papillary muscle instead of the usual three to four smaller muscles.

congestive heart failure. The physical examination reveals a holosystolic murmur heard best over the affected valve area and at the apex (the sternum in cats with mitral dysplasia) (see Figure 74–45 and Table 74–3). Less commonly, a soft diastolic rumble is auscultated over the inflow tract of the ventricle. A loud gallop may be evident.[111] Right, left, or biventricular congestive heart failure may be evident from examination and radiography. Atrial arrhythmias, especially atrial fibrillation, are common. An ECG may also indicate atrial and ventricular enlargement, findings that are substantiated by thoracic radiography and echocardiography (Figures 74–46 to 74–51). Ventricular conduction disturbances are very common in dogs with tricuspid dysplasia.

Definitive diagnosis requires echocardiography and possibly cardiac catheterization and angiocardiography. Abnormal location, shape, motion, or attachment of the valve apparatus is observed by echocardiography (Figures 74–46 and 74–49). Doppler studies document a regurgitant jet or valvular stenosis. At the catheterization table, the ventricular injection of contrast material outlines a dilated ventricle, regurgitant valve orifice, and a huge atrium (Figures 74–47 and 74–51). Clearance of

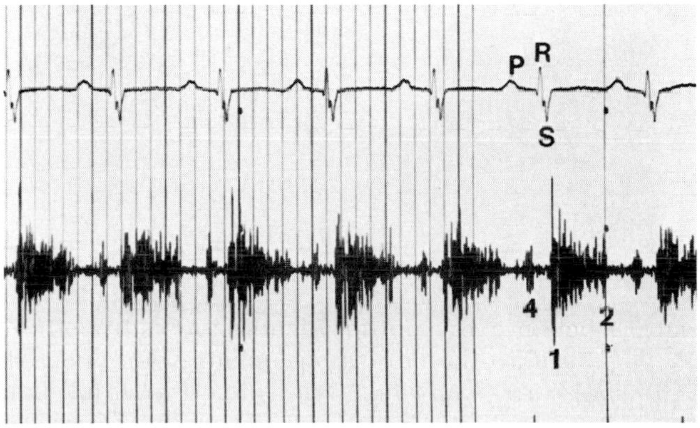

FIGURE 74–45. Phonocardiogram from a cat with mitral regurgitation due to dysplasia of the mitral valve. An S-4 gallop (4) is evident as well as a systolic murmur between the first and second heart sounds.

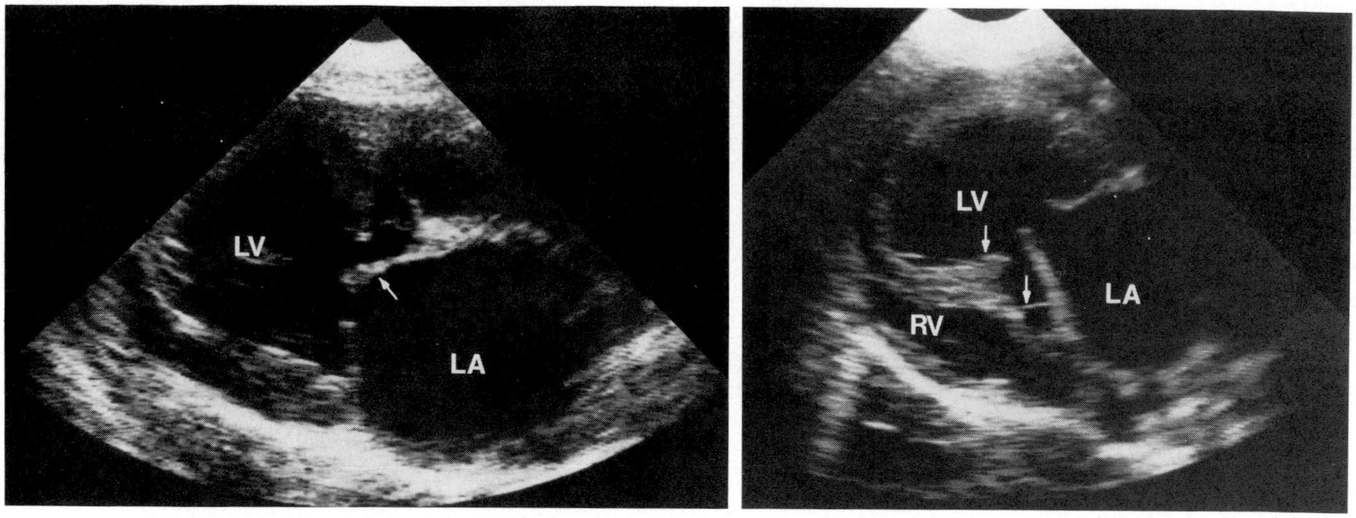

FIGURE 74–46. Cross sectional echocardiograms from a dog with mitral valve dysplasia with mitral stenosis and subaortic stenosis. The dysplastic mitral valve is characterized in the left panel by a marked thickening of the cranioventral leaflet (arrow). There is also left atrial (LA) dilation. LV = left ventricle. The right panel was obtained from the left hemithorax and shows the left atrium, left ventricle (LV), and right ventricle (RV). The mitral valve opening was maximal at this point and it is markedly narrowed when compared to normal dogs. The subaortic obstruction is also evident here (upper arrows) well below the aortic valve proper (lower arrow).

contrast is markedly delayed. Global ventricular muscle function is much better than that observed in cases of idiopathic dilated cardiomyopathy.[115] Potential catheterization abnormalities have been discussed previously.

Clinical Management. The natural history of atrioventricular valve dysplasia is often one of progressive valve dysfunction, cardiomegaly, heart failure, and death. While only the most severely affected animals are likely to be described in clinical reports, it is emphasized that heart failure and atrial arrhythmias often develop within the first year of life.[114, 119] Cats with mitral dysplasia may live normally for a number of years before developing heart failure, or may never develop clinical signs at all. When significant cardiomegaly is evident, the prognosis is guarded to poor.

The therapy of atrioventricular malformation is supportive. Surgical replacement of valves has been done only under experimental conditions. It is conceivable that a stenotic valve could be surgically opened or dilated with a balloon valvuloplasty catheter. Treatment of congestive heart failure, if present, and management of atrial fibrillation are required in advanced cases (Table 74–5).

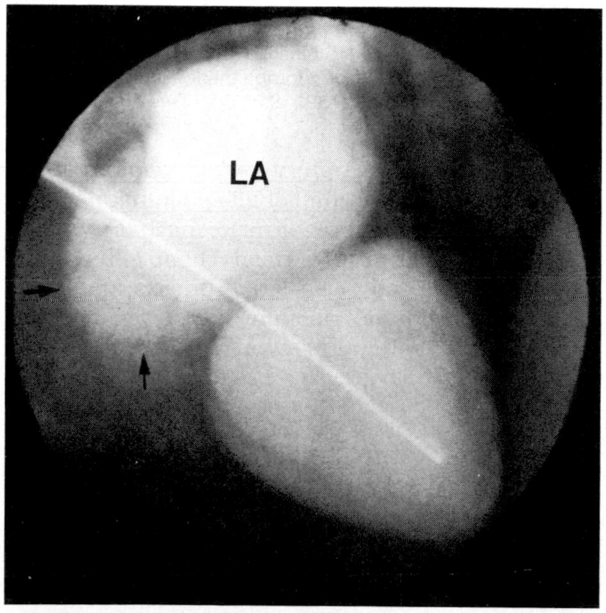

FIGURE 74–47. Angiocardiogram from a cat with mitral valve dysplasia. Following injection of contrast into the left ventricle, there is opacification of the dilated left atrium (LA) and the left auricular appendage (arrows). The left ventricle is significantly enlarged.

LESIONS CAUSING RIGHT TO LEFT SHUNTING: CYANOTIC HEART DISEASE

The term "cyanotic congenital heart disease" is both useful and misleading. While most clinicians immediately think of lesions that cause pulmonary to systemic shunting, such as the tetralogy of Fallot, a wide variety of malformations can induce arterial hypoxemia and cyanosis. Moreover, when congenital heart malformations of any type lead to congestive heart failure with pulmonary dysfunction, cyanosis can develop. Thus, the pup or kitten with left to right shunting PDA, left ventricular overload, pulmonary edema, and ventilation/perfusion inequality is as likely to be blue as the pup with the tetralogy. Still, cyanotic heart disease is a useful designation for classifying a variety of conditions that result in systemic arterial desaturation.[122–147] Since the pathophysiology and clinical signs of these conditions are similar, they will be considered as a group. Only the most important defects are discussed to illustrate the clinical syndrome common to these conditions.

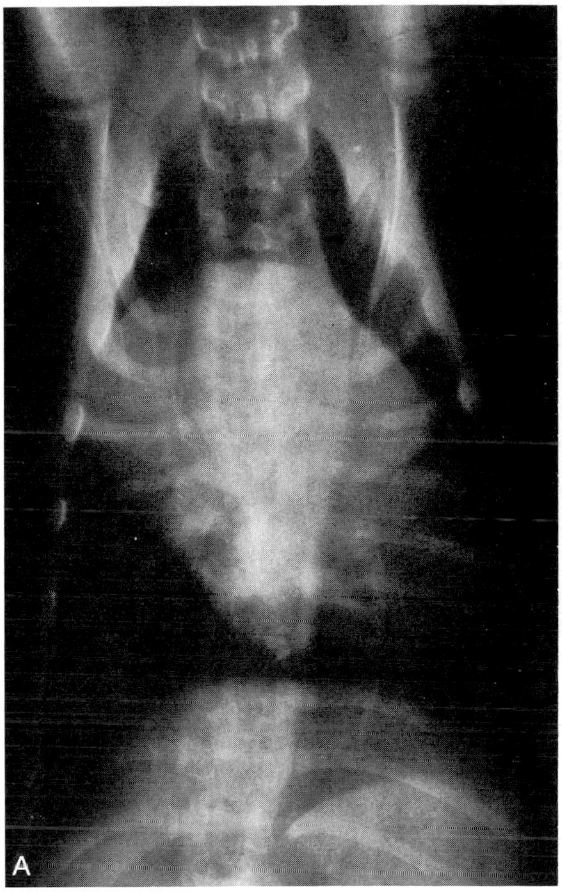

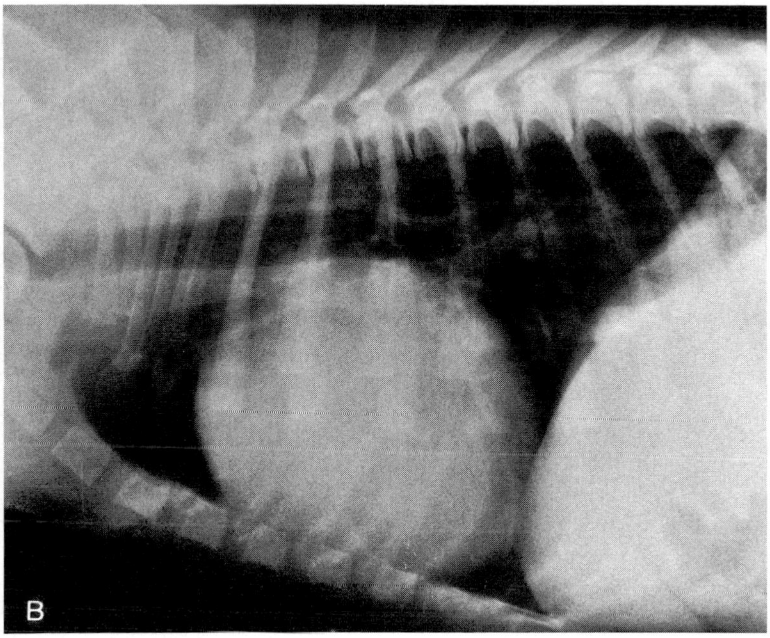

FIGURE 74–48. Dorsoventral and lateral radiographs from a dog with tricuspid valve dysplasia. The ventrodorsal film shows marked dilation of the right atrium with displacement of the cardiac apex to the left. The lateral film shows generalized rounding of the cardiac silhouette and slight attenuation of pulmonary vascularity.

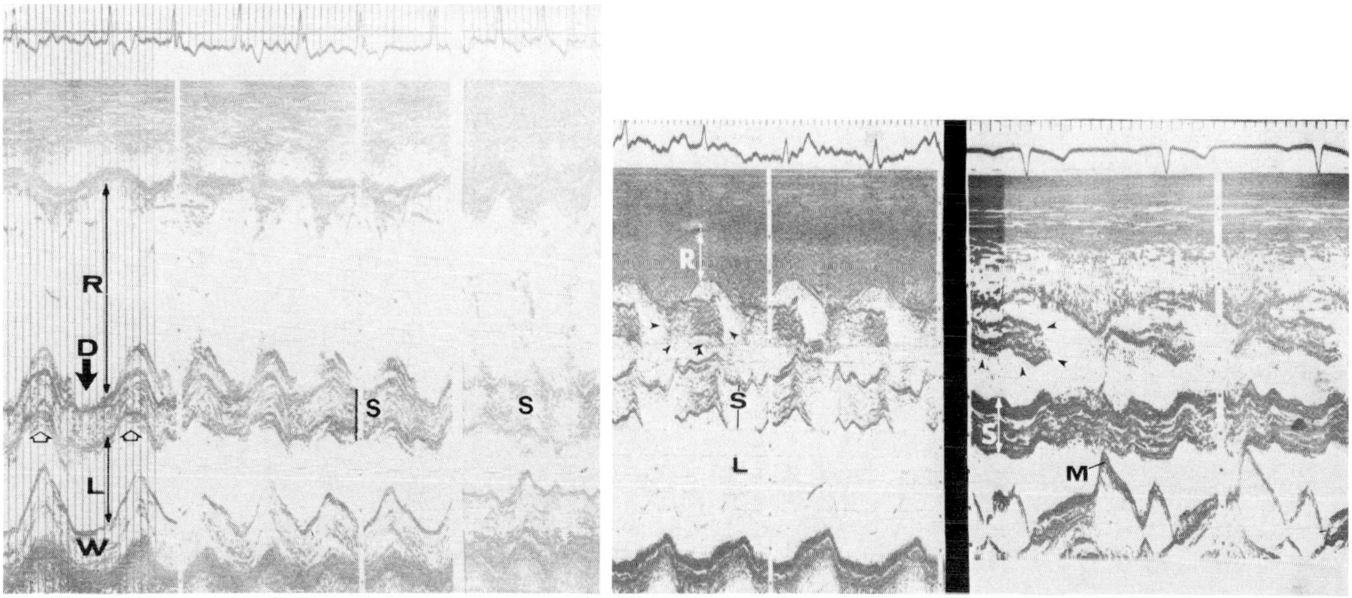

FIGURE 74–49. M-mode echocardiograms from dogs with tricuspid valve dysplasia. The left panel shows marked dilation of the right ventricle (R) when compared to the left ventricle (L). There is also diastolic displacement of the ventricular septum into the left ventricle as a result of volume overloading of the right side of the heart (D arrow). Paradoxical septal motion is also evident (open arrows). The ventricular septum (S) and left ventricular free wall (W) are noted. In the right panel, the dysplastic tricuspid valve is evident as a mass of echoes (arrowheads) within the right ventricle. The abnormal motion and filling slope of the tricuspid valve are easily seen when compared to that of the normal mitral valve (M) below.

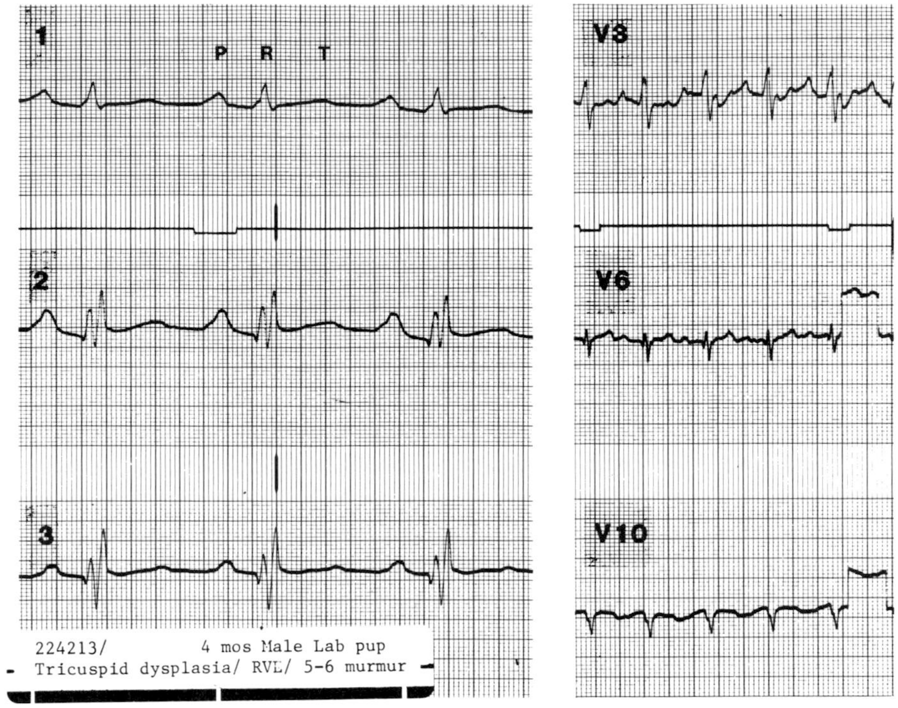

FIGURE 74–50. Electrocardiogram obtained from a pup with tricuspid valve dysplasia. Widening of the P-waves is characteristic of atrial enlargement. The P-wave amplitude is also prominent. An intraventricular conduction disturbance is not uncommonly found in dogs with tricuspid dysplasia, but the left chest lead (V_3) shows a prominent S-wave compatible with right ventricular enlargement. Standard calibration; paper speed = 100 mm per second for left panel and 50 mm per second for right panel.

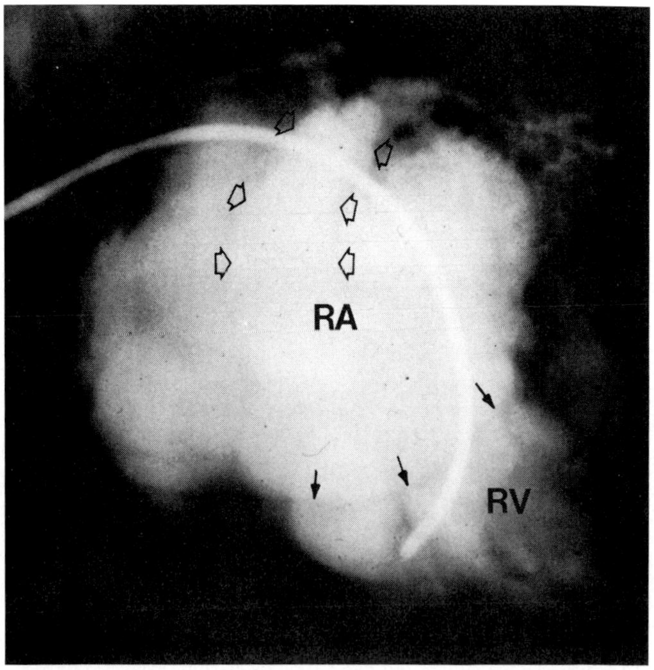

FIGURE 74–51. Angiocardiogram from a dog with tricuspid dysplasia. Following injection of contrast into the right ventricle (RV), there is marked regurgitation into the right atrium (RA). The tricuspid annulus and ventral extent of the right atrium are shown (arrows). The right atrium is massively dilated. The pulmonary artery, demarcated by the open arrows, is superimposed on the RA.

UNDERSTANDING CLINICAL MANIFESTATIONS OF CYANOTIC HEART DISEASE

Mechanisms of Right to Left Shunting. In order for desaturated venous blood to shunt into the systemic arteries there must either be a transposition of the great vessels or systemic veins, or there must be a defect between pulmonary and systemic circulations and a mechanism to raise pressure on the right side of the circulation. For example, if the aorta exits from the right ventricle, as it does in transposition of the great vessels, only desaturated blood will perfuse the body and the patient will succumb shortly after birth. On the other hand, if in this case a portion of the systemic pulmonary venous return shunts through an ASD into the right atrium, then desaturated venous blood will mix with oxygenated blood from the pulmonary veins. This patient also will develop arterial hypoxemia, cyanosis, and clinical signs from tissue hypoxia, but is likely to survive for some time.

As mentioned in the section on Cardiac Catheterization, a septal defect between the atria, ventricles, or aorticopulmonary trunk permits blood to flow from the path of greatest to least resistance and pressure. Accordingly, right to left shunting generally will not develop unless there is an obstruction to blood flow on the right side of the circulation or there is a substantial increase in pulmonary vascular resistance. Tricuspid stenosis (or atresia) and pulmonic stenosis (or atresia) are examples of obstructive right heart lesions. The term Eisenmenger's physiology (or syndrome) has already been used to define a situation where a left to right shunt reverses to right to left in response to marked increases in pulmonary vascular resistance (Figures 74–15, 74–16, 74–17, and 74–23).[148–150] The factors underlying the development of pulmonary hypertension are incompletely understood in children and in animals.[15, 49, 60, 148, 150] Clinical cardiologists are aware of the association between large bore defects and pulmonary vascular disease. Reversed shunting has been observed with PDA, aorticopulmonary communication, ventricular septal defect, and atrial septal defect. Moreover, Eisenmenger's physiology develops rapidly in small animals (almost always before six months of age).

The anatomic changes in the muscular and small pulmonary arteries observed in dogs and cats with Eisenmenger's physiology are similar to those of humans as described by Edwards and Heath and recently amended by Roberts.[15, 148] Intimal thickening, medial hypertrophy, and plexiform lesions are the salient abnormalities in most cases. The plexiform lesion is considered irreversible; consequently, neither medical therapy nor closure of the shunt will effectively improve the condition once these lesions have developed. In fact, surgical closure of the shunt pathway forces the right ventricle to work against a tremendous resistance, since the systemic circulation, which acts as a "pop-off" valve, can no longer be accessed. Such closure will cause a marked decline in cardiac output and right ventricular failure. Thus, the dictum: one does not surgically close a reversed PDA.

Effects of Hypoxemia. Systemic hypoxemia can be detected with an arterial blood gas obtained while the animal breathes room air. Providing the patient 100 per cent oxygen to breathe neither significantly improves the hypoxemia nor the cyanosis in most cases of right to left shunting.[15] Clinical signs of cyanotic heart disease are a result of tissue hypoxia and include stunting, weakness, anxiety, syncope, and seizures.[5–9, 15, 59, 137–139] Since systemic hypoxemia increases plasma erythropoietin concentrations, secondary polythemia develops in cyanotic heart disease. When the PCV exceeds the 65 to 68 per cent range, hyperviscosity can predispose to thrombosis and microvascular complications.[15, 148] Metabolic acidosis is another potential complication of protracted hypoxemia.[15, 59]

Systemic:Pulmonary Resistance. The magnitude of right to left shunting fluctuates with the systemic vascular resistance or the ratio of pulmonary to systemic resistance.[15] Exercise may promote vasodilation, decrease the systemic/pulmonary resistance ratio, and increase the right to left shunt. Tachycardia or elevated sympathetic tone may cause difficulties in cases of right ventricular hypertrophy, since ventricular outflow obstruction may increase, pulmonary flow diminish, and right to left shunting worsen.[15] This is one of the suggested reasons for using β-blockers, like propranolol, in some types of cyanotic heart disease.[139, 140] Anemia or even relative anemia (normal hematocrit in a hypoxemic patient) can result in a decline in the ratio of systemic to pulmonary resistance when the pulmonary resistance is a fixed lesion such as pulmonic valve stenosis.[138] Therefore, therapeutic phlebotomy in cyanotic patients not only decreases oxygen content per dl blood, but also decreases systemic vascular resistance, increasing the arterial hypoxemia. The relative impact on systemic/pulmonary resistance of reducing hematocrit in animals with pulmonary hypertension has not been reported.

Additional Circulatory Factors. Right to left shunting leads to compensatory increases in nutritive blood flow to the lung via the bronchial arteries. These tortuous systemic collateral vessels are easily recognized at angiography (see Figure 74–56) ventral to the descending aorta. Blood from these vessels may return via pulmonary veins and increase venous admixture. While uncommon, it is possible for these vessels to rupture, leading to hemoptysis.

Another potential problem in right to left shunting is paradoxical embolization. This is defined as a venous to systemic embolus. Normally, the canine and feline pulmonary vasculature filters systemic venous emboli before they can reach the left side of the circulation. With reversed shunting, the possibility of coronary, cerebral, or other systemic emboli must always be considered, particularly when venipunctures or IV catheters are used. Clots, bacteria, or air may gain access to vital organs by this mechanism.

CLINICAL EVALUATION OF THE CYANOTIC HEART DISEASE PATIENT

History and Physical Examination. Most cases of cyanotic congenital heart disease encountered in veterinary medicine are associated with pulmonic stenosis, pulmonary hypertension, or tricuspid valve disease. In the last case, shunting is invariably across an ASD or patent foramen ovale. Historical complaints include failure to grow, cyanosis, shortness of breath, exercise intolerance, weakness, syncope, and seizures. Affected animals often have a gasping pattern of ventilation when stressed. Arterial PO_2 and PCO_2 are decreased. These animals may develop adverse reactions (particularly bradycardia) to sedatives and tranquilizers, and may not improve appreciably following administration of supplemental oxygen. Most cases are polycythemic, but the hemoglobin concentration must be compared to age-matched normal animals.[128]

Clinical features of Eisenmenger's physiology tend to be similar, regardless of the underlying lesions, while reversed shunting associated with tetralogy of Fallot differs in some important ways.[8, 9, 128] One important auscultatory feature of Eisenmenger's syndrome is the loud or split second heart sound of pulmonary hypertension. This may be the only auscultatory abnormality and it is lacking in tetralogy of Fallot. An ejection sound with a soft, short, systolic murmur also may be evident at the left base in dogs with Eisenmenger's physiology. Diastolic murmurs of pulmonic insufficiency are rare in the author's experience.

Additional Studies. Cyanotic heart disease (tricuspid atresia and anomalous systemic venous return are exceptions) is characterized by right ventricular hypertrophy, which is evident on echocardiograms, ECG, and the thoracic radiograph. However, it is stressed that marked cardiomegaly is NOT typical of many cyanotic cardiac conditions, and the heart may not appear enlarged on survey films. As a general rule, the lungs appear underperfused in cyanotic heart diseases.[24] The main pulmonary artery and proximal lobar arteries are dilated when Eisenmenger's physiology is the basis for reversed shunting, but are not enlarged in tetralogy of Fallot or tricuspid atresia with ASD.

Echocardiography. The echocardiogram is very helpful in assessing the cyanotic patient since most large defects can be visualized, the right ventricular inflow and outflow regions can be evaluated, and the site of right to left shunting identified through echocontrast or Doppler studies (Figures 74–23 and 74–55). Detailed ultrasound studies may render cardiac catheterization unnecessary, unless surgery is contemplated and pulmonary hypertension (as opposed to pulmonic stenosis) cannot be otherwise ruled out. If pulmonic valve insufficiency is observed by Doppler echocardiography, the velocity of the regurgitant jet should be measured. A peak velocity of <2 m/s argues against a diagnosis of pulmonary hypertension.

Cardiac Catheterization. Cardiac catheterization is a definitive study for identifying pulmonary hypertension (Figure 74–5) and outlining anatomic defects, pulmonary artery size, and shunting. Angiocardiograms in cyanotic heart disease can be very confusing. It is helpful to include a vena caval and possibly a right atrial injection in the angiographic series. The cardiologist must also study abnormal catheter positions as a clue to large septal defects and vessel transpositions. Aortic injections invariably demonstrate prominent bronchoesophageal collaterals.

It is essential to know if pulmonary hypertension is or is not present prior to cardiac or vascular surgery in a patient with cyanotic heart disease. When pulmonary vascular resistance is normal, pulmonary flow can be augmented and systemic hypoxemia improved by creation of the shunt between a systemic and a pulmonary artery.[15, 128, 136, 141] Elevated pulmonary vascular resistance negates the usefulness of such surgery since left to right shunting is unable to occur.

TETRALOGY OF FALLOT

Components of the tetralogy are right ventricular outflow obstruction (pulmonic stenosis), secondary right ventricular hypertrophy, a subaortic ventricular septal defect, and overriding aorta (Figure 74–52). When pulmonary atresia occurs owing to grossly unequal partitioning of the truncus, the term "pseudotruncus arteriosus" has been used.

Pathogenesis. Tetralogy of Fallot is a genetically transmitted disorder in some breeds, propagated as a polygenic trait. Patterson and colleagues studied this malformation in the Keeshond breed and observed a spectrum of lesions, ranging from the subclinical to the clinically complicated.[124–127] They hypothesized that malformation of the conotruncal system, swellings responsible for partitioning of the truncus arteriosus into the aorta and pulmonary artery and the conus into right and left ventricular outflow tracts, are influenced by multiple alleles. Their breeding studies in the Keeshond indicated that increasing the genetic liability for conotruncal malformation, the "dose of abnormal genes," resulted in progressive severity of congenital heart disease.[4]

Patterson et al. graded the conotruncal defects pathologically as follows: grade 1: persistence of the conus septum fusion line, aneurysm of the ventricular septum, and absence of the papillary muscle of the conus. These represent subclinical malformations. Grade 2: pulmonic stenosis or ventricular septal defect plus the grade 1 lesions. Grade 3: tetralogy of Fallot: pulmonic stenosis, ventricular septal defect, and dextropositioned aorta (with secondary right ventricular hypertrophy), plus grade 1 lesions. Additional abnormalities found in some dogs included dilated and tortuous ascending aorta, pulmonary atresia, hypoplasia of the crista supraventricularis, and anomalies of the aortic arch system. The reader is referred to the excellent studies of Patterson et al. for further detail.[4, 124–127]

Pathophysiology. As with other right to left shunts, the essential components are the increased right-sided resistance and pressure, and the communication between pulmonary and systemic circulations (Figures 74–52 and 74–53). Owing to the high resistance RV outlet and elevated right ventricular pressure (RVP), desaturated blood shunts through the septal defect to mix with blood coming from the left ventricle.[122–123] Pulmonary arterial flow and venous return are scant, the left atrium (LA) and left ventricular cavities remain small, and the significant contribution of right ventricular blood to systemic blood flow causes hypoxemia, decreased he-

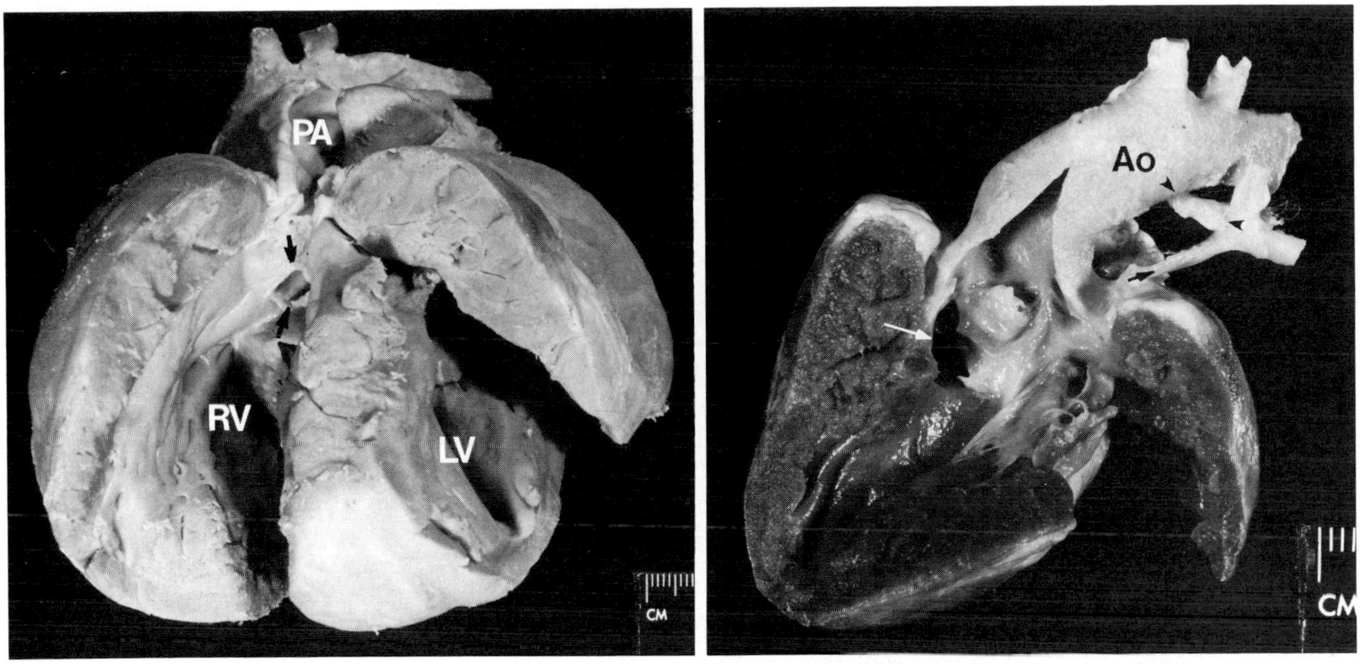

FIGURE 74–52. Tetralogy of Fallot. Left panel is from a dog and is cut to show the ventricular septal defect from the open right ventricle (RV). The defect is high in the septum (arrows) but below the pulmonary valve. The right ventricular wall is markedly hypertrophied, equal in thickness to the left ventricle (LV). PA = pulmonary artery. The right panel is from a cat with tetralogy of Fallot and pulmonary artery atresia (pseudotruncus arteriosus). The left ventricle has been opened to expose the large ventricular septal defect (white arrow), the hypoplastic pulmonary artery (small arrow), and the dilated aorta (Ao). Pulmonary flow was through the ductus arteriosus, the origin and termination of which are shown by arrowheads. While the lobar pulmonary arteries were patent, almost no blood was found in the main pulmonary artery.

moglobin oxygen saturation (O_2 sat.), cyanosis, and secondary polycythemia.

Right ventricular hypertrophy (RVH) can be detected by clinical means, such as electrocardiography. Cardiac murmurs are usually evident, attributed to high velocity flow across the pulmonic stenosis or possibly to shunting across the usually large and nonrestrictive VSD. Systemic collateral circulation increases via the bronchial arterial system. Other aspects of clinical pathophysiology have been previously described (see Understanding Clinical Manifestations of Cyanotic Heart Disease).

Clinical Findings. Tetralogy of Fallot is common in the Keeshond, English bulldog, and in some families of other breeds and is recognized in the cat.[9] Presenting complaints and clinical complications are similar to those previously described for cyanotic heart disease. While the ejection murmur of pulmonic stenosis is the most common auscultatory abnormality, it is not uncommon to identify a sternal border murmur that may indicate radiation of the PS or shunting into the septal defect. Some dogs have no obvious murmur, related to pulmonary atresia and/or polycythemia with hyperviscosity (which decreases turbulence) and ejection across a large, nonrestrictive VSD. Cyanosis is typical, but acyanotic cases are not uncommon. Exercise or excitement may induce cyanosis by accentuating right to left shunting.

Radiography usually shows a normal-sized heart with rounding of the right ventricular border (Figure 74–54).

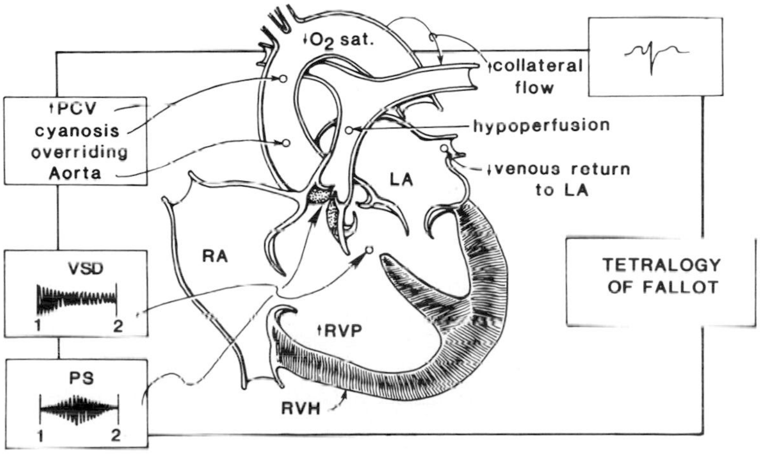

FIGURE 74–53. Schematic illustration demonstrating the pathophysiology of tetralogy of Fallot. See text for details. (By permission from Bonagura, JD: Congenital heart disease. *In* Bonagura, JD (ed): Cardiology. New York, Churchill Livingstone, 1987.)

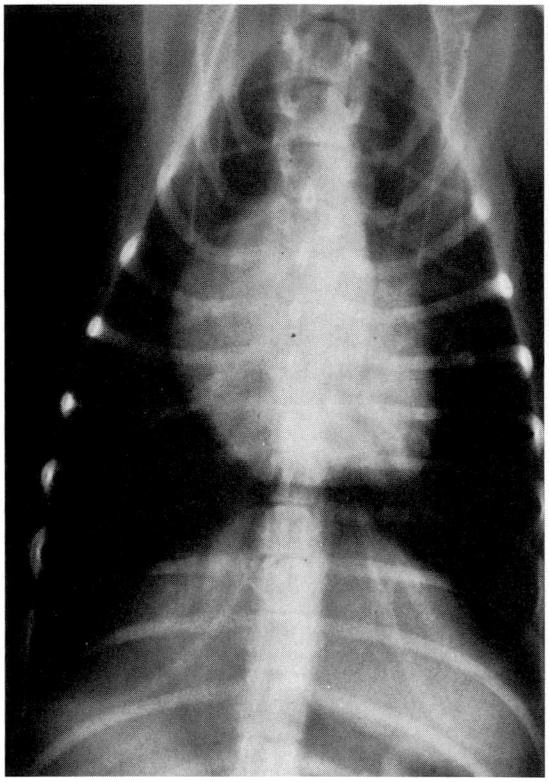

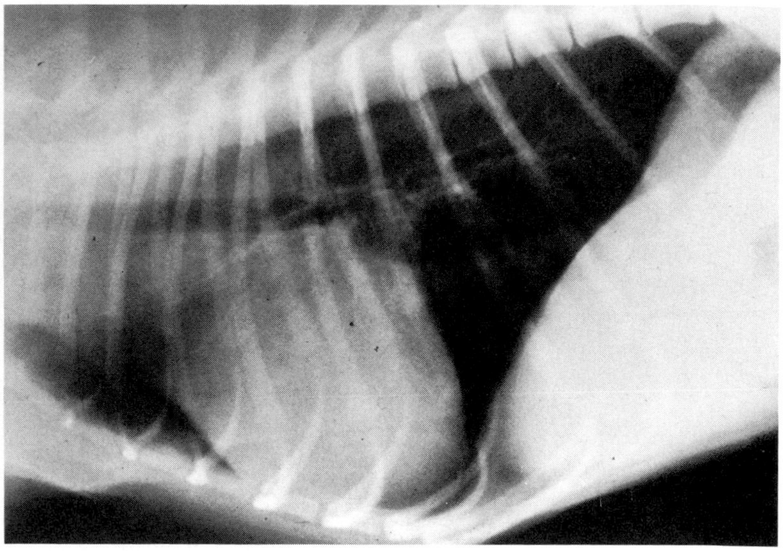

FIGURE 74–54. Ventrodorsal and lateral radiographs from a dog with tetralogy of Fallot. The ventrodorsal film shows mild rounding of the right side of the heart, but overall, the heart is minimally enlarged. The lungs are hypolucent. The lateral film shows some widening of the cranial mediastinum, which may be the result of an abnormal aortic arch. Pulmonary vascularity is markedly reduced.

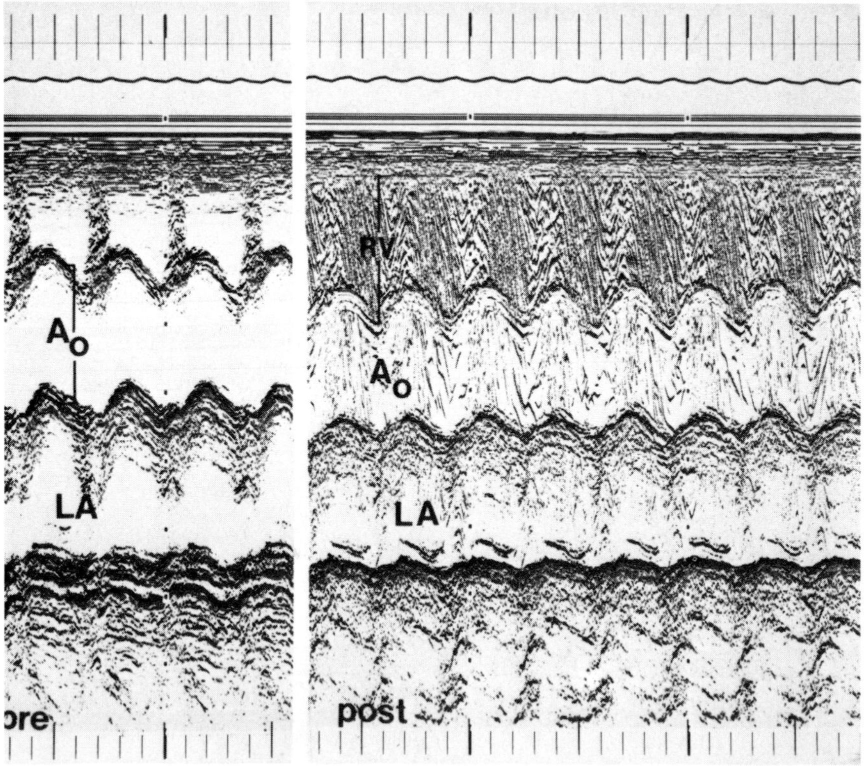

FIGURE 74–55. Contrast echocardiogram obtained from a dog with tetralogy of Fallot. Following an injection of saline into the cephalic vein, the right ventricle (RV) is opacified, as well as the aorta (Ao), compatible with right to left shunting. Notice the streaming effect of the echocontrast in the right ventricle. During diastole the bubbles enter in an almost linear fashion. During systole, the RV echo pattern is deranged and there is increased evidence of echocontrast within the aortic root, a finding compatible with systolic shunting of blood.

The main pulmonary artery is not enlarged, in contrast to the usual case of PS with intact ventricular septum. Pulmonary circulation is diminished and the left auricle may be inconspicuous subsequent to decreased venous return. While the ECG usually exhibits a right axis deviation, a left or cranial axis may be found in some cats.[129] The Doppler echocardiogram reveals right ventricular hypertrophy, small left chamber dimensions, the large subaortic VSD, and right ventricular outflow obstruction. Bubble (or Doppler) studies (Figure 74–55) document right to left shunting at the ventricular outflow level.[130]

Cardiac catheterization demonstrates virtual equilibration of left and right ventricular systolic pressures in most cases, compatible with a large VSD.[128] An oxygen step-down is recorded at the left ventricular outflow level and the aortic blood is relatively desaturated. Angiocardiography reveals right ventricular hypertrophy, pulmonic stenosis with minimal poststenotic dilatation, a large subaortic VSD, a small, dorsally displaced left ventricle, a widened ascending aorta, and prominent bronchial circulation (Figure 74–56).[124–128] Either valvular or subvalvular PS, or both, may be found. Bidirectional shunting across the VSD is common in the anesthetized animal. Anticoagulation therapy (e.g., heparin) should be used to prevent cerebral embolization during and for 3–5 days after cardiac catheterization.

Clinical Management. The *natural history* of tetralogy

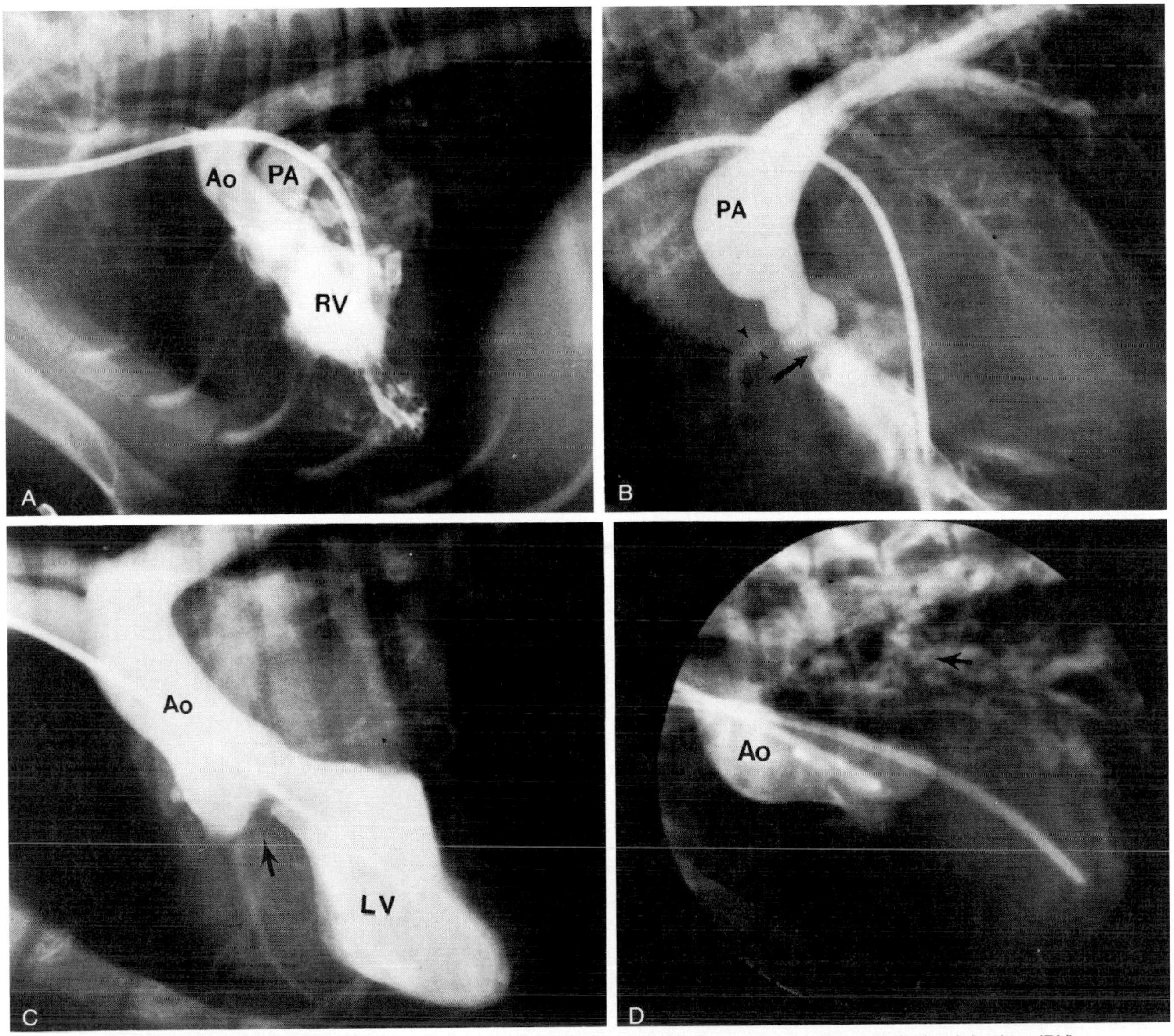

FIGURE 74–56. Angiocardiograms from animals with tetralogy of Fallot. *A,* A right ventricular injection (RV) documents simultaneous opacification of both the pulmonary artery (PA) and the aorta (Ao) in this dog. The right ventricular wall is hypertrophied. *B,* A right ventriculogram from a dog documents a subvalvular pulmonic stenosis (arrow) and normally formed, but relatively small, pulmonary valve sinuses above the arrow. There is mild poststenotic dilation of the main pulmonary artery and slight opacification of the ascending aorta cranial to the pulmonary artery. A dilated right coronary artery is shown (arrowheads). *C,* Left ventricular injection showing overriding of the aorta (arrow). *D,* Aortic injection in a cat with tetralogy of Fallot. The aorta is slightly widened and there is marked increase in collateral circulation via the bronchoesophageal system (arrow). The tortuous nature of these vessels is typical of collateral flow in right to left cardiac shunting.

of Fallot, like other causes of cyanotic heart disease, is that the defect can be tolerated for years, provided pulmonary blood flow is maintained and hyperviscosity is controlled. In cases of pulmonary atresia, pulmonary blood flow must be derived from the ductus arteriosus (which must maintain patency) or from a bronchial artery. Sudden death is common, related to complications of hypoxia, hyperviscosity, or cardiac arrhythmia. Unlike PS with intact ventricular septum, congestive heart failure is very unlikely to develop.

Both medical and surgical *therapy* can be employed in the management of tetralogy of Fallot. While definitive correction of the defect (closing the VSD and removing or bypassing the PS) can be done under cardiopulmonary bypass, such surgery is rarely performed in animals. It is emphasized that the PS should not be relieved if the VSD cannot be closed because marked left to right shunting with subsequent left ventricular failure may develop.[128]

Surgical palliation through the creation of a systemic to pulmonary shunt can be quite rewarding (Figure 74–57).[128, 141] Subclavian to pulmonary artery (Blalock-Taussig), ascending aorta to pulmonary artery (Potts), and aorta to right pulmonary artery (Waterston-Cooley) connections have been made in dogs and cats. By increasing pulmonary venous return, left heart size increases, and there is a greater contribution of oxygenated blood to the systemic circulation. The size of the shunt must be controlled to prevent overloading of the diminutive left ventricle and subsequent pulmonary edema. The extent to which these shunts remain patent postoperatively has not been addressed.

Adjunctive therapy includes phlebotomy to control the PCV between 62 and 68 per cent (in the normally hydrated patient), which appears satisfactory for most cases. As mentioned above, excessive bleeding should not be done and the blood volume should be replaced with crystalloid fluids to maintain cardiac output and tissue oxygen delivery.[138] As discussed earlier, some children with tetralogy of Fallot benefit from β-blockade with propranolol; however, the clinical efficacy of this treatment in animals has not undergone controlled studies.[139, 140] Severe hypoxic spells are treated with cage rest, oxygen, morphine sulfate, and sodium bicarbonate (if metabolic acidosis is evident). Drugs with marked systemic vasodilating properties should be avoided.

OTHER CAUSES OF CYANOTIC CONGENITAL HEART DISEASE

Other causes of cyanotic congenital heart disease include Eisenmenger's syndrome secondary to PDA, atrioventricular septal defects, and aorticopulmonary window.

Tricuspid Valve Dysplasia. Tricuspid valve dysplasia, particularly atresia or stenosis of the valve, can cause cyanosis since the elevated right atrial pressure behind the obstruction may maintain patency of the foramen ovale or an ASD.[117] The right ventricle is small or hypoplastic unless there is an associated VSD, in which case there may be a functional remnant of the ventricular outflow tract. The combination of PS with an ASD also can result in cyanosis subsequent to increased diastolic pressures in the right heart.

Double Outlet Right Ventricle. Double outlet right ventricle, wherein both great vessels exit from the right ventricle, has been reported in the dog and cat.[146, 147] A VSD provides the left ventricle an avenue for outflow into the great vessels. Pulmonary overcirculation is present unless there is pulmonic stenosis or pulmonary hypertension develops. Cyanosis is likely based on the origin of the aorta and is most severe if there is PS or pulmonary hypertension.

Transposition of the Great Arteries. In uncorrected transposition of the great arteries, the aorta originates from the right ventricle and the pulmonary trunk from the left ventricle.[15, 145] In the pure case, two independent circulations exist and the systemic arteries never receive oxygenated blood. Survival of the animal depends on the presence (or production) of shunts between the two

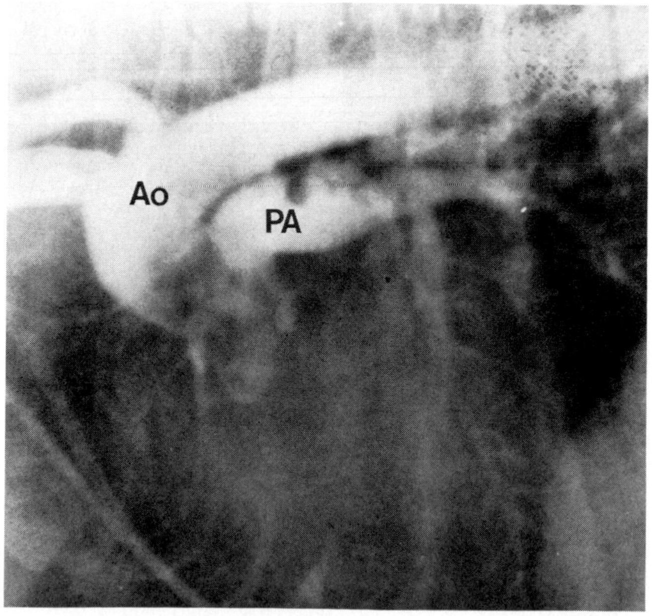

FIGURE 74–57. Successful systemic to pulmonary shunt used to palliate the tetralogy of Fallot. Following injection of contrast into the aorta, the pulmonary artery is also opacified. A filling defect (above the A in PA) is a result of surgical scarring.

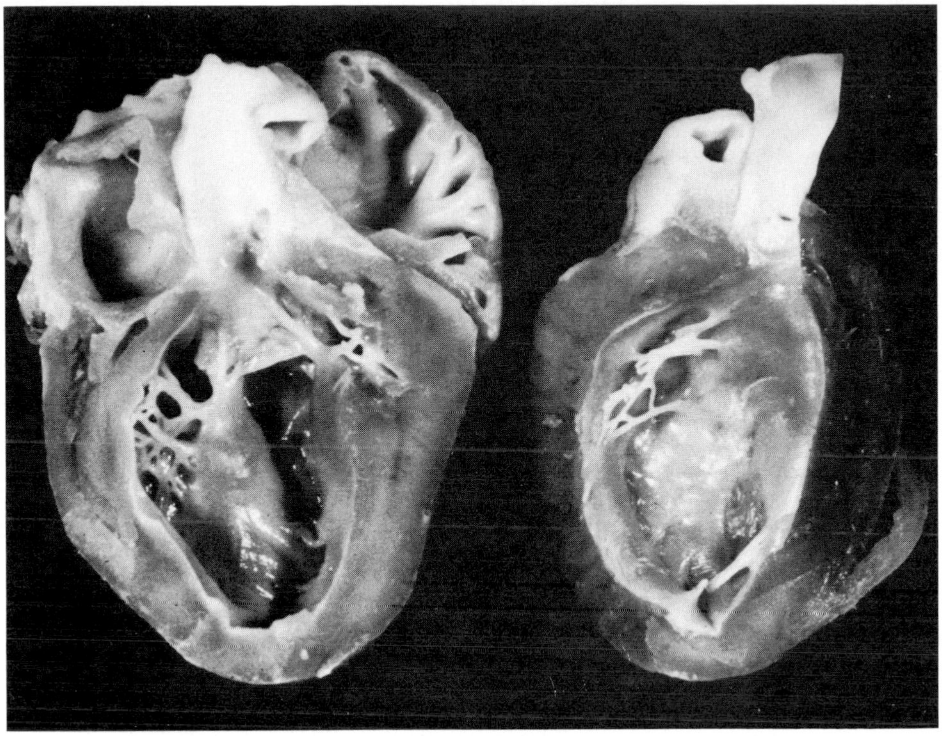

FIGURE 74–58. Open left ventricle from a Burmese cat with endocardial fibroelastosis. The left ventricle is dilated and there is marked thickening of the subendocardium. (Courtesy of Dr. Robert Hamlin, The Ohio State University.)

circulations to allow for mixing of blood to prevent fatal hypoxemia. These defects are complex, generally lethal, and probably underdiagnosed in animals, relative to children, since neonatal care is not supervised by veterinarians.

Pulmonary Atresia. Pulmonary atresia with ventricular septal defect is essentially the exaggerated form of tetralogy of Fallot, and causes severe right to left shunting across a large VSD. With persistent *truncus arteriosus*, the failure of partitioning of the fetal truncus, there is a large VSD and the single large vessel originates from both ventricles.[144] Ventricular blood mixes within the common artery prior to distribution to the body and pulmonary vessels.

MISCELLANEOUS CARDIAC DEFECTS

The potential for different anatomic forms and physiologic variants of congenital heart disease is tremendous, and it is beyond the scope of this chapter to discuss rare malformations. The following section summarizes clinically relevant aspects of cardiac and pericardial defects not yet discussed.

Endocardial Fibroelastosis

Endocardial fibroelastosis has been reported in the dog and cat and is probably familial in some families of Burmese and Siamese cats.[12, 13, 36, 151–155] The gross anatomic findings include left ventricular and left atrial dilatation, with severe endocardial thickening characterized grossly by diffuse, white, opaque thickening of the luminal lining (Figure 74 58). Histologic lesions in the cat include diffuse hypocellular, fibroelastic thickening of the endocardium with layering of thin, randomly organized collagen and elastic fibers.[151, 153] Edema of the endocardium with dilation of lymphatics is prominent and there is no evidence of myocardial inflammation or necrosis.

The diagnosis of primary endocardial fibroelastosis is, at times, tenuous, inasmuch as chronic left ventricular dilatation may lead to similar changes, particularly in the setting of mitral dysplasia and aortic stenosis. Dogs with endocardial fibroelastosis often have thickening of the mitral valve leaflets and mitral regurgitation.[154, 155] Similar difficulties in diagnosis exist in children with this disorder.[15]

The clinical features of endocardial fibroelastosis include early development of left or bi-ventricular failure, generally before six months of age. Mitral regurgitation may be evident. Left ventricular and atrial dilation are evident on radiographs and on the ECG. Limited echocardiographic studies performed to this date suggest reduction of left ventricular myocardial function, as opposed to pure valvular disease in which shortening fraction tends to be normal or increased.[155] Left ventricular diastolic pressures are elevated at catheterization, compatible with ventricular stiffness, ventricular failure, or volume overload from mitral regurgitation.[155]

Principal differential diagnoses include neonatal myocarditis, atrioventricular valve dysplasia, and critical aortic stenosis. Affected animals do poorly. Medical treatment of congestive heart failure may be effective in prolonging life, but recovery is unlikely in actual cases of endocardial fibroelastosis.

Other Congenital Defects

Anomalous development of the atria has been recognized in small animals. Cor triatriatum has been reported in a cat, and the author and others have observed cor triatriatum dexter (termed "triple atria") and saccular anomalies of the caudal right atrium in dogs and cats.[156–158] In cor triatriatum the venous drainage enters an additional, accessory atrial chamber, which is separated from the true atrium by a membrane. When the membrane is obstructive, dilation of the venous chamber and the entering veins is evident and congestion develops in the lungs, or in the case of a right atrial membrane, in the liver. Affected animals are examined for signs attributable to pulmonary edema or (with cor triatriatum dexter) for ascites. The author has also seen three cats with saccular dilation of the caudal right atrium that protruded into the left hemithorax but did not cause clinical signs. Treatment for these conditions would require surgical breakdown or bypass of the obstruction. We have been unsuccessful thus far in dilating the membrane with a balloon catheter but were successful in surgically correcting the obstruction.

Multiple cardiac anomalies have been described in kittens and in pups by a number of authors.[159–162] Pyle and Patterson studied a family of boxer dogs with multiple defects in which secundum-type atrial septal defects were prominent.[161] Other abnormalities included right and left ventricular outflow tract obstruction and persistent fetal elements of the right atrium. Ogburn et al.[162] described multiple defects in a family of Saluki dogs that included PDA, tricuspid and pulmonic abnormalities, and mitral insufficiency. This isolated situation emphasizes the genetic basis of many congenital defects and documents the need for counseling breeders to successfully prevent the propagation of these anomalies.

Peritoneopericardial Diaphragmatic Hernia

Congenital peritoneopericardial diaphragmatic hernia is a relatively common developmental anomaly of the dog and cat.[163–170] While not representative of a true cardiac anomaly, this condition can be confused with other congenital and acquired conditions. In the typical case, abdominal viscera are found within the pericardial sac. This malformation probably represents abnormal development of the septum transversum or pleuroperitoneal folds in the fetus.[167] Defects range from mild cases with only omentum and a lobe of liver within the hernia sac, to the presence of multiple organs and intestinal loops adjacent to the heart. The condition can be confusing in the cat, since gas-filled intestinal loops are found less often than in puppies, and the clinician may misdiagnose the condition as cardiomegaly from another cause (Figure 74–59).

The clinical signs of peritoneopericardial hernia are variable, ranging from respiratory distress, wheezing, and colic to vomiting. Cats frequently reach maturity without apparent symptoms. Physical examination indicates an abnormal position of the cardiac apex or inability to auscultate the heart sounds in the usual location. A soft systolic murmur may be evident, but the genesis of this is unknown. Borborygmus may be evident over the heart. A palpable defect at the caudoventral midline or a malformation of the xiphoid is present in some cases.

Thoracic radiography demonstrates enlargement and altered contour of the cardiac silhouette, lack of the normal separation between the pericardial shadow and the diaphragm, and inhomogeneity of the apparent cardiac density. Gas may be found within the pericardium. A soft tissue density situated ventral to the caudal vena cava on the lateral view usually represents the dorsal extent of the hernia. Anomalous development of the sternum is quite suggestive of the hernia in suitable clinical circumstances. Barium shows the position of the stomach and intestines, whereas a nonselective angiocardiogram (Figure 74–59) may demonstrate asymmetry of cardiac position and the presence of a filling defect and/or fluid within the pericardial sac. Cross-sectional echocardiography also can be used to substantiate the diagnosis, particularly when hepatic lobes are identified within the hernia sac.

Therapy involves surgical reduction of the hernia and replacement of abdominal contents in the peritoneal space. Such surgery may decrease clinical signs and prevent herniation of an abdominal organ.[36]

VASCULAR ANOMALIES

Vascular anomalies can be classified based on their location within the vascular system. A number of vascular malformations have been reported.[49, 50, 171–196] Patent ductus arteriosus represents the most important of the vascular malformations, and has been discussed. Peripheral vascular disorders, including abnormal abdominal and hepatic venous drainage and arteriovenous fistulas, are detailed in their respective chapters. Unilateral atresia of a pulmonary artery has been described in a cat with respiratory difficulty.[185] Coronary arteries can develop anomalously, but rarely cause documented clinical disease. Other major vascular defects center about the aorta and the systemic venous drainage, and these will be briefly addressed.

AORTIC ANOMALIES

Persistent Right Aortic Arch. Persistence of the right, as opposed to the left, fourth aortic arch causes regurgitation in weanlings (Figures 74–9 and 74–60).[49, 50, 171–183] Vascular ring anomalies include this common malformation, and other total or partial ring anomalies such as those formed by retroesophageal subclavian arteries and double aortic arch.[177, 179, 180, 184] The cardinal feature of these defects is regurgitation of solid food due to obstruction of the esophagus. Occasionally, other cardiac defects are present, including PDA. This condition is described more fully in Chapter 83.

Aorticopulmonary Septal Defect (Window). As opposed to the PDA, this persistent aorticopulmonary communication is caused by failure of the truncus arteriosus to differentiate.[188–191] Subsequently, shunting develops between the ascending aorta and pulmonary

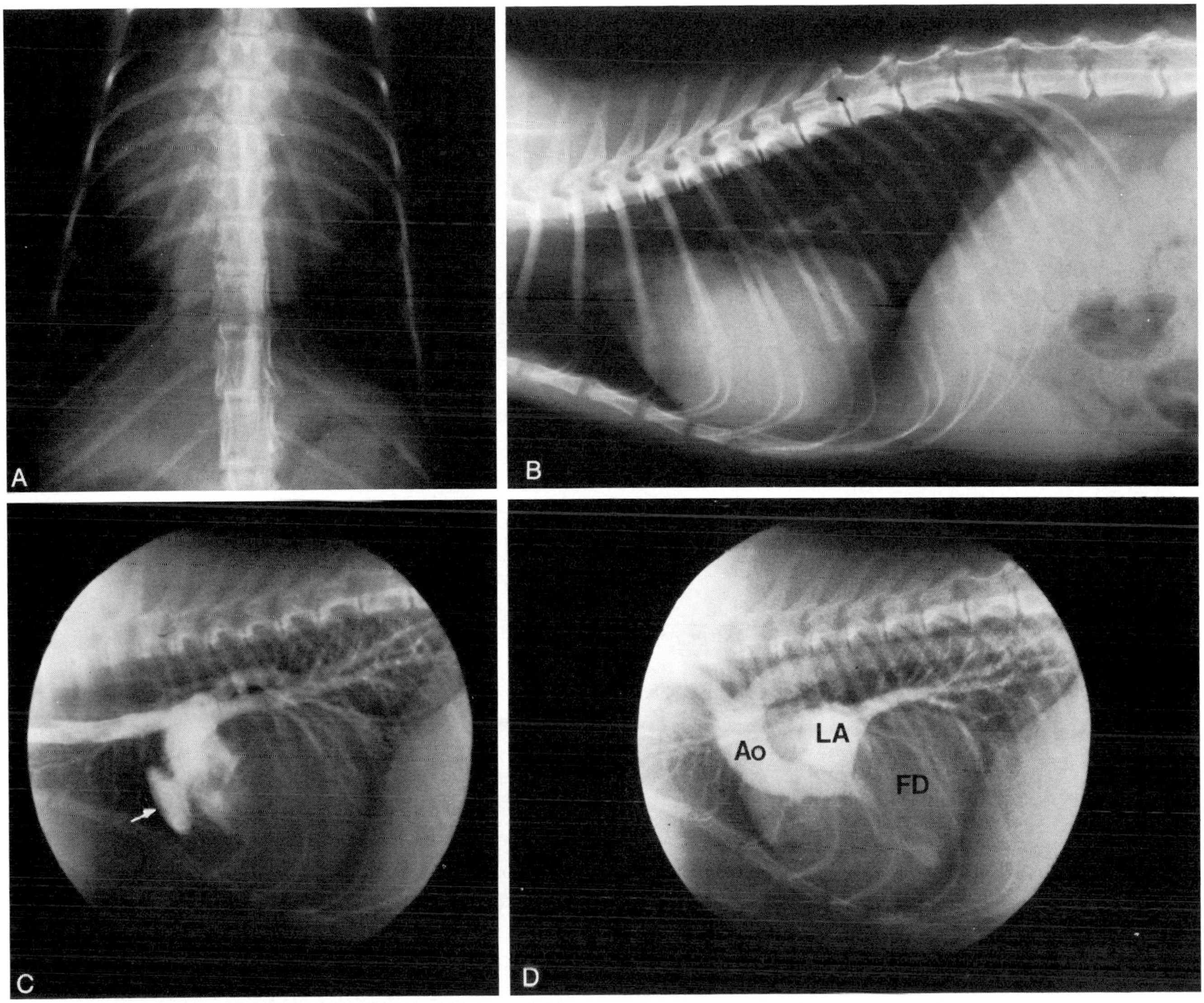

FIGURE 74–59. Peritoneopericardial hernia in a cat. *A,* The dorsoventral radiograph shows apparent enlargement of the cardiac silhouette but continuity between the pericardium and diaphragm. *B,* The lateral radiograph shows a misshapen cardiac silhouette with variability in density within the pericardial sac. The caudal vena cava is the most dorsal fluid density connecting the heart and abdomen. *C,* Following injection of contrast into the cephalic vein, the right side of the heart is opacified. The cranial vena cava, right atrium, right auricle (arrow), a portion of the right ventricle, and the pulmonary artery system are opacified. Note the tremendous distance between the ventral border of the apparent cardiac silhouette and the endocardial surface. *D,* Following return of contrast through the lungs, the pulmonary veins, left atrium (LA), a small portion of the left ventricle, and the aorta (Ao) are opacified. A large fluid density filling defect (FD), evident caudal to the heart, is very typical of peritoneopericardial hernia in the cat.

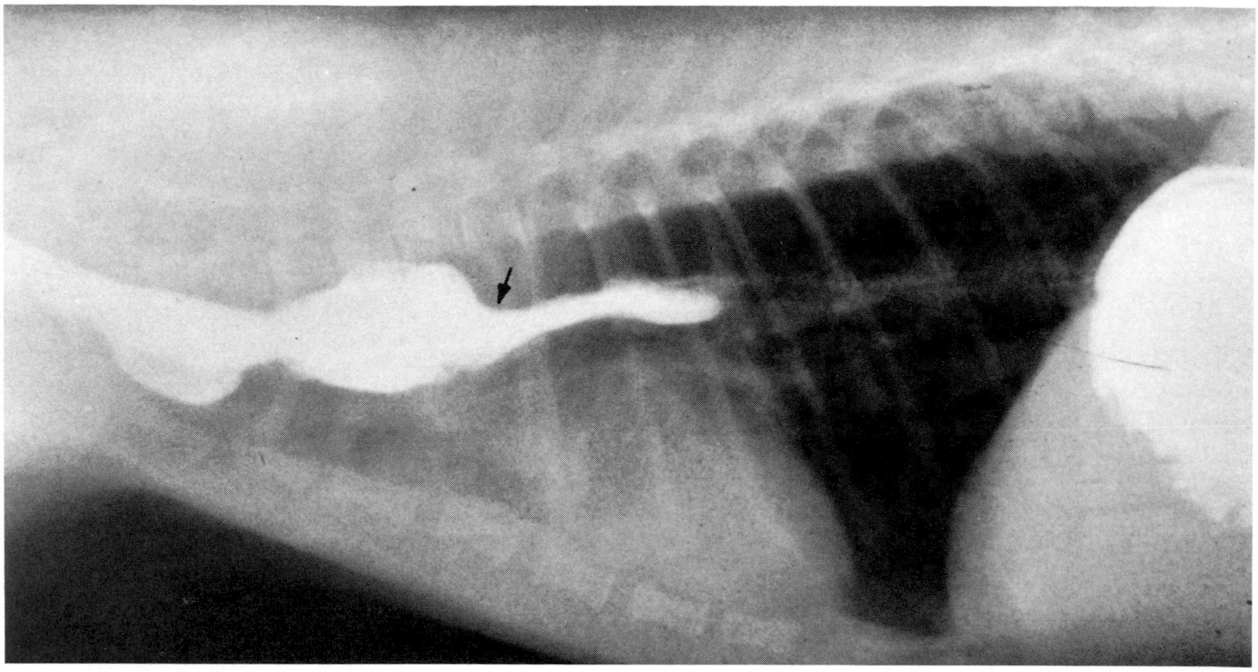

FIGURE 74–60. Persistent right aortic arch in a cat. The barium swallow indicates constriction of the esophagus at the base of the heart (arrow).

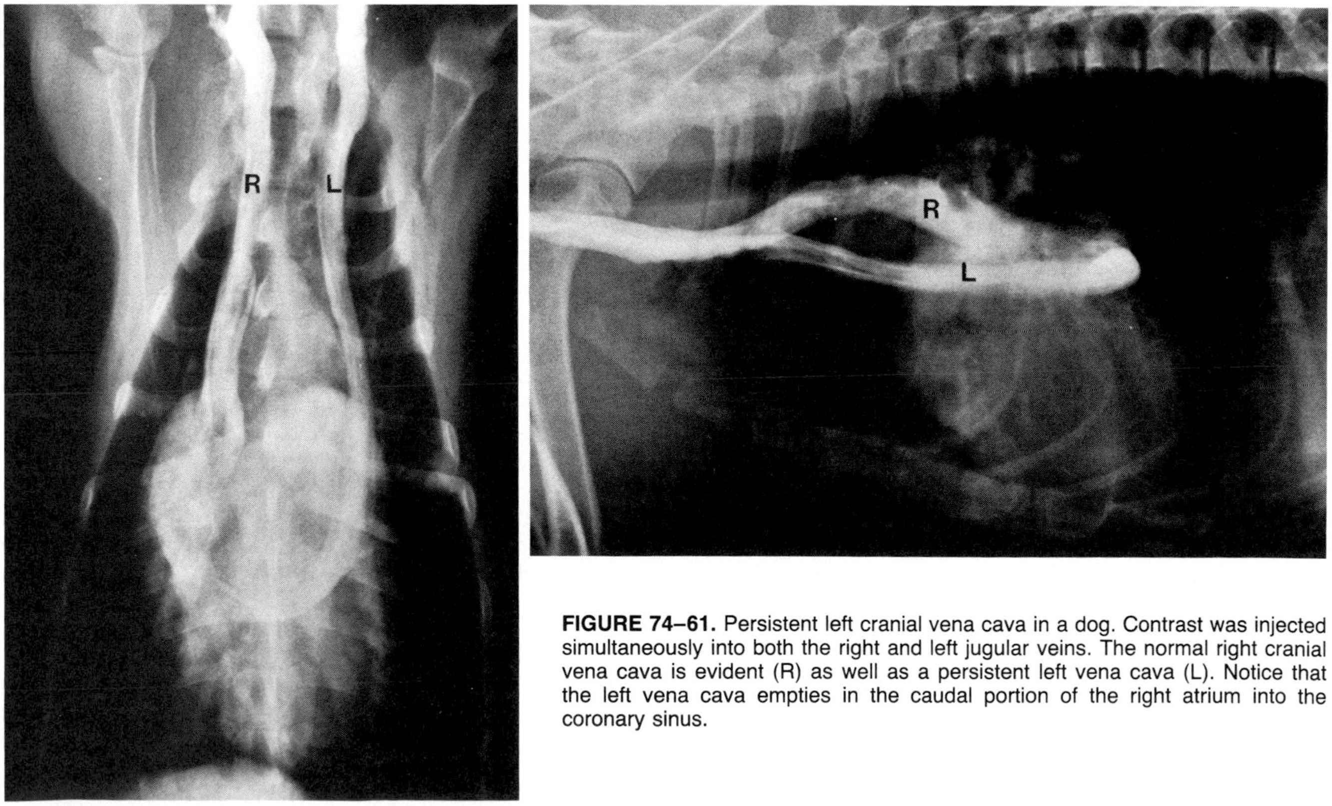

FIGURE 74–61. Persistent left cranial vena cava in a dog. Contrast was injected simultaneously into both the right and left jugular veins. The normal right cranial vena cava is evident (R) as well as a persistent left vena cava (L). Notice that the left vena cava empties in the caudal portion of the right atrium into the coronary sinus.

artery. While a clinical condition similar to that of PDA potentially could develop, the author's experience and that reported in the literature suggests that pulmonary hypertension develops during the first year of life and that clinical signs are similar to those in dogs that develop Eisenmenger's physiology due to other defects. Management is similar to that for a reversed PDA. Surgery is difficult without cardiopulmonary bypass and should not be attempted if pulmonary vascular resistance is markedly elevated. This defect is not synonymous with a short, wide PDA that sometimes is referred to as a "window."

Coarctation of the Aorta. This is a rare defect in the dog and is characterized by narrowing of the aorta distal to the subclavian artery, adjacent to the ductus arteriosus. A case reported by Eyster had systolic and diastolic murmurs and left ventricular failure.[192] The clinical features of coarctation in children are well described and in many ways are similar to this case.[15]

Aortic interruption in a dog[193] and a case of tubular hypoplasia of the ascending aorta in a dog[194] also have been described. While these lesions differ from coarctation, they are additional examples of malformation of the aorta in small animals.

VENOUS ANOMALIES

Thoracic venous anomalies rarely cause cardiac problems in small animals. Total or partial anomalous pulmonary venous return has been reported in a dog and behaves functionally as a left to right shunt at the atrial level.[80] Abnormalities of abdominal venous drainage, such as patent ductus venosus, can induce hepatic encephalopathy. A relatively common venous abnormality of clinical significance during thoracic surgery is the persistent left cranial vena cava.[195] This vessel, normally present in the fetus as part of the left cardinal venous system, may persist and drain into the embryologically related coronary sinus in the caudal aspect of the right atrium (Figure 74–61). Persistent left cranial vena cava may interfere with surgical exposure, particularly during surgical treatment of persistent right fourth aortic arch, but otherwise it is of no known functional significance. As with right fourth aortic arch, this vascular anomaly is common in German shepherds, and has been reported in other canine breeds as well as in cats.[133, 195] Division of this vessel generally poses no clinical problem provided the normal right cranial vena cava is also present.

References

1. Patterson, DF: Congenital heart disease in the dog. Ann NY Acad Sci 127:541, 1965.
2. Patterson, DF: Epidemiologic and genetic studies of congenital heart disease in the dog. Circ Res 23:171, 1968.
3. Patterson, DF, et al.: Hereditary cardiovascular malformation of the dog. The Clinical Delineation of Birth Defects. Birth Defects 8:160, 1972.
4. Patterson, DF: Congenital defects of the cardiovascular system of dogs: Studies in comparative cardiology. Adv Vet Sci Comp Med 20:1, 1976.
5. Ettinger, SJ and Suter, PF (eds): Canine Cardiology. Philadelphia, WB Saunders, 1970.
6. Ettinger, SJ and Suter, PF: Congenital Heart Disease. *In* Ettinger, SJ (ed): Textbook of Veterinary Internal Medicine. Philadelphia, WB Saunders, 1975.
7. Pyle, RL: Common Congenital Heart Defects. *In* Kirk, RW (ed): Current Veterinary Therapy VI. Philadelphia, WB Saunders, 1977.
8. Pyle, RL: Congenital Heart Disease. *In* Ettinger, SJ (ed): Textbook of Veterinary Internal Medicine, 2nd ed. Philadelphia, WB Saunders, 1983, p 933.
9. Thomas, WP: Congenital Heart Disease. *In* Kirk, RW (ed): Current Veterinary Therapy VIII. Philadelphia, WB Saunders, 1986, p 301.
10. Tashjian, RJ, et al.: Studies on cardiovascular disease in the cat. Ann NY Acad Sci 127:581, 1965.
11. Severin, GA: Congenital and acquired heart disease. JAVMA 151:1733, 1967.
12. Liu, SK: Pathology of feline heart disease. Vet Clin North Am 7:323, 1977.
13. Bolton, GR and Liu, SK: Congenital heart diseases of the cat. Vet Clin North Am 7:341, 1977.
14. Detweiler, DK, Patterson, DF: The prevalence and types of cardiovascular disease in dogs. Ann NY Acad Sci 127:481, 1965.
15. Friedman, WF: Congenital heart disease in infancy and childhood. *In* Braunwald, E (ed): Heart Disease, 2nd ed. Philadelphia, WB Saunders, 1984, p 941.
16. Van Mierop, LSH: Pathology and pathogenesis of the common cardiac malformations. Cardiol Clin 2:28, 1970.
17. Detweiler, DK: Genetic aspects of cardiovascular diseases in animals. Circulation 30:114, 1964.
18. Shive, RJ, et al.: Chromosome studies in dogs with congenital cardiac defects. Cytogenetics 4:340, 1965.
19. Patterson, DF, et al.: Congenital malformations of the cardiovascular system associated with chromosomal abnormalities. Zentralbl Vet Med 13:669, 1966.
20. Patterson, DF: Canine congenital heart disease: Epidemiology and etiological hypotheses. J Small Anim Pract 12:263, 1971.
21. Kalter, H and Warkany, J: Congenital malformations: Etiologic factors and their role in prevention. Part I and II. N Engl J Med 308:424, 1983.
22. Suter, PF: The radiographic diagnosis of canine and feline heart disease. Comp Cont Educ Pract Vet 3:441, 1981.
23. Myer CW and Bonagura, JD: Survey radiography of the heart. Vet Clin North Am 12:213, 1982.
24. Suter, PF and Lord, PF: Thoracic radiography of the dog and cat. Wettswill, Switzerland, 1984.
25. Buchanan, JW and Patterson, DF: Selective angiocardiography in dogs with congenital cardiovascular disease. J Am Vet Radiol Soc 6:21, 1965.
26. Bonagura, JD, et al.: Angiocardiography. Vet Clin North Am 12:239, 1982.
27. Bonagura JD and Herring, DS: Echocardiography II: Congenital heart disease. Vet Clin North Am 15:1195, 1985.
28. Weyman, AE: Cross-sectional echocardiography. Philadelphia, Lea and Febiger, 1982.
29a. Valdes-Cruz, LM, et al.: Validation of a Doppler echocardiographic method for calculating severity of discrete stenotic obstructions in a canine preparation. Circulation 69:1177, 1984.
29b. Hatle, L and Angelsen, B: Doppler Ultrasound in Cardiology, second edition. Philadelphia, Lea and Febiger, 1985.
29c. Perez, JE: Doppler echocardiography. New York, McGraw-Hill, 1987.
29d. Kisslo, J: Doppler Color-Flow Imaging. Philadelphia, WB Saunders, 1988.
30. Bonagura, JD and Pipers, FS: Diagnosis of cardiac lesions by contrast echocardiography. JAVMA 182:396, 1983.
31. Trautvet, E, et al.: Evolution of the electrocardiogram in young dogs with congenital heart disease leading to right ventricular hypertrophy. J Electrocardiology 14:275, 1981.
32. Hill, JD and Moore, EN: Epicardial excitation studies in dogs with congenital right ventricular hypertrophy. Circ Res 20:649, 1967.
33. Barry, WH and Grossman, W: Cardiac catheterization. *In* Braunwald, E (ed): Heart Disease, 2nd ed. Philadelphia, WB Saunders, 1984, p 279.
34. Buchanan, JW and Pyle, RL: Cardiac tamponade during catheterization of a dog with congenital heart disease. JAVMA 149:1056, 1966.

35. Morady, F, et al.: Rapid method for determination of shunt ratio using a thermodilution technique. Am Heart J 106:369, 1983.
36. Harpster, NK: The cardiovascular system. *In* Holzworth, J (ed): Disease of the Cat: Medicine and Surgery. Philadelphia, WB Saunders, 1986, p 820.
37. Patterson, DF and Detweiler, DK: Hereditary transmission of patent ductus arteriosus in the dog. Am Heart J 74:289, 1967.
38. Patterson, DF: Animal models of congenital heart disease (with special reference to patent ductus arteriosus in the dog). Nat Acad Sci, No. 1594, 1968, p 131.
39. Patterson, DF, et al.: Hereditary patient ductus arteriosus and its sequelae in the dog. Circ Res 28:1, 1971.
40. Patterson, DF: Patent Ductus Arteriosus. *In* A Manual of Clinical Cardiology. AAHA 1972.
41. Gittenberger-de-Groot, et al.: Histologic studies on normal and persistent ductus arteriosus in the dog. JAAC 6:394, 1985.
42. House, EW and Ederstrom, HE: Anatomical changes with age in the heart and ductus arteriosus in the dog after birth. Anat Rec 160:289, 1968.
43. Heymann, MA: Pharmacologic use of prostaglandin E1 in infants with congenital heart disease. Am Heart J 101:837, 1981.
44. Ackerman N, et al.: Patent ductus arteriosus in the dog: a retrospective study of radiographic, epidemiologic, and clinical findings. Am J Vet Res 39:1805, 1978.
45. Cohen, JS, et al.: Patent ductus arteriosus in five cats. JAAHA 11:95, 1975.
46. Jeraj, K, et al.: Patent ductus arteriosus with pulmonary hypertension in a cat. JAVMA 172:1432, 1978.
47. Smetzer, DL and Breznock, EM: Auscultatory diagnosis of patent ductus arteriosus in the dog. JAVMA 160:80, 1972.
48. Jones, CL and Buchanan, JW: Patent ductus arteriosus: anatomy and surgery in a cat. JAVMA 179:364, 1981.
49. Reed, JH and Bonasch, H: The surgical treatment of a persistent right aortic arch and patent ductus arteriosus in a dog. Canad Vet J 5:240, 1964.
50. Buchanan, JW: Symposium: Thoracic surgery in the dog and cat, III. Patent ductus arteriosus and persistent right aortic arch surgery in dogs. J Small Anim Pract 9:409, 1968.
51. Breznock, EM, et al.: A surgical method for correction of patent ductus arteriosus in the dog. JAVMA 158:753, 1971.
52. Bojrab, MJ: Current Techniques in Small Animal Surgery. Philadelphia, Lea and Febiger, 1972.
53. Eyster, GE, et al.: Patent ductus arteriosus in the dog: characteristics of occurrence and results of surgery in one hundred consecutive cases. JAVMA 168:435, 1976.
54. Buchanan, JW, et al.: Patent ductus arteriosus surgery in small dogs. JAVMA 151:701, 1967.
55. Atwell, RB: Patent ductus arteriosus in a dog—attempted medical closure. Vet Record 101:425, 1977.
56. Linde, LM, et al.: Effect of acetyl strophanthidin on pulmonary circulation of a dog with patent ductus arteriosus. Am J Vet Res 30:1057, 1969.
57. Eyster, GE, et al.: Recanalized patent ductus arteriosus in the dog. J Small Anim Pract 16:743, 1975.
58. Weirich, WE, et al.: Late consequences of patent ductus arteriosus in the dog: a report of six cases. JAAHA 14:40, 1978.
59. Legendre, AM, et al.: Secondary polycythemia and seizures due to right-to-left shunting patent ductus arteriosus in a dog. JAVMA 164:1198, 1974.
60. Pyle, RL, et al.: Patent ductus arteriosus with pulmonary hypertension in the dog. JAVMA 178:565, 1981.
61. Turk, JR, et al.: Necrotizing pulmonary arteritis in a dog with patent ductus arteriosus. J Small Anim Pract 22:603, 1981.
62. Hamlin, RL, et al.: Ostium secundum type interatrial septal defects in the dog. JAVMA 143:149, 1963.
63. Eyster, GE, et al.: Surgical repair of atrial septal defect in a dog. JAVMA 169:1081, 1976.
64. Troy, GC and Turnwald, GH: Atrial fibrillation and abnormal ventricular conduction presented as right bundle branch block in a dog with an atrial septum primum defect. JAAHA 15:417, 1979.
65. Jeraj, K, et al.: Atrial septal defect (sinus venosus type) in a dog. JAVMA 177:342, 1980.
66. Liu, SK and Ettinger, S: Persistent common atrioventricular canal in two cats. JAVMA 153:556, 1968.
67. Farrow, CS: Atrial septal defect in a kitten. Mod Vet Pract 65:281, 1984.
68. Hamlin, RL, et al.: Interventricular septal defect (Roger's disease) in the dog. JAVMA 145:331, 1964.
69. Clark, DR, et al.: Imperforate cardiac septal defect in a dog. JAVMA 156:1020, 1970.
70. Gelatt, KN and McGill, LD: Clinical characteristics in microphthalmia with colobomas of the Australian shepherd dog. JAVMA 162:393, 1973.
71. Breznock, EM: Spontaneous closure of ventricular septal defects in the dog. JAVMA 162:399, 1973.
72. Okubo, S, et al.: Relevance of location of defect and pulmonary vascular resistance to the intracardiac pattern of left to right shunt flow in dogs with experimental ventricular septal defect. Circulation 73:775, 1986.
73. Nakai, M, et al.: Quantitative evaluation of the pattern of shunt flow in the right ventricle and pulmonary artery of dogs with experimental ventricular septal defect. J Clin Invest 72:779, 1983.
74. Sheridan, JP, et al.: Pulmonary artery banding in the cat: a case report. J Small Anim Pract 12:45, 1971.
75. Eyster, GE, et al.: Pulmonary artery banding for ventricular septal defect in dogs and cats. JAVMA 170:434, 1977.
76. Breznock, EM, et al.: Surgical correction, using hypothermia, of an interventricular septal defect in the dog. JAVMA 158:1391, 1971.
77. Braden, TD, et al.: Correction of a ventricular septal defect in a dog. JAVMA 161:507, 1972.
78. Lister, G, et al.: Physiologic effects of increasing hemoglobin concentration in left-to-right shunting in infants with ventricular septal defects. N Engl J Med 306:502, 1982.
79. Synhorst, DP, et al.: Hemodynamic effects of vasodilator agents in dogs with experimental ventricular septal defects. Circulation 54:472, 1976.
80. Hilwig, RL and Bishop, SP: Anomalous pulmonary venous return in a Great Dane. Am J Vet Res 36:299, 1975.
81. Tashjian, RJ, et al.: Isolated pulmonic valvular stenosis in a dog. JAVMA 135:94, 1959.
82. Custer, MA, et al.: Correction of pulmonic stenosis. JAVMA 139:565, 1961.
83. Hamlin, RL, et al.: Atypical clinical findings in a dog with pulmonic stenosis. JAVMA 142:520, 1963.
84. Weirich, WE, et al.: Myocardial infarction and pulmonic stenosis in a dog. JAVMA 159:315, 1971.
85. Lowensohn, HS, et al.: Phasic right coronary artery blood flow in conscious dogs with normal and elevated right ventricular pressure. Circ Res 39:760, 1976.
86. Patterson, DF, et al.: Hereditary dysplasia of the pulmonary valve in beagle dogs. Am J Cardiol 47:631, 1981.
87. Eyster GE: Pulmonic stenosis. *In* Bojrab, MJ (ed): Current Techniques in Small Animal Surgery, 2nd Ed. Philadelphia, WB Saunders, 1983, p 462.
88. Fingland, RB, et al.: Pulmonic stenosis in the dog. JAVMA 189:218, 1986.
89. Hawe, RS: Pulmonic stenosis in a cat. JAAHA 17:777, 1981.
90. Hembrough, FB, et al.: Cardiovascular dynamics of surgically prepared pulmonary stenosis. Am J Vet Res 32:793, 1971.
91. Ford, RB, et al.: Use of an extracardiac conduit in the repair of supravalvular pulmonic stenosis in a dog. JAVMA 172:922, 1978.
92. Whiting, PG, et al.: Double outlet right ventricle for relief of pulmonic stenosis in dogs. An experimental study. Vet Surg 13:64, 1984.
93. Breznock, EM and Good, GL: A patch-graft technique for correction of pulmonic stenosis in dogs. JAVMA 169:1090, 1976.
94a. Kan, JS, et al.: Percutaneous balloon valvuloplasty: a new method for treating congenital pulmonary valve stenosis. N Engl J Med 307:539, 1982.
94b. Bright JM, et al: Percutaneous balloon valvuloplasty for treatment of pulmonic stenosis in a dog. JAVMA 191:995, 1987.
94c. Sisson, DD and MacCoy, DM: Treatment of congenital pulmonic stenosis in two dogs by balloon valvuloplasty. J Vet Int Med 2:92, 1988.
95. Eyster, GE and Keller, WF: Congenital pulmonic valve insufficiency in a dog. JAVMA 164:599, 1974.
96. Polzin, DJ and Ogburn, P: Isolated pulmonary valvular insufficiency in a dog. JAAHA 17:301, 1981.
97. Patterson, DF and Detweiler, DK: Predominance of German

shepherd and boxer breeds among dogs with congenital subaortic stenosis. Am Heart J 65:429, 1963.
98. Patterson, DF and Flickinger, GL: Subaortic stenosis in a Boxer. Clinico-Pathologic Conference. JAVMA 145:363, 1964.
99. Pyle, RL: Aortic stenosis. *In* A Manual of Clinical Cardiology. JAAHA, 1972.
100. Pyle, RL, et al.: The genetics and pathology of discrete subaortic stenosis in the Newfoundland dog. Am Heart J 92:324, 1976.
101. Liu, S: Supravalvular aortic stenosis with deformity of the aortic valve in a cat. JAVMA 152:55, 1968.
102. Bohn, FK, et al.: Supravalvular Aortenstenose beim Hund. Zentralbl Vet Med 14:85, 1967.
103. Flickinger, GL and Patterson, DF: Coronary lesions associated with congenital subaortic stenosis in the dog. J Path Bact 93:133, 1967.
104. Pyle, RL, et al.: Left circumflex coronary artery hemodynamics in conscious dogs with congenital subaortic stenosis. Circ Res 33:34, 1973.
105. Rogers, WA, et al.: Experimental production of supravalvular aortic stenosis in the dog. J Appl Physiol 30:917, 1971.
106. Wingfield, WE, et al.: Echocardiographic assessment of congenital aortic stenosis in dogs. JAVMA 183:673, 1983.
107. Breznock, EM, et al.: Valved apico-aortic conduit for relief of left ventricular hypertension caused by discrete subaortic stenosis in dogs. JAVMA 182:51, 1983.
108. Eyster, GE, et al.: Aortic regurgitation in the dog. JAVMA 168:138, 1976.
109. Carmichael, JA, et al.: A case of canine subaortic stenosis and aortic valvular insufficiency, with particular reference to diagnostic technique. J Small Anim Pract 9:213, 1968.
110. Frater, RWM and Ellis, FH: The anatomy of the canine mitral valve. J Surg Res 1:171, 1961.
111. Hamlin, RL, et al.: Congenital mitral insufficiency in the dog. JAVMA 146:1088, 1965.
112. Hamlin, RL and Harris, SG: Mitral incompetence in Great Dane pups. JAVMA 154:790, 1969.
113. Dear, MG: Mitral incompetence in dogs of 0-5 years of age. J Small Anim Pract 12:1, 1971.
114. Liu, SK and Tilley, LP: Malformation of the canine mitral valve complex. JAVMA 167:465, 1975.
115. Lord, PF, et al.: Left ventricular angiocardiography in congenital mitral valve insufficiency of the dog. JAVMA 166:1069, 1975.
116. Ljunggred, G, et al.: Four cases of congenital malformation of the heart in a litter of eleven dogs. J Small Anim Pract 7:611, 1966.
117. Lord, PF, et al.: Congenital tricuspid stenosis with right ventricular hypoplasia in a cat. JAVMA 153:300, 1968.
118. Weirich, WE, et al.: Congenital tricuspid insufficiency in a dog. JAVMA 162:1025, 1974.
119. Liu, SK and Tilley, LP: Dysplasia of the tricuspid valve in the dog and cat. JAVMA 169:623, 1976.
120. Eyster, GE, et al.: Ebstein's anomaly: a report of 3 cases in the dog. JAVMA 170:709, 1977.
121. Tilley, LP and Liu, SK: Letter to the editor. JAVMA 170:798, 1977.
122. Hamlin, RL, et al.: Antemortem diagnosis of tetralogy of Fallot in a dog. JAVMA 140:948, 1962.
123. Clark, DR, et al.: Tetralogy of Fallot in the dog. JAVMA 152:462, 1968.
124. Patterson, DF, et al.: Hereditary defects of the conotruncal septum in Keeshond dogs: pathologic and genetic studies. Am J Cardiol 34:187, 1974.
125. Van Mierop, et al.: Hereditary conotruncal septal defects in Keeshond dogs: Embryologic studies. Am J Cardiol 40:936, 1977.
126. Patterson, DF and Medway, W: Hereditary diseases of the dog. JAVMA 149:1741, 1966.
127. Patterson, DF: Tetralogy of Fallot. *In* A Manual of Clinical Cardiology. JAAHA, 1972.
128. Ringwald RE and Bonagura, JD: Tetralogy of Fallot in the dog: Clinical findings in 13 cases. JAAHA, in press.
129. Bolton, GR, et al.: Tetralogy of Fallot in three cats. JAVMA 160:1622, 1972.
130. Bush, M, et al.: Tetralogy of Fallot in a cat. JAVMA 161:1679, 1972.
131. Kirby, D and Gillick, A: Polycythemia and tetralogy of Fallot in a cat. Can Vet J 15:114, 1974.
132. Eyster, GE, et al.: Tetralogy of Fallot in a cat. JAVMA 171:280, 1977.
133. Lombard, CW and Twitchell, MJ: Tetralogy of Fallot, persistent left cranial vena cava and retinal detachment in a cat. JAAHA 14:624, 1978.
134. Hawe, RS, et al.: Tetralogy of Fallot in a 5-year old cat. JAAHA 15:329, 1979.
135. van Heerden, J and Lourens, DC: Tetralogy of Fallot in a two and one half year old cat. JAAHA 17:129, 1981.
136. Miller, CW, et al.: Microsurgical management of tetralogy of Fallot in a cat. JAVMA 186:708, 1985.
137. Voncoldi, JH, et al.: Effects of chronic right to left cardiac shunt on hypoxic sensitivity of mongrel dogs. J Appl Physiol 58:1767, 1985.
138. Beekman, RH and Tuuri, DT: Acute hemodynamic effects of increasing hemoglobin concentration in children with a right to left ventricular shunt and relative anemia. J Am Coll Cardiol 5:357, 1985.
139. Garson, A, et al.: Propranolol: the preferred palliation for tetralogy of Fallot. Am J Cardiol 47:1098, 1981.
140. Eyster, GE, et al.: Beta adrenergic blockades for management of tetralogy of Fallot in a dog. JAVMA 169:637, 1976.
141. Stephenson, LW, et al.: Staged surgical management of tetralogy of Fallot in infants. Circulation 58:837, 1978.
142. Herrtage, ME, et al.: Surgical correction of the tetralogy of Fallot in a dog. J Small Anim Pract 24:51, 1983.
143. Downey, RS and Liptrap, RM: An unusual congenital cardiac defect in a dog. Can Vet J 7:233, 1966.
144. Buergelt, CD, et al.: Persistent truncus arteriosus in a cat. JAVMA 153:548, 1968.
145. Straw, RC, et al.: Transposition of the great arteries in a cat. JAVMA 187:634, 1985.
146. Jeraj, K, et al.: Double outlet right ventricle in a cat. JAVMA 173:1356, 1978.
147. Turk, JR, et al.: Double outlet right ventricle in a dog. JAAHA 17:789, 1981.
148. Roberts, WC: A simple histologic classification of pulmonary arterial hypertension. Am J Cardiol 58:385, 1986.
149. Feldman, EC: Eisenmenger's syndrome in the dog: Case reports. JAAHA 17:477, 1981.
150. Nimmo-Wilhie, JS and Feldman, EG: Pulmonary vascular lesions associated with congenital heart defects in three dogs. JAAHA 17:485, 1981.
151. Eliot, TS, Jr, et al.: First report of the occurrence of neonatal endocardial fibroelastosis in cats and dogs. JAVMA 133:271, 1958.
152. Bohn, FK, et al.: Clinico-pathologic conference case presentation. JAVMA 157:1360, 1970.
153. Paasch, LH and Zook, BC: The pathogenesis of endocardial fibroelastosis in Burmese cats. Lab Invest 42:197, 1980.
154. Krahwinkel, DJ and Coogan, PS: Endocardial fibroelastosis in a Great Dane pup. JAVMA 159:328, 1971.
155. Lombard, CW and Buergelt, CD: Endocardial fibroelastosis in four dogs. JAAHA 20:271, 1984.
156. Gordon, B, et al.: Pulmonary congestion associated with cor triatriatum in a cat. JAVMA 180:75, 1982.
157. Alboliras, ET, et al.: Cor triatriatum dexter: two-dimensional echocardiographic diagnosis. J Am Coll Cardiol 9:334, 1987.
158. Linde-Sipman, JS and Stokhof, AA: Triple atria in a pup. JAVMA 165:539, 1974.
159. Perkins, RL: Multiple congenital cardiovascular anomalies in a kitten. JAVMA 160:1430, 1972.
160. Dear, MG: An unusual combination of congenital cardiac anomalies in a cat. J Small Anim Prac 11:37, 1970.
161. Pyle, RL and Patterson, DF: Multiple cardiovascular malformations in a family of boxer dogs. JAVMA 160:965, 1972.
162. Ogburn, PN, et al.: Multiple cardiac anomalies in a family of Aluke dogs. JAVMA 179:57, 1981.
163. Detweiler, DK, et al.: Diagnosis and surgical correction of peritoneopericardial diaphragmatic hernia. JAVMA 137:177, 1960.
164. Baker, GJ and Williams, CSF: Diaphragmatic pericardial hernia in the dog. Vet Rec 78:578, 1966.
165. Clinton, JM: A case of congenital pericardioperitoneal communication in a dog. J Am Vet Radiol Soc 8:57, 1967.
166. Atkins, CE: Suspect congenital peritoneopericardial diaphragmatic hernia in an adult cat. JAVMA 165:175, 1974.

167. Evans, SM and Biery, DW: Congenital peritoneopericardial diaphragmatic hernia in the dog and cat: a literature review and 17 additional case histories. Vet Radiol 21:108, 1980.
168. Willard, MD and Aronson, E: Peritoneopericardial diaphragmatic hernia in a cat. JAVMA 178:481, 1981.
169. Eyster, GA, et al.: Congenital pericardial diaphragmatic hernia and multiple cardiac defects in a litter of collies. JAVMA 170:516, 1977.
170. Van der Gaag, I and Van Der Luer, RJT: Eight cases of pericardial defects in the dog. Vet Pathol 14:14, 1977.
171. Detweiler, DK and Alam, MW: Persistent right arch with associated esophageal dilatation in dogs. Cornell Vet 45:209, 1955.
172. Kealy, JK: Persistent right aortic arch in the Greyhound. Irish Vet J 15:197, 1961.
173. Imhoff, RK and Foster, WJ: Persistent right aortic arch in a ten-year-old dog. JAVMA 143:599, 1963.
174. Coward, TG: Persistent right aortic arch in two Great Dane littermates. J Small Anim Prac 5:245, 1964.
175. Lawson, DD and Pirie, HM: Conditions of the canine oesophagus—II. Vascular rings, achalasia, tumours and peri-oesophageal lesions. J Small Anim Prac 7:117, 1966.
176. Van Den Ingh, TSGAM and Van Der Linde-Sipman, JS: Vascular rings in the dog. JAVMA 164:939, 1974.
177. Helphrey, ML: Vascular ring anomalies in the dog. Vet Clin North Am 9:207, 1979.
178. Shires, PK and Liu, W: Persistent right aortic arch in dogs: a long term follow-up after surgical correction. JAAHA 17:773, 1981.
179. Ultman, SH, et al.: Double aortic arch and persistent right aortic arch in two littermates: surgical treatment. JAAHA 16:533, 1980.
180. Martin, DG, et al.: Double aortic arch in a dog. JAVMA 183:697, 1983.
181. Pobisch, R and Eisenmenger, E: Osophagusdilatation infolge Rechtsaorta und Abschnurung durch das Lig. arteriosum beim Hund. Wien Tierarztl Monatschr 53:147, 1966.
182. Berry, AP, et al.: Persistent right aortic arch in a kitten. Vet Rec 114:336, 1984.
183. Wheaton, LG, et al.: Persistent right aortic arch associated with other vascular anomalies in two cats. JAVMA 184:848, 1984.
184. Andli, IA, et al.: Unusual vascular ring in a cat: left aortic arch with right ligamentum arteriosum. Vet Rec 114:338, 1984.
185. Hawe, RS, et al.: Congenital unilateral absence of a pulmonary artery in a cat. JAAHA 21:111, 1985.
186. Vitums, A: Anomalous origin of the right subclavian and common carotid arteries in the dog. Cornell Vet 42:5, 1962.
187. Day, SB: A left coronary artery originating from a single coronary stem in a dog. Anat Rec 134:55, 1959.
188. Will, JW: Subvalvular pulmonary stenosis and aorticopulmonary septal defect in the cat. JAVMA 135:913, 1969.
189. Eyster, GE, et al.: Aorticopulmonary septal defect in a dog. JAVMA 167:1094, 1975.
190. Lombard, CW, et al.: Clinico-pathologic conference. JAVMA 172:75, 1978.
191. Nelson, AW: Aorticopulmonary window in a dog. JAVMA 188:1055, 1986.
192. Eyster, GE, et al.: Coarctation of the aorta in a dog. JAVMA 169:426, 1976.
193. Nichols, JB, et al.: Aortic interruption in a dog. JAVMA 174:1091, 1979.
194. Sandusky, GE, et al.: Tubular hypoplasia of the ascending aorta and patent ductus arteriosus in a dog. JAVMA 176:536, 1980.
195. Buchanan, JW: Persistent left cranial vena cava in dogs: angiocardiography, significance, and coexisting anomalies. J Am Vet Radiol Soc 4:1, 1963.
196. Wallace, CR: Absence of posterior vena cava in a dog. JAVMA 136:27, 1960.

DRUG INDEX

Digoxin (Lanoxin, Cardoxin)	0.002–0.005 mg/lb	orally	q12h	Positive inotropic drug Decreases heart rate
Furosemide (Lasix)	0.25–1 mg/lb	orally, SQ, IM, IV	q8–12h	Diuretic
Hydralazine (Apresoline)	0.25–1 mg/lb	orally	q12h	Vasodilator Decreases mitral regurgitation and L ⟶ R shunting
Propranolol (Inderal)	0.25–0.5 mg/lb	orally	q8–12h	?Decreases dynamic outflow obstruction Decreases myocardial O_2 consumption Slows heart rate Antiarrhythmic

75 VALVULAR HEART DISEASE

STEPHEN J. ETTINGER

THE MITRAL COMPLEX

The term *mitral complex* refers to the following anatomic structures: leaflets (the septal and lateral leaflets), the mitral valve annulus, the left atrium, the chordae tendineae, the papillary muscles, and the left ventricular muscle wall.[1, 2] The mitral valve components are the structures most commonly affected in both canine and feline heart disease.

Acquired mitral valvular stenosis has been reported but is a most unusual condition. Mitral valvular regurgitation occurs quite commonly. Mitral valvular insufficiency may be due to disease affecting any or all of the components of the mitral complex. This section deals with diseases resulting in valvular leaflet fibrosis, ruptured chordae tendineae, left atrial tear, and bacterial endocarditis resulting in valvular deformity. Ventricular muscle dysfunction associated with cardiomyopathy is discussed in Chapter 77. Atrial dysrhythmias and asynchronous ventricular contractions due to ventricular arrhythmias are discussed in Chapter 76.

CHRONIC MITRAL VALVULAR INSUFFICIENCY (CMVI)

Chronic mitral valvular pathology resulting in mitral insufficiency is the most frequent cause of congestive heart failure in the dog. It occurs in the feline but much less commonly than in dogs. Names used to describe this disease have been summarized.[3] Numerous clinical studies have determined an 8 to 42 per cent incidence of this condition in dogs. These figures vary, with lower percentages representing a general clinical population and the higher percentages indicating the frequency recognized at necropsy. Male cocker spaniels are more prone to congestive heart failure from this disease than are females.[4] The disease is recognized far more commonly in small and medium-sized canine breeds. Mitral valvular insufficiency in the large and giant breeds is usually related to myocardial disease, as it is in the cat.

Clinical Signs. The clinical course of chronic mitral valvular insufficiency due to valve leaflet pathology is usually progressive over a period of weeks to years. Exacerbations and remissions of heart failure in the clinical disease usually occur. Table 75–1 lists the clinical signs and a description of the four phases of heart disease reported.[3] In phase one, the patient is without clinical signs and remains for an indefinite period in a state of satisfactory cardiac compensation.

As the disease progresses to phase two, signs of early decompensation develop. A deeply resonant cough is the most common sign of disease at this time. In most cases, the cough is reported to be nocturnal, often starting during the night or in the early morning hours. A small amount of white or blood-tinged phlegm may be expectorated at the end of the coughing paroxysm. Often, the sudden onset of the first coughing episode makes the owner believe that the pet has swallowed a bone.

The dog may also be presented for episodes of difficult breathing (dyspnea) or rapid breathing (tachypnea). Respiratory signs are frequently associated with the cardiac cough. Often the cough is so severe that the owner ignores the presence of respiratory distress, although the tachypnea is evident.

As the disease progresses to phase three, coughing becomes more frequent, occurring in paroxysms throughout the day. The history may suggest that coughing is induced when the animal is excited, pulls on a leash, or drinks water.

Phase three progresses to phase four in a variable manner. In both states, orthopnea (an inability to breathe while lying down) may be reported by the owner. It is also apparent that the patient is restless at night. Paroxysmal pulmonary edema is associated with extreme restlessness at night. Often, because edema is paroxysmal in nature, the clinical signs subside before the animal is seen by the emergency veterinarian.

When the heart and lungs are no longer able to compensate for the disease, gross pulmonary edema occurs and becomes progressively more severe in phase four. Associated signs of right-sided heart failure, such as peripheral venous engorgement, hepatomegaly, ascites, and subcutaneous edema, may develop. Increased pressure backing up from the left side of the heart increases pulmonary vascular pressure and ultimately strains the right ventricle until it, too, finally fails.

Syncope is reported in some dogs with chronic mitral valvular insufficiency. It may be associated with atrial

TABLE 75–1. CLINICAL AND RADIOGRAPHIC DESCRIPTION OF THE PHASES OF CHRONIC MITRAL VALVULAR FIBROSIS*

Phase	Description	Clinical Signs	Radiographic Signs† Dorsoventral View	Radiographic Signs† Lateral View
1.	Compensated mitral valvular insufficiency	Murmur only; no signs of pulmonary or systemic disease related to mitral insufficiency; normal exercise tolerance	Slightly enlarged left auricle; left ventricle unremarkable	Slightly enlarged left atrium; left ventricle unremarkable; the lung fields are clear
2.	Early phase of decompensating chronic mitral insufficiency, confined to left side (prodromal stage)	Occasional cough or respiratory embarrassment referable to mild degree of pulmonary congestion occurs after strenuous exertion; only left heart involved, and systemic signs are not present	Left ventricular enlargement‡ which may obscure enlargement of the left auricle; apex becomes rounded; dense and dilated pulmonary veins join the left atrium	Left atrial enlargement eliminates distal bend of trachea at the base of the heart; left ventricle enlarges; angle of trachea with thoracic spine decreases; caudal waist stretched; pulmonary veins approximate density of arteries and may be slightly dilated at junction with left atrium; lung field remains clear
3.	Cardiac dysfunction and decompensation; increased load on right ventricle and pulmonary hypertension may result in impending right ventricular disease	Signs of cough and pulmonary congestion present after exercise and at night; strain on right ventricle may produce signs of right heart failure	Left auricle may be visible again on left border; left atrium tends to force the main stem bronchi apart; ventricular enlargement progresses to general cardiac enlargement; pulmonary interstitial edema is present	Marked left atrial enlargement; craniocaudal diameter increases markedly owing to right ventricular enlargement; intrapulmonary vascular structures blurred in hilar and middle zones of lung field, which appears hazy; intrapulmonary arteries and/or veins accentuated; occasional liver enlargement
4.	Congestive heart failure with left or left and right heart decompensation	Pulmonary edema, often with signs of severe right heart failure such as ascites, pleural effusion, and liver enlargement; signs develop in dogs at rest and are exaggerated by even minimal exercise	Left auricle visible at left border; left atrium forces main stem bronchi apart; pulmonary congestion and pulmonary alveolar edema; occasionally pleural and pericardial effusion	Large to very large left atrium displacing left main stem bronchus dorsally; moderate to extreme enlargement of cardiac silhouette; pulmonary alveolar edema (air bronchograms, mottling); dense pulmonary arteries; occasionally large caudal vena cava; pleural and/or pericardial effusion; ascites; hepatomegaly

*The radiographic classification is based on that originally proposed by Hamlin (1968). The number of radiographic signs has been expanded and includes both lateral and dorsoventral views because the presence or absence of a single sign in one view, no matter how pronounced, may be deceiving. Radiographic signs compatible with pulmonary or systemic circulatory failure have also been included since they may be of help in proving the presence of heart failure.

†See Figures 75–3 to 75–5, which illustrate the phases.

‡Before assessing enlargement, shifting of the cardiac apex must be considered.

Table modified from Table 13–1 in Ettinger, S. J., and Suter, P. F.: Canine Cardiology. Philadelphia, W. B. Saunders Company, 1970.

premature beats or paroxysmal atrial tachycardia. An important cause of syncope is tussive fainting (see Chapters 11 and 18). This may be the most common cause of fainting in association with valvular insufficiency in small and medium-sized breeds. A significant percentage of patients with mitral valvular fibrosis are presented initially for signs associated with syncope, with or without associated seizure activity. This subset of patients often has no pulmonary signs secondary to cardiac dysfunction early in the course of the syncope. This changes, however, as the disease progresses.

Clinical Course. Chronic mitral valvular insufficiency becomes apparent pathologically in young animals at two or three years of age. Systolic murmurs usually become audible in patients between five and seven years of age. Although the onset of clinical signs is variable, many patients begin to develop signs of some cardiac decompensation after eight or nine years of age. The patient often compensates satisfactorily and may live for years with only occasional cardiac signs.

In general, serious pathophysiologic manifestations of chronic valvular insufficiency appear to be more frequent in the small and medium-sized dogs. The reason for the prevalence of this disease in these breeds is not clear.

Physical Examination. Depending on the state of decompensation, examination of the dog varies considerably. Coughing and respiratory distress may be observed while the history is being taken. In most cases of mitral valvular insufficiency, coughing can be elicited by the veterinarian by gentle tracheal palpation at the thoracic inlet. Panting must be critically evaluated, since it is a frequent manifestation of anxiety in both the dog and the cat during the visit to the hospital.

In compensated cardiac patients, the color of the mucous membranes is usually unremarkable. An injected appearance with a muddy color may be noticed in dogs with advanced stages of this disease. Cyanosis is recognized only in advanced cases when there is peripheral stasis of the blood or when the severity of pulmonary edema actually interferes with gaseous exchange in the lung parenchyma.

Dental and periodontal disease is often present in older patients presented with chronic valvular disease. However, there is no indication that this disease and chronic valvular heart disease are otherwise related. Chronic dental disease may be associated with regional lymph node enlargement. This may be responsible for pharyngeal irritation and coughing.

Palpation of the thorax reveals a precordial thrill when the intensity of the systolic murmur is a grade five or six out of six. The thrill is palpable over the point of maximal intensity at the left caudal sternal border. It may radiate over the entire precordium in dogs with intensely severe murmurs. A left ventricular heave or apical thrust may be obvious at the caudal sternal border in dogs with advanced valvular heart disease. Unless right-sided heart failure accompanies this disease, the abdomen is unremarkable in most instances. Severe chronic coughing may be responsible for the appearance of a hard, tense abdominal muscle wall. Other abdominal organ abnormalities may be noted when there is more than one disease present at the time of the examination.

Subcutaneous edema is unusual even in advanced cases of chronic valvular insufficiency. When it does occur, it always accompanies ascites. Abdominal enlargement due to right-sided heart failure always develops before subcutaneous edema when due to heart disease in the dog.

Palpation of the femoral pulse provides important diagnostic clues to the state of the heart disease. In normal and asymptomatic dogs, the pulse is usually slow and strong. As the disease becomes more severe, the pulse becomes rapid and jerky. Atrial premature contractions, ventricular premature contractions, paroxysmal tachycardias, and atrial fibrillation may induce a pulse deficit.

Auscultation. The murmur associated with early chronic mitral valvular insufficiency is a soft, early systolic murmur. As the disease progresses, the sound becomes more intense and holosystolic (Figure 75–1). The murmur is a mixture of high- and low-frequency sounds, although on occasion a high-frequency musical whoop or seagull-type murmur may be auscultated. This cardiac bruit is most intense at the left caudal sternal border; when severe, it radiates cranially, dorsally, and to the right hemithorax.

The intensity of the first heart sound is initially increased in dogs with this disease, although it may later be reduced in intensity. Should pulmonary hypertension develop, the intensity of the second heart sound may also be increased. Low-frequency, third, or fourth heart sounds result from a rapid inflow of blood from the left atrium into the left ventricle during diastole. They are not normally heard, however. These sounds become much louder and more audible in animals with heart failure. When an intense holosystolic murmur obscures the second heart sound, the pronounced third heart sound may be mistaken for the second sound. The presence of an audible third or fourth heart sound is referred to as a gallop sound. This indicates the presence of congestive heart failure (Figure 75–2). Such low-frequency heart sounds are most clearly heard over the mitral valve region with the bell of the stethoscope. This is in contrast to the second heart sound, a high-frequency sound that is auscultated best with the diaphragm over the left cranial thoracic region. When mitral valvular insufficiency is intense, the sounds radiate to the right and mimic, or may be associated with, chronic tricuspid valvular insufficiency.

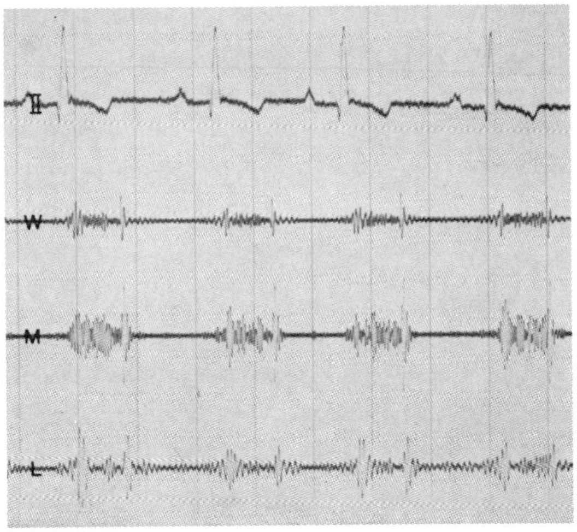

FIGURE 75–1. Systolic murmur of mitral insufficiency due to chronic mitral valvular fibrosis (endocardiosis). This phonocardiogram demonstrates an electrocardiographic lead II (top line) recorded simultaneously with three channels of heart sounds at high- (50 to 500 cycles per second), medium- (100 to 200 cps), and low- (50 to 100 cps) frequency bands. This is a mixed-frequency murmur, holosystolic in nature. Note that the murmur begins with the first heart sound and continues through systole to the second heart sound.

The intensity and rhythm of the heart sounds in this disease are usually constant unless a cardiac arrhythmia is present. Often, normal sinus arrhythmia may be responsible for moderate variations in the heart sounds. Premature contractions produce early heart sounds. In such cases, the intensity of the murmur is usually diminished or absent, and the second heart sound may also be absent. When paroxysmal tachycardias develop, the normal sinus rhythm is periodically disrupted by bursts of rapid beats, which begin and end abruptly. If atrial fibrillation develops, the heart rate is rapid and usually irregular. The first heart sound then is variable in intensity, as are the holosystolic murmur and the second heart sound.

Radiographic Examination. The radiographic appearance of chronic valvular insufficiency varies with the phase and severity of the condition. Left atrial and left and right ventricular enlargement are associated with mitral insufficiency. The result is characteristic changes in the cardiac silhouette and the pulmonary lung field. It is not possible to radiographically differentiate the etiologic basis of the mitral insufficiency. Nevertheless, the radiographic evaluation is the most sensitive clinical indicator of pulmonary hemodynamics. It permits the visualization of small changes involving the interstitium, the alveolar spaces, and venous congestion.

Left atrial enlargement is one of the earliest and most

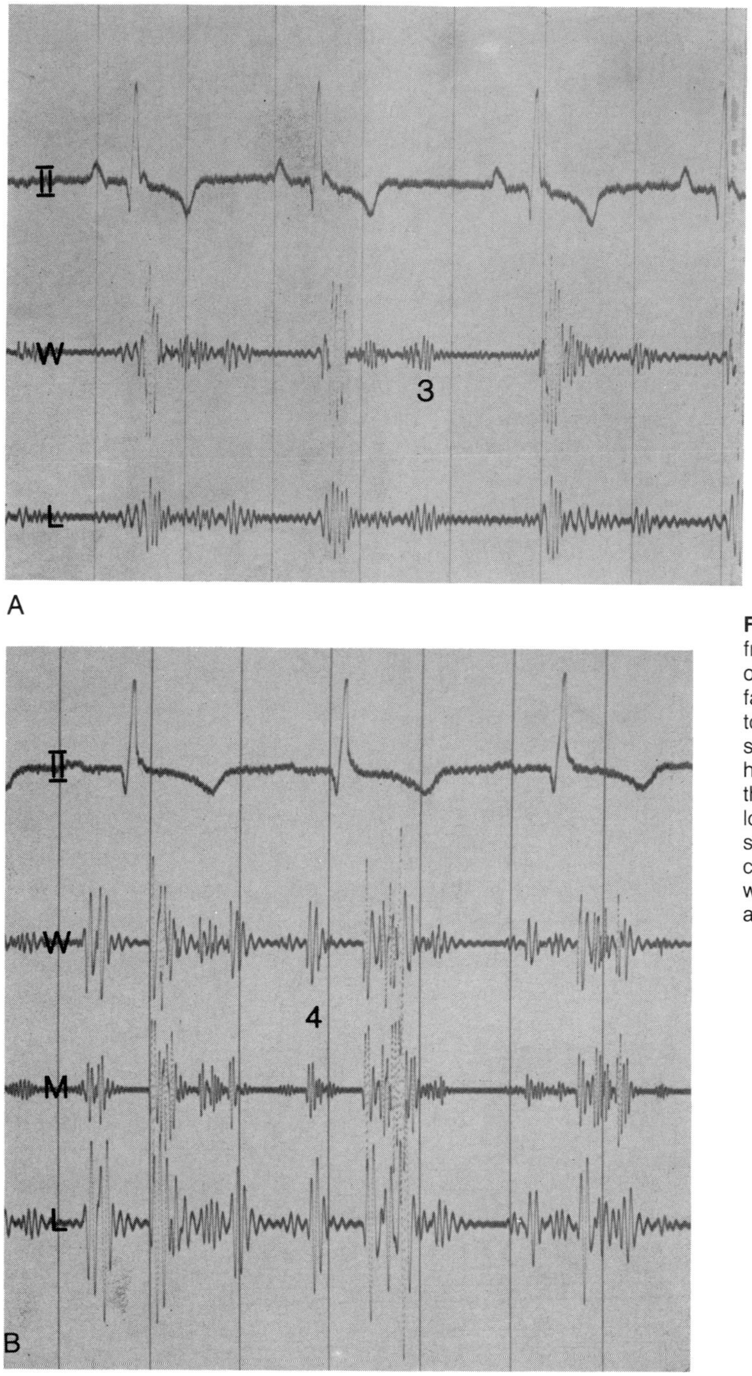

FIGURE 75–2. A holosystolic murmur is recorded on several frequency band ranges simultaneously with a lead II electrocardiogram. *A,* This patient was presented with acute congestive heart failure and has a loud protodiastolic gallop which is often referred to as a third heart sound (3). Often the third heart sound is sufficiently loud that it may be confused with the normal second heart sound. *B,* A presystolic gallop or S_4 rhythm (4) is present on this tracing. The presystolic gallop is loudest on the wide (W) and low (L) bands of this tracing because this is a low-frequency heart sound. The presence of a presystolic or S_4 gallop rhythm denotes congestive heart failure. The S_4 accentuated sound is associated with a strong atrial contraction moving a column of blood into an already overfilled ventricle.

consistent features of mitral valvular insufficiency. As the left atrium enlarges, it elevates the trachea and diminishes the angle between the trachea and thoracic spine on the lateral view. Simultaneously, it eliminates the ventral bend in the distal extremity of the trachea. When severely dilated, the left atrium extends as a wedge-shaped density into the diaphragmatic lung field. This represents extension of the pulmonary veins joining the atrium. In the hilar region, the dilated veins may appear as dense oval masses when seen on end and may easily be mistaken for enlarged hilar lymph nodes or tumor masses.

Dorsoventral compression of the main stem bronchi occurs with marked atrial involvement. Normally superimposed on each other, the lucent main stem bronchi, when divided, form a V-shaped structure that opens caudally. In cases of advanced valvular insufficiency, the left bronchus is displaced dorsally and appears flattened on the lateral projection.

On a laterally viewed projection, dilatation of the left atrium is responsible for disappearance of the caudal cardiac waist and straightening of the caudal cardiac border. The latter may occasionally merge with the silhouette of the diaphragm.

An early and characteristic sign of mitral valvular insufficiency is protrusion of the enlarged left atrium over the left heart border of the dorsoventral radiograph. As left ventricular enlargement progresses, there is increased rounding of the left cardiac border. Ventricular enlargement results in displacement to the left of the cardiac border and gives the cardiac apex a widened and rounded appearance. In such cases, the enlarged ventricular border may obscure the protrusion of the left atrium. In advanced cases, a dense, well-defined mass within the caudal half of the cardiac silhouette represents the dilated central portion of the left atrium. Dilatation of the left atrium forces the main stem bronchi apart and changes their angle from acute to obtuse.

Secondary to the changes described in the left side of the heart, right ventricular enlargement and enlargement of the right cardiac border occur. The transverse diameter of the cardiac silhouette in the dorsoventral projection then increases significantly.

Venous structures may be recognized by their confluence at the dilated left atrium in this disease. Dilated pulmonary veins indicate backing up of blood owing to left-sided heart failure. The dilated pulmonary veins are usually well outlined in the dorsoventral view. In a group of experimental dogs with surgically induced insufficiency of the mitral valve, a consistent feature was localized dilatation of the main pulmonary artery.[5]

As congestive heart failure develops, the extracardiac or pulmonary signs become evident radiographically. Venous congestion develops initially as the pressure from the left atrium backs up into the pulmonary veins. The central veins dilate and distend and become more evident in the peripheral lung fields. The dilated veins are both denser and larger than the corresponding pulmonary arteries.

Venous congestion progressively develops into interstitial and finally alveolar lung edema. Interstitial edema is recognized by poorly outlined pulmonary vessels, by accentuation of the bronchial wall (since the fluid around the bronchi makes the air-filled structures more apparent), and by a generalized increase in the density of the pulmonary parenchyma. Alveolar pulmonary edema often is first seen in the right caudal lobe and the perihilar regions. It is characterized by confluent areas of fuzzy, indistinct, "cloud-like" radiodensities and air bronchograms.

Signs of right-sided heart failure are likely to develop when advanced left-sided congestive heart failure is present.

The clinical and radiographic findings in the four phases of chronic mitral valvular fibrosis are summarized in Table 75–1. Representative radiographs of this disease are seen in Figures 75–3 through 75–5.

Electrocardiography. Electrocardiographic findings in mitral valvular insufficiency vary from normal tracings to those with marked abnormalities of the rate, rhythm, or configuration of complexes. Of significant importance is the sequential recording of electrocardiographic tracings in patients from the early to the more advanced stages of valvular insufficiency. Noting significant changes in serial electrocardiograms may be beneficial in suggesting treatment and a prognosis for this condition.

Most electrocardiographic abnormalities associated with mitral valvular fibrosis are the result of accentuations of the normal electrocardiogram (ECG). The mean electric axis in the frontal plane usually remains between 40 and 100 degrees. Occasionally, left axis deviation develops with marked left ventricular hypertrophy (left hemibranch or fascicular bundle branch block has been coined to identify this alteration; however, this term may not be correct). Even when the axis is shifted to the left, left ventricular hypertrophy may not be present. The axis is not likely to be less than −30 degrees. Normal sinus rhythms (including sinus rhythm, sinus arrhythmia, and wandering pacemaker) are expected in dogs with this disease. Cats usually maintain only a sinus rhythm although atrial fibrillation and/or ventricular ectopy are recognized as the disease progresses. Compensatory sinus tachycardia develops when the cardiac function is decreased. Supraventricular arrhythmias (atrial and atrioventricular or junctional premature contractions) may develop. Occurring less frequently than single premature contractions are paroxysmal supraventricular tachycardias, ventricular premature beats, and paroxysmal ventricular tachycardia.

Evaluation of 24-hour ECG ambulatory monitoring indicates that a significant number of canine patients exhibit simple atrial and ventricular ectopy and some also exhibit nonsustained ventricular tachycardia. Sudden death reported by owners of pets with mitral valve disease is likely to be due to such arrhythmias. Cardioactive therapeutic agents, electrolyte-depleting diuretics, and hypotension from vasodilator therapy could complicate such unrecognized arrhythmias. Diuretic agents used therapeutically may activate the renin-angiotensin and sympathetic nervous systems. These drugs promote the renal loss of both potassium and magnesium, which substantially increase the frequency and complexity of malignant ventricular arrhythmias. Although not usually observed in routine serum electrolyte determinations, these alterations may contribute to the progressive deterioration of cardiac function or the occurrence of sudden death.[6] Atrioventricular dissociation and ventricular tachycardia occur in advanced and terminal mitral valvular disease. Quite often, atrial fibrillation is recognized late in this disease and is almost always associated with combined left and right heart failure. It is more commonly observed in the male dog, but females are also affected. Atrial fibrillation is seen, but as noted, with less frequency, in the feline. ECGs of such cardiac arrhythmias are included in Chapter 76.

Left atrial enlargement, represented by widening of the P wave over 0.04 second (P mitrale), is common in dogs with moderate to severe mitral valvular insufficiency. Left ventricular hypertrophy in dogs is recognized on the ECG by prolongation of the QRS complex (greater than 0.05 second in small and medium-sized breeds or 0.06 second in larger breeds); increased amplitude of the QRS complex in leads II, III, and aVF (R wave greater than 2.5 to 3.0 mV; left axis deviation in the frontal plane; and the presence of S-T repolarization changes (Figure 75–6). In the cat, left ventricular hypertrophy may be suspected when the P wave exceeds 0.03 second in duration and the QRS complex is wider than 0.03 second and taller than 0.7 mV in leads II and aVF.

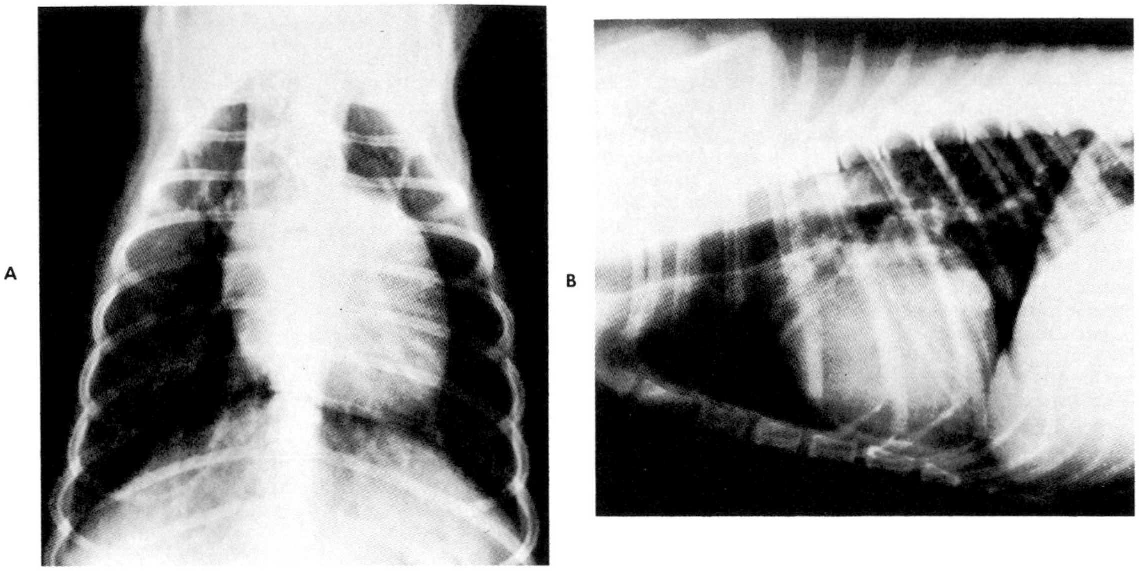

FIGURE 75–3. Dorsoventral and lateral projections of the thorax. This patient is in an early phase of disease due to chronic mitral valvular fibrosis or endocardiosis. Notice the evidence of early cardiac enlargement. *A,* The increased size of the right ventricle is apparent on the dorsoventral projection at the level of 5 to 11 o'clock. *B,* The increased size of the right ventricular border is especially noted by increased sternal contact on the lateral projection. The cranial and caudal waists are indistinct on the lateral projection. There is early separation of the left and right main stem bronchi due to left atrial enlargement.

As mitral insufficiency progresses, pulmonary lesions develop and ultimately impair right-sided heart function. When the right side of the heart is sufficiently stressed, right atrial strain is indicated by increased amplitude of the P waves greater than 0.4 mV (P pulmonale). In the dog, prolongation of the initial forces to the right (greater than 0.01 second) may suggest right ventricular hypertrophy in association with left-sided heart enlargement. Other indications of right ventricular hypertrophy in association with left-sided heart disease due to mitral insufficiency are the presence of deep Q waves in leads II, III, and aVF (all three together); the presence of an S wave in lead I; the presence of a deep S wave in lead V_4 or right axis deviation in the frontal plane.

S-T and T wave changes reflect the presence of ventricular hypertrophy. They must be distinguished from ischemic changes and from electrolyte and drug alterations.

Vectorcardiograms demonstrate an increase in initial forces to the right in the frontal and horizontal planes. There is an overall increase in the magnitude of the vector loop. Terminal forces in the horizontal plane are

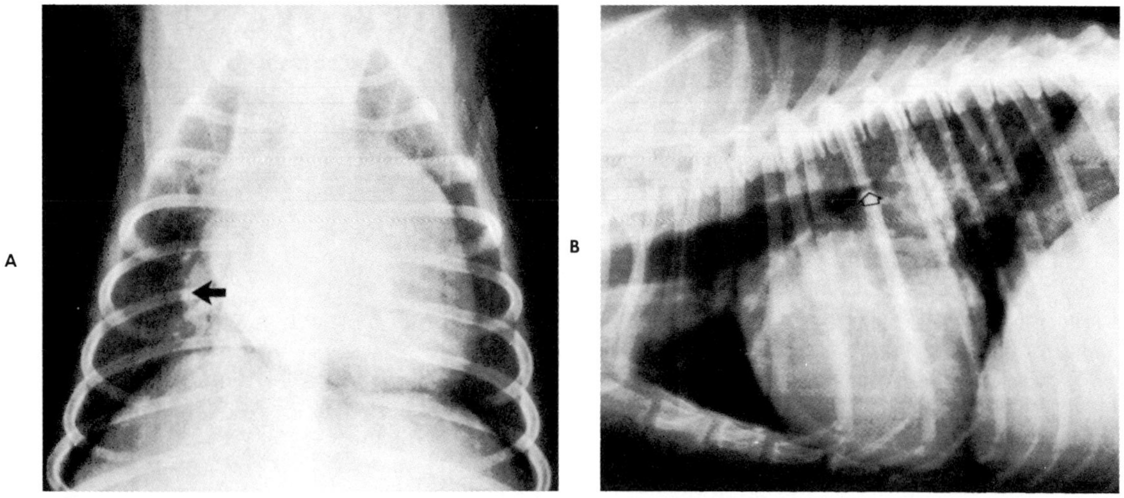

FIGURE 75–4. The same patient as in Figure 75–3, radiographed two years later when heart failure developed. The right and left ventricles are enlarged. *A,* The entire cardiac silhouette on the dorsoventral view is proportionately greater. The lung fields show evidence of hilar congestion and small air bronchograms are evident centrally (solid arrow). *B,* There is elevation of the trachea, and the left main stem bronchus (open arrow) is elevated and compressed dorsoventrally on the lateral view. There is continued right ventricular encroachment on the sternal region.

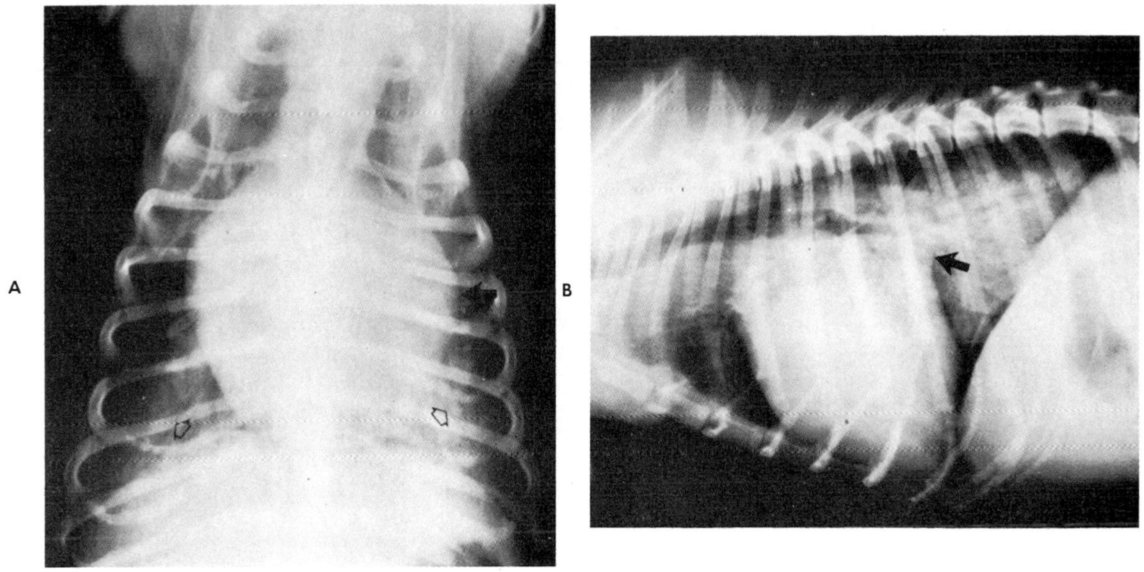

FIGURE 75–5. Patient with pulmonary edema secondary to advanced chronic mitral valvular fibrosis (endocardiosis). The cardiac silhouette is greatly enlarged; the left atrium bulges on both the dorsoventral *(A)* and lateral *(B)* projections (arrows). The lung fields are dense with alveolar and interstitial fluid. Air bronchograms extend from the hilar region to the periphery and are particularly obvious in the diaphragmatic lobes (open arrows). There is elevation of the trachea, which is indicative of cardiac enlargement. Right heart failure is evidenced by an increased postcaval size and marked hepatomegaly.

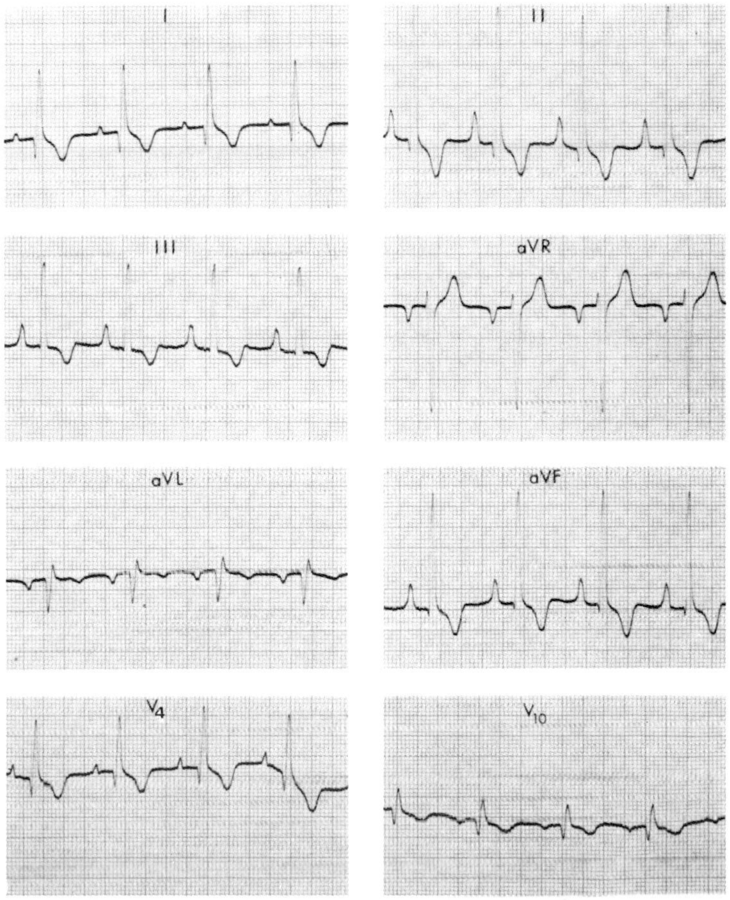

FIGURE 75–6. A representative eight-lead electrocardiogram from a dog with chronic mitral valvular insufficiency. The dog is in a sinus rhythm; the electric axis in the frontal plane is 70 degrees; and P mitrale, P pulmonale, and signs of left ventricular hypertrophy are present.

directed leftward but may be prolonged terminally, especially in the dorsal direction. Often the loop fails to close (S-T depression or elevation).

Laboratory Findings. In the absence of concurrent disease, hematologic values are normal in dogs and cats with chronic valvular insufficiency. Occasionally, the white blood cell count is elevated, reflecting a bronchopneumonia, a severe stress state, or a systemic infectious process. Moderate prerenal azotemia occurs, and elevated liver-enzyme levels are indicative of chronic hepatic congestion.

Biochemical changes within the heart continue to receive attention in an effort to appreciate cellular relationships in heart failure. An understanding of these changes (see Chapters 71 and 72) is important in the development and use of therapeutic agents to treat heart failure. Depletion of cardiac norepinephrine stores in heart-failure patients has been documented. This is of physiologic importance because in heart failure, appropriate inotropic and chronotropic responses do not occur with stimulation of the cardiac sympathetic nerves.[7] Changes include a decrease in myosin ATPase activity, a decrease in calcium transport by the sarcoplasmic reticulum, and a significant decrease in β-adrenergic receptor density in failing left ventricular tissue. This is likely the result of chronic exposure to high concentrations of circulating catecholamines. Mean arterial plasma norepinephrine concentrations in human patients with cardiac failure have been shown to be significantly elevated when compared to levels in normal individuals without heart failure.[8]

Although cardiac output and contractility studies may appear normal, these often fail to take into consideration the effects of both forward and reverse output of blood. Likewise, there is a diminished ability of the heart muscle to shorten and develop force with a given velocity under loading conditions. These factors result in a downward and rightward shift of the ventricular function curve associated with heart failure. Ventricular diastolic dysfunction then becomes a major contributor to the high pulmonary and venous pressures that contribute to the development of congestive heart failure.[7]

As the severity of the mitral regurgitation increases, left atrial pressures increase. These may be recorded by cardiac catheterization. Elevated left atrial pressures due to mitral insufficiency are characterized by large V waves with a prominent Y descent. In most cases, left ventricular pressures remain normal, although the end diastolic pressure exceeds 10 mm Hg when heart failure develops. In advanced mitral insufficiency, the right ventricular and pulmonary systolic pressures elevate modestly. Right ventricular end-diastolic pressures remain normal until right-sided heart failure occurs.

Indicator-dilution curves demonstrate that dye is not ejected from the ventricle as a bolus. Instead, the dye gradually becomes diluted owing to constant regurgitation from the ventricle into the atrium. In a series of dogs with chronic valvular insufficiency, the end-diastolic volumes were markedly increased and the systolic volume was slightly increased, while the stroke volume was markedly increased when compared with that of normal dogs.[9] The ejection fraction was slightly higher than normal, and the cardiac output was grossly increased over that of normal dogs. These findings are consistent with a volume-overload syndrome.

Echocardiographic Examination. Echocardiography is a noninvasive clinical tool that greatly enhances the clinician's ability to accurately identify, describe, and follow the progress of many cardiac diseases. Valvular insufficiency in dogs is being extensively studied. Echocardiography (along with Doppler echocardiography) is especially useful in the serial follow-up and management of patients with mitral regurgitation.

The clinician and client are provided with a clear, descriptive picture of the severity of the disease process. In addition, echocardiography provides valuable information regarding the quantity of regurgitation and end-diastolic and end-systolic volumes of the left ventricle, as well as indices of left ventricular systolic and diastolic function.[10] Serial, noninvasive evaluations of the regurgitant fraction, left ventricular function, and left atrial size are useful in evaluation of therapeutic interventions.[11]

Characteristic findings on 2-D and M-mode echocardiographic studies of dogs (and less commonly, cats) with mitral valvular incompetence include thickening to a variable degree of the septal (anterior) leaflet of the mitral valve, thickening to a lesser degree of the free wall (lateral) leaflet, mitral valve fluttering into the LV during diastole, and marked "flail" into the left atrium during ventricular systole. Often a large incompetent valve annulus is observed. The left atrial size progressively enlarges, dilating well beyond the approximately normal 1:1 ratio between it and the aortic outflow tract.

Left ventricular contractility remains vigorous to increased (over 40 per cent); the ejection fraction is apparently not diminished except for the physiologic finding of both forward and backward flow of blood from the heart. The left ventricular cavity progressively dilates; the chordae tendineae, when seen, vary with the stage of the disease from thickened and shortened to elongated or fractured. Tricuspid insufficiency with right atrial and ventricular enlargement does occur.

Measurements for the normal dog and cat, while not yet standardized, have been summarized by the author.[12, 13] Representative echocardiographic abnormalities seen in mitral valvular insufficiency are displayed in Figure 75–7.

Differential Diagnosis. The differential diagnoses for chronic valvular insufficiency are complicated by the fact that many dogs over five to seven years of age presented for examination have murmurs over the left sternal border. It is paramount to auscultate all murmurs and to associate the clinical signs with the severity of the cardiac disease. Often, concurrent disease states may be present. Not uncommonly, the degree of valvular insufficiency is minimal, and heart function is quite well compensated.

The major differential diagnostic considerations of chronic mitral valvular disease include pneumonia, acute and chronic pulmonary diseases, tracheal collapse, stertorous breathing of brachycephalic dogs, chronic tricuspid valvular insufficiency, acute rupture of the chordae tendineae, moderate to marked anemia, idiopathic congestive cardiomyopathy, and congenital cardiovascular conditions, including ventricular septal defect and aortic stenosis.

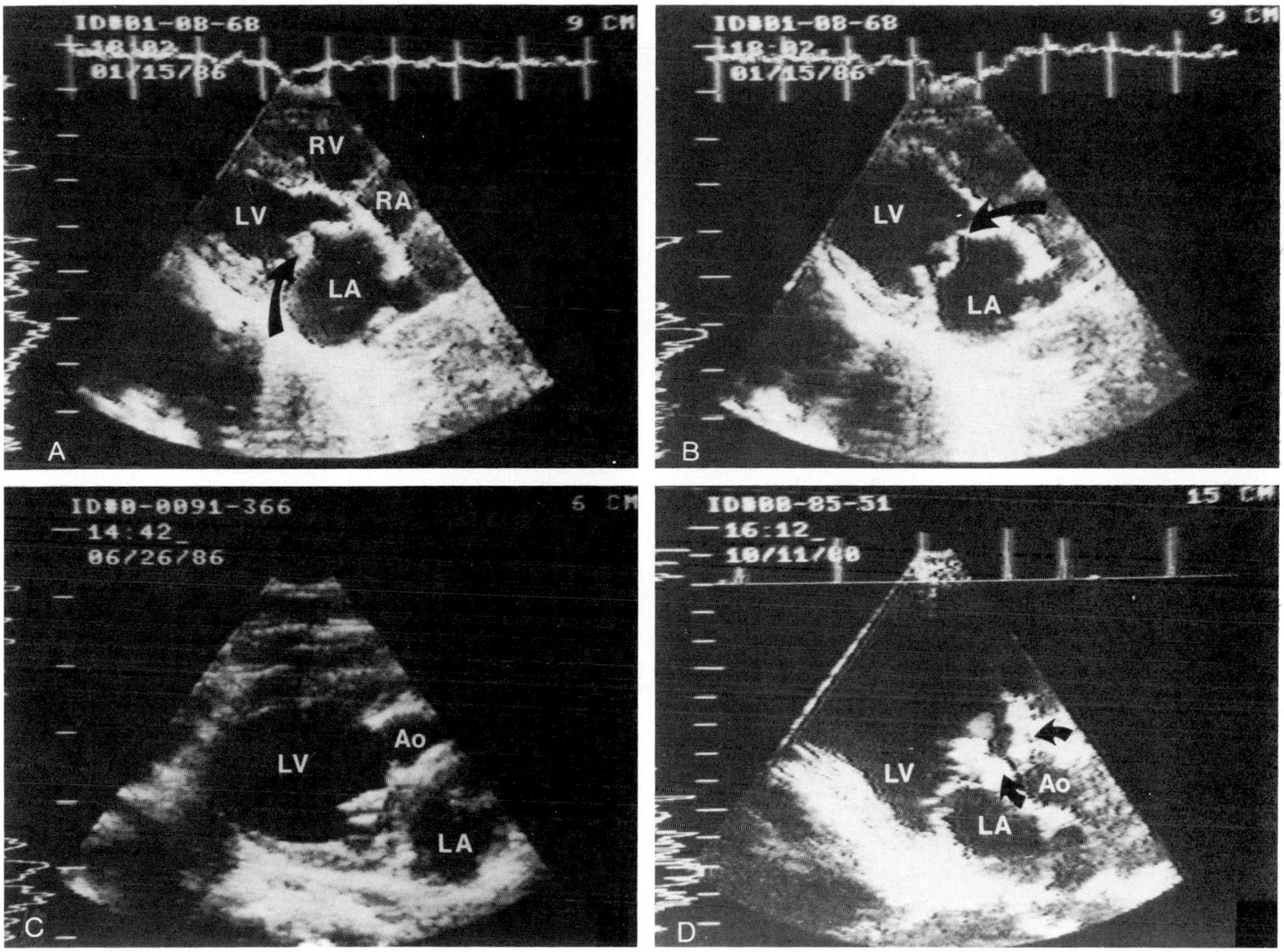

FIGURE 75–7. Echocardiograms from dogs and cats with valvular heart disease. *A,* Right long-axis parasternal view from a dog with chronic mitral valvular fibrosis. The four chambers are identified and are dilated. The mitral valve leaflets (arrow) are thickened and insufficient. *B,* Same dog and orientation showing a flail mitral valve (arrow). The entire septal leaflet is beyond the A-V ring within the left atrium. *C,* Cat with congestive cardiomyopathy and mitral insufficiency secondary to mitral annular ring dilation. The cardiac chambers are dilated and the LV wall is very thin. The LA diameter exceeds that of the aortic root in contrast to the normal 1:1. *D,* Canine with calcific aortic valvular insufficiency due to aortic valvular endocarditis. The area of the aortic root (arrows) is thickened and calcific. The valves obstruct the outflow tract and are insufficient, allowing the leaflets to flail backward into the LV cavity. The LV is also dilated due to the severe aortic regurgitation.

Prognosis. Dogs with chronic mitral valvular insufficiency remain compensated and asymptomatic throughout most of their lives (while in phase one). Congestive heart failure or cardiac dysfunction may or may not develop but usually progresses slowly and insidiously. Therapy is often helpful in delaying further circulatory imbalance in the early stages of this disease (phases two and three). Even as the disease progresses to overt congestive heart failure (phase four), therapeutic methods may be successful in relieving the clinical signs and providing an additional period of comfortable, quality life for the dog.

Although, as veterinarians, it is appropriate to enthusiastically encourage treatment of the symptoms, it is only proper to point out the reality and grave severity of the disease to owners whose pets are in an advanced degree of failure. The veterinarian should not ignore the fact that the mortality of patients with signs of congestive heart failure remains extremely high. Symptoms and discomfort may be alleviated, but no therapeutic interventions have yet been shown to significantly improve long-term survival in humans or pets.[6] Although not directly transferable to the canine, the prognosis of heart failure in human patients remains dismal; less than 50 per cent of patients survive a five-year period.[14] Dogs with early (phase one) disease may never develop clinical signs. However, some patients deteriorate and the disease process takes an inexorably progressive course. Treatment of signs (see below) of phases two and three is often very rewarding, and the pet may be expected to remain comfortable, leading a good-quality, although more sedate, lifestyle. Once overt heart failure develops, life expectancy is often reduced to four to eight months. Treatment in humans as well as the canine and feline species has for years consisted of rest, diuretic agents, cardiac glycosides, dietary sodium restriction, and more recently, manipulation of cardiac preload and afterload performance with vasodilating agents. New inotropic agents, many still in the research and development phase, remain on the horizon. Despite such approaches, many patients remain symptomatically compromised and the prognosis remains very poor. Treatment may extend comfortable life in some cases for several years. Sudden death or acute intractable congestive failure may develop at any time regardless of therapeutic interventions. The course of the disease in the cat is less rapid and requires differentiation from other causes of myocardial failure (see Chapter 77).

A realistic discussion of prognosis, lifestyle, costs, and reasonable alternatives should be properly outlined to the client at this time. Client rejection of a frank discussion may occur, and the practitioner should be prepared to discuss the problem with the client more than once, with a strong regard for the psychological reaction of the family to the prognosis. Referral to a specialist may be of benefit to the owner and pet at this time.

Therapy. Treatment for chronic valvular insufficiency is usually symptomatic. Although therapeutic measures may improve circulatory function, the etiologic inciting factors are not controlled. Medical care cannot directly prevent further pathology from developing. The long-term prognosis for dogs in phases one and two heart disease is variable to good; in phase three it is poor—often only months to a year; and in phase four it is dismal, regardless of therapy, if one looks at the long-term picture. Traditionally, the treatment of congestive heart failure is based on the use of rest, diuretics, cardiac glycosides, and restriction of dietary sodium. Adjunctive therapy includes the use of preload and afterload vasodilating agents.[19] Generally, therapy is initiated according to the phase of the clinical disease. Most physicians believe that drug therapy in CHF is effective in relieving symptoms and improving exercise tolerance, but they do not believe that such therapy actually improves survival.[14]

Asymptomatic dogs (phase one) require neither therapy nor restriction of exercise. Sodium need not be restricted in the diet, although foods excessively high in salt and poor-quality proteins should be avoided. Dogs that are clinically asymptomatic and that have no radiographic and/or electrocardiographic findings of significant cardiac enlargement do not require a low-sodium diet. Prophylactic digitalization is advised only in selected cases, as is the use of vasodilating agents.

In a large-scale survey among physicians treating patients with heart failure, most regarded diuretics as their first line of treatment. In part, this is done to allow a more liberal diet (an important point in small animal medicine as well). Only seven per cent of those surveyed used digitalis alone, but virtually all included this drug in the regimen of patients with moderate to severe congestive heart failure. The tendency to reserve digitalis stems from its potentially toxic side effects. Very few of those surveyed used vasodilators as part of their initial protocol for heart failure and only 50 per cent of the patients classified as being in phase three heart failure were maintained on vasodilator therapy.[14] Although veterinary medical practice differs from human medicine, the comparisons regarding diagnosis and treatment are significant.

In dogs with early signs of congestive heart failure (phase two), restriction of strenuous exercise and excitement, as well as restriction of sodium and caloric intake, may suffice. Occasional episodes of dyspnea, coughing, and fatigue, before heart failure develops, are usually well controlled by dietary sodium restriction combined with the administration of bronchodilators, diuretics, and, occasionally, sedatives. Because most cases do not progress beyond this stage, the importance of such therapy should not be underestimated. Bronchodilation is effectively accomplished with drugs listed in Table 75–2.

For patients with advanced signs of congestive heart failure (phases three and four), the proper use of cardiac glycosides still has no single substitute. Cardiac glycosides are used for the treatment of heart failure; recommended dosages in dogs and cats have been described (see Chapter 73).

Digitalis prolongs diastole, thus improving diastolic filling. This permits the heart to improve cardiac output through the Frank-Starling curve. In chronic congestive heart failure, this has been proposed as the principal long-term benefit of the cardiac glycosides. The reduction of the cardiac ventricular rate is sufficiently important to recommend continued use of medications used in treating congestive heart failure.[7] Even when diuretics and systemic vasodilators eliminated signs of heart failure, the additional administration of digoxin further improved cardiac function in humans with congestive heart failure.[15]

Diuretics are useful alone or in combination with cardiac glycosides to mobilize excess sodium and water retained by the body (see Chapter 73). While diuretic agents may effectively control abnormal fluid collection, they should not be considered substitutes for or alternatives to cardiac glycosides in the treatment of advanced congestive heart failure. Sudden, unexpected death in congestive heart failure occurs often. It is suggested that electrolyte deficits, activation of neurohormonal mechanisms, and drug therapy may account for some of the arrhythmogenic factors. Of all the treatment modalities recommended for congestive heart failure, the diuretic agents are most likely to promote the renal loss of potassium and magnesium. Reduction of electrolyte levels is thought to result in elevation of circulating catecholamines and aldosterone. Thus the beneficial effects of the diuretics must be weighed against their potential serious adverse effects.

When congestive heart failure is present, therapy with digitalis and diuretics should be supplemented by restricted sodium intake. Some dogs refuse all low-sodium diets. In such cases, it is preferable to allow these patients to eat moderately low-sodium-content foods such as K/D or home-prepared diets and to use diuretic therapy to eliminate excessive quantities of salts retained by the body. During periods of heart failure, exercise should be completely restricted. Hospitalization is the best means of accomplishing exercise restriction. In addition, the cardiac output of patients undergoing cage rest is enhanced.

When heart failure is refractory to diuretic and/or digitalis therapy, drugs that reduce venous return to the heart (preload and afterload reducing agents) allow the

TABLE 75–2. ANTITUSSIVE AND BRONCHODILATOR-ANTITUSSIVE COMBINATION MEDICATIONS

Generic Name and Preparation		Trade Name	Dosage
Aminophylline 1½ gm (100 mg) tablets		—	5 mg/lb q6–12h as needed
Theophylline (elixir 80 mg/Tbls) (capsules 100 & 200 mg)		Elixophyllin, Theolixir	5 mg/lb q6–12h as needed
Oxtriphylline 400 or 600 mg SA tablets		Choledyl SA	Similar to aminophylline; reported to cause fewer GI problems
Theophylline with glyceryl guaiacolate: 150 mg theophylline + 90 mg glyceryl guaiacolate per capsule or Tbls		Quibron	1 capsule q8–12h for larger dogs; ¼ to 1 Tbls elixir q8–12h for smaller dogs and cats
Aminophylline with ¼ or ½ gm phenobarbital		—	½ to 1 tablet q6–12h
Theophylline 130 mg Ephedrine HCl 24 mg Phenobarbital 8 mg		Tedral tablets	¼ to 1 tablet q8–12h
Hydrocodone bitartrate 5 mg Homatropine methylbromide 1.5 mg	per tablet or per 5 cc	Hycodan	½ to 1 tablet (or teaspoon) q6–24h as needed; may increase dosage if sedative effect does not occur
Hydrocodone 5 mg Phenyltoloxamine 10 mg	per tablet or per 5 cc	Tussinex	½ to 1 tablet (or teaspoon) q6–24h as needed; may increase dosage if sedative effect does not occur
Butorphanol tartrate 5, 10, 25 mg tablets		Torbutrol	0.25 mg/lb q6–12h; may cause sedation
Prednisone 2 mg Trimeprazine 5 mg	per tablet or spansule	Temaril-P	1 tablet per 20 lbs q12h; good for allergic and noninfectious inflammatory coughing (i.e., tracheal collapse)
Guaifenesin 100 mg Dextromethorphan 15 mg	per 5 cc	Robitussin-DM	Non-narcotic; OTC preparation; for temporary antitussive effect. Dosage similar to that for adults and children

ventricles to become more compliant and thus improve cardiac output. Afterload reducing agents such as hydralazine decrease peripheral vascular resistance, increase atrial compliance, and improve ejection characteristics. One study that reported on a small number of dogs with mitral regurgitation suggested that there were improved hemodynamics and clinical benefits following hydralazine treatment along with conventional cardiac drugs.[16] Vasodilators such as hydralazine and mixed vasovenodilators such as prazosin may be used (see Chapter 73). Since these agents may result in dizziness, loss of appetite, increased heart rate, and hypotension when given in excess, and because they tend to have a sedative effect, the author prefers initially to use a low dose once or twice daily and then increase the dosage weekly as required. Controlled clinical studies using placebos and these products in dogs have not been reported. Many human and veterinary cardiologists appear to favor the angiotensin-converting enzyme inhibitors because it is recognized that the renin-angiotensin system contributes to systemic vasoconstriction in congestive heart failure patients. Inhibition of the angiotensin-converting enzyme has been shown to result in the improvement of both resting and exercise cardiac function as a result of vasodilation.[17]

Despite the known beneficial effects of these competitive enzyme inhibitors, a substantial percentage of human patients with refractory heart failure do not exhibit a beneficial response or they discontinue the drug due to the serious side effects.[18] The same experience has been found in dogs and cats given both captopril and enalapril.

For this reason, this author prefers to begin therapy in dogs and cats with congestive heart failure at the lowest dosage and increase the drug according to response, if needed. Captopril, while suggested as a t.i.d. medication, is often not tolerated more than twice daily in dogs. In cats it may be tolerated only once daily. Enalapril is usually given only once daily in dogs and cats (see Chapter 73 for recommended dosages, precautions, and additional information). Once begun, the drugs are continued indefinitely when favorable results occur. If the pet is also receiving digitalis and loss of appetite develops, the clinician must decide which drug is responsible for the problem.

Other agents used in treating the clinical signs resulting from mitral valvular insufficiency include antitussives such as dihydrocodeinone, torbutaline HCL, phenobarbital, and mild oral tranquilizers. It should be understood that these agents are not substitutes for appropriate cardiac therapy. They may be used in conjunction with the previously mentioned drugs to make the patient more comfortable.

In acute heart failure, a reduction in central venous return is also achieved by using nitroglycerin topical ointment, which is transcutaneously absorbed. It is applied (using a finger cot or a rubber glove) to the inguinal region, ear pinna, or other nonhairy area of the body. It may be reapplied every four to six hours.

Phlebotomy and rotating tourniquet are techniques

that are rarely used in medicine today. When effectively used, the end result is peripheral venous pooling and a reduction in the return of blood to the right side of the heart.

Oxygen therapy provided in a cool, humidity-controlled environment may be of benefit, but one must recall that severe pulmonary edema blocks an oxygen-enriched air supply.

A significant amount of evidence now demonstrates that myocardial catecholamine levels are often reduced in the presence of severe congestive heart failure. It is hypothesized that this is the result of chronic increased sympathetic activity. When β-blockers are administered to heart failure patients, hemodynamic deterioration occurs. This indicates that the autonomic nervous system assumes an important role in the myocardial performance of heart failure patients.[19]

Some of the newer positive inotropic agents used to treat heart failure are based on the concept of catecholamine depletion. Dobutamine, a synthetic sympathomimetic amine, exerts a potent positive inotropic action on the heart. Dobutamine has only minimal effects on vascular tone and exposes the patient to fewer arrhythmias and less tachycardia than do some of its precursors. Due to its availability in injectable form only, it is not useful for the long-term treatment of heart failure. Its short-term administration may result in long-term functional improvement in patients with severe heart failure.[19] Long-term use, i.e., more than 48 hours, results in the rapid induction of tolerance to all of the sympathomimetic amines.

Phosphodiesterase inhibitors increase intracellular cAMP by inhibiting the breakdown of cAMP. These drugs, acting as inotropic-vasodilating agents, are often useful in reversing the hemodynamic abnormalities of congestive heart failure. Theophylline, a frequently used drug in veterinary medicine, exerts at least part of its effect in this manner. In addition, a number of newer bipyridine derivatives have been developed that when given intravenously or orally produce a marked beneficial hemodynamic response in the patient with severe heart failure.

The oral products are not yet available commercially in the United States, and amrinone (Inocor) is useful intravenously in some heart failure patients (see Chapter 73). Although highly touted as being the newest modality of therapy, it is of significance to recognize that the prognosis for patients treated with these agents remains poor, although there is likely to be early clinical symptomatic improvement.[20, 21]

In an important review article, it has been observed in human beings that both symptomatic and hemodynamic improvement occurs during short-term use of these drugs. Long-term use may not always be benign; the prognosis remains poor and it is not yet clear whether such therapy delayed, had no effect on, or perhaps even hastened the demise of the patient.[22]

Since oral bipyridine compounds, considered to be much more potent than the IV amrinone product, are not yet commercially available, their use except under experimental situations cannot be recommended. A report of success with oral milrinone at 0.16 mg/lb (0.34 mg/kg) in 13 dogs with congestive cardiomyopathy suggests that the drug may be quite effective in improving contractility and hemodynamics. Improved contractility was considered responsible for the improvement in seven of the dogs, while vasodilation appeared to be the major source of benefit in three dogs, and a combination of both in three others.[23] These drugs are usually given along with other conventional compounds and methods used to treat congestive heart failure. Injectable infusion of milrinone into patients with advanced heart failure in a large multicenter human study proved effective and safe for 48 hours.[24]

The author's experience with injectable amrinone has been good in some acute cases of canine congestive heart failure. It has reversed the clinical signs in a number of dogs presented with congestive cardiomyopathy and chronic mitral valvular heart disease. Given initially over five minutes as a bolus, using 0.35 mg/lb,

TABLE 75–3. THERAPEUTIC APPROACH TO CONGESTIVE HEART FAILURE

Phase of Heart Disease	Digitalis	Diuretics	Bronchodilators	Exercise Restriction	Low-Sodium Diet	Vasodilators	Other
I/IV	No	No	No	No	No	No	No
II/IV	No	No	As needed	Restrict hunting and excessive running	No. Consider geriatric diet	No	No
Early III/IV	Yes	Initially yes. Later, only as required	Yes	Yes, but brief running OK Walking is good	Yes, to moderate level	Maybe	May require cough suppressants
Late III/IV	Yes	Yes, regularly	As needed	Yes. Restrict to brief activity only	Yes, to level of 6–10 mg/lb	Yes	Cough suppressants (?). Rapid digitalization if acute; may use aldosterone-inhibiting agents. New inotropic agents may be of benefit
IV/IV	Yes	Yes	Yes, oral or by injection	Yes. Restrict to cage	Yes. Use approximately 6 mg/lb	Yes, by IV infusion; oral or ointment	Narcotic sedatives, oxygen therapy, phlebotomy; tourniquets (?)

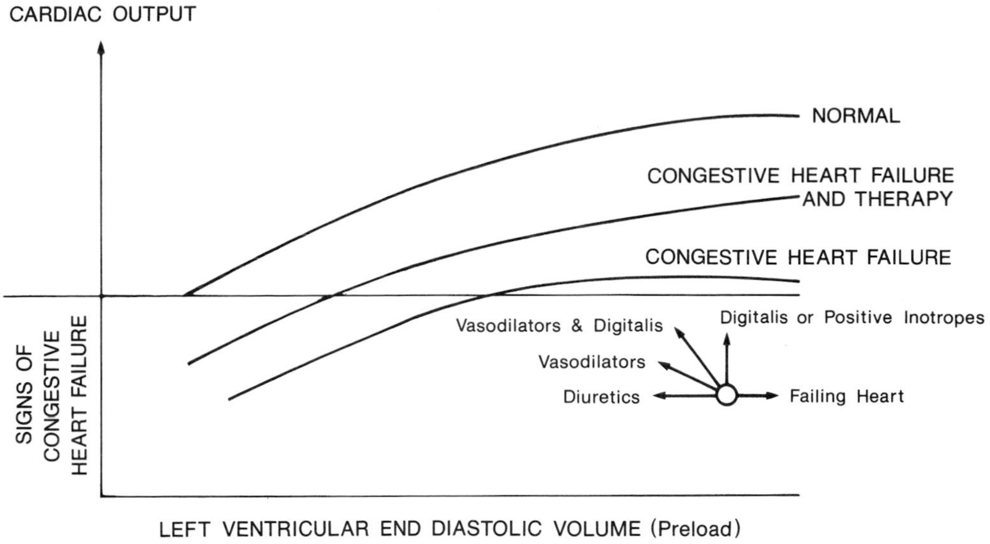

FIGURE 75–8. A conceptual graph describing the effects of therapeutic modalities on cardiac output and left ventricular preload.

it is then administered in a lactated Ringer's solution and given as a continuous infusion at 5 to 10 mcg/lb/min. The drug has reversed the signs of heart failure in some of the patients and in those with treatable congestive cardiomyopathy was considered life-saving. Due to the fluid volumes required, it has not been given to cats in heart failure.

Atrial natriuretic polypeptide is a cardiac hormone with fluid volume–reducing and vasodilating activities.[25] Continued research and investigation in this area is likely to result in an entirely new approach to congestive heart failure treatment in the upcoming years.

Table 75–3 summarizes the options for cardiac therapy based on the clinical phase of the disease. Figure 75–8 summarizes the effects of various modalities of therapy in heart failure.

Surgical Correction. Surgical correction of mitral valve disease in dogs and cats is not a recognized therapeutic modality. In humans, where mitral incompetence is the result of myxomatous degeneration of the valve, especially when the chordae are shortened or elongated, valve repair is not possible and replacement of the valve is usually considered as the only acceptable alternative.[26]

Pathology of Chronic Valvular Disease. Numerous authors have described the gross pathologic findings in this disease.[3] The mitral valve appears grossly thickened with grayish-white nodules on the leaflet edges. The leaflets are contracted to a variable degree, depending on the stage of the disease process (Figure 75–9). The valve leaflet commissures are not fused. Although the chordae tendineae are unlikely to be fused, they are usually thickened. In some cases, there is fibrosis where the chordae tendineae attach to the papillary muscles.[27] The mitral annulus is usually dilated, thus adding to the mitral incompetency.

Whitney divided the valvular processes into four types.[28] In Type I, small nodules are present on the free edges of the valve, there is some opacity at the basal portion of the leaflet, and the chordae tendineae (CT) are normal. Type II valves have large, coalescing, and occasionally multiple nodules, while the leaflet opacity becomes more infiltrative but the CT remain normal. Type III valves have larger coalescing nodules, plaque-like deformities at the points of nodular contact, irregular opacity and thickening at the valve base, and a thickened valve with decreased flexibility and insufficiency. Hemorrhage and calcification may be seen within the valve; the CT are thickened where they meet the valve leaflet. In Type IV the valves are grossly deformed by coalescing nodules and plaque-like elevations. The cusps are contracted with rolled-in margins and the CT are thick, irregular, and, on occasion, ruptured.

In another study of 64 cases, a similar report described three groups of canine patients: those with small discrete lesions with or without large nodules, those with extensive thickening throughout the rough valve zone, and those with thickened valve leaflets and ruptured chordae tendineae. As the disease progressed histologically, the leaflets became more redundant and the chordae tendineae more elongated.[29]

Although the mitral valve is usually the most commonly affected, other cardiac valves may be similarly affected. The mitral valve is affected most commonly, followed by the mitral and tricuspid valves together, and

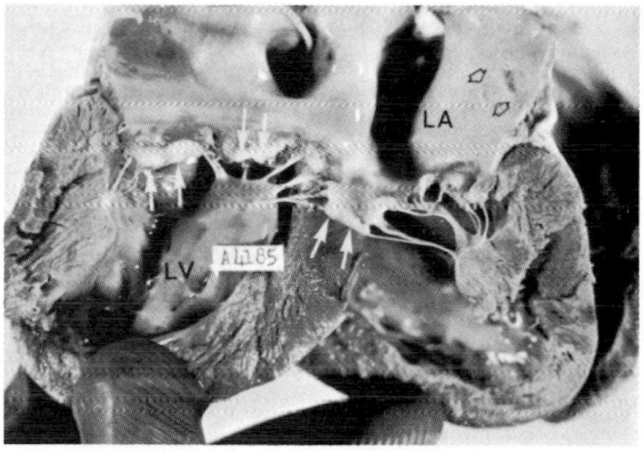

FIGURE 75–9. Postmortem specimen of opened left ventricle (LV) and left atrium (LA). The left ventricular wall is thickened, and the mitral valve leaflets are grossly thickened and contracted, with grayish-white nodules rolling in the free edges (white arrows). The valve leaflets are not fused, and the chordae tendineae appear normal. Jet lesions present on the left atrial wall (between open arrows) result when the regurgitant streams of blood from the left ventricle continuously strike the atrial wall. (Courtesy of Dr. S.-K. Liu, The Animal Medical Center, New York.)

then by tricuspid valve fibrosis only.[30] The aortic valve, the pulmonic valve, and other combinations of valves are affected. Detweiler and colleagues reported the microscopic findings as ". . . collagen and elastic fibrosis, edema, increased ground substance, and sometimes amyloid deposition and hemorrhage."[31] Other authors found amyloid deposits in five of 80 dogs with endocardiosis.[32] They reported that the characteristic fibrillar structure found in amyloid deposits was seen by electron microscopy. In a more complete study of valvular amyloidosis, it was noted that the average diameter of the amyloid fibrils was 100 A.[33] There was a close relationship of amyloid deposits to active fibroblasts, collagen fibers, and macrophages. Senile valvular amyloidosis may occur without other organ involvement. The earliest changes in the connective tissue ground substance were reported to be a result of the accumulation of water and stainable acid mucopolysaccharides.[34]

The morphologic picture of this disease was further described as dystrophic and proliferative processes within the spongiosa and fibrosa of the valve.[29, 35] Histochemically, hyaluronidase-susceptible acid mucopolysaccharides of the hyaluronic acid, chondroitin sulfate types were found. Fibrosis and metaplastic formation of cartilage and adipose tissue, as well as fragmentation of elastic fibers, were recognized in the spongiosa. Dystrophic changes were also seen in the fibrosa. These authors further reported, on the basis of electrophoretic studies of aqueous extracts of canine heart valves, that such changes represent noninflammatory atrophic processes.[35]

This description of the valvular changes is summarized as a noninflammatory, dystrophic process, referred to as endocardiosis.[36] Another author prefers the terms myxomatous transformation or mucoid degeneration, which are more precise than the term fibrosis, applied by Ettinger and Suter and by this author in the first edition of this textbook.[3, 37]

Regardless of the name given to the changes that occur in the mitral valve leaflet, it is important to recognize the multiplicity of problems that together cause the pathophysiology of this disease. In addition to the complications of simple valvular insufficiency, there may well be one or more of the following abnormalities: changes in the intramural coronary arteries; ventricular and/or atrial muscle ischemia; cardiac arrhythmias; damaged chordae tendineae, papillary muscles, and left atrial endocardium; mitral ring annular dilatation; and pulmonary and/or peripheral circulatory irregularities. It is the complex of these problems that accounts for the disease process thus described.

Microscopic intramural myocardial infarction (MIMI) is often an accompanying factor with chronic valvular heart disease in the dog. This is discussed under Ischemic Myocardial Disease (see Chapter 77).

Grossly, dilatation of the left atrium is followed by eccentric hypertrophy and dilatation of the left ventricle. Right ventricular involvement may occur as left A-V valvular insufficiency becomes more severe and additional strain is placed on the right side of the heart. As pulmonary hypertension and tricuspid insufficiency develop, the right ventricle enlarges and the right atrium may also dilate.

On the intimal surface of the left atrium, roughened fibrous plaques (referred to as "jet lesions") develop. These lesions result from the forceful regurgitation of blood from the ventricle back into the atrium. Owing to the chronic increasing atrial volume, that chamber dilates and thickens gradually to an enormous size. Splitting of the left atrial endocardium may occur at the site of the jet lesions.

Extracardiac lesions develop as the severity of mitral valvular insufficiency increases and circulatory failure occurs. The most significant of the extracardiac lesions is pulmonary edema. As the lung loses its spongy texture and becomes fibrous, hyperemic, and congested, clinical signs of respiratory difficulty become apparent. Alveolar and interstitial pulmonary edema are two of the end results of advanced chronic valvular heart disease.

Another cause of mitral valvular insufficiency is congenital mitral valve dysplasia. This condition occurs clinically in young dogs and is associated with progressive left-sided heart failure; its clinical signs are indistinguishable from those of other causes of mitral insufficiency. This condition and the valvular abnormalities are discussed in Chapter 74. Other causes of mitral insufficiency are outlined in the discussion of the mitral complex in the initial paragraphs of this chapter.

Etiology of Valvular Fibrosis (Endocardiosis). The etiology of chronic valvular fibrosis (endocardiosis) in dogs is still unknown. Numerous theories have been suggested. Viral valvulitis, prior bacterial endocarditis, autoimmune disease, hemodynamic alterations, and age-related alterations of collagen tissue are a few of the theories expressed. These theories have been discussed.[3] At this time, there are no additional clues to the exact etiology of this disease. It would appear that prior bacterial endocarditis or viral valvulitis are not likely causes of this problem.

Senile valvular amyloidosis is most likely due to synthesis by valvular stromal cells such as fibroblasts and macrophages.[33]

One group of authors suggested that stress and possible nutritional factors may cause endocrine dysfunctions responsible for chronic valvular fibrosis.[38] They produced similar lesions in 17 young dogs by giving multiple injections of ACTH and desoxycorticosteroids.

ENDOCARDIAL SPLITTING AND LEFT ATRIAL RUPTURE

Endocardial splitting of the left atrial wall is a complication of chronic mitral valvular insufficiency, rather than a separate disease. Occasionally, the medial wall of the atrium ruptures, although the caudal wall is more commonly affected by this disease.

Pathologically, the lesion begins as an incomplete split of the endocardium over which fibrin deposits. The rupture may heal or occasionally may re-rupture completely, resulting in hemopericardium. Usually the rupture is recognized at the point of a prior jet lesion. Healed splits are in the form of depressed scars, whereas jet lesions are plaque-like proliferations rising over the endocardial surface.[39] This disease has been described in the dachshund and cocker spaniel; however, it is seen in other breeds as well, including poodles.[37] The disease is seen with greater frequency in male dogs. Endocardial splitting of the interatrial septum may result in an acquired atrial septal defect. Left atrial tear also occurs secondarily to congenital patent ductus arteriosus. This author has observed left atrial tears in dogs with idiopathic congestive cardiomyopathy and rarely in cats with cardiomyopathy and aortic embolism.

Cardiovascular Examination. Generally, the history and physical examination of animals with endocardial splitting of the left atrial wall do not differ from those of patients with chronic mitral valvular insufficiency. These diseases are usually recognized in middle-aged or older animals. As described previously, they occur with greater frequency in the chondrodystrophic breeds and are seen most often in male dogs.

A mixed-frequency holosystolic murmur is best heard over the left caudal sternal region and usually radiates dorsally, cranially, and to the right. In most cases, the murmur is loud and produces a palpable precordial thrill. Arrhythmias (most often supraventricular premature contractions or atrial fibrillation) are common. In dogs with normal sinus rhythms, the diastolic gallop sound, when present, is associated with congestive heart failure. In most cases, dogs developing hemopericardium secondary to left atrial tear do not have obviously muffled heart sounds. When one has the opportunity to examine the dog just before and immediately after a left atrial tear, there is an obvious decrease in the intensity of the cardiac murmur and heart sounds.

The radiographic signs of endocardial splitting and left atrial tear depend upon the presence or absence of hemopericardium. If hemopericardium has not occurred, thoracic radiographs are similar to those of dogs with phase three or phase four heart failure due to mitral valvular insufficiency. Extreme left atrial enlargement, indicated by a triangular extension of the cardiac silhouette into the diaphragmatic lobes, is recognized. The left ventricular border remains straight on the lateral radiograph. Thus, the cardiac silhouette is dissimilar in the lateral and dorsoventral views. When hemopericardium develops, the cardiac silhouette appears moderately to greatly enlarged and is globular in both views. Roentgen signs of left-sided heart failure are usually present, although pulmonary edema is absent.

Atrial rupture should be considered when a dog with radiographic signs of advanced chronic mitral valvular fibrosis suddenly develops a globular cardiac silhouette. This is often associated clinically with an episode of syncope and, occasionally, with seizure activity. When positioning the dog for radiographic examination, extreme care is essential if a left atrial rupture is suspected. An imminent tear may be provoked by forcing the dog to lie and struggle in an uncomfortable position. In some cases, only the slightest exertion may result in exacerbation of the left atrial tear.

The ECG recorded is usually consistent with that observed for chronic mitral valvular fibrosis. The P wave is prolonged and the QRS complex is likely to have features of ventricular hypertrophy. Dissecting hemorrhage results in myocardial changes, which are likely to cause the dysrhythmias associated with left atrial rupture.[40] Arrhythmias recognized include supraventricular premature beats, paroxysmal and persistent atrial fibrillation, and ventricular extrasystoles. Decreased ECG amplitudes and electrical alternans are infrequent.

Evidence of pericardial effusion is suggested radiographically but is best demonstrated by echocardiographic examination. Rarely is the tear observed, but effusion is apparent. In such cases, pericardiocentesis may be performed. Whole blood with a normal clotting time may be withdrawn from the pericardial sac. If hemopericardium has been present for any significant length of time and no new hemorrhage has occurred, then only a serous or serosanguineous fluid is removed. Clots may form in the pericardial sac, and the remainder of the blood is defibrinated so that it will not clot when removed.

In most cases, when pericardial effusion is recognized in dogs with this syndrome, it is associated with acute exacerbations of heart failure or syncopal episodes or both. In such cases, the clinical distress of the patient precludes performing a pericardiocentesis at that time.

Differential Diagnosis. The differential diagnosis of endocardial rupture includes chronic congestive heart failure due to mitral valvular disease, as well as acute rupture of the chordae tendineae. Pericardial effusion due to pericarditis, neoplastic invasion of the pericardium, or other causes must be considered (see Chapter 78). Peritoneal-pericardial diaphragmatic hernias are usually seen in younger dogs but may occur in older animals.

Treatment. Since cardiac tamponade develops rapidly, treatment of acute rupture of the left atrium with severe hemopericardium is usually not successful. Once the clinician is familiar with this disease syndrome, the disease usually can be diagnosed on the basis of the loud or acutely altered valvular heart murmur, supraventricular arrhythmias, the history of rapid onset of heart failure, and the peripheral venous engorgement. The globular silhouette apparent on both lateral and dorsoventral radiographic views of the thorax also helps to confirm the diagnosis.

Withdrawal of pericardial whole blood may temporarily improve cardiac function; however, hemorrhage is likely to continue. If one is certain that the bleeding has stopped and the pericardial fluid has clotted, then withdrawal of some pericardial fluid to reduce cardiac tamponade improves cardiac function. If complete rupture of the atrium is suspected and hemorrhagic pericardial effusion is present, then blood should not be removed following pericardiocentesis, since it is likely to enlarge the size of the tear and produce further pericardial blood accumulation. Treatment of the chronic mitral valvular insufficiency and arrhythmias is advised.

RUPTURE OF THE CHORDAE TENDINEAE

The chordae tendineae are fibrous collagen bands that extend from the papillary muscles to the edges of the atrioventricular valve leaflets. Their function, in part, is to prevent eversion of the valve leaflets into the atria during ventricular systole. Eversion of the valve leaflet results in marked valvular incompetency. The syndrome of rupture of the chordae tendineae in the dog has been classified as an acute, subacute, or chronic disease.[41]

It has not been described in the cat. The acute syndrome is clinically characterized by sudden onset of severe congestive heart failure. The acute syndrome occurs when a first order chorda tendinea ruptures, resulting in sudden, massive mitral or tricuspid insufficiency.[5, 41, 42] Global left ventricular systolic performance is markedly impaired when there is disruption of the chordal attachments to the mitral valve.[43] Dogs succumbing to this syndrome have massive pulmonary edema with a large amount of frothy blood-tinged fluid pouring from the oral and nasal cavities after death. The subacute form of the disease develops in association with protracted mitral valvular insufficiency. Dogs with chronic rupture of chordae tendineae do not have symptomatic cardiac disease, and the condition is recognized incidentally at necropsy. Since the subacute and chronic forms of this disease are clinically indistinguishable from chronic mitral valvular insufficiency, the following discussion describes only an acute rupture of a primary or first-order chorda tendinea.

The etiology of rupture of the chorda tendinea is unknown. Bacterial endocarditis, trauma, and other obvious causes were ruled out in a study of 28 cases.[41] The degree of associated chronic valvular disease has also been recorded by these authors. Of seven dogs with acute rupture, two had marginal fibrosis and five had fibrosis that was not severe enough to be considered advanced chronic valvular heart disease. Experience with additional dogs since the publication of this first report continues to indicate that chronic valvular heart disease is not a primary finding at the time of postmortem. One author reported that some normal-appearing chordae tendineae had severe degenerative histologic changes, and others reported foci of changes within ruptured human chordae that were part of the general myxomatous degeneration occurring in the mitral valve.[37, 44]

Cardiovascular Examination. The dog is presented with extreme pulmonary edema, severe respiratory distress, cyanosis due to pulmonary embarrassment, and marked venous engorgement. Protracted dyspnea, orthopnea, and cardiac coughing have not been present in the prior medical history of the patient. In most cases, clinical signs became apparent only in the previous 12 to 24 hours. Dogs with severe respiratory distress stand with the forelimbs abducted and the head and neck distended. This syndrome is recognized most often in poodles, although other breeds are affected.

Generally, the dog is in good physical condition, although clinically it is experiencing severe respiratory distress. A precordial thrill is readily palpated and a jerky pulse is felt bilaterally. Marked venous (jugular) engorgement and a jugular pulse are noted upon careful examination of the cervical region.

A harsh holosystolic murmur, usually loud enough to produce a precordial thrill, is auscultated at the left caudal sternal border. The murmur radiates over the entire thorax and in most instances is so loud that it may be auscultated over most portions of the body. Because of gross pulmonary edema and bubbling rales, a state of congestive heart failure usually is diagnosed without the aid of a stethoscope. The heart sounds are rapid and may be difficult to differentiate from the lung sounds when respiratory distress is acute. If the heart sounds are distinguishable, a gallop rhythm due to volume overload of the left atrium may be present.

The radiographic feature of mottling of the peripheral lung field in dogs with this syndrome is similar to that found in chronic mitral valve disease with severe left-sided heart failure. It is advised that radiographs not be taken when positioning of the patient will cause further respiratory embarrassment. In some cases, one radiographic view of the thorax taken in a position in which the dog is comfortable may aid in the clinical diagnosis.

When radiographs are obtained, pulmonary alveolar edema is recognized, along with slight to moderate left atrial enlargement. Unlike chronic valvular heart disease, generalized cardiac enlargement may not be as apparent.

Echocardiographic examination rarely demonstrates the chordal tear. Signs of left atrial enlargement, mitral valvular disease, and occasionally a flail mitral valve leaflet are observed.

One report of a dog with a ruptured chorda tendinea has been described using M-mode echocardiography. These authors demonstrated the left atrial echogram with the flail mitral valve cusp or its attached chordal remnant protruding into the left atrium during early ventricular systole. An attempt to correct the problem surgically was not successful.[45]

Electrocardiograms are difficult to obtain from patients with severe pulmonary distress. Because it is necessary to determine the nature of the cardiac rhythm for drug therapy, an ECG should be taken. Using as little restraint as possible, attach the leads to the dog in the usual manner. The ECG should be recorded in any position the dog assumes without discomfort. The electrocardiographic tracing indicates the cardiac rate and rhythm and may suggest other abnormalities. If the condition can be therapeutically controlled, a complete ECG may be taken in the normal position at a later time. In most patients, a sinus rhythm or a sinus tachycardia is present. Arrhythmias are occasionally present.

Left atrial dilatation (P mitrale) is usually not as evident in this syndrome as it is in chronic mitral valvular insufficiency. P pulmonale, indicative of right atrial strain, is often present.

Cardiac Catheterization. Elevation of the left atrial V waves, followed by a precipitous descent of the left atrial pressure curve, has been recorded with experimentally induced chordae tendineae rupture. One study induced chordae tendineae rupture in a group of normal dogs.[5] In dogs demonstrating signs similar to those described previously, there was a rise in the mean left atrial and main pulmonary artery pressures.[41, 42] In such cases, the large C wave usually fused with the V component. The major difference between the acute chordae tendineae rupture and a chronic mitral valvular fibrosis with insufficiency is the sudden hemodynamic overload placed on the left atrium and pulmonary vascular bed. In chronic valvular heart disease, the left atrium has time to compensate for increased pressure by dilatation and hypertrophy. In acute rupture of the chordae tendineae, the clinical syndrome is directly related to an inability of the left atrium to tolerate the burden of an acute hemodynamic overload.

Differential Diagnosis. The major diagnostic differentiations include acute volume overload of the left side of the heart, progressive chronic valvular insufficiency, left atrial tear or rupture, bronchopneumonia, electric shock, heat prostration, and adult pulmonary distress syndrome or severe high-permeability pulmonary edema of toxic, infectious, or central nervous system origin.

The history, age, access to toxins, and other cardinal noncardiac signs, as well as breed and size of dog, help to distinguish these problems. A chronic cardiac history suggests a left atrial tear or progressive disease, while a loud murmur of sudden onset is consistent with this diagnosis.

Treatment. Treatment for acute rupture of one or more primary chordae tendineae has usually been unsuccessful. Despite therapy, the signs of this disease advance rapidly, and death occurs from pulmonary edema. The prognosis is grave; however, attempts at therapy should include all those methods outlined in Table 75–3 for phase four heart disease. Occasionally, a dog does well with such therapy, but the owner must be aware that reoccurrence of the heart failure within a short period is a distinct possibility.

OTHER VALVULAR HEART DISEASES

TRICUSPID INSUFFICIENCY

Fibrosis (endocardiosis) of the tricuspid valve leaflets results in a tricuspid valvular insufficiency, a disease similar to that affecting the mitral valve leaflets. In the majority of cases, chronic mitral disease and tricuspid valvular disease in the dog occur concurrently. Tricuspid insufficiency is also associated with rupture of a tricuspid leaflet chorda tendinea,[42] bacterial endocarditis, heartworm disease, and dilatation of the tricuspid valve annulus in idiopathic congestive cardiomyopathy. Tricuspid valvular insufficiency occurs with congenital cardiac malformations such as Epstein's anomaly, tricuspid valve dysplasia, tricuspid atresia, advanced patent ductus arteriosus, or pulmonic stenosis, and atrioventricular canal. Chronic tricuspid valvular fibrosis or endocardiosis also occurs as an isolated disease entity. It has been recognized by this author most frequently in the dachshund and cocker spaniel, although it is also observed in other breeds. It has not been described in the feline as caused by valvular fibrosis or endocardiosis, but it commonly occurs secondary to tricuspid annular dilatation due to congestive cardiomyopathy.

Cardiovascular Examination. In most cases, dogs with tricuspid valvular insufficiency are presented with signs of respiratory distress owing to the primary disease, chronic mitral valvular insufficiency. The signs referable to tricuspid insufficiency are progressive abdominal distention, anorexia, weight loss, and, occasionally, vomiting and diarrhea. The latter is likely the result of congestion and edema of the liver, spleen, and gastrointestinal tract (*cardiac cachexia*). The signs of right-sided heart failure predominate clinically, unless signs of left-sided heart failure are very advanced. Systolic jugular pulsations and venous engorgement of the superficial and jugular veins are usually evident. Hepatic enlargement due to venous congestion may be responsible for abdominal tenderness. A positive hepatojugular reflex is present. The jugular venous pressure increases and the veins distend when pressure is applied over the liver. This occurs when overfilling of the hepatic sinusoids is relieved by applying pressure to the abdomen and forcing the blood into the jugular veins.

Peripheral edema is a sign of right-sided heart failure in human beings. However, it does not occur in dogs and cats during heart failure, unless ascites is also present. In more advanced cases of right-sided heart failure, pleural or pericardial effusion or both may develop. General anasarca is an uncommon finding even with advanced right-sided heart failure.

A holosystolic mixed-frequency murmur similar to that which is auscultated with mitral valvular insufficiency is auscultated at the right third to fifth intercostal space along the midthoracic wall when there is a defect in the valve leaflets. If the murmur is extremely loud, it may radiate to the left thoracic wall. In such cases, it is difficult to differentiate the disease from combined mitral and tricuspid insufficiency. Atrial fibrillation, if present, results in a variable-intensity murmur, an irregular rhythm, and a pulse deficit.

In most cases, the electrocardiographic examination does not provide evidence of chronic tricuspid valvular heart disease. If the right atrium is enlarged and strained, P pulmonale and prolongation of the P-R interval may occur. There is usually no alteration in the mean frontal plane electric axis. Most often, signs of left ventricular hypertrophy and left atrial enlargement predominate on the ECG since the left-sided heart disease is quite severe.

Radiographically, it is usually difficult to distinguish chronic tricuspid valvular heart disease from chronic mitral valvular insufficiency unless signs of advanced right-sided heart failure are present.

When moderate to massive right atrial enlargement occurs, it is indicated on the lateral radiograph by a slight dorsal deviation of the trachea cranial to the carina. The caudal vena cava may appear displaced dorsally and is denser than normal, which allows it to be seen within the cardiac silhouette. The elevation of the trachea cranial to the carina results in a reversed (upside-down) V sign. Marked right atrial enlargement may induce a bulge in the cranial quadrant of the cardiac silhouette. On the dorsoventral view, the cranial vena cava may curve to the right before it enters the right atrium, if an enlarged right atrium is present. There may be a bulge in the cranial right quadrant due to the enlarged right atrium.

Right ventricular enlargement does occur with chronic tricuspid valvular insufficiency. It is not distinguishable, however, from the dilatation that is usually associated with chronic mitral valvular insufficiency. Signs of left-sided heart failure are likely to be present when there is concurrent right and left ventricular enlargement.

The secondary signs of right-sided heart failure, when present, are important in suggesting the diagnosis of chronic tricuspid valvular insufficiency. Hepatomegaly and congestion with enlargement of the abdominal organs follow the onset of the right-sided heart failure. Pleural and pericardial effusion as well as ascites may be indicative of advanced right-sided heart failure.

Ultrasound examination with right heart failure mimics, and often is associated with, left A-V valvular insufficiency. Marked dilatation of the right ventricle occurs, along with a widely dilated right atrium. Tricuspid valvular insufficiency is apparent; there may be abnormal valvular fluttering and/or flail valve syndrome. Dilated vena cava entering the right atrium is likely to accentuate the apparent size of the right atrium. Right heart failure signs result in pleural effusion, ascites, and hepatic venous engorgement.

Aspiration of the ascitic or pleural fluid reveals a thin, straw-colored to blood-tinged modified transudate with a specific gravity that is usually between 1.018 and 1.025 and contains small numbers of both red and white blood cells. In long-standing cases, the fluid becomes bloodier and the specific gravity increases further owing to protein and cellular components. Mesothelial cells are present as a result of chronic inflammation of the cavity walls. If a secondary infection is present, the number of white blood cells in the fluid is increased. Not infrequently, the mesothelial cells are classified as being reactive. They must not be misinterpreted as being neoplastic, since carcinoma is in the differential diagnosis.

In the presence of chronic passive liver congestion, liver-enzyme levels are moderately elevated. Retention of bromsulphalein dye may be increased and serum bile acids are increased modestly. Icterus and bilirubinemia are unlikely sequelae to tricuspid valvular insufficiency. Moderate elevations of renal function tests are anticipated.

Differential Diagnosis. Chronic mitral valvular insufficiency with radiation of the murmur to the right thoracic wall represents the major differential diagnostic problem for this disease. In addition, heartworm disease may cause signs of right-sided heart failure. When a compensated heart condition is present, concurrent primary abdominal lesions, such as neoplasia or hepatic dysfunction, may require differentiation. Restrictive pericarditis results in some similar clinical signs (see Chapter 78). Other noncardiac causes of ascites have been discussed in Chapter 28. In young and middle-aged dogs with loud murmurs over the cranial to mid-right thoracic wall, a congenital defect such as a ventricular septal defect or a pulmonic or an aortic stenosis should be considered. In the larger breeds of dogs, idiopathic congestive cardiomyopathy may result in similar clinical signs. In cardiomyopathy, however, there is usually no significant murmur of tricuspid valvular insufficiency.

Treatment. Patients with chronic valvular insufficiency are likely to respond to the usual techniques applied in the treatment of congestive heart failure. Digitalization, combined multiple diuretic therapy, vasodilator therapy, and low-sodium diets are indicated. When extreme abdominal distention is present, abdominal paracentesis may be necessary. The technique for abdominal drainage has been described (Chapter 28). When ascites is marked, a large amount of fluid must be removed before an adequate response to therapeutic agents will occur.

AORTIC VALVE DISEASE

As an acquired cardiovascular condition in the dog or cat, valvular aortic stenosis is uncommon. In the cat, and rarely in the dog, obstructive cardiomyopathy is a cause of a subvalvular aortic obstruction. This is the result of left ventricular papillary muscle hypertrophy with subsequent left ventricular outflow tract obstruction (see Chapter 77). It does occur as a congenital lesion (see Chapter 74). Aortic valvular insufficiency, either acquired or congenital, is also recognized infrequently in both species. When it does occur, it results in diastolic overloading of the left ventricle. As a disease entity, aortic valvular insufficiency usually develops in dogs secondary to bacterial endocarditis (Chapter 79). It has been reported to occur secondary to trauma of an aortic valve leaflet following cardiac catheterization, after repeated cardiac punctures, or following rupture of the sinus of Valsalva associated with aortic valvular bacterial endocarditis;[46] it is at times associated with congenital cardiac defects.[3, 47]

Cardiovascular Examination. Unless cardiac decompensation or emboli result, aortic valvular insufficiency does not cause clinical signs. When signs do develop, dullness, lethargy, and weight loss become apparent. In cases of bacterial endocarditis, a recurrent fever and intermittent lameness develop. As the degree of left ventricular hypertrophy increases, a prominent left ventricular heave is observed over the left cardiac apex. A pulse that rises and falls sharply is characteristic of aortic insufficiency and is referred to as a thready, bounding, or water-hammer pulse. This pulse develops because of the rapid diastolic run-off associated with the insufficient valve.

When associated with active bacterial endocarditis, emboli originating from the endocardium may lodge elsewhere in the body, producing clinical signs of organ dysfunction and septicemia. A decrescendo diastolic murmur that begins with the second heart sound is auscultated at the aortic valve region. This murmur is described as a blowing, high-frequency sound of low intensity (Figure 75–10). A systolic murmur is usually present too. In cases with marked left ventricular en-

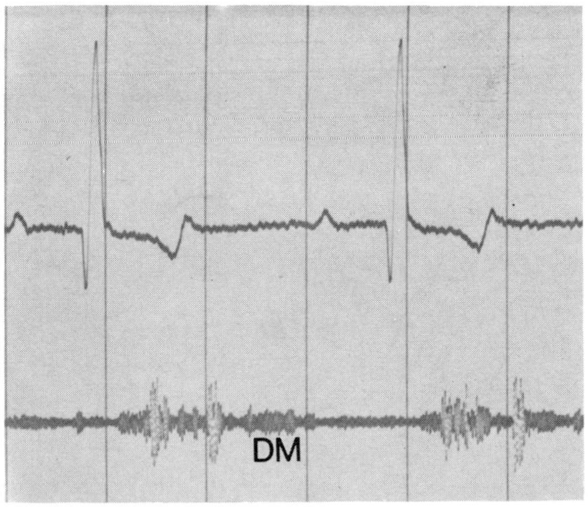

FIGURE 75–10. Note the diastolic murmur (DM) in this Boxer with aortic valvular insufficiency. In addition, a systolic murmur is present. This patient had calcific aortic insufficiency (demonstrated in Figure 75–11).

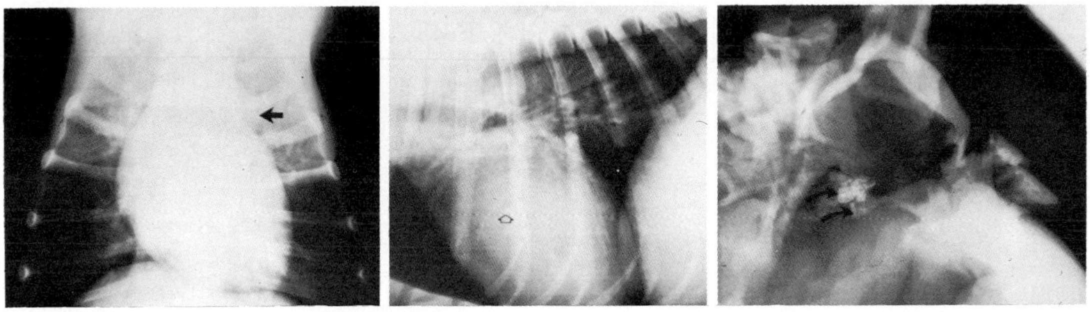

A B C

FIGURE 75–11. Aortic insufficiency. Dorsoventral and lateral radiographic projections of a three-year-old Boxer. The dog had progressive heart failure associated with a systolic and loud decrescendo diastolic murmur (see Fig. 75–10). The cardiac silhouette appears somewhat elongated in the dorsoventral position on the lateral projection. *A,* There is minimal bulging of the initial portion of the descending aortic arch (arrow) on the dorsoventral projection. *B,* A small band of calcified material on the lateral projection (open arrow) indicates the position of the pathologically calcified aortic valve. *C,* Postmortem radiograph of the opened left ventricular cavity. The calcified aortic valve leaflets are more apparent in this position (curved arrows). The final diagnosis was calcific aortic insufficiency secondary to chronic bacterial endocarditis.

largement, the ECG indicates signs of left ventricular hypertrophy and P mitrale. Ventricular arrhythmias are often observed when the etiology involves an active endocarditis due to microabscessation of the myocardium.

In uncomplicated cases of aortic valvular insufficiency, the radiographs are unlikely to be diagnostic. Isolated left ventricular enlargement resulting from this disease is difficult to clearly assess unless secondary left atrial enlargement is present. When aortic insufficiency occurs secondary to other congenital or acquired heart diseases, the roentgen signs attributable to the primary disease predominate. If calcific aortic valvular insufficiency is present, a calcified aortic valve may be recognized (Figure 75–11).

Echocardiography. Cardiac ultrasound examination of the dog or cat with suspected aortic valve disease is the preferred clinical method of examination today. It noninvasively, safely, and quickly demonstrates pathologic abnormalities and provides a definitive diagnosis as well as exhibiting the severity of the pathology involved.

Echocardiographic findings with valvular endocarditis (see Chapter 74 for congenital defects and Chapters 77 and 79 for other acquired problems) include one or more of the following: irregularities and thickening of the valve leaflets, multiple irregularities in the aortic root, valve prolapse into the left ventricle during diastole signaling aortic regurgitation, and diastolic fluttering of a torn aortic valve (see Figure 75–7 and 75–11).[48]

Ultrasound examination also demonstrates the degree of left ventricular dilatation, diastolic fluttering of the mitral valve, premature closing of the mitral valve, and left ventricular hyperkinesia.

Treatment. When aortic insufficiency is recognized and diagnosed as a secondary feature of bacterial endocarditis, the patient should be treated for that disease (see Chapter 79). When heart failure occurs, the usual methods of therapy, which include digitalization, diuretics, vasodilators, low-sodium diet, and restricted exercise, should be employed. Surgery could be performed, although reports of such treatment for this disease are not available. Appropriate antiarrhythmic therapy, along with antimicrobial agents, is life-supporting. Infarction, sepsis, and renal failure may develop.[49]

PULMONIC INSUFFICIENCY

Pulmonic insufficiency is a rare condition that occurs secondary to heartworm disease and patent ductus arteriosus with pulmonary hypertension.[50] It has also been reported in dogs that had a surgical correction for heartworm removal. In the latter situation, apparent trauma to the pulmonic valve leaflets occurred. A dog with iatrogenic pulmonic insufficiency following cardiac catheterization has been described.[51] Pulmonic insufficiency is an unusual condition that generally is not hemodynamically significant.

MITRAL STENOSIS

Mitral stenosis is a rare disease entity that has been described in several dogs. It is associated with left atrial dilatation, cardiac arrhythmias, left atrial mural thrombi, and a diastolic rumbling murmur. Reports of the medical care of patients with this syndrome are very infrequent.

References

1. Silverman, M and Hurst, WJ: The mitral complex. Am Heart J 76:399, 1968.
2. Fenoglio, JJ, et al.: Canine mitral complex. Circ Res 31:417, 1972.
3. Ettinger, SJ and Suter, PF: Canine Cardiology. Philadelphia, WB Saunders, 1970.
4. Detweiler, DK and Patterson, DF: The prevalence and types of cardiovascular diseases in dogs. Ann NY Acad Sci 127:481, 1965.
5. Bousfield, WED, and Bowden, NLR: Observations on surgically induced insufficiency of the canine mitral valve. Br Vet J 128:567, 1972.
6. Packer, M: Sudden unexpected death in patients with congestive heart failure: a second frontier. Circulation 72(4):681, 1985.
7. McCall, D and O'Rourke, RA: Congestive heart failure. Mod Conc Cardio Dis 54:55, 1985.

8. Hasking, GJ, et al.: Norepinephrine spillover to plasma in patients with congestive heart failure: evidence of increased overall and cardiorenal sympathetic nervous activity. Circulation 73(4):615, 1986.
9. Lord, PF: Left ventricular volumes of the diseased canine heart. Am J Vet Res 35:493, 1974.
10. Schlant, RC: The management of chronic mitral regurgitation. Counc Clin Cardiol News 12(1):1, 1986.
11. Blumlein, S, et al.: Quantitation of mitral regurgitation by Doppler echocardiography. Circulation 74(2):306, 1986.
12. Ettinger, SJ and Lusk, RH: Echocardiographic techniques in the dog and cat. *In* Schapira, J, et al. (eds): Two-dimensional Echocardiography.
13. Lusk, RH and Ettinger, SJ: Echocardiographic techniques in the dog and cat. Personal observation.
14. Hlatky, MA, et al.: Physician practice in the management of heart failure. J Am Coll Cardiol 8(4):966, 1986.
15. Gheorghiade, M, et al.: Hemodynamic effects of intravenous digoxin in patients with severe heart failure initially treated with diuretics and vasodilators. J Am Coll Cardiol 9(4):849, 1987.
16. Kittleson, MD, et al.: Oral hydralazine therapy for chronic mitral regurgitation in the dog. JAVMA 182(11):1205, 1983.
17. Creager, MA, et al.: Acute and long-term effects of enalapril on the cardiovascular response to exercise tolerance in patients with congestive heart failure. J Am Coll Cardiol 6(1):163, 1985.
18. Walsh, J and Greenberg, B: Results of long-term vasodilator therapy in patients with refractory congestive heart failure. Circulation 64(3):499, 1981.
19. Colucci, W, et al.: New positive inotropic agents in the treatment of congestive heart failure. N Engl J Med 314(5):290, 1986.
20. Baim, DS, et al.: Survival of patients with severe congestive heart failure treated with oral milrinone. J Am Coll Cardiol 7(3):661, 1986.
21. Simonton, CA, et al: Milrinone in congestive heart failure: Acute and chronic hemodynamic and clinical evaluation. J Am Coll Cardiol 6(2):453, 1985.
22. Braunwald, E: Newer positive inotropic agents. Circulation 73:236, 1986.
23. Kittleson, MD, et al.: The acute hemodynamic effects of milrinone in dogs with severe idiopathic myocardial failure. J Vet Int Med 1:121, 1987.
24. Anderson, JL, et al.: Efficacy and safety of sustained (48 hour) intravenous infusions of milrinone in patients with severe congestive heart failure: A multicenter study. J Am Coll Cardiol 9(4):711, 1987.
25. Saito, Y, et al.: Clinical application of atrial natriuretic polypeptide in patients with congestive heart failure: beneficial effects on left ventricular function. Circulation 76(1):115, 1987.
26. Kirklin, JW: Mitral valve repair for mitral incompetence. Mod Conc Cardio Dis 56(2):7, 1987.
27. Das, KM and Tashjian, RJ: Chronic mitral valve disease in the dog. Vet Med 60:1209, 1965.
28. Whitney, JC: Observations on the effects of age on the severity of heart valve lesions in the dog. J Sm Anim Pract 15:511, 1974.
29. Kogure, K: Pathology of chronic mitral valvular disease in the dog. Jap J Vet Sci 42(3):323, 1980.
30. Bretschneider, J: Zur Pathologie und Pathogenese der sog. Endocarditis Valvularis Chronica Fibrosa des Hundes. Inaug Diss, Univ Giessen, 1962.
31. Detweiler, DK, et al.: The natural history of acquired cardiac disability of the dog. Ann NY Acad Sci 147:318, 1968.
32. Schneider, P, et al.: Amyloidose der Herzklappen beim Hund. Vet Pathol 8:130, 1971.
33. Ernst, E, et al.: Elektronen mikroskopische Untersuchungen über die Amyloidose der Atrioventrikularklappen des Hundes. Beitr Pathol 152:361, 1974.
34. Wagner, B: Myocardial disease in man and dog, some properties. Ann NY Acad Sci 147:354, 1968.
35. Sokkar, SM and Trautwein, G: Die Endokardiose der Atrioventrikularklappen des Hundes. Zentralbl Veterinaermed (A) 17:757, 1970.
36. Sokkar, SM and Trautwein, G: Endocardiosis in the dog. Zentralbl Veterinaermed (A) 18:1, 1971.
37. Buchanan, JW: Valvular disease (endocardiosis) in dogs. Adv Vet Sci Comp Med 21:75, 1979.
38. Schneider, V, et al.: Experimentelle, durch ACTH und DOC induzierte Herzklappenendokardiose bei Hunden. Endokrinologie 62:202, 1963.
39. Stunzi, H and Mann, M: Rupture of the atrium. Zentralbl Veterinaermed (A) 20:409, 1973.
40. Buchanan, JW, and Kelly, AM: Endocardial splitting of the left atrium in the dog. J Am Vet Rad Soc 5:28, 1964.
41. Ettinger, SJ and Buergelt, CD: Ruptured chordae tendineae in the dog. JAVMA 155:535, 1969.
42. Ettinger, SJ and Buergelt, CD: Atrioventricular dissociation (incomplete) with accrochage in a dog with ruptured chordae tendineae. Am J Vet Res 29:1499, 1968.
43. Hansen, DE, et al.: Valvular-ventricular interaction: importance of the mitral apparatus in canine left ventricular systolic performance. Circulation 73(6):1310, 1986.
44. Caulfield, JB, et al.: Connective tissue abnormalities in spontaneous rupture of chordae tendineae. Arch Pathol 91:537, 1971.
45. Olivier, NB, et al.: M-mode echocardiography in the diagnosis of ruptured mitral chordae tendineae in a dog. JAVMA 184(5):588, 1984.
46. Kleine, LJ, et al.: Rupture of the aortic sinus and aortic insufficiency in a dog. JAVMA 149:1050, 1966.
47. Eyster, GE, et al.: Aortic regurgitation in the dog. JAVMA 168:138, 1976.
48. Bonagura, JD and Pipers, FS: Echocardiographic features of aortic valve endocarditis in a dog, a cow, and a horse. JAVMA 182:595, 1983.
49. Sisson, D and Thomas, WP: Endocarditis of the aortic valve in the dog. JAVMA 184(5):570, 1984.
50. Detweiler, DK and Patterson, DF: A phonograph record of heart sounds and murmurs of the dog. Ann NY Acad Sci 127:322, 1965.
51. Hamlin, RL, et al.: Iatrogenic pulmonic insufficiency in a dog. JAVMA 141:725, 1962.

76 CARDIAC ARRHYTHMIAS

STEPHEN J. ETTINGER

An arrhythmia is a deviation from the normal cardiac rate or rhythm, site of origin of the cardiac impulse, or sequence of activation of the atria and ventricles. In both the cat and dog, specific anatomic pathology that correlates with the observed arrhythmias often is not obvious in the myocardium. However, advances in electrophysiology and cardiac mapping have demonstrated abnormalities that correlate with some of the arrhythmias. Still, a significant percentage of arrhythmias occur in the absence of detectable anatomic pathology; conversely, even in the presence of marked pathology, arrhythmias may be absent.[1,2] Arrhythmias can be considered to ". . . result from functional derangements rather than from pathologic alterations."[2]

The text to follow describes the nature of the arrhythmias, their clinical features, and specific information concerning drug therapy. Table 76–1 represents a compilation of antiarrhythmic agents currently useful in treating canine and feline arrhythmias.

NORMAL ELECTROPHYSIOLOGY

In the quiescent state, the resting heart muscle cell has an electric potential of about 90 millivolts across the cell membrane. The interior of the cell is negative with respect to the exterior. This so-called *resting membrane potential* (RP), −80 to −90 millivolts, is altered by electrical currents and chemical mediators, which act on the cell to change the membrane potential. When the membrane potential reaches another critical point, referred to as the *threshold membrane potential* (TP) (usually approximately −60 millivolts), an action potential or spike occurs. This represents depolarization and then the subsequent repolarization of the cell. The electrical gradient across the cell wall rises to about 20 millivolts following depolarization, when the positively charged sodium ions flow into the cell across the semipermeable cell membrane and reverse the polarity of the stimulated portion of this membrane. The action-potential spike spreads to adjacent cells by generating electrotonic currents, which results in a sequence of depolarization of excitable cells. Contraction of cardiac muscle cells occurs when there is a spike or action potential in cardiac cells that contain myofibrils (unspecialized myocardial fibers). The cell contracts when it is adequately stimulated to depolarize, as calcium defuses into the myofibrils along with sodium and catalyzes *excitation-contraction coupling* events.

The electrical activity of the cardiac cell may be divided into five phases (Figure 76–1). Phase zero is the period of rapid depolarization, during which reversal of polarity of the cell membrane occurs as sodium suddenly enters the cell. During phase zero, depolarization with a positive overshoot occurs. The spike is then followed by an initial rapid return toward the resting potential (phase one). Phase zero depolarization results from the opening of a specialized membrane channel, the fast channel through which sodium ions pass rapidly. After the upstroke of the action potential, the fast sodium current ceases to flow as the sodium channels inactivate and the membrane potential begins to return to the resting level during phase one. A smaller and slower secondary inward current referred to as the slow Ca^{++} channel, carries sodium and calcium ions during phases one and two, thus slowing the return of the action potential to the resting level. This period of rapid repolarization is followed by a slow period of repolarization (phase two) and then a more rapid stage (phase three). The delayed efflux of the potassium ion brings the cell back to the resting membrane level at −80 to −90 millivolts and results in the repolarization (phases one, two, and three) of the action-potential spike. During phase four, the membrane potential has returned to the resting potential. This is a period during which the cardiac cell restores its ionic composition in preparation for the next action-potential spike. Figure 76–1 is a diagram of the transmembrane action potential and unipolar electrocardiogram of a cardiac muscle fiber. Following phase zero, repolarization of the cell occurs, and the physiologic feature of cell excitability is gradually recovered. Figure 76–2 is a graphic representation of a normal transmembrane action potential and of the responses elicited by stimuli applied during various stages of repolarization. In addition, the usual relationships between transmembrane potentials and cathodal excitability are provided.

Undifferentiated myocardial cells usually demonstrate a stable resting potential of −90 millivolts. The sinoatrial node (S-A node), some atrial fibers, the bundle

TABLE 76–1. DRUGS USED FOR THE TREATMENT OF CARDIAC ARRHYTHMIAS

Generic Name	Trade Name	Administration Route	Common Indications	Dosage	Comments
Amiodarone	Cordarone	Oral	Recurrent ventricular fibrillation; recurrent hemodynamically unstable ventricular tachycardia	2–4 mg/lb q12h	Side effects include proarrhythmias, pulmonary fibrosis, hypothyroidism, liver necrosis, photosensitivity and others. Minimum use in veterinary medicine at this time
Atenolol	Tenormin	Oral	Same as propranolol	0.2–1.0 mg/lb q24h	Weakness; depression; hypotension; bradycardia
Atropine Tablets Injectable		 Oral IV, IM, SQ	1. Hyperactive carotid sinus reflex (S-A arrest) 2. A-V block (2nd and 3rd degree)	0.6–2.0 grain q2–6h or 0.1–0.3 mg/lb IV, IM, SQ	1. Do not use in states of heart failure 2. Do not administer when bronchial tree secretions are a problem 3. Used infrequently in heart block
Digoxin Tablets Elixir Injectable	Lanoxin Cardoxin	 Oral Oral IV	1. Congestive heart failure 2. Supraventricular premature contractions, atrial tachycardia, atrial fibrillation, and sinus tachycardia	0.005–0.01 mg/lb daily divided AM and PM as maintenance dosage; double dosage initially first 24–48 hrs for rapid effect; lower dosage in large and giant breeds of dogs	1. Digitalize cautiously 2. Monitor with ECG 3. All doses are approximate and the patient must be monitored frequently 4. Side effects—malaise, anorexia, vomiting, diarrhea
Diltiazem	Cardizem	Oral	?Supraventricular arrhythmias; reported useful in feline HOCM	0.2–0.7 mg/lb q8h in dogs 0.7 mg/lb q8h in cats	Side effects include bradycardia, hypotension, collapse, and severe weakness
Disopyramide	Norpace	Oral	Ventricular arrhythmias	5–10 mg/lb q8h (q12h using long-acting product)	May be used in conjunction with quinidine or procainamide
Encainide	Enkaid	Oral	Sustained life-threatening ventricular arrhythmias	0.2–0.5 mg/lb q8h	Proarrhythmic effects occur; may aggravate CHF and COCM; not widely studied or used clinically in dogs or cats at time of publication
Flecainide	Tambocor	Oral	Sustained life-threatening ventricular arrhythmias	0.5–3 mg/lb q8–12h	Proarrhythmic effects may occur; no experience in cats
Isopropamide	Darbid	Oral	1. Sinoatrial arrest 2. Sick sinus syndrome 3. Incomplete AV block 4. Complete AV block	2.5–5.0 mg q8–12h	May induce kerato-conjunctivitis sicca; possibly switch to propantheline if ineffective
Isoproterenol Injectable	Isuprel Injectable	IM, IV, SC	1. Advanced 2nd degree and 3rd degree heart block 2. S-A arrest 3. Sinus bradycardia(?) 4. Cardiac arrest	For arrhythmias: 1 mg/200 cc D5W IV to increase heart rate, use to effect 0.1–0.2 mg SQ or IM, q4h for heart block	May be used on temporary basis parenterally until conduction improves or a pacemaker is implanted
Lidocaine 2% without epinephrine	Xylocaine	IV only	1. Life-threatening arrhythmias 2. To suppress arrhythmia formation during cardiac catheterization or surgery	1. 2–4 mg/lb IV slow bolus over 2 min or until arrhythmia controlled 2. 1 mg/lb IV slowly, then 20–30 mcq/lb/min continuous infusion 3. For cats use 400 mg/L drip to effect	1. Reserve for serious arrhythmias 2. Toxicity includes convulsions and respiratory arrest 3. Single IV dose lasts 15 to 20 min only

TABLE 76–1. DRUGS USED FOR THE TREATMENT OF CARDIAC ARRHYTHMIAS *Continued*

Generic Name	Trade Name	Administration Route	Common Indications	Dosage	Comments
Mexiletine	Mexitil	Oral	Suppression of symptomatic ventricular arrhythmias	1–4 mg/lb q8–12h (dogs)	Few side effects; may be used with digoxin and Class I antiarrhythmic agents
Phenytoin Capsules Injectable	Dilantin	 Oral IV	1. Some ventricular arrhythmias 2. May be useful in treating arrhythmias due to digitalis overdose	5–8 mg/lb q8h	Infrequently used as an antiarrhythmic drug
Procainamide Capsules Tablets Injectable	Pronestyl Pronestyl-SR Procan-SR Pronestyl	Oral Oral Oral IV	1. Ventricular premature contractions 2. Ventricular tachycardia	1. 3–10 mg/lb q4h (to 8h sustained release form) 2. 3–4 mg/lb IV over 5 min, then infuse 5–18 mcq/lb/min	1. IV effect is brief, and oral maintenance dose must be given q4h 2. Oral forms available in sustained release tablets may not be absorbed
Propranolol Tablets Injectable	Inderal	 Oral IV	1. Sinus tachycardia 2. Atrial tachycardia 3. To slow ventricular rate in atrial fibrillation or to distinguish the latter from ventricular tachycardia 4. Arrhythmias of digitalis intoxication 5. Preexcitation atrial syndromes 6. Some ventricular arrhythmias, when other agents fail	Oral: general 0.2–0.5 mg/lb q8h. 2.5–20 mg/lb q8–12h small dogs. 10–40 mg q8–12h medium and large dogs. 40–80 mg q8–12h large and giant dogs. 2.5 mg q12–24h cats. 0.25–0.5 mg IV no more frequently than q1–3 min; administer until rate slows or toxicity occurs. Cats 0.25–0.5 mg IV	1. Use with caution; as a negative inotropic agent it may induce congestive heart failure 2. Excessive dosage causes reduction in cardiac rate and prolongation of P-R and Q-T intervals 3. Can partially antagonize with IV atropine
Quinidine gluconate Injectable Tablets	Quinidine gluconate Injectable Quinaglute Quinidex	IM Oral	Same as quinidine sulfate	3 to 10 mg/lb q2–4h by injection. Delayed release forms are same dosage but given q8–12h	Same as quinidine sulfate
Quinidine sulfate Tablets	Quinidine sulfate	Oral	1. Ventricular premature contractions 2. Ventricular tachycardia	3 to 10 mg/lb q6–8h may be given q2h until loading dose controls arrhythmia or induces toxicity	1. Do not use in presence of congestive heart failure unless this is being treated simultaneously 2. Toxicity results in increased heart rate and prolongation of the ECG intervals 3. Often effective in lower doses when used with procainamide
Tocainide	Tonocard	Oral	Suppression of symptomatic ventricular arrhythmias	7–50 mg/lb q8–12h (dogs)	May need to use with other Class I antiarrhythmic agents for better effect
Verapamil	Isoptin	Oral IV	Conversion of rapid supraventricular tachycardia—especially pre-excitation type	0.5–2.0 mg/lb/os q8–12h. 0.05–0.15 mg/lb IV slowly	Side effects are weakness, collapse, bradycardia. Contraindicated in shock, heart block, SSS, CHF, V tachycardia

of His and its branches, and the Purkinje fibers differ from other cardiac tissue in that their cells are capable of spontaneous or automatic discharge. These cells normally undergo slow depolarization during phase four (diastole). Cells that undergo slow depolarization during phase four elicit an action potential when the resting transmembrane potential is reduced to the threshold potential at about ± 60 millivolts.

Cells that have the unique electrophysiologic property of spontaneous discharge are said to possess *automaticity*. Automatic cells within the heart that are capable of spontaneous discharge are called *pacemaker cells*. These cells either act directly as the cardiac pacemaker or have the potential for such action. The fibers with the most rapid rate of spontaneous discharge, or automaticity of the cell membrane, assume the function of the cardiac pacemaker (normally the sinoatrial node). Automaticity of certain cardiac fibers results in a regularity of muscle

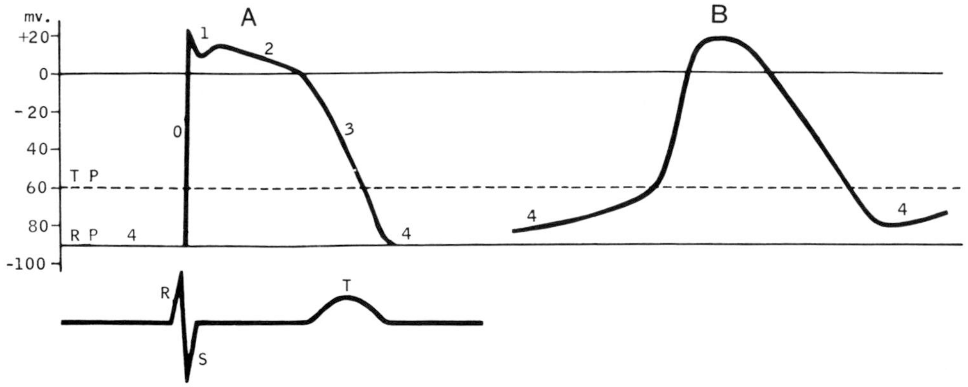

FIGURE 76–1. *A* is a diagrammatic drawing of action potential and electrocardiogram of cardiac muscle fiber. *B,* Depolarization and action potential of pacemaker fiber. RP, resting membrane potential; TP, threshold potential at which pacemaker spontaneously fires its action potential; 0, depolarization with positive overshoot (intrinsic deflection of R wave); 2, plateau; 3, corresponds to T wave; 4, diastole during which pacemaker undergoes spontaneous slow depolarization until it reaches threshold potential and fires. (From Friedberg, CK: Diseases of the Heart, 3rd ed. Philadelphia, WB Saunders, 1966.)

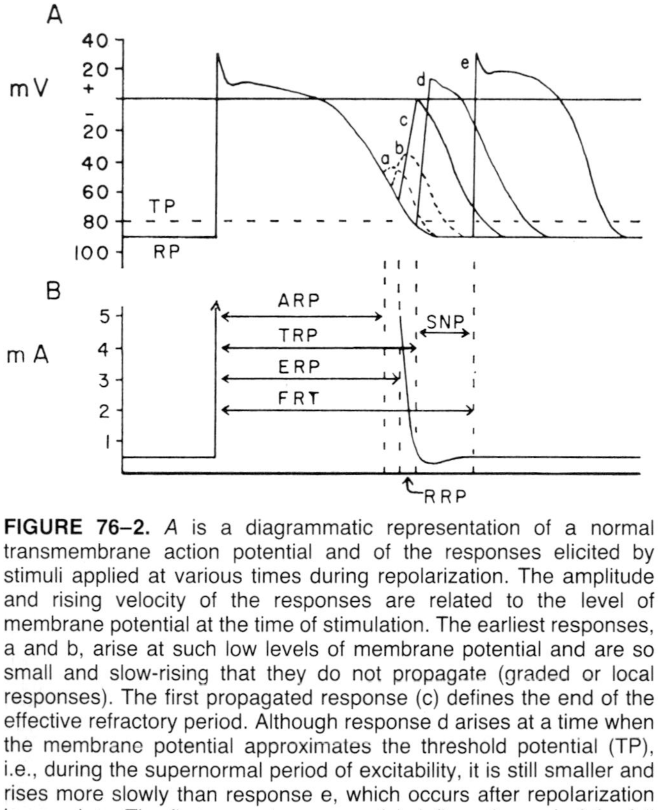

FIGURE 76–2. *A* is a diagrammatic representation of a normal transmembrane action potential and of the responses elicited by stimuli applied at various times during repolarization. The amplitude and rising velocity of the responses are related to the level of membrane potential at the time of stimulation. The earliest responses, a and b, arise at such low levels of membrane potential and are so small and slow-rising that they do not propagate (graded or local responses). The first propagated response (c) defines the end of the effective refractory period. Although response d arises at a time when the membrane potential approximates the threshold potential (TP), i.e., during the supernormal period of excitability, it is still smaller and rises more slowly than response e, which occurs after repolarization is complete. The first normal response (e) defines the end of the full recovery time. *B* is a schematic representation of the usual relationships between transmembrane potentials and cathodal excitability. The changes in threshold are related to an arbitrary scale of recurrent strength. The fiber becomes inexcitable coincident with the inscription of phase 0 of the action potential. Recovery of excitability, as indicated by changes in threshold, progresses slowly during phase 3. The terminal portion of phase 3 is associated with a period of supernormal exitability. The diagram also illustrates the approximate duration of the absolute refractory period (ARP), the effective refractory period (ERP), relative refractory period (RRP), total refractory period (TRP), full recovery time (FRT), and the period of supernormal excitability (SNP). (From Singer, DH and Hoffman, BF: Progr Cardiovasc Dis 7:231, 1964.)

excitation and subsequent contraction. It is an important basis for the continuity and normal regularity of the heart.

The normal sinus pacemaker depresses the automaticity of other cardiac fibers with potential pacemaker function through overdrive suppression. This suppression reduces the likelihood of escape or ectopic impulse formation from fibers below the S-A node.[3]

Detailed description of electrophysiologic testing in the diagnosis and treatment of cardiac arrhythmias is very complex but well studied. The American Heart Association monograph on this subject may be of interest to those requiring more detailed electrophysiologic descriptions of arrhythmias.[4]

THE ELECTROCARDIOGRAM

The electrocardiogram (ECG) is a graphic record of the voltage produced by the cardiac muscle cells during their depolarization and repolarization. Voltage on the vertical axis is plotted against time on the horizontal axis. The ECG yields information concerning the time required for electrical conduction through various parts of the heart, as well as the course of the electrical activation of the heart and the presence or absence of arrhythmias. Figure 76–3 is a tracing of a lead II electrocardiogram from a normal canine heart. It demonstrates the periods of activation at the various levels of cardiac conducting tissue. Tables 76–2*A* and 76–2*B* present the normal criteria for the canine and feline electrocardiogram.

PHYSIOLOGIC PROPERTIES OF NORMAL HEART MUSCLE

The four fundamental characteristics of cardiac tissue are automaticity (rhythmicity), conductivity, excitability, and contractility.

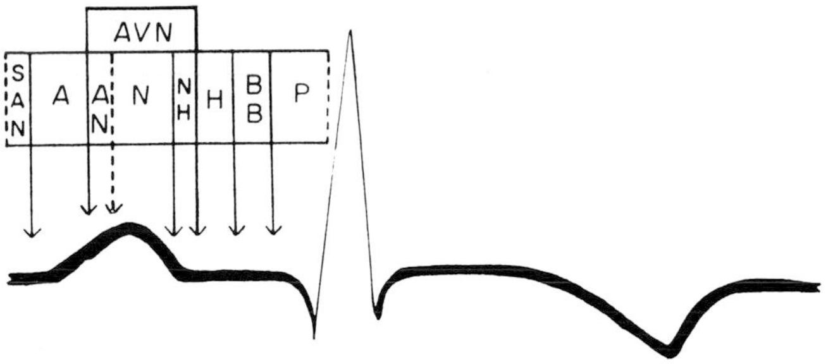

FIGURE 76–3. Tracing of the lead II electrocardiogram of the canine heart showing the time of activation of the various specialized cardiac tissues. SAN, sinoatrial node; A, atrium; AVN, atrioventricular node; H, His bundle; BB, bundle branches; and P, peripheral Purkinje fibers. The subdivisions of the atrioventricular node represent the atrionodal junction (AN), the middle node (N), and the transition from node to His bundle (NH). (From Hoffman, BF and Singer, DH: Progr Cardiovasc Dis 7:266, 1964.)

AUTOMATICITY

The sinoatrial node is established as the dominant pacemaker in the normal heart because it manifests a slow diastolic depolarization (phase four) that is steeper than that of other cardiac tissue. If, for some reason, the sinoatrial node is depressed, then other automatic tissue of lower independent rates of automaticity takes over as the pacemaker, temporarily or permanently. When the sinoatrial node is depressed, a passive ectopic rhythm results. In such cases, the activity of a lower group of automatic cells is enhanced and it assumes the pacemaking function of the heart. In contrast, an active ectopic rhythm results when enhanced automaticity of cells outside the sinoatrial node causes an increased rate of automaticity. In such cases, the ectopic rhythm is usually more rapid than the rhythm of the basic sinoatrial node that normally controls the heart rate.

Two major factors modify the cycle length of automatic fibers, the slope of diastolic depolarization and the difference between the threshold potential and the maximum diastolic potential that is present at the end of repolarization. The site of impulse formation thus depends upon the speed with which phase four depolarization reaches the threshold potential in different fiber groups.[5]

The nervous system, concentrations of various metabolites, electrolytes, hormones in the blood, and cardioactive drugs are clinically important in influencing the rate of firing of pacemaker cells. The following factors may increase automaticity: (1) increased sympathetic activity, (2) hypokalemia, (3) hypercalcemia, (4) decreased parasympathetic activity, (5) hypoxia, (6) hyperthermia, (7) hypercapnia, (8) acidosis, (9) mechanical effects, such as stretching, and (10) specific drugs, such as the cardiac glycosides.[2] Factors that decrease automaticity of cells include (1) decreased sympathetic activity, such as that produced by β-blocking agents, (2) increased parasympathetic tone, produced by the use of drugs such as acetylcholine, (3) hypocalcemia, (4) decreased P_{CO_2}, (5) hyperkalemia, (6) increased P_{O_2}, (7) hypothermia, (8) alkalosis, (9) reduced stretching of fibers, and (10) the effects of certain drugs such as antiarrhythmic agents such as quinidine, procainamide, and phenytoin.[2]

TABLE 76–2A. CRITERIA FOR THE NORMAL CANINE ELECTROCARDIOGRAM

Heart rate—60 to 160 beats per minute for adult dogs; up to 180 beats per minute in toy breeds, and 220 beats per minute for puppies.
Heart rhythm—Normal sinus rhythm; sinus arrhythmia; and wandering sinoatrial pacemaker.
P wave—Up to 0.4 millivolt in amplitude; up to 0.04 second in duration; always positive in leads II and aV_F; positive or isoelectric in lead I.
P-R interval—0.06 to 0.14 second duration.
QRS complex—Mean electric axis, frontal plane, 40 to 100 degrees.
Amplitude—Maximum amplitude of R wave 2.5 to 3.0 millivolts in leads II, III, and aV_F. Complex positive in leads II, III, and aVF; negative in lead V_{10}.
Duration—To 0.05 second (0.06 second in dogs over 40 lb).
Q-T—0.15 to 0.22 second duration.
S-T segment and T wave—S-T segment free of marked coving (repolarization changes).
S-T segment depression not greater than 0.2 millivolt.
S-T segment elevation not greater than 0.15 millivolt.
T wave negative in lead V_{10}.
T wave amplitude not greater than 25 per cent of amplitude of R wave.

EXCITABILITY

Excitability refers to the ability of living tissue to respond to stimulation by propagation of the stimulating impulse. When a low-intensity stimulus is followed by a response, the tissue is considered to have a relatively high level of excitability; when even high intensity stimulation fails to elicit a response, that tissue is considered to be relatively inexcitable.

Excitability is increased during the phase of supernormal excitability in the cardiac cycle (Figure 76–2), increased sympathetic tone, decreased parasympathetic tone, hypokalemia, hypercalcemia, depressed automaticity, and some arrhythmias. Decreased excitability occurs during the absolute and relative refractory periods of the cardiac cycle (Figure 76–2), decreased

TABLE 76–2B. CRITERIA FOR THE NORMAL FELINE ELECTROCARDIOGRAM

Heart rate—240 beats per minute maximum.
Heart rhythm—Normal sinus rhythm or, infrequently, sinus arrhythmia.
P wave—Positive in leads II and aV_F; may be isoelectric or positive in lead I; should not exceed 0.03 second in duration.
P-R interval—0.04 to 0.08 second duration (inversely related to the heart rate).
QRS complex—More variable than in the canine; the mean electric axis in the frontal plane is often insignificant. Often the QRS complex is nearly isoelectric in all frontal plane limb leads (so-called horizontal heart).
The amplitude of the R wave is usually low; marked amplitude of R waves (over 0.8 millivolt) in the frontal plane leads may suggest ventricular hypertrophy.
Less than 0.04 second in duration.
Q-T segment—0.16 to 0.18 second duration.
S-T segment and T wave—S-T segment and T wave should be small and free of repolarization changes as well as marked depression or elevation.

sympathetic tone, increased parasympathetic tone, hyperkalemia, ischemia, enhanced automaticity resulting in a relative decrease in the resting membrane potential, and the use of antiarrhythmic drugs, such as quinidine, procainamide, and digitalis.[2]

CONDUCTIVITY

Tissue composed of a series of individual cells is said to possess conductivity when the cells can propagate an impulse. Conductivity is related to the excitability of the cells. The rate of rise of phase zero depolarization, i.e., the rapid phase (Figure 76–1), determines the conduction velocity. During the period of the spike action potential, there is an influx of sodium (fast channels) into the cells and a rapid change in the transmembrane potential and the inscription of the waves of depolarization on the electrocardiogram (i.e., the P wave and QRS complex). When conductivity is low, the rapid phase of the action potential is slower and of lower amplitude. Action potentials generated by the continued propagation of a subnormal amplitude are characterized by a slow upstroke, small amplitude, and low speed of conduction.

Within the heart, conductivity is most rapid within the specialized conduction fibers and less rapid in the myocardium and in the region of the A-V node. The following factors enhance conductivity: (1) large intercalated discs and nexus structures within the cell, (2) a period of supernormal excitability during early diastole, (3) increased sympathetic tone and circulating catecholamines, (4) decreased parasympathetic tone, (5) decreased automaticity, (6) shortened refractory period, (7) hypokalemia, and (8) hypercalcemia.[2] Conversely, conductivity is decreased with (1) cardiac refractory periods, (2) decreased sympathetic tone, (3) increased parasympathetic tone, (4) increased automaticity, (5) tachycardia, (6) hypoxia, (7) myocardial disease, and (8) the use of cardiac drugs such as quinidine, procainamide, and digitalis.

CONTRACTILITY

Increased or decreased cardiac contractile states may predispose the patient to arrhythmias. The use of clinical therapeutic agents for the control of arrhythmias may further alter cardiac contractility. It is generally believed that calcium is stored in the sarcoplasmic reticulum and is released in response to an action potential. The intracellular concentration of free calcium increases and then alters the rate of ATP splitting and subsequent tension development. This then stimulates the process of excitation-contraction coupling. Chapter 73 discusses the effects of digitalis in greater detail.

The following factors may be associated with increased levels of cardiac contractility: (1) hypervolemia, (2) increased venous return to the heart, (3) anemia, (4) hypothermia, (5) exercise, (6) emotions, (7) hyperthyroidism, (8) hypercalcemia, (9) digitalis, and (10) sympathomimetic amines. Long periods of bed rest, generalized myocardial disease, shock, hypothyroidism, hypocalcemia, and the use of most antiarrhythmic drugs may decrease cardiac contractility.

THE FUNDAMENTAL MECHANISMS OF CARDIAC ARRHYTHMIAS

Disturbances in two basic processes, impulse formation and impulse conduction (either alone or in combination), may be the cause of a cardiac arrhythmia. Disturbances or abnormalities of *impulse formation* are considered the result of altered automaticity. Passive ectopic arrhythmias are the result of depression of the sinoatrial node and its normal rate of automaticity. In such cases, lower tissues that have the physiologic property of automaticity assume the pacemaking function on a temporary or permanent basis. Active ectopic rhythms develop when increased automaticity occurs in a region of the heart other than the normal sinoatrial tissue.

It is thus clear that changes in the maximum diastolic potential and/or the rate of depolarization may affect the rate of automatic activity. This factor involving altered transmembrane potentials is responsible for most of the cardiac arrhythmias that occur. In addition to altered automaticity, abnormal impulse generation may occur when *triggered impulses* or *afterdepolarizations* develop. This occurs when, at some point after repolarization has started, a second depolarization arises. Early and late afterdepolarizations have been described[6] and are reported to be due to exposure to catecholamines, cardiac glycosides, hypoxia, hypercarbia, rheumatic heart disease, and cardiomyopathy. Triggered arrhythmias differ from simple automatic rhythms only in that the abnormal impulse or repetitive activity results from either an automatic or stimulated action potential. Once an afterdepolarization occurs it can attain threshold and initiate another response. This may result in a self-sustaining rhythm.[7]

Disturbances in *cardiac conduction*, such as conduction delay or block, may occur in the presence of refractory tissue, decremental conduction, or inhomogeneous conduction. Local block with *reentry* is often postulated as a cause of conduction disturbances with arrhythmia formation. The abnormal impulse travels over the pathway in a circular fashion. Reentry should be considered whenever ectopic premature systoles occur at a fixed time interval after the dominant beat (also referred to as fixed coupling).

When an impulse lingers long enough in some part of the heart as a result of slowing of conduction, it may then reexcite other portions of the heart after they have recovered excitability. If the slowed conduction is accompanied by *unidirectional block*, reentrant excitation occurs.[8] Reentry is favored by decreased conduction velocity, a short refractory period, and unidirectional block. The basic requirements for reentry are an area of one-way block, a circumscribed pathway over which the impulse can travel, and conduction that is so slow that the travel time in the pathway is longer than the effective refractory period of the fibers proximal to the region of the unidirectional block.[7] Figure 76–4 demonstrates two classic schematic representations of reentry in cardiac fibers. Drugs used to treat reentrant arrhythmias do so either by improving conduction in the depressed region of the block or by depressing further conduction to the point of complete block.

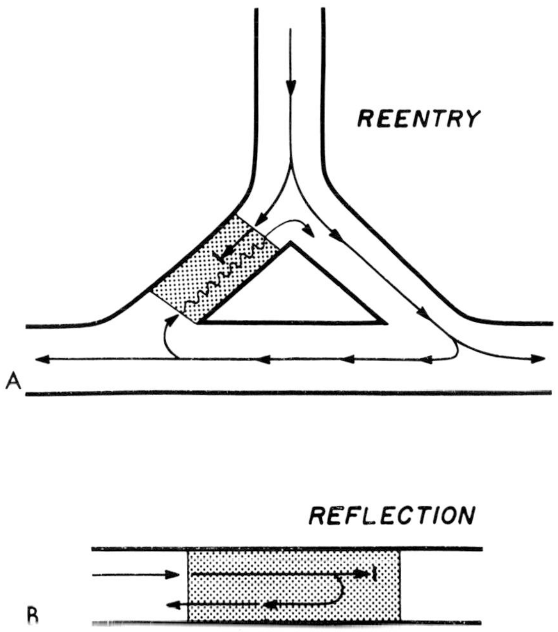

FIGURE 76–4. Two models of reentry according to Schmitt and Erlanger. *A* is a diagram showing a loop of cardiac fibers that could represent either a terminal branch of a Purkinje fiber ending on ventricular muscle or a loop of the Purkinje syncytium. In this case, one-way block and slow conduction permit reentry. *B* is a linear strand of cardiac muscle showing a depolarized zone in a portion of its cross section. One-way block occurs in the depolarized zone, permitting the propagating impulse to reflect back in the direction from which it came. (From Bigger, JT: Mechanisms and Diagnosis of Arrhythmias. *In* Braunwald E (ed): Heart Disease: A Textbook of Cardiovascular Medicine, 1st ed. Philadelphia, WB Saunders, 1980.)

Finally, it is difficult to determine in every cardiac arrhythmia whether the underlying disorder involves impulse formation or impulse conduction. In many arrhythmias, it is apparent that combined disturbances of impulse formation and conduction are present.

THE HEMODYNAMIC CONSEQUENCES OF ARRHYTHMIAS

The hemodynamic consequences of cardiac arrhythmias depend on at least ten factors: (1) the ventricular rate, (2) the duration of the abnormal rate, (3) the temporal relationship between the atria and ventricles, (4) the sequence of ventricular activation, (5) the functional cardiac status, (6) the cycle length irregularity, (7) drug therapy, (8) other disease, (9) preservation of the functional state of the motor system, and (10) the anxiety associated with the irregularity.[9]

Sinus bradycardia usually causes no problems unless the stroke volume is limited by significant cardiac disease, such as myocardial infarction. Sinus bradycardia of sick sinus syndrome is associated with signs of asthenia and occasionally syncope. In advanced states of heart block, there usually is a reduced cardiac output.

Atrial fibrillation is usually associated with a decreased cardiac output, even when the ventricular rate does not exceed the original cardiac rate. Initially, ventricular tachycardia may have no significant effect on the cardiac output. When prolonged or when associated with other problems, the arrhythmia becomes more significant. Ventricular tachycardia may be associated with a significantly reduced cardiac output if there is systemic hypotension and decreased cerebral, coronary, and renal blood flow.

Other organ systems may also be affected. Cerebral blood flow is reduced as much as 8 to 12 per cent by premature beats. Rapid supraventricular tachycardia reduces cerebral blood flow by as much as 14 per cent, atrial fibrillation by 23 per cent, and ventricular tachycardia by 40 to 75 per cent. Splanchnic and renal circulation is reduced by 20 to 40 per cent in the presence of tachyarrhythmias. Coronary circulation is reduced by 5 per cent following supraventricular premature contractions and by up to 25 per cent following frequent supraventricular premature beats.[2] Paroxysmal atrial tachycardia may reduce the coronary circulation by 35 per cent, and atrial fibrillation or rapid ventricular rates may reduce it by 40 per cent.

Ventricular tachycardia may lower coronary blood flow by as much as 60 per cent. The ECG shows ischemic changes when the coronary blood flow is reduced by 25 per cent or more.

THE CLINICAL APPROACH TO ARRHYTHMIAS

RECOGNITION

Recognizing the cardiac arrhythmia requires a thorough physical examination, which includes auscultation of the heart, examination of the venous return and mucous membranes, and palpation of the arterial pulse. An irregular cardiac rate and/or pulse rate, variable intensity of the heart sounds, a cardiac murmur, reduced intensity of the cardiac sounds, and abnormal splitting of the first or second heart sounds may suggest a cardiac disturbance. The presence of an abnormality at the time of the physical examination is an indication for a more detailed cardiovascular examination. An irregular pulse or a pulse deficit is further evidence of a cardiac disturbance and suggests the need for an electrocardiographic examination.

The electrocardiogram is an integral part of the examination of older patients, of patients with suspicious physical findings, of animals with suspected cardiac arrhythmias, and in undiagnosed cases presented for general evaluation with nonspecific clinical signs.

HISTORY

Some arrhythmias occur in otherwise normal hearts. Sinus arrhythmia and wandering pacemaker are the most common benign arrhythmias; others include prolonged sinoatrial pause, low grade A-V block, right bundle-branch block, occasional ventricular premature contractions, and supraventricular tachycardia. When an arrhythmia other than one due to respiration is recognized, organic heart disease must be considered. Attempts to determine the etiology should be undertaken.

Primary cardiac disease is often responsible for cardiac

irregularities, including arrhythmias due to bacterial or viral infections involving the heart muscle, progressive congenital cardiac disease (subvalvular aortic stenosis), and degenerative myocardial disease (microscopic intramural myocardial infarction). Paroxysmal atrial tachycardia and atrial fibrillation are both associated with mitral valvular disease. Congestive heart failure and inadequate coronary circulation may result in ventricular tachycardia, which may be prefibrillatory in nature.

Functional or organic diseases of other organ systems may affect the cardiovascular system and may be responsible for the genesis of cardiac arrhythmias. Psychogenic central nervous system stimulation, trauma, and organic brain disease may cause sympathetic or vagal stimulation, which can induce an arrhythmia. Pulmonary disease with hypoxemia and right-sided heart strain may induce an irregularity of the cardiac rhythm. Hyperthyroidism and hypothyroidism and other endocrinopathies with secondary electrolyte disturbances (such as an addisonian crisis or Cushing's disease) may have arrhythmogenic effects. Chronic vomiting or diarrhea caused by gastrointestinal disease may result in fluid loss and electrolyte disturbances. These disorders, as well as the vagal reflexes resulting from pain associated with chronic or acute gastrointestinal disease, may alter cardiac rhythm. One consistent cause of sinus tachycardia in the dog is pain, such as that due to fractures or acute pancreatitis.[10] Disease affecting the urinary system can be associated with systemic hypertension, fluid loss, and electrolyte disturbances.

Generalized diseases such as infections and toxemias may induce irregularities of the cardiac rate. Fever and anemia are responsible for an increased heart rate in both the dog and cat. Regardless of the etiology, acid-base disturbances associated with fluid imbalances and electrolyte disturbances may result in cardiac rhythm irregularities. Primary or metastatic cardiac neoplasia is another cause of arrhythmias. This is particularly important when considering such neoplasms as heart-base tumors and carotid body tumors and hemangiosarcomas.

The use of proarrhythmic agents, potassium-depleting diuretic agents, sympathomimetic amines, amphetamines, caffeine and theophylline preparations, as well as atropine or thyroid preparations may be responsible for iatrogenic cardiac arrhythmias. The withdrawal of such agents may abolish the arrhythmia.

CLINICAL SIGNS

The clinical signs of arrhythmias are often subjective in humans. Anxiety, palpitations, faintness, dizziness, light-headedness, syncope, fatigue, exertional intolerance, shortness of breath, and seizures are associated with arrhythmias. In veterinary medicine, the clinician must be alert to the objective signs that are reported by the animal's owner. Signs suggestive of arrhythmias include weakness, exercise intolerance, fainting, shortness of breath, and congestive heart failure. One common term used by animal owners to indicate paroxysmal episodes of cardiac arrhythmias is "falling over."

The objective signs used by veterinarians to recognize arrhythmias include variations in the cardiac rate, either above or below the normal limits, and paroxysmal or persistent irregularity of the cardiac rhythm.

ELECTROCARDIOGRAPHY AND ECHOCARDIOGRAPHY

The electrocardiogram should be considered an integral part of the diagnosis of arrhythmias. The information obtained from the electrocardiogram is essential in determining the appropriate treatment for cardiac arrhythmias. Noninvasive means are still the nearly universal method for recognizing, identifying, and treating arrhythmias in small animal medicine. Electrophysiologic programmed stimulation is not a clinically applicable technique at this time. Twenty-four–hour continuous ambulatory ECG monitoring is one effective method of determining the severity of cardiac rhythm disturbances. Using specialized monitoring equipment, usually provided by the laboratory for the duration of the testing period, the dog or cat has several chest leads attached without discomfort to the skin. These leads are connected to the small tape monitor, which is inserted into a "doggie" backpack pocket. The backpack is kept on the pet for 24 hours. The pet rarely objects to the backpack or the monitor. The detection and quantitation of brady- or tachyarrhythmias are significantly enhanced using this technique. Tracings along with readouts from the computer are usually returned one to two days after completing the testing.

It is important to properly assess the presence or absence of an arrhythmia as well as to determine the potential significance, if any, of the irregularity. Aberrant ventricular conduction resulting in bundle branch block patterns is an example of possible innocent irregularities that could easily be mistaken for an arrhythmia.

Echocardiography, both M-mode and two-dimensional ultrasound, is a useful noninvasive method of evaluating cardiac function. In addition to identifying anatomic abnormalities, it is helpful in evaluating atrial and ventricular function in the presence of arrhythmias. Drugs may be chosen based on the identification of ventricular dysfunction. Prior to pacemaker insertion, ultrasound provides important information regarding cardiac chamber size and function. The author has found Table 76–3 useful in approaching cardiac rhythm disturbances.

LABORATORY STUDIES

The minimum laboratory tests required for understanding and treating cardiac arrhythmias include a complete blood count, the blood urea nitrogen (BUN) level, serum electrolyte levels, and a urinalysis. Because arrhythmias are only part of the overall disease being studied, it is recommended that these individual studies be performed as part of a more complete multiphasic screening panel. Electrolyte disturbances due to drugs or disease are a major consideration whenever arrhythmias occur.

TREATMENT

The therapeutic approach to cardiac arrhythmias requires an understanding of the primary or secondary

TABLE 76–3. APPROACH TO THE RECOGNITION OF CARDIAC RHYTHM DISTURBANCES

Rhythm	*Regular*	Fast (>180/min)	Sinus tachycardia	
			Supraventricular tachycardia	
			Ventricular tachycardia	
		Normal (70–160 [180])	Normal sinus rhythm	
		Slow (<70/min)	Sinus bradycardia	
			Second- and third-degree heart block	
	Irregular	Rhythmic or occasionally erratic	Premature beats	Supraventricular
				Ventricular
			Sinus arrhythmia	
		Irregularly irregular	Atrial fibrillation	
			Atrial tachycardia with block	
			Ventricular tachycardia	
			Advanced second-degree heart block	
			Sick sinus syndrome	

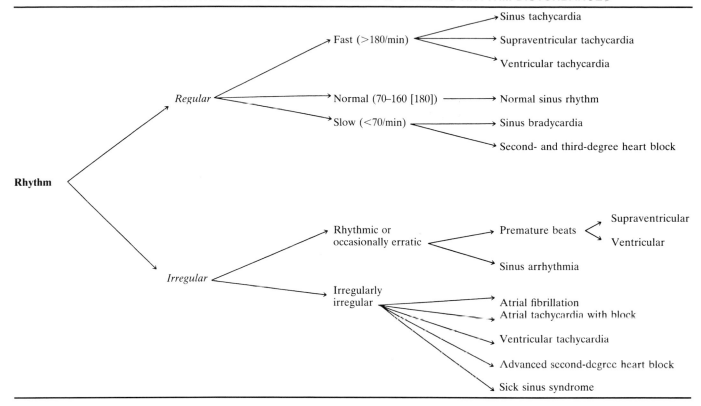

nature of the rhythm disturbance. It may be necessary to treat an underlying disease as well as a cardiac arrhythmia. Attempting to treat cardiac arrhythmias without understanding or evaluating the patient in detail only leads to frustration and ultimate therapeutic failure.

THE CLASSIFICATION OF ANTIARRHYTHMIC AGENTS

AGENTS THAT REMOVE OR SUPPRESS PRECIPITATING FACTORS

Hypoxia, acidosis, electrolyte disturbances, bradycardia, and abnormal sympathetic stimulation may be responsible for the production of cardiac arrhythmias. Oxygen, digitalis, diuretics, and β-adrenergic stimulating agents may all increase contractility and coronary blood flow. They may disperse refractoriness and restore membrane potentials. As a result, these agents may be indicated in patients with hypoxemia or enlarged dilated hearts with a low cardiac output.[11]

Acidosis may be effectively counteracted with the proper use of sodium bicarbonate. Correction of acidosis increases the threshold to ventricular fibrillation. Because hypokalemic states enhance automaticity, this electrolyte disturbance requires correction to prevent potential arrhythmia development. β-Adrenergic blockade is of value in the suppression of arrhythmias associated with hyperexcitability and general anesthesia. Atropine, β-adrenergic blocking agents, and implantation of cardiac pacemakers may counter the bradyarrhythmia by increasing the heart rate or reversing the process or cause of the arrhythmia.

Psychological stress has been demonstrated to significantly enhance vulnerability to ectopic ventricular arrhythmias. Cardiac arrhythmias following coronary artery ligation were significantly reduced when intravenous diazepam at 0.4 mg/lb (1 mg/kg) or chlordiazepoxide at 4.5 mg/lb or 10 mg/kg was used first.[12, 13] These and other studies suggest that suppression of the central nervous system may be one effective method of treating some ventricular arrhythmias.

AGENTS THAT INCREASE AUTOMATICITY

Agents that increase automaticity are especially indicated for the treatment of the bradyarrhythmias. These agents may be useful in treating symptomatic slow heart rates that are associated clinically with fainting, weakness, hypotension, sinus pauses, or periods of cardiac arrest. Such therapeutic agents include the sympathomimetic amines, such as isoproterenol and epinephrine. Parasympathetic blocking agents (such as atropine) and alkalinizing agents (such as molar sodium lactate or sodium bicarbonate) increase automaticity, especially in slow heart rates due to hyperkalemia, hypoxia, or acidosis, and in repeated Stokes-Adams attacks with episodes of cardiac arrest. Another therapeutic mechanism that increases automaticity is the cardiac pacemaker. This device is being used more often in veterinary medicine.

ELECTROPHYSIOLOGIC CLASSIFICATION OF ANTIARRHYTHMIC DRUGS

During the last decade a classification system has been developed that is regarded as the standard nomenclature for antiarrhythmic drugs.[14] Antiarrhythmic drugs are grouped into four classes, each class having one predominant effect on the cardiac action potential. See Table 76–4 and the following discussion of specific drugs.

Many of the drugs identified fit into a category at one dosage rate but would perhaps be more correctly identified in multiple categories. Similarly subclassification still does not really help in choosing effective drug therapy for a specific patient. Drugs are still chosen on the basis of effectiveness, side effects, and ease of administration. Of greater clinical relevance is the growing trend to use drugs in combination. These permit the use of lower dosages of each agent, thus limiting side effects. No one combination of antiarrhythmic agents is superior and an empirical approach is still used to select therapeutic agents.[14a]

In choosing therapeutic agents to control arrhythmias the clinician should be aware that ± 30 per cent of ventricular arrhythmias may disappear in patients given placebo therapy only. Alternatively, many antiarrhythmic agents have specific proarrhythmic tendencies. Thus, careful monitoring of the pet is required when such drugs are administered.

Table 76–1 is a compilation of therapeutic agents currently in clinical use in treating canine and feline arrhythmias.

CLASS I DRUGS

The electrophysiologic effect of Class I agents is to slow the maximal rate of phase zero depolarization of the cardiac action potential. Drugs in this group have a direct membrane-stabilizing or local anesthetic action due to the selective blocking of Na^+ influx through the fast Na^+ channels of the cell membrane. The reduction in the rate of phase zero depolarization is associated with a decrease in impulse conduction velocity, an increase in the threshold of excitability, and an inhibition of spontaneous depolarization of pacemaker cells. Within this class are three subgroups, each having its own electrophysiologic and antiarrhythmic differences.

Class IA. Antiarrhythmic Class IA drugs markedly depress phase zero action potentials, depress the conduction of electrical impulses throughout the heart, and slow cardiac repolarization. These effects are observed electrocardiographically as widening of the QRS complex and prolongation of the Q-T interval. Quinidine, procainamide, and disopyramide are drugs in this class.

Class IB. Class IB drugs shorten the action potential duration and cardiac repolarization, but increase the electrical stimulus required to produce fibrillation.[15] Lidocaine, phenytoin, tocainide, and mexiletine are examples of drugs in this group.

Class IC. Class IC drugs, like class IA, markedly depress the rate of phase zero depolarization and conduction velocity. They exert little effect on refractoriness or action potential duration. Flecainide and encainide are examples of drugs in this category.

TABLE 76–4. CLASSIFICATION OF ANTIARRHYTHMIC AGENTS FOR USE IN SMALL ANIMALS

Class I Antiarrhythmic Drugs		Effect is to decrease membrane conduction of sodium
Type IA	Quinidine	
	Procainamide	
	Disopyramide	
Type IB	Lidocaine	
	Tocainide	
	Mexiletine	
	Phenytoin	
Type IC	Encainide	
	Flecainide	
Class II Antiarrhythmic Drugs		Effect is to reduce sympathetic excitation of the heart
	Propranolol	
	Atenolol	
	Metoprolol	
	Nadolol	
	Pindolol	
	Timolol	
	Esmolol	
	Sotalol	
Class III Antiarrhythmic Drugs		Effect is to lengthen action potential durations and thus increase refractoriness
	Amiodarone	
	Bretylium	
Class IV Antiarrhythmic Drugs		Effect is to decrease the slow inward Ca^{++} currents into the cells
	Verapamil	
	Diltiazem	
	Nifedipine	

CLASS II DRUGS

This group of drugs inhibit sympathoadrenal excitation of the heart through blockade of the cardiac β_1 receptors or by interfering with the release of norepinephrine from sympathetic nerves. β-Blockers suppress tachyarrhythmias and ectopic pacemakers arising from sympathetically mediated increases in automaticity. They also slow A-V conduction, which is effective in reducing the ventricular rate response to supraventricular tachyarrhythmias. Propranolol and atenolol are but two of the many β-blockers now available.

CLASS III DRUGS

These drugs specifically prolong the action potential duration and extend the refractory period. They are capable of increasing the atrial and ventricular fibrillatory threshold. Bretylium and amiodarone are antiarrhythmic drugs in this category. Their use in dogs and cats has been limited to date.

CLASS IV DRUGS

This group of drugs, referred to as the calcium channel blockers, exert little effect on the fast Na^+ responses but have a relatively specific inhibitory effect on transmembrane Ca^{++} influx during phases one and two. Clinically, these drugs are useful to suppress supraventricular and nodal reentrant tachycardias, thereby slowing the sinus rate and prolonging A-V conduction. Verapamil, diltiazem, and nifedipine are examples of drugs in this group. The use of these agents for atrial fibrillation and sustained ventricular arrhythmias is not recommended in dogs or cats in large part because they exert a marked negative inotropic effect.

SPECIFIC CLASS IA DRUGS

Quinidine. Quinidine prolongs conduction in the His-Purkinje system and the ventricular myocardium, increases the diastolic threshold of excitability in the atria and ventricles, and prolongs the effective refractory period. Quinidine depresses the rate of spontaneous diastolic depolarization in pacemaker fibers, decreases the rate of depolarization of the action potential that arises from the resting potential, and shifts the membrane responsiveness curve to the right. Thus it is the prototype Class IA antiarrhythmic drug.

The depression of myocardial excitability following quinidine administration provides a partial explanation of the drug's ability to abolish or depress formation of ectopic impulses. In addition, the velocity of conduction is uniformly decreased, and this in turn is responsible for prolongation of both the P-R interval and the QRS complex.

Because quinidine causes prolongation of the effective refractory period of cardiac fibers, the time during which cardiac fibers may be excited by an electrical impulse is shorter than normal. This important feature effectively abolishes a considerable amount of ectopic activity resulting from repetitive electrical stimulation (reentry). By decreasing the slope of the curve of slow diastolic depolarization, quinidine also reduces the frequency of spontaneous discharge of pacemaker tissue.

Clinically effective doses of quinidine may prolong the P-R interval, widen the QRS complex, and prolong the Q T interval. Quinidine need not be discontinued when these electrocardiographic changes occur. When further changes develop, such as prolongation of the QRS complex by 25 per cent or more, the drug should be discontinued, since more serious arrhythmias may result. The antivagal and anticholinergic effects of quinidine may result in an increased cardiac rate.

In the dog and, at times, the cat, quinidine therapy may be indicated for the treatment of ventricular premature contractions, ventricular tachycardia, and atrial fibrillation after the rapid ventricular rate has been slowed with digitalis. Quinidine may also be effective for the treatment of some paroxysmal supraventricular tachycardias. Quinidine is less effective in the conversion of atrial fibrillation to normal sinus rhythm in the dog than it is in humans. Quinidine may cause atrial fibrillation to revert to a sinus rhythm, but this usually occurs only after very high dosages, often approaching toxic levels. In addition, it is the rare dog that benefits from such reversion, and almost universally, conversion back to atrial fibrillation occurs quite quickly. Thus, the drug is rarely used for this purpose in dogs or cats, unless the arrhythmia is of recent onset due to thoracic trauma or anesthesia. There is little experience with quinidine in atrial fibrillation in the cat. It is likely that features similar to those in the dog exist and there appears to be little reason for its use in such cases.

Quinidine is available as quinidine sulfate in three-grain, 200 mg tablets. It is also available as an injectable preparation, quinidine gluconate injection, 80 mg/ml. In addition, quinidine is available in several slow-release formulations, combining quinidine polygalacturonate, quinidine gluconate, or quinidine sulfate. By using the principle of delayed absorption, these products may be administered less frequently, thereby improving owner compliance.

There is no fixed dosage for quinidine preparations. Clinical experience suggests that high doses are often necessary for favorable results.

Quinidine sulfate is administered orally at the level of 3 to 10 mg/lb in the dog. It may be administered in consecutive doses every two hours if the urgency of the arrhythmia indicates such therapy. Then it is administered every six to eight hours to control the cardiac irregularity. Delayed release forms are dosed every 8 to 12 hours.

Quinidine gluconate should not be administered by intravenous injection in order to avoid circulatory depression and overdosage. If oral medication is not possible or if the clinician is concerned about a lack of adequate oral absorption of the drug, quinidine gluconate may be administered by deep intramuscular injection. The dosage for intramuscular quinidine is 3 to 10 mg/lb every three to six hours.

In the cat, quinidine is usually given in a sustained-release form using approximately one-quarter tablet twice daily. The dosage is titrated to effect, thus avoiding the undesirable side effects of anorexia and vomiting.

Quinidine is contraindicated in patients with idiosyncratic reactions to the drug and in cases of complete heart block. It should be used with caution in patients with incomplete heart block. Caution is particularly advised in cases of congestive heart failure because of the negative inotropic effects of the agent. It should not be used to treat arrhythmias arising from digitalis intoxication.

The principal side effects of quinidine overdosage in dogs are gastrointestinal, but neurologic signs (confusion and seizures) may also develop. Microsomal enzyme inducers increase the rate of excretion of quinidine. Quinidine increases serum digoxin levels and caution is advised when the drugs are administered concurrently. Where possible, the drugs should not be used together. If they must, careful attention to serum digoxin levels is advised. Reducing the dosage of digoxin by half is often recommended. The use of alternative antiarrhythmic agents such as procainamide or mexiletine is suggested instead.

Procainamide (Pronestyl). The effects of procainamide on the heart are similar to those of quinidine, another class IA antiarrhythmic. The antivagal and anticholinergic effects of procainamide are less intense than quinidine and rarely result in an increase in the cardiac rate.

When high doses of procainamide are administered, the electrocardiogram indicates prolongation of the P-R and Q-T intervals and the QRS complex. In addition to prolongation of the electrocardiographic intervals, the other major side effect of procainamide is hypotension. This occurs most frequently when the product is given intravenously.

Procainamide, like quinidine, is used to suppress premature ventricular contractions and ventricular tachycardia. It may be used with quinidine; when used together, both drugs are given at lower dosages to induce the desired clinical effects. This approach is safer, since lower total dosages may be used for each drug and fewer side effects are encountered. Because procainamide clinically causes fewer gastrointestinal side effects in dogs, this author prefers it to quinidine in cases of postgastric torsion arrhythmias.

Procainamide is contraindicated and should be discontinued when complete heart block, prolongation of the QRS complex, or anorexia, nausea, and vomiting develop. Hypotension should be corrected prior to the administration of procainamide.

Procainamide hydrochloride is available in 250 mg, 375 mg, and 500 mg strength capsules or tablets. It is also available in sustained release 250, 375, and 500 mg tablets. The bioavailability is lower than that of the standard formulation. These tablets may be poorly absorbed, and the clinician should evaluate stool samples to ascertain that the tablets are not being excreted intact after administration. It is also available as procainamide hydrochloride injection in 100 mg/ml vials.

The suggested initial dosage is 3 to 10 mg/lb body weight orally or intramuscularly. This dose may be repeated (or increased) every two hours until the arrhythmia is abolished or toxic effects are observed. The drug is then given every eight hours, using the sustained release form or every four to six hours with the standard preparation.

Intravenously, for the treatment of ventricular tachycardia, a loading dose of 3 to 4 mg/lb is given over five minutes, followed by an infusion at the rate of 5 to 18 mcg/lb/min.[16] Hypotension can be a significant clinical side effect of this agent. After conversion of the cardiac arrhythmia with intravenous medication, oral maintenance doses are administered.

Disopyramide (Norpace). Disopyramide has many electrophysiologic effects similar to quinidine and procainamide. It is useful in the treatment of some refractory ventricular arrhythmias or when toxic reactions to other antiarrhythmic agents suggest a change of drug. The author has used this drug alone and in combination with lowered dosages of quinidine or procainamide with some success, but it is not considered a first-line therapeutic product.

The drug is contraindicated for use in animals with uncontrolled congestive heart failure, pulmonary edema, glaucoma, urinary retention, advanced A-V block, and sinus node dysfunction. The drug is less hazardous when there is no left ventricular dysfunction. Hyperkalemia accentuates its depressant myocardial effect and hypokalemia reduces its therapeutic effect.

Disopyramide is well-absorbed orally but has a very short serum half-life. It is available in a sustained-release form. It is excreted primarily through the kidneys, although there is also some hepatic degradation.

Side effects are principally anticholinergic, including dryness of the mucous membranes and mouth, as well as fecal and urinary retention. Abdominal distress and nausea are less common than with quinidine.

The drug is presently not recommended for use in cats because of lack of clinical experience. In dogs, 5 to 10 mg/lb are administered every eight hours. Higher dosages may be required but have not been used by this author.

SPECIFIC CLASS IB DRUGS

Lidocaine (Xylocaine). Lidocaine, a class IB antiarrhythmic, is more effective for the treatment of ventricular arrhythmias than for the supraventricular arrhythmias. Clinically useful doses of lidocaine produce no significant alterations of the QRS duration or A-V conduction time.

Lidocaine decreases the action potential amplitude, its duration, and the maximum slope of phase zero depolarization. It shortens the effective refractory period, depresses automaticity, and suppresses accelerating ectopic foci.[17] The drug significantly increases the threshold to ventricular fibrillation in the dog.[18]

Although lidocaine decreases ventricular excitability and conductivity at therapeutic dosages, it is not likely to affect myocardial contractility, systemic arterial blood pressure, or the absolute refractory period when given in therapeutic dosages.

Lidocaine is effective in controlling ventricular arrhythmias and is indicated for the control of acute ventricular arrhythmias associated with cardiac surgery, cardiac catheterization, and angiocardiography, as well as life-threatening ventricular arrhythmias resulting from cardiac disease and occasionally, digitalis intoxication. Lidocaine is contraindicated and not useful for sinoatrial, atrioventricular, and intraventricular block. Lidocaine is available as a 2 per cent solution for intravenous injection. It is a drug with a short duration of activity and it is usually cleared from the bloodstream within 20 minutes. Intravenous use is presently indicated for the control of life-threatening cardiac arrhythmias.

The usual dosage of lidocaine is 2 to 4 mg/lb, intravenously as a slow bolus, half given initially and the balance slowly over three to five minutes. Continuous electrocardiographic monitoring is essential with lidocaine therapy. Its effects may last for 10 to 20 minutes. Some clinicians prefer a lower loading dosage of 1 mg/lb given as a slow bolus, followed by a 20- to 30- mcg/lb/min continuous infusion.

There are reports of sudden death in four of seven cats given lidocaine.[19] Conduction disturbances and bradyarrhythmias were recorded when less than 0.45 mg/lb (1 mg/kg) was used.[19] When given to effect by a slow intravenous drip containing 400 mg/liter of fluid (20 ml, 2 per cent solution), other clinicians have not experienced the same problems in the cat.

Lidocaine should be administered according to the recurrence of the arrhythmia as indicated by electrocardiographic monitoring. Following cessation of the arrhythmia, longer-acting antiarrhythmic agents should be substituted for lidocaine.

The sign of Lidocaine intoxication, caused by excessive dosage, is convulsions. Such convulsions usually subside shortly after discontinuance of therapy. Short-acting intravenous barbiturates or diazepam may be necessary to control the seizures, and endotracheal intubation is in order if respiratory arrest occurs.

Hepatic disease, chloramphenicol, propranolol, and norepinephrine may all delay metabolic degradation of lidocaine. Hepatic microsomal enzyme inducers and isoproterenol enhance degradation, necessitating careful monitoring when these drugs are used concurrently.

A number of new drugs similar to lidocaine in structure or action, but which can be administered effectively by the oral route, have become available recently. The major pharmacokinetic advantage of these products is the increased half-life following oral administration. This feature permits administration once or twice a day, a particularly advantageous feature in veterinary medicine. Drugs such as tocainide and mexiletine are examples.

Tocainide. Tocainide is a structured congener of lidocaine, sharing the same electrophysiologic properties. Its advantage is that it is an oral preparation with a long plasma concentration effect, permitting it to be used every 8 to 12 hours. Although scattered reports of its effectiveness in dogs from 7 to 50 mg/lb two to three times daily are mentioned, this author has been very disappointed in the clinical antiarrhythmic effects of tocainide. Reports of its effectiveness when combined with propranolol require further documentation. The author has not used the drug in cats. In one large study of humans, when mexiletine and tocainide were compared clinically it was determined that they have different clinical effects.[20]

Mexiletine. Another newly approved Class IB drug with electrophysiologic effects similar to those of lidocaine, but which is given orally, is mexiletine. Its greatest usefulness is in the treatment of ventricular arrhythmias, many of which are nonresponsive to conventional therapy. The drug has no significant negative inotropic effect, and side effects, which are reversible, usually involve gastrointestinal and CNS reactions. It may also be used with digoxin, since it does not increase serum digoxin levels as quinidine does. The drug has been safely employed in association with β-blockers and other Type I antiarrhythmic agents. It appears to be well-suited for patients with compromised cardiac function, which extends its therapeutic efficacy.

Well absorbed from the intestinal tract after oral administration, its first pass hepatic extraction is generally low. It is metabolized in the liver and liver impairment prolongs the effective half-life.

Available in 150, 200, and 250 mg capsules, mexiletine is given orally two to three times daily. The author usually doses initially at 1 to 4 mg/lb twice daily and increases these levels if necessary. Clinical experience with canine ventricular arrhythmias treated with mexiletine to date has been very favorable.

SPECIFIC CLASS IC DRUGS

Encainide and Flecainide. Several Class IC antiarrhythmic agents are available. These drugs display the Na^+ conductance blocking ability of Class I drugs but are distinct from the others in that they do not prolong the refractory period. Their use in the treatment of cardiac arrhythmias is principally in treating ventricular premature contractions (VPCs) and ventricular tachycardia.

Flecainide may induce, aggravate, or worsen pre-existing heart failure.[21] As with other antiarrhythmic agents, it may have deleterious proarrhythmic effects in some patients. Although it is an effective antiarrhythmic agent, its efficacy is limited to a subgroup of patients. The reported oral dosage in dogs ranges from 0.5 to 3 mg/lb two to three times daily. Using 50 to 100 mg twice daily in average-sized dogs, the author is not favorably impressed with the drug when compared to using Type IB mexiletine for severe refractory arrhythmias.

Encainide is a t.i.d. product in the same class, indicated for the treatment of sustained ventricular tachycardia. Its effects are similar to those of flecainide and it appears to have many of the same contraindications. It may have an additional indication in the treatment of chronic atrial tachycardia. Further studies are required in small animal cardiology regarding the dosage, effectiveness, and recommendations for this product.

SPECIFIC CLASS II DRUGS

Propranolol (Inderal). Propranolol is a β-adrenergic blocking agent. It reduces or abolishes increased chronotrope and inotrope by reducing S-A node activity. It also decreases conduction velocity, automaticity (quinidine-like effect), and the ventricular rate, while increasing the A-V nodal refractory period. It results in a decreased heart rate at rest and with exercise, a reduced cardiac output and left ventricular work, while reducing myocardial oxygen consumption. The dextro-isomer component decreases automaticity, and the levo-isomer is the β-blocker at the receptor sites in the heart. Bronchial smooth muscle constriction is an important undesirable effect that may occur. Electrophysiologically, its antiarrhythmic effects are due to a reduction in the resting membrane potential and spontaneous diastolic depolarization. Conduction velocity and membrane responsiveness are slowed.

Although propranolol is well-absorbed orally, there is a large but variable first pass elimination via the liver and portal circulation. In addition, plasma protein binding is variable, and occasionally, active metabolites have similar antiarrhythmic effects. The effective half-life of orally administered propranolol in dogs is three to six hours, but antiarrhythmic effects often persist beyond this period. Using increased oral dosages less frequently (e.g., twice daily) on a chronic basis often provides effective therapeutic levels of the drugs. Propranolol is available in tablet form (10, 20, 40, 60, 80, and 90 mg) as well as in long-acting capsules (60, 80, 120, and 160 mg) and injectable ampules (1 mg/ml).

Propranolol is indicated for both dogs and cats in the treatment of supraventricular tachycardia, pre-excitation syndrome or accelerated conduction tachycardias, atrial flutter, and atrial fibrillation. Its role in the therapy of ventricular premature contractions and tachycardias is usually in association with a Class I antiarrhythmic agent when the arrhythmia is refractory to single drug therapy.

It is usually combined with digoxin therapy in treating atrial fibrillation. Both drugs are administered initially, there being no benefit in achieving the positive inotropic effects of digitalis first, since control of the ventricular rate is also important, especially in dogs.

Propranolol is also used to treat some cases of digitalis intoxication, although phenytoin, lidocaine, or potassium chloride may be of greater benefit. Combined with quinidine, procainamide, or disopyramide, the drug has been found by the author to be useful in controlling recurrent atrial tachycardia or ventricular arrhythmias otherwise found to be refractory to drug therapy. Its role in the treatment of systemic hypertension is now recognized in veterinary medicine (see Chapter 109). It has been successfully used in the management of feline hypertrophic cardiomyopathy because it assists in reducing intraventricular outflow tract obstruction and decreases the cardiac rate and myocardial oxygen consumption while increasing myocardial compliance. The drug has also been used in cats with thyrotoxicosis prior to surgical removal of thyroid adenoma(s) or in conjunction with oral antithyroid drugs.

Propranolol is usually contraindicated in the bradycardia-tachycardia syndrome, in heart block, and in patients with asthma. Congestive heart failure and hypotension should be considered as relative contraindications to its use. Owing to the points discussed previously with respect to the pharmacokinetics of propranolol, the dosage rate is quite variable and must be individually titrated. Oral dosages vary from 2.5 to 20 mg for smaller dogs and 20 to 40 mg for larger dogs, either two or three times daily. An approximate initial dosage, titrated to effect is 0.2 to 0.5 mg/lb q8h in the dog. It is rarely necessary to give 80 mg/dose to giant breeds except for the first few dosages to reduce the heart rate. Use of the long-acting form may allow for easier therapy and owner compliance in larger dogs. The 60-mg capsule is approximately equal when given once daily to 20 mg given t.i.d. Dosage retitration is required when switching to the long-acting formulation. Cats usually require 2.5 mg twice daily, although once daily administration of the drug is often necessary due to the undesirable side effects from twice daily administration.

Intravenous therapy is reserved for acute arrhythmia therapy, especially anesthetic-induced atrial tachycardia and spontaneous atrial tachyarrhythmias associated with the Wolff-Parkinson-White (WPW) pre-excitation syndrome. Increments of 0.25 to 0.5 mg are given every one to three minutes up to a maximum of 3 to 5 mg in dogs. Dosages of 0.05 to 0.1 mg are given to cats intravenously. Electrocardiographic monitoring throughout is essential. Acute heart failure or hypotension may develop when administering the drug, but this is unusual.

The most frequently encountered side effects in dogs and cats following oral use include lethargy, fatigue, depression, anorexia, and on occasion, vomiting and diarrhea. Adverse reactions include hypotension, heart failure, and heart block. After prolonged usage the drug should be slowly withdrawn, since acute withdrawal may be associated with arrhythmia formation.

Other β-blocking agents are marketed and may be of additional value, since the frequency of dosage may be decreased. To date, experience with atenolol and nadolol has not been more positive than that with propranolol.

CLASS III ANTIARRHYTHMIC DRUGS

Two drugs in this group with no direct effect on normal fast Na^+ conductance or that lack β-blocking properties are bretylium and amiodarone. Bretylium has been used for refractory ventricular arrhythmias and recurrent ventricular fibrillation in humans. Clinical experience is limited in dogs and the drug is currently not included in the usual schedule of antiarrhythmic agents. Amiodarone prolongs the duration of the action potential and increases the refractory period, both without altering the rate of depolarization. By relaxing vascular smooth muscle, it reduces afterload and does not diminish LV ejection fraction. Its principal use is for the treatment of refractory ventricular arrhythmias. The drug is not without serious side effects, including pulmonary fibrosis, liver damage, possible exacerbation of the arrhythmia, or induction of heart block, as well as photosensitization and hyper- or hypothyroidism.

Due to the long half-life of amiodarone, caution is required in its administration. Loading doses may be given, but reduction to once daily administration soon after is suggested.

Amiodarone increases serum digoxin levels so that the digoxin dosage should be reduced by 50 per cent or more when therapy is started. Quinidine and procainamide levels are also elevated and reducing the dosage or discontinuing the drug is suggested.

There is little experience with this drug in small animals and its use should be limited to patients with life-threatening arrhythmias and in situations when close supervision and continuous monitoring are possible. A dosage of 2 to 4 mg/lb q12h may be evaluated.

CLASS IV ANTIARRHYTHMIC DRUGS

The calcium channel blocking agents have previously been described. Although a number of products are used in humans, only verapamil has been used widely by veterinary cardiologists in dogs and cats.

In humans, the drug is used for several reasons, including its vasodilating effect, for anti-anginal therapy, and for controlling supraventricular tachycardia. Although the vasodilating action may be of some benefit in congestive heart failure, the negative inotropic effects of the drugs preclude their use as first-line therapy in heart failure patients.[21]

In veterinary small animal medicine verapamil is principally used for slowing the heart rate in WPW pre-excitation cases and in some other supraventricular tachycardias. It slows the sinus rate, prolongs A-V nodal impulse conduction, and reduces the ventricular rate in atrial fibrillation or flutter, although it is not uniformly successful and may induce ventricular arrhythmias in these cases.

Verapamil is currently recommended for use only in supraventricular tachycardia and WPW syndromes without atrial fibrillation in both dogs and cats. It may be given slowly IV at 0.05 to 0.15 mg/lb, repeating the dose twice if favorable effects do not occur. Acute hypotension, collapse, and hypocalcemia can be serious life-threatening side effects of verapamil overdosage. Orally, the dosage is 0.5 to 2.0 mg/lb, usually two or three times daily.[23]

Diltiazem is another calcium channel blocking agent used in humans for the treatment of angina. It has had little recorded use in dogs or cats to date. Suggestions for its use with supraventricular arrhythmias are questionable. Alone or combined with β-blocking agents it may depress ventricular function and/or prolong A-V nodal conduction time. It may be useful in the management of feline hypertrophic cardiomyopathy at a dosage rate of 0.7 mg/lb q8h. Incidental reports of its use in dogs for supraventricular arrhythmias suggest a range of 0.2 to 0.7 mg/lb q8h.

PREMATURE ECTOPIC BEATS

Premature ectopic cardiac rhythms arise from a supraventricular or ventricular focus. Supraventricular ectopic beats may be classified as atrial or junctional rhythms. This latter classification relates only to the electrocardiographic appearance and, in fact, may be electrophysiologically inaccurate in describing the origin of the premature beat.

Ectopic premature foci interrupt the normal cardiac rhythm in one or more of the following sequences: resetting, resetting with pause, compensatory pause, and interpolation. Resetting results in the formation of an entirely new cardiac rhythm. As a result, the period from the ectopic P wave to the next normal P wave is that of the regular rhythm. In resetting with pause, the ectopic beat temporarily depresses the sinoatrial node. Consequently, the sinus beat following the premature beat is slightly delayed, and the pause is greater than one normal P-P interval but less than two normal P-P intervals. Generally, resetting and resetting with pause are associated with supraventricular premature arrhythmias. Compensatory pause and interpolation are more commonly associated with ventricular arrhythmias. In compensatory pause, the sinus impulse that follows the ectopic beat fails to initiate a regular ventricular beat because the ventricle is still in the absolute refractory period as a result of the ectopic rhythm. Then there is a prolonged interval between the ectopic beat and the next normal beat. The interval between the normal beat preceding the ectopic beat and the sinus beat following

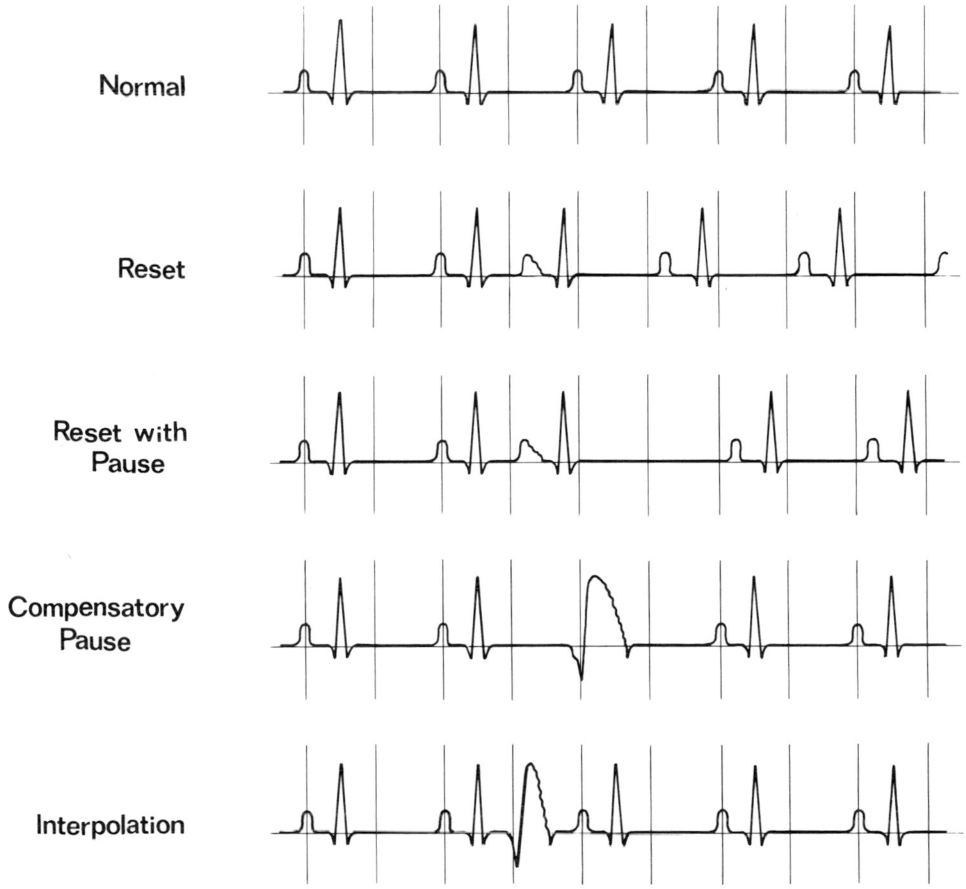

FIGURE 76–5. Schematic representations of normal sinus rhythm and premature complexes. *Normal sinus rhythm:* The heart rate remains constant, and the interval from P to P or from R to R does not change. *Resetting:* An atrial premature contraction (beat 3) resets the sinus rhythm, so the period from the beginning of the premature P wave to the next normal P wave is equal to exactly one P-P interval. *Resetting with pause:* The atrial premature contraction (beat 3) is followed by a pause greater than one P-P interval but less than two P-P intervals. *Compensatory pause:* The ventricular premature contraction (beat 3) is followed by a compensatory pause; that is, the period from the normal P wave in the beat preceding the ventricular premature contraction to the normal P wave of the beat following the ventricular premature contraction is equivalent to exactly two P-P intervals. The sinus P wave occurs on time, but it is not conducted through the atrioventricular node to the ventricle, which is in a refractory state due to the ventricular premature contraction. *Interpolation:* A ventricular premature contraction (beat 3) occurs between two normal sinus complexes without disrupting normal rhythm. Interpolated beats are unusual in dogs. (From Ettinger, SJ and Suter, PF: Canine Cardiology. Philadelphia, WB Saunders, 1970.)

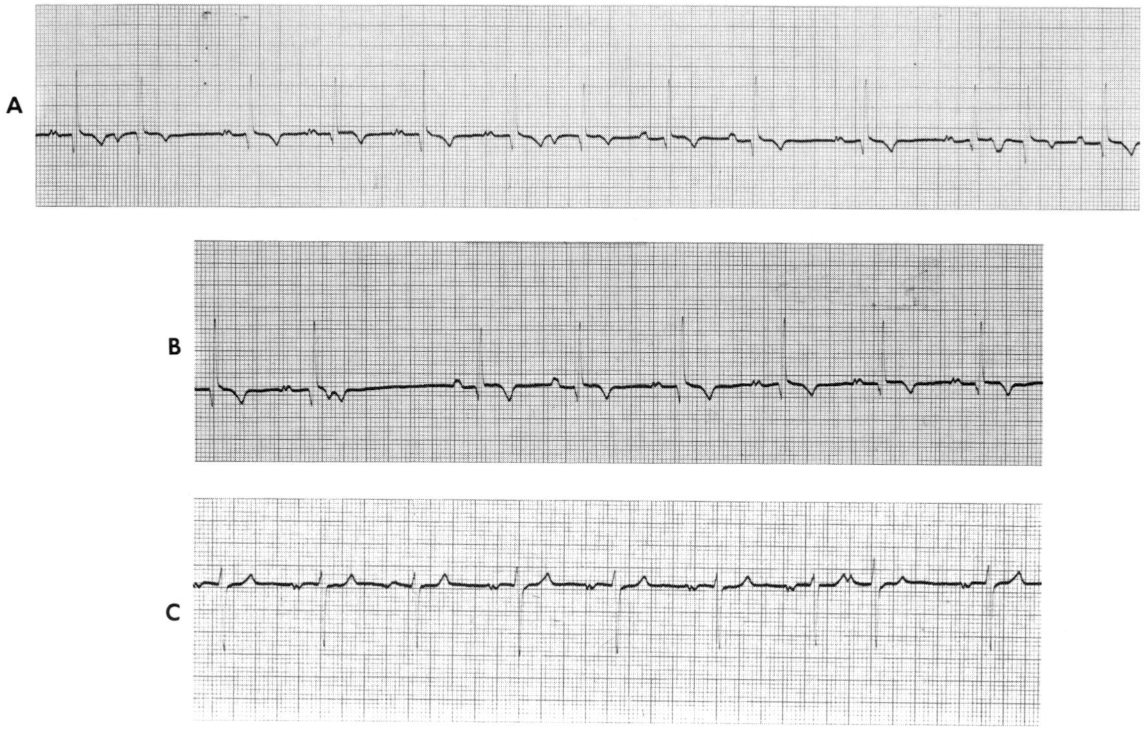

FIGURE 76–6. Supraventricular premature contractions. *A* is a lead II electrocardiogram from a dog with chronic mitral valvular fibrosis and congestive heart failure. The heart rate is 160 beats per minute. Beats number 2, 7, and 12 are supraventricular premature contractions. Note the negative P waves of the abnormal beats. They are premature, the P-R interval is longer than normal, and the premature P waves are followed by normal QRS complexes. There is resetting with pause after the first premature contraction and resetting without pause after the second and third premature beats. *B* and *C* are lead II tracings from a dog with syncopal episodes. In *B*, the second full complex is followed by a blocked atrial premature beat. This is within the T wave, distorting its appearance in contrast with the other more normal T waves. Because the P occurs too early to depolarize the ventricles, the remainder of the beat is blocked. A pause follows the blocked beat, much as if the entire complex occurred, since the premature P wave further suppresses the A-V node. *C* shows the same dog as *B* and demonstrates another supraventricular premature beat in the next-to-last complex. Again, the P wave is intermixed with the T wave of the preceding beat. This distorts both waves, but note that the QRS complex occurs early and is followed by resetting with pause.

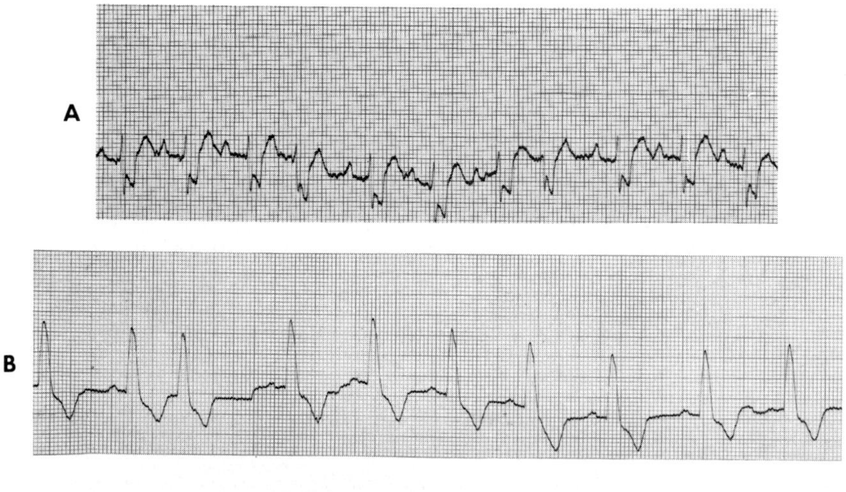

FIGURE 76–7. Supraventricular premature contractions in a cat. *A,* Lead II from a cat with hypertrophic cardiomyopathy and an irregular rhythm. The QRS complexes are bizarre in form because of a ventricular conduction abnormality and delay but most are preceded by P waves and followed by T waves. The fourth and eighth beats occur early and premature P waves are lost in the preceding T waves. These supraventricular premature beats are followed by QRS complexes just as all the others are and resetting with pause (beat 4) and without a pause (beat 8) is present. *B* shows supraventricular premature contraction present in a cat with left ventricular enlargement and left bundle branch block. The third complex occurs early and is followed by resetting with pause. This a lead I tracing.

the ectopic beat is equal to twice the normal P-to-P interval. Occurring less commonly in small animal electrocardiography is interpolation. An interpolated beat is a complete extra complex occurring between two normal cycles. The interpolated beat does not interrupt the normal rhythm (Figure 76–5).

Supraventricular Premature Contractions

Ectopic foci resulting in premature rhythms that arise from tissue above the ventricles, including the region of the S-A node, right and left atria, A-V node, and the junctional tissue, are referred to as supraventricular premature contractions (Figures 76–6 and 76–7). These cardiac arrhythmias are characterized electrocardiographically by premature P waves that are different in configuration and/or size from the normal P wave. This reflects electrical conduction across the atria. Because the P wave arises above the ventricular tissue, the conduction across the common bundle of His and into the ventricles is normal. As a result, the pattern of ventricular conduction is usually unaffected. Supraventricular premature contractions that arise from tissue high in the atria usually result in a prolonged P-R interval because the atrial impulse reaches the A-V node during the relative refractory phase. The P wave thus remains in the A-V node longer, prolonging the P-R interval. Supraventricular premature beats with shorter P-R intervals are more likely to be associated with aberrant QRS complexes as a result of regular and rapid conduction across the A-V node and into a partially refractory ventricle. Occasionally, the premature P wave occurs so early that the impulse is blocked in the A-V node because the latter is in a state of absolute refractoriness from a previous conduction. In such cases, atrial premature contractions are blocked and a P wave that occurs early in the sequence is not followed by a QRS complex but rather by a long pause (Fig. 76–6*B*).

Supraventricular premature contractions are most often associated with resetting or resetting with pause. For purposes of identification, supraventricular premature contractions may be designated atrial or junctional. Atrial premature contractions are considered to arise higher in the atrial tissue. They are characterized by premature P waves that are abnormal in size and configuration and are usually associated with a prolonged P-R interval and a normal QRS-T complex following the premature beat. Junctional premature beats (also referred to as atrioventricular or nodal beats) are considered to result when the impulse arises from the region of the coronary sinus or the junctional A-V tissue. Although this is not always anatomically correct, electrocardiographically these junctional rhythms may be differentiated from atrial premature beats.

The clinical significance of both atrial and junctional premature beats is the same. The only valid reason to continue to identify these rhythms as such is to more readily identify abnormal configurations. Junctional premature contractions are characterized by negative P waves in leads II, III, and aVF; P waves that are premature and that are usually followed by a prolonged P-R interval; and a QRS-T complex that appears normal. The P-R interval may be shorter because of the shorter distance the impulse travels to the A-V node. In these instances, the P wave may occur before, during, or after the QRS complex. This may occur because retrograde conduction across the atrium is actually slower than the antegrade conduction of that impulse through the ventricle.

Supraventricular premature contractions are associated with atrial dilatation and atrial myocarditis. They have been reported to occur in cats with hyperthyroidism.[24] These contractions may precede the onset of established atrial fibrillation. They are generally considered a result of atrial irritability due to diseases such as valvular disease, pericarditis, endocarditis, atrial tumors, and heartworms. Supraventricular premature contractions also result from digitalis intoxication, sympathomimetic amines, some anesthetic agents, toxic agents affecting the S-A node, hypoxia, hypokalemia, and decreased vagal tone with increased irritability in the area of the atrioventricular node.

Clinical Signs. Generally, animals are asymptomatic, although signs such as syncope and paroxysms of weakness may accompany frequent premature contractions. During auscultation of the heart, the premature beats occur early and are generally followed by a pause. When the ectopic contraction occurs, the intensity of the heart sounds is often different from that of the normal beat. A pulse deficit may be associated with premature contractions. Since premature beats result in early contractions of the ventricle, the period of atrial systole may be incomplete. This may result in a temporary diminished intensity of murmurs otherwise present. The beat following the premature beat may be correspondingly louder owing to additional filling of the ventricle and a subsequently increased myocardial contraction. When no murmurs are present, a premature beat may cause a slight murmur owing to temporary A-V valvular incompetency. Supraventricular premature contractions will be at times associated with splitting of the second heart sound.

Treatment is not usually indicated for occasional supraventricular premature contractions. When this rhythm disturbance occurs, atrial disease is considered likely and signs of heart failure may be present. In such cases, digitalization improves cardiac function by increasing the strength of muscular contraction and slowing atrioventricular conduction. B blocking agents such as propranolol are used when frequent supraventricular premature beats occur. This drug slows A-V nodal conduction and may help to reduce the frequency of such beats. It is usually given along with digitalis but may be used alone if heart failure or insufficiency is not a problem. Refractory cases are rarely treated with quinidine to decrease the frequency of the abnormal contractions. Calcium channel blockers such as verapamil may occasionally be used (see Antiarrhythmic Agents).

Ventricular Premature Contractions

Ectopic foci that arise anywhere within the ventricles and result in premature depolarization and contraction of the ventricle are ventricular premature contractions (VPC) (premature ventricular contractions, PVC; ventricular premature beat, VPB) (Figures 76–8 and 76–9). The closer the ectopic impulse is to the bundle of His, the more normal the ventricular complex will be. The ventricular premature contraction may be conducted through the myocardium at a slower than normal rate. This results in a wide and aberrant QRS complex. Ventricular premature beats are usually followed by a compensatory pause and/or less commonly, appear in the interpolated form (see Figure 76–5). Resetting and resetting with pause following an ectopic ventricular rhythm are unusual.

Because the S-A node continues to discharge at its normal rate and because impulses arising from the ventricle are not usually conducted in a retrograde manner to the atria, normal sinus P waves occur at their regular interval. The normal P wave is not always clearly observed, since it may occur during the period of the aberrant QRS complex. The compensatory pause following a ventricular premature contraction occurs because the sinus P waves reach the A-V node while that node is refractory, owing to partial but incomplete retrograde conduction from the ventricular premature contraction. Thus, the interval from the P wave of the normal beat preceding the ventricular premature contraction to the P wave in the next normal cycle, following the ectopic rhythm, is exactly that of two normal P-P intervals.

Ventricular premature contractions are beats occurring with a premature, prolonged, and bizarre-appearing QRS-T complex. The P wave is unrelated to the abnormal QRS-T complex. Occasionally, the QRS-T complex appears normal or nearly normal because the ectopic rhythm arose near the common bundle of His. In such cases, impulse conduction is through normal ventricular conduction pathways, which then results in a normal to slightly modified ventricular complex.

Ventricular premature contractions (and ventricular tachycardia) are associated with almost all cardiovascular diseases when the heart muscle is damaged, irritated, or made hypoxic; with myocardial fibrosis and mechanical irritation; and with drug intoxications involving, for example, digitalis, antiarrhythmic agents, ingested poisons, chemotherapeutic agents, and following intravenous anesthetic administration of the short-acting barbiturates and some narcoleptic agents, such as xylazine. Toxemia due to noncardiac medical problems may be associated secondarily with VPC formation. The toxemia may be caused by renal failure, gastric dilatation-volvulus complex, snake bites, and some cancerous conditions, to name but a few. Anxiety, stress, severe pain, cardiac catheterization, and manipulation of the heart during surgery are other causes. A list of individual causes of ventricular premature beats is beyond the scope of this chapter; suffice it to say that disease, drugs, hyperthyroidism, and physical irritants are all capable of inducing arrhythmias. A thorough search of all sys-

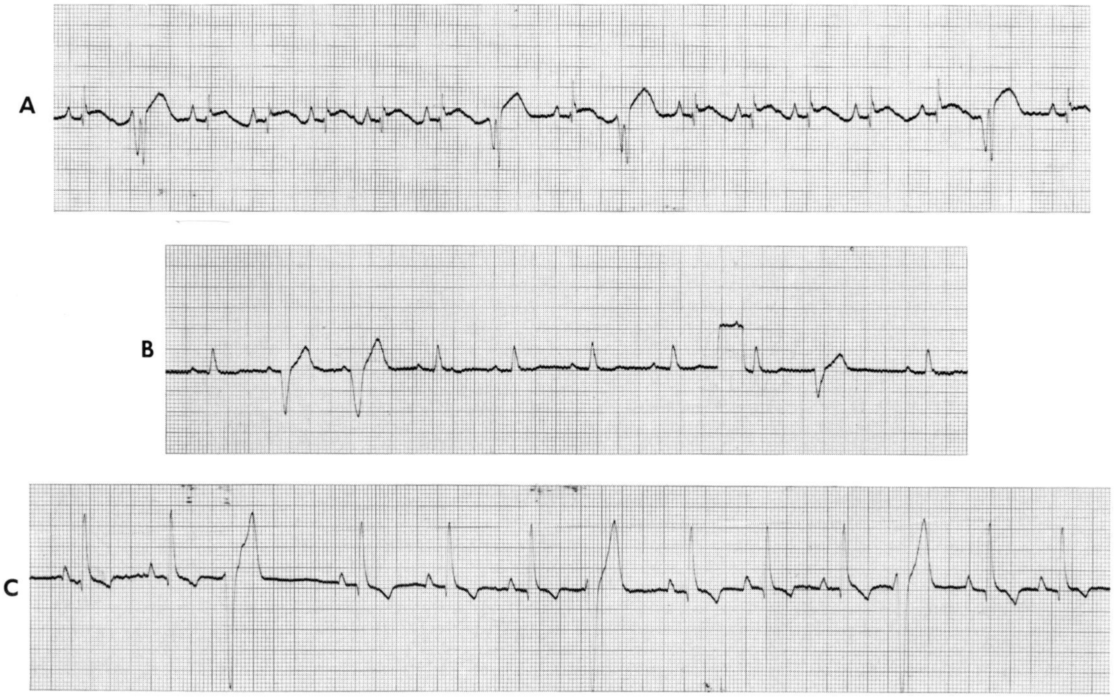

FIGURE 76–8. Ventricular premature contractions. *A* shows that the normal rhythm of this cat in lead II is interrupted by single ventricular premature contractions. The VPCs occur slightly prematurely and are without normal P waves, and the QRS complexes are aberrant in nature. At postmortem examination there were large areas of myocardial fibrosis involving both ventricles. *B*, The lead II tracing of this cat indicates a normal sinus rhythm interrupted by a pair of ventricular premature beats and later in the tracing, by a single ventricular premature contraction. The abnormal beats occur prematurely, although P waves occur in their normal interval during the first two premature beats. The ventricular premature beats were the result of active leukemia affecting the myocardium. These were controlled with antiarrhythmic agents during the initial phases of therapy. *C* shows ventricular premature beats interrupting the rhythm (lead III electrocardiogram) of a Boston bulldog. The abnormal beats are characterized by being premature and aberrant in form. The normal rhythm is not grossly interrupted by the beats. This arrhythmia was associated with a nonspecific myocarditis and was controlled with antiarrhythmic agents.

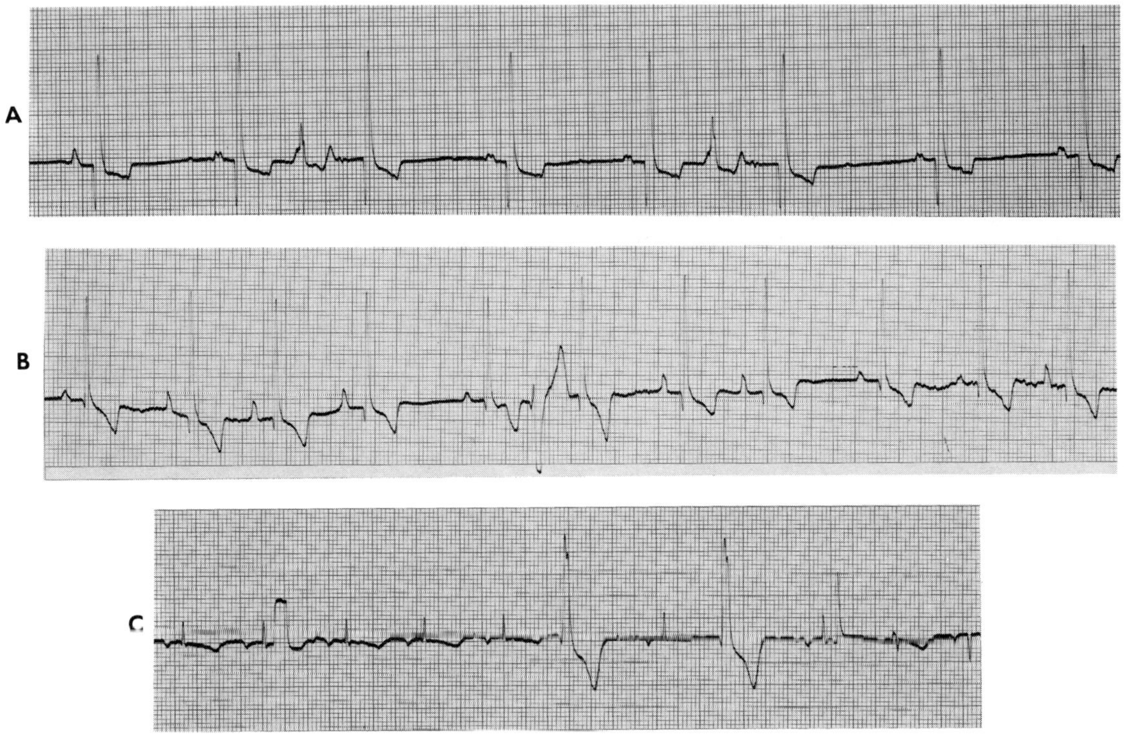

FIGURE 76–9. Ventricular premature contractions. *A* demonstrates an interpolated ventricular premature contraction characterized by a premature beat occurring between two normally placed electrocardiographic complexes. The premature beats (3 and 7) do not interfere with the sinus arrhythmia in this lead II tracing from a dog. In *B,* an interpolated ventricular premature contraction is noted in the tracing of lead II. Note that the T wave for the complex following the premature beat appears to be buried in the T wave of the interpolated beat. There is slight aberrancy of the QRS complex following the ectopic beat as demonstrated by a slightly irregular T wave. *C* shows ventricular premature beat present in a cat with a thyroid adenoma. The cat was placed on propranolol therapy, surgery was performed, and repeat electrocardiographic tracings over the next year did not demonstrate any further arrhythmias.

tems and exogenous causes is necessary whenever such a problem is recognized. Ectopic beats are considered very serious when they occur frequently, when they are multifocal, or when two or more occur in a row. The presence of premature ventricular contractions in the dog is generally considered to be pathologic.[1, 25] The presence of frequent VPCs suggests the need for antiarrhythmic therapy. Five to ten abnormal beats per minute should be considered a guideline rather than a definitive level at which therapy is indicated. At times, it may be desirable to treat even fewer VPCs per minute if symptomatology is suspected.

Clinical Signs. Single ventricular premature contractions usually do not cause clinical symptoms. Multiple premature contractions may result in syncope, spells of weakness or faintness, and occasionally, seizure-like activity. During auscultation of the heart, the ectopic contraction occurs early and the beat is usually associated with a lower intensity cardiac sound than normal. It is usually followed immediately by a more intense sound, since additional time has allowed blood to fill the ventricle more completely. A pulse deficit is usually associated with ventricular premature contractions.

Ventricular premature contractions may be the result of digitalis intoxication, and in such cases, digitalis should be discontinued. Antiarrhythmic agents may be used when ventricular premature contractions are not drug-induced. When decreased cardiac efficiency results in ventricular premature contractions, the use of cardiac glycosides may be indicated. In such cases, the digitalis agent should used with electrocardiographic and close clinical supervision.

Dogs and cats with atrial fibrillation and reduced myocardial performance, such as caused by congestive cardiomyopathy, frequently develop ventricular premature contractions. Therapeutic digitalization often diminishes the frequency of these beats. Cats suffering from congestive cardiomyopathy at times have ventricular arrhythmias present that also respond to digitalis therapy along with diuretics and β-adrenergic blockade. Premature beats associated with short-acting barbiturate anesthetics occur quite frequently soon after anesthetic induction. These usually do not require medical treatment unless they fail to resolve after 15 to 20 minutes or there is associated organic heart disease, attacks of paroxysmal atrial tachycardia, the presence of the "R on T" phenomenon, accelerating repetitive extrasystoles, multifocal ventricular arrhythmias, or digitalis intoxication.[26]

CLASSIFICATION OF PREMATURE CONTRACTIONS

Premature contractions that arise from a single ectopic focus, that are constant in form, and that have either a regular P-P (supraventricular premature contractions) or R-R interval (ventricular premature contractions) are referred to as coupled beats or unifocal premature

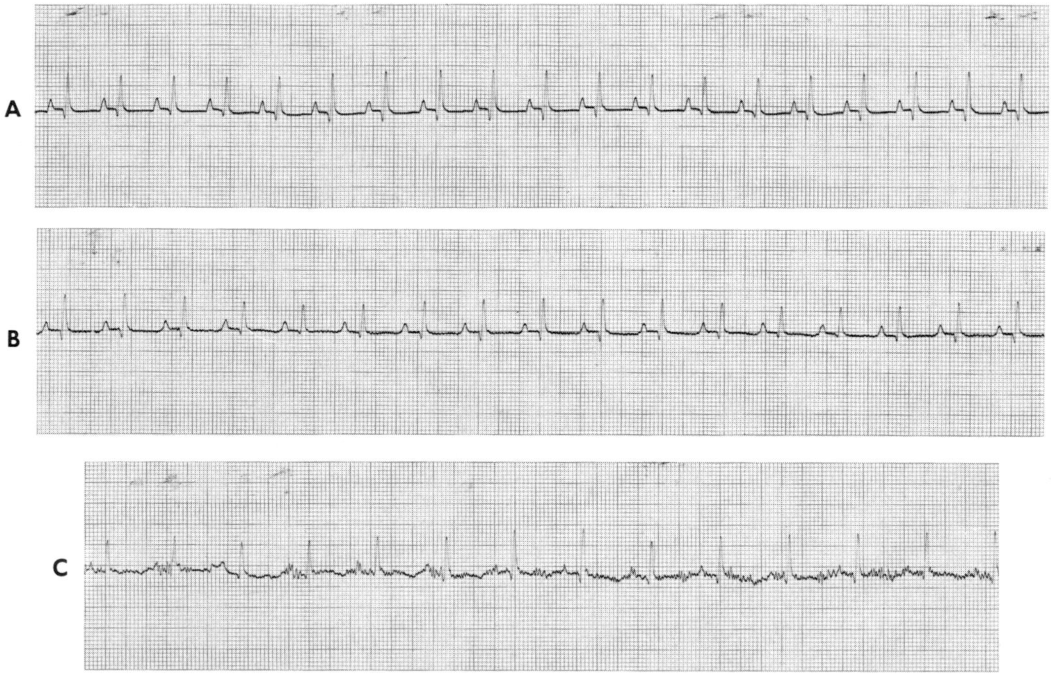

FIGURE 76–10. *A* shows supraventricular tachycardia occurring during anesthesia. A heart rate of 240 beats per minute occurred when the patient was monitored shortly after induction of anesthesia. This increased rate continued for several minutes. 0.15 mg of Inderal was administered intravenously, and the heart rate slowed immediately to 200 beats per minute *(B)* and shortly thereafter to 180 per minute *(C)*. The surgical procedure was uneventful and the patient recovered normally.

contractions. When multifocal (more than one focus is present), the P-P or R-R interval may vary, and the premature beats vary in form.

Premature beats may occur singly, irregularly, or in repetitive patterns. When two premature beats occur in sequence, they are referred to as a pair; three are a run and four or more compose a tachycardia. Paroxysmal tachycardia indicates bursts of four or more abnormal beats, initially preceded by a premature contraction.

Bigeminy describes a normal beat followed by a single premature contraction; trigeminy refers to a premature contraction occurring after two normal beats. The terminology of pairs, runs, tachycardia, bigeminy, trigeminy, and so on is used for both supraventricular and ventricular rhythms.

THE TACHYCARDIAS

The normal heart rate in medium-sized and large breeds of dogs should not exceed 160 beats per minute. The heart rate in the toy breeds and in young dogs may be as high as 180 beats per minute. In cats and puppies, the normal heart rate may be as high as 220 or 230 beats per minute. When rates exceed these limits, the term tachycardia is appropriate. A tachycardia refers to bursts of the cardiac rhythm at an abnormally rapid rate, either in paroxysms (four or more in sequence) or as a continuous rhythm.

Tachycardias are classified as supraventricular or ventricular in origin. Supraventricular tachycardias (Figures 76–10 through 76–12), like the supraventricular premature beat, include those thought to arise from the atria as well as those thought to arise from the region of atrioventricular junctional tissue. Ventricular tachycardias are associated with bundle of His or idioventricular rhythms occurring paroxysmally or continuously.

Supraventricular Tachycardia

The most common tachycardia arising within the supraventricular tissue is sinus tachycardia (Figure 76–10). In this condition, the heart rate exceeds the upper limits of normal. The electrocardiographic complexes are usually normal, although occasionally tall P waves occur in association with a rapid cardiac rate. A variable or regular P-P wave is present. Significant sinus arrhythmia usually disappears during periods of more rapid cardiac rhythm. When the heart rate is so rapid that the period of electrical diastole is shortened, there may be superimposition of the T and P waves. Sinus tachycardia usually slows when vagal maneuvers are performed, although the rate increases after the maneuvers are stopped.

In contrast to sinus tachycardia, atrial tachycardia (Figure 76–11) occurs as either a paroxysm or a continuous rhythm (Figure 76–12). In this rhythm, the abnormal focus is in the atrium. There is a perfectly regular cardiac rate with a regular R-R interval. Usually the P wave is different from that of the normal sinus P wave. The abnormal P wave may be buried within the previous T wave in very rapid rate disturbances. Vagal maneuvers usually break paroxysmal atrial tachycardia.

When the rapid cardiac rate is associated with QRS

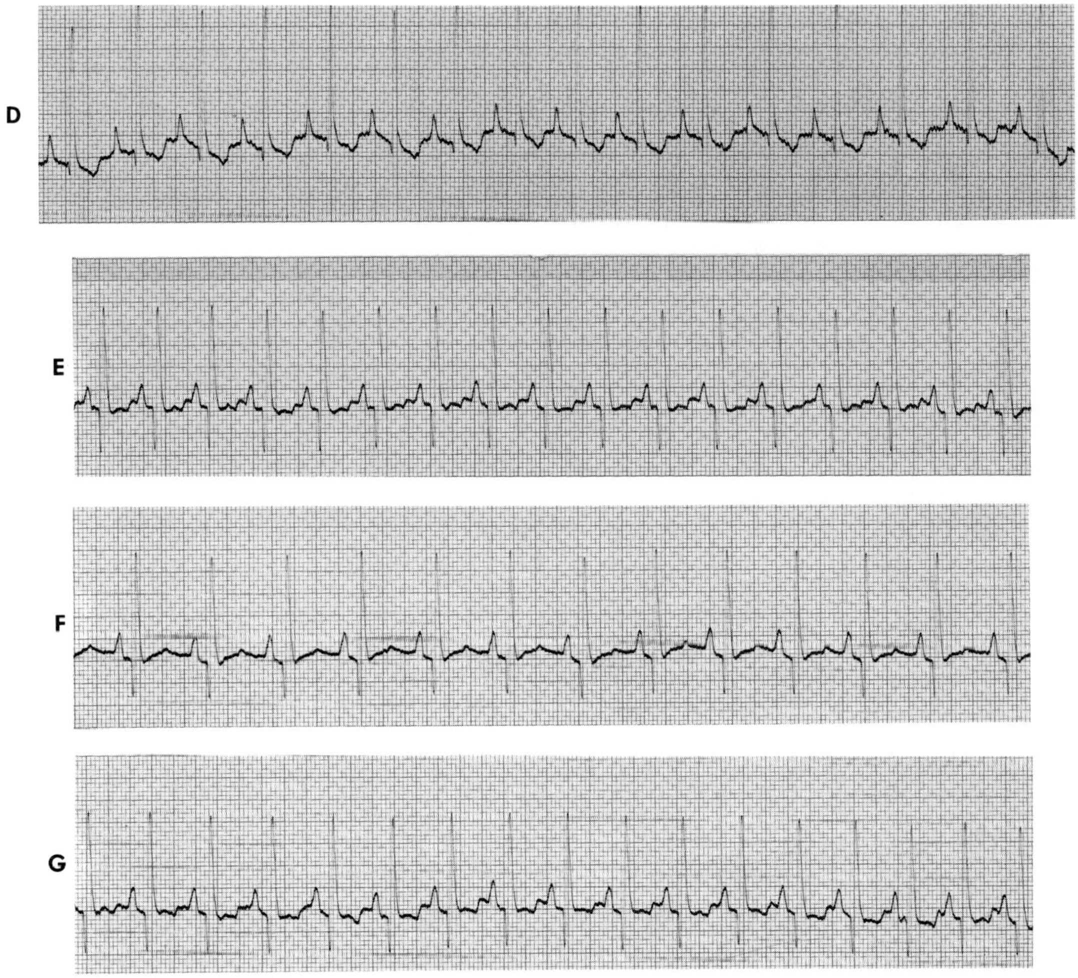

FIGURE 76–10 *Continued D* shows sinus tachycardia in a dog with congestive heart failure. The rate is rapid, between 210 and 220 per minute with slight R-R variations (14 or 15 boxes). Often when the rate increases significantly, P pulmonale or an increase in height of the P waves occurs, suggesting right atrial strain. *E, F,* and *G* are lead II tracings from a dog with sinus tachycardia presented for episodic weakness. These recurring episodes were of uncertain etiology but could be controlled with mild tranquilization. Note the rapid rate in *E* and *G*, which slowed only temporarily when ocular pressure was gently applied in strip *F*.

complexes that are preceded by negative P waves or by P waves occurring within the QRS complex, the rhythm is said to arise from the coronary sinus or the region of atrioventricular junctional tissue. This descriptive terminology merely helps to identify the appearance of the abnormal electrocardiographic findings. It is important to define the origin of the rhythm, since rapid rhythms occurring with normal QRS complexes but without associated P waves may arise from or near the bundle of His and may be ventricular rather than supraventricular in origin.

Usually in supraventricular tachycardia, the ventricular complexes are normal in appearance. This may be modified, however, by aberrancy or bundle-branch block.

Supraventricular tachycardias are recognized in nervous patients; in those with fever, anemia, toxemia, congestive heart failure, and hyperthyroidism; following electric shock, snake bites, and some poisonings; in hypercalcemic states; and in other medical states, especially those associated with pain. These rhythms may occur in association with atrial disease and often are associated with chronic mitral valvular insufficiency, cardiomyopathies, and many congenital heart defects. Electrophysiologic abnormalities and concurrent alterations in the cell structure were reported to be involved in feline atrial tachyarrhythmias induced by cardiomyopathy.[27] Infiltrative atrial diseases and atrial myocarditis due to other causes may also be responsible. Supraventricular tachycardias may be induced during cardiac catheterization, as well as during general surgery. A supraventricular tachycardia associated with inhalation anesthesia may occur. This most often arises when preanesthetic agents other than atropine are omitted.

Clinical signs. Although the pulse rate and the heart sounds are rapid and regular, murmurs are not usually present unless there is underlying cardiac disease responsible for the hemodynamic disturbance. Murmurs are usually auscultated when anemia is responsible for the rapid cardiac rate or when congestive heart failure is associated with anatomic intracardiac pathology. Murmurs are less obvious when excessively rapid rates occur and when marked pulmonary pathology, such as pulmonary edema, is present.

Fainting, with or without incontinence and occasionally, with convulsions, is one of the major clinical

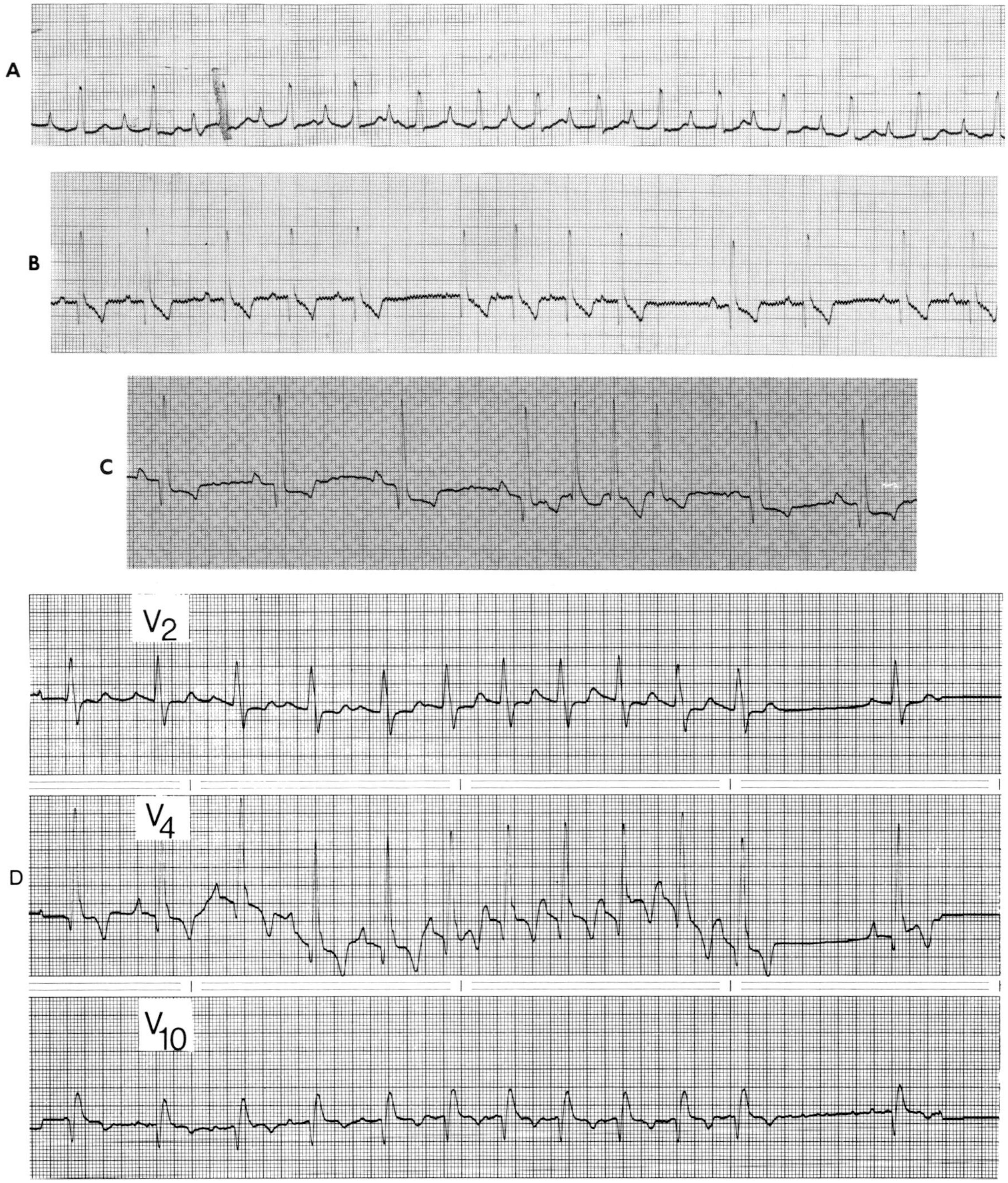

FIGURE 76–11. Supraventricular tachycardia. *A* shows a paroxysmal atrial tachycardia. The third complex is a supraventricular premature beat with an early and irregular P wave. It is followed by a run of nine regular beats arising from irritable atrial foci. The paroxysms with a rate of 180 per minute break after the tenth beat in the run, and the heart returns to a slower sinus rhythm of 143 beats per minute. The atrial tachycardia was associated with weakness, crying, and occasional brief seizures. The prolonged P-R interval, 0.16 second, was present prior to any therapy and suggests severe atrial enlargement and conduction delay. *B* shows a burst of paroxysmal supraventricular tachycardia that occurred in this Boston terrier with chronic mitral valvular disease. The patient was experiencing periodic episodes of syncope. Note the regularity of the R to R interval during the paroxysm of four beats. The heart rate at the time was momentarily 200 beats per minute. These episodes could be terminated by inducing vagal pressure by pressing on the eyeballs. *C* is a rhythm strip that demonstrates a burst of paroxysmal atrial tachycardia initiated by a supraventricular premature contraction (beat 4). The atrial tachycardia is brief, three beats only, and then the rhythm returns to its more normal state. During such paroxysms, the owner may be aware of weakness, staggering, or syncope in the pet. *D* is a simultaneous lead V_2, V_4, and V_{10} tracing from a dog during a syncopal episode. This standard poodle had congestive cardiomyopathy. The tracing demonstrates left atrial and left ventricular enlargement. The fourth beat is an atrial premature beat that begins the paroxysmal tachycardia. The tachyarrhythmia ends with an 0.84-second pause before a sinus beat occurs.

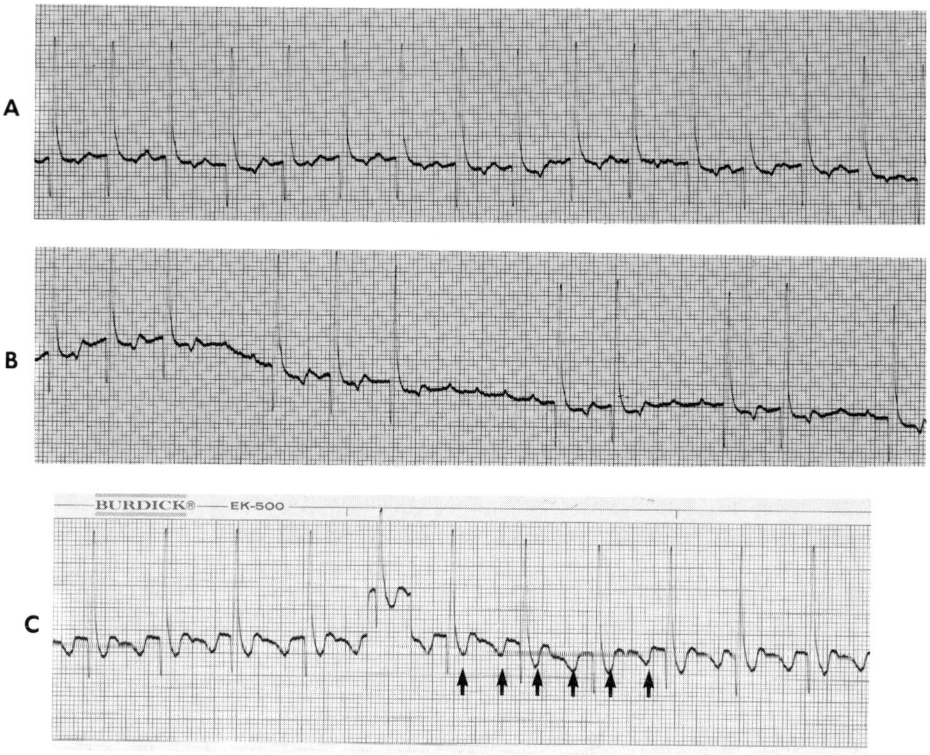

FIGURE 76–12. Atrial tachycardia. *A* shows a poodle with chronic mitral valve disease, coughing, and weakness with a rapid heart rate of 240 per minute. Gentle ocular pressure caused the persistent atrial tachycardia *(A)* to break, and paroxysmal atrial tachycardia *(B)* with varying degrees of block resulted. Note the regularity of the P waves and its continuity, indicating regular rapid atrial rhythm with block at or below the level of the A-V node. Digoxin therapy was begun, the dog improved clinically, and the ventricular rate *(C)* slowed to about 200 per minute, but a persistent 2:1 block was present. Note the negative P waves occurring at a regular interval during the latter portion of the QRS and early T waves, as well as just preceding each QRS complex (arrows). A standardization impulse during beat 5 is present in this tracing.

findings in chronic mitral valvular fibrosis associated with paroxysmal atrial tachycardia. Occasionally, the owner may report episodes of weakness and disorientation in the pet. Many of these episodes are presumed to be due to paroxysmal supraventricular tachycardia. The presence of frequent supraventricular premature contractions on the electrocardiogram and fainting or weakness in the history permit a presumptive diagnosis of paroxysmal atrial tachycardia as the cause of syncope or spells of weakness, or both (see Chapter 11).

Treatment. For the temporary relief of supraventricular tachycardia, carotid sinus or ocular pressure increases vagal tone enough to depress the ectopic atrial pacemaker. Intravenous vasopressors are rarely necessary to induce vagal cardiac stimulation.

In patients with congestive heart failure, therapeutic digitalization may be indicated to terminate such an arrhythmia. When the arrhythmia is not due to cardiac failure, the β-adrenergic blocking agent propranolol (Inderal) is useful, especially for anesthesia-induced supraventricular tachyarrhythmias. Direct-current cardioversion is another effective method for restoring a slower sinus rhythm.

Atrial dysrhythmias are often observed in dogs following the gastric dilatation-volvulus syndrome, usually in association with various ventricular rhythm disturbances.

ACCELERATED CONDUCTION TACHYARRHYTHMIAS (PRE-EXCITATION SYNDROMES)

An uncommon arrhythmia with dramatic clinical and electrocardiographic findings is observed when a sinus impulse is conducted through the atria and into the ventricles by way of an accessory conduction pathway before the impulse can be conducted through the normal A-V nodal conduction system.

Three types of accessory tract atrioventricular conduction have been described.[28] In the WPW syndrome the right lateral (Kent) bundle(s) connect the right atrium and ventricle. Another pathway uses the James fibers (posterior internodal tract), while a third type, called the Mahaim type, has abnormal beats that originate below the region of normal delay in the A-V conduction system. The Kent and James types have short P-R intervals, a delta wave in the QRS complex, and normal to prolonged QRS complexes. The Mahaim type of accessory conduction has a normal P-R interval and a long QRS with a delta wave.

Dysrhythmias involving pre-excitation in both dogs and cats, while unusual, have been described.[19, 28–30] The overall incidence of the problem is unknown. In humans there is a significant incidence of tachyarrhythmias associated with pre-excitation syndromes. Most often paroxysmal supraventricular tachycardia is observed, although other arrhythmias may also be observed. Chaotic rhythms with extremely rapid and aberrant ventricular rates may develop, perhaps owing to atrial fibrillation and antegrade conduction over the accessory pathway.

Clinical signs are usually absent unless a tachyarrhythmia is present. In the few clinical cases seen in dogs and cats where signs do occur, weakness, syncopal episodes, and congestive heart failure were the predominant clinical features. Cardiomegaly has been a finding uniformly present in dogs and cats observed by the author with these arrhythmias. Murmurs are variably present, and gallop sounds occur during the periods of slower rates in those animals demonstrating congestive heart failure.

The electrocardiograms are variable, probably because of the variety of accessory conduction pathways that are factors. The P-R intervals vary from short to normal; delta waves appear either just before or within the initial period of ventricular conduction. The QRS complexes vary from normal with a delta wave, to normal in appearance, though wide, to aberrant and prolonged (Figures 76–13 and 76–14).

Treatment is aimed principally at preventing or controlling tachyarrhythmias. Vagal stimulation and valsalva maneuvers are used for humans with this disorder, but in small animals drug therapy appears to be required in most cases. In acute cases, intravenous and oral verapamil, a slow-channel blocking agent, is now considered the first line of therapy for terminating the circus tachycardia. It must be cautiously administered intravenously, slowly over a three-minute period. If the animal is already on β-blocking agents, the dosage should be further reduced since bradycardia and hypotension are likely to develop.[31] Quinidine, procainamide, and propranolol either alone or in combination have been successfully used to increase the refractory period of the accessory pathway so that reentry becomes impossible, thereby permitting normal antegrade A-V nodal conduction to take place. Other drugs useful in humans with WPW tachycardia include tensilon, disopyramide, encainide, and amiodarone (see Table 76–1 for more specific information). Electrical DC cardioversion is rarely available at most veterinary hospitals, but it, too, provides an effective means of treating the dysrhythmia, particularly if atrial fibrillation is present. Caution is required when administering any of these drugs, because adverse effects can develop. Digitalis is at times avoided, since it may depress normal A-V conduction and accelerate the anomalous conduction.[32] Surgical interruption of the anomalous pathway(s) is being used in some humans who have been drug-resistant, but this possibility has not been explored in veterinary medicine.

ATRIAL FIBRILLATION

Atrial fibrillation (Figure 76–15) is characterized by the absence of an atrial systole. Instead, the atria transmit numerous rapid, irregular, and fractionated impulses to the A-V node. Many impulses excite the A-V node. Some enter the node but fail to emerge; others emerge at an irregular rate. Atrial fibrillation is thought to result from multiple and concurrent circulating reentrant excitation wave fronts.[33] Consequently, the ventricular rate that follows is both rapid and irregular. The normal atrial P waves are replaced by baseline undulations (F waves) on the electrocardiogram. Normal to slightly aberrant ventricular complexes occur irregularly and usually at a rapid rate. Because atrial fibrillation is often associated with cardiomegaly, a left bundle branch block pattern, producing additional QRS aberrancy, may be observed on the ECG tracing. Right bundle branch block and atrial fibrillation have been observed by the author in both congenital and acquired cardiac disorders (Figure 76–15). This gives the ECG a particularly aberrant pattern. When the ventricular rate is

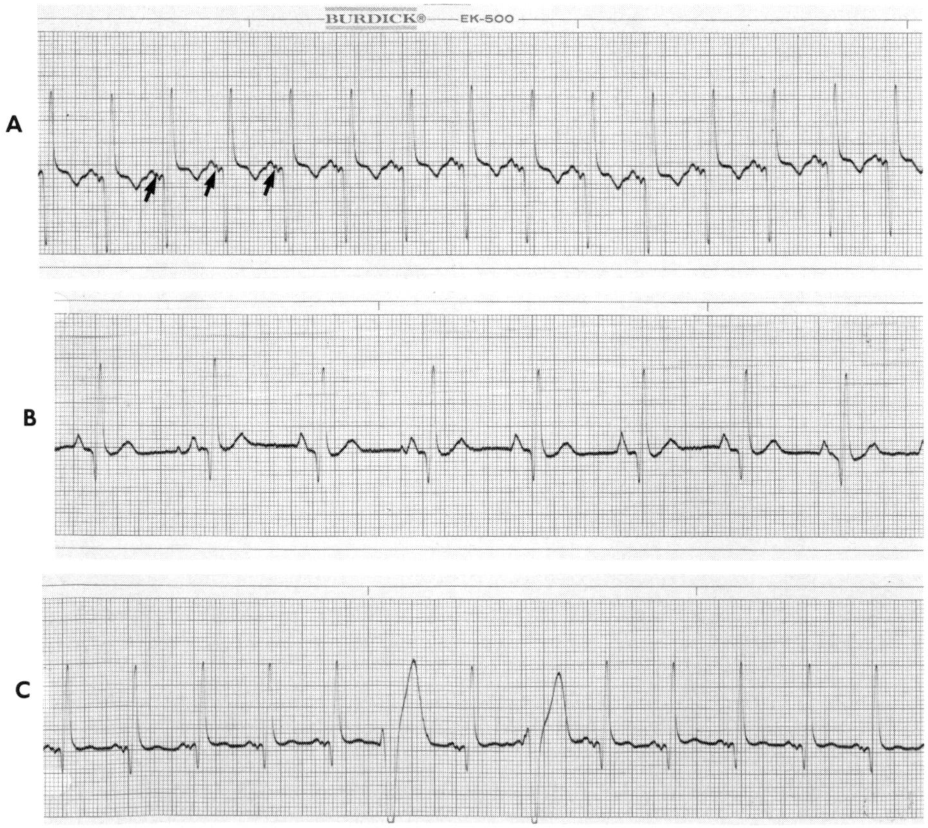

FIGURE 76–13. Accelerated conduction syndrome. This middle-aged Doberman pinscher was presented with congestive heart failure with a rapid regular heart rate and pulse. Previous symptomatology was absent. *A* is a lead II tracing with a short P-R interval (0.07 sec) and a rapid heart rate (222 per minute). A delta wave appears in the P-R segment (arrow). IV propranolol *(B)* slowed the rate and prolonged the P-R interval, but the arrhythmia returned *(C)* after six minutes, along with occasional ventricular premature contractions. The rhythm was ultimately controlled only with the combined therapy of quinidine, procainamide, and propranolol given orally. Treatment had been successful for over one year when the animal suddenly developed acute pulmonary edema and died.

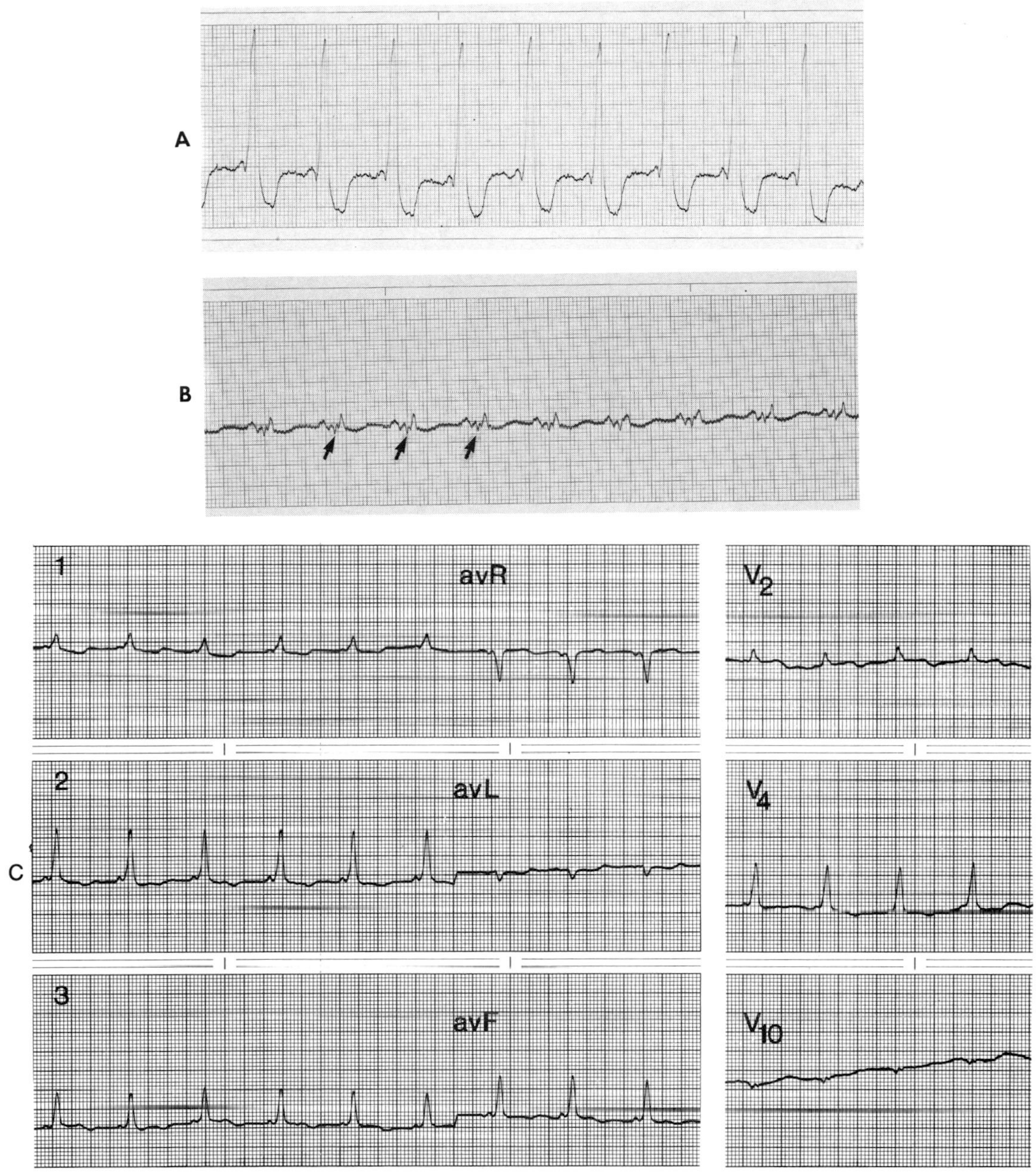

FIGURE 76–14. Accelerated conduction syndrome in a cat. *A* is a lead II tracing at twice normal amplitude. The short P-R interval and wide, slightly aberrant QRS complexes were present when the cat was seen with marked respiratory distress. Digoxin and diuretic therapy controlled the symptomatology. *B,* The P waves are followed by a biphasic wave (delta wave, arrow) in the P-R segment just at the initiation of the QRS complex. This tracing was taken while the cat was in clinical remission during drug therapy. *C* represents a nine lead electrocardiogram from a cat with an accelerated conduction abnormality. The cat periodically has rapid tachycardia, severe dyspnea, and anxiety. This tracing was taken after the rhythm was slowed with oral verapamil. The P-R interval is abbreviated, there is a hint of a delta wave, and the QRS is prolonged.

either extremely rapid or slow, the marked irregularity of the rhythm may be less obvious during auscultation. Concealed conduction refers to incomplete penetration of the A-V junction by an atrial impulse. This may delay formation or conduction of a subsequent impulse. Concealed conduction is an important factor in the sporadically irregular ventricular rate associated with atrial fibrillation.[2]

Atrial fibrillation should be considered a serious disturbance of the cardiac rhythm. It is almost invariably associated with significant and advanced cardiac disease. It is generally associated with considerable enlargement of one or both atria.

Atrial fibrillation has been reported to occur predominantly in the male dog and published studies have been reviewed.[34, 35] The condition is associated with both congenital and acquired cardiac diseases. It may also occur in association with noncardiac diseases that result in electrolyte disturbances with secondary cardiac manifestations.

Atrial fibrillation is unusual in dogs that weigh less than ten pounds and in cats (Figure 76–16), although it

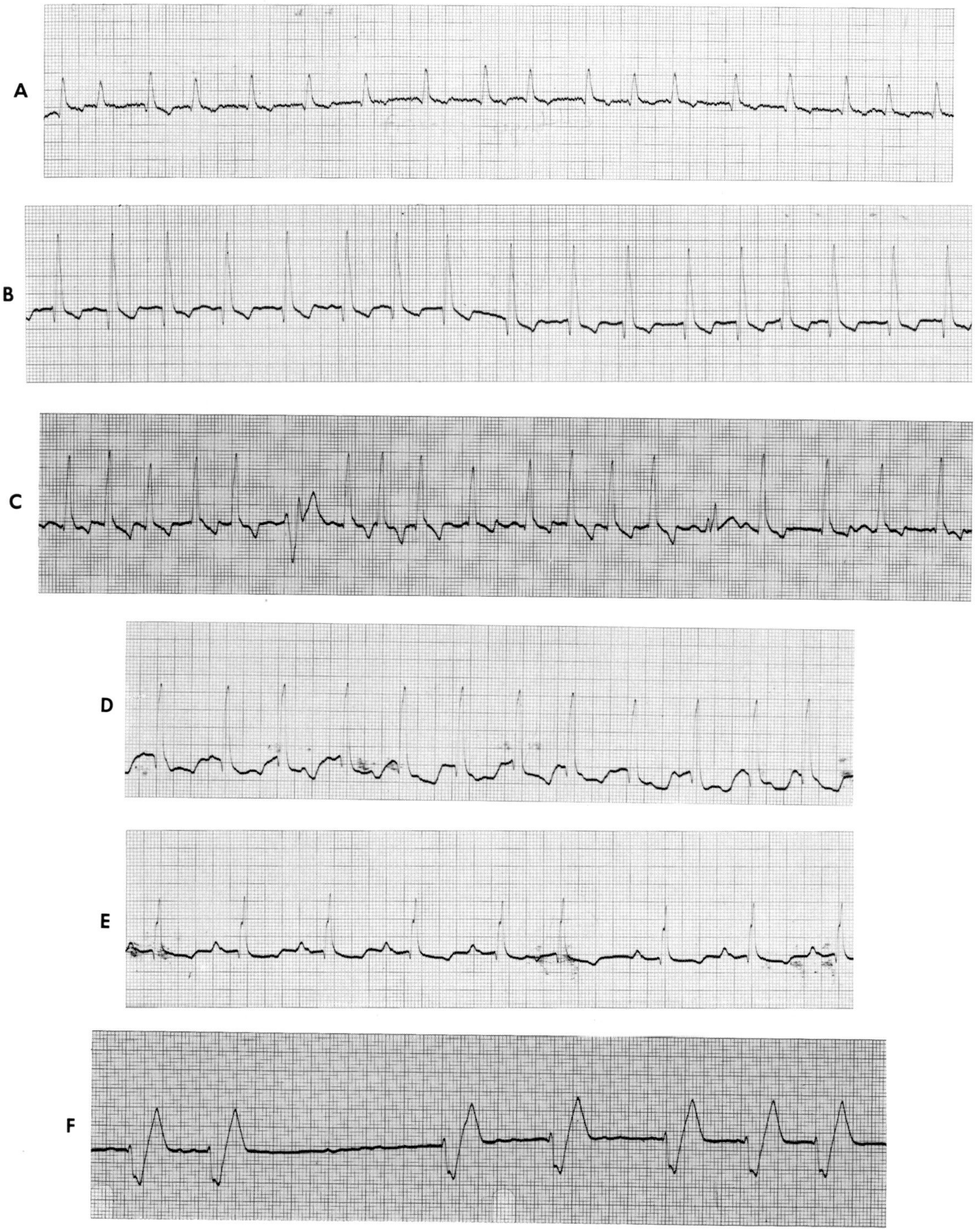

FIGURE 76–15 *See legend on opposite page*

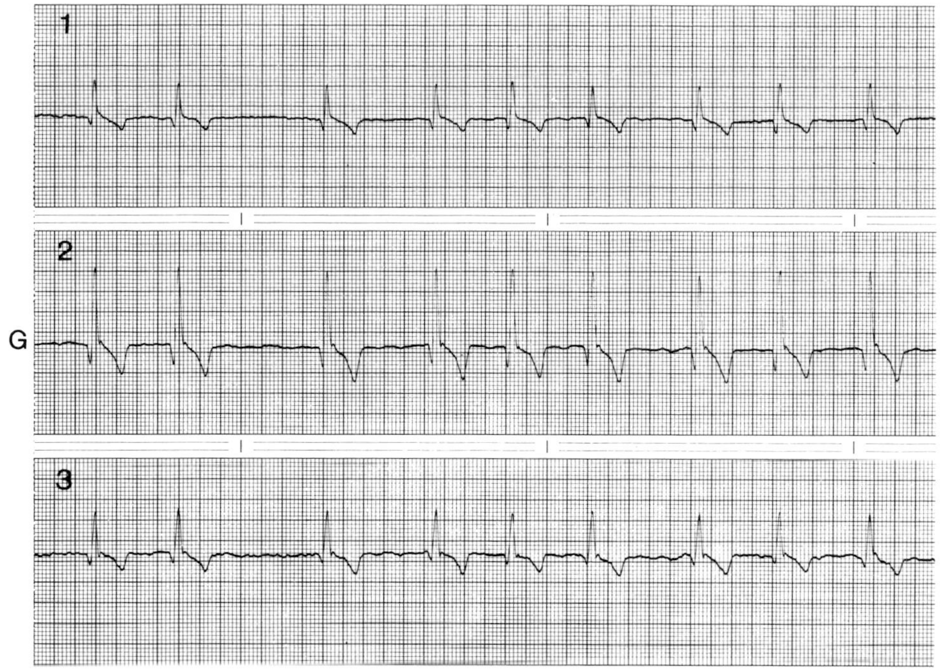

FIGURE 76–15. Atrial fibrillation. *A* is a lead II tracing from a Great Dane presented for coughing, respiratory distress, and weight loss. The heart rate was rapid and irregular, and there was a marked pulse deficit on physical examination. The heart rate varied from 190 to 200 beats per minute. There are no P waves on the electrocardiogram; instead, there is an irregular undulating baseline. The QRS complexes occur irregularly and are somewhat variable in appearance owing to slight ventricular aberrancy. The patient had idiopathic congestive cardiomyopathy. *B,* A lead II tracing from a dog with congestive heart failure secondary to patent ductus arteriosus. The heart rate of 180 beats per minute was rapid and irregular. The electrocardiogram demonstrates atrial fibrillation with absent P waves and an irregular baseline. The QRS complexes occur irregularly and are wide, indicating left ventricular hypertrophy. The atrial fibrillation returned to normal sinus rhythm, without electrical or drug therapy, after the ductus was ligated. *C* is a lead II tracing of a dog with a chronic mitral valve disease, an enlarged left atrium, and a rapid, irregular cardiac rate with pulse deficit. This tracing demonstrates atrial fibrillation and intermittent ventricular premature contractions. Although the baseline occasionally suggests atrial activity, regularly spaced P waves are in fact absent. The irregular ventricular rate strongly supports the diagnosis clinically and the ECG confirms the arrhythmia. *D* is a lead II tracing of a dog with atrial fibrillation secondary to chronic mitral valvular disease. The heart rate of 180 beats per minute was rapid and irregular. A 100 watt-second cardioverting shock was administered transthoracically. Normal sinus rhythm returned *(E)*. The sixth beat of tracing E demonstrates a junctional (supraventricular) premature contraction, which frequently is associated with chronic atrial enlargement and atrial irritability immediately following cardioversion. *F* shows a slow ventricular rate in a Newfoundland with medically stabilized congestive cardiomyopathy and right bundle branch block. Note the absence of P waves in this lead II tracing, the irregular baseline, and the irregular ventricular rate. Right bundle branch block was confirmed by the delayed rightward depolarization pattern in the other leads as well. *G* is a three-channel simultaneously recorded electrocardiogram from a German shepherd in atrial fibrillation associated with congestive cardiomyopathy. The baseline undulates irregularly and the ventricular complexes occur irregularly in sequence. P waves are absent and signs of left heart enlargement are present.

has been seen and described in both instances.[36] The disorder occurs primarily in the larger breeds, most often in association with idiopathic congestive cardiomyopathy (see Chapter 77). In one study, atrial fibrillation occurred 40 times more often in giant breeds than in other dogs.[35] In this author's experience, atrial fibrillation is observed most often in dogs with large left atria associated with idiopathic congestive cardiomyopathy, chronic mitral valvular fibrosis and insufficiency, and complicated patent ductus arteriosus. Its occurrence in association with pericardial and heartworm diseases is infrequent. In the cat, it is almost always observed in cardiomyopathy of either the congestive or hypertrophic form. It is rarely seen with other feline problems.

Nonprimary cardiac diseases such as pneumonia, pulmonary emboli, thoracic trauma, hypoadrenocorticism, mediastinal carcinoma, and lymphoma, as well as thoracic surgery, hyperthyroidism, and severe colic, have the potential of inducing atrial fibrillation.

Clinical Signs. The clinical signs of left- and/or right-sided heart failure are usually associated with atrial fibrillation in both the dog and cat. Other frequently associated clinical signs are syncope, weakness, weight loss, and ascites.

The heart rate is irregular and rapid, and a pulse deficit is apparent when the ventricular rate is rapid. The intensity of the heart sounds and murmurs is variable. The first heart sound varies in intensity; the second heart sound may be variably absent. Systolic murmurs also vary in both intensity and duration. In idiopathic congestive cardiomyopathy, systolic murmurs are usually absent. Not infrequently, the presence of gallop rhythms or accentuated diastolic heart sounds makes it difficult to interpret the heart sounds by auscultation alone.

Atrial fibrillation must be differentiated clinically from supraventricular premature contractions, ventricular premature contractions, atrial tachycardia, atrial flutter, and paroxysmal ventricular tachycardia.

Paroxysmal atrial fibrillation (Figure 76–17) has been

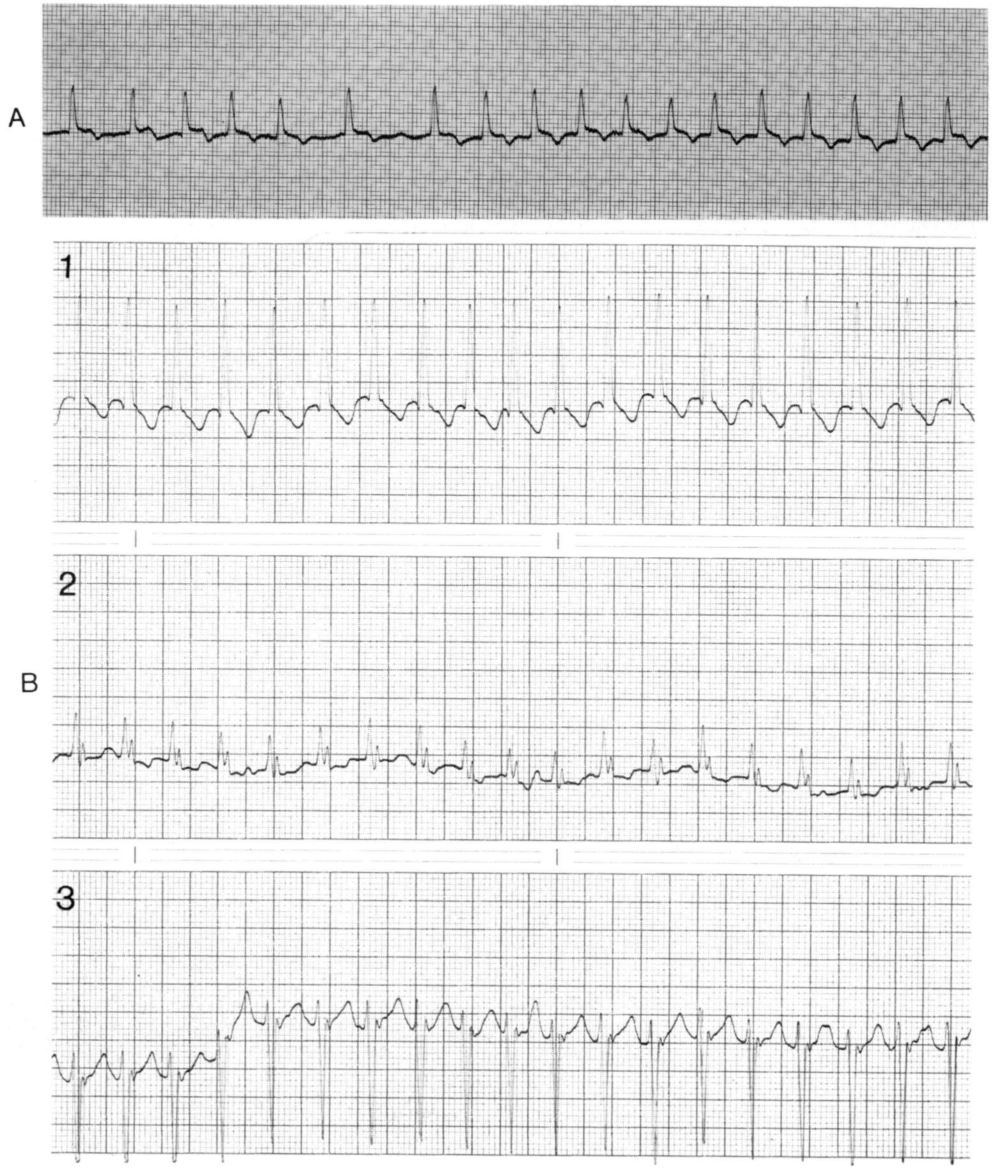

FIGURE 76–16. *A*, Atrial fibrillation in a cat. This is an infrequently recognized dysrhythmia, perhaps because atrial fibrillation is more common when the heart mass is greater. The characteristic features are similar to those of dogs. The height of the QRS complexes in this lead II tracing also suggests left heart enlargement, which was due to congestive cardiomyopathy. *B*, Leads 1, 2, and 3 recorded simultaneously from a cat with echocardiographically demonstrated hypertrophic cardiomyopathy. Atrial fibrillation was suspected when a rapid but slightly irregular rhythm was auscultated. In addition to an alteration in the electrical axis and normal QRS appearance, the ventricular complexes are slightly irregular in rhythm and P waves are absent.

reported.[30] Although established atrial fibrillation was not present in these cases, all of the patients had signs of significant cardiac disease, and established atrial fibrillation did develop in three of five reported cases after several months. In two dogs with paroxysmal atrial fibrillation, one was associated with pericardial effusion that resolved after pericardiocentesis and the second occurred in a dog with focal myocardial abnormalities.[37] It was reported to be due to myocardial irritability following trauma in another dog.[38]

Treatment. Because atrial fibrillation is commonly associated with signs of congestive heart failure, medical therapy should be instituted as soon as the clinical diagnosis is established.

Therapy for atrial fibrillation is generally the same as for other forms of congestive heart failure. The primary function of medical therapy is to slow the ventricular rate. Therefore, use of either digitalis or β-adrenergic blocking agents is initially suggested. Electrical DC cardioversion is an option rarely available to most practicing veterinarians.

Digitalis slows the ventricular rate through both vagal and extravagal influences by increasing the effective refractory period of the atrioventricular transmission

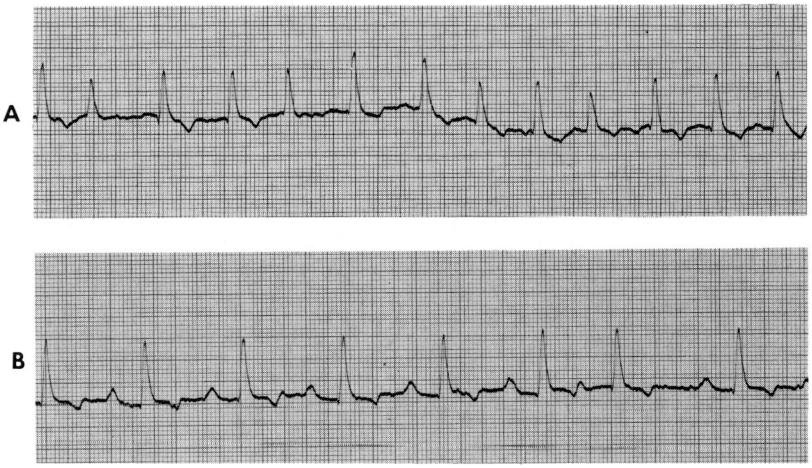

FIGURE 76–17. Paroxysmal atrial fibrillation. The rapid and irregular (220 ±) heart rate *(A)* of atrial fibrillation was noted when this dog was presented with signs of heart failure. While diagnostic studies were being completed, the rate slowed and became more regular *(B)*. *B* shows an enlarged left atrium, a prolonged P-R conduction time, and a supraventricular premature beat (beat 7). The dog was digitalized, and a sinus rhythm persisted for several months before atrial fibrillation once again recurred.

system and by increasing the atrial frequency. The latter increases the degree of A-V nodal concealed conduction, thus favorably slowing the ventricular rate. Digoxin is recommended for this purpose in both dogs and cats. Digitoxin has not been found to be effective in this condition by this author and others.[39] Toxic levels of digoxin may develop prior to adequate ventricular rate reduction. It is not wise to push digoxin levels, since dangerously high levels may develop. The best approach to follow is to administer digoxin in judicious amounts. When the heart fails to slow adequately, other forms of therapy, especially β-blocking agents or DC cardioversion, should be considered.

Propranolol (a β-adrenergic blocking agent) given orally is an effective therapeutic adjunct for slowing the ventricular rate. The negative inotropic effects of β-blocking agents should be considered when administering such drugs to patients in congestive heart failure, particularly those that have not been protected by therapeutic digitalization. This author usually administers digoxin and propranolol simultaneously to patients with atrial fibrillation. Since slowing of the ventricular rate effectively improves cardiac output, there appears to be little need for concern about the possible negative inotropism that could develop.

Quinidine may be used to convert atrial fibrillation to a normal sinus rhythm. The success rate in converting this arrhythmia to a normal sinus rhythm varies among clinicians. Regardless of medical conversion, the great likelihood of toxic side effects, the potential of inducing or aggravating congestive heart failure, and the extremely high return rate of atrial fibrillation within a very short period following quinidine therapy generally dictates that this drug not be used for this purpose in dogs or cats. An exception to this is atrial fibrillation of recent onset. Animals developing this rhythm after thoracic trauma or anesthesia may permanently convert to sinus rhythm after only a few doses of quinidine.

Direct-current cardioversion is a rapid and consistently effective method of restoring a normal sinus rhythm in atrial fibrillation in human beings.[40] Its use in dogs has also been demonstrated.[34, 41] Cardioversion depolarizes the entire heart momentarily. This allows the sinoatrial node to resume its normal pacemaking function. Cardioversion is performed in patients that have been removed from oral digitalis therapy for at least 24 hours. It is important to control congestive heart failure prior to cardioversion. Frequently, the rhythm returns to atrial fibrillation after a variable period of time. Cardioversion is generally recommended when the left atrium and general heart size are not too large or the disease process is not far advanced. In cases of longstanding, severe left atrial enlargement, cardioversion is either unlikely to occur or normal rhythm is only briefly restored. The benefits of cardioversion must be weighed against the danger of sedation and the struggle of the procedure itself.

Atrial fibrillation should be considered a serious arrhythmia. It is usually associated with significant cardiac disease. While this author enjoys a slightly increased therapeutic record, others observed that three-quarters of their dogs with atrial fibrillation died or were euthanatized within three months of the diagnosis.[35] Only 7 per cent of that series survived 12 months.

ATRIAL FLUTTER

An uncommon electrocardiographic finding in dogs is atrial flutter. It is considered even rarer in cats. In general, atrial flutter is found in heart disease associated with atrial enlargement, myocardial disease, cardiac catheterization, and developing supraventricular tachyarrhythmias or atrial fibrillation. Clinical signs are those associated with the diseases mentioned. Usually, the arrhythmia is distinguished only by electrocardiographic monitoring. The electrocardiogram reveals a regular, rapid atrial rhythm with normal atrial activation, resulting usually in a rapid but more regular ventricular rate than in atrial fibrillation (see Figure 76–18). Atrial flutter is normally a sign of progressive serious cardiac disease in the dog. Treatment may include attempts at drug (quinidine) cardioversion, or most likely, control of the ventricular rate with digoxin and propranolol. DC cardioversion is not likely to be any more successful than it is in dogs with chronic atrial fibrillation. Usually, atrial flutter reverts spontaneously to a sinus rhythm or it progresses to atrial fibrillation.

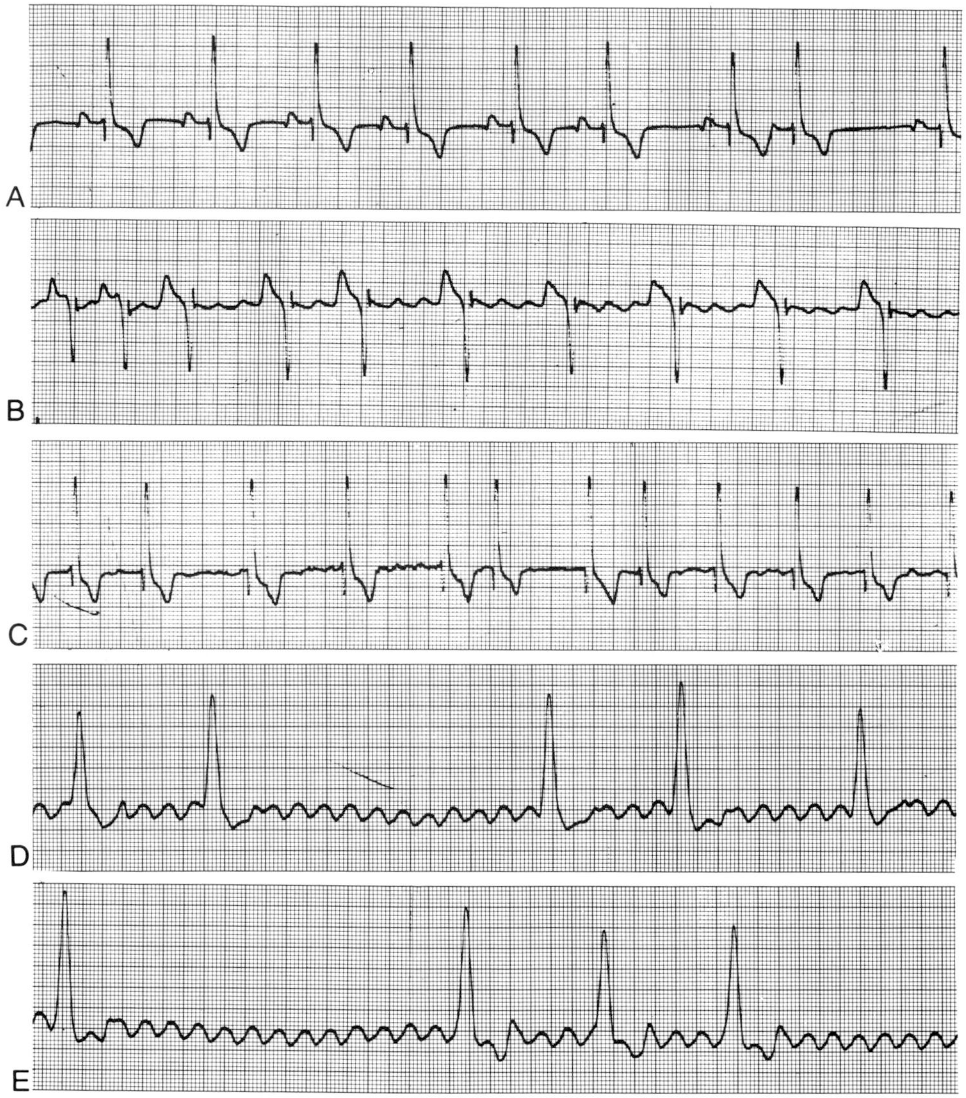

FIGURE 76–18. Progression of occasional atrial premature beats *(A)* in a dog with chronic mitral valvular heart disease to atrial flutter *(B)* during digitalization for heart failure. The atrial flutter waves in *B* occur regularly although the ventricular response is slightly irregular. Strip *C* demonstrates full progression to atrial fibrillation in the same dog. *D* and *E* is a continuous lead II electrocardiogram from a dog with atrial flutter and complete heart block. The idioventricular rhythm is slow and irregular with wide aberrant QRS complexes occurring at 50 beats per minute. The atrial flutter rate is 480 per minute. Note the sawtooth appearance of the atrial rhythm.

Ventricular Tachycardia and Atrioventricular Dissociation

In ventricular tachyarrhythmias (Figures 76–19 through 76–21), the impulse arises within the tissue of the ventricle. Depending upon the proximity of the impulse origin to the common bundle of His, the appearance of the beat varies from that of a nearly normal QRS complex to that of a wide, aberrant complex. The latter results from slow muscle fiber to muscle fiber conduction, whereas the former is due to rapid Purkinje-fiber-system network conduction. The dominant rhythm is ventricular, while the atrial pacemaker still continues to fire, although at a slower rate than the more dominant focus in the ventricle. Since ventricular beats do not usually traverse the A-V node via retrograde conduction, the electrocardiogram is characterized by both an atrial focus and a ventricular focus. In order for the ventricular rhythm to remain dominant, the ventricular rate must be as rapid as, or even faster than, the atrial rate.

Ventricular tachycardia (VT) by definition means a series of three or more consecutive beats, which arise from the ventricular conduction system distal to the bundle of His or the ventricular muscle. The QRS complex is wide during the VT. *Sustained VT* is prolonged and requires drug or electrical cardioversion therapy whereas *nonsustained VT* has short bursts of irregular rhythms that terminate spontaneously.[41a]

The atrium is depolarized when the P wave begins in the S-A node and travels across the atrial myocardium to the A-V node. In most cases, the P wave is blocked at the level of the lower A-V junctional tissue as a result of the latter's refractoriness from partial retrograde conduction of the ventricular beat. This P wave is referred to as an *interfered P wave*. Occasionally, the P wave reaches the A-V node and bundle of His sufficiently early in the time sequence. Then the ventricle

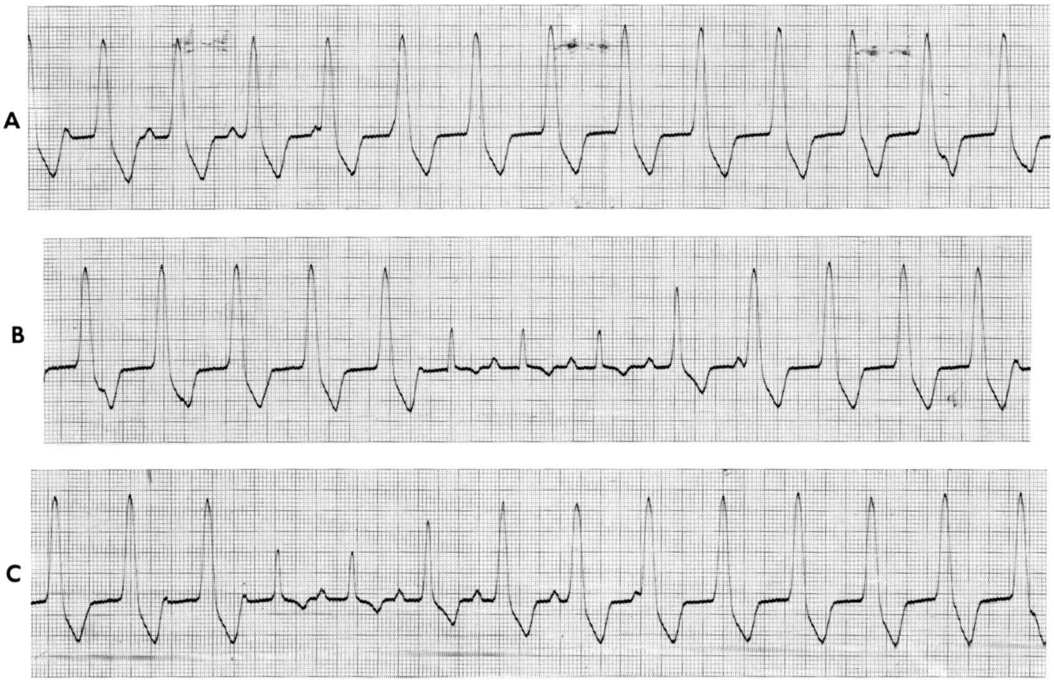

FIGURE 76–19. *A, B,* and *C* show ventricular tachycardia. Lead II electrocardiograms recorded from an Afghan hound presented in collapse. The heart sounds were variable on auscultation, and a pulse deficit was palpated. Tracing *A* demonstrates the ventricular tachycardia recorded at the time of entry. This arrhythmia was considered life-threatening, and the patient was started on intravenous lidocaine. In tracing *A,* the P waves occur just prior to the ventricular complexes at the beginning of the tracing and work their way into the ventricular complexes. This occurs because the independent ventricular rate is faster than the sinus rate. The ventricular rate is 166 beats per minute, and the atrial rate is 150 beats per minute. Following intravenous lidocaine, slowing of the ventricular response occurred *(B).* As the atrial and ventricular responses approximate each other, the sinus P waves intermittently capture the rhythm, resulting in normal beats in the middle of the tracing. Tracing *C* represents the reappearance of the P waves when they occur early enough to capture the rhythm. The rhythm was entirely controlled shortly thereafter with intravenous therapy after which an oral antiarrhythmic agent was used.

Illustration continued on following page

has not been made refractory by a prior idioventricular beat. At such times, the P wave is conducted through the normal ventricular conduction system, and a normal QRS complex associated with a P wave occurs. The latter beat is referred to as a *capture beat,* in contrast to the *idioventricular beat* that has been dominant. When the P waves occur and stimulate the ventricular myocardium at or near the same time as the idioventricular focus, a QRS-T complex results that is similar to, but not the same as, a normal capture beat. This QRS-T complex beat is referred to as a *fusion beat.* The fusion beat has an appearance that combines features of the ventricular and sinus beats.

In order for ventricular tachycardia to be present, the idioventricular rhythm must develop at the same rate as, or at a faster rate than, the atrial rhythm. The QRS complexes vary in appearance from normal to wide and aberrant. The presence of capture and fusion beats verifies the diagnosis of ventricular tachycardia. This is actually an incomplete form of atrioventricular dissociation, because the atrioventricular node is capable of impulse transmission, if it is not in a refractory state.[42] *Isorhythmic dissociation, accrochage,* or *synchrony* refers to the presence of an atrial rhythm that is electrically related in some uncertain manner to the idioventricular rhythm. The ventricle then maintains the dominant rhythm, and the atrial rate is electrically associated with the dominant rhythm.[34]

The main characteristic of a ventricular tachycardia is a rapid, irregularly appearing QRS complex (normal in appearance if the origin of the beat is close to the common bundle of His). The complexes are associated with a uniform R-R interval. The latter is not true when capture and fusion beats interrupt the predominant ventricular rhythm or when multiple foci are responsible for the arrhythmia.

Supraventricular tachycardia with aberrancy must be distinguished from ventricular tachycardia for therapeutic and prognostic purposes. Ventricular tachycardia is usually recognized by careful analysis of the QRS complex form, the rate and regularity of the rhythm, and the relationship of atrial to ventricular activity.

Even with careful attention to these points it is often difficult to be completely certain of the diagnosis. In such cases in humans, the diagnosis is made by analysis of the depolarization of the bundle of His to both atrial and ventricular potentials.[43]

Ventricular tachycardia should be considered a serious and possibly prefibrillatory rhythm. Ventricular tachycardia and A-V dissociation are essentially the same rhythm. The only difference between the two is the ventricular rate. When the idioventricular rate exceeds 100 beats per minute, the rhythm is called a ventricular tachycardia. If it is slower than that, the term A-V dissociation is used.

Ventricular tachyarrhythmias are associated with car-

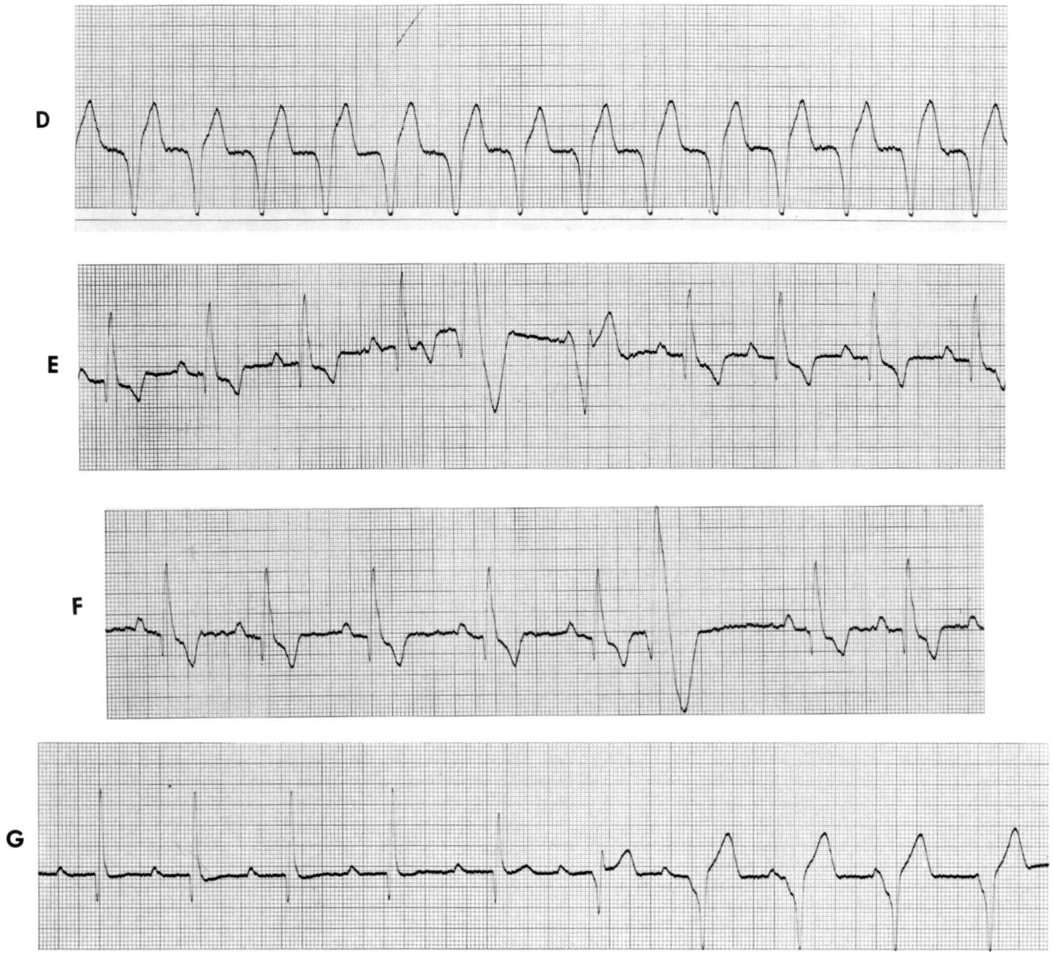

FIGURE 76–19 *Continued D, E, F,* and *G* are electrocardiographic tracings from a Doberman pinscher presented after an acute episode of collapse. The initial tracing *(D)* indicated persistent ventricular tachycardia at the rate of 187 beats per minute. Oral antiarrhythmic therapy was started while other evaluations of the patient were being made. The laboratory and clinical studies did not reveal a cause for this disease. The condition was considered to be the result of degenerative myocardial disease. The arrhythmia was controlled using a combination of quinidine and procainamide. Eight weeks after the acute episode, the rhythm strip *(E)* demonstrated two premature ventricular contractions within an otherwise normal rhythm. The patient was acting normally and was continued on antiarrhythmic agents. Seven months after the onset of the arrhythmia, the tracing *(F)* demonstrated only one ventricular premature contraction over a 60-second period. The patient died several months later after therapy was discontinued. The post-mortem examination revealed nonspecific degenerative myocarditis. *G,* Ventricular tachycardia due to digitalis intoxication. Lead II tracing demonstrating a normal sinus rhythm initially followed by ventricular tachycardia. This patient was on high levels of digoxin and potassium-depleting diuretics. Note the prolonged P-R interval, 0.19 second, during the sinus rhythm phase of this tracing. Digoxin was discontinued temporarily, and potassium replacement was completed. The dog returned to a normal sinus rhythm.

diomyopathies, myocarditis, advanced congestive heart failure with myocardial anoxia, and intramural coronary arteriosclerosis (microscopic intramural myocardial infarction, MIMI). Dilated (congestive) cardiomyopathy has been demonstrated to be associated with a very high incidence of ventricular arrhythmias in humans[44] and the author's experience in dogs and cats is in clinical concordance with this. Drug intoxications such as excesses of the digitalis glycosides, antiarrhythmic agents, sympathomimetics, and atropine may be responsible for ventricular tachycardia. Also associated with inducing this arrhythmia is manipulation of the heart during cardiac catheterization and surgery, as well as manipulation of other body organs during surgical techniques. Electrolyte disturbances (especially hypokalemia), hypoxia, endocarditis, infiltrative myocardial diseases, cardiomyopathies, heartworm disease, and advanced congenital cardiac defects may all be associated with ventricular rhythms and ventricular tachycardia.

Ventricular tachycardia occurs in many clinical situations in which advanced disease is present. This may be a direct or indirect effect of that disease process. Ventricular tachycardia should signal the need for immediate and serious attention to both the cardiac problem and the primary disease. One example of this situation is the gastric dilatation-volvulus complex, in which it is thought that alterations in gas exchange result in tissue hypoxia, electrolyte and pH changes, and cell death. Most dogs with this problem develop cardiac arrhythmias during surgery or up to 48 hours postoperatively.[45] While treatment is often successful, there remains a high mortality, which is even greater in those animals that do not receive medical attention for the rhythm disturbance.

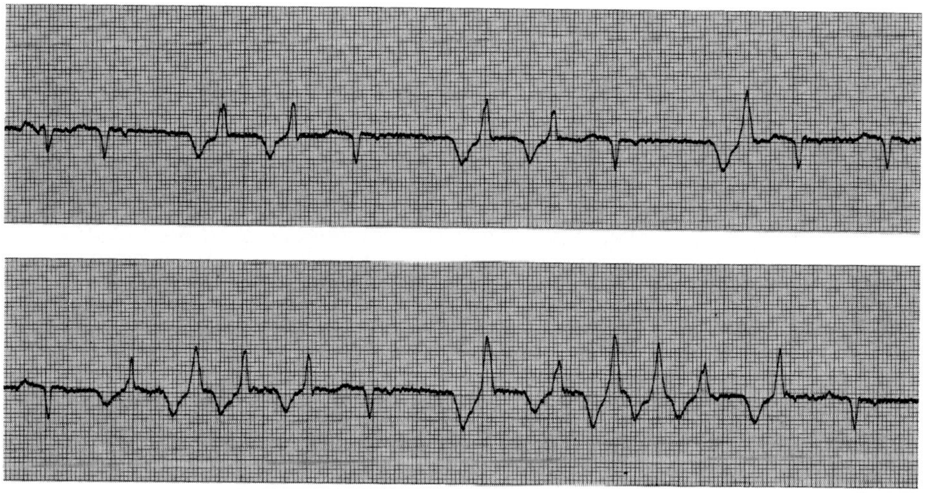

FIGURE 76–20. Ventricular tachycardia in a cat. Lead II continuous tracing. This cat was presented for lethargy and hiding as well as weight loss. Despite vigorous therapy, death ensued and at necropsy an enlarged, dilated heart was found. Ventricular tachycardia is not often encountered in cats and is always considered to be a serious sign.

A

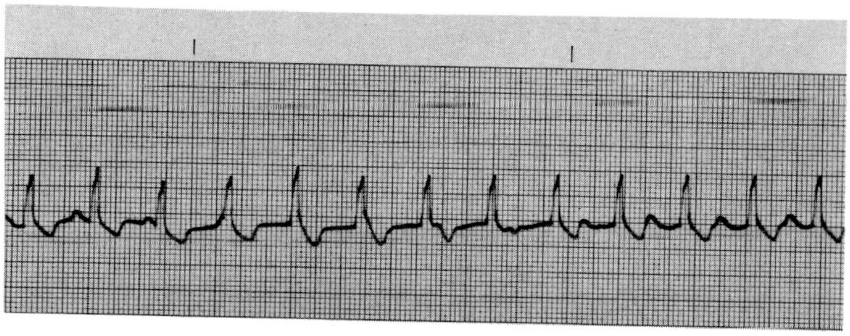

B

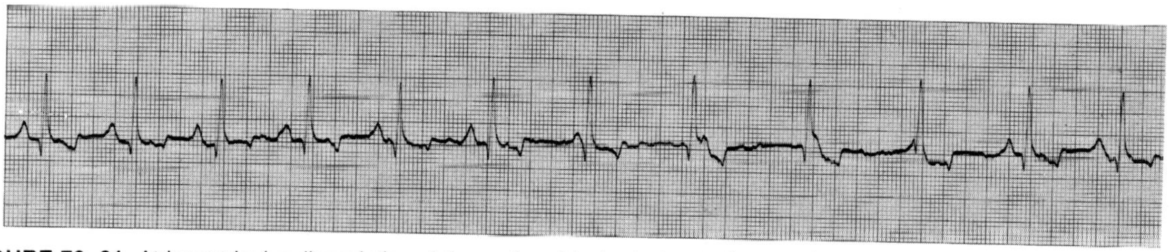

FIGURE 76–21. Atrioventricular dissociation. A form of ventricular tachycardia associated with rapid or normal atrial and ventricular rhythms that occur independently of each other is referred to as A-V dissociation. When complete in form there is no capture or fusion. The first ECG *(A)* demonstrates a rapid irregular rhythm, which this five-year-old Samoyed had had for several years. Note that the P waves are independent of the ventricular complexes and that the atrial rhythm (P-P interval) is slightly slower than the ventricular rhythm. Treatment for this condition is not immediately essential, although cautious digitalization may delay or retard the ultimate development of congestive heart failure (which usually will develop). The ECG shown in *B* is from another Samoyed dog, which developed congestive heart failure after several years of the arrhythmia. Digoxin therapy sustained the dog for an additional 18 months after the first bout of heart failure occurred. Note that the atrial rate is related to the ventricular rate, with the P waves occurring either before or after each QRS complex.

Ventricular tachycardia has been observed in both dogs and cats following nonpenetrating thoracic trauma. Once again, treatment first requires recognition of the arrhythmia, which may be overlooked in light of the other problems being considered following such trauma. One study in dogs suggested that careful monitoring of dogs for 24 to 48 hours after thoracic trauma was indicated, due to the often delayed onset of ventricular arrhythmias. Shock and myocardial ischemia due to hemorrhage and necrosis, as well as neurogenic factors, are possible causes of dysrhythmias following thoracic trauma.[46]

Alkalosis, acidosis, endotoxemia, and exogenous toxemias are other, often overlooked conditions that, when severe, are likely to cause ventricular rhythm disturbances. One of these problems may be the cause of sudden death in a patient that otherwise appears to be medically stable.

Clinical signs. Dyspnea, weakness, fainting, and collapse are signs associated with ventricular tachycardia. Congestive heart failure may be present or may develop if the arrhythmia is prolonged.

Owing to variable filling of the ventricle, the heart sounds may appear diminished or are variable in intensity. A rapid rhythm may be auscultated, and occasionally a pulse deficit is present. Cardiac murmurs are associated with specific cardiac pathology. In shorthaired dogs and cats and in those animals with clipped jugular regions, cannon "A" waves are seen in jugular veins. These result when the atria contract against a closed A-V valve, causing blood to travel retrograde from the atrium back into the jugular veins.

Treatment. To treat or not to treat is the question in patients with ventricular arrhythmias. Several studies in human beings have suggested that ventricular arrhythmias in the asymptomatic patient with well-preserved ventricular function need not be treated.[47] When heart failure is present and the arrhythmias are not symptomatic, therapy may worsen pump function.[48] Still, even with initial normal cardiac function, others have shown an increased frequency of sudden death in patients not treated.[49]

Often in small animal practice, it is difficult to establish the severity of symptoms unless they are very apparent or advanced. Thus, the veterinarian must use clinical judgement along with diagnostic data (including ECG, echocardiography, radiographs, 24-hour ambulatory ECG monitoring) to determine if therapy is indicated.

Certain facts assist the clinician in deciding whether to treat or not. Sustained ventricular arrhythmias are more serious than nonsustained rhythms. Malignant rhythms with greater than five to ten VPCs per minute are usually regarded as more serious than single, occasional ectopic beats. Ventricular tachycardia associated with known heart disease or other diseases is likely to be a serious and life-threatening problem. Occasional unifocal beats are usually of less significance than more frequent multifocal rhythms. When drugs such as digitalis, quinidine, or other cardiac agents are being used and a ventricular tachycardia is recognized, it is generally wise to discontinue the drug until the origin of the arrhythmia has been established. It must be clearly determined that the drug presently being used is not responsible for the clinical condition of the patient. In general, antiarrhythmic agents are used in small animals to control such cardiac arrhythmias (see the section entitled Classification of Antiarrhythmic Agents).

Although most antiarrhythmic agents available for use in humans have been used to treat canine ventricular dysrhythmias, there is a paucity of knowledge regarding their use in the feline. Many cats react adversely to some of the drugs. Experience with ventricular arrhythmias in cats presently leads this author to the conclusion that only quinidine and propranolol are safe and effective. Lidocaine may in special cases also be administered (see Specific Class IB Drugs). Other drugs may prove to be effective, but until studies to this effect are available they probably should not be used as first line agents to treat ventricular arrhythmias.

In addition, direct-current cardioversion may be used to reset the cardiac rhythm. Cardiac glycosides should be considered when a ventricular arrhythmia is present in association with congestive heart failure. The clinician must attempt to determine if the cardiac arrhythmia is the result of heart failure. In cases of heart failure, cardiac glycosides are indicated, whereas in cases of digitalis intoxication or marked ventricular muscle irritability, cardiac glycoside therapy is contraindicated.

Until the nature of the underlying disease responsible for the rhythm is recognized and the rhythm is controlled, the prognosis for patients with ventricular tachycardia must remain guarded. Multifocal ventricular arrhythmias should be considered more serious than arrhythmias that are unifocal in origin.

VENTRICULAR FIBRILLATION

Ventricular fibrillation (Figure 76–22) is characterized by a complete lack of well-defined QRS complexes. The waveforms appear as low-voltage, irregular undulations that are generally larger than those recognized in the course of atrial fibrillation.

Hemodynamically, ventricular fibrillation is equivalent to cardiac arrest. The ventricular twitching is rapid, irregular, and uncoordinated. Heart sounds, pulse, and blood pressure are clinically nonexistent.

Ventricular fibrillation, like cardiac arrest, is a serious disturbance. In order to be successful, therapy must be instituted immediately. Endotracheal intubation must be performed first to maintain a patent airway. Simultaneously, a sharp blow is made to the precordium, followed by external cardiac massage. Oxygen is administered by mouth via tube until a mechanical respirator can be attached. If a defibrillator is available, external cardiac defibrillation should be performed without hesitation, using maximum strength impulses. The administration of 0.1 ml epinephrine, isoproterenol, or norepinephrine intracardially is indicated immediately following the recognition of ventricular fibrillation. This is followed by continuous cardiac massage, artificial respiration, and defibrillation. If the patient does not respond immediately, continuous intravenous fluids and sodium bicarbonate are administered, and vasopressor agents are administered intermittently. This is continued until a regular cardiac rate, associated with satisfactory

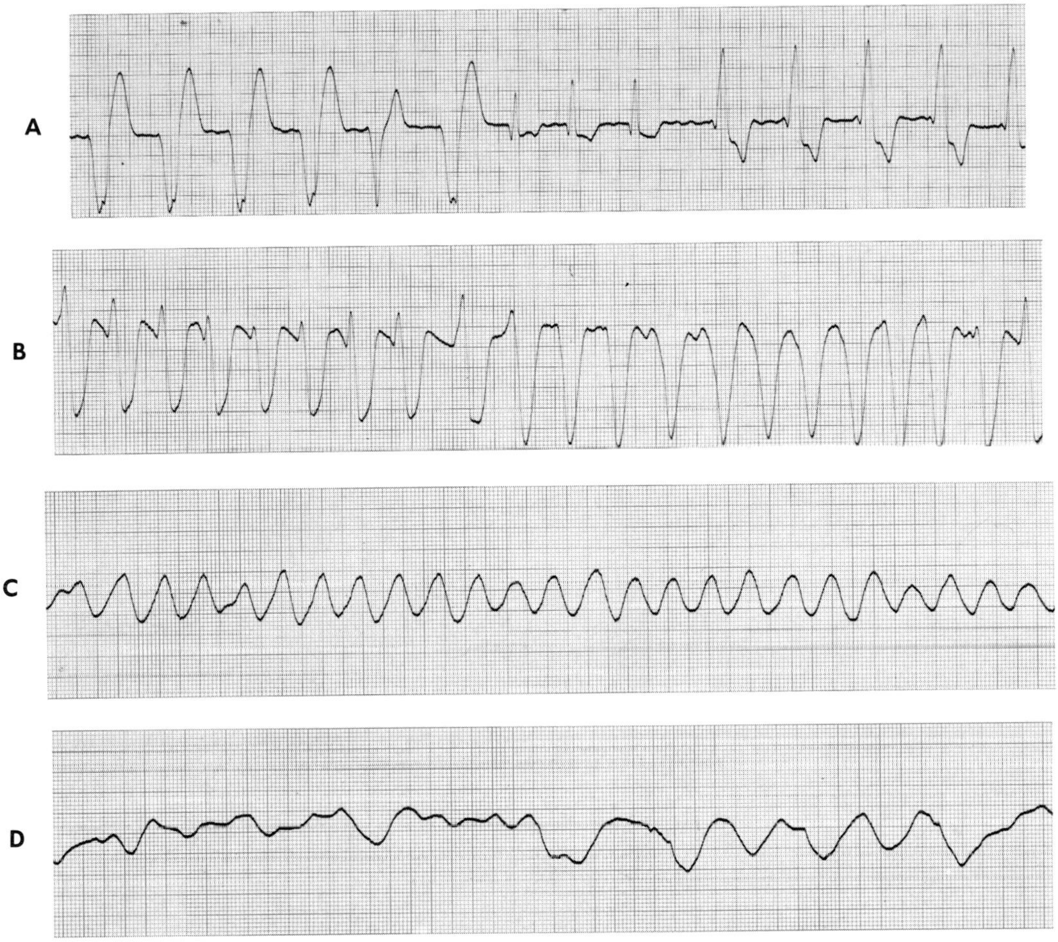

FIGURE 76–22. Electrocardiographic tracings of a dog presented in acute collapse. There was marked abdominal pain on physical examination. Tracing *A* demonstrates ventricular tachycardia, multifocal in origin, and an apparent absence of P waves. The patient's condition rapidly deteriorated, and ventricular tachycardia occurred *(B)*. This progressed to ventricular flutter *(C)* and ultimately ventricular fibrillation *(D)*. Attempts at resuscitation were unsuccessful. The patient had splenic and gastric torsion at necropsy.

blood pressure levels and voluntary respiration, occurs. Cardiopulmonary arrest beyond two to three minutes is usually irreversible.

Many drugs exert a protective influence on the threshold for ventricular fibrillation. Those with protective effects that are often used clinically include propranolol (0.2 mg/lb or 0.5 mg/kg), acetylpromazine (0.4 mg/lb or 1 mg/kg), and chlorpromazine (1 mg/lb).[50] Other agents have proven experimentally useful but have little clinical applicability. In general, prevention is the best method of treatment.

THE BRADYARRHYTHMIAS

SINUS BRADYCARDIA

Sinus bradycardia (Figure 76–23) is characterized by normal electrocardiographic complexes occurring in either a sinus rhythm or sinus arrhythmia in which the heart rate is less than 60 beats per minute. This condition is seen most frequently as a normal, nonpathologic finding in larger animals, athletic animals, highly trained animals, and occasionally normal patients without clinical signs. Clinically, these patients usually exhibit no abnormal findings other than a slow heart rate. The femoral pulses of patients with sinus bradycardia are remarkably slow but strong. It is usually this full and bounding pulse wave that draws the clinician's attention to the cardiac irregularity.

Occasionally, if the heart rate is too slow, the patient may appear lethargic or may be reported to have episodes of weakness and/or syncope. Generally, treatment of this condition is unnecessary. Patients that develop a normal cardiac rate in response to the administration of atropine, or that can increase their cardiac rate merely with exercise, usually require no therapeutic assistance. In those patients that exhibit clinical signs that are referable to the slower cardiac rate, the use of atropine-like drugs in time-release capsule form (isopropamide, Darbid) or the implantation of a cardiac pacemaker may be necessary.

One form of sinus bradycardia that is clinically significant relates to the sick sinus syndrome complex. In this problem there may be a slow cardiac rate, weakness, and occasionally syncope. Affected animals (frequently schnauzers) may have signs of mitral valvular heart disease as well as a sinus bradycardia. Supraventricular arrhythmias, sinus arrest, and escape rhythms may be

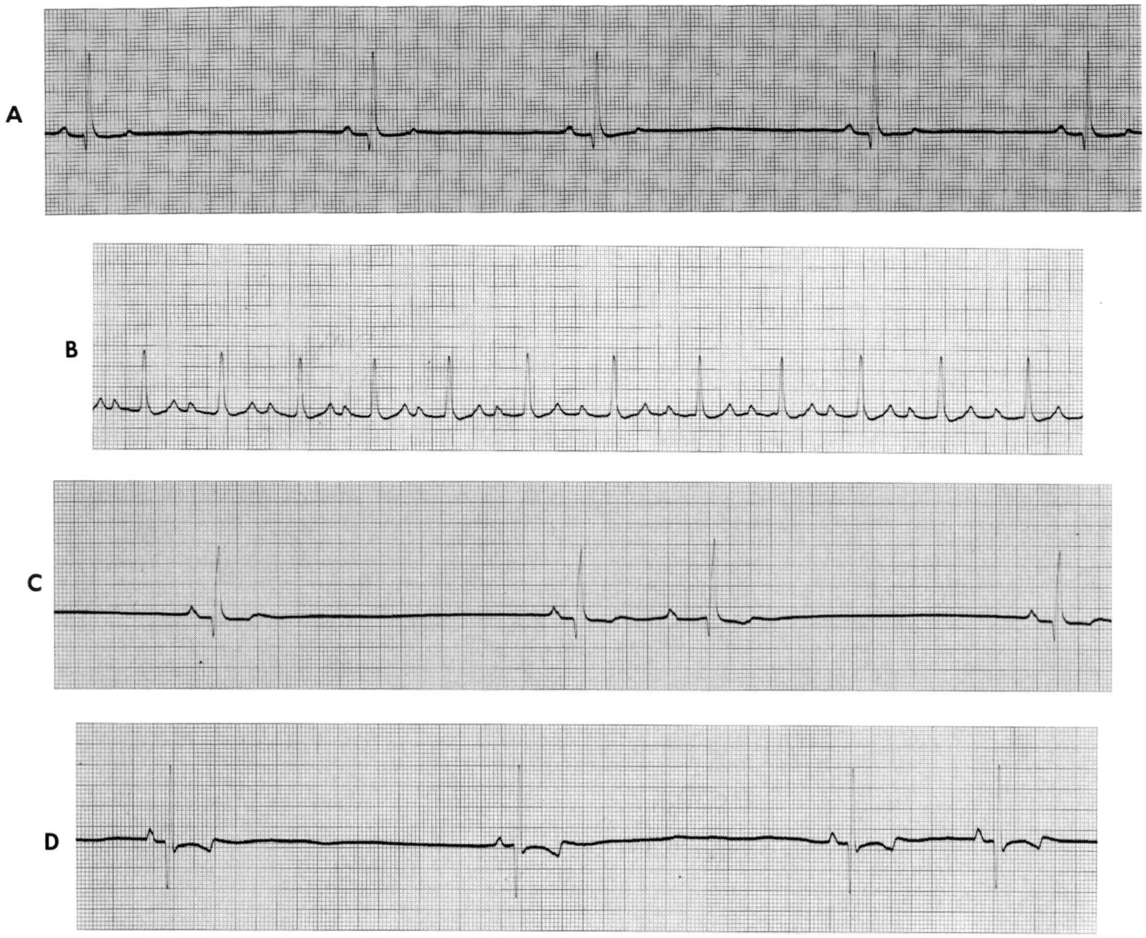

FIGURE 76–23. *A* demonstrates sinus bradycardia. Tracing *A* is a lead II tracing from a dog referred for evaluation of a slow cardiac rate. There were no abnormal clinical signs and the pulse was strong. The electrocardiogram demonstrates a sinus arrhythmia with pronounced bradycardia. The ventricular rate was approximately 55 beat per minute. There were no significant electrocardiographic abnormalities. Following atropine administration, the cardiac rate increased to 140 beats per minute *(B)*. *B,* because the patient was asymptomatic, no therapy was suggested and the patient continued satisfactorily without drug therapy. This could be a form of athletic heart with a normal sinus bradycardia. *C* shows an electrocardiogram taken several days following patent ductus arteriosus surgery. The cardiac rate in this dog was very slow. The third electrocardiographic complex is associated with marked prolongation of the P-R interval. There were no other abnormalities found, and the patient was normal. The heart rate returned to normal later in the postoperative period. *D* is an electrocardiographic tracing taken from a dog with abdominal lymphosarcoma. The cardiac rate in this patient was very slow, and the electrocardiogram revealed a marked sinus arrhythmia and sinus bradycardia. Because of the lack of symptoms, therapy was not recommended. The patient was not expressing signs of clinical disease.

part of this syndrome. Treatment is outlined in the section describing this disease.

SINOATRIAL (S-A) ARREST (PROLONGED SINUS PAUSE)

When the sinoatrial node fails to generate an impulse, the next regularly scheduled atrial depolarization does not follow (Figure 76–24). Thus, the P wave and its accompanying QRS-T complex do not occur. In such cases, the duration of the P-P interval is equal to at least twice that of the dominant P-P interval. Often when the sinoatrial node is this depressed, the junctional nodal tissue or the Purkinje fibers temporarily assume the pacemaking function. This results in the generation of either junctional or ventricular escape beats.

Usually sinoatrial arrest is not a clinically significant finding. It may result from excessive vagal stimulation, such as occurs with ocular or carotid sinus pressure or disease, some pharyngeal lesions, and digitalis, quinidine, or other drug intoxication. Pathologic conditions of the atrial myocardium, such as dilatation or fibrosis, may be associated with this irregularity.

This arrhythmia is observed most frequently, but not exclusively, in the brachycephalic breeds. In these breeds, the cardiac rhythm is regularly and markedly slowed during expiration. The sinus arrest that occurs is then an extreme accentuation of sinus arrhythmias. Thus, the condition is more correctly termed prolonged sinus pause.

Clinical Signs. Signs that occur with this condition are usually those of weakness, wobbling, stumbling, or syncope associated with temporary asystole. Syncopal episodes without Stokes-Adams seizures may occur. Sinoatrial syncope was described first in the schnauzer breed.[51] All dogs were between six and ten years of age

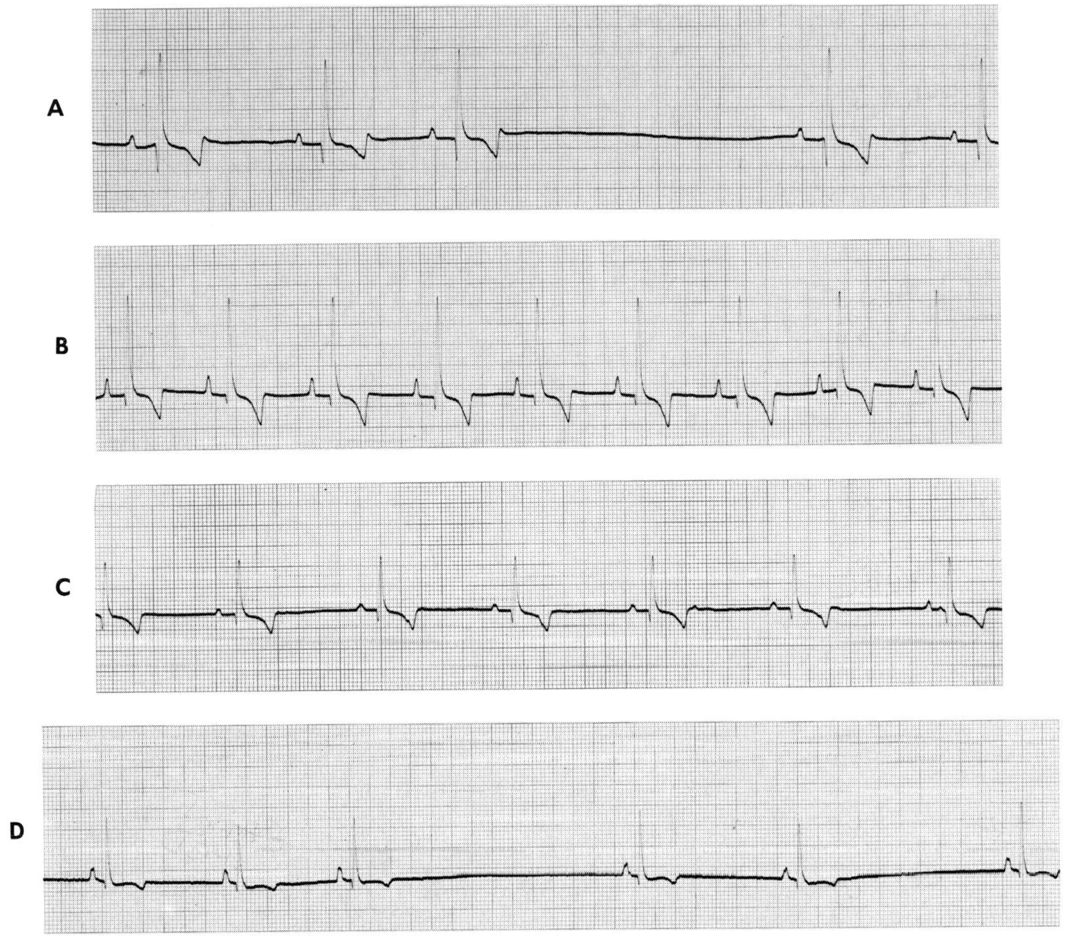

FIGURE 76–24. Sinoatrial arrest. *A* is from a cocker spaniel, 11 years old, presented to the hospital for evaluation of several syncopal attacks. The heart rate was slow with intermittent long pauses. The electrocardiogram *(A)* demonstrated sinoatrial arrest of 1.8 seconds. Tracing *B* demonstrates the electrocardiogram following the administration of atropine intravenously. The rhythm was sinus in origin and the heart rate 125 beats per minute. The dog was given an atropine-like substance usually reserved for the treatment of gastrointestinal disorders (Darbid). The patient experienced no further problems while on medication. Tracing *C* represents the rhythm after three weeks of this drug. The therapy was continued for three months and then slowly discontinued. The patient has not experienced problems since. *D* is from a dog with chronic mitral valvular fibrosis presented with a history of chronic coughing. The electrocardiogram revealed episodes of marked sinus arrhythmia. Because the pause is greater than two normal P to P intervals, this may be interpreted as temporary sinoatrial arrest. The condition is usually insignificant, unless the patient is symptomatic. In this case it could be considered an accentuated sinus arrhythmia. The dog was digitalized without complication, because of signs of heart failure.

and exhibited clinical signs similar to those described previously. In this group, the signs did not progress and the condition was considered to be more of a nuisance than life-threatening. Atropine injections (0.4 mg subcutaneously) increased the heart rate temporarily in some of the dogs. Disease in this latter group is probably better classified as part of the sick sinus syndrome.

Treatment. Adrenergic-stimulating agents, such as epinephrine or isoproterenol, are useful for increasing the cardiac rate and speeding atrioventricular conduction. Parasympathetic blocking agents, such as atropine or atropine-like derivatives, may also be beneficial. Many dogs with the condition have been successfully managed with time-release preparations of isopropamide (Darbid or Darbazine), which has an anticholinergic effect. This atropine-like effect increases the heart rate.

Several reports of specific breeds with atrial conduction disturbances, weakness, syncope, and occasionally, death are available. A strain of purebred pugs was shown to have intermittent sinus pauses and paroxysmal second degree heart block.[52] Clinically, collapse occurred after excitement and hyperactivity. The condition, assumed to be a hereditable autosomal recessive trait, was characterized histologically by narrowing and fibrosis of the midportion of the bundle of His. Dalmatians may be similarly affected as a result of disease of the sinus node and multiple atrial arteries, resulting in abnormalities of the sinus rhythm. Doberman pinschers occasionally die suddenly, and histopathology reveals A-V nodal and His bundle disease consequent to local ischemia. The common findings in these dogs are atrial arrhythmias and often sinoatrial arrest, syncope, and at times, sudden death. The diseases relate to vascular abnormalities of the S-A and A-V nodal regions.

When an electrolyte imbalance or a toxic response to drug therapy is the cause of S-A arrest, the causative factors should be eliminated if possible. Treatment in such cases is that required to increase cardiac conductivity for a temporary period.

ATRIAL STANDSTILL

An uncommon problem that deserves mention is complete atrial standstill. The condition is recognized when P waves are absent from the ECG in all beats, as well as on intracardiac electrograms. The ventricular complexes appear normal, the heart rate fails to increase or show P waves (ECG) after exercise or atropine, the atria remain immobile when observed fluoroscopically or by echocardiography, and the atria fail to respond to electrical stimulation.[53]

Cardiac causes include Springer spaniel muscular dystrophies, chronic dilated cardiomyopathies, and atrial myocarditis.

The condition is due to marked sinus bradycardia, digitalis, quinidine, or antiarrhythmic drug toxicity, CO_2 poisoning, hyperkalemia, and open heart surgery, and also occurs prior to ventricular arrest and death and when there is irreversible and extensive atrial disease (Figure 76–25).[54]

These animals may show no signs of the primary disease, or their cardiac symptomatology may include weakness, wobbliness, and syncope. Treatment is directed at correcting the cause.

ATRIOVENTRICULAR BLOCK

Atrioventricular block indicates either a partial delay or complete blockage of impulse conduction from the atria to the ventricles. There are three major categories of atrioventricular block that are recognized: first, second, and third degree.

First degree atrioventricular block is also known as partial or incomplete heart block (Figure 76–26). In first degree atrioventricular block, the P-R interval is greater than 0.14 second in the dog and 0.08 second in the cat. Each P wave is followed by the normal QRS-T complex, the cardiac rhythm is normal, and the condition can be factually determined only by an electrocardiographic tracing.

Second degree atrioventricular heart block is another partial or incomplete heart block (Figure 76–27). The P waves and the QRS complexes bear a continuous relationship until a ventricular beat is periodically dropped. In this category, the Wenckebach phenomenon (Mobitz type I A-V block) refers to the fact that the P-R interval progressively increases until a P wave occurs and the QRS complex is dropped. This suggests a conduction delay in the A-V node. In Mobitz type II A-V block, the P-R interval remains unchanged and the dropped beat occurs without prior electrocardiographic abnormalities. This is likely to result when the block is in the bundle of His or its branches. Second degree heart block may also be simple or advanced. In the latter, the ventricle responds only to every second, third, or fourth P wave. In more advanced second degree heart block (with incomplete A-V dissociation), the ventricular response is greater than 40 beats per minute, but there is no relationship between the P waves and QRS-T complexes unless an occasional capture beat occurs. Electrophysiologic studies show that Mobitz type I A-V block

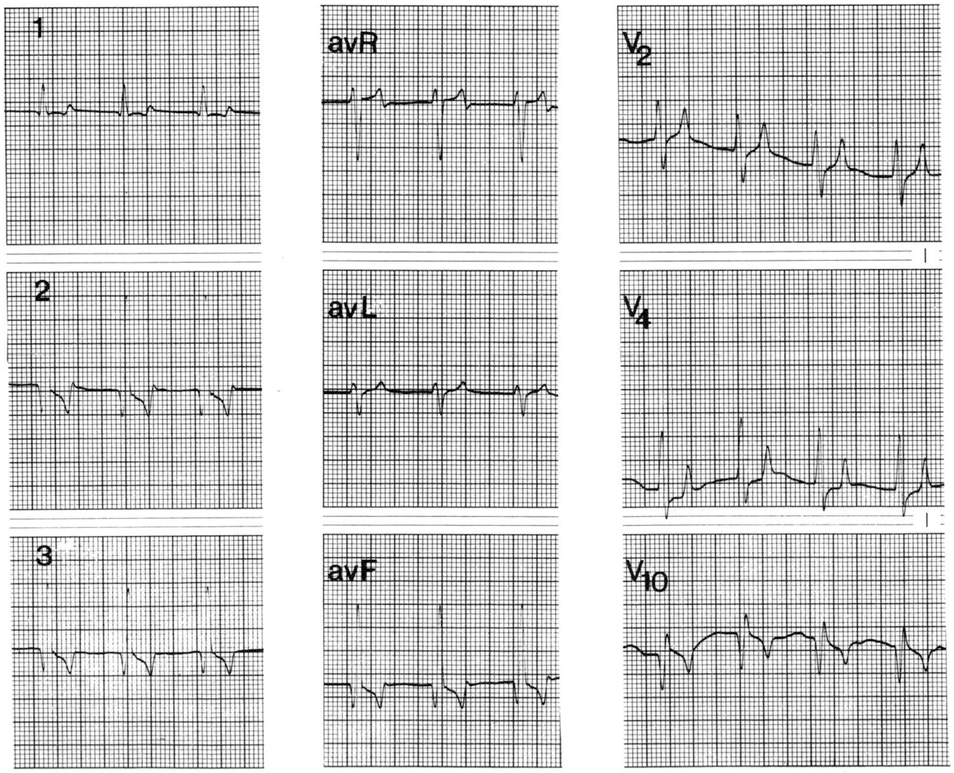

FIGURE 76–25. Atrial standstill in a dog with long-standing treated Addison's disease. The potassium level was 7.8 mEq when the dog was presented with marked malaise. The P waves are absent, the baseline is flat and the ventricular rate regular. Normal sinus rhythm resumed hours after increased cortisols were administered orally.

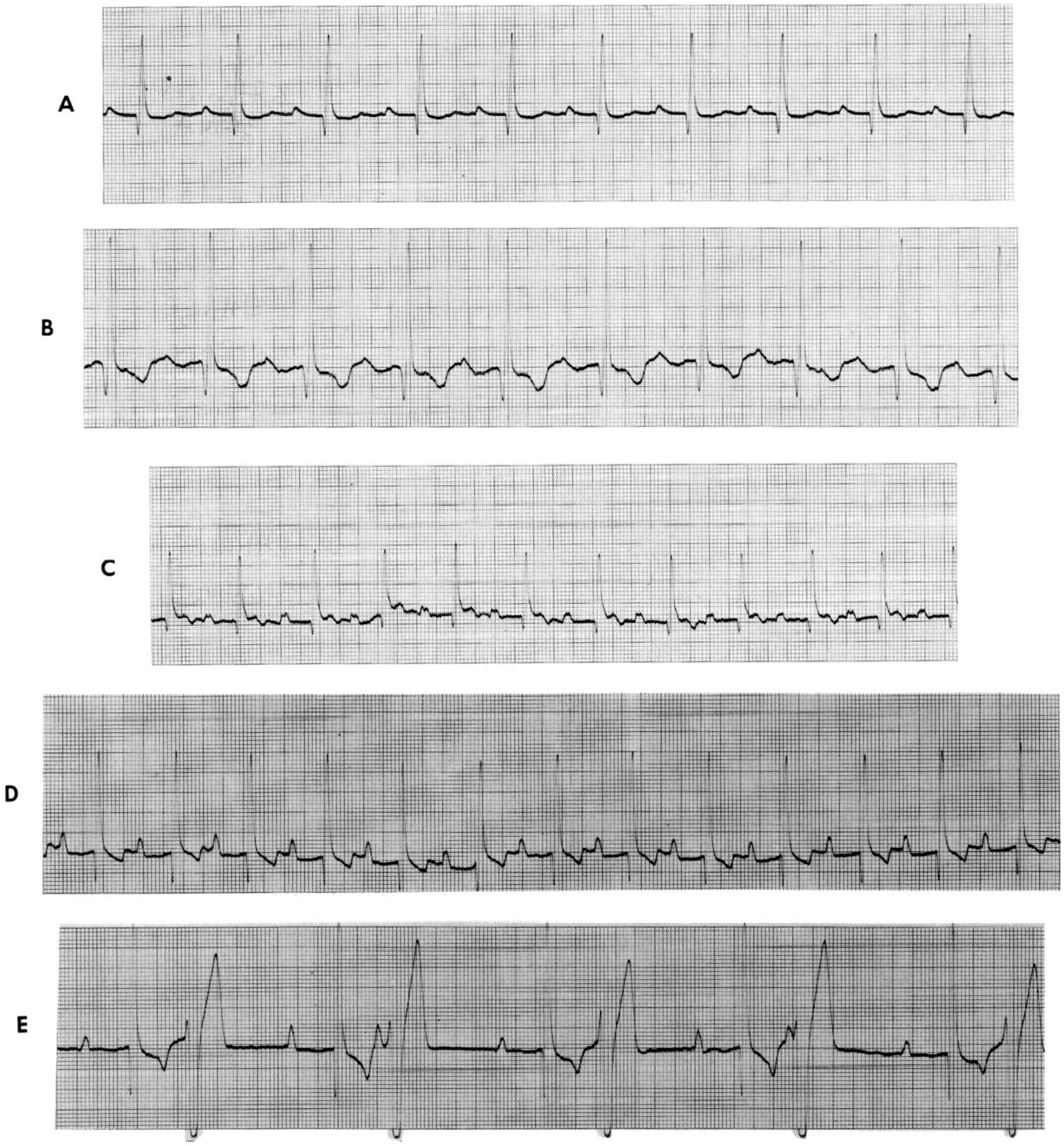

FIGURE 76–26. First degree heart block. Tracing *A* represents a dog with a P-R interval of 0.14 second and an otherwise normal cardiac rate and rhythm. This patient had evidence of marked left atrial disease and was not on medication at the time of the electrocardiographic tracing. Tracings *B* and *C* represent two patients showing signs of digitalis intoxication. The P-R intervals are prolonged to 0.20 second and 0.16 second, respectively. These patients had clinical signs of digitalis intoxication necessitating reduction of the dosage of digoxin. *D* is from a dog with a prolonged P-R interval, which had not been on therapy but was in heart failure and had very large atria, accounting for the prolonged P-R interval of 0.16 second. When therapeutic digoxin levels were exceeded *(E),* the P-R interval prolonged to 0.22 second and ventricular bigeminy resulted. Digoxin levels were reduced and the condition was temporarily stabilized.

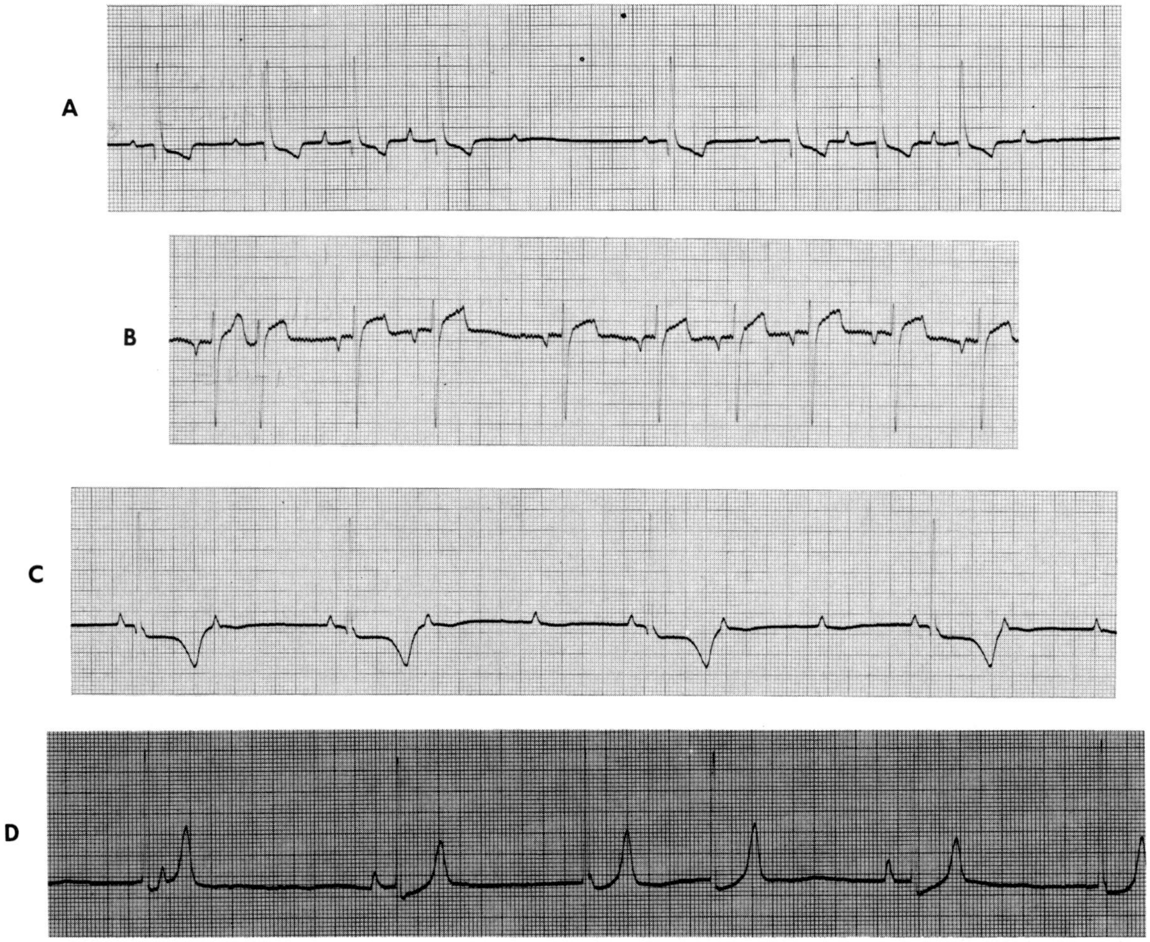

FIGURE 76–27. Second degree heart block. Tracing *A* demonstrates second degree heart block in a dog with digoxin intoxication. There is progressive P-R prolongation until second degree heart block occurs. This blockage occurs twice on the lead II strip. Cardiac medication was discontinued temporarily. Tracing *B* represents the electrocardiogram taken one week later. There is an atrial premature contraction at the beginning of this tracing. The P-R interval has returned to normal, and the patient was started on a lower level of digitalis. Advanced second degree heart block is seen in tracing *C*, representing a dog with 2:1 and 3:1 A-V block. Note that the P-R interval prior to the QRS complexes is the same, indicating that second degree heart block is present since some A-V conduction does occur. The ventricular response is frequently blocked. The P-P interval varies as a result of sinus arrhythmia. *D* shows a tracing from a West Highland white terrier with advanced second degree heart block. Although the atria and ventricles are dissociated, electrocardiographically the ventricular rate is greater than 40 beats per minute, thereby differentiating this from complete heart block. This dog responded well for more than two years with regular Darbid therapy. At times the electrocardiogram demonstrated lower degrees of second degree, and occasionally, first degree heart block.

usually occurs at the A-V node, whereas Mobitz type II A-V block is usually an infra-His bundle phenomenon.[55]

Third degree or *complete heart block* occurs when atrial conduction does not proceed through the A-V node and/or the ventricular conducting system. In such cases, the atrial rate is rapid and independent of the idioventricular rate. By definition, the ventricular rate in complete heart block is lower than 40 beats per minute (Figure 76–28). The nonconducted P waves are at times blocked distal to the bundle of His, indicating that bilateral bundle branch block is present.[55]

Atrioventricular block is associated with such cardiac conditions as enlarged atria, fibrosis of the atria and/or A-V junctional tissue, congenital defects, invasive myocardial growths, myocardial trauma (iatrogenic or natural), and occasionally, heartworm disease. Bacterial endocarditis is an underlying cause in some animals with heart block.[56] Infectious processes, toxemias, vagal stimulation, and hypoxia are other causes. Hyperkalemia is a cause for complete heart block and atrial arrest. In some brachycephalic breeds and smaller toy breeds (especially the Chihuahua), occasional second degree heart block occurs without clinical significance. Second degree heart block was observed to occur three times per hour in very young normal dogs and increased to 18 times per hour in puppies 10 to 11 weeks of age. It then decreased in frequency to less than once per hour in adult dogs in one study.[57] Therapeutic agents such as digitalis, quinidine, xylazine, and doxorubicin must always be considered when heart block is observed.

There have now been many reports of complete heart block in both dogs and cats. In some cases the animals are less than two years old, and it is hypothesized that a congenital lesion is present. The latter is not known with certainty. Histopathology, when available, usually suggests A-V nodal or His bundle vascular disease, fibrosis, or pathology.

Clinical Signs. First degree heart block is usually without clinical signs unless the disorder is associated with digitalis intoxication. In the latter case, depression, anorexia, vomiting, and diarrhea are anticipated. Usually, the clinical signs of digitalis intoxication and first degree heart block are associated with a reduction in the congestive failure symptomatology.

Second degree heart block may exhibit the same clinical signs as first degree block if digitalis intoxication is the cause. Usually a slower cardiac rate is auscultated and regular dropping of the ventricular complexes occurs. In more advanced forms of second degree A-V block that are unrelated to drug intoxication, the rhythm is slow and irregular. Heart sounds may vary in intensity owing to variations in ventricular filling. Low-frequency atrial sounds may be heard at the cardiac apex between the ventricular sounds. Frequent dropping of ventricular complexes may be associated with weakness or syncopal episodes. No clinical signs are observed in dogs showing intermittent second degree block associated with respiratory cardiodepression unless the frequency of the heart block interferes with a normal cardiac output. Dogs being treated with digitalis but without toxic signs may have high vagal tone and occasional second degree block (Wenckebach type). These animals are without clinical signs.

Advanced second degree and complete A-V heart block (third degree) are more likely to be associated with clinical signs than are the less severe forms of heart block. Decreased exercise tolerance, listlessness, and panting are usually associated with syncopal episodes. The latter occur without provocation or following exercise and may be associated with brief seizure activity. Syncopal episodes with or without convulsive seizures due to A-V block have been referred to as Stokes-Adams seizures.[34] Prolonged advanced second degree and third degree complete A-V block often result in the clinical features of bilateral congestive heart failure.

Treatment. When heart block of any degree is due to drug toxicity (especially digitalis products), the treatment includes immediate withdrawal of the drug. Supportive electrolyte and fluid therapy should be used as necessary.

First degree heart block due to atrial dilatation need not be considered significant except as it relates to the underlying cardiac disease. When a high-normal to mild P-R prolongation develops with digitalis therapy, first degree heart block may be present without clinical signs of intoxication. No efforts should be made to control this P-R prolongation. Likewise, second degree A-V heart block unassociated with signs of digitalis intoxication need not be a reason to reduce the dosage of the glycoside if the animal is faring well and the owner is made aware of the clinical signs that might develop. Serum digoxin levels may be necessary to distinguish normal from near-toxic patients. Isoproterenol may be the initial drug of choice for the treatment of advanced heart block when severe clinical signs are present.

Isoproterenol is a catecholamine that produces a β-adrenergic response. It increases atrioventricular impulse conduction and ventricular excitability. In addition to the positive cardiac stimulation from this drug, isoproterenol also induces bronchial smooth muscle relaxation and peripheral vascular dilatation. Isoproterenol is administered in an intravenous infusion with dextrose and water (1 mg per 200 cc) to effect a ventricular rate of 80 to 120 beats per minute. It may be continuously infused IV if an infusion device and monitoring equipment are available. Alternatively, isoproterenol may be given every four hours at the rate of 0.1 to 0.2 mg intramuscularly or subcutaneously until rate and rhythm control have been established. Sustained-acting forms of oral isoproterenol tablets are no longer available. Sublingual forms do not provide an effect for prolonged use. Elixir forms of isoproterenol are not useful for the treatment of atrioventricular block in the dog or cat. Isoproterenol may provide temporary relief for A-V heart block until a transvenous temporary or permanent pacemaker can be implanted.

Atropine reduces secretions produced in the upper and lower respiratory tracts. It provides bronchial dilatation but makes respiratory tract secretions more viscid and difficult to remove. Because atropine inhibits salivation and secretions of the respiratory tract as well as vagovagal reflexes during anesthesia and surgery, it is used in most patients as a preanesthetic agent.

The specific use of atropine in cardiac disease is limited to the treatment of hyperactive carotid sinus reflexes and bradycardia associated with syncope. Its

A

B

C

D

E

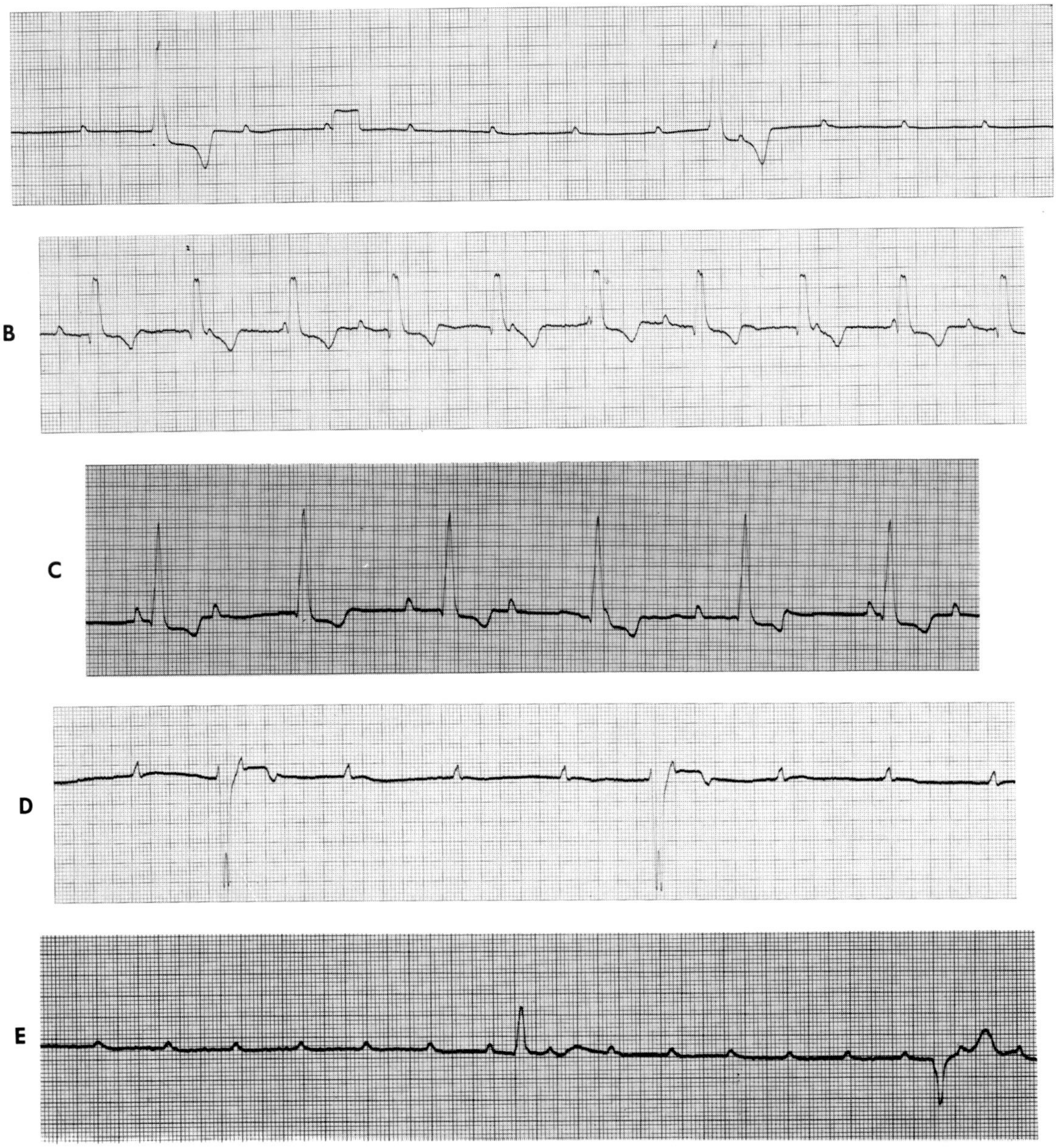

FIGURE 76–28. Complete heart block. Tracing *A* is a lead III electrocardiogram (half amplitude) of a patient with complete heart block. The atrial rate is 136 beats per minute, and the ventricular rhythm varies between 20 and 30 beats per minute. After the patient was started on an isoproterenol drip *(B)* the ventricular response increased to 120 beats per minute. Complete A-V dissociation was present in this patient. Tracing *C* represents another patient with an idioventricular rhythm and complete heart block. Note the varying P-R intervals that result from A-V dissociation. There are two independent pacemakers, one in the atrium and one in the ventricle. The P waves and T waves must be separated from each other to interpret the electrocardiogram. Tracing *D* represents another patient with complete (third degree) heart block. An idioventricular rhythm occurs, which bears no relationship to the P waves. In both QRS complexes, P waves are superimposed on the S-T segment. *E* shows a three-year-old cat presented for evaluation of syncope with a slow irregular cardiac rate and a pounding pulse upon physical examination. Complete heart block with an atrial rate of over 200 per minute and a slow idioventricular rate was recorded electrocardiographically. The cause of the heart block was thought to be fibrosis in the region of the bundle of His associated with cardiomyopathy.

use for sinoatrial arrest and atrioventricular block is recommended at the rate of 0.6 to 2.0 mg subcutaneously or orally, repeated every two to four hours. Atropine by injection is used most frequently as a provocative test to determine if the sinus rate can be increased or the heart block abolished. Thereafter, oral forms of atropine-like drugs are most often used. Isopropamide sustained-release drugs, used most commonly in dogs as anticholinergic agents (Darbid, Darbazine), are often effective in treating various forms of heart block. These are administered on a weight basis while observing for the side effects of dryness of the mucous membranes, pupillary dilatation, and constipation. Other atropine-like products may be similarly used. Often there is an adequate but small increase in the cardiac rate and decreased symptomatology with these preparations.

Complete heart block of a persistent nature is most properly treated with implantation of a cardiac pacemaker. While generally beyond the financial capacity of clients, costs have been reduced so that in selected cases such treatment by a regional referral center is no longer impractical. Most pacemakers employed in small animals are demand-type units providing for a basal rate in the range of 90 to 110 beats per minute (Figure 76–29). Rates can be adjusted from the outside after implantation in some of the modern units.

Permanent implanted pacemaker therapy works well in dogs. Transvenous placement of the pacing lead into the right ventricle requires fluoroscopic control in order to pass the lead and place it properly in the ventricle. The lead is transfixed to the jugular vein and sternothyreoideus muscle. A subcutaneous tunnel is created to bring the lead to the pacemaker, which is implanted subcutaneously in the dorsolateral aspect of the neck. Depending on the patient, the technique may be performed under local anesthesia, narcotic sedation, or a general anesthetic.[58]

An alternative therapy reportedly successful in older dogs uses a temporary transvenous pacemaker while the animal is anesthetized and a ventral abdominal, transdiaphragmatic approach is used to implant the permanent pacemaker. The pacing lead is screwed into the LV apex and led out of the thorax through a small incision in the diaphragm. The lead is then attached to the pacemaker, which is allowed to float freely in the abdominal cavity. A double pursestring suture is placed around the wire in the diaphragm to stabilize it and prevent it from being pulled out.[59] Other surgical techniques include a lateral thoracotomy or sternotomy, with placement of the pacemaker itself in the flank or abdominal cavity.

Pacemakers, while expensive, are often available through cardiologists, pathologists, or morticians. They should be examined for battery life and then resterilized for use in the dog. New pacing wires are still required and must be purchased from the pacemaker company. At the time of this writing, the Academy of Veterinary Cardiology was distributing pacemakers at a reduced cost.

SICK SINUS SYNDROME (BRADYCARDIA-TACHYCARDIA SYNDROME)

When the sinoatrial node is unable to generate an impulse and there is a failure to develop an ectopic pacemaker or the rhythm produced is a tachyarrhythmia, clinical cardiac (rate and rhythm) and neurologic (syncope and weakness) signs may appear. This condition, termed the sick sinus syndrome, may be character-

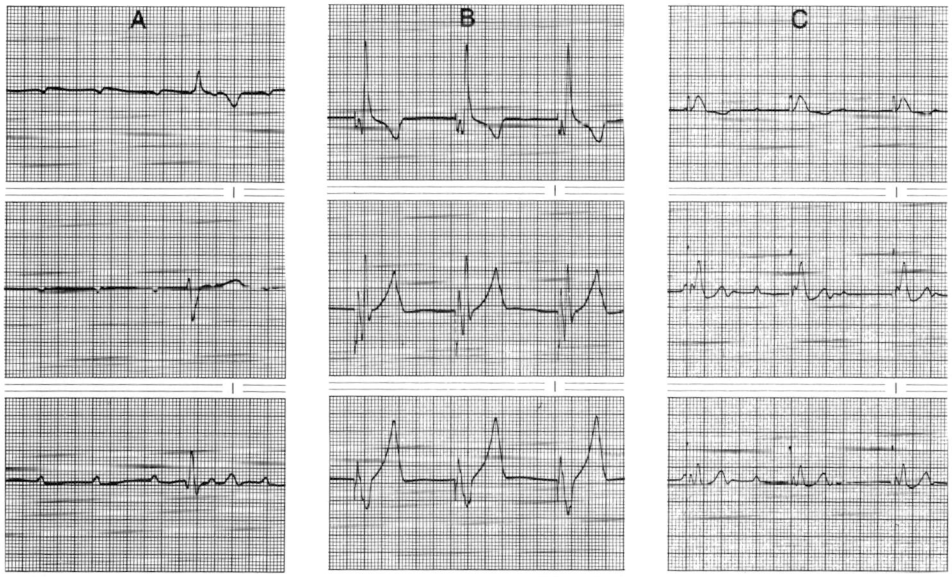

FIGURE 76–29. Pacemaker implantation. These tracings are simultaneously recorded leads I, II, and III taken at 50 mm per second. *A* represents a cocker spaniel in complete heart block. The ventricular rate was 32 per minute when the dog was presented for syncopal episodes. A pacemaker was implanted transvenously into the RV cavity. *B* demonstrates the ECG of dog *(A)* during pacing. The heart rate is 100 per minute. Notice the "pacemaker spikes" preceding each ventricular complex, which represent the electrical stimulus provided to the ventricle by the pacemaker. The ventricular complexes occur at the same rate in dogs *B* and *C* but they appear different due to variable ventricular conduction. *C* is from a dog with heart block in which a pacemaker was implanted. P waves are present but are not conducted. The pacemaker spikes are positive in all three leads preceding the ventricular complex.

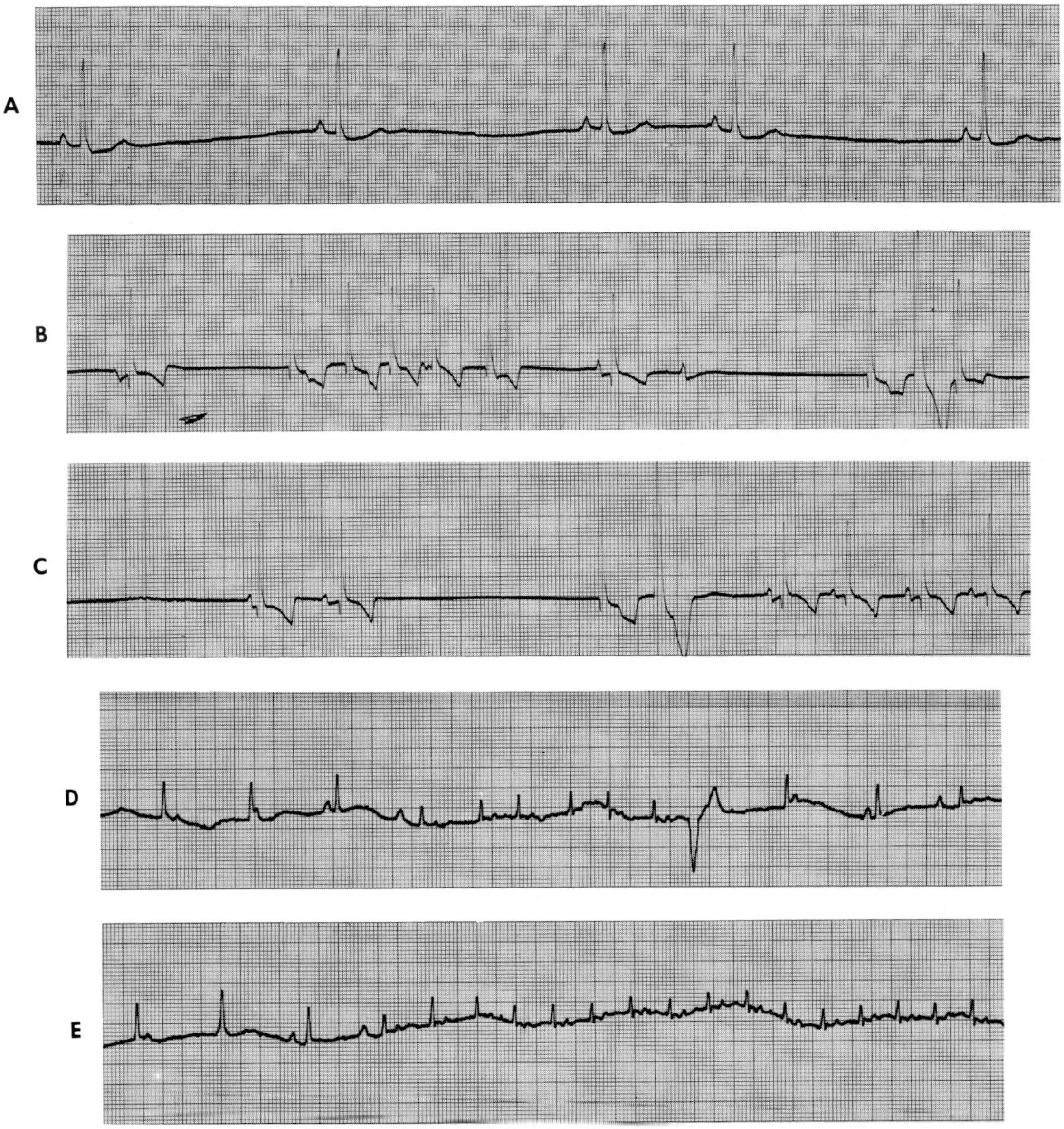

FIGURE 76–30. Sick sinus syndrome. *A* is a lead II tracing from a schnauzer bitch with signs of weakness, syncope, and heavy breathing. The heart rate is variable but always slow. There are occasional long pauses without cardiac activity. Anticholinergic-type drugs were helpful in controlling the symptoms, along with diuretic agents. *B* and *C* are lead II strips from a seven-year-old Chihuahua with frequent syncopal attacks not associated with excitement, coughing, or exertion. Electrocardiographic features of sick sinus syndrome or bradycardia-tachycardia include a burst of atrial tachycardia *(B),* second degree heart block *(B),* atrial or sinus pause *(C),* junctional escape beats (*B* and *C*), and ventricular premature contractions (*B* and *C*). This animal responded reasonably well to digoxin therapy only, although some episodes of syncope continued to occur. The dog died at home nearly one year later, during one of the attacks. *D* and *E* are representative tracings from a cat with the tachycardia-bradycardia syndrome. Although sinus arrest is not present, periods of slower heart rate, bursts of tachycardia, premature beats, and escape rhythms are all present.

ized by one or more of the following ECG rhythms: sinus bradycardia, sinoatrial block, sinus arrest, and alternating brady- and tachyarrhythmias.

Although there are few detailed pathologic descriptions of this syndrome in veterinary medicine, the human literature describes a multitude of problems involving the region of the sinoatrial node, including vascular, degenerative, inflammatory, and infiltrative lesions. It has been emphasized that this condition has a vascular basis because the sinoatrial node region is supplied by only a single vessel and this vessel has frequently been implicated as being abnormal.[60]

Although not often reported in cats, the condition occurs in many canine breeds. The female miniature schnauzer is the dog most commonly affected, and the boxer, dachshund, and pug are also singled out in several reports. In this author's experience, the condition is observed most often among schnauzers, but many other breeds are also affected. Although any age animal may develop this problem, the condition usually occurs in middle-aged to older dogs.

Affected animals are presented for evaluation of weakness, ataxia, and occasional confusion, with or without syncopal episodes. When present, syncope may be accompanied by a brief seizure (see Chapter 11).

The individual electrocardiographic features have been described in the preceding sections, but when multiple arrhythmias coexist, this syndrome is then recognized (Figure 76–30). The most characteristic feature, other than persistent sinus bradycardia, occurs when sinus arrest followed by supraventricular or ventricular escape or premature beats initiates paroxysms of supraventricular or ventricular tachycardia.

While standard electrocardiographic equipment may provide excellent tracings and diagnoses, occasionally one may need to employ ECG telemetry, continuous ECG ambulatory (Holter type) monitoring, exercise stress testing, drugs (isoproterenol, atropine), and vagal maneuvers, and occasionally, atrial pacing and sinus node recovery time (SNRT) measurements, in order to obtain a diagnosis. Monitoring permits the recognition of arrhythmias that do not occur continuously. Drugs (atropine) and vagal maneuvers demonstrate the response to stimuli, which is usually incomplete or inappropriate in the disease and the SNRT is prolonged when compared with that of normal dogs.[61, 62]

Noninvasive evaluation of sinus node function includes carotid sinus massage, exercise testing, drug testing (atropine, isoproterenol, propranolol), and measurement of the heart rate. Abnormal responses occur in most cases of sinus node dysfunction.[63]

Treatment. Unfortunately, drug therapy alone is not likely to be entirely successful. Drugs used to treat tachyarrhythmias may aggravate the bradyarrhythmia component and vice versa. The long-term pharmacologic success in the treatment of bradyarrhythmias is limited. Drug therapy for this condition may be associated with undesirable side effects such as dryness of the mouth, persistent pupillary dilatation, and chronic constipation.[64] Permanent pacemaker implantation affords the greatest likelihood for successful therapy. Over half of all pacemakers placed in human beings at this time are for the treatment of the sick sinus syndrome.

When pacemaker therapy is not feasible, this author has had a moderate degree of success with drug therapy. Atropine-like derivatives used for bradyarrhythmias and heart block, digitalis and furosemide for heart failure, and occasionally quinidine, procainamide, disopyramide, and propranolol for tachyarrhythmias are required. Digoxin does not exert negative chronotropic effects and can safely be used to treat pump failure or to control tachyarrhythmias in sick sinus syndrome.[65] On occasion, this author has used a combination of digoxin, diuretics, and atropine-like agents to treat the symptoms of the tachycardia-bradycardia complex of this disease. More often, the tachycardia or bradycardia portion of the syndrome predominates, and thus, attention is directed toward that problem. As stated earlier, pacemaker therapy, preferably the demand-type unit, is the method of choice for treating the sick sinus syndrome.

The prognosis for long-term survival is poor, but extended life expectancy of good quality has been observed with both conventional drug therapy and pacemaker implantation. Death, when it occurs, may be sudden and is associated with the onset of an acute arrhythmia, or it may be related to chronic congestive heart failure unresponsive to supportive therapy.

References

1. Detweiler, DK, et al.: Diseases of the Cardiovascular System. *In* Catcott, EJ (ed): Canine Medicine. Santa Barbara, American Veterinary Publications, Inc, 1968.
2. Bellet, S: Essentials of Cardiac Arrhythmias. Philadelphia, WB Saunders, 1972.
3. Cranefield, PF, et al.: Genesis of cardiac arrhythmias. Circulation 47:190, 1973.
4. American Heart Association: State of the art consensus on electrophysiologic testing in the diagnosis and treatment of patients with cardiac arrhythmias. Circulation Supplement 75(4):1, 1987.
5. Vera, Z and Mason, DT: Reentry versus automaticity: role in tachyarrhythmia genesis and antiarrhythmic therapy. Am Heart J 101:329, 1981.
6. Wit, AL and Rosen, MR: Cellular electrophysiology of cardiac arrhythmias. Mod Conc Cardio Dis 50:1, 1981.
7. Hoffman, BF and Rosen, MR: Cellular mechanisms for cardiac arrhythmias. Circ Res 49:1, 1981.
8. Rosen, MR and Hoffman, BF: Mechanism of action of antiarrhythmic drugs. Circ Res 32:1, 1973.
9. Samet, P: Hemodynamic sequelae of cardiac arrhythmias. Circulation 47:399, 1973.
10. Hamlin, RL, et al.: Clinical relevancy of heart rate in the dog. JAVMA 151:60, 1967.
11. Gettes, LS: The electrophysiologic effects of antiarrhythmic drugs. Am J Cardiol 28:526, 1971.
12. Muir, WW, et al.: Antiarrhythmic effects of diazepam during coronary artery occlusion in dogs. Am J Vet Res 36:1203, 1975.
13. Gillis, RA: Antiarrhythmic properties of chlordiazepoxide. Circulation 49:272, 1974.
14. Adams, HR: New perspectives in cardiology: pharmacodynamic classification of antiarrhythmic drugs. JAVMA 189(5):525, 1986.
14a. Zipes, DP: A consideration of antiarrhythmic therapy. Circulation 72:949, 1985.
15. Muir, WW: Pharmacology of antiarrhythmic drugs used in dogs and cats. Proceed ACVIM, 1987, p 254.
16. Novotny, MJ and Adams, HR: New perspectives in cardiology: recent advances in antiarrhythmic drug therapy. JAVMA 189(5):533, 1986.
17. Rosen, MR, et al.: The effects of lidocaine on the canine ECG

and electrophysiologic properties of Purkinje fibers. Am Heart J 91:191, 1976.

18. Gerstenblith, G, et al.: Quantitative study of the effect of lidocaine on the threshold for ventricular fibrillation in the dog. Am J Cardiol 30:242, 1972.
19. Tilley, LP and Weitz, J: Pharmacologic and other forms of medical therapy in feline cardiac disease. Vet Clin North Am 74:425, 1977.
20. Hession, M, et al.: Mexiletine and tocainide: does response to one predict response to the other? J Am Coll Cardiol 7(2):338, 1986.
21. Angelo, AV, et al.: Influence of left ventricular dysfunction on flecainide therapy. J Am Coll Cardiol 9(1):163, 1987.
22. O'Rourke, RA: Calcium-entry blockade: basic concepts and clinical implications. Circulation 75(5):1, 1987.
23. Allert, JA and Adams, HR: New Perspectives in Cardiovascular Medicine: The Calcium Channel Blocking Drugs. JAVMA 190(5):573, 1987.
24. Peterson, ME, et al.: Electrocardiographic Findings in 45 Cats With Hyperthyroidism. JAVMA 180(8):934, 1982.
25. Lannek, N: A clinical and experimental study on the electrocardiogram in dogs. Thesis, Stockholm, 1949.
26. Muir, WW: Thiobarbiturate-induced dysrhthmias: the role of heart rate and autonomic imbalance. Am J Vet Res 38:1377, 1977.
27. Boyden, PA, et al.: Mechanisms for Atrial Arrhythmias Associated with Cardiomyopathy: A Study of Feline Hearts with Primary Myocardial Disease. Circulation 69(5):1036, 1984.
28. Boineau, JP and Moore, EN: Evidence for propagation of activation across an accessory atrioventricular connection on types A and B pre-excitation. Circulation 41:375, 1970.
29. Ogburn, PN: Ventricular pre-excitation (Wolff-Parkinson-White Syndrome) in a cat. JAAHA 13:171, 1977.
30. Bolton, GR and Ettinger, SJ: Paroxysmal atrial fibrillation in the dog. JAVMA 158:64, 1971.
31. Wellens, H: Wolff-Parkinson-White Syndrome. Mod Con Cardio Dis 52(12):57, 1983.
32. Chung, EK: Tachyarrhythmias in Wolff-Parkinson-White syndrome; antiarrhythmic drug therapy. JAMA 237:376, 1977.
33. Olshansky, B and Waldo, AL: Atrial fibrillation: update on mechanism, diagnosis and management. Mod Con Cardio Dis 56(5):23, 1987.
34. Ettinger, SJ and Suter, PF: Canine Cardiology. Philadelphia, WB Saunders, 1970.
35. Bohn, FK, et al.: Atrial fibrillation in dogs. Br Vet J 127:485, 1971.
36. Buchanan, JW: Spontaneous arrhythmias and conduction disturbances in domestic animals. Ann NY Acad Sci 127:224, 1965.
37. Bohn, FK: Paroxysmales Vorhofflimmern Bei Hunden. Dtsch Tierarztl Wochenschr 76:198, 1969.
38. Madewell, BR, et al.: Paroxysmal atrial fibrillation associated with trauma in a dog. JAVMA 171:273, 1977.
39. Bohn, FK: Behandlung von Hunden mit Vorhofflimmern. Tierarztl Prax 59:184, 1978.
40. Friedberg, CK: Diseases of the Heart. Philadelphia, WB Saunders, 1966.
41. Ettinger, S: Conversion of spontaneous atrial fibrillation in dogs using direct current synchronized shock. JAVMA 152:41, 1968.

41a. McGovern, BA and Ruskin, JN: Ventricular tachycardia: Initial assessment and approach to treatment. Mod Con Cardio Dis 56:13, 1987.

42. Ettinger, SJ and Buergelt, DC: Atrioventricular dissociation (incomplete) with accrochage in a dog with ruptured chordae tendineae. Am J Vet Res 29:1499, 1968.
43. Kastor, JA, et al.: Clinical electrophysiology of ventricular tachycardia. N Engl J Med 304:1004, 1981.
44. Brandenburg, RO: Cardiomyopathies and their role in sudden death. J Am Coll Cardiol 5(6):185B, 1985.
45. Muir, WW and Lipowitz, AJ: Cardiac dysrhythmias associated with gastric dilation-volvulus in the dog. JAVMA 181:363, 1978.
46. Macintire, DK and Snider, TG: Cardiac arrhythmias associated with multiple trauma in dogs. JAVMA 184(5):541, 1984.
47. Surawicz, B: Prognosis of ventricular arrhythmias in relation to sudden cardiac death: therapeutic implications. J Am Coll Cardiol 10(2):435, 1987.
48. Wilson, JR: Use of antiarrhythmic drugs in patients with heart failure: clinical efficacy, hemodynamic results, and relation to survival. Circulation 75(4):4, 1987.
49. Deal, BJ, et al.: Ventricular Tachycardia in a Young Population Without Overt Heart Disease. Circulation 73(6):1111, 1986.
50. Clayborn, A and Szabunwiewicz, M: Am J Vet Res Vol. 34, 1973.
51. Hamlin, RL, et al.: Sinoatrial syncope in miniature schnauzers. JAVMA 161:1022, 1972.
52. James, TN, et al.: Clinicopathologic correlations—De subitaneis mortibus XV. Hereditary stenosis of the His bundle in pug dogs. Circulation 52:1152, 1975.
53. Tilley, LP and Liu, SK: Persistent atrial standstill in the dog with muscular dystrophy. ACVIM Ann Meeting Abstracts, Seattle, Washington, 1979.
54. Jeraj, K, et al.: Atrial standstill, myocarditis and destruction of cardiac conduction system. Am Heart J 99:185, 1980.
55. Castellanos, A, et al.: Contribution of His bundle recordings to the understanding of clinical arrhythmias. Am J Cardiol 28:499, 1971.
56. Robertson, BT and Giles, HD: Complete heart block associated with vegetative endocarditis in a dog. JAVMA 161:180, 1972.
57. Branch, CE, et al.: Frequency of second-degree atrioventricular heart block in dogs. Am J Vet Res 36:925, 1975.
58. Sisson, D: Permanent transvenous pacemaker implantation in the dog. ACVIM 13:101, 1986.
59. Fox, PR, et al.: Ventral Abdominal, Transdiaphragmatic Approach for Implantation of Cardiac Pacemakers in the Dog. JAVMA 189(10):1303, 1986.
60. James, TN: The sinus node. Am J Cardiol 40:965, 1977.
61. Clark, DR, et al.: Artificial pacemaker implantation for control of sinoatrial syncope in a miniature schnauzer. Southwest Vet 28:101, 1975.
62. Padilla, J: The sick sinus syndrome in the dog. Submitted for publication, 1982.
63. Crossen, KJ and Cain, ME: Assessment and management of sinus node dysfunction. Mod Con Cardio Dis 55(9):43, 1986.
64. Chung, EK: Sick sinus syndrome: Current views. Mod Con Cardio Dis 49:67, 1980.
65. Mason, DT and Awan, NA: Recent advances in digitalis research. Am J Cardiol 43:1056, 1979.
66. Bigger, JT: Management of Arrhythmias. *In* Braunwald, E (ed): Heart Disease. Philadelphia, WB Saunders, 1980.

77 MYOCARDIAL DISEASES

PHILIP R. FOX

The term cardiomyopathy denotes structural or functional abnormalities of the myocardium. Primary cardiomyopathy excludes diseases resulting from congenital, ischemic, hypertensive, vascular, pulmonary parenchymal, acquired valvular, or other cardiovascular disorders.[1, 2]

Various schemes used to classify myocardial diseases are based on physiologic, pathologic, or clinical characteristics: primary or "idiopathic" (describes the myocardium as the sole source of disease whose etiology is unknown), secondary (relates the myocardial disorder to identifiable systemic or metabolic disease), etiology (e.g., taurine deficiency cardiomyopathy), pathology (e.g., infiltrative cardiomyopathy), clinical presentation (e.g., congestive cardiomyopathy), myocardial structure (e.g., hypertrophic or dilated cardiomyopathy), and myocardial function (e.g., systolic or diastolic failure).[1-26] No single method completely defines all salient features or variables and strict categorization is not always possible. Intergrade and merging forms of myocardial disease are common in cats and progressive alterations in cardiac chamber morphology and function may occur. Functional and structural categories may overlap. Echocardiography has greatly advanced the characterization of cardiomyopathies. With ultrasonic evaluation the older clinical approach of pigeon-holing feline myocardial disease into a pure classification of hypertrophic or dilated cardiomyopathy is changing. Current concepts favor integration of cardiac performance (e.g., systolic versus diastolic dysfunction) with structure.[14, 22-26] Causes and classification of diseases affecting the myocardium of dogs and cats are listed in Table 77–1.

INCIDENCE

Cardiomyopathies comprise the majority of feline cardiovascular diseases. Necropsy has reported an incidence of 8.5 per cent of 4933 cats autopsied during 1962 to 1976 at The Animal Medical Center.[7] The clinical incidence has been estimated at 12 to 15 percent when secondary cardiomyopathies are taken into consideration.[14]

Canine myocardial disease comprises a smaller percentage of cardiovascular disorders. Specific clinical or necropsy incidence has not been reported. There appears to be less functional and structural heterogeneity in canine cardiomyopathies than feline cardiomyopathies, although several canine breeds display notable variation with respect to pathophysiology and clinical presentation.

DIAGNOSTIC STRATEGIES

Therapy has historically been based upon structural classification inferred from history, physical examination, electrocardiography, and plain film radiography. While this is often sufficient for diagnosing canine dilated cardiomyopathy (i.e., systolic dysfunction), it is insufficient for accurate classification of feline myocardial disorders. Nonselective angiocardiography provides additional structural information (e.g., cardiac chamber morphology) and may suggest abnormal hemodynamic changes (e.g., circulation time).[27-29] However, such functional assessments are often inaccurate in all but classic forms of cardiomyopathy. Angiocardiography is also associated with significant morbidity and mortality in decompensated patients, or when arrhythmias are present. Echocardiography provides advantages of a rapid, noninvasive technique for assessing cardiac structure and function.[30-33]

When combined with the above data base, heart failure may be clinically approached as a syndrome of systolic or diastolic dysfunction associated with morphologic cardiac changes (Tables 77–2 to 77–4). Congestive signs and related hemodynamic abnormalities caused by primary or secondary myocardial disorders can then be appropriately treated.

PRIMARY CARDIOMYOPATHIES

HEART FAILURE DUE TO SYSTOLIC DYSFUNCTION ("PUMP FAILURE")

Systolic (i.e., myocardial or pump) failure results when the ventricles fail to generate normal contractile force. Examples include primary (idiopathic) dilated cardiomyopathy or secondary dilated cardiomyopathy

TABLE 77–1. CAUSES OF MYOCARDIAL DISEASE

- I. Primary (Idiopathic) Cardiomyopathies
  - A. Hypertrophic
  - B. Dilated (congestive)
  - C. Restrictive
  - D. Intermediate or Intergrade
- II. Secondary Cardiomyopathies
  - A. Metabolic
    - 1. Endocrine
      - Thyrotoxicosis
      - Acromegaly
      - Pheochromocytoma
      - Hyperadrenocorticism (Cushing's disease)
      - Uremia (?)
      - Hypothyroidism (?)
    - 2. Nutritional
      - Selenium/Vitamin E deficiency
      - Taurine deficiency
      - Carnitine deficiency
      - Obesity
  - B. Infiltrative
    - Neoplasia
    - Glycogen storage diseases
    - Mucopolysaccharidosis (?)
  - C. Fibroplastic
    - Endomyocardial fibrosis
    - Endocardial fibroelastosis
  - D. Hypersensitivity
  - E. Physical agents
    - Hyperpyrexia
    - Hypothermia
  - F. Toxic
    - Doxorubicin
    - Cobalt
    - Catecholamines
    - Lead
    - Ethanol
  - G. Inflammatory
    - 1. Infectious
      - Viral
      - Bacterial
      - Parasitic
      - Fungal
      - Algal
    - 2. Noninfectious
      - Collagen diseases
  - H. Genetic
    - Hypertrophic cardiomyopathy (?)
    - Dilated cardiomyopathy (?)
    - Endocardial fibroelastosis
  - I. Miscellaneous
    - Ischemia
    - Muscular dystrophy
    - Conduction system disorders
    - Excessive left ventricular moderator bands

resulting from toxins (e.g., doxorubicin), infection (e.g., canine parvovirus), or inflammation (e.g., physical agents).[1, 2, 34] In the classic form, all four cardiac chambers are severely dilated. This is associated with reduced cardiac output, increased end-systolic and end-diastolic ventricular volumes, and excessive wall tension. Congestive heart failure results from both depressed contractility and failure (or overcompensation) of neuroendocrine, hepatorenal, and peripheral vascular compensatory mechanisms. Systolic dysfunction may range from mild to severe contractile impairment coupled with heterogeneous structural variations. Prognosis is not always directly related to indices of contractility, especially in cats with taurine deficiency.

TABLE 77–2. CLINICAL CHARACTERISTICS OF HEART FAILURE DUE TO SYSTOLIC (PUMPING) DYSFUNCTION

- I. Forward Heart Failure (i.e., decreased cardiac output, reduced tissue perfusion)
  - Weakness
  - Lethargy
  - Depression
  - Exercise intolerance
  - Anorexia
  - Weak cardiac apex beat
  - Soft heart sounds
  - Hypokinetic femoral pulses
  - Hypothermia
- II. Backward Heart Failure (i.e., elevated venous pressures behind the failing ventricles)
  - Dyspnea
  - Muffled heart/lung sounds (effusions)
  - Hepatomegaly
  - Hydroperitoneum
  - Peripheral edema
- III. Other Findings
  - S_3 gallop rhythm

DILATED (CONGESTIVE) CARDIOMYOPATHY (DCM)

Etiology. Dilated cardiomyopathy is the most common canine myocardial disorder.[12, 18, 19, 26, 34, 61–69] The reported feline incidence varies from approximately 17 to 20 per cent of necropsies[7, 35] to about 40 per cent in clinical studies.[16] This difference may be attributable to different criteria for classification, changes in causative factors, or regional population differences. Since early 1988, however, the feline incidence has been sharply reduced, correlating with dietary taurine fortification by commercial feline pet food manufacturers.[69a]

The etiology of primary (idiopathic) DCM is unknown. It may represent the end-stage result of myocardial injury caused by various metabolic, toxic, or infectious agents.[1, 2, 36, 51] Myocardial toxins including anthracyclines (especially doxorubicin)[34, 37, 38] and cyclophosphamide[39] have induced DCM in humans and animals. Microvascular hyperreactivity with myocytolysis, reactive hypertrophy, and progressive systolic dysfunction has been demonstrated in the Syrian hamster.[40] Familial transmission in humans is considered rare.[1, 2, 41] Metabolic deficiencies have been demonstrated in human familial DCM including carnitine deficiency.[42, 43] Carnitine-linked defects of myocardial metabolism have

TABLE 77–3. CLINICAL CHARACTERIZATION OF HEART FAILURE DUE TO DIASTOLIC DYSFUNCTION (DECREASED VENTRICULAR COMPLIANCE)

- I. Forward Cardiac Output Usually Adequate
- II. Backward Heart Failure (i.e., elevated venous pressures behind failing ventricle)
  - Dyspnea (acute)
  - Tachypnea
  - Pulmonary rales/rhonchi
  - Normal heart sounds (unless effusions)
  - Normal or accentuated cardiac apex beat
  - Normal femoral pulses
  - Hypothermia (cats)
- III. Other Findings
  - S_4 gallop rhythm

TABLE 77–4. STRUCTURAL AND FUNCTIONAL CHARACTERISTICS OF THE CARDIOMYOPATHIES

	Left Ventricle							Left Atrium		Congestive Heart Failure	
Type	*Shape*	*Dilatation*	*Hypertrophy*	*Systolic Volume*	*Diastolic Volume*	*Systolic Function*	*Diastolic Function*	*Size*	*Mitral Regurgitation*	*Left Sided*	*Right Sided*
Primary											
Dilated (congestive)	Globular	+ + +	0 or +	↑↑	↑↑	↓↓↓	N or ↓	+	+	+	+ + +
Hyper-trophic	Slitlike	0	+ + +	↓	N or ↓	↑↑; cavity elimination; gradients	Abnormal relaxation & filling	+ + or + + +	+ or + +	+ + +	+; (+ + + late)
Restric-tive	Irregular (intra-cavity fibrosis)	0 or +	+ + or + + +	N or ↓	N or ↓	N or ↓	Cavity restriction (early) or oblitera-tion (late)	+ + or + + +	+ + or + + +	+ +	+; + + + (late)
Secondary											
Thyrotox-icosis	Variable	0 or +	+ +	N or ↓	N or ↑	↑↑	N or ↓	+ +	+ or + +	+	0 to + +
Doxo-rubicin	Similar to dilated cardiomyopathy										

0 = absent; + = mild; + + = moderate; + + + = severe; ↓ = reduced; ↑ = increased; N = Normal
From Fox, PR: Feline cardiomyopathy. *In* Bonagura, JD (ed): Contemporary Issues. Small Animal Practice: Cardiology. Vol 7. New York, Churchill Livingstone, 1987, p 157.

been demonstrated in association with canine DCM.[44] Infective (probably viral) and immunologic factors have been implicated in some cases of DCM based upon myocardial nuclear changes, high viral antibody titers in some affected people, circulating immune complexes in cases of human myocarditis-associated DCM, and immunoregulatory defects.[44–47] Selenium deficiency has been associated with DCM in humans (Keshan disease)[48–49] and animals,[34, 50]although it has not been proven to be the sole cause of myocardial disease.

Taurine deficiency has recently been associated with reversible myocardial failure in felines.[51] It is not clear whether low plasma taurine causes dilated cardiomyopathy or if it facilitates action of other etiologic factors in the genesis of this disease.

Abnormal Physiology. The principal functional defect of DCM is depressed ventricular contractile performance (i.e., systolic or pump dysfunction).[1, 2] Cardiac chamber dilatation may be present prior to clinical signs if stroke volume is maintained by sympathetic, renal, hormonal, and increased end-diastolic fiber length (i.e., compensatory mechanisms). Sinus tachycardia may contribute to maintain cardiac output in canine DCM, but this finding is uncommon with feline DCM. Elevated ventricular end-diastolic pressures may result from reduced systolic emptying and increased end-systolic residual volume. These pressures represent additional compensatory mechanisms, which temporarily maintain cardiac output. Alterations in left ventricular relaxation and diastolic compliance coexist with impaired contractile function and contribute to elevated filling pressures.[52, 53] Ventricular dilatation causes geometric distortion of the atrioventricular valve apparatus causing mitral regurgitation.[7, 16, 24, 34, 54] This further reduces forward stroke volume and contributes to left atrial dilatation. The latter predisposes to atrial arrhythmias, especially atrial fibrillation.[55, 56] Sudden arrhythmias often herald acute cardiac decompensation. Resultant loss of atrial contribution and reduced time for diastolic filling markedly decreases cardiac output. Inadequate forward flow produces clinical signs of low-output failure as muscles and organs become poorly perfused. Decreased renal perfusion stimulates the renin-angiotensin-aldosterone system, which increases preload and afterload. Enhanced sympathetic activity contributes to increased preload and peripheral vascular resistance. The latter further reduces cardiac output.[1, 2] Ventricular hypertrophy may occur as a compensatory mechanism to reduce wall tension and pressure according to the law of Laplace.[57] Congestive signs ultimately develop.

Pathology. Post-mortem examination discloses a globular-shaped heart with severe dilatation of all four cardiac chambers (Figure 77–1). Heart weights are significantly greater than normal. Ventricular walls become abnormally thin, although various degrees of compensatory hypertrophy may be present, especially in cats. Papillary muscles and trabeculae are atrophied. Focal endocardial fibrosis may be present. Atrioventricular valve circumference is usually enlarged, but valve leaflets are normal. Cardiac muscle cells may display vari-

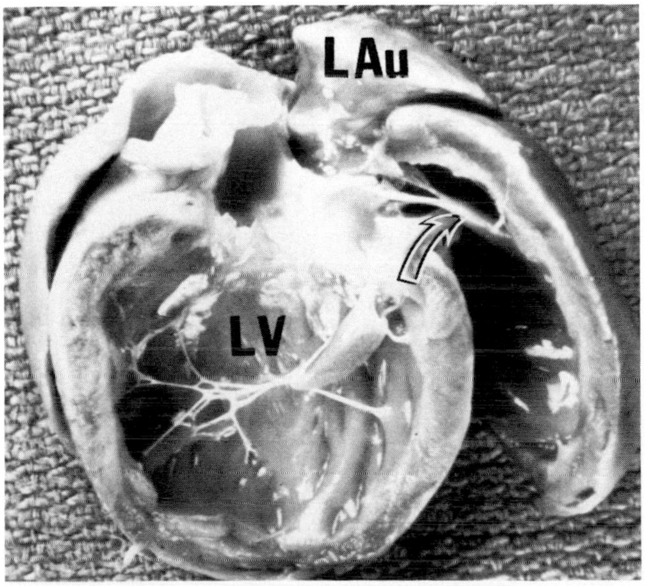

FIGURE 77–1. Heart from a six-year-old male Siamese with dilated cardiomyopathy. The left ventricle (LV) is severely dilated. Papillary muscles (arrow) are atrophic and thin. The left auricle (LAu) is enlarged. A small network of aberrant moderator bands appears as thread-like strands across the mid left ventricle.

ous degrees of degeneration ranging from coagulation, granulation, and sarcoplasmic vacuolization to myocytolysis.[1–8, 11, 12, 16, 19, 20, 24–26, 34, 35, 61]

CLINICAL MANIFESTATIONS

Feline DCM. Signalment suggests young to middle-aged cats (range, 5 months to 16 years with a mean of about 7 1/2 years).[8, 16] All breeds are affected, although Siamese, Abyssinian, and Burmese breeds display a particularly high incidence. Reports of sex predisposition vary from male preponderance,[8] slight female predominance,[16] or relatively equal distribution.[23, 25]

Presenting clinical signs are usually vague. They include anorexia, dyspnea, lethargy, or emesis for one to three days' duration. Paresis of a front or rear leg results from acute embolization. Syncope is rare.[16, 17, 23–25]

Physical examination reveals lethargy, depression, and dehydration (usually 5 to 8 per cent). Hypothermia is usually present or is recorded shortly after admission. Auscultation may reveal a gallop rhythm (usually S_3) and a left and/or right apical systolic heart murmur. Lung sounds may reveal "crackles" due to pulmonary edema. Alternatively, or in addition, heart and lung sounds may be muffled if significant pericardial or pleural effusion is present. The left cardiac apex beat (precordial impulse) and femoral arterial pulse are weak. Hydroperitoneum and hepatomegaly can occur if right-sided heart failure is present (Table 77–2).

Electrocardiography displays normal sinus rhythm in about one-half of affected cats, while bradycardia is recorded in less than one-quarter. The reported incidence of left ventricular enlargement (R wave in lead II greater than 0.9 mV, or QRS complex duration greater than 0.04 sec) is 25 to 39 per cent.[16, 25] Ventricular premature complexes have been recorded in almost one-half of affected cats in one study,[16] but less commonly by other investigators.[5, 24, 25] Various other arrhythmias are occasionally detected.

Radiographs classically display generalized, severe cardiomegaly, which is often silhouetted by pleural effusion (Figure 77–2). Pulmonary venous congestion or mild pulmonary edema may be present concurrently, but this is often obscured by the effusion. A characteristic round, globoid-shaped ventricular apex may be evident in the ventrodorsal view. A dilated caudal vena cava, hepatomegaly, and hydroperitoneum may be present.[5, 6, 10–12, 14, 16, 17, 23–25, 29, 54, 58]

Nonselective angiocardiography may display moderate left atrial enlargement, severe left and right ventricular dilatation, atrophic papillary muscles, reduced aortic diameter, and slow circulation time (see Table 77–4 and Figure 77–3).[11, 14, 16, 27–29] Hazards associated with angiocardiography are due to tranquilizer-related arrhythmias and adverse reactions to contrast medium.[28] Thus, it should not be performed in severely decompensated animals.

Echocardiography provides rapid, safe, and reliable noninvasive evaluation of cardiac function, as well as structure (Figure 77–4). Diagnostic features include greatly enlarged ventricular end-diastolic and end-systolic dimensions; significantly depressed indices of left ventricular contractility (e.g., decreased left ventricular ejection time, prolonged pre-ejection period, decreased fractional shortening and velocity of circumferential fiber shortening; aortic root, interventricular septal, and left ventricular free wall hypokinesis); moderate left atrial and severe right ventricular dilatation.[14, 16, 17, 23–25, 30–33] Left ventricular free wall and interventricular septal thickness may be reduced or appear normal if compensatory hypertrophy has occurred.

Clinical laboratory abnormalities are common. Most

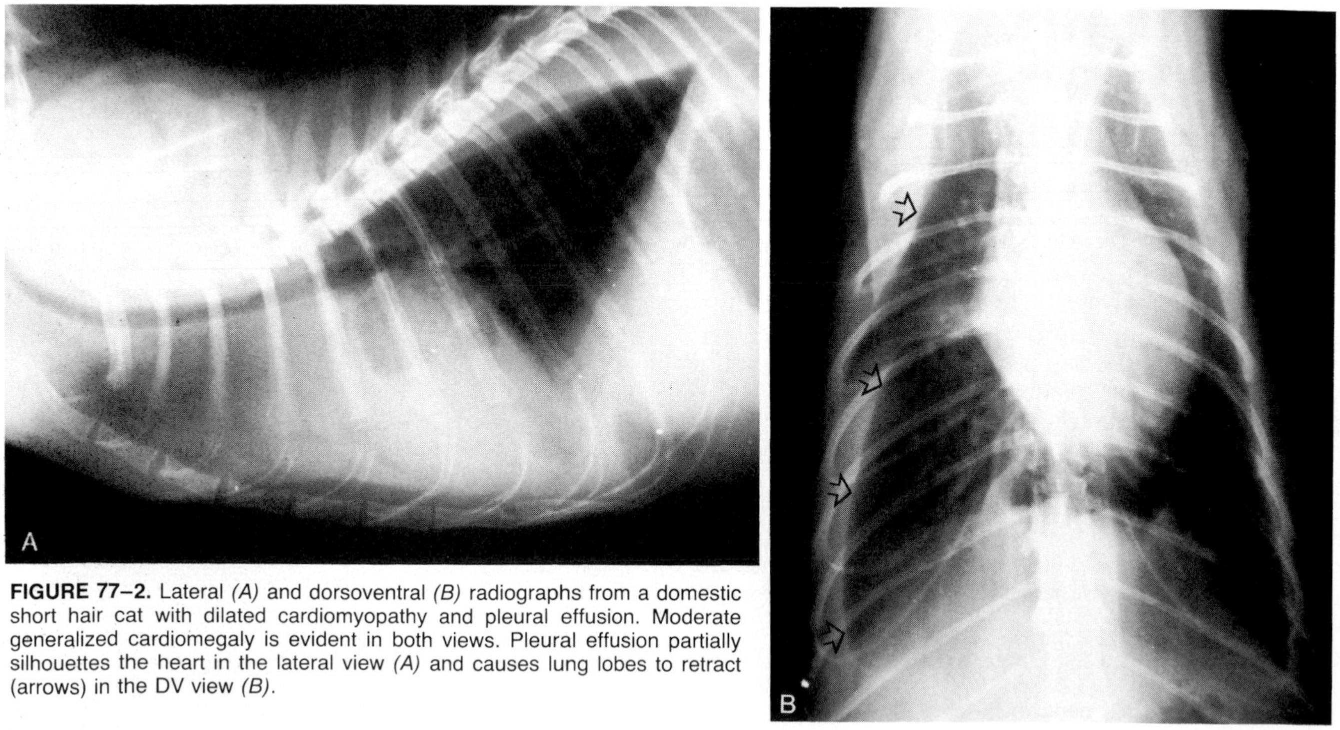

FIGURE 77–2. Lateral *(A)* and dorsoventral *(B)* radiographs from a domestic short hair cat with dilated cardiomyopathy and pleural effusion. Moderate generalized cardiomegaly is evident in both views. Pleural effusion partially silhouettes the heart in the lateral view *(A)* and causes lung lobes to retract (arrows) in the DV view *(B)*.

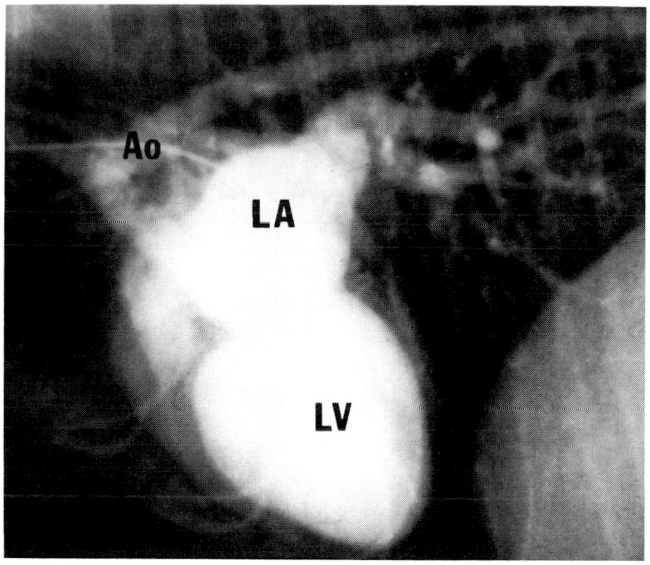

FIGURE 77–3. Nonselective angiocardiogram from a three-year-old female domestic short hair cat with dilated cardiomyopathy. The left ventricle (LV) is severely dilated. Moderate left atrial (LA) enlargement is present. Papillary muscles are thin and barely visible. The aorta (Ao) is poorly opacified, suggesting reduced forward stroke volume and poor cardiac output.

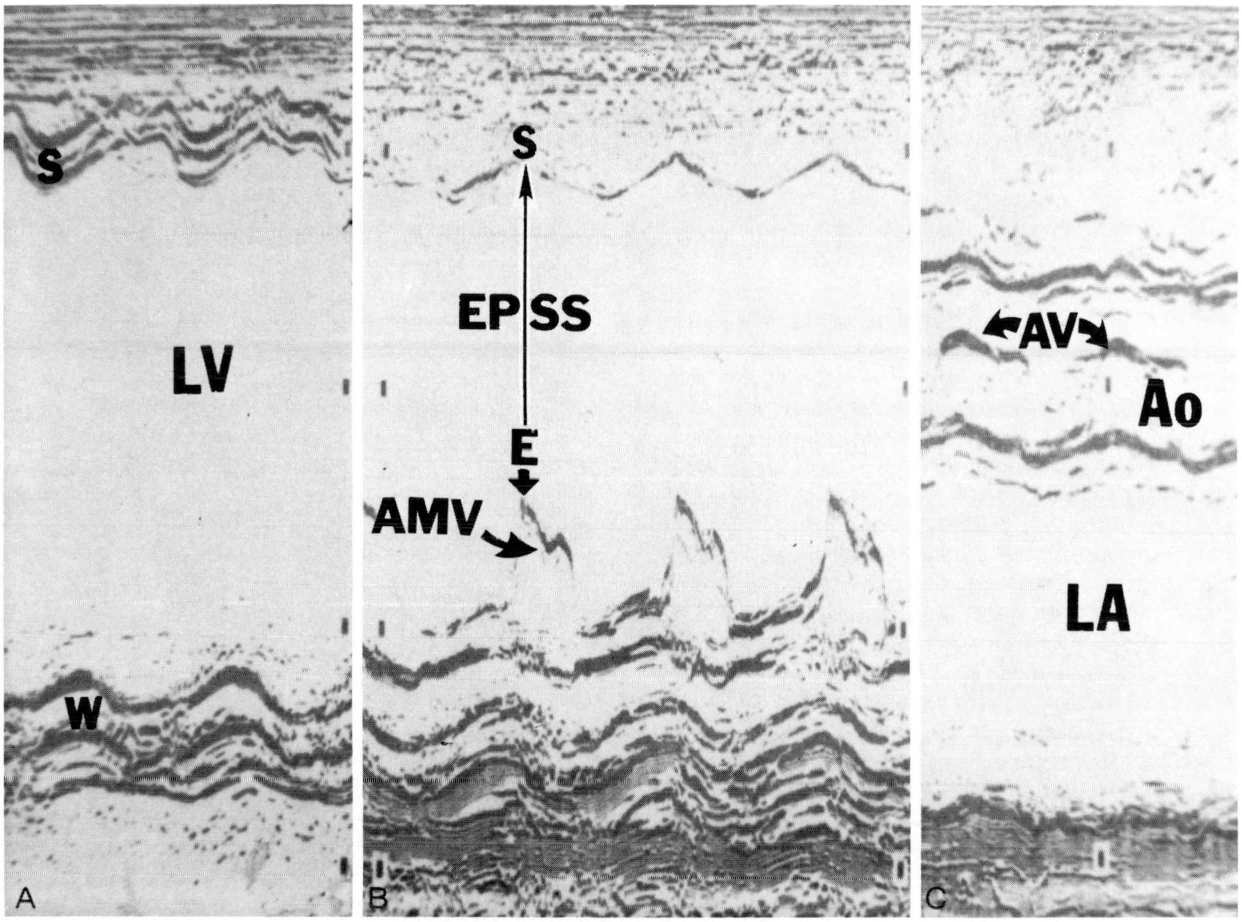

FIGURE 77–4. M-mode echocardiogram from a five-year-old male Abyssinian cat with dilated cardiomyopathy illustrating the heart from the three standard echocardiographic positions. *A*, Echogram obtained from the ventricular level just below the mitral valve. Severe dilatation of the left ventricle (LV) during systole and diastole is evident. Both the interventricular septum (S) and left ventricular posterior wall (W) are thinner than normal. There is slight paradoxic motion of the interventricular septum. *B*, Echogram from the mitral valve level. The E-point (E) of the anterior mitral valve (AMV) is widely separated from the interventricular septum (S). This E-point septal separation (EPSS) denotes severe LV dilatation. *C*, Echogram obtained at the aortic root level. The left atrium (LA) is greatly dilated. AO = aortic root; AV = aortic valve.

cats are azotemic (e.g., blood urea nitrogen, 35 to 60 mg/dl; normal, 20 to 30 mg/dl) resulting from reduced cardiac output, decreased water consumption, anorexia, and fluid sequestration (effusions). Low plasma taurine levels (less than 20 μM/dl[51, 51a] occur in cats fed taurine deficient diets.[51] Mild hyperglycemia may be present.[10, 11, 23–25] With thromboembolic disease, coagulopathies are common. Disseminated intravascular coagulation may occur in association with consumptive coagulopathy, in liver-mediated coagulopathy, or from effects of thromboembolism. In addition, elevations in serum lactic acid dehydrogenase, creatinine phosphokinase, alanine aminotransferase, and aspartate aminotransferase are recorded during thromboembolism.[59, 60]

Differential diagnosis includes other causes of congestive heart failure. Congenital cardiac anomalies must be strongly considered in young cats, especially lesions causing volume overload (e.g., ventricular septal defect, atrioventricular valve dysplasia, common atrioventricular canal). Some cats with congenital mitral valve malformation survive into middle and old age until they develop severe atrial and ventricular dilatation and myocardial failure. Pericardiodiaphragmatic hernia may cause generalized, severe cardiomegaly. Acquired valvular disease and endocarditis are rare. All causes of pleural effusion must be considered since right-sided heart failure is usually common with decompensated DCM. Thyrotoxicosis and hypertrophic or restrictive cardiomyopathy may cause right-sided failure as well. Since cardiogenic shock may dominate the clinical presentation with systolic failure, diseases inducing a shock-like state must be considered.

Canine DCM. The signalment typically describes young, predominantly male, large and giant breed dogs.[8, 12, 18–20, 26, 61–72] Reported age of onset ranges from 6 months to 14.5 years, with a mean age of about four to six years.

Clinical signs may occur acutely (over one to three days). They include dyspnea, coughing, syncope, exercise intolerance, or abdominal distention. In others, more subtle subacute changes occur over five to seven days, such as partial anorexia, weight loss (often pronounced), and mild to moderate lethargy.

Physical examination reveals abnormalities consistent with low cardiac output, left-sided heart failure (e.g., pulmonary edema), or right-sided heart failure (e.g., pericardial, pleural, abdominal effusions). Biventricular failure may sometimes coexist. The patient may be weak with prolonged capillary refill time, pale mucous membranes, and hypokinetic femoral arterial pulses. Jugular venous distention or pulsations, abdominal distention (ascites), and hepatosplenomegaly may be detected. Auscultation often reveals a left or right apical murmur of mild to moderate intensity from atrioventricular valvular insufficiency due to altered atrioventricular valve complex geometry. A rapid, irregular heart rate and an S_3 gallop rhythm may be present. Muffled heart and lung sounds may be due to diminished contractility or the damping effects of pericardial and pleural effusion. Increased bronchovesicular sounds and inspiratory crackles may be evident. Weight loss may be obvious resulting in accentuated ribs and dorsal spinous vertebral processes.[18–20, 26, 62]

Electrocardiography usually suggests left heart enlargement and often displays arrhythmias.[12, 18–20, 26, 62, 63, 65, 67, 71] The most common arrhythmia is atrial fibrillation (Figure 77–5*A*), a rapid, irregularly irregular supraventricular tachycardia without P waves. It is usually detected during initial physical examination or develops during early stages of treatment. Less frequently, paroxysmal atrial tachycardia or sinus tachycardia (Figure 77–5*B*) (often with atrial premature complexes) is recorded. Sinus rhythm is seen consistently only with DCM in Doberman pinschers (Figure 77–5*C*) and English cocker spaniels. Ventricular arrhythmias (Figure 77–5*D*) may be present or coexist with supraventricular rhythm disorders as singles, pairs, or triplets of ventricular premature complexes. Occasionally, paroxysmal or sus-

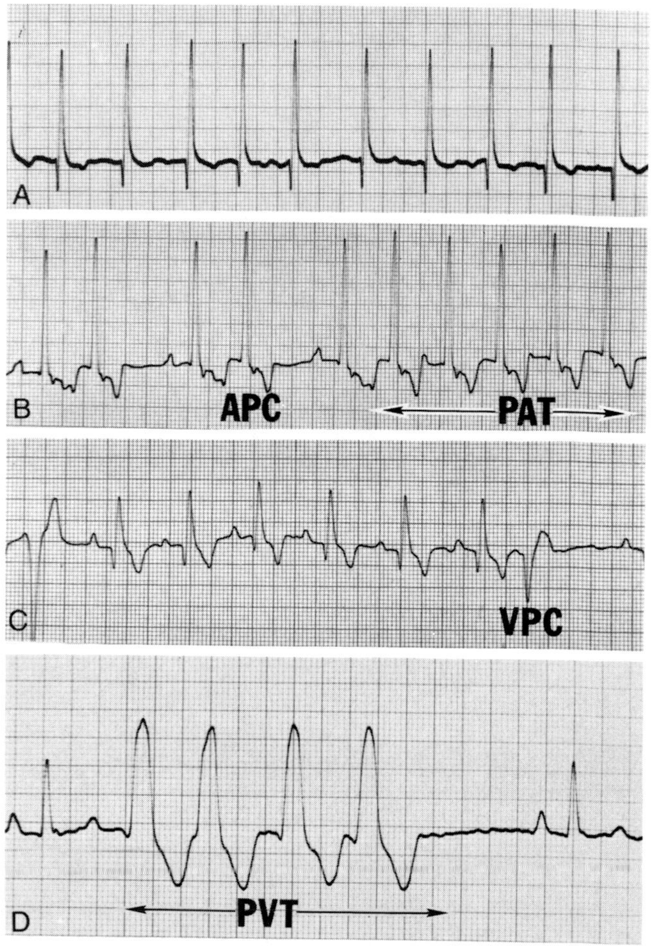

FIGURE 77–5. Electrocardiograms (lead II, 50 mm/sec, 1 mV = 1 cm) recorded from dogs with cardiomyopathy. *A*, Atrial fibrillation in a three-year-old male Great Dane with dilated cardiomyopathy. The rhythm is totally irregular and P waves are absent. *B*, Paroxysmal atrial tachycardia and atrial premature complexes in a four-year-old male St. Bernard with dilated cardiomyopathy. P waves are wide and R waves are tall suggesting left atrial and ventricular enlargement, respectively. *C*, Sinus tachycardia in a six-year-old male Doberman pinscher with dilated cardiomyopathy. The QRS complexes are wide (0.07 second or greater) suggesting left bundle branch block. Occasional ventricular premature complexes are present. *D*, Paroxysmal ventricular tachycardia in an eight-year-old female boxer with "boxer cardiomyopathy." The ventricular ectopic impulses have a left bundle branch block pattern (wide and upright). P waves are wide suggesting left atrial enlargement. VPC = ventricular premature complex; APC = atrial premature complex; PAT = paroxysmal atrial tachycardia; PVT = paroxysmal ventricular tachycardia.

tained ventricular tachycardia is recorded. Left ventricular enlargement is often present (R wave in lead II taller than 3.0 mV or QRS duration wider than 0.065 sec with ST-T segment "slurring"). With severe pericardial or pleural effusion, R waves may be small (less than 1.0 mV). Left atrial enlargement (P mitrale) is often present unless atrial fibrillation or sustained ventricular tachycardia occurs. P mitrale is indicated by P wave duration greater than 0.04 sec.

Radiographs display characteristic generalized cardiomegaly.[12, 18–20, 26, 29, 62, 67] The heart may appear rounded and globoid, especially if pericardial effusion is present (Figure 77–6). Some breeds, such as the Doberman pinscher, may display only left atrial enlargement. An interstitial and alveolar pulmonary pattern consistent with pulmonary edema may be seen in the perihilar region (i.e., dorsally and caudally) or diffusely, if severe left-sided heart failure occurs (especially in Doberman pinschers and English cocker spaniels) (Figure 77–7). Pleural effusion may obscure the cardiac silhouette. Hydroperitoneum and hepatosplenomegaly may be present.

Echocardiography displays changes similar to those described under feline DCM (see Figure 77–8).[19, 20, 26, 31, 66, 69] Clinical laboratory abnormalities include prerenal azotemia, elevated serum ALT (SGPT), and reduced serum protein levels. Gross and ultrastructural altera-

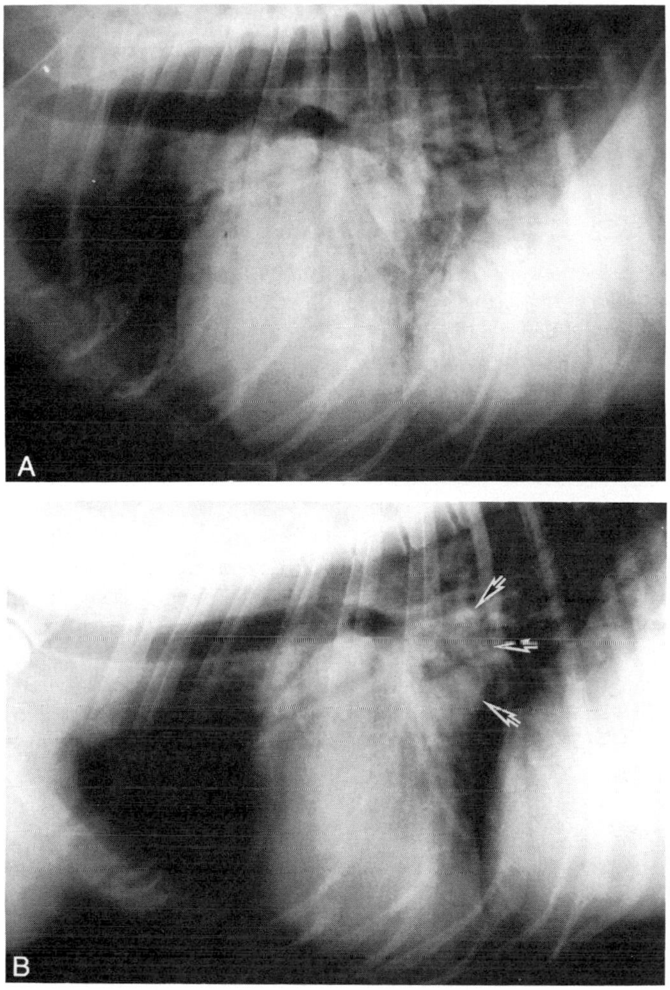

FIGURE 77–7. Lateral thoracic radiographs from a three-year-old male Doberman pinscher with dilated cardiomyopathy and acute pulmonary edema. *A*, Pretreatment radiograph shows an increased interstitial and alveolar pulmonary pattern dorsal and caudal to the heart. This is compatible with pulmonary edema. *B*, Two days after therapy pulmonary infiltrates have cleared. There is severe left atrial enlargement (arrows) with only mild generalized cardiomegaly.

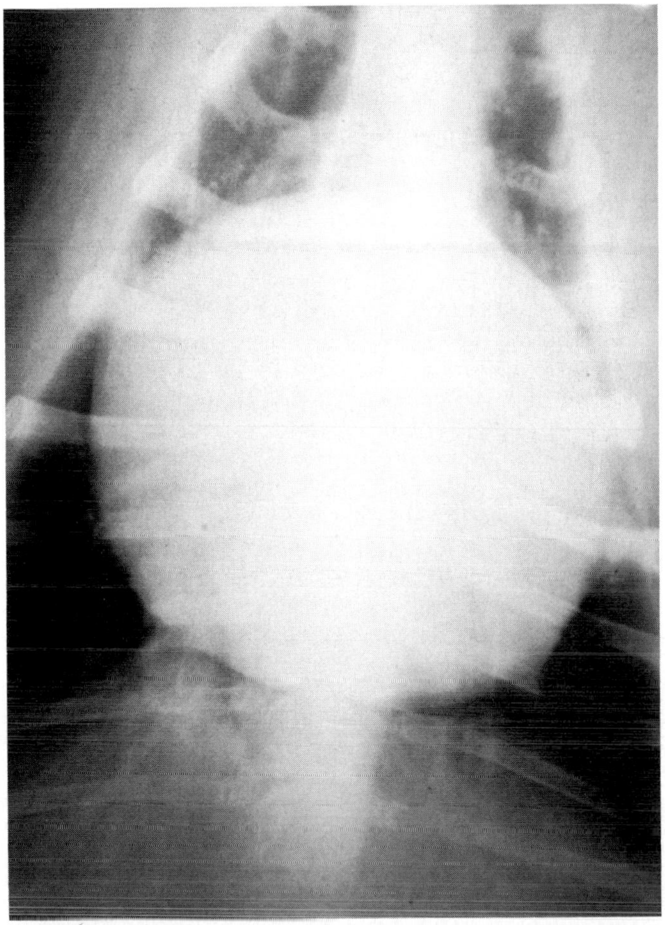

FIGURE 77–6. Dorsoventral thoracic radiograph from a four-year-old male German shepherd dog with dilated cardiomyopathy. Severe pericardial effusion is present, which confers a round shape to the cardiac silhouette.

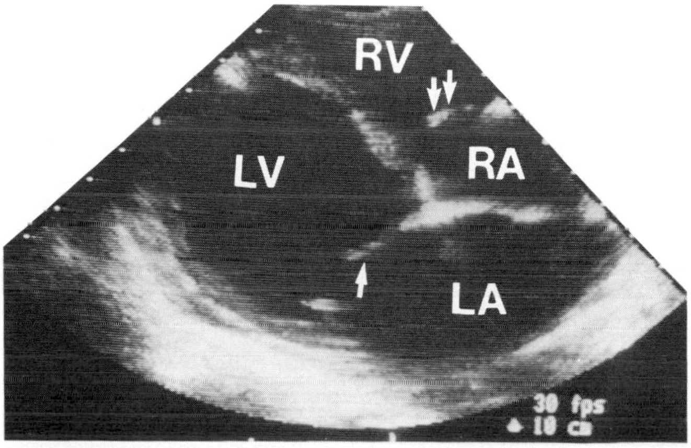

FIGURE 77–8. Two-dimensional echocardiogram of a one-year-old greyhound showing a modified four-chamber view. There is severe dilatation of the left atrium (LA), left ventricle (LV), right ventricle (RV), and right atrium (RA). Systolic function was greatly reduced. Arrows point to the mitral and tricuspid valves.

tions are similar to those described in cats with the exception of thromboembolic disease.[34, 35, 61]

Dilated cardiomyopathy in *Doberman pinschers* may resemble the classic form of giant breed idiopathic cardiomyopathy described above. A large subset, however, displays clinical features that differ consistently from the "classic" form with respect to radiographic changes, electrocardiographic findings, and prognosis.[18–20, 26, 61–66] While severely reduced left ventricular contractility (systolic dysfunction) and typical historical and physical examination abnormalities are typically present, radiographs often show left atrial enlargement rather than generalized cardiomegaly (Figure 77–7). The most common radiographic extracardiac signs of heart failure are alveolar pulmonary edema and enlargement of the right cranial lobar pulmonary vein. Pulmonary edema may be diffuse rather than confined to dorsal and caudal lung regions. Pleural effusion, when present, is usually mild.[62, 63] Electrocardiographic changes typically show sinus rhythm with left ventricular enlargement or left bundle branch block pattern (QRS duration greater than 0.07 sec) (Figure 77–5*C*) and ventricular arrhythmias. Ventricular arrhythmias usually persist throughout the course of treatment. Less frequently, these dogs present with or develop atrial fibrillation. Prognosis is grave with most Dobermans dying within six weeks of diagnosis.[62, 63, 66]

Occasionally, some clinically normal Dobermans are identified with only mild to moderate radiographic left atrial enlargement, and moderately to slightly reduced myocardial function. These dogs may develop acute left-sided congestive heart failure 1 to 15 months later and respond poorly to therapy.[66]

Pathologic findings in Doberman DCM include atrial and ventricular dilatation, reduced left ventricular wall thickness, myocyte degeneration, fatty infiltration, and myocardial fibrosis.[34, 35, 62–64]

Boxer cardiomyopathy describes a primary myocardial disorder in the boxer breed distinguished by extensive histologic myocardial changes, absence of severe atrial or ventricular dilatation, and usually ventricular arrhythmias.[67] Affected dogs range from 1 to 15 years of age (average, 8.2 years; median, 8.5 years). Males are affected slightly more often and there has been a greater prevalence in some breeding lines. Clinical features may be divided into three nearly equal categories: syncope or episodic weakness, left-sided congestive heart failure (sometimes, biventricular failure), and asymptomatic with cardiac arrhythmias. Murmurs of mitral insufficiency are recorded in about one-half of the cases. Thoracic radiographic findings are variable. In most asymptomatic dogs and in about one-half of syncopal animals, no significant abnormalities are present. Cardiomegaly and pulmonary edema accompany cases of advanced heart failure. Pleural effusion is uncommon. Electrocardiographic changes are quite characteristic for boxer cardiomyopathy. Ventricular premature complexes occurring singly, in pairs, or in runs are most common in incidence, followed by paroxysmal ventricular tachycardia. Ventricular ectopias characteristically arise from the right ventricle and demonstrate a left bundle branch pattern (i.e., wide, bizarre, upright QRS complexes in leads I, II, III, aVF) (Figure 77–5*D*). Supraventricular tachyarrhythmias are occasionally recorded. During normal sinus rhythm, P, QRS, and T complexes are usually unremarkable.[26, 67]

Prognosis for long-term survival in boxers with ventricular arrhythmias and heart failure is usually less than six months. Boxers in the other categories without congestive heart failure may survive up to two years in some cases. Sudden death is common. Post-mortem findings may reveal mild left ventricular hypertrophy and dilatation, left atrial dilatation, and thickened, nodular mitral (and occasionally, aortic or tricuspid) valves. Histologically, active myocardial changes (e.g., focal myocytolysis, myofiber degeneration, and mild mononuclear cellular infiltration) and chronic alterations (e.g., myofiber atrophy, fibrosis, and fatty change) are routinely present. The chronic changes are more common.[67] Myocardial carnitine deficiency has been demonstrated in some affected dogs.[44]

In small breed dogs, dilated cardiomyopathy has been described in the *English cocker spaniel*.[68–71] Affected dogs ranged from two to nine years of age (mean, 5.8 years), with approximately equal sex distribution. A familial predisposition has been suggested.[68, 71] Clinical signs most commonly included acute dyspnea and sudden death. Physical examination typically disclosed auscultatory abnormalities (rales, murmurs). The most notable electrocardiographic changes included left ventricular enlargement (tall R waves in lead II and ST segment "slurring") with sinus rhythm. Deep Q waves may be commonly recorded. Radiographic changes include pulmonary edema and biventricular enlargement.[68] Echocardiographic characterization included increased end-systolic and usually end-diastolic dimensions. Depressed myocardial function was recorded by echocardiography in only 75 per cent of affected dogs.[69]

Based on a limited number of animals studied, dilated cardiomyopathy in English cocker spaniels may differ from that in large and giant breed dogs in the following ways: (1) the disease is often typified by a long asymptomatic period; (2) early ECG abnormalities (especially left ventricular enlargement) may be recorded during the asymptomatic period; (3) myocardial function may be less depressed than in other breeds with dilated cardiomyopathy; (4) congestive heart failure usually results from progressive systolic dysfunction.[69] English cocker spaniels, as other small breed dogs, may be affected with chronic acquired valvular disease.

ENDOCARDIAL FIBROELASTOSIS

This rare anomaly is characterized by diffuse endocardial thickening by fibrous and elastic tissues, which are thicker and more organized adjacent to the myocardium.[34] It has been reported from a few unrelated dogs[72] and as a primary inherited congenital anomaly in Burmese cats.[73] Structural and functional features are similar to those observed with dilated cardiomyopathy (severe cardiac chamber dilatation, systolic dysfunction) except for the presence of pronounced, diffuse endocardial fibroelastosis. The clinical distinction between this syndrome and DCM is often blurred. Treatment is therefore similar to that described for systolic dysfunction below.

TREATMENT OF HEART FAILURE DUE TO SYSTOLIC DYSFUNCTION

Ideally, management of heart failure due to systolic dysfunction involves the following: treat causative or associated factors (e.g., taurine deficiency in cats), avoid cardiotoxic or cardiosuppressive agents, augment cardiac contractility, reduce or eliminate congestive signs, treat arrhythmias, and administer special drugs when indicated (e.g., aspirin). Since etiology or contributory factors are usually obscure, standard therapy relies on inotropic agents to enhance contractility, diuretics to reduce congestive signs, vasodilators to promote ventricular unloading, antiarrhythmic drugs, exercise restriction, and dietary modification.[1, 2, 10–12, 14, 16–20, 22 26, 37, 42, 44, 51, 62, 67, 74–76] Overall therapeutic goals to reduce congestion and improve exercise tolerance are directed to optimize cardiac output by pharmacologic manipulation of the four major determinants of left ventricular performance: preload (ventricular filling pressure), afterload (arterial pressure and resistance to ventricular emptying), myocardial contractility, and heart rate and rhythm.[73]

Since congestive heart failure is caused by impaired ventricular systolic function, inotropic agents are used to stimulate the depressed myocardium. This is based on the presumption of adequate contractile reserve or residual myocardial function.[77–79] However, global cardiac performance and systemic perfusion must sufficiently improve in order for an inotropic agent to be clinically beneficial. This depends, in part, on the severity, chronicity, and etiology of heart failure, as well as limits imposed by the toxic/therapeutic ratio of the inotrope.[74] Recent developments in positive inotropic drugs appear promising, especially the phosphodiesterase inhibitors such as amrinone and milrinone.[80]

Diuretics have been standardly employed to reduce signs of congestion by inhibiting renal tubular reabsorption of sodium or its accompanying anions.[81] Efficacy depends upon drug potency to inhibit electrolyte reabsorption, site of drug action in the nephron, and ultimately, homeostatic factors (e.g., aldosterone, antidiuretic hormone), which increase renal sodium and water reabsorption and diminish diuretic action.[82]

Vasodilator therapy is often used to reduce resistance to left ventricular ejection, and thereby improve cardiac performance. The injured myocardium may lose the ability to maintain cardiac output in the face of increased outflow resistance (i.e., afterload). Ventricular performance becomes inversely related to this impedance.[83] An "afterload mismatch" may develop caused by the increased level of vascular resistance and inability of the heart to eject an appropriate quantity of blood.[84] Vasodilator therapy clearly improves signs of congestion and may enhance long-term survivability. They are undergoing wider use as adjuvant therapy.

THERAPY OF FELINE DILATED CARDIOMYOPATHY

Cardiogenic shock is common in decompensated cats. Contributing factors are low cardiac output and impaired tissue perfusion due to severely reduced myocardial contractility, diminished cardiac preload from anorexia, vomiting and extravascular fluid accumulation (effusions), and increased afterload. Arrhythmias are sometimes present. This syndrome is rapidly progressive and potentially lethal. Prompt treatment is necessary.

Immediate Therapy. Mechanical fluid removal by thoracocentesis should be performed when auscultation reveals muffled heart and lung sounds associated with dyspnea. This reduces the physical constraint on lung expansion, thereby improving ventilation. One to three hundred milliliters of pleural effusion may be removed in this fashion without tranquilization or untoward effects. A mild pneumothorax may result if the needle punctures a lung, but this rarely seems to pose a clinical problem. A 19 to 21 gauge, 1.9 cm long, butterfly needle is preferred for this technique. Further diagnostic tests (e.g., ECG, radiographs) may then be safely performed.

Diuretics are administered as a next step to reduce edema or effusion. Furosemide, a potent loop diuretic, is most commonly selected. Cats are highly sensitive to its effects. It is initially dosed at 0.5 mg/lb (1.1 mg/kg) IV or IM q12h. Diuresis may occur within 30 min. For cats previously receiving oral maintenance furosemide, this dose is sometimes increased to 1.0 mg/lb (2.2 mg/kg) q8h to q12h. Overzealous administration, however, may severely reduce ventricular filling (preload), cause azotemia and electrolyte abnormalities, reduce cardiac output, and prolong renal clearance of certain drugs (e.g., digoxin).[10–12, 14, 16, 17, 23–25, 81, 82]

Positive inotropic agents are administered to stimulate the depressed myocardium. Classically, digoxin has been utilized. Intravenous digitalization has been advocated in severely affected cats, employing a total calculated dose of 0.0025 mg/lb (0.005 mg/kg) lean body weight. One-half of the dose is injected, followed one hour later by one-quarter of the total calculated dose. The last one-quarter of the dose is repeated but may be omitted if ECG evidence of digitalis toxicity (progressive bradycardia, development of atrioventricular block, or other arrhythmia) occurs.[10, 23–25]

Synthetic sympathomimetic amines provide greater inotropic activity than digoxin and provide a finer control for acute management of cardiogenic shock. Dopamine, a norepinephrine precursor, directly stimulates cardiac β_1-adrenergic receptors, as well as causing release of myocardial stores of norepinephrine.[85] The latter may limit the efficacy of dopamine if such stores are depleted.[86] At lower doses, it stimulates renal dopaminergic receptors, promoting renal cortical blood flow and diuresis. At high doses, it stimulates α_1-adrenergic receptors, resulting in increased systemic arterial and venous pressures.[87, 88] This vasoconstrictor activity is undesirable, as it increases impedance to ventricular ejection. Tachycardia, arrhythmias, and increased myocardial oxygen demand are other potential adverse effects. Recommended dose is 1 to 2.2 μg/lb/min (2 to 5 μg/kg/min) administered by constant-rate infusion.

Dobutamine exerts its positive inotropic effects through stimulation of myocardial α and β receptors.[79, 89, 90] It has little effect on heart rate or blood pressure when administered at doses between 2.0 and 5 μg/lb/min (5 to 10 μg/kg/min), exerts a lesser effect on the sinoatrial node (and therefore heart rate) than on myocardial tissue, and does not stimulate renal dopaminergic receptors.[74, 80, 91] Attenuation of hemodynamic effects have been reported in humans requiring upward dose titration.[92] However, improved exercise performance and functional classification have also been noted with short-term dobutamine administration.[93, 94] This effect has yet to be established in veterinary medicine. A common adverse side effect in cats is seizures.[23–25] These are typically focal facial in nature but occasionally become generalized. They have been observed at infusion rates as low as 2.5 μg/lb/min (5 μg/kg/min). Seizures abate as soon as the dobutamine infusion is stopped and they often do not recur when the dose is reduced by 50 per cent. If seizures continue at reduced dosage, dobutamine should be discontinued and dopamine substituted.

Dramatic improvements in myocardial function and reduction in congestive signs have been described with oral taurine supplementation.[51] Studies are currently in progress to evaluate dietary taurine concentrations, taurine blood levels, and the role of taurine in the therapeutic management of DCM. Oral taurine should be administered (250 mg q12h) to cats suspected of being taurine deficient during the acute period, in addition to the aforementioned therapies.

A new class of potent inotropic drugs has emerged whose action involves inhibition of cardiac phosphodiesterase F-III. These nonadrenergic, nonglycoside inotropes possess mild to moderate arteriolar dilating properties.[80] Amrinone for short-term support of myocardial failure has been used in dogs at 0.5 to 1.5 mg/lb (1 to 3 mg/kg) as an IV bolus followed by a constant rate infusion of 5 to 50 μg/lb/min (10 to 100 μg/kg/min). The dose in cats may be similar but pharmacokinetics have not been reported. Milrinone, a derivative of amrinone, has been studied experimentally but is not yet commercially available. It has been shown to improve left ventricular contractile force in cats when infused at 0.5 μg/lb/min (1 μg/kg/min). An oral dose of 0.25 to 0.5 mg/lb (0.5 to 1.0 mg/kg) q12h has proven effective in dogs, but similar studies have not been completed in cats.[95]

Beneficial effects have been reported with β-adrenergic blocking drugs in human dilated cardiomyopathy.[96, 97] Protection against increased sympathetic tone accompanying heart failure has been the suggested rationale for use. However, lack of improvement has been reported by others[98] as well as deterioration with withdrawal of β-blocking therapy.[99] β-adrenergic blocking drugs (e.g., propranolol) are most commonly used to slow the ventricular rate when supraventricular tachyarrhythmias are unresponsive to digoxin or for management of ventricular arrhythmias.[10, 12, 16, 23–25] Their use in situations where heart rate and rhythm are controlled is speculative and potentially deleterious.

Judicious fluid therapy is beneficial to combat the effects of shock and circulatory failure. Intravenous fluid supplementation helps prevent severe reduction in preload (and cardiac output) and reduces vascular volume contraction caused by diuretics, anorexia, and shock. A mixture of 0.45 per cent NaCl (or half strength lactated Ringer's solution) with 2.5 per cent dextrose in water is given at a submaintenance dose of 10 to 20 ml/lb/day (22 to 44 ml/kg/day), slowly IV, in two to three divided doses. Potassium chloride must often be supplemented (e.g., 5 to 7 mEq for each 250 ml of fluids). Serum electrolytes should be monitored. The infusion rate and dose vary with each patient and must be balanced to optimize cardiac output without exacerbating pulmonary edema or effusions.[10, 23–25] Central venous pressure (CVP) monitoring may provide a helpful guide to gauge infusion rate. Increases in CVP exceeding 2 to 5 cm H_2O within 30 min may be suggestive of hypervolemia.[100] In such situations, the fluid infusion rate should be reduced by 50 per cent, or temporarily discontinued. If pulmonary edema develops, prompt discontinuation of fluids should be followed by an intravenous bolus of furosemide, 0.5 mg/lb (1.1 mg/kg). Subcutaneous fluid administration may then be substituted for the intravenous route.

Vasodilators are theoretically useful adjuncts in the treatment of DCM. They should not be given if hypotension or cardiogenic shock is present unless blood pressure can be maintained with other agents (e.g., dopamine). Their place in the therapeutic strategy of this disease has not yet been clearly defined and efficacy is still undetermined. Nevertheless, several agents have been advocated based upon subjective clinical experience. Two per cent nitroglycerin ointment has profound venodilating effects and lesser action on arteriolar beds. It has significant action on cutaneous and skeletal muscle beds with lesser activity in visceral organs.[101] However, the venodilating action may actually reduce cardiac output in heart failure states where ventricular filling pressures are not elevated.[102] Hydralazine, an arteriolar dilator, has been used, 0.25 to 0.4 mg/lb (0.5 to 0.8 mg/kg) q12h, with subjective improvement in a small number of cats.[17] Captopril, an angiotensin enzyme converting inhibitor, is a balanced vasodilator with actions on both arterial and venous beds. Its efficacy in treating heart failure has been well documented in humans.[103, 104] In cats, it has been dosed at 3.12 to 6.25 mg q8h to q12h. Anorexia and hypotension (manifested as weakness and lethargy) are the most common side effects.[23–25]

Since hypothermia is common during the decompensated state, external environmental heating is an important adjunct to therapy. This is easily accomplished using a heat lamp placed at an appropriate distance to avoid thermal burns. Supplemental environmental heating should be continued until a compensated state is achieved.

Maintenance Therapy. If cardiogenic shock can be reversed and the heart failure state compensated, oral drug maintenance may be instituted. Furosemide is initially dosed at 0.5 to 1 mg/lb (1.1 to 2.2 mg/kg) q12h to q24h. Higher doses of 1.0 to 2.0 mg/lb (2.2 to 4.4 mg/kg) q8h to q12h may be required for management of recurrent heart failure or in refractory cases.[10, 23–25] The combination drug, hydrochlorothiazide/spironolactone has also been used at 1.0 to 2.0 mg/lb (2.2 to 4.4 mg/kg) for chronic maintenance,[16, 17] although the thiazide may be ineffective in the presence of renal dysfunction. Since prerenal azotemia is common in affected cats, furosemide is often preferred. Diuretic dosage must be specifically tailored to individual needs and administration should be temporarily discontinued if anorexia, azotemia, or dehydration occurs.

Digoxin may be given in pill or elixir form. Although higher plasma levels and more accurate dosing can be achieved with the elixir,[106, 107] this preparation is more unpalatable to cats. The 0.125 mg tablet is readily tolerated, but its small size makes it difficult to accurately divide into doses less than one-quarter of a tablet (0.031 mg).[10] Males may develop higher serum levels than females at the same body weight, and food administered in conjunction with digoxin may decrease drug absorption.[106, 107] However, digoxin toxicity is a greater clinical problem than is under-digitalization. Anorexia and depression are early signs of digoxin toxicity.[10, 11, 14, 23–25] Vomiting accompanies more severe intoxication. Clinical illness in normal cats given toxic doses may last up to 96 hours.[106, 107] The biologic half-life of digoxin in healthy cats given a single IV injection is 33.3 ± 9.5 hours. The mean half-life during a three-day period after chronic oral administration of elixir 0.025 mg/lb (0.05 mg/kg) q12h was 79 hours (range, 33 to 202 hours),[108] indicating that digoxin elimination is capacity-limited in the cat. In cardiomyopathic cats with reduced cardiac output and renal insufficiency, digoxin toxicity may persist up to seven days.[25] Toxic plasma concentrations in healthy cats ranged from 2.4 to 2.9 ng/ml,[108] but some cardiomyopathic cats display clinical signs of toxicity at half this level.[109] The most striking ECG evidence of digoxin toxicosis in one study was ST segment elevation, and PQ interval prolongation may be noted at nontoxic concentrations.[108] Thus, the maintenance dose is highly individualized and may vary with disease progression. Based on a calculated dose of 0.0025 to 0.005 mg/lb (0.005 to 0.01 mg/kg) lean body weight and normal renal function, the following guidelines are suggested: cats weighing 3 to 7 lb (1.9 to 3.2 kg), 1/4 of 0.125 mg digoxin tablet every two to three days; 7 to 12 lb (3.2 to 6.0 kg), 1/4 tablet daily or every other day; cats weighing more than 12 pounds (6.0 kg), 1/4 tablet daily.[10, 23–25]

Vasodilator drugs have been used for maintenance therapy in compensated cats unable to tolerate digoxin, or where a significant component of mitral insufficiency is suspected. Captopril dosed at 3.12 to 6.25 mg (1/8 to 1/4 of a 25 mg tablet) q8h to q12h has been tolerated in this setting for long periods.

Dietary modifications should include elimination of foods with high sodium content. Prescription diets for sodium restriction (Feline h/d) may be tried, or home preparation formulas used.[110] More importantly, new evidence suggests beneficial effects of oral taurine supplementation (250 mg q12h) for cats on taurine-deficient diets or when plasma taurine is less than 20 nmol/ml.[51, 51a] Avoidance of low taurine diet is essential.

Prognosis during the period of initial management (cardiogenic shock) is generally guarded to poor, but has improved during the last decade. This is due to advances in diagnostic recognition (especially by echocardiography), refinements in therapeutic protocols, and taurine supplementation. Mortality is highest during the first five to seven days. If extracardiac signs of edema or effusions can be controlled and hydration maintained, many cats resume eating and prognosis improves. Thromboembolic disease is a grave complication and affected cats seldom survive. Cardiogenic shock confers a poor prognosis, although some cats will respond to aggressive therapy. Clinical signs improve by two weeks post therapy. Echocardiography changes (e.g., left ventricular end-diastolic and end-systolic dimensions, fractional shortening) may improve within three or four weeks.[51] In some individuals, systolic function may dramatically improve and cardiac chamber dilatation become reduced during the course of chronic therapy.[23–25, 51] Structural and functional characteristics may occasionally become dramatically altered over time, resulting in an intermediate or intergrade form of cardiomyopathy. Survival for longer than four years has been observed.

CANINE DILATED CARDIOMYOPATHY

Immediate Therapy. Initial treatment is based upon the severity, progression, and type of congestive heart failure.[12, 18–20, 26, 62, 63, 67] Rapid and fatal decompensation and disease progression are possible, especially when arrhythmias are present. Stressful diagnostic procedures may need to be temporarily postponed, pending aggressive emergency treatment (e.g., intravenous furosemide, cutaneous nitroglycerin ointment, supplemental oxygen administration).

Therapeutic thoracocentesis is performed in dyspneic animals when heart and lung sounds are muffled and thoracic percussion indicates effusion. Occasionally, severe ascites must be drained if it impairs respiration. This causes no untoward effects, even when three or four liters are removed.

Diuretics are initially given in high doses. Furosemide is utilized for its quick onset of action, marked potency, and steep dose-response curve, even in the presence of impaired renal function.[81] When administered intravenously, its onset of action and peak effect are rapid (5 and 30 minutes, respectively).[105] Furosemide may also cause venodilatation and preload reduction even before its diuretic effects,[111, 112] which helps relieve dyspnea from pulmonary edema. Therefore, in severely dyspneic states, furosemide is administered IV or IM 1.0 to 2.0 mg/lb ([2.2 to 4.4 mg/kg] q8h to q12h).

If additional preload reduction is deemed necessary due to life threatening pulmonary edema, venodilatation can be significantly increased with topical, cutaneous application of 2 per cent nitroglycerin ointment. Some afterload reduction is produced as well.[102] Dosage is 1/4 to 1 inch applied to the axilla, ear pinna, or a shaved skin region every four to six hours. Care should be taken to avoid contact with human skin.

Inotropic support is required to stimulate the depressed myocardium. Digitalis has been most commonly used.[12, 18–20, 26, 62, 63] Maintenance oral digitalization is usually sufficient. The dose is 0.005 to 0.007 mg/lb (0.01 to 0.015 mg/kg) of lean body weight PO divided q12h (not to exceed 0.75 mg/day in giant breed dogs). Some animals, especially the Doberman pinscher breed and dogs with impaired renal function, are very sensitive to the effects of digitalis. In these situations, the dose is reduced (e.g., 0.25 to 0.375 mg divided twice daily).[19, 26] A loading dose (i.e., twice the oral maintenance dose in two divided doses) during the first day is occasionally advocated to achieve digoxin blood levels more quickly.[12, 18–20] However, this increases the likelihood of digoxin toxicity. Intravenous digitalization with 0.005 to 0.01 mg/lb (0.01 to 0.02 mg/kg) in two to four divided doses, given over four hours, has been suggested by some authors when heart rates due to atrial fibrillation exceed 230 bpm.[19]

Unfortunately, clinical response to digoxin and serum blood levels are variable, inconsistent, and unpredictable. For example, digoxin administered to ten dogs with DCM (0.22 mg/m^2 of body surface area q12h) in one study was efficacious in only four cases. Positive inotropic effects could not be predicted by clinical criteria, echocardiographic base line shortening fraction, heart rate, or jugular PVO_2.[113] In another study of 81 dogs with atrial fibrillation, there was only a weak correlation between serum digoxin dosage and serum digoxin concentration.[114] Heart failure related alterations in renal function, volume of distribution, and drug absorption may be causative in this disease.

Digitalization must therefore be individualized and guided by serum digoxin concentrations. Electrolyte levels, blood urea nitrogen, and creatinine levels should be monitored periodically, since azotemia and hypokalemia predispose to digoxin toxicity.[102] Biologic half-life is normally 20 to 35 hours. Therapeutic levels after five to seven days of therapy fall between 1.0 and 2.5 ng/ml, when assessed 8 to 12 hours after the last oral dose.[19, 115–118] The ECG should be monitored regularly if isolated ventricular premature complexes (VPCs) are detected during digitalization. Digoxin may be temporarily withdrawn and antiarrhythmic treatment initiated if more than 25 VPCs/min or ventricular tachycardia occurs. Lidocaine has minimal adverse hemodynamic effects and is given as an IV bolus at 1 to 2 mg/lb (2 to 4 mg/kg), repeated up to a maximum of 4 mg/lb (8 mg/kg) or as a constant rate infusion, 12 to 35 μg/lb/min (25 to 75 μg/kg/min). Quinidine should be avoided, since it may increase serum digoxin levels by decreasing its renal clearance and predispose to digoxin toxicity.[119] Quinidine's vagolytic effect may also accelerate atrioventricular conduction and thereby increase the ventricular rate in atrial fibrillation. Procainamide can be used instead, 3 to 10 mg/lb (6 to 20 mg/kg) q6h to q8h IM or PO.

If significant renal disease or renal insufficiency is present, digitoxin may be substituted for digoxin. Digitoxin is rapidly cleared by the liver (rather than by the kidney) and is highly protein bound. It has a lesser parasympathetic effect than digoxin and therefore may be less effective in controlling supraventricular arrhythmias.[117, 120] Its half-life is approximately 8 to 12 hours. The recommended dosage of digitoxin is 0.02 to 0.04 mg/lb (0.04 to 0.08 mg/kg) divided q8h to q12h. Therapeutic serum concentration is 15 to 35 ng/ml when measured six to eight hours after the last oral dose.[115–118]

A more potent inotropic drug may be desired for acute, short-term management when systolic function (contractility) is extremely poor, if cardiogenic shock is present, or if Doberman pinschers are affected. Two sympathomimetic amines have been used for this purpose. Dopamine 1 to 2.5 μg/lb/min (2 to 5 μg/kg/min) produces inotropic effects, partly by direct myocardial stimulation and partly by release of myocardial stores of norepinephrine. At higher dosages (2.5 to 7.0 μg/lb/min or 5 to 15 μg/kg/min), it may cause vasoconstriction (α-adrenergic stimulation), increase heart rate and/or myocardial oxygen demand, and cause ventricular arrhythmias.[85, 87, 88] Dobutamine 1 to 5 μg/lb/min (2 to 10 μg/kg/min) causes direct myocardial stimulation with minimum effect on heart rate or α-adrenergic vasoconstriction. It may, therefore, be more useful in the management of severe heart failure.[89–91] In addition, long-term hemodynamic benefits have resulted in humans with even brief infusion intervals.[93, 94]

Currently, interest has focused on a new class of inotropic agents having both positive inotropic and vasodilatory effects. These nonglycoside, nonsympathomimetic positive inotropes selectively inhibit cyclic AMP–specific cardiac phosphodiesterase F-III.[80] Amrinone can substantially augment performance of the failing heart,[121] although reports of limited efficacy and side effects in humans have surfaced.[122] In dogs with induced myocardial failure, amrinone infusions increased contractility 40 to 200 per cent above base line, increasing cardiac output by 80 per cent. This drug is not routinely used except for short-term administration in severe, refractory heart failure; initial dose is 0.5 to 1.5 mg/lb (1 to 3 mg/kg) (slow IV bolus) followed by 5 to 50 μg/lb/min (10 to 100 μg/kg/min) constant rate infusion.[95, 123]

Milrinone, a bipyridine derivative closely related to amrinone, has similar pharmacologic and hemodynamic effects. It is approximately 15 times more potent on a per milligram basis[124] and has less side effects than amrinone.[73] When milrinone was used as the sole therapeutic agent in dogs with myocardial failure, left ventricular function improved in all animals. A small number experienced worsening of ventricular arrhythmias. An oral dose of 0.25 to 0.5 mg/lb (0.5 to 1.0 mg/kg) q12h is effective in increasing myocardial contractility.[125] The half-life in dogs is two to three hours and positive inotropic effect was 75 per cent of maximum five to seven hours after administration. Milrinone may be required every six to eight hours in some dogs.[126] This drug is not yet marketed, but is expected for release in the future.

Vasodilator drugs have been used to reduce venous congestion and improve cardiac performance by reducing resistance to left ventricular ejection (i.e., afterload).[76] Several findings provide additional rationale for their use. Inappropriate afterload elevation, for example, has been demonstrated to be an important factor in human dilated cardiomyopathy.[84] In addition, a large percentage of people with systolic dysfunction have clinically relevant mitral regurgitation. Forward cardiac output has been enhanced when regurgitation was reduced by vasodilator therapy.[127] Mitral regurgitation is also common with canine dilated cardiomyopathy.[12, 18–20, 26] Various drugs have been used including balanced vasodilators (captopril, 0.25 mg/lb (0.5 mg/kg) q8h to q12h; prazosin, 1 to 2 mg q8h to q12h), arteriolar dilators (hydralazine, 0.5 to 1 mg/lb or 1 to 2 mg/kg q12h) and venodilators (2 per cent nitroglycerin ointment, 1/2 to 1 inch cutaneously q4h to q6h). However, controlled veterinary clinical trials to support efficacy have not been reported. Potential hazards of vasodilator decreased preload and cardiac output, vomiting and diarrhea (especially captopril), and reflex sinus tachycardia (especially hydralazine). Moreover, small hearts without mitral regurgitation may respond poorly.

Maintenance Therapy. Fluid therapy is sometimes required after aggressive diuresis to expand a vascular compartment contracted by nonalimentation and diuretic agents. Fluid dosage and administration rate must be individualized based upon phase of heart failure, hydration status, and serum protein, electrolyte, creatinine, and blood urea nitrogen concentrations. Submaintenance doses are advocated.

Lactated Ringer's solution or a mixture of lactated Ringer's and 5 per cent dextrose in water may be infused at 10 to 20 ml/lb/day (22 to 44 ml/kg/day) divided in two or three doses. Potassium chloride may be added, according to serum deficits or empirically supplemented in fluids (5 to 7 mEq per 250 ml). If pulmonary edema is present, fluid administration should be discontinued. Central venous pressure (CVP) measurements may help indicate the heart's ability to pump the fluids being returned to it. Normal CVP is between 0 and 5 cm H_2O; measurements in the 15 to 20 cm H_2O range are too high and indicate that fluid administration should be interrupted.[128]

In most breeds (except boxers and Doberman pinschers), atrial fibrillation is present at or near the time of cardiac decompensation. Because severe atrial enlargement or irreversible morphologic alterations in atrial tissue cause or contribute to this arrhythmia,[56, 129, 130] conversion to sustained sinus rhythm is usually not possible. Therefore, therapeutic goals focus upon reducing the ventricular rate below 140 bpm to allow sufficient ventricular diastolic filling. Digitalis glycosides are utilized to slow conduction through the atrioventricular node.

The oral maintenance dose of digoxin for large and giant breed dogs is 0.005 to 0.007 mg/lb (0.01 to 0.015 mg/kg) divided q12h (loading dose schedules routinely produce toxic serum concentrations). Therapeutic digoxin levels have been achieved in 2 to 4.5 days using oral maintenance digitalization.[131] When digitalized, some dogs with atrial fibrillation undergo ventricular rate slowing below 150 bpm, although less than 20 per cent may respond in this fashion.[114]

β-Adrenergic blocking agents are usually required to further reduce the ventricular rate in atrial fibrillation when unresponsive to digoxin. Propranolol, a nonspecific β-adrenergic blocker, has been used most commonly after the animal has been digitalized for two to three days.[12, 18–20, 26] Starting dose is 0.22 mg/lb (0.5 mg/kg) PO divided q8h. If needed, daily increments of 10 mg q8h are added to this dose—maximum daily dose, 0.45 mg/lb (1.0 mg/kg) q8h until the resting heart rate is 100 to 140 bpm. Other β-blocking drugs may allow longer dosing intervals such as nadolol dosed at 0.12 to 0.2 mg/lb (0.25 to 0.4 mg/kg) q12h, titrated to effect. Drugs with greater cardioselectivity (i.e., β_1-adrenoceptor selectivity) include metoprolol dosed at 6 to 12 mg/lb (12.5 to 25 mg/kg) q8h to q12h and atenolol, 0.12 to 0.5 mg/lb (0.25 to 1.0 mg/kg) PO q12h to q24h, to effect.

The calcium channel antagonist diltiazem is proving useful to control the ventricular rate in supraventricular arrhythmias, especially atrial fibrillation. It has a mild negative inotropic effect and causes peripheral vasodilation. Given at 0.2 to 0.4 mg/lb (0.5–1.0 mg/kg) PO q8h, it may replace the need for β-adrenergic blockers.[132a]

Boxer cardiomyopathy usually requires a therapeutic approach modified toward management of resistant ventricular arrhythmias. Commonly used antiarrhythmic drugs include procainamide, 3 to 10 mg/lb (6 to 20 mg/kg) q6h, or quinidine, 3 to 10 mg/lb (6 to 20 mg/kg) q8h; propranolol may need to be added, 0.25 to 0.5 mg/lb (0.5 to 1.0 mg/kg) q8h. Supraventricular arrhythmias and congestive heart failure are treated in the manner similar to that described above. Prednisolone, 0.5 mg/lb (1 mg/kg) q12h, are occasionally given when arrhythmias are refractory to antiarrhythmic therapy.

Most dogs may be maintained with digoxin, furosemide, and a β-blocking drug or diltiazem. Exercise should be restricted to reduce cardiac work load. Dietary sodium should be reduced using a commercial prescription diet (h/d) or home preparation. Cardiac cachexia is a common occurrence and diets should provide adequate protein, vitamins, minerals, and calories.[110] Optimal digitalization can be facilitated by serum digoxin evaluations to help verify toxic doses or identify subtherapeutic levels. Digoxin dosages must often be reduced if severe weight loss or azotemia develops. Biochemical profiles should be performed to evaluate electrolyte and renal status whenever anorexia or vomiting occurs. The ECG and thoracic radiograph should be reevaluated immediately if clinical signs suggest decompensation (e.g., dyspnea, syncope, exercise intolerance, abdominal enlargement).

In dogs with demonstrated myocardial L-carnitine deficiency (via endomyocardial biopsy), or with low plasma carnitine concentrations, oral supplementation with L-carnitine, 2 g q8h, is recommended.

Diuretic agents must often be increased or modified over time when disease progression and homeoregulatory mechanisms reduce their efficacy. Furosemide may be increased 2.0 to 3.0 mg/lb (4.4 to 6.6 mg/kg) PO q8h as needed. The addition of another diuretic drug acting at a different site in the nephron or at a similar site by a different mechanism of action may enhance natriuresis and diuresis.[103, 132] Diuretic drugs used for this purpose include: hydrochlorothiazide, 1 to 2 mg/lb (2 to 4 mg/kg) PO q12h; hydrochlorothiazide/spironolactone combined product, 0.5 to 2 mg/lb/day (1 to 4 mg/kg/day) PO; spironolactone, 1 to 2 mg/lb/day (2 to 4 mg/kg/day) PO; triamterene, 1 to 2 mg/lb/day (2 to 4 mg/kg/day) PO. The last two drugs are potassium sparing agents. They may be selected if hypokalemia has resulted from anorexia or large doses of potent loop diuretics. In general, hypokalemia and metabolic alkalosis are rare. Hyperkalemia is a potential side effect when potassium sparing diuretics are used in the presence of renal disease, potassium supplementation or cotherapy with angiotensin converting enzyme inhibitors (e.g., captopril, enalapril).[1, 2, 102] A relatively new loop diuretic, bumetanide, is 40 to 70 times more potent than furosemide. Potential side effects include ototoxicity and electrolyte imbalance.[133, 134] This drug has not yet been carefully evaluated for use in treating canine dilated cardiomyopathy.

The prognosis is guarded in canine dilated cardiomyopathy. Atrial fibrillation is associated with a poor outcome with a reported six month mortality rate of 74 to 85 per cent.[114, 135, 136] Dogs with atrial fibrillation that demonstrate a positive inotropic response to digoxin (i.e., increased shortening fraction echocardiographically) may live longer than those who do not. Heart rate is probably not a reliable predictor of digoxin response or life expectancy.[113] Boxers with congestive heart failure and ventricular arrhythmias and Doberman pinschers have the worst prognosis. Sudden death is common. Progressive right-sided heart failure is an ominous sign.

Many dogs become compensated on medication and may survive up to two years. Overall mean survival is approximately six months. Death is associated with congestive heart failure or arrhythmias.

HEART FAILURE DUE TO DIASTOLIC DYSFUNCTION

Ventricular hypertrophy or fibrosis may result from various primary or secondary myocardial disorders, especially in cats.[3–20, 23–26, 34] In humans, these processes decrease left ventricular compliance (i.e., increase myocardial stiffness) and impede diastolic filling. Systolic (pumping) function is usually adequate but clinical signs result from diastolic dysfunction. Associated causes include impaired ventricular relaxation, myofibrillar architectural disarray, abnormal ventricular cavity shape, endomyocardial fibrosis, and ventricular cavity distortion.[1, 2, 137, 138] Diastolic dysfunction in animals has been less well characterized than in humans with hypertrophic and restrictive cardiomyopathy. However, these diseases in animals appear to similarly decrease ventricular filling, resulting in hemodynamic impairment and congestive heart failure.

Left ventricular hypertrophy is an important compensatory response to chronic left ventricular pressure or volume overload.[139] It may be observed with various systemic, metabolic, and infiltrative diseases or in athletic individuals, or it may be idiopathic. Hypertrophy represents an appropriate, adaptive response or is associated with depressed cardiac function and structural changes.[1, 2, 13, 15, 25, 34] The clinical significance of left ventricular hypertrophy and its therapeutic and prognostic implications are dependent upon accurate characterization of causative factors and their correction, where possible. Echocardiography is the most accurate noninvasive method to detect hypertrophy. All potential identifiable causes of left ventricular hypertrophy (e.g., thyrotoxicosis, renovascular hypertension, pressure overload) should be investigated. Angiographic or echocardiographic evidence of left ventricular hypertrophy does not, therefore, automatically equate with a diagnosis of idiopathic hypertrophic cardiomyopathy.

HYPERTROPHIC CARDIOMYOPATHY (HCM)

Etiology. Hypertrophic cardiomyopathy represents a common feline myocardial disorder with a heterogeneous morphologic expression. In dogs, it is rare by comparison, although popularization of cardiac ultrasound may uncover a higher incidence than detected by previous catheterization techniques.

The etiology in dogs and cats is unknown. Human studies have demonstrated familial transmission with an autosomal dominant mode of inheritance, as well as nonfamilial varieties of HCM.[140–142] Other possible etiologies include enhanced myocardial responsiveness to circulating catecholamines or excessive catecholamine production, abnormal compensatory hypertrophy resulting from myocardial ischemia or fibrosis, and a primary collagen abnormality with secondary ventricular hypertrophy.[143–145] It may be possible that HCM is not a single disease but represents a group of etiologically different disorders.[142]

Abnormal Physiology. Morphologically heterogeneous, HCM characteristically represents increased muscle mass due to a hypertrophied, nondilated left ventricle. The principal pathophysiologic consequence is elevated left ventricular end-diastolic pressure in the face of a normal or reduced end-diastolic volume.[1, 2, 5, 142] Global left ventricular diastolic function is adversely affected through several interrelated abnormalities.[142, 146–148] Decreased early, rapid diastolic filling results from reduced ventricular distensibility (i.e., compliance) and prolonged (or incomplete) relaxation.[146, 147] Increased muscle stiffness may be caused by fibrosis or cell disorganization,[149] while ventricular chamber stiffness results from increased muscle stiffness and muscle mass (hypertrophy).[142] Mitral regurgitation develops from distortional changes in the mitral valve apparatus (resulting from ventricular hypertrophy), or possibly from interference with normal mitral valve closure due to anterior motion of the mitral valve during mid-systole.[142, 150] The left atrium dilates in response to increased end-diastolic pressures, and pulmonary venous pressures eventually become elevated.

Left ventricular function is hyperdynamic.[151] Ventricular ejection may be nearly completed during the first third of the systolic ejection period.[150, 152] Development of an intraventricular pressure gradient (i.e., dynamic subaortic obstruction to left ventricular outflow) has received much attention in human HCM[142] and has been demonstrated in the cat[5] and dog.[153] Affected individuals may exhibit anterior motion of the mitral valve leaflet across the outflow tract to the ventricular septum during early systole. This may cause mechanical impedance to left ventricular ejection and increase systolic intraventricular pressures, myocardial wall stress, and oxygen demand.[142] The clinical incidence and role of dynamic subaortic pressure gradients in dogs and cats, however, are unknown.

Pathology. The principal pathologic features of primary (idiopathic) HCM are abnormal left ventricular hypertrophy and increased ventricular muscle mass in the absence of a causative systemic or cardiac disease. A number of nonspecific but predictable characteristics may be present. Left ventricular hypertrophy is a hallmark and may vary in pattern and extent in humans[142] and animals.[5, 7, 8, 34, 153–159] In dogs, disproportionate thickening of the ventricular septum (asymmetric septal hypertrophy) is the rule.[153, 155–157] The ventricular septal–free wall thickness ratio exceeds 1.1 in most dogs[153, 155–157] and six out of ten had ratios greater than or equal to 1.3 (although both the septum and free wall are hypertrophied).[155, 157] In cats, about two-thirds to three-quarters have symmetric left ventricular hypertrophy.[157, 158] Ventricular septal disorganization (greater than 5 per cent of the tissue section) has been reported in 20 per cent of affected dogs[155 157] and 27 per cent of affected cats.[157, 158] In cats, this occurred only in those with asymmetric septal hypertrophy. Fibrous connective tissue may be present focally or diffusely in the endocardium,[7, 156–159] conduction system,[158] or myocardium.[7, 159] Narrowed, small intramural coronary arteries are recognized histologically[142, 159] and may be components of the hypertrophied ventricle.[160] Heart weight/body weight ratio is increased.[157] Decompensated animals may display evidence of left and/or right-sided congestive heart failure, although the former is more common in cats.[155–159] Thromboembolic disease frequently accompanies cardiac decompensation in felines but not canines.

Clinical Manifestations

Feline HCM. The signalment describes a wide age range (5 months to 17 years)[7, 15, 157, 158] with a mean age of 4.8 to 7 years.[157] Because these cases were largely collected before clinical recognition of diseases causing secondary ventricular hypertrophy (e.g., thyrotoxicosis, renovascular hypertension), the upper age range may include cats with "secondary" hypertrophic cardiomyopathy. Domestic short hair cats are most frequently reported followed by the domestic long hair. The Persian breed may be predisposed.[5, 8] This disease is rare in the Siamese, Burmese, and Abyssinian breeds, which are predisposed to dilated cardiomyopathy. Males are more commonly affected; studies have reported 23 to 87 per cent of cases occurring in males.

A presenting clinical sign usually is acute dyspnea associated with pulmonary edema or biventricular failure. Anorexia and vomiting may precede clinical signs by one or two days. Paresis of a front leg or posterior paralysis may result from thromboembolic disease. Sudden death may occur.[1, 6, 16, 17, 23–25]

Auscultation may disclose a diastolic gallop rhythm (usually S_4), rales, soft systolic murmurs (I-II/VI) over the mitral and/or tricuspid valve areas, and arrhythmias. Heart and lung sounds will be muffled if significant pleural or pericardial effusion is present. The left precordial apex beat is usually palpably normal or hyperdynamic. Paresis and absence of femoral arterial pulses accompany distal aortic thromboembolism (Table 77–3).[6, 10–12, 14, 16, 17, 23–25]

Electrocardiographic abnormalities have been recorded in 35 to 70 per cent of affected cats.[5, 17] The most commonly reported findings are conduction disturbances, of which only left anterior fascicular block is most consistent. The latter is rare in other forms of primary myocardial diseases. Left ventricular enlargement patterns (QRS greater than 0.04 ms; R waves in lead II greater than 0.9 mV) are present in some cats, but are not diagnostic for HCM. Arrhythmias occur in one-quarter to one-half of affected cats, with ventricular premature complexes predominating.

Plain film radiography may show mild to moderate left ventricular enlargement with moderate to severe left atrial enlargement. The latter is particularly obvious on the dorsoventral view. Pulmonary venous congestion, interstitial and/or alveolar pulmonary densities (suggesting pulmonary edema), and occasionally, slight pleural effusion occur most commonly (Figure 77–9). Pulmonary edema in cats may be patchy and focal rather than located in the perihilar region as with dogs. Severe, diffuse edema is rarely seen with systolic failure but is common with diastolic dysfunction (e.g., hypertrophic or restrictive cardiomyopathies). With chronic or advanced HCM, cardiomegaly may be generalized, accompanied by extracardiac signs of severe biventricular failure (e.g., pleural, pericardial, or abdominal effusion, hepatosplenomegaly, pulmonary edema).[10, 11, 14, 16, 17, 23–25]

Nonselective angiocardiography discloses left ventricular free wall hypertrophy, severe reduction of the left ventricular chamber (often slit-like in appearance), and extremely hypertrophied papillary muscles (Figures 77–10 and 77–11). The left atrium is moderately to severely dilated. Pulmonary veins may be tortuous due to elevated left ventricular end-diastolic pressure. Circulatory transit time may be normal or accelerated (Table 77–4). Ball thrombi may occasionally be present in the left atrium or ventricle.[10, 11, 14, 16, 23–25, 27–29]

Echocardiography is the most sensitive technique for evaluation of hypertrophy (Figure 77–12) and noninvasively allows assessment of myocardial function. It illustrates hypertrophy of the ventricular septum and left ventricular free wall, decreased internal dimensions, normal to elevated fractional shortening and right ventricular dilatation (late in the disease course of some cases) may be evident. Left atrial enlargement is often marked. Pericardial or pleural effusion or left heart ball thrombi may be imaged. Occasionally, systolic anterior motion of the mitral valve and partial systolic closure of the aortic valve may be noted.[14, 16, 18, 23–25, 30]

Differential diagnosis must include all causes of left ventricular hypertrophy. Congenital aortic stenosis,[161] thyrotoxicosis,[13] restrictive and infiltrative cardiomyopathy[7, 23–26] and systemic hypertension should be considered.[15, 162] Since right-sided congestive heart failure may be present, congenital and acquired heart diseases, as well as extracardiac causes of effusions must be considered. Pericardial effusion may occasionally be pronounced with HCM. Pericardial diseases and feline infectious peritonitis constitute other sources of pericardial effusion.[16, 163]

Canine HCM. This disease has been insufficiently studied in dogs to allow a characteristic clinical description. Canine hypertrophic cardiomyopathy has been reported in 13 dogs ranging from 10 weeks to 13 years of age.[153–157] Various breeds were reported, with the German shepherd recorded four times. Males were predominantly affected. The etiology is unknown.

Clinical history is variable, ranging from asympto-

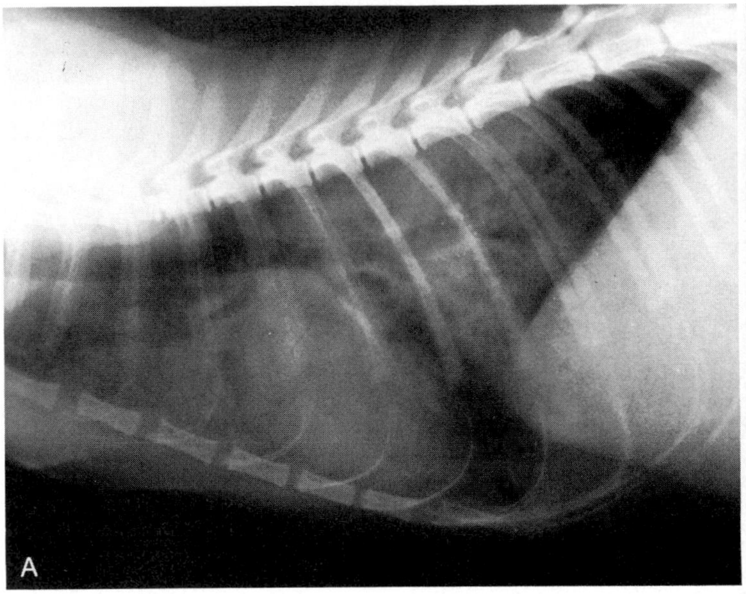

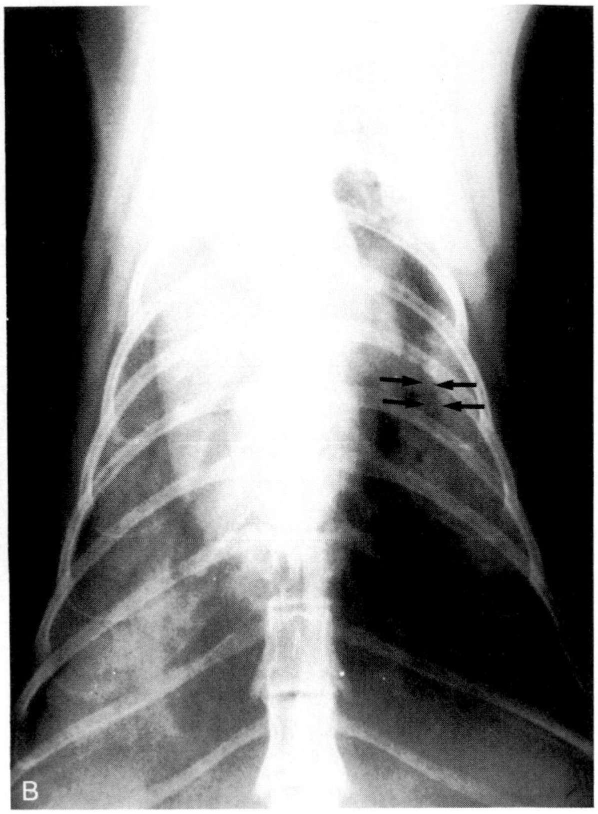

FIGURE 77–9. Lateral *(A)* and dorsoventral *(B)* thoracic radiographs from a seven-year-old male domestic short hair cat with decompensated hypertrophic cardiomyopathy. There is an alveolar infiltrate which has a focal, patchy distribution compatible with pulmonary edema. Air bronchograms are present (arrows). Pulmonary infiltrates resolved after two days of furosemide administration.

matic to sudden, unexplained death. The latter represented causes of mortality in eight out of ten awake or anesthetized dogs studied retrospectively.[155, 156] Evidence of heart failure (e.g., syncope, exercise intolerance, coughing, dyspnea, ascites, hepatomegaly, pleural effusion) were recorded in four out of 12 dogs.[153–156] Heart murmurs were present in two young, asymptomatic dogs, although auscultatory results were not recorded in the larger post-mortem retrospective study. In affected humans, a late onset systolic murmur located between the left apex and base is usually evident when a dynamic subaortic pressure gradient (associated with systolic anterior motion of the mitral valve) is present.[74, 150] The dynamic obstruction and murmur may be enhanced by factors that increase contractility (e.g., isoproterenol, ventricular premature complexes), or decrease arterial pressure (e.g., sodium nitroprusside). Factors decreasing contractility (e.g., β-adrenergic blocking drugs) or increasing arterial blood pressure (e.g., phenylephrine, methoxamine) may reduce or abolish the dynamic obstruction or associated heart murmur.[142, 153]

Radiographic findings may be unremarkable or display moderate left atrial and ventricular enlargement with extracardiac signs of congestive heart failure.

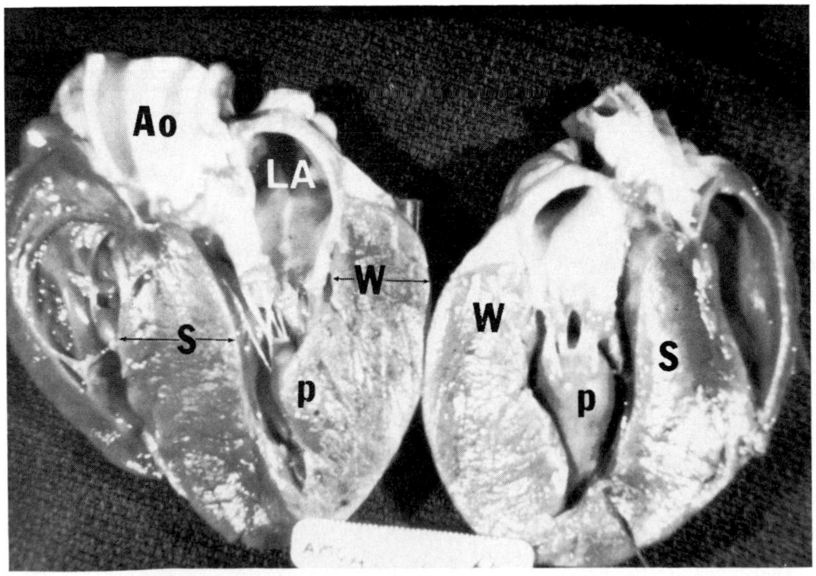

FIGURE 77–10. Heart from an adult male domestic short hair cat with hypertrophic cardiomyopathy. Severe hypertrophy of the left ventricular posterior wall (W), interventricular septum (S) and papillary muscles (p) is evident. Compare pathologic changes with angiocardiographic correlates in Figure 77–11. LA = left atrium; Ao = aorta. (Courtesy of Dr. S. K. Liu.)

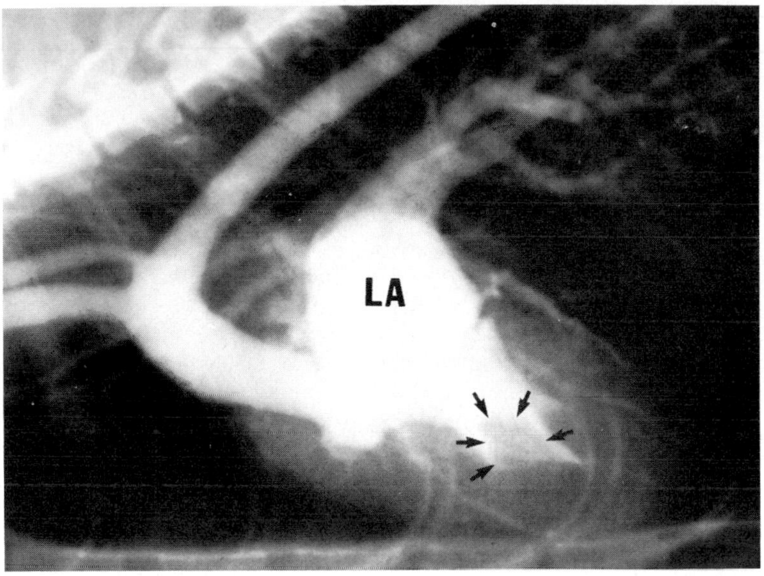

FIGURE 77–11. Nonselective angiocardiogram from an adult male domestic short hair cat with hypertrophic cardiomyopathy. The left ventricular cavity is severely reduced due to myocardial hypertrophy. Papillary muscles are hypertrophied (arrows). The left atrium (LA) is moderately enlarged.

Electrocardiograms recorded in seven dogs showed a high incidence of conduction abnormalities (e.g., first- and third-degree atrioventricular block, bifascicular and right bundle branch block). Depression or slurring of the ST segment was noted in two animals with normal rhythms.[153–155] In humans, characteristic features include increased QRS voltage, left anterior hemiblock, ST and T wave abnormalities, prominent abnormal Q waves (suggesting ventricular septal hypertrophy) in leads II, III, aVF, or V_4–V_6, and ventricular arrhythmias. However, the ECG is often unremarkable.[1, 2, 164–166]

Echocardiographic characterization is similar to that described for feline HCM. Because asymmetric septal hypertrophy was a dominant feature of necropsied cases,[155–157] this may be an expected finding in affected dogs assessed by ultrasound.

Angiographic changes (left ventricular hypertrophy, decreased left ventricular end-systolic volume, mild mitral regurgitation, systolic anterior motion of the mitral valve, and variable dynamic subaortic gradient) have been demonstrated in one dog.[153]

Differential diagnosis is complicated by the small number of reported cases. Congenital aortic stenosis causes left ventricular hypertrophy and systolic anterior motion of the mitral valve. Athletic working or hunting dogs may display compensatory left ventricular hypertrophy. Systemic or metabolic causes of conduction system abnormalities should be investigated when A-V nodal block or bundle branch block are detected.

RESTRICTIVE CARDIOMYOPATHY (RCM)

When diastolic ventricular volume and stretch (i.e., compliance) is impaired by endocardial, subendocardial, or myocardial fibrosis or infiltrative disease, restrictive cardiomyopathy is said to be present. It is characterized

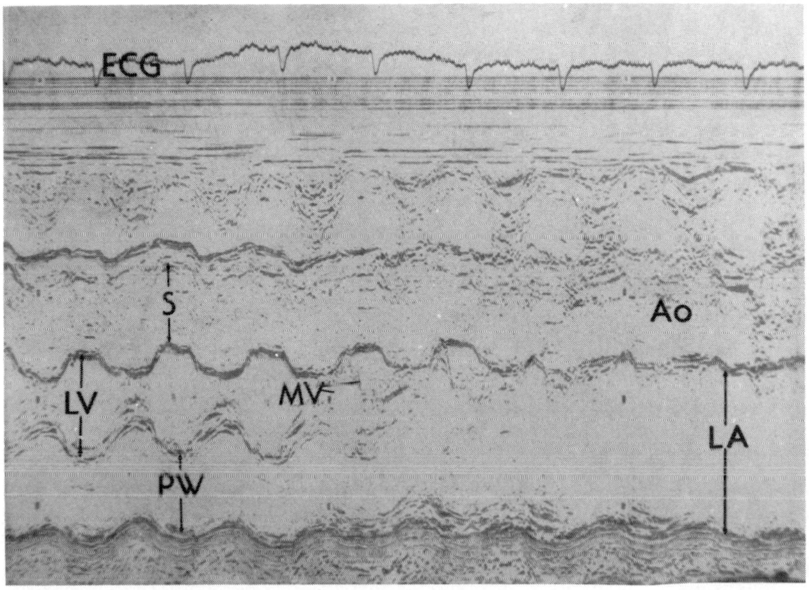

FIGURE 77–12. M-mode echocardiogram recorded just below the mitral valve from a female, three-year-old domestic short hair cat with hypertrophic cardiomyopathy. There is severe thickening of the interventricular septum (S) and left ventricular posterior wall (PW). LV = left ventricle; MV = mitral valve; Ao = aortic root; LA = left atrium.

by elevated ventricular filling pressures with normal or near normal systolic function.[1, 2, 166, 167] Hemodynamically, it resembles restrictive pericarditis. Limitation of ventricular filling reduces preload and ultimately, cardiac output. In cases of extensive endomyocardial fibrosis, the left ventricular chamber may become obliterated (Table 77–4).

Confusion regarding terminology may occur since some literature has designated restrictive cardiomyopathy under the terminology of "intermediate" cardiomyopathy.[16, 17] While mild, diffuse, or focal fibrosis may accompany all forms of myocardial diseases, the fibrosis does not constitute the predominant morphologic abnormality, nor does it significantly impair diastolic function. The term intermediate cardiomyopathy is better reserved for morphologic disorders characterized by ventricular dilatation with or without hypertrophy, often with mild to moderate reduction in systolic function.[23–25]

Feline RCM. Restrictive cardiomyopathy is the least common of the feline primary (idiopathic) myocardial disorders.[7, 8, 71] Primary RCM is not reported in the dog. Endocardial fibrosis without eosinophilia is the predominant form of primary feline RCM. Secondary causes are rare and result from infiltrative neoplastic or infectious disorders.[7, 8, 10–12, 15, 23–25, 34, 170] Etiology of the primary disease is unknown.

Reported ages vary from 8 months to 19 years.[7, 8, 16, 17, 169, 170] There is no particular breed predisposition. A male predominance was reported at one institution[7, 8, 169] and an approximately equal sex distribution at another.[16, 17]

Clinical signs are quite variable and include left-sided failure (pulmonary edema), right-sided failure (pleural, pericardial, or abdominal effusion), or biventricular failure. There is a high incidence of thromboembolic disease. Anorexia and vomiting may be present for a short but variable period of time. Clinical signs usually worsen or develop acutely.[7, 8, 16, 17, 23–25, 169, 170]

Physical examination findings usually include dyspnea, paresis (from thromboembolism), and hypothermia. Auscultatory abnormalities include muffled heart and lung sounds (from pleural effusions), rales (from pulmonary edema), gallop heart rhythms, mild to moderate intensity systolic murmurs at the left and/or right cardiac apex, and irregularities in heart rate and rhythm. Femoral arterial pulse deficits and occasionally, hepatomegaly or ascites may be palpated.[8, 16, 17, 23–25]

Electrocardiographic abnormalities have been recorded in 31 to 70 per cent of affected cats.[8, 17] Left atrial and ventricular enlargement patterns are common. Ventricular and supraventricular arrhythmias are frequently recorded.

Plain radiographs usually display an interstitial and alveolar pattern (pulmonary edema) or moderate to severe pleural effusion. A globoid cardiac silhouette occasionally results from pericardial effusion. If effusion is absent or minimal, dramatic left atrial enlargement may be evident. This is typified on the lateral view by a large left atrial bulge elevating the trachea over the heart base and on the dorsoventral view by pronounced left auricular enlargement. The left ventricle may be enlarged on both views. Pulmonary veins are often prominent and tortuous. Hepatomegaly and mild to moderate ascites may be present.[16, 17, 23–25, 169]

Nonselective angiocardiography has provided the most sensitive means of clinical diagnosis (Table 77–4), although it is associated with slight morbidity and mortality. Characteristic changes include left ventricular hypertrophy with an irregular, often obliterated left ventricular cavity, severe left atrial enlargement, and tortuous pulmonary veins. Left atrial or ventricular thrombi may be present (Figure 77–13).[8, 10, 11, 16, 17, 23–25, 28]

Catheterization has demonstrated mitral regurgitation, left ventricular filling defects, and morphologic mid–left ventricular stenosis. Intraventricular pressure gradients correlating with these structural alterations have been demonstrated.[8, 54]

Echocardiography may demonstrate hypertrophy of the left ventricular septum and free wall, severe left atrial enlargement, normal to mildly depressed indices of left ventricular performance (e.g., fractional shortening, velocity of circumferential fiber shortening), and occasionally, abnormal or depressed motion of the ventricular septum or left ventricular free wall. The left ventricular internal dimensions are usually reduced. With M-mode echocardiography, a sweep from the apex to mitral valve position often discloses an irregular ventricular chamber filled with extraneous echoes. These are associated with extensive fibrosis and occasionally, cavity obliteration. Two-dimensional echocardiography confers the ability to better visualize loss of normal left ventricular chamber symmetry and allows visualization of distorted, fused papillary muscles. Increased endocardial echogenicity has been observed. Right ventricular dilatation is often evident.

Gross pathologic findings include a heart weight to body weight ratio greater than normal due to increased left ventricular mass (hypertrophy). Extreme left atrial and auricular enlargement is common. Hypertrophy of the left ventricle with pronounced, diffuse endocardial thickening and myocardial fibrosis is the pathologic hallmark. Fibrous adhesions between the papillary muscles and myocardium, distortion and fusion of chordae tendineae, and mitral valve leaflets may be seen. Aortic or cardiac chamber thromboemboli may occur.[7, 8, 169, 170]

Differential diagnosis must include all forms of heart disease that result in ventricular hypertrophy and congestive heart failure. Since left ventricular hypertrophy is a dominant feature of RCM and older cats are often affected by this disease, thyrotoxicosis and systemic hypertension must be considered. Secondary causes of increased endomyocardial echogenicity and left ventricular chamber obliteration must include neoplastic and infectious diseases. Constrictive pericarditis may clinically resemble RCM.

TREATMENT OF HEART FAILURE ASSOCIATED WITH DIASTOLIC DYSFUNCTION

The basic underlying disease process of hypertrophic cardiomyopathy may progress along several pathways: diastolic dysfunction (the most common), dynamic subaortic obstruction (uncommon), myocardial fibrosis and ischemia, and a "burn-out" phase resulting in end-stage

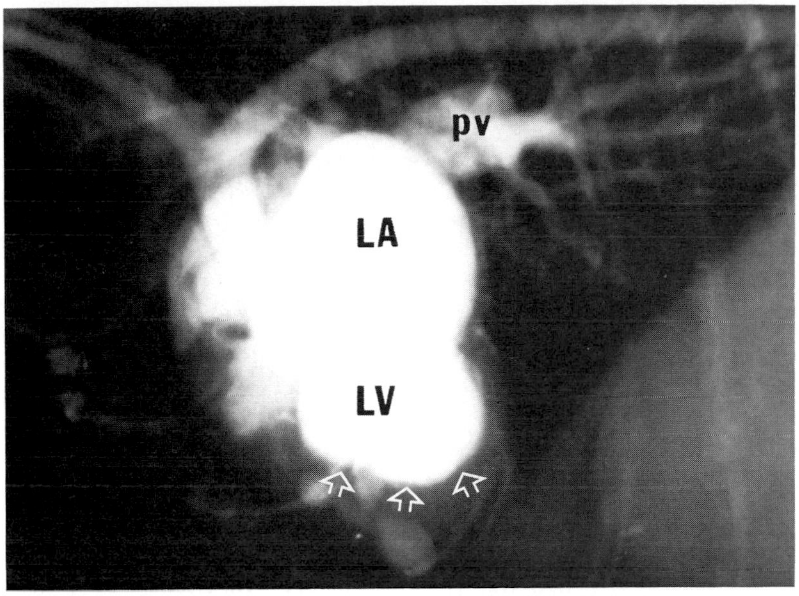

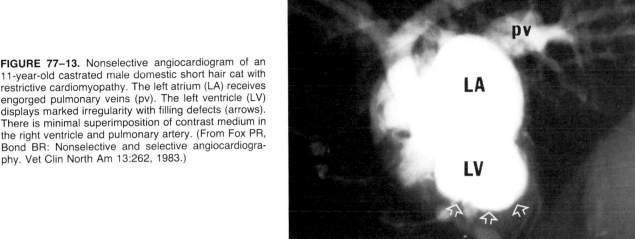

FIGURE 77–13. Nonselective angiocardiogram of an 11-year-old castrated male domestic short hair cat with restrictive cardiomyopathy. The left atrium (LA) receives engorged pulmonary veins (pv). The left ventricle (LV) displays marked irregularity with filling defects (arrows). There is minimal superimposition of contrast medium in the right ventricle and pulmonary artery. (From Fox PR, Bond BR: Nonselective and selective angiocardiography. Vet Clin North Am 13:262, 1983.)

depression of ventricular contractility. Thus, clinical signs may be due to one or more of these factors to which therapy must be appropriately tailored. Therapy for heart failure resulting from hypertrophic or restrictive cardiomyopathy employs strategies directed toward eliminating pulmonary edema or effusions, managing arrhythmias, and modifying factors contributing to diastolic dysfunction.[1, 2] Diastolic dysfunction may be reduced by interventions or drugs that decrease ventricular contractility, increase left ventricular filling, expand the left ventricular outflow tract, and enhance ventricular distensibility (i.e., compliance).[74, 142, 166]

HYPERTROPHIC CARDIOMYOPATHY

Treatment recommendations are hindered by lack of controlled clinical trials involving cats and by absence of reports describing therapy in dogs. Therapeutic strategies have therefore been modified for cats from human protocols.[1, 2, 10–12, 14, 16, 17, 23–25, 75, 142, 166] Responses to pharmacologic agents are variable and therapy must be adjusted individually. Diuretics and β-adrenergic blockade have long been the cornerstone of medical therapy in cats.

Diuretics represent the initial therapeutic step. Mild to moderately severe pulmonary edema is very responsive to furosemide, 0.5 mg/lb (1.1 mg/kg) IV or IM q8h to q12h, which reduces left ventricular end-diastolic, mean left atrial, and pulmonary capillary pressures. After 24 to 36 hours, administration frequency may be decreased to q12h or q24h and administered orally. Thereafter, furosemide is gradually reduced to the lowest effective maintenance dosage. Some cats remain stable on 0.5 mg/lb (1.1 mg/kg) given every other day. Alternatively, maintenance therapy with a hydrochlorothiazide/spironolactone combination drug may be used (1.0 mg/lb or 2.2 mg/kg daily).[16, 17]

With disease progression, left-sided heart failure may worsen and right-sided heart failure develop. This requires upward dose titration of furosemide (1.0 to 2.0 mg/lb or 2.2 to 4.4 mg/kg q8h). Refractory right-sided heart failure may respond to the addition of a second diuretic agent acting at a different site in the nephron. Hydrochlorothiazide has been used for this purpose, 0.5 to 1 mg/lb (1 to 2 mg/kg) PO q12h. While furosemide rarely causes electrolyte imbalance, combination diuretic therapy must be monitored closely for azotemia, hyponatremia, or hypokalemia.[23–25]

In cases of severe, fulminating pulmonary edema, the initial furosemide dosage may be increased to 1.0 mg/lb (2.2 mg/kg) IV or IM q8h or q12h. Supplemental oxygen therapy (40 to 60 per cent oxygen-enriched inspired gas) may be beneficial to improve pulmonary gas exchange by increasing the driving force for oxygen diffusion into alveolar capillaries. Preload reduction can be enhanced with 2 per cent nitroglycerin ointment (1/8 to 1/4 inch applied cutaneously to the ear pinna every four to six hours for 24 to 36 hours).[10, 23–25]

β-Adrenergic blockade with propranolol has been the mainstay of medical treatment for human HCM. It inhibits sympathetic cardiac stimulation and diminishes myocardial oxygen requirements by reducing heart rate, left ventricular contractility, and systolic myocardial wall stress.[171–173] Left ventricular diastolic compliance may improve indirectly through reduction of heart rate or myocardial ischemia.[166, 174] While similar beneficial effects have not been proven with feline HCM, propranolol is still advocated for these reasons. Oral dosage is 2.5 mg q8h to q12h in cats weighing less than 13 lb (6 kg) and 5 mg q8h to q12h in cats weighing more than 13 lb (6 kg). Propranolol is usually administered 24 to 36 hours after diuretic therapy is initiated unless sinus tachycardia or ventricular arrhythmias are present. In the latter case, it is coadministered with diuretics. The question of whether prophylactic therapy for asymptomatic patients is warranted has not been answered.

Calcium-channel blockers, especially verapamil, have been shown to be effective in management of human HCM. Multiple factors contribute to clinical response to verapamil, including reduction in heart rate, blood pressure, a mild negative inotropic effect (reducing myocardial oxygen consumption),[175] and improvement of rapid diastolic ventricular filling.[176] Unfortunately, clinical trials with this drug are lacking in cats and until further research is completed, verapamil cannot be recommended. Diltiazem, however, has been used in affected cats with atrial fibrillation (3.75 to 15 mg q8 to 12 hours)[176a] and in place of propranolol in a small number of cats with HCM.[176b]

Certain drugs have been considered to be harmful in human hypertrophic cardiomyopathy based on their propensity to increase dynamic left ventricular outflow obstruction. They include drugs that increase contractility (digitalis), lower arterial pressure, or decrease ventricular volume (overdiuresis, vasodilators).[1, 2, 142, 166] In certain clinical conditions, however, use of these drugs may be considered. Severe right-sided heart failure unresponsive to diuretics and dietary sodium restriction may require digitalis as may supraventricular tachycardias. Vasodilators (e.g., captopril) have also been used for refractory right-sided failure. Untoward effects have not been clinically observed by the author with these drugs.

Prognosis is guarded to good depending upon disease progression, concomitant arrhythmias, and development of thromboembolic disease. Atrial fibrillation or severe, refractory right-sided congestive heart failure confers a poor prognosis. Thromboemboli may be associated with acute decompensation. If the heart failure state can be successfully managed, distal aortic embolism and associated signs may resolve. Repeated embolic episodes, however, usually follow. Sudden death may occur but survival exceeding six years has been observed.

RESTRICTIVE CARDIOMYOPATHY

Treatment in cats often involves managing pulmonary edema and/or pleural, pericardial, or abdominal effusions, as well as serious ventricular or supraventricular arrhythmias. Therapeutic strategies are similar to those listed for hypertrophic cardiomyopathy. Treatment is most successful with uncomplicated left-sided failure. Success may be short-lived due to thromboembolic disease, exacerbation of heart failure, or malignant arrhythmias.

In dogs, restrictive cardiomyopathy is rare. When it occurs, it usually results from infiltrative processes (e.g., neoplasia). Treatment is usually unsuccessful.

HEART FAILURE ASSOCIATED WITH MYOCARDIAL DISEASES OF UNSPECIFIED OR MIXED MYOCARDIAL DYSFUNCTION

INTERGRADE OR INTERMEDIATE CARDIOMYOPATHIES

Myocardial diseases are often labile. At any point in time they may exhibit various structural alterations (e.g., dilatation and hypertrophy) within one or both functional categories of systolic or diastolic dysfunction. The cardiomyopathic process may not be clearly definable from history, physical examination, radiographic, or angiocardiographic findings. Variable states of compensation and heart failure may develop over time,[23–25] similar to myocardial diseases in humans.[1, 2] Intergrade or intermediate cardiomyopathies occur commonly in cats. Occasionally they are observed in dogs, especially the Doberman pinscher[62, 66] and English cocker spaniel breeds.[68, 69]

Because the natural history of myocardial disease is labile and variable, compensation, deterioration, and structural or functional change may manifest acutely or develop over extended periods of time. Thus, frequent diagnostic reevaluations, especially with echocardiography, are often required for accurate and timely characterization of the disease state. Serum taurine levels should be checked in cats. Taurine-deficient cats with structural and functional characteristics intermediate between the dilated and normal state have occasionally been detected.

EXCESSIVE LEFT VENTRICULAR MODERATOR BANDS AND HEART FAILURE IN CATS

In cats, a pathologic syndrome has been described in which morphologically distinct changes in cardiac structure have been associated with heart failure. These changes relate to abnormal moderator band networks bridging the left ventricular septum, free wall, or papillary muscles. The heart weight to body weight ratios in these cats are lower than those of other forms of primary cardiomyopathies.[9, 170]

Normally, moderator bands are present in the right ventricle of cats, monkeys, sheep, pigs, and oxen,[177] in both canine ventricles,[178] and in the left ventricle of humans.[179] They transport Purkinje fibers from the atrioventricular bundle.[180] Abnormal, diffuse networks have been identified in cats in association with congestive heart failure and myocardial structural changes.[9] Since they have been identified in kittens as young as one day of age, in some cases at least, aberrant moderator bands may represent a congenital form of heart disease.[170] In other cats, individuals up to 13 years old have been identified with abnormal moderator band networks, cardiac dilatation or hypertrophy, and congestive heart failure.[9]

There is no breed predisposition and the reported sex distribution is approximately equal. Moreover, there is extreme variation in gross structure and density of excessive moderator band networks (e.g., from a complex "spider-web" pattern to a single aberrant thread) (Figure 77–14). This heterogeneity may cause a spectrum of pathophysiologic consequences. Thus, the direct and indirect relationship of abnormal moderator bands to heart disease and potential association with cardiomyopathic disorders is unclear.

In humans, they are termed false tendons, false chordae tendineae, or aberrant bands. They have been noted as incidental findings at necropsy,[179] have been associated with precordial murmurs[181] and premature ventricular contractions,[182] and mimic more important pathologic entities.[183]

In affected cats clinical findings are quite variable and

include anorexia, dyspnea, hypothermia, left- and/or right-sided congestive heart failure, gallop rhythms, systolic heart murmurs, thromboembolic disease, and arrhythmias. Electrocardiographic changes in 21 reported cases included right bundle branch block in six cats, left anterior fascicular block in four, first and third degree A-V block in three, and sinus bradycardia in four cats. Cardiomegaly was a consistent radiographic finding. Cardiac catheterization in two cats revealed normal systolic but elevated left ventricular end-diastolic pressure (30 to 40 mm Hg). Necropsies reveal a tendency for left ventricular hypertrophy in younger cats (mean age, four years) or dilatation in older cats (mean age, nine years). Microscopic myocardial changes were similar to those recorded with dilated and hypertrophic forms of cardiomyopathy.[9, 170]

Diagnosis is often difficult based on the heterogeneous nature of clinical and structural abnormalities. Nonselective angiocardiography has been largely insensitive for identifying moderator band networks. Recently, M-mode and two-dimensional echocardiography have facilitated moderator band recognition and provide valuable information about cardiac structure and function. Moderator bands may be imaged in the left ventricular cavity, traversing the ventricular septum and free wall (Figure 77–15).[24, 25]

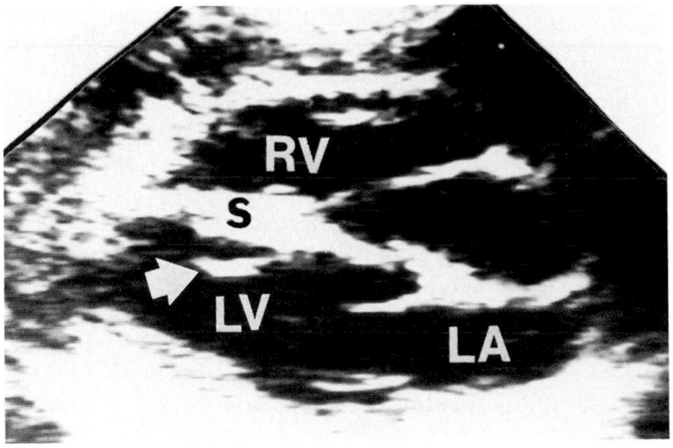

FIGURE 77–15. Two-dimensional echocardiogram recorded at the right intercostal position of a mature domestic short hair cat. In this long axis view aberrant moderator bands (arrow) may be visualized in the left ventricle (LV). LA = left atrium; S = interventricular septum; RV = right ventricle.

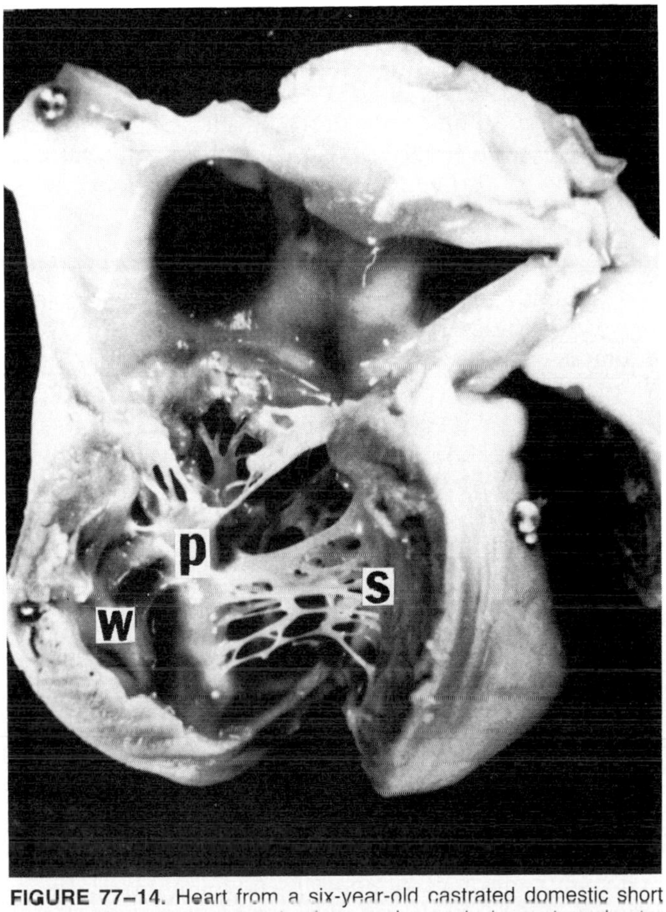

FIGURE 77–14. Heart from a six-year-old castrated domestic short hair cat. There is a network of excessive and aberrant moderator bands adhered to the ventricular septum (s), posterior papillary muscle (p), and left ventricular posterior wall (w). Dilatation and hypertrophy of the left atrium is evident. (From Liu SK, Fox PR, Tilley LP: Excessive left ventricular moderator bands in the left ventricle of 21 cats. JAVMA 180:1215, 1982.)

Differential diagnoses include aortic or mitral valve vegetations, flail aortic or mitral valves, pedunculated thrombi, or tumors.[184] Other forms of primary or secondary myocardial disease may mimic the heart failure state associated with this abnormality.

TREATMENT OF HEART FAILURE ASSOCIATED WITH INTERMEDIATE CARDIOMYOPATHY (MIXED MYOCARDIAL DYSFUNCTION)

Many feline myocardial disorders display myocardial hypertrophy, dilatation, and slight reduction in contractile performance. Furosemide is administered 0.5 to 0.8 mg/lb (1.1 to 1.6 mg/kg) IV or IM to alleviate extracardiac manifestations of congestive failure (pulmonary edema, effusions). Digoxin is added (as described under feline DCM) if severe right-sided heart failure or supraventricular tachyarrhythmias are present. Lidocaine (0.10 to 0.45 mg/lb or 0.25 to 1.0 mg/kg IV over 5 min) or propranolol (2.5 to 5 mg PO q8h to q12h) is administered for serious ventricular arrhythmias such as frequent or multifocal ventricular premature contractions or ventricular tachycardia. Oral taurine supplementation and dietary change are necessary in taurine deficient cats.

Cases of canine myocardial diseases in which myocardial function is mildly depressed or where coexisting acquired chronic valvular disease is present should be similarly approached. Drug doses listed previously may be employed.

Therapy in affected dogs and cats must be individualized and governed by predominant disease stages and pathophysiologic manifestations. Reversible or contributory factors (e.g., thyrotoxicosis) should be detected and corrected.

THROMBOEMBOLIC DISEASE ASSOCIATED WITH CARDIOMYOPATHY

Thromboembolism is a well-recognized syndrome associated with feline myocardial disorders.[3–12, 14, 16, 17, 23–25,

[29, 34, 57, 59, 60, 185] Thrombosis is formation of a clot within a cardiac chamber or vessel lumen. Embolization occurs when a clot or other foreign material enlodges within a vessel. At necropsy thromboembolism has been reported in up to 48 per cent of myopathic cats.[9] The overall clinical incidence of feline thromboembolism, however, is less than indicated by autopsy data.

Distal aortic (saddle) embolization occurs in more than 90 per cent of cats affected with thromboembolic disease. The brachial artery may sometimes be occluded and mural thrombi are occasionally present in the left atrium or ventricle.[7] Various other organs may become embolized. Reports of thromboembolism associated with canine myocardial disease are lacking.

PATHOPHYSIOLOGY

Pathogenesis of thrombosis involves a combination of three factors:[186, 187] local vessel or tissue injury, circulatory stasis, and altered blood coagulability. These factors may be variably present in cardiomyopathic cats, thereby promoting thromboembolic disease.

Pathologic changes involving atrial and ventricular endothelial surfaces may present reactive surfaces to circulating blood. This may trigger a thrombotic process by inducing platelet adhesion and aggregation with subsequent activation of the intrinsic clotting cascade. Endocardial thickening may occur with all myocardiopathies and is most common with the restrictive and hypertrophic forms.[7] Structural changes are patchy, focal, or diffuse and are composed of hyaline, fibrous, and granulation tissue with collagenous fibers.

Blood flow may be altered in myopathic hearts. Left atrial and auricular enlargement results from mitral regurgitation or elevated end-diastolic pressure. Regional circulatory stasis may ensue. Intracavitary stasis may follow functional or anatomic midventricular stenosis (especially in the apical region),[53] or accompany chronic heart failure.[188] Abnormal left ventricular moderator bands may contribute to altered circulation.[9]

Hypercoagulable states commonly accompany thromboembolic disease in cardiomyopathic cats. Disseminated intravascular coagulation associated with consumptive coagulopathy, with liver-mediated coagulopathy, or from thromboembolism was present in more than 75 per cent of affected cats in one study.[59] Moreover, feline platelets are very reactive and responsive to serotonin-induced aggregation.[189] Serotonin is a vasoactive amine released from platelets during the platelet release reaction and is present in high concentration in feline platelets.[190]

Collateral circulation plays an important role in clinical thromboembolic disease. Experimental distal aortic ligation does not duplicate the clinical syndrome caused by a saddle embolus. However, with experimentally induced aortic thromboembolism, the naturally occurring syndrome is simulated.[191, 192] This underscores the importance of vasoactive substances (e.g., serotonin) elaborated by the clot and their effects on collateral circulation.[193] Other chemicals such as thromboxane A_2 cause vasoconstriction[194] and can be reduced by antiprostaglandin drugs such as aspirin.[195]

Ischemic neuromyopathy of peripheral skeletal muscles and nerves is a predictable consequence of arterial occlusion and in particular, of clot-associated inhibition of collateral circulation.[196] Ischemia abolishes fast axoplasmic flow causing conduction failure. This becomes irreversible after five or six hours. With saddle embolization, nerve lesions start at the midthigh region. The majority of nerve fibers display wallerian-type degeneration, while some show damage to the myelin sheath only. In clinical cases of spontaneous aortic thromboembolism, duration of initial ischemia is sufficient to cause loss of peripheral nerve function and induce pathologic changes. Distal limbs below the stifle are especially injured after saddle embolization of the distal aorta. Cranial tibial muscles are more severely affected than gastrocnemii. Focal necrosis, myophagia, and architectural changes may be evident histologically.[196] This inhibits hock flexion more than extension while hip flexion and extension are maintained. Distal limb sensation is severely affected.[59]

CLINICAL MANIFESTATIONS

Clinical signs (e.g., dyspnea, weakness) are attributable to congestive heart failure or result from affected organs and extent of thromboembolism (e.g., myocardial or renal infarction). Most cats present with a lateralizing paraparesis due to saddle embolus at the distal aortic trifurcation. Acute occlusion causes pain, pallor of affected paws, paresthesia, paralysis, cyanotic nail beds, absence of femoral arterial pulses, and cold extremities. These cats can flex or extend the hips but not the hocks, resulting in a dragging motion of affected limbs. Anterior tibial and gastrocnemius muscles are often firm or become hard by 12 to 18 hours after embolization due to ischemic myopathy. Occasionally, a single brachial artery is embolized, causing monoparesis. Renal, mesenteric, or pulmonary embolization may cause death. Intermittent claudication is occasionally the only clinical complaint and may herald severe thromboembolism.[59]

DIAGNOSTIC EVALUATION

If thromboembolism is suspected based on history and clinical signs, a minimum data base should be generated. This includes thoracic radiographs, an electrocardiogram, a biochemical profile, and a feline leukemia virus test.

Approximately one-half of affected cats have heart murmurs or gallop rhythms. Common electrocardiographic abnormalities include supraventricular arrhythmias, cardiac chamber enlargement (especially left atrium and ventricle), and left anterior fascicular block. Most affected cats appear clinically dehydrated. This is usually reflected by mild prerenal azotemia. Serum concentrations of alanine aminotransferase (formerly SGPT) and aspartate aminotransferase (formerly SGOT) are elevated by about 12 hours and peak by 36 hours post-embolization, indicating hepatic and skeletal muscle inflammation and necrosis. Lactic dehydrogenase (LDH) and creatinine phosphokinase (CPK) enzymes are greatly increased shortly after embolization, indicating widespread cellular injury. They may remain elevated for weeks. Hyperglycemia, mature leukocytosis, and lymphopenia may be present.[59]

Thoracic radiographs typically display cardiac chamber enlargement. Most affected cats have associated extracardiac signs of congestive heart failure (e.g., pulmonary edema, pleural effusion).

Echocardiography provides rapid, noninvasive assessment of cardiac structure and function and detects intracardiac thrombi when present (Figure 77–16). This allows early, accurate characterization of the cardiomyopathic disorder to facilitate appropriate therapy.

Nonselective angiocardiography in the stabilized patient facilitates diagnosis if echocardiography is not available. It provides additional information by determining the anatomic extent of thromboembolism (Figure 77–17), and assessing collateral flow.

Differential diagnoses for acute posterior paresis should include trauma, intervertebral disc extrusion, spinal lymphosarcoma, and fibrocartilaginous infarction. Additional diagnostic procedures may therefore be required. However, physical examination findings coupled with the presence of a gallop rhythm, arrhythmia, or radiographic evidence of heart failure are often diagnostic.

TREATMENT

Therapy is directed toward managing the heart failure state as previously discussed. Propranolol should be avoided since it has no demonstrated antithrombotic effects[197] and may enhance peripheral vasoconstriction through β-adrenergic receptor blockade.

Surgical embolectomy is contraindicated in view of decompensated heart failure, hypothermia, and disseminated intravascular coagulation, which accompanies thromboembolism.[10, 23–25, 59, 60] Moreover, significant ischemic neuromyopathy has already occurred preoperatively in most instances. It is not surprising that results of embolectomy have been poor. Results of embolectomy catheters have been unfavorable.[16]

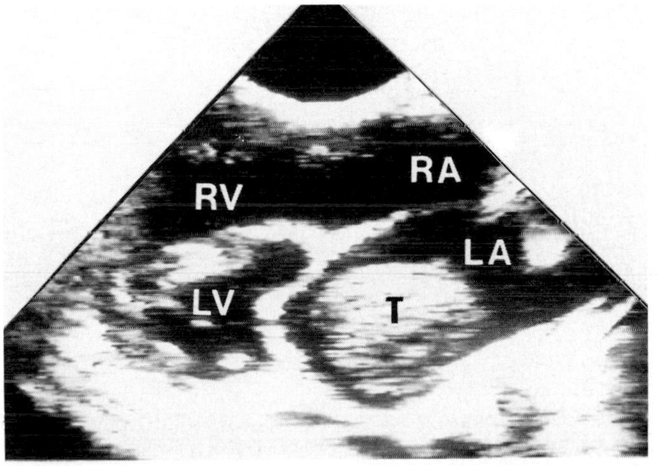

FIGURE 77–16. Two-dimensional echocardiogram recorded at the right intercostal position from a 13-year-old male castrated domestic short hair cat. In this long axis view of the heart a large ball thrombus (T) is visible in the left atrium (LA). LV = left ventricle; RV = right ventricle; RA = right atrium.

Various medical treatments have been used for acute and chronic management of thromboembolic disease, although most are empirical. Arteriolar dilatation with acetylpromazine maleate and hydralazine has been proposed to improve collateral circulation.[16] However, vasodilatation resulting from hydralazine is not uniform. Splanchnic, coronary, cerebral, and renal blood flow, for example, is increased but flow to muscle beds is not dramatically altered.[199–201] Moreover, it has not been demonstrated that hydralazine or acetylpromazine alters platelet-induced reduction of collateral flow caused by vasoactive substances such as serotonin.

Thrombolytic agents have been widely used in humans but are only recently being investigated in cats. Streptokinase administered to cats in a model of experimentally induced aortic thromboembolism failed to produce significant improvement as measured by venous angiograms or thermal circulatory indices.[202] Some of these agents (e.g., streptokinase, urokinase) act by generating the nonspecific proteolytic enzyme plasmin through conversion of the proenzyme plasminogen. This causes a generalized lytic state with the incipient hazard of bleeding complications.[203] More ideal thrombolytic agents such as human tissue plasminogen activator have higher specificity and safety.[204] Currently they are prohibitively expensive.

Anticoagulants (e.g., heparin) have no effect on established thrombi. Their use has been based on the premise that by retarding clotting factor synthesis or accelerating their inactivation, thrombosis from activated blood clotting pathways can be prevented. Heparin acts by binding to antithrombin III, enhancing its ability to neutralize activated factors XII, XI, X, IX, and thrombin.[205] This prevents activation of the coagulation process. It is administered as an initial IV dose of 1000 USP units, followed three hours later by 25 USP units/lb (50 USP units/kg) subcutaneously, which is repeated at six to eight hour intervals.[16] The dose is then adjusted to prolong clotting time two or two and one half times the pretreatment baseline index value. Bleeding is a major complication.

The coumadin drug warfarin has been proposed for chronic oral maintenance in cats surviving an embolic episode.[16] It impairs metabolism of hepatic vitamin K, a vitamin necessary for synthesis of procoagulants (factors II or prothrombin, VII, IX, and X).[206] The initial dosage (0.5 to 1.0 mg daily) is adjusted to prolong the prothrombin time to twice the normal value.[16] Beneficial clinical results await documentation.

Antiplatelet aggregating drugs are theoretically beneficial during and after a thromboembolic episode to prevent further embolic events. Aspirin induces a functional defect in platelets by inactivation, through acetylation, of cyclooxygenase, an enzyme critical in thromboxane A_2 synthesis.[207, 208] The latter is an arachidonic acid derivative, which induces platelet activation. This occurs mainly through platelet adenosine diphosphate release, the common pathway in platelet aggregation.[186] Vasoconstriction results from released platelet thromboxane A_2 and serotonin.[143, 206] Aspirin dosed at 1.25 mg per cat (about 10 mg/lb or 25 mg/kg) effectively inhibits platelet function for three to five days.[197, 209] Collateral circulation has been demonstrated to improve in aspirin-

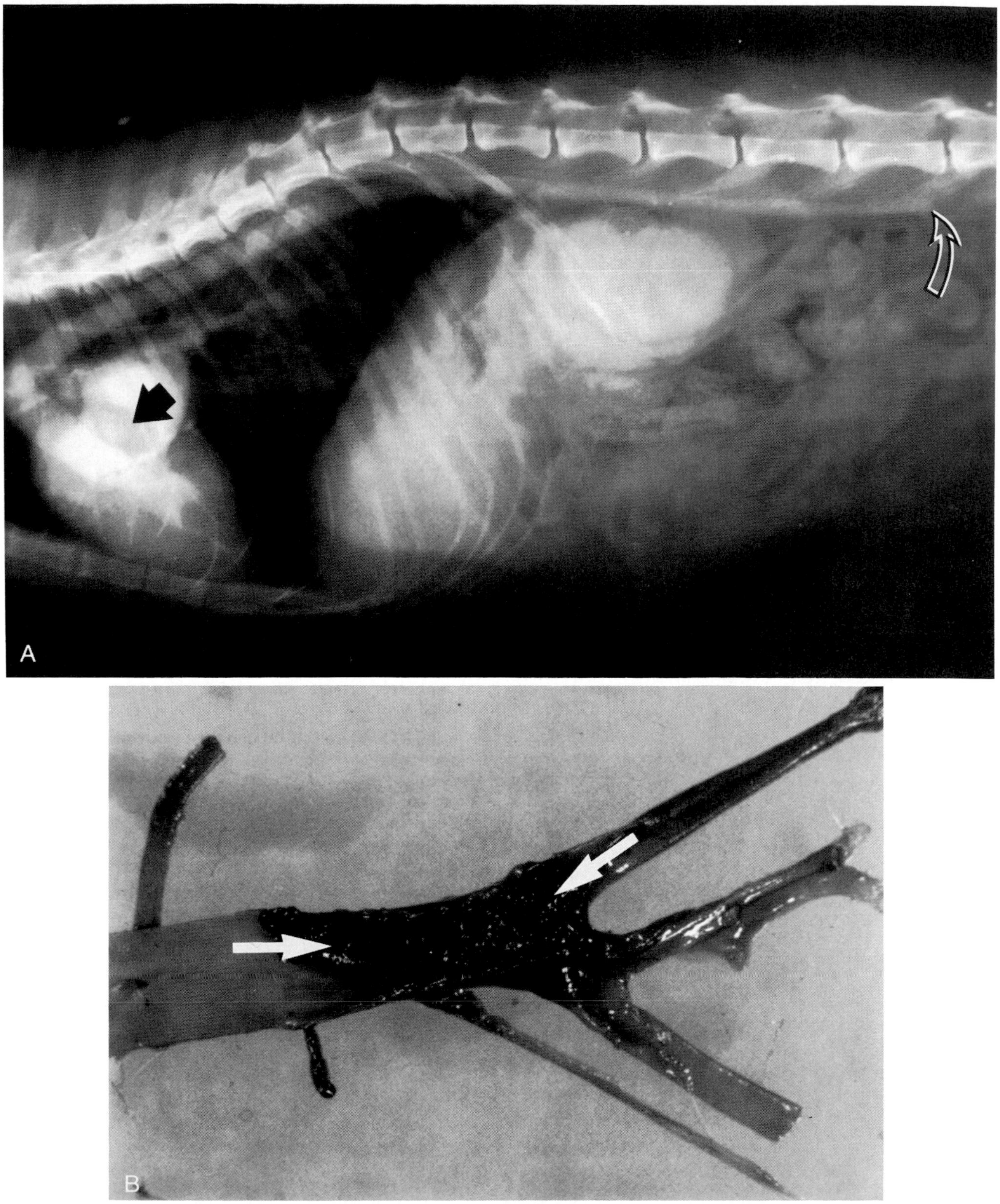

FIGURE 77–17. *A*, Nonselective angiocardiogram of a seven-year-old female domestic short hair cat with hypertrophic cardiomyopathy and thromboembolic disease. There is a ball thrombus in the left atrium (closed arrow) and a saddle embolism in the distal aorta (open arrow). *B*, Distal aorta of same cat illustrating the saddle embolus between the arrows.

treated cats with experimentally induced aortic thrombosis.[195] The recommended dose is one-quarter of a five grain tablet every second to third day.[10, 195, 197, 209]

Much concern exists regarding potential inhibition of prostacyclin synthesis by aspirin.[210] Prostacyclin, the major cyclooxygenase product in vascular endothelium, causes vascular vasodilatation[211] and inhibition of platelet aggregation.[212] The optimal aspirin dose that inhibits thromboxane A_2 production but spares vascular endothelial prostacyclin synthesis has not yet been demonstrated for cats.

With successful management of the heart failure state, motor ability may begin to return within 10 to 14 days. By three weeks, significant motor function (i.e., hock extension and flexion) has often returned, typically better in one leg than the other.[23–25, 59] Recovery may be due to remyelination of nerves injured by ischemia. Ischemic myopathy affects the cranial tibial muscles more severely than others, which appears to correlate with later clinical return of hock flexional ability. Motor function may be completely normal by four to six weeks, although a conscious proprioceptive deficit or conformational abnormality (e.g., extreme hock flexion) may persist in one leg. Complete reinnervation of damaged nerves may require more time.

PROGNOSIS

Short-term prognosis depends upon the nature and responsiveness of the underlying myocardial disorder and heart failure state. The majority of affected cats incur other thromboembolic episodes although survival of four years has been observed post embolization.

SECONDARY CARDIOMYOPATHIES, MYOCARDITIS, AND MYOCARDIAL INJURY

Secondary cardiomyopathy designates myocardial structural or functional alterations resulting from known systemic or metabolic abnormalities (Table 77–1). Overlap may occur between functional and structural categories. For example, neoplastic or fungal myocardial infiltration may cause secondary restrictive cardiomyopathy and diastolic dysfunction; doxorubicin toxicity and feline taurine deficiency may result in systolic dysfunction and dilated cardiomyopathy.[10–20, 23–26, 34, 43–46, 48–51, 213–217] As offending stimuli or etiologies become identified, the primary (idiopathic) cardiomyopathies will eventually be classified as secondary myocardial disorders. This should enable a more rational and effective approach toward prevention, treatment, or potentially, cure. Hyperthyroidism and thyrocardiac disease is a classic example.

NONINFECTIOUS CAUSES OF MYOCARDIAL DISEASE

Many noninfectious agents may directly or indirectly damage the myocardium.[1, 2, 15, 34] Injury may be acute or chronic, transient or permanent, dose- or rate-limited. Inflammation (myocarditis) may or may not be present. Stimuli for myocardial injury may involve drugs, chemicals, toxins, physical agents (radiation, excessive heat), nutritional disorders, and a variety of systemic and metabolic diseases.[1, 2, 15, 34]

Hyperthyroidism (Thyrotoxic Myocardial Disease). Hyperthyroidism is a polysystemic disorder resulting from excessive levels of the thyroid hormones, thyroxine (T_4) and triiodothyronine (T_3). It is one of the most common feline endocrine disorders with a reported incidence at one institution of approximately 1 out of every 300 cats.[213–216] Functional thyroid adenoma (adenomatous hyperplasia) involving one or both thyroid lobes is the most common cause. Thyroid carcinomas in cats are rare, constituting one to two per cent of feline thyroid tumors.[213–216] In dogs, functional thyroid tumors are uncommon.

Pathophysiologic changes relate to the polysystemic nature of thyrotoxicosis. Excess thyroid hormones increase energy metabolism and heat production, causing increased appetite, weight loss, muscle wasting, weakness, and slightly elevated body temperature.[218] Alterations in cardiovascular hemodynamics are secondary to direct effects of thyroid hormone on the heart and increased adrenergic stimulation.[218–220] Enhanced metabolic rate elevates oxygen consumption and decreases peripheral vascular resistance. Increased sympathetic drive causes hyperexcitability and tachycardia. A hyperkinetic state may result with ensuing high output heart failure.[213, 218–225]

FELINE HYPERTHYROIDISM. Middle-aged to older cats are affected, ranging from 6 to 20 years of age. There is no breed or sex predisposition. Clinical signs include weight loss, polyuria, polydipsia, polyphagia, hyperactivity, vomiting, diarrhea, and panting. Mature leukocytosis, eosinopenia, and increased mean corpuscular volume are common hematologic findings. Additional laboratory abnormalities include elevated serum alanine aminotransferase, aspartate aminotransferase, and alkaline phosphatase. Cardiovascular abnormalities include tachycardia, soft to moderate intensity systolic murmurs, gallop rhythms, dyspnea, and arrhythmias.[213–216, 222–225]

Numerous electrocardiographic changes have been recorded.[16, 213, 215, 216, 222–225] Sinus tachycardia and increased R wave amplitude in lead II are the most common. Supraventricular and ventricular arrhythmias and conduction abnormalities are often present.

Cardiomegaly is a common feature of hyperthyroid cats with reported incidences of 40[225, 226] to 49[213] per cent. Radiographic evidence of heart failure (e.g., pulmonary edema and/or pleural effusion) was observed in 16 out of a series of 82 cats.[213] One-quarter of affected cats had pulmonary edema while three-quarters displayed pleural effusion or edema and effusion.

Echocardiographic abnormalities of hyperthyroid cats are common and distinctive.[223–229] In a series of 103 untreated hyperthyroid cats, the most frequently detected changes included hypertrophy of the left ventricular posterior wall (72 per cent), interventricular septum (40 per cent), increased aortic root (18 per cent) and left atrial (70 per cent) diameters, and left ventricular end-diastolic dimension (46 per cent). Fractional shortening and velocity of circumferential fiber shortening were enhanced in 21 and 15 per cent, respectively.[228] Some of these changes are similar to those observed with hypertrophic cardiomyopathy. The two disorders may be differentiated in that hyperthyroid cats have normal or increased ventricular wall amplitude, aortic amplitude, or percentage of thickening of the left ventricular wall and interventricular septum.[225]

Many cardiovascular abnormalities are reversible once successful treatment to establish euthyroidism has been accomplished. Heart murmur intensity may diminish, arrhythmias and ECG evidence of left ventricular chamber enlargement may resolve, congestive signs may be eliminated, and radiographic reduction of cardiomegaly usually occurs.[16, 24, 25, 222–224, 226–228] Echocardiography has demonstrated reduction in left ventricular hypertrophy, shortening fraction, and velocity of circumferential fiber shortening in many cats, although one or more echocardiographic mensurals may remain abnormal after treatment.[226, 228]

Gross pathologic cardiac changes include a reduced body weight, increased heart weight to body weight ratio, left atrial enlargement, and left ventricular hypertrophy (usually symmetric). Histologic cardiac abnormalities include large, hyperchromatic nuclei, interstitial fibrosis, endocardial fibroplasia, fibrosis of the atrioventricular node, and myocardial cellular disorganization.[13]

Treatment may be instituted using chronic administration of an antithyroid drug, surgical thyroidectomy, or radioactive iodine (^{131}I).[215, 216] Most commonly, therapeutic protocols utilize short-term preoperative treatment (three to six weeks) with antithyroid drugs to inhibit thyroid hormone synthesis and effect a euthyroid state. Methimazole is recommended (5 mg q8h) over propylthiouracil (50 mg q8h) because of its lower incidence of side effects.[216, 230] After about two weeks of therapy, T_4 values usually decline into a normal range. At this time, surgical thyroidectomy can be performed.[231] If congestive heart failure accompanies the thyrotoxic state, methimazole should be started and furosemide added, 0.5 mg/lb (1.1 mg/kg) q8h to q12h. If hyperthyroid cats cannot tolerate antithyroid drugs, or if significant ventricular or supraventricular arrhythmias occur, propranolol should be administered for 7 to 14 days preoperatively (2.5 to 5 mg q8h as required to control tachyarrhythmia). In the presence of severe congestive heart failure, propranolol must be used very cautiously since its negative inotropic action may depress contractility. Its use in this state is usually reserved for tachyarrhythmias, which may contribute to heart failure by inhibiting diastolic ventricular filling, or with sustained ventricular tachycardia.[25, 26, 216, 222, 223]

Alternatively, radioactive iodine provides a safe and effective therapeutic modality.[215, 216, 232] Morbidity and mortality are less than with surgery, but nuclear medicine facilities are required.

Prognosis is good with surgical thyroidectomy or radioactive iodine therapy, although the former is associated with significant morbidity and mortality.[215, 216, 231] Cardiomyopathy induced by thyrotoxicosis is largely reversible.

Canine hyperthyroidism. In contrast to those in felines, canine thyroid tumors are more frequently malignant (adenocarcinoma) than benign (adenoma), and clinical hyperthyroidism is rare. Neoplasia of thyroid origin accounts for up to two per cent of canine neoplasms.[217] There is no sex predilection, but boxers are more commonly affected. In one series of 55 dogs with thyroid tumors, approximately 33 per cent were capable of radioiodine uptake and about 20 per cent exhibited signs of hyperthyroidism.[217, 233] It has been estimated that only one-fourth of clinically detected thyroid tumors (usually, carcinomas) secrete sufficient thyroid hormone to cause hyperthyroidism.[234]

Canine thyrotoxicosis may display great clinical variability. Onset may be abrupt or insidious. Signs may be mild or severe. Polydipsia and polyuria are the most frequent abnormalities and often the first to develop. Other signs occur in proportion to severity and duration of the thyrotoxic state. They include excessive panting, restlessness, fatigue and weakness, polyphagia, hyperdefecation, and weight loss (in advanced cases). Physical examination findings include hyperkinetic femoral arterial pulses and precordial apex beats.[217, 233–235] Heart rates seldom exceed the normal range (in contrast to feline hyperthyroidism), although ECG evidence of left ventricular enlargement (tall R waves) may be present.[235] Plasma levels of thyroid hormones are elevated in hyperthyroid dogs.

Treatment involves prompt surgical thyroidectomy. Metastasis may occur in 40 per cent of adenocarcinomas by the time of clinical examination and has been detected in up to 80 per cent of affected dogs at necropsy. Total volume of tumor mass may correlate with metastasis. Preoperative use of antithyroid drugs should probably be used as described in feline hyperthyroidism. However, surgery without such preparation has been described without untoward effects[234] (possibly due to more rapid rates of deiodination and excretion of T_3 and T_4 in canines). Chemotherapy or radiotherapy may be used in dogs with inoperable or disseminated disease.

Prognosis for dogs with malignant tumors is variable. Early detection and resection greatly benefit some animals. With tumors greater than 5 cm in diameter, however, long-term prognosis is poor.[217]

Toxins, Chemicals, and Physical Agents. Cardiotoxicity is common following certain chemotherapeutic protocols for neoplastic diseases. The highest incidence follows use of anthacyclines, especially doxorubicin. Arrhythmias (ventricular, supraventricular, and conduction abnormalities), dilated cardiomyopathy, and congestive heart failure are documented in dogs receiving cumulative doses ranging from greater than 240 mg/m^2 to 150 mg/m^2 or less.[236, 237] Acute cardiotoxicity may also occur after initial therapy.[238] Characteristic pathologic findings in chronic toxicity include cardiac chamber dilatation, systolic (myocardial) failure, myocyte degeneration and atrophy (myofibrillar loss, cytoplasmic vacuolization and myocytolysis), myocardial interstitial fibrosis, and edema.[236, 237] Pathogenesis of doxorubicin-induced myocardial injury is controversial, although it probably does not relate to the drug's anti-tumor effect. The time of onset of heart failure from the last doxorubicin treatment is quite variable. Serial ECGs and M-mode echocardiograms are unreliable in demonstrating doxorubicin-induced cardiomyopathy before congestive heart failure has become clinically evident.[237] Resultant heart failure is usually refractory to therapy.

Cats appear more resistant to cardiotoxic effects of doxorubicin than dogs. A chronic cumulative dose of 100 to 125 mg/m^2 did not result in cardiotoxicity when studied in 30 cats[239] and arrhythmias were recorded in only 1 out of 14 cats receiving up to 180 mg/m^2.[240] In another feline study, three cats receiving higher doses (265 to 320 mg/m^2) displayed histologic cardiac lesions but no clinical signs of heart failure.[241]

Other agents causing myocardial injury include hydrocarbons, carbon monoxide, mercury, arsenic, spider stings, and selenium deficiency. Physical agents, such as heat stroke and hypothermia, blunt or penetrating trauma, electric shock, or hypersensitivity reactions may also be injurious.[1, 2, 34]

ISCHEMIA AND OTHER CAUSES OF MYOCARDIAL DYSFUNCTION

Although approximately one-third of all human deaths in the United States are due to ischemic heart disease (one-half attributable to acute myocardial infarction resulting from atherosclerosis),[242] coronary artery insufficiency is not a singularly significant cause of morbidity and mortality in canines and felines. However, atherosclerosis (degenerative coronary artery disease), embolism, coronary vasoconstriction, or other causes of reduced coronary perfusion may impair removal of metabolites, alter cellular physiology, affect contractility, and cause cellular death.

Microscopic myocardial infarction is rare, but can occur from infective endocarditis-induced coronary embolism,[243, 244] or from emboli from septic, neoplastic, or thrombotic diseases.[19, 20] Sudden development of pronounced (i.e., greater than 0.5 mV) ST-T deviation on the ECG should prompt suspicion of myocardial infarction. Antiarrhythmic therapy and treatment of the underlying condition is required.

Microscopic focal myocardial infarction is a common finding in older dogs. It is often associated with mitral valve myxomatous degeneration and insufficiency (endocardiosis). Myocardial lesions are related to arteriosclerotic vascular lesions (hyalinosis, amyloidosis, thickening of musculoelastic fibers, and microthombi).[245, 246] Specific effects of these lesions are unclear, although they may contribute to the process of heart failure.

Myocardial necrosis may result from a variety of noncardiac factors. Coronary vasoconstriction secondary to increased sympathetic traffic may be associated with central nervous system trauma,[247] acute gastric dilatation-volvulus,[248] high levels of circulating catecholamines,[249] digitalis toxicity,[250] atherosclerosis (especially with severe hypothyroidism and hypercholesterolemia),[251] and pancreatitis.

Abnormalities in potassium, calcium, and acid-base status may result from a variety of systemic and metabolic diseases. They may directly cause cellular injury, arrhythmias, and myocardial dysfunction, or contribute to those effects caused by the underlying disease. In this fashion, various endocrine disorders (e.g., acromegaly, hypothyroidism, uremia, hyperadrenocorticism, pheochromocytoma, diabetes mellitus), obesity, and hematologic diseases adversely affect myocardial structure and function.[1, 2, 15, 253]

NEOPLASTIC AND INFILTRATIVE MYOCARDIAL DISEASE

Cardiac neoplasia may be associated with a number of extracardiac (i.e., systemic) abnormalities, depending upon whether the heart is affected primarily or secondarily (i.e., due to metastasis). Fever, cachexia, lethargy, anemia, leukocytosis, thrombocytopenia, and systemic embolization may represent clinical findings. Cardiac manifestations include disturbances of conduction or rhythm, congestive heart failure, pericardial effusion or tamponade, and syncope. Specific signs are closely related to anatomic location of the tumor.[252]

Secondary cardiac neoplasms greatly outnumber primary heart tumors in the dog and cat.[253–260] Hemangiosarcoma is the most common primary cardiac tumor, although it commonly arises from noncardiac sites. Cardiac origin has been recorded in 3 per cent,[255] 40 per cent,[256] and 50 per cent[257] of affected dogs at necropsy. German shepherd dogs accounted for about one-third of recorded cardiac cases. Affected dogs ranged in age from 2 to 15 years (mean, 10 years) with no sex predilection.[256–258] In cats, the heart is the most common site of hemangiosarcoma metastasis,[259] but primary right atrial origin is rare.[254]

Canine chemodectomas are predominantly aortic body tumors with a predilection for brachycephalic breeds (boxers, Boston terriers) in the 6 to 14 year range. They usually originate at the base of the aorta and/or pulmonary artery. Small tumors are well-defined but large neoplasms may infiltrate the atria, ventricles, and surrounding tissues. Metastasis occurs one-fifth to one-quarter of the time but local invasion is common.[260] This tumor is rare in cats.

Lymphosarcoma occasionally infiltrates the myocardium. Approximately 10 to 15 per cent of feline lymphosarcoma cases have histologic evidence of myocardial infiltration with neoplastic or atypical lymphocytes. This percentage increases to about 20 per cent when cases of leukemia with lymphoma are considered.[261]

Myocarditis. Myocarditis denotes inflammation of myocytes, interstitium, or vascular structures. It may be due to a host of factors affecting the heart muscle primarily or secondarily, may be an acute or chronic process, and may completely resolve or result in irreversible morphologic changes and congestive heart failure. Clinical expression is variable, ranging from asymptomatic focal inflammation to generalized myocarditis with fatal arrhythmias and congestive heart failure. Myocarditis or clinical signs may occur from direct invasion and cellular damage by the infectious agent or result from toxic, allergic, or hypersensitivity response by the host from the inciting stimulus.[1, 2, 262]

Etiologic diagnosis is usually difficult and must often be implied from extracardiac manifestations of the disease process. Clinical features of the systemic disease are often dominant, overshadow cardiac signs, and facilitate etiologic identification.

Clinical abnormalities (when present) vary greatly, depending upon the site and extent of cardiac involvement, nature, and severity of associated systemic illness. Electrocardiographic changes may be nonspecific (such as ST and T wave alterations), transient, or sustained, or display atrial and ventricular arrhythmias and conduction disturbances. Arrhythmias may be present during the height of infection or occur after clinical signs have subsided. Radiographic examination may be unremarkable or disclose marked cardiomegaly with pulmonary congestion or pleural effusion. Laboratory tests, such as cardiac serum enzyme elevations (e.g., LDH, SGOT), are usually of little help. Serodiagnostic tests for specific diseases (e.g., trypanosomiasis, toxoplasmosis, parvovirus) may be valuable to establish a diagnosis when combined with the other data. Therapy is usually supportive and tailored to treat the dominant systemic disease or its metabolic sequelae. Congestive heart failure or arrhythmias are treated in standard fashion.

Viral Myocarditis. Canine parvovirus (a small, single-stranded DNA virus) was recognized in 1978 for its world-wide disease pandemic lasting for several years.[34, 169, 170, 263–270] The myocardial manifestation usually occurred without concurrent enteritis. It was initially expressed as a peracute fatal myocarditis affecting robust, healthy pups during the first three to eight weeks of life that were born into a contaminated environment without sufficient maternal antibody protection. Clinical signs included sudden hyperpnea, dyspnea, crying, cyanosis, and unexpected death from pulmonary edema within minutes to hours. Arrhythmias, tachycardia, left apical systolic murmurs, gallop rhythms, pulmonary edema, and cardiomegaly were clinical features. Most cases died before therapy could be instituted or despite therapy. Post-mortem findings included enlarged, dilated hearts, often with pale myocardial streaks. Histologic hallmarks were large basophilic or amphophilic intranuclear inclusion bodies (Figure 77–18). A focal mononuclear cell infiltrate was variably present. This syndrome is now rarely encountered, perhaps because of widespread development of protective maternal antibody through viral exposure and vaccination.

A second clinical form occurs in which nonfatal neonatal parvovirus myocarditis results in dilated cardiomyopathy with congestive heart failure in young adults (typically, five or six months of age).[19, 20, 26, 34, 169, 170, 268, 270] Grossly, distinctive streaks from myocardial scarring (fibrosis) are diffusely present without histologic evidence of inflammation.[20, 34, 169] Experimental in utero infection with parvovirus has also demonstrated myocardial disease in dogs ranging from 3 to 14 weeks of age.[271] These findings suggest a relationship between viral myocarditis and dilated cardiomyopathy. Viral myocarditis from parvovirus in adult dogs is rarely observed but has been reported.[272]

Canine distemper virus causes myocarditis in puppies infected experimentally at five to seven days of age but not in those infected at 10 to 21 days of age.[273] Myocardial lesions in the younger group were present by 16 days of age. Lesions consisted of multifocal myonecrosis,

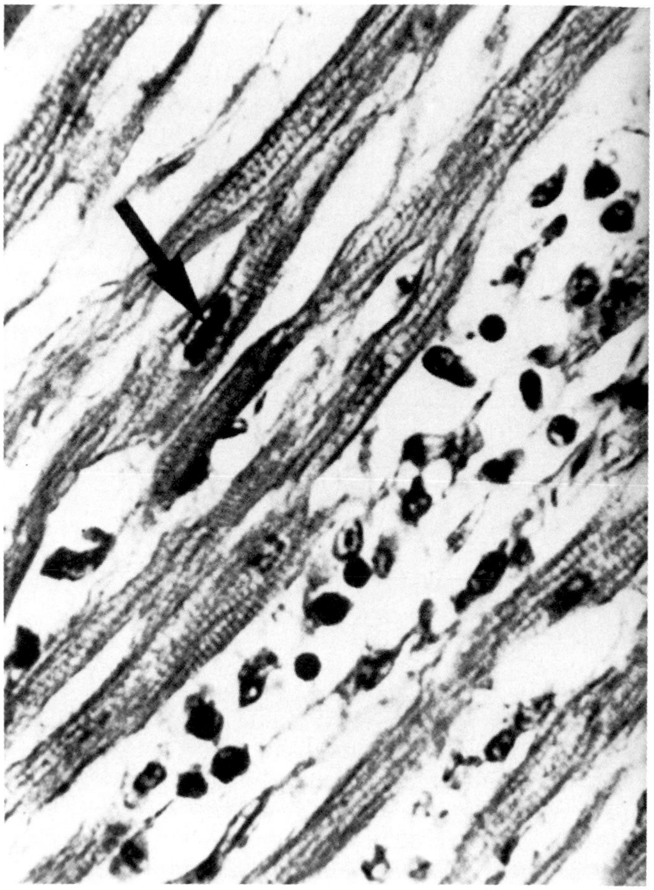

FIGURE 77–18. Photomicrograph of the left ventricular myocardium, showing a myocardial cell nucleus containing a basophilic inclusion body (arrow) and mononuclear cell infiltration between myofibers. H & E stain; X 400. (From Jezyk PF, Haskins ME, Jones CL: Myocarditis of probable viral origin in pups of weaning age. JAVMA 174:1204, 1979.)

minimal inflammatory cell response, mineralization, and fibrosis.

Canine herpesvirus experimentally used to infect puppies during the second trimester of pregnancy has resulted in fetal and perinatal death with necrotizing myocarditis and intranuclear inclusion bodies.[274] The potential role of these viruses in development of myocardial disease in naturally infected dogs has not been established.

Myocarditis of suspected viral origin was recorded in 25 cats.[169] Twenty-one had an acute clinical course composed of dyspnea, depression, and leukocytosis for one to two days prior to death. Subendocardial petechia or diffuse hemorrhage, endomyocardial infiltration with lymphocytes and plasma cells, and myocytolysis were common findings. Other cats with chronic endomyocarditis and restrictive cardiomyopathy died of congestive heart failure. Severe, diffuse endocardial fibrosis was the prominent feature; endomyocardial fibrosis and arteriosclerosis was marked in advanced cases.

Protozoal Myocarditis. Trypanosomiasis (Chagas' disease) has been reported in young dogs less than two years of age from the southeastern United States (Louisiana, Texas).[275–278] Males are more commonly affected. The protozoan *Trypanosoma cruzi* is enzootic among wild animals and dogs in that region.[276, 279] It is spread by reduviid blood sucking insects and causes an acute syndrome characterized by cardiac abnormalities (tachycardia, weak atrial pulses, arrhythmias, cardiomegaly, hepatomegaly, pulmonary edema, ascites) and systemic signs (weight loss, diarrhea, lethargy, anorexia, lymphadenopathy, sudden death). Granulomatous myocarditis associated with amastigotes of *T. cruzi* (predominantly within myocytes) is the hallmark feature. The right atrium and ventricle are dilated and most severely affected. Lesions also appear in the left heart.[275, 278] With experimentally induced chronic Chagas' disease, lesions were detected both within the conducting system, as well as the myocardium.[280] Ante-mortem diagnosis is possible using blood culture techniques and serologic testing. Because of public health significance, treatment is generally not undertaken.

Toxoplasmosis caused by the obligate intracellular coccidian parasite, *Toxoplasma gondii,* occurs in a wide variety of birds and mammals. Occasionally, it can cause myocarditis as part of a polysystemic process or in immunosuppressed animals. Slowly dividing, long-lived bradyzoites may encyst in myocardium, and produce a chronic infection. They may rupture (excyst) and proliferate (tachyzoites), causing a hypersensitivity reaction and necrosis. Immune-suppression from drugs or disease (e.g., feline leukemia virus) may cause released bradyzoites to rapidly proliferate and exacerbate myocarditis.[281] Neonatal toxoplasmosis and myocarditis (multifocal necrosis with tachyzoites) have been reported in 18 and 32 day old kittens.[282] Death was probably due to pneumonia. In a group of 20 cats with toxoplasmosis, histologic lesions were found in 12 but were only severe in 1 cat. Cysts and bradyzoites were rare in these lesions and clinical signs of heart disease were usually absent.[16] Thus, toxoplasmosis-induced myocarditis is apparently overshadowed in most cases by more dominant systemic effects.

Hepatozoon canis may penetrate the myocardium during its life cycle (schizogony),[283, 284] and has been reported in the Texas Gulf coast.[284, 285] Nonsuppurative interstitial myocarditis containing *Hepatozoon*-like schizonts was detected in 42 per cent of 50 apparently healthy cats necropsied in Israel[286] and *Hepatozoon* has been reported in a North American cat.[287] The brown dog tick, *Rhipicephalus sanguineus*, is the definitive host of *H. canis*. Dogs become infected by ingesting a tick containing sporulated oocysts. Clinical systemic signs include anorexia, fever, stiffness, neutrophilic leukocytosis, and periosteal new bone reaction.[285] Because of the wide distribution of the brown dog tick and mobile pet population, this disease may spread to other locations.

Bacterial Myocarditis. Bacterial myocarditis can result from sepsis, bacterial endocarditis, or pericarditis.[288] Pathologic bacteremia occurs when systemic venous or lymphatic drainage of an infected tissue seeds the blood stream. Abscessation or focal suppurative myocarditis may result. Fever and arrhythmias provide clinical suspicion. Serial blood cultures should be taken in an attempt to identify the causative organism and provide information regarding antibiotic sensitivity. Two-dimensional echocardiography can occasionally detect myocardial abscesses.

Mycoses and Algae. Myocardial infection by fungi or algae is usually a secondary manifestation of the disseminated disease process associated with reduced host defense or immunosuppressive therapy. Aortic valvular endocarditis and endomyocarditis were observed in a dog with generalized cryptococcosis *(Cryptococcus neoformans).*[289] Coccidioidal dissemination *(Coccidioides immitis)* has been reported to affect the heart.[290, 291] Disseminated aspergillosis *(Aspergillus terreus)* was found in suppurative myocardial foci[292] and in nonsuppurative granulomatous endomyocardial foci[293] in dogs. *Paecilomyces varioti* was identified from myocardial granulomas in dogs with systemic paecilomycosis.[294] Algae-like organisms, *Prototheca wickerhamii, P. zopfi,* and other *Prototheca* spp., have been associated with granulomatous myocarditis and disseminated protothecosis in four dogs.[295-298] In this species, disseminated protothecosis is hypothesized to develop after colonic infection. Treatment of disseminated mycosis or algal infections has been largely unrewarding.

Miscellaneous Myocardiopathies. Persistent atrial standstill associated with a facioscapulohumeral-like skeletal muscular dystrophy has been reported in dogs (especially English spaniels)[299, 300] and with dilated cardiomyopathy in cats (especially Siamese).[300] Greatly enlarged, paper-thin atria are usually present. Myocardial fibrosis and focal myocarditis and necrosis are sometimes evident. Pacemaker therapy has successfully controlled clinical signs due to the bradyarrhythmia in dogs.[301, 302]

Glycogen storage diseases leading to glycogen accumulation are heritable disorders of connective tissue. Cardiovascular abnormalities may occur as part of polysystemic changes. A type II glycogen storage disease (Pompe's disease) was suspected in four Lapland dogs with cardiomegaly, electrocardiographic and radiographic abnormalities, and myocardial glycogen infiltration.[303] Biochemical identification of α-glucosidase deficiency, an enzyme responsible for glycogen metabolism was found in one dog. Glycogenic cardiomegaly was proposed from another Lapland dog.[304] Two subclasses of genetic mucopolysaccharidoses (MPS), diseases resulting from defects in glycosaminoglycan metabolism, have been reported from cats—MPS I (Hurler's syndrome) in domestic short hair cats[305] and MPS VI (Maroteaux-Lamy syndrome) in Siamese cats.[306] Cardiac involvement has not been significant in these cases, although it has been important in their human counterparts.[307]

Inflammatory and degenerative lesions have been demonstrated in the conducting system of dogs displaying syncope and sudden death. His bundle stenosis, fibrosis, and degeneration have been described in related pug dogs.[308] Luminal narrowing of small arteries in the region of the His bundle was described as a probable cause of His bundle degeneration in a group of dogs (mostly Doberman pinschers) with sudden death.[309] Atrioventricular bundle fibrosis was noted in 12 dogs who died unexpectedly.[310] Ten of these dogs were male, five were Dobermans. Some dogs displayed sudden episodes of viciousness or seizures. All had hypoxic-type degeneration in the hippocampus and dorsal half of the midpoint of the cerebral cortex suggesting possible association between arrhythmias and hypoxia.

References

1. Wenger, NK, et al.: Cardiomyopathy and myocardial involvement in systemic disease. *In* Hurst JW (ed): The Heart. New York, McGraw-Hill Book, 1986, p 1181.
2. Wynne, JW and Braunwald, E: The cardiomyopathies and myocarditides. *In* Braunwald E (ed): Heart Disease, 2nd ed. Philadelphia, WB Saunders, 1984, p 1399.
3. Tilley, LP and Liu, SK: Cardiomyopathy and thromboembolism in the cat. Fel Pract 5:32, 1975.
4. Liu, SK, et al.: Feline cardiomyopathy. Recent Adv Stud Card Struct Metab 10:627, 1975.
5. Tilley, LP, et al.: Primary myocardial disease in the cat: A model for human cardiomyopathy. Am J Pathol 87:493, 1977.
6. Harpster, N: Feline cardiomyopathy. Vet Clin North Am 7:355, 1977.
7. Liu, SK: Pathology of feline heart diseases. Vet Clin North Am 7:323, 1977.
8. Liu, SK and Tilley, LP: Animal models of primary myocardial diseases. Yale J Biol Med 53:191, 1980.
9. Liu, SK, et al.: Excessive moderator bands in the left ventricle of 21 cats. JAVMA 180:1215, 1982.
10. Fox, PR: Feline myocardial diseases. *In* Kirk RW (ed): Current Veterinary Therapy VIII. Philadelphia, WB Saunders, 1983, p 337.
11. Fox, PR, et al.: The Cardiovascular System. *In* Pratt PW (ed): Feline Medicine. Santa Barbara, CA, American Veterinary Publ, 1983, p 249.
12. Tilley, LP, et al.: Myocardial disease. *In* Ettinger SJ (ed): Textbook of Veterinary Internal Medicine, 2nd ed. Philadelphia, WB Saunders, 1983, p 1029.
13. Liu, SK, et al.: Hypertrophic cardiomyopathy and hyperthyroidism in the cat. JAVMA 185:52, 1984.
14. Bond, BR and Fox, PR: Advances in feline cardiomyopathy. Vet Clin North Am 14:1021, 1984.
15. Fox, PR: Cardiovascular disorders in systemic diseases. *In* Tilley LP and Owens JM (eds): Manual of Small Animal Cardiology. New York, Churchill Livingstone, 1985, p 265.
16. Harpster, NK: The cardiovascular system. *In* Holzworth J (ed): Diseases of the Cat. Philadelphia, WB Saunders, 1986, p 820.
17. Harpster, NK: Feline myocardial diseases. *In* Kirk RW (ed): Current Veterinary Therapy IX. Philadelphia, WB Saunders, 1986, p 380.
18. Wood, GL: Canine myocardial diseases. *In* Kirk RW (ed): Current Veterinary Therapy VIII. Philadelphia, WB Saunders, 1983, p 321.
19. Ware, WA and Bonagura, JD: Canine myocardial diseases. *In* Kirk RW (ed): Current Veterinary Therapy IX. Philadelphia, WB Saunders, 1986, p 370.
20. Thomas, WP: Myocardial diseases of the dog. *In* Bonagura JD (ed): Contemp Issues Small Anim Pract: Cardiology. Vol 7. New York, Churchill Livingstone, 1987, p 117.
21. Report of the WHO/ISFC task force on the definition and classification of cardiomyopathies. Br Heart J 44:672, 1980.
22. Goodwin, JF: Congestive and hypertrophic cardiomyopathies. A decade of study. Lancet 1:731, 1970.
23. Fox, PR: Feline myocardial diseases—A clinical approach. Proc 9th Annu Kal Kan Symp, Vernon, Calif, 1986, p 57.
24. Fox, PR: Feline myocardial diseases. *In* Fox PR (ed): Textbook of Canine and Feline Cardiology. New York, Churchill Livingstone, 1988, p 435.
25. Fox, PR: Feline cardiomyopathy. *In* Bonagura JD (ed): Contemp Issues Small Anim Pract: Cardiology. Vol 7. New York, Churchill Livingstone, 1987, p 157.
26. Fox, PR: Canine myocardial diseases. *In* Fox PR (ed): Textbook of Canine and Feline Cardiology. New York, Churchill Livingstone, 1988, p 467.
27. Owens, JM and Twedt, DC: Nonselective angiocardiography in the cat. Vet Clin North Am 7:309, 1977.
28. Fox, PR and Bond, BR: Nonselective and selective angiocardiography. Vet Clin North Am 13:259, 1983.
29. Suter, PF: Thoracic Radiography. A Text Atlas of Thoracic Diseases of the Dog and Cat. Wettswil, Switzerland, Peter F. Suter, 1984.
30. Pipers, FS and Hamlin, RL: Clinical use of echocardiography in the domestic cat. JAVMA 176:57, 1980.
31. Bonagura, JD: M-mode echocardiography: Basic principles. Vet Clin North Am 13:299, 1983.
32. Soderberg, SF, et al.: Echocardiography as a diagnostic aid for feline cardiomyopathy. Vet Radiol 24:66, 1983.
33. Bonagura, JD and Herring, DS: Echocardiography: Acquired heart disease. Vet Clin North Am 15:1209, 1985.
34. Van Vleet, JF and Ferrans, V: Myocardial diseases of animals. Am J Pathol 124:98, 1986.
35. Liu, SK: Pathology of feline heart disease. *In* Kirk RW (ed): Current Veterinary Therapy V. Philadelphia, WB Saunders, 1974, p 341.
36. Adelman, AG, et al.: Current concepts of primary cardiomyopathy. Cardiovasc Med 2:495, 1977.
37. Greene, HL, et al.: How to minimize doxorubicin toxicity. Cardiovasc Med 7:306, 1982.
38. Ferrans, VJ: Overview of cardiac pathology in relation to anthracycline cardiotoxicity. Cancer Treat Rep 62:955, 1978.
39. Gottdiener, JS, et al.: Cardiotoxicity associated with high dose cyclophosphamide therapy. Arch Intern Med 141;758, 1981.
40. Factor, SM, et al.: Microvascular spasm in the cardiomyopathic Syrian hamster: A preventative cause of focal myocardial necrosis. Circulation 66:342, 1982.
41. Berko, B and Swift, M: X-linked dilated cardiomyopathy. N Engl J Med 316:1186, 1987.
42. Waber, LJ, et al.: Carnitine deficiency presenting as familial cardiomyopathy: a treatable defect in carnitine transport. J Pediatr 101:700, 1982.
43. Rebouche, CJ and Engel, AG: Carnitine metabolism and deficiency syndromes. Mayo Clin Proc 58:533, 1983.
44. Keene, BW, et al.: Carnitine-linked defects of myocardial metabolism in canine dilated cardiomyopathy. Proc Fourth Annu Vet Med Forum, Vol II (Abstr)14:54, 1986.
45. Dec, GW, et al.: Active myocarditis in the spectrum of acute dilated cardiomyopathies. N Engl J Med 312:885, 1985.
46. Maisch, B, et al.: Diagnostic relevance of humoral and cytotoxic immune reactions in primary and secondary dilated cardiomyopathy. Am J Cardiol 52:1072, 1983.
47. Unverferth, DV: The etiology of idiopathic dilated cardiomyopathy. *In* Unverferth DV (ed): Dilated Cardiomyopathy. Mount Kisco, NY, Futura, 1985, p 213.
48. Editorial: Selenium in the heart of China. Lancet 2:889, 1979.
49. Johnson, RA, et al.: An occidental case of cardiomyopathy and selenium deficiency. N Engl J Med 304:1210, 1981.
50. Hsu, FS and Du, SJ: Cardiac diseases in swine. *In* Roberts HR, Dodds WJ (eds): Pig Model for Biomedical Research. Pig Research Inst, Taiwan, Republic of China, 1982, p 134.
51. Pion, PD, et al.: Myocardial failure associated with low plasma taurine levels in cats and its reversal with oral taurine. Science 237:764, 1987.
51a. Fox PR, et al.: Plasma taurine concentrations in cats with acquired and congenital heart disease. (Abstr 71). Proc 6th Annu ACVIM Forum, 1988, p 758.
52. Grossman, W, et al.: Alterations in left ventricular relaxation and diastolic compliance in congestive cardiomyopathy. Cardiovasc Res 13:514, 1979.
53. Lord, PF: Left ventricular diastolic stiffness in dogs with congestive cardiomyopathy and volume overload. Am J Vet Res 37:953, 1976.
54. Lord, PF, et al.: Radiographic and hemodynamic evaluation of cardiomyopathy and thromboembolism in the cat. JAVMA 164:154, 1974.
55. Boyden, PA, et al.: Effects of left atrial enlargement on atrial transmembrane potentials and structure in dogs with mitral valve fibrosis. Am J Cardiol 49:1896, 1982.
56. Boyden, PA, et al.: Mechanisms for atrial arrhythmias associated with cardiomyopathy: a study of feline hearts with primary myocardial disease. Circulation 69:1036, 1984.
57. Benjamin, IJ, et al.: Cardiac hypertrophy in idiopathic dilated congestive cardiomyopathy: A clinicopathologic study. Circulation 64:422, 1981.
58. Suter, PF: The radiographic diagnosis of canine and feline heart disease. Comp Cont Ed Pract Vet 3:441, 1981.
59. Fox, PR: Feline thromboembolism associated with cardiomyopathy. Proc 5th Annu Vet Med Forum, 1987.
60. Fox, PR and Dodds, WJ: Coagulopathies observed with spontaneous aortic thromboembolism in cardiomyopathic cats. Proc Am Coll Vet Intern Med (Abstr.) 1982, p 83.

61. Van Vleet, JF, et al.: Pathologic alterations in congestive cardiomyopathy of dogs. Am J Vet Res 42:416, 1981.
62. Calvert, CA, et al.: Congestive cardiomyopathy in Doberman pinscher dogs. JAVMA 181:598, 1982.
63. Calvert, CA: Dilated (congestive) cardiomyopathy in Doberman pinschers. Comp Cont Ed Pract Vet 6:417, 1986.
64. Hazlett, MJ, et al.: A retrospective study of heart disease in Doberman pinscher dogs. Can Vet J 24:205, 1983.
65. Hill, BL: Canine idiopathic congestive cardiomyopathy. Compend Cont Ed 3:615, 1981.
66. Calvert, CA and Brown, J: Use of M-mode echocardiography in the diagnosis of congestive cardiomyopathy in Doberman pinschers. JAVMA 189:293, 1986.
67. Harpster, NK: Boxer cardiomyopathy. *In* Kirk RW (ed): Current Veterinary Therapy VIII. Philadelphia, WB Saunders, 1983, p 329.
68. Staaden, RV: Cardiomyopathy of English cocker spaniels. JAVMA 178:1289, 1981.
69a. Fox PR: Unpublished data, 1988.
69. Gooding, JP, et al.: Echocardiographic characterization of dilatation cardiomyopathy in the English cocker spaniel. Am J Vet Res 47:1978, 1986.
70. Fox, PR: Unpublished data, 1988.
71. Gooding, JP, et al.: A cardiomyopathy in the English cocker spaniel: a clinico-pathological investigation. J Small Anim Pract 23:133, 1982.
72. Lombard, CW and Buergielt, CD: Endocardial fibroelastosis in four dogs. JAAHA 20:271, 1984.
73. Zook, BC and Paasch, LH: Endocardial fibroelastosis in Burmese cats. Am J Pathol 106:435, 1982.
74. Maskin, CS, et al.: Inotropic drugs for treatment of the failing heart. Cardiovasc Clin 14:1, 1984.
75. Goodwin, JF: The frontiers of cardiomyopathy. Br Heart J 48:1, 1982.
76. Spodick, DH: Effective management of congestive cardiomyopathy. Arch Intern Med 142:689, 1982.
77. Sonnenblick, EH: Force-velocity relations in mammalian heart muscle. Am J Physiol 202:931, 1962.
78. Dyke, SE, et al.: Detection of latent function in acutely ischemic myocardium in dogs: Comparison of pharmacologic inotropic stimulation and post extrasystolic potentiation (PESP). Circ Res 36:490, 1975.
79. Spann, JF, Jr, et al.: Contractile performance of the hypertrophied and chronically failing cat ventricle. Am J Physiol 223:1150, 1972.
80. Colucci, WS, et al.: New positive inotropic agents in the treatment of congestive heart failure. Mechanisms of action and recent clinical developments. N Engl J Med 314:349, 1986.
81. Opie, LH and Kaplan, NM: Diuretic therapy. *In* Opie LH (ed): Drugs for the Heart. Orlando, Grune & Stratton, 1987, p 111.
82. Brest, AN: Clinical pharmacology of diuretic drugs. Cardiovasc Clin 14:31, 1984.
83. Cohn, JN: Vasodilator therapy for heart failure: The influence of impedance on left ventricular performance. Circulation 48:5, 1973.
84. Hirota, Y, et al.: Mechanisms of compensation and decompensation in dilated cardiomyopathy. Am J Cardiol 54:1033, 1984.
85. Goldberg, LI: Cardiovascular and renal actions of dopamine: Potential clinical implications. Pharmacol Rev 24:1, 1972.
86. Chidsey, CA, et al.: Catecholamine excretion and cardiac stores of norepinephrine in congestive heart failure. Am J Med 39:442, 1965.
87. Beregovich, J, et al.: Dose-related hemodynamic and renal effects of dopamine in congestive heart failure. Am Heart J 87:550, 1974.
88. Goldberg, LI: Dopamine–clinical uses of endogenous catecholamine. N Engl J Med 291:707, 1984.
89. Kenakin, TP: An in vitro quantitative analysis of the α adrenoceptor partial agonist activity of dobutamine and its relevance to inotropic selectivity. J Pharmacol Exp Ther 216:210, 1981.
90. Ruffolo, RR Jr, et al.: α- and β-adrenergic effects of the stereoisomers of dobutamine. J Pharmacol Exp Ther 219:447, 1981.
91. Kittleson, MD: Dobutamine. JAVMA 177:642, 1980.
92. Unverferth, DV, et al.: Tolerance to dobutamine after a 72 hour continuous infusion. Am J Med 69:262, 1980.
93. Unverferth, DV, et al.: The hemodynamic and metabolic advantages gained by a three-day infusion of dobutamine in patients with congestive cardiomyopathy. Am Heart J 106:29, 1983.
94. Liang, C, et al.: Sustained improvement of cardiac function in patients with congestive heart failure after short-term infusion of dobutamine. Circulation 69:113, 1984.
95. Kittleson, MD: Management of heart failure: Therapeutic strategies and drug pharmacology. *In* Fox PR (ed): Textbook of Canine and Feline Cardiology. New York, Churchill Livingstone, 1988, p 171.
96. Swedberg, K, et al.: Beneficial effects of long-term β-blockade in congestive cardiomyopathy. Br Heart J 44:117, 1980.
97. Waagstein, F, et al.: β-Blockers in dilated cardiomyopathies: They work. Europ Heart J 4:173, 1983.
98. Ikram, H and Fitzpatrick, MA: β blockade for dilated cardiomyopathy: The evidence against therapeutic benefit. Eur Heart J 4:179, 1983.
99. Swedberg, K, et al.: Adverse effects of β-blockade withdrawal in patients with congestive cardiomyopathy. Br Heart J 44:134, 1980.
100. Booth, HW, Jr, et al.: Cardiovascular effects of rapid infusion of crystalloid in the hypovolemic cat. J Small Anim Pract 26:477, 1985.
101. Vatner, SF, et al.: Effects of nitroglycerin on cardiac function and regional blood flow distribution in conscious dogs. Am J Physiol 234:H-244, 1978.
102. Smith, TW and Braunwald, E: The management of heart failure. *In* Braunwald E (ed): Heart Disease. Philadelphia, WB Saunders, 1984, p 503.
103. Captopril Multicenter Study Group: A placebo trial of captopril in refractory chronic congestive heart failure. J Am Coll Cardiol 2:755, 1983.
104. Levine, E, et al.: Acute and long-term response to an oral converting enzyme inhibitor, captopril, in congestive heart failure. Circulation 62:35, 1980.
105. Frazier, HS and Yager, H: Drug therapy: The clinical use of diuretics. N Engl J Med 288:246, 1973.
106. Erichsen, DF, et al.: Therapeutic and toxic plasma concentrations of digoxin in the cat. Am J Vet Res 41:2049, 1980.
107. Erichsen, DF, et al.: Plasma levels of digoxin in the cat: some clinical applications. JAAHA 14:734, 1978.
108. Bolton, GR and Powell, AA: Plasma kinetics of digoxin in the cat. Am J Vet Res 43:1994, 1982.
109. Fox, PR: Unpublished data.
110. Ralston, SL and Fox, PR: Dietary management, nutrition and the heart. *In* Fox PR (ed): Textbook of Canine and Feline Cardiology. New York, Churchill Livingstone, 1988, p 219.
111. Biddle, TL and Yu, PN: Effect of furosemide on hemodynamics and lung water in acute pulmonary edema secondary to myocardial infarction. Am J Cardiol 43:86, 1979.
112. Bourland, WA, et al.: The role of the kidney in the early nondiuretic action of furosemide to reduce elevated left atrial pressure in the hypervolemic dog. J Pharmacol Exp Ther 282:222, 1977.
113. Kittleson, MD, et al.: Efficacy of digoxin administration in dogs with idiopathic congestive cardiomyopathy. JAVMA 186:162, 1985.
114. Bonagura, JD and Ware, WA: Atrial fibrillation in the dog: Clinical findings in 81 cases. JAAHA 22:111, 1986.
115. Kittleson, ME: Drugs used in the management of heart failure. *In* Kirk RW (ed): Current Veterinary Therapy VIII. Philadelphia, WB Saunders, 1983, p 285.
116. Breznock, EM: Application of canine plasma kinetics of digoxin and digitoxin to therapeutic digitalization in the dog. Am J Vet Res 34:993, 1973.
117. Hamlin, RL: Basis for selection of a cardiac glycoside for dogs. Proc First Symp Vet Pharmacol Ther, 1978, p 241.
118. DeRick, A, et al.: Plasma concentrations of digoxin and digitoxin during digitalization of healthy dogs and dogs with cardiac failure. Am J Vet Res 39:811, 1978.
119. Rameis, H: Quinidine-digoxin interaction: are the pharmacokinetics of both drugs altered? Int J Clin Pharmacol Ther Toxicol 23:145, 1985.
120. Runge, TM: Clinical implications of differences in pharmacodynamic action of polar and nonpolar cardiac glycosides. Am Heart J 93:248, 1977.
121. Benotti, JR, et al.: Effects of amrinone on myocardial energy metabolism and hemodynamics in patients with severe heart failure. Circulation 62:29, 1980.
122. Franciosa, JA: Intravenous amrinone: an advance or a wrong step? Ann Intern Med 102:399, 1985.

123. A summary of laboratory and clinical data on Inocor (brand of amrinone). Sterling Winthrop Research Institute, Rensselaer, NY, 1980.
124. Alousi, AA, et al.: Cardiotonic activity of milrinone, a new and potent bipyridine, on the normal and failing heart of experimental animals. J Cardiovasc Pharmacol 5:792, 1983.
125. Kittleson, MD, et al.: Echocardiographic and clinical effects of milrinone in dogs with myocardial failure. Am J Vet Res 46:1659, 1985.
126. Kittleson, MD and Knowlen, GG: Positive inotropic drugs in heart failure. *In* Kirk RW (ed): Current Veterinary Therapy IX. Philadelphia, WB Saunders, 1986, p 323.
127. Weiland, DS, et al.: Contribution of reduced mitral regurgitant volume to vasodilator effect in severe left ventricular failure secondary to coronary artery disease or idiopathic dilated cardiomyopathy. Am J Cardiol 58:1046, 1986.
128. Haskins, SC: Shock (the pathophysiology and management of the circulatory collapse states). *In* Kirk RW (ed): Current Veterinary Therapy VIII. Philadelphia, WB Saunders, 1983, p 2.
129. Trautwein, W, et al.: Electrophysiologic study of human heart muscle. Circ Res 10:306, 1962.
130. Garber, EB, et al.: Left atrial size in patients with atrial fibrillation: an echocardiographic study. Am J Med Sci 272:57, 1976.
131. Pedersoli, WM: Serum digoxin concentrations in healthy dogs treated without a loading dose. J Vet Pharmacol Ther 1:279, 1978.
132. Wollam, GL, et al.: Diuretic potency of combined hydrochlorthiazide and furosemide therapy in patients with azotemia. Am J Med 72:929, 1982.
132a. Hamlin, RL: Clinical use of diltiazem for dogs in atrial fibrillation (Abstr 73). Proc 6th Annu ACVIM Forum, 1988, p 759.
133. Asbury, MJ, et al.: Bumetanide: Potent new "loop" diuretic. Br Med J 1:211, 1972.
134. Brater, DC, et al.: Bumetanide and furosemide. Clin Pharmacol Ther 34:207, 1983.
135. Bohn, FK, et al.: Atrial fibrillation in dogs. Br Vet J 127:485, 1971.
136. Thomas, RE: Atrial fibrillation in the dog: A review of eight cases. J Small Anim Pract 25:421, 1984.
137. Braunwald, E, et al.: Idiopathic hypertrophic subaortic stenosis. Arc 29/30:4, 1, 1964.
138. Sanderson, JE, et al.: Left ventricular filling in hypertrophic cardiomyopathy: an angiographic study. Br Heart J 39:661, 1977.
139. Panidis, IP, et al.: Development and regression of left ventricular hypertrophy. J Am Coll Cardiol 3:1309, 1984.
140. Ciro, E, et al.: Heterogeneous morphologic expression of genetically transmitted hypertrophic cardiomyopathy. Circulation 67:1227, 1983.
141. Maron, BJ and Mulvihill, JJ: The genetics of hypertrophic cardiomyopathy. Ann Intern Med 105:610, 1986.
142. Maron, BJ, et al.: Hypertrophic cardiomyopathy. Interrelations of clinical manifestations, pathophysiology and therapy. N Engl J Med 316:780, 1987.
143. Perloff, JK: Pathogenesis of hypertrophic cardiomyopathy: hypothesis and speculation. Am Heart J 101:219, 1981.
144. Goodwin, JF: Prospects and predictions for the cardiomyopathies. Circulation 50:210, 1974.
145. James, TN and Marshall, TK: De subitaneis mortibus. XII. Asymmetrical hypertrophy of the heart. Circulation 51:1149, 1975.
146. Stewart, S, et al.: Impaired rate of left ventricular filling in idiopathic subaortic stenosis and valvular aortic stenosis. Circulation 37:8, 1968.
147. Gaasch, WH, et al.: Left ventricular compliance: mechanisms and clinical implications. Am J Cardiol 38:645, 1976.
148. Hanrath, P, et al.: Left ventricular relaxation and filling pattern in different forms of left ventricular hypertrophy: an echocardiographic study. Am J Cardiol 45:15, 1980.
149. St. Johns, et al.: Histopathological specificity of hypertrophic obstructive cardiomyopathy; myocardial fibre disarray and myocardial fibrosis. Br Heart J 44:433, 1980.
150. Wigle, ED, et al.: Hypertrophic cardiomyopathy: the importance of the site and the extent of hypertrophy: a review. Prog Cardiovasc Dis 28:1, 1985.
151. Pouleur, H, et al.: Force-velocity-length relations in hypertrophic cardiomyopathy: evidence of normal or depressed myocardial contractility. Am J Cardiol 52:813, 1983.
152. Grose, R, et al.: Angiographic and hemodynamic correlations in hypertrophic cardiomyopathy with intracavitary systolic pressure gradients. Am J Cardiol 58:1085, 1986.
153. Thomas, WP, et al.: Hypertrophic obstructive cardiomyopathy in a dog: clinical, hemodynamic, angiographic and pathologic studies. JAAHA 20:253, 1984.
154. Swindle, MM, et al.: Mitral valve prolapse and hypertrophic cardiomyopathy in a pup. JAVMA 184:1515, 1984.
155. Liu, SK, et al.: Hypertrophic cardiomyopathy in the dog. Am J Pathol 94:497, 1979.
156. Liu, SK, et al.: Canine hypertrophic cardiomyopathy. JAVMA 174:708, 1979.
157. Maron, BJ, et al.: Spontaneously occurring hypertrophic cardiomyopathy in dogs and cats: A potential animal model of a human disease. *In* Kaltenbach M, Epstein SE (eds): Hypertrophic Cardiomyopathy. Berlin, Springer-Verlag, 1982, p 73.
158. Liu, SK, et al.: Feline hypertrophic cardiomyopathy: Gross anatomic and quantitative histologic features. Am J Path 102:388, 1981.
159. Van Vleet, J, et al.: Pathologic alterations in hypertrophic and congestive cardiomyopathy of cats. Am J Vet Res 41:2037, 1980.
160. Maron, BJ, et al.: Intramural ("small vessel") coronary artery disease in hypertrophic cardiomyopathy. J Am Coll Cardiol 8:545, 1986.
161. Fox, PR: Congenital feline heart diseases. *In* Fox PR (ed): Textbook of Canine and Feline Cardiology. New York, Churchill Livingstone, 1988.
162. Cowgill, LD and Kallet AJ: Systemic hypertension. *In* Kirk RW (ed): Current Veterinary Therapy IX. Philadelphia, WB Saunders, 1986, p 360.
163. Rush, JE, et al.: Retrospective study of pericardial disease in cats. Proc Fifth Annu Vet Med Forum. Am Coll Vet Intern Med (Abstr), 1987.
164. Savage, DD, et al.: Electrocardiographic findings in patients with obstructive and nonobstructive hypertrophic cardiomyopathy. Circulation 58:402, 1978.
165. Frank, S and Braunwald, E: Idiopathic hypertrophic subaortic stenosis: clinical analysis of 126 patients with emphasis on natural history. Circulation 37:759, 1968.
166. Maron, BJ, et al.: Hypertrophic cardiomyopathy. Interrelations of clinical manifestations, pathophysiology, and therapy. N Engl J Med 316:844, 1987.
167. Benotti, JR, et al.: Clinical profile of restrictive cardiomyopathy. Circulation 61:1206, 1980.
168. Chew, CYC, et al.: Primary restrictive cardiomyopathy: Nontropical endomyocardial fibrosis and hypereosinophilic heart disease. Br Heart J 39:399, 1977.
169. Liu, SK: Myocarditis and cardiomyopathy in the dog and cat. Heart Vessels 1 (Suppl 1):122, 1985.
170. Liu, SK: Cardiovascular pathology. *In* Fox PR (ed): Textbook of Canine and Feline Cardiology. New York, Churchill Livingstone, 1988, p 641.
171. Cohen, LS and Braunwald, E: Amelioration of angina pectoris in idiopathic hypertrophic subaortic stenosis with β-adrenergic blockade. Circulation 35:847, 1967.
172. Thompson, DS, et al.: Effects of propranolol on myocardial oxygen consumption, substrate extraction and haemodynamics in hypertrophic obstructive cardiomyopathy. Br Heart J 44:488, 1980.
173. Flamm, MD, et al.: Muscular subaortic stenosis: prevention of outflow obstruction with propranolol. Circulation 38:846, 1968.
174. Hess, OM, et al.: Diastolic function in hypertrophic cardiomyopathy: effects of propranolol and verapamil on diastolic stiffness. Eur Heart J 4:47, 1983.
175. Rosing, DR, et al.: Use of calcium-channel blocking drugs in hypertrophic cardiomyopathy. Am J Cardiol 55:185, 1985.
176. Bonow, RO, et al.: Verapamil-induced improvement in left ventricular diastolic filling and increased exercise tolerance in patients with hypertrophic cardiomyopathy: short- and long-term effects. Circulation 72:853, 1985.
176a. Fox, PR: Unpublished data, 1988.
176b. Bright, JM, and Golden, L: The use of calcium channel blockers in cats with hypertrophic cardiomyopathy. Proc 6th Annu ACVIM Forum, 1988, p 184.
177. Truex, RC and Warshow, LJ: The incidence and size of the moderator band in man and in mammals. Anat Rec 82:361, 1942.

178. Miller, ME, et al.: Anatomy of the Dog, 2nd ed. Philadelphia, WB Saunders, 1964, p 641.
179. Turner, Sir W: A human heart with moderator bands in the left ventricle. J Anat Physiol 27:19, 1893.
180. Sandusky, GE and White, SL: Scanning electron microscopy of the canine atrioventricular bundle and moderator band. Am J Vet Res 46:249, 1985.
181. Roberts, WC: Anomalous left ventricular band: an unemphasized cause of a precordial musical murmur. Am J Cardiol 23:735, 1969.
182. Michihiro, S, et al.: Incidence of the coexitence of left ventricular false tendons and premature ventricular contractions in apparently healthy subjects. Circulation 70:793, 1984.
183. Choo, MH, et al.: Anomalous chordae tendineae: a source of echocardiographic confusion. Angiology 33:756, 1982.
184. Feigenbaum, H: Echocardiography, 4th ed. Philadelphia, Lea & Febiger, 1986.
185. Flanders, J: Feline aortic thromboembolism. Compend Cont Ed 8:473, 1986.
186. Furster, V and Chesebro, JH: Antithrombotic therapy: Role of platelet-inhibitor drugs. I. Current Concepts of thrombogenesis: Role of platelets. Mayo Clin Proc 56:102, 1981.
187. Hirsch, J: Hypercoagulability. Semin Hematol 14:409, 1977.
188. Edwards, WD: Aneurysms and mural thrombi of the left ventricle. Mayo Clin Proc 56:129, 1981.
189. Weiser, MG and Kociba, GJ: Platelet concentration and platelet volume distribution in healthy cats. Am J Vet Res 45:518, 1984.
190. Dodds, WJ: Platelet function in animals: species specificities. *In* de Gaetano G, Garattini S (eds): Platelets: A Multidisciplinary Approach. Raven Press, New York, 1978, p 45.
191. Imhoff, RK: Production of aortic occlusion resembling acute aortic embolism syndrome in cats. Nature 192:979, 1961.
192. Schaub, RG, et al.: Inhibition of feline collateral vessel development following experimental thrombolic occlusion. Circ Res 39:736, 1976.
193. Schaub, RG, et al.: Serotonin as a factor in depression of collateral blood flow following experimental arterial thrombosis. J Lab Clin Med 90:645, 1977.
194. Grygleski, RJ: Prostaglandins, platelets and atherosclerosis. CRC Crit Rev Biochem 7:291, 1980.
195. Schaub, RG, et al.: Effect of aspirin on collateral blood flow after experimental thrombosis of the feline aorta. Am J Vet Res 43:1647, 1982.
196. Griffiths, IR and Duncan, ID: Ischaemic neuromyopathy in cats. Vet Rec 104:518, 1979.
197. Allen, DG, et al.: Effects of aspirin and propranolol alone and in combination on hemostatic determinants in the healthy cat. Am J Vet Res 46:660, 1985.
198. Buchanan, JW, et al.: Aortic embolism in cats: prevalence, surgical treatment and electrocardiography. Vet Rec 79:496, 1966.
199. Schneeweiss, A: Drug Therapy in Cardiovascular Diseases. Philadelphia, Lea & Febiger, 1986, p 52.
200. Freis, ED: Changing attitudes to hypertension. Ann Intern Med 78:141, 1973.
201. Oblad, B: A study of the mechanism of the hemodynamic effects of hydralazine in man. Acta Pharmacol Toxicol 20:1, 1963.
202. Killingsworth, CR, et al.: Streptokinase treatment of cats with experimentally induced aortic thrombosis. Am J Vet Res 47:1351, 1986.
203. Kaplan, AP, et al.: Molecular mechanisms of fibrinolysis in man. Thromb Haemost 39:263, 1978.
204. Sherry, S: Tissue plasminogen activator (t-PA). New Engl J Med 313:1014, 1985.
205. Rosenberg, RD and Lam, L: Correlation between structure and function of heparin. Proc Natl Acad Sci USA 76:1218, 1979.
206. Bell, RW: Metabolism of Vitamin K and prothrombin synthesis: anticoagulants and the vitamin K-epoxide cycle. Fed Proc 37:2599, 1978.
207. Roth, GJ, et al.: Acetylation of prostaglandin synthesis by aspirin. Proc Natl Acad Sci USA 72:3073, 1975.
208. Hamberg, M, et al.: Thromboxanes: A new group of biologically active compounds derived from prostaglandin endoperoxides. Proc Natl Acad Sci USA 72:299, 1975.
209. Greene, CE: Aspirin and feline platelet aggregation. JAVMA 188:1820, 1985.
210. Preston, FE, et al.: Inhibition of prostacyclin and platelet thromboxane A2 after low dose aspirin. N Engl J Med 304:76, 1981.
211. Moncada, S, et al.: An enzyme isolated from arteries transforms prostaglandin endoperoxides to an unstable substance that inhibits platelet aggregation. Nature 263:663, 1976.
212. Armstrong, JM, et al.: Comparison of the vasopressor effects of prostacyclin and 6-oxoprostaglandin Fl-α with those of prostaglandin E2 in rats and rabbits. Br J Pharmacol 62:125, 1978.
213. Peterson, ME, et al: Feline hyperthyroidism: pretreatment clinical and laboratory evaluation of 131 cases. JAVMA 183:103, 1983.
214. Hoenig, M, et al.: Toxic nodular goiter in the cat. J Small Anim Pract 23:1, 1982.
215. Peterson, ME: Feline hyperthyroidism. Vet Clin North Am 14:809, 1984.
216. Peterson, ME and Turrel, JM: Feline hyperthyroidism. *In* Kirk RW (ed): Current Veterinary Therapy IX. Philadelphia, WB Saunders, 1986, p 1026.
217. Loar, AS: Canine thyroid tumors. *In* Kirk RW (ed): Current Veterinary Therapy IX. Philadelphia, WB Saunders, 1986, p 1033.
218. Ingbar, SH and Woeber, KA: The thyroid gland. *In* Williams RH (ed): Textbook of Endocrinology, 6th ed. Philadelphia, WB Saunders, 1981, p 117.
219. Klein, I and Levey, GS: New perspectives on thyroid hormone, catecholamines, and the heart. Am J Med 76:167, 1984.
220. Forfar, JC and Caldwall, GC: Hyperthyroid heart disease. Clin Endocrinol Metab 14:491, 1985.
221. Grossman, W, Braunwald, E: High cardiac output states. *In* Braunwald E (ed): Heart Disease, 2nd ed. Philadelphia, WB Saunders, 1984, p 807.
222. Bond, BR: Hyperthyroid heart disease in cats. *In* Kirk RW (ed): Current Veterinary Therapy IX. Philadelphia, WB Saunders, 1986, p 399.
223. Bond, BR: Hyperthyroidism and other high cardiac output states. *In* Fox PR (ed): Textbook of Canine and Feline Cardiology. New York, Churchill Livingstone, 1988, p 255.
224. Jacobs, G, et al.: Congestive heart failure associated with hyperthyroidism in cats. JAVMA 188:52, 1986.
225. Moise, NS, et al.: Echocardiography, electrocardiography, and radiography of cats with dilatation cardiomyopathy, hypertrophic cardiomyopathy and hyperthyroidism. Am J Vet Res 47:1476, 1986.
226. Moise, NS and Dietze, AE: Echocardiographic, electrocardiographic, and radiographic detection of cardiomegaly in hyperthyroid cats. Am J Res 47:1487, 1986.
227. Peterson, ME, et al.: Electrocardiographic findings in 45 cats with hyperthyroidism. JAVMA 180:934, 1982.
228. Bond, BR, et al.: Echocardiographic findings in 103 cats with hyperthyroidism. JAVMA 192:1546, 1988.
229. Bond, BR, et al.: Echocardiographic evaluation of 45 cats with hyperthyroidism. J Ultrasound Med Suppl 2:184, 1983.
230. Peterson, ME, et al.: Propylthiouracil-associated hemolytic anemia, thrombocytopenia and antinuclear antibodies in cats with hyperthyroidism. JAVMA 184:806, 1984.
231. Birchard, SJ, et al.: Surgical treatment of feline hyperthyroidism: results of 85 cases. JAAHA 20:705, 1984.
232. Meric, SM, et al.: Serum thyroxine concentrations after radioactive iodine therapy in cats with hyperthyroidism. JAVMA 188:1038, 1986.
233. Rijnberk, A: Iodine metabolism and thyroid disease in the dog. Utrecht, The Netherlands, Drukkerij Elinkwijk, 1971.
234. Belshaw, BE: Thyroid diseases. *In* Ettinger SJ (ed): Textbook of Veterinary Internal Medicine, 2nd ed. Philadelphia, WB Saunders, 1983, p 1592.
235. Rijnberk, A and Leav, I: Thyroid tumors. *In* Kirk RW (ed): Current Veterinary Therapy VI. Philadelphia, WB Saunders, 1977, p 1020.
236. Van Vleet, JF, et al.: Cardiac disease induced by chronic Adriamycin administration in dogs and an evaluation of vitamin E and selenium as cardioprotectants. Am J Pathol 99:13, 1980.
237. Loar, AS and Susaneck, SJ: Doxorubicin-induced cardiotoxicity in five dogs. Semin Vet Med Surg 1:68, 1986.
238. Kehoe, R, et al.: Adriamycin-induced cardiac dysrhythmias in an experimental dog model. Cancer Treat Rep 62:963, 1978.
239. Mauldin, N, et al.: Efficacy and toxicity of doxorubicin and cyclophosphamide used in the treatment of selected malignant tumors in 23 cats. JVIM 2:60, 1988.

240. Jeglum, KA, et al.: Chemotherapy of advanced mammary adenocarcinoma in 14 cats. JAVMA 187:157, 1985.
241. Cotter, SM, et al.: Renal disease in five tumor-bearing cats treated with Adriamycin. JAAHA 21:405, 1985.
242. Alpert, JS and Braunwald, E: Acute myocardial infarction: Pathological, pathophysiological and clinical manifestations. *In* Braunwald E (ed): Heart Disease. Philadelphia, WB Saunders, 1984, p 1262.
243. Nielson, SW and Nielson, LB: Coronary embolism in valvular bacterial endocarditis in two dogs. JAVMA 125:376, 1954.
244. Sisson, D and Thomas, WP: Endocarditis of the aortic valve in the dog. JAVMA 184:570, 1984.
245. Detweiler, DK, et al.: The natural history of acquired cardiac disability of the dog. Ann NY Acad Sci 147:318, 1968.
246. Johnsson, L: Coronary arterial lesions and myocardial infarcts in the dog. A pathologic and microangiopathic study. Acta Vet Scand Suppl 38:1, 1972.
247. King, JM, et al.: Myocardial necrosis secondary to neural lesions in domestic animals. JAVMA 180:144, 1982.
248. Muir, WW and Weisbrode, SE: Myocardial ischemia in dogs with gastric dilatation-volvulus. JAVMA 181:363, 1982.
249. Van Vleet, PD, et al.: Focal myocarditis associated with pheochromocytomas. N Engl J Med 274:1102, 1966.
250. Bourdios, PS, et al.: The sub-acute toxicology of digoxin in dogs: clinical chemistry and histopathology of heart and kidneys. Arch Toxicol 51:273, 1982.
251. Liu, SK, et al.: Clinical and pathologic findings in dogs with atherosclerosis: 21 cases (1970-1983). JAVMA 189:227, 1986.
252. Colucci, WS and Braunwald, E: Primary tumors of the heart. *In* Braunwald E (ed): Heart Disease. Philadelphia, WB Saunders, 1984, p 1457.
253. Fox, PR and Nichols, R: Cardiovascular involvement with systemic and metabolic diseases. *In* Fox PR (ed): Textbook of Canine and Feline Cardiology. New York, Churchill Livingstone, 1988, p. 565.
254. Tilley, LP, et al.: Cardiovascular tumors in the cat. JAAHA 17:1009, 1981.
255. Brown, NO, et al.: Canine hemangiosarcoma. JAVMA 186:56, 1985.
256. Pearson, CR and Head, KW: Malignant hemangioendothelioma (angiosarcoma) in the dog. J Small Anim Pract 17:737, 1976.
257. Klein, LJ, et al.: Primary cardiac hemangiosarcoma in dogs. JAVMA 157:326, 1970.
258. Aronsohn, M: Cardiac hemangiosarcoma in the dog: A review of 38 cases. JAVMA 187:922, 1985.
259. Patnaik, AK and Liu, SK: Angiosarcomas in cats. J Small Anim Pract 18:191, 1977.
260. Patnaik, AK, et al.: Canine chemodectoma (extra-adrenal paragangliomas)—a comparative study. J Small Anim Pract 16:785, 1975.
261. Patnaik, AK: Personal communication, 1987.
262. Wenger, NK, et al.: Myocarditis. *In* Hurst JW (ed): The Heart, 6th ed. New York, McGraw-Hill Book, 1985, p 1158.
263. Hayes, MA, et al.: Sudden death in young dogs with myocarditis caused by parvovirus. JAVMA 174:1197, 1979.
264. Jezyk, PF, et al.: Myocarditis of probable viral origin in pups of weaning age. JAVMA 174:1204, 1979.
265. Carpenter, JL, et al.: Intestinal and cardiopulmonary forms of parvovirus infection in a litter of pups. JAVMA 176:1269, 1980.
266. Robinsin, WF, et al.: Canine parvoviral myocarditis: A morphologic description of the natural disease. Vet Pathol 17:282, 1980.
267. Lenghans, C and Studdert, MJ: Generalized parvovirus disease in neonatal pups. JAVMA 181:41, 1982.
268. Kramer, JM, et al.: Canine parvovirus: Update. VM/SAC 75:1541, 1980.
269. Atwell, RB and Kelly, WR: Canine parvovirus: a cause of chronic myocardial fibrosis and adolescent congestive heart failure. J Small Anim Pract 21:609, 1980.
270. Lenghaus, C and Studdert, MJ: Animal model of human disease: acute and chronic viral myocarditis; acute diffuse nonsuppurative myocarditis and residual myocardial scarring following infection with canine parvovirus. Am J Pathol 115:316, 1984.
271. Lenghaus, C, et al.: Acute and chronic canine parvovirus myocarditis following intrauterine inoculation. Aust Vet J 56:465, 1980.
272. Ilgen, BE and Conroy, JD: Fatal cardiomyopathy in an adult dog resembling parvovirus-induced myocarditis: A case report. JAVMA 18:613, 1982.
273. Higgens, RJ, et al.: Canine distemper virus-associated cardiac necrosis in the dog. Vet Pathol 18:472, 1981.
274. Hashimoto, A, et al.: Experimental transplacental transmission of canine herpes virus in pregnant bitches during the second trimester of gestation. Am J Vet Res 44:610, 1983.
275. Williams, GD, et al.: Naturally occurring trypanosomiasis (Chagas' disease) in dogs. JAVMA 171:171, 1977.
276. Tomlinson, MJ, et al.: Occurrence of antibody to *Trypanosoma cruzi* in dogs in the southeastern United States. Am J Vet Res 42:1444, 1981.
277. Tippit, TS: Canine trypanosomiasis. Southwest Vet 31:97, 1978.
278. Snider, TG, III: Myocarditis caused by *Trypanosoma cruzi* in a native Louisiana dog. JAVMA 173:247, 1980.
279. Woody, NC and Woody, HB: American trypanosomiasis. I. Clinical and epidemiologic background of Chagas' disease in the United States. J Pediatr 58:568, 1961.
280. Andrade, ZA, et al.: Damage and healing in the conducting tissue of the heart (an experimental study in dogs infected with *Trypanosoma cruzi*). J Pathol 143:93, 1984.
281. Jacobson, RH: Toxoplasmosis - Feline infections and their zoonotic potential. *In* Kirk RW (ed): Current Veterinary Therapy VII. Philadelphia, WB Saunders, 1980, p 1307.
282. Dubey, JP and Johnstone, I: Fatal neonatal toxoplasmosis in cats. JAAHA 18:461, 1982.
283. McCully, RM, et al.: Observations on naturally acquired hepatozoonosis of wild carnivores and dogs in the Republic of South Africa. Onderstepoort J Vet Res 42:117, 1975.
284. Craig, TM, et al.: Diagnosis of *Hepatozoon canis* by muscle biopsy. JAAHA 20:301, 1984.
285. Craig, TM, et al.: *Hepatozoon canis* infection in dogs: clinical, radiographic and hematologic findings. JAVMA 173:967, 1978.
286. Nobel, TA, et al.: Histopathology of the myocardium in 50 apparently healthy cats. Lab Anim 8:119, 1974.
287. Ewing, GO: Granulomatous cholangiohepatitis in a cat due to a protozoan parasite resembling *Hepatozoon canis*. Feline Pract 7:37, 1977.
288. Calvert, CA: Endocarditis and bacteremia. *In* Fox PR: Textbook of Canine and Feline Cardiology. New York, Churchill Livingstone, 1988.
289. Edwards, NJ and Rebhum, WC: Generalized cryptococcosis: A case report. JAAHA 15:439, 1979.
290. Maddy, KT: Disseminated coccidioidomycosis of the dog. JAVMA 132:483, 1958.
291. Reed, RE: Diagnosis of disseminated canine coccidioidomycosis. JAVMA 128:196, 1956.
292. Wood, GH, et al.: Disseminated aspergillosis in a dog. JAVMA 172:704, 1978.
293. Mullaney, TP, et al.: Disseminated aspergillosis in a dog. JAVMA 182:516, 1983.
294. Patnaik, AK, et al.: Paecilomycosis in a dog. JAVMA 161:806, 1972.
295. Tyler, DE, et al.: Disseminated protothecosis with central nervous system involvement in a dog. JAVMA 176:987, 1980.
296. Moor, FM, et al.: Unsuccessful treatment of disseminated protothecosis in a dog. JAVMA 186:705, 1985.
297. Gaunt, SD, et al.: Disseminated protothecosis in a dog. JAVMA 8:906, 1984.
298. Merideth, RE, et al.: Systemic protothecosis with ocular manifestations in a dog. JAAHA 20:153, 1984.
299. Jeraj, K, et al.: Atrial standstill, myocarditis and destruction of cardiac conduction system: clinicopathologic correlation in a dog. Am Heart J 99:185, 1980.
300. Tilley, LP and Liu, SK: Persistent atrial standstill in the dog and cat. Proc Am Coll Vet Intern Med (Abstr), 1983, p 43.
301. Tilley, LP: Essentials of Canine and Feline Electrocardiography, 2nd ed. Philadelphia, Lea & Febiger, 1985.
302. Schollmeyer: Pacemaker therapy. *In* Fox PR (ed): Textbook of Canine and Feline Cardiology. New York, Churchill Livingstone, 1988, p 625.
303. Walvoort, HC, et al.: Canine glycogen storage disease type II: a clinical study of four affected Lapland dogs. JAAHA 20:279, 1984.
304. Mostafa, IE: A case of glycogenic cardiomegaly in a dog. Acta Vet Scand 11:197, 1970.
305. Haskins, ME, et al.: Mucopolysaccharidosis in a domestic shorthaired cat: A disease distinct from that seen in the Siamese cat. JAVMA 175:384, 1979.
306. Haskins, ME, et al.: The pathology of feline arylsulfatase B deficient mucopolysaccharidosis. Am J Pathol 101:657, 1980.

307. Renteria, VG, et al.: The heart in the Hurler syndrome: Gross, histologic and ultrastructural observations in five necropsy cases. Am J Cardiol 38:487, 1976.
308. James, TN, et al.: Hereditary stenosis of the His bundle in pug dogs. Circulation 52:1152, 1975.
309. James, TN and Drake, EA: Sudden death in Doberman pinschers. Ann Intern Med 68:821, 1968.
310. Meierhenry, EF and Liu, SK: Atrioventricular bundle degeneration associated with sudden death in the dog. JAVMA 172:1418, 1978.

DRUG INDEX

Drug	Use	Canine	Feline
Positive Inotropic Agents			
Amrinone (Inocor)	Short-term inotropic support	0.5–1.5 mg/lb IV bolus 5–50 mcg/lb min CRI	
Digoxin (Lanoxin)	Life-threatening supraventricular arrhythmias	Rapid IV: 0.005 to 0.01 mg/lb divided in 2–4 doses	Rapid IV: 0.002 mg/lb IV divided (half initially, then ¼ of total calculated dose at ½ to 1 hr intervals)
	Maintenance inotropic support	Maintenance (oral) 0.005–0.007 mg/lb PO q12h (max, 0.75 mg divided)	Maintenance (oral): 4–7 lb 0.015 mg (i.e., ¼ of 0.062 mg tab) q48–72h; 7–13 lb—0.015 mg q24–48h; 13+ lb—0.015 mg q12–24h
Digitoxin (Crystodigin)	Maintenance inotropic support	0.02 to 0.04 mg/lb divided q8–12h	
Dobutamine (Dobutrex)	Short-term inotropic support	1–5 mcg/lb/min IV CRI	1–5 mcg/lb/min IV CRI
Dopamine (Intropin)	Same	1–2.5 mg/lb/min IV CRI	1–2.5 mcg/lb/min IV CRI
Milrinone (experimental)	Maintenance inotropic support	0.25–0.5 mg/lb q12h PO	
Diuretics	Reduce congestion, effusions		
Furosemide (Laxis)		1.1–2.2 mg/lb IV PO, IM q6-12h	0.5 to 2.2 mg/lb IV, IM, PO q8–24h
Hydrochlorthiazide-spironolactone (Aldactazide)			1.1 to 2.2 mg/lb PO, q12h
Hydrochlorthiazide (Hydrodiuril)		1–2 mg/lb PO q12h	1 to 2 mg/lb PO q12h
Spironolactone (Aldactone)		1–2 mg/lb PO daily	
Triamterene (Dyrenium)		1–2 mg/lb PO daily	
Vasodilators	Ventricular unloading		
Captopril (Capoten)	Balanced vasodilator	0.25–0.5 mg/lb PO q8–12h	0.25 to 0.75 mg PO q8-24h
Hydralazine (Apresoline)	Arterial dilation	0.5–1 mg/lb q12h	0.25 to 0.4 mg/lb q12h
Prazosin (Minipress)	Balanced vasodilator	0.5–1 mg PO q8–12h	
2% nitroglycerin ointment (Nitro-Bid)	Venous vasodilator	¼ to 1 inch cutaneously q4–6h	⅛ inch cutaneously q4–6h
Isosorbide dinitrate (Isordril)	Venous vasodilator	0.25 to 1.0 mg/lb PO q18–12h	
Beta-adrenergic Blockers	Slow ventricular rate Protect against catecholamine-induced arrhythmias Promote diastolic compliance		
Propranolol (Inderal)	Same	0.1–0.5 mg/lb PO q8h	1.25–2.5 mg PO q8-12h
Atenolol (Tenormin)	Same Cardioselective	0.25–0.5 mg/lb PO q12-24h	
Nadolol (Corgard)	Same	0.12–0.2 mg/lb PO q12h	
Metoprolol (Lopressor)	Same Cardioselective	12.5–25 mg PO q8–12h	
Ventricular Antiarrhythmics	Control ventricular arrhythmias		
Lidocaine (Xylocaine)		1–2 mg/lb IV bolus (max, 4 mg/lb) over 10 min; 12.5–37.5 mcg/lb IV CRI	0.12–0.5 mg/lb IV over 10 minutes
Procainamide (Pronestyl, Procan)		3–4 mg/lb IV over 5 min. (beware of hypotension); 4 to 10 mg/lb PO, IM q6–8h	
Quinidine (Quiniglute Duratabs, Cardioquin)		3–10 mg/lb q6h IM (gluconate) or PO (many preparations)	
Propranolol (Inderal)		0.01–0.03 mg/lb IV slowly; 0.01–0.5 mg/lb PO q8h	1.25–2.5 mg/lb PO q8–12h
Tocainide (Tonocard)		12.5 mg/lb PO q6h	

78 PERICARDIAL DISORDERS

WILLIAM P. THOMAS

Cardiac diseases primarily affecting the pericardium constitute a relatively small but distinctive percentage of the clinically important cardiovascular diseases of dogs.[1-5] Although much less prevalent than acquired valvular and myocardial diseases, pericardial disease, especially pericardial effusion, is one of the most common causes of right heart failure in dogs.[2] In contrast, all types of pericardial disease are considered very uncommon in cats.[6-11] Although pericardial disorders are sometimes misdiagnosed as other cardiac and extracardiac diseases, the combined findings from physical examination and routine diagnostic tests are usually sufficiently characteristic to allow a presumptive or definitive diagnosis to be made, particularly as echocardiography has become more commonly used in veterinary cardiology. Because the signs of pericardial disease can vary from subclinical to life-threatening, and because the pathophysiology and treatment of these conditions are very different from those of most other common cardiac disorders, it is important for veterinary clinicians to understand their principal clinical manifestations and the role of various diagnostic examinations in their recognition, evaluation, and treatment.

PERICARDIAL ANATOMY AND NORMAL FUNCTION

The pericardium is a thin, translucent serofibrous membrane that "double-envelopes" the heart and the proximal portions of the great vessels as a thin, serous visceral pericardium (epicardium) tightly adherent to the surface of the myocardium, and a thicker, serofibrous parietal pericardium (the pericardial sac). The fibrous portion of the parietal pericardium blends into the adventitia of the great vessels, while the double serous layer encloses a potential pericardial space containing up to 15 ml (mean, 1 to 2.5 ml) of clear, lymph-like serous fluid in the dog.[12] While the pericardium is clearly not essential for life, it serves several physical functions, including (1) a ligamentous function, stabilizing the heart in an optimum functional position; (2) a membrane function, lubricating and protecting the beating heart against external friction and inflammation from the contiguous pleura and lung; and (3) a mechanical function, maintaining optimum functional cardiac geometry, balancing transmural pressure, ventricular compliance, and left and right ventricular outputs, and limiting acute ventricular dilatation.[12, 13]

Although a large number of specific local or systemic disorders can affect the pericardium, it is diagnostically useful to group these conditions according to their primary effect on the pericardium, since this determines the physiologic consequences and clinical manifestations that allow their recognition. On this basis, the acquired pericardial diseases can be classified as causing pericardial effusion, pericardial fibrosis, or space-occupying pericardial masses. During the following discussion of these major classes, it should be understood that they often coexist (e.g., pericardial fibrosis with effusion, pericardial mass with effusion or fibrosis).

Reported causes of pericardial disease in dogs[14-19] and cats[11, 17, 20, 21] are listed in Table 78–1. More complete lists of conditions known to cause pericardial disease in humans (and potentially in animals) can be found in the references.[22-24]

PATHOPHYSIOLOGY OF PERICARDIAL DISEASE

The effects of pericardial disease on the circulation result mainly from compression (restriction) of the ventricles. Unlike most other types of cardiac disease, which cause impairment of systolic ventricular function by reducing ventricular contractility primarily (dilated cardiomyopathy) or secondarily (acute or chronic pressure or volume overload states), in most cases pericardial disease does not significantly affect ventricular contractility and the systolic pumping ability of the heart. Instead, because of the contribution of the pericardium to diastolic ventricular compliance and its relative nondistensibility, the most important hemodynamic effect of pericardial disease is to decrease diastolic ventricular compliance, impair ventricular filling, and thereby limit diastolic ventricular volume and cardiac output, despite markedly elevated diastolic ventricular, atrial, and venous pressures.[25-27]

TABLE 78–1. PERICARDIAL DISEASES OF THE DOG AND CAT

Congenital Disorders
Pericardial defects
Peritoneopericardial hernia
Pericardial cyst (?)
Acquired Disorders
Pericardial effusion
Transudate (hydropericardium)
Congestive heart failure
Hypoalbuminemia
Peritoneopericardial hernia
Exudate (pericarditis)
Infection–bacterial, fungal
Sterile–idiopathic, uremia, other infectious diseases (FIP), other (?)
Hemorrhage (hemopericardium)
Neoplasia–hemangiosarcoma, heart base tumor, mesothelioma, lymphosarcoma, other
Trauma–iatrogenic, external
Cardiac rupture, especially left atrium
Idiopathic (pericarditis)
Constrictive pericarditis
Idiopathic pericarditis
Infection–bacterial (actinomycosis, nocardiosis, tuberculosis), fungal (coccidioidomycosis)
Pericardial foreign body (metal)
Neoplasia–heart base tumor, mesothelioma
Intrapericardiac masses (± effusion/fibrosis)
Pericardial cyst
Neoplasm
Granuloma–actinomycosis, coccidioidomycosis
Pericardial abscess

PERICARDIAL EFFUSION WITH TAMPONADE

The normal pericardium provides little resistance to ventricular diastolic expansion unless the ventricles are dilated.[12] If ventricular compliance is normal and pericardial pressure is low, normal transmural pressure and ventricular filling occur at low atrial and ventricular diastolic (filling) pressures. When pericardial fluid accumulates and raises pericardial pressure above atmospheric pressure, the transmural pressure gradient and ventricular filling require elevated atrial and ventricular diastolic pressures. As pericardial pressure continues to rise, increasing venous pressure results in systemic congestion and edema (ascites, pleural effusion) and stroke volume is reduced (cardiac tamponade is present), resulting in signs of fatigue, weakness, azotemia, and diminished arterial pulses. Because of equal pressure on both ventricles, ventricular, atrial, pulmonary, and systemic venous diastolic pressures equilibrate with pericardial pressure (Figure 78–1*A*). However, the thinner right ventricle is more susceptible to compression than the thicker left ventricle, resulting in signs mainly of right heart failure, with the left heart and lungs protected from developing pulmonary edema by diminished right heart output.[25–27]

The clinical signs of cardiac tamponade depend on the rate of fluid accumulation and the severity of the resulting cardiac compression. The parietal pericardium is capable of limited acute stretching, allowing accumulation of a small volume of pericardial fluid with little increase in pericardial pressure. As its elastic limit is reached, however, addition of a small additional fluid volume causes a large increase in pericardial pressure and cardiac compression. In the dog, a rapidly developing effusion of only 50 to 100 ml (e.g., left atrial perforation) can cause severe cardiac tamponade, decreased cardiac output, cardiogenic shock without signs of congestive heart failure, and death. If the effusion develops gradually, however, the pericardium can stretch to accommodate 1000 ml or more before signs of cardiac tamponade develop. In this case, systemic compensatory mechanisms increase plasma volume and venous pressure, support blood pressure and cardiac output, and allow development of signs of congestive heart failure rather than shock. The severity of signs in each case is therefore not directly related to the quantity of pericardial fluid, which is determined by the rate of fluid accumulation and the compliance of the pericardium. Pericardial fibrosis limits its ability to stretch, allowing cardiac tamponade to occur with a smaller volume of effusion.

PERICARDIAL FIBROSIS WITH CONSTRICTION

The pathophysiology of constrictive pericarditis is similar to cardiac tamponade in that the main effect is limitation of diastolic ventricular volume, elevation of ventricular, atrial, and venous diastolic pressures, and development of signs of congestive heart failure.[25, 26] Since this process takes time, patients develop signs of right heart failure rather than cardiogenic shock. The pericardium may be greatly thickened in infective pericarditis, or may be only 1 to 2 mm thick in idiopathic cases. The hemodynamics of pericardial constriction differ from cardiac tamponade mainly by a more prominent early diastolic (y) descent. This occurs because the fibrous pericardial shell allows relatively normal, rapid, early diastolic ventricular filling to occur. However, its elastic limit is reached in early diastole, terminating ventricular filling and causing a rapid rise in diastolic ventricular and atrial pressures to a plateau (Figure 78–1*B*). The abrupt end of the rapid filling period may be accompanied by an early diastolic sound ("pericardial knock") analogous to the third heart sound. In pericardial effusion with tamponade, resistance to ventricular filling occurs throughout diastole, resulting in more gradual filling, a less prominent y descent (Figure 78–1*A*), and absence of a pericardial knock. In both cases, however, systemic and pulmonary venous pressures are usually greatly elevated.

In constrictive pericarditis it is important to understand the "bilayered" nature of the pericardium. Since either or both of the parietal and visceral (epicardial) layers may be affected, surgical treatment may require either only simple parietal pericardiectomy or more complicated epicardial stripping to obtain hemodynamic and symptomatic relief.

INTRAPERICARDIAC MASSES

The hemodynamic effects and clinical signs of an intrapericardiac mass are influenced by its nature and etiology (e.g., infection, neoplasia), the size and location of the lesion, and the presence of accompanying pericardial effusion and/or fibrosis. Small masses (e.g., heart base tumors) may be clinically silent. Larger masses

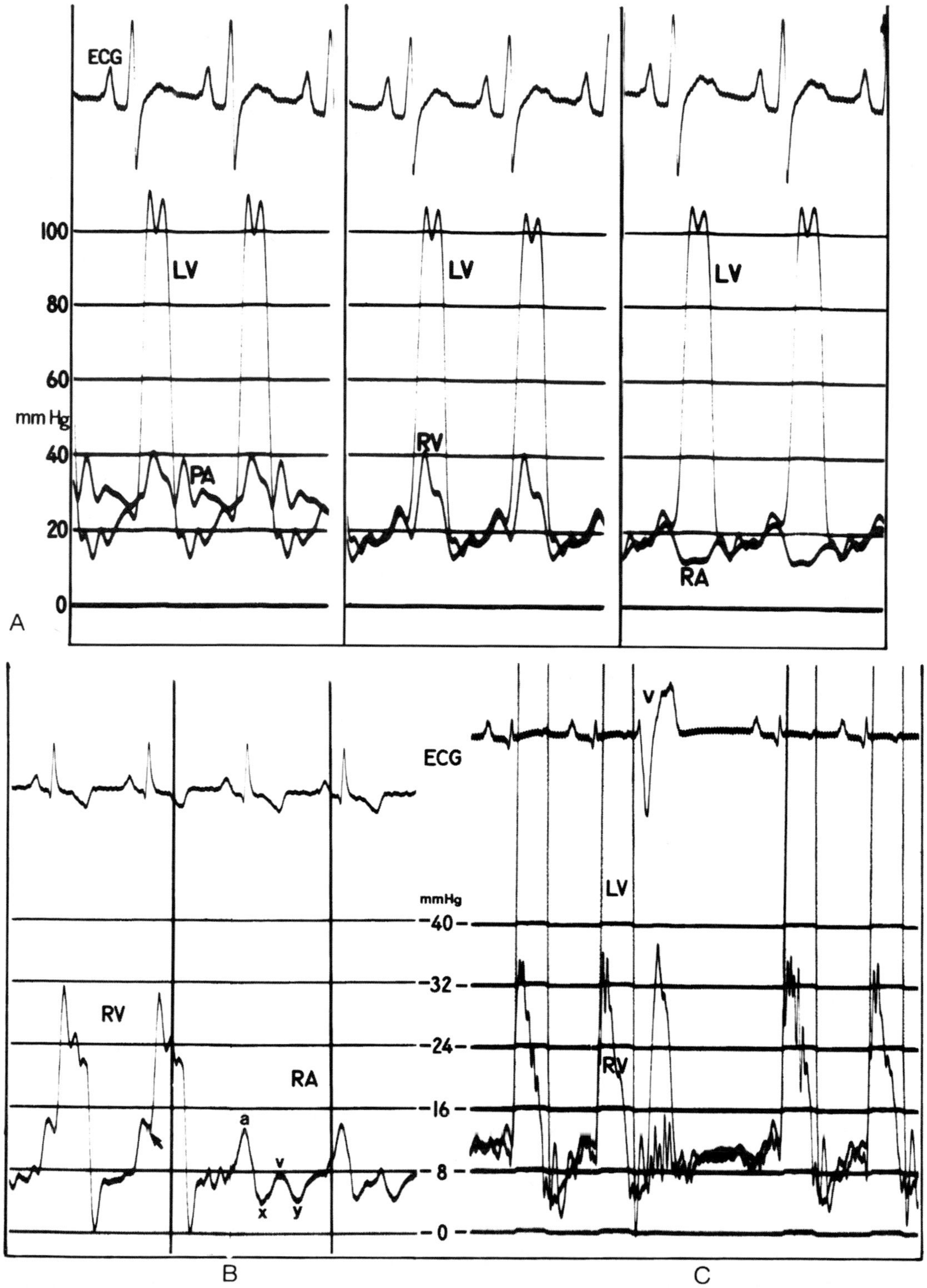

FIGURE 78–1. Hemodynamics of pericardial disease. *A,* Intracardiac pressures from a dog with pericardial effusion and cardiac tamponade. There is elevation (20 to 25 mmHg) and equilibration of end-diastolic pressures and superimposition of diastolic tracings in the left ventricle (LV), pulmonary artery (PA), right ventricle (RV), and right atrium (RA). The early diastolic (y) descent on the atrial and ventricular tracings is not prominent. *B,* Right ventricular (RV) and right atrial (RA) pressures from a dog with constrictive pericarditis. There is an early diastolic dip and mid-diastolic plateau on the ventricular tracing, the RV end-diastolic pressure is elevated to 14 mmHg (arrow), and the RA a wave and x and y descents are prominent. *C,* Right (RV) and left (LV) ventricular pressures from a dog with constrictive pericarditis show mild elevation (12 mmHg) of end-diastolic pressures, a prominent early diastolic descent, and mid-diastolic plateau, seen best during the pause following a premature ventricular complex (V). (From Thomas, WP, et al.: Constrictive pericardial disease in the dog. JAVMA 184:546, 1984.)

may cause clinical signs by invasion or compression and obstruction of cardiac chambers or great vessels (e.g., heart base tumor invasion of cranial vena cava, right atrium, or pulmonary artery). The most common cause of clinical signs in such cases, however, is concurrent pericardial effusion or fibrosis, the mass lesion being discovered during investigation of the generalized pericardial disorder.

CONGENITAL PERICARDIAL DISORDERS

Although small, subclinical pericardial defects may be more common, peritoneopericardial hernia is the only congenital pericardial disorder that often produces clinical signs in dogs and cats.[14–17]

PERICARDIAL DEFECTS

Very few cases of congenital pericardial defects have been reported in dogs and cats.[28–33] Most (including eight dogs in one report[28]) were diagnosed incidentally during necropsy examination for other disorders. Most of the defects involved the left side as round or oval openings with part of the heart protruding through the defect. Trauma as the underlying cause could not be excluded in most cases. Congenital complete absence of the pericardium is very rare.[29] Although most such defects are clinically silent, electrocardiographic or radiographic abnormalities may occur, and herniation and strangulation of part of an atrium or ventricle may rarely occur, although ante-mortem diagnosis of cardiac incarceration has not been reported in dogs or cats.[30, 31]

PERITONEOPERICARDIAL HERNIA

Incomplete development of the ventral diaphragm (the embryologic septum transversum) and failure of fusion of the pleuropericardial membranes result in a persistent communication between the peritoneal and pericardial cavities. This allows herniation of abdominal organs into the pericardial sac, while the pleural space remains intact. The size of the defect, degree of herniation, and resulting stretching of the pericardium vary from a small hernia involving only omentum, which is clinically silent and detected at necropsy,[32] to a very large hernia variably involving liver, spleen, stomach, and small and large bowel within a greatly dilated pericardial sac (Figure 78–2). Defects of the cranioventral abdominal wall and/or caudal sternebrae may accompany the pericardial defect.[32] A predisposition for the Weimaraner breed has been suggested.[34] Coexisting cardiac or other congenital defects have also been reported in a few cases.[35–37]

Although most patients with this defect develop clinical signs and are recognized in the first year of life, some remain clinically normal for several years or are diagnosed incidentally at necropsy.[34] Clinical signs are most often respiratory (dyspnea, tachypnea, cough) or gastrointestinal (vomiting, diarrhea) in origin, but weight loss, anorexia, abdominal discomfort or enlargement, shock, and collapse have been reported. Physical examination may be unremarkable or may reveal diminished or displaced cardiac impulse and heart sounds. In cats, an apical systolic murmur is sometimes audible. With large hernias the abdomen may feel small and devoid of normally palpable organs, and cranial abdominal discomfort may occur if the small bowel or a liver lobe becomes strangulated. Cardiac tamponade and physical signs of right heart failure may also occur, especially when a liver lobe becomes incarcerated by the defect.

The electrocardiogram is usually not diagnostic, although diminished voltages or axis deviation (due to cardiac displacement) may occur. The diagnosis is usually suspected or confirmed by radiographic examination.[37] Survey thoracic radiographs show cardiomegaly, the extent of which depends on the extent of the herniation. The cardiac shadow is usually rounded or ovoid, and there is silhouetting between the cardiac silhouette and the ventral diaphragm, seen best on the lateral view. Cranial displacement of abdominal organs, especially the liver and stomach, and the presence of gas or fecal-filled bowel loops within the cardiac shadow confirm the diagnosis (Figure 78–2). With smaller hernias involving omentum and mesentery, a fat density may be visible around the denser heart shadow within the enlarged, inhomogeneous cardiac silhouette. Herniated bowel may be outlined by upper GI contrast (barium) administration. In equivocal cases, fluoroscopy, nonselective angiocardiography, tomography, positive or negative contrast peritoneography, pneumopericardiography, or echocardiography[38] may be used to help confirm the diagnosis.[32]

Although the occasional patient that develops cardiac tamponade may benefit temporarily from pericardiocentesis, this defect is surgically correctable via laparotomy or thoracotomy.[34, 38] Correction is recommended in almost all cases, even those found incidentally, and the prognosis is usually excellent.

ACQUIRED PERICARDIAL DISORDERS

PERICARDIAL EFFUSION

By far the most common clinical pericardial disorder in dogs and cats is pericardial effusion with cardiac tamponade and congestive heart failure.[1–11] Because the common causes of clinically significant pericardial effusion produce similar clinical signs of cardiac tamponade, it is appropriate to discuss these disorders as a syndrome with a variety of possible specific etiologies.

Causes and Types of Effusions. The causes of pericardial effusion are often subdivided into groups based on the laboratory characteristics of the fluid (Table 78–1). On this basis, most fluids may be classified as a transudate (or modified transudate), exudate (inflammatory), or hemorrhage (sanguineous or serosanguineous). A chylous (or pseudochylous) effusion may also rarely occur with some conditions. A transudate or modified transudate is commonly found in the pericar-

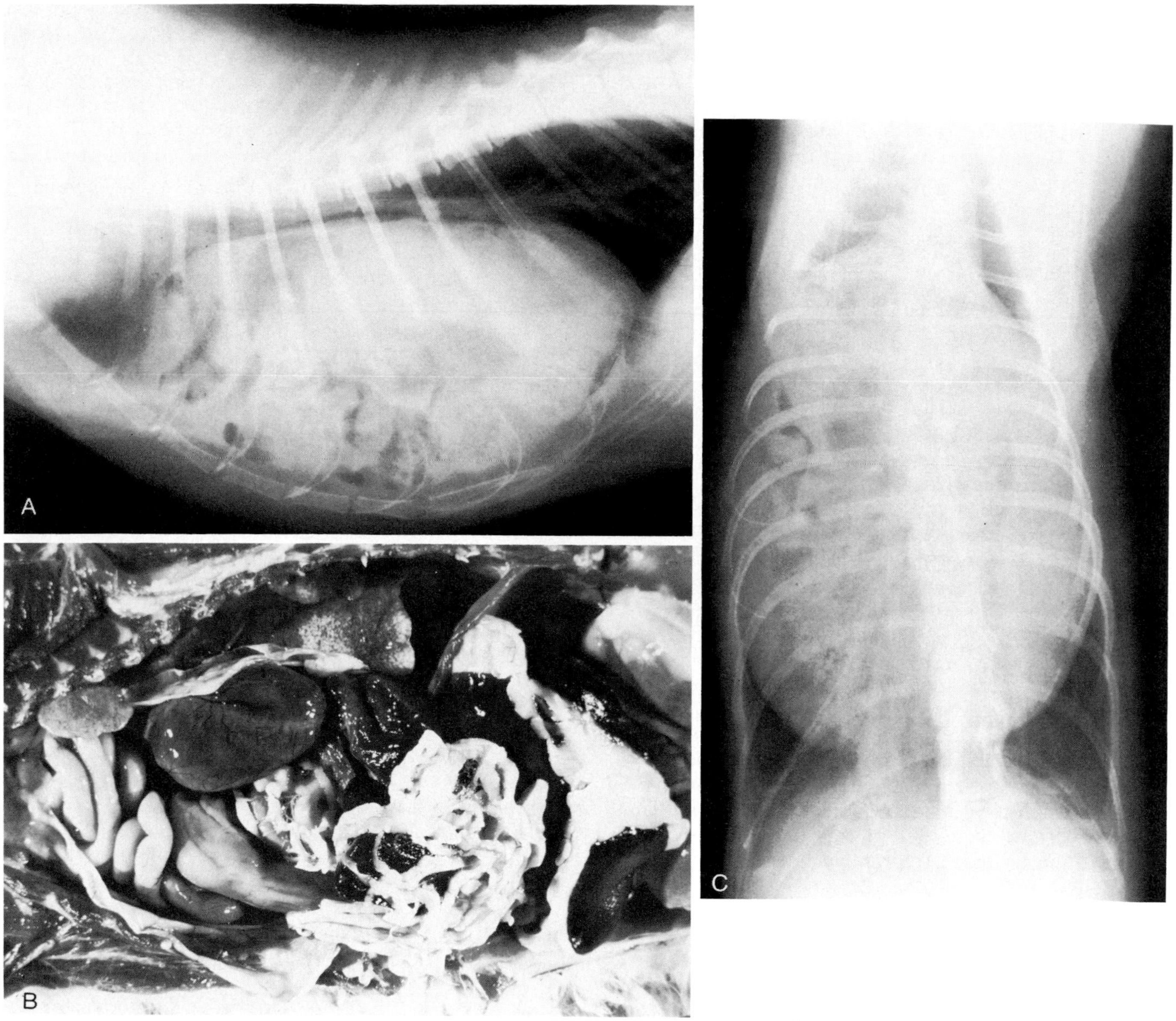

FIGURE 78–2. Peritoneo-pericardial hernia in a two-year-old cat. Radiographs *A* (lateral) and *B* (dorsoventral) show a greatly enlarged, rounded cardiac silhouette. Gas-filled and fecal-filled bowel loops are visible within the cardiac shadow, and there is silhouetting of the cardiac shadow with the ventral diaphragm. At necropsy *(C),* the hernia consisted of small and large bowel, omentum, and a portion of the liver. The heart is displaced dorsally by the herniated abdominal organs.

dial sac of patients with right heart or biventricular failure from any cause, in those with hypoalbuminemia, and in some patients with peritoneopericardial hernia, usually when a section of liver is involved. Except for the latter disorder, the volume of effusion is usually small and causes few hemodynamic or clinical consequences, being detected by echocardiography or at surgery or necropsy. Such subclinical effusions may, however, influence the radiographic size and shape of the cardiac silhouette and its apparent change following medical therapy.[32]

Exudative (inflammatory) pericardial effusions are diagnosed infrequently in dogs because infective pericarditis and other noninfectious causes of pericarditis are uncommon.[14–19] Symptomatic pericardial effusion is very uncommon in cats, but infection is one of its most common causes.[11, 17, 20, 21] Infective exudates are usually purulent, serofibrinous, or serosanguineous, and cytology indicates an inflammatory process with numerous degenerating neutrophils and variable numbers of reactive mesothelial cells. The causative organism(s) are sometimes seen in the fluid, but identification requires aerobic and anaerobic culture. In dogs and cats, infective pericarditis has been reported due to tuberculosis, coccidioidomycosis, actinomycosis, nocardiosis, and other bacteria, including *Pasteurella multocida.*[39–43] Clinically significant, bacteriologically sterile inflammatory effusions have also been reported secondary to feline infectious peritonitis in cats,[44] and small effusions may be found in other infectious diseases, such as leptospirosis and canine distemper in dogs.[14–19] A sterile, inflammatory serofibrinous or serosanguineous effusion can also be caused by chronic uremia (extremely rare in dogs and cats)[11, 17, 45] and other collagen vascular diseases, following myocardial infarction or pericardiotomy for cardiac surgery in humans.[22–24]

The majority of the clinically significant pericardial effusions in dogs (i.e., those that cause cardiac tamponade) are sanguineous (hemorrhagic) or serosanguineous, noninflammatory or mildly inflammatory, and nonseptic. The most common causes are cardiac or extracardiac neoplasms within the pericardial sac, and idiopathic pericarditis.[14–19] Other reported but much less common causes include left atrial perforation secondary to chronic mitral regurgitation,[46, 47] external or iatrogenic trauma,[48, 49] pericardial cysts[50] or other pericardial masses, and uremia.[45] Traumatic pericardial hemorrhage has been reported in dogs due to gunshots[48] and right ventricular perforation during cardiac catheterization.[49] It may also occur from coronary or cardiac laceration during pericardial or pleural paracentesis. In cats, the most commonly reported causes of pericardial effusion are feline infectious peritonitis, bacterial infection, and neoplasia.[11, 17, 20, 21]

Spontaneous left atrial perforation is a well-recognized but infrequent complication of chronic myxomatous degeneration and regurgitation of the mitral valve.[46, 47] Severe dilatation of the left atrium causes endocardial tears that often do not perforate but heal spontaneously (Figure 78–3*D*). When a tear perforates the atrial wall, acute hemopericardium and cardiac tamponade cause sudden hypotension and acute death, or an acute exacerbation of previous signs of heart disease (cough, dyspnea) if the hemorrhage is not fatal. Small dog breeds are mainly affected by this type of valvular disease, and a predisposition to this complication has been reported in the poodle, dachshund, and cocker spaniel breeds, especially in males.[46]

Neoplasms are the most frequent cause of sanguineous and serosanguineous pericardial effusion in dogs and cats.[14–21] In dogs, the most common tumors are hemangiosarcoma and heart base neoplasms, although mesothelioma, lymphosarcoma, and rarely, other sarcomas or metastatic tumors have been reported.[14–19] The same types of tumors occur in the cat, but lymphosarcoma is more common, while heart base tumors and hemangiosarcoma are rare.[11, 17, 20, 51] In the dog, hemangiosarcoma (hemangioendothelioma, angiosarcoma) occurs as a primary tumor of the spleen, liver, lung, other soft tissue, and the wall of the right atrium, auricle, or rarely, the right ventricle, with a predilection for the German shepherd breed.[52–57] Hemangiosarcoma is a rare tumor of the heart of cats.[58, 59] Clinical signs when the heart is involved usually result from metastatic lesions or from cardiac tamponade. This tumor tends to metastasize early, especially to lung (Figure 78–3*A*), and can cause acute, rapidly recurring hemopericardium. Consequently, the prognosis for animals with this tumor is always very guarded to poor, even when surgical removal is attempted.

Heart base tumors are neoplasms of several histologic types arising at the heart base in proximity to and usually attached to the ascending aorta (Figure 78–3*B*).[60–71] They are one of the most common causes of serosanguineous pericardial effusion in the dog, but are rare in cats.[51, 71] Depending on the pathologic study, the most common histologic types in dogs are the chemodectoma (chemoreceptor cell tumor, nonchromaffin paraganglioma, aortic body tumor), which arises from chemoreceptor cells around the base of the aorta,[60–64] and ectopic thyroid adenocarcinoma.[65–67] Other less common types include parathyroid or connective tissue tumors. Since the different types are clinically indistinguishable, the generic term heart base tumor is probably most appropriate. The chemodectoma has a predilection for brachycephalic breeds of dogs (boxer, bulldog, Boston terrier), and an association between aortic body tumors and interstitial cell testicular tumors in male boxers has been reported.[62] Heart base tumors tend to be locally invasive but slow to metastasize. Clinical signs may be caused by space occupation or invasion of the cranial vena cava, right atrium, or pulmonary artery (rare), but most often result from pericardial effusion. Noneffusive heart base tumors are occasionally diagnosed by echocardiography or at necropsy in older dogs.

Mesothelioma, an uncommon neoplasm arising from the mesothelial layer of serous membranes of the thorax and abdomen, occasionally affects the pericardium of dogs and cats as a diffuse granular or fibrous-appearing thickening, causing pericardial effusion or, rarely, effusive-constrictive pericarditis (Figure 78–3*C*).[72–75] Other neoplasms have been reported as rare, isolated cases in both dogs and cats.

Idiopathic hemorrhagic pericarditis (also called idiopathic hemorrhagic or benign pericardial effusion) is a common condition of uncertain etiology that typically occurs in medium to large breed, young to middle-aged dogs.[76–78] The effusion is sanguineous (hemorrhagic), serosanguineous, or rarely, serous or serofibrinous.[78] It is nonseptic and cytologically mildly inflammatory or noninflammatory, and pericardial histology shows variable mononuclear inflammation, congestion, and fibrosis.[77] This effusion may be self-limiting, with spontaneous resolution following one or two pericardiocenteses, or may reoccur rapidly or as long as several years after initial diagnosis.

Of considerable practical clinical importance is the fact that most pericardial effusates in dogs are sanguineous or serosanguineous, have variable and overlapping laboratory characteristics, and are therefore usually not etiologically distinguishable.[79–81] Neoplastic cells and reactive mesothelial cells are difficult or impossible to distinguish microscopically, and review of effusates of several etiologies has demonstrated the wide range of values for total and differential cell counts for each cause.[80] Of the most common causes in dogs, heart base tumors tend to cause more serous, less cellular effusates than hemangiosarcomas or idiopathic pericarditis, but this is not reliable for definitive diagnosis. A sanguineous or serosanguineous effusion should always prompt consideration of a neoplastic etiology. However, neither the age and breed of dog nor the gross appearance of the fluid should be used to diagnose neoplastic pericardial

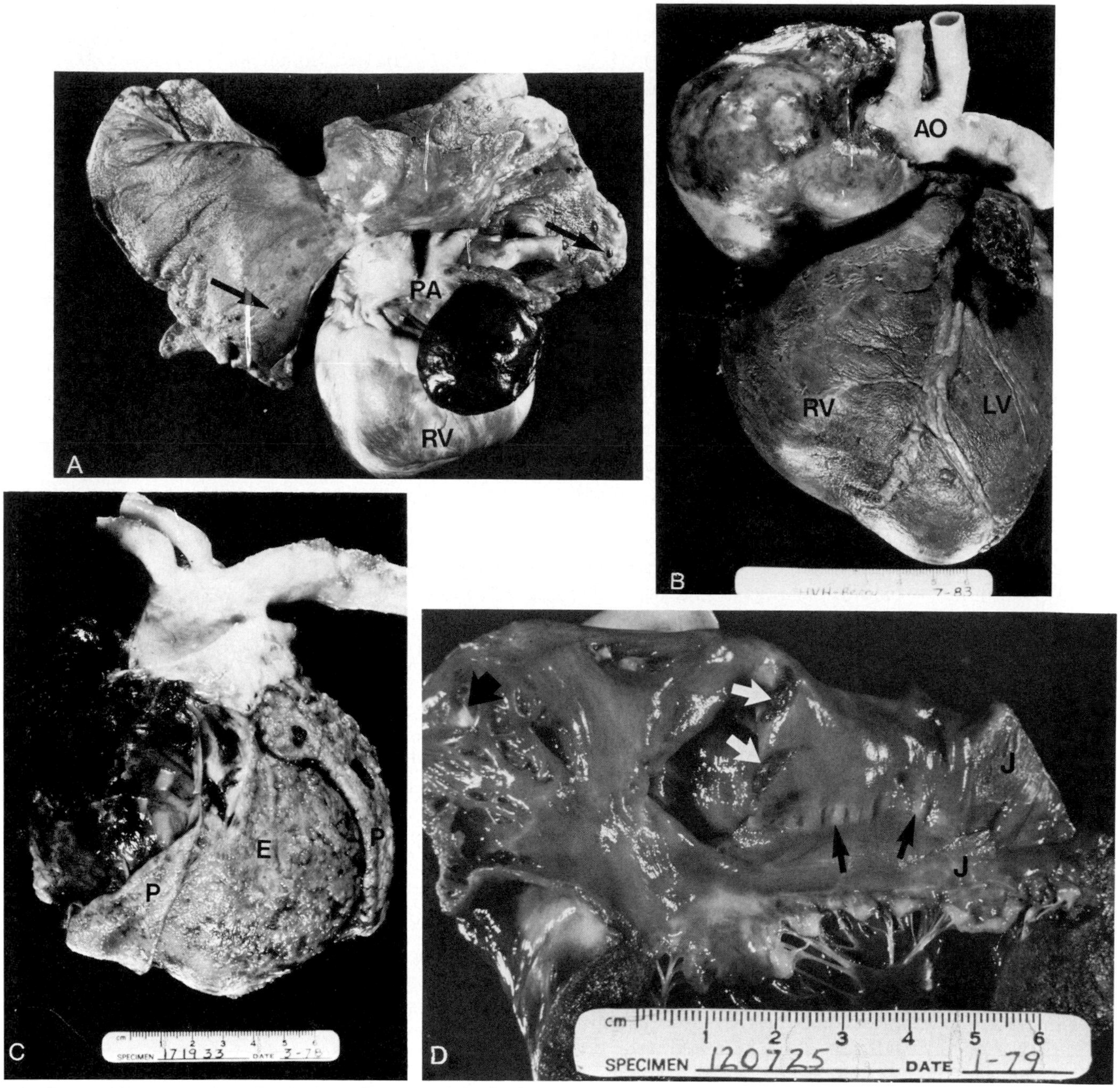

FIGURE 78–3. Pathology of pericardial effusion in the dog. *A,* Heart and lungs of a six-year-old bull mastiff with hemangiosarcoma originating from the right auricle. Multiple small pulmonary metastases are seen in the lungs (arrows). RA = right atrium, RV = right ventricle. *B,* Heart from a nine-year-old Labrador retriever with a heart base tumor (chemodectoma) arising from the region of the ascending aorta. AO = aorta, RV = right ventricle, LV = left ventricle. *C,* Pericardial mesothelioma in a ten-year-old Afghan. Both epicardium (E) and the thickened parietal pericardium (P) show granular proliferation. Effusive-constrictive pericarditis was present. *D,* Open left heart from a 12-year-old poodle that died suddenly from acute hemopericardium with cardiac tamponade. There is myxomatous degeneration of the mitral valve, and in the left atrium there are fibrous endocardial jet lesions (J) due to chronic mitral regurgitation, fresh (small black arrows) and thrombosed, older (white arrows) endocardial tears, and the perforation (large black arrow) that caused the acute pericardial hemorrhage.

effusion without a more definitive diagnosis established by special studies, especially two-dimensional echocardiography, or histologic confirmation.

History and Clinical Signs. Small pericardial effusions and some slowly developing larger effusions produce no clinical signs of cardiac compression. Signs related to the primary etiology (infection, trauma, neoplasia) are variable and nonspecific. Clinical signs of pericardial effusion result mainly from cardiac compression. Acute cardiac tamponade causes rapid development of weakness, dyspnea, collapse (cardiogenic shock), or sudden death. Most effusions, however, develop gradually enough to cause signs of chronic cardiac tamponade. Except for a recognized predilection for occurrence in older animals and certain dog breeds, especially German shepherds, there is usually no relevant past medical history. Common presenting complaints include lethargy, respiratory problems (tachypnea, cough), abdominal enlargement, weakness, and syncope.

Physical Diagnosis. Small effusions are usually not detectable by routine examination. Larger effusions often cause diminished, dull heart sounds on both sides of the thorax. The palpable precordial impulse may also be diminished. These same findings may also occur in patients with pleural effusion or intrathoracic masses, low cardiac output, or simple obesity. Cardiac arrhythmias are sometimes detected but, in most cases, except dogs with mitral regurgitation, murmurs and gallops characteristic of other disorders are not heard. Dogs with left atrial perforation have a systolic murmur that may be diminished in intensity from previous examinations.[46] Diminished heart sounds are most significant when accompanied by physical signs of cardiac compression, including resting tachycardia, peripheral venous hypertension (jugular vein distention/pulse, CVP often greater than 15 cm H_2O), and arterial hypotension or diminished pulse strength. Pulsus paradoxus, a palpable or measurable variation in arterial pressure characterized by an exaggerated decrease in systolic and mean pressure (greater than 10 mmHg), and decreased pulse pressure, is strongly suggestive of cardiac tamponade (Figure 78–4). Other signs of chronic cardiac tamponade include signs of right heart failure, including ascites, hepatomegaly, and pleural effusion. In particular, the three signs of jugular venous distention, a weak and variable arterial pulse, and diminished heart sounds are strongly suggestive of pericardial effusion with tamponade.[23, 24]

Electrocardiography. Although there are no pathognomonic electrocardiographic findings in pericardial disease, several findings support the diagnosis of pericardial effusion (Figure 78–5).[82, 83] Diminished QRS voltages are a common finding (50 to 60 per cent), especially if a prior tracing is available for comparison. In dogs, QRS amplitudes less than 1.0 mV in limb and thoracic leads are considered diminished.[82] Other causes include pleural effusion, other thoracic masses, and obesity. Low amplitudes are occasionally recorded in otherwise normal dogs. The low QRS amplitudes often recorded from normal cats make recognition of diminished amplitudes very difficult.[82] Nonspecific ST segment deviation is common but usually mild, and the cardiac rhythm is usually sinus tachycardia, although supraventricular and ventricular arrhythmias are recorded in many dogs (40 per cent).[17] Electrical alternans of the QRS-T complexes (due to physical swinging of the heart) is often visible (50 per cent) in carefully recorded and examined tracings.[17, 83] Although not highly sensitive, this finding is very suggestive of pericardial effusion in the right clinical setting. Care must be taken not to misinterpret respiratory QRS variations as electrical alternans.

Radiography. Small effusions may cause no recognizable change on survey thoracic radiographs. As fluid increases and the pericardium dilates, the cardiac silhouette becomes enlarged and spherical in shape, with loss of normal chamber contours (Figure 78–6).[32] The exception is left atrial perforation from mitral regurgitation, in which left atrial enlargement is still visible.[46]

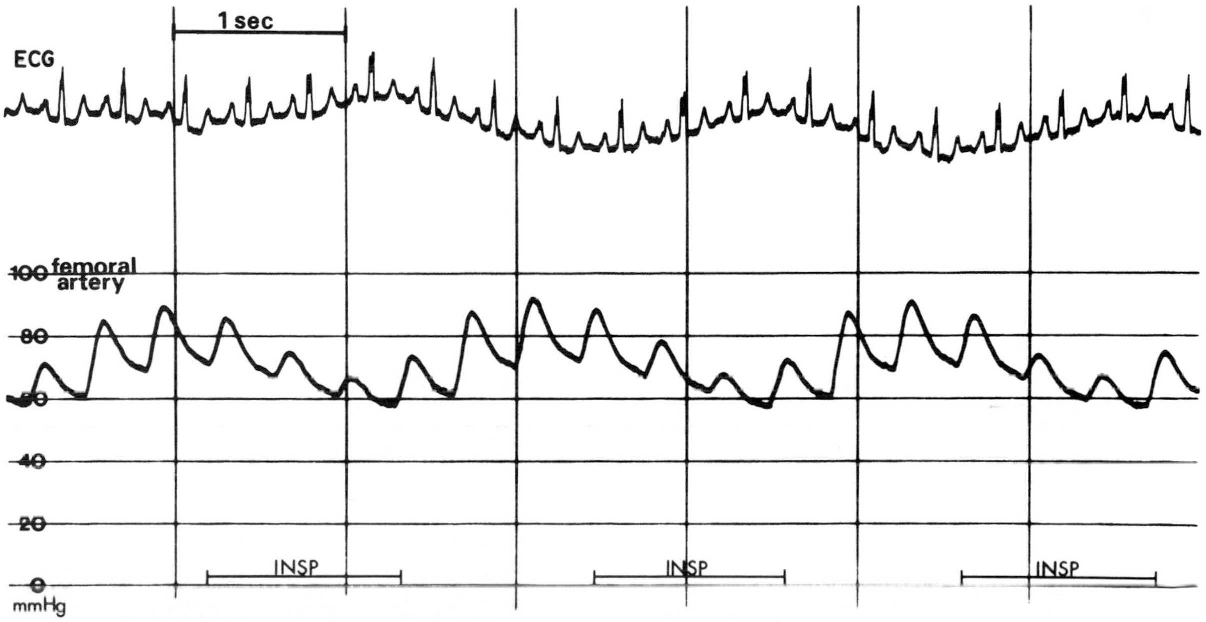

FIGURE 78–4. Pulsus paradoxus in a dog with cardiac tamponade. This direct femoral artery pressure tracing shows an exaggerated fall in arterial systolic and mean pressures (15 to 20 mmHg) and a markedly decreased pulse pressure during inspiration (INSP).

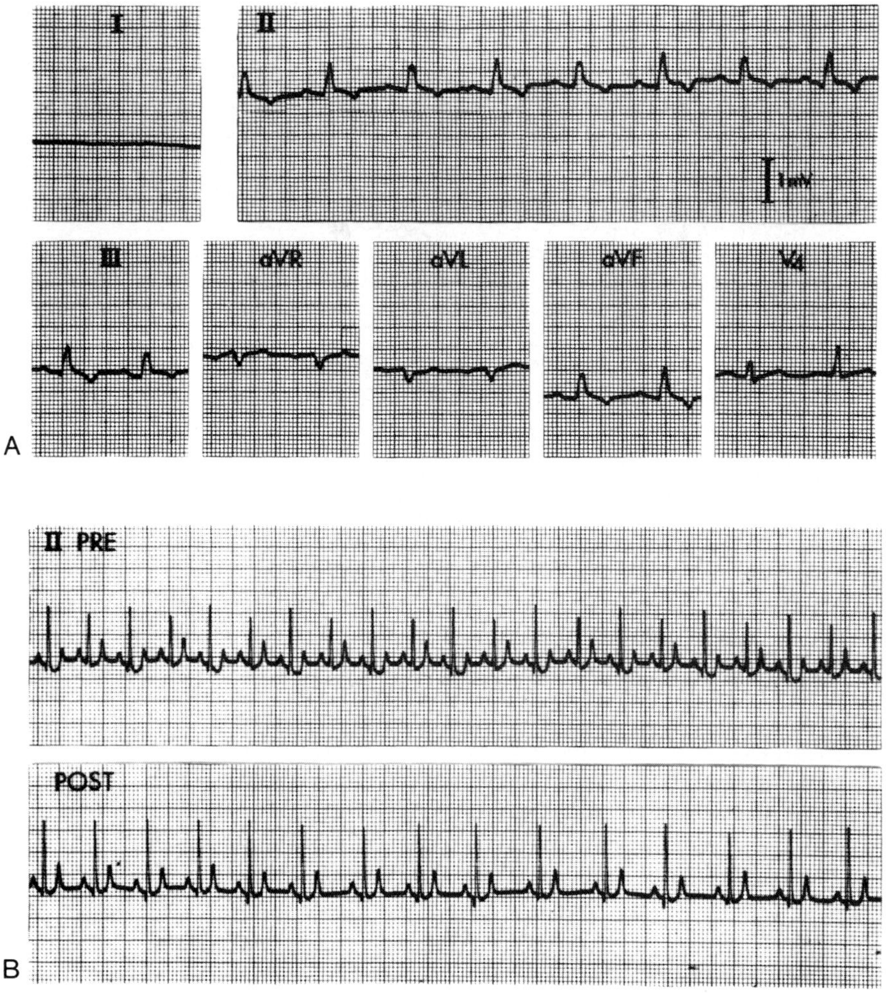

FIGURE 78–5. Electrocardiographic features of pericardial effusion in the dog. *A,* Decreased QRS voltages (less than 1.0 mV) are present in all leads. Electrical alternans of the QRS-T complexes can be seen, especially in leads II, III, and V4 (CV_6LU). Paper speed = 50 mm/sec. *B,* Electrical alternans. Before pericardiocentesis (PRE), alternating QRS-T amplitudes with no change in PR interval is present in lead II. After pericardial drainage (POST), alternation is abolished, QRS amplitude has increased, and heart rate has decreased. Paper speed = 25 mm/sec.

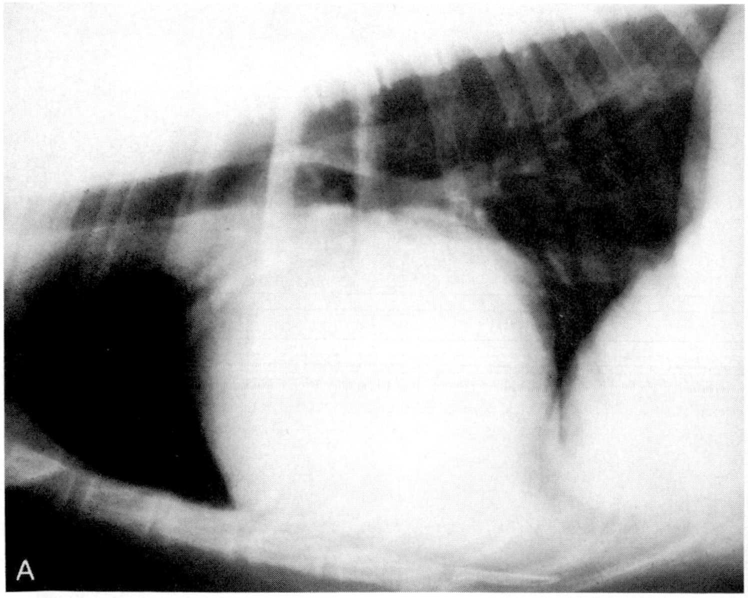

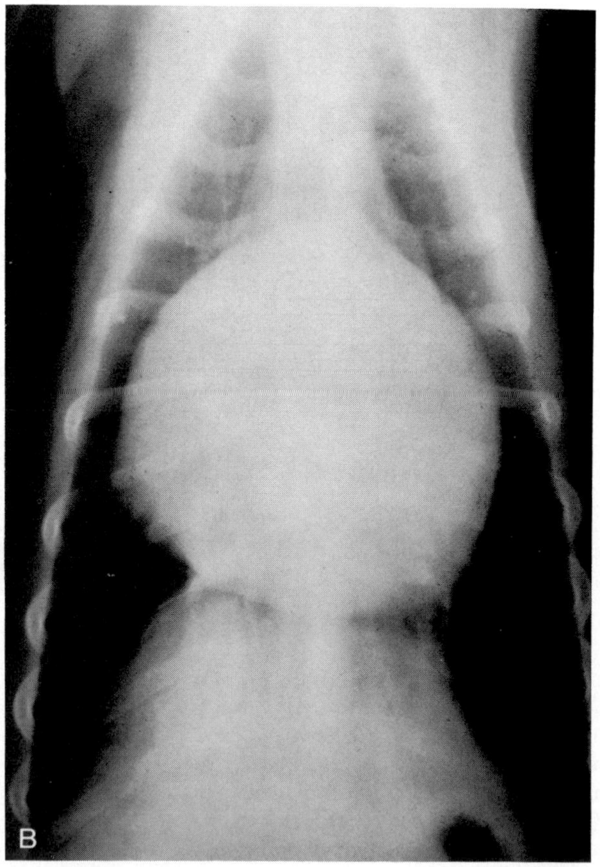

FIGURE 78–6. Radiographic features of pericardial effusion in the dog. Lateral *(A)* and dorsoventral *(B)* radiographs show a moderately enlarged, rounded cardiac silhouette in a dog with a moderate pericardial effusion.

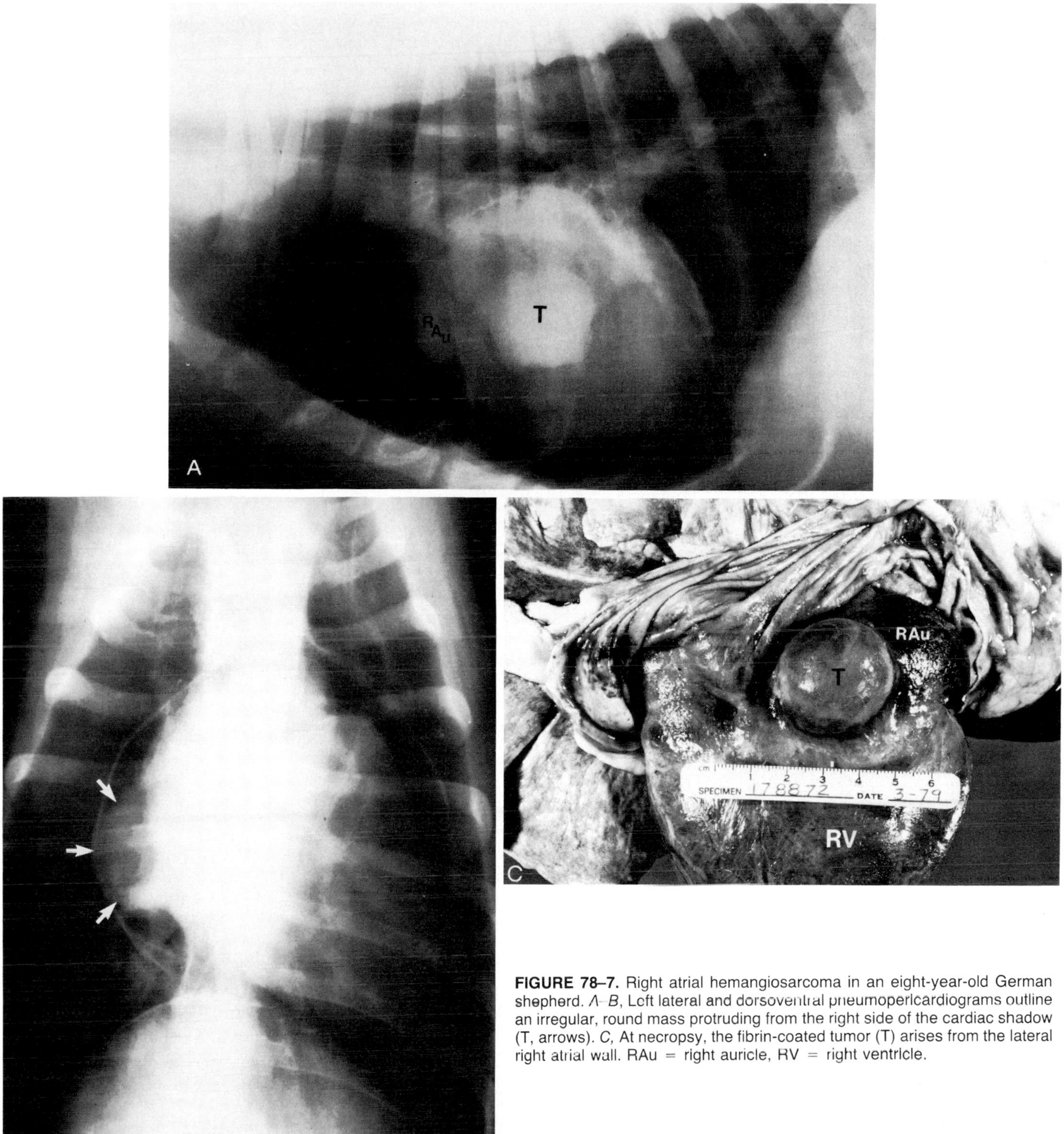

FIGURE 78–7. Right atrial hemangiosarcoma in an eight-year-old German shepherd. *A–B*, Left lateral and dorsoventral pneumopericardiograms outline an irregular, round mass protruding from the right side of the cardiac shadow (T, arrows). *C*, At necropsy, the fibrin-coated tumor (T) arises from the lateral right atrial wall. RAu = right auricle, RV = right ventricle.

The degree of cardiomegaly depends on the rate of development and volume of effusion, so that the *size* of the cardiac shadow is less important than its *shape* in recognizing pericardial effusion. Other changes that may be present include widening of the caudal vena cava, and pleural effusion, which may prevent accurate interpretation of the cardiac silhouette. Occasionally a tumor or other mass may produce a bulge in the cardiac outline, and heart base tumors sometimes displace the trachea dorsally at the cranial heart base. Other cardiac disorders that occasionally produce a rounded cardiac silhouette and simulate pericardial effusion include dilated cardiomyopathy and congenital tricuspid valve dysplasia with massive right atrial dilatation.[2, 32]

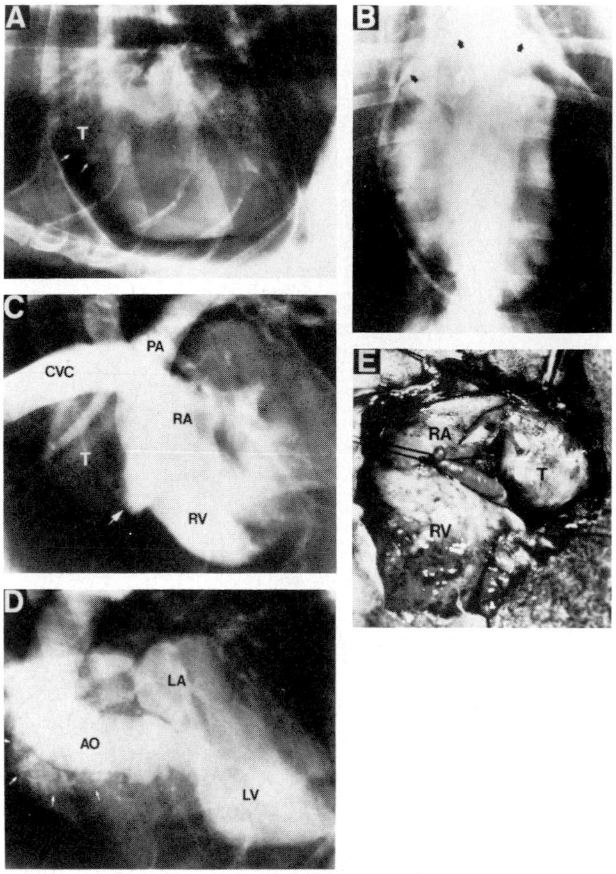

FIGURE 78–8. Heart base tumor (chemodectoma) in an 11-year-old Samoyed. *A,* Right lateral pneumopericardiogram shows a tumor mass (T) preventing gas from outlining the cranial heart base region above the right auricle (arrows). *B,* Dorsoventral pneumopericardiogram also shows failure of gas to reach the cranial heart base (arrows). *C,* Nonselective angiocardiogram shows a nonopacified soft tissue mass (T) cranial to the right atrium (RA) and right auricle (arrow). CVC = cranial vena cava, RV = right ventricle, PA = pulmonary artery. *D,* Later in the series, during left heart opacification, the circular tumor mass (arrows) causes a vascular blush adjacent to the ascending aorta (AO). LA = left atrium, LV = left ventricle. *E,* At surgery the tumor (T) was adherent to the ascending aorta medial to the right auricle (retracted by suture). (From Thomas, WP, et al.: Diagnostic pneumopericardiography in dogs with spontaneous pericardial effusion. Vet Radiol 25:2, 1984.)

Other radiographic procedures that may supplement survey radiography include fluoroscopy, pneumopericardiography, and angiocardiography. Fluoroscopy shows an enlarged, "quiet" heart with nearly motionless cardiac borders except at the heart base. Pneumopericardiography, performed immediately following pericardiocentesis, has been shown to outline normal cardiac borders and heart base structures,[84] and to outline intrapericardiac mass lesions, including right atrial hemangiosarcomas (Figure 78–7), heart base tumors (Figure 78–8), and pericardial cysts (see below).[85, 86] Nonselective angiography may be used to demonstrate normal cardiac chambers dorsally displaced within the enlarged heart shadow. Angiography may also be used to outline cardiac masses, especially right atrial or heart base tumors.[68, 69, 87, 88] Right atrial hemangiosarcomas occasionally displace contrast within the right atrium. Heart base tumors may produce displacement or compression of the cranial vena cava, right or left atria, or pulmonary artery. In addition, a well-vascularized heart base tumor may be outlined as a vascular blush following left heart opacification (Figure 78–8).[86]

Echocardiography. The most important new development in the diagnosis of pericardial disease and its causes has been M-mode and two-dimensional echocardiography.[89–93] Echocardiography is the most sensitive and specific method available for detecting and quantifying pericardial effusion, even in patients with very small, subclinical effusions. The M-mode echocardiogram shows the echo-free pericardial effusion space between the ventricular walls and pericardium on both sides of the heart (Figures 78–9*A* and *B*). It also may demonstrate swinging of the heart within the pericardial effusion space, and compression and collapse of the right atrium or ventricle with cardiac tamponade.[93] The two-dimensional echocardiogram can rapidly demonstrate the volume and distribution of the effusion around the heart (Figures 78–9*C* and *D*). In addition, it has been shown to accurately identify and localize pericardial and cardiac masses, including right atrial and heart base tumors, much more accurately than other techniques.[91, 92] Using two-dimensional echocardiography, hemangiosarcomas are imaged as soft tissue masses arising from the right atrium or auricle (Figure 78–10), while heart base tumors are attached to, and move with, the ascending aorta (Figure 78–11). Intrapericardiac metastatic lesions may also be seen in some cases.[91]

Pericardiocentesis. The definitive diagnosis of pericardial effusion, if echocardiography is not available, is established by pericardiocentesis and fluid removal. It is indicated in all cases of cardiac tamponade to reduce pericardial pressure, improve cardiac filling, and relieve clinical signs, at least temporarily. It is also indicated in cases of asymptomatic pericardial effusion of uncertain origin. Aseptic samples should be collected for physical, cytologic, and microbiologic evaluation, followed by complete pericardial drainage (unless acute, continuous hemorrhage is occurring).

Pericardiocentesis, properly performed, is a simple and safe procedure.[14, 94] The author's preferred technique uses a 14 to 16 gauge, 5 to 6 inch, over-the-needle radiopaque catheter with one to three extra side holes cut near the tip. The patient, usually unsedated and with the electrocardiogram being monitored, is positioned in left lateral recumbency on the x-ray table, and an area of the right precordium (4th to 6th intercostal spaces) is chosen to avoid the large extramural coronary arteries on the left side. After the area is surgically prepared and infiltrated with local anesthetic, the needle-catheter combination is inserted through a small stab incision and advanced slowly toward the heart. When fluid is obtained, the catheter is advanced over the needle, which is then removed. All pericardial fluid is removed, gently altering the patient's position if necessary, and samples are submitted for analysis.

Serious complications from pericardiocentesis, performed as described, are rare. Perforation of the right ventricle is not usually serious, but coronary laceration or penetration of a hemangiosarcoma may cause acute, even fatal pericardial hemorrhage, which requires repeat centesis. Ventricular arrhythmias are common if the epicardium is contacted, but these usually subside

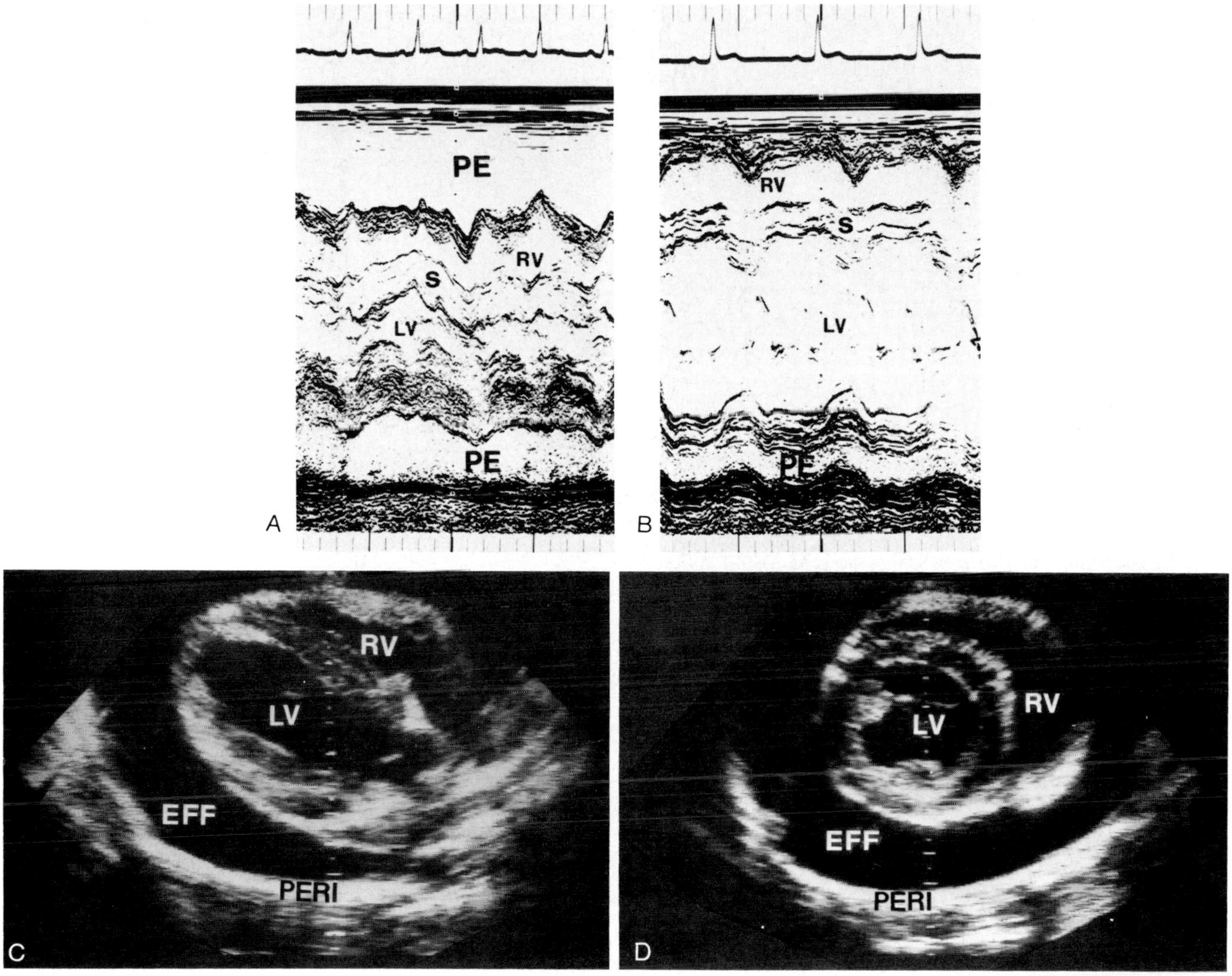

FIGURE 78–9. Echocardiographic features of pericardial effusion in the dog. *A–B,* M-mode echocardiograms recorded before *(A)* and after *(B)* pericardiocentesis in a dog with a large pericardial effusion. In *A,* the effusion (PE) is recognized as an echo free space between the chest wall and right ventricle (RV) proximally, and between the pericardium and left ventricle (LV) distally. The internal dimension of the left ventricle is greatly reduced. In *B* the effusion has been almost completely removed, leaving only a small residual effusion (PE). The left ventricular chamber dimension has increased to normal. S = ventricular septum. *C–D,* Long-axis and short-axis two-dimensional echocardiograms from a dog with a moderate idiopathic pericardial effusion. The anechoic effusion space (EFF) surrounds the heart within the pericardium (PERI). No masses are seen.

quickly if the needle is withdrawn slightly. Cardiac motion is not felt when the pericardium is penetrated, while epicardial contact can be recognized by a scratching or bouncing sensation through the needle that should prompt slight needle retraction. If there is doubt regarding the origin of a hemorrhagic fluid (cardiac versus pericardial), it may be compared with a peripheral blood sample. Hemorrhagic pericardial effusates, if not caused by acute hemorrhage, usually do not clot, and have a different PCV than peripheral blood and xanthochromic serum following centrifugation. Following pericardiocentesis, the patient should be monitored for arrhythmias or hemorrhage for a few hours.[17]

Pneumopericardiography. If two-dimensional echocardiography is not available, then pneumopericardiography should be performed immediately after pericardial drainage to identify any intrapericardiac mass lesions. Approximately three-quarters of the removed fluid is replaced with CO_2 or room air, and radiographs are obtained in right lateral, left lateral, dorsoventral, and ventrodorsal positions.[84–86] The lateral views are most informative, and positional horizontal beam views may be used to better visualize specific areas. Particular attention is paid to the areas of the right atrium and heart base, and care must be taken not to misinterpret normal structures as abnormal masses. Hemangiosarcomas are usually outlined with the right atrium or auricle on the left lateral view (Figure 78–7), while heart base tumors are variably outlined near the ascending aorta on either lateral or dorsoventral views (Figure 78–8).

Differential Diagnosis. The differential diagnosis of pericardial effusion includes other causes of right heart or biventricular failure, such as dilated cardiomyopathy,

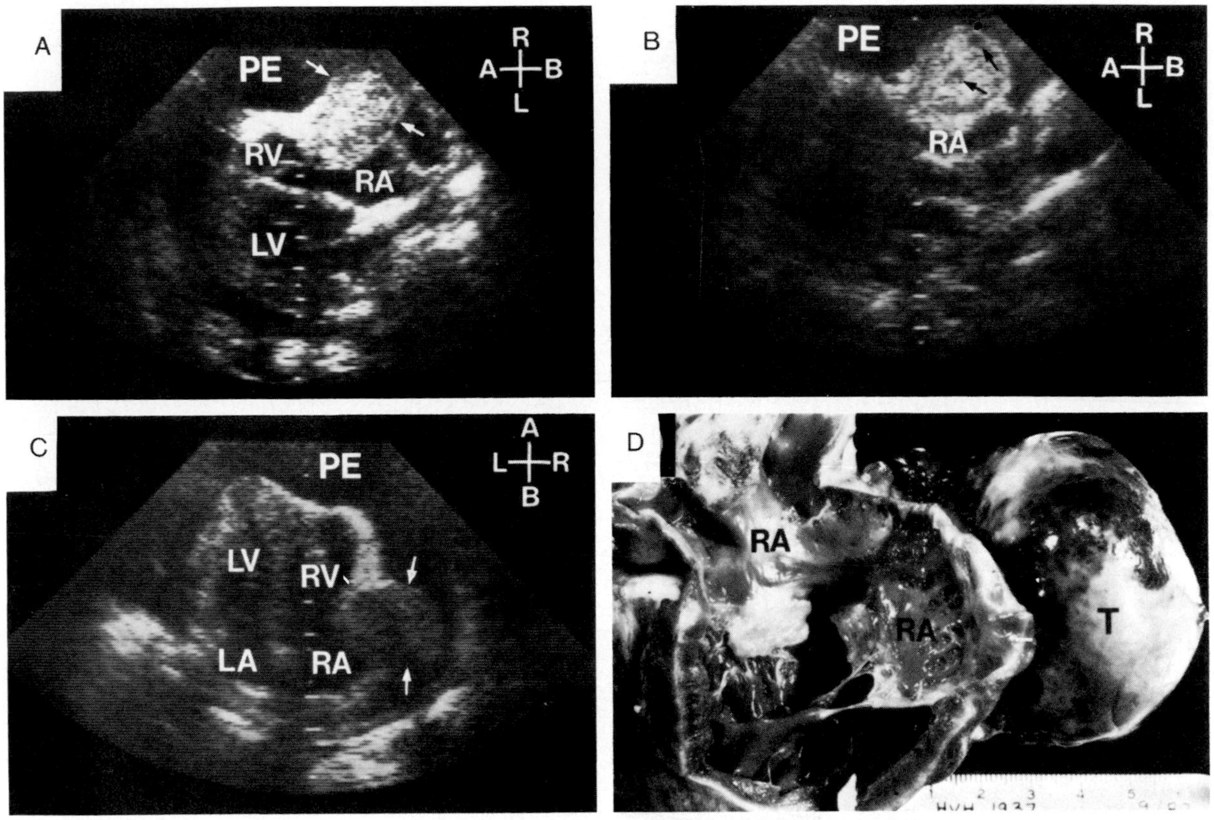

FIGURE 78–10. Right atrial hemangiosarcoma and pericardial effusion in a dog. *A,* Right intercostal long-axis view shows ovoid tumor mass (arrows) arising from right atrial wall. *B,* Similar view shows small hypoechoic areas within the tumor (arrows). *C,* Left intercostal four chamber view shows the tumor (arrows) indenting the right heart near the atrioventricular junction. *D,* Necropsy specimen one month later shows the tumor (T) protruding from the epicardial surface of the right atrium. A = apex, B = base, R = right, L = left, PE = pericardial effusion, RV = right ventricle, RA = right atrium, LV = left ventricle, LA = left atrium. (From Thomas, WP, et al.: Detection of cardiac masses in dogs by two-dimensional echocardiography. Vet Radiol 25:65, 1984.)

congenital or acquired tricuspid regurgitation, and cor pulmonale, and other disorders that may cause abdominal or pleural effusion, diminished heart sounds, or similar radiographic changes.

TREATMENT. The most important initial therapy of pericardial effusion with tamponade is pericardiocentesis. Most patients with cardiac tamponade experience rapid improvement in signs following pericardial drainage. Subsequent treatment depends on the confirmed or suspected underlying disorder. In most cases, medical therapy is of limited value. Small effusions secondary to other disorders (e.g., congestive heart failure, infectious diseases) usually decrease if the primary disorder is successfully treated. If signs of congestive heart failure are present, it may be tempting to institute aggressive medical treatment with diuretics and/or vasodilators to control ascites. However, because elevated venous pressure is critical for maintaining transmural filling pressure in the compressed ventricles, such therapy, by lowering venous pressure, may dramatically diminish stroke volume and cardiac output, causing weakness or even collapse.[25–27] Caution is therefore advised in administration of diuretics and vasodilators to dogs and cats suspected of having cardiac tamponade.

Infective pericarditis should be aggressively treated with antimicrobial drugs selected by results of culture and sensitivity. Continuous or intermittent pericardial drainage using an indwelling pericardial catheter may be indicated and, because of the potential for marked pericardial fibrosis and constriction, pericardiectomy is almost always indicated.[23, 24]

Acute hemopericardium from trauma or left atrial perforation should be relieved by pericardiocentesis if cardiac tamponade is present. Continuous or recurrent bleeding is an indication for surgical exploration.[46–48]

In patients with sanguineous or serosanguineous pericardial effusion, treatment following initial pericardiocentesis is based on the probable etiology, as defined by fluid analysis, pneumopericardiography, or echocardiography (and, rarely, angiography), as outlined in Figure 78–12.[14–17] If no mass lesion is identified, a diagnosis of idiopathic pericarditis is made and a conservative approach is recommended, consisting of follow-up examination for recurrence (ECG, radiography, echocardiography) and one additional pericardiocentesis, if necessary. About 50 per cent of dogs with idiopathic hemorrhagic pericarditis recover following pericardiocentesis alone. In the remainder, effusion may recur within days or up to several years later. For recurrent idiopathic effusions, use of oral, parenteral, or intrapericardiac corticosteroids has been recommended in humans,[24] but their efficacy has not been

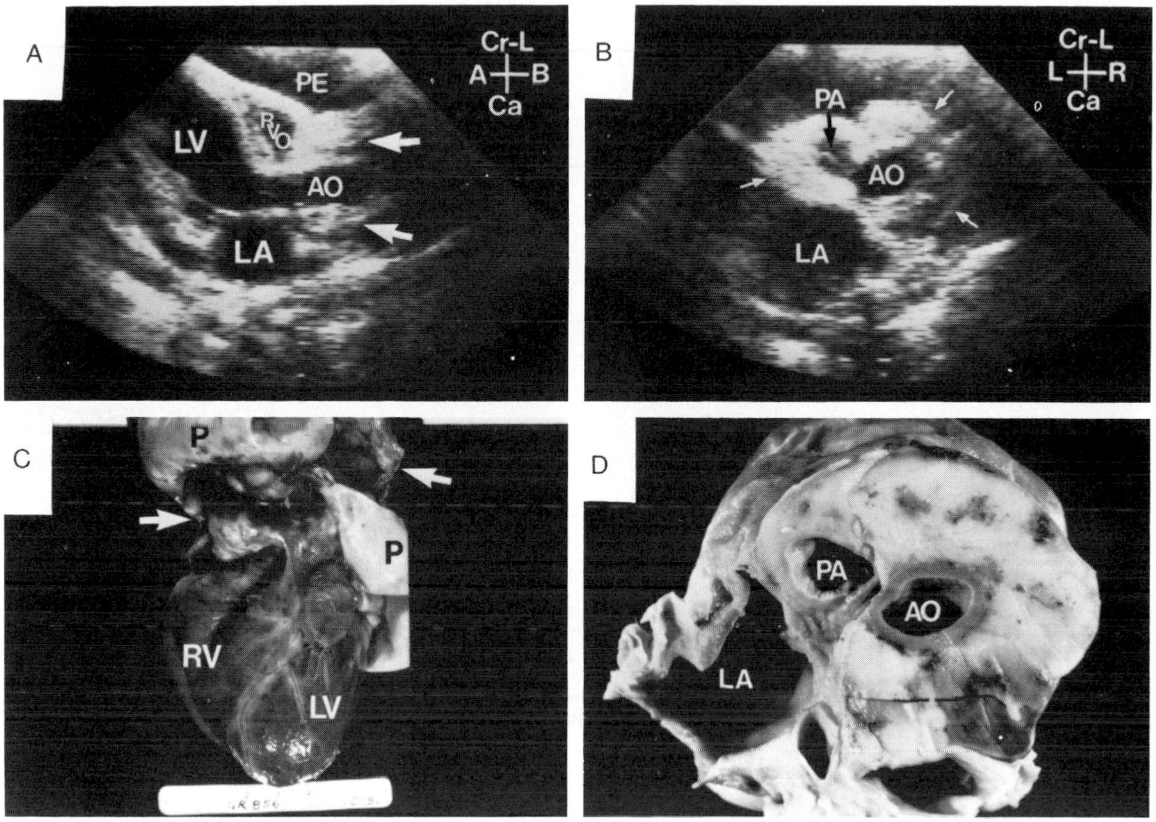

FIGURE 78–11. Heart base tumor (chemodectoma) and pericardial effusion in a dog. *A,* Left intercostal long-axis view shows a soft tissue mass on both sides of the ascending aorta (arrows). *B,* Left intercostal short-axis view shows tumor (white arrows) surrounding the aorta and pulmonary artery. *C–D,* Necropsy specimen shows intra- and extrapericardial portions of the tumor (arrows) and infiltration around both great vessels as seen in *B.* (From Thomas, WP, et al.: Detection of cardiac masses in dogs by two-dimensional echocardiography. Vet Radiol 25:65, 1984.)

evaluated in dogs and cats in this setting. Such effusions can usually be permanently prevented by subtotal parietal pericardiectomy.[17, 19, 76, 77, 95] The risk of pericardial fibrosis and constriction from idiopathic pericarditis in dogs appears to be low.

If a mass lesion is identified as the cause of the effusion, at least three treatment options should be considered. The most aggressive approach involves thoracotomy, parietal pericardiectomy, and an attempt to resect the mass. This approach has been successful in most patients with nonneoplastic masses (cyst, abscess, granuloma),[96] partially successful with certain accessible heart base tumors,[96, 97] and uniformly unsuccessful with right atrial hemangiosarcomas, which have usually spread within the pericardium or metastasized to the lungs by the time the diagnosis is made. The author therefore advocates a conservative approach to almost all patients with right atrial masses. There are no available reports of the effects of chemotherapy or radiotherapy of these tumors in dogs and cats.

In animals with recurrent effusion caused by a nonresectable heart base tumor, subtotal parietal pericardiectomy has shown gratifying results in preventing cardiac tamponade and allowing comfortable survival up to four years after the initial diagnosis. Because many heart base tumors grow slowly, metastasize late, and do not bleed, pericardiectomy is a reasonable alternative to euthanasia or repeated pericardiocentesis in some animals. Because of the metastatic behavior and bleeding potential of hemangiosarcomas, the author does not recommend pericardiectomy for these patients.

The prognosis for dogs and cats with pericardial effusion and cardiac tamponade clearly depends on the underlying etiology. In dogs, idiopathic pericarditis and pericardial cysts have an excellent prognosis with treatment, infective pericarditis and potentially resectable heart base or other neoplasms have a very guarded prognosis, and hemangiosarcoma or nonresectable heart base or other neoplasms have a guarded short-term and poor long-term prognosis.

CONSTRICTIVE PERICARDITIS

The syndrome of diastolic restriction with accompanying clinical signs can be caused by loss of pericardial compliance from pericardial fibrosis (constrictive pericarditis) without any pericardial effusion, or by a combination of fibrosis and a small pericardial effusion (effusive-constrictive pericarditis). Although much less common than pericardial effusion alone, constrictive (or effusive-constrictive) pericarditis has been reported in dogs due to a variety of causes, including recurrent idiopathic hemorrhagic pericarditis, metallic foreign bodies, bacterial or fungal infections, neoplasms such as mesothelioma and heart base tumors, and as an idiopathic disorder (Table 78–1)(Figure 78–13).[98–101] It has also been produced in dogs following traumatic pericardial hemorrhage.[102] Many other less common causes

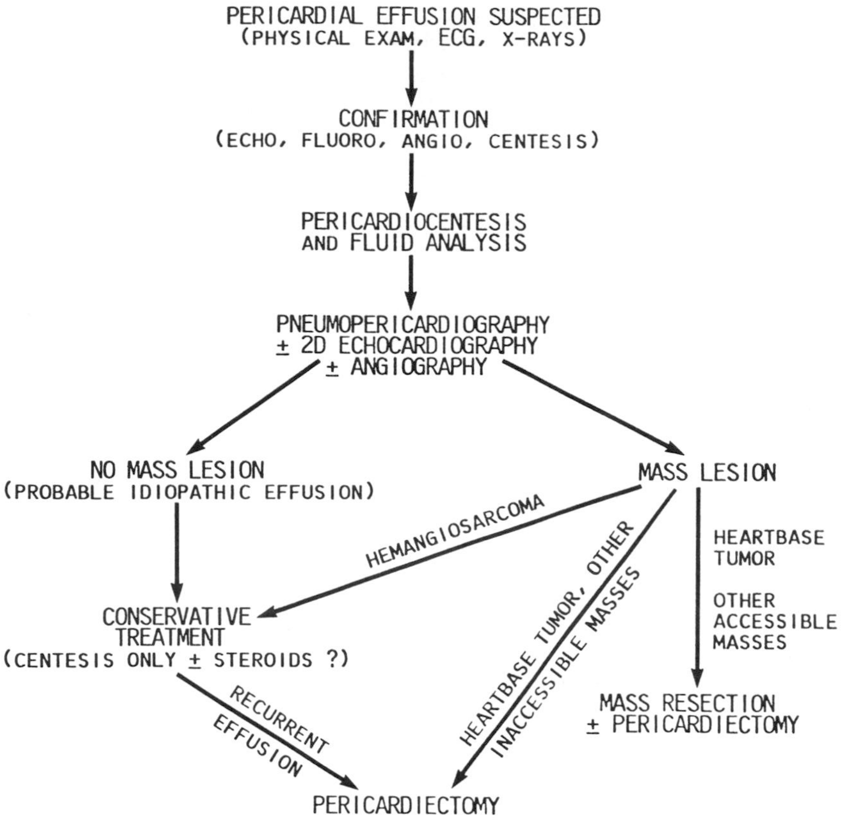

FIGURE 78–12. Flow chart for the diagnosis and treatment of sanguineous pericardial effusion in the dog.

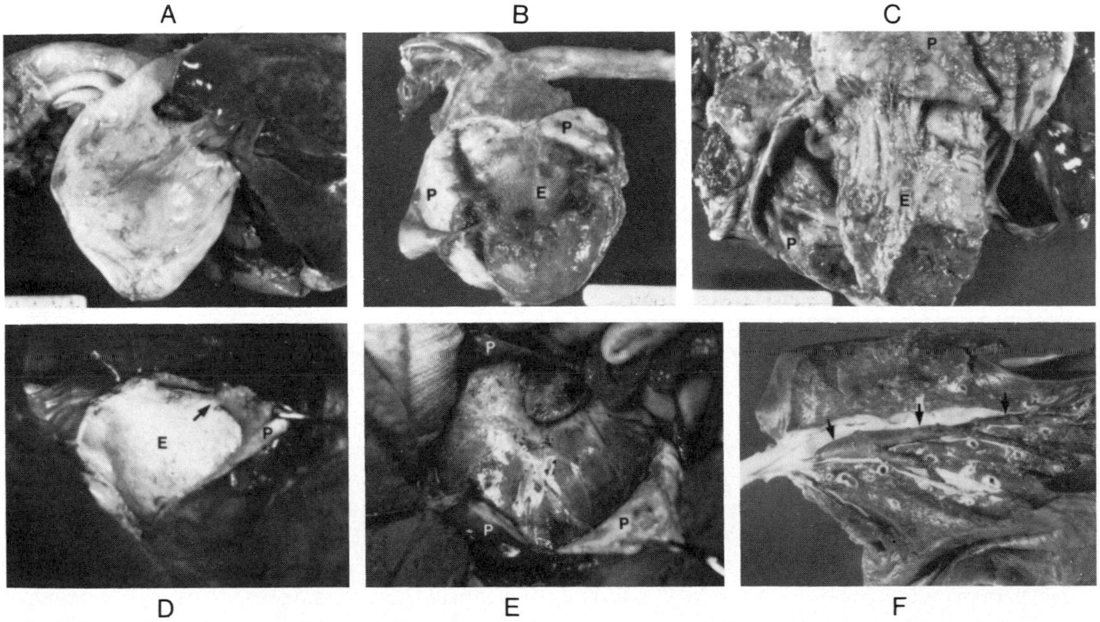

FIGURE 78–13. Pathology of constrictive pericarditis in the dog. *A–B,* Heart showing thickened, opaque pericardium surrounding the heart. The parietal pericardium (P) is thickened, there is epicardial fibrosis (E) over the lateral left ventricle, and epipericardial adhesions are present. *C,* Actinomycotic pericarditis. A layer of fibrin coats the epicardium (E) and reflected pericardium (P). The dark area at the apex was an area of pericardial adhesion. *D,* Heart viewed during surgery. The parietal pericardium (P) has been partially resected, revealing marked epicardial fibrosis (E) and an area of pericardial adhesion (arrow). *E,* Similar surgical view in another dog shows thickening of the reflected parietal pericardium (P), but minimal epicardial involvement and no adhesions. *F,* Left caudal lung lobe from a dog that died several days after pericardiectomy. A large thrombus is present in the lobar pulmonary artery and its branches (arrows). (From Thomas, WP, et al.: Constrictive pericardial disease in the dog. JAVMA 184:546, 1984.)

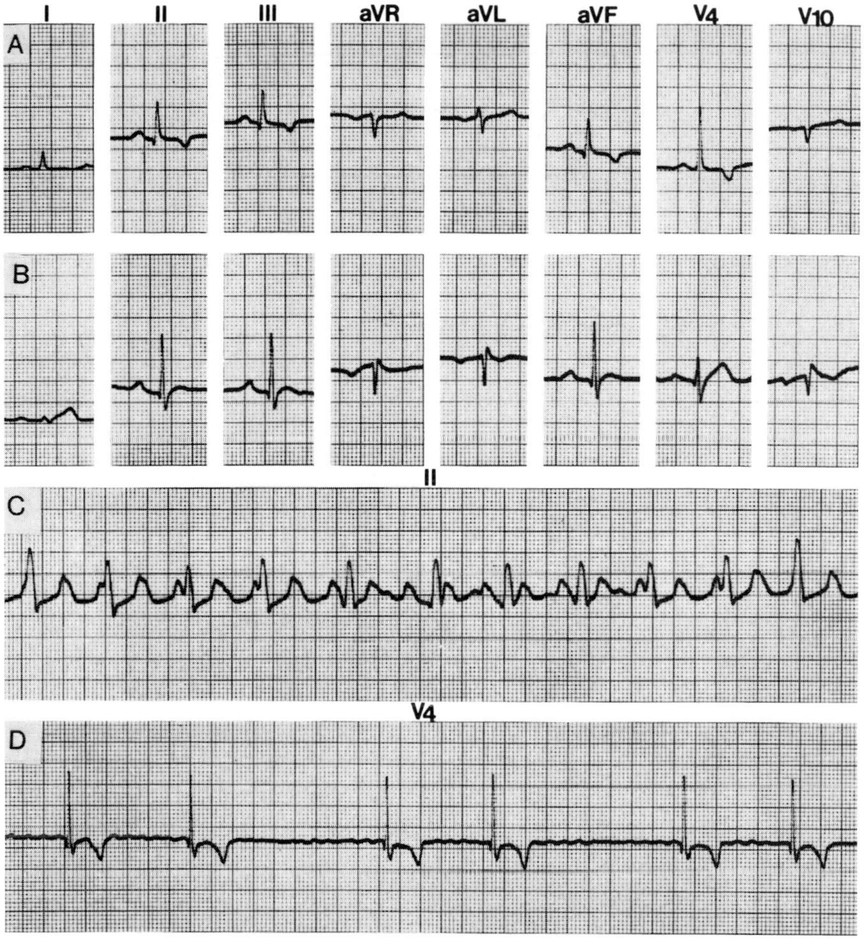

FIGURE 78–14. Electrocardiographic features of constrictive pericarditis in four dogs. *A,* The P wave is prolonged (60 msec) and QRS voltages are diminished in all leads except V4. *B,* The P wave is prolonged (60 msec) but QRS voltages are not clearly diminished. The S waves in leads I, II, and III and the S wave nearly equal to the R wave in lead V4 are suggestive of right ventricular enlargement. *C,* Paroxysmal supraventricular tachycardia with 2:1 A-V block recorded during cardiac catheterization. *D,* Atrial fibrillation with a slow ventricular rate (55 to 65/min) recorded during cardiac catheterization. Calibration 1 cm = 1 mV. Paper speed = 50 mm/sec in A, B, and C, 25 mm/sec in D. (From Thomas, WP, et al.: Constrictive pericardial disease in the dog. JAVMA 184:546, 1984.)

have been reported in humans.[22–24] Although infection is one of the most common causes of pericardial disease in the cat, a proven ante-mortem diagnosis of constrictive pericarditis has not been reported in the cat.[11, 17, 20, 21]

History and Clinical Signs. Presenting history and clinical signs are often similar to those in patients with pericardial effusion. Most commonly affected are dogs of large breeds, both sexes, and dogs over four years of age.[101] The most common owner complaint is abdominal enlargement (ascites). Other common complaints include lethargy, weight loss, exertional fatigue or weakness, tachypnea, and syncope, all of which are related to restricted cardiac output and development of signs of right heart failure. Although these signs may develop rapidly (in less than one week) in effusive-constrictive pericarditis, most dogs have clinical signs from 1 to 12 months prior to diagnosis, usually due to associated subtle or misinterpreted physical and laboratory findings.

Diagnosis. Findings on noninvasive examinations may be suggestive of the diagnosis but are often subtle and not specific. On physical examination jugular venous distention and ascites are consistent findings. The jugular venous pulse may be prominent, and the arterial pulse is weak in about 50 per cent of dogs, but pulsus paradoxus is absent. Heart sounds are often diminished, but an early diastolic pericardial knock, which is common in humans, is heard infrequently in dogs.[98, 101]

The electrocardiogram (Figure 78–14) shows prolonged P wave duration (more than 45 msec) in most cases and diminished QRS voltages in about 50 per cent, but electrical alternans is absent. Sinus rhythm is usually present but supraventricular tachyarrhythmias, especially atrial fibrillation, are common, especially during anesthesia.[101] Radiographs characteristically show variable pleural effusion, mild to moderate cardiomegaly, rounding of part of the cardiac shadow in one or both views, and widening or distortion of the caudal vena cava (Figure 78–15). Fluoroscopy shows diminished motion of the cardiac borders in most dogs, but angiocardiography is either normal or shows only atrial and vena caval dilatation or distortion and variably increased endocardial-pericardial distance along the right heart border (Figure 78–15). Echocardiograms may detect any pericardial effusion and may help rule out other types of heart disease, but they do not allow recognition of pericardial thickening in most dogs.

In summary, constrictive pericarditis should be considered in a dog or cat with signs of right heart failure (especially jugular venous distention/pulse) not caused by other congenital or acquired valvular or myocardial disease. Although noninvasive studies may be supportive, reliable preoperative diagnosis requires cardiac

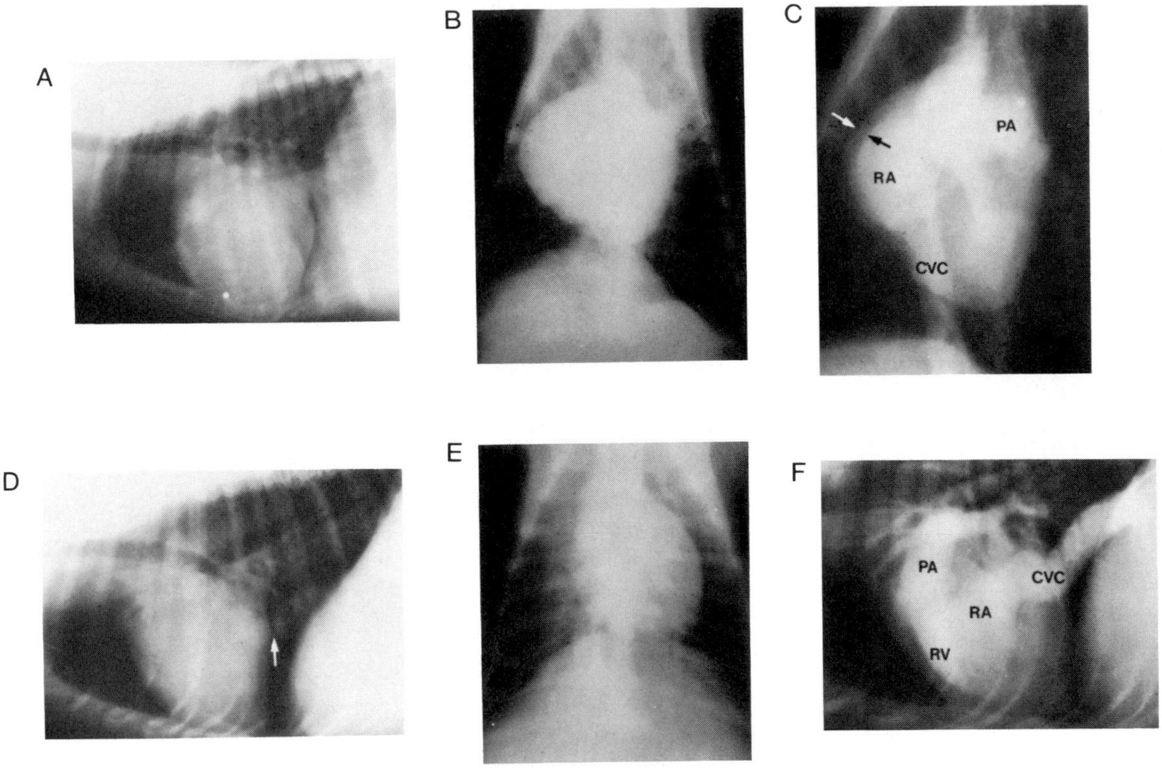

FIGURE 78–15. Radiographic-angiographic studies in two dogs with constrictive pericarditis (*A–C* = dog 1, *D–F* = dog 2). *A–B,* Lateral and DV views of dog 1 show rounding of the caudal and right borders of the cardiac shadow. A radiopaque pellet is seen near the cardiac apex. *C,* Right heart angiocardiogram following caudal vena caval (CVC) injection (DV view) shows right atrial (RA) dilatation and increased endocardial-pericardial thickness (7 to 8 mm, arrows). The mobile intrapericardiac pellet lies near the pulmonary artery (PA). *D–E,* Lateral and DV views of dog 2 show normal heart size, rounding of the cardiac shadow (DV), and a ventral deflection of the caudal vena cava (arrow). *F,* Right heart angiocardiogram following caudal vena caval (CVC) injection shows the tortuous course of the vena cava near the right atrium (RA). The right ventricle (RV) and pulmonary artery (PA) appear normal. The endocardial-pericardial thickness is not clearly increased, and the left heart study also appeared normal. (From Thomas, WP, et al.: Constrictive pericardial disease in the dog. JAVMA 184:546, 1984.)

catheterization and demonstration of elevation and equilibration of atrial and ventricular diastolic pressures (Figure 78–1).

Treatment. Medical treatment is of little value in constrictive pericarditis. Although diuretic and venodilator therapy may help control signs of right heart failure, the benefits are usually temporary. Constrictive pericarditis is a surgical disorder that is treated by pericardiectomy. It is not possible prior to surgery to assess the relative degree of epicardial versus parietal pericardial involvement, although both are usually affected with infective pericarditis. Subtotal parietal pericardiectomy alone is usually successful if there is minimal epicardial fibrosis (Figure 78–13). Epicardial stripping, a technically more difficult and risky procedure, is required if there is epicardial involvement, and recurrence of epicardial constriction is common. Parietal pericardiectomy has been successful in about 75 per cent of reported cases in dogs.[98, 101]

INTRAPERICARDIAC MASSES

Mass lesions within the pericardial sac most often arise from a cardiac structure (e.g., atrium, great vessel) and are usually diagnosed when there is associated pericardial effusion or fibrosis. As shown in Table 78–1, such lesions include pericardial cysts, neoplasms (especially right atrial hemangiosarcoma and heart base neoplasms), infective granulomas, and abscesses. Occasionally such lesions cause clinical signs by space occupation, compression, or obstruction of a cardiac chamber or vessel (e.g., atrial, cranial vena caval, or pulmonary artery invasion by heart base neoplasms). Signs vary with the nature and location of the mass. Although these lesions may occasionally be suspected from abnormalities found on survey thoracic radiographs, special radiographic procedures (pneumopericardiography, angiography) or echocardiography are usually required for their diagnosis. In particular, two-dimensional echocardiography has greatly improved the clinician's ability to identify and localize intracardiac and intrapericardiac masses, allowing more rapid and accurate diagnosis, prognosis, and prediction of successful surgical intervention.[91] Two-dimensional echocardiographic examination (or pneumopericardiography, if echo is not available) is strongly indicated in all patients with pericardial effusion, to detect such mass lesions for possible surgical treatment. Although a guarded prognosis is warranted in patients with neoplasms, abscesses and granulomas, pericardial cysts are usually readily resected with a very good long-term prognosis.

References

1. Detweiler, DK and Patterson, DF: The prevalence and types of cardiovascular disease in dogs. Ann NY Acad Sci 127:481, 1965.
2. Ettinger, SJ and Suter, PF: Canine Cardiology. Philadelphia, WB Saunders, 1970.
3. Zook, BC: Some spontaneous cardiovascular lesions in dogs and cats. Adv Cardiol 13:148, 1974.
4. Detweiler, DK, et al.: The cardiovascular system. *In* Catcott, EJ (ed): Canine Medicine, 4th ed. Santa Barbara, American Veterinary Publications, 1979, p 813.
5. Darke, PGG: Cardiovascular system. *In* Chandler, EA, et al. (eds): Canine Medicine and Therapeutics, 2nd ed. Oxford, Blackwell Scientific Publ, 1984, p 1.
6. Liu, SK: Acquired cardiac lesions leading to congestive heart failure in the cat. Am J Vet Res 31:2071, 1970.
7. Liu, SK, et al.: Congestive heart failure in the cat. JAVMA 156:1319, 1970.
8. Harris, SG and Ogburn, PN: The cardiovascular system. *In* Catcott, EJ (ed): Feline Medicine and Surgery, 2nd ed. Santa Barbara, American Veterinary Publications, 1975, p 195.
9. Harpster, NK: Cardiovascular diseases of the domestic cat. Adv Vet Sci Comp Med 21:39, 1977.
10. Fox, PR, et al.: The cardiovascular system. *In* Pratt, PW (ed): Feline Medicine, 1st ed. Santa Barbara, American Veterinary Publications, 1983, p 249.
11. Harpster, NK: The cardiovascular system. *In* Holzworth, J (ed): Diseases of the Cat. Medicine and Surgery. Philadelphia, WB Saunders, 1987, p 820.
12. Holt, JP: The normal pericardium. Am J Cardiol 26:455, 1970.
13. Spodick, DH: The pericardium: structure, function, and disease spectrum. Cardiovasc Clin 7:1, 1976.
14. Thomas, WP: Pericardial disease. *In* Ettinger, SJ (ed): Textbook of Veterinary Internal Medicine, 2nd ed. Philadelphia, WB Saunders, 1983, p 1080.
15. Lombard, CW: Pericardial disease. Vet Clin North Am 13:337, 1983.
16. Reed, JR: Pericardial diseases of the dog and cat. *In* Bonagura, JD (ed): Cardiology. Contemporary Issues in Small Animal Practice. Churchill Livingstone, New York, 1987, p 177.
17. Harpster, NK: The pericardium. *In* Gourley, IM and Vasseur, PB (eds): General Small Animal Surgery. JB Lippincott, Philadelphia, 1985, p 837.
18. Jones, CL: Pericardial effusion in the dog. Comp Cont Ed Pract Vet 1:680, 1979.
19. Berg, RJ and Wingfield, W: Pericardial effusion in the dog: a review of 42 cases. JAAHA 20:721, 1984.
20. Owens, JM: Pericardial effusion in the cat. Vet Clin North Am 7:373, 1977.
21. Rush, JE, et al.: Retrospective study of pericardial disease in cats (abstract). Proc 5th Annu Vet Med Forum :922, 1987.
22. Roberts, WC and Spray, TL: Pericardial heart disease: a study of its causes, consequences, and morphologic features. Cardiovasc Clin 7:11, 1976.
23. Shabetai, R: The Pericardium. New York, Grune & Stratton, 1981.
24. Lorell, BH and Braunwald, E: Pericardial disease. *In* Braunwald, E (ed): Heart Disease. A Textbook of Cardiovascular Medicine, 2nd ed. Philadelphia, WB Saunders, 1984, p 1470.
25. Spodick, DH: Pathophysiology of disorders of the pericardium. *In* Levine, HJ (ed): Clinical Cardiovascular Physiology. New York, Grune & Stratton, 1976, p 621.
26. Shabetai, R: The pathophysiology of cardiac tamponade and constriction. Cardiovasc Clin 7:67, 1976.
27. Shabetai, R: Changing concepts of cardiac tamponade. Mod Conc Cardiovasc Dis 52:19, 1983.
28. van der Gaag, I and van der Luer, RJT: Eight cases of pericardial defects in the dog. Vet Pathol 14:14, 1977.
29. Detweiler, DK: Wesen und Haufigkeit von herzkrankheiten bei hunden. Zbl Veterinarmed 9:317, 1962.
30. van den Ingh, TSGAM: Perikarddefekt mit einklemmung des herzens bei einem hund. Schweiz Arch Tierheilk 119:473, 1977.
31. Milli, UH and Unsuren, H: Incarceration of the heart resulted from pericardial rupture in a dog. Veterinar Fakultesi Dergisi Ankara Universitesi 29:214, 1982.
32. Suter, PF: Thoracic Radiography. A Text Atlas of Thoracic Diseases of the Dog and Cat. Wettsweil, Switzerland, Peter F Suter, 1984, p 194.
33. Patterson, DF: Canine congenital heart disease: epidemiology and etiological hypotheses. J Sm Anim Pract 12:263, 1971.
34. Evans, SM and Biery, DN: Congenital peritoneopericardial diaphragmatic hernia in the dog: a literature review and 17 additional case histories. Vet Radiol 21:108, 1980.
35. Butler, HC: Congenital diaphragmatic hernia and umbilical hernia in a dog. JAVMA 136:559, 1960.
36. Eyster, GE, et al.: Congenital pericardial diaphragmatic hernia and multiple cardiac defects in a litter of collies. JAVMA 170:516, 1977.
37. Rendano, VT and Parker, RB: Polycystic kidneys and peritoneopericardial diaphragmatic hernia in the cat: a case report. J Sm Anim Pract 17:479, 1976.
38. Schulman, AJ, et al.: Congenital peritoneopericardial diaphragmatic hernia in a dog. JAAHA 21:655, 1985.
39. Fisher, EW and Thompson, H: Congestive cardiac failure as a result of tuberculous pericarditis. J Sm Anim Pract 12:629, 1971.
40. Chastain, CB, et al.: Pericardial effusion from granulomatous pleuritis and pericarditis in a dog. JAVMA 164:1201, 1974.
41. Lorenzana, R, et al.: Infectious pericardial effusion in a dog. JAAHA 21:725, 1985.
42. Price, PM: What is your diagnosis (mineralizing pericarditis)? JAVMA 188:1447, 1986.
43. Blunden, AS: Traumatic pericarditis in the cat (letter). Vet Rec 101:433, 1977.
44. deMadron, E: Pericarditis with cardiac tamponade secondary to feline infectious peritonitis in a cat. JAAHA 22:65, 1986.
45. Madewell, BR and Norrdin, RW: Renal failure associated with pericardial effusion in a dog. JAVMA 167:1091, 1975.
46. Buchanan, JW and Kelly, AM: Endocardial splitting of the left atrium in the dog with hemorrhage and hemopericardium. J Am Vet Radiol Soc 5:28, 1964.
47. Stunzi, H and Ammann-Mann, M: Nicht-traumatische Rupturen des Herzvorhofs beim Hund. Zbl Vet Med A 20:409, 1973.
48. Shaw, BE, et al.: Traumatic pericarditis in a dog. JAVMA 174:501, 1979.
49. Buchanan, JW and Pyle, RL: Cardiac tamponade during catheterization of a dog with congenital heart disease. JAVMA 149:1056, 1966.
50. Marion, J, et al.: Pericardial effusion in a young dog. JAVMA 157:1055, 1970.
51. Tilley, LP, et al.: Cardiovascular tumors in the cat. JAAHA 17:1009, 1981.
52. Kleine, LJ, et al.: Primary cardiac hemangiosarcomas in dogs. JAVMA 157:326, 1970.
53. Pearson, GR and Head, KW: Malignant hemangioendothelioma (angiosarcoma) in the dog. J Sm Anim Pract 17:737, 1976.
54. Oksanen, A: Haemangiosarcoma in dogs. J Comp Pathol 88:585, 1978.
55. Ng, CY and Mills, JN: Clinical and haematological features of haemangiosarcoma in dogs. Aust Vet J 62:1, 1985.
56. Brown, NO, et al.: Canine hemangiosarcoma: retrospective analysis of 104 cases. JAVMA 186:56, 1985.
57. Aronsohn, M: Cardiac hemangiosarcoma in the dog: a review of 38 cases. JAVMA 187:922, 1985.
58. Patnaik, AK and Liu, SK: Angiosarcoma in cats. J Sm Anim Pract 18:191, 1977.
59. Scavelli, TD, et al.: Hemangiosarcoma in the cat: retrospective evaluation of 31 surgical cases. JAVMA 187:817, 1985.
60. Nilsson, T: Heart-base tumours in the dog. Acta Pathol Microbiol Scand 37:385, 1955.
61. Jubb, KVF and Kennedy, PC: Tumors of the nonchromaffin paraganglia in dogs. Cancer 10:89, 1957.
62. Johnson, KH: Aortic body tumors in the dog. JAVMA 152:154, 1968.

63. Hayes, HM, Jr: An hypothesis for the etiology of canine chemoreceptor system neoplasms, based upon an epidemiological study of 73 cases among hospital patients. J Sm Anim Pract 16:337, 1975.
64. Patnaik, AK, et al.: Canine chemodectoma (extra-adrenal paragangliomas)—a comparative study. J Sm Anim Pract 16:785, 1975.
65. Thake, DC, et al.: Ectopic thyroid adenomas at the base of the heart in the dog: ultrastructural identification of dense tubular structures in endoplasmic reticulum. Vet Pathol 8:421, 1971.
66. Cheville, NF: Ultrastructure of canine carotid body and aortic body tumors: comparison with tissue of thyroid and parathyroid origin. Vet Pathol 9:166, 1972.
67. von Bomhard, D, et al.: Zur histogenese der herzbasistumoren beim hund. Eine histologische, histolchemische und electronenmikroskopische studie. Zbl Vet Med A 21:208, 1974.
68. Cantwell, HD, et al.: Angiographic diagnosis of heart base tumor in the dog. JAAHA 18:83, 1982.
69. Grain, E, and Evans, JE, Jr: What is your diagnosis (heart base tumor)? JAVMA 186:1327, 1985.
70. Bhargava, AK: Diagnosis of mediastinal and heart base tumors in dogs using contrast pleurography. J Am Vet Radiol Soc 11:56, 1970.
71. Buergelt, CD and Das, KM: Aortic body tumor in a cat. A case report. Pathol Vet 5:84, 1968.
72. Brunner, P: Papillary-polypous mesothelioma of the pericardium of a dog (at the same time a contribution to the question as to primary tumours arising from serous cover cells). Virchows Arch Abt A Path Anat 357:275, 1972.
73. Tilley, LP, et al.: Pericardial mesothelioma with effusion in a cat. JAAHA 11:60, 1975.
74. Thrall, DE and Goldschmidt, MH: Mesothelioma in the dog: six case reports. J Am Vet Radiol Soc 19:107, 1978.
75. Ikede, BO, et al.: Pericardial mesothelioma with cardiac tamponade in a dog. Vet Pathol 17:496, 1980.
76. Gibbs, C, et al.: Idiopathic pericardial haemorrhage in dogs: a review of fourteen cases. J Sm Anim Pract 23:483, 1982.
77. Berg, RJ, et al.: Idiopathic hemorrhagic pericardial effusion in eight dogs. JAVMA 185:988, 1984.
78. Chen, KY: Idiopathic serofibrinous pericarditis and pleuritis with bilateral congestive heart failure in a young dog. J Chinese Soc Vet Sci 10:99, 1984.
79. Wilkins, RJ: Evaluation of thoracic, pericardial and abdominal effusions. *In* Kirk, RW (ed): Current Veterinary Therapy VI. WB Saunders, Philadelphia, 1977, p 321.
80. Sisson, D, et al.: Diagnostic value of pericardial fluid analysis in the dog. JAVMA 184:51, 1984.
81. Edwards, NJ, et al.: The diagnostic value of pericardial fluid pH determinations. Proc 4th Annu Vet Med Forum II:13/111, 1986.
82. Tilley, LP: Essentials of Canine and Feline Electrocardiography: Interpretation and Treatment. Lea & Febiger, Philadelphia, 1985.
83. Bonagura, JD: Electrical alternans associated with pericardial effusion in the dog. JAVMA 178:574, 1981.
84. Reed, JR, et al.: Pneumopericardiography in the normal dog. Vet Radiol 24:112, 1983.
85. Ticer, JW and Ettinger, SJ: Pneumopericardiography. *In* Ticer, JW (ed): Radiographic Technique in Small Animal Practice. WB Saunders, Philadelphia, 1975, p 302.
86. Thomas, WP, et al.: Diagnostic pneumopericardiography in dogs with spontaneous pericardial effusion. Vet Radiol 25:2, 1984.
87. Buchanan, JW: Selective angiography and angiocardiography in dogs with acquired cardiovascular disease. J Am Vet Radiol Soc 6:5, 1965.
88. Bohn, FK and Rhodes, WH: Angiograms and angiocardiograms in dogs and cats: some unusual filling defects. J Am Vet Radiol Soc 11:21, 1970.
89. Christensen, EF and Bonte, FJ: The relative accuracy of echocardiography, intravenous CO_2 studies, and blood-pool scanning in detecting pericardial effusions in dogs. Radiology 91:265, 1968.
90. Bonagura, JD and Pipers, FS: Echocardiographic features of pericardial effusion in dogs. JAVMA 179:49, 1981.
91. Thomas, WP, et al.: Detection of cardiac masses in dogs by two-dimensional echocardiography. Vet Radiol 25:65, 1984.
92. Trautvetter, E and Bob, M: Zur diagnose des perikardergusses beim hund mit hilfe der zweidimensionalen echokardiographie. Berl Munch Tierarztl Wschr 99:308, 1986.
93. Feigenbaum, H: Echocardiography, 4th ed. Lea & Febiger, Philadelphia, 1986, p 548.
94. Ettinger, SJ: Pericardiocentesis. Vet Clin North Am 4:403, 1974.
95. Matthieson, DT and Lammerding, J: Partial pericardiectomy for idiopathic hemorrhagic pericardial effusion in the dog. JAAHA 21:41, 1985.
96. Wagner, SD and Breznock, EM: Surgical management of pericardial and intramyocardial diseases including chemodectomas. *In* Bojrab, MJ (ed): Current Techniques in Small Animal Surgery, 2nd ed. Philadelphia, Lea & Febiger, 1983, p 470.
97. Brownlie, SE and Clayton Jones, DG: Successful removal of a heart base tumour in a dog with pericardial haemorrhagic effusion. J Sm Anim Pract 26:191, 1985.
98. Schwartz, A, et al.: Constrictive pericarditis in two dogs. JAVMA 159:763, 1971.
99. Ader, P and Hansen, J: Constrictive pericarditis in a dog. Canine Pract 7:16, 1980.
100. Neer, TM: Chronic constrictive pericarditis in an American staffordshire. JAAHA 18:595, 1982.
101. Thomas, WP, et al.: Constrictive pericardial disease in the dog. JAVMA 184:546, 1984.
102. Sbokos, CG, et al.: Traumatic hemopericardium and chronic constrictive pericarditis. Ann Thorac Surg 23:225, 1977.

79 INFECTIVE ENDOCARDITIS

J. A. WOODFIELD and DAVID SISSON

Infections of the valves and endocardial lining of the heart are commonly referred to as "infective endocarditis." This term is preferable to the old terms "acute or subacute bacterial endocarditis," since microorganisms other than bacteria may cause endocarditis. The most common location for infection is the heart valves, although it may originate in other areas, including the mural endocardium, septal defects, patent ductus arteriosus, or arteriovenous shunts. The first recorded reference to infective endocarditis in humans was made in 1646 by Rivière.[1] One of the first descriptions of its occurrence in animals was made by Schornagel in 1936.[2]

Prior to the use of antibiotics, people survived serious systemic bacterial infections. However, survival rarely occurred with infective endocarditis. Since host defense mechanisms had little effect on its elimination, the disease was virtually fatal.[3] Only since the introduction of proper antibiotic therapy has the prognosis for infective endocarditis dramatically improved.

In humans and animals, infective endocarditis is a serious cardiac disorder that may be overlooked due to systemic manifestations in other organ systems. Therefore, it is imperative that a complete understanding of infective endocarditis be developed to facilitate the accurate diagnosis and treatment of patients with this disorder. It is only by the proper (1) recognition of the clinical manifestations, (2) identification of the infectious agent by blood cultures, (3) instigation of appropriate antimicrobial therapy, (4) recognition and management of complications, and (5) institution of prophylactic measures that the management of infective endocarditis can be successful.

INCIDENCE AND DISTRIBUTION

The true prevalence of infective endocarditis in dogs and cats in the clinical setting is unknown.[4,5] Review of canine necropsy studies indicates that the incidence of endocarditis may be as low as 0.06 per cent or as high as 6.6 per cent.[2,6–12] Specific breed predilections have not been identified; however, there is a higher incidence of endocarditis in German shepherd dogs and possibly in Boxers.[7,8,11–13] It is reported to frequently occur in medium to large-breed male dogs over four years of age.[7,8,11,12,14] Infective endocarditis has been reported to occur with higher frequency in association with congenital heart defects.[11,12,15,16] However, most affected dogs had no evidence of pre-existing congenital or acquired heart disease.[2,7–14,17,18] Only in two studies was a higher incidence of endocarditis identified with congenital heart defects. These were in dogs affected with fibrous subaortic stenosis.[12,17] No relationship between degenerative valve disease and infective endocarditis has been identified in the dog, which is contrary to what is found in humans.[11,19,20]

ETIOLOGY AND PATHOPHYSIOLOGY

Acute versus Subacute Forms

Historically, infective endocarditis has been divided into acute and subacute forms, based on the progression of untreated infections. In human patients, acute infective endocarditis was caused by severe infections from *Staphylococcus aureus, Streptococcus pneumoniae*, or *Neisseria gonorrhoeae*.[3,21] These bacteria can initiate virulent infections that may end in death within a few days to weeks. Typically, the acute form has a higher incidence of invading normal heart valves. In contrast, the subacute form is usually preceded by an endocardial lesion and has a prolonged and progressive course. In most cases, viridans streptococci or enterococci are the causative agents associated with subacute infective endocarditis in humans.[3,21] The clinical differentiation of acute and subacute infective endocarditis can be helpful in the initial management of the disease; however, there are many incidents in which the clinical progression has had no relationship to the initiating agent.[22,23] Some investigators have recommended elimination of the older terms *acute* and *subacute*.[24] This is suggested because acute infective endocarditis may become subacute with proper treatment, whereas the subacute form may convert to a life-threatening condition. Although these terms are useful in understanding the etiology and pathogenesis of infective endocarditis, classification based on the etiologic agent is more beneficial in the management of infective endocarditis.[3]

Etiology

Almost any microorganism is capable of causing infective endocarditis. In dogs with infective endocarditis, *Streptococcus* spp., *Staphylococcus* spp., *Escherichia coli, Corynebacterium* spp., *Pseudomonas aeruginosa, Erysipelothrix rhusiopathiae*, and *Aerobacter aerogenes* are commonly isolated.[2, 5, 7–14, 18, 25–28] Other aerobic and anaerobic gram-positive and gram-negative bacteria have also been reported to cause infective endocarditis.[12, 13, 29] In addition to bacteria, organisms such as fungi, *Rickettsia*, and *Chlamydia* have been reported to cause infective endocarditis in humans.[30–32] However, nonbacterial infective endocarditis has not been documented in dogs or cats. Although *Streptococcus* spp. have historically been the most commonly incriminated bacteria associated with infective endocarditis, recent investigations have identified a more variable distribution.[12, 18, 29] The reason for this discrepancy is unknown; however, in human patients the spectrum of causative agents in infective endocarditis has changed during the antibiotic era.[22, 23, 33–35]

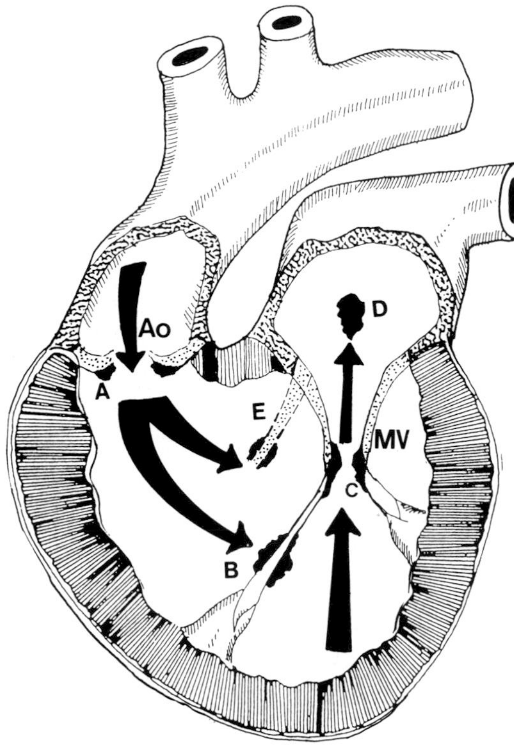

FIGURE 79–1. Site of infective endocarditis within the left ventricle of dogs and cats. Arrows at the aortic valve (Ao) indicate the development of the Venturi effect when blood from a high pressure source (aorta) flows through the aortic valves into a low pressure sink (the ventricle is in diastole) during aortic regurgitation. The vegetative lesions originate on the ventricular surface of the aortic valve leaflets when the Venturi effect drives bacteria into this area (A). A similar effect is seen with mitral regurgitation. The regurgitant stream (arrows on the right) will pass from the ventricle (high pressure) through the mitral valves (MV) to the low pressure sink within the left atrium during systole, thus depositing bacteria on the atrial surface of the mitral valve (C). High velocity regurgitant jets may also produce satellite infections on the chordae tendineae (B) from aortic regurgitation or within the left atrium (D) from mitral regurgitation. The ventricular surface of the anterior mitral valve (E) may also become infected because of its contact with the aortic regurgitant jet during ventricular diastole. (Adapted from Robard, SL: Blood velocity and endocarditis. Circulation 27:18, 1963, by permission of the American Heart Association, Inc.)

Pathogenesis

ABNORMAL VALVE

The factors leading to infective endocarditis vary depending on whether the affected valve is normal or abnormal. Based on the results in animals with experimental infective endocarditis and in reviewing the findings in both veterinary and human medicine, at least five factors have been proposed that interact to initiate infective endocarditis on abnormal valves.[3, 21, 29, 36, 37] These include hemodynamic factors, nonbacterial thrombus formation, transient bacteremia, microorganism thrombotic interaction, and immunologic factors.

Hemodynamic Factors. Robard showed how the Venturi effect can distribute a high-pressure infected stream into a low pressure sink and establish a characteristic colony distribution. Consistently, the colonies appeared just beyond the orifice, within the low pressure area.[38] This finding is easily demonstrated when infective endocarditis is associated with the high-pressure gradients seen with either aortic or mitral regurgitation (Figure 79–1). Typically, the bacteria colonize the lower pressure atrial surface of the mitral valve and the ventricular surface of the aortic valve. It is thought the Venturi effect causes a decrease in the lateral pressure and possibly a decrease in intimal perfusion immediately within the low pressure sink from the regurgitant flow, thus predisposing these areas to bacterial colonization. Similarly, a higher incidence of infective endocarditis is seen associated with those congenital heart defects having high pressure and velocity gradients (small ventricular defects and patent ductus arteriosus); this can be attributed to the Venturi effect. In addition, this may explain why infective endocarditis is uncommon with cardiac defects with low pressure gradients or low flow, such as large ventricular or atrial septal defects.

Besides the Venturi effect, high-velocity regurgitant jets from the turbulent stream can cause mechanical damage to the valvular endocardial surface and may also damage cardiac structures downstream (Figure 79–1).[39] These satellite areas are usually where the jet contacts the endocardial surface. With mitral regurgitation, damage is within the left atrial wall. When associated with aortic regurgitation, the chordae tendineae are affected. In humans with congestive heart failure, the incidence of infective endocarditis is much less common. This is thought to be caused by changes in the Venturi effect and decreases in the velocities of the regurgitant jets from diminished left ventricular function.[40]

Platelet-Fibrin Thrombus. Trauma to the endocardial surface from turbulence and jet effects of regurgitant flow may result in the exposure of collagen. This initiates a series of events similar to the platelet plug seen in other systemic vascular injuries. The end result is the deposition of a sterile platelet-fibrin thrombus. In experimental animals it is difficult to produce infective endocarditis without the initiating endocardial trauma and thrombus formation.[36, 41] The significance of the platelet-fibrin thrombus is that it may originate from any number of stresses or injuries to the endocardium.

Bacteremia. Bacteremias may occur at any time; they are a common occurrence, associated with numerous procedures. Most involve some manipulation that causes the intermittent release of bacteria. In humans, such procedures include dental work, bronchoscopy, endoscopy, chewing, and many others.[21, 42] Portals of entry in animals have been associated with dental work and routine extracardiac infections involving the skin, bone, lung, tonsils, intestine, urogenital tract, and prostate.[5, 7, 8, 9, 11, 25, 43–46] The severity of the bacteremia is low, with counts less than ten colony units/ml and they are of short duration, with a bacteremia of less than 30 minutes. Most transient bacteremias are of little clinical importance even when a platelet-fibrin thrombus is present. The failure of such organisms to implant on the thrombus is related to their very low numbers and low invasiveness.

Microorganism-Valve Interaction. The ability of some bacteria to adhere to the platelet-fibrin thrombus increases their pathogenicity in infective endocarditis. One study demonstrated that those organisms common in infective endocarditis adhered more readily to normal canine aortic leaflets in vitro than did organisms not commonly associated with infective endocarditis.[47] It has been shown that the adherence of some bacteria may depend on their ability to produce a complex extracellular polysaccharide called dextran. Dextran produced by some streptococcal organisms within the oral flora helps them adhere to the dental enamel and plays an important role in dental caries. This adhering ability of dextran-producing bacteria may also be an important factor in the pathogenesis of infective endocarditis.[48, 49]

The platelet aggregating ability of some of the bacteria may be a factor in the pathophysiology of infective endocarditis. Some of the staphylococcal and streptococcal bacteria aggregate platelets to a greater extent than do others.[50] In one study, very low numbers of platelets increased the adherence of streptococci to fibrin.[49] It is possible these bacteria have a greater affinity for the platelet-fibrin thrombi formed on damaged valves and endocardium.

Once bacteria have colonized an abnormal valve, deposition of fibrin and platelets and bacterial growth continues. As the thrombus enlarges, it serves as a protective barrier to natural host defenses. The uninhibited bacteria grow rapidly and large colony counts may develop within the vegetation. The effects of antimicrobial agents may be impaired by decreased metabolism of bacteria deep within the thrombus.[51]

Immunologic Factors. The role of circulating antibodies in the formation of infective endocarditis is still controversial. Circulating antibodies, particularly agglutinins, may cause accumulation of bacteria to a critical level, allowing replication sufficient to initiate adherence and infection on the platelet-fibrin thrombus.[3, 21, 52] However, in a recent study, the circulating antibodies are thought to be more protective by decreasing the number of circulating bacteria. Some strains of bacteria are eliminated by antibodies, complement, and other bactericidal factors, preventing the development of experimental infective endocarditis.[53]

NORMAL VALVE

The specific factors that lead to the infection of a normal valve are not completely understood. The development of the platelet-fibrin thrombus is probably not involved in the etiology of infective endocarditis on normal valves.[3, 21] However, transient bacteremia may play a more important role. A greater degree of bacteremia and the high virulence of the invading organism may allow only small numbers of bacteria to infect a normal valve.[21]

In addition, other factors may be involved that modify host resistance and play an important role in the establishment of infective endocarditis on normal valves. Additional factors include treatment with immunosuppressive agents, neoplasias, inappropriate antimicrobial therapy, and possibly, indwelling catheters.[11, 29, 37, 46]

PATHOLOGY

Cardiovascular Pathology

Vegetative thrombi of infective endocarditis develop mainly on the commissures of the mitral and/or aortic valves in dogs and cats.[2, 5, 7–14, 17, 18] Infections involving the valves of the right heart or mural endocardium are rare.[2, 7–14] The size and number of lesions are quite variable. They may be single or multiple and vary from a few millimeters to large vegetative lesions that impair normal valve function (Figure 79–2). Variation depends on the duration of the infection and virulence of the organism. Valvular destruction can be rapid with an acute virulent infection. Histologically, in acute infections many bacteria and polymorphonuclear leukocytes infiltrate the valve stroma, which become necrotic. Platelet-fibrin thrombus then covers the developing lesion.[3, 21] In fresh, subacute infections, which develop more slowly, three distinct layers can be identified: first, a superficial fibrin layer; second, a middle layer composed primarily of bacteria; and last, a deep layer of platelets, erythrocytes, leukocytes, and fewer bacteria.[3, 21] In contrast to the more ulcerative acute infections, the leukocytes in subacute infective endocarditis are usually histiocytes and lymphocytes, with fewer polymorphonuclear cells. The underlying valve stroma may also show evidence of repair with fibroplasia and capillary development.[21] Older vegetations may be more organized, with a layer of dense fibrous tissue, hyalinization, and possibly, calcification. Due to tissue organization, older vegetations tend to be less friable.[21, 54]

Prolapse or perforation of the valve may occur if necrosis and destruction are severe.[21, 37] In advanced infections the chordae tendineae may also be involved, leading to rupture and acute mitral regurgitation. Rapid

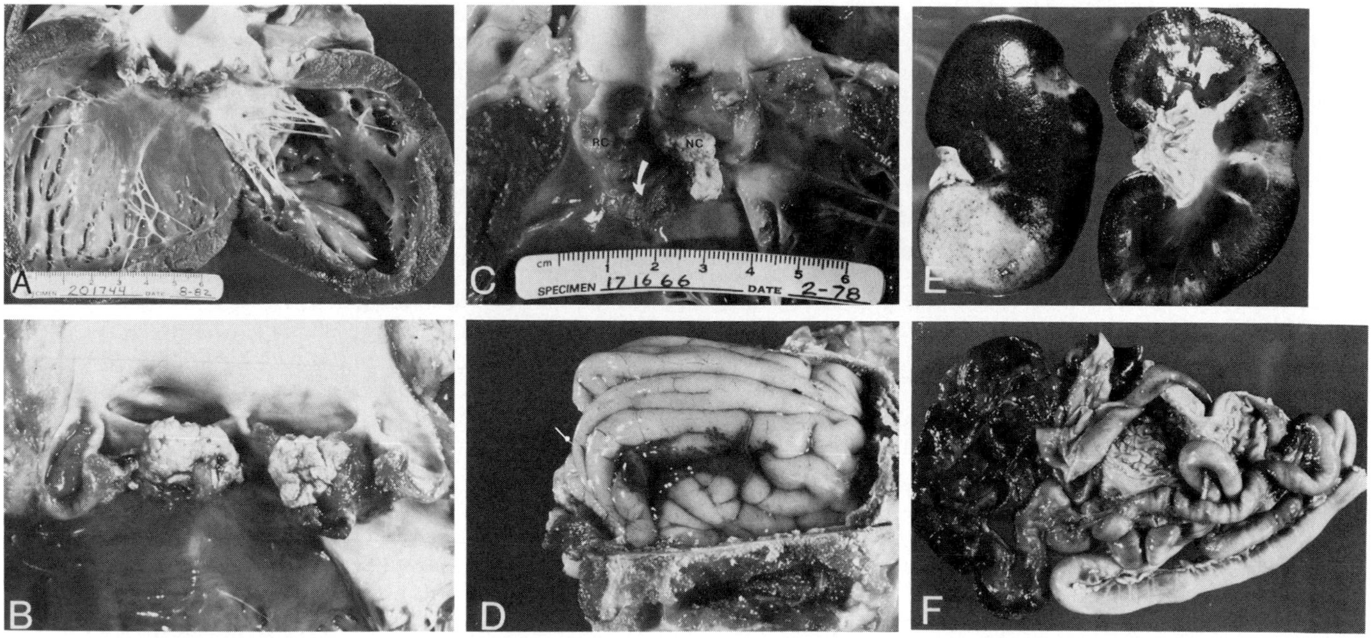

FIGURE 79–2. Pathologic findings in infective endocarditis. *A*, Left ventricular dilatation with aortic valve vegetative lesions in a dog. *B*, Large vegetative lesions associated with the ventricular surface of thickened aortic valve leaflets. *C*, Destruction of the right coronary cusp (RC) and avulsion of the noncoronary cusp (NC) resulting in aortic regurgitation. The arrow indicates a contact lesion where the flailed aortic leaflet impacted the ventricular septum just below the valve. Systemic embolization and infarction of the brain *(D)*, kidneys *(E)*, and mesenteric arteries to the small intestine *(F)* are common sequelae to infective endocarditis. (From Sisson, D and Thomas, WP: Endocarditis of the aortic valve in the dog. JAVMA 184:570, 1984.)

valve dysfunction with regurgitation can result in left heart failure and is a frequent occurrence in dogs dying of either aortic or mitral valve infective endocarditis.[11, 12, 25]

Once the valvular infection has been established, it may spread rapidly and involve the sinus of Valsalva, mural endocardium, valve annulus, pericardium, or myocardium. Various manifestations of the spreading infection have been reported. It may result in abscess formation, myocarditis, pericarditis, and possible involvement of the conduction system, causing any number of different arrhythmias.[11, 12, 37]

Extracardiac Pathology

Beeson demonstrated that bacteria are released from the vegetative thrombus at a relatively constant rate.[55] The predilection of infective endocarditis for the aortic and mitral valves and the development of friable vegetations can lead to systemic embolization, infarction, and metastatic infection. These factors are important in the pathogenesis of the clinical manifestation of systemic infective endocarditis. From studies reviewing necropsies, the kidney and spleen are the most commonly affected organs, but the heart, brain, intestine, and other organs may be affected as well (Figure 79–2).[8, 11–14, 17] Effects of embolization depend on the sizes of emboli, the organ affected, the amount of vascular obstruction, and the collateral circulation.[29, 37] Effects may be nonclinical, such as those in the spleen, or may result in serious organ impairment if the kidney or brain is involved.[12, 29, 56–59] Infections may be primary or secondary (metastatic). Therefore, the relative importance of septic arthritis, discospondylitis, and urinary tract infections is uncertain.[12, 29] The presence of rheumatoid factor, anti-nuclear antibodies, and circulating immune complexes can contribute to the development of renal glomerulonephritis, myocarditis, and polyarthritis associated with infective endocarditis in both animals and humans.[11, 12, 60–62]

CLINICAL MANIFESTATIONS

The diagnosis of infective endocarditis is often complicated by systemic involvement. Infective endocarditis invariably presents with a wide range of clinical signs that often mimic other diseases. Clinical manifestations may involve any organ system and can arise from four major processes. Interaction of the primary infected valve, embolization, secondary bacteremia, and abnormal globulin deposition can all lead to the clinical syndrome associated with infective endocarditis.

History and Clinical Signs

Most signs are nonspecific and often suggest systemic or extracardiac infection rather than primary cardiac disease. Weakness, lethargy, lameness, anorexia, and weight loss are the most common presenting complaints reported by owners.[11, 12] Lameness may be intermittent or continuous and may shift from one limb to another. Less common complaints, including vomiting, diarrhea, hemi- or paraparesis, seizures, and blindness, have also been described.[29] In some patients a history of surgery, dental work, immunosuppressive therapy, intravenous drug therapy, trauma, or a prior infection has been noted.[29, 46] Owners may observe cardiac signs (labored breathing, coughing, exercise intolerance) in addition to signs associated with other organ systems. Dogs with aortic rather than mitral valve involvement tend to show signs of congestive heart failure more frequently.[12] If tachyarrhythmias or heart block develops, then syncope or collapse may also be seen. Unfortunately, the history may lack evidence of a previous infection, an identifiable port of entry, or a pre-existing cardiac abnormality that may have initiated the infective endocarditis.[11, 12, 14, 18]

Physical Examination

Dogs with infective endocarditis usually have recurrent or persistent fever.[11] However, if the patient has a chronic infection, heart failure, or previous history of antibiotic or corticosteroid treatment, fever may not be present.[21] In one study it was shown that fever was more common in dogs with mitral infective endocarditis than in those with aortic infective endocarditis.[12]

Infective endocarditis should always be suspected in any patient in which an organic murmur develops rapidly. Systolic murmurs are commonly heard in both aortic and mitral infective endocarditis (Figure 79–3).[3, 11, 12, 21] These murmurs must be differentiated from physiologic murmurs of anemia or fever. In addition, murmurs from congenital or acquired heart disease must be identified, especially in older small-breed dogs, in which murmurs of mitral regurgitation are common. The significance of a rapidly changing and developing murmur has been exaggerated as an important indicator of the presence of infective endocarditis. In one study of infective endocarditis in dogs, only 65 per cent of the affected dogs had a murmur, whereas murmurs were detected in 95 per cent of the affected dogs in another study.[11, 12] In humans, up to 30 per cent of patients with acute and 10 per cent of those with subacute valvular infective endocarditis did not have murmurs at presentation.[21, 63, 64] Identification of a diastolic murmur in association with hyperkinetic pulses strongly indicates infective endocarditis with aortic regurgitation (Figure 79–3).[12, 20] Besides early diastolic murmurs, mid to late diastolic (Austin Flint type) murmurs may be heard in dogs.[12] An Austin Flint murmur is thought to originate from a functional mitral stenosis when the regurgitant stream of aortic insufficiency hits the anterior mitral valve leaflet, causing a premature closure of the mitral valve and simulating an organic mitral obstruction.[65, 66] In addition, S_3 gallop sounds are commonly heard, particularly when left heart failure is present. Several arrhythmias resulting from myocarditis, heart failure, myocardial infarction, or conduction system involvement can be auscultated as well.[12]

Hyperkinetic arterial pulses caused by a wide pulse pressure may be associated with aortic infective endocarditis and regurgitation. Two factors are responsible for the wide pressure difference. First, the lower diastolic pressure results from retrograde flow into the less resistant left ventricle and dilated peripheral arterioles. Second, the systolic pressure is elevated from the rapid ejection of a larger stroke volume.[67, 68] If the aortic regurgitation is severe, the head and extremities may "bob" (DeMussett's sign) with each contraction, due to the severely widened pulse pressure.[67] The severity of the hemodynamic effects of aortic regurgitation can be documented by obtaining direct or indirect measurement of arterial blood pressure (Figure 79–4).

The physical manifestations of systemic embolization, metastatic infection, and immune complex interaction are varied. Retinal hemorrhage, petechiation, hyphema, or epistaxis may occur.[29] Cold extremities, necrotic skin associated with pain, and cyanosis are strongly suggestive of peripheral arterial embolization. Septic or immune-mediated arthritis may be present, especially if shifting leg lameness, joint pain, or joint stiffness is noted. In two reported cases, the lameness was due to hypertrophic osteopathy secondary to infective endocarditis.[69, 70] In addition, a variety of neurologic signs may be present if the spinal cord or brain is involved.

DIAGNOSTIC TESTING

Blood Cultures

One of the most important diagnostic tests for the diagnosis and treatment of infective endocarditis is iso-

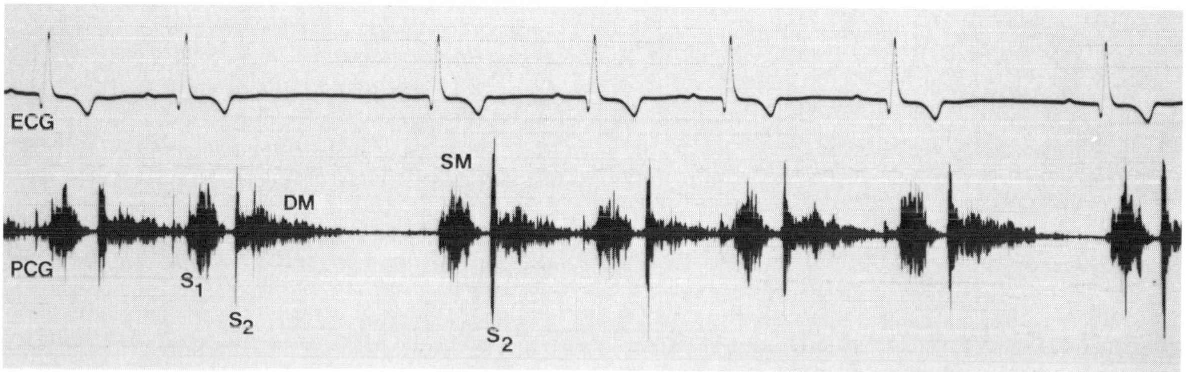

FIGURE 79–3. Phonocardiogram (PCG) and electrocardiogram (ECG) recorded at the left cardiac base from a dog with aortic endocarditis. A systolic murmur (SM) and an early decrescendo diastolic murmur (DM) are present. S_1 = first heart sound, S_2 = second heart. (From Sisson, D and Thomas, WP: Endocarditis of the aortic valve in the dog. JAVMA 184:570, 1984.)

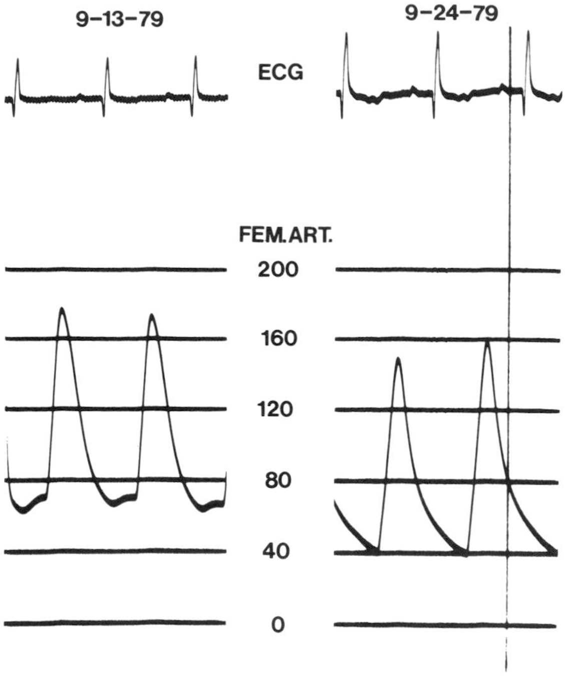

FIGURE 79–4. Direct femoral artery pressure measured in a dog with aortic regurgitation from infective endocarditis. On admission (left tracing) the systolic arterial pressure was elevated (170 mm Hg) and the diastolic arterial pressure was decreased (65 mm Hg), resulting in hyperkinetic pulses (pulse pressure = 105 mm Hg). As the aortic regurgitation and congestive heart failure progressed (right tracing 11 days later), the diastolic arterial pressure declined to 40 mm Hg and the pulse pressure increased to 120 mm Hg. (From Sisson, D and Thomas, WP: Endocarditis of the aortic valve in the dog. JAVMA 184:570, 1984.)

lation of the causative microorganism from blood cultures.[3, 21, 29, 37] Several investigators have demonstrated a continuous bacteremia associated with infective endocarditis.[55, 71, 72] Weiss showed that bacteremic showers correlated with increases in body temperature, but this was not documented in other studies.[73, 74] Most bacterial counts seen with infective endocarditis are low, with counts usually around 100 colonies/ml.[74, 75] Beeson and associates showed higher counts could be obtained by arterial samples, but counts were not significantly different from venous samples.[55] Therefore, most studies in humans have documented that the bacteremia of infective endocarditis is constant rather than intermittent and taking arterial samples at the time of fever does not necessarily increase the yield of positive cultures.

TECHNIQUE

Various protocols have been used to increase the yield of positive blood cultures in both humans and animals.[71, 76] Successful isolation depends on the number of samples, the volume of blood used in the inoculate, and the laboratory technology. Most protocols are designed around a few important concepts. After sterile preparation of the venipuncture site (jugular vein), two to three separate blood samples should be collected within a 24-hour period. The interval between samples should be greater than one hour, but in severe cases can be as frequent as every five minutes.[3] If antibiotics have been used, minimizing their effect can be achieved by (1) a 1:10 dilution of the sample to the culture broth, (2) adding sodium polyanetholsulfonate, which inactivates aminoglycosides (usually in commercial broths), and (3) using antimicrobial removal devices.[71] Studies have shown strong correlation of the volume of blood cultured to positive culture results.[77] Ideally, a minimum of 10 ml should be used for each sample in dogs or cats. In humans, 30 ml samples are routinely used.[71]

PROCESSING

Various blood culture media containing tryptic soy or biphasic broth are commercially available. The commercial media are designed for the cultivation of anaerobic bacteria, and unless vented will not permit the growth of pseudomonads or yeasts. Routinely, each sample is divided into equal amounts for both anaerobic and aerobic cultivation. Each is inoculated into two tryptic soy broth media and one is vented for aerobic growth. Some microbiologists even recommend using a third bottle of biphasic media to increase yield.[71] Most clinically important bacteria can be isolated within seven days.[74] However, fastidious, slow-growing bacteria may need 7 to 23 days to become evident. Because of this, blood cultures should be allowed to incubate for at least three weeks before being discarded.

Blood cultures are considered positive if the same organism is cultured in two or more different samples. In dogs with infective endocarditis, 75 per cent had positive blood cultures.[12] In spite of the rigorous technique, culture-negative infective endocarditis may still occur. Factors that may lead to culture-negative infective endocarditis include recent antibiotic therapy, uremia, chronic endocarditis, and nonbacterial or noninfective endocarditis.[3, 21]

Electrocardiography

The electrocardiogram is typically abnormal in dogs with infective endocarditis but usually indicates nonspecific findings (Figure 79–5).[5, 11–13] Chamber enlargement may be evident, especially if the infection is longstanding and congestive heart failure is present. Arrhythmias and conduction defects may be seen in up to 75 per cent of the affected dogs.[11, 12] If aortic infective endocarditis invades the upper septal myocardium, the A-V node or conduction system may be involved, leading to various A-V blocks, branch blocks, or arrhythmias. S-T segment elevation or depression consistent with hypoxia from coronary embolism or myocardial infarction may also be noted. In one study in humans, evidence of heart block and infarction carried a poorer prognosis.[78] Serial electrocardiograms may be helpful in assessing the progression of infective endocarditis in dogs.

Radiography

Radiographic changes with infective endocarditis are nonspecific, reflecting changes associated with chamber

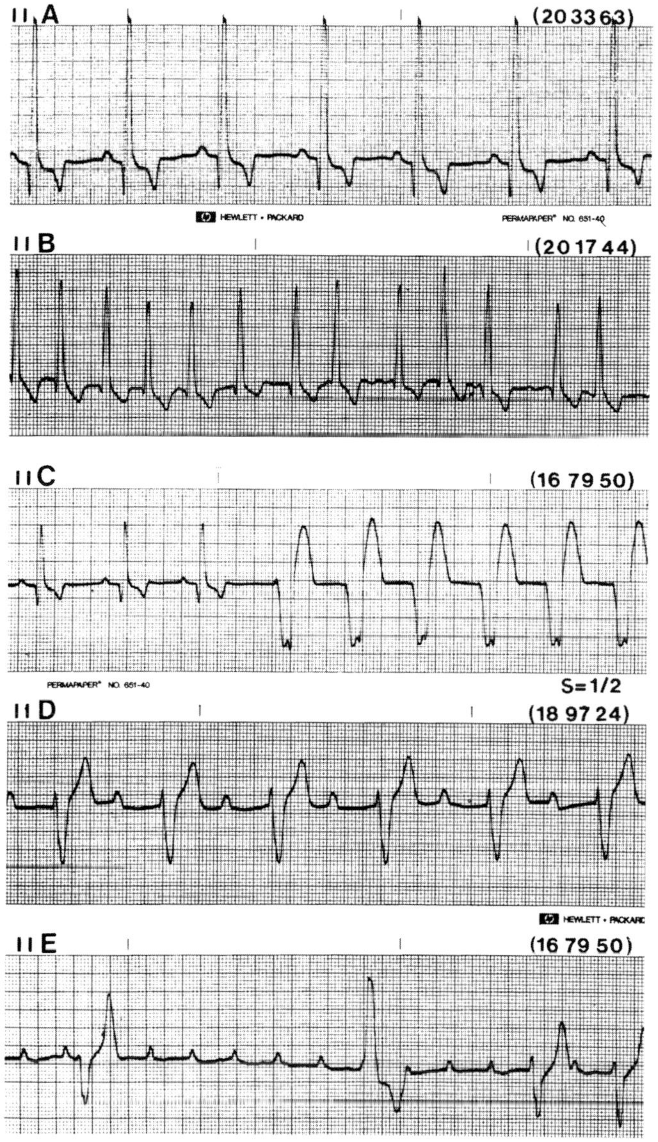

FIGURE 79–5. Common electrocardiographic abnormalities associated with infective endocarditis. *A*, Indicates increased P wave duration and QRS amplitude consistent with left atrial and ventricular enlargement recorded in a six year old female Labrador Retriever. A variety of arrhythmias may arise from infective endocarditis. *B*, Demonstrates atrial fibrillation in a seven year old male Doberman Pinscher with aortic endocarditis. *C*, Demonstrates ventricular tachycardia in a five year old male Boxer. If the infective lesion involves the conduction system, then various conduction abnormalities may develop. *D*, Shows a seven-year-old male German shepherd dog with first degree AV block and right bundle branch block. *E*, Tracing from the same dog in (C) recorded after progression of the endocarditis. Tracing demonstrates the development of complete AV block in addition to the ventricular arrhythmias. These arrhythmias may occur especially if the AV node is involved. Paper speed = 50 mm/sec. Sensitivity 1 cm = 1 mV except where indicated. (From Sisson, D and Thomas, WP: Endocarditis of the aortic valve in the dog. JAVMA 184:570, 1984.)

enlargement and signs related to congestive heart failure. Radiographs may help stage the severity of congestive heart failure and aid in the prognosis of dogs or cats with infective endocarditis. In some cases, cardiac catheterization and angiocardiography assist in the assessment of hemodynamic changes and provide more definitive assessment of left ventricular function (Figure 79–6).[37]

Echocardiography

Echocardiography has been a valuable diagnostic tool in the evaluation of patients suspected of having infective endocarditis. Its use in animals has been reported on several occasions.[12, 37, 25, 79–82] The advantage of M-mode and two-dimensional echocardiography results from its ability to noninvasively image internal cardiac structures, to detect vegetative lesions, and to indirectly determine abnormal hemodynamic parameters (Figure 79–7).[83–85] Echocardiography is particularly beneficial in infective endocarditis patients that are culture-negative or do not have a suspicious murmur; however, it is not an alternative to properly performed blood cultures. Echocardiography may detect vegetative lesions as small as two millimeters and allows visualization of cardiac complications such as ventricular dilatation, flailed leaflets, and ruptured chordae tendineae. Aortic valve vegetations are readily imaged, but it is difficult to distinguish mitral vegetations from myxomatous degeneration. M-mode examination of infective endocarditis reveals multiple linear echoes, usually seen only during diastole.[83] M-mode also allows for indirect assessment of aortic regurgitation by evaluating mitral valve function and movement. These changes are seen as mitral valve flutter and premature closure of the mitral valve in advanced cases of aortic regurgitation. Two-dimensional echocardiography gives a better picture of the spatial relationship of affected valves and allows estimation of leaflet involvement, mobility, and shape. Echocardiography can yield information that provides prognostic indications for infective endocarditis. In humans, it has been suggested that those cases of infective endocarditis with vegetations have a poorer prognosis than those without lesions, and patients with aortic infective endocarditis carry a poorer prognosis than those with mitral infective endocarditis.[86, 87] Echocardiography enables indirect determination of left ventricular function for use in monitoring the severity and progression of infective endocarditis.

Laboratory Findings

Fifty to sixty per cent of dogs with infective endocarditis have a mild normocytic, normochromic anemia similar to anemias occurring with infection or chronic disease.[11, 12] Affected dogs may have a leukocytosis with a left shift. Leukocytosis is present in 80 per cent or more of dogs with infective endocarditis. In most cases this is due to a relative neutrophilia and monocytosis.[11, 12] Left shift may only be noted in later stages of infective endocarditis if there is significant systemic involvement. The blood urea nitrogen is frequently elevated and may reflect renal changes associated with infarction, glomerulonephritis, or embolization. Pyuria, hematuria, and proteinuria detected on urinalysis may represent primary renal involvement. Urine cultures can be misleading and should not be substituted for blood

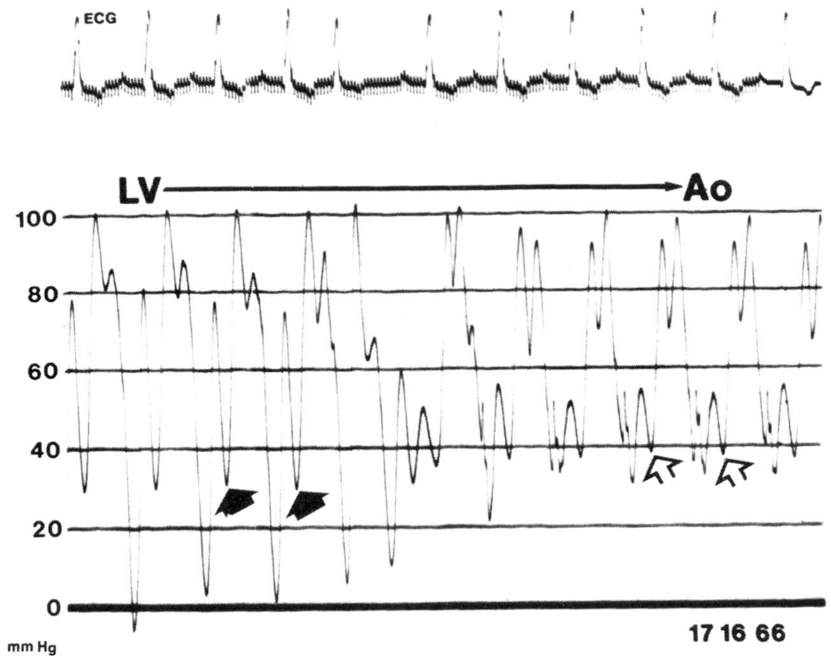

FIGURE 79–6. Left ventricular catheterization from the left ventricle (LV) to the aorta (Ao) in a dog with severe aortic regurgitation from infective endocarditis. The left ventricular end diastolic pressures are increased (closed arrows), consistent with left ventricular failure. The arterial diastolic pressures (open arrows) are decreased and approach the left ventricular end diastolic pressures indicating severe aortic regurgitation. The exact pressures are difficult to determine due to catheter whip artifact. (From Sisson, D and Thomas, WP: Endocarditis of the aortic valve in the dog. JAVMA 184:570, 1984.)

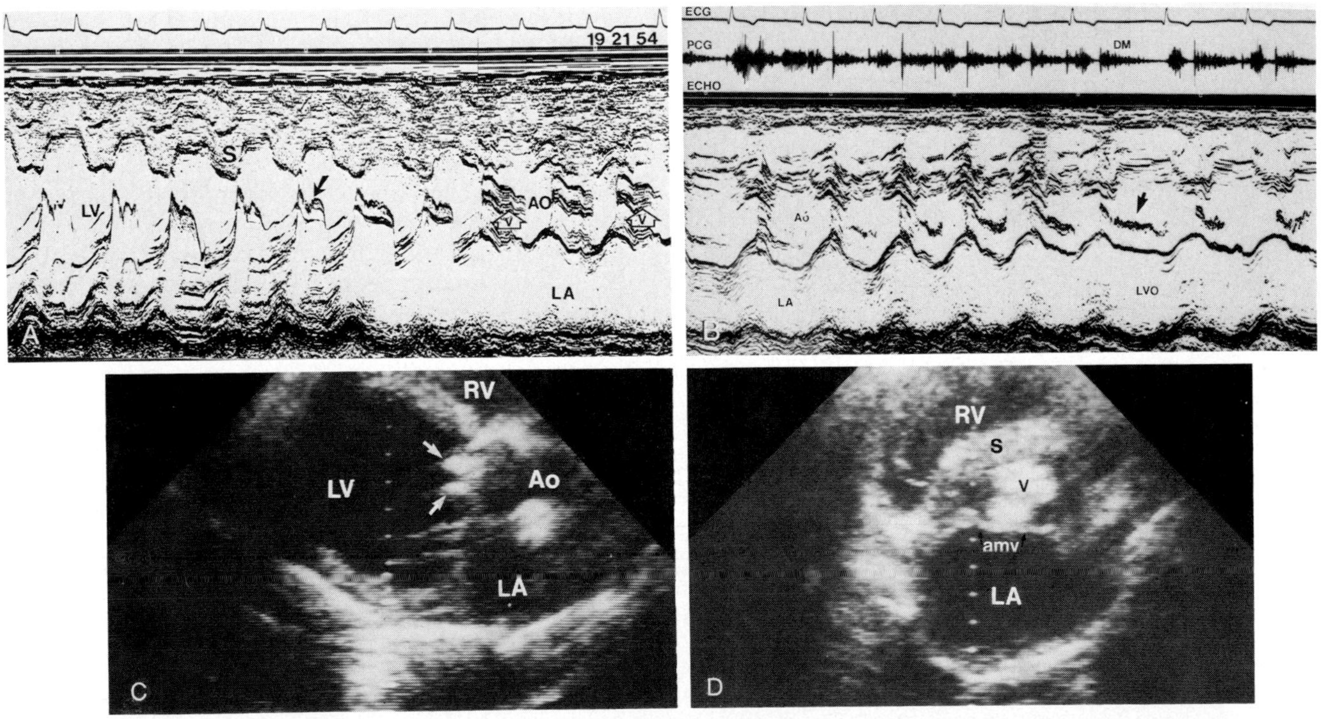

FIGURE 79–7. M-mode and two-dimensional echocardiography in infective endocarditis. *A*, M-mode echocardiogram showing multiple parallel linear echos (enclosed V) in the aortic root (Ao) during diastole. The findings are typical of aortic valve vegetations. Diastolic fluttering of the mitral valve (closed arrow) reflects aortic regurgitation. *B*, M-mode echocardiogram recorded simultaneously with an electrocardiogram (ECG) and phonocardiogram (PCG). A thickened flailed leaflet (closed arrow) is present in the left ventricular outflow tract (LVO). Note the association of the flailed leaflet during diastole with the pronounced diastolic murmur (DM) on the PCG. *C*, A long-axis two-dimensional echocardiogram recorded in the right parasternal view. Large aortic valve vegetations (arrows) are seen prolapsing into the left ventricle (LV). The left ventricle is also dilated from the volume overload of aortic regurgitation. *D*, A short-axis view 90° perpendicular to *C*. The large vegetative lesions (V) are seen in the left ventricular outflow tract between the anterior mitral valve (amv) and the ventricular septum (S). LV = left ventricle, LA = left atrium, S = ventricular septum, Ao = aorta, RV = right ventricle. M-mode echocardiograms recorded at a paper speed of 50 min/sec and depth markers (1 cm) are shown at 1 second intervals. Two-dimensional echocardiograms show 1 cm depth markers in the center of the images. (Figures *A*, *C*, and *D* from Sisson, D and Thomas, WP: Endocarditis of the aortic valve in the dog. JAVMA 184:570, 1984.)

cultures. A variety of other abnormal laboratory tests have been related to infective endocarditis, including positive anti-nuclear antibodies and Coombs' test. In addition, cytological analysis of joint fluid and cerebral spinal fluid may reveal septic or nonseptic inflammation.[11, 37, 62]

Diagnosis

A definitive diagnosis of infective endocarditis can be made when a positive blood culture is seen with evidence of cardiac involvement, i.e., a new murmur, hyperkinetic pulses, signs of congestive heart failure, and especially, echocardiographic visualization of vegetative lesions. Signs of systemic embolization also support the diagnosis. If blood cultures are negative, then the diagnosis must be made based on the combination of cardiac signs with evidence of systemic infection and/or signs of embolization. It is particularly difficult to separate mitral infective endocarditis from acquired mitral regurgitation with concurrent bacteremia. In most instances, if clinical signs suggest cardiac infection, then a tentative diagnosis of infective endocarditis should be made until proven otherwise.

MANAGEMENT

Therapy

The major goals in treatment of infective endocarditis are to arrest and control the progression of valvular damage and cardiac complications, to eliminate the primary infection, and to prevent systemic involvement and embolization. Each case is unique, and proper management dictates individualized therapy. All factors must be taken into account when recommending a therapeutic regimen. Treatment should be aggressive and intense with frequent reassessments to maximize conditions for a favorable response. Recommendations for the treatment of animals are adapted from human treatments for the management of infective endocarditis.[3, 88]

ANTIMICROBIAL THERAPY

Most patients have been ill for extended periods, and the time required to obtain blood cultures will not alter the course of the disease significantly. In fact, failure to identify the causative agent can result in improper antibiotic therapy, prolonged treatment and recovery, increased risk of complications, progressive valvular destruction and heart failure, and relapse of infection. Once the organism has been identified, antimicrobial sensitivity and minimum inhibitory concentrations (MIC) should be performed. In addition, minimum bactericidal concentrations (MBC) and serum bactericidal titers (SBT) are helpful for optimal antibiotic therapy.

Antimicrobial therapy should not be delayed while waiting for culture and sensitivity results. Empirical therapy should be started after blood cultures have been obtained. Ideally, initial choices include a combination of bactericidal antibiotics sensitive to potential penicillin-resistant staphylococci and gram-negative bacteria. Once the infective agent has been identified, the initial regimen should be modified to reflect sensitivities, MIC, MBC, and SBT.

Ability to penetrate fibrin thrombi is an important factor in selecting an appropriate antimicrobial drug. Antibiotics used can be given safely at doses higher than serum concentrations and greater than the MBC (Table 79–1). Following initial antibiotic administration, SBT may be useful in measuring the patient's serum bactericidal effectiveness. Penicillin or synthetic penicillins are usually effective against streptococci and anaerobes. Gram-negative bacteria typically respond to aminoglycosides, and sometimes ampicillin and cephalosporins. Staphylococcal infections should be treated with cephalosporins or penicillinase-resistant penicillins. Culture-negative infective endocarditis is treated as if a *Pseudomonas, E. coli*, or penicillin-resistant staphylococci were present. This routinely requires the combination of a penicillin or cephalosporin and an aminoglycoside.

Antibiotics should be administered intravenously rather than orally. Absorption from the gastrointestinal tract is variable and unpredictable. Antibiotics should be given for four to six weeks. Unfortunately, long-term parenteral therapy is impractical for most veterinary patients. One alternative is to administer antibiotics intravenously for 7 to 14 days in the hospital. If the patient responds favorably, then parenteral administration can be followed by oral medication for an additional three to four weeks. If aminoglycoside therapy is instituted, renal function should be routinely evaluated. Amikacin is used by the authors if renal function is compromised or if long-term aminoglycoside therapy is indicated.

TREATMENT OF OTHER FACTORS

All patients should be evaluated for a source of the infection. Concurrent infections reported in animals with infective endocarditis include periodontal disease, prostatitis, pneumonia, abscesses, urinary tract infections, and discospondylitis.[29] Any extracardiac infections should be aggressively treated by either medical or surgical means. Systemic embolization and infarctions are difficult to manage. Anticoagulants have not been shown to reduce systemic complications, and severe hemorrhage may result.[21]

Cardiac complications should be treated aggressively. If congestive heart failure is present, appropriate management should begin using cardiac glycosides, diuretics, and vasodilators (see Chapter 73). The patient should be monitored for severe tachyarrhythmias as well. Sustained supraventricular tachycardias, multifocal ventricular premature contractions, or ventricular tachycardia requires appropriate antiarrhythmic therapy (see Chapter 76). Conduction abnormalities may also occur. If severe bradycardias or heart block are present, then pacemaker implantation (temporary or permanent) may be indicated.

TABLE 79–1. ANTIMICROBIAL THERAPY FOR INFECTIVE ENDOCARDITIS

Organism	First Choice	Alternative	Resistance
Staphylococcus	CEP, PEN, or AMP* OXA†	GEN or CHPC‡	PEN, AMP
β-Hemolytic streptococcus	PEN or AMP	CEP, CHPC‡, or ERY‡	GEN, AMK
E. coli	AMP,* GEN, or AMK	AMP* or TIC	PEN, AMP, CEP
Pseudomonas	GEN or AMK CARB + GEN	TIC, CARB	PEN, AMP, CEP
Klebsiella	GEN or AMK	CEP or TIC	PEN, AMP CHPC
Corynebacterium	PEN or AMP	CEP or ERY	—
Erysipelothrix	PEN or AMP	CEP	—
Anaerobes	PEN or AMP	CEP, CHPC‡, or CLIN‡	GEN
Culture negative	PEN + GEN OXA + GEN	CEP +/− GEN or AMK	—

AMK	= amikacin	5 mg/kg	IV, IM, SC	q 8 h
AMP	= sodium ampicillin	10 mg/kg	IV, IM, SC	q 6 h
CARB	= disodium carbenicillin	15–50 mg/kg	IV	q 6–8 h
CEP	= cephalothin	33 mg/kg	IV, IM	q 8 h
CHPC	= chloramphenicol	45–60 mg/kg	IV, IM, SC	q 8 h
CLIN	= clindamycin	10 mg/kg	PO	q 12 h
ERY	= erythromycin	5–20 mg/kg	PO	q 8 h
GEN	= gentamicin	2–4 mg/kg	IV, IM, SC	q 8 h
OXA	= oxacillin	8–15 mg/kg	IV, IM, SC	q 6 h
PEN	= sodium penicillin G	20,000 U/kg	IV, IM, SC	q 6 h
TIC	= ticarcillin	35 mg/kg	IV, IM, SC	q 6 h

*Only if sensitive.
†Only if resistant to CEP, PEN, and AMP.
‡Use only after parenteral therapy with clinical response.

VALVE REPLACEMENT

In humans, patients with acute onset aortic infective endocarditis and concurrent congestive heart failure undergo emergency valve replacement to avoid a fatal outcome. Ideally, valve replacement in animals would be the treatment of choice to properly control severe cases of infective endocarditis. However, because of economic and technical limitations, valve replacement is not a viable option for most veterinary patients. One of the authors has attempted valve replacements in two dogs with severe aortic infective endocarditis. Both died immediately following surgery from a combination of problems related to the underlying disease and surgical complications.

REEVALUATION

Patients should be monitored daily during treatment. Performing a complete physical and cardiac examination may detect subtle changes that may precede an acute hemodynamic decompensation. In addition, routine laboratory tests should be performed to assess renal and hepatic function. Follow-up blood cultures at two days, and at one and two months following initiation of therapy should be obtained to assess efficacy of treatment and to detect relapse.

Prophylaxis

Prevention of infective endocarditis requires identification of susceptible individuals and knowledge of procedures or circumstances that may precipitate transient bacteremias. Use of prophylaxis in humans and animals is still controversial. Recommendations are based on adaptation of protocols from human medicine, limited experimental studies in animals, and one report of bacteremia-associated dental management in dogs.[3, 21, 43, 89, 90] The American Heart Association recommends chemoprophylaxis in patients with underlying cardiac disease undergoing dental manipulation, or surgical or diagnostic procedures involving the respiratory, urogenital, or gastrointestinal tracts.[91] General guidelines include using a broad spectrum antibiotic (cephalosporin, ampicillin, erythromycin) 1 to 2 hours before the procedure, followed by appropriate dosing for an additional 12 to 24 hours. In dogs and cats with pre-existing heart disease, particularly fibrous subaortic stenosis, ampicillin and gentamicin given 1 hour before and continued for an additional 24 hours have been recommended as prophylactic measures.[29]

PROGNOSIS

Long-term prognosis for infective endocarditis in dogs is extremely poor. Most die from sepsis, systemic embolization, renal failure, arrhythmias, or congestive heart failure. Congestive heart failure is the single most reported cause of death in dogs with infective endocarditis.[12] In most cases, congestive heart failure progressed until it became unresponsive to medical management or severe arrhythmias developed. The survival times ranged from a few days to almost two years, but the majority of patients died or were euthanized within six months of diagnosis.

Prognosis is influenced by the virulence of the causative agent, hemodynamic consequences, development of congestive heart failure, and severity of the extracardiac complications. A more favorable prognosis may occur if aggressive therapy is begun before severe valvular damage and systemic complications develop.[12] Unexplained fever in association with other nonspecific systemic signs necessitates a high index of suspicion of infective endocarditis.

References

1. Rivière, L: Cited by Major RH: Notes on the history of endocarditis. Bull Hist Med 17:351, 1945.
2. Schornagel, H: Endocarditis. Tijdschr Diergeneeskd 63:57, 143, 1936.
3. Wilson, WR, et al.: Infective endocarditis. *In* Brandenburg RO, et al. (eds): Cardiology: Fundamentals and Practice. Chicago, Yearbook Medical Publishers, 1987, p 1504.
4. Ettinger, SJ and Suter, PF: Canine Cardiology. Philadelphia, WB Saunders, 1970.
5. Murdoch, DB and Baker, JR: Bacterial endocarditis in the dog. J Sm Anim Pract 18:687, 1977.
6. Jones, TC and Zook, BC: Aging changes in the vascular system of animals. Ann NY Acad Sci 127:671, 1965.
7. Lundh, T: Fibrinous endocarditis in dogs. Acta Vet Scand 5:17, 1964.
8. Shouse, C and Meier, H: Acute vegetative endocarditis in the dog and cat. JAVMA 129:278, 1956.
9. Detweiler, DK, et al.: The prevalence of spontaneously occurring cardiovascular disease in dogs. Am J Public Health 51:228, 1961.
10. Winquist, G: Topografisk och etiologisk sammanstallning de fibrinosa och ulcerosa endokarditerna hos en del av vora husdjur. Skand Vet Tidskr 35:575, 1945.
11. Calvert, CA: Valvular bacterial endocarditis in the dog. JAVMA 180:1080, 1982.
12. Sisson, D and Thomas, WP: Endocarditis of the aortic valve in the dog. JAVMA 184:570, 1984.
13. Drazner, FH: Bacterial endocarditis in the dog. Comp Cont Ed Prac Vet 1:918, 1979.
14. Anderson, CA and Dubielzig, RR: Vegetative endocarditis in dogs. JAAHA 20:149, 1984.
15. Gelfman, R and Levine, SA: The incidence of acute and subacute bacterial endocarditis in congenital heart disease. Am J Med Sci 204:324, 1942.
16. Johnson, CM and Rhodes, HK: Pediatric endocarditis. Mayo Clin Proc 57:86, 1982.
17. Muna, WFT, et al.: Discrete subaortic stenosis in Newfoundland dogs: Association of infective endocarditis. Am J Cardiol 41:746, 1978.
18. Calvert, CA, et al.: Cardiovascular infections in dogs: Epizootiology, clinical manifestations, and prognosis. JAVMA 187:612, 1985.
19. Buchanan, JW: Valvular disease (endocardiosis in dogs). Adv Vet Sci Comp Med 21:75, 1979.
20. Lunginbuhl, H and Detweiler, DK: Cardiovascular lesions in dogs. Ann NY Acad Sci 127:5, 1965.
21. Weinstein, L: Infective endocarditis. *In* Braunwald E (ed): Heart Disease, A Textbook of Cardiovascular Medicine, 3rd ed. Philadelphia, WB Saunders, 1988, p 1093.
22. Uwaydah, MM and Weinberg, AN: Bacterial endocarditis—a changing pattern. N Engl J Med 273:1231, 1965.
23. Kaye, D, et al.: Bacterial endocarditis: the changing patterns since introduction of penicillin therapy. *In* Antimicrobial Agents and Chemotherapy. Washington DC, American Society of Microbiology, 1961, p 37.
24. Lerner, PI and Weinstein, L: Infective endocarditis in the antibiotic era. N Engl J Med 274:199, 1966.
25. Lombard, CW and Buergelt, CD: Vegetative bacterial endocarditis in dogs; echocardiographic diagnosis and clinical signs. J Sm Anim Pract 24:325, 1983.
26. Hoenig, M and Gillette, DM: Endocarditis caused by *Erysipelothrix rhusiopathiae* in a dog. JAVMA 176:326, 1980.
27. Henik, RA, et al.: Endocarditis caused by *Corynebacterium* sp. in a dog. JAVMA 189:1458, 1986.
28. Eriksen, K, et al.: Endocarditis in two dogs caused by *Erysipelothrix rhusiopathiae*. J Sm Anim Prac 28:117, 1987.
29. Sisson, D: Acquired valvular heart disease in dogs and cats. *In* Bonagura JD (ed): Contemporary Issues in Small Animal Practice—Cardiology, vol 7. New York, Churchill Livingstone, 1987, p 59.
30. Scheld, WM and Sande, MA: Endocarditis and intravascular infections. *In* Mandell GL, et al. (eds): Principles and Practice of Infectious Diseases, 2nd ed. New York, John Wiley and Sons, 1985, p 504.
31. Applefeld, MM, et al.: Q fever endocarditis—a case occuring in the United States. Am Heart J 93:669, 1977.
32. Jones, RB, et al.: Subacute chlamydial endocarditis. JAMA 247:655, 1982.
33. Brandenburg, RO, et al.: Infective endocarditis—a 25 year overview of diagnosis and therapy. J Am Coll Cardiol 1:280, 1983.
34. Wilson, WR and Washington, JA II: Infective endocarditis—a changing spectrum? (Editorial). Mayo Clin Proc 52:254, 1977.
35. Tompsett, R: Bacterial endocarditis: Changes in the clinical spectrum. Arch Intern Med 119:329, 1967.
36. Wright, AJ and Wilson, WR: Experimental animal endocarditis. Mayo Clin Proc 57:10, 1982.
37. Bonagura, JD: Bacterial endocarditis. *In* Ettinger SJ (ed): Textbook of Veterinary Internal Medicine, 2nd ed. Philadelphia, WB Saunders, 1983, p 1052.
38. Robard, S: Blood velocity and endocarditis. Circulation 27:18, 1963.
39. Lepeschkin, E: On the relation between the site of valvular involvement in endocarditis and the blood pressure resting on the valve. Am J Med Sci 224:31, 1952.
40. Allen, AC: Mechanism of localization of vegetative of bacterial endocarditis. Arch Pathol 27:399, 1939.
41. Angrist, AA, et al.: Experimental endocarditis. *In* Kaye D (ed): Infective Endocarditis. Baltimore, University Park Press, 1976, p 11.
42. Everett, ED and Hirschman, JV: Transient bacteremias and endocarditis: a review. Medicine 56:61, 1977.
43. Black, AP: Bacteremia during ultrasonic teeth cleaning and extraction in the dog. JAAHA 16:611, 1980.
44. Eyster, GE, et al.: Aortic regurgitation in the dogs. JAVMA 168:138, 1976.
45. Dear, MG: Bacterial endocarditis. *In* Kirk RW (ed): Current Veterinary Therapy VI. Philadelphia, WB Saunders, 1977, p 357.
46. Calvert, CA and Greene, CE: Bacteremia in dogs: diagnosis, treatment, and prognosis. Comp Cont Ed Prac Vet 8:179, 1986.
47. Gould, K, et al.: Adherence of bacteria to heart valves in vitro. J Clin Invest 56:1364, 1975.
48. Holmes, RK and Ramirez-Rhonda, CH: Adherence of bacteria to the endothelium of heart valves. *In* Infective Endocarditis, an American Heart Association Monograph, No 52:12, 1977.
49. Scheld, WM, et al.: Bacterial adherence in the pathogenesis of endocarditis: Interaction of bacterial dextran, platelets, and fibrin. J Clin Invest 61:1394, 1978.
50. Clawson, CC, et al.: Platelet interaction with bacteria. IV. Stimulation of the release reaction. Am J Pathol 81:411, 1975.
51. Durack, DT and Beeson, PB: Experimental bacterial endocarditis. II. Survival of bacteria in endocardial vegetations. Br J Exp Pathol 53:50, 1972.
52. Wadsworth, AB: A study of the endocardial lesions developing during pneumococcus infection in horses. J Med Res 34:279, 1919.
53. Durack, DT, et al.: Effect of immunization on susceptibility to experimental *Streptococcus mutans* and *Streptococcus sanguis* endocarditis. Infect Immunol 22:52, 1978.
54. Durney, ER and Phil, MB: Endocarditis. *In* Hurst JW, et al. (eds): The Heart, Arteries and Veins, 6th ed. New York, McGraw-Hill, 1986, p 1130.
55. Beeson, PB, et al.: Observations on the sites of removal of bacteria from the blood in patients with bacterial endocarditis. J Exp Med 81:9, 1945.
56. Knight, DN, et al.: Clinico-pathologic conference (chronic endocarditis in dogs). JAVMA 160:212, 1972.

57. Neilson, SW and Neilson, LB: Coronary embolism in valvular bacterial endocarditis in the dog. JAVMA 125:376, 1954.
58. Fregin, GF, et al.: Myocardial infarction in a dog with bacterial endocarditis. JAVMA 160:956, 1972.
59. Swanwick, RA and Williams, OJ: Fatal myocardial infarct in a greyhound. J Small Anim Pract 23:451, 1982.
60. Phair, JP and Clarke, J: Immunology of infective endocarditis. Prog Cardiovasc Dis 22:137, 1979.
61. Bayer, AS, et al.: Circulating immune complexes in infective endocarditis. New Engl J Med 27:1500, 1977.
62. Bennett, D, et al.: Bacterial endocarditis with polyarthritis in 2 (Alsatian) dogs associated with circulating autoantibodies. J Sm Anim Pract 19:185, 1978.
63. Weinstein, L and Rubin, RH: Infective endocarditis—1973. Progr Cardiovasc Dis 16:239, 1973.
64. Weinstein, L: Modern infective endocarditis: Past, present and future. JAMA 233:260, 1975.
65. Perloff, JK: Systolic, diastolic and continuous murmurs. *In* Hurst JW (ed): The Heart, 4th ed. New York, McGraw-Hill, 1978, p 268.
66. Craige, E: Echophonocardiography and other noninvasive techniques to elucidate heart murmurs. *In* Braunwald E (ed): Heart Disease, A Textbook of Cardiovascular Medicine, 3rd ed. Philadelphia, WB Saunders, 1988, p 65.
67. Braunwald, E: The physical examination. *In* Braunwald E (ed): Heart Disease, A Textbook of Cardiovascular Medicine, 3rd ed. Philadelphia, WB Saunders, 1988, p 13.
68. Johnson, AD, et al.: The medical and surgical management of patients with aortic valve disease. A symposium—University of California, San Diego, and San Diego Veterans Administration Hospital (Specialty Conference). West J Med 126:460, 1977.
69. Brodey, RS: Hypertrophic osteoarthropathy in the dog. A clinicopathologic survey of 60 cases. JAVMA 159:1242, 1971.
70. Vulgamott, JC and Clark, RG: Arterial hypertension and hypertrophic pulmonary osteopathy associated with aortic valvular endocarditis in a dog. JAVMA 177:243, 1980.
71. Washington, JA II: The role of the microbiology laboratory in the diagnosis and antimicrobial treatment of infective endocarditis. Mayo Clin Proc 57:22, 1982.
72. Mallèn MS, et al.: Comparative study of blood cultures made from artery, vein, and bone morrow in patients with subacute bacterial endocarditis. Am Heart J 33:692, 1947.
73. Weiss, H and Ottenberg, R: Relation between bacteria and temperature in subacute bacterial endocarditis. J Infect Dis 50:61, 1932.
74. Wright, HD: The bacteriology of subacute infective endocarditis. Pathol Bacteriol 28:541, 1925.
75. Werner, AS, et al.: Studies on the bacteremia of bacterial endocarditis. JAMA 202:199, 1967.
76. Hirsh, DC, et al.: Blood culture of the canine patient. JAVMA 184:175, 1984.
77. Washington, JA II: The Detection of Septicemia. West Palm Beach, Florida, CRC Press, 1978.
78. Miller, MH and Casey, JI: Infective endocarditis: New diagnostic technique. Am Heart J 96:123, 1978.
79. Bonagura, JD and Pipers, FS: Echocardiographic features of aortic valve endocarditis in a dog, a cow, and a horse. JAVMA 182:595, 1983.
80. Pipers, FS, et al.: Echocardiographic diagnosis of endocarditis in a bull. JAVMA 172:1313, 1978.
81. Ware, WA, et al.: Echocardiographic diagnosis of pulmonic valve vegetative endocarditis. JAVMA 188:185, 1986.
82. Lacuata, AO, et al.: Electrocardiographic and echocardiographic findings in four cases of bovine endocarditis. JAVMA 176:1355, 1980.
83. Feigenbaum, H: Echocardiography, 4th ed. Philadelphia, Lea and Febiger, 1986.
84. Wann, IS, et al.: Echocardiography in bacterial endocarditis. N Engl J Med 295:135, 1976.
85. Roy, P, et al.: Spectrum of echocardiographic findings in bacterial endocarditis. Circulation 53:474, 1976.
86. Young, JB, et al.: Prognostic significance of valvular vegetations identified by M-mode echocardiography in infective endocarditis. Circulation 58:11, 1978.
87. Come, PC, et al.: Diagnostic accuracy of M-mode echocardiography in active infective endocarditis and prognostic implications of ultrasound-detectable vegetations. Am Heart J 103:839, 1982.
88. Wilson, WR, et al.: General considerations in the diagnosis and treatment of infective endocarditis. Mayo Clin Proc 57:81, 1982.
89. Chadwick, EG and Stanford, ST: Prevention of infective endocarditis. Mod Concepts Cardiovasc Dis 55:11, 1986.
90. Keys, TF: Antimicrobial prophylaxis for patients with congenital or valvular heart disease. Mayo Clin Proc 57:171, 1982.
91. Kaplan, EL, et al.: Prevention of bacterial endocarditis. Circulation 56:139A, 1977.

80 HEARTWORM DISEASE

CLARENCE A. RAWLINGS and CLAY A. CALVERT

EPIZOOTIOLOGY

Heartworm disease is distributed widely in the United States. Few veterinarians practice in areas where heartworm disease is not considered as a cause for cardiopulmonary disease, is not routinely monitored, and is not prevented by regular medication. Infection rates up to 45 per cent are reported as occurring within 150 miles of the Atlantic coast from Texas to New Jersey and along the Mississippi River and its major tributaries. Most of the remainder of the United States and southern Canada have infection rates up to 5 per cent. States with infrequently diagnosed heartworm infections include Washington, Utah, Idaho, Nevada, and Montana.[1] Heartworm infection is spread throughout much of the tropical world. Endemic areas in Japan and Australia have both presented a major challenge to veterinarians and contributed much to the understanding of heartworm disease and its management.[2]

Frequency of infection as related to signalment and lifestyle has been studied in several surveys. Male dogs are more frequently infected than female dogs. This ratio has been found to be as high as 4:1 and is greater in the respective populations at risk.[3] The age at which heartworm infection is most frequently diagnosed varies with the local infection rate and the age of dogs at risk. Endemic regions will have heartworm infection diagnosed as early as one year, whereas infection in most areas is diagnosed between 3 and 15 years of age.[4] Dogs housed outside are four to five times more likely to be infected than indoor dogs. Large dogs are more susceptible than small dogs and haircoat does not appear to affect the probability of infection.[3] The more commonly exposed breeds such as the German shepherd, English pointer, setters, retrievers, and beagles are the most commonly infected. Boxers have been reported as having an unusually high incidence.[5] Review of epidemiologic studies may be for academic curiosity, as individual female dogs, dogs that live mostly indoors, dogs that are small, and dogs that have long hair are susceptible and have been infected with heartworms. In regions where heartworms are common, all dogs should be considered at risk and be placed on surveillance/preventive programs.[2]

CARDIOPULMONARY DISEASE DEVELOPMENT

Life Cycle. Heartworm infection is spread by many different species of mosquitoes and the geographic extent of the disease is probably directly related to that of susceptible mosquitoes. Female mosquitoes serve as the intermediate host and obtain a blood meal from a dog with circulating *Dirofilaria immitis* microfilariae. The microfilariae develop over two months and are capable of infecting another dog within 2 to 2.5 weeks.[6,7] The infective larva enters the skin via the bite wound on the next dog and migrates through body tissues for the next 100 days. At that time, young adults (or L_5) enter the vascular system and travel to the small pulmonary arteries. Approximately six months after the infective larvae enter their new host, microfilaremia occurs and their numbers usually increase markedly over the next six months. Subsequently, the microfilarial concentration frequently declines in dogs with a one-time infection.[2]

Disease severity and onset are partially a reflection of the number of adult heartworms, which may vary from 1 to over 250 per dog.[8] Until the heartworm number exceeds 50 in a 50-lb dog (25 in a 25-kg dog) nearly all of the heartworms reside in the caudal pulmonary arteries. As the number increases even more, they move to the right ventricle. The right atrium frequently contains heartworms when their number exceeds 50 and even higher numbers of heartworms result in extension into the vena cava.[9]

Response to Live Heartworms. Heartworms within the pulmonary arteries damage the endothelial lining with changes being seen by scanning electron microscopy as early as three days after heartworm transplantation. Pulmonary arteries in dogs with transplanted adult heartworms have endothelial swelling, widened intercellular junctions, sloughing of longitudinal strips of endothelium, and adhesion of many activated leukocytes and platelets to the damaged area. Damage of the endothelium increases its permeability to serum proteins and water.[10,11] Both leak into the perivascular interstitium. Trophic factors appear to be released by the activated platelets and leukocytes. These factors (such as platelet derived growth factor or PDGF) stimulate migration and multiplication of smooth muscle cells within the tunica media. When examined as early as three weeks after heartworm transplantation, the rapidly dividing smooth muscle cells have migrated from the media to the intima, where they continue to rapidly multiply. Pathognomonic villi of heartworm disease consist of these rapidly dividing smooth muscle cells and the collagen produced by them. The villi have some areas of damaged endothelium, but most of the surface is covered by an abnormal endothelial type of cell. Villi may become quite complicated and range in size from a few microns to several millimeters. Just as the heartworms are distributed to the caudal and accessory lung lobes, so are the endothelial damage and villi.[10–13] Within four to six weeks of adulticide treatment, the movement of heartworms away from the large pulmonary arteries permits resolution of their surface changes[4] (Figure 80–1).

Arteriographic abnormalities can be seen within weeks of heartworm transplantation into dogs. Arteries to the caudal and accessory lung lobes dilate, become tortuous, develop aneurysms, and lose their normal tapering arborization. Arteries with a diameter smaller than the adult heartworms frequently appear to be abruptly pruned. Blood flow is frequently obstructed and diverted to nonaffected lung lobes. In dogs treated with thiacetarsamide to reduce the number of adult heartworms, the dilatation and tortuosity decrease within a few months.[14] Pulmonary hypertension has been observed to resolve after elimination of adult heartworms.[15] The central lesions resolve more completely than peripheral arterial changes. Some residual fibrosis can remain about the distal arteries, but proximal arteries return more toward normalcy as evaluated by hemodynamic function, scanning electron microscopy, and arteriography.[10, 14–16] Much of the decreased diameter of

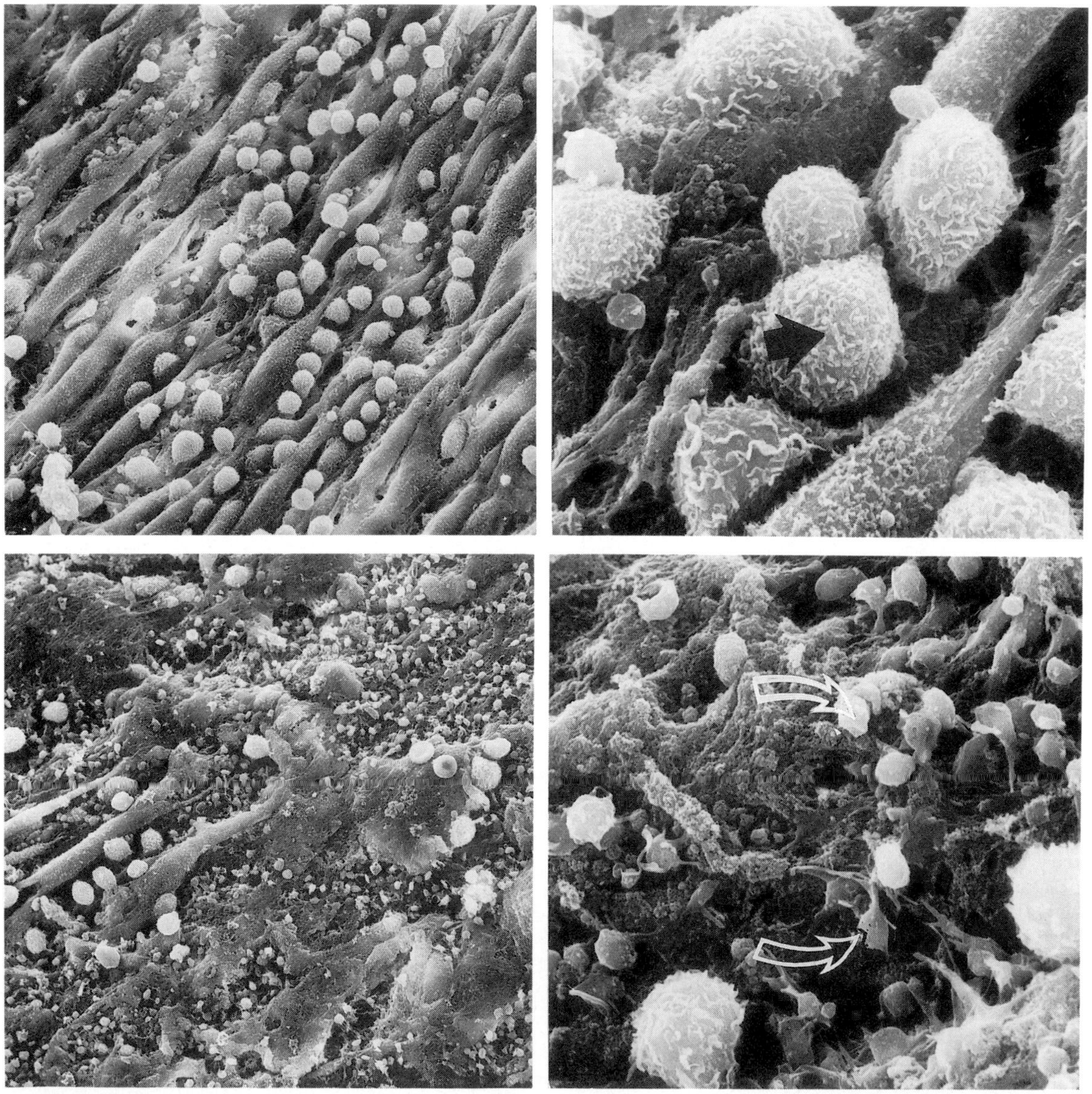

FIGURE 80–1. Scanning electron micrographs (magnifications of × 400 to 2000) of pulmonary arterial surfaces, four days following heartworm transplantation. These samples were selected from areas with uptake of Evan's blue dye. Swollen, edematous endothelial cells are present, and many leukocytes (solid arrow) are adhered to the disrupted surface. Some areas have lost their endothelial cover, and activated platelets (open arrows) have adhered to the exposed subendothelium. (From Schaub, RG et al.: Platelet adhesion and myointimal proliferation in canine pulmonary arteries. Am Assoc Pathol 104:13–22, 1981.)

the large pulmonary arteries is probably due to the decreased pulmonary arterial pressure and the greater amount of elasticity in the large pulmonary arteries.[2]

Increased permeability of the vascular surfaces produces perivascular edema, which can be seen as consolidation of an alveolar pattern on radiographs. An interstitial pattern is frequently seen.[16] This interstitial pattern is probably a combination of vascular disease, perivascular fluid leakage, and inflammatory fluids. The alveolar signs can resolve rapidly with appropriate treatment, whereas the interstitial lesions may persist even after elimination of adult heartworms[2] (Figure 80–2).

The mechanisms of platelet involvement in producing arterial disease have been blocked in several studies using inhibiting drugs such as aspirin in dosages as low as 2.0 mg/lb q12h (5 mg/kg).[17] Nonsteroid anti-inflammatory drugs, such as aspirin, reduce platelet adhesion, increase platelet life span, decrease the villus proliferation, and decrease arterial disease. When dogs were permitted to develop arterial disease during sustained heartworm infection, aspirin arrested the disease sequence so successfully that arterial disease resolved during continued heartworm infection.[17] Resolution of disease has been observed in clinical patients in similar fashion to that observed in research dogs. Clinical patients with congestive heart failure and with enlarged pulmonary arteries have had their clinical response markedly improved with aspirin and cage confinement.[18] In addition to blocking the progression of arterial disease, elimination of heartworms by arsenical treatment is essential for severely ill clinical patients to have long-term improvement.

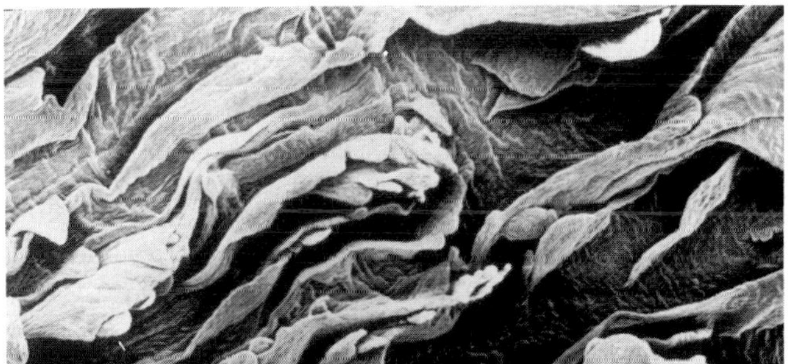

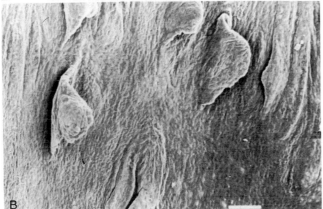

FIGURE 80–2. *A*, Scanning electron micrograph (× 100) from a caudal pulmonary arterial surface of a dog transplanted with 28 adult heartworms one year previously. The surface is extensively involved with rugous and villous proliferations. *B*, Scanning electron micrograph (× 100) from a caudal pulmonary arterial surface similar to Figure 80–2*A*. This dog was from a group treated with 7 mg/kg aspirin throughout the one-year heartworm infection. The villi are fewer and smaller than in the nontreated control dog. Dogs that were treated for only the final six months of the one-year infection had pulmonary arteries that were similar to those of dogs treated with aspirin for the entire year. (From Rawlings, CA, et al.: Effect of acetylsalicylic acid on pulmonary arteriosclerosis induced by a one year *Dirofilaria immitis* infection. Arteriosclerosis 5:355–365, 1985.)

Response to Dead Heartworms. The worst disease is that seen after adult heartworms have died and their fragments have been swept distally into the small pulmonary arteries. The response at the pulmonary arterial surface is an exacerbation of that seen to live heartworms. Villous proliferation is exuberant and there are also thrombi and a granulomatous inflammatory reaction about the dead heartworms.[19] Blood flow becomes severely impaired, sometimes with no flow going to the caudal lung lobes.[20] The caudal lung lobes frequently develop severe consolidation and fail to function for either blood gas exchange or blood flow. Severe coughing, dyspnea, and even hemoptysis may develop. The increased vascular resistance (after-load) can produce acute cardiac failure, especially in the compromised right ventricle.[2] When aspirin treatment is started concurrently with thiacetarsamide, aspirin markedly reduces the severity of arterial disease and impaired blood flow. In contrast, anti-inflammatory dosages of corticosteroids increase arterial disease and prolong the presence of heartworm fragments within the pulmonary arteries.[20–22] Corticosteroids can be effective in reducing the acute pulmonary congestion produced by heartworm death, but are indicated only for the treatment of significant clinical signs such as dyspnea, severe coughing, and hemoptysis[2] (Figure 80–3).

Clinical Signs as a Reflection of the Response to Heartworms. Clinical signs are a reflection of the number of infecting heartworms, the duration of infection, and the response of the canine host. Most dogs are asymptomatic. Coughing and dyspnea are the most common signs and are usually associated with parenchymal disease of caudal lung lobes. This disease is focused about the pulmonary arteries with edema and inflammatory fluids accumulating due to increased vascular permeability to serum proteins and fluids. The inflammatory reaction, especially that to dead heartworms, surrounds the small airways and could provide the stimuli for coughing. Some dyspnea may be associated with the difficulty of propelling pulmonary blood flow through a highly resistant arterial system.

Decreased ability to exercise and the sequence of right ventricular dilation, hypertrophy, and failure are the response to the fixed vascular resistance and pulmonary hypertension of arterial disease. This fixed resistance impedes arterial flow and increases the work of the right ventricle. Severe disease restricts the ability to recruit arteries to transport the high blood flow needed for exercise.[15] This decreases the dog's ability to exercise. This resistance to flow is complicated by heartworm-infected dogs' having an exaggerated hypertensive response to alveolar hypoxia.[23] The increased pumping work of perfusing the diseased arterial system produces

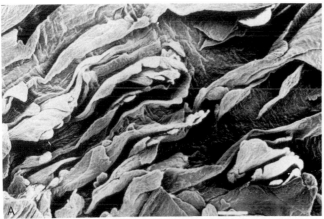

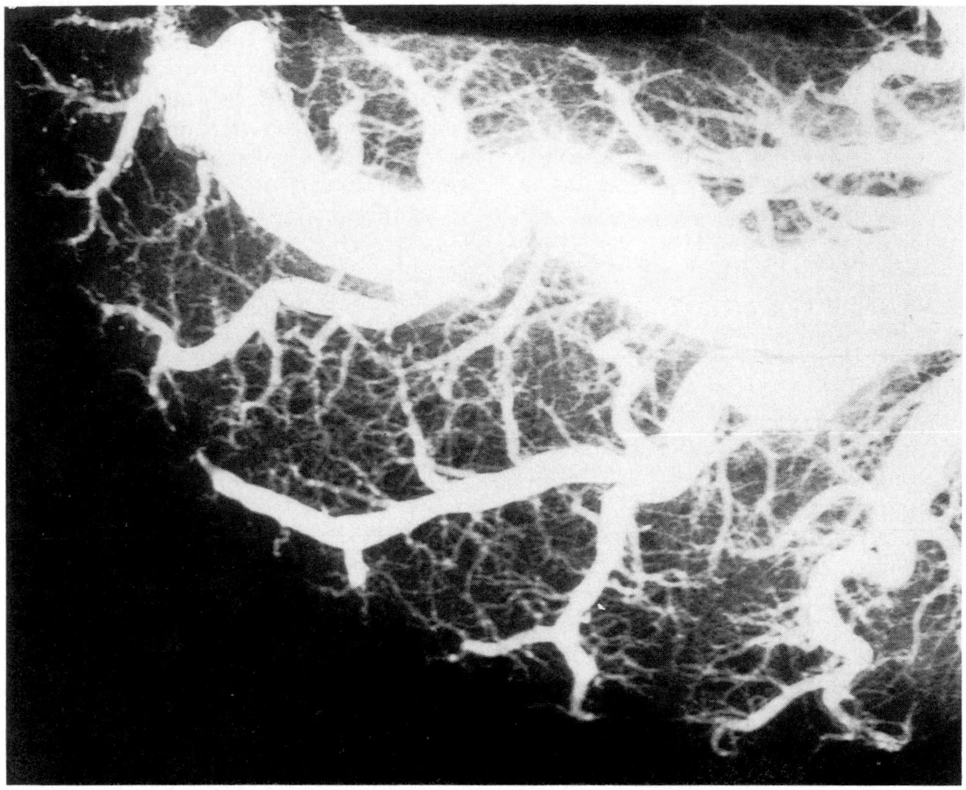

FIGURE 80–3. Postmortem arteriogram from a dog with a naturally contracted and severe heartworm infection. The dog was heparinized prior to euthanasia, the pulmonary vasculature was flushed to clear residual blood, the airways were inflated, and the arteries were injected with a combination of barium sulfate and gelatin. When the gelatin had hardened, a radiograph of the right caudal lung lobe was taken. The caudal lobar artery is dilated and mildly tortuous. Arterial branches from the lobar artery are also dilated and these arterial branches abruptly terminate or are "pruned." Arteries with dilatations have lumens sufficient to provide residences for adult heartworms. Intimal lesions involve those arteries that are dilated. (From Rawlings, CA: Heartworm Disease in Dogs and Cats. Philadelphia, WB Saunders, 1986.)

a sequence of right ventricular dilation, hypertrophy, and right-sided congestive heart failure. Heart failure patients frequently have had increased exercise and/or excitement of variable duration before presentation with overt signs of heart failure. Failing patients most typically present with ascites and an enlarged liver. Cardiac cachexia develops as the disease progresses.

Hemoptysis occasionally occurs, especially after the heartworms have been killed by thiacetarsamide, and is the result of vascular and airway wall ruptures. This blood loss normally starts in the caudal lung lobes in an area of severe vascular and parenchymal disease. A combination of vascular wall disease and coughing trauma probably produces the ruptures of vascular and airway walls.

PRETREATMENT EVALUATION

Adulticide treatment should be started after the patient has been evaluated and treated symptomatically for disease complications. This evaluation should provide a means of developing an intelligent prognosis and modifying the supportive treatment approach.

History and Physical Examination. The historical questions should be both general and specific relating to heartworm infection and cardiopulmonary disease. General questions include (1) the dog's age, (2) previous residences and travel, (3) trends in appetite, body condition, and activity, (4) water consumption and urination habits, (5) vomiting, regurgitation, and diarrhea, and (6) other diseases and medical therapy. Specific questions should be directed toward detecting cardiopulmonary disease. These signs include decreased exercise tolerance, coughing, dyspnea, sneezing, hemoptysis, epistaxis, fainting, collapse, and wasting of general body condition.

Microfilarial Detection and Differentiation. The least desirable microfilarial diagnostic procedures are the nonconcentration tests, which are frequently falsely negative and not specific for differentiating *Dirofilaria immitis* from *Dipetalonema reconditum*. The wet smear with a drop of freshly drawn venous blood can be used to detect microfilaria gyrating among the red blood cells. Differentiation of the species of microfilaria is based on the facts that *Dipetalonema* microfilariae advance across the slide and *Dirofilaria* tend to gyrate in place. *Dirofilaria* microfilariae are also larger, being at least as wide as the red blood cells. This size criterion is difficult to assess with active microfilaria. Another nonconcentration test is the examination of the buffy coat of a microhematocrit tube[2] (Table 80–1).

The concentration tests (filter or Knott's) should be done when conducting annual or semiannual health maintenance tests, examining dogs with signs typical of heartworm infection, and determining the efficacy of microfilaricide treatments. Concentration techniques are

TABLE 80–1. DIFFERENTIATION OF MICROFILARIAE OF *DIROFILARIA IMMITIS* AND *DIPETALONEMA RECONDITUM*

Characteristic	*D. immitis*	*D. reconditum*
Length (Knott)	>290 μm	<275 μm
Width (Knott)	>6 μm	<6 μm
Length (Wet smear)	>310 μm	<290 μm
Length (Filter)	>240 μm	<240 μm
Motility (Wet smear)	Sluggish	Active
Head shape (Knott, filter)	Tapered	Blunt
Cephalic hook (Knott)	Absent	Present
Posterior extremity hook (Knott)	Absent	Present
Body shape (Knott)	Straight	Crescent
Acid phosphatase	Two distinct zones	Dispersed

more likely to identify circulating microfilariae, as the volume of blood is greater (1 milliliter versus 1 drop). Selection of a concentration test is a matter of personal choice, as their accuracy is similar and very good. The cheapest is the modified Knott's test, which requires more time to perform than the filter techniques (Evsco and PitmanMoore). Both types of filter tests lyse the red blood cells and fix the microfilaria. Differentiation of microfilaria by size (*Dirofilaria immitis* microfilariae being greater than 290 μm in length and 6 μm in width and *Dipetalonema reconditum* being less than 275 μm in length and less than 6 μm in width) is based on the Knott's test. These size criteria are smaller for microfilariae in the filter lysate than when the microfilariae are preserved in the two per cent formalin of the Knott's test. *Dirofilaria immitis* microfilariae have tapered heads with neither a cephalic nor posterior extremity hook.[2]

Even concentration tests fail to detect microfilaria in 10 to 67 per cent of the dogs with adult heartworm infection. Before a diagnosis of occult infection is made, microfilarial concentration tests should be negative on at least two or three occasions. Microfilaria concentrations are lower in the winter months and there is a diurnal cycle for individual dogs. Circulating microfilariae may be eliminated by an immune response, which identifies and destroys microfilariae in the lung. Other etiologies of occult infections are unisexual heartworm populations, sterile heartworms, and immature or prepatent adult infections. Immunodiagnostic tests have been developed to identify these microfilaria-negative infections.[2]

Radiology. Since radiographic abnormalities develop early, thoracic radiographs are the diagnostic procedures most useful in characterizing the severity of heartworm infection. Typical changes include right ventricular enlargement, increased prominence of the main pulmonary artery, enlarged lobar pulmonary arteries, enlargement and then obstruction of the peripheral pulmonary arteries, and perivascular parenchymal disease. Arterial lesions and the associated parenchymal disease tend to be more severe in the caudal lung lobes.[2, 16]

Proper positioning is critical in obtaining consistently diagnostic thoracic radiographs. The ventrodorsal projection is preferred for assessment of right ventricular and main pulmonary arterial size while the dorsoventral projection is better for measuring the caudal lobar arteries. We feel that the ventrodorsal view is easier to consistently align correctly. The diagnosis of right ventricular and main pulmonary arterial enlargement is subjective, as the silhouette size varies with the breed of the dog. Dogs with narrow upright chests tend to have a more upright heart and smaller cardiac silhouettes, in contrast to breeds with a rounder thorax, such as beagles, which normally have more prominent right hearts and main pulmonary arteries. Over-interpretation of right ventricular enlargement in round-chested dogs is common and can increase the tendency to falsely diagnose heartworm infection. The lateral radiograph is used to measure the right cranial lobar artery and to characterize the parenchymal pattern in the caudal lung lobes. The diameter of the right cranial lobar artery at its intersection with the right fourth rib should not exceed the narrowest diameter of the fourth rib and the diameter of the caudal lobar arteries at their intersection with the ninth rib should be no larger than the narrowest diameter of the ninth rib.[2]

Several studies have determined the frequency of radiographic abnormalities in dogs with heartworm infection. In one study, 86 per cent of 200 microfilaria-positive dogs had radiographic changes typical of heartworm infection. Approximately 60 per cent had right ventricular enlargement, 20 per cent of those with severe enlargement.[24] Another study identified 72 per cent as having enlarged right ventricles.[25] These percentages vary with the severity of infection typically seen in a practice area. Dogs that are more heavily infected with heartworms have more severe radiographic signs. Approximately the same percentage of infected dogs with enlarged right ventricles also have enlargement of the main pulmonary artery. Lobar arterial disease (enlargement and/or tortuosity) is present in approximately one-half of our cases. When lobar arteries have a measured increase in their diameters, the likelihood of heartworm infection is very high.

The worst parenchymal disease is seen when dead heartworms move distally in the pulmonary arteries following adulticide treatment. Parenchymal signs include alveolar and interstitial roentgen signs. Some dogs develop similar signs prior to adulticide treatment. The alveolar signs have ill-defined fluffy margins, coalescence of densities, air bronchograms, lobar distribution of infiltrates, central location of the infiltrate, and peribronchiolar nodules. These changes are most common about the lobar pulmonary arteries in the two caudal and the intermediate lung lobes.[19, 21] Some parenchymal signs are interstitial and indicate fibrosis produced by chronic disease. Alveolar signs usually regress rapidly with no treatment and if clinical signs are present, the signs can be reduced more quickly with corticosteroid treatment.[21]

Clinical Pathology. In contrast to the pathognomonic lesions seen with thoracic radiographs, no similar changes are present in the complete blood count, serum chemistry profile, and urinalysis of dogs with heartworm disease. Studies have been done to compare heartworm-infected dogs with non-infected dogs. Likewise, dogs have been studied before and after experimentally induced infections. Heartworm-induced changes are inconsistent and even when present, they usually do not lead to a diagnosis of heartworm infection.[2] Much of the rationale for doing these procedures is to detect coexistent disease.

Eosinophilia and basophilia are the most consistently observed changes during heartworm infection and other more common parasitic infections. *Dipetalonema reconditum* infection produces an eosinophilia of even greater magnitude than *Dirofilaria immitis* infection.[26] We consider eosinophilia (>1,500 cells/mm^3) and basophilia to be supportive of, but not diagnostic for heartworm infection. Segmented neutrophil and monocyte concentrations frequently increase after adulticide treatment. Approximately 1 in 10 of the authors' patients have a mild regenerative anemia of 27 to 36 per cent. This is probably produced by increased hemolysis and is present in only the more severely affected dogs. Thrombocytopenia is common, as the activation and adhesion of platelets to the damaged endothelium increases their consumption and shortens their life span.[2, 4]

Heartworm-infected dogs can have an increased total protein concentration, as the globulin concentrations are frequently increased. Hypoalbuminemia is present in some severely affected dogs, usually as a result of renal glomerular disease or hepatic insufficiency. Increased concentrations of liver enzymes are present in at least 10 per cent of our patients. Increased enzyme concentrations have not proven predictive of treatment complications and most dogs have a return to normal liver enzyme concentration within weeks of adulticide treatment. Some of these dogs also have evidence of decreased liver function (increased retention of Bromosulphalein dye), especially those with congestive heart failure. Azotemia may occur, but is not common.[2, 4]

Some dogs have abnormalities on urinalysis, but these are not usually produced by the heartworm infection. Proteinuria occurs infrequently as a heartworm-initiated glomerulopathy.

Immunodiagnostic Tests. The indirect fluorescent antibody absorption test has proven very useful in the diagnosis of occult heartworm disease in which there are high concentrations of antibodies to the microfilariae. It has decreased in popularity because the newer ELISA-antigen tests are more versatile and appear to be both more sensitive and specific for heartworm infection. For the indirect fluorescent antibody test, microfilariae are incubated in serum from a dog with suspected heartworm infection. The microfilariae are then washed, placed with rabbit anti-dog IgG fluorescein isocyanate, and then examined with an ultraviolet microscope. Fluorescence on the microfilarial surface is a positive test result. Cross-reactivity with *Dipetalonema* and intestinal parasites has not been detected. This test is limited in application to those dogs with immune-mediated disease and requires sophisticated laboratory technique and equipment.

The antibody response to adult heartworms was the basis for several enzyme-linked immunosorbent assay tests marketed during the early 1980s. These were unsatisfactory as they frequently yielded false-positive test results.

Tests using monoclonal culture-produced antibodies to circulating adult antigens have proven successful during the mid-1980s. Their technology has proven to be much more specific than the tests for antibodies to adults. These enzyme-linked immunosorbent assays for adult antigens (ELISA Ag) most often appear to test for antigens of female uterine origin. Protocols vary and the manufacturer's directions should be followed for each test kit. Positive and negative control tests are included. The tests include Filarochek (Mallinckrodt), Dirochek (Synbiotics Corp), and CITE-Heartworm (AgriTech Systems Inc). The Dirochek has been modified slightly and is currently marketed as ClinEase CH (Norden Laboratories). All kits are designed for use in the practitioner's laboratory. Initial data have shown these tests to be both sensitive and specific. Cross-reactivities with *Dipetalonema* and intestinal parasites have not been detected. False-positive test results appear to be infrequent. False-negative test results can be produced by infections of few heartworms, especially infections of predominantly male heartworms. With each test, the clinician should request documentation of its specificity and sensitivity. Test results must be interpreted with respect to other clinical data. Since the tests are based upon detection of heartworm antigen, these have been used successfully to diagnose heartworm infection in cats. Occasionally, cats with infections consisting of only one or two heartworms have false-negative tests results.[2]

Electrocardiography. The electrocardiogram (ECG) of most dogs with heartworm infection is normal. Right ventricular hypertrophy (RVH) and cardiac rhythm disturbances are infrequent.[27] For these reasons the ECG is not a component of the minimum data base (MDB).

The most common ECG abnormality associated with heartworm infection is RVH and occurs only in dogs with severe pulmonary hypertension resulting from pulmonary arterial disease. Electrocardiographic evidence of RVH has been correlated to increased right-ventricular weights and chronic pulmonary hypertension with peak systolic pressures of at least 50 mmHg and a mean pressure of 30 mmHg.[28, 29] The absence of ECG evidence of RVH does not preclude the presence of pulmonary hypertension. The distinction between RVH and right-ventricular dilatation also should be appreciated. Right-ventricular dilatation, evidenced by right ventricular enlargement on thoracic radiographs, is common in heartworm-infected dogs that lack ECG evidence of RVH.[27] The right ventricle dilates before hypertrophy occurs and the ECG is not sensitive to right ventricular dilatation.[7, 30]

Heartworm-infected dogs with severe pulmonary arterial disease without ECG evidence of RVH develop exercise-exacerbated pulmonary hypertension. Telemetric or Holter ECG recordings reflect S-wave, ST-segment, and T-wave changes consistent with acute cor pulmonale.[31]

Some dogs with radiographic evidence of severe pulmonary arterial disease and most dogs with these findings and associated right-sided congestive heart failure have ECG evidence of RVH.[27] When there is ECG evidence of RVH, there is always radiographic evidence of severe pulmonary arterial disease.[27] If ascites occurs in a dog with heartworm infection and ECG evidence of RVH is absent, the cause of the ascites is often another disorder. The existence of another disorder is further indicated if radiographic evidence of severe pulmonary arterial disease is absent.[27] Right-sided congestive heart failure is seldom present or imminent if either radiographic evidence of severe pulmonary arterial disease or ECG evidence of RVH is absent.

The ECG criteria of RVH have been well defined and verified.[28, 29] The most accurate ECG correlation of RVH is afforded by the presence of three or more of the signs of RVH.[27, 29, 32] When RVH is present in heartworm-infected dogs, excessive S-wave voltages are present in leads V_2 (CV_6LL) and V_4 (CV_6LU) and three or more criteria of RVH are present in more than 75 per cent of all instances.[27] When radiographic evidence of right ventricular enlargement is absent or minimal, abnormalities of leads V_{10}, II, I, and the mean electrical axis in the frontal plane occur in less than ten per cent of heartworm-infected dogs.[27]

In heartworm-infected dogs, the presence of a positive T wave was highly specific for RVH but this criterion was not sensitive. A similar degree of specificity was found for excessive S-wave voltage in lead II and abnormal mean electrical axis of the transverse plane. However, over one-third of dogs with radiographic evidence of severe right ventricular enlargement and three or more ECG criteria of RVH lacked these criteria. The specificities and sensitivities of abnormalities in leads V_2, V_4, and the frontal plane mean electrical axis were each 75 per cent or greater.[27]

Right atrial enlargement is uncommonly associated with heartworm disease–induced cor pulmonale. In our experience, P pulmonale (P_{II} or P_{aVF} greater than 0.4mv) occurs in less than one per cent of heartworm-infected dogs and in less than ten per cent of dogs with severe pulmonary arterial disease.

Although numerous types of cardiac rhythm disturbances have been observed in heartworm-infected dogs, such abnormalities are uncommon.[33] The most common rhythm disturbances observed by us are atrial premature contractions and atrial fibrillation, which are associated with radiographic evidence of severe pulmonary arterial disease. The incidence of abnormal heart rhythms is probably underestimated since only short-term, static ECGs are normally recorded.

The Minimum Data Base. There is not a uniformity of opinion about the minimum data base (MDB) for dogs with heartworm infection. Furthermore, the MDB should be determined, in part, by the history, age, and severity of disease. In general, young asymptomatic dogs, especially those tested annually for *Dirofilaria immitis* microfilariae, do not require an extensive MDB. A complete blood count, BUN, urinalysis, and thoracic radiographs are sufficient, provided a thorough history and physical examination indicates that severe pulmonary disease is unlikely.

Middle-aged and old dogs, dogs not tested annually, symptomatic dogs, and those with proven or suspected occult infections require an extended data base. Under these circumstances a complete blood count, serum chemistry profile, urinalysis, and possibly a platelet count (at least a platelet estimation) are indicated.

Thoracic radiographs are singularly the most informative, practical tests of the severity of heartworm disease. Thoracic radiographs should be evaluated primarily in two regards: pulmonary arterial disease and pulmonary parenchymal disease, which is usually secondary to the former. Although right ventricular enlargement is associated with heartworm disease, this abnormality is an inconsistent finding, is highly breed or confirmation variable, and is subject to errors in interpretation resulting from incorrect patient positioning.

The ECG is not an integral component of the MDB. Most dogs with heartworm infection have a normal ECG. The most common ECG abnormality, RVH, is only associated with pulmonary arterial disease severe enough to cause severe pulmonary hypertension. Cardiac rhythm disturbances are not commonly associated with heartworm disease.[27, 33]

The ECG may be included in an extended data base when there is radiographic and clinical evidence of either congestive heart failure or severe pulmonary arterial disease. If there is strong ECG evidence of RVH, then overt right-sided congestive heart failure is usually present or imminent.[27] In many instances, ascites and evidence of elevation of the central venous pressure (distended jugular veins, jugular pulses) are already present. If ascites is present in the absence of ECG evidence of RVH, cytologic analysis of the ascitic fluid is imperative because the absence of RVH suggests the possibility of another disorder being the cause of the ascites.

Ascites due to heartworm infection is usually produced by severe pulmonary arterial disease and pulmonary hypertension.[18] Ascitic patients should have a paracentesis so that cytology and chemical analysis may be performed. The fluid is usually serosanguineous or amber in appearance. Ascitic fluid resulting from right-sided congestive heart failure, being of post-sinusoidal origin, is a high protein (greater than 2.5 mg/dl) modified transudate consisting predominantly of erythrocytes and normal-appearing lymphocytes with fewer numbers of non-degenerate neutrophils. Depending on the duration of the effusion, macrophages and reactive mesothelial cells may be present in variable, but usually low percentages. If analysis indicates that the effusion is a pure transudate or exudate, the presence of other abnormalities must be considered.

Hypoalbuminemia is an uncommon sequela to heartworm disease but when present is usually associated with clinical and/or radiographic evidence of severe heartworm disease. Hypoalbuminemia may result from either a protein-losing glomerulopathy or hepatic insufficiency. If ascites and/or icterus is also present, the prognosis is poor. In the presence of hypoalbuminemia, multiple urinalyses are recommended in order to better define the presence of proteinuria. In addition, hepatic function tests, such as bile acid levels or an ammonia tolerance test or BSP retention should be performed.

In one study, 79 of 102 dogs (78 per cent) with heartworm infection had renal lesions.[31] Most dogs with subclinical heartworm disease do not have significant proteinuria.[35] However, dogs with severe pulmonary arterial disease, especially right-sided congestive heart failure often have significant proteinuria, presumably resulting from glomerular disease.[36]

Proteinuria, when of a significant degree and when associated with hypoalbuminemia, indicates severe glomerular disease. A 24-hour quantitation of proteinuria may be indicated in order to quantitate the protein loss. The severity and specific diagnosis of a glomerulopathy can be accomplished only by renal biopsy. Quantitation of proteinuria and renal biopsy are not necessary if the BUN, creatinine, and serum albumin concentrations are within normal limits.

Azotemia is an uncommon complication of heartworm disease and, when present, is usually of pre-renal or renal origin. Azotemia associated with a urine specific gravity of greater than 1.030 and minimal proteinuria is most likely of pre-renal origin. Azotemia associated with a urine specific gravity of greater than 1.030 and significant proteinuria may be the result of a glomerulopathy. A 24-hour quantitation of proteinuria and/or a renal biopsy may be indicated in the latter circumstances, particularly if hypoalbuminemia coexists. Mild azotemia (BUN, 40 to 100 mg/dl) associated with normoalbuminemia and no, minimal, or moderate proteinuria is not a contraindication to heartworm treatment, provided that fluid therapy is administered and improvement of azotemia ensues.

Icterus is an uncommon complication of heartworm disease. When present, icterus is associated with either the vena cava syndrome or severe pulmonary arterial disease with hemoglobinuria and/or right-sided congestive heart failure. In the presence of icterus, hepatic function should be assessed by the evaluation of the BUN, serum albumin concentration, bile acid level, and possibly an ammonia tolerance test.

Hemoglobinuria is an uncommon complication of heartworm disease and is associated with either the vena cava syndrome or severe pulmonary arterial disease and concomitant thromboembolism. In the presence of hemoglobinuria, a platelet count, activated clotting time, and possibly a coagulogram should be procured.

Liver enzyme activity (SGPT and SAP) is usually of limited importance as a component of the MDB. Most heartworm-infected dogs have normal or only slightly elevated serum liver enzyme activity.[36] Up to ten-fold increased serum liver enzyme activity has not been associated with an increased incidence of acute thiacetarsamide Na toxicity, mortality, or treatment failures.[36] BSP retention is mildly increased in approximately 20 per cent of heartworm-infected dogs and approximately 50 per cent of dogs with concomitant right-sided congestive heart failure. Retention of 8 to 15 per cent of the BSP at 30 minutes is not associated with an increased risk of thiacetarsamide Na toxicity, mortality, or treatment failures.[36] In fact, thiacetarsamide efficacy is increased in dogs with reduced hepatic function.[37]

It is the author's opinion that up to ten-fold increased liver enzyme activity alone is not an indication to delay or abort adulticide treatment. Serum enzyme activity and BSP retention are usually improved or normal within six weeks following thiacetarsamide Na treatment in dogs with abnormal pre-treatment values.[36]

In summary, there is no known laboratory test or tests that are predictive of acute thiacetarsamide toxicity.[38, 39]

CLINICAL SYNDROMES (DIAGNOSIS AND TREATMENT)

Asymptomatic Patients. Dogs that are determined to be asymptomatic based upon the history, physical examination, and the appropriate minimum data base should be treated with an adulticide and microfilaricide soon after the diagnosis of circulating *Dirofilaria immitis* microfilariae. It is difficult to imagine an asymptomatic heartworm-positive dog that should not be treated to eliminate the heartworms and then be placed on a preventive program. Few dogs develop complications during treatment, but no pre-treatment diagnostic maneuvers predict thiacetarsamide adverse reaction nor consistently predict which dogs will suffer from thromboembolic disease.

We recommend no supplemental therapy in addition to good nutrition and the standard adulticide and microfilaricide treatment. Routine use of corticosteroids is probably contraindicated as they have been shown to reduce thiacetarsamide efficacy. Aspirin could be rationalized as being beneficial for all dogs being challenged by heartworm death, but we prefer to restrict aspirin's use to those dogs with severe arterial disease, many of which have congestive heart failure.

Dogs should be hospitalized and treated with a standard four injections of thiacetarsamide given over two days (refer to section on Adulticide Treatment). The dog should be confined and observed closely for at least three weeks. Microfilaricide treatment should be initiated in three to six weeks, with the earlier time being for those dogs having no problems before or during treatment. When the dogs are microfilaria negative, a preventive program should begin if the heartworm season is present. Dogs should be retested for microfilariae once or twice a year, depending on the duration of the potential infective period of the year and local frequency of heartworm disease.

Patients with Pulmonary Disease. Thromboembolic and parenchymal disease most frequently develops following death of the adult heartworms, especially after adulticide treatment. Severe parenchymal disease may be the reason for signs prior to adulticide treatment. The parenchymal disease from either heartworm etiology is treated in similar fashion. Coughing and dyspnea with tachypnea are the typical presenting signs. Other signs are fever and hemoptysis. Auscultation may reveal the presence of crackles and areas of decreased air sounds. These signs frequently develop acutely and are most prone to develop within the first three weeks of adulticide administration. Some dogs have such severe thromboembolic disease that they present with tachycardia, pale mucous membranes, and a weak femoral pulse.

The most useful diagnostic tool, after a good physical examination, is the thoracic radiograph. Other useful procedures include complete blood count, platelet count, activated clotting time, coagulation tests, transtracheal wash, and arterial blood gases. The complete blood count may be consistent with either a stress leukogram or a severe inflammatory response. Thrombocytopenia is typical and reflects platelet consumption on the injured arterial surfaces and dead heartworm fragments. A few dogs have prolonged clotting times. A transtracheal wash for cytology and culture may reveal inflammation with eosinophils. It is seldom indicative of bacterial infection. Arterial blood gases in the dyspneic animal reflect hypoxemia. The carbon dioxide partial pressure varies with the disease severity. The dyspneic dog is usually hypocarbic as the animal is ventilating excessively in response to the hypoxemia, but some are so ill that even the carbon dioxide is not effectively exchanged and thus accumulates. Many dogs with parenchymal disease produced by heartworms have occult infections. These dogs should have repeated microfilarial examinations followed by an immunodiagnostic (ELISA Ag) test.

A mixed alveolar and interstitial pattern is typically found around the lobar arteries of the caudal and accessory lung lobes. The caudal lobar distribution of an alveolar pattern in mature dogs living in heartworm endemic areas is strongly suggestive of heartworm disease. The alveolar pattern is probably produced by the increased vascular permeability. These alveolar signs are frequently responsive to treatment, in contrast to the interstitial pattern, which is a reflection of more chronic and fibrotic changes. Dead heartworms move distally into the smaller pulmonary arteries where the vascular injury initiates an exaggerated response similar to that seen to live heartworms. In addition to the exuberant villous proliferation, thrombosis and inflammation are initiated by the dying heartworms. The increased vascular permeability permits serum and proteins to leak into the perivascular parenchyma. Pulmonary compliance decreases, which leads to an increase in respiratory effort. The decreased gas exchange (ventilation-perfusion mismatching), along with a decreased compliance, produces dyspnea. Since these dogs are hypoxemic, some of their dyspnea may be related to a hypoxia-mediated pulmonary hypertension. The inflammatory changes are probably the stimulus to coughing. Dogs with severe vascular injury may cough up blood that has left the vascular system and entered the airways.

When the lungs are examined in the dog with thromboembolic disease, the caudal lung lobes are heavy with edema and hemorrhage. The arteries to these caudal lung lobes are frequently totally obstructed with villous proliferation and thromboembolism. The arteries are surrounded by chronic granulomatous inflammation. Proximate to the dead heartworm fragments may be areas of acute inflammation.

Treatment is strict cage confinement and anti-inflammatory dosages of daily corticosteroid treatment (prednisolone or prednisone at 0.5 to 1 mg/lb (1 to 2 mg/kg). The corticosteroid treatment may only require a couple of days to a week of administration and it should be discontinued as soon as significant clinical and radiographic improvements are detected. Animals with cardiovascular collapse should be treated judiciously with intravenous fluids.

Occult Heartworm Infections. The presence of adult heartworms in the absence of detected microfilaremia was first documented a half century ago.[40] This syndrome is often referred to as occult heartworm disease or infection. The incidence of occult infections among dogs harboring adult heartworms varies by geographic region from 5 to 67 per cent.[40–46] In general, the prevalence of occult heartworm disease in the continental United States is thought to be 10 to 20 per cent of all heartworm infections. Occult heartworm infection may result from unisex infections, prepatent infections, drug-induced sterility, and immune-mediated elimination of microfilariae. Prepatent and unisex infections have accounted for 57 to 85 per cent of occult infections in various locations in the United States, Australia, and Japan.[40–46] Prepatent infections with immature (L_5) worms in the pulmonary arteries or heart are particularly likely in the colder months of the year when dogs have been infected during the previous summer.

Drugs such as stibophen, levamisole, and ivermectin (at high dosages) can result in abortion and sterility or depressed reproductive function of female heartworms.[47–58] Thus, incomplete or ineffective adulticide could lead to an occult infection.

Occult heartworm infection may also result, particularly in highly endemic regions, from depression of microfilaria production or microfilarial destruction via immune mechanisms. One of the first effects of developing immunity against intestinal nematodes is reduced fecundity.[53, 54] As the number of adult heartworms increases, the number of microfilariae produced by each female decreases.[40]

Some clinicians prefer to limit the term "occult heartworm infection" to immune-mediated destruction of microfilariae.[55] Immune-mediated occult infections result from host hypersensitization to microfilarial antigens.[55, 56] Excess microfilaria-specific humoral antibody (IgG) exists in these occult infections. When patency exists, there is a state of antigen excess and humoral antibody is consumed.[56–59]

Antibody-dependent leukocyte adhesion to microfilariae in the pulmonary circulation results in subsequent entrapment of microfilariae in the pulmonary capillaries.[56, 60, 61] Microfilaria-leukocyte (neutrophils, eosinophils) complexes may be engulfed by phagocytic cells of the reticuloendothelial system within the lungs. Many dead microfilariae are found surrounded by a granulomatous inflammation. Once microfilariae disappear from the circulation, they usually do not reappear.[28]

Immune mediated occult infections are associated with a higher prevalence of severe pulmonary disease than microfilaremic infections. The age, size, and sex of dogs with occult infections are not different from those of dogs with patent infections.[18, 62] Approximately 70 to 80 per cent of dogs with severe pulmonary arterial disease seen by the authors have occult infections.[18, 62] Allergic pneumonitis and pulmonary eosinophilic granulomatosis are also usually associated with occult infections.[62–64] The relatively high prevalence of severe complications associated with occult infections is related to host-parasite interactions and increased adult worm burden. Chronicity is probably not a factor since the ages of dogs with severe pulmonary arterial disease, both occult and microfilaremic, are not different from those of dogs with patent infections and minimal disease.

The treatment of dogs with occult infections varies from that of patent infections in several regards. Since microfilaremia is absent, microfilaricide drugs are not required. Also, diethylcarbamazine may be prescribed immediately in order to prevent re-infection. Special treatment regimens are indicated for dogs with complications of occult infection such as severe pulmonary arterial disease, with or without right-sided congestive heart failure; allergic pneumonitis, and pulmonary eosinophilic granulomatosis.

Severe Pulmonary Arterial Disease. The severity of heartworm disease is usually directly related to the severity of pulmonary arterial disease. Severe pulmonary arterial disease is associated with platelet consumption, fibrin deposition, thromboembolism, pulmonary hypertension, right-sided congestive heart failure, hemolysis, hemoglobinuria, and secondary parenchymal lung disease.[7, 8, 10, 12, 14–16, 19, 65, 66]

The severity of pulmonary arterial disease can be assessed by thoracic radiographs (Figure 80–4). The diameters of the caudal lobar pulmonary arteries should not normally exceed those of the ninth ribs at their points of superimposition on the ventro-dorsal or dorsoventral projection.[67] The lobar arteries of severely affected dogs are usually 2.5 to 3.5 times the diameters of the ninth ribs and may be 4 to 5 times as large.[62] The cranial lobar pulmonary arteries, as viewed on the lateral projection, are normally no wider than the corresponding veins or the proximal portions of the fourth ribs.[63] Severe heartworm disease produces cranial lobar arterial diameters that are at least 1.2 times the diameters of the corresponding veins (Figure 80–4).[62] Approximately 10 per cent of heartworm-infected dogs seen by the authors have clinical and radiographic evidence of severe pulmonary arterial disease. Affected dogs are usually 4 to 7 years of age and middle- to large-sized, and approximately 70 per cent have occult infections.[62]

Clinical signs commonly associated with severe pulmonary arterial disease are coughing, exercise intolerance, syncope, weight loss, and right-sided congestive heart failure. Parenchymal lung disease often occurs secondary to severe pulmonary arterial disease (Figure 80–5). Associated clinical signs are coughing, pyrexia, crackles, and hemoptysis. Parenchymal lung complications may be present at the time of diagnosis but are more common one to three weeks following thiacetarsamide Na treatment (Figure 80–6).

Hemoglobinuria is an occasional complication of severe pulmonary arterial disease, is associated with thrombocytopenia and regenerative anemia, and may occur prior to or following thiacetarsamide Na treatment. Hemoglobinuria results from hemolysis, which is the result of erythrocyte trauma caused by endothelial damage, fibrin production, and thromboembolism.[65, 68] Although heartworm-infected dogs may have positive Coombs' test reactions, the presence of immunoglobulin and complement on the erythrocytes does not seem to be related to anemia.[68]

Since platelet adhesion and activation are involved in the pathogenesis of pulmonary arterial disease, drugs that modify platelet function can be beneficial.[7, 10–12, 69, 70] Heartworm-infected dogs treated with aspirin have less platelet adhesion, vascular damage, and villous proliferation than heartworm-infected dogs not given aspirin.[11, 12, 17, 71]

Cage confinement and aspirin treatment are recommended for dogs with severe pulmonary arterial disease.[11, 18, 21, 62, 69] Affected dogs should be cage confined and receive aspirin treatment 2.2 to 3.0 mg/lb (5 to 7 mg/kg) daily for two to three weeks prior to, during, and for three to four weeks following thiacetarsamide Na treatment.

Approximately 50 per cent of dogs with severe pulmonary arterial disease have overt evidence of right-sided congestive heart failure.[18, 62, 72] Affected dogs have evidence of elevated central venous pressure (jugular pulses, distended jugular veins) and ascites. The effusion is a high protein (greater than 2.5 mg/dl) modified transudate that is either serosanguineous or amber in appearance.

In addition to cage confinement and aspirin treatment, dogs with right-sided congestive heart failure should be treated with conservative dosages of diuretics and a low-sodium diet. Paracentesis is not recommended unless the degree of ascites is such that the patient cannot lie down or sleep comfortably because of fluid pressure on the diaphragm. Excessive paracentesis contributes to hypoalbuminemia, which is already a problem in some dogs.

Digoxin is not recommended, has been shown to be unnecessary, and often results in digoxin toxicity.[18, 62] The relatively large size of many heartworm-infected dogs, decreased volume of distribution due to cachexia, and overestimation of lean body weight due to the effect of ascites probably accounts for the relatively high incidence of digoxin toxicity.

During the pre-adulticide period of cage confinement and aspirin treatment, concomitant problems may develop or be discovered. Parenchymal lung disease secondary to arterial disease should be suspected if dyspnea, crackles, pyrexia, or hemoptysis occur. Thoracic radiographs are indicated under these circumstances in order to determine the degree of parenchymal disease (Figure 80–8). If parenchymal disease is confirmed, corticosteroid hormones such as prednisone at 0.5 to 1 mg/lb (1 to 2 mg/kg) daily are recommended until there is clinical and radiographic evidence of its resolution, usually three to seven days.

Hemoglobinuria may occur and is associated with anemia, thrombocytopenia, and a leukocytosis, usually with a left shift. Most patients with large pulmonary arteries and hemoglobinuria have a normal or nearly normal activated clotting time, a normal coagulogram, and an absence of signs of bleeding or hemorrhage. Heparin 70 to 110 U/lb (150 to 250 U/kg) SQ, q8h is an effective treatment and thrombocytopenia and hemoglobinuria usually resolve within one to three days. Heparin treatment should be continued until the platelet count is over 150,000/mm^3.

Following at least one week of aspirin and cage confinement and the resolution of parenchymal lung complications, thiacetarsamide Na treatment is given in the standard fashion.

The most common and severe complication of adulticide therapy is pulmonary thromboembolism. Dogs with severe pulmonary arterial disease are at increased risk of this complication from 7 to 30 days post-adulticide, the greatest risk occurring between 10 to 17 days post-adulticide. Thrombocytopenia is associated with pulmonary arterial thromboembolism and the platelet count should be monitored periodically throughout the treatment period.

Dogs with severe pulmonary arterial disease, with or without overt right-sided congestive heart failure have a significantly greater chance of survival when treated with protracted cage confinement and aspirin than when these

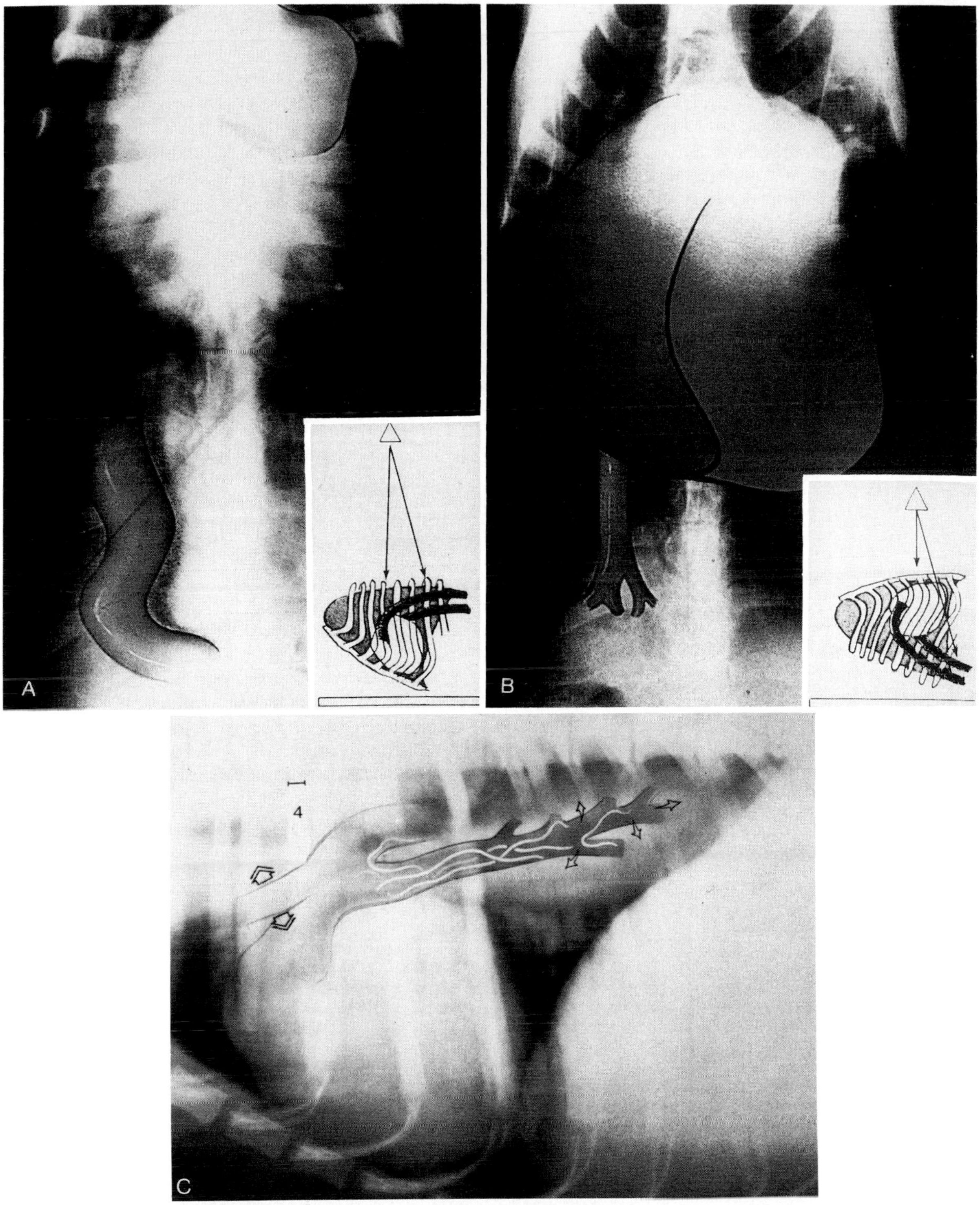

FIGURE 80–4. *A,* The dorsoventral position is the natural one for imaging the thorax. Owing to their greater distance from the cassette, the main pulmonary artery and caudal lobar arteries are magnified more than the right ventricle. The magnification of the main and caudal lobar arteries can be seen on the radiograph, and the reason for this magnification is demonstrated in the inset. *B,* We prefer the ventrodorsal position because we believe we can more consistently align dogs properly in this position. This position does magnify the right ventricle, in contrast to that seen in the dorsoventral position. *C,* An illustrated radiograph of the lateral view of the thorax. The alveolar pattern is frequently associated with an enlarged caudal lobar artery or an aneurysm. The increased parenchyma may compound the problem of determining the extent of the lobar arteries and of the heart. The lesions are markedly increased by the thromboembolism produced by dying heartworms. The diameter of the right cranial lobar artery also exceeds the diameter of the fourth rib, as measured just below the vertebrae. (From Rawlings, CA, et al.: Development and resolution of pulmonary disease in heartworm infection: Illustrated review. J Am Anim Hosp Assoc 17:711–720, 1981.)

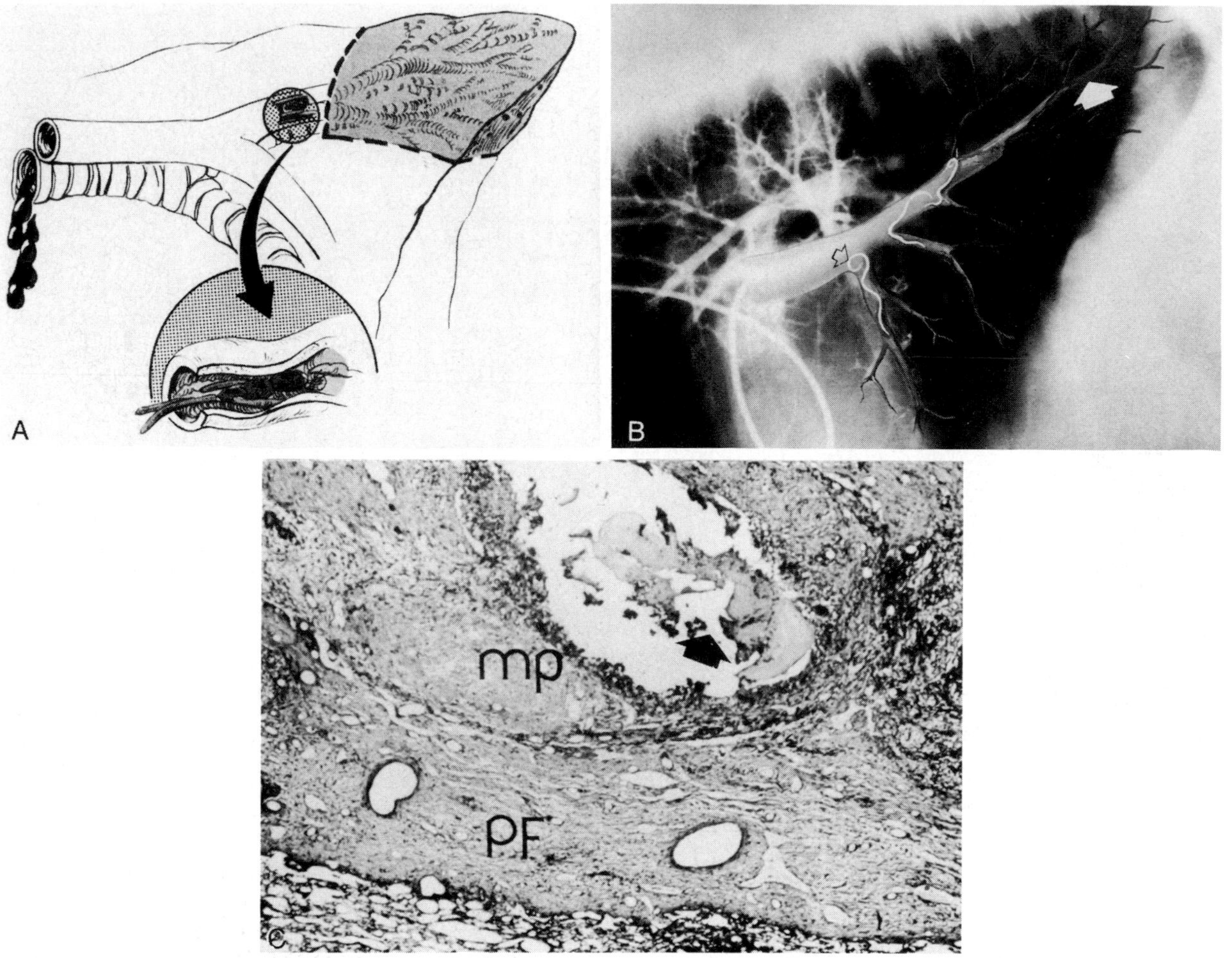

FIGURE 80–5. *A,* When adult heartworms die, the caudal lobar arteries frequently become obstructed with thrombi, and their arterial walls develop severe intimal proliferation, fibrosis, and granulomatous inflammation. The darker area of lung distal to the arterial disease (see illustration) produces the clinical signs (coughing, dyspnea, hemoptysis, and so forth) and a radiographic pattern of increased density in the lung field. Hemoptysis may develop when blood leaks into the airway and initiates coughing. This response may be massive if many heartworm adults are killed by an adulticide, or it may be insidious if the heartworms gradually die naturally. (From Rawlings, CA, et al.: The response of the canine's heart and lungs to *Dirofilaria immitis*. J Am Anim Hosp Assoc 14:17–32, 1978.) *B,* Illustrated right pulmonary arteriogram demonstrating the obstructed caudal lobar arteries. Blood flow is diverted toward the cranial pulmonary arteries. Dead or dying heartworms ("crumpled," white curvilinear silhouettes at the open dark arrow) and mural thrombi (white arrow) are illustrated within the distal caudal pulmonary arteries. This type of obstruction is typical following death of heartworms. Although this dog had severe obstruction of blood flow, clinical signs of pulmonary disease were not detected, probably as it was confined after thiacetarsamide treatment. With either exercise or stress, overt cardiopulmonary disease would have likely resulted. (From Rawlings, CA, et al.: Development and resolution of pulmonary disease in heartworm infection: Illustrated review. J Am Anim Hosp Assoc 17:711–720, 1981.) *C,* Micrograph of the cross section of a caudal lobar artery obtained four weeks after thiacetarsamide treatment. In addition to the expected inflammatory response to dying parasites (arrow), the vascular response includes myointimal proliferation (mp) and periarterial fibrosis (PF). (From Keith, JC, Jr, et al.: Treatment of canine dirofilariasis: Pulmonary thromboembolism caused by thiacetarsamide-microscopic changes. Am J Vet Res 44:1272–1277, 1983.)

provisions are not provided. Approximately 80 per cent of affected dogs survive treatment and return to a functional status. The survival percentages for dogs with severe pulmonary arterial disease with and without right-sided congestive heart failure are nearly identical.[18, 62] Whether hunting and working dogs return to full capabilities has not been determined.

Protracted aspirin therapy is associated with 10 to 15 per cent incidence of significant gastrointestinal bleeding.[62] For this reason the packed cell volume should be monitored. Melena is not a sensitive indicator of early bleeding. Cimetidine, protectants or emollients may be administered prophylactically but do not eliminate the possibility of bleeding complications.[62] Anorexia and depression may be associated with gastrointestinal bleeding. If additional evidence of bleeding, such as decreasing packed cell volume, hematemesis or melena occur, aspirin treatment should be stopped for several days. Cimetidine, sucralfate, and protectants are generally recommended.

The authors feel that both cage confinement and aspirin treatment are important aspects of the treatment of severe pulmonary arterial disease. However, thromboembolic complications are not eliminated. The presence of right-sided congestive heart failure in this group of dogs is of no additional prognostic importance. Most

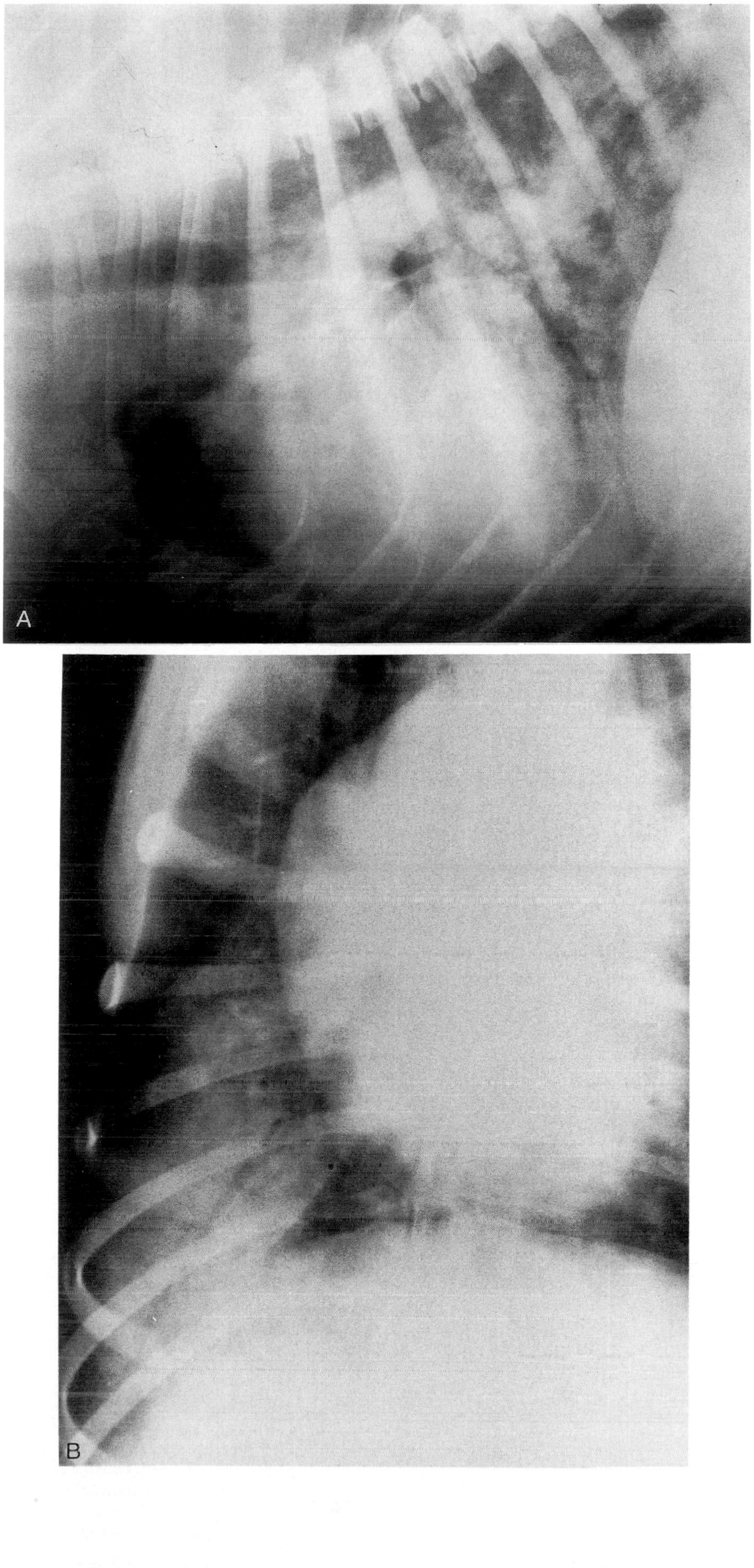

FIGURE 80–6. Thoracic radiographs of dog with severe parenchymal disease developing after adulticide treatment. The dog was dyspneic and coughing. Alveolar disease, with air bronchograms, is present in the caudal lung lobes. On the lateral view *(A)*, one can obtain the impression of enlarged and tortuous right cranial and left caudal lobar pulmonary arteries. Arterial margins are difficult to define because of the surrounding parenchymal disease. The caudal ventral portion of the ventrodorsal thoracic radiograph *(B)* has evidence of severe alveolar disease in the right caudal lobe. Treatment should include anti-inflammatory dosages of corticosteroids, cage confinement, and when the arterial partial pressure of oxygen is less than 70 mmHg, nasal administration of oxygen. Bronchodilators may be beneficial and cough suppressants are only used if the coughing is violent.

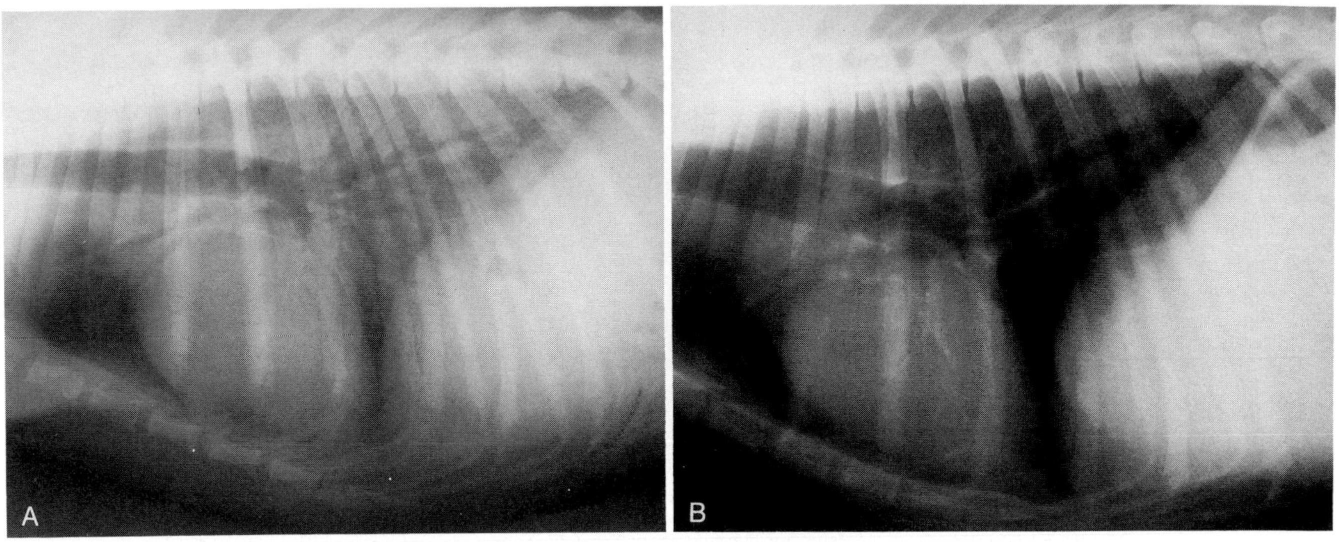

FIGURE 80–7. *A*, Thoracic radiographs of a dog with allergic pneumonitis induced by occult heartworm disease. Alveolar disease is present throughout the lung with widespread distribution of air bronchograms. It is difficult to evaluate the vascular structures until this pneumonitis has been reduced. An ELISA-antigen test is very useful in developing a clinical diagnosis of occult heartworm disease, treated with corticosteroids and supportive care. *B*, Thoracic radiograph of the pneumonitis case in *A* three days later after treatment with prednisone and cage confinement. In this case the lungs cleared and there was little evidence of heartworm infection as viewed with radiographs.

dogs free of clinical signs of pulmonary hypertension six months following treatment will remain so.

Occult Heartworm Disease Pneumonitis. A hypersensitivity type of pneumonitis develops in approximately 10 to 15 per cent of dogs with immune-mediated occult heartworm infections.[73] Heartworm pneumonitis is a type of pulmonary infiltrate with eosinophilia (PIE) syndrome. This syndrome resembles tropical eosinophilia (pulmonary eosinophilia), a microfilarial disease of human beings.[74–78] Occult heartworm disease results from antibody-dependent leukocyte adhesion to microfilariae and their subsequent entrapment within the pulmonary capillaries.[56, 60, 61] The inflammatory reaction includes neutrophils and eosinophils. The pneumonitis syndrome occurs when a hypersensitivity develops and is characterized by an unusually high number of eosinophils in the inflammatory response.[60, 61]

Affected dogs experience respiratory distress of variable severity and duration. In general, clinical signs are progressive over a period of a few weeks to six months or longer.[73] Coughing and dyspnea are the predominant clinical signs but severely affected dogs may experience mild cyanosis, anorexia, and weight loss. Bilateral, diffuse "crackles" can be ausculted over the areas of the caudal lung lobes.

Clinical signs of occult heartworm pneumonitis resemble those of other cardiopulmonary disorders such as left-sided congestive heart failure, pulmonary manifestations of systemic mycoses, severe pulmonary hypertension, and others. The differential diagnosis is based on the epizootiology, thoracic radiographic abnormalities, clinical pathology data, and serodiagnostic tests.

The typical dog with occult heartworm-induced pneumonitis is three to seven years of age, is of medium to large size, does not have a heart murmur, spends considerable time out of doors, and is not receiving prophylaxis against heartworm infection. Such epizootiologic criteria are usually different from those of dogs with left-sided congestive heart failure (excepting dilated cardiomyopathy), pneumonia, chronic lower airway disease, and metastatic neoplasia.

The thoracic radiographic abnormalities associated with heartworm pneumonitis are somewhat uniform and characteristic (Figure 80–7). There are diffuse, bilateral linear interstitial and alveolar infiltrates of the caudal lung lobes. The characteristics of these infiltrates most nearly resemble those of pulmonary blastomycosis and neurogenic pulmonary edema. The pattern is not typical of cardiogenic pulmonary edema.

The clinical pathology abnormalities associated with heartworm pneumonitis are variable eosinophilia, basophilia, and hyperglobulinemia. Transtracheal lavage cytology consists of a sterile, eosinophilic exudate with some nondegenerate neutrophils and macrophages. The indirect fluorescent antibody test for microfilarial cuticular antigen and adult *D. immitis* antigen serologic tests are usually positive.

Corticosteroid hormone treatment of heartworm pneumonitis is indicated and highly effective. Most dogs experience a rapid and complete resolution of clinical and radiographic abnormalities within three to five days of treatment. In some instances, clinical improvement is seen within 24 hours. Prednisone or prednisolone at 0.5 to 1 mg/lb (1 to 2 mg/kg) daily is the most often employed corticosteroid hormone. Dexamethasone (0.1 to 0.2 mg/lb or 0.2 to 0.4 mg/kg) has also been effective. Treatment is usually given orally but may be administered intravenously or intramuscularly to severely affected dogs in order to achieve more rapid and higher blood levels. Corticosteroid hormone treatment is stopped when there is both clinical and radiographic evidence of maximum resolution of the pulmonary infiltrates. Thiacetarsamide Na treatment should be initiated as soon thereafter as feasible.

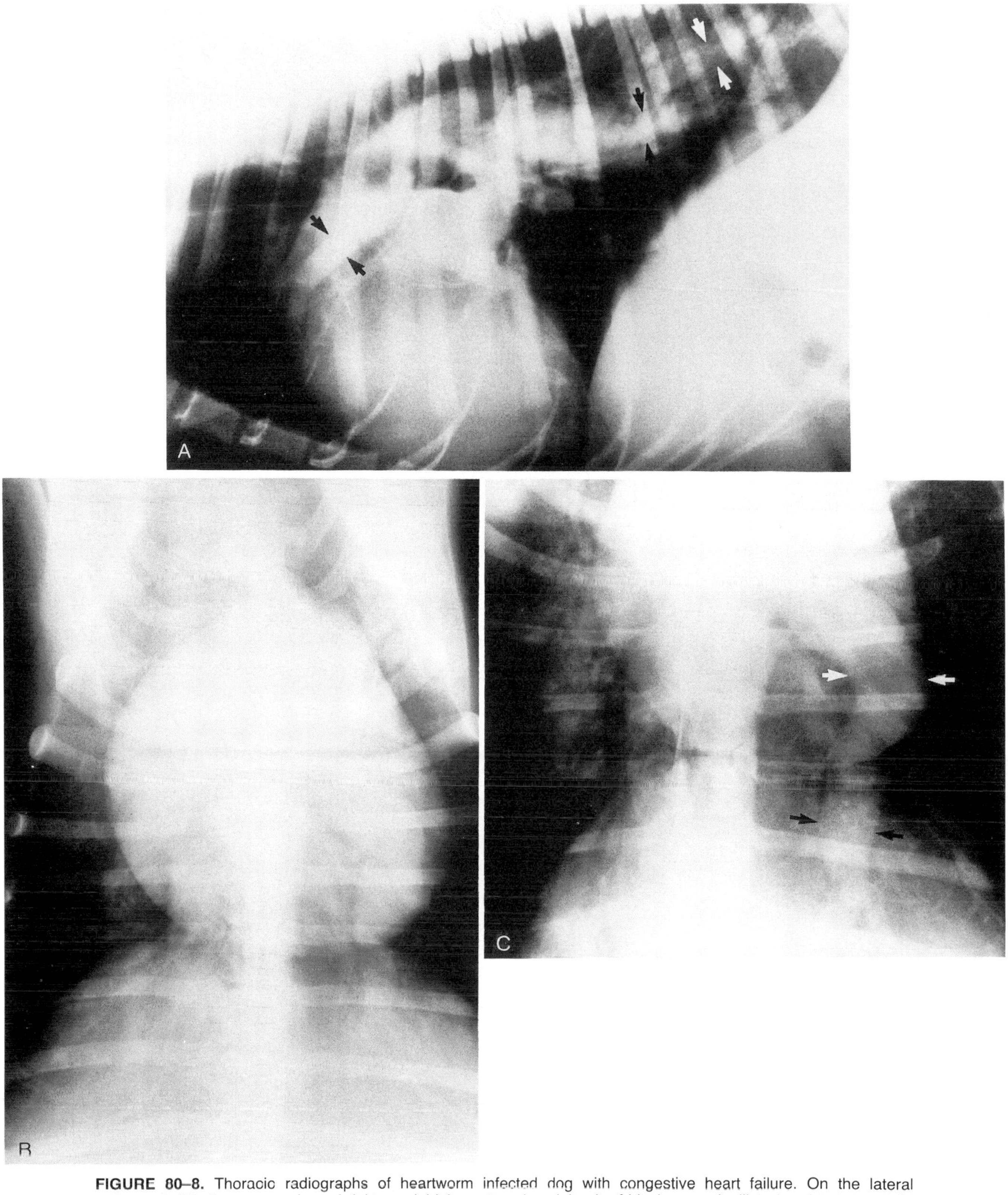

FIGURE 80–8. Thoracic radiographs of heartworm infected dog with congestive heart failure. On the lateral radiograph *(A)*, there are enlarged right cranial lobar artery (cranial pair of black arrows), dilated and tortuous right (caudal pair of black arrows) and left (white arrows) caudal lobar arteries, and increased sternal contact of the dilated right ventricle. On the ventrodorsal view *(B)*, the right artery appears (white and black arrows) even larger on the dorsoventral view *(C)*. Electrocardiograms of these dogs usually have signs of right ventricular hypertrophy. Many of these dogs are amicrofilaremic. Treatment is normally cage confinement, judicious dosages of furosemide, and aspirin followed by adulticide treatment in one or two weeks when failure signs resolve.

HEARTWORM INFECTION TREATMENT AND PREVENTION

ADULTICIDE TREATMENT

The recommended treatment regimen for dogs with subclinical or mildly or moderately clinical heartworm disease has not changed during the past quarter of a century.[79] The treatment of dogs with severe pulmonary arterial disease and complications of heartworm disease are discussed elsewhere.

Only the organoarsenic compounds belonging to the phenylarsenoxides are effective adulticide agents. Only thiacetarsamide is sufficiently stable in aqueous solution for storage in multiple dose vials. The steep dose-response curve and narrow therapeutic index produce variable efficacy and frequent toxicity.

Thiacetarsamide should be stored under refrigeration (2 to 8° C). The expiration time of the amber-colored, sealed vials under refrigeration is 15 months. At room temperature, when exposed to light, and when air enters the vials, the deterioration time is significantly shorter. Deterioration is indicated by precipitation and a yellow-orange discoloration.

The mechanism of the adulticidal effect of thiacetarsamide has not been determined. The half-life of the drug following intravenous administration is approximately 43 minutes and more than 85 per cent of the administered arsenic is eliminated during the first 48 hours.[37, 80–82] The highest tissue concentrations are found in the liver and, to a lesser extent, the kidneys.

Following each injection of thiacetarsamide, similar peak concentrations of arsenic occur in the blood. However, the post-distribution concentration increases with each dose.[81] Arsenic may be detectable in the blood in low concentrations for up to 12 days following the standard treatment regimen.[81]

The concentration of arsenic in the blood after 36 hours was higher for the ensuing two weeks in dogs wherein all heartworms were killed as compared to dogs wherein adulticide was incomplete. There is also a direct correlation between the arsenic content of adult heartworms and drug efficacy.[37] The duration of exposure to the minimum effective concentration of arsenic appears to be the factor most important to efficacy.[81]

Indications and Contraindications. Treatment of *D. immitis* infection is indicated in most heartworm infected patients. The success rate of treatment in dogs with subclinical and mildly clinical infections is very high. Even dogs with moderate and severe disease can be effectively treated; however, post-adulticide complications and mortality are greater.[18, 62]

Treatment may not be necessary in old dogs with subclinical or mildly clinical infections. This is particularly true in regions with a low incidence of heartworm infection. In such regions, the average worm burden of infected dogs tends to be lower than that of highly endemic regions and worm burden is a factor influencing the severity of pulmonary arterial disease.

The existence of concomitant, life-threatening diseases constitutes a relative contraindication to heartworm treatment. A thorough evaluation of concomitant problems is necessary in order to determine prognosis and whether or not effective treatment is feasible. Diseases such as neoplasia, renal failure, and cardiomyopathy may complicate or preclude heartworm therapy.

Various sequelae of chronic heartworm disease may exist at the time of diagnosis and some contraindicate heartworm treatment. Severe renal failure, most often resulting from a glomerulopathy and including the nephrotic syndrome, is an occasional complication of heartworm disease. The irreversibility of such renal disease precludes the long-term survival of affected dogs. Hepatic insufficiency characterized by hypoalbuminemia; abnormal function tests, such as BSP retention and ammonia tolerance; and icterus may coexist with right-sided congestive heart failure. Renal failure may also be present in such cases. Heartworm treatment in such instances is not indicated.

Indications to Interrupt Treatment. Vomiting, lethargy, and anorexia are common complications of thiacetarsamide treatment and are most often encountered following the first or second drug injections. One or two episodes of vomiting are not an indication to abort therapy provided that the patient's overall demeanor has not deteriorated and anorexia is absent. Repetitive or protracted vomiting is associated with lethargy and anorexia and is an indication to abort treatment.

Icterus, an uncommon complication of thiacetarsamide toxicity, is always an indication to abort therapy. Unfortunately, this complication cannot be accurately predicted. Careful observation of the patient and examination of the urine for the presence of bilirubin prior to each treatment may reveal early signs of hepatotoxicity. Marked bilirubinuria following the first treatment is an indication to proceed with caution.

Azotemia is an uncommon complication of thiacetarsamide treatment provided that an adequate MDB has been procured and properly evaluated. If azotemia is discovered during the course of treatment, treatment is interrupted only if the BUN is moderately to severely elevated. Treatment can usually be completed without complication if the BUN is less than 100 mg/dl, provided that intravenous balanced electrolyte solutions are administered during and for several days following thiacetarsamide treatment.

Whenever the adulticide regimen is interrupted, the entire regimen should be repeated in approximately four weeks. In all but the most severely affected dogs, a delay in treatment of this duration is of no consequence.

Thiacetarsamide should be injected at intervals of not less than 8 hours or longer than 15 hours. The recommended dosage is 1.0 mg/lb (0.10 ml/lb) or 2.2 mg/kg (0.22 ml/kg) BID for two days, intravenously. Although slightly higher dosages may be more efficacious, the risk of toxicity is also increased.[81, 83, 84] Likewise, increasing the treatment schedule to three days (six injections) is not recommended because increased efficacy has not been demonstrated, but more severe post-treatment lung complications result.[85]

After an initial dose of thiacetarsamide Na, arsenic is detectable in the blood for one week or longer. There is a direct relationship between blood arsenic concentrations and drug efficacy. Prolonged exposure of heartworms to arsenic appears to be a factor determining efficacy.[82, 86] It is apparent that the dosage regimen more than the total dosage of thiacetarsamide is critical to drug efficacy.[79, 80, 83] Dogs that rapidly metabolize and/or excrete thiacetarsamide from the blood may be more likely to have decreased adulticide efficacy than dogs that eliminate the drug more slowly.[82] There is currently no method for determining this prior to treatment.

Each injection should be administered in a peripheral vein as distally as feasible. Each injection should be given at a different location, although the same vein may be used for two injections. Thiacetarsamide may be given via either a two syringe and needle or two syringe and "butterfly" catheter technique. Indwelling catheters are not necessary nor recommended. The drug should never be injected unless there is absolute certainty of proper cannulation of the vein. Once proper cannulation is assured, the drug should be injected at an expeditious but not rapid rate so that the risk of patient movement is minimized.

Thiacetarsamide directly damages the endothelium of veins at the injection site. When multiple injections are given at or near the same site the possibility of drug leakage is increased. Likewise, vascular damage created by indwelling catheters may predispose to drug extravasation. If a jugular catheter is in place, any or all injections may be given by this route.

It should not be expected that thiacetarsamide will kill every heartworm in every treated dog. There is variation in efficacy among individual dogs. Immature worms, especially female worms, are more resistant. When corticosteroid hormones are administered during and immediately following thiacetarsamide treatment, fewer female heartworms are killed.[20, 21, 87] Essentially 100 per cent of male heartworms are killed by thiacetarsamide at two months, six months, one year, and two years post-L_3 inoculation. At approximately four months post-infection, approximately 40 per cent of the young adult (L_5) male worms in the heart are killed.[88] Thiacetarsamide is less effective against female *D. immitis*. Kill rates of approximately 100 per cent, 20 per cent, 40 per cent, 25 per cent, and 75 per cent have been estimated against worms 2, 4, 6, 12, and 24 months post-L_3 inoculation, respectively.[88] It should be emphasized that these figures are estimates. It is not necessary, however, to kill 100 per cent of adult heartworms in order to reduce significant resolution of pulmonary arterial disease.

Before each dosage of thiacetarsamide, the authors recommend that the patient be examined, rectal temperature taken, and be fed one-half hour prior to treatment. In addition, a urine sample can be obtained and examined for the presence of bilirubinuria, the earliest laboratory sign of hepatoxicity.

Thiacetarsamide Na Toxicity. Major organs of elimination of thiacetarsamide are the liver and kidneys.[80] The dose should be calculated accurately with adjustments for variations in patient size. Hepatic or renal insufficiency probably reduces the rate of drug excretion and increases the risk of drug toxicity. If, for any reason, the treatment schedule is disrupted, the entire regimen must be repeated at a later date. The risk of toxicity associated with subsequent treatments is decreased.

Most dogs that experience acute reactions to thiacetarsamide do so following the first or second dosages.[39] For this reason, patients should be observed closely during this time. Vomiting and anorexia are the most common signs of thiacetarsamide toxicity and can be expected in 10 to 15 per cent of treated dogs.[39] One or two episodes of vomiting following an injection of adulticide is common and of no particular concern provided that the dog's overall demeanor and appetite do not deteriorate.

Repetitive vomiting, lethargy, and anorexia are the most common, serious clinical signs of toxicity and under no circumstances should treatment be continued. The patient should be given balanced electrolyte solutions if necessary to maintain or reestablish hydration. Vitamins and so-called liver-sparing drugs containing methionine, inositol, and choline are of no documentable value.

Dogs experiencing toxicity should be fed a high-carbohydrate, low-fat diet for several days or longer and exercise should be severely restricted for four weeks. After three to four weeks, adulticide treatment should be reinstituted with further toxicity problems being uncommon.

The earliest laboratory sign of hepatic toxicity is bilirubinuria. However, bilirubinuria alone is not an indication to abort treatment. Marked or gross bilirubinuria after the first or second treatment, while unusual, is cause for concern. The patient should be observed closely but if persistent or repetitive vomiting, anorexia, and lethargy are absent, treatment can be continued. When severe bilirubinuria occurs following the first or second treatment, some dogs are already experiencing overt signs of toxicity, while others will do so following the next injection. Bilirubinuria is a common finding following the third and fourth injections, but is cause for concern only if the dog is clinically sick.

Icterus occurs in less than five per cent of treated dogs; is usually associated with vomiting, anorexia, and lethargy;[39] and is always an indication to stop treatment. There is no specific treatment for hepatoxicity resulting in icterus other than maintenance or reestablishment of hydration, restricted activity, and a high-carbohydrate, low-fat diet. Occasionally icterus and severe illness develop several days following completion of treatment and some of these patients die. Whether or not this type of complication can be prevented is uncertain. In some cases, however, clinical or laboratory evidence of impending toxicity is overlooked.

Serum liver enzyme activity commonly increases during thiacetarsamide treatment. There is no consistent correlation of rising enzyme activity and impending toxicity. Likewise, pre-treatment serum liver enzyme activity is not related to thiacetarsamide toxicity.[39] For these reasons, it is not necessary to monitor serum liver enzyme activity during treatment. By six weeks post-treatment, serum liver enzyme activity is usually normal or decreased in comparison to pre-treatment values.

Drug-Resistant Infections. Thiacetarsamide does not eradicate all heartworms in every dog treated. Young worms are more difficult to kill; male worms 4 months post-L_3 infection and female worms 4 to 12 months post-infection are difficult to eradicate.[88] In instances where infected dogs have not been tested annually, the ages of offending heartworms are uncertain. In many instances, dogs have probably been infected more than once so that there is more than one worm population. The worm population is young in infected dogs that had been confirmed negative by prior annual testing.

When microfilaremia persists after thiacetarsamide and microfilaricide treatment, a second attempt at microfilaricide is usually recommended. If ivermectin was the drug used, the treatment should be repeated. If another microfilaricide was used initially, then ivermectin is the best choice for the second treatment.

If a second course of microfilaricide treatment fails to clear the microfilariae, some clinicians prefer to repeat the entire course of heartworm treatment. An alternative is to perform an adult antigen test at 60 days post-thiacetarsamide.[89] A negative post-treatment test result indicates that no or few adult heartworms are present and that microfilaricide treatment failed. A positive test result indicates persisting adult worms. Retreatment with adulticide should be considered. If the heartworm infection has occurred during the past year, immediately repeating thiacetarsamide treatment is not likely to eradicate the young female worms. In this circumstance, the dog may be placed on ivermectin prophylaxis (0.003 mg/lb or 0.006 mg/kg, monthly) to prevent superinfection and adulticide treatment planned for one year hence. Since some worms are killed by initial thiacetarsamide treatment, pulmonary arterial disease does not worsen markedly during the ensuing year. If arterial disease is present, aspirin given daily at 2.0 mg/lb (5 mg/kg) would be beneficial.

If persisting adult worms of an unknown age distribution are suspected, a second course of thiacetarsamide and microfilaricide (preferably ivermectin) may be given. If microfilaremia is not eradicated by this course of treatment, then ivermectin should be prescribed and re-treatment planned for one year later.

When dithiazanine or levamisole is administered as a microfilaricide, a concentration test is performed immediately after a certain number of days of treatment. The microfilaria count may be drastically reduced by these drugs even if adult, gravid female worms have survived. Thus a negative concentration test is possible even though adulticide has not been complete. Although the microfilaria concentration will rapidly increase after the microfilaricide treatment is stopped, this will not be detected unless a second concentration test is performed after one to several weeks.

When ivermectin is employed successfully as a microfilaricide, at least 90 per cent of dogs are cleared by 21 days post-treatment. If a concentration test is performed at four weeks post-ivermectin, microfilaria recrudescence due to persisting gravid female worms will be detected.

MICROFILARICIDE TREATMENT

Although dithiazanine, levamisole, fenthion, and ivermectin are variably effective microfilaricide drugs, only dithiazanine is approved by the FDA. The most effective microfilaricide is ivermectin. Microfilaricide treatment is given three to six weeks post-thiacetarsamide treatment. Although microfilarial numbers are quickly reduced, they are often difficult to eliminate. All microfilaricide drugs are given to effect with extension of the treatment schedule when necessary.

Dithiazanine should be administered at a dosage range of 3.0 to 5 mg/lb (7 to 11 mg/kg) for 7 to 10 days. After five to seven days, microfilarial counts are usually reduced by 90 per cent, but low concentrations (less than 10/ml) often persist, even though all adult worms are eliminated. After seven days, a microfilaria concentration test is performed. If microfilariae are detected and adverse reactions are absent, the dose may be continued or increased to 5 to 7 mg/lb (11 to 15 mg/kg), daily for an additional week. If adverse reactions have occurred, an alternate drug is selected.

Adverse reactions caused by dithiazanine are usually vomiting, diarrhea, anorexia, and occasionally, weakness. Reactions are more commonly associated with higher dosages. Vomiting may be prevented by dividing the dosage and administering the drug after a small meal or by the administration of an antiemetic. Vomitus and feces of dogs receiving dithiazanine are stained purple and will irreversibly stain fabrics that they contact.

Ivermectin is a highly effective microfilaricide that is also not FDA approved for this purpose. Current knowledge indicates that a dosage of 20 μg/lb (0.020 mg/lb) (50 μg/kg [0.05 mg/kg]), one dose, administered four weeks post-thiacetarsamide is a very effective regimen. One ml of Ivomec is diluted in 9 ml of propylene glycol, USP and administered at a dosage of 1 ml/44 lb (1 ml/20 kg).[90, 91] When used, this regimen is administered in the morning and the dog observed throughout the day for evidence of adverse reactions. The dog is discharged in the later afternoon. Until further information and testing are available, ivermectin should not be administered to collie and collie-mix dogs.

A microfilaria concentration test is performed three to four weeks post-ivermectin. If microfilaremia persists, the regimen is repeated. If microfilaremia is detected three to four weeks following the second dose of ivermectin, adult heartworms probably remain. These dogs should be tested by an antigen ELISA test two to three months after the adulticide treatment.

Adverse reactions associated with ivermectin are of three types.[90] The first type is not necessarily associated with high concentrations of microfilariae and has been seen mostly in collies. It is characterized by the acute onset of ataxia, mydriasis, weakness, seizures, coma, and often, death. Other types of adverse reactions are associated with high concentrations of circulating microfilariae. In less than five per cent of treated dogs, adverse reactions of variable severity occur beginning one to two hours post-administration. Lethargy and vomiting are usually the extent of the reaction. Tachypnea, tachycardia, weakness, pale mucous membranes, and shock are uncommon extensions of such a reaction. The patient is observed for such reactions and supportive intravenous fluid therapy and soluble corticosteroid hormones are administered at appropriate dosages when indicated. Deaths due to this type of reaction are rare unless the patient is not closely observed, shock occurs, and the irreversible phase is reached before therapy is initiated. Occasionally, lethargy and anorexia are reported to occur one to two days post-treatment.

Although microfilarial counts are not routinely performed, the incidence of the latter two types of adverse reactions could be reduced if ivermectin were not administered when high concentrations of microfilariae were detected.

Levamisole is not FDA approved for use in dogs but is, nonetheless, a commonly employed microfilaricide. Levamisole eliminates microfilariae in approximately 90 per cent of affected dogs when administered at a dosage of 4.5 to 5.0 mg/lb (10 to 11 mg/kg), daily for 7 to 14 days. A concentration test is performed after seven days, and if positive, the treatment is continued for five to seven additional days.

The therapeutic index of levamisole is narrow and variation from the recommended dosage is to be avoided. Vomiting is the most common adverse reaction but the incidence of vomiting can be diminished by administering levamisole after a small meal. In fact, levamisole should never be administered to a dog that has not recently eaten. Vomiting can also be diminished by prophylactic antiemetic treatment. Although not tested under controlled conditions, dividing the daily dosage also diminishes the incidence of adverse reactions while efficacy may be maintained. Lethargy, diarrhea, nervousness, and muscle stiffness or tremors are less common, but are more significant adverse effects that necessitate withdrawal of levamisole treatment. If microfilariae persist after two weeks of treatment, an alternate drug is chosen.

Levamisole eliminates microfilariae, kills some male adult heartworms, and may sterilize adult female worms. Thus it is possible that adult heartworms can survive thiacetarsamide and levamisole treatment, even though circulating microfilariae are absent.[92, 93] Such an eventuality can be detected if an adult antigen test remains positive several months following completion of levamisole treatment.

Fenthion has been employed as a microfilaricide even though it is not FDA approved for that purpose in dogs. Fenthion (13.8 per cent or 20 per cent solution) is administered topically, once weekly, at a dosage of 7 mg/lb (15 mg/kg) beginning 4 to 6 weeks post-thiacetarsamide treatment. Microfilariae are usually cleared after two to three treatments. If microfilaremia persists, an alternate drug is chosen. Although uncommon, clinical signs of organophosphate toxicity may occur following fenthion administration. The subcutaneous administration of fenthion is not recommended.

When microfilaremia has been eliminated by any of the aforementioned drugs, prophylactic therapy should be initiated at the appropriate time, that is, immediately if reinfection is an immediate possibility. Several weeks following the apparent elimination of microfilariae, another concentration test is recommended in order to detect recrudescence resulting from persisting adult heartworms. This is particularly recommended when dithiazanine or levamisole has been administered. When microfilariae are eradicated, concentration tests are recommended at 6- or 12-month intervals.

IATROGENIC OCCULT INFECTIONS

Occult infection can be produced if certain variations from the recommended treatment occur. Levamisole is an undependable adulticide drug. It may kill some or all adult male worms but seldom eradicates all of the female worms.[94] However, levamisole may sterilize the females and following microfilaricide treatment the infection may be mistakenly assumed to have been eradicated.

Ivermectin, when administered at high dosage (0.1 to 0.2 mg/lb or 0.2 to 0.5 mg/kg) prior to adulticide treatment, can suppress subsequent microfilaria production. Even if subsequent adulticide treatment is incomplete, microfilaria concentrations in the peripheral blood may be low and difficult to detect for weeks.[95–98]

DIETHYLCARBAMAZINE (DEC) AND MICROFILAREMIA

Diethylcarbamazine treatment should never be initiated in a microfilaremic dog. However, if a dog is already receiving daily DEC treatment and is found to be microfilaremic, DEC may be continued. It is imperative that the client understand that the drug must be continued on a daily basis. If, for any reason, DEC is not administered for several days or longer, re-institution may produce an adverse reaction.

Microfilaremia can occur in dogs receiving DEC under several circumstances. Failure of the client to administer the drug faithfully may result in infection. Recrudescence of microfilariae following incomplete adulticide treatment may not be detected unless a concentration test is performed one or more weeks after the completion of dithiazanine or levamisole treatment. Low concentrations of microfilariae often remain following dithiazanine treatment and may not be detected on an initial concentration test. It is possible, however, that this low level microfilaremia may be detected on a subsequent test.

DIETHYLCARBAMAZINE AND OCCULT INFECTIONS

Diethylcarbamazine for prophylaxis may be initiated as soon as occult infection is diagnosed. Likewise, prophylaxis should be continued when occult infection is discovered in a dog already receiving the drug. Since microfilaremia is absent, adverse reactions do not occur.

PROPHYLAXIS AND MICROFILAREMIA

If a delay in adulticide treatment is necessary, the possibility of superinfection exists. Such a delay might be the result of young, female worms that have not been eradicated by thiacetarsamide. A treatment delay might be necessitated by concomitant problems. Under these circumstances ivermectin (0.003 mg/lb or 0.006 mg/kg) may be administered until adulticide treatment is repeated.

PREVENTION OF HEARTWORM INFECTION

Heartworm infection has been effectively prevented by daily treatment of diethylcarbamazine since it was introduced in the early 1960s. Ivermectin, which has been a very effective preventive in laboratory and field studies, has recently been approved by the FDA. Another approved program is the semiannual administration of thiacetarsamide.

Diethylcarbamazine at 1.1 to 1.3 mg/lb (2.5 to 3.0 mg/kg) has been tested by many investigators and consistently found to prevent adult infections in dogs inoculated with infective larvae. Several products are available and seem to be equally effective. Occasional development of one or two adult heartworms has occurred in individual dogs during experimental infections. In addition, some clients apparently forget to give their dog its daily preventive dose and these dogs can develop infections. Since diethylcarbamazine probably effects a molting stage, such as the L_3 to L_4 at 9 to 12 days after infection, it should be started prior to the mosquito season.[21]

All dogs in endemic areas should be on a heartworm preventive program. We recommend that they be started on a program at the time that they are being administered their puppy immunizations. In seasonal and non-endemic areas, diethylcarbamazine may be stopped one month after the first frost and begun again one month prior to the spring mosquito season. Before a six-month-old dog is placed on the diethylcarbamazine program, a concentration test for microfilaria should be determined to be negative.[99]

Diethylcarbamazine has proven to be a very safe drug when given to heartworm-negative dogs. Although there have been field reports of male sterility, repeated studies have failed to document any decreased reproductive function in male dogs during chronic administration. In both people and dogs, diethylcarbamazine has been given continuously over several generations without any apparent effect on reproduction. Some dogs vomit and appear to be depressed after starting diethylcarbamazine treatment. This subtle response seems to be rare.

Heartworm-positive dogs should not be given diethylcarbamazine as some dogs develop adverse reactions of variable severity, including death. Dogs with less than 50 microfilariae/ml seldom develop reactions.[100] In dogs with a higher concentration of microfilaria, the percentage of adverse reactions ranges from 15 to 86 per cent. These reactions can usually be detected within the first hour of treatment. During the initial phase of the reaction, dogs become depressed, lethargic, and less responsive to stimuli. Vomiting, defecation, and diarrhea may develop. During the next phase, cardiovascular signs of bradycardia, soft heart sounds, and weak femoral pulse can be detected. In the third phase, shock is present as characterized by pale, cool, and tacky mucous membranes, prolonged capillary refill time, decreased arterial pulse, tachycardia, and tachypnea. The dogs salivate, become recumbent, develop hepatomegaly, and die.[101–103] Other typical findings include increased liver enzyme concentrations, thrombocytopenia, and a leukocyte response. Treatment is to administer shock dosages of corticosteroids and intravenous fluids.

Ivermectin has proven to be very effective in preventing infection in dogs experimentally inoculated with infective larvae and those naturally exposed to mosquitoes bearing infective larvae.[104, 105] It is marketed such that one of three different tablet sizes is used for any size of dog. The dosage is either a 68-μg tablet for a 1- to 25-pound dog, a 136-μg tablet for a 26- to 50-pound dog, and a 272-μg tablet for a 51- to 100-pound dog. Dogs over 100 pounds are given multiple tablets. The minimum dosage is 2.5 μg/lb (5.98 μg/kg), a dosage that has proven highly efficacious and is twice the dosage that has generally been effective in preventing heartworm infections.

Toxicity has occurred in heartworm-positive dogs when ivermectin was used at higher dosages in collies and to eliminate microfilaria. Dogs with high microfilarial concentrations given ivermectin at 90 μg/lb (200 μg/kg) have had reactions characterized by lethargy, vomiting, anorexia, shock, and death, which developed within one hour to two days of treatment. Collies given a similar dosage have had ataxia, mydriasis, weakness, seizures, coma, and deaths.[90] Similar reactions have not been seen in the studies evaluating ivermectin efficacy as a preventive. The drug insert approved by the Food and Drug Administration states that, "Clients should be advised to observe collies closely for at least eight hours after treatment and to contact their veterinarian if any toxic signs are noted" (FDA insert on Heartgard 30). Despite ivermectin's apparent safety in experimental and field prophylaxis studies, widespread clinical use may result in detection of idiosyncratic reactions in collie-type dogs.

Ivermectin's advantages over diethylcarbamazine are that dogs do not need to be free of heartworms for a preventive program to be started and larvae infecting the dog as many as two months previously are prevented from developing into adults. If ivermectin is given as a microfilaricide, infections contracted during the previous two months should be blocked. Another potential use of ivermectin might be in senile and debilitated dogs in which the decision is made to delay or not treat with adulticide. These dogs might be placed on a combination of ivermectin, aspirin, strict confinement, and good supportive care in order to prevent further infection, to reduce arterial disease, and to reduce further cardiopulmonary stress. An evaluation months later might also indicate that the patient has improved sufficiently to be treated with the standard adulticide and microfilaricide protocol.

With both diethylcarbamazine and ivermectin preventive programs, dogs should be tested annually unless they live in a highly endemic area where the testing should be done every six months.

If dogs in endemic areas are being evaluated for heartworm infection during prepurchase examination, veterinarians should consider using both microfilarial concentration tests and the immunodiagnostic tests for circulating antigens. Since both ivermectin and levamisole can be obtained "over-the-counter," it is possible for owners to temporarily clear a heartworm-infected dog of microfilaria. Since the ELISA tests for adult antigens seldom have false results, an adult infection, particularly of many female heartworms, would likely produce a positive test result. Additional diagnostic information could be obtained with a thoracic radiograph.

References

1. Heartworm Infection Incidence Map 1986. Proc Heartworm

Symp. Washington, DC, Amer Heartworm Soc, 1986, inside cover.

2. Rawlings, CA: Heartworm disease in dogs and cats. Philadelphia, PA, WB Saunders, 1986.
3. Lewis, RE, Losonsky, JM: Sex and age distribution of dogs with heartworm disease. *In* Otto, GF (ed): Proc Heartworm Symp, 1977, Bonner Springs, KS, Vet Med Pub Co, 1977.
4. Calvert, CA and Rawlings, CA: Canine heartworm disease. *In* Kirk, RW (ed): Current Veterinary Therapy VIII. Philadelphia, WB Saunders, 1983, p 348.
5. Wallenstein, WL, Tibola, BJ: Survey of canine filariasis in Maryland area—Incidence of *Dirofilaria immitis* and *Dipetalonema*. JAVMA 137:712, 1960.
6. Orihel, TC: Morphology of the larval stages of *Dirofilaria immitis* in the dog. J Parasit 47:251, 1961.
7. Rawlings, CA, et al.: The response of the canine's heart and lungs to *Dirofilaria immitis*. JAAHA 14:17, 1978.
8. Rawlings, CA, et al.: Development and resolution of pulmonary disease in heartworm infection: Illustrated review. JAAHA 17:711, 1981.
9. Jackson, RF, et al.: Distribution of heartworms in the right side of the heart and adjacent vessels of the dog. JAVMA 149:515, 1966.
10. Schaub, RG, Rawlings, CA: Pulmonary vascular response during phases of canine heartworm disease: A scanning electron microscopic study. Am J Vet Res 41:1082, 1980.
11. Schaub, RG, et al.: Platelet adhesion and myointimal proliferation in canine pulmonary arteries. Am J Pathol 104:13, 1981.
12. Keith, JC, et al.: Early arterial injury-induced myointimal proliferation in canine pulmonary arteries. Vet Res 44:181, 1983.
13. Adcock, JL: Pulmonary arterial lesions in canine dirofilariasis. Am J Vet Res 22:655, 1961.
14. Rawlings, CA, et al.: Post-adulticide changes in *Dirofilaria immitis* infected beagles. Am J Vet Res 44:8, 1983.
15. Rawlings, CA, et al.: Development and resolution of pulmonary arteriographic lesions in heartworm disease. JAVMA 16:17, 1980.
16. Rawlings, CA: Cardiopulmonary function in the dog with *Dirofilaria immitis*: During infection and after treatment. Am J Vet Res 41:319, 1980.
17. Rawlings, CA, et al.: Development and resolution of radiographic lesions in canine heartworm disease. JAVMA 178:1172, 1981.
18. Rawlings, CA, et al.: Effect of acetylsalicylic acid on pulmonary arteriosclerosis induced by a one year *Dirofilaria immitis* infection. Arteriosclerosis 5:355, 1985.
19. Calvert, CA, Thrall, DE: Treatment of canine heartworm disease coexisting with right-side heart failure. JAVMA 180:1201, 1982.
20. Rawlings, CA, et al.: Aspirin and prednisolone modification of post-adulticide pulmonary arterial disease in heartworm infection: Arteriographic study. Am J Vet Res 44:821, 1983.
21. Rawlings, CA, et al.: Aspirin and prednisolone modification of radiographic changes caused by adulticide treatment in dogs with heartworm infection. JAVMA 182:131, 1983.
22. Keith, JC, et al.: Pulmonary thromboembolism during therapy of dirofilariasis with thiacetarsamide modificator with aspirin or prednisolone. Am J Vet Res 44:1278, 1983.
23. Rawlings, CA, et al.: Susceptibility of dogs with heartworm disease to hypoxia. Am J Vet Res 38:1365, 1977.
24. Losonsky, JM, et al.: Thoracic radiographic abnormalities in 200 dogs with spontaneous heartworm infections. Vet Radiol 24:120, 1983.
25. Lewis, RE, Losonsky, JM: The frequency of roentgen signs in heartworm disease. Proc Am Heartworm Soc 77:73, 1977.
26. Rawlings, CA, et al.: Eosinophilia and basophilia in *Dirofilaria immitis* and *Dipetalonema reconditum*. JAAHA 16:699, 1980.
27. Calvert, CA, et al.: Comparisons of radiographic and electrocardiographic abnormalities in canine heartworm disease. Vet Radiol 27:2, 1986.
28. Knight, DH: Heartworm disease. Adv Vet Sci Comp Med 1:107, 1977.
29. Hill, JD: Electrocardiographic diagnosis of right ventricular enlargement in dogs. J Electrocardiol 4:347, 1971.
30. Rawlings, CA, Lewis, RE: Right ventricular enlargement in heartworm disease. Am J Vet Res 38:1801, 1977.
31. Miller, MS: The electrocardiogram of dogs with heartworm infection. Clinical report and review of the literature. Sem Vet Med Surg 2:28, 1987.
32. Wallace, CR, Hamilton, WF: Study of spontaneous congestive heart failure in the dog. Circ Res 11:301, 1962.
33. Ogburn, PN, et al.: Electrocardiographic and phonocardiographic alterations in canine heartworm disease. *In* Otto, GF (ed): Proc Heartworm Symp, 1977, Bonner Springs, KS, Vet Med Pub Co, 1978, pp 67–72.
34. Shirota, K, et al.: Canine interstitial nephritis with special reference to glomerular lesions and filariasis. Jap J Vet Sci 41:119, 1979.
35. Barsanti, JA: Serum and urine proteins in dogs infected with *Dirofilaria immitis*. *In* Otto, GF (ed): Proc Heartworm Symp, 1977, Bonner Springs, KS, Vet Med Pub Co, 1978, p 53.
36. Calvert, CA, Rawlings, CA: Diagnosis and treatment of canine heartworm disease. *In* Kirk, RW (ed): Current Veterinary Therapy VIII. Philadelphia, WB Saunders, 1985, p 348.
37. Holmes, RA, et al.: Thiacetarsamide sodium: pharmacokinetics and the effects of decreased liver function on efficacy against *Dirofilaria immitis* in dogs. *In* Otto, GF (ed): Proc Heartworm Symp, 1986, Washington, DC, Amer Heartworm Soc, p, 57.
38. Hoskins, JD, et al.: Heartworm disease in dogs from Louisiana: pretreatment clinical and laboratory evaluation. JAAHA 20:205, 1984.
39. Hoskins, JD, et al.: Effects of thiacetarsamide sodium in Louisiana dogs with naturally-occurring canine heartworm disease. Proc Am Heartworm Soc 83:134, 1983.
40. Otto, GF: The significance of microfilaremia in the diagnosis of heartworm infection. *In* Otto, GF (ed): Proc Heartworm Symp, 1977, Bonner Springs, KS, Vet Med Pub Co, 1978, pp 22–30.
41. Hinman, EH: Studies on the dog heartworm, *Dirofilaria immitis* with special reference to periodicity. Am J Trop Med 15:371, 1935.
42. Carlisle, CH: The incidence of *Dirofilaria immitis* in dogs in Queensland. Austral Vet J 45:535, 1969.
43. Kume, S: Canine Heartworm Disease, A Discussion of the Current Knowledge. Gainesville, FL, Univ of Florida Press, 1970, p 44.
44. Watson, AD, et al.: A survey of canine filariasis in Sydney. Austral Vet J 49:31, 1973.
45. Streitel, RH, et al.: Prevalence of *Dirofilaria immitis* infections in dogs from a humane shelter in Ohio. JAVMA 170:720, 1977.
46. Jackson, RF: A study on the filter techniques for the detection and identification of canine microfilariae. *In* Otto, GF (ed): Proc Heartworm Symp, 1971, Bonner Springs, KS, Vet Med Pub Co, 1978, p 31.
47. Anaataphruty, M, et al.: Studies on chemotherapy of parasitic helminths. Efficacy of ivermectin on the circulating microfilaria and embryonic development in the female worm of *Dirofilaria immitis*. Jap J Parasit 31:517, 1982.
48. Knight, DH, et al.: Microfilaricidal efficacy of ivermectin in adulticide treated and untreated heartworm infected dogs. *In* Otto, GF (ed): Proc Heartworm Symp 1986. Washington, DC, Amer Heartworm Soc, 1986, p 19.
49. Wright, WH, Underwood, PC: A survey of 1,000 dog heartworm cases treated with firadin. N Am Vet 17:39, 1936.
50. Foley, RJ: The treatment of canine filariasis. Vet Med 45:485, 1950.
51. Jackson, RF, Otto, GF: Thiacetarsamide reevaluation. *In* Otto, GF (ed): Proc Heartworm Symp 1980. Bonner Springs, KS, Vet Med Pub Co, 1981, p 137.
52. Rawlings, CA, et al.: Four types of *Dirofilaria immitis* infections in dogs. JAVMA 180:1323, 1982.
53. Barth, EE, et al.: Studies on the mechanism of the self-cure action in rats infected with *Nippostrongylus brasiliensis*. Immunology 10:459, 1966.
54. Chandler, AC: Studies on the nature of immunity to intestinal nematodes. Am J Hyg 23:1, 1936.
55. Knight, DH: Heartworm disease. *In* Ettinger, SJ (ed): Textbook of Veterinary Internal Medicine. Philadelphia, WB Saunders, 1983, p 1097.
56. Wong, MM: Studies on microfilaremia in dogs. II. Levels of microfilaremia in relation to immunologic responses of the host. Am J Trop Med Hyg 13:66, 1964.
57. Pacheco, G: Progressive changes in certain serological responses

to *Dirofilaria immitis* infection in the dog. J Parasitol 52:311, 1966.
58. Bradley, RE, Alfort, BT: Efficacy of levamasole resinate against *Dirofilaria immitis* in dogs. Mod Vet Pract 58:518, 1977.
59. Wong, MM, Suter, PF: Indirect fluorescent antibody test in occult dirofilariasis. Am J Vet Res 10:414, 1979.
60. Wong, MM, et al.: Dirofilariasis without circulating microfilariae: A problem in diagnosis. JAVMA 163:133, 1973.
61. Wong, MM: Experimental occult dirofilariasis in dogs with special reference to immunological responses and its relationship to "eosinophilic lung" in man. Southeast Asian J Trop Med Public Hlth 5:480, 1974.
62. Calvert, CA, et al.: Therapy of canine heartworm disease with concomitant severe pulmonary arterial disease. Comp Cont Educ.
63. Calvert, CA, Losonsky, JM: Occult heartworm disease associated allergic pneumonitis. JAVMA 186:1097, 1985.
64. Calvert, CA, Rawlings, CA: Pulmonary manifestations of heartworm disease. Vet Clin North Am 15:991, 1985.
65. Confer, AW, et al.: Four cases of pulmonary nodular eosinophilic granulomatosis in dogs. Cornell Vet 73:41, 1983.
66. Ishahara, K, et al.: Clinicopathological studies in canine dirofilarial hemoglobulinuria. Jap J Vet Sci 40:525, 1978.
67. Clemmons, RM, et al.: The interaction between heartworms and platelets. *In* Otto, GF (ed): Proc Heartworm Symp, 1983, Edwardsville, KS, Vet Med Pub Co, 1983.
68. Thrall, DE, Losonsky, JM: A method of evaluating canine pulmonary circulating dynamics from survey radiographs. JAAHA 12:457, 1976.
69. Werner, LL, et al.: The incidence of positive Coombs' antiglobulin reactions in heartworm infected and non-infected dogs. *In* Otto, GF (ed): Proc Heartworm Symp, 1983, Edwardsville, KS, Vet Med Pub Co, 1983, p 21.
70. Schaub, RG, et al.: Effect of long term aspirin treatment on platelet adhesion to chronically damaged canine pulmonary arteries. Thromb Haemostasis 46:680, 1981.
71. Schaub, RG, et al.: The effect of aceylsalicylic acid on vascular damage and myointimal proliferation in canine pulmonary arteries subjected to chronic injury by *Dirofilaria immitis* infection. Am J Vet Res 44:449, 1983.
72. Rawlings, CA, et al.: An aspirin prednisolone combination to modify postadulticide lung disease in heartworm infected dogs. Am J Vet Res 45:2371, 1984.
73. Calvert, CA, et al.: Comparison of radiographic and electrocardiographic abnormalities in canine heartworm disease. Vet Radiol 27:2, 1986.
74. Wong, MM, Guest, MF: Filarial antibodies and eosinophilia in human subjects in an endemic area. Trans R Soc Trop Med Hyg 63:796, 1969.
75. Weingarten, RJ: Tropical eosinophilia. Lancet 1:103, 1943.
76. Van der Sar, S and Hartz, H: The syndrome, tropical eosinophilia and microfilaria. Amer J Trop Med Hyg 25:83, 1945.
77. Liebow, AA and Hannum, CA: Eosinophilia, ancylostomiasis, and strongyloidosis in the South Pacific area. Yale J Biol Med 18:381, 1976.
78. Raich, RA and Gleason, DF: Pulmonary symptoms and eosinophilia due to filariasis. Tubercle 40:462, 1959.
79. Donohugh, DL: Tropical eosinophilia. An etiologic inquiry. N Engl J Med 269:1357, 1963.
80. Jackson, RF: Two day treatment with thiacetarsamide for canine heartworm disease. JAVMA 142:23, 1963.
81. Drudge, JH: Arsenamide in the treatment of canine filariasis. Am J Vet Res 13:220, 1952.
82. Sundlof, SF, et al.: Pharmacokinetics of thiacetarsamide in relationship to therapeutic efficacy. *In* Otto, GF (ed): Proc Heartworm Symp, 1986, Washington, DC, Vet Heartworm Soc, 1986, p 65.
83. Holmes, RA, et al.: Thiacetarsamide in dogs. Disposition, kinetics, and correlations with selected indocyanine green kinetic values. Am J Vet Res 47:1338, 1968.
84. Otto, GF, Maren, TH: Possible use of an arsenical compound in the treatment of heartworm in dogs. Vet Med 42:128, 1947.
85. Courtney, CH, et al.: New dose schedule for the treatment of canine dirofilariasis with thiacetarsamide. *In* Otto, GF (ed): Proc Heartworm Symp. Washington, DC, Amer Heartworm Soc, 1986, p 49.
86. Jackson, RF, Otto, GF: Thiacetarsamide reevaluation. *In* Otto, GF (ed): Proc Heartworm Symp 1980. Bonner Springs, KS, Vet Med Pub Co, 1981.
87. Eagle, H: The minimal effective concentrations of *I. palladum in vitro* in relation to the therapeutic dose. Am J Syph Gonor Ven Dis 23:310, 1939.
88. McCall, JW, et al.: Re-evaluation of thiacetarsamide as an adulticidal agent against *Dirofilaria immitis* in dogs. *In* Otto, GF (ed): Proc Heartworm Symp 1980. Bonner Springs, Kansas, Vet Med Pub Co, 1982, p 141.
89. Blair, LS, et al.: Efficacy of thiacetarsamide in experimentally infected dogs at 2, 4, 6, 12, or 24 months post-infection with *Dirofilaria immitis*. *In* Otto, GF (ed): Proc Heartworm Symp 1983. Edwardsville, KS, Vet Med Pub Co, 1983, p 130.
90. Atwell, RB, et al.: The use of antigen test for diagnosis as an indicator of filarial numbers, and for assessing filarial mortality following thiacetarsamide therapy. *In* Otto, GF (ed): Proc Heartworm Symp 1986. Washington, DC, Amer Heartworm Soc, p 71.
91. Lambert, G, et al.: Evaluation of a new microfilaricide in dogs. Vet Med Sm Anim Clinic 65:676, 1970.
92. Jackson, RF: Ivermectin again. Am Heartworm Soc Bull 10:9, 1984.
93. Chaikin, RJ: Levamisole as a simultaneous microfilaricidal adulticide in canine heartworm disease. Canine Pract 6:32, 1979.
94. Rawlings, CA, et al.: Four types of occult *Dirofilaria immitis* infection in dogs. JAVMA 180:1323, 1982.
95. Jackson, RF: The activity of levamisole against the various stages of *Dirofilaria immitis* in the dog. *In* Otto, GF (ed): Proc Heartworm Symp 1977. Bonner Springs, KS, Vet Med Pub Co, 1981, p 137.
96. Campbell, WC, Blair, LS: Efficacy of avermectin against *Dirofilaria immitis* in dogs. Helminthology 52:308, 1978.
97. Blair, LS, Campbell, WC: Efficacy of avermectin B_{1a} against microfilariae of *Dirofilaria immitis*. Am J Vet Res 40:1031, 1979.
98. Pleu, RE, et al.: Clearance of *Dirofilaria immitis* microfilaria in dogs using 200 mcg/kg ivermectin subcutaneously. *In* Otto, GF (ed): Proc Heartworm Symp 1983. Edwardsville, Kansas, Vet Med Pub Co, 1983, p 153.
99. Knight, DL, et al.: Microfilaricidal efficacy of ivermectin in adulticide treated and untreated heartworm infected dogs. *In* Otto GF (ed): Proc Heartworm Symp 1986. Washington, DC, Amer Heartworm Soc, 1986, p 19.
100. Recommended procedures for the management of canine heartworm disease. Proc Am Heartworm Symp 1986. Washington, DC, Amer Heartworm Soc p 203.
101. Rawlings, CA, et al.: Diethylcarbamazine adverse reaction and relationship to microfilaremia. *In* Otto, GF (ed): Proc Heartworm Symp 1986. Washington, DC, Amer Heartworm Soc, 1986, pp 143–148.
102. Palumbo, NE, et al.: Preliminary observations on adverse reactions to diethylcarbamazine (DEC) in dogs infected with *Dirofilaria immitis*. *In* Otto, GF (ed): Proc Heartworm Symp 1977. Bonner Springs, Kansas, Vet Med Pub Co, 1977, pp 97–103.
103. Powers, DG, et al.: *Dirofilaria immitis*. I. Adverse reactions associated with diethylcarbamazine therapy in microfilaremic dogs. *In* Otto, GF (ed): Proc Heartworm Symp 1977. Bonner Springs, Kansas, Vet Med Pub Co, 1977, p 108.
104. Atwell, RB, Boreham, PFL: Studies on the adverse reactions following diethylcarbamazine to microfilaria-positive *(D. immitis)* dogs. *In* Otto, GF (ed): Proc Heartworm Symp 1983. Edwardsville, KS, Vet Med Pub Co, 1983, p 105.
105. Campbell, WC, et al.: Ivermectin vs. heartworm: The present status. *In* Otto GF (ed): Proc Heartworm Symp, 1983. Edwardsville, KS, Vet Med Pub Co, 1983, p 83.
106. McCall, JW, et al.: Prevention of natural acquisition of heartworm infection in dogs by monthly treatment with ivermectin. *In* Otto, GF (ed): Proc Heartworm Symp 1983. Edwardsville, KS, Vet Med Pub Co, 1983, p 83.

81 PERIPHERAL VASCULAR DISEASE

PETER F. SUTER

The peripheral vessels, including arteries, arterioles, capillaries, venules, veins and lymphatics, play an important role in almost every type of disease. The peripheral vessels may be involved primarily and initiate changes in the surrounding tissues (primary vascular disease). A disease may start in the tissues and involve the vessels secondarily (secondary vascular disease) or disease processes may affect tissues and vessels simultaneously. A substantial number of the peripheral vascular diseases that occur in humans also occur in dogs and cats, but significant clinical signs are often milder or uncommon when compared with their severity and prevalence in human medicine. A classification based on the vessel type involved is proposed in Table 81–1.

TABLE 81–1. PERIPHERAL VASCULAR DISEASES

- Diseases of Arteries and Arterioles
  - Organic Forms
    - Occlusive diseases
      - Arterial embolism
      - Arterial thrombosis
      - Angiitis, vasculitis
      - Post-traumatic vascular disorders
      - Diabetic arteropathy
    - Nonocclusive diseases
      - Arteriovenous fistula
      - Arterial aneurysm
      - Arterial calcification
      - Arteriosclerosis, hyalinosis, amyloidosis
      - Atherosclerosis, atheromatosis angiitis, vasculitis
  - Functional Forms
    - Vasospasm, traumatic, toxic
- Diseases of Veins
  - Phlebectasia
  - Varicosis
  - Phlebitis
  - Thrombophlebitis
- Diseases of Capillaries
- Diseases of Lymphatics
  - Lymphangitis
  - Lymphatic atrophy
  - Lymphedema
  - Lymphangiectasia
  - Hypoplasia, aplasia, hyperplasia
- Tumors of Peripheral Blood Vessels
  - Angioma, hemangioma, vascular hamartoma
  - Hemangiosarcoma

OCCLUSIVE ARTERIAL DISEASES, ARTERIAL THROMBOEMBOLISM

Arterial occlusion can be caused by organic (morphologic) obstruction including post-traumatic disorders, thrombosis, embolism, arteritis and degenerative arterial wall lesions such as atherosclerosis. Mural or extramural hematomas, extramural masses (neoplasms, abscesses), and increased pressure of the surrounding tissue, such as compartmental syndrome or intimal tears forming valve like structures, can acutely or gradually occlude the arterial lumen and stop blood flow. Clinically significant consequences of complete arterial occlusion are tissue hypoxemia, ischemia, neuropathy and eventually tissue necrosis (infarction). Infarcts are uncommon, when compared to the high frequency of vascular injuries in traumas. The rich supply of collateral vessels to organs and limbs accounts probably for the rarity with which infarcts are encountered.[1] The exceptions are organs (kidneys) or regions supplied by endarteries that have no connections to a collateral vascular bed.

Arterial Thromboembolism in Cats

(See Chapter 77)

Arterial Thrombosis and Thromboembolism in Dogs

A thrombus is an aggregation of blood factors, primarily platelets, and fibrin with entrapment of blood cell elements. Thrombosis is the formation or presence of a thrombus. It implies a clinical and pathologic state in which the blood supply to tissue is interrupted by a blood clot formed in a major vessel. Early in the thrombus formation in veins or in the heart, a clot or pieces thereof may break off and may be carried by the blood stream as emboli. Emboli can also consist of tissue particles, gas, clumps of bacteria, fat droplets, parasites, foreign bodies such as pieces of catheters, hairs and any other type of particle that may be brought into the bloodstream. Emboli that are trapped in an artery can start thrombus formation. Vascular occlusion can occur at the site of the thrombus formation or at a distant site where an embolus carried in the bloodstream gets caught at a vascular bifurcation or becomes wedged in a narrowing artery (thromboembolism).

For thrombosis or thromboembolism to occur, a local or/and generalized predisposition for clot formation and/or a deficit in clot lysis have to be present. Major preconditions that promote arterial thrombosis are: (1) damage to the vascular endothelium, (2) sluggish blood flow, namely prestasis or stasis and/or an altered blood flow pattern, and (3) changes in the constituents of the blood, mainly platelets, coagulation proteins and/or inhibitors of the coagulation, causing a state of hypercoagulability.

In Table 81–2 the predisposing factors and conditions associated with thrombosis and thromboembolism have been compiled. Inflammation due to infections, bacterial endocarditis, trauma and aberrant location of parasites in epidemic heartworm areas arc among the most common causes for thrombosis initiated by vascular endothelial damage. Inflammation and trauma commonly lead to platelet disruptions and promote clotting. Immunologic mechanisms such as in autoimmune diseases or hypersensitivity reactions play an important role in thrombus formation. In the majority of thrombotic and thromboembolic events a combination of several factors is at work. DIC (disseminated intravascular coagulation or consumptive coagulopathy), a sequela to many disease processes, is associated with hypercoagulability and mainly microvascular thrombus formation.

In some cases thrombosis is secondary to disease processes occurring in the immediate vicinity of an artery, i.e., a tumor.[2] In other cases the thrombosis-initiating disease is located in a distant organ such as in the kidneys (glomerulopathy), the adrenals (Cushing's syndrome), or the intestine (protein-losing enteropathy).[3–7] Thrombosis can also occur with drug therapy (L-asparaginase).[8]

TABLE 81–2. CAUSES AND PREDISPOSING FACTORS OF THROMBOSIS AND THROMBOEMBOLISM

Vascular Diseases, endothelial and/or wall damage
Arteriosclerosis (hyalinosis, amyloidosis)
Atherosclerosis
Vasculitis (angiitis), phlebitis, arteritis
Suppurative, septicemic, or granulomatous processes
Parasitosis (dirofilariasis)
Trauma, contusion, crushing injury, catheterization, indwelling catheters
Injection of irritating or hypertonic substances
Neoplastic invasion
Slowing of Blood Flow
Hypovolemia, shock
Cardiac insufficiency
Incarceration of blood vessels
Compression of blood vessels
Hypercoagulability
Increase in coagulation proteins or inadequate removal of activated coagulation factors
Deficiency of antithrombin III-factor
Disturbed fibrinolysis
Platelet disorders, thrombocytosis
Dehydration and/or hyperviscosity
Thromboembolic Events
Pieces breaking off from clots in veins, at heart valves or from atrial thrombi
Introduction of foreign material into the heart or veins, i.e., hairs, gun pellets, fat tissue from fractures, pieces of indwelling catheters
Aberrant location of parasites

It is beyond the scope of this chapter to discuss the interrelationship between arterial disease, hypercoagulability and thrombosis of internal organs. The following paragraphs will be confined to the clinical problems associated with systemic arterial thrombosis and thromboembolism. Systemic thromboembolism is less common in dogs than in cats, in which cardiomyopathies are the major cause of thromboembolism.

Clinical History. The great variety of diseases that can induce arterial thrombosis and thromboembolism provides for a diversified clinical history. Fairly commonly the first clue to the diagnosis may come from a carefully collected history.

Clinical Signs. It is a fair assumption that most thromboembolic events cause little or no clinically noticeable signs. Particularly after trauma or surgery thrombus formation is common, but due to rapid clot lysis and abundant collateral circulation, signs are usually transitory. In complete thrombotic arterial occlusion, ischemic injury begins within minutes, but the effect may not be evident for days and sometimes months (post-ischemic muscle fibrosis and muscle contracture).[1]

Because of the secondary nature of most thrombotic events and because thrombi can form simultaneously anywhere in the body the clinical picture is varied. It often represents an admixture of signs due to the underlying primary disease (i.e., endocarditis, dirofilariasis, renal disease) combined with signs caused by the occlusion of arteries to the limbs (in particular the hind limbs) or/and arteries to organs (in particular the kidneys and guts).

Arterial occlusion in the central nervous system is rarely diagnosed. For signs to occur, several arteries have to be occluded simultaneously as in severe atherosclerosis or with embolization following arterial catheterization.

Type and severity of the clinical signs depend on: (1) location, size and number of thrombi, (2) completeness and time frame within which the obstruction occurs, (3) age, composition and organization of the thrombus, (4) infection or sterility of the clot, (5) whether it is a single or repeated event, (6) the compensatory mechanisms elicited such as the opening up of collaterals, clot lysis and restoration of blood flow, (7) the complications that develop (tissue necrosis, local infection, hyperesthesia), and (8) the age of the animal. Thromboxane A2 and serotonin released from platelets may cause vasospasm impairing the opening up of collateral arteries as is known to occur in cats.

Thrombosis is a dynamic process. Thrombi undergo constant structural changes because deposition and lysis of fibrin take place concurrently. Later on, thrombi can become organized and may permanently block an artery. Most often, however, the fibrin is lysed spontaneously by plasmin and phagocytized by leukocytes. These processes reduce the size of the clot and break off material from the thrombus. Reducing the size of the thrombus leads to thromboemboli gradually moving peripherally and lodging in smaller, more peripheral vessels.

In humans, the classical signs of a sudden complete obstruction of a major limb artery are the signs of the seven "Ps," namely pain, paleness, paresthesia, pulselessness, polar (cold), paresis/paralysis, and prostration. The signs occurring in animals are similar. The so-called saddle thrombus formation at the trifurcation of the distal aorta extending into the two external iliac arteries and the common origin of the internal iliacs is the most frequently diagnosed peripheral thrombosis in dogs. It is found in dogs with bacterial endocarditis.[9, 10] In heartworm-infested areas it is often due to an aberrant location of adult worms.[11–13]

With a partial and/or a slow-onset arterial occlusion signs may be absent or the dog owner may observe an unsteady gait or lameness progressing to stumbling, weakness or even collapse in the hindquarters if the blood flow to both limbs is impaired. Following a short period of rest, the dogs often behave normally again. Some owners reported that their dog had lost weight and stamina. Others noticed licking or chewing at the hindlimbs or hypersensitivity over the lumbosacral region and the hindlimbs.

With an acute complete arterial occlusion, dogs may be unable to rise, may show extreme pain in the hindlimbs, and may be in severe general distress.

On clinical examination one often notices cool distal limbs and swollen muscles. The segmental and pedal reflexes may be depressed. Occasionally, hypersensitivity over the lumbar spine exists. A slow onset and progression of a peripheral neuropathy following trauma may be associated with ischemia of peripheral nerves.[1]

Thrombosis of front limb arteries also occurs, but the signs are usually less dramatic and unilateral. Cerebrovascular occlusions may lead to sudden disorientation, weakness, anisocoria, and hemiamaurosis.

With endocarditis, emboli break off continuously and lead to multiple thrombotic events involving the abdominal organs in particular kidneys and small intestines. Every complete occlusion of a renal artery invariably causes a renal infarct because renal arteries are endarteries with no collateral circulation. Clinically, the dogs are depressed and show reduced activity, an arched back, sublumbar pain on palpation, and hematuria. Acute occlusion of several mesenteric arteries initially induces intestinal hyperactivity followed by ileus and sometimes intestinal infarction. The owner notices sudden anorexia, vomiting, bowel evacuation, and signs of abdominal pain of variable intensity. The feces may contain blood. With bowel infarction severe signs of an acute abdomen and shock develop.

Cardiac murmurs with a maximum intensity over the aortic valve can be auscultated in thromboembolic disease due to endocarditis. In dirofilariasis a split second heart sound may be present (for additional signs see Chapter 80).

Diagnosis. In all dogs with peripheral arterial thrombosis a survey radiograph of the thorax should be made. It serves to evaluate cardiac size and shape and to recognize pulmonary signs of edema, thrombosis or dirofilariasis. Further, radiographs of the pelvic and hind limb region are indicated to rule out masses exerting pressure on the aorta and for periosteal reactions in the sublumbar area. Occasionally, a radiopaque foreign body such as a gun pellet flushed from the heart to the caudal aorta is observed.[14]

Laboratory data are often noncontributory to the final diagnosis. However, laboratory abnormalities may provide valuable information regarding underlying primary diseases (renal, pancreatic or hepatic conditions). Sometimes serum fibrinogen levels are increased. Shortened test times for routine coagulograms (APTT, PT and TT, spontaneous clotting time) are compatible with hypercoagulability. Leukocytosis is common. AST (SGOT) and creatinine kinase are often elevated. The content of fibrin degradation products can also be increased. Several hypercoagulable states (glomerulopathies, hypoproteinemias) are associated with reduced levels of antithrombin III (AT III).[15]

A minimal data base for the recognition of renal or hepatic disease is advisable. A Knott's test or serology for the detection of dirofilariasis should be performed in endemic areas. Repeated blood cultures and/or echocardiography are indicated if endocarditis is a tentative diagnosis.

Confirmation of the diagnosis requires the proof of a vascular occlusion, which can be gained from an aortogram (Figure 81–1). The aortogram demonstrates the exact location and extent of the vascular occlusion and the formation, if any, of a collateral vascular bed. Radiolucent emboli such as heartworms may be outlined (longitudinal filling defects). The assessment of the extent of the formation of collateral circulation is important for the selection of the most appropriate therapy.

Aortography is performed by injecting 0.2 to 0.5 ml/lb (0.5 to 1 ml/kg) of meglumine diatrizoate or a similar iodine containing contrast medium through a catheter placed in the abdominal aorta. The cutdown for the introduction of the catheter can be located in a carotid artery or in the uninvolved femoral artery. Several VD radiographs should be exposed approximately two seconds after the beginning of the injection of the contrast medium. Alternate diagnostic methods not usually avail-

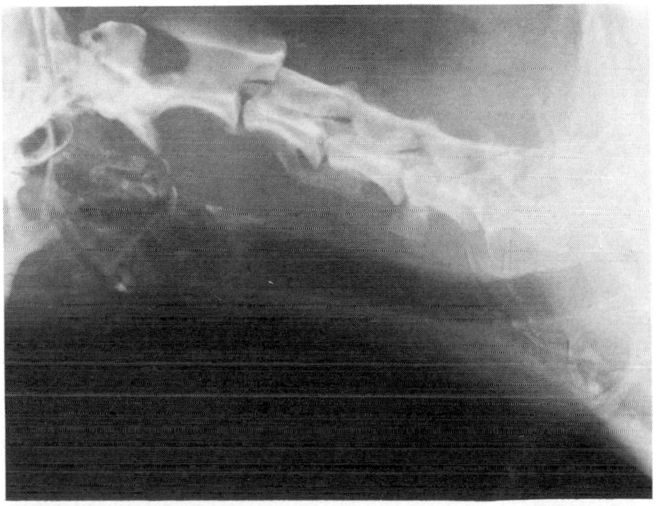

FIGURE 81–1. Calcification of the arterial walls in a seven-year-old toy poodle with left heart failure, chronic cough, and cyanosis. In addition to the calcification of the arterial walls depicted on this radiograph, there was calcification of the coronary arteries, renal arteries, several branches of the abdominal aorta, and the iliac arteries.

able in practice are thermography, perfusion scans, ultrasonography and the use of a Doppler probe.[16]

The differential diagnoses include trauma, brachial plexus neuropathy, spinal or pelvic tumors, infections such as canine distemper or toxoplasmosis, old dog myelopathy, disk protrusion and the cauda equina compression syndrome.

The prognosis depends upon the etiology, the severity of the signs and the presence or absence of local complications (ulcers, muscular fibrosis), and concurrent embolization to visceral organs. Even in cases with spontaneous recovery, relapses must be expected. Rapid diagnosis of a complete arterial occlusion and treatment are essential to avoid irreversible tissue damage.

Treatment. Treatment should be directed against the underlying disease or cause of the thrombosis and should attenuate the clinical signs until the clot is dissolved or removed, or until collateral circulation is sufficient.

The thrombus, when diagnosed early and located precisely, can be removed surgically by embolectomy or resection anastomosis or with an embolectomy catheter as in cats.[1, 17, 18] Both conservative and surgical treatment should be started by giving analgesics and heparin, 100 IU/lb IV and by keeping the dog in a quiet and warm place. Electrolyte solutions should be given to correct dehydration and dilute the blood. Dextran products, 5 to 10 ml/lb IV, can further improve on the rheology of the blood and reduce platelet aggregation. The additional treatment modalities are directed against the inciting pathologic conditions (hypercoagulability, reduction of coagulation proteins, replacement of AT III and albumin).

Heparin therapy needs to be adapted to the case. The goal is to stop the growth of the thrombus with a dose that causes no hemorrhage. It is advisable to start with a small dose and increase it until the APTT is prolonged from two to two and one-half normal.[19] Heparin cannot dissolve clots. In the event of hemorrhaging, heparin can be neutralized by giving protamine sulfate. After three to five days of treatment, the heparin dose is gradually reduced over 48 to 72 hours (abrupt stoppage could cause a rebound hypercoagulability) and the dog is put on an increasing dose of an oral anticoagulant (coumarins are preferable to indanediones).[19] The initial dosage is 0.5 to 2.5 mg/lb q24h of a coumarin preparation such as warfarin sodium (Coumadin). The appropriate dose must be found by "titration" using the ACT test or PT. Aspirin renders the platelets nonfunctional by preventing their aggregation. The dosage is 1.5 to 2.5 mg/lb PO q24h to q48h.

Streptokinase, urokinase and TPA (tissue plasminogen activator) are potent activators of fibrinolysis by transforming plasminogen to plasmin. All three drugs are very expensive and have led to uncontrolled bleeding in humans. The dosage of streptokinase in dogs has not been determined. Killingworth et al. concluded that in cats a loading dose of 90,000 IU of streptokinase IV over 20 to 30 min followed by three maintenance doses of 45,000 IU/h produced systemic fibrinolysis. However, dog plasminogen is less easily activated than cat plasminogen.[20, 21]

Following surgery streptokinase should be used carefully. For monitoring fibrinolysis and detecting hemostatic abnormalities prior to the use of streptokinase, thrombin clotting time or APTT should be run.[19]

NONOCCLUSIVE ARTERIAL DISEASES

Nonocclusive arterial diseases include traumas, arterial aneurysms, arteriovenous fistulas, arteriosclerosis, angiitis (vasculitis) and functional abnormalities. Some of the nonocclusive diseases can secondarily become occlusive diseases, e.g., arteriosclerosis. Degenerative arterial wall abnormalities can occur secondary to metabolic, traumatic, toxic or infectious conditions. A slight to moderate degree of degenerative arterial wall changes is regularly detectable in old dogs and cats.

Arterial Aneurysm

An arterial aneurysm is defined as a sac formed by the dilatation of the wall of an artery. Aneurysms are rare in dogs and are unknown in cats. Most aneurysms are detected incidentally at necropsy. Aneurysms can be subdivided into three major types: true aneurysm (aneurysma verum), dissecting aneurysm (aneurysma dissecans), and false or spurious aneurysm (aneurysma spurium).

TRUE ANEURYSM

A true aneurysm is a vascular dilatation caused by a weakening of the arterial wall (or venous wall) and subsequent widening of the vascular lumen. Aneurysms are formed by destruction of the media and/or the elastic fibers of large arteries by inflammatory or degenerative processes or they are due to spontaneous or iatrogenic traumas (arterial surgery or puncture). In dogs most aneurysms are found in the aorta and are due to migrating larvae of *Spirocerca lupi*.[22, 23] Furthermore, aneurysms are well known to occur in areas with turbulent blood flow such as in arteriovenous fistulas or in the aorta near the opening of the patent ductus arteriosus. In humans, congenital aneurysms are encountered with Marfan's disease.

Peripheral aneurysms present as soft, warm, pulsating bulges over which a machinery murmur can be auscultated occasionally (see arteriovenous fistulas). The signs of aortic aneurysms rarely permit a diagnosis while the patient is alive. They are either absent or vague. Only if a spontaneous rupture of an aneurysm takes place will there be pain, signs of anemia and shock, or a pleural or mediastinal effusion. Exsanguination due to an aneurysmal rupture is rare, however, and has only been reported once.[24]

SPURIOUS ANEURYSMS

Traumatic spurious aneurysms (arterial lacerations that fail to heal) are probably more common than is usually realized. The resulting local hematoma and subsequent circulatory disturbances are probably falsely attributed to infection or venous obstruction.[25] An aneurysma spurium in the hindlimb of a dog resulted from a gunshot wound.[25] A similar case has been described under the designation of traumatic arteriovenous fistula.[26] The lesion of this dog seemed to have characteristics of both spurious aneurysm and arteriovenous fistula.

The clinical signs are lameness, persistent pain and deep muscular swelling that do not respond to local therapeutic measures and systemic therapy with antibiotics or glucocorticoids. Pitting peripheral edema can also be present. Neither blood nor pus can be aspirated from the swelling. On survey radiographs one notices soft tissue swelling. On rare occasions a foreign body such as a gun pellet is responsible for the arterial laceration.

The diagnosis of spurious aneurysm requires confirmation by an angiographic study. A suitable contrast medium is injected intra-arterially, proximal to the swelling, and a series of radiographs is obtained. At the area of the arterial defect, a nodular exudation of contrast medium can be seen. The differential diagnosis includes chronic infection, obstruction of a deep vein or abscessation. In spurious aneurysm, no temperature elevation or neutrophilia is encountered. The prognosis is favorable if the artery is sutured.

Functional Forms of Arterial Diseases

It is well known to anyone doing catheterizations in dogs and cats that arteries may go into spasm when handled or traumatized. Vasospasm occurs regularly both in blunt and perforating traumas. Perivascular injection of irritating substances commonly initiates vasospasm. Vasospasm and the associated damages to the surrounding tissue can be minimized or avoided by local infiltration with procaine hydrochloride or lidocaine. Vasospasm also occurs if an artery ruptures spontaneously, e.g., in a rupture of a cerebral aneurysm (stroke) in humans. Experiments done by this author suggest that the same may occur in dogs. Spontaneous conditions of this sort are rarely diagnosed clinically because angiography required to confirm the diagnosis is not routinely available.

Vasospasm may also be elicited by exotoxins. The best known example is ergotism. The differential diagnosis is thrombosis due to vasculitis (see later in this chapter).

Arteriovenous Fistulas (Arteriovenous Malformations)

An arteriovenous fistula (A-V fistula) or malformation is an abnormal communication between an artery and vein that bypasses the capillary network. A-V fistulas are uncommon in dogs and rare in cats. The true incidence of the condition is unknown. A-V fistulas can be of central location such as an intracardiac defect (ventricular septal defect) or an extracardiac defect (patent ductus arteriosus) and are discussed in Chapter 74. In this section only peripheral A-V fistulas will be discussed. The A-V fistulas that have been reported in the veterinary literature are of congenital or acquired origin.[27] Acquired A-V fistulas are always localized, i.e., confined to one area connecting an artery to a vein, whereas congenital A-V malformations may be localized or multiple. Multiple A-V malformations are very rare and consist of several poorly defined small A-V communications that seldom cause clinical problems. They may be incompletely outlined with arteriography.

In human medicine, a confusing array of names has been used in the past to designate congenital A-V fistulas (hemangioma racemosum, Park-Weber syndrome, hemangioma cavernosum, strawberry birthmark, nevus angiectasis, cirsoid aneurysm, congenital A-V aneurysm).[28]

Congenital A-V fistulas are due to an arrest or a misdirection of the embryologic differentiation process at various stages of the development of the vascular system. The persistence of the primitive equipotential capillaries (primary anlage) and the subsequent failure of the existing anastomotic embryologic channels to differentiate into arteries or veins is responsible for the persistence of abnormal communications between arteries and veins.

The most common cause of an acquired A-V fistula is blunt or penetrating trauma including iatrogenic trauma such as veni-puncture and accidental perivascular injection of an irritating substance (thiobarbiturates).[27, 29–32] Further causes are neovascularization with tumors of the neck area (carotid body tumor, thyroid tumor).[27, 33] Additional causes cited in the human medical literature are spontaneous aneurysmal rupture, ligature in mass of arteries and veins and erosion of contiguous walls of two vessels by infection or arteriosclerosis. While uncommon, most A-V fistulas involve the extremities.[26, 27, 29–32, 34, 35] They may, however, occur anywhere in the body, the neck, spinal cord, flank, head, brain, abdomen, liver, and lung.[27, 33, 37–47] Irrespective of cause and location the altered flow dynamics induced by A-V fistulas are similar and may act as a potent stimulus for the development of an extensive collateral circulation. The responses of the heart and peripheral circulation to the altered flow dynamics have been studied extensively in experimental dogs.[49, 50]

With the formation of an A-V fistula two competing circulatory pathways exist: the normal arterial-capillary-venous system and a new system that acts as a short-cut with a reduced peripheral vascular resistance. Blood follows the path of least resistance and robs the normal pathway of its flow. Because of the rapid runoff of the blood through the A-V fistula into the capacitant venous circulation, turbulence and vascular vibrations occur. The venous pressure, the oxygen saturation of the venous blood, and the diameter and number of the anastomotic arteries and veins increase. Eventually an ectasia of the feeding artery and aneurysmal sacs in the venous area of the A-V communications may develop. Furthermore, histologic changes take place in the affected vessels. Arteries begin to look more like veins (venification) and veins like arteries (arterialization).

Blood flow through a large fistula can be so intense as to cause retrograde flow from the distal artery into the fistula. Arterial blood supply to the tissues distal to the A-V fistula may thus be compromised owing to the competition with the fistula and secondary venous hypertension or even reversal of blood flow in the dilated veins. Local edema and ischemia followed by tissue necrosis, ulceration or organ dysfunction may ensue. In large and mostly centrally located fistulas the central blood dynamics become also affected. A large flow across the A-V fistula compromises the blood supply to other regions of the body by shifting blood into the capacitant venous circulation. Owing to compensatory reactions, blood volume, heart rate and contraction increase. The augmented cardiac output and the gradual expansion of the blood volume to 30 per cent or more above the prefistula value restores normal blood supply to the deprived areas. Eventually, however, the increased venous return (increased preload) and the elevated cardiac workload may induce high output heart failure.[43]

The magnitude of the A-V fistula's effects, i.e., shunting of blood and degree of collateral development, is closely related to its location in the vascular tree, to the caliber of the vessels involved, to the duration of the shunt flow (collateral development is a continuous process), and to the number and distensibility of the vessels. The vessels from which the collateral circulation develops are mostly pre-existing unused arterial communications. Morbidity is greatest for centrally located A-V fistulas, for fistulas that cause organ dysfunction and/or for massively shunting lesions that induce a high output state.

Clinical history and signs vary according to the location, size, duration, etiopathology and topography of the fistula. Small A-V fistulas of the extremities are noticed by the owners as painless, easily compressible warm bulges or may be detected incidentally on routine clinical examination. With medium size or large fistulas of the extremities a continuous palpable thrill and pulsation, along with a machinery murmur, can be detected on examination of the bulge. The leg or part of the body distal to the fistula may be swollen, warmer or colder than the proximal area, painful, and affected by pitting or secondary inflammatory edema. Lameness, cyanosis and/or therapy-resistant ulcers at the toes,[30] scab formation or even gangrene can occur distally to the fistula because of severe local ischemia. In the dilated superficial veins a faint pulsation may be felt.

Pulse and heart rate are increased in medium to large size fistulas. In the feeding arteries a water-hammer pulse is often present. In animals with high-output heart failure one may be able to auscultate flow murmur or a pathologic mitral murmur due to secondary mitral insufficiency and moist lung sounds indicating pulmonary edema.

When firm pressure is applied proximal to the A-V fistula or if the feeding artery is compressed, the thrill and bruit disappear and pulse and heart rate may drop, as a result of a diminished venous return and reduced cardiac output. When noticed clinically, this sign is referred to as Branham's bradycardia sign. This test is called Branham's or Nicoladoni-Branham's test and together with the local thrill or fremitus and the bruit is pathognomonic for A-V fistulas.

Other signs may be present, depending on the location and the circumstances of the A-V fistula. An A-V fistula in the orbit caused exophthalmus.[38] Recurrent bleeding from the mouth was observed in an A-V fistula of the tongue.[41] Restless behavior and lethargy followed by progressive seizures and hemiparesis were present in a ten-year-old mixed breed dog with a subcortical cerebral A-V malformation.[42] The tentative diagnosis was a well-circumscribed mass compressing the brain. An A-V fistula of the spinal cord at the thoracolumbar junctions in a ten-month-old female Australian shepherd dog caused a deteriorating hind limb ataxia, difficulty in getting up and down, hypersensitivity over the lumbosacral region, and after three months urinary incontinence.[36] A-V fistulas in tumors can be recognized because of the strong pulsation and fremitus detectable during palpation of the tumor mass.[27] When auscultating the tumor mass a machinery-type murmur or bruit may be heard.[33]

A-V fistulas of the liver connect the hepatic artery to the portal vein and cause portal hypertension or even reversal of the blood flow in the portal vein. Abdominal distention due to low protein ascites is a major clinical sign.[44–47] Furthermore, as a result of a hepatofugal blood flow, portosystemic collateral vessels and signs of hepatoencephalopathy may develop.[46] Some of these A-V fistulas turn out to be hamartomas.[51]

Pulmonary A-V fistulas can lead to respiratory distress and cyanosis.[48] On survey radiographs of the thorax of animals with large fistulas one may see cardiomegaly, a prominent aortic arch, a hypervascular lung field, and an increased interstitial or patchy pulmonary radiodensity indicating pulmonary congestion or edema respectively. Confirmation of the clinical diagnosis of a peripheral A-V fistula is based on the presence of a soft mass, which adheres to the underlying tissue and in which a thrill or fremitus can be palpated and/or a murmur can be auscultated. A positive Branham's test is pathognomonic for an A-V fistula but it is present only in large lesions.

For a preoperative investigation of the topography and extent of the fistula, angiography is very useful. Based on the angiograms a decision about prognosis and operability can be made and a detailed planning of surgery is possible. This information is helpful in preserving an adequate arterial blood supply and proper venous drainage to the region distal to the fistula following radical excision of the lesion. Survey radiographs of the region of the fistula rarely provide additional information such as local periosteal reaction or bony rarefication in the vicinity of the fistula. For A-V fistulas located in the distal two thirds of a limb, the contrast medium is injected into the brachial or femoral artery respectively.

Following a small cutdown over the artery a catheter or a suitable needle-catheter combination is placed in the vessel. If the fistula is located in the proximal third of the limb or in the trunk or an internal organ, a selective catheterization of the feeding vessel at its origin from the aorta or the carotid artery should be attempted. This needs to be done under image intensified fluoroscopic control. The correct position of the catheter is checked with a test injection of 2 to 5 ml of a contrast medium. A suitable contrast medium (meglumine iothalamate, Conray 60 per cent; meglumine diatrizoate, Hypaque R 50 or Renografin R 60 or megluminioglicate) is then injected. For small fistulas 3 to 4 ml and for large fistulas 15 to 20 ml of contrast medium are needed. If possible several radiographs should be made in rapid sequence beginning at the time of the contrast medium injection to outline both arteries and veins. Application of a tourniquet may facilitate the outlining of multiple congenital small fistulas at different locations of the limb.

The absence of a normal capillary phase and the premature outlining of the veins are typical for shunting lesions. It is important to try to identify the barely visible distal continuation of the artery feeding the fistula. The differential diagnoses of A-V fistulas include neoplasms, varices, abscesses, cystic skin lesions, aneurysms, lymphedema and scars.

The prognosis in small A-V fistulas is good. In large fistulas or for those located in areas that are difficult to reach for corrective surgery, the prognosis is usually poor. There is an inherent tendency of the collateral flow to continuously increase.[52] Congenital A-V fistulas usually have a poorer prognosis than acquired ones.

The treatment of A-V fistulas is surgical or in inaccessible areas by vascular embolization, except for small lesions that can be controlled temporarily by pressure wraps. Careful ligation of all proximal and distal arteries feeding the fistula, ligation of the draining veins (so-called quadruple ligation) and complete excision of the arteriovenous collaterals with the venous aneurysmal sacs is the only adequate method to guarantee lasting success.[40] The surgical reanastomosing of the affected artery to its distal normal continuation is usually not critical in small animals because of their well-developed collateral circulation. In relapses after an initial careful resection or if multiple fistulas are present, a wide excision of the involved area(s) or limb amputation may be the only alternative. Animals with large A-V fistulas may have a substantially increased blood volume. A sudden closure of the shunt will be followed by an immediate increase in blood pressure and a vagally mediated bradycardia. Therefore one should be cautious in administering fluids intravenously to these animals.

In human medicine the arteriographic embolization technique has been used successfully when a surgical approach was technically difficult, mutilating or too hazardous for the patient.[53] Embolization was achieved with the selective or superselective injection of biodegradable substances (muscle tissue, gelatine sponge) or nonresorbable material (silicone microspheres, polyvinyl alcohol foam, isobutyl-z-cyanoacrylate or wool-tufted wire coils).

Arteriosclerosis and Atherosclerosis

Arteriosclerosis is defined as chronic arterial change consisting of hardening, loss of elasticity and luminal narrowing resulting from proliferative and degenerative, not inflammatory, changes of the wall. Atherosclerosis is considered a form of arteriosclerosis in which the inner portions of the arterial wall (intima and inner portions of media) are thickened by deposits (plaques) containing cholesterol, lipoid material and lipophages. Arteriosclerotic lesions are common in old dogs and cats. The lesions are usually mild, but even moderately severe lesions are unimportant to health and survival. The only exception is hyaline degeneration of the intramural coronary arteries, which can be associated with arterial stenosis, occlusion, and focal myocardial infarction. Intramural coronary artery fibrosis, hyalinosis and amyloidosis were found in 26.4 percent of old dogs necropsied.[54] The intramural arteriosclerotic processes are particularly common in dogs with heart failure due to endocardiosis. Endothelial plaque formation in the aorta due to arteriosclerosis was present in 77.8 per cent of 58 dogs brought to a small animal clinic in Helsinki for euthanasia.[55] Some of the arteriosclerotic changes in this study were associated with clinical signs. A predilection of the renal vessels for arteriosclerosis was found in 15- to 20-month-old greyhounds.[56]

The risks of arterial occlusion are highest in arteries containing lipoid plaques (atheromas). Atheromas, however, are only rarely formed in dogs with arteriosclerosis. They are, however, a feature of atherosclerosis, sometimes referred to as arterial xanthomatosis, and are almost exclusively found in dogs with atrophy of the thyroid.[57, 58] The expression atherosclerosis will be used as defined by Liu et al., namely as a thickening of the inner arterial wall in association with lipid deposits.[58]

Atherosclerosis has not been described in cats. Contrary to the disease in humans, extensive plaque formation and arterial calcification (Figure 81–2) are uncommon in atherosclerosis of dogs.

A predisposition for spontaneous atherosclerosis has been found in old (nine years and older) obese dogs with atrophied thyroid glands and hypothyroidism.[57–59] This observation is in accordance with experiments in which atherosclerosis could be induced in thyroidectomized dogs fed large quantities of cholesterol or cholic acids.[60, 61] The spontaneous disease mainly affects male dogs and spayed female dogs. An increased prevalence rate in miniature schnauzers, Doberman pinschers, and Labrador retrievers has been observed.[58] Hypertension due to renal disease seems to be able to accelerate the development of stenotic lesions.[55]

The stenosing lesions develop in all segments of the arterial tree. They are most common and most severe in the extramural and intramural coronary arteries where they might be associated with infarcts. Other commonly affected areas are the carotid and the renal arteries. Severe lesions associated with infarcts can also be found in the cerebral arteries.[62] The distribution and severity of the lesions and the thyroid atrophy correspond well with the clinical signs most often observed, namely lethargy, anorexia, weakness, dyspnea, collapse, heart failure, vomiting, disorientation, blindness, circling and coma.[58, 62] Electrocardiographic abnormalities are atrial fibrillation, notched QRS complexes, and ST segment elevation that can also be found in myocardial infarction.

Laboratory abnormalities include hypercholesterolemia, hyperlipidemia, low T3 and T4 values, elevated BUN and liver enzymes and high values for α_2 and β

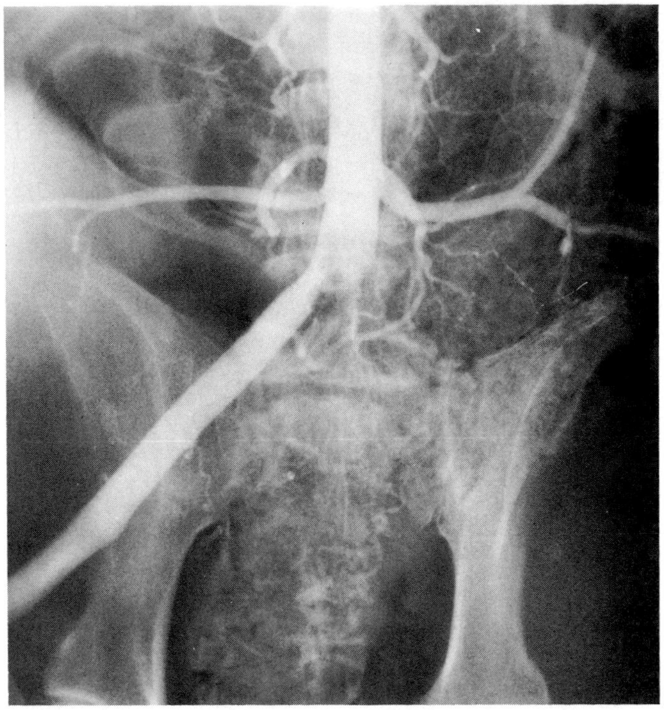

FIGURE 81–2. Aortogram of a seven-year-old Saint Bernard dog with a saddle thrombus at the aortic trifurcation associated with a chondrosarcoma located in the vicinity of the terminal aorta. The owner had observed four episodes of pain and weakness in the hindlimbs that developed gradually when the dog was taken for a walk. At the beginning of the walk, the dog was normal. If the dog was forced to continue walking after the signs of pain and lameness had appeared, it collapsed. After resting for a few moments the dog was able to walk again. On clinical examination the femoral pulse was difficult to feel and the periphery of the hindlimbs was cool. Pain could be elicited when the pelvic area was palpated. Aortography was performed and a radiograph was taken at four seconds after the beginning of the injection of contrast medium. On the aortogram the common origin of the internal iliac arteries and the left external iliac artery contain no contrast medium, suggesting that they have been occluded completely. A partial occlusion has reduced the flow of contrast medium into the right external iliac artery. Some collateral blood supply to the hind limbs probably occurs via the seventh lumbar artery. Anticoagulation therapy was instituted, but it failed to provide relief and the dog was euthanatized at the request of the owner.

fractions in the protein electrophoresis. Hyperamylasemia in association with pancreatitis may also occur. The lipidemia might play a major role in the pathogenesis of pancreatitis. The BUN elevation is often associated with renal infarcts.

Not all dogs with hypothyroidism develop atherosclerosis. Only those referred to as hyper-responders in which increased levels of very low-density β-lipoproteins are found are prone to develop atherosclerosis and plaques. In these dogs the blood levels of the low-density lipoproteins are probably increased because of a reduction of lipoprotein receptors and a reduction of lipoid removal by the tissues. The increased lipoprotein levels account for the lipoid deposits in the arteries.

In cases with necrosis and calcification of the arterial walls hypervitaminosis D has to be considered as a differential diagnosis.[63, 64]

The prognosis of dogs with clinical signs of stenosing atherosclerosis is poor due to the irreversibility of the underlying lesions and the fact that no methods exist for an early diagnosis. Presently no therapy for dogs with atherosclerosis has been developed. However, prophylactically one may attempt in high risk dogs to treat for hypothyroidism and give antihypertensive and blood cholesterol-reducing medications. Furthermore, a diet low in cholesterol may be indicated.

Vasculitis, Angiitis

Vasculitis or angiitis are synonymous terms for a clinicopathologic process or a syndrome characterized by inflammation and necrosis of blood vessels. Vasculitis is a common occurrence in a wide variety of inflammatory and toxic conditions and is of major importance in the pathogenesis of a substantial number of diseases of dogs and cats. It involves arteries and veins of different sizes and locations.

Vasculitis may develop from within the vessel, or from the outside by extension of inflammation from neighboring tissues. In the first case the endothelial surface of the vessel gets damaged by infectious agents, by endotoxins or exotoxins, or by immune reactions. At the swollen and/or disrupted endothelial surface negatively charged carboxyl groups of collagens of the vessel wall become exposed and initiate activation of the Hageman factor. Consequently activation of complement, kinin and plasmin systems, and increased vascular permeability and acute inflammation occur.[65] Polymorphonuclear and other white blood cells may be attracted and cellular infiltration of the vascular wall takes place. The cells release their intracytoplasmic lysosomal enzymes, causing further damage and necrosis of the vessel wall. Polymorphonuclear cells may also be attracted by antigen-antibody complexes (immune complexes) deposited in the vessel wall. Furthermore some immunopathogenetic mechanisms initiated in the blood vessel wall may be cell mediated.[66] The disruption of the endothelial surface and the inflammation of the vessel wall predispose to thrombosis and occlusion of the lumen and may be accompanied by hemorrhage and ischemic changes in the surrounding tissues. Particularly in chronic cases a granulomatous type reaction of the vessel wall can dominate.

Difficulties and confusion have plagued efforts to classify the clinical entities in the broad spectrum of vasculitides in humans.[66] Even greater problems exist in veterinary medicine because the histopathologic criteria and type of inflammation are infrequently characterized, a large number of vasculitides are of unknown origin, and often different names are used for the same disease entities. For practical clinical purposes it is probably most convenient to differentiate between primary and secondary vasculitides. The etiology of the secondary vasculitides is known and thus poses little classification problems. They are found in infectious diseases such as feline infectious peritonitis, coronavirus infection of dogs, Rocky Mountain spotted fever, and dirofilariasis, and may also occur in immunopathogenetic connective collagen diseases, such as systemic lupus erythematosus and rheumatoid arthritis. These and other secondary vasculitides are dealt with throughout this textbook. The following paragraphs will be limited to the basic concepts and clinical manifestations of primary and idiopathic vasculitides.

HYPERSENSITIVITY VASCULITIS

The designation hypersensitivity vasculitis (HV) or hypersensitivity angiitis refers to a large and heterogeneous group of clinical syndromes with multisystemic necrotizing vasculitis. HV is the most common angiitis in animals. Etiologically the hypersensitivity vasculitides in dogs and cats encompass a yet undetermined number of primary and secondary vascular diseases. Most primary hypersensitivity vasculitides are of unknown origin. In humans, HV has been commonly associated with infections, drug reactions, toxins, chronic neoplasia and immune-mediated diseases (lupus erythematosus, rheumatoid arthritis).

The lesions of HV affect mainly arterioles, capillaries and venules and are uniform in nature, suggesting an acute episodic pathogenesis rather than a continuous exposure to drugs, microbial antigens or immune complexes. Most often HV results from deposition of immune complexes within vessel walls. This leads among other changes (fibroproliferation, thrombosis) to infiltration of neutrophils in and around the vessel wall and to leukocytoclasis (deposition of nuclear debris or nuclear dust in the vessel wall). HV is thus often referred to as leukocytoclastic vasculitis.[67] Another name that is used occasionally is allergic vasculitis. In cell-mediated or delayed-hypersensitivity immune diseases lymphocytes and other mononuclear cells, rather than neutrophils, are found in the blood vessels affected by HV.[68]

With HV the lesions are usually less extensive than in polyarteritis nodosa and the organ distribution is slightly different.[65] In HV the most commonly affected organ is the skin. However, mucous membranes, renal glomeruli, lungs and the central nervous system may also be involved.[65]

Clinically HV is accompanied by systemic signs such as phasic pyrexia, listlessness, and anorexia. In some cases lymphadenopathy, myalgia, epistaxis, drooling, sneezing or arthralgia have been observed. In addition to the generalized signs manifestations of organ lesions will be present. Most common are skin lesions such as wheals, urticaria, purpura, nodules, bullae, crusty lesions, necrosis and ulcers. In many cases the skin lesions are associated with pain and/or pruritus.[67, 69] Somewhat less common are ulcers at the mucocutaneous junctions or of the mucous membranes, and pitting edemas of the dependent areas such as limbs, ventral trunk, head and scrotum. The preferred locations of ulcers are the head, namely external ear canal and pinnae, the face, the bony prominences of the limbs and the footpads. Skin and renal lesions rarely occur together in the same patient.

HV of internal organs is often not diagnosed, because the clinical signs are vague due to the simultaneous involvement of more than one organ system or the organ manifestations are confused with infectious, degenerative or traumatic conditions, e.g., pneumonia, pulmonary thrombosis, occult dirofilariasis, lupus erythematosus, glomerulonephritis, myositis or spinal paralysis.[70, 71]

The clinicopathologic findings of primary HV vary according to severity, duration and organ involvement. Lymphopenia, eosinopenia, hypoalbuminemia, hyperglobulinemia and hyperfibrinogenemia are common. Leukocytosis with a left shift or leukopenia, neutropenia, monocytosis, a mild normocytic normochromic anemia, and thrombocythemia are less consistent findings. Serum liver enzymes and triglycerides are often elevated.

The diagnosis is confirmed by histologic examination of biopsy specimens of the skin or the lymph nodes and by excluding other immune-mediated diseases based on negative Coombs', ANA and rheumatoid factor tests. Special immunologic tests have been recommended to prove a low concentration of complement and elevated levels of circulating immune complexes.[72] The history is helpful if drug hypersensitivity is suspected.

In the differential diagnosis one has to rule out pemphigus vulgaris and foliaceus, bullous pemphigoid, systemic lupus erythematosus, dirofilariasis, specific infectious diseases, chronic neoplasia, and cold hemagglutination disease. The prognosis is usually good.

A variety of therapeutic agents have been advocated. In all cases with HV unnecessary drugs should be discontinued. In many cases immunosuppressive dosages of prednisolone with or without an antibiotic have been used successfully. In cases of failure cyclophosphamide has been advocated. In dogs with lesions involving the skin only dapsone (Avlosulfon), 0.5 mg/lb q8h PO for the first two weeks, 0.5 mg/lb q12h for another two weeks, followed by 0.5 mg/lb daily after clinical improvement, has been used successfully.[69] To prevent relapses 0.5 mg/lb of dapsone was then given three times weekly for four months.[69] In dogs treated with dapsone the blood picture has to be monitored regularly. As an alternative to dapsone, sulfasalazine (Azulfidine) at an initial dosage of 22 mg/lb q8h PO has been recommended.[67] After the lesions had improved the dosage intervals were first increased to 12 and later on to 24 hrs. Dogs receiving sulfasalazine should be watched for side effects, e.g., fever, keratoconjunctivitis sicca or abnormalities of the blood picture.

POLYARTERITIS NODOSA

Polyarteritis nodosa (PAN) is a very rare polysystemic disease associated with a necrotizing vasculitis of unknown cause. In humans, PAN is classified among the immune-mediated collagen disorders. The disease affects predominantly segments and bifurcations of small- and medium-sized muscular arteries; it occurs in dogs and cats. In humans, PAN has its name from purpural lesions that are palpable in the subcutaneous tissue. Palpable nodules are, however, no regular feature of PAN in animals. The vascular lesions consist of intimal proliferation, vessel wall degeneration, necrosis, and thrombosis in all stages of development. PAN leads to a loss of the integrity of the vessel wall, petechial and ecchymotic hemorrhages, focal areas of tissue infarction and necrosis, aneurysm formation, and nodular swelling and thickening of the major arteries. The target tissues of PAN in dogs are the kidneys, skin, mucous membranes, adrenals, meninges, gastrointestinal tract, connective tissue and myocardium.[73] The lungs are usually spared.

The clinical picture comprises systemic signs, such as pyrexia, lethargy, reluctance to walk, vague pain and/or weight loss, and a wide spectrum of manifestations of organ system lesions including linear skin ulceration, ulceration of mucous membranes, nasal discharge, spinal pain, and signs of cardiac and/or renal failure.[73] The clinicopathologic findings may include leukocytosis with left shift and proteinuria.

The differential diagnosis is hypersensitivity angiitis. The diagnosis is confirmed by histologic examination of biopsy specimens of the skin.

The prognosis is uncertain to poor. Treatment schedules include glucocorticoids and/or cyclophosphamide.

LYMPHOMATOID GRANULOMATOSIS AND MISCELLANEOUS VASCULITIDES

Lymphomatoid granulomatosis and other nonclassified vasculitides are characterized by a polymorpholymphocytoid, plasmacytoid and histiocytoid granulomatous infiltration around blood vessels. Nodular lesions of variable size due to lymphomatosis have been first described in the lungs of dogs.[74] The nodular lesions are grossly indistinguishable from secondary lung tumors or lymphosarcomatous nodular lesions. In some of the masses infarction with necrosis and cavitation takes place. The bronchial lymph nodes can be slightly to greatly enlarged and pulmonary thrombosis is common. The etiology of this rare condition is unknown. Occasionally, similar lesions are associated with eosinophilic pneumonitis seen in occult dirofilariasis, however, they can also occur outside of endemic areas of dirofilariasis.[75, 76] An immune-mediated cause is likely because in some cases large amounts of immunoglobulin G and M can be demonstrated in plasma cells and macrophages.[76] Efforts to identify an antigen have been unsuccessful so far.

The differential diagnosis is primary or secondary neoplasia with which this condition is often confused and hypersensitivity angiitis of the lung, which has been encountered in a cat by this author. The diagnosis is rarely made clinically and requires histologic examination of biopsy material.

The prognosis is usually poor. In some of the patients multicentric lymphosarcoma may develop at a later date. Therapy with glucocorticoids and cytotoxic immunosuppressive drugs is only temporarily effective.

DISEASES OF VEINS

Diseases of the venous system are few. They are considered of minor importance in dogs and cats in spite of the fact that veins are commonly affected by or involved in trauma, thromboembolism, edema formation, local inflammation, and septic processes. Disorders of the venous system include injuries, superficial and deep phlebitis and thrombosis (thrombophlebitis), pulmonary embolism, venous compression syndromes, varices, and ulcers.

Varicosis and ulceration are rare in dogs and cats. Varicosis can accompany arteriovenous fistulas. Cutaneous phlebectasia is a benign lesion sometimes erroneously called telangiectasia. It has been reported to occur almost exclusively in dogs with spontaneous or iatrogenic Cushing's syndrome.[77] Phlebectasia is an abnormal dilatation, extension, or reduplication of veins or capillaries, or a combination of these changes and is referred to in humans as cherry angioma. No specific treatment is required.

Perforation or blunt trauma to veins is usually well tolerated. In perforations clotting usually occurs rapidly and occludes the damaged vein. Occlusion or severance of veins, even large ones, leads only temporarily to edema and cyanosis because of the existence of a large collateral system. If all veins draining an area are compromised, edema and cyanosis and sometimes even necrosis ensue. Fat tissue is particularly vulnerable and necrosis easily occurs.

Spontaneous venous thrombosis is rare in dogs and cats. Thrombosis following blunt trauma and perforating injuries, in particular venipuncture or long-time venous catheterization, is common. Stasis, hypercoagulability, and intimal damage (Virchow's triad) are the major initiators of thrombosis. Phlebitis is a major cause of intimal damage. The thrombosis is usually of little consequence locally. However, emboli may break off from the thrombus as clot lysis takes place. The emboli are carried to the lung where they can cause thrombosis of the pulmonary vascular tree if favorable circumstances exist, i.e., sluggish circulation, hypercoagulability, and a reduced ability to lyse the clot. In most animals blood clots carried to the lung are rapidly lysed and cause no problems. However, in animals with inflammatory diseases, dehydration and heart failure, clot formation may continue in the pulmonary vessels and lead to vascular occlusion, severe dyspnea, and pain. In thrombophlebitis due to microorganisms the infection is carried with the emboli to the lung where it causes a thromboembolic pneumonia.

Phlebitis can occur by extension of an inflammatory process from the surrounding tissue to the vein. Phlebitis can also start from an intimal lesion. Common causes are the injection of irritating drugs, the infusion of large amounts of fluid, and the long-term use of intravenous catheters.[78] Infusion-related phlebitis occurs in three forms: chemical (injury of vein by irritating drugs), physical (traumatization of intima by catheters, needles, hypertonicity or particulate matter in fluids infused), and microbial (infection by agents present in the infused fluid, in the skin or at the catheter tip).[79] These physiochemical and biological interactions at the cannula-vein junction not only cause phlebitis but also induce thrombosis. The resulting thrombophlebitis, sterile or septic, usually remains a local process with little or no systemic consequences. Only in patients with serious illnesses or with a compromised immune system will septic complications such as thromboembolic pneumonia or endocarditis develop.

In venous occlusion and in compression syndromes the clinical signs depend on the anatomic location and the extent of the obstructive process. The acute obstruction of centrally located and deep veins causes edema, cyanosis, discomfort and venous dilatation distal to the obstruction site. Obstruction of the central portion of the cranial vena cava causes edema in the neck, ventral head, dependent portions of the chest wall and the front limbs. Sometimes these signs are associated with pleural effusion. Obstructions in the renal or pelvic area cause edema of the hind limbs and the scrotum. The severity and duration of the clinical signs depends on the availability and the opening up of collateral veins and on the reserve capacity of the regional lymph system. Besides thrombosis common causes of venous obstruction are invasive malignant processes and the compression of the veins by abscesses, big hematomas, tumor masses, and enlarged lymph nodes. Tumors with a great tendency to invade veins are chemodectomas and adrenal tumors.

The prognosis and therapy of venous obstruction depend on the primary disease.

DISEASES OF THE PERIPHERAL LYMPHATICS

The lymphatic system comprises highly specialized tissues that are interconnected by a widespread system of lymph vessels. It is closely associated functionally, anatomically, and embryologically with the venous system. The lymph vessels originate in the perivascular spaces. They form an anastomotic capillary system that serves to transport excessive fluid, proteins, solutes, and macromolecular particles from the body tissues to the lymph nodes and eventually back into the venous system. Lymphatics contain valves that favor unidirectional, centripetal lymph flow, which is maintained by outside pressure on lymphatics by pulsating arteries and muscle contraction. The collection of lymph fluid occurs by osmosis, diffusion, and filtration. The lymph system maintains the fluid and protein balance between extravascular and intravascular fluid pools and acts as a safety valve between them. In addition to its function as a transport system, the lymph system also has a major role in the body's defense. It is a filtering system that impedes the spread of microorganisms and neoplastic cells. The cellular components, in particular the lymphocytes, are indispensable for immunologic reactions and antibody formation.

The importance of the transport function of the lymph system is often underestimated. The clinical signs of disease are usually dominated by the deficits in the specific functions of the tissue in which the dysfunction of the lymph system occurs, such as lymphedema of the extremities, enteropathy in intestinal lymphangiectasis, or restrictive respiratory disease in lymph fistula (chylothorax) of the pleural space. Lymphatic disorders can be subdivided into those of internal organs, such as intestinal lymphangiectasis and peripheral lymphatic disorders. In Table 81–3, the types and causes of peripheral lymphatic disorders are summarized.

Extensive functional and morphologic studies of lymph system disorders have been performed in experimental dogs.[80] Lymphography has been used to study the morphology of spontaneous congenital anomalies and acquired obstruction of the lymph system.[81–84]

TABLE 81–3. CAUSES OF PERIPHERAL LYMPHATIC DISORDERS

Lymphangitis, Lymphangiopathy, Lymphadenitis, Lymphadenopathy
Infection
Neoplasia
Reactive hyperplastic disease
Granuloma
Lymphedema
Primary—Developmental Abnormality of Lymph Vessels
Hypoplasia
Aplasia
Lymphangiectasia
Hyperplasia
Secondary—Acquired Occlusion or Loss of Lymphatic Pathways
Surgical excision of lymphatics or lymph nodes
Post-traumatic lymphangiopathy
Neoplastic invasion or extrinsic compression of lymph tissue
Acute obstructive lymphadenitis and lymphangitis
Chronic sclerosing lymphangitis and lymphadenitis
Lymphatic atrophy with interstitial fibrosis
Radiation therapy
Lymphocysts
Cystic hygroma, lymphoceles or pseudocysts
Lymphangiomas

Inflammatory Lymphatic Disorders (Lymphangitis and Lymphadenitis)

Lymphangitis and lymphadenitis are common secondary to local infection of skin, mucosal membranes, and subcutaneous tissue due to skin scarifications, licking, juvenile pyoderma, foreign bodies buried in the subcutaneous tissue, and superficial granulomatous lesions.

Lymphangitis can be of bacterial (streptococci, staphylococci) or fungal origin. As the lymphatics drain inflammatory agents and their products from tissue spaces they can become inflamed and occluded. In the lymph nodes microorganisms are phagocytized and inactivated or killed by humoral and cellular mechanisms. During this process lymph nodes may become obstructed, enlarged and hot and painful to palpation.

Lameness and a warm, painful local swelling accompany lymphangitis of the limbs. Most animals are febrile, some are also anorectic and depressed. With acute lymphangitis, the white blood cell counts are elevated.

Whether or not the lymphangitis leads to abscessation depends on the drainage capacities of the lymphatics. Lymphangitis may become chronic if it is associated with a granulomatous or chronic lesion such as with a hidden foreign body, or an unsuccessfully treated acute inflammation. The persistence of an inflammatory edema results in mesenchymal cell proliferation, which in turn can cause local induration and irreversible thickening of skin and subcutis.

Prognosis is favorable if lymphangitis is treated early and appropriately. Therapy consists of moist, warm local compresses or soaks to reduce swelling and promote drainage. Aggressive local antimicrobial therapy and systemic use of antibiotics for four to seven days in animals with fever and anorexia usually leads to a rapid recovery. If the lymphangitis fails to respond to treatment, a bacterial culture and sensitivity testing should be performed. Surgical exploration is indicated if fistulous tracts or abscesses are present or if a foreign body might have caused the lymphangitis.

Lymphedema

The term *lymphedema* refers to a swelling of some part of the body due to a mechanical failure of lymphatic drainage.[80] This term should not be used for other forms of edema, such as circulatory edema due to venous obstruction, or generalized edema due to hypoproteinemia. Lymphedemas are best subdivided into primary and secondary forms. Primary edema refers to a lymphatic obstruction with no underlying lymphatic disease. In secondary lymphedema there is a well-defined disease process that has damaged or obstructed the lymphatics or the lymph nodes.

PRIMARY LYMPHEDEMA

Primary lymphedema in humans has been subdivided into nonhereditary and hereditary (Nonne-Milroy-Meige disease).[80] According to morphologic criteria the primary lymphedemas are further subdivided into aplasia, hypoplasia, and hyperplasia.[85] In aplasia the lymph vessels are absent. In hypoplasia they are deficient in size and number and in hyperplasia a diffuse increase in their size and number exists. The abnormalities are confined to the cutis and subcutis and leave the deeper areas free of changes.

Hereditary lymphedema is often congenital. Congenital hereditary lymphedema similar to Milroy's disease in humans has been reported in dogs.[82, 84, 86, 87]

Edema due to aplasia or hypoplasia of the proximal lymph channels and/or the popliteal lymph nodes of an extremity is most often encountered in the hindlimbs of young dogs. The edema can be transient and is only seen during the juvenile period or it can become permanent. In mild cases it is restricted to the hindlimbs; in severe cases it progresses to whole body edema and can lead to premature death.

Usually the owner reports that a swelling of one or several limbs had existed since birth or that an edema had appeared after a mild trauma. The swelling consists of a painless, neither excessively warm nor cool, pitting edema of varying extent. The edema is not accompanied by lameness, and many have been treated unsuccessfully with pressure wraps, glucocorticoids, and/or antibiotics. Growth and activity of the affected dogs are normal. The distribution of the edema over the body regions varies. One or both hindlimbs are usually affected, with the forelimbs less so. In 24 affected offspring of six matings among affected and normal dogs, some had edema of the hindlimbs only, some had all four limbs involved, and some had edema of all four limbs, trunk, and tail.[82] In some of the dogs, the lymph nodes were barely palpable or absent, and the total plasma protein values, serum protein electrophoretic pattern, blood cell count, and blood chemistry were all normal.

The diagnosis of primary lymphedema is based on history and clinical signs. In doubtful cases visual or radiographic lymphography may be needed to confirm the diagnosis. Radiographic lymphography is also helpful in determining the morphology of the anomalous lymphatic system.

Radiographic lymphography is performed by selective cannulation of a peripheral lymph vessel and subsequent injection of a radiopaque dye.[81, 83] The cannulation of a lymphatic channel is easy if lymphangiectases have formed. In the other cases vital dyes, such as 0.5 per cent Evans blue or patent blue violet 11 per cent, are injected subcutaneously into the webs of the foot. By selective resorption of these dyes the main lymphatic channels dorsal to the metacarpus or metatarsus become outlined and can be cannulated with a 26-gauge needle, a small plastic tubing or a special lymphatic cannula after a local cutdown. An iodine containing soluble contrast medium such as sodium and meglumine diatrizoate (Renografin, Hypaque) is then injected slowly and radiographs of the region of interest are made as soon as possible. Water-soluble contrast media rapidly diffuse through the walls of the lymphatic channels into the surrounding tissue, which causes the radiographic details to be blurred unless the radiographs are taken shortly after the injection of the dye.

In primary lymphedema hypoplasia of the lymphatics of the proximal limb and aplasia of the lymph nodes may be seen. Some lymphatics end blindly; others lead into collateral vessels around instead of into the lymph nodes or the area where they are found normally. The failure to outline a lymph node is not absolute proof of its absence. The abnormalities of the lymphatics in the proximal limb region may or may not cause marked dilatation of the distal lymphatics (lymphangiectases). In some cases the lymphatics are hypoplastic throughout their course. In aplasia it may be impossible to find lymphatics that are suitable for cannulation and injection of radiographic dye. Following the cutdown, the abnormal nature of these vessels that have taken up some of the vital dye injected into the webs of the foot is easily recognized.

In dogs with the lymphedema confined to one limb five differential diagnoses have to be considered: inflammatory edema, trauma, venous obstruction, secondary lymphedema, and arteriovenous fistula. If the edema involves both forelimbs, the differential diagnosis is thrombosis of the cranial vena cava or compression or invasion of the vein by a mediastinal mass. With mediastinal masses the edema usually involves also the head and neck area. Bilateral hindlimb edema can be due to an obstruction of the sublumbar lymph nodes by neoplastic infiltration (see Secondary Lymphedema). Lymphedema due to hypoproteinemia should be considered as a differential diagnosis if all four limbs are involved.

The prognosis of congenital lymphedema, as far as reversibility of the condition is concerned, is guarded. A few dogs with hindlimb edema during the neonatal period may improve spontaneously. Dogs with severe edema of the limbs and the trunk often succumb during the first few weeks after birth.[82] In longstanding untreated lymphedema a mesenchymal response leads to a permanent induration of the edematous region. Longstanding edema also exposes the area to complications, such as abrasions and infection, which can be difficult to treat.

Therapeutic relief can be obtained in some dogs by long-term (several months) bandaging in Robert-Jones splints. Diuretics and glucocorticoids may enhance the effect of the bandages. If bandaging does not improve the condition, surgical excision of the subcutaneous edematous tissue and the superficial fascia can bring lasting improvement.[84] Corrective surgery has to be performed in two steps, thus preserving the viability of the skin. The objectives of surgery are (1) to remove permanently the stagnant pool of osmotically active proteinaceous subcutaneous fluid, (2) to reduce the potential space for fluid accumulation, (3) to increase tissue tension, thus reducing filtration and forcing fluids back into the venous capillary bed, and (4) to improve drainage via the deep tissue planes.

It is advisable to recommend that dogs with primary lymphedema should not be used for breeding. Test matings of dogs with congenital lymphedema support the hypothesis of an autosomal dominant inheritance with variable expressivity of the morphogenesis of the lymphatics. The latter explains the wide variations in severity and extent of the edema among carriers.[82] Continued morphogenesis of lymph vessels after birth, with formation of abnormal lymph channels, was suspected to occur in some carriers with functional adequate lymph drainage later in life.

SECONDARY LYMPHEDEMA

Persistent lymphedema only occurs after a considerable number of major lymph channels (sometimes all channels) or several sequential lymph nodes and their afferent or efferent lymphatics have been excised or blocked. The rapid opening up of collaterals, the rerouting of lymph flow through peripheral lymphaticovenous anastomosis, dermal lymphatics or tissue spaces (so-called paralymphatic routes of lymph drainage), and an increased fluid uptake by the veins can delay or prevent edema formation. Concurrent impairment of both venous and lymphatic drainage, however, leads rapidly to edema formation. Secondary lymphedema is often due to a combination of venous and lymphatic obstruction. Obstruction of the veins increases the flow in the lymph channels by disturbing Starling's equilibrium of tissue fluid formation and overloads the lymph channels.

Several causes of secondary lymphedema have been summarized in Table 81–3. Most common are posttraumatic or postsurgical interruption of lymphatics, excision of lymph nodes containing neoplastic metastases, and blockage of lymph nodes and lymph vessels by compression of invasive neoplasms. Lymphedema secondary to local neoplasia is usually a sign of a widely disseminated and highly invasive malignant process. Atrophy of the lymphatics associated with progressive interstitial fibrosis due to high protein content edema or infection is a rare cause of secondary lymphedema.[88]

Secondary lymphatic blockage or combined lymphatic and venous obstruction causes dilatation and increased permeability of the distally located lymphatics. Due to distention of the lymph channels valvular competency is lost, resulting in stagnation of lymph flow, mural insufficiency and accumulation of proteinaceous fluid in the subcutaneous tissues. Sometimes the direction of lymph flow is even reversed. The location and severity of the obstruction determines the extent of the edema formation. Sublumbar or intrapelvic obstruction induces bilateral hindlimb edema and edema of the thighs and external genitalia. Mediastinal masses and thrombosis of the cranial vena cava induce bilateral edema of the front limbs, and edema ventral to the thorax, the neck, and the head.

Secondary lymphedema is more common than primary lymphedema. It can, however, be difficult to determine its cause without a good history. In some cases the owners are able to relate to a previous trauma, infection or surgery. It is essential to know that lymphedema can often occur months or even years after the initial insult. The initial complaints of the owner vary depending on the underlying primary disease from an intermittent or gradually increasing localized pitting edema, which can be associated with signs ranging from lameness to signs of systemic illness.

The clinical signs vary depending on the cause of the lymphedema. Lymphedema may be confined to the periphery of a limb or it may extend all the way to the trunk. It can be confined to one extremity or sometimes, depending on the location of the interruption of the lymph system, both limbs can be involved. It is very important to carefully check all palpable lymph nodes for enlargement and pain. In the front limbs the subscapular region should also be examined. With bilateral hindlimb edema rectal or abdominal palpation of the sublumbar lymph nodes is essential. In male dogs the prostate and anal area, and in female dogs the mammary glands, the perianal region and the vagina should be carefully inspected in order to detect neoplasms, which can lead to obstructive intrapelvic processes. Intrapelvic masses should be suspected in all dogs with hindlimb edema and vague signs of sublumbar pain, discomfort when walking downstairs and/or difficulties with defecation or urination.

Depending on the type and extent of the lesion the limb edema may be the only detectable abnormality, or systemic signs such as fever, anorexia and weight loss may also be present.

The clinicopathologic findings depend on the underlying primary disorder and can be very varied.

If no definitive diagnosis can be made based on history and clinical examination, a radiograph of the region where the presumptive obstruction might be located, mostly the pelvic and the cranial thoracic area, should be taken. In a substantial number of cases soft tissue masses or destructive bony lesions can be detected radiographically. In cases with negative survey radiographs or if the diagnosis is still unclear a suitable contrast study is indicated. Lymphography is rarely needed; a less specific study such as an arteriography or a venography will often suffice. In cases with front limb edema valuable information can be gained about the mediastinal region by performing an esophography. Valuable information on the pelvic region can be obtained by performing an excretory urography or a cystography and urethrography, by insufflating air into the rectum or by doing a barium enema. With these studies the size of the sublumbar lymph nodes can be assessed more accurately than on survey radiographs.

Lymphograms of secondary lymphedema often show an increased number of tortuous and/or dilated lymphatics. The incompetency of the valves leads to stasis or even centrifugal instead of centripetal flow of the injected dye outlining dermal lymph capillaries (dermal backflow). In cases with a blockage of the lymph nodes by inflammation or metastasizing tumor cells the normal lymph channels may not be outlined. Sometimes collaterals are seen coursing around instead of into the lymph nodes. The abnormal lymph nodes appear either as enlarged nodular structures with filling defects (areas that contain no contrast medium) or they are not seen at all. The filling defects represent nodal areas occluded by inflammatory reaction or by tumor emboli. Sometimes contrast medium oozes spontaneously from a dilated lymph channel into the surrounding tissue, or a rupture of a lymphatic occurs when the contrast medium is injected with excessive pressure. The contrast medium that has leaked from the lymphatics may later be seen in interstitial tissue spaces, which can be mistaken for lymph vessels.

The differential diagnosis of secondary lymphedema includes primary lymphedema, low protein edema due to hypoalbuminemia, regional venous obstruction, cellulitis and phlebitis. The close association of lymphatic and venous structures can make it difficult to distinguish between lymphatic and venous obstruction. As mentioned previously the two often occur together. Ulceration, dermatitis, cyanosis, weeping varices, and/or fat necrosis are signs of venous obstruction rather than of lymph stasis. Local hematomas due to clotting disorders can sometimes be confused with secondary lymphedema.

The prognosis of secondary lymphedema depends on the underlying primary disease, the location and severity of the obstruction and the systemic status of the patient. In general a blockage located in a central region, such as in the axillary or sublumbar area, or an obstruction of the lymph nodes by tumor metastases has a poor prognosis.

Treatment depends on a precise diagnosis of the underlying cause. Anti-inflammatory medication, bandaging, diuretics, and gentle physical therapy are helpful in most traumatic and postsurgical edemas. Infectious disorders require long-term antimicrobial therapy. With neoplastic conditions, anti-inflammatory medication or cytostatic drugs or both can provide temporary relief. Reconstructive surgery with establishment of alternative lymphatic drainage has not been attempted in dogs and cats with secondary lymphedema.

LYMPHANGIOMA

Lymphangiomas are benign tumors of lymphatic capillaries and are thought to develop when primitive lymphatic sacs fail to establish venous communication.[89] The lesions present as large, fluctuant masses in the subcutaneous, fascial, mediastinal, and retroperitoneal space. They consist of dilated cystic, fluid-filled cavities lined by flattened endothelial cells and focal lymphoid aggregates, and subdivided by multiple septae. They are bound externally by a fairly thick connective tissue wall and are filled with translucent or blood-tinged, sterile fluid with a variable protein content (1.3 to 4.5 gm/dl and a specific gravity of 1.009 to 1.014).

Lymphangiomas are often noticed incidentally. Sometimes lymphangiomas exert pressure on surrounding structures and may interfere with muscle function, breathing (compression of the trachea), urination, or with the normal functioning of the gastrointestinal canal. The differential diagnoses include other types of space-occupying masses such as abscesses, enlarged lymph nodes, neoplasms and congenital cysts of non-lymphogenic origin. Prognosis is usually good. Treatment is surgical either by excision or marsupialization.

References

1. MacCoy, DM and Trotter, EJ: Brachial paralysis subsequent to traumatic partial occlusion of the right subclavian artery. JAAHA 13:625, 1977.
2. Parker, AJ, et al.: Iliac artery thrombosis and osteosarcoma in a dog. JAAHA 8:254, 1972.
3. Slauson, DO and Gribble, DH: Thrombosis complicating renal amyloidosis in dogs. Vet Pathol 8:352, 1971.
4. DiBartola, SP and Meuten, DJ: Renal amyloidosis in two dogs presented for thromboembolic phenomena. JAAHA 16:129, 1980.
5. Diener, R and Langham, R: Cushing's disease in the canine. Small Anim Clin 1:274, 1961.
6. Burns, MG, et al.: Pulmonary artery thrombosis in three dogs with hyperadrenocorticism. JAVMA 178:388, 1981.
7. Finco, DR, et al.: Chronic enteric disease and hypoproteinemia in nine dogs. JAVMA 163:262, 1973.
8. Green, RA: Clinical implications of Antithrombin III deficiency in animal diseases. Comp Contin Ed 6:537, 1984.
9. Kraft, CG and Kraft, AM: Thromboembolic occlusion of the iliac arteries in dogs. JAVMA 147:944, 1963.
10. Ettinger, SJ and Suter, PF: Canine Cardiology. Philadelphia, WB Saunders, 1970.
11. Liu, SK, et al.: Adult *Dirofilaria immitis* in the arterial system of a dog. JAVMA 148:1501, 1966.
12. Knight, DH: Heartworm heart disease. Adv Vet Sci Comp Med 21:107, 1977.
13. Stuart, BP, et al.: Ischemic myopathy associated with systemic dirofilariasis. JAAHA 14:36, 1978.
14. Wade, P, et al.: Surgical removal of an aortic foreign body. Iowa State University Vet 35:7, 1973.
15. Green, RA, et al.: Hypoalbuminemia-related platelet hypersensitivity in two dogs with nephrotic syndrome. JAVMA 186:485, 1985.
16. Kraus, KH, et al.: Use of thermography in the diagnosis of aortic thrombosis in a dog. JAAHA 22:489, 1986.
17. Denholm, TC: Thrombosis of the femoral artery in a dog. Vet Rec 75:970, 1963.
18. Crowe, DT: Peripheral vessels. *In* Bojrab, MJ (ed): Current Techniques in Small Animal Surgery. Philadelphia, Lea & Febiger, 1983, p 476.
19. Feldmann, BF: Thrombosis—diagnosis and treatment. *In* Kirk, RW (ed.). Current Veterinary Therapy IX. Philadelphia, WB Saunders, 1986, p 505.
20. Killingworth, CR et al.: Streptokinase treatment of cats with experimentally induced aortic thrombosis. Am J Vet Res 47:1351, 1986.
21. Wulf, R and Mertz, E: Studies on plasminogen. VIII. Species specificity of streptokinase. Can J Biochem 47:927, 1969.

Nonocclusive Arterial Diseases, Peripheral Arteriovenous Fistula

22. Bailey, WS: Epizootiology of cancer in animals. Ann NY Acad Sci 108:890, 1963.
23. Bohn, FK and Rhodes, WH: Angiograms and angiocardiograms in dogs and cats: Some unusual filling defects. J Am Vet Rad Soc 11:21, 1970.
24. Ivoghli, B: Fatal aortic aneurysm and rupture caused by *Spirocerca lupi* in a dog. JAVMA 170:834, 1977.

25. Hauser, P: A case of a spurious aneurysm in a dog which was diagnosed radiographically and treated successfully by surgery (German). Schweiz Arch Tierheilk 116:95, 1974.
26. MacCoy, DM: Traumatic arteriovenous fistula and major arterial injury from a gunshot wound in a dog. JAAHA 13:158, 1977.
27. Bouayad, H, et al.: Peripheral acquired arteriovenous fistula: a report of four cases and literature review. JAAHA 23:205, 1987.
28. Szilagyi, DE, et al.: Peripheral congenital arteriovenous fistulas. Surgery 57:61, 1965.
29. Ettinger, et al.: Peripheral arteriovenous fistula in a dog. JAVMA 153:1055, 1968.
30. Slocum, B, et al.: Acquired arteriovenous fistula in two cats. JAVMA 162:271, 1973.
31. Furneaux, RW, et al.: Arteriovenous fistulation following dewclaw removal in a cat. JAAHA 10:569, 1974.
32. Turner, BM: Acquired arteriovenous fistula in a dog following perivascular injection of thiopentone sodium. J Small Anim Pract 28:301, 1987.
33. Hopper, PE, et al.: Carotid body tumor associated with an arteriovenous fistula in a dog. Comp Cont Ed 5:68, 1983.
34. Clayton-Jones, DG, et al.: Arteriovenous fistula in the metatarsal pad of a dog: a case report. J Small Anim Pract 22:635, 1981.
35. Harari, J, et al.: Recurrent peripheral arteriovenous fistula and hyperthyroidism in a cat. JAAHA 20:760, 1984.
36. Cordy, DR: Vascular malformations and hemangiomas of the canine spinal cord. Vet Pathol 16:275, 1979.
37. Butterfield, AB, et al.: Acquired peripheral arteriovenous fistula in a dog. JAVMA 176:445, 1980.
38. Rubin, LF and Patterson, DF: Arteriovenous fistula of the orbit in a dog. Cornell Vet 55:471, 1965.
39. Kealy, JK, et al.: Arteriovenous fistula in the ear of a dog: a case report. J Small Anim Pract 11:15, 1970.
40. Suter, PF, et al.: Arteriovenous fistula of the temporal branches of the external carotid artery in a dog. JAVMA 158:349, 1971.
41. Franczuski, D and Gabbert, NH: Arteriovenous fistula in the tongue of a dog: a case report. JAAHA 22:355, 1986.
42. Hause, WR, et al.: Cerebral arteriovenous malformation in a dog. JAAHA 18:601, 1982.
43. Bolton, GR, et al.: Arteriovenous fistula of the aorta and caudal vena cava causing congestive heart failure in a cat. JAAHA 12:463, 1976.
44. Easley, JC and Carpenter, JL: Hepatic arteriovenous fistula in two Saint Bernard pups. JAVMA 165:167, 1975.
45. Legendre, AM, et al.: Ascites associated with intrahepatic arteriovenous fistula in a cat. JAVMA 168:589, 1976.
46. Rogers, WA, et al.: Intrahepatic arteriovenous fistulae in a dog resulting in portal hypertension, portacaval shunts, and reversal of portal blood flow. JAAHA 13:470, 1977.
47. Landers, EA and Mitten, RW: Intrahepatic arteriovenous fistula with portosystemic communications: a case report. J Am Vet Rad Soc 19:70, 1978.
48. Njoku, CO, et al.: Pulmonary vascular hamartoma in a dog. JAVMA 161:378, 1972.
49. Holman, E: Abnormal Arteriovenous Communications, 2nd ed. Springfield, Ill, Charles C Thomas, 1968.
50. Holman, E: Reflections on arteriovenous fistulas. Am Thor Surg 11:176, 1971.
51. McGavin, MD and Henry, J: Canine hepatic vascular hamartoma associated with ascites. JAVMA 160:864, 1972.
52. Holling, HE: Peripheral Vascular Diseases. Philadelphia, JB Lippincott, 1972.
53. McNeese, S, et al.: Definitive treatment of selective vascular injuries and posttraumatic arteriovenous fistulas by arteriographic embolization. Am J Surg 140:252, 1980.
54. Jonsson, I: Coronary arterial lesions and myocardial infarcts in the dog. Acta Vet Scand Suppl 38:1972, and Acta Vet Scand 15: 206, 1974.
55. Valtonen, MH and Oksanen, A: Cardiovascular disease and nephritis in dogs. J Small Anim Pract 13:687, 1972.
56. Bjotvedt, G: Spontaneous renal arteriosclerosis in Greyhounds. Canine Practice 13:26, 1986.
57. Wissler, RW: Comparative Atherosclerosis. *In* Roberts, JC and Strauss, R (eds) New York, Harper & Row, 1965, p 342.
58. Liu, SK, et al.: Clinical and pathologic findings in dogs with atherosclerosis: 21 cases (1970-83). JAVMA 189:227, 1986.
59. Luginbühl, H, et al.: Comparative atherosclerosis. Adv Vet Sci and Comp Med 21:421, 1977.
60. McAllister, WB and Waters, LL: Vascular lesions in the dog following thyroidectomy and viosterol feeding. Yale J Biol Med 22:651, 1950.
61. Rogers, WA, et al.: Lipids and lipoproteins in normal dogs and in dogs with secondary hyperlipoproteinemia. JAVMA 166:1092, 1975.
62. Patterson, JS, et al.: Neurologic manifestations of cerebrovascular atherosclerosis associated with primary hypothyroidism in a dog. JAVMA 186:499, 1985.
63. Aegerter, EE and Kirkpatrick, JA: Orthopedic Diseases. Physiology, Pathology, Radiology, 3rd ed. Philadelphia, WB Saunders, 1968.
64. Suter, PF: Zur Gefahr der Ueberdosierung von Vitamin-D Proparaten. Schweiz Arch Tierhk 99:421, 1957.
65. Easley, JR: Necrotizing Vasculitis: An overview. JAAHA 15:207, 1979.
66. Fauci, SA et al.: The spectrum of vasculitis. Clinical, pathologic, immunologic, and therapeutic considerations. Ann Int Med 89(Part I):660, 1978.
67. Fadok, VA and Barrie, J: Sulfasalazine responsive vasculitis in the dog: A case report. JAAHA 20:161, 1982.
68. Wiggins, RC and Cochrane, CG: Immune-complex mediated biological effects. N Engl J Med 304:518, 1981.
69. Manning, TO and Scott, DW: Cutaneous vasculitis in a dog. JAAHA 16:61, 1980.
70. Hoff, EJ and Vandevelde, M: Case report: Necrotizing vasculitis in the central nervous systems of two dogs. Vet Pathol 18:219, 1981.
71. Meric, SM, et al.: Necrotizing vasculitis of the spinal pachyleptomeningeal arteries in three Bernese mountain dogs. JAAHA 22:459, 1986.
72. Randell, MG and Hurvitz, AI: Immune-mediated vasculitis in five dogs. JAVMA 183:207, 1983.
73. Kelly, DF, et al.: Polyarteritis in the dog: A case report. Vet Rec 92:363, 1973.
74. Lucke, VM, et al.: Lymphomatoid granulomatosis of the lung in young dogs. Vet Path 16:405, 1979.
75. Suter, PF and Lord, PF: Thoracic Radiography, Text atlas. Chapter II. Suter, PF, 8908 Wettswil, Switzerland, 1984, p 625.
76. Von Rotz, A, et al.: Eosinophilic granulomatous pneumonia in a dog. Vet Rec 118:631, 1986.
77. Scott, DW: Cutaneous phlebectasias in cushingoid dogs. JAAHA 21: 351, 1985.
78. Burrows, CF: Techniques and complications of intravenous and intraarterial catheterization in dogs and cats. JAVMA 163:1357, 1973.
79. Friedland, G: Infusion related phlebitis—is the in-line filter the solution? Editorial. New Engl J Med 312:113, 1984.

Diseases of Peripheral Lymphatics

80. Földi, Diseases of Lymphatics and Lymph Circulation. Springfield, Ill, Charles C Thomas, 1969.
81. Skelley, JF, et al.: Applications of direct lymphangiography in the dog. Am J Vet Res 25:747, 1964.
82. Patterson, DF, et al.: Congenital hereditary lymphedema in the dog. Part. I Clinical and genetic studies. J Med Genet 4:145, 1967.
83. Suter, PF: Die Lymphography beim Hund, eine Röentgenologische Methode zur Diagnose von Veränderungen am Lymphsystem. Habilitationsschrift. Juris Verlag, Zurich, Switzerland, 1969.
84. Leighton, RL and Suter, PF: Primary lymphedema of the hindlimb in the dog. JAVMA 175:369, 1979.
85. Kinmonth, JB: Primary lymphedema of the lower limb. Proc Roy Soc Med 58:1021, 1965.
86. Luginbühl, H, et al.: Congenital hereditary lymphedema in the dog. Part II, Pathological studies. J Med Genet 4:153, 1967.
87. Griffin, CE and MacCoy, DM: Primary lymphedema: A case report and discussion. JAAHA 14:375, 1978.
88. Carmichael, NG, et al.: Secondary lymphedema in a dog. J Small Anim Pract 27:335, 1986.
89. Chait, D, et al.: Management of cystic hygromas. Surg Gynecol Obstet 139:55, 1974.
90. Stambaugh, JE, et al.: Lymphangioma in four dogs. JAVMA 173:759, 1978.

INDEX

INDEX

Note: Page numbers in *italics* refer to illustrations; page numbers followed by the letter t refer to tables.

Abdomen, enlargement of, 131–138
ascites and, 133–135
canine Cushing's syndrome and, 138
carcinomatosis and, 136–137
chylous peritonitis and, 136
feline infectious peritonitis and, 137
hemoperitoneum and, 136
hepatomegaly and, 137
in canine hyperadrenocorticism, 1727, *1727*
peritoneal surface and, 131
peritonitis and, 135
pneumoperitoneum and, 136
recognizing peritoneal disease and, 131–133, 132t, *133*, 134t
renomegaly and, 137
splenomegaly and, 137
evaluation of, anorexia and, 16
polyphagia and, 16
gastric dilatation-volvulus-torsion syndrome and, 1279
pain in, 131
hematuria and, 161–162
palpation of, 1399
respiratory disease and, diagnosis of, 749
surgery and, pleural effusion caused by, 881
Abdominocentesis, in heart failure therapy, 967
Abducens nerves, focal diseases of, 715–716
Abortion, 1803
Abscess(es), 275
carnassial, 1211–1212, *1214*
definition of, 126
intracranial, *604*, 604–605
of lung, pneumothorax and, 885
periodontal, 1223, *1224*
prostatic, 1873–1874
pulmonary, 847
retropharyngeal, 1237, *1237*
Absorption, large intestinal, 1398
small intestinal, tests of, 1338–1339
small intestine and, 1324–1327, *1325*
Acanthamebiasis, brain and, 606
Acanthocyte-like cells, 2150, *2154*
Accelerated conduction tachyarrhythmias, 1073–1074, *1074*, *1075*
Accrochage, 1081
Acetaminophen intoxication, 479
differentiation of, 459t, 465t, 479
Achalasia, cricopharyngeal, 787
Achondrodysplasia, 2383
Acid-base balance, in hypoadrenocorticism, 1761t, 1762
in pulmonary edema, 862
physiology of, 440t, 440–443
acid-base disturbances and, 442–443, 443t
blood sample collection and, 442
buffer systems and, 440–441
carbon dioxide control and, 441
plasma bicarbonate control and, 441–442, *442*
lower respiratory disease and, 820
regulation of, chronic renal failure and, 1922–1923
Acid-base disorders, 440–443, 443t
brain and, 616–617
drug index for, 449t
in liver disease, 1461–1462
mixed, 443t, 446–447
Acidosis. *See also* Metabolic acidosis; Respiratory acidosis.
in insulin antagonism/resistance, 1702
renal tubular, 2026t, 2026–2027
Acne, in canine hyperadrenocorticism, 1727
Acquired tolerance, immune system and, 2292
Acromegaly, 1600–1602
diagnosis of, 1601, *1602*
historic findings and clinical signs in, in dogs, *1600*, 1600–1601, *1601*
treatment of, 1601–1602, *1603*
ACTH. *See* Adrenocorticotropic hormone.
Actinic dermatitis, of pinna, 249
Actinomycosis, 271–272
osteomyelitis and, 2380
Action potential, gastric, 1293
of cardiac cell, 1051, *1054*
Activated coagulation time, 2250–2251
Acupressure, 492
Acupuncture, 484–496, *485*
acupuncture points and, 494–495
expected results and, 494–495
selection of, 494
attitudes toward, 495
efficacy of, clinical evidence for, 486
research on, 486
historical background of, 484–486
indications for, 491
information and education about, 496
legal and ethical implications of, 496
modes of action of, 486–491
autonomic theories of, 487, *489*
bioelectrical theory of, 488–489, 491
combination theory of, 488, *490*
gate theory of, 487, *488*
humoral theories of, 487–488, *489*
inhibitory surround theory of, 487
precautions with, 491
sequelae of, 491
techniques for, 492–494
acupressure and, 492
aquapuncture and, 493
cupping and, 492
electroacupuncture and, 493, *493*
implantation and, 493
laserpuncture and, 493–494
needles and, *485*, 492
temperature variation and, 492–493
ultrasound and, 493
traditional Oriental medicine and, 491
Adenine nucleotides, platelets and, 2266
Adenocarcinoma, from anal sac apocrine glands, hypercalcemia and, 1613t, 1613–1614, *1614*, *1615*
in dogs, 83
prostatic, 1816, *1875*, 1875–1876, *1876*
small intestinal, *1376*, 1376–1377, *1377*
Adenohypophysis, functional corticotropic adenoma of, hypercortisolism associated with, 1591–1592, *1592*
Adenoma, chromophobe, endocrinologically inactive, in pars distalis, 1591, *1591*
corticotropic, functional, of adenohypophysis, hypercortisolism and, 1591–1592, *1592*
hepatocellular, 1513
of adrenal gland, pathology of, 1725
of pars intermedia, *1593*, 1593–1600
growth hormone excess and, 1596, *1596*, *1597*
growth hormone–induced diabetes mellitus and, 1594–1596
growth hormone–induced glucose intolerance and, pathogenesis of, 1596–1597
hyperglycemia and glucose intolerance recognition and, 1597
Adenoma *(Continued)*
of pars intermedia, hypopituitarism and, diagnosis of, 1593
insulin treatment of, *1598*, 1598–1600, *1599*
ovariohysterectomy and, 1597–1598
pituitary impairment and, by drugs, 1593–1594, *1594*, *1595*
treatment of, 1597
of perianal gland, 1572, *1572*
of pituitary, pathology of, 1724
ADH. *See* Antidiuretic hormone.
Adhesion, of platelets, 2266, 2277
defects of, 2268–2271
Adrenal diseases. *See also* Hyperadrenocorticism; *specific diseases*.
neoplastic, pathology of, 1725
pathophysiology of, 1723, *1724*
polycythemia and, therapeutic principles for, 104
Adrenalectomy, in feline hyperadrenocorticism, 1756
in pituitary-dependent hyperadrenocorticism, 1747
β-Adrenergic agonists, in hyperkalemia, in acute renal failure, 1977
β-Adrenergic blockers, in heart failure therapy, 963–964
Adrenergic response, gastric dilatation-volvulus-torsion syndrome and, 1279
Adrenergic stimulation, cardiopulmonary response to, 176–177
Adrenocortical hyperplasia, nodular, bilateral, pathology of, 1724–1725
simple bilateral, pathology of, 1724
Adrenocorticotropic hormone (ACTH), ectopic ACTH syndrome and, pathophysiology of, 1724
endogenous concentrations of, in hyperadrenocorticism, 1741–1743, *1743*
glucocorticoid secretion and, 1721–1723
biosynthesis and, 1721–1722
function and, 1722
neuroendocrine control and, 1722–1723
neuroendocrine function and, 1587–1588
pituitary-hypothalamic diseases and, 1579
plasma, endogenous, in feline hyperadrenocorticism, 1756
in hypoadrenocorticism, 1766–1767, *1771*
Adrenocorticotropic hormone (ACTH) stimulation test, dexamethasone suppression test and, functioning adrenocortical tumors and, 1737–1738, *1739*
iatrogenic, 1738, *1738*
in hyperadrenocorticism, 1741
in feline hyperadrenocorticism, 1755
in hyperadrenocorticism, 1737–1738
in hypoadrenocorticism, 1766
in normal dogs, 1737, *1738*
misleading results and, 1738
theory and, 1737
Adverse reactions. *See* Drug reactions, adverse.
Aelurostrongylus abstrusus, 836
diagnosis of, 836, *837*
Afghan hounds, hereditary myelopathy of, 660–661
Afterdepolarizations, cardiac arrhythmias and, 1056
Afterload, cardiac output and, 905, *906*
heart failure therapy and, 941
in heart failure, reduction of, *919*, 919–920
Agalactia, 1833
Age, adverse drug reactions and, 500
alopecia and, 114

Age *(Continued)*
anemia and, 92
cyanosis and, 97
pain and, 20
pruritus and, 122
thyroid hormone metabolism and, in dog, 1640
tremor and, 54–55
Agglutination, immune-mediated, 2150, *2152*, *2153*
Aggregation, of platelets, 2266–2267, 2267t, 2276–2277
deficiencies of, 2271–2272
Aggression, 72
behavioral signs and, 70–71
in cats, 236–237
intraspecific, 236
toward people, 236–237
in dogs, 232–235
dominance, 232–233
fear-induced, 234
interfemale, 233–234
intermale, 233
pain-induced, 234
parental, 234
pathophysiologic disorders and, 235
predatory behavior and, 234–235
pseudocyesis and, 234
territorial/protective, 234
Airway, cardiopulmonary resuscitation and, 174
humidification of, lower respiratory disease and, 819
Alanine aminotransferase, in canine hyperadrenocorticism, 1731
in liver disease, 1436–1437
Albumin, hypoalbuminemia and, causes of, 14t
in nephrotic syndrome, 2020–2021
nephrotic syndrome and, 1941–1942
synthesis and regulation of, in liver disease, 1433–1434
Alcohol intoxication, 459t, 460t, 481
Aldosterone, heart failure and, 909
Algae, myocarditis and, 1125
ocular manifestations of, *78*, 81–82
Alkaline phosphatase, abnormal values of, causes of, 13t
in canine hyperadrenocorticism, 1731
in liver disease, 1438–1439
Alkalosis. *See* Metabolic alkalosis; Respiratory alkalosis.
Alkylating agents, in cancer chemotherapy, 532–533
Allergic contact dermatitis, 2316–2317
Allergic otitis, 257
Allergy(ies). *See also* Hypersensitivity reactions.
alopecia and, 120
to drugs, 501–504
adverse reactions resembling, 504–505
clinical manifestations of, 502–504
diagnosis of, 504
immunologic mechanisms and, 501–502
response characteristics and, 501
Alloploidy, 184
Alloxan, insulin-secreting tumors and, 1715
Alopecia, 113–121
cicatricial, 113
congenital, of pinna, 247
definition of, 113, 119
diagnostic plan for, 119
historical findings in, 114–115, 117
in canine hyperadrenocorticism, 1727, *1728*
noncicatricial, 113
normal hair growth and structure and, 113
outcome in, 121
pathophysiology of, 113–114, 114t–118t
periodic, of pinna, 249
physical examination in, 117–119
primary skin lesions and, 117–118
secondary lesions and, 119
pruritus and, 116–117
signalment in, 114
testosterone- and estrogen-responsive, 6
treatment goals for, 119–120
Alpha-chain disease, paraproteinemias and, 2309
Alpha-fetoprotein, hepatic, abnormalities of, causes of, 1442–1443
Alphanaphthylthiourea (ANTU) intoxication, 465t, 467
Alternate-day therapy, with corticosteroids, 422
Altitude, polycythemia and, 102
Alveoli, diagnostic approach to, 752
pattern of, radiographic interpretation and, 757, *757*, 758t
Amblyopia, hereditary, in Irish setter, 597
Amebiasis, 286, 1412
Amino acids, aromatic, hepatic encephalopathy and, 1464
regulation of, in liver disease, 1435–1436
Aminoglutethimide, in canine hyperadrenocorticism, 1753–1754
Aminoglycosides, 396–398
action of, 396
activity spectrum of, 396–397, 397t
clinical pharmacology of, 397
dosage modification and, 398, 409t–410t
resistance to, 397
toxicity of, 397–398
Aminopenicillins, 388–389
activity spectrum of, 388–389
clinical pharmacology of, 389
4-Aminopyridine. *See* Avitrol intoxication.
Ammonia, hepatic encephalopathy and, 1463–1464
metabolism of, in liver disease, 1451, 1453–1456, *1454*
Ammonia challenge test, tubular function and, 1900
Ammonia tolerance testing, in liver disease, 1455–1456
Ammoniagenesis, renal, renal failure and, 1990
Ammonium urate calculi, in liver disease, 1456
Ammonium urate crystalluria, in liver disease, 1456
Ammonium urate urolithiasis. *See* Urolithiasis.
Amrinone, actions of, 953
in heart failure therapy, 953–954
indications for, 953
toxicity and interactions of, 954
Amylase, abnormal values of, causes of, 12t
Amyloidosis, hepatic manifestations of, 1511
in nephrotic syndrome, 2012–2013
etiology of, 2013
renal, 2012–2013
pathogenesis of, 1939, 1941, 1941t
renal, prognosis of, 2016
treatment of, 2019
Anal diseases, 1567–1574
anatomy and, 1559–1560, *1560*
defecation and, physiology of, 1560–1561
fecal incontinence and, 1573t, 1573–1574
history and physical examination in, 1561
special examination in, 1561
Anal foreign bodies, 1567
Anal sac, apocrine glands of, adenocarcinoma from, hypercalcemia and, 1613t, 1613–1614, *1614*, *1615*
Anal sac disease, in cat, 1572
in dog, 1570–1572
diagnosis of, 1571
history and clinical signs in, 1571
treatment of, 1571–1572
Anal strictures, 1567
Anal tumors, 1572–1573
malignant, 1572–1573
of perianal gland, 1572, *1572*
Analgesics, in idiopathic lower urinary tract disease, 2079
in liver failure, 1516
Anamnesis, in diabetes mellitus, 1682
insulin-secreting tumors and, 1708t, 1709
Anatomic barriers, of lower urinary tract, 2115
Anatomic disorders, urinary incontinence and, 149–150
Anatomic shunts, central cyanosis and, 96
Anconeal process, ununited, in chondrodystrophic breeds, *2350*, 2353, *2354*
Ancylostomiasis, in developing countries, 221
Andersonstrongylus milksi, 838
Androgens, in nonregenerative anemia, in chronic renal failure, 2003–2004, 2004t
Anemia, 91–94, 2159–2176, *2160*
aplastic, 2173–2174
drug reactions and, 507, 507t
Anemia *(Continued)*
aplastic, treatment of, 2174
as paraneoplastic syndrome, 518–519
definition of, 91
diagnostic plan for, 93–94
extra-marrow, 2171–2173
chronic disease and, 2171–2172
endocrine failures and, 2172
non-regenerative, feline leukemia virus and, *2172*, 2172–2173
renal failure and, 2172
hemolytic, 2163–2171
cold-agglutinin disease and, 2166
copper toxicity and, 2171
drug-related, 2165–2166
erythrocyte oxidative injury and, *2168*, 2168–2170
erythroparasitic organisms and, 2166–2168
immune-mediated, 2163–2166, 2299–2303
immunohemolytic, *2163*, 2163–2165
inherited metabolic disorders and, 2170–2171
microangiopathic, 2171
neonatal isoerythrolysis and, 2166
hemorrhage and, 2160–2163
coagulation biochemistry defects and, 2161
iron deficiency and, *2161*, 2161–2163, *2162*
thrombocytopenia and, 2160–2161
trauma/lacerations and, 2160
historical findings in, 92
hypochromic, 91
intra-marrow, *2173*, 2173–2176
chloramphenicol toxicity and, 2176
lymphoproliferative disorders and, 2176
myeloaplasia and, 2173–2174
myelodysplasia and, 2174–2175, *2175*
myelofibrosis and, 2176
myeloproliferative, 2175–2176, *2176*
osteosclerosis and, 2176
iron deficiency, hemorrhage and, *2161*, 2161–2163, *2162*
liver disease and, 1484
treatment of, 1521
macrocytic, 91
marrow response to, kinetics of, 2157–2158
microcytic, 91
myelophthisic, 92
nonregenerative, 91–92
in chronic renal failure, 2002–2004, 2003t
androgens and, 2003–2004, 2004t
recombinant human erythropoietin in, 2004
transfusion therapy in, 2004
normochromic, 91
normocytic, 91
ocular manifestations of, 79
outcome in, 94
pathophysiology of, 91–92
nonregenerative anemia and, 92
regenerative anemia and, 91–92
physical findings in, 92–93
regenerative, 91, 92
renal failure and, 1918
weakness and, 47
Anesthetics, emergency medicine and, 215–216
in feline hyperthyroidism, 1665
in liver failure, 1516
inhalant, hepatic toxicity of, 1497
local, otitis externa and, 255
thyroid hormone metabolism and, in dog, 1640
Anestrus, canine, 1782–1783
in hyperadrenocorticism, 1729–1730
feline, 1787
Aneuploidy, 184
Aneurysm, arterial, 1188–1189
spurious, 1188–1189
true, 1188
Aneurysmal bone cyst, 2394
Angiitis. *See* Vasculitis.
Angiocardiography, in congenital heart disease, 980, 982
Angioedema, 118
Angiography, in peripheral edema, 44
in renal disease, 1913, *1913*
Angiostrongylus vasorum, 838
Angiotensin, heart failure and, 909

Angiotensin-converting enzyme inhibitors, in heart failure therapy, 961–963
Animal-facilitated therapy, 241–242
Anodontia, 1209
Anorexia, 15–17
diagnostic plan for, 16
history in, 15–16
in chronic renal failure, diet therapy and, 1995–1996
pathophysiology of, 15
physical findings in, 16
therapeutic goals in, 16–17
Anotia, 247
Anoxia, cerebral, 599–600
Antacids, gastric ulceration and, 1310
Anterior tibialis reflex, testing for, 569, *571*
Anthrax, 273
Antianxiety agents, 229–230
Antiarrhythmic agents, electrophysiologic classification of, 1060t, 1060–1065
in gastric dilatation-volvulus-torsion syndrome, 1286–1287
increasing automaticity, 1059
removing or suppressing precipitating factors, 1059
Antibacterial agents, in idiopathic lower urinary tract disease, 2079
in otitis externa, 255
Antibiotics, cell wall–active, 394
cephalosporin, hematopoietic stem cell death and, 2199
in cancer chemotherapy, 533
in exocrine pancreatic insufficiency, 1548
in liver failure, 1516
β-lactam, 386–387
nonclassical, 393 394
thrombocytopathies induced by, 2275
Antibodies, anti-insulin, insulin antagonism/resistance and, 1702–1703
chimeric, 2289
immune response and, 2283
Antibody class, incomplete, in immune-mediated hemolytic anemia, 2300
Anticholinergic drugs, in acute gastritis, 1302
Anticholinesterase intoxication, 466
Anticoagulants, in glomerulonephritis, 2018–2019
renal failure and, 1991
Anticonvulsants, 68–69
hepatopathy associated with, 1495–1496
in liver failure, 1516
Antidiuretic hormone (ADH), heart failure and, 910
in polyuria and polydipsia, 140
Antidotes, 457, 461t–464t. *See also* Toxicology.
Antiemetic drugs, in acute gastritis, 1302
Antifungal drugs, activity spectrum of, 395–396
clinical pharmacology of, 396
toxicity of, 396
Antigen(s), cross-reacting, 2297
hidden, 2297
nature of, 2283
self, alteration of, 2297
Antigen-specific receptors, structure and function of, 2285–2287
Antigenic determinants, 2283
Antigenic stimulation, chronic, lymphocytosis secondary to, 2208
Anthelmintics, 1342t–1343t
hepatitis associated with, 1496–1497
Antihormonal therapy, insulin-secreting tumors and, 1714–1715
Anti-infectives, for urinary tract, 404
Anti-inflammatory agents, corticosteroids as, 419
in idiopathic lower urinary tract disease, 2080
in otitis externa, 255
nonsteroidal, thrombocytopathies induced by, 2274, 2274t
Anti-insulin antibodies, in insulin antagonism/resistance, 1702–1703
Antimetabolites, in cancer chemotherapy, 533
Antimicrobial drugs, 381–410
action of, 383 386
bacterial sensitivity and, 383–385
Antimicrobial drugs *(Continued)*
action of, distribution and, 385
environmental conditions and, 385–386
canine urinary tract infections and, 382
cell wall synthesis inhibiting, 386–394
clinical applications of, 404–408
antimicrobial selection and, 405–408, 409t–410t
therapeutic approach and, 404–405
in chronic inflammatory bowel disease, 1407–1408
in infective endocarditis, 1159, 1160t
in urinary obstruction, 2035
microbial cell wall labilizing, 395–396
microbial intermediate metabolism inhibiting, 402–404
microbial nucleic acid synthesis inhibiting, 401–402
prophylactic use of, 408, 410
protein synthesis inhibiting, 396–398
bacteriostatic, 398–401
selection of, 381–382
sensitivity testing and, 384–385
therapeutic approach and, 382
treatment role of, 383
Antimycotic agents, in otitis externa, 255
Antineoplastic chemotherapy. *See* Cancer, chemotherapy in.
Antinuclear antibody tests, in systemic lupus erythematosus, 2310–2312, *2311*
Antiparasitic agents, in otitis externa, 255
Anti-platelet therapy, in glomerulonephritis, 2018–2019
Antiseptics, in idiopathic lower urinary tract disease, 2079
Antispasmodics, in idiopathic lower urinary tract disease, 2079–2080
Antithyroid drugs, in feline hyperthyroidism, 1661–1664, 1662t, *1662–1664*, 1663t
ANTU. *See* Alphanaphthylthiourea intoxication.
Anus. *See also headings beginning with term* Anal.
imperforate, 1569–1570
diagnosis of, 1569, *1569*, 1570
history and clinical signs in, 1569
treatment of, 1569–1570
Anxiety. *See* Separation anxiety.
Aorta, coarctation of, 1027
Aortic arch, right, persistent, 1024, *1026*
Aortic regurgitation, 1011
heart failure and, 914
Aortic stenosis, 1004, 1007–1011
clinical findings in, 1008–1010, *1009*, *1010*
clinical management of, 1007t, 1011
natural history of, 1010–1011
pathogenesis of, 1004, 1007, *1008*
pathophysiology of, 1007–1008, *1008*
Aortic valve disease, 1048–1049
cardiovascular examination in, *1048*, 1048–1049, *1049*
echocardiography in, 1049, *1049*
Aorticopulmonary septal defect, 1024, 1027
Aplastic anemia, 2173–2174
drug reactions and, 507, 507t
treatment of, 2174
Apocrine glands, of anal sac, adenocarcinoma from, hypercalcemia and, 1613t, 1613–1614, *1614*, *1615*
Apodia, 2384
Appetite, 31–32
Aquapuncture, 493
Aqueous vasopressin test, tubular function and, 1900
Arginase, in liver disease, 1437–1438
Arrhythmias. *See* Cardiac arrhythmias.
Arsenic intoxication, 470–471
differentiation of, 459t, 470
Arterial blood gases, cyanosis and, 99
Arterial diseases, nonocclusive, 1188–1194
functional forms of, 1189
occlusive, 1185–1188
Arterial thrombosis. *See* Thrombosis, arterial.
Arteries, great, transposition of, cyanotic heart disease and, 1022–1023
Arteriography, cerebral, 579–580, 582, *582*
Arteriosclerosis, 1191–1192
Arteriovenous fistulas, 1189–1191
hepatic, 1506–1507
Arthritides, drug-induced, 2371
immuno-mediated, treatment of, 2372–2373
Arthritis, crystal-induced, 2373
enteropathic, 2371
treatment of, 2373
infectious, 2362–2366
bacterial, 2362–2363, *2364*
bacterial L-forms and, 2363
fungal, 2365–2366
mycoplasmal, 2363–2364
protozoal, 2366
rickettsial, 2364–2365
spirochetal, 2365
viral, 2365
noninfectious, 2366–2373
apparent immunologic cause and, 2366–2367
crystal-induced, 2373
rheumatoid, 2313–2314
of dogs, 2366–2367, *2367*, *2368*
treatment of, 2373
Arthropathy(ies), developmental, 2346–2359
dietary, 2361
inborn errors of metabolism and, 2359–2361
neoplastic, 2361–2362
neuropathic, 2345–2346
Arthropod bites or stings, 474–475
differentiation of, 467t, 473t, 475
therapy of, 461t–464t, 475
Articular cartilage, damage to, 2337, *2337*
enchondral cores and, retained, 2395–2396, *2396*
exostoses and, multiple, 676, 2383–2384, *2384*
Ascarids, small bowel diarrhea and, 1342t–1343t, *1345*, 1345–1346, *1346*
Ascending pathways, pain and, 19
Ascites, 133–135
differential diagnosis of, *133*, 134
history and physical examination in, 134
portal hypertension and, 1458–1459, *1459*
radiographic examination in, *133*, 134
treatment of, 134–135, 1520–1521
weakness and, 47
Aseptic meningitis. *See* Meningitis, corticosteroid-responsive.
Aseptic necrosis, of femoral head, 2359, *2360*, *2361*
Aspartate aminotransferase, in liver disease, 1437
Aspergillosis, 359–362
clinical manifestations of, 359–360
in aspergillus osteomyelitis, 360
in canine disseminated aspergillosis, 359–360
in canine nasal aspergillosis, 359
in feline aspergillosis, 360
diagnosis of, 360–361
aspergillus osteomyelitis and, 360–361
canine disseminated aspergillosis and, 360–361
feline aspergillosis and, 361
nasal aspergillosis and, 360, *360*, *361*
etiology and epizootiology of, 359
osteomyelitis and, 2381
pathogenesis of, 359
prognosis in, 362
pulmonary manifestations of, 835
treatment of, 361–362
Aspiration, prostatic, *1866*, 1866–1867
splenic, splenomegaly and, 2242
Aspirin intoxication, 478–479
differentiation of, 459t, 465t, 479
Asthenia. *See also* Weakness.
definition of, 46
Asthma, feline. *See* Bronchitis, allergic, feline.
Ataxia, 57–58
cerebellar, 58
differential diagnosis of, *58*, 59t, 60
hereditary, in terrier, 599
in hound, 661
in Jack Russell terriers, 660
in smooth-haired fox terriers, 660
sensory, 57
toxicity and, 614 615
truncal, 57
vestibular, 57t, 57–58

Atelectasis, 847
Atherosclerosis, 1191–1192, *1192*
Atlantoaxial subluxation, 634–637
clinical findings in, 635, *635*
diagnosis of, 635–636, *636*
etiology and pathogenesis of, 634–635
treatment of, 636–637
Atopy, 2314–2316
diagnosis of, 2315
pathophysiology of, 2314–2315, *1315*
prognosis of, 2316
treatment of, 2316
Atrial fibrillation, 1074–1075, *1076–1078*, 1077–1079
clinical signs of, 1077–1078, *1079*
treatment of, 1078–1079
Atrial flutter, 1079, *1080*
Atrial natriuretic hormone, heart failure and, 910
Atrial pressure, right heart evaluation and, *933*, 933–934, *934*
Atrial septal defects. *See* Atrioventricular septal defects.
Atrial standstill, 1087–1088, *1088*
Atrial wall, left, endocardial splitting of, 1044–1045
rupture of, 1044–1045
Atrioventricular block, 1088–1093
clinical signs of, 1092
first degree, 1088, *1089*
second degree, 1088, *1090*
third degree, 1088, *1091*, 1092
treatment of, 1092–1093, *1093*
Atrioventricular dissociation, 1079–1084, *1081–1083*
Atrioventricular septal defects, 993–1000
clinical findings in, 997–998
atrial defects and, *995–998*, 997–998
ventricular defects and, *989*, *990*, *997*, 998, *999*
clinical management of, 998, 1000, 1007t
heart failure and, 914
natural history of, 998
pathogenesis of, 993, *993*, *994*
pathophysiology of, 993, *994*, 995–996
atrial defects and, 995, *995*, *996*
Eisenmenger's physiology and, 996, *996*
ventricular defects and, *994*, 995–996
Atrioventricular valve dysplasia, 1011–1014
clinical findings in, 1011, 1013–1014, *1013–1016*
clinical management of, 1007t, 1014
pathogenesis of, 1011, *1012*, *1013*
pathophysiology of, 1011
Atrium(a), anomalous development of, 1024
Atropine, cardiopulmonary response to, 176
Attention-getting phenomena, learned, 72
Attitudinal reactions, in neurologic examination, 558–559
Attrition, of teeth, 1211, *1212*, *1213*
Audiometry, impedance, brain disease diagnosis and, 588
Aujeszky's disease, 603
Auricular dermatosis, marginal, 247, 249
Auscultation, cyanosis and, 97–98
in chronic mitral valvular insufficiency, 1033, *1033*, *1034*
Autoagglutinins, in-saline acting, in immune-mediated hemolytic anemia, 2300, *2300*
Autodigestion, defenses against, 1529t, *1530*, 1530–1531, *1531*, 1531t
Autoimmune disorders, cutaneous manifestations of, 9
oral lesions and, 1229
pleural effusion and, 880–881, *881*
Autoimmunity, 2294
allergic drug reactions and, 503–504
Automaticity, of heart muscle, 1053, 1054–1055
agents increasing, 1059
Autonomic theories, acupuncture and, 487, *489*
Avitrol intoxication, 467–468
differentiation of, 460t, 468
Avulsion, of teeth, 1211, *1212*
Axial-atlantal-occipital malformations, 2343, *2343*
Azathioprine, in chronic inflammatory bowel disease, 1408–1409
Azotemia, 1893
causes of, 14t
characterization of, 1915–1916, 1916t
Azotemia *(Continued)*
postrenal, 1893, 1965, 1965t
localization of, 1971
prerenal, 1893, 1964–1965, 1965t
localization of, 1970–1971

B lymphocytes, regulators of, 2284
structure and function of, 2285–2287, *2286*
T cell cooperation with, 2291
Babesiosis, 287–288, 2167, *2167*
cutaneous manifestations of, 8
Babinski reflex, testing for, 573
Bacillus piliformis, small bowel diarrhea and, 1357
Bacteremia, infective endocarditis and, 1153
Bacteria, in urine, dysuria and, 164
Bacterial culture, large intestinal disease and, 1400
Bacterial endocarditis. *See* Infective endocarditis.
Bacterial flora, normal, of penis, 1881, 1882t
Bacterial infections, 265–276
alopecia and, 120
arthritis and, 2362–2363, *2364*
chronic inflammatory bowel disease and, 1404
cutaneous manifestations of, 7
diarrhea and. *See* Diarrhea, small bowel, bacterial.
diabetes mellitus and, 1705–1706
drugs for. *See* Antibiotics; Antimicrobial drugs.
in developing countries, 222
infertility and, in bitch, 1843–1845, 1844t
lymphadenitis and, 2229–2230
idiopathic lymphadenopathies and, 2230
puppy strangles and, 2229–2230
streptococcal, contagious, 2229
mediastinal, granulomatosis with, 892
myocardial, 1125
ocular manifestations of, 81
of brain, 604–605
abscess and, *604*, 604–605
of external ear canal, 256
of intestinal tract, 267–269
of large intestine, 1413–1415
of lower urinary tract, 2114–2123
anatomic barriers and, 2115
chemical defense and, 2115, 2116
consequences of, 2114
definitions and, 2111t, 2114
diabetes mellitus and, 2116
excess glucocorticoids and, 2116
host defense compromise and, 2116
immunology and, 2116
microflora and, 2115
normal defense mechanisms and, 2114–2115
urine flow and, 2115
of lower urinary tract. *See* Urinary tract infections.
of respiratory tract, 265–267, 830–832
prostatic, 1869–1874
systemic, 269–274
rhinitis and, 778, *779*
zoonotic, 191–192
Bacterial L-forms, arthritis and, 2363
Bacterial meningomyelitis. *See* Meningomyelitis, bacterial.
Bacterial overgrowth, 269
small intestinal, 1373–1375
clinical signs of, 1374
diagnosis of, 1339, 1374
pathogenesis of, 1373–1374
treatment of, 1374–1375
Bacterial products, in cancer therapy, 537–538
Bacterial sensitivity, to antimicrobial drugs, 383–385
BAER. *See* Brain stem auditory evoked responses.
Balanoposthitis, 1886, *1887*
Balantidiasis, 286–287, 1412
Barium enema, 1402–1404, 1403t
Basenji, hypertrophic gastritis of, 1306
immunoproliferative enteropathy of, 1364–1365
Basic Life Support, in cardiopulmonary resuscitation, 173–174
Basophil(s), 2211–2217
basophilia and, 2212t, 2212–2213
Basophil(s) *(Continued)*
leukemias and myeloproliferative syndromes and, 2213t, 2213–2214, 2214t
incidence and etiology of, 2214, 2216
lymphoproliferative disorders and, 2217
morphology of, 2211–2212, *2212*
myeloproliferative disorders and, 2216–2217
production and kinetics of, 2212
stippling of, 2147, *2149*
Basophilia, 2212t, 2212–2213
Bedlington terrier, copper-associated hepatitis in, 1488–1491, *1489*
Behavioral disorders, 227–237, 228t
in cats, 235–237
in dogs, 228–235
Behavioral signs, 70–74, 71t
client relations and, 72–73
diagnosis of, 70–72, 71t
diagnostic goals for, 73
pain and, 20
specific disease states and, 71t, 73–74
Behavioral therapy, for fears and phobias, 228
Benign monoclonal gammopathy, paraproteinemias and, 2308–2309
Benign prostatic hyperplasia, 1867–1868
clinical signs in, 1867–1868
diagnosis of, 1868
pathophysiology of, 1867
treatment of, 1868
Bentiromide, in exocrine pancreatic insufficiency, 1543, *1544*
Bernard-Soulier syndrome, 2270–2271
Besnoitia, 282
Bicarbonate, plasma, renal control of, acid-base and, 441–442, *442*
Biceps reflex, testing for, 567, 569, *569*
Bile, production of, 1424, 1425t
Bile acids, in liver disease, 1449t, 1449–1451, *1450*, *1452*, *1453*
Biliary system, 1424, 1425t
Biliary tract disease, diagnosis of, *1555*, 1555–1556, *1556*
nonobstructive, 1556t, 1556–1557
intraluminal, *1556*, 1556–1557, 1557t
mural, 1557
neoplastic, 1512–1513, 1557
obstructive, 1556t, 1557–1558
extramural, 1558
intraluminal, 1557
mural, 1557
rupture and, 1558
traumatic, 1484
Bilirubin, abnormal values of, causes of, 13t
in urine, renal disease and, 1904
metabolism of, liver disease and, 1443–1446, *1444*, 1446t, *1447*, 1448
Biochemical tests, fecal, 1337
in diabetes mellitus, 1685t, 1685–1686
large intestinal disease and, 1400
nutritional assessment and, 451
serum, in canine hypothyroidism, 1642t, 1644–1645
in feline hyperthyroidism, 1658
in feline panleukopenia, 316
lymphadenopathy and, 2228
splenomegaly and, 2241, 2241t
Bioelectrical theory, acupuncture and, 488–489, 491
Biopsy, gastric, 1298–1299, *1299*
hepatic, in hyperadrenocorticism, 1741
in liver disease, 1469t, 1469–1470
in small bowel diarrhea, 1340–1341
of bladder, in lower urinary tract disease, 2113
of large intestine, techniques for, 1402, *1402*
of lung, open lung, 766
percutaneous fine needle aspiration, *764*, 764–765, *765*
pleural disorders and, 874
of lymph nodes, in lymphadenopathy, 2229
oral cavity diseases and, 1208
peripheral nerve disorders and, 714
pleural, 874, *874*
prostatic, *1866*, 1867, *1867*
renal, in nephrotic syndrome, 2014–2016
in primary renal failure, 1973

Biopsy *(Continued)*
renal, in renal disease, 1914–1915, *1915*
spinal cord tumors and, 680–681
thyroid, in canine hypothyroidism, 1649
transbrachial, *763*, 763–764, *764*
urethral, in lower urinary tract disease, 2113
Biotin deficiency, brain and, 616
Biotoxins, 472–478
Bipyridine derivatives, in heart failure therapy, 954
Birman cat neutrophil granulation anomaly, 2188, *2188*
Bites, arthropod, 474–475
differentiation of, 467t, 473t, 475
therapy of, 461t–464t, 475
inflicted on humans, 192–193
prevention of, 192–193
of poisonous lizards, 475–476
rabies and, animal management and, 300
Bladder, anatomic defects of, 2113
atony of. *See also* Urinary retention.
definition of, 155
treatment of, 164
hematuria and, 162
hypotonic, urethral obstruction and, 2075–2076
neoplasia of, 2123–2128
biologic behavior and tumor types and, 2124, 2124t
diagnosis and clinical staging of, 2125–2127, *2126*
epithelial, 2124
etiology of, 2125
nonepithelial, 2124–2125
treatment of, 2127–2128
pelvic, 2133
ruptured, emergency treatment of, 2132
size of, dysuria and, 164
Blastomycosis, 341–346
clinical manifestations of, 342t, 342–343
diagnosis of, 343–344
epizootiology of, 341, *341*
etiology of, 341
hypercalcemia and, 1619
ocular manifestations of, 81–82
osteomyelitis and, 2380
pathogenesis of, 341–342
public health considerations and, 346
pulmonary manifestations of, 834
diagnosis of, 834, *835*
treatment and prognosis in, 344–346
Bleeding disorders, 105–107. *See also* Coagulopathies; Hemorrhage.
clinical approach in, 106
coagulation factor levels and, 106
coma and stupor and, 63
in canine hypothyroidism, adult-onset, 1643–1644
laboratory approach in, *106*, 106–107, 107t
paraproteinemias and, 2306
platelet levels and, 105–106
Bleeding time, platelet function and, 2276
Blepharitis, ocular manifestations of, 76
Block vertebrae, etiology and pathogenesis of, 646
Blood. *See also* Hematology; Hemoglobins; Hemostasis; Hemostatic disorders; *specific blood components.*
diseases of. *See specific diseases.*
erythropoiesis and, 2145, *2146*
in stools, diarrhea and, 34
in urine. *See also* Hematuria.
occult, renal disease and, 1903–1904
loss of, in anemia, regenerative, 91
pancreatic enzymes in, 1531
Blood chemistry, in lower urinary tract disease, 2109
in small bowel diarrhea, 1334t, 1334–1335
Blood coagulation profile, coma and stupor and, 63–64
Blood cultures, in infective endocarditis, 1155–1156
Blood flow. *See* Circulation
Blood glucose. *See* Glucose.
Blood neutrophil pools, 2193–2194, *2194*
Blood pressure. *See also* Hypertension.
central venous, in peripheral edema, 44–45
in canine hyperadrenocorticism, 1732
measurement of, *2052*, 2052–2053, *2053*, 2053t
Blood pressure *(Continued)*
normal determinants of, 2047–2048
Blood samples, collection of, 2181–2182, 2249
Blood supply, of pituitary, 1582, *1583*
to liver, 1422
Blood transfusion, 2176–2178
canine, 2177
feline, 2177–2178
in nonregenerative anemia, in chronic renal failure, 2004
Blood urea nitrogen (BUN), glomerular function and, 1896, 1897, *1897*
in hypoadrenocorticism, 1761, 1761t, 1762t
Blood values, abnormal, tables of, as guide to disease syndromes, 11t–14t
Blood volume, conservation of, gastric dilatation-volvulus-torsion syndrome and, 1279–1280
depletion of, heart failure and, 918, *918*
Blood-brain barrier, hepatic encephalopathy and, 1465
Body fluid compartments, physiology of, *429*, 429–431, *430*
Body weight. *See headings beginning with term* Weight.
Bone cysts, *2393*, 2393–2394
Bone disease. *See also* Skeletal diseases; *specific diseases.*
hypercalcemia and, 1618–1619
Bone infarct, *2394*, 2394–2395
Bone marrow. *See also* Anemia.
examination of, 2183, 2184t, 2185
anemia and, 93–94
lymphadenopathy and, 2228
reference intervals and, 2185t, 2185–2186, 2186t
necrosis of, neutropenia and, 2200
Bone marrow aspirate, polycythemia and, 103
Bone marrow pools, neutrophil production and kinetics and, 2193
Border collie, cerebellar degeneration in, 598
Bordetellosis, 265–266
Borreliosis, 271
Botulism, 274
Bowel habits, changes in, 72
Boxer, dilated cardiomyopathy in, 1104
neuropathy in, 724
Brachial plexus, avulsion or stretch of, 712t, 720–721, *721*
neuritis and, 727
Bradyarrhythmias, 1085–1095
atrial standstill and, 1088, *1088*
atrioventricular block and, 1088–1093
clinical signs of, 1092
first degree, 1088, *1089*
second degree, 1088, *1090*
third degree, 1091, *1092*
treatment of, 1092–1093, *1093*
sick sinus syndrome and, 1093, *1094*, 1095
sinoatrial arrest and, 1086–1088, *1087*
sinus bradycardia and, 1086, *1086*
Bradycardia-tachycardia syndrome, 1093, *1094*, 1095
Brain. *See also* Central nervous system; *headings beginning with terms* Cerebellar, Cerebral.
resuscitation of, 179
Brain diseases, 578t, 578–619
cerebrovascular, 599–601
congenital, 591–592
cranial trauma and, 612–613, *613*, 613t, *614*
degenerative, 592–599
developmental, 588–592
diagnosis of, 578–588, 579t
brain scans in, 584
brain stem auditory evoked responses in, 588
cavernous sinus venography and, 582, *583*
cerebral angiography and, 579–580, 582, *582*
cerebrospinal fluid and, 578
computerized axial tomography in, 584
electroencephalography in, 584–585, *585–587*
electromyography in, 588
evoked potentials in, 585, 588
impedance audiometry in, 588
nuclear magnetic resonance imaging in, 584
survey radiography and, 578–579, *579–581*
Brain diseases *(Continued)*
diagnosis of, ultrasonography in, 584
ventriculography and, 582–583, *584*
visual evoked responses in, 588
inflammatory, 601–609
metabolic, 615–619
neoplastic. *See* Tumor(s).
toxicologic, 613–615
Brain scans, 584
Brain stem auditory evoked responses (BAER), brain disease diagnosis and, 588
Brain stem dysfunction, paresis and paralysis and, 59
Breathing, cardiopulmonary resuscitation and, 174
Breed(s). *See also specific breeds.*
adverse drug reactions and, 500
alopecia and, 114
anemia and, 92
chondrodystrophic, ununited anconeal process in, *2350*, *2354*, 2354–2355
cyanosis and, 97
pain and, 20
pruritus and, 122
Breeding season, 1779. *See also* Estrous cycle.
Bromocriptine, in canine hyperadrenocorticism, 1753
Bronchi, diagnostic approach to, 751–752
distribution of, radiographic interpretation and, 758
Bronchial compression, 829
Bronchial disease, cough suppression and, 821
foreign bodies and, 828–829
parasitic, 829
Bronchial mineralization, 829
Bronchiectasis, 827–828
diagnosis of, 828, *828*
Bronchitis, allergic, canine, 825
allergic, feline, 822–825
diagnosis of, 823, *823*, *824*
presentation of, 822–823
prognosis in, 825
treatment of, 823–825
chronic, 825–827
presentation of, 826, *826*
prognosis in, 827
treatment of, 826–827
Bronchodilation, in heart failure therapy, 967
in pulmonary edema, 861
lower respiratory disease and, 820
Bronchoesophageal fistulas, 829
Bronchoscopy, 761–764
bronchoscopes and, 761
examination by, 760t, *762*, 762–763, *763*
indications for, 761–762
specimens for, 763
transbrachial biopsy and, *763*, 763–764, *764*
Brucellosis, canine, 270–271
in humans, 191–192
prevention of, 191–192
infertility and, in bitch, 1842–1843
Brucellosis canis, cutaneous manifestations of, 7
Bruisability, in canine hyperadrenocorticism, 1730
BSP retention test, in canine hyperadrenocorticism, 1732
Buffer systems, in extracellular fluid, acid-base and, 440–441
Buffy coat smears, 2185
quantitative, *2182*, 2183
Bull mastiff, cerebellar degeneration in, 598
Bulla, 118
Bullous diseases, pulmonary, 845
Bullous pemphigoid, oral lesions and, 1229
Bumetanide, in heart failure therapy, 956
Bumps. *See* Tumor(s).
BUN. *See* Blood urea nitrogen.
Burn(s), of oral cavity, 1231
poisoning and, 467
Burst therapy, with corticosteroids, 422
Butterfly vertebrae, etiology and pathogenesis of, 646

Cachexia, as paraneoplastic syndrome, 519
cardiac, dietary management and, 965–966

Calcification, ectopic, in canine hyperadrenocorticism, 1730, *1731*
meniscal, 2344–2345
Calcinosis, periarticular, multicentric, 2360–2361
Calcium. *See also* Hypercalcemia; Hypocalcemia.
abnormal values of, causes of, 13t
in hypoadrenocorticism, electrolyte imbalance and, 1768
serum levels of, in hypoadrenocorticism, 1761t, 1762
Calcium antagonists, in heart failure therapy, 964–965
Calcium chloride, cardiopulmonary response to, 176
Calcium gluconate, in hyperkalemia, in acute renal failure, 1977
Calcium oxalate urolithiasis. *See* Urolithiasis.
Calcium phosphate deposition disease, in Great Dane, 640
Calcium phosphate urolithiasis. *See* Urolithiasis.
Calcium supplementation, in chronic renal failure, divalent ion imbalances in, 2001–2002
oral, in hypocalcemia, 1628–1629, 1629t
parenteral, in hypocalcemia, 1626t, 1628
Calcivirus, feline, 319–320
acute, 319–320
carrier state of, 320
pulmonary manifestations of, 830
Calories, recommended intake of, in chronic renal failure, 1994
Campylobacter infections, 268
in humans, 192
of large intestine, 1413–1414
small bowel diarrhea and, *1356*, 1356–1357
Cancer. *See also* Tumor(s).
abdominal carcinomatosis and, 136–137
biologic therapy and, 536t, 536–540
bacterial products and, 537–538
chemical immunomodulators and, 538–539
cytokines and, 539
future perspectives for, 540
lymphokines and, 539
monoclonal antibodies and, 539–540
serum factors and, 540
tumor cell vaccines and, 539
tumor immunology and, 537
cellular biology of, 515–516
cell cycle and, 516, *516*
cell surface and cytoplasmic alterations and, 515, 515t
differentiation and de-differentiation and, 515
chemotherapy and, 530–536
biologic basis for, 530
corticosteroids and, 419
drugs used in, 532–533, 534t–536t, 535–536
guidelines for, 532
insulin-secreting tumors and, 1715
pharmacologic factors and, 530–532
thyroid tumors and, in dog, 1669–1670
diagnosis of, 527–529
diagnostic tests in, 527–529
history in, 527
physical examination in, 527
gastric, 1317–1318, *1318*
hypercalcemia and, 1610–1615
hyperthermia and, 542–543
biologic considerations and, 542–543
metastasis and, 516–517
multimodality therapy and, 543–544
of chest wall, metastatic, 871
primary, 871, *871*
radiation therapy and, 540–541
biologic considerations and, 540–541
practical considerations and, 541, 542t
surgical treatment of, 529–530
weight loss and, 4
Candida, urinary tract infection and, 2123
Canine. *See under specific disorder*; e.g., Parvovirus, canine.
Capillaria aerophila, 836–837
Capillaria feliscati, 2114
Capillaria plica, 2113
Captopril, actions of, 961–962
in heart failure therapy, 961–962
Captopril *(Continued)*
indications for, 962
toxicity and interactions of, 962
Capture beat, 1080
Carbapenems, 393–394
activity spectrum of, 393–394
clinical pharmacology of, 394
Carbohydrate(s), digestion and absorption of, 1326
metabolism of, corticosteroids and, 416
in liver disease, 1431
Carbon dioxide, respiratory control of, acid-base and, 441
Carcinoma(s). *See also specific carcinomas*.
cholangiocellular, 1512–1513
hepatocellular, 1511–1512, *1512*
of adrenal gland, pathology of, 1725
scirrhous, 894–895
thyroid, 893–894
transitional cell, of lower urinary tract, 2128, 2129t
prostatic, *1876*, 1877
Carcinomatosis, abdominal, 136–137
differential diagnosis of, 136–137
history and physical examination in, 136
laboratory examination in, 136
radiographic examination in, 136
Cardiac arrhythmias, 1051–1095
antiarrhythmic agents and, classification of, 1059
electrophysiologic classification of, 1060t, 1060–1065
in gastric dilatation-volvulus-torsion syndrome, 1286–1287
increasing automaticity and, 1059
removing or suppressing precipitating factors of, 1059
bradyarrhythmias and, 1085–1095
atrial standstill and, 1087–1088, *1088*
atrioventricular block and, 1088–1093, *1089–1091*, *1093*
sick sinus syndrome and, 1093, *1094*, 1095
sinus, 1085, *1086*
cardiopulmonary arrest and, 172–173
clinical signs of, 1058
drugs used in, 1052t–1053t
echocardiography and, 1058, 1059t
electrocardiogram and, 1054, *1055*, 1055t
electrocardiography and, 1058
hemodynamic consequences of, 1057
history and, 1057–1058
laboratory studies in, 1058
mechanisms of, 1056–1057, *1057*
normal electrophysiology and, 1051, 1053–1054, *1054*
normal heart muscle and, 1054–1056
automaticity and, 1055
conductivity and, *1054*, 1056
contractility and, 1056
excitability and, *1055*, 1055–1056
premature ectopic beats and, *1065*, 1065–1070
classification of, 1069–1070
supraventricular, *1066*, 1067
ventricular premature contractions and, *1065*, 1067–1070, *1068*, *1069*
recognition of, 1057
tachycardias and, *1070–1073*, 1070–1085
accelerated conduction in, 1073–1074, *1074*, *1075*
atrial fibrillation and, 1074–1075, *1076–1078*, 1077–1079
atrial flutter and, 1079, *1080*
supraventricular, *1070–1073*, 1070–1079
ventricular fibrillation and, 1084–1085, *1085*
ventricular, atrioventricular dissociation and, 1079–1084, *1081–1083*
treatment of, 1058–1059
Cardiac cachexia, dietary management and, 965–966
Cardiac catheterization, in chordae tendinae rupture, 1046
in congenital heart disease, 982, *983*, 984, *984*
in cyanotic heart disease, 1018
Cardiac conduction, *1054*, 1056
cardiac arrhythmias and, 1056
Cardiac contractility, 1056
cardiac output and, 905–907, *906*
heart failure therapy and, 940–941
Cardiac disease. *See* Cardiac valvular disease; Cardiomyopathy; Heart disease; Heart failure; Heart murmur; *specific diseases*.
Cardiac dysrhythmias, in gastric dilatation-volvulus-torsion syndrome, 1285–1286
Cardiac evaluation, 923–936
evolution of, 923
of left heart, 923–932
alternate methods for, 932
cardiac output measurement and, 926–927, 927t
left ventricular contractile indices and, 929t, 929–932, *930–932*
left ventricular pressures and, 928–929
pulmonary venous pressure and, 927–928
size and morphology and, 923–926, *924*, 924t, *925*
of right heart, 933–935
invasive hemodynamic evaluation and, 935
right atrial pressure and, *933*, 933–934, *934*
right ventricular performance and, 934–935
size and morphology and, 933
Cardiac gland region, of stomach, 1290
Cardiac imaging, in congenital heart disease, 977–980
Cardiac output, detriments of, 900–907, 901t, *902*
afterload and, 905, *906*
contractility and, 905–907, *906*
heart rate and, 901, *902*
preload and, 901–902, *903*, 904, *904*
gastric dilatation-volvulus-torsion syndrome and, 1250
measurement of, 926–927, 927t
Cardiac tamponade, pericardial effusion with, 1133, *1134*
Cardiac valve(s), malformation of, 1000–1014
aortic regurgitation and, 1011
aortic stenosis and, 1004, 1007–1011
atrioventricular valve dysplasia and, 1011–1014
in infective endocarditis, 1152–1153
pulmonic insufficiency and, 1004, *1006*
pulmonic stenosis and, 1000–1004, *1019*
microorganism interaction with, in infective endocarditis, 1153
normal, in infective endocarditis, 1153
replacement of, in infective endocarditis, 1160
Cardiac valvular disease, 1031–1049
aortic valve and, 1048–1049
fibrotic, etiology of, 1044
mitral complex and, 1031–1047
chordae tendinae rupture and, 1045–1047
chronic mitral valvular insufficiency and, 1031–1044
endocardial splitting and left atrial rupture and, 1044–1045
mitral stenosis and, 1049
pulmonic insufficiency and, 1049
tricuspid insufficiency and, 1047–1048
Cardiomyopathy, 1097–1125, 1098t
bacterial myocarditis and, 1125
congestive. *See* Cardiomyopathy, dilated.
diagnostic strategies for, 1097, 1098t, 1099t
diastolic dysfunction and, 1110–1114
treatment of, 1114–1116
dilated, 1098–1100
canine, clinical manifestations of, *1102*, 1102–1104, *1103*
in boxer, 1104
in Doberman pinscher, 1104
in English cocker spaniel, 1104
treatment of, 1107–1110
etiology of, 1098–1099
feline, clinical manifestations of, 1098t, 1099t, 1100, *1100*, *1101*, 1102
treatment of, 1105–1107
pathology of, *1099*, 1099–1100
physiology of, 1099
drugs used in, 1131t
excessive left ventricular moderator bands and, in cats, 1116–1117, *1117*
hypertrophic, 1110–1113

Cardiomyopathy *(Continued)*
hypertrophic, abnormal physiology in, 1110
canine, clinical manifestations of, 1111–1113
etiology of, 1110
feline, clinical manifestations of, 1111, *1112*, *1113*
pathology of, 1110–1111
treatment of, 1115–1116
incidence of, 1097
inflammation and, 1123–1124
intermediate, 1116
treatment of, 1117
ischemia and, 1123
neoplastic, 1123
primary, 1097–1104
systolic dysfunction and, 1097–1098
protozoal myocarditis and, 1124–1125
restrictive, 1113–1114, *1115*
treatment of, 1116
secondary, 1121–1123
systolic dysfunction and, 1097–1098
treatment of, 1105–1110
thromboembolic disease associated with, 1117–1121
clinical manifestations of, 1118
diagnosis of, 1118–1119, *1119*, *1120*
pathophysiology of, 1118
prognosis in, 1121
treatment of, 1119, 1121
viral myocarditis and, 1124, *1124*
Cardiopulmonary arrest, 171–173
clinical signs of, 171–173
electrocardiography and, *172*, 172–173, *173*
risk for, 171
Cardiopulmonary resuscitation (CPR), 172, 173–180
ABCs of, 173, 174
advanced life support and, 175
basic life support and, 173–174
blood flow during, 174–175
brain resuscitation and, 179
closed chest, 175
diagnosis and defibrillation step in, 175–176
emergency drugs and, 176–177
fibrillation treatment and, 178–179
intensive care and, 179
open chest, 175
patient response to, gauging, 179
prolonged life support and, 179
Cardiopulmonary system, uremia and, 1920
Cardiovascular disease, polycythemia and, 102
protozoal, 287–292
Cardiovascular system, allergic drug reactions and, 504–505
corticosteroids and, 416
gastric dilatation-volvulus-torsion syndrome and, 1279
in canine hypothyroidism, adult-onset, 1642t, 1643
in feline hyperthyroidism, 1657t, 1657–1658
weakness and, 47
Caries, dental, 1210–1211, *1211*
Carnassial abscess, 1211–1212, *1214*
Carpal joint, luxations and subluxations of, 2339
Carriers, 2283
Cartilage, damage to, 2337, *2337*
enchondral cores and, retained, 2395–2396, *2396*
exostoses of, multiple, 676, 2383–2384, *2384*
Castration, penile anatomy and physiology and, 1882–1883
Casts, dysuria and, 164
in urinary sediment, 1905–1907, *1906*, *1908*
urinary, 2031–2032
Cat. *See under disease or disorder*; e.g., Peritonitis, infectious, feline.
Cat scratch disease, in humans, 192
prevention of, 192
Cataracts, diabetes mellitus and, 1704–1705
Catecholamines, in heart failure therapy, 948
Catheters. *See also* Cardiac catheterization.
central venous, pleural effusion caused by, 883
urethral obstruction and, 2075
urinary tract infection and, 2116–2117
Caudal cervical instabilities, 2343–2344, *2344*
Caudal vena cava, gastric dilatation-volvulus-torsion syndrome and, 1279
Caustic poisoning, 467t, 481
Cavernous sinus venography, 582, *583*
CBC. *See* Complete blood count.
Cell(s), in urinary sediment, renal disease and, 1904t, 1904–1905, 1905t
Cell cycle, cancer and, 516, *516*
Cell wall synthesis, inhibitors of, 386–394. *See also specific drugs.*
Cell-mediated immunity, 2284
uremia and, 1918–1919
Central nervous system. *See also* Brain; Spinal cord; Spinal cord diseases; *headings beginning with terms* Cerebellar, Cerebral.
degenerations of, behavioral signs of, 74
in canine hyperadrenocorticism, 1736
o,p′-DDD therapy and, 1751–1752
pesticides affecting, intoxication by, 459–460, 460t, 464–466, 465t
reticulosis of, behavioral signs of, 73
Central venous catheters, pleural effusion caused by, 883
Central venous pressure, in peripheral edema, 44–45
Cephalic phase, of gastric secretion, 1291
Cephalosporins, 391–393
activity spectrum of, 393, 394t
clinical pharmacology of, 393
first-generation, for oral use, 392
activity spectrum of, 392
clinical pharmacology of, 392
first-generation, for parenteral use, 391–392
activity spectrum of, 391, 392t
clinical pharmacology of, 391–392
hematopoietic stem cell death and, 2199
second-generation, 392–393
activity spectrum of, 392–393
clinical pharmacology of, 393
third-generation, 393
Cerebellar ataxia, 58
Cerebellar degeneration, 591–592, 597–598
in border collie, 598
in bull mastiff, 598
in Gordon setter, 597–598
in Kerry blue terrier, 597
in rough coated collie, 598
Cerebellar malformation, 591, *592*
Cerebellar tremor, 56
Cerebral anoxia, 599–600
Cerebral arteriography, 579–580, 582, *582*
Cerebral dysfunction, paresis and paralysis and, 59
Cerebral hypoxia, 599–600
behavioral signs of, 73
Cerebral sensitivity, hepatic encephalopathy and, 1465
Cerebrospinal edema, reduction of, corticosteroids and, 419–420, 420t
Cerebrospinal fluid (CSF), analysis of, spinal cord disease and, 627
spinal cord tumors and, 679
collection of, 575–576
coma and stupor and, 64
evaluation of, 576–577
brain disease and, 578
Cerebrovascular accidents, metabolic, 62
Cerebrovascular diseases, of brain, 599–601
Ceroid lipofuscinosis, 594
Ceruminolytic agents, otitis externa and, 255
Ceruminous otitis, 257
Cervical spondylomyelopathy. *See* Spondylomyelopathy, cervical.
Cervix, tumors of, 1819
Cestodes, intestinal, cutaneous manifestations of, 8
Chagas' disease. *See* Trypanosomiasis.
Chédiak-Higashi syndrome, 2271
cutaneous manifestations of, 5
ocular manifestations of, 77
Cheilitis, 1232, *1233*
Chemical(s), anemia and, 92
myocardial disease and, 1122–1123
toxic polyneuropathies and, 726t, 726–727
Chemical burns, of oral cavity, 1231
Chemical defense, of lower urinary tract, 2115, 2116
Chemical defibrillation, 179
Chemistry profile, in feline hyperadrenocorticism, 1755
in glomerular disease, 1944
Chemodectoma, 894
Chemoreceptor trigger zone (CTZ), vomiting and, 27–28
Chemotherapy. *See also* Drug(s).
aplastic anemia and, 2174
cancer and. *See* Cancer, chemotherapy and.
hematopoietic stem cell death and, 2198
Chest wall, blunt trauma and, 869–870, *870*
masses and infiltrative disorders of, 870–872
infectious, 871–872
metastatic, 871
primary tumors and, 871, *871*
treatment of, 871
thoracic wall deformity and, 870
Chewing, self-mutilation and, 71
Chimeric antibodies, 2289
Chlamydial diseases, 276–281
ocular manifestations of, 82–83
Chlamydiosis, feline. *See* Pneumonitis, feline.
Chloramphenicol, 399–400
action of, 400
activity spectrum of, 399–400
clinical pharmacology of, 400
toxicity of, 400
anemia and, 2176
hematopoietic stem cell death and, in cats, 2198
Chloride, abnormal values of, causes of, 13t
Chocolate intoxication, 460t, 481
Cholangiocellular carcinoma, 1513
Cholangitis-cholangiohepatitis syndrome, in cats, 1480–1483
biliary cirrhosis and, 1482–1483
lymphocytic, chronic, 1482
suppurative, 1480–1482
Cholecystitis, 1557
Cholelithiasis, *1556*, 1556–1557
Cholephilic dyes, organic ion, in liver disease, 1448–1449, 1449t
Cholestasis, jaundice versus, 108
Cholesterol, 203
abnormal values of, causes of, 13t
diagnostic tests for, 199
hypercholesterolemia and, 203. *See also* Hyperlipidemia.
causes of, 13t
in canine hyperadrenocorticism, 1731–1732
Chondrodysplasia puncta, 2383
Chondrodystrophic breeds, ununited anconeal process in, *2350*, *2354*, 2354–2355
Chondrodystrophy, 2346
zinc-responsive, 2387
Chondromas, in dog, 2389
Chondrosarcoma, in dog, 2389, *2389*
Chordae tendinae, rupture of, 1045–1047
cardiac catheterization in, 1046
cardiovascular examination in, 1046
differential diagnosis of, 1047
treatment of, 1042t, 1047
Chow chow, myotonia of, 738
Chromogenic substrates, in coagulation assays, 2252
Chromophobe adenoma, endocrinologically inactive, in pars distalis, 1591, *1591*
Chromosomal abnormalities, congenital defects and, 184–185
Chronic mitral valvular insufficiency. *See* Mitral valve insufficiency, chronic.
Chronic obstructive pulmonary disease (COPD), 847
polycythemia and, 102
therapeutic principles for, 103
CHV. *See* Herpesvirus, canine.
Chylomicron(s), 203
hyperchylomicronemia and, idiopathic, canine hyperlipidemia and, 207
inherited, in cat, *200*, 200t, 200–202, *201*
polyneuropathy with, 725
Chylomicron test, 199, 206

Chylothorax, 884, 884t
Chyme, 1289
Cigarette poisoning, 459t, 460t, 481
Ciliary dyskinesia, primary, 827
Circling, 72
in neurologic examination, 557, *557*
Circulation, cardiopulmonary resuscitation and, 174–175
enterohepatic, 1425
gastric mucosal injury and, 1300–1301
Circulatory failure, 899
Cirrhosis, 1497–1499
biliary, in cats, 1482–1483
Citrates, in canine calcium oxalate urolithiasis, 2102
Cleaning agents, otitis externa and, 255
Clearance, of drugs, 380
Clearance ratios, tubular function and, 1900
Cleft palate, 771, *773*, 1231, *1232*
Client relations, behavioral signs and, 72–73
emergency medicine and, 209–210
Clitoral hypertrophy, in canine hyperadrenocorticism, 1729–1730
Clone(s), forbidden, 2297
immune response and, recognition in, 2284
Clostridia, small bowel diarrhea and, 1357–1358
Clostridium botulinum, toxic polyneuropathy and, 727
Clot retraction, platelet function and, 2276
Coagulation factors, bleeding disorders and, 106
laboratory studies and, *106*, 107, 107t
Coagulation system. *See also* Platelet(s).
in canine hypothyroidism, adult-onset, 1643–1644
platelets and, 2267
Coagulation tests, 2250–2252
Coagulopathies, 2252–2261
hemorrhage and, 2161
hereditary, 2258–2261
clinical signs of, 2259–2260
laboratory aspects of, 2259t, 2260
pathophysiology of, 2258–2259, 2259t
therapy of, 2260–2261
liver disease and, 2256–2258
clinical aspects of, 2257
laboratory aspects of, *2255*, 2257–2258
pathophysiology of, 2256–2257
treatment of, 2258
ocular manifestations of, 79–80
vitamin K deficiency and, antagonism and, 2252–2254
clinical signs of, 2253–2254
pathophysiology of, 2252–2253
therapy of, 2254
Coat, color of, alopecia and, 114
in canine hypothyroidism, adult-onset, 1642t, 1642–1643
Cobalt irradiation, in feline hyperadrenocorticism, 1756
Coccidial diseases, 281–285
small bowel diarrhea and, 1348–1349
Coccidioidomycosis, 346–351
clinical manifestations of, 347
diagnosis of, 347–349, *348–350*
etiology and epizootiology of, *341*, 346–347
ocular manifestations of, 82
pathogenesis of, 347
prognosis in, 350–351
public health significance of, 351
pulmonary manifestations of, 834
systemic, osteomyelitis and, 2379–2380, *2380*
treatment of, 349–350
Cocker spaniel, English, dilated cardiomyopathy in, 1104
Coenurosis, cerebral, 607
Colchicine, in liver disease, 1517
Cold. *See also* Hypothermia.
acupuncture and, 493
Cold agglutinin disease, 2166
cutaneous manifestations of, 9
Colibacillosis, 267–268
Colitis, definition of, 36
eosinophilic, 1409–1410
Histoplasma, 1412
protothecal, 1413
pseudomembranous, 1415
Colitis *(Continued)*
ulcerative, histiocytic, 1410
Collie, border, cerebellar degeneration in, 598
rough coated, cerebellar degeneration in, 598
Collie sheep dog, neuroaxonal dystrophy in, 599
Colon. *See also* Intestine(s), large.
ascending, 1397
Colonoscopy, flexible, 1402
large intestine and, chronic inflammatory bowel disease and, *1401*, 1406
Coma, ancillary diagnostics in, 63–64
blood tests in, 63
definition of, 61
hepatic, treatment of, 1517–1520, 1518t
history in, 62–63
myxedema, in canine hypothyroidism, 1644
neurologic examination in, 63
physical examination and, 63
rule-outs for, 61–62
toxicity and, 614–615
treatment of, 64–65
emergency, *64*, 64–65
maintenance, 65
urinalysis in, 63
Coma scale, 64, 64t
Combination theory, acupuncture and, 488, *490*
Comedo, 119
Complement cascade, B lymphocytes and, 2286
Complete blood count (CBC), anemia and, 93
in canine hyperadrenocorticism, 1730
in canine hypothyroidism, 1642t, 1644
in feline hyperadrenocorticism, 1755
in feline hyperthyroidism, 1658
large intestinal disease and, 1400
polycythemia and, 103
Compound 1080/1081 intoxication, 465–466
Computed tomography (CT), 584
in hyperadrenocorticism, 1743, *1744*
Conductivity, of heart muscle, *1054*, 1056
cardiac arrhythmias and, 1056
Conformation, lameness and, in dogs, 166
Confrontational abnormalities, 2346
Congenital abnormalities, 183–186, 591–592
cytoplasmic inclusions in, 2191–2192, *2192*
exocrine pancreatic insufficiency and, 1539
causes of, 184–186
coma and stupor and, 62
esophageal, 1261
frequency of, 183
infertility and, in bitch, 1050–1051
lameness and, in cats, 169
nature and effect of, 183–184
of bladder, 2113
of foramen magnum, 592
of heart. *See* Cardiac valve(s), malformation of; Heart disease, congenital.
of lips, 1231, *1232*
of nervous system, 554
of odontoid process, 634–637, *635*, *636*
of pinnae, 247
of teeth, 1209–1210
of tongue, 1233
pericardial, 1135
pulmonary, 846
uterine, 1801
vaginal, 1807–1809, *1808*
vertebral, 645–647
clinical findings in, 646
diagnosis of, 646–647, *647*
etiology and pathogenesis of, 645–646
treatment of, 647
Congestive cardiomyopathy. *See* Cardiomyopathy, dilated.
Congestive heart failure, 900
in canine hyperadrenocorticism, 1735
liver disease and, 1484
pleural effusion due to, 877
Congestive splenomegaly, pathogenesis of, 2238t, 2239–2240
Conjunctivitis, 274–275
Consciousness, 61–65. *See also* Coma; Stupor.
functional states of brain and, 61
normal, 61
wakefulness and, maintenance of, 61
Constipation, definition of, 36
diagnostic procedures in, 38
historical findings in, 36
outcome in, 39–40
pathophysiology of, 36, 37t, *38*, *39*
physical examination and, 37–38
treatment goals in, 38–39, *40*
Contact dermatitis, allergic, 2316–2317
Contractility, of heart muscle, 1056
cardiac output and, 905–907, *906*
heart failure therapy and, 940–941
Contusions, of penis, 1885–1886
pulmonary, 840–841
Coombs' test, direct, in immune-mediated hemolytic anemia, 2302
COPD. *See* Chronic obstructive pulmonary disease.
Copper toxicity, hemolytic disease and, 2171
Cor pulmonale, 847–848
Corgi, Pembroke Welsh, telangiectasia of, 2030
Corneal reflex, testing for, 564
Coronavirus, canine, diarrhea and, 1353
gastroenteritis and, 308–309
clinical signs of, 308–309
diagnosis of, 309
epizootiology of, 308
etiology of, 308
treatment and prevention of, 304t, 309
feline, 330–338. *See also* Peritonitis, infectious, feline.
enteric, 331, 1354
viruses and, 330–331, 331t
Coronavirus-like particles, 331
Coronoid process, hypoplasia of, 2355, *2356*
medial, fragmented, *2351*, 2351–2354, *2352*
Corticosteroids, 413–426, 428t
administration frequency and duration and, 421–422
alternate-day therapy and, 422
burst therapy and, 422
daily oral therapy and, 422
administration method and, 420–421
local, 420–421
systemic, 421
adverse effects of, 424–426
iatrogenic hyperadrenocorticism-like disease as, 423t, *423–425*, 425–426
iatrogenic secondary hypoadrenocorticism as, *423*, 424–425
management of, 426
anti-inflammation and, 419
antineoplastic chemotherapy and, 419
cerebrospinal edema and, 419–420, 420t
reduction of, 419–420, 420t
endogenous deficiency of, treatment of, 419
eosinopenia associated with, 2210–2211
excess of, hyperlipidemia and, canine, 207
immunosuppression and, 419
in chronic inflammatory bowel disease, 1408
in glomerulonephritis, 2017–2018
lymphopenia associated with, 2208–2209
meningitis responsive to. *See* Meningitis, corticosteroid-responsive.
natural, 413t, 413–414, *414*
action of, duration of, 415, 416t
relative potency of, *414*, 414t, 414–415, *415*
neutrophilia associated with, 2195, *2195*
physiologic and pharmacologic effects of, 415–418
carbohydrate metabolism and, 416
cardiovascular system and, 416
detoxification and, 417
electrolytes and, 416
endocrine system and, 417–418, *418*
fat metabolism and, 416
fetal development and, 418
gastrointestinal tract and, 416
hematolymphatic system and, 417
immunity and, 417
lactation and, 417
liver and, 416
musculoskeletal system and, 417
nervous system and, 417
pregnancy and, 417
protein metabolism and, 416

Corticosteroids *(Continued)*
physiologic and pharmacologic effects of, trace minerals and, 416
water distribution and, 416
precautions with, 422–424
synthetic, action of, duration of, 415, 416t
relative potency of, *414*, 414t, 414–415, *415*
urinary, in hyperadrenocorticism, 1736
Corticotropic adenoma, functional, of adenohypophysis, hypercortisolism and, 1591–1592, *1592*
Corticotropin-releasing hormone (CRH), glucocorticoid secretion and, 1721
Corticotropin-releasing hormone (CRH) stimulation test, in hyperadrenocorticism, 1743
Cortisol, adenohypophysis and, 1591–1592, *1592*
hypercortisolism and, functional corticotropic adenoma, 1591–1592, *1592*
in hyperadrenocorticism, 1736–1737
in hypoadrenocorticism, 1766
Cough(ing), 85–87, 86t. *See also* Tracheobronchitis, infectious.
cyanosis and, 97, 98
definition of, 85
diagnostic approach to, 85–87
polycythemia and, 102
regurgitation and, 31
suppression of, in heart failure therapy, 967
lower respiratory disease and, 820–829
expectorants and, 821
medication nebulization and, 821
treatment goals and, 86t, 87, 87t
Counterconditioning, for fears and phobias, 228
CPR. *See* Cardiopulmonary resuscitation.
Cranial muscles, symmetry of, testing for, 564
Cranial nerve(s), examination of, 559–561
peripheral, focal diseases of, 715–719
Cranial nerve function testing, 561–566
cranial muscle symmetry and, 564
facial reflexes and, 564, *565*
gag reflex and, 564, 566
menace response and, *560*, 561, *561*
ocular motility and, 563–564
ocular position and, 563, *563*
oral cavity and, 564, 566, 566t
pathologic nystagmus and, 564
pupil size and, 563
pupillary light reflex and, 561, *562*, 563
pupillary symmetry and, 563
Cranial polyneuropathy, 727–728
Craniomandibular osteopathy, 2393, *2393*
Craniopharyngioma, 1592, *1592*, *1593*
Creatinine, abnormal values of, causes of, 14t
clearance of, 1896t, 1897–1898
serum levels of, glomerular function and, 1896–1897, *1897*
Creatinine kinase, abnormal values of, causes of, 13t
Crenation, 2150, 2153
Crensoma vulpis, 838
CRH. *See* Corticotropin-releasing hormone.
Cricopharyngeal achalasia, 787
Cromolyn sodium, in chronic inflammatory bowel disease, 1409
Cross linking antigen, 2287
Crossed extensor reflex, testing for, 573, *573*, 574t
Crust, 119
Crying, pain and, 20
Cryptococcosis, canine, clinical manifestations of, 355
feline, clinical manifestations of, 354–355, *355*
ocular manifestations of, 81
osteomyelitis and, 2380
pulmonary manifestations of, 834–835
Cryptosporidiosis, in humans, 190
Cryptosporidium, 283
small bowel diarrhea and, 1349
Crystal(s), dysuria and, 164
in urinary sediment, 1907, *1907*
Crystalluria, canine urolithiasis and, 2086
CSF. *See* Cerebrospinal fluid.
CT. *See* Computed tomography.
CTZ. *See* Chemoreceptor trigger zone.
Culture, of uroliths, 2087
Cupping, acupuncture and, 492
Curettage, periodontal disease and, 1225
Cushing's syndrome. *See* Hyperadrenocorticism.
Cutaneous larval migrans, in humans, 189
prevention of, 189
Cutaneous lupus erythematosus, 2312–2313
diagnosis of, 2313
pathology of, 2312–2313, *1213*
prognosis of, 2313
treatment of, 2313
Cutaneous manifestations. *See also* Dermatologic disease; Skin.
allergic drug reactions and, 504
of food hypersensitivity, 194–196
diagnosis of, 195–196
historical findings in, 195
long-term nutritional management of, 196
pathogenesis of, 194–195
Cutaneous reflex, testing for, 569, 573
Cuterebriasis, brain and, 607
Cyanosis, 95–100
cardiopulmonary arrest and, 172
central, 95–96
definition of, 95
diagnostic plan for, 98–99
historical findings in, 97
in heart disease. *See* Heart disease, congenital and cyanotic.
pathophysiology of, 95t, 95–97
central cyanosis and, 95–96
peripheral cyanosis and, 96–97
peripheral, 95, 96–97, 100
physical findings in, 97–98
polycythemia and, 103
treatment goals in, 99t, 99–100
Cyclic neutropenia, 5
Cyclooxygenase deficiency, 2271
Cyclophosphamides, cyclic neutropenia induced by, 2201
cystitis and, 2123
Cyproheptadine, in canine hyperadrenocorticism, 1753
Cyst(s), 117
arachnoid, spinal, 686–687, *688*
epidermoid, 682–683
hepatic, congenital, 1510
mediastinal, 894
of bone, *2393*, 2393–2394
ovarian, persistent estrus and, *1792*, 1792–1795, 1793t
paraprostatic, 1869, *1869*
pathophysiology of, 127
pilonidal, 682–683
pulmonary, 845
pneumothorax and, 885, *886*
renal, 2024–2025
Cystic endometrial hyperplasia (CEH), 1798–1801, 1799t
Cystic mucinous hypertrophy, 1557
Cystine urolithiasis. *See* Urolithiasis.
Cystinuria, 2027
canine, in cystine urolithiasis, 2097–2098
Cystitis, 275–276
cyclophosphamide and, 2123
emphysematous, 2122
proliferative, *2122*, 2122–2123
Cystocentesis, urethral obstruction and, 2073–2074
Cystometry, in lower urinary tract disease, 2113
Cytauxzoonosis, 288–289, 2167–2168
Cytoisospora, 282
Cytokines, 2291
in cancer therapy, 539
Cytology, in lower urinary tract disease, 2110
Cytoprotective agents, gastric ulceration and, 1310
Cytotoxic agents, canine mammary gland tumors and, 1823
in chronic inflammatory bowel disease, 1409
Cytotoxic cells, 2284

Dachshund, sensory neuropathy of, 724
Dalmatian, leukodystrophy in, 596
urolithiasis in, uric acid and ammonium urate, 2093–2094
Dancing Doberman disease, 74, 724–725, *725*
Darkroom procedure, radiography and, 753
Deafness, inner ear disease and, 260
Deciduous teeth, retained, 1209, *1209*
Decompression, in gastric dilatation-volvulus-torsion syndrome, 1284
Decorticate behavior, coma and stupor and, 63
Defecation behavior problems, in cats, 236
in dogs, 231, 232
Defibrillation, cardiopulmonary resuscitation and, 175–176
chemical, 179
Deficiency syndromes, anemia and, 92
oral lesions and, 1228
Deforming arthritis, 2366–2367
Degenerative joint disease, lameness and, in cats, 169
Dehydration, diarrhea and, 34
Delirium, definition of, 61
Dementia, behavioral signs and, 70
Demodicosis, cutaneous manifestations of, 7
Demyelinating myelopathy, of miniature poodles, 596
Dental disease, rhinitis due to, 776
Dental structures, 1203–1207, *1204*, *1205*
Dentistry, restorative, 1214–1215
Depression, definition of, 61
toxicity and, 614–615
Dermatitis, actinic, of pinna, 249
contact, allergic, 2316–2317
fly strike, of pinna, 249
herpetiform, canine, 2318
of lip folds, chronic, 1232, *1233*
Dermatologic disease. *See also* Cutaneous manifestations; Skin; *specific diseases*.
allergic, ocular manifestations of, 75–76
immune-related, 2314–2324
ocular manifestations of, 75–76
in developing countries, 220t, 223–224
infectious, antimicrobial selection for, 407, 407t
ocular manifestations of, 76–77
Dermatomycosis, in humans, 192
Dermatomyositis, 5, 740–741
canine, 2317–2318
of pinnae, 251
Dermatophytosis, of pinna, 249
Dermatosis, auricular, marginal, 247, 249
vitamin A–responsive, 8
zinc-responsive, 8
of pinnae, 251
Dermoid sinus, 682–683
Desoxycorticosterone (DOCA), in hypoadrenocorticism, electrolyte imbalance and, 1768
Destructive behavior, in cats, 237
Detoxification, corticosteroids and, 417
Detrusor muscle, bladder atony and, 155–156
treatment of, 164
Developing countries, 217–225
diagnostic aids in, 224
drugs in, 224
infectious diseases in, *221*, 221–223, *222*
medical, dermatologic, and surgical disorders in, 220t, 223–224
neoplasia in, *223*, 224
nutritional disorders in, 218
parasitic infestations in, 218–219, *219*, *220*, 220t
pet-owner relationships in, 218
preventive medicine in, 224
socioeconomic factors in, 217–218
veterinary education in, 224–225
Development, fetal, corticosteroids and, 418
sexual, disorders of, infertility and, in bitch, 1848–1849
Developmental disorders, 588–592. *See also* Congenital abnormalities.
lameness and, in cats, 169
Dexamethasone screening test, in hyperadrenocorticism, 1738–1740
feline, 1756
in normal dogs, *1739*, 1739–1740, *1740*
misleading results of, *1738*, 1740
protocol for, 1739, *1740*
theory and, 1738–1739, *1739*

Dexamethasone suppression test, adrenocorticotropic hormone stimulation test and, in hyperadrenocorticism, 1741
in hyperadrenocorticism, *1742*, 1742–1743, *1743*
Dextrans, thrombocytopathies induced by, 2274–2275
Diabetes insipidus, central, polyuria and polydipsia and, 142–143
nephrogenic, 2028
polyuria and polydipsia and, 143
pituitary, 1605–1606, *1606*
treatment of, 1606
Diabetes mellitus, 1676–1707
anamnesis and, 1682
bicarbonate therapy in, 1691
biochemical panel in, 1685t, 1685–1686
complications of, 1704–1706
cutaneous manifestations of, 7
diagnosis of, 1683–1684, *1684*
dietary therapy in, in nonketotic diabetes, 1693–1696, *1694–1696*, 1696t
etiology and pathogenesis of, *1676*, 1676–1678
fluid therapy in, *1686*, 1686–1689
composition and rate in, 1686–1687
glucose supplementation in, 1688–1689
patient monitoring and, 1689
phosphate supplementation and, 1688
potassium supplementation and, *1687*, 1687–1688, 1688t
glycosylated hemoglobin and, 1697
growth hormone–induced, 1594–1596
hemogram in, 1685
home management of, in nonketotic diabetes, 1696–1697
hyperadrenocorticism and, treatment of, 1750
hyperlipidemia and, canine, 206
feline, *199*, 199–200
insulin therapy in, 1689–1691
alternative approaches for, 1690–1691
complications of, 1697–1704
in nonketotic diabetes, 1692, *1693–1696*, 1693t, 1694–1696, 1696t
intermittent intermuscular regimen for, 1690
islet cell transplantation in, 1706–1707
ketoacidosis and, treatment of, 1686, 1691–1692
nonketotic, treatment of, 1692–1697
ocular manifestations of, 77
oral lesions and, 1228
pancreatic enzymes in, 1686
pathophysiology of, 1678–1682
hyperosmolar nonketotic diabetes mellitus and, 1680–1682
ketoacidosis and, 1678–1680, *1679–1681*
nonketotic diabetes mellitus and, 1678
patient evaluation in, 1684–1685
ketoacidosis and, 1685
nonketotic diabetes mellitus and, 1684–1685
physical examination in, 1682–1683, *1683*
polyneuropathy in, 725, *726*
polyuria and polydipsia and, 142
signalment and, 1682
thrombocytopathies associated with, 2276
urinalysis in, 1686
urinary tract infection and, 2116
Dialysis, in acute renal failure, 1981
nondialytic management versus, 1979
Diaphragmatic displacement, 867–869
bilateral, 867
unilateral, 867
Diaphragmatic eventration, 867
Diaphragmatic hernia, *868*, 868–869
history and, 868
management of, 868–869
pericardial, peritoneal, 869, *869*
peritoneopericardial, 1024, *1025*
pleural effusion caused by, 883
Diaphragmatic paralysis, 867–868
Diarrhea, 33–35
diagnostic plan for, 34–35, *35*
historical findings in, 34
large bowel, small bowel diarrhea differentiated from, 1332–1334, 1333t
mechanisms of, 33–34
outcome in, 35
Diarrhea *(Continued)*
pathophysiology of, 33–34
physical findings in, 34
small bowel, bacterial, 1354–1359
Bacillus piliformis and, 1357
Campylobacter and, *1356*, 1356–1357
canine hemorrhagic enteritis and, 1358
Clostridia and, 1357–1358
Escherichia coli and, 1357
Mycobacteria and, 1358–1359
Salmonella and, 1355–1356
Shigella and, 1359
staphylococci and, 1359
Yersinia and, 1357
bacterial overgrowth and, 1373–1375
clinical signs in, 1374
diagnosis of, 1374
pathogenesis of, 1373–1374
treatment of, 1374–1375
chronic inflammatory small bowel diseases and, 1362–1367
diagnosis of, 1330t–1332t, 1330–1341
bacterial overgrowth and, 1339
biopsy in, 1340–1341
digestive and absorptive function tests in, 1338–1339
endoscopy in, 1339–1340
fecal examinations in, 1335t, 1335–1338
hematology and blood chemistry in, 1334t, 1334–1335
history in, 1331–1332
large bowel diarrhea versus, 1332–1334, 1333t
physical examination in, 1334, 1334t
radiography in, 1339, *1340*
therapeutic response and, 1340
ultrasonography in, 1339
dietary, 1341, 1344
drug and toxin-induced, 1344
exudative, mechanisms of, 1329–1330
mechanisms of, 1328–1330
deranged motility and, 1330
osmotic diarrhea and, 1328–1329, 1329t
permeability diarrhea and, 1329–1330
secretory diarrhea and, 1329
mycotic, 1359–1362
intestinal histoplasmosis and, 1359–1361, *1360*
phycomycosis and, *1361*, 1361–1362, *1362*
osmotic, mechanisms of, 1328–1329, 1329t
parasitic, 1341, 1341t–1343t, 1344–1350, *1345*
ascarids and, 1342t–1343t, *1345*, 1345–1346, *1346*
coccidia and, *1345*, 1348–1349
Giardia and, *1345*, 1349–1350
hookworms and, 1342t–1343t, *1345*, 1346–1347
metazoan parasites and, 1348
Pentatrichomonas and, 1350
protozoan, 1350
Strongyloides and, 1347–1348
tapeworms and, 1342t–1343t, 1348
whipworms and, 1347
permeability, mechanisms of, 1329–1330
protein-losing enteropathy and intestinal lymphangiectasia and, 1367–1370
clinical signs in, 1368–1369
diagnosis of, *1368–1370*, 1369–1370
pathogenesis of, 1367–1368, *1368*
treatment of, 1370, *1371*
rickettsial, 1359
secretory, mechanisms of, 1329
short bowel syndrome and, 1375
thyroid-related, 1375–1376, *1376*
treatment of, 1385–1389
acute diarrhea and, 1385, 1386t
chronic diarrhea and, 1385, 1387t, 1388t, 1388–1389
villous atrophy and, 1370–1373
idiopathic, 1371–1372
wheat-sensitive enteropathy and, 1372–1373
viral, 1350–1354, *1351*
canine coronavirus and, 1353
canine parvovirus and, 1351–1353, *1352*
Diarrhea *(Continued)*
small bowel, viral, canine rotavirus and, 1353–1354
feline panleukopenia virus and, 1354
feline rotavirus and, 1354
therapeutic goals in, 35
Diastolic dysfunction, heart failure associated with, treatment of, 1114–1116
Diastolic mechanical inhibition, heart failure and, 915
Diazoxide, insulin-secreting tumors and, 1714–1715
DIC. *See* Disseminated intravascular coagulopathy.
Diestrus, canine, 1785
Diet, alopecia and, 115
anemia and, 92
anorexia and, 16
arthropathies and, 2361
calculolytic, canine struvite urolithiasis and, infection-induced, 2091
in canine struvite urolithiasis, sterile, 2092
in canine uric acid and ammonium urate urolithiasis, 2095
diarrhea and, 34
small bowel, 1341, 1344
in canine calcium oxalate urolithiasis, 2100–2101
in canine cystine urolithiasis, 2098
in chronic inflammatory bowel disease, 1406–1407
liver failure and, 1514–1516
nutritional support and, 453
polyphagia and, 16
pruritus and, 122–123
Diet therapy. *See also* Nutritional support.
in acute gastritis, 1302
in chronic renal failure, complications of, 1994–1996
in diabetes mellitus, nonketotic, 1693–1694, *1694*
in exocrine pancreatic insufficiency, 1547
in heart failure, 965–966
cardiac cachexia and, 965–966
sodium restriction and, 965
renal failure and, 1991–1996
benefits of, 1992–1993
canine protein requirements and, 1993
indications for, 1993
rationale for, 1991t, 1991–1992
recommendations for, 1993–1994
reduced protein diets and, 1992, *1992*
Diethylcarbamazine, in heartworm disease, 1181
Differential count, 2183, 2184
Differentiation, cellular, cancer and, 515
Differentiation markers, lymphocyte differentiation and, 2285
Diffusion, impairment of, central cyanosis and, 96
Digestion, autodigestion and, defenses against, 1529t, *1530*, 1530–1531, *1531*, 1531t
enzymes in, 1529t, 1529–1530
small intestine and, 1324–1327, *1325*
tests of, 1338–1339
Digital compression, urethral obstruction and, 2073
Digitalis, actions of, 943–944
in heart failure therapy, 943–948
in pulmonary edema, 862
indications for, 945–947
pharmacokinetics of, 944–945
toxicity and interactions of, 947–948
Dilated cardiomyopathy. *See* Cardiomyopathy, dilated.
Dimethylsulfoxide (DMSO), in idiopathic lower urinary tract disease, 2080
Dioctophyma renale, 2114
Diphallia, 1884–1885, *1885*
Dipylidiasis. *See* Tapeworms.
Diquat intoxication, 467
differentiation of, 459t, 465t, 467, 467t
Direct immunofluorescence test, in bullous pemphigoid, 2323
in immune-mediated thrombocytopenia, 2304
Dirofilariasis. *See* Heartworm disease.
Discoid lupus erythematosus. *See* Cutaneous lupus erythematosus.
Discoid meniscus, 2345
Disinfectant poisoning, 467t, 481

Diskospondylitis, 650–654
diagnosis of, 651–652, *652*, *653*
etiology and pathogenesis of, 650
clinical findings in, 650–651
treatment of, 652–654
Disopyramide (Norpace), 1062
Disorientation, behavioral signs and, 71t, 71–72
severe, 72
Disseminated intravascular coagulopathy (DIC), 2254–2256
as paraneoplastic syndrome, 520–521
clinical signs of, 2254–2255, *2255*
laboratory evaluation of, 2255
pathophysiology of, 2254
therapy of, 2255–2256
Distal denervating disease, 729
Distal symmetrical polyneuropathy, 729
Distemper, canine, 301–303, 601–602
clinical signs of, 301–302
diagnosis of, 302
epizootiology of, 301
etiology of, 301
in developing countries, 222
ocular manifestations of, 82
pulmonary manifestations of, 829–830
treatment and prevention of, 302–303, 304t
Distemper myelitis, in dogs, 654
Distemper myoclonus, 655
Disuse osteoporosis, 2396
Diuretics, in heart failure therapy, 954–957
loop diuretics and, 955–956
potassium-sparing diuretics and, 957
thiazide diuretics and, 956–957
in oliguria, 1978–1979
in pulmonary edema, 861
in urinary obstruction, 2035–2036
thiazide, in canine calcium oxalate urolithiasis, 2101–2102
Diurnal variation, neuroendocrine control and, 1722
Divalent ion imbalances, therapy of, 1999t, 1999–2002
oral calcium supplementation in, 2001–2002
phosphate restriction in, 1999–2001
vitamin D and metabolites in, 2002
Diversity, immune system and, *2286*, 2287–2289, *2288*, *2289*
Diverticula, esophageal, 1272–1273, *1272–1274*
vesicourachal, function and dysfunction and, 2076–2077
macroscopic, *2077*, 2077–2078
microscopic, *2077*
treatment of, 2078
DMSO. *See* Dimethylsulfoxide.
Doberman pinscher, chronic hepatitis in, 1491
dancing Doberman disease in, 74, 724–725, *725*
dilated cardiomyopathy in, 1104
Dobutamine, actions of, 951–952
in heart failure therapy, 951–953
indications for, *950–951*, 952
toxicity and interactions of, 952–953
DOCA. *See* Desoxycorticosterone.
Dog. *See under specific disorder*; e.g., Parvovirus, canine.
Dog pox, 1567
Domains, B lymphocytes and, 2286
Dominance, genetic, 185–186
incomplete, 186
Dopamine, actions of, 949
in heart failure therapy, 949
indications for, 949
toxicity and interactions of, 949
Dose-response relationship, drug action and, 376
Dosing rate, drugs and, 380t, 380–381
Drooling, 1242, *1247*
Dropped jaw, 1215–1216
Drug(s). *See also specific drugs and drug types.*
absorption and disposition of, 376–378
administration routes and, 376
bioavailability and, 376–377, 377t
distribution and, 377
elimination processes and, 377–378
acid-base disorders and, 449t
acquired immunodeficiencies and, 2299
Drug(s) *(Continued)*
action of, dose-response relationship and, 376
pharmacologic basis of, 375–376
site and mechanisms of, 375–376
administration routes for, 177
endotracheal, 177
intracardiac, 177
intraosseous, 177
intravenous, 177
adverse reactions to. *See* Drug reactions, adverse.
alopecia and, 117
anemia and, 92
cancer chemotherapy and. *See* Cancer, chemotherapy and.
cardiac arrhythmias and, 1052t–1053t
chronic renal failure and, 2004–2005, 2005t
clearance of, 380
congenital heart disease and, 1030t
cyanosis and, 97
diarrhea and, 34, 1344
disordered micturition and, 153t, 153–154
disposition of, *378*, 378–379, 381
distribution of, volume of, 379, 379t
dosing rate and, 380t, 380–381
emergency medicine and, 212, 214t
endocrine pancreatic disorders and, 1720t
esophageal diseases and, 1277t
esophageal responses to, 1257–1258
feline viral diseases and, 340t
for improving cardiac contractility, 942–953
for pain, 22t
gastric motility disorders and, 1313
gastric ulceration and, 1308
half-life of, 379–380, 380t
heart failure therapy and, 975t
hematopoietic stem cell death and, 2198
hemolytic anemia and, 2165–2166
hepatic fibrosis and, 1517
hypersensitivities to, 2324–2326
diagnosis of, 2326
pathophysiology of, *2325*, 2325t, 2325–2326
prognosis of, 2326
therapy of, 2326
hypertensive disease and, 2056t
immunologic disorders and, 2328t
in developing countries, 224
interactions of, adverse drug reactions and, 500
kidney and ureteral disorders and, 2046t
large intestinal disease and, 1420t
liver disease caused by, 1493t, 1493–1497
anticonvulsants and, 1495–1496
antihelmintics and, 1496–1497
glucocorticoids and, 1494–1495, *1496*
inhalant anesthetics and, 1497
liver failure and, 1516–1517
nebulization of, lower respiratory disease and, 821
otitis externa and, 255
ototoxic, vestibulocochlear nerve and, 718
pancreatitis and, 1534
pituitary impairment by, 1593–1594, *1594*, *1595*
plasma concentrations of, monitoring, 381
poisoning and, 461t–464t
polyuria and polydipsia and, 141t, 144
skeletal diseases and, 2399t
thiol-containing, in canine cystine urolithiasis, 2098
thrombocytopathies induced by, 2274–2275
thyroid hormone metabolism and, in dog, 1639–1640
toxic polyneuropathies and, 726t, 726–727
tremor induced by, 56
urinary retention and, 159, 159t
weakness related to, 48
Drug eruption, 9
Drug fever, allergic drug reactions and, 505
Drug reactions, adverse, 499–509
allergic, 501–504
characteristics of, 501
clinical manifestations of, 502–504
diagnosis of, 504
immunologic mechanisms and, 501–502
development of, 499–501
Drug reactions *(Continued)*
adverse, development of, age and, 500
breed characteristics and, 500
disease and, 500
drug factors and, 499–500
drug interactions and, 500
environmental factors and, 500–501
habitus and, 500
immunologic status and, 500
pregnancy and, 500
sex and, 500
species and, 500
management of, 508–509
pinnae and, 250
prevention of, in acute renal failure, 1980–1981
resembling allergy, 504–505
cardiovascular, 504–505
drug fever and, 505
hematologic, 505
timing of, 501
toxic, 505–508
aplastic anemia and, 507, 507t
kidneys and, 505, 506t
liver and, 505–507, 506t
medication errors and, 507–508
Drying agents, otitis externa and, 255
Duct obstruction, pancreatitis and, 1534
Duodenal reflux, pancreatitis and, 1534
Dural ossification, 655, *656*
Dyschezia, definition of, 36
diagnostic procedures in, 38
diarrhea and, 34
historical findings in, 37
pathophysiology of, 36, *37*, *38*
physical examination in, 37–38
treatment goals in, 39
Dyschondrosteosis, 2383
Dysgenesis, sacrocaudal, in Manx cats, 685
Dysostoses, 2384
Dysphagia, 32, 1236–1237
clinical findings in, 32
definition of, *27*, *32*
diagnostic plan for, 32
glossopharyngeal or vagus nerve lesions and, 719
mediastinal disorders and, 887
Dysplasia, of atrioventricular valves. *See* Atrioventricular valve dysplasia.
of hip, 2355–2358, *2357*, *2358*
of shoulder, 2358
of tricuspid valve, cyanotic heart disease and, 1022
Dyspnea, 88–90
cyanosis and, *97*, *98*
diagnosis of, 89t, 90, 752
nocturnal, paroxysmal, in heart failure, 916
pathophysiology of, 88–90
lower airway problems and, 89
pleural diseases and, 89
reduced hemoglobin states and, 89
upper airway problems and, 88t, 88–89
polycythemia and, 102
regurgitation and, 31
treatment of, 89t, 90
Dysproteinemia, platelet dysfunction in, 2272
Dystocia, 1829–1831
Dystrophy, neuroaxonal, of Rottweilers, 682
Dysuria, 163–164
definition of, 163
diagnostic approach to, 163–164
hematuria and, 161
pathophysiology of, 163, 163t
treatment goals in, 164
vesicourachal diverticula and, treatment of, 2078

Ear canal, cleaning of, 254–255
Ear diseases, 246–261. *See also* Otitis externa; Otitis interna; Otitis media.
anatomy and, 260
hearing and, 260
history and, 246
of external ear canal, 252–258
anatomy and, 252
bacterial, 256

Ear diseases *(Continued)*
of external ear canal, causes of, 254
epizootiology of, 253
examination and, 253–254
pathophysiology of, 252–253
treatment of, 254–256
yeast, 256
of middle ear, 258–259
anatomy and, 258
of pinnae, 247–252
acquired diseases and, 247, *248*, 249–252
anatomy and, 247
congenital defects and, 247
examination and, 247
parasitic, 256–257
allergic, 257
neoplastic, 257–258
surgical management of, 258
physical examination and, 246
Ear mites, 256–257
Eating, vomiting and, time relationship of, 28–29
Eating behavior problems. *See also* Polyphagia.
in cats, 237
Eccentrocytes, 2150, *2151*
Ecchymoses, polycythemia and, 103
ECF. *See* Extracellular fluid.
ECG. *See* Electrocardiography.
Echinococcosis. *See* Tapeworms.
Echocardiography, cardiac arrhythmias and, 1058, 1059t
in chronic mitral valvular insufficiency, 1038, *1039*
in congenital heart disease, 978–980, *979*
in cyanotic heart disease, 1018, *1020*
in infective endocarditis, 1157, *1158*
Eclampsia, hypocalcemia and, 1625–1626
Ectoparasitic diseases, zoonotic, 191
Ectopic ACTH syndrome, pathophysiology of, 1724
Ectopic beats, premature, *1065*, 1065–1070
classification of, 1069–1070
supraventricular, *1066*, 1067
ventricular, *1065*, 1067–1070, *1068*, *1069*
Ectopic calcification, in canine hyperadrenocorticism, 1730, *1731*
Ectrodactyly syndrome, 2384
Edema, cerebrospinal, reduction of, corticosteroids and, 419–420, 420t
in nephrotic syndrome, 2021–2022
treatment of, 2021–2022
lameness and, in dogs, 166
liver failure and, treatment of, 1520–1521
mediastinal, 889
nephrotic syndrome and, 1942, *1942*
peripheral, 41–45
ancillary diagnostic aids for, 43–45
clinical pathology of, 43–44, 44t
diagnostic approach to, *44*, 45
history and physical examination in, 43
localized and generalized, 45
localized versus generalized, 42t, 42–43
pathophysiology of, *41*, 41–42, 42t
pulmonary. *See* Pulmonary edema.
Education, about acupuncture, 496
in developing countries, 224–225
EEG. *See* Electroencephalography.
Effector systems, immune response and, 2283
Ehrlichiosis, canine, 277–279
anemia and, 92, 2174
hematopoietic stem cell death and, 2200
in developing countries, 222–223
platelet dysfunction in, 2273
ocular manifestations of, 81
Eisenmenger's physiology, atrioventricular septal defects and, 996, *996*
Ejaculation, antegrade, failure to achieve, 1887–1888
physiology of, 1881–1882
retrograde, treatment of, 1857
Elbow joint, dysplasia of, *2349–2352*, 2350–2354
fragmented medial coronoid process and, *2351*, 2351–2354, *2352*
osteochondritis dissecans and, of medial condyle, of humerus, 2354, *2355*
Elbow joint *(Continued)*
dysplasia of, ununited anconeal process and, in nonchondrodystrophic breeds, *2353*, 2354, *2354*
luxations and subluxations of, 2338, *2338*, *2339*
Electric burns, of oral cavity, 1231
Electrical countershock, fibrillation and, 178–179
Electroacupuncture, 493, *493*
Electrocardiography (ECG), 1054, *1055*, 1055t
cardiac arrhythmias and, 1058
cardiopulmonary arrest and, *172*, 172–173, *173*
cyanosis and, 99
in chronic mitral valvular insufficiency, 1035–1036, *1037*, 1038
in congenital heart disease, 980, *980–982*
in heartworm disease, 1168–1169
in hypoadrenocorticism, 1763–1766
hyperkalemia and, 1763–1764, *1765*, 1766
in infective endocarditis, 1156, *1157*
in peripheral edema, 44–45
in pulmonary edema, 859
pericardial effusion and, 1139, *1140*
Electrodiagnostics, coma and stupor and, 64
Electroencephalography (EEG), 584–585, *585–587*
coma and stupor and, 64
Electrolyte(s), corticosteroids and, 416
gastric secretion of, 1291–1292
serum levels of, in canine hyperadrenocorticism, 1732
in hypoadrenocorticism, 1762–1763
Electrolyte disturbances, brain and, 616–617
in hypoadrenocorticism, treatment of, 1767–1768
in liver disease, 1459–1461
weakness and, 48, 48t, 49t
Electromechanical dissociation, cardiopulmonary arrest and, 172, *173*
Electromyography (EMG), brain disease diagnosis and, 588
in canine dermatomyositis, 2318
peripheral nerve disorders and, 711–714
needle electromyography and, 712–713, *713*
nerve stimulation and, 713–714, *714*, 715t
Electronic particle counters, 2182–2183
Electrophoresis, lipoproteins and, 199
Electrophysiology, spinal cord disease and, 628
Elimination, of drugs, 377–378
Elimination behavior problems, in cats, 235–236
in dogs, 231–232
Embolism. *See also* Thromboembolic disease.
fibrocartilaginous, ischemic myelopathy due to, 670–671
pulmonary, pleural effusion caused by, 883
Emergencies, in acute renal failure, 1969–1970
Emergency medicine, 209–216
emergency classification and, 209–211
client relations and, 209–210
evaluation and triage in, 209
history and physical examination in, 210–211
future directions for, 216
standards for, 211–216
anesthesia and, 215–216
equipment, drugs, and supplies and, 212, 213t, 214t
ethicolegal considerations and, 216
extended management and, 215
monitoring and supportive care and, 214–215, 215t
patient care and, 214
personnel and, 211–212
physical plant and, 211, *212*
radiography and, 216
records and, 214
referring veterinarians and, 214
support services and, 212–214
ultrasonography and, 216
EMG. *See* Electromyography.
Emphysema, 847
subcutaneous, cyanosis and, 98
Emphysematous cystitis, 2122
Empyema, pleural effusion and, 879–880
Enalapril, actions of, 962–963
in heart failure therapy, 962–963
Enamel hypoplasia, 1210, *1210*
Encainide, 1063
Encephalitis, behavioral signs of, 73
in pugs, 608–609
postvaccinal, brain and, 603–604
Encephalitozoonosis, 291–292
canine, 606
Encephalopathy, hepatic, 1462–1466, *1463*
ammonia and, 1463–1464
aromatic amino acids and, 1464
behavioral signs and, 73
behavioral signs of, 73
blood-brain barrier and, 1465
cerebral sensitivity and, 1465
false neurotransmitters and, 1465
glutamate and, 1464
glutamine and, 1464
hypoglycemia and, 1465–1466
inhibitory neurotransmitters and, 1465
α-ketoglutarate and, 1464
mercaptans and, 1464
methionine and, 1464
neuroreceptor alterations and, 1465
neurotransmitters and, 1465
short-chain fatty acids and, 1464
ischemic, feline, 600–601
metabolic, coma and stupor and, 62
Enchondral cartilage cores, retained, 2395–2396, *2396*
End-stage kidney, 1985
Endocardial fibroelastosis, 1023, *1023*, 1104
Endocardiosis, etiology of, 1044
Endocarditis, infective. *See* Infective endocarditis.
Endocrine disorders, anemia of, 2172
as paraneoplastic syndrome, 520
brain and, 617
cutaneous manifestations of, 6–7
pinnae and, 251
secondary hypertension and, 2050–2051
weakness and, 48
weight loss and, 4
Endocrine function, of small intestine, 1328
Endocrine system, corticosteroids and, 417–418, *418*
in canine hypothyroidism, adult-onset, 1644
uremia and, 1920
Endodontic disease, 1212–1214, *1214*
Endometritis, chronic, infertility and, 1845
Endoparasitic diseases, in developing countries, 221
Endoscopy, esophageal diseases and, 1260–1261, *1261*
gastric disease and, 1297–1298, *1298*
in lower urinary tract disease, 2111
in small bowel diarrhea, 1339–1340
of large intestine, 1400–1402
biopsy techniques and, 1402
flexible colonoscopy and, 1402
proctoscopy and, 1400–1402
Energy metabolism, nutritional assessment and, 451–452
of platelets, 2266
English cocker spaniel, dilated cardiomyopathy in, 1104
English pointer, sensory neuropathy of, 724
Enteritis, granulomatous, 1366–1367, *1367*
hemorrhagic, canine, 1358
lymphocytic-plasmacytic, 1362–1364
clinical signs of, 1363
diagnosis of, 1363, *1363*
treatment of, 1363–1364
parvoviral, hematopoietic stem cell death and, 2199
Enterohepatic circulation, 1425
Enteropathies, chronic, diarrhea and, 1362–1376
immunoproliferative, of Basenji dogs, 1364–1365
protein-losing, 1367–1370
clinical signs of, 1368–1369
diagnosis of, *1368–1370*, 1369–1370
pathogenesis of, 1367–1368, *1368*
treatment of, 1370, *1371*
wheat-sensitive, 1372–1373
clinical signs of, 1372
diagnosis of, 1372–1373
treatment of, 1373
Enterosystemic cycle, diarrhea and, 33

Enterotoxigenic diarrhea. *See* Diarrhea, small bowel, bacterial.
Enuresis. *See also* Urinary incontinence.
  definition of, 148
Environmental factors, adverse drug reactions and, 500 501
  alopecia and, 115
  anemia and, 92
  coma and stupor and, 62
  congenital defects and, 184
  coughing and, 86–87
  diarrhea and, 34
  pruritus and, 123
  stress and. *See* Stress.
Enzymes, deficiencies of, cutaneous manifestations of, 5
  digestive, 1529t, 1529–1530
  hepatic, abnormalities of, causes of, 1441–1443
    in liver disease, 1436t, 1436–1441
  pancreatic, activity of, in exocrine pancreatic insufficiency, 1542
    in blood, 1531
    in diabetes mellitus, 1686
  replacement of, in exocrine pancreatic insufficiency, 1546–1547
Eosinopenia, 2210–2211
  causes of, 12t
  corticosteroid-associated, 2210–2211
Eosinophil(s), 2209–2210
  morphology of, *2209*, 2209–2210
  production and kinetics of, 2210
  response patterns of, 2210–2211
    eosinopenia and, 2210–2211
    eosinophilia and, 2210, 2211t
Eosinophilia, 2210, 2211t
  causes of, 12t
  hypereosinophilic syndromes and, 2210
  hypersensitivity reactions and, 2210
  inflammation and, 2210
  noninfectious granulomatous disorders with, mediastinal, 892, *893*
  parasitism and, 2210
  pleural effusion with, 883–884
  tumor-associated, 2210
Eosinophilic colitis, 1409–1410
Eosinophilic diseases. *See also* Gastritis, eosinophilic; *specific diseases.*
  pulmonary, 838–839
Eosinophilic gastroenteritis, canine, 1365–1366
Eosinophilic granuloma, 1305–1306
Eosinophilic leukemia, 2216
Epidermal collarettes, 119
Epidermoid cyst, 682–683
Epilepsy. *See also* Seizure(s).
  definition of, 66
Epinephrine, cardiopulmonary response to, 176
  in heart failure therapy, 948–949
  in insulin antagonism/resistance, 1702
  indications for, 948–949
Epiphysiolysis, 2347
Epistaxis, polycythemia and, 103
Epulis, 1230, *1230*
Equipment, emergency medicine and, 212, 213t
Erection, failure to achieve, 1887
  persistent, 1888
  physiology of, 1881–1882
Erosion, 119
Erosive arthritis, 2366–2367
Erythema multiforme, 9
Erythemic myelosis, 2216
Erythrocyte(s), biochemistry of, 2158–2159
    hemoglobins and, 2158
    metabolism and, *2158*, 2158–2159
  fragility and deformability of, 2154–2156, *2155*
  fragmentation of, 2150, *2153*
  immunoglobulin and complement detection on, 2154
  in hypoadrenocorticism, 1760
  kinetics of, 2157–2158
    anemia and, marrow response to, 2157–2158
    senescence and, 2157
    survival and, 2157
  morphology of, on Wright's stained blood films, 2147–2153, *2148*
Erythrocyte(s) *(Continued)*
  nucleated, 2147, *2148*
    leukocyte count correction for, 2183
  oxidative injury to, anemia and, *2168*, 2168–2170
  punched out, 2150, 2153
  reference values for, 2156–2157
    neonatal and juvenile, 2156–2157
  sizing of, automated cell counting and, *2146*, 2146–2147, *2147*
Erythrocytosis, primary, 2216
Erythroleukemia, 2216
Erythroparasitic organisms, hemolytic anemias due to, 2166–2168
Erythropoiesis, 2145, *2146*
Erythropoietin, depression of, 2171–2173
    chronic disease and, 2171–2172
    endocrine failures and, 2172
    renal failure and, 2172
  polycythemia and, 103
Escherichia coli infections, of large intestine, 1414–1415
  small bowel diarrhea and, 1357
Esophageal diseases, congenital, 1261–1266
  diagnosis of, 1258–1261
    clinical signs and, 1258–1259
    history and, 1259
    physical examination and, 1259, 1264t
    radiology in, 1259–1261, *1261*
  drugs used in, 1277t
  foreign bodies and, 1268–1270
    clinical signs of, 1269
    diagnosis of, 1269
    treatment of, 1269–1270, *1269–1271*
  motility abnormalities and, 1264t, 1266
  neoplastic, 1273–1275
  obstructive, 1271–1272, *1272*
  vascular ring abnormalities and, *1266*, 1266–1267
Esophageal diverticuli, 1272–1273, *1272–1274*
Esophageal fistula, 1274
Esophageal hiatus, disorders of, 1274
Esophageal rupture, pleural effusion caused by, 882, *882*
Esophageal sphincters, lower, anatomy of, 1256, *1256*
  pharmacologic responses of, 1257–1258
  upper, anatomy of, 1255 1256
Esophagitis, *1267*, 1267–1268, *1268*
Esophagraphy, esophageal diseases and, 1259–1261
Esophagus, anatomy of, 1255–1257
    lower sphincter and, 1256, *1256*
    physiology of swallowing and, 1256–1257, *1258*
    upper sphincter and, 1255–1256
  pharmacologic responses of, 1257–1258
  strictures of, 1270–1271, *1271*
Estrogens, abnormal metabolism of, bone disorders and, 2396
  in persistent estrus, 1796
  hematopoietic stem cell death and, in dogs, 2198
  toxicity of, aplastic anemia and, 2174
Estrous cycle, canine, 1782–1785, *1784*
    anestrus and, 1782–1783
    diestrus and, 1785
    estrus and, 1784–1785
    proestrus and, 1783–1784
  feline, 1787–1788
    anestrus and, 1787
    estrus and, 1787–1788, *1788*
      induction of, 1049–1050, 1050t
      split periods of, 1796, *1844*, 1847
    interfollicular stage and, 1788
    metestrus and, 1788
    pregnancy and, 1788
    proestrus and, 1787
  persistent estrus and, 1792–1796
    estrogen therapy and, 1796
    liver disease and, 1796
    ovarian cysts and, *1792*, 1792–1795, 1793t
      diagnosis of, 1793t, 1793–1794
      treatment of, *1794*, 1794–1795
    ovarian tumors and, *1795*, 1795t, 1795–1796
    split estrus periods and, 1796
Ethacrynic acid, in heart failure therapy, 956
Ethicolegal concerns, acupuncture and, 496
  emergency medicine and, 216
Ethyl alcohol intoxication, 459t, 460t, 481
Ethylene glycol intoxication, 457–459
  differentiation of, 458, 459t, 460t
  therapy of, 458–459, 461t–464t
Euploidy, 184
Euthanasia, human-pet bonds and, 243
"Euthyroid sick" syndrome, canine, thyroid hormone metabolism and, 1638–1639
Eventration, diaphragmatic, 867
Evoked potentials, brain disease diagnosis and, 585, 588
Evoked responses, auditory, brain stem, 588
  visual, 588
Excitability, of heart muscle, *1055*, 1055–1056
Excitation-contraction coupling events, 1051
Excoriation, 119
Excretory urography, in renal disease, 1911t, 1911–1912
Exocrine pancreatic insufficiency. *See* Pancreatic insufficiency, exocrine.
Exogenous vasopressin test, tubular function and, 1899–1900
Exostoses, cartilaginous, multiple, 2383–2384, *2384*
Expectorants, lower respiratory disease and, 821
Exposure, pruritus and, 123
Exposure time, radiography and, 752–753
Extended care, emergency medicine and, 215
Extensor carpi radialis reflex, testing for, 567, *568*
External beam irradiation, thyroid tumors and, in dog, 1670
Extracellular fluid (ECF), buffer systems in, acid-base and, 440–441
Extremities, examination of, cyanosis and, 98
Eye(s). *See also headings beginning with term* Ocular.
  in canine hypothyroidism, adult-onset, 1643
  in neurological examination, 702t, 702–707
  respiratory disease and, diagnosis of, 750
  systemic disease and, 75–84
    canine ocular tumors and, 83–84
    dermatologic, 75–76
      infectious, 76–77
    diagnostic principles and, 75
    feline ocular tumors and, 84
    inborn errors of metabolism and, 79, 79t
    infectious, in cat, 82–83
      in dog, 79t, 80–82
    integumentary, congenital and hereditary, 77
    lipid metabolism disorders and, 77, *78*
    lipid storage disease and, 79
    metabolic, 77
    nutritional disorders and, 80
    vascular, 79–80
  therapeutic principles and, 75
Eye position, coma and stupor and, 63
Eyelid, third, in neurological examination, 706

Facial nerves, focal diseases of, *717*, 717–718
  paralysis of, idiopathic, 717–718
Facial reflexes, testing for, 564, *565*
Facial rubbing syndrome, 74
Facial sensory examination, 564, *565*
Facial sinus, 1211–1212, *1214*
Failure to cycle, in canine hyperadrenocorticism, 1729
Failure to thrive, polycythemia and, 103
Fanconi syndrome, 2027
Fasting blood ammonia, in liver disease, 1455–1456, *1456*, *1457*
Fat, digestion and absorption of, 1325–1326
  metabolism of, corticosteroids and, 416
  reserves of, nutritional assessment and, 451
Fatigue. *See also* Weakness.
  definition of, 46
Fatty acids, 203
  short-chain, hepatic encephalopathy and, 1464
Fear, aggression induced by, in cats, 236
  behavioral signs and, 71t, 71–72
  elimination behavior problems and, in dogs, 231
  in dogs, 228–229
    aggression and, 234
Fecal examination, diarrhea and, 35
  in exocrine pancreatic insufficiency, 1545–1546

Fecal examination *(Continued)*
in small bowel diarrhea, 1335t, 1335–1338
fecal biochemistry determinations and, 1337
for infectious agents, 1336
for parasites, 1335t, 1335–1336
microscopic, *1336*, 1336–1337, *1337*
protein loss and, 1337–1338
Fecal flotation, 1399
Fecal incontinence, 1573t, 1573–1574
Fecal occult blood, large intestinal disease and, 1400
Fecal sedimentation, 1399
Fecal smears, direct, 1399
Fecal staining, 1399
Feces. *See also* Constipation; Diarrhea.
anemia and, 92
gross examination of, 1399
Fecoliths, feline, 1573
Feedback, neuroendocrine system and, 1580
Feline. *See under disease or disorder*; e.g., Peritonitis, infectious, feline.
Feline lymphosarcoma leukemia complex, 84
FeLV. *See* Leukemia(s), feline.
Female(s), 1777–1788
breeding season and puberty in, 1779, *1782*
canine estrous cycle and, 1782–1785, *1784*
anestrus and, 1782–1783
diestrus and, 1785
estrus and, 1784–1785
proestrus and, 1783–1784
feline estrous cycle and, 1787–1788
anestrus and, 1787
estrus and, 1787–1788, *1788*
interfollicular stage and, 1788
metestrus and, 1788
pregnancy and, 1788
proestrus and, 1787
infertility in. *See* Infertility, in bitch.
ovarian cycle in, 1779–1782, *1782*, *1783*
parturition and, 1786–1787
pregnancy and, in bitch, 1785–1786, *1786*
structural peculiarities of, *1777*, 1777–1778, *1778*
vagina in, hormonally induced changes in, 1778–1779, *1780–1781*
Femoral head, aseptic necrosis of, 2359, *2360*, *2361*
Femoral nerve injury, *722*, 723
Fetal development, corticosteroids and, 418
Fetal resorption, 1845
Fever, *24*, 24–26. *See also* Hyperthermia.
anemia and, 93
as paraneoplastic syndrome, 519
clinical presentation of, 24–25
diarrhea and, 34
drug, allergic drug reactions and, 505
hematuria and, 161–162
pathogenesis of, 24, *25*
treatment of, 25–26, 26t
weakness and, 48
weight loss and, 4
Fibrillation, treatment of, 178–179
Fibrin(ogen) degradation products assay, 2252
Fibrinogen assays, 2251–2252
Fibrinoid leukodystrophy, 596
Fibrinolysis, 2248–2249, *2249*
primary, *2249*, 2256
Fibroelastosis, endocardial, 1023, *1023*, 1104
Fibrosarcoma, in dog, 2389
Fibrosis, hepatic, drug control of, 1517
hepatoportal, chronic hepatitis associated with, in dogs, 1492
of cardiac valves, etiology of, 1044
pericardial, with constriction, 1133, *1134*
Fibular nerve injury, 722–723
Filariasis, ocular, 81
Filaroides hirthi, 837–838
Filaroides osleri, tracheal disease due to, 798–799, *800*
Filtration, splenic, 2235–2236
FIP. *See* Peritonitis, infectious, feline.
Fistula(s), arteriovenous, 1189–1191
hepatic, 1506–1507
bronchoesophageal, 829
esophageal, 1274
perianal, 1567–1569

Fistula(s) *(Continued)*
perianal, differential diagnosis of, 1568
history and physical findings in, 1568, *1568*
treatment of, *1568*, 1568–1569
rectovaginal, *1568*, 1570, *1570*
urethral, 2135
Flank-sucking, 74
Fleas, in humans, 193
plague and, 191
Flecainide, 1063
Fleet-like enema intoxication, 459t, 460t, 480
Flexor reflexes, testing for, 569, *572*
Flooding, for fears and phobias, 228
Fluid disorders, in chronic renal failure, therapy for, 1996
in liver disease, 1459–1461
Fluid therapy, general guidelines for, 431, 432t
in acute gastritis, 1302
in acute renal failure, 1974–1976
in diabetes mellitus, *1686*, 1686–1689
composition and rate and, 1686–1687
glucose supplementation and, 1688–1689
patient monitoring and, 1689
phosphate supplementation and, 1688
potassium supplementation and, *1687*, 1687–1688, 1688t
in heart failure therapy, 967
Flukes, in gallbladder, 1557, 1557t
in lung, 835–836
diagnosis of, 836, *837*
pancreatic, in cats, 1549
Flushing, urethral obstruction and, 2074, 2074t
Fly strike dermatitis, of pinna, 249
Folate, serum, in small bowel diarrhea, 1339
Follicle-stimulating hormone (FSH), neuroendocrine function and, 1587
Food hypersensitivity, 194–197
cutaneous manifestations of, 8–9, 194–196
diagnosis of, 195–196
historical findings in, 195
long-term nutritional management of, 196
pathogenesis of, 194–195
gastrointestinal syndromes associated with, 196–197
Foramen magnum, congenital malformation of, 592
Foreign bodies, anal, 1567
bronchial, 828–829
esophageal, 1268–1270
clinical signs of, 1269
diagnosis of, 1269
treatment of, 1269–1270, *1269–1271*
in larynx, 790
in oral cavity, 1231
in pharynx, 783–784
in rhinarium, 772–773
in trachea, 808, 810
rectal, 1567
Fox terrier, smooth-haired, hereditary ataxia in, 660
Fractional clearances, tubular function and, 1900
Fracture
healing of, osteomyelitis and, 2381, *2381*
of os penis, 1886
of teeth, 1211, *1211–1213*
Frenulum, penile, persistent, 1884, *1884*
Frostbite, of pinna, 249–250
FSH. *See* Follicle-stimulating hormone.
Fucosidosis, 594–595
Fulminant hepatic failure, treatment of, 1521t, 1521–1522
Function tests, diarrhea and, 35
Fundic gland region, of stomach, 1290
Fungal infections, alopecia and, 120
antifungal drugs and, activity spectrum of, 395–396
clinical pharmacology of, 396
toxicity of, 396
arthritis and, 2365–2366
cutaneous manifestations of, 7
mediastinal, 891–892, *892*
ocular manifestations of, *78*, 81–82
of large intestine, 1412–1413
pulmonary, 833–838
rhinitis and, 778–780, *780*

Fungal meningomyelitis. *See* Meningomyelitis, fungal.
Furosemide, actions of, 955
in heart failure therapy, 955–956
in oliguria, 1978–1979
indications for, 955
toxicity and interactions of, 955–956
Fusion beat, 1081

Gag reflex, testing for, 564, 566, 566t
Gait. *See also* Ataxia.
cyanosis and, 97
in neurologic examination, 558
lameness and, in dogs, 166
Galactostasis, 1834
Gallbladder disease, diagnosis of, *1555*, 1555–1556, *1556*
nonobstructive, 1556t, 1556–1557
intraluminal, *1556*, 1556–1557, 1557t
mural, 1557
obstructive, 1556t, 1557–1558
extramural, 1558
intraluminal, 1557
mural, 1557
Gallbladder sediment, *1556*, 1556–1557
Gallop rhythm, in heart failure, 916
Gamma-glutamyl transferase, in liver disease, 1439–1441, *1440*
Ganglioradiculitis, 727–728
Gangliosidosis, 593–594
ocular manifestations of, 79
Garbage poisoning, 460t, 478
Gastric dilatation-volvulus-torsion syndrome (GDVT), 1278–1287
cardiac dysrhythmias in, 1285–1286
clinical signs and diagnosis of, 1281
definition of, 1278, *1279*, *1280*
emergency preoperative treatment for, 1281
incidence and breed susceptibility and, 1278
pathophysiology of, 1278–1281
other organ systems and, 1279–1281
postoperative care in, 1286–1287
antiarrhythmic therapy in, 1286–1287
antibiotics in, 1287
feeding in, 1287
fluid therapy in, 1287
recurrence and prevention of, 1287
surgical decisions regarding, 1281–1285, *1282–1286*
Gastric diseases, 1294–1319. *See also specific diseases.*
clinical evaluation in, 1294–1299, *1295*, *1297–1299*
gastric mucosal injury and, 1299–1301, *1300*
neoplastic, 1317–1319
Gastric emptying, 1292–1293, *1293*
Gastric filling, 1291
Gastric fluid analysis, 1295–1296
Gastric motility, 1292–1293, *1293*
disorders of, 1312–1314
diagnosis of, 1314
etiology of, 1313t, 1313–1314
idiopathic, 1313
treatment of, 1314
Gastric mucosal injury, 1299–1301
mechanisms of, 1299–1301
agents and, 1300
blood flow alterations and, 1300–1301
endogenous factors in, 1301
gastric mucosal barrier and, 1299–1300, *1300*
Gastric outlet obstructions, 1310–1312
clinical findings in, 1311
diagnosis of, 1311–1312, *1312*
etiology of, 1311
pathophysiology of, 1311
treatment of, 1312
Gastric phase, of gastric secretion, 1291
Gastric secretion, 1291–1292
hydrochloric acid production and, 1291, *1292*
of acid, 1291
of electrolytes, 1291–1292
of gastrin, 1292, *1292*, 1292t
of mucus, 1292

Gastric secretion *(Continued)*
of pepsin, 1292
testing of, 1299
Gastric stasis, 1313, 1313t
Gastric ulceration. *See* Ulcer(s), gastric.
Gastrin, gastric secretion of, 1292, *1292*, 1292t
Gastrinoma, 1314–1317
clinical findings and, 1315
diagnosis of, 1315–1317, *1316*
etiology of, 1315
pathophysiology of, 1315, *1315*
treatment of, 1317
Gastritis, acute, 1301–1303
diagnosis of, 1302
etiology of, 1301
pathophysiology of, 1301
treatment of, 1302–1303
chronic, 1303–1305
atrophic, 1304
clinical findings in, 1304
diagnosis of, 1304
etiology of, 1303
granulomatous, 1304
pathophysiology of, 1303–1304
superficial, 1304
treatment of, 1304–1305
eosinophilic, 1305–1306
clinical findings in, 1305
diagnosis of, 1305–1306
pathophysiology of, 1305
treatment of, 1306
hypertrophic, of basenji dogs, 1306
reflux, 1314
Gastrocnemius reflex, testing for, 569
Gastroenteritis, eosinophilic, canine, 1365–1366
viral, 306–310
canine coronavirus and, 308–309
canine herpesvirus and, 309
canine parvovirus and, 306 308
pseudorabies and, 310
Gastrointestinal diseases. *See also* Gastric diseases; *specific diseases*.
associated with food allergy, 196–197
poisoning and, 459t
protozoal, 285–287
weight loss and, 4
Gastrointestinal tract. *See also specific organs*.
bacterial infections of, 267–269
corticosteroids and, 416
gastric dilatation-volvulus-torsion syndrome and, 1281
in canine hypothyroidism, adult-onset, 1643
in feline hyperthyroidism, 1655t, 1656
lesions of, 895
mushroom poisoning and, 459t, 460t, 469t, 477
poisoning and, 467
uremia and, 1919–1920
Gastropathy(ies), hypertrophic, 1306–1308
clinical findings in, 1307
cystic, focal, 1306
diagnosis of, 1307, *1307*
glandular, 1306
of Basenji dogs, 1306
pathophysiology of, 1306–1307
pyloric, chronic, 1307
treatment of, 1307–1308
Gastropexy, in gastric dilatation-volvulus-torsion syndrome, 1284–1285, *1285*, *1286*
Gate control theory, of pain, 19
acupuncture and, 487, *488*
GDVT. *See* Gastric dilatation-volvulus-torsion syndrome.
Genetic disorders, congenital, 185–186
lameness and, in cats, 169
of bone, 2383–2385
oral lesions and, 1228
Genetic factors, alopecia and, 113, 119
congenital defects and, 184–186
exocrine pancreatic insufficiency and, 1539
pancreatitis and, 1535
Genitalia. *See also* Female(s); Male(s); *specific organs*.
dysuria and, 164
Genodermatoses, 5
Geotrichosis, ocular manifestations of, 82
German shepherd, hypopituitarism in, 1588–1589, *1589*, 1589t, *1590*
Gestation, prolonged, 1828
GH. *See* Growth hormone.
GH-RH. *See* Growth hormone-releasing hormone.
Giant axonal neuropathy, 725
Giardiasis, 285–286, 1411
in humans, 190
prevention of, 190
small bowel diarrhea and, *1345*, 1349–1350
Gingival hyperplasia, *1219*, 1220–1221
Gingivitis, 1217–1220
clinical manifestations of, 1217–1218, *1218*, *1219*
etiology of, 1217, *1217*, *1218*
histopathology of, 1218–1219, *1219*
treatment of, 1219, *1220*
ulcerative, necrotizing, 1219–1220
Globoid cell leukodystrophy, 596, 656–657, 724
Globulin(s), synthesis and regulation of, in liver disease, 1434t, 1434–1435
Glomerular disease, diagnosis of, 1943–1945
laboratory findings in, 1943–1945
pathophysiology of, 1937–1943
amyloidosis and, 1939, 1941, 1941t
glomerulonephritis and, *1938*, 1938–1939, 1939t, *1940*, 1940t
nephrotic syndrome and, 1941–1943
normal glomerular structure and function and, 1937–1938, *1938*
Glomerular filtration rate, decreased, *1930*, 1930–1931
hyperfiltration and, renal failure and, 1988–1990
Glomerular function, evaluation of, 1896t, 1896–1898
blood urea nitrogen and, 1896, 1897, *1897*
creatinine clearance and, 1896t, 1897–1898
radioisotope studies and, 1898
renal clearance and, 1897
serum creatinine and, 1896–1897, *1897*
sodium sulfanilate half-life and, 1898
Glomerular sclerosis, 2011
Glomerulonephritis, etiology of, 2011–2012, 2012t
glomerular injury in, *1938*, 1938–1939, 1939t, *1940*, 1940t
pleural effusion caused by, 882
prognosis of, 2016
treatment of, 2017–2019
anticoagulant and anti-platelet therapy in, 2018–2019
corticosteroid and immunosuppressive therapy in, 2017–2018
eliminating causative factors in, 2017
Glomerulonephropathies, in nephrotic syndrome, 2009t, 2009–2010, *2010*
membranoproliferative, 2011
membranous, 2011
morphologic forms of, 2010–2011
proliferative, 2011
Glossitis, 1234–1236, *1235*, *1236*
Glossopharyngeal nerves, focal diseases of, 719
Glucagon, in insulin antagonism/resistance, 1702
Glucagon tolerance test, in hyperadrenocorticism, 1740–1741
Glucocerebrosidosis, 594
Glucocorticoids, excess, infertility and, in bitch, 1848
urinary tract infection and, 2116
hepatopathy associated with, 1494–1495, *1496*
in exocrine pancreatic insufficiency, 1548
in hyperadrenocorticism, 1741, 1749–1750
in hypoadrenocorticism, 1758–1759, *1759*, 1770
hypovolemia and, 1767
in idiopathic lower urinary tract disease, 2080
in insulin antagonism/resistance, *1701*, 1701–1702
in liver failure, 1517
insulin secreting tumors and, 1714
secretion of, regulation of, 1721–1723
adrenocorticotrophic hormone and related peptides and, 1721–1723
corticotropin-releasing hormone and, 1721
Glucose, abnormal values of, causes of, 13t
blood levels of, in canine hyperadrenocorticism, 1730
in feline hyperadrenocorticism, 1755
determination of, insulin-secreting tumors and, 1710–1711
in hyperkalemia, in acute renal failure, 1977
in hypoadrenocorticism, electrolyte imbalance and, 1768
in urine, renal disease and, 1903
serum levels of, in hypoadrenocorticism, 1761, 1761t, 1762t
Glucose intolerance, exocrine pancreatic insufficiency and, 1540
growth hormone-induced, pathogenesis of, 1596–1597
recognition of, 1597
treatment of, 1597
insulin and, *1598*, 1598–1600, *1599*
ovariohysterectomy and, 1597–1598
Glucose supplementation, in diabetes mellitus, 1688–1689
Glucose tolerance test, in exocrine pancreatic insufficiency, 1545
Glucose-insulin ratios, insulin-secreting tumors and, 1711
Glutamate, hepatic encephalopathy and, 1464
Glutamine, hepatic encephalopathy and, 1464
Glycogen metabolism disorders, 738–739
Glycogen storage diseases, 1511
Glycogenosis, 595
Glycoproteinosis, 595
Glycosuria, renal, 2027–2028
polyuria and polydipsia and, 144
Glycosylated hemoglobin, in diabetes mellitus, 1697
Gonadal hormone abnormalities, cutaneous manifestations of, 6
Gonadotropin-releasing hormone (GnRH), 1583
Gordon setter, cerebellar degeneration in, 597–598
Gout, 2373
Graft-versus-host disease (GVHD), cutaneous manifestations of, 9
Granulocytic leukemia, *2215*, 2216
Granuloma(s), definition of, 126
eosinophilic, 1305–1306
labial, 1232–1233, *1234*
Granulomatosis, bacterial infection associated with, mediastinal, 892
lymphomatoid, 1194
noninfectious, with eosinophilia, mediastinal, 892, *893*
Granulomatous diseases. *See also specific diseases*.
disseminated, neutropenia and, 2200
pulmonary, 839–840
treatment of, 840, *840*, *841*
Granulomatous enteritis, 1366–1367, *1367*
Granulomatous gastritis, 1304
Granulomatous meningoencephalitis, 607–608, 657–658, *657–659*
coma and stupor and, 62
Granulopoiesis, immune suppression of, 2201
Gray platelet syndrome, 2271
Great arteries, transposition of, cyanotic heart disease and, 1022–1023
Great Dane, calcium phosphate deposition disease in, 640
Griseofulvin, 402
Grooming, excessive, 72
in cats, 237
Growth factor, insulin-like, in pituitary-hypothalamic disease, 1602–1603, *1604–1606*
Growth hormone (GH), deficiency of, bone abnormalities and, 2385
in mature dog, 1589–1590, *1590*, *1591*
diabetes mellitus induced by, 1594–1596
excess of, in cats, 1602, *1603*, *1604*
in dogs, historic signs and laboratory findings in, 1596, 1596, *1597*
glucose intolerance induced by, pathogenesis of, 1596–1597
in insulin antagonism/resistance, 1702, *1702*, *1703*
pituitary-hypothalamic diseases and, 1579

Growth hormone (GH) *(Continued)*
secretion of, in canine hyperadrenocorticism, 1734–1735, 1735t
Growth hormone dependent syndromes, cutaneous manifestations of, 7
Growth hormone-releasing hormone (GH-RH), 1583
GVHD. *See* Graft-versus-host disease.

Habitus, adverse drug reactions and, 500
Half-life, pharmacokinetics and, 379–380, 380t
Hallucinogens, behavioral signs of, 73
Hammondia, 282
Haploidy, 184
Haptens, 2283
Harelip, 771, *773*, 1231, *1232*
HDL. *See* Lipoprotein(s), high density.
Head, evaluation of, anorexia and, 16
polyphagia and, 16
respiratory disease and, diagnosis of, 749–750
Head trauma, coma and stupor and, 62, 63
Head-bobbing, 74
Hearing, inner ear disease and, 260
Heart. *See also entries beginning with* Cardiac.
cardiopulmonary arrest and, 171–173
cardiopulmonary resuscitation and, 172, 173–180
hypertrophy of, heart failure and, 910–911, *911*
hypokalemia and, physiology of, 1763–1764, *1765*, 1766
radiographic interpretation and, in respiratory disease, 758, *759*
Heart block, complete, 1088, *1091*, 1092
Heart disease. *See also* Cardiac valvular disease; Cardiomyopathy; Heart failure; Heart murmur; *specific diseases.*
congenital, 976–1027
cardiac valve malformation and, 1000–1014
causes of, 977t, 985–986
classification of, 986
clinical evaluation of, 976–984
angiocardiography in, 980, 982
cardiac catheterization in, 982, *983*, 984, *984*
cardiac imaging in, 977–980, *979*
electrocardiography in, 980, *980–982*
history and physical examination in, 976t, 976–977
cyanotic, 1014, 1017–1023
clinical evaluation of, 1017–1018
clinical manifestations of, 1017
double outlet right ventricle and, 1022
pulmonary atresia and, 1023
tetralogy of Fallot and, 1018–1022, *1019*
transposition of great arteries and, 1022–1023
tricuspid valve dysplasia and, 1022
drugs used in, 1030t
malformations causing systemic to pulmonary shunting and, 986–1000
prevalence of, 985t, 985–986
vascular anomalies and, 1024, 1027
aortic, 1024, *1026*, 1027
venous, *1026*, 1027
polycythemia and, therapeutic principles for, 103–104
syncope due to, 52–53
Heart failure, 899t, 899–921
acute, 900
backward, 900
causes of, 899t, 911–915
diastolic mechanical inhibition as, 915
pressure overloading as, *912*, *913*, 913–914
systolic mechanical overload as, 913
ventricular contractility and, *912*, 912–913, *913*
chronic, 900
circulatory, 899
classification and staging of, 942
clinical manifestations of, *912*, *913*, 915t, 915–917
compensated, 900
compensatory mechanisms and, *907*, 907–911
cardiac hypertrophy and, 910–911, *911*
renal-adrenal-pituitary interactions and, 908–910, *909*

Heart failure *(Continued)*
compensatory mechanisms and, sympathetic nervous system and, 907–908, *909*, *910*
congestive, 900
in canine hyperadrenocorticism, 1735
liver disease and, 1484
pleural effusion due to, 877
decompensated, 900
detriments of cardiac output and, 900–907, 901t, *902*
afterload and, 905, *906*
contractility and, 905–907, *906*
heart rate and, 901, *902*
preload and, 901–902, *903*, 904, *904*
forward, 900
functional classification of, 899t, 917, 917t
generalized, 900
high output, 900
left-sided, 900
myocardial, 899
refractory, 900
right-sided, 900
treatment of, 917–920, 939–969
β-adrenergic blockers in, 963–964
afterload and, 941
ancillary therapy in, 966–967
angiotensin-converting enzyme inhibitors in, 961–963
arteriolar vasodilation and, 918–919, *919*
bipyridine derivatives in, 953–954
blood volume depletion and venodilation and, 918, *918*
calcium antagonists in, 964–965
contractility and, 940–941
dietary, 965–966
cardiac cachexia and, 965–966
sodium restriction and, 965
diuretics in, 954–957
loop, 955–956
potassium-sparing, 957
thiazide, 956–957
drugs used in, 975t
heart rate and, 942
increased contractility and afterload reduction and, *919*, 919–920
integrated therapeutic strategies and, 967–969
myocardial oxygen demand and, 942
positive inotropic drugs in, 942–953
preload and, 941
vasodilators in, 957–961
Heart murmur, cyanosis and, 97–98
polycythemia and, 103
Heart muscle, automaticity of, 1053, 1054–1055
agents increasing, 1059
conductivity of, *1054*, 1056
cardiac arrhythmias and, 1056
contractility of, 1056
cardiac output and, 905–907, *906*
heart failure therapy and, 940–941
diseases of. *See* Cardiomyopathy; *specific diseases.*
excitability of, *1055*, 1055–1056
Heart rate, cardiac output and, 901, *902*
heart failure therapy and, 942
Heartworm disease, 1163–1182
adulticide treatment of, 1178–1180
drug-resistant infections and, 1179–1180
indications and contraindications for, 1178
interruption of, 1178–1179
thiacetarsamide toxicity and, 1179
brain and, 606
cutaneous manifestations of, 8
diagnosis and treatment of, asymptomatic patients and, 1170
occult heartworm disease pneumonitis and, 1176, *1176*
occult infections and, 1171
pulmonary disease and, 1170–1171
severe pulmonary artery disease and, 1171–1172, *1173–1177*, 1174, 1176
diethylcarbamazine and, 1181
epizootiology of, 1163–1177
cardiopulmonary disease development and, 1163–1166

Heartworm disease *(Continued)*
epizootiology of, pre-treatment evaluation and, 1166–1170
iatrogenic occult infections and, 1181
in humans, 190
prevention of, 190
microfilaremia and, 1181
microfilaricide treatment and, 1180–1181
prophylaxia and, 1181–1182
treatment and prevention of, 1178–1182
Heat. *See also* Estrous cycle.
silent, 1848
Heavy metals, toxic polyneuropathies and, 726t, 726–727
Heinz bodies, 2147, *2149*, 2150, *2155*
Helminth infestations, in developing countries, 221
Hemagglutinins, cold, in immune-mediated hemolytic anemia, 2300
Hemangiomas, splenic, 2237–2238
Hemangiosarcomas, splenic, 2237–2238
Hematochezia, definition of, 36
diarrhea and, 34
Hematocrit, cyanosis and, 98
Hematologic disorders, immunologic, 2299–2305
in liver disease, 1427–1428, *1428*
oral lesions and, 1228
Hematologic manifestations, allergic drug reactions and, 503–504, 505
Hematology. *See also* Erythrocytes.
erythrocyte evaluation and, reference values for, 2156–2157
in feline panleukopenia, 316
in lower urinary tract disease, 2109
in small bowel diarrhea, 1334t, 1334–1335
lymphadenopathy and, 2228
splenomegaly and, 2241, 2241t
techniques for, 2181–2182
blood sample collection and, 2181–2182
technological considerations in, 2145–2156
automated cell counting and, *2146*, 2146–2147, *2147*
erythrocyte fragility and deformability and, 2154–2156, *2155*
erythrocyte morphology and, on Wright's stained blood films, 2147–2153, *2148*
immunoglobulin and complement detection and, 2154
reticulocyte counting and, 2153–2154, *2154*, *2155*
sizing erythrocytes and, *2146*, 2146–2147, *2147*
Hematolymphatic system, corticosteroids and, 417
Hematomas, auricular, of pinna, 251–252
definition of, 126
mineralizing, in dog, 2389
pathophysiology of, 127
splenic, 2238
Hematopoiesis, 2186, *2187*
cyclic, canine, 2200–2201
spleen and, 2235
Hematopoietic space, reduced, neutropenia and, 2200
Hematuria, 160–163, 2028–2031, 2029t
diagnostic approach to, 161t, 161–163
dysuria and, 164
iatrogenic, 160
lower urinary tract, 160
occult blood and, renal disease and, 1903–1904
pathophysiology of, 160–161, 161t
pigmenturia differentiated from, 160
polycythemia and, 102
renal, 2029–2031
idiopathic, in dogs, 2030
renal parasites and, 2030–2031
renal parenchymal, 160
systemic disease and, 160–161
telangiectasia and, in Pembroke Welsh corgis, 2030
treatment goals in, 163
ureteral, 2029–2030
vesicourachal diverticula and, treatment of, 2078
Hemihopping, in neurologic examination, 559, *559*
Hemistanding, in neurologic examination, 559, *559*
Hemivertebrae, etiology and pathogenesis of, 645–646

Hemiwalking, in neurologic examination, 559, *559*
Hemobartonellosis, 276–277, *2166*, 2166–2167
Hemodynamic evaluation, invasive, right heart evaluation and, 935
Hemodynamics, cardiac arrhythmias and, 1057
in infective endocarditis, 1152, *1152*
Hemoglobins, 2158
glycosylated, in diabetes mellitus, 1697
reduced, definition of, 95
dyspnea and tachypnea and, 89
Hemogram, cyanosis and, 98
in diabetes mellitus, 1685
Hemolysins, intravascular, in immune-mediated hemolytic anemia, 2300
Hemolysis, 2168–2170
anemia and. *See* Anemia, hemolytic.
canine, 2168–2169, *2169*
feline, 2169–2170
in anemia, regenerative, 91–92
poisoning and, 469t
treatment of, 2170
Hemoperitoneum, 136
Hemophilia A, arthropathy due to, 2359–2360
Hemorrhage. *See also* Bleeding disorders.
anemia and, 93, 2160–2163
coagulation biochemistry defects and, 2161
iron deficiency, *2161*, 2161–2163, *2162*
thrombocytopenia and, 2160–2161
trauma/lacerations and, 2160
gastrointestinal, 1462
intracerebral, 600
liver failure and, treatment of, 1521
mediastinal, 889, *889*
of spinal cord, 658, 660
Hemostasis
in liver disease, 1428t, 1428–1430, 1430t
laboratory evaluation of, 2249–2252
activated coagulation time and partial thromboplastin time and, 2250–2251
chromogenic substrates and, 2252
fibrin(ogen) degradation products assay and, 2252
fibrinogen assays and, 2251–2252
one-stage prothrombin time and, 2251
quality control and sample collection and, 2249–2250
thrombin time and, 2251
von Willebrand's factor assay and, 2252, 2253t
physiology of, *2246*, 2246–2249, *2247*
fibrinolysis and, 2248–2249, *2249*
hemostatic modulation and, 2248, *2249*
Hemostatic disorders, 2246–2262. *See also* Bleeding disorders; Coagulopathies.
in uremia, 1918
Hepatic coma, treatment of, 1518–1520, 1518t
Hepatic cysts, congenital, 1510
Hepatic disease. *See also specific diseases.*
cutaneous manifestations of, 9
platelet dysfunction in, 2272–2273
pleural effusions associated with, 881
Hepatic encephalopathy. *See* Encephalopathy, hepatic.
Hepatic fibrosis, drug control of, 1517
Hepatic insufficiency, brain and, 618
Hepatic lipidosis, diabetes mellitus and, 1705
Hepatitis, anthelmintic-associated, 1496–1497
chronic, 1484t, 1484–1492
active, 1484–1485
in dogs, 1484t, 1487–1492
copper-associated, in Bedlington terriers, 1488–1491, *1489*
copper-associated, in West Highland white terriers, 1491–1492
dissecting, lobular, 1492
hepatoportal fibrosis and, 1492
in Doberman pinschers, 1491
infectious hepatitis-associated, 1492
leptospirosis-associated, 1492
lobular, 1485
persistent, 1485
infectious, canine, 303–305
clinical signs of, 304–305
diagnosis of, 305
epizootiology of, 303–304
Hepatitis *(Continued)*
infectious, etiology of, 303
ocular manifestations of, 82
treatment and prevention of, 305
Hepatocellular adenoma, 1513
Hepatocellular carcinomas, 1511–1512, *1512*
Hepatomegaly, 137–138
in canine hyperadrenocorticism, 1729
Hepatopathy, anticonvulsant, 1495–1496
glucocorticoid, 1494–1495, *1496*
Hepatoportal fibrosis, chronic hepatitis associated with, in dogs, 1492
Hepatotoxicity, drug reactions and, 505–507, 506t
Hepatozoonosis, 290–291
Hereditary ataxia, in terriers, 599
Heredity. *See* Genetic factors.
Hernia, diaphragmatic, *868*, 868–869
history and, 868
management of, 868–869
pericardial, peritoneal, 869, *869*
peritoneopericardial, 1024, *1025*
traumatic, pleural effusion caused by, 883
perineal, 1561–1563
history and presenting signs in, 1562, *1562*, *1563*
incidence and etiology of, 1561–1562
treatment of, 1562–1563
peritoneopericardial, 1135, *1136*
Herpesvirus, brain and, 6403
canine, gastroenteritis and, 309
feline, ocular manifestations of, *78*, 83
Herpetiform dermatitis, canine, 2318
Heteroploidy, 184
Hickey-Hare test, tubular function and, 1899
Hip joint, dysplasia of, 2355–2358, *2357*, *2358*
luxations and subluxations of, 2340, *2341*
Histiocytic ulcerative colitis, 1410
Histoplasma colitis, 1412
Histoplasmosis, 351–354
clinical manifestations of, 351–352, 354–355
cryptococcosis and, canine, 355
feline, 354–355, *355*
in cats, 351–352
in dogs, 352
diagnosis of, *352*, 352–353, *353*, *355*, 355–356, *356*
etiology and epizootiology of, *341*, 351
intestinal, 1359–1361, *1360*
ocular manifestations of, 82
osteomyelitis and, 2380
pathogenesis of, 351, 354
prognosis in, 356
pulmonary manifestations of, 833–834
treatment of, 353–354, 356
Hookworms, in developing countries, 221
small bowel diarrhea and, 1342t–1343t, *1345*, 1346–1347
Hopping, in neurologic examination, 559, *560*
Hormone(s). *See also* Pituitary-hypothalamic diseases; *specific hormones.*
acquired immunodeficiencies and, 2299
alopecia and, 120
anemia and, 92
canine mammary gland tumors and, 1824
growth. *See* Growth hormone.
hypophysiotropic, 1583
in cancer chemotherapy, 533, 535
metabolism of, liver disease and, 1426, 1426t
pituitary, 1584, 1584–1585
vaginal changes induced by, 1778–1779, *1780–1781*
Host, modification of, 2295
Host defense, of lower urinary tract, compromise of, 2116
Hound ataxia, 661
Housebreaking, of dogs, 231
Howell-Jolly bodies, 2150
H_2-receptor antagonists, gastric ulceration and, 1310
Human(s), aggression toward, in cats, 236–237
alopecia and, 115
attitudes of, 239–240
bites and, animal management and, 300
Human(s) *(Continued)*
owner management problems and, infertility and, in bitch, 1050, 1840–1842, *1842–1844*, 1846–1847
pruritus and, 123
rabies vaccination for, 300
zoonoses and, 188–193, 189t
bacterial, 191–192
ectoparasitic, 191
mycotic, 192
parasitic, 188–190
Human-animal bond, 239–244
animal-facilitated therapy and, 241–242
euthanasia and, 244
pet ownership and, 239–240
pets' roles and, 240t, 240–241, 241t
veterinarians and, 242–243
breaking bonds and, 243
maintaining bonds and, 242–243
making bonds and, 242
Humerus, medial condyle of, osteochondritis dissecans of, 2354, *2355*
Humoral immunity, 2284
Humoral theories, acupuncture and, 487–488, *489*
Hydatidosis, in developing countries, 221
Hydralazine, actions of, 958
in heart failure therapy, 958–959
indications for, 958–959
toxicity and interactions of, 959
Hydranencephaly, 591
Hydration, respiratory disease and, diagnosis of, 749
Hydrocephalus, 588–591
behavioral signs of, 74
clinical signs of, *584*, *587*, 588–590, *589*, *590*
treatment of, 590–591
Hydrochloric acid, gastric secretion of, 1291
production of, 1291, *1292*
Hydrocortisone, in hypoadrenocorticism, electrolyte imbalance and, 1768
Hydromyelia, 692–693, *693*
Hyperadrenocorticism, 739–740
bone disease and, 2382
canine, 1721
complications of, 1735–1736
differential diagnosis of, 1735t, 1736
history in, 1725–1729
in-hospital evaluation of, 1730–1735
o,p'-DDD therapy in, 1750–1753
pathophysiology of, 1723, *1724*
physical examination in, 1729–1730
pituitary tumors in, treatment of, 1754
pituitary-adrenocortical axis evaluation in, 1736–1745
computed tomography and, 1743
CRH stimulation test and, 1743
discrimination tests and, 1741–1743
general approach to, 1736
metyrapone testing and, 1745
radioisotope imaging and, 1745
screening tests and, 1736–1741
ultrasonography and, 1743, *1744*
signalment and, 1725, *1726*
spontaneous remission of, 1754–1755
treatment of, 1745–1753
adrenal tumor hyperadrenocorticism and, *1745*, 1745–1747, *1746*
aminoglutethimide in, 1753–1754
bromocriptine in, 1753
cyproheptadine in, 1753
ketoconazole in, 1754
metyrapone in, 1754
pituitary-dependent hyperadrenocorticism and, 1747
trilostane in, 1753
using o,p'-DDD, 1747–1751, *1749*, *1751*, 1752
cutaneous manifestations of, 6
feline, 1755–1756
history and physical examination in, 1755, 1755t
in-hospital examination and, 1755–1756
signalment and, 1755
treatment of, 1756

Hyperadrenocorticism *(Continued)*
lymphocytosis and, 2208
polycythemia and, 102
polyuria and polydipsia and, 141–142
thrombocytopathies associated with, 2276
Hyperadrenocorticism-like disease, iatrogenic, corticosteroids and, 423t, *423–425*, 425–426
Hyperbilirubinemia. *See also* Jaundice.
causes of, 13t
Hypercalcemia, 1610–1621
blastomycosis and, 1619
bone disease and, 1618–1619
brain and, 616
causes of, 13t
general considerations in, 1610, *1611*, 1611t
hypervitaminosis D and, 1619
hypoadrenocorticism and, 1615
hypophosphatemia and, 1612
malignancy and, 1610–1615
pancreatitis and, 1534
patient evaluation in, 1611t, 1619–1620, 1620t
polyuria and polydipsia and, 143
primary hyperparathyroidism and, 1616–1618, *1617*
renal disease and, 1615–1616
treatment of, 1620–1621
weakness and, 48, 48t
Hypercalciuria, hypercalcemic, in canine calcium oxalate urolithiasis, 2099
normocalcemic, in canine calcium oxalate urolithiasis, 2099–2100
Hyperchloremia, causes of, 13t
Hypercholesterolemia, 203. *See also* Hyperlipidemia.
causes of, 13t
Hyperchylomicronemia, idiopathic, hyperlipidemia and, canine, 207
inherited, in cat, *200*, 200t, 200–202, *201*
polyneuropathy with, 725
Hypercoagulation, nephrotic syndrome and, 1942–1943, *1943*
testing for, 2277, 2277t
thrombocytopathies associated with, 2275–2276
Hypercortisolism, functional corticotropic adenoma and, of adenohypophysis, 1591–1592, *1592*
Hyperemia, polycythemia and, 103
Hypereosinophilic syndromes, eosinophilia and, 2210
feline, 1366
Hyperesthenuria, 1899
Hyperesthesia syndromes, canine, 729
feline, 729
behavioral signs of, 73
Hyperfiltration, of glomerular capillaries, renal failure and, 1988–1990
Hyperglycemia, causes of, 13t
insulin-induced, 1698, *1698*, *1699*
recognition of, 1597
Hyperinsulinism polyneuropathy, 725, *726*
Hyperkalemia, 439–440
brain and, 616
causes of, 13t
clinical signs and diagnosis of, 440
etiology of, *437*, 438t, 439–440
in acute renal failure, 1969
treatment of, 1976–1977
in chronic renal failure, therapy for, 1997
in hypoadrenocorticism, causes of, 1763, 1764t
physiology of, heart and, 1763–1764, *1765*, 1766
treatment of, 440
weakness and, 48, 48t, 49t
Hyperkinesis, 74
Hyperlipemia, drug-induced, in cat, 200
nephrotic syndrome and, 1941
Hyperlipidemia, canine, 203–208
clinical recognition of, 205–206
clinical investigation tools and, 206
clinical signs and, 205
laboratory tests and, 205–206
diseases associated with, 206–207
lipid physiology and, 203–205
treatment of, 207t, 207–208
feline, 198–202
diagnosis of, 199, 199t
Hyperlipidemia *(Continued)*
feline, diagnostic tests and, for cholesterol and triglycerides, 199
lipid transport and, lipoproteins in, 198
lipoprotein metabolism and, 198
primary, 200–202
secondary, 199–200
in nephrotic syndrome, 2022
Hyperlipoproteinemia, idiopathic, hyperlipidemia and, canine, 207
pancreatitis and, 1534
Hypernatremia, 436–437, 1603–1605
brain and, 617
causes of, 14t
clinical signs and diagnosis of, 437
etiology of, 435t, 436–437
signs and symptoms of, 1605
treatment of, 437, 1605
with hypovolemia, 617
Hyperoxaluria, in canine calcium oxalate urolithiasis, 2100
Hyperparathyroidism, nutritional, bone disease and, 2382, *2382*
primary, bone disease and, 2382
hypercalcemia and, 1616–1618, *1617*
renal, bone disease and, 2381–2382
secondary, nutritional, 2361
chronic renal failure and, 1923–1924, 1024t
Hyperphosphatemia, causes of, 14t
minimizing, in acute renal failure, 1981
Hyperpigmentation, 119
in canine hyperadrenocorticism, *1728*, 1729
Hyperplasia, adrenocortical, pathology of, 1724–1725
fibrous, periodontal, 1230, *1230*
gingival, *1219*, 1220–1221
nodular, hepatic, 1513
of pituitary, pathology of, 1724
oral, 1230, *1230*
prostatic, benign, 1867–1868
splenomegaly and, pathogenesis of, 2239
vaginal, 1811, *1811*
Hyperploidy, 184
Hyperproteinemia, causes of, 14t
Hypersegmentation, nuclear, of neutrophils, *2189*, 2189–2190
Hypersensitivity diseases, pulmonary, 838–839
Hypersensitivity reactions, *2293*, 2293–2294. *See also* Allergy(ies).
delayed, ocular manifestations of, 76
eosinophilia and, 2210
immediate, allergic drug reactions and, 502–503
ocular manifestations of, 76
to drugs, 2324–2326
diagnosis of, 2326
pathophysiology of, *2325*, 2325t, 2325–2326
prognosis of, 2326
therapy of, 2326
to food. *See* Food hypersensitivity.
type I, 2325, *2325*, 2293
type II, 2325, 2293
type III, 2325–2326, 2293
type IV, 2326, 2294
vasculitis and, 1192–1193
Hypertension, 2047–2054
blood pressure measurement and, *2052*, 2052–2053, *2053*, 2053t
clinical consequences of, *2051*, 2051–2052, *2052*
in chronic renal failure, 2005–2006
in nephrotic syndrome, 1942, *1942*, 2022
normal blood pressure determinants and, 2047–2048
of glomerular capillaries, renal failure and, 1988–1990
pathophysiology of, 2948–2051, 2049t
primary hypertension and, 2048–2049
secondary hypertension and, 2049–2051
portal, 1456–1459, 1457t, *1458*
ascites and, 1458–1459, *1459*
pulmonary, patent ductus arteriosus with, 991, *991*, *992*
systemic, ocular manifestations of, *78*, 79
therapy for, 2053–2054
drugs for, 2056t
Hyperthermia, 23–24, *24*. *See also* Fever.
brain and, 618–619
in cancer therapy, 542–543
biologic considerations and, 542–543
treatment of, 26
Hyperthyroidism, canine, thyroid neoplasia and, 1667–1671
clinical features of, 1668
diagnosis of, 1668–1669
pathology of, 1667t, 1667–1668
prognosis of, 1670–1671
treatment of, 1669–1670
feline, 1654–1667
apathy in, 1658
causes of, 1654–1655
clinical manifestations of, 1655–1658
liver disease and, 1484
screening laboratory tests in, 1658
thyroid function tests and, 1658–1661
treatment of, 1661–1667, 1662t
antithyroid drugs in, 1661–1664, 1662t
radioactive iodine in, 1666–1667
surgical, 1664–1666
myocardial disease and, 1121–1122
in cats, 1121–1122
in dogs, 1122
pleural effusion caused by, 883
polyuria and polydipsia and, *139*, *140*, 144
Hypertriglyceridemia, 203. *See also* Hyperlipidemia.
Hypertrophic cardiomyopathy. *See* Cardiomyopathy, hypertrophic.
Hypertrophic gastropathies. *See* Gastropathy(ies), hypertrophic.
Hypertrophic neuropathy, 725
Hypertrophic osteodystrophy, 2391–2392, *2392*
Hypertrophic osteopathy, 2395, *2395*
as paraneoplastic syndrome, 519–520
Hypertrophy, cardiac, heart failure and, 910–911, *911*
mucinous, cystic, 1557
Hyperuricuria, in canine calcium oxalate urolithiasis, 2100
Hypervariable regions, 2287
Hyperviscosity, as paraneoplastic syndrome, 520–521
paraproteinemias and, 2306
Hypervitaminosis A, arthropathy due to, 2361
bone disorders and, 2387
brain and, 616
of cats, 661
Hypervitaminosis D, bone disorders and, 2385, 2387
hypercalcemia and, 1619
Hypoadrenocorticism, 1756–1771
clinical pathology of, 1760–1763
electrocardiogram in, 1763–1766
etiology of, 1757–1758
primary adrenocortical failure and, 1757
secondary adrenocortical failure and, 1757–1758
feline, *1770*, 1771, *1771*
history and, 1760, 1760t
hormone studies and, 1766–1767
hypercalcemia and, 1615
pathophysiology of, 1758–1759
glandular destruction and, 1759
glucocorticoids and, 1758–1759, *1759*
mineralocorticoids and, 1758, *1758*
sex hormones and, 1759
physical examination in, 1760
polyuria and polydipsia and, 143–144
primary, in dog, treatment of, 1769t, 1769–1770
prognosis of, 1770–1771
radiology in, 1763
secondary, iatrogenic, corticosteroids and, *423*, 424–425
in dog, treatment of, 1770
signalment and, 1759–1760
treatment of, 1767–1770, 1768t
acidosis and, 1768–1769
electrolyte imbalance and, 1767–1768
hypovolemia and, 1767, 1768t
maintenance therapy and, 1769t, 1769–1770
response to, 1769

Hypoalbuminemia, causes of, 14t
in nephrotic syndrome, 1941–1942, 2020–2021
Hypocalcemia, 1621–1629
brain and, 616
causes of, 13t
eclampsia and, 1625–1626
general considerations in, *1611*, 1621t, 1621–1622
hypoparathyroidism and, *1617*, 1623, *1624*, 1625, 1626t, 1627t
treatment of, 1627t, 1629
pancreatitis and, 1627
primary renal disease and, 1622, *1623*, *1624*
symptomatic, 1621
treatment of, 1628–1629
oral therapy in, with vitamin D and calcium, 1628–1629, 1629t
parenteral calcium therapy in, 1626t, 1628
weakness and, 48, 48t
Hypochloremia, causes of, 13t
Hypochondrodysplasia, 2383
Hypochromic cells, 2150, *2153*
Hypofibrinogenemia, hereditary, 2272
Hypogammaglobulinemia, transient, of infancy, 2299
Hypoglossal nerves, focal diseases of, 719
Hypoglycemia, acute, insulin-secreting tumors and, medical therapy for, 1713–1714
brain and, 617
causes of, 13t
chronic, insulin-secreting tumors and, medical therapy for, 1714–1715
hepatic encephalopathy and, 1465–1466
insulin therapy and, 1703–1704
parturition and, 1832–1833
Hypogonadism, hypogonadotrophic, treatment of, 1856–1857
Hypokalemia, 438–439
brain and, 616
causes of, 13t
clinical signs and diagnosis of, 438–439
etiology of, 438, 438t
in acute renal failure, treatment of, 1977
in chronic renal failure, therapy for, 1997–1998, *1998*
polyuria and polydipsia and, 144
treatment of, 439, *439*
weakness and, 48, 48t, 49t
Hypoluteoidism, infertility and, 1845–1846
Hypomyelination, tremor and, 55
Hypomyelinogenesis, 592, *592*
Hyponatremia, 435–436
brain and, 616–617
causes of, 14t
clinical signs and diagnosis of, 436
etiology of, 435t, 435–436
in hypoadrenocorticism, causes of, 1763, 1764t
treatment of, 436
with hypovolemia, 616–617
Hypoparathyroidism, primary, hypocalcemia and, *1617*, 1623, *1624*, 1625, 1626t, 1627t
treatment of, 1627t, 1629
secondary, hypocalcemia and, treatment of, 1629
Hypoperfusion, acute renal failure caused by, *1934–1936*, 1935–1937
Hypophosphatemia, causes of, 14t
hypercalcemia and, 1612, 1616
Hypophysectomy, in pituitary-dependent hyperadrenocorticism, 1747
Hypophysiotropic cells, neurotransmitter regulation of, 1583
Hypophysiotropic concept, 1580–1581
Hypopituitarism, 1588, 1588t
diagnosis of, 1593
in German shepherd, 1588–1589, *1589*, 1589t, *1590*
pituitary tumors and, 1590–1591
Hypoplasia, of coronoid process, 2355, *2356*
of enamel, 1210, *1210*
of trachea, 804–806, 808
features of, 805–806, *806–807*, 808
prognosis and therapy of, 804–806, 808
penile, 1883
Hypoploidy, 184
Hypoproteinemia, causes of, 14t
weight loss and, 4
Hyposegmentation, nuclear, of neutrophils, 2188–2189, *2189*
Hyposensitization, in atopy, 2316
Hypospadias, *1883*, 1883–1884, *1884*, 2135
Hyposthenuria, 1899
Hypothalamic-hypophyseal connections, 1582, *1584*
Hypothalamic-pituitary-thyroid-extrathyroid axis, thyroid hormone secretion and, *1636*, 1637, *1637*
Hypothalamus. *See also* Pituitary-hypothalamic diseases.
anatomy of, 1582
Hypothermia. *See also* Cold.
brain and, 618
cardiopulmonary arrest and, 171–172
treatment of, 26
Hypothyroidism, brain and, 617
canine, 1641–1643
adult-onset, clinical signs in, 1642–1644
secondary hypothyroidism and, 1644
causes of, 1641–1642
congenital hypothyroidism and, 1641
hypothalamic hypothyroidism and, 1642
pituitary hypothyroidism and, 1641–1642
thyroidal hypothyroidism and, 1641
congenital, clinical signs in, 1644
diagnosis of, therapeutic trial for, 1653
iatrogenic, 1641
screening laboratory tests and, 1644–1645
thyroid function tests and, 1645–1649
treatment of, 1649–1653
monitoring therapy and, 1653
therapeutic failure and, 1653
thyroid hormone preparations and, 1650–1652
bioavailability and efficacy of, 1649–1650
dosage of, 1652
overdosage of, 1652–1653
congenital, bone abnormalities and, 2385
cutaneous manifestations of, 6
feline, 1653–1654
causes of, 1653–1654
clinical signs of, 1654
diagnosis of, 1654
treatment of, 1654
hyperlipidemia and, canine, 206–207
feline, 199
myopathy and, 739, *739*
polyneuropathy and, 725
Hypotrichosis, 113
Hypoventilation, alveolar, central cyanosis and, 96
polycythemia and, 102
Hypovitaminosis A, bone disorders and, 2387
brain and, 615
Hypovitaminosis B, brain and, 615–616
Hypovitaminosis C, bone disorders and, 2387
Hypovitaminosis D, bone disorders and, 2387
Hypovolemia, hypernatremia with, 617
hyponatremia with, 617
in hypoadrenocorticism, treatment of, 1767, 1768t
Hypoxemia, arterial, central cyanosis and, 95–96
definition of, 95
cyanosis and, 99–100
in cyanotic heart disease, 1017
Hypoxia, cerebral, 599–600
behavioral signs and, 73
Hysteria, 72

Icterus. *See* Jaundice.
Idiotype network, immune system and, 2292
Idiotypic determinants, immune system and, 2292
Idioventricular beat, 1080
Ileocecal sphincter, 1397
Illness(es), chronic, anemia and, 92
coma and stupor and, 63
infertility and, in bitch, 1848
thyroid hormone metabolism and, 1637–1638
Imidazoles. *See* Antifungal drugs.
Immotile cilia syndrome. *See* Ciliary dyskinesia, primary.
Immune function, of spleen, 2236–2237
small intestine and, 1328
Immune response, 2283–2289
antigen and, 2283
antigen-specific receptors and, 2285–2287
B lymphocytes and, 2285–2287, *2286*
Ig isotype function and, 2287
Ig specificity and, 2287
T lymphocytes and, 2287
TCR and, 2287
cellular interactions in, 2289–2295
diversity and, generation of, *2286*, 2287–2289, *2288*, *2289*
immune system features and, 2283
labor division and, 2283–2284
lymphocyte differentiation and, 2285, *2286*
major histocompatibility complex gene products in, 2289–2293, *2290*
immune system regulation and, 2292–2293
T cell activation and, *2290*, 2291
T-B cell cooperation and, 2291
T-T interactions and, 2291–2292
manipulation of, 2294–2295
host modification and, 2295
vaccination and, 2294–2295
memory and specificity and, 2284, *2284*
primary, 2284
recognition in, *2284*, 2284–2285
secondary, 2284
Immune status, nutritional assessment and, 451
Immune system, abnormalities of, oral lesions and, 1228–1229
regulation of, 2292–2293
Immune-mediated arthritides, treatment of, 2372–2373
Immune-mediated etiology, in chronic inflammatory bowel disease, 1404–1405
Immune-mediated hemolytic anemia, 2299–2303
diagnosis of, 2301–2302
pathophysiology of, 2299–2301
prognosis of, 2303
treatment of, 2302–2303, 2303t
Immune-mediated neutropenia, 2202
Immune-mediated orchitis, treatment of, 1857
Immune-mediated thrombocytopenia, diagnosis of, 2304
pathophysiology of, 2303–2304
prognosis of, 2305
treatment of, 2304–2305
Immunity, cell-mediated, 2284
uremia and, 1918–1919
corticosteroids and, 417
humoral, 2284
Immunodeficiency diseases, 2294, 2298–2299
primary, 2298–2299
combined, 2298
selective IgA deficiency and, 2298–2299
secondary, 2299
Immunodiagnostic tests, in heartworm disease, 1168
Immunodominant sites, 2285
Immunofluorescence test, direct, in bullous pemphigoid, 2323
in immune-mediated thrombocytopenia, 2304
indirect, in systemic lupus erythematosus, *2311*, 2311–2312
Immunogen, 2283
Immunoglobulin(s), fine specificity of, 2287
immune response and, 2285
Immunoglobulin isotypes, 2287
Immunohemolytic anemia, *2163*, 2163–2165
Immunologic diseases, 2293–2294, 2297–2326. *See also specific diseases.*
alopecia and, 120
autoimmunity and, 2294
cross-reacting antigens and, 2297
dermatologic, 2314–2324
drug hypersensitivities and, 2324–2326
drugs for, 2328t
forbidden clone and, 2297
hidden antigens and, 2297
hypersensitivity responses and, *2293*, 2293–2294
immunodeficiency and, 2294, 2298–2299
immunohematologic, 2299–2305
immunoregulatory failure and, 2297–2298, 2298t

Immunologic diseases *(Continued)*
lameness and, in cats, 169
paraproteinemias and, *2305*, 2305–2309
pulmonary, 838–839
pustular and ulcerative, of pinnae, 250
rheumatoid, 2309–2314
self antigens and, alteration of, 2297
Immunologic mechanisms, allergic drug reactions and, 501–502
Immunologic status, adverse drug reactions and, 500
Immunology, 2283–2295
arthritis and, 2366–2367
of lower urinary tract, abnormal, 2116
normal, 2116
of tumors, biologic therapy and, 537
scope of, 2283
Immunomodulators, in cancer therapy, 538–539
Immunoproliferative enteropathy, of Basenji dogs, 1364–1365
Immunoreactivity, serum trypsin-like, in exocrine pancreatic insufficiency, 1542–1543, *1543*
Immunoregulation, failure of, 2297–2298, 2298t
Immunostimulants, canine mammary gland tumors and, 1824
Immunosuppression, corticosteroids and, 419
in chronic inflammatory bowel disease, 1408–1409
in glomerulonephritis, 2017–2018
in granulopoiesis, 2201
Immunotherapy, canine mammary gland tumors and, 1824
Impaction, dental, 1209–1210
Impedance audiometry, brain disease diagnosis and, 588
Impulse formation, cardiac arrhythmias and, 1056
Inborn errors of metabolism, ocular manifestations of, 79
Incisura angularis, 1289
Incontinence, fecal, 1573t, 1573–1574
urinary. *See* Urinary incontinence.
Inderal. *See* Propranolol.
Indirect immunofluorescence test, in systemic lupus erythematosus, *2311*, 2311–2312
Indocyanine green, in liver disease, 1448–1449, 1449t
Infarct, of bone, *2394*, 2394–2395
Infarction, cerebral, 600
Infection(s). *See also* Abscess(es).
acquired immunodeficiencies and, 2299
acute, eosinopenia and, 2211
lymphopenia in, 2209
antimicrobial drugs in, 383. *See also specific drugs*.
bacterial. *See* Bacterial infections.
canine struvite urolithiasis induced by, prevention of, 2093
chronic, weakness and, 47
dermatologic, antimicrobial selection for, 407, 407t
fungal. *See* Fungal infections.
hepatic, inflammatory, 1479–1483, *1481*
in developing countries, *221*, 221–223, *222*
intracytoplasmic inclusions in, 2190–2191, *2191*
in acute renal failure, 1970
lameness and, in cats, 169
laryngeal, 790
liver failure and, treatment of, 1521
mycobacterial, mediastinal, 892
ocular manifestations of, 81
pulmonary, 832
small bowel diarrhea and, 1358–1359
neutrophilia associated with, *2195*, 2195–2196
of chest wall, 871–872
of inner ear, vestibulocochlear nerve and, 718, *718*
of middle ear, facial nerve disorders and, 717
of urinary tract. *See* Urinary tract infections.
orthopedic, antimicrobial selection for, 407–408
pancreatitis and, 1534
pharyngeal, 784
pulmonary, 829–838
bacterial, 830–832
fungal, 833–838
Infection(s) *(Continued)*
pulmonary, pleural effusion associated with, 879
protozoal, 832–833
viral, 829–830
struvite urolithiasis induced by, 2064t, 2068, 2088, 2090t, 2090–2092, 2091t
systemic, antimicrobial selection for, 408
viral. *See* Viral diseases.
weight loss and, 4
Infectious agents, fecal examinations for, 1336
Infectious arthritis. *See* Arthritis, infectious.
Infectious canine hepatitis. *See* Hepatitis, infectious, canine.
Infective endocarditis, 1151–1161
acute versus subacute forms of, 1151–1152
clinical manifestations of, 1154–1155
history and clinical signs and, 1154–1155
physical examination and, 1155, *1155*, *1156*
diagnosis of, 1155–1159
blood cultures in, 1155–1156
echocardiography in, 1157, *1158*
electrocardiography in, 1156, *1157*
laboratory findings in, 1157, 1159
radiography in, 1156–1157, *1158*
etiology of, 1152
incidence and distribution of, 1151
management of, 1159–1160
antimicrobials in, 1159, 1160t
valve replacement in, 1160
pathogenesis of, *1152*, 1152–1153
pathology of, 1153–1154
cardiovascular, 1153–1154, *1154*
extracardiac, 1154, *1154*
prognosis for, 1160–1161
prophylaxis for, 1160
Infertility, 1838–1857
in bitch, 1838–1851
apparent, 1842
bacterial infections and, 1843–1845, 1844t
Brucella infection and, 1842–1843
Brucella-negative bitch and, 1840–1842
general health and, 1842
male and, 1840, *1842*
owner management practices and, 1840–1842, *1843*, *1844*
chronic endometritis and, 1845
early fetal resorption and, 1845
failure to cycle and, 1848–1850
estrus induction and, 1049–1050, 1050t
glucocorticoid excess and, 1848
premature ovarian failure and, 1849
primary versus secondary failure to cycle and, 1849
sexual development disorders and, 1848–1849
silent heat and, 1848
surgical diagnosis of, 1849
underlying disease and, 1848
failure to permit breeding and, 1050–1051
behavior and, 1050
congenital anomalies and, 1050–1051
mismanagement and, 1050
history and, 1838, 1839t–1840t
hypoluteoidism and, 1845–1846
miscellaneous causes of, 1846
physical examination and, 1838, 1840, *1841*
uterine or oviduct occlusion and, 1846
with prolonged interestrus intervals, 1847–1848
in-hospital evaluation and, 1847–1848
owner management practices and, *1842*, 1847
with shortened interestrus intervals, 1846–1847
owner management problems and, 1846–1847
physiopathology of, *1842*, 1846
split heats and, *1844*, 1847
treatment of, 1847
in male, 1851–1857
classification of, 1851, 1851t
diagnosis of, 1840, *1842*, 1851, 1853, *1853–1855*
history and, 1851, 1852t
physical examination and, 1851
treatment of, 1853, 1855–1857
hypogonadotrophic hypogonadism and, 1856–1857
Infertility *(Continued)*
in male, treatment of, immune-mediated orchitis and, 1857
Leydig cell failure and, 1855–1856
primary spermatogenesis failure and, 1853, 1855
primary testicular failure and, 1853
retrograde ejaculation and, 1857
Infiltrative splenomegaly, pathogenesis of, 2240
Inflammation. *See also* Inflammatory diseases; *specific diseases*.
alopecia and, 114, 120
anti-inflammatory agents and, corticosteroids as, 419
in idiopathic lower urinary tract disease, 2080
in otitis externa, 255
nonsteroidal, thrombocytopathies induced by, 2274, 2274t
chronic, weakness and, 47
coma and stupor and, 62
eosinophilia and, 2210
gastric motility disorders and, 1313
neutrophilia associated with, *2195*, 2195–2196
of gallbladder and bile ducts, 1557
of nervous system, 554
of salivary glands, 1251, *1251*
pathophysiology of, 126–127
Inflammatory bowel disease, chronic, diarrhea and, 1362–1367
idiopathic, 1404–1409
clinical findings in, 1405
colonoscopic findings in, *1401*, 1406
etiology of, 1404–1405
histologic findings in, 1406
laboratory findings in, 1405
pathophysiology of, 1405
prognosis of, 1409
radiographic findings in, 1406
treatment of, 1406–1409
liver disease and, 1483–1484
Inflammatory diseases, hepatic, 1479–1499
infectious, 1479–1483, *1481*
noninfectious, 1483
primary, 1484t, 1484–1499
secondary, 1483–1484
of bone, 2378–2379
of brain, 601–609
bacterial, 604–605
mycotic, 605–606
of unknown cause, 607–609
parasitic, metazoal, 606–607
protozoal, 606
rickettsial, 604
viral, 601–604
of large intestine, 1404–1415
Inflammatory splenomegaly, pathogenesis of, 2238t, 2238–2239
Infundibular process, 1582
Ingestive behavior problems. *See also* Polyphagia.
in cats, 237
vomiting and, time relationship of, 28–29
Inhibitory surround theory, acupuncture and, 487
Injuries. *See also* Trauma.
anal, 1573
categorization and prioritization of, 210–211
to lips and cheeks, 1231–1232, *1232*
to salivary glands, 1242, *1247–1250*, 1249, 1251
to tongue, 1233–1234, *1234*, *1235*
Inner ear, infections of, vestibulocochlear nerve and, 718, *718*
Inotropes, positive, 942–953
Insecticide intoxication, 466
Insulin, antagonism/resistance and, 1700, 1700t, *1701*
acidosis and, 1702
anti-insulin antibodies and, 1702–1703
epinephrine and, 1702
glucocorticoids and, *1701*, 1701–1702
growth hormone and, 1702
norepinephrine and, 1702
progesterone and, 1700–1701
renal failure and, 1702
subcutaneous degradation and, 1703, *1704*

Insulin *(Continued)*
basal, determination of, insulin-secreting tumors and, 1710–1711, 1711t
glucose intolerance and, 1598, 1598–1600, *1599*
in hyperkalemia, in acute renal failure, 1977
in hypoadrenocorticism, electrolyte imbalance and, 1768
plasma levels of, in canine hyperadrenocorticism, 1730
rapid metabolism of, *1699*, 1699–1700, *1700*
Insulin therapy, 1689–1691
alternative approaches for, 1690–1691
complications of, 1697–1704
dietary therapy in, nonketotic diabetes and, 1694–1696, *1694–1696*, 1696t
intermittent intramuscular regimen for, 1690
in nonketotic diabetes, 1692, *1693*, 1693t
Insulin-glucose ratios, insulin secreting tumors and, 1711
Insulin-like growth factors, 1585, *1586*, 1587
in pituitary-hypothalamic disease, 1602–1603, *1604–1606*
Intact nephron hypothesis, chronic renal failure and, 1921
Integumentary disorders, congenital and hereditary, ocular manifestations of, 77
Intensive care, cardiopulmonary arrest and, 179
Interfered P wave, 1080
Interfollicular stage, feline, 1788
Intermittent therapy, with corticosteroids, 422
Intersexuality, infertility and, 1849
Interstitial cell tumors, 1815
Intervertebral disk disease, 661–670
clinical findings in, 663–664
diagnosis of, 664–666, *665–668*
etiology and pathogenesis of, 661–663, *662*
treatment of, 666–669
chemonucleolysis and, 670
type I disk extrusion and, 666–669, 668t
type II disk protrusion and, 669
Intestinal lymphangiectasia. *See* Lymphangiectasia, intestinal.
Intestinal phase, of gastric secretion, 1291
Intestine(s). *See also* Anal diseases; Gastrointestinal diseases; Gastrointestinal tract; Rectal diseases; *specific diseases.*
large, bacterial infections of, 1413–1415
drugs for, 1420t
eosinophilic colitis and, 1409–1410
evaluation of, 1398–1404
endoscopy in, 1400–1402
examination and laboratory evaluation of, 1399–1400
history and clinical signs in, 1398, 1399t
radiography in, 1402–1404
fungal infections of, 1412–1413
histiocytic ulcerative colitis and, 1410
idiopathic chronic inflammatory bowel disease and, 1404–1409
clinical findings in, 1405
colonoscopic findings in, *1401*, 1406
etiology of, 1414–1405
histologic findings in, 1406
laboratory findings in, 1405
pathophysiology of, 1405
prognosis of, 1409
radiographic findings in, 1406
treatment of, 1406–1409
idiopathic megacolon and, 1415–1416
injury to, 1416–1417
intussusception and, 1416
irritable bowel syndrome and, 1416
neoplasia of, 1417–1418, 1565–1566
diagnosis of, 1566, *1566*
history and physical findings in, *1565*, 1565–1566, *1566*
treatment of, 1566
normal function of, 1397–1398
absorption and, 1398
microflora and, 1398
motility and, 1397–1398
secretions and, 1398
normal structure of, 1397
parasitic diseases of, 1410–1412
Intestine(s) *(Continued)*
motility of, 1327–1328, 1330, 1397–1398
diarrhea and, 33
small, anatomy of, 1323–1324, *1324*
diarrhea and. *See* Diarrhea, small bowel.
digestion and absorption and, 1324–1327, *1325*
diseases of, neoplastic, 1376–1379
treatment of, 1385–1389
duodenal ulcers and, 1379–1380, *1380*
endocrine function and, 1328
microflora of, exocrine pancreatic insufficiency and, 1540
motility of, 1327–1328
deranged, diarrhea caused by, 1330
mucosa of, exocrine pancreatic insufficiency and, *1539*, 1539–1540
obstruction of, 1380–1381, *1380–1384*, 1385
water and solute transport and, 1327
Intracytoplasmic inclusions, in congenital diseases, 2191–2192, *2192*
in infectious diseases, 2190–2191, *2191*
Intradermal skin test, in atopy, 2315
Intrapericardiac masses, 1133, 1135, 1149
Intravenous fluids, cardiopulmonary response to, 177
Intravenous pyelography. *See* Excretory urography.
Intussusception, 1416
Iodine, metabolism of, thyroid gland and, *1633*, 1633–1634
radioactive, in feline hyperthyroidism, 1666–1667
thyroid tumors and, in dog, 1670
Ion imbalances, divalent. *See* Divalent ion imbalances.
Irish setter, hereditary quadriplegia and amblyopia in, 597
Iron deficiency anemia. *See* Anemia, iron deficiency.
Iron intoxication, 479–480
differentiation of, 459t–464t, 467t, 480
Irritable bowel syndrome, 1416
Irritation, poisoning and, 467
Ischemia, acute renal failure caused by, *1934–1936*, 1935–1937
myocardial dysfunction and, 1123
pain from, 19
pancreatitis and, 1535
Ischemic encephalopathy, feline, 600–601
Ischemic myelopathy, due to fibrocartilaginous embolism, 670–671
Ischemic neuropathies, 723
Ischemic tubular necrosis, 1965t, 1965–1966, 1966t
Islet cells, transplantation of, in diabetes mellitus, 1706–1707
tumors of. *See* Tumor(s), islet cell.
Isoerythrolysis, neonatal, 2166
Isoproterenol, cardiopulmonary response to, 177
in heart failure therapy, 949
indications for, 949
Isorhythmic dissociation, 1081
Isospora, small bowel diarrhea and, *1345*, 1348–1349
Isosthenuria, 1899
Isotypes, 2286
of immunoglobulins, 2287
Itching. *See also* Pruritus.
Ito cells, 1424

Jack Russell terrier, hereditary ataxia in, 660
Jaundice, 108–112
anemia and, 93
cholestasis versus, 108
definition of, 108
detection of, 108
diagnostic approach to, *110*, 111
pathophysiology of, 108–111, *109*
treatment of, 111–112
Jaw(s), 1215–1216
dropped, 1215–1216
malocclusion of, 1215, *1215*, *1216*
mandibular neuropraxia and, 1215–1216
masticatory muscle myositis and, 741–742
clinical features of, 741–742
management of, 742
Jaw(s) *(Continued)*
masticatory muscle myositis and, pathogenesis of, 741, *742*
rubber, renal failure and, 1982
temporomandibular joint abnormalities and, 1207, 1216
Jaw-champing, 74
Joint diseases, 2329–2373, 2330t. *See also* Arthritis; Arthropathy(ies).
degenerative, 2329–2336
clinical signs of, 2331
pathologic findings in, *2333–2335*, 2333–2336
primary, 2329–2331
radiographic sings of, 2331–2333, *2332*
secondary, 2331, 2331t
treatment of, 2336
developmental, 2346–2359
confrontational abnormalities and, 2346
physeal disorders and, 2346–2347
dietary, 2361
inborn errors of metabolism and, 2359–2361
inflammatory, 2362–2373
infectious, 2362–2366
noninfectious, 2366–2373
meniscal, 2344–2345
calcification and, 2344–2345
tears and, 2344
neoplastic, 2361–2362
neuropathic arthropathy and, 2345–2346
noninflammatory, 2329–2362
sesamoid bone and, 2345
traumatic, 2336–2344
articular cartilage damage and, 2337, *2337*
luxations and subluxations and, 2337–2343
soft tissue damage and, 2337
spinal articular instabilities and, 2343–2344
temporomandibular instabilities and, 2343
Junctional diversity, 2288

Kennel cough. *See* Bordetellosis; Tracheobronchitis, infectious.
Keratoconjunctivitis sicca, ocular manifestations of, 76
Kerry blue terrier, cerebellar degeneration in, 597
Ketoacidosis, diabetes mellitus and, 1705
pathophysiology of, 1678–1680, *1679,* 1681
patient evaluation in, 1685
therapy and, 1686
treatment of, 1691–1692
Ketoconazole, in canine hyperadrenocorticism, 1754
in feline hyperadrenocorticism, 1756
α-Ketoglutarate, hepatic encephalopathy and, 1464
Ketones, in urine, renal disease and, 1903
Kidney. *See also headings beginning with term* Renal.
end-stage, 1985
polycystic, 2024–2025, *2025*
Killer cells, 2284
Kindling, seizures and, 67
Krabbe type leukodystrophy. *See* Leukodystrophy, globoid cell.
Kupffer cells, 1423–1424

Labor. *See also* Parturition.
early onset of, 1828
Laboratory studies, cardiac arrhythmias and, 1058
gastric disease and, 1294–1296, *1295*
hemostasis and. *See* Hemostasis, laboratory evaluation of.
in canine hypothyroidism, 1644–1645
in chronic inflammatory bowel disease, 1405
in chronic mitral valvular insufficiency, 1038
in chronic renal failure, 1926, 1981–1983, *1982*
in congenital heart disease, 977
in exocrine pancreatic insufficiency, 1542–1546
in feline hyperthyroidism, 1658
in feline panleukopenia, 316
in glomerular disease, 1943–1945
in hyperlipidemia, canine, 205–206
feline, 199
in infective endocarditis, 1157, 1159

Laboratory studies *(Continued)*
in liver disease, 1421–1422
in nephrotic syndrome, 2007–2009
in pancreatitis, 1535–1536, *1536*
in urinary tract infection, bacterial, 2117, 2118
Labrador retriever, type 2 myofiber deficiency of, 738
Lacerations, hemorrhage and, anemia and, 2160
β-Lactamase inhibitors, 390–391
activity spectrum of, 390–391
clinical pharmacology of, 391
Lactate dehydrogenase, abnormal values of, causes of, 13t
Lactation, 1833–1834
agalactia and, 1833
corticosteroids and, 417
inadequate, 1833–1834
mammary congestion and, 1834
mastitis and, 1834
Lameness, in cats, 169–170
evaluation of, 170
pathophysiology of, 169–170, 170t
in dogs, 165–168
evaluation of, 166t, 166–168
pathophysiology of, 165, 165t
Large intestines. *See* Intestine(s), large.
Larval migrans, brain and, 607
cutaneous, in humans, 189
prevention of, 189
visceral, in humans, 188
prevention of, 188
Larynx, collapse of, 791–792, *792*, *793*
diagnostic approach to, 751
disorders of, 789–793
diagnosis of, 788–789, *789*
foreign bodies in, 790
infection of, 790
neoplasia of, 792–793
paralysis of, *790*, 790–791, *791*
paresis or paralysis of, glossopharyngeal or vagus nerve lesions and, 719
spasm of, 790
structure and function of, 788
trauma to, 789
Laserpuncture, 493–494
Lassitude. *See also* Weakness.
definition of, 46
LDL, 204
Lead intoxication, 469–470
bone disorders and, 2396
differentiation of, 459t, 460t, 470
Legal considerations, acupuncture and, 496
Leiomyomas, gastric, *1299*, 1317
Leishmaniasis, 289–290
cutaneous manifestations of, 7–8
ocular manifestations of, 81
Lentivirus infection, hematopoietic stem cell death and, 2200
Leptocytosis, 2150, 2153
Leptomeningeal cysts, 686–687, *688*
Leptospirosis, 269–270
chronic hepatitis associated with, in dogs, 1492
in humans, 192
prevention of, 192
Lethargy. *See also* Weakness.
behavioral signs and, 71t, 71–72
definition of, 46
in canine hyperadrenocorticism, 1727
polycythemia and, 102
Leukemia(s), basophilic, 2216
basophils and, 2213–2214
clinical signs and physical findings in, 2214
eosinophilic, 2216
erythemic myelosis and, 2216
erythroleukemia and, 2216
feline, 324–330
aplastic anemia and, 2174
control of, 329–330
diagnostic tests for, 328–329
diseases associated with, 328, 328t
etiology of, 324–325
hematopoietic stem cell death and, 2199
immunosuppression induced by, 327
latent infections and, 327–328, 328t
Leukemia(s) *(Continued)*
feline, neutropenia and, 2201
non-regenerative anemia associated with, *2172*, 2172–2173
oncogenesis and, 327
pathogenesis of, 326–328
stages and, 326t, 326–327
persistent viremia and, consequences of, 327
prevalence of, 326
pulmonary manifestations of, 830
structural proteins in, 325
transmission of, 326
treatment of, 329
virus subgroups and, 325–326
granulocytic, *2215*, 2216
incidence and etiology of, 2214
lymphocytic, *2215*, 2217
mast cell, 2216
megakaryocytic, 2216–2217
monocytic, *2215*, 2216
myelomonocytic, *2215*, 2216
plasma cell, *2215*, 2217
polycythemia vera and, 2216
Leukemoid reactions, neutrophilia associated with, 2196–2197
Leukocyte(s), 2181–2217. *See also* Basophil(s); Eosinophil(s); Lymphocyte(s); Monocyte(s); Neutrophil(s).
bone marrow examination and, 2183, 2184t, 2185
buffy coat smears and, 2185
hematology techniques and, 2181–2182
hematopoiesis and, 2186, *2187*
in hypoadrenocorticism, 1760–1761
reference intervals and, 2185t, 2185–2186, 2186t
Leukocyte count, correction of, for nucleated erythrocytes, 2183
differential, 2183, 2184t
estimation of, 2182
quantitative, 2182–2183
electronic particle counters and, 2182–2183
manual, 2182
quantitative buffy coat analysis and, *2182*, 2183
Leukocyte esterase, in urine, renal disease and, 1904
Leukocytosis, neutrophilic, extreme, 2196–2197
Leukodystrophy, Dalmatian, 596
fibrinoid, 596
globoid cell, 596, 656–657, 724
Krabbe type. *See* Leukodystrophy, globoid cell.
metachromatic, 596
Leukoencephalomyelopathy, of Rottweilers, 597, 671–672
Leukograms, interpretation of, absolute cell counts for, 2183
Leydig cell failure, treatment of, 1856
Leydig cell tumors, 1815
LH. *See* Luteinizing hormone.
Lichenification, 119
Licking, self-mutilation and, 71
Lidocaine (Xylocaine), 1062–1063
cardiopulmonary response to, 177
Limb(s), disuse of, pain and, 20
Limb posture, in neurologic examination, 557, *558*
Limb shortening, 2347–2348
Lincosamides, 400t, 400–401
action of, 401
activity spectrum of, 400t, 400–401
clinical pharmacology of, 401
Linear tomography, spinal cord disease and, 628
Lip(s), cheilitis and, 1232, *1233*
congenital anomalies of, 1231, *1232*
dermatitis of, 1232, *1233*
granuloma of, 1232–1233, *1234*
injuries of, 1231–1232, *1232*
neoplasms of, 1233
Lipid(s). *See also* Hyperlipidemia.
in canine hyperadrenocorticism, 1731–1732
metabolism of, disorders of, ocular manifestations of, 77, *78*
in liver disease, 1431–1432
plasma, in liver disease, 1432–1433
platelets and, 2266
renal failure and, 1990–1991
Lipid storage disease, ocular manifestations of, 79
Lipidosis, hepatic, 1507–1510, *1509*
diabetes mellitus and, 1705
Lipofuscinosis, ceroid, neuronal, ocular manifestations of, 79
Lipoprotein(s), 203–208, *204*, 205t. *See also* Hyperlipoproteinemia.
abnormal, 205
high density (HDL), 204–205
in lipid transport, 198
low density (LDL), 204
metabolism of, 198
plasma, in liver disease, 1432–1433
very low density (VLDL), 203–204
Lipoprotein lipase activity, 199
β-Lipotropic hormone (β-LPH), function of, 1722
Lissencephaly, 591, *591*
Litter box, elimination behavior problems and, in cats, 236
Liver. *See also headings beginning with term* Hepatic.
biopsy of, in hyperadrenocorticism, 1741
corticosteroids and, 416
functions of, 1421t
hematologic and hemostatic functions of, 1427
intermediary metabolism and, 1426, 1426t, 1427t
physioanatomic features of, 1422–1425
anatomy and, 1422–1424, *1423*
biliary system and bile production and, 1424, 1425t
blood supply and, 1422
enterohepatic circulation and, 1425
hepatic regeneration and, 1424–1425
hepatic size alterations and, 1425, 1425t
trauma to, 1484
Liver disease, 1421–1470, 1479–1522. *See also specific diseases.*
acid-base disorders and, 1461–1462
amino acid regulation and, 1435–1436
ammonia and urea metabolism and, 1451, 1453–1456, *1454*
fasting blood ammonia and ammonia tolerance testing and, 1449t, 1455–1456, *1456*, *1457*
ammonium urate crystalluria or calculi and, 1456
bile acids and, 1449t, 1449–1451, *1450*, *1452*, *1453*
bilirubin metabolism and, 1443–1446, *1444*, 1446t, *1447*, 1448
carbohydrate metabolism and, 1431
cholestatic, hyperlipidemia and, canine, 207
coagulopathy in, 2256–2258
clinical aspects of, 2257
laboratory aspects of, 2257–2258
pathophysiology of, 2256–2257
treatment of, 2258
drug-induced, 1493t, 1493–1497
anticonvulsants and, 1495–1496
anthelmintics and, 1496–1497
glucocorticoids and, 1494–1495, *1496*
inhalant anesthetics and, 1497
gastrointestinal ulceration and hemorrhage and, 1462, *1462*
hematologic abnormalities in, 1427–1428, *1428*
hemostasis and, 1428t, 1428–1430, 1430t
hepatic biopsy and, 1469t, 1469–1470
hepatic encephalopathy and, 1462–1466, *1463*
ammonia and, 1463–1464
aromatic amino acids and, 1464
blood-brain barrier and, 1465
cerebral sensitivity and, 1465
false neurotransmitters and, 1465
glutamate and, 1464
glutamine and, 1464
hypoglycemia and, 1465–1466
inhibitory neurotransmitters and, 1465
α-ketoglutarate and, 1464
mercaptans and, 1464
methionine and, 1464
neuroreceptor alterations and, 1465
neurotransmitters and, 1465
short-chain fatty acids and, 1464
in persistent estrus, 1796
inflammatory, 1479–1499
infectious, 1479–1483, *1481*
noninfectious, 1483

Liver disease (Continued)
inflammatory, noninfectious, primary, 1484t, 1484–1499
secondary, 1483–1484
laboratory diagnosis of, 1421–1422
lipid metabolism and, 1431–1432
liver enzymes and, 1436t, 1436–1441
abnormalities of, causes of, 1441–1443
alanine aminotransferase and, 1436–1437
alkaline phosphatase and, 1438–1439
alpha-fetoprotein and, 1442–1443
arginase and, 1437–1438
aspartate aminotransferase and, 1437
gamma-glutamyl transferase and, 1439–1441, *1440*
neoplastic, 1511–1513
metastatic, 1513
nonepithelial, 1513
primary tumors and, 1511t, 1511–1513
noninflammatory, 1499–1511
vascular, 1499–1507
organic anion cholephilic dyes and, 1448–1449, 1449t
plasma electrolyte, fluid, and renal disorders and, 1459–1461
plasma lipids and lipoproteins and, 1432–1433
polyuria and polydipsia and, *139*, 142
portal hypertension and, 1456–1459, 1457t, *1458*
ascites and, 1458–1459, *1459*
protein synthesis and regulation and, 1433–1435
albumin and, 1433–1434
serum globulins and, 1434t, 1434–1435
radiography and, 1466–1467, *1467*
toxic injury and, 1492–1493
treatment of, 1513–1522
hepatic failure and, 1514, 1517–1522
supportive and symptomatic, 1514–1517
ultrasonography and, 1467–1469, *1468*, 1468t, *1469*
uric acid and, 1456
Liver failure, complications of, treatment of, 1517–1522
drugs in, 1516–1517
fulminant, treatment of, 1521t, 1521–1522
specific therapy for, 1514
supportive and symptomatic therapy for, 1514–1517
Lizards, poisonous, 475–476
Lobar consolidation, 847, *848*
β-LPH, function of, 1722
Lumbosacral joint, instabilities of, 2344, *2345*
Lumbosacral plexus injury, *722*, 723
Lumps. *See* Tumor(s).
Lung(s), abscesses of, pneumothorax and, 885
gastric dilatation-volvulus-torsion syndrome and, 1280–1281
Lung flukes, 835–836
diagnosis of, 836, *837*
Lung sounds, harsh, expiratory, polycythemia and, 103
Lung torsion, pleural effusion caused by, 883
Lung worms, 835, 836–838
in cats, 836
diagnosis of, 836, *837*
tracheal disease due to, 798–799, *800*
Lupus erythematosus cell test, in systemic lupus erythematosus, 2310–2311, *2311*, *2312*
Luteinizing hormone (LH), neuroendocrine function and, 1587
Luxations, 2337–2343
of carpal joint, 2339
of elbow joint, 2338, *2338*, *2339*
of hip joint, 2340, *2341*
of shoulder joint, 2338
of stifle joint, 2340–2343
of tarsal joint, 2339–2340
of temporomandibular joint, nontraumatic, 2343
patellar, 2358–2359, *2359*, *2360*
Lyme disease, cutaneous manifestations of, 7
in humans, 191
Lymph nodes, 2225–2233
anatomy, histology, and physiology of, 2225, *2226*
aspirate of, in lymphadenopathy, 2228–2229, *2229*
Lymph nodes (Continued)
biopsy of, in lymphadenopathy, 2229
lymphadenopathy and. *See* Lymphadenopathy.
respiratory disease and, diagnosis of, 749
Lymphadenectasis, definition of, 126
Lymphadenitis, 1195, 2226
bacterial, 2229–2230
idiopathic lymphadenopathies and, 2230
puppy strangles and, 2229–2230
streptococcal, contagious, 2229
Lymphadenopathy, 2225–2230
anemia and, 93
definitions and, 126, 2225–2226
disorders associated with, 2229–2230
idiopathic, 2230
infiltrative, 2226
mediastinal, benign, 891, *892*
metastatic, 893
neoplastic, 893, *894*
pathogenesis of, 2226, 2227t
pathophysiology of, 127
patient evaluation and, 2226–2229
bone marrow evaluation in, 2228
hematologic and serum biochemical findings in, 2228
history and physical findings in, 2226–2228, 2227t
lymph node aspirate in, 2228–2229, *2229*
lymph node biopsy in, 2229
radiography and ultrasonography in, 2228
reactive, 2226
Lymphangiectasia, intestinal, 1367–1370
clinical signs of, 1368–1369
diagnosis of, *1368–1370*, 1369–1370
pathogenesis of, 1367–1368, *1368*
treatment of, 1370, *1371*
Lymphangioma, 1198
Lymphangitis, 1195
Lymphatic disorders, peripheral, 1195t, 1195–1198
inflammatory, 1195
Lymphedema, 1196–1198
primary, 1196
secondary, 1197–1198
Lymphocyte(s), 2205–2207. *See also* B lymphocytes; T lymphocytes.
differentiation of, 2285, *2286*
immune response and, 2283
lifespan of, 2207
morphology of, 2205–2206, *2206*
production, recirculation, and kinetics of, 2206–2207
response patterns of, 2207–2209
lymphocytosis and, 2207–2208, 2208t
lymphopenia and, 2208t, 2208–2209
Lymphocytic leukemia, *2215*, 2217
Lymphocytic thyroiditis, canine hypothyroidism and, 1641
Lymphocytic-plasmacytic enteritis, 1362–1364
clinical signs of, 1363
diagnosis of, 1363, *1363*
treatment of, 1363–1364
Lymphocytosis, 2207–2208, 2208t
causes of, 12t
chronic antigenic stimulation and, 2208
hypoadrenocorticism and, 2208
lymphoid neoplasia and, 2208
physiologic, 2207–2208
Lymphoid organs, primary, 2285
secondary, 2285
Lymphokines, 2284
in cancer therapy, 539
Lymphoma, canine, 2232t–2234t, 2233
malignant, ocular, 83–84
feline, 2230–2233
alimentary form of, 2231
mediastinal form of, 2230–2231
multicentric form of, 2231
therapy for, 2231–2233, 2232t
Lymphomatoid granulomatosis, 1194
Lymphopenia, 2208t, 2208–2209
causes of, 12t
corticosteroid-associated, 2208–2209
in acute infection, 2209
Lymphopenia (Continued)
lymphocyte-rich lymph and, loss, sequestration, or blockage of, 2209
Lymphopoiesis, 2206–2207, *2207*
Lymphoproliferative disorders, 2176, 2217
Lymphoreticular tumors, in cat, 2390
Lymphosarcoma, 2362
hypercalcemia and, 1612–1613, *1613*
pulmonary, 853, *853*, *854*
small intestinal, 1377–1379, *1377–1379*
staging of, 523t
Lysodren, in hyperadrenocorticism, 1748–1749

Macroadenomas, of pituitary, pathology of, 1724
Macroglobulinemia, primary, paraproteinemias and, 2308
Macrolides, 400t, 400–401
action of, 401
activity spectrum of, 400t, 400–401
clinical pharmacology of, 401
Macrophages, 2292
Macule, 117
Major histocompatibility complex (MHC) gene products, and immune response. *See* Immune response, major histocompatibility complex gene products and.
Malabsorption, liver failure and, treatment of, 1521
Malar abscess, 1211–1212, *1214*
Male(s), 1788–1790
functional capacity of, 1790
infertility in. *See* Infertility, in male.
structural peculiarities of, 1788–1789
testicular descent and, 1790
testicular function and, 1789–1790
Malformations. *See* Congenital abnormalities.
Malignancy. *See* Cancer; Tumor(s).
Malnutrition, alopecia and, 113
protein-calorie, exocrine pancreatic insufficiency and, 1541
thyroid hormone metabolism and, 1637–1638
Malocclusion, 1215, *1215*, *1216*
Mammary congestion, lactation and, 1834
Mammary gland tumors, canine, 1820–1824
biologic behavior and clinical features of, 1820–1821, *1821*, 1821t
feline, 1824
Mandibular gland, injury to, 1242
Mandibular neuropraxia, 1215–1216
Mange, notoedric, of pinna, 250
sarcoptic, of pinna, 250
Mannitol, in oliguria, 1979
Mannosidosis, 595
Manx cats, sacrocaudal dysgenesis in, 685
Massage, prostatic, 1863, *1863*
urethral obstruction and, 2073
Masses. *See* Tumor(s).
Mast cell leukemia, 2216
Mast cell tumors, small intestinal, 1379
Masticatory muscle myositis, 741–742
clinical features of, 741–742
management of, 742
pathogenesis of, 741, *742*
Mastiff, bull, cerebellar degeneration in, 598
Mastitis, lactation and, 1834
Mastocytosis, systemic, gastric ulceration and, 1309
Maternal behavior, abnormal, 1834–1835
Mean corpuscular hemoglobin concentration, 91
Mean corpuscular volume, 91
Median nerve injury, *721*, 722
Mediastinal disorders, 886–895, *887*
diagnosis of, 888–889
edema and, 889
hemorrhagic, 889, *889*
history and, 887
physical findings in, 887, *888*
widening and, 889
Mediastinitis, 889–890
acute, 889, *890*
chronic, 889
treatment of, 889–890
Mediastinoscopy, pleural disorders and, 877
Medical disorders, in developing countries, 220t, 223–224

Medical emergencies, in acute renal failure, 1969–1970
Medication(s). *See* Drug(s).
Medication errors, drug reactions and, 507–508
Megacolon, definition of, 36
  idiopathic, 1415–1416
Megaesophagus, 1261t, 1261–1266
  clinical signs of, 1263
  differential diagnosis of, 1263–1264, 1264t
  epidemiology of, 1263
  glossopharyngeal or vagus nerve lesions and, 719
  idiopathic, cause and pathophysiology of, 1261–1262
  prognosis in, 1265–1266
  regurgitation and, 30–31
  secondary, cause and pathophysiology of, 1262t, 1262–1263
  treatment of, 1264–1265
Megakaryocytic leukemia, 2216–2217
Melanoma, ocular, primary, in dogs, 83
Membrane potential, resting, 1051
  threshold, 1051
Membrane transport defects, uremia and, 1918
Memory, immune response and, 2284
Menace response, coma and stupor and, 63
  test of, 560, 561, *561*, 702–703, *703*
Meningeal cysts, 686–687, *688*
Meningitis, aseptic. *See* Meningitis, corticosteroid-responsive.
  corticosteroid-responsive, 609, 647–648
    clinical findings in, 647–648
    diagnosis of, 648
    etiology and pathogenesis of, 647
    treatment of, 648
  feline infectious peritonitis and, 655–656
Meningoencephalitis, granulomatous, coma and stupor and, 62
Meningoencephalomyelitis, granulomatous, 607–608, 657–658, *657–659*
  pyogranulomatous, 608, 685
Meningomyelitis, 637–640
  bacterial, diagnosis of, 638–639
    treatment of, 639–640
  etiology and pathogenesis of, 637
  fungal, clinical findings in, 637
    diagnosis of, *638*, 638–639
    treatment of, 640
  protothecal, clinical findings in, 638
    diagnosis of, 639
    treatment of, 640
  rickettsial, clinical findings in, 637–638
    diagnosis of, 639
    treatment of, 640
Meniscal calcification, 2344–2345
Meniscal tears, 2344
Meniscus, discoid, 2345
Mental lapse aggression syndrome, 74
Mental status evaluation, 556–557, *557*
Mercaptans, hepatic encephalopathy and, 1464
Mercury intoxication, 460t, 467t, 472
Metabolic acidosis, 443–445
  clinical signs and diagnosis of, *437*, 443–444
  compensation and, 443, 443t
  etiology of, *437*, 443, 443t
  in acute renal failure, 1969–1970
    treatment of, 1977–1978
  in chronic renal failure, 1998–1999
    pathophysiology of, 1998
    treatment of, 1998–1999
  in hypoadrenocorticism, treatment of, 1768–1769
  treatment of, *437*, 444–445
Metabolic alkalosis, 445
  clinical signs and diagnosis of, 445
  compensation and, 443t, 445
  etiology of, 445
  treatment of, 445
  ocular manifestations of, 77
Metabolic disorders, gastric motility disorders and, 1313
  gastric mucosal injury and, 1301
  gastric ulceration and, 1308–1309
  hemolytic disease associated with, 2170–2171
  lameness and, in cats, 169–170
  of brain, 615–619
Metabolic disorders *(Continued)*
  of brain, endocrine, 617
    mineral, electrolyte, and acid-base disturbances and, 616–617
    nutritional, 615–616
    polysystemic, 617–619
  parturition and, 1831–1833
  syncope and, 53
  weakness and, 48–49
Metabolic encephalopathies, coma and stupor and, 62
Metabolic injuries, to nervous system, 553
Metabolic rate, decreased, in canine hypothyroidism, 1642, 1642t
Metabolic storage diseases, 592–596, 593t
Metabolism, alopecia and, 113, 120
  inborn errors of, arthropathies due to, 2359–2361
    ocular manifestations of, 79
  intermediate, microbial, inhibitors of, 402–404
  of ammonia, in liver disease, 1451, 1453–1456, *1454*
  of bilirubin, liver disease and, 1443–1446, *1444*, 1446t, *1447*, 1448
  of carbohydrates, corticosteroids and, 416
    in liver disease, 1431
  of energy, nutritional assessment and, 451–452
    of platelets, 2266
  of erythrocytes, *2158*, 2158–2159
  of estrogen, abnormal, 2396
  of fat, corticosteroids and, 416
  of glycogen, disorders of, 738–739
  of hormones, liver disease and, 1426, 1426t
  of insulin, rapid, *1699*, 1699–1700, *1700*
  of iodine, thyroid gland and, *1633*, 1633–1634
  of lipids, in liver disease, 1431–1432
  of lipoproteins, 198
  of protein, corticosteroids and, 416
  of thyroid hormone. *See* Thyroid hormone, metabolism of.
  of urea, in liver disease, 1451, 1453–1456, *1454*
  of vitamins, liver disease and, 1426, 1427t
  of water. *See* Water, metabolism of.
  stress and, 450
  uremia and, 1920
Metachromatic leukodystrophy, 596
Metaldehyde intoxication, 466
Metallosis, osteomyelitis and, 2381
Metaplasia, squamous, of prostate, 1868
Metastasis(es), 514, 516–517
  in hyperadrenocorticism, surgery and, 1747
  to bone, 2390
  to liver, 1513
  to mediastinal lymph nodes, 893
  to prostate, 1877
Metestrus, feline, 1788
Methemoglobinemia, *2168*, 2168–2170
  canine, 2168–2169
  central cyanosis and, 96
  cyanosis and, 100
  feline, 2169–2170
  treatment of, 2170
Methenamine, 404
Methimazole, in feline hyperthyroidism, 1661–1664, 1662t, *1662–1664*, 1663t
    adverse effects associated with, 1663t, 1663–1664, *1664*
Methionine, hepatic encephalopathy and, 1464
Methoxamine, cardiopulmonary response to, 176
Metritis, 275, 1801
Metronidazole, 402
  action of, 402
  activity spectrum of, 402
  clinical pharmacology of, 402
  in chronic inflammatory bowel disease, 1407–1408
Metyrapone, in canine hyperadrenocorticism, 1754
  in feline hyperadrenocorticism, 1756
Metyrapone testing, in hyperadrenocorticism, 1745
Mexiletine, 1063
Microadenomas, of pituitary, pathology of, 1724
Microbiology, renal disorders and, 1907–1911, 1909t
Microflora, in urinary sediment, renal disease and, 1905
Microflora *(Continued)*
  large intestinal, 1398
  of lower urinary tract, abnormal, 2115
    normal, 2115
  small intestinal, exocrine pancreatic insufficiency and, 1540
Micturition. *See also* Urinary retention; Urination.
  abnormal, 149
  definition of, 148
  dysuria and, 164
  normal, 148–149
Middle ear, infections of, facial nerve disorders and, 717
Milrinone, actions of, 954
  in heart failure therapy, 954
  indications for, 954
Mineral disturbances, brain and, 616–617
Mineralization, bronchial, 829
  pulmonary, 846–847
  renal, renal failure and, 1990
Mineralocorticoids, in hyperadrenocorticism, 1749–1750
  in hypoadrenocorticism, 1758, *1758*
Miniature poodles, demyelinating myelopathy of, 596, 649–650
Minimum data base, in heartworm disease, 1169–1170
Mites, ears and, 256–257
  in humans, 193
Mitral complex, 1031–1047
  chordae tendinae rupture and, 1045–1047
  chronic mitral valvular insufficiency and, 1031–1044
  endocardial splitting and left atrial rupture and, 1044–1045
Mitral regurgitation, heart failure and, *912*, 914
Mitral stenosis, 1049
Mitral valve insufficiency, chronic, 1031–1044
    auscultation in, 1033, *1033*, *1034*
    clinical course of, 1032
    clinical signs of, 1031–1032, 1032t
    differential diagnosis of, 1038
    echocardiography in, 1038, *1039*
    electrocardiography in, 1035–1036, *1037*, 1038
    laboratory findings in, 1038
    pathology of, 1043–1044, *1043*
    physical examination in, 1032–1033
    prognosis in, 1039–1040
    radiographic examination in, 1032t, 1033–1035, *1036*, 1037
    surgical correction of, 1043
    therapy of, 1040–1043, 1041t, 1042t, *1043*
Moderator bands, left ventricular, excessive, heart failure and, 1116–1117, *1117*
Monitoring, emergency medicine and, 214–215, 215t
Monobactams, 394
Monoclonal antibodies, immune response and, 2285
  in cancer therapy, 539–540
Monoclonal gammopathy, benign, paraproteinemias and, 2308–2309
Monocyte(s), 2203–2204
  morphology of, 2204, *2204*
  production and kinetics of, 2204
  response patterns of, 2204–2205
    monocyte-macrophage system disorders and, 2205
    monocytopenia and, 2205
    monocytosis and, 2204–2205, 2205t
Monocyte-macrophage system, disorders of, 2205
Monocytic leukemia, *2215*, 2216
Monocytopenia, 2205
Monocytosis, 2204–2205, 2205t
  causes of, 12t
Mononuclear diseases, pulmonary, 839–840
    treatment of, 840, *840*, *841*
Morphine, in heart failure therapy, 966
Mothball poisoning, 469t, 480–481
Motility, gastric. *See* Gastric motility.
  of large intestine, 1397–1398
  of small intestine, 1327–1328
    deranged, diarrhea caused by, 1330
Motility modifiers, in chronic inflammatory bowel disease, 1409

Motor neuron disease, cervical disease of, 59–60
Movement, voluntary, spinal cord disease and, 629
Mucocele, salivary, 1242, 1249, *1249*, *1250*
management of, 1249, 1251
Mucopolysaccharidoses, 595–596, 675
arthropathy due to, 2360
cutaneous manifestations of, 5
type I, 2384–2385
type VI, 2385, *2386*
type VII, 2385
Mucosa, gastric, injury of, 1299–1301
agents and, 1300
blood flow alterations and, 1300–1301
endogenous factors in, 1301
gastric mucosal barrier and, 1299–1300, *1300*
small intestinal, exocrine pancreatic insufficiency and, *1539*, 1539–1540
Mucous membranes, hematuria and, 162
Mucus, gastric secretion of, 1292
Multicentric periarticular calcinosis, 2360–2361
Multimodality therapy, in cancer, 543–544
Muscle(s), atrophy of, lameness and, in dogs, 166
spinal cord disease and, 630
cranial, symmetry of, testing for, 564
detrusor, bladder atony and, 155–156
treatment of, 164
heart. *See* Heart muscle.
in canine hypothyroidism, adult-onset, 1643
in feline hyperthyroidism, 1656
masticatory, myositis of, 741–742
clinical features of, 741–742
management of, 742
pathogenesis of, 741, *742*
skeletal, disorders of. *See* Skeletal muscle disorders.
weakness of, in canine hyperadrenocorticism, 1727
Muscle tone, spinal cord disease and, 630
Muscular dystrophy, 739
Musculoskeletal system. *See also* Muscle(s); Skeletal muscle disorders; *headings beginning with term* Bone.
corticosteroids and, 417
respiratory disease and, diagnosis of, 749
Mushroom poisoning, 476–477
symptomatology of, 459t, 460t, 469t, 477
MVO_2. *See* Myocardial oxygen demand.
Myasthenia gravis, 735–737
acquired, *736*, 736–737
management of, 736–737
as paraneoplastic syndrome, 520–521
congenital, 737
feline, 737
pathophysiology of, 735
Mycobacterial infections, mediastinal, 892
ocular manifestations of, 81
pulmonary, 832
small bowel diarrhea and, 1358–1359
urinary tract infection and, 2123
Mycoplasma felis, ocular manifestations of, 83
Mycoplasma gatae, ocular manifestations of, 83
Mycoplasmas, arthritis and, 2363–2364
lower urinary tract disease and, in cats, 2063
Mycoses, cutaneous manifestations of, 7
myocarditis and, 1125
systemic, 605
osteomyelitis and, 2379–2381
Mycotic diseases, deep, 341–367
antimycotic agents and, in otitis externa, 255
diarrhea and. *See* Diarrhea, small bowel, mycotic.
lower urinary tract disease and, in cats, 2063
of brain, 605–606
stomatitis and, *1229*, 1229–1230
zoonotic, 192
Mycotoxins, 459t, 477–478
Myelitis, distemper, in dogs, 654
feline infectious peritonitis and, 655–656
protozoal, 684–685
Myeloaplasia, 2173–2174
treatment of, 2174
Myelodysplasia, 676–677, 2174–2175, *2175*
neutropenia and, 2200
Myelofibrosis, 2176
neutropenia and, 2200
Myelography, spinal cord disease and, 627–628, *628*
spinal cord tumors and, 679–680, *681*
Myeloid leukemia, *2215*, 2216
Myeloma, multiple, of chest wall, 871
paraproteinemias and, 2306–2308
Myelomalacia, hemorrhagic, progressive, *683*, 683–684
of Afghan hounds, 660–661
Myelomonocytic leukemia, *2215*, 2216
Myelopathy, degenerative, of cats, 649
of dogs, 648–649
demyelinating, of miniature poodles, 596, 649–650
ischemic, due to fibrocartilaginous embolism, 670–671
Myelophthisic anemia, 92
Myeloproliferative disorders, 2175–2176, *2176*, 2216–2217
basophils and, 2213–2214
platelet dysfunction in, 2273
Myelosis, erythemic, 2216
megakaryocytic, 2216–2217
Myocardial depressant factor, gastric dilatation-volvulus-torsion syndrome and, 1281
Myocardial diseases. *See* Cardiomyopathy; *specific diseases.*
Myocardial failure, 899
Myocardial oxygen demand (MVO_2), heart failure therapy and, 942
Myocarditis, 1123–1125
algae and, 1125
bacterial, 1125
mycoses and, 1125
protozoal, 1124–1125
viral, 1124, *1124*
Myoclonus, distemper, 655
Myopathy, hypothyroid, 739, *739*
necrotizing, of Afghan hounds, 660–661
nemaline, 739
of skeletal muscles, 734–742, 735t
Myositis, of masticatory muscle, 741–742
clinical features of, 741–742
management of, 742
pathogenesis of, 741, *742*
Myotonia, *737*, 737–738
human, 738
in canine hyperadrenocorticism, 1729
of chow chow dogs, 738
of Labrador retriever dogs, type 2 myofiber deficiency and, 738
pathophysiology of, 737–738
Myxedema coma, in canine hypothyroidism, adult-onset, 1644

Nares, congenital stenosis of, 771–772
Nasal cavity, diagnostic approach to, 751
foreign body rhinitis and, 774–775, *775*
neoplasia of, *780*, 780–782, *781*
rhinitis and, bacterial, 778, *779*
dental disease and, *776*
fungal, 778–780, *780*
palatine defects and, 775–776, *775–778*
parasitic, 780
viral, 776–778, *779*
trauma to, 774
Nasopharyngeal polyps, 784, *784*
Natural killer cells, 2292
Nausea, definition of, 27
Near-drowning, 843
Neck, evaluation of, anorexia and, 16
polyphagia and, 16
Necrosis, aseptic, of femoral head, 2359, *2360*, *2361*
bone marrow, neutropenia and, 2200
of pulmonary neoplasia, pneumothorax and, 885
tubular. *See* Tubular necrosis, acute.
Necrotizing ulcerative gingivitis, 1219–1220
Necrotizing vasculitis, 677
Needles, acupuncture and, *485*, 492
Nemaline myopathy, 739
Nematodes, intestinal, cutaneous manifestations of, 8
Nematodiasis, spinal, 687
Neoplasia. *See* Cancer; Tumor(s).
Neoplastic cells, dysuria and, 164
Nephritis, acute renal failure caused by, 1937
chronic interstitial, 1985
Nephrological syndromes, 1962, 1962t–1964t
Nephrons, adaptation in, chronic renal disease and, *1921*, 1921–1922, 1922t
Nephropathy, diabetes mellitus and, 1706
Nephrosis, acute renal failure caused by, 1928–1930, *1929*
Nephrotic range proteinuria, 2007
Nephrotic syndrome, 2006–2024
causes of, 2009–2013
amyloidosis and, 2012–2013
glomerulonephropathies and, 2009t, 2009–2012, *2110*
clinical and laboratory characteristics of, 2007–2009
definition and clinical implications of, 2006–2007
diagnosis of, 2013–2016
syndrome analysis and, 2014t, 2014–2016, 2015t, *2016*
syndrome identification and, 2013t, 2013–2014
hypercoagulability and, 1942–1943, *1943*
hyperlipemia and, 1941
hyperlipidemia and, in cat, 199
hypoalbuminemia and, 1941–1942
pathophysiology of, 1941–1943
prognosis of, 2016
sodium retention, hypertension, and edema and, 1942, *1942*
thrombocytopathies associated with, 2275
treatment of, 2016–2024
amyloidosis and, 2019
glomerulonephritis and, 2017–2019
symptomatic and supportive, 2020–2024
Nephrotoxic acute tubular necrosis, 1966–1967, 1967t
Nephrotoxicity, drug reactions and, 505, 506t
acute renal failure caused by, 1931, *1932*, 1933–1935
Nervous system. *See also* Central nervous system; Sympathetic nervous system.
corticosteroids and, 417
in canine hypothyroidism, adult-onset, 1643
in feline hyperthyroidism, 1656
Neuritis, brachial plexus, 727
Neuro-ophthalmology, 702t, 702–707
menace response and, 702–703, *703*
nystagmus and, 707
palpebral fissure and, 706
palpebral reflex and, 707
pupil size and, *704*, 704–706, 705t
pharmacologic testing of, 705–706
pupillary light response and, 703–704, *704*
strabismus and, 706–707
third eyelid and, 706
Neuroaxonal dystrophy, 598–599
feline, 598
of Rottweilers, 682
Neuroendocrine control, adrenocorticotropic hormone and related peptides in, 1722–1723
diurnal variation and, 1722
physiologic factors and, 1722
stress and, 1723
Neuroendocrine function. *See* Pituitary-hypothalamic diseases, endocrine rhythms and neuroendocrine function and.
Neurogenic disorders, urinary incontinence and, 149
Neurohypophysis, history of, 1580
pituitary-hypothalamic diseases and, 1580
Neurologic complications, of uremia, 1919
Neurologic disorders, gastric ulceration and, 1308
weakness and, 49
Neurologic evaluation, *549*, 549–577
anorexia and, 16
history taking and, 549–554
disease categories and, 553–554
information collection and, 550–552, *550–552*
organizing information and, 552–553, *553*

Neurologic evaluation *(Continued)*
neurologic examination and, 554–557, 555t, *556*
polyphagia and, 16
Neurologic examination, 554–557, 555t, *556*
attitudinal and postural reactions and, 558–559, *558–560*
cranial nerve exam and, 559–561
cranial nerve function testing and, *560–563*, 561–566, *565*, 566t
cyanosis and, 98
eye in, 702t, 702–707
general observations and, 556–557
pain and, 21
peripheral nerve disorders and, 711, 711t, 712t
spinal cord diseases and, 626
spinal segmental reflexes and, 566–577, *567–575*, 574t
technique for, 555–556
Neurologic inhibition, gastric motility disorders and, 1313
Neurologic theories, of acupuncture, 487
Neuromuscular diseases, weakness and, 49
Neuronal ceroid lipofuscinosis, ocular manifestations of, 79
Neuropathic arthropathy, 2345–2346
Neuropathy, diabetes mellitus and, 1706
giant axonal, 725
hypertrophic, 725
ischemic, 723
of Boxer dogs, 724
peripheral. *See* Peripheral neuropathies.
sensory, 729
in dachshunds, 724
of English pointer, 724
of short hair pointer, 724
trigeminal, idiopathic, 716, *716*
sensory, 716–717
vestibular, idiopathic, 718–719
Neuropraxia, mandibular, 1215–1216
Neuroreceptors, hepatic encephalopathy and, 1465
Neurotransmitters, false, hepatic encephalopathy and, 1465
hepatic encephalopathy and, 1465
hypophysiotropic cell regulation by, 1583
inhibitory, hepatic encephalopathy and, 1465
Neutropenia, 2194t, 2197, *2197*
causes of, 12t
cyclic, 5
cyclophosphamide-induced, 2201
immune-mediated, 2202
reduced survival, 2201–2202
Neutrophil(s), 2186–2187
morphology of, 2187–2193
cytoplasmic, in disease, 2190–2193
in health, 2188, *2188*
nuclear, in disease, 2188–2190
in health, 2187–2188
production and kinetics of, 2193–2194
response patterns of, 2194–2203
cyclic stem cell input or proliferation and, 2200–2201
defective production and, 2197, *2197*
functional abnormalities and, *2202*, 2202–2203, 2203t
granulopoiesis and, immune suppression of, 2201
hematopoietic stem cell death and, 2197–2200
neutropenia and, 2194t, 2197, *2197*
neutrophilia and, 2194t, 2194–2197
prognosis of, 2202
reduced hematopoietic space and, 2200
reduced survival neutropenia and, 2201–2202
tissue demand for, increased, 2202
Neutrophil function, uremia and, 1918–1919
Neutrophilia, 2194t, 2194–2197
causes of, 11t
corticosteroid-associated, 2195, *2195*
inflammation and infection associated with, *2195*, 2195–2196
leukemoid reactions and, 2196–2197
leukocytosis and, 2196–2197
physiologic, 2194–2195, *2195*
Neutrophilic leukemia, *2215*, 2216
Niacin deficiency, brain and, 616
Nitrofurantoin, 404
action of, 404
activity spectrum of, 404
clinical pharmacology of, 404
toxicity of, 404
Nitroglycerin, actions of, 959
in heart failure therapy, 959–960
indications for, 959–960
toxicity and interactions of, 960
Nocardiosis, 272
osteomyelitis and, 2380–2381
Nociceptive evaluation, 573
of reflexes, 569, 573
Nocturia. *See also* Urinary incontinence.
definition of, 148
Nodular hyperplasia, hepatic, 1513
Nodule, 117, 514. *See also* Tumor(s).
density of, radiographic interpretation and, in respiratory disease, 758
Nonagglutinins, cold-acting, in immune-mediated hemolytic anemia, 2300–2301
Nonoliguric acute tubular necrosis, sequential phases of, 1968
Nonsteroidal anti-inflammatory agents, thrombocytopathies induced by, 2274, 2274t
Norepinephrine, in insulin antagonism/resistance, 1702
Norpace. *See* Disopyramide.
Nose, disorders of, 768–782
diagnosis of, 769–771
history in, 769
physical examination in, 769–770, *770*
radiography in, 770–771, *770–773*
of nasal cavity, 774–782, *775–781*
of paranasal sinuses, 782, *782*, *783*
of rhinarium, 771–773, *773*, *774*
structure and function of, 768–769, *769*
Nuclear hypersegmentation, of neutrophils, *2189*, 2189–2190
Nuclear hyposegmentation, of neutrophils, 2188–2189, *2189*
Nuclear magnetic resonance imaging, 584
Nuclear maturation, asynchronous, of neutrophils, 2189, *2189*
Nuclear medicine, in renal disease, 1914
Nucleic acid synthesis, microbial, inhibitors of, 401–402
Nutrition. *See also* Diet; Diet therapy; Malnutrition; Nutritional support.
alopecia and, 120
exocrine pancreatic insufficiency and, 1541
pancreatitis and, 1534
Nutritional disorders, cutaneous manifestations of, 8–9
in developing countries, 218
ocular manifestations of, 80
of bone, 2385, 2387
of brain, 615–616
of nervous system, 553
weakness and, 49–50
Nutritional management, in acute renal failure, 1980
Nutritional support, 450–454. *See also* Diet therapy.
brief, nonstressed starvation and, 450
diets and, 453
indications and contraindications for, 452
nutritional assessment and, 451–452
biochemical parameters and, 451
energy metabolism and, 451–452
fat reserves and, 451
immune status and, 451
protein status and, 451
nutritional plan and, 452
stress and, 450
total parenteral nutrition and, 453–454
tube feeding and, 452–453
Nystagmus, coma and stupor and, 63
in neurological examination, 707
pathologic, testing for, 564
Obesity, in canine hyperadrenocorticism, 1728
polycythemia and, 103
pulmonary manifestations of, 846
thyroid hormone metabolism and, in dog, 1640
Observation, pain and, 20
poisoning and, 457
Obstipation, definition of, 36
Obturator nerve injury, *722*, 723
Occult blood, in urine, renal disease and, 1903–1904
large intestinal disease and, 1400
Ocular filariasis, ocular manifestations of, 81
Ocular motility, test for, 563–564
Ocular position, test for, 563, *563*
Ocular tumors, canine, 83–84
feline, 84
Oculomotor nerves, focal diseases of, 715–716
Odontoid process malformations, 634–637
clinical findings in, 635, *635*
diagnosis of, 635–636, *636*
treatment of, 636–637
Odynophagia, definition of, 27
Olfactory nerves, focal diseases of, 715
Oliguria, converting to nonoliguria, 1978–1979
detection of, 1971–1972
Oliguric acute tubular necrosis, sequential phases of, 1967–1968
o,p′-DDD, in feline hyperadrenocorticism, 1756
in hyperadrenocorticism, 1747–1753
diabetes mellitus and, 1750
failure of, 1750
glucocorticoids and, 1749–1750
improvement with, 1750, *1751*, *1752*
initiating therapy and, 1748, *1749*
maintenance therapy and, 1750–1751
mineralocorticoids and, 1749–1750
monitoring and, 1748, *1749*
pretreatment assessments and, 1747
therapeutic goals and, 1748, *1749*
Ophthalmologic changes, mediastinal disorders and, 887
Ophthalmomyiasis, ocular manifestations of, 81
Optic nerves, focal diseases of, 715
Oral cavity, 1203–1207
anatomy and function of, 1203
dental structures and, 1203–1207, *1204*, *1205*
occlusion and articulation and, *1206*, 1206–1207
temporomandibular joint and, 1207
tooth eruption and, *1205*, 1205t, 1205–1206
diseases of, affecting tooth structure, 1209–1215
burns and, 1231
foreign body injury and, 1231
history and examination in, 1207–1209, *1208*
hyperplastic and neoplastic, *1230*, 1230–1231
immune system abnormalities and, 1228–1229
jaws and, 1215–1216
lips and cheeks and, 1231–1233
local diseases causing, 1229–1230
local therapy in, 1231
oropharyngeal, neoplastic, *1238*, 1238–1241, *1239*, 1240t
periodontal, 1216–1227
pharyngeal, 1236–1238
salivary glands and, 1241–1252
systemic disease causing, 1228
tongue and, 1233–1236
neurologic examination and, 564, 566
oropharynx and, 1207, *1207*
Oral hygiene, 1223, *1224*, 1225
Oral hypoglycemic agents, in nonketotic diabetes mellitus, 1692
Oral protectants, in acute gastritis, 1302–1303
Orchiectomy, testicular tumors and, 1815
Orchitis, immune-regulated, treatment of, 1857
Organophosphate intoxication, 466
Oriental medicine, traditional, 491
Oropharynx, 1207, *1207*
neoplasia of, *1238*, 1238–1241, *1239*, 1240t
management of, 1239, *1240*
tonsils and, 1239, 1240t, 1241, *1241*
Orthopedic infections, antimicrobial selection for, 407–408

Orthopnea, 86
Oslerus osleri, 837
Osmolality, of urine, tubular function and, 1898–1899
Osmotic fragility test, in immune mediated hemolytic anemia, 2302
Ossification, dural, 655, *656*
Ossification centers, ectopic, 2355, *2356*, *2357*
Osteoarthritis. *See* Joint diseases, degenerative.
Osteoarthrosis. *See* Joint diseases, degenerative.
Osteochondritis, *2348*, 2348–2350, *2349*
Osteochondritis dissecans, of medial condyle, of humerus, 2354, *2355*
Osteochondrodysplasias, 2383–2384
Osteochondromas, in cat, 2390, *2390*
  in dog, 2389
Osteochondromatosis, 871
Osteochondrosis, *2348*, 2348–2350, *2349*
Osteodystrophy, chronic renal failure and, 1923–1924, 1024t
  hypertrophic, 2391–2392, *2392*
Osteogenic sarcoma, 2362
Osteomas, in cat, 2390
  in dog, 2389
Osteomyelitis, aspergillus, clinical manifestations of, 360
    diagnosis of, 360–361
  nonsuppurative, 2379–2381
    fracture healing and, 2381, *2381*
    metallosis and, 2381
    systemic mycoses and, 2379–2381
  suppurative, 2378, *2378*, *2379*
  vertebral. *See* Diskospondylitis.
Osteopathy, craniomandibular, 2393, *2393*
  hypertrophic, 2395, *2395*
    as paraneoplastic syndrome, 519–520
Osteopetrosis, neutropenia and, 2200
Osteoporosis, 2382–2383
  disuse, 2396
Osteosarcoma, in cat, 2390
  in dog, 2387–2389, *2388*
  parosteal, in cat, 2390
Osteosclerosis, 2176
Otitis, allergic, 257
  ceruminous, 257
Otitis externa, 275
  causes of, 254
  epizoology of, 253
  examination and, 253–254
  pathophysiology of, 252–253
  surgical management of, 258
  treatment of, 254–256
    cleansing and, 254–255
    medications and, 255
Otitis interna, 260–261, 275
Otitis media, 258–259, 275
  clinical signs and findings in, 259
  diagnosis of, 259
  etiology and pathogenesis of, 258–259
  treatment of, 259
Otocephalic syndrome, 591
Otoscope, 253
Outlet resistance, urinary retention and, 156
Ovarian cycle, 1779–1782, *1782*, *1783*
Ovarian cysts, persistent estrus and, *1792*, 1792–1795, 1793t
    diagnosis of, 1793t, 1793–1794
    treatment of, *1794*, 1794–1795
Ovarian failure, premature, 1849
Ovarian tumors, 1818–1819
  persistent estrus and, *1795*, 1795t, 1795–1796
Ovariohysterectomy, glucose intolerance and, 1597–1598
Overactivity, in cats, 237
  in dogs, 232
  weakness and, 50
Overdominance, 186
Overnutrition, of growing dog, bone disorders and, 2387
Overwork, weakness and, 50
Oviducts, occlusion of, infertility and, 1846
Owners. *See* Human(s).
Oxygen. *See also* Hypoxemia.
  cerebral anoxia and, 599–600
Oxygen *(Continued)*
  cerebral hypoxia and, 599–600
    behavioral signs and, 73
  in pulmonary edema, 862
Oxygen demand, myocardial, heart failure therapy and, 942
Oxygen therapy, in heart failure therapy, 966–967
Oxygenation, lower respiratory disease and, 816–818

Pacemaker cells, 1053
Pacing, 72
Pain, 18–22
  abdominal, 131
    hematuria and, 161–162
  acute versus chronic, 20
  aggression induced by, 234
  cutaneous, 165
  cyanosis and, 97
  deep, 165
  diagnostic plan for, 21
  differential diagnosis of, 19–20
  exaggerated responsiveness to, 573
  historic findings in, 20
  lameness and, in dogs, 165
  medications for, 22t
  pathophysiology of, 18–19
    ascending pathways and, 19
    ischemic pain and, 19
    pain theory and, 19
    primary afferent neuron and, 18–19
  physical findings in, 20–21
  treatment goals for, 21, 22t
  treatment outcome and, 21–22
Pain perception, loss of, 573, *574*
Palate, cleft, 771, *773*, 1231, *1232*
  defects of, rhinitis due to, 775–776, *775–778*
  soft, defects of, 784–786, *785*, *786*
Pallor, poisoning and, 469t
Palpation, abdominal, 1399
  constipation and, 37
  cyanosis and, 98
  diarrhea and, 34
  dyschezia and, 37
  pain and, 20–21
  prostatic, 1862
  rectal, 1399
  tenesmus and, 37
Palpebral fissure, in neurological examination, 706
Palpebral reflex, testing for, 564, *565*
  testing of, 707
Pancreas, endocrine, disorders of. *See also* Diabetes mellitus.
    drugs used for, 1720t
    neoplastic, 1707–1716
  exocrine, 1528t, 1528–1549
    anatomy of, *1528*, 1528–1529
    biochemistry and physiology of, 1529–1531
      autodigestion and, defenses against, 1529t, *1530*, 1530–1531, *1531*, 1531t
      digestive enzymes and, 1529t, 1529–1530
      pancreatic enzymes and, in blood, 1531
      secretion and, regulation of, 1531
    diseases of, 1531–1549
      neoplastic, 1548
      parasitic, 1549
Pancreatic acinar atrophy, 1538
Pancreatic disease, cutaneous manifestations of, 9
Pancreatic enzymes, in diabetes mellitus, 1686
Pancreatic insufficiency, exocrine, 1538–1548
    diagnosis of, 1541–1546
    etiology of, 1538–1539
    pathophysiology of, 1539–1541
    prognosis of, 1548
    treatment of, 1546–1548
Pancreatitis, 1531t, 1531–1538
  acute, liver disease and, 1483
  chronic, 1538–1539
  diabetes mellitus and, 1705
  diagnosis of, 1535–1536
    history and clinical signs in, 1535
    laboratory studies in, 1535–1536, *1536*
    radiographic signs in, 1535
Pancreatitis *(Continued)*
  etiology of, 1534–1535
  hyperlipidemia and, canine, 206
  hypocalcemia and, 1627
  pathophysiology of, *1530–1533*, 1531t–1533t, 1532–1534
  platelet dysfunction in, 2273
  pleural effusions associated with, 881
  prognosis of, 1538
  treatment of, 1536–1538
Panhypopituitarism, bone abnormalities and, 2385
Panleukopenia, feline, 314–317
    clinical signs of, 315–316
      in-utero infections and, 315
      older kittens and adult cats and, 315–316
    diagnosis of, 316
    diarrhea and, 1354
    differential diagnosis of, 316
    epizootiology of, 314
    etiology of, 314
    hematopoietic stem cell death and, 2199
    laboratory diagnosis of, 316
    pathogenesis of, 314–315
      early neonatal infections and, 315
      in-utero infections and, 315
      older kittens and, 315
    prevention of, 317
    treatment of, 316–317
Panniculus reflex, testing for, 569, 573
Panosteitis, 2360, 2391, *2391*
Pansteatitis, cutaneous manifestations of, 8
Panting, in canine hyperadrenocorticism, 1728–1729
Pantothenic acid deficiency, brain and, 616
Papillomatosis, oral, 1230
Papule, 117, 514
Paracentesis, abdominal, techniques of, 132–133, 134t
Paragonimum kellicotti, 835–836
  diagnosis of, 836, *837*
Paralysis, brain stem dysfunction and, 59
  cerebral dysfunction and, 59
  cervical spinal cord disease and, 59–60
  diaphragmatic, 867–868
  differential diagnosis of, *58*, 59t, 60
  laryngeal, *790*, 790–791, *791*
  lower motor neuron disease and, 59–60
  of facial nerve, idiopathic, 717–718
  of hindlimbs, cyanosis and, 97
  pharyngeal, 786–787
Paranasal sinuses, disorders of, 782, *782*, *783*
Paraneoplastic polyneuropathy, 725–726
Paraneoplastic syndromes, 518–521, 519t
Paraphimosis, 1886–1887
Parapneumonic effusion, 879
Paraprostatic cysts, 1869, *1869*
Paraproteinemias, *2305*, 2305–2309
  clinical diseases associated with, 2306–2309
  clinical manifestations of, 2306
Paraquat intoxication, 467
  differentiation of, 459t, 465t, 467, 467t
Parasitic diseases, alopecia and, 120
  antiparasitic agents and, in otitis externa, 255
  bronchial, 829
  cutaneous manifestations of, 7–8
  dermatologic, ocular manifestations of, 76–77
  diarrhea and. *See* Diarrhea, small bowel, parasitic.
  eosinophilia and, 2210
  fecal examinations for, 1335t, 1335–1336
  hepatic, 1483
  in developing countries, 218–219, *219*, *220*, 220t
  intestinal migration of, 838
  lower urinary tract disease and, in cats, 2063
  metazoal, brain and, 606–607
  ocular manifestations of, in dog, 80–81
  of external ear, 256–257
  of gallbladder, 1557, 1557t
  of large intestine, 1410–1412
  of lower urinary tract, 2113–2114
  of pinnae, 251
  pancreatic, in cats, 1549
  renal, 2030–2031
  rhinitis and, 780
  zoonotic, 188–190

Parathyroid disease, hypercalcemia and, 1610–1621
blastomycosis and, 1619
bone disease and, 1618–1619
general considerations in, 1610, *1611*, 1611t
hyperadrenocorticism and, 1615
hypervitaminosis D and, 1619
malignancy and, 1610–1615
patient evaluation in, 1611t, 1619–1620, 1620t
primary hyperparathyroidism and, 1616–1618, *1617*
renal disease and, 1615–1616
treatment of, 1620–1621
hypocalcemia and, 1621–1629
eclampsia and, 1625–1626
general considerations in, *1611*, 1621t, 1621–1622
hypoparathyroidism and, *1617*, 1623, *1624*, 1625, 1626t, 1627t
pancreatitis and, 1627
primary renal disease and, 1622, *1623*, *1624*
treatment of, 1627–1629
Parental aggression, 234
Paresis, 58–60
brain stem dysfunction and, 59
cerebral dysfunction and, 59
cervical spinal cord disease and, 59–60
differential diagnosis of, *58*, 59t, 60
lower motor neuron disease and, 59–60
toxicity and, 614–615
Parotid gland, injury to, 1242, *1247*, *1248*
Pars distalis, endocrinologically inactive chromophobe adenoma arising in, 1591, *1591*
Pars intermedia, adenoma of. *See* Adenoma, of pars intermedia.
anatomy of, 1581–1582
Partial pressure, definition of, 95
Partial thromboplastin time, 2250–2251
Parturition, 1786–1787
abnormal, 1828–1831
delayed, 1828
dystocia and, 1829–1831
early onset and, 1828
prolonged, 1828–1829
abnormal maternal behavior and, 1834–1835
disorders of, drugs used in, 1836t–1837t
hypoglycemia and, 1832–1833
lactation problems and, 1833–1834
normal, 1826–1828
puerperal tetany and, 1831–1832
Parvovirus, canine, brain and, 603
clinical signs in, 1351
diagnosis of, 1351–1352, *1352*
diarrhea and, 1351–1353
gastroenteritis and, 306–308
clinical signs of, 307
diagnosis of, 307
epizootiology of, 307
etiology of, 306–307
treatment and prevention of, 304t, 307–308
in developing countries, 222
prevention of, 1353
prognosis and complications of, 1352–1353
treatment of, 1252
hematopoietic stem cell death and, 2199
Pasteurellosis, 266–267
Patch, 117
Patch skin test, in allergic contact dermatitis, 2317
Patella, luxation of, 2358–2359, *2359*, *2360*
Patellar reflex, testing for, 569, *571*
Patent ductus arteriosus, 986–992, *987*
clinical findings in, 988, 991–992
left to right shunting and, *987*, 988, *989*, *990*, 991
pulmonary hypertension and, 991, *991*, *992*
clinical management of, 992, 1007t
heart failure and, 914
natural history of, 991–992
pathogenesis of, 986
pathophysiology of, 986, 988, *988*
reversed, 992
Patient care, emergency medicine and, 214
Patient monitoring, in acute renal failure, 1974, 1975t
in chronic renal failure, 2006
Peak level, drug administration and, 68
Pelger-Huët anomaly, 2187–2188, *2188*
Pelvic bladder, 2133
Pelvic limb reflexes, testing for, 569, *570*
Pemphigoid, 2323–2324
bullous, 2323–2324, *2324*
oral lesions and, 1229
Pemphigus, 2318–2322
diagnosis of, 2319t, 2320
pathophysiology of, 2319, *2319*
treatment and prognosis of, 2321–2322
types of, 2319–2321
Pemphigus erythematosus, 2320–2321
Pemphigus foliaceous, 2319–2321
clinical signs of, 2319
diagnosis of, 2319–2321, *2320*
Pemphigus vegetans, 2321, *2322*
Pemphigus vulgaris, 773, *774*, 2321
oral lesions and, 1229
D-Penicillamine, in liver failure, 1517
Penicillin(s), 386–387
action of, 386
activity spectrum of, 386
aminopenicillins and, 388–389
activity spectrum of, 388–389
clinical pharmacology of, 389
antipseudomonal, 389–390, 390t
activity spectrum of, 389–390, 390t
clinical pharmacology of, 390
antistaphylococcal, 388
activity spectrum of, 388
clinical pharmacology of, 388, 409t–410t
natural, 387–388
activity spectrum of, 387
clinical pharmacology of, 387–388
resistance mechanisms and, 386–387, *387*
Penis, acquired morphologic disorders of, 1885–1887
anatomy and physiology of, 1881–1883
balanoposthitis and, 1886, *1887*
castration and, 1882–1883
congenital morphologic disorders of, 1883–1885
congenital preputial stenosis and, with phimosis, 1884, *1885*
contusion or injury of, 1885–1886
duplication of, 1884–1885, *1885*
fracture of, 1886
frenulum persistence and, 1884, *1884*
functional disorders of, 1887–1888
hypoplasia of, 1883
hypospadias and preputial defects of, *1883*, 1883–1884, *1884*
neoplasia of, 1816, 1887
normal bacterial flora of, 1881, 1882t
paraphimosis and, 1886–1887
urethral prolapse and, 1885, *1885*
Pentatrichomonas, small bowel diarrhea and, 1350
Pepsin, gastric secretion of, 1292
Peptides, regulatory, pancreatic, exocrine pancreatic insufficiency and, 1540
Percutaneous fine needle aspiration lung biopsy, *764*, 764–765, *765*
Perforation, of large intestine, nontraumatic, 1416–1417
Perianal fistula, 1568–1569
differential diagnosis of, 1568
history and physical findings in, 1568, *1568*
treatment of, *1568*, 1568–1569
Perianal gland adenomas, 1572, *1572*
Pericardial effusion, 1135–1145
causes of, 1135–1138, *1138*
differential diagnosis of, 1143–1144
echocardiography in, 1142, *1143–1145*
electrocardiography in, 1139, *1140*
history and clinical signs of, 1138–1139
pericardiocentesis in, 1142–1143
physical diagnosis of, 1139, *1139*
pneumopericardiography in, *1141*, *1142*, 1143
radiography in, 1139, *1140–1142*, 1141–1142
treatment of, 1144–1145, *1146*
types of, 1135–1138, *1138*
with tamponade, 1133, *1134*
Pericardial fibrosis, with constriction, 1133, *1134*
Pericardiocentesis, pericardial effusion and, 1142–1143
Pericarditis, constrictive, 1145, *1146*, 1147–1148
diagnosis of, *1147*, 1147–1148, *1148*
history and clinical signs in, 1147
treatment of, 1148
Pericardium, anatomy and normal function of, 1132, 1133t
diseases of, 1132–1148
acquired, 1135–1148
congenital, 1135
pathophysiology of, 1132–1135
Periesophageal obstructions, 1271–1272, *1272*
Perineal hernia, 1561–1563
history and presenting signs in, 1562, *1562*, *1563*
incidence and etiology of, 1561–1562
treatment of, 1562–1563
Perineal reflexes, testing for, 569, *572*
Periodontal abscess, 1223, *1224*
Periodontal disease, 1216–1227
in cats, 1226–1227, *1227*
Periodontal fibrous hyperplasia, 1230, *1230*
Periodontal therapy, 1223, 1225–1226
curettage and, 1225
extraction and, 1226
oral hygiene and, 1223, *1224*, 1225
scaling and root planing and, 1225, *1225*
surgical pocket elimination and, *1223*, *1224*, 1225–1226
Periodontitis, 1221–1227
clinical manifestations of, *1221*, 1221–1222
etiology of, 1221
histopathology of, 1222
radiographic manifestations of, 1222, *1222*
treatment of, 1222, *1223*, *1224*
Peripheral nerve disorders, 708–729, *709*
clinical evaluation of, 710–714
diagnostic aids in, 711–714
history in, 710–711
neurologic, 711, 711t, 712t
drugs for, 732t
focal, of cranial nerves, 715–719
of spinal nerves, 719–724
multifocal, 724–729
physiology and pathophysiology of, 708–710, *709*, *710*, 710t
neoplasia of, 723–724, *724*
Peripheral neuropathies, traumatic, 719–723
brachial plexus avulsion or stretch and, 712t, 720–721, *721*
diagnosis, therapy, and prognosis of, 719–720, 720t
femoral nerve injury and, *722*, 723
lumbosacral plexus injury and, *722*, 723
median and ulnar nerve injury and, *721*, 722
peroneal or fibular nerve injury and, *722*, 722–723
pudendal nerve injury and, 723
radial nerve injury and, *721*, 722
sciatic nerve injury and, 722, *722*
suprascapular nerve injury and, *721*, 721–722
tibial nerve injury and, *722*, 723
Peripheral vascular disease, 1185t, 1185–1198
arterial, nonocclusive, 1188–1194
occlusive, 1185–1188
lymphatic, 1195t, 1195–1198
venous, 1194–1195
Perirenal pseudocysts, feline, 2025–2026
Peritoneopericardial hernia, 1135, *1136*
Peritoneum, disease of. *See also* Peritonitis.
recognition of, 131–133, 132t, *133*, 134t
surface of, 131
Peritonitis, 135
chylous, 136
differential diagnosis of, 135
infectious, 137, 602–603
cats at risk and, 333
clinical manifestations of, 333–337
neurologic, 335, *336*
ocular, 334–335, *335*
clinical signs in, 137
control of, in catteries, 337–338
diagnosis of, 336–337
differential diagnosis of, 137, 336

Peritonitis *(Continued)*
infectious, effusive, 333–334
laboratory examination in, 137, 336
noneffusive, 334, *334*
meningitis and myelitis and, 655–656
ocular manifestations of, 83
pathogenesis of, 331–333, *332*
pulmonary manifestations of, 830
radiographic examination in, 137
transmission of, 331
treatment of, 337
viruses and, 330–331, 331t
laboratory examination in, 135
physical examination in, 135
radiographic and ultrasound examinations in, 135
treatment of, 135
Peroneal nerve injury, *722*, 722–723
Personality changes, behavioral signs and, 72
Personnel, emergency medicine and, 211–212
Pesticide intoxication, affecting central nervous system, 459–460, 464–466
differentiation of, 460t, 465, 465t
coagulopathy caused by, 468–469
differentiation of, 459t, 465t, 469, 469t
Pet(s), as companions, 241–242
Pet ownership, 239–240
in developing countries, 218
Petroleum product poisoning, 459t, 460t, 465t, 467t, 473t, 481
pH, of urine, renal disease and, 1903
Pheohyphomycosis, 606
Phagocytosis, spleen and, 2235–2236
Pharmacodynamics, of antimicrobial drugs, 385–386
Pharmacokinetics, 378–381. *See also* Drug(s).
clearance and, 380
disposition curve and, *378*, 378–379
distribution volume and, 379, 379t
dosing rate and, 380t, 380–381
drug disposition and, alterations in, 381
half-life and, 379–380, 380t
of antimicrobial drugs, 385
plasma concentrations and, monitoring, 381
Pharmacology, 375–382. *See also* Drug(s).
antimicrobial therapy and, 381–382
drug absorption and disposition and, 376–378
drug action and, 375–376
pharmacokinetics and, 378–381
Pharyngitis, 1236
Pharyngostomy intubation, 787
Pharynx, cricopharyngeal achalasia and, 787
diagnostic approach to, 751, 783
dysphagia and, 1236–1237
foreign bodies in, 783–784
infection of, 784
nasopharyngeal polyps and, 784, *784*
neoplasia of, *787*, 787–788, *788*
paralysis of, 786–787
pharyngitis and, 1236
pharyngostomy intubation and, 787
retropharyngeal abscess and, 1237, *1237*
soft palate defects and, 784–786, *785*, *786*
structure and function of, 782–783
tonsillitis and, 1237–1238, 1238t
trauma to, 783–784
Phenolsulfonphthalein half-life, tubular function and, 1900
Phenylbutazone toxicity, aplastic anemia and, 2174
hematopoietic stem cell death and, in dogs, 2198–2199
Pheochromocytoma, cutaneous manifestations of, 7
polyuria and polydipsia and, 144
Phimosis, congenital preputial stenosis and, 1884, *1885*
Phobias, in dogs, 228–229
Phosphate, abnormal values of, causes of, 14t
dietary, renal failure and, 1990
serum levels of, in canine hyperadrenocorticism, 1732
Phosphate retention, effects of, 1999–2000
treatment of, 1999t, 2000t, 2000–2001
Phosphate supplementation, in diabetes mellitus, 1688
Phosphofructokinase deficiency, hemolytic disease associated with, 2171
Phospholipids, 203
Phosphorus intoxication, 468
differentiation of, 459t, 465t, 468
Phycomycosis, 362–364, *1361*, 1361–1362, *1362*
clinical manifestations of, 362–363
diagnosis of, 363–364
epizootiology of, 362
etiology of, 362
pathogenesis of, 362
treatment and prognosis in, 364
Physeal disorders, 2346–2347
radioulnar, 2346–2347, *1247*
Physical agents, myocardial disease and, 1122–1123
Physical examination, ear disease and, 246
emergency medicine and, 210–211
spinal cord diseases and, 626
Physical plant, emergency medicine and, 211, *212*
Physiotherapy, lower respiratory disease and, 819–820
Pickwickian syndrome, pulmonary manifestations of, 846
Pigmentary disorders, congenital and hereditary, ocular manifestations of, 77
Pigmenturia, hematuria differentiated from, 160
Pilonidal cyst, 682–683
Pilonidal sinus, 682–683
Pinna erythema, 250
idiopathic, 250
Pinnae, diseases of, 247–252
acquired diseases and, 247, *248*, 249–252
anatomy and, 247
congenital defects and, 247
examination and, 247
Pituitary gland, anatomy of, 1581–1582, *1582*
drug impairment of, 1593–1594, *1594*, *1595*
hyperplasia of, pathology of, 1724
macroadenomas of, pathology of, 1724
malformation of, canine hypothyroidism and, 1642
microadenomas of, pathology of, 1724
tumors of. *See* Tumor(s), pituitary.
vascularization of, 1582, *1583*
Pituitary hormones, *1584*, 1584–1585
measurement of, in dog, 1588
Pituitary-adrenocortical axis, evaluation of, in hyperadrenocorticism, 1736–1745
computed tomography in, 1743
CRH stimulation test in, 1743
discrimination tests and, 1741–1743
general approach to, 1736
metyrapone testing in, 1745
radioisotope imaging in, 1745
screening tests and, 1736–1741
ultrasonography in, 1743, *1744*
Pituitary-dependent hyperadrenocorticism. *See* Hyperadrenocorticism, canine.
Pituitary-hypothalamic diseases, 1579–1606
anatomy and, 1581–1582
developmental, 1581
hypothalamic-hypophyseal connections and, 1582
hypothalamus and, 1582
macroscopic, 1581
pituitary and, 1581–1582
endocrine rhythms and neuroendocrine function and, 1584–1606
acromegaly and, 1600–1602
adrenocorticotropic hormone and, 1587–1588
chromophobe adenoma and, endocrinologically inactive, 1591, *1591*
craniopharyngioma and, 1592, *1592*, *1593*
follicle-stimulating hormone and, 1587
functional corticotropic adenoma and, 1591–1592, *1592*
growth hormone deficiency and, in mature dog, 1588–1590, *1590*, *1591*
hypernatremia and, 1603–1605
hypopituitarism and, 1588, 1588t
in German shepherd, 1588–1589, *1589*, 1589t, *1590*
pituitary tumors and, 1590–1591
insulin-like growth factors and, 1585, *1586*, 1587, 1602–1603, *1604–1606*
luteinizing hormone and, 1587
Pituitary-hypothalamic diseases *(Continued)*
endocrine rhythms and neuroendocrine function and, pars intermedia adenoma and, *1593*, 1593–1600
pituitary diabetes insipidus and, 1605–1606, *1606*
pituitary hormone measurement and, in dog, 1588
pituitary hormones and, *1584*, 1584–1585
prolactin and, 1587
thyroid-stimulating hormone and, 1587
feedback and, 1580
historic background of, 1579–1580
adrenocorticotrophic hormone and, 1579
growth hormone and prolactin and, 1579
neurohypophysis and, 1580
thyroid-stimulating hormone and, 1580
hypophysiotropic concept and, 1580–1581
hypophysiotropic hormones and, 1583
neurotransmitter regulation and, 1583
Plague, in humans, 191
prevention of, 191
Plant(s), poisonous, 459t, 473t, 476
Plant alkaloids, in cancer chemotherapy, 533
Plant awn stomatitis, 1231
Plaque, 117
Plasma cell leukemia, *2215*, 2217
Plasma insulin, in canine hyperadrenocorticism, 1730
Plasma turbidity test, in exocrine pancreatic insufficiency, 1543–1545
Plasmacytic-lymphocytic synovitis, 2371
treatment of, 2372–2373
Plasmapheresis, canine mammary gland tumors and, 1824
Platelet(s), 2265–2267
adhesion of, 2266, 2277
aggregation of, 2266–2267, 2267t, 2276–2277
anatomy and biochemistry of, 2265
biochemistry of, 2266
bleeding disorders and, 105–106
laboratory studies and, 107
coagulation and, 2267
control of, 2267
counting, 2276
organelle zone of, 2266, 2266t
peripheral zone of, 2265
physiology of, 2266
platelet function assessment and, 2276–2277
release reaction and, 2267
sol-gel zone of, 2265
Platelet dysfunction, 2265–2277
adhesion defects and, 2268–2271
aggregation deficiencies and, 2271–2272
drug-induced, 2274–2275
hypercoagulation-associated, 2275–2276
release reaction deficiencies and, 2271
secondary, 2272–2274
Platelet factor–3 test, in immune-mediated thrombocytopenia, 2304
Platelet plug, dissolution of, 2248–2249, *2249*
Platelet-fibrin thrombus, in infective endocarditis, 1152–1153
Play, aggression induced by, in cats, 236–237
problems of, in dogs, 230–231
Pleura, anatomy and physiology of, 872
Pleural disorders, 872–895
diagnosis of, 873–877
diagnostic approach and, 873
diagnostic thoracocentesis and, 875–876, *876*
identification of pleural effusion and, 873–874
mediastinoscopy in, 877
open biopsy and, 874
pleural biopsy and, 874, *874*
therapeutic thoracocentesis and, 876–877
thoracic radiography in, 873
thoracoscopy and, 875, *875*
dyspnea and tachypnea and, 89
history and physical findings in, 872
Pleural effusion, abdominal surgery and, 881
autoimmune disorders associated with, 880–881, *881*
central venous catheters and, 883
clinical manifestations of, 872–873
congestive heart failure and, 877

Pleural effusion *(Continued)*
diagnostic approach to, 752
diagnostic procedures causing, 882
empyema and, 879–880
esophageal rupture and, 882, *882*
glomerulonephritis and, 882
hepatic disorders and, 881
hyperthyroidism and, 883
identification of, 873–874
lung torsion and, 883
neoplastic, 878–879
of undetermined etiology, 883–884
eosinophilia and, 883–884
pancreatitis and, 881
parapneumonic effusion and, 879
postpartum status and, 882–883
pulmonary infection and, 879
pulmonary thrombosis or embolism and, 883
pyometra and, 882–883
trauma and, 883
traumatic diaphragmatic hernia and, 883
Pneumocolon, 1404
Pneumocystosis, 291, 833
Pneumomediastinum, 890–891, *891*
causes of, 890t
clinical manifestations of, 891
treatment of, 891
Pneumonia, aspiration, 841–843
diagnosis of, 842, *842*
presentation of, 842
prevention of, 843
prognosis in, 843
treatment of, 842–843
bacterial, 830–832
diagnosis of, 831
presentation of, 830–831
prognosis in, 832
treatment of, 831t, 831–832
streptococcal, 267
viral, canine, 830
Pneumonitis, feline, 276
heartworm disease and, occult, 1176, *1176*
Pneumopericardiography, pericardial effusion and, *1141*, *1142*, 1143
Pneumoperitoneum, 136
Pneumothorax, 884–886, *885*
diagnosis of, 886
iatrogenic, 885
lung abscesses producing, 885
pulmonary cysts and, 885, *886*
pulmonary neoplastic necrosis producing, 885
spontaneous, 885
traumatic, 885
treatment of, 886
Pointer, English, sensory neuropathy of, 724
short hair, sensory neuropathy of, 724
Poisoning. *See* Toxicology.
Polioencephalomalacia, 600
Polioencephalomyelitis, feline, 656
idiopathic, 608
Pollakiuria, 163
Polyarteritis nodosa, 1193–1194, 2371–2372
Polyarthritis, idiopathic, treatment of, 2372–2373
nondeforming, neoplasia and, 2371
of greyhounds, 2367
progressive, feline, 2367–2372
Polychromatophilic cells, 2147, *2148*
Polycystic kidneys, 2024–2025, *2025*
Polycythemia, 101–104
definition of, 101
diagnostic plan for, 103, *104*
etiopathogenesis of, 101t, 101–102
appropriate secondary polycythemia and, 101–102
inappropriate secondary polycythemia and, 102
historical findings in, 102–103
ocular manifestations of, 80
pathophysiology of, 102
physical findings in, 103
primary, 101, 2216
therapeutic principles for, 103
prognosis for, 104
secondary, 101
therapeutic principles for, 103t, 103–104
Polycythemia vera, 101, 2216
therapeutic principles for, 103
Polydactyly, 2384
Polydipsia, *139*, 139–147, *140*
chronic renal failure and, 1922, 1922t
diagnostic approach to, 144t, 144–145, 145t, *146*, 147
diarrhea and, 34
etiology of, 141t, 141–144
history in, *140*, 140–141
in canine hyperadrenocorticism, 1725–1726
pathophysiology of, 139–140
Polymorphism, 2290
Polymyositis, 740
Polymyxins, 395
activity spectrum of, 395
Polyneuritis, chronic progressive, 728–729
chronic relapsing, 728–729
feline, 729
Polyneuropathies, cranial, 727–728
diabetic, 725, *726*
distal symmetrical, 729
familial, 724–725
hyperinsulinism, 725, *726*
hypothyroid, 725
inflammatory and immune-mediated, 727–729
metabolic, 725–726
paraneoplastic, 725–726
toxic, 726t, 726–727
weakness and, 49
with inherited hyperchylomicronemia, in cats, 725
Polyp(s), adenomatous, benign, 1317
nasopharyngeal, 784, *784*
Polyphagia, 15–17
diagnostic plan for, 16
history in, 15–16
in canine hyperadrenocorticism, 1726–1727
pathophysiology of, 15
physical findings in, 16
therapeutic goals in, 16–17
Polyploidy, 184
Polyradiculoneuritis, acute, 728, *728*
chronic progressive, 728–729
chronic relapsing, 728–729
Polysystemic disorders, brain and, 617–619
Polyuria, *139*, 139–147, *140*
chronic renal failure and, 1922, 1922t
diagnostic approach to, 144t, 144–145, 145t, *146*, 147
dysuria and, 163
etiology of, 141t, 141–144
history in, *140*, 140–141
in canine hyperadrenocorticism, 1725–1726
pathophysiology of, 139–140
Poodle, miniature, demyelinating myelopathy of, 596, 649–650
Porencephaly, 591
Porphyria, feline, 2171
Portal hypertension, 1456–1459, 1457t, *1458*
ascites and, 1458–1459, *1459*
Portal systemic shunts, 1499–1506, *1500*, *1501*, *1503–1505*
Portal vascular abnormalities, uric acid and ammonium urate urolithiasis and, in dogs, 2094, 2096
Portal vein, gastric dilatation-volvulus-torsion syndrome and, 1279
Positioning, radiography and, 753–754, *755*
Postictal phase, seizures and, 68
Post-ingestion distress, 31
Postpartum status, pleural effusion caused by, 882–883
Postural reactions, in neurologic examination, 558–559
Posture, coma and stupor and, 63
lameness and, in dogs, 166
Potassium. *See also* Hyperkalemia; Hypokalemia.
abnormal values of, causes of, 13t
physiology of, *437*, 437–438
serum levels of, in hypoadrenocorticism, 1761t, 1762
Potassium imbalance, 437–440
hyperkalemia and, *437*, 438t, 439–440
hypokalemia and, 438t, 438–439
Potassium imbalance *(Continued)*
in chronic renal failure, therapy for, 1997–1998
potassium physiology and, *437*, 437–438
Potassium supplementation, in diabetes mellitus, *1687*, 1687–1688, 1688t
Prazosin, actions of, 961
in heart failure therapy, 961
indications for, 961
toxicity and interactions of, 961
Prealbumin, thyroxine binding, serum, in canine hypothyroidism, 1648–1649
Predatory behavior, 234–235
Pre-excitation syndromes, 1073–1074, *1074*, *1075*
Pregnancy, adverse drug reactions and, 500
corticosteroids and, 417
feline, 1788
in bitch, 1785–1786, *1786*
Preictal phase, seizures and, 68
Preload, cardiac output and, 901–902, *903*, 904, *904*
heart failure therapy and, 941
reduction of, in pulmonary edema, 862
Premature contractions, classification of, 1069–1070
supraventricular, *1066*, 1067
ventricular, *1065*, 1067–1070, *1068*, *1069*
Prepuce, congenital stenosis of, with phimosis, 1884, *1885*
defects of, 1883–1884
normal bacterial flora of, 1881, 1882t
tumors of, 1817
Pressure overloading, heart failure and, *912*, *913*, 913–914
Preventive medicine, in developing countries, 224
Priapism, 1888
Primary afferent neuron, pain and, 18–19
Procainamide (Pronestyl), 1061–1062
Proctitis, 1567
definition of, 36
Proctoscopy, 1400–1402
complications of, 1402
equipment for, 1400, *1400*
indications for, 1400
technique for, 1400–1402, *1401*
Proestrus, canine, 1783–1784
feline, 1787
Profilmetry, urethral, in lower urinary tract disease, 2113
Progesterone, in insulin antagonism/resistance, 1700–1701
Progressive hemorrhagic myelomalacia (PHM), *683*, 683–684
Projectile vomiting, 29
Prolactin, 1583, 1587
pituitary-hypothalamic diseases and, 1579
Proliferative cystitis, *2122*, 2122–2123
Prolonged sinus pause, 1085–1087, *1087*
Pronestyl. *See* Procainamide.
Prophylaxis, antimicrobial drugs in, 408, 410
Propranolol (Inderal), 1063–1064
in heart failure therapy, 963–964
indications for, 963–964
toxicity and interactions of, 964
Proprioceptive positioning, in neurologic examination, *558*, 559
Proprioceptive reflexes, testing for, 566–569
Prostate, adenocarcinoma of, 1816
canine diseases of, 1859–1877, *1860*
bacterial, 1869–1874
clinical signs in, 1860–1861, *1861*, 1861t
cystic, 1869
diagnosis of, 1861–1867
history in, 1861–1862
palpation in, 1862
prostatic aspiration in, *1866*, 1866–1867
prostatic biopsy in, *1866*, 1867, *1867*
prostatic massage and, 1863, *1863*
radiography in, 1863–1865, *1864*, *1865*
semen evaluation and, *1862*, 1862–1863, *1863*
ultrasonography in, 1865–1866, *1866*
urethral discharge and, 1862
hyperplastic, 1867–1868
metaplastic, 1868
multiple, 1877
neoplastic, 1874–1877

Prostatitis, abscessation and, 1873–1874
acute, 1870
bacterial, 1869–1874
chronic, 1870–1873
clinical signs in, 1870
diagnosis of, 1870–1871
pathophysiology of, 1870
treatment of, *1871*, 1871–1873, 1871t–1873t, *1872*
pathophysiology of, 1869–1870
Protective aggression, 234
Protein, canine requirement for, 1993
digestion and absorption of, 1326–1327
in urine, renal disease and, 1903
loss of, gastrointestinal, fecal tests and, 1337–1338
metabolism of, corticosteroids and, 416
recommended intake of, for cats, in chronic renal failure, 1994
for dogs, in chronic renal failure, 1993–1994
reduction of, in chronic renal failure, 1992, *1992*
regulation of, in liver disease, albumin and, 1433–1434
serum globulins and, 1434t, 1434–1435
synthesis of, bacteriostatic inhibitors of, 398–401
in liver disease, 1433–1435
albumin and, 1433–1434
serum globulins and, 1434t, 1434–1435
urinary, concentration of, in glomerular disease, 1943–1944
loss of, in glomerular disease, 1944, 1944t
Protein malnutrition, in chronic renal failure, diet therapy and, 1994–1995
Protein status, nutritional assessment and, 451
Protein-calorie malnutrition, exocrine pancreatic insufficiency and, 1540
Protein-losing enteropathies. *See* Enteropathies, protein-losing.
Proteinuria, 2031
dysuria and, 164
in glomerular disease, classification and localization of, 1943
in nephrotic syndrome, 2020–2021
modifying magnitude of, 2020–2021
nephrotic range, 2007
Proteolytic activity, fecal, in exocrine pancreatic insufficiency, 1545–1546, *1546*
Prothrombin time, one-stage, 2251
Prototheca, ocular manifestations of, 82
Protothecal colitis, 1413
Protothecal meningomyelitis. *See* Meningomyelitis, protothecal.
Protothecosis, 365–367, 605–606
clinical manifestations of, 366
diagnosis of, 366, *366*, *367*
etiology and epizootiology of, 365
pathogenesis of, 366
prognosis in, 367
Protozoal diseases, 281–292
arthritic, 2366
cardiovascular and visceral, 287–292
coccidial, 281–285
enteric, 285–287
in developing countries, 222
myocardial, 1124–1125
of brain, 606
pulmonary, 832–833
Protozoal myelitis, 684–685
Provocative testing, insulin-secreting tumors and, 1711–1712
Pruritus, 122–125
alopecia and, 116–117
definition of, 122
diagnostic plan for, 123, 125
historical findings in, 122–123
pathophysiology of, 122
physical findings in, 123, 124t
therapeutic goals for, 125
PRV. *See* Pseudorabies virus.
Pseudoachondrodysplasia, 2383
Pseudochylothorax, 884, 884t
Pseudocoprostasis, 1573
Pseudocyesis, 234
Pseudocysts, perirenal, feline, 2025–2026
Pseudogout, 2373
Pseudomembranous colitis, 1415
Pseudomyotonia, in canine hyperadrenocorticism, 1729
Pseudorabies virus (PRV), gastroenteritis and, 310
Psychogenic factors, alopecia and, 120
polydipsia and, 142
Psychological factors, weakness and, 50
Puberty, 1779
Pudendal nerve injury, 723
Puerperal tetany, 1831–1832
hypocalcemia and, 1625–1626
Pug encephalitis, 608–609
Pulmonary abscesses, 847
Pulmonary atresia, cyanotic heart disease and, 1023
Pulmonary contusions, 840–841
Pulmonary crackles, cyanosis and, 98
Pulmonary density, radiographic interpretation and, 754, 758–759
Pulmonary disease. *See* Respiratory disease.
Pulmonary edema, 853–863
clinicopathology of, 857
differential diagnosis of, 855t, 860–861
electrocardiography in, 858
etiology and pathophysiology of, 854–856, 855t
history and clinical signs in, 856–857
poisoning and, 465t
radiographic examination in, 858–860, *858–860*
treatment of, 861–863
acid-base balance in, 862
bronchodilating agents in, 861
digitalis in, 862
diuretics in, 861
oxygen in, 862
preload reduction in, 862
sedation in, 861–862
Pulmonary embolism, pleural effusion caused by, 883
Pulmonary hypertension, patent ductus arteriosus with, 991, *991*, *992*
Pulmonary infection, pleural effusion associated with, 879
Pulmonary mineralization, 846–847
Pulmonary pattern, radiographic interpretation and, 754, 756, *756*, *757*, 758t
Pulmonary resistance, in cyanotic heart disease, 1017
Pulmonary thrombosis, pleural effusion caused by, 883
Pulmonary venous pressure, left heart evaluation and, 927–928
Pulmonic insufficiency, 1004, *1006*, 1049
Pulmonic stenosis, 1000–1004, *1019*
clinical findings in, 1000, *1002–1006*, 1003
clinical management of, 1003–1004, *1005*, 1007t
natural history of, 1003
pathogenesis of, 1000, *1001*
pathophysiology of, 1000, *1002*
Pulse, absence of, cardiopulmonary arrest and, 172
Pump failure, 1097–1098
Pupil size, coma and stupor and, 63
testing for, 563, *704*, 704–706, 705t
pharmacologic, 705–706
symmetry and, 563
Pupillary light reflex, coma and stupor and, 63
testing for, 561, *562*, 563, 703–704, *704*
Puppy strangles, 2229–2230
Pustule, 117
Pyelography, intravenous. *See* Excretory urography.
Pyelonephritis, 1945, 1947, *1947*
clinical and laboratory findings in, 2037–2038
diagnosis of, 1952–1953, 2038
in canine hyperadrenocorticism, 1735
prognosis of, 2038
treatment of, 2038
urinary tract infection and, 2036–2037
Pyloric dysfunction, gastric motility disorders and, 1313–1314
Pyloric gastropathy, hypertrophic, chronic, 1307
Pyloric gland region, of stomach, 1290
Pyloric stenosis, 1311
Pyloromyotomy, in gastric dilatation-volvulus-torsion syndrome, 1284
Pylorus, 1289
Pyoderma, 274
Pyogranulomatous meningoencephalomyelitis, 608, 685
Pyometra, 1798–1801, 1799t
pleural effusion caused by, 882–883
polyuria and polydipsia and, 143
Pyridylium herbicide intoxication, 467
differentiation of, 459t, 465t, 467, 467t
Pyruvate kinase deficiency, hemolytic disease associated with, 2170–2171
Pyuria, dysuria and, 164

Quadriplegia, hereditary, in Irish setter, 597
Quinidine, 1061
Quinolones, 401–402
action of, 401
activity spectrum of, 401
clinical pharmacology of, 401–402
toxicity of, 402

Rabies, 601
animals exposed to, management of, 300–301
canine, 298–301
clinical signs of, 299
diagnosis of, 299
epizootiology of, 298–299
etiology of, 298
treatment and prevention of, 299–300
feline, 322–324
clinical signs of, 323–324
furious phase and, 323–324
paralytic phase and, 324
prodromal phase and, 323
control of, 324
vaccination and, 324
differential diagnosis of, 324
epizootiology of, 322–323
etiology of, 322
laboratory diagnosis of, 324
pathogenesis of, 323
public health aspects of, 323
transmission of, 323
human bites and, animal management and, 300
human rabies vaccination and, 300
in developing countries, 221–222
in humans, 193
prevention of, 193
Radial nerve injury, *721*, 722
Radiation, hematopoietic stem cell death and, 2197–2200
Radiation therapy, 540–541
biological considerations and, 540–541
canine mammary gland tumors and, 1824
in feline hyperadrenocorticism, 1756
practical considerations and, 541, 542t
thyroid tumors and, in dog, 1670
Radioactive iodine, in feline hyperthyroidism, 1666–1667
thyroid tumors and, in dog, 1670
Radiography, canine urolithiasis and, 2086t, 2086–2087
coma and stupor and, 64
emergency medicine and, 216
esophageal diseases and, 1259–1261
technique with, 1259–1261
gastric disease and, 1296–1297, *1297*
in canine hyperadrenocorticism, 1732–1734
abdominal, *1731*, 1733, *1733*, *1734*
general approach to, 1732–1733
thoracic, 1733–1734
in chronic mitral valvular insufficiency, 1032t, 1033–1035, *1036*, 1037
in chronic renal failure, 1926
in congenital heart disease, 977–978
in degenerative joint disease, 2331–2333, *2332*
in feline hyperadrenocorticism, 1755
in hypoadrenocorticism, 1763
in infective endocarditis, 1156–1157, *1158*
in large intestinal disease, 1402–1404
barium enema and, 1402–1404, 1403t
pneumocolon and, 1404
survey abdominal radiographs and, 1402

Radiography *(Continued)*
in liver disease, 1466–1467, *1467*
in lower urinary tract disease, 2111, *2112*
in pancreatitis, 1535
in periodontitis, 1222, *1222*
in peripheral edema, 44–45
in prostatic disease, 1863–1865, *1864*, *1865*
in pulmonary edema, 858–860, *858–860*
in small bowel diarrhea, 1339, *1340*
in urinary tract infection, bacterial, 2118–2119
insulin-secreting tumors and, 1710
large intestine and, chronic inflammatory bowel disease and, 1406
lymphadenopathy and, 2228
mediastinal disorders and, 888
nasal disorders and, 770–771, *770–773*
oral cavity diseases and, *1208*, 1208–1209
pericardial effusion and, 1139, *1140–1142*, 1141–1142
polycythemia and, 103
renal disorders and, 1911–1915
excretory urography and, 1911t, 1911–1912
survey radiographs and, 1911
respiratory disease and, 752–759
interpretation and, 754–759, *755–757*, 758t, *759*
technical quality and, 752–754, *753–755*
spinal cord tumors and, 679, *679*, *680*
splenomegaly and, 2241–2242
survey, of skull, 578–579, *579–581*
thoracic, cyanosis and, 99
pleural disorders and, 873
urinary tract infection and, bacterial, 2117
vertebral, noncontrast, spinal cord disease and, 627
Radioisotope studies, of adrenals, 1745
of thyroid, in canine hypothyroidism, 1649, *1650*
in feline hyperthyroidism, *1660*, 1660–1661, *1661*
Radionuclide imaging, glomerular function and, 1898
splenomegaly and, 2241–2242
Recognition, immune response and, *2284*, 2284–2285
Recombinant human erythropoietin, in nonregenerative anemia, in chronic renal failure, 2004
Records, emergency medicine and, 214
Rectal aplasia, 1569–1570
diagnosis of, 1569, *1569*, 1570
history and clinical signs in, 1569
treatment of, 1569–1570
Rectal diseases, 1561–1567
anatomy and, 1559–1560, *1560*
defecation and, physiology of, 1560–1561
history and physical examination in, 1561
neoplastic, 1565–1566
diagnosis of, 1566, *1566*
history and physical findings in, *1565*, 1565–1566, *1566*
treatment of, 1566
special examination in, 1561
Rectal foreign bodies, 1567
Rectal palpation, 1399
Rectal prolapse, 1563–1565
history and resulting signs in, 1563
physical findings in, 1564, *1564*
postoperative care and, 1565
prognosis of, 1565
treatment of, 1564–1565
Rectal strictures, 1567
Rectovaginal fistula, *1568*, 1570, *1570*
Red blood cell morphology, cyanosis and, 98
Red cell aplasia, feline leukemia virus and, 92
idiopathic, 92
Red pulp, of spleen, 2234
Reentry, cardiac arrhythmias and, 1056
REF. *See* Renal erythropoietic factor.
Referrals, emergency medicine and, 214
Reflex(es), anterior tibialis, testing for, 569, *571*
Babinski, testing for, 573
biceps, testing for, 567, 569, *569*, 574t
corneal, testing for, 564
crossed extensor, testing for, 573, *573*, 574t
extensor carpi radialis, testing for, 567, *568*

Reflex(es) *(Continued)*
flexor, testing for, 569, *572*, 574t
gag, testing for, 564, 566
gastrocnemius, testing for, 569
nociceptive, testing for, 569, 573
palpebral, testing for, 564, *565*, 707
panniculus, testing for, 569, 573
patellar, testing for, 569, *571*, 574t
pelvic limb, testing for, 569, *570*
perineal, testing for, 569, *572*, 574t
proprioceptive, testing for, 566–569
pupillary light, testing for, 561, *562*, 563
testing of, 703–704, *704*
retractor oculi, testing for, 564
spinal, spinal cord disease and, 629–630
thoracic limb, testing for, 567–569, *567*
triceps, testing for, 567, *568*, 574t
Reflex dyssynergia, urethral obstruction and, 2075–2076
Reflux, definition of, 30
duodenal, pancreatitis and, 1534
vesicoureteral, urinary tract infection and, 2036–2037
Reflux gastritis, 1314
Regeneration, hepatic, 1424–1425
Regurgitation, 30–32, 31t
clinical features of, 31–32
definition of, 30
diagnostic plan for, 32
pathophysiology of, 31
physical findings in, 32
vomiting differentiated from, 27
Release reaction, deficiencies of, 2271
platelets and, 2267
Renal-adrenal-pituitary interactions, heart failure and, 908–910, *909*
Renal biopsy, in nephrotic syndrome, 2014–2016
indications for, 2009t, 2014–2015
methods for, 2015–2016, *1016*
Renal clearance, 1897
Renal control, of plasma bicarbonate, acid-base and, 441–442, *442*
Renal cysts, 2024–2025
Renal damage, poisoning and, 460t
Renal disease, 1893–1953
clinical evaluation of, 1894–1896
glomerular function and, 1896t, 1896–1898
history and, 1894–1895
physical examination in, *1895*, 1895–1896
signalment and, 1894
tubular function and, 1898t, 1898–1900
urinalysis and, 1900–1907
cutaneous manifestations of, 9
drugs for, 2046t
hypercalcemia and, 1615–1616
in liver disease, 1459–1461
microbiology and, 1907–1911, 1909t
polycythemia and, 102
primary, hypocalcemia and, 1622, *1623*, *1624*
radiology in, 1911–1915
excretory urography and, 1911t, 1911–1912
survey radiographs and, 1911
secondary hypertension and, 2049–2050
Renal erythropoietic factor (REF), in polycythemia, 101
Renal failure, 1893
acute, 1926–1937, 1927t, 1928t, 1962–1981
causes of, 1963–1968, 1965t
postrenal, 1965, 1965t
prerenal, 1964–1965, 1965t
primary, 1965t–1967t, 1965–1968
chronic renal failure versus, 1926, *1926*, 1927t, 1972
decreased glomerular filtration rate and, *1930*, 1930–1931
definition and clinical characteristics of, 1962–1963
diagnosis of, 1937, 1968–1973
syndrome analysis and, 1968–1973, 1969t
syndrome identification and, 1966t, 1968
ischemia and, *1934–1936*, 1935–1937
nephritis and, 1937
nephrosis and, 1928–1930, *1929*
nephrotoxins and, 1931, *1932*, 1933–1935

Renal failure *(Continued)*
acute, prognosis of, 1973–1974
reduced urine flow and, *1930*, 1930–1931
treatment of, 1974t–1976t, 1974–1981, *1980*
minimizing hyperphosphatemia and, 1981
preventing adverse drug reactions and, 1980–1981
anemia and, 92, 1918, 2172
chronic, 1920–1926, 1981–2006
acute failure differentiated from, 1926, *1926*, 1927t, 1972
clinical characteristics of, 1981–1983, *1982*, 1982t
definition and clinical significance of, 1981
diagnosis of, 1926, 1983–1985, 1984t, 1985t
early detection in, 1983–1984
syndrome analysis in, 1984t, 1984–1985, 1985t
syndrome identification in, 1983
pathophysiology of, 1920–1926
acid-base balance regulation and, 1922–1923
disease progression and, 1924–1926, *1925*
intact nephron hypothesis and, 1921
osteodystrophy and, 1923–1924, 1924t
polyuria/polydipsia and, 1922, 1922t
renal secondary hyperparathyroidism and, 1923–1924, 1924t
residual neuron adaptation and, *1921*, 1921–1922, 1922t
trade-off hypothesis and, 1922
urinary concentrating defects and, 1922
prognosis of, 1985–1986
treatment of, 1986–2006
diet therapy in, 1991t, 1991–1996, *1992*
divalent ion imbalances and, 1999t, 1999–2002, 2000t
drug therapy in, 2004–2005, 2005t
electrolyte disorders and, 1996–1998
fluid disorders and, 1996
hypertension and, 2005–2006
medical, conservative, 1986t, 1986–1987
metabolic acidosis and, 1998–1999
modifying progression and, 1987–1991, *1988*, *1989*
nonregenerative anemia and, 2002–2004, 2003t, 2004t
patient monitoring and, 2006
urinary tract infection and, 2006
in insulin antagonism/resistance, 1702
in nephrotic syndrome, symptomatic and supportive treatment of, 2020
neoplastic, polycythemia and, therapeutic principles for, 104
primary. *See* Tubular necrosis, acute.
progression of, 1987–1988, *1988*, 2006
causes of, 1988–1991
Renal glycosuria, 2027–2028
Renal insufficiency, 1893
Renal system, in feline hyperthyroidism, 1655t, 1656–1657
Renal tubular acidosis, 2026t, 2026–2027
Renal tubular disease, polyuria and polydipsia and, *139*, 141
Renal tubular function. *See* Tubular function.
Renomegaly, 137–138
Repetitive behaviors, 72
Repositol vasopressin test, tubular function and, 1900
Reproductive system, in canine hypothyroidism, adult-onset, 1643
Reservoir function, spleen and, 2235–2236
Resorption, of teeth, 1211
Respiration, pattern of, cyanosis and, 97, 98
Respiratory acidosis, 445–446
clinical signs of, 446, 446t
compensation and, 443t, 446
treatment of, 446
Respiratory alkalosis, 446
compensation and, 443t, 446, 446t
Respiratory control, of carbon dioxide, acid-base and, 441
Respiratory disease, arterial, heartworm disease and, 1171–1172, *1173–1177*, 1174, 1176
therapeutic principles for, 103

Respiratory disease *(Continued)*
chronic obstructive, 847
polycythemia and, 102
therapeutic principles for, 103
diagnosis of, 747t, 747–766
alveoli and, 752
bronchoscopy in, 760t, 761–764, *762–764*
dyspneic patient and, 752
history and, 747–749, 748t
nasal cavity and sinuses and, 751
nondyspneic patient and, 750–751, 751t
open lung biopsy in, 766
percutaneous fine needle aspiration lung biopsy in, *764*, 764–765, *765*
pharynx and larynx and, 751
physical examination and, 749–750
pleural effusions and, 752
radiography in, 752–759
trachea and bronchi and, 751–752
transtracheal aspiration in, 759–761, *760*, 760t, *761*
heartworm disease and, 1170–1171
lower, 816–863
acid-base balance in, 820
airway humidification in, 819
bronchodilation in, 820
cough suppression in, 820–829
expectorants and, 821
medication nebulization and, 821
cystic-bullous, 845
hypersensitivity and immune-mediated, 838–839
infectious, 829–838
bacterial, 830–832
fungal, 833–838
protozoal, 832–833
viral, 829–830
management of, 816–820
mononuclear, 839–840
neoplastic, 848–853
non-neoplastic, 829
oxygenation and ventilation in, 816–819, 817t
physiotherapy in, 819–820
sequelae to, 847–848
traumatic, 840–845
polycythemia and, 102
weakness and, 50
viral, feline, 317–322
clinical findings in, 318–320
control of, 321
differential diagnosis of, 320
etiology of, 317
laboratory diagnosis of, 320–321
predisposing factors and, 317–318
transmission of, 318
treatment of, 321
vaccination for, 322
Respiratory distress, definition of, 85
poisoning and, 465t
Respiratory phase, radiography and, 752, *753*
Respiratory system, antimicrobial selection for, 406t, 406–407
bacterial infections of, 265–267
in feline hyperthyroidism, 1655
Rest, in heart failure therapy, 966
Resting membrane potential, 1051
Restraint, external ear canal examination and, 254
urethral obstruction and, 2073
Restrictive cardiomyopathy. *See* Cardiomyopathy, restrictive.
Retching, definition of, 27
Reticulocytes, 91
counting, 2153–2154, *2154–2155*
Reticuloendothelial diseases, oral lesions and, 1228
Reticulosis. *See* Meningoencephalomyelitis, granulomatous.
Retinopathy, diabetes mellitus and, 1705
Retractor oculi reflex, testing for, 564
Retriever, Labrador, type 2 myofiber deficiency of, 738
Retroperitoneal masses, polycythemia and, 103
Retropharyngeal abscess, 1237, *1237*
Rhabdomyosarcoma, treatment of, 2128, 2129t
Rheumatoid arthritis, 2313–2314
of dogs, 2366–2367, *2367*, *2368*
treatment of, 2373
Rheumatoid diseases, 2309–2314
Rhinarium, disorders of, 771–773, *773*, *774*
Rhinitis, bacterial, 778, *779*
dental disease and, 776
foreign body, 774–775, *775*
fungal, 778–780, *780*
palatine defects and, 775–776, *775–778*
parasitic, 780
viral, 776–778, *779*
Rhinosporidiosis, 364–365
clinical manifestations of, 365, *365*
diagnosis of, 365
etiology and epizootiology of, *364*, 364–365
treatment and prognosis of, 365
Rhinotracheitis, viral, feline, 318–319
acute, 318, *318*
carrier state of, 318–319
chronic sequelae to, 318, *319*
Riboflavin deficiency, brain and, 616
Rickettsial diseases, 276–281
arthritic, 2364–2365
cutaneous manifestations of, 8
diarrhea and, 1359
of brain, 604
pulmonary manifestations of, 830
Rickettsial meningomyelitis. *See* Meningomyelitis, rickettsial.
Risk factors, for lower urinary tract disease, in cat, 2058, 2059t
Rocky Mountain spotted fever (RMSF), 280–281, brain and, 604
in humans, 191
prevention of, 191
ocular manifestations of, 81
Root planing, of teeth, 1225
Rotavirus, canine, diarrhea and, 1353–1354
feline, diarrhea and, 1354
Rottweiler, leukoencephalomyelopathy of, 597, 671–672
neuroaxonal dystrophy in, 598–599, 682
Rough-coated collie, cerebellar degeneration in, 598
Rouleaux formation, 2150, *2153*
Roundworms. *See* Larval migrans.
Rubber jaw syndrome, in chronic renal failure, 1982
Rubbing, self-mutilation and, 71
Rupture, of biliary tract, 1558

Sacrocaudal dysgenesis, in Manx cats, 685
Salicylates, thrombocytopathies induced by, 2274, 2274t
Saline, in hypoadrenocorticism, electrolyte imbalance and, 1767–1768
Salivary glands, 1241–1252
anatomy and physiology of, 1241
drooling and, 1242, *1247*
history and examination of, 1241–1242, *1243–1246*
inflammatory diseases of, 1251, *1251*
injuries to, 1242, 1247–1250, 1249, 1251
neoplasia of, 1251–1252
Salivary mucocele, 1242, 1249, *1249*, *1250*
management of, 1249, 1251
Salmon poisoning disease, 277, 1359
Salmonella infections, 268–269
in humans, 192
of large intestine, 1414
small bowel diarrhea and, 1355–1356
Salt supplementation, in hypoadrenocorticism, 1770
Sarcocystis, 282–283
Sarcoma, osteogenic, 2362
synovial cell, 2361–2362
Scabies, of pinna, 250
Scale(s), 118–119
Scaling, of teeth, 1225, *1225*
Scar, 119
Sciatic nerve injury, 722, *722*
Scirrhous carcinoma, 894–895
Sclerosis, glomerular, 2011
Scratching, self-mutilation and, 71
Screening tests, for hyperadrenocorticism, 1736–1741
Scrotal tumors, 1817
Secretion(s), gastric. *See* Gastric secretion.
large intestinal, 1398
pancreatic, regulation of, 1531
Secretory component, 2287
Sedatives, in liver failure, 1516
in pulmonary edema, 861–862
Seizure(s), 66–69
behavioral signs of, 73
coma and stupor and, 63
definition of, 66
diagnostic plan for, 67–68
focal, 66
generalized, 66
historical findings in, 67
outcome and, 69
pathophysiology of, 66–67
physical findings in, 67
toxicity and, 614–615
treatment goals for, 68–69
Seizure focus, 66
Self-mutilation, 71, 72
Self-non-self discrimination, immune response and, 2284
Semen, prostatic disease and, *1862*, 1862–1863, *1863*
Seminomas, 1815
"Senile" brain, behavioral signs of, 74
Sensitivity, cerebral, hepatic encephalopathy and, 1465
Sensory ataxia, 57
Sensory dysfunction, spinal cord disease and, 630
Sensory trigeminal neuropathy, 716–717
Separation anxiety, in dogs, 229–230
antianxiety medication and, 229–230
Septal defects, aorticopulmonary, 1024, 1027
atrioventricular. *See* Atrioventricular septal defects.
Serology, in feline panleukopenia, 316
Sertoli cell tumors, 1815
cutaneous manifestations of, 6
Serum biochemistries, in canine hypothyroidism, 1642t, 1644–1645
in feline hyperthyroidism, 1658
in feline panleukopenia, 316
lymphadenopathy and, 2228
splenomegaly and, 2241, 2241t
Serum enzymes, abnormal values of, causes of, 12t–14t
Serum factors, in cancer therapy, 540
Serum phosphate, in canine hyperadrenocorticism, 1732
Serum proteins, abnormal values of, causes of, 14t
Serum sickness, allergic drug reactions and, 503
Serum tests, in exocrine pancreatic insufficiency, 1542–1545
Serum trypsin-like immunoreactivity, in exocrine pancreatic insufficiency, 1542–1543, *1543*
Sesamoid bone disorders, 2345
Setter, Gordon, cerebellar degeneration in, 597–598
Irish, hereditary quadriplegia and amblyopia in, 597
Sex. *See also* Female(s); Male(s).
adverse drug reactions and, 500
alopecia and, 114
pain and, 20
pruritus and, 122
Sex hormones. *See also* Androgens; Estrogens; Testosterone.
in hypoadrenocorticism, 1759
Sexual data, pruritus and, 123
Sexual development, disorders of, infertility and, in bitch, 1848–1849
Sexual history, alopecia and, 115
Sheep dog, collie, neuroaxonal dystrophy in, 599
Shigella, small bowel diarrhea and, 1359
Shivering. *See* Tremor.
Shock, gastric dilatation-volvulus-torsion syndrome and, 1250
liver disease and, 1484

Short bowel syndrome, 1375
Short haired pointer, sensory neuropathy of, 724
Shoulder joint, dysplasia of, 2358
luxations and subluxations of, 2338
Shunts, anatomic, central cyanosis and, 96
SIADH. *See* Syndrome of inappropriate secretion of antidiuretic hormone.
Sick sinus syndrome, 1093, *1094*, 1095
Silent heat, infertility and, 1848
Sinoatrial arrest, 1085–1087, *1087*
Sinus(es), diagnostic approach to, 751
facial, 1211–1212, *1214*
paranasal. *See* Paranasal sinuses.
Sinus bradycardia, 1085, *1086*
SIPS. *See* Subinvolved placental sites.
Skeletal diseases, 2378–2396
drugs for, 2399t
extraskeletal system disturbances and, 2385
genetic, 2383–2385
inflammatory, 2378–2381
metabolic, 2381–2383
neoplastic, 2387–2391
in cat, 2389–2390
in dog, 2387–2389
metastatic, 2390
nutritional, 2385, 2387
of undetermined etiology, 2391–2393
Skeletal muscle disorders, 733–742
drugs for, 744t
historical perspective on, 733
muscle structure and, *733*, 733–734, 734t, *735*
myopathy and, 734–742, 735t
physiology and, 734
Skin. *See also* Dermatologic disease; *headings beginning with term* Cutaneous; *specific diseases.*
as sensor of internal disorders, 5–10, 6t
autoimmune disorders and, 9
bacterial infections and, 7
congenital-hereditary syndromes and, 5
endocrinopathies and, 6–7
fungal infections and, 7
hepatic disease and, 9
neoplasia and, 10
nutritional disorders and, 8–9
pancreatic disease and, 9
parasitic diseases and, 7–8
renal disease and, 9
thallium toxicosis and, 9
bacterial infections of, 274
care of, pruritus and, 123
hematuria and, 162
in canine hyperadrenocorticism, 1727–1728
in canine hypothyroidism, adult-onset, 1642t, 1642–1643
respiratory disease and, diagnosis of, 749
Skull, survey radiography of, 578–579, *579–581*
SLE. *See* Systemic lupus erythematosus.
Sleep disorientation aggression, 74
Small intestines. *See* Intestine(s), small.
Smoke inhalation, 844–845
Smooth-haired fox terriers, hereditary ataxia in, 660
Snake venom poisoning, 472–473
differentiation of, 473, 473t
polyneuropathy and, 727
Socioeconomic factors, in developing countries, 217–218
Sodium. *See also* Hypernatremia; Hyponatremia.
abnormal values of, causes of, 14t
disorders of, in chronic renal failure, therapy for, 1996–1997
restriction of, heart failure therapy and, 965
retention of, nephrotic syndrome and, 1942, *1942*
serum levels of, in hypoadrenocorticism, 1761t, 1762
total body, disorders of, 431–435
physiology and, 431
volume contraction and, 432t, 432–434, 434t
volume expansion and, 434t, 434–435
Sodium bicarbonate, cardiopulmonary response to, 176–177
in hyperkalemia, in acute renal failure, 1976–1977
Sodium bicarbonate *(Continued)*
in hypoadrenocorticism, electrolyte imbalance and, 1768
Sodium nitroprusside, actions of, 960
in heart failure therapy, 960–961
indications for, 960
toxicity and interactions of, 960–961
Sodium sulfonilate, half-life of, 1898
Soft palate defects, 784–786, *785*, *786*
Soft tissue, supporting joints, damage to, 2337
Solute, intestinal transport of, 1327
Somatic mutation, immune system and, 2288
Somatostatin, 1583
Somogyi overswing, 1698, *1698*, *1699*
Spasm, laryngeal, 790
Species, adverse drug reactions and, 500
Specific gravity, of urine, renal disease and, 1904
tubular function and, 1898–1899
Specificity, immune response and, 2284, *2284*
Specula, external ear canal examination and, 253–254
Spermatogenesis, primary failure of, treatment of, 1853, 1855
Spherocytes, 2150, *2151*
Sphincter, esophageal, lower, 1256, *1256*
pharmacologic responses of, 1257–1258
upper, 1255–1256
ileocecal, 1397
Sphingomyelinosis, 594
Spina bifida, 685–686, *686*
Spinal accessory nerves, focal diseases of, 719
Spinal arachnoid cysts, 686–687, *688*
Spinal articulations, instabilities of, 2343–2344
Spinal cord. *See also* Central nervous system.
acute injury of, clinical findings in, 689
diagnosis of, 689–690
etiology and pathogenesis of, 688–689, *689*
treatment of, 690–691
chronic compression of, clinical findings in, 689
diagnosis of, 690
etiology and pathogenesis of, 689
treatment of, 691
trauma to, 687–691
Spinal cord diseases, 624–694, 625t, 626t
cervical, 632t, 633
cervical enlargement and, 633
lumbar enlargement and, 634
paresis and paralysis and, 59–60
thoracolumbar, 633–634
clinical signs of, 629–630
diagnosis of, 625–629
ancillary diagnostic investigations and, 627–629
differential, 617
history and, 625–626
minimum data base and, 617
neurologic examination and, 626
physical examination and, 626
problem list and, 626–627
signalment and, 625
localization of, 625t, 626t, 630–634, *631*, 632t
mechanisms of, 624–629
diagnostic approach and, 625–629
Spinal muscular atrophy, progressive, 724
Spinal nematodiasis, 687
Spinal nerve root disorders, 719
Spinal nerves, focal diseases of, obturator nerve injury and, *722*, 723
peripheral, 719–724
Spinal reflex(es), spinal cord disease and, 629–630
Spinal reflex examination, 566–577
interpretation of, 574–577, *575*
nociceptive, 569, *572*, 573
nociceptive evaluation and, 573, *574*
proprioceptive, 566–569, *567–571*
special reflexes and, 573, *573*, 574t
Spirochetal arthritis, 2365
Spleen, 2232–2242
anatomy and histology of, 2234–2235
enlargement. *See* Splenomegaly.
gastric dilatation-volvulus-torsion syndrome and, 1279
masses of, 2237–2238
definitions and nomenclature for, 2237–2238
Spleen *(Continued)*
physiology of, 2235–2237
filtration, phagocytosis, and reservoir function and, 2235–2236
hematopoiesis and, 2235
immunologic function and, 2236–2237
Splenectomy, in gastric dilatation-volvulus-torsion syndrome, 1284
Splenomegaly, 137–138, 2238–2242
anemia and, 93
definitions and, 2238
pathogenesis of, 2238t, 2238–2240
congestive splenomegaly and, 2238t, 2239–2240
hyperplastic splenomegaly and, 2239
infiltrative splenomegaly and, 2240
inflammatory splenomegaly and, 2238t, 2238–2239
patient evaluation in, 2240–2242
aspiration in, 2242
hematologic and serum biochemical findings in, 2241, 2241t
history and physical findings in, 2240–2241
imaging in, *2241*, 2241–2242
surgical, 2242
polycythemia and, 103
Spondylitis. *See* Diskospondylitis.
Spondyloepiphyseal dysplasia tarda, 2383
Spondylomyelopathy, cervical, 640–645
clinical findings in, 641–642, *643*, *644*
etiology and pathogenesis of, 640–641
treatment of, 642–645
Spondylosis deformans, 691–692, *692*
Spongiform degeneration, 596–597
Sporotrichosis, 356–359
clinical manifestations of, 357–358
cutaneous manifestations of, 7
diagnosis of, 358
epizootiology of, 357
etiology of, 356–357, *357*
in humans, 192
pathogenesis of, 357
prognosis in, 358–359
public health aspects of, 359
treatment of, 358
Squamous metaplasia, prostatic, 1868
Staging, of neoplasms, clinical, 522t, 522–523, 523t
Staining, of fecal smears, 1399
Stanguria, 163
Staphylococcal infections, cutaneous manifestations of, 7
dermatologic, ocular manifestations of, 76
small bowel diarrhea and, 1359
Starch tolerance test, in exocrine pancreatic insufficiency, 1545
Starvation, brief, nonstressed, effects of, 450
Status epilepticus, definition of, 66
Steatorrhea, examination for, in exocrine pancreatic insufficiency, 1545, *1545*
Stem cell(s), 2285
cyclic input or proliferation of, 2200–2201
death of, 2197–2200
canine ehrlichiosis and, 2200
cephalosporins and, 2199
chemotherapy drugs and, 2198
chloramphenicol toxicity and, in cats, 2198
estrogen toxicity and, in dog, 2198
feline leukemia virus infection and, 2199
lentivirus infection of, in cats, 2200
parvovirus infections and, *2197*, 2199
phenylbutazone toxicosis and, in dogs, 2198–2199
radiation effects and, 2197–2198
Stenosis, aortic. *See* Aortic stenosis.
congenital, preputial, with phimosis, 1884, *1885*
mitral, 1049
of nares, 771–772
pulmonic. *See* Pulmonic stenosis.
pyloric, 1311
tracheal, segmental, 804, *805*
urethral, 2135–2136
of vertebral canal. *See* Vertebral canal stenosis.
Steroids, androgenic, anabolic, in liver failure, 1516–1517
urinary, in hypoadrenocorticism, 1766

Stifle joint, luxations and subluxations of, 2340–2343
Stings. *See also* Bites.
  arthropod, 474–475
    differentiation of, 467t, 473t, 474
    therapy of, 461t–464t, 475
Stomach. *See also headings beginning with term* Gastric.
  anatomy of, 1289–1290
    functional, *1289*, 1289–1290
    microscopic, 1290, *1290*
  physiology of, 1290–1293
    gastric filling and, 1291
    gastric motility and emptying and, 1292–1293, *1293*
    gastric secretion and, 1291–1292
Stomach torsion. *See* Gastric dilatation-volvulus-torsion syndrome.
Stomatitis, 1227–1231
  diagnosis of, *1227*, 1228
  of unknown origin, 1231
  plant awn, 1231
Stool. *See* Constipation; Diarrhea; Feces; *headings beginning with term* Fecal.
Storage diseases, metabolic, 592–596, 593t
Storage pool disease, 2271
Strabismus, in neurological examination, 706–707
Streptococcal lymphadenitis, contagious, 2229
Streptozotocin, insulin-secreting tumors and, 1715
Stress, 73
  eating disorders and, 16
  gastric mucosal injury and, 1301
  gastric ulceration and, 1308
  management of, in heart failure therapy, 966
  metabolic response to, 450
  neuroendocrine control and, 1723
  o,p′-DDD therapy and, 1752
Stricture(s), anal, 1567
  esophageal, 1270–1271, *1271*
  rectal, 1567
  urethral, 2135–2136
Stridor, cyanosis and, 97, 98
Stroke(s), behavioral signs of, 73–74
Strongyloides, small bowel diarrhea and, 1347–1348
Struvite urolithiasis. *See* Urolithiasis, struvite.
Strychnine intoxication, 465
Stunting, polycythemia and, 103
Stupor, ancillary diagnostics in, 63–64
  blood tests in, 63
  definition of, 61
  history in, 62–63
  neurologic examination in, 63
  physical examination and, 63
  rule-outs for, 61–62
  treatment of, 64–65
    emergency, *64*, 64–65
    maintenance, *65*
  urinalysis in, 63
Subcutaneous degradation, in insulin antagonism/resistance, 1703, *1704*
Subinvolved placental sites (SIPS), 1802
Sublingual gland, injury to, 1242, 1249, 1249, *1250*
Subluxations, 2337–2343
  atlantoaxial subluxation, 634–637
    clinical findings in, 635, *635*
    diagnosis of, 635–636, *636*
    etiology and pathogenesis of, 634–635
    treatment of, 636–637
  of carpal joint, 2339
  of elbow joint, 2338, *2338*, *2339*
  of hip joint, 2340, *2341*
  of shoulder joint, *2338*
  of stifle joint, 2340–2343
  of tarsal joint, 2339–2340
Sulfasalazine, in chronic inflammatory bowel disease, 1407
Sulfobromophthalein, in liver disease, 1448–1449, 1449t
Sulfonamides, 403
  action of, 403
  activity spectrum of, 403
  clinical pharmacology of, 403
Supernumerary teeth, 1209, *1210*
Supplies, emergency medicine and, 212, 213t
Support services, emergency medicine and, 212–214
Suprascapular nerve injury, *721*, 721–722
Supraventricular premature contractions, *1066*, 1067
Supraventricular tachycardia, *1070–1073*, 1070–1079
  clinical signs of, 1071, 1073
  treatment of, 1073
Surgery, abdominal, pleural effusion caused by, 881
  canine mammary gland tumors and, 1822–1823
  gastric ulceration and, 1310
  in cancer, 529–530
  in feline hyperthyroidism, 1664–1666
    anesthesia for, 1665
    complications of, 1666
    long-term management and, 1666
    preoperative preparation for, 1664–1665
  in gastric dilatation-volvulus-torsion syndrome, 1281–1285, *1282–1286*
  in hyperadrenocorticism, adrenal tumor, *1745*, *1746*, 1745–1747
    pituitary-dependent, 1747
  in otitis externa, 258
  in peripheral edema, 44–45
  in urolithiasis, indications for, 2104
  infertility and, diagnosis of, 1849
  insulin-secreting tumors and, 1712–1713, *1713*
  ovarian tumors and, 1818
  periodontal disease and, *1223*, *1224*, 1225–1226
  splenomegaly and, 2242
  thyroid hormone metabolism and, in dog, 1640
  thyroid tumors and, in dog, 1669
  vaginal and vulvar tumors and, 1819–1820
Surgical disorders, within developing countries, 220t, 223–224
Swallowing, physiology of, 1256–1257, *1258*
Sympathetic nervous system, heart failure and, 907–908, *909*, *910*
Sympathomimetic amines, in heart failure therapy, 953
Synchrony, 1081
Syncope, 50–53, 51t, 52t
  cardiac dysfunction and, 52–53
  clinical summary of, 50–51
  cyanosis and, 97
  definition of, 46
  iatrogenic causes of, 53
  in normal heart, with peripheral vascular dysfunction, 51–52
  metabolic disturbances associated with, 53
  miscellaneous causes of, 53
  tussive, 53
Syndactyly, 2384
Syndrome of inappropriate secretion of antidiuretic hormone (SIADH), 616–617
Synovial cell sarcoma, 2361–2362
Synovitis, plasmacytic-lymphocytic, 2371
  treatment of, 2372–2373
  villonodular, 2362
Syringomyelia, 692–693
Systematic desensitization, for fears and phobias, 228
Systemic lupus erythematosus (SLE), 2309–2312, 2370
  clinical signs of, 2309
  cutaneous manifestations of, 9
  diagnosis of, 2309–2312, *2311*
    antinuclear antibody tests in, 2310–2312, *2311*
  pathophysiology of, 2309, *2310*, *2311*
  treatment of, 2312, 2372–2373
Systemic mastocytosis, gastric ulceration and, 1309
Systolic dysfunction, heart failure due to, 1097–1098
  treatment of, 1105–1110
Systolic mechanical overload, heart failure and, 913

T lymphocytes, activation of, 2291
  B cell cooperation with, 2291
  cytotoxic, 2291
  regulators of, 2284
  structure and function of, 2287
  suppressor cells and, 2291–2292
  T cell interactions of, 2291–2292
T_3 concentration, serum, in canine hypothyroidism, 1645, 1647
T_4 concentration, serum, in canine hypothyroidism, 1645, 1647
Tachyarrhythmias, accelerated conduction, 1073–1074, *1074*, *1075*
Tachycardias, *1070–1073*, 1070–1085
  accelerated conduction, 1073–1074, *1074*, *1075*
  atrial fibrillation and, 1074–1075, *1076–1078*, 1077–1079
    clinical signs of, 1077–1078, *1079*
    treatment of, 1078–1079
  atrial flutter and, 1079, *1080*
  supraventricular, *1070–1073*, 1070–1079
    clinical signs of, 1071, 1073
    treatment of, 1073
  ventricular, atrioventricular dissociation and, 1079–1084, *1081–1083*
  ventricular fibrillation and, 1084–1085, *1085*
Tachypnea, 88–90
  diagnosis and treatment of, 89t, 90
  pathophysiology of, 88–90
    lower airway problems and, 89
    pleural diseases and, 89
    reduced hemoglobin states and, 89
    upper airway problems and, 88t, 88–89
Tail chasing, 72
Tapeworms, in humans, 189, 190
    prevention of, 189, 190
  small bowel diarrhea and, 1342t–1343t, 1348
Tarsal joint, luxations and subluxations of, 2339–2340
Taurine deficiency, ocular manifestations of, *78*, 80
Technique charts, radiography and, 753, *754*
Teeth, caries and, 1210–1211, *1211*
  carnassial abscess and, 1211–1212, *1214*
  congenital anomalies of, 1209–1210
  deciduous, retained, 1209, *1209*
  diseases affecting structure of, 1209–1215
  enamel hypoplasia and, 1210, *1210*
  endodontic disease and, 1212–1214, *1214*
  eruption of, *1205*, 1205t, 1205–1206
  extraction of, in periodontal disease, 1226
  impaction of, 1209–1210
  occlusion and articulation of, *1206*, 1206–1207
  restorative dentistry and, 1214–1215
  root planing of, 1225
  scaling, 1225, *1225*
  supernumerary, 1209, *1210*
  tetracycline staining of, 1210, *1210*
  trauma to, 1211, *1211–1213*
Telangiectasia, of Pembroke Welsh corgis, 2030
Telogen effluvium, alopecia and, 120
Temperature. *See also* Cold; Fever; Hyperthermia; Hypothermia.
  pain and, 21
Temperature variation, acupuncture and, 492–493
Temporomandibular joint (TMJ), 1207
  abnormalities of, 1216
  instabilities of, 2343
TEN. *See* Toxic epidermal necrolysis.
Tenesmus, definition of, 36
  diagnostic procedures in, 38
  diarrhea and, 34
  historical findings in, 36
  pathophysiology of, 36, 37t
  physical examination in, 37–38
  treatment goals in, 39
Terminal retch, 86
Terrier, Bedlington, copper-associated hepatitis in, 1488–1491, *1489*
  fox, smooth-haired, hereditary ataxia in, 660
  hereditary ataxia in, 599
  Jack Russell, hereditary ataxia in, 660
  Kerry blue, cerebellar degeneration in, 597
  West Highland white, copper-associated hepatitis in, 1491–1492
Territorial aggression, 234
  in cats, 236, 237
Testicular atrophy, in canine hyperadrenocorticism, 1729–1730
Testicular descent, 1790
Testicular failure, primary, treatment of, 1853
Testicular function, 1789–1790

Testicular tumors, 1814–1816
clinical features of, 1814–1815
Leydig cell, 1815
seminomas and, 1815
Sertoli cell, 1815
treatment and prognosis of, 1815–1816
Testosterone, polycythemia and, 102
Tetanus, 273–274
brain and, 605, *605*
Tetany, puerperal, 1831–1832
hypocalcemia and, 1625–1626
Tetracyclines, 398–399
action of, 399
activity spectrum of, 399
clinical pharmacology of, 399
resistance to, 399
teeth stained by, 1210, *1210*
Tetralogy of Fallot, 1018–1022, *1019*
clinical findings in, 1019, *1020*, 1021, *1021*
clinical management of, 1021–1022, *1022*
pathogenesis of, 1018
pathophysiology of, 1018–1019, *1019*
Tetraparesis, cyanosis and, 97
Tetraplegia, cyanosis and, 97, 98
Thallium intoxication, 471–472
cutaneous manifestations of, 9
differentiation of, 459t, 460t, 465t, 467t, 471
Thermal burns, of oral cavity, 1231
Thermoregulation, 23t, 23–26. *See also* Fever; Hyperthermia; Hypothermia.
fever and, 24, *24*
pathogenesis of, 24, *25*
hyperthermia and, 23–24, *24*
clinical presentation of, 24–25
Thiacetarsamide, in heartworm disease, 1178–1179
toxicity of, 1179
Thiamine deficiency, brain and, 615–616
ocular manifestations of, 80
Thoracic cavity, evaluation of, anorexia and, 16
polyphagia and, 16
Thoracic limb reflexes, testing for, *567*, 567–569
Thoracic wall deformity, 870
Thoracocentesis, diagnostic, 875–876, *876*
in heart failure therapy, 967
therapeutic, 876–877
Thoracoscopy, pleural disorders and, 875, *875*
Thorax, respiratory disease and, diagnosis of, 750, 751t
Threshold membrane potential, 1051
Thrombasthenia, 2271
Thrombasthenic-thrombopathia, canine, 2271
Thrombin time, 2251
Thrombocythemia, canine, 2273
Thrombocytopathies, acquired, 2272–2276
hereditary, 2268–2272
Thrombocytopenia, 105
cyclic, infectious, of dogs, 279–280
hemorrhage and, anemia and, 2160–2161
immune-mediated, 2303–2305, *2304*
diagnosis of, 2304
pathophysiology of, 2303–2304
prognosis of, 2305
treatment of, 2304–2305
Thromboembolic disease. *See also* Embolism.
cardiomyopathy and, 1117–1121
clinical manifestations of, 1118
diagnosis of, 1118–1119, *1119*, *1120*
pathophysiology of, 1118
prognosis in, 1121
treatment of, 1119, 1121
pulmonary, 845–846
in canine hyperadrenocorticism, 1735–1736
Thrombopathia, canine, 2271–2272
Thrombosis, 2261–2262
arterial, in dogs, 1185–1188, 1186t
clinical signs of, 1186–1187
diagnosis of, *1187*, 1187–1188
history in, 1186
treatment of, 1188
clinical signs of, 2261
diagnosis of, 2261–2262
pulmonary, pleural effusion caused by, 883
therapy of, 2262
Thrombotic diathesis, in nephrotic syndrome, 2023t, 2023–2024
treatment of, 2023t, 2023–2024
Thromboxane synthetase deficiency, 2271
Thymoma, 895
Thyroglobulin, circulating antibodies to, in canine hypothyroidism, 1648
Thyroid carcinoma, 893–894
Thyroid diseases, 1632–1671. *See also* Hyperthyroidism; Hypothyroidism; *specific diseases*.
diarrhea and, 1375–1376, *1376*
drugs used in, 1675t
neoplastic. *See* Tumor(s), thyroid.
Thyroid function tests, in canine hyperadrenocorticism, 1734, *1734*
in canine hypothyroidism, 1645–1649
in feline hyperthyroidism, 1658–1661
Thyroid gland, anatomy of, 1632–1633
in cats, 1633
in dogs, 1632–1633
microstructure and, 1633, *1633*
idiopathic atrophy of, canine hypothyroidism and, 1641
in feline hyperthyroidism, 1656
neoplastic destruction of, canine hypothyroidism and, 1641
physiology of, 1633–1637
iodine metabolism and, *1633*, 1633–1634
plasma hormone binding and, 1635–1637, *1636*
thyroid hormone metabolism and, *1633*, 1634–1635, *1635*, *1636*
thyroid hormone secretion and, regulation of, *1636*, 1637, *1637*
thyroid hormone synthesis and secretion and, *1633*, 1634
thyroid hormone action and, *1636*, 1640–1641
thyroid hormone metabolism and, 1637–1640
age effects on, in dog, 1640
canine "euthyroid sick" syndrome and, 1638–1639
drugs effects on, in dog, 1639–1640
illness and malnutrition and, 1637–1638
obesity and, in dog, 1640
surgery and anesthesia and, in dog, 1640
Thyroid hormone, action of, *1636*, 1640–1641
metabolism of, *1633*, 1634–1635, *1635*, *1636*
age and, in dog, 1640
canine "euthyroid sick" syndrome and, 1638–1639
drugs and, in dog, 1639–1640
illness and malnutrition and, 1637–1638
obesity and, in dog, 1640
plasma hormone binding of, 1635–1637, *1636*
preparations of, 1650–1652
bioavailability and efficacy of, determinants of, 1649–1650
diagnostic use of, 1653
dose of, factors affecting, 1652
monitoring therapy with, 1653
overdose of, signs of, 1652–1653
therapeutic failure with, 1653
resting serum concentrations of, in feline hyperthyroidism, 1658–1659, *1659*
secretion of, regulation of, *1636*, 1637, *1637*
synthesis and secretion of, *1633*, 1634
Thyroid hormone autoantibodies, circulating, in canine hypothyroidism, 1648
Thyroid hormone binding ratio, in canine hypothyroidism, 1648
Thyroid hormone suppression test, in feline hyperthyroidism, 1659
Thyroid stimulating hormone (TSH), deficiency of, canine hypothyroidism and, 1642
endogenous serum concentrations of, in canine hypothyroidism, 1649
neuroendocrine function and, 1587
pituitary-hypothalamic diseases and, 1580
Thyroid stimulating hormone (TSH) response test, in feline hyperthyroidism, 1659–1660
Thyroid-stimulating hormone (TSH) stimulation test, in canine hypothyroidism, 1645–1646, *1646*
Thyroiditis, lymphocytic, canine hypothyroidism and, 1641
Thyrotoxic myocardial disease, 1121–1122
Thyrotoxicosis, signs of, 1652–1653
Thyrotropin. *See* Thyroid stimulating hormone.
Thyrotropin-releasing hormone (TRH), 1583
Thyrotropin-releasing hormone (TRH) stimulation test, in canine hypothyroidism, *1637*, *1646*, 1646–1647
Thyroxine, synthetic, 1650–1652, *1651*
Thyroxine binding prealbumin, serum, in canine hypothyroidism, 1648–1649
Tibial nerve injury, *722*, 723
Tick infestations, ears and, 257
in developing countries, 219, *219*, *220*, 220t
polyneuropathy and, 727
Tissue perfusion, gastric dilatation-volvulus-torsion syndrome and, 1250
TMJ. *See* Temporomandibular joint.
TNM system, 128
Toad poisoning, 473–474
differentiation of, 467t, 473, 474
Tocainide, 1063
Tomography, linear, spinal cord disease and, 628
Tongue, congenital anomalies of, 1233
glossitis and, 1234–1236, *1235*, *1236*
injuries of, 1233–1234, *1234*, *1235*
neoplasia of, 1236
Tonsillitis, 1237–1238, 1238t
Tooth. *See* Teeth.
Total parenteral nutrition (TPN), 453–454
Toxic change, of neutrophils, *2189*, 2190, *2190*
Toxic epidermal necrolysis (TEN), 9
Toxicity. *See also* Toxicology.
of chloramphenicol, hematopoietic stem cell death and, 2198
of copper, hemolytic disease associated with, 2171
of estrogen, hematopoietic stem cell death and, 2198
of phenylbutazone, hematopoietic stem cell death and, 2198–2199
oral lesions and, 1228
phenylbutazone, aplastic anemia and, 2174
Toxicology, 456–481
acetaminophen and, 479
differentiation of, 459t, 467t, 479
alopecia and, 120
alpha-naphthylthiourea and, 465t, 467
anticholinesterase and, therapy of, 466
arsenic and, 470–471
differentiation of, 459t, 470
arthropod bites or stings and, 474–475
differentiation of, 467t, 473t, 475
therapy of, 461t–464t, 475
aspirin and, 478–479
differentiation of, 459t, 465t, 479
avitrol and, 467–468
differentiation of, 460t, 468
behavioral signs of, 73
biotoxins and, 472–478
brain effects and, 613–615
signs of, 614t, 614–615
caustics and, 467t, 481
chloramphenicol, anemia and, 2176
chocolate and, 460t, 481
cigarettes and, 459t, 460t, 481
coma and stupor and, 62
compound 1080/1081 and, therapy of, 465–466
disinfectants and, 467t, 481
estrogen, aplastic anemia and, 2174
ethyl alcohol and, 459t, 460t, 481
ethylene glycol and, 457–459
clinical signs of, 458
differentiation of, 458, 459t, 460t
laboratory information and, 458
therapy of, 458–459, 461t–464t
toxicological analysis and, 458
Fleet-like enema preparations and, 459t, 460t, 480
garbage and, 460t, 478
insecticides and, therapy of, 466
iron and, 479–480
differentiation of, 459t–464t, 467t, 480
lead and, 469–470
differentiation of, 459t, 460t, 470

Toxicology *(Continued)*
- liver injury and, 1492–1493
- lizards and, 475–476
- mercury and, 460t, 467t, 472
- metaldehyde and, therapy of, 466
- mothballs and, 469t, 481
- mushrooms and, 476–477
  - symptomatology of, 459t, 460t, 469t, 477
- mycotoxins and, 459t, 477–478
  - moldy walnuts and, 460t, 478
- nervous system and, 553
- organophosphate and, therapy of, 466
- pesticides causing coagulopathy and, 468–469
  - differentiation of, 459t, 465t, 469, 469t
- petroleum products and, 459t, 460t, 465t, 467t, 473t, 481
- phosphorus and, 468
  - differentiation of, 459t, 465t, 468
- plants and, 459t, 473t, 476
- polyneuropathies and, 726t, 726–727
  - chemical agents and, 726t, 726–727
  - *Clostridium botulinum* toxin and, 727
  - drugs and, 726t, 726–727
  - heavy metals and, 726t, 726–727
  - snake venom neurotoxin and, 727
  - tick neurotoxin and, 727
- pesticides affecting central nervous system and, 459–460, 464–466
  - clinical signs of, 460, 464–465
  - differentiation of, 460t, 465
  - laboratory information and, 465
  - therapy of, 465–466
  - toxicological analysis and, 465
- pyridylium herbicides and, 467
  - differentiation of, 459t, 465t, 467, 467t
  - therapy of, 459t, 465t, 467, 467t
- snake venom and, 472–473
  - differentiation of, 473, 473t
- strychnine and, therapy of, 465
- thallium and, 471–472
  - differentiation of, 459t, 460t, 465t, 467t, 471
- toad poisoning and, 473–474
  - differentiation of, 467t, 473t, 474
- treatment principles and, 456–457
  - antidotes and, 457
  - life-threatening conditions and, 456
  - patient observation in, 457
  - poison removal and, 456–457
  - supportive and symptomatic care in, 457
- walnuts and, moldy, 460t, 478
- zinc and, 471
  - differentiation of, 459t, 460t, 469t, 471
- zinc phosphide and, 466–467
  - differentiation of, 459t, 460t, 465t, 467
  - laboratory information and, 466
  - therapy of, 467
  - toxicological analysis and, 466–467

Toxicosis, thyroid, 1652–1653

Toxin(s), acute renal failure caused by, 1931, *1932*, 1933–1935
- diarrhea induced by, 1344
- hepatic encephalopathy and, pathogenesis of, 1463–1466
- myocardial disease and, 1122–1123
- tremor induced by, 56
- uremic, 1917t, 1917–1918

Toxoplasmosis, 283–285
- brain and, 606
- in humans, 190
  - prevention of, 190
- myositis due to, 740, *740*
- ocular manifestations of, 80–81
- pulmonary manifestations of, 832–833

TPN. *See* Total parenteral nutrition.

Trace elements, exocrine pancreatic insufficiency and, 1541

Trace minerals, corticosteroids and, 416

Trachea, collapsed, 799–804
  - additional examinations in, 801
  - differential diagnosis of, 801, 804
  - etiology of, 800
  - features of, 800–801
  - radiography in, *801–803*, 801–804
  - treatment of, 799t, 804

Trachea *(Continued)*
- foreign bodies in, 808, 810
- trauma to, 813–814
  - radiographic examination and, *805*, 813–814, *814*
  - treatment of, 814

Tracheal diseases, 795–814
- clinicopathology of, 796
- diagnosis of, 751–752, 795–796
- history and common associations of, 795
- hypoplastic, 804–806, 808
  - features of, 805–806, *806–807*, 808
  - prognosis and therapy of, 804–806, 808
- neoplastic, 810, 812
  - features of, 810
  - radiographic examination of, 810
  - treatment of, 810, 812
- obstructive, 808, 810
  - features of, 808
  - radiographic examination in, 808, *809*, 810, *811–813*
  - treatment of, 810, 812
- physical examination and, 795
- radiographic examination and, 796–797

Tracheal stenosis, segmental, 804, *805*

Tracheitis, 797–798
- diagnostic aids for, 798
- differential diagnosis of, 798
- etiology of, 798
- features of, 797–798
- therapy of, 798, 799t

Tracheobronchitis, infectious, 305–306
- canine, 821–822
  - clinical signs of, 306
  - diagnosis of, 306, 821–822
  - epizootiology of, 305
  - etiology of, 305
  - presentation of, 821
  - prevention and control of, 306, 822
  - prognosis in, 822
  - treatment of, 306, 822

Trade-off hypothesis, chronic renal failure and, 1922

Traditional Chinese Medicine, 491

Transfusion therapy, 2176–2178
- in cats, 2177–2178
- in dogs, 2177
- in nonregenerative anemia, in chronic renal failure, 2004

Transitional cell carcinoma, of lower urinary tract, treatment of, 2128, 2129t
- prostatic, *1876*, 1877

Transitional vertebrae, etiology and pathogenesis of, 646

Transmissible venereal tumor, canine, 1816–1817

Transport, intestinal, of water and solute, 1327

Transtracheal aspiration, 759–761
- complications of, 761
- method for, 759–760, *760*
- preparation for, 759, 760t
- results of, 761
- specimens for, 760–761, *761*

Trauma, alopecia and, 120
- cranial, 612–613, *613*, 613t, *614*
- hemorrhage and, anemia and, 2160
- lameness and, in cats, 170
- laryngeal, 789
- pain and, 20
- pancreatitis and, 1534
- peripheral neuropathies and. *See* Peripheral neuropathies, traumatic.
- peritoneal disease and, 132
- pleural effusion caused by, 883
- pneumothorax and, 885
- to chest, 869–870, *870*
- to facial nerve, 717
- to hypoglossal nerve, 719
- to large intestine, 1416
- to liver and bile ducts, 1484
- to lower urinary tract, 2130–2132
  - clinical signs of, 2130
  - diagnosis of, 2130
  - emergency treatment of, 2131–2132
  - physical examination in, 2130–2131

Trauma *(Continued)*
- to lungs, 840–845
- to nasal cavities, 774
- to nervous system, 553–554
- to pharynx, 783–784
- to rhinarium, 772–773
- to teeth, 1211, *1211*
- to trigeminal nerve, 716, *716*
- tracheal, 813–814
  - radiographic examination and, *805*, 813–814, *814*
  - treatment of, 814

Traumatic joint disease, 2336–2344
- articular cartilage and, 2337, *2337*
- luxations and subluxations and, 2337–2343
- soft tissue and, 2337

Tremor, 54–56

Tremor(s), acquired, 599
- cerebellar, 56
- drug- and toxin-induced, 56
- hypomyelination and, 55
- in white dogs, 55–56
- pathophysiology of, 54
- senile, 54–55
- toxicity and, 614–615

TRH. *See* Thyrotropin-releasing hormone.

Triage, emergency medicine and, 209

Triceps reflex, testing for, 567, *568*

Trichomoniasis, 286, 1411–1412

Trichuriasis, 1410–1411

Tricuspid insufficiency, 1047–1048

Tricuspid valve dysplasia, cyanotic heart disease and, 1022

Trigeminal nerves, focal diseases of, *716*, 716–717
- neoplasia of, 716
- trauma to, 716, *716*

Trigeminal neuropathy, idiopathic, 716, *716*
- sensory, 716–717

Triggered impulses, cardiac arrhythmias and, 1056

Triglycerides, 203
- diagnostic tests for, 199

Triiodothyronine, synthetic, *1651*, 1652

Triiodothyronine resin uptake, in canine hypothyroidism, 1648

Triiodothyronine suppression test, in feline hyperthyroidism, 1659

Trilostane, in canine hyperadrenocorticism, 1753

Trituration, 1293

Trochlear nerves, focal diseases of, 715–716

Trough level, drug administration and, 68

Truncal ataxia, 57

Trypanosomiasis, 1124–1125
- American, 289
- in developing countries, 222

TSH. *See* Thyroid-stimulating hormone.

Tube feeding, 452–453

Tuberculosis, 267
- ocular manifestations of, 81

Tubular defects, 2024–2028
- anatomic, 2024–2025, *2025*
- definition and identification of, 2024, 2024t
- functional, 2026–2028

Tubular function, clinical evaluation of, 1898–1900
  - ammonia challenge test and, 1900
  - exogenous vasopressin test and, 1899–1900
  - fractional clearances and, 1900
  - Hickey-Hare test and, 1899
  - phenolsulfonphthalein half-life and, 1900
  - urine specific gravity and osmolality and, 1898–1899
  - water deprivation test and, 1899

Tubular necrosis, acute, 1965–1968
  - causes of, determining, 1972–1973
    - localization of, 1970–1971
  - definition of, 1965, 1965t
  - ischemic, 1965t, 1965–1966, 1966t
  - nephrotoxic, 1966–1967, 1967t
  - nonoliguric, sequential phases of, 1968
  - oliguric, sequential phases of, 1967–1968

Tularemia, 272–273
- in humans, 191
  - prevention of, 191

Tumor(s), 117, 126–130
- adrenal, in feline hyperadrenocorticism, 1756

Tumor(s) *(Continued)*
adrenal, pathophysiology of, 1723, *1724*
alopecia and, 113–114, 120
anal, 1572–1573
malignant, 1572–1573
of perianal gland, 1572, *1572*
arthropathy due to, 2361–2362
metastatic, 2362
primary, 2361–2362
biliary, 1557
bone, 2387–2391
in cat, 2389–2390
in dog, 2387–2389
metastatic, 2390
cervical, 1819
colonic and rectal, 1565–1566
diagnosis of, 1566, *1566*
history and physical findings in, *1565*, 1565–1566, *1566*
treatment of, 1566
coma and stupor and, 62
cutaneous manifestations of, 10
definition of, 126, 514
diagnostic plan for, 128–130
doubling time and, *515*, 515
eosinophilia associated with, 2210
esophageal, 1273–1275
expansiveness of, 514
fulminant, 514
gastric, 1317–1319
benign, 1317
clinical findings and, 1318
diagnosis of, 1318
malignant, 1317–1318, *1318*
treatment of, 1318–1319
hepatic, 1511–1513
metastatic, 1513
nonepithelial, 1513
primary, 1511t, 1511–1513
historical findings and, 127
immunology of, biologic therapy and, 537
in developing countries, *223*, 224
intrapericardiac, 1133, 1135, 1148
invasiveness of, 514
islet cell, insulin-secreting, 1707–1716
anamnesis and, 1708t, 1709
clinical pathologic abnormalities in, 1709t, 1710
confirmation of, 1710–1712
differential diagnosis of, 1709t, 1709–1710, 1710t
medical therapy and, acute hypoglycemic crisis and, 1713–1714
chronic hypoglycemia and, 1714–1715
physical examination and, 1709
prognosis of, 1715–1716
radiography in, 1710
surgical therapy in, 1712–1713, *1713*
ultrasonography in, 1710
lameness and, in cats, 170
laryngeal, 792–793
latent period and, 514
lymphoid, lymphocytosis and, 2208
lymphoreticular, in cat, 2390
mammary, canine, 1820–1824
adjuvant therapy for, 1823–1824
biologic behavior and clinical features of, 1820–1821, *1821*, 1821t
histopathology of, 1821–1822, 1822t
surgical therapy of, 1822–1823
feline, 1824
mediastinal, 893–895, *894*
lymphadenopathy and, 893, *894*
mobility of, 514
myocardial dysfunction and, 1123
neutropenia and, 2200
nondeforming polyarthritis associated with, 2371
ocular, canine, 83–84
feline, 84
of adrenal gland, pathology of, 1725
of brain, 609–612, 610t
behavioral signs of, 73
clinical signs of, 612
diagnosis of, 612
incidence of, 609–611, 610t, *611*, 611t

Tumor(s) *(Continued)*
of brain, pathogenesis of, 609
prognosis and treatment of, 612
of exocrine pancreas, 1548
of external ear canal, 257–258
of facial nerve, 717
of hypoglossal nerve, 719
of large intestine, 1417–1418
clinical findings in, *1401*, 1417
incidence of, 1417
treatment of, 1417–1418
of lips and cheeks, 1233
of nasal cavities, *780*, 780–782, *781*
of nervous system, 554
of peripheral nerves, 723–724, *724*
of pinnae, 251
of prepuce, 1817
of rhinarium, 773, *774*
of salivary glands, 1251–1252
of spinal cord, 677–682
clinical findings in, 678–679
diagnosis of, 679–681
etiology and pathogenesis of, 677–678
treatment of, 681–682
of thoracic wall, 870–872
metastatic, 871
primary, 871, *871*
treatment of, 871
of tongue, 1236
of trigeminal nerve, 716
of urinary bladder, 2123–2128
biologic behavior and types of, 2124, 2124t
diagnosis and clinical staging of, 2125–2127, *2126*
epithelial, 2124
etiology of, 2125
nonepithelial, 2124–2125
treatment of, 2127–2128
oral, 1230–1231
oropharyngeal, *1238*, 1238–1241, *1239*, 1240t
management of, 1239, *1240*
tonsils and, 1239, 1240t, 1241, *1241*
outcome in, 130
ovarian, 1818–1819
persistent estrus and, *1795*, 1795t, 1795–1796
pancreatic, 1314–1317
pathophysiology of, 126–127
pedunculated, 514
penile, 1816, 1887
pharyngeal, *787*, 787–788, *788*
physical findings and, 127–128
pituitary, canine hypothyroidism and, 1641–1642
hypopituitarism caused by, 1590–1591
in hyperadrenocorticism, surgery and, 1747
surgery and, 1747
treatment of, 1754–1755
pleural effusion and, 878–879
post-diagnosis delay and, 514–515
pre-diagnosis period and, 514
progressive, 514
prostatic, 1816, 1874–1877
pulmonary, 848–853
metastatic, 851–853
diagnosis of, *851*, 851–852, *852*
presentation of, 851
prognosis in, 853
treatment of, 852–853
necrosis of, pneumothorax and, 885
primary, 848–851
diagnosis of, *848*, 849–850, *850*
presentation of, 849
prognosis in, 851
treatment of, 850–851
quiescent, 514
reproductive, prevention of, 1824–1825
scrotal, 1817
sessile, 514
small intestinal, 1376–1379
mast cell, 1379
splenic, 2237–2238
stable, 514
superficial, in pharyngeal area, 1252
testicular, 1814–1816
clinical features of, 1814–1815

Tumor(s) *(Continued)*
testicular, Leydig cell, 1815
seminoma and, 1814–1815
Sertoli cell, 1814–1815
treatment and prognosis of, 1815–1816
therapeutic goals for, 130
thyroid, canine, clinical features of, 1667t, 1668
diagnosis of, 1668–1669
hypothyroidism and, 1641
pathology of, 1667t, 1667–1668
prognosis of, 1670–1671
treatment of, 1669–1670
TNM system and, 128
tracheal, 810, 812
features of, 810
radiographic examination of, 810
treatment of, 810, 812
urethral, 2128–2130
diagnosis of, 2129–2130, *2130*
uterine, 1803, 1819
vaginal, 1809, 1811, 1819–1820
vascular, benign, of spinal cord, 693–694
venereal, canine transmissible, 1816–1817
clinical features of, 1816–1817
diagnosis of, 1817
treatment of, 1817
venereal cell, transmissible, 1230–1231
vulvar, 1819–1820
weakness and, 49
Tumor biology, 513–523, *514*
cell cycle and, 516, *516*
cell surface and cytoplasmic alterations and, 515, 515t
clinical staging and, 522t, 522–523, 523t
describing neoplasia and, 513–515
physical characteristics and, 514
subjective descriptions and, 514
temporal measures and, 514–515
differentiation and de-differentiation and, 515
metastasis and, 516–517
paraneoplastic syndromes and, 518–521, 519t
pathologic diagnosis and grading and, 521t, 521–522
tumor heterogeneity and, 517–518
Tumor cell vaccines, in cancer therapy, 539
Tussive syncope, 53
Tylosin, in chronic inflammatory bowel disease, 1408
Tyrosinemia, cutaneous manifestations of, 5
Tyzzer's disease, 269

Ulcer(s), duodenal, 1379–1380, *1380*
gastric, 1308–1310
clinical findings in, 1309
diagnosis of, 1309
etiology of, 1308, 1308t
pathophysiology of, 1308–1309
treatment of, 1309–1310
gastrointestinal, in liver disease, 1462, *1462*
on skin, 119
Ulcerative colitis, histiocytic, 1410
Ulnar nerve injury, *721*, 722
Ultracentrifugation, lipoproteins and, 199
Ultrasonography, 584
abdominal, 132, 132t, *133*
acupuncture and, 493
canine urolithiasis and, 2086t, 2086–2087
emergency medicine and, 216
in hyperadrenocorticism, 1743, *1744*
in liver disease, 1467–1469, *1468*, 1468t, *1469*
in lower urinary tract disease, 2111, *2113*
in prostatic disease, 1865–1866, *1866*
in renal disease, 1912–1913
in small bowel diarrhea, 1339
insulin-secreting tumors and, 1710
lymphadenopathy and, 2228
splenomegaly and, 2241, *2241*
Unconsciousness, coma and stupor and, 63
Unidirectional block, cardiac arrhythmias and, 1056
Upper airway obstruction, 88–89
Upper respiratory infection, feline, ocular manifestations of, 82–83
Urachal remnant, 2133

Urea, metabolism of, in liver disease, 1451, 1453–1456, *1454*
Urea cycle enzyme deficiencies, 1510
Urea nitrogen, abnormal values of, causes of, 14t
Ureaplasmas, lower urinary tract disease and, in cats, 2063
Urease inhibitors, canine struvite urolithiasis and, infection-induced, 2091–2092
Uremia, 1893
brain and, 617–618
cardiopulmonary complications in, 1920
gastrointestinal complications in, 1919–1920
management of, 1979–1980
dietary, 1979
infection prevention and, 1980–1981
nutritional, 1980
vomiting and, 1979–1980, *1980*
metabolic and endocrine complications in, 1920
neurologic complications in, 1919
oral lesions and, 1228
pancreatitis and, 1534
pathophysiology of, 1916–1920
hemostatic defects and, 1918
membrane transport defects and, 1918
neutrophil function and cell-mediated immunity and, 1918–1919
renal failure and, 1918
toxins and, 1917t, 1917–1918
platelet dysfunction in, 2272
Ureters, ectopic, 2133
disorders of, drugs for, 2046t
Urethra, normal bacterial flora of, 1881, 1882t
prolapse of, 1885, *1885*
ruptured, emergency treatment of, 2132
Urethral discharge, prostatic disease and, 1862
Urethral disease, 2134–2136
acquired, 2135–2136
congenital/hereditary, 2135
diagnosis of, 2134–2136
neoplastic, 2128–2130
diagnosis of, 2129–2130, *2130*
Urethral fistulae, 2135
Urethral incompetence, idiopathic, canine, 2133
Urethral plugs, prevention of, 2076
struvite, 2068, 2069t
treatment of, 2072–2076
hypotonic urinary bladders and reflex dyssynergia and, 2075–2076
immediate aftercare and, 2074–2075
indwelling urinary catheters and, 2075
medical treatment and, 2072
reestablishing urethral patency and, 2072–2074
Urethral prolapse, 2136
Urethral stenosis, 2135–2136
Urethral stricture, 2135–2136
Urethritis, 2135
therapy of, 2135
Urethrocystitis, 2135
Uric acid, in liver disease, 1456
Uric acid urolithiasis. *See* Urolithiasis.
Urinalysis, in canine hyperadrenocorticism, 1732
in diabetes mellitus, 1686
in feline hyperadrenocorticism, 1755
in glomerular disease, 1943
in hypoadrenocorticism, 1761
in lower urinary tract disease, *2109*, 2109–2110, *2110*
large intestinal disease and, 1400
renal disorders and, 1900–1907
chemical properties and, 1903–1904
performance and interpretation of, 1901
physical properties and, 1903
sediment and, microscopic evaluation of, 1904t, 1904–1907
urine collection and, 1901, *1902*
urinary tract infection and, bacterial, 2117–2118
Urinary abnormalities, asymptomatic, 2028–2032
definition and identification of, 2028
Urinary bladder. *See* Bladder.
Urinary casts, 2031–2032
Urinary habits, changes in, 72
Urinary incontinence, 148–154
complications of, 150
management of, 154
Urinary incontinence *(Continued)*
definition of, 148
diagnostic plan for, 151–153, *152*
diseases associated with, 2132–2134
dysuria and, 163
idiopathic, feline, 2133
management of, 153–154
pathophysiology of, 148–150
recognition of, 150–151
Urinary obstruction, 2032–2036
clinical signs and symptoms of, 2032–2033
definition and clinical significance of, 2032
diagnosis of, 2033–2034
prognosis of, 2034
treatment of, 2034–2036
antimicrobial therapy in, 2035
obstruction relief in, 2035
postobstructive diuresis and, 2035–2036
therapeutic goals and priorities of, 2034–2035
Urinary retention, 155–159
complications of, 156
management of, 159
definition of, 155
diagnostic plan for, 158
management of, 158–159
pathophysiology of, 155–156
recognition of, 156–158, *157*
Urinary tract, lower. *See also* Bladder; Urethra.
anatomy and physiology of, 2108
Urinary tract defenses, 1947–1953
infection initiation and maintenance and, 1948, *1949–1950*, 1950–1952
normal voiding and, 1948
urinary antibacterial properties and, 1947–1948
Urinary tract disorders, 2108–2136
anatomic defects and, of bladder, 2113
anti-infectives for, 404
bacterial. *See* Urinary tract infections.
candidal, 2123
clinical signs of, 2108
diagnosis of, 2108–2113
bladder/urethral biopsy in, 2113
bladder/urethral endoscopy in, 2111
cystometry and urethral profilmetry in, 2113
cytology in, 2110
hematology/blood chemistry values in, 2109
radiography in, 2111, *2112*
ultrasonography in, 2111, *2113*
urinalysis in, *2109*, 2109–2110, *2110*
urine culture in, 2110–2111, 2111t
feline, 2057–2080
anatomic abnormalities and, *2076*, 2076–2078
bacteria and, 2062–2063
diagnosis of, 2061t, 2062, 2062t
etiopathogenesis of, 2061t, 2062
treatment of, 2062t, 2062–2063
drugs for, 2082t
epidemiologic studies of, 2057
idiopathic, 2079–2080
etiopathogenesis of, 2079
treatment of, 2079–2080
incidence and proportional morbidity of, 2057–2058
mycoplasmas and ureaplasmas and, 2063
mycotic agents and, 2063
parasites and, 2063
risk factors for, 2058, 2059t
terminology for, 2057, 2058t
viruses and, 2058–2062
clinical studies of, 2059–2060, *2060*
diagnosis of, 2060–2061, 2061t
experimental studies of, 2058–2059
treatment of, 2061t, 2061–2062
mycoplasmic, 2123
neoplastic, 2123–2130
parasitic, 2113–2114
traumatic, 2130–2132
urethral, 2134–2136
urinary incontinence and, 2132–2134
diagnosis of, 2133–2134, *2134*
Urinary tract infections, 161, 2036–2038
bacterial, 2114–2123
complicated acute, treatment of, 2120
definitions and, 2111t, 2114
Urinary tract infections *(Continued)*
bacterial, diagnosis of, 2061t, 2062, 2062t, 2117–2119
emphysematous cystitis and, 2122
etiopathogenesis of, 2061t, 2062
in cats, 2062–2063
localization of, 2118–2119
persistent, 2119
treatment of, 2121, 2129t
proliferative cystitis and, *2122*, 2122–2123
recurrent, 2119
treatment of, 2120–2121
reinfections and, 2119
treatment of, 2120–2121
simple acute, treatment of, 2120
treatment of, 2062t, 2062–2063, 2119t, 2119–2122
vesicourachal diverticula and, treatment of, 2078
candidal, 2123
canine, antimicrobial therapy and, 382
struvite urolithiasis and, 2090–2091
clinical and laboratory findings in, 2037–2038
control of, in canine uric acid and ammonium urate urolithiasis, 2096
cyclophosphamide cystitis and, 2123
definition and clinical significance of, 2036
detection and management of, in chronic renal failure, 2006
diagnosis of, 2038
mycoplasmal, 2123
preventing, 1980–1981
prognosis of, 2038
treatment of, 2038
upper, 1945, 1947, *1947*
diagnosis of, 1952–1953
vesicoureteral reflux and pyelonephritis and, 2036–2037
Urination. *See also* Dysuria; Hematuria.
behavior problems and, in cats, 236
in dogs, 231–232
definition of, 148
excitement, in dogs, 232
normal, as urinary tract defense, 1948
submissive, in dogs, 231–232
Urine. *See also* Hematuria; Polyuria; Proteinuria.
alkalinization of, in canine cystine urolithiasis, 2098
in canine uric acid and ammonium urate urolithiasis, 2096
anemia and, 92
antibacterial properties of, 1947–1948
concentration of, chronic renal failure and, 1922, 1922t
corticosteroids in, in hyperadrenocorticism, 1736
oliguria and, converting to nonoliguria, 1978–1979
detection of, 1971–1972
osmolality of, tubular function and, 1898–1899
specific gravity of, renal disease and, 1904
tubular function and, 1898–1899
steroids in, in hypoadrenocorticism, 1766
volume augmentation of, in canine uric acid and ammonium urate urolithiasis, 2096
Urine acidifiers, canine struvite urolithiasis and, sterile, 2092
Urine culture, in lower urinary tract disease, 2110–2111, 2111t
urinary tract infection and, bacterial, 2118, 2129t
Urine flow, 2115
reduced, *1930*, 1930–1931
Urine marking, in dogs, 231
Urocystoliths, vesicourachal diverticula and, treatment of, 2078
Urogenital system, antimicrobial selection for, 405t, 405–406
Urography, excretory, in renal disease, 1911t, 1911–1912
Urolithiasis, 2036, 2063–2069
ammonium urate, 2065t, 2068–2069
treatment and prevention of, 2072
calcium oxalate, 2065t, 2069
treatment and prevention of, 2072
calcium phosphate, 2065t, 2069
canine, 2083–2104

Urolithiasis *(Continued)*
canine, calcium oxalate, 2098–2102
biological behavior of, 2100
etiopathogenesis of, 2099–2100
medical treatment and prevention of, 2100–2102, 2101t
mineral composition and, 2099
calcium phosphate, 2102–2103
etiopathogenesis of, 2102
medical treatment and prevention of, 2102–2103
mineral composition and, 2102
chemical and physical characteristics of, 2083–2087, 2084t
matrix composition and, 2083, 2085
mineral composition and, 2083, 2084t
names and, 2083, 2084t
cystine, 2097–2098
biological behavior of, 2098
etiopathogenesis of, 2097
in dogs, 2097–2098
medical management of, 2098
mineral composition and, 2097
prevention of, 2098
detection of, 2085t, 2085–2087
crystalluria and, 2086
radiography and ultrasonography and, 2086t, 2086–2087
urolith analysis and, 2087
urolith culture and, 2087
etiopathogenesis of, 2085
silica, 2103–2104
biological behavior of, 2103
etiopathogenesis of, 2103
medical management and prevention of, 2103t, 2103–2104
mineral composition and, 2103
struvite, 2087–2093
biological behavior of, 2089
etiopathogenesis of, 2088–2089
infection-induced, 2088, 2090t, 2090–2092, 2091t
prevention of, 2093
medical treatment of, 2089–2093
mineral composition and, 2087–2088
monitoring therapeutic response and, 2092
precautions for, 2092–2093
prevention of, 2093
sterile, 2088–2089
prevention of, 2093
treatment of, 2090t, 2091t, 2092
surgical management of, indications for, 2104
uncommon, 2104
uric acid and ammonium urate, 2093–2097
biological behavior of, 2094–2095
etiopathogenesis of, 2093–2094
medical management of, 2095–2096
mineral composition and, 2084t, 2093
monitoring therapeutic response and, 2096–2097
portal vascular anomalies and, 2094
prevention of, 2097
urolith initiation and growth and, 2085
diagnosis of, 2058t, 2061t, 2064, 2070t
struvite, 2064–2068, 2065t, *2066*, 2066t
experimental studies of, 2065t, 2066–2067, *2067*
naturally occurring infection-induced uroliths and, 2064t, 2068
naturally occurring sterile uroliths and, 2064t, 2065t, 2067–2068
naturally occurring urethral plugs and, 2068, 2069t
terminology for, 2063–2064, 2064t–2066t, *2065*
treatment and prevention of, 2070–2072, 2071t
ammonium urate uroliths and, 2072
calcium oxalate uroliths and, 2072
struvite uroliths and, 2070–2072, 2071t
Urological syndromes, 1962, 1962t–1964t
feline. *See* Urinary tract disorders, feline.
Urothelial debridement, in idiopathic lower urinary tract disease, 2080
Uterine diseases, 1797–1804
drugs used in, 1805t
Uterine diseases *(Continued)*
neoplastic, 1803, 1819
Uterine torsion, 1801
Uterus, abortion and, 1803
anatomy and physiology of, 1797–1798
congenital anomalies of, 1801
occlusion of, infertility and, 1846
primary inertia of, 1802
prolapse of, 1801–1802
rupture of, 1802–1803
subinvolved placental sites and, 1802
Uveitis, 76, 76t
Uveodermatologic syndrome, ocular manifestations of, 76

Vaccination, 2294–2295
coma and stupor and, 62
for feline viral diseases, 313t, 313–314
for rabies, in cats, 324
for upper respiratory disease, feline, 322
human, for rabies, 300
Vaccines, tumor cell, in cancer therapy, 539
Vacuum therapy, acupuncture and, 492
Vagina, anatomy and physiology of, 1806–1807, *1810*
anomalies of, 1807–1809, *1808*
congenital abnormalities of, infertility and, 1050–1051
hormonally induced changes in, 1778–1779, *1780–1781*
lacerations of, 1812
prolapse of, 1811–1812, *1812*
tumors of, 1819–1820
Vaginal disorders, 1806–1812
hyperplastic, 1811, *1811*
neoplastic, 1809, 1811
Vaginitis, 275, 1809, *1810*
Vagus nerves, focal diseases of, 719
Valves. *See* Cardiac valve(s), malformation of.
Vascular anomalies, 1024, 1027
aortic, 1024, *1026*, 1027
of spinal cord, 693–694
venous, *1026*, 1027
Vascular disease, arterial, nonocclusive, 1188–1194
functional forms of, 1189
occlusive, 1185–1188
coma and stupor and, 62
lameness and, in cats, 170
mediastinal, 895
ocular manifestations of, 79–80
peripheral, 1185–1198
arterial, nonocclusive, 1188–1194
occlusive, 1185–1188
lymphatic, 1195t, 1195–1198
syncope and, 51–52
venous, 1194–1195
Vascular injuries, to nervous system, 554
Vascular ring abnormalities, esophagus and, *1266*, 1266–1267
Vasculitides, 1194
Vasculitis, hypersensitivity, 1193
necrotizing, 677
of pinnae, 250–251
Vasodilation, arteriolar, in heart failure, 918–919, *919*
in heart failure therapy, 957–961
in oliguria, 1979
Vasopressin, exogenous, tubular function and, 1899–1900
Vena cava, gastric dilatation-volvulus-torsion syndrome and, 1279
Venodilation, heart failure and, 918
Venography, cavernous sinus, 582, *583*
Venoms, poisoning and, 472–476
Venous anomalies, *1026*, 1027
Venous diseases, 1194–1195
Ventilation(s), absence of, cardiopulmonary arrest and, 172
lower respiratory disease and, 816–817, 818–819
Ventilation-perfusion mismatch, central cyanosis and, 96
Ventricle, right, double outlet, cyanotic heart disease and, 1022
Ventricular asystole, cardiopulmonary arrest and, 172, *172*
Ventricular contractility, in heart failure, *919*, 919–920
left heart evaluation and, 929t, 929–932, *930–932*
primary reduction of, heart failure and, *912*, 912–913, *913*
Ventricular fibrillation, cardiopulmonary arrest and, 172, *173*
Ventricular performance, right heart evaluation and, 934–935
Ventricular premature contractions, *1065*, 1067–1070, *1068*, *1069*
Ventricular pressures, left heart evaluation and, 928–929
Ventricular septal defects. *See* Atrioventricular septal defects.
Ventricular tachycardia, atrioventricular dissociation and, 1079–1084, *1081–1083*
nonsustained, 1080
sustained, 1080
Ventriculography, 582–583, *584*
VER. *See* Visual evoked responses.
Vertebrae, block, etiology and pathogenesis of, 646
butterfly, etiology and pathogenesis of, 646
transitional, etiology and pathogenesis of, 646
Vertebral canal stenosis, lumbosacral, 672–675
clinical findings in, 672–673
diagnosis of, 673, *674*, *675*
etiology and pathogenesis of, 672, 672t
treatment of, 673–675
Vertebral segmentation defects, 2384
Vesicle, 118
Vesicourachal diverticula, 2076–2078
function and dysfunction and, 2076–2077
macroscopic, *2077*, 2077–2078
microscopic, 2077
treatment of, 2078
Vesicoureteral reflux, urinary tract infection and, 2036–2037
Vestibular ataxia, 57t, 57–58
Vestibulocochlear nerves, congenital and familial diseases of, 718
focal diseases of, *718*, 718–719
Veterinarians, human-animal bonds and, 242–243
breaking bonds and, 243
maintaining bonds and, 242–243
making bonds and, 242
referring, emergency medicine and, 214
Veterinary education, in developing countries, 224–225
Villonodular synovitis, 2362
Villous atrophy, 1370–1373
idiopathic, 1371–1372
clinical signs of, 1371
diagnosis of, 1371–1372
treatment of, 1372
wheat-sensitive enteropathy and, 1372–1373
clinical signs of, 1372
diagnosis of, 1372–1373
treatment of, 1373
Vinca alkaloids, in cancer chemotherapy, 533
Viral diseases, arthritic, 2365
canine, 298–310
diarrhea and. *See* Diarrhea, small bowel, viral.
feline, 312–338
infertility and, 1844–1845
myocardial, 1124, *1124*
ocular manifestations of, 82
of brain, 601–604
predisposing factors and, 312–314, 313t
cattery cats and, 313
disease control and, 312–313
vaccination and, 313t, 313–314
pulmonary, 829–830
rhinitis and, 776–778, *779*
stomatitis and, *1227*, 1229
treatment of, drugs used in, 340t
Virus(es), isolation of, in feline panleukopenia, 316
lower urinary tract disease and, in cats, 2058–2062
clinical studies of, 2059–2060, *2060*
diagnosis of, 2060–2061, 2061t
experimental studies of, 2058–2059

Visceral diseases, protozoal, 287–292
Visceral larval migrans, in humans, 188
prevention of, 188
ocular manifestations of, 81
Visual evoked responses (VER), brain disease diagnosis and, 588
Vitamin(s), exocrine pancreatic insufficiency and, 1541
in exocrine pancreatic insufficiency, 1547–1548
metabolism of, liver disease and, 1426, 1427t
water-soluble, recommended intake of, in chronic renal failure, 1994
Vitamin A, deficiency of, ocular manifestations of, 80
hypervitaminosis A and, arthropathy due to, 2361
bone disorders and, 2387
brain and, 616
of cats, 661
recommended intake of, in chronic renal failure, 1994
Vitamin A–responsive dermatosis, 8
Vitamin B_{12}, deficiency of, brain and, 616
in small bowel diarrhea, measurement of, 1339
Vitamin D, hypervitaminosis D and, bone disorders and, 2385, 2387
hypercalcemia and, 1619
in chronic renal failure, divalent ion imbalances in, 2002
oral, in hypocalcemia, 1628–1629, 1629t
recommended intake of, in chronic renal failure, 1994
Vitamin E deficiency, ocular manifestations of, 80
Vitamin K deficiency, coagulopathy and. *See* Coagulopathies, vitamin K deficiency and, antagonism and.
VLDL. *See* Lipoprotein(s), very low density.
Vocalization, aimless, 72
excessive, in cats, 237
in dogs, 237
Voiding. *See* Urination.
Volume contraction, 432–434
clinical signs of, 432, 434t
etiology of, 432, 432t
treatment of, 432t, 432–434
composition and, 432t, 433–434
rate and, 433
volume and, 432–434
Volume depletion, in acute renal failure, 1970
Volume expansion, 434–435
clinical signs and diagnosis of, 434t, 434–435
etiology of, 434
treatment of, 435
Volume overloading, heart failure and, *912*, 913–914
Volvulus. *See also* Gastric dilatation-volvulus-torsion syndrome.
Vomiting, 27–30
chronic, intermittent, 29
clinical features of, 28t, 28–29
definition of, 27
diagnostic plan for, 30
diarrhea and, 34
pathophysiology of, 27–28
physical examination and, 29–30
projectile, 29
regurgitation differentiated from, 27
treatment of, 30
uremic, prevention of, 1979–1980, *1980*
Vomiting center, 27–28
Vomitus, content of, 29
Von Willebrand's disease, 2258–2261, 2268t, 2268–2270
canine, 2269–2270
clinical signs of, 2259–2260
human, 2267
laboratory aspects of, 2259t, 2260
laboratory evaluation in, 2268–2269, 2269t
pathophysiology of, 2258–2259, 2259t
therapy of, 2260–2261
Von Willebrand's factor assay, 2252, 2253t
Vulva, congenital abnormalities of, infertility and, 1050–1051
tumors of, 1819–1820

Waldenstrom's macroglobulinemia, paraproteinemias and, 2308
Walnuts, moldy, poisoning by, 460t, 478
Wasting, chronic, weakness and, 47
Water, distribution of, corticosteroids and, 416
intestinal transport of, 1327
metabolism of, disorders of, 435–437
hypernatremia as, 435t, 436–437
hyponatremia as, 435t, 435–436
physiology and, 435
physiology of, 435
Water deprivation test, tubular function and, 1899
Weakness, 46–50
causes of, 47t, 47–50
cyanosis and, 97
drug-related, 48
history in, 46
laboratory tests in, 46–47, 47t
lameness and, in dogs, 165
physical examination in, 46
regurgitation and, 31
Weight changes, hematuria and, 161
Weight gain, 3. *See also* Obesity.
polyphagia and, 16
Weight loss, 3
anorexia and, 16
diagnostic approach to, 4
diarrhea and, 34
pathophysiology of, 4
polyphagia and, 16
regurgitation and, 31
West Highland white terrier, copper-associated hepatitis in, 1491–1492
Wheal, 117–118
Wheat-sensitive enteropathy, 1372–1373
clinical signs of, 1372
diagnosis of, 1372–1373
treatment of, 1373
Wheel barrowing, in neurologic examination, 559, *559*
Whining, pain and, 20
Whipworms, 1410–1411
small bowel diarrhea and, 1347
White coat, in dogs, tremor and, 55–56
White pulp, of spleen, 2234

Xanthine oxidase inhibitors, in canine uric acid and ammonium urate urolithiasis, 2095–2096
Xerostomia, 1229
XO syndrome, infertility and, 1849
XXY syndrome, infertility and, 1848–1849
Xylocaine. *See* Lidocaine.
Xylose absorption test, small bowel diarrhea and, *1338*, 1338–1339

Yeast infections, of external ear canal, 256
Yersinia infections, 269
of large intestine, 1414
small bowel diarrhea and, 1357

Zinc intoxication, 471
differentiation of, 459t, 460t, 469t, 471
Zinc phosphate intoxication, 466–467
differentiation of, 459t, 460t, 465t, 467
Zinc-responsive dermatosis, 8
Zoonoses, 188–193, 189t
bacterial, 191–192
ectoparasitic, 191
mycotic, 192
parasitic, 188–190